FOURTH EDITION

ROGERS' TEXTBOOK OF PEDIATRIC INTENSIVE CARE

FOURTH EDITION

ROGERS' TEXTBOOK OF PEDIATRIC INTENSIVE CARE

Editor

David G. Nichols, MD, MBA
Professor
Department of Anesthesiology and
　Department of Critical Care
　Medicine and Pediatrics
Vice Dean for Education
The Johns Hopkins University
　School of Medicine
Baltimore, Maryland

Section Editors

Alice D. Ackerman, MD, FAAP, FCCM
Andrew C. Argent, FCPaeds (SA), MMed(Paeds)
Katherine Biagas, MD
Joseph A. Carcillo, Jr., MD
Heidi J. Dalton, MD
Z. Leah Harris, MD
Niranjan "Tex" Kissoon, MD, FPAP, FRCP(C),
　FCCM, FACPE, CPE
Patrick M. Kochanek, MD
Keith C. Kocis, MD, MS
Jacques Lacroix, MD, FRCPC
Duncan J. Macrae, BMSc, MBChB, FRCA, FRCPCH
Vinay M. Nadkarni, MD
Murray Pollack, MD, MBA
Charles L. Schleien, MD
Donald H. Shaffner, MD
Sunit C. Singhi, MB, BS, MD
Robert C. Tasker, MB, BS, MD, FRCP
Robert D. Truog, MD
Hans-Dieter Volk
Edwin van der Voort, MD
Randell C. Wetzel, MB, BS, MSBus, FAAP, FCCM
Hector R. Wong, MD
Myron Yaster, MD

Wolters Kluwer | Lippincott Williams & Wilkins
Health
Philadelphia · Baltimore · New York · London
Buenos Aires · Hong Kong · Sydney · Tokyo

Acquisitions Editor: Brian Brown
Managing Editor: Nicole Dernoski
Developmental Editor: Molly Connors
Project Manager: Nicole Walz
Manufacturing Manager: Benjamin Rivera
Marketing Manager: Angela Panetta
Cover Designer: Larry Didona
Design Coordinator: Terry Mallon
Production Services: Aptara, Inc.

© 2008 by LIPPINCOTT WILLIAMS & WILKINS, a Wolters Kluwer business
© 1996 by WILLIAMS & WILKINS
530 Walnut Street
Philadelphia, PA 19106

Printed in the United States of America.

Library of Congress Cataloging-in-Publication Data

Rogers' textbook of pediatric intensive care / editor, David G. Nichols: section editors, Alice D. Ackerman . . . [et al.]. — 4th ed.
    p. ;   cm.
  Rev. ed. of; Textbook of pediatric intensive care / editor, Mark C. Rogers; associate editor, David G. Nichols; section editors, Alice D. Ackerman . . . [et al.]. 3rd ed. © 1996
  Includes bibliographical references and index.
  ISBN 978-0-7817-8275-3
  ISBN 0-7817-8275-9
  1. Pediatric intensive care.   I. Nichols, David G. (David Gregory), 1951-   II. Rogers, Mark C.
III. Textbook of pediatric intensive care.   IV. Title: Textbook of pediatric intensive care.
  [DNLM: 1. Intensive Care.   2. Child.   3. Infant. WS 366 R729 2008]
RJ370.T49 2008
618.92′0028—dc22

2007046976

The creation of the *Textbook of Pediatric Intensive Care* was originally done with an eye both toward what should be in it and how it would be perceived by practitioners of other specialties in Pediatrics. What was this new specialty really about? The problem was really how to define the specialty and its literature so that a fellow who was studying to be a Pediatric Intensive Care physician would be able to rely mostly on the *Textbook Pediatric Intensive Care* for information on any patient. We did not want anyone to have to go, too early or too often, through textbooks of other specialties to find answers to problems being encountered with patients in the PICU. As a result of this philosophical choice, this textbook grew to be an enormous undertaking. Although books on the PICU did exist when the first edition of this textbook was written, they were either paperback outlines or largely concerning the cardiopulmonary aspects of PICU care.

On the other hand, we were determined to cover all systems (including infectious disease, nutrition, and metabolic problems), to educate the fellows on the principles and electronics of sophisticated monitoring equipment on which they were relying, to highlight psychological and ethical problems in the PICU, etc. All relevant physiology and pharmacology would be included. Any disease that we thought was going to constitute a meaningful patient population in the PICU—from rhabdomyolysis to kyphoscoliosis—would be included.

The Hopkins faculty and fellows performed herculean work on the book. It took 18 months to write, and it grew from one volume to two, as our knowledge of the new field grew with it. The faculty and fellows helped to define the field, as they wrote truly comprehensive reviews in their chapters. I remain in awe and in debt of what they accomplished.

Of all of the reviews that we received, the one that gave us the most pleasure called the book "The Bible of Pediatric Intensive Care." That description gave our faculty and fellows recognition that I knew they had worked so hard to achieve.

The *Textbook of Pediatric Intensive Care*, and its associated *Handbook of Pediatric Intensive Care*, co-edited by Mark Helfaer (a former Hopkins fellow and faculty member now Director of the PICU at the Children's Hospital in Philadelphia), have been translated into Japanese, Russian, Spanish, and Portuguese. The original contributors set a very high standard, but I am highly confident that it is one that the present authors and editors of the fourth edition, under the enormously capable leadership of David Nichols, will only exceed.

Mark C. Rogers, MD

CONTRIBUTORS

Nicholas S. Abend, MD
Department of Neurology
University of Pennsylvania School of Medicine
Philadelphia, Pennsylvania

Mateo Aboy, PhD
Department of Electronics Engineering & Technology
Oregon Institute of Technology
Portland, Oregon

Kareem Abu-Elmagd, MD
Thomas E. Starzl Transplantation Institute
University of Pittsburgh
Pittsburgh, Pennsylvania

Alice D. Ackerman, MD, FAAP, FCCM
Department of Pediatrics
Carilion Clinic/Roanoke Memorial Hospital
Roanoke, Virginia

Meredith L. Allen, MB, BS, FRACP, PhD
Portex Department of Anaesthesia, Intensive Therapy,
    and Respiratory Medicine
Institute of Child Health, University College
London, United Kingdom

Andrew C. Argent, FCPaeds(SA), MMed(Paeds)
School of Child and Adolescent Health
University of Cape Town
Cape Town, South Africa

John H. Arnold, MD
Department of Anaesthesia (Pediatrics)
Harvard Medical School
Boston, Massachusetts

Stephen Ashwall, MD
Department of Pediatrics
Loma Linda University School of Medicine
Loma Linda, California

John Scott Baird, MD
Department of Pediatrics
Columbia University, College of Physicians and Surgeons
New York, New York

Aristides Baltodano, MD
Departamento de Pediatriay Cuidados Criticos
Universidad de Costa Rica, Escuela de Medicina
San José, Costa Rica

Kenneth J. Banasiak, MD
Department of Pediatrics
Yale University School of Medicine
New Haven, Connecticut

Arun Bansal, MD
Department of Pediatrics
Postgraduate Institute of Medical
    Education and Research
Chandigarh, India

Jeffrey S. Barrett, PhD, FCP
Department of Pediatrics
University of Pennsylvania School of Medicine
Philadelphia, Pennsylvania

Heather Woods Barthel, BA
Government, Community, and Public Affairs
The Johns Hopkins Institutions
Baltimore, Maryland

Hülya Bayir, MD
Departments of Critical Care Medicine and
Environmental and Occupational Health
University of Pittsburgh School of Medicine
Pittsburgh, Pennsylvania

Robert A. Berg, MD, FAAP, FCCM
Department of Pediatrics
The University of Arizona College of Medicine
Tucson, Arizona

Ivor D. Berkowitz, MBBChir
Department of Anesthesiology & Critical Care Medicine
The Johns Hopkins University School of Medicine
Baltimore, Maryland

Katherine Biagas, MD
Department of Pediatrics
Columbia University, College of Physicians and Surgeons
New York, New York

Michael T. Bigham, MD
Pediatric Critical Care Medicine
Cincinnati Children's Hospital Medical Center
Cincinnati, Ohio

Mark S. Bleiweis, MD
Departments of Surgery and Pediatrics
University of Florida College of Medicine
Gainesville, Florida

Jeffrey L. Blumer, PhD, MD
Department of Pediatrics
Case Western Reserve University
Cleveland, Ohio

Clifford W. Bogue, MD
Department of Pediatrics
Yale University School of Medicine
New Haven, Connecticut

Geoffrey J. Bond, MD, FRACS
Department of Pediatrics
University of Pittsburgh School of Medicine
Pittsburgh, Pennsylvania

M. Brigid Bradley, MD
Department of Pediatrics
Columbia University, College of Physicians and Surgeons
New York, New York

Kenneth M. Brady, MD
Department of Anesthesiology & Critical Care Medicine
The Johns Hopkins University School of Medicine
Baltimore, Maryland

Ewa B. Brandys, MD
Department of Physical Medicine & Rehabilitation
The Johns Hopkins University School of Medicine
Baltimore, Maryland

John Philip Breinholt, III, MD
Department of Pediatrics
Baylor College of Medicine
Houston, Texas

Richard J. Brilli, MD
Department of Pediatrics
University of Cincinnati College of Medicine
Cincinnati, Ohio

Deborah L. Brown, MD
Department of Pediatrics
The University of Texas School of Medicine
Houston, Texas

Werther Brunow de Carvalho, MD
Departamento de Pediatria
Universidade Federal de São Paulo
Escola Paulista de Medicina
São Paulo, Brasil

Timothy E. Bunchman, MD
Department of Pediatric Nephrology
Michigan State University, College of Human Medicine
East Lansing, Michigan

Warwick W. Butt, MB, BS, FRACP, FJFICM
Department of Pediatrics
Melbourne University, Faculty of Medicine, Dentistry,
    and Health Sciences
Melbourne, Victoria, Australia

Mitchell S. Cairo, MD
Department of Pediatrics
Columbia University, College of Physicians and Surgeons
New York, New York

James D. Campbell, MD, MS
Department of Pediatrics
Center for Vaccine Development
University of Maryland School of Medicine
Baltimore, Maryland

Michael F. Canarie, MD
Department of Pediatrics
Yale University School of Medicine
New Haven, Connecticut

G. Patricia Cantwell, MD
Department of Critical Care Medicine
University of Miami, Miller School of Medicine
Miami, Florida

Joseph A. Carcillo, MD
Departments of Critical Care Medicine
    and Pediatrics
University of Pittsburgh School of Medicine
Pittsburgh, Pennsylvania

Todd Carpenter, MD
Department of Pediatrics
University of Colorado at Denver and
    Health Sciences Center
Denver, Colorado

Thomas O. Carpenter, MD
Department of Pediatrics
Yale University School of Medicine
New Haven, Connecticut

Ira M. Cheifetz, MD, FCCM, FAARC
Department of Pediatrics
Duke University School of Medicine
Durham, North Carolina

James R. Christensen, MD
Departments of Physical Medicine & Rehabilitation
    and Pediatrics
The Johns Hopkins University School of Medicine
Baltimore, Maryland

Wendy K. Chung, MD, PhD
Departments of Pediatrics and Medicine
Columbia University, College of Physicians
    and Surgeons
New York, New York

Robert S.B. Clark, MD
Departments of Pediatrics and Critical Care Medicine
University of Pittsburgh School of Medicine
Pittsburgh, Pennsylvania

Steven A. Conrad, MD, PhD, FCCM
Departments of Pediatrics, Medicine, Emergency
    Medicine, and Anesthesiology
Louisiana State University Health Sciences Center
Shreveport, Louisiana

Arthur Cooper, MD, MS
Department of Surgery
Columbia University, College of Physicians and Surgeons
New York, New York

Mehrengise K. Cooper, MD, FRCPCH
Department of Paediatrics
Imperial College School of Medicine
London, United Kingdom

Ashraf H. Coovadia, MD
Department of Paediatrics and Child Health
University of The Witwatersrand
Johannesburg, Gauteng, South Africa

Jose A. Cortes, MD
Departments of Pediatrics and
    Anesthesiology & Critical Care Medicine
The University of Texas School of Medicine
Houston, Texas

Mary K. Dahmer, PhD
Department of Molecular Sciences
University of Tennessee Health Science Center
Memphis, Tennessee

Heidi J. Dalton, MD
Department of Pediatrics
George Washington University School of Medicine
    and Health Sciences
Washington, DC

Sally L. Davidson Ward, MD
Department of Pediatrics
University of Southern California, Keck School of Medicine
Los Angeles, California

Allan de Caen, MD, FRCPC
Department of Pediatrics
University of Alberta, Faculty of Medicine & Dentistry
Edmonton, Alberta, Canada

Susan W. Denfield, MD
Department of Pediatrics
Baylor College of Medicine
Houston, Texas

Denis J. Devictor, MD, PhD
Département de Pédiatrie
Université Paris-Sud 11
Le Kremlin-Bicêtre, France

Troy E. Dominguez, MD
Department of Anesthesiology and Critical Care
University of Pennsylvania School of Medicine
Philadelphia, Pennsylvania

Aaron J. Donoghue, MD, MSCE
Departments of Anesthesiology and Critical Care
    and Pediatrics
University of Pennsylvania School of Medicine
Philadelphia, Pennsylvania

Lesley Doughty, MD
Department of Pediatrics
University of Cincinnati School of Medicine
Cincinnati, Ohio

William J. Dreyer, MD
Department of Pediatrics
Baylor College of Medicine
Houston, Texas

Jonathan Duff, MD, FRCPC
Pediatric Intensive Care Unit
Stollery Children's Hospital
Edmonton, Alberta, Canada

Trevor Duke, MD, FRACP
Department of Pediatrics
University of Melbourne School of Medicine
Parkville, Victoria, Australia

R. Blaine Easley, MD
Department of Anesthesiology and
    Critical Care Medicine
The Johns Hopkins University School of Medicine
Baltimore, Maryland

Ori Eyal, MD
Pediatric Endocrinology and Diabetes Unit
The Chaim Sheba Medical Center
Tel Aviv University Sackler School of Medicine
Tel Hashomer, Israel

Edward Vincent S. Faustino, MD
Department of Pediatrics
Yale University School of Medicine
New Haven, Connecticut

Kathryn A. Felmet, MD
Department of Critical Care Medicine
University of Pittsburgh School of Medicine
Pittsburgh, Pennsylvania

Pamela Feuer, MD
Department of Pediatrics
Columbia University, College of Physicians and Surgeons
New York, New York

Alan I. Fields, MD, FCCM
Departments of Pediatrics and
    Anesthesiology & Critical Care Medicine
The University of Texas School of Medicine
Houston, Texas

Jeffrey R. Fineman, MD
Department of Pediatrics
Cardiovascular Research Institute
University of California, San Francisco
San Francisco, California

Ericka L. Fink, MD
Department of Critical Care Medicine
Children's Hospital of Pittsburgh
Pittsburgh, Pennsylvania

George L. Foltin, MD
Departments of Pediatrics and Emergency Medicine
New York University School of Medicine
New York, New York

Marcelo Cunio Machado Fonseca, MD
Departamento de Pediatria
Universidade Federal de São Paulo
Escola Paulista de Medicina
São Paulo, Brasil

Alain Fraisse, MD, PhD
Départment de Cardiologie
Université de la Méditerranée
Marseille, France

Philippe S. Friedlich, MD, Ms, Epi, MBA
Department of Pediatrics
University of Southern California, Keck School of Medicine
Los Angeles, California

Muraya Gathinji, MS
The Johns Hopkins University School of Medicine
Baltimore, Maryland

Jonathan Gillis, MB, BS, PhD, FRACP, FJFICM
Department of Paediatric Intensive Care
Children's Hospital at Westmead
Sydney, New South Wales, Australia

Brahm Goldstein, MD, FCCM
Novo Nordisk, Inc.
Princeton, New Jersey

Salvatore R. Goodwin, MD
Department of Anesthesiology & Critical Care
Mayo Clinic, College of Medicine
Rochester, Minnesota

Ana Lia Graciano, MD, FAAP
Department of Pediatrics
University of California at San Francisco
Fresno, California

Alan Graham, MD
Department of Pediatrics
Oregon Health & Science University
Portland, Oregon

Philip L. Graham III, MD, MSc
Department of Pediatrics
Columbia University College of Physicians and Surgeons
New York, New York

Bruce M. Greenwald, MD
Department of Pediatrics
Weill Medical College of Cornell University
New York, New York

Brandt P. Groh, MD
Department of Pediatrics
Penn State College of Medicine
Hershey, Pennsylvania

Anne-Marie Guerguerian, MD, FRCPC, FAAP
Departments of Critical Care Medicine and Pediatrics
University of Toronto, Faculty of Medicine
Toronto, Ontario, Canada

Richard Hackbarth, MD
Department of Pediatrics and Human Development
Michigan State University, College of Human Medicine
East Lansing, Michigan

Gabriel G. Haddad, MD
Departments of Pediatrics and Neurosciences
University of California, San Diego, School of Medicine
San Diego, California

Mark W. Hall, MD
Department of Pediatrics
The Ohio State University College of Medicine
Columbus, Ohio

Gillian C. Halley, MBChB
Paediatric Intensive Care Unit
Royal Brompton Hospital
London, United Kingdom

Donna S. Hamel, RRT, RCP, FAARC
Department of Pediatric Critical Care Medicine
Duke University Medical Center
Durham, North Carolina

Yong Y. Han, MD
Department of Pediatrics and Communicable Diseases
University of Michigan Medical School
Ann Arbor, Michigan

George E. Hardart, MD
Department of Pediatrics
Columbia University, College of Physicians and Surgeons
New York, New York

Z. Leah Harris, MD
Department of Anesthesiology & Critical Care Medicine
The Johns Hopkins University School of Medicine
Baltimore, Maryland

A. Marc Harrison, MD
Pediatric Critical Care
Children's Hospital, Cleveland Clinic
Cleveland, Ohio

Abeer Hassoun, MD
Department of Pediatrics
Columbia University, College of Physicians and Surgeons
New York, New York

Jan A. Hazelzet, MD, PhD, FCCM
Pediatric Intensive Care Unit
Sophia Childrens Hospital, Erasmus Medical Center
Rotterdam, The Netherlands

Mary Fran Hazinski, RN, MSN, FAAN
Departments of Surgery and Pediatrics
Vanderbilt University School of Medicine
Nashville, Tennessee

Gregory P. Heldt, MD
Department of Pediatrics
University of California, San Diego, School of Medicine
San Diego, California

Mark A. Helfaer, MD
Departments of Anesthesiology and Critical Care
University of Pennsylvania School of Medicine
Philadelphia, Pennsylvania

Mark J. Heulitt, MD
Departments of Pediatrics, Physiology and Biophysics
University of Arkansas for Medical Sciences,
    College of Medicine
Little Rock, Arkansas

Siew Yen Ho, MD
Imperial College, National Heart & Lung Institute
London, United Kingdom

Julien I. Hoffman, MD
Department of Pediatrics
University of California, San Francisco
San Francisco, California

Joy D. Howell, MD
Department of Pediatrics
Weill Medical College of Cornell University
New York, New York

Elizabeth A. Hunt, MD, MPH
Department of Anesthesiology & Critical Care Medicine
The Johns Hopkins University School of Medicine
Baltimore, Maryland

S. Adil Husain, MD
Department of Surgery
University of Indiana
Indianapolis, Indiana

Tomas Iölster, MD
Departamento de Pediatria
Universidad Austral School of Medicine
Pilar, Buenos Aires, Argentina

Ronald Jaffe, MD
Department of Pathology
University of Pittsburgh School of Medicine
Pittsburgh, Pennsylvania

M. Jayashree, MB, BS, MD
Department of Pediatrics
Advanced Pediatric Centre
Post Graduate Institute of Medical Education and Research
Chandigarh, India

John Lynn Jefferies, MD, MPH
Department of Pediatrics
Baylor College of Medicine
Houston, Texas

Larry W. Jenkins, PhD
Departments of Neurological Surgery and Neurobiology
Safar Center for Resuscitation Research
University of Pittsburgh School of Medicine
Pittsburgh, Pennsylvania

Sachin S. Jogal, MD
Department of Pediatric Hematology/Oncology/
    Bone Marrow Transplantation
Medical College of Wisconsin
Milwaukee, Wisconsin

Cíntia Johnston, RRT
Departamentos da Medicina e Pediatria
Universidade Federal de São Paulo
Escola Paulista de Medicina
São Paulo, Brasil

Phillippe Jouvet, MD, PhD
Department of Pediatrics
University of Montreal, Faculty of Medicine
Montreal, Quebec, Canada

Sushil K. Kabra, MD, DNB
Department of Pediatrics
All India Institute of Medical Sciences
New Delhi, India

Jonathan R. Kaltman, MD
Department of Cardiology
University of Pennsylvania School of Medicine
Philadelphia, Pennsylvania

Thomas G. Keens, MD
Departments of Pediatrics, Physiology and Biophysics
University of Southern California, Keck School of Medicine
Los Angeles, California

Lisa K. Kelly, MD
Department of Pediatrics
University of Southern California, Keck School of Medicine
Los Angeles, California

Andrea Kelly, MD
Department of Pediatrics
University of Pennsylvania School of Medicine
Philadelphia, Pennsylvania

Sudha Kilaru V. Kessler, MD
Department of Neurology
University of Pennsylvania School of Medicine
Philadelphia, Pennsylvania

Alka Khadwal, MD
Department of Pediatrics
Postgraduate Institute of Medical Education & Research
Chandigarh, India

Praveen Khilnani, MD, FCCM
Department of Pediatrics
Ipapollo Hospital
New Delhi, India

Jeffrey J. Kim, MD
Department of Pediatrics
Baylor College of Medicine
Houston, Texas

Carroll J. King, MD
Departments of Pediatrics and
    Anesthesiology & Critical Care Medicine
The University of Texas School of Medicine
Houston, Texas

Fenella Kirkham, MBBChir
Neurosciences Unit
Institute of Child Health, University
    College London
London, United Kingdom

Niranjan "Tex" Kissoon, MD, FAAP, FRCP(C),
FCCM, FACPE, CPE
Department of Pediatrics
University of British Columbia, Faculty of Medicine
Vancouver, British Columbia, Canada

Nigel J. Klein, MB, BS, MD
Infectious Diseases and Microbiology Unit
Institute of Child Health
London, United Kingdom

Monica E. Kleinman, MD
Department of Anaesthesia
Harvard Medical School
Boston, Massachusetts

Patrick M. Kochanek, MD
Safar Center for Resuscitation Research
Departments of Critical Care Medicine,
    Anesthesiology, and Pediatrics
University of Pittsburgh School of Medicine
Pittsburgh, Pennsylvania

Keith C. Kocis, MD, MS
Department of Pediatric Critical Care Medicine
The University of North Carolina
Chapel Hill, North Carolina

Karen L. Kotloff, MD
Department of Pediatrics
University of Maryland School of Medicine
Baltimore, Maryland

Sheila S. Kun, RN, BSN, MS
Division of Pediatric Pulmonology
Childrens Hospital Los Angeles
Los Angeles, California

Jacques Lacroix, MD, FRCPC
Département de pédiatrie
Université de Montréal, Faculté de Médicine
Montréal, Quebec, Canada

Jos M. Latour, RN, MSN
Department of Pediatrics
Erasmus Medical Center
Rotterdam, The Netherlands

Miriam K. Laufer, MD
Department of Pediatrics
Center for Vaccine Development
University of Maryland School
    of Medicine
Baltimore, Maryland

Matthew B. Laurens, MD, MPH
Department of Pediatrics
University of Maryland School of Medicine
Baltimore, Maryland

Heitor Pons Leite, MD, PhD
Departamento de Pediatria
Universidade Federal de São Paulo
Escola Paulista de Medicina
São Paulo, Brasil

Daniel L. Levin, MD
Departments of Pediatrics and Anesthesia
Dartmouth Medical School
Hanover, New Hampshire

Daniel J. Licht, MD
Department of Neurology
University of Pennsylvania School of Medicine
Philadelphia, Pennsylvania

Rakesh Lodha, MD
Department of Pediatrics
All India Institute of Medical Sciences
Ansari Nagar, New Delhi, India

David M. Loeb, MD, PhD
Departments of Pediatrics and Oncology
The Johns Hopkins University School of Medicine
Baltimore, Maryland

Anne Lortie, MD
Department of Pediatrics
University of Montreal, Faculty of Medicine
Montreal, Quebec, Canada

Naomi L.C. Luban, MD
Departments of Pediatrics and Pathology
George Washington University School of Medicine
    and Health Sciences
Washington, DC

Robert Luten, MD
Department of Emergency Medicine
University of Florida College of Medicine
Jacksonville, Florida

Duncan J. Macrae, BMSc, MBChB, FRCA, FRCPCH
Department of Pediatrics
University of London, Imperial College
London, United Kingdom

Mioara D. Manole, MD
Department of Pediatrics
University of Pittsburgh School of Medicine
Pittsburgh, Pennsylvania

Bruno Maranda, MD, MSc
Service of Medical Genetics
Ste. Justine Hospital
Montreal, Quebec, Canada

Bradley S. Marino, MD, MPP, MSCE
Department of Pediatrics
University of Cincinnati College of Medicine
Cincinnati, Ohio

M. Michele Mariscalco, MD
Department of Pediatrics
Baylor College of Medicine
Houston, Texas

Barry P. Markovitz, MD, MPH
Departments of Anesthesiology and Pediatrics
University of Southern California, Keck School of Medicine
Los Angeles, California

Dolly Martin, RN
Intestinal Rehabilitation and Transplant Center
Thomas E. Starzl Transplantation Institute
Pittsburgh, Pennsylvania

Norma Maxvold, MD
Department of Pediatric Critical Care
DeVos Children's Hospital
Grand Rapids, Michigan

George V. Mazariegos, MD, FACS
Department of Pediatrics
University of Pittsburgh School of Medicine
Pittsburgh, Pennsylvania

Jennifer A. McArthur, DO
Department of Pediatrics
Medical College of Wisconsin
Milwaukee, Wisconsin

Kathleen L. Meert, MD, FCCM
Department of Pediatrics
Wayne State University School of Medicine
Detroit, Michigan

Rodrigo Mejia, MD, FAAP
Departments of Pediatrics and
    Anesthesiology & Critical Care Medicine
The University of Texas School of Medicine
Houston, Texas

Jon N. Meliones, MD
Department of Pediatric Critical Care
Duke University School of Medicine
Durham, North Carolina

Jessica Mesman, RN, PhD
Department of Technology and Society Studies
Maastricht University
Maastricht, The Netherlands

David Joshua Michelson, MD
Department of Pediatrics, Division of Child Neurology
Loma Linda University School of Medicine
Loma Linda, California

Johnny Millar, MBChB, PhD
Pediatric Intensive Care Unit
Royal Children's Hospital
Melbourne, Australia

Katsuyuki Miyasaka, MD, PhD, FAAP, FCCP
Nagano Children's Hospital
Toyoshina, Nagano, Japan

Vicki L. Montgomery, MD, FAAP, FCCM
Department of Pediatrics
University of Louisville School of Medicine
Louisville, Kentucky

Wynne E. Morrison, MD
Department of Anesthesiology and Critical Care
University of Pennsylvania School of Medicine
Philadelphia, Pennsylvania

Thomas Moshang, Jr., MD
Department of Pediatrics
University of Pennsylvania School of Medicine
Philadelphia, Pennsylvania

M. Michele Moss, MD
Department of Pediatrics
University of Arkansas for Medical Sciences
Little Rock, Arkansas

Simon Nadel, FRCP
Paediatric Intensive Care Unit
Department of Paediatrics
St. Mary's Hospital
London, United Kingdom

Vinay M. Nadkarni, MD
Departments of Anesthesiology & Critical Care
    and Pediatrics
University of Pennsylvania School of Medicine
Philadelphia, Pennsylvania

David P. Nelson, MD
Department of Pediatrics
Baylor College of Medicine
Houston, Texas

Kristen L. Nelson, MD
Department of Anesthesiology & Critical Care Medicine
The Johns Hopkins University School of Medicine
Baltimore, Maryland

Charle RJC Newton, MBChB, MD, MRCP, FRCPCH
Department of Neurosciences
University College of London
London, United Kingdom

David G. Nichols, MD
Departments of Anesthesiology & Critical Care Medicine
    and Pediatrics
The Johns Hopkins University School of Medicine
Baltimore, Maryland

Sharon E. Oberfield, MD
Department of Pediatrics
Columbia University, College of Physicians
    and Surgeons
New York, New York

George Ofori-Amanfo, MD
Department of Pediatrics
Columbia University, College of Physicians and Surgeons
New York, New York

Peter E. Oishi, MD
Department of Pediatrics
University of California, San Francisco
San Francisco, California

Richard A. Orr, MD
Departments of Critical Care Medicine and Pediatrics
University of Pittsburgh School of Medicine
Pittsburgh, Pennsylvania

John Pappachan, MA, MBBChir, FRCA
Paediatric Intensive Care Unit
Southampton University Hospitals Trust
Southampton, England

Robert I. Parker, MD
Department of Pediatrics
SUNY at Stony Brook School of Medicine
Stony Brook, New York

Mark J. Peters, MD, PhD
Portex Unit
Institute of Child Health
London, United Kingdom

Frank S. Pidcock, MD
Departments of Physical Medicine & Rehabilitation
   and Pediatrics
The Johns Hopkins University School of Medicine
Baltimore, Maryland

Murray Pollack, MD, MBA
Phoenix Children's Hospital
Phoenix, Arizona

Steven Pon, MD
Department of Pediatrics
Weill Medical College of Cornell University
New York, New York

Frank L. Powell, PhD
Department of Medicine
University of California, San Diego, School of Medicine
San Diego, California

Jack F. Price, MD
Department of Pediatrics
Baylor College of Medicine
Houston, Texas

Michael Quasney, PhD, MD
Department of Pediatrics
University of Tennessee Health Science Center
Memphis, Tennessee

Gerardo Quezada, MD, FAAP
Department of Pediatrics
The University of Texas School of Medicine
Houston, Texas

Elisabeth L. Raab, MD
Department of Pediatrics
University of Southern California, Keck School of Medicine
Los Angeles, California

Surender Rajasekaran, MD, MPH
Department of Pediatrics
University of Tennesse Health Science Center
Memphis, Tennessee

Rangasamy Ramanathan, MD, FAAP
Department of Pediatrics
University of Southern California, Keck School
   of Medicine
Los Angeles, California

Suchitra Ranjit, MD, DCH
Pediatric Intensive Care Unit
Apollo Hospitals
Chennai, India

Thyyar M. Ravindranath, MD
Department of Pediatrics
Columbia University, College of Physicians and Surgeons
New York, New York

Chitra Ravishankar, MD
Department of Pediatrics
University of Pennsylvania
Philadelphia, Pennsylvania

Antonio Rodriguez-Nuñez, MD, PhD
Department of Pediatrics
University of Santiago de Compostela
Santiago de Compostela, Spain

Mark C. Rogers, MD, MBA
Department of Anesthesiology & Critical Care Medicine
The Johns Hopkins University School of Medicine
Baltimore, Maryland

Lewis H. Romer, MD
Departments of Anesthesiology & Critical Care Medicine,
   Pediatrics, and Cell Biology
The Johns Hopkins University School of Medicine
Baltimore, Maryland

Susan R. Rose, MD
Division of Pediatric Endocrinology
University of Cincinnati College of Medicine
Cincinnati, Ohio

Joseph W. Rossano, MD
Department of Pediatrics
Baylor College of Medicine
Houston, Texas

Daniel Russo, MD
Departamento de Pediatria
Universidad Austral School of Medicine
Pilar, Buenos Aires, Argentina

Monique M. Ryan, MB, BS, MMed, FRACP
Department of Paediatrics
Royal Children's Hospital
Parkville, Victoria, Australia

Michael E. Rytting, MD, FAAP
Department of Pediatrics
The University of Texas School of Medicine
Houston, Texas

Cristina Sadowsky, MD
Department of Physical Medicine & Rehabilitation
The Johns Hopkins University School of Medicine
Baltimore, Maryland

Cynthia F. Salorio, PhD
Department of Physical Medicine & Rehabilitation
The Johns Hopkins University School of Medicine
Baltimore, Maryland

Stephen M. Schexnayder, MD
Department of Pediatrics
University of Arkansas College of Medicine
Little Rock, Arkansas

Charles L. Schleien, MD
Departments of Pediatrics and Anesthesiology
Columbia University, College of Physicians and Surgeons
New York, New York

Eduardo Schnitzler, MD
Departamento de Pediatria
Universidad Austral School of Medicine
Pilar, Buenos Aires, Argentina

Steven M. Schwartz, MD
Department of Pediatrics
University of Toronto
Toronto, Ontario, Canada

Istvan Seri, MD
Professor of Pediatrics
University of Southern California, Keck School of Medicine

Donald H. Shaffner, MD
Department of Anesthesiology & Critical Care Medicine
The Johns Hopkins University School of Medicine
Baltimore, Maryland

Thomas P. Shanley, MD
Department of Pediatrics and Communicable Diseases
University of Michigan Medical School
Ann Arbor, Michigan

R. Lara Shekerdemian, MBChB, MD, MRCP (UK), FRACP, FRCPCH
Paediatric Intensive Care Unit
The Royal Children's Hospital
Melbourne, Victoria, Australia

Naoki Shimizu, MD, PhD
Department of Anaesthesia and Intensive Care
National Centre for Child Health and Development
Tokyo, Japan

Jakub Simon, MD
Department of Pediatrics
University of Maryland School of Medicine
Baltimore, Maryland

Shari Simone, MS, APRN, CPNP-AC
Department of Pediatrics
University of Maryland School of Medicine
Baltimore, Maryland

Rakesh Sindhi, MD, FACS
Department of Pediatrics
University of Pittsburgh School of Medicine
Pittsburgh, Pennsylvania

Sunit C. Singhi, MB, BS, MD
Department of Pediatrics
Postgraduate Institute of Medical Education and Research
Chandigarh, India

Pratibha D. Singhi, MB, BS, MD
Department of Pediatrics
Postgraduate Institute of Medical Education and Research
Chandigarh, India

Peter W. Skippen, MD, FANZCA, FJFICM, FRCPC
Department of Pediatrics
University of British Columbia
Vancouver, British Columbia, Canada

Zdenek Slavik, MD, DM, FRCPCH
Department of Pediatrics
Charles University
Pilsen, Czech Republic

Arthur Smerling, MD
Departments of Pediatrics and Anesthesiology
Columbia University, College of Physicians and Surgeons
New York, New York

Kyle A. Soltys, MD
Department of Pediatrics
University of Pittsburgh School of Medicine
Pittsburgh, Pennsylvania

F. Meridith Sonnett, MD
Department of Pediatrics
Columbia University, College of Physicians and Surgeons
New York, New York

Robert H. Squires, Jr., MD
Department of Pediatrics
University of Pittsburgh School of Medicine
Pittsburgh, Pennsylvania

Kimberly D. Statler, MD, MPH
Departments of Pediatrics and Neurology
University of Utah School of Medicine
Salt Lake City, Utah

Kurt R. Stenmark, MD
Department of Pediatric Critical Care
Developmental Lung Biology Laboratory
University of Colorado at Denver and Health Sciences Center
Denver, Colorado

Caron Strahlendorf, MD
Divisions of Hematology, Oncology,
   & Bone Marrow Transplantation
University of British Columbia
Vancouver, British Columbia, Canada

John P. Straumanis, MD
Department of Pediatrics
University of Maryland School of Medicine
Baltimore, Maryland

Kevin J. Sullivan, MD
Department of Anesthesiology & Critical Care
Mayo Clinic, College of Medicine
Rochester, Minnesota

Stacy J. Suskauer, MD
Department of Physical Medicine & Rehabilitation
The Johns Hopkins University School of Medicine
Baltimore, Maryland

William V. Tamborlane, MD
Department of Pediatrics
Yale University School of Medicine
New Haven, Connecticut

Robert F. Tamburro, MD, MSc
Department of Pediatrics
Pennsylvania State University College of Medicine
Hershey, Pennsylvania

Ronn E. Tanel, MD
Department of Pediatrics
University of Pennsylvania School of Medicine
Philadelphia, Pennsylvania

Robert C. Tasker, MB, BS, MD, FRCP
Department of Paediatrics
Cambridge University, School of Clinical Medicine
Cambridge, United Kingdom

David F. Teitel, MD
Department of Pediatrics
Cardiovascular Research Institute
University of California, San Francisco
San Francisco, California

Neal J. Thomas, MD, MSc
Pediatrics and Health Evaluation Sciences
Pennsylvania State University College of Medicine
Hershey, Pennsylvania

James A. Thomas, MD
Department of Pediatrics
University of Texas Southwestern Medical School
Dallas, Texas

Ann E. Thompson, MD
Department of Critical Care Medicine
University of Pittsburgh School of Medicine
Pittsburgh, Pennsylvania

James Tibballs, BMedSc, MB, BS, MEd, MBA, MD, FANZCA, FJFICM, FACTM
Australian Venom Research Unit
University of Melbourne
Melbourne, Victoria, Australia

Shane M. Tibby, MBChB, MRCP, MSc
Department of Paediatric Intensive Care
Evelina Children's Hospital
Guy's and St. Thomas' NHS Foundation Trust
London, United Kingdom

Pierre Tissières, MD, MSc
Départment de Pédiatrie
Hôpital de Bicêtre
Le Kremlin-Bicêtre, France

Joseph D. Tobias, MD
Department of Anesthesiology
University of Missouri School of Medicine
Columbia, Missouri

Philip Toltzis, MD
Department of Pediatrics
Case Western Reserve University
Cleveland, Ohio

Jeffrey A. Towbin, MD
Department of Pediatrics
Baylor College of Medicine
Houston, Texas

Melissa K. Trovato, MD
Department of Physical Medicine & Rehabilitation
The Johns Hopkins University School of Medicine
Baltimore, Maryland

Robert D. Truog, MD
Departments of Social Medicine & Anaesthesia
Harvard Medical School
Boston, Massachusetts

Vinay Vaidya, MB, BS
Department of Pediatrics
University of Maryland School of Medicine
Baltimore, Maryland

Edwin van der Voort, MD
Department of Pediatrics
Erasmus MC-Sophia Children's Hospital
Rotterdam, The Netherlands

Colin B. Van Orman, MD
Department of Pediatrics
University of Utah School of Medicine
Salt Lake City, Utah

John S. Venglarcik, III, MD
Department of Pediatrics
Northeastern Ohio Universities, College of Medicine
Rootstown, Ohio

Shekhar T. Venkataraman, MD
Departments of Critical Care Medicine and Pediatrics
University of Pittsburgh School of Medicine
Pittsburgh, Pennsylvania

Kathleen M. Ventre, MD
Department of Pediatrics
University of Utah School of Medicine
Salt Lake City, Utah

Prof.-Dr. med. Hans-Dieter Volk
Charité Institut für Medizinische Immunologie
Berlin, Germany

Steven A. Webber, MBChB, MRCP
Department of Pediatrics
University of Pittsburgh School of Medicine
Pittsburgh, Pennsylvania

Stuart A. Weinzimer, MD
Department of Pediatrics
Yale University School of Medicine
New Haven, Connecticut

Richard S. Weisman, PharmD, ABAT
Department of Pediatrics
University of Miami, Miller School of Medicine
Miami, Florida

David L. Wessel, MD
Division of Critical Care Medicine
Children's National Medical Center
Washington, DC

Randall C. Wetzel, MB, BS, MS Bus., FAAP, FCCM
Departments of Pediatrics and Anesthesiology
University of Southern California, Keck School of Medicine
Los Angeles, California

Derek S. Wheeler, MD
Department of Pediatrics
University of Cincinnati Medical Center
Cincinnati, Ohio

Michael Wilhelm, MD
Department of Pediatrics
Columbia University, College of Physicians and Surgeons
New York, New York

Kenneth D. Winkel, MB, BS, PhD
Australian Venom Research Unit
Department of Pharmacology
University of Melbourne
Melbourne, Australia

Gerhard K. Wolf, MD
Department of Anaesthesia
Harvard Medical School
Boston, Massachusetts

Edward C.C. Wong, MD
Departments of Pediatrics and Pathology
George Washington University School of Medicine
    and Health Sciences
Washington, DC

Hector R. Wong, MD
Department of Pediatrics
University of Cincinnati College of Medicine
Cincinnati, Ohio

Angela T. Wratney, MD, MHSc
Department of Pediatrics
George Washington University School
    of Medicine
Washington, DC

Myron Yaster, MD
Department of Anesthesiology & Critical Care Medicine
The Johns Hopkins University School of Medicine
Baltimore, Maryland

Roger W. Yurt, MD
Department of Surgery
Weill Medical College of Cornell University
New York, New York

Arno L. Zaritsky, MD
Department of Pediatrics
University of Florida College of Medicine
Gainesville, Florida

David Zideman, QHP(C), BSc, MB, BS, FRCA, FIMC
Department of Anaesthetics
Hammersmith Hospital
London, United Kingdom

Basilia Zingarelli, MD, PhD
Deparment of Pediatrics
University of Cincinnati College of Medicine
Cincinnati, Ohio

Athena F. Zuppa, MD, MSCE
Department of Anesthesiology and Critical Care
University of Pennsylvania School of Medicine
Philadelphia, Pennsylvania

The first edition of the *Rogers' Textbook of Pediatric Intensive Care*, through the vision of Mark Rogers, set out to codify the existing knowledge of a new specialty with scientific rigor, a comprehensive scope, and a dedication to the well-being of the sick child. Twenty years later, the world of pediatric intensive care is virtually unrecognizable, even compared to the last edition, which was published in 1996. While the traditions of the *Rogers' Textbook* endure in this fourth edition, the authors and editors have also sought to capture the changed world in which pediatric clinicians care for their patients.

All of medicine is in transition from a view that emphasizes pathophysiologic mechanisms to one that emphasizes genetic variability and molecular interactions. Therefore, this textbook presents pediatric intensive care from both perspectives. The new one, emphasizing genetic variability and molecular biology, is covered in individual chapters and in a special section entitled "Basic Concepts of Pediatric Critical Care."

The care delivery system has also evolved, with far greater emphasis on the scientific principles of quality improvement, patient safety, evidence-based medicine, technology, and biomedical informatics. Yet, these tools do not benefit the sick child fully without the leadership of the pediatric intensivist, as detailed in the sections concerning "Professionalism, Leadership, and Systems-based Practice" and "Life Support Technologies."

Nevertheless, the care of the sick child and his or her family remain the focus of this edition. Sections on diseases related to each organ system, on "Initial Stabilization," and on "Ethical and Compassionate Care of the Sick Child" remain the heart of the book.

The first edition of the *Rogers' Textbook* was compiled almost entirely by the faculty of the Johns Hopkins PICU. The current edition reflects the involvement of nearly 300 authors and editors from 16 different countries. Pediatric intensive care is now decidedly global in scale, yet closely integrated, with experts from every country sharing knowledge and contributing to this project. The advent of the World Federation of Pediatric Intensive and Critical Care Societies (WFPICCS), with its quadrennial World Congresses and of our specialty journal, *Pediatric Critical Care Medicine*, has immensely fostered this global integration. The fourth edition of the *Rogers' Textbook* becomes a partner in this effort by serving as the official WFPICCS textbook and by the publishing of regular updates in *Pediatric Critical Care Medicine*.

Every comprehensive medical text requires an enormous investment of time, energy, and expertise by its contributors. This text would not have been possible without the dedication and diligence of the authors and editors represented in its pages. Our managing editor, Tzipora Sofare, has looked after the myriad of tasks necessary to produce such a text and somehow managed to keep this large group of talented and busy people focused. On behalf of the editorial board, I express our gratitude for her dedication, fine attention to detail, and passion for the written word. Lippincott Williams & Wilkins, our publisher, has been unfailingly supportive of this project. We thank Brian Brown for his encouragement, Molly Connors for her advice, and Wendy Beth Jackelow for her artistic renderings.

I am deeply grateful and enormously indebted to all of those involved in this project. Moreover, we as a group owe a debt of gratitude to all of the physicians, nurses, technicians, and other caregivers who have supported us, participated in shaping this specialty, and provided excellent care to our patients. If just one critically ill child is saved because of these efforts, then that dividend will be sufficient.

David G. Nichols, MD
Baltimore, MD, USA

■ FOREWORD

Tell me, and I will forget
  Show me, and I will remember
  Involve me, and I will understand
  —Chinese proverb

The publication in 1988 of the first edition of the *Rogers' Textbook of Pediatric Intensive Care* was a significant moment in the evolution of pediatric intensive care (PIC). It marked the first comprehensive published review that consolidated and defined the body of science of this new, emerging specialty. With subsequent updated editions, it is still considered by many as the standard reference source for pediatric critical care medicine. Almost 2 years later, the launch of the fourth edition marks another significant milestone in the international growth and expansion of this increasingly complex specialty.

The formative years of PIC focused on establishing new clinical techniques, adapting new technology, and creating mostly unproven theories for understanding evolving clinical practice. With the application of vigorous scientific principles, a period of reevaluation and exploration followed that generated a legitimate body of science unique to this specialty. Those of us who were trained and mentored three decades ago by the pioneers of our specialty have been fortunate to observe from the beginning the maturation of PIC, including an extraordinary acceleration in growth of new knowledge created worldwide by an enthusiastic and expanding international group of highly trained clinical scientists.

Original scientific enquiry into the mysteries of PIC now involves research groups from around the world. The rate of transformation and the increasing sophistication of acquiring new knowledge reflect the growth and richness of problem solving by today's generation of international specialists, many of whom have contributed to this textbook. These leaders have accepted with gusto the truism attributed to John Updike that "problems that have solutions are not problems."

Each new generation of specialists builds upon the past and has increasingly powerful scientific tools and innovative statistical techniques to problem solve. Sophisticated design and development of complex studies are increasingly focused on revealing the fundamental basis of disease and disease processes that create life-threatening illness in children. The international depth and quality of the body of scientific knowledge captured in the new edition is extraordinary. It also provides a glimpse for the future through discussions of new developments in genomic medicine, microcellular responses to stress, and molecular bases of multiple-organ interaction, including sepsis and a host of other fundamental but complex molecular and micro responses to current disease and physiologic processes.

An even more striking and pleasing observation of this edition is the significant diversity of backgrounds and experiences of those from this expanding, multidisciplinary, international community who contribute as authors.

The World Federation of Pediatric and Intensive Care Societies (WFPICCS) was formally established at an inaugural Board meeting in Paris in 1997. It arose from the vision of a few world leaders in pediatric critical care who believed that together they could create something greater than their individual efforts. All shared a vision to create a global environment in which all children with potential life-threatening illnesses would have access to an appropriate high standard of intensive care that would be made possible through the promotion of research and education and the distribution of knowledge across international borders.

The collective wisdom of the inaugural Board of WFPICCS determined as a high priority a specific objective to promote international education programs through the active dissemination of scientific information relevant to the specialty worldwide. An important contribution to that process was achieved at the WFPICCS World Congress in Montreal in the year 2, when the definitive WFPICCS international PIC journal, *Pediatric Critical Care Medicine*, was launched. This journal now has over 2, subscribers worldwide, receives over 3 submissions for publication each year, is indexed by ISI, and regularly publishes abstracts in 6 languages, including abstract supplements for prestigious international symposia and congresses.

The publication of the fourth edition of the *Rogers' Textbook on Pediatric Intensive Care* marks another milestone for the international PIC community. WFPICCS has endorsed this edition as the official textbook of the World Federation. Contributions from all regions of the world make it an invaluable resource for PIC specialists and others worldwide. The launch of this WFPICCS international textbook also creates an exciting and innovative link with its highly successful international journal. This collaboration provides a unique, ongoing, and timely opportunity to refresh the textbook's content through regularly published, targeted updates of individual sections of the textbook within the journal.

During an informal discussion among a group of international leaders at the 2 WFPICCS Congress, a prominent North American leader was overheard saying, "We were not aware that there were so many pediatric critical care specialists outside of our country doing such outstanding [academic] work."

In Thomas Friedman's book, *The World is Flat*, the author reminds us that international creativity exploded "when the walls came down and the windows went up" through globalization of products and services. Friedman refers to the new technologies of personal computers, fiberoptic cables, and freely available shared software that have shrunk the business world and empowered individuals to collaborate in ways that are still evolving and yet to be discovered. Health care knowledge and clinical practice are not immune to this change. The rate of growth of new knowledge worldwide, and its distribution and dissemination create new and exciting challenges, particularly to editors of health care textbooks and journals.

The traditional openness of PIC specialists to share new knowledge cuts across borders and melts away cultural and other differences. It reflects our shared humanity. A child whose life is threatened by reversible disease should not be denied access to appropriate support through ignorance caused by delays or failure to transfer accumulated wisdom, knowledge, and experiences among specialists worldwide. The international PIC community now has many opportunities for rapidly communicating scientific findings and experiences. The ultimate benefactors are seriously ill infants and children worldwide.

The launch of the fourth edition *of Rogers' Textbook of Pediatric Intensive Care* as the official textbook for the World Federation and the international success of the WFPICCS journal, *Pediatric Critical Care Medicine*, confirms the vision of the inaugural Board of WFPICCS and reinforces the importance of maintaining strong international leadership, collaboration, and involvement within our specialty.

Although many new and exciting challenges lie ahead as we learn and adapt to the new flat world of globalization of healthcare, the launch of this fourth edition marks another significant step forward for our profession and, ultimately, our patients and their families.

Geoffrey A. Barker, MD, FRCP
Inaugural President, World Federation
of Pediatric Intensive & Critical Care Societies
Professor, Critical Care, Anesthesia, and Pediatrics
Hospital for Sick Children
University of Toronto

■ CONTENTS

PART ONE ■ CRITICAL CARE INTEGRATION

SECTION I ■ INTRODUCTION TO THE PRACTICE OF PEDIATRIC CRITICAL CARE

SECTION II ■ PROFESSIONALISM, LEADERSHIP, AND SYSTEMS-BASED PRACTICE

SECTION II ■ ENVIRONMENTAL CRISES

SECTION III ■ LIFE-SUPPORT TECHNOLOGIES

PART THREE ■ CRITICAL CARE ORGAN SYSTEMS

SECTION I ■ RESPIRATORY DISEASE

SECTION VIII ■ RENAL, ENDOCRINE, AND METABOLIC DISORDERS

SECTION IX ■ ONCOLOGIC AND HEMATOLOGIC DISORDERS

A SELECTED GLOSSARY OF ABBREVIATIONS

AACT	American Academy of Clinical Toxicology
AAMC	American Association of Medical Colleges
AB	acute bronchiolitis
ABCD	amphotericin B colloidal dispersion
ABI	acquired brain injury
ABIM	American Board of Internal Medicine
ABLC	amphotericin B lipid complex
ABP	American Board of Pediatrics
ABRT	activity-based restoration therapy
ACCM	American College of Critical Care Medicine
ACCP	American College of Chest Physicians
ACGME	Accreditation Council of Graduate Medical Education
AchR	acetylcholine receptor
ACP-ASIM	American College of Physicians-American Society of Internal Medicine
ACS	abdominal compartment syndrome
ACS	acute chest syndrome
AD	autonomic dysreflexia
AD	autosomal dominant
ADA	adenosine deaminase
ADEM	acute disseminated encephalomyelitis
AED	automated external defibrillator
AFB	acid-fast bacillus
AG	anion gap
AHA	American Heart Association
AI	adrenal insufficiency
AICDA	activation-induced cytidine deaminase
AIDP	acute inflammatory demyelinating polyradiculopathy
AIF	apoptosis-inducing factor
AIP	acute intermittent porphyria
AIS	arterial ischemic stroke
ALA	5-aminolevulinic acid
ALC	absolute lymphocyte count
ALCAPA	anomalous left coronary artery from the pulmonary artery
ALL	acute lymphoblastic leukemia
AlloSCT	allogeneic stem cell transplantation
ALTE	apparent life-threatening event
AMAN	acute motor axonal neuropathy
AML	acute mylelocytic leukemia
AMSAN	acute motor and sensory axonal neuropathy
ANC	absolute neutrophil count
ANF	atrial natriuretic factor
ANOVA	analysis of variance
ANP	A-type natriuretic peptide, atrial natriuretic peptide
ANT	adenine nucleotide translocator
AP-1	activator protein-1
APA	antiphospholipid antibodies
APACHE	Acute Physiology and Chronic Health Evaluation
APAS	antiphospholipid antibody syndrome
APL	acute promyelocytic leukemia
APR	all-patient redefined
APRV	airway pressure release ventilation
AR	autosomal recessive
ARPANET	Advanced Research Projects Agency Network
ARR	absolute risk reduction
ARVD	arrhythmogenic right ventricular dysplasia
ASA	acetylsalicylic acid
ASC	acute splenic sequestration crisis
ASIA	American Spinal Injury Association
ASO	allele-specific oligonucleotide
ATC	automatic tube compensation
ATN	acute tubular necrosis
ATRA	all-trans retinoic acid
AUC	area under the curve
AutoSCT	autologous stem cell transplantation
AVNRT	atrioventricular nodal reentrant tachycardia
AVP	arginine vasopressin
AVRT	atrioventricular reciprocating tachycardia
BAEP	brainstem auditory-evoked potential
BCAA	branched-chain amino acids
BDG	bidirectional Glenn shunt
BDNF	brain-derived neurotrophic factor
bHLH	basic helix-loop-helix
BIP	bleomycin-induced pneumonitis
BIS	bispectral index
BLI	blast lung injury
BNP	B-type natriuretic peptide, brain natriuretic peptide
BO	bronchiolitis obliterans
BOOP	bronchiolitis obliterans with organizing pneumonia
BPD	bronchopulmonary dysplasia
BPI	bactericidal/permeability-increasing protein
BT	Blalock-Taussig
BTK	Bruton's tyrosine kinase
C1-INH	C1 esterase inhibitor
CAM	cell adhesion molecule
CAMTS	Commission on Accreditation of Medical Transport Systems
CARS	compensatory anti-inflammatory response syndrome
CASR	calcium-sensing receptor
CAVH	continuous arteriovenous hemofiltration
CCAM	congenital cystic adenomatoid malformation
CCHS	congenital central hypoventilation syndrome
CCI	corrected count increment
CDC	Centers for Disease Control and Prevention
CDH	congenital diaphragmatic hernia
CDSR	Cochrane Database of Systematic Reviews
CEI	cholinesterase inhibitors
CFU	colony-forming units
CGD	chronic granulomatous disease
cGVHD	chronic graft-versus-host disease
Cho	choline and phosphatidylcholine
CID	combined immune deficiencies
CIM	critical illness myopathy

CIMNA	critical illness neuromuscular abnormality
CIN	contrast medium-induced nephropathy
CIP	critical illness polyneuropathy
CM	cerebral malaria
CMAP	compound muscle action potentials
CML	chronic myelogenous leucemia
CMO I/II	corticosterone methyloxidase I/II
CMRGlu	cerebral metabolic rates for glucose
CMS	Centers for Medicare and Medicaid Services
CNP	c-type natriuretic peptide
CoBaTrICE	Competency-based Training programme in Intensive Care Medicine for Europe
COMT	catechol-O-methyltransferase
COPE	Creating Opportunities for Parent Empowerment
CPD	citrate-monobasic sodium phosphate-dextrose
CPDA-1	citrate-monobasic sodium phosphate-dextrose-adenine
CPK	creatine phosphokinase
CPOE	computerized physician order entry
CPT	current procedural terminology
CPT	chest physiotherapy
CQI	continuous quality improvement
CR	complement receptor
CRBSI	catheter-related bloodstream infection
CRH	corticotrophin-releasing hormone
CRIB	Clinical Risk Index for Babies
CRP	C-reactive protein
CRRT	continuous renal replacement therapy
CRT	capillary refill time
CRT	cardiac resynchronization therapy
CSE	convulsive status epilepticus
CSW	cerebral salt wasting
CTL	cytotoxic T lymphocyte
CTX	ciguatoxin
CV	coefficient of the variation
CVA	cerebrovascular accident
CVB	coxsackievirus B
CVD	cerebrovascular disease
CVID	common variable immunodeficiency
CVVH	continuous venovenous hemofiltration
CVVHD	continuous venovenous hemodialysis
CVVHDF	continuous venovenous hemodiafiltration
DBD	donation after brain death
DC	dendritic cell
DCD	donation after cardiac death
DCM	dilated cardiomyopathy
DDAVP	1-deamino(8-D-arginine) vasopressin
DF	dengue fever
DGS	DiGeorge syndrome
DHA	docosahexaenoic acid
DHCA	deep hypothermic circulatory arrest
DHEAS	dehydroepiandrosterone sulfate
DHF	decompensated heart failure
DHF	dengue hemorrhagic fever
DI	diabetes insipidus
DIC	disseminated intravascular coagulation
DIT	diiodotyrosine
DKA	diabetic ketoacidosis
DMD	Duchenne muscular dystrophy
DMSO	dimethyl sulfoxide
DORV	double-outlet right venticle
DPF	differential pathlength factor
DPI	dry-powder inhaler
DPPC	dipalmitoylphosphatidylcholine
DRG	diagnosis-related group
DSS	dengue shock syndrome
dTc-p	central-to-peripheral temperature gradient
dTp-a	peripheral-to-ambient temperature gradient
DWI	diffusion-weighted imaging
EAAs	excitatory amino acids

EAPCCT	European Association of Poisons Centres and Clinical Toxicologists
EAT	ectopic atrial tachycardia
EBM	evidence-based medicine
ECF	extracellular fluid
ECLS	extracorporeal life support
ECM	extracellular matrix
ECPR	extracorporeal cardiopulmonary resuscitation
EDH	epidural hematoma
EDHF	endothelial-derived hyperpolarizing factor
EEE	Eastern equine encephalitis
EELV	end-expiratory lung volume
EFE	endocardial fibroelastosis
EGFR	epidermal growth factor receptor
EIA	enzyme immunoassay
ELBW	extremely low birth weight
ELISA	enzyme-linked immunosorbent assay
ELSO	Extracorporeal Life Support Organization
EMG	electromyography
EMR	electronic medical record
EMS-C	emergency medical services for children
EMT	epithelial-mesenchymal transdifferentiation
EMTALA	Emergency Medical Transportation and Labor Act
ENaCs	epithelial sodium channels
EPA	eicosapentaenoic acid
ER	endoplasmic reticulum
ERK	extracellular receptor kinase
ERK 1/2	extracellular signal-regulated kinase 1 and 2
ESRD	end-stage renal disease
ET	endothelin
ETC	electron transport chain
ETI	endotracheal intubation
ETT	endotracheal tube
FAOD	fatty acid oxidation disorder
FAST	focused assessment by sonography in trauma
FDP	fibrin degradation products
FGF	fibroblast growth factor
FHF	fulminant hepatic failure
FISH	fluorescence in situ hybridization
FLAIR	fluid-attenuated inversion recovery
FMEA	failure modes and effects analysis
FOT	forced oscillation technique
FRC	functional residual capacity
FTC	fiberoptic transducer-tipped catheter
FWD	free water deficit
G6PD	glucose-6-phosphate dehydrogenase
GAS	group A *Streptococcus*
GAβHS	group A β hemolytic streptococcal disease
GBS	group B *Streptococcus*
GBS	Guillain-Barré syndrome
GCSE	generalized convulsive status epilepticus
GCSF	granulocyte colony-stimulating factor
GHB	gamma hydroxybutyrate
GLA	gamma-linoleic acid
Gln	glutamine
Glu	glutamic acid
GLUT	glucose transporter protein
GM-CSF	granulocyte-macrophage colony-stimulating factor
GN	glomerulonephritis
GRE	gradient-recalled echo
GSD	glycogen-storage disease
GSH	glutathione
GSSG	oxidized and inactive form of glutathione
GVHD	graft-versus-host disease
HAART	highly active antiretroviral therapy
HAE	hereditary angioedema
HAS	human albumin solution
HAT	human African trypanosomiasis
HC	heparin cofactor

hCG	human chorionic gonadotropin
HCM	hypertrophic cardiomyopathy
HDi	intermittent hemodialysis
HELLP	hemolysis, elevated liver enzymes, and low platelets
HFJV	high-frequency jet ventilation
HFRS	hemorrhagic fever with renal syndrome
HFV	high-frequency ventilation
HGF	hepatocyte growth factor
HHS	hyperglycemic hyperosmolar syndrome
HI	hyperinsulinism
Hib	Haemophilus influenzae type b
HIE	hypoxic-ischemic encephalopathy
HIF	hypoxia inducible factor
HIPAA	Health Insurance Portability and Accountability Act
HIT	heparin-induced thrombocytopenia
HLA	human leukocyte antigen
HLA	histocompatibility leukocyte antigen
HLH	hemophagocytic lymphohistiocytosis
HMGB1	high mobility group box 1
hMPV	human metapneumovirus
HO	heme oxygenase
HPA	hypothalamic-pituitary-adrenal
HPC	hematopoietic progenitor cell
HPE	homeostatic peripheral expansion
HPS	Hantavirus pulmonary syndrome
HRE	hypoxia response elements
HSCT	hematopoietic stem cell transplant
HSE	herpes simplex encephalitis
HSF	heat shock factor
HSP	heat shock protein
HTIG	human tetanus immunoglobulin
HUS	hemolytic uremic syndrome
IABP	intra-aortic balloon pump
IAH	intra-abdominal hypertension
IART	intra-atrial reentrant tachycardia
ICAM	intercellular adhesion molecule
ICD	International Classification of Disease
ICD	implantable cardioverter-defibrillator
ICOS	inducible T-cell costimulator gene
IEM	inborn errors of metabolism
IF	intrinsic factor
IgSF	immunoglobulin superfamily
IKK	inhibitor κB kinase
IMCI	integrated management of childhood illness
IMV	intermittent mandatory ventilation
iNO	inhaled nitric oxide
IO	intraosseous
IOM	Institute of Medicine
IP	ischemic preconditioning
IP3	inositol 1,4,5-triphosphate
IPA	invasive pulmonary aspergillosis
IPEX	immune deficiency, polyendocrinopathy, X-linked
IQR	interquartile range
IRAK	IL-1 receptor-associated kinase
IRF	interferon regulatory transcription factor
iTBI	inflicted traumatic brain injury
ITP	idiopathic thrombocytopenic purpura
JCAHO	Joint Commission on Accreditation of Healthcare Organizations
JE	Japanese encephalitis
JET	junctional ectopic tachycardia
JMG	juvenile myasthenia gravis
JNK	c-jun kinase
K_{ATP}	ATP-sensitive potassium
KGF	keratinocyte growth factor
LAD-1	leukocyte adhesion deficiency-1
LamB	liposomal amphotericin B
LBP	LPS-binding protein
LCMRg	local cerebral metabolic rate for glucose
LCOS	low cardiac output syndrome
LCT	long-chain triglycerides
LDF	laser-Doppler flowmetry
LFA	lymphocyte function-associated antigen
LGMD	limb-girdle muscular dystrophies
LHR	lung-head ratio
LIP	lower inflection point
LIP	lymphocytic interstitial pneumonitis
LMA	laryngeal mask airway
LMWH	low-molecular-weight heparin
LOCHS	late-onset central hypoventilation syndrome
LODS	Logistic Organ Dysfunction Score
LPR	lactate-to-pyruvate ratio
LQTS	long QT syndrome
LRR	leucine-rich repeat
LTA	lipoteichoic acid
LTD	long-term depression
LTP	long-term potentiation
LVNC	left ventricular noncompaction
MAC	membrane attack complex
MAC	mean alveolar concentration
MAC	*Mycobacterium avium* complex
MALDI-TOF	matrix-assisted laser desorption ionization-time of flight
MANOVA	multivariate analysis of variance
MAO	monoamine oxidase
MAPK	mitogen-activated protein kinase
MARS	molecular absorbent recirculating system
MAS	meconium aspiration syndrome
MAS	macrophage activation syndrome
MASPs	MLB-associated serine-proteases
MAST	military anti-shock trousers
MAT	multifocal atrial tachycardia
MBL	mannose-binding lectin
MCHC	mean corpuscular hemoglobin concentration
M-CSF	macrophage colony-stimulating factor
MCT	medium-chain triglycerides
MCV	mean cell volume
MDA	methylenedioxyamphetamine
MDI	metered-dose inhaler
MDS	myelodysplastic syndrome
MELAS	mitochondrial encephalopathy, lactic acidosis, and stroke
MERRF	mitochondrial encephalopathy with ragged red fibers
MH	malignant hyperthermia
MHC	major histocompatibility complex
MHLS	malignant hyperthermia-like syndrome
mI	myoinositol
MIC	minimum inhibitory concentration
MIF	macrophage migration inhibitory factor
MIP	maximum intensity projections
MIT	monoiodotyrosine
MLC	myosin light chain
MLCK	myosin light-chain kinase
MMPs	matrix metalloproteinases
MOC	maintenance of certification
MPS	mucopolysaccharidoses
MRP1	multidrug resistance-associated protein 1
MRS	MR spectroscopy
MSAF	meconium-stained amniotic fluid
MSE	mean squared error
MSUD	maple syrup urine disease
MYPT	myosin phosphatase target subunit
NA	neuraminidase
NAA	N-acetyl aspartate
NAC	N-acetylcysteine
NADPH	nicotinamide adenine dinucleotide phosphate
NAHI	nonaccidental head injury
NALPs	NACCHT-, LRR-pyrin domain (PYD)-containing proteins

NAPQI	N-acetyl-p-benzoquinone-imine
NASCIS	National Acute Spinal Cord Injury Studies
NAVA	neurally adjusted ventilatory assist
NCC	neurocysticercosis
NCRSE	nonconvulsive refractory status epilepticus
NCSE	nonconvulsive status epilepticus
NCX	Na^+/Ca^{2+} exchanger
NEC	necrotizing enterocolitis
NEI	neuroendocrine-immune
NEMO	nuclear factor κB essential modulator
NI	neuraminidase inhibitors
NIPPV	noninvasive positive-pressure ventilation
NIV	noninvasive ventilation
NMBA	neuromuscular blocking agents
NMS	neurolept malignant syndrome
NNIS	National Nosocomial Infections Surveillance
NNRTI	non-nucleoside reverse transcriptase inhibitors
NOD	nucleotide-binding oligomerization domain
NPPV	noninvasive positive-pressure ventilation
NPV	negative predictive value
NRCPR	National Registry of Cardiopulmonary Resuscitation
NRTI	nucleoside reverse transcriptase inhibitors
NSE	neuron serum enolase
NT	neurotrophin
NTI	nonthyroidal illness
NT-proBNP	N-terminal pro-brain natriuretic pepetide
NTR	neurotrophin receptor
ONOO	peroxynitrite
OPA	oropharyngeal airway
OPO	Organ Procurement Organization
OPS	orthogonal polarization spectral
OPTN	Organ Procurement and Transplantation Network
OSAS	obstructive sleep apnea syndrome
PAC	pulmonary artery catheter
PAF	platelet-activating factor
PAH	pulmonary artery hypertension
PAI-1	plasminogen activator inhibitor 1
PAMP	pathogen-associated molecular pattern
PAPVC	partial anomalous pulmonary venous connection
PARP	poly(ADP-ribose) polymerase
PAV	proportional-assist ventilation
PBB	protected bronchial brush
PBC	pre-Botzinger Complex
PBEF	pre-B-cell colony-enhancing factor
PBG	porphobilinogen
PBI	primary blast injury
PBMC	peripheral blood monocytes
PBP	penicillin-binding protein
PC	pressure control/pressure-controlled
PC	phosphatidylcholine
PC	protein C
PCA	patient-controlled analgesia
PCD	programmed cell death
PCP	paramethoxyamphetamine, phencyclidine
PCP	pneumocystis pneumonia, *Pneumocystis carinii* pneumonia, *Pneumocystis jiroveci* (previously *P. carinii*) pneumonia
PCPC	Pediatric Cerebral Performance Category
PD	peritoneal dialysis
PDA	personal digital assistant
PDA	patent ductus arteriosus
PDE	phosphodiesterase
PEA	pulseless electrical activity
PECAM	platelet-endothelial cell adhesion molecule
PEEPi	intrinsic positive end-expiratory pressure
PEG-ES	polyethylene glycol electrolyte solutions
PELOD	Pediatric Logistic Organ Dysfunction
PEMOD	Pediatric Multiple Organ Dysfunction
PEP	post-exposure prophylaxis

PET	partial exchange transfusion
PFI	peripheral perfusion (flow) index
PGIS	prostacyclin synthase
PI	protease inhibitors
PI3K	phosphatidylinositol-3-kinase
PICO	*p*opulation, *i*ntervention, *c*omparison, *o*utcomes
PIE	pulmonary interstitial emphysema
PIM	Pediatric Index of Mortality
PIRO	*p*redisposing conditions, *i*nsult, *r*esponse, *o*rgan dysfunction
PKA	protein kinase A
PKB	protein kinase B
PKC	protein kinase C
PLEDS	periodic lateralized epileptiform discharges
PMC	pseudomembranous colitis
PMN/PMNL	polymorphonuclear leukocyte, polymorphonuclear neutrophil
PMV	prolonged mechanical ventilation
POPC	pediatric overall performance category
PPE	personal protective equipment
PPHN	persistent pulmonary hypertension of the newborn
PPRs	pattern recognition receptors
PPV	positive predictive value
PPV	positive-pressure ventilation
PRISM	Pediatric Risk of Mortality
PRSL	potential renal solute load
PRTH	pituitary resistance to thyroid hormone
PRVC	pressure-regulated volume control
PS	phosphatidylserine
PSI	Physiologic Stability Index
PSV	pressure-support ventilation
PTA	posttraumatic amnesia
PT-GVHD	posttransfusion graft-versus-host disease
PTHrP	parathyroid hormone-related peptide
PTLD	posttransplantion lymphoproliferative disorder
PTU	propylthiouracil
PUFA	polyunsaturated fatty acid
pVHL	von Hippel-Landau protein
PYD	pyrin domain
Q10	ubiquinone
QI	quality improvement
RA	retinoic acid
RAAS	renin-angiotensin-aldosterone system
RACHS-1	Risk-adjusted Classification System for Congenital Heart Surgery
RAR	retinoic acid receptor
RAS	reticular activating system
rBPI	recombinant bactericidal/permeability-increasing protein
RCM	restrictive cardiomyopathy
RCP	respiratory care practitioner
RCPCH	Royal College of Paediatrics and Child Health
RCT	randomized, controlled trial
RDS	respiratory distress syndrome
R-ECMO	resuscitation extracorporeal membrane oxygenation
REE	resting energy expenditure
REM	rapid-eye movement
RFLPs	restriction fragment length polymorphisms
rFVIIa	recombinant factor VIIa
RHAMM	receptor for hyaluronic acid-mediated motility
rhAPC	recombinant human activated protein C
rhF.VIIa	activated recombinant human factor VII
rhGCSF	recombinant human granulocyte colony-stimulating factor
ROC	receiver operating characteristic
ROI	return on investment
ROM	range of motion
RONS	reactive oxygen and nitrogen species
ROSC	return of spontaneous circulation

RPLS	reversible posterior leukoencephalopathy
RQ	respiratory quotient (CO_2 production/O_2 consumption)
RRR	relative risk reduction
RSE	refractory status epilepticus
RSI	rapid-sequence intubation
RSL	renal solute load
RSV	respiratory syncytial virus
RT	reactive (or secondary) thrombocytosis
RTH	resistance to thyroid hormone
RVU	relative value unit
RXR	retinoid X receptor
RyR	ryanodine receptor
S1P	sphingosine-1-phosphate
SAM	surface-active material
SAMPLE	*symptoms, allergies, medications, past illnesses, last meal, events* and environment
SAP	simplified acute physiology
SBECD	sulphobutylether-beta-cyclodextrin sodium
SCA	sickle cell anemia
SCCM	Society of Critical Care Medicine
SCD	sickle cell disease
SCD	sudden cardiac death
SCI	spinal cord injury
SCID	severe combined immunodeficiency disease
SCIWORA	spinal cord injury without radiographic abnormality
sCR1	soluble complement receptor type 1
SCUT	slow continuous ultrafiltration
SDH	subdural hemorrhage
SE	spin echo
SE	status epilepticus
SERCA	sarcoplasmic/endoplasmic reticulum Ca^{2+}-ATPase
SFD	solute fluid deficit
sGC	soluble guanylate cyclase
SIADH	syndrome of inappropriate antidiuretic hormone
SIMV-PC	synchronized, intermittent mandatory ventilation-pressure control
SLE	systemic lupus erythematosus
SMA 1	spinal muscular atrophy type 1
SMS	superior mediastinal syndrome
SNAP	Score for Neonatal Acute Physiology
SNARE	soluble N-ethylmaleimide-sensitive factor attachment protein receptor
SND	sinus node dysfunction
SNP	single nucleotide polymorphism
SNP	sodium nitroprusside
SNS	sympathetic nervous system
SOC	store-operated calcium
SOD	superoxide dismutase
SOFA	sequential organ failure assessment
SOJIA	systemic onset juvenile idiopathic arthritis
SR	sarcoplasmic reticulum
SRBD	sleep-related breathing disorders
SS	serotonin syndrome
SSI	surgical-site infection
SSPE	subacute sclerosing panencephalitis
StAR	steroidogenic acute regulatory protein
STSS	streptococcal toxic shock syndrome
SVCS	superior vena cava syndrome
SVDK	snake venom detection kit
SVT	supraventricular tachycardia
SWI	susceptibility-weighted imaging
T&A	adenotonsillectomy
TA	truncus arteriosus
TACI	transmembrane activator and calcium-modulating and cyclophilin ligand interactor
TAFI	thrombin-activatable fibrinolysis inhibitor
TAI	traumatic axonal injury
TAMOF	thrombocytopenia-associated multiple organ failure

TAPVC	total anomalous pulmonary venous connection
TBG	thyroxine-binding globulin
TBM	tubercular meningitis
TBSA	total body surface area
TBW	total body water
TCA	tricarboxylic acid cycle
TCD	transcranial Doppler
TFPI	tissue factor pathway inhibitor
TGA	transposition of the great arteries
TGF	transforming growth factor
THAM	tromethamine
TIR	Toll/IL-1 receptor
TISS	Therapeutic Intervention Scoring System
TK	thymidine kinase
TLR	Toll-like receptor
TLS	tumor lysis syndrome
TM	tympanic membrane
TM	toxic megacolon
TMP-SMX	trimethoprim-sulfamethoxazole
TMP-SMZ	trimethoprim-sulfamethoxazole
TOI	tissue oxygenation index
tPA	tissue plasminogen activator
TR	thyroid hormone receptors
TRAF	TNF receptor-associated factor
TRALI	transfusion-related acute lung injury
TRBC	(99m)Tc (Technetium)-labelled red blood cells
TRH	thyrotropin-releasing hormone
TRP	tubular reabsorption of phosphate
TRPC	transient receptor potential channels
TSH	thyroid-stimulating hormone
TSST	toxic shock syndrome toxin
TTN	transient tachypnea of the newborn
TTP	thrombotic thrombocytopenic purpura
TTX	tetrodotoxin
TXA_2	thromboxane
UGT	glucuronosyltransferase
UH	unfractionated heparin
UIP	upper inflection point
UNOS	United Network for Organ Sharing
V/Q	ventilation/perfusion
VAP	ventilator-associated pneumonia
VC	volume control/volume-controlled
VC	vital capacity
VCAM	vascular cell adhesion molecule
VDR	vitamin D receptor
VE-cadherin	vascular endothelial-cadherin
VEGF	vascular endothelial growth factor
VEP	visual-evoked potential
VF	ventricular fibrillation
VHF	viral hemorrhagic fevers
VICAM-1	vascular cellular adhesion molecule-1
VILI	ventilator induced lung injury
VLBW	very low birth weight
VNTRs	variable number of tandem repeats
VOC	vaso-occlusive crisis
VOD	veno-occlusive disease
VoIP	Voice-over Internet protocol
VTE	venous thromboembolism
WASP	Wiscott-Aldrich syndrome protein
WBGT	wet bulb globe temperature
WFPCCS	World Federation of Pediatric Critical Care Societies
WNND	West Nile neuroinvasive disease
WNV	West Nile virus
WPW	Wolff-Parkinson-White
XDH	xanthine dehydrogenase
XLA	X-linked agammaglobulinemia
XLP	X-linked lymphoproliferative disease
XO	xanthine oxidase
XOR	xanthine oxidoreductase

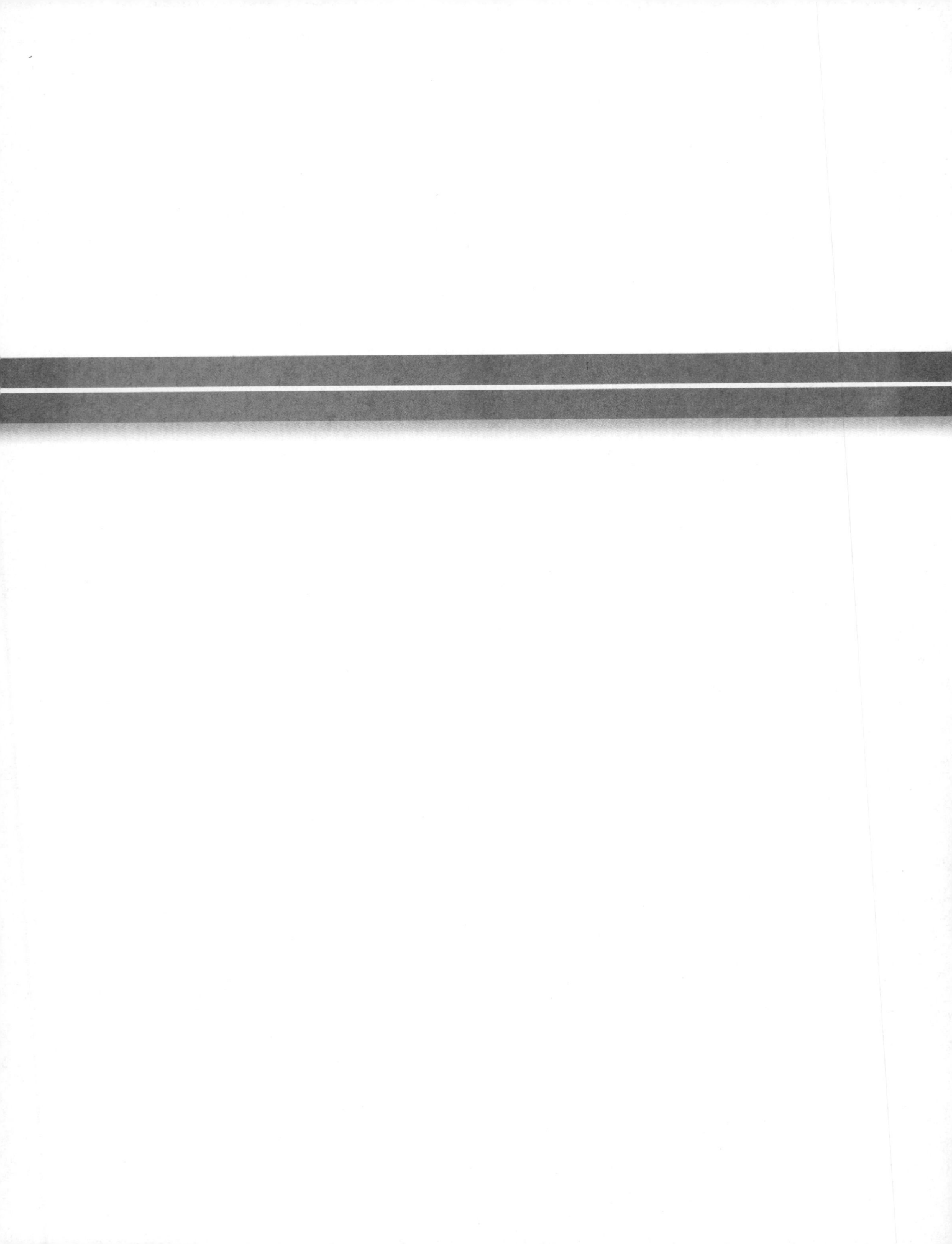

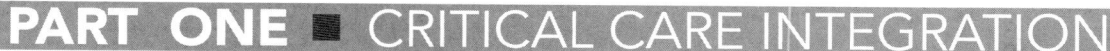

PART ONE ▪ CRITICAL CARE INTEGRATION

CHAPTER 1 ■ THE HISTORY OF PEDIATRIC INTENSIVE CARE AROUND THE WORLD

MARK C. ROGERS

This chapter provides a history of the development of Pediatric Intensive Care as a specialty. Told in the "first person" by those involved, it represents a unique view of how the many early pioneers and developers of the Pediatric Intensive Care field contributed to its creation.

The contributors of this chapter wrote their own stories, largely unedited and deliberately without references. These are personal stories of the struggle to create such a field, to develop standards for the field, to envision a mechanism by which to pay for patient care, and to evolve a political basis to underpin the documentation and regulation of practitioners in the specialty.

Although many countries are represented, the list of potential contributors is greater than the list of actual contributors. I attempted to contact far more people than could be reached and, as a result, some people who deserve to be included have unfortunately been omitted. Because this "living history" will be updated with each edition of the *Textbook of Pediatric Intensive Care*, more histories can and will be included in the future. In the meantime, here are the stories of the men and women making important contributions to the field of Pediatric Intensive Care.

THE HISTORY OF PEDIATRIC INTENSIVE CARE AT JOHNS HOPKINS

Mark C. Rogers, MD[1]

On August 1, 1969, one month out of medical school and one month into an internship in Pediatrics at Harvard Medical School's Massachusetts General Hospital (MGH) and the Boston Children's Hospital, I arrived for my newborn experience at the Boston Lying-In Hospital. This was the obstetrics and gynecology teaching hospital for Harvard, and I was supposed to attend deliveries in order to resuscitate newborns if needed and to be responsible at night for all newborns, both in the well-baby nurseries (there were several) and in the ICU, which had approximately 30 critically ill newborns.

On arrival, I was met by the junior resident, who happened to have been a fraternity brother of mine several years earlier, when I was an undergraduate at Columbia University. After a brief hello, we toured the facility and made rounds with the attending physician, who was there only during the daytime. I learned where the delivery rooms were and met the nurses in the rather rudimentary ICU. I also learned that, during the

day, radiologists were available to read films but that, at night, not only did they go home, they shut down the automatic developer to ensure that the trainees did not break it. I would be responsible for doing old-fashioned "hand-dipping" of x-rays that I then would have to read.

All of this was overwhelming, but not as big a shock as when my fellow resident announced around 4 p.m. that he had been up for 36 hours and would be going home in a few hours. The attending had left to conduct research in the basic science building several hours before, and a neonatal research fellow was supposed to be on call, but I could not count on him arriving for several hours. There were no cell phones, and beepers outside of the hospital were unreliable. An intern for a month, I found myself alone with massive responsibilities for which I felt unprepared.

This frightening circumstance was organized as it was because no effective facilities existed for ventilating newborns or even for getting blood gases. A neonate had to live 36 hours before being put on a small-animal ventilator, and blood gases were limited to only one or two sets per night for the entire nursery because it was necessary to call in the fellow or the technician from home, and they were only required to do one, or perhaps two, per night.

This "primitive" state of intensive care for newborns was somewhat different from how care was being provided to other young infants and children at the Boston Children's Hospital and the MGH. Those institutions had relatively new neonatology support but not yet enough to support the Lying-In Hospital. Older infant and child critical care was developing rapidly out of the need to care for critically ill children in the postoperative period. This was the era of major advances in pediatric surgery, especially pediatric cardiac surgery and the pediatric anesthesia that went along with it. Critical care was largely a continuation of intraoperative and postoperative care. The anesthesiologists, with a new group being dedicated as pediatric anesthesiologists, worked alongside interested pediatricians, largely derived from pediatric pulmonologists and cardiologists. Together, they would care for postoperative patients in the postop recovery room. This system was also being duplicated for critically ill children who had not undergone surgery, sometimes in the postop recovery room and sometimes, but rarely, in a separate area of the general pediatric ward.

Barriers to the Organization of the Pediatric Intensive Care Unit

At this point, small and local attempts to provide this postoperative and medical intensive care of infants and children were being made in several centers around the US and the rest of the world. They were all running into similar problems that represented barriers to the growth of the field. Among these problems were different perspectives for the pediatrician, for the surgeon, and for the anesthesiologist.

The concern for general pediatricians was that "their" patient was "their responsibility," even when they were practicing at offices miles from the hospital. There also was the belief that some patients were "too sick to touch"—an actual quote from 25 years ago from an eminent professor of pediatrics in a prestigious British university. This same man was in the audience of the first Grand Rounds that I presented at Johns Hopkins, at which he strenuously objected to my description of how to obtain arterial blood gases from an infant or child. The surgeons had general anxiety about maintaining control of their surgical patients, even when they wanted to spend all their time operating. This anxiety commonly resulted in the assignment of the ICU responsibilities to the most junior (nonoperating) member of the surgical team, often a junior intern, and sometimes even to a senior medical student. The anesthesiologists had a traditional interest in the cardiorespiratory care of patients but needed to grow toward a more broad-based pathophysiologic approach that embraced nutrition, infectious disease, and metabolic issues if they wanted to be fully involved in intensive care.

Reimbursement for time devoted to intensive care was virtually nonexistent and was also a real problem. In fact, my initial primary appointment at Johns Hopkins was in Pediatrics but was changed to Anesthesiology when, on arrival at Hopkins in July 1977, I advertised in the *Journal of Pediatrics* for fellows for July 1978. The administrator of the Department of Pediatrics objected because he did not want the department to risk the salary of two fellows ($15,000 each in that era) when the department was financially in trouble. However, the Department of Anesthesiology was willing to stand behind the financial commitment and, as a result, my primary and secondary appointments were switched. The Department of Pediatrics was not swayed by the argument that the PICU would end up making more money than any division of Pediatrics, which turned out to be true.

Nursing was the next barrier. Although medical care for critically ill children was making progress, the organization of nursing care would be vital. The skills, both technical and psychological, required to deal with critically ill and dying children comprise such a special set that it would be impossible to rotate nurses from regular wards in and out of the ICU. Nevertheless, for an undeveloped field such as Pediatric Intensive Care, it was difficult for nursing leaders to justify such an organization, staffing pattern, and training program and have it supported by a hospital administration always short of funds. As a result, growth would come from the increasing need for postoperative care for children with congenital defects, congenital heart disease, and trauma. The nurses would often start with a pediatric surgical background and evolve into more generalized PICU nurses. Around the world, many institutions and many individuals were trying to come to grips with these problems, and one of them was Johns Hopkins.

Arrival at Johns Hopkins University School of Medicine

Despite my horrifying lack of preparation for the ICU, not even 10 years later, in 1977, I joined the faculty of the Johns Hopkins University School of Medicine as the director of the

PICU, an embryonic but growing separate facility within the Children's Center. My recruitment was led by J. Alex Haller, Jr., MD, Professor of Pediatric Surgery, and my selection probably resulted from the eclectic and unusual background that I had for that era.

During medical school, I had become fascinated with the new cardiac care units that were devoted to the new physiology and pharmacology for cardiac arrhythmias. I volunteered to go to medical school for 5 years, spending 6 months of each year under a National Institutes of Health (NIH) fellowship studying "the theoretical model of the T wave" of the EKG with J. A. Abildskov, a famous arrhythmia expert at the Upstate Medical Center in Syracuse, New York. He encouraged me to study how the central nervous system altered sympathetic tone and, therefore, cardiac innervation and the electrocardiogram. It was a prescient choice, as that was a fascinating way to study problems that would occur repetitively in the ICU. In fact, Dr. Julius Richmond, later to be Surgeon General of the US, was dean of my medical school and a mentor who saw much of my work in the context of his research in sudden infant death syndrome.

As I was fortunate to be able to use the fellowship to study at several institutions, I spent two summers at the University of Minnesota, studying under Dr. Howard Burchell, editor of the leading cardiac journal of the era, *Circulation*. He asked me write a paper on the T wave, which he published in *Circulation* just as I was graduating in 1969 and beginning my internship at the MGH and pediatric residency at the Children's Hospital. At those institutions, I saw the beginnings of intensive care, particularly at the MGH. At that institution, I can well remember spending the night of the Apollo 11 moon walk in the "special care area," a designated area in the Burnham (Children's) Building. During this period, I developed the habit of writing up interesting cases and even had them published in journals such as the *New England Journal of Medicine* and the *Journal of Pediatrics*. Several years later, when I returned as a resident in anesthesia to the unit at the MGH, it was organized under Drs. Daniel Shannon and David Todres, and I used the writing skills that I had honed earlier to write multiple papers with them.

For training in pediatric cardiology, I studied at Duke under Dr. Madison Spach and discovered that the natural clinical area of interest for me was not in the cath lab but in caring for patients in the postop period. Many postoperative complications occurred during that era, but the surgery was new and exciting, and few surgeons wanted to spend their time in the ICU. Encouraged by Drs. David Sabiston and Merel Harmel, respectively Chairs of Surgery and Anesthesiology, I decided to look into intensive care. As I saw no training programs applicable in Pediatrics, I chose Anesthesiology—at that time, not an entirely popular choice.

I arrived back at the MGH for my anesthesia residency in the department of Dr. Richard Kitz and realized very quickly that experiences in adult respiratory care with Dr. Henning Pontoppidan and in cardiovascular anesthesia with Dr. Myron Laver would be enormously helpful. In Pediatrics, as previously mentioned, Drs. Shannon and Todres were very helpful in my education, and we had the opportunity to write multiple papers together, making possible my ultimate recruitment to begin my career as Director of Pediatric Intensive Care as my very first academic position.

I arrived at Hopkins to find a small, largely open, six- to eight-bed facility with a few truly dedicated nurses, especially Mary Cronin, RN, and, later, Dottie Lappie, RN. While not guaranteed, it was possible to have a vision that this would evolve into a large, modern facility with full-time faculty and with dedicated full-time nurses. It was also possible to dream about a training program for fellows, a textbook defining the field, a subspecialty designation with boards, and even the far-out thought of a World Congress in Pediatric Intensive Care in the years ahead. That vision was palpable and real to me because, as a person trained in pediatric cardiology, I had seen these same stages in the growth of that field. I "knew" that a parallel path would eventually occur in Pediatric Intensive Care and that Hopkins could be a platform to accomplish those goals. It was quite a hubristic vision for a 36-year-old but, with the help of Dr. Steven Nugent, whom I recruited from the Children's Hospital in Philadelphia (CHOP), and Dr. James Robotham, who was then in the pediatric pulmonary group and available to us part-time, we began the Hopkins PICU. Many outstanding faculty members, a large number of whom came from our own fellowship program, followed, and all contributed their talents as the unit grew to 14 beds and a full clinical and research program within a few years. Dr. John Downes of CHOP was always helpful to me and available if I wanted to ask for advice.

In the first year, we were able to recruit our first three fellows: Drs. Greg Stidham (now director of the PICU at the University of Tennessee in Memphis), Frank Gioia (then a resident in Pediatrics at the University of Louisville), and Donna Caniano, a surgical resident from Albany who was interested in pediatric intensive care. They began a series of truly outstanding fellows who, among other things, became faculty at Hopkins and ultimately my successors. Hopkins has had over 60 fellows over the years; approximately two dozen former fellows run PICUs in the US, and a similar number run units throughout the world. Perhaps the most important decision that we made in the development of the fellowship was to model it on a 2- to 3-year Pediatric subspecialty program, with 1 year clinical and 1 to 2 years of research rather than the traditional 1-year Anesthesiology clinical-research program. This innovation enabled us to easily approach future issues, such as training for the intensive care boards and related certification, because virtually all our people were certified in Pediatrics and had full research experience, even if a fair number of them were trained in Anesthesiology as well.

With regard to research, Dr. Richard Traystman was Director of Research in the newly created Department of Anesthesiology and Critical Care Medicine to which I was promoted and simultaneously chaired as Professor of Anesthesiology and Pediatric Intensive Care a short 2 years later. His recruitment to the department and dedication to research education of the fellows were singularly responsible for the stream of Hopkins PICU fellows who succeeded with presentations, publications, and NIH grants. Our interest in a research base for the specialty was both a strategic decision and a practical decision to differentiate our program from many others that did not have Dr. Traystman or the resources to support basic research.

One additional advantage that I had in the PICU at Hopkins was created by Dr. Haller, who headed Pediatric Surgery. He had the foresight to get the Johns Hopkins Children's Center designated as the state trauma center for children, including a helicopter system with a helipad. It was not difficult, with that trauma system as a base, to expand the helicopter coverage to include infants and children who had medical and surgical conditions inappropriate for care at local hospitals and who required emergency evacuation to major PICUs. As a result, the concept of having dedicated and even designated PICUs became the norm, and the standards for such units (medical coverage, nursing coverage, facilities, associated operating rooms, emergency transport, etc.) became possible. The establishment of these standards made it difficult for a PICU to develop in any but the most sophisticated medical centers. In Maryland, we were the only PICU for a decade until one of our fellows, Dr. Alice Ackerman, started one at the University of Maryland.

The History of "The Boards" in Pediatric Intensive Care

To paraphrase John F. Kennedy after the unsuccessful "Bay of Pigs" invasion of Cuba, "Success has many fathers, while failure is an orphan."

At the beginning, no one wanted to be responsible for pediatric intensive care. For most departments of Pediatrics, it was a financial burden that they could ill afford. Nevertheless, a few departments persisted, hired faculty, and built units. For most departments of Surgery and for Pediatric Surgery, all income was derived in the operating room, and it was inappropriate to spend enormous resources on the postoperative care of the children, as residents could do this and care could be supervised at a distance. The situation was largely to stay this way for more than the next decade. For most departments of Anesthesiology, it might be challenging, but it was not possible to get out of doing all of the cases, because the operating room was the primary responsibility. Of all of these specialties, however, Anesthesiology had the most flexibility, as the specialty was in an enormous growth phase, both financially and in manpower. Anesthesiology had the resources to invest and the intellectual need to grow into a major force in the field, and it became very involved in Pediatric Intensive Care in the formative years of the field. That development raised the political questions of how the field would develop and who would control the developing certification criteria and boards.

While the original desire of the American Board of Pediatrics throughout the 1970s and 1980s was to resist new boards, it was becoming difficult to defend that position. The number of physicians concentrating in areas such as Pediatric Intensive Care and Pediatric Emergency Care was growing and, unless Pediatrics developed a home for them, there was a possibility that they would ultimately drift away to Anesthesiology and to the new specialty of Emergency Medicine.

While Anesthesiology was particularly aggressive in developing a field of Critical Care and developing standards for certification in a subspecialty of Critical Care (combining both adult and pediatrics), Pediatrics ultimately decided, through the American Board of Pediatrics, that new specialties should be established in a number of fields, including Pediatric Intensive Care. They were insistent, however, that the entry criteria would require certification in Pediatrics, with sufficient additional training in intensive care to sit for the boards. However, a number of pediatricians had dual-trained in Anesthesiology and some had triple-trained in pediatric cardiology, or pulmonology, or the like. The American Board of Pediatrics finally had to construct an initial sub-board for Pediatric Intensive Care composed of pediatricians with ICU experience, pediatric pulmonologists with ICU experience, pediatric cardiologists with ICU experience, neonatologists with PICU experience, and pediatricians with Anesthesiology and ICU experience. The debate as to what was sufficient ICU experience, how much time was required in other subspecialties, and other issues took a year to resolve. Individuals representing each group were selected and spent approximately 6 months constructing an examination, so that the first Board exam was administered in 1991. Interestingly, no one who participated in constructing the questions had to take an official exam. As young as we all were, we were "grandfathered" in. I never did take an examination!

The First World Congress of Pediatric Intensive Care and Formation of the International Pediatric Intensive Care Organizations

With Pediatric Intensive Care developing around the world, it was natural that the specialty would work toward developing a World Congress. The problem in doing so was not that representatives of the specialty throughout the world who wanted to hold such a meeting did not exist: Having been the recipient of many, many invitations to visit units around the world (many run by individuals who are contributing to this chapter), I knew that such individuals and such units existed. The problem was financial. Many of the individuals in units around the world who should attend such a Congress could not afford to do so. What would be the point of organizing a Congress that would be attended only by physicians and nurses from the US and other rich, Western countries, but not from sections of the world with real problems to solve and few resources? The solution was simple but revolutionary. Because the PICU at Hopkins was part of a very well supported Department of Anesthesiology and Critical Care, the department would use its resources to support the effort.

With the capable help of Ms. Peggy Riley, who was administrator for the Congress, the department allocated $250,000 from its endowment to underwrite the Congress, which was held in Baltimore in 1992. The money paid for registration fees and accommodations for those who could not afford them and even to pay for the travel for participants from such countries as the Former Soviet Union and parts of South America. Events such as a group visit to a Baltimore Orioles baseball game were free, and some of the new textbooks were donated to units that needed them but could not afford them.

Several hundred attendees came from over 50 countries, including Asia, South America, Europe, Africa, and Australia. One of the more interesting anecdotes from the meeting was a visit to my office from the Federal Bureau of Investigation representatives who were inquiring about how we chose attendees (we didn't) because one of them (never identified) was considered an undesirable by the agency. One of the many beneficial outcomes of this first World Congress was a self-perpetuating committee structure by the time of the second World Congress in Rotterdam, which led to the formation of the World Federation of Pediatric Critical Care Societies (WFPCCS).

DEVELOPMENT OF PEDIATRIC CRITICAL CARE MEDICINE AT THE CHILDREN'S HOSPITAL OF PHILADELPHIA

John J. Downes, MD[2]

The evolution of Pediatric Critical Care Medicine and creation of a PICU at the CHOP proceeded gradually during the early and middle 1960s, with help from several sources. The development in 1962 of a 14-bed medical neonatal intensive care unit (NICU) at the Pennsylvania Hospital by Thomas Boggs, MD, head of neonatology at CHOP and the Pennsylvania Hospital, and of a 12-bed surgical NICU at CHOP by C. Everett Koop, MD, the Chief of Surgery, established the concept and proved the value of a discrete area for providing special care to critically ill patients.

Leonard Bachman, MD, Chief of Anesthesiology at CHOP, collaborated with Dr. Koop in providing tracheal intubation and mechanical ventilation for those "surgical" infants with respiratory failure, created a "stat team" to perform cardiopulmonary resuscitation throughout the hospital, and founded an "Inhalation Therapy Service" (the predecessor of today's respiratory therapy) with technicians whom he trained. On occasion, he and his colleagues assisted in the care of a child in respiratory failure due to a severe asthmatic episode using tracheal intubation and prolonged ether or halothane anesthesia in the operating room. Also, in the early 1960s, Drs. Rachael Ash, Chief of Cardiology at CHOP, and William Rashkind (later the inventor of the balloon atrial septostomy and father of interventional cardiology) established a discrete section of the surgical ward that was staffed by a special team of nurses to provide 24-hour care for postoperative cardiac surgical patients. The anesthesiologists usually supervised their respiratory care and participated in all resuscitations.

My initial experiences were as a rotating pediatric anesthesiology resident at CHOP from the Penn program in June and July 1960, complemented by learning fundamentals about the support of the postoperative neonate from Dr. Koop and his chief resident and the basic care of the child with severe cardiac disease from Dr. Rashkind. Following my completion of a research fellowship in pharmacology at Penn in 1962 and 1963, Dr. Bachman offered and I accepted a staff position in anesthesiology at CHOP. At that time, Dr. Boggs and I applied for an NIH grant to study the efficacy of a protocol of mechanical ventilation and acid-base management in preterm infants with very severe respiratory distress syndrome (RDS). To our surprise, we were awarded the funds to begin the study in January 1964 at Pennsylvania Hospital's new NICU. Through Len Bachman's fundraising, we purchased ultra-micro blood gas equipment, established a blood gas laboratory adjacent that served the entire hospital, and soon had a technician 24 hours per day. We subsequently procured similar equipment using our NIH grant for use at Pennsylvania's NICU. That put the diagnosis of respiratory failure as well as severe acid-base disturbances on a rational basis.

At the time that I began on staff at CHOP, David Anthony ("Tony") Nightingale joined us as a fellow from the Alder Hey Children's Hospital in Liverpool. Tony already had 2 years of experience as a registrar at Alder Hey with G. Jackson Rees, the founder of the first PICU in the UK. Based on his experience and skill, Tony should have been the attending staff and I the fellow, but that soon proved irrelevant, as we worked together in harmony. He introduced us to the use of chest physiotherapy in infants, and to the Mapelson-D ventilating system, which quickly became the standard device for manual ventilation throughout CHOP.

In 1964, we developed a respiratory care service staffed by Len Bachman, David Wood, an experienced pediatric allergist/pulmonologist, with me to provide respiratory evaluation and assisted ventilation when needed anywhere in the hospital.

We applied for an NIH research grant to study the pathogenesis of respiratory failure in infants and children with asthma, bronchiolitis, and pneumonia; this was funded in early 1965 and enabled us to hire a fellow to work on our "service" to obtain data and help care for patients. Our first fellow was Theodore "Ted" Striker, who had just finished an anesthesiology residency at Penn and who later became Chair of Anesthesiology at Cincinnati Children's Hospital (1976–2000). He had ideas, enthusiasm, and boundless energy for our projects. Also joining us in 1964 was Sylvan Stool, a pediatric otolaryngologist from Denver, later to become internationally renowned for his work with hearing disorders in children and children with upper airway anomalies.

In January 1964, I visited the new NICU at Toronto's Hospital for Sick Children, spending several days with Paul Swyer, the Director of Neonatology, and his fellows, Maria Delivoria (who later came to Penn) and Henry Levison. They were the first group to achieve success in treating a series of severely asphyxiated preterm infants with RDS using mechanical ventilation. Also during 1964 and 1965, I visited MGH, learning from Henning Pontoppidan and Mike Laver in their respiratory ICU. In 1965, I visited Paris and the 16-bed PICU and the NICU at St. Vincent de Paul Children's Hospital. There, two pioneers in Neonatal and Pediatric Intensive Care in Europe, G. Huault and J.B. Joly, received me warmly, and I spent time with them in their PICU, which had opened in 1963.

In 1966, John Waldhausen, a Hopkins- and Penn-trained cardiovascular surgeon, joined CHOP as the first full-time Chief of Cardiothoracic Surgery. From John and Bill Rashkind, we all learned about the modern care of the infant with congenital heart disease. That same year, Honorato Nicodemus, a Penn-trained anesthesiologist originally from the Philippines, became our fellow for a very productive 2-year period. He later became the ranking anesthesiologist in the US Navy and personal anesthesiologist for President Ronald Reagan when he had colon surgery.

Also in 1966, Len Bachman and I, with the support of our colleagues, began pushing hard with the leadership of the medical staff and the hospital administration for creation of a discrete PICU. Once the Chair of Pediatrics, Alfred Bongiovanni, a pre-eminent endocrinologist, and Erna Goulding, the Director of Nursing, understood and embraced the concept of a PICU, and with advocacy from Drs. Koop, Rashkind, and Waldhausen, the Medical Staff Executive Committee and the hospital administrator agreed to proceed with establishing a PICU under the leadership of the Division of Anesthesiology. However, the location remained problematic in our old, crowded hospital building that dated back to 1916. Harry Bishop, a senior surgeon and president of the medical staff at the time, devised a plan of bed exchanges, and we were able to get adequate space.

In January 1967, the PICU opened and was immediately full. We cared for over 600 infants and children that first year, approximately 150 of whom were cardiac surgical patients. I served as medical director, and one of our four pediatric anesthesiology fellows was assigned to the unit for a week at a time. Our three anesthesiology staff members rotated on-call duties for the operating room and the PICU. We had three to four fellows, all anesthesiology trained, spending 1 or occasionally 2 years in pediatric anesthesia and Pediatric Critical Care Medicine (PCCM). Most pursued academic careers, usually in pediatric anesthesiology, with PCCM as an alternative interest.

In May 1967, because our PICU accepted nonsurgical neonates, I admitted a 34-week-old, 2,500-g, newborn boy with acute respiratory failure due to RDS. After 2 weeks of mechanical ventilation, one cardiac arrest, and several pneumothoraces, he developed a chest x-ray with fibrosis and small cysts, much worse than the Wilson-Mikity syndrome pictures we had previously seen in a few RDS survivors. He required a tracheostomy and long-term mechanical ventilation, because no end was in sight and the parents were fully committed to an all-out effort. A few weeks later, an article by Northway and Rosan appeared in the *New England Journal of Medicine* that described a new disorder, bronchopulmonary dysplasia. Our baby's condition now had a name. Finally in July, after nearly 2 months, we were able to liberate him from mechanical ventilation and discharge him home with the tracheostomy that was finally removed at age 18 months. Thus began our experience in caring for children with chronic respiratory failure and with home care. This boy thrived, graduated from college, and has a lovely family living in upstate Pennsylvania.

In 1968, Russ Raphaely returned from serving with the US Navy in Vietnam; after completing a fellowship year at CHOP, he joined our staff with a focus on cardiac anesthesia and pediatric intensive care. Also in 1969, Stephan Kampschulte, a native of Munich who had trained in anesthesia and critical care medicine (CCM) with Peter Safar in Pittsburgh, spent 4 months with us in the PICU. He then returned to Pittsburgh Children's Hospital to be director of their new PICU. He was our first PCCM leader export.

In January 1972, Len Bachman left CHOP to become Pennsylvania's Secretary of Health, and I became his successor. I negotiated for 6 months with the CHOP Board for department status and for their commitment to more appropriate staff compensation and adequate clinical, administrative, and training budgets.

In 1974, CHOP moved, and we opened a brand new PICU with 14 open-ward beds and six isolation rooms, but we outgrew our space within a year, in part due to children with long-term critical care needs, especially mechanical ventilation. Critical care had taken on a new dimension—chronic care. We opened an "intermediate" unit of 10 beds, called the "PICI," adjacent to the acute unit. The focus shifted from acute care to maintaining ventilation, achieving growth and development, and preparing families to take a partially disabled infant or child home. We discharged our first ventilator-dependent infant home with her parents in late 1975. Over the next 4 years, several other families went home with infants on mechanical ventilation but with limited nursing care or other support. In July 1979, we obtained a contract from the State Department of Health for a statewide home-care program that included both medical and nursing oversight. It was run by Bob Kettrick of our department until he left in 1987 and, since then, by me.

Our training program in PCCM began admitting pediatricians without Anesthesiology training in 1975 with Steve Nugent, who performed extraordinarily well and was one of the first staff in the new PICU at Johns Hopkins Hospital. However, we encouraged interested students and pediatric residents to also train in anesthesiology prior to their PCCM fellowship, as many did during the 1970s and early 1980s. Most of our new staff had such training. When, in the late 1980s, the American Board of Pediatrics required 3 years of training for program approval and sub-board certification, and the Health Care Financing Administration rules made dual residencies difficult to finance, the numbers of physicians pursuing that course plummeted. However, PCCM has thrived and remains allied to its pediatric anesthesiology roots in most leading programs.

PEDIATRIC INTENSIVE CARE AT THE MASSACHUSETTS GENERAL HOSPITAL

I. David Todres, MD,[3] and Daniel C. Shannon, MD[4]

The development of the NICU and PICU at the MGH came about as a result of the insight and efforts of the Chief of Pediatrics, Dr. Nathan Talbot. Dr. Talbot was deeply sensitive to the need for personalized, dedicated facilities for high-risk children as a result of the death of two infants from chemotherapy overdose. Dr. Talbot then worked with Dr. Henning Pontoppidan, Chief of the Respiratory ICU (RICU), to have critically ill children in need of mechanical ventilation cared for in the RICU while preparations were being made for the development of a separate NICU and PICU. Dr. Daniel Shannon assumed the primary role of caring for the pediatric patients admitted to the RICU. Dr. Talbot converted one of the general pediatric floors to a 7-bed PICU, a 12-bed NICU, and an 8-bed step-down unit. The step-down unit was one of the earliest to be developed in the country and cared for children who were recovering from critical illness but required a level of care that could not be provided on the general pediatric floor. These new units were established in 1971, with Dr. Shannon appointed as director of the three units. Dr. John Herrin, a pediatric nephrologist, joined Dr. Shannon as associate director, and Dr. David Todres was recruited as associate director through the Department of Anesthesia, then under the direction of Dr. Richard Kitz. Dr. Todres' experience in postoperative care of cardiac patients was gained from training in Britain. When Dr. Shannon later became Director of the Pediatric Pulmonary Unit, Dr. Todres assumed leadership of the three units.

In addition to the pediatric residents at MGH, residents from Children's Hospital and the MGH Department of Anesthesia rotated through the PICU and NICU to gain experience in managing critically ill infants and children. Fellows began training in 1972, and formed the first generation of ICU staff at the MGH and directors of other major units across the US.

Crucial to the care of these critically ill children was the development of an ICU laboratory to provide data on blood gases, electrolytes, and drug levels. The blood gas laboratory for the RICU, under the directorship of Dr. Myron Laver, was helpful in guiding the development of the PICU micro-sample laboratory, located adjacent to the ICU units. He also taught us about vasopressors and muscle relaxants in newborns and, in general, had a brilliant, far-sighted vision.

The units soon established a national and international reputation through a number of studies and publications. Dr. Shannon's work on congenital central hypoventilation (Ondine curse) was among the earliest in this rare and life-threatening condition. Other contributions included the appreciation that critical illness in the child affects not only the child, but also the immediate family, a report of the first use of methylxanthine (theophylline) to treat and prevent apnea/bradycardia of prematurity, a demonstration that chemical regulation of

breathing was defective in "near-SIDS" babies, cardiorespiratory monitors to digitize the signal and identify abnormal cardiac and respiratory waveforms that could be compared to events witnessed by nurses in the ICU and parents at home, and the use of ^{133}Xe to measure regional lung function in critically ill children and infants in the ICU. We also produced some of the pioneering work on newborn intraventricular hemorrhage and its sequelae. Finally, Dr. Jay Roberts, working in the Department of Anesthesia and the NICU, successfully treated the first infant in the world with inhaled nitric oxide.

The ICUs produced outstanding graduates from its fellowship program. Among them was Dr. Robert Crone, who is now Director of the International Health Program at Harvard Medical School. Dr. Mark Rockoff became nationally known for his expertise in neurologic intensive care and anesthesia and is currently Director of Operating Room Services at Children's Hospital in Boston.

ORIGINS OF A PEDIATRIC INTENSIVE CARE UNIT IN CANADA

A.W. Conn, MD, FRCPC[5]

During the 50 years following World War II, the Hospital for Sick Children in Toronto, underwent almost continuous expansion. During that period, the bed capacity was enlarged from approximately 250 to 815 beds, with all of the ancillary services increasing proportionately. My association with all of the changes was first as an anaesthetic resident, then as Chief of Anaesthesia (1960–1971), and finally as Director of Paediatric Intensive Care (1971–1981).

The expansion was created by the increasing numbers of "sicker" patients in both paediatrics and surgery, but especially in the anaesthetic world, by the major advances in the cardiovascular and neurosurgical fields. In the 1950s, major postoperative patients were sent to isolated beds scattered throughout the hospital and cared for by nurses who had no special training (in the time-honoured tradition). Change began with the creation of a recovery room that operated on an 8-hour daytime shift. Soon it was obvious that some cases were not ready to disappear into the wards, so they had to remain in the recovery room overnight. Later, some cases had to remain several days, curtailing space for the next day's postop patients. By 1960, an eight-bed separate unit was established for long-term use under the aegis of Anaesthesia for administration and respiratory care (respirators were coming into general use). Pressures for more space continued, and planning began for larger quarters, including a small laboratory, isolation beds, specialized equipment, and most importantly, full-time medical coverage and specialized intensive care nurses. In 1969, a whirlwind tour was conducted of 26 different ICUs in six major centres by a SickKids team that included nurses, surgeon, anaesthetist, architect, and administrator, to get the latest "gen" before finalizing our own plans.

In 1971, the R.S. McLaughlin PICU was formally opened, funded by a $2 million bequest from the McLaughlin Foundation. This 22-bed unit was complete with laboratory, isolation rooms, sophisticated equipment, and full-time medical and nursing staff. Its purpose was to provide a multidisciplinary service to a wide variety of life-threatening conditions (multiple trauma, near-drownings, epiglottitis, maxillofacial injuries, as well as the major cardiac, neural, and general surgical cases, pulmonary and cerebral oedema, poisonings, burns, etc.). Between 1,300 and 1,400 cases were admitted per year, providing a great training centre for paediatric trainees of all disciplines. Costs for monitoring equipment approached $100,000 per bed, while daily rates were triple those of general ward care. Administratively, the unit was under the director, who had direct access to the CEO of the hospital and appointments to most clinical services. Each patient remained under the overall control of the referring paediatrician or surgeon, although in practice, responsibility was shared. Initially, such sharing was quite a novelty to some, but the good results overcame such qualms! The nursing service remained under the head of nursing, and very few problems were encountered—in fact the PICU was a "happy ship."

In 1971, on my retirement, Dr. Geoff Barker was appointed director and, shortly thereafter, in keeping with tradition, began planning a much larger and more spacious unit (doubled in size), with ever-more expensive equipment requirements. This superb unit, which was incorporated into a brand new wing of the hospital, opened in February 1993 and was named the Critical Care Medicine ward. It continues to make remarkable advances in paediatric treatment and research.

HISTORY OF PAEDIATRIC INTENSIVE CARE—PERSONAL EXPERIENCES

Duncan Matthew, MB CHB, FRCP, FRCPCH, DCH[6]

Having trained in Scotland, I began my paediatric intensive care journey in 1969, when I was a houseman/intern at the Royal Hospital for Sick Children in Edinburgh. A desperately ill 8-year-old with severe diabetic ketoacidosis was admitted to our general paediatric ward. An attempt was made to resuscitate her in the ward's treatment room, where, despite our best efforts, she died. We had rather basic resuscitation skills and no intensive care team or unit. Critically ill children, including those who required ventilation, were managed on the ordinary wards. I was aware that we should have done better and that ICUs had recently become available in the UK for adults, so the question immediately arose, "why not for children?" Next came my involvement in the management of the first premature baby to be ventilated for RDS in Edinburgh. Unfortunately, the Bird 7 ventilator decided that it would only provide inspiration if its manual breath button was pressed, and this became my job—60 times per minute for the next 15 hours until intraventricular haemorrhage intervened—a truly Scandinavian apprenticeship!

At that time, some paediatric centres had developed special facilities for the postoperative management of children following cardiac surgery, but, in the UK, only Alder Hey Children's Hospital had a general PICU. It had been opened in 1964, and was led by Drs. G. Jackson Rees and Dick Jones. Although there was no recognition of the subspecialty, no training program, and no such unit in Scotland, I was determined to make paediatric intensive care my future.

Three years later, after a self-constructed training programme of paediatric neurology, pulmonology, nephrology, cardiology, general paediatrics, and adult intensive care, I was on hand when Dr. Hamish Simpson returned from a Neonatal Research Fellowship at the Cardiovascular Research Institute in San Francisco, determined to open a PICU at Sick Kids, Edinburgh. This he succeeded in doing, with the help of two paediatric anaesthetists, Drs. Donald Grubb and Dick Burtles. He took me in tow, and the unit opened in 1972 with all of two beds. Hamish had the novel conviction that children on ventilators should have their arterial blood gases monitored. We responded to this, but it was to be some years before intra-arterial cannulae could be inserted percutaneously into small children; so, we became masters of the arterial stab, and our patients became pin cushions.

My first winter of intensive care involved continuous 24/7 on-call and certainly provided a steep learning curve. Two years later, I was about to broaden my experience with a year's training in paediatric anaesthesia, when Dr. Edmund Hey, the eminent neonatologist at Great Ormond Street (GOS) Children's Hospital, recruited me to help in setting up a general PICU. I recruited a fellow Scot, Dr. Bob Dinwiddie, recently back from the CHOP, to help run the unit and the annual St Andrew's night party!

At GOS, a post-cardiac surgery unit had been set up by Mr. David Waterston and Dr. Dick Bonham Carter, but other critically ill children were cared for and ventilated on their own wards, using the enormous industrial washing machine-like Engstrom ventilators, otherwise known as medical students. The new unit was to be run by paediatricians, with some assistance from the anaesthetists. This was an important decision, as it moved paediatricians into the front line of delivery of care to critically ill children, which had previously been mostly the preserve of paediatric and adult anaesthetists. The new 10-bed PICU opened in 1975 and, along with its sister unit at Guy's Hospital, provided most of the general paediatric intensive care for the children of the South East of England for the next 10 years.

I soon made a pilgrimage to Alder Hey Children's Hospital to meet one of the true pioneers of paediatric intensive care in the UK, Dr. Dick Jones. He had already established an efficient regional service and had written, with Dr. J.B. Owen Thomas, the seminal book *The Care of the Critically Ill Child*. Dick's lucid challenge was forthright: "The management of cardiorespiratory failure is in the main easy—sort out brain failure!" Responding to this, the main area of research of the PICU at GOS over the next decade was in neurointensive care with pioneering work by Dr. Robert Tasker. Respiratory failure was not entirely ignored; Drs. Peter Helms and Rob Ross Russell produced important work on regional ventilation (good lung up) and on diaphragmatic failure.

By 1993, Paediatric Intensive Care in the UK had become recognised. The Paediatric Intensive Care Society for nurses, anaesthetists, paediatricians, surgeons, and others involved in providing intensive care for children had been formed. At GOS, a purpose-built, 30-bed PICU had been opened and, with the Institute of Child Health, an academic department under Professor David Hatch had been created. The British Paediatric Association developed a report in 1993, "The Care of Critically Ill Children," which highlighted the deficiencies and specified the changes needed, urging the government to act. It found that only 51% of children who required paediatric intensive care received it in PICUs. Unfortunately, the government shelved the issue. Fortunately, there was a happy ending, albeit delayed. In 1997, the new working party, The National Coordinating Group on Paediatric Intensive Care, produced "A Framework for the Future," which, at long last, produced action and funding.

HISTORY OF PAEDIATRIC INTENSIVE CARE—SPAIN

Francisco Ruza, MD, PhD[7]

I started my career in Paediatric Intensive Care in the late 1960s, having newly finished my paediatric residency at the Children's Hospital La Paz (HILP). I was given the task of managing the paediatric part of a new surgical NICU, which was part of the paediatric surgical department, dedicated to the attention of the newborn children and infants who required surgical treatment. This unit constituted the germ of what, years later, would become the PICU.

It soon became clear that there was a need to treat in an organized way all critically ill children, regardless of the kind of pathology they had. At that time, the HILP had an enormous clinical load, as it was the first of a series of big paediatric hospitals that were being built in Spain. The need was growing because of the medical pathology seen with alterations of metabolism frequently associated with severe dehydration and acute renal failure. Dr. Francisco Rodrigo and I organized a young team of paediatricians for the continuous and well-standardized treatment of severe dehydration. We established the original therapeutic patterns needed for aggressive and individualized treatment of intravenous electrolytic alteration. Importantly, we were able to develop reliable, early diagnosis of acute renal failure and particularly of renal venous thrombosis. The evidence of improved outcome that we achieved accelerated the creation of a multidisciplinary PICU for all children, regardless of their age and illness.

To plan and organise the unit, I visited many of the existing PICUs in the US and in some European countries, compiling as many documents as possible. This information, allied with a lot of will and a certain amount of imagination, made possible the development of a PICU that was truly functional. The creation of diagnostic and therapeutic protocols constituted a hard and exciting job that reminded me of the words of the Spanish poet: "Walker, there's no path; the path is made by walking."

I remember that period as the most creative and exciting that I have ever lived. We were starting a specialty that constituted an authentic revolution in clinical care in the paediatric hospitals. The opening of the PICU drastically changed the organization of our hospital, as all of the critical patients were concentrated in a specific physical area of the hospital, moving them away from the general hospitalization halls.

Another important challenge associated with these organizational and physical changes in the paediatric hospitals was the education and training of the doctors and nurses in the techniques and protocols of intensive care. Publication of our courses was the origin of our series of books. Right from the beginning, we had a great number of applications from paediatricians who wanted to train in Paediatric Intensive Care and wanted to work in our PICU. A great number

of paediatric intensivists achieved their training in full or in part in our PICU, and they now work in numerous PICUs in Spain, Central and Latin America, several European countries, and Russia.

A special problem that we had in the early days was how the PICUs would be structured within the organizations inside the hospital. Adult intensive care, Anaesthesia, and Paediatrics worried about them. Times of turbulence finally resolved in the most rational way when the PICUs were organized with Paediatrics. Very dynamic protocols were established with general paediatrics and with the medical and paediatric surgical subspecialties. The organization of the PICUs as multidisciplinary medical-surgical units provided the best solution to appropriate organizational demands.

Nowadays, the outlook of the specialty has radically changed. In Spain, an authentic network of PICUs covers almost the entire country. The number of paediatric intensivists is large, and the demand for education in the field is very great. The fellowship programs now provide physicians in training with a well-planned and organized training program, with wide and varied sources of information, structure, and resources to make advances in the field. To a great extent, this is the best legacy that the veterans leave to the new generations of paediatric intensivists.

The specialty has now become a full member of the university educational program, integrating teaching programs in Paediatrics with the doctorate and master's programs. This guarantees a serious and well-established teaching program. We have created the Spanish Society of Paediatric Intensive Care (SECIP), with great scientific activity, congresses, and reunions. We are now positioned to properly train new generations of doctors and nurses who can contribute to research to sustain the progress that has been made.

When I contemplate the evolution that the specialty has had and the huge work accomplished by many people since the beginning, I feel an earnest satisfaction, knowing that the progress made has positively influenced the quality of care of critically ill children.

THE PEDIATRIC INTENSIVE CARE UNIT IN AUSTRALIA

Frank Shann, MB, BS, FRACP, MD, FJFICM[8]

In 1970, not long after I graduated from medical school, I was working as a junior doctor in the Emergency Department of the Royal Children's Hospital (RCH) in Melbourne. A child was brought in with severe hypovolemia, and the senior medical staff was unable to insert an intravenous cannula. They pressed the emergency button, which summoned the intensive care consultant. Geoff Mullins strode into the resuscitation room, picked up a large-bore catheter (not one of those wimpy, fine-bore ones) and popped it in at the first attempt. I was watching breathlessly from the back row and, when The Great Man walked past me on the way out, I murmured, "That was fantastic!"—to which he replied, in an off-handed fashion, "I remember almost missing one of those once." Clearly, I had to work in intensive care. But I didn't get there straight away. I finished training as an internist in adult medicine, spent a year in Africa, and then trained for 2 years in general paediatrics at the RCH. Only then did I work in the ICU as a senior resident, in 1976.

The ICU at the RCH began in 1963, so it was one of the first paediatric ICUs in the world. It started in part of the post-operative recovery room, and all of the doctors were from the anaesthetic department. The first paediatricians to work in the unit were Peter Loughnan, in 1973, and me, in 1976. The first paper describing prolonged endotracheal intubation in children was published from Melbourne (*Brit J Anaesth*. 1965; 37:161–73). Tracheostomy had a very high complication rate in small children. Dr. Bernard Brandstater, an Australian working at the American University Hospital in Beirut, demonstrated (1959–1962) that polyvinyl chloride nasotracheal tubes could be used instead of tracheostomy tubes. Because polyvinyl chloride tubes soften at body temperature, they do not cause sub-glottic stenosis if tubes of the correct size are used—unlike rubber or metal tubes. This seemingly trivial observation enabled the development of modern neonatal and paediatric intensive care, because it allowed prolonged mechanical ventilation in children. Dr. Brandstater's original report, at a meeting in Vienna in 1962, was an extraordinary document. It spelled out all of the important principles of endotracheal intubation in children: The tube must fit easily through the cricoid ring, it must be firmly fixed in place with the tip in the mid-trachea, meticulous humidification and suction are essential, and the tube should be changed only if there are signs of obstruction.

Do you remember your first anxious night alone in charge of an ICU? In 1976, in Melbourne, there was only one doctor in the unit at night (expertly supervised by a superb team of experienced nurses). At approximately 3 a.m. on my first night, I had to ring the consultant on call. The phone was answered by his wife. "It's Frank Shann here, from Intensive Care at the Royal Children's. Is Dr. Mullins there?" "Just a minute; I'll see if he's the man in bed next to me." A short pause. "That is my wife's idea of a joke."

After spending 1976 in the ICU at the RCH, I worked as the only paediatrician in the highlands region of Papua New Guinea, serving a population of approximately 1.5 million people. In 1982, I returned to Melbourne as a senior resident in intensive care at the RCH. I was appointed as a consultant in 1983, as director of the unit in 1986, and as Professor of Critical Care at the University of Melbourne in 1995.

The ICU at the RCH is the only specialist paediatric ICU for the whole of Victoria, Tasmania, and southern New South Wales—an area approximately the size of California, but with a total population of only approximately 6 million people. Because we are the only specialist ICU for the region, we never refuse an admission, and we take a close interest in public health issues that affect children in our area. For example, three ICU consultants are members of a statutory committee that investigates the cause of every child death in Victoria. In 1979, the unit established a transport service for critically ill children. For many years, all of the transports were done by the ICU consultant on duty, but now almost all of the approximate 300 transports per year are done by a senior resident and a nurse from the unit, many of them by fixed-wing aircraft or helicopter.

Regionalizing paediatric critical care has many advantages. Large units have more experience with difficult or uncommon problems, they can be staffed by full-time specialists in paediatric critical care, and they can provide a high-quality emergency transport service at little extra cost. An important benefit from regionalization is that the unit feels responsible for all children in the region—for the provision of critical care, for teaching, and for public health issues.

I conclude with the two Golden Rules of paediatric critical care. *Rule 1. The most important thing is to get the basics exactly right all of the time:* airway (the right size tube in the right place, properly secured, with good humidification and suction), breathing (the right Po_2 and Pco_2), and circulation (a euvolemic patient with good myocardial contractility). *Rule 2. Organizational issues are crucially important:* We need large PICUs responsible for *all* of the children in a region (with a population of approximately 1 million children), staffed by doctors and nurses who are full-time specialists in paediatric critical care, with a properly funded transport service for critically ill children.

ORIGINS OF THE PICU AT YALE

George Lister, MD[9]

My interest in critical care medicine arose somewhat precipitously when I found myself working as a resident in an area referred to as the "croup room," which I thought resembled Loch Ness; the fog was so dense that one could not see the patients but could only locate them by sound. Some of my other patients with serious cardiac or respiratory disorders were clustered close by but, fortunately, were not subjected to the thick air of anonymity bestowed by the mist. Our program had a neonatal special care unit, originally designed by one of the fathers of neonatology, Lou Gluck, but older children with critical illness were more scattered and had no single individual or group to champion their needs. Needless to say, this left us residents to rely on a mixture of nervousness and inventiveness to find assistance when our responsibility exceeded our skills and knowledge. I awoke one morning, just prior to a visit to Yale by Abe Rudolph, who was scheduled to be the Grover Powers Lecturer, with the idea that I wished to gain the background to take care of critically ill children and develop a curriculum to get an education to prepare me—although I had no clue whether this was possible. I must admit that, when I expressed this interest, one of my attendings quipped that I would soon enter a field of tertiary or quaternary pediatrics in which I would only be taking care of sick machines. Others advised that this was not a field for a pediatrician. Others simply gave me bewildered looks. But, I also received plenty of support and assistance for taking a novel path.

By the time of my residency, I had already developed a deep interest in cardiorespiratory physiology by virtue of some serendipitous events. As part of my education as a medical student, I was required to complete a thesis. During my pediatric clerkship, I participated in the transport of a neonate with total anomalous pulmonary venous return (i.e., I went along for the ride while trying to write a history and physical without getting nauseated in a cramped, hot ambulance). When we arrived, I asked if I could observe the emergency cardiac catheterization. Although the infant had a tragic outcome, I took interest in the data and the physiologic interpretation and asked the attending cardiologist, Michael Berman, if he would check my calculations of blood flows, which were riddled with erroneous assumptions. I am deeply grateful to him because he took the time and interest to teach me and then suggested that I take an elective in pediatric cardiology. I followed his advice and, in so doing, met one of my lifelong mentors and friends, Norman Talner, Chief of Pediatric Cardiology.

Although I began a research project in cardiology that could serve as my thesis, Norman suggested that I apply for a Bay Area Heart Association Fellowship because he thought that one of the preceptors, Julien Hoffman, would be a terrific teacher and that the environment in San Francisco would be ideal for a student with my interests. I was awarded the fellowship during my fourth year of medical school and, in the process, met the most remarkable group of physician-scientists imaginable at the Cardiovascular Research Institute (CVRI) of the University of California at San Francisco (UCSF). Having Julien as a preceptor was the most fortunate event in my professional career. I arrived in San Francisco, he handed me a huge stack of papers, presented a problem related to the error in estimating oxygen consumption when calculating blood flow in infants, and suggested that I figure out how to solve it. I will not recount the details, but in the course of this all-too-brief fellowship, I was able to complete the project; develop a system for measuring oxygen consumption; submit my first manuscript, which was published with an editorial; initiate an enduring friendship with two great teachers, Julien Hoffman and Abe Rudolph; and launch a sustaining career interest in oxygen transport.

Thus, when Abe Rudolph visited New Haven during my residency, I was given the opportunity to meet with him and discuss my career options. Brash as I was and somewhat oblivious to barriers, I asked if I might take a trip to UCSF and meet with him, the head of neonatology (Rod Phibbs), and the head of pulmonology (Bill Tooley) to see if a program could be fashioned to prepare me to take care of critically ill children. Remarkably, I visited and was given a schedule to meet with each of these individuals and an offer to try to fulfill my wild and overly ambitious plans. With such an invitation and 2 years as a pediatric intern and resident under my belt, I loaded my car and headed for California. I started my odyssey as a fellow in cardiology for 6 months, then spent 6 months in neonatology, and returned to cardiology the following summer.

After I learned a bit more about the opportunities at UCSF, I arranged a meeting with Hillary Don, the director of the adult ICU, and asked if I might spend a month working there so that I could begin to learn about the management of critically ill adults. For many years, the pediatric cardiac surgical patients had been cared for in the NICU because of the commitment and talents of such individuals as George Gregory, who attended there and had extensive experience in managing such patients. When Paul Ebert (Chairman of Surgery and renowned pediatric cardiac surgeon) arrived at UCSF a few years earlier, the volume of cardiac surgery increased so much that it created a need to have some of the children cared for in the adult unit. Hence, my inquiry was well received, because of the supposition that I might even be useful in the care of those "babies" with heart disease. The experience proved to be invaluable to me. And, shortly after I finished and much to my surprise, Bill Hamilton, Chairman of Anesthesiology, asked if I would take a faculty position to work in the adult (and pediatric) ICU, which was under the aegis of Anesthesiology. A subsequent meeting was arranged with Bill Hamilton, Mel Grumbach (Chairman of Pediatrics), and Abe Rudolph to work out the details. We

agreed that I would finish the planned rotations I had arranged during my second year as a fellow, continue with my research, and start on the faculty at UCSF in July—as a Pediatric Intensive Care physician. Perhaps one more element helped to accelerate my education. After I was on the faculty only a few months, the director of the ICU had a serious medical condition (from which he fortunately fully recovered); in very short order, I found myself as a codirector of an adult-pediatric ICU—an experience that might be viewed as a baptism by fire, but one that served as another opportunity to learn.

After remaining on the faculty at UCSF for approximately 18 months, I decided that I should leave because it was time for me to see if I could develop my own research directions and perhaps create a program for others who were interested in Pediatric Intensive Care. Following this, a few other accidents helped to launch my career. Before leaving UCSF, I was speaking at a seminar on cardiovascular care when I met a cardiac anesthesiologist from Johns Hopkins who heard my presentation on postoperative care of the child. He subsequently invited me to speak at Hopkins, where I met Mark Rogers, which initiated a long-time friendship and professional interaction. Soon after taking a faculty position at Yale, as I was struggling to get my laboratory off the ground, I received a phone call on a Saturday afternoon from two friends and collaborators whom I had met at research meetings: Doug Jones and Mike Simmons, the codirectors of the neonatal nursery at Johns Hopkins. They announced to me that they had a fellow for me; I stated that I did not have a training program, to which they responded, *"Now* you do." Thus began a fellowship program at Yale and the start of recruitment of additional faculty to develop that program.

THE BEGINNINGS OF PAEDIATRIC INTENSIVE CARE IN FRANCE

Gilbert Huault, MD[10]

The beginning of paediatric intensive care in France owes much to accidental circumstances.

As I was trained both in adult intensive care and paediatrics during my residency, I initiated paediatric intensive care in the stream of other pioneers in adult intensive care medicine. Besides my paediatric duties, I spent many nights on call in the first unit of medical transports that was created by Dr. Maurice Cara at Necked Hospital in Paris. I also spent 1 year of my residency in the first unit of adult intensive care medicine created in the early 1950s by Professor Pierre Collaret, the inventor of the concept of "coma depose" (later "brain death"), at Claude Bernard Hospital in Paris. There, the young resident that I was dared once to transfer an adult patient with very severe pulmonary tuberculosis (who was being cared for by the Assistant Professor) into another department that I judged much more appropriate for the patient. This was, of course, not at all appreciated by the Assistant Professor, and all of my hopes of a career in adult intensive care medicine suddenly vanished, as it was the only adult intensive care department at that time in France. Dr. Jean-Jacques Pocatello, one of the pioneers in adult intensive care medicine in France (not a physician, but a pharmacist who developed the technique of blood gases in the department), had the final word in the dispute when he said to the young resident, "It's never wise to tell a husband that he is cuckold...! Why won't you practice intensive care medicine in children?"

As I had practiced paediatrics before, I decided to spend 6 months in the paediatric neurology department, which was created by Professor Stephanie Thieffry at l'Hôpital des Enfants Malades (The Hospital for Sick Children) in Paris. This department was taking care of all children with poliomyelitis or tetanus using iron lungs, swivel beds, and, sometimes, the Engstrom adult respirator. Because I was very shocked to have to refuse all of the demands to take care of distressed newborns, I decided as a resident to accept a newborn from a French province who was suffering tetanus, on July 14 (the French independence day), 1963. A bit anxious, I phoned Jean-Jacques Pocidalo, who spent most of his professional life in the Claude Bernard Hospital adult ICU. He pointed me toward a recent paper from South Africa that described how to treat neonatal tetanus using muscle paralysis and mechanical ventilation. The newborn was cured after 3 weeks of mechanical ventilation using a very original respirator, called "R.P.R.," which was actually developed by a submarine engineer in 1940. This case report was the subject of my medical thesis. Then, the respirator was developed by an industrial man and commercialised in France, where it was the only ventilator in use for newborns and children for almost 20 years.

At the end of my semester in neuropaediatrics, I severely criticized the organisation of the department openly with the chief of the department. Once again, my total lack of diplomacy was about to make me definitely renounce my career as an intensivist, when several months later, I was suddenly called on by Professor Thieffry. He explained to me that he was leaving for another institution and would be transferring the poliomyelitis unit. "You severely criticized my unit," he said, "I now want you to run it. We will see how well you manage it!"

It was, indeed, a real challenge, as the new hospital, Saint Vincent de Paul in Paris, had minimal access to modern techniques. I prepared by living in the hospital and learning as much as I could and, finally, with the help of colleagues of the Cara's team, 18 children, supported either by iron lungs or by positive ventilation, were transferred within a single day. The unit was opening, although to much skepticism.

The equipment was at first very archaic. Then, the unit started to use a new device for measuring blood gases and stepwise acquired the first cardio monitors in use in France. In the unit, we performed the first peritoneal dialyses, conceived the first kits adapted to chest drainage, put in practice the first total parenteral nutrition techniques, and performed the first defibrillations ever made in children in France.

On May 8, 1965 (Victory Day in France), Professor Jean-Paul Binet, a famous French cardiac surgeon, operated on an infant who was suffering from an abnormal vascular ring. The occurrence of two cardiac arrests in the operating theatre convinced him that the infant was going to die. He was very surprised to learn 3 days later that the child was doing fine and was ultimately discharged from the unit. He suddenly realised the great importance of paediatric intensive care to congenital cardiopathies, in which the postsurgical mortality was very high. Thus, within the 10 subsequent years or so, approximately 1,500 cardiac children were operated on.

Of course, I could not do everything on my own. Over time, a team was structured around me (including an energetic and powerful head nurse), which constituted a group of high-quality nurses and highly enthusiastic fellows who were seduced by this new type of medicine. At the end of the 1960s, the unit was covered by the so-called "Four Musketeers": Jean-Bernard Joly, Jean Kachaner, Jacques Saint-Martin, and Gilbert Huault. Within a few years, the unit served as a teaching and training centre for new physicians and nurses interested in this new type of practice in paediatrics. Quite quickly, the "hive" spread: Michel Cloup opened up a new unit in Les Enfants Malades Hospital in Paris, as did Jean Laugier in Tours, in 1968. François Beaufils created another unit at Bretonneau Hospital in Paris, in 1971. Michel Dehan started a NICU in the brand new hospital built in Clamart (in the environs of Paris). Nowadays, approximately 50 NICUs and 35 PICUs can be found in France, including overseas territories. This is a nice outcome for what began as an accidental circumstance.

THE DEVELOPMENT OF PEDIATRIC INTENSIVE CARE IN ISRAEL

Zohar Barzilay, MD[11]

I went to London (Imperial College) in 1974, during the First World Congress on Intensive Care, to meet with Peter Safar, then program director at Presbyterian Hospital in Pittsburgh and Chairman of the Department of Anesthesiology and Critical Care at the University of Pittsburgh. Peter interviewed me in London and accepted me for his fellowship program in Pittsburgh, a leading center for intensive care.

In December 1974, I began a rotation at the Montefiore Hospital Surgical ICU (SICU) with Dr. Arnold S. Sladen for 3 months, working with Dennis Greenbaum. Subsequently, I rotated through various units with the well-known faculty in adult critical care, including Drs. Ake Grenvik and Jim Snyder, for 3 months (adult MICU, SICU). It was only after completing that training that I spent 12 months with Bob Binda and David Ryan at Children's Hospital in Pittsburgh (including rotations in pediatric cardiology and in neonatology at The Magee Woman's Hospital).

Upon returning to Israel in late 1976, I first joined the adult ICU team but gradually took on more and more pediatric patient responsibilities at Sheba Medical Center. In November 1977, we finally organized and opened the first PICU in the country. The head nurse at the time, Ms. De-boer, had also completed 6 months of training at the Children's Hospital in Pittsburgh. Apart from organizing the physical facility (the actual unit), we had to train nurses and residents in pediatric critical care medicine. The first PICU was a five-bed unit, attended by eight nurses and two physicians. Word of our capabilities spread through the medical community, and we began teaching and training medical students, physicians, nurses, and paramedics. In addition to more traditional training, we provided training in cardiopulmonary resuscitation and in advanced cardiac life support.

In 1982, I went on a sabbatical in Anesthesiology and Critical Care Medicine with Dr. Mark Rogers at the Johns Hopkins Medical Center in Baltimore, Maryland. This was my first organized exposure to a well-manned, well-equipped, and functioning multidisciplinary PICU that was part of a distinguished department. The research that I conducted with

Dr. Richard Traystman, Director of Research in the Department, also became an unforgettable experience and a milestone in my future career. Upon returning to Sheba in 1983, many procedures and therapeutic modalities were adjusted according to my experiences at Hopkins. By now, Israel had four PICUs, and four more were in the planning stage.

In contrast to adult critical care medicine in Israel, which is organized in Anesthesiology, PICU physicians are mostly pediatricians who become interested in critical care medicine. This is probably true because Pediatric Anesthesiology was nonexistent in Israel in the era in which Pediatric Intensive Care developed as a specialty. Today, we have approximately 120 PICU beds and in 12 PICUs in the country, and fellowship training, including board certification, is available in Pediatric Critical Care Medicine.

In 1984, the PICU at Sheba was renovated and expanded to include patients coming from all disciplines of medicine. We began caring for children in Israel and those from neighboring countries. Most major PICU physicians and nurses in Israel completed their critical-care rotations at Sheba. Among them were G. Hauser of Georgetown in Washington, D.C.; M. Sagy-Schneider, now in New York; and N. Noviski, who went to the MGH in Boston. In the mid-1980s, we trained four Palestinian physicians (two pediatricians) for 2 years. They later established the ICU and PICU in the Gaza Strip. Our PICU continues to be home for most transferees from Gaza, mostly patients in need of cardiac surgery, treatment for cancer, or rehabilitation.

The PICU had become a department, the Department of Pediatric Critical Care. It is the largest PICU in the country and has approximately 1,000 patients per year; they are admitted for trauma, sepsis, congenital anomalies, cardiac surgery, neurosurgery, and respiratory failure. Care is administered in an 18-bed facility, with 10 ICU beds and 9 step-down beds uniquely designed as 10 and 8 separate patient rooms located in 2 circles around central halls. In addition, the department has a small operating room, an extracorporeal membrane oxygenation room, and 2 sleep-study rooms with electroencephalogram capability (located in the Safra Children's Hospital at the Chaim Sheba Medical Center, a tertiary care center that serves a population of approximately 1 million). Ours is one of the few PICU facilities that also does sleep studies. The 3 full-time faculty, 37 nurses, and the fellowship program are all certified in Pediatric Critical Care Medicine.

HOW I BECAME INTERESTED IN INTENSIVE CARE IN AUSTRIA

George Simbruner, MD[12]

Interest in a field arises from being confronted with needs and from meeting people. Pediatric care, in its wider meaning, includes newborns and children. Freshly graduated from Vienna University, I started to work at the University of Stellenbosch, Tygerberg Hospital, in Cape Province, South Africa. Professor Victor Harrison and his team at Groote Schuur Hospital were the first to intubate and ventilate newborn infants with RDS. In Tygerberg Hospital, we used the negative-pressure ventilator (air-shields) to ventilate premature infants. After my return to Vienna in 1972, I got fully involved in neonatal intensive care. My first statistics about survival of ventilated newborns

were shocking. Only 1 out of 100 ventilated newborns had survived in 1973. The ventilator in use was a bulky respirator constructed for adult patients and badly adapted for prematures. I decided to construct a new, modern ventilator, bought fluidic elements from Corning, New York, and assembled a fluidic-controlled, jet-stream respirator that allowed ventilation with frequencies up to 5 Hz. Testing this apparatus and studying lung mechanics with a Beckman Amplifier got me more and more involved in respiratory intensive care.

During early 1980s, I was asked to set up a PICU at Vienna's Children's Hospital. I probably had never met Professor Mark Rogers in person before but knew about him from reading his standard book on Pediatric Intensive Care (the "Red Book," but 10 times larger than Mao's). I decided to invite this famous professor as guest professor to visit and lecture at our new PICU. I knew that he was engaged in improving the PICU in Ljubljana, Slovenia, and that he would fly there in the near future. Encouraged by a vision, I wrote a letter (e-mail had not yet been invented) to invite him to stop over in Vienna on his way to Ljubljana. Professor Rogers, open to all interested in PICU, agreed. I took him to the most distinguished old pubs and to a small-orchestra performance in a small room of the famous concert hall, "Musikvereinssaal." When I realized his enthusiasm for the site, I proposed to him to come for a month to Vienna. During that time, we could also attend a concert in the large, beautiful hall of the "Musikvereinssaal," where the famous New Year's Concert was performed. Thus, in 1986, Professor Rogers spent a month in Vienna, lectured on intensive care, and helped to set up the PICU. He stimulated and helped us to fully develop intensive care techniques. Due to this personal encounter with Dr. Rogers as teacher and, later, friend, I participated as an invited lecturer in the first World Congress on Pediatric Intensive Care held in Baltimore. As a young doctor, I was very proud to be among the founding members of the WFPCCS.

This experience also fostered my personal view that teaching intensive care medicine was an important and very rewarding task. I remained in the field of intensive care but focused on neonatal intensive care, became editor of the section on "Neonatal and Pediatric Intensive Care" in the journal *Intensive Care Medicine*, and developed a worldwide postgraduate teaching enterprise named IPOKRaTES. Those early days of Pediatric Intensive Care were dominated by one person, Dr. Mark Rogers. In this historical review, it is appropriate to acknowledge his enormous contributions to the development of Pediatric Intensive Care, particularly in Europe.

THE HISTORY OF PEDIATRIC INTENSIVE CARE IN THAILAND

Subharee Suwanjutha, MD, FCCP[13]

Pediatric Intensive Care has received special recognition as a new specialty over the past 25 years. Thailand also recognized its need for an organized area to deliver specialized care and to train individuals devoted to the care of critically ill children. This need led to the development of PICUs in several hospitals in both urban and rural areas.

The NIH in the US regards the PICU as an area where assigned, full-time personnel—qualified physicians and nurses—are available 24 hours per day. In Thailand, before the year

1980, only a few teaching hospitals were qualified with these criteria, because resources were limited.

The first PICUs were established at Chulalongkorn Medical School in 1968, at Siriraj Medical School in 1970, and at Ramathibodi Medical School in 1973. At present, Thailand has a total of 12 medical schools: eight in Bangkok and the vicinity and four in rural areas. Each of these medical schools has its own PICU. In hospitals under the control of the Ministry of Public Health, 21 medical centers and hospitals are under the responsibility of the "Office of Rural Doctor Production." All of these medical centers are affiliated with five medical schools, and most of them have their own PICU.

Personnel Development in Pediatric Intensive Care

An inadequate pediatric intensive care background among ICU personnel prompted the establishment of an organized pediatric intensive care training program. The Department of Pediatrics of Ramathibodi Hospital was one of the earliest groups to develop such a program. The group is comprised of a pediatric pulmonologist, cardiologist, neurologist, infectious disease specialist, nephrologist, and other subspecialists in critical care. These individuals are knowledgeable in the application of new technology and practical management of patients with multisystem involvements. The four leading problems in our PICU during that period of time were respiratory, neurologic, cardiac, and gastrointestinal diseases. During the pediatric intensive care training program's inception, a group of pediatric pulmonologists and pediatric anesthesiologists made a strong effort to incorporate both fields into the care of critically ill children. In 1980, this group started the first organized critical care team and, subsequently, the first national training program in Pediatric Intensive Care for physicians and nurses at the national level. This course included 2 weeks of clinical training and, for nurses, an additional 2 weeks of ward practice. Since 1980, physicians have sent ICU and respiratory care nurses into the program for 2 weeks of practical training.

In 1982, a nationwide training course in Pediatric Intensive Care at the international level was organized by the respiratory care committee members of Ramathibodi Hospital. I was assigned by the committee to be the coordinator of the program and to submit a proposal to the World Health Organization requesting the sponsorship of an overseas adviser for the course. The adviser approved by the World Health Organization was Professor Mark Rogers, who was then the Chairman of the Department of Anesthesiology and Critical Care Medicine at the Johns Hopkins University Hospital in Baltimore. All participants in the course were physicians and nurses actively involved in the care of critically ill children in provincial and large general hospitals throughout Thailand. The program was very successful, and the event was the beginning of a new era in Pediatric Intensive Care in Thailand. Since then, more pediatricians and pediatric nurses have gone abroad for further training in pediatric pulmonology and critical care. After 1982, three of the staff members from the faculty of medicine at Ramathibodi Hospital, including two physicians (Drs. Teerachai Chantarojanasiri and Aroonwan Preutthipan) and one intensive care nurse (Mrs. Suparat Vaicheeta) went to the US for further training in pediatric critical care and pulmonology at the Johns Hopkins University Hospital through the kind support and collaboration of Professor Rogers.

In 1988, a fellowship training program for the subspecialty of pediatric pulmonology and critical care for board-certified pediatricians was approved by the Medical Council of Thailand, and I was appointed chairperson of this subspecialty board. Ramathibodi and Chulalongkorn University Hospitals were the first two medical centers approved by the medical council of Thailand to be institutes for training in pediatric pulmonology and critical care. The first two fellows received their sub-board certification in June 1992. At this writing, 23 clinical fellows have received sub-board certification in pediatric pulmonology and critical care.

Progress and Development of PICU in Thailand over the Past 25 Years

Since the introduction of the specialty of pediatric pulmonology and critical care medicine, the mortality rate of the nation's critically ill children has been reduced. However, the morbidity rate of chronic illness or disability due to the intensive management of chronic pulmonary problems and impaired neurologic function has increased. Many patients cannot be discharged due to the need for chronic respiratory therapy that requires more sophisticated equipment. One way to lessen the problem of prolonged hospitalization, especially ICU care, and to speed up the turnover rate, was to establish a respiratory home-care program, which has been successfully developed. This program was introduced at Ramathibodi Hospital in 1995. Other initiated programs include the creation of extended ward-care facilities and a training course for respiratory care nurse specialists in 2004. In 2006, the first national seminar for pediatric critical care nurses was organized by the faculty of medicine at Ramathibodi Hospital. More than 250 nurses participated in the course. A program for the training of pediatric critical care nurse specialists is being planned for the near future.

Organization of the Thai Critical Care Society

It is evident at present that Thailand and other developing countries are facing the problem of financing a good healthcare program. PICU specialists must be aware that the goal of this specialty is not only to save lives or to improve the care of critically ill children, but also to maintain a good quality of life. The fact that many colleagues in other PICUs around the country were involved in the care of children generated great enthusiasm and led to the successful founding of the Thai Society of Critical Care Medicine in 1984. This society became a member of the Western Pacific Association for Critical Care Medicine and successfully organized the Sixth Congress of the Western Pacific Association for Critical Care Medicine in Bangkok in December 1991. More than 800 participants joined the Congress, including experts from all over the world, who not only contributed current knowledge in this field but also created a better understanding among critical care specialists. The success of this meeting and its repercussions was greater than expected.

The Thai Society for Pediatric Respiratory and Critical Care Medicine was founded in 1998. As a president of the society, I was honored to be one of the founding members of the World Federation of Pediatric Intensive and Critical Care Societies, which was successfully organized under the leadership of Professor Geoffrey A. Barker in 1998.

Conclusion

Since 1982, considerable progress has been made in pediatric critical care in Thailand. The Thai Society for Pediatric Respiratory and Critical Care Medicine, with approximately 400 members comprised of physicians and nurses from hospitals throughout the country, has successfully organized the national conference, seminars, workshops, and short-course training for physicians and nurses who care for critically ill children. We hope that the continued cooperation and collaboration among the intensive care specialists and societies at the national and international levels will make available a high standard of pediatric intensive and critical care to all children of the world.

THE DEVELOPMENT OF NEONATAL AND PEDIATRIC INTENSIVE CARE IN GUAYAQUIL, ECUADOR

Jose Fernando Gomez-Rosales, MD, FAAP[14]

Our hospital was inaugurated as the Hospital Gineco-Obstetrico Enrique C. Sotomayor in September 1948, and in 1950, we started a premature babies department to try to help those very tiny babies to live. We confronted the usual problems of that time: Rh incompatibility, hyaline membrane disease, kernicterus, sepsis, immaturity, and the like using four incubators in a small room. Dr. Manuel Ignacio Gomez-Lince was the first director of the department and was in charge of the newborns of the hospital. He created a group of physicians who wanted to work with neonates and begin this new specialty. Support for this effort came in an unusual manner.

The H. Junta de Beneficencia de Guayaquil is a central charitable institution that was created to help the very poor people of the country. It supports the four biggest hospitals in each field in Ecuador, including the Children's Hospital "Roberto Gilbert," with 342 beds, and the Maternity Hospital "Enrique C. Sotomayor," with 320 beds. Currently, we have between 32,000 and 40,000 births every year at the Maternity Hospital. We deliver approximately 80% of the babies born in our province. Our history, like many others, was to begin in Neonatal Intensive Care and to grow into Pediatric Intensive Care.

As the maternity hospital grew, it was necessary to increase the area for premature babies, and in 1981, the H. Junta de Beneficencia de Guayaquil decided to create our NICU, because the small prematures needed respiratory assistance and we did not have ventilators or experience in this field. So, in 1982, I went to the Ochsner Clinic in New Orleans to spend some time in their NICU with Dr. Jay P. Goldsmith to learn mainly the management of respiratory problems of premature infants.

We started in 1983 as a small unit with three open incubators, ventilators, and monitors; this area grew to 10 places in 1988 to service the need. In that year, we also started the postgraduate course in Pediatrics in the Children's and the Maternity Hospitals. At that time, mortality was very high, but we cut it by nearly 50% by 1993.

After the first international congress that our department held in 1989, Dr. Mark Rogers, one of our guests—who was subsequently nominated as the international coordinator for all our Congresses—awarded a fellowship for one of our doctors. We sent Dr. Guillermo Munoz, who spent 6 months in the NICU and PICU at Hopkins.

One of the events that brought us national attention occurred in 1993, when sextuplets were born in our hospital at 26 weeks of gestation. Unfortunately, we lost one after 29 days

of fighting with many complications. We ultimately ended up with four healthy children, all of whom are now normal adolescents and good students with normal neuromuscular and brain function.

After we increased our beds, Discovery Laboratories of Pennsylvania approached us and proposed testing Surfaxin, an artificial surfactant, in our patients in a U.S. Federal Drug Administration-approved trial. In turn, they provided us with a new set of eight beds for the unit; when we finished the work, we consolidated both areas and now are working with a total of 18 beds. By 1980, the interest in improving the care of critically ill children had grown from its neonatal beginnings into interest in Pediatric Intensive Care. The H. Junta de Beneficencia started a seven-bed PICU with Dr. Ines Zavala in charge at the Children's Hospital Roberto Gilbert. Dr. Cecilia Masache started a separate NICU in 2000. The unit now has 19 beds in the PICU and 22–26 beds in the NICU. Dr. Ines Zavala is in charge of the PICU, and Dr. Marisol Kittyle is in charge of the NICU. The NICU receives babies who are born in small clinics in the city and mainly babies who are born out of the city in small towns or in the country. The children in the PICU can be postoperative or brought to the Children's Hospital with all of the conditions that are seen in similar PICU environments throughout the world.

THE DEVELOPMENT OF PEDIATRIC INTENSIVE CARE IN BRAZIL

Jefferson Pedro Piva, MD, PhD,[15] and Pedro Celiny R Garcia, MD, PhD[16]

In the early 1970s, several epidemic disease outbreaks occurred in Brazil. Some of them (measles, poliomyelitis, diphtheria, diarrhea, and meningococcal disease) had remarkable mortality rates and represented a big challenge to Brazilian general pediatricians. Most of the referral hospitals (general and pediatrics) created small units for better isolating these infected patients and providing better care. The skilled staff members (medical staff and nurses) and the limited available technical resources were concentrated in these units. At the same time, the neonatal mortality rate in Brazil was very high because of infections, and the model of caring for premature and sick newborns in closed units was immediately adopted and extended to those pediatric units for infected patients. This was the birth of Pediatric Intensive Care in our country.

Rapidly, the concept of PICU was consolidated and adopted in large hospital centers of Brazil. The leaders of this movement were: (a) in São Paulo, Anthony Wong, Mario Telles, Jr., Werther Carvalho, and Mario Hircheimer; (b) in Curitiba, Izrail Cat and Ismar Strachman; (c) in Porto Alegre, Pedro Celina Garcia, Paulo Carvel, and Jefferson Piva; (d) in Belo Horizonte, Julio Sena and Waldemar Fernal. During the early 1980s, looking forward to the growth of Pediatric Intensive Care in Brazil, this group identified that it would be imperative to organize the new specialty, disseminate the knowledge throughout our country, interact with outside centers of pediatric intensive care, and promote research development in this area.

In this era, Jefferson Piva and Pedro Celiny Garcia, who were two pediatric intensivists working in Porto Alegre (southern Brazil), assumed their leadership in this process. Dr. Piva was the director of the PICU at Hospital Santo Antonio, a large university-affiliated children's hospital, and Dr. Celiny Garcia was the director of the PICU at Hospital São Lucas, a university-affiliated general hospital located in the same city.

Although working in two different PICUs, Piva and Celiny Garcia joined efforts in the development and organization of the specialty. In particular, they worked inside the Brazilian Pediatric Society and the Brazilian Critical Care Association and held relevant positions on the executive board of both organizations, which contributed to creating more opportunities for this new specialty. As a result of these and other actions, the Brazilian Pediatric Society and the Brazilian Critical Care Association, in 1990, formalized joint board certification in Pediatric Intensive Care. Since then (nearly 16 years ago), more than 1,200 pediatric intensivists have been board certified in Brazil.

Drs. Piva and Celiny Garcia published the first edition of their book in 1985, which is now in its fourth edition. With each new edition, they incorporate a broad spectrum of authors from diverse regions of Brazil and different parts of the world. Their book, *Medicinal Intensive me Pediatric* (*Critical Care in Pediatrics*) is considered one of most important and relevant books in the Brazilian intensive care field, with over 10,000 copies in circulation in Brazil and South America. The last edition (5th) of this book was published in 2005.

In 1986, Piva and Celiny Garcia promoted the first meeting, enrolling all of the South American Pediatric intensivists. It was at this meeting that the Latin American Committee of Pediatric Intensive Care was created; it later became the Latin American Society of Pediatric Intensive Care (SLACIP). During the first World Congress on Pediatric Intensive Care in Baltimore (1992), the first SLACIP meeting was organized as a pre-congress meeting, a practice that has continued at all subsequent World Congresses.

In 1996, Dr. Piva moved to the Hospital São Lucas (PUCRS University) to work in the same PICU with Dr. Celiny Garcia. A new, modern PICU was created, and the pediatric emergency department was incorporated under their leadership.

THE HISTORY OF PEDIATRIC INTENSIVE CARE IN THE PHILIPPINES

Mae Ouano, MD[17]

Herminia L. Cifra, MD, known as the mother of Pediatric Critical Care Medicine in the Philippines, graduated from the University of the Philippines Medical School in 1972. After graduation, she trained in Pediatrics at the University of the Philippines-Philippine General Hospital (UP-PGH). Subsequently, she started formal training in pediatric critical care and spent time at the Royal Alexandra Hospital in Australia. For many years, her work focused on training nurses and doctors in pediatric critical care.

At her PICU at the Philippine Children's Medical Center, she eventually had 10 PICU beds and six intermediate beds. An additional nine beds were located at the UP-PGH. In 1990, Dr. Cifra founded the Philippine Society of Critical Care Medicine, an integrated society for both adult and pediatric critical care specialists. By 1997, a total of 11 Pediatric Intensive Care fellows had graduated from the pediatric critical care training program that she pioneered. This significant milestone prompted the need to form a separate pediatric intensive care society. In the same year, Dr. Cifra formed the Society of Pediatric Critical Care Medicine Philippines and held the position of founding president, with other founding officers from around the country.

Dr. Cifra remained the driving force and inspiration behind Philippine Critical Care Medicine, especially in Pediatrics, until her untimely death in 2005.

Affiliations

1. Founder, Pediatric Intensive Care Unit, Johns Hopkins Hospital.
2. Founder, Pediatric Intensive Care Unit, Children's Hospital of Philadelphia.
3. Associate Director of Pediatric Intensive Care, Massachusetts General Hospital.
4. Founder of Pediatric Intensive Care, Massachusetts General Hospital.
5. Founder, Pediatric Intensive Care Unit, Hospital for Sick Children, Toronto.
6. Formerly, Director of Intensive Care, Great Ormond Street Children's Hospital, London. Founding Chairman of the Paediatric Intensive Care Society.
7. Founding Director, PICU and Emergency Service Hospital Infantil La Paz, Professor in Pediatrics, Universidad Autónoma Madrid.
8. Founding Director and Professor, Intensive Care, Royal Children's Hospital, Melbourne.
9. Founding Director, Pediatric Intensive Care Unit, Yale University.
10. Founding Director, Pediatric Intensive Care Unit, Saint Vincent de Paul Hospital, Paris.
11. Founding Director of Pediatric Critical Care Medicine, Sheba Medical Center, Israel.
12. Professor of Pediatrics and Neonatology, Med University Innsbruck, Austria.
13. Founder, Pediatric Intensive Care, Ramathibodi Hospital. Honorary advisor of PICU Committee, Ramathibodi Hospital. President of the Thai Society for Pediatric Respiratory and Critical Care Medicine, Thailand.
14. Hospital Gineco-Obstetrico Enrique C. Sotomayor.
15. Associate Professor of Pediatrics at the School of Medicine at PUCRS University and the School of Medicine at UFRGS University. Associate Director of PICU, Hospital São Lucas da PUCRS. Member of the Executive Board of the World Federation of Pediatric Intensive and Critical Care Societies (WFPICC). Associate Editor of *Pediatric Critical Care Medicine*.
16. Associate Professor of Pediatrics, School of Medicine PUCRS University. Director of PICU, Hospital São Lucas da PUCRS, Associate Editor, *Jornal de Pediatria* (Brazil).
17. Former fellow of Dr. Herminia L. Cifra.

CHAPTER 2 ■ PEDIATRIC INTENSIVE CARE: A GLOBAL PERSPECTIVE

TREVOR DUKE • NIRANJAN KISSOON • EDWIN VAN DER VOORT

During the last 100 years, Western countries have seen dramatic reductions in child mortality and overall improvements in child health, resulting from economic development, public health interventions, improved nutrition and maternal health, increased immunization and education, and advances in health techno-logy and curative care. In the UK, North America, Australia, New Zealand, Japan, the Scandinavian countries, and Western Europe, child mortality rates fell from over 100 per 1000 live births at the end of the 19th century to less than 10 per 1000 live births at the beginning of the 21st century.

Pediatric intensive care played a small but significant role in these remarkable outcomes, although the majority of reductions in child mortality occurred long before the first use of prolonged per-laryngeal intubation of infants via polyvinyl chloride tubes in the early 1960s—the signal event that allowed children to be mechanically ventilated for prolonged periods without tracheostomy and thus heralded the development of PICUs (40). From 1960 through 1964, the under-5 mortality rate for 21 countries in Europe, North America, Australasia, and Asia that would go on to develop modern PICUs was 29 per 1000 live births [interquartile range (IQR), 24–34]. By 1999, the under-5 mortality rate for these countries was 7 per 1000 live births (IQR, 5.5–8) (1).

Despite these advances in rich countries, 90% of the world's children, the majority of whom live in developing countries and in the poorer areas of countries with mixed economies, have not shared in this remarkable prosperity and progress. The World Health Organization (WHO) estimates that, every year, more than 10 million children die; 99% of these deaths occur in developing countries (24,48). **Figure 2.1** shows the distribution of child mortality globally, with the majority of under-5 deaths occurring in sub-Saharan Africa and South Asia. In 2001, 47 countries had child mortality rates >100 per 1000 live births. Ten countries—eight in sub-Saharan Africa—had mortality rates of >200 per 1000 live births.

For most children throughout the world, access to intensive care is nonexistent, and access to even basic healthcare is a challenge. In developing countries, most of the care of seriously ill children is provided by nurses, paramedic workers, and non-specialist doctors in rural or remote hospitals or overcrowded urban hospitals. In most such hospitals, resources are inadequate, access to evidence and information is poor, and ongoing professional development and staff training are minimal (6,9). These basic deficiencies affect the lives of millions of children each year and are the backdrop to any consideration of the appropriate role of intensive care.

In an ideal world, good-quality intensive care would be available to all children. However, in those countries with limited resources, the provision of intensive care that will bene-fit only a few must be weighed against the greater needs of the many. Attending to less costly, but vitally important, basic healthcare needs reduces global inequity and may decrease the need for intensive care resources. An examination of the causes of global childhood mortality underscores this point.

CAUSES OF GLOBAL CHILD MORTALITY

The major causes of death globally in children under 5 years of age are listed in **Table 2.1** (48). Although not shown in the table, the proportions of deaths associated with these diseases are region specific, with skewed distribution on the African continent. For example, 94% and 89% of the world's malaria and HIV/AIDS deaths, respectively, occur in Africa.

More than 50% of children who die in developing countries have moderate or severe malnutrition, and malnutrition is implicated in deaths from diarrhea (61%), malaria (57%), pneumonia (52%), and measles (45%). Nearly 75% of the world's malnourished children live in 10 countries, and more than 99% live in developing countries (**Fig. 2.2**). Although children often present with a single condition (e.g., acute respiratory infection), those who are most likely to die often have experienced several other infections in recent months, have more than one current infection (e.g., pneumonia and diarrhea, or pneumonia and malaria), *and* have malnutrition with micronutrient (such as iron, zinc, or vitamin A) deficiency.

THE WORLD HEALTH ORGANIZATION'S APPROACH TO GLOBAL CHILD MORTALITY

In 2003, *Lancet* published a series on child survival, outlining the evidence for effective interventions in reducing child mortality. Twenty-three interventions (15 preventative and eight curative) that aimed at the commonest causes of child mortality had high-grade evidence for effectiveness, through large randomized trials or systematic reviews (24). These interventions were selected for being low cost and having potential for implementation at near universal scale in low-income countries. Some interventions protect against deaths from many causes. For example, breast-feeding protects against deaths from diarrhea, pneumonia, and neonatal sepsis; insecticide-treated materials (bed nets, sheets, etc.) protect against deaths from malaria and reduce deaths from preterm delivery. However, with the exception of breast-feeding (estimated global

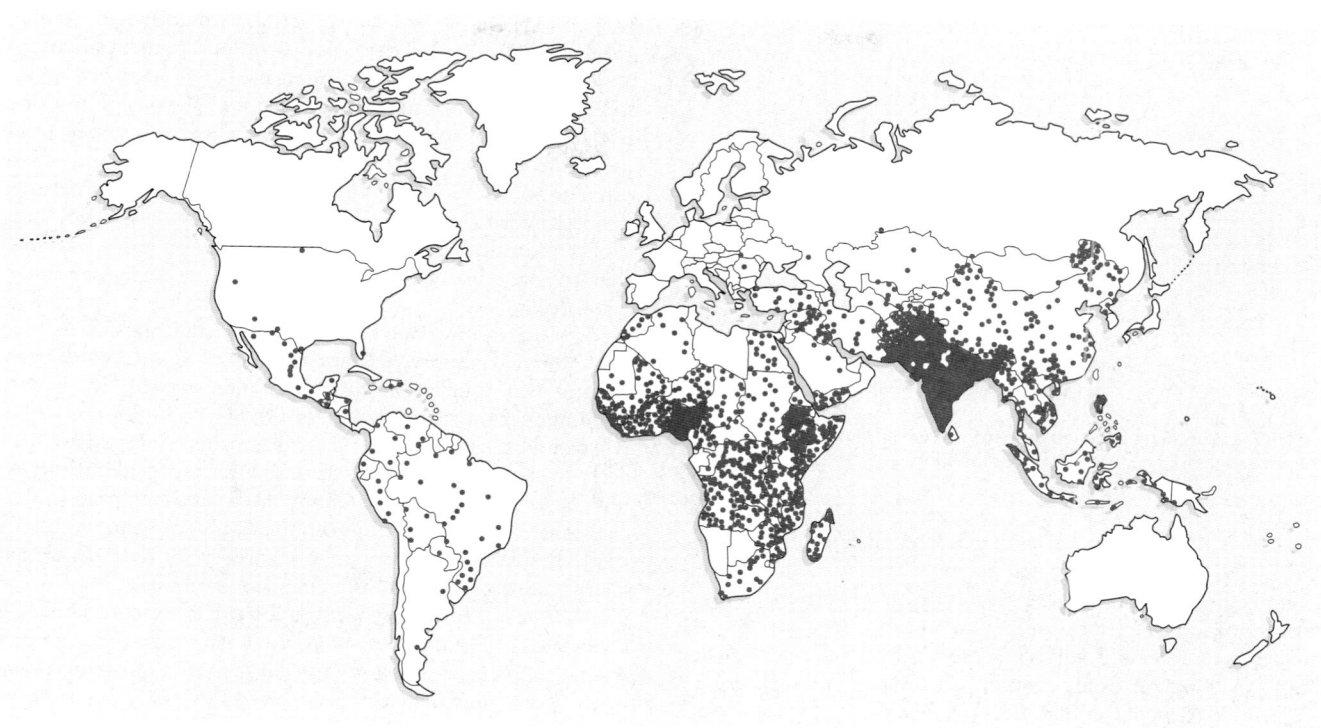

FIGURE 2.1. The distribution of global child mortality. 1 dot = 5000 annual deaths. Adapted from Black RE, Morris SS, Bryce J. Where and why are 10 million children dying each year? *Lancet.* 2003;361:2226–2234, with permission.

TABLE 2.1

THE MAJOR CAUSES OF DEATHS IN CHILDREN UNDER 5 YEARS OF AGE GLOBALLY, WITH ESTIMATES FOR 2000–2003

Causes of death	Number of deaths (1,000s)	% of Total annual global deaths
IN CHILDREN Mo–5 Yrs		
Acute respiratory infections	2,027	19
Diarrheal diseases	1,762	17
Malaria	853	8
Measles	395	4
HIV/AIDS	321	3
Injuries	305	3
Others	1,022	10
	6,685	64
IN NEONATAL CHILDREN		
Preterm birth	1,083	10
Severe infection	1,016	10
Birth asphyxia	894	8
Congenital anomalies	294	3
Neonatal tetanus	257	2
Diarrheal diseases	108	1
Other	258	2
	3,910	36
Total	10,595	100

From: World Health Report 2005—Make every mother and child count. Statistical annex, p. 190. http://www.who.int/whr/2005/en/ (accessed July 2006).

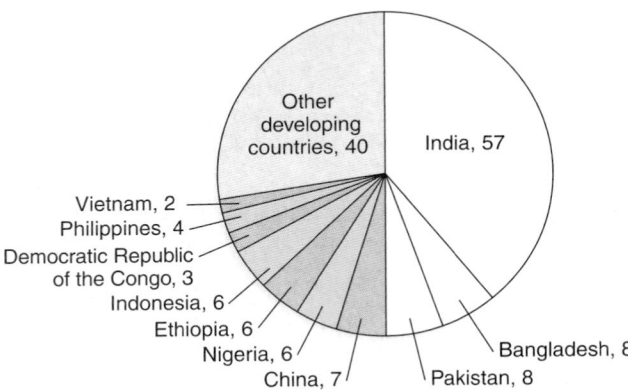

FIGURE 2.2. Nearly three-quarters of the world's underweight children live in just 10 countries. (values in millions).

coverage of 90%), the global coverage of basic interventions for reducing child deaths from common conditions is low. The WHO/UNICEF Child Survival Strategy aims for the universal implementation of a basic package of interventions, along with advocacy for better health financing and a better political environment for child survival. The United Nations Millennium Development Goals contain benchmarks and targets for countries in reducing child mortality rates, with most countries aiming for a two-thirds reduction in under-5 mortality from the 1990 national figure, by 2015 (42).

A part of the Child Survival Strategy is *integrated case management*. To promote a comprehensive model of care for the sick child in 1995, WHO developed the Integrated Management of Childhood Illness (IMCI). IMCI focuses on primary healthcare workers managing the most important causes of childhood illness, including identification and treatment of children with multiple pathologies. An evaluation of IMCI in Bangladesh and Tanzania showed improvements in the quality of case management; now, over 90 countries have adopted the strategy, albeit often in pilot projects or with moderate coverage.

In recognizing the need for effective referral services, WHO has produced complementary guidelines on pediatric care for district or provincial hospitals (47). These guidelines emphasize that diagnosis and drug treatment are not in themselves sufficient for the optimal care of the seriously ill child, but that triage, emergency care, supportive care (including oxygen, nutrition, safe administration of IV fluids), monitoring, discharge planning, and follow-up are also essential. These processes of care were found to be deficient in audits of practice in many developing and transitional countries (8,11,32). Increasing evidence demonstrates that triage and emergency care (29), as well as standardized management of severe malnutrition (2,36,45), severe pneumonia (7), and neonatal conditions (10), can reduce in-hospital mortality.

Standardized management includes high-dependency care and general intensive care with capability for postoperative surgical management of children (46).

ETHICS OF PROVIDING PEDIATRIC INTENSIVE CARE IN DEVELOPING COUNTRIES

When countries have child mortality rates of >30 per 1000 live births, a major proportion of child deaths will be preventable or treatable by simple measures, such as immunization, primary care, and basic curative services in hospitals. In these situations, expending vast resources on intensive care in tertiary institutions accessible to only a small proportion of children does not make sense when simpler and cheaper life-saving treatments are not available to a substantial proportion of the child population. Moreover, child mortality rates are not evenly distributed: Within most countries, some regions or districts have higher mortality rates and others have lower mortality rates than the national average. The factors behind such uneven distribution of mortality rates include poverty, lack of access to services, minority groups, and geographical isolation.

An ethical approach to intensive care is, therefore, problematic. Is it appropriate to provide intensive care to children in middle-class urban areas that have low child mortality rates when children in remote rural areas or urban slums do not have access to basic health interventions? Ethical considerations are not constrained by national boundaries, although practical decisions of resource distribution invariably are. Should a child in a rich Western country receive surgery for hypoplastic left heart syndrome when children in poor developing countries do not have access to surgery for simple cardiac anomalies, such as a ventricular septal defect, or do not have access to antibiotics when they have pneumonia? To a large extent, questions of equity of access and disparity between countries are tempered by practical realities. If children in Western countries were *not* offered palliative surgery for complex cardiac disease, this would not mean that children in developing countries would necessarily be more likely to receive surgery for cardiac defects with better prognoses. These ethical dilemmas will remain as long as vast income inequity and extreme poverty exist in the world, but they can be partially addressed through greater global cooperation and collaboration between child health institutions and through greater generosity by rich governments in the provision of overseas developmental aid.

The main argument against providing intensive care in high-mortality areas is that doing so would divert scarce resources away from more effective low-cost interventions. Following the principles of equity, countries should ensure that highly cost-effective health interventions that will reduce mortality are available to *all* children, *before* funding intensive care services. In very poor countries, evidence of extremely high mortality rates and low occupancy rates (because of inability to pay) in adult ICUs emphasizes the limited value of intensive care services to population health in these settings (33).

Based on the principle of distributive justice, some authors have argued for defining, based on the nation's resources, a minimum level of care that must be available for all children (38). In India, for example, it has been suggested that oxygen, intravenous access and fluid resuscitation, antibiotics, and non-invasive application of continuous positive airway pressure in a clean environment be considered the minimum level of intensive care support that should be made available to all children (38). In South Africa, the HIV epidemic has placed a large burden on pediatric intensive care (23,49) and raised complex ethical issues. Some authors have suggested a utilitarian approach, whereby it is ethically defensible to refuse to ventilate children with severe HIV-associated pneumonia if the resources for doing so are redirected toward programs aimed at preventing mother-to-child transmission (22). Such decisions can never be made over an individual case, but rather can only be decided after consideration of the issues of justice and broader health policies.

Good practical and ethical arguments exist for providing selective and limited postoperative intensive care services, even where national or regional mortality rates are high. Many patients who have undergone surgery die for lack of appropriate supportive care, including mechanical ventilation, in the first 24 postoperative hours. WHO suggests that facilities for intensive care should be available in any hospital where surgery and anesthesia are performed, and it has published standards for PICUs in large referral hospitals, district/provincial hospitals, and small hospitals in developing countries (46). These standards outline conditions that should be able to be managed, procedures that should be able to be performed, and personnel, drugs, and equipment that are necessary. Where mechanical ventilation is available, there is a good basis for providing intensive care for a few selected other nonsurgical conditions, particularly neuromuscular paralysis after snake bite, which is time limited and likely to result in a good outcome if appropriate supportive care is provided.

Intensive care engenders major dilemmas in expectations of survival and extent of treatment. In developing countries, parents often have more conservative attitudes toward withdrawal of life support than do the treating clinicians, who in general have a more utilitarian attitude to resource allocation, with emphasis toward avoidance of significant handicap (44). Limitation of treatment is the most commonly reported mode of death in PICUs in developing countries, and active withdrawal is not widely practiced (18). These issues present ethical as well as resource implications and must be considered when planning pediatric intensive care services for areas with limited human, technical, and financial resources.

In providing equitable pediatric intensive care, indications for admission should be severity of illness and likelihood of a good outcome, and admission or access to treatment should not be limited by inability to pay. In developing countries, serious childhood illness is a major economic burden on many families, especially if care for the child is provided away from the community. The need to cease work and to pay for transport, admission, and expensive prolonged treatment can lead to a cycle of poverty and poor health that affects the entire family.

EXPERIENCES OF PEDIATRIC INTENSIVE CARE IN TRANSITIONAL OR MIXED ECONOMIES

Transitional countries in Asia and the Americas, as well as South Africa, which has a wide range of economic and health development, have introduced pediatric intensive care services during the last two decades. The limiting factors to quality of care that were identified in South America included inadequate interdepartmental organization, lack of treatment protocols, too few pediatric intensivists, inferior equipment, lack of qualified technicians, and lack of training and recognition of pediatric intensive care nurses. A standard of quality in the PICU was proposed, with highest priority given to the training and certification of intensive care specialists, nurses, and residents; administration; supervision; protocol development; and upgrading of equipment (13). The development of pediatric intensive care has also been well documented in Malaysia (16,17). In Kuala Lumpur, introduction of 24-hour staffing by

critical care physicians reduced the case-mix–adjusted mortality. Each of these structural and organizational issues was considered to be far more important than was invasive hemodynamic monitoring or costly drugs and equipment.

Nosocomial sepsis is an ever-present danger in PICUs, and has been a feature of pediatric and neonatal ICUs in developing countries (21,25,28,31). Strictly applied evidence-based antibiotic policies, hand washing, and other infection-control procedures are vital to ensure patient safety, and these should be cornerstones of intensive care. However, studies have shown that it is difficult to directly implement and sustain Western guidelines for the prevention of nosocomial infections in PICUs in developing countries; they have further shown that adapted, locally appropriate guidelines should be further studied and that the importance of institutional commitment to infection control and microbiology services should be emphasized (4,37).

Models of pediatric intensive care in developing and industrialized countries that are designed to minimize risk should include the use of safe and simple procedures for appropriate periods, with particular attention to drug prescribing and selection of appropriate aims and modes of therapy, including noninvasive methods (12).

Regionalization or Decentralization

Strong evidence from Western countries demonstrates that the centralization of pediatric intensive care services results in lower mortality than do decentralized or fragmented services (35). However, several prerequisites accompany centralized services, including transportation to a tertiary hospital from peripheral facilities and appropriate pretransport management (14). In many developing countries, roads are poor, appropriate vehicles are often not available, and fuel costs are prohibitive (5). Families may be required to pay fuel costs or a transportation fee—another impediment to access. If transportation is not freely available, pediatric intensive care will not fulfill the principle of equity, because it will not be accessible to a large portion of the population. Furthermore, children from remote areas may die in transit as their families attempt to transport them to the hospital themselves. Appropriate pretransport management requires good communication infrastructure and, for peripheral hospitals in many countries, improved quality of basic emergency care. Both needs should be addressed before, or in parallel with, the development of pediatric intensive care services.

In Malaysia, the outcome for children transferred from community hospitals by nonspecialized transport was no different from that of children directly admitted to the PICU from within the tertiary institution (15), but this study did not take into account the critically ill children who never reached the tertiary center. In the same country, the outcome from major trauma managed in district hospitals is significantly worse than the outcome from major trauma in adults and children managed in tertiary centers, emphasizing the benefit of centralized management of acute severe illness, when possible, *and* the importance of improving the quality of care in district hospitals, regardless of whether care is regionalized or decentralized (39). Planning for intensive care should take into consideration the entire spectrum of services necessary to care for the critically ill (26), including prehospital resuscitation, transport, and subspecialty support services.

NEONATAL MORTALITY

More than one-third of deaths in the under-5 age group occur during the first month of life (see Table 2.1), and the majority of neonatal deaths occur within the first few days of birth. Most of the 3.9 million annual neonatal deaths occur in socioeconomic deprivation in developing countries. Programs to improve neonatal survival focus on supervised clean deliveries, essential care of the newborn (early breast-feeding, skin-to-skin warmth), steroids for preterm labor, antibiotics for premature rupture of membranes, maternal tetanus toxoid to prevent neonatal tetanus, prevention of mother-to-child transmission of HIV, and identification of sick neonates who require referral to hospitals.

Recently, the WHO produced guidelines for the management of seriously ill neonates in hospitals in developing countries (47). Hospital care for seriously ill neonates should focus first on high-dependency care, including evidence-based antibiotic prescribing, prevention of nosocomial infections, enteral nutrition, safe use of oxygen and intravenous fluids, staff training, audit, and management (10). Where staff resources are limited, involving mothers in high-dependency care has been shown to be highly effective (3). When these interventions are conducted optimally, the introduction of nasal continuous positive airway pressure may be the most effective initial approach to ventilatory support (27). The literature contains many reports concerning neonatal intensive care in developing countries (20,41,43) and the debate about regionalization of care (34), but these are beyond the scope of this chapter.

As neonatal mortality falls, resources must be available to deal with the increased morbidity that will occur in survivors, including malnutrition, chronic lung disease, and neurologic disease among survivors of prematurity. These morbidities have implications for pediatric services, including intensive care.

THE ROLE OF PEDIATRIC INTENSIVE CARE IN COMPLEX EMERGENCIES

Complex emergencies are identified as acute situations that involve excess mortality (>1 death per 10,000 per day). They may be due to natural (e.g., earthquake, floods, tsunami) or unnatural (war, famine) disasters, or both. Complex emergencies are dynamic, with variable durations, recovery, resettlement, rehabilitation, and development phases. After the initial disaster, high mortality rates are usually due to diarrheal disease (including cholera and dysentery), measles, malaria, meningococcal disease, tuberculosis, neonatal causes, trauma, malnutrition, and micronutrient deficiency (30). The United Nations High Commission for Refugees estimates that such circumstances affect up to 10 million people per year.

Many factors impede the delivery of healthcare in such situations, including lack of human resources and referral services, security constraints, poor supervision and coordination, and failure of integration with local health services or transition to a sustainable health system. In addition, lack of evidence-based, locally adapted guidelines limit the effectiveness of healthcare in these situations and contribute to the chaos (30). The first priority in complex emergencies will be management of the initial casualties, for which good emergency care systems and trauma management are vital (19), and intensive care, especially for postoperative management, is optimal. After the immediate emergency phase, high mortality rates in complex emergencies will be addressed through public health measures and developing basic services.

CONCLUSIONS AND FUTURE DIRECTIONS

The development of pediatric intensive care services should take into account the level of preventative and basic curative treatment available to all children in the subject country, as well as the national and regional mortality rates. Preexisting conditions for pediatric intensive care are good vaccine services, good-quality primary and first-referral level care, under-5 mortality rates of <30 per 1000 live births, availability of transportation, good access for the majority of the population, and sufficient human resources. Some form of intensive care, with capacity for management of children after surgery, should be available in any hospital where surgery and anesthesia are performed.

Hospitals should be recognized by governments and communities as core social institutions. The quality of care provided in hospitals—and the nature of interactions between health systems, patients, and their families—have major consequences for child health and survival, human rights, poverty alleviation, and development. In developing and transitional countries, pediatric intensive care specialists possess the potential to improve the management of seriously ill children throughout their countries by training staff in smaller hospitals, by encouraging the building of effective emergency health systems for children, and by providing high-quality clinical care in tertiary settings that have PICUs.

KEY POINTS

- Throughout the world, approximately 10 million children die annually, with 99% of these deaths occurring in developing countries. If countries could achieve universal coverage for basic preventative and curative interventions, 5.5 million of these deaths could be prevented.
- In the 1960s, countries that went on to develop pediatric intensive care services achieved average under-5 mortality rates of 29 per 1,000 live births. In the following 40 years, this decreased to an average of 7 per 1,000 live births.
- Preexisting conditions for pediatric intensive care are good vaccine services, good-quality primary and first-referral level care, under-5 mortality rates of <30 per 1,000 live births, availability of transportation, good access for the majority of the population, and sufficient human resources.
- The WHO has established guidelines for the optimal care of critically ill children in hospitals in which resources are limited, including recommendations on triage, emergency care, supportive care (including oxygen, nutrition, safe administration of intravenous fluids), monitoring, discharge planning, and follow-up. The WHO also has established guidelines for general ICUs with capability for the postoperative management of children. Some form of intensive care, with capacity for the postoperative management of children, should be available in any hospital where surgery

and anesthesia are performed. These curative services should be widely available before countries invest in PICUs.

■ The development of pediatric intensive care services should take into account the level of preventative and basic curative treatment available to all children in the particular country, and the national and regional child mortality rates.

■ In developing countries, pediatric intensive care raises many ethical issues, particular issues of resource distribution, equity, and access.

■ Positive experiences of pediatric intensive care have been described in several transitional or mixed-economy countries, including Malaysia, Singapore, South Africa, and countries in Latin America.

References

1. Ahmad OB, Lopez AD, Inoue M. The decline in child mortality: A reappraisal. *Bull World Health Organ* 2000;78:1175–91.
2. Ahmed T, Ali M, Ullah MM, et al. Mortality in severely malnourished children with diarrhoea and use of a standardised management protocol. *Lancet* 2001;353:1912–22.
3. Arif MA, Arif K. Low birthweight babies in the third world: Maternal nursing versus professional nursing care. *J Trop Pediatr* 2006;45:278–80.
4. Berg DE, Hershow RC, Ramirez CA, et al. Control of nosocomial infections in an intensive care unit in Guatemala City. *Clin Infect Dis* 1995;32:953–8.
5. Duke T. Transport of seriously ill children: a neglected global issue. *Intensive Care Med* 2003;29:1414–6.
6. Duke T. Clinical care for seriously ill children in district hospitals: A global public health issue. *Lancet* 2004;363:1922–3.
7. Duke T, Frank D, Mgone J. Hypoxaemia in children with severe pneumonia in Papua New Guinea. *Int J TB Lung Dis* 2000;5:511–9.
8. Duke T, Keshishiyan E, Kuttumuratova A, et al. The quality of hospital care for children in Kazakhstan, Republic of Moldova and Russia. *Lancet* 2006;367:919–25.
9. Duke T, Tamburlini G, The Paediatric Quality Care Group. Improving the quality of paediatric care in peripheral hospitals in developing countries. *Arch Dis Child* 2003;88:563–5.
10. Duke T, Willie L, Mgone JM. The effect of introduction of minimal standards of neonatal care on in-hospital mortality. *PNG Med J* 2000;43:127–36.
11. English M, Esamai F, Wasunna A, et al. Assessment of inpatient paediatric care in first referral level hospitals in 13 districts in Kenya. *Lancet* 2004;363:1948–53.
12. Frey B, Argent A. Safe paediatric intensive care. Part 1: Does more medical care lead to improved outcomes? *Intensive Care Med* 2004;30:1041–6.
13. Garcia PC. International standard of quality in the paediatric intensive care unit: A model for paediatric intensive care units in South America. *Crit Care Med* 1993;9 Suppl:S409–10.
14. Goh AY-T, Abdel-Latif ME. Transport of critically ill children in a resource-limited setting: Alternatives to a specialized retrieval team. *Intensive Care Med* 2004;30:339.
15. Goh AY-T, Abdel-Latif ME-A, Lum LC-S, et al. Outcome of children with different accessibility to tertiary pediatric intensive care in a developing country: A prospective cohort study. *Intensive Care Med* 2003;29:97–102.
16. Goh AY-T, Lum LC, Abdel-Latif ME. Impact of 24-hour critical care physician staffing on case-mix adjusted mortality in paediatric intensive care. *Lancet* 2006;357:445–6.
17. Goh AY-T, Lum LC, Chan PW. Paediatric intensive care in Kuala Lumpur, Malaysia: A developing subspecialty. *J Trop Pediatr* 1999;45:362–4.
18. Goh AY-T, Lum LC, Chan PW, et al. Withdrawal and limitation of life support in paediatric intensive care. *Arch Dis Child* 1999;80:424–8.
19. Goosen J, Mock C, Quansah R. Preparing and responding to mass casualties in the developing world. *Int J Inj Contr Saf Promot* 2005;12:115–17.
20. Grupo Colorativo Neocosur. Very-low-birth-weight infant outcomes in 11 South American NICUs. *J Perinatol* 2003;22:2–7.
21. Jeena P, Thompson E, Nchabeleng M, et al. Emergence of multi-drug resistant Acinetobacter anitratus species in neonatal and paediatric intensive care units in a developing country: concerns about antimicrobial policies. *Ann Trop Paediatr* 2001;21:245–51.
22. Jeena PM, McNally LM, Stobie M, et al. Challenges in the provision of ICU services to HIV infected children in resource poor settings: A South African case study. *J Med Ethics* 2005;31:226–30.
23. Jeena PM, Wesley AG, Coovadia HM. Admission patterns and outcomes in a paediatric intensive care unit in South Africa over a 25-year period (1971–1995). *Intensive Care Med* 2006;25:88–94.
24. Jones G, Steketee RW, Black RE, et al. How many child deaths can we prevent this year? *Lancet* 2003;362:65–71.
25. Khuri-Bulos NA, Shennak M, Agabi S, et al. Nosocomial infections in the intensive care units at a university hospital in a developing country: Comparison with National Nosocomial Infections Surveillance intensive care unit rates. *Am J Infect Control* 1999;27:547–52.
26. Kissoon N. Child with absent vital signs. *Indian J Pediatr* 2001;68:278.
27. Koyamaibole L, Kado J, Qovu JD, et al. An evaluation of bubble-CPAP in a neonatal unit in a developing country: Effective respiratory support that can be applied by nurses. *J Trop Pediatr* 2005; e-publication December 2, 2005:1–5.
28. Merchant M, Karnad DR, Kanbur AA. Incidence of nosocomial infections in a medical intensive care unit and general medical ward in a public hospital in Bombay, India. *J Hosp Infect* 2006;39:143–8.
29. Molyneux E, Ahmad S, Robertson A. Improved triage and emergency care for children reduces inpatient mortality in a resource-constrained setting. *Bull World Health Organ* 2006;84:319.
30. Moss WJ, Ramakrishnan M, Storms D, et al. Child health in complex emergencies. *Bull World Health Organ* 2006;84:64.
31. Musoke RN, Revathi G. Emergence of multidrug-resistant gram-negative organisms in a neonatal unit and the therapeutic implications. *J Trop Paediatr* 2000;46:86–91.
32. Nolan T, Angos P, Cunha AJLA, et al. Quality of hospital care for seriously ill children in less developed countries. *Lancet* 2001;357:106–10.
33. Ouedraogo N, Niakara A, Simpore A, et al. Intensive care in Africa: A report of the first two years of activity of the intensive care unit of Ouagadougou national hospital (Burkina Faso). *Sante* 2002;12:375–82.
34. Paul VK, Singh M. Regionalized perinatal care in developing countries. *Semin Neonatol* 2004;9:117–24.
35. Pearson G, Shann F, Barry P, et al. Should paediatric intensive care be centralised? Trent verses Victoria. *Lancet* 1997;349:1213–7.
36. Puoane T, Sanders D, Chopra M, et al. Evaluating the clinical management of severely malnourished children- a study of two rural district hospitals. *S Afr Med J* 2001;91:137–41.
37. Rhinehart E, Goldmann DA, O'Rourke EJ. Adaption of Centres for Disease Control guidelines for the prevention of nosocomial infection in a pediatric intensive care unit in Jakarta, Indonesia. *Am J Med* 1991;91 (3B):213–20S.
38. Sarnaik AP, Daphtary K, Sarnaik AA. Ethical issues in paediatric intensive care in developing countries: Combining Western technology and Eastern wisdom. *Indian J Pediatr* 2005;72:339–42.
39. Sethi D, Aljunid S, Saperi SB, et al. Comparison of the effectiveness of major trauma services provided by tertiary and secondary hospitals in Malaysia. *J Trauma* 2002;53:516.
40. Shann FA, Duncan AW, Brandstater B. Prolonged per-laryngeal endotracheal intubation in children: 40 years on. *Anesth Intensive Care* 2003;31:663–6.
41. Singh M, Deorari AL, Paul VK, et al. Three-year experience with neonatal ventilation from a tertiary care hospital in Delhi. *Indian Pediatr* 1993;30:783–9.
42. The World Bank Group. Millennium Development Goals. http://www.developmentgoals.org/Child·Mortality.htm (accessed April 2006).
43. Trotman H, Barton M. The impact of the establishment of a neonatal intensive care unit on the outcome of very low birthweight infants at the University Hospital of the West Indies. *West Indian Med J* 2005;54:297–301.
44. Wainer S, Khuzwayo H. Attitudes of mothers, doctors, and nurses towards neonatal intensive care in a developing society. *Pediatrics* 1993;91:1171–5.
45. Wilkinson D, Scrace M, Boyd N. Reduction in in-hospital mortality of children with malnutrition. *J Trop Pediatr* 1996;42:114–5.
46. World Health Organization. Anaesthetic infrastructure and supplies. In: *Surgical Care at the District Hospital*. Geneva: WHO; 2003: 15–1–15–12.
47. World Health Organization. Hospital Care for Children: Guidelines for the management of common illnesses with limited resources. http//www.who.int/child-adolescent-health/publications/CHILD_HEALTH/PB.htm (accessed July 2006). Geneva: WHO, ISBN 92 4 154670 0.
48. World Health Organization. Statistical annex. In: *World Health Report 2005: Make every mother and child count*. p. 190. http://www.who.int/whr/2005/en/ (accessed July 2006).
49. Zar HJ, Apolles P, Argent A, et al. The etiology and outcome of pneumonia in human immunodeficiency virus-infected children admitted to intensive care in a developing country. *Pediatr Crit Care Med* 2001;2:108–12.

CHAPTER 3 ■ IMPACT OF PEDIATRIC CRITICAL CARE ON THE FAMILY, COMMUNITY, AND SOCIETY

LEWIS H. ROMER • DAVID G. NICHOLS • HEATHER WOODS BARTHEL • JOS M. LATOUR • JESSICA MESMAN

The acute and comprehensive nature of the care provided in the PICU has made it a frequent point of entry into the hospital system and a highly visible contact point for many types of emergency services for children. The circumstances that bring children and their families to the PICU often involve crises that summon the attention of entire families and have ripple effects throughout their communities. Care of the critically ill child therefore has a high impact factor with regard to society at large. Additionally, as a consequence of this important role, the PICU care team may have opportunities to interface with a large number of diverse perspectives and venues. If they are performed skillfully, these interface functions can have a positive impact on the care of children, both within and outside the walls of the PICU.

The goals of this chapter include the enhancement of sensitivity, efficiency, and effectiveness in the PICU professional's interactions with the families that they serve. The major focus points are the initial establishment of a working relationship, process points for difficult segments of the hospital course, dealing with disability and death, and functions that the PICU practitioner may have in increasing societal awareness of child health and safety.

ORIENTING THE FAMILY TO THE PICU ENVIRONMENT

The admission of a critically ill child to a PICU initiates a unique relationship—the PICU care team cares not only for the child, but also for the parents, siblings, grandparents, and significant others of that child. This "additional" family-centered care is now recognized worldwide and has become standard practice in the PICU. The needs of parents may vary by country or even within a country due to ethnic, social, cultural, or personal differences. Therefore, the context of family-centered care should be based on the individual needs and requirements of the whole family. Knowledge of both specific parental needs and salient features of past parental experiences in the PICU environment is crucial for healthcare workers to set common goals for the process of guiding the parents through the intensive-care period and beyond.

Changes in Family Structure

The values and norms of many regions in the world are changing rapidly, and these changes impact upon the family structure. Traditionally, a family is a two-parent unit in which the mother is the caretaker of the children and the household and the father is the breadwinner. Databases from the US and Europe provide evidence that the nontraditional family structure is becoming more common. The prevalence of divorce among American families increased from 8.3% in 1990 to 10.2% in 2003 (Table 3.1). In the 25 countries of the European Community, the number of divorces has almost doubled in the past 30 years (Table 3.2). The consequences of these changes include an increase in single-parent families and a shift in the socioeconomics of family structure. Many mothers do not stay at home full-time, but participate in the working environment. Many become the head of the household, and some may have sole legal responsibility for their children.

Another type of major demographic change in family structure is exemplified by China, the country with one quarter of the world's population. The one-child policy introduced in China in 1979 affected family composition dramatically (16). The Chinese government claimed that this was a short-term measure to achieve a voluntary small-family structure, but the regulation still exists. This kind of family planning might directly influence parental psychologic and socioeconomic well-being when a child becomes critically ill. One recurrent observation of parents who find themselves suddenly and unexpectedly thrust into the crisis of their child's critical illness in the PICU is that this situation threatens the reversal of the expected natural order: Children are supposed to care for aging parents and "carry the baton" into the next generation. Worldwide family demographics that indicate a smaller number of offspring per family may intensify the poignancy of the reversal of this dynamic. Regardless of ethnicity and the reasons for changes in family structure, parental coping with a critically ill child is fundamentally based on the individual family's values, norms, behaviors, and attitudes.

These changing and diverse aspects of family life increase the need for healthcare workers to understand the individual family structure of each child admitted to a PICU. Assessment of family structure and functioning on a child's admission is prerequisite to guiding the parents during and after the intensive-care period. Specific factors of a family assessment that should be considered include current marital relationship(s), parental roles, communication and coping patterns, religious background, cultural values, and factors that identify this child as unique (e.g., only child, only son, only daughter, youngest, or eldest). Knowledge of family-coping style and modes of function provides essential insights for multidisciplinary, psychosocial intervention for the child and family throughout the hospital admission period.

MARITAL STATUS OF THE US POPULATION FROM 1990 TO 2004

Marital status	1990		1995		2000		2004	
	n	%	*n*	%	*n*	%	*n*	%
Never married[a]	40.4	22.2	43.9	22.9	48.2	23.9	53.2	24.8
Married[a]	112.6	61.9	116.7	60.9	120.1	59.5	125.8	58.5
Widowed[a]	13.8	7.6	13.4	7.0	13.7	6.8	13.8	6.4
Divorced[a]	15.1	8.3	17.6	9.2	19.8	9.8	21.8	10.3
Total[a]	181.8		191.6		201.8		214.5	

[a]In millions (181.8 represents 181,800,000); persons ≥18 years old of age. Excludes members of the Armed Forces, except those living off-post or with their families on post. Beginning 2001 population controls based on Census 2000 and an expanded sample of households. Data from US Census Bureau: www.census.gov/compendia/statab/population/. Accessed January 2007.

Creating a Therapeutic Alliance

Parental participation is a widely accepted part of PICU care. It is believed that the child benefits from the presence of his parents, and some argue that parental participation positively influences the outcome of a child's illness. Conversely, Pochard et al. found a high incidence of depression and other major emotional disorders among family members of (French) ICU patients. Emotional issues may block the family's receptivity to information or requests for participation in decision making (29).

The level of detail initially supplied and the care team's expectations of family cooperation must depend on parental needs, preferences, and reaction styles (28). Therefore, physicians and nurses must evaluate the knowledge and receptiveness of the parents so that common goals can be set for the care of their child. Family-centered care goes well beyond the very important process of informing parents about the condition of their child. The goal is to forge a collaborative relationship based on mutual respect and open communication between the healthcare professionals and the parents—*the therapeutic alliance*. The foundation of this alliance rests on the consensus that the best interest of the child is of fundamental importance. At stressful interludes that test communication skills, reminders about the collaborative nature of care are very effective reinforcements for cooperation between the child's family and the PICU staff. This alliance provides a shared context for the team–family communications that are essential to care (38). It is also a framework for additional conflict-resolution and consensus-building measures (**Table 3.3**).

Recognition of Parental Needs

The needs and preferences of the parents must be discovered and factored into the care plan. PICU staff members must take a leading role in supporting parents during the PICU admission of their child. Several studies have been conducted to gain an understanding of parental experiences during a child's critical illness (11,13,21,35,41). The priorities that emerge from these studies are consistent over time and are mostly related to information given to parents by the professionals and the proximity of parents to their child (**Table 3.4**).

Studies that focused on parental experiences during the PICU admission identify that PICU parents experience less reassurance at admission due to the high level of acuity and the need for urgent medical interventions (10). As the PICU course continues, interaction with the medical team is a barrier for some parents and can eventually become a source of stress and anxiety. Minor failings in the discharge process generate increased anxiety in PICU parents, although they are generally satisfied with the aftercare. Fathers and mothers may respond to stressors differently in the PICU. Thus, fathers reported that the major stressors were witnessing technical procedures that their children required and trying to maintain a parental role during the PICU course. Surprisingly, professional staff communication was experienced as less of an issue (4). Every PICU team should carefully assess its own professional approaches to parental guidance.

Family-centered Care

In pediatric critical care, the philosophy of family-centered care is a well-known concept. However, the elements of family-centered care are not always clearly understood. This confusion has led to wide variation in practice and results (1,18). The most comprehensive description of family-centered care is based on six dimensions, which are related to the roles of the professionals and the parents (**Table 3.5**). Pediatric critical care physicians and nurses must emphasize effective interventions for the improvement of family-centered care.

Regarding the *respect for the child and family*, global attention to equity in healthcare for all children and parents is

NUMBER OF DIVORCES IN THE EUROPEAN UNION FROM 1973 TO 2003

Years	European Union (25 countries)
1973	503,842
1983	718,318
1993	742,294
2003	955,688

Data from Eurostat: http://epp.eurostat.ec.europa.eu. Accessed January 2007.

TABLE 3.3

STRATEGIES FOR RESOLUTION OF TEAM-FAMILY CONFLICT

Sources of conflict	Strategies for resolution
Uncertainty regarding reversibility of condition and potential for improvement	Determine parents' understanding of likelihood that care will influence outcome Provide support, data, and perspective
Suboptimal communication or multiple sources of care-provider input	Encourage questions Conduct family and team meetings Incorporate major consultants' input into family meeting Provide unified message from a single care provider
Parental concerns over invasive monitoring and/or therapy	Explain downside of avoiding monitoring or therapy Explain the need to balance multiple risks in the quest for optimal long-term outcome Explore sources of parental anxiety
Setbacks or complications in the child's clinical course	Focus on long view and the fact that inconsistent progress is typical of a complex PICU course Explain time-limited trials of new therapies Obtain subspecialty consultation
Feelings of powerlessness	Emphasize parents' role on the care team Clarify parental expectations regarding their role in decision making Reassure parents regarding the essential role of parental love, support, and encouragement
Concerns regarding pain	Ensure parental involvement in pain score assessments and patient-, parent-, or nurse-controlled analgesia
Fear regarding possible death of the child	Validate risk of death and provide context Explain aspects of integrative view of multisystems management—care of the whole child Encourage parents to articulate their personal and family experiences with loss

a critical priority. Inconsistencies in the approach to children and parents that are related to recurrent discrimination result in inconsistent access to healthcare and differential treatment. Children from ethnic minorities may experience significant difficulties in accessing healthcare, compared with children from majority groups. Disparities in access to care and quality of service may arise from differences in insurance coverage, economic means, language barriers, cultural competency, geography, or ongoing internecine conflict. Healthcare professionals must be aware of the barriers faced by parents and respect the cultural diversity of their patients.

As detailed in the previous section, providing *information and education* to parents builds a basis for collaboration in the care of the critically ill child. Effective and understandable

TABLE 3.4

PARENTAL NEEDS IN THE PICU

Knowing how the child is treated
Being with the child
Feeling that hope exists
Participating in the care
Unrestricted visiting
Receiving honest answers from the healthcare team
Receiving understandable information
Receiving daily information
Having a place to rest near the PICU
Receiving empathy from professionals

communication between parents and professionals decreases parental stress and anxiety and fosters trust.

Coordination of care in a PICU entails collaboration with other departments, such as the emergency room and the pediatric wards. A PICU is by nature a transitional unit, with admissions and discharges frequently having other addresses within the medical center. The PICU team must carefully coordinate transfers to precisely address multiple facets of care, such as basic daily care, diagnostic tests, procedures, and consultations. For parents, the continuity of these processes becomes visible only when communications from the professionals are timely, accurate, and linked to a planned time schedule.

Parents are, by nature, concerned about *physical support* to their child with regard to pain and comfort, and this concern influences parental equilibrium. Incomplete communication about either anticipated painful procedures or needed pain control increase parental stress. The explanation and transparent use of validated pain and comfort assessment instruments can improve the recovery of the critically ill child and the well-being of the parent (6).

Emotional support to parents hinges upon recognition of the traumatic stress symptoms that are common among parents in the PICU. Parent educational and support programs may be valuable in the PICU for both short- and long-term improvement of parents' mental health. Although identification of parental stress and coping strategies in the PICU has been studied extensively, effective interventions to reduce stress are limited in scope. An effective example is the COPE program—Creating Opportunities for Parent Empowerment—which uses

TABLE 3.5

SIX DIMENSIONS OF FAMILY-CENTERED CARE

Respect for the child and family	Respect of multicultural and diversity issues, such as race, ethnicity, rituals, norms, values, beliefs, and socioeconomics
Information and education	Communication and teaching in an understandable language
Coordination of care	Timely and accurate coordination of care within a single unit and between units
Physical support	Prevention of suffering from pain and discomfort
Emotional support	Support that facilitates the family's emotional and spiritual needs
Involvement of parents	An open and flexible organization that facilitates parental participation in decision making and care based on the needs of child and family

educational media about the emotions and behaviors of sick children to improve the psychosocial outcomes of critically ill children and their mothers (24). This educational-behavioral intervention may decrease the incidence of posttraumatic stress disorder among mothers 1 year after PICU admission of their child.

The *involvement of parents* in PICU care is widely considered best practice. Physicians and nurses should provide open visiting hours, participation in care, and parental involvement in decision making. Parental presence during invasive procedures and medical rounds should be considered.

The current multicultural changes in communities and societies require professionals to be aware of the cultural diversity in the functioning of the family. Knowledge and understanding of various religions and beliefs are necessary to provide the best possible family-centered care. Family-centered care should not be practiced from a general viewpoint but should always be based on individual needs and preferences of the child, parents, and family members.

RECOVERY AND REINTEGRATION AFTER CRITICAL ILLNESS

Although discharge from the hospital after critical illness is a joyous occasion, the challenges for the child and family may continue if the child has a chronic illness or was left with sequelae after a prolonged PICU stay. These challenges are often physical, psychosocial, educational, and financial in nature. Preparing the family for reintegration into family and community life requires an action plan that the PICU team must set in motion.

Discharge Planning

Discharge planning represents the process by which parents are given an integrated package of instructions for disposition, medications, medical equipment, diet, and medical follow-up that will facilitate further recovery and health maintenance for the child. Although the effectiveness of discharge planning in reducing readmission rates or mortality is controversial, parents desire an integrated process by which to incorporate the

vast amount of information required to care for a child with a chronic illness after intensive care (30). The discharge planning process is more likely to be successful from the parent's perspective if it is coordinated by a single person or through a single source. That person is often a nurse who combines an understanding of the disease process and the patient's hospital course with an intimate knowledge of community resources that the patient will need in the future. Some of the major objectives of discharge planning are listed in **Table 3.6**.

Physical Aspects of Recovery and Reintegration

At the most basic level, the child returning home after a prolonged PICU stay has several physical needs. Prolonged mechanical ventilation (>1 week) increases the risk for weakness secondary to critical illness polyneuropathy or myopathy (5). Such patients may still be weak at the time of discharge to home. In addition to good nutrition, family members can provide physical therapy, which serves both to improve mobility and strength and provide an opportunity for bonding and

TABLE 3.6

DISCHARGE PLANNING OBJECTIVES

Determine best practical disposition (rehabilitation hospital versus home).

Help parents gain access to insurance programs and other financial services for children with chronic illnesses.

Ensure that parents are trained in cardiopulmonary resuscitation and the use of relevant medical technology.

Arrange for home nursing.

Arrange for a medical technology company to service medical equipment in the home.

Instruct parents on discharge medications and work with physician staff to simplify the medication list where possible.

Connect the parents with support and patient advocacy groups.

Give the family a realistic understanding of the challenges they face.

Spread hope and optimism to the child and family.

renewing alliances with the child. Newborns and infants may be malnourished after a prolonged PICU stay but recover quickly by 6 months (17). With proper attention to nutritional support during the PICU stay, older children generally avoid malnutrition altogether. Nevertheless, parents require very specific instructions on proper diet for the returning child. When possible, oral feeding should be encouraged, because it also provides an opportunity for parent-child bonding. However, some children, especially those with severe neurologic disability, require tube feedings to maintain adequate caloric intake. Conversely, a small subset of patients with morbid obesity and upper airway obstruction requires caloric restriction as part of the home therapeutic plan.

Technologic Aspects of Recovery and Reintegration

Numerous technologic devices now support care in the home. In fact, they have become so ubiquitous that physicians might automatically assume that every family can simply adapt to their usage. These devices range from mechanical ventilators to feeding tubes, dialysis machines, infusion pumps, and monitoring devices. In addition, many children have implanted devices (defibrillators, ventriculoperitoneal shunts, etc.). Although these devices may not require active parental intervention, they may nevertheless fail, making it imperative that parents understand the signs and symptoms of device failure so that they may obtain prompt medical intervention. Most devices have achieved a remarkable safety record and are clearly beneficial in extending the lives of chronically ill children outside of the hospital (2,37). However, parents must understand the technology and its use with their child, know how to troubleshoot problems, and have adequate backup supplies and a backup power source. Adequate preparation in these areas will maximize both the safety of the child and the psychologic health of the parents.

Most families develop rather astounding mastery of the technical details. The far greater challenge is to adapt to the disruption of "normal" family life that occurs during the care of technology-dependent children. Alarms ring. Interventions must be performed on schedule. Changes in the child's condition require parental adaptation. These three events will inevitably stress the normal rhythm of family life. Parental sleep deprivation often results (15). A physician's responsibility is to help the parents decide whether their family unit has the strength and resilience to cope with the technology-dependent child in their home. If the answer is yes, then parents and medical professionals should work together to devise a reasonable care schedule that draws on the strengths and skills of all members of the immediate family, supported by visiting nurses and other medical professionals. Such a schedule should allow for respite for each member in the immediate family. If the answer is no, then the physician should assist the family in finding a pediatric chronic care hospital.

Psychologic Aspects of Recovery and Reintegration—The Child

A short visit to the doctor may frighten a child. A prolonged stay in a PICU marked by vital-organ failure, invasive pro-

TABLE 3.7

DIAGNOSTIC CRITERIA AND MANAGEMENT OF POSTTRAUMATIC STRESS DISORDER

Diagnostic criteria
History: Extreme traumatic stress (may occur during PICU stay)   **Symptoms:** Fear, agitation, recurrent intrusive thoughts, aggressive behaviors, avoidance of stimuli associated with the trauma (or generalized withdrawal), persistent physiologic arousal (hypertension, tachycardia) for >1 month after PICU stay   **Management Strategy**   Screening for symptoms prior to hospital discharge   Explanation and counseling for the parents   Psychiatric evaluation of the child (for possible cognitive or pharmacotherapy)   Notification of the primary care physician and the school*   Development of specialized support and team approach*
*If authorized by the parents.

cedures, and separation from family and familiar surroundings may lead to lasting neuropsychiatric damage in the form of posttraumatic stress disorder (PTSD, **Table 3.7**). The *Diagnostic and Statistical Manual of Mental Disorders (DSM IV)* defines PTSD as a clinical syndrome following extreme traumatic stress that is accompanied by fear, agitation, recurrent intrusive thoughts, avoidance of stimuli associated with the trauma (or generalized withdrawal), and persistent physiologic arousal for >1 month after the traumatic event (3). If symptoms occur within 1 month after the traumatic event, they are labeled "acute stress disorder" and predict later PTSD. This type of reaction appears to be associated with the severity of the critical illness and with the number of invasive procedures (33). However, the origins of this disorder are not fully understood, because it may occur among children who appear to have been adequately sedated for invasive procedures. Yet, the consequences of PTSD are quite clear in the form of diminished intellectual and social functioning, heightened parental stress, and even decreased immunocompetence (39). Up to 62% of children who survive critical illness will have symptoms of posttraumatic stress, and 10% will carry the clinical diagnosis of PTSD.

The pathobiology of PTSD appears to involve disordered emotional memory consolidation in the amygdala during a highly stressful event. Acute stress leads to a surge in catecholamine and glucocorticoid release. Data from experimental animals reveal that catecholamines activate adrenergic receptors in the amygdala and play a critical role in memory consolidation (12). Similarly, direct injection of a glucocorticoid agonist into the basolateral amygdala enhances memory consolidation (34).

Given the prevalence and destructive impact of PTSD, the authors recommend that every child who has endured a prolonged critical illness undergo screening for this disorder. The parents should be screened as well. If a diagnosis of PTSD is established, a simple explanation and demystification of the symptomatology opens the door for cognitive or pharmacologic therapy for the child and/or parents, a context in which to understand the next stage of recovery, and empowerment of the family. The primary care physician and appropriate school officials should also be alerted. Without these interventions, the family is faced with a bewildering symptom complex.

Psychologic Aspects of Recovery and Reintegration—The Family

Even in the absence of a formal diagnosis of PTSD, the parents and siblings experience stress as they attempt to reintegrate the now chronically ill child after a PICU stay. Carnevale et al. identified six principal themes of this stress: (a) the reality of overwhelming parental responsibility, (b) the intense desire for a "normal" family life that seems no longer attainable, (c) confrontation with the outside world that seems to devalue the life of the chronically ill child, (d) social isolation, (e) uncertainty about the child's (or sibling's) feelings, and (f) a sense of unfairness and helplessness in the face of a moral order that allows child and family suffering. Despite the complex tensions produced by these feelings, most families also report a sense of enrichment by the presence of the injured or chronically ill child who is so demanding of their care (7).

Families need not be helpless in the face of this stress. The management strategy begins in the hospital with an explanation about the nature of the stress and reassurance that their response is common and expected under the circumstances. The next steps involve teaching parents about the behaviors and emotions that their child may display after hospitalization and fostering parental involvement in the child's physical and emotional care. Formal stress management techniques may also be beneficial. Such an approach is associated with reduced depression and stress among parents (24).

The financial burdens associated with the care of a PICU survivor may also be substantial if the child is left with chronic disability. Adequate health insurance is a tremendous help for these families, but out-of-pocket finances are still necessary for care, as indicated by the greater financial burden that low-income families assume even after controlling for insurance status (27). In the US and in some European countries, most families with a ventilator-dependent child can receive at least 8 hrs of in-home nursing assistance if federal support programs are utilized properly. A social worker or other medical professional knowledgeable in federal assistance programs for children with chronic disabilities should counsel the parents. The immediate family (as opposed to extended family or healthcare professionals) is the unit responsible for the delivery of the child's healthcare, and this formidable challenge is added to all the other responsibilities of a normal family. Healthcare professionals must therefore ensure that as much attention is directed toward fostering optimal functioning of the family unit as is directed to the child's medications (31).

Reintegration into the Community

The return to school exemplifies the milestone of reintegration into the community for the child. This milestone implies that major physiologic changes in the child are unlikely during the school day and that the child is mobile either via ambulation or wheelchair. While necessary, those conditions are hardly sufficient. Parents must educate teachers, the principal, and the school nurse about medications, medical equipment, behavior patterns, and special needs. Equally important is the parent's role as a relentless advocate for the child to receive the specialized services necessary to enhance his chances for learning and social adaptation. The primary care pediatrician must support the parents in this advocacy role and serve as a resource for the school in the individual child's case, and more generally by providing guidance on the proper nurturing of the disabled child within the school system.

PREPARING FOR AND RESPONDING TO DEATH

When a child's life comes to a premature end in the context of a PICU course, the hope and expectations that accompanied the entry into PICU care also end, and the reverberations in the lives of the child's family and community, and the lives of the PICU staff, cannot be overestimated.

Through the child who is the shared focus of their hopes and energies, parents and staff become part of a shared social order. Families, with their individual views and backgrounds, and staff members, with their various specific rules and rituals, meet each other around the bed of the dying child. To cope with the death of their child, parents need support from their relatives, friends, and the involved staff members. The staff has its own responsibilities, and a PICU should have a clear policy about how to act, what information is needed, how tasks are distributed among clinicians and parents, and sensitivity toward matters that may affect the end-of-life care, such as sociocultural specificities. In this section, some aspects of end-of-life care in the PICU will be discussed, with particular emphasis on parents and families.

Anticipating Loss

Whether a child dies suddenly and unexpectedly due to an accident or at the end of a long illness, the question remains: Can one ever be prepared?

Unexpected death shortly after admission complicates the supportive role of the PICU team as they struggle to care for a shattered family in shock. In the first busy moments of the child's PICU stay, no relationship exists between staff and family. They meet for the first time in one of the most tragic moments of life. Considering the overwhelming situation, it is helpful if one team member stays with the parents to explain the course of events and to outline necessary medical and legal procedures. In a case in which child abuse is suspected, parents have not only lost their child but have also become part of a police investigation. Even in this challenging situation, PICU caregivers must strive to remain supportive to parents, while providing appropriate medical information to child protective authorities and the police. If emotions threaten to overwhelm the PICU team attending the death of a child abuse victim, it may be useful for specific team members to focus on parental support while others interface with government authorities.

Not every child dies suddenly. In cases of a severe chronic illness such as cancer, the process of dying may be dreaded but anticipated for some time. When death is expected, the staff have the opportunity to prepare parents for the process of dying. In anticipation of the loss of their child, parents will experience pain and sorrow.

Although one may recognize similar patterns of grief and distress in families of different backgrounds, each situation requires an individual approach. After all, parents do not leave everything behind in the airlock; they come in with their hopes, emotions, expectations, cultural rituals, and expressions of grief. Each parent must find or be given a role in the end-of-life care of the dying child. The PICU team helps parents to develop their roles by listening, understanding, and helping them to interpret the unfolding events. Sometimes disagreements arise between the team and the family over end-of-life care. The resolution of these frictions may require support from a third party, often another professional member of the PICU team. The role of a social worker in the care and aftercare of parents is particularly useful in these situations.

Parents should be prepared for the changing appearance of the child, including gasping and other potential responses of the dying body. The appearance of a dying child may provoke not only grief, but also fear, alarm, and even revulsion among some family members.

The family should also be given advice on pragmatic issues, such as access to external support networks, funeral arrangements, death registration, and postmortem examination. Informing family is crucial, but generally, other details are as important. The staff must seek out insights into the specific questions, wishes, fears, and expectations that parents might have. Some parents want to take their child home before dying or initiate religious or spiritual rituals. These requests may require planning and communication with other parties or authorities.

In case of active withdrawal of life support, most children die within minutes or hours, but it does not always happen this way. Nor does the decision to limit life support always end the process swiftly. It can be decided to switch to a nonreanimation (or do not resuscitate) policy that includes continued maintenance care. With this decision, the staff enters a new treatment trajectory, usually without laboratory tests or frequent checking of vital signs. While the nursing care remains central, the medical technology is relegated to the margin. This trajectory calms hectic activity around the child but also marks the beginning of a period of anxious waiting for the parents. After all of the intense activity and exhaustion of the previous weeks or even months, time slows, and getting through the day becomes a different sort of challenge, one that may be best filled by family members bonding with each other—around and with the dying child.

Modes of Death

Modern technology has multiplied the modes of death in a PICU. Possible modes of death in the PICU include death despite active treatment, brain death, limitation of critical care (nontreatment), or active withdrawal of life support. Each of these modes of death occurs within a specific sociocultural context. Goh et al. stress the fact that limitation of critical care as a common mode of death is based on a Western ethical frame of justification and may therefore be inappropriate for people with other cultural backgrounds (14). An increasing cultural diversity in most societies makes it important to

take these cultural differences into account. [For an extensive discussion on the implications of cultural differences in end-of-life care, see appendix D, pp. 509–552, of the Institute of Medicine publication *When Children Die* (22)]. Factors in planning for the mode of death extend beyond medical considerations and include the family's social relations, religion, and responsibilities, as well as the previous personal experiences of the physicians—relationships and factors that explain some of the various modes of death chosen within the context of Western medicine (14). The death of a child in a PICU in Anglo-Saxon–influenced countries is the outcome of decision making that includes a deliberative process in which the parents participate. In the more Greek/Latin-influenced part of Europe, most children in the PICU die despite active treatment (9). In Europe, clinicians do not give away the final authority over withdrawal of life support. In Islamic culture, withdrawal of life support may not be an option. At the other end of the spectrum, the Dutch parliament recently passed a law specifically allowing various categories of physician-assisted dying for children over 12 years of age (40). Despite these evident differences, every parent is unique and acts accordingly, and these actions may occur despite a specific cultural attitude to the contrary.

Decision Making and End-of-life Care

The physician usually initiates the discussion regarding discontinuation of treatment, which does not imply that parents do not think about this option. Many times, they consider this possibility even before the physician raises the issue (25). The choice between withdraw and limitation of life support is not always clear for parents. To them, every option may carry too much guilt to allow a choice: If they choose continuation of care, they might keep their child alive longer, but this time might be filled with suffering; if they decide to withdraw treatment, they may have the sense that something could have been done after all and that they took that chance away. Although at this juncture some parents defer to physicians, they must live with the ultimate decision for years to come. Therefore, involvement of families in this decision-making process should be standard of care.

Notwithstanding the requirement of parental consent, it is the medical team that takes the ultimate responsibility. Leaving the decision entirely up to the parents is impossible in light of the fact that they often lack the knowledge to correctly interpret all of the information. Additionally, the stressful circumstances in which parents must face these issues may hamper objectivity. Therefore, most PICU teams attempt to find a position that respects parental authority without leaving parents alone in the decision. Approaches to parental responsibility then become the crux of the matter.

To be able to participate effectively in the decision-making process, parents must be well informed about their child's condition, level of discomfort, prognosis, and available treatments and their consequences. Information about resources for additional advice and support should be clear. Evidence suggests that most parents prefer full disclosure of information. For many, being fully informed helps them to comprehend and give meaning to the situation and to participate in the decision-making process. After listening carefully and understanding the parental and family circumstances, the medical staff should advise parents gently, yet clearly, about the best option in their medical opinion. Parental assessment of the child's physical and emotional suffering plays an important role in the decision about the continuation of life support (25). It should be clear for parents that palliative care, with its focus on prevention and relief of physical and emotional suffering, is a major part of the overall care policy throughout the remainder of the child's life and that it does not necessarily preclude curative or life-prolonging care (22).

Practice patterns regarding the involvement of the child in the decision-making process vary widely and depend on their age, knowledge, level of understanding, and physical condition, which does not imply neglect of the child's wishes or refusal to tell them about their condition. Where possible, children should be informed about their condition, and their wishes should be respected.

Nurses are often the team members who are most involved in the care of the child and the support of parents throughout the PICU stay. They instruct the family about their child's treatment, show them around the PICU, inform them in everyday language about the child's condition, and function as their touchstone. Despite the primacy of this relationship, many studies show that bedside nurses are under-represented in decision-making meetings (22).

Death and Dying

The death of a child is a devastating experience for the family and particularly for the parents. It shatters the ground on which they have built their lives and challenges their personal cosmic order. Parents try to preserve the relationship with their dying child by being present and by touching and talking to their child. The need to be in the immediate presence of the child before, during, and after death may also be based on a need to maintain connection with the child (23). In times of existential need, people tend to search for the meaning of life and death. Meert et al. stress that a spiritual element is associated with the efforts of parents to stay connected with their child. Memories of specific events, such as holding the child on their lap, or tangible mementoes can be considered in the light of the search for meaning and the need to be connected that ensue over the months following the death of a child. Other related imperatives include the parents' acceptance of the child's death and their perception that care of their child has been given with compassion and respect and that the ultimate trust invested in the care team has been upheld. Ideally, families should be offered a "family advocate"—someone separate from the PICU team whose sole function is to comfort and advocate on behalf of the family. The parents might prefer the presence of a pastoral care provider as their advocate, especially when rituals such as praying and reading sacred texts are vital elements that strengthen the family through hope and faith. The PICU team should know the parents' religious affiliation and avoid misunderstandings by first checking to determine if specific pastoral care is desired. Awareness of conflicting needs between parents may avoid friction that exacerbates negative affects at the most difficult of times.

In cases in which it is age appropriate, sibling involvement in end-of-life care is an important part of their bereavement process. Their grief and their capability to help or understand should not be dismissed. However, young children are not always able to comprehend the situation or to interpret the intense grief of their parents, and it is essential to regularly reevaluate their emotional and intellectual capacity to deal with the situation.

Forms of Support

During the process of dying, the staff carefully tries to deal with the needs of children and their families. The family tries to cope with their situation by finding meaning in what is happening and by living day to day (22). Through a constant redefinition of the situation they are confronting, parents try to prepare for death and, at the same time, preserve their relationship with their child. Involvement of family in the end-of-life care of their child is a way to endorse the parental role as being the child's original caregiver, provider of love, and decision maker (26). Marginalization of parents in the process of care will result in feelings of helplessness. Preservation of the child-parent relationship is an important parental coping mechanism, and fathers and mothers may exhibit different types of coping mechanisms. If one parent (often the father) withdraws when he knows his child is dying, the reasons should be explored and an opportunity provided to include the withdrawn parent in the planning of care, if possible.

Some studies reveal that parents experience communication with staff as problematic (26). They feel that seeking information about their child's condition is time consuming and that they have lost control over their child. It is important that staff members endeavor to gauge the appropriate level of medical specificity when they communicate with parents. Some parents prefer detailed information about every lab test result and ventilator setting, but too much detail and technical information can confuse parental perceptions of the child's overall condition and experience.

Staff members are an important part of the support network of families. In addition to providing them information, they offer emotional care as well. By listening to the hopes and fears of parents, staff members create room for parents' emotional expressions in which they can foster strength and trust. Some studies show that parents desire a certain level of reciprocity in emotional expression (26). Staff members who are willing to show their own feelings of consideration are perceived as more authentic and easier to turn to than those who do not allow themselves to express their feelings of empathy. If a primary nurse has been assigned to the child during the entire admission, she is likely to best know the patient and family. The primary nurse can help to explain the family members' style of emotional expression to the other caregivers. A style of communication that is informed by these insights is an important resource. Additionally, open admission of sorrow for the loss can be helpful for parents, allowing them to perceive that their child is not just a "routine case" for staff members (20).

Responding to Loss

After the death of a child, the equipment is turned off and the monitor falls silent, but not all is yet said and done. Once again, those involved change their frame of reference and switch to the set of priorities appropriate after a child has died. These actions are marked by doing things in slow motion, by respect, and by enhancing the language of compassion while diminishing technical data. Now, the toiling ventilators, blinking monitors, and beeping alarms are silenced. There is only tranquility, and all technology is brushed aside. If the child's life in the PICU was always entwined with the technology around his bed, these ties can be severed after death, ending a "hybrid" existence and leaving only the child again.

Coping Strategies

The emotional bond between parent and child lingers after a child's death. Staff members aid parents in coping with their loss by helping them toward the recognition that strengthening the emotional bond with their child helps them to integrate the loss. Good contact—even after their child has died—reduces parents' sense of guilt and improves their self-worth. After their child's death, parents are allowed to spend as much time alone with their child as they wish and bid farewell in quietude. In addition to privacy, social and religious rituals may be important parts of the bereavement process. Physical care, such as touching, bathing, and dressing their child after death, may be an important part of the bereavement process. These activities can act as a corridor for the (nursing) staff in their effort to help parents with their grief. With this aim in mind, some medical centers offer to photograph the child after death. If parents do not wish to have these photographs immediately, they may be stored in the record for future availability. Other mementoes, such as a footprint or a lock of hair, may be offered as helpful keepsakes during the grieving process and beyond.

It is important to create a space of privacy for everyone involved when a child is dying. However, a separate room is not always available. Closed curtains do not act as walls. The limited space makes it impossible for the staff to shield other parents from unforeseen emergencies. As such, the death of a child in the PICU is an event that also concerns other families on the ward. They are aware of what is happening, death and grief are right in front of them, and this can catalyze anxiety and despair, because the situation of another family represents a possible personal future that they dare not consider. The PICU team should counsel parents to avoid identifying their child's condition with those of other patients (20).

Follow-up Meetings—Moments of Reflection

Follow-up meetings are crucial to help parents deal with the loss of their child. They are equally important for parents who lose a child suddenly and for those for whom the child's death was expected. Bereavement meetings offer the opportunity for reflection on the death of the child in several ways, and Cook et al. propose some key elements to be included in them (8). The staff can explain in more detail what has happened on the basis of all of the available information. The parents can use this meeting to express their concerns and ask for clarification. To accomplish these objectives, a follow-up meeting should be delayed for at least 8 weeks, which allows the staff to collect relevant information (including postmortem results when available) and affords families the time to reflect on what has happened and to prepare their questions. Having knowledge of how a life ended makes a world of difference. In their looking back on their child's treatment and death, the parents and staff reflect on the interventions applied and the decisions made. What was once an erratic series of events is now a logical story that is subject to interpretation. A visit to the PICU where the child died can be a crucial element of the follow-up

and helpful in the grieving process but must be done on a voluntary basis only. Follow-up meetings are specifically aimed at a form of retrospection that allows parents to move on with their lives.

The Supportive Network

It is important to ensure that adequate support is available in addition to the PICU team. Indeed, some investigators express their concern about the dominance of staff members as the primary support network during the process of dying (25). They stress the need for families to also maintain and strengthen their private support network. Contact with staff will decrease dramatically after the child has died, whereas friends, family, and community may be supportive throughout the entire bereavement process. For families that have them, networks of family members and close friends can be considered central actors in the care of parents and siblings. It is also advisable to facilitate the involvement of other support networks, such as religious communities, palliative care programs, and local or national support networks, to establish continuity of care after death. In addition to this web of support, the availability of specific community services should be communicated to the parents.

Grief Experiences of PICU Staff

Staff members will experience a wide range of emotions while caring for a dying child. When a child's stay in the PICU lasts several months, the emotional bonding process may cause staff members to identify with the parents (28). Caring for a chronically ill child frequently leads to a high level of attachment. Strong emotional engagement does not always distort professional judgment—it may cause staff to better relate to families' responses. Nor is emotional detachment always a virtue, given that it can blind people's awareness of suffering and lead to medical decisions that are insensitive to parents' needs. Furthermore, parents understand the genuine emotional expressions of staff as supportive, which helps them in their process of grief.

Considering the high level of involvement of PICU staff in the dying process and their exposure to many deaths, careful attention to their grief experience is also necessary. PICU staff members face a difficult task, considering the fact that they will be confronted with the intimate and intense emotions of families. More than casual and occasional support from colleagues, family, and friends is needed to help staff through these cases. A study of the grief experiences of PICU nurses describes how the intensity and duration of their grief are related to personal experiences and to their relationships with the child and his family (32). High levels of attachment to the child and/or the family affect the depth and duration of feelings of sadness. More-experienced nurses feel less overwhelmed by their feelings of sadness and anger than do their less-experienced colleagues. Ideal notions about why a child should die, in what way, and with what type of involvement from the PICU staff may clash painfully with the reality of the situation. Some argue that situations of dissonance have a strong effect on grief responses (32). In other words, managing one's own grief is an ongoing learning process, and more-experienced colleagues can play a supportive role in this process. To cope with their own feelings of grief, some PICU nurses share their feelings with colleagues, whereas others prefer a more private sphere in which to express their sadness. Other coping strategies are self-nurturing, maintaining a balance between involvement and detachment while the child is dying, and seeking closure of the relationship with the family after the child has died.

PICU staff benefit greatly from an understanding of the relational dynamics among family and staff. Moments of reflection, embedded in a structured way in the PICU practice, can act as a space in which to resolve the difficulties and intense emotions that PICU staff experience during end-of-life care. Although relief sometimes prevails after the death of a child, informal discussion can also trigger questions about the management of the PICU course that require a multidisciplinary meeting. Retrospective multidisciplinary deliberations in which the entire PICU team reviews the cases of children who have died are essential forums and should not be swept aside. However, these moments of reflection tend to be sacrificed in the hectic rhythm of the PICU, a circumstance that can make nurses and residents feel that possibilities do not exist for the presentation and processing of their views on specific treatment policies. Obviously, efforts should be made so that this situation is avoided.

THE ROLE OF THE PEDIATRIC CRITICAL CARE PROFESSIONAL IN SOCIETAL RESPONSES TO CHILD MORBIDITY AND MORTALITY

Modeling Advocacy

The PICU provides willing observers with a unique window on society: Themes and patterns of childhood illness and injury can be indicators of shortcomings in public policy. Despite these insights, the pressures of patient care, institutional and academic responsibilities, and professional development leave little time in the work life of the critical care practitioner for the pursuit of child advocacy. Moreover, most healthcare professionals are not conversant with the process and bureaucracy of legislative bodies and human-service delivery systems. These realities are powerful supporters of the status quo. However, strategies for the reduction of preventable disease and injury are essential elements of our commitment to the improvement of child health and safety. Furthermore, each publicly visible effort that the pediatric critical care community makes in this regard has the potential to inspire the next generation of PICU professionals and child health advocates.

Three of this chapter's authors were presented with an opportunity to "act locally" in this regard. During the 2004–2005 heating season, the Johns Hopkins PICU treated seven children who were burned as a result of the use of open-flame heat sources in homes in which power had been disconnected following lapses in payment of utility bills. Five of these seven children died. In several instances, the families were in the process of applying for funds through the Maryland Energy Assistance Program when their power was turned off. One of the PICU attending physicians mobilized an energy task force within the medical center to address utility company policy. These efforts focused on the process of power termination in homes with small children. The energy task force included a second PICU attending physician, the medical director of the pediatric burn center, the pediatric trauma coordinator, the medical center's vice president and general counsel, a social worker from the institution's child injury prevention center, and public affairs and government relations staff. They met serially for several months

with the Maryland Department of Human Resources, the Public Service Commission, and the utility companies to ensure that applications for energy assistance would be processed in a timely manner to avoid unnecessary power termination. When a bill to revise the Energy Assistance Program Act was introduced in the state legislature, one of the intensivists seized the opportunity to provide testimony at the hearing and proposed an amendment to give special consideration to low-income households with children. Both the Department of Human Resources and the Senate Finance Committee looked favorably on this amendment. The bill, with this amendment included, passed both the state Senate and House on a unanimous vote (Chapter 119 of Senate Bill 129 of the 2005 Legislative Session of the Maryland General Assembly).

Passage of that bill was a catalyst that led to the formation of a formal work group that met to address power terminations to homes with children. It was an inclusive work group that included the Johns Hopkins energy task force, the Office of Home Energy Programs, the Public Service Commission, the Office of Peoples Council, and utility companies from across the State. It was a difficult and, at times, contentious process that required the skills, insights, and energies of every member of the Hopkins task force. However, in the end, all parties were able to reach a binding, nonregulatory settlement agreement to minimize the possibility of power termination. Elements of this amended agreement included expansion of the hours for energy-assistance inquiries and of payment plan options, as well as a 55-day grace period. At the time of this writing, the incidence of pediatric burn injuries following energy shut-offs has fallen dramatically in the State of Maryland, and the energy task force is currently monitoring the situation for signs that the system is in need of further adjustment.

The Challenge

Society entrusts pediatric critical care providers with the care of its sickest children. An extension of that trust is the confidence that caring professionals will act on opportunities for responsible citizenship by working toward the improvement of child health and safety through legislative process when necessary.

Toward this end, it is important to remember that preventable injury continues to be a leading cause of childhood death (19). Head injuries and multiple trauma cases that result from motor vehicle collisions, bicycle accidents, and other vehicular mishaps are regular features in the PICU census and remain far too common contributors to death and disability in childhood [State Legislative Report for 2005 of the American Academy of Pediatrics (AAP), available at www.aap.org/advocacy.html]. Data on the progress of three types of child safety legislation have been abstracted from this AAP report and presented in summary graphic form in **Figure 3.1**. The incomplete status of several legislative agendas may resonate with series of patients that present to any major pediatric center. Although seat belts and infant seats are required throughout the US, booster seats are on the law books in only 33 states and the District of Columbia. Bicycle helmets are required in only 26 states (and the District), and the containment of firearms is mandated in only 18 states. Legislative agendas on these and other topics for localities in the US may be tracked via listings at www.aap.org/advocacy/sgalinks.htm.

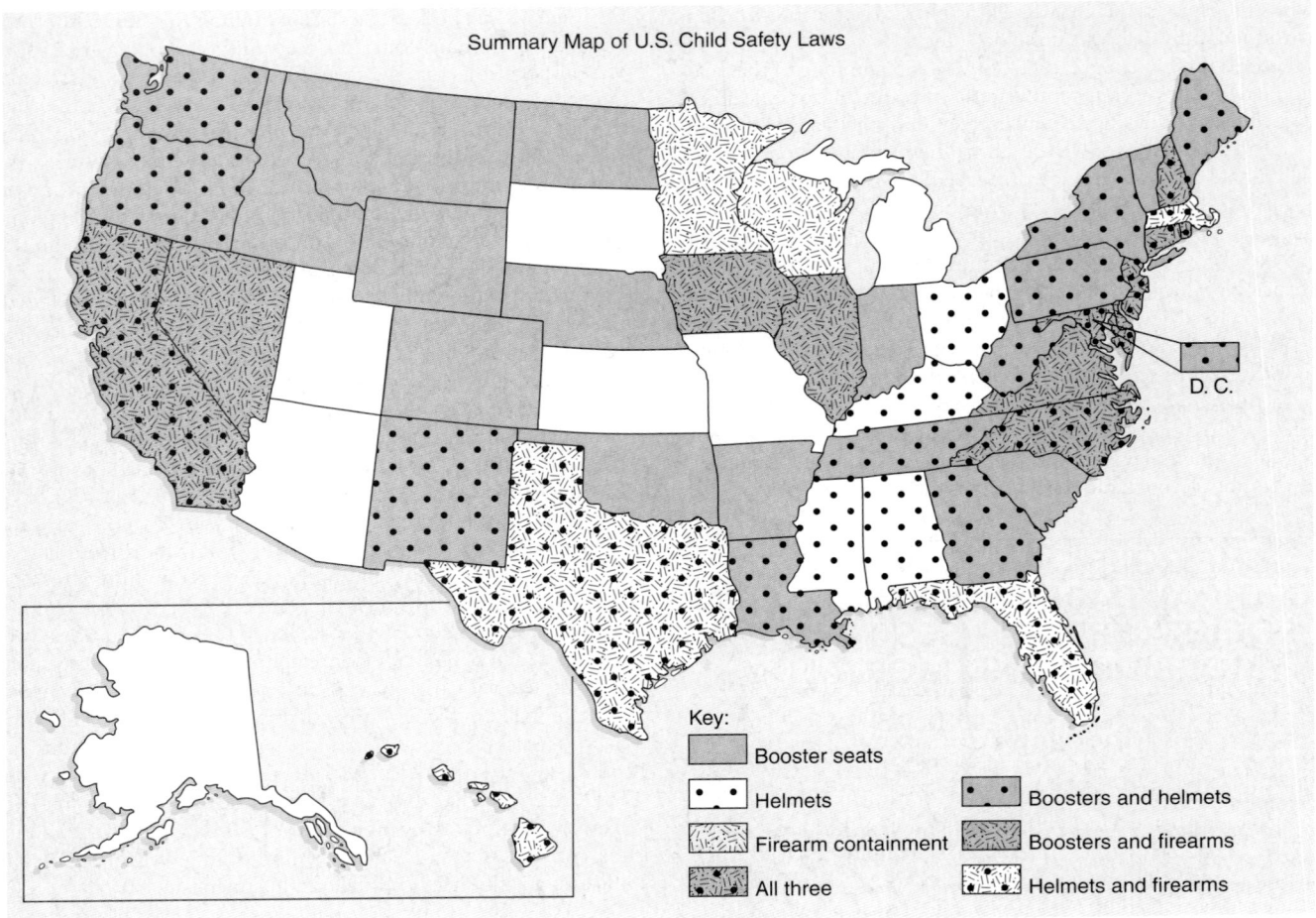

FIGURE 3.1. Summary map of US child safety laws. The presence or absence of laws requiring three key initiatives for child safety is coded according to the key (*lower right*) for the 50 United States and the nation's capitol, the District of Columbia (DC). White signifies the absence of laws mandating action on any of these key. Other codes denote the existence of these laws individually in pairs, or altogether. Data have been abstracted from the American Academy of *Pediatrics*. 2005 State Legislation Report. Legislation pending at the end of the 2005 legislative sessions is not included in this figure. Map template downloaded from www.infoplease.com, accessed January 2007.

CONCLUSIONS AND FUTURE DIRECTIONS

Research into the impact of the PICU over the past 5 years has yielded important indicators of difficulty with communication and adaptation in the PICU environment. The next step includes the development and testing of templated benchmarks and maintenance programs that can be used to improve the management of PICU stressors for both families and PICU staff. Reduction in the incidence of psychosocial sequelae for our patients may require the development of multidisciplinary PICU follow-up programs that include the critical care team. The challenge of PTDS should be addressed similarly through integrated strategies for the prevention, early detection, and treatment of graded severities of this disorder. Specific data are needed regarding the association of PTSD with specific sedative and analgesic strategies during invasive procedures in the PICU (33).

PICU care at the end-of-life could be improved by developing the broad implementation of training and team building for care providers, using real-time interaction with standardized patients (36). These efforts must encompass the entire family of PICU professionals, including all practitioner- and student-level front-line personnel: physicians, nurses, respiratory therapists, extracorporeal membrane oxygenation specialists, social workers, psychologists, and pastoral care providers.

Finally, a coordinated and broadly based effort is necessary to more effectively and immediately channel awareness of pressing child health-related issues into legislative action.

KEY POINTS

- PICU care involves multiple interfaces with the child, family, and community.
- The model of family-centered care includes the specific context and needs of the family in the care plan.
- Early planning for disposition and special needs, including counseling, teaching, and training, is required to optimally provide for care beyond the PICU.

- Posttraumatic stress disorder is a widely pervasive sequel of critical care that requires early intervention and long-term follow-up.
- Skillful direction of care in the terminal scenario requires the empathetic anticipation of the needs of family and staff.
- PICU practice offers the opportunity for patient advocacy beyond the walls of the hospital to decrease the incidence of childhood disease and injury.

ACKNOWLEDGMENTS

The authors thank Drs. Jason Custer, Jamie Schwartz, and Hal Shaffner for helpful discussions.

References

1. American Academy of *Pediatrics*. CoHC. Family-centered care and the pediatrician's role. *Pediatrics* 2003;112:691–7.
2. Amin RS, Fitton CM. Tracheostomy and home ventilation in children. *Semin Neonatol* 2003;8:127–35.
3. Association AP. *The Diagnostic and Statistical Manual of Mental Disorders, 4th ed., Text Revision*. Washington, DC: American Psychiatric Association, 2000.
4. Board R. Father stress during a child's critical care hospitalization. *J Pediatr Health Care* 2004;18:244–9.
5. Bolton CF. Neuromuscular manifestations of critical illness. *Muscle Nerve* 2005;32:140–63.
6. Brinker D. Sedation and comfort issues in the ventilated infant and child. *Crit Care Nurs Clin North Am* 2004;16:365–77, viii–ix.
7. Carnevale FA, Alexander E, Davis M, et al. Daily living with distress and enrichment: The moral experience of families with ventilator-assisted children at home. *Pediatrics* 2006;117:e48–60.
8. Cook P, White DK, Ross-Russell RI. Bereavement support following sudden and unexpected death: Guidelines for care. *Arch Dis Child* 2002;87:36–8.
9. Devictor DJ, Nguyen DT. Forgoing life-sustaining treatments in children: A comparison between Northern and Southern European pediatric intensive care units. *Pediatr Crit Care Med* 2004;5:211–5.
10. Diaz-Caneja A, Gledhill J, Weaver T, et al. A child's admission to hospital: A qualitative study examining the experiences of parents. *Intensive Care Med* 2005;31:1248–54.
11. Farrell MF, Frost C. The most important needs of parents of critically ill children: Parents' perceptions. *Intensive Crit Care Nurs* 1992;8:130–9.
12. Ferry B, McGaugh JL. Clenbuterol administration into the basolateral amygdala post-training enhances retention in an inhibitory avoidance task. *Neurobiol Learn Mem* 1999;72:8–12.
13. Fisher MD. Identified needs of parents in a pediatric intensive care unit. *Crit Care Nurse* 1994;14:82–90.
14. Goh AY, Lum LC, Chan PW, et al. Withdrawal and limitation of life support in paediatric intensive care. *Arch Dis Child* 1999;80:424–8.
15. Heaton J, Noyes J, Sloper P, et al. Families' experiences of caring for technology-dependent children: a temporal perspective. *Health Soc Care Community* 2005;13:441–50.
16. Hesketh T, Lu L, Xing ZW. The effect of China's one-child family policy after 25 years. *N Engl J Med* 2005;353:1171–6.
17. Hulst J, Joosten K, Zimmermann L, et al. Malnutrition in critically ill children: from admission to 6 months after discharge. *Clin Nutr* 2004;23:223–32.
18. Hutchfield K. Family-centred care: A concept analysis. *J Adv Nurs* 1999;29:1178–87.
19. Joffe AR, Lalani A. Injury admissions to pediatric intensive care are predictable and preventable: A call to action. *J Intensive Care Med* 2006;21:227–34.
20. Johnson AH. Death in the PICU: Caring for the "other" families. *J Pediatr Nurs* 1997;12:273–7.
21. Kirschbaum MS. Needs of parents of critically ill children. *Dimens Crit Care Nurs* 1990;9:344–52.
22. Field MJ, Behrman RE. *When Children Die: Improving Palliative and End-of-Life Care for Children and Their Families*. Washington, DC: The National Academies Press; 2004:671.
23. Meert KL, Thurston CS, Briller SH. The spiritual needs of parents at the time of their child's death in the pediatric intensive care unit and during bereavement: A qualitative study. *Pediatr Crit Care Med* 2005;6:420–7.
24. Melnyk BM, Alpert-Gillis L, Feinstein NF, et al. Creating opportunities for parent empowerment: Program effects on the mental health/coping outcomes of critically ill young children and their mothers. *Pediatrics* 2004;113:e597–607.
25. Meyer EC, Burns JP, Griffith JL, et al. Parental perspectives on end-of-life care in the pediatric intensive care unit. *Crit Care Med* 2002;30:226–31.
26. Meyer EC, Ritholz MD, Burns JP, et al. Improving the quality of end-of-life care in the pediatric intensive care unit: Parents' priorities and recommendations. *Pediatrics* 2006;117:649–57.
27. Newacheck PW, Inkelas M, Kim SE. Health services use and health care expenditures for children with disabilities. *Pediatrics* 2004;114:79–85.
28. Peebles-Kleiger MJ. Pediatric and neonatal intensive care hospitalization as traumatic stressor: Implications for intervention. *Bull Menninger Clin* 2000;64:257–80.
29. Pochard F, Azoulay E, Chevret S, et al. Symptoms of anxiety and depression in family members of intensive care unit patients: Ethical hypothesis regarding decision-making capacity. *Crit Care Med* 2001;29:1893–7.
30. Rahi JS, Manaras I, Tuomainen H, et al. Meeting the needs of parents around the time of diagnosis of disability among their children: Evaluation of a novel program for information, support, and liaison by key workers. *Pediatrics* 2004;114:e477–82.
31. Raina P, O'Donnell M, Rosenbaum P, et al. The health and well-being of caregivers of children with cerebral palsy. *Pediatrics* 2005;115:e626–36.
32. Rashotte J. Dwelling with stories that haunt us: Building a meaningful nursing practice. *Nurs Inq* 2005;12:34–42.
33. Rennick JE, Morin I, Kim D, et al. Identifying children at high risk for psychological sequelae after pediatric intensive care unit hospitalization. *Pediatr Crit Care Med* 2004;5:358–63.
34. Roozendaal B, McGaugh JL. Glucocorticoid receptor agonist and antagonist administration into the basolateral but not central amygdala modulates memory storage. *Neurobiol Learn Mem* 1997;67:176–9.
35. Scott LD. Perceived needs of parents of critically ill children. *J Soc Pediatr Nurs* 1998;3:4–12.
36. Serwint JR. The use of standardized patients in pediatric residency training in palliative care: Anatomy of a standardized patient case scenario. *J Palliat Med* 2002;5:146–53.
37. Srinivasan S, Doty SM, White TR, et al. Frequency, causes, and outcome of home ventilator failure. *Chest* 1998;114:1363–7.
38. Studdert DM, Burns JP, Mello MM, et al. Nature of conflict in the care of pediatric intensive care patients with prolonged stay. *Pediatrics* 2003;112:553–8.
39. Surtees P, Wainwright N, Day N, et al. Adverse experience in childhood as a developmental risk factor for altered immune status in adulthood. *Int J Behav Med* 2003;10:251–68.
40. Vrakking AM, van der Heide A, Arts WF, et al. Medical end-of-life decisions for children in the Netherlands. *Arch Pediatr Adolesc Med* 2005;159:802–9.
41. Ward K. Perceived needs of parents of critically ill infants in a neonatal intensive care unit (NICU). *Pediatr Nurs* 2001;27:281–6.

CHAPTER 4 ■ PROFESSIONALISM, SIMULATION TRAINING, AND LEADERSHIP IN PEDIATRIC CRITICAL CARE

ALICE D. ACKERMAN • ELIZABETH HUNT • VINAY NADKARNI

The goals of this chapter are to elucidate some of the important concepts of professionalism and leadership as they apply to the everyday lives of pediatric intensive care practitioners and to emphasize how utilizing these concepts can make the practice of pediatric intensive care more effective, more efficient, more patient centered, and more rewarding. The focus is on aspects of professionalism and leadership as they pertain *mostly* to the physician and relies upon literature primarily from North American and European sources, which in no way is intended to exclude other intensive care professionals or suggest that the primarily Western views described are the only valid concepts guiding our behavior. Because the notion of "professionalism" has become enmeshed within our training programs with how we teach our trainees, much of this chapter also focuses on the educational approach to both professionalism and leadership. Material presented in this chapter, when understood in the context of the other chapters in this section, helps to complete the discussion of the "core competencies" beyond the cognitive knowledge base required of our practitioners.

PROFESSIONALISM

Historical Background

Origins of Professionalism

The Western understanding of the medical professional originated with Hippocrates in the 4th century, BCE. The oath that bears his name is a very personal commitment to use one's ability for the good of patients. It gives honor to the teachers and mentors of the medical profession. It specifically prohibits the physician from performing euthanasia. It speaks to the morals of the physician, in connection with her medical practice and with everyday life. It requires the physician to maintain patient confidentiality and allows the physician to garner the respect of society as long as she upholds the oath. It has guided our expectations of physician ethical and moral behavior for over 2000 years. Most medical students in the US recite this or a similar oath at their graduation, prior to receiving their degrees. If all physicians continued to live and practice in line with the simple requirements of this oath, chapters such as this would not be included in such textbooks. However, the growing number of committees established to manage "code of professional conduct" issues in medical schools and hospitals attests to the unavoidable fact that physicians, among other healthcare professionals, do not always uphold the most basic of rules. In addition, our understanding and expectation of professionalism has changed over the past centuries.

Professionalism in the 20th Century

Starting in the mid-1900s, the definition of a profession assumed the more societal reflection that it maintains today, compared to the individual focus predominant in the 19th and early 20th centuries. Modern society expects and demands that members of a profession be formally trained to gain a specific knowledge base. It allows the profession to be largely self-regulating with regard to standards of education, performance, and disciplinary mechanisms. A member of the profession is expected to be more oriented toward public service than to individual profit and to behave according to a code of ethics. In exchange, society accords members of the profession a relatively high stature and respect.

More recently, changes in society and within medicine itself have led to concerns about the medical profession as a whole, as well as the behavior of individual members of the profession in particular. Skyrocketing healthcare costs, the impact of managed care limiting physician reimbursement and independence, and an ever-increasing technologic complexity have affected the internal and the external perceptions of what constitutes appropriate professional behavior.

Professionalism Today

New standards of the Accreditation Council of Graduate Medical Education (ACGME) require that professionalism be taught to residents and fellows, and the new standards for maintenance of certification (MOC) of the American Board of Pediatrics (ABP) require evidence of ongoing professional behavior in its diplomates. Other requirements for MOC include excellence in patient care, evidence of practice-based learning and improvement, evaluation of interpersonal and communication skills, and demonstration of the understanding of the components of systems-based practice, in addition to satisfactory completion of the traditional standardized secure examination.

TABLE 4.1

COMMITMENTS OF THE MEDICAL PROFESSIONAL

Commitment	Examples
Professional competence	Engage in life-long learning; maintain necessary skills for self and team; ensure that all members of the profession remain competent
Honesty with patients	Inform patients truthfully; acknowledge errors
Patient confidentiality	This may not be possible if patient poses a risk to society.
Maintaining appropriate relationships with patients	Includes the avoidance of sexual relationships, using patients for financial gain, etc.
Improve quality of care	At both an individual and systems-wide level, participate in mechanisms that encourage continuous improvement in care delivery
Improve access to care	Promote public health, preventive medicine, and patient advocacy; eliminate discrimination within physician's own system of practice
Ensure just distribution of resources	Provide cost-effective care; use evidence-based guidelines
Further scientific knowledge	Uphold scientific standards, promote research, create new knowledge; ensure its integrity
Manage conflicts of interest	Full disclosure
Professional responsibilities	Work collaboratively with others; discipline those who fail to uphold professional standards; develop new standards and train new members appropriately

Adapted from Medical Professionalism Project. Medical professionalism in the new millennium: A physician charter. *Ann Intern Med.* 2002; 136:243–246.

As discussed next, the components of MOC revolve around a new definition of medical professionalism.

Professionalism and the "Core Competencies." In 2003, the Institute of Medicine (IOM) (11) declared that today's medical professional should be able to provide patient-centered care, work in interdisciplinary teams, employ evidence-based principles, apply quality-improvement methodologies, and utilize informatics in the practice of medicine. These are the five noncognitive "core competencies" that the physician of the new millennium is expected to possess. They were adopted by the ACGME in the form that is probably more familiar to both trainees and practicing intensivists: patient care, practice-based learning and improvement, interpersonal communication skills, professionalism, and systems-based practice (1). These competencies form the core but not the entirety of our professional behavior. Clearly, each identified competency includes a multitude of specific knowledge points and behavioral characteristics. How are the IOM's competencies related to professionalism?

Professionalism and the "Physician Charter." The relationship between the core competencies and medical professionalism was addressed in part by the American Board of Internal Medicine (ABIM) Foundation, working in conjunction with the American College of Physicians-American Society of Internal Medicine (ACP-ASIM) Foundation and the European Federation of Internal Medicine in the 2002 publication, "Medical Professionalism in the New Millennium: A Physician Charter," which appeared simultaneously in the *Annals of Internal Medicine* (24) and the *Lancet*. This publication was the out-

come of a summit of numerous medical societies throughout the US and Europe, an attempt to call to action physicians throughout the world to develop a renewed sense of professionalism. The charter set forth 10 commitments (**Table 4.1**) of the professional once she has acknowledged the guiding ethical principles of the primacy of patient welfare, patient autonomy, and social justice. The items listed in the Physician Charter represent a potentially desired outcome; however, the roadmap for how to reach this proposed optimal state of the medical professional is not inherent in the charter.

In 2002, the Royal College of Paediatrics and Child Health (RCPCH) in the UK published a statement on the duties and responsibilities of pediatricians, entitled "Good Medical Practice in Paediatrics and Child Health." This document defines the ways in which the "good-enough doctor" can be recognized and unacceptable behavior or performance can be identified. It focuses on many of the same areas as does the ABIM Foundation Charter, but it is specific to those who care for children, and it provides concrete examples of acceptable and unacceptable practice. The Royal College identifies actions and behaviors that could cause the pediatrician in the UK to lose his registration with the General Medical Council. The individual examples of unacceptable behavior are elucidating. Overall, the document lists 59 duties and responsibilities, divided into the following eight major areas: Good medical practice (professional competence); good clinical care (the practice of competent care, ensuring appropriate access to care); maintaining good medical practice (keeping abreast of current medical knowledge and maintaining performance); teaching and training, appraising and assessing; conducting relationships with patients (consent, confidentiality, trust, communication, and terminating physician-patient relationships); dealing with problems in professional practice (conduct and performance of colleagues, complaints, and malpractice insurance); working with colleagues (treating colleagues fairly, working in and leading teams, arranging cover, accepting appointments, sharing information, and delegation and referral); and finally, a section entitled "probity," which deals with conflicts of interest, research, personal health, financial interests, and related issues. It also addresses the seeming paradox that arises when one is encouraged to participate as a member of an interdisciplinary team, yet professionalism demands that one take personal accountability for one's professional conduct and the care provided. Readers are encouraged to obtain this document, which is available at www.rcpch.ac.uk/publications/recent_publications/GMP.pdf (26).

The CoBaTrICE (Competency-based Training programme in Intensive Care Medicine for Europe) collaboration published a list of competencies expected of adult intensive care physicians based on consensus developed over a 3-year period. Professionalism is one of the 12 "domains" listed and was weighted heavily in importance by the majority of the participants in the Delphi processes (22) used to develop consensus. Within the professionalism domain, CoBaTrICE includes the following competencies: communication skills; professional relationships with patients, relatives, and other members of the healthcare team; and "self governance" (5).

Personal Attributes of the Medical Professional. These descriptions of professionalism place a great deal of emphasis on the outward, measurable or observable conduct of the physician but pay little attention to the intrinsic attributes that identify a physician as a true professional. The American Association of Medical Colleges (AAMC) has determined that the medical professional in today's society should be knowledgeable, skillful, altruistic, and dutiful, and has encouraged schools of medicine to incorporate teaching of professional attitudes and behaviors into their curricula (15). Others add qualities such as compassion, integrity, fidelity, and self-effacement as important in the "good" doctor (7). Gregory Larkin, who writes about how to model and mentor students in professionalism, suggests that we first map virtues and vices in professional practice. He has identified "four valences" of professional behavior in order of best to worst: ideal, desired, unacceptable, and egregious (19). For example, ideal behaviors would include showing altruism toward others and having humility regarding one's own achievements. Desired behaviors would be acting in the best interest of the patient and arriving on time for work. On the negative side of the spectrum, unprofessional behaviors would include arriving late or breaching confidentiality, while egregious behaviors would include lying, falsifying medical records, and engaging in substance abuse.

Teaching Professionalism

Once we understand what actions, behaviors, and attributes are consistent with professionalism, the next question becomes: "How do we teach this?" The answer is both simple and complex. Although the most important aspect of learning to act as a professional appears to be having the appropriate role models (7,15), we nonetheless must find a way to help our students and trainees understand the relationship between such ideal attributes as altruism and the behaviors—good and bad—that they observe daily at patients' bedsides. Many schools of medicine have developed courses on professionalism or humanism, yet students today are graduating with a cynicism that they did not have 40 years ago. Why?

Dichotomy between Ideal Behavior and Reality. Students learn in the clinical setting by observing the behavior of many individuals with whom they interact. It is not just the wise professor, who embodies all of the desired virtues of the physician, who will affect those most likely to be influenced. Rather, it appears that students are most influenced by those with whom they spend the most time. The influence of residents and fellows on the attitudes of medical students has probably been underestimated. Students and trainees not only hear what we say, but note what we do; in a significant number of cases, the two are diametrically opposed. We are, in fact, teaching cynicism (7,15). Critical care clinicians must find a way to stay centered on the core values of the medical profession as we care for patients and as we train our students and residents/fellows. Schools of medicine, while stating that they wish faculty to exhibit professional behavior and serve as role models for students, residents, and fellows, may not reward the outstanding clinician-teacher role model as well as or as overtly as they reward the successful researcher-academician (19). The gap between what we say we want and what we reward must be closed or at least diminished if medicine wishes to make professionalism a reality and to establish those physicians who embody professionalism as revered role models.

Impact of Burnout on Professional Behavior. Trainees themselves often do not realize their impact on students or other trainees. A significant percentage of residents may suffer from burnout (a syndrome of emotional exhaustion, depersonalization, and a sense of low personal accomplishment), and this can easily be transmitted to the students and colleagues with whom they work. Burnout among internal medicine residents was associated with self-reported unprofessional behavior in a recent study (27). Critical care units are stressful places; black humor and occasional disdain for the patient have been noted to occur. Burnout is a major problem among residents, fellow, and attending physicians (4,21,25). The risk of unintentionally teaching unprofessional behavior through our actions is, therefore, great under these circumstances. Residents, fellows, and students will more readily emulate our actions than our teachings.

Reflective Learning. Much has been written on how to overcome the tension between the "overt" and "covert" curricula in medical education as it pertains to professionalism. It has been suggested that the culture in today's hospitals and in many medical systems is antithetical to the development of the virtuous healthcare practitioner (6). One approach, applicable to practicing intensivists as well as trainees, is to develop a more reflective approach to ongoing behavioral learning (7). In this way, we acknowledge when our behavior is different from what is optimal, and we can identify reasons for that difference. Bringing this acknowledgment into our consciousness may prevent the discrepancy between the ideal and the real from turning into cynicism. As we become more reflective, we can utilize the stories that surround our involvement with our patients to help identify emotional issues in our own responses to them or their situations.

A specific approach, termed "narrative-based professionalism," presents the opportunity to rectify the tension between tacit and explicit values (7); for example, between altruism and self-interest. In this scheme, young professionals are immersed in a wide array of narratives or stories that help to develop role modeling, self-awareness, narrative competence, and community service. In addition, the ACGME has offered some suggestions for teaching and assessing professionalism that may be found on their web site, where one can find access to numerous web-based resources for education, assessments (including 360-degree evaluations), and references (2). The ABP web site lists guidelines for how to evaluate professionalism of pediatric residents. One way to approach the teaching of professionalism and the core competencies is through simulation.

Professionalism Training Addressed through Simulation

As mentioned throughout this chapter, various scientific and regulatory bodies are becoming more interested in ensuring that physicians are *intentionally* trained in various aspects of professionalism. As a medical community, we are no longer content to assume that traditional training *should* result in physicians who are competent at procedures, effective and compassionate communicators, able to function as team leaders, and able to practice per consensus statements or evidence-based guidelines. The aviation, defense, and nuclear energy industries have a history of success in safety and skill-based performance improvement using simulation interventions in training. In 1999, the IOM specifically called for establishment of interdisciplinary team-training programs that incorporate efficient training methods, including simulation (18). Thus, interest has dramatically increased in identifying innovative mechanisms (such as simulation) to enhance traditional training methods and to measure the effectiveness of those methods.

Simulation training has the potential to contribute to professionalism through a variety of mechanisms. First, following the credo of the Hippocratic Oath, our first obligation to our patients is to "Do no harm." Effectively, this means that we must find methods to optimize our training; that is, to be the best doctors we can be and avoid "practicing" on our patients. One example is methods used to train how to perform procedures. The old mantra of "see one, do one, teach one" does a disservice both to the patient *and* to the physician in training. A growing number of published controlled trials demonstrate that physicians randomized to training programs that utilize simulation perform "better" (defined variably as faster completion of surgery, fewer errors made during a procedure, etc.) than those trained through usual programs, including those for laparoscopic surgery, vascular catheterizations, and early airway management (3,10,23). An example of a pediatric critical care procedure that could be practiced prior to performing on a live patient is placement of a central venous catheter. A new fellow could practice the myriad steps involved in successfully performing this procedure from beginning to end, including the steps that require communication with others. She could obtain informed consent, address whether or not the family should be present for the procedure, establish a sterile field, use ultrasound guidance to identify the vessel, practice the Seldinger technique, secure and dress the catheter, and document the procedure in the medical record. Increasing evidence demonstrates that simulation can shorten the time to competence and increase the likelihood that, when a physician is performing a procedure for the first time, the patient is safer than if the physician did not have simulation training.

Another important way in which simulation can be used to enhance professionalism is through various exercises focused on improving communication. One study utilized standardized patients with multidisciplinary intensive care teams to practice talking to families about issues such as delivering bad news, discussion of brain death, and approaching the family about organ donation (30). A national body funded this study, in which the exercise was well received by participants. The intervention was associated with increased organ donation rates, presumably due to more effective communication postintervention. Other types of communication that could be practiced using a standardized patient to enhance communication with a real patient or family member include: obtaining consent, discussion of withdrawal of care, request for autopsy, disclosure of errors, and delivering an apology.

Simulation can be used to diagnose deficiencies in team management of critical care issues and then, ideally, to address the issues identified in subsequent exercises. For example, mock codes have been used to identify deficiencies in the management of simulated pediatric trauma victims in the trauma bay and in simulated medical emergencies (8,14). These interdisciplinary exercises are a powerful means of observing team dynamics and assessing complex issues, such as leadership, communication, and adherence to important protocols (e. g., the American Heart Association's Basic, Pediatric, and Advanced Life Support algorithms).

Simulation can also be used to help assess competency. Most believe that it would be unwise to tightly link or require simulation performance to accreditation because little investigation has been conducted on the correlation between competent performance on a simulator, competent operational performance on real patients, and patient outcomes. However, it is already possible and advisable to assess whether a physician can adhere to accepted protocols as part of a training program. For example, programs can create scenarios with a high-fidelity simulator to test whether participants are able to follow consensus protocols on the management of cardiopulmonary arrest, difficult airway, shock, or traumatic brain injury with elevated intracranial pressure. Deviation from clinical protocols can be identified and addressed to improve protocol understanding and compliance and to employ a "train-to-success" approach.

The approach to simulation training has been categorized based on the different types of simulations used in the training. Simulation modalities can be categorized in a number of ways, one example of which is presented in **Table 4.2**. In addition to this type of categorization, the simulation community often uses the phrases "high-fidelity" and "low-fidelity" simulation. These terms have no universally accepted definitions. However, most would agree that "high-fidelity" simulators are more sophisticated and interact in some way with the user; for example, if the user delivers a medication to a "high-fidelity mannequin," a computer can be programmed to have the mannequin's monitor respond appropriately, thus helping to "suspend disbelief."

TABLE 4.2

TYPES OF SIMULATION—EXAMPLES FROM PEDIATRIC CRITICAL CARE

Type of simulation	Examples from pediatric critical care practice
Standardized patients	Training toward effective and compassionate communication: end-of-life discussions, autopsy, organ donation, obtaining consent, disclosure of errors, offering apologies, HIV exposure
High-fidelity mannequin	Team training—cardiopulmonary resuscitation, difficult airway scenarios, shock management, elevated intracranial pressure management
Virtual reality	Bronchoscopy, endoscopy, endovascular procedures
Partial-task trainer	Airway trainers—bag-valve-mask ventilation and nasal and oral tracheal intubation, central-line chests, lumbar-puncture trainers, arterial-line trainers
Screen-based microsimulation	Advanced Cardiac Life Support, trauma management, critical care scenarios

However, the impact of the fidelity intensity (realism) of simulated scenarios on outcome is unknown and is an area for further study.

In creating a simulation program, it is important to match the type of simulation with the goals and objectives of the educational experience. Arguably, the most important component of simulation is the feedback. Corrective and directive feedback should be timely, constructive, and specific and may "slow the decay of acquired skills and allow learners to self-assess and monitor their progress toward skill acquisition and maintenance" (16). Ideally, if mistakes are made, the physician should be allowed to practice again until she achieves the expected outcome. Rather than walking away feeling deflated, she feels empowered.

LEADERSHIP

As mentioned earlier, one of the elements that can be taught through simulation is leadership. Leadership training is another way in which professionalism can be addressed and taught. Fellows entering pediatric critical care and pediatric anesthesiology training at a large children's hospital were evaluated on their knowledge of the "core competencies" (20). After investigators discovered that first-year fellows had a limited knowledge and understanding of the meaning and importance of the core competencies, they developed an educational program to teach the components of leadership that would help fellows to become competent in systems-based practice, professionalism, and communication skills. They discovered that (a) although fellows were willing to try to learn the material, they were not willing to devote much time to it, and (b) faculty members found it difficult to deliver the competencies within the existing structure. It also became clear to the investigators that faculty are not prepared to teach the competencies beyond the didactic level.

Other institutions are developing similar programs to address the competencies and help their fellows and faculty to develop stronger leadership skills. Such training differs from the standard "professional development" courses traditionally offered at schools of medicine, which are geared specifically to competency in research and teaching methods and to prepare for promotion. Although important for success within the medical school hierarchy, this traditional training may not be sufficient to improve clinical outcomes or to develop the kind of skills necessary to prepare trainees and practitioners to lead the diverse and rapidly changing subspecialty of pediatric critical care into the future.

What Is a Leader?

The definition of a leader can be complex. Most simply, it can be said that a leader is the person who "gets things done." Achieving results is what we do in the ICU. It is also what we need to do in the meeting room if we expect to convince the hospital to buy that piece of equipment for our patients or in the unit if we want the resident to accomplish something in particular. Leadership is the way in which we achieve results. It is the way we empower others—and ourselves—and it is the way we ensure a better future for our profession.

The Joint Commission on Accreditation of Healthcare Organizations (JCAHO) in the United States has published revisions of its standards that pertain to physician leaders in American hospitals. These are separate from the requirements it makes of medical staff in general (12). The new requirements are based on JCAHO's understanding of the relationship between leadership and the provision of quality healthcare, with an emphasis on patient safety. The medical staff of the hospital is identified as one of three components of hospital leadership, the other two being the governing body (such as the board of directors) and the management (also known as the administration). Medical staff must become intimately involved with developing the mission and vision of the institution, participate in developing safety and quality goals, and become involved in the budgeting process and interpretation of financial statements. The medical staff is expected to be knowledgeable about the population served by the institution, about applicable laws and regulations, and about their own individual and shared responsibilities and accountabilities.

Hospitals are responsible for orienting the medical staff leaders to these areas. In addition, each institution is expected to provide training for all leaders in conflict management, systems-based practice, team structure and function, evidence-based decision making, and development of mutual respect between disciplines. Each hospital that seeks accreditation will be expected to monitor the effectiveness of its leadership groups and to engage outside expertise (consultants) if adequate expertise does not reside within the institution for training and performance of the leadership tasks identified above.

These requirements will lead institutions to incorporate physicians into the overall leadership structure of the hospital to a much greater extent than most have done so far. With the growing need for physician leaders at all levels, the pediatric intensivist will have much to offer in terms of her understanding of patient needs, quality, patient flow, resuscitation, and other issues. The physician who has the proper training in several areas of management and leadership, who can apply systems-based ideals, develop evidenced-based medical practices, and oversee quality initiatives will be highly desired by those institutions striving to embrace these standards. Other valuable skills will clearly be effective communication and conflict management.

Leadership Training

Leadership training teaches individuals multiple skills, including time-management, effective communication, program development, visioning, and team development and leadership, to name but a few. Participants are helped to understand their "leadership style" through a number of possible mechanisms. Much of current leadership training is based on the development of what has been termed "emotional intelligence" by Daniel Goleman, a noted leader in executive development (9). Emotional intelligence is composed of four fundamental components: self-awareness, self-management, social awareness, and social skill. Each of these areas contains specific competencies to be developed. Different styles of leadership emphasize different patterns of emotional intelligence and, therefore, competencies. Because competencies can be taught and learned, it follows that effective leaders can be developed.

Most pediatric critical care fellows and junior faculty report that they have not received any formal training in management or leadership. They feel particularly unprepared to handle stress, manage conflict (within their own team or with other groups), manage time, and evaluate team performance (28). Leadership training is therefore clearly needed.

Leadership training exists in many forms and may be accessed in a variety of ways. Readers are encouraged to seek training at the local level when available. Numerous web-based programs are also available. One example is the leadership training presented by the American Academy of Pediatrics (AAP) and the Pediatric Leadership Alliance. AAP members can pay a fee and have access to this online training for a period of 3 years. It is available through the *PediaLink* Learning center found at www.aap.org. Another source of physician leadership information is the American College of Physician Executives (www.acpe.org). They provide quality publications and courses and can be helpful to those physicians who seek advanced degrees in management. Such individual courses that teach communication skills, management of conflict, and dealing with disruptive physician behavior can be accessed. Readers should not exclude attending seminars or lectures aimed at business professionals, because the basic concepts of communication, time management, stress management, and conflict management are applicable, regardless of specific work setting.

Numerous books have been written on the topics of leadership and management. One should decide whether she wants to develop personal leadership qualities or to learn more about organizational behavior and how to develop an organization (ICU, critical care division, family). A few recommended references are listed in **Table 4.3**. In no way can this list be exhaustive or even inclusive of the best in the field. Each "expert" in leadership development has her favorites. This list is therefore biased toward the interests of the authors. Absence from this list does not imply lack of value. New or trendy resources that might become outdated have intentionally been omitted.

Practicing Leadership through Management of Interdisciplinary Teams

To achieve a positive change in the medical society requires the physician to be both a "team player" and a "team leader." Learning to work as part of an interdisciplinary team may be difficult for the physician, who is traditionally taught to function alone and assume individual responsibility. The fact that the interdisciplinary team is proving to be the best method to ensure that patients receive coordinated, appropriate care is recognized by practitioners of primary care, internal medicine, geriatrics, and other specialties. In an interdisciplinary team, members from various disciplines coordinate their efforts, communicating with each other directly, for the benefit of the patient and to achieve optimal patient outcomes (13). Pediatric critical care has long embraced the notion of the interdisciplinary healthcare team. We may therefore consider our subspecialty one of the "early adopters" and leaders within medicine. Our challenge now is to leverage our relatively loosely defined teams into highly functional teams that will achieve specific purposes.

Definition of Teams

Most of us think of a team as a "group of people working together," usually with a common goal. However, recent business literature has defined a team more rigorously. A team is not just a committee or a working group. It is not a collection of individuals who want to "be a team." An effective team is a group of individuals working toward a particular performance goal—a group of individuals more committed to team outcome than individual performance. An effective team functions with rigor and discipline. Its members have complementary skills, and they agree upon a common approach, while holding each other mutually accountable for their performance. The leader of the team does not direct the activities of the other members but works to build commitment, fill gaps, shift the leadership role as appropriate, and do real work beyond decision making (17). Unfortunately, the word "team" has become a buzzword in today's medical management literature as well as in everyday life, thereby losing some of its impact.

Functional Teams

The functional team we experience as we perform work rounds has a performance goal: evaluating the patients in as expeditious a fashion as possible, enabling patient care decisions to

TABLE 4.3

SUGGESTED SOURCES FOR LEADERSHIP EDUCATION

Web sites		
Web site/URL	**Title/Description**	**Limitations**
American Academy of Pediatrics (AAP) www.AAP.org/ pedialink	Pediatric Leadership Alliance Provides education on leadership styles, issues facing leaders, spends lots of time on team development and management; interactive; content is available for 3 years	Cost to access the educational materials; available to both members and nonmembers; lower cost to members
www.Keirsey.com	Temperament Sorter Temperament test based on the book *Please Understand Me II*; provides an interactive test to gauge personality types based on observable behavior patterns	No cost, but registration may be required
www.personalitypage.com	The Personality Page Provides access to simplified Myers-Briggs Type Indicator (MBTI) test on line	Cost to register, $5; lots of additional links
http://typelogic.com	Read about different personality types after taking the MBTI test or investigating your type some other way	No cost; lots of links

Books		
Author	**Title/Publisher**	**Description**
Allen, D	*Getting Things Done: The Art of Stress-free Productivity.* New York: Penguin Putnam Inc., 2001	A not-so-basic introduction to time management and goal setting
Blanchard K, Zigarmi P, and Zigarmi D	*Leadership and the One-Minute Manager: Increasing Effectiveness through Situational Leadership.* New York: William Morrow and Company, 1985	Easy steps to take to achieve leadership effectiveness in daily life and work situations
Blanchard K, Oncken W, Burrows H	*The One-Minute Manager Meets the Monkey.* New York: William Morrow and Company, 1989	How to manage time, how to delegate, how to coach, and how to achieve efficiency and effectiveness
Collins, J	*Good to Great.* New York: Harper Collins Publishers, Inc., 2001	Among other topics, looks at the qualities of leaders that allow some companies to make a leap into greatness
Covey SR	*The 7 Habits of Highly Effective People: Powerful Lessons in Personal Change.* New York: A Fireside Book, 1989	The book that started it all; easy to read, discusses personal characteristics and their relationship to effectiveness at work as well as at home
Covey SR	*Principle-centered Leadership.* New York: Free Press, 2002	Applying the principles of the *7 Habits* to leadership and organizations
Covey SR	*The 8th Habit: From Effectiveness to Greatness.* New York: Free Press, 2004	The way to "find your voice and inspire others to find theirs" and become a great leader
Fisher R, Ury W, Patton B	*Getting to Yes: Negotiating Agreement without Giving In.* New York: Penguin Books, 1991	Every significant piece of communication can be a negotiation; this book shows how to do so effectively
Johnson S	*Who Moved My Cheese?* New York: GP Putnam & Sons, 2002	Easy-to-read book that addresses how we do (or don't) embrace change
Katzenbach JR, Smith DK	*The Wisdom of Teams: Creating the High-Performance Organization.* New York: Harper Collins, 2003	Discussion of how teams function and how to make them function better
Phillips DT	*Lincoln on Leadership: Executive Strategies for Tough Times.* New York: Warner Books, Inc., 1992	Entertaining yet poignant examples of leadership choices culled from the life of Abraham Lincoln
Senge PM	*The Fifth Discipline: The Art and Practice of the Learning Organization.* New York: Currency Doubleday, 1994	How leadership can help guide your organization to change; includes a discussion on "team learning"
Ury W	*Getting Past No: Negotiating Your Way from Confrontation to Cooperation.* New York: Bantam Books, 1993	More strategies on getting others to agree with you, and finding the best solution to avoid or manage conflict

be made with the optimal amount of information and with appropriate attention to detail to prevent medical error. The overall goal of the team is to assist patients to recover from illness, injury, or operation so that they can leave the ICU at the optimal time. Each member participates by contributing her particular expertise. This is a team in which specific members are routinely assigned, not specifically chosen for their particular competencies. However, the leaders of the unit (medical and nursing directors) usually choose the general roles needed by the team.

By default, the team leader during rounds is generally the attending physician or the most experienced physician available. However, the team is much more effective if, at various points during the rounding process, the direct input of various members is fostered. The bedside nurse may be the most competent member to assess the level of the patient's pain over the course of the shift. The physical therapist is probably the most competent to assess the patient's likelihood of walking that day. The social worker is likely best equipped to address the needs of the family as they cope with the illness of the child, and so on. Input from all members of the team may be crucial when making certain decisions, such as whether to extubate the patient, transfer to the ward, or perform a tracheotomy. The child and the family will be the most important members of the team when considering end-of-life decisions in conjunction with the rest of the medical team.

In critical care, we cannot envision working without the interdisciplinary healthcare team. It has become a routine part of our practice. Unfortunately, in the health-professions literature, the value of health teams has been described and evaluated more in the primary care, elderly, and end-of-life settings and not in the critical care setting, suggesting that our subspecialty might be able to add considerably to the medical leadership literature.

Care must be taken to avoid confusing the *interdisciplinary* team with a *multidisciplinary* team. A clear hierarchy categorizes the latter; normally, the physician is the permanent leader, and most, if not all communication flows through the physician. Little direct interaction occurs between team members. The *interdisciplinary* team, on the other hand, functions by enabling and empowering each member of the team to interact with the others; it allows and encourages all members to contribute their expertise to the overall good. Direct and open communication occurs between and among the various disciplines, and each discipline respects and involves the others.

Units with a team-oriented culture appear to perform better, with shorter lengths of stay, better quality of patient care, and lower nursing turnover (28), but identifying such units may not be simple, because impressions of team culture differ between the physician and nursing staffs in a unit (29).

Developing a Functional Team

How does one go about turning the typical working group into a highly functional team? Many potential avenues are available. The remainder of this discussion focuses on recommendations from the business literature—specifically, issues identified by Katzenbach and Smith (17). Not all suggestions can be followed in every activity, but these authors provide numerous insights that may be applied successfully to the medical

field. The authors identify the "team basics" that define the discipline required for optimal team performance. The team should be composed of a small number of individuals, usually fewer than 12. These individuals should possess complementary skills to ensure success for the task at hand. The team members must share a common purpose, a common set of specific performance goals, and a commonly agreed-upon working approach. Last, team members should hold each other mutually accountable for the performance of the entire team. The single, most important factor that guides team success seems to be a "clear and compelling performance challenge." Sometimes, this performance challenge can be developed by the team members; at other times, it is defined by an outside individual, such as the hospital administrative officer. The role of the team leader has been identified as important but not critical. However, the leader's major goal should be to build commitment among all team members, fill gaps in knowledge or skills as necessary, shift the leadership role to other members as appropriate, and contribute real work in reaching team outcomes.

The overall performance ethic of the team often determines the difference between a team that consistently achieves its goals and one in which only random team successes are noted.

In many organizations, the significant danger exists of teams developing without the requisite discipline and rigor to ensure and sustain success. It is up to the team leaders as well as the organization's leaders to ensure that the discipline needed for team success is identified and supported.

In forming a highly effective team, it is necessary that the leader establish both the urgency and the direction of the team. All team members must believe that the team has an urgent and worthwhile purpose. Expectations should be clear. Members should be selected based on skills possessed and not on personalities. Katzenbach and Smith identify three categories of skills: technical and functional, problem-solving, and interpersonal. Sometimes, it is more useful to choose at least a few members who have the potential to develop the skills required if the rest of the team is willing to invest the time and energy necessary to help them to gain those skills. This is obviously true in the typical healthcare team scenario in which residents and students, novice nurses, and others are welcomed onto the team and assisted in learning the particular skills they need to ensure team success. The team should be challenged with a few immediate performance-oriented tasks and goals (getting the patient extubated, solving the problem of ventilator-associated pneumonia, enrolling patients in a new unit-based research study). The performance goals must include a clear "stretch" component, so that the team members strive for the desired result (such as eliminating catheter-related bloodstream infections or ventilator-associated pneumonia). Data must be made available to team members on a regular basis, so that they can benchmark their progress and degree of success. The team should congratulate itself when performance goals are met. Even though the team should be focused on communal success, it is important to acknowledge the individual contributions of each team member in allowing that success.

Teams sometimes get "sick." A sick team can be diagnosed by a loss of energy or enthusiasm; a sense of helplessness; a lack of purpose or identity; presence of nonproductive conversations, cynicism, and mistrust; interpersonal attacks made secretively and to outsiders; and lots of defused responsibility when things go wrong. Team members may place blame on top management, on the remainder of the organization, or on the "system." When these symptoms of a sick team are recognized, the following treatment options are available:

1. Revisit the basics; reestablish the purpose of the team.
2. Go for small wins—pick a few important items that are relatively easy to achieve (the proverbial "low-hanging fruit" often mentioned by executives) and give members a sense of accomplishment.
3. Bring in new information and approaches, such as external benchmarks or examples of other units that have achieved a goal similar to that on which you are working.
4. Take advantage of facilitators and training.
5. Change the team's membership, perhaps even the leader.

CONCLUSIONS AND FUTURE DIRECTIONS

Professionalism is an area of today's medicine to which attention must be paid, both in the clinical arena and in the classroom. Only by paying attention to the development of renewed professionalism will our field and our subspecialty be able to thrive in the future. Research is necessary to determine the best methods by which to teach professionalism to our students and trainees and to evaluate the level of professionalism among practicing intensivists. However, use of role modeling, simulation, and leadership training is likely to be among our approaches to this very important task.

Leadership development and training is important to enhance professional development, improve patient care, and engage in systems-based practice. The core competencies become increasingly important as more attention is paid to these issues in credentialing, certification, and maintenance of certification. Leadership can be learned. Effective means of teaching leadership techniques have been developed by business, and these can be adapted to medicine. Additional research should be targeted toward assessing the effectiveness of the growing number of educational opportunities in this area.

The subsequent chapters in this section focus on many topics and skills that contribute to the development of effective leadership. The section editors and the authors of each of the chapters hope that the reader will find useful information and develop a working knowledge base of the competencies that will define the pediatric critical care *professional* in the 21st century.

KEY POINTS

- Although the notion of the medical professional originated with Hippocrates in the 4th century BCE, it has evolved over the succeeding centuries.
- Many "prescriptions" for professional physician behavior are available.
- These prescriptions mostly relate to the newly developed "core competencies" of the ACGME.

- Teaching professionalism demands attention to both the overt and covert curricula and may be most effectively approached through reflective learning.
- Simulation is a useful approach to teach needed skills, assess competencies, and enhance professionalism.
- Leadership skills can be learned.
- One key skill in today's medical environment is the leadership of, and participation in, teams.
- To be functional, a team must have a clear purpose and specific performance goals and utilize a commonly agreed-upon approach. Team members must demonstrate mutual respect.

References

1. ACGME. Outcome Project, 1999.
2. ACGME. Advancing education in medical professionalism. An educational resource from the ACGME outcome project: Accreditation Council for Graduate Medical Education, 2004.
3. Chaer R, Derubertis B, Lin S, et al. Simulation improves resident performance in catheter-based intervention: results of a randomized, controlled study. *Ann Surg* 2006;244:343–52.
4. Chen SM, McMurray A. "Burnout" in intensive care nurses. *J Nurs Res* 2001;9:152–64.
5. CoBaTrICE. *Development of Core Competencies for an International Training Programme in Intensive Care Medicine* Intensive Care Med. Berlin: Springer-Verlag, 2006.
6. Connelly JE. The other side of professionalism: Doctor to doctor. *Camb Q Healthc Ethics* 2003;12:178–83.
7. Coulehan J. Viewpoint: Today's professionalism: Engaging the mind but not the heart. *Acad Med* 2005;80:892–8.
8. DeVita M, Schaefer J, Lutz J, et al. Improving medical emergency team (MET) performance using a novel curriculum and a computerized human patient simulator. *Qual Saf Health Care* 2005;14:326–31.
9. Goleman D. Leadership that gets results. *Harvard Business Review* 2000: 78–90.
10. Grantcharov T, Kristiansen V, Bendix J, et al. Randomized clinical trial of virtual reality simulation for laparoscopic skills training. *Br J Surg* 2004; 91:146–50.
11. Greiner AC, Knebel E. *Health Professions Education: A Bridge to Quality*. Washington, DC: National Academies Press, 2003.
12. Hakim A. JCAHO standards up the ante for leadership. *Physician Executive* 2006;32:30–3.
13. Hall P, Weaver L. Interdisciplinary education and teamwork: A long and winding road. *Med Educ* 2001;35:867–75.
14. Hunt E, Hohenhaus S, Luo X, et al. Simulation of pediatric trauma stabilization in 35 North Carolina emergency departments: Identification of targets for performance improvement. *Pediatrics* 2006;117: 641–48.
15. Inui TS. *A Flag in the Wind: Educating for Professionalism in Medicine*. Washington, DC: Association of American Medical Colleges, 2003.
16. Issenberg S, McGaghie W, ER P, et al. Features and uses of high-fidelity medical simulations that lead to effective learning: A BEME systematic review. *Med Teach* 2005;27:10–28.
17. Katzenbach JR, Smith DK. *The Wisdom of Teams: Creating the High-performance Organization*. New York: Harper Collins, 2003.
18. Kohn L. To err is human: An interview with the Institute of Medicine's Linda Kohn. *Jt Comm J Qual Improv* 2000;26:227–34.
19. Larkin GL. Mapping, modeling and mentoring: Charting a course for professionalism in graduate medical education. *Camb Q Healthc Ethics* 2003;12:167–77.
20. Lattore P, Wetzel RC, Yanofsky SD. Professionalism, interpersonal communications, and leadership in anesthesiology. Annual Meeting of the Association of University Anesthesiologists and Anesthesia Education Foundation.Tuscon, Arizona, 2006.
21. Levi BH, Thomas NJ, Green MJ, et al. Jading in the pediatric intensive care unit: Implications for healthcare providers of medically complex children. *Pediatr Crit Care Med* 2004;5:275–7.
22. Linstone HA, Turoff M. *The Delphi Method: Techniques and Applications*. Boston: Addison-Wesley, 2002.
23. Mayo P, Hackney J, Mueck J, et al. Achieving house staff competence in emergency airway management: Results of a teaching program using a computerized patient simulator. *Crit Care Med* 2004;32: 2422–7.
24. Medical Professionalism Project. Medical professionalism in the new millennium: A physician charter. *Ann Intern Med* 2002;136:243–6.

25. Meier DE, Back AL, Morrison RS. The inner life of physicians and care of the seriously ill. *JAMA* 2001;286:3007–14.
26. Royal College of Paediatrics. *Good Medical Practice in Paediatrics and Child Health: Duties and Responsibilities of Paediatricians.* London: Royal College of Paediatrics and Child Health, 2002.
27. Shanafelt TD, Bradley KA, Wipf JE, et al. Burnout and self-reported patient care in an internal medicine residency program. *Ann Intern Med* 2002;136:358–67.
28. Stockwell DC, Pollack MM, Turenne WM, et al. Leadership and manage-

ment training of pediatric intensivists: How do we gain our skills? *Pediatr Crit Care Med* 2005;6:665–70.
29. Thomas EJ, Sexton JB, Helmreich RL. Discrepant attitudes about teamwork among critical care nurses and physicians [see comment]. *Crit Care Med* 2003;31:956–9.
30. Williams M. Interdisciplinary experiential training for end-of-life care and organ donation. National Consent Conference on Organ Donation. Orlando, FL, April 2003.

CHAPTER 5 ■ PHYSICAL DESIGN AND PERSONNEL ORGANIZATION OF THE PICU

M. MICHELE MOSS • SHARI SIMONE

PICU ORGANIZATION

Optimal care for the unique needs of the seriously ill pediatric patient occurs best in an ICU specifically designed for children and separate from adult or neonatal facilities. During the 1970s, as technology advanced in the care of critically ill patients, healthcare professionals recognized that specialized units were needed for this specific group of patients. The first recognized ICU was developed in the 1950s, in Copenhagen, Denmark (24), with the primary purpose of caring for victims of the poliomyelitis epidemic (36). In the US, ICUs for predominantly adult patients were developed in the 1960s; shortly thereafter, the earliest NICUs were formed (24).

The first PICU in the US was opened in 1967 at Children's Hospital of Philadelphia by Dr. John Downes (24). PICUs initially developed as free-standing units within hospitals during the late 1960s and early 1970s but were mostly found in large, metropolitan areas at large, free-standing children's hospitals or within large, usually university-affiliated medical centers. During the 1980s, PICUs proliferated to essentially all freestanding children's hospitals. During the 1990s, a survey of hospitals (51) with PICUs revealed that these units had a variety of sizes and staffing. Few units—6%—had more than 18 beds, whereas >40% had only 4–6 beds. At the time, most of the PICUs were affiliated with medical schools and were in hospitals that were the primary teaching program sites for pediatrics. A 2001 survey of PICUs (54) revealed that 41% were in private or community hospitals and 43% were in university hospitals or tertiary-level medical centers. From 1995 to 2001, the number of PICUs increased 13.7%, with a corresponding 23.9% increase in the number of beds. The mean number of PICU beds per pediatric population in the US in 2001 was 1:18,542. The distribution of PICUs was similar by regions, but the individual states varied in number of PICU beds. Wyoming was listed as the only state without PICU beds (54).

The development of PICUs in Europe predated the US experience, with the first PICU being founded at Childrens' Hospital in Goteburg, Sweden, in the 1950s in response to the poliomyelitis epidemic that also resulted in the formation of the ICU in Copenhagen (36). PICUs proliferated in Europe as in the US, with most being located within large multidisciplinary hospitals. By 2000, Spain had 34 PICUs, all linked to the Public Health System (37). All were combined medical and surgical units, and 12 were combined pediatric and neonatal units. The size of the units varied; 15 had fewer than 7 beds, 8 units had between 7 and 12 beds, and another 8 units had between 13 and 18 beds.

In Latin America, the first PICUs were developed in 1972 in Peru and Venezuela followed by Brazil in 1974 (15). The current distribution of PICUs in South America reflects "a strong relationship between the financial stability of each region and the complexity and quality of pediatric intensive care" (50). Most PICUs are located in the more developed countries of Brazil, Uruguay, Venezuela, and Argentina (15). In Sao Paulo, Brazil, in 2004, 107 NICUs and PICUs were serving a pediatric population of approximately 2.6 million (20). In a survey of these units with an approximate 80% return rate, 1067 beds were identified. The PICUs were associated with philanthropic organizations (15%), private institutions (46%), and public institutions (46%) with the number of operational beds varying between 2 and 60 (20). Many units are staffed by neonatologists rather than by pediatric intensivists. Interestingly, geographic areas with the least population had the greatest number of beds.

In India, the first PICUs were established at Chennai, Chandigarh, in New Delhi during the 1990s (30). The number of PICUs in India has grown, with most being located in private hospitals and a few in teaching hospitals. Despite a pediatric population in excess of 300 million, India lags behind in pediatric critical care services because government financial support has in the past been directed toward higher-yield preventive health strategies.

Because of extremely limited resources in Africa, PICU beds are rare and extremely limited, as are ICU beds for adults (11). The patterns of disease caused by lack of basic public health services led to a high mortality rate for largely preventable diseases and an overburdened intensive care system. For example, in Zimbabwe, infant respiratory distress syndrome has a 46% mortality rate (33). The HIV epidemic in sub-Saharan Africa has overburdened an already stretched system, and pediatric patients with advanced disease have a poor outcome. A review of diagnoses in the PICU at King Edward Hospital, Durban, KwaZulu Natal, South Africa, noted that admissions due to diseases preventable by immunizations, such as measles, diphtheria, tetanus, and poliomyelitis, drastically decreased between 1971 and 1995 (31). However, the epidemics of HIV and *Shigella dysenteriae* type I and its association with hemolytic uremic syndrome have become more common diagnoses at time of admission. The PICU is a 12-bed unit serving the province of KwaZulu Natal and its pediatric population of 3–4 million. The major admission criterion is need for mechanical ventilation, with half of the beds dedicated to neonatal patients and half to older children.

In the early 1990s, the two major organizations that served pediatric critical care medical specialists [the Section on Critical Care and Committee on Hospital Care of the American

Academy of Pediatrics (AAP) and the Section on Pediatrics of the Society of Critical Care Medicine (SCCM)], jointly developed criteria for categorizing PICUs. The impetus was to better define the optimal staffing, design, equipment, and support services required for seriously and critically ill and injured pediatric patients. In the initial guidelines, PICUs were categorized into three levels of care, but in the revision published in 2004, they were categorized into Level I and Level II units (56). Level I units have staffing, facilities, and equipment to provide optimal care to the most severely ill or injured patients. The staffing of a Level I unit includes pediatric intensivists, nurses with extensive training in pediatric critical care, respiratory therapy staff primarily dedicated to the PICU, and immediate access to a broad range of pediatric medical and subspecialists, including but not limited to, anesthesiologists, surgeons, cardiac surgeons, neurologists, cardiologists, otolaryngologists, and radiologists. Level II units are staffed by pediatric intensivists, but other pediatric specialty physician support may be less readily available than in Level I units.

In 1997, the Intensive Care Chapter of the Indian Academy of Pediatrics was formed, followed by the formation of the Pediatric Section of the Indian Society of Critical Care Medicine in 1998. In 2002, these two groups published consensus guidelines for PICUs in India (34). As in the AAP/SCCM guidelines, unit design, necessary equipment, and staffing were among the areas addressed. Additionally, admission and discharge criteria for Level 3, or tertiary level units, and Level 2, or step-down level units, are discussed. Nursing staff recommendations include one nurse for each intubated patient and as many as two nurses for very unstable patients. More stable patients may share a nurse with another stable patient.

REGIONALIZATION OF PEDIATRIC CRITICAL CARE SERVICES

The resources required to support the demanding staffing and highly technical needs of critically ill and injured pediatric patients are often unevenly proportioned due to multiple factors, including population disparities, geographic limitations, and financial constraints. Regionalization is defined in a statement from the AAP (4) as "a process for organizing resources within a geographic region to ensure access to medical care within a level appropriate to a patient's needs. . . " In Pediatrics, regionalization of critical care services was developed initially for NICUs, such that the more critical and complex neonates were transported and cared for in those NICUs with the most sophisticated equipment and broader support staff. This concept spread with the advent of PICUs in the 1970s. Considering the relatively few critical or potentially unstable children with illness or injuries as compared to adults, and the broader range of diseases and injuries, the concept of regionalization makes even more sense for the pediatric population. Government or financial entities can mandate regionalization, but more commonly, regionalization has developed due to geographic constraints and well-developed referral patterns.

Studies (55,63) have supported the concept of regionalization (often called *centralization* in Europe) with their demonstration of better patient outcomes. A study that compared a centralized system in Australia with a noncentralized system in England projected that more than half of risk-adjusted mortal-

ities occur in the centralized system compared with the noncentralized system (48). Regionalization or centralization was supported by a study that showed an inverse relationship of the volume of PICU patients to the risk-adjusted mortality and length of stay (60). Regionalization has also been supported for pediatric cardiac surgery by a study that showed less mortality in centers with the highest volumes (32).

In the US, three geographic models of regionalization have been described (65). The first are regions comprised of large geographic areas, as seen in largely rural settings, with only one or two large urban centers that are able to support a high-level PICU. Such examples are found mostly in the western and southern states such as New Mexico or Arkansas. In this model, the geographic area is large but often not highly populated, so that few critically ill children are spread over large distances. The transport of patients to the appropriate PICU requires preparation and well-developed transport services.

The second model is a large geographic area that is both rural and suburban, with multiple urban centers capable of housing an upper-level PICU. Often, considerable overlap of services is found in these areas, such that referral patterns may not be the most geographically logical. "Competition" for patients may exist in these areas, and financial referral patterns are often seen. Illinois is an example of a state that has urban, suburban, and large rural areas and multiple PICUs.

The third type of geographic referral area is seen in the more populated eastern states. This model is a relatively small geographic area with a large population and, frequently, multiple PICUs. New York City is an example. Rather than geographic area, the local referral patterns and financial constraints define regionalization.

Regionalization of pediatric critical care includes both the PICU and the continuum of services from prehospital care, hospital-based emergency care, intensive care, and specialized services to rehabilitation services. Even the prehospital education components of injury prevention, recognition of serious and critical illness and injury, and accessing the total healthcare system available are parts of this continuum. Emergency medical services for children are part of this continuum and have been studied and supported by grants from Maternal and Child Health. In 1993, the Institute of Medicine recognized the importance of the development of this pediatric continuum in its report *Emergency Medical Services for Children*, which argued that "society has a special obligation to address the needs of children" (26). Often, pediatric services are buried within adult services, and adequate training and experience are lacking for caregivers to deliver optimal care to children. Training for prehospital and primary hospital caregivers is crucial to provide the best care and outcomes for children. Safe and efficient transport (again, with adequate training of the caregivers) to higher levels of care must also be provided for a system to be appropriate.

The state of California had early experience in the regionalization of pediatric critical care services. In 1981, the Pediatric Intensive Care Network of Northern and Central California was formed by the medical directors of the 10 PICUs that existed at that time (65). They undertook a study that examined pediatric intensive care resources and, from that, developed a model of regionalization. An extensive effort was undertaken to outline where patients who "could benefit from PICU intervention" were receiving their care. During the study in 1984, 3889 patients were admitted to one of the existing

PICUs, with a 5.8% rate of death and an average length of stay of 4.9 days (65). During the same period, 3,066 patients, ranging in age from 7 days to 18 years, were admitted to community hospitals that did not have designated PICUs. Due to a marked discrepancy in the severity of illness, the PICUs had a higher rate of death than did the community hospitals. Using this data and with a grant from the Division of Maternal and Child Health of the Department of Health and Human Services, a model for regionalization in northern California was developed. A networking process among the PICUs in the region resulted in cooperative data collection, educational programs, and development and review of statewide standards for PICUs (65).

Countries outside of the US have also struggled with the issues surrounding regionalization. Sweden undertook the task of centralizing pediatric cardiac surgery from four centers to two during the 1990s, resulting in a reduction in mortality rate from 9.5% to 1.9% over a 5-year period (38). The need for regionalization of pediatric care in India was recognized in an editorial in *Indian Pediatrics* that called for development of a four-tier system that would provide low-cost interventions and technology to children throughout the country and not just in the high-population and higher-income areas (30). The author proposed that caregivers able to recognize the need for urgent referral and access to oxygen, intravenous/intraosseous fluids, and antibiotics would be available at Primary Health Centers throughout the country. Level 1 hospitals would be able to handle serious pediatric illness, whereas Level 2 hospitals would have small, 4–6-bed PICUs that would function as Level 2 PICUs, according to guidelines for PICUs developed in India. Level 3 hospitals would be major teaching institutions located in each state and would have a tertiary PICU capable of state-of-the-art pediatric critical care. Embedded in the mission of these tertiary PICUs would be education of physicians, nurses, and healthcare workers, as well as research. A strong transport system would have to be developed throughout the country to address the need to move patients along the levels of care (30).

PICU POPULATION

Patients admitted to PICUs represent a broad range of age groups and disease states. Generally, NICUs admit newborns who have complications of prematurity or delivery or who have congenital anatomic defects. PICUs admit patients from the neonatal period through adolescence. Additionally, because patients with chronic "pediatric" diseases are now living into adulthood, many of those critically ill patients are cared for in PICUs. The most common example would be adults with congenital heart diseases who need further congenital heart surgery and the expertise of a congenital heart surgeon and pediatric cardiologist. Postoperatively, they are often cared for in PICUs or in pediatric cardiac ICUs.

Admission criteria for PICUs have been defined by the Society for Critical Care Medicine and the AAP (3). In general, admission to a PICU requires acute respiratory, neurologic, or hemodynamic instability; some other specific organ dysfunction; or the imminent risk of instability. Often, the patients are postoperative patients who are at risk for respiratory or hemodynamic instability or specific organ dysfunction. Usually, patients require specific technologic intervention that can

only be performed in an intensive care setting with its increased nursing staff. In the US, most patients cared for in PICUs in 2001 (54) were medical, with approximately one-third being surgical and another 10% being cardiac medical or surgical patients. In developing countries with limited resources, the admission criterion for a PICU is often the need for mechanical ventilation. Other types of intensive care, such as dialysis or close monitoring of vital signs in unstable patients, may occur outside the PICU, if at all.

Specialized PICUs have been developed in areas with large referral bases, such as pediatric burn ICUs, or, more commonly, pediatric cardiac ICUs. The latter have been proliferating since the mid-1990s, although several large programs have had dedicated cardiac ICUs since the 1980s. One perceived advantage of the separate pediatric cardiac ICU is that the staff training and experience are focused on cardiac medical and postoperative issues, allowing for more standardized practice and efficient care. Because the technology required to support these patients becomes increasingly complex with the proliferation of mechanical support devices and complex pharmacologic strategies, additional, extensive staff training is required.

The cardiac ICU patient management team is composed of nurses; respiratory therapists; mid-level practitioners, such as advanced practice nurses (APNs) or physician assistants (PAs); and physicians, including intensivists, pediatric cardiologists, pediatric cardiovascular surgeons, and pediatric cardiac anesthesiologists. Residents in pediatrics and cardiac surgery and fellows in critical care and cardiology play varying roles in these cardiac ICUs. The intensive care patient management is generally led by pediatric intensivists, pediatric cardiac anesthesiologists, pediatric cardiologists with intensive care experience, or physicians dually trained and board certified in pediatric critical care and cardiology. Currently, postgraduate fellowship programs exist that are generally 1 year in length and provide additional training in pediatric cardiac intensive care. These programs are not recognized by the Accreditation Council for Graduate Medical Education (ACGME) at this time, and board certification or special competency is not currently available in the discipline of pediatric cardiac intensive care.

Specialized PICUs are less common outside of the US and Europe, mostly because of limited resources. Pediatric burn patients in Russia, for example, are referred to the national burn hospital but are admitted to the general PICU (23).

PICU PERSONNEL AND STAFFING MODELS

Optimal care for seriously ill and injured pediatric patients requires coordinated multidisciplinary care by physicians, nurses, respiratory therapists, and others, including pharmacists, child-life specialists, social workers, chaplains, nutritionists, and physical, occupational, and speech therapists. Pediatric intensivists should coordinate patient care among the pediatric medical and surgical subspecialists, physicians in training, and primary care physicians.

The development of the discipline of pediatric critical care medicine paralleled the development of PICUs. Care of the critically ill adult patient initially focused on organ-specific failure, and care was provided by a specialist; for example, a pulmonologist cared for patients with respiratory failure, or a cardiologist managed patients with acute cardiac conditions. With the advent of neonatal intensive care, a new model of care developed. Premature and other seriously ill newborns were cared for by pediatricians who oversaw the complete patient, recognizing that all of the organs were at risk during critical illness. The model of the neonatologist was then translated into the pediatric intensivist model.

Intensivists

The pediatric intensivist oversees the "total" patient, with training in both specific organ failure and the interaction of whole-body systems. Training programs in pediatric critical care management initially developed from anesthesiology training programs and ultimately from pediatric training programs. Early on, anesthesiologists applied their intraoperative experience in caring for the whole patient with the need for extensive monitoring to the intensive care environment. Pediatricians, emulating both the anesthesiology and the neonatology model, progressed to the current pediatric intensivist model.

In 1985, the American Board of Pediatrics (ABP) led the recognition for the Pediatric Critical Care Medicine subspecialty and offered the first board exam in 1987. The first accreditation of postgraduate fellowship programs followed in 1990, with recognition by the Residency Review Committee of the Accreditation Council for Graduate Medical Education. Nursing also recognized pediatric critical care as a special entity. In 1986, the American Association of Critical Care Nurses offered a certification program in pediatric critical care and, in 1999, a program for clinical nurse specialists in pediatric critical care.

Currently, certification by the ABP for pediatric intensivists requires completion of 3 years of pediatric residency training with certification by the ABP in general pediatrics, and completion of 3 years of pediatric critical care fellowship training in an ACGME-approved training program. Certification is time limited, and the practitioner must be recertified every 7 years. The recertification process, overseen by the ABP, is changing toward an ongoing process that addresses the "Six Core Competencies" promoted by the ACGME, which include patient care, medical knowledge, practice-based learning and improvement, interpersonal skills and communication, professionalism, and systems-based practice. Pediatric anesthesiologists and pediatric surgeons can earn a certificate of Special Competency in Critical Care.

Worldwide certification in intensive care, and particularly pediatric intensive care, is varied and often not available. For some countries, intensive care is certified through specialty boards such as internal medicine or surgery. In Spain, Switzerland, Australia, New Zealand, and Hong Kong, for example, critical care is a primary specialty with separate certification (10). Training requirements vary throughout the world. Because of this variability and despite some similarities in curricula, a process was undertaken by the *competency-based training* program in *intensive care* medicine in *Europe* (CoBaTrICE) collaboration to develop core competencies for an international training program in adult critical care. This collaboration is composed of physicians from Europe, Asia, North America, South America, and Africa and is supported by various organizations, including the European Society of Inten-

sive Care Medicine and the Society of Critical Care Medicine. Currently, no process is underway for an international training program in pediatric critical care. In many locations, physicians who practice in PICUs are pediatricians with special interest in intensive care who have been unable to train in an organized training program.

In addition to the expanding workload in PICUs due to pharmacologic and technologic advances, pediatric intensivists have a variety of other work-related activities. Because most PICUs are associated with pediatric and/or pediatric critical care training programs, most pediatric intensivists have teaching commitments for a variety of audiences, including residents, critical care fellows, nursing staff, and other medical caregivers. Additionally, many pediatric intensivists are members of an academic faculty, which means they also have research and administrative responsibilities such as medical direction of code teams, medical emergency teams, and transport systems. The clinical arena for the pediatric intensivist has broadened to include coordinating sedation programs for patients who need procedures outside of the operating room and participating in palliative care programs. In addition, due to the multidisciplinary roles in the PICU, pediatric intensivists actively participate in hospital and university committees. The 2003 Future of Pediatric Education II Survey of Sections project (8) revealed that, overall, pediatric intensivists devote ~15% time to teaching across all age groups. Younger intensivists (<40 years old) spend 14% of their time in research, whereas intensivists 40–49 years of age spend 10%, and those ≥50 years old spend 7%. Intensivists who are >50 years old spend approximately 20% of their time on administrative duties as compared to intensivists who are <40 years old, who spend on average ~12% of their time on administrative duties.

Physicians

Multiple staffing models exist for PICUs throughout the world. In the US, most PICUs are staffed by ABP-certified or ABP-eligible pediatric intensivists (54). From 1995 to 2001, the number of PICUs staffed by pediatric intensivists rose from ~90% to 94% (54). Intensivists provide care through different staffing patterns, and most frequently, the intensivists are the primary physicians or they co-attend with a medical or surgical specialty service. In another model, intensivists serve as primary attendings on a small number of patients but consultants on all PICU patients. In the US, pediatric intensivists control most PICU admissions. Patient coverage in the PICU frequently involves residents or fellows in addition to the pediatric intensivists.

The effect of training programs on mortality has been shown to vary. One study suggested a higher risk of mortality when PICUs were staffed by residents alone and a much lower risk when staffed by intensive care fellows (51). Larger PICUs in the US more commonly than smaller units have 24-hour, in-house, attending-level coverage, with as many as 40% of those with >20 beds having attending-level, in-house coverage. A study in Malaysia showed that having pediatric intensivists in-house around the clock rather than only during the day, with the night time covered by general pediatricians, lowered standardized mortality ratios and decreased lengths of stay (29). Pediatric hospitalists who work with pediatric intensivists have also helped to improve outcomes (59).

Nurses

Pediatric critical care nurses provide unique contributions to the delivery of care for medically unstable and vulnerable infants and children. The critical care nurse performs continuous, vigilant, compassionate care that is based on the needs and characteristics of the patient and family and that allows for ongoing physiologic patient assessments, implementation and evaluation of responses to the treatment plan, and assessment and development of plans to meet the needs of the family. An essential skill of the critical care nurse is the ability to effectively communicate with all members of the healthcare team and maintain ongoing dialog to ensure rapid responses to changes in the child's condition.

The current healthcare situation of a nurse shortage and an aging nurse workforce is a common experience worldwide and has created unique challenges in providing comprehensive care that optimizes patient outcomes. Nursing leadership has been challenged to develop innovative staffing and nursing care models to maintain a high quality of care. Adequate nurse staffing is critical to the delivery of quality patient care and directly influences the rate of preventable adverse events (43,53). In a study of unplanned extubations in a children's hospital PICU in the US, a patient-to-nurse ratio of 1:1 was significantly associated with a decrease in unplanned extubations (39). Not surprising, the presence of the nurse at the patient's bedside is essential to ensure patient safety.

A study conducted in Hong Kong found that 51% of incidents were detected by direct observation versus 27% by monitor detection (13). The investigators concluded that, despite advances in technology, there was no substitute for the expertise of the nurse providing direct patient care.

Nurse-to-patient ratios in ICUs are primarily based on patient census and acuity and may range from 1:3 to 2:1 (44). However, other factors must be considered in determining staffing needs, including the level of experience of the nurses who are providing the care, available technology, unit layout, and support staff. In addition, because the condition of critically ill children can rapidly change, maintaining flexibility in nursing staff is imperative.

Critical care nursing organizations such as the American Association of Critical Care Nurses, the Australian College of Critical Care Nurses, and the British Association of Critical Care Nurses have developed ICU nursing workforce position statements that outline nurse staffing standards based on best practice evidence; these statements are available at their respective websites. In addition, the World Federation of Critical Care Nurses, an organization comprised of over 20 critical care nursing associations, has developed minimum workforce requirements that can be adapted to meet the nursing staff and system requirements of a particular country or jurisdiction (64).

Care Delivery Models

Nursing care delivery models continue to evolve with the changing critical care environment; these models include an emphasis on the patient-family relationship, customer-focused behaviors, process improvement, safety, and achieving high-quality clinical and behavioral outcomes. Since 1990, the Magnet Nursing Services Recognition Program for Excellence in Nursing Services of the American Nurses Credentialing Center has honored national and international organizations that demonstrate excellence in nursing practice with Magnet status. Magnet hospitals have demonstrated higher-than-average nurse recruitment and retention rates, as well as other indicators of quality (1). One important component evaluated is the effective use of a patient care delivery model that promotes nursing responsibility, authority, and autonomy and one in which best practices are utilized. Nursing departments are charged to shape a patient care delivery model that fits the individual organization's core values and to design a structural framework that will help to operationalize those values through the delivery of quality patient care. Recent studies have reported improved patient outcomes within hospital environments that support professional nursing practice (2,27).

Expanded nursing roles have also been developed in response to changes in the healthcare system. In the United States, the role of nursing case management has greatly impacted discharge planning of medically complex patients. In other nations, similar specialist roles (i.e., liaison nurses) have been created to streamline ICU transitional care and reduce the impact and potential complications associated with transferring patients within the healthcare system (16).

Leadership

Effective nursing leadership has been shown to be a key component in the retention of hospital nurses (12). The leadership characteristics of the nurse manager greatly affect the work environment of critical care nurses. Therefore, desirable qualifications of the nurse manager include substantial pediatric expertise and completion of a master's degree in nursing administration. The nurse manager must have a vision for the unit, which is a realistic and attractive future for the organization, the skills and expertise to lead the team, the trust of employees, and ongoing dialog with the PICU team.

Other nursing leadership roles that may have differing titles but similar functions around the world include clinical nurse specialists and critical care nurse consultants. The qualifications required for these advanced practice nursing roles include a master's degree in nursing and extensive expertise in pediatric critical care. The clinical nurse specialist in the US and Canada incorporates the roles of expert clinician, consultant, educator, and researcher. The roles of the nurse consultant in the UK parallel those of the clinical nurse specialist in the US and Canada, with the addition of functioning as a transformational leader who influences both organizational and educational development (18).

Professional Development

The professional development of the nursing staff in the PICU is the responsibility of experienced staff members, unit educators, mentors, and advanced practice nurses, including a clinical nurse specialist. The process is ideally coordinated by the pediatric clinical nurse specialist or similar advanced-practice nurse who holds a master's degree in nursing and has substantial pediatric critical care expertise. Staff education begins with a didactic and clinical orientation program that provides a foundation for novice nurses to safely care for critically ill children. In addition, designing a professional development program that outlines a realistic advancement plan and identifies those strategies necessary to achieve goals is an important responsibility of the PICU leadership team. Benner's model of knowledge and skill acquisition is a useful framework for identifying how a nurse progresses from novice to expert practitioner (28). The characteristics of each of these levels of clinical expertise can be incorporated to meet the educational needs and promote successful advancement of the individual.

As the novice staff nurse gains expertise, the professional development plan should specify the education, mentoring, and skill acquisition required to prepare the novice to take on additional roles. Examples include charge nurse responsibilities, arrest team member, transport team member, trauma team member, preceptor for newly hired nurses, and mentor for nurses following orientation. Other important requirements to ensure mastery of skills include completion of pediatric advanced life support provider certification and an annual review of high-risk, low-volume therapies and patient-specific core competencies. Obtaining pediatric critical care nursing certification is desirable (6). The critical care registered nurse certification distinguishes nurses who have obtained an advanced body of knowledge necessary to care for critically ill patients.

Participation in ongoing educational programs specific to pediatric critical care is essential for nurses to build on previously acquired knowledge and skills. Continuing nursing education requirements are broadly defined by state nursing legislation, regulations, and professional organizations. Nursing education programs span the spectrum from unit-based in-services, hospital workshops, local seminars, and regional conferences, to national and international nursing conferences. All provide unique opportunities for nurses to expand knowledge and skills, exchange ideas, network, identify best practices from other institutions, and share information with the health care team.

The nursing staff is also responsible for participating in those unit functions necessary to support and improve the delivery of quality patient care. Activities include, but are not limited to, quality improvement programs; the development of policies, procedures, standards of care, critical pathways, and guidelines; and the evaluation of practice outcomes.

Mid-level Practitioners

Nurse practitioners (NPs) and PAs have become integral members of the PICU multidisciplinary team, primarily in the US. The emergence of these roles in the PICU environment was largely a result of pediatric residency curriculum changes combined with increasing PICU demands (22,41,62). In July 2003, all residency programs in the US were subject to the ACGME's new restriction in duty hours. PICU resources have been further impacted by the aging nurse workforce and the increasing complexity of patient care, coupled with the demands for improved patient and PICU outcomes. These changes have propelled modifications in traditional physician staffing patterns and have led to the addition of NPs and PAs to provide continuity and quality care to critically ill children.

Varieties of PICU collaborative practice models have been reported in which physicians, in combination with NPs and/or PAs, collectively use knowledge and skill sets to enhance patient care (21,22,40–42,62). In university-affiliated teaching hospitals, the traditional medical team of intensivists, fellows, and residents now includes NPs and PAs. Examples of patient care models in large PICUs include staffing two complete teams, one composed of residents and the other composed of NPs; a combined team of residents and NPs; a combined team of

residents, PAs, and NPs; or a team of only NPs. Separate NP and resident teams allow faculty to provide education that is directed toward the specific needs of the group. For example, educational rounds for rotating residents may include a discussion of the evidence-based management for patients with status asthmaticus. In comparison, educational rounds for seasoned NPs may include a discussion on evidence-based therapies for acute respiratory failure when conventional management fails. Tailoring educational needs and clinical skills may result in improved satisfaction for NPs and rotating residents. However, teams composed of residents, NPs, and/or PAs provide unique leadership and mentoring opportunities for practitioners. Staffing patterns in smaller PICUs include various combinations of residents, NPs, and PAs. The team composition affects the distribution of responsibilities given to NPs and PAs, but in general, the primary focus involves managing a daily caseload of patients and often supplementing the 24-hour on-call coverage previously filled by residents and fellows. In centers without fellowship programs, NPs play a greater role in supervising resident teams. In community hospitals, the numbers of NPs and PAs in critical care are substantially greater, because more positions are required to provide daily 24-hour coverage.

Since the emergence of pediatric acute care and critical care NP programs during the early 1990s, the number of NPs in the PICU has increased exponentially. The differences and similarities between NPs and PAs are listed in **Table 5.1**. The educational preparation and clinical expertise of NPs and PAs differ; therefore, the clinicians' contributions to the delivery of care in the PICU are unique. PICU NPs are nurses who have typically completed a graduate program with a pediatric acute care or critical care emphasis; some may have completed a pediatric primary care program. All PICU NPs have pediatric clinical expertise prior to entering the graduate program, but the breadth of clinical expertise will vary. In comparison, PAs complete 2 years of college courses in basic science and behavioral sciences before entering a PA program that averages 26 months and consists of an intense curriculum with both clinical and didactic components. PAs are educated in the medical model, which is designed to complement physician training. They often have previous healthcare experience as emergency medical technicians or paramedics.

Published reports describe the NP and PA scope of practice and the debate surrounding best-practice models in the PICU setting (5,21,25,40–42,62). Two national surveys that describe the functions of pediatric and adult critical and acute practitioners demonstrate that the NP provides aspects of care that are reflective of advanced-practice nursing in addition to direct patient management responsibilities (35,62). Global responsibilities include providing comprehensive patient management combined with consultation, education, research, quality improvement, and leadership activities.

In contrast to the NP role, the PA philosophical basis mimics the medical model and is disease focused. PAs are licensed to practice medicine with physician supervision. In the PICU setting, PAs perform direct patient management, including conducting physical exams, diagnosing and treating patients, ordering and interpreting tests, and performing duties that require advanced technical skills. Few publications exist on the role of the PA in pediatric critical care (41). However, the literature describes the success of the PA in specialty care settings (14,46).

TABLE 5.1

SCOPE OF PRACTICE OF NURSE PRACTITIONERS AND PHYSICIAN ASSISTANTS

Responsibilities	Nurse practitioners	Physician assistants
Patient management		
Assessment	Comprehensive and problem-specific model of care	Problem-specific model of care
Diagnosis and treatment	Diagnosis rendered independently with awareness of the entire system and the patient's response to illness	Diagnosis rendered under direct supervision of physician
Procedures	Proficient to perform procedures to support/monitor patient condition, treat acute problems, or prevent complications independently by practice agreement	Proficient to perform procedures under direction of physician
Prescription and documentation	Full prescriptive authority, independent documentation	Requires cosignature for prescription and documentation of practice
Education		
Patient education	Promotes health maintenance	Provides health education specific to medical treatment plan
Staff mentoring	Mentors nurses, nurse practitioners, residents, and students	Mentors physician assistants, residents, and medical students
Consultant	Serves as a consultant for variety of nursing care issues	May participate in unit-specific activities
	Participates on hospital committees as advanced nurse practitioner representative	Primary role is direct patient management
	Participates in development of policies/standards/ competencies for pediatric critical care	
Research	Advances pediatric nursing knowledge by contributing to evidence-based practice	May participate in research in a variety of roles
System management	Advanced nursing skills promote system evaluation and efforts to improve care delivery	No specific training in this area, but impacts care system

The first study to examine the use of NPs and PAs in pediatric critical care surveyed medical directors of PICUs in the US and found that 62.8% of responding institutions employed physician extenders (19). The physician respondents reported a skill level of NPs and PAs that was comparable to second- or third-year residents.

Since this early study, emerging research examines the quality of care administered by NPs and PAs in comparison to residents. An exploration of outcomes of patients who were cared for by NPs, PAs, or resident physicians revealed comparable results for each group (57). Similar findings were reported upon an examination of the trends in care by nonphysician clinicians, including NPs and PAs, over a 10-year span (25). Research specifically examining the effect of NP and PA care on patient and system outcomes is favorable. Beneficial outcomes include decreased lengths of stay, decreased costs of care, decreased adverse complications, enhanced communication and collaboration, parental and staff satisfaction, and continuity of care (17,40,45).

Because most nations of the world are experiencing rising healthcare costs and a shortage of healthcare providers, the need for alternative healthcare practitioners has resulted in the development of NP and PA roles in primary care settings since the early 1990s (47). These roles are rapidly evolving in acute care areas but remain in infancy in pediatric critical care. International colleagues may gain insight by examining the successes and mistakes of the US, because the advanced practice issues faced in role development and implementation, including educational standards, credentialing, licensure, titling, prescribing medications, liability, and reimbursement, are common to all.

Respiratory Therapists

Respiratory therapists are an integral part of the bedside care of the pediatric intensive care patient. Respiratory disease in most PICUs is the most common diagnosis, and the impairment of respiratory function complicates many other diseases. In addition to their expertise in mechanical ventilators, respiratory therapists provide pulmonary treatments, including inhaled medications, and they should be trained in pediatric modalities of aerosol delivery and mechanical ventilation. For all levels of PICUs, the American College of Critical Care Medicine of the SCCM recommends that an in-house respiratory therapist who is experienced in pediatric respiratory failure be available at all times (56). Frequently, respiratory therapists have expanded duties, including sampling and running blood gases and other bedside laboratories, participating in patient transport both intra- and interfacility, and participating in extracorporeal membrane oxygenation support. Their participation in the care of the PICU patient is crucial for optimal outcomes. In many countries outside the US, appropriately trained bedside nurses may provide a similar function to the respiratory therapist.

Other Ancillary Personnel

Multiple other personnel are required for the best care of the PICU patient. Pharmacists are an integral part of the PICU team. A satellite pharmacy should be close to the PICU; in lieu of that, a system must be available to allow immediate dispensing of medications. Additionally, the presence of a clinical pharmacologist helps in the management of patients with complex medication regimens and variable pharmacokinetics. Nutritionists, physical therapists, occupational therapists, speech therapists, and social workers also play significant roles in the care of the PICU patient; consequently, they should have training in pediatric environments. Child life and play therapists also have an important role in helping patients and their families to adjust to critical illness. Chaplains and bereavement teams can also be instrumental in assisting a family to cope with the death of their child.

PHYSICAL DESIGN

Environment of Care

When designing a PICU, several aspects must be taken into account, including regulations from oversight institutions such as government agencies and the Joint Commission, available physical space and location, expertise and needs to the PICU personnel, and pediatric patient- and family-centered concepts. The American College of Critical Care Medicine published guidelines for ICU design in 1995 (58). As in PICU patient care, a multidisciplinary approach was suggested that involves ICU leaders, including the nurse manager, medical director, architects, engineering staff, and hospital administration. Additionally, family, interior designers, nursing staff, physician staff, respiratory therapy staff, and others involved in patient care should be asked for design input.

The American College of Critical Care Medicine also included the environment of care as an important component to patient- and family-centered care in their Clinical Practice Guidelines for Support of the Family in the Patient-Centered ICU (7). The environment of care has been shown in multiple studies to have an impact on patient outcome. In addition to the design affecting infection control and improving patient outcomes by limiting spread of infections, it can affect other aspects of the patient experience. Initially, PICUs were of large, ward-type designs. Today, the recommendation is for individual rooms designed in such a way that the risk of infection is decreased, the staff can adequately visualize the patient and monitors, and the patient and family have privacy. Each room must be large enough to comfortably accommodate the patient's bed, increasingly complex types of medical equipment, and power and vacuum sources. The minimum recommended area for pediatric patients is 250 square feet (~23 square meters) per bed space (56). Because of the importance of family presence in the care of pediatric patients in the PICU setting, larger rooms are being designed to accommodate sleeping and private spaces for parents.

Unit Architectural Design

Individual Rooms

Infection is spread by both direct contact and airborne routes; having separate rooms for each bed space in the PICU minimizes direct-contact spread. Multiple numbers of sinks placed in easily accessible areas for handwashing also decreases infection spread by direct contact. Individual rooms can have specific air-flow patterns to prevent infection. Patients who are im-

munocompromised should be in rooms with positive air flow; i.e., the air in the room is sent out and not pulled in. Patients with potentially communicable diseases, including being colonized with resistant organisms, should be in rooms in which the air is pulled in and not sent out. Some systems allow the flow patterns to be changed depending on the type patient in the room.

Noise

ICUs of all types can be noisy environments because of the amount of equipment, alarms, and staff necessary for patient care and safety. Excessive noise has been shown to have a negative effect on patients, as noted by decreased oxygen saturations, decreased sleep, and increased blood pressure and heart rate (61). Ambient noise levels in hospitals may run as high as 45 to 70 dB; the World Health Organization recommendation is that ambient noise not exceed 35 dB (9). The multiple hard surfaces (e.g., floors and cabinetry) in hospitals and ICUs can accentuate noise levels. The use of various materials for floor coverings and ceilings can abate the noise level, while maintaining easy cleaning and infection control. Glass doors and counters can also reduce noise levels.

Lighting

Lighting has also been shown to impact patient outcome. Most studies, which have evaluated adult patients, have shown that patients who are exposed to natural sunlight have decreased lengths of stay and improved mental status (61). Many state health departments stipulate that each ICU bed must have a window or, at the very minimum, a skylight. Some guidelines also recommend that the level of lighting for patient rooms not exceed 30 fc (foot candles), with the ability to dim the level to as low as 6.5 fc at night (58). Adequate lighting must be available for charting and for emergencies and procedures, thereby requiring lighting systems with multiple types of lights.

Electrical Requirements

Each room or bed space must have ample electrical power, oxygen, compressed air, and vacuum outlets. The SCCM (58) recommendation is for at least 16 electrical outlets and two each for oxygen and compressed air. A minimum of three vacuum outlets is required. Units with high levels of acuity may need more of those outlets, as well as outlets for nitrogen. Electrical outlets should be placed at the head of the bed and 36 inches (1 meter) above ground for easy access. Other outlets may be necessary in other parts of the room. The electrical power to the PICU should be delivered by a feeder separate from other parts of the hospital. Additionally, power should be connected to an emergency power source.

The PICU should have adequate hard-wire support, so that computers can be placed at each bedside, charting area, and other workspaces. Wireless connection to the Internet should be available in the PICU for both staff and families. Each PICU should have an area for viewing radiographic studies; it should also be equipped with digital radiograph viewing equipment, a personal computer for viewing outside studies on CD or DVD, and possibly digital ultrasound viewing equipment, especially if the unit has a high number of cardiac patients.

Emergency Power

The emergency power source for the hospital should be safe from the effects of potential disaster situations. For example, emergency generators should not be in the basement of a hospital if the area is at any risk of flooding (49). Life-support equipment, such as extracorporeal membrane oxygenation circuits or mechanical ventilators, should be on outlets that are connected to emergency generator power, whereas other less critical pieces of equipment may be connected to outlets not supported during power shortages. Water must be available in each room for handwashing and other uses. If hemodialysis is to be performed at the bedside, the water source must be certified.

Central Areas

Central areas should have adequate visualization of the patient rooms and adequate desk space for all caregivers, including nurses, physicians, respiratory therapists, consultants, social workers, pharmacists, and others. A centralized monitoring system should be nearby.

Storage

In addition to the centralized charting and monitor areas, storage for emergency equipment and ventilators must be within the unit. Each unit should have "dirty" and "clean" utility areas as well as food and formula preparation areas. A satellite pharmacy is best for the PICU; in lieu of that, medication storage and preparation areas, with refrigeration and locked areas as indicated, should be available.

Family and Caregiver Areas

In addition to the patient rooms, the overall PICU should be designed to allow for optimal patient care and support for the caregivers. The unit should have an entry primarily for family and visitors that can be controlled for security. Another entry should be available for patient transport and medical personnel.

Further family-support areas (in addition to family space within the patient's room) are important. They should have a waiting room with seating for approximately two family members per patient. Waiting areas can include nourishment-support areas with refrigerators and microwaves, laundry support, access to telephones, and diversions, such as television, video games, and aquariums. Conference areas for private conferences between medical caregivers, social workers, and family should be available. A private area for lactation equipment should be available.

Additional Considerations

Age-appropriate diversion equipment, such as televisions, video game and DVD players, and music systems should be available in each patient room. Other age-appropriate toys that are easily disinfected can be provided as needed. An easily readable clock should be in each patient room. Twenty-four-hour atomic clocks are easily seen and can help to decrease time variability on documentation.

CONCLUSIONS AND FUTURE DIRECTIONS

The primary objective of pediatric intensive care is to provide specialized care to patients ranging in age from neonates to adolescents. Seriously ill pediatric patients are best cared for in ICUs designed for them, and the physical design of the facility and personnel organization are integral components of PICUs. In the US, pediatric intensive care resources are regionalized into three models: large geographic areas that encompass rural areas, rural and suburban areas, and small geographic areas that house large populations. Healthcare providers in the PICU include multidisciplinary teams of intensivists, physicians, nurse practitioners, physician assistants, nurses, pharmacists, therapists, and others. These health professionals provide a care-delivery model focused on beneficial clinical and behavioral outcomes, patient-family relationships, and safety. Government and accreditation agencies regulate PICU physical design, including room design, noise level, and lighting and electrical requirements. Evidence suggests that the current model of pediatric intensive care provides unparalleled healthcare to a vulnerable patient population.

Because of the aging and limited workforce, the future of the field is challenged by the need for more physicians, nurses, mid-level practitioners, and other healthcare providers who are specialized in pediatric intensive care. As technology becomes more complicated, both staffing and unit design must adjust to meet the needs of the newer technologies. Additionally, the focus of the PICU, both in design and in treatment, must be the patients and their families.

KEY POINTS

- Seriously and critically ill and injured pediatric patients are best cared for in PICUs separate from adult or neonatal ICUs.
- Because of the uneven distribution of resources, the regionalization of PICUs is often recommended.
- PICU design should be multidisciplinary and include members of the healthcare team, architects, engineers, hospital administration, and family.
- Optimal care is provided by a multidisciplinary team that includes physicians, nurses, respiratory therapists, pharmacists, and others.
- Various staffing patterns exist, depending on acuity of patients in the PICU and availability of support staff.

References

1. Aiken LH, Havens DS, Sloane DM. The Magnet Nursing Services Recognition® program: A comparison of two groups of magnet hospitals. *Am J Nurs* 2000;100(3):26–30.
2. Allen DE, Vitale-Nolen RA. Patient care delivery model improves nurse job satisfaction. *J Cont Educ Nurs* 2005;36:277–82.
3. American Academy of Pediatrics, Committee on Hospital Care and Section on Critical Care and Society of Critical Care Medicine, Pediatric Section Admission Criteria Task Force. Guidelines for developing admission and discharge policies for the pediatric intensive care unit. *Pediatrics* 1999;103(4):840–2.
4. American Academy of Pediatrics, Committee on Pediatric Emergency Medicine and American College of Critical Care Medicine and Society of Critical Care Medicine, Pediatric Section, Task Force on Regionalization of Pediatric Critical Care. Consensus report for regionalization of services for critically ill or injured children. *Pediatrics* 2000;105(1):152–5.
5. American Academy of Pediatrics, Committee on Pediatric Workforce. Scope of practice issues in the delivery of pediatric health care. *Pediatrics* 2003;111(2):426–35.
6. American Association of Critical Care Nurses. Critical Care workforce position statement. Accessed from http://www.aacn.org/aacn/pnbpolicy.nsf/wdoc/pmp. Accessed on December 12, 2006.
7. Davidson JE, Powers K, Hedayat KM, et al. American College of Critical Care Medicine Task Force 2004–2005, Society of Critical Care Medicine. Clinical practice guidelines for support of the family in the patient-centered ICU. *Crit Care Med* 2007;35(2):605–22.

8. Anderson MR, Jewett EA, Cull WL, et al. Practice of pediatric critical care medicine: Results of the future of Pediatric Education II Survey of Sections project. *Pediatr Crit Care Med* 2003;4(4):412–7.

9. Berglund B, Lindvall T, Schwela DH, eds. Guidelines for Community Noise. World Health Organization 1999: http://www.who.int/docstore/peh/noise/guidelines2.html. Accessed on January 26, 2007.

10. Besso J, Bhagwanjee S, Takezawa J, et al. A global view of education and training in critical care medicine. *Crit Care Clin* 2006;22:539–46.

11. Bhagwanjee S. Critical care in Africa. *Crit Care Clin* 2006;22:433–8.

12. Boyle DK, Bott MJ, Hansen HE, et al. Managers' leadership and critical care nurses' intent to stay. *Am J Crit Care* 1999;8:361–71.

13. Buckley T, Short T, Rowbottom Y, et al. Critical incident reporting in the intensive care unit. *Anaesthesia* 1997;52(5):403–9.

14. Carzoli RP, Martinez-Cruz M, Cuevas LL, et al. Comparison of neonatal nurse practitioners, physician assistants, and residents in the neonatal intensive care unit. *Arch Pediatr Adolesc Med* 1994;148:1271–6.

15. Celis-Rodriquez E, Rubiano S. Critical care in Latin America: Current situation. *Crit Care Clin* 2006;22:439–63.

16. Chaboyer W, Foster MM, Kendall E. The intensive care unit liaison nurse: Towards a clear role description. *Int Crit Care Nurs* 2004;20(2):77–86.

17. Christmas AB, Reynolds J, Hodges S, et al. Physician extenders impact trauma systems. *J Trauma* 2005;58(5):917–20.

18. Dawson D, McEwen A. Critical care without walls: The role of the nurse consultant in critical care. *Int Crit Care Nurs* 2005;21(6):334–43.

19. DeNicola L, Kleid D, Brink L, et al. Use of pediatric physician extenders in pediatric and neonatal intensive care units. *Crit Care Med* 1994;22(11):1856–64.

20. de Souza DC, Troster EJ, de Carvalho WB, et al. Availability of pediatric and neonatal intensive care units in the city of São Paulo. *J Pediatr (Rio J)* 2004;80(6):453–60.

21. Delametter GL. Advanced practice nursing and the role of the pediatric critical care nurse practitioner. *Crit Care Nurs Q* 1999;21(4):16–22.

22. Derengowski SL, Irving SY, Koogle PV, et al. Defining the role of the pediatric critical care nurse practitioner in a tertiary care center. *Crit Care Med* 2000;28(7):2626–30.

23. DiCarlo JV, Zaitseva TA, Khodateleva TV, et al. Comparative assessment of pediatric intensive care in Moscow, the Russian Federation: A prospective, multicenter study. *Crit Care Med* 1996;24(8):1403–7.

24. Downes JJ. The historical evolution, current status, and prospective development of pediatric critical care. *Crit Care Clin* 1992;8(1):1–22.

25. Druss BG, Marcus SC, Olfson M, et al. Trends in care by nonphysician clinicians in the United States. *N Engl J Med* 2003;348(2):130–7.

26. Durch JS, Lohr KN. *Emergency Medical Services for Children* Washington, DC: National Academy Press, 1993.

27. Foley BJ, Kee CC, Minick P, et al. Characteristics of nurses and hospital work environments that foster satisfaction and clinical expertise. *J Nurs Admin* 2002;5:273–81.

28. Gatley EP. From novice to expert: The use of intuitive knowledge as a basis for district nurse education. *Nurse Educ Today* 1992;12(2):81–7.

29. Goh AY-T, Lum LC-S, Abdel-Latif ME-A. Impact of 24-hour critical care physician staffing on case-mix-adjusted mortality in paediatric intensive care. *Lancet* 2001;357:445–6.

30. Govil YC. Pediatric intensive care in India: Time for introspection and intensification. *Indian Pediatr* 2006;43:675–6.

31. Jeena PM, Wesley AG, Coovadia HM. Admission patterns and outcomes in a paediatric intensive care unit in South Africa over a 25-year period (1971–1995). *Intensive Care Med* 1999;25:88–94.

32. Jenkins KJ, Newburger JW, Lock JE, et al. In-hospital mortality for surgical repair of congenital heart defects: Preliminary observations of variation by hospital caseload. *Pediatrics* 1995;95(3):323–30.

33. Kambarami R, Chidede O, Chirisa M. Neonatal intensive care in a developing country: Outcome and factors associated with mortality. *Cent Afr J Med* 2000;46(8):205–7.

34. Khilnani P, Udani S, Singhi S, et al. Consensus guidelines for pediatric intensive care units in India. *Indian Pediatr* 2002;39:43–50.

35. Kleinpell R, Gawlinski A. Assessing outcomes in advanced practice nursing practice: The use of quality indicators and evidence-based practice. *AACN Clin Issues* 2005;16(1):43–57.

36. Lassen HC. A preliminary report on the 1952 epidemic of poliomyelitis in Copenhagen with special reference to the treatment of acute respiratory insufficiency. *Lancet* 1953;1(1):37–41.

37. López-Herce J, Sancho L, Martinó JM. Study of paediatric intensive care units in Spain. *Intensive Care Med* 2000;26:62–8.

38. Lundstrom NR, Berggren H, Björkhem G, et al. Centralization of pediatric heart surgery in Sweden. *Pediatr Cardiol* 2000;21:353–7.

39. Marcin JP, Rutan E, Rapetti PM, et al. Nurse staffing and unplanned extubation in the pediatric intensive care unit. *Pediatr Crit Care Med* 2005;6:254–7.

40. Martin SA. The pediatric critical care nurse practitioner: Evolution and impact. *Pediatr Nurs* 1999;25(5):505–17.

41. Mathur M, Rampersad A, Howard K, et al. Physician assistants as physician extenders in the pediatric intensive care unit setting—a 5-year experience. *Pediatr Crit Care Med* 2005;6(1):14–9.

42. Molitor-Kirsch S, Thompson L, Milonovich L. The changing face of critical care medicine. *AACN Clin Issues* 2005;16(2):172–7.

43. Needleman J, Buerhaus P, Mattke S, et al. Nurse-staffing levels and the quality of care in hospitals. *N Engl J Med* 2002;346:1715–21.

44. Odetola FO, Clark, SJ, Freed GL, et al. A national survey of pediatric critical care resources in the United States. *Pediatrics* 2005;115:382–6.

45. Oswanski MF, Sharma OP, Shekhar SR. Comparative review of use of physician assistants in a level I trauma center. *Am Surg* 2004;70(3):272–9.

46. Ottley RG, Agbontaen JX, Wilkow BR. The hospitalist PA: An emerging opportunity. *JAAPA* 2000;13(11):21–8.

47. Pearson A, Peels S. Advanced practice in nursing: International perspective. *Int J Nurs Pract* 2002;8(2):S1–S4.

48. Pearson G, Shann F, Barry P, et al. Should paediatric intensive care be centralized? Trent versus Victoria. *Lancet* 1997;349(9060):1213–7.

49. Perrin K. A first for this century: Closing and reopening of a children's hospital during a disaster. *Pediatrics* 2006;117(5):381–5.

50. Piva JP, Schnitzler E, Garcia PC, et al. The burden of paediatric intensive care: A South American perspective. *Paediatr Respir Rev* 2005;6:160–5.

51. Pollack MM, Cuerdon TC, Getson PR. Pediatric intensive care units: Results of a national survey. *Crit Care Med* 1993;21(4):607–14.

52. Pollack MM, Patel KM, Ruttimann UE. Pediatric critical care training programs have a positive effect on pediatric intensive care mortality. *Crit Care Med* 1997;25(10):1637–42.

53. Potter P, Barr N, McSweeney M, et al. Identifying nurse staffing and patient outcome relationships: A guide for change in care delivery. *Nurs Economics* 2003;21:158–66.

54. Randolph AG, Gonzales CA, Cortellini L, et al. Growth of pediatric intensive care units in the United States from 1995 to 2001. *J Pediatr* 2004;144:792–98.

55. Richardson DK, Reed K, Cutler C, et al. Perinatal regionalization versus hospital competition: The Hartford example. *Pediatrics* 1995;96:417–23.

56. Rosenberg DI, Moss MM. American College of Critical Care Medicine of the Society of Critical Care Medicine. Guidelines and levels of care for pediatric intensive care units. *Pediatrics* 2004;114(4):1114–25.

57. Rudy EB, Davidson LJ, Daly B, et al. Care activities and outcomes of patients cared for by acute care nurse practitioners, physician assistants, and resident physicians: A comparison. *Am J Crit Care* 1998;7(4):267–81.

58. Society of Critical Care Medicine. Guidelines/Practice Parameters Committee of the American College of Critical Care Medicine. Guidelines for intensive care unit design. *Crit Care Med* 1995;23(3):582–8.

59. Tenner PA, Dibrell H, Taylor RP. Improved survival with hospitalists in a pediatric intensive care unit. *Crit Care Med* 2003;31(3):847–52.

60. Tilford JM, Simpson PM, Green JW, et al. Volume-outcome relationships in pediatric intensive care units. *Pediatrics* 2000;106(2):289–94.

61. Ulrich R, Quan X, Zimring C, et al. The role of the physical environment in the hospital of the 21st century: A once-in-a-lifetime opportunity. http://www.rwjf.org/publications/otherlist.jsp. Accessed on August 29, 2006.

62. Verger JT, Marcoux KK, Madden MA, et al. Nurse practitioners in pediatric critical care: Results of a national survey. *AACN Clin Issues* 2005; 16(3):396–408.

63. West JG, Cales RH, Gazzaniga AB. Impact of regionalization. *The Orange County experience. Arch Surg* 1983;118(6):740–4.

64. World Federation of Critical Care Nurses. http://www.wfccn.org/index.html. Accessed on January 22, 2007.

65. Yeh TS. Regionalization of pediatric critical care. *Crit Care Clin* 1992; 8(1):23–35.

CHAPTER 6 ■ PRACTICE MANAGEMENT: THE BUSINESS OF PEDIATRIC CRITICAL CARE

ALICE D. ACKERMAN • J. MARC HARRISON

The business of critical care has become increasingly complex. Managing that business requires intimate knowledge of the field, understanding of the environment, and the ability to converse with hospital and system administrators in a way that enables the physician or other healthcare provider to accomplish necessary actions on behalf of the patient. Attention to the business of practicing critical care is exceedingly important. Much like the discussion of leadership in Chapter 4, the rudiments of business planning and management must be understood by all practitioners hoping to develop an effective and efficient PICU. Although the term "practice management" for physicians in outpatient settings revolves around maximizing practice income and managing staff, in the hospital-based setting of the PICU, the areas of interest are similar, but in many ways distinct. This chapter addresses the financing of PICUs and critical care practices, as well as issues of billing and coding, physician compliance, recruitment and retention of critical care practitioners, performance evaluation, and productivity measurement. In addition, some aspects of new program development, including the basics of how to write a business plan, are discussed. The chapter is necessarily limited in scope and serves more as a reference to additional materials than as a definitive work in and of itself.

FINANCING THE UNIT AND THE PRACTICE

Hospital Costs and Billing

Much attention has been paid in the American and European literature to the costs of critical care. The US spent $5267 per capita on healthcare services in 2002, over $3000 more than the median of the 30 countries that participate in the Organization for Economic Cooperation and Development; healthcare spending accounted for 14.6% of the US gross domestic product (8). Switzerland, the next in line, spent 11.2% of its gross domestic product, or the equivalent of $3446 per capita. Identifying the ways in which healthcare dollars are spent reveals that critical care accounts for ~20% of inpatient costs, or 0.9% of the gross domestic product (17) in the US. Although efforts at controlling costs in adult ICUs have been given significant attention in the medical, economic, and quality-care literature, little is known about the costs of pediatric critical care globally. The ICU is a cost-intensive environment, and it is therefore important for the practitioner to remain cost conscious while providing pediatric and neonatal critical care services. However, given the relatively small size of the PICU population compared to that of adult ICU users, the overall impact of reducing pediatric critical care costs will be much less important to a nation's overall healthcare expenditures. In the US, however, this fact has not prevented government officials from making cuts in aid programs such as Medicaid, which specifically, although unintentionally, harm children disproportionately to adults (3). We must therefore strive to be cost conscious and cost efficient while we provide the best care possible to our patients.

Internationally, PICUs are funded in many different ways. Whether they and their medical and nursing staffs are funded by the government, private organizations, or by a mechanism of private/public healthcare insurance, financial issues are important. Financing the hospital-based costs (equipment, space, nursing, ancillary personnel) is often different from financing the costs of the attending physicians. The costs of graduate medical education may also play a significant role in the various systems.

An exhaustive review of the financing, cost, and structure of pediatric critical care services worldwide is beyond the scope of this chapter. The authors have concentrated on the situation in the US, due to the paucity of comparable international data.

In the US, most hospital services are funded through a diagnosis-related group (DRG)-based system, although the specific nature of this scheme varies from state to state. Hospitals receive funding in a prospective manner as determined by the Centers for Medicare and Medicaid Services (CMS). The DRG system for calculating prospective payments to hospitals for inpatient services began in 1983 and has undergone only minor changes to date. In general, it establishes norms for lengths of stay for groups of diagnoses, and hospitals are paid for the average length of stay for a particular diagnosis, regardless of how long the patient actually remains in the hospital. Various comorbidities may increase the weight of the DRG for any particular patient, leading to higher-than-average reimbursement. The average weight of all DRGs for an individual hospital is known as the *case-mix index*. In addition, most payers, including CMS, have a mechanism to identify "outliers" and can reimburse differently for such patients.

New changes planned for FY 2007 and beyond will alter the way the federal government calculates the prospective payment based on these codes. The changes are being initiated due to perceived inequities in the current system. CMS alleges that certain poorly reimbursed but highly needed services are unavailable, whereas other potentially less-needed but better-reimbursed services are overly available. The changes will occur in two areas. One is predicted to change the case-mix index of medical, compared to surgical, patients. The other is anticipated to shift payments between hospitals. It will change payments based on severity of illness (6). Therefore, hospitals with a higher proportion of critically ill patients are likely to receive additional reimbursement.

The effectiveness of such a program will depend on appropriate International Classification of Disease (ICD)-9 coding and complete physician documentation. A larger number of diagnostic groups will be recognized by the new system. It is likely to be more useful in pediatrics than is the current DRG system used by CMS. Additionally, CMS is undertaking an evaluation of potential alternatives to the current DRG severity system (6).

Some states' Medicaid programs use a DRG system with a pediatric modification to determine reimbursements to children's hospitals and large pediatric services within general hospitals (24). Although it is more closely reflective of actual pediatric length of stay data, it is not universally accepted by all states or payers.

Physician Billing and Compliance

With apologies to the international community, the information in this section refers exclusively to billing and compliance in the US. In the US, physician or other provider billing is separate from hospital billing. Physicians generate charges based on codes [current procedural terminology (CPT) codes] that describe work done and justify these charges, in part, by the use of ICD-9 codes that indicate why the patient needed the medical care. It bears noting that, while the US is still using the ninth version of ICD, most of the rest of the world is using the tenth version (ICD-10).

Historical Perspective

Most of the rules for billing and coding were developed by CMS, which was originally known as the Healthcare Financing Administration (HCFA). HCFA/CMS was born in 1977 and is an agency of the US Department of Health and Human Services. CMS oversees many programs, including Medicare, Medicaid, the State Children's Health Insurance Program, the provisions under the Health Insurance Portability and Accountability Act (HIPAA), and clinical laboratory improvement amendments. CMS is powerful because it is the single largest purchaser of healthcare in the US. Approximately one in every four Americans receives some CMS-related benefit, totaling more than 71.2 million beneficiaries. One of every three dollars spent on healthcare in the US comes through CMS. Because of the enormity of the cost implications, CMS is focused on making certain that dollars spent on healthcare are medically necessary and meet certain criteria for payment.

Fraud and Abuse

HIPAA, in 1996, and the Balanced Budget Act of 1997 gave CMS new tools and resources for "stepping up program integrity activities" to deter and detect fraud, waste, and abuse within the system. Because funding for the detection activities is self-perpetuating, the agency has financial motivation to recover funds from fraudulent activities. CMS directs physicians to use certain codes to indicate services and disease states so that it can better track the utilization of medical care and provision of payments. All payers in the US now use the same coding systems. Therefore, all providers who intend to bill for medical services in the US must use the appropriate codes and are obligated to understand and obey the rules regarding medical necessity, billing, and coding.

Coding Systems

Current Procedural Terminology. Current procedural terminology was developed in 1966 by the American Medical Association (AMA) as a means of assisting physicians in identifying certain procedures that they perform for patients. The first stand-alone version of CPT was written in 1977. Since then, it has gone through several major and yearly minor revisions. The version in use at this writing is CPT-4, with CPT-5 expected since 2003, but not yet published. (It is important to use the revision for the current year, indicated as CPT-200X.) The use of CPT is mandated by CMS for clinicians to describe services rendered to patients. It is a collaborative effort of the AMA and CMS. The yearly additions, deletions, and revisions to descriptions of services and procedures are overseen by the AMA CPT editorial panel, with input from the CPT advisory committee. The CPT editorial panel is comprised of 17 members. Eleven of these are physicians suggested by various medical specialty societies (therefore, a pediatrician is not always on the panel); the other members represent CMS, Blue Cross and Blue Shield, the American Hospital Association, America's health insurance plans, performance measures development organizations, and the CPT advisory committee. The CPT advisory committee is a 90-member group with representation from the majority of major physician organizations, such as the American Academy of Pediatrics (AAP) and the Society of Critical Care Medicine. Member organizations must be members of the AMA house of delegates or the Healthcare Professionals Advisory Committee.

CPT is divided into six sections of 5-digit codes. The sections that pertain most to pediatric critical care practitioners are found in: "Evaluation and Management (E and M)," which has no procedures but describes most of what we do; "Surgery," which includes some of the procedures we perform; "Medicine," listing most of our common procedures; and "Anesthesia," which is used by some individuals in some states to bill for sedation services beyond moderate sedation. Each section of the book is preceded by written guidelines that contain the rules that the clinician must follow to bill and document correctly and to avoid being charged with fraud and abuse. Each section is further divided into subsections. For example, the E and M section contains (among others) the following subsections: office and outpatient services, hospital services, consultations, emergency department, critical care services, and neonatal intensive care. Any practitioner who is planning to bill for services must be acquainted with the content of those areas that pertain to her practice. It would be impractical to reiterate all of the rules in this chapter, although the major issues for pediatric critical care will be discussed. Because a new version of CPT, with the potential for new rules included, is published each year, *the clinician must seek out the most current version available on a yearly basis.* Although the AMA owns the copyright for CPT, books describing the codes and the rules that govern their use may also be obtained from other sources.

Relationship of Current Procedural Terminology to Clinician Reimbursement. CPT codes are related to reimbursement for clinical services through a mechanism known as the *resource-based relative value scale,* which assigns a relative value unit (RVU) to each item that has a CPT code. This scale was developed by the Harvard School of Public Health in the mid-1980s, under a government mandate. It was introduced into clinical practice in 1992, the year that CPT codes for E and M services were introduced, and detailed instructions for using the codes were added to the CPT book. Each CPT code is assigned a number of RVUs that are used to determine payment through Medicare, but they may be used by other payers as well. RVUs are reviewed by the AMA/Specialty Society Relative Value Scale Update Committee. This committee advises CMS on what value should be associated with each CPT code. However, CMS is not obligated to follow the advice provided. Three components comprise an RVU: physician work (PW), practice expense (PE), and professional liability (PL). In addition, a geographical variation is provided to accommodate the variations in the cost of living in different regions of the country. This variation is linked to the geographical consumer-price index (GCPI). The general formula for calculating reimbursement under Medicare is:

$$\text{Payment} = [(\text{RVU}_{work} \times \text{GPCI}_{work}) + (\text{RVU}_{expense} \\ \times \text{GCPI}_{expense}) + \text{RVU}_{malpractice} \\ \times \text{GCPI}_{malpractice})] \times \text{CF(conversionfactor)}$$

The conversion factor (CF) is necessary to convert the general formula to the actual dollars paid per service. The CF must be changed yearly to maintain what is known as "budget neutrality" in case any changes in the codes, valuations, or numbers of Medicare recipients would result in a total increase of more than $20 million in any one year. For calendar year 2007, however, the formula contains a new factor, the budget neutrality (BN) adjustment, which has the effect of decreasing Medicare physician reimbursements by ~10% (7). The 2007 payment formula is:

$$\text{Payment} = [(\text{RVU}_{work} \times \text{GPCI}_{work} \times \text{BN}) + \\ (\text{RVU}_{expense} \times \text{GCPI}_{expense}) + \\ \text{RVU}_{malpractice} \times \text{GCPI}_{malpractice})] \times \text{CF}$$

The value of BN for calendar year 2007 is 0.8994. CMS chose to apply the BN adjustor instead of adjusting the CF downward because the potential budget overrun was due to changes in physician work RVUs. If the CF had been changed, it would have had the effect of decreasing all elements in the reimbursement equation by ~5%. Many physician organizations are pressing Congress to revise the general formula for reimbursement, citing problems of access to care for Medicare and Medicaid recipients. As reimbursement per RVU falls, physicians are increasingly unwilling to provide care for these patient populations.

Revisions to RVU assignment can be made yearly, but they *must* be made at least every 5 years. Each year, in late November or early December, the RVUs for new, revised, and ongoing codes as of January 1 of the following year are published in the Federal Register. This publication also describes any new documentation requirements and changes to definitions of the CPT codes. The most recent physician work RVUs for some common pediatric and neonatal CPT codes are listed in **Table 6.1** (7).

Although CMS oversees Medicaid and Medicare, it does not set the actual reimbursement rates for Medicaid, because this decision is left to the states. Consequently, the system contains a potential inequity, in that, in most states, the actual Medicaid reimbursement for any given CPT code is lower than the Medicare reimbursement for the same code. A 2007 report by the Public Citizen Health Research Group revealed that the average Medicaid reimbursement to physicians is only 69% of that paid by Medicare (25) and that the quality of care, scope of services, eligibility requirements, and reimbursements vary tremendously from state to state. The state and federal governments support Medicaid jointly, whereas Medicare is totally federally funded. Therefore, whereas the published RVUs and reimbursement formulas presented above are used as absolute reimbursement standards for Medicare, they are only used as guidelines for Medicaid, and private payers are not obligated to abide by the CMS guidelines at all.

TABLE 6.1

RVUs FOR COMMONLY USED CPT CODES IN PEDIATRIC CRITICAL CARE

CPT code	Descriptor	Work RVUs
99291	Hourly critical care, first 30–74 mins	4.5
99292	Hourly critical care, each additional 30 mins	2.25
99293	Pediatric critical care (29 days—24 months), initial day	15.98
99294	Pediatric critical care (29 days—24 months), subsequent days	7.99
99295	Neonatal critical care (less than 29 days), initial day	18.46
99296	Neonatal critical care (less than 29 days), subsequent days	7.99
99289	Pediatric critical care transport, up to 24 months of age, first 30–74 mins	4.79
99290	Pediatric critical care transport, up to 24 months of age, each additional 30 mins	2.40
99221	Inpatient care, initial, lowest level	1.88
99222	Inpatient care, initial, moderate level	2.56
99223	Inpatient care, initial, highest level	3.78
99231	Inpatient care subsequent, lowest level	0.76
99132	Inpatient care subsequent, moderate level	1.39
99233	Inpatient care subsequent, highest level	2.0
99440	Newborn resuscitation	2.93

Data from Centers for Medicare and Medicaid Services. Medicare program: Revision to payment policies; final rule. *Federal Register.* 2006;71:69624–70251.

To determine how much a provider will be paid under non-Medicare plans, a request should be made for a payment schedule from the local carriers, including Medicaid and the Medicaid health maintenance organizations (HMOs), as well as the primary private insurers in the area. The AAP and other child-friendly organizations have launched a campaign to educate legislators about the inequity in access to healthcare that arises due to poor Medicaid reimbursement rates. Many state AAP chapters are active in discussions with local legislators. Because most of this activity occurs at a state level, pediatric critical care practitioners are encouraged to work with their state governments toward ensuring that all children have access to the highest quality pediatric critical care possible by advocating adequate reimbursement to providers.

Coding for Diseases and Diagnoses

ICD-9 coding. By choosing the appropriate ICD code, the healthcare provider tells the payer *why* the service associated with the CPT code indicated on the bill was provided. The international classification of diseases was developed by the World Health Organization for the storage and retrieval of diagnostic data for statistical and epidemiologic use. In 1950, the US Public Health Service and the Veteran's Administration tested the classification scheme for possible clinical use. In 1979, the then-current version (ICD-9) was introduced for use by hospitals and states for tracking data on discharge diagnoses and other topics. In 1988, the Medicare Catastrophic Coverage Act required physicians by law to submit diagnostic codes for Medicare reimbursement, effective April 1, 1989. CMS (then HCFA) designated ICD-9-Clinical Modification (-CM) as the required coding system. The next numbered version of ICD (ICD-10) was developed by the World Health Organization in 1993 and is in use in most countries but on hold in the US. It contains at least 5500 more codes, with new diagnoses, and is more user-friendly (more consistent with medical care and the way clinicians think about diagnoses). ICD-10 is alphanumeric and will require major changes to US computer systems, which will be very costly. Hence, although the lack of ICD-10 data limits the US in being able to compare its diagnoses with those of the rest of the world, the change is unlikely to occur until it is mandated by legislation. ICD-9-CM lists of diagnoses are published yearly, with changes taking effect on October 1 of the year before the designated year of the codes. For example, the 2007 version of ICD-9 took effect October 1, 2006. Recent additions pertinent to critical care include diagnoses such as severe sepsis and systemic inflammatory response syndrome. The 2007 edition, which represents the ninth version of ICD-9-CM, included over 300 total additions and revisions. Most of the time, the revisions are made to stay in line with current medical terminology. For instance, in 2007, the title for the diagnostic group for epilepsy (category 345.xx) was changed to epilepsy and recurrent seizures (5). This slight change may seem unimportant; however, medical personnel often use the term "seizure disorder" when describing a patient with epilepsy. In the past, if one documented "seizure disorder," the diagnosis code would yield a term that was considered nonspecific by the payers and create a risk of nonpayment.

Most physicians and other providers receive very little training in diagnostic coding for the purpose of billing. Some basic guidelines can help the clinician to be more successful in clearly communicating the reasons for the provision of critical care or performance of specific procedures. In general, the *first* diagnosis reported should be the diagnosis primarily responsible for *why that child needed that service on that day*. It should be specific to the service provided by that subspecialty, especially if other physicians will submit a bill for an encounter on the same day. When choosing a code, the clinician should think as specifically as possible and imagine an auditor for the payer looking at the CPT charge, for example, for the first hour of critical care for that day. A primary diagnosis should be chosen that explains why the clinician needed to provide critical care that day. For example, the patient with sickle cell disease, suffering from acute chest syndrome in the PICU on a ventilator because of hypoxemia, should have a primary diagnosis that is specific to critical care. In this case, the authors would choose "acute respiratory failure" from the list of all possible diagnoses and document that diagnosis in the chart. Based on medical training, the inclination is to list the underlying disease, such as sickle cell anemia, as the primary diagnosis. However, in justifying the need for medical care, the underlying diagnosis should be listed *last*, if at all. Currently, up to four diagnostic codes per patient per day can be listed on the form that is submitted to the payers. The most acute and most specific codes should be listed first.

Of equal importance is how the provider documents the diagnostic information in the chart. It is helpful to use language that can be directly translated to one of the ICD-9 codes. This is especially true when others are performing chart abstraction to obtain billing information and the provider is not actually choosing the codes. The abstractor can only choose a code based on what is written in the chart note for that day by the attending physician or by the resident and attending together (see below for a discussion of teaching physician rules in documentation). Therefore, if the patient has epilepsy, it should not be recorded as "seizures" or "convulsions," because these are separate diagnoses. As noted earlier, however, the term *recurrent seizures* is now considered equivalent to epilepsy. Epilepsy is considered more specific than either convulsions or seizures and should therefore be used whenever appropriate to the child's condition. In addition, the provider should try to be as specific as possible in describing the condition. Without this information, the abstractors will be forced to resort to a nonspecific descriptor, and the true nature of the patient's severity of illness will be lost. In the epilepsy example, one would need to indicate whether the epilepsy is focal or generalized, intractable or not, and the like. It is useful, even in an abstraction situation, for the clinician to review the ICD-9 codes for commonly seen diagnoses to become familiar with the language used.

Some Specific Current Procedural Terminology Codes for E and M Services in the PICU

In 2005, a new code was introduced for billing pediatric critical care. However, the majority of pediatric critical care billing still utilizes the original hourly critical care code. Situations under which the provider should utilize each of the possible critical care codes will be reviewed in this section. In-patient hospital care codes are not discussed, although usually, a subset of patients in the ICU should more appropriately be billed with those codes. In addition, "bundling" will be discussed but not the specifics of the procedure codes that are or are not bundled with the various critical care codes. Any provider who is billing for any service must become familiar with the rules and guidelines provided in the most current CPT book.

The major determinant of critical care billing in the US is the *condition of the patient*. Regardless of which code is used, the patient must meet the definition of critical care. For the purposes of CPT coding, a patient is considered to be critically ill if he has a life-threatening illness or injury and if some treatment option is being exercised to prevent worsening of that life-threatening condition. Patients may be critically ill and stable, but the physician must take care to document how the provision of care under the physician's direction is sustaining that stability. Patients who are in ICUs for monitoring purposes only and do not require interventions do not meet the definition of being critically ill. The mere presence of a patient in the ICU does not qualify that patient for consideration as critically ill. Patients may be critically ill for many days; they may be critically ill even if they have a do-not-resuscitate order. The definition of critical care has evolved somewhat over the years; the most current definition will be found in the current version of the CPT coding book (4). In addition to the requirement for the patient's condition to meet the definition of critical illness, the practitioner must be providing critical care. It is not adequate that the physician visits a patient for 5–10 mins, makes no changes in their life-sustaining therapy, and thinks that critical care has been provided to that patient.

Three basic coding families are used to indicate services provided to patients in the PICU; they depend on the patient's age and location (**Table 6.2**). Although they all depend on the patient meeting the criteria for critical illness just described, the requirements for physician attention vary by code; therefore, the physician's documentation should be completed accordingly.

The Hourly Critical Care Code. The basic hourly critical care codes, 99291 and 99292, are used to bill critical care services for patients older than 24 months through adulthood. These codes may be used in any location and are the *only* codes that can be used in an outpatient setting (such as the emergency department). The rules for using these codes are the same, whether

TABLE 6.2

AGE AND LOCATION RELATIONSHIP TO SPECIFIC CRITICAL CARE CODES

Code	Location	Age
99289–99290	Transport, requires direct face-to-face presence of the attending physician	0–24 months
99291–99292	Outpatient	Any
99291–99292	Any	>24 months
99293–99294	Inpatient	29 days–24 months
99295–99296	Inpatient	0–28 days
99298–99300	Inpatient	Weight-based

Data from American Medical Association. *Current Procedural Terminology: CPT 2007: Professional Edition.* Chicago: American Medical Association, 2006;696.

the code is used in adults or children. Specifically, direct time spent by the attending physician is counted (time spent by a resident or fellow *alone* does not count). The practitioner who is billing must give her full attention to that patient for that period of time and therefore cannot provide care to other patients at the same time.

The time spent with the patient includes time spent reviewing labs and radiographs (as long as this is done in the unit), time discussing the case with other physicians (not residents or fellows), and time performing documentation, in addition to the examination and treatment. Although it is an hourly code, the physician should document and bill for a total amount of time spent with that patient on that day. The CPT guidelines specify how the time is to be counted. For example, the first 30 to 74 mins constitutes the first "hour" of critical care. Charts of how to count and bill critical care time are available in every CPT book. Any patient who requires less than 30 mins of critical care should be billed using regular inpatient hospital care codes.

Some procedures are bundled into the code and cannot be billed for separately. Bundled codes are codes for which a separate bill cannot be generated because it has been determined that they occur so often together; the RVUs for the main code have already been adjusted to account for them. For example, for 99291, the first hour of critical care, the procedures that are bundled when performed during the critical period include such activities as interpretation of cardiac output measurements, placement of nasogastric and orogastric tubes, and ventilatory management. For the procedures that are not bundled, such as placement of a percutaneous central venous catheter, the time it takes to do the procedure cannot count as both critical care time and procedure time. The provider's note should include a specific statement such as, "I spent X time providing critical care to this patient, not including time spent performing procedures." Any unbundled procedures should then be billed separately. The use of modifiers will not be discussed in this chapter. However, the reader should note that in the situation just described, the proper billing of both an E or M code (critical care time) and a procedure code on the same day requires the use of modifier "-25" (4).

Time spent with family under this code requires careful justification—the accompanying note must specify that the time spent with family was because the patient was incompetent *and* that the discussion was directly related to the decision making for that day. Giving an update to family members, unless medical decision making occurs during that update, does not count toward the time. Time off of the floor or unit, even if it is directly related to the patient, also cannot be counted in the time calculation. The reason for this policy is that if the physician is away from the floor or unit, she cannot be immediately available to the patient.

The Global Codes. The codes for pediatric and neonatal critical care (99293–99296) are considered global codes and are billed once per patient per day. These codes require that the patient resides in an inpatient setting (usually the PICU or the NICU) and meets the same definition of critical illness as listed earlier. They differ somewhat from the hourly codes in the requirement for physician interaction with the patient and, therefore, in documentation. The global codes require that the physician provide "personal direct supervision of the healthcare team in the performance of cognitive and procedural

TABLE 6.3

REFERENCES AND ADDITIONAL READINGS FOR CRITICAL CARE BILLING AND CODING

AMA CPT 2006, 2007, etc.	American Medical Association	2005, 2006, etc.
AMA ICD-9	American Medical Association	2005, 2006, etc.
Coding for Pediatrics	American Academy of Pediatrics	Yearly
Billing and Coding in Critical Care	Society of Critical Care Medicine	2006, every 2–3 years

activities." These codes have more procedures bundled into them than do the hourly codes. They are divided into two families—one for pediatric (99293, 99294) and one for neonatal (99295, 99296) critical care. In each case, the first code listed is to be used for the first day of critical care, and the second code is used for subsequent days. It should be noted that, because 99295 and 99296 are for use in neonates, patients who are 29 days of age or older must be billed using 99293 or 99294. If a patient is in the hospital and is being billed using 99296 (neonatal critical care, subsequent days) for the first 28 days of life, on the day that the patient becomes 29 days of age, the provider must switch codes and bill under 99294 (pediatric critical care, subsequent days). If one continues to submit a bill for this patient using 99296 after the 28th day of life, most third-party payers will reject the claim.

Additional global codes that cover pediatric patients between the ages of 2 and 5 years and between 5 and 12 years have been proposed. Acceptance of these additional codes would require a complete renumbering of the sequence of critical care codes. The earliest a practitioner might see the new codes would be in 2009.

The practitioner should be aware of many more issues concerning billing for critical care services prior to submitting any bills. Additional reference materials are listed in **Table 6.3**.

Putting It All Together—The Superbill

To tell CMS or another payer both what service(s) were performed on a particular day and why the clinician provided that service, the provider must be able to code for both CPT and ICD-9. It is convenient to have a pre-made form holding most of the useful codes for that particular unit or group of practitioners on which the provider can easily check off what was done and why, thus requiring less work and time in finding the correct codes to meet coding standards. Such a form is generally referred to as a "superbill." In some practices, it might be called an "encounter form." The provider completes the form and gives it to the person or organization that will complete the official billing instrument that will be sent to the payers. Electronic methods, some handheld, are also available to permit comprehensive billing and coding for physicians (see Chapter 11). Of all approaches, a knowledgeable person or group of certified coders who provide chart abstraction will save the provider the most time, capture all documented services, and avoid problems with billing and coding compliance. An example of a 2005 superbill used in a PICU where the physicians are responsible for choosing correct CPT and ICD-9-CM codes is presented in **Figure 6.1**. The form is double-sided; **Figure 6.1A** represents the front of the form, with room for the patient identifier. It lists the commonly used CPT codes for 1 week's worth of interactions. All physicians in the group can bill using the same sheet

for the week. At the bottom of the first page, space is provided for the patient ICD-9-CM diagnoses codes, which are obtained from the back of the form (**Fig. 6.1B**). The diagnostic codes are numbered, usually from 1 through 4, and those numbers are transcribed to the front of the sheet for that day. Because a patient's illness evolves over time, the order of the diagnoses as well as which are chosen for a particular day, usually change as the week progresses.

Compliance refers to the provider's understanding of and complying with all billing and coding rules, especially teaching-physician rules for those who work in an academic institution. Failure to meet compliance standards can lead to charges of fraud and abuse. Hence, chart documentation becomes critically important. The provider must document the patient's condition, the thought process that accompanied the evaluation, and the indications for any procedures that were performed. For hourly critical care services, it is essential for the attending physician to indicate, using the word "I," how much time was spent providing critical care. For the global pediatric and neonatal services, no specification of time spent is necessary, because the physician is stating in her note the direct supervision of the healthcare team. Any diagnoses that will be coded by ICD-9 should also be mentioned in the chart.

Routine internal audits of physician billing activity can identify the need for additional education in billing and coding practices and should be performed routinely by the billing group. Routine audits and training will prepare physicians and other practitioners should an external audit ever be conducted. If internal issues are found and attempts at educating providers about correct coding are documented, external auditors will be more likely to classify identified problems as individual error rather than systematic attempts at fraud.

RECRUITMENT AND RETENTION OF INTENSIVISTS

Building an ICU service requires staff. Chapter 5 identifies various members of the healthcare team who are important in providing appropriate care for patients in PICUs. This section is concerned with general approaches to hiring and mentoring individuals. It speaks mostly of physicians, but the principles are similar regardless of the type of healthcare provider being recruited. Physician leaders of critical care units must be cognizant of human resource issues when recruiting individuals to work in their units. Because hiring laws differ by country and region, and because of cultural differences between various places in the world, some of this discussion must be relatively nonspecific. When possible, appropriate references or

PEDIATRIC CRITICAL CARE MEDICINE

| 2005 |

PRIMARY SERVICE:_____

PRIMARY ATTENDING:_____

DATE RANGE:_____

CODE	DESCRIPTION	MON	M	TUES	M	WED	M	THURS	M	FRI	M	SAT	M	SUN	M
	EVALUATION & MANAGEMENT														
99221 - 23	INITIAL HOSPITAL CARE	1 2 3		1 2 3		1 2 3		1 2 3		1 2 3		1 2 3		1 2 3	
99231 - 33	SUBSEQUENT HOSPITAL CARE	1 2 3		1 2 3		1 2 3		1 2 3		1 2 3		1 2 3		1 2 3	
99238 - 39	HOSPITAL DISCHARGE (30 or 60 MINS)	38 39		38 39		38 39		38 39		38 39		38 39		38 39	
99291	CRIT CARE - 1ST HOUR OVER 24 MONTHS														
99292	CRITICAL CARE- ADDITIONAL 30 MIN														
99293	PED CRIT CARE - INIT 29 DAYS - 24 MONTHS														
99294	PED CRITICAL CARE- SUBS														
99295	NEO INTENSIVE CARE - INITIAL 0-28 DAYS														
99296	NEO INTENSIVE CARE- SUBSEQUENT														
	PROCEDURES		Dx		Dx		Dx		Dx		Dx		Dx		Dx
31500 ‡	ENDOTRACHEAL INTUBATION Ø														
31525	DIRECT LARYNGOSCOPY (DIAGNOSTIC)														
32000	THORACENTESIS Ø														
32002	CHEST TUBE (pneumothorax)														
32020	CHEST TUBE (fluid)														
33010	PERICARDIOCENTESIS - INTIAL														
33011	PERICARDIOCENTESIS - SUBS														
33015	pericardial TUBE														
36450	EXCHANGE TRANSFUSION (NEWBORN)														
36455	EXCHANGE TRANSFUSION (NON-NEWBORN)														
36555	CVP < 5 yr old														
36556	CVP >= 5 yr old														
36568	PICC < 5 yr old														
36569	PICC >= 5 yr old														
36580	line replacement same site														
36620 ‡	ARTERIAL CATHETER, PERCUTANEOUS														
36680	insert intraosseous														
36800	insert hemodialysis catheter														
92950	CPR														
33960	ECMO, 1st 24 hrs														
33961	ECMO, subsequent days														
	MODIFIERS	**USE MODIFIER 25 FOR SEPARATELY IDENTIFIABLE E&M ON DAY YOU PERFORM A PROCEDURE**													
	DIAGNOSES														
DOCUMENTATION ATTACHED															
		‡ CANNOT BILL WITH CODES 99293, 99294, 99295, 99296							Ø = modifier 51 EXEMPT						

Attending Signature:

DOCTOR 1	DOCTOR 2	DOCTOR 3

DOCTOR 4	DOCTOR 5	DOCTOR 4	DOCTOR 7

FIGURE 6.1. Example of a superbill from the year 2005 showing how billing and coding in the PICU can be facilitated by creation of a one-page instrument. Because of yearly modifications in both CPT and ICD-9-CM codes, this is only an example and cannot be used to actually bill. **A:** Front of bill, containing patient identifier information, CPT codes, and a place to indicate which diagnoses (from the back) are being used on that day. Physicians initial the specific charges and then sign at the bottom of the sheet. *(continued)*

PEDIATRIC CRITICAL DIAGNOSES 2005

INFECTIOUS DISEASES

	005. 1	Botulism
	008. 45	C. difficile colitis
	008. 61	Rotavirus
	033. ___	Whooping cough_____
	036. ___	**Meningococcal infections**
	038. ___	**septicemia**_____
	040. 82	**toxic shock syndrome**
	041. ___	bacterial infection in diseases classified elsewhere
	042. xx	HIV disease - AIDS (symptomatic)
	047. ___	viral meningitis_____
	052. ___	Chickenpox/varicella_____
	054. ___	herpes simplex_____
	066. 4	West Nile virus
	070. ___	viral hepatitis_____
	078. 3	Cat-scratch disease
	079. ___	viral infection in conditions classified elsewhere _____
	112. 5	**systemic candidiasis**
	112. ___	other candidal infections_____
	136. 3	Pneumocystis pneumonia
	___ ___	_____

NEOPLASMS

	___ ___	_____
	___ ___	_____

ENDOCRINE, NUTRITIONAL, METABOLIC, IMMUNITY

	250. 11	**Diabetes (type I) with ketoacidosis**
	250. 31	**type I diabetes with coma**
	250. 8__	diabetes with hypoglycemia/hypoglycemic shock
	251. ___	hypoglycemia _____
	253. 2	panhypopituitarism (non-iatrogenic)
	253. 7	iatrogenic pituitary disorders
	253. 5	Diabetes insipidus
	253. 6	SIADH
	255. 4	adrenocortical insufficiency
	275. 2	hyper/hypo-magnesemia
	275. 41	hypocalcemia
	275. 42	hypercalcemia
	276. 0	hyperosmolality/hypernatremia
	276. 1	hypo-osmolality/hyponatremia
	276. 2	acidosis (metabolic OR respiratory)
	276. 3	alkalosis (metabolic OR respiratory)
	276. 4	mixed acid-base disturbance
	276. 5	volume depletion-hypovolemia
	276. 6	fluid overload/fluid retention
	276. 7	hyperkalemia
	276. 8	hypokalemia
	278. 01	morbid obesity
	279. ___	Immune disorders (not HIV) _____
	___ ___	_____

BLOOD AND BLOOD-FORMING ORGANS

	285. 9	anemia, NOS
	280. 9	iron deficiency anemia, NOS
	285. 1	acute posthemorrhagic anemia (not post-op)
	285. 21	anemia in end-stage renal disease
	285. 22	anemia in neoplastic disease
	282. 61	sickle cell anemia **WITHOUT** crisis
	282. 62	sickle cell **WITH** crisis
	282. 63	Hb S/Hb C **WITHOUT** crisis
	282. 64	Hb S/Hb C **WITH** crisis
	283. 11	HUS (hemolytic uremic syndrome)
	286. 6	defibrination syndromes (DIC)
	286. 7	acquired coagulation factor deficiency
	289. 7	methemoglobinemia
	287. 4	secondary thrombocytopenia
	288. 0	neutropenia

MENTAL & PSYCHOLOGICAL DISORDERS

	292. 0	drug withdrawal syndrome
	315. 9	developmental delay (NOS)
	319. xx	mental retardation NOS

NERVOUS SYSTEM AND SENSE ORGANS

	320. ___	bacterial meningitis_____
	323. ___	encephalitis, myelitis, encephalomyelitis (includes ADEM and cat-scratch)_____
	348. 30	encephalopathy, NOS
	324. ___	intracranial and intraspinal abscess_____
	326. xx	late effects of pyogenic intracranial infection
	331. 4	obstructive hydrocephalus (acquired)
	337. 3	autonomic dysreflexia

NERVOUS SYSTEM AND SENSE ORGANS (CONT)

	325. xx	thrombosis of intracranial venous sinuses-**pyogenic**
	437. 6	intracranial venous sinus thrombosis-**non-pyogenic**
	343. 9	cerebral palsy NOS
	345. ___	**Epilepsy (Need type and whether intractable)** _____
	345. 3	**Grand mal status**
	348. 1	anoxic brain damage
	348. 4	brain herniation
	348. 5	cerebral edema
	357. 0	Guillain-Barre syndrome
	357. 82	critical illness polyneuropathy
	359. 81	critical illness myopathy

CIRCULATORY SYSTEM

	401. 0	Essential hypertension-malignant
	401. 1	Essential hypertension-benign
	405. 01	secondary hypertension-malignant renovascular
	405. 09	secondary hypertension-malignant other
	405. 11	benign renovascular
	405. 19	benign other
	415. 0	Acute cor pulmonale
	416. 0	Primary pulmonary hypertension
	416. 9	Cor pulmonale, NOS (non-acute)
	420. ___	Acute pericarditis_____
	421. ___	Acute/subacute endocarditis _____
	422. ___	Acute myocarditis_____
	425. ___	Cardiomyopathy_____
	426. ___	conduction disorders (blocks)_____
	427. ___	Dysrhythmias_____
	427. 5	Cardiac arrest
	428. 0	congestive (right) heart failure
	428. 1	Left heart failure (pulmonary edema)
	428. 3__	diastolic heart failure
	428. 9	heart failure, unspecified
	458. 0	**Hypotension/orthostatic**
	458. 1	hypotension/chronic
	458. 2	hypotension/iatrogenic (post-operative)
	458. 9	Hypotension NOS

CEREBROVASCULAR DISEASE

	430. xx	subarachnoid hemorrhage (non-traumatic)
	431. xx	Intracerebral hemorrhage (non-traumatic)
	432. ___	Other non-traumatic intracranial hemorrhage
	437. 2	Hypertensive encephalopathy

RESPIRATORY SYSTEM

	464. 10	Acute **tracheitis** without obstruction
	464. 11	Acute **tracheitis** with obstruction
	464. 20	Acute **laryngotracheitis** without obst
	464. 21	Acute **laryngotracheitis** with obstruction
	464. 4	croup syndrome
	465. 9	acute URI, NOS
	466. 11	**RSV bronchiolitis**
	466. 19	non-RSV bronchiolitis
	478. 3__	paralysis of vocal cords_____
	480. ___	viral pneumonia _____
	481. xx	**pneumococcal pneumonia**/lobar infiltrate NOS
	482. ___	other bacterial pneumonia_____
	483. 0	mycoplasma pneumonia
	486. xx	pneumonia, org unspecified
	487. ___	Influenza (note manifestation)_____
	493. 00	**ASTHMA WITHOUT STATUS**
	493. 01	**STATUS ASTHMATICUS**
	493. 02	**ACUTE ASTHMA EXACERBATION**
	507. 0	aspiration pneumonia
	510. ___	empyema_____
	511. ___	Pleurisy (non-traumatic)_____
	512. 0	pneumothorax-spontaneous tension
	512. 1	pneumothorax-iatrogenic (post-operative)
	512. 8	pneumothorax-other spontaneous
	514. xx	pulmonary edema (chronic-NOS)
	518. 4	pulmonary edema (acute **without** heart failure)
	518. 0	atelectasis (pulmonary collapse)
	518. 1	mediastinal emphysema
	518. 5	**pulmonary insufficiency following trauma and surgery**
	518. 81	**Acute respiratory failure**
	518. 82	**ARDS NEC** (use 518.5 if post-op/post-trauma)
	518. 83	chronic respiratory failure
	518. 84	**acute on chronic respiratory failure**
	519. 4	paralysis of diaphragm
	___ ___	_____

PERINATAL CONDITIONS

	770. 7	BPD
	362. 21	retinopathy of prematurity
	772. 1__	IVH (grade_____)

DIGESTIVE DISEASES

	530. 81	Gastroesophageal reflux
	564. 00	Constipation
	567. ___	peritonitis_____
	578. 0	hematemesis
	578. 1	melena
	578. 9	GI-Bleed, NOS

GENITOURINARY SYSTEM

	581. ___	nephrotic syndrome_____
	584. ___	acute renal failure_____
	585. xx	Chronic renal failure
	586. xx	uremia/renal failure, NOS
	590. 1__	acute pyelonephritis_____
	599. 0	UTI, NOS

CONGENITAL ANOMALIES

	745. 2	tetralogy of fallot
	745. 5	ASD (secundum)
	745. 4	VSD
	747. 1__	coarctation of aorta
	741. ___	spina bifida (Hydrocephalus ? Yes___ No___)
	758. 0	Down syndrome
	___ ___	_____

SYMPTOMS, SIGNS & ILL-DEFINED CONDITIONS

	780. 01	coma
	780. 02	transient
	780. 09	other_____
	780. 31	febrile seizure
	780. 39	other convulsions
	780. 53	sleep apnea (with hypersomnia)
	780. 59	sleep apnea unspecified
	780. 6	fever
	782. 5	cyanosis (not newborn)
	783. 41	failure to thrive
	785. 50	**SHOCK** unspecified
	785. 51	**SHOCK** cardiogenic
	785. 52	**SHOCK** septic (must code 995.92 first)
	785. 59	**SHOCK** other (hypovolemic)
	786. 01	hyperventilation (not psychogenic)
	786. 03	apnea (not sleep apnea, NOT newborn)
	786. 06	tachypnea (not TTN)
	786. 09	respiratory distress/insufficiency
	786. 1	stridor
	786. 3	hemoptysis
	787. 91	diarrhea
	788. 5	oliguria and anuria
	789. 0_	Abdominal pain (specify site)_____
	790. 7	bacteremia (no signs of clinical infection)
	798. 0	SIDS
	798. 2	Death in less than 24 hr, cause unknown
	799. 0	asphyxia/hypoxia/anoxia
	799. 1	respiratory arrest

INJURY AND POISONING

ACUTE TRAUMA/POISONING

	958. 4	Traumatic shock
	994. 1	drowning and near drowning
	995. 5__	child maltreatment syndrome
	995. 9__	**Systemic inflammatory response syndrome**
	___ ___	_____

OMPLICATIONS OF PROCEDURES & DEVICES

	996. 63	VP shunt infection
	996. 75	VP shunt malfunction
	997. 1	**cardiac insufficiency during or from a procedure**
	995. 4	**shock due to anesthesia**
	998. 0	**post-operative shock (hypovolemic, septic)**
	998. 11	Post-procedure hemorrhage
	___ ___	_____

OTHERS

	V15. 81	Non-compliance with medical care
	___ ___	_____

FOR DX #	USE E-CODE:

FIGURE 6.1. (*continued*) **B:** List of commonly used ICD-9-CM codes. These codes may be chosen and numbered, then the numbers transferred to the front of the sheet. Bold font indicates common critical care diagnoses; shaded boxes indicate nonspecific diagnoses that should not be used as primary diagnoses.

recommendations for additional reading are provided. The principles discussed here can be adapted based on the perspective of the country, region, or institution involved. No part of the following discussion is meant to suggest that national, regional, or institutional processes are incorrect; rather, we have tried to focus on best practices when available.

New intensivists are recruited for one of two reasons: either additional staff are necessary due to program growth, or the program has sustained the loss of one or more intensivists. This loss may be due to a number of reasons, such as illness, retirement (becoming a more frequent issue due to the number of pediatric intensivists over the age of 50), or relocation due to family considerations. However, occasionally, the necessity to recruit is caused by a failure to retain a valuable member of the staff, generally due to unhappiness on the part of the physician caused by some component of lack of fit—whether on the basis of salary, job description, lifestyle, or dissatisfaction with the division head or chair (15). Because retention strategies seem costly, some groups, units, or universities do not engage in them as much as they should. However, the recruitment of new physicians is even more costly, especially when it occurs because of the failure to retain experienced, highly functioning members of the team. The cost of recruiting and training new faculty has been estimated to be one-and-a-half times the first year's salary (12). Therefore, plans for the retention of valuable physicians should be in place even before the recruitment begins. Successful recruitment begins well before an employment ad is created or a candidate is interviewed. Suggested steps in the recruitment process are indicated in **Figure 6.2**.

Establish the Need

To establish the need for the desired recruitment requires completing at least the rudiments of a business plan, the components of which will be discussed in a later section. The position must have a clear purpose, and the job duties must be elucidated. A source of funding must be established, as well as a salary range, which will vary by experience and specific job title. Will the person be doing anything other than clinical care? How much time is the candidate expected to spend on the job? Will the individual have leadership and administrative duties? What are the teaching commitments? Is research activity ex-

pected? If so, how is it to be funded? What will be the criteria against which the unit or department will measure success? It is wise to prepare a written, prioritized list of duties, expected outcomes, and desirable traits of the successful candidate before the recruitment begins. The unit or division director must also be aware of any specific rules for hiring physicians in the home institution. Most public institutions in the US, for example, are bound by strict human resources guidelines regarding gender and racial discrimination, as well as established guidelines regarding salary, benefits, title, and other issues. Failure to comply with human resources guidelines could invalidate a recruitment process. In many cases, specific permission must be obtained to "open" a position.

The Search Committee

Many intensive care unit directors, when faced with the need to recruit staff members, believe that it is not necessary to establish a search committee—that one is needed only for high-level recruitments. However, the authors suggest that having a search committee, even if it is only an informal committee, will help to establish the seriousness with which the search is undertaken and keep the process moving forward. We recommend establishing membership of the committee before the position is posted or advertised. Members of the committee should be involved in determining criteria and priorities in advance. The leader of the search (usually the unit or division director) should communicate his vision for the position to the committee. What type of candidate is being sought? What is this job? All major stakeholders should be involved in the committee; it should be comprised of most of the individuals who will be involved in interviewing the candidates.

A good committee contains individuals with different perspectives and areas of expertise. We recommend the PICU physician recruitment search committee contain representatives from the attending physician group (both prospective colleagues of the candidate and physician users of the PICU), nursing personnel, representatives from hospital or department administration, PICU fellows, and others as deemed appropriate. It is important for candidates to be given the opportunity to meet a wide and representative group of individuals, yet the number should not be so overwhelming that they are left

The Recruitment Process

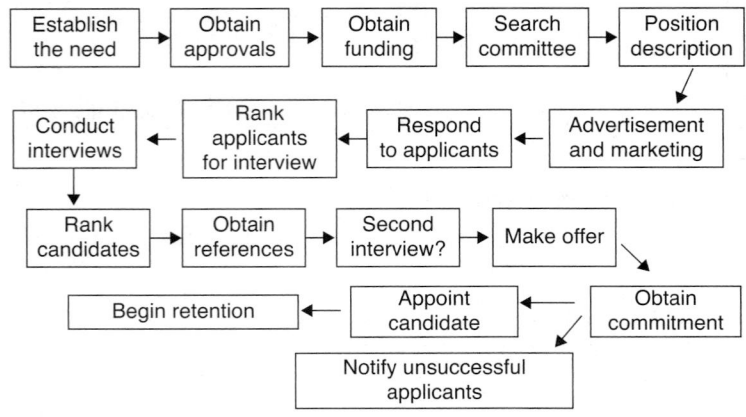

FIGURE 6.2. Algorithm of sequential steps in the recruitment and retention process.

confused at the end of the day. However, broad-based input will be most helpful in finding the right candidate who is the best fit for the institution and the particular situation.

Another issue important to recruiting the best candidate is ensuring appropriate diversity on the committee. This includes race and gender as well as position and role.

The search committee should meet to discuss the needs of the unit or division and to establish the position description. They should then formulate a timeline, working "backward" from the desired start date to allow enough time to obtain licensure, help with relocation, and attend to other related issues. Often, the need is immediate, necessitating that searches begin as soon as the opening is identified. The committee should decide on selection criteria, how candidates will be evaluated, and how feedback will be given to the committee chair. How will different qualifications be weighted? Will the position be advertised and, if so, where and how?

Using a Professional Search Firm

Increasingly, medical searches are being conducted by professional search firms. Sometimes, it is necessary or desirable to utilize one of these firms, especially if the position is one with significant leadership or extremely specialized expertise requirements. In addition, if the position is critical or has proved difficult to fill, the services of a search firm may be helpful. However, search firms are relatively expensive. Many require the payment of a flat fee that generally runs in the thousands of dollars, while others require some percentage of the first year's salary. Using a firm can be very helpful, but it does not absolve the person leading the search of all responsibilities. However, if the institution is inexperienced or if the physician leader does not have the time necessary to attend to all the detailed steps listed in **Figure 6.2**, using a firm may be the best use of available resources. Once the position has been advertised and responses have been received, some fraction of candidates will be invited to interview.

The Interview

The interview has three purposes: (a) it gives the search leader and committee a chance to evaluate the candidate, (b) it allows one to "sell" the division/unit and hospital or medical school to the candidate and, most importantly, (c) it provides the opportunity to test how well the candidate will fit with the culture of the institution or group that he will be joining. Failure to use the interview for all three purposes is a common mistake and one that may lead to hiring the wrong person. The "selling" of the institution or group is exceedingly important and must start before the candidate sets foot in the institution. Initial interactions with support personnel are important. The individual who handles the logistics of the proposed trip has a profound impact on the candidate, especially if things go wrong. The schedule must be comprehensive but not overwhelming. It is important to include time for breakfast, lunch, and dinner and to plan for some breaks in the schedule, allowing the candidate time to freshen up, collect his thoughts, make a phone call, and the like. The interview day should include a tour of the facilities. It is important to maintain clarity throughout the process. Everyone who is meeting the candidate should under-

stand the position and why this candidate is being evaluated. They should be knowledgeable enough to answer basic questions and should know what to do with questions that they are unable to answer.

The interview day should be organized in a sensible fashion. A model agenda is listed in **Table 6.4**. In general, the day should begin with clear instructions on how the candidate will arrive at the medical center or ICU. We find it useful to have the division director meet the candidate in the morning for breakfast, to start the day on an informal note and to provide an overview of the program, the position, and the day. Efforts should be made to remain on schedule; hence, it is useful to plan some time between appointments, especially if the candidate is expected to travel from one office or building to another. One member of the host division or department should be identified to guide the candidate from place to place; alternatively, the candidate can be assigned to a conference room or open office, and those doing the interviewing can be asked to meet him there. The total length of the first visit can be from 1 to 1.5 days and should include dinner on either the night before the formal interviews or the night between the days. Because the candidate will not have his spouse or partner present at the first interview, the dinner participants should be comprised of representatives of the search committee. Often, the dinner is a good time to check for "fit" with the host division. A "wrap-up" session with the division head or unit director (whoever is leading the search) should be scheduled at the conclusion of the entire visit to establish next steps, obtain first impressions, and to give both parties the opportunity to ask any questions that may have arisen during the visit. The candidate should leave with the knowledge of how to obtain more information and answers to any questions that have not been addressed. It is also useful to clarify whether the candidate has specific time-sensitive issues that might affect his decision-making process. Any issues relating to spouse or family members should be discussed at this point (spouse must find a job, children must be enrolled in school, etc.). The leader must always keep in mind, however, that some questions should not be asked, because they might lead to suggestions of discrimination in the future, depending on the laws of the home country. Checking with the human resources office prior to conducting the interview can provide guidance on topics that may be considered "off limits."

Making a Decision

Following the visit, efforts should be made to receive feedback from the members of the search committee and others who met with the candidate. A specific feedback form that is developed by the search committee and is specific to this particular position should be used; an example is provided in **Figure 6.3**. At this point, if numerous candidates seem appropriate to your needs, a second visit might be scheduled. However, this is not always necessary.

Once a tentative decision has been made, but before making an official offer, the candidate's references should be checked. It is useful if the division head or unit director conducts the reference checks by phone, even though the institution will most likely require written letters of recommendation to meet hiring, appointment, or credentialing standards. Checking of references must be done religiously. It is useful to call a variety

TABLE 6.4

POTENTIAL AGENDA FOR AN INTERVIEW DAY

Time	Meet with	Reason
7:30–8:30	Division head over breakfast	Discuss overview of position, institution, and location. Provide orientation to the day, explain who the candidate is meeting and why
8:35–9:30	Join work rounds in PICU	Obtain a glimpse of the way the team operates in action, see a cross-section of the types of patients in the ICU
9:35–10:00	Senior nursing members	Chance to interact with nonphysician members of the team and interact with a group
10:10–10:30	Junior faculty member	Obtain additional viewpoints, learn about how newly recruited members are treated, discuss items that might be important from a personal, social standpoint
10:35–11:00	Division administrator	Review departmental/divisional support, benefits, etc.
11:10–11:50	Research faculty member	Learn about research opportunities, obtain additional information
12:00–1:00	Nurse practitioners over lunch	Learn about the nurse practitioner program, add another component to the team members
1:10–1:35	Non-PICU department of Pediatrics faculty member	Learn perspective of outsider to how PICU functions
1:40–2:10	PICU fellowship director	Discuss fellowship issues and obtain further insight into how the ICU works
2:15–2:45	Cardiac surgeon	Discuss perspectives from a nonintensivist who utilizes intensive care services and is part of the team
3:00–3:30	Pediatric department chair (can sometimes wait for second visit)	Obtain overview of department, learn what is needed for promotion and tenure if in an academic setting
3:35–4:00	PICU fellows	Obtain perspective of trainees
4:00–5:00	Division head	Wrap up, answer any questions, determine next steps and time frame. Share first impressions
5:00–6:00	Break	Someone can drive candidate back to the hotel for rest and freshening up before dinner
6:00–8:00	Division members over dinner	Time to test the "fit" of the candidate with the rest of the group. Will the candidate be comfortable with the culture and dynamics of the team?

of individuals at the candidate's home institution or others who have worked with the candidate in a prior position. They should represent as diverse a group of individuals as the candidate is likely to work with in the new job. Calls should be made to the person's immediate supervisor, colleagues, and subordinates. At least one evaluation should be obtained from a nurse or allied healthcare worker.

Once the references have been called, it is important to reevaluate the committee's decision. Does this individual have all of the qualifications that were decided upon prior to the search? If not, what aspects take priority? Although the clinical needs might be significant, a person who is a poor fit will not be of value in the long run. The leader should be certain that both the candidate and the committee are clear on the candidate's capabilities and the needs of the job. Any areas of disconnect should be identified and addressed prior to moving forward. The most important question from the standpoint of the prospective boss should be, "Will this individual enhance the team already in place?"

Making an Offer

Making the offer can be the most difficult part of the process for both candidates and their prospective supervisors. It is very important for both parties to be sincere, open, and straightfor-

ward. Supervisors should not make promises that cannot be kept and should not make the job seem easier than it is. It is crucial that, at this juncture, the candidate have a clear understanding as to the expected on-call duties or likely number of hours worked per week. The candidate must be able to trust the information provided by the supervisor. An employee who arrives to find that work expectations are considerably higher than presented will soon develop mistrust and resentment. If the truth will dissuade the chosen individual from accepting the offer, it is better for the division head or unit director to know that and move on to another candidate. Likewise, candidates should not misrepresent their interests or willingness to perform tasks that they would rather not do in an effort to obtain the position.

In most cases, a verbal offer should be followed by a written letter or contract, which should include a statement of expectations for job performance. The letter or contract should identify all sources of support for the physician—not only the salary. In most cases, it is also important to document the expectations for "citizenship" in the group as well as specific responsibilities. Depending on the local rules or customs, the contents of the offer letter/contract may be predetermined, and the boss may have little ability to craft it. In that case, it may be helpful to write an addendum that includes all of these details. Legal advice may be necessary before any written document is sent to the candidate.

PEDIATRIC CRITICAL CARE
FACULTY CANDIDATE EVALUATION FORM

Date _____ Candidate _____ Interviewer _____

On a scale of 1-5 with **5 being the best,** please rate the candidate on the following characteristics:

---

1.   **Clinical training and experience** (i.e. junior/senior clinician). Rate candidate's perceived ability to care for the most difficult pediatric critical care patients, serve as a regional resource. Note any special or advanced skills. Note any interest in specific patient populations (i.e. neuro, cardiac).

    1   2   3   4   5

Comments:

---

2.   **Research training and experience** if applicable. Identify types of mentoring needed, and whether candidate is at an independent research stage. Name potential collaborators.

    1   2   3   4   5

Comments:

---

3.   **Personality and warmth.** Please rate how well this candidate will interact with other faculty, staff and students.

    1   2   3   4   5

Comments:

---

4.   **Teaching interest, experience and ability.** Does the candidate have a documented track record in teaching others? How does the candidate see his/her role in training others, including non-physicians?

    1   2   3   4   5

Comments:

---

5.   **Quality of ideas** for building and sustaining a solid pediatric critical care program. This can be focused in patient care, education or research, depending upon the current needs of the program and the candidate's experience and expertise.

    1   2   3   4   5

Comments:

---

6.   **Perceived interest by the candidate in this position.** Is the candidate prepared to move if selected? Are there specific impediments to relocation? Time constraints? Please note any special issues or concerns

    1   2   3   4   5

Comments:

FIGURE 6.3. Example of a typical faculty candidate evaluation form.

Retention

Once the preferred candidate is identified, recruited, and hired, the process must begin to develop and maintain job satisfaction for the employee. In academic medical centers, physician retention and faculty development are synonymous. The tech-niques developed in academic medical centers may be useful in other practice situations. In general, physicians are seeking a supportive environment, with transparent operations, in which data are shared. They want their contributions to be recognized. Salary, although important, is not the most critical factor in providing for faculty satisfaction. Trust and communication

TABLE 6.5

DIFFERENCES BETWEEN "BABY-BOOMERS" AND "GENERATION-X"

	Generation Xers	Boomers
Work–life balance	Willing to work hard but only if balance can be achieved	Work hard out of loyalty
Relationship to job/Institution	Expect to change jobs frequently	Expect long-term job security
Recognition of need to "pay dues"	Not felt to be relevant to future career development	Expect to do this for success
Willingness for self-sacrifice	Will endure this occasionally	See self-sacrifice as virtue
Response to authority	Question authority	Respect authority

Adapted from Bickel J, Brown A. Generation X: Implications for faculty recruitment and development in academic health centers. *Acad Med.* 2005;80:205–210.

with the immediate supervisor in the academic medical center are important (15) and, similar to studies of worker satisfaction in other industries, barriers to effective communication should be identified and removed.

Mentoring enhances retention; this is especially the case in the academic center but can be equally important in the practice setting. Mentoring establishes a welcoming environment for the newly hired, helps them to feel that they are part of the community, and fosters their ability to develop a career while more rapidly learning the culture and norms of the group. Increasingly, however, mentoring and coaching techniques that worked "in the old days" are proving to be no longer effective, as organized medicine deals with the impact of the "generation Xer." The term "generation-X" refers to the cohort of individuals born between 1963 and 1981. This is the generation of most newly trained individuals and junior- to mid-level faculty. Certain qualities have been identified that distinguish the generation-X members from the "baby boomers" (born between 1945 and 1962), who still hold most of leadership positions within the field of medicine (12). Major differences exist between these two groups in attitudes toward work-life balance, importance of the job or institution to the individual's sense of overall well-being, willingness for self-sacrifice, recognition of the need to pay one's dues, and response to authority (**Table 6.5**). If mentors (who are generally in the baby-boomer group) are unaware of these characteristics of the generation-X individuals whom they are trying to mentor, the relationship may not be as productive or as helpful as it could otherwise be.

The International Campaign to Revitalize Academic Medicine has identified a crisis in academic medicine in Great Britain and Europe (18,29), as well as in developing countries, due to physicians' desire for flexible schedules, among other things. The retention of physicians in high-stress, high-demand subspecialties such as pediatric critical care will depend on our ability to meet the needs of this group of young physicians. Both how our jobs are structured and the mentoring and other support offered to physicians must take these differences and requirements into account.

PHYSICIAN PRODUCTIVITY

Historically, pediatric critical care evolved in the world of academic medicine. Until recently, the approach of many aca-

demic medical centers toward practice management and fiscal responsibility was laissez faire. Issues related to business—contracting, coding, billing, malpractice—are still not routinely taught in pediatric critical care fellowship programs. It is still quite possible for a fellow to complete training and remain unfamiliar with the issues described in this chapter.

Improvements in information technology and a highly demanding reimbursement environment have made attention to clinical productivity both possible and necessary for pediatric intensivists. More hands-on care is provided by attending academic intensivists at the bedside now than was the case at the time that this text was last published. As the style of their practice has changed, academicians have adopted an interest in coding and reimbursement that used to be the sole purview of those in private practice. To justify additional intensivists, adequate salaries, and productivity-based reimbursement to medical and administrative leadership, pediatric intensivists should be conversant in the language of productivity and tools to ensure its optimization.

Defining Clinical Productivity

Demographics

Perhaps the simplest method of defining an intensivist's productivity is a volumetric measurement of clinical activity. A director of a PICU should be able to describe the activity of the unit as a whole, and of individual intensivists specifically, in terms of admissions, procedures, average daily census, average length of stay, resource utilization (e.g., extracorporeal membrane oxygenation, ventilators, and inotropic support), risk of mortality (PRISM III or PIM2), and similar topics. Daily entry of patient information into an institutional and/or multicenter database, such as the Virtual Pediatric Intensive Care Unit, provides a tremendously valuable source of data that is highly understandable to medically savvy and lay people alike.

Professional activity is usually described in terms of a fraction of a full-time equivalent (FTE), whereby a 1.0 FTE is carrying a "full" clinical load. Because the standards for "full time" work vary by institution, other useful descriptors include time on-service, frequency of night and weekend call, and clinical hours worked per week. Because much of an intensivist's practice occurs when colleagues from other specialties are out of the hospital and asleep, these facts may be persuasive during attempts to justify additional FTEs.

Billing

When a patient's bill is generated, the amount of the charge is recorded by the billing agents and may be reported to the physicians on a weekly, monthly, quarterly, and/or yearly basis. The actual amount billed is arbitrary and may be set by the physician group or administrators; therefore, it does not directly relate to the amount of work performed by the intensivists. Collections are generally counted on monthly, quarterly, and yearly bases. Dividing the total amount received by the total amount billed determines the *gross collection rate*. This parameter is only a weak measure of productivity for a number of reasons. To a large extent, the price paid is at the discretion of the third-party payer or is determined by CMS, as described earlier. The *net collection rate* takes into account contractual relationships with third-party payers and patient demographics (self-pay, commercial insurance, government programs). Contracted reimbursement is often negotiated and based on a multiple (or fraction) of the current Medicare reimbursement for an RVU. The net collection rate will almost always be higher than the gross collection rate. The net collection rate is calculated by dividing the amount received by the amount that should have been collected for that time period. Efficient billing processes will yield net collection rates in excess of 90%–95%, meaning that the office is collecting almost every dollar that is allowable by the particular payer. Patients without insurance are known as "self-pay patients" and are unlikely to be able to pay the entire amount billed for a stay in the PICU. Therefore, a high percentage of self-pay patients will significantly decrease the net collection rate, unless the bill is determined to be uncollectible and is officially written off. The net collection rate, although a good estimate of the effectiveness of the billing office, is a poor measure of physician productivity. However, for physicians in practice who receive no subsidies from the hospital, the various collection rates are very important. *Net revenue*, or the amount of money remaining after all practice costs have been considered, will be the best measure of productivity in this situation. However, for physicians in hospitals and academic medical centers, other, more reliable measures of productivity have been developed.

Relative Value Units

As noted in the section on billing and coding, every CPT code is assigned a value by the CMS that is described in terms of RVUs. In theory, complex medical decision making and technically difficult procedures are tied to higher RVUs (1,2). Given the consistency of work RVUs across settings, this measure is typically used to benchmark and describe productivity. It is important to note that RVUs do not necessarily translate directly to revenue. As also noted in the section on billing and coding, CMS annually assigns a uniform national conversion factor (in dollars) to the reimbursement formula. For non-Medicare insurers, payment is set at the payer's discretion. Most third-party reimbursement is negotiated as a percentage of the value of an RVU (16,19).

Benchmarking Productivity through Measurement of Relative Value Units. Work RVUs are the most commonly used unit of productivity for benchmarking physician clinical activity. Benchmark figures are available through professional organiza-

tions (e.g., American Association of Medical Colleges) and private consulting companies. Benchmarking is usually reported in terms of upper and lower quartiles and the median for a 1.0 FTE. Consulting firms will provide information that categorizes performance based on unit characteristics—number of beds, number of intensivists, academic versus community setting, and the like. Given the relatively small number of PICUs nationally, it is common for external benchmarking to inaccurately describe a particular practice's patient population.

For example, pediatric intensivists may staff two 10-bed PICUs in the same city. One unit may care for a robust neonatal cardiac surgery population, while the other has an active bone marrow transplant program. The cardiac unit may generate more RVUs per patient day because of the relatively high RVUs associated with the global CPT codes used in patients <2 years of age. A comparison of the RVUs produced by a cardiac intensivist versus one who works primarily in the oncologic ICU could be misleading in terms of clinical effort.

Additionally, because the benchmark data available are presented normalized to 1.0 FTE, certain elements of error may be introduced in the calculations. The definition of how much work is performed by a full-time intensivist (1.0 FTE) varies from center to center. It is not possible to compare the effort based on hours per week, weeks of service per year, or other terms, because a clinical service can be organized in many different ways. The addition of trainees and students may alter the relative time one spends in direct patient care but may make this a parameter that is difficult to adequately measure.

Experience has shown that the most useful benchmark for productivity is within each institution. One of the authors (JMH) has developed an internal approach to benchmarking that has enhanced productivity at his institution. In this system, each pediatric intensivist's RVU production is benchmarked against the others and against the individual's performance over the previous 2 years. This approach is described in more detail here.

Maximizing Productivity at One Institution

Timely Billing. Pediatric intensivists bill for a wide variety of services in different circumstances—global critical care, time-based critical care, procedures, sedation, transport, dialysis, extracorporeal membrane oxygenation, etc. The clinical pace and patient turnover is frantic in most PICUs, and it is very easy for the attending intensivist to forget what services were provided to each patient on a given day. When the author's (JMH) institution implemented a *mandatory daily billing* strategy, physician RVU production rose by 10%.

Concurrent Coding. Daily review of the medical record, in conjunction with timely billing, increases measured productivity. In the just-mentioned approach, a coder, rounding daily to compare documentation in the medical record with physician billing, has the ability to identify clinical activity that the physician neglects to bill, find inadequate documentation (e.g., time not noted) to substantiate a code, and identify patients for whom the intensivist forgot to bill altogether. The initiation of this program increased RVU production by an additional 10%, decreased the denial rate from 5% to <1%, and decreased the overtime hours in the billing department.

Information Sharing. Physicians are goal-oriented, data-driven, and competitive. Sharing comparative productivity data within a group of intensivists can be a highly productive or destructive experience. Punitive use of this data can destroy trust and collegiality within a group. The author (JMH) developed a mechanism by which this information is shared in the form of individualized charts on a quarterly basis. Each intensivist is able to identify her performance, while her colleagues' data is de-identified. The experience in this situation was that variance between high and low performers narrowed at the same time that overall productivity increased.

Correct Coding

In some circles, "correct coding" is synonymous with maximizing productivity. It is crucial that physicians, coders, and billing personnel receive regular updates on relevant CPT codes and their correct use. Both systematic undercoding and overcoding are unethical and illegal.

Aligned Incentives

Monetary bonuses based on productivity have proved to increase billing and RVU generation in a number of settings (5). If this strategy is employed, even greater attention to detail than normal must be paid to ensure that coding is in compliance with national standards. Nonmonetary incentives for productivity can be effective. These can include additional nonclinical time, hiring mid-level providers to support clinical activities, or purchasing an interesting but nonessential technology for the PICU.

Nontraditional Measures of Productivity

Historically, discussions of physician productivity were linked exclusively to professional revenue/RVUs. It is increasingly apparent that physicians in general, and intensivists in particular, make tremendous contributions to their hospitals. Clinical and financial symbiosis between pediatric intensivists and hospitals has spawned a number of creative measures of productivity. Pediatric intensivists are indispensable for clinical program development and financial health in modern children's hospitals or departments of pediatrics within general medical centers. As such, it is justifiable for pediatric intensivists to negotiate for financial support from their hospital in excess of professional revenue.

Contribution to Hospital Revenue

As mentioned earlier, in the discussion on billing and coding, in general, hospitals are paid a fixed amount for an admission based on the DRG associated with the patient's illness. The hospital is paid the same amount regardless of whether the admission is 2 days or 2 weeks. A hospital's economic survival is usually based on razor-thin margins of 3%–5%. Intensivists who provide efficient management that decreases length of stay and cost per case can make the difference between a positive or negative contribution to the organization.

Investigators found that an academic, adult ICU accounted for 24% of the institutional profit margin (11). At the Children's Hospital of the Cleveland Clinic, the contribution margin for admissions to the PICU is four times greater than for admissions to a regular nursing floor.

Some third-party payers have begun to pay hospitals more for more complex cases. All-patient redefined (APR) DRG severity-adjusted indicators (complexity, concurrent diagnoses, length of stay, cost per case, readmission rate) are used to justify higher levels of payment. Accurate calculation of APR DRG severity depends on accurate physician (intensivist) documentation. Physicians who are motivated to fully document their patient's condition contribute substantially to the hospital's financial health.

Quality Improvement Activity

Hospitals are motivated to provide safe, high-quality care for humanitarian reasons. They will also be increasingly financially driven to do so. In 2003, the CMS initiated a demonstration project that financially rewarded hospitals for excellence in five areas (10). This trend, termed "pay for performance," will play a prominent role in healthcare reimbursement for the foreseeable future. Intensivists can have a significant effect on hospital quality (14). Our specialty's contribution to the "quality" movement may rank as a uniquely important form of productivity.

Subsidy for Vital but Poorly Compensated Services

Pediatric intensivists are uniquely qualified to provide procedural services that are clinically vital but not necessarily well compensated in professional revenue. Vascular access and procedural sedation are prime examples of these services. Hospitals may choose to recognize and encourage these activities by pediatric intensivists for a number of reasons—dedication to a pain-free environment, technical revenue associated with these services, or freeing other physicians (primarily anesthesiologists and surgeons) to engage in very lucrative activities. It would be reasonable for an intensivist leader to expect institutional financial support for his group to provide a very poorly compensated but necessary activity.

Productivity Related to the Academic Mission

Intensivists who practice in academic medical centers have more missions than the clinical one described earlier. Measures of productivity must therefore take into consideration the teaching, research, and administrative roles held by these physician-faculty members. Various schools of medicine have developed paradigms to identify and track faculty productivity based on hours of teaching, size of grants awarded, numbers of papers published in peer-reviewed publications, and similar parameters. The term *mission-based management* has been coined to describe the alignment of how faculty members spend their time with how they generate income and how they are paid. It developed during the late 1980s and early 1990s as a way to identify the financial sustainability of academic medical centers in the face of falling clinical reimbursements, increased government regulations, and diminishing support for the teaching and administrative missions within schools of medicine (22). In the academic medical center setting, productivity and performance must be based on more than a physician's clinical activity and an estimate by the physician as to time spent teaching, conducting research, and performing administrative duties. Various approaches to measuring productivity in these areas have been developed. They are not simple, and must be crafted to meet the needs of individual centers and to support the specific cultures of those centers. Because of the complexity of this issue and the wide interest on the part of chairs and deans in further developments in this area, the Association of American Medical Colleges, in 2002, produced a management series on mission-based management, which is available free of charge on the Internet at www.academicmedicine.org/pt/re/acmed/mbm.htm.

PERFORMANCE EVALUATION AND FEEDBACK

Earlier sections addressed issues of recruiting and retaining physicians as well as ways to measure physician productivity. Another major area of great importance to the longevity of any division or unit is the method used to evaluate the performance of the intensivists. Many approaches can be taken but, in general, an evaluation process must be initiated that is fair, comprehensive, and conducted on a routine basis. Just as productivity should be measured according to the physician's various activities, the performance evaluation should include all areas in which the physician participates. Best practices suggest that goals and objectives for performance should be established at the beginning of the period, that these goals be given weights and priorities, and that the person being reviewed be aware of and help to develop the performance review criteria in advance.

Areas to be evaluated should be tied to the job or position description whenever possible, emphasizing the need to make the job description truly descriptive of how the individual will spend his time. If the physician is to be evaluated on the success of a new program he was to develop, program development should be in the job description. Establishing clear expectations helps to improve performance. In the business world, much is made of the inclusion of "stretch" goals to push individual productivity and performance to the greatest possible heights (26). A stretch goal might revolve around program development, meeting specific safety objectives, or obtaining a certain amount of research funding. Whatever is determined to be appropriate for the individual should be identified, with clear parameters and metrics provided so that the intensivist can know whether or not the goal was met. Participation in quality-improvement activities, such as Six Sigma (21), involves setting stretch goals and finding ways to meet them.

Increasingly, organizations are utilizing the "balanced scorecard" approach to evaluate individual and team performance. This technique combines different types of indicators of performance into an overall snapshot of the individual's contributions to the organization's well-being. Other organizations are relying increasingly on 360-degree feedback to evaluate the individual's perceived strengths and weaknesses by obtaining input from peers, trainees, supervisors, patient's parents, and allied healthcare workers.

Regardless of the format for formal performance review, it is essential that the individual be given feedback concerning how he is doing. The leader must strive to do this regularly and objectively. Although the meetings need not be formal, they should be conducted in a professional manner. Constructive feedback should be provided. This is important for new members of the group as well as for those who are more seasoned. This is a challenging aspect of leadership for many medical directors and division heads, but if it is done routinely and in the fashion described, it need not lead to anxiety and agitation.

Providing feedback on an ongoing schedule is a much better practice than providing it once per year, when the performance review (and potential salary) is being discussed. In addition, it helps to establish an appropriate relationship between the physician and the leader.

DEVELOPING NEW PROGRAMS: WRITING A BUSINESS PLAN

An essential component of any business is growth; it is therefore imperative that medical professionals develop a clear sense of how to propose new programs and see them through to completion. Most often, administrators and chairs will request a business plan when a faculty member suggests starting a new program or project, such as developing a transport team, starting a sedation service, or hiring new or additional staff.

The purpose of a business plan is to elucidate the reasons to institute the program, identify the costs (in time, financial and human resources, and space), and calculate projected benefits. Although the simplest of plans can be communicated verbally, under most circumstances, the plan should be written, presenting the appropriate substantiating data and references or resources from which assumptions were made. Being asked to prepare a business plan should not induce fear. One does not need a business education to write a viable business plan. However, the use of some standard business approaches may make it easier to communicate needs and expected benefits more clearly to nonclinical individuals who may hold the key to obtaining approval or funds for the program. If pediatric intensivists want to effectively compete for their department's, school's, or hospital's limited available investment dollars, the business planning must be convincing and carefully done. Data and business information are important but should not overshadow the *ideas* on which the plan is based. Although the numbers are essential to demonstrate that the physician has a concept of what is achievable and how much it will cost, the numbers alone are unlikely to be the critical determinant of whether the proposal will gain acceptance.

The *why* of the proposal is at least as important as the *how* or the *how much*. Key investors (chair, chief executive officer, dean) will need to understand the importance of the project and to be convinced that it is necessary; as well, they will have to be convinced why a particular person or team should be managing the project. What historical factors point to one's ability to take responsibility for a project like this and succeed? Looking at the project and the proposal from the perspective of what an outside investor might want to see will help to clarify and crystallize the major points. The following suggestions will increase effectiveness and creativity of thought and presentation.

Planning

The most important piece of the business plan is the *planning* that happens before any words, tables, or figures appear on paper. The starting point of the planning must allow the planner to answer the questions "What do you want to do?" "Why and how do you plan to accomplish it?" and "How much will it cost?"

The answers to these questions should be based in the organization's or unit's strategic plan. The strategic goals should be aligned with those of the parent organization (hospital, group practice, or medical school) in which the unit or group exists. If the goals are not aligned, the plan is unlikely to achieve buy-in from the upper-level decision makers. Therefore, the plan must start with a clear and compelling mission, vision, and goals. These should be in writing and should reflect input from the appropriate team members and other stakeholders. The plan being proposed must support the mission and vision of the unit/group and must clearly relate to the accomplishment of at least one of the stated strategic goals of the unit/group.

The proposed project must be important if significant resources are being requested to make it happen. The more expensive it is expected to be, the more important it should be to the organization. How do you identify what is important? As mentioned earlier, alignment with the organization's strategic plan is the first step. If the proposed project supports a local, regional, national, or international need, especially one endorsed by a prominent organization, it rises in importance. If local supporters are vocal in identifying the need, the organization's leaders will be more inclined to listen.

A good plan starts with a good idea—one that is either unique in its approach to the problem being addressed or provides "a better mousetrap." "Better" can mean "cheaper," but this does not necessarily have to be the case. If it is not cheaper, it must have a better *return on investment* (ROI). What will the parent organization get for its investment in resources (human resources, space, capital)? A commonly sought ROI might be market share or revenue, but these alone will not be enough. Will you be meeting or exceeding published benchmarks in serving a particular patient population? Will you be delivering a new service that does not currently exist in your community? How big is the need for that service/unit in the community? Will you be competing with other units or institutions to provide this service, or will the new service bring you into a "blue ocean" (20), where you can operate away from the competition?

Occasionally, the business plan is required for relatively mundane reasons, such as the need to hire an additional physician for the group. In this case, approval is usually (but not always) assured, and the sponsoring organization simply needs to "see the numbers" to understand the costs involved. However, even here, approval will be much more likely if the stated plan can align the proposed recruitment with overall organizational strategy and highlight how the recruitment will add value to the group. Is there a particular skill that would be useful for your group to possess? Does this relate to changing patient characteristics (such as the care of patients receiving a new service—for example, liver transplantation) or evolution of the standard of care? It is useful in such situations to identify how the field has changed since the last recruitment was undertaken and to explain why this new expertise is required to continue to provide state-of-the-art care for the children who are admitted to the unit.

One should never take for granted that resources will be made available for any project, even replacement recruitments. The authors believe that, to be successful, every request for resources must be accompanied by a well-thought-out, written plan that carefully articulates the need, the reason, the method, and the expected ROI. The plan should include a method by which to monitor or judge success. It should include a parameter or parameters that are straightforward and easy to measure. The general expectation is that at least a one-for-one

ROI will be appreciated by the end of a 3- to 5-year period, although these expectations vary with the particular circumstances. Sometimes a service is necessary but will not lead to enough specific direct increase in revenue to achieve the stated goal. In cases such as these, it may be useful to look at "downstream" revenue, or the ripple effect of the proposed program on admissions for other services, the enhancement of research opportunities, improved educational experiences, and similar issues. Because these metrics can be difficult to measure, some indicator of success should be agreed on prior to the start of the project.

Obtaining the necessary data to include in a winning business plan can be difficult. It is usually necessary to partner with a representative of the hospital's or medical school's finance or marketing office, so that a baseline can be obtained for market share, length of stay, profit and loss, or whatever parameter one is planning on improving with the proposed program. Having appropriate baseline data is essential. Chief executive officers, department chairs, and deans will want to know the source of the data, how the competitive analysis was performed and which assumptions were used, and how the proposed program metrics will demonstrate success. The more succinctly and directly these questions can be addressed, the greater the likelihood that the upper-level decision makers will be able to accept the plan as presented.

For areas in which data may not be readily available or the data are unable to prove the point, obtaining buy-in and written testimonials of support from appropriate stakeholders will be essential. Even if the data are available, the use of strategic stories can be very helpful (23). The multinational company, 3M (creator of the Post-it note, among other innovations), developed the art of "strategic story telling" into a corporate cultural approach to business planning (27). They believe that the ability to tell a compelling story in narrative instead of bullet points requires the author to understand the strategic logic of the proposal in intimate detail. This, in turn, allows the reader to understand in more depth the entire business situation. The following components are further suggested to produce a well-executed strategic story (27): First, set the stage by describing the current situation, the details of the status quo, who the players are, and what relationships exist in the field. Next, introduce the dramatic conflict. In this section, the author identifies the challenges faced by the group or unit and the critical issues that are obstacles to success. Finally, the story must reach resolution by following a logical argument that is specific to the current situation. If the plan is written well, the reader will be able to understand the vision of the author and her group. The intentions and the markers of success will be clear.

Writing the Plan

Regardless of the approach taken to writing the business plan, the outcome must be a document that is clear, easy to read, logical, and can stand alone in support of the proposal. One potential format for organizing a written business plan is presented in **Table 6.6**. The components are described in more detail here.

The Executive Summary

The executive summary will be the first thing the reader sees and probably the only part that the reader remembers. It might

TABLE 6.6

A POTENTIAL APPROACH TO ORGANIZING A WRITTEN BUSINESS PLAN

Component	Purpose
Executive summary	Makes the case for whatever is being proposed in a one- or two-page summary. May be the only part read by the main decision maker.
Introduction and overview	Introduces reader to the PICU and the topic. Provides a glimpse into benchmarking this PICU against others in the city, region, or nation.
Business concept	Presents the project the author wants to do. Ties the proposal to the strategic goals of the unit and the institution.
Market analysis	Provides an understanding of how many children may need the service being proposed. Describes the current demand and the likely supply over time.
Competitive analysis	Identifies the internal and external competitors. Demonstrates author's understanding of the entire field and potential problems.
Business strategy	Shows how the author plans to overcome the competitive threats and meet the identified needs. Provides metrics to determine success.
Financial plan	Provides a clear estimate of the financial resources required to initiate and complete the plan, as well as an estimate of the return on investment for the institution or backer.
Operations plan	Indicates the operating capacities of the leader to achieve the stated goals. Identifies additional personnel and space required. Has a clear demonstration of author's responsibility to the project.
Summary	Provides a concluding statement pulling together the initial vision with the proposed outcome. States clearly what the proposal will accomplish for whom and in what manner.
Tables and graphs	Presents substantiating data that is not needed within the body of the proposal but might be needed to justify issues raised.

Adapted from Cohn KH, Schwartz RW. Business plan writing for physicians. *Am J Surg.* 2002;184:114–120.

be the only part of the written plan to be read by a busy chief executive officer, department chair, or dean. It therefore must be a well-written, one- or two-page (the shorter, the better) summary of the salient features from the other sections of the plan. Because of its importance, it should probably be the last thing written. It must be consistent with the entire plan and make the case for the project being proposed.

Introduction and Overview

The Introduction and Overview is a relatively short section of the written plan that describes the unit or group and its history. One can include statistics on recent growth, current staff members, and, most importantly, the mission, vision, and goals of the group. The introduction sets the stage for the rest of the plan and helps to tell the reader why this team is in a position to determine the needs of the community. Although boasting is not recommended, the plan can be strengthened by highlighting recent accomplishments by the physician or nursing staff, awards received, and similar achievements. It may be useful to provide some data that benchmark the unit with other PICUs in the city, state, region, or nation. Does this PICU serve a specific niche population? Are there specific geographic issues to consider? How is this unit of value to the rest of the organization?

The Business Concept

The Business Concept section is the heart of the proposal. What is the author planning to do and why (for example, beginning a sedation service)? What is the evidence for an unmet need in the community or patient population (for example, long waits for pediatric MRIs, frequently canceled tests, and unhappiness on the part of referring physicians, radiologists, and parents)? What is the value of what is proposed? (How much time can

be saved from being able to do these tests smoothly? How many more patients might come to the institution if the process were more patient friendly?) Who will receive the value (faculty members, referring physicians, the institution, other services, patients, etc.)?

Market Analysis

The Market Analysis may tie into the introductory remarks concerning the position/status of the unit in the world of pediatric critical care. This section contains an overview of the local market so that the reader understands which other institutions are also attempting to provide the same or similar services to patients in the general area. An assessment of the current market share for a particular service should be included and can usually be obtained from the hospital's marketing, planning, or finance office. Analysis of population trends and any epidemiologic data that will help to support the request should be included in this section. For example, if the proposal is to develop a specialized trauma response team within the hospital, the plan must provide narrative and supporting data on the numbers of children of various ages who have been involved in trauma. Is the number increasing? Are the types of trauma changing so that a different subset of individuals must be available to care for the patients? Has the time of day or time of year in which trauma victims are admitted to the institution changed? Are other nearby hospitals decreasing their ability to care for the same patient population?

The plan must identify why this unit or division is the appropriate group to receive the support to develop the service being proposed. For a sedation team, why PICU and not anesthesia? For trauma, how will this service incorporate surgical members?

Competitive Analysis

The Competitive Analysis section identifies any direct and indirect competitors, both external (other hospitals) and internal (other services or individuals). How difficult or easy will it be to accomplish the stated goals? How will potential difficulties be overcome? It is useful to clearly identify these obstacles, in that it demonstrates a complete knowledge of the competitive environment and should provide some assurances to the reader that the author has considered methods to overcome the most significant competitive barriers to success. Approaches to overcoming potential barriers are developed in the business strategy section.

Business Strategy

The Business Strategy section contains the description of how the plan will be achieved. It describes how the group will overcome the competitive forces identified in the preceding section. It may include such elements as a marketing plan—how to reach referring physicians, referring hospitals, primary care clinicians, or patients—the volume of services anticipated over a period of time, how the provision of the new service will foster long-term growth for the unit, and similar issues. It will explain how this unit will be differentiated from all other units and why it will become the unit of choice for this particular service. If the unit is not in a heavily competitive environment externally, the business strategy must identify what the benefit will be to the unit's further success. It must also identify why the PICU should receive the resources when other departments or units are simultaneously requesting support for something that they consider equally as important.

Financial Plan

The financial plan will be scrutinized by the administrative staff and must be compiled in a professional fashion, although it is not intended to meet formal accounting standards. It is useful to obtain assistance in composing this section. In short, the financial plan should identify the proposed revenues and costs associated with the program described in the plan. In a hospital setting, the identification of revenues may not always be straightforward, and one must look at all revenues related to the patient population when appropriate. For example, if the leader were proposing to hire a pediatric intensivist who was also a neurologist, revenues that the hospital would derive from additional electroencephalograms and neurologic imaging might be included, even though those revenues might not normally be attributed to the PICU. Similarly, in identifying costs, care must be taken to reflect the total costs that might be attributable to the patient population.

Institutions are particularly interested in the "marginal" costs and revenues associated with a new program. The term *marginal* can be loosely defined as describing the cost or revenue associated with the next patient. Marginal costs are distinguished from fixed costs, such as the cost of electricity and other things that would be spent even if the additional patient were not there. For example, the cost of drugs used to treat a particular patient is a marginal cost. The costs of nursing care and the costs of other staff can be difficult to assign as marginal or fixed. If another nurse is needed on a shift because of a particular patient, the cost of the nurse is a marginal cost. If the nurse was already there, being paid a full salary even without the patient, then the nurse's salary for that day is fixed. As noted in the earlier section on productivity, decreasing the length of stay for a patient because of a new program will, in essence, decrease marginal costs and potentially result in a net positive financial balance for the institution.

Justifying projects that will have a net negative financial impact is clearly more difficult than if the project will potentially provide a significant new source of revenue or save a significant percentage of current costs. Even if the financial plan indicates a negative impact, however, the proposal may still be supportable if it meets a significant enough need or can yield a significant improvement in quality. It is necessary to acknowledge the negative financial impact in these situations and to identify how the financial burden to the institution will be lessened over time. For example, a proposal to hire enough additional pediatric intensivists to allow the unit to have 24-hr, on-site intensivist coverage 7 days per week might not in itself yield a financial benefit to the institution. However, if the patient population requires this level of attention, the enhanced physician services will improve patient safety and outcomes, in addition to improving night-time teaching and supervision of residents and fellows. These improvements may provide adequate rationale to allow the additional hires, despite the increase in marginal cost.

Operations Plan

In the Operations Plan, the need for additional staff, space, equipment, and similar items is identified. What are the optimal conditions to enable the stated goals to be met? If the entire package cannot be funded, what are the minimal requirements necessary? Sometimes providing the reader the ability to partially fund the request will mean the difference between receiving a portion of what was requested and receiving nothing. It can therefore be useful to make the various operations of the plan contingent on various levels of funding, being clear about what the expected outcomes at each level will be.

The reader also must be confident that any resources provided to the project will be well spent. Therefore, this section should also identify how the project will be implemented: Who will be responsible for project oversight? What milestones will be tracked? When will the leader know if something is not going according to plan, and what will be done about it? A timeline of activities and expected outcomes is helpful in this section. Last, quality management and patient safety issues should be discussed as part of the operations and implementation plan.

Summary

The summary section should not repeat the contents of the Executive Summary, but rather should be more of a concluding statement that succinctly integrates the initial vision with the proposed outcome, leaving out most of what is between. It should be no longer than one paragraph and should end on a positive note, reiterating what the proposal will accomplish, for whom, and in what manner.

BUSINESS EDUCATION FOR PEDIATRIC INTENSIVISTS

Many educational options exist for pediatric intensivists who wish to learn more about business. The choices are as wide ranging as the needs of the individuals seeking information. They range from 1-day Practice Management courses sponsored by the American Academy of Pediatrics' (www.aap.org) section on Pediatric Critical Care, to Internet-based or live Master's of Business Administration programs, to a variety of courses and graduate degrees available through the American College of Physician Executives (www.acpe.org). Additional sources for information and training are listed in Chapter 4.

A Master's of Business Administration or Master's in Medical Management may be most relevant to intensivists who are interested in hospital administration. According to the American College of Physician Executives, hospital physician medical directors and chief executive officers with graduate degrees earn more than those without graduate degrees.

CONCLUSIONS AND FUTURE DIRECTIONS

Historically, financial savvy has not been a prerequisite for achievement in academic medicine. Many teaching institutions now require a more rigorous level of financial accountability from their faculty (9,28). It is not uncommon for academic practices to reward clinical productivity with increased income or the opportunity to engage in discretionary spending. In this era of fiscal responsibility, the ability to prospectively model and retrospectively analyze the impact of new codes or billing practices is a necessity for physician leaders. The ability of critical care division leaders to appropriately recruit, mentor, and retain expensive faculty is equally important. Knowing how to obtain the resources necessary to start new programs or develop new services is crucially important. Designers of fellowship programs may wish to include practice management topics in their program curricula.

KEY POINTS

- Critical care is expensive. Knowledge of how PICUs are financed can help to identify areas for improved efficiency.
- Physicians in the US must understand the rules for billing and coding.
- CPT codes are used to identify what the provider of service did for the patient. ICD-9-CM codes are used to identify why the service was needed by the patient.
- A superbill can be helpful in presenting all of the codes together on one page to make billing more streamlined.
- The recruitment of physicians and other healthcare providers is critical to the well-being of the subspecialty.
- Retention is facilitated by mentoring. Approaches to mentoring must change to be consistent with the needs of the generation-X individuals now in the workforce.
- Performance evaluation and timely feedback are part of the retention plan and can support maintenance of excellence
- Numerous ways exist to measure physician productivity. Clinically, the most widely used method is RVU tracking. Academic medical centers have developed mission-based methods to monitor overall productivity.
- The growth of pediatric critical care services requires knowledge of business planning and skills in writing a formal business plan.

- Fellowship training programs may want to include business education and practice management topics in their curricula.

References

1. American Academy of Pediatrics Resource-Based Relative Value Scale Project Advisory Committee. Issues in the application of the resource-based relative value scale system to pediatrics: A subject review. *Pediatrics* 1998;102:996–8.
2. American Academy of Pediatrics. Committee on Coding and Nomenclature. Application of the resource-based relative value scale to pediatrics. *Pediatrics* 2004;113:1437–40.
3. American Academy of Pediatrics. National child health advocates urge congress to reject harmful cuts to medicaid in administration's budget proposal. Elk Grove Village, IL: American Academy of Pediatrics, 2005:2.
4. American Medical Association. *Current Procedural Terminology: CPT 2007: Professional Edition.* Chicago: American Medical Association, 2006:696.
5. American Medical Association. *Physician ICD-9-CM 2007, Volumes 1 and 2.* Chicago: Ingenix, Inc., 2006.
6. Centers for Medicare and Medicaid Services. FY 2007 Inpatient prospective payment system final rule: Gradual implementation of improved accuracy in diagnosis-related group payments. http:www.cms.hhs.gov/apps/media/press/release.asp?Counter=122. Fact Sheet. Washington, DC: U.S. Department of Health and Human Services, 2006.
7. Centers for Medicare and Medicaid Services. Medicare program: Revision to payment policies; final rule. *Federal Register* 2006;71:69624–70251.
8. Anderson GF, Hussey PS, Frogner BK, et al. Health spending in the United States and the rest of the industrialized world. *Health Aff* (Millwood) 2005;24:903–14.
9. Andreae MC, Freed GL. A new paradigm in academic health centers: Productivity-based physician compensation. *Med Group Mgt* 2001;48:44–50.
10. Anonymous. Looking at lessons on quality from the Medicare pay-for-performance hospital demonstration. *Quality Letter for Healthcare Leaders* 2005;17:2–3;5–13.
11. Bekes CE, Dellinger RP, Brooks D, et al. Critical care medicine as a distinct product line with substantial financial profitability: The role of business planning. *Crit Care Med* 2004;32:1207–14.
12. Bickel J, Brown A. Generation X: Implications for faculty recruitment and development in academic health centers. *Acad Med* 2005;80:205–10.
13. Cohn KH, Schwartz RW. Business plan writing for physicians. *Am J Surg* 2002;184:114–20.
14. Curtis JR, Cook DJ, Wall RJ, et al. Intensive care unit quality improvement: A "how-to" guide for the interdisciplinary team. *Crit Care Med* 2006;34:211–8.
15. Demmy T, Kivlahan C, Stone T, et al. Physicians' perceptions of institutional and leadership factors influencing their job satisfaction at one academic medical center. *Acad Med* 2002;77:1235–40.
16. Fernandez R, Crane B, Reed J. Know when to hold 'em, fold 'em. A tool to project expected provider pay from contracts. MGMA Connex. 2004;4:48–52.
17. Gilmer T, Schneiderman LJ, Teetzel H, et al. The costs of nonbeneficial treatment in the intensive care setting. *Health Aff* (Millwood) 2005;24:961–71.
18. Gray S, Alexander K, Eaton J. Equal Opportunity for all? Trends in flexible training 1995–2001. *Med Teach* 2004;26:256–9.
19. Guglielmo W. How well is it working? Medicare's formula has revolutionalized the way you're paid, and not just by the feds. *We took a look at the pros and cons 10 years after its birth. Med Econ* 2002;79:69–73.
20. Kim WC, Mauborgne R. *Blue Ocean Strategy: How to Create Uncontested Market Space and Make the Competition Irrelevant.* Boston: Harvard Business School Press, 2005.
21. Lazarus IR, Novicoff WM. Six Sigma enters the healthcare mainstream: Performance-improvement technique has proven its worth and staying power. *Managed Healthcare Executive* 2004: 26–32.
22. Mallon WT. Introduction: The history and legacy of mission-based management, Academic Medicine Management Series: Mission-Based Management. American Association of Medical Colleges, 2002. www.academicmedicine.org/pt/re/acmed/mbm.htm. Accessed April 2007.
23. McKee R. Storytelling that moves people. A conversation with screenwriting coach Robert McKee. *Harv Bus Rev* 2003;81:51–5.
24. Payne SM, Schwartz RM. An evaluation of pediatric-modified diagnosis-related groups. *Health Care Financ Rev* 1993;15:51–70.
25. Ramirez de Arellano AB, Wolfe SM. Unsettling scores: A ranking of state Medicaid programs. Public Citizen Health Research Group, 2007. www.citizen.org/medicaid. Accessed April 2007.
26. Roach DW, Troboy LK, Cochran LF. The effects of humor and goal setting

on individual brainstorming performance. *J Am Acad Bus, Cambridge* 2006;10:31–6.

27. Shaw G, Brown R, Bromiley P. Strategic Stories: How 3M is rewriting business planning. *Harv Bus Rev* 1998;76:41–50.

28. Tarquinio GT, Dittus RS, Byrne DW, et al. Effects of performance-based compensation and faculty track on the clinical activity, research portfolio, and teaching mission of a large academic department of medicine. *Acad Med* 2003;78:690–701.

29. Tugwell P. Campaign to revitalise academic medicine kicks off. *Br Med J* 2004;328:597.

CHAPTER 7 ■ RESEARCH DESIGN AND STATISTICAL ANALYSIS

WYNNE E. MORRISON • ELIZABETH A. HUNT • ANNE-MARIE GUERGUERIAN

Research in pediatric critical care is challenging, partly because of the wide variety of diseases treated in the typical multidisciplinary pediatric unit and the resultant rarity of any one process in a single practitioner's or center's experience. Critically ill children also have a lower mortality rate than do adults admitted to intensive care, which can make extrapolating results from adult studies problematic and frequently requires the assessment of outcomes other than mortality in pediatric studies to avoid impossibly large sample-size requirements. In addition, research in the PICU by definition involves vulnerable subjects, which leads to special ethical and regulatory requirements.

Yet, patient-based research remains vitally important, both to critically examine the dogma of usual practice and to determine which therapies are appropriate to adapt from adults to children. Sixty years ago, the highest possible concentration of oxygen was presumed to be best for neonates (47), the toxic effects of which are now well recognized. Similarly, much of our vigorously defended current standard of care will someday fall by the wayside as we continue to study and learn from past errors. If data from adults could be universally applied to children, extracorporeal life support would have been abandoned as a therapy (3), and we would have no concerns about the use of drotrecogin alfa in pediatrics (12).

This chapter focuses predominantly on clinical research rather than basic science or translational research, although many of the statistical methods can apply to all types of research. Funding issues are not addressed and have been recently summarized elsewhere (36). We also do not address the ethics and regulation of research, monitoring of trials, or database management and, instead, focus on basic methods in clinical trial design and statistical analysis. This brief overview is in no way a substitute for collaboration with experts in statistics and trial design, and many common mistakes and much wasted effort can be avoided by the involvement of those with appropriate expertise in the earliest planning phases of a study.

STUDY DESIGN

Defining the Research Question

The first step of a study is to define the research question. A well-constructed question will delineate the important components of a study. There is a difference between asking "Does insulin use in the PICU reduce mortality?" and asking "Does targeted glucose control with an insulin infusion versus placebo reduce 30-day mortality in PICU patients younger than 18 years who are mechanically ventilated or receiving vasoactive infusions?" In the latter question, it is clear that the *study subjects* are children who are ventilated or on vasoactive infusions. The *study site* is the PICU. The *intervention* is glucose control with an insulin infusion. The *alternative* is placebo. Both groups will receive *standard therapy*. The *outcome* of interest is 30-day mortality. A precise question also helps determine to which groups of patients your results are applicable.

The question should contain the *primary outcome measure* or *dependent variable*—the variable that is dependent on intervention, explicitly stated. It should also contain the primary *independent variable* being studied. This will be something to which the subjects are exposed, either intentionally, as during a *randomized, controlled trial* (RCT), or as part of their everyday life, as during a *cohort study*. The independent variable is also referred to as the *exposure variable* and may be a potential risk factor or an intervention.

The Research Team

Meinert emphasizes the importance of explicitly assigning tasks to specific members of the research team at the beginning of a study (29). Consider inviting an epidemiologist or someone trained in study design to be on the team. Whereas the clinician-scientist will have clinical expertise about the subject, the epidemiologist can address study design, power calculations, and issues related to limiting bias (Table 7.1) (27).

Someone with biostatistics training should be consulted early to ensure that data collection and the database format facilitate analysis and enable the answering of the research question. The data set collected should be as parsimonious as possible, focusing closely on variables required to answer the study question and avoiding variables that do not help in answering the question. Excessive data collection will take time, be distracting, may diminish the overall quality of data collection, and may tempt you to overstep your conclusions if the extra data are not related to the original hypothesis.

Finally, research assistants serve an integral role on a study team, but they must be properly trained. It is a shame to discover that, after 100 or 200 chart reviews, they have been using the wrong definition for your primary outcome measure!

Choosing a Study Design

Once the question is clear, the best possible design to answer it can be determined. The investigator should ask, "If I had unlimited resources, how would I design my study to have the best chance of answering the question?" and then balance this ideal with a study design that can be feasibly conducted using

TABLE 7.1

DEFINITIONS

> *Bias* – Deviation of results or inferences from the truth, or processes leading to such deviation. Any trend in the collection, analysis, interpretation, publication, or review of data that can lead to conclusions that are systematically different from the truth (27).
>
> *Confounder* – A situation in which a measure of the effect of an exposure on risk is distorted because of the association of exposure with other factor(s) that influence the outcome of the study (27).
>
> *Interaction* – Differences in the effects of one or more factors according to the level of the remaining factor(s), also called *effect modification* (27).
>
> *Equipoise* – A state of genuine uncertainty about the benefits or harms that may result from each of two or more regimens. A state of equipoise is an indication for a randomized controlled trial, because there are no ethical concerns about one regimen being better for a particular patient (27).
>
> *Stratified randomization* – A randomization procedure in which strata are identified and subjects randomly allocated within each (27).
>
> *Blinded study* – A study in which observer(s) and/or subjects are kept ignorant of the group to which the subjects are assigned, as in the experiment, or of the population from which the subjects come, as in the nonexperimental study. The intent of keeping subjects and/or investigators blinded (i.e., unaware of knowledge that might introduce bias) is to eliminate the effect of such biases (27).
>
> *Quasi-experiment* – A situation in which the investigator lacks full control over the allocation and/or timing of intervention but nonetheless conducts the study as if it were an experiment, allocating subjects to groups (27).
>
> *Misclassification* – The erroneous classification of an individual, a value, or an attribute into a category other than that to which it should be assigned. The probability of misclassification may be the same in all study groups (nondifferential misclassification) or may vary between groups (differential misclassification) (27).
>
> *Publication bias* – A delay in publication or nonpublication of studies with small treatment effects or negative results (9,12,38).

available resources. Possible resource limitations that may ultimately affect the study design include money, time, and available subjects with the exposure or outcome of interest. Each study design has specific limitations and potential biases that can be anticipated and perhaps minimized.

Observational versus Experimental Studies

Studies are either observational or experimental. *Observational studies* observe nature as-is, with no manipulation or interventions. Investigators note whether subjects were exposed to the independent variable of interest and whether they developed the outcome of interest; however, the investigator does not control if the subject is exposed to the independent variable or putative risk factor (42). In any study, other factors associated with the dependent variable should be identified, especially those that may serve as *confounders* or *interact* with the exposure of interest (see **Table 7.1**) (27). A limitation of observational studies is the uncertainty of whether the association between the independent and dependent variables was because of the relationship of interest or because of unmeasured exposures (15). Examples of observational study designs include case-control studies, pre-postinterventional studies, and cohort studies.

In an *experimental study*, the investigator controls which study group the patient will join. Ideally, enrollment into a particular study arm is by random assignment. If any other factor, such as age, gender, socioeconomic status, or severity of disease, influences the chances that a subject will be assigned to a particular study arm, the study arms will not be equivalent in all respects. One will be less sure that associations between the independent and dependent variables are *because* of the independent variable as opposed to the factor that influenced group assignment. For example, in a pre-postintervention trial, the period in which a subject was enrolled dictates his study group and intervention, which makes it an observational study.

Differences between groups could be due to the independent variable of interest or due to other factors that varied between the periods.

Rothman and Greenland state that the "ideal experiment would create a set of circumstances across which only one factor affecting the outcome of interest would vary," that is, the independent variable of interest (42). The impossible ideal would be to enroll a group of subjects, observe their baseline characteristics, and then observe how many of the subjects develop the outcome of interest when exposed to a placebo. The next key step would be to go back in time and enroll the *same* group of subjects into the other study arm so that differences in baseline characteristics could not be a factor, and then have every single aspect of their treatment be identical, except they would be treated with the study intervention rather than placebo.

This impossible scenario would allow us to isolate the effect of the independent variable of interest, with no concern about whether the results we see are due to differences in the study groups or differences in the way we treat them. The idea of having an imaginary study group that is identical in every way to a placebo group except for the independent variable of interest is counter to fact, and thus we refer to this argument as the *counterfactual* (35,42). In that the counterfactual state cannot be achieved, clinical investigators should always be aware of this limitation and attempt to conduct the best study that most reliably estimates the isolated effect of the independent variable of interest.

Randomized, Controlled Trial

A prospective RCT is considered the highest quality experimental clinical study type and the closest design to the counterfactual ideal. Randomization attempts to make study groups as similar as possible. If, for example, one study group is older than the other, and older subjects are more likely to develop the outcome of interest, then the true relationship between the independent and dependent variables may be obscured. In this case, age either may act as a confounder or may interact with the exposure variable. In either case, randomization provides the highest likelihood of ensuring an equal balance of known and unknown confounders between the study groups.

Multiple quality issues must be considered to achieve a well-designed and conducted RCT, the first issue being the randomization process. Mechanisms such as the use of random digit tables, opaque envelopes, and central data centers, exist to ensure that assignment *remains* completely random and to prevent manipulation of the process. Imagine that a clinician believes that an intervention is effective and would prefer that particularly sick patients get the intervention rather than placebo (which suggests an ethical problem with *equipoise* going into the study) (see **Table 7.1**). If the physician is able to hold the envelopes up to light and sort through them to identify one in the desired group, the process is no longer random. A truly concealed randomization process provides the best possible chance of balancing known and unknown confounders between the study groups.

Another issue to consider during the design phase is whether randomization should be stratified or blocked. Consider the implications if older children are known to have a higher likelihood of a bad outcome than are infants for a particular disease and, by chance, most of the older children in a study are randomized to the placebo arm and most of the infants are randomized to the intervention arm. If the results show that those in the placebo arm do worse than those in the intervention arm, it will be difficult to discern whether this difference is because of the intervention or because of the age difference of the study groups. This situation can be avoided by performing *stratified randomization* at the beginning of the study to ensure that the age distribution between the study groups will be as similar as possible (see **Table 7.1**) (27).

Block randomization is a means by which to ensure that an equal number of patients will be in each study arm at the end of prespecified enrollment periods or blocks. This process is especially valuable when conducting a relatively small study. For example, if a sample size calculation reveals the need to enroll 20 patients in a study but, due to chance, 18 of the patients were randomized to intervention and 2 to placebo, the question at hand would not be answered. If patients had been randomized into blocks of 4, investigators would know that for every 4 patients enrolled, 2 would be in the intervention arm and 2 would be in the placebo arm, and that, ultimately, 10 patients would be in the intervention arm and 10 in the study arm. A downside to block randomization is that, if the process is transparent, a clinician may be able to predict to which arm the next subject would be enrolled and thus have the potential to manipulate the randomization process. This shortcoming can be overcome by varying the size of the blocks in a random order so that it is no longer predictable at which point the blocks become even.

Another important feature of a controlled trial is *blinding*, or *masking* (see **Table 7.1**) (27,29). The purpose of blinding is to attempt to eliminate or reduce the chances that a subject will be treated differently or diagnosed differently merely because of the study group to which he has been assigned. Language referring to blinding—single, double, and the like—is not used consistently. However, groups that may be blinded to maintain

validity of the study include (a) study subjects, (b) clinicians who are treating the study subjects, (c) investigators who are assessing whether or not the subject developed the outcome of interest, and (d) statisticians who are performing analysis of the results. The consensus is that, to maintain the highest likelihood that study results will remain valid, it is best to blind the first three groups; however, debate continues regarding whether the statistician should be blinded, and most agree that members of the Data and Safety Monitoring Board should not be (39).

High-quality studies include a proper power calculation during the design phase and proper maintenance of group assignment, including attention to attrition, crossovers, adherence, and contamination (15). If the study groups become incomparable for any reason, it is no longer certain that an association seen between the intervention and the outcome of interest is because of the intervention, although statistical methods, such as multivariate regression analysis, can sometimes be used to account for known confounders. A well-conducted, prospective, blinded RCT is the closest to the counterfactual experiment possible and thus provides the highest chance of obtaining valid and reliable results.

Although an RCT may be ideal, occasionally, this study design is not feasible and/or ethical. RCTs are expensive in terms of cost, number of patients, and time required to obtain a valid answer. Also, ethically, subjects cannot be randomized to study interventions or placebos that are believed to be harmful. For cases in which an RCT is not appropriate, the highest quality nonrandomized, controlled trial or observational study method possible should be chosen.

Nonrandomized, Controlled Trials

Not all experimental clinical studies are RCTs. As long as the investigator is able to assign the study group to which an individual will be enrolled, the study is still considered experimental. However, some refer to studies in which factors other than randomization influence the study arm to which a subject is assigned as *quasi-experimental* (27,42). The lack of true randomization introduces possible bias.

Observational Studies

We will briefly review several types of observational studies. Being familiar with the strengths and limitations of each one allows the researcher to make the best choice of study design possible.

Case Report

A *case report* is an account of an interesting observation in a single patient and can be a valuable addition to the literature. Examples of useful case reports would be those that inform the medical community about a new pathogen or genetic variant or that demonstrate a new procedure or use of a medication. The problem with case reports is that they may lead the reader to conclude causality when none exists. For example, if an author reports that he performed a new procedure and the patient recovered, we will never know if the patient would also have recovered *without* the procedure. The counterfactual cannot occur, so it is prudent to be wary of drawing conclusions, particularly regarding causal relationships, from a single case report.

Case Series

A *case series* is a report of a number of patients with a similar presentation, diagnostic test, therapeutic maneuver, or outcome. Valid conclusions are more likely to be drawn from a case series if the reported cases represent consecutive cases or a random sampling of all cases. If all cases of a particular disease are identified, valuable statistics can be calculated, such as the *case fatality rate,* which is the proportion of patients with a disease who die from that disease (27). Also, details regarding the demographics of cases can be reported. Although valuable lessons can be learned from the experience of others, definitive conclusions regarding the observations are impossible, because no control group is provided for comparison.

A recent example is a prospective case series of 89 consecutive patients treated with a helium-oxygen mixture (heliox) in the ICUs of an academic center (5). The authors report that children ≤18 years of age accounted for 72.8% of use, and the indication was upper airway disease 47% of the time and lower airway disease 53% of the time. Investigators can report interesting information using the denominator of 89 consecutive patients. However, without controls, they cannot comment about the effect of the heliox, good or bad. They also cannot calculate whether a higher proportion of patients treated with heliox avoided intubation than those treated with conventional oxygen therapy. The information gleaned from case series can be informative and can help to provide preliminary statistics useful for designing future studies, such as planning enrollment rates or power calculations, but these reports provide little evidence that a particular treatment is more effective than another or placebo.

Case-Control Study

Some observational studies utilize a control population and move closer to the counterfactual ideal by including a comparison group. In a *case-control study,* an investigator compares patients who have the outcome of interest (cases) to those who do not (controls) and measures any significant difference in the proportion of each who were exposed to the independent variable of interest. The beauty of the case-control study is that it is a very efficient study design in that it can be completed in a relatively short period and few study personnel are needed; thus, it is relatively inexpensive to perform.

The key component of case-control studies is that cases are identified before controls. The number of cases can be the most important limiting resource. Increasing the number of cases is the most effective method of increasing the power of the study; thus, financial and personnel resources should be concentrated on identifying as many additional cases as possible. It is also possible to increase the power of a study by choosing more than one control per case. Depending on the limitations set on the type of control for the study, it would theoretically be possible to choose an unlimited number of controls per case. However, expenses in terms of both time and money are associated with each enrollment; thus, a point of diminishing return is reached. It is generally accepted that enrolling more than four controls per case does not significantly improve power (15,49). Using a larger number of controls makes sense only when minimal excess resources are expended (e. g., secondary analysis of data from a database).

Case-control studies are ideal in two scenarios. The first situation occurs when the study must be completed in a short time, such as during a suspected infectious disease outbreak. The other situation is for the study of rare diseases. If an investigator tries to conduct an RCT or cohort study for a rare disease or outcome of interest, a great deal of time and money would have to be expended, perhaps enrolling thousands of patients, in an effort to enlist a sufficient number of cases for analysis. However, if a registry of cases of the rare disease exists, a case-control study could capitalize on such a resource.

Potential problems are associated with case-control studies. It is possible that controls are actually latent cases not yet identified or that those identified as exposed were not actually exposed. Either type of error would be referred to as *misclassification* (**Table 7.1**) (27). Such an *information bias* can affect the validity the conclusions. Another limitation of case-control studies is that they cannot demonstrate *temporality.* Data on both cases and controls are gathered at the same time (*cross-sectional*), so that it is generally difficult to prove that the subject was first exposed to the putative risk factor and subsequently developed the outcome of interest. Conclusions about causality will be much stronger if investigators develop methods to assess the timing of exposure in relation to when the disease or outcome of interest developed.

Another potential misclassification problem is *recall bias.* Once cases and controls are identified, the investigator attempts to ascertain whether the subjects were "exposed." A risk does exist that patients who have developed a disease have been pondering how they did so and thus are more likely to recall that they have been exposed. Such differences in recall would tend to overestimate the effect of the exposure on the likelihood of developing the outcome. Finally, in that cases and controls are chosen rather than being randomly sampled from the source population, the possibility of *selection bias* does exist.

Because randomization is not an option, confounders must be dealt with during either the design or analysis phases of the study. During the design phase, *matching* can be used to try to force patients to have similar baseline characteristics. Care must be taken to avoid matching on the exposures being studied, because such matching will preclude analysis. If matching on any variable, an appropriate matched analysis must be performed (42), and consulting a statistician is strongly advised. An alternative to matching is to perform stratified analysis at the end of the study or use regression to adjust for confounders.

Pre-Postintervention Study

A pre-postintervention study uses historical controls and is often utilized for health services research. Data are collected on a patient population prior to a change in practice, and these are compared to data collected after the change in practice. Ideally, the study is designed before the intervention or change in practice is in place. Data should be collected on potential confounding variables, including severity of illness indices and therapies that might affect outcomes. It is important to keep other components of care as similar as possible. Unfortunately, any changes in practice over time, including improved care due to experience of the healthcare team, will make the groups less comparable. A common problem occurs when data collection for the post-intervention period are prospective, while those for the pre-intervention period are retrospective. Retrospective data collection is often less detailed and less reliable.

Cohort Study

To study potentially harmful exposures for which randomization would be unethical, a *cohort* study may be the best option. For a cohort study, patients are enrolled and information is collected on exposures. Some of the exposures will be the subject of the study, and others will be potential confounders. The participants are then followed over time and observed to see who will develop the outcome. The relationship between the independent and dependent variables can be studied in patients who begin the study free of the outcome of interest by comparing those who are not exposed and others who are either (a) naturally exposed or (b) choose to be exposed. Because the subjects begin disease free, the disease incidence rate for the exposed group can ultimately be compared to that for the unexposed group; this is the *relative risk*.

A well-conducted prospective cohort study is generally considered the strongest type of observational study. In terms of being able to make causal inferences, its main strength is demonstration of *temporality*. If the subjects are disease free upon enrollment, it can at least be demonstrated that the exposure came before the outcome, which is a necessary but not sufficient component for proving causality.

Unfortunately, prospective cohort studies are very resource intensive, including time, money, and subjects. Efficiency can be increased by performing a *retrospective cohort*, which entails going back in time, collecting data on a defined population, and determining whether each subject subsequently developed the outcome of interest. Although data will be collected on as many known confounders as possible, it will not be possible to collect data on *unknown* confounders.

Systematic Reviews and Meta-Analysis

Synthesizing data in the form of a review that incorporates new knowledge within a larger body of available evidence has been part of healthcare research and education for over a century. Specific terms and definitions have emerged to characterize the different approaches and methods used to prepare a systematic review.

Traditional reviews or overviews are *narrative reviews*, which usually contain noncomprehensive synthesis of data, nonsystematic searching and evaluation of the literature, and expert opinion, without specific attention to the research design of the published studies. These sometimes include simple methods to summarize findings across studies. *Systematic reviews* use a pre-established methodology to comprehensively describe and summarize a body of research. They are prepared using a systematic approach, incorporated into a protocol and detailed in a methods section. Like most experimental designs, systematic reviews specifically intend to minimize bias and random errors (11,20).

A systematic review may or may not contain a *meta-analysis*. A meta-analysis is a statistical analysis designed to synthesize the data from two or more *independent* studies toward answering a specific research question. A systematic review should respond to uncertainty surrounding a question; for example, when many studies have shown small effects, when larger trials may be impossible to perform, when studies have apparently conflicting results, when a clinical practice is not supported by empirical evidence, or when the importance of the evidence is not appreciated. Systematic reviews may justify pursuing (or not) a clinical trial and help to avoid pitfalls in designing a new trial.

The quality of studies examined in a systematic review determines the quality of the review. Biases in the original studies will not disappear, and the validity of results will not improve in a systematic review. Heterogeneity between studies limits the ability to produce valid summaries when combining studies. Systematic reviews attempt to minimize *selection bias* by adopting a systematic, unbiased method to include or exclude studies. However, as published data are usually relied upon, *publication bias* (see **Table 7.1**) is unavoidable.

A systematic review should be approached like any well-designed experiment. The QUOROM (30,46) and MOOSE (48) Groups have produced recommendations for the reporting of systematic reviews and meta-analyses; others offer specific approaches, methods, and templates, such as the Cochrane Collaboration Systematic Reviews (30). These guidelines are intended to strengthen and homogenize the quality and reporting of systematic reviews.

The first step in designing a systematic review is to clearly formulate a question or hypothesis that is answerable, clinically relevant, and both focused and generalizable. A team of experts on both the subject and methodology is necessary. The research design and methods should be comprehensive, transparent, reproducible, and detailed a priori in a protocol. The setting is the literature; the study population or sample is each independent study. Selection criteria with search terms, inclusion and exclusion criteria, and methods for critical appraisal should be detailed, with explicit methods for data extraction. Inclusion criteria might specify each individual study's subjects, design (e.g., only RCTs), setting, intervention, controls, date of publication, language, or type of journal in which published.

An outcome and follow-up period must be defined across studies. In-depth analyses should include both an assessment of the quality of the studies and a quantitative assessment of the data. Omitting the qualitative assessment may lead to a cookbook approach that fails to identify important sources of bias or heterogeneity between studies; determining the minimal acceptable methodologic quality a priori maintains the quality of the review.

The methods used to locate studies should be well described, including search terms used, databases searched (e.g., Medline, Embase, Psychinfo, Cochrane), whether references were hand searched, and if a reference was the result of a personal communication with experts. Final eligibility of studies should be determined by more than one team member, with processes for maintaining a log of included and excluded studies and resolving disagreements. A checklist should be developed to determine which studies meet inclusion criteria; quality scales for inclusion have been developed by several authors (9,19,20,23,31,45).

Data presentation and a meta-analysis require choosing a common summary statistic and units of measurement, because the individual studies may not have reported the treatment effect in the same format. Summary plots can illustrate trends, differences, and commonalities between studies. Forrest plots (**Fig. 7.1**) and L'Abbé plots (**Fig. 7.2**) help investigators to compare the treatment effect and relative weight of each study in the overall analysis. Other methods (e.g., *sensitivity analyses*) can be used to detect an overwhelming effect of one study on the combined analysis. The assistance of an experienced

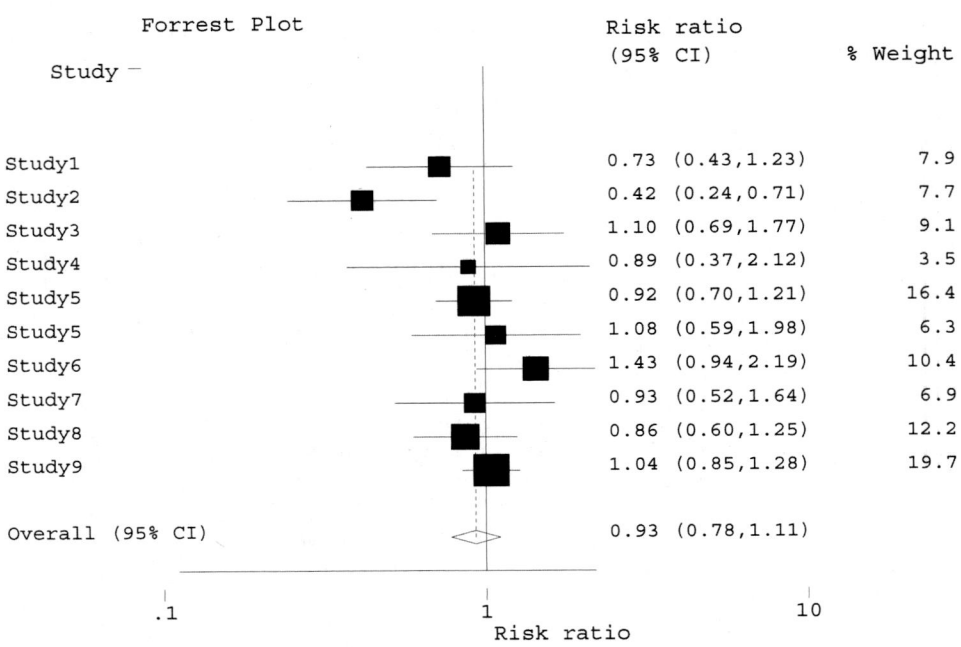

FIGURE 7.1. A Forrest plot visually compares studies in a meta-analysis. Studies with greater patient numbers have larger boxes, and the precision of the confidence intervals is represented by the length of the horizontal bars. Positive and negative effects are indicated by whether the central point of the line falls to the left or right of the vertical bar. The confidence intervals for the risk ratio for almost all the studies shown here include 1, as does the overall estimate, leading to an acceptance of the null hypothesis of no treatment effect.

methodologist is essential in choosing a valid summary statistic and computing a combined treatment effect. The choice of the summary statistic will influence the test of homogeneity used to analyze whether the treatment effect is similar in all studies.

Meta-analysis can legitimately proceed (11) if the individual studies are not qualitatively or quantitatively heterogeneous. Software is available—some at no cost, such as Review Manager (RevMan) from Cochrane, and some commercially—for performing meta-analyses.

Qualitative Research

The term *qualitative research* is generally used to describe a group of techniques that have been adapted from the social

sciences and applied to healthcare. The research is often exploratory and observational and typically deals more with the cultural aspects of medicine and the personal experience of healthcare providers, patients, and families. Qualitative studies are not necessarily subject to randomization or the experimental method of altering one variable while keeping all others stable, because the complexity of the real world does not usually allow such control (40); such studies are often described as *inductive* rather than *deductive*. Yet, this very fact allows examination of those issues and questions that do not lend themselves to interventional trial design; quantitative and qualitative methods should, therefore, be complementary and each implemented where appropriate to the research question.

A variety of techniques can fall under the label "qualitative." Examples include in-depth interviews, focus groups, textual analysis, or observation of behaviors. Recent qualitative

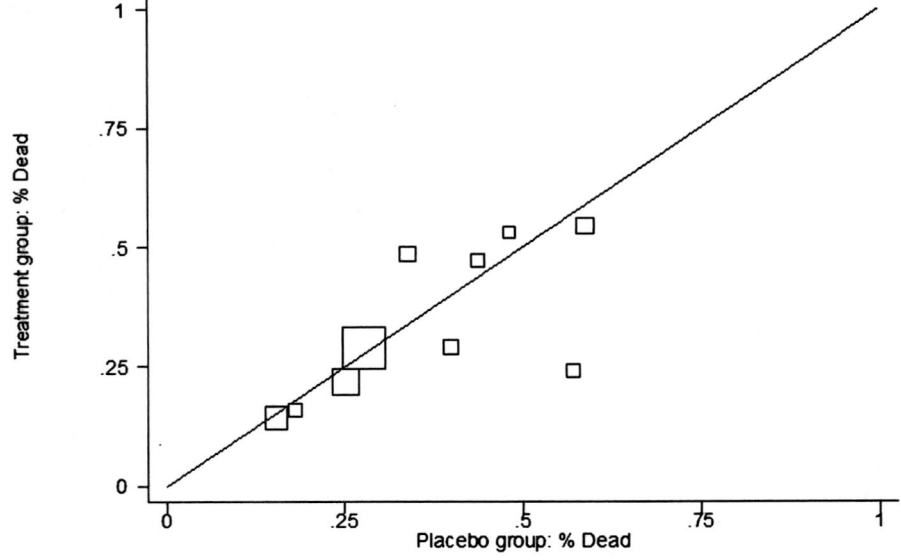

FIGURE 7.2. A L'Abbé plot of the same studies shown in **Figure 7.1** shows each study as a box. Larger boxes indicate studies with larger sample sizes. The diagonal line is the "line of no effect," with an equal proportion of deaths in the treatment and placebo groups. Boxes falling predominantly to one side of the line would indicate either a treatment effect or publication bias.

studies in pediatric critical care demonstrate how such methods can be used to explore complex topics. Meert, et al. (28) interviewed parents regarding their spiritual needs following a child's death. They describe themes that recur in the interviews, such as a need to maintain a connection with the child during the illness and after death. Although the information obtained is not easily amenable to statistical comparisons, it is still useful to practitioners who are trying to understand the family's experience. Another study used focus groups to explore parent and healthcare worker opinions regarding an exception from informed consent for an RCT of therapeutic hypothermia following pediatric cardiac arrest (32), illustrating that a thorough exploration of a research question may require a combination of qualitative and quantitative methods.

A well-done qualitative analysis is just as rigorous as any study (16). A well-formulated research question, clear methods, and an assessment of validity and reliability are essential. Not all results will be generalizable, but the population should be described well enough that it is apparent when they are not. Standard methods include using multiple investigators to code themes so that their results can be compared and "member checking" by taking results back to interviewees or group attendees to confirm if the formal description adequately reflects their experience. Sample size is often not determined a priori; rather, data collection continues until no new themes are identified (*thematic saturation*) (43).

STATISTICAL ANALYSIS

Introduction

Statistics is a science of probability, not certainty. For any clinician who is either performing research or hoping to apply the results of research in the care of patients, it is important to understand what conclusions can be drawn from statistical tests, what the limitations are, and what common mistakes investigators make in the analysis and presentation of data. Although computerized software packages can perform the calculations required for most statistical analyses, computers are unable to judge the accuracy, validity, or importance of the data they are given. Computers will faithfully provide an answer, even when asked the wrong question. Both a clinician's insight into the problem and a statistician's input into choosing an appropriate test are invaluable. The following is a brief primer on statistical methods, from a clinician's perspective, with a focus more on vocabulary, context, and concepts than on equations.

Definitions

The first step on the road to learning statistics is a familiarity with the language. Methods generally involve collecting and analyzing information on a *sample* of a population and making inferences about the population as a whole. *Population* does not necessarily imply individuals; examples of populations could be "all children younger than 2 years with traumatic brain injury," "all academic medical centers in the United States," etc. Whether a sample is chosen appropriately will have a tremendous effect on whether the results can be meaningfully interpreted (33). For example, a proven intervention for in

patients at an academic center (those at the severe end of the disease spectrum) may not be applicable to outpatients with the same disease. The difference between population and sample statistics leads to the confusing habit of having two symbols for most summary statistics; for example, s^2 and σ^2 for the sample and population variance, respectively.

Types of Data

Different tests are appropriate for different types of data (39). *Nominal* or *categorical* variables fall into categories without a specific order (e.g., race, car color, blood type). A *dichotomous* or *binary* variable has only two categories (e.g., gender, mortality). Summary statistics for categorical variables are usually expressed as proportions; "30% female" makes more sense than an "average" gender. An *ordinal* variable is a categorical variable that is ranked (e.g., grade in school, Glasgow outcome scale). These are all *discrete* variables, meaning that gaps exist between possible values (e.g., the Glasgow outcome scale does not include a score of 2.6). For a *continuous* variable, any value can be taken along a scale with infinite possible values (e.g., weight). Some technically discrete variables can be statistically treated as if they are continuous if a sufficient number of possible ranked values exist (e.g., Pediatric Risk of Mortality score).

Descriptive Statistics

The *distribution* of a variable refers to a frequency plot in which the data fall. Several summary statistics can be applied to a distribution. It is good practice to develop the habit of looking at data graphically rather than relying solely on summary statistics to describe the data; surprising patterns can emerge. Statistics that somehow describe the "middle" of the data are called *measures of central tendency*. The *mode* is the most common value of the variable. A bimodal distribution has two "most common" values. The *median* is the middle value when the values are ranked. The *mean* (average) is the sum of the values divided by the number of measurements.

The dispersion or variability of data should also be described. A *range* is simply the difference between the largest and smallest values. A *percentile* refers to the value in the data that is larger than a given percent of observations when they are ranked. Thus, the 90th percentile would be the observation larger than 90% of observations. The 50th percentile is the same as the median. *Quartile* refers to dividing the data into quarters—with the lowest quartile, therefore, being all observations below the 25th percentile. The interquartile range (IQR) is the difference between the 25th and 75th percentiles and contains the middle 50% of data.

The *variance* (s^2) is more informative about variability in the sample.

$$s^2 = \frac{\sum_{i=1}^{n}(x_i - \overline{x})^2}{n - 1}$$

The steps to solve this equation are:

1. Calculate the mean.

2. For each individual observation, square the difference between that observation and the mean (to get rid of negative numbers).
3. Add all of the squared results together.
4. Divide by the *degrees of freedom*, which for this equation is 1 less than the total number of observations (once the mean is known, only $n - 1$ observations are truly independent).

The *standard deviation* is the square root of the variance, which is a more intuitively meaningful number, because the units are the same as the original observations (e.g., years rather than years²).

The *standard error of the mean* (SEM) is sometimes confused with the standard deviation (SD). If a sample of "n" randomly selected observations is repeatedly taken from a population, the SEM is the variability of the *means* of those repeated samples. It is obtained by dividing the SD by the square root of the sample size (n). The SD should be used when describing the variability of a sample; the SEM, instead, is a description of the precision of an estimate of the population mean. The SEM is always smaller than the SD, and authors sometimes make their data appear less variable than it truly is by inappropriately presenting the SEM rather than the SD when simply describing the sample.

Normal Distribution

Continuous data often tend to take the shape of a *normal distribution*, which is a typical bell-shaped curve (**Fig. 7.3**), in which the mean, mode, and median are the same and the frequency of each value decreases the farther away it is from that mean. The distribution is symmetric above and below the mean and is predictable (95% of observations are within 1.96 standard deviations of the mean). Many physiologic variables behave in a somewhat normal fashion; for example, an "average" blood pressure is far more common than an extremely high or low one. Some statistical tests (e.g., Student's *t* test; analysis of variance, ANOVA) assume that a continuous outcome variable follows a fairly normal distribution. A distribution is *skewed* when the values are not symmetric around the mean (**Fig. 7.4**). A median and IQR are better descriptors of highly skewed data than are the mean and the SD. Extreme outliers will pull the mean in their direction but have little effect on the median, as the outlier only counts as a "high" or "low" value in choosing a median rather than contributing numerically to the calculation (1). For example, if a billionaire moved into my neighborhood, the mean income would increase dramatically; in contrast, the median would change minimally, if at all.

Skewed Data and Transformation

What if the data are not normally distributed? A possible solution is to *transform* the data so that it appears normal. Probably the most commonly used transformation is a logarithmic transformation, as it tends to take data that are highly positively skewed and pull the extreme values closer to the center (**Fig. 7.5**) (21). Each value is replaced with the log of the value, and the statistical test is run on the transformed data. Many other transformations can be used, from square or cube roots, to reciprocals, to some combination of the above. For some statistical tests, the goal of transformation is to achieve equality of variances rather than a specific distribution of the outcome. In some ways, transforming data seems like cheating, but it is usually a valid solution that has the advantage of mathematically preserving the relationships of the original data. One caveat is that it is important to present results in the original units, which will make more intuitive sense than "log-days," for instance. Nonparametric tests (tests designed for non-normally distributed data; discussed later) are another option; these tests, however, lose some of the information contained in the original data.

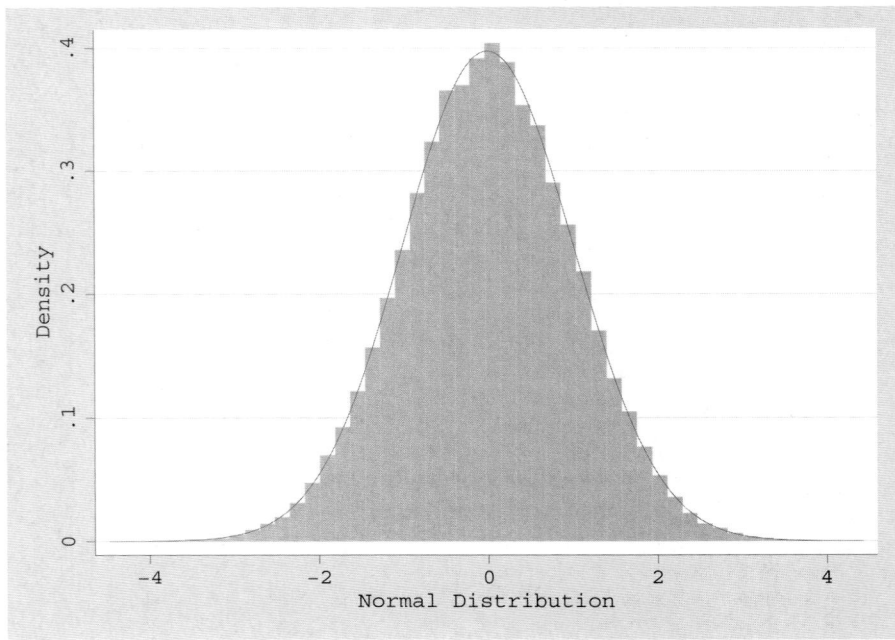

FIGURE 7.3. Standard normal distribution. The mean is both the most common value and the median. The distribution is symmetric on either side of the mean, with more extreme values becoming progressively less frequent.

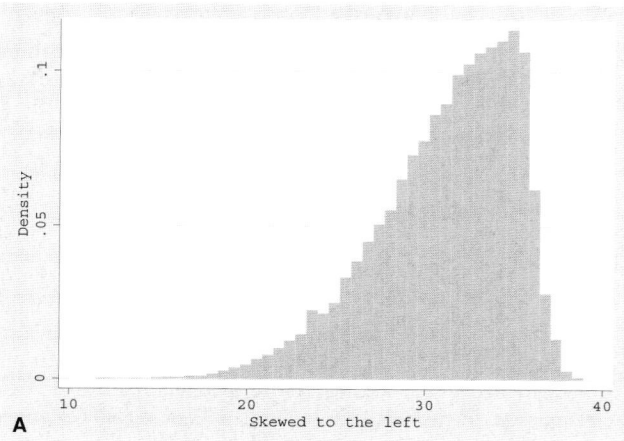 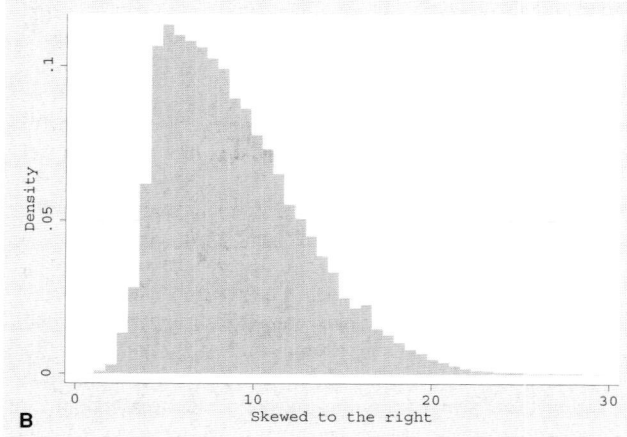

FIGURE 7.4. Skewness. A distribution that is skewed to the left has outliers that are much smaller than the median, which will pull the mean lower than the median. A distribution that is skewed to the right has outliers that are much higher than the median, pulling the mean up.

Confidence Intervals and Hypothesis Testing

Hypothesis Testing

Hypothesis testing refers to using statistics to either accept or reject a hypothesis; it is never possible to *prove* a hypothesis, only accept or reject it to some degree of certainty. The *null hypothesis* is the assumption that no difference exists between the result and the true population parameter (or, when comparing two samples, that no difference exists between them). The *alternative hypothesis* is that a difference really exists. *Equivalency* trials are becoming more common, however, in which the null hypothesis is actually that a difference *does* exist between groups.

It is possible to be wrong when you accept or reject a hypothesis. Two types of errors exist:

■ Type I error [alpha error (α), false positive]: The null hypothesis is incorrectly rejected (e.g., it is concluded that two therapies are different when really they are the same).

■ Type II error [beta error (β), false negative]: The null hypothesis is incorrectly accepted (e.g., no difference is found between two therapies when in reality a difference does exist).

Investigators decide what level of α and β error they are willing to accept. The α level is typically set at 0.05 (meaning a 5%, or 1-in-20 chance of a Type I error) and the β level is often set at 0.1 to 0.2. In general, the less willing one is to mistakenly accept the null hypothesis, the more one must be willing to mistakenly reject it. The only way to decrease the chances of both an α and β error is to increase the sample size (see discussion on power analysis and sample size calculation later in the chapter).

The "0.05" α cutoff is familiar to clinicians as the most commonly accepted level of *statistical significance*. The *p value* was originally developed by Fisher during the 1920s as a scale for assessing strength of evidence, and it was not intended to provide a definitive "accept" or "reject"; it is defined as the *probability*, under the assumption of no true difference (i.e., the null hypothesis is correct), of obtaining—due to chance alone—a

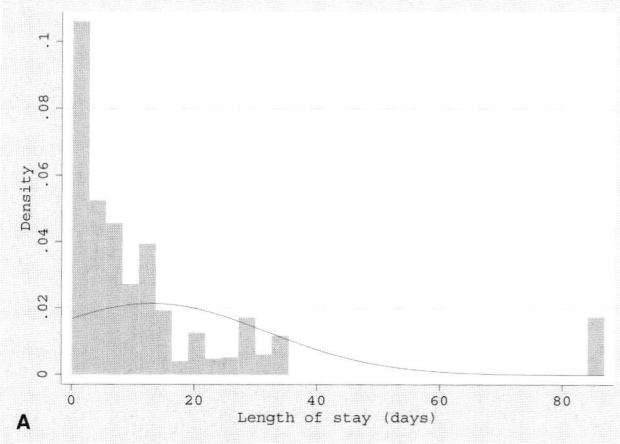 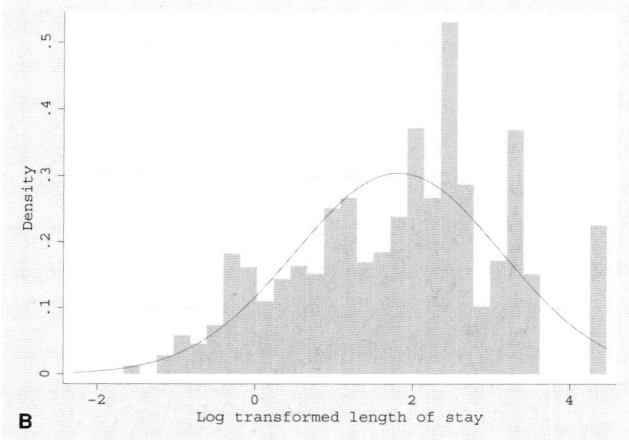

FIGURE 7.5. Data transformation. (**A**) Length of stay (usually highly skewed to the right) of children admitted to a PICU over 1 year. (**B**) A natural log transformation often helps right-skewed data to better approximate a normal distribution.

result equal to or more extreme than the one seen. As often used today, the null hypothesis (no difference demonstrated) is accepted if $p \geq 0.05$ and the null hypothesis (difference demonstrated) is rejected if $p < 0.05$. Many different statistical tests can generate a p value. The cutoff is arbitrary; some conclusions may be drawn from $p = 0.07$ (most commonly "a larger study is indicated"!), and $p = 0.001$ is more convincing than $p = 0.04$. Presenting exact p values, which computers make possible, is more useful than stating only a range.

A p value reflects only the strength of the data used to compute it; it does not take into account any prior evidence (other studies, lab data, physiologic reasoning) that might affect interpretation of the data. *Bayesian* theory refers to using the results of any study to adjust the *pre-test probability* of a certain belief, rather than drawing potentially incorrect conclusions by making each study stand completely on its own (13). A discussion of the methods is beyond the scope of this chapter; however, an interesting example has been published that illustrates the use of adult data and a Bayesian analysis to design a trial of IV immune globulin versus plasmapheresis in children with Guillain-Barré syndrome (14).

It is also important not to confuse statistical significance with *clinical importance*. Especially in trials employing large numbers, it is possible to find a statistically significant result in which the magnitude of the difference shown is so small that it is really not relevant in the real world. The same thing can happen when the outcome chosen is not important in the long run. This type of mistake does not fall into the realm of Type I or Type II error, because the mathematical/statistical conclusions are perfectly valid, but it is a mistake nonetheless. A hypothetical example would be enrolling 2000 patients in a trial of Vitamin E for bronchiolitis and showing that the average oxygen saturation in the intervention versus control group was 95% versus 94%, with $p = 0.02$. Regardless of the p value, this difference is nothing to get excited about.

Confidence Intervals

Many statisticians and investigators are uncomfortable with the "yes/no" results obtained with typical hypothesis testing and feel that confidence intervals are a much more informative way to present data. A *95% confidence interval* (CI) is the mathematical corollary of a p value of 0.05. As an example, if investigators decided to study platelet counts in the PICU and, after evaluating 50 patients, found that the mean platelet count was 242, with a 95% CI range of 206 to 277, they would be 95% certain that the true population value (mean platelet count for *all* similar children) fell within that range. After evaluating 500 children, they found a mean of 236, with a 95% CI of 226 to 245. The larger the sample size, the narrower the CI becomes (the estimate is more precise). CIs can be obtained for any estimate: a difference between two groups, odds ratios from regression, etc. If a 95% CI for a difference between two means includes 0, then by definition, the p is not <0.05. Presenting the data this way gives a more useful representation of the precision of the estimate and potential size of a treatment difference (55). The range obtained can be particularly useful in negative studies to help a reader determine whether a clinically important difference might be detectable using larger numbers.

Multiple Comparisons

Problems arise if investigators make many different comparisons and state that they are willing to accept a 1 in 20 chance of a Type I error for each. It makes sense that, if 100 different comparisons are made, a statistically significant result (in this case, a false positive) would be found, on average, in five of them by chance alone. The overall risk of a Type I error may become unacceptably high. A particular problem occurs in *data dredging* or extensive subgroup analysis, in which investigators examine large amounts of data looking for significant relationships that were not anticipated a priori—inevitably, significant but erroneous results will be found (26). Statistical methods exist, such as the *Bonferroni procedure*, which adjust for multiple comparisons by setting a more stringent α cutoff for each comparison to decrease the overall risk of error. Of course, being too strict can increase the chance of missing important relationships. The same reasoning applies to the practice of setting a lower p value for stopping a trial early due to an *interim analysis*. Examining the data too often increases the chance of making a Type I error, so that such analyses should be planned prospectively in such a way that the risks are understood. An extreme example of this mistake would be an investigator who keeps adding 5 more patients to the study until the desired answer is statistically significant (which is almost certain to occur, by chance, at some point) and then stops enrollment.

Power Analysis and Sample Size Calculations

Choosing an appropriate sample size is essential to good study design (25). A study that is too large wastes time and resources and unnecessarily exposes too many patients to the risks of randomization by continuing to assign patients to placebo or treatment groups when a therapy could have been proven helpful/harmful/useless at an earlier point. A study that is too small fails to conclusively answer a question and is also ultimately wasteful. Sample size and power calculations are always, however, approximations (39).

The *power* of a study is defined as 1 minus β, or 100% minus the risk of making a Type II error. Thus, a study with 80% power accepts a Type II error of 0.2; a study with 90% power accepts a β of 0.1. Equations for sample size calculations vary, depending on what type of outcome is chosen (e.g., continuous vs. dichotomous data) and what type of statistical analysis is planned (e.g., univariate comparisons vs. multiple regression vs. survival analysis). An example of a specific calculation (for comparing means from two groups with equal variances and equal numbers of subjects in each group) is useful to show what information may be used for a typical calculation. The key items an investigator needs to estimate a sample size for a comparative trial are the type of outcome variable, the desired detectable difference in outcome between two groups, the anticipated precision or variability in the measurement of the outcome, and the acceptable levels of α and β:

$$N = [(z_{\alpha/2} + z_\beta)^2 * 2\sigma^2]/\Delta 2$$

N is the required number of subjects per study arm; z is a statistic derived from the normal distribution based on the α and β errors that are believed acceptable. z becomes larger for a smaller α or β, therefore increasing the sample size required if the researcher wants a lower risk of a Type I or Type II error.

σ reflects the variability in the population; a greater variability in the outcome requires more subjects. The only variable in the denominator is Δ, which is the difference in outcome between the two groups, and a larger number of subjects is required to detect a smaller difference between groups. A large anticipated difference (or treatment effect) would not require as large a sample. Looking for small differences requires very large numbers. The equations do not account for dropouts or study logistical issues; these problems should be anticipated, and they often increase the enrollment goal by 10%–30%.

Some information, such as the precision or variability in the outcome to be measured, may not be reliably known before beginning the study. Investigators often obtain this information from published studies in similar patient populations, from their own pilot data, or by making an educated guess.

In attempting to design a feasible study, investigators may use various strategies to try to decrease the required sample size, some of which are more legitimate than others (44). Accepting a slightly higher risk of a Type I or Type II error or anticipating a greater treatment effect may be reasonable if the trade-offs are well understood. Choosing a more common surrogate end point (e.g., ventilator-free days rather than mortality) may allow for a smaller study, but care must be taken to ensure that clinically relevant outcomes are still considered. If possible, using a more precise outcome and minimizing variability is helpful.

Using a "1-tailed" versus "2-tailed" α will greatly decrease the required numbers, but is usually not appropriate (51). Using a "2-tailed" or "2-sided" test means understanding that the intervention could either improve or worsen the outcome—it is hardly ever the case that one can be certain that the effect will only be in one direction (the above equation includes "$\alpha/2$," assuming a 2-tailed α).

Although it is best to perform a power analysis in the planning stages of a study, it is also possible to do a "post hoc" analysis using the data actually obtained (whether it is appropriate to do so is controversial). In this case, the sample size is known, and the size of the difference that could have been detected, given the sample size, acceptable error rate, and actual variability observed, is calculated.

Sensitivity and Specificity

Sensitivity and specificity are important in evaluating diagnostic tests, but similar concepts can apply when considering the association of a certain risk factor with a disease. The best way to remember the definitions is to visualize them on a 2×2 table:

	DISEASE	
	Present	Absent
TEST		
Positive	TP	FP
Negative	FN	TN

Columns represent the true disease state or the best approximation—a *gold standard* test. Rows represent the test being evaluated. TP = true positive, FP = false positive, FN = false negative, TN = true negative. Sensitivity and specificity are obtained by adding down columns. *Sensitivity* is the probability that a test is positive given that the disease is truly present—TP/(TP + FN). *Specificity* is the probability that the test is negative given that the disease is truly absent—TN/(TN + FP). In the clinical situation, it is usually not known beforehand if the disease is present or not; therefore, *predictive values* (the rows) are relevant, rather than sensitivity and specificity. If a test is positive, the *positive predictive value*—PPV = TP/(TP + FP)—is the probability that the disease is really present. Conversely, if a test is negative, the *negative predictive value*—NPV = TN/(TN + FN)—is the probability that the disease is truly absent. The problem with the PPV and NPV is that these values vary with the prevalence of disease.

As an example, suppose investigators develop a rapid bedside test for respiratory syncytial virus (RSV), and they evaluate house staff use of the test one winter in 138 infants who present with lower respiratory tract symptoms. Their 2×2 table comparing the new test to the gold standard respiratory syncytial virus direct fluorescent antibody shows:

	DISEASE		
	Present	Absent	
TEST			
Positive	61	5	66
Negative	6	66	72
	67	71	138

The sensitivity of the test is, therefore, 61/67 (91%), and the specificity is 66/71 (93%). The PPV is 61/66 (92%), and the NPV is 66/72 (92%). The disease *prevalence* in this case is 67/138 (49%). The investigators are excited, and decide to put the test into clinical use. They train the incoming interns in July by having them try the test on all patients admitted that month, regardless of the presenting symptoms. The prevalence of the disease has changed dramatically—only 1% of 1,000 patients admitted have RSV. The table now looks as follows:

	DISEASE		
	Present	Absent	
TEST			
Positive	9	69	78
Negative	1	921	922
	10	990	1000

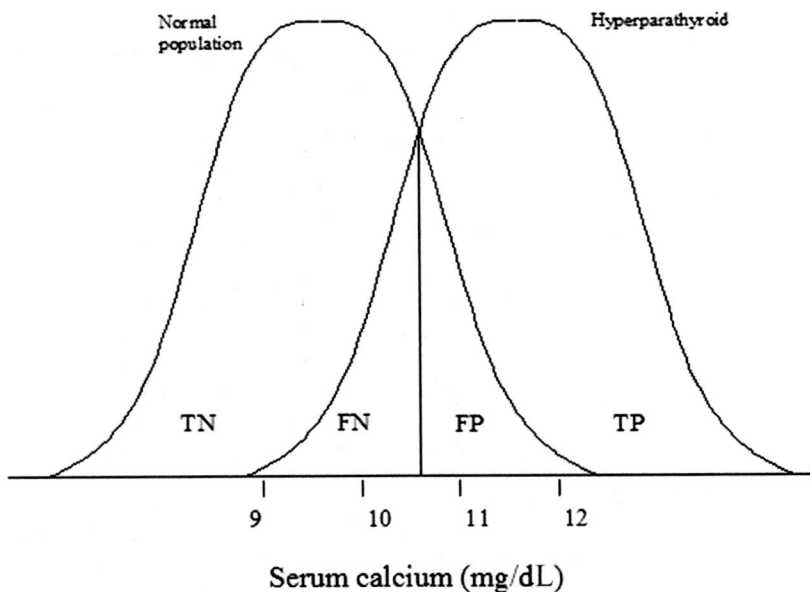

FIGURE 7.6. Overlapping curves of calcium values in normal and hyperparathyroid patients illustrate tradeoffs in sensitivity and specificity, with varying cutoff points for what is considered an "abnormal" test. TN, true negative; FN, false negative; FP, false positive; TP, true positive.

Although the sensitivity and specificity are not affected by prevalence, the PPV is now 9/78 (12%) and the NPV is 921/922 (99.9%), and false positives now outnumber true positives. This example illustrates the same point stressed in the earlier discussion of Bayesian analysis—that knowledge of the pre-test probability of disease before performing the test (or study!) will inevitably affect interpretation of the results. This is a frequently encountered problem when an attempt is made to adapt a test or therapy proven useful in one population to a population in which it has not been evaluated.

When a continuous variable is being evaluated as a diagnostic test, a balance between sensitivity and specificity must be achieved in setting a cutoff point for diagnosing a disease. As an example, consider two hypothetical overlapping curves along the range of serum calcium levels for patients with and without hyperparathyroidism (**Fig. 7.6**). If serum calcium level

were used as a diagnostic test for this disease, setting a lower cutoff (e.g., 9 mg/dL) would be an overly sensitive test. Most patients with the disease would have a positive test, but many without would as well. Setting a higher cutoff (e.g., 12 mg/dL) would conversely be overly specific. This method would render very few false positives, but many potential cases (true positives) would be missed. Choosing a different, more *accurate* test (i.e., one with less overlap between the two curves) would be the only way to improve both sensitivity and specificity.

Receiver Operating Characteristic Curves

Receiver operating characteristic (ROC) curves are often presented when comparing the performance of diagnostic tests, risk factors, or scales to predict dichotomous outcomes (**Fig. 7.7**). The curve is obtained by plotting sensitivity on the y-axis versus 1 – specificity (1 minus specificity) on the x-axis

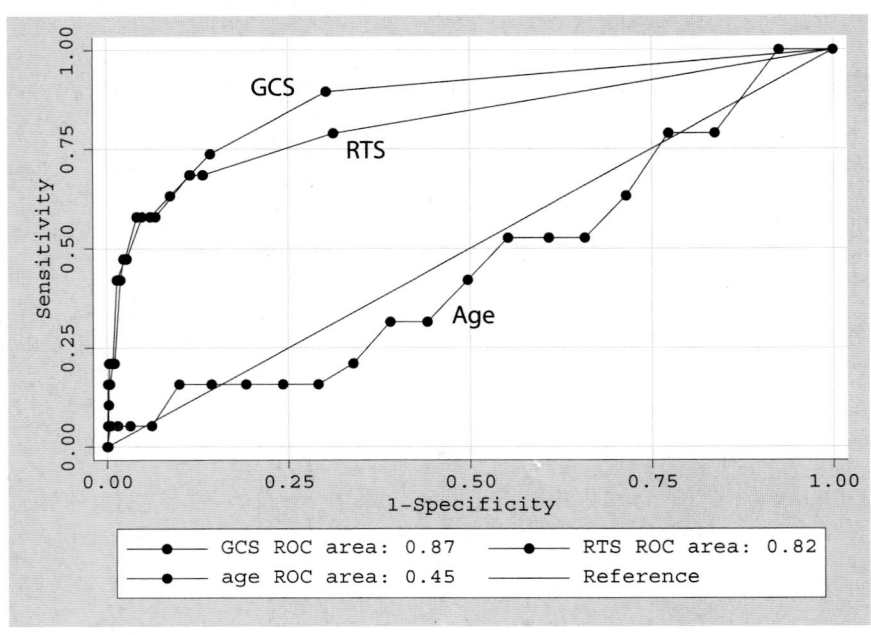

FIGURE 7.7. Receiver operating characteristic curve, evaluating Glasgow coma scale (GCS), revised trauma score (RTS), and age as predictors of mortality.

for various cutoff points of a diagnostic test. The *area under the curve* (AUC) is calculated as a measure of the discriminatory power of the test. A perfect test (sensitivity and specificity of 100% at all points) would be a right angle, with the apex at the upper left corner, and it would have an AUC of 1.0. A test no better than chance would fall on the diagonal line and have an AUC of 0.5 (see Chapter 9). The best cutoff point for the diagnostic test falls at the point along the curve closest to the upper left corner.

Figure 7.7 illustrates the use of the Glasgow coma scale (GCS), revised trauma score (RTS), and age as predictors of mortality in over 11,000 patients with traumatic brain injury. GCS appears to be the best predictor (AUC = 0.87) versus RTS (AUC = 0.82). Age is no better than chance, with an AUC = 0.45, despite the fact that younger age was a highly significant predictor of greater mortality (not shown); it is still a very poor *discriminatory* test for giving a "cutoff" point. Additionally, even though GCS is the best predictor of the three, its best cutoff point reaches a sensitivity of 75% and specificity of 90%, making it not very useful as a diagnostic test. The example also illustrates that, when evaluating a potential diagnostic test, it does not necessarily help to say, "A statistically significant difference in GCS is observed between survivors and nonsurvivors," because doing so begins with the result and looks backward. Rather, the predictive power of different cutoff points should be examined, such as by using an ROC curve, to determine sensitivity and specificity, and it should be determined if the test performs adequately with a given prevalence of disease.

Specific Statistical Tests

The following is a brief overview of several statistical tests that provides some guidance on choosing the correct test to use; more detailed references and software are available for guidance on performing each test (7,17,34,41). The list is not exhaustive, but it presents some of the most commonly encountered methods. The choice of test depends on the type of outcome to be analyzed, number of different groups to be compared, size of the sample, variability of data, and nature of the question.

Student's *t* test

Student's *t* test can be used to compare means of continuous data. It is possible to compare a single mean to a population parameter (i.e., normal value) or to compare *two* means. If the two values are related (e.g., before and after measurement on the same patient), it is necessary to use a *paired t* test. The formulae vary based on whether the test is paired and whether variances are equal, but all generate a "*t* statistic," which is compared to a standard curve or table to generate a *p* value; in other words, the proportion of time that a difference as extreme as the one seen or greater would occur by chance alone. The curve used depends on the degrees of freedom, so that a larger sample results in a narrower curve and, hence, a lower *p* value. One of the assumptions of the *t* test is that the continuous outcome follows a roughly normal distribution; large numbers allow for some deviation from this requirement.

Analysis of Variance

The ANOVA is used to compare the mean of a continuous outcome from *more than two groups*. This tool is useful when comparing several groups to avoid starting with repeated *t* tests between pairs of groups, which can lead to the problem of multiple comparisons. ANOVA examines the variability in the observations between the groups and compares this to the variability within the groups. Significantly more variability "between" than "within" the groups suggests that a real difference exists between them. ANOVA generates a *variance ratio* or *F statistic* from the ratio of between and within group sums of squared deviations from the mean, adjusted for the degrees of freedom. Standard tables then provide the risk that such a difference could be seen by chance.

Like the *t* test, ANOVA assumes that the outcome is roughly normally distributed, with greater deviations from normality allowed as the numbers get larger. Other assumptions are that the groups have fairly equal variances. A very important assumption is that the values are independent of each other; classical ANOVA analysis cannot be used to compare multiple measurements on single individuals.

One-way ANOVA refers to models with only one independent variable. An example would be a study of time that physicians spend talking with families based on the families' educational levels (time would be the continuous outcome; educational level—high school, college, graduate school—would be the categorical independent variable). *Two-way ANOVA* refers to an analysis with two factors as independent variables. An example might be looking at the effect of race and gender on blood pressure. *Repeated-measures ANOVA* is the counterpart of the paired *t* test and is used when the measurements are somehow connected, such as a series of measurements on individual patients.

Nonparametric Tests

What should be done if an investigator wants to compare the means of two or more groups, and the outcome is not even close to normally distributed? The first step is to see if a transformation will work (see the earlier discussion). If not, it is possible to use a *nonparametric test*. Nonparametric tests make no assumptions about the distribution of data and are typically appropriate in the same cases in which a median should be used rather than a mean as a descriptive statistic. The most common method is to replace the actual values in the data with *ranks* so that, instead of comparing actual blood pressure measurements, for example, the difference in blood pressure between two groups is decided based on whether the higher values are predominantly in one group and the lower values are in the other. Ranking solves the problem of highly skewed or variable data and extreme outliers because a value that is far out of range of all the others becomes simply the "highest" value. The problem is that some of the information contained in the original data is lost by converting it to ranks. The nonparametric equivalents of paired and unpaired *t* tests are the *Wilcoxon rank sum* and the *Mann-Whitney U*, respectively. The *Kruskal-Wallis test*, the nonparametric equivalent of ANOVA, is used for comparing medians of more than two groups. The *Friedman test* is the nonparametric equivalent of 2-way or repeated measures ANOVA.

Chi Squared and Fisher's Exact Test

The chi-squared (χ^2) test is used to compare *counts* or *proportions* obtained with nominal or categorical data. Data of this sort are often presented in 2×2 (or 2×3, etc.) *contingency tables*. As a hypothetical example, comparison of mortality among male and female infants born at 23 weeks' gestation might appear as follows.

	Died	Survived
Male	53 (56%)	42 (44%)
Female	34 (41%)	48 (59%)
Total	87	90

The χ^2 statistic is calculated by comparing the observed to expected values in each cell (the expected value would be that obtained if the percentage of males and females who died was exactly the same percent). The formula is:

$$\text{Chi squared} = \sum \frac{(O - E)^2}{E}$$

The result is then compared to a χ^2 table for the appropriate degrees of freedom (larger values of this statistic indicate a greater deviation from expected results) to yield a percent of time that such a result would be obtained by chance alone. A "2-tailed" χ^2 test does not exist; because all values are squared, the distribution falls entirely above 0. The χ^2, as opposed to a *t* test, can also be used for more than two groups. *McNemar's test* is the equivalent of χ^2 for paired data. Using a *kappa* statistic is an example of applying a similar analysis of observed and expected values to evaluate agreement between two observers, or *interrater reliability*.

The χ^2 approximation runs into difficulty when small numbers are expected. Any time that the expected frequency for a cell is ≤ 5, it is better to use *Fisher's exact* test. Fisher's exact test can also be used with larger numbers; however, the calculations are far more laborious than they are for the χ^2 test (which is, of course, made less of a problem with computers).

Correlation

Correlation is one way to examine a relationship between two variables. *Pearson's correlation coefficient (r)* (also known as *sample correlation coefficient* or *product-moment correlation coefficient*) evaluates a linear relationship between two continuous variables. The result obtained is a number somewhere between -1 and 1. A result of r = 1.0 would indicate a perfect positive correlation, r = 0 would be no correlation (or no relationship between the variables), and r = -1.0 would be a perfect negative correlation. In real life, such absolute numbers are rarely obtained. Because the test can detect only *linear* relationships, it is important to examine data to ensure that other, nonlinear, relationships are not missed (**Fig. 7.8**). A visual observation also helps to detect outliers that may pull the slope of the line in their direction. As is the case with most statistical

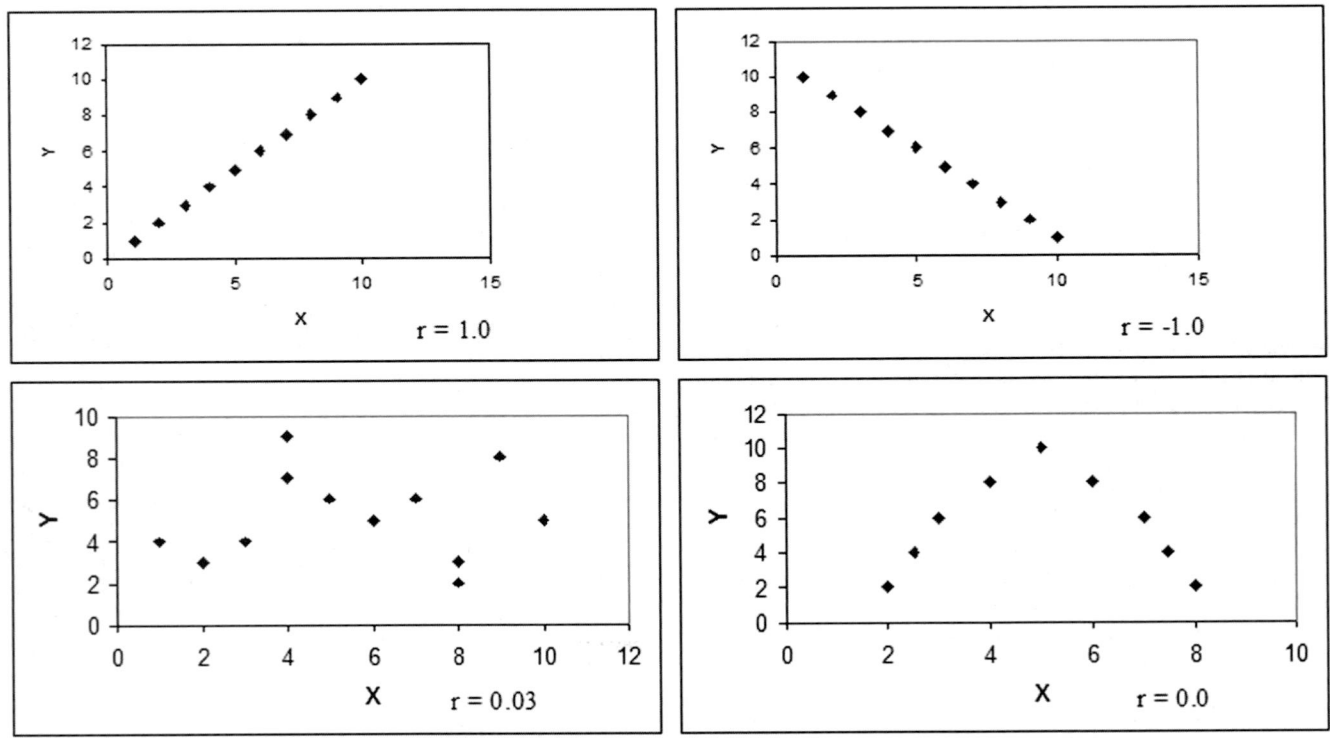

FIGURE 7.8. Pearson's correlation coefficient (r) is shown for each of the above graphs, with perfect linear relationships shown with r = 1.0 and r = −1.0 and almost no relationship shown with r = 0.03. The bottom right graph illustrates that the test is sensitive only to linear relationships; r = 0, which would imply no relationship, but it is obvious from looking at the data that a relationship actually exists between x and y.

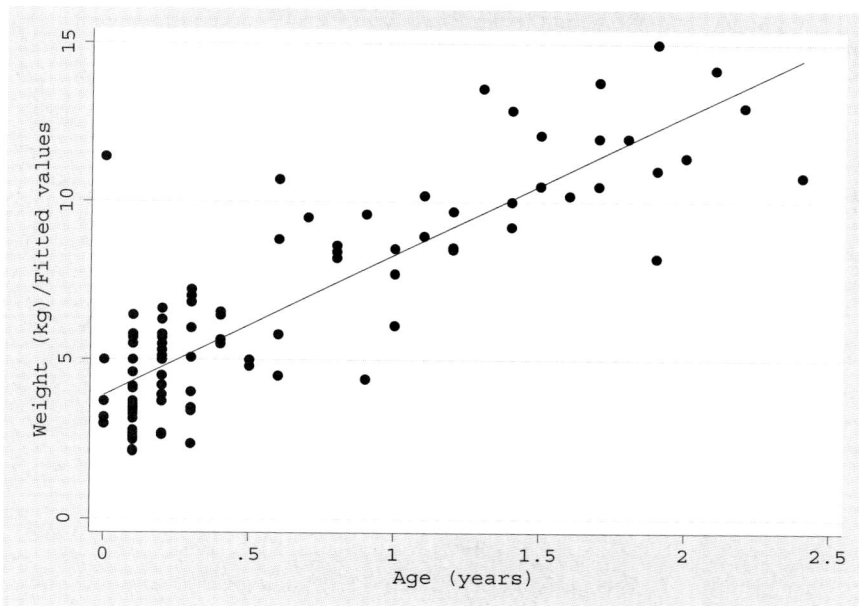

FIGURE 7.9. A scatterplot of age and weight of children <2.5 years of age on admission to a PICU. The line represents the *best fit* line determined by a regression equation generated to predict weight from age. *Residuals* are the distances between the predicted weight (*the line*) and each actual weight (*individual points*).

tests, even a very strong relationship indicates an association only, and not causality. Confidence intervals or a *p* value can accompany the correlation coefficient and give an idea of the estimate's precision. For a curve of a similar shape (and hence similar r), a greater number of measurements results in a lower *p* value. Yet, if a significant *p* value is obtained, but the correlation coefficient shows only a weak relationship (e.g., r = 0.1, *p* <0.01), the low *p* value should not be interpreted as an important finding—only a weak relationship has been demonstrated. Pearson's assumes that the data are fairly normally distributed. The nonparametric equivalent is *Spearman's rho* (ρ).

The square of the correlation coefficient (r^2) is called the *coefficient of determination* and is an indication of how the extent to which the variability in the y variable is explained by the variability in the x variable. r^2 ranges from 0 to 1 and becomes much more meaningful when used in the context of multiple regression.

Regression

Regression is a technique that is being used more and more frequently in epidemiology and clinical studies, and a discussion of the intricacies is far beyond the scope of this chapter (6,18,24,52). As opposed to correlation, in which the x and y variables are basically interchangeable, regression involves *predicting* an outcome variable based on one or more other variables. The *predictor variable* can also be known as the *explanatory variable* or *independent variable*. The *outcome variable* can also be called the *response variable* or *dependent variable*. Whereas in correlation both variables must be continuous, in regression, it is possible to have other variable types (dichotomous, categorical) as predictors. Although the terms *prediction* and *predictor* are commonly used, any relationship between predictor and outcome variables cannot be proven causative, but merely statistically associated.

Linear regression is used when the outcome variable is a continuous measurement, such that the predictive equation is mathematically the equation of a line:

$$y = a + b_1x_1 + b_2x_2 \ldots + e$$

Where:

y = outcome variable
x = predictor variable(s)
a = y-intercept, or value of y when x = 0 (often not a meaningful number)
b = change in y for each unit change in x (often called the *coefficient*, *beta*, β, or *slope*)
e = error (variability in y not accounted for by the equation = *residual*)

Simple linear regression refers to a model with one predictor variable; *multiple linear regression* means that more than one predictor is present. A simple regression model can be visualized graphically (**Fig. 7.9**). The computer estimates the coefficient for the variable (i.e., slope of the line) by finding the line that minimizes the total distance of each individual point from that line. The *residual* value is the difference between the actual value (the point) and the predicted value (the line) from the equation. *Residual analysis* examines patterns found in the residuals; a random scatter about the line provides reassurance that the model has a good fit. An equation with multiple predictors cannot be visualized; statistically, a "line" is generated with a coefficient for each predictor variable that yields the best prediction of the outcome variable. Such an analysis can be used to *adjust* for possible *confounders* or other variables that are anticipated to affect the outcome of interest. For example, in the example shown in **Figure 7.9**, gender or race might be entered into the equation used to predict weight from age. Another frequently used technique is to adjust for a severity of illness measure (see Chapter 9) when assessing the impact of a variable of interest on an outcome. Any coefficient derived can be tested for statistical significance (generating a *p* value or 95% CI for the true value of the coefficient). For linear regression, a 95% CI that includes 0 would be equivalent to a *p* value >0.05. In the simple regression model shown in the graph (sometimes called *univariate* analysis), each increase in age by 1 year is associated with a 4.4-kg increase in weight (95% CI, 3.9–5; *p* <0.0005). As seen in this example, an equation derived from one population should not be applied to a dissimilar group, as such a rapid yearly increase in weight would not be expected in teenagers.

When presenting regression data, it is important to report how the variables have been defined. In the example, the coefficient would be different if age had been entered in months rather than in years. In addition, if gender were entered into the equation, stating that the coefficient for gender is "+0.2 kg" makes no sense, unless the readers know that gender has been coded as 0 for females and 1 for males (in which case males would, on average, weigh 0.2 kg more than females *of the same age* in this dataset). r^2 is similar to the coefficient of determination mentioned under correlation. It is an indicator of the amount of variability in the outcome variable that is accounted for by the variability in all the predictors. r^2 will usually increase, even if only slightly, for every variable added to the model; the goal is to achieve a model that is as *parsimonious* as possible, meaning that it has a reasonably high r^2 with the fewest possible predictors.

Logistic regression is a similar technique that is used when the outcome is dichotomous, such as survival or mortality. When coefficients are obtained for a logistic regression equation, their interpretation is less intuitive than for linear regression, because the numbers must be entered into a logarithmic equation to calculate a predicted proportion with the outcome. For this reason, many investigators will present results of a logistic regression analysis as an *odds ratio* (OR) rather than give the coefficients themselves. The OR is defined as the odds of the outcome event occurring (with the predictor variable present) divided by the odds of it occurring if the predictor is absent (for continuous or ordinal predictors, the ratio is the increase in odds for each unit increase in the predictor). **Table 7.2** presents ORs for predicting death in patients who were admitted to a PICU after trauma, based on a regression equation including the gender, age, and whether the injury was in a motor vehicle crash. In this example, which includes only three predictors in the equation, gender appears to have no significant effect on mortality, as the 95% CI for the OR includes 1 (0.92–1.21). Increasing age is significantly associated with a lower risk of death (OR, 0.96; 95% CI, 0.95–0.97 for each increase in age by 1 year), and having a motor vehicle crash as the mechanism of injury increases the odds of mortality (OR, 1.8; 95% CI, 1.61–2.13).

Pitfalls of regression include trying to fit too many variables into an equation when the numbers are relatively small—called *overfitting*. Sample size calculations are possible but complicated. A general rule of thumb is that 10 times as many subjects must be included as predictor variables. For logistic regression,

more than 10 *outcome events* (e.g., deaths) must be included for each predictor (6). Automated methods also exist (e.g., stepwise regression) to generate a model by using a cutoff level of significance to include or exclude predictor variables from among multiple candidate variables. Caution with these methods is appropriate, as the computer has no appreciation for biologic rationale or the relationships between the variables. In addition, if two *collinear* predictor variables (i.e., they tend to vary together) are included, a meaningful relationship with the outcome may be obscured, as significant contributions to the outcome's variability will be divided between them. As an example, it would be problematic to include both systolic blood pressure and mean blood pressure in an equation used to predict outcome after trauma. Special methods (see the following sections) are also required if repeated measurements are performed on individuals or if the subjects are somehow grouped (e.g., if 1000 students are studied, the fact that they cluster into three different schools must be considered).

Longitudinal Data

In *cross-sectional studies*, each subject gives rise to one response or a single outcome. The response variable is measured once or is an irreversible end point (e.g., death from acute respiratory distress syndrome). In *longitudinal studies*, the investigator examines a sample of subjects over time. When the response of interest involves not only whether or not the event occurs once, but more importantly, the interval of time between a baseline landmark and when the event occurs (i.e., the *time to the event*), methods collectively known as *survival analysis* are used to analyze the results. When the response or outcome of interest is measured in the same subject repeatedly over time (e.g., seizures, blood pressure, oxygen index, serum sodium), a different approach using *longitudinal data analysis methods* should be used (50,56,57). If these methods are not used, the assumptions of basic statistical techniques reviewed earlier (in which all observations in a study sample are independent of each other) are violated. Repeated measurements in a subject are correlated, and this correlation must be taken into account to avoid making erroneous estimates. The simplest example of a continuous outcome measured twice (e.g., blood pressure before and after an intervention) can be compared using a paired *t* test. More than two measurements warrant different methods. The type of outcome (continuous, dichotomous, or counts) determines the type of longitudinal analysis method.

Multivariate analysis of variance (MANOVA) can be used when multiple dependent as well as multiple independent variables exist. This method can also be used to compare groups over time; however, the intervals of time must be weighted

---

TABLE 7.2

ODDS RATIOS FOR DEATH AMONG CHILDREN ADMITTED TO A PICU FOLLOWING TRAUMA

	Odds ratio	95% Confidence interval	*p* Value
Gender (0 = M, 1 = F)	1.06	0.93–1.21	0.391
Age (years)	0.96	0.95–0.97	<0.001
MVC (0 = No, 1 = Yes)	1.80	1.61–2.13	<0.001
MVC, motor vehicle crash			

equally. To examine an outcome measured repeatedly over time using several predictor variables, more complex techniques of longitudinal analysis, called *generalized estimating equations* (GEE) or mixed random effects model, are required (10). Computers are generally unable to tell when these methods are required and will simply produce wrong estimates. Examining the data graphically can assist in the choice of the best model. These methods can also be used to account for *clustering* within certain subgroups.

Survival Analysis

Survival analysis methods relate to the analysis of data for which the *time to an event* (e.g., time to death, time to graft failure, time to extubation, time to developing an infection, time to wean off extracorporeal membrane oxygenation) is the outcome of interest; the term *survival time* is often used whether the event is death or not. Event-time methods take into account *censoring*, which refers to the possibility that some subjects will not experience the event of interest by the end of the observation period. Censoring also occurs when some subjects are followed for different periods of time than others, or lost to follow-up entirely. These data must be considered in the analysis; using a *t* test to compare the average time until patients develop an outcome if they are followed for different lengths of time would ignore important information and introduce bias.

In survival analysis or event-time methods, two fundamental data must be known for each subject. The first is the interval of *time at risk*, also called the *exposure* time. The second indicator must report whether the event occurs or if censoring occurs (no event by the end of the exposure time). The basic notation for survival analysis uses the survival function at time t, $S(t)$, which is the probability of being event-free beyond time t. The cumulative incidence function at time t, denoted as $F(t) = 1 - S(t)$, is the complementary probability that the event has occurred by time t. The *Kaplan-Meier estimator* is a nonparametric estimator of the survival function, $S(t)$ that can be computed to estimate and illustrate the probability of survival. The hazard function $h(t)$ is the instantaneous event rate of subjects who have not experienced the event yet or who have survived to time t. The hazard ratio will be the ratio of two hazards and relies on the assumption that this ratio is constant over time—the *proportional hazards assumption*. Cox proportional hazard regression is a tool for assessing the relationship of multiple predictors for event-time studies. Finally, if more than two exclusive end points for a single event are possible (e.g., in congenital heart disease repair, there could be survival with re-operation, survival after one operation, or death), different methods must be used, such as competing risks analysis methods (2).

A hypothetical data set that evaluates central line–related infections in jugular compared to femoral lines can illustrate the Kaplan-Meier estimator, which uses the series of conditional probabilities for each subject of being infection free on day $t + 1$ if the subject was infection free on day t (**Table 7.3** and

---

TABLE 7.3

HYPOTHETICAL DATA FOR CENTRAL LINE INFECTIONS IN TWO GROUPS OF 10 CHILDREN AFTER CARDIAC SURGERY WITH FEMORAL VERSUS JUGULAR LINES

Line inserted	Time day of follow-up	Number at risk (n_i)	Number infected (y_i)	Number censored: transferred from ICU	Conditional probability of being free of infection $(n_i - y_i)/n_i$	Survival function: Kaplan-Meier estimator of the probability of being free of infection
Jugular	1	10	0	0	(10 – 0)/10 = 1	1
	2	10	0	0	(10 – 0)/10 = 1	1 × 1 = 1
	3	10	1	1	(10 – 1)/10 = 0.9	0.9 × 1 = 0.9
	4	8	0	0	(8 – 0)/8 = 1	1 × 0.9 = 0.9
	5	8	2	0	(8 – 2)/8 = 0.75	0.75 × 0.9 = 0.675
	6	6	1	1	(6 – 1)/6 = 0.83	0.83 × 0.675 = 0.56
	7	4	1	0	(4 – 1)/4 = 0.75	0.75 × 0.56 = 0.42
	8	3	1	0	(3 – 1)/3 = 0.66	0.66 × 0.42 = 0.27
	9	2	1	1	(2 – 1)/2 = 0.5	0.5 × 0.27 = 0.13
	10	1	0	0	(1 – 0)/1 = 1	1 × 0.13 = 0.13
Femoral	1	10	1	0	(10 – 1)/10 = 0.9	0.9
	2	9	2	0	(9 – 2)/9 = 0.78	0.78 × 0.9 = 0.69
	3	7	1	1	(7 – 1)/7 = 0.85	0.85 × 0.69 = 0.59
	4	5	3	0	(5 – 3)/5 = 0.4	0.4 × 0.59 = 0.236
	5	2	1	0	(2 – 1)/2 = 0.5	0.5 × 0.236 = 0.12
	6	1	1	0	(1 – 1)/1 = 0	0 × 0.12 = 0
	7	None				
	8	None				
	9	None				
	10	None				

Numbers of infections, as well as number of children transferred (censored), are noted. Those who have been discharged are no longer followed for infections; therefore, the conditional probability of being infection free at each time period is based only on those children who have neither failed (infection) nor been censored (transferred).

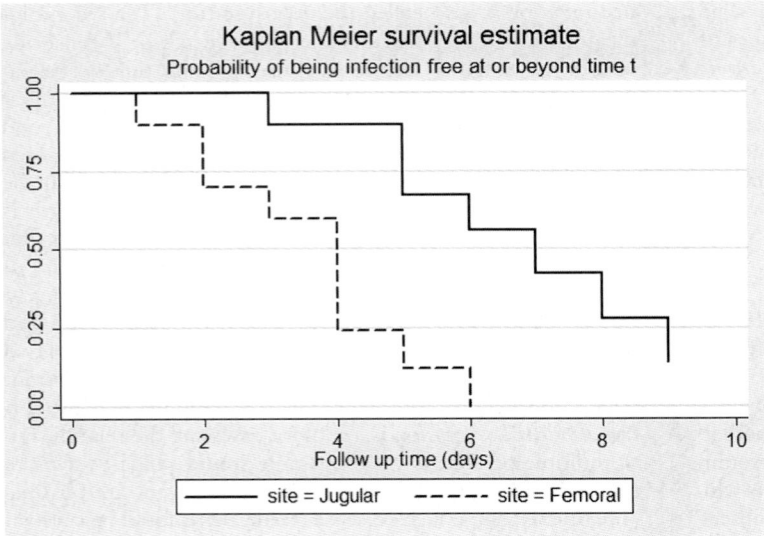

FIGURE 7.10. Plot of the Kaplan-Meier estimate of the survival function, S(t), of the probability of being infection free by time, t, from the example shown in **Table 7.3**. On visual inspection, the probability of being infection free at a given time seems greater in the group with jugular lines. Formal statistical testing with the log rank test provides a p value $= 0.002$.

Fig. 7.10). The log-rank test allows a comparison of both curves by setting the null hypothesis of no difference between curves at all follow-up times and the alternative that the curves differ at one or more times. The aim is to compare the probability of being event free (infection free) at time t between groups. The calculations take into account both whether an infection occurred and whether the patient was discharged (censored) without having to exclude patients because their follow-up period was short.

REPORTING RESULTS

Standards for preparing, analyzing, and reporting research results exist. Multidisciplinary research teams, including methodologists such as biostatisticians, epidemiologists, and clinical trialists, improve the quality of the design and analysis and should be involved in the preparation of the results and their interpretation to minimize bias in the inferences and interpretation of the evidence. Certain organizations and journals have proposed guidelines to improve the quality of the reporting of RCTs (4) or surveys (22) that are useful for investigators. Although pediatric critical care investigators cannot be expert in all domains of the analysis, as principal investigators or coinvestigators, they remain responsible for the preparation of the manuscripts and of the message disseminated by the reports.

CONCLUSIONS AND FUTURE DIRECTIONS

The tremendous complexity of the care provided by pediatric intensivists in an era of rapidly changing technology continuously provides investigators with fruitful questions and a desperate need for their insight and hard work. The importance of collaboration among centers is becoming more and more obvious, recently evidenced by the work being produced by the Pediatric Acute Lung Injury and Sepsis Investigators (PALISI) network (37) and Collaborative Pediatric Critical Care Research

Network (54); others are working on better ways to manage and evaluate the tremendous amount of data that intensivists process daily (53). Just as the demand for expert clinicians in the field is increasing, the need will increase for those who can undertake and interpret complex research and translate it into patient care. Skill in both arenas is necessary to provide the best possible care to children and their families.

KEY POINTS

Study Design

- Defining a clear, detailed, answerable research question is the first step in beginning a project.
- Involving experts in statistics and study design during the first planning phases of a study will save much wasted effort.
- A well-designed RCT is the gold standard of clinical trials, but is resource intensive and impossible in some situations.
- Other observational studies (case-control, pre-post intervention, cohort studies) can be very helpful if their limitations are understood.
- A systematic review/meta-analysis cannot improve the quality of the data from the individual trials included.
- Qualitative research includes a variety of observational and exploratory techniques. Methods in these studies should be just as rigorous as in quantitative studies.

Statistical Analysis

- Computers are an invaluable tool for performing statistical analyses, but they cannot determine if the right question has been asked or if the appropriate test has been used.
- The type of statistical test chosen depends on the type of data, distribution of the data, total number of subjects, number of groups involved, number of measurements per subject, whether measurements are made over time, and what question is asked.

- Visually inspecting patterns in the data before running any statistical test will aid in detecting unexpected patterns and choosing the appropriate test.
- Investigators choose the amount of risk of reaching a wrong conclusion that they are willing to accept. Cutoffs, such as an α level of 0.05, are arbitrary and established by convention.
- CIs are often a more informative tool with which to describe the precision of an estimate, rather than looking for definitive yes/no answers from a p value.
- Trials that are either far too large or far too small are both wasteful and potentially unethical if subjects are exposed to unnecessary risks. Proper planning using available information before beginning the trial can sometimes prevent these errors.

ACKNOWLEDGMENT

The authors would like to acknowledge the debt owed to the faculty of the Johns Hopkins Bloomberg School of Public Health, particularly Scott Zeger, PhD, Marie Diener-West, PhD, Leon Gordis, MD, DrPH, and Steven Goodman, MD, PhD, on whose lectures and class notes we relied heavily for the content of this chapter.

References

1. Altman DG, Bland JM. Detecting skewness from summary information. *Br Med J* 1996;313:1200.
2. Amark KM, Karamlou T, O'Carroll A, et al. Independent factors associated with mortality, reintervention, and achievement of complete repair in children with pulmonary atresia with ventricular septal defect. *J Am Coll Cardiol* 2006;47:1448–56.
3. Bartlett RH. Extracorporeal life support: History and new directions. *Semin Perinatol* 2005;29:2–7.
4. Begg C, Cho M, Eastwood S, et al. Improving the quality of reporting of randomized controlled trials. The CONSORT statement. *JAMA* 1996;276:637–9.
5. Berkenbosch JW, Grueber RE, Graff GR, et al. Patterns of helium-oxygen (heliox) usage in the critical care environment. *J Intensive Care Med* 2004;19:335–44.
6. Concato J, Feinstein AR, Holford TR. The risk of determining risk with multivariable models. *Ann Intern Med* 1993;118:201–10.
7. Dawson B, Trapp RG. *Basic & Clinical Biostatistics*. New York: Lange Medical Books/McGraw-Hill, 2004.
8. Dickersin K. The existence of publication bias and risk factors for its occurrence. *JAMA* 1990;263:1385–9.
9. Dickersin K, Berlin JA. Meta-analysis: State-of-the-science. *Epidemiol Rev* 1992;14:154–76.
10. Diggle P, Diggle P. *Analysis of Longitudinal Data*. Oxford, New York: Oxford University Press, 2002.
11. Egger M, Smith GD, Altman DG. *Systematic Reviews in Health Care: Meta-Analysis in Context*. London: BMJ Publishing Group, 2001.
12. Goldstein B, Nadel S, Peters M, et al. ENHANCE: Results of a global open-label trial of drotrecogin alfa (activated) in children with severe sepsis. *Pediatr Crit Care Med* 2006;7. Epub Ahead Of Print.
13. Goodman SN. Introduction to Bayesian methods I: Measuring the strength of evidence. *Clin Trials* 2005;2:282–90; discussion 301–4, 64–78.
14. Goodman SN, Sladky JT. A Bayesian approach to randomized controlled trials in children utilizing information from adults: The case of Guillain-Barré syndrome. *Clin Trials* 2005;2:305–10; discussion 64–78.
15. Gordis L. *Epidemiology*. Philadelphia: Saunders, 2004.
16. Green J, Britten N. Qualitative research and evidence based medicine. *Br Med J* 1998;316:1230–2.
17. Hassard TH. *Understanding Biostatistics*. St. Louis: Mosby Year Book, 1991.
18. Hosmer DW, Lemeshow S. *Applied Logistic Regression*. New York: Wiley, 2000.
19. Jadad AR, McQuay HJ. Meta-analyses to evaluate analgesic interventions: A systematic qualitative review of their methodology. *J Clin Epidemiol* 1996;49:235–43.
20. Juni P, Altman DG, Egger M. Systematic reviews in health care: Assessing the quality of controlled clinical trials. *Br Med J* 2001;323:42–6.
21. Keene ON. The log transformation is special. *Stat Med* 1995;14:811–9.
22. Kelley K, Clark B, Brown V, et al. Good practice in the conduct and reporting of survey research. *Int J Qual Health Care* 2003;15:261–6.
23. Khan KS, Daya S, Jadad A. The importance of quality of primary studies in producing unbiased systematic reviews. *Arch Intern Med* 1996;156:661–6.
24. Kleinbaum DG, Kleinbaum DG. *Applied Regression Analysis and Other Multivariable Methods*. Pacific Grove: Duxbury Press, 1998.
25. Lachin JM. Introduction to sample size determination and power analysis for clinical trials. *Control Clin Trials* 1981;2:93–113.
26. Lagakos SW. The challenge of subgroup analyses—Reporting without distorting. *N Engl J Med* 2006;354:1667–69.
27. Last JM, International Epidemiological Association. *A Dictionary of Epidemiology*. New York: Oxford University Press, 2001.
28. Meert KL, Thurston CS, Briller SH. The spiritual needs of parents at the time of their child's death in the pediatric intensive care unit and during bereavement: A qualitative study. *Pediatr Crit Care Med* 2005;6:420–7.
29. Meinert CL, Tonascia S. *Clinical Trials: Design, Conduct, and Analysis*. New York: Oxford University Press, 1986.
30. Moher D, Cook DJ, Eastwood S, et al. Improving the quality of reports of meta-analyses of randomised controlled trials: The QUOROM statement. Quality of Reporting of Meta-analyses. *Lancet* 1999;354:1896–1900.
31. Moher D, Jadad AR, Tugwell P. Assessing the quality of randomized controlled trials. Current issues and future directions. *Int J Technol Assess Health Care* 1996;12:195–208.
32. Morris MC, Nadkarni VM, Ward FR, et al. Exception from informed consent for pediatric resuscitation research: Community consultation for a trial of brain cooling after in-hospital cardiac arrest. *Pediatrics* 2004;114:776–81.
33. Moye LA, Deswal A. Perils of the random experiment. *Am J Ther* 2003;10:112–21.
34. Myers JL, Well A. *Research Design and Statistical Analysis*. Mahwah, NJ: Lawrence Erlbaum Associates, 2003.
35. Newman SC. *Biostatistical Methods in Epidemiology*. New York: John Wiley & Sons, 2001.
36. Nicholson CE, Wetzel RC. Research in Pediatric Critical Care. In: Fuhrman BP, Zimmerman J, eds. *Pediatric Critical Care*. Philadelphia: Mosby-Elsevier, 2006:29–57.
37. PALISI network. Website:http://pedsccm.wustl.edu/research/palisi/palisi.html. Accessed April 17, 2006.
38. Peters JL, Sutton AJ, Jones DR, et al. Comparison of two methods to detect publication bias in meta-analysis. *JAMA* 2006;295:676–80.
39. Piantadosi S. *Clinical Trials: A Methodologic Perspective*. Hoboken, NJ: Wiley-Interscience, 2005.
40. Pope C, Mays N. Opening the black box: An encounter in the corridors of health services research. *Br Med J* 1993;306:315–8.
41. Rosner B. *Fundamentals of Biostatistics*. Belmont, CA: Thomson-Brooks/Cole, 2006.
42. Rothman KJ, Greenland S. *Modern Epidemiology*. Philadelphia: Lippincott-Raven, 1998.
43. Sandelowski M. Sample size in qualitative research. *Res Nurs Health* 1995;18:179–83.
44. Scales DC, Rubenfeld GD. Estimating sample size in critical care clinical trials. *J Crit Care* 2005;20:6–11.
45. Schulz KF, Chalmers I, Hayes RJ, et al. Empirical evidence of bias. Dimensions of methodological quality associated with estimates of treatment effects in controlled trials. *JAMA* 1995;273:408–12.
46. Shea B, Moher D, Graham I, et al. A comparison of the quality of Cochrane reviews and systematic reviews published in paper-based journals. *Eval Health Prof* 2002;25:116–29.
47. Silverman WA. A cautionary tale about supplemental oxygen: The albatross of neonatal medicine. *Pediatrics* 2004;113:394–96.
48. Stroup DF, Berlin JA, Morton SC, et al. Meta-analysis of observational studies in epidemiology: A proposal for reporting. Meta-analysis of observational studies in epidemiology (MOOSE) group. *JAMA* 2000;283:2008–12.
49. Szklo M, Nieto FJ. *Epidemiology: Beyond the Basics*. Sudbury, MA: Jones and Bartlett, 2004.
50. Twisk JWR. *Applied Longitudinal Data Analysis for Epidemiology: A Practical Guide*. Cambridge NY: Cambridge University Press, 2003.
51. United States Food and Drug Administration (FDA). International Conference on Harmonization. Statistical principles for clinical trials. E9, 1998.
52. Vittinghoff E. *Regression Methods in Biostatistics: Linear, Logistic, Survival, and Repeated Measures Models*. New York: Springer, 2005.
53. Wetzel RC. The virtual pediatric intensive care unit. Practice in the new millennium. *Pediatr Clin North Am* 2001;48:795–814.
54. Willson DF, Dean JM, Newth C, et al. Collaborative Pediatric Critical Care Research Network (CPCCRN). *Pediatr Crit Care Med* 2006;7:301–7.
55. Young KD, Lewis RJ. What is confidence? Part 1: The use and interpretation of confidence intervals. *Ann Emerg Med* 1997;30:307–10.
56. Zeger SL, Liang KY. Longitudinal data analysis for discrete and continuous outcomes. *Biometrics* 1986;42:121–30.
57. Zeger SL, Liang KY, Albert PS. Models for longitudinal data: A generalized estimating equation approach. *Biometrics* 1988;44:1049–60.

CHAPTER 8 ■ EVIDENCE-BASED MEDICINE

BARRY P. MARKOVITZ • KATHLEEN L. MEERT

CASE SCENARIOS

Case 1

A 5-year-old boy is admitted to the PICU following an unintentional hanging injury. He was found apneic and bradycardic after an indeterminate time period. His mother, a pediatric ER nurse, administered rescue breaths; his heart rate improved, and spontaneous, irregular respirations ensued. Emergency medical services (EMS) arrived shortly thereafter, intubated his trachea, and initiated manual ventilation. He arrives in the PICU with stable hemodynamics, but still unconscious. The parents ask if anything can be done to improve their son's chance of a favorable neurologic recovery. They specifically mention hearing that hypothermia may be useful in this situation.

Case 2

A 6-month-old girl is being treated in the PICU for pneumococcal sepsis. She is on full mechanical ventilatory support and requires dopamine and epinephrine to maintain a satisfactory blood pressure, despite aggressive fluid resuscitation. The medical student on the service, having just completed an adult ICU rotation, asks if her adrenal function has been evaluated. She states that, in adults, adrenal insufficiency in septic shock portends a very poor outcome. An adrenocorticotropic hormone stimulation test is performed using 250 mcg corticotropin. The patient's serum cortisol concentration increases from 15 mcg/dL at baseline to 20 mcg/dL 60 mins after receiving corticotropin. What does this mean?

Case 3

A 7-year-old, developmentally delayed boy is admitted to the PICU with aspiration pneumonitis. He is tachypneic with labored breathing, anxious but alert. On a non-rebreather face mask, his oxygen saturations are 90%. His chest radiograph demonstrates diffuse airspace disease. With his progressive course, preparations are made to intubate and initiate mechanical ventilation. The parents ask if any other means of respiratory support is available so that invasive ventilation can be avoided.

INTRODUCTION

As intensivists in our PICUs, we are faced with the above situations and questions daily. How would such questions be addressed at the time of the first edition of this textbook? We would have relied on a combination of our experience, discussions with colleagues, textbooks, or memory of a study in the medical literature. In this "classic" paradigm, few qualms were expressed about our reliance on unsystematic, anecdotal observations to draw conclusions. We believed that a thorough grounding in pathophysiology should usually enable us to determine the proper management of patients and that common sense was sufficient to adequately evaluate new therapies and diagnostic tests. Guidelines could be developed based on the "expertise" of content knowledge and clinical experience. This approach was not considered "anti-intellectual." Indeed, the more experience one had, the more wisdom one acquired, and great respect has always been (and should always be) afforded to the wise among us. However, the learning curve associated with gaining such wisdom was long and not very steep.

Beginning formally in 1992, the paradigm shifted. Guyatt et al. coined the term *evidence-based medicine* (EBM) and formed the Evidence-Based Medicine Working Group (4). EBM "is the conscientious, explicit, and judicious use of current best evidence in making decisions about the care of individual patients" (15). EBM involves the integration of this evidence with clinical experience and each patient's preferences and values. Instinct, experience, knowledge of disease mechanisms, and common sense are necessary but insufficient to properly evaluate and apply new therapies, diagnostic modalities, or prediction tools. Rules of evidence interpretation must be learned to practice EBM; the rules were developed and disseminated during more than a decade of publishing in the *Journal of the American Medical Association (JAMA)* in what has become the living handbook of EBM: *The Users' Guides to the Medical Literature* (11). Now available in print (5,17), on the web (3), and as an interactive textbook online (19), these guides outline core methods for the critical appraisal of evidence (Step 3 below).

Five steps are involved in the EBM approach to patient care:

1. Framing the sometimes nebulous need for information into a structured "clinical question."
2. Tracking down the available evidence to answer the question through a focused search of the medical literature.
3. Critically appraising the evidence identified for its validity (degree of freedom from bias), results (magnitude of effect), and applicability to the patient.
4. Integrating the appraised evidence with our experience and the patient's unique situation and values.
5. Self-appraising of our effectiveness in steps 1–4.

EBM's roots extend into the 1980s, when the science of clinical epidemiology was codified by Sackett et al. at McMaster University in Hamilton, Ontario. Their landmark text, *Clinical Epidemiology: A Basic Science for Clinical Medicine,* published in 1985, described the quantitative tools that would become the "acronym soup" of EBM: RR (relative risk), RRR (relative risk reduction), NNT (number needed to treat), etc. (14). From just two citations in the National Library of Medicine's PubMed (MEDLINE) in 1992 to 2977 in 2005, EBM has grown to a worldwide phenomenon, to the extent that the basic paradigm is now rarely questioned. Although many now espouse its value, in assessing its impact, it is difficult to submit EBM to the same rigorous methodology that it requires of the questions that it is used to answer. Furthermore, EBM has several clear limitations.

Some critiques can be answered readily:

- EBM has been pejoratively labeled "cookbook medicine." EBM explicitly calls for the integration of the uniqueness of each patient—both their pathophysiology and their values—in determining how to apply evidence from clinical research.
- EBM has been maligned as a tool of administrators determined to cut costs by refusing to pay for therapies not "proven effective" by EBM standards. EBM, however, is just as likely to proffer support for very expensive interventions as it is for low-cost care.

EBM engenders more troublesome questions. Despite a huge increase in the publication of well-designed and clinically meaningful research studies over the past several decades, many questions remain for which valid evidence simply does not exist. In our field of Pediatric Critical Care in particular, it has been difficult to conduct the type of definitive, randomized, controlled trials that should form our evidence base. Two suggested solutions are: (a) This deficiency can often be addressed by careful consideration of trials in other populations, such as neonates or adults; and (b) this reality should, and indeed has, spurred our community to aggressively form networks and seek funding to conduct the multicentered trials necessary to address this void.

Another concern, given the often hectic nature of our practice, asks how one should find the time to create clinical questions, search for trials, properly and critically appraise them, and apply them judiciously to our patient care—in "real time?" The criticism has been leveled, therefore, that EBM is an "ivory tower" exercise and that it is unrealistic to expect busy practitioners to accomplish regularly. This criticism is also not easily deflected, because practicing EBM "by the book" does require additional time. Two answers to this concern are: (a) Many of our patients have similar conditions, so that once we learn the "correct" answers to our clinical questions the first time, we need not reinvent the wheel with each subsequent patient (although we must remain attuned to possible changes from new research findings); and (b) "shortcuts" do exist, such as tapping into preappraised sources of evidence, so that all that needs to be critically considered is the applicability of the evidence to each individual patient (see "Secondary Evidence Sources").

GETTING STARTED: THE CLINICAL QUESTION

The first step in the EBM approach to obtain focused evidence involves creating a structured "clinical question," which usually takes the "PICO" format: *Population, Intervention, Comparison* (if applicable), and *Outcomes.* Thus, a well-designed clinical question for our first case scenario might

read: In children with acute hypoxic-ischemic encephalopathy (population), does hypothermia (intervention), compared to standard supportive care (comparison), reduce mortality and improve neurologic recovery (outcome)? A poorly phrased clinical question for this case might read: What is the role of hypothermia in the PICU? Or, Is hypothermia neuroprotective? These make for nice (nonsystematic) review article titles, but their lack of focus leads us on an unnecessarily inefficient literature search. The importance of focus and the need for efficiency will be clear shortly.

TYPES OF EVIDENCE

Before we begin to search for evidence to answer our questions, we must clearly define the types of evidence available. Although several classification schemes could be considered, we will simply refer to the evidence sources as "primary" or "secondary."

Primary evidence refers to individual, or original, clinical research trials that report the findings of therapeutic intervention studies, tests of new diagnostic technology or prediction tools, and the like. These original trials form the base of an evidence pyramid (**Fig. 8.1**). They are the foundation of whether and how we can and/or should draw conclusions about the validity, results, and applicability of the best available evidence from clinical research. The pure EBM paradigm has the modern clinician searching for, identifying, and then critically appraising an original research study to decide the best care for his patient.

In many cases, however, trials are not particularly well designed or executed, leaving serious validity questions. Ultimately, if a trial is truly so potentially biased that we should not trust the results (which should be discernible from a critical appraisal of the trial), the results should not influence us in either direction. However, other problems are associated with using original trials in the practice of EBM.

Sometimes clinical trials have too few subjects to detect a treatment difference (inadequate "power"); such "negative"

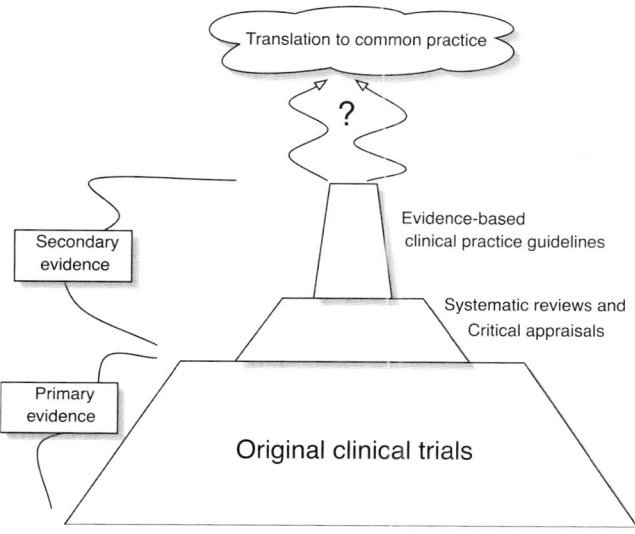

FIGURE 8.1. The evidence pyramid.

trials also do not help our decision making, because they do not rule in or out a significant treatment effect. In addition, several trials may be published on a given question, and reading, appraising, and integrating them all would clearly constitute an improbable bedside exercise. What is the solution to these issues?

Secondary evidence sources include preappraised evidence, systematic reviews, and evidence-based clinical practice guidelines. The busy clinician may not need to perform a rigorous critical appraisal of a primary research paper if such an appraisal has already been performed and published. In our field, for example, since 1997, the PedsCCM Evidence-based Journal Club has posted hundreds of critical appraisals of relevant studies, all easily accessible on the PedsCCM web site (PedsCCM.org). Many other such "journal clubs" exist on the web and serve as one of the "shortcuts" to practicing EBM.

Systematic reviews represent the next and even more valuable level of secondary evidence, depending on the question at hand. A systematic review, unlike a typical general topic review, is focused on a defined clinical question and follows a rigorous (and reproducible) methodology in searching for, including and excluding, assessing, and summarizing original clinical trials. A systematic review would (or should) almost certainly never be entitled: "Myocarditis in 2006: A Review." However, an overview (synonymous term for systematic review) could well carry the title: "Immunoglobulin Therapy for Myocarditis: A Systematic Review." When specific quantitative analysis is undertaken to pool the results of numerous trials in a systematic review, it constitutes a *meta-analysis*. All meta-analyses are systematic reviews, but the converse is not necessarily the case. In a properly completed systematic review, a large amount of evidence is filtered, appraised, and summarized.

The third and highest level of secondary evidence can be found as evidence-based *clinical practice guidelines*. Organizations, hospitals, and government agencies may have already undertaken a full evidence-based review of a clinical question and appraised and synthesized the results as a practice guideline. The strength of the recommendations flows from the strength of the evidence. Inconsistent systems have been used to grade evidence and recommendations, but it is hoped that a more consistent toolset will be adopted in time (2).

To add yet another level, *users' guides* are also available for systematic reviews (10) and clinical practice guidelines to enable us to appraise secondary evidence sources (8,20).

SEARCHING FOR THE EVIDENCE

MEDLINE from the National Library of Medicine is the premiere database of citations and abstracts of the biomedical literature and is freely available online via PubMed (**Table 8.1** provides a list of resources and URLs). The built-in EBM filters, accessible from the "clinical queries" link, are particularly helpful for focusing searches in this huge database. These filters allow very focused searching for study type (e.g., therapy, diagnosis, etc.) as well as the ability to set the search to be very sensitive or more specific. Limits are easily defined to find results based on systematic reviews, age groups, and other search criteria. PubMed's LinkOut service provides direct links from the abstracts to a manuscript's full-text version, usually on the publisher's web site. (Accessing the full-text version often requires a personal or institutional subscription to the journal.)

The *Cochrane Collaboration* is an international organization dedicated to producing and maintaining a database of systematic reviews on virtually every aspect of healthcare. The Cochrane Database of Systematic Reviews (CDSR) is its primary product and should be part of the repertoire of all EBM practitioners. Although the CDSR is now indexed in MEDLINE, a personal or institutional subscription is necessary to access the full reviews.

Evidence-based clinical practice guidelines can be found via MEDLINE searches if they have been published in cited journals. Organizations, such as the Society of Critical Care Medicine and the American Academy of Pediatrics offer their guidelines freely online. The National Guideline Clearinghouse is a valuable service of the US Department of Health and Human Services.

An increasing number of hybrid subscription products can be found online that offer a range of evidence types, obscuring the boundary between primary and secondary sources. MEDLINE can also be searched from proprietary interfaces, such as those provided by OVID, SkolarMD, or MD Consult. These subscription products offer many other features, including full-text journal and textbook access, as well as the ability to search across different types of resources. Many also offer unique EBM filter tools, similar to the "clinical queries" feature of PubMed noted earlier. Focused and succinct, evidence-based topic summaries can also be found in Clinical Evidence and UptoDate Online.

APPRAISING AND APPLYING THE EVIDENCE

The core exercise of EBM is the critical appraisal of evidence, and the handbook (some would say "bible") of critical appraisal is the *JAMA* series noted earlier: *The Users' Guides to the Medical Literature*. Although different evidence types require different specific criteria, all can be organized into three major questions: Is the study valid? What are the results? Are the results applicable to my patient? Let us address the three case scenarios presented at the beginning of the chapter as exercises in formulating clinical questions, searching for, appraising, and applying the evidence.

Therapy Article Appraisal

In Case 1, to respond to the parents' question regarding the use of hypothermia in their son with nonintentional hanging injury, the following focused clinical question would be formulated: In children with hypoxic-ischemic encephalopathy, does hypothermia improve outcome? A MEDLINE search using the key words "hypothermia" and "hypoxic-ischemic encephalopathy," limiting the search to randomized, controlled trials, produced seven studies, all conducted in neonates. Retrieving and reviewing the most recent trial, "Whole-Body Hypothermia for Neonates with Hypoxic-Ischemic Encephalopathy," published by the NICHD Neonatal Research Network (16), showed that the objective of the study was to determine whether whole-body cooling initiated before 6 hrs of age and continued for 72 hrs in term infants with moderate to severe encephalopathy would reduce death or disability at 18 to 22 months of age, as compared with usual care. As outlined in the

TABLE 8.1

DATABASES AND EBM RESOURCES ON THE WORLDWIDE WEB

Resource type	Name	URL	Notes
MEDLINE	PubMed	http://www.pubmed.gov	See clinical queries tool
	OVID*	http://www.ovid.com/	Textbooks, EBM filters
	MD Consult*	http://www.mdconsult.com	Textbooks, other tools
	SkolarMD*	http://md.skolar.com/	Textbooks, EBM resources
Users' guides to the medical literature	Users' Guides Interactive*	http://www.usersguides.org	Interactive features complement original articles
	Canadian Centre for Health Evidence	http://www.cche.net/usersguides/main.asp	
Systematic reviews	Cochrane Collaboration	http://www.cochrane.org	Full-text requires subscription
Evidence-based reviews	Clinical evidence*	http://www.clinicalevidence.com/	
	UptoDate*	http://www.utdol.com	
EB Journal Club	PedsCCM EBJC	http://pedsccm.org	
Clinical practice guidelines	National Guideline Clearinghouse	http://www.guidelines.gov	
	American Academy of Pediatrics	http://aappolicy.aappublications.org/	Also policy statements, clinical reports
	Society of Critical Care Medicine/American College of Critical Care Medicine	http://www.sccm.org	
Search tools/ directories	Google Scholar	http://scholar.google.com	
	HealthLinks University of Washington	http://healthlinks.washington.edu/hsl/liaisons/schnall/pediatrics.html	
Diagnostic decision support	Isabel*	http://www.isabelhealthcare.com	
EBM tools/Resources	Centre for Evidence Based Medicine	http://www.cebm.utoronto.ca/dev/ebmcalc1_7/ebmcalc_v1_7.html	Online and PDA versions
	Netting the Evidence	http://www.shef.ac.uk/scharr/ir/netting/	
	WWWeb Epidemiology and EBM Sources	http://www.vetmed.wsu.edu/courses-jmgay/EpiLinks.htm	Very comprehensive resource list
	Resources for practicing EBM	http://pedsccm.org	
Online EBM tutorial	Introduction to EBM	http://www.hsl.unc.edu/services/tutorials/ebm/index.htm	From Duke University and UNC-Chapel Hill

*Subscription (institutional or personal) required.

Users' Guides to the Medical Literature series, you undertake a critical appraisal of this study. The three major steps of the appraisal are (a) determining the study's validity, (b) summarizing the results, and (c) determining the applicability of the results to your patient.

Are the Results of the Study Valid?

Validity is a measure of how well the results of a study represent the true magnitude and direction of the treatment's effect, free from a number of potential sources of bias. For example, many factors in addition to total-body cooling are likely to influence the outcome of patients with hypoxic-ischemic encephalopathy. For the study results to be valid, the study must be designed in such a way as to prevent these other factors from confounding patient outcomes in a systematic way. Several questions can be asked to help assess the validity of the hypothermia trial (6):

Was the Assignment of Patients to Treatments Randomized? Random assignment to treatment and control groups makes it more likely that factors known to influence outcome (e.g., severity of illness) and unknown factors will be evenly distributed between the two groups at the start of the trial. Infants enrolled in the hypothermia study were randomly assigned to whole-body cooling to 33.5°C for 72 hrs or normothermia.

Were All Patients Who Entered the Trial Properly Accounted for and Attributed at Its Conclusion? Follow-up was achieved in all patients in the hypothermia group (100%) and in all but 3 of the patients in the normothermia group (96.5%). Patients lost to follow-up may have different outcomes than do those remaining in a trial. For example, if patients lost to follow-up in the normothermia group failed to keep their appointments because they had recovered completely, and if these patients were dropped from the analysis, the lack of follow-up would cause the normothermia group to appear to have a worse outcome than if the lost patients had been included. Keeping patients in the groups to which they were randomized, rather than excluding those who were noncompliant with therapy or lost to follow-up is referred to as an *intention-to-treat analysis*.

Were Patients, Health Workers, and Study Personnel Blind to Treatment? Blinding helps to prevent researchers' opinions about the experimental treatment from influencing their assessment of patient outcomes. In the hypothermia trial, caregivers were not blinded, but those who assessed patient outcomes were unaware of the group assignments.

Were the Groups Similar at the Start of the Trial? As mentioned, many factors other than the experimental therapy can influence patient outcomes. Ideally, these other factors should be similar between groups at the start of the trial. Randomization helps to ensure a balance of baseline patient characteristics between groups in large clinical trials. However, if specific patient characteristics are known or suspected to be important confounding variables, the investigators should demonstrate that the treatment and control groups were similar with respect to these variables. In the hypothermia trial, both groups were similar in such baseline characteristics as age, sex, weight, and severity of illness.

Aside from the Experimental Intervention, were the Groups Treated Equally? Cointerventions may also confound patient outcomes. In some trials, explicit treatment protocols for major cointerventions are employed. Major cointerventions and their use should at least be described. Particularly in nonblinded studies, the differential use of cointerventions between groups can confound results. In the hypothermia trial, infants in the two groups received the same monitoring of vital signs and surveillance for organ dysfunction. Protocols for the use of oxygen, mechanical ventilation, sedation, and other treatments were not explicitly mentioned.

What Were the Results?

An excellent review of how to evaluate results is available from Guyatt et al. (7).

How Large was the Treatment Effect? Death or moderate-to-severe disability occurred in 45 of 102 (44%) infants in the hypothermia group, compared with 64 of 103 (62%) in the control group. Dichotomous outcomes (i.e., survived vs. died) can be best described in terms of the absolute risk reduction (ARR), RR, RRR, and NNT. ARR is the arithmetic difference in rates of poor outcomes between the treatment and control groups. In this study, the ARR is 62%–44%, or 18%. RR can otherwise be defined as the ratio of risk between treated group: control group; here, the RR is 44/62, or 0.71. RRR is the proportional reduction in the rates of bad outcomes between treatment and control groups. In the study under consideration, the RRR is (62 – 44)/62, or 0.29. The NNT is the number of patients who need to be treated to achieve one additional favorable outcome; NNT is calculated as 1/ARR. Here, the NNT is 1/0.18, or 6 (the NNT is, by convention, typically rounded up to the next whole number). An advantage of ARR and NNT is that these metrics take into account the prevalence rate in untreated patients, whereas RR and RRR do not. For example, if death or disability occurred in 4.4% of hypothermia-treated patients and in 6.2% of controls, the RR and RRR would remain as 0.71

and 0.29, respectively. However, ARR would be markedly decreased to 6.2% to 4.4%, or 1.8%, and NNT would increase to 60.

How Precise was the Estimate of the Treatment Effect? The magnitude of the treatment effect reported in a study is really an estimate of the true effect based on the sample of patients included in the trial. Confidence intervals (CIs) help us to evaluate how precise that estimate is. In the hypothermia trial, the 95% CI for ARR for death or disability is 4%–31%. The true ARR may be as low as 4% or as high as 31%, but we can be 95% sure that the true value for ARR lies within this range. The 95% CIs for RR, RRR, and NNT are 0.54–0.95, 0.05–0.46, and 3–22, respectively. Although these ranges are rather wide, indicating a lack of precision, the lower 95% CI of the ARR is greater than zero, enabling us to conclude that a "statistically significant" difference exists in rates of poor outcomes between the two groups. We must then decide whether such a small difference is worth the burden of therapy. It may seem "worth it" to treat as few as three infants with hypothermia to prevent one poor outcome, but is it still "worth it" if we must treat 22 infants?

Will the Results Help Me in Caring for My Patient?

Can the Results be Applied to My Patient Care? Patients to whom we intend to apply the results of a trial should be similar to the patients included in the trial. We must consider how similar the boy with nonintentional hanging injury is to the patients enrolled in the hypothermia study. Study patients were infants of at least 36 weeks' gestational age, <6 hrs old, with severe acidosis or perinatal complications, who underwent resuscitation at birth and who had moderate-to-severe encephalopathy. Our patient is older, and the mechanism of injury is different. Whether the results can be applied to our patient is unknown.

Were All Clinically Important Outcomes Considered? Many clinical trials only evaluate physiologic markers as outcomes. Unless strong evidence supports the use of such markers as good surrogates for the outcomes that are important to patients, families, and physicians (e.g., mortality, disability), such studies should be viewed with caution. The medical literature is replete with examples of how a particular therapy was shown to improve a physiologic marker, only to be later shown to increase morbidity or mortality. In the hypothermia trial, several secondary outcomes were considered, including disabling cerebral palsy, blindness, and hearing impairment. Applying a neuroprotective strategy may be associated with a risk of reducing mortality while increasing the number of survivors with disabilities. However, both mortality and disabilities tended to decrease in hypothermia-treated infants.

Are the Likely Treatment Benefits Worth the Potential Harms and Costs? This question takes into consideration not only the risks and benefits of therapy, but also the patient's and family's preferences and values. In the hypothermia trial, infants who received the therapy had better outcomes, whereas the incidence of serious adverse events was similar between groups. However, because the applicability of these findings to our patient is unknown, treatment with hypothermia may or may not be indicated.

Scenario Resolution

Based on a review of this valid and meaningful randomized, controlled trial, the boy undergoes total body cooling in the PICU. Because a question remains regarding the applicability of the results to this patient, the practitioner should explain to the parents that cooling may or may not improve the boy's chance of survival or reduce disabilities.

Prediction Article Appraisal

Regarding the case of the 6-month-old girl with pneumococcal sepsis (Case 2), the physician is unsure of how to answer the medical student's question and asks her to look up the answer and present it to the team. The physician helps the student to formulate the following focused clinical question: Does adrenal insufficiency predict mortality in children with septic shock? The student, pressed for time, goes directly to PedsCCM.org to try to find an existing critical appraisal on the topic (18). Using the search term "adrenal insufficiency," she finds two articles that have been reviewed. She downloads the article that includes "children" in the title and presents it to the group. The article, "Absolute and Relative Adrenal Insufficiency in Children with Septic Shock" by Pizarro et al., aims to evaluate the incidence of adrenal insufficiency and determine the relationship between adrenal function, the development of catecholamine-resistant septic shock, and outcome in children (12).

Are the Results of the Study Valid?

Prognosis refers to the possible outcomes of a disease and their frequency. Prognostic factors are patient characteristics such as symptoms, signs, or laboratory tests that can be used to predict outcome. Combinations of prognostic factors, or prediction tools, can be developed to categorize heterogeneous groups of patients into different levels of risk for a specified outcome. In the septic shock study by Pizarro et al., several factors, including corticotropin response, are evaluated as potential predictors of two outcomes—the development of catecholamine-resistant shock and mortality. To assess the validity of a prediction tool, the following questions must be answered (13):

Was a Representative Group of Patients Completely Followed-up? Prediction tools may perform well in one population and poorly in another. Therefore, the population studied must be representative of the target population to which the tool will be applied. Consecutive or random inclusion of patients helps to prevent selection bias. The septic shock study included 57 children consecutively admitted to the PICU who met criteria established by the American College of Critical Care Medicine (ACCM) for the diagnosis of septic shock. All patients were followed until death or PICU discharge. Such complete follow-up is important because if patients lost to follow-up have a better or worse outcome than other study patients, the prediction tool may not perform as well when applied in another population.

Were All Potential Predictors Included? Investigators must decide which variables to test as potential predictors of an outcome. In general, the more relevant the variables included, the more likely a satisfactory prediction tool will result. In the septic shock study, patients were categorized

into four groups based on their baseline cortisol level and response to corticotropin as follows: (a) absolute adrenal insufficiency (baseline cortisol <20 mcg/dL, with increase ≤9 mcg/dL), (b) relative adrenal insufficiency (baseline cortisol ≥20 mcg/dL with increase ≤9 mcg/dL), (c) adequate adrenal response with elevated baseline cortisol (baseline cortisol ≥20 mcg/dL, with increase >9 mcg/dL), and (d) adequate adrenal response without elevated baseline cortisol (baseline cortisol <20 mcg/dL, with increase >9 mcg/dL). Patients were also categorized into three groups based on their need for cardiovascular support: (a) fluid-responsive shock, (b) fluid-refractory dopamine/dobutamine-responsive shock, and (c) catecholamine-resistant shock. Other potential predictors assessed were the presence of chronic disease and multiple organ failure.

Did the Investigators Test the Independent Contribution of Each Predictor Variable? Clinical variables are often correlated with each other. To show that a variable is an independent predictor of outcome, its predictive power must remain when other potential predictors are taken into consideration. For example, the presence of catecholamine-resistant shock was associated with death when evaluated as a single variable using univariate statistics. However, when chronic disease, multiple organ failure, and catecholamine-resistant shock were evaluated using multiple regression analysis, catecholamine resistance was no longer a significant predictor of mortality. The independence of a predictor variable is a function of the set of variables with which it is being evaluated. For example, catecholamine resistance might be an independent predictor of mortality if evaluated as part of a completely different set of variables.

Were Outcome Variables Clearly and Objectively Defined? For patient outcomes to be reliably assessed, outcomes should be clearly and objectively defined. Also, knowledge of the presence or absence of predictors in individual patients may lead to bias in the assessment of outcomes. In the septic shock study, two outcomes were considered. The first outcome, catecholamine-resistant shock, was defined using ACCM criteria. The second outcome, mortality, was obvious and objective. Clinicians were blinded to the results of the corticotropin stimulation test until after study completion.

What Are the Results?

Prediction tools with a few easily assessed predictor variables that place patients into clear outcome categories are most useful.

What are The Prediction Tools? Two prediction tools were reported. First, corticotropin response (≤9 mcg/dL) and multiple organ failure independently predicted catecholamine-resistant shock. Second, chronic illness and multiple organ failure independently predicted mortality. Importantly, corticotropin response did not predict mortality on univariate or multivariate testing.

How Well does the Model Categorize Patients into Different Levels of Risk? The four categories of adrenal response placed patients into four categories of risk for catecholamine-resistant shock. Of those patients with absolute adrenal insufficiency, 100% had catecholamine-resistant shock. Of those with relative adrenal insufficiency, 80% had catecholamine-resistant shock. Of those with adequate adrenal response and elevated baseline cortisol, 60% had catecholamine-resistant shock. Of those with adequate adrenal response without elevated baseline cortisol, 30% had catecholamine-resistant shock. When patients with absolute and relative adrenal insufficiency were combined (corticotropin response ≤9 mcg/dL) and compared with those having adequate response (>9 mcg/dL), the RR of catecholamine-resistant shock was 1.88 (95% CI, 1.26–2.79).

Patients with absolute and relative adrenal insufficiency tended to have higher mortality (50% and 53%, respectively), compared with those having adequate adrenal response, with or without elevated baseline cortisol (33% and 24%, respectively); however, the relationship was not significant. The RR of death for patients with adrenal insufficiency compared with those having adequate adrenal response was 1.72 (95% CI, 0.97–3.06).

What is the Confidence Level in the Estimates of Risk? The precision of the estimates of relative risk are again reflected in the CIs. The relative risk of developing catecholamine-resistant shock for septic patients with adrenal insufficiency may be as low as 1.26 or as high as 2.79, based on a 95% CI. The RR of death for patients with adrenal insufficiency may be as low as 0.97 or as high as 3.06. Of note, a CI for relative risk that includes 1 indicates that no statistically significant difference in outcome between groups is observed. Given that the lower limit of the CI for mortality is <1 in this sample, confirmation of the study's findings in another sample of pediatric patients with septic shock appears warranted before widespread application of these findings in clinical practice.

Can You Apply the Prediction Tool in Your Patient Care?

Does the Tool Maintain its Predictive Power in a New Sample of Patients? Prediction tools are derived using one sample of patients and, ideally, are tested in another sample. If the prediction tool maintains its accuracy in the new sample, confidence in the tool's usefulness increases. In the septic shock study, the predictors were not tested in a new sample of patients, leaving uncertainty in the tool's validity.

Are Your Patients Similar to Those Used in Deriving and Validating the Tool? If the patient populations used to derive and validate the prediction tool differ greatly from your patient population, the tool may not perform well in your patients. For example, chronic disease was present in 74% of patients in the septic shock study, with the most frequent diagnoses being malignancy (16%), hepatic failure (14%), and neurologic illness (11%). Therefore, the prediction tool may not perform well for the previously healthy pediatric patient presenting with septic shock.

Does the Tool Improve Your Clinical Decisions? Prediction tools are most useful if they can be shown to improve decision making beyond clinician judgment. The septic shock study provides evidence that adrenal insufficiency is common in children with septic shock (i.e., 44% of patients) and that it is associated with catecholamine-resistant shock. Whether hydrocortisone replacement will reduce catecholamine-resistant shock or mortality in septic patients cannot be answered from this study.

Scenario Resolution

The patient has catecholamine-resistant shock and absolute adrenal insufficiency based on the definitions used in this study. Based on the literature review, the physician suspects that her chance of mortality is high. Therapy is initiated with hydrocortisone, with uncertainty as to whether it will improve her outcome. Practicing EBM at the bedside does not always result in definitive answers. Clinicians must continue to incorporate pathophysiology and clinical experience into the decisions they make.

Systematic Review Appraisal

In the case of the 7-year-old, developmentally delayed boy with respiratory failure (Case 3), the following focused clinical question can be formulated: In children with hypoxemic respiratory failure, does noninvasive ventilation (compared to invasive ventilation) result in improved outcomes? A PubMed search, using the key words "noninvasive ventilation" and "acute hypoxemic respiratory failure," produces 47 articles on the subject. Rather than reviewing all of the articles, the search strategy is limited to include "reviews" only. The limit setting for "meta-analysis" on PubMed is occasionally too restrictive and will not include all systematic reviews. The article by Keenen et al., "Does noninvasive positive pressure ventilation improve outcome in acute hypoxemic respiratory failure? A systematic review" (9) is chosen. The objective of the article is to systematically review the randomized, controlled trials of patients with acute hypoxemic respiratory failure unrelated to cardiogenic pulmonary edema, to determine the effect of the addition of noninvasive positive-pressure ventilation (NPPV) to standard therapy on endotracheal intubation, ICU and hospital lengths of stay, and mortality. A critical appraisal of the review is undertaken that assesses the validity, results, and applicability in a manner similar to the therapy and prediction appraisals described earlier (11) and notes the direct parallel of these questions to similar assessments of primary trials.

Are the Results of the Overview Valid?

Did the Overview Address a Focused Clinical Question? The objective of a systematic review should be clearly stated so that the reader can know whether the review is applicable to the clinical question he is trying to answer. As demonstrated by the Keenan review, study objectives are often best stated in terms of the relationship between an exposure (i.e., NPPV), and one or more outcomes (i.e., endotracheal intubation, ICU days, hospital days, and mortality) in a specific population (i.e., patients with noncardiogenic acute hypoxemic respiratory failure).

Were the Criteria used to Select Articles for Inclusion Appropriate? The criteria used to select articles for inclusion in an evidence-based review should be explicitly described, analogous to the inclusion and exclusion criteria for patients in a primary clinical trial. Criteria for including trials in a review may include the exposures, outcomes, patients, and methodologic standards for each individual trial. Defining the inclusion criteria helps to prevent investigators from choosing studies that support their own opinions. In the NPPV review, selection criteria were well suited to answer the clinical question. Selection criteria were (a) comparison of NPPV and standard therapy to standard therapy alone, (b) outcomes of need for endotracheal intubation, length of ICU and hospital stay, and mortality, (c) study populations comprised mostly of patients with acute hypoxemic respiratory failure not associated with cardiogenic pulmonary edema or chronic obstructive pulmonary disease (COPD) and not requiring immediate ventilator support, and (d) randomized, controlled trials.

Is It Unlikely that Important Relevant Studies Were Missed? Searching several bibliographic databases and reference lists of identified articles and using personal communications are ways to ensure that relevant studies are not missed in a review. US physicians should appreciate that a minority of biomedical publications are cited in MEDLINE and that high-quality trials from around the world (not cited in MEDLINE) are rapidly increasing in volume. Personal communications with investigators in the field of inquiry can help to identify published trials that may otherwise have been missed, as well as studies that are still in press or otherwise unpublished. The analogy to primary clinical trials here is the recruitment strategy. For example, just as using a convenience sample of patients (i.e., only those admitted between 9 a.m. and 5 p.m.) may bias a primary study, searching only for published trials in MEDLINE may bias a systematic review. In the NPPV review, the authors searched MEDLINE, EMBASE, and the Cochrane Library. They searched abstracts from key professional meetings, reference lists from all identified studies, and contacted the first-named authors of some studies to help to identify studies not otherwise retrieved by their search strategy.

Was the Validity of the Included Studies Appraised? It is important to know whether or not the individual studies included in the review are of good quality. If the individual studies are not valid, confidence in the overall results of the review should be limited. Validity of the individual studies can be assessed by asking questions similar to those described earlier for therapy and prediction tools. The parallel between appraising systematic reviews and primary clinical trials here is obvious but more complex. No standards exist by which individual trials in a systematic review are measured, which leads to a varying quality of trials included in most reviews. In the NPPV review, the authors appraised the individual trials using 11 validity criteria. These included: randomization, concealment, blinding, patient selection, comparability of groups at baseline, treatment protocols, confounders, cointerventions, outcome definitions, extent of follow-up, and intention-to-treat analysis.

Were Assessments of Studies Reproducible? Authors of reviews must make many decisions, such as which trials to include, how valid the trials are, and what data to abstract from them. Knowing that these types of decisions were made independently by more than one author, and that they were agreed upon, increases our confidence in the results. The parallel issue here to the clinical trial is whether the clinical trial reported reproducibility of assessments between observers who made subjective measurements (i.e., radiographic assessments). Clinical trials often report agreement coefficients, such as kappa (κ) scores, or mention independent assessors and agreement by consensus. In the NPPV review, data abstractions and validity assessments were performed by two of the authors independently and in duplicate. Differences in opinion were resolved by consensus or by consulting a third investigator.

Were the Results Similar from Study to Study? We would have greater confidence in the results of a systematic review if we knew that the individual studies included in the review showed treatment effects that were all going in the same direction. In other words, if each of the individual studies showed a treatment benefit, we would have more confidence than if some studies showed benefit and others did not. Lack of consistency between studies can be due to differences in exposures, outcomes, patients, or study design, or can be due to chance alone. Statistical tests of homogeneity tell us whether differences in results between studies are likely due to chance or other study factors. In the NPPV review, significant heterogeneity between studies (differences likely not due to chance) was demonstrated for the effect of NPPV on endotracheal intubation rates. Statistically significant heterogeneity was not demonstrated for the other outcomes assessed. However, Keenan et al. suspected that clinically important heterogeneity was present, based on visual inspection and comparison of the plotted ARRs and CIs for each of the studies. Differences between studies were attributed primarily to differences in the study populations. It is important to regard quantitative results (i.e., meta-analyses) with suspicion if significant heterogeneity is identified. It may not be appropriate to combine such trials.

What Are the Results?

What are the Overall Results of the Overview? A systematic review attempts to provide an overall average effect of a therapy, prediction tool, or other exposure. The overall results are considered in the same way that the results from individual studies are considered. Systematic reviews should present results using summary measures that clearly show the clinical importance of the result. For example, for systematic reviews of a therapy, these measures would include ARRs, RRs, and NNTs. Some authors may weight individual studies included in the review according to their sample size or validity, with larger, more valid studies contributing more weight to the overall result. In the NPPV review, 763 studies were identified in the initial search. Of these, eight randomized, controlled trials with a total of 366 patients met the authors' inclusion criteria. Six of the trials included patients with COPD or cardiogenic pulmonary edema; however, the authors were able to obtain patient-specific data on patients without these diagnoses. Overall, NPPV was associated with a significantly lower rate of endotracheal intubation than standard therapy (ARR, 23%; 95% CI, 10%–35%), a reduction in ICU length of stay (1.9 days; 95% CI, 1–2.9 days), an increase in length of hospital stay (2.8 days; 95% CI, 0.9–4.7 days), and a reduction in ICU mortality (ARR, 17%; 95% CI, 8%–26%), with a trend toward lower hospital mortality (ARR, 10%; 95% CI, −7% to 27%). Subgroup analyses of trials that excluded patients with COPD or cardiogenic pulmonary edema showed similar results.

How Precise were the Results? CIs can be calculated to demonstrate the range of the average treatment effect across studies. In the NPPV study, the 95% CIs for the ARR for endotracheal intubation and ICU mortality are relatively wide; however, their lower limits still represent important clinical effects (i.e., ARR of 8% for ICU mortality). The 95% CI for ARR for hospital mortality includes zero, suggesting that hospital mortality may increase or decrease with the use of NPPV.

Will the Results Help Me in Caring for My Patients?

Can the Results be Applied to my Patient Care? An advantage of systematic reviews is that they typically include large numbers of patients with diverse clinical characteristics. If the results of individual studies included in the review are consistent, it is more likely that the overall results of the review will be applicable to your patient. However, in the NPPV study, we found important heterogeneity in the results between studies, probably due to differences in patient populations. For example, of the eight trials included in the review, two focused on immunocompromised patients, one on surgical patients after lung resection, one on community-acquired pneumonia, one on postextubation respiratory failure, and three on more diverse groups of patients. Also, all of the study patients were adults. Therefore, any application of the results to our patient should proceed with caution.

Were all Clinically Important Outcomes Considered? Although focused systematic reviews, like focused clinical trials, are more likely to demonstrate valid results, important clinical outcomes should not be ignored. In the NPPV study, such outcomes as cost, complications, and patients' comfort and sedation requirements were not considered.

Are the Benefits Worth the Costs and Potential Harm? Valid overviews can provide strong evidence regarding the effect of a therapy or other exposure on patient outcomes. In the NPPV study, however, a determination of overall benefit is difficult to make because of heterogeneity between included studies and the lack of information on such outcomes as complications and cost. Heterogeneity between studies suggests that specific populations may derive benefit from the application of NPPV, whereas others may not. When deciding to apply a therapy, clinicians must take patient and family preferences and concerns into consideration.

Scenario Resolution

Based on critical appraisal, it is explained to the parents that the risks and benefits of NPPV in children with aspiration pneumonitis are not known. The parents request that NPPV be tried because they are unsure as to whether endotracheal intubation is in the best interest of their child in light of his severe developmental delay. NPPV is instituted, and the boy's oxygen saturations increase to 98%. The physician and the parents then discuss options for care and decide on a further course of action should the boy's condition deteriorate.

BRINGING IT ALL TOGETHER

Evidence-based medicine is part of mainstream healthcare. The skills involved are core competencies for postgraduate medical training, as part of "practice-based learning" (1). Subspecialty residents (fellows) in pediatric critical care medicine training programs across the country (and internationally) are submitting critical appraisals to the PedsCCM Evidence-based Journal Club, in part, to fulfill these requirements. The challenge, then, is the consistent practice of EBM in the PICU over time.

Some challenges to practicing EBM in the PICU in real time have already been addressed. In addition to some of the solutions offered, the staff of each PICU—physicians and nurses—should consider a regular process of reviewing evidence with the goal of creating local evidence-based policies and procedures for sets of conditions for which national or international guidelines do not exist, thus accomplishing three objectives: (a) establishment (or reaffirmation) of the multidisciplinary approach to patient care in the PICU, (b) engagement all the key stakeholders in the PICU in the EBM process, and (c) establishment of a growing local library of care protocols and pathways to optimize consistency across providers. Although it has been difficult to prove in pediatric critical care, consistency of care in virtually every other aspect of healthcare has been shown to be synonymous with improved quality of care. This process may also serve to address the little-discussed fifth step of EBM—self-appraisal of effectiveness in practicing EBM.

Other "holes" in the EBM paradigm have no easy solutions. What if multiple primary studies exist with no systematic review to combine (if appropriate) the results? What happens when a large randomized, controlled trial is published that contradicts findings of an existing systematic review? How, exactly, should we apply the results of studies in adults to children? There are no pat answers to these difficult questions. We are left, ultimately, with recognizing EBM for what it truly is—a set of tools to supplement our clinical skills. EBM cannot and should not replace clinical judgment. It is not a cookbook to be blindly followed. Like any tool, sometimes it is very useful, and sometimes it is not.

CONCLUSIONS AND FUTURE DIRECTIONS

EBM requires ready access to evidence. It is almost quaint to read the early *Users' Guides to the Medical Literature*, which describe residents going to the medical library to search MEDLINE and photocopy studies from print journals. Computing power and networking capabilities have advanced exponentially in a decade. The tools to enable the practice of "point-of-care" evidence-based medicine are already here. Many PICUs have Internet-enabled wired or wireless workstations at the patient's bedside to enable direct database searching. Primary and secondary evidence sources can be accessed around the clock. Handheld devices and cell phones can either carry databases (a downloadable handheld version of the PedsCCM Evidence-based Journal Club is available) or connect to them. Limitations to evidence are no longer physical, but temporal. It still takes precious time to search, read, appraise, and apply evidence. Perhaps someday in the not-too-distant future, we will be able to make a call from our cell phones and have the evidence downloaded directly to our cerebrums, as "Trinity" does when she "learns" to fly a military helicopter with just a brief fluttering of her eyelids in the 1999 motion picture *The Matrix*. Until such time, EBM's role is much like Morpheus' guiding of Neo in the same movie: It can show us the door, but we have to walk through it.

KEY POINTS

■ Five steps are involved for the practitioner in the EBM approach to patient care: (a) framing a structured clinical question, (b) conducting a focused search of the literature to find the answer to the question, (c) appraising the evidence for its validity, results, and applicability to the patient, (d) integrating the evidence with practitioner's experience and patient's unique situation, and (e) the practitioner self-appraising his effectiveness in Steps a through d.

- A structured clinical question usually takes the PICO format: population, intervention, comparison, and outcomes.
- Types of evidence consist of primary sources (individual clinical research trials) and secondary sources (preappraised evidence, systematic reviews, and evidence-based clinical practice guidelines).
- Sources for the evidence include the National Library of Medicine (PubMed), the Cochrane Collaboration, and MEDLINE.
- The handbook of critical appraisal of evidence is *The Users' Guides to the Medical Literature.*
- The three question categories that all evidence must meet are: Is the study valid? What are the results? Are the results applicable to the patient? Specific subquestions differ based on the type of evidence being appraised.
- The skills involved in EBM are now among the core competencies for postgraduate medical training.

References

1. Accreditation Council for Graduate Medical Education. Common Program Requirements. (*Pediatrics*, February 2004). Available at: http://www.acgme.org/acWebsite/dutyHours/dh_dutyHoursCommonPR.pdf. Accessed March 28, 2006.
2. Atkins D, Best D, Briss PA, et al. GRADE Working Group. Grading quality of evidence and strength of recommendations. *Br Med J* 2004;328(7454):1490.
3. Centre for Health Evidence. Users' Guides to Evidence-Based Practice. Available from: http://www.cche.net/usersguides/main.asp. Accessed February 14, 2006.
4. Evidence-Based Medicine Working Group. Evidence-based medicine. A new approach to teaching the practice of medicine. *JAMA* 1992;268(17): 2420–5.
5. Guyatt G, Drummond R, eds. *Users' Guides to the Medical Literature: A Manual for Evidence-Based Clinical Practice.* Chicago: AMA Press, 2002.
6. Guyatt GH, Sackett DL, Cook DJ. Users' guides to the medical literature. II. How to use an article about therapy or prevention. A. Are the results of the study valid? Evidence-Based Medicine Working Group. *JAMA* 1993;270:2598–2601.
7. Guyatt GH, Sackett DL, Cook DJ. Users' guides to the medical literature. II. How to use an article about therapy or prevention. B. What were the results and will they help me in caring for my patients? Evidence-Based Medicine Working Group. *JAMA* 1994;271:59–63.
8. Hayward RSA, Wilson MC, Tunis SR, et al. Users' guides to the medical literature. VIII. How to use clinical practice guidelines A. Are the recommendations valid? *JAMA* 1995;274(7):570–4.
9. Keenan SP, Sinuff T, Cook DJ, et al. Does noninvasive positive pressure ventilation improve outcome in acute hypoxemic respiratory failure? A systematic review. *Crit Care Med* 2004;32:2516–23.
10. Oxman AD, Cook DJ, Guyatt GH. Users' guides to the medical literature. VI. How to use an overview. Evidence-Based Medicine Working Group. *JAMA* 1994;272(17):1367–71.
11. Oxman AD, Sackett DL, Guyatt GH. Users' guides to the medical literature. I. How to get started. The Evidence-Based Medicine Working Group. *JAMA* 1993;270(17):2093–5.
12. Pizarro CF, Troster EJ, Damiani D, et al. Absolute and relative adrenal insufficiency in children with septic shock. *Crit Care Med* 2005;33:855–9.
13. Randolph AG, Guyatt GH, Calvin JE, et al. Understanding articles describing clinical prediction tools. Evidenced Based Medicine in Critical Care Group. *Crit Care Med* 1998;26:1603–12.
14. Sackett DL, Haynes RB, Tugwell P, eds. *Clinical Epidemiology: A Basic Science for Clinical Medicine.* Boston: Little Brown, 1985.
15. Sackett DL, Rosenberg WM, Gray JA, et al. Evidence based medicine: What it is and what it isn't. *Br Med J* 1996;312(7023):71–2.
16. Shankaran S, Laptook AR, Ehrenkranz RA, et al. Whole-body hypothermia for neonates with hypoxic-ischemic encephalopathy. NICHHD Neonatal Research Network. *N Engl J Med* 2005;353:1574–84.
17. Straus SE, Richardson WS, Glasziou P, et al., eds. *Evidence-based Medicine: How to Practice and Teach EBM.* London: Elsevier, 2005.
18. The PedsCCM Evidence-Based Journal Club. Available from: http://pedsccm.org. Accessed February 14, 2006.
19. Users' Guides Interactive. Available from: http://www.usersguides.org. Accessed February 14, 2006.
20. Wilson MC, Hayward RSA, Tunis SR, et al. Users' guides to the medical literature. VIII. How to use clinical practice guidelines B. What are the recommendations and will they help you in caring for your patients? *JAMA* 1995;274(20):1630–2.

CHAPTER 9 ■ SEVERITY-OF-ILLNESS SCORING SYSTEMS

MURRAY M. POLLACK

Many issues face pediatric critical care that can be influenced by a severity-of-illness assessment. These include defining, measuring, and improving quality; understanding the importance of structures and processes of care; applying appropriate risk adjustment for both research and administrative studies; and aiding clinical decision making. Scoring systems, especially those that measure acuity or severity of illness, help in understanding and even solving many of these issues by assimilating and quantifying clinical data that are otherwise difficult to objectively summarize. Most scoring systems objectively measure severity of illness, either directly through derangements in physiologic status or indirectly through surrogate markers, such as therapies or diagnoses, and the many scoring systems calibrate these quantitative observations to a risk of a particular outcome, usually survival or death.

SCIENTIFIC FOUNDATIONS

Historic Perspective

The "modern" history of PICU scoring systems started with the Clinical Classification Scoring System, a subjective categorization of a patient's anticipated clinical needs, ranging from routine ward care (Category 1) to frequent physician and nursing assessments and therapeutic interventions (Category 4). Although the methodology is simple by today's standards, it established the basis of severity of illness as a concept related to both physiologic instability and amount of therapy. The Clinical Classification system was quickly followed by the Therapeutic Intervention Scoring System (TISS) (2). The fundamental concept underlying the TISS score was that, as sick patients worsened, they received more therapy, such as mechanical ventilation or vasoactive agent infusions; thus, the number and sophistication of therapies served as a surrogate for severity of illness. Initially, 76 therapies and monitoring techniques were graded from 1 to 4 based on the complexity, skill, and cost required to provide these modalities. The quantity of therapy (TISS points) was also significantly correlated to daily and total PICU cost. Both of these scoring systems were used in pediatric critical care evaluations. The TISS score still exists today, although the number of therapies have been reduced and objectivity has been added to the score (19). The TISS score is still useful as a means of tracking and quantifying the relative amount of therapy and costs and as a surrogate measure of severity of illness.

The concepts of sequential and multiple organ system failures (MOSF) were also important in the development of the concepts of severity of illness (1). The earliest reports of MOSF focused on patients who had undergone emergency thoraco-abdominal operations or who sustained multiple traumas. Importantly, the concepts of severity of illness were advanced by noting that mortality rates increased as the number of failed organ systems increased. Some researchers even suggested that the number of failed organ systems and the duration of organ system failures could be applied to individual patients, perhaps even defining a state of futility (10). Higher physiologic instability on admission was also correlated with a higher risk of developing MOSF. The MOSF syndrome was initially described in children in 1986 (40). Organ system failure has continued to be an important concept, with evolving pediatric methods to track the number, duration, and resolution of organ system failures (5).

Organ system failures have recently been proposed as an outcome measure. In that death is a relatively uncommon occurrence in PICUs, it is appealing to postulate that the number of organ failures or the temporal resolution of these organ failures could be a practical and more plentiful outcome variable. This is the conceptual approach taken by the Pediatric Logistic Organ Dysfunction (PELOD) score (13). Unfortunately, some of the validation data of the PELOD score required retraction, and the utility of the score at this time is in question (12).

Physiologic status was the conceptual basis for MOSF and the TISS score. Physiologic instability was the reason for the therapeutic needs, and physiologic status and therapeutic needs comprised the underlying bases of the definition of organ system failure. Conceptually, severity of illness may be considered a continuous variable with extremes of outcomes (survival, death) that occur at low and high values. The threshold value that determines the outcome is unknown and may vary from patient to patient. Intermediate outcomes may occur at intermediate points between intact survival and death; the elucidation of this issue represents, perhaps, the next breakthrough in severity-of-illness research. This concept of severity of illness has been exceptionally productive in pediatric, neonatal, and adult intensive care, using such scores as the Pediatric Risk of Mortality (PRISM), Score for Neonatal Acute Physiology (SNAP), Acute Physiology and Chronic Health Evaluation (APACHE), and many others. These scoring systems have become so common and useful in critical care literature that a PubMed search for any one of them generates literally thousands of references.

Development of Scoring Systems

Important steps in the development of a severity-of-illness scoring system include defining a clear and relevant outcome (dependent variable) and adhering to well-defined methodologic standards (15). The most commonly measured PICU outcomes are mortality, organ dysfunction, length of stay, and functional outcome.

The second step in developing a scoring system is to identify the predictor (independent) variables. To minimize observation bias, data elements used to create a score should be selected a priori and collected in a blinded manner from the outcome. The final selection of predictor variables and their relative weights or importance is accomplished statistically from candidate variables using a combination of expert opinion and statistical analyses. For example, in selecting predictor variables for a mortality prediction score, such variables as blood pressure, heart rate, temperature, mental status, and creatinine levels should be seriously considered because expert opinion determines their importance. These predictor variables must be available and reliably measured. Reliability may be assessed in two ways: when a measurement that one observer obtains for a predictor variable is remeasured by the same person (intraobserver reliability) or when it is remeasured by a different person (interobserver reliability). The different statistical measures of reliability depend on whether the variable is nominal [kappa (κ) statistic], ordinal (weighted κ statistic), or continuous (intraclass correlation coefficient). An example of a potentially unreliable variable is the Po_2/Fio_2 ratio because the actual or tracheal Fio_2, when delivered by face mask, is only an estimate, and children frequently do not have their face masks appropriately situated to reliably estimate the Fio_2.

The statistical methods for score development have become relatively routine. In the *univariate* step, the contribution of each variable or each variable range is tested for its relationship to the outcome without the effect of other variables. *Multivariable analysis* is the current statistical standard for both variable selection as well as the determination of the relative weights or variable coefficients in a prediction model. Variables that are significant in the univariate steps are combined in the multivariate step. Usually, rather liberal statistical criteria for inclusion of variables from the univariate analyses are used (e.g., $p < 0.30$). Multivariable logistic regression is most often utilized for dichotomous outcomes (including survival and death), multivariable linear regression analysis is most often utilized for continuous variables (e.g., length of stay), and multivariable linear analysis or quadratic discriminant function analysis is most often used for categorical outcomes (e.g., diagnoses) (6). The coefficients for the independent variables may be converted into the scoring system. Neural networks generally can only be used as prediction models and not scoring systems, because it is difficult to use neural networks to generate the weights needed to create a score. Other statistical techniques include recursive partitioning or classification trees, especially if particular variable thresholds or "cut points" are a priority in nonlinear and complex associations among the variables.

The univariate stage of the analysis provides useful insights for understanding the contribution of a single variable toward mortality risk (27). Listed in **Table 9.1** are the odds of dying (mortality odds ratio) for patients whose worst physiologic variable value is in the indicated range, compared with patients whose worst value falls in the midrange of survivors (40th–60th percentile) when no other information is known. Compare the relative importance of these variables to their relative importance in the PRISM III score, which has undergone

TABLE 9.1		

RELATIVE MORTALITY RISKS OF PHYSIOLOGIC ABNORMALITIES

Physiologic variable	Range	Mortality odds ratio
Respiratory rate (breaths/min)	>100	2.50
Heart rate (beats/min)	<75	3.49
Creatinine (mg/dL)	>0.90	14.59
Blood urea nitrogen (mg/dL)	>20	11.34
Total CO_2 (mmol/L)	<5	21.30
pH (units)	<7	30.89
Hemoglobin (g/L)	<6	6.87
Leukocytes (cells/mm^3)	>40,000	4.16
Glucose (mg/dL)	>400	12.79
Sodium (mmol/L)	>150	17.21
Pupils	Fixed and dilated	112.55
Coma	GCS score <8	19.11

The relative mortality risks for extremes of physiologic dysfunction of variables are shown without regard to other information (univariate analysis). Mortality odds ratio is the odds of dying for infants whose worst physiologic variable value (during the first 12 hrs of PICU care) falls in the range, compared to the odds of dying for patients whose worst value falls in the midrange of PICU survivors (40th–60th percentiles) when no other information is known. Data are shown for selected physiologic variable ranges. Data from Pollack MM, Patel KM, Ruttimann UE. The Pediatric Risk of Mortality III-Acute Physiology Score (PRISM III-APS): A method of acessing physiologic instability for pediatric intensive care unit patients. *J Pediatr* 1997;131:575–581.

the multivariate analysis step (**Table 9.2**) (26). Some variables, such as respiratory rate and hemoglobin, are not included because they lose significance in the multivariate analysis. Such variables as fixed and dilated pupils are almost four times more "predictive" than severe acidosis in the univariate analysis, but less than twice as "predictive" as severe acidosis in the multivariate analysis. Also note that some variables used for literally decades in severity scores (i.e., platelets, glucose) are intermittently "discovered" for their association to outcome, usually in a univariate analysis.

Care must be taken when developing a score or risk prediction model using multivariate analyses to avoid "overfitting"; that is, the creation of a model fitted to idiosyncrasies (noise) of the data. The likelihood that overfitting will occur is highest when the number of variables included in the analysis or in the score is relatively large compared to the size of the database. A common rule suggests that at least 10 outcome events (e.g., deaths) per independent variable be included in the analysis (more stringent) or prediction rule (less stringent). Data reduction techniques, including deleting variables known to have high measurement error, analyzing principal components, deriving summary indices, and clustering variables, have been described to avoid overfitting.

Internal validation, or validation of the score in population subset(s) from which the score was derived, is usually performed first because poor internal validation often predicts a model's failure to validate to an external data set. The three common methods for internal validation are data-splitting, cross-validation, and bootstrapping. In *data-splitting*, a random portion of the sample is used for the model development

TABLE 9.2

PRISM III SCORE

Cardiovascular and neurologic vital signs		
Systolic blood pressure (mm Hg)	Score = 3	Score = 7
Neonate	40–55	<40
Infant	45–65	<45
Child	55–75	<55
Adolescent	65–85	<65
Temperature	Score = 3	
	<33°C or >40°C	
Mental status	Score = 5	
	Stupor/coma or GCS <8	
Heart rate (beats per minute)	Score = 3	Score = 4
Neonate	215–225	>225
Infant	215–225	>225
Child	185–205	>205
Adolescent	145–155	>155
Pupillary reflexes	Score = 7	Score = 11
	One fixed	Both fixed

Acid–base, blood gases		
Acidosis (pH or total CO_2)	Score = 2	Score = 6
pH	7–7.28	<7
CO_2	5–16.9	<5
PCO_2 (mm Hg)	Score = 1	Score = 3
	50–75	>75
Alkalosis: Total CO_2 (mmol/L)	Score = 4	
	>34	
PaO_2 (mm Hg)	Score = 3	Score = 6
	42–49	<42

Chemistry tests	
Glucose	Score = 2
	>200 mg/dL or >11 mmol/L
Potassium (mmol/L)	Score = 3
	>6.9
Blood urea nitrogen (BUN)	Score = 3
Neonate	>11.9 mg/dL or >4.3 mmol/L
All other ages	>14.9 mg/dL or >5.4 mmol/L
Creatinine	Score = 2
Neonate	>0.85 mg/dL or >75 mcmol/L
Infant	>0.90 mg/dL or >80 mcmol/L
Child	>0.90 mg/dL or >80 mcmol/L
Adolescent	>1.30 mg/dL or >115 mcmol/L

Hematology tests			
White blood cell count (cells/mm^3)	Score = 4		
	<3,000		
Platelet count ($\times$ 10^3 cells/mm^3)	Score = 2	Score = 4	Score = 5
	100–200	50–99	<50
Prothrombin time (PT) or			
Partial thromboplastin time (PTT)	Score = 3		
Neonate	PT >22 or PTT >85		
All other ages	PT >22.0 or PTT >57.0		

Compare to Table 9.1 for the changing relative importance of physiologic abnormalities after multivariate statistical analysis. Other factors that contribute to mortality risk include nonoperative cardiovascular disease, chromosomal anomaly, cancer, previous PICU admission, pre-ICU CPR, postoperative, acute diabetes (e.g., DKA), and admission from an inpatient unit. GCS, Glasgow Coma Scale.

(training set), and the remainder is used for the model validation (validation set). *Cross-validation* is repeated data-splitting, which generates many training and validation data sets, and this technique is superior to data-splitting for small data sets. *Bootstrapping* involves testing the performance of the model on a large number of samples randomly drawn from the original sample, with replacement.

Ideally, the score should be validated in an independent (external) data set. However, when the scoring system is used to assess an issue such as "quality of care," there is no assurance that the external data set will have the identical quality of care as the data set used for model development. In these cases, internal validation may be the best that can be expected.

For scoring systems that predict a dichotomous outcome (e.g., survival, death), important measures of performance are the sensitivity, specificity, and positive and negative predictive values. For scoring systems that generate ordinal or continuous outcomes (e.g., probability of death), two essential and objective measures of a score's performance are discrimination and calibration. *Discrimination*, or the ability of a model to distinguish between outcome groups, is most often assessed by the area under the receiver operating characteristic (ROC) curve. This measure is also commonly referred to as the "c-statistic." The ROC area is a measure of how well a model separates those predicted to experience the outcome from those predicted not to experience the outcome. For example, the ROC for the PRISM score approximates 0.9 in most data sets. If all of the PRISM scores of survivors were placed in one bucket, all of the PRISM scores of deaths were placed in another bucket, and scores were randomly picked from each bucket, an ROC of 0.9 would mean that 90% of the time, the PRISM score of the death would be higher than that of the survivor. Chance performance results in an ROC of 0.5.

The *calibration* of a model is a comparison of the number of predicted outcomes with the number of actual outcomes for a range of prediction intervals. The most accepted method for measuring calibration is the goodness-of-fit statistic proposed by Lemeshow and Hosmer. Although the calibration of a scoring system is necessary in the data used to develop the score, deviations from calibration in independent data sets are more difficult to evaluate. Often, deviations from predicted are expected in independent datasets because of real differences between performances of the independent dataset and the reference dataset from which the model was developed.

An important concept during this era, when very large databases are common, is that scoring systems and their prediction algorithms are based on past data. At their very best, they are accurate for the time period that generated the data in the institution(s) that contributed the data. However, the future never exactly mirrors the past; as the databases get larger and larger, assessments of the differences between the numbers of predicted and expected outcomes will often be statistically significantly different. This difference may be caused by relatively insignificant differences in care that become evident only in very large data sets.

Scoring Systems

Neonatal PICU Severity Scores

Currently, two well-established neonatal scores are used for assessing severity of illness and mortality risk. The Clinical Risk Index for Babies (CRIB) was developed in the UK for infants with birth weights of <1,500 g (38). It is composed of only six variables: birth weight, gestational age, presence of congenital anomalies, highest and lowest appropriate inspired oxygen, and the worst base deficit collected in the first 12 hrs after birth. The SNAP was originally based on the pediatric Physiologic Stability Index (PSI), the first severity score of the PRISM series. SNAP II is a second-generation, physiology-based score for neonatal severity of illness developed from a very large multi-institutional group of NICUs in the US and Canada (31). SNAP II measures severity of illness in infants by utilizing physiologic data collected during the first 12 hrs of care. It consists of six items, including lowest mean blood pressure, lowest temperature, lowest pH, lowest PaO_2/FiO_2 ratio, urine output, and the presence of multiple seizures. SNAP II has also been modified for use as a mortality prediction model (SNAPPE II) by including birth weight, small-for-gestational age, and low Apgar Scores.

PICU Severity Scores

The acuity scoring systems most commonly used to predict mortality are the PRISM score (29), the PRISM III score (26), and the Pediatric Index of Mortality, second version (PIM II) (34).

The PRISM score initially started as the PSI, a quantitative score developed from the subjective assessments of intensivists concerning the importance of physiologic status. The PSI was simplified and objectivity was added, resulting in the PRISM score. PRISM III (see **Table 9.2**), the third generation of this scoring system, was a total revision of the physiologic variables and their ranges based on statistical criteria. It was originally developed on 11,165 patients from 32 different PICUs in the US. The mortality prediction algorithms are routinely updated, the last update being completed on over 19,000 patients. It is unique among pediatric scoring systems in that it is also central to methods to predict length of stay (32). PRISM III mortality risk assessments are made using the first 12 hrs of PICU care. Twelve hours of data collection ensures that over 90% of all laboratory tests collected will be captured at least once in the first 24 hrs after admission.

The PIM II scoring system was developed from 14 ICUs and PICUs from Australia, New Zealand, and the UK. PIM II requires 10 variables collected from the time of initial patient contact by the ICU team (which could also include the emergency department stay or transport time) up to the first hour after ICU admission. Compared to PRISM III, PIM II is less likely to be biased by the quality of treatment after admission to the PICU, as variables are collected within the first hour after admission. However, it may be more biased by such issues as time spent in the emergency department and on transport, as the observation period in which to collect physiologic data is potentially different for each patient. PIM also includes a therapy (mechanical ventilation) as an important predictor variable, a variable that is clearly biased by prehospital care, care in the emergency department, care in the PICU, and healthcare systems. At this time, PIM II has not been extensively tested in the US.

Functional Status Scores

The Pediatric Cerebral Performance Category (PCPC) and the Pediatric Overall Performance Category (POPC) are the only measures of functional outcome widely used in pediatric intensive care (3). They are functional outcome scores developed from the Glasgow Outcome Scales to assess the short-term functional outcome of pediatric intensive care. The scales can be used to assess changes in cognitive (PCPC) and physical (POPC) disabilities. Unfortunately, they are very dependent on the clinical projection of the outcome by the healthcare provider. These scales will need extensive validation, as children are often in a naturally dependent state during growth and development and because providers, especially PICU providers, have very limited experience with confirming their projections with a large number of follow-ups. The scales correlate with a higher severity of illness (higher PRISM scores), longer lengths of stay, and, more importantly, with the Stanford-Binet Intelligence Scale-IV (measured at hospital discharge), the Bayley Scales of Infant Development-II (measured at hospital discharge), and the Vineland Adaptive Behavior Scales (measured at 1 month and 6 months after discharge). Unfortunately, the large standard deviations in the score categories imply that they are not suitable for individuals and that very large samples would be needed if they were used in large epidemiologic outcome studies.

Other Scores

Other specialized scores are often used in intensive care patients. The Pediatric Trauma Score is a complicated version of the adult Revised Trauma Score (36). Scores also exist for croup, asthma, and pediatric respiratory failure. Scores for meningococcemia are of particular interest to pediatric intensivists in Europe (4,20). Recent interest and effort have focused on scores for pediatric cardiac surgery. These methods assess outcome from the entire hospital stay, including non-ICU outcomes from surgery and routine care. However, because these patients are tightly integrated into the ICU, they are of interest to intensivists. A consensus process was used to categorize operative procedures into six risk categories to develop the Risk-Adjusted Classification System for Congenital Heart Surgery (RACHS-1), and mortality rates were then observed for the risk categories from independent data sets (9). RACHS-1 has been used in multiple peer-reviewed publications that involve cardiovascular surgery quality factors. The Aristotle method, which is being developed by congenital heart surgery groups in the US and Europe, is comprised of basic and complex evaluation techniques that were initially subjectively derived, with objectivity added with the development of large data sets (11). At this time, these methodologies have not been adequately statistically validated in peer-reviewed literature.

APPLICATIONS TO PEDIATRIC INTENSIVE CARE

Conceptually, severity-of-illness scores are frequently central to the investigations of intensive care. Importantly, their use serves to impart a practical advantage of enhancing the credibility and acceptability of research and administrative studies by helping to ensure appropriate case-mix adjustment—controlling for physiologic status, diagnoses, age, operative status, and other factors. For example, recommendations for use of the intensivist model of care provision were based on research that

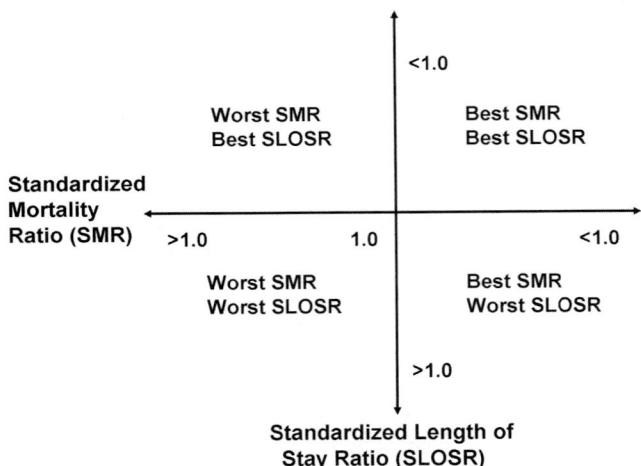

FIGURE 9.1. Quality and efficiency assessments using standardized mortality ratios (SMRs) and standardized length-of-stay ratios (SLOSRs). SMRs and SLOSRs are determined using severity of illness-based methodologies. SMRs and SLOSRs <1 indicate better-than-predicted performance, and those ratios >1 indicate worse-than-predicted performance.

required severity-of-illness scores to promote appropriate case-mix adjustment (21).

A major use for these scores is *benchmarking*, a process through which performance levels of organizations are observed and compared to standards. Benchmarking is usually either external, through comparison to a concurrent sample from other institutions or a historic sample through the use of prediction algorithms or historic data, or internal, self-comparison (of a person, department, or institution) during different time periods. External or "competitive" benchmarking allows for direct comparisons between individual hospitals or ICUs. The observed mortality rate divided by the expected mortality rate (standardized mortality ratio) and the observed length of stay divided by the expected length of stay (standardized length-of-stay ratio) have become standards for benchmarking ICU performance and quality (**Fig. 9.1**). Internal benchmarking enables doctors, ICUs, hospitals, or health systems to compare performance measures within their own practice, typically over time. For example, standardized ICU length-of-stay ratios can be compared for all patients or for those with a specific condition longitudinally with the same or different care practices and practitioners.

Use of the framework of the Institute of Medicine's (IOM) quality initiative provides a fruitful effort to review the many aspects of care that include severity-of-illness scoring systems. After releasing its report on patient safety, *To Err Is Human,* the IOM produced a safety report entitled *Crossing the Quality Chasm* (7,8). In the latter, a mandate is proposed for improvement in six dimensions of healthcare performance: safety, effectiveness, patient-centeredness, timeliness, efficiency, and equity. Generally, these aims are applied to relatively large healthcare organizations, such as hospitals or healthcare networks. Recently, it has been argued that such individual care units as ICUs may also be appropriate care areas that may embrace the IOM's quality aims (35). The utility of pediatric intensive care severity-of-illness scores is well represented in their ability to promote the IOM's quality initiative.

Safety

The IOM's report on medical errors and patient safety brought considerable attention to the problem of iatrogenic injury suffered by hospitalized patients. Adverse events, including medication errors, are increased in settings (such as the PICU) in which the healthcare provided is complex because of the patient population, and the use of acuity scores is important in this documentation. Specific examples of adverse events are nosocomial infections and unplanned extubations, which are important contributors to PICU morbidity and mortality. Severity of illness influences the risk of these adverse events; benchmarking the rates of nosocomial infections (33) and unplanned extubations (17) is best done when adjusted for severity of illness of the populations.

Effectiveness

A common theme of the last two decades of pediatric critical care research is that pediatric critical care medicine is highly variable between practitioners and institutions. The most fundamental variability among PICUs is, perhaps, the variability in patient acuity reflected in many aspects of care, including mortality rates, efficiency rates, and the use of therapeutic and monitoring modalities (18,23,24,28,39). The credibility of studies that focus on variability requires scientifically valid methods to adjust for acuity. Studying variability using scientifically valid acuity methods to adjust for case-mix differences has led to many recommendations about the delivery of pediatric critical care, including such basic premises in the organization and structure of care as the use of pediatric intensivists (23), fellows (25), and regionalization of care in pediatric centers (22). Arguably, the overall structure of pediatric intensive care in many nations has been shaped by studies that require severity-of-illness scores.

Patient Centeredness

Patients and families have become more actively involved in their own healthcare decisions. At present, the odds are stacked against physicians to perform as excellent prognosticators under situations of life and death (21). Medical school and clinical textbooks do not provide the appropriate training and information. Physicians are not taught the appropriate skill sets to constantly record and evaluate their own performance. They are sometimes rewarded for using heuristics when they are correct, but their correct assessment is merely a statistical chance, not necessarily a validation of a heuristic. Remarkably, few, if any, reports exist of educational efforts to improve a physician" prognostication skills, even though these skills are central to the physician's ability to choose appropriate therapies for physiologic dysfunction and to counsel patients and families. A family is often given firm opinions by a physician without knowing how much faith to place in these predictions, and they may give more credibility to the physician's predictions than is warranted. If the predictions are proven wrong, the patient's and family's trust in their physician may be reduced. More importantly, when an active decision concerning withdrawals and limitations of care is needed, their trust (or lack of trust) in their physician's prognostic abilities may be misplaced.

In the PICU, substantial disparity is seen between providers' prognostication estimates (30). Early identification of patients in the PICU for whom further curative, life-prolonging, or life-sustaining therapies are futile or very unlikely to be beneficial could help with difficult decisions, obviate undue patient suffering, and help to direct scarce resources to more cost-effective uses. It is not surprising that some have suggested that acuity scores could be used to aid in these decisions. However, organizations, such as the Society of Critical Care Medicine's Ethics Committee, have warned that prognostication scores should be used with caution in individuals, emphasizing that probability of death is only one of the factors pertinent to decision making (37).

Among the pediatric acuity scores, only PRISM has been tested for its ability to aid in decision making for individual patients. Unfortunately, the practicality of using severity-of-illness scores for this purpose is limited. First, the group that can be identified with zero survivors (no false positives) is very small. In a sample of 10,608 patients from 32 PICUs, of whom 571 died, the observed survivors and sample sizes for the three highest scores of PRISM III > 28, PRISM III > 35, and PRISM III > 42 were 10/158, 3/57, and 0/21, respectively. Thus, in a multi-institutional sample of over 10,000 patients, only one small group of 21 patients (0.19% of the sample) could be detected with zero survivors. Second, and probably more important, the statistical reliability and, therefore, the clinical reliability of predicting outcome in small groups of patients will limit the clinical utility of these methods (16).

Timeliness

Timeliness is a marker of the adequacy of processes to achieve acceptable outcomes. Although in some environments, timeliness is conceptualized with a "customer service" focus (e.g., timely and effective communication, wait times), in the PICU, it is more appropriate to conceptualize it as resource availability. PICU outcomes have been associated with specific personnel availability, including the presence of intensivists and critical care fellows. These studies required acuity scores (23,25).

Efficiency

An important goal is to deliver quality care in a cost-effective and efficient manner. Acuity scores are common and important methods by which to provide controls for case-mix variables and, thus, allow for standardized comparisons. One of the most important aspects of variability among PICUs is in the delivery of efficient care (18,24,32). The standardized length-of-stay ratio is the ratio of observed-to-predicted lengths of stay, where predicted length of stay depends on the case-mix and the diagnostic and physiologic status (32). The standardized length-of-stay ratio can be used to compare a particular unit over time on this element of resource use, but it can also be used to determine if a particular PICU's resource use is above or below that of similar PICUs. It has become standard in benchmarking PICU performance and quality (see **Fig. 9.1**). PRISM III is the only pediatric severity-of-illness score that has been used in efficiency evaluations.

Equity

The goal of equity is to provide impartial care for populations and for individuals, free from bias related to race, ethnicity, insurance status, income, or gender. Several studies in the US have found application to this issue and have depended on acuity scoring systems (14). One regional study found that emergency PICU admissions from lower socioeconomic strata had higher severity of illness, which is consistent with a lack of prehospital care (20). Data collected from three large PICUs in the US suggested that, after adjusting for severity of illness, no differences in standardized mortality ratios or resource use could be attributed to race, gender, or insurance status (40).

CONCLUSIONS AND FUTURE DIRECTIONS

The number of severity-of-illness systems has increased dramatically in the past 20 years. The number of uses for clinicians, clinical and health services researchers, and those involved in quality improvement efforts has increased. In particular, methodologies based on severity-of-illness scoring systems have become the standard for PICU outcome and efficiency benchmarking. As other efforts (such as the IOM's quality initiative) develop, severity-of-illness scoring systems will likely be part of the process. If the care for PICU patients is to be fundamentally improved, an understanding of the current care environment, existing evidence base, opportunities for improvement, and documentation of the improvements must be realized. Severity-of-illness scoring systems are fundamental to the methodology that will advance this effort.

KEY POINTS

- Severity scoring systems are ubiquitous in pediatric critical care. They are involved in quality and efficiency assessments and case-mix adjustments in research, and they provide important information, even in administrative databases. Severity scores may be general, such as PRISM and PIM, or may be relevant only to specific diseases or conditions, such as trauma and meningococcemia.

- Physiology-based severity systems are based on the concept of a multiple-organ system. Increasing physiologic derangements are associated with increasing mortality risk.

- The development and validation of severity scoring systems follow well-established statistical techniques. Users should evaluate the performance of such scores carefully and base their decisions on statistical criteria. In particular, this includes the definition of the outcome, clarity, and applicability of the specific predictor (dependent) variables and the performance of the overall score in terms of calibration and validation.

References

1. Baue AE. Multiple, progressive or sequential systems failure: A syndrome of the 1970s. *Arch Surg* 1980;115:136–40.

2. Cullen DJ, Civetta JM, Briggs BA, et al. Therapeutic intervention scoring system: A method for quantitative comparison of patient care. *Crit Care Med* 1974;2:57–60.

3. Fiser DH, Long N, Roberson PK, et al. Relationship of pediatric overall performance category and pediatric cerebral performance category scores at pediatric intensive care unit discharge with outcome measures collected at hospital discharge and 1- and 6-month follow-up assessments. *Crit Care Med* 2000;28:2616–20.

4. Flaegstad T, Kaaresen PI, Stokland T, et al. Factors associated with fatal outcome in childhood meningococcal disease. *Acta Paediatr* 1995;84:1137–42.

5. Graciano AL, Balko JA, Rahn DS, et al. The pediatric multiple organ dysfunction score (P-MODS): Development and validation of an objective scale to measure the severity of multiple organ dysfunction in critically ill children. *Crit Care Med* 2005;33:1484–91.

6. Hand DJ. Statistical methods in diagnosis. *Stat Methods Med Res* 1992;1:49–67.

7. Institute of Medicine: Committee on Quality of Health Care in America. *To Err Is Human: Building a Safer Health System.* Washington, DC: National Academy Press, 2000.

8. Institute of Medicine: Committee on Quality of Health Care in America. *Crossing the Quality Chasm: A New Health System for the 21st Century.* Washington, DC: National Academy Press, 2001.

9. Jenkins KJ, Gauvreau K, Newburger JW, et al. Consensus-based method for risk adjustment for surgery for congenital heart disease. *J Thor Cardiovasc Surg* 2002;123:110–8.

10. Knaus WA, Draper EA, Wagner DP, et al. Prognosis in acute organ system failure. *Ann Surg* 1985;202:685–93.

11. Lacour-Gayet F, Clarke DR, Aristotle Committee. The Aristotle method: A new concept to evaluate quality of care based on complexity. *Curr Opin Pediatr* 2005;17:412–7.

12. Leteurtre S, Duhamel A, Frandbastien B, et al. Paediatric logistic organ dysfunction (PELOD) score. *Lancet* 2003;367:897.

13. Leteurtre S, Martinot A, Duhamel A, et al. Validation of the paediatric logistic organ dysfunction (PELOD) score: Prospective, observational, multicentre study. *Lancet* 2003;236:192–7.

14. Lopez AM, Tilford JM, Anand KJ, et al. Variation in pediatric intensive care therapies and outcomes by race, gender, and insurance status. *Pediatr Crit Care Med* 2006;7:2–6.

15. Marcin JP, Pollack MM. Review of the methodologies and applications of scoring systems in neonatal and pediatric intensive care. *Pediatr Crit Care Med* 2000;1:20–7.

16. Marcin JP, Pollack MM, Patel KM, et al. Decision support issues using a physiology based score. *Intensive Care Med* 1998;24(12):1299–304.

17. Marcin JP, Rutan E, Rapetti PM, et al. Nurse staffing and unplanned extubations in the pediatric intensive care unit. *Pediatr Crit Care Med* 2005;6:254–7.

18. Marcin JP, Slonim AD, Pollack MM, et al. Long-stay patients in the pediatric intensive care unit. *Crit Care Med* 2001;29:652–7.

19. Miranda DR, de Rijk A, Schaufeli W. Simplified therapeutic intervention scoring system: The TISS-28 items: Results from a multicenter study. *Crit Care Med* 1966;24:64–73.

20. Naclerio AL, Gardner JW, Pollack MM. Socioeconomic factors and emergency pediatric ICU admissions. *Ann NY Acad Sci* 1999;896:379–82.

21. Pollack MM. "Prognostication Scores." Appendix in: Field MJ, Behrman R, eds. *When Children Die. Improving Palliative and End-of-Life Care for Children and Their Families.* Institute of Medicine of the National Academies. Available at: www.nap.edu/catalog/1039.html. Accessed 2003.

22. Pollack MM, Alexander SR, Clarke N, et al. Improved outcomes from tertiary center pediatric intensive care: A statewide comparison of tertiary and nontertiary care facilities. *Crit Care Med* 1991:19150–9.

23. Pollack MM, Cuerdon TT, Patel KM, et al. Impact of quality-of-care factors on pediatric intensive care unit mortality. *JAMA* 1994;272:941–6.

24. Pollack MM, Getson PR, Ruttimann UE, et al. Efficiency of intensive care. A comparative analysis of eight pediatric intensive care units. *JAMA* 1987;258:1481–86.

25. Pollack MM, Patel KM, Ruttimann E. Pediatric critical care training programs have a positive effect on pediatric intensive care mortality. *Crit Care Med* 1997;25:1637–42.

26. Pollack MM, Patel KM, Ruttimann UE. PRISM III: An updated pediatric risk of mortality score. *Crit Care Med* 1996;24:743–52.

27. Pollack MM, Patel KM, Ruttimann UE. The Pediatric Risk of Mortality III—Acute Physiology Score (PRISM III-APS): A method of assessing physiologic instability for pediatric intensive care unit patients. *J Pediatr* 1997;131:575–81.

28. Pollack MM, Ruttimann UE, Getson PR. Accurate prediction of the outcome of pediatric intensive care. A new quantitative method. *N Engl J Med* 1987;316:134–9.

29. Pollack MM, Ruttimann UE, Getson PR. Pediatric Risk of Mortality (PRISM) score. *Crit Care Med* 1988;16:1110–16.

30. Randolph AG, Zollo MB, Egger JM, et al. Variability in physician opinion on limiting life support. *Pediatrics* 1999;103:E46.

31. Richardson DK, Gray JE, McCormick MC, et al. Score for neonatal acute physiology: A physiologic severity index for neonatal intensive care. *Pediatrics* 1993;91:617–23.

32. Ruttimann UE, Patel KM, Pollack MM. Length of stay and efficiency in pediatric intensive care units. *J Pediatr* 1998;133:79–85.

33. Singh-Naz N, Sprague BM, Patel KM, et al. Risk factors for nosocomial infection in critically ill children: A prospective cohort study. *Crit Care Med* 1996;24:875–8.

34. Slater A, Shann F, Pearson G. PIM2: A revised version of the paediatric index of mortality. *Intensive Care Med* 2003;29:278–85.

35. Slonim AD, Pollack MM. Integrating the Institute of Medicine's six quality aims into pediatric critical care: Relevance and applications. *Pediatr Crit Care Med* 2005;6:264–9.

36. Tepas JJ, Ramenofsky ML, Mollitt DL, et al. The pediatric trauma score as a predictor of injury severity: An objective assessment. *J Trauma* 1988;28:425–9.

37. The Ethics Committee of the Society of Critical Care Medicine. Consensus statement of the society of critical care medicine ethics committee regarding futile and other possibly inadvisable treatments. *Crit Care Med* 1997;25:987–91.

38. The International Neonatal Network: The CRIB (Clinical Risk Index for Babies) score: A tool for assessing initial neonatal risk and comparing performance of neonatal intensive care units. *Lancet* 1993;342:193–8.

39. Tilford JM, Simpson PM, Yeh TS, et al. Variation in therapy and outcome for pediatric head trauma patients. *Crit Care Med* 2001;29:1056–61.

40. Wilkinson JD, Pollack MM, Ruttimann UE, et al. Outcome of pediatric patients with multiple organ system failure. *Crit Care Med* 1986;14:271–4.

CHAPTER 10 ■ QUALITY IMPROVEMENT, PATIENT SAFETY, AND MEDICAL ERROR

ANDREW C. ARGENT • VICKI L. MONTGOMERY

Historically, intensivists have been committed to improving the quality of care provided to their patients. A number of processes can contribute to the ultimate goal of improving outcomes for patients admitted to the PICU, including defining the goals and standards to be achieved in conjunction with the resources available; addressing the issues associated with provision of safe care (or avoiding harm); responding appropriately to potential or actual adverse events; monitoring the standards, processes, and outcomes of pediatric intensive care; learning from the available data; developing and implementing strategies to improve delivery of quality care; evaluating the initiatives; and reiterating the process from the beginning.

The object of this chapter is to provide the pediatric intensivist with (a) an overview of patient safety, including common definitions; (b) an approach to continuous quality improvement, working within teams and systems; (c) principles of human factors engineering; and a discussion of practical responses to, and legal implications of, adverse events in the PICU.

Since the 1960s, authors have focused attention on the fact that quality of healthcare delivery can be improved by understanding the processes of providing care and by applying principles that have been developed in other industries to improve quality (13). During the 1990s, various authors started to focus on errors in medicine and helped to develop an understanding of factors that contribute to adverse events in healthcare (32). During the same period, a number of publications identified the extent of adverse events in healthcare and the possible ramifications in terms of human life and costs, with 44,000–98,000 Americans dying each year as a result of medical error (42) and costs associated with preventable adverse events in healthcare estimated at $17 billion (22). At the beginning of the 21st century, a number of landmark reports were published, such as the Institute of Medicine's (IOM) *To Err is Human: Building a Safer Health System* (22) and the United Kingdom National Health Service's *An Organisation with a Memory* (14). These publications and similar works in Australia prompted an escalation in patient safety initiatives at local and national levels in many countries throughout the world. The public developed an unprecedented awareness of medical error and the harm that might be experienced as a result of entering the healthcare system.

The true scope of morbidity related to medical error, particularly in infants and children, is unknown. Error rates in hospitalized children have been estimated to range from 1.81 to 2.96 per 100 discharges (38). Although the incidence of error in the PICU is unknown, most reports suggest that more errors, particularly medication errors, occur in the PICU than in any other location in the hospital. There is much room for improving safety. However, before the risk of error in the PICU can be reduced, the language of patient safety must be understood and a deeper understanding must be developed of the principles of systems analysis, work models, and other problem-solving tools and skills frequently used in other industries to minimize the risks of adverse events.

DEFINITIONS

The National Patient Safety Foundation defines *patient safety* as the avoidance, prevention, and amelioration of adverse outcomes or injuries stemming from the processes of healthcare (1). The IOM defines patient safety simply as "freedom from accidental injury" (22). Although other definitions exist, this simple definition is the essence of a long-standing tenet of medical care that originated with Hippocrates: "First do no harm." Patients expect to receive healthcare without experiencing preventable harm.

An *adverse event* is an injury caused by medical management rather than by the underlying condition of the patient (22). Some adverse events are not preventable and are not classified as errors (a patient with no known drug allergies develops urticaria while receiving penicillin), while others are considered preventable and result from medical error (a patient with a penicillin allergy receives ampicillin and develops anaphylaxis).

Medical error is the failure of a planned action to be completed as intended (sometimes referred to as *an error in execution*) or the use of a wrong plan to achieve an aim (sometimes referred to as *an error of planning*) (22,32). An example of an error in execution is intubating the esophagus when the intent was to intubate the trachea and failing to recognize the malposition. Failure to perform a procedure according to policy is another example. Treating a patient who has *Enterobacter* pneumonia with a drug that only covers gram-positive organisms illustrates an error of planning.

James Reason, a noted expert on human factors and error, further categorizes medical error into narrower categories that are important for understanding the role that humans have in error and guiding the development of strategies to prevent the same error from occurring in the future (32). Slips and lapses are errors in execution. A *slip* is an observable action that deviates from what was planned (the wrong drug is programmed into an IV pump or ordered from a drop-down menu), whereas a *lapse* represents a memory failure (a nurse placing a nasogastric tube fails to follow all of the steps of the policy, and placement in the trachea is unrecognized until respiratory distress develops). A *mistake* is a knowledge-based failure: A plan is carried out correctly, but the planned action was wrong for the situation. *Active errors* (also referred to as *sharp-end errors*) typically occur in a patient care area by a front-line provider, and the effect is almost immediately apparent. *Latent errors* (also referred to as *blunt errors*) are usually system-based problems and may relate to poor design, incorrect installation, look-alike packaging, sound-alike names, faulty maintenance, and bad management decisions. Latent errors are usually more difficult to identify than active errors and may have occurred days, weeks, months, or years before the accident. These errors are typically hard to recognize and may be hidden within the structure of the organization, the computer program, or care process. Workers in healthcare frequently develop "work arounds" for these remote system problems, which leads to generalized acceptance that the "work around" is normal. However, fully investigating and uncovering latent errors is more likely to result in the development of a better system than is focusing on active errors.

Work models provide a conceptual framework for investigating events and processes so that all contributing factors are evaluated. Many versions exist. Plan–Do–Check–Act is commonly used. Another model for investigating events include Design, Equipment, Procedures, Operators, Supplies and Materials, and Environment (DEPOSE) (22). The premise of all work models is that an organized, systematic approach to event investigation results in reliable data that can be used to develop a new system.

A *system* is "a set of interdependent human and nonhuman elements interacting to achieve a common aim" (22). A system can be a unit or department within a hospital, an entire hospital, or many hospitals. Systems can be simple (linear) or complex, loosely or tightly coupled, and isolated or overlapping with other systems. Healthcare is considered a complex, tightly coupled system. In the PICU, the system elements include the people (patients, healthcare providers, environmental services, visitors, etc.), equipment (monitors, devices, computers, and other communication tools), environment (lighting, noise, lack of standardization, high acuity, staffing), and decision making (complex, multiple data sources, frequent interruptions).

The process of improving care in healthcare is generally referred to as *continuous quality improvement* (CQI), which is a continual process of reviewing and improving the practices and procedures associated with providing goods or services (10). CQI programs may evaluate structure, process, or outcome, either as independent components of the CQI process or, more commonly, all simultaneously, because considerable overlap exists between the components and quality of care. Structure is essentially the people, physical layout, management, and equipment. Factors such as adequate staffing for patient acuity levels, the right equipment at the right time, and involvement of an intensivist in the care of all critically ill patients are ways that structure influences quality. Processes refer to how care is delivered: Are policies routinely followed, are evidenced-based medicine guidelines routinely followed, does transfer of patients occur in an organized manner? Outcomes summarize the effectiveness of care, including adverse events. Common outcome measures include risk-adjusted mortality, hospital-acquired infections, and adverse medication errors. In healthcare, CQI should lead to improved patient safety and better outcomes (10). However, because many physicians and other healthcare professionals lack formal training in CQI

and other concepts such as the use of work models, human factors engineering, and understanding systems, progress has been slow compared to non-healthcare industries.

MEDICAL ERROR: HUMAN ERROR AND SYSTEMS

Rarely does medical error result from a healthcare worker intentionally inflicting harm on a patient. More commonly, medical error results when the healthcare worker fails to perform perfectly (active errors) and the system does not have adequate redundancy or layers to prevent the error from reaching the patient. Reason's book, *Human Error*, provides an easy-to-read, in-depth discussion of human error (32). In it, he dissects the etiology of human errors and factors necessary for developing processes that will minimize the risk that human error will result in harm. After all, active errors will always occur because of limitations inherent to humans, which include the impact of emotions, perceptions, stress, fatigue, cognition, and the environment on performance and decision-making abilities. Stated another way, error occurs when cognitive processes converge with three other elements: nature of the task and its environmental circumstances, the mechanisms that govern performance, and the nature of the individual who produced the failure (32). Thus, reduction and elimination of medical error in the PICU must take into account these elements as well as other principles of systems analysis and event investigation.

The healthcare system, whether referring to a single ICU, hospital, state, or nation, is a complex, tightly coupled system. A complex system contains many components that interact with many other components in both predictable and unexpected ways, are specialized and interdependent, and serve multiple functions. Tightly coupled systems have no buffer between actions and are more difficult to change than loosely coupled systems. In tightly coupled systems, one action quickly gives rise to other actions such that it is nearly impossible to recognize failure or intercede and prevent the failure from reaching a patient. The "Swiss Cheese Model" described by Reason is a conceptual framework for thinking about error prevention in complex systems (32). In this model, each layer has associated potential failures that represent "holes" in the layers. When multiple holes line up, the downstream effect is that failure happens. In the case of patient care, a medical error occurs. However, complex, tightly coupled systems can be made safer, as demonstrated by successes in the aviation and nuclear energy industries. Within medicine, the field of Anesthesiology has had success in improving safety. Characteristics of safe, complex systems include simplification when possible, standardization of processes, redundancy and back-up, many checks and balances, and automation whenever possible so that error does not result in an inferior product or service—or, in the case of healthcare, patient harm. Unfortunately, healthcare has developed as individual pieces rather than a cohesive system. Device and technology manufacturers, the pharmaceutical industry, and competition for patients contribute to the complexity of the system, particularly in the area of standardization. It is common in pediatric intensive care to have multiple brands of IV infusion devices, ventilators, monitors, and central-line products within the same unit.

Safety is not the responsibility of a single person, device, or department within a system, but rather the product of the interactions of components of the system (22). Leaders in PICUs should strive to find ways to simplify and standardize care. For example, PICUs that have instituted central-line bundles, ventilator-weaning protocols, and sedation guidelines for intubated patients have had success in decreasing hospital-acquired infections and unplanned extubations.

THE PICU ENVIRONMENT

Complexity of the Environment

The physical and psychologic milieu of the PICU contributes to the risk for medical error. During any given day in the PICU, the number and types of healthcare providers and patient acuity and census may significantly and unexpectedly change. To make the best decisions possible for the patients, much data, multiple assessments, and opinions from physician and non-physician caregivers must be analyzed in a quick, organized manner. Decision making is complex and involves interpreting multiple pieces of data in a short amount of time in an environment that frequently requires multitasking. Frequently, patient care must be triaged, as it is impossible to be at the bedside of more than one patient at a time. Intensivists routinely discuss death, withdrawal or limitation of care, and life-altering consequences of a critical illness or injury with parents and other family members. Intensivists must have a working knowledge of many types and brands of equipment. The environment is noisy, full of distractions, and lacks standardization and ergonomic design. It is rare for a task to progress to completion without at least one interruption. All of these characteristics contribute to the complexity of the PICU environment and have the potential to negatively impact patient safety.

Impact of the PICU Environment on Human Error

Understanding how we interact with our environment is essential to developing processes and systems that improve safety in the PICU. The study of the interactions between humans, the tools that they use, and the environment in which they live and work is referred to as *human factors engineering* (22,44). Evaluating human factors to provide insight into where and why systems or processes break down has been applied in other industries for years. For example, investigation of aviation accidents demonstrated that take-offs and landings were the times of highest risk during flight. The concept of the "sterile" cockpit developed because factors contributing to human error, such as stress, authority gradients, and distractions, were identified as playing a role in crashes. During take-offs and landings, a detailed checklist is used and only conversation related to these activities is allowed. Distractions are minimized, and roles are well defined.

Human performance is influenced by the psychologic limits of the individual, training and education, knowledge, fatigue, communication, and perceptions. In the PICU, the high acuity of illness, constant exposure to death and to grieving parents, fatigue, inappropriate staffing (numbers and skill set),

an ever-changing body of knowledge, lack of equipment standardization, multiple simultaneous demands, and the use of many interventions associated with narrow therapeutic windows all affect human performance. A commentary published by the Agency for Healthcare Research and Quality in 2005 highlights the impact of working conditions (such as interruptions and keeping pace with the changing needs of patients) on the clinical decision-making abilities of nurses (19). A study by Grayson found that errors tend to occur within 30 mins after sudden changes in patient needs in an environment that is dominated by distractions and interruptions (17). Given that patient status and census are constantly changing and that multitasking is normal in ICUs, it is easy to understand why they are among the most error-prone areas in hospitals. Overall, compared to other industries, little is known about human factors and the ICU environment, but recent studies related to increased workload, fatigue, and emotional stress clearly demonstrate the influence of human factors on patient (and healthcare provider) safety (2,4,6,7,23,26,33).

Work Load and Fatigue

It is clear from the sleep literature that acute and chronic sleep deprivation negatively impact performance and place sleep-deprived practitioners at risk for personal injury, mood disturbances, and stress-related illnesses (19,43). The extent to which fatigue-related errors actually contribute to patient harm is largely unknown, although fatigue is identified as a factor in root-cause analysis investigations of events. Sleep research conducted in laboratory and clinical settings suggests that fatigue significantly impairs the performance of healthcare providers.

Cumulative sleepiness, mood disturbance, and psychomotor vigilance performance decreases during a week of sleep restricted to 4–5 hrs per night (12). Interns made significantly more serious medical and diagnostic errors during the critical-care rotation when the schedule (traditional) included call every third night and extended (>24 hrs) shifts (23). In another study that used a similar design, interns who were working a traditional schedule had more attentional failures during the night (26). Although increasing data describe the benefit of decreasing sleep deprivation and fatigue, the increased number of patient handovers has become a new source of error. As staff changes occur, with handover of information from one group of caregivers to another, valuable patient information may not be communicated. New strategies for improving teamwork and access to patient information are necessary to minimize the occurrence of handover-related errors.

Unfortunately, many physicians underappreciate the affect of fatigue and stress on performance and do not perceive that inadequate rest or stressful situations contribute to medical error. These attitudes differ substantially from those in other industries. In a direct comparison of the aviation industry and medicine in terms of attitudes toward teamwork, perceptions of stress and fatigue, and error, results showed that, compared to pilots, physicians underplay the importance of fatigue and workload on error (37). When trained observers rated the function of the team, the aviation team routinely received standard or higher ratings (85% of the time, a standard or higher rating was assigned) compared to surgical, anesthetic, and surgical-anesthetic teams (30%–50% of the time, a poor-to-minimal rating was assigned). The aviation industry has had considerable success in improving passenger safety, largely because of advances in addressing fatigue, stress, and need for teamwork.

The need for adequate rest and appropriate staffing levels is also important for nurses (24,40). Lower patient-to-nurse staffing ratios (fewer patients assigned to one nurse) have been associated with a lower risk of adverse events, such as urinary tract infections and decubitus ulcers (24,7). Having nurses with the appropriate skill set (education and training) and adequate rest at the bedside is also important for outcomes (6,7,24,33). ICU nurses complete many tasks during a shift. The higher the acuity, the more tasks a nurse must complete during a shift. These tasks include direct patient care activities, documentation, and discussions with physicians, therapists, and families. It is unknown how many actions can be completed by one nurse in the ICU environment before the risk of error increases. Pediatric intensivists, particularly those who function as medical directors, should advocate for appropriate staffing levels, orientation and ongoing education, and rewards for staff nurses.

Communication

Effective communication is another area that is essential to improving safety. Communication between all members of the healthcare team is crucial to safe patient handovers. The Joint Commission on Accreditation of Healthcare Organizations (JCAHO) has noted that poor communication is a factor in the majority of sentinel events. The 2006 JCAHO national patient safety goals include several requirements for improving communication throughout the hospital.

Patients in the PICU move throughout the hospital to have specialized procedures and diagnostic testing, and providers from multiple disciplines enter the PICU to care for these patients. In an ideal system, information should flow easily between all team members without regard to professional stature, seniority, discipline, expertise, or authority. Patient data should be available, legible, timely, and complete. A specific structure for sharing patient information, particularly at the time of patient handovers, facilitates good communication, as has been demonstrated by the use of daily goals (31). For critically ill infants and children, communication is fundamental to ensuring that patients receive appropriate care, whether the handover is between nurses, physicians in the PICU, physicians in different areas of the hospital, or physicians involved in the transport of a patient from one facility to another.

The ideal communication system is difficult to achieve in healthcare for several reasons, including authority gradients, time and physical restraints, technology limitations, and a perception that teamwork is not essential to good patient outcomes. The negative impact of authority gradients on safety was first noted in the aviation industry. Investigation of events demonstrated that effective communication between pilots and copilots was negatively impacted if a significant difference existed in their experience, perceived expertise, or authority. Authority gradients affect the ability of the lower-ranking person to voice concern and the ability of the higher-ranking person to accept and act on the concern. The concept of authority gradients was introduced to medicine in the 2000 IOM report (22). The traditional hierarchical approach to patient care in medicine hinders effective and timely communication be-

tween attending physicians and trainees, physicians and nurses, and administration and staff. A technique called *S*ituation, *B*ackground, *A*ssessment, and *R*ecommendation (SBAR) has been introduced to the healthcare field as a method by which to improve communication between team members and to overcome perceived and real restrictions related to hierarchy. This technique provides the healthcare worker with a framework for communicating a concern about a patient or situation and empowers the worker to move up the authority gradient if the concern is not addressed in a professional or timely manner. Another communication tool, "PASS the BATON," developed by the Defense Department to comply with a JCAHO patient-safety goal, provides structure for transferring patient care from one individual to another regardless of the disciplines involved. The acronym provides prompts for relaying *P*atient data, such as name, age, sex, and location; *A*ssessment, such as chief complaint, vital signs, active problems, signs and symptoms; *S*ituation, which includes current status and circumstances; *S*afety concerns, including critical lab values and reports, allergies; *B*ackground, which includes pertinent past medical history and current medications; *A*ctions, including what has been done and what needs to be done; *T*iming of care-related activities, including urgent matters and prioritization; *O*wnership (nurse, physician, therapist) of specific care issues; and *N*ext, which details anticipated changes in condition and any plans or contingency plans to manage changes.

ERROR PREVENTION: SAFETY CULTURE, REPORTING, SYSTEMS ANALYSIS, CONTINUOUS QUALITY IMPROVEMENT, AND TECHNOLOGY

If the ICU environment is a complex system with ample opportunity for medical error to occur, how does the intensivist develop a safer PICU? Conceptually, intensivists should work to develop an environment that allows the investigation of actual and averted (near-miss) events and that learns from errors. Four subculture attributes are necessary for supporting an environment in which learning from errors is embraced: reporting, just, flexible, and learning (34). In a *reporting culture*, members of the staff are actively engaged in reporting accidents and near misses. Various assurances exist that reporting of events is not handled in a punitive manner. The aviation industry has had great success with creating and maintaining a reporting culture. In a *just culture*, safeguards exist that allow the identification of individuals who repeatedly fail to follow policies or who act with malicious intent, while protecting those who report errors and near misses. The willingness and competence to correctly interpret safety data, form correct conclusions, and implement new processes describes features of a *learning culture*. Perhaps the most difficult culture to develop is that of flexibility. In a *flexible culture*, individuals must be willing to move between a traditional, hierarchical structure to a flatter, professional structure so that individuals with expertise in an area may investigate and design solutions.

To identify ways to improve patient safety in the PICU, an error-reporting system(s) must be in place. Identification of adverse events is the only way to know that issues exist. Types of reporting systems include voluntary reporting, mandatory reporting, concurrent surveillance, automated surveillance (e.g., an order for naloxone triggers a concurrent review of a patient's record to evaluate for error), and chart review (3). Automated and concurrent surveillance methods generally detect more events than does voluntary self-reporting. Automated surveillance is ideal for detecting events that require antidotes or specific laboratory monitoring. For example, an order for naloxone would trigger an investigation as to whether an error involving an opioid occurred. Concurrent surveillance is more suited for identifying errors manifested by changes in signs and symptoms (3).

Voluntary and mandatory reporting systems of actual events generally underdetect error and are, by definition, reactionary, because a report is generated after an event has occurred. Historically, many barriers have impeded the reporting of errors in medicine. These barriers include the negative emotional impact that disclosure has on the person (people) involved, risk of disclosure on medical malpractice, and risk of job loss or other punitive acts. To maximize the effectiveness of self-reporting systems, leaders must avoid blaming the involved staff for the error and demonstrate that reports generate changes in practice. Successful reporting systems are user friendly and readily accessible. Allowing anonymous reporting also improves reporting rates and helps to foster the concept of a "just culture." Some institutions choose to start with the reporting of averted or near-miss events, as actual patient harm does not occur in these instances and the individuals involved perceive less threat to self. Identifying averted errors is a proactive, rather than reactive, approach to improving patient safety because events that could lead to patient harm are evaluated before actual harm occurs. Once an area of concern is identified, the process must be scrutinized so that each component is identified and evaluated for its contribution to the event. Applying work-model principles is integral to beginning and completing the process in a manner that leads to adequate safeguards for preventing an error from reaching a patient. If only the most obvious link to the error is recognized, the same error will likely occur again, because other aspects of the process that contributed to the original event are not recognized. The trialing and redesigning phases help to ensure that the final product is a good solution and provides a clearly defined end point to the project.

When an event occurs or an opportunity to improve safety is prospectively identified, a team is assembled to design a new process. The team should include representation from any area or service that had a role in the care of the patient. Including the appropriate people helps to ensure that a thorough planning stage occurs. Once the team is assembled, the current process should be diagrammed so that each component of the process is articulated, and people from areas not on the team should be interviewed. These steps will provide the basis for identifying where failure is likely to occur, developing an alternative process, trialing the new process, evaluating the new process, and redesigning as needed. Essentially, these steps encompass the basis of systems analysis, human factors engineering, and CQI. Pronovost et al. detailed how to apply processes for improving patient safety in an ICU by describing an incident that occurred in an adult ICU, how it was investigated, and the steps that were taken to prevent it from happening again (30).

Various work models exist that provide a template for ensuring a logical, thoughtful, and inclusive process for revising a current process or developing a new one. A frequently used

work model is "Plan, Do, Check, Act" (22). Using a work model is key to fully appreciating the successes and limitations of the current process, identifying why error occurred, and developing an alternative system that eliminates current limitations and has minimal risk of introducing new sources of error.

Minimizing the risk of new error or evaluating current processes for sources of error can be accomplished by using an organized approach to evaluate where failure may occur and its significance if the error occurs. A commonly used failure analysis tool is Failure Modes and Effects Analysis (FMEA). In performing an analysis using FMEA, a specific procedure and tool are used to identify possible failures of a product or service and to determine the frequency and impact of the failure. Information about this tool and how to use it can be found at several web sites (15). The information learned from an FMEA provides valuable data for designing a safer process, as failures are anticipated and solutions for preventing failures from causing patient harm are built into the process.

Intensivists function within teams on a daily basis. However, few intensivists have any formal training in leading teams and understanding how teams function. Additional reading and training on these topics, especially for those who aspire to leadership roles in the ICU, should be obtained. In a study that distributed the Intensive Care Unit Management Attitudes Questionnaire (which was adapted from the Flight Management Attitudes Questionnaire) to 226 physicians and 324 nurses from ICUs in six hospitals, physician members of teams perceived the function of the team differently from other members of the team (37,41). In general, the physicians rated the quality of collaboration and communication much higher than the nurses did. Unfortunately, this finding is not unique to this study. Physicians tend to perceive teamwork and communication as being better than do the nonphysician members of the team. This discrepancy contributes to the slower progress in safety initiatives in medicine compared to other industries and to the disconnect that occurs between physicians and nurses in the daily care of patients.

Preexisting attitudes, whether held by physician or nonphysician staff, can lead to failure of even the best-investigated and designed projects. Introducing change and providing education is fundamental to success. Such strategies as mass mailings of educational materials or conducting conferences are least likely to effect changes in physician practice. Multiple small sessions, individualized audits and feedback, informal and formal sessions directed by local opinion leaders, and frequent reminders and prompts (preprinted order sets, pop-up windows) are all necessary to bring success to project implementation and long-term sustainability.

The introduction of new technology in the PICU should undergo the same scrutiny that other processes do. That is, to maximize the successes and minimize the risk of failures, the technology should be assessed for potential advances in care as well as potential failures. Prior to purchase and implementation, a detailed process for use and a sound educational program are essential to achieve success with the new technology. Also, assessment of the technology should include assignment of value, because technology is usually a significant financial investment for a hospital. Value can be demonstrated in a variety of ways, including showing savings, improved market advantage, improved efficiency, improved customer satisfaction, and improved patient safety.

On the surface, it seems intuitive that technology should contribute to advances in patient safety (5). The rapidly expanding body of knowledge to be mastered, the need to simultaneously monitor many parameters of patient status, the multiple team members involved in a patient's care, and the complexity of the system are reasons that technology could be beneficial. Information technology can facilitate better communication by allowing on-site and remote access to patient records and providing a foundation for patient handovers. Access to reference materials, policies, evidence-based medicine guidelines, and databases is easier and wider using modern technology than it has been at any time in the history of medicine.

In addition, information technology has allowed the introduction of computerized physician order entry (CPOE) and clinical-decision support systems. The use of CPOE, combined with clinical-decision support, has led to decreases in some types of medication errors, particularly those related to calculations, prescribing drugs for which the patient has an allergy, and ordering drugs contraindicated based on organ dysfunction or drug-drug interactions. The use of *forcing functions*—automatic prompts that appear when preprogrammed rules are violated—is known to decrease errors and improve compliance with treatment guidelines. Monitoring trends in vital signs and laboratory data by computer programs can provide early warning to staff about worrisome patient changes and allow appropriate interventions before an adverse event occurs. "Smart pump" technology is another application aimed at decreasing the number of errors related to continuous drug infusions. These pumps allow the selection of a drug from a library. During the pump-programming phase, prompts and alarms help to minimize the risk of the wrong drug dose being entered.

Although advances in technology have decreased the frequency of error in some areas, other types of error have not been reduced, and new types of error have been introduced. The selection of the wrong drug during CPOE and ignoring forcing functions or alerts because too many appear are two types of actions demonstrating that technology can contribute to error. Selection of the wrong patient has also occurred during CPOE, so that medications are ordered on the wrong patient. Increases in mortality and adverse drug events have been reported post-implementation of CPOE programs. The development of computer programs by independent vendors or practitioners has led to new communication problems. The lack of standardization or "talk" between proprietary programs limits the sharing of patient information, which may lead to duplication of work (physician enters a drug, but the CPOE program does not interface with the pharmacy program, requiring the drug order to be entered a second time). Most computerized systems have not resulted in decreases in documentation time. Physicians and other providers now spend more time interfacing with various types of technology. This increase in time generally has led to decreased time for direct contact with patients and families and dissatisfaction among practitioners. The lack of integration among various programs within hospitals, between hospitals, and between inpatient and outpatient facilities is a source of error and frustration.

Despite some of the limitations that still exist, decreasing medical error in the PICU is achievable. Since 2000, the results from several studies performed in PICUs show that decreases in medical error can occur with or without the introduction of new technology. The use of work models allowed investigators at two institutions to decrease the rate of unplanned extubations (29,36). A study conducted by one of the groups illustrated the application of CQI methodology to reduce an event associated with patient harm (36). In their PICU, a multidisciplinary team was formed to evaluate unplanned extubations using the institution's CQI model of "Plan, Do, Check, Act." The team reviewed all unplanned extubation events to identify areas in which the care of intubated patients could be altered. Inadequate sedation and an unorganized approach to weaning and extubating patients were identified as factors that contributed to unplanned extubations. In the "Do, Check, Act" phases, processes were added and refined to address these factors, and the incidence of unplanned extubations decreased.

Both of these studies demonstrate important principles for embarking on CQI projects. The project must have relevance to the unit. If the unit has a very low incidence of unplanned extubations but a high incidence of catheter-related bloodstream infections, the staff is more likely to become vested in a project to decrease catheter-related infections than in one to decrease unplanned extubations. The project must be feasible—a key aspect when introducing CQI. It is much easier to change culture and develop a cohesive team if early projects have short timelines and achieve success. Early CQI activities are also beneficial if noncontroversial projects are chosen. The development of guidelines and pathways is another strategy by which to apply CQI to improve or standardize a procedure or practice. The team should understand that CQI is not a fast process. The project to reduce unplanned extubations described here occurred over several years. The time invested allows the team to study the process and develop solutions that are likely to improve the process with minimal risk of introducing new sources of error.

MEDICAL ERROR AND THE PICU ENVIRONMENT

The IOM's report "Crossing the Quality Chasm" (20) recommended six aims for improvement: safety, effectiveness, equity, timeliness, patient-centeredness, and efficiency. These aims may be used as a framework for specific areas of intervention to advance quality of care in the PICU (39) (**Table 10.1**).

Intensive care is provided within the wider environment of hospitals and healthcare systems. The aims are applicable to the healthcare system in its entirety, as well as within the particular context of the PICU, but achieving these aims in the larger environment may depend on achieving them first in areas such as the PICU.

A number of studies have clearly demonstrated that specific organizational structures for pediatric critical care within a healthcare system are associated with better outcomes (28). It is also useful to evaluate the specific activities within the PICU in terms of the aims described here.

QUALITY MANAGEMENT AND RESOURCE ALLOCATION

It is clear that resources must be allocated to the process of quality management and that a linkage exists between the overall

TABLE 10.1

SPECIFIC AREAS OF INTERVENTION TO ADVANCE QUALITY OF CARE IN THE PICU

Aims for improvement	Categories and definitions	Potential monitoring and intervention
Patient safety	Diagnostic errors	Autopsies Morbidity and mortality discussions
	Treatment errors, including: Medication errors	Regular review of prescriptions and drug administration by pharmacy staff
	Nosocomial infections Procedures	Monitoring of nosocomial infections in the PICU Monitoring of incidents such as accidental extubation, complications of vascular access
	Prevention	Ensuring that preventative policies are clear-cut and regularly implemented
	Other	
Effectiveness	Evidence-based practice based on sound research evidence	Implementation of clinical guidelines where possible and focus on collection of appropriate data to inform decisions
Equity	Access to appropriate care for all regardless of factors such as race, ethnicity, financial status, gender etc.	Regular review of patient population and identification of disparities in care between various groupings of people
Timeliness	Timely provision of care and information Timely transmission of information	Monitoring of time taken for care and intervention Focus on optimal transmission of information between members of the PICU team
Patient-centeredness		Use of validated surveys of families
Efficiency	Efficient and cost-effective utilization of resources Appropriate planning of intensive and high care bed numbers	Cost per patient Severity of illness and acuity of care scoring Monitoring of "nonintensive care" activities

resources available to a PICU and the standards that can realistically be achieved in that unit. In all contexts, but particularly in those in which healthcare resources are limited, the need exists for a definition of the standards and goals of treatment to be offered in the PICU, reasonable allocation of resources, appropriate management of those resources, accountability for the use of those resources, and ongoing feedback to the stakeholders.

Involving all of the stakeholders, including patients and families, healthcare workers, hospital managers, and funders of health services, is fundamental to the process of setting standards and goals of therapy. Failure to involve all stakeholders almost inevitably leads to problems of communication and failure of clinical services, as documented in the inquiry into pediatric cardiac services in Bristol in the UK (25).

Both the process of setting standards and goals and that of resource allocation inevitably require the use of rationing. *Rationing* refers to the process of allocating scarce resources; it differs from eliminating waste, optimizing expenditures, and withholding inappropriate therapy. Rationing itself may happen at a number of levels, including at the bedside (clinician making a decision about whether to admit a child), at the institutional level (managers allocating resources to the PICU), and at higher levels (national or provincial allocation of health budgets). It is frequently done implicitly, but ideally should be done explicitly, with accountability for the decisions taken. Rationing includes the process of making rational, defensible, and ethical decisions about *which beneficial interventions to withhold* from which patients so that *resources can be allocated toward other (possibly more) beneficial activities.*

Although it may be difficult to establish a system for fair allocation of resources, the concept of accountability for reasonableness (A4R) is one model that facilitates the process (11). The A4R concept includes:

- Relevance: Decisions should be made on the basis of reasons that are relevant under the circumstances.
- Publicity: Decisions and the processes by which they are reached should be transparent and publicly available.
- Revision: Opportunities should be available to alter those decisions in the light of further information or argument.
- Enforcement: Either voluntary or public regulation of the process should be possible to ensure that the first three conditions are actually met.

Others have described rationing resources on the basis of concepts such as autonomy, utility, and equity (9).

Ideally, the therapy and interventions offered in the PICU should be evidence based (although data are limited in many situations), and measurement of the standards and goals that are achieved should be required to provide motivation or justification to the resources allocated to the services. Stakeholders should agree both on the treatment to be offered in the PICU and on the measurable standards and goals of the service. As described above, these measurements must be relevant to the clinical service, accurate, reproducible, and doable. It is particularly important that measured outcomes are relevant to all healthcare services—not just to the PICU (e.g., measuring the overall outcome of congenital heart disease in a region and measuring the postoperative mortality of pediatric cardiac surgery may differ considerably). The processes of measuring risk-adjusted morbidity and mortality are relevant to this process and are discussed in detail in Chapter 7.

The body of evidence from adult intensive care on the outcomes of triage decisions made by intensivists is ever increasing (21). Intrinsic to this literature is the fact that the quality of intensive care services cannot be fully assessed solely from data on patients admitted to the ICU. It is essential to collect and appropriately interpret data regarding the outcomes of patients who were either refused or not offered admission to the ICU.

In the light of current concerns about avian influenza and the possibility of large outbreaks of communicable disease, or of large numbers of casualties from disasters of other kinds, the potential for expanding current intensive care services to deal with such events should also be considered. This marker of resource allocation has rarely been considered until very recently (16). The legal standing of admission and discharge criteria for the PICU has rarely been challenged, but it is likely that courts would sympathetically view criteria that have been established using the A4R principles.

LEGAL ISSUES AND QUALITY CONTROL IN THE PICU

The legal issues that relate to the practice of pediatric intensive care vary throughout the world. However, a number of themes are common to most systems: the recognition of criminal intent, negligence, and malpractice; identification of "truth"; issues related to compensation of anyone who suffers an adverse event while in the PICU; and the use of the legal system to enforce quality of healthcare.

It is generally agreed that the vast majority of healthcare workers do not harbor criminal intent toward their patients; however, rare incidents have been reported in which nurses or doctors have set out to harm patients, and such instances must be guarded against.

Most legal processes are designed to apportion blame and appropriate retribution. In addition, compensation may be provided to victims of adverse events and their families. A variety of systems exist throughout the world, including factors such as no-fault compensation, tort (or allocation of blame) litigation, availability of mediators, structured settlements, capped awards, and open disclosure. The particular system applicable has significant implications for legal processes. In Scandinavian countries, where most healthcare needs are automatically covered by the state, claims for compensation are significantly reduced. In the US, compensation is provided by the tort system, but the process is expensive and a number of studies have shown that the system serves a tiny proportion of people who have been harmed (35).

Ideally, information required for the allocation of blame and assessment of damages (i.e., data that can be used in the legal process) should be separate from information required for the improvement and development of healthcare services (which should be confidential and legally privileged). Unfortunately, few countries in the world allow such a separation (35).

Negligence has been defined as a failure to maintain the standard expected of a reasonably careful and knowledgeable practitioner acting in a similar situation (27). In many countries, the standard is that of "current practice." Recently, courts

in the United States have moved away from this definition of standard care to a "reasonableness test," and this may happen with regard to adoption of new technology (27), clinical practice guidelines, and informed consent. In the area of new technology, the test entails an evaluation of the costs and benefits of specific technology, particularly regarding patient safety. Authoritative and evidence-based guidelines for clinical practice can also be used as criteria for the evaluation of negligence, and this has implications for healthcare providers and for the organizations that establish clinical practice guidelines. In many countries, guidelines for clinical practice are increasingly being provided at the national level. Finally, regarding consent for procedures, some courts have held that fully informed consent includes providing information about the location of recognized centers of care for the particular conditions involved. The Bristol Royal Infirmary inquiry also highlighted the need for parents to be given full information and an appropriate length of time in which to make decisions about consent for major surgical interventions (25).

It is clear that litigation will more likely ensue when families have a sense that they have not received full information about an event. Some families have even made it clear that their reason for litigation was to discover the "truth." Much litigation could be avoided if full and appropriate information were provided to families by the team responsible for the care of their child. In fact, evidence suggests that courts in a number of countries believe that doctors particularly have a positive legal duty to inform the patient and his family of the facts surrounding an error (18).

Recommendations for appropriate responses to adverse events have recently been reviewed (45) and include:

- Managing the patient and the family. The problem must be handled, and any further threats to patient safety must be eliminated. The patient and the family must be informed that a problem has occurred. The exact timing of this process will depend on the child's condition and the family but should ideally occur within a maximum of 24 hrs from the event. The most senior person available at the time should do the informing, and the physician responsible for the patient's care should also be informed immediately and should personally speak with the family as soon as possible. The process should include providing information about what happened, accepting responsibility, apologizing for the event, and advising what has been done to prevent further adverse events. Follow-up meetings to provide information should be scheduled as appropriate and should be attended by appropriate representatives from the hospital management. Support for the patient and the family (including attention to billing issues) must be provided. It seems that early discussion of possible compensation is appropriate and helpful.
- Ensure that PICU personnel involved in the adverse event receive appropriate support, adequate time to recover from the effects of the incident, and ongoing support in dealing with the process. Clearly, this requires established training programs and support systems. If the primary care provider is not able to function normally and effectively, a replacement must be found (and the family must be informed of the change).
- Ensure that everything possible is done to preserve the evidence and information that may be required to understand exactly what happened. The lengths taken must relate to the

severity of the episode (or near miss). In some circumstances, it may be appropriate to seal the area in which the incident took place until it has been fully evaluated.

- The process by which to investigate the incident and provide clarity about the event must be established and come into action immediately. The sooner the process is enacted, the more effective it is likely to be. In constituting the group of people who will undertake the investigation, it is advisable to involve those who have an understanding of the clinical context, functioning of PICU systems, implications of the event for the patient and the family, and potential financial and other implications of the event; they should also be independent from the personal aspects of the problems.
- All aspects of this process should be appropriately and carefully documented.
- The events should be reported to the appropriate authorities within the hospital and the health system.

The available evidence suggests that, at least in the US, this process is associated with reduced litigation and associated costs, reduced claims for compensation, and significant improvements in relationships between healthcare systems and patients. However, it also appears that, rather than the occurrence of an adverse event, or an adverse event due to negligence, the severity of the patient's disability is more likely to determine the size of the payment to the plaintiff (8).

CONCLUSIONS AND FUTURE DIRECTIONS

Much can be done to improve the quality of care of patients in pediatric intensive care and to reduce the risks of adverse events and errors. The quality of care that can be provided in a particular situation is limited by the resources available, but resources should always be allocated to the specific task of identifying areas of concern and developing ways of improving care. It is essential that comprehensive team- and systems-based approaches are employed to improve care and limit errors. The ongoing measurement and assessment of systems is an essential component of quality improvement.

Legal systems can be developed to aid in improving the quality of medical care, although current systems in many parts of the world are particularly expensive and relatively ineffective in improving the quality of care.

KEY POINTS

- Medical error is associated with high morbidity, mortality, and costs.
- Patient safety is defined as the avoidance, prevention, and amelioration of adverse outcomes or injuries that stem from the processes of healthcare.
- Improving quality of care and patient safety requires an understanding of factors within the PICU environment that may contribute to the occurrence of adverse events.
- Both actual and potential adverse events must be documented in a systematic way and considered in their full context to allow the development of realistic and appropriate responses to limit further problems.

- Institutions must develop structured and appropriate responses to adverse events to ensure that the harmful effects are minimized and that future problems are averted.
- Most legal systems require that the facts regarding adverse events be honestly and fully presented to the family and individuals affected.
- Changes in legal definitions of "reasonable care" may potentially affect the way in which institutions are held liable for adverse events that occur.

References

1. Agenda for Research and Development in Patient Safety. National Patient Safety Foundation at the AMA, http://www.ama-assn.org/med-sci/npsf/research/research.htm. Accessed on May 24, 1999.
2. Aiken LH, Clarke SP, Sloane DM, et al. Hospital nurse staffing and patient mortality, nurse burnout, and job dissatisfaction. *JAMA* 2002;288:1987–93.
3. Aspden P, Corrigan JM, Wolcott J, eds. *Patient Safety: Achieving a New Standard for Care.* Washington, DC: The National Academies Press, 2004.
4. Bartel P, Offermeier W, Smith F, et al. Attention and working memory in resident anaesthetists after night duty: Group and individual effects. *Occup Environ Med* 2004;61:167–70.
5. Bates DW, Gawande AA. Patient safety: Improving safety with information technology. *N Engl J Med* 2003;348:2526–34.
6. Blegen MA, Goode C, Reed L. Nurse staffing and patient outcomes. *Nurs Res* 1998;47:43–50.
7. Blegen MA, Vaughn T. A multisite study of nurse staffing and patient occurrences. *Nurs Econ* 1998;16:196–203.
8. Brennan TA, Sox CM, Burstin HR. Relation between negligent adverse events and the outcomes of medical-malpractice litigation. *N Engl J Med* 1996;335:1963–7.
9. Cook D, Giacomini M. The sound of silence: Rationing resources for critically ill patients. *Crit Care* 1999;3:R1–R3.
10. Counte MA, Meuer S. Issues in the assessment of continuous quality improvement implementation in health care organizations. *Int J Qual Health Care* 2001;13:197–207.
11. Daniels N, Sabin J. The ethics of accountability in managed care reform. *Health Aff* 1998;17:50–64.
12. Dinges DF, Pack F, Williams K, et al. Cumulative sleepiness, mood disturbance and psychomotor vigilance performance decrements during a week of sleep restricted to 4–5 hours per night. *Sleep* 1997;20(4):267–77.
13. Donabedian A. Quality assessment and monitoring. Retrospect and prospect. *Eval Health Prof* 1983;6:363–75.
14. Donaldson L. *An Organisation with a Memory: Report of an Expert Group on Learning from Adverse Events in the NHS Chaired by the Chief Medical Officer.* London: The Stationery Office, 2000.
15. Failure Mode and Effects Analysis. http://www.isixsigma.com/tt/fmea/, http://www.isixsigma.com/offsite.asp?A=Fr&Url=http://www.fmeainfocentre.com, http://www.ihi.org/ihi/workspace/tools/fmea/, http://www.va.gov/ncps/SafetyTopics/HFMEA/HFMEAIntro.pdf. Accessed on February 23, 2007.
16. Gomersall CD, Tai DY, Loo S, et al. Expanding ICU facilities in an epidemic: Recommendations based on experience from the SARS epidemic in Hong Kong and Singapore. *Intensive Care Med* 2006;32:1004–13.
17. Grayson D, Boxerman S, Potter P, et al. Do transient working conditions trigger medical errors? In: Henrikson K, Battles JB, Marks ES, et al., eds. *Advances in Patient Safety: From Research to Implementation Vol. 1, Research Findings.* Rockville, MD: Agency for Healthcare Research and Quality; 2005:53–64. AHRQ publication 05-0021-1.
18. Hébert CP, Levin AV, Robertson G. Bioethics for clinicians: 23. Disclosure of medical error. *CMAJ* 2001;164:509–13.
19. Hughes RG, Clancy CM. Working conditions that support patient safety. *J Nurs Care Qual* 2005;20:289–92.
20. Institute of Medicine Committee on Quality of Health Care in America. Crossing the Quality Chasm: A New Health System for the 21st Century. Washington DC, National Academy Press, 2001.
21. Joynt GM, Gomersall CD. Is "more" always "better"? Moving towards optimal utilization of and high dependency and intensive care beds by selecting the right patients for admission. *Anaesth Intensive Care* 2006;34:423–5.
22. Kohn LT, Corrigan JM, Donaldson MS, eds. *To Err is Human: Building a Safer Health System.* Washington, DC: National Academy Press, 2000.
23. Landrigan CP, Rothschild JM, Cronin JW, et al. Effect of reducing interns' work hours on serious medical errors in intensive care units. *N Engl J Med* 2004;351:1838–48.
24. Lankshear AJ, Sheldon TA, Maynard A. Nurse staffing and healthcare outcomes: A systematic review of the international research evidence. *Adv Nurs Sci* 2005;28:163–74.

25. Learning from Bristol: The report of the public inquiry into children's heart surgery at the Bristol Royal Infirmary 1984–1995. Command Paper: CM 5207. Published by the Bristol Royal Infirmary Inquiry, July 2001.
26. Lockley SW, Cronin JW, Evans EE, et al. Effect of reducing interns' weekly work hours on sleep and attentional failures. *N Engl J Med* 2004;351: 1829–37.
27. Mello MM, Studdert DM, Brennan TA. The Leapfrog standards: Ready to jump from marketplace to courtroom? *Health Aff* 2003;22:46–59.
28. Pearson G, Shann F, Barry P, et al. Should paediatric intensive care be centralized? Trent versus Victoria. *Lancet* 1997;26:1213–7.
29. Popernack ML, Thomas NJ, Lucking SE. Decreasing unplanned extubations: Utilization of the Penn State Children's Hospital sedation algorithm. *Pediatr Crit Care Med* 2004;5:58–62.
30. Pronovost PJ, Wu A, Sexton JB. Acute decompensation after removing a central venous line: Practical approaches to increasing patient safety in an intensive care unit. *Ann Intern Med* 2004;140:1025–33.
31. Pronovost P, Berenholtz S, Dorman T, et al. Improving communication in the ICU using daily goals. *J Crit Care* 2003;18:71–5.
32. Reason J. *Human Error*. Cambridge: Cambridge University Press, 1990.
33. Rogers AE, Hwang W, Scott LD, et al. The working hours of hospital staff nurses and patient safety. *Health Aff* 2004;23:202–12.
34. Ruchlin HS. Role of leadership in instilling a culture of safety: Lessons from the literature. *J Healthc Manag* 2004;49:47–58.
35. Runciman WB, Merry A, Tito F. Error Blame and the law in health care—an Antipodean perspective. *Ann Intern Med* 2003;138:974–9.
36. Sadowski R, Dechert RE, Bandy KP, et al. Continuous quality improvement: Reducing unplanned extubations in a pediatric intensive care unit. *Pediatrics* 2004;114:628–32.
37. Sexton JB, Thomas EJ, Helmreich RL. Error, stress, and teamwork in medicine and aviation: Cross-sectional surveys. *British Med J* 2000;320: 745–7.
38. Slonim AD, LaFleur BJ, Ahmed W, et al. Hospital-reported medical errors in children. *Pediatrics* 2003;111:617–21.
39. Slonim AD, Pollack MM. Integrating the Institute of Medicine's six quality aims into pediatric critical care: Relevance and applications. *Pediatr Crit Care Med* 2005;6:264–9
40. Sochalski J. Quality of care, nurse staffing, and patient outcomes. *Policy Polit Nurs Pract* 2001;2:9–18.
41. Thomas EJ, Sexton JB, Helmreich RL. Discrepant attitudes about teamwork among critical care nurses and physicians. *Crit Care Med* 2003;31:956–9.
42. Thomas, EJ, Studdert DM, Newhouse JP, et al. Cost of medical injuries in Utah and Colorado. *Inquiry* 1999;36:255–64.
43. Van Drogen HPA, Dinges DF. Circadian rhythms in fatigue, alertness, and performance. In: Kryger MH, Roth T, Dement WC, eds. *Principles and Practice of Sleep Medicine*, 3rd ed. Philadelphia: WB Saunders, 2000:391–399.
44. Weinger MB. Incorporating human factors into the design of medical devices. *JAMA* 1998;280:1484.
45. When things go wrong. Responding to adverse events. A consensus statement of the Harvard hospitals. Massachusetts Coalition for the Prevention of Medical Errors, 2006.

CHAPTER 11 ■ INFORMATION TECHNOLOGY IN THE PICU

VINAY VAIDYA • STEVEN PON

The use of information technology has become just as ubiquitous and commonplace in the healthcare environment as it has in our personal lives. Today, the answer to any question that the mind can conceive is only a few mouse clicks and milliseconds away, thanks to the Internet and search engines, which have made available the collective wisdom and cumulative knowledge of mankind like nothing else has before. Yet, physicians as a group and the healthcare field in general have been slow to embrace technology when compared with other large industries, such as aviation, banking, and travel. Paradoxically, medicine is perhaps one of the most information-rich fields, and its practice is entwined with the management of information. The average physician has thousands of facts at his fingertips, and the Medline database has more than 16 million articles. Medical care has become so complex that it far exceeds the capacity of the human mind to implement it without the help of information technology. Clearly, computers have altered the way in which we deliver patient care to the point where we have come to depend on information technology in all aspects of medical care.

The focus of this chapter is on those information technologies and applications that have demonstrated a significant impact on healthcare delivery or those that have the potential to do so. The electronic medical record (EMR), computerized physician order entry (CPOE), clinical decision-support systems (DSSs), the Internet, telemedicine, and handheld computers are some of the technologies that have the potential of reducing errors, improving efficiency and quality of care, and reducing healthcare costs.

THE ELECTRONIC MEDICAL RECORD

Increasing numbers of personal health records are now stored in electronic form and are accessed and updated across communications networks. These databases comprise the EMR, or computer-based patient record. Its potential and real benefits include improved quality of care, cost savings, higher productivity, and easier aggregation and analysis of health data. The quality of care can be improved by more timely, more complete, and better-organized information delivery to the healthcare provider. Clinical decisions can also be supported through quantitative analysis of past experience; development of clinical rules, alerts, and protocols; and ready access to relevant reference materials. Eliminating duplicate testing and reducing lengths of stay by improving the quality of care can reduce costs. Making patient information more accessible to multiple users simultaneously, improving the continuity of care, creat-ing more consistent and comprehensive content, and reducing practice variation can enhance the productivity of healthcare workers. Finally, the EMR can facilitate research, education, quality improvement, outcomes assessment, and strategic planning.

While comprehensive implementations remain rare or nonexistent, some consensus does exist regarding the content and scope of the EMR. The three principle functions of this or any database are: data acquisition, data access, and data storage.

Data Acquisition

The complete EMR acquires data from a variety of sources, including hospital registration, nurse and physician input, laboratory services, radiology and other test interpretations, therapist and nutrition services, monitoring devices, and physicians' orders. The most important system that feeds the database is the "enterprise-wide master patient index" that ensures that each patient is identified properly and uniquely. Every other system must have the correct identifier to deliver its data to the correct patient record. A multimedia database can include images from such platforms as radiographs, electrocardiograms, fetal monitors, sonography, MRIs, CTs, and even paper-based documents, such as consent forms, questionnaires, and sometimes, handwritten notes and hand-drawn diagrams. Data acquisition is organized in a manner that minimizes duplicative effort and maximizes data consistency (7).

One of the significant challenges to any implementation of an EMR is engineering the interfaces between it and the host of systems that feed it data. The challenge is all the more daunting when it involves two-way interfaces, as with CPOE. Considering that a data element passes from one of several feeder systems through different computers, with possible transformations of that data element along the way, and considering the possibilities of lost transmissions, computer downtimes, and network interruptions, consistent error-free data feeding would seem a virtual miracle. In a high-volume environment, a centralized interface engine that routes and converts transaction messages from disparate feeder systems can solve many of the interface issues.

The capture of textual information such as progress notes, nursing assessments, or even radiology reports can present particular challenges. For the most part, text is entered via a keyboard, but alternatives include voice recognition, handwriting recognition, or handheld or wireless devices. Semiautomated text entry, with menu systems that feed structured or unstructured forms, is inconsistently successful. Although menu-driven systems do not have the same expressivity of free text, they lend themselves to the capture of text as data. Collecting data better allows for future analysis; however, despite this significant advantage over collecting bland text, these systems tend to be rigid, can make the unusual virtually impossible to enter, generally require more time to use, and may be a significant source of frustration for the clinician. The decision to pursue data rather than text requires an institutional commitment to the philosophy that data are more valuable and worth the difficulties that capturing can present.

Data Access

The EMR serves as the focal point for most healthcare professionals. It might be accessed at inpatient sites, in emergency departments, nursing facilities, physician offices, clinics, laboratory facilities, and, possibly, the home of a patient receiving home health services. The ideal computerized patient record is available when and where it is needed. However, databases with sensitive information must be controlled to prevent unauthorized use or alteration. These systems must satisfy five requirements: access control, authentication, confidentiality, integrity, and attribution/nonrepudiation. *Access control* means that only authorized persons are allowed access for authorized uses. *Authentication* refers to confirmation that a person granted access is, in fact, who they purport to be. *Confidentiality* prevents unauthorized disclosure of information. *Integrity* ensures that information content remains unalterable except under authorized circumstances. *Attribution/nonrepudiation* means that all actions taken (access, data entry, and data modification) are reliably traceable.

Much has been written about the interface through which most healthcare providers interact with the EMR. It should be user friendly and intuitive. Most clinicians have little time or patience to sit through tedious training sessions, and once trained, few clinicians will recall more than the minimum required to complete their immediate, routine tasks. The EMR should be capable of providing a full, seamless view of the patient over time and across points of care. Views should be configurable so that a given user's information needs and workflow can be accommodated. Both detailed and summary views that juxtapose relevant data allow the clinician to acquire the information required to optimize expedient decision making. Displays should be configured to highlight key information while suppressing clutter but, at the same time, making all pertinent data readily accessible. Dynamic linkages should exist between the EMR and supporting functions, such as expert systems, clinical pathways, protocols, and reference material. Response times must be sufficiently speedy, and workstations should be conveniently accessible to the point of care. Mobile connections would be a bonus, but access of patient data via wireless connections and portable devices must overcome usability and security hurdles before it can be fully implemented. The patient database also supports many areas of research, education, decision support, and external reporting. Thus, data in aggregate must be accessible by personnel in administration, finance, quality assurance, and research areas. Critical issues of patient information confidentiality are discussed later, under Health Insurance Portability and Accountability Act (HIPAA) regulations. The security of the database includes physical security, prevention of unauthorized access, and protection from malicious software.

Data Storage

The multimedia data of the comprehensive EMR are stored on media that allow for long-term storage and for searches and rapid retrieval of enormous volumes of data. The specific type of medium is not as important as ready availability of the data. The database must be updated in a way that ensures that it is current, complete, and consistent. Data, once entered, should be modifiable only in accordance with strict rules that ensure data integrity.

All databases must be backed-up periodically to protect against data loss. The strategy for doing so as seamlessly as possible, along with establishing a clear and workable recovery strategy, is absolutely imperative with an EMR.

Stored data should be marked with time stamps. Although the data can be modified, both the original and the revised versions should be maintained using appropriate time stamping. Appropriate safeguards must ensure database integrity—that its pieces do not lose their links and that the data are not subject to unauthorized modification. Supplanting the paper record with the EMR as the official medical record requires thoughtful consideration of the limitations of paper copies to accurately reflect the electronic record. Sanctioned hard copies of the patient record will be necessary for sharing with other healthcare institutions or with the legal system.

Whereas a clinical *data repository* is a database optimized to retrieve data on individual patients, a *data warehouse* is a database designed to support data analysis across individuals. This function can be distinguished from a simple archival function. The warehouse structure is designed to support a variety of analyses, including elaborate queries on large amounts of data. The data are generally static and updated intermittently in batches rather than continuously.

Hospitals can use data warehouses to perform financial analyses or quality assessments. With decision support tools, they can be useful in negotiating managed care contracts or distributing resources to clinical or ancillary services. Subsets of a data warehouse that are structured to support a single department or function are called *data marts* and are designed to perform periodic analyses or to produce standard reports run repeatedly, such as monthly financial statements or quality measurements. Some decision-support databases can be partially digested for more rapid analysis. In finance and administration, they can assist in strategic planning and, with appropriate modeling, can predict the impact of decisions before they are made. In medicine, data marts can take the form of a clinical database to support evidence-based decisions. *Data mining* applications can sift through mountains of data in the warehouse and run complex algorithms to find obscure patterns. However, as with any database, the questions must be defined as precisely as possible and the database must be designed appropriately to render meaningful results.

Clinical Decision-support Systems

Clinical DSSs are an integrated set of programs and databases that provide users with the ability to interrogate those databases and analyze information, retrieving data from external sources if necessary, to assist in decision making. Most medical DSSs are designed to improve the process and the outcome of clinical decision making. They can yield most of the benefit of clinical-information systems by helping to implement shortened inpatient lengths of stay, decreasing adverse drug interactions, improving the consistency and content of medical records, improving continuity of care and follow-up, and reducing practice variation.

Retrospective decision-support tools can be applied to aggregate patient data to find historic patterns. Real-time DSSs can be passive or active. Passive systems are activated when clinicians request help. Such assistance can come as reference material, automated calculations, or data review. Active systems include alerts and reminders that are triggered by pre-programmed rules. A warning displayed when penicillin is ordered for a patient known to be allergic is an example of an active DSS.

An effective DSS must have accurate and complete data, a user-friendly interface, a reliable knowledge base, and a good inferencing mechanism. The knowledge base can include information regarding risks, costs, disease states, clinical and laboratory findings, and clinical guidelines. The inference engine determines how and when the appropriate knowledge is applied.

Implementation

The implementation of an EMR system requires an investment of additional staff, hardware, software, and an expanded communications infrastructure or network. For large hospital networks, the costs can be exorbitant.

Developing an EMR requires careful planning and phased implementation. The specific needs of the institution must be examined, particularly with regard to the existing technology and practices. The process should be viewed as an opportunity to enhance care rather than simply to replace paper records, and it requires a reassessment of existing practices and re-engineering of healthcare delivery. As each incremental phase of implementation is approached, the focus should be on overcoming specific barriers to care rather than on the nebulous goal of "creating a paperless process."

The first phase generally provides a patient-centric repository of clinical test results, including laboratory, radiology, pathology, and other textual data. A subsequent phase can include capture of paper document images, radiology images, and other nontextual data. A key phase is the capture of clinical data at the point of care, including vital signs, intake and output, nursing documentation, and physician notes. The implementation of a physician order-entry system is another key phase that requires careful coordination among services and interdigitating systems.

Ensuring that the EMR satisfies every need involves considerable planning, designing, and testing. Even well-designed, off-the-shelf EMR systems can satisfy only 80% of the complex requirements of any multipractitioner organization. The remainder must be either adapted from other content or created from scratch. Substantial "expert" direction from teams of physicians, nurses, other allied healthcare providers, and medical records and financial staff is required to assist in developing the design and implementation of all EMRs. If clinicians abdicate their responsibility in participating in this tedious process, they are virtually ensuring that the resulting system will fail to satisfy their needs. Physician acceptance and participation can be enhanced by acknowledging the importance of physicians in the process, training them early and often, frequently and routinely eliciting their feedback, and demonstrating responsiveness to their needs and concerns.

Clinical information technology specialists generally interpret the requests from clinicians for configuration. A dedicated technical staff must also ensure instantaneous access to, and constant availability of, patient information. As the size and variety of information systems increase, enterprises will find it necessary to implement a "help desk" service.

Promises and Limitations

Information technology in the form of an EMR promises improved patient care. Potential benefits of information technology include providing rapid access to integrated clinical data and extant medical knowledge, eliminating illegibility, improving communication, and issuing applicable reminders and checks for appropriate medical actions.

A number of studies show that information technology can provide various benefits, including increasing adherence to guidelines (particularly in the outpatient arena) and decreasing some medication errors. However, most of these studies come from a very small number of institutions with home-grown clinical-information systems that were developed by devoted groups of clinicians. Very few studies show that the commercially available systems confer similar benefits and, even if they do, it is unclear that their success can be migrated from one implementation to another. In fact, any benefit may be outweighed by new problems introduced by the systems themselves. In effect, one set of problems may be traded for another (3).

Despite considerable progress, the sentiment expressed by G. Octo Barnett in 1966 is often echoed today, "It is frustrating to meet with repeated disappointments when the objectives are superficially so simple" (1). The medical information space is vastly more complicated than it seems at first. EMR software programs are enormously complex, are built by large teams of programmers with input by numerous clinicians, demand high-speed processors and high-bandwidth networks, and rely on often fragile interfaces with other hospital systems. Their implementation currently requires tremendous effort by both clinicians and technical specialists to configure these systems according to the specific needs of an institution and in ways that will enhance care rather than impede it. An often-unappreciated complicating factor is that the technology does not simply replace paper; it also reengineers care—deliberately or not.

Errors can and do occur in programming or configuration. Many programming deficiencies can be detected and corrected with thorough testing, preferably in a development environment that does not affect real patients; however, some of these problems will only become apparent under unique circumstances that are presented by patient care. Indefatigable vigilance for these errors is essential.

Numerous other unintended consequences result from implementing an EMR, including creation of new kinds of errors, increase in work for clinicians, untoward alteration of workflow and change in communication patterns, increase in system demands, continuation of the persistence of paper use, and fostering of potential overdependence on the technology.

New Kinds of Errors

Although some errors can be avoided by using an EMR with CPOE, other errors may be created or propagated. Many "new" errors are a result of poorly designed interfaces. Clinicians can easily make "juxtaposition errors," intending to select one item but selecting another close to it. Long, dense pick lists in a small font exacerbate this problem. A similar kind of error is mistaking an open chart of one patient to be that belonging to another, or picking the wrong patient from a long list of patients.

Interfaces between electronic systems are particularly vulnerable and can cause various new kinds of errors. Patients who have been physically transferred but remain, disembodied, in their previous electronic location may have all of their care suspended pending completion of the electronic transfer. Worse, should electronic transfers be delayed, medications may be delivered to a patient's former room and administered to a different patient admitted to that room. Allergies may be entered in the bedside system, but interface problems can prevent that information from reaching the pharmacy or nutrition systems. Occasionally, laboratory results can be inserted into the wrong medical record because of interface issues.

Rigid interpretation of policies and procedures can be configured into the EMR but may lead to difficulties in clinical practice when dealing with ambiguous circumstances and exceptions. Sometimes the process of care is incompletely understood, and codification can be disastrous. Policies at most institutions include automatic stop orders that require rewriting medication orders within a specified time frame. Compliance to this rule can be forced through programming, but implementing this rule without safeguards could lead to automatic discontinuation of medications and missed doses.

The benefit of legibility in electronically written notes can be outweighed by novel problems. Overuse of copy-paste functions can result in repetitive, monotonous, and loquacious notes punctuated by the sin of repeating erroneous text verbatim. The automatic transcription of data such as laboratory results or vital signs often bypasses cognition, something that does not happen when data are transcribed by hand.

Increased Work for Clinicians

Although transcription errors can be eliminated by computerized order entry, it often falls to clinicians to shoulder the added burden of what might otherwise be considered clerical functions. Documentation in a structured format rather than as free text can enhance completeness and facilitate later data retrieval; however, it can also increase work by forcing the clinician to find ways to fit round pegs into square holes. Similarly, rigidly structured order input can force clinicians to waste time trying different ways to order nonstandard tests or therapies—with little guarantee that these orders will actually be executed.

Clinical alerts can help clinicians make decisions—for example, when penicillin is mistakenly ordered for an allergic patient—but persistent interruptions of work by alerts can increase the workload of the clinician who must decipher their meaning and assess the risk in each specific circumstance. The frequency of these alerts can become intolerable when they are not delivered to the right clinician with the right information and at the right time and place. When these alerts become too frequent and too predictable, clinicians might adapt by "response chaining": dismissing the alerts with rote keystrokes

much as a pianist plays a familiar tune. Alerts that evoke this response cannot be effective.

Poorly integrated clinical-information systems cause clinicians to access many different sources for information to solve a clinical problem, thereby increasing work. Similarly, users should not be required to input the same bit of data in multiple locations in different systems.

Another time-consuming feature of the EMR, perhaps the most exasperating, is the loss of data. Workstation or interface crashes, network collisions, or other system failures can be the culprit. System delays from a wide variety of causes also waste valuable time, as does having to hunt for an available workstation because those installed are insufficient in number or inconveniently placed.

Unfavorable Alteration of Workflow

The introduction of an EMR system significantly alters the sociotechnologic milieu. Previously well-functioning medical practices may become entirely dysfunctional. The implementation of an EMR requires work processes modeling, but can sometimes result in ossifying those processes to something too inflexible for efficient and effective patient care.

Patients expected to be emergently admitted to the PICU but still in transit often have medications and urgent therapies ordered and prepared before arrival. A CPOE system may prohibit the ordering or dispensing of medications for patients who have not yet been admitted. In a paper environment, nurses arrange dosing schedules based on the ordered frequency and other ordered medications. However, in many CPOE systems, medication orders go direct to the pharmacy and bypass the bedside nurse. Physicians are then saddled with picking the specific times of administration, only to have that schedule revised later by the nurse.

Sometimes, well-defined manual processes can be implemented in more than one way electronically. Without the clear delineation of an institutionally sanctioned method, confusion and catastrophe can result. Transferring patients from one unit to another or to the operating room typically requires the discontinuation and reinitiation of all orders, including medications. With implementation of CPOE, clinicians without proper direction could suspend rather than discontinue the old orders. Reactivation of suspended orders could result in duplication and double-dosing of medications ordered on transfer.

Redundant orders are sometimes facilitated by CPOE. The gate-keeping function of clerical personnel processing orders for routine radiographs or laboratories is bypassed. Remote access by multiple physicians acting on the same bit of new information can also generate duplicate orders.

Untoward Changes in Communication Patterns

Many care providers blame clinical-information systems for unsatisfactory reductions in face-to-face communication. Some users complain that the EMR creates an "illusion of communication" (2), in which users believe that information entered into the system will be somehow communicated to the relevant personnel. This assumption can result in the missed or delayed execution of orders or failure to appreciate the recommendations of a consultant. Users may erroneously assume that allergies entered into the system will adequately protect patients from receiving offending food or drugs.

Because of the time-consuming nature of CPOE and because workstations are not always available at the bedside, orders are often written after work rounds. In teaching hospitals, order writing is often delegated to the least experienced individual, such as the first-year resident. Residents may not readily appreciate the nuances of an order until they are confronted with an order screen that demands numerous inputs. By that time, the other members of the care team have disbanded, and clarification of the order requires tracking down and reconsulting the relevant personnel.

High System Demands and Frequent Changes

No installed EMR can remain static for long. Maintenance, revisions, and upgrades of both software and hardware contribute to constant flux. Consequences should be expected with every change, and many changes require testing that can become onerous. Although minor changes can occur without supplemental training of personnel, failure to provide training for some changes can cause significant user frustration and errors. Some configuration changes requested by one group may also adversely affect other users in unexpected ways. Mechanisms must be developed to resolve conflicts of this nature. As clinicians become increasingly dependent on the system, pressure to keep the system operational mounts, requiring around-the-clock technical support. One poignant analogy likened system maintenance to "repairing a jet engine in flight" (2).

Persistence of Paper

Anecdotally, the installation of an EMR is associated with an increase in consumption of paper towels: clinicians often jot vital signs and other data on any scrap of paper available, to be entered into the EMR at a later, more convenient time. Whereas "going paperless" is an often-stated goal, the elimination of this most versatile recording device is unlikely. An EMR changes the pattern of paper consumption: a higher proportion of pulp is sent to the shredder rather than to medical records. Reports are printed in the process of caring for patients and are often discarded at the end of a shift. Some institutions also regularly print worksheets as backup in the event that the system experiences unscheduled downtime.

A more insidious problem of persisting paper can arise when the patient chart is divided between paper and an electronic version, particularly when one medical service writes notes in one medium and another service uses the other. Splitting physician documentation can result in breakdowns in communication, with serious consequences. Delineation of the exact constituents of the legal medical record is also a necessary exercise, one that must be repeated as the systems change.

Overdependence on Technology

As the EMR becomes more integrated into clinical practice, downtime becomes more onerous to the users. Prolonged failures can even cripple an organization by causing delays, diminishing capacity, and limiting capabilities. Although backup systems can never quite replace the fully functioning system, contingencies for downtime must be developed, and users must be adequately trained to execute these plans efficiently.

Clinical DSSs can enhance the educational value of interactions with the EMR. They can also increase reliance on the information presented, without providing significant learning, thereby precipitating uncertainty and paralysis in practitioners who encounter situations in which decision support is not available. The danger also exists that clinicians will accept advice rendered by clinical DSSs in circumstances when they should not.

Human-factors Engineering

Cognitive science, computer science, and human-factors engineering are among the many disciplines that can facilitate the development of a successful EMR system. Human-factors engineering investigates human capabilities and limitations and applies that knowledge in the design of systems, software, environments, training, and personnel management. The application of human-factors considerations in developing an EMR, particularly regarding CPOE, can maximize the successful design and implementation of these systems. Some human-factors principles may seem self-evident but can be overlooked when not approached systematically. Developers must understand the users, must undertake detailed task analyses, and must assess computer-supported cooperative work—the study of how people work within organizations and how technology affects them and their work. Three principles of this study that may improve clinical-information systems are accounting for incentive structures, understanding workflow, and promoting awareness of the activities of other group members. Institutional and personal incentives for using an EMR differ, but only the latter will effectively influence use. Awareness of the roles played by other team members enhances collaboration. Improving collaboration may decrease the incidence of medical errors (13).

Another important area of human-factors engineering relates to interface design. Interfaces should be simple and consistent, with important data highlighted, such as the patient name or weight. "Progressive disclosure" means that commonly used and important functions should be presented first and in a logical order, whereas infrequently used functions should be hidden but available. Minimizing "human memory load" can be accomplished by displaying all relevant information together. Potential user errors should be anticipated, and easy error recovery should be designed into the system. Error messages should be informative and could include advice about error recovery. Other feedback should be provided to acknowledge user actions, particularly when the system appears frozen. Given the chaotic healthcare environment, the interface should also be designed to forgive interruptions, allowing work to be saved and resumed later.

User satisfaction is an important predictor of system success. Satisfaction is enhanced when the systems are designed with the users' needs and preferences in mind. Peers who serve as advocates for their groups during development, and subsequently teach other users, generally increase acceptance of the systems. Ease of use, rapid response times, flexibility and customizability, mobile workstations, implementation of effective decision-support tools, access to reference information, and adequate training and support are all important factors in enhancing both user satisfaction and system success.

HEALTH INSURANCE PORTABILITY AND ACCOUNTABILITY ACT

The Health Insurance Portability and Accountability Act (HIPAA) was intended to protect health insurance coverage for workers and their families if they changed or lost their jobs. While attempting to decrease the administrative burdens of healthcare delivery (administrative simplification), a number of important issues were raised about patient privacy. Examination of the full impact of HIPAA is well beyond the scope of this chapter, but some elements are particularly relevant to a discussion of the EMR.

The Security Standards of the Act mandate safeguards for the physical storage and maintenance of, and access to, patient data. The Privacy Rule protects confidentiality and privacy of protected health information. The intent of these regulations was not to prevent legitimate access to information but to put limits on uses of patient information beyond patient care or business activities directly related to patient care. Specifically, the Privacy Rule (a) limits the nonconsensual use and release of private health information, (b) gives patients new rights to access their medical records and to know who has accessed them, (c) restricts most disclosures of health information to the minimum needed for the intended purpose, (d) establishes new criminal and civil sanctions for improper use or disclosure, and (e) establishes new requirements for access to records by researchers and others.

Specific implementation of these rules depends on the circumstances of each organization. Hospitals with computer networks must have security measures to permit appropriate access. Regardless of the specifics, institutional policies must be established and followed. In the past, employees who violated these policies, including sharing personal access (e.g., passwords) or accessing information to which the employee had no right, were punished by official reprimand or, at worst, dismissal. Under the new rules, violators may also face criminal or civil penalties.

The Privacy Rule also has a significant impact on research as it relates to (a) obtaining consent paperwork that safeguards the privacy of participating patients, (b) simplifying guidelines regarding the limited circumstances in which patient health information may be used for research purposes without authorization by the research subject, and (c) clarifying methods by which protected patient health information can be identified so that such information can be disclosed freely. Although the intent of HIPAA policies was not to limit research, evidence suggests that HIPAA-mandated authorizations discourage patients from participating (9).

THE INTERNET

The Internet has undergone phenomenal growth in the last decade and has transformed the very nature of information transactions. It is estimated that the number of Internet users will exceed 1 billion by 2008. The influence of this exponential growth has often been compared to the revolution engendered by Gutenberg's invention of the printing press in the 15th century. In contrast to such traditional information as libraries, the Internet provides instant access to vast amounts of information on any subject, anywhere, at anytime, to anyone with a computer and Internet access. For the healthcare worker, it has become both a vast repository of clinical and research knowledge and a tool used in day-to-day practice. The Internet is a loosely defined aggregate of global computers connected in a network that is constantly evolving. Wikipedia (www.wikipedia.com), the largest online Internet encyclopedia, defines the Internet as:

> The worldwide, publicly accessible network of interconnected computer networks, a "network of networks" that consists of millions of smaller domestic, academic, business, and government networks which together carry various information and services, such as electronic mail, online chat, file transfer, and the interlinked Web pages and other documents of the World Wide Web.

Often, the terms *Internet* and *World Wide Web* (WWW) are mistakenly interchanged, but the two are not synonymous. The Internet is a collection of interconnected computer networks, whereas the WWW is a collection of interconnected documents, linked by hyperlinks. The *intra*net is an internal network that uses Internet technologies and is often used by organizations to provide a secure network to support internal exchange of information. Web pages are accessed through applications known as *browsers*, such as Internet Explorer, Netscape, Mozilla Firefox, and others, whereas information on the WWW is searched via search engines such as Google. Common methods of Internet access include dial-up, broadband cable, Wi-Fi, and cell phones. Wi-Fi provides wireless access to computer networks and to the Internet. Wi-Fi hotspots are local areas where wireless coverage is provided either free of charge or for a fee, allowing users with mobile computers to access the Internet. Many universities and hospitals provide wireless access throughout their campuses.

The Internet, which began in the in late 1960s as a US military application, was designed to provide a communications network that would work even if some of the nodes were destroyed by possible nuclear attacks. The Advanced Research Projects Agency Network (ARPANET), developed by the Department of Defense, was the precursor of the global Internet. From its humble beginnings, the system grew steadily during the 1980s into a network of global computers. It extended beyond military use into the academic environment, where it was mainly used for e-mails and file transfers. Subsequent growth was exponential, with the introduction of the WWW, allowing its spread beyond academic boundaries into general public and commercial use. The WWW provided a simple and easy way to search and find documents on the Internet, which in turn, fueled the rapid explosion of accessible information that was placed on the web. The next phase ushered in the development of commercial use of the Internet to serve a multitude of functions, from booking airline tickets to accessing medical records, from e-commerce to e-health.

Internet Communication Services

The Internet supports various forms of communication services and protocols that allow information to flow from point to point, including e-mail, newsgroups, LISTSERVs, file transfer protocols, streaming media, voice-over-Internet protocols, and others.

E-mail communication was among the initial and most widely used Internet services. Although it is extensively used by almost all healthcare workers to communicate among themselves, recent trends include e-mails between physicians and patients, which increases opportunities for patient access to care, education, and the potential for increased compliance to therapy. Both healthcare providers and patients must be aware of the limitations and hazards posed by this means of communication. E-mail is vulnerable to being intercepted, read, or even modified by unauthorized parties. As has been well demonstrated, e-mail has been used effectively by unscrupulous individuals for the mass dissemination of computer viruses. Measures such as encryption, electronic signature, and virus scanning can improve the safety of e-mail communications but may not totally eliminate all of the hazards.

Newsgroups and LISTSERVs

As an extension of e-mail communications, groups with common interests form a common e-mail group known as a LISTSERV or a mailing list. The e-mails that originate from any member of the group are directed to all members and serve to generate ongoing discussion on any given topic of interest. For example, healthcare workers exchange ideas on pediatric intensive care–related topics via the PICU LISTSERV.

Newsgroups are similar to mailing lists, where members of the newsgroup post and respond to messages. Unlike the mailing list, where e-mails are sent to all members, newsgroup messages are posted on a news server from which members can access and respond to the postings. Newsgroup software allows users to search for a topic of interest or to follow all messages in a single discussion thread. Many patients who share a common diagnosis (e.g., Down syndrome) often join newsgroups to communicate with other patients and families with similar medical conditions.

File transfer protocol (FTP) allows files to be transferred and retrieved between computers connected over the Internet. Documents, images, sound, and video files can all be transferred via this protocol. Digitized radiology files are often transmitted using these protocols.

Streaming media such as *webcasts* permit the broadcast of audio and visual data to any remote computer that is connected to the Internet. It may be used to broadcast medical conference proceedings, either live or from archived files, to a large number of participants who may otherwise not have been able to attend in person. Webcasts of talks from nationally and internationally renowned scientists can thus be made available to remote users at any time. Although webcasts are primarily one-way presentations to an audience that does not communicate with the presenter, *web conferences* are smaller, more interactive meetings that enable two or more participants to simultaneously view and hear the same content in real time on remote computers connected via the Internet. Thus, web conferences allow professionals to communicate effectively through virtual interactive meetings over the Internet, thereby reducing the travel time and expenses involved in face-to-face meetings.

Podcasting is a variation of a webcast that contains only audio material. Podcasts can be easily downloaded to portable digital audio players and listened to on the move. The Society for Critical Care Medicine offers iCritical Care podcasts (http://www.sccm.org/SCCM/Publications/iCritical+Care/) that allow listeners to keep up-to-date with the latest topics in critical care. Users can download and listen to audio content on mobile digital audio players. New content is automatically downloaded to users' desktop computers and synchronized with their audio devices whenever these devices are connected to the computers. Many of the podcasts provide continuing medical education credits.

Webcasts and podcasts can be created relatively easily by anyone using simple equipment. Webcams can be used to create low-budget webcasts or, more commonly, live video communications. For example, Internet users can watch live surgery anywhere in the world. Voice-over-Internet protocol (VoIP), which allows voice to travel over the Internet, either free of charge or at a much reduced cost compared to a normal telephone call, has made real-time audio and video conferencing relatively easy and affordable.

Internet Searching Tips and Resources for Providers

Search engines enable users to rapidly pinpoint the information of interest from among billions of websites and documents available on the WWW. To produce relevant search results, the Google search engine uses a mathematical formula to rank pages based on the frequency with which they have been cited by other sites.

Although searching the web has become second nature to most healthcare workers, the use of certain advanced search techniques can help to improve the sensitivity and specificity of any given search. Frequently visited websites can be bookmarked for easy future access. Placing quotation marks around search words in Google ensures that all of the words within the quotation are searched together as a single phrase; for example, entering the search term "toxic shock syndrome" ensures that all three words are searched together as a single phrase rather than each word being searched separately. A minus sign placed before a word ensures that the particular word is excluded from the search; for example, entering the search term, "immunodeficiency –HIV" ensures that the search filters out all results that contain the term "HIV," thus returning results only pertaining to immunodeficiency disorders not related to HIV. A specific term can be searched within a specific website; for example, "stroke site:http://medschool.umaryland.edu" will search for all web pages within the University of Maryland School of Medicine's website that contain the word "stroke." Other advanced search strategies can be accessed from the Google search page by clicking on the link, "Advanced Search."

The Google search engine includes a simple calculator and a conversion calculator that healthcare providers may find useful. Entering the term "5 × 10" in the search box, returns the calculated value of 50, while entering the term "98 F to C" returns the value "36.6 degrees Celsius" by converting 98 degrees Fahrenheit to Celsius.

A recent addition is the Google Scholar Beta search engine at www.scholar.google.com, which is Google's effort to index scholarly literature. Google Scholar allows users to conduct a comprehensive search of scholarly literature that includes peer-reviewed papers, abstracts, and articles, as well as theses and books from academic publishers, professional societies, preprint repositories, universities, and other scholarly organizations. The results are thus more extensive than those obtained by searching the Medline database through PubMed. Results are sorted by the frequency with which each article is cited in other scholarly literature. Each search result contains bibliographic information, such as the title, author name, and source of publication, as well as the availability of the article from local academic libraries. The Google Scholar search engine also permits searching by author, title, and publication.

In addition to the PubMed and Google Scholar search engines for journal articles and scholarly work, a number of websites are particularly useful to pediatric critical care practitioners. The Pediatric Critical Care Medicine website at http://www.PedsCCM.org is a comprehensive website dedicated to the specialty. It contains many useful clinical and research resources, evidence-based medicine journal club discussions, conference and continuing medical education (CME) information, job listings, and links to other useful websites.

The Virtual PICU website at http://www.vpicu.org provides a common space for the sharing of information by the international community that provides care for critically ill children. It offers the Virtual PICU software, a clinical database for standardized data collection, analysis, and comparative reports among PICUs. Participants can collect information on patient and hospital measures, diagnoses, interventions, discharges, organ donations, and pediatric severity of illness and mortality scores. This data can be used for internal research, multisite research, and benchmarking measures. The Virtual PICU also hosts the PICUList, an e-mail mailing list for the discussion of PICU issues.

Some other useful medical reference websites include www.emedicine.com, a web-based electronic textbook; UptoDate Online at www.utdol.com, a subscription-based comprehensive electronic textbook to which many academic institutions subscribe; www.mdconsult.com and www.merckmedicus.com, both of which offer similar services that include journal articles, electronic textbooks, drug references, and patient education material. Many of these websites provide CME courses that can be completed online. Features include the ability to search for CME by specialty, to receive e-mail alerts of new CME courses that match areas of interest, to automatically log and track CME activities completed, and to view a list of CME requirements for each state. Many of the CME courses are available in Webcast format that simulates the conference environment by displaying the speaker and the slides. For those who prefer to attend live, in-person CME courses, www.findthatce.com allows users to locate CMEs, searchable by geographic location and topic of interest. Users can even specify details such as the distance they would drive to attend a live CME program and a variety of other options. A number of services provide e-mail delivery of tables of contents from various journals, which is yet another way the Internet can help practitioners to keep up with current medical literature.

Healthcare on the Internet for Consumers

The Internet provides an ideal media for meeting consumer healthcare needs, as large volumes of frequently updated medical information can be published rapidly, cheaply, and efficiently. Using the Internet to obtain health information regarding diagnosis, treatment, and drug medications is one of the most popular consumer uses of the Internet. Users can access this information from the privacy and convenience of their homes. Patients who share common health problems have formed numerous online communities that provide peer support, information on the latest research, and an exchange of personal experiences. A 2002 study by the California Healthcare Foundation found that 70% of consumers reported that the information found on the Internet influences their treatment decisions. The Internet empowers consumers, who can now easily learn where physicians trained, if they have any outstanding lawsuits, and how a particular hospital ranks relative to other hospitals.

Although the Internet can provide convenient access to a large body of useful healthcare information, consumers must be aware of the quality and authenticity of this information before they use it to make critical decisions affecting their healthcare. Many publications on the Internet lack the peer-review process associated with printed publications. An Australian study in 2003 found that many consumers do not properly interpret the healthcare information they find on the Internet and that this, in turn, could lead to anxiety and poor compliance with therapy (11). Healthcare professionals should guide and teach consumers on how to find reliable healthcare information on the Internet, emphasizing the variable quality of such information. Because anyone can host a website cheaply and quickly, the Internet is open to the use of unscrupulous individuals. The publication of medical information that ranges from incorrect to outright dangerous and the sale of illicit drugs via the Internet are some examples of the misuse of this technology. A 2004 study found that information on the Internet regarding medical emergencies was often incomplete and, in some cases, potentially dangerous (15).

A wide range of high-quality websites is available for consumer health information. The Medline Plus website (http://medlineplus.gov) is the consumer version of the National Library of Medicine's Medline database and includes consumer healthcare information on more than 700 topics, drug information for patients, a medical encyclopedia, interactive tutorials and videos, and links to ClinicalTrials.gov, which provides information about clinical research trials in human volunteers. New features enable consumers to register for e-mail updates and to download the *Medline Plus* magazine. Medline Plus also links to many other useful healthcare sites that meet a certain standard. The website of the Centers for Disease Control and Prevention (http://www.cdc.gov) contains information that supports the goal of promoting health and quality of life by preventing and controlling disease, injury, and disability. It contains information on topics such as environmental health, emergency preparedness and response, health promotion, traveler's health, vaccines, and immunizations. Other commercial and pharmaceutical websites that are geared toward consumer health information include www.WebMD.com, www.Intelihealth.com, and www.DrKoop.com. Many medical societies (e.g., the American Diabetic Association) also provide consumer health information on their websites, as do healthcare insurance organizations.

Physicians and the Internet

Physicians, while being among the highest users of e-mail for personal use, have often been reluctant to use the Internet for patient interactions. On the other hand, patients are eager for electronic communications with their physicians. Many patients feel more comfortable communicating via e-mail than discussing their questions in person. A 2002 Harris Interactive study found that 90% of surveyed Americans said that they would like to be able to contact their physician on the Internet; 40% said that they would pay for this access, and 77% said that they would like to be able to ask questions online rather than visit the doctor's office. A study by Blue Shield and ConnectiCare found that they could provide online health visits for much less money than in-office visits and compensate the physicians fairly. However, doctors are reluctant to provide this service. Many doctors consider e-mail communications with patients as an additional burden on an already overcrowded schedule and have concerns regarding liability, privacy, and re-imbursement issues.

Internet and Security

Although the Internet is geared toward providing open access to publicly stored information, it is equally important to safe-guard transactions related to healthcare and e-commerce from unauthorized access. This protection is achieved either by the encryption of data as it is transmitted over the Internet to pre-vent its interception or by limiting access to data by placing it on secure internal networks and providing access through authenticated user accounts and passwords.

As the Internet evolves and continues to provide increased connectivity among healthcare providers, healthcare institu-tions, and consumers at ever-increasing speeds, we should be able to harness its power for patient care, safety, improved ef-ficiencies, and cost savings. All aspects of healthcare, including medical education, research, and clinical practice will continue to be transformed as the power of the Internet unfolds in the coming years. The day is not far off when individual medi-cal records will be universally accessible online not only for providers but also for patients.

HANDHELD COMPUTERS

Point-of-care computing, also known as *mobile computing*, is a fast-emerging technology that allows users to access infor-mation resources at the point of care and at the time of care. Thanks to advances in wireless networks, hardware, and pro-cessor speeds, mobile computing is making major inroads into the healthcare environment. Small, portable, handheld com-puters, also known as *personal digital assistants* (PDAs) are powerful enough to meet most of the information needs of to-day's healthcare workers. The newer Smartphones combine a cellular phone with a PDA, thus increasing utility while elim-inating the need to carry two separate devices. With a wide array of devices from which to choose and the rapid growth in development of medical software, PDAs come very close to replacing the functionality found in laptop computers. More and more practitioners are depending on these valuable de-vices, which fit comfortably in their coat pockets as well as in their hands. Perhaps it may not be too farfetched to imagine the day when PDAs may well replace the stethoscope as the physi-cian's primary tool. The earliest PDAs were mainly designed as electronic replacements for the paper-based organizer and the personal phone book. Today, the PDA offers much more functionality than the original basic electronic organizer. It can be used as a phone, a pager, an e-mail and text-messaging de-vice, an MP3 player for listening to professional educational material or to music, a voice recorder for patient documenta-tion, a camera for personal or professional pictures, a medical textbook or drug reference source, a newspaper, a radio, a tele-vision, a PALS handbook, an electronic book reader, a GPS de-vice, a wireless web browser, a device for medical billing or to print patient handouts, a patient database to review laboratory values and order medications—the list of uses seems endless.

Whether used to research the latest evidence-based citation on MEDLINE or the location of the nearest sushi restaurant in a new city, PDAs can provide today's healthcare workers with a wide array of information when and where it is needed. The PDA's compact form factor and wireless connectivity result in unparalleled convenience and ease of use.

Hardware and Software

PDAs are available in two broad categories: those based on the Palm operating system and those based on the Windows mo-bile operating system. Initially, the Palm-based PDAs were less expensive and had a greater choice of software titles, making them the preferred option for many users. However, the dif-ference between the two platforms is shrinking, both in price and the software availability; therefore, choosing between them is mainly based on user preference. An ever-increasing variety of medical software programs, both free and commercial, is available for downloading from the WWW. These programs, designed for various healthcare tasks, enhance the usefulness of PDAs by meeting the specific needs of healthcare practition-ers. One of the most comprehensive sources of information in pediatrics available for handheld computers is the Pediatrics on Hand website at http://www.dcchildrens.com/pdas/home.aspx. This site has information that ranges from how to buy a PDA to an extensive list of carefully reviewed software targeted at the pediatric healthcare provider. The website is maintained by Dr. David C. Stockwell, a PICU physician at Children's Na-tional Medical Center in Washington, DC. A categorized list of software that PICU practitioners may find useful is shown in **Table 11.1**.

Useful Services for Handheld Computers

A number of websites provide useful medical services specifi-cally geared for use on PDAs. MD on Tap (http://mdot.nlm.nih .gov/proj/mdot/mdot.php) is an application that allows mobile healthcare professionals to search and retrieve MEDLINE ci-tations directly from their handheld devices, through a wire-less connection to the Internet. Healthcare professionals can thus wirelessly access the entire MEDLINE database, with its more than 16 million citations, at the point of care, while they are away from their desktop computers. This accessibility is a distinct advantage over other similar services that provide ac-cess to MEDLINE citations but require users to synchronize their handhelds to their desktops to retrieve the search results. An alternate way to access the MEDLINE database via PDA is the PubMed website, http://pubmedhh.nlm.nih.gov/nlm/, which has been specifically optimized for searching the MED-LINE database via mobile handheld devices. The *MerckMedi-cus PDA tools* include useful downloads, such as the Pocket Guide to Diagnostic Tests; Asthma Guidelines from the Na-tional Heart, Lung, and Blood Institute; and other DSS tools. *Mobile MerckMedicus* provides citations and abstracts for the current issues of over 200 medical journals. Abstracts from selected journals are downloaded to the PDA during synchro-nization with a desktop computer and can be viewed on the PDA at any time. *MD Consult Mobile* is a PDA companion to the web-based MD Consult service that allows users to read medical news, drug updates, and tables of contents from

TABLE 11.1

MEDICAL SOFTWARE FOR HANDHELD COMPUTERS

Drug References
Pediatric Lexi-Drugs is the handheld version of the standard pediatric drug reference book that is by far the most comprehensive and widely used pediatric drug reference. *ePocrates Rx* is another drug reference available for free downloading to PDAs. It contains adult and pediatric dosing information. *Epocrates Essentials* is a suite of applications available for an annual paid subscription. In addition to the free drug reference, it includes a differential diagnosis guide, a disease reference guide, a laboratory guide, and many other features.

Medical References
Some of the commonly used pediatric reference textbooks available in the handheld format include the *American Academy of Pediatrics Red Book 2006*, *The Harriet Lane Handbook*, the *5-Minute Pediatric Clinical Consult*, and the *Washington Manual Pediatrics Survival Guide*. *UptoDate*, the popular evidence-based information resource, is also available for use on PDAs running the Windows mobile operating system.

Medical Calculators and Utilities
ER and ICU Toolbox is a useful suite of applications geared toward emergency and ICU care. Useful modules include PALS protocols, code medications and drip calculators, a drug calculator, an antibiotic guide, a toxicology guide, and many more.
PICU Tools (free) is similar software application that consists of many useful calculators, such as a blood gas calculator, Swan-Ganz calculator, and other reference materials that are useful in the PICU environment. It is written and maintained by Dr. Michael J. Verive, a PICU physician.
Documents to Go is a suite of programs equivalent to desktop Microsoft Office Suite software; it allows Word, Excel, and PowerPoint documents to be seamlessly viewed, edited, and saved on the PDA and synchronized with corresponding files on the desktop. PowerPoint presentations, lecture notes, abstracts of MEDLINE citations, educational handouts, policy manuals, procedure note templates, and Excel files with research data are some examples of files that can be easily stored and accessed from the PDA using Documents to Go.

Patient Databases
PatientKeeper is a popular patient database program that integrates with clinical-information systems to provide ready access to test results, medication histories, allergies, vital signs, and other clinical information through handheld computers at the point of care.

Billing and Coding Software
Numerous software products are available for use on PDAs to assist with billing and coding, including *PatientKeeper Charge Capture*, Skyscape's *ICD-9 CM*, *ZapMed*, *BluefishRx*, and others that enable providers to look up and select ICD-9 codes, CPT codes, and evaluation and management codes, and to wirelessly transmit the billing data to appropriate sites.

---

journals on their PDAs. *AvantGo* is a free, mobile content service that synchronizes mobile versions of favorite websites, called "channels," to users' PDAs or Smartphones. AvantGo offers medical channels, along with channels in many other categories, such as news, weather, sports, and education.

Limitations and the Future of Handheld Computers

Although PDAs hold great promise as innovative productivity tools for healthcare practitioners, they are associated with certain limitations. The small screen size limits the amount of information that can be viewed in one screen, and the display can sometimes be visually challenging. Although the compact form factor makes PDAs portable and convenient to carry, the chance of damage from inadvertently dropping these small mobile devices is increased. Unlike desktop computers, PDAs can be easily misplaced or stolen, and because PDAs can store relatively large amounts of patient data, loss or theft of the device may potentially jeopardize the confidentiality of protected health information. Many healthcare software applications include data encryption technology to ensure HIPAA compliance and safeguard against such loss. Healthcare workers should be educated about these risks and reminded to keep careful physical custody of their devices and to use passwords to prevent unauthorized access. In spite of some of the inherent limitations, the future for PDA usage among healthcare workers is bright. A 2006 meta-analysis of surveys revealed clear evidence of an increasing trend in PDA usage by healthcare professionals. The overall adoption rate by individuals ranged between 45% and 85%, indicating a high but somewhat variable adoption (5). This adoption rate represents the highest rate of increase, according to a commonly accepted model that is used to measure the diffusion of any new technology. These trends indicate that, without doubt, PDAs or "peripheral brains," as they are commonly called, will continue to enjoy increasing popularity and acceptance among PICU and other healthcare providers.

TELEMEDICINE

Although the term *telemedicine* conjures up futuristic visions, such as robotic surgery, it has been used universally for decades in the form of simple telephone communications between healthcare providers and patients. Although telemedicine often implies healthcare provided by physicians, *telehealth* covers a much broader scope to include healthcare provided by nurses and pharmacists, as well as healthcare education provided to medical practitioners. The Office for the Advancement of Telehealth describes telemedicine as "the use of electronic information and telecommunication technologies to support long-distance clinical healthcare, patient and professional health-related education, public health, and health administration" (10).

One of the early examples of use of groundbreaking telemedicine service occurred during the 1960s, when the University of Nebraska provided remote telemedicine psychiatric services to a state hospital located more than 100 miles away. Another example occurred when a physician on an Antarctica research expedition in 1999 found a lump in her breast but was unable to leave the expedition for 8 months due to winter weather conditions. Via remote consultation, she performed a biopsy on herself, and her colleagues received instructions on how to make pathology slides and transmit the pictures to physicians in the US via satellite. A diagnosis of breast cancer was made, and chemotherapeutic agents available at the research station were used until the physician could be flown back to the US. Although this represents a rather dramatic example, telemedicine is more commonly used to ensure equitable access to expert medical care in remote and underserved areas, provide remote patient and provider education, reduce travel requirements, improve patient care, and reduce costs. It can improve the collaboration and sharing among distant providers, and it permits experts to deliver state-of-the-art care to many more patients in resource-limited areas than would be possible via traditional face-to-face encounters. Technologies that are commonly used to provide live, interactive communications between linked sites, making telemedicine feasible, include videoconferencing, Internet communications, store-and-forward imaging, streaming media, and land-line and wireless communications.

Several studies have demonstrated that full-time intensivist coverage in ICUs results in a significant reduction in ICU mortality, lengths of stay, and resource utilization (6). Yet, the national shortage of intensivists and the high cost associated with 24-hr intensivist coverage are barriers that preclude hospitals from providing such services. The application of telemedicine in ICUs is ideally suited to address this shortfall by allowing off-site intensivists to monitor and care for many more ICU patients than is possible with direct hands-on care. Initial studies of remote ICU monitoring conducted at the Johns Hopkins University demonstrated a reduction in severity-adjusted ICU mortality by 68% and a 44% reduction in the incidence of ICU complications. ICU lengths of stay and ICU costs were also decreased (12). A commercial remote ICU telemedicine company, VISICU, evolved from this research and offers continuous management of ICU patients by providing off-site remote monitoring to augment the on-site care provided by local healthcare providers. Although remote ICU care via telemedicine will not replace on-site care, it can supplement the level of care by improving the level of expert physician coverage.

Preliminary studies of telemedicine applications have demonstrated successful live, interactive consultations provided by regional PICU experts for critically ill children being cared for in adult ICUs in remote communities (8). Although these are examples of successful telemedicine applications, systematic reviews of telemedicine projects have shown mixed to negative results. The outcomes most often studied include user satisfaction, financial benefits, and clinical outcomes. A systematic review of more than 600 telemedicine cost-benefit studies found that <10% of the studies met the criteria for good economic analysis. Of the 24 studies included in the review, many were small-scale or short-term projects, leading the authors to conclude that the current evidence did not conclusively demonstrate a cost-benefit advantage from telemedicine projects (14). Similarly, a Cochrane review in 2000 that evaluated clinical outcomes identified seven telemedicine trials and concluded that evidence from these trials failed to show unequivocal clinical benefits (4). The strongest evidence of clinical benefit is from home-based telemedicine projects for chronic disease management and diagnostic telemedicine projects in psychiatry and dermatology.

Although telemedicine has the potential to ensure quality healthcare to remote and underserved populations, reduce costs, and address the national shortage of healthcare providers, its widespread progress has been hampered by a number of constraints. For telemedicine to succeed, both providers and end users must "buy in." Many practitioners often resist new technology due to real or perceived concerns that it may reduce their autonomy. Reimbursement guidelines must be created to ensure that providers are compensated for services rendered. Current licensures are state based, making it difficult to provide care across state boundaries. Sustained funding is necessary for the initial setup and for ongoing support and maintenance. As solutions to these challenges continue to evolve, telemedicine will play in increasing role in the ICU of the future. Large-scale, good-quality research trials that compare telemedicine directly with conventional, face-to-face, traditional healthcare should be conducted to convincingly demonstrate the benefits of this modality.

CONCLUSIONS AND FUTURE DIRECTIONS

In this chapter, we have discussed some representative applications and information technologies that are reshaping the way in which medical care is being delivered now and will be delivered in the future. Although the use of information technology in healthcare has been gathering rapid momentum, its widespread implementation and uniform utilization are still a dream that has not been fully realized. Technology will undoubtedly continue to play a greater role in all aspects of health delivery, including clinical practice, research, and education. However, technology by itself is not a panacea, and it will never replace compassionate patient care and human contact. Experience has clearly shown that the improper selection and implementation of technology in the healthcare arena will produce negative results instead of bringing about improvement in safety, efficiency, and costs. Certainly, transitioning from a traditional, paper-based healthcare system to a digital one is a change of gargantuan proportions. To successfully make this transition, organizations must be committed to innovation, progress, and change. Administrators and clinicians must work in harmony during the selection, implementation, and evaluation phases of any major technologic change and must be prepared to deal with the positive and negative impact of such a change. Individuals and organizations that are most adaptive to this changing healthcare climate brought on by increasing use of information technology will emerge successful. In the famous words of Charles Darwin, "It is not the strongest of the species that survive, nor the most intelligent, but the one most responsive to change."

KEY POINTS

- Potential and real benefits of the EMR include improved quality of care, cost savings, higher productivity, and easier aggregation and analysis of health data. The EMR can facilitate research, education, quality improvement, outcomes assessment, and strategic planning.
- Clinical DSSs are an integrated set of programs and databases that provide users with the ability to interrogate those databases and analyze information, retrieving data from external sources if necessary, to assist in decision making.
- Medical DSSs can use clinical-information systems to shorten inpatient lengths of stay, decrease adverse drug interactions, improve the consistency and content of medical records, improve continuity of care and follow-up, and reduce practice variation.
- The Security Standards and Privacy Rule of the HIPAA are particularly relevant to the use of an EMR system.
- The Internet is a collection of interconnected computer networks, whereas the WWW is a collection of interconnected documents, linked by hyperlinks. The *intranet* is an internal network that uses Internet technologies and is often used by organizations to provide a secure network to support internal exchange of information.
- Web pages are accessed through applications known as *browsers*, such as Internet Explorer, Netscape, Mozilla Firefox, and others, whereas information on the WWW is searched via search engines such as Google.
- The Internet supports various forms of communication services and protocols, including e-mail, newsgroups, LISTSERVs, file transfer protocols, streaming media, voice-over-Internet protocols, and others.
- The Google Scholar Beta search engine allows users to conduct a comprehensive search of scholarly literature that includes peer-reviewed papers, abstracts, and articles, as well as theses and books from academic publishers, professional societies, preprint repositories, universities, and other scholarly organizations.
- The Pediatric Critical Care Medicine website (http://www.PedsCCM.org) is a comprehensive website dedicated to the specialty; it contains many useful clinical and research resources, evidence-based medicine journal club discussions, conference and CME information, job listings, and links to other useful websites.
- The Virtual PICU website at http://www.vpicu.org provides a common space for the sharing of information by the international community that provides care for critically ill children.
- A wide range of high-quality websites is available for consumer health information, including http://medlineplus.gov, www.ClinicalTrials.gov, www.cdc.gov, www.WebMD.com, www.Intelihealth.com, and www.DrKoop.com.
- The PDA can be used as a phone, a pager, an e-mail and text-messaging device, an MP3 player for listening to professional educational material or music, a voice recorder for patient documentation, a camera for personal or professional pictures, a medical textbook or drug reference source, a newspaper, a radio, a television, a PALS handbook, an electronic book reader, a GPS device, a wireless web browser, a device for medical billing or to print patient handouts, a patient database to review laboratory values and order medications, etc.
- A number of websites provide useful medical services specifically geared for use on PDAs; among them are MD on tap, MerckMedicus PDA tools, Mobile Merck Medicus, MD Consult Mobile, and AvantGo.
- Telemedicine is commonly used to ensure equitable access to expert medical care in remote and underserved areas, provide remote patient and provider education, reduce travel requirements, improve patient care, and reduce costs. Technologies that are commonly used to provide live, interactive communications between linked sites, making telemedicine feasible, include videoconferencing, Internet communications, store-and-forward imaging, streaming media, and land-line and wireless communications.

References

1. Barnett GO. Report to the National Institutes of Health Division of Research Grants Computer Research Study Section on computer applications in medical communication and information retrieval systems as related to the improvement of patient care and the medical record–September 26, 1966. *J Am Med Inform Assoc* 2006;13(2):127–35; discussion 136–7.
2. Campbell EM, Sittig DF, Ash JS, et al. Types of unintended consequences related to computerized provider order entry. *J Am Med Inform Assoc* 2006;13(5):547–56.
3. Chaudhry B, Wang J, Wu S, et al. Systematic review: Impact of health information technology on quality, efficiency, and costs of medical care. *Ann Intern Med* 2006;144(10):742–52.
4. Currell R, Urquhart C, Wainwright P, et al. Telemedicine versus face-to-face patient care: Effects on professional practice and health care outcomes. *Cochrane Database Syst Rev* 2000;(2):CD002098.
5. Garritty C, El Emam K. Who's using PDAs? Estimates of PDA use by health care providers: A systematic review of surveys. *J Med Internet Res* 2006;8(2):e7.
6. Hanson CW, 3rd, Deutschman CS, Anderson HL, 3rd et al. Effects of an organized critical care service on outcomes and resource utilization: A cohort study. *Crit Care Med* 1999;27(2):270–4.
7. Institute of Medicine: *Crossing the Quality Chasm: A New Health System for the 21st Century*. Washington, DC: National Academy Press 2001:164–180.
8. Marcin JP, Schepps DE, Page KA, et al. The use of telemedicine to provide pediatric critical care consultations to pediatric trauma patients admitted to a remote trauma intensive care unit: a preliminary report. *Pediatr Crit Care Med* 2004;5(3):251–6.
9. Nosowsky R, Giordano TJ. The Health Insurance Portability and Accountability Act of 1996 (HIPAA) privacy rule: Implications for clinical research. *Annu Rev Med* 2006;57:575–90.
10. The Office for the Advancement of Telehealth (OAT). HRSA—U.S Department of Health and Human Services, Health Resources and Service Administration. Available at http://www.hrsa.gov/telehealth/. Accessed January 28, 2007.
11. Peterson G, Aslani P, Williams KA. How do consumers search for and appraise information on medicines on the Internet? A qualitative study using focus groups. *J Med Internet Res* 2003;5(4):e33.
12. Rosenfeld BA, Dorman T, Breslow MJ, et al. Intensive care unit telemedicine: Alternate paradigm for providing continuous intensivist care. *Crit Care Med* 2000;28(12):3925–31.
13. Saathoff A. Human factors considerations relevant to CPOE implementations. *J Healthc Inf Manag* 2005;19(3):71–8.
14. Whitten PS, Mair FS, Haycox A, et al. Systematic review of cost effectiveness studies of telemedicine interventions. *Br Med J* 2002;324(7351):1434–1437.
15. Zun LS, Blume DN, Lester J, et al. Accuracy of emergency medical information on the web. *Am J Emerg Med* 2004;22(2):94–7.

CHAPTER 12 ■ PAIN AND SEDATION MANAGEMENT IN THE CRITICALLY ILL CHILD

MYRON YASTER • R. BLAINE EASLEY • KENNETH M. BRADY

> We must all die. But that I can save (a person) from days of torture, that is what I feel as my great and ever new privilege. Pain is a more terrible lord of mankind than even death itself.
>
> *Albert Schweitzer*

The treatment and alleviation of pain is a basic human right for everyone, regardless of age (55,74). Unfortunately, however, even when their pain is obvious, children frequently receive no treatment or inadequate treatment for pain and painful procedures, with newborn and critically ill children being especially vulnerable. The conventional "wisdom" that children neither respond to nor remember painful experiences to the same degree that adults do is simply untrue. Indeed, all of the nerve pathways essential for the transmission and perception of pain are present and functioning by 24 weeks of gestation (38). Recent research in newborn animals has revealed that the failure to provide analgesia for pain results in a "rewiring" of the nerve pathways responsible for pain transmission in the dorsal horn of the spinal cord and in increased pain perception for *future* painful insults. This finding confirms human newborn research, in which the failure to provide anesthesia or analgesia for newborn circumcision resulted in both short-term physiologic perturbations and longer-term behavioral changes, particularly during immunization (65).

The PICU poses unique challenges. Hospitalization in general and admission to the PICU in particular are frightening and painful experiences for children and their families. Pain in the PICU can be the result of the primary illness, trauma, or disease process, or it can be the result of medical interventions such as laryngeal intubation and mechanical ventilation, placement of invasive monitors, and other procedures. In addition, pain can be exacerbated by emotional distress and anxiety, two common ingredients of the PICU stay. Distress and anxiety may be the result of separation from parents and family, being surrounded by unfamiliar people and smells, loss of day and night awake and sleep cycles, and the fear of pain, loss of control, and even death. Thus, not only is pain control important in the critically ill, but so too is the need for sedation.

Nonpharmacologic measures such as open communication, reassurance, parental presence, and psychologic interventions are helpful and essential in basic management. Nevertheless, many critically ill patients need pharmacologically induced sedation to facilitate respiratory management and treatment of multiorgan system dysfunction or for the performance of invasive procedures. Regardless of the methods used, the goals of sedation are to provide anxiolysis, loss of consciousness, cooperation, amnesia, and immobility.

The past 15 years have seen an explosion in research and interest in pediatric pain management and an increase in the development of pediatric pain services, primarily under the direction of pediatric anesthesiologists. The pain service teams provide pain management for acute, postoperative, terminal, neuropathic, and chronic pain. In this chapter, we have attempted to consolidate in a comprehensive manner some of the recent advances in pain and sedation management in an attempt to provide a better understanding of how to manage pain and sedation in the critically ill child.

PAIN AND SEDATION ASSESSMENT

The International Association for the Study of Pain defines pain as "an unpleasant and emotional experience associated with actual or potential tissue damage, or described in terms of such damage" (44). Pain is a subjective experience; operationally, it can be defined as "what the patient says hurts" and exists "when the patient says it does." Infants, preverbal children, and children between the ages of 2 and 7 (Piaget's "preoperational thought stage") may be unable to describe their pain or their subjective experiences, which has led many to conclude incorrectly that children do not experience pain in the same way that adults do. Clearly, children do not have to know (or be able to express) the meaning of an experience to have the experience. On the other hand, because pain is essentially a subjective experience, it is becoming increasingly clear that the child's perspective of pain is an indispensable facet of pediatric pain management and an essential element in the specialized study of childhood pain. Indeed, pain assessment and management are interdependent, and one is essentially useless without the other. The goal of pain assessment is to provide accurate data about the location and intensity of pain and the effectiveness of measures used to alleviate or abolish it.

Instruments currently exist to measure and assess pain in children of all ages, although few work well or have been validated for patients admitted to the PICU. The sensitivity and specificity of these instruments has been widely debated and has resulted in a plethora of studies to validate their reliability and validity. The most commonly used instruments measure the quality and intensity of pain and are "self-report measures" that make use of pictures or word descriptors to describe pain. Pain intensity or severity can be measured in children as young as 3 years of age by using either the Oucher scale (developed by Dr. Judy Beyer), a two-part scale with a vertical numeric scale

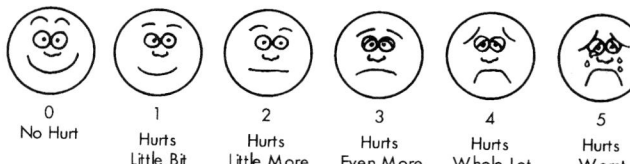

FIGURE 12.1. Six-face pain scale for use with children.

(0–100) on one side and six photographs of a young child on the other, or a visual analog scale, a 10-cm line with a smiling face on one end and a distraught, crying face on the other. In fact, the Oucher scale has even been validated by sex and race! Because of its simplicity, the authors primarily use a simplified six-face pain scale originally developed by Dr. Donna Wong and modified by others (61) (**Fig. 12.1**). This scale is attached to the vital sign record, and nurses are instructed to use it or a more age-appropriate self-report measure whenever vital signs are taken. Alternatively, color, word-graphic rating scales, and poker chips have been used to assess the intensity of pain in children. Obviously, these self-report measures are impossible to use in intubated, sedated, and paralyzed patients.

In infants and newborns, pain has been assessed by measuring physiologic responses to a nociceptive stimulus such as blood pressure and heart rate changes (observational pain scale, or OPS) or by measuring levels of adrenal stress hormones (23). Obviously, scales that rely on physiologic parameters can be misleading in an ICU setting, where alterations in vital signs can occur unrelated to the level of sedation. Additionally, patients with cardiovascular dysfunction requiring vasoactive medications may not develop tachycardia and hypertension despite severe agitation or pain. Alternatively, behavioral approaches have utilized facial expression, body movements, and the intensity and quality of crying as indices of response to nociceptive stimuli (37).

Sedation assessment has been much more difficult. The most commonly used procedural sedation assessment tool is the University of Michigan Sedation Scale (41). The COMFORT scale (5,8) is another commonly used PICU pain and sedation tool that utilizes both behaviors and physiologic parameters (**Table 12.1**); it relies on the measurement of five behavioral variables (alertness, facial tension, muscle tone, agitation, movement) and three physiologic variables (heart rate, respiration, blood pressure). Each is assigned a score ranging from 1 to 5, to give a total score ranging from 8 (deep sedation) to 40 (alert and agitated). A modified COMFORT scale that eliminates physiologic parameters has also been developed (34).

Other scoring systems, such as the Sedation-Agitation Scale, also eliminate the use of physiologic parameters and visually assess the level of the patient's comfort, grading it from 1 (nonarouseable) to 7 (dangerous agitation such as pulling at the endotracheal tube) (59). A commonly used sedation scale in the adult ICU population, the Ramsay sedation score (**Table 12.2**), was designed for use in the postanesthesia care unit (50). It assigns a value based on observation of the patient and includes a tactile stimulus provided to the patient (in this case, a glabellar tap). The Hartwig score also uses a visual assessment of the patient, but the stimulus is tracheal suctioning (31). Scales that assess response to a tactile stimulus require disturbing the patient to differentiate between the deeper levels of sedation. Obviously, scales that involve evaluating a patient's

response to a stimulus or observing their behavior are not valid during the use of neuromuscular blocking agents that prevent patient movement.

Our need to measure a "number" and the intensivist's love of gadgets and technology have led many to advocate the use of the bispectral index monitor (BIS monitor, Aspect Medical, Newton, MA) as a means of assessing the depth of sedation without the necessity of stimulating the patient and without relying on physiologic parameters. The BIS is a modified electroencephalographic monitor that uses a preset algorithm to evaluate the electroencephalogram. The BIS number is determined from three primary factors, including the frequency of the electroencephalographic waves, the synchronization of low- and high-frequency information, and the percentage of time in burst suppression. Part of the simplicity and attraction of the BIS monitor is that the depth of sedation/anesthesia is displayed numerically, ranging from 0 to 100, with 40 to 60 being a suitable level of surgical anesthesia. First developed for use in adults undergoing isoflurane general anesthesia, its use has spread to patients of all ages who are undergoing sedation, from moderate to general anesthesia utilizing IV sedatives and hypnotics. Several studies have compared BIS to the COMFORT scales (68). Unfortunately, the meaning of the BIS monitor measures and the numbers that it generates in a healthy versus critically ill child being sedated using a myriad of IV drugs remains anecdotal and is unclear.

Therefore, despite several options, the optimal means of evaluating the depth of sedation in many PICU patients remains elusive. Better (and validated) assessment tools for both pain and sedation management in the critically ill are desperately needed (5,34,68). The State Behavioral Scale, which takes advantage of a progression of observations, has been validated for sedation management in the PICU (18). The patient's graded response to progressive levels of stimuli (voice, touch, noxious stimuli) helps to establish the overall level of sedation (**Table 12.3**). The lack of formal pain and sedation scoring as a means of titrating medication often results in both overdosing and underdosing of the drugs used to provide analgesia and sedation (5,15). The implications are obvious: Failure to provide adequate pain and sedation can be devastating and lead to posttraumatic stress disorder, whereas overdosing leads to rapid development of tolerance and excessive drug delivery.

PAIN AND SEDATION MANAGEMENT— GENERAL PRINCIPLES

Physiologic Changes That Affect Pharmacokinetics in the Critically Ill Patient

Very few studies have evaluated the pharmacokinetic and pharmacodynamic properties of drugs in critically ill patients. Most pharmacokinetic studies are performed using healthy adult volunteers, adult patients who are only minimally ill, or adult patients in a stable phase of chronic disease. These data are then extrapolated to infants, children, adolescents, and to both adult and pediatric critically ill patients. So little pharmacokinetic and pharmacodynamic testing has been performed in children

TABLE 12.1

COMFORT SCALE

Alertness		Calmness/Agitation		Respiratory response		Physical movement	
Deeply asleep	1	Calm	1	No coughing and no spontaneous respiration	1	No spontaneous movement	1
Lightly asleep	2	Slightly anxious	2	Spontaneous respiration minimal response to vent	2	Occasional slight movement	2
Drowsy	3	Anxious	3	Occasional cough or resistance to vent	3	Frequent, slight movement	3
Fully awake and alert	4	Very anxious	4	Actively breathes against vent or coughs regularly	4	Vigorous movement, extremities only	4
Hyper-alert	5	Panicky	5	Fights vent, coughing, or choking	5	Vigorous movement, including torso and head	5

Mean arterial blood pressure		Heart rate		Muscle tone		Facial tension	
Any observation LO	1	Any observation LO	1	Totally relaxed, no tone	1	Facial muscles totally relaxed	1
All six observations within baseline range	2	All six observations within baseline range	2	Reduced tone	2	Facial muscle tone normal, no tension evident	2
One to three of six observations HI	3	One to three of six observations HI	3	Normal tone	3	Tension evident in some facial muscles	3
Four to five of six observations HI	4	Four to five of six observations HI	4	Increased tone with flexion of fingers and toes	4	Tension evident throughout facial muscles	4
All six observations HI	5	All six observations HI	5	Extreme rigidity and flexion of fingers and toes	5	Facial muscles contorted and grimacing	5

Review the medical record for heart rate and blood pressure data recorded over the 24-hr period prior to initial COMFORT score determination. Using the following data and equations, calculate the baseline range limits (e.g., HI, LO), and record where appropriate.

Heart Rate:
1. Range of Normal Values

Age (years)	Rate (beats/minute)
0–1	120–180
>1–2	100–130
>2–4	90–120
>4–8	80–110
>8	70–100

2. Study Limit Calculations
Observed baseline heart rate = lowest heart rate within the range of normal values charted over the 24-hr period preceding observation #1 = _____

LO limit heart rate = Observed baseline − (Observed baseline × 0.15) = _____
HI limit heart rate = Observed baseline + (Observed baseline × 0.15) = _____

Mean arterial pressure (MAP):

1. Range of Normal Values

Age (years)	Pressure (mm Hg)
0–1	47–82
>1–5	60–90
>5–7	60–93
>7–10	67–100
>10–12	68–102
>12–14	72–107

2. Study Limit Calculations
Observed Baseline MAP = lowest MAP within the range of normal values charted over the 24-hour period preceding observation #1 = _____

LO limit MAP = Observed baseline − (Observed baseline × 0.15) = _____
HI limit MAP = Observed baseline + (Observed baseline × 0.15) = _____

Adapted from Ambuel B, Hamlett KW, Marx CM, et al. Assessing distress in pediatric intensive care environments: The COMFORT scale. *J Pediatr Psychol* 1992;17:95–109.

TABLE 12.2

MODIFIED RAMSAY SEDATION SCORE

1. Awake—Anxious, agitated, restless
2. Awake—Eyes open, cooperative, oriented, tranquil
3. Asleep—Responds (opens eyes) only to command, light touch, normal tone of voice
4. Asleep—Brisk response to light glabellar tap or loud noise/voice
5. Asleep—Sluggish response to light glabellar tap or loud noise/voice
6. Asleep—No response to light glabellar tap or loud noise/voice

Adapted from Ramsay MA, Savage TM, Simpson BR, Goodwin R. Controlled sedation with alphaxalone-alphadolone. *Br Med J* 1974;2:656–9.

that they are often considered "therapeutic orphans." To help remedy this situation, the US Food and Drug Administration (FDA) has mandated pediatric pharmacokinetic and dynamic studies in all new drugs that enter the American marketplace. Unfortunately, the critically ill will have no such future protection. Unstable patients often present with significant hemodynamic alterations and organ dysfunction, which may significantly alter drug absorption, transport, metabolism, and excretion of drugs. Studies performed in healthy patients may offer little insight into how these drugs perform in the critically ill.

Absorption

Virtually all drugs used in current practice are delivered to their site of action by the blood. *Pharmacodynamics* describes the relationship between the concentration of drug at the site of action and the physiologic response. The way in which drugs get into the blood and the amount that gets to the site of action depend on *pharmacokinetics*—that is, the study of drug disposition in the body over time. Pharmacokinetics includes the route of administration, absorption, distribution, and elimination of drug molecules by the body over time.

In healthy patients, the enteral (oral and, occasionally, rectal) route of drug administration is most common and is the most widely studied. Enterally administered drugs must pass through the cells that line the mucosal surface of the gastrointestinal (GI) tract to enter the bloodstream. Drainage of intestinal blood flow into the portal system presents the drug to the liver for metabolism before the drug can be distributed throughout the body. This process leads to the first-pass effect seen with many oral drugs—much of the absorbed drug is taken directly to the liver via the portal circulation and is rapidly metabolized and "lost" before it ever reaches the systemic circulation. Alteration of venous blood flow that cause the drug to bypass the liver could result in significantly higher serum drug levels after oral absorption and lead to clinical sequelae. Absorption from the GI tract may be reduced in ICU patients for several reasons, including altered GI motility and peristalsis (ileus, recent GI surgery), reduced gut function and absorptive surface area (pancreatitis, recent GI surgery), reduced GI blood flow (shock), and physical removal of drug by nasogastric suc-

tioning. Because of this, enteral administration of drugs may not be possible in the critically ill. Additionally, the oral dosage forms of some drugs may prevent their use in the critically ill patient, even when these other factors are not in play. For example, sustained-release tablet preparations of opioids, such as OxyContin and MS Contin, must be swallowed whole and cannot be crushed or given via a nasogastric tube. Obviously, young children, infants, and the critically ill will not be able to do this. On the other hand, as a patient's condition improves overall, gut function also improves, and the enteral route may be considered as a viable route of drug administration. Transmucosal drug delivery, which uses rapidly disintegrating tablet formulations, is a new method of drug delivery and absorption that may be of importance in the near future.

Parenteral [intravenous (IV), intramuscular (IM), and subcutaneous (SQ)] drug administration is most common in the critically ill. Intravenous administration deposits drug directly into the bloodstream and is therefore the preferred route of drug administration in the ICU. Intramuscular, transdermal, and subcutaneous injections are rarely used in the critically ill because drug absorption from muscle or through skin or subcutaneous tissue may be decreased due to decreased tissue perfusion and decreased movement of drug through edematous tissue. However, as patients improve, the transdermal route (e.g., using fentanyl, clonidine) may become useful, particularly when IV access becomes a severe problem.

Distribution

Distribution describes the transportation and movement of a drug throughout the body. Several factors associated with critical illness can potentially affect the distribution of drugs in the body. Poor perfusion is often a factor that limits distribution of a drug to its target tissue. Altered receptor binding as a result of edema, malnutrition, uremic toxins, and downregulation will also change the amount of drug attached to tissue. Many analgesic drugs are transported through the body attached to the serum proteins albumin and γ-globulin. The extent of protein binding varies considerably among analgesic drugs, from 7% for codeine to 93% for sufentanil (20). The extent of protein binding may decrease in critical illness, causing elevated free levels of drug and possible toxicity. Additionally, third-spacing of fluid may result in additional volume into which the drug can distribute.

Metabolism and Elimination

Metabolism is the physical and chemical alteration of drug molecules for the purposes of detoxifying parent molecules and rendering fat-soluble chemicals more water soluble. Drugs or their metabolites are then eliminated by the kidneys. Any disease that affects hepatic or renal function or causes hypoperfusion of the liver or kidneys may diminish metabolism and elimination of the drug, possibly resulting in drug accumulation and toxicity. It is common for ICU patients to have some degree of either renal or hepatic functional impairment. Furthermore, many critically ill children and newborns have diseases in which intra-abdominal pressure is significantly increased (necrotizing enterocolitis, severe ileus, recent GI surgery), which will impair both portal and renal blood flow. In critically ill patients with

TABLE 12.3

STATE BEHAVIORAL SCALE/MODIFIED MOTOR ACTIVITY ASSESSMENT SCALE

>−3	Unresponsive	No spontaneous respiratory effort No cough, or coughs only with suctioning No response to noxious stimuli Unable to pay attention to care provider Does not distress with any procedure (including noxious) Does not move
−2	Responsive only to noxious stimuli[a]	Spontaneous yet supported breathing Coughs with suctioning/repositioning Responds to noxious stimuli Unable to pay attention to care provider Will distress with a noxious procedure Does not move/occasional movement of limbs or shifting of position
−1	Responsive to touch or name	Spontaneous but ineffective nonsupported breaths Coughs with suctioning/repositioning Responds to touch/voice Able to pay attention but drifts off after stimulation Distresses with procedures Able to calm with comforting touch or voice when stimulus is removed Occasional movement of limbs or shifting of position
0	Calm and cooperative	Spontaneous and effective breathing Coughs when repositioned/occasional spontaneous cough Responds to voice/no external stimulus is required to elicit response Spontaneously pays attention to care provider Distresses with procedures Able to calm with comforting touch or voice when stimulus is removed Occasional movement of limbs or shifting of position/increased movement (restless, squirming)
+1	Restless and cooperative	Spontaneous effective breathing/having difficulty breathing with ventilator Occasional spontaneous cough Responds to voice/no external stimulus is required to elicit response Drifts off/spontaneously pays attention to care provider Intermittently unsafe Does not consistently calm, despite 5-min attempt/unable to console Increased movement (restless, squirming)
+2	Agitated	May have difficulty breathing with ventilator Coughing spontaneously No external stimulus required to elicit response Spontaneously pays attention to care provider Unsafe (biting endotracheal tube, pulling at catheters, cannot be left alone) Unable to console Increased movement (restless, squirming, or thrashing side-to-side, kicking legs)

[a]Noxious stimuli, endotracheal tube suctioning, or 5 secs of nail bed pressure.
From Curley MA, Harris SK, Fraser KA, et al. State Behavioral Scale: A sedation assessment instrument for infants and young children supported on mechanical ventilation. *Pediatr Crit Care Med* 2006;7:107–14, with permission.

organ dysfunction, the clinician must expect the unpredictable metabolism and elimination of drugs and must monitor for therapeutic outcomes and possible adverse effects.

The liver is the major route for drug metabolism and detoxification for a wide variety of analgesic and sedative drugs, the majority of which are lipid soluble compounds. This lipid solubility enhances their passage through the blood-brain barrier (BBB) and preselects the liver as the organ of elimination (because renal physiology requires drugs to be water soluble to be filtered and excreted). Some degree of hepatic dysfunction is present in many ICU patients and may result in reduced drug clearance because of decreased hepatocellular enzyme activ-ity or reduced hepatic blood and/or bile flow. Most, but not all, drugs are metabolized in a two-part process, the goal of which is to change fat-soluble, active, unexcretable drug into water-soluble, inactive drug that can be excreted in the bile or by the kidneys (**Fig. 12.2**). The first phase of metabolism (phase I) commonly involves the cytochrome P450 (CYP) system, which is a large family of hemoproteins involved in the metabolism of drugs and in the manufacture of steroids. Phase I metabolism usually involves oxidation, hydroxylation, hydrolysis, or reduction. Phase I reactions are listed in **Table 12.4**. The metabolites of these reactions may be less active or highly reactive and even toxic. The phase I metabolite is then

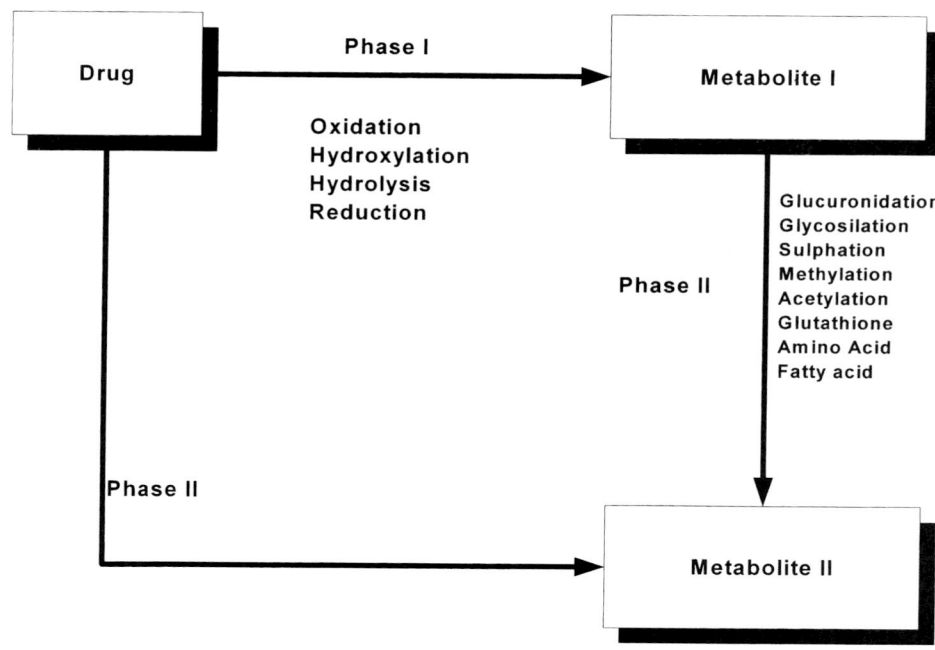

FIGURE 12.2. The two-part process by which most drugs are metabolized, the goal of which is to change fat-soluble, active, unexcretable drugs into water-soluble, inactive drugs that can be excreted in the bile or by the kidneys.

metabolized further by a phase II enzyme that conjugates it with either a glucuronide, a sulfide group, an amino acid, or glutathione (see **Fig. 12.2**). Some drugs are metabolized directly by phase II enzymes (e.g., morphine). A third metabolic pathway is becoming increasingly important: metabolism by blood and tissue esterases. These enzymes are ubiquitous and are found in large supply in the blood and elsewhere. Drugs metabolized by esterases, such as remifentanil, are unlikely to be affected by disease.

Most pain and sedation medications used in the critically ill are metabolized by phase I or phase II reactions in the liver. In general, the metabolism of opioid analgesics is very effective and is limited more by blood flow to the liver than by the inherent ability of the hepatocyte enzymes. The CYP microenzyme system is significantly altered in critical illness, thus decreasing phase I oxidative metabolism (48). One of the CYP enzymes, CYP2D6, is subject to genetic polymorphism and does not function in 10% of the population, even in normal conditions. This enzyme metabolizes codeine to morphine. In patients who lack a functioning CYP2D6, either genetically or because of liver disease, codeine will be a poor or ineffective analgesic (14). In addition to the reduction in the CYP enzyme system, phase II conjugation pathways, such as glucuronidation, may also be impaired in ICU patients, particularly if the liver is subjected to low blood flow, hypoxia, and/or stress.

Chronic liver disease selectively impairs oxidative pathways, leaving glucuronidation intact.

The kidneys are responsible for clearing both the parent drug and metabolites produced by the liver. In renal failure, both the parent drug and metabolites may accumulate and result in toxicity. Morphine is metabolized to morphine-3-glucuronide and morphine-6-glucuronide. Morphine-3-glucuronide does not have analgesic activity, whereas morphine-6-glucuronide is an active metabolite eliminated by the kidneys. In renal failure, morphine-6-glucuronide may accumulate, and it has been associated with toxicity. Meperidine is metabolized to the metabolite normeperidine, which is renally cleared. In renal failure, normeperidine may accumulate and cause central nervous system (CNS) excitability and possible seizures.

Analgesics in the PICU

The basic principles of pain management—believing the patient (and when possible, listening to what patient or family are saying), utilizing pain scores to guide management, providing for sleep, and rapidly delivering analgesics when they are needed—are the building blocks of pain management in young and/or critically ill patients. A surprising issue is the enormous variation in dosing and the rapid development of tolerance that may occur in the critically ill and very young. It is common for patients in the ICU to require enormous doses of analgesics and sedatives—doses so high that, to an outsider, they seem preposterous, if not dangerous. In general, practitioners use medications as needed and titrate to effect. Furthermore, a multimodal approach to therapy is advocated, in which different families of drugs, as well as cognitive and alternative approaches (music therapy, light touch, etc.), are utilized from the initiation of therapy. In the next sections, the pharmacology, pharmacokinetics, and special issues unique to the use of analgesic and sedative drugs in critically ill children will be reviewed.

TABLE 12.4

PHASE I REACTIONS

Cytochrome P450 system
Alcohol dehydrogenases
Aldehyde dehydrogenases
Amine oxidases
Xanthine oxidases
Aromatase

ANALGESICS WITH ANTIPYRETIC ACTIVITY OR NONOPIOID ("WEAKER") ANALGESICS

The "weaker" or "milder" analgesics with antipyretic activity, of which acetaminophen (paracetamol), salicylate (aspirin), ibuprofen, naproxen, and diclofenac are the classic examples, comprise a heterogenous group of nonsteroidal anti-inflammatory drugs (NSAIDs) and nonopioid analgesics (9) (Table 12.5). They provide pain relief primarily by blocking peripheral and central prostaglandin production by inhibiting cyclooxygenase (COX) types 1, 2, and 3. These analgesic agents are administered enterally via the oral or, on occasion, the rectal route and are particularly useful for inflammatory, bony, or rheumatic pain. Parenterally administered NSAIDs, such as ketorolac, are available for use in children in whom the oral or rectal routes of administration are not possible. Unfortunately, regardless of dose, the nonopioid analgesics reach a "ceiling effect" above which pain cannot be relieved using these drugs alone. Consequently, these weaker analgesics are often administered in oral combination forms with opioids, such as codeine, oxycodone, or hydrocodone.

Aspirin, one of the oldest and most effective nonopioid analgesics, has been largely abandoned in pediatric practice because of its possible role in Reye syndrome, its effects on platelet function, and its gastric irritant properties. Despite these problems, choline-magnesium trisalicylate (Trilisate) is increasingly being used in our pediatric pain management practice, particularly in the management of postoperative pain and in the child with cancer. Choline-magnesium trisalicylate is a unique aspirin-like compound that does not bind to platelets and therefore has minimal, if any, effects on platelet function. It is a convenient drug to give to children because it is available in both liquid and tablet form, and is administered either twice per day or every 6 hrs. The association of salicylates with Reye syndrome will limit its use, even though the risk of developing this syndrome postoperatively or in cancer is extremely unlikely.

The most commonly used nonopioid analgesic in pediatric practice remains acetaminophen (paracetamol). Unlike aspirin and the other NSAIDs, acetaminophen works primarily centrally (COX 3) and has minimal, if any, anti-inflammatory activity. When administered in normal doses (10–15 mg/kg, orally), acetaminophen is extremely safe and has very few serious side effects. It is an antipyretic and, like all enterally administered NSAIDs, takes approximately 30 mins to provide effective analgesia. Several investigators have reported that acetaminophen should be administered rectally in significantly higher doses than previously recommended (10). They recommend doses as high as 30–40 mg/kg when the drug is administered rectally as a single (loading) dose. Follow-up rectal doses are 30 mg/kg every 8 hrs. Regardless of the route of delivery, the daily maximum acetaminophen doses in the preterm, term, and older child are 60, 80, and 90 mg/kg, respectively (see Table 12.5).

The discovery of at least two peripheral COX isoenzymes, COX-1 and COX-2, has updated our knowledge of NSAIDs. The two COX isoenzymes share structural and enzymatic similarities but are specifically regulated at the molecular level and may be distinguished in their functions. Protective prostaglandins, which preserve the integrity of the stomach lining and maintain normal renal function in a compromised kidney, are synthesized by COX-1. COX-2 is inducible, and the inducing stimuli include proinflammatory cytokines and growth factors, implying a role for COX-2 in both inflammation and control of cell growth. In addition to the induction of COX-2 in inflammatory lesions, it is present constitutively in the brain and spinal cord, where it may be involved in nerve transmission, particularly that for pain and fever. Prostaglandins made by COX-2 are also important in ovulation and in the birth

---

TABLE 12.5

ORAL DOSING GUIDELINES FOR COMMONLY USED NONOPIOID ANALGESICS

Drug	Dose (mg/kg) (<60 kg)	Dose (mg) (>60 kg)	Interval (hours)	Daily maximum dose (mg/kg) (<60 kg)	Daily maximum dose (mg) (>60 kg)	Side effects
Acetaminophen	10–15[a]	650–1000	4	100[a]	4000	Toxic doses—hepatotoxicity; lacks anti-inflammatory activity
Ibuprofen	5–10	400–600[c]	6	40[b,c]	2400[c]	GI irritation, bronchospasm, interferes with platelet function, hematuria
Naproxen	5–6[c]	250–375[c]	12	24[b,c]	1000[c]	See ibuprofen
Aspirin[d]	10–15[c,d]	650–1000[c]	4	80[b,c,d]	3600[c]	Reye syndrome[d], see ibuprofen
Choline Mg Tri-Salicylate[e] (Trilisate)	7.5–15[b,c]	500–1000[c]	4–8	80[b,c,d]	3600[c]	See aspirin

[a]Maximum daily doses for acetaminophen should be reduced to 80 mg/kg in term neonates and infants and to 60 mg/kg in preterm neonates. Supplied in multiple liquid formulations ranging from 20–100 mg/mL, making accidental overdosage easy. Rectal suppositories are available, dosing 25–40 mg/kg every 6 hrs.
[b]Dosing guidelines for neonates and infants have not been established.
[c]Higher doses may be used in selected cases for treatment of rheumatologic conditions in children.
[d]Aspirin carries a risk of provoking Reye syndrome in infants and children. If other analgesics are available, aspirin use should be restricted to indications in which antiplatelet or anti-inflammatory effect is required, rather than as a routine analgesic or antipyretic in neonates, infants, or children. Dosing guidelines for aspirin in neonates have not been established.
[e]Aspirin-like compound that does not affect platelet adhesiveness or aggregation
Adapted from Berde CB, Sethna NF. Analgesics for the treatment of pain in children. *N Engl J Med* 2002;347:1094–103.

process. The discovery of COX-2 has made possible the design of drugs that reduce inflammation without removing those protective prostaglandins in the stomach and kidney that are made by COX-1. In fact, developing a more specific COX-2 inhibitor was the "Holy Grail" of drug research because this class of drug would have all the anti-inflammatory and analgesic properties desired in a drug and none of the GI and antiplatelet side effects. Unfortunately, the growing controversy regarding the potential adverse cardiovascular risks of prolonged use of the COX-2 inhibitors has dampened much of the enthusiasm for these drugs and has led to the removal of rofecoxib from the market by its manufacturer (35). Finally, many orthopedic surgeons are concerned about the negative influence of all NSAIDs, both selective and nonselective COX inhibitors, on bone growth and healing (19). Thus, most pediatric orthopedic surgeons have recommended that these drugs not be used in their patients during the postoperative period.

OPIOID ANALGESICS

Historically, opium and its derivatives (e.g., paregoric, morphine) were used for the treatment of diarrhea (dysentery) and pain. The beneficial psychologic and physiologic effects of opium, as well as its toxicity and potential for abuse, have been well known to physicians and the public for centuries. On the other hand, many physicians through the ages have underutilized opium when treating patients in pain for fear that their patients would be harmed by its use. In the present era, addiction is particularly feared. Opium's easy availability, despite every effort by the government to control it, has resulted in a scourge of addiction that has devastated large segments of the population. Until and unless opium's dark consequences (yin) can be separated from its benefits (yang), innumerable numbers of patients will suffer unnecessarily.

Opioid Receptors

Over the past 30 years, multiple opioid receptors and subtypes have been identified and classified. An understanding of the complex nature and organization of these multiple opioid receptors is essential for an adequate understanding of the response to, and control of, pain (52). The CNS contains four primary opioid receptor types, designated μ (for morphine), κ, δ, and σ. Recently, the μ, κ, and δ receptors have been cloned and have yielded invaluable information on receptor structure and function (51).

The differentiation of agonists and antagonists is fundamental to pharmacology. A neurotransmitter is defined as having agonist activity, whereas a drug that blocks the action of a neurotransmitter is an antagonist. By definition, receptor recognition of an agonist is "translated" into other cellular alterations (that is, the agonist initiates a pharmacologic effect), whereas an antagonist occupies the receptor without initiating the transduction step (that is, it has no intrinsic activity or efficacy). The intrinsic activity of a drug defines the ability of the drug–receptor complex to initiate a pharmacologic effect. Drugs that produce less than a maximal response have a lowered intrinsic activity and are called *partial agonists*. Partial agonists also have antagonistic properties because, by binding the receptor site, they block access of full agonists to it. Morphine and related opiates are μ agonists, and drugs that block the effects of opiates at the μ receptor, such as naloxone, are designated *antagonists*.

The μ, κ, and δ receptors are unique but produce analgesia primarily by inhibiting synaptic transmission in the CNS and myenteric plexus. They are usually found on the presynaptic nerve terminal, and they decrease the release of excitatory neurotransmitters from terminals that carry nociceptive stimuli. As a result, neurons are hyperpolarized, which suppresses spontaneous discharge and evoked responses. These receptors are coupled to guanine nucleotide-binding regulatory proteins (G proteins) and regulate transmembrane signaling by regulating adenylate cyclase (cyclic AMP), various ion (K, Ca, Na) channels and transport proteins, and phospholipases C and A_2 (diacylglycerol and inositol triphosphate activation of protein kinase C) (16).

Drug Selection

The opioids most commonly used in the management of pain are μ agonists (**Table 12.6**). These include morphine, meperidine, methadone, codeine, oxycodone, and the fentanyls. In the PICU, fentanyl and morphine are the most commonly utilized opioids. Mixed agonist-antagonist drugs act as agonists or partial agonists at one receptor and antagonists at another receptor. Mixed (opioid) agonist-antagonist drugs include pentazocine, butorphanol, nalorphine, dezocine, and nalbuphine; these are agonists or partial agonists at the κ and δ receptors and antagonists or partial agonists at the μ receptor. These drugs are being increasingly used, as is low-dose naloxone, to tame or prevent some opioid-induced side effects such as pruritus and nausea (43). Buprenorphine is considered a partial agonist at the μ and κ receptors and may have a role in the prevention or treatment of patients who will or have become dependent on opioids.

At equianalgesic doses, the pharmacodynamic effects of all of the μ-opioid agonists are similar and include analgesia, respiratory depression, sedation, nausea and vomiting, pruritus, constipation, miosis, tolerance, and physical dependence. Although the opioids may cause some sedation, they are not amnestic agents and, in the PICU, are often coadministered with anxiolytic and amnestic medications such as benzodiazepines (midazolam, diazepam, and lorazepam) or ketamine. Which opioid to use in the PICU may be determined by differences in pharmacokinetic, pharmacodynamic, and physiochemical properties, all of which may affect the latency, potency, and duration of analgesic action. In many classes of drugs, drug selection is based on pharmacokinetic parameters such as half-life. With the opioids, the terminal or β-phase half-life alone is not an appropriate measure for drug selection, because the onset and duration of effect with a single dose may have more to do with distribution and redistribution of the drug into and out of the brain than with elimination half-life. Opioid distribution into the brain is based partially on the lipid solubility of the drug. The more lipid-soluble the drug, the faster its penetration into the brain, and the quicker the response. For example, fentanyl, a very lipid-soluble drug, has a rapid onset and short duration of action following a single bolus dose because of the rapid redistribution of drug out of the brain, not because of a short elimination half-life. Continuous long-term opioid administration may be associated with the

TABLE 12.6

OPIOID ANALGESIC INITIAL DOSAGE GUIDELINES

Drug	Equianalgesic dose (mg) IV, IM, SC	Equianalgesic dose (mg) oral	Usual starting IV (SC) doses and intervals <50 kg	Usual starting IV (SC) doses and intervals >50 kg	Parenteral/oral ratio	Usual starting oral doses and intervals <50 kg	Usual starting oral doses and intervals >50 kg
Codeine	120	200	NA	NA	1:2	0.5–1 mg/kg every 3–4 hrs	30–60 mg every 3–4 hrs[a]
Fentanyl	0.1	NA[b]	**Bolus:** 0.5–1 mcg/kg every 0.5–2 hrs **Infusion:** 0.5–2 mcg/kg/hr	**Bolus:** 25–50 mcg every 1–2 hrs **Infusion:** 25–100 mcg/hr	NA	NA	NA
Hydrocodone	NA	10–20	NA	NA	NA	0.1 mg/kg every 3–4 hrs	5–10 mg every 3–4 hrs[a]
Hydromorphone	1.5–2	3–5[c]	**Bolus:** 0.02 mg/kg every 0.5–2 hrs **Infusion:** 0.004 mg/kg/hr	**Bolus:** 1 mg every 0.5–2 hrs **Infusion:** 0.3 mg/hr	1:2 1:4[c]	0.03–0.08 mg/kg every 3–4 hrs	2–4 mg every 3–4 hrs
Meperidine[d]	75–100	150–200	**Bolus:** 1 mg/kg every 2–3 hrs	**Bolus:** 50–100 mg every 2–3 hrs	1:2	1–2 mg/kg every 3–4 hrs	100–150 mg every 3–4 hrs
Methadone	10	10–20	0.1 mg/kg every 4–8 hrs	5–10 mg every 4–8 hrs	1:2	0.2 mg/kg every 4–8 hrs	10 mg every 4–8 hrs
Morphine	10	30–50	**Bolus:** 0.1 mg/kg every 0.5–2 hrs **Infusion:** 0.025 mg/kg/hr	**Bolus:** 5–10 mg every 0.5–2 hrs **Infusion:** 2 mg/hr	1:3 chronic 1:5 single	**Immediate Release:** 0.3 mg/kg every 3–4 hrs **Sustained Release:** 20–35 kg: 10–15 mg every 8–12 hrs 35–50 kg: 15–30 mg every 8–12	**Immediate Release:** 15–20 mg every 3–4 hrs **Sustained Release:** 30–45 mg every 8–12 hrs
Oxycodone	NA	10–20	NA	NA	NA	0.1 mg/kg every 3–4 hrs	5–10 mg every 3–4 hrs[a,e]

[a]Commercial preparations are often combined with acetaminophen or ibuprofen; must be converted to morphine by CYP2D6 for analgesic effect.

[b]Oral transmucosal form available (Actiq): dose 10–15 mcg/kg.

[c]The equianalgesic oral dose and parenteral/oral dose ratios are not well established.

[d]Also called pethidine. Meperidine should generally be avoided if other opioids are available, especially with chronic use, because its metabolite, normeperidine, can produce seizures.

[e]A sustained-release preparation is available.

Adapted from Berde CB, Sethna NF. Analgesics for the treatment of pain in children. *N Engl J Med* 2002;347:1094–103.

accumulation of the drug in fat tissue. As a result, duration of action may be affected more by the redistribution of drug out of fat tissue than by the elimination half-life. An understanding of the pharmacokinetic, pharmacodynamic, and physiochemical properties of each opioid is essential, as each drug has unique characteristics.

Morphine

Morphine is the gold standard μ agonist, and it can be administered in the critically ill patient using the IV, epidural, intrathecal, oral, IM, and rectal routes, for both analgesia and sedation. It is a moderately potent opioid and is commonly administered IV in doses of 0.1 mg/kg (see **Table 12.6**). Obviously, this dose must be modified based on the patient's age and disease state. To minimize the complications associated with IV morphine (or any opioid) administration, it is recommended that *the dose be titrated at the bedside* until the desired level of analgesia is achieved. When administered by the oral route, morphine has an IV:oral-dose ratio of ~1:3 (0.1 mg/kg IV morphine = 0.3 mg/kg oral morphine). This ratio reflects the high first-pass effect rather than the extent of absorption, which is nearly 100%. In healthy children, the terminal elimination half-life (t1/2) is 2–3 hrs. Peak effect occurs within 20 mins, with a duration of action of 2–7 hrs following IV administration. Compared to fentanyl, because morphine is less lipid soluble, it has a slower onset of action and a longer duration. Due to its lower lipid solubility, it also has a smaller volume of distribution than does fentanyl. In adults, morphine has a serum minimum effective analgesic concentration of ~10 to 50 L.

The liver is the major site of biotransformation for most opioids, and the major metabolic pathway is oxidation. The exceptions are morphine and buprenorphine, which primarily undergo glucuronidation, and remifentanil, which is cleared by ester hydrolysis. Many of these reactions are catalyzed in the liver by microsomal mixed-function oxidases that require the CYP system, nicotinamide adenine diphosphate (NADPH), and oxygen. The CYP system is very immature at birth and does not reach adult levels until the first or second month of life (29). The immaturity of this hepatic enzyme system may explain the prolonged clearance or elimination of some opioids during the first few days to weeks of life. On the other hand, the CYP system can be induced by various drugs (phenobarbital) and substrates, and it matures regardless of gestational age. Thus, it may be the age from birth—and not the duration of gestation—that determines how premature and full-term infants metabolize drugs. Indeed, it has been demonstrated that sufentanil is more rapidly metabolized and eliminated in 2- to 3-week-old infants than in newborns <1 week old (27).

Morphine is primarily glucuronidated into two forms: an inactive form, morphine-3-glucuronide, and an active form, morphine-6-glucuronide. Both glucuronides are excreted by the kidney. In patients with renal failure or with reduced glomerular filtration rates (e.g., neonates), morphine-6-glucuronide can accumulate and cause toxic side effects, including respiratory depression, an important consideration both when prescribing morphine and when administering other opioids that are metabolized into morphine, such as methadone and codeine.

The pharmacokinetics of opioids in patients with liver disease and in critically ill patients requires special attention. Many disease states common in ICU patients may alter the metabolism and elimination of morphine. Severe cirrhosis, septic shock, and renal failure decrease the clearance of morphine and its metabolites, resulting in prolonged duration and possible toxicity. The oxidation of opioids is reduced in patients with cirrhosis, resulting in decreased drug clearance (e.g., meperidine, dextropropoxyphene, pentazocine, tramadol, alfentanil) and/or increased oral bioavailability, which is caused by a reduced first-pass metabolism (e.g., meperidine, pentazocine, dihydrocodeine). Although glucuronidation is thought to be less affected in cirrhosis, the clearance of morphine is decreased and oral bioavailability increased. The consequence of reduced drug metabolism is the risk of accumulation in the body, especially with repeated administration. Lower doses or longer administration intervals should be used to minimize this risk. Meperidine poses a special concern because it is metabolized into normeperidine, a toxic metabolite that, in liver disease, causes seizures and accumulates. On the other hand, drugs such as codeine, which are inactive but are metabolized in the liver into active forms, may be ineffective in patients with liver disease. Finally, the disposition of a few opioids, such as fentanyl, sufentanil, and remifentanil, appears to be unaffected in liver disease, and these drugs are used preferentially in managing pain in patients with liver disease (66).

Fentanyl(s)

Because of its rapid onset (usually <1 min) and brief duration of action (30–45 mins), fentanyl has become a favored analgesic for short procedures, such as bone marrow aspirations, fracture reductions, suturing lacerations, endoscopy, and dental procedures, as well as for patients admitted to the PICU. Fentanyl is ~100 times more potent than morphine (the equianalgesic dose is 1 mcg/kg) and is largely devoid of hypnotic or sedative activity (see **Table 12.6**). Sufentanil is a potent fentanyl derivative and is ~10 times more potent than fentanyl. It is most commonly used as the principal component of cardiac anesthesia and is administered in doses of 15–30 mcg/kg. Alfentanil is ~5–10 times less potent than fentanyl and has an extremely short duration of action, usually <15–20 mins. Remifentanil is a μ-opioid receptor agonist with unique pharmacokinetic properties. It is ~10 times more potent than fentanyl and must be given by continuous IV infusion because it has an extremely short half-life (26).

Fentanyl is considered to be the most hemodynamically stable opioid, and it has become the opioid of choice for critically ill patients. Nevertheless, the principles of careful monitoring and titration to effect also apply to fentanyl, particularly in the hypovolemic patient. Furthermore, in addition to its ability to block the systemic and pulmonary hemodynamic responses to pain, fentanyl prevents the biochemical and endocrine stress (catabolic) response to painful stimuli that may be detrimental in the seriously ill patient. Fentanyl does have some serious side effects, such as the development of glottic and chest wall rigidity following rapid infusions of ≥5 mcg/kg and the development of bradycardia. The etiology of the glottic and chest wall rigidity is unclear, but its implications are not—it may make ventilation difficult or impossible. Chest wall rigidity can be treated with either neuromuscular relaxants or naloxone.

In adults, the serum minimum effective analgesic concentration of fentanyl is ~0.5–2.5 mcg/L. Fentanyl, like morphine, is primarily glucuronidated into inactive forms that are excreted by the kidney. It is highly lipid soluble and is rapidly distributed to tissues that are well perfused, such as the brain and the heart. Normally, the effect of a single dose of fentanyl is terminated by rapid redistribution to inactive tissue sites, such as fat, skeletal muscles, and lung, rather than by elimination. This rapid redistribution produces a dramatic decline in the plasma concentration of the drug. In this manner, its very short duration of action is akin to other drugs, such as thiopental, the action of which is terminated by redistribution. However, following multiple or large doses of fentanyl (e.g., when it is used as a primary anesthetic agent or when used in high-dose or lengthy continuous infusions), prolongation of effect will occur because elimination and not distribution will determine the duration of effect.

It is clear that the duration of drug action for many drugs is not solely the function of clearance or terminal elimination half-life, but rather reflects the complex interaction of drug elimination, drug absorption, and rate constants for drug transfer to and from sites of action ("effect sites"). The term *context-sensitive half-time* refers to the time it takes for drug concentration at idealized effect sites to decrease by half (32). The context-sensitive half-time for fentanyl increases dramatically when it is administered by continuous infusion (32). In newborns who received fentanyl infusions for >36 hrs, the context-sensitive half-life was >9 hrs following cessation of the infusion (53). Even single doses of fentanyl may have prolonged effects in the newborn, particularly those neonates with abnormal or decreased liver blood flow following acute illness or abdominal surgery. Additionally, certain conditions that may raise intra-abdominal pressure may further decrease liver blood flow by shunting blood away from the liver via the still patent ductus venosus.

Fentanyl and its structurally related relatives sufentanil, alfentanil, and remifentanil are highly lipophilic drugs that rapidly penetrate all membranes, including the BBB. Following an IV bolus, fentanyl is rapidly eliminated from plasma as the result of its extensive uptake by body tissues. The fentanyls are highly bound to α-1 acid glycoproteins in the plasma, which are reduced in the newborn. The fraction of free, unbound sufentanil is significantly increased in neonates and children who are <1 year of age (19.5 $\pm$ 2.7% and 11.5 $\pm$ 3.2%, respectively) compared with older children and adults (8.1 $\pm$ 1.4% and 7.8 $\pm$ 1.5%, respectively), and this correlates to levels of α-1 acid glycoproteins in the blood.

The pharmacokinetics of remifentanil are unique and characterized by small volumes, rapid clearances, and low variability compared to other IV anesthetic drugs. The drug has a rapid onset of action (half-time for equilibration between blood and the effect compartment = 1.3 min) and a short, context-sensitive half-life (3–5 mins). The latter property is attributable to hydrolytic metabolism of the compound by nonspecific tissue and plasma esterases. The pharmacokinetics of remifentanil suggests that, within 10 mins of starting an infusion, remifentanil will nearly reach steady state. Thus, changing the infusion rate of remifentanil will produce rapid changes in drug effect. The rapid metabolism of remifentanil and its small volume of distribution mean that remifentanil will not accumulate. Discontinuing the drug rapidly terminates its effects regardless of how long it was being administered (32). Finally, the primary metabolite has little biologic activity, making it safe even in patients with renal disease.

Fentanyl is metabolized by the liver to inactive metabolites that are eliminated by the kidney. Due to its rapid penetration into the brain, it has an onset of effect within 30 secs and a

peak effect occurring in 5–15 mins following IV administration. It has a relatively short duration of action, 30–60 mins, due to redistribution out of the brain as a result of its high lipid solubility. Compared to morphine, fentanyl has a larger volume of distribution, slower clearance, and a longer terminal half-life of ~8 hrs. Although renal failure does not significantly alter the pharmacokinetics and pharmacodynamics of fentanyl in most patients, a few studies have demonstrated increases in the volume of distribution and elimination half-life in those critically ill patients with renal failure who receive continuous fentanyl infusions. A study in patients who had renal failure and received kidney transplants found a decrease in fentanyl clearance associated with prolonged ventilatory depression.

The metabolism of fentanyl is determined primarily by liver perfusion. Diseases associated with decreased liver blood flow, such as cardiac failure, may decrease the clearance of fentanyl. Long-term, continuous infusions of fentanyl may result in a prolonged elimination 1/2 and duration of action as a result of drug accumulation in peripheral tissues. Administering fentanyl by continuous infusion requires frequent titration, as the terminal t1/2 may be as long as 16 hrs in this setting. Unlike morphine, fentanyl is not associated with mast-cell histamine release, and it may be preferred in patients who are susceptible to the cardiovascular effects of morphine.

Hydromorphone

Hydromorphone, a derivative of morphine, is an opioid with appreciable selectivity for μ opioid receptors. It is noted for its rapid onset and 4- to 6-hr duration of action. It differs from its parent compound, morphine, in that it is five times more potent and 10 times more lipid soluble and does not have an active metabolite (see **Table 12.6**). Its half-life of elimination is 3–4 hrs and, like morphine and meperidine, it shows very wide intrasubject pharmacokinetic variability. Hydromorphone is less sedating than morphine and is thought by many to be associated with fewer systemic side effects. Hence, it is often used as an alternative to morphine in IV patient-controlled analgesia (PCA) or when the latter produces too much sedation, nausea, or itching. Additionally, hydromorphone is receiving renewed attention as an alternative morphine for the treatment of prolonged, cancer-related pain because it can be prepared in more concentrated aqueous solutions than morphine.

Hydromorphone is effective when administered IV, subcutaneously, epidurally, or orally. The IV route of administration is the most commonly used technique in the ICU. Following a loading dose of 5–20 mcg/kg, a continuous infusion ranging between 3 and 5 mcg/kg/hr is started. Supplemental boluses of 3–5 mcg/kg are administered either by the nurse or by the patient as needed. When administered epidurally, either continuous infusions of 2–4 mcg/kg/hr (the adult dose is 0.15–0.3 mg/hr) or continuous infusions with patient-controlled boluses of 1–3 mcg/kg per bolus (the adult dose is 0.15–0.3 mg/bolus) can be used.

Methadone

Primarily thought of as a drug to treat or wean opioid-addicted or opioid-dependent patients, methadone is increasingly being used for postoperative pain relief and for the treatment of intractable pain. It is noted for its slow elimination, very long duration of effective analgesia, and high oral bioavailability (see **Table 12.6**). Methadone is metabolized extremely slowly and has a very prolonged duration of action, based in part on the fact that its principal metabolite is morphine. The elimination half-life of methadone averages 19 hrs, and clearance averages 5.4 mL/min/kg in children 1–18 years of age.

Methadone has the longest elimination half-life of any of the commonly available opiates, and it may provide 12 to 36 hrs of analgesia following a single IV or oral dose. Pharmacokinetically, children are indistinguishable from young adults. Because a single dose of methadone can achieve and sustain a high drug plasma level, it is a convenient way to provide prolonged analgesia without requiring an IM injection. When administered either orally or intravenously, it may be viewed as an alternative to the use of continuous IV opioid infusions (a "poor man's" PCA). Some recommend loading patients with an initial dose of IV methadone, 0.1–0.2 mg/kg, and then titrating in 0.05 mg/kg increments every 10 to 15 mins until analgesia is achieved (57). Supplemental methadone can be administered in 0.05–0.1 mg/kg increments administered by slow IV infusion every 4–12 hrs as needed. The use of small incremental doses administered by "sliding scale" have also been reported (57). Using this method, small increments of methadone are administered IV over 20 mins every 4 hrs via a "sliding" scale on a "reverse p.r.n." (the nurse asks the patient) basis: 0.07–0.08 mg/kg for severe pain, 0.05–0.06 mg/kg for moderate pain, 0.03 mg/kg for little or no pain if the patient is alert, and no drug if the patient has little pain and is "somnolent." The influence of pathophysiology on the pharmacokinetics and pharmacodynamics of methadone are unknown, primarily because its use as an analgesic is a relatively recent phenomenon. Dosing decisions must be made conservatively in the very young and in patients with various end-organ diseases.

Additionally, we and others use methadone to wean patients who have become physically dependent on opioids following prolonged analgesic therapy (63,67,73). When used to treat dependence and withdrawal symptoms, clonidine, an α_2 agonist, can be concomitantly administered in doses of 5 mcg/kg to significantly reduce withdrawal symptomatology. Finally, because methadone is extremely well absorbed from the GI tract and has a bioavailability of 80%–90%, it is extremely easy to convert IV dosing regimens to oral regimens. The conversion dose of morphine to methadone has been challenged. Traditionally, it was thought that the ratio of morphine to methadone was ~1:1; it now appears that it is closer to 1:0.25, or even 1:0.1. Underestimating methadone's potency substantially increases the risk of potential life-threatening toxicity. Methadone may provide analgesia even when patients become tolerant to other opioids, sometimes referred to as *incomplete cross-tolerance*. Incomplete cross-tolerance for methadone may be due in part to its antagonist actions at the *N*-methyl-D-aspartate (NMDA) receptor.

Patient- and Surrogate (Parent, Nurse)-Controlled Analgesia

Because of the enormous individual variations in pain perception and opioid metabolism, fixed doses and time intervals make little sense. Based on the pharmacokinetics of the opi-

oids, it should be clear that it may be necessary to give IV boluses of morphine at intervals of 1–2 hrs to avoid marked fluctuations in plasma drug levels. Continuous IV infusions can provide steady analgesic levels and are preferable to IM injections. Continuous infusions have been used with great safety and effectiveness in children and are commonly used in the PICU. (Common opioid infusion regimens are presented in **Table 12.7**.) However, they are not a panacea, because the perception and intensity of pain is not constant. For example, a postoperative patient may be very comfortable resting in bed and may require little adjustment in pain management. This same patient may experience excruciating pain when coughing, voiding, or getting out of bed. Thus, rational pain management requires some form of titration to effect whenever any opioid is administered. Demand-analgesia, or PCA, devices have been developed to give patients and, in some cases, parents and nurses, some measure of control over their or their children's pain therapy. The device is a microprocessor-driven pump with a button that the patient presses to self-administer a small dose of opioid.

PCA devices allow patients to administer small amounts of an analgesic whenever they feel a need for more pain relief. The dosage of opioid, number of boluses per hour, and the time interval between boluses (the "lock-out period") are programmed into the equipment by the pain service physician to allow maximum patient flexibility and sense of control with minimal risk of overdosage. Generally, because older patients know that if they have severe pain they can obtain relief immediately, many prefer dosing regimens that result in mild-to-moderate pain in exchange for fewer side effects such as nausea or pruritus. The most commonly prescribed opioids for IV PCA are morphine, hydromorphone, and fentanyl.

The PCA pump computer stores within its memory the number of boluses the patient has received and the number of attempts the patient has made at receiving boluses. This information allows the physician to evaluate how well the patient understands the use of the pump and facilitates programming the pump more efficiently. Many PCA units allow low "background" continuous infusions (morphine, 20–30 mcg/kg/hr; hydromorphone, 3–4 mcg/kg/hr; fentanyl, 0.5 mcg/kg/hr) in addition to self-administered boluses, sometimes called "PCA-Plus." A continuous background infusion is particularly useful at night and often provides more restful sleep by preventing the patient from awakening in pain. It also increases the potential for overdosage (45). Although the adult literature on pain does not support the use of continuous background infusions, it has been our experience that continuous infusions are essential for both the patient and the physicians (fewer phone calls, problems, etc.). In our practice, we almost always use continuous background infusions when prescribing IV (or epidural) PCA.

PCA requires a patient with enough intelligence and manual dexterity and strength to operate the pump. Thus, it was initially limited to adolescents and teenagers, but the lower age limit for patients in whom this treatment modality can be used continues to fall. In fact, it has been observed that any child able to play computerized games can operate a PCA pump (ages 5–6). Allowing surrogates (parents, nurses) to initiate a PCA bolus is very controversial. Some centers empower nurses and parents to initiate PCA boluses, and use this technology in children who are even <1 year of age. The incidence of common opioid-induced side effects is similar to that observed in older patients (45). Interestingly, respiratory

TABLE 12.7

COMMON OPIOID INFUSION RATES IN THE PICU

Agent	Load/p.r.n.	Infusion range	Comments
Fentanyl	1 mcg/kg	1–5 mcg/kg/hr	Extensive clinical experience Relatively stable hemodynamic effects Blunts the stress response Pharmacology similar to morphine after prolonged infusion (>18 hrs)
Morphine	0.05–0.1 mg/kg	0.05–0.1 mg/kg/hr	Inexpensive Extensive clinical experience Histamine release and venodilation may cause hypotension
Hydromorphone	0.015 mg/kg	10–15 mcg/kg/hr	Fewer opioid-induced side effects such as pruritus and histamine release More expensive than morphine
Remifentanil	0.5–1 mcg/kg	0.1–0.5 mcg/kg/min	Short duration of infusion Rapid development of tolerance Esterase metabolism rapid breakdown and no analgesia after 10 min Expensive

These are suggested boluses and initiation ranges, and their effect must be titrated for each patient to the appropriate level of analgesia. p.r.n., as needed.

depression is very rare but does occur, reinforcing the need for close monitoring and established nursing protocols. Difficulties with PCA include its increased costs, patient age limitations, and the bureaucratic (physician, nursing, and pharmacy) obstacles (protocols, education, storage arrangements) that must be overcome prior to its implementation. Contraindications include inability to push the bolus button (weakness, arm restraints), inability to understand how to use the machine, and a patient's desire not to assume responsibility for his own care.

Preventing Opioid-induced Side Effects

Regardless of the method of administration, all opioids produce unwanted side effects, such as pruritus, nausea and vomiting, constipation, urinary retention, cognitive impairment, tolerance, and dependence. Many patients suffer needlessly because they would rather experience pain than these opioid-induced side effects. In a randomized, controlled, clinical trial in non–critically ill children and adolescents, it was demonstrated that low-dose naloxone infusions (0.25–1 mcg/kg/hr) can significantly reduce opioid-induced side effects without affecting opioid-induced analgesia (43). This study has changed our practice, but has left unanswered many new questions that are the basis of much of our current research.

LOCAL ANESTHETICS

Local anesthetics are drugs that reversibly block the conduction of neural impulses along central and peripheral nerve pathways (62,72). To be effective, local anesthetics must be physically deposited, usually by needles or by indwelling catheters, in the immediate vicinity of the nerves to be blocked (6). In

this way, local anesthetics are unlike virtually all other drugs used in modern medicine, which, regardless of their means of entry into the body, are delivered to their site of action by a carrier—namely, the blood. Removal of local anesthetics from the neural tissue results in spontaneous and complete return of nerve conduction, with no evidence of structural damage to nerve fibers as a result of the drugs' effects.

Procedure-related pain is that pain inflicted on patients in the course of their medical or surgical treatment. It is also among the most difficult form of pain to handle—by both the patient experiencing it and the healthcare professionals who must inflict it. Examples of procedure-related pain include that caused by insertion of an arterial or IV catheter (e.g., routine percutaneous IV access or cardiac catheterization), bone marrow aspiration, thoracostomy tube placement, lumbar puncture, and repair of minor surgical wounds (traumatic lacerations or deliberate incisions, e.g., prior to a cutdown for venous access). Unfortunately, the most frequent response of physicians to procedure-related pain is denial. This "turning away" is uniquely easy when dealing with pediatric patients because children can be physically restrained, are not routinely asked if they are in pain, and are usually unable to withdraw their consent. Fortunately, the appropriate use of local anesthesia can abolish much of this pain.

Additionally, because regional anesthesia produces profound analgesia with minimal physiologic alterations, it is increasingly being used in children as a component of intraoperative, postoperative, and posttraumatic pain management, and for pain that is difficult to treat with systemic narcotics. For example, children who cannot tolerate opioids because of opioid-induced ventilatory depression or who have become tolerant to the analgesic effects of opioids can be made completely pain free with the use of local anesthetic techniques. Prolonged analgesia can also be provided by continuously administering local anesthetic agents by way of indwelling catheters placed in the epidural, intrathecal, intercostal, intrapleural, or other spaces (6,12). Because of these myriad benefits and because of our ability to overcome many of the technical difficulties that limited the use of local anesthetics in the past, local anesthetics and regional anesthetic techniques have become an essential component in the armamentarium of managing childhood pain.

Less local anesthetic is necessary to block the transmission of pain than is necessary to produce muscle paralysis. Thus, pain sensation can be blocked without blocking motor function by using dilute concentrations of local anesthetics, sometimes referred to as *differential nerve block*. In fact, concentrated local anesthetic solutions (e.g., 2% lidocaine vs. 1.0%) increase the quality of sensory blockade only minimally. On the other hand, a concentrated local anesthetic will increase the incidence of motor blockade and systemic toxicity. To minimize this effect, concentrated solutions of local anesthetics can be diluted with preservative-free normal saline. Interestingly, when this is done in clinical practice, differential conduction blockade is often misinterpreted by patients as failure of the local anesthetic to produce adequate anesthesia because the patient may continue to perceive proprioception and light touch or have motor function even though pain is completely blocked.

Other factors influence the quality and duration of a nerve block, such as the addition of a vasoconstrictor to the anesthetic mixture, the use of mixtures of local anesthetics, and the site of drug administration. Vasoconstrictors, particularly epinephrine, are frequently added to local anesthetic solutions. Epinephrine decreases the rate of vascular absorption of local anesthetic from the site of administration, thereby increasing the time that the local anesthetic is in contact with nerve fibers, particularly for drugs, such as lidocaine, that are poorly lipid soluble. This addition lengthens the duration of sensory blockade for lidocaine by almost 50% and decreases peak plasma local anesthetic concentrations by one-third. More lipid-soluble agents, such as bupivacaine, ropivacaine, and etidocaine, are less affected by the addition of epinephrine (33).

By causing local vasoconstriction, epinephrine reduces bleeding at sites of injury. Interestingly, epinephrine also improves the intensity of anesthesia and increases the effectiveness of dilute concentrations of local anesthetics. Epinephrine-containing solutions should never be injected into areas supplied by end arteries, such as the penis or digits. Injection of an epinephrine-containing solution into these areas may lead to tissue ischemia or necrosis. Epinephrine is often added to local anesthetic solutions in concentrations of 5 to 10 mcg/mL (1:200,000–100,000). Higher epinephrine concentrations offer no advantage in further reducing peak plasma local anesthetic concentrations and may, in fact, produce adverse systemic hemodynamic effects.

The systemic toxic effects of local anesthetics are determined by the total dose of drug administered, protein binding, the rapidity of absorption into the blood, and the site of injection. Toxicity primarily occurs by unintended IV administration or by accumulation of excessive amounts of drug administered either by repeated bolus dosing or by continuous infusion, therefore belying the idea of accepted "maximum" doses of these drugs, because even small fractions of the accepted "maximum" dosages of local anesthetics will produce toxic systemic effects if the local anesthetic is injected intra-arterially, intravenously, or into any highly vascular location (**Table 12.8**). In general, the peak absorption of local anesthetic depends on the site of the block, because the site of injection influences the rate of plasma uptake by the vascularity of the tissues. The more vascular the site of injection, the more readily uptake can occur and the more sudden and intense system toxic effects will be. The order of absorption from highest to lowest is: intercostal, intrapleural, intratracheal > caudal/epidural > brachial plexus > distal peripheral > subcutaneous > fat. Bupivacaine toxicity is the most feared because the electrical asystole it produces has been refractory to treatment and has often resulted in death. In the past, some patients have been saved from bupivacaine-induced cardiac arrest by being placed on cardiopulmonary bypass. Recently, IV intralipid, acting as a sponge or sink to "soak up" bupivacaine, has been used successfully (69). Finally, lidocaine is the only local anesthetic that is used intravenously and orally (mexiletine) as an antiarrythmic and as a method of treating neuropathic pain (4,25). In neuropathic pain states, lidocaine blocks conduction of sodium channels in peripheral and central neurons and thereby dampens both peripheral nociceptor sensitization and, ultimately central nervous system hyperexcitability.

TABLE 12.8

MAXIMUM LOCAL ANESTHETIC DOSING GUIDELINES

Drug	Dose (mg/kg) without epinephrine	Dose (mg/kg) with epinephrine	Duration (hours)	Contraindications	Comments
Bupivacaine[a]	2	3	3–6		Reduce dose by 50% in neonates
Chloroprocaine[b]	8	10	1	Plasma cholinesterase deficiency	Short-acting, rapid metabolism; useful in neonates and patients with seizures or liver disease
Lidocaine	5	7	1		
Ropivacaine	2	3	3–6		Less cardiotoxicity than bupivacaine

[a]When given by epidural continuous infusion: 0.2–0.4 mg/kg/hr.
[b]In neonatal epidural continuous infusion: 10–15 mg/kg/hr. Ropivacine, a stereoselective enantiomer is less toxic than bupivacaine (28).

EPIDURAL ANESTHESIA/ANALGESIA

The deposition of local anesthetics, opioids, α_2 agonists (clonidine), midazolam, steroids, and/or ketamine can be used to palliate acute pain and is most commonly used in pediatrics for the management of postoperative pain and traumatic pain.

Complications are rare. In adults, hypotension is the most often noted complication during bolus dosing, and the higher thoracic level blocks increase the risk for these events. However, in children <8 years of age, hypotension is extremely rare even with higher-level blocks. However, as in adults, if hypotension does occur, it is often related to sympathetic blockade and systemic absorption of local anesthetic into the bloodstream. Aside from the potential for local anesthetic toxicity from continuous infusions into the epidural space or direct intravascular injection, other reported complications are urinary retention, site infection, chemical meningitis, and inadvertent spinal anesthesia. Epidural insertion is contraindicated in patients with coagulation disorders and the presence of infection at the intended site of insertion.

Local Anesthetic Dosage for Epidural Analgesia

Bupivacaine and lidocaine are the most commonly used agents for epidural analgesia. Many techniques facilitate the initiation and maintenance of epidural anesthesia and analgesia. Typical practice is to load with a dose of 1 mL/kg of either 0.125% or 0.25% bupivacaine (maximum 20 mL), followed 45–90 mins later with a continuous infusion of a 0.1% (1 mg/mL) solution at a dose not to exceed 0.4 mg/kg/hr. For lidocaine, a concentration of 0.1%–0.5% (1–5 mg/mL) can be used. In neonates and infants, lidocaine is preferred because it is less toxic, and unlike bupivacaine, plasma lidocaine levels can be measured and used to guide therapy. In neonates, a 1-mg/mL lidocaine solution is used and infusions are started at 0.8 mL/kg/hr.

Adjuvants Used in Epidural Analgesia

In addition to local anesthetics, agents have been added to regional and neuraxial blocks to augment the duration and intensity of analgesia. The most common and effective adjuvants are opioids and the α_2 agonist clonidine. Less commonly used adjuvants include ketamine, midazolam, and steroids. Unlike local anesthetics, which are primarily active on the spinal cord and nerve roots, both opioids and α_2 agonists have a substantial amount of systemic absorption and central activity that are perhaps greater than their local effect. Although these central effects are perhaps their most important site of action, they are the source of complications that should be recognized by the PICU clinician when evaluating patients with epidural analgesia that may contain these agents.

Regardless of the opioid used in the epidural space, a regular system of monitoring for respiratory depression is required. Clinical signs that predict impending respiratory depression include somnolence, small pupils, and small tidal volumes. The authors also use and recommend oxygen-saturation monitoring in all patients with opioids in the epidural space, particu-larly within the first 24 hrs of instituting therapy. Adverse (or desired) effects of α_2 agonists include somnolence, sedation, and hypotension.

SEDATION IN THE PICU

Anxiety, fear, a sense of helplessness, and lack of sleep will potentiate pain and, if left untreated, can lead to psychosis in critically ill patients. "ICU (-induced) psychosis" is a well-described phenomenon in adult patients that typically occurs 3–5 days after admission to the ICU. This syndrome is caused by a combination of factors that include the patient's premorbid personality (attitude toward illness, age, and defense mechanisms), psychologic disturbances, the environment (frightening atmosphere, unusual and disturbing sounds, lack of windows, deprivation of day-night cycles, etc.), and lack of sleep. Furthermore, the failure to provide adequate sedation, analgesia, and amnesia can lead to the development of posttraumatic stress syndrome. Sleep and the restorative effects of normal sleep are essential in all humans. A variety of factors prevent sleep in critically ill patients. Patients are subjected to constant light, noise, rounds, visitors, anxious family, pain, procedures, blood sampling, and more often than not, an endotracheal tube. Children are frightened by the machines in the PICU and usually misinterpret staff conversations heard from around the bed. Further, many of the drugs that produce sedation may interfere with normal sleep architecture, thereby paradoxically increasing the need for more sedation.

Sedation for patients who require prolonged immobility may last for days or even weeks (**Table 12.9**). Alternatively, sedation for painful or nonpainful procedures may be brief, lasting <30–60 mins. Indeed, procedural sedation is an increasingly important function of the ICU and its staff. In many institutions, because of their airway, monitoring, and rescue skills, intensivists provide pediatric procedural sedation for both critically ill patients and for healthy children who are undergoing scheduled procedures such as diagnostic imaging studies, bone marrow aspirations, and endoscopy. In choosing a technique for procedural sedation, it is first essential to clearly identify the goals of the sedation plan and to differentiate between sedation and analgesia. Not all procedures or clinical situations demand both, and commonly, one is needed more than the other.

Procedural sedation exists across a continuum that varies from a state of wakefulness, to anxiolysis, to moderate sedation ("conscious sedation"), to deep sedation, to general anesthesia (1,2). The drugs chosen and the underlying condition of the patient may make this transition more or less likely, and individual variations in drug response are not always predictable. Thus, physicians must always be prepared for the common possibility that the patient may pass into a greater depth of sedation than initially planned, and she must be able to manage the consequences.

Benzodiazepines

The benzodiazepines comprise a family of drugs that are the most important sedative/hypnotic/anxiolytic drugs currently used in clinical practice. Diazepam, midazolam, triazolam, and lorazepam are members of this family (**Table 12.10**). These

TABLE 12.9

COMMON INITIATION RANGES FOR SEDATIVE INFUSIONS IN THE PICU

Agent	Load/p.r.n.	Infusion range	Comments
Midazolam	0.05–0.1 mg/kg	0.05–0.1 mg/kg/hr	Commonly used sedative Extensive clinical experience Metabolism via cytochrome P450
Lorazepam	0.05–0.1 mg/kg	0.025–0.05 mg/kg/hr	Less clinical experience Polyethylene glycol preservative; watch for osmolar gap and acidosis Metabolized via glucuronyl transferase Maximum p.r.n. dose, 2 mg
Pentobarbital	0.5–1 mg/kg	1–2 mg/kg/hr	Negative inotropic effect Can monitor levels
Propofol	2–3 mg/kg	75–250 mcg/kg/min	Rapid emergence Short procedural sedation only! Contraindicated for prolonged infusions in children secondary to lethal propofol infusion syndrome
Dexmedetomidine	0.3–1 mcg/kg	0.25–0.7 mcg/kg/hr	Adverse bradycardia and hypotension during loading Limited clinical experience in children
Ketamine	1–2 mg/kg	1–2 mg/kg/hr	Increased heart rate and blood pressure secondary to catecholamine release; bronchodilator May need supplemental benzodiazepine and antisialagogue

These are suggested boluses and initiation ranges, and their effect must be titrated for each patient to the appropriate level of sedation.

drugs are extremely potent amnestics, anticonvulsants, sedatives, hypnotics, and skeletal muscle relaxants and are effective whether given parenterally or enterally. *They have no analgesic properties.* They work by augmenting γ-aminobutyric acid (GABA) and glycine transmission. GABA is the major inhibitory neurotransmitter within the brain, whereas glycine is an inhibitory neurotransmitter in the spinal cord and brainstem. Binding of a benzodiazepine to its receptor on the α subunit of the GABA transmembrane receptor facilitates the binding of GABA to the β subunit (shifts the dose response to the left) and allows extracellular chloride to enter into a cell, causing membrane hyperpolarization and resistance to neuronal excitation and resulting in sedation, anxiolysis, muscle relaxation, and anticonvulsant activity. Alternatively, the binding of an antagonist such as flumazenil does not alter GABA synaptic transmission efficiency but competitively blocks the actions of agonist agents.

Within the CNS, the benzodiazepines reduce cerebral metabolism and blood flow. They alter consciousness along a dose-dependent continuum that ranges from anxiolysis to general anesthesia, but they do not produce normal sleep; indeed, they may interfere with normal sleep architecture. The

TABLE 12.10

COMMONLY USED BENZODIAZEPINES

Generic	Brand	How supplied		Active metabolite	Equipotent IV dose (mg/kg)
Diazepam	Valium	Parenteral: Tablet: Oral solution:	5 mg/mL 2, 5, 10 mg 1, 5 mg/mL	Yes	0.1–0.2
Lorazepam	Ativan	Parenteral: Tablet: Oral solution:	2, 4 mg/mL 0.5, 1, 2 mg 2 mg/mL	No	0.03–0.05
Midazolam	Versed	Parenteral: Oral solution:	1, 5 mg/mL 2 mg/mL	Yes	0.05–0.1
Oxazepam	Serax	Tablet: Capsule:	15 mg 10, 15, 30 mg	No	NA
Triazolam	Halcion	Tablet:	0.125, 0.25 mg	No	NA

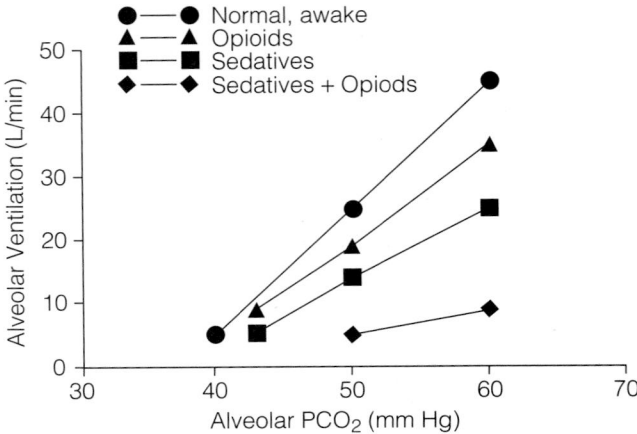

FIGURE 12.3. The relationship between ventilation and carbon dioxide is represented by a family of curves. Each curve has two parameters (an intercept and slope). Sedatives and opioids shift the position and slope to the right. The combination of drugs produces the most profound effects. From Yaster M, Nichols DG, Deshpande JK, Wetzel RC. Midazolam-fentanyl intravenous sedation in children: Case report of respiratory arrest. *Pediatrics.* 1990;86:463–467, with permission.

benzodiazepines are potent anticonvulsants and impair the acquisition of new information (anterograde amnesia) without affecting previously stored information (retrograde amnesia). The latter attribute is quite useful to the intensivist because often a patient is too hemodynamically unstable to adequately sedate (e.g., cardioversion, intubation). Benzodiazepines, by providing intense anterograde amnesia, can prevent a patient from remembering a painful or unpleasant procedure.

Benzodiazepines produce dose-dependent depression of breathing and affect the ventilatory responses to both hypoxia and hypercapnia. In small doses, the benzodiazepines minimally affect minute ventilation. In higher doses, however, they can blunt or abolish the respiratory responses to both hypercarbia and hypoxia. Drug-induced respiratory depression is quantified by the ventilatory response to inhaled or rebreathed CO_2 (75) (**Fig. 12.3**). The depressant drug may either reduce the slope of the CO_2 response curve or shift the x-intercept to the right. A reduced slope implies a diminished ventilatory response at any given arterial $Paco_2$ level. The x-intercept of the curve, known as the *apneic threshold,* indicates relative position of the curve and is defined as that $Paco_2$ threshold value required to stimulate spontaneous respiration. The benzodiazepines produce hypoventilation primarily by decreasing tidal volume, which is manifested by a reduction of the slope of the CO_2 response curve without a change in the x-intercept (see **Fig. 12.3**). The depressant effect of the benzodiazepines begins within 1–4 mins of an IV injection and lasts for at least 30 mins.

The benzodiazepine-induced decrease in the ventilatory response to hypoxia is particularly dangerous, as the hypoxic drive is the "backup" system in the control of ventilation. Drug-induced hypoventilation rapidly decreases alveolar and arterial oxygen saturation. In unmedicated persons, the hypoxic ventilatory drive provides some protection from hypoventilation-induced hypoxia. If both the hypoxic and hypercarbic drive to breath are blunted or blocked by the benzodiazepines, apnea and death may result from their use. Furthermore, the respi-

ratory depression seen with the benzodiazepines is potentiated with the concomitant administration of any opioid (75), requiring a reduction in the dose of both drugs when they are administered together and underscoring the need for very close observation and monitoring of patients who receive these drugs. The risk of using these drugs may be significantly increased in children with chronic CO_2 retention, who are <1–2 months of age, are chronically dependent on the hypoxic drive to ventilate, and who are receiving opioids concomitantly. Finally, the respiratory depression produced by the benzodiazepine agonists can be antagonized by flumazenil.

The benzodiazepines produce variable cardiovascular effects. They reduce both preload and afterload; arterial blood pressure and cardiac output are minimally affected. However, in the presence of hypovolemia or catecholamine depletion, the benzodiazepines, like virtually all other sedatives, may produce significant hypotension and must, therefore, be administered with great caution, particularly if administered by a rapid bolus injection. Benzodiazepines significantly affect blood pressure and cardiac output when combined with opioids and are therefore more dangerous when combined than when either is given alone.

The use of continuous infusion versus intermittent dosing of benzodiazepines is debatable. The advantages of continuous infusion, namely, stable blood levels and clinical effects without "peaks and valleys," may be counterbalanced by an increased risk for drug accumulation and the more rapid development of tolerance. Interestingly, the use of continuous infusions in patients following cardiac surgery has resulted in depression of cardiac output by >20% (58). In general, the use of continuous infusions is most common when shorter-acting agents, such as midazolam, are used. Long-term infusions and altered metabolism secondary to illness increase the risk for drug accumulation and modified pharmacokinetics, even when short-half-life drugs are used. Longer-acting agents (e.g., lorazepam, diazepam) may be less likely to induce tolerance, allow sedation to be interrupted for patient evaluation, and are often significantly cheaper than continuous infusions (40). Because of this, it is our practice to preferentially use intermittent dosing.

Diazepam

Diazepam, once the most commonly used benzodiazepine, has been largely replaced in clinical practice by midazolam and lorazepam. Diazepam is poorly water soluble, and the solvent vehicle for parenteral administration contains several organic solvents such as propylene glycol and sodium benzoate, both of which are toxic in the newborn. Its poor water solubility makes absorption from an IM site erratic and incomplete. Thus, the oral or IV route of administration is preferred. Unfortunately, even the IV route is problematic because diazepam is painful when administered IV and causes thrombophlebitis. Following absorption, diazepam is very slowly N-demethylated in the liver into two active metabolites, desmethyl diazepam and oxazepam. Desmethyldiazepam is metabolized even more slowly than diazepam and has a half-life of elimination of 48–96 hrs. Oxazepam is rapidly glucuronidated and excreted in the urine. The presence of these active metabolites explains, in part, the very long duration of action of diazepam and why it has largely been replaced by midazolam. On the other hand, the prolonged sedation may be a desired effect in patients who require extended sedation.

Dosage and Route of Administration

Diazepam is an effective sedative, anxiolytic, and amnestic when administered orally, rectally, or intravenously. When administered IV, 0.05–0.1 mg/kg, it rapidly allays anxiety and apprehension and can be titrated to effect. Additionally, this same dose can be used as an anticonvulsant to temporarily stop seizure activity. The oral dose is two to three times the IV dose and takes 30–90 mins to produce similar hypnotic effects.

Midazolam

Midazolam is a water-soluble benzodiazepine that is four times more potent than diazepam and is well absorbed via IM, oral, rectal, or transmucosal routes of administration. Unlike diazepam, midazolam can be administered IV and rarely causes thrombophlebitis. Although manufactured as an acid to make it water soluble at physiologic pH, midazolam becomes highly lipophilic and rapidly crosses the BBB to gain access to the benzodiazepine receptors in the CNS, which accounts for its dramatic clinical effect. It has a relatively large volume of distribution, short elimination half-life, and high clearance, and it is hydroxylated in the liver into inactive metabolites. It is characterized by rapid onset, short duration of action following a single parenteral dose, and little accumulation following repeated or continuous infusion dosing. When administered enterally, usually for procedural sedation, <50% of the administered dose is bioavailable because of extraction by the liver ("first pass").

Dosage and Route of Administration

When used for sedation prior to procedures or as a premedication, midazolam can be administered IV (0.05–0.1 mg/kg), IM (0.1 mg/kg), rectally (0.3–1.0 mg/kg), orally (0.5–1.0 mg/kg; maximum dose 20 mg), or nasally (0.2 mg/kg). Obviously, IV administration produces the most rapid onset of effect and therefore must be titrated with continuous cardiorespiratory monitoring. It also produces the shortest duration of effect. When administered rectally, midazolam takes ~10 mins to produce its effect, whereas when administered orally, it takes 20–30 mins to achieve adequate sedation.

Midazolam is commonly administered in the ICU by continuous IV infusion for prolonged sedation. Several dosing regimens are available. Silvasi and Rosen recommend starting with a loading dose of 0.2 mg/kg, followed by a continuous infusion of 0.4–0.6 mcg/kg/min (58). On the other hand, Booker et al. required 2–6 mcg/kg/min to achieve adequate sedation in postoperative cardiac patients using the same loading dose as Silvasi and Rosen (11). Tolerance and dependence will develop to prolonged midazolam infusions and, if stopped suddenly, will result in severe withdrawal symptoms. Benzodiazepine-withdrawal symptoms are similar to withdrawal alcohol (delirium tremens) and will occur when cumulative midazolam dosing exceeds 60 mg/kg (21). Clonidine, 3–5 mcg/kg, administered orally or transdermally may ameliorate many of these withdrawal symptoms. Alternatively, patients should be weaned slowly by gradual tapering of the dosage, rather than by abrupt discontinuance of these drugs.

Lorazepam

Lorazepam is a relatively inexpensive, water-soluble benzodiazepine that is increasingly being used to sedate patients in the PICU. The duration of action of lorazepam (2–4 hrs) is longer than that of midazolam, allowing intermittent, on-demand administration. Unlike midazolam, lorazepam is metabolized by glucuronyl transferase and not by the CYP system. Thus, it is less affected by liver disease and by other drugs that are metabolized by the CYP system, such as anticonvulsants, rifampicin (rifampin), and cimetidine. Additionally, unlike diazepam, lorazepam has no active metabolites. As with all benzodiazepines, tolerance develops with its use, and abrupt cessation results in symptoms of withdrawal (21).

Dosage and Route of Administration

Lorazepam is an effective sedative, anxiolytic, and amnestic when administered orally or intravenously. When administered IV, 0.05–0.1 mg/kg (maximum dose, 2 mg), it rapidly allays anxiety and apprehension and should be titrated to effect. Additionally, this same dose can be used as an anticonvulsant to stop seizure activity. The oral dose is twice the IV dose, and is often used to wean benzodiazepine-dependent patients slowly.

BARBITURATES

The barbiturates have been greatly supplanted by the benzodiazepines for the treatment of insomnia both in and out of the ICU. These drugs are neither anxiolytics nor analgesics; rather, they globally depress the CNS to various degrees and produce effects that range from sedation to general anesthesia in a dose-dependent manner. When managing patients in pain, caution must be exercised in the use of barbiturates because, in small doses, they increase the perception of pain and cause excitement rather than sedation ("antanalgesia"). However, when barbiturates are given in doses high enough to produce general anesthesia, pain perception, in addition to consciousness, is obliterated. Thus, a dose-dependent continuum of CNS effects exists following barbiturate administration. At lower doses, barbiturates produce sleep; at higher doses, they produce general anesthesia. Infrequently, barbiturates produce an idiosyncratic, hyperkinetic reaction in children that is characterized by agitation, incoherence, disorientation, and tantrums. All but methohexital are potent anticonvulsants and can be used acutely and chronically for this purpose. Additionally, they reduce cerebral blood flow and cerebral metabolism in proportion to their degree of cerebral depression and are often used for this purpose in the ICU following head injury. Thus, thiopental is often used to treat spikes of intracranial pressure by producing unconsciousness, thereby reducing cerebral blood flow. However, these drugs are of no prophylactic value in preventing or minimizing secondary brain injury in patients with elevated intracranial pressure. Indeed, the use of barbiturate-induced coma for this purpose has largely been abandoned.

The barbiturates have significant effects on the cardiovascular system. They must be given with great caution in hemodynamically unstable patients. All of the barbiturates directly depress the myocardium and the arterial vascular tree and cause significant hypotension. If the baroreceptor compensatory system is intact, hypotension results in a reflex tachycardia that may help to restore blood pressure. When barbiturates are given to patients with minimal compensatory reserves, such as patients who are catecholamine or volume depleted, profound hypotension and even cardiac arrest can occur. The dose of ultra-short-acting barbiturates (e.g., thiopental) needed to induce unconsciousness in hypovolemic patients for intubation should be reduced by 75% or entirely eliminated.

The barbiturates are generally classified into long-, medium-, and ultra-short-acting agents based on their pharmacokinetic and pharmacodynamic profiles. Phenobarbital is a long-acting barbiturate with a half-life of elimination of 24–96 hr. It is most commonly used as an anticonvulsant in doses of 10–20 mg/kg; rarely is it used to produce sleep. In fact, its very long duration of action and very slow onset time make it an inappropriate hypnotic agent in any medical setting. Pentobarbital and secobarbital are medium-acting barbiturates with half-lives of elimination that range between 20 and 45 hrs. Sleep is induced within 10–15 mins of an IV or IM bolus injection and will last ~2–6 hrs. It may also be administered orally or rectally. Pentobarbital is generally used to produce sleep, immobility for diagnostic imaging studies, and long-lasting sedation, and is administered in doses that range between 2 and 6 mg/kg, with a maximum dose of 150 mg. IV thiopental, 4–7 mg/kg, and methohexital, 1–2 mg/kg, are ultra-short-acting agents (i.e., they produce unconsciousness for <10 mins) despite having elimination half-lives of 4–24 hrs. Recovery from the effects of IV thiopental and methohexital has nothing to do with their biotransformation and elimination from the body. Rather, their effects are terminated by redistribution from the brain to other body tissue compartments, which has very important clinical implications. If, for example, thiopental is given by repeated intermittent doses or by a prolonged IV infusion (e.g., in head trauma), prolongation of effect will occur because elimination, not distribution, will determine the duration of the drug's effect. The ultra-short-acting agents are generally used to induce general anesthesia IV, particularly prior to tracheal intubation. The dose of thiopental, for example, is reduced to 1–2 mg/kg rather than 4–7 mg/kg when it is given to hemodynamically unstable patients. Because it has a pH >10, thiopental can produce catastrophic damage if it is injected intra-arterially. Thus, one must be certain of the functionality of an IV catheter before this drug is injected. Thiopental and methohexital may also be administered rectally (20–30 mg/kg) to produce immobility for nonpainful diagnostic imaging procedures. The resulting sedation lasts for 60–90 mins.

PROPOFOL

Propofol, 2,6-diisopropylphenol, is an alkylphenol IV general anesthetic widely used in the operating room and in adult ICUs (60). It is unrelated to other general anesthetics and is formulated as a 1% (10 mg/mL) solution in 10% soybean oil, 2.25% glycerol, and 1.2% egg phosphatide. The lipid component is essentially identical to that used for parenteral nutrition (10% Intralipid). The drug's rapid onset of action, its dose-proportional sedative/anesthetic effects, and its rapid dissipation of clinical effects after discontinuance of drug administration are responsible for its widespread acceptance as a general anesthetic and for its potential use as a sedative to facilitate mechanical ven-

tilation in critically ill patients. Propofol, like barbiturates and other general anesthetics, appears to bind to the GABA receptor, namely, the A subunit (GABA$_A$), which potentiates GABA-mediated synaptic inhibition within the CNS.

The pharmacokinetics of propofol after bolus doses or following continuous infusions has been studied extensively in healthy children and adults (60). The drug's disposition profile is best characterized by a three-compartment pharmacokinetic model (56). After IV administration, propofol rapidly distributes from the central compartment (blood) into two additional compartments: a larger, rapidly equilibrating compartment and an enormous, slowly equilibrating third compartment. Clearance from the central compartment is very rapid, exceeding total hepatic blood flow, and results in rapid recovery of consciousness. This rapid clearance from the central compartment, rather than metabolism, is responsible for its short duration of effect. Propofol undergoes hepatic metabolism by conjugation, and the resultant water-soluble compounds are excreted in the kidney. Complete elimination from the body may take many hours or even days, despite minimal blood concentrations.

Although their actions are similar, propofol is chemically unrelated to the barbiturates. Like the barbiturates, it has negative inotropic properties and is a potent vasodilator. It is a rapid-acting sedative/amnestic agent without analgesic properties that also allows rapid recovery. Because of its rapid onset, rapid recovery time, and lack of active metabolites, it has largely replaced thiopental as the most commonly used IV general anesthetic induction agent in the operating room. Additionally, it is commonly given by infusion in combination with short-lived opioids (e.g., fentanyl) to produce general anesthesia for short procedures such as bronchoscopy and endoscopy. In the PICU, it is used to produce unconsciousness prior to intubation and, in the adult ICU, to produce prolonged, continuous sedation and to treat refractory status epilepticus. The latter effect is interesting because, at low doses, propofol may actually be proconvulsant, and propofol administration has been associated with abnormal, "herky-jerky" (myotonic) movements. However, this concern has probably been overemphasized, because no true electroencephalographic evidence of seizure activity has ever been documented with propofol administration.

Propofol is manufactured in a lipid emulsion derived from egg whites, which both causes pain on injection and makes the solution an ideal culture media for bacterial growth. The pain on injection can be prevented by pretreatment with IV lidocaine, fentanyl, or ketamine. Many practitioners mix lidocaine (10–20 mg) or ketamine (1–2 mg/mL) into the propofol solution to prevent injection pain and to provide analgesia for the procedure. The risk of bacterial contamination of the solution can be prevented by meticulous aseptic technique. Once a vial is opened, the unused content should be disposed of promptly and not saved for later use. If an infusion is being used, the syringe and tubing should be dated, timed, and changed every 6 hrs.

Unlike in the operating room, where propofol is given to relatively healthy patients for periods that range from minutes to hours, patients in the ICU are by definition critically ill and may receive propofol for days. Therefore, insignificant effects during anesthesia may become very important in the critically ill. The literature contains many reports of unexpected fatal lactic acidosis in critically ill children who were sedated for prolonged periods with propofol (propofol infusion syndrome) (13,17). Although this association has been disputed (64), it underscores the importance and need for pharmacokinetic and dynamic studies in critically ill children. Some studies do demonstrate uncoupling of oxidative phosphorylation in mitochondria and inhibition of CYP isoenzymes. Nevertheless, why propofol would produce lactic acidosis and liver dysfunction following prolonged use and how it can be prevented are unclear. Until these issues are resolved, prolonged (>6 hrs) propofol infusions in critically ill children should be avoided.

Dosing and Route of Administration

When given in the ICU to induce deep sedation/general anesthesia for intubation or other painful procedures such as cardioversion, 2–3 mg/kg of propofol is given by IV push. Because of the effects of myocardial depression and decreased systemic vascular resistance, caution must be taken when giving this drug in this way to already compromised children. If sustained procedural general anesthesia/deep sedation is desired, an infusion of undiluted propofol can be given at 150–250 mcg/kg/min. This infusion rate is titrated up and down based on the level of procedural stimulation. In some patients, infusion rates as high as 400–500 mcg/kg/min are required. At the conclusion of the procedure, the infusion can be stopped suddenly or titrated down in anticipation of its end. Return to a preprocedural state of consciousness is rapid and depends on dose and duration of the propofol infusion. Finally, older patients typically report a pleasant feeling on awakening.

INHALATIONAL ANESTHETICS

Inhalational anesthetic agents are commonly used in the operating room to provide general anesthesia (amnesia, immobility, loss of consciousness, and analgesia) for surgery. Although their mechanism of action is unknown, volatile general anesthetics are predictable, have a rapid onset and emergence, and are easily titratable to effect. These features are appealing for use in the ICU. However, costs, variability in clinician and nursing credentialing and comfort with this class of drug, and the logistic issues of administering a volatile anesthetic gas for extended periods of time in the ICU have prevented their widespread use. Reported usage in the PICU has most often been for sedation failures, detoxification following prolonged use of other sedatives and opioids, and in the treatment of status asthmaticus (7).

Isoflurane

Although all of the volatile general anesthetic agents have been used in the PICU, discussion here focuses on isoflurane because it is the oldest, cheapest, and most commonly used. Isoflurane is a halogenated ether compound that, when vaporized, has a pungent, caustic odor (it smells like "dry-cleaning fluid") that may induce laryngospasm and bronchospasm. These characteristics are very different from sevoflurane, which has a pleasant, almost sweet aroma and can be used to treat bronchospasm. As a patient breathes the vaporized gas, general anesthesia is produced. Isoflurane, like all volatile general anesthetics, has a very narrow therapeutic index; the end-tidal concentration required to produce general anesthesia is 1.2%, and the lethal end-tidal concentration is 4%. The drug is dispensed via a vaporizer that converts liquid isoflurane into a gas. Adjusting the dial of the vaporizer allows a greater concentration of volatile anesthetic to be taken into the inhaled gas mixture breathed by the patient. Unlike nitrous oxide (N_2O), volatile anesthetics do not lower the fraction of inspired oxygen.

An understanding of the primary physiologic effects of the vapor anesthetics is essential for the intensivist. Isoflurane is a negative inotrope and vasodilator, and increasing its concentration (and anesthetic depth) produces a progressive depression in the myocardial contractile state of the heart and in peripheral vasodilation, which results in hypotension and a compensatory increase in heart rate. Volatile anesthetics are potent respiratory depressants and decrease minute ventilation by >30%. They primarily do this by decreasing tidal volume and by altering the respiratory center's hypoxic and hypercarbic drive to breathe. Yet, patients breathing spontaneously on a vapor anesthetic appear to be tachypneic, with respiratory rates as high as 40 breaths/min. This increase in respiratory rate is an ineffective compensation for the profound decrease in tidal volume that these drugs produce. Anesthetized patients breathing spontaneously will have end-tidal CO_2 levels in the mid 50-mm Hg range. Finally, once general anesthesia is induced, isoflurane, like all other vapor anesthetics, is among the most potent bronchodilators known in medicine. Many patients in status asthmaticus who are unresponsive to any other form of treatment will "break" when anesthetized with isoflurane.

Isoflurane causes a decrease in cerebral metabolic rate and increases in cerebral blood flow, cerebral vasodilation, and possibly, intracranial pressure (although this is blunted with hyperventilation). This uncoupling of cerebral metabolic rate to cerebral blood flow precludes the use of isoflurane in patients with increased intracranial pressure. Finally, isoflurane is a potent anticonvulsant and is occasionally used in the treatment of refractory status epilepticus.

Sedative effects from isoflurane can be observed at exhaled concentrations of 0.3%–1%. Analgesic and general anesthetic effects are often observed at end-tidal concentrations of 1%–1.2% and higher. It should be noted that the longer the gas is inhaled, the greater the amount of volatile agent distributed and stored in fat-soluble compartments. Thus, the duration of agent administration and the size of the patient are important factors in achieving adequate sedation, analgesia, and anesthesia, and in wake-up and recovery.

In addition to concerns with volatile anesthetic usage in altered intracranial compliance, volatile agents are contraindicated in those patients with a history of malignant hyperthermia or in those who are at risk of developing malignant hyperthermia, such as patients with Duchenne muscular dystrophy. Additionally, like N_2O, the use of isoflurane is limited by institutional and nursing credentialing, availability of specialized delivery and monitoring equipment, and the ability to scavenge exhaled gas.

KETAMINE

Structurally related to phencyclidine (PCP), ketamine is an NMDA antagonist that produces an altered state of consciousness (hallucinations), amnesia, and analgesia (71). Ketamine is most commonly manufactured as a racemic mixture that contains both chiral S+ and R− enantiomers. These stereoisomers have different anesthetic potency (4:1, respectively) but have similar kinetics, and are both metabolized by hepatic N-methylation to norketamine, which is further metabolized by hydroxylation and ultimately excreted in the urine. Norketamine retains reduced analgesic and sedative properties (approximately one-third of the parent compound). Because the pharmacokinetics of ketamine rely on both hepatic metabolism and renal excretion, its duration of action and dose effect will be altered in many critically ill patients.

Pharmacokinetic data in pediatric patients is limited. Ketamine and norketamine half-life elimination in postoperative cardiac patients has been described to be 3.1 hrs and 6 hrs, respectively (30). Although tolerance has been reported, the literature contains no clinical reports of dependence or withdrawal following ketamine administration. The minimal respiratory depressant effects and relatively stable hemodynamics associated with its use make this an appealing drug for procedural sedation in the PICU.

In addition to its binding to the NMDA receptor, ketamine causes an increase in catecholamine release and cholinergic receptor stimulation, resulting in bronchodilation and an increase in systemic vascular resistance, heart rate, and cardiac output. Thus, ketamine is often used in asthmatic patients and in hemodynamically unstable patients or patients with congenital heart disease (71). Nevertheless, it is important to realize that ketamine is actually a negative inotrope, and it is this catecholamine release that helps to support blood pressure. This relationship is important when ketamine is administered to patients who are catecholamine-depleted because ketamine can cause profound hypotension and shock in these patients. Other adverse effects of ketamine include hallucinations, myotonic jerking movements, and excessive salivation. Ketamine also raises cerebral blood flow and cerebral oxygen consumption and should be avoided in patients with, or at risk for, increased intracranial pressure. Recent reports of a single enantiomer form (S+ enantiomer) have demonstrated fewer side effects, more rapid onset, and faster recovery compared to the racemic mixture (49). Because of the psychomotor agitation, vocalization, and salivation, coadministration of glycopyrrolate (0.03 mg/kg) and midazolam (0.1 mg/kg), either intravenously or orally, helps to reduce these adverse symptoms.

Other adverse effects remain controversial and include the occurrence of apnea in infants, a possible increased incidence of laryngospasm, lowering of the seizure threshold, and elevation of intracranial pressure. These are infrequent events but should be considered by the practitioner. Certainly, they emphasize the need for strict fasting guidelines, careful monitoring during and after usage, and availability of additional or alternative agents in case adverse events occur.

Dosage and Route of Administration

Ketamine can be administered for procedural sedation by nasal, oral, IV, and IM routes with good results. With IV administration, onset of action and recovery are relatively rapid (1–2 mins and 30–60 mins, respectively) but can be quite variable. Further, when given in rapid IV doses of 4 mg/kg, ketamine induces general anesthesia and can be used for rapid sequence induction (71). Like all IV sedatives, ketamine is titrated in aliquots of 0.5 to 1 mg/kg every 2–3 mins until an adequate level of sedation/analgesia is achieved. For induction of anesthesia, typically 4 mg/kg is administered IV. Intramuscular administration can be used if IV access is unavailable. Typically, 3–5 mg/kg

is coadministered in one syringe with atropine and midazolam (0.01 and 0.1 mg/kg, respectively). Similarly, ketamine can be given orally (5 mg/kg) and coadministered with atropine (0.02 mg/kg) and midazolam (0.5–1 mg/kg). For patients who require nonprocedural sedation, ketamine infusions have been used with mixed success. Typically, a loading dose of 1 to 2 mg/kg is followed by a continuous infusion ranging between 1 and 4 mg/kg/hr. Issues of tolerance and withdrawal symptoms have been raised following prolonged infusions, and patients should be closely monitored following discontinuation of prolonged ketamine exposure. Experimental data in animals suggest that ketamine promotes apoptosis in the developing brain, raising caution about prolonged ketamine use in the infant. However, at this writing, no human data support this concern.

α_2 ADRENERGIC AGONISTS IN SEDATION AND PAIN

α_2Agonists exert their effects by activating α_2 adrenergic receptors throughout the body. Three subtypes of this G-protein-coupled receptor have been characterized. The α_{2A} adrenoceptor mediates sedation, sleep, analgesia, and sympatholysis, whereas the α_{2B} adrenoceptor mediates vasoconstriction, anti-shivering, and endogenous analgesia. Both clonidine and dexmedetomidine belong to the imidazoline class of α_2 adrenergic agonists. Drugs from this class have a variety of physiologic effects on the heart, brain, lungs, kidneys, and on hormonal regulation, and they are used clinically for their antihypertensive and sedative/analgesic effects.

Clonidine

Clonidine is an imidazole α_2 agonist that binds to α_2:α_1 receptors in a ratio of 200:1. Clonidine is moderately lipid soluble and is almost completely absorbed following an oral dose. Peak serum levels occur at 1–3 hrs and in as little as 15–20 mins following epidural or spinal administration. Because of its large volume of distribution, clonidine has a long half-life of elimination of 12–24 hrs. It has little if any ventilatory depressant effects and best achieves analgesia when administered epidurally. Sedation, sleep, and the treatment of withdrawal symptomatology (from opioids, benzodiazepines, etc.) are the result of activation of α_2 receptors in the locus caeruleus. α_2 receptors, when centrally stimulated, prevent the presynaptic release of norepinephrine in the sympathetic nervous system (negative feedback loop) and account for clonidine's antihypertensive effects. Of note, the rebound hypertension seen with abrupt discontinuation of clonidine is thought to be from removal of the central inhibition of sympathetic activity. Interestingly, direct action on peripheral α_2 receptors results in peripheral vasoconstriction. Finally, adult studies have demonstrated clonidine to be an effective antishivering drug. The mechanism of this effect is thought to be through central thermoregulatory inhibition rather than peripherally on the muscles' thermogenic activity.

Because of its bioavailability, clonidine has been administered by almost every route. It can be given subcutaneously, orally, intravenously, transdermally, intranasally, and rectally. For sedation in the PICU and operating rooms, oral sedative doses of 2–5 mcg/kg are given every 4–6 hrs. This dose of the oral (neuraxial or crushed tablets) solution has also been given rectally. When given intranasally, the neuraxial solution should be used at the same dose. In patients with prolonged opioid and benzodiazepine exposure, clonidine patches of 100 to 300 mcg are frequently used. Typically, we start with the lower patch (2–4 mcg/kg/hr) and titrate up over 3–4 days. For treatment of shivering, an IV dose of 1.5 mcg/kg can be given. Because the IV solution is not available in the US, the neuraxial solution is often used. Although the concerns over rebound hypertension from clonidine are always present, we have been able to stop clonidine after 3–4 days of use without problem. If using a patch, step-down typically occurs over 2–3 weeks, once weaning from other agents has been completed.

Dexmedetomidine

Dexmedetomidine is an imidazole α_2 agonist that is similar to clonidine but with an even higher $\alpha_2:\alpha_1$ specificity ratio of 1600:1 (vs. 200:1). The drug's half-life of elimination is 1.5 to 3 hrs, and half of the drug is excreted unchanged in the urine. Biotransformation of the remaining drug is through the CYP2A6 system. Dexmedetomidine is highly lipid soluble and quickly crosses the BBB. Its primary CNS effect is to stimulate receptors in the vasomotor center of the medulla, which decreases sympathetic tone. It also stimulates central parasympathetic outflow and decreases sympathetic outflow from the locus caeruleus of the brainstem, a relay station that has long been implicated in the sleep–wake cycle. The decreased outflow from the locus caeruleus allows for increased activity of the inhibitory GABA neurons, which cause sedation, analgesia, and natural REM sleep. The sedative effects of α_2 agonists is antagonized by α_1 agonists and explains why drugs with a relatively low $\alpha_1:\alpha_2$ ratio, such as clonidine, are less effective at producing sleep and sedation.

Dexmedetomidine is approved for the sedation of intubated, ventilated, adult patients in the ICU but not in children. When administered in clinical doses (0.2–0.7 mg/kg/hr), dexmedetomidine produces dose-dependent sedation with minimal respiratory depressant effects. Patients appear to be calm and relaxed, breathe spontaneously, and are easy to arouse. In the heart, α_2 agonists decrease tachycardia through blockade of the cardioaccelerator nerve and produce bradycardia through vagomimetic action. In the peripheral vasculature, they exhibit both vasodilatory action through sympatholysis and vasoconstriction through direct action on the α_2 adrenoceptors on the smooth muscle cells. Thus, bolus dosing can cause rapid changes in heart rate and blood pressure, necessitating a slow initiating infusion (10–30 mins), followed by a maintenance infusion. When given in the recommended doses, dexmedetomidine decreases blood pressure and heart rate in adults and is given cautiously in patients with preexisting bradycardia, arteriovenous conduction defects, hypotension, and decreased cardiac output. The use of dexmedetomidine in an anesthesiology-supervised sedation service for radiologic imaging studies was prospectively evaluated (42). Sixty-two patients aged 6 months to 10 years were loaded with dexmedetomidine (2 mcg/kg) over 10 mins until sedated; an infusion of 1 mcg/kg/hr was then begun. Heart rate and blood pressure decreased 15%. No significant changes in respiratory rate or end-tidal CO_2 were observed. Mean recovery time was 32 mins. Although these results are preliminary, dexmedetomidine may provide safe se-

dation for procedures with minimal effect on the airway and breathing and herald a new era in procedural sedation.

THE PROBLEM PATIENT

Infants and children who require prolonged (days to weeks) sedation and immobility often require prodigious amounts of sedation. For those patients who have failed routine sedative and analgesic approaches, we usually begin with an augmented sedation regimen in which a benzodiazepine (usually diazepam or lorazepam) is alternated with an antihistamine (e.g., diphenhydramine) or a κ-opioid receptor mixed agonist-antagonist (e.g., butorphanol or nalbuphine) on an every 4- to 6-hr basis. In this way, each medicine is given 4–6 times per day, but the interval between receiving a medication to help with sedation is reduced to every 2–3 hrs. If response is good but the timing seems too far apart, we favor more frequent dosing at the same dose, rather than giving higher doses infrequently. This rationale is chosen because it helps to maintain a more even sedation and analgesic level. Alternative sedatives are listed in **Table 12.11**. Although patients who are difficult to sedate are a frequent problem in the PICU, clear communication with family and staff and emphasis on a team solution to the problem will address many of the issues that an improved and rational pharmacologic approach to sedation cannot.

NEUROMUSCULAR BLOCKADE

The principal pharmacologic effect of neuromuscular blocking agents is to interrupt the transmission of nerve impulses to the neuromuscular junction. These drugs have no analgesic or sedative properties and must always be administered after adequate sedation has been achieved. However, the clinical need for immobility in mechanically ventilated children occasionally necessitates neuromuscular blockade. Based on their mechanism of action, these drugs can be divided into two types: depolarizing (mimic the action of acetylcholine) and nondepolarizing (competitively block the actions of acetylcholine) agents. These drugs can also be subdivided into short- (succinylcholine, mivacurium), intermediate- (atracurium, vecuronium, rocuronium, cisatracurium), and long- (pancuronium, doxacurium, pipecuronium) acting drugs (**Table 12.12**). The onset of neuromuscular blockade is more rapid and less intense at the laryngeal muscles (vocal cords) than at the peripheral muscles. Further, the diaphragm is the muscle most resistant to paralysis; twice the dose is required to paralyze the diaphragm than is needed to paralyze the adductor pollicis muscle. Neuromuscular blocking agents are large, highly charged, water-soluble particles at physiologic pH. Thus, they are limited to the extracellular volume and cannot cross the BBB, placenta, or GI epithelium. Therefore, these drugs have no CNS or analgesic effects, cannot be given orally and, when given to pregnant women, do not affect the fetus.

The principal use of neuromuscular blocking agents in the ICU is to provide paralysis to facilitate tracheal intubation and to improve the conditions needed to mechanically ventilate patients or to keep patients immobile. The choice of drug is influenced by the speed of onset, duration of action, method of excretion (kidney, liver, or plasma), and the drug's side effect profile. The fastest paralytic agent is succinylcholine; it achieves

TABLE 12.11

ALTERNATIVE SEDATIVE AGENTS IN THE PICU

Drug	Dose (mg/kg)	Route	Interval (hrs)	Comments
Diphenhydramine	0.5–1	PO, IV, IM	4–6	Antihistamine; provides sedation and is antipruritic and antiemetic Adverse effects include dry mouth, tachycardia, and respiratory depression
Butorphanol	0.01–0.02	IV	4–6	Mixed opioid agonist/antagonist; risk of reversing analgesic effects of μ-agonist opioids
	0.05	PO		Weak analgesic with minimal respiratory depressive effects
Promethazine	0.5–1	IV, PO, PR, IM	6–8	Phenothiazine commonly used as an antiemetic Risk of causing extrapyramidal reactions and neuroleptic malignant syndrome
Haloperidol	0.01–0.02	IV, IM	8–12	Antipsychotic; can have dystonic reactions and neuroleptic malignant syndrome
	0.1–0.2	PO		Not for p.r.n. use
Chloral hydrate	50–100	PO, PR	24	Aliphatic alcohol, unknown mechanism of action Not to be used repetitively or in prolonged fashion Unpredictable onset and duration of sedative effects GI irritant No analgesic effects
Clonidine	0.002–0.005	PO	4–6	α_2 adrenergic agonist Possible hypotension Potentiates sedative/analgesic effects of other agents Available in transcutaneous patches of 0.1, 0.2, 0.3 mg, which are changed every 7 days

total paralysis in <1 min and has a very brief duration of action (3–5 mins). The only nondepolarizing agent that comes close to the onset of time of succinylcholine-induced paralysis is rocuronium. Rocuronium takes 1 to 2 mins to achieve paralysis, but its duration of action is significantly longer than that of succinylcholine (45–90 min). Regardless of the drug used to achieve paralysis, the degree of neuromuscular blockade is best evaluated by monitoring the evoked skeletal responses produced by an electrical stimulus delivered percutaneously to the ulnar or facial nerves by a peripheral nerve stimulator.

The only depolarizing agent in current use is succinylcholine. Succinylcholine mimics acetylcholine in its structure, binding to the acetylcholine receptor at the motor endplate in a noncompetitive fashion, resulting in depolarization, which is manifest in older children and adults by a phase of muscular fasciculation. Muscle fasciculations increase intragastric, intraocular, and intracranial pressure. They may also be associated with the development of the myalgias that are quite common after succinylcholine administration. Interestingly, children under the age of 4 years may not fasciculate. The disappearance of muscle fasciculation heralds the onset of a brief period of profound neuromuscular paralysis, as succinylcholine continues to occupy the receptor. Succinylcholine subsequently diffuses off the receptor and is metabolized by plasma and hepatic pseudocholinesterase. Newborn infants are relatively resistant to the effects of succinylcholine when dose requirements are compared with adults on a milligram-per-kilogram basis, probably due to their increased volume of distribution. In fact, the neonate requires approximately twice as

TABLE 12.12

COMPARATIVE PHARMACOLOGY OF NONDEPOLARIZING NEUROMUSCULAR BLOCKING DRUGS

Drug	ED95 (mg/kg)	Intubating dose (mg/kg)	Onset to maximum twitch depression (min)	Duration to return to 25% control twitch height (min)	Duration to return to train of four >0.9 (min)	Continuous infusion (mcg/kg/min)
Pancuronium	0.05	0.1	3–5	60–90	120–220	NA
Doxacurium	0.03	0.06	4–6		NA	NA
Vecuronium	0.05	0.1	3–5	20–35	50–80	1
Rocuronium	0.3	0.6–1.2	1–2	20–35	50–80	3–10
Cis-atracurium	0.05	0.1	3–5	20–35	60–90	0.4–4
Mivacurium	0.1	0.2–0.3	2–3	12–20	25–40	3–15

much succinylcholine (2 mg/kg) as does the adult (1 mg/kg) to facilitate tracheal intubation.

Redistribution and metabolism of succinylcholine determine the duration of its neuromuscular blockade. Despite a lower plasma concentration of pseudocholinesterase in infancy, the redistribution of succinylcholine from a relatively small muscle mass to a large extracellular fluid compartment quickly terminates the neuromuscular blocking effects. With prolonged or repeated exposure to succinylcholine, the membrane repolarizes but remains refractory to subsequent depolarization by acetylcholine. A so-called "phase II block" results, the clinical characteristics of which resemble a nondepolarizing block. The exact mechanism of this block has not been elucidated.

The neuromuscular blockade following succinylcholine can be prolonged if the patient has an abnormal, genetically derived variant of pseudocholinesterase. The diagnosis of this disorder relies on a clinical history of prolonged neuromuscular blockade following standard doses of succinylcholine and may be substantiated by assaying the plasma pseudocholinesterase inhibition by dibucaine. A positive family history is supportive evidence for the diagnosis. Management should consist of controlled ventilation with sedation until the block spontaneously dissipates. Although the administration of blood or plasma has been advocated for the treatment of this disorder, it cannot be recommended because of the inherent risks involved with this approach. Hepatic dysfunction, hypermagnesemia, and pregnancy are also associated with a prolonged block following succinylcholine administration.

Because a variety of side effects accompanies the administration of succinylcholine, including potentially lethal hyperkalemia, it is no longer recommended for routine use prior to intubation. Patients with muscular dystrophy, acute denervation injury that leads to skeletal muscle atrophy (e.g., spinal cord trauma), demyelinating diseases, and those with third-degree, unhealed burns are most at risk for life-threatening hyperkalemia (potassium concentrations >10 mEq/L). Interestingly, succinylcholine produces a rise in potassium (0.5 mEq/L), even in normal patients. Additional side effects of succinylcholine include severe bradycardia and other dysrhythmias; myalgia; myoglobinuria; increased gastric, intraocular, and intracranial pressure; and sustained skeletal muscle contractions, particularly of the masseter muscles. It is also a profound trigger of malignant hyperthermia in susceptible patients. Because of the risk of giving succinylcholine to males with undiagnosed muscular dystrophy, the FDA has issued a black-box warning concerning its use. Because of the myriad problems associated with this drug, many pediatric anesthesiologists no longer use it for routine (non–rapid-sequence) intubation.

Finally, succinylcholine stimulates all cholinergic autonomic receptors: nicotinic receptors of both sympathetic and parasympathetic ganglia and muscarinic receptors in the sinus node of the heart. This stimulation results in negative inotropic and chronotropic effects following an initial dose. In children, in whom the parasympathetic tone predominates, severe bradycardia and even sinus arrest may occur. The bradycardia occurs with greater frequency and severity following a second dose of succinylcholine in older children and adults. It *can* be effectively prevented by pretreatment with atropine (0.02 mg/kg, minimum dose 0.15 mg) or glycopyrrolate (0.01 mg/kg).

Nondepolarizing muscle relaxants competitively occupy the postsynaptic nicotinic acetylcholine receptor without causing a change in the configuration of the receptor. Occupancy of 65% of these receptors by nondepolarizing muscle relaxants does not produce any evidence of weakness or paralysis. Neuromuscular transmission falls when 80% of the receptors are occupied. Interestingly, when 95% of receptors are occupied, patients cannot swallow, cough, or protect their airways, but they can achieve normal tidal volumes and even vital capacity breaths. It is therefore wise to monitor weakness and recovery with blockade monitors. Prolonged use in the ICU may result in muscular weakness on recovery ("critical illness myopathy"). Choosing a nondepolarizing muscle relaxant is based on differences in onset time, duration of action, method of metabolism and excretion (kidney vs. liver vs. plasma), and cardiovascular side effect profile. Nondepolarizing muscle relaxants exert cardiovascular effects via blockade of cardiac muscarinic receptors (e.g., pancuronium produces tachycardia) and via histamine release (e.g., mivacurium produces mild hypotension).

Several drugs, events, and medical conditions unrelated to drug therapy may enhance the neuromuscular block produced by nondepolarizing muscle relaxants, including the concomitant use of aminoglycoside antibiotics, volatile anesthetic agents, high-dose furosemide, magnesium and lithium therapy, and cyclosporine. Hypercarbia and hypothermia potentiate the neuromuscular blockade produced by nondepolarizing muscle relaxants. The former is particularly pernicious; with muscle weakness, one breathes less, which produces hypercarbia, which in turn potentiates the paralysis, which weakens the diaphragm, and the circle continues. Finally, burn injuries and female gender are also associated with enhanced neuromuscular blockade.

Anticholinesterase Drugs— Reversal of Paralysis

Anticholinesterase drugs, such as neostigmine (0.07 mg/kg), edrophonium (0.5–1 mg/kg), and pyridostigmine (0.2 mg/kg), are often administered to antagonize the paralysis produced by nondepolarizing muscle relaxants. These drugs inhibit acetylcholinesterase, which is normally responsible for the rapid hydrolysis of acetylcholine into choline and acetic acid at the neuromuscular junction. The inhibition of acetylcholine hydrolysis by the esterase allows more acetylcholine to be available at the neuromuscular junction, thereby allowing return of muscle function. It also allows more acetylcholine to be available at muscarinic and nicotinic acetylcholine receptors, thereby producing bradycardia, salivation, miosis, and hyperperistalsis, as well as the desired return of neuromuscular function. Thus, whenever giving an anticholinesterase to reverse nondepolarizing muscle relaxants, one must always preadminister an anticholinergic such as atropine (0.02 mg/kg; minimum dose, 0.15 mg) or glycopyrrolate (0.01 mg/kg) to prevent adverse muscarinic effects such as bradycardia and hypersalivation.

The presence of residual neuromuscular blockade can be evaluated by using a peripheral nerve stimulator. The poles of the stimulator are placed over the peripheral nerve, usually the ulnar nerve at the wrist or elbow, and an impulse is applied. The twitch response of the adductor pollicis and flexor digitorum muscles to specific types of electrical stimulation gives clues to the presence or absence of blockade. The nondepolarizing neuromuscular blockade is characterized by (a) decreased contraction to a single impulse, (b) unsustained response to tetanic stimulation of 50 Hz at 2.5 sec; (c) diminution of the fourth-twitch response compared with the first-twitch response of >70% following four 2-Hz stimuli (train of four), (d) facilitation of the contractile response following tetanic stimulation, and (e) antagonism by acetylcholinesterase inhibitors. Abolition of the fourth-twitch response of the train of four correlates with a 75% reduction in standard-twitch tension. It must be remembered, however, that the magnitude and duration of the impulse influence the twitch response and that twitch response is not altered until >75% of the receptors are blocked. On the other hand, abolition of a single twitch on a train of four corresponds to 95% receptor blockade.

WEANING OF OPIOIDS/SEDATIVES

Dependence and Prevention of Withdrawal

Tolerance and *physical dependence* with repeated opioid and sedative administration is a common phenomenon in the PICU. The most studied and characteristic features are described in all μ-agonist opioids. *Tolerance* is the development of a need to increase the dose of an opioid or benzodiazepine agonist to achieve the same analgesic or sedative effect previously achieved with a lower dose. Tolerance to the analgesic effects of opioids usually develops following 10–21 days of morphine administration. However, patients rarely develop tolerance to the constipating effects of opioids. Additionally, cross-tolerance develops between all of the μ-opioid agonists. In that this cross-tolerance is rarely complete, opioid rotation—that is, changing from one opioid to another, can be helpful in preventing a continuous escalation in analgesic dosing. When it is necessary to switch—careful consideration must be given to the choice of opioid, dose, and degree of cross-tolerance. When switching opioids in tolerant patients, the equianalgesic dosing should be conservatively underestimated by a factor of 2.

Physical dependence, sometimes referred to as "neuroadaptation," is caused by repeated administration of an opioid, which necessitates the continued administration of the drug to prevent the appearance of a withdrawal or abstinence syndrome that is characteristic for that particular drug (47). It usually occurs after 2 to 3 weeks of morphine administration but may occur after only a few days of therapy. Very young infants treated with very high-dose fentanyl infusions following surgical repair of congenital heart disease and/or who require extracorporeal membrane oxygenation have been identified to be at particular risk.

Physical dependence must be differentiated from *addiction* (47). *Addiction* is a term used to connote a severe degree of drug abuse and dependence that is an extreme of behavior, in which drug use pervades the total life activity of the user and of the range of circumstances in which drug use controls the user's behavior. In a sense, addiction is a subset of physical dependence. Anyone who is addicted to an opioid is physically dependent; however, not everyone who is physically dependent is addicted. Patients appropriately treated with morphine and other opioid agonists for pain can become tolerant and physically dependent. They rarely, if ever, become psychologically dependent or addicted.

When physical dependence has been established, sudden discontinuation of an opioid or benzodiazepine agonist produces a *withdrawal* syndrome within 24 hrs of drug cessation. Symptoms reach their peak within 72 hrs and include abdominal cramps, vomiting, diarrhea, tachycardia, hypertension, diaphoresis, restlessness, insomnia, movement disorders, reversible neurologic abnormalities, and seizures.

Clinical and experimental data suggest that the duration of receptor occupancy is an important factor in the development of tolerance and dependence. Thus, continuous infusions may produce tolerance more rapidly than intermittent therapy (36), and this is particularly true for fentanyl. Tolerance and dependence *predictably* develop following only 5–10 days (2.5 mg/kg total fentanyl dose) of continuous fentanyl infusions, but may develop more rapidly in some patients. Nevertheless, prolonged therapy (>10 days), even by intermittent bolus administration, should be *expected* to produce opioid dependence.

Withdrawal Scales and Weaning Strategies

In the PICU, opioid and benzodiazepine withdrawal are common iatrogenic complications of the necessary analgesic and sedative strategies used to care for critically ill children. Just as the judicious monitoring and administration of these agents correlate with improved care, appropriate assessment tools to recognize and treat withdrawal symptoms must be utilized, as well as strategies developed to effectively wean those patients who are at risk for withdrawal symptoms.

Withdrawal/Abstinence Scales for Infants and Children in the PICU

In the NICU, withdrawal scores were originally developed to care for infants born to drug-addicted mothers. Neonatal, like adult, opioid withdrawal is a disorder characterized by generalized irritability, respiratory distress, GI distress, autonomic overactivity, and even seizures. Similar symptoms and degree of severity are seen in iatrogenic abstinence from opioids and are less well described but attributable to other sedatives/analgesics such as benzodiazepines.

The most widely used tool to assess neonatal abstinence is the Finnegan scale (**Table 12.13**). However, it has never been validated for use in evaluating infants and children outside the newborn period. Further, it has never been standardized for withdrawal symptoms characteristic of ex utero exposure. Although commonly used, the Finnegan scale involves a complicated assessment and has a high degree of inter-rater variability. The American Academy of Pediatrics (AAP) committee on drug usage reviewed this issue and published their recommendation in 1998 (3). Their consensus statement recommended that each institution adopt an abstinence scoring method to measure the severity of withdrawal. They felt that evidence indicated that abstinence scoring provided a consistent means of quantifying signs of psychomotor behavior and correlating them with severity of withdrawal to provide the best decision about the institution of pharmacologic therapy. Further, the study section suggested that the evidence for a combined approach would be more objective and would facilitate a quantitative strategy

TABLE 12.13

THE FINNEGAN NEONATAL ABSTINENCE SCORE

Sign/Symptoms	Score
Cry	
Excessive	2
Continuous	3
Sleep (# hours after feeding)	
<1 hr	3
<2 hrs	2
<3 hrs	1
Moro reflex	
Hyperactive	2
Markedly hyperactive	3
Tremors	
Mild	1
Moderate-severe	2
Moderate-severe when undisturbed	3
Increased tone	2
Frequent yawning	2
Sneezing	1
Nasal congestion	1
Nasal flaring	2
Respiratory rate	
>60 bpm	1
>60 bpm with retractions	2
Excoriation	1
Seizures	5
Sweating	1
Fever	
100–101°F	1
>101°F	2
Mottling	1
Excessive sucking	1
Poor feeding	2
Regurgitation	2
Projectile vomiting	3
Stooling	
Loose	2
Watery	3

Scores are interpreted as follows: 0–7, mild symptoms of withdrawal; 8–11, moderate withdrawal; 12–15, severe withdrawal.
bpm, breaths per minute.
Adapted from Finnegan LP. Neonatal Abstinence. In: Nelson NM, ed. *Current Therapy in Neonatal-Perinatal Medicine* Toronto, Ontario: BC Decker;1985:262–70.

toward increasing or decreasing dosing. Interestingly, they favored the Lipsitz scale (**Table 12.14**) over the more widely used Finnegan tool (39). The Lipsitz tool offers the advantage of being a relatively simple numeric system with a reported 77% sensitivity that uses a value >4 as an indication of significant signs of withdrawal. These properties contrast with the Finnegan scale, which uses a weighted scoring of 31 items and may be too complex for routine use on a busy clinical service.

When pharmacologic treatment is chosen, the AAP recommends that tincture of opium be the preferred drug for neonatal opiate withdrawal. For sedative-hypnotic withdrawal, phenobarbital is the agent of choice. Despite clear, evidence-based recommendations from the AAP, the management of the newborn with psychomotor behavior consistent with withdrawal varies widely. A survey of neonatal withdrawal treatment found inconsistent policies, scale utilization, and treatment regimens between institutions and individual physicians (54). These findings reflect similar findings of earlier studies and reemphasize the disparity between the published evidence/recommendations that support the use of withdrawal scoring and current clinical practice for neonatal withdrawal treatment.

As mentioned, neonatal assessment tools for withdrawal continue to be applied to infants and children beyond the newborn period, despite the lack of validation for use in this age range. Franck investigated the use of an adapted neonatal assessment tool in older children (24). This 21-item checklist was initially used for opioid weaning and modified for the evaluation of opioid and benzodiazepine withdrawal symptoms (24). Their small study demonstrated good inter-rater and content validity of the tool, as well as its applicability to a wide range of ages (6–28 months). This withdrawal scale, the opioid and benzodiazepine withdrawal score (OBWS), has the potential to guide the tapering of sedatives and analgesic agents inside and outside of the ICU across a wide range of ages.

Adult withdrawal assessment tools are often individual-based and involve personal reporting of symptoms by the patient. A clinician-administered tool (clinical opiate withdrawal scale, COWS) was developed to provide a simplified, 11-question score to assess withdrawal symptoms, and its application in iatrogenic and abuse-related opioid withdrawal scenarios was reviewed (70). Although simple and promising, its applicability to other agents (such as benzodiazepines) and to the pediatric age group is unknown.

Weaning Strategies in Infants and Children with Critical Illness

Tolerance and physical dependence are the consequences of the duration and quantity of opioid and sedative use in the ICU. As discussed earlier, tolerance will develop to some degree following opioid and benzodiazepine use of 3–5 days. When the risk for withdrawal symptoms is increased, the preference is to wean patients from their opioids and sedatives rather than abruptly stop therapy (73,74). This is a more appropriate clinical strategy than one designed to treat the symptoms of withdrawal and is akin to the therapeutic strategy used in weaning patients from other drugs (e.g., steroids), when abrupt cessation can be catastrophic. Unfortunately, abrupt withdrawal of opioids and sedatives to facilitate extubation and transfer of patients out of the PICU is common experience. If sedative/opioid usage has been short (i.e., <72 hrs), discontinuation is an option but may be inappropriate for some patients. However, our practice for infusions or frequent administration of an agent for >5 days is to develop an agent-specific weaning strategy. Shorter intervals of exposure facilitate more aggressive weaning strategies, whereas durations of exposure >10 days require a more cautious weaning strategy (**Tables 12.15 and 12.16**).

To simplify the weaning process, we make every effort to convert the patient from IV to oral therapy and from continuous infusions to intermittent bolus therapy (73,74). This strategy makes the care of the patient significantly easier, and allows for the final tapering and weaning to be accomplished in an outpatient setting. In most cases, the same opioid can be used in weaning that was used therapeutically. For practical reasons, however, it may be necessary to change from one opioid to another because of ease of administration, duration of action, and ability to taper the dose.

TABLE 12.14

LIPSITZ ABSTINENCE WITHDRAWAL SCALE

Signs	Score			
	0	1	2	3
Tremors (muscle activity of limbs)	Normal	Minimally increased when hungry or disturbed	Moderate or marked increase when undisturbed; subside when fed or held snugly	Marked increase or continuous, even when undisturbed; going onto seizure-like movements
Irritability (excessive crying)	None	Slightly increased	Moderate to severe when disturbed or hungry	Marked even when undisturbed
Reflexes	Normal	Increased	Markedly increased	—
Stool	Normal	Explosive, but normal frequency	Explosive, >8 days	—
Muscle tone	Normal	Increased	Rigidity	—
Skin abrasions	No	Redness of knees and elbows	Breaking of the skin	—
Respiratory rate/min	<55	55–75	76–95	—
Repetitive sneezing	No	Yes	—	—
Repetitive yawning	No	Yes	—	—
Vomiting	No	Yes	—	—
Fever	No	Yes	—	—

Scores are interpreted as follows: 0, no withdrawal symptoms; 1–2, mild withdrawal; 2–3, moderate withdrawal; >4, severe withdrawal.
Adapted from Lipsitz PJ. A proposed narcotic withdrawal score for use with newborn infants. A pragmatic evaluation of its efficacy. *Clin Pediatr* 1975;14:592–4.

On changing from one opioid to another, equianalgesic dosing is mandatory. Additionally, to avoid over- or underdosing when converting from one drug to another, conservative action and titration of the dosage downward to achieve the desired clinical effect are recommended. Furthermore, the calculated conversion should be given for 24–48 hrs before any attempt at weaning is made. Once this is accomplished, the drugs should be administered on a 6-hr (morphine) or 12-hr (methadone), around-the-clock basis, and weaning is begun. The patient's drug regimen is decreased by 10%–20% of the original total opioid dose per day. When the lowest doses are reached, usually in 5–7 days, the interval of drug dosing is increased from

TABLE 12.15

OPIOID AND BENZODIAZEPINE TAPERING GUIDELINES

If opioids or benzodiazepines have been in use for 3–5 days, consider the following:
1. Initiate withdrawal assessment tool every 4–6 hrs and continue for 1–2 days after cessation of all opioids/sedatives.
2. Reduce opioid/benzodiazepine administration by 20% of pre-taper dose every day.
3. If withdrawal symptoms develop, stop weaning for 24 hrs.
4. If withdrawal symptoms/scores do not improve or worsen:
   a. Increase opioid/benzodiazepine to previous dose.
   b. Consider adding clonidine, especially if symptoms do not improve.
   c. Consult pain service.

If opioids or benzodiazepines in use >10 days, consider the following options:
1. Follow above guidelines.
2. Reduce opioid/benzodiazepine slowly. Perform a reduction of 10% of pretapered dose every day. If patient is on multiple agents, alternate between agents for reduction, effectively reducing each agent every other day.
3. If withdrawal symptoms develop, stop weaning for 24 hrs.
4. If withdrawal symptoms/scores do not improve or worsen:
   a. Increase last agent weaned to previous dose.
   b. Add or increase clonidine.
   c. Consult pain service.

Adapted from Franck LS, Naughton I, Winter I. Opioid and benzodiazepine withdrawal symptoms in paediatric intensive care patients. *Intensive Crit Care Nurs* 2004; 20:344–51.

TABLE 12.16

CONVERSION STRATEGIES FOR WEANING FROM COMMONLY USED SEDATIVES AND ANALGESICS

Benzodiazepines (IV midazolam to oral lorazepam):
1. Calculate the total daily dose being provided to the patient by infusion and any additional daily "as-needed doses" of midazolam.
2. Calculate the total midazolam dose (in milligrams) and divide by 8. Result will be the milligrams of lorazepam to be given orally per day. This lorazepam amount should be divided and dosed every 4–6 hrs.
3. After the second oral lorazepam dose, reduce the midazolam infusion by 50%.
4. After the third oral lorazepam dose, reduce the midazolam infusion by 50%.
5. After the fourth lorazepam dose, discontinue IV midazolam.

Opioid (IV fentanyl to oral methadone):
1. Calculate the total daily dose being provided to the patient by infusion and any additional daily "as-needed doses" of fentanyl.
2. Calculate the total fentanyl dose (in milligrams). Because of the off-setting effects of bioavailability, potency, and half-life, an equivalent oral methadone dose can be administered. Divide this methadone dose every 12 hrs.
3. After the second oral methadone dose, reduce the fentanyl infusion by 50%.
4. After the third oral methadone dose, reduce the fentanyl infusion by 50%.
5. After the fourth oral methadone dose, discontinue IV fentanyl.
6. Over next 24 hrs, rescue doses of morphine (0.05 mg/kg IV or oral) are provided for withdrawal symptoms. The total morphine dose administered is calculated and added to the total daily methadone dose. This new total daily methadone dose is divided and dosed every 12 hrs for the next day.
7. Repeat step 6 until a stable methadone dose is achieved.

Barbiturate (IV pentobarbital to oral phenobarbital):
1. Stop the pentobarbital infusion and convert to IV phenobarbital as follows:

Pentobarbital Infusion (mg/kg/hr)	Phenobarbital loading dose (mg/kg)
1–2	8
2–3	15
3–4	20

2. Six hours later, administer half of the loading dose of phenobarbital IV over 1 hr.
3. Six hours later, infuse second half of phenobarbital loading dose over 1 hr.
4. Six hours later, administer first maintenance phenobarbital dose (1/3 of initial loading dose) IV and repeat every 12 hrs.
5. If evidence of withdrawal is observed during this conversion, provide additional maintenance dose of phenobarbital IV and continue IV dosing every 12 hrs.
6. After a 24-hr period of maintenance IV phenobarbital, with minimal or no withdrawal symptoms, and no additional doses of phenobarbital, change to oral phenobarbital at same 12-hr interval.
7. Maintenance oral phenobarbital dosing is then weaned 10%–20% every week from the preweaning dosage.

Adapted from Tobias JD. Tolerance, withdrawal, and physical dependency after long-term sedation and analgesia of children in the pediatric intensive care unit. *Crit Care Med* 2000;28:2122–32.

every 6, 8, or 12 hrs, to once per day. Therapy is then stopped completely. We believe that this schedule should be strictly adhered to. If symptoms of withdrawal develop, they are treated with clonidine 2–4 mcg/kg every 4–6 hrs on an as-needed basis. The α_2 adrenergic agents prevent or mitigate the occurrence of drug withdrawal syndrome symptomatology regardless of the drug that is causing addiction or dependence. We have used clonidine in treating infants born to drug-addicted mothers and in patients who have become opioid dependent secondary to pain and sedation therapy. Additionally, the literature contains anecdotal case reports of using dexmedetomidine to prevent withdrawal symptoms in patients who are dependent on opioids and sedatives (22,46), which we suspect will become an important new tool in the future.

CONCLUSIONS AND FUTURE DIRECTIONS

We have attempted to consolidate in a comprehensive manner much of the available information on pain management in crit-

ically ill children. All children, even the newborn and critically ill, require analgesia for pain and for painful procedures. Unrelieved pain interferes with sleep, leads to fatigue and a sense of helplessness, and may result in increased morbidity and/or mortality. Sedation practices in critically ill patients have been shown to alter the duration of mechanical ventilation and affect care in adult patients. Future research that evaluates sedation practices in children who are critically ill and in those who require sedation will advance the development and implementation of new tools and new sedative agents. The driving force and ultimate goal of pain and sedation treatment must be to improve the quality of life for these children. Leaving these issues unaddressed will undermine part of our fundamental humanity and our roles as healers and physicians.

KEY POINTS

- The treatment and alleviation of pain is a basic human right for everyone, regardless of age.
- Pain is a subjective experience; pain and sedation assessment and management are interdependent, and one is

- essentially useless without the other. The most commonly used assessment instrument in the PICU is the COMFORT scale.
- Very few studies have evaluated the pharmacokinetic and pharmacodynamic properties of analgesic and sedative drugs in critically ill patients. Most of the recommendations in this chapter are based on experience and best practice, rather than on evidence-based medicine.
- Sedatives and analgesics are given by titration to effect. Many PICU patients require enormous doses of analgesics and sedatives, doses so high, that to an outsider they seem preposterous if not dangerous.
- The most commonly used nonopioid analgesic in pediatric practice remains acetaminophen (paracetamol). Regardless of route of delivery, the daily maximum acetaminophen doses in the preterm, term, and older child ares 60, 80, and 90 mg/kg, respectively.
- Opioids bind to G-protein-coupled receptors and regulate transmembrane signaling by regulating adenylate cyclase (cyclic AMP), various ion (K, Ca, Na) channels and transport proteins, and phospholipases C and A_2.
- The opioids most commonly used in the management of pain are μ agonists. These include morphine, meperidine, methadone, codeine, oxycodone, and the fentanyls. At equianalgesic doses, the pharmacodynamic effects of all of the μ-opioid agonists are similar and include analgesia, respiratory depression, sedation, nausea and vomiting, pruritus, constipation, miosis, tolerance, and physical dependence.
- Fentanyl is 50 to 100 times more potent than morphine and has become the most commonly used analgesic for procedures and pain control in the PICU. It is short-acting following single doses (redistribution) but long-acting ("context-sensitive half-life") following infusions.
- Methadone can be used to treat pain very effectively and to wean patients who have become physically dependent on opioids following prolonged analgesic therapy.
- Procedure-related pain is that which is inflicted on patients in the course of their medical or surgical treatment and is best treated with local anesthetics; drugs that reversibly block conduction of neural impulses along central and peripheral nerve pathways.
- The systemic toxic effects of local anesthetics are determined by the total dose of drug administered, protein binding, the rapidity of absorption into the blood, and the site of injection. Bupivacaine toxicity is the most feared.
- Deposition of local anesthetics, opioids, α_2 agonists (clonidine), midazolam, steroids, and/or ketamine into the epidural space via indwelling catheters can be used for postoperative and traumatic pain.
- Anxiety, fear, a sense of helplessness, and lack of sleep will potentiate pain and, if left untreated, can lead to psychosis in critically ill patients.
- Procedural sedation exists across a continuum, varying from a state of wakefulness, to anxiolysis, to moderate sedation ("conscious sedation"), to deep sedation, to general anesthesia.
- Most sedatives, such as the benzodiazepines, chloral hydrate, and the barbiturates, and all neuromuscular blocking agents, have no analgesic properties and may actually exacerbate pain.

- The benzodiazepines are extremely potent amnestics, anticonvulsants, sedatives, hypnotics, and skeletal muscle relaxants, are effective whether given parenterally or enterally, and produce dose-dependent depression of breathing.
- Benzodiazepine-withdrawal symptoms are similar to withdrawal from alcohol (delirium tremens).
- Unexpected fatal lactic acidosis in critically ill children who are sedated for prolonged periods with propofol (propofol infusion syndrome) precludes prolonged (>6 hrs) use in the PICU.
- The use of inhalational anesthetic agents (N_2O, isoflurane) in the PICU is limited by institutional and nursing credentialing, availability of specialized delivery and monitoring equipment, and the ability to scavenge exhaled gas.
- α_2 Agonists, particularly dexmedetomidine, are a new tool in the sedation of ventilated and nonventilated patients in the PICU.
- Neuromuscular blocking agents have no analgesic or sedative properties and must never be given until adequate sedation and amnesia have been achieved. They are not substitutes for pain control.
- Succinylcholine is no longer recommended for routine use in children. It is still available for emergency use during a rapid-sequence induction.
- When physical dependence has been established, sudden discontinuation of an opioid or benzodiazepine agonist produces a withdrawal syndrome within 24 to 72 hrs of drug cessation. A simplified, clinician-administered tool (clinical opiate withdrawal scale, COWS) is recommended to assess withdrawal symptoms and guide therapy.

References

1. American Academy of Pediatrics. Committee on Drugs. Guidelines for monitoring and management of pediatric patients during and after sedation for diagnostic and therapeutic procedures. *Pediatrics* 1992;89:1110–5.
2. American Society of Anesthesiologists Task Force on Sedation and Analgesia by Non-Anesthesiologists. Practice guidelines for sedation and analgesia by non-anesthesiologists. *Anesthesiology* 1996;84:459–71.
3. American Academy of Pediatrics. Committee on Drugs. Neonatal drug withdrawal. *Pediatrics* 1998;101:1079–88.
4. Abdi S, Lee DH, Chung JM. The anti-allodynic effects of amitriptyline, gabapentin, and lidocaine in a rat model of neuropathic pain. *Anesth Analg* 1998;87:1360–6.
5. Ambuel B, Hamlett KW, Marx CM, et al. Assessing distress in pediatric intensive care environments: The COMFORT scale. *J Pediatr Psychol* 1992;17:95–109.
6. Aram L, Krane EJ, Kozloski LJ, et al. Tunneled epidural catheters for prolonged analgesia in pediatric patients. *Anesth Analg* 2001;92:1432–8.
7. Arnold JH, Truog RD, Rice SA. Prolonged administration of isoflurane to pediatric patients during mechanical ventilation. *Anesth Analg* 1993;76:520–6.
8. Bear LA, Ward-Smith P. Interrater reliability of the COMFORT Scale. *Pediatr Nurs* 2006;32:427–34.
9. Berde CB, Sethna NF. Analgesics for the treatment of pain in children. *N Engl J Med* 2002;347:1094–103.
10. Birmingham PK, Tobin MJ, Henthorn TK, et al. Twenty-four-hour pharmacokinetics of rectal acetaminophen in children: an old drug with new recommendations. *Anesthesiology* 1997;87:244–52.
11. Booker PD, Beechey A, Lloyd-Thomas AR. Sedation of children requiring artificial ventilation using an infusion of midazolam. *Br J Anaesth* 1986;58:1104–8.
12. Bosenberg AT, Bland BA, Schulte-Steinberg O, et al. Thoracic epidural anesthesia via caudal route in infants. *Anesthesiology* 1988;69:265–9.
13. Bray RJ. Propofol infusion syndrome in children. *Paediatr Anaesth* 1998;8:491–9.
14. Caraco Y, Sheller J, Wood AJ. Impact of ethnic origin and quinidine coadministration on codeine's disposition and pharmacodynamic effects. *J Pharmacol Exp Ther* 1999;290:413–22.
15. Courtman SP, Wardurgh A, Petros AJ. Comparison of the bispectral index

monitor with the Comfort score in assessing level of sedation of critically ill children. *Intensive Care Med* 2003;29:2239–46.

16. Crain SM, Shen KF. Modulation of opioid analgesia, tolerance and dependence by Gs- coupled, GM1 ganglioside-regulated opioid receptor functions. *Trends Pharmacol Sci* 1998;19:358–65.

17. Cray SH, Robinson BH, Cox PN. Lactic acidemia and bradyarrhythmia in a child sedated with propofol. *Crit Care Med* 1998;26:2087–92.

18. Curley MA, Harris SK, Fraser KA, et al. State Behavioral Scale: A sedation assessment instrument for infants and young children supported on mechanical ventilation. *Pediatr Crit Care Med* 2006;7:107–14.

19. Dahners LE, Mullis BH. Effects of nonsteroidal anti-inflammatory drugs on bone formation and soft-tissue healing. *J Am Acad Orthop Surg* 2004;12:139–43.

20. Davies G, Kingswood C, Street M. Pharmacokinetics of opioids in renal dysfunction. *Clin Pharmacokinet* 1996;31:410–22.

21. Dominguez KD, Crowley MR, Coleman DM, et al. Withdrawal from lorazepam in critically ill children. *Ann Pharmacother* 2006;40:1035–9.

22. Finkel JC, Elrefai A. The use of dexmedetomidine to facilitate opioid and benzodiazepine detoxification in an infant. *Anesth Analg* 2004;98:1658–9.

23. Franck LS, Miaskowski C. Measurement of neonatal responses to painful stimuli: A research review. *J Pain Symptom Manage* 1997;14:343–78.

24. Franck LS, Naughton I, Winter I. Opioid and benzodiazepine withdrawal symptoms in paediatric intensive care patients. *Intensive Crit Care Nurs* 2004;20:344–51.

25. Galer BS, Harle J, Rowbotham MC. Response to intravenous lidocaine infusion predicts subsequent response to oral mexiletine: A prospective study. *J Pain Symptom Manage* 1996;12:161–7.

26. Glass PS, Gan TJ, Howell S. A review of the pharmacokinetics and pharmacodynamics of remifentanil. *Anesth Analg* 1999;89:S7–14.

27. Greeley WJ, de Bruijn NP. Changes in sufentanil pharmacokinetics within the neonatal period. *Anesth Analg* 1988;67:86–90.

28. Habre W, Bergesio R, Johnson C, et al. Pharmacokinetics of ropivacaine following caudal analgesia in children. *Paediatr Anaesth* 2000;10:143–7.

29. Hakkola J, Tanaka E, Pelkonen O. Developmental expression of cytochrome P450 enzymes in human liver. *Pharmacol Toxicol* 1998;82:209–17.

30. Hartvig P, Larsson E, Joachimsson PO. Postoperative analgesia and sedation following pediatric cardiac surgery using a constant infusion of ketamine. *J Cardiothorac Vasc Anesth* 1993;7:148–53.

31. Hartwig S, Roth B, Theisohn M. Clinical experience with continuous intravenous sedation using midazolam and fentanyl in the paediatric intensive care unit. *Eur J Pediatr* 1991;150:784–8.

32. Hughes MA, Glass PS, Jacobs JR. Context-sensitive half-time in multicompartment pharmacokinetic models for intravenous anesthetic drugs. *Anesthesiology* 1992;76:334–41.

33. Hurley RJ, Feldman HS, Latka C, et al. The effects of epinephrine on the anesthetic and hemodynamic properties of ropivacaine and bupivacaine after epidural administration in the dog. *Reg Anesth* 1991;16:303–8.

34. Ista E, van Dijk M, Tibboel D, et al. Assessment of sedation levels in pediatric intensive care patients can be improved by using the COMFORT "behavior" scale. *Pediatr Crit Care Med* 2005;6:58–63.

35. Johnsen SP, Larsson H, Tarone RE, et al. Risk of hospitalization for myocardial infarction among users of rofecoxib, celecoxib, and other NSAIDs: A population-based case-control study. *Arch Intern Med* 2005;165:978–84.

36. Katz R, Kelly HW, Hsi A. Prospective study on the occurrence of withdrawal in critically ill children who receive fentanyl by continuous infusion. *Crit Care Med* 1994;22:763–7.

37. Krechel SW, Bildner J. CRIES: A new neonatal postoperative pain measurement score. Initial testing of validity and reliability. *Paediatric Anaesthesia* 1995;5:53–61.

38. Lee SJ, Ralston HJ, Drey EA, et al. Fetal pain: A systematic multidisciplinary review of the evidence. *JAMA* 2005;294:947–54.

39. Lipsitz PJ. A proposed narcotic withdrawal score for use with newborn infants. A pragmatic evaluation of its efficacy. *Clin Pediatr* 1975;14:592–4.

40. Lugo RA, Chester EA, Cash J, et al. A cost analysis of enterally administered lorazepam in the pediatric intensive care unit. *Crit Care Med* 1999;27:417–21.

41. Malviya S, Voepel-Lewis T, Tait AR, et al. Depth of sedation in children undergoing computed tomography: Validity and reliability of the University of Michigan Sedation Scale (UMSS). *Br J Anaesth* 2002;88:241–5.

42. Mason KP, Zgleszewski SE, Dearden JL, et al. Dexmedetomidine for pediatric sedation for computed tomography imaging studies. *Anesth Analg* 2006;103:57–62.

43. Maxwell LG, Kaufmann SC, Bitzer S, et al. The effects of a small-dose naloxone infusion on opioid-induced side effects and analgesia in children and adolescents treated with intravenous patient-controlled analgesia: A double-blind, prospective, randomized, controlled study. *Anesth Analg* 2005;100:953–8.

44. Merskey H, Albe-Fessard DG, Bonica JJ. Pain terms: A list with definitions and notes on usage. Recommended by the IASP Subcommittee on Taxonomy. *Pain* 1979;6:249–52.

45. Monitto CL, Greenberg RS, Kost-Byerly S, et al. The safety and efficacy of parent-/nurse-controlled analgesia in patients less than six years of age. *Anesth Analg* 2000;91:573–9.

46. Multz AS. Prolonged dexmedetomidine infusion as an adjunct in treating sedation-induced withdrawal. *Anesth Analg* 2003;96:1054–1055.

47. O'Brien CP. Drug Addiction and Drug Abuse. In: Hardman JG, Limbird LE, eds. *Goodman and Gilman's the Pharmacological Basis of Therapeutics.* New York: McGraw-Hill; 1996:557–578.

48. Park GR. Molecular mechanisms of drug metabolism in the critically ill. *Br J Anaesth* 1996;77:32–49.

49. Pees C, Haas NA, Ewert P, et al. Comparison of analgesic/sedative effect of racemic ketamine and S(+)-ketamine during cardiac catheterization in newborns and children. *Pediatr Cardiol* 2003;24:424–9.

50. Ramsay MA. Measuring level of sedation in the intensive care unit. *JAMA* 2000;284:441–2.

51. Raynor K, Kong H, Chen Y, et al. Pharmacological characterization of the cloned kappa-, delta-, and mu-opioid receptors. *Mol Pharmacol* 1994;45:330–4.

52. Sabbe MB, Yaksh TL. Pharmacology of spinal opioids. *J Pain Symptom Manage* 1990;5:191–203.

53. Santeiro ML, Christie J, Stromquist C, et al. Pharmacokinetics of continuous infusion fentanyl in newborns. *J Perinatol* 1997;17:135–9.

54. Sarkar S, Donn SM. Management of neonatal abstinence syndrome in neonatal intensive care units: A national survey. *J Perinatol* 2006;26:15–7.

55. Schechter NL, Berde CB, Yaster M. *Pain in Infants, Children, and Adolescents.* Baltimore: Williams and Wilkins, 1993.

56. Schuttler J, Ihmsen H. Population pharmacokinetics of propofol: A multicenter study. *Anesthesiology* 2000;92:727–38.

57. Shannon M, Berde CB. Pharmacologic management of pain in children and adolescents. *Pediatr Clin North Am* 1989;36:855–71.

58. Silvasi DL, Rosen DA, Rosen KR. Continuous intravenous midazolam infusion for sedation in the pediatric intensive care unit. *Anesth Analg* 1988;67:286–8.

59. Simmons LE, Riker RR, Prato BS, et al. Assessing sedation during intensive care unit mechanical ventilation with the Bispectral Index and the Sedation-Agitation Scale. *Crit Care Med* 1999;27:1499–504.

60. Smith I, White PF, Nathanson M, et al. Propofol. An update on its clinical use. *Anesthesiology* 1994;81:1005–43.

61. Spagrud LJ, Piira T, von Baeyer CL. Children's self-report of pain intensity. *Am J Nurs* 2003;103:62–4.

62. Strichartz GR. Neural Physiology and Local Anesthetic Action. In: Cousins MJ, Bridenbaugh PO. *Neural Blockade in Clinical Anesthesia and Management of Pain.* Philadelphia: Lippincott-Raven; 1998:35–54.

63. Suresh S, Anand KJ. Opioid tolerance in neonates: Mechanisms, diagnosis, assessment, and management. *Semin Perinatol* 1998;22:425–33.

64. Susla GM. Propofol toxicity in critically ill pediatric patients: Show us the proof. *Crit Care Med* 1998;26:1959–60.

65. Taddio A, Katz J, Ilersich AL, et al. Effect of neonatal circumcision on pain response during subsequent routine vaccination. *Lancet* 1997;349:599–603.

66. Tegeder I, Lotsch J, Geisslinger G. Pharmacokinetics of opioids in liver disease. *Clin Pharmacokinet* 1999;37:17–40.

67. Tobias JD. Tolerance, withdrawal, and physical dependency after long-term sedation and analgesia of children in the pediatric intensive care unit. *Crit Care Med* 2000;28:2122–32.

68. Tobias JD. Monitoring the depth of sedation in the pediatric ICU patient: Where are we, or more importantly, where are our patients? *Pediatr Crit Care Med* 2005;6:715–8.

69. Weinberg GL, Ripper R, Murphy P, et al. Lipid infusion accelerates removal of bupivacaine and recovery from bupivacaine toxicity in the isolated rat heart. *Reg Anesth Pain Med* 2006;31:296–303.

70. Wesson DR, Ling W. The clinical opiate withdrawal scale (COWS). *J Psychoactive Drugs* 2003;35:253–9.

71. White PF, Way WL, Trevor AJ. Ketamine—its pharmacology and therapeutic uses. *Anesthesiology* 1982;56:119–36.

72. Wilder RT. Local anesthetics for the pediatric patient. *Pediatr Clin North Am* 2000;47:545–58.

73. Yaster M, Kost-Byerly S, Berde C, et al. The management of opioid and benzodiazepine dependence in infants, children, and adolescents. *Pediatrics* 1996;98:135–40.

74. Yaster M, Krane EJ, Kaplan RF, et al. *Pediatric Pain Management and Sedation Handbook.* St. Louis: Mosby Year Book, Inc., 1997.

75. Yaster M, Nichols DG, Deshpande JK, Wetzel RC. Midazolam-fentanyl intravenous sedation in children: Case report of respiratory arrest. *Pediatrics* 1990;86:463–7.

CHAPTER 13 ■ REHABILITATION OF CHILDREN WITH CRITICAL ILLNESS

MELISSA K. TROVATO • FRANK S. PIDCOCK • CRISTINA L. SADOWSKY • EWA B. BRANDYS •
STACY J. SUSKAUER • CYNTHIA F. SALORIO • JAMES R. CHRISTENSEN

The rehabilitation needs of a child with critical illness may not be apparent or may be difficult to prioritize while a child is receiving intensive care. As medical care advances, children are increasingly surviving severe injuries and illnesses. The survival of critical injury or illness may be associated with acquired disability of either a transient or permanent nature. Following the onset of disability, rehabilitation services help to maximize the function of a child in his home, school, and community.

This chapter focuses on those principles of rehabilitation of interest to healthcare providers in a PICU and provides general recommendations for the prevention of secondary impairments due to bed rest and immobility. Topics discussed include (a) basic concepts of rehabilitation, (b) the importance of early rehabilitation, (c) prevention and treatment of clinical complications, and (d) the rehabilitation treatment and management of specific illnesses.

BASIC CONCEPTS OF REHABILITATION

Rehabilitation is the process of maximizing function and independence in an individual with a disability. The World Health Organization's International Classification of Functioning, Disability, and Health (ICF) provides structure for discussing the sequelae of disease based on an individual's function at the levels of impairment, activity, and participation (53). *Impairment* is defined as a disturbance at the organ level (e.g., muscle weakness or contracture); limitation in *activity* is a disturbance at the person level (e.g., the inability to walk), and limitation in *participation* (e.g., a wheelchair user's inability to attend a school in a nonaccessible building) involves how an individual interacts with her community and society. Rehabilitation professionals evaluate an individual's function at the impairment, activity, and participation levels and subsequently design a program of care to maximize the child's participation at home, at school, and in the community.

Rehabilitation in the PICU

During the course of critical illness, the rehabilitation team should be considered an important contributor to a child's care. Consultation with the rehabilitation team early during a hospitalization allows for monitoring for secondary impairments while maximizing preventative efforts, ensures the appropriate advancement of rehabilitation treatments as soon as the child is medically ready, and facilitates discharge planning.

The rehabilitation team is led by a physiatrist, who is a physician specializing in physical medicine and rehabilitation. The physiatrist has been trained in a broad range of medical and functional problems that are associated with illness and injury. Training includes a minimum of 4 years of a postdoctoral residency, comprised of 1 year of internship and 3 years of specialty training. A pediatric physiatrist may have also completed a pediatric residency and/or pediatric rehabilitation fellowship. Additional physiatric subspecialty fellowship training is available in musculoskeletal care, traumatic brain injury, spinal cord injury, and pain management.

While a child is in the PICU, the physiatrist serves as a link between the rehabilitation and PICU teams; the physiatrist's role includes monitoring the child's medical status and initiating appropriate rehabilitation services when appropriate, as well as coordinating the rehabilitative care program. The rehabilitation team may be comprised of physical therapists, occupational therapists, speech and language pathologists, as well as psychologists and therapeutic recreation specialists, depending on the institution. Ideally, the rehabilitation and PICU teams work together to prevent complications of bed rest, such as contractures, so that when a child is ready for more aggressive rehabilitation services, secondary impairments that might impede functional progress have been limited or prevented.

PALLIATIVE CARE AND REHABILITATION

Rehabilitation and palliative care are not mutually exclusive. Palliative care "seeks to prevent or relieve the physical and emotional distress produced by a life-threatening medical condition or its treatment, to help patients with such conditions and their families live as normally as possible" (21). The American Academy of Pediatrics supports offering the components of palliative care at the time of diagnosis and continuing throughout the course of illness, regardless of whether the outcome ends in cure or death (1). Conditions appropriate for pediatric palliative care are those for which symptom control and maintenance of function are central aspects of the treatment plan and include (a) conditions for which curative treatment is possible but may fail; (b) conditions that require intensive, long-term treatment aimed at maintaining quality of life; (c) progressive conditions in which treatment is exclusively palliative after diagnosis; and (d) conditions that involve severe, nonprogressive disability and cause extreme vulnerability to health complications (5). Thus, palliative care is not limited to those children who are thought to be in the active process of dying, and it can be provided concurrently with curative and life-prolonging interventions. Depending on the child's primary diagnosis, comorbidities, family circumstances, values, and resources, the pathway of care, or the "mix of curative or life-prolonging care and palliative care" services, will vary (21).

Although much attention has been directed to pain and symptom management in children receiving palliative care, less awareness has been directed toward preservation and recovery of function for this population, in part because of the previously held notion that palliative care was reserved for those actively dying. With the increased focus on delivering palliative care services to an expanded group of children, attention should be directed not only to symptom management but also toward maintaining function and age-appropriate independence. Interventions by the physical medicine and rehabilitation team play a critical role in accomplishing these goals.

Rehabilitation is a symptom-oriented process in which a multidisciplinary team works together to creatively empower the child and family to improve quality of life by maintaining and enhancing functional skills. Although rehabilitation may result in functional benefit at any point in the child's illness trajectory, the child and family benefit most when rehabilitative efforts are introduced once the acute medical issues have been stabilized and the child tolerates positioning and handling. A consult may be obtained prior to this point for assistance with prognosis and discussion with the family, as needed. Delivery of services may occur in the acute/PICU setting, rehabilitation setting, home, outpatient, or school settings. The specific goals of rehabilitation will vary depending on the wishes of child and family, the child's clinical status, treatment plan, resources, and values. Common goals of rehabilitation include minimizing the effects of motor deficits, sensory deficits, cerebellar dysfunction, cranial nerve deficits, oral motor deficits, cognitive dysfunction, and deconditioning (12). Ideally, for children who receive palliative care services, rehabilitation would focus on preserving and maximizing skills to prevent or slow the progression of disability. As the child's disease progresses, rehabilitative efforts build on previously learned strategies to mitigate symptoms of weakness and fatigue by making environmental modifications and introducing compensatory measures and assistive devices so that the child can maintain independence as long as possible. Rehabilitation strategies also focus on family and caregiver education—teaching strategies that will ease the burden of care. Thus, palliative care services and rehabilitation services aim to "add life to the child's years, not simply years to the child's life" (1).

REHABILITATION CONTINUUM OF CARE

Critical care physicians must advocate for optimal rehabilitation services for their patients; to do this, they must understand the key elements that comprise a model pediatric rehabilitation system. These elements are discussed below.

The ideal characteristics of a rehabilitation system include (a) adjacency to an acute medical center (enabling close cooperation between the acute care and rehabilitation teams); (b) continuity of rehabilitation care throughout the acute and rehabilitation hospitalizations; (c) a full complement of rehabilitation professionals and services available to meet the needs

of the patients, working together as a coordinated, interdisciplinary team with common goals; (d) specialized expertise for specialized problems (such as cognitive and behavioral rehabilitation for patients with brain injury or intense motor therapy for patients with spinal cord injury); (e) early transfers to the rehabilitation setting, where certain problems (e.g., the agitated patient with posttraumatic brain injury) are better managed by an experienced interdisciplinary team; (f) a continuum of services flexibly provided in a range of environments to best meet the individual needs of the children and their families; and (g) resources to facilitate and optimize community/school reintegration (10).

Related to the principle that specialized populations require specialized programs, children and adolescents are best served by specialized pediatric rehabilitation programs, thereby ensuring the provision of essential components of care, including (a) expertise in the rehabilitation of children, taking into account the growth and development of the child; (b) developmentally appropriate treatments and environment; (c) a family-centered approach; and (d) attention to the education of the child as well as the reintegration of that child into the educational system. Concerning accreditation of rehabilitation programs, the Commission on Accreditation of Rehabilitation Facilities has clinically relevant accreditation guidelines that help ensure that a program meets standards specific for pediatric rehabilitation, as well as for subspecialty programs, such as for brain injury.

An essential component of a pediatric rehabilitation program is the family-centered approach, which recognizes the child and the family as the most important and unchanging members of the rehabilitation, medical, and educational teams. Family-centered programs appreciate that the family can ultimately be the most effective case manager. As such, the family is actively involved in defining the rehabilitation goals for the child. It is also important that family members learn self-advocacy skills.

Ideally, a rehabilitation system should provide a continuum of services, allowing the appropriate intensity and type of rehabilitation to be delivered in the most efficacious and least restrictive setting. In that the goal of rehabilitation is to improve function (cognitive, behavioral, motor, social, etc.) and, in some conditions (such as traumatic brain injury), function does not generalize well from one setting to another, it is often most efficacious for patients to learn new skills and strategies in the actual environment in which they will need to perform. Consequently, although an acute inpatient rehabilitation program that can provide constant medical and nursing care and intense rehabilitation may be the best place for the initial rehabilitation, an alternate setting might be the best way to complete the rehabilitation. The rehabilitation system at the Johns Hopkins/Kennedy Krieger Institute provides such a flexible continuum, with an acute rehabilitation umbrella that includes an inpatient hospital unit, a day hospital (also licensed as a school), and an in-the-home/community program—all of which have dedicated interdisciplinary teams—as well as appropriate outpatient services. This system provides rehabilitation in the setting that best matches the patient's needs and abilities as well as the family's resources.

The last and arguably most important step in rehabilitation is community reintegration and, for children, this includes the critical step of return to school. Education (along with play) is the work of children, and consequently it is necessary for all programs that deliver rehabilitation to children and adolescents to provide educational resources during rehabilitation and to assist in school reintegration. Considerable care and effort is required to optimize this process. The assistance that the child will need to facilitate the transition from the rehabilitation to the educational system will vary based on the disability, ranging from problem solving with regard to architectural barriers for a student with orthopedic impairments to developing a totally new placement to accommodate the cognitive, behavioral, and motor impairments of a child with brain injury. In facilitating this process, it is important to know that, as required by law, all students are guaranteed free access to state-of-the-art public education that is individualized to meet their needs in the least restrictive setting (46).

PREVENTION AND TREATMENT OF CLINICAL COMPLICATIONS THAT AFFECT THE CRITICALLY ILL CHILD

Effects of Inactivity and Bed Rest

The body's response to inactivity and bed rest has been well studied. Many anatomic and physiologic changes are known to occur within the musculoskeletal, cardiovascular, and pulmonary systems in response to bed rest, including diminished muscle mass, decreased muscle strength, muscle shortening, osteoporosis, and cardiovascular and pulmonary deconditioning (24). In addition, inactivity puts the skin at risk for breakdown.

Musculoskeletal Complications

Bed rest results in generalized atrophy that is more prominent in those muscles that provide antigravity strength, such as the gastrocnemius-soleus. Atrophy occurs through a decrease in cross-sectional muscle mass and shortening of muscle fibers. In addition, the synthesis of intramuscular collagen fibers is reduced during immobility, resulting in an increased amount of noncontractile intramuscular tissue, which further negatively impacts the mechanical properties of the muscles. The amount of atrophy that occurs in a given muscle directly correlates to the loss of strength and reduced endurance in that muscle. During strict bed rest, muscle strength is reduced by up to 15% of baseline strength per week; a plateau in loss of function is reached at 25% to 40% of baseline strength. It may take 2 to 3 weeks to recover strength lost during 1 week of bed rest. Stretching of a muscle during periods of inactivity may reduce atrophy and maintain contractile properties by holding the muscle in a lengthened position and slowing the formation of noncontractile proteins (26). Stretching will also prevent muscle shortening or contracture formation.

Musculoskeletal contractures and peripheral nerve injuries are insidious, potentially debilitating, and preventable complications of immobility in the intensive care setting. Disease-related changes in muscle tone, limb restraints, and awkward positions are factors that predispose the pediatric patient in the PICU to these problems. Protracted abnormal limb and joint position in the absence of active movements can rapidly progress to muscle contractures and limitation in joint range of motion (ROM), especially noted in the ankles, knees, and hips,

but possibly involving any area. A goal of early rehabilitation intervention in the PICU is to preserve ROM in weight-bearing joints in the lower extremity for ambulation and in the manipulative joints of the upper extremity for self-care and fine-motor activities.

The mainstay of treatment to preserve ROM and to prevent muscle contractures is moving the limbs. Acceptable parameters for performing these movements should be established in conjunction with the PICU staff. Some factors that limit the ability to perform these exercises include increased intracranial pressure, skin grafts across joints, wound dressings, intravascular lines or endotracheal tubes, and hemodynamic instability.

A ROM program is usually developed by either a physical or occupational therapist. The therapist determines the type, duration, and frequency of the exercises and is responsible for teaching the program to the staff and family members. A schedule that includes the details of desired movements is usually placed at the bedside.

Plastic splints designed to hold a joint in an antideformity position are commonly used to provide a static stretch of muscles that cross joints to minimize the development of muscle contractures. The ankles and wrists are the most common joints on which these splints are used. The splints hold the joints as close to the neutral anatomic position as possible. Some models of ankle splints also have a "kick stand" that prevents lateral rotation of the foot and leg. Skin breakdown caused by unrelieved pressure is a complication of these splints. They require careful application and consistent skin checks to ensure that decubitus ulcers do not form, which is especially important if the patient is insensate or unable to communicate discomfort or pain.

Peripheral nerve compression is another preventable musculoskeletal complication that may occur in the PICU. The peroneal and ulnar nerves are at high risk for nerve impingement due to their exposure at the knee and elbow, respectively. The brachial plexus is susceptible to stretch injury from interventions that require wide abduction or external rotation of the shoulders. Appropriate positions to avoid nerve injuries are listed in **Table 13.1**. Although critical illness polyneuropathy or myopathy may also cause limb weakness in the PICU setting, it is important to consider a mononeuropathy as the cause of weakness.

Bed rest also results in reduced bone mineral density. Stimulation to bones from weight bearing, gravity, and muscle activity are necessary to maintain adequate bone health, and these forces are significantly diminished during bed rest. Disuse osteopenia is typically noted in the subperiosteal region of the bones. Bone density can decrease by 40% after 12 weeks of bed rest, resulting in osteoporosis (37). Bone resorption during immobility can result in symptomatic hypercalcemia, particularly in adolescent males following trauma (33).

Cardiovascular Complications

The cardiovascular system also becomes deconditioned with inactivity. Stroke volume at rest decreases, whereas cardiac output is not significantly changed. Resting heart rate increases, as well as heart rate following submaximal exercise. Orthostatic hypotension may develop because the body has difficulty readjusting to the upright position due to impaired venous response. In otherwise healthy subjects, the cardiovascular response has

TABLE 13.1

PROPER POSITIONING TO AVOID NERVE COMPRESSION

Nerve	Anatomy	Avoid	Intervention
Peroneal nerve	Compression at the head of the fibula	Hip and knee flexion Foot inversion	Knees in extension and feet in dorsiflexion
		Heavy or bulky dressings just below the knee	Windowing of dressing over the fibular head
		Prolonged side lying	Alternate sides and position in bed
Ulnar nerve	Compression in the cubital tunnel	Elbow flexion and pronation	Elbow extended, forearm supinated
Brachial plexus	Decreased distance between the clavicle and the first rib	Shoulder abduction greater than 90 degrees with the arm in external rotation	Limit abduction to no more than 90 degrees and allow 30 degrees of horizontal adduction

From Gaebler-Spira D, Uellendahl J. Pediatric Limb Deficiencies. In: Molnar GA, Alexander MA, eds. *Pediatric Rehabilitation,* 3rd ed. Philadelphia: Hanley & Belfus, Inc.; 1999:331–50, with permission.

been completely lost following 3 weeks of bed rest. Three to 5 weeks of therapy may be required for the body to redevelop compensatory responses to change in positioning. Prevention of, and early treatment for, cardiovascular deconditioning may include early mobilization, including ROM exercises, isometric and/or isotonic strengthening exercises, upright positioning in bed (as able), and standing (when appropriate). A tilt-table may be necessary to gradually reintroduce upright positioning if standing is not tolerated.

Pulmonary Complications

Weakness of the diaphragm, intercostals, and abdominal muscles caused by bed rest contribute to pulmonary deconditioning. Resulting changes in respiratory function may include reduced tidal volume, minute volume, vital capacity, and maximum voluntary ventilation. When appropriate, preventative measures should be instituted, such as early mobilization and good pulmonary hygiene, including frequent position changes, deep-breathing exercises, incentive spirometry, and chest percussion (if necessary).

Decubitus Ulcers

Skin is also at risk with immobilization. Decubitus ulcers result from prolonged pressure applied externally over a specific area. Skin breakdown occurs frequently in individuals who are insensate, such as persons with spinal cord injury, and in those with a reduced level of alertness, including individuals with brain injuries and those receiving sedating and/or paralyzing medications. The duration of unrelieved pressure over an area of skin is the most significant contributing factor to skin breakdown. Other risk factors that predispose skin to breakdown include the presence of shearing forces, friction, moisture, and increased body temperature (39). Poor nutritional status also contributes to skin breakdown and delayed healing. The most common sites of decubitus ulcers are the ischia, sacrum, greater trochanters, and heels. In the PICU, the occiput is also a common location for skin breakdown, due to prolonged supine positioning. The Braden scale and Norton scale are tools available to assess a patient's risk for decubitus

ulcers (15,38). Prevention of ulcers should be an important part of PICU care. A patient's skin should be examined at each shift change for areas of redness, blisters, rashes, bruises, or skin breaks. The mainstay of preventative skin care in immobile patients is repositioning every 2 hrs, with care to relieve areas of concentrated pressure. When transferring the patient, shearing forces should be avoided by minimizing the dragging of any body parts across a surface. Pressure-reducing mattresses and seating systems should be used when appropriate. The treatment of skin breakdown requires the reduction/elimination of pressure over the wound, restoring or maintaining adequate nutrition, and caring for local wounds, as directed by depth and size of the wound.

Venous Thrombosis

The rates of diagnosis of venous thromboembolism (VTE) in the pediatric population are highest in infants (1–23 months of age) and teenagers (15–17 years of age), but VTEs also occur in the 2- to 14-year-old age group (49,16). The rate of occurrence in the infant population is comparable to the rate of occurrence in the teenage populations (49). Venous catheter use has been reported as the most common predisposing factor for VTE, followed by surgery and trauma; pregnancy and spinal cord injury also increase the risk for VTE (49,16). Prophylaxis for VTE using mechanical or pharmacologic interventions should be considered for PICU patients.

Gastrointestinal Complications

Gastritis and gastrointestinal (GI) ulceration can result from imbalances that occur within the GI system due to physiologic stress (14). Risk factors for gastritis and GI ulceration include severe head injury, severe burn injury, respiratory failure, coagulopathy, Pediatric Risk of Mortality score >10, risk for hypoxia to GI tract, and exposure to medications known to compromise GI tract integrity; pharmacologic GI prophylaxis should be considered for children who meet these criteria and for other critically ill pediatric patients on a case-by-case basis.

Psychological Issues Surrounding Intensive Care Admissions

Critically ill children who are admitted to the intensive care setting are frequently exposed to highly invasive procedures. In addition, the environment of the PICU can be fast-paced, loud, and confusing and, as such, can potentially be extremely stressful for children and their families. The compounded stressors of the illness or trauma itself and the subsequent hospitalization can put children at high risk for acute distress, adverse psychological outcomes, and poor adjustment following discharge. Therefore, it is important to identify potential psychological stressors for a child during intensive care treatment and take steps to diminish their impact whenever possible.

Children in the PICU often demonstrate sleep disturbances, both due to their primary medical condition and/or exacerbated by the constant light and sound in the PICU. Additionally, they are exposed to unfamiliar situations and procedures and may experience sensory overload or deprivation due to the lights and sounds of the machines combined with the lack of movement and relative monotony of the environmental stimuli. Medications, particularly those with paralytic or sedative qualities, can also lead to sensory changes and distortions in body sensation or cognitive awareness (6). Therefore, children are at risk for what has been termed in adults as "ICU syndrome" or "ICU psychosis." Children may experience acute periods of confusion, disorientation, delirium, or even exhibit delusions or illusions/hallucinations. Whereas the presence of these symptoms were once thought to be related to the presenting illness or medication effects, it is now known that the environment of the PICU itself can produce or exacerbate them due to the atypical sensory environment and disruption to sleep. These episodes can be frightening for both the children and parents (19).

Although the psychological response to hospitalization for critical illness has not been extensively studied in the pediatric population, growing evidence suggests that children exhibit symptoms of psychological distress during and following a PICU admission. Furthermore, they appear to be particularly vulnerable to a range of negative psychological and behavioral manifestations, including posttraumatic stress disorder, which may persist long after discharge and may warrant psychiatric intervention. For example, studies that examined acute stress and coping during hospitalization showed that children in the PICU are more likely than other hospitalized children to show signs of anxiety, depression, posttraumatic stress symptoms, fearfulness, restlessness, withdrawal, and angry or hostile behaviors (28). Children, particularly very young children, may not have developed the range of psychological responses necessary to cope effectively with the stress and disruption in routine caused by the experience of a critical illness, the impact of pain and invasive procedures, and the potentially frightening environment of the intensive care setting (17).

Children who are younger, are more critically ill, have a longer hospital stay, and endure more invasive procedures appear to demonstrate significantly more medical fears and ongoing posttraumatic stress symptoms (including increased anxiety, nightmares, recurrent intrusive thoughts about their hospital experience, and a lower sense of control over their health) for 6 months after hospital discharge (44,45). The number of invasive procedures has been shown to be the strongest predictor of adverse psychological outcome following PICU stay (45). In addition, children with more severe illness, who are therefore more likely to be medicated with sedatives and analgesics, have more adverse psychological symptoms, including intrusive memories about specific procedures they experienced. Although clinical lore has assumed that children do not tend to recall their PICU experiences, evidence suggests that children may, in fact, remember intensive care procedures and hospitalization, and that these memories are present even in those children who were given sedating medications (6,45).

The parents' psychological response to having a critically ill child has also been examined. The parents of critically ill children are at risk for developing anxiety, depression, and other emotional disturbances, including symptoms of posttraumatic stress disorder (30). One study evaluated the utility of an educational and behavioral intervention program (Creating Opportunities for Parent Empowerment, or COPE) that provided education and parent–child coping activities at three time points: during the early stages of PICU admission, following transfer to the general medical setting, and following discharge home (35). The researchers found that the intervention resulted in a large reduction in adverse outcomes in both the mothers and children, compared to a group provided with education alone. Mothers in the COPE group reported less stress during hospitalization and less depression and posttraumatic stress symptoms after hospitalization. Additionally, the children in the COPE group exhibited fewer withdrawal symptoms, negative behavioral symptoms, and externalizing behaviors at 6 months and 12 months after discharge, and they were rated as having less hyperactivity and troublesome behavior by parents.

Results of the studies to date highlight the importance of minimizing the psychological trauma of PICU hospitalization, particularly when it comes to invasive procedures. In addition, the pediatric medical psychology literature highlights the need for adjusting the environment and providing information developmentally and cognitively appropriate to the child (43). Consistent reassurance and explanation of procedures in a developmentally appropriate manner is important in providing children with a sense of control and safety. For example, providing an explanation for the reason for the procedure, what to expect, and how it might feel can increase a child's sense of control over his environment. Rasnake and Linscheid noted that the use of standardized, developmentally appropriate information in preparing children for medical procedures (as opposed to standard information) resulted in reduced anxiety and fewer distress behaviors during the procedures in those who received the modified information and preparation (43).

Several strategies can be implemented to minimize the impact of the PICU environment and potential for distress in children who require intensive care hospitalization for critical illness (6). For example, frequent orientation to the time, day, and place, and implementation of a normal day/night routine will reduce the potential for disorientation. When possible, providing familiar objects and child-friendly stimuli, as well as allowing frequent visits from family members will reduce the anxiety and general apprehension that children feel in the unfamiliar PICU environment. Therapeutic touch, provided by parents or nurses, has been shown to reduce stress and provide comfort to children during critical illness. Developmentally appropriate medical play and the provision of behavioral coping strategies and supportive psychological intervention as early as feasible can potentially reduce the long-term impact of the illness and hospitalization (30). In addition, studies have demonstrated the positive impact on the child and parent when the parent is present and frequently participates in the child's care (35).

In summary, children hospitalized in the intensive care setting are at risk for acute distress and adverse psychological symptoms that can potentially persist long after discharge. Young children who are exposed to numerous invasive procedures appear to be most at risk. It is important that steps be taken to minimize the development of these symptoms as early as possible. Modification of the environment to promote day/night routines, availability of child-friendly stimuli, and provision of therapeutic information in a developmentally appropriate manner, as well as encouraging parents to assist in their child's care and coping, appear to be most beneficial in reducing psychological distress and promoting positive adjustment after a PICU hospitalization.

REHABILITATION OF SPECIFIC CRITICAL ILLNESSES

To complement this general information on rehabilitation, this section addresses specific disorders that require specialized acute and long-term rehabilitation. We will highlight the acute medical and rehabilitation management applicable to the PICU setting, as well as the long-term outcome and management necessary to assist the PICU physician in providing guidance to patients and families.

Acquired Brain Injury

Acquired brain injury (ABI) has many etiologies, including trauma, infection, hypoxia and ischemia, genetic metabolic disorders, tumors, and vascular disorders. Trauma is the most common etiology of ABI; the incidence of mild to severe traumatic brain injury (TBI) varies from 100 to 400 per 100,000 children per year. Consequently, much of this chapter focuses on TBI.

Classification of Severity of Injury

TBI severity is classified by clinical markers, reflecting the initial severity of injury and the trajectory of recovery. The Glasgow Coma Scale (GCS) is used as an "up-front" marker of severity. Length of coma (absence of spontaneous eye opening), time to follow commands (TFC), and length of posttraumatic amnesia (PTA, a period following injury when memory for new information is impaired) are used to reflect the trajectory of recovery. These markers of severity are known to correlate with long-term outcome.

Mild TBI is defined by an initial GCS of 13 to 15, loss of consciousness for <1 hr (but usually absent or transient), and PTA for ≤1 hr. If these criteria are met, but a focal lesion is seen on CT scan or a focal neurologic deficit is observed, the injury is reclassified as either a complicated mild or moderate TBI. Moderate TBI is defined by a GCS of 9 to 12 or loss of consciousness for 1 to 24 hrs. Severe TBI is defined by a GCS of 3 to 8, loss of consciousness for ≥24 hrs, or PTA for ≥24 hrs (in adults) or ≥1 week (in children). It is important to recognize that PTA criteria can stand alone when classifying severity of injury.

Medical Issues after Acquired Brain Injury

After acute injury to the brain, almost every system in the body is affected. Some of these effects are isolated to the acute period, while others are not. Elsewhere in this chapter, we have covered many medical issues that are applicable to the brain-injured patient: effects of bed rest, musculoskeletal disorders, deep venous thrombosis, and chronic ventilator management. Other medical issues after ABI/TBI, by system, include the following.

Cardiovascular. Autonomic instability can present with hypertension, tachycardia, hyperthermia, tachypnea, and hypertonia and decerebrate posturing in the very severely injured. This condition is associated with dysfunction of the thalamus or hypothalamus and the connections to the cortical, subcortical, and brainstem areas that mediate autonomic functions. Bromocriptine, propranolol, clonidine, lorazepam, dantrolene, and morphine sulfate have been used for treatment (8).

Infectious Disease/Immune System. Acute depression of cell-mediated immunity, including suppression of T-cell function and cytokine production, occurs after severe TBI, and a high incidence of infection is reported (36).

Nutrition/Gastrointestinal System. The delivery of adequate enteral nutrition may be complicated by early feeding intolerance due to altered gastric motility (delayed emptying in first week, gastric dysrhythmias), gastroesophageal reflux, and dysphagia (necessitating clinical evaluation +/− modified barium swallow to safely guide oral feeding). A hypermetabolic/hypercatabolic period occurs early after ABI (initial 1–2 weeks), and early intervention is important to ensure appropriate nutrition (42).

Neurologic System. Posttraumatic seizures are classified as immediate (first 24 hrs), early (days 2–7), or late (after the first 7 days). Unlike early and late seizures, immediate posttraumatic seizures do not have significant prognostic utility. Risk of posttraumatic epilepsy increases with increasing severity of injury (0.5% for mild, 1.2% for moderate, and 10% for severe TBI) and with certain types of injuries (e.g., skull fracture and contusion with subdural hematoma) (3). Anticonvulsant prophylaxis with phenytoin (Dilantin) has been shown to be efficacious only for the first week postinjury (51). Posttraumatic hydrocephalus is most commonly a result of cortical atrophy, but progressive hydrocephalus must be ruled out. The risk of hydrocephalus increases with longer duration of coma, increased age, and decompressive craniotomy (34). Sensory deficits are not uncommon after TBI and include hearing impairments and visual impairments of many etiologies. The "sinking skin flap syndrome" can occur after decompressive craniectomy. Symptoms include headaches, dizziness, lethargy, as well as neurologic deterioration with mental status changes and progressive motor impairments, such as hemiplegia. These symptoms are likely related to the effect of atmospheric pressure on the brain and possibly to the in-and-out movement of the brain through the skull defect. Repair of the craniotomy can result in increased cerebral blood flow, decreased symptoms, and improved neurologic function (47).

Agitation is a natural phase of recovery from TBI. Generally, sedating medications should be avoided during recovery from

TBI. However, if the agitated stage of recovery occurs in the PICU setting, medication to calm the patient may be necessary for safety reasons. Spasticity and movement disorders may be an early or late manifestation of ABI. Typically, tone problems are managed with medication only after failing positional and orthotic management.

Urinary and Bowel Incontinence. Incontinence is common after moderate and severe neurologic injuries and may be due to cognitive/behavioral issues, frontal lobe injury, associated injury to the spinal cord, or direct bladder/bowel injury. Medical management during the acute period is important to prevent urinary retention and constipation.

Endocrine. Endocrine abnormalities may occur transiently during the acute period, are linked to the severity of injury, and include the syndrome of inappropriate antidiuretic hormone secretion, diabetes insipidus (which may rarely persist after the acute period), hypogonadism, cortisol hyporesponsiveness, and hypothyroidism (18).

Prognostic Factors

A child's prognosis following ABI is influenced by several different factors. Qualities inherent to the individual child and her family can impact the outcome. In addition, the etiology of injury and severity of injury are useful to consider in predicting recovery. A child's age and premorbid deficits and the family's function and access to resources impact recovery from ABI. The effect of the child's age depends on the type of ABI. The younger brain has increased plasticity, which results in better outcome after focal injuries (strokes). However, with TBI, younger children (<5–8 years of age) have worse outcomes than older children and adolescents, a finding that appears to be related to increased susceptibility of the younger brain to trauma and to the long-term effect of decreased ability to learn new information and skills. An increased incidence of premorbid learning and behavioral problems is seen among children with TBI; generally, learning and behavioral problems will be exacerbated with ABI. Concerning family factors, it is well known in all types of brain injury (congenital and acquired) that children have better outcomes if their families have more resources, are under less stress, and are more "structured and organized" in their daily life.

The etiology of ABI is prognostically important, because the etiology dictates the distribution, type, and severity of injury. Most children, especially those with focal injuries and isolated traumatic injuries, can be expected to make considerable neurologic recovery. One of the major exceptions is children with hypoxic-ischemic injury who have severe neurologic deficits, such as those that occur with near-drowning or prolonged cardiac arrest. It is also important to consider whether a secondary injury is associated. For example, if a child with TBI has a secondary injury, such as a stroke related to a herniation syndrome or a hypoxic-ischemic injury from shock, his outcome will be worse.

Severity-of-injury factors are very useful in predicting general categories of outcome, which helps to guide recommendations for appropriate medical and rehabilitation management. Children and adolescents with mild TBI usually do well, although they may have postconcussion symptoms (e.g., headache, fatigue, sleep disturbances, balance deficits, lightheadedness, dizziness, inattention, memory deficits, slowed response time, and lability of affect) for which the family will benefit from prospective guidance. As they return to their normal activities at home and school, the primary physician should monitor these children for new learning or behavioral problems.

With both moderate and severe TBI, children can be expected to have persisting neurobehavioral, academic, and "real-world" deficits; within this range of severity, a strong correlation exists between severity and outcome (27). For children with moderate-to-severe TBI, ongoing cognitive and behavioral changes from the child's individual baseline should be expected, even though cognitive testing may remain or return to within the normal range. This group benefits from evaluation, guidance, and appropriate treatment from experienced clinicians.

For children with the most severe TBIs, significant long-term cognitive and behavioral problems, as well as possible motor impairments, can be expected. Nevertheless, one should remain optimistic that meaningful recovery will occur. In a very severely injured cohort of children in whom the median TFC was 5 to 6 weeks, 73% regained independence in ambulation and self-care, and 10% remained partially dependent in self-care and achieved limited ambulation. If the TFC was <6 weeks, 94% of the patients had the better outcome (9).

Outcome

Focal neurologic deficits, while not typical in developmental disabilities, are seen in children with ABI. For example, children with strokes may acquire an aphasia or hemiplegia. As previously discussed, plasticity of the young brain with focal injuries will aid in the recovery of these impairments. Unlike an adult, a child under 5 to 8 years of age with a new left middle cerebral artery stroke associated with aphasia can be expected to recover a significant amount of speech and language. A neonate with a similar stroke might have early delays in speech and language acquisition but should eventually demonstrate abilities within the normal range.

After TBI, children's deficits are related to the distribution of their injury; both contusions and diffuse axonal injury must be considered. It is important to remember that the full extent of diffuse axonal injury may not be appreciated on clinical CT or MRI. The frontal lobes are frequently injured, resulting in cognitive and behavioral deficits. It is usual to recover general intellectual abilities within the normal range after TBI (exceptions are the very young and the extremely severely injured). However, specific neuropsychological deficits are frequently present and debilitating, including impairments of memory, attention, speed (of processing and output), and executive function (the organizational and planning abilities that allow success in achieving goals). Communication disorders also occur, and symptoms such as word-finding problems are common. Behavioral and psychiatric disorders are common after TBI; problems stemming from disinhibition, such as secondary attention deficit hyperactivity disorder, are most notable.

Behavioral and cognitive impairments are seen as the most problematic for patients with TBI and their families; however, motor impairments occur and their effects should not be minimized. Even for those who have a good recovery, motor speed and high-level coordination are usually diminished. For the smaller subset of patients with continuing severe motor disabilities, impairments include disorders of tone (spasticity, rigidity, dystonia), balance, coordination, ataxia, and tremors.

These impairments are usually associated with deep injuries to the basal ganglia, thalamus, brainstem, and cerebellar outflow tracts. Also, peripheral nerve injuries are common.

Recovery and Rehabilitation after Acquired Brain Injury

As a general rule, most of the recovery after ABI occurs within the first year, and the majority of that recovery usually occurs within the first 3 to 6 months. However, it is important to recognize that spontaneous recovery is known to occur years after injury. Although late changes may be small, they can greatly impact quality of life (e.g., a small improvement in memory may translate into significantly increased independence at home or work). With therapeutic interventions, improvements in function can occur years after injury, even though the patient's function has been stable for years.

Rehabilitation in the PICU. Early rehabilitation is known to decrease the length of total hospitalization after TBI. Rehabilitation should begin early in the PICU course, with the initial goal of preventing those secondary impairments that are known to impede recovery. Initially, even before the child is medically stable, "preventive maintenance" should begin, including attention to positioning and splinting to prevent contractures, peripheral nerve injuries, and decubitus ulcers. When the child is more stable and tolerates handling, a passive ROM program can be started. As recovery continues, the child becomes a more active participant in rehabilitation.

Cognitive and behavioral recovery after TBI occurs in a relatively predictable manner, as described by the Rancho Los Amigos Scale of Cognitive Functioning (**Table 13.2**), which helps staff and families understand the expected progression of recovery. Behavioral/environmental guidelines should be provided as appropriate for the child's stage of recovery. For example, during Levels I and II (no response and generalized response), a family's stress can be lessened by offering suggestions for how they can talk to their child and participate in their child's care. When the child progresses to Level IV (confused and agitated), it is important that staff and family recognize this as an improvement in the child's mental status, because this knowledge helps all to tolerate this difficult stage. However, it is also important to institute environmental and behavioral strategies to minimize agitation. The basic goal is to minimize sensory overload (which is difficult in the PICU), yet at the same time provide enough familiar sensory input so that the

patient can be as oriented as possible. Manipulating the environment and schedule to allow for distinction between day and night and promoting appropriate sleep are beneficial. Further strategies should be individualized after careful observation of the child; these might include treating pain appropriately, providing the comforting voice of a family member (in person or in a recording), asking visitors to leave the room if agitation is increasing, turning off the TV, removing items from the room that appear to increase agitation, removing noxious stimuli promptly (such as a soiled diaper), and facilitating communication (which might include a picture board for an intubated patient who cannot speak).

Rehabilitation after the PICU. The need for continuing brain injury rehabilitation will be determined by the number, type, and severity of impairments that affect the child's ability to communicate, perform activities of daily living, and ambulate. The need for medical and nursing care and for safety-related supervision, as well as the age and size of the patient, family resources, and available rehabilitation resources will also factor into the decision. As a general rule, acute, intense, interdisciplinary rehabilitation is justifiable if the patient has multiple impairments and will benefit from a minimum of 3 hrs of therapy per day. It is the obligation of the acute medical system to identify these functional impairments and the need for rehabilitation and to make certain that appropriate rehabilitation services are arranged.

Acquired Spinal Cord Injuries

Spinal cord injuries (SCIs) occur in children as a result of trauma, infection, mass lesion, vascular event, autoimmune disease, or as a complication of spine procedures. Spinal cord dysfunction can compromise the function of multiple body systems; thus, it is important for the pediatric critical care team to understand physiologic changes that occur in the child with SCI and for rehabilitation efforts to be initiated during a child's PICU stay. Key points regarding the epidemiology, evaluation, and treatment of a child with SCI are summarized below.

Of the approximately 11,000 new traumatic SCIs that occur yearly in the United States, 3.7% occur in children younger than 16 years of age and 20.3% occur in individuals younger than 20 (4). Based on unique anatomic and biomechanical differences in the cervical spine between younger and older children, different patterns of traumatic SCI are seen in children ages 0 to 8 years and those ages 9 to 19 years. In young children, neural damage can occur even without radiographic (x-ray, CT) evidence of spinal column injury. This phenomenon is termed *spinal cord injury without radiographic abnormality*, or SCIWORA, and is presumed to occur secondary to an increased elasticity of the spine that results in transient subluxation of the spinal column and causes the cord to stretch. In children, a latent period from 30 min to 4 days between injury and onset of paralysis has been reported after SCIWORA. After major trauma in young children, any worsening on serial neurologic examination should prompt efforts to rule out spinal cord lesion. MRI techniques are helpful for detailing soft-tissue injury in 65% of children with SCIWORA and may reveal abnormalities that include rupture of anterior or posterior longitudinal ligaments, endplate fractures, intradisk abnormalities,

RANCHO LOS AMIGOS SCALE OF COGNITIVE FUNCTIONING

Level	Clinical description
Level I	No response
Level II	Generalized response
Level III	Localized response
Level IV	Confused, agitated response
Level V	Confused, nonagitated response
Level VI	Confused, appropriate response
Level VII	Automatic, appropriate response
Level VII	Purposeful, appropriate response

and spinal cord changes ranging from edema or hemorrhage to complete transection (41).

Acute intervention to treat the SCI itself is limited. Until recently, corticosteroid administration has been advocated in adults within the first 8 hrs after injury, but recent data does not support this treatment. Corticosteroid administration in children <13 years of age has not been studied. Spine immobilization is important in limiting further injury. Younger children have proportionally larger heads, necessitating thoracic elevation or/and occipital recess to prevent flexion of the head and neck and to best align the cervical spine during spine immobilization. The need for, and timing of, surgical intervention depends on the type of injury and neurologic findings.

Medical Issues after Spinal Cord Injuries

A systematic approach to medical management of children with SCI in the PICU is advocated.

Respiratory. The primary respiratory dysfunction in children with SCI is restrictive respiratory insufficiency induced by muscle paralysis. A smaller obstructive component exists in children with high cervical injuries due to unbalanced vagal nerve activity, predisposing to airway hyper-reactivity. Patients with C1 to C3 injury are usually dependent on mechanical ventilation. During initial hospitalization, pneumococcal vaccine should be given to children >2 years of age with respiratory dysfunction, and influenza vaccination should be administered yearly to children who are >6 months (52).

Cardiovascular. Venous thromboembolism occurs in 1.1% of children 13 years or younger with SCI, compared with 4.4% among those 14 to 19 years old (29). Recommendations for prophylaxis and treatment for VTE in children over the age of 14 with SCI are similar to those for adults (13); because of the low incidence of VTE in children <14, case-by-case consideration of the actual risk is advised (29).

Autonomic dysreflexia (AD), a phenomenon unique to persons with injury at T6 level or above, manifests with sweating, facial flushing, headaches, piloerection, and hypertension; hypertension can result in cerebral hemorrhage. The mechanism for AD is postulated to be an accumulation of substance P and a deficiency of inhibitory neurotransmitters (e.g., norepinephrine, GABA, 5HT) below the level of injury, with resultant supersensitivity of spinal α- and peripheral adrenoreceptors. The carotid sinus and aortic arch baroreceptors are less sensitive to very high or very low blood pressure values (<60 or >160 mm Hg), thus limiting their ability to respond during AD. The treatment of AD is symptomatic. The patient should be positioned upright, thus producing an orthostatic decrease in blood pressure. The precipitating factor should be identified and removed. Lower urinary tract irritants account for 75% to 85% of AD episodes and anorectal stimulation for 13% to 19%; thus, the bladder should be catheterized or indwelling catheter should be checked for dysfunction and/or replaced, and the bowel program should be performed using lidocaine gel to prevent noxious stimuli. Other GI factors, cutaneous stimuli, trauma, fracture, and deep venous thrombosis should also be considered. For individuals who present with high blood pressure and do not respond to conservative measures, the use of antihypertensive medications with rapid onset and short half-life (e.g., nitroglycerin SL/paste/IV, clonidine PO, hydralazine IV) should be considered.

Fever. Fever is common in the acute and subacute phase of SCI. Differential diagnoses include infection, VTE, pressure ulcer, and heterotopic ossification/myositis ossificans (periarticular bone-like formation in the muscle tissue that occurs below neurologic injury level, most commonly in the hips, knees, elbows, and shoulders). In 8% to 11% of hospitalized adolescents and adults with SCI, no etiology for fever is found, and the fever is presumed to be secondary to thermoregulatory abnormalities (7).

Gastrointestinal. Because gastrointestinal dysfunction is multifactorial in individuals with SCI, the early establishment of a bowel regimen that ensures complete and regular emptying is important. Stool softeners, rectal stimulation, and laxatives are the mainstays of therapy. Initiation of GI prophylaxis with H_2 blockers is advocated due to high incidence of stress ulcer formation.

Hypercalcemia. Hypercalcemia of immobility can occur in 10% to 23% of individuals with SCI, mostly adolescents and young males (33). The elevation in calcium can occur at as early as 2 weeks following the spinal cord injury, but is most common 4 to 8 weeks after injury. Management includes hydration, furosemide, and biphosphonates, such as pamidronate.

Genitourinary. Genitourinary system manifestations in the acute phase consist mainly of urinary retention secondary to nervous system dysfunction and urinary tract infections related to bladder instrumentation. In the PICU, rapidly transitioning from the use of an indwelling device to a program of intermittent catheterization will limit infection.

Dermal. In a patient with neurologic deficits, skin ulcerations or pressure sores can occur after only 1 to 2 hrs of immobilization on a backboard. Proper positioning and frequent position changes, along with the use of pressure-relieving materials and devices, are the mainstays of skin care in individuals with limited mobility and insensate skin.

Soft Tissue and Joints. Soft tissue and joint contractures are frequent complications in children with SCI. ROM in the upper and lower extremities can be preserved by starting early and aggressive rehabilitation and by using adequate splinting (i.e., resting hand splints, ankle-foot orthosis).

Muscular. Within 1 month of SCI, muscle fiber cross-sectional area declines and muscle fibers are smaller, have less contractile protein, produce lower peak contractile forces, and have decreased resistance to fatigue. Stretching and strength training of the spared muscles during bed rest prevent atrophy and loss of strength and contractile proteins. Electric neuromuscular stimulation of the paralyzed muscles may provide similar benefits.

Prognostic Factors and Outcome after Spinal Cord Injury

Clinicians should avoid extremes of offering false hope or false pessimism when talking with patients with SCI and their families. Most who survive SCI do not experience complete severance of their spinal cords. An accurate neurologic examination aids in predicting recovery; however, any prognostication should be made cautiously early after injury, because spinal shock and other confounding variables (very young age, difficulty following instructions, head injury, mechanical ventilation, intoxication, severe multiple injuries) may interfere with the neurologic examination (11). Patients with MRI findings of hemorrhage or extensive segments of edema will have less motor recovery in comparison with patients with small, nonhemorrhagic lesions, although MRI itself is not as accurate a predictor as the physical examination (31). The most utilized neurologic assessment in SCI is based on the Standards of the American Spinal Injury Association (ASIA) Impairment Scale (AIS) and, if confounders are carefully considered, it is the best tool for early prognostication. An accurate classification of impairment after SCI requires thorough understanding of the Standards of AIS and careful neurologic examination. Details of the examination and scoring method can be found in the booklet that describes the standards (2).

Elements of ASIA Standard assessment consist of manual strength testing of 10 key muscles on each side of the body, light touch and pinprick sensation testing in 28 dermatomes (from C2 to S5, with the S4–5 taken as one level) on each side of the body, and digital rectal exam for S4 to S5 motor function (voluntary anal sphincter contraction) and presence of any anal sensation. Other sensory modalities, motor testing of the other muscle groups, and detailed neurologic exam are also required but do not alter the results of ASIA standard classification. If the patient has some sacral sparing (partial function in the most caudal, S4–S5, spinal cord segments), by ASIA Standards, she is classified as having *incomplete injury*. If no sacral sparing is present, the injury is classified as *complete* even if function is partially preserved below the level of injury.

The AIS consists of five grades: A, complete; B, sensory incomplete; C and D, motor incomplete; and E, normal motor and sensory function (**Table 13.3**). The standard ASIA examination also defines motor, sensory, and neurologic levels of injury, as well as motor, light touch, and pin prick scores. ASIA motor level is highly correlated with functional recovery in adults (31). Prognosis may be more accurate if based on ASIA examination 72 hrs after the acute injury rather than on the initial emergency room evaluation (11). If the child is in spinal shock, the examination should be repeated once the child emerges from spinal shock. Various criteria have been used to indicate resolution of spinal shock, with the return of bulbocavernosus reflex (segmental spinal reflex supplied by the S3–S4 sacral nerves) as the most commonly accepted clinical sign. (22). Caution should be exercised when the ASIA terminology of completeness of injury is discussed with the family. "Complete injury," ASIA-A, indicates lack of sacral sparing, but does not necessarily indicate lack of function below the level of injury and does not mean that no axons cross the injury site. Because young children often cannot follow instructions to cooperate with the rigorous testing of the ASIA exam, this examination may not be as useful for prognostication, and clinical judgment should be exercised in interpreting a child's function.

Conversion from complete to incomplete SCI has been reported at as late as 2.5 years after injury in adults (31). In all SCI patients, the occurrence of conversion from complete to incomplete has been reported from 4.1% to 25.3%, with the rate of distal motor function recovery from 2.5% to 15.5% (22). Because the timing of initial classification of completeness in

---

TABLE 13.3

ASIA IMPAIRMENT SCALE (AIS) CLASSIFICATION

AIS	Clinical description
A Complete	No motor (tested as voluntary external anal sphincter contraction during digital rectal exam) or sensory function is preserved in the sacral segments S4–S5.
A Complete with ZPP	No motor or sensory function is preserved in the sacral segments S4–S5, but some motor or sensory function is present below the neurologic level and represents zone of partial preservation (ZPP).
B Sensory incomplete	Some sensory but no motor function is preserved in the S4–S5 segments, and no motor function is preserved more than three levels below the motor level on a given side.
C Motor incomplete	Motor function is present in the S4–S5 segments; OR only some sensory function is present in the S4–S5 segments, along with some motor function preserved more than three levels below the motor level on a given side. *And* More than half of the key muscles below the neurologic level have a muscle grade less than 3 (0–2).
D Motor incomplete	Motor function is present in the S4–S5 segments; OR only some sensory function is present in the S4–S5 segments, along with some motor function preserved more than three levels below the motor level on a given side *And* At least half of the key muscles below the neurologic level have a muscle grade of 3 or better (3–5).
E Normal	Normal motor and sensory function; AIS E is used in follow-up assessment in individuals who have recovered from a documented SCI. If, on initial evaluation, no deficits are present, the individual is neurologically intact and the AIS does not apply.

Adapted from American Spinal Injury Association. *International Standards for Neurological Classification of SCI*, revised 2000. Chicago, IL: American Spinal Injury Association, 2000.

these studies varies from 1 day to several months after injury, and due to methodologic differences, it is difficult to interpret this literature.

The majority of neurologic recovery in complete SCI occurs during the first 6 to 9 months (11). Studies have shown that considerable potential for recovery of the damaged human spinal cord continues for years after injury. In patients with complete tetraplegia, every motor level regained has significant functional implications and correlates with self-care function. Patients with injuries at C1 to C4 who are classified as AISA-A are dependent for self-care and transfers and are independent with power wheelchair mobility with specialized controls; those with functional levels of C8 to T1 are independent in ADLs, transfers, and bed mobility, and are able to use a manual wheelchair. Studies of adults revealed that those with complete tetraplegia typically gain an additional motor level in the upper extremity within 1 year after injury. Those with complete paraplegia rarely demonstrate change in neurologic level between 1 month and 1 year postinjury. Patients with complete SCI rarely walk, although those with incomplete injuries have a more favorable prognosis for community ambulation (11).

Rehabilitation after Spinal Cord Injury

Consultation from a pediatric physiatrist and rehabilitation services will provide a baseline motor-sensory and functional assessment, initiate a rehabilitation plan, help to outline prognosis, and facilitate transition from an intensive care setting to a rehabilitation phase that is focused on recovery and maximizing function of the injured child. Physical and occupational therapy will provide assistance with positioning and bracing, introduce exercises, and begin mobilization and functional training. Appropriate positioning is indicated to prevent skin breakdown, compression neuropathy, contractures, and increased spasticity. Patients with high cervical cord injuries benefit from speech pathology evaluation and therapy to assist with communication (augmentative technology, speaking valves) and with swallow evaluation in patients with tracheostomy. For ventilator-dependent patients, the ability to direct others in how to assist them is important.

Traditional rehabilitation is focused on improving the strength of spared muscles and teaching alternative compensation patterns to substitute for the paralyzed muscles, with the goal of achieving maximum functional independence. Newer rehabilitation approaches have been emerging, along with intensive research on treatments for SCI. Activity-based restoration therapy (ABRT) utilizes technologically advanced equipment, modalities, and training paradigms based on principles of motor learning. For example, electrical stimulation is used to generate muscle contractions in paralyzed muscle groups to produce functionally useful sequential patterns. For all persons with SCI, this electrical stimulation prevents muscle atrophy and cardiovascular compromise. Additionally, for young children who are injured before growth stops and whose motor-sensory development is incomplete, ABRT provides an opportunity for practicing activities never experienced prior to injury. ABRT is delivered most comprehensively and intensively during inpatient rehabilitation; however, when the child is ready for discharge from the inpatient program, ABRT therapies are transitioned to the child's home for long-term treatment.

Amputations

The child with an acquired amputation often requires intensive care due to the circumstances involved with the loss of limb. Trauma is the leading cause of amputation in childhood, with etiologies varying depending on region of the country and age of the child (23). Traumatic amputations are twice as frequent as disease-related amputations, which are typically due to either tumor or infection. A single limb is involved in more than 90% of cases of pediatric amputation. Multiple limb involvement secondary to autoamputation is most commonly seen in cases that result from septic emboli, purpura fulminans, or disseminated intravascular coagulopathy.

During the acute postamputation period, rehabilitation goals include pain control, positioning to prevent loss of ROM, maintenance of strength and flexibility, and emotional support. In addition to adequate analgesic intervention, a skin desensitization program that consists of gentle tapping, massage, and soft tissue and scar mobilization can be an important part of treatment for phantom sensations and phantom pain (20).

Positioning the residual limb to prevent the development of flexion contractures is critical, especially in lower limb amputations, when walking with a prosthesis is usually the ultimate goal. Common contractures that must be avoided include hip flexion, hip abduction, hip external rotation, and knee flexion. Procedures and positions to prevent these complications include lying with the hip positioned neutrally or in extension (often aided by prone positioning), facilitating neutral rotation of the leg at the hip, and early ambulation. Positions to avoid include propping the residual limb with pillows, prolonged sitting, and lying with the leg positioned in flexion, abduction, and external rotation. In upper limb amputations, mobilization exercises for the shoulder and scapulae should be performed to prevent contracture formation that would limit the ability to move an upper limb prosthesis through space. A consult by the physical medicine and rehabilitation team may be beneficial to help with prosthesis prescription, recommendations about residual limb preparation, and family counseling regarding anticipated progress with functional use of the prosthetic limb.

As the patient's condition improves, attention should be given to the child's potential to develop psychological and social adjustment problems. This process begins in the PICU by assessing family interactions, temperament, coping style, and planning skills. Medical social workers play an instrumental role in helping families to obtain supportive community services. Psychosocial intervention may be as important as optimal wound healing and residual limb care with regard to the long-term function of the child and family. Successful reintegration into the community and school will in part depend on self-esteem, motivation, and family support. It is not too early to start addressing these issues in the PICU.

Rehabilitation Care for Critically Ill Children with Burns

The rehabilitation management of burns in the PICU focuses on the prevention of secondary complications that impair function following medical stabilization. In children with severe burn

TABLE 13.4

POSITIONING THE PEDIATRIC BURN PATIENT

Area of burn	Contracture risk	Contracture prevention
Anterior neck	Flexion	Extension, no pillows
Anterior axilla	Shoulder adduction	90 degrees abduction with neutral rotation
Posterior axilla	Shoulder extension	Shoulder flexion
Elbow/forearm	Flexion/pronation	Elbow extended, forearm supinated
Wrists	Flexion	15–20 degrees extension
Metacarpophalangeals	Hyperextension	70–90 degrees flexion
Interphalangeals	Flexion	Full extension
Palmar burn	Finger flexion, thumb opposition	All joints full extension, thumb radially abducted
Chest	Lateral/anterior flexion	Straight, no lateral or anterior flexion
Hips	Flexion, adduction, external rotation	Extension, 10 degrees abduction, neural rotation
Knees	Flexion	Extension
Ankles	Plantar flexion	90 degrees dorsiflexion

Adapted from Taggart P, Haining R. Rehabilitation of Burn Injuries. In: Molnar GE, Alexander MA, ed. *Pediatric Rehabilitation*, 3rd ed. Philadelphia: Hanley & Belfus, Inc.; 1999:351–64.

injury, early rehabilitation goals include prevention of predictable deformities and secondary injuries through a program of positioning and splinting plus ROM exercises. Another early priority should be to establish a long-term relationship between the patient and family and the rehabilitation team to facilitate continuation of, and compliance with, therapies after discharge from the PICU (48).

Even in the early phase of burn treatment, general positioning guidelines within the constraints required for graft healing and fluid management have an important role in decreasing contractures and subsequent deformity. Unfortunately, the position of comfort may not be the optimal position to prevent contractures. Guidelines for positioning based on the area of the burn (**Table 13.4**) should be posted, reviewed, and adjusted by the burn therapists and communicated to the nursing staff on a daily basis (50).

Special attention should be given to the lower extremities, because flexion contractures are common, especially in young children. In preambulatory infants, the development of contractures in these areas can adversely affect the development of walking ability. Positioning in prone, if tolerated, can prevent hip flexion contractures, and the use of knee immobilizers is helpful for decreasing knee flexion contractures. The frequency and duration of specialized positioning is determined by the patient's medical needs, ability to tolerate the interventions, and skin integrity. In sedated, immobile patients, a pressure-relief mattress or overlay should be used in combination with repositioning and turning at least every 2 hrs to prevent skin breakdown from unrelieved pressure. Proper positioning can also help in the control of edema. The elevation of hands and feet for edema control should be instituted during the first 72 hrs following a burn injury.

Splints provide a static stretch in a desired position over time and are a useful addition to the positioning program. Splinting should be instituted when skin tightness is noticed or preemptively in cases of large body-surface burns that involve the neck, axilla, hands, or feet (50). Flexion deformities of the neck can be minimized with the judicious use of thermoplastic neck splints and positioning in slight neck extension if the patient is unable to tolerate a neck collar. Ankle plantar flexion contractures commonly develop with prolonged bed rest and should be treated with the use of an ankle splint that blocks plantar flexion. Careful application of these splints, with attention to pressure points at the heel and metatarsal heads, is necessary so that skin breakdown does not occur in these areas.

During the acute period of treatment for a severe burn injury, ROM exercises may be limited by the requirements for immobilization during the process of skin grafting. However, if joints are not moved through their ROM for a prolonged period, contraction of joint capsules and shortening of tendon and muscles that cross joints can occur rapidly. Therefore, clear communication between therapists and physicians as to when it is appropriate to perform ROM exercises is an integral part of ensuring optimal results from the grafting procedures. Range of motion exercises should generally occur during twice-a-day therapy sessions that are coordinated with the PICU staff's routines and schedules. Ideally, these sessions should be scheduled during times of planned analgesia or anesthesia to allow more aggressive joint movements. Often, it is practical to schedule ROM exercises during dressing changes so that stretching can occur once bulky dressings have been removed. Therapists should set a goal of moving all joints through a full ROM while paying attention to factors (including anxiety, wound status, extremity perfusion, and security of the patient's airway and vascular access devices) that may concurrently compromise the patient's medical stability (48).

In addition to maintaining soft tissue and joint ROM, the rehabilitation interventions just described can also decrease the risk of secondary neurologic and skin injuries associated with prolonged immobility. Although fairly common, weakness and sensory deficits due to peripheral neuropathies unrelated to direct burn injury are easily overlooked, particularly in a critically ill child (25). Although a generalized peripheral neuropathy syndrome is the neuromuscular abnormality most frequently diagnosed in association with burn injuries, localized neuropathies due to compression or stretch injuries also occur. Focal neuropathies may by prevented through meticulous attention to proper positioning, splint checks for

TABLE 13.5

COMPONENTS OF A PEDIATRIC MEDICAL VENTILATION WEANING PROGRAM

Multidisciplinary evaluations to facilitate the weaning process	Evaluation team should include: physician (including physiatrist), nurse, pulmonary specialist, registered dietitian, physical therapist, occupational therapist, speech/language pathologist, child life/therapeutic recreation specialist, education specialist, psychologist, pharmacist, social worker
Readiness to wean: Initial evaluation tailored to the child's underlying conditions and comorbidities	Evaluation tests should include: chest films, blood gas (correlate with SaO_2, $ETCO_2$), tracheostomy culture/Gram stain, pulmonary function tests, secretion management evaluation, airway clearance capacity, bronchoscopy, test of strength and function of muscles involved in inspiration and exhalation, posture analysis
Establishment of a therapy program designed to meet the goals of the patient, the family, and the rehabilitation team	Program should accomplish the following: ■ Initiate rehabilitation interventions to increase inspiratory/expiratory muscle strength and endurance, increase chest wall movement, maximize skeletal muscle strength and endurance, maximize mobility, decrease spasticity, increase independence in activities of daily living, enhance vocal quality and oropharyngeal function, improve communication skills (verbal and nonverbal), promote cognitive development ■ Manage anxiety and compliance with therapy program and weaning from ventilation ■ Maximize nutritional status ■ Manage secretion and airway clearance through positioning, bronchodilators, chest physiotherapy, breathing exercises, suctioning, assistive cough, mechanical insufflation-exsufflation, oscillatory devices, speaking valves. ■ Establish a patient-driven weaning process that considers the energy expended for breathing and exercise, monitors the child's physiologic and psychologic response to weaning, decreases support by either increasing the length of time off of the ventilator or gradually decreasing the pressure or number of assisted breaths. ■ Plan for discharge and community reintegration.

Adapted from MacIntyre NR, Epstein SK, Carson S, et al. Management of patients requiring prolonged mechanical ventilation: Report of a NAMDRC consensus conference. *Chest* 2005;128:3937–54.

appropriate fit, and skin checks for early sign of pressure damage.

REHABILITATION AND WEANING FROM PROLONGED MECHANICAL VENTILATION

Prolonged mechanical ventilation (PMV) is defined as the need for mechanical ventilation for greater than 21 days for at least 6 hrs per day (32). In the pediatric population, systemic factors, mechanical factors, iatrogenic factors, complications of long-term hospitalization, and psychological factors may all contribute to the need for PMV (32). Determining which of these factors contributes to a particular child's need for PMV is critical in designing a customized weaning plan for that child.

The ideal environment for weaning children from PMV is a setting that offers a multidisciplinary coordinated team approach that can meet the following goals: (a) include the child and family as active team participants, (b) wean the child from mechanical ventilation and/or provide the least restrictive and invasive form of ventilation, (c) prevent/minimize secondary medical complications, (d) promote family–child interactions, (e) facilitate the growth and development of the child, (f) educate the family to care for the child at home, and (g) identify community resources to support the child and family at discharge (32). Common components of a pediatric ventilator weaning program that can be used in the rehabilitation setting are outlined in **Table 13.5** (40).

CONCLUSIONS AND FUTURE DIRECTIONS

Children admitted to the PICU for a variety of diagnoses and mechanisms of injury can benefit from rehabilitation services. Ideally, provided services should begin with a rehabilitation consult, where available, so that the physiatrist may direct the rehabilitation care with the team. A rehabilitation consult is best sought early in the course of treatment so that appropriate interventions, such as positioning and splinting, may be initiated to prevent muscle shortening, contractures, and other problems. Preventing complications when possible will make for a smoother recovery and, possibly, shorter rehabilitation course. Rehabilitation services are appropriate not only for children who are expected to recover but may also be useful in cases in which palliative care is the goal. Acute rehabilitation stays can help with family adjustment and training in caring for the child's needs and appropriate use of equipment prior to discharge home. Currently, intensivists and physiatrists are collaborating to examine various PICU interventions to understand their impact on long-term outcomes, such as neurologic recovery following ABI or SCI. Future efforts could be directed toward optimizing rehabilitation interventions to decrease such sequelae of critical illness as complications of prolonged bed rest.

KEY POINTS

■ A physiatrist should be consulted early in the course of the illness.

■ Positioning is important for the prevention of contractures and decubitus ulcers.

■ Prolonged bed rest negatively impacts multiple systems.

■ Bowel and bladder programs should be initiated in the PICU.

■ Palliative care and rehabilitation are not mutually exclusive.

■ Children with ABI or SCI often have related dysfunction in multiple other systems.

References

1. American Academy of Pediatrics. Committee on Bioethics and Committee on Hospital Care. Palliative Care for Children. *Pediatrics* 2000;106(2): 351–7.
2. American Spinal Injury Association. *International Standards for Neurological Classification of SCI*, revised 2000. Chicago, IL: American Spinal Injury Association, 2000.
3. Annegers JF, Hauser WA, Coan SP, et al. A population-based study of seizures after traumatic brain injuries. *N Engl J Med* 1998;338(1):20–42.
4. Annual Statistical Report, July 2005. National Spinal Cord Injury Statistical Center, University of Alabama at Birmingham. Facts and figures at a glance, at http://www.spinalcord.uab.edu.
5. Association for Children with Life Threatening or Terminal Conditions and their Families, Royal College of Paediatrics and Child Health. *A Guide to the Development of Children's Palliative Care Services.* London, 1997.
6. Baker C. Preventing ICU syndrome in children. *Paediatric Nurs* 2004; 16(10):32–5.
7. Beraldo PS, Neves EG, Alves CM, et al. Pyrexia in hospitalized spinal cord injury patients. *Paraplegia* 1993;31(3):186–91.
8. Blackman JA, Patrick PD, Buck ML, et al. Paroxysmal autonomic instability with dystonia after brain injury. *Arch Neurol* 2004;61:321–8.
9. Brink JD, Imbus C, Woo-Sam J. Physical recovery after severe closed head trauma in children and adolescents. *J Pediatr* 1980;97:721–7.
10. Burke DC. Review of subject: Models of brain injury rehabilitation. *Brain Inj* 1995;9:735–43.
11. Burns AS, Ditunno JF. Establishing prognosis and maximizing functional outcomes after spinal cord injury. *Spine* 2001;26(24S):S137–145.
12. Cheville A. Rehabilitation of patients with advanced cancer. *Cancer* 2001;92(4):1039–48.
13. Consortium for Spinal Cord Medicine. Prevention of thromboembolism in spinal cord injury. *J Spinal Cord Med* 1997;20:259–83.
14. Crill CM, Hak EB. Upper gastrointestinal tract bleeding in critically ill pediatric patients. *Pharmacotherapy* 1999;19(2):162–80.
15. Curley MA, Razmus IS, Roberts KE, et al. Predicting pressure ulcer risk in pediatric patients: The Braden Q scale. *Nurs Res* 2003;53:22–33.
16. Cyr C, Michon B, Pettersen G, et al. Venous thromboembolism after severe injury in children. *Acta Haematol* 2006;115:198–200.
17. Davies A. Psychological stress in critical care. *Paediatr Nurs* 1998; 10(2):24–6.
18. Dimopoulou I, Tsagarakis S, Theodorakopoulou M, et al. Endocrine abnormalities in critical care patients with moderate to severe head trauma: Incidence, pattern and predisposing factors. *Intensive Care Med* 2004;30: 1051–7.
19. Dyer I. Intensive care unit syndrome. *Nurs Times* 1996;92(35):58–9.
20. Esquenazi A. Upper Limb Amputee Rehabilitation and Prosthetic Restoration. In: Braddom RL, ed. *Physical Medicine & Rehabilitation*, 1st ed. Philadelphia: W.B. Saunders Company; 1996:275–88.
21. Field MJ, Behrman BE, eds. *When Children Die: Improving Palliative and End-of-Life Care for Children and Their Families.* Washington, DC: National Academic Press, 2003.
22. Fisher CG, Noonan VK, Smith DE, et al. Motor recovery, functional status, and health-related quality of life in patients with complete spinal cord injuries. *Spine* 2005;30(19):2200–7.
23. Gaebler-Spira D, Uellendahl J. Pediatric Limb Deficiencies. In: Molnar GA, Alexander MA, eds. *Pediatric Rehabilitation*, 3rd ed. Philadelphia: Hanley & Belfus; 1999:331–50.
24. Halar EM, Bell K. Immobility and inactivity: Physiological and functional changes, prevention and treatment. In: DeLisa JA, Gans BM, Walsh NE, et al., *Physical Medicine and Rehabilitation: Principles and Practice*, 4th ed., Vol. 2. Philadelphia: Lippincott Williams and Wilkins, 2005:1447–67.
25. Helm PA, Pandian G, Heck E. Neuromuscular problems in the burn patient: Cause and prevention. *Arch Phys Med Rehabil* 1985;66:451–53.
26. Herbert RD, Balnave RJ. The effect of position of immobilization on resting length, resting stiffness, and weight of the soleus muscle of the rabbit. *J Orthop Res* 1993;11(3):358–66.
27. Jaffe KM, Polissar NL, Fay GC, et al. Recovery trends over three years following pediatric traumatic brain injury. *Arch Phys Med Rehabil* 1995;76:17–26.
28. Jones SM, Fiser DH, Livingston RL. Behavioral changes in pediatric intensive care units. *Am J Dis Child* 1992;146(3):375–79.
29. Jones T, Ugalde V, Franks P, et al. Venous thromboembolism after spinal cord injury: Incidence, time course and associated risk factors in 16,240 adults and children. *Arch Phys Med Rehabil* 2005;86:2240–47.
30. Kazak AE, Boeving CA, Alderfer MA, et al. Posttraumatic stress symptoms during treatment in parents of children with cancer. *J Clin Oncol* 2005;23(30):7405–10.
31. Kirshblum SC, O'Connor KC. Predicting neurologic recovery in traumatic cervical spinal cord injury. *Arch Phys Med Rehabil* 1998;79:1456–66.
32. MacIntyre NR, Epstein SK, Carson S, et al. Management of patients requiring prolonged mechanical ventilation: Report of a NAMDRC consensus conference. *Chest* 2005;128:3937–54.
33. Maynard FM. Immobilization hypercalcemia following spinal cord injury. *Arch Phys Med Rehabil* 1986;67:41–4.
34. Mazzini L, Campini R, Angelino E, et al. Post-traumatic hydrocephalus: A clinical, neuroradiologic and neuropsychologic assessment of long-term outcome. *Arch Phys Med Rehabil* 2003;84:1637–41.
35. Melnyk BM, Alpert-Gillis L, Feinstein NF, et al. Creating opportunities for parent empowerment: program effects on the mental health/coping outcomes of critically ill young children and their mothers. *Pediatrics* 2004;113(6):597–607.
36. Miller CH, Quattrocchi KB, Frank EH, et al. Humoral and cellular immunity following severe head injury: Review and current investigations. *Neurol Res* 1991;13(2):117–24.
37. Minare P. Immobilization osteoporosis: A review. *Clin Rheumatol* 1989; 8:95–103.
38. Norton D. Calculating the risk: Reflections on the Norton Scale. *Decubitus* 1989;2:24–31.
39. O'Connor K. Pressure Ulcers. In: DeLisa JA, Gans BM, Walsh NE, et al., *Physical Medicine and Rehabilitation: Principles and Practice*, 4th ed., Vol. 2. Philadelphia: Lippincott Williams and Wilkins, 2005:1605–18.
40. Padman R, Alexander M, Thorogood C. Respiratory management of pediatric patients with spinal cord injuries: Retrospective review of the duPont experience. *Neurorehabil Neural Repair* 2003;17:32–6.
41. Pang D. Spinal cord injury without radiographic abnormalities in children, two decades later. *Neurosurgery* 2004;55(6):1325–43.
42. Pepe JL, Barba CA. The metabolic response to acute traumatic brain injury and implications for nutritional support. *J Head Trauma Rehabil* 1999;14(5):462–74.
43. Rasnake LK, Linscheid TR. Anxiety reduction in children receiving medical care: Developmental considerations. *J Dev Behav Pediatr* 1989;10:169–75.
44. Rennick JE, Johnston CC, Dougherty G, et al. Children's psychological responses after critical illness and exposure to invasive technology. *J Dev Behav Pediatr* 2002;23(3):133–44.
45. Rennick JE, Morin I, Kim D, et al. Identifying children at high risk for psychological sequelae after pediatric intensive care unit hospitalization. *Pediatr Crit Care Med* 2004;5(4):358–63.
46. Savage R. Identification, classification, and placement issues for students with traumatic brain injuries. *J Head Trauma Rehabil* 1991;6:1–9.
47. Schiffer J, Gur R, Nisim U, et al. Symptomatic patients after craniectomy. *Surg Neurol* 1997;47(3):231–37.
48. Sheridan RL. Burn Rehabilitation. *eMedicine*, http://www.emedicine.com/pmr/topic163.htm, Accessed July 18, 2006.
49. Stein P, Kayali F, Olson R. Incidence of venous thromboembolism in infants and children: data from the national hospital discharge survey. *J Pediatr* 2004;145:563–65.
50. Taggart P, Haining R. Rehabilitation of Burn Injuries. In: Molnar GE, Alexander MA, ed. *Pediatric Rehabilitation*, 3rd ed. Philadelphia: Hanley & Belfus; 1999:351–64.
51. Temkin NJ, Dikmen SS, Wilensky AJ, et al. A randomized, double-blind study of phenytoin for the prevention of post-traumatic seizures. *N Engl J Med* 1993;323:497–502.
52. Waites KB, Canupp KC, Edwards K, et al. Immunogenicity of pneumococcal vaccine in persons with spinal cord injury. *Arch Phys Med Rehabil* 1998;79(12):1504–9.
53. World Health Organization. International Classification of Functioning, Disability, and Health: ICF. Geneva: World Health Organization, 2001.

CHAPTER 14 ■ ETHICS

GEORGE E. HARDART • DENIS J. DEVICTOR • ROBERT D. TRUOG

Today's practicing pediatric intensivist is likely to face ethically challenging situations with regularity. The climate of the PICU is charged with forces that cause such situations to occur with much greater frequency than in general medical practice. These forces include the availability, power, and cost of life-sustaining technology, the fast pace and inherent uncertainty of treatment decisions, the common occurrence of end-of-life decisions and care, and the subtleties of surrogate decision making for children, particularly as they approach the age at which they can begin to decide for themselves.

This chapter begins with an introduction to the history of medical ethics and an overview of the ethical theories that are useful in understanding and framing moral dilemmas, followed by a discussion of informed consent and surrogate decision making. Mastery of these essential concepts is perhaps the most important tool for effectively managing ethically challenging situations. Finally, the chapter includes a comprehensive section on end-of-life care in the PICU. In that one of the most important duties of the pediatric intensivist is to assist patients and families through the dying process, a thorough understanding of this complex issue is required for all who teach and practice pediatric critical care.

THE FOUNDATION OF MEDICAL ETHICS

The terms "ethics" and "morality" are often used interchangeably, but most philosophers draw a subtle distinction between the two. *Morality* consists of social norms of behavior, and often varies dramatically between cultures. The discipline of *ethics*, on the other hand, involves the development of philosophic reasons for or against a set of moral judgments. Usually, the latter effort attempts to articulate and justify principles that form the foundation for rules of conduct and decision making in the face of competing moral claims.

Medical ethics is the discipline devoted to the identification, analysis, and resolution of value-based problems that arise in the care of patients. It is a special kind of ethics only insofar as it relates to the peculiar dilemmas that arise in medicine, not because it embodies or appeals to some special moral principles or methodology. The term "bioethics" is often used interchangeably with "medical ethics," although the former has a slightly broader meaning, including ethical problems that arise outside of the area of medicine (e.g., issues surrounding research on animals). In summary, the practice of medical ethics seeks to identify and resolve competing moral claims among patients, their families, healthcare professionals, healthcare institutions, and society at large.

The Development of Medical Ethics

Concern for ethical issues in medicine dates back at least to the time of Hippocrates. Nevertheless, until the middle of the 20th century, little additional thought was given to the unique problems that arise within the context of clinical practice and medical research. The revelations of the Nazi atrocities after World War II led to the reaffirmation of the importance of ethics in medicine and research and were directly responsible for the formulation of codes of ethics pertaining to research on human subjects (e.g., the Nuremberg Code in the late 1940s, followed by the declaration of Helsinki in 1964).

In the decades following World War II, the development of antibiotics, vaccines, and effective diagnostic and therapeutic technologies transformed medicine from a profession that focused on caring to one that focused on curing. The expectations of physicians and patients have grown considerably; yet, medical advances have brought with them ethical dilemmas that increasingly find their way into public and professional consciousness.

Publication of a 1962 *LIFE* magazine article entitled, "They Decide Who Lives, Who Dies," presented such an event. The article described the efforts of a committee of ordinary citizens, not physicians, in Seattle, who were charged with the task of allocating access to hemodialysis therapy (then a scarce resource) for critically ill patients who would die without it. The committee disbanded itself after it realized that its selection process was influenced by its own middle-class values, rather than by an objectively fair allocation procedure. Public—and then Congressional—dismay at the reality of scarce but effective medical technology led to the 1973 passage of the end-stage renal disease program. Under this legislation, the Federal Medicare Program assumed responsibility for anyone in need of chronic dialysis, regardless of socioeconomic status. Like many federal initiatives in the 1960s and 1970s, this program has proven to be far more costly than initially expected and serves as a lasting illustration of the pitfalls inherent with using governmental assurances of payment as a means for solving problems of medical scarcity (28).

The medical profession's attention to these issues was further heightened by a 1973 article in the *New England Journal of Medicine* that described the decision by physicians and parents to withhold treatment from 43 critically ill infants in the neonatal intensive care unit at Yale-New Haven Hospital (19). This account was among the first to bring attention to the fact that medical technology had reached a point at which the decision to end life had to be made deliberately by physicians and families.

Perhaps no event captured the importance of public and professional attention to these difficult issues more than the 1976 New Jersey Supreme Court Decision on Karen Ann Quinlan.

On the night of April 15, 1973, this 21-year-old woman experienced a respiratory arrest that left her in a persistent vegetative state. Her father petitioned the court for authority to be named as her guardian and for permission to discontinue the ventilator. His request was opposed by her doctors, the hospital, and the prosecutors for the local county and the state of New Jersey. The New Jersey Supreme Court ruled that the patient had a constitutional "right to privacy" to be removed from the ventilator if the family, the physicians, and the hospital ethics committee agreed. Despite the prevailing opinion of her doctors, she did not die when removed from the ventilator, but lived for almost another decade. This was the first of many cases that helped to shape our current views about the withdrawal of life-sustaining treatments.

Overview of Ethical Theories

Broadly speaking, two ethical theories—*utilitarianism* and *deontology*—have dominated Western intellectual tradition. Both theories attempt to provide a set of "first principles" for approaching ethical conflict. More recently, a number of alternative theories—some ancient and some new—have emerged as useful tools for analyzing complex ethical decisions. Perhaps the best known of these has come to be known as *principlism*, but several other theories offer unique and powerful perspectives and will be described in this section.

The Utilitarian and Deontological Theories

The utilitarian philosophy was developed in the 18th and 19th centuries by English philosophers Jeremy Bentham and John Stuart Mill. *Utilitarianism* is rooted in the thesis that an action or practice is right (when compared to any alternative action or practice) if it leads to the greatest possible balance of good consequences or the least possible balance of bad consequences in the world as a whole. According to this view, moral codes and traditions are designed to promote human welfare by maximizing benefits and minimizing harm.

The other dominant ethical theory, *deontology*, was heavily influenced by the writings of the philosopher Immanuel Kant. According to this approach, consequence is rejected as the first principle; Kant argued that actions should be guided by generalizable moral obligations or duties, regardless of consequences.

The ongoing debate about euthanasia illustrates the differences between these approaches. Utilitarians may argue, for example, that when a terminally ill patient requests to be killed, the consequences of complying with that request are favorable for everyone concerned. The patient's desires are satisfied, the physician can rest assured that the act was in the patient's best interest (as defined by the patient), and even society may benefit by not incurring the expenses associated with a prolonged dying process. Deontologists, on the other hand, feel that the prohibition against killing should stop us from taking the life of another, regardless of the consequences. Under this approach, euthanasia is always wrong, even if we are convinced that carrying it out does not harm anyone's interest. Some deontologists base their beliefs upon a religious perspective (the Ten Commandments are a typical list of deontologic principles), whereas others derive a set of duties and obligations by theoretical analysis. Even utilitarians often agree that rules have an important place in ethics, if only because of the inherent difficulties involved in predicting the consequences of our actions. To use the euthanasia example again, a deontologist might argue that, even though performing euthanasia does not *appear* to harm anyone's interest, the *long-term* consequences of permitting this act might be diminishment of our respect for human life and possible eventual erosion of the core values of the medical profession. This argument would be a reason to oppose euthanasia, even by the utilitarian standard.

Principlism

In reality, few people are pure deontologists or consequentialists. Most of us blend these two perspectives (as well as others) in our reasoning about ethical issues. In the search for practical guidance to moral dilemmas, therefore, leading ethical theorists over the last 30 years have turned instead to a "principles approach" to moral reasoning. For example, in what is widely regarded as a classic textbook on modern medical ethics, Tom Beauchamp and James Childress advocate four principles on which to base ethical analysis: respect for autonomy (self-determination), beneficence (doing good), nonmaleficence (avoiding harm), and justice (fair distribution) (8). When faced with a moral dilemma, the task is to identify the relevant ethical principles that bear on the case, which will suggest a set of rules that are pertinent to the situation. From these rules, the proper judgment regarding the particular case should be discernible.

The problem with this approach is that, because more than one principle may have bearing on any given case, conflicting rules and judgments may be the fruit of deliberation. Because principlism does not rank the four principles in order of priority, this approach falls short of comprehensively resolving many ethical dilemmas that arise in clinical practice. Nevertheless, a principles approach is often very useful for identifying the most salient ethical issues that arise in challenging clinical scenarios.

Other Ethical Theories

Virtue-based ethics represents perhaps the most ancient medical ethical theory, and it dominated Eastern and Western medical ethics until the 20th century. Although now overshadowed by the language of principles, duties, and rights, virtue ethics is reemerging as an important approach to thinking about moral issues in medicine (36). The basic premise of virtue ethics is that the character and motives of moral agents, such as physicians, matter greatly. Fidelity, truthfulness, compassion, justice, temperance, integrity, and fortitude are some of the moral virtues that are highly valued in physicians. Proponents of virtue ethics do not argue that it could replace or make unnecessary rules and principles: In a pluralistic society such as ours, minimum expectations must be established, and even the most virtuous person is capable of performing wrong actions. Conversely, a role for virtue in practice is made apparent through the recognition that it is not difficult for doctors to evade a set of rules if they are intent on doing so. Finally, a virtue-ethics approach may be particularly valuable when conflicts among principles arise; moral virtues can play a role in guiding the balancing of principles and arriving at morally acceptable resolutions.

Proponents of *case-based reasoning*, or *casuistic analysis*, argue that a principles-based approach is too indeterminate and abstract to be of much help with real-life dilemmas (29). They advocate instead for the use of *paradigmatic cases*, that is, real cases about which a consensus currently exists. As new cases arise, they are analyzed in terms of how they are similar to, or different from, the paradigmatic cases, a method referred to as *moral triangulation*. For example, since the "Baby Doe" episode in 1984, general agreement exists in medicine, law, and ethics that babies with Down syndrome and correctable surgical anomalies should undergo surgical repair of their conditions and not be allowed to die from them. Similarly, general agreement also prescribes that babies with Trisomy 13 or 18 who have potentially lethal congenital defects need not be offered life-prolonging therapies, but may ethically be treated with only comfort care. When faced with the problem of how to treat a newborn with congenital anomalies intermediate between those of Trisomy 21 and 13/18, a proponent of the case-based approach might attempt to address the question by first exploring the ways in which the child is more like an infant with Down syndrome or more like an infant with Trisomy 13/18. In combination with such factors as the severity of the defects and the preferences of the family, this approach would attempt to "triangulate" toward the most reasonable solution.

An alternative theory that has arisen from the feminist movement is an approach based on the primacy of "caring" (13). In its more radical form, this perspective minimizes the importance of ethical theory and principles and seeks resolutions to difficult cases that best preserve the relationships involved. As opposed to a principle-based approach, this perspective is less concerned with maintaining internal consistency and the observance of formal rules. When confronted with a case about whether to allow a small child to donate a kidney to a sibling, for example, a proponent of the "caring" approach would ask which of the alternative options would best promote the well-being of the relationships among the family and others involved.

Finally, a perspective that has developed within the fields of literature and the humanities focuses on the value of "narrative (14)." Unlike the terse case histories that tend to be favored in the busy hospital setting, this approach emphasizes the importance of understanding cases in all their detail and complexity. Rather than attempting to "shrink" cases to their essential elements and then apply a specific "rule" or "principle," the proponent of the narrative approach insist that only by analyzing cases in all their richness and texture can we hope to arrive at solutions that are sufficiently nuanced and sophisticated. Indeed, this approach hearkens back to the admonitions of many of the great medical clinicians who emphasized the overriding importance of careful history taking. These giants of medicine would undoubtedly be just as critical of our overreliance on invasive technology and imaging studies as the proponent of narrative is critical of "principles."

Applications and Limitations of Theories

It can be safely stated that no single "correct" ethical theory exists. When subjected to intense analytic scrutiny, all ethical theories have shortcomings and imperfections. The descriptions of the major ethical theories offered in this section are not intended to serve as a menu from which the reader should choose their favorite theory and apply it in their clinical practice. Rather, it is likely that knowledge of all these ethical theories will enhance moral decision making as it occurs at the bedside. It may be that, in discussions of rationing, utilitarian arguments are most appropriate for framing the issues, whereas in intrafamilial conflicts about treatment choices, it is possible that feminist ethics reasoning will be most helpful in resolving a dilemma. Finally, it should be noted that, more often than not, the application of each of these theories to individual cases will ultimately lead to similar moral conclusions; such convergence serves to strengthen our moral judgments.

Ethics and the Law

Physicians generally have one of two attitudes toward the law. Either they claim to be unconcerned about legal precedent and only interested in practicing "good medicine," or they are fearful of making any decision or taking any action without first learning whether it is "legal." Both extreme views could lead to naïve or imprudent decisions about difficult ethical dilemmas in clinical practice.

First, when considering legal precedents in ethical decision making, it is important to keep in mind that no single, monolithic statement can be made about the "law" in most ethical controversies. The body of law that supports the American legal system is actually the product of many factors. For example, legislative mandates or court decisions in one state do not hold as precedent or law in any other state. Superimposed on state law and legislation is the federal system, with its own jurisdictions, which can also disagree concerning key points.

Second, whereas both ethics and the law are concerned with identifying which actions are acceptable within a given society, they remain fundamentally distinct. Acting in accordance with the law is no guarantee that one is acting ethically, as emphasized by the Nuremberg Court in evaluating the actions of the Nazi concentration camp guards. Law, as it relates to morality, usually represents the minimum requirements regarding moral duties and rights for a given society. Law represents the floor, and not the ceiling, for standards about morality.

ESSENTIAL ELEMENTS OF MEDICAL DECISION MAKING

Informed Consent

Although the practice of obtaining informed consent is second nature to today's physicians, many view it as a burden imposed by lawyers. Viewed in this way, the communication process is reduced to the physician's effort to avoid a lawsuit. A more constructive mindset is that the informed consent process can actually help strengthen and improve communications in the physician–patient relationship. As noted by Gutheil and colleagues:

> Informed consent is not an empty gesture toward liability reduction, but an interaction between physician and patient, a dialogue intended not only to satisfy their legal requirements, but to do more as well. The real clinical opportunity offered by informed consent is that of transforming uncertainty from a threat into the very basis on which an alliance can be formed. (24)

From this perspective, it becomes clear that an understanding and appreciation of the role of informed consent is central to sound and ethical medical practice.

Many people are surprised that the idea that the patient should be the primary source of decision-making power in the physician–patient relationship is a very recent development, at least in historic terms. Dating from the age of Hippocrates until the very recent past, most decisions were the sole prerogative of the physician. This approach to medical care can no longer be justified, however, because it fails to respect the fundamental importance of the patient's values and goals by placing the clinician's value structure ahead of that of the patient. The ascendancy of respect for patient autonomy and the right to self-determination has become paramount only in the last several decades, yet the roots of this transformation are much deeper. The philosophic and ethical basis for self-determination can be found among the Medieval and Renaissance thinkers, who so greatly influenced the framers of the American Constitution and Bill of Rights. Philosophers such as John Locke, Edmund Burke, and Immanuel Kant, among others, articulated the intellectual foundation for the notion that it is not the State but the individual who is sovereign. In its modern form, informed consent must satisfy four requirements: competency, disclosure, understanding, and voluntariness.

Competency

A competent individual has the capacity to *understand* the therapy in question, *consider* the risks and benefits, *decide* upon a course of action, and *appreciate* the consequences of the choice (6). Although adults are generally presumed to be legally competent, children are considered incompetent in the United States until the age of 18 or 21, depending on the jurisdiction. In both ethics and law, however, this arbitrary age cutoff is overly simplistic. Two major exceptions deserve mention. *Emancipated minors* are deemed to be competent on the basis of legal definitions, whereas *mature minors* are competent on the basis of a judicial decision in a particular case. For example, many states define emancipated minors as those who are pregnant or a parent, those serving in the armed forces, or those living independent of guardians. Alternatively, minors who are not emancipated may nevertheless be deemed competent by a judge to make medical decisions on their own, which may occur, for example, when a judge determines that a minor's Jehovah's Witness religious beliefs are sufficiently mature and considered that the patient may legally refuse blood products, despite the wishes of his parents or caregivers.

Although physicians implicitly assess their patient's competence during virtually all their encounters, questions of competence typically arise when the patient's behavior is unusual, when "clearly beneficial" treatment is refused, or when decisions with serious consequences (such as end-of-life decisions) are being made. When faced with such questions, it is sometimes helpful to draw a distinction between competence and decision-making capacity. A thorough evaluation can determine that a patient who was formerly granted the legal presumption of competence has been incapacitated by medical illness or mental disorder and has forfeited his decision-making authority. Conversely, it is possible to have decision-making capacity—the ability to understand medical information, reason about risks and benefits, appreciate consequences, and make stable choices—but still be considered legally incompetent. This point is most strikingly displayed in the case of adolescents.

The legal age of majority is an oversimplification of the maturational and developmental process in children. Children as young as 6 or 7 years of age are often able to have reasoned opinions about certain aspects of their care, and most adolescents have views and perspectives that deserve serious consideration. The fact that parents must give legal consent for medical treatments performed on minor children does not mean that the opinions of the children and adolescents should be considered irrelevant or ignored. In 1995, the Committee on Bioethics of the American Academy of Pediatrics issued a statement that advocated a dramatic broadening of the authority ceded to minor patients in medical decision making (1). In this statement, they recommended that, for older school-aged children (e.g., 9–12 years old), physicians should seek the patient's assent for proposed tests and treatments in developmentally appropriate situations, such as an orthopedic device to manage scoliosis in an 11-year-old. However, they did note that, "in situations in which the patient will have to receive medical care despite his or her objection, the patient should be told that fact and should not be deceived." For adolescent patients (e.g., 14–17 years old) the committee encouraged physicians to obtain informed consent for a broad range of tests and treatments, provided the patient has decisional capacity and law permits it. They did, however, encourage parental involvement in such cases. These recommendations have proved to be controversial in theory and challenging to implement in practice. It has been argued that these recommendations go too far, and that it is ultimately in the best interest of minor patients that parents retain final decision-making authority (38).

Disclosure

The concept of disclosure (of information) has been, and remains, a central component of the doctrine of informed consent. The question of what constitutes "sufficient information" to ensure a truly informed consent has been addressed by the courts. Until recently, the accepted practice held physicians to the *professional standard*, which required physicians to disclose only that information that would be customarily disclosed by their colleagues. However, in the pivotal 1972 case of *Canterbury v. Spence*, the Federal Appeals Court in Washington, DC, established the *reasonable person standard*, which holds that the degree of disclosure should be determined by the information that a reasonable person (or reasonable group of persons, such as a jury) would require to make a decision regarding medical therapy.

Understanding

The inclusion of understanding in the definition of informed consent addresses one of the historic concerns about disclosure as the sole determinant of informed consent. One can easily imagine situations in which understanding does not occur despite a *competent* decision maker and full *disclosure* of information. If the physician uses excessive medical jargon or the patient is ignorant of "basic" medical concepts, then understanding is unlikely. Similarly, because of the effects of illness or the stress of an illness in a loved one, a patient or family member may not "hear" what is said, in which case understanding is not achieved. How can the physician ensure that the decision maker fully understands the nature, implications, and extent of the therapy under consideration? The answer is that the physician cannot *guarantee* complete understanding, but has an obligation to try to establish an adequate level of understanding for the decision at hand. This shifts the paradigm of informed consent away from a one-sided disclosure of information by the physician, to a two-way communication process, whereby the physician and decision maker ask questions of each other and learn about one another. Misconceptions are exposed, pockets of ignorance are addressed, and trust is established. Through this process, understanding is maximized.

Voluntariness

An action is voluntary when it is free from the coercive and manipulative influences of others. Coercive influences are those for which the weight of the influence is derived from a credible threat, such as when revocation of privileges is used to "encourage" prisoners to consent to medical research. Influences may be manipulative if a physician takes advantage of the unequal distribution of information and knowledge in the physician–patient relationship to "nonpersuasively" influence the outcome of a decision. Such influences may be subtle or blatant, ranging from the withholding or de-emphasizing of information that might affect the patient's decision, to outright lying in deliberations with patients. However, the obligation to avoid coercion and manipulation does not alleviate the professional obligation to exert *persuasive* influence over patients when one course of action is clearly indicated, through the use of persistent and rational argument (for example, when a competent patient refuses to undergo an appendectomy for simple appendicitis).

Exceptions to Informed Consent

Several exceptions to informed consent have traditionally been recognized. The first, and least controversial, is the *emergency exception*, which allows a physician to treat a patient when significant harm is imminent, when the patient is incapable of consenting, and when no surrogate is immediately available.

More controversial is the *therapeutic privilege exception*. Under this exception, physicians may forgo attempts to obtain informed consent when they believe that the patient will experience more harm than benefit from the disclosure. Recently, the tendency in law and ethics has been to constrain this exception because it assumes that the physician knows what is best for the patient. This assumption violates the general view that patients themselves provide the most reliable information about what is in their best interest; it also ignores a body of empirical evidence that indicates that physicians systematically underestimate the desire of patients to know their diagnosis and to be involved in decision making (5).

The use of placebos is a tempting application of the therapeutic privilege exception that is almost always unjustified. For example, the secret administration of a placebo rather than an active agent to a patient with substance abuse problems may be thought to be justified as being in the patient's best interests in overcoming addiction, but the loss of trust that occurs when the patient realizes that he has been tricked almost always leads to more harm than good.

Finally, the "waiver" exception arises when patients choose to relinquish decisional authority to the physician. Although the legitimacy of waivers is generally accepted, some do express concern that widespread use of waivers could have a negative effect on the general practice of informed consent.

Proxy Decision Making

Medical decisions for patients who are incompetent must be made by proxy, or surrogate, decision makers. The justification for proxy decisions depends on whether the patient was formerly competent or never competent. For formerly competent patients, decisions are based on the principle of respect for autonomy, just as for competent patients. However, in the case of never-competent patients who have, therefore, never been autonomous decision makers, decisions must be justified through appeal to the principles of beneficence (the provision of benefits) and nonmaleficence (the avoidance of harm), which direct proxies to choose the course that is "best" for the patient.

The Substituted Judgment Standard

The formulation for decision making when the patient was formerly competent is called *substituted judgment*. Under this approach, proxies are asked to discern the course of action that is most consistent with the patient's longstanding wishes, beliefs, values, and life goals. In other words, an attempt is made to preserve the patient's autonomy by reconstructing, as precisely as possible, his subjective beliefs. Although this approach is sound in theory, it becomes difficult and imprecise when put into practice. Is the surrogate close enough to the patient to truly reconstruct his values and preferences? Did the patient discuss these preferences frankly, or is the surrogate merely imagining what the patient would have wanted? Is the decision partially based on the surrogate's own interests in the outcome of the decision, or solely on the patient's interests?

Despite its shortcomings, however, the substituted judgment standard remains the accepted approach for formerly competent patients. Some have proposed that this approach be abandoned in favor of others that address its shortcomings, such as approaches that provide better approximations of the patient's preferences (e.g., advanced directives) and those that rely on more objective criteria for decisions (e.g., the best-interests standard).

The Best-Interests Standard

If patients have never expressed preferences, beliefs, and values, it naturally follows that these cannot be used as a basis for proxy decision making. Such is the case for never-competent persons, such as young children and mentally retarded adults. In these cases, in which subjective information is unavailable, more objective strategies must be utilized to make medical decisions on their behalf. The best-interests standard asks decision makers to perform an analysis of the benefits and burdens of a medical situation and arrive at the decision that maximizes the benefit-to-burden ratio for the patient. This standard, although being the age-old modus operandi for parental decision making, also faces many hurdles in application. Whereas in its ideal state it is an objective criterion, in practice it is open to value judgments on many levels. The personal preferences of the decision maker, which should not be considered in the benefit-versus-burden analysis, may enter into the decision about whether the life is "meaningful" or is "worth living." Additionally, the "social worth" of the patient and the burdens of the patient on the family and society may slip into the benefit-versus-burden analysis. Surrogates are, therefore, admonished to weigh the burdens and benefits from the patient's perspective—never from their own.

Advance Directives

In response to the shortcomings of proxy decision making, advance directives that attempt to preserve the patient's subjective values during times of legal incompetence have been developed. The ideal advance directive would be readily available in emergencies, frequently updated to reflect a person's current preferences and values, broad enough to be useful in a multitude of situations, and specific enough to provide clear guidance in decision making.

Most states now have legislation that recognizes the legality of certain advance directives. Written and oral instructions, often called *living wills*, contain treatment directives to be followed if and when a patient becomes incapable of making treatment decisions. These documents have been criticized as being too ambiguous in many critical decisions, because no one could possibly anticipate every potential occurrence.

In an attempt to approach the ideal advance directive, the *healthcare durable power of attorney* has emerged as an increasingly popular and available alternative to living wills. Unlike living wills, which specify treatment decisions in advance, the healthcare proxy establishes a decision-making process. Healthcare proxy laws permit patients to delegate the authority for their medical treatment decisions in the event of incapacity. Under these circumstances, many of the theoretical problems with proxy decision making evaporate, because the individual has voluntarily transferred the right to decide to another. The Patient Self-Determination Act, passed by Congress in 1991, requires that all Medicare/Medicaid participating institutions inform patients of their rights to formulate advance directives upon admission.

SPECIAL TOPICS IN MEDICAL DECISION MAKING

Religious Beliefs in the Decision-Making Process

Although the courts have acknowledged the virtually unlimited right of competent adults to refuse medical treatment, they have been much more protective of children. The threshold for overriding parents' wishes depends on an objective assessment of the risks to the child. In general, if the circumstances do not involve life-threatening choices or certain risks of substantial harm to the child, the physician is obligated to respect the decisions of the parents, even when the physician strongly disagrees with the choice. In some jurisdictions, for example, parents are permitted the right to refuse standard immunizations for religious reasons.

However, as the threat to the child increases and the benefits of treatment are more certain, actions to override parental choices are not only legally supported, but, in most jurisdictions, required. Numerous court opinions have upheld the notion, first articulated in the 1944 case of *Prince* v. *Massachusetts*, that a parent may make a martyr of himself because of religious convictions, "but he is not free to make a martyr of his child." In numerous decisions since then, courts have upheld the right of physicians to override parental refusal of transfusions or other accepted therapy when a child's life is at risk. Court-ordered blood transfusions for the children of Jehovah's Witness parents have become perhaps the best-known and most frequent example of this type of judicial involvement.

Uncertainty

Physicians (and patients, as well) virtually never make decisions without some degree of uncertainty. Decisions are based on probabilities, intuition, clinical experience, and medical knowledge. Even the most "scientific" of these, medical knowledge, can rarely be said to be certain. The knowledge of medicine is based on information derived from experiments, and these experiments are based on probabilistic estimates of their chances of revealing "truth." In other words, physicians are constantly making decisions based on a less-than-ideal amount of information, and they cannot predict with certainty the consequences of their decisions. Given that uncertainty is an essential part of decision making for physicians, the degree of uncertainty will vary from decision to decision, as will the magnitude of the consequences of those decisions. Almost 50 years ago, Renée Fox identified three sources of uncertainty in physician practice: (a) insufficient mastery of available knowledge, (b) limitations of available knowledge, and (c) physician difficulty in distinguishing personal ignorance from limitations in available knowledge.

With regard to decisions involving life and death in the PICU, uncertainty is frequently high and the consequences extreme. Despite uncertainty, however, decisions must be made, and physicians respond in different ways. Although many of their responses are predictable and understandable, one noteworthy tendency is a reluctance on the part of physicians to disclose uncertainty to the patient and family and, sometimes, to disregard altogether the uncertainty inherent in the decision-making process. In fact, Fox observed that, as physicians moved from theoretical discussions about uncertain decisions to actual clinical encounters, their disregard for any element of uncertainty became highly pervasive. This disregard for uncertainty frequently is translated into certainty about the proper course of action when discussing the situation with the patient and family. Although this aura of certainty may have positive effects (maintaining trust in the physician–patient relationship, avoidance of stress within the patient and family, timeliness of decisions, etc.), it has been argued that this "mask of infallibility" also serves to maintain professional control over decision making and to exclude the patient and family from meaningful participation in the decision-making process (30).

Rationing

American society is acutely aware that the financial costs of the US healthcare system are staggering, and this reality is naturally transmitted to clinicians, who feel a sense of duty to use healthcare dollars efficiently in treating patients. This pressure is intensified by the prevalence of managed care organizations that routinely track the money that clinicians spend in treating patients and frequently equate good performance with low cost. Ethical issues are raised by the possibility that bedside physicians might "microallocate" resources (i.e., refrain from providing potentially beneficial treatment based on monetary cost or other limitations). Traditionally, physicians have had fiduciary relationships with their patients that obligate them to serve the patient's health interests without compromise. This traditional approach has come under increasing attack as financial pressures on physicians and hospitals have mounted.

In allocating *absolutely* scarce resources, such as ICU beds, physicians have long been responsible for triaging the recipient of the resource, based on need, ability to benefit, or the principle of "first come, first served." On the other hand, a healthcare budget represents a *relatively* scarce resource; if the patient, insurance company, or society were willing to pay the price, then the treatment could be provided. Until recently, physicians have considered it unethical to deny patients any treatment that is only relatively scarce (i.e., to deny a treatment on purely financial grounds). As we increasingly acknowledge that the healthcare budget is not infinite, however, this old dichotomy is breaking down, and both clinicians and ethicists are exploring ways to ration resources that are only relatively scarce in an open and equitable manner. This new development is not without its critics, who hold that doctors must uncompromisingly make the welfare of their individual patients their primary objective. They further argue that, while healthcare costs to the nation are high, resources in this country are plentiful, and it is a fiction to suppose that the money saved through cheaper medical care would be diverted to nobler purposes in society. More likely, those dollars will go toward the profit margin of an institution or toward a societal expenditure with no relationship to healthcare. To quote Marcia Angell, "Doctors should continue to care for each patient unstintingly, even while they join with other citizens to devise a more efficient and just health care system." (4)

Family Interests in Medical Decision Making

Surrogate decision makers are usually family members or others with close, intimate relationships to the patient that give the surrogates' decisions legitimacy, because presumably they know the patient's preferences very well and are motivated by close emotional ties to act in the patient's best interest. Paradoxically, one of the main criticisms of proxy decision making is that family members may be *too close* to act as proxies and may make decisions based on their own lives and interests and not truly on those of the patient; it is possible that the broad range of acceptable options available to proxies will make detection of these conflicts very difficult. Others feel that this is an oversimplified conception of the physician–patient relationship that does not acknowledge the complexity of family relationships and the interdependency of individual and family interests. For example, imagine a young woman who is a loving mother, sister, and daughter. It is extremely unlikely that she would make any important decision, such as taking a new job in a different city, without considering how the decision would impact her family. It is argued that this woman would obviously want family interests considered in her important healthcare decisions, and that to think of this as a conflict of interest, with herself and her family as adversaries, would be inaccurate and a disservice to all involved (26). Supporting this view, a recent study of adult intensivists, pediatric intensivists, and neonatologists found that a majority of all three groups believed that family interests are legitimate considerations in medical decision making and that the physician–patient relationship is not exclusive (25).

The parent–child relationship represents a very special type of surrogate decision-making role. Traditionally, the parent–child relationship is one of the few situations in which the state grants authority to one individual over another. Furthermore, unlike the state, parents are not bound by the best-interests criterion when dealing with their children. For example, consider such common parental decisions as placing children in daycare or in the hands of a teenage baby-sitter, or requiring them to do household chores. It would be difficult to argue that exposing children to the countless microbes in daycare or to an inexperienced caregiver is strictly in their best interests. Despite this, parents daily make decisions such as these for their children. Such decisions—and parental authority in general—are justified by an appeal to family welfare and character, recognizing that children, as family members, have certain responsibilities to the family. Thus, in our society and law, the greatest latitude is given to parents in making healthcare decisions for their minor children. Significantly less leeway is given to families in deciding for adult family members and, when the state is called upon to decide, it must strictly adhere to the best-interests standard.

Consent for Practicing Procedures on Newly Deceased Patients

The use of dead patients for teaching purposes has been a source of controversy that dates back at least to the Middle Ages. Some have argued that it is ethically justifiable to perform practice procedures on the newly dead without permission from the family, because these procedures cannot harm the deceased, substantial social benefit is to be gained, and families could not realistically be expected to discuss consent at such a difficult time (35). Indeed, a recent study showed that 39% of training programs in emergency and critical care medicine use newly dead patients to teach various resuscitation procedures (for example, endotracheal intubation, central line placement, and pericardiocentesis). Few of these programs obtain either verbal or written consent from the families (10).

Despite the frequency of this practice without consent, some have argued that teaching procedures on newly deceased patients is ethical only when permission is first obtained from the family. In addition, given its sensitive nature, this teaching technique should be reserved only for those who truly need to master the skills and only as the culmination of a structured learning sequence, not a haphazard event (10).

ESSENTIAL ELEMENTS OF END-OF-LIFE CARE

The Goals of Care

Approximately 50,000 children die in the United States each year; 20%–25% of these deaths occur in the PICU. These statistics, coupled with the fact that the death of a child is always extraordinarily tragic, highlight the critical role that pediatric intensivists play in end-of-life care. In this section, issues pertaining to the dying process in the PICU and the healthcare team's role in that process will be addressed. These issues have the most relevance for those patients whose goals of care have been redirected from life-sustaining, curative goals to comfort-ensuring goals, usually patients with terminal illnesses or other conditions for which the benefits of further life-sustaining therapy are in question (e.g., neurologically devastated patients).

Implicit in the phrase "redirecting the goals of care" is that care is never withdrawn from a patient, only life-sustaining treatment. Although this is arguably a semantic point, studies have shown that physicians actually spend less time caring for patients with do-not-resuscitate (DNR) orders than they spend caring for patients without them. Indeed, the withdrawal of care is one of the greatest fears of patients and families in these situations. Thinking in terms of the goals of care for an individual patient can aid the physician in discussions with the healthcare team and the family when making or revising a management plan.

Delivering Bad News

Effective communication is particularly important when dealing with critically ill patients and their families. Unfortunately, doctors receive limited training in communicating with patients. Studies show that patients, families, nurses, social workers, and chaplains often complain of the brevity and poor choice of words doctors use in these settings (23). Although the approach to each meeting in which bad news is conveyed must be individualized, several strategies may prove helpful for the pediatric intensivist:

- *Prepare in advance.* Know who will be in the meeting and their relationship to the patient before entering the room. Anticipate questions and prepare answers that will be clear, direct, and understandable to the family.
- *Have everyone seated.* Studies have shown that families like to be seated near the door when receiving bad news, so as to reduce the feeling of being trapped. Do not stand during the conversation. Families find this particularly offensive, and it has been shown that people consistently think the doctor spent less time with them when the physician was standing during the conversation. Introduce yourself and all your colleagues by title and name. Although many families cannot remember anyone's name after hearing tragic news, they appreciate the personal connection that the formal introduction establishes.
- *Avoid jargon.* Doctors and nurses easily slip into the jargon associated with the intensive care culture, but these loose terms only confuse families or lead to misconceptions that can be difficult to resolve.
- *Talk less.* Studies show that family satisfaction with meetings is inversely correlated to the percentage of time occupied by physician speech (34). Avoid opening meetings with a long monologue. Use the beginning of meetings to determine the family's level of understanding, specific areas of concern, and desire for information.
- *Show compassion.* Although most physicians believe that they show appropriate compassion, families consistently believe the opposite after they receive bad news. Many want to hear an expression of sorrow by the healthcare team as an affirmation of their grief. They also wish to be allowed time to talk and express their feelings.
- *Avoid distractions.* To the extent possible, physicians should establish a therapeutic environment in which to share the sensitive information. They should leave pagers outside the room, position someone near the door to avoid interruptions, and ensure follow-up, both immediately and in the following days and weeks with appropriate counselors (40).

The manner in which difficult news is conveyed can leave a lasting impression; physicians, especially critical care physicians, would be well served to master these skills as well as they do some of the more technical aspects of practice.

Do-Not-Resuscitate Orders

Until 1976, no hospital in the United States publicly acknowledged that it provided care that was not intended to prolong and preserve life. In that year, both the Massachusetts General Hospital and Boston's Beth Israel Hospital acknowledged their use of DNR orders in the *New England Journal of Medicine.* Since that time, DNR orders have become commonplace; in fact, the Joint Commission on Accreditation of Healthcare Organizations now requires hospitals to have DNR policies. Although they are ubiquitous, DNR orders and policies are not without problems in theory and implementation.

For example, the name itself implies that the choice is whether to resuscitate or not, implying that resuscitation is possible, but will not be attempted. For many dying patients, the outcomes from resuscitation are dismal. This problem has been reinforced on television and in the movies, where high rates of successful resuscitation have generated false expectations among the public at large (18). For these reasons, many hospitals have adopted a new terminology, referring instead to "do-not-attempt-resuscitation," or DNAR. This conveys to families that, even if resuscitation is attempted, the results may be uncertain at best.

In addition, DNR orders are often vague and open to interpretation, leaving substantial opportunity for miscommunication and error. Does "resuscitation" refer to treatment of an acute cardiac arrest (intubation and ventilation, chest compressions, cardioversion, and medications), or does it also mean "do-not-intubate" for such conditions as respiratory failure secondary to pneumonia? Should patients with DNR orders receive suctioning for airway secretions, be treated with antibiotics, or be given tube feedings? Should they be excluded from the ICU or denied palliative surgery? Such difficulties in implementation have led to the development of novel approaches to DNR policies, such as procedure-specific DNR policies and goal-directed DNR orders.

Finally, DNR orders are unique in that they focus exclusively on what will *not* be done, rather than what will be done. In this sense, they address only a small fraction of the issues that arise in the care of seriously ill patients. As such, patients with DNR orders often feel that they have been abandoned by their caregivers. Indeed, as previously mentioned, studies have shown that physicians do, in fact, spend less time caring for patients who have DNR orders. This is unfortunate, because patients with DNR orders often need more attention in the form of aggressive palliative care than do patients who are not imminently dying. Many hospitals now recognize this adverse effect of DNR orders and have responded with the development of palliative care services that focus on what can be done for the dying patient, rather than what will be withheld.

Forgoing Life-Sustaining Treatments

The rights of patients or their surrogates to refuse or remove unwanted medical treatment, even if such a decision involves life-sustaining therapy, have been supported by the United States Supreme Court, a special Presidential Commission, and in policy statements by the American Medical Association, the Society for Critical Care Medicine, and the American Thoracic Society.

In discussions about whether or not to provide life-sustaining therapies, several issues arise commonly, including the distinction between ordinary and extraordinary treatments, the distinction between withholding a treatment and withdrawing a treatment, the appropriate role of sedatives and analgesics in the care of the dying, and whether artificial nutrition and hydration ("tube" feedings) may ever be forgone. These issues are discussed below.

The Ordinary/Extraordinary Distinction

One of the most commonly used justifications for withholding "high-tech" therapy from patients is the belief that "extraordinary" treatments are not ethically mandatory. For example, one study showed that 74% of physicians and nurses think that the ordinary/extraordinary distinction is helpful in resolving ethical dilemmas (43). Although this terminology is still used in the writings of some religious traditions, clinicians should understand that the distinction between ordinary and extraordinary treatments is not considered to be helpful when attempting to reason through the ethical aspects of difficult decisions. Consider two alternative interpretations of the ordinary/extraordinary distinction. One interpretation would be that ordinary treatments are *customarily* performed, whereas extraordinary treatments are not. Clearly, however, a simple appeal to what is customary cannot suffice as a justification for what is morally required. In addition, from a legal perspective, the courts have explicitly rejected the view that any relationship exists between what is "customary" and what is "legal." Another interpretation of the ordinary/extraordinary distinction would hold that ordinary treatments are morally required, whereas extraordinary treatments are morally optional. However, this is essentially a circular argument, because it claims that ordinary treatments are morally required because they are ordinary, and extraordinary treatments are morally optional because they are extraordinary.

In a study that asked pediatricians about their views on the repair of duodenal atresia in healthy babies and in babies with Down syndrome, most pediatricians said that duodenal atresia was an "ordinary" procedure in the case of healthy infants but an "extraordinary" procedure in the case of babies with Down syndrome (41). In that the procedure was the same in each case, the use of the terms "ordinary" and "extraordinary" served to mask the ethical judgments that were being made about the nature of the clinical condition.

A much more legitimate and useful approach to thinking about whether a procedure is ethically required is to inquire about the balance of the benefits versus the burdens for a particular procedure in a particular patient. In other words, rather than relying on such terminology as ordinary and extraordinary to decide whether a treatment should be offered, it should be considered whether the proposed benefits exceed the burdens. If, for example, a child with a malignancy is very

unlikely to survive even with the administration of highly toxic chemotherapy, then the burdens of that therapy clearly exceed the benefits. On the other hand, physicians and society now generally agree that the benefits of repairing duodenal atresia in patients with Down syndrome exceed the burdens, and thus the procedure is morally required.

The Withholding/Withdrawing Distinction

Is there a difference between stopping a treatment once it is started and not starting it in the first place? In other words, is there an ethical difference between deciding not to intubate a patient because we do not think that he will recover, and extubating a patient who has failed to recover despite a period of ventilation? Surveys have repeatedly shown that physicians believe a difference does exist. For example, a 1993 study reported that 66% of physicians and nurses discern an ethical difference between withdrawing and withholding a treatment, and nearly half agreed with the statement "there is an emerging consensus. . . that withdrawing a treatment is ethically different from withholding or not starting it" (43). In another survey of 360 attending physicians, house staff, and medical students, 73% felt that withdrawing is different from withholding (11). These reports indicate that physicians are much more comfortable in withholding treatments than in withdrawing them.

It is interesting that this strong opinion reported among clinicians is strikingly at odds with the prevailing view among ethicists and lawyers. Legal scholars and ethicists have been quite consistent in expressing the opinion that doctors should not differentiate between decisions to withhold or withdraw medical treatments. In the landmark *Cruzan* case, for example, justices from the US Supreme Court wrote that doctors should consider decisions to withhold and withdraw as equivalent, to ensure that patients receive adequate trials of therapy. A typical example occurs in the delivery room, when the viability of premature babies is often difficult to assess in the moments immediately following birth. The Supreme Court's decision implies that physicians should deal with this uncertainty by proceeding with resuscitation, but that they should be willing to withdraw the life-sustaining treatment if, after a trial of therapy, further support is no longer justified. Despite these opinions from law and philosophy, clinicians persist in believing that these two actions are differentiated. Part of the reason is clearly psychological. Physicians feel more responsible for the death of a patient when it results from the withdrawal of a therapy than they do when it results from the withholding of a therapy. This psychological distinction is important and cannot be made to disappear by legal or philosophic reasoning, no matter how persuasive. Nevertheless, when confronted with these situations, physicians should consider the perspectives from law and philosophy, because in many cases adoption of these views will lead to better clinical decision making.

Medical Nutrition and Hydration

Should techniques for providing medical nutrition and hydration (intravenous fluids, parenteral nutrition, tube feedings, etc.) be considered medical treatments? If so, can they then be ethically withdrawn by the same process and criteria that are used for other types of medical treatment? In other words, if it is ethically acceptable to withdraw a ventilator from a terminally ill patient, is it also ethically acceptable to withdraw medically provided nutrition and hydration? (Note that this question does not propose withholding oral feedings from patients who want to eat or drink.) A gradually emerging consensus in both law and ethics answers these questions in the affirmative (33). A large number of court decisions, including that in the above-mentioned *Cruzan* case, concluded that medically provided nutrition and hydration should be considered medical treatments and that patients or their surrogates should have the right to refuse them. The decision of whether or not to administer this therapy should be based on the same criteria outlined earlier for other treatments; that is, an analysis of the balance between the benefits and burdens of providing the therapy. This consensus was recently challenged in the highly publicized case of Terry Schiavo, a 41-year-old woman in a persistent vegetative state, whose husband and parents were locked in a decade-long legal duel over the husband's decision as legal surrogate to withdraw medical nutrition and hydration from his wife. Despite her parents' attempts—through the courts, the political process, and involvement of the national media—to stop the withdrawal of nutrition and hydration, the courts consistently decided in favor of the husband as legal surrogate, and she died after withdrawal of nutrition and hydration in March 2005. Although this case did not seriously challenge the legal status of medical nutrition and hydration as medical interventions that can be refused or withdrawn, it did expose a public rift in the moral acceptance of this practice (37).

Many clinicians have been reluctant to accept the withdrawal of medical nutrition and hydration, at least in part because "feeding" seems to be such a basic and fundamental aspect of the care they provide to their patients. In the terminology of the distinction discussed earlier, it seems so "ordinary." However, this provides yet another example of the inadequacies of the ordinary/extraordinary distinction, because for certain patients, particularly those who are permanently unconscious or imminently dying, medically administered feedings can no longer provide any benefit.

Pediatricians have been particularly slow to acknowledge this emerging consensus (21) for several reasons. First, prognoses are often more uncertain in children, given their remarkable ability to recover from injury. Second, even normal newborns need assistance with feedings, so pediatricians are less likely to see artificial feedings as a "medical" treatment. Third, whereas the hospice experience shows that refusal of food and water is frequently seen in elderly patients who are dying a natural death, the death of a child is never a "natural" event, and caregivers are reluctant to accept it with apparent passivity. Nevertheless, the principles that have evolved in governing the administration or withdrawal of medically provided feedings in adults are equally applicable in children, and no reason is justifiable to treat the pediatric population differently.

Sedatives and Analgesics in the Care of the Dying

Physicians who care for patients in a PICU will be called upon to discontinue life support from dying patients. In these tragic circumstances, the question then becomes how best to manage the patient during the dying process. Some erroneously believe that no sedatives or analgesics should be given in these situations, based on their belief that it is important both ethically and legally that the patient die from his underly-

ing disease, without any contribution from the respiratory or cardiac depression that are frequent side effects of these medications.

The reluctance of many physicians to aggressively treat the pain and suffering experienced by the terminally ill has been one of the most powerful forces driving the movement in favor of euthanasia and physician-assisted suicide. Individuals who have watched loved ones die without adequate pain relief have spearheaded this movement, firm in the belief that patients should have the opportunity to commit suicide if their suffering is unbearable, particularly when physicians seem unwilling to do whatever is necessary to control the suffering. This unwillingness on the part of the physician is unfortunate, particularly as nothing in the law, ethics, or any of the major religious traditions precludes physicians from aggressively treating the pain and suffering of the terminally ill, even when such treatment may hasten a patient's demise. Nevertheless, it has been shown that as many as 40% of doctors and nurses give inadequate pain medication, most often out of fear of hastening a patient's death (43).

The ethical principle that is relevant to this question is the *Doctrine of Double Effect*, originally developed within the Catholic tradition but now widely acknowledged in other religious traditions, as well as in law and philosophy. The doctrine states that when an action has two effects, one of which is inherently good and the other inherently bad, it can be justified if certain conditions are met (**Fig. 14.1**). For example, the administration of morphine to a dying patient produces both a good effect (relief of pain and suffering) and the potential for a bad effect (hastening the patient's death through respiratory depression). The conditions that must be satisfied in order for the action to be justified are:

- *The action in itself must be good or, at least, morally indifferent.* (Administration of the morphine itself is morally indifferent.)
- *The agent must intend only the good effect and not the evil effect. The evil effect is foreseen, not intended. It is allowed, not sought.* (In the case of administering morphine to a terminally ill patient, the physician must intend only the relief of the patient's pain and suffering. Respiratory depression and the potential for an earlier death is a foreseen complication, but is not sought.)
- *The evil effect cannot be a means to the good effect.* (If the physician administers a bolus of potassium chloride instead

1. Act—morally good or neutral
2. Good effect is intended
3. Bad effect merely foreseen
4. Bad effect not the means to the good effect
5. Proportionality—good must outweigh the bad

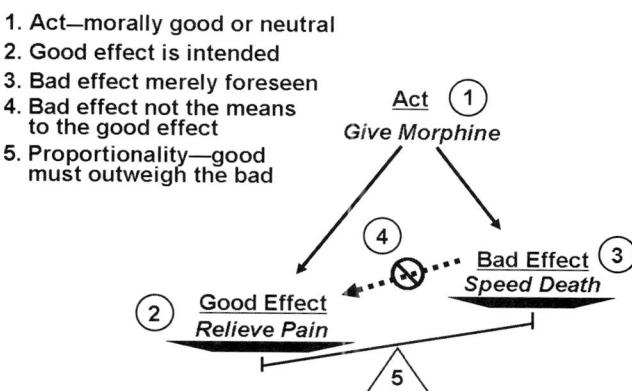

FIGURE 14.1. The Doctrine of Double Effect.

of morphine, this condition would be violated. By administering potassium chloride, the evil effect [death] becomes the means to the good effect [relief from suffering]. By contrast, morphine does not depend on the side effect of death to effectively relieve pain.)

- *The good intended must outweigh the evil permitted.* In the case of an imminently dying patient, the benefit of pain relief clearly outweighs the risk of death. This would not be true if the patient were not terminally ill. For example, if an otherwise healthy patient required so much morphine for pain control that he developed serious respiratory depression, he should be placed on a ventilator and not allowed to die.

In summary, despite the beliefs of many clinicians, no moral, legal, or religious reasons justify withholding adequate pain relief from dying patients. Pain and suffering should always be adequately treated, even if the treatment results in a foreseen but unintended hastening of death.

What is the difference between currently accepted practice and the performance of euthanasia? The key difference lies in the *intention* of the physician. As long as the physician's intention is treatment of the patient's pain and suffering, the administration of analgesics and sedatives is noncontroversial. When the physician's intention is to kill the patient, then the line between accepted practice and euthanasia has been crossed.

SPECIAL TOPICS IN END-OF-LIFE CARE

Futility

The extraordinary advances in life-sustaining therapies that have developed during the last few decades have spawned a new type of ethical conflict between physicians and families over decisions to continue or forgo life-support therapy. Intensivists can expect to face situations in which they believe that further treatment for a given patient is "futile," while the patient's family feels strongly that the treatment must continue. In fact, over 80% of ICU physicians reported having withdrawn support from patients on the grounds of futility, and at least sometimes this was done over the objections of the family (7). The potential for these conflicts has led to the development of approaches to the problem of futility that seek to resolve conflicts between physicians and families and justify difficult decisions in these troublesome cases.

The earliest approach to the futility debate was to attempt to define futility. These definitions largely rely on either quantitative or qualitative criteria. Quantitative definitions attempt to attach "hard" statistical prognostications to treatment decisions. For example, Schneiderman suggested that if "in the last 100 cases a medical treatment has been useless, [physicians] should regard that treatment as futile (39)." Qualitative definitions attempt to identify specific clinical outcomes (such as the persistent vegetative state), in which life-sustaining treatments would not provide benefit and, therefore, should not be offered. Ultimately, attempts to resolve futility disputes through the use of definitions were not successful, because it was recognized that the conflict in such cases does not typically revolve around the medical facts, statistics, and definitions of the case; instead, the crux of the dispute is almost always a conflict of values and a disagreement over whether the treatment in question is "worth it."

More recently, *fair process-based* approaches to futility have been developed and advocated by hospitals and by the American Medical Association in a 1999 report (3); in 1999, Texas became the first state to enact a law that establishes a statewide fair-process approach to futility cases based this report. Experience with the Texas legislation is still limited, but one hospital reported 47 futility consultations over a 2-year period. In 43 of these cases, the ethics committee agreed that further treatment was futile, and in 37 of these, the families agreed to withdrawal of life-sustaining treatment. In six cases, however, the families disagreed with the determination of futility. In three cases, the families agreed within a few days, in two cases the patients died during the 10-day waiting period mandated by the legislation, and in one case, the patient died awaiting transfer to an alternate provider who had agreed to provide treatment (20).

Whereas this legislation and other procedural approaches do give weight to the subjective determination by the patient or the patient's surrogate of what constitutes a worthwhile outcome, they also clearly allow for the possibility that the process will result in a unilateral decision by the institution to not offer the treatment in question. Such approaches, if they are to be successful, must honor the value system of the patient and family, protect the integrity of the medical professionals involved, and function in an open and fair manner that maximizes the chances for an acceptable resolution. The elements of such a procedural approach appear in **Table 14.1.**

Baby Doe

Baby Doe was an infant born in Indiana in 1982 with Down syndrome and esophageal atresia. He was allowed to die without surgical intervention, and his death sparked a legal and political controversy that subsequently led to the development of the "Baby Doe regulations." In 1985, Congress passed amendments to the Child Abuse and Treatment Act that designated the "withholding of medically indicated treatment" from children as child abuse. "Medically indicated treatment" is defined as any treatment (including nutrition and hydration) likely to ameliorate life-threatening conditions, although three situations are given under which treatment (other than appropriate nutrition, hydration, or medication) is optional:

- If the infant is chronically and irreversibly comatose
- If the treatment would merely prolong dying, and would not be effective in ameliorating or correcting all the infant's life-threatening conditions
- If the treatment would be virtually futile in terms of the survival of the infant, and the treatment itself under such circumstances would be inhumane

These regulations, which are still in effect today, specify the legislation that states must have in their child abuse laws to qualify for federal funds.

The intention of these regulations is to protect disabled infants with life-threatening conditions; however, they have drawn sharp criticism from many, including the American Medical Association, and have been poorly accepted by neonatologists. The debate over these regulations and the treatment of handicapped infants in the ICU touches on many of the ethical issues discussed in this chapter. How should parents and

TABLE 14.1

KEY ELEMENTS OF A HOSPITAL POLICY ON POTENTIALLY FUTILE TREATMENT

Hospital policy should be "bilateral," addressing overtreatment by both clinicians and families.
- Families can request a consult if they believe clinicians are demanding "overtreatment."
- Clinicians can request a consult when they believe families are demanding "overtreatment."

Efforts to achieve resolution with the patient and family must be clearly documented, emphasizing that limiting the use of life-sustaining treatments will not lead to abandonment.

If sustained and repeated efforts fail, the case is referred to the institutional Ethics Advisory Committee.

Three-phase consultation process:
- Phase 1: Meeting with committee and clinical team. The purpose is to present the medical perspective on the case.
- Phase 2: Meeting with committee and the patient or family. The purpose is to allow the patient or family to "tell their story."
- Phase 3: The committee meets alone. The purpose is to make a determination of whether further use of life-sustaining treatment is inappropriate or harmful.

If the committee supports the caregivers' assessment, then four options should be considered:
- Clinicians may pursue further attempts at consensus with the patient or surrogate, but only when clear avenues for negotiation exist that have not already been explored.
- Clinicians may attempt to transfer care to another physician within the hospital or to another hospital, which serves as a check on the system and provides evidence of community consensus.
- The hospital administration could seek a judicial resolution to the conflict, on grounds that the patient's surrogate is not acting in the patient's best interest.
- The hospital administration could sanction the unilateral forgoing or removal of life-sustaining treatments. Such action should occur only after informing the patient or surrogate decision maker of the plan and only after giving them sufficient opportunity to seek alternate medical care, legal advice, and, possibly, judicial involvement, if desired.

physicians justify decisions for these severely handicapped children? What role, if any, should family interests play in these decisions? How should medical uncertainty regarding the infant's outcome factor into the equation? How is "futile" treatment determined for these patients? Is the withholding or withdrawing of medical nutrition and hydration from these babies ever allowable?

The Baby Doe regulations have not provided answers to any of these difficult questions. Additionally, the regulations themselves have little direct authority over physicians and parents. They do not create federally mandated standards of care for the treatment of infants. Nor do they authorize legal penalties for individuals or hospitals who are involved in forgoing medical treatment of an infant. They become an issue only if someone reports the forgoing of life-support from an infant as child abuse or neglect.

The Use of Neuromuscular Blocking Agents during Withdrawal of Life Support

As outlined in the section on the use of sedatives and analgesics, the use of opioids, benzodiazepines, and even barbiturates is justified if intended to alleviate the patient's suffering during the dying process. Neuromuscular blocking agents (NMBA) cannot serve this purpose, because they have no analgesic, anxiolytic, or sedative effect; their sole effect is chemical paralysis. The use of these agents may even serve to mask the presence of treatable suffering, which is less likely to be diagnosed due to lack of patient communication and movement. Nevertheless, it has been reported that anywhere from 6%–12% of intensive care physicians have used NMBAs during withdrawal of life support. Although some justify the use of these drugs as useful in reducing the suffering experienced by family members who witness agonal movements, the Ethics Committee of

the Society of Critical Care Medicine recommends that these drugs not be used during withdrawal of life support, stating that "the best way to relieve their suffering is by reassuring them of the patient's comfort through the use of adequate sedation and analgesia (45)." Consequently, the best course of action is to ensure the absence of pharmacologic paralysis before withdrawal of ventilator support.

A rare but difficult dilemma can arise when the pharmacologic effects of the NMBAs are not reversible (due to overdosage or renal/hepatic failure) for days or weeks. Under these unusual circumstances it may be permissible to proceed with ventilator withdrawal provided that (a) it is highly certain that the patient cannot survive without the ventilator, (b) the patient's comfort is carefully managed with sufficient dosages of sedatives and analgesics, and (c) it is determined that the benefits of waiting for the return of neuromuscular function (e.g., interaction with family members before death) do not outweigh the burdens (45).

International Perspectives on End-of-life Care

Although this section on end-of-life care has largely been written from a North American perspective, important international differences exist in end-of-life practices in the ICU (15,17,44,47,48). As might be expected, marked variability in end-of-life practice is seen around the world, but it is interesting that a substantial amount of variability is also seen within countries (31). Variability has been documented in all aspects of decision making, including the range of acceptable practices, the decision-making participants, and the frequency of limitations of life-sustaining therapies.

Perhaps the most salient international differences in end-of-life care relate to questions of decision-making participation and authority. Fundamental differences in end-of-life decision making for competent and formerly competent adults have been well documented across country and culture. In pediatric critical care, the situation is further complicated by the fact that the patient is typically not a competent decision maker. The American standard for decision making for critically ill children, described by The American Academy of Pediatrics, is that parents are granted decision-making authority for their children, and informed parental permission is required for treatment decisions (2). In essence, the presumption is that parents are the best custodians of their child's best interests, and, consequently, their participation is obligatory. This parental autonomy can be overridden in rare instances through the judicial process, but even when the courts become involved, wide latitude is generally granted to parents. Studies show that European attitudes differ. For example, French physicians—not parents—have a dominant role in medical decisions. The justification for this practice is that French intensivists believe that parental autonomy in intensive care is an illusion, because parents do not possess the knowledge or experience necessary to make truly informed decisions. Further, French pediatric intensivists believe that this practice protects parents from the responsibility and guilt of making tragic decisions for their child (16). This paternalistic attitude is firmly contested by North American intensivists (22,27).

Substantial variability has also been reported among countries regarding decisions to forgo life support. In the United States, 53%–58% of patients who die in the PICU do so after decisions to withhold or withdraw life-sustaining therapy (9,46). In Brazil, the percentage of patients who die following a decision to withhold or withdraw life-sustaining treatment is 18%, with family participation in the decision-making process occurring in 36% of deaths (31). Significant variability has also been reported across the European continent. For example, the incidence of withdrawal of life-sustaining treatment ranged from 47% in the north to 30% in the south of Europe (17). With regard to parental participation in the process, less variability was evident. In both the north and south of Europe, senior clinicians are the main decision makers, and family input carries significantly less weight. Parents were present during their children's deaths in 69% of northern and 49% of southern European PICUs.

In a survey of European neonatologists, the frequency of withdrawal of mechanical ventilation was highest in the Netherlands, the United Kingdom, and Sweden; it was intermediate in France and Germany, and lowest in Spain and Italy (15). In only the Netherlands and France did a substantial proportion of respondents report the administration of drugs in hopeless cases with the purpose of ending the patient's life. Physicians more likely to agree with ideas consistent with preserving life at all costs were from Hungary, Estonia, Lithuania, and Italy, whereas those more likely to agree with statements that quality of life must be taken into account were from the United Kingdom, the Netherlands, and Sweden.

With regard to end-of-life issues, the ethical climate in Europe appears to be evolving. The European Commission has ruled that the patient has the right to self-determination, including the right to refuse unwanted therapies. Recently, laws pertaining to patient rights have also been adopted in France and Belgium; they explicitly state that doctors must respect the refusal of treatment expressed by a competent patient, even if his life is threatened. These laws concern autonomous patients,

mainly adults; they do not concern neonates and children in the settings of neonatal or pediatric intensive care.

Although it is easy to document differences among countries, it is more difficult to explain them. Diverse cultural, religious, philosophic, legal, and professional attitudes may be involved. European cultures are not static or homogeneous. Even within a particular ethnic group, significant differences may exist, depending on country of residence, gender, age, education, social circumstances, generation, and assimilation into the host society (12). For example, significant differences have been found in end-of-life decision-making styles between Japanese living in Japan, and Japanese-speaking and English-speaking Japanese Americans in California. Interestingly, the differences were greatest between the Japanese-speaking Japanese Americans and the other two groups (32). Religion also influences decision making. Some surveys, for example, have shown that Catholic clinicians in Europe are less likely to withhold or withdraw treatment than are their Protestant or agnostic counterparts (47). Other factors may influence the approach to end-of-life care, such as organizational factors, patient reimbursement status, the role of ethics committees, and the consultants' legal environment in the country (12).

In many Western countries, national and supranational legal authorities have begun debating the issue, and quality care at the end of life is recognized as a global problem for public health and health systems (42). The international community has begun the process of measuring, analyzing, and debating the differences among cultures and countries with regard to end-of-life treatment, because it is recognized that studying international practices may lead to opportunities to improve the quality of end-of-life care across borders. A convergence of opinion about good practice appears to be developing among professional societies in Europe and in the United States (12). That end-of-life care is now a well-recognized field of investigation and the scientific literature on the subject is now considerable has led to a common language between pediatric intensivists, allowing them to compare their practices. End-of-life issues are becoming an essential topic at international congresses, and international consensus meetings have been organized on the subject (12). This emerging international dialog will likely lead to a deeper understanding of, and appreciation for, the many differences found in the practice of end-of-life care and—it is hoped—to incremental improvement in the field.

CONCLUSIONS AND FUTURE DIRECTIONS

Medical ethics is a relatively young area of active inquiry and research. Most of the early work has been done in North America and Western Europe and has been based on the philosophic methods traditionally dominant in those cultures. Although beneficial in the sense of bringing many previously taboo subjects to light for vigorous discussion and debate, this Western focus has resulted in a disproportionate emphasis on a narrow range of intellectual and cultural background. Increasingly, globalization is changing the fundamental fabric of social practices throughout the world, and medicine is at the heart of this evolution. Over the next decades, we can anticipate research that will provide empirical descriptions of how bioethical dilemmas are managed in different countries and cultures, and we will benefit from the input of other philosophic, religious, and intellectual perspectives as we grapple with these exceedingly difficult and important aspects of the practice of pediatric critical care medicine.

KEY POINTS

- Knowledge of ethical theory is necessary to construct coherent justifications for dilemmas in clinical decision making. Foundational ethical theories include those based on consequences, such as *utilitarianism*, and those based on duties, such as *Kantianism*.

- Legal considerations provide a general framework for decision making but rarely provide a definitive answer to complex ethical questions. The law typically represents the floor, not the ceiling, of standards of morality.

- Informed consent is a process, not an event, and it has four key requirements: competency, disclosure, understanding, and voluntariness.

- Competency involves the capacity to *understand* the therapy in question, *consider* the risks and benefits, *decide* on a course of action, and *appreciate* the consequences of the choice.

- Minors may be legally empowered to make their own decisions if they are deemed *emancipated* by state law or determined to be a *mature minor* by a judge.

- The two main standards for *surrogate decision making* are the *substituted judgment standard* (choosing what the patient would have chosen, if still competent) and the *best-interest standard* (choosing what seems to be objectively best for the patient). The former is used for patients who were once competent and who expressed preferences, whereas the latter is used for patients who have never been competent, including children.

- Currently, two types of advance directives are used: *living wills* specify the treatments that a patient wants in certain clinical circumstances, while the *healthcare durable power of attorney* names a surrogate to make decisions if and when the patient lacks decisional capacity.

- Clinicians should refrain from speaking about withdrawal of care. Although treatments may be withdrawn, *care is never withdrawn*. Care may be redirected from a focus on cure to a focus on comfort.

- Distinguishing between treatments that are *ordinary* versus *extraordinary* is rarely helpful, because determination of whether to withdraw a treatment should made be based on the balance of benefits and burdens, as perceived by the patient, rather than upon any particular feature of the treatment itself (e.g., ECMO may be "ordinary" in one context and "extraordinary" in another).

- Although clinicians are generally more comfortable *withholding* a treatment (e.g., tracheal intubation) than *withdrawing* it, better decisions are made if these events are seen as equivalent; for example, allowing patients to receive trials of therapy with the understanding that the treatment may be withdrawn later if it is not sufficiently beneficial.

- *Medical nutrition and hydration* (e.g., tube feedings and intravenous fluids) are legally regarded as medical treatments and may be withheld or withdrawn by the same criteria used for other medical treatments, such as dialysis or mechanical ventilation.

- Sedatives and analgesics should be administered to dying patients, even if they hasten the patient's death, as long as they are *titrated* to the level of the patient's distress and are administered with the *intention* of relieving the patient's pain and suffering, not with the intention of causing death.

- Clinicians should be cautious when judging medical treatments to be futile, because these decisions are rarely based entirely on medical factors and usually involve value judgments. Determinations of futility should only be made in the context of a *carefully defined procedure* that assures due process for the patient and his family.

- *Neuromuscular blocking agents* should never be administered at the end of life to patients who have not been receiving them for therapeutic purposes. When life support is withdrawn from patients who are therapeutically paralyzed, the paralytic effects should generally be allowed to wear off before life support is withdrawn.

- Ethical and legal standards show important international variation. For example, paternalistic practices are more common in Europe than in North America. In addition, practices around the withdrawal of life support vary substantially around the world.

References

1. Informed consent, parental permission, and assent in pediatric practice. Committee on Bioethics, American Academy of Pediatrics. *Pediatrics* 1995; 95:314–7.
2. Ethics and the care of critically ill infants and children. American Academy of Pediatrics Committee on Bioethics. *Pediatrics* 1996;98:149–52.
3. Medical futility in end-of-life care: Report of the Council on Ethical and Judicial Affairs. *JAMA* 1999;281:937–41.
4. Angell M. The doctor as double agent. *Kennedy Inst Ethics J* 1993;3: 279–86.
5. Annas GJ. Informed consent, cancer, and truth in prognosis. *N Engl J Med* 1994;330:223–25.
6. Appelbaum PS, Grisso T. Assessing patients' capacities to consent to treatment. *N Engl J Med* 1988;319:1635–8.
7. Asch DA, Hansen-Flaschen J, Lanken PN. Decisions to limit or continue life-sustaining treatment by critical care physicians in the United States: Conflicts between physicians' practices and patients' wishes. *Am J Respir Crit Care Med* 1995;151:288–92.
8. Beauchamp TL, Childress JF. *Principles of Biomedical Ethics*, 5th ed. New York: Oxford University Press; 2001:454.
9. Burns JP, Mitchell C, Outwater KM, et al. End-of-life care in the pediatric intensive care unit after the forgoing of life-sustaining treatment. *Crit Care Med* 2000;28:3060–6.
10. Burns JP, Reardon FE, Truog RD. Using newly deceased patients to teach resuscitation procedures. *N Engl J Med* 1994;331:1652–5.
11. Caralis PV, Hammond JS. Attitudes of medical students, housestaff, and faculty physicians toward euthanasia and termination of life-sustaining treatment. *Crit Care Med* 1992;20:683–90.
12. Carlet J, Thijs LG, Antonelli M, et al. Challenges in end-of-life care in the ICU. Statement of the 5th International Consensus Conference in Critical Care: Brussels, Belgium, April 2003. *Intensive Care Med* 2004;30: 770–84.
13. Carse AL. The "voice of care": Implications for bioethical education. *J Med Philos* 1991;16:5–28.
14. Coles R. *The Call of Stories: Teaching and the Moral Imagination*. Boston: Houghton Mifflin, 1989.
15. Cuttini M, Nadai M, Kaminski M, et al. End-of-life decisions in neonatal intensive care: Physicians' self-reported practices in seven European countries. EURONIC Study Group. *Lancet* 2000;355:2112–8.
16. Devictor DJ, Nguyen DT. Forgoing life-sustaining treatments: How the decision is made in French pediatric intensive care units. *Crit Care Med* 2001;29:1356–9.
17. Devictor DJ, Nguyen DT. Forgoing life-sustaining treatments in children: A comparison between Northern and Southern European pediatric intensive care units. *Pediatr Crit Care Med* 2004;5:211–5.
18. Diem SJ, Lantos JD, Tulsky JA. Cardiopulmonary resuscitation on television. Miracles and misinformation. *N Engl J Med* 1996;334:1578–82.
19. Duff RS, Campbell AG. Moral and ethical dilemmas in the special-care nursery. *N Engl J Med* 1973;289:890–4.

20. Fine RL, Mayo TW. Resolution of futility by due process: Early experience with the Texas Advance Directives Act. *Ann Intern Med* 2003;138:743–6.

21. Frader J. Forgoing life-sustaining food and water: Newborns. In: Lynn J, ed. *By No Extraordinary Means: The Choice to Forgo Life-Sustaining Food and Water.* Bloomington: Indiana University Press; 1989:180–5.

22. Frader JE. Forgoing life support across borders: Who decides and why? *Pediatr Crit Care Med* 2004;5:289–90.

23. Greenberg LW, Jewett LS, Gluck RS, et al. Giving information for a life-threatening diagnosis. Parents' and oncologists' perceptions. *Am J Dis Child* 1984;138:649–53.

24. Gutheil TG, Bursztajn H, Brodsky A. Malpractice prevention through the sharing of uncertainty. Informed consent and the therapeutic alliance. *N Engl J Med* 1984;311:49–51.

25. Hardart GE, Truog RD. Attitudes and preferences of intensivists regarding the role of family interests in medical decision making for incompetent patients. *Crit Care Med* 2003;31:1895–1900.

26. Hardwig J. What about the family? *Hastings Cent Rep* 1990;20:5–10.

27. Hoehn KS, Nelson RM. Parents should not be excluded from decisions to forgo life-sustaining treatments! *Crit Care Med* 2001;29:1480–1.

28. Iglehart JK. The American health care system. The End-Stage Renal Disease Program. *N Engl J Med* 1993;328:366–71.

29. Jonsen AR, Toulmin S. *The Abuse of Casuistry: A History of Moral Reasoning.* Los Angeles: University of California Press; 1988:420.

30. Katz J. Why doctors don't disclose uncertainty. *Hastings Cent Rep* 1984; 14:35–44.

31. Kipper DJ, Piva JP, Garcia PC, et al. Evolution of the medical practices and modes of death on pediatric intensive care units in southern Brazil. *Pediatr Crit Care Med* 2005;6:258–63.

32. Matsumura S, Bito S, Liu H, et al. Acculturation of attitudes toward end-of-life care: A cross-cultural survey of Japanese Americans and Japanese. *J Gen Intern Med* 2002;17:531–9.

33. McCann RM, Hall WJ, Groth-Juncker A. Comfort care for terminally ill patients. The appropriate use of nutrition and hydration. *JAMA* 1994;272: 1263–6.

34. McDonagh JR, Elliott TB, Engelberg RA, et al. Family satisfaction with family conferences about end-of-life care in the intensive care unit: Increased proportion of family speech is associated with increased satisfaction. *Crit Care Med* 2004;32:1484–8.

35. Orlowski JP, Kanoti GA, Mehlman MJ. The ethics of using newly dead patients for teaching and practicing intubation techniques. *N Engl J Med* 1988;319:439–41.

36. Pellegrino ED, Thomasma DC. *The Virtues in Medical Practice.* New York: Oxford University Press, 1993.

37. Quill TE. Terri Schiavo – A tragedy compounded. *N Engl J Med* 2005;352:1630–3.

38. Ross LF. Health care decision making by children. Is it in their best interest? *Hastings Cent Rep* 1997;27:41–45.

39. Schneiderman LJ, Jecker NS, Jonsen AR. Medical futility: Its meaning and ethical implications. *Ann Intern Med* 1990;112:949–54.

40. Sharp MC, Strauss RP, Lorch SC. Communicating medical bad news: Parents' experiences and preferences. *J Pediatr* 1992;121:539–46.

41. Shaw A, Randolph JG, Manard B. Ethical issues in pediatric surgery: A national survey of pediatricians and pediatric surgeons. *Pediatrics* 1977; 60:588–99.

42. Singer PA, Bowman KW. Quality end-of-life care: A global perspective. *BMC Palliat Care* 2002;1:4.

43. Solomon MZ, O'Donnell L, Jennings B, et al. Decisions near the end of life: Professional views on life-sustaining treatments. *Am J Public Health* 1993; 83:14–23.

44. Sprung CL, Eidelman LA. Worldwide similarities and differences in the foregoing of life-sustaining treatments. *Intensive Care Med* 1996;22:1003–5.

45. Truog RD, Cist AF, Brackett SE, et al. Recommendations for end-of-life care in the intensive care unit: The Ethics Committee of the Society of Critical Care Medicine. *Crit Care Med* 2001;29:2332–48.

46. Vernon DD, Dean JM, Timmons OD, et al. Modes of death in the pediatric intensive care unit: Withdrawal and limitation of supportive care. *Crit Care Med* 1993;21:1798–1802.

47. Vincent JL. Forgoing life support in western European intensive care units: The results of an ethical questionnaire. *Crit Care Med* 1999;27:1626–33.

48. Yaguchi A, Truog RD, Curtis JR, et al. International differences in end-of-life attitudes in the intensive care unit: Results of a survey. *Arch Intern Med* 2005;165:1970–5.

CHAPTER 15 ■ ORGAN DONATION

KRISTEN L. NELSON • IVOR D. BERKOWITZ

Since the first successful organ transplant more than 50 years ago, organ donation has saved several hundred thousand lives. In 2005 alone, more than 28,000 solid organs were transplanted in the US, resulting in an average of 76 organs being transplanted each day. Of these, 1960 transplants were performed in pediatric patients. To date, over 19,000 pediatric donors <18 years of age have donated over 67,000 organs, a process which has allowed other children to live longer and better-quality lives (based on Organ Procurement and Transplantation Network, OPTN, data as of August 25, 2006).

The kidneys, heart, liver, lungs, intestine, and pancreas are transplantable organs. These organs come to be donated through donation after brain death (DBD), donation after cardiac death (DCD), and living donation. The first two pathways will be discussed in some detail in this chapter. Currently, most transplanted organs come from deceased donors who have been declared brain dead. However, an increasing number of organs is being obtained by living donation and DCD. Indeed, in 2001, for the first time in transplant history, the number of living donors exceeded the number of deceased donors. Furthermore, the number of DCD organs donated has continued to increase each year.

However, a marked imbalance remains between the supply of organs for transplantation and the demand for transplantable organs. As of 2006, more than 90,000 people are awaiting transplantation. Of these, almost 2200 are <18 years of age. The greatest number of adult patients on the waiting list requires kidney transplantation, followed by those who require lung and liver transplantations. For patients <18 years old, the greatest numbers are waiting for a liver, followed by those waiting for kidney and heart transplantation (**Fig. 15.1**). In 2005, more than 7000 patients with various types of organ failure died while waiting for an organ to become available, an average of almost 20 people per day (based on OPTN data of August 25, 2006). A specific challenge in pediatric transplantation is the need to match the size of the donor organ to the size of the recipient. Whereas most organs must be transplanted intact, necessitating close size matching, the liver and lungs can be transplanted into smaller children as a segment of a larger organ, thereby increasing transplantation options.

Perhaps the most important factor accounting for the widening gap between the demand for organs and their supply is the failure to obtain consent for organ donation from the families of potential organ donors. Rates of consent vary widely among geographic areas of the country and among racial groups. Two reasons explain most of the unrealized donor potential of brain-dead individuals. The first reason is that many families of brain-dead eligible donors are not given the option of donation, either because potentially eligible donors are not identified or consent for donation is not requested. Race, level of education, and prejudice may contribute to the perception that some families would probably not be interested in donation. The families of donor-eligible, brain-dead African American donors are less likely to be offered the option of donation than are Caucasian families. The second reason is that, often, >50% of donor-eligible families who are asked for permission for donation decline consent, even though public opinion surveys show that >75% of individuals would donate organs if asked. Several factors have been defined that appear to contribute to this discrepancy between what individuals say they would do and how families really decide. The hospital experiences of families substantially influence whether they consent for the organ donation of a deceased family member. Families who refuse consent are less satisfied with their hospital experiences, especially with the quality of care received by their loved ones, than are donor families. They are also less satisfied with the donor process. They are less likely to believe that they had adequate time and privacy to decide about donation. Families who decline donation are also less likely to have a clear understanding of brain death (43,44). Indeed, a majority of these family members believed that a brain-dead person would recover. On the other hand, donor families were much more likely to understand the concept of brain death and were satisfied with the care received by their loved ones and with the process of request. A wide variation in consent rates is also found among transplant centers across the country, with some centers obtaining consent as often as 90% of the time.

Several prominent organizations and government departments, including but not limited to the Institute of Medicine, the Department of Health and Human Services, and the United Network for Organ Sharing (UNOS), have realized that changes can be made in the process of organ donation to maximize the numbers of organs donated and subsequently transplanted, while ensuring comfort to the donors, recipients, the families of all involved. The systems changes that will be necessary to save the lives of those on the waiting list require collaboration with all involved organizations and healthcare employees—including the pediatric intensivists, who will play a pivotal role.

HISTORY OF ORGAN DONATION

The first successful organ transplantation, in which a kidney was transplanted from one identical twin to another, took place in Boston in 1954. Over the next 15 years, other organs were successfully procured from non–beating heart donors and transplanted into nonrelated individuals. As transplant techniques and technology improved, so did the interest in easily identifying those who were in need of a transplant. In 1968, the Southeast Organ Procurement Foundation was formed as

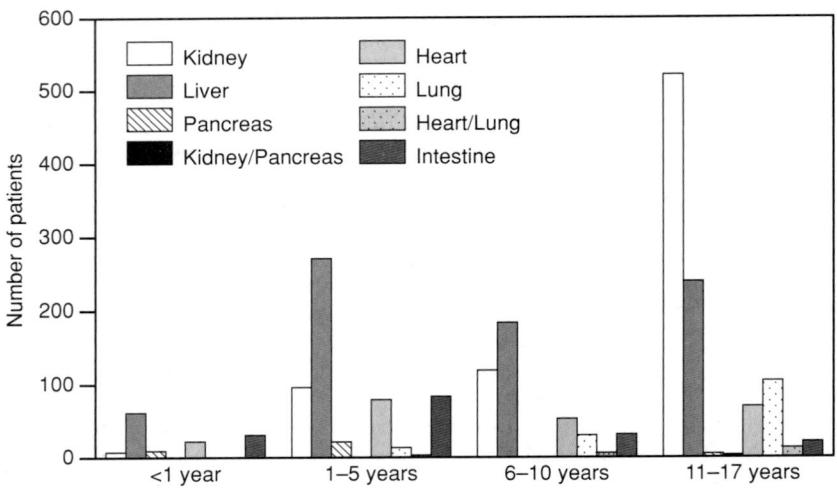

FIGURE 15.1. Pediatric waiting list for organs by age. Note the high overall demand for liver, kidneys, and heart and peak pediatric demand for kidney transplantation in adolescence. Based on OPTN data as of August 25, 2006.

an organization for transplant professionals and, in 1977, implemented the first computer-based organ matching system, known as the UNOS. UNOS became an independent nonprofit organization in 1984 and received the first federal contract to operate the OPTN. This contract is still held by UNOS today. Members of the OPTN include transplant hospitals and organ procurement organizations (OPOs). OPOs are nonprofit organizations responsible for the coordination of processes involving the organ donor and her family, transplant hospitals, and potential transplant recipients, all in an effort to ensure that the organ donor process is maximized and that all involved are emotionally and ethically comfortable with the process.

Public awareness for the need for organ donors was also expanded by the Uniform Anatomical Gift Act, enacted in 1968, which gave individuals 18 years of age and older the right to donate organs and tissues. This act is operative in all states in the US. The wish to donate organs is expressed by individuals on a donor card or driver's license.

ORGAN DONATION AFTER BRAIN DEATH

In 1967, the first organ transplantation from a brain-dead patient occurred, and several age-old ethical issues related to the declaration of death again received national attention. The Harvard criteria for brain death were published in 1968 and subsequently modified by specialist professional societies. *Brain death* refers to complete and irreversible cessation of brain function, and its declaration is a topic of complex medical, legal, ethical, and religious import (see Chapter 61).

In 1987, a task force that consisted of representatives from the American Academy of Pediatrics and the American Academy of Neurology, as well as representatives from several other professional medical and legal societies, proposed guidelines for the determination of brain death in children in the US (9). By the 1980s, determination of death by brain-death criteria was accepted in all states in the US, including the District of Columbia.

At present, most organ transplants come from brain-dead donors, although donation through living donation consti-

tutes a significant proportion of the donations, and donation through DCD is increasing.

Mandatory seat belt laws have resulted in a reduction in the number of individuals who sustain severe head injuries during motor vehicle accidents. Furthermore, improvement in the management of severely brain-injured patients has played a role in decreasing the number of brain-dead donors. Currently, approximately only 55% of all brain-dead children become organ donors (41). Because some organs cannot be transplanted from living donors, and the number of people awaiting organ transplants continues to significantly outweigh the number of donors, DCD and other alternative sources of organ donation are being explored.

Process

Once a potential organ donor has been identified, meticulous care must be delivered to these patients to maintain organ viability. The process begins with early recognition of brain death and early referral to the OPO to maximize the number of transplantable organs. Efficient time management is essential, because delays >72 hrs (from time of event that led to brain death to aortic cross-clamp) have been associated with poor outcomes in cardiac transplantation.

Several ethical issues exist surrounding the process of organ donation. It is important to understand these issues, because the intensivist plays a vital role in the identification of donors, in the family discussions concerning organ donation consent, and in the management of organ donors and recipients.

The ethical framework for organ donation in the US is based on two primary principles. The first is the "dead donor rule," which explicitly states that organ removal must not be the proximate cause of death. This is the case for both brain-dead and DCD cases. Second is the principle of autonomy, as it is applied to the potential donor and her family. The patient's or the patient's family's wishes regarding donation must be honored. The implication of this principle is that every family must be asked about their loved one's wishes— and their own wishes when a minor is involved. Indeed, US legislation now mandates that patients' families be asked about organ and tissue donation after brain-death declaration.

Medical staff may no longer make subjective judgments as to which families they believe will consent to organ donation. All families must be asked so that the decision to donate their loved ones' organs rests with them.

Based on these principles, it becomes clear that the role is complex for physicians who care for profoundly brain-damaged children who might progress to brain death (49). On the one hand, they must advocate for the best medical care for their patients. On the other, they must, at appropriate times, raise the concern and even the likelihood of progression to neurologic devastation, a hopeless prognosis, and even the progression to brain death; as well, they must refer such patients to the OPO. Increasingly, US society is exposed by public media to the issues and concepts of brain death. Nevertheless, brain death is a concept that is poorly understood by the lay public (43). It is very difficult for a family to believe that their child is dead when the child is warm to the touch, the monitor displays a heart beat, the chest moves with each ventilator breath, and urine collects in the bladder catheter tubing. It is the task of the pediatric intensivist caring for a neurologically devastated patient who might progress to brain death to begin to educate the family about brain death, what it is, and its significance. The second responsibility of the physician in attempting to maximize the likelihood of organ donation is to make an early referral to the regional OPO if progression to brain death appears likely, enabling the OPO to better begin the process of determining transplant eligibility. Many ICUs in the US use a Glasgow Come Scale score of 3 to 5 as an indicator to notify their local OPO (22).

Dealing with the grieving families of previously healthy children who are now faced with issues of brain death is an emotionally difficult and wrenching experience for caretakers, who possibly harbor feelings of guilt and failure at not being able to save the life of an injured child. These feelings may be compounded when the caretakers are placed in the trying ethical situation of caring for a potential organ donor and a possible recipient, a situation that may arise in multidisciplinary ICUs.

After the declaration of brain death, this information is conveyed to the family of the brain-dead child in a kind, compassionate, yet clear and decisive fashion, without the use of euphemisms to describe the fact that the child has died. Current recommendations are that the request for organ donation be temporally separated from the meeting at which the family is informed of the death of the patient. This "decoupling" can be accomplished by a subsequent meeting with the family, at which point organ donation and other post-death issues, including request for autopsy and funeral information, can be discussed. Decoupling has been shown to increase consent rates.

An often-raised concern is who should discuss the issue of donation with the family—the child's physician, who has an established clinical relationship with them, or the OPO representative, a stranger to them (52). In 1998, the US Health Care Financing Administration, now the Centers for Medicare and Medicaid services, changed the Federal Conditions of Participation, mandating that hospitals notify their local OPO when a patient's death is "imminent," so that families can be approached and the option of organ and tissue donation can be discussed. The legislation was aimed at increasing rates of organ donation. Physicians perceived this as excluding them from the care and counseling of their patients, especially at such a devastating time for their patients' families. The Conditions of Participation were subsequently revised and clarified; they

now require collaboration between the hospital and the OPO staffs and suggest that, ideally, the OPO and hospital together decide how and by whom the family will be approached. Organ donor consent rates are highest when the families are approached jointly by members of the healthcare team and the OPO. Family support from patient advocates, social workers, nurses, and physicians must remain a priority during both the dying process and after the declaration of death, when the child remains in the PICU before going to the operating room for organ removal (52).

ORGAN DONATION AFTER CARDIAC DEATH

Organ donation from patients who have experienced "cardiac death," or organ DCD, began in the 1960s, preceding the practice of donation following brain death. The technologies of intensive care medicine that appeared during the 1950s and 1960s, particularly mechanical ventilation and inotropic support, meant that many patients who would have died were able to be resuscitated and kept alive, but without neurologic function. It was realized that such severely brain-injured patients often progressed to brain death and that intensive-care management of these brain-dead patients allowed for adequate perfusion of organs (kidney, liver, heart, lungs, intestine, and pancreas) for potential organ procurement. Interest in DCD subsequently diminished.

Resurgence of interest in DCD began in 1997, with the Executive Summary of the Institute of Medicine (IOM) on "Non–Heart Beating Organ Transplantation: Medical and Ethical Issues in Procurement." This report was prompted by the imbalance between the number of potential organ donors and the number of those awaiting transplantation, and reflected an effort to explore other options to expand the donor pool (11). The expression of family autonomy in demanding that institutions abide by their wishes to donate the organs of their neurologically devastated but not brain-dead family members also stimulated medical institutions to develop policies for DCD. "organ donation after cardiac death" has currently replaced the phrase "non–heart beating organ donation" used in the IOM report. DCD refers to the donation of organs (usually kidneys and, less frequently, liver, pancreas, and lungs) from organ donors who have been declared dead on the basis of cardiorespiratory criteria; that is, a documented cessation of both cardiac and respiratory function. Only extremely rarely has cardiac transplantation occurred after DCD.

Two main categories of DCD have been subsequently described: (a) DCD after uncontrolled death, and (b) DCD after controlled death. In the first case, death occurred in an uncontrolled fashion, often in an emergency room, and organs, usually only kidneys, were rapidly removed. This was the mode of obtaining cadaveric organs before 1968, when brain death was defined and began to be accepted. Uncontrolled DCD is currently a rarely used modality in the US, although it is used as a mode of obtaining donor organs in other countries in which DBD and controlled DCD are not widely accepted (11). Controlled DCD is, on the other hand, becoming an increasingly common mode for obtaining organs for donation and will be the mode of DCD referred to in the remainder of this chapter.

Candidates

Patients who may qualify as DCD donors are those for whom the decision has been made to withdraw life-sustaining therapy (mechanical ventilation and vasopressor support). Most of the children who undergo DCD have sustained a profound, irreversible neurologic injury (head injury, hypoxic ischemic encephalopathy, or stroke) but do not meet the criteria for brain death. A few children have other single-organ, noncerebral, life-threatening medical problems from which they will not recover, such as respiratory failure secondary to progressive spinal muscular atrophy or dependence on extracorporeal membrane oxygenation for irreversible cardiac or respiratory failure.

Process

The decision to withdraw life-sustaining measures must be made completely independently of consideration of donation. A decision to withdraw therapy is based on consideration of the patient's and surrogate's wishes, after considering the prognosis, burden and benefits of continued therapy, issues of futility of future medical treatment, and goals of care.

To ensure the absence of any coercion and appearance or perception that the healthcare team is withdrawing life-sustaining therapy and hastening death to obtain organs, it is imperative that the emphasis be on making the decision to withdraw life-sustaining therapy before raising the issue of organ donation with the family. This priority is even more important, and perhaps even ethically tenuous, when the staff in a multidisciplinary ICU—who may also be caring for potential organ recipients—is also responsible for the care of children who may become organ donors. Indeed, some intensivists, in an effort to avoid the perception that life-sustaining therapy has been withdrawn to obtain organs, feel that the care of the dying child and the discussion about organ donation should not be carried out by the same physicians who might be involved with the care of an organ recipient. Involving other physicians to participate in this process may be logistically difficult. To further ensure the integrity of the DCD process, particularly the absence of family coercion, some institutions have mandated a formal ethics committee consultation with the family and healthcare team. Prior to approaching the family about DCD, the local OPO must be notified, and the child must be evaluated for donation eligibility. It is devastating for a family to be approached for DCD and to give consent only later to discover that the child is not an appropriate donor candidate.

Several ethical issues surrounding the concept of DCD obviously exist. To address these issues, the IOM published criteria that should be followed by hospitals that wish to implement DCD. All OPOs should discuss the option of DCD with local hospitals, healthcare professionals, and the community, and a protocol should be in place for DCD to occur. Importantly, organ procurement must not hasten death, and the entire process should focus on the patient and the family (11).

It is important to realize that the process of controlled DCD differs in some important ways from DBD, and these differences must be carefully explained to the donors' families. The withdrawal of life-sustaining therapies from a DCD donor involves the cessation of vasopressors and mechanical ventilation, either through disconnecting the ventilator or extubations, and this usually occurs in the operating room or an adjacent room. Withdrawal may occur in the ICU, but transport time to the operating room can be prolonged and increases organ ischemia. Most extrarenal organs are recovered for transplantation from DCD donors who had support withdrawn in the operating room. However, the location of the withdrawal should ensure the comfort of the donor and the family. Family members, if they wish, should be permitted to accompany the patient to the operating room and remain with the patient until the onset of pulselessness, at which point the family leaves and preparation begins for organ recovery. Death is declared later, usually after an interval of 2–5 mins. Regardless of the site of withdrawal of life-sustaining therapy, support for the family must continue to be provided by the ICU medical and nursing staff, family advocates, and clergy staff. Appropriate comfort care and symptom management must remain a priority.

Implicit in DCD is the necessity for indisputable evidence of death prior to declaration of death and organ removal (the "dead donor" rule). The determination of death by cardiorespiratory criteria necessitates determination of *cessation* of both cardiorespiratory function and *irreversibility* (4,11). Cessation of respiratory function is determined by absence of breathing. Cessation of cardiac function is determined, under the time constraints of DCD, by the absence of electrical activity of a contracting heart (asystole or fibrillation), together with the absence of ventricular ejection, which can be demonstrated by the absence of pulsatility on an arterial line tracing or by Doppler flow study. Although the 1997 IOM report suggested that asystole be present, because the criteria for cardiac death is absent circulation, documentation of lack of cardiac ejection is definitive.

The issue of the "irreversibility" component in the definition of cardiorespiratory criteria for death is addressed by including in the DCD protocol a time period of circulatory cessation that will exclude the possibility of "autoresuscitation"; this is the phenomenon of spontaneous restoration of cardiac contractility and ejection that can occur after a period of absent ejection. Most institutions incorporate into their DCD protocols the declaration of death after 5 mins of documented absence of cardiac ejection and absence of circulation. The Society of Critical Care Medicine has recommended that "at least two minutes of observation is required and more than five minutes is not recommended (7)."

Another issue that must be explained to donor families is the maximal time window for natural death to occur after withdrawal of life support. To reduce warm ischemia time to a minimum, most transplant centers will only procure organs from a DCD donor if the patient dies within 1 hr of discontinuation of life-sustaining therapies. It must be explained to the family that if death does not ensue within that hour, their loved one will be returned to the ICU for continuation of comfort care.

To avoid creating false hope for families that their loved one will indeed become an organ donor, the option of DCD should only be offered for patients who, in the best judgment of their physicians, will die within 1 hr of discontinuation of life support. However, it is often difficult to ascertain with complete certainty that this will occur. Investigators at the University of Wisconsin have developed an adult scoring system that helps to predict the likelihood that potential DCD patients will die within 2 hrs of withdrawal of life support. This evaluation is based on the patient's age, body mass index, oxygen saturation level, level of spontaneous ventilation, requirement and dosage of vasopressors, and mechanical ventilation indices. Based on this tool, an accurate prediction of death within 1–2 hrs after extubation was achieved in >90% of patients (16). Although most transplant teams require that organs be procured within 1 hr after extubation, organs that can withstand longer ischemic times, such as kidneys, may still be procured within a 2-hr window. UNOS has also developed a set of criteria to aid in identifying those patients who may become DCD candidates. Such predictive information is not available for pediatric patients.

The administration of drugs to the organ donor that can potentially reduce ischemia–reperfusion injury to the transplanted organs has generated ethical tension in the ICU and transplant community. Clinical and experimental evidence supports the use of the premortem administration of heparin for its protective effect on vascular endothelium and for preventing thrombosis in the donor organs. Administration of heparin does improve the function of organs removed by DCD. Phentolamine, an α-blocker vasodilator, is also used by some OPOs to improve donated organ function. The ethical concern about the administration of these drugs is that no benefit accrues to the patient and, indeed, these drugs may be harmful and perhaps even hasten death by causing bleeding or hypotension, in the case of heparin and phentolamine, respectively. A recent consensus report of a national conference on DCD stated that no evidence exists that heparin causes bleeding of a magnitude that will hasten death after the withdrawal of life-sustaining therapy. It is recommended that heparin be administered to the organ donor following withdrawal but only after consent for administration has been obtained from the family. The indications for the use of phentolamine and antioxidants (e.g., N-acetyl cysteine and vitamin E) are not clear, and their use depends on individual OPO and hospital DCD policies (4,11).

The coordination of the DCD process may take as long as 24 hrs, and this must be carefully and sensitively explained to the families so that they can be prepared to allow the process to occur. This waiting period can be difficult for any family, but it is especially important to inform the families that the legacy of their family member can live on as a gift of life to several people who are waiting for an organ transplant.

Organs that have been successfully transplanted after cardiac death include kidneys, livers, pancreata, lungs, and even a heart. (This DCD heart transplant was performed under a research protocol, and minimal information is available on the recipient. The patient is alive at this writing. Hearts from DCD donors are not currently available for transplantation into recipients, but research is on-going to determine the viability of DCD hearts for transplantation.)

EVALUATION OF DONOR ELIGIBILITY

No tests specific to organ donation, such as viral serologic tests or tissue typing, should be obtained from a patient prior to obtaining family consent for donation; this applies in cases of both DBD and DCD. The serologic testing to be performed once consent has been obtained includes testing for human im-

munodeficiency virus (HIV), human T-cell lymphotrophic virus (HTLV), venereal disease (VDRL test), and cytomegalovirus (CMV), as well as hepatitis B core antibody, hepatitis B surface antigen, and hepatitis C antibody. Liver and renal function tests are usually already available. Blood, urine, and sputum cultures should be obtained from each potential donor.

Two-dimensional echocardiography is helpful to initially assess cardiac-loading conditions and contractility and to serially reevaluate the effects of management. Bronchoscopy is often required to assess anatomic variations and injuries to each lung. Other evaluations and laboratory tests to be performed can be found in the UNOS Critical Pathway for the Pediatric Organ Donor (**Fig. 15.2**).

Contraindications to Organ Donation

Relatively few absolute contraindications exist to organ transplantation, and often these absolutes become relative, based on the degree of organ failure in the individual potential recipient (**Table 15.1**). The ultimate decision concerning whether an organ should be transplanted lies with the transplant surgeon, based on the information gathered by the OPO and intensive care team, as well as by visual inspection of the organ at the time of procurement. The surgeon and the transplant team must decide if the risks to the potential recipient of continuing to wait for a transplant outweigh the risks of transplantation with a "less than ideal" organ. This approach has been encompassed in one of the "best practice" principles adopted by organized groups of transplant hospitals and OPOs (known collectively as organ transplant breakthrough collaboratives) and is known as the "rule-in" philosophy: "Refer and evaluate every donor, every time," regardless of the medical status of the donor (26). The goals of the collaboratives are discussed later in this chapter.

Infections

Untreated, overwhelming sepsis usually precludes organ donation, but bacteremia and fungemia are not absolute contraindications. Although the aggressive treatment of infections is critical in donors, recipient outcomes do not significantly differ between selected infected and noninfected bacteremic donors. Furthermore, organ donation can often proceed with treatment of sepsis and meningitis after 24 hrs of appropriate antibiotics.

Potential organ donors infected with hepatitis B or C may be eligible to donate organs to those infected with the same virus and may even donate to noninfected recipients in extreme cases. Patients with HIV infection remain a controversial issue. Many of these patients are living longer lives due to the efficacy of protease inhibitors. However, transplantation from HIV-positive donors is currently contraindicated. Transplantation from HIV-positive donors to positive recipients, as in the case of hepatitis B and C, is frequently debated. Regardless, all patients should be referred to the OPO for discussion with the transplant team.

The CMV status of the donor and recipient is extremely important, because of the risk of infection in the immunosuppressed recipient, especially in those with a negative CMV status. Ganciclovir prophylaxis of CMV-negative recipients who receive organs from CMV-positive donors has greatly reduced the morbidity and mortality associated with CMV infection in these patients.

Critical Pathway for the Pediatric Organ Donor

Patient Name _____

UNOS ID Number _____

Collaborative Practice	Phase I Identification and Referral	Phase II Declaration of Brain Death and Consent	Phase III Donor Management	Phase III Donor Evaluation	Phase IV Organ Recovery Phase
The following professionals may be involved to enhance the donation process. Check all that apply. ○ Physician / Intensivist ○ Primary Care Physician ○ Critical Care RN ○ Nurse Supervisor ○ Organ Procurement Organization (OPO) ○ OPO Coordinator (OPC) ○ OPO Family Services Coor. ○ Medical Examiner ○ Respiratory Therapy ○ Laboratory ○ Radiology ○ Anesthesiology ○ OR/Surgery Staff ○ Clergy ○ Social Worker ○ Pharmacist ○ Child Life Specialist	○ Identify all patients who may be potential organ and/or tissue donors. ○ Initial call to OPO to notify of potential donor with devastating neurological injury (organ donor) or patient with grave prognosis (tissue donor) after consultation with treating physician. ○ Formal contact and referral to OPO when first brain death exam anticipated. ○ OPC on site and begins evaluation. ○ Notify charge nurse and intensivist/attending MD of presence on unit. Time _____ Date _____ Ht ____ Wt ____ ABO confirmed by blood bank ____ ○ Identify legal guardian/next-of-kin (NOK). ○ Notify ME/Coroner's office of impending death.	○ Brain death documented per hospital protocol. Time _____ Date _____ ○ Complete appropriate forms (death certificate, release of remains, etc.). ○ If patient does not meet brain death criteria, reevaluate after observation interval. ○ If withdrawal of life support is anticipated, consider donation after cardiac death (DCD) protocol. In all cases consider tissue donation. ○ Collaborative plan for family approach with ICU and OPO staff. ○ Identify/offer support services for family (primary physician, clergy, social worker, etc.). ○ MD notifies family of death. ○ OPO/hospital staff talks to family about donation. ○ NOK consents to donation ○ OPO staff obtains signed consent and medical/social history. Time _____ Date _____ ○ ME/Coroner formal notification. ○ ME/Coroner releases body for donation.	○ New orders written in collaboration with intensivists and OPO staff ○ Begin organ allocation ○ OPC sets tentative OR time ○ Ensure adequate IV/arterial access for support and procurement	○ Obtain blood/lymph nodes for tissue typing and cross-match ○ Obtain pre/post transfusion blood for serology testing per OPO protocol and communicate results when available. ○ Notify the following of pending case: • OR/anesthesiology • Procurement surgeons • House supervisor • Tissue typing labs ○ Cardiology/pulmonary and other specialty consults as requested by OPC ○ Lung measurements per CXR by OPC ○ Organ recovery process discontinued if donor organs unsuitable for transplantation after evaluation	○ Notification of OR for needed equipment, time, and organs to be recovered ○ Pre-op checklist ○ Communicate appropriate test results to recipient centers ○ Collaborate with accepting recipient centers on OR time ○ Procurement supplies present in OR ○ Prepare patient for transport to OR ____ IV ____ O_2 ____ PEEP ____ Pumps ○ Transport to OR Time _____ Date _____ ○ OR nurse confirms completion of all required documentation to include consent and brain death documentation. ○ OR nurse checks patient identification.
	○ OPC determines suitability of donor following chart review. *Stop Pathway – If not suitable for organ and tissue donation.*	○ *Family/ME/Coroner denies donation – Stop pathway – initiate post-mortem protocol – support family*			
Labs and Diagnostics	○ Per ICU protocol	○ Review lab results ○ Review hemodynamics	○ Determine need and write orders for ongoing lab testing ○ Same as adult except for H & H after transfusion, if necessary	○ Blood chemistry ○ CBC with diff ○ UA ○ UA for C & S ○ PT, PTT ○ ABO ○ A Subtype ○ Liver function tests ○ Blood culture × 2 / 15 minutes to 1 hour apart, different sites ○ Sputum Gram stain and C & S ○ Type & cross-match ____ # units PRBCs ○ CXR ○ ABGs ○ EKG ○ Echo ○ Bedside diagnostic/therapeutic bronchoscopy	○ Labs drawn in OR as per surgeon or OPC request ○ Communicate with pathology – arrange for pathology testing ○ BX liver and/or kidneys as indicated
Cardiopulmonary Care	○ Pt maintained on ventilator		○ Optimize ventilator settings to achieve SaO_2 >95% ○ O_2 challenge for lung placement PEEP = 5 cm, FiO_2 @ 100% 20 min, obtain ABG ○ ABGs as ordered ○ VS PRN ○ Pulmonary toilet (bronchial drainage, percussion, turning and suctioning, vest when appropriate)	○ Monitor and maintain the following age specific parameters ____ BP ____ HR ____ CVP ____ PaO_2 ____ SaO_2 >95% ____ pH 7.35–7.45	○ Portable O_2 @100% FiO_2 for transport to OR ○ Ambu bag and PEEP valve ○ Move to OR

FIGURE 15.2. UNOS critical pathway for the pediatric organ donor. From United Network for Organ Sharing. Available at: http://www.unos.org/SharedContentDocuments/Crit_Pathway_Pediatric_04.pdf. Accessed March 26, 2007. (*Continued*)

Critical Pathway for the Pediatric Organ Donor

Patient Name _____

UNOS ID Number _____

Collaborative Practice	Phase I Identification and Referral	Phase II Declaration of Brain Death and Consent	Phase III Donor Management	Donor Evaluation	Phase IV Organ Recovery Phase
Treatments/Ongoing Care	○ ICU staff responsible for maintaining normal hemodynamic parameters, normothermia, and ventilatory support as per ICU protocol		○ NG tube placed and functioning ○ Maintain temperature >36.5°C and <38°C ○ Eye care		○ Set OR temp as directed by OPC ○ Bronchoscopy as per lung recovery team ○ Post-mortem care
Medications	○ Continue as per ICU protocol/care plan		○ DC former meds except pressors and antibiotics ○ Initiate broad-spectrum antibiotic if not previously administered ○ Maintain age-specific parameters for: BP, HR, urine output, electrolytes, glucose, temperature, PT/PTT, CBC ○ See age-specific donor management recommendations ○ Medication as requested by OPC		○ Management of antidiuretics, diuretics, and heparin per transplant surgeon
Optimal Outcomes	Potential donor is identified, and a referral is made to OPO	Family offered the option of organ/tissue donation, and their decision is supported.	Optimize organ function	The donor is evaluated and found to be suitable for donation.	All suitable, consented organs are recovered for transplant.

This work supported by HRSA contract 231-00-0115.

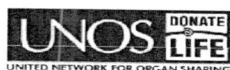

FIGURE 15.2. (*Continued*)

Malignancies

Most active malignancies represent a contraindication to donation, with the exception of some low-grade brain tumors and nonmelanomatous skin cancer. The malignancies seen most frequently in the pediatric patient—leukemia, lymphoma, and often high-grade brain tumors—represent a barrier to donation because they have a potential high rate of recurrence in recipients. Controversy exists regarding the "safe" period of cancer-free time (remission or cure) that potential donors must demonstrate before becoming eligible donors.

Medical Examiner Cases

Annually, nearly 180 potential deceased donors are prevented from donating viable organs by coroners or medical examiners, which translates to a loss of several hundred organs. Due in part to the growing organ waiting list and the shortage of

---

TABLE 15.1

CONTRAINDICATIONS TO ORGAN DONATION

Category	Contraindications
Infectious	HIV with specified conditions or positive serology or viral culture; any retroviral infection (including HTLV); tuberculosis; prion diseases (Creutzfeldt-Jacob); herpetic septicemia; rabies; hepatitis B surface antigen positive; fungal and viral meningitis; viral encephalitis (including West Nile virus)
Neoplasm	Active malignancies, including Hodgkin disease, leukemia, and multiple myeloma Note: Non-melanoma skin carcinoma and certain low-grade brain tumors are eligible.
Hematologic conditions	Aplastic anemia, agranulocytosis
Other conditions	Gangrene of bowel, extreme prematurity

Relatively few "absolute" contraindications exist today, and every potential donor should be referred, even if they have one of the above conditions.
HTLV, human T-cell lymphotrophic virus
From Organ Donation Breakthrough Collaborative. Best practices evaluation final report. Available at: http://www.organdonor.gov/bestpractice2005.htm. Accessed September 1, 2006.

organ supply, as well as to the heroic efforts of the organ transplant breakthrough collaboratives, the National Association of Medical Examiners has adopted a goal of "zero rejection" of potential donor cases referred to them, even though many pediatric patients who die from causes with legal implications, such as motor vehicle accidents or child abuse, must be referred to the medical examiner for autopsy. However, an autopsy does not preclude organ donation per se. Visual inspection of the body and organs, complemented by medical photography by the medical examiner, who is present in the operating room prior to organ removal, provides sufficient legal evidence. Occasionally, certain organs may be precluded from transplantation (40).

PHYSIOLOGIC CONSIDERATIONS AND MEDICAL MANAGEMENT OF THE PEDIATRIC ORGAN DONOR

Physicians who care for patients eligible for organ donation following brain death must work together as a team with the OPO coordinator, ICU nurses, respiratory therapists, clergy, social workers, family advocates, and medical examiners (in some cases) to optimize therapy and maintain the viability of potential donor organs. Today, most OPOs and ICUs utilize a standardized donor management protocol. UNOS has published such a protocol, known as the Critical Pathway for the Organ Donor, with separate pathways for adult and pediatric donors (see **Fig. 15.2**)

General

To effectively manage pediatric organ donors, an intensivist must be able to anticipate and recognize the multitude of physiologic derangements that occur, specifically with brain death (**Figs. 15.3 and 15.4**).

Hemodynamic changes may occur in brain-dead patients that may ultimately affect the potential transplantability of other organs. The severity of these changes has some relation to the time course of progression of the brain injury, with more rapid increases in elevated intracranial pressure (ICP) and subsequent brain death often resulting in more extensive pathophysiologic changes (39).

Although the physiologic changes that occur with brain death have been studied for many years, the interactions and mechanisms that underlie this process remain incompletely understood. The classic studies of Novitzky and colleagues in the 1980s, using a baboon model of brain death, have provided important information about this complex process. In these experimental models, as progressive elevation of ICP developed prior to brain death, cerebral ischemia occurred in a craniocaudal direction. Initially, brainstem ischemia resulted in vagal activation, with resultant bradycardia. As the ischemia progressed to involve the pons, the well-known Cushing response occurred with hypertension (due to sympathetic stimulation) and bradycardia (due to continued vagal stimulation). Progressive ischemia of the vagal nucleus in the medulla oblongata then led to cessation of its function, resulting in uncontrolled sympathetic stimulation—the "catecholamine storm" (18,23). A period of intense vasoconstriction occurs due to an increase

in systemic and, to a lesser degree, in pulmonary vascular resistance, resulting in systemic hypertension, tachycardia, and possibly tissue ischemia. The duration and severity of this catecholamine storm varies and may be related to the rapidity of onset of brain death. Pituitary hormone depletion also often accompanies this storm, associated with ischemia of the anterior and posterior pituitary.

On a cellular level, elevated catecholamine levels during this period lead to activation of second-messenger systems, which result in accumulation of intracellular calcium. Elevated intracellular calcium results in activation of proteases, lipases, endonucleases, oxygen reactive species, and free radicals, which culminates in mitochondrial dysfunction, DNA injury, and cell death, potentially affecting cells in all organs. The loss of high-energy phosphates upon cell death results in decreased production of ATP. Without the necessary energy provided by ATP for ion channel regulation, the sarcoplasmic reticulum cannot take up or release cytosolic calcium, perpetuating the intracellular calcium–induced injury, which occurs at the peak of increase in the systemic vascular resistance (SVR) (24,46).

Within hours of this process, catecholamine depletion occurs, with a significant generalized vasodilation, culminating in hemodynamic collapse (24). The free radical formation that is initiated during the period of intense vasoconstriction now continues with the reperfusion that occurs during this vasodilatory period. The injury of ischemia–reperfusion is due in large part to the production of free radicals and reactive oxygen species (32,45).

Currently, as many as 25% of potential organ donors are lost due to the hemodynamic instability that accompanies this vasodilatory phase. It is imperative for the ICU team and OPO coordinator to anticipate and manage these changes to maximize organ retrieval and survival. The time frame of donor management may vary from a few hours to 24 hrs and sometimes longer. After the declaration of brain death, the team must transition the goal of care from cerebral-protective strategies to those that optimize organ donation management.

Cardiovascular Pathophysiology

Catecholamine Storm

Once brain death occurs, the cardiovascular consequences of brain death are multiple and may stem from several mechanisms. The catecholamine storm, as previously described, often results in severe hypertension and tachycardia. The levels of endogenous epinephrine, norepinephrine, and dopamine may be increased several 100-fold during this storm (24,39). Generalized vasoconstriction occurs as a result of the increased catecholamine levels, with subsequent increased myocardial oxygen demand and calcium-induced injury that can affect all blood vessels, including the coronary arteries. The increase in myocardial oxygen demand in the setting of limited oxygen supply results in a shift from aerobic to anaerobic metabolism. The overall result may be subendocardial ischemia and, during this catecholamine storm, electrocardiographic changes suggestive of ischemia may be seen. Experimentally, ischemic changes are predominantly seen in the left ventricle, resulting in decreased left ventricular cardiac output (CO), despite the increase in contractility induced by the catecholamine storm (24). At the point of maximal SVR, a discrepancy occurs in CO, with

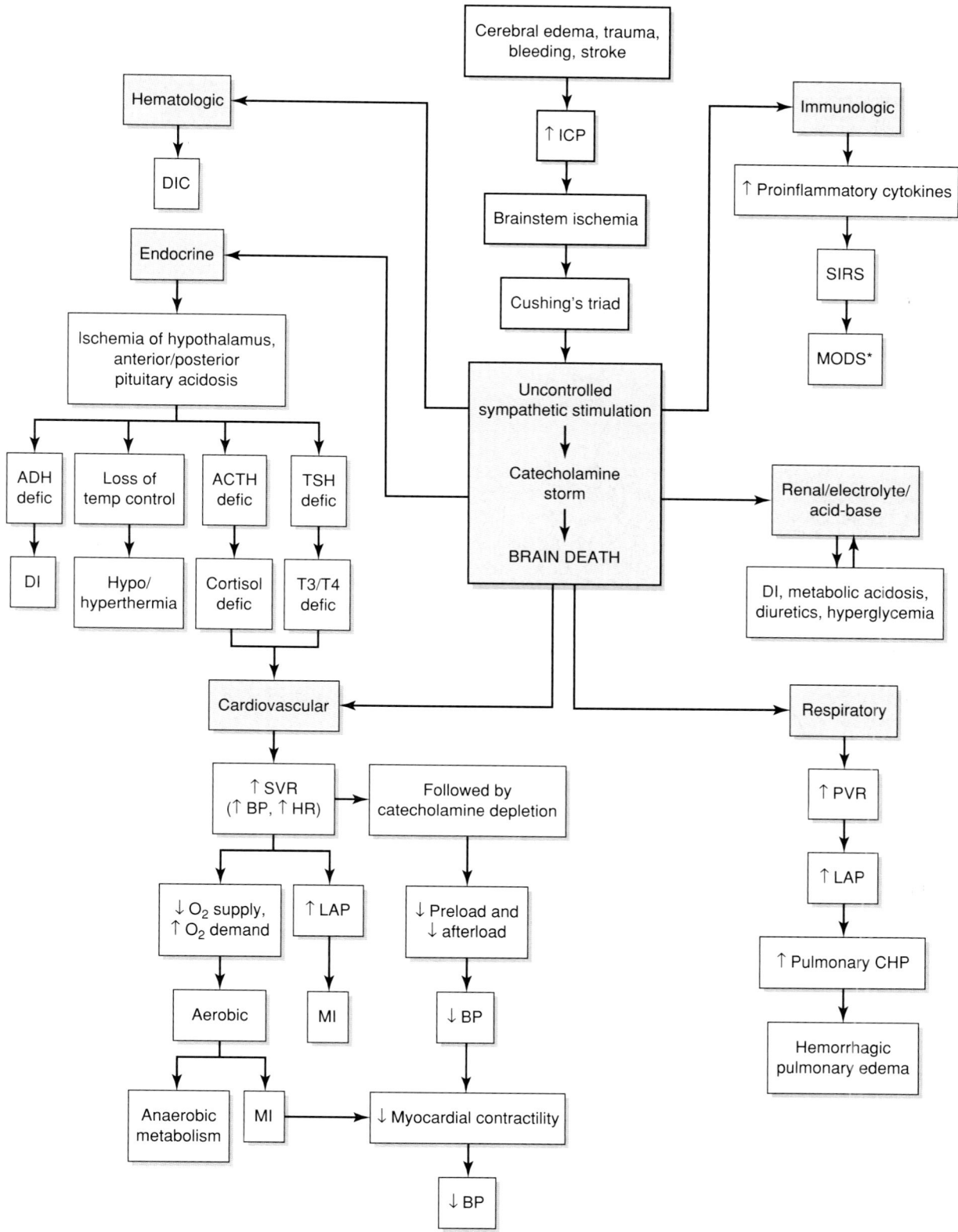

FIGURE 15.3. Physiologic events associated with brain death. Brain death has physiologic consequences for multiple organ systems that translate to complex medical management. DIC, disseminated intravascular coagulopathy; ICP, intracranial pressure; SIRS, systemic inflammatory response syndrome; MODS, multiple organ dysfunction syndrome; DI, diabetes insipidus; ACTH, adrenocorticotropic hormone; TSH, thyroid-stimulating hormone; ADH, antidiuretic hormone; SVR, systemic vascular resistance; BP, blood pressure; HR, heart rate; LAP, left atrial pressure; MI, myocardial ischemia; PVR, peripheral vascular resistance; CHP, capillary hydrostatic pressure.
*The systemic inflammatory response elicited by brain death may ultimately contribute to organ dysfunction in the heart, lungs, kidneys, and liver.

A. Cardiovascular, Fluid/Electrolyte and Hematologic Abnormalities
1. Assess blood pressure, heart rate, peripheral perfusion, urine output
2. Maintain normothermia
3. Obtain labs (CMP with Mg, Phos, CBC, PT/INR, PTT, FBG, ABG, cardiac enzymes)
4. Hemodynamic, fluid resuscitation, and hematologic goals

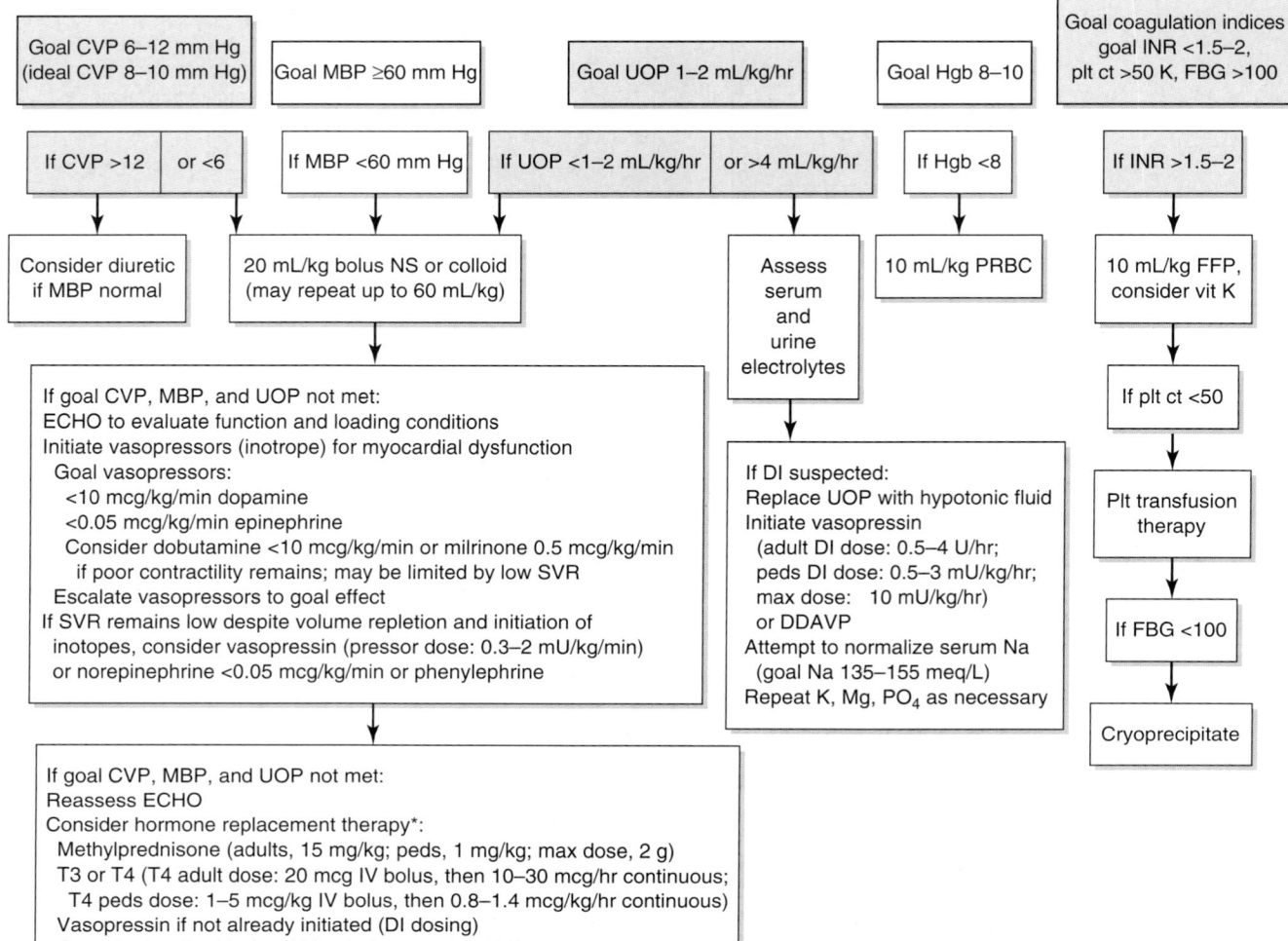

B. Respiratory Abnormality (multifactorial)
1. Mechanical ventilation goals
   a. FiO$_2$ 40%
   b. PEEP 5 cm H$_2$O
   c. Peak inspiratory pressure or plateau pressure <30–35 mm Hg
   d. Tidal volume (if volume control) 8–10 mL/kg; 6–8 mL/kg if ARDS
   e. Normal pH and pCO$_2$
   f. PaO$_2$ >100 or sats >95%, PaO$_2$:FiO2 ratio >300
2. Evaluate anatomy, injury, infection with bronchoscopy and serial chest x-ray if needed
   a. Obtain sputum for Gram stain, culture
3. Hypoxia or other injury (contusion, edema, pneumonia)
   a. Mechanical ventilation adjustment (i.e., increase FiO$_2$, PEEP)
   b. Consider diuretics if pulmonary edema noted if MBP normal, especially if CVP >8
   c. Consider methylprednisone if not previously administered
   d. Consider naloxone 8 mg IV

FIGURE 15.4. The management of the potential pediatric organ donor is often complex and involves frequent reassessment and adjustments in care. Management of these patients should be done in conjunction with the local OPO. CMP, comprehensive metabolic panel; UOP, urine output; CVP, central venous pressure; Hgb, hemoglobin; INR, international normalized ratio; plt, platelet; FBG, fibrinogen; MBP, mean blood pressure; NS, normal saline; PRBC, packed red blood cells; FFP, frozen fresh plasma; DI, diabetes insipidus; DDAVP,1-deamino(8-D-arginine) vasopressin; ARDS, acute respiratory distress syndrome; PEEP, positive end-expiratory pressure.
*Some institutions and OPOs may institute hormone replacement therapy earlier.

right ventricular CO now exceeding left ventricular CO. The effect of this discrepancy is an accumulation of blood in the lungs with a resultant significant elevation in left atrial pressure that temporarily exceeds mean pulmonary artery pressure and contributes to the formation of neurogenic pulmonary edema (discussed later) (18). Subendocardial ischemia also affects the papillary muscles at this point, resulting in mitral insufficiency and further increasing the left atrial pressure.

Although the shift to anaerobic metabolism is in large part due to significant ischemia with lack of energy stores, it may also be due in part to relative thyroid deficiency, which is discussed in more detail later. The final result of this shift to anaerobic metabolism often manifests as decreased contractility, usually within a few hours after brain death has occurred (24).

Cardiac arrhythmias may also occur due to necrosis of the conduction system or irritable myocardium due to ischemia during this vasoconstrictive period. Bradyarrhythmias and supraventricular and ventricular arrhythmias have all been documented (54).

Generalized Vasodilation

Hypotension is the most common problem encountered by physicians who care for pediatric organ donors. Once ischemia progresses to involve the cervical medulla, depletion of catecholamine stores occurs, resulting in generalized vasodilation. Significant decreases in preload and afterload often then predominate, contributing to cardiac dysfunction by the Frank-Starling mechanism. Loss of sympathetic vasomotor tone results in a dramatic decrease in afterload and leads to relative intravascular hypovolemia and decreased preload. One study revealed that, although contractility was reduced in brain-dead subjects, this event developed over 3–4 hrs, whereas the decrease in systemic vascular resistance or afterload occurred within 15 mins after brain death (39). The decrease in afterload also leads to a decrease in aortic pressure, with a subsequent decrease in coronary artery perfusion pressure and the development of myocardial ischemia. Therefore, it appears that the altered loading conditions—a decrease in afterload and preload—may play a central role in cardiac dysfunction in the brain-dead patient and may often be a reversible phenomenon if recognized and treated early and aggressively (47,51).

Although loss of vasomotor tone related to catecholamine depletion is a major cause of hypotension, many other factors also play a role. These include hypovolemia caused by fluid restriction or the use of diuretics (such as mannitol and furosemide) administered for cerebral edema management, as well as excessive urine losses due to diabetes insipidus (DI) and an osmotic diuresis from hyperglycemia. Hypothermia, occurring either after brain death or cardiac arrest, may also induce a diuresis. Other causes of hypotension include abnormal function of the hypothalamic-pituitary axis due to pituitary hormone depletion and potentially massive cytokine release, both of which are discussed in further detail in subsequent sections.

Evaluation and Management of Cardiovascular Abnormalities

General

The duration of the catecholamine surge is variable and unpredictable, but animal studies have shown that this period may last 15 mins (24,54). Because this phenomenon appears to be relatively short-lived and may indeed have occurred before the patient was even evaluated in the emergency room or PICU, many physicians choose not to treat the hypertension. However, short-acting β-blockers, such as esmolol, may be used to treat this centrally mediated hypertension and/or tachycardia. Esmolol has the advantage of being a continuous, titratable infusion. If bradyarrhythmias develop, epinephrine is often the drug of choice, because the heart in a brain-dead patient is essentially denervated and no longer responsive to atropine.

On the other hand, the vasodilatory phase and resultant hypotension frequently require medical management. Initial therapy consists of restoration of intravascular volume followed, if necessary, by vasopressor therapy. Assessment and maintenance of adequate intravascular volume can be difficult in brain-dead patients. Central venous pressure (CVP) measurement can provide helpful information. Optimal CVP is between 8 and 10 mm Hg. Measurements above that have been associated with increases in the arterial–alveolar gradient and hypoxia, which would potentially affect the transplantability of organ donor lungs (28,51). On the other hand, CVP of <8 mm Hg may adversely affect transplantable livers and kidneys, which require higher arterial pressures for adequate perfusion (6). Pulmonary artery catheters may be utilized in organ donors to assess CO and other hemodynamic parameters. Their use in the pediatric population is uncommon and can, in almost all cases, be replaced with two-dimensional echocardiography (ECHO) and CVP measurements.

Even in cases of poor myocardial contractility, volume infusion is often initially indicated, because the decreased contractility may be secondary to diminished preload. CVP monitoring and serial ECHOs may be helpful to evaluate loading conditions and contractility. The choice of fluids for intravascular volume expansion includes isotonic crystalloid solutions (normal saline) or colloid solutions (5% albumin). Packed red blood cell transfusions may be indicated if the hematocrit is <25%–30%.

If hypotension persists despite volume replacement, evaluation of cardiac function and possible initiation of inotrope therapy are indicated. ECHO is the best clinically available method for imaging a potential heart donor and may be performed at the bedside via either the transthoracic or transesophageal routes. If the ventricular ejection fraction is <45%, or if regional wall motion abnormalities are seen, aggressive cardiac resuscitation may be needed before such a heart is suitable for transplantation. Correction of loading conditions and factors, such as acidosis, hypoxia, hypercarbia, electrolyte abnormalities, anemia, dehydration, and/or overhydration, that may result from, or exacerbate, decreased preload and afterload may result in an improvement in ejection fraction and suitability for transplantation (34,51). Most acute deaths following cardiac transplantation are caused by right ventricular failure as a result of elevated pulmonary vascular resistance in the recipient or decreased contractility in the donor. Treatment of the impaired contractility in the donor may also partially ameliorate right ventricular failure and prolong the graft life in the recipient. An electrocardiogram should also be obtained to determine potential injury. Serial ECHOs reveal substantial improvement in cardiac contractility after the above-mentioned adverse conditions have been reversed. In a study performed by the California Transplant Donor Network,

16 donor patients whose hearts had been declined by regional transplant centers based on initial ECHO findings underwent repeat ECHOs after optimizing loading and metabolic conditions as well as infusion of IV steroids, usually within 10 hrs after the initial cardiac ECHO. An improvement in left ventricular ejection fraction was noted, and 12 of the 16 donor hearts were transplanted, with a 92% survival rate at an average follow-up of 16 months (55).

Vasopressors

The use of vasopressor agents to maintain blood pressure in organ donors is often required after adequate intravascular volume replacement in order to improve cardiac function, if myocardial dysfunction is present, or to increase SVR in cases of severe vasodilation. Dopamine has been the vasopressor most commonly used in organ donors, because renal and splanchnic blood flow can often be maintained at dosages of <10 mcg/kg/min. Low-dose epinephrine or norepinephrine (≤0.05 mcg/kg/min) may be instituted as second-line inotropes. However, administration of exogenous catecholamines, agents with both α- and β-agonist action (such as dopamine, epinephrine, and norepinephrine) may further deplete myocardial ATP stores and downregulate β-receptors, both of which may adversely affect post-transplantation cardiac function in the recipient (46). Norepinephrine use in the donor has been shown to be associated with increased post–renal transplant acute tubular necrosis and dialysis requirements in recipients. It has also been associated with reduced myocardial function after cardiac transplantation, but its use does not appear to compromise transplanted livers (36,37). In contrast, epinephrine in modest doses has been shown in animal models to maintain renal perfusion while simultaneously improving cardiac function.

Patients who have experienced significant or prolonged hypotension, hypoxia, and/or ischemia are at particular risk for myocardial dysfunction that may require additional inotropic therapy. Dobutamine, a pure β-agonist, may be needed in such cases. However, peripheral vasodilation usually limits its use in these patients due to the diminished SVR already present. Furthermore, because β-receptor downregulation may occur in these patients, dobutamine may not be as effective. Although evidence for its use is lacking, milrinone, a phosphodiesterase inhibitor, may be instituted in cases where dobutamine is not tolerated but cardiac dysfunction exists.

The prolonged use of catecholamine vasopressor agents has been inconsistently associated with poor or delayed organ function and survival but may preclude the viability of some organs for transplantation. In the past, transplant centers often considered a donor heart to be unsuitable for transplantation if the dopamine requirement or its equivalent exceeded 10–15 mcg/kg/min. High doses of both endogenous catecholamines, as seen with the catecholamine storm, as well as exogenous catecholamine administration, can lead to a downregulation in β-receptors on cardiac myocytes, as previously stated, and can cause myocardial hemorrhage and contraction band necrosis. However, a retrospective study that evaluated the effect of donor catecholamine use on graft survival revealed that, in over 2400 transplanted kidneys, the 4-year renal graft survival was >75% (36). Further support of this potential effect of donor catecholamine use on kidney transplant recipients was revealed in a case-controlled study that found a significant decrease in rejection and increase in graft survival in donors who were treated with catecholamine, compared to those who were not (37). Catecholamines have also been shown to downregulate adhesion molecules, which may at least partially explain some of the positive effects seen with catecholamine administration. Adhesion molecules are postulated to play an important adverse role in recipient rejection of transplanted organs.

Despite volume replacement and inotropic therapy, some patients may continue to have hypotension associated with severe vasodilation and reduced SVR. Agents with pure α-agonist function, such as phenylephrine or norepinephrine, may be required in such cases. However, the vasoconstriction associated with α-adrenergic agents may compromise the perfusion of potential donor organs, particularly the kidneys, liver, and heart.

The use of vasopressin in this setting of hemodynamic instability associated with vasodilation and low SVR has recently received increased attention. Although vasopressin is used primarily to control DI in the brain-dead organ donor, through its effect on the V_1 receptor, it also functions as a vasoconstrictor through V_2-receptor effects. A defect in the baroreceptor reflex-mediated secretion of vasopressin from the posterior pituitary results in brain-dead patients developing exquisite sensitivity to the vasoconstrictive effects of vasopressin, even without the presence of DI. The attraction of vasopressin as a pressor lies in its ability to act synergistically with catecholamines, often resulting in a much reduced need for the catecholamines (35). In a retrospective review of critically ill children who were undergoing evaluation for brain death and potential organ recovery, those children who had been treated with vasopressin were seven times more likely to be weaned from α-agonist vasopressors, compared to age-matched controls. Furthermore, the graft function of transplanted livers, kidneys, and hearts was good and was not sufficiently different in the vasopressin-treated group (13). Good graft function in transplanted livers, kidneys, and hearts has also been shown in a randomized, controlled study of vasopressin versus saline (27). The usual pediatric vasopressor dose range of vasopressin is 0.3–2 mU/kg/min (0.0003–0.002 U/kg/min).

At present, due to improved critical care management and the significant deficiency of available organs, if a donor does require high doses of vasopressors, the organs may still be considered for transplantation, albeit at a potentially higher risk for delayed graft function and failure in the recipient.

Hormone Replacement

If significant intravascular volume has been restored and inotropes and vasopressors have been initiated but hypotension persists, pituitary hormone depletion should be suspected. The loss of an intact hypothalamic-pituitary neuroendocrine axis may result in cardiovascular derangements and temperature instability, presumably due to deficiency of hypothalamic and pituitary hormones. Deficiency of adrenocorticotropic hormone and thyroid-stimulating hormone (TSH), in particular, will produce cortisol and thyroid hormone deficiency, respectively, both of which can play important roles in hemodynamic stability. Clinical clues of hormone deficiency will be those symptoms of myocardial dysfunction, because these hormones are normally involved in maintaining myocardial contractility. Intractable hypotension despite increasing vasopressor doses should raise the suspicion of hormone deficiency, and replacement with thyroid hormone and corticosteroids should be strongly considered. Today, many transplant centers and OPOs routinely administer triiodothyronine (T_3) or thyroxine (T_4) in addition to methylprednisolone, vasopressin, and, often, insulin to unstable brain-dead donors. In a classic study, hormone replacement therapy consisting of T_3, cortisol, and insulin was evaluated in brain-dead donors compared with those who did not receive replacement therapy. The hormone-replacement group had a significant decrease in vasopressor requirement, with an increase in mean arterial blood pressure and CO, compared with the nontreated group [25]. A retrospective study of the effects of hormone replacement therapy in the form of methylprednisolone, vasopressin, and/or T_3 or T_4 administered to brain-dead donors compared with those who did not receive hormone replacement showed that 1-month organ recipient survival in the triple hormone replacement group was significantly increased, whereas early graft dysfunction was decreased [35]. However, other studies have revealed no beneficial effect [31]. It is hoped that ongoing clinical trials in this area will clarify the use of hormone replacement in brain-dead donors. Currently, many OPOs, supported by UNOS/OPTN, recommend the administration of these hormones, particularly to hemodynamically unstable donors.

In that many brain-dead donors do develop hemodynamic instability, it is important to evaluate donor suitability in terms of potential for successful organ resuscitation and subsequent donation, as opposed to simply relying on the initial assessment of organ function alone. Investigators evaluated 150 potential adult multiorgan donors, of which 35% (52 patients) were initially deemed unacceptable donors based on vasopressor requirements that averaged the equivalent of 25 mcg of dopamine per kg/min and mean arterial blood pressures <55 mm Hg, despite the pressor support and other hemodynamic parameters. After the institution of methylprednisolone, vasopressin, T_3, and insulin combined with glucose as necessary, organs from >80% of these patients were successfully retrieved and transplanted [51].

Respiratory Pathophysiology

The greatest discrepancy between supply and demand in organ donation is for lungs, with only 7%–22% of potential lung donors deemed suitable for donation. Furthermore, >30% of the lungs deemed potentially suitable are not transplanted due to brain-death–associated lung injury, which includes neurogenic pulmonary edema and a systemic inflammatory response associated with cytokine and thromboxane release and adhesion molecule upregulation [3,19].

Brain-dead patients may develop neurogenic pulmonary edema, requiring mechanical ventilation support at high ventilator settings. The mechanisms responsible for neurogenic pulmonary edema include vasoconstriction that leads to elevated systemic vascular resistance associated with the catecholamine surge, which results in a shift of a large volume of blood away from the peripheral circulation toward the central circulation, particularly the right side of the heart. This shift results in an increase in left atrial pressure, with subsequent increased pulmonary capillary hydrostatic pressure culminating in hemorrhagic pulmonary edema. Concomitantly, increased capillary permeability occurs due to the local release of norepinephrine and neuropeptide Y during the catecholamine surge [18].

Other causes of respiratory insufficiency may result from direct injury due to pulmonary contusions, mucus plugging, pulmonary microemboli, or aspiration, and from the aggressive fluid resuscitative efforts often required for brain-dead patients caused by the hemodynamic changes described earlier. Ventilation-perfusion defects may also occur due to the vasodilation that follows catecholamine depletion, because some lung areas may not be effectively perfused [3]. Lung injury in the donor is common and is the main reason for the underutilization of this organ for transplant.

Evaluation and Management of Respiratory Abnormalities

High levels of positive end-expiratory pressure (PEEP) may be required to maintain oxygenation and prevent atelectasis. High ventilatory pressures may initially be required to obtain and maintain adequate lung recruitment and relative hypocarbia as treatment for elevated ICP. With progression to brain death, carbon dioxide production, as a by-product of cerebral metabolism, becomes minimal, with substantially reduced total-body carbon dioxide production. Minute ventilation can then be greatly reduced in these patients, thereby permitting the lowering of ventilatory pressures and preserving viable lung tissue for potential transplantation. Common mechanical ventilation goals implemented by OPOs exist, but no conclusive evidence supports these ventilation parameters. To address this issue, a multicentered, randomized, controlled study is being conducted to determine the optimal protective ventilatory strategies in organ donors. The current recommendations are usually to maintain a normal pH of 7.35 to 7.45, with normocapnia, and tidal volumes of 8 to 12 mL/kg for volume-ventilated patients with normal lungs or 6 to 8 mL/kg in the presence of diffuse lung disease such as acute respiratory distress syndrome (ARDS). Because research in ARDS has shown benefit with low-tidal volume strategies, the use of higher tidal volumes in potential organ donors may play a role in the exacerbation of inflammatory lung injury. For volume-ventilated adult patients, peak airway pressure should not exceed 40 to 45 cm H_2O, while plateau pressure should not exceed 30 to 35 cm H_2O. If a difference of >10 cm H_2O exists between the peak and plateau pressures, increased resistance may be the problem, and suctioning and bronchodilators may be the solution. If the difference is <10 cm H_2O, decreased compliance may be the problem, and treatment of the underlying cause, such as pulmonary edema or ARDS, may diminish the potential for barotrauma. If peak pressures remain high, switching to pressure ventilation, which is used commonly in pediatric patients, may be appropriate. For pressure-ventilated patients, peak inspiratory pressure, which represents the peak airway pressure, should be maintained at <30–35 cm H_2O. PEEP should continue to allow lung expansion to be maintained at or above functional residual capacity to prevent atelectasis, and inspired oxygen concentration of ≤40% should be used if possible, while maintaining oxygen saturations of at least 92% to 95% and a Pa_{O_2} of at least 100 mm Hg. High concentrations of inspired oxygen diminish the alveolar nitrogen content and result in "resorption atelectasis," potentially creating or worsening ventilation-perfusion defects and hypoxemia [21,30]. The maneuvers to decrease resistance or increase compliance may improve lung function and potential transplantability. However, if the pulmonary abnormality cannot be reversed, the lungs will not be suitable for transplantation. In such cases, altering mechanical ventilation settings to provide lower tidal volumes or lower peak inspiratory pressures may still preserve the viability of other organs through diminishing the systemic inflammatory response associated with high ventilating pressures.

A tracheal Gram stain and aspirate should be obtained to identify any potential infectious process. Serial chest radiographs may be required as surveillance for the development of infiltrates, atelectasis, and pneumothoraces. A unilateral infiltrate does not exclude donation. Bronchoscopy without lavage may also be required to evaluate the airway for secretions and aspirated contents and to obtain cultures, because tracheal cultures obtained from the endotracheal tube may not reflect lower-airway flora. Antibiotic coverage in recipients of a transplanted lung should be based on positive cultures and sensitivities obtained from the donor during bronchoscopy. Aggressive pulmonary toilet, with frequent suctioning, repositioning of the donor, and chest physiotherapy when appropriate, is vital to maintaining suitability of the lungs for transplantation.

A bolus dose of methylprednisolone (usual dose: 15 mg/kg in adults, 1 mg/kg in children; maximum dose, 2 g) given to the brain-dead donor is often used to decrease the systemic inflammatory effect in the donor and to potentially decrease the possibility of rejection following lung transplantation. Steroid administration may also result in better oxygenation, especially when given early after brain death, and may result in an increase in transplantable lungs (8).

Although little supportive efficacy data exist, some investigators have advocated for the use of a single bolus dose of naloxone to be given as a component of a lung management strategy. The precise mechanism of naloxone's action in this role is unknown, but free radical scavenging has been proposed (10).

An oxygen challenge test is often performed to assess lung function and transplantability. The lowest possible level of PEEP is used for the test, often 4 to 5 mm Hg, and the inspired oxygen is then increased to 100%. Following a 5- to 10-min period for equilibrium, an arterial blood gas is obtained. A PaO_2 on 100% oxygen or a PaO_2 –>-to-FiO_2 ratio $\geq$300 mm Hg often signifies lung viability for transplantation (18). Although the use of high ventilator settings to improve this ratio may increase lung transplantability, preliminary evidence suggests that such settings may increase the systemic inflammatory response in the liver, kidneys, and heart, potentially diminishing their transplantability.

Immune System Pathophysiology

Following brain death, increased secretion of proinflammatory cytokines, chemokines, and adhesion molecules occurs in most organs, released in response to stress and resulting in a systemic inflammatory response (15). Free radical formation associated with brain death results in the increased production of nuclear factor κB, which then controls the secretion of acute phase cytokines, such as tumor necrosis factor (TNF)-α and interleukin (IL)-2 (32,45). Some of these cytokines may contribute to cell apoptosis and may lead to further vasodilation and increased

vessel capacitance, exacerbating the injury associated with the catecholamine surge and subsequent hypotension (15). This inflammatory upregulation may also adversely affect organ function post-transplantation and may increase the likelihood of rejection in transplant recipients (3).

Although the exact mechanisms associated with this inflammatory cytokine release are not completely understood, it appears that a hemodynamic mechanism is at least partially responsible. It has been shown in a rat animal model that brain death resulted in increased serum levels of IL-1β and TNF-α. Pretreatment of the animals with phentolamine, an α-adrenergic antagonist, prevented the hypertensive crisis seen with the catecholamine surge and resulted in lower serum levels of these cytokines and better oxygenation. Furthermore, norepinephrine treatment of the hypotension following catecholamine depletion also decreased serum cytokine levels (3).

Steroids have been shown to decrease the systemic inflammatory response as well, presumably because of the decrease in cytokine production. In a prospective study of cytokine expression in both living and brain-dead donors, cytokine levels were significantly increased in brain-dead donors compared with the living donor controls. In contrast, the brain-dead donors who were given steroids prior to organ harvesting had cytokine levels comparable to the living donors (14).

Endocrine Pathophysiology

Diabetes Insipidus

DI due to destruction of the posterior pituitary results in central antidiuretic hormone deficiency and is a common endocrinologic complication encountered in severely brain-injured and particularly in brain-dead patients. The development of DI should, in fact, alert the physician that brain death may be developing. DI results from the inability of the kidney tubules to reabsorb water in the absence of antidiuretic hormone. Left untreated, this condition may lead to severe dehydration, hypotension, and hypernatremia.

Evaluation and Management of Diabetes Insipidus. Clinical signs of DI include polyuria, with a urine osmolarity often <200 mOsm/L and serum hypernatremia, often with a serum sodium >150 mEq/L.

The treatment of DI often includes vasopressin supplementation. Vasopressin is often instituted as a continuous infusion, with a usual starting dose of 0.5 mU/kg/hr. Because fluid loss in DI can be profound, adjustments in vasopressin therapy may have to be made as frequently as every 10 mins until the desired effect is achieved, usually with urine output in the range of 2 to 4 mL/kg/hr. If the desired output is not achieved, the rate of the vasopressin infusion may be doubled, usually up to 2 to 3 mU/kg/hr, with the current suggested maximum pediatric dose for DI being 10 mU/kg/hr. It is important to remember the vasoconstrictive effects of vasopressin, especially at higher doses, which may lead to increased vasomotor tone and hypertension, potentially impairing perfusion to other organs. Desmopressin acetate, on the other hand, is essentially devoid of vasopressor effects. However, it has a long half-life, with effects lasting an average of 12 hrs, and is therefore difficult to titrate (18).

In some cases of DI in brain-dead patients, until urine output can be effectively controlled with vasopressin replacement, fluid replacement may be necessary to prevent excessive fluid loss and resultant dehydration. This process can be particularly harmful in brain-dead patients who already often have diminished preload from a variety of other sources, as previously described (17,18). Urine output can, in fact, be as high as 10 mL/kg/hr, such that rapid dehydration and hypotension can develop and be difficult to control in such patients without fluid replacement. Fluid replacement is usually in the form of hypotonic IV fluids, often 0.25%–0.5% normal saline, in an attempt to match the ongoing hypotonic urine losses. Glucose-containing replacement IV fluids should be avoided, because hyperglycemia will lead to further urine loss through an osmotic diuresis. Frequent assessment of volume hemodynamic status and electrolyte concentration is imperative in patients with DI to prevent dehydration, as well as overhydration and possible hyponatremia (53). Once urine output of 2 to 4 mL/kg/hr has been achieved, fluid replacement can be discontinued to prevent overhydration and edema.

Other electrolyte abnormalities often accompany DI due to polyuria; these include hypokalemia, hypocalcemia, hypophosphatemia, and hypomagnesemia.

Adrenal Dysfunction

Adrenocorticotropic hormone deficiency may occur in brain-dead patients secondary to anterior pituitary necrosis, with consequent adrenal dysfunction and low cortisol levels; in addition, it may contribute to myocardial dysfunction (24,46). A relative adrenal insufficiency has been described in trauma and critically ill patients; this may result in higher requirements for vasopressors. However, the data supporting cortisol replacement therapy in brain-dead patients remain controversial, but most OPO donor management protocols do call for a steroid bolus dose, usually in the form of methylprednisolone, in addition to the other hormone replacements previously discussed. Steroids may decrease the systemic inflammatory response effect and reduce the need for vasopressor support, as previously discussed (8). A bolus dose of methylprednisolone 15 mg/kg in adults and 1 mg/kg in children, with a maximum dose of 2 g is often used.

Thyroid Dysfunction

Thyroid deficiency may follow brain death and may result in a shift toward anaerobic metabolism, exacerbating hemodynamic instability and resulting in elevated serum lactate levels.

The normal physiologic effects of thyroid hormone are probably due to T_3, of which 80% is formed in peripheral nonthyroid tissue by conversion from T_4. The remaining percentage of T_3 is released from the thyroid gland itself. Low T_3 and T_4 with normal TSH levels and elevated reverse T_3 levels are often noted in critically ill adults and children, often representing the "sick euthyroid" state. Three stages of "sick euthyroid" state have been described in critical illness, and these may represent a progression in severity. Initially, with critical illness, T_3 levels may be decreased, with an increase in reverse T_3 levels, while the remainder of thyroid testing is normal. As the illness becomes more severe or prolonged, T_4 levels may decrease. The most severe form of "sick euthyroid" state is represented by a concomitant decrease in TSH. The use of cer-

tain vasopressors, such as dopamine and possibly dobutamine, may create or aggravate the sick euthyroid syndrome by decreasing the secretion of TSH from the pituitary. This effect would presumably be minimal in brain-dead patients because of pituitary necrosis.

Evaluation and Management of Thyroid Dysfunction. Thyroid hormone replacement has been studied in critical illness, including following cardiopulmonary bypass, as well as in brain-dead donors. The studies have produced varied results, and more definitive studies are necessary. However, in brain-dead donors, supplementation of T_3 or T_4 may result in improved myocardial function and lower vasopressor requirements, with improved blood pressure and CO. A shift back to aerobic metabolism may also occur, with improved organ perfusion and a decrease in lactic acidosis. Most data on the replacement of thyroid hormone are in the adult transplantation literature. Data on this topic in pediatric brain-dead donors are limited. The effects of T_4 infusion alone on vasopressor support in brain-dead children were retrospectively evaluated. T_4 administration was associated with decreased vasopressor requirements in such children, after adjusting for steroid use, fluid status, and baseline vasopressor need prior to T_4 administration (56). The usual adult bolus dose of T_4 is 20 mcg IV, followed by a continuous infusion of 10 mcg/hr IV; in children, the bolus dose is 1 to 5 mcg/kg/hr, with a continuous-infusion dose of 0.8 to 1.4 mcg/kg/hr (31,42).

Hyperglycemia and Insulin

Hyperglycemia occurs frequently in brain-dead patients. The catecholamine surge that occurs with brain death invariably contributes to this hyperglycemia. Initially, elevated glucose levels represent an appropriate physiologic response to stress, supplying the brain and other organs with the energy necessary for increased metabolic demands. Catecholamines are known to result in insulin resistance, thus inhibiting glucose uptake. If the physiologic stress is not lessened or removed, hyperglycemia continues. The adverse effects of hyperglycemia and the mechanisms responsible for these effects in critically ill adults continue to be intensely studied. In a prospective, randomized, controlled study of critically ill patients in a surgical ICU who were treated with either conventional or intensive insulin therapy, in addition to other positive findings, the need for vasopressors decreased in the intensively treated group (50). Controlled study must be conducted in brain-dead donors to determine if similar glucose management is necessary.

Complications associated with hyperglycemia in brain-dead donors include an osmotic diuresis, which can further exacerbate the hemodynamic instability associated with catecholamine depletion. An insulin infusion to maintain serum glucose levels in the range of 120–180 mg/dL should correct the diuresis associated with hyperglycemia. Furthermore, studies have shown that hyperglycemia in brain-dead organ donors may impair subsequent liver (48) and pancreatic dysfunction in transplant recipients (29). However, hyperglycemia is not usually thought to be due to primary endocrine insufficiency and should not be used as a marker of pancreatic function. Hyperglycemia also induces the formation of oxygen radicals and thereby produces an inflammatory effect (45). The exact consequences of hyperglycemia on recipient organ function have yet to be elucidated.

Temperature Instability

Temperature instability is often one of the first clinical signs that neurologic injury has progressed to brain death. This lack of temperature control and subsequent poikilothermia is ultimately due to loss of hypothalamic-pituitary control, as well as hormone deficiency, as described earlier. Hyperthermia may initially be noted as a result of vasoconstriction associated with the catecholamine surge; hypothermia may follow as intense vasodilation occurs. The large surface area-to-mass ratio contributes to the child's predisposition for heat loss through the skin. Vasoconstriction of the peripheral blood vessels occurs in an attempt to reduce this heat loss. The ability to shiver is lost once brain death occurs, thereby preventing heat generation. Thyroid hormone deficiency potentially exacerbates the lack of temperature control.

Complications of hypothermia may develop in the brain-dead donor and include a "cold diuresis"; coagulopathy, resulting in an increased risk of bleeding and thrombosis; and neutrophil dysfunction, potentially predisposing the donor to infection. In addition, hypothermia shifts the oxygen dissociation curve to the left, further decreasing the supply of oxygen to tissues and exacerbating the metabolic acidosis that often develops from the vasoconstriction associated with hypothermia.

Management of Temperature Regulatory Abnormalities. To maintain the body temperature of organ donors, the environmental temperature must be maintained and heat loss must be minimized. Radiant heat warmers, thermal mattresses, heated inspired ventilation gases, and warm IV fluids can be used to maintain body temperature. Ideally, core body temperature should be maintained in the normal range. Thyroid hormone replacement may also improve temperature regulation.

Renal, Electrolyte, and Acid–Base Disorders

Several metabolic derangements frequently develop in the critically ill and are often exacerbated in brain-dead patients. The hypernatremia that accompanies brain death is multifactorial. Often caused by DI, it is also due to the management of elevated ICP with hypertonic saline and diuretics. Indeed, hypernatremia and hyperosmolarity are goals of therapy when managing elevated ICP. However, hypernatremia can adversely affect potentially transplantable organs, especially the liver. A study that examined the effect of donor serum sodium concentration on the postoperative function of liver transplants demonstrated that serum sodium values > 155 mEq/L adversely affected graft survival and was an independent predictor of early graft loss in the recipient (48).

Metabolic acidosis may also occur due to numerous factors such as myocardial dysfunction and low CO, renal insufficiency, and hypothermia. Evaluation and treatment of the underlying cause is vital to maintenance of organ suitability. Hyperkalemia associated with metabolic acidosis may predispose to arrhythmias in an already irritable myocardium. Hyperkalemia may also be due in part to the hyperglycemia that frequently accompanies brain death. With appropriate treatment of hyperglycemia, potassium levels should be routinely monitored as potassium begins to enter the cells.

Several other electrolyte abnormalities may occur that include hypokalemia, hypophosphatemia, hypocalcemia, and hypomagnesemia, all of which may contribute to myocardial dysfunction and should be appropriately supplemented.

Coagulopathy

Severely brain-injured patients may frequently develop a significant disseminated intravascular consumptive coagulopathy, which may result from release of thromboplastin and tissue plasminogen from injured and necrotic brain tissue (18). Aggressive fluid resuscitation with colloid, crystalloid, and blood products may result in dilution of platelets and circulating clotting factors. Hypothermia may also result in disseminated intravascular coagulopathy and increased platelet aggregation. The platelet count should be maintained at $\geq 50,000$, while fibrinogen should be at least 100 mg/dL. Coagulopathy should be corrected with fresh frozen plasma, cryoprecipitate, and platelets, as necessary.

ORGAN RECOVERY AND SURVIVAL RATES

Currently, an overall average of 3.06 organs is successfully retrieved from each donor. Because nine organs (if donor liver is split for two separate donations) can potentially be retrieved from DBD donors and eight can be retrieved from DCD donors, the management and ultimate procurement of organs can be greatly improved upon (1).

Recipient survival is highest in those who have received an organ through living donation. For organs obtained from deceased donors, kidneys obtained through DCD often demonstrate graft survival rates comparable to those organs obtained through DBD, even though DCD kidneys often have a higher rate of delayed graft function (4). Early investigators also found significantly more delayed graft function and primary nonfunction in the recipients of kidneys from DCD donors. However, many of these organs were obtained through uncontrolled DCD. Furthermore, the difference in primary nonfunction became nonsignificant after 1998, presumably due to controlled DCD, different techniques, preservation fluids, and better immunosuppression. Acute kidney rejection and graft survival at 1, 5, and 10 years was also not significantly different between DCD and DBD donors (2). Livers obtained through DCD often have higher rates of graft failure, compared to those obtained through DBD (4). However, in a series of liver transplants obtained through controlled DCD, 100% recipient and organ survival at an average of 18 months was observed. No events of primary nonfunction were reported, but 75% of recipients developed acute rejection at some point during this follow-up. All episodes of rejection responded to steroid administration, and no episodes of chronic rejection occurred (33). Furthermore, an analysis of OPTN data revealed that, when low-risk recipients receive low-risk DCD livers, defined by warm ischemia time of <30 mins and cold ischemia time of <10 hrs, the graft survival rates are comparable to those obtained from DBD donors (20). Today, over 160,000 people are living with a functioning transplanted organ, an increase of 100% over the past decade (38).

CONCLUSIONS AND FUTURE DIRECTIONS

Several prominent healthcare and governmental organizations have realized the urgent need for improvement in the organ donor process, extending from how team members approach donors and their families to the management of the organ donor after consent has been obtained. The IOM issued a follow-up report in May 2006 that called for improvements in the current system of organ procurement. This report highlights the efforts of the Health Resources and Services Administration in the formation of a series of organ donation breakthrough collaboratives (12). The first collaborative was convened in April 2003 and involved 95 hospitals and OPOs, although no children's hospitals were included. In the second collaborative, launched in 2004, 11 children's hospitals participated in an effort to help focus on pediatric organ donation "best practices." The goal of these collaboratives is to create a systematic national program to spread these accepted "best practices" of the organ procurement process to the nation's largest hospitals in order to achieve organ donation rates >75%. To date, participating hospitals have achieved major increases in *conversion rates*, the term applied to consent for organ donation, which has also led to increases on a national level (5,26). With the continued joint efforts of the of the ICU staff and the OPO members who are involved in the management of potential organ donors, and with additional collaboratives to spread the "best practices" and promote public awareness, it is hoped that many more waiting recipients will receive a transplant, not only saving lives, but also improving the quality of those lives.

KEY POINTS

- Options for organ donation include DBD, DCD, and living donation.
- Organs most in demand for pediatric patients on the transplant waiting list are liver, followed by kidney and heart.
- The demand for organs currently far exceeds the available supply for several reasons. Approximately 50% of family members currently refuse to give consent for organ donation from their deceased loved ones. Other reasons include the failure to identify eligible donors and failure to give families the option of donation.
- In cases of DBD, request for organ donation should be "decoupled" from informing the family of the death.
- Organ donation from patients who have experienced "cardiac death," or DCD, began in the 1960s, preceding the practice of donation following brain death. Resurgence of DCD began again in 1997, with the IOM report, prompted by the extreme shortage of available organs and family wishes to be able to donate organs of neurologically devastated but not brain-dead family members.
- In cases of DCD, the decision to withdraw care must always have been made prior to discussing organ donation.
- Often, kidneys that can be retrieved through the DCD process have comparable graft survival rates to those obtained through DBD.

- Relatively few absolute contraindications are associated with organ transplantation, and often these absolutes become relative based on the individual recipient.
- Today, most OPOs and ICUs utilize a standardized donor management protocol. UNOS has published such a protocol, known as the Critical Pathway for the Organ Donor.
- Brain-dead donor management requires a change in the goal of care from cerebral-protective strategies to organ-donor–supportive strategies.
- Several hemodynamic changes may occur in brain-dead patients that may ultimately affect the potential transplantability of other organs.
- Brainstem ischemia proceeds in a craniocaudal direction, ultimately involving the vagal nucleus in the medulla oblongata, resulting in uncontrolled sympathetic stimulation—the "catecholamine storm."
- Shortly thereafter, catecholamine depletion occurs, with a significant generalized vasodilation, culminating in hemodynamic collapse from reduced preload and afterload. As many as 25% of potential donors are lost due to this hemodynamic instability.
- Hypotension is the most common problem encountered by physicians who care for pediatric organ donors; it can be caused by vasodilation, hypovolemia (due to diuretic use, DI, osmotic diuresis, and hypothermia), and myocardial dysfunction.
- Optimal CVP for managing brain-dead organ donors is between 8 and 10 mm Hg.
- Myocardial dysfunction is multifactorial and may be due to altered loading conditions, ischemia, acidosis, hypoxia, massive cytokine release that results in a systemic inflammatory state and abnormal function of the hypothalamic-pituitary axis that results in pituitary hormone depletion.
- Dopamine has been the vasopressor most commonly used in organ donors, because renal and splanchnic blood flow can often be maintained at levels <10 mcg/kg/min.
- The vasoconstriction associated with α-adrenergic agents, such as phenylephrine, epinephrine, and norepinephrine, must be taken into account, because perfusion to organs may be compromised, particularly the kidneys, liver, and heart.
- Vasopressin is becoming a favored vasopressor for management of hypotension that is neither fluid nor inotrope responsive. It acts synergistically with catecholamines, often resulting in a much reduced requirement for catecholamines.
- Intractable hypotension should raise the suspicion of hormone deficiency, and replacement with thyroid hormone and corticosteroids should be strongly considered.
- Currently, most transplant centers and OPOs routinely administer T_3 or T_4, in addition to methylprednisolone, vasopressin, and, often, insulin to brain-dead donors to improve or prevent the deterioration in myocardial function.
- Potential donor lungs may be compromised by neurogenic pulmonary edema, pneumonia, and the systemic inflammatory response associated with brain death.
- A P_{AO_2} on 100% oxygen or a P_{AO_2}-to-F_{IO_2} ratio ≥ 300 mm Hg often signifies lung viability for transplantation.
- Hypernatremia in the brain-dead donor due to hypertonic saline administration, DI, or osmotic diuresis can adversely affect potentially transplantable organs, especially the liver.

- The treatment of DI often includes vasopressin supplementation. However, in the initial phase of management until urine output can be effectively controlled with vasopressin, fluid replacement may be necessary to prevent dehydration.
- Severely brain-injured patients may frequently develop a significant disseminated intravascular consumptive coagulopathy, which may result from the release of thromboplastin and tissue plasminogen from injured and necrotic brain tissue.
- Currently, an overall average of 3.06 organs is successfully procured from each donor.
- The IOM issued a report in May 2006 that called for improvements in the current system of organ procurement and highlights the efforts of the Health Resources and Services Administration (HRSA) in the formation of a series of organ donation breakthrough collaboratives.
- The goal of these collaboratives is to create a systematic, national program to spread the "known best practices" of the organ procurement process to the largest hospitals in the US, to achieve organ donation rates >75% in these hospitals.

ACKNOWLEDGMENTS

Regarding all OPTN data, this work was supported in part by Health Resources and Services Administration contract 231-00-0115. The content is the responsibility of the authors alone and does not necessarily reflect the views or policies of the Department of Health and Human Services, nor does mention of trade names, commercial products, or organizations imply endorsement by the US Government.

References

1. 2005 Annual Report of the U.S. Organ Procurement and Transplantation Network and the Scientific Registry of Transplant Recipients: Transplant data 1994–2004. Department of Health and Human Services, Health Resources and Services Administration, Healthcare Systems Bureau, Division of Transplantation, Rockville, MD; United Network for Organ Sharing, Richmond, VA; University Renal Research and Education Association, Ann Arbor, MI.
2. Alonso A, Fernandez-Rivera C, Villaverde P, et al. Renal transplantation from non-heart-beating donors: A single-center 10-year experience. *Transplant Proc* 2005;37:3658–60.
3. Avlonitis VS, Wigfield CH, Kirby JA, et al. The hemodynamic mechanisms of lung injury and systemic inflammatory response following brain death in the transplant donor. *Am J Transplant* 2005;5:684–93.
4. Bernat JL, D'Alessandro AM, Port FK, et al. Report of a national conference on donation after cardiac death. *Am J Transplant* 2006;6:281–91.
5. Bratton SL, Kolovos NS, Roach ES, et al. Pediatric organ transplantation needs: Organ donation best practices. *Arch Pediatr Adolesc Med* 2006;160:468–72.
6. Brockmann JG, Vaidya A, Reddy S, et al. Retrieval of abdominal organs for transplantation. *Br J Surg* 2006;93:133–46.
7. Ethics Committee, American College of Critical Care Medicine, Society of Critical Care Medicine. Recommendation for nonheartbeating organ donation. A position paper by the Ethics Committee, American College of Critical Care Medicine, Society of Critical Care Medicine. *Crit Care Med* 2001;29:1826–31.
8. Follette DM, Rudich SM, Babcock WD. Improved oxygenation and increased lung donor recovery with high-dose steroid administration after brain death. *J Heart Lung Transplant* 1998;17:423–9.
9. Guidelines for the determination of brain death in children. Task force for the determination of brain death in children. *Neurology* 1987;37:1077–8.
10. Improvement in pulmonary function following administration of naloxone in brain dead patients. *Transplantation* 2006;82:439–40.
11. Institute of Medicine, National Academy of Sciences. *Non-heart-beating Organ Transplantation: Medical and Ethical Issues in Procurement*. Washington DC: National Academy Press, 1997.
12. Institute of Medicine. Organ donation: Opportunities for action. May 2006. Available at: http://www.nap.edu/catalog/11643.html. Accessed on February 8, 2007.
13. Katz K, Lawler J, Wax J, et al. Vasopressin pressor effects in critically ill children during evaluation for brain death and organ recovery. *Resuscitation* 2000;47:33–40.
14. Kuecuek O, Mantouvalou L, Klemz R, et al. Significant reduction of proinflammatory cytokines by treatment of the brain-dead donor. *Transplant Proc* 2005;37:387–8.
15. Land WG. The role of postischemic reperfusion injury and other nonantigen-dependent inflammatory pathways in transplantation. *Transplantation* 2005;79:505–14.
16. Lewis J, Peltier J, Nelson H, et al. Development of the University of Wisconsin Donation after Cardiac Death Evaluation Tool. *Prog Transplant* 2003;13:265–73.
17. Lugo N, Silver P, Nimkoff L, et al. Diagnosis and management algorithm of acute onset of central diabetes insipidus in critically ill children. *J Pediatr Endocrinol Metab* 1997;10(6):633–9.
18. Lutz-Dettinger N, de Jaeger A, Kerremans I. Care of the potential pediatric organ donor. *Pediatr Clin North Am* 2001;48:715–49.
19. Mascia L, Bosma K, Pasero D, et al. Ventilatory and hemodynamic management of potential organ donors: An observational survey. *Crit Care Med* 2006;34:321–7.
20. Mateo R, Cho Y, Singh G, et al. Risk factors for graft survival after liver transplantation from donation after cardiac death donors: An analysis of OPTN/UNOS data. *Am J Transplant* 2006;6(4):791–6.
21. Matuschak GM. Optimizing ventilatory support of the potential organ donor during evolving brain death: Maximizing lung availability for transplantation. *Crit Care Med* 2006;34:548–9.
22. Metzger RA, Taylor GJ, McGaw LJ, et al. Research to practice: A national consensus conference. *Prog Transplant* 2005;15(4):379–84.
23. Novitzky D. Donor management: State of the art. *Transplant Proc* 1997; 29:3773–5.
24. Novitzky D. Detrimental effects of brain death on the potential organ donor. *Transplant Proc* 1997;29:3770–2.
25. Novitzky D, Cooper DK, Morrell D, et al. Brain death, triiodothyronine depletion, and inhibition of oxidative phosphorylation: Relevance to management of organ donors. *Transplant Proc* 1987;19:4110–11.
26. Organ Donation Breakthrough Collaborative. Best practices evaluation final report. Available at: http://www.organdonor.gov/bestpractice2005.htm. Accessed September 1, 2006.
27. Pennefather SH, Bullock RE, Mantle D, et al. Use of low dose arginine vasopressin to support brain-dead organ donors. *Transplantation* 1995;59:58–62.
28. Pilcher DV, Scheinkestel CD, Snell GI, et al. High central venous pressure is associated with prolonged mechanical ventilation and increased mortality after lung transplantation. *J Thorac Cardiovasc Surg* 2005;129:912–8.
29. Powner DJ. Donor care before pancreatic tissue transplantation. *Prog Transplant* 2005;15:129–36.
30. Powner DJ, Darby JM, Stuart SA. Recommendations for mechanical ventilation during donor care. *Prog Transplant* 2000;10:33–8.
31. Powner DJ, Hernandez M. A review of thyroid hormone administration during adult donor care. *Prog Transplant* 2005;15:202–7.
32. Pratschke J, Tullius SG, Neuhaus P. Brain death associated ischemia/reperfusion injury. *Ann Transplant* 2004;9:78–80.
33. Reich DJ, Munoz SJ, Rothstein KD, et al. Controlled non-heart-beating donor liver transplantation: A successful single center experience, with topic update. *Transplantation* 2000;70:1159–66.
34. Rosendale JD, Chabalewski FL, McBride MA, et al. Increased transplanted organs from the use of a standardized donor management protocol. *Am J Transplant* 2002;2:761–8.
35. Rosendale JD, Kauffman HM, McBride MA, et al. Hormonal resuscitation yields more transplanted hearts, with improved early function. *Transplantation* 2003;75:1336–41.
36. Schnuelle P, Berger S, de Boer J, et al. Effects of catecholamine application to brain-dead donors on graft survival in solid organ transplantation. *Transplantation* 2001;72:455–63.
37. Schnuelle P, Lorenz D, Mueller A, et al. Donor catecholamine use reduces acute allograft rejection and improves graft survival after cadaveric renal transplantation. *Kidney Int* 1999;56:738–46.
38. Scientific Registry of Transplant Recipients. People living with a functioning graft at year end by organ, 19952005. Available at: http://www.ustransplant.org/. Accessed September 1, 2006.
39. Sebening C, Hagl C, Szabo G, et al. Cardiocirculatory effects of acutely increased intracranial pressure and subsequent brain death. *Eur J Cardiothorac Surg* 1995;9:360–72.
40. Shafer TJ, Schkade LL, Evans RW, et al. Vital role of medical examiners and coroners in organ transplantation. *Am J Transplant* 2003;4:160–8.
41. Sheehy E, Conrad SL, Brigham LE, et al. Estimating the number of potential organ donors in the United States. *N Engl J Med* 2003;349:667–74.
42. Shemie SD, Ross H, Pagliarello J, et al. Organ donor management in Canada: Recommendations of the forum on medical management to optimize organ potential. *CMAJ* 2006;174:S13–30.
43. Siminoff LA, Mercer MB, Arnold R. Families' understanding of brain death. *Prog Transplant* 2003;13:218–24.

44. Siminoff LA, Gordon N, Hewlett J, et al. Factors influencing families' consent for donation of solid organs for transplantation. *JAMA* 2001;286:71–7.

45. Singer P, Shapiro H, Cohen J. Brain death and organ damage: The modulating effects of nutrition. *Transplantation* 2005;80:1363–8.

46. Smith M. Physiologic changes during brain stem death – lessons for management of the organ donor. *J Heart Lung Transplant* 2004;23:S217–22.

47. Szabo G. Physiologic changes after brain death. *J Heart Lung Transplant* 2004;23:S223–6.

48. Totsuka E, Fung U, Hakamada K, et al. Analysis of clinical variables of donors and recipients with respect to short-term graft outcome in human liver transplantation. *Transplant Proc* 2004;36:2215–8.

49. Truog RD, Christ G, Browning DM, et al. Sudden traumatic death in children: "We did everything, but your child didn't survive." *JAMA* 2006; 295:2646–54.

50. van den Berghe G, Wouters P, Weekers F, et al. Intensive insulin therapy in the critically ill patients. *N Engl J Med* 2001;345:1359–67.

51. Wheeldon DR, Potter CD, Oduro A, et al. Transforming the "unacceptable" donor: Outcomes from the adoption of a standardized donor management technique. *J Heart Lung Transplant* 1995;14:734–42.

52. Williams MA, Lipsett PA, Rushton CH, et al. The physician's role in discussing organ donation with families. *Crit Care Med* 2003;31:1568–73.

53. Wise-Faberowski L, Soriano SG, Ferrari L, et al. Perioperative management of diabetes insipidus in children. *J Neurosurg Anesthesiol* 2004;16(3): 220–5.

54. Wood KE, Becker BN, McCartney JG, et al. Care of the potential organ donor. *N Engl J Med* 2004;351:2730–9.

55. Zaroff JG, Babcock WD, Shiboski SC, et al. Temporal changes in left ventricular systolic function in heart donors: Results of serial echocardiography. *J Heart Lung Transplant* 2003;22:383–8.

56. Zuppa AF, Nadkarni V, Davis L, et al. The effect of a thyroid hormone infusion on vasopressor support in critically ill children with cessation of neurologic function. *Crit Care Med* 2004;32:2318–22.

CHAPTER 16 ■ GENOMIC MEDICINE

MARY K. DAHMER • MICHAEL QUASNEY

During the last 15 years, advances, such as the sequencing of the human genome, high-throughput genotyping, microarrays, and proteomic analyses, have altered the vision of how medicine will be practiced in the future. These advances have rapidly expanded the understanding of specific diseases and treatments. Although the initial impact of these advances has primarily involved inherited diseases and cancers, other areas within the practice of medicine are now being affected, including the area of pediatric critical care. This chapter will describe these new techniques and how they can be used to answer critical questions in medicine, and will provide examples in which the techniques have been used to study critical illnesses.

TECHNOLOGIC ADVANCES

Genotyping DNA Polymorphisms

The sequencing of the human genome has revealed that many genes are polymorphic; that is, small differences exist in DNA sequences among individuals. Polymorphic genes are those in which variation at a specific nucleotide site is found in greater than 1% of the general population and, in some instances, in as much as 50% of the population. Such sites are referred to as *polymorphic sites* (by contrast, *mutations* are considered to be sites at which variation occurs in less than 1% of the population). Polymorphic sites within a gene do not necessarily affect the expression or function of the gene product. Polymorphisms that occur in a noncoding region of the gene not involved with the regulation of transcription of mRNA from a DNA template or with processing or stability of the mRNA transcript will have no effect on gene expression. Even polymorphisms in the coding region of a gene may not affect the function or stability of the gene's protein product if they do not change the encoded amino acid (a silent substitution), or if the amino acid substitution does not affect the stability or function of the protein. However, in many instances, polymorphic sites affect the expression (by altering noncoding regulatory regions of the gene) or function (by altering the amino acid sequence) of the protein product. Polymorphisms that result in alterations in levels or in functioning of proteins are responsible for the genetically determined variation in our physical characteristics, our physiology, and our personality traits. Genetic variability also appears to explain part of the variability seen in patient populations with regard to susceptibility to disease, severity of disease, and response to treatment. Polymorphisms are not only of interest because of the subset responsible for genetic variability but also because they occur fairly frequently in the human genome and can be used as markers to map genes involved with disease to specific regions of the genome. To be used as a marker, a polymorphism does not have to change the expression or function of a protein product; rather, it only needs to be linked to the gene involved with the disease of interest.

Polymorphisms in the DNA sequence may exist in several forms, with the most frequent form being a single nucleotide polymorphism (SNP) due to a base pair substitution. In addition, polymorphisms within genes may be due to insertions or deletions of fragments of DNA or to the presence of a variable number of tandem repeats (VNTRs) of short, repetitive DNA sequences. Although a number of approaches have been used to identify genetic polymorphisms, currently the most frequently used method is simply to sequence and compare the gene of interest in a number of individuals. Because individuals have two copies of each gene, at any given polymorphic site, an individual can be either heterozygous or homozygous for one, or the other, polymorphism found at that site. Once a polymorphic site within a gene is identified, a number of methods can be used to determine the genotype of individuals having that polymorphic site.

Almost all genotyping techniques require amplification of the fragment of DNA that contains the site of interest by the polymerase chain reaction (PCR) technique. This technique allows for the amplification of a specific region of the genome (in this case the region that contains the polymorphic site). It uses as primers for the PCR small pieces of single-stranded DNA that are complementary to regions that flank the polymorphic site. For most insertions or deletions and VNTRs, the genotype can be determined by examining the size of the PCR products using gel electrophoresis. Such an approach can also be used to genotype SNPs present in restriction enzyme recognition sites, so called restriction fragment length polymorphisms (RFLPs). Restriction enzymes recognize and cut DNA at specific nucleotide sequences, and a polymorphism in such a site alters the enzyme's ability to recognize and cut the DNA (**Fig. 16.1**). Many early studies that examined the association of polymorphisms with disease examined polymorphisms that resulted in differences in the size of the DNA fragment(s) seen either after PCR (insertions or deletions of a section of DNA or VNTRs) or after PCR and restriction digests (RFLPs), because the presence of such sites could be easily determined using gel electrophoresis. However, such techniques are not useful for the many SNPs that are not located in restriction sites; consequently, other techniques have been developed to genotype such sites.

One such technique is allele-specific PCR (**Fig. 16.2**). Copies of DNA with different nucleotides at a specific polymorphic site are considered to be different alleles of the gene. Allele-specific

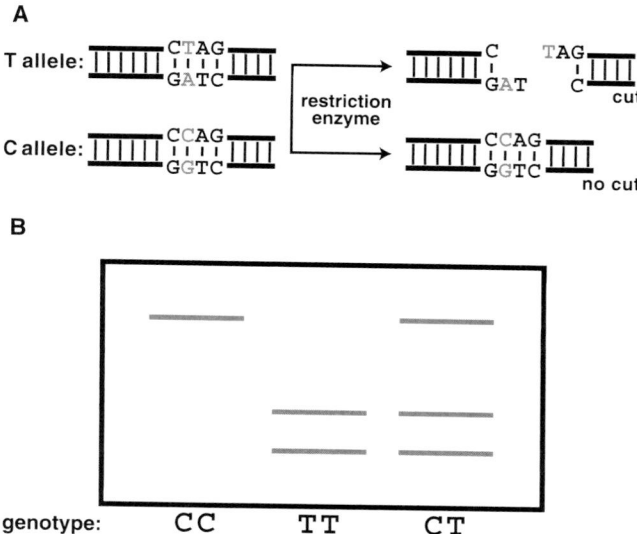

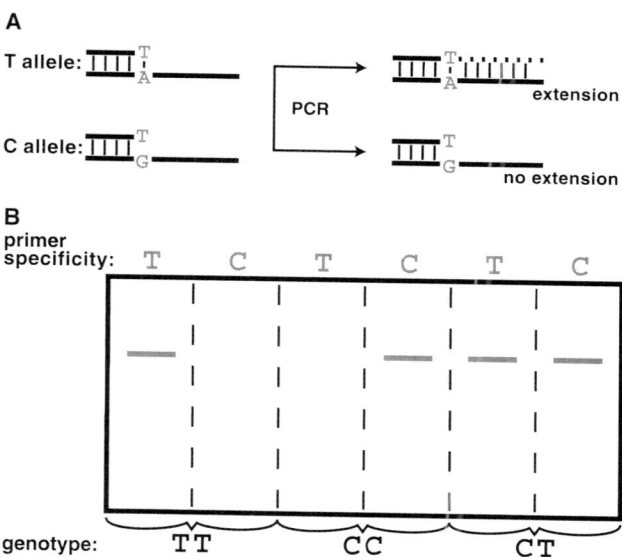

FIGURE 16.1. Genotyping a restriction site polymorphism. **A:** The nucleotide at the indicated polymorphic site is either a thymine (T) or a cytosine (C). When T is present, a restriction enzyme recognition site is formed, which is cleaved in the presence of the restriction enzyme. If C is present, the restriction enzyme does not cut. **B:** After incubation with the restriction enzyme, cleavage of the DNA is determined by gel electrophoresis. The expected results are shown for three individuals homozygous for T, for C, or heterozygous for T and C are shown.

FIGURE 16.2. Genotyping by allele-specific PCR. Two separate reactions are used to genotype each individual. Reactions contain a common primer and one of two allele-specific primers, each of which end with one of the two nucleotides found at the polymorphic site. **A:** In the example, the allele-specific primer shown is for the T allele (only extension from the allele-specific primer, not the common primer is shown). If either copy of the patient's DNA has the T allele at this site, the last nucleotide will hybridize and extension will occur, allowing a productive PCR reaction. If either copy of the patient's DNA contains the C allele, the last nucleotide of the primer cannot hybridize, and extension does not occur, thus resulting in no PCR product. **B:** The presence or absence of a PCR product for each reaction is determined by gel electrophoresis. The expected results are shown for three individuals homozygous for T, for C, or heterozygous for T and C.

primers that are identical except for the last nucleotide are used in the PCR reactions. PCR reactions generate new pieces of DNA through the addition of nucleotides to the 3′ end of a primer hybridized to the DNA of interest, which acts as a template. To genotype an individual using the allele-specific PCR technique, two different PCR reactions are performed, each with a different allele-specific primer and a second primer common to both reactions. If the individual has a copy of the allele of interest, the last nucleotide of the allele-specific primer will hybridize to it and a PCR product will be generated. If no match is located at the 3′ end of the primer, extension by the polymerase is so inefficient that no detectable PCR product is formed. Presence or absence of the PCR product can be determined using gel electrophoresis or by other methods more amenable to high-throughput techniques.

Another technique often used to genotype SNPs is based on hybridization with allele-specific oligonucleotide (ASO) probes labeled so that they can be detected (**Fig. 16.3**). Such probes differ only by a single nucleotide (the polymorphic site, which is generally in the middle of the ASO). To genotype an individual, a separate assay is performed with each ASO probe. In the simplest of these types of assays, hybridization conditions are chosen such that each ASO hybridizes only to its specific allele. The presence of one mismatched nucleotide is enough to prevent annealing under the hybridization conditions used.

More recently, with the increased interest in SNPs as tools for mapping genes and for candidate-gene association studies, techniques for high-throughput SNP genotyping have been developed. These techniques include some that are performed in solution and others that are solid-phase reactions performed on supports, such as beads or DNA microarrays. The underlying strategies for the newer, high-throughput techniques are similar to the older more labor-intensive techniques, but these new

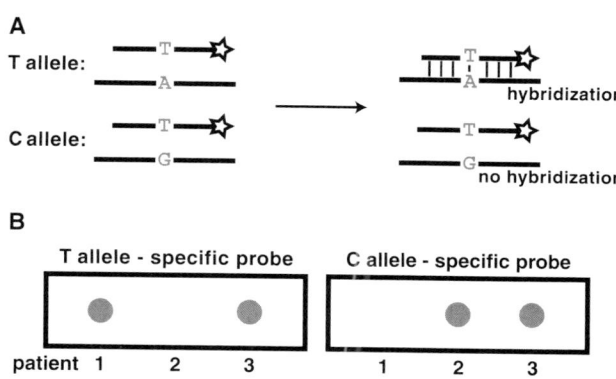

FIGURE 16.3. Genotyping by allele-specific hybridization. Two allele-specific oligonucleotide (ASO) probes are made and are identical except for the polymorphic site. The probes are tagged for visualization, as indicated by the star. **A:** The allele-specific probe for only the T allele is shown. This ASO will hybridize only to the DNA that contains a perfectly matched complementary sequence—in this case, the T allele. Although only one reaction is shown (containing the ASO that contains T), two reactions, each containing one of the two different ASOs, are performed for each patient sample. **B:** Hybridization can be visualized in a variety of ways, depending on the tag used. The expected results are shown for three individuals homozygous for T, for C, or heterozygous for T and C.

techniques allow for the simultaneous detection of hundreds of SNPs. Discriminating which allele is present is often accomplished using hybridization, single base-pair extension ("mini-sequencing"), or allele-specific PCR. Detection techniques used include fluorescence, fluorescence polarization, and mass spectrometry. The various techniques available and their advantages and disadvantages have been reviewed elsewhere (11). It is not yet known which of these techniques will prove the most reliable and cost effective.

DNA Microarrays and Gene Expression

During the last 10 years, DNA microarrays have become a popular tool because they provide the ability to examine subtle differences in the sequence or expression of tens of thousands of genes at one time. A DNA microarray is a platform (usually a glass slide, nylon membrane, or silicon chip) to which thousands of specific single-stranded fragments of DNA have been attached to specific areas. In a sample, the presence of DNA or cDNA that is complementary to the DNA fragments attached to the support is identified by allowing hybridization to occur and then visualizing hybridized DNA, usually through fluorescence detection. The DNA sequences that attach to the platform are determined by the kind of information the user wants from the DNA microarray. For example, the DNA fragments may have been chosen to examine genotypes at many different SNP sites in the genome or to examine mRNA expression from many, or all, genes in the genome (expression profiling). The most common and established uses for DNA microarrays are genotyping and expression profiling; however, more recently microarrays have been used for a number of other purposes.

Interest has increased in using DNA microarrays for gene expression studies because the comparison of gene expression for all genes in normal versus diseased cells, or untreated versus treated cells, can be examined relatively quickly and easily (30). Such an approach may lead to the discovery of new proteins or classes of proteins involved with the pathology or treatment of a disease, or even to the identification of novel pathways involved with disease progression or treatment. Because DNA microarrays are most commonly used for examining gene expression, this technique will be described in more detail. Other uses of DNA microarrays involve adapting the basic technique or combining it with other techniques.

Microarrays have proven most useful for comparing differences in gene expression (levels of mRNA) rather than absolute levels of expression. Usually, the comparison is between normal and diseased, or untreated and treated, samples. Such studies have been used to examine certain aspects of critical illness in tissue culture and animal models, as well as in patients. The general approach to expression profiling is shown in **Figure 16.4.** Basically, normal and diseased or untreated and treated cells or tissues from humans or animal models are obtained, and mRNA is prepared. Because mRNA is not very stable, it is converted to complementary DNA (cDNA) using the enzyme reverse transcriptase, thus generating cDNA copies that originated only from mRNA; consequently, only cDNA from genes that are expressing mRNA is present in the sample. During the reverse transcription, fluorophore-labeled nucleotides are incorporated into the cDNA, with a different fluorophore incorporated into each of the two samples (often fluorophores that fluoresce green or red are used). The cDNA from the two

samples is then mixed and allowed to hybridize to the single-stranded DNA present on the microarray. The microarray may contain DNA probes for a subset of genes that are of particular interest to the investigator, or they may contain probes for all genes identified in the genome. The presence of hybridization is visualized via the fluorescent labels. For the example shown in **Figure 16.4,** if the gene is expressed only in the normal sample, the spot will be green (indicated by nucleotides within black circles); if it is only expressed in the diseased sample, the spot will be red (indicated by nucleotides within black triangles); and if mRNA for the given gene is expressed equally in both samples, the spot will be yellow (indicated by a mixture of nucleotides within black circles and black triangles). The relative ratio of mRNA can also be determined by gradations in the color. Results obtained using microarrays that indicate differences in mRNA expression must be confirmed using more classical techniques, such as Northern blotting or real-time PCR. In addition, one must consider that an increase in mRNA does not always translate into an increase in protein levels. Consequently, it is also useful to confirm the results by determining whether increased levels of the protein product are also observed for those genes that show increased gene expression in DNA microarray analyses.

The huge amounts of data generated by microarrays and other high-throughput technologies have proved difficult to analyze, and a new field of study, bioinformatics, has arisen in part from the need to analyze such data. Bioinformatics has been defined as research, development, or application of computational tools to be used for acquiring, storing, organizing, archiving, analyzing, or visualizing large amounts of data. The field of bioinformatics is now grappling with finding new and useful ways to analyze the data that are generated by gene expression profiling and genotyping using microarrays. Such analyses may be used to identify the pathways involved in those disease or gene expression profiles associated with clinical outcome.

Proteomics

The field of proteomics is the study of the proteome, which comprises all the proteins present in a cell or tissue, and is essentially the protein complement of the genome. The proteome will differ between different cell types or tissues because a unique set of proteins is expressed in each. The proteome of a particular cell or tissue can also change. Differentiation, development of disease, and response to extracellular signals or drugs will modify the proteome. Proteomics is aimed at studying global differences in protein populations, including changes in levels of specific proteins, post-translational modifications, and protein–protein interactions. Study of the proteome is particularly important because it has become clear that levels of mRNA often do not correspond to levels of the protein product (49). In addition, although it appears that more than 100,000 mRNA transcripts exist (from ~30,000 genes), it is estimated that over 1 million proteins exist, suggesting that substantial protein processing and modification are involved in generating the proteome (55). Clearly then, studying the proteins expressed in the cell is advantageous in addition to studying the genome and gene expression (mRNA) via DNA microarrays. The drawback of studying the proteome is that it is much more difficult than studying gene sequences or mRNA expression

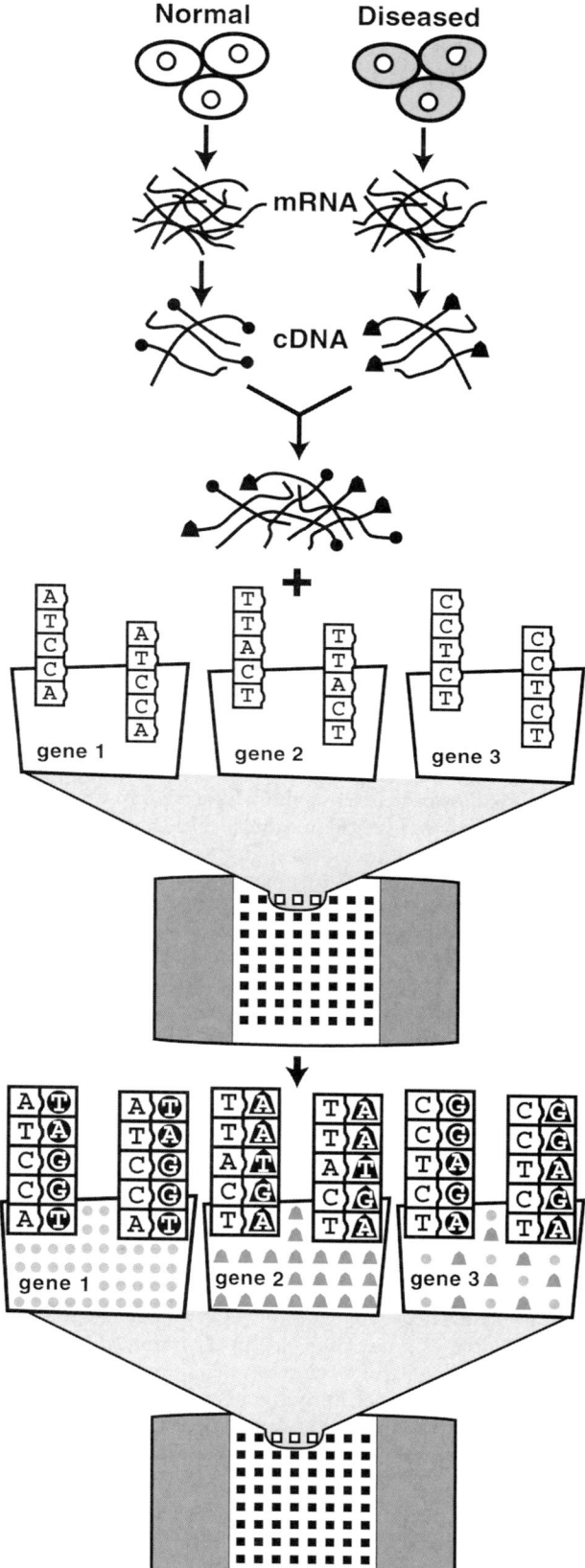

due to the diversity of protein physical characteristics and limitations of the currently available techniques (49,55). However, great strides have been made in the field of proteomics, and a number of new techniques are being developed to enhance the ability to use proteomics to study disease (55).

The proteomic strategies most applicable to medicine are those that examine differences in protein expression either between normal and diseased or between untreated and treated cells or tissues. The goal of such experiments is to identify biomarkers associated with disease or to identify novel targets for drug development.

The proteomic studies used to identify proteins differentially expressed during disease or treatment generally use high-resolution, two-dimensional gel electrophoresis to separate proteins and examine differences in expression levels, followed by mass spectrometry to identify the individual proteins (55). In two-dimensional electrophoresis, proteins are first separated by isoelectric focusing, which separates proteins on the basis of their intrinsic charge (determined by the relative contents of acidic and basic residues). In the second dimension, the proteins that are previously separated via charge are further separated based on mass. Proteins are then visualized and quantitated by staining, as is shown in **Figure 16.5**. A significant limitation of this technique is that only 1,000 to 2,000 of the most abundant proteins can be resolved.

After two-dimensional electrophoresis, mass spectrometry is used to identify proteins of interest, generally those that are differentially expressed when normal and diseased samples or untreated and treated samples are compared. The region of the gel containing the protein of interest is cut from the gel and digested with a protease, generally trypsin. The peptides generated are then analyzed by mass spectrometry to determine the mass of each peptide. Matrix-assisted laser desorption ionization-time of flight (MALDI-TOF) mass spectrometry is often used because it is sensitive, accurate, and can be automated for high-throughput uses (55). The peptide mass map generated after mass spectrometry of the peptides that result from proteolysis can, in turn, be used to search a database that contains the predicted proteins of all identified genes, as well as the predicted mass of all proteolytic peptide products from these genes. Comparison of the peptide mass map with the database allows identification of the proteins of interest. Other types of mass spectrometry can be used if MALDI-TOF mass spectrometry does not allow identification of the proteins (55).

The field of proteomics is just beginning to have an impact on the practice of medicine. Proteomic approaches are being used to characterize changes in the proteome associated with

FIGURE 16.4. Expression profiling of normal and diseased tissue using a DNA microarray. mRNA is purified from normal and diseased cells and converted to cDNA by use of reverse transcriptase and labeled nucleotides that fluoresce either green (indicated by nucleotides within black circles) or red (indicated by nucleotides within black triangles), respectively. The cDNA samples are mixed and hybridized to a DNA microarray composed of single-stranded oligonucleotides from genes of interest attached to specific spots on the array. If a gene is expressed only in normal tissue, the spot on the array will fluoresce green (gene 1); if it is expressed only in diseased tissue, it will fluoresce red (gene 2); and if it is expressed equally in both, it will fluoresce yellow (gene 3). The example shows differential expression of gene 1 and gene 2 in normal and diseased cells. Gene 1 is expressed only in normal cells, gene 2 is expressed only in diseased cells, and gene 3 is equally expressed in both types of cells.

Adult Urine

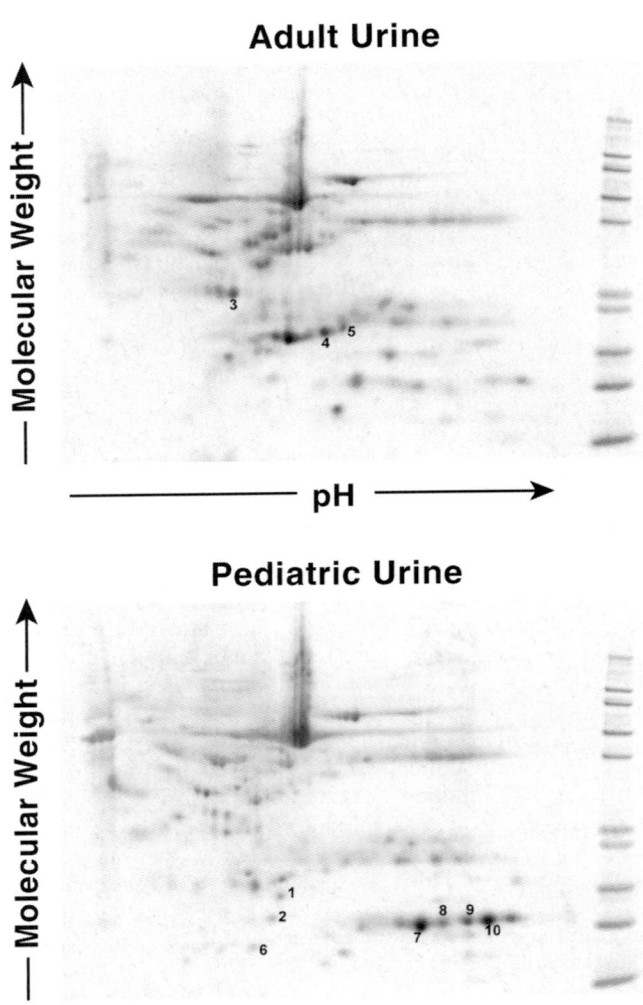

Pediatric Urine

FIGURE 16.5. Two-dimensional polyacrylamide gel electrophoresis of urine samples from adults and children suffering a similar degree of blunt traumatic injury. The gels are representative of the proteomic signatures of three adults and three children. The numbers indicate examples of proteins that appear to be relatively unique in the respective urine samples of adults and children with blunt traumatic injury. (Courtesy of H. Wong).

cancer development and prognosis. In addition, proteomic approaches have been recognized as useful strategies for identifying novel drug targets and for evaluating mechanisms of action, as well as the potential toxicity, of new drugs. Recent studies have also examined differences in the proteome of bronchoalveolar lavage (BAL) fluid in patients with various lung diseases (6,59,63), as well as changes in the proteome of alveolar macrophages during disease or after exposure to various agents (62).

In summary, the sequencing of the human genome has driven the development of high-throughput analysis of the genome, the transcriptome (mRNA expression analysis via DNA arrays), and the proteome. The data generated by these approaches have resulted in the development of the field of bioinformatics, which is necessary to process, store, and analyze the massive amount of data generated by these new approaches. It is clear that, for the medical field, the most useful

information will be obtained by integrating these approaches to provide the most accurate understanding of disease states, thereby providing new markers for disease and new drug targets for novel treatments.

APPLICATIONS IN CRITICAL CARE

Genetic Polymorphisms

An individual's response to critical illness or injury—and to treatment—is highly variable and involves a highly integrated, dynamic, and complex system that includes multiple organ systems, cell types, and molecular pathways. It has been difficult to study the host response and explain the clinical phenotypes in part because of the complexity of the response and the number of variables involved. However, such recent advances in technologies as those described in the previous section have allowed the development of research efforts aimed at examining these complex biologic responses. This section focuses on accumulating evidence that indicates that genetic variability in individuals can affect the disease process and the response to treatment in patients suffering from critical illnesses.

Pharmacogenetics

A number of studies indicate that genetic variation can be an important consideration in the pharmacologic treatment of individuals, including critically ill children. Polymorphisms in genes coding for proteins involved with drug transport, signal transduction pathways, and metabolic pathways appear to alter drug response. For a number of drugs, convincing evidence suggests that the variability in response is due to genetic polymorphisms present in the patient, and these cases are perhaps the best example of how genetic variability can impact patient care. The concept that genetic variation can influence drug action in a clinically significant way and affect the treatment of critically ill patients can be illustrated with several drugs used in the PICU (**Table 16.1**). Several examples in which polymorphisms are found in drug receptors, drug transporters, or enzymes involved in drug metabolism are discussed here.

β_2-Adrenergic receptor (β_2-AR) agonists are potent bronchodilators and are the primary treatment for exacerbations of asthma. β_2-Agonists activate the β_2-AR, which leads to increased intracellular production of cyclic AMP (cAMP), the relaxation of the smooth muscle that lines the small bronchiolar airways, and bronchodilation. Multiple genetic variations exist in the regulatory and coding regions of the β_2-AR gene; these are associated with receptor expression, function, and bronchodilator response. One such polymorphism results in either a glutamine (Gln) or glutamic acid (Glu) at amino acid position 27 in the β_2-AR. Recently, an association between the Gln27Glu genotype in African American children with status asthmaticus and the need for aminophylline treatment has been described (19).

Aminophylline inhibits phosphodiesterase, the enzyme responsible for degradation of cAMP, and results in higher levels of β_2-AR-stimulated cAMP. Interestingly, the Glu27 variant is in complete linkage disequilibrium with an SNP in the promoter region of the gene (18) associated with decreased levels of receptor expression (39). Together, these observations suggest that the need for aminophylline treatment in African

TABLE 16.1

GENES WITH POLYMORPHISMS THAT ALTER DRUG EFFECTS

Gene	Specific drug or drug class	Consequence of polymorphism
Butyrylcholinesterase	Succinylcholine	Prolonged paralytic effect
N-acetyltransferase	Procainamide	Altered serum levels and potential variable toxicities
β_2-adrenergic receptor	Albuterol, terbutaline	Altered desensitization and decreased bronchodilation
β_1-adrenergic receptor	β_1-agonists	Decreased cardiovascular response to β_1-agonists
G_s protein α	β-blockers	Decreased antihypertensive effect
CYP2C9	Warfarin, phenytoin, nonsteroidal anti-inflammatories	Increased anticoagulant effects of warfarin
CYP2D6	Antidepressants, codeine, β-blockers	Decreased codeine analgesia, increased antidepressant toxicity
CYP3A4/3A5/3A7	Midazolam, steroids, calcium channel blockers	Altered clearance of midazolam and steroids
CYP2C19	Omeprazole	Altered peptic ulcer response to omeprazole

American patients with status asthmaticus and the Gln27Glu genotype may be due to reduced receptor levels and cAMP production because of the presence of the Glu27 gene variant. In such patients, the addition of aminophylline treatment may be required to increase cAMP levels to clinically efficacious levels, representing an example in which children with a particular genotype may respond more effectively when a treatment is targeted at "compensating" for a specific genetic variation.

Another example of genetic variation in receptors for common drugs used in the PICU involves the α_{2c}-adrenergic and β_1-adrenergic receptors. Diminished cardiac contractility and refractoriness to vasoactive agents are commonly observed in critically ill children. Cardiac contractility is mediated in part via catecholamines through binding to α_{2c}-adrenergic and β_1-adrenergic receptors. A polymorphism that results in a deletion of four amino acids in the α_{2c}-adrenergic receptor (Del322–325) is associated with development of congestive heart failure in African Americans (52). A glycine-to-arginine substitution at amino acid position 389 in the β_1-adrenergic receptor acts synergistically with the polymorphism in the α_{2c}-adrenergic receptor to increase the risk of heart failure in this population.

Examples of polymorphisms that influence the metabolism of drugs commonly used in the PICU also exist. Succinylcholine continues to be used in some circumstances as a rapid onset, short-duration, depolarizing muscle relaxant. Several studies have described genetic polymorphisms associated with decreased activity in the gene coding for butyrylcholinesterase, an enzyme involved in the hydrolysis of succinylcholine to its inert form. Individuals with polymorphic forms of the gene associated with decreased activity of butyrylcholinesterase exhibit a prolonged paralytic effect of succinylcholine (5). Another example is N-acetyltransferase, an enzyme involved in the metabolism of the anti-arrhythmic drug procainamide. Several genetic polymorphisms influence the rate at which procainamide is acetylated, thereby influencing serum procainamide levels (43) and drug-associated toxicities. Finally, many genetic variations have been described in the gene coding for cytochrome P450, which is involved in the metabolism of a large number of drugs commonly used in the PICU setting, including proton pump inhibitors, antiepileptics, angiotensin II blockers, β-blockers, and nonsteroidal anti-inflammatory agents. Further studies are needed to better identify those polymorphisms that may have a significant influence on the ther-

apies used to treat critically ill children. Knowledge of these genetic variations may provide opportunities to refine treatment strategies and enhance medication efficacy and safety. Although the list of genetic polymorphisms in the genes that influence drug action is large, additional studies are necessary before such information can be used in PICUs to refine treatment strategies.

Genetic Variation and Sepsis

Sepsis is perhaps the best example of an illness commonly seen in the PICU in which genetic polymorphisms appear to influence susceptibility to, or outcome from, disease. Individuals are known to respond to infections in a highly variable fashion. Whereas most patients will recover and do well, a significant portion will develop severe sepsis and may develop multiorgan system failure, refractory hypotension, and die. This individual variability in the susceptibility to, and outcome from, sepsis has been attributed to a number of factors, including virulence and pathogen load. Data from recent studies suggest that an individual's genetic makeup also plays an important role in his variable response to infection and sepsis.

The host response to a pathogen first requires recognition of pathogen-associated products (e.g., endotoxin), followed by a cascade of mediators (e.g., cytokines) that result in the biologic response. The initial recognition and the resultant response require numerous cellular proteins, many of which are highly polymorphic, and this variation may influence the overall response to the infection. In this section, the evidence that indicates that genetic variability in specific genes plays a role in development of sepsis and its outcome will be discussed. The focus will be on genes that exhibit the strongest evidence for a role for human genetic variation in severity of infection or the development of sepsis. However, the possible association of other polymorphic genes with sepsis is an active area of research (15).

Receptors. The inflammatory response to gram-negative bacterial infections involves recognition of lipopolysaccharide (LPS) by a cell surface receptor complex composed of at least three proteins: TLR4, CD14, and MD-2. A number of human and animal studies suggest that variations in the *TLR4* gene can generate variability in susceptibility and/or response to infection. A single amino acid change can significantly reduce response to LPS in mice (48) and enhance susceptibility to infection. Two SNPs identified in the human *TLR4* gene result in the replacement of an aspartic acid at amino acid position 299 with glycine (Gly299) and a threonine at amino acid position 399 with an isoleucine (Ile399). Studies have demonstrated an association of the Gly299Ile399 haplotype with a reduced response to LPS, as determined by examining airway reactivity or systemic cytokine response to inhaled LPS (3). An association of the *TLR4* Gly299Ile399 variant with gram-negative bacterial infections and septic shock (1,33) and mortality in systemic inflammatory response syndrome (12) has also been demonstrated in humans.

Recognition of bacterial infections also involves a number of Fcγ receptors located on the cell surface of leukocytes that bind to the constant region of immunoglobulin G (IgG) and are involved in the phagocytosis of IgG-coated bacteria and subsequent stimulation of the inflammatory response. Genetic polymorphisms have been identified in the genes coding for (a) the FcγRIIIa receptor, which alters the affinity of the receptor for IgG_1, IgG_3, and IgG_4; (b) the FcγRIIIb receptor, which alters the opsonization efficiency required for phagocytosis; and (c) the FcγRIIa receptor, which alters the affinity of the receptor for the Fc portion of IgG_2. Reduced phagocytosis of IgG_2 opsonized particles has been demonstrated in cells from individuals homozygous for the FcγRIIa-R131 variant, compared with cells from individuals homozygous for the more common FcγRIIa-H131. IgG_2 is the main antibody subtype produced against encapsulated bacteria, such as *Streptococcus pneumoniae*, *Haemophilus influenzae* type b, and *Neisseria meningitides*, and it plays an important role in their phagocytosis. Association studies have examined whether individuals with these variant Fcγ receptors have increased susceptibility to, or worse outcome from, infections, particularly meningococcal disease, and most studies have demonstrated an association between infection and/or sepsis and the FcγRIIa and FcγRIIIb polymorphisms. For example, higher frequencies of the FcγRIIa-R131/R131 or FcγRIIIb-Na2/Na2 genotypes have been found in patients with meningococcal disease (8,16,46,47,57), particularly in patients with severe meningococcal disease (46,47) or fulminant meningococcal septic shock (8,16), when compared with a healthy control population.

Cytokines. A cascade of mediators follows host recognition of pathogen-associated products. This cascade of mediators begins with proinflammatory cytokines, such as tumor necrosis factor (TNF)-α and interleukins (ILs), such as IL-1 and IL-6, which are produced and secreted within minutes of a pathogenic stimulus and lead to the secretion of many other cytokines and chemokines. This reaction is balanced by the subsequent release of anti-inflammatory cytokines, such as IL-10 and IL-1_{RA}. The current theory is that an overexaggerated proinflammatory response that results in an imbalance between the proinflammatory and anti-inflammatory cytokines leads to the clinical manifestation of severe sepsis and septic shock. Why this imbalance occurs and leads to an exaggerated response is largely unknown, as is whether certain individuals are more prone to develop an overly exaggerated response. Genetic variability within genes coding for the proinflammatory and anti-inflammatory cytokines might influence this balance and could potentially influence the overall susceptibility to, and outcome from, sepsis.

The primary proinflammatory cytokine TNF-α plays a key role in the activation of the inflammatory response. TNF-α is also believed to play an important role in the development of the harmful effects of the systemic inflammatory response, such as capillary leak, hypotension, acute respiratory distress syndrome (ARDS), and multiple organ system failure. Thus, overproduction of TNF-α may be one of the mechanisms that contribute to an imbalance between proinflammatory and anti-inflammatory cytokines. Several SNPs that influence TNF-α production have been identified within the regulatory region of the gene coding for TNF-α (2,34,38,54). In vitro studies that use LPS-stimulated macrophages have demonstrated that the rarer TNF-α-308A allele is associated with increased transcription (61) and increased secretion of TNF-α (34), compared with the more common TNF-α-308G allele. Another polymorphism associated with higher levels of TNF-α is located approximately 250 base pairs downstream from the transcriptional start site for the gene coding for lymphotoxin alpha (LT-α, also known as TNF-β). This site (also referred to as the TNFB allele, LT-α+250, and the TNF-β+252 site; LT-α+250 site will be used in this chapter) is approximately 3.2 kilobases upstream from the *TNF-α* gene.

Many studies have demonstrated an association between the *TNF-α* polymorphisms and the clinical presentation and/or outcome in patients with bacterial infections (2,36,38,40, 41,54,58). For example, the frequency of the TNF-α-308A allele is higher in adults who died from septic shock (40) and in children who died from meningococcal disease, compared with controls (41). Even those children who were heterozygous at this position (TNF-α-308 G/A) were at increased risk for more fulminant meningococcal disease and death, compared with those children who were homozygous for the wild-type genotype (TNF-α-308 G/G). The A/A genotype at the LT-α+250 site in adults with community-acquired pneumonia is associated with a greater risk of sepsis, compared with adults with the other genotypes (58). Adult patients in postoperative and trauma ICUs who developed sepsis and were homozygous for the LT-α+250 A allele had higher levels of TNF-α and a higher mortality (35,53,54). Similarly, an association between the LT-α+250 A allele, higher serum levels of TNF-α, and higher mortality in bacteremic children has been observed (38). Thus, an association appears to exist between certain genotypes in the regulatory region of the gene coding for TNF-α, levels of TNF-α production, and mortality in patients with sepsis.

The effects of the proinflammatory cytokines are counterbalanced by anti-inflammatory cytokines, such as IL-1_{RA}, such that it would be reasonable to suggest that low anti-inflammatory cytokines could also lead to an overzealous proinflammatory response. IL-1_{RA} is a competitive inhibitor of IL-1. Polymorphisms in the gene coding for IL-1_{RA} include one in which a variable number of repeats occur for an 86-base pair sequence. This polymorphism is found in intron 2 and appears to be associated with variable levels of IL-1_{RA}.

The various alleles of the *IL-1_{RA}* gene have been the most extensively examined variations of the *IL-1* gene family for association with susceptibility to, and outcome from, sepsis. A higher frequency of the A2 allele has been demonstrated in Caucasian adults with severe sepsis, compared with the frequency of the A2 allele in a healthy Caucasian population, but no association with mortality was observed within the population with sepsis (21), suggesting that individuals with the A2 allele are at increased risk for the development of severe sepsis but not at increased risk of worse outcome once sepsis has developed. In contrast to these studies, while no increased susceptibility to the development of sepsis was demonstrated in adults (4) or children with meningococcal disease (10), the presence of the A2 allele in adults with severe sepsis was associated with an increased risk for mortality (4). Thus, genetic variability in the IL-1 locus, particularly the IL-1$_{RA}$ A2 allele, appears to place patients with infections at greater risk for the development of severe sepsis and perhaps at greater risk for mortality once sepsis has developed.

Other Mediators. A variety of proteins other than cytokines play important roles in the pathogenesis of sepsis, and the influence of genetic variation in the genes coding for these proteins on the susceptibility to, and outcome from, sepsis has also been investigated. For example, the pathogenesis of multiorgan system failure is thought to involve endothelial dysfunction and an imbalance between inhibitors of fibrinolysis and endogenous anticoagulants. Plasminogen activator inhibitor 1 (PAI-1) inhibits the potent fibrinolytic, plasminogen activator; elevated plasma concentrations of PAI-1 have been observed in sepsis (44) and severe meningococcal disease (7), and high concentrations are correlated with worse outcome. A single-nucleotide insertion/deletion polymorphism exists within the promoter region of the gene coding for PAI-1 that is associated with variable amounts of PAI-1 production; individuals homozygous for the 4G/4G genotype produce more PAI-1 than either individuals heterozygous (4G/5G) or homozygous for five guanines (5G/5G) (20). Children with meningococcal disease who had the 4G/4G genotype had higher plasma levels of PAI-1 (28) and an increased risk of death from sepsis, compared with children with either the 4G/5G or 5G/5G genotypes (23,26,28). Thus, a strong association appears to exist between the PAI-1 4G/4G genotype, high plasma concentrations of PAI-1, and worse outcome in critical illness.

Angiotensin I–converting enzyme (ACE) polymorphisms have also been evaluated in patients with acute lung injury (ALI) and ARDS. ACE is primarily responsible for converting angiotensin I to angiotensin II but also appears to be involved in the metabolism of chemotactic peptides. ACE is present in all tissues, including the pulmonary endothelium. Individuals have variable plasma and tissue levels of ACE, and genetic variation appears to account for a substantial amount of this variation. A polymorphism that consists of an insertion (I)/deletion (D) of a 287–base-pair repeat sequence in intron 16 of the gene coding for ACE is associated with variable plasma levels; individuals with the DD genotype have higher plasma and tissue levels of ACE compared with individuals who are heterozygous or are homozygous for the insertion sequence (56). In adults with ARDS, ACE concentrations in BAL fluid are elevated, raising the possibility that a genetic predisposition may exist for the development of more severe lung injury in those individuals with the D/D genotype. An association between the D allele and ARDS has been observed in adults (37). A higher percentage of adults with ARDS had the D/D genotype, compared with adults who were at risk for the development of ARDS, including those who had undergone coronary artery bypass graft surgery or were in the ICU with other diagnoses. Interestingly, the D/D genotype is associated with more severe meningococcal disease in children, as measured by a higher predicted risk of mortality, greater prevalence of inotropic support and mechanical ventilation, and longer PICU stay (27). Thus, the genetic

variation in the *ACE* gene may be associated with more severe lung injury in certain types of lung injury or infection.

Genetic polymorphisms have also been extensively studied in the genes coding for four major surfactant proteins: A, B, C, and D, which exhibit a variety of functions, including a role in host defenses in the lung and the reduction of surface tension at the air–liquid interface. Several SNPs within intron 2, exon 4, and the 5′ and 3′ flanking regions of the gene coding for surfactant protein-B (SP-B) have been identified. A C/T nucleotide variation at position 1580 in exon 4 changes amino acid 131 from threonine to isoleucine (31), altering a site for N-linked glycosylation and perhaps the processing and/or function of SP-B, resulting in decreased functional SP-B. Deficiency in, or impaired activity of, SP-B is implicated in a variety of interstitial pulmonary diseases, including acute respiratory failure and death in newborns and mice (31), and ARDS (24,25,32). In addition, lower levels of surfactant proteins and a diminished ability of surfactant to lower surface tension have been found in BAL fluid obtained from patients with ARDS (25,45). Genetic variations in the regulatory or functional regions of the gene encoding for SP-B may, therefore, influence susceptibility to, and outcome from, severe lung injury and respiratory failure. An association between the SP-B+1580 polymorphism, specifically, the CC genotype, and severe lung injury has been described (50).

Limitations

Several limitations to genetic association studies should be noted. First, such studies should not be performed by grouping subjects from different ethnic groups. It is well known that the frequency of many of these polymorphisms varies between ethnic groups and that, therefore, comparisons should only be made within ethnic groups. A second limitation is that the specific nucleotide variation being investigated may, in fact, not be involved but, rather, may be closely linked to the actual genetic variation causing the association. For example, the genes coding for TNF-α and LT-α lie on chromosome 6 within the major histocompatibility complex near the human leukocyte antigen (HLA) loci and are in strong linkage disequilibrium with several HLA alleles that may be involved in controlling TNF-α secretion. Last, care must be taken in choosing the appropriate control group. In many studies, the frequency of the polymorphism in a group of hospitalized patients is compared with the frequency of the polymorphism in a healthy control population. However, the control population may not have been exposed to the same pathogens to which the hospitalized patients are exposed. Rather, a more appropriate control group for comparison would be a group of hospitalized patients who do not develop infection or a group with a similar infection who did not develop sepsis.

Expression Profiling

Research in areas relevant to critical care that uses expression profiling with DNA microarrays has primarily focused on studies of the host inflammatory response to various types of injury and medications. For example, the use of DNA microarrays in cell culture models has demonstrated differential responses to LPS, TNF-α, and stretch in alveolar epithelial cells (17). Gene expression profiles of traumatic, thermal, or sepsis injury models in mouse leukocytes have demonstrated that the majority of the leukocyte mRNAs expressed among the models were unique to the mechanism of injury (9). However, several mRNAs were upregulated or downregulated in a similar fashion, suggesting a common transcriptional response to injury regardless of the inciting stimulus. Many of these mRNAs were identified as coding for components of various pathways involved in either the immune response or cell death.

DNA microarrays have also been used in a number of animal models of critical illness. Organ-specific transcriptional response has been demonstrated in both rat (13) and mouse (14) cecal ligation and puncture models of sepsis. Increased expression of mRNAs for proinflammatory and anti-inflammatory cytokines, antiproteases, antioxidants, cytokine receptor antagonists, tissue and vascular permeability factors, and apoptotic factors were observed. The use of DNA microarrays has also identified the expression of a large number of inflammatory genes and transforming growth factor (TGF)-β in LPS-(29) and nickel-induced (60) models of lung injury in mice.

Last, DNA microarrays have been used to analyze gene expression in critical illness in humans. Elevated levels of mRNA coding for pre–B-cell colony-enhancing factor (PBEF) have been observed in BAL fluid from humans with ALI (64). PBEF protein levels were also elevated in BAL fluid and serum from patients with ALI, compared with healthy controls. Cardiopulmonary bypass is associated with a profound systemic inflammatory response, and DNA microarrays have been used to examine leukocyte mRNA isolated from adults who underwent cardiopulmonary bypass (51). Quantitative changes were observed in a number of mRNA transcripts, including the metalloproteinase kinase MAP4K1, an activator of proinflammatory and proapoptotic pathways. It remains to be determined how these varied transcript levels translate into specific protein levels and how they function.

Proteomic Analyses

In the area of proteomics, two-dimensional polyacrylamide gel electrophoresis and mass spectrometry have identified quantitative changes in a number of proteins, including cytokines, chemokines, signaling molecules, and cytoskeletal components in LPS-stimulated human neutrophils (22). Proteomic techniques have been used to compare BAL fluid and plasma in healthy adults and adults with ALI (6). Albumin, transferrin, IgG, and clusterin were demonstrated to be increased in the BAL fluid relative to plasma levels of adults with ALI. This finding is consistent with the theory that ALI is characterized by an increase in the permeability of pulmonary capillaries. Interestingly, surfactant protein A was absent in the BAL fluid from many of the patients with ALI, in contrast to BAL fluid from healthy volunteers. These techniques have also been employed using BAL fluid from patients with other pulmonary disease processes, including asthma, cystic fibrosis, bacterial pneumonia, and other infections (42,59).

CONCLUSIONS AND FUTURE DIRECTIONS

The recent development of new technologies has provided new tools to (a) examine the "global" molecular response to injuries or illnesses seen in the PICU, and (b) examine the role that genetic variation may play in influencing an individual's susceptibility to, and outcome from, critical illnesses, such as sepsis and ARDS. Such studies will provide new insight into the pathogenesis of various critical illnesses and, potentially, new treatment strategies. In addition, future genetic studies that use these types of technologies will someday enable physicians to provide critically ill children with a more individualized approach to treatment.

KEY POINTS

■ New techniques developed in genomics and proteomics have allowed for better understanding of the pathophysiology of critical illnesses.

■ Individual genetic variation may influence susceptibility to, and outcome from, illnesses common in PICUs, such as sepsis and ARDS.

■ The response to medications may be influenced by the individual's genetic makeup. These variations may involve drug transporters, receptors, components of signal transduction pathways, and proteins involved in drug metabolism.

■ Genetic variation in the ability of an individual to recognize pathogenic signals and activate signal transduction pathways may also influence the degree of susceptibility to, and outcome from, illnesses common in PICUs.

■ Of particular interest is the effect of genetic variation on the extent of the inflammatory reaction in response to infection and trauma; individuals genetically predisposed to a more exaggerated inflammatory response due to an imbalance in their proinflammatory and anti-inflammatory cytokines may have a poorer outcome.

■ Genetic variation within a number of other mediators may also influence the degree of lung injury in response to bacterial and viral infections, as well as other types of injury that can result in ARDS.

■ In the future, genomic medicine will allow for treatments specifically tailored to an individual's genetic makeup.

References

1. Agnese DM, Calvano JE, Hahm SJ, et al. Human toll-like receptor 4 mutations but not CD14 polymorphisms are associated with an increased risk of gram-negative infections. *J Infect Dis* 2002;186:1522–5.
2. Appoloni O, Dupont E, Vandercruys M, et al. Association of tumor necrosis factor-2 allele with plasma tumor necrosis factor-alpha levels and mortality from septic shock. *Am J Med* 2001;110:486–8.
3. Arbour NC, Lorenz E, Schutte BC, et al. TLR4 mutations are associated with endotoxin hyporesponsiveness in humans. *Nat Genet* 2000;25:187–91.
4. Arnalich F, Lopez-Maderuelo D, Codoceo R, et al. Interleukin-1 receptor antagonist gene polymorphism and mortality in patients with severe sepsis. *Clin Exp Immunol* 2002;127:331–6.
5. Barta C, Sasvari-Szekely M, Devai A, et al. Analysis of mutations in the plasma cholinesterase gene of patients with a history of prolonged neuromuscular block during anesthesia. *Mol Genet Metab* 2001;74:484–8.
6. Bowler RP, Duda B, Chan ED, et al. Proteomic analysis of pulmonary edema fluid and plasma in patients with acute lung injury. *Am J Physiol Lung Cell Mol Physiol* 2004;286:L1095–104.
7. Brandtzaeg P, Joo GB, Brusletto B, et al. Plasminogen activator inhibitor 1 and 2, alpha-2-antiplasmin, plasminogen, and endotoxin levels in systemic meningococcal disease. *Thromb Res* 1990;57:271–8.
8. Bredius RG, Derkx BH, Fijen CA, et al. Fc gamma receptor IIa (CD32) polymorphism in fulminant meningococcal septic shock in children. *J Infect Dis* 1994;170:848–53.
9. Brownstein BH, Logvinenko T, Lederer JA, et al. Commonality and differences in leukocyte gene expression patterns among three models of inflammation and injury. *Physiol Genomics* 2006;24:298–309.
10. Carrol ED, Mobbs KJ, Thomson AP, et al. Variable number tandem repeat

polymorphism of the interleukin-1 receptor antagonist gene in meningococcal disease. *Clin Infect Dis* 2002;35:495–7.

11. Chen X, Sullivan PF. Single nucleotide polymorphism genotyping: Biochemistry, protocol, cost, and throughput. *Pharmacogenomics J* 2003;3:77–96.

12. Child NJ, Yang IA, Pulletz MC, et al. Polymorphisms in Toll-like receptor 4 and the systemic inflammatory response syndrome. *Biochem Soc Trans* 2003; 31:652–3.

13. Chinnaiyan AM, Huber-Lang M, Kumar-Sinha C, et al. Molecular signatures of sepsis: Multiorgan gene expression profiles of systemic inflammation. *Am J Pathol* 2001;159:1199–209.

14. Cobb JP, Laramie JM, Stormo GD, et al. Sepsis gene expression profiling: Murine splenic compared with hepatic responses determined by using complementary DNA microarrays. *Crit Care Med* 2002;30:2711–21.

15. Dahmer MK, Randolph A, Vitali S, et al. Genetic polymorphisms in sepsis. *Pediatr Crit Care Med* 2005;6:S61–73.

16. Domingo P, Muniz-Diaz E, Baraldes MA, et al. Associations between Fc gamma receptor IIA polymorphisms and the risk and prognosis of meningococcal disease. *Am J Med* 2002;112:19–25.

17. dos Santos CC, Han B, Andrade CF, et al. DNA microarray analysis of gene expression in alveolar epithelial cells in response to TNFalpha, LPS, and cyclic stretch. *Physiol Genomics* 2004;19:331–42.

18. Drysdale CM, McGraw DW, Stack CB, et al. Complex promoter and coding region b2-adrenergic receptor haplotypes alter receptor expression and predict in vivo responsiveness. *Proc Natl Acad Sci USA* 2000;97:10483–8.

19. Elbahlawan L, Binaei S, Christensen ML, et al. Beta2-Adrenergic receptor polymorphisms in African American children with status asthmaticus. *Pediatr Crit Care Med* 2006;7(1):87–9.

20. Eriksson P, Kallin B, van't Hooft FM, et al. Allele-specific increase in basal transcription of the plasminogen-activator inhibitor 1 gene is associated with myocardial infarction. *Proc Natl Acad Sci USA* 1995;92:1851–5.

21. Fang XM, Schroder S, Hoeft A, et al. Comparison of two polymorphisms of the interleukin-1 gene family: Interleukin-1 receptor antagonist polymorphism contributes to susceptibility to severe sepsis. *Crit Care Med* 1999; 27:1330–4.

22. Fessler MB, Malcolm KC, Duncan MW, et al. A genomic and proteomic analysis of activation of the human neutrophil by lipopolysaccharide and its mediation by p38 mitogen-activated protein kinase. *J Biol Chem* 2002;277:31291–302.

23. Geishofer G, Binder A, Muller M, et al. 4G/5G promoter polymorphism in the plasminogen-activator-inhibitor-1 gene in children with systemic meningococcaemia. *Eur J Pediatr* 2005;164:486–90.

24. Greene KE, Wright JR, Steinberg KP, et al. Serial changes in surfactant-associated proteins in lung and serum before and after onset of ARDS. *Am J Respir Crit Care Med* 1999;160:1843–50.

25. Gregory TJ, Longmore WJ, Moxley MA, et al. Surfactant chemical composition and biophysical activity in acute respiratory distress syndrome. *J Clin Invest* 1991;88:1976–81.

26. Haralambous E, Hibberd ML, Hermans PW, et al. Role of functional plasminogen-activator-inhibitor-1 4G/5G promoter polymorphism in susceptibility, severity, and outcome of meningococcal disease in Caucasian children. *Crit Care Med* 2003;31:2788–93.

27. Harding D, Baines PB, Brull D, et al. Severity of meningococcal disease in children and the angiotensin-converting enzyme insertion/deletion polymorphism. *Am J Respir Crit Care Med* 2002;165:1103–6.

28. Hermans PW, Hibberd ML, Booy R, et al. 4G/5G promoter polymorphism in the plasminogen-activator-inhibitor-1 gene and outcome of meningococcal disease. Meningococcal Research Group. *Lancet* 1999;354:556–60.

29. Jeyaseelan S, Chu HW, Young SK, et al. Transcriptional profiling of lipopolysaccharide-induced acute lung injury. *Infect Immun* 2004;72:7247–56.

30. King HC, Sinha AA. Gene expression profile analysis by DNA microarrays: Promise and pitfalls. *JAMA* 2001;286:2280–8.

31. Lin Z, deMello DE, Wallot M, et al. An SP-B gene mutation responsible for SP-B deficiency in fatal congenital alveolar proteinosis: Evidence for a mutation hotspot in exon 4. *Mol Genet Metab* 1998;64:25–35.

32. Lin Z, Pearson C, Chinchilli V, et al. Polymorphisms of human SP-A, SP-B, and SP-D genes: Association of SP-B Thr131Ile with ARDS. *Clin Genet* 2000;58:181–91.

33. Lorenz E, Mira JP, Frees KL, et al. Relevance of mutations in the TLR4 receptor in patients with gram-negative septic shock. *Arch Intern Med* 2002;162:1028–32.

34. Louis E, Franchimont D, Piron A, et al. Tumour necrosis factor (TNF) gene polymorphism influences TNF-alpha production in lipopolysaccharide (LPS)-stimulated whole blood cell culture in healthy humans. *Clin Exp Immunol* 1998;113:401–6.

35. Majetschak M, Flohe S, Obertacke U, et al. Relation of a TNF gene polymorphism to severe sepsis in trauma patients. *Ann Surg* 1999;230:207–14.

36. Majetschak M, Obertacke U, Schade FU, et al. Tumor necrosis factor gene polymorphisms, leukocyte function, and sepsis susceptibility in blunt trauma patients. *Clin Diagn Lab Immunol* 2002;9:1205–11.

37. Marshall RP, Webb S, Bellingan GJ, et al. Angiotensin converting enzyme insertion/deletion polymorphism is associated with susceptibility and outcome in acute respiratory distress syndrome. *Am J Respir Crit Care Med* 2002;166:646–50.

38. McArthur JA, Zhang Q, Quasney MW. Association between the A/A genotype at the lymphotoxin-alpha+250 site and increased mortality in children with positive blood cultures. *Pediatr Crit Care Med* 2002;3:341–4.

39. McGraw DW, Forbes S, Kramer L, et al. Polymorphisms of the 5′ leader cistron of the human β2-adrenergic receptor regulate receptor expression. *J Clin Invest* 1998;102:1927–32.

40. Mira JP, Cariou A, Grall F, et al. Association of TNF2, a TNF-alpha promoter polymorphism, with septic shock susceptibility and mortality: A multicenter study. *JAMA* 1999;282:561–8.

41. Nadel S, Newport MJ, Booy R, et al. Variation in the tumor necrosis factor-alpha gene promoter region may be associated with death from meningococcal disease. *J Infect Dis* 1996;174:878–80.

42. Neumann M, von Bredow C, Ratjen F, et al. Bronchoalveolar lavage protein patterns in children with malignancies, immunosuppression, fever and pulmonary infiltrates. *Proteomics* 2002;2:683–9.

43. Okumura K, Kita T, Chikazawa S, et al. Genotyping of N-acetylation polymorphism and correlation with procainamide metabolism. *Clin Pharmacol Ther* 1997;61:509–17.

44. Paramo JA, Perez JL, Serrano M, et al. Types 1 and 2 plasminogen activator inhibitor and tumor necrosis factor alpha in patients with sepsis. *Thromb Haemost* 1990;64:3–6.

45. Pison U, Bock JC, Pietschmann S, et al. The adult respiratory distress syndrome: Pathophysiological concepts related to the pulmonary surfactant system. In: Robertson BTH, ed. *Surfactant Therapy for Lung Disease.* New York: Marcel Dekker; 1995:167–97.

46. Platonov AE, Kuijper EJ, Vershinina IV, et al. Meningococcal disease and polymorphism of FcgammaRIIa (CD32) in late complement component-deficient individuals. *Clin Exp Immunol* 1998;111:97–101.

47. Platonov AE, Shipulin GA, Vershinina IV, et al. Association of human Fc gamma RIIa (CD32) polymorphism with susceptibility to and severity of meningococcal disease. *Clin Infect Dis* 1998;27:746–50.

48. Poltorak A, He X, Smirnova I, et al. Defective LPS signaling in C3H/HeJ and C57BL/10ScCr mice: Mutations in Tlr4 gene. *Science* 1998;282:2085–8.

49. Pradet-Balade B, Boulme F, Beug H, et al. Translation control: Bridging the gap between genomics and proteomics?. *Trends Biochem Sci* 2001;26:225–9.

50. Quasney MW, Waterer GW, Dahmer MK, et al. Association between surfactant protein B + 1580 polymorphism and the risk of respiratory failure in adults with community-acquired pneumonia. *Crit Care Med* 2004;32:1115–9.

51. Seeburger J, Hoffmann J, Wendel HP, et al. Gene expression changes in leukocytes during cardiopulmonary bypass are dependent on circuit coating. *Circulation* 2005;112:I224–8.

52. Small KM, Wagoner LE, Levin AM, et al. Synergistic polymorphisms of beta1- and alpha2C-adrenergic receptors and the risk of congestive heart failure. *N Engl J Med* 2002;347:1135–42.

53. Stuber F, Petersen M, Bokelmann F, et al. A genomic polymorphism within the tumor necrosis factor locus influences plasma tumor necrosis factor-alpha concentrations and outcome of patients with severe sepsis. *Crit Care Med* 1996;24:381–4.

54. Stuber F, Udalova IA, Book M, et al. −308 tumor necrosis factor (TNF) polymorphism is not associated with survival in severe sepsis and is unrelated to lipopolysaccharide inducibility of the human TNF promoter. *J Inflamm* 1995;46:42–50.

55. Stults JT, Arnott D. Proteomics. *Methods Enzymol* 2005;402:245–89.

56. Tiret L, Rigat B, Visvikis S, et al. Evidence, from combined segregation and linkage analysis, that a variant of the angiotensin I-converting enzyme (ACE) gene controls plasma ACE levels. *Am J Hum Genet* 1992;51:197–205.

57. van der Pol WL, Huizinga TW, Vidarsson G, et al. Relevance of Fcgamma receptor and interleukin-10 polymorphisms for meningococcal disease. *J Infect Dis* 2001;184:1548–55.

58. Waterer GW, Quasney MW, Cantor RM, et al. Septic shock and respiratory failure in community-acquired pneumonia have different TNF polymorphism associations. *Am J Respir Crit Care Med* 2001;163:1599–604.

59. Wattiez R, Falmagne P. Proteomics of bronchoalveolar lavage fluid. *J Chromatogr B Analyt Technol Biomed Life Sci* 2005;815:169–78.

60. Wesselkamper SC, Case LM, Henning LN, et al. Gene expression changes during the development of acute lung injury: Role of transforming growth factor beta. *Am J Respir Crit Care Med* 2005;172:1399–411.

61. Wilson AG, Symons JA, McDowell TL, et al. Effects of a polymorphism in the human tumor necrosis factor alpha promoter on transcriptional activation. *Proc Natl Acad Sci USA* 1997;94:3195–9.

62. Wu HM, Jin M, Marsh CB. Toward functional proteomics of alveolar macrophages. *Am J Physiol Lung Cell Mol Physiol* 2005;288:L585–95.

63. Wu J, Kobayashi M, Sousa EA, et al. Differential proteomic analysis of bronchoalveolar lavage fluid in asthmatics following segmental antigen challenge. *Mol Cell Proteomics* 2005;4:1251–64.

64. Ye SQ, Simon BA, Maloney JP, et al. Pre-B-cell colony-enhancing factor as a potential novel biomarker in acute lung injury. *Am J Respir Crit Care Med* 2005;171:361–70.

CHAPTER 17 ■ INNATE IMMUNITY AND INFLAMMATION

JAMES A. THOMAS

ICU patients fall into three classes, based on their capacity to mount an inflammatory response: effective responders, ineffective responders, and dead. Effective responders focus an intense, localized reaction that destroys and removes microbial invaders and dead and dying tissue while preventing the activation of similar processes at remote, unaffected locations. Ineffective responders, on the other hand, lack the wherewithal to localize the injury, muster sufficient destructive intensity at the injury site, or contain the reaction locally. Dead patients are either effective responders with an overwhelming injury or infection or ineffective responders who cannot be saved by ICU care.

To understand inflammation is, in some respects, to grasp the breadth of human disease. Premature neonates stressed by cold, infection, or formula feeding can develop necrotizing enterocolitis; infants with respiratory syncytial virus (RSV) suffer bronchiolitis; children admitted after open-heart surgery exhibit signs of systemic activation of an inflammatory cascade. Different injuries provoke distinct manifestations of the inflammatory response. A complex host can generate many more reactions—foreign body, granulomatous, suppurative, hypersensitivity, immune complex, toxic, or septic shock—than can one with a simpler genome. Although a comprehensive categorization of different inflammatory processes exceeds the scope of this chapter, the following sections outline some elements of an ancient system that has evolved to protect the host from insults to its integrity—the innate immune system.

The survival of a species depends on its ability to perpetuate itself. To accomplish this, members must succeed at three fundamental activities. First, they must generate adequate nutrition to reach reproductive age. Moreover, organisms that nurture their young must do the same for the next generation until the latter achieves independence. The second essential task is to avoid becoming another organism's food source. This direct competitive pressure between genomes, whether in predator–prey or parasite–host relationships, has selected for behavioral and physiologic adaptations that favor survival to reproductive age. Finally, organisms must ensure the passage of their genetic information to the next generation and the survival of this new generation to reproductive age.

The struggle to achieve these ends is fraught with danger. During the course of activities to develop, survive, and reproduce, organisms encounter forces and agents that compromise their integrity and threaten their biologic quest. Gravity can hurl bodies from trees during food foraging, and bacteria can gain access to the warm, humid, and nutrient-rich subepithelium via abrasions or puncture wounds. Most major injuries or infections, such as those treated in modern ICUs, would be nonsurvivable without antibiotics, antiseptic surgery, and modern nursing care. To maintain a competitive advantage and survive minor-to-moderate threats, however, most species have evolved a repertoire of behavioral and physiologic responses to help them avoid, or defend themselves against, threats to their integrity. These countermeasures include mechanisms to limit secondary injury or microbial dissemination if an initial attack succeeds and primary (epithelial) defenses are breached. Finally, with the threat contained, successful defenses modulate the intensity of the reaction and commence repairing the damage occasioned by the insult and the reaction to it. Defects that impair any of these three responses hamper the host's survival chances.

The aggregate of early physiologic responses that detect and respond to injury are loosely referred to as *innate immunity*, whereas the inflammatory response represents innate immunity at work. The history of our evolving understanding of host defense and inflammation is summarized in this chapter. Major concepts associated with innate immunity and the inflammatory response are defined, and the current thinking regarding the nature of injury signals, the acute cellular and systemic responses to injury, and their regulation and overall impact are reviewed.

HISTORY OF KNOWLEDGE OF INFLAMMATION AND INNATE IMMUNITY

The concept of innate immunity is more modern than the notion of inflammation (4,25,35,42,44). Early Mesopotamian caregivers were familiar with the signs and symptoms of inflammation, but as an early codifier of medical knowledge, Hippocrates (460–377 BC) receives credit for both documenting the early vocabulary associated with the inflammatory response and recognizing it as a prerequisite for the healing process.

The Roman encyclopedist Aulus Cornelius Celsus (~35–50 BC) is the second ancient Westerner whose contribution to the study of inflammation survives. In his treatise, *De Medicina*, he coined the initial four cardinal signs of inflammation: calor (heat), dolor (pain), tumor (swelling), and rubor (redness or erythema). The fifth sign, *functio laesa* (dysfunction of inflamed organs) was attributed to the Greek physician Galen of Pergamon (129–200 AD), whose writings dominated Western medical thought until the European Renaissance. According to some scholars, Galen's influence over the practice of medicine in Europe stifled observation and empiricism, whereas medieval Muslim physicians in Spain, North Africa, and the Middle

East contributed more to the understanding and treatment of inflammation than did their European counterparts during this period.

Beutler identifies two threads in what would now be called the history of inflammation research. The first focuses on characterizing what is sensed or what triggers the inflammatory response. Before Koch promulgated his postulates, investigators attempted to purify toxins from putrid meat to better understand why the same process in a patient's injured leg triggered severe side effects, including gangrene, shock, and death. These studies ultimately gave way to the isolation and characterization of microbial toxins, such as lipopolysaccharide (LPS), peptidoglycan, and lipoteichoic acid.

The second line of inquiry concentrated on describing the response to infection and invasion. The famous Scottish surgeon John Hunter (1728–1793) first recognized leukocytes at the site of inflammation and was one of the first to describe the inflammatory response as a form of host defense and not a disease process. Moreover, as light microscopy improved during the 18th and 19th centuries, investigators such as Dutrochet, Virchow, Waller, and Addison described inflammatory leukocyte morphology and the loose association of some with the vessel wall, the firm adherence of others to the wall, and the extravasation of other cells beyond the vessel confines. Cohnheim detailed the stepwise events of leukocyte rolling, adhesion, and diapedesis and speculated that changes in vascular wall properties promoted this process. Schultze's descriptions of different leukocyte morphologies preceded Elie Metchnikov's observations of phagocytosis in macrophages and granulocytes that led to the formulation of his cellular theory of immunity in 1884. Paul Erlich's identification and analysis of antibodies and complement gave rise to the concept of humoral immunity and opened the era of functional studies that have characterized subsequent studies of immunity and inflammation.

Since the early 20th century, efforts to unravel the adaptive immune response eclipsed study of innate immunity. However, description of the first genetic defect underlying chronic granulomatous disease (in the 1960s); isolation and characterization of cytokines, receptors, and signaling molecules critical to inflammation; recognition that adaptive immunity depends on innate immunity to function; and the sequence information windfall from the Human Genome Project have helped to fuel resurgent interest in understanding the depth and complexity of innate immunity.

Recognizing the relationship between inflammation and the neuroendocrine system has coalesced more recently than investigators' comprehension of leukocyte biology, soluble mediators, and the vascular system. Investigation into the stress response has also highlighted the importance and interdependence of the central nervous system (CNS) and the hypothalamic-pituitary axis in preparing complex hosts to defend themselves against various threats.

DEFINITIONS AND GENERAL CONCEPTS

Innate Immunity

As Beutler observes, "it is sometimes difficult to decide where the innate immune system ends and the rest of the host begins"

(4). The statement reflects the difficulty inherent in attempting to distinguish one physiologic system from another in an organism that functions as an integrated whole. Although the host's innate response to injury or infection employs specialized cells and macromolecules to defend itself, any body tissue may become infected, traumatized, or deprived of blood flow. Therefore, tissues considered "nonimmune" must be able to detect and respond to an insult before the microbial load overwhelms or the host exsanguinates. Thus, the entire host participates in innate immunity.

Defining the limits of the innate immune system may be futile, but characterizing core features and functions of innate immunity is possible. First, it is old—much older than adaptive (lymphocyte-based) immunity. In fact, it most likely developed in parallel with early metazoans more than 600 million years ago (3). Moreover, elements of immunity shared by plants, invertebrates, and vertebrates alike, such as intracellular kinases critical to disease resistance and pathogen recognition, are older than components found only in vertebrates. Second, like the nervous system with which it is tightly linked, innate immunity has both afferent and efferent limbs, suggesting that the two systems may have evolved from a common ancestral threat-sensing and response system (4). Third, the cellular receptors for sensing invasion or injury are encoded in the germline of the host, signifying that they have evolved to recognize something essential and therefore invariant in either microbes or the host and that they can be mobilized quickly.

Three essential functions of innate immunity deserve mention here, two of which will be discussed further. Pathogen or injury recognition is the first and most important of these. Without the ability to recognize pathogens or injury, the host is immunologically blind to the threats that surround it. The second function of innate immunity is response to the threat. Doing so effectively requires mechanisms to assess the magnitude, localization, and type of insult, and to match, coordinate, and regulate the response to that threat. Finally, and as an integral component of its response to microbial invasion, innate immunity instructs the adaptive immune response as to the identity of the invader, and it provides additional information about the preferred adaptive effector response (B-cell versus T-cell–mediated). The *adaptive immune response* is noted in this chapter and treated in depth elsewhere in the text.

What, then, is *innate immunity*? The term refers to the cells, subcellular elements, and molecules that act to eliminate invading pathogens and limit the spread of tissue damage. The cells involved include leukocytes, particularly polymorphonuclear cells (neutrophils, basophils, eosinophils); mast cells; and mononuclear phagocytes (monocytes, tissue macrophages, dendritic cells), as well as lymphocytes, natural killer cells, neurons, and neuroendocrine cells. Platelets are the major subcellular element and are essential to coagulation. Molecular mediators of innate immunity range from major antimicrobial proteins (complement, defensins, cathelicidins, lysozyme, and lactoferrin) to pro- and anti-inflammatory cytokines and chemokines (tumor necrosis factor [TNF]-α, interleukin [IL]-1β, IL-8, IL-6, interferon [IFN]-γ, IL-10), to neurotransmitters involved in neurogenic inflammation (substance P, calcitonin gene-related peptide, epinephrine, serotonin). The mechanisms by which some of these components cooperate to protect the host following injury will be the focus of the remainder of this chapter.

Adaptive Immunity

In contrast to the notion of preset responsiveness inherent in innate immunity, adaptive immunity denotes the ability to vary an immune response depending on the received stimulus. The existence of this adaptability implies two additional qualities: the capacity to distinguish among different stimuli, and a pre-existing pool of effectors capable of responding to almost any molecular motif. The nearly unlimited repertoire of lymphocytes, generated by somatic recombination and hypermutation of the genes that code for their antigen receptors, nonetheless arises from the interaction between innate immune cells (antigen-presenting cells) and lymphocytes (T-helper cells). Although adaptive immunity is a more recent and restricted system of host defense than is innate immunity, it remains dependent on its evolutionary predecessor (innate immunity) for proper function.

Inflammation

Defining inflammation is also complex because it comes in many guises. A peritonsillar abscess and necrotizing bacterial pneumonia, lupus nephritis, and acute tubular necrosis that leads to renal failure, and the cerebral responses to trauma and viral encephalitis are all inflammatory conditions. These reactions share elements in common but also have unique aspects that are determined by the injury itself, the tissue(s) involved, and the overall state of the host at the time of insult. The inflammatory response, broadly defined, is: a localized reaction elicited by microbial invasion or tissue injury that serves to destroy, dilute, or sequester both the injurious agent and injured tissue and to initiate the healing process.

An intact inflammatory response is essential for host survival, performing at least three critical functions. First, it prevents disease extension. Through a variety of strategies, including extravasation of serum proteins, migration of leukocyte effectors, and local thrombosis, innate immunity contains invading microbes and delineates boundaries between viable and nonviable tissue. Second, the response is critical for the development of adaptive immunity against infectious organisms. Its "adjuvant effect" on antigen presentation to T cells instructs them to respond to the antigen as an invader. Finally, control and resolution of the inflammatory response promotes eventual healing, with a combination of regeneration, remodeling, and scarring.

Several general concepts about inflammation deserve mention. First, when it functions appropriately, the inflammatory response is a localized phenomenon. The reaction may occur within either a microscopic domain, such as Ghon complex within a lymph node, or it may occupy an entire body cavity, as occurs during peritonitis. Although the extent of the response is much broader in the second example, the host has evolved measures to contain inflammatory mediators within the focus and prevent their systemic spillover (34). A second, related idea is that generalized activation of even a single component of the inflammatory response can be lethal to the host. A ruptured appendix, for example, may trigger pulmonary endothelial activation, neutrophil influx into remote alveoli, and the development of acute respiratory distress syndrome (ARDS), a nonsurvivable condition without inten-

sive care. The third notion is that the acute inflammatory response is invariant and stereotyped. Whereas the extent and intensity of the reaction vary considerably, depending on the degree of insult, in general, the host's innate immunity uses the same mechanisms and kinetics to sense and respond to repeated injuries.

Inflammation is also an integrated biologic response, the overall control of which is still poorly understood. Most attempts at comprehensive descriptions of the host response to infection and injury remain phenomenologic, and only recently have investigators applied a more systems-oriented approach toward understanding aspects of innate immunity (e.g., the monocyte-phagocyte system or neutrophil biology) (16,51).

Finally, different schemata have evolved to categorize inflammation. We distinguish between acute, subacute, and chronic inflammation to group inflammatory responses according to onset and duration. Effector mechanisms based on pathologic description of an inflammatory lesion (neutrophilic infiltrative, caseating, necrotizing, histiocytic) provide another basis for distinction. We also describe inflammatory responses based on the inciting injury mechanisms, such as infectious, immune complex, trauma, hypoxic–ischemic, although these descriptors provide little insight into the type of specific inflammatory response they trigger.

Essential Functions and Components of a Physiologic Host Defense System

A host response to insult must accomplish a minimum of four functions. It must first detect the injury or microbial invasion and alert the appropriate effectors, both local and distant from the lesion. This sensing function constitutes the afferent limb of the response. Second, in the efferent arm, the response must contain the injury or infection, minimizing the chances that microbes, the contents of necrotic cells, or the toxic endogenous mediators elaborated at the site of inflammation spill into the blood and lymph or spread throughout natural cavities or along tissue planes. Third, the response should eliminate the invading organism and/or damaged or dead tissue. Fourth, it must be able to turn itself off and initiate the healing process. Vertebrates have also evolved the ability to prevent productive reinfection via lymphocyte-mediated immunologic memory, a fifth function absent in most other multicellular organisms. Innate immunity is critical to each of these functions, but it collaborates with adaptive immunity in eliminating some pathogens and in the generation of a memory response.

The necessary components of a physiologic host defense system must subserve these four functions, possessing, at minimum, three capabilities. The first is an injury-sensing apparatus. Without the ability to sense damage to its integrity, the host cannot engage in responses to prevent further injury and repair the primary injury. Second, such a system must be able to initiate local protective responses and recruit distant support to reinforce the local response. Finally, it must incorporate controls that modulate the type, intensity, and timing of responses. The next section discusses the nature of injury signals, followed by an examination of how the mammalian host protects itself against infections and other injuries.

Injury Signals

The term *injury signal* carries inherent ambiguity. It could signify a stimulus that causes injury or a marker that host tissue has been injured or invaded. The following discussion refers to the second meaning of the term—the indicator that signifies damage. A distinction should be made between primary and secondary injury signals. Primary signals are generated or liberated by an insult that threatens the host. They can be molecules or forces (such as bacterial endotoxin, products of necrotic cell death, or thermal injury) that in turn generate endogenous, secondary signals (e.g., cytokines or neurotransmitters) that extend, amplify, propagate, or terminate primary signals.

Background

In *Lives of the Cell*, Lewis Thomas commented on the symbolic importance of injury sensing, hinting at the existence of an injury language:

> It is the information carried by the bacteria that we cannot abide. The gram-negative bacteria are the best examples of this. They display lipopolysaccharide endotoxin in their walls, and these macromolecules are read by our tissues as the very worst of bad news. When we sense lipopolysaccharide, we are likely to turn on every defense at our disposal.... There is nothing intrinsically poisonous about endotoxin, but it must look awful, or feel awful, when sensed by cells (52).

Early attempts to understand illness recognized the association between rotting or putrefaction and its toxic effects on different hosts (4). By the mid-19th century, investigators had begun to isolate activities from dead bacteria that could sicken animals immunized against infection with them, suggesting that an inanimate property of a formerly live organism encoded a threat. Subsequent work on the lymphocyte recognition of pathogens led Burnet, Lederburg, and others to propose a dichotomous antigen-sensing system in which lymphocytes that sensed self-antigens were suppressed, while those that recognized non–self-antigens persisted (7,23). The limitations of this "either–or" code and the acknowledgment that effective vaccines required inflammation-causing adjuvants to ensure specific immunity prompted Janeway to propose that innate immunity recognized invariant attributes specific to classes of pathogens (pathogen-associated molecular patterns) via a germline-encoded sensory system (pattern-recognition receptors) (18). This "stranger theory" failed to account for certain phenomena, such as autoimmunity and the temporary tolerance of the pregnant female to the foreign fetus within her body. Matzinger later articulated the "Danger Theory," which proposed that the presence or threat of injury determined responsiveness more than the foreignness of the stimulus (31). Her "hyppo hypothesis," in which normally occult *hydrophobic portions* (hyppo) within activators and sensors are exposed by injury and subsequently interact to trigger an innate immune response, offers a physicochemical basis for injury signaling that, while intriguing, remains unproven (45).

Current Knowledge

Despite knowledge about the major injury mechanisms and their consequences, little is known about the molecular char-

acter of the injury signals they generate. The consequences of physical/mechanical (burn/scald, temperature extreme, electrical, radiation, atmospheric pressure), toxic (metabolic poison, free radical), ischemia–reperfusion, autoimmune, and infectious injuries have been extensively documented in clinical and experimental literatures. Many of these injuries can cause extensive tissue destruction, which, in itself, can pose a threat to survival through secondary injury, such as exsanguinating hemorrhage, unconsciousness, airway obstruction, or critical organ dysfunction (e.g., status epilepticus, myocardial depression, renal failure). With the exception of microbial invasion and infection, however, the molecular identity of primary signals produced by these injuries remains elusive. So, precisely what is known about primary injury signals, what is suspected, and what remains speculative?

Many injury signals from bacteria, fungi, and viruses have been isolated and chemically characterized. Although Janeway referred to them as "patterns," they are, above all, molecules or domains within molecules (4), and they belong to most major macromolecular classes, including carbohydrates, lipids, nucleic acids, proteins, and compound macromolecules, such as glycolipids, lipopeptides, and glycoproteins. Lipopolysaccharide, for example, is a complex, phosphorylated glycolipid that composes approximately 75% of the outer leaflet of the outer membrane of gram-negative bacteria. Although different species have varying patterns of LPS acylation and glycosylation, the lipid A moiety activates the innate immune system (41,53). Moreover, the facultative anaerobic gram-negative commensal species in the human gastrointestinal and respiratory tracts synthesize similar hexacylated, lipid A- and lipid-containing polysaccharides and oligosaccharides, putative "mucosal" LPSs (33) that are best recognized by the CD-14/Toll-like receptor (TLR)-4/MD2 receptor apparatus. As discussed in the following section, different signals activate overlapping, sometimes identical signaling pathways (TLR/IL-1 signaling and nuclear factor [NF]-κB translocation) and cellular responses (cytokine and chemokine production and cell surface marker changes).

The existence of primary injury signals of endogenous origin has been postulated, but their exact identity has been difficult to document. Several reports offer evidence that necrotic cells trigger an injury response (11,26,46,47). Identifying the molecule(s) that precipitate the response has nonetheless proved difficult. In one instance, the signal appeared transiently following physical cell disruption, but it has defied efforts to assign its subcellular origin (26). The possible role of heat shock proteins (Hsps) highlights the challenges to those seeking endogenous injury signals. This topic is reviewed by Wallin (55). Early reports implicated mammalian Hsps as activators of the innate immune response. These studies have been plagued, however, by the specter of LPS contamination. Despite the application of standard controls to rule out LPS contamination in these systems, innate immune activation resembled the response to LPS stimulation. Moreover, Hsps purified from mouse liver in an LPS-free process failed to stimulate innate immunity, casting doubt on the ability of these molecules to act as endogenous injury signals.

The most convincing demonstration to date of an endogenous injury signal has been the biochemical purification of a low molecular-weight activity from dying cells that augments an adaptive immune response (46). Investigators fractionated the cytosol from cells killed by ultraviolet irradiation and assayed the ability of fractions to prime a T-cell response (a read-out of intact innate immune function). Mass spectrometry of the isolated low molecular-weight activity matched the spectrum of uric acid (a common product of purine catabolism, present in high intracellular concentrations in injured and dying cells), and uricase or allopurinol treatments abolished the ability of this fraction and dying cells to boost the T-cell response in vitro and in vivo. Moreover, the uric acid concentrations that stimulated dendritic cell maturation fell within the range of crystal formation, and uric acid crystals (and not soluble uric acid) exhibited immunostimulatory behavior. Together, these data suggest that a phase transition from soluble to insoluble (associated with supersaturated concentrations of uric acid at the site of cellular disruption) may convert a normal component of both the intracellular and extracellular milieus into an injury signal (46).

Extracellular matrix degradation products may also function as primary injury signals. Separate investigative groups identified the immunostimulatory potential of soluble hyaluronic acid fragments—the breakdown products of solid-phase polymeric hyaluronic acid (38,50)—later demonstrating TLR4- and TLR2-dependent signal transduction (19,49). The extra domain A of fibronectin, the product of an alternatively spliced exon produced in response to tissue injury and essential to wound healing, also triggers an inflammatory response through TLR4. Thus, injury-dependent alterations of the extracellular matrix, which is normally immunologically silent, may convert these macromolecules into injury signals.

Additional candidate primary injury signals include the chromatic-associated protein high mobility group box 1 (HMGB1) and extracellular ATP. HMGB1 is an ancient DNA-binding protein that stabilizes nucleosomes and functions as an activating transcription factor. More recent studies demonstrate its secretion from activated macrophages and dendritic cells, interaction with the receptor for advanced glycation end products, and localized inflammation, thus conferring a cytokine function for HMGB1. However, demonstration of its release from necrotic cells and TLR2- and TLR4-dependent initiation of an innate immune response also suggest a role for HMGB1 as a primary injury signal (28).

ATP accumulates in the extracellular space following tissue injury and appears to mediate at least an adjunctive function to primary injury signals. For example, it is a key factor in the release of mature IL-1β. Synthesized as a pro-molecule, this proinflammatory cytokine must undergo caspase-1–mediated cleavage to become active and be secreted. Following LPS stimulation, macrophages accumulate large amounts of intracellular pro–IL-1β, but ATP acting on the P2X$_7$ receptor leads to massive release of mature IL-1β.

Summary of Current Knowledge

Although our present knowledge of microbial molecules that trigger innate immune responses exceeds current understanding of endogenous injury signals, ignorance regarding both abounds. For example, although genetic evidence supports the notion that the TLR4/MD2 receptor complex recognizes LPS, how the latter physically interacts with the receptor complex still eludes description. Moreover, the concentration of a particular signal dictates the host response to it. Picogram quantities of LPS trigger inflammatory responses, while milligram

amounts of uric acid are required for its crystallization to an activating form in physiologic solutions. Finally, the identity, characterization, and classification of novel injury signals may uncover unexpected strategies used by the host to distinguish normal homeostasis from a threat, some of which may represent minute deviations from the range of normal concentration or activity. For example, the mammalian equivalent of the plant "guard hypothesis"—in which intracellular sentinels targeted by viral proteins are under the surveillance of proteins that can detect viral modifications and mount a resistance response when these changes are detected—has yet to be described.

Cellular Recognition and Response to Injury Signals

Our understanding of how cells sense and respond to injury has expanded during the last decade. As often occurs in science, developments in apparently unrelated fields fueled this growth. Findings that stem from Nobel-prize winning work on the genetics of *Drosophila* embryogenesis provided an initial glimpse of the receptor and intracellular signaling molecules for injury signals (56). The Human Genome Project provided the sequence information that identified the first human TLRs. In addition, The Human Genome Project provided the technology that allowed multiple investigative groups to implicate the TLR family in the innate immune response (32) and, using positional cloning, to subsequently identify the murine homolog of TLR4 as the mammalian LPS sensor (40). The emerging picture, while far from complete, represents a significant advance over our knowledge at the end of the last century.

Essential Characteristics of an Injury-Sensing Apparatus

The first required component of a defense system, an injury sensing apparatus, must have several characteristics to protect the host. First, it must be widely distributed, with components either present or rapidly inducible in all tissues. Second, the sensory machinery must be sensitive, with a low activation threshold, a requirement that favors the initiation of responses at low-injury burden.

A third characteristic, that injury sensors be promiscuous (capable of detecting more than a single signal), is neither required nor universal but would be selected for to maximize genetic economy. TLR2, for example, senses lipoteichoic acid, porins, and lipoarabinomannan in bacteria; zymosan and phospholipomannan in fungi; tGPI-mutin in trypanosomes; and measles virus hemagglutinin protein (2). This ability to recognize more than one activator, particularly when coupled with the ability to associate with different family members (e.g., when TLR2 and TLR6 combine to detect lipoteichoic acid), provides the host with an extended recognition spectrum using a limited number of genes.

A final, required feature of the host sensory apparatus is the sequestration of sensors from signals in the uninjured state. Nature accomplishes this separation through different strategies. Epithelial barriers, for example, constitute the most effective means of partitioning microbial invaders and their sensors, but plasma membranes accomplish the same purpose at a cellular level, particularly if intracellular molecules signal cellular injury when released. The break-down products of extracellular matrix, prevalent in some rheumatic diseases, may also be recognized as injury, while the polymeric forms are immunologically inert (49). The rationale for this sequestration requirement is obvious. Signal and sensor in continuous contact would either maintain the system in a state of constant activation, or the organism would develop a damping mechanism ("tolerance") to render it insensitive to real injury or infection.

Current Knowledge

Mammalian hosts have evolved multiple means of recognizing injury, depending on the type, location, and severity. Pyogenic extracellular bacteria and herpes viruses can both kill the undefended host, albeit through different mechanisms. In fact, the distinct strategies employed by mammals results from eons of coexisting with commensal bacteria and viruses, keeping them at bay or quiescent, and quickly containing them following the breaching of barriers or suppressed immune surveillance. Opportunistic infections occur when commensals and nonpathogenic organisms exploit the weakened host, while pathogens have evolved mechanisms to circumvent intact defenses.

Cataloging all injury sensors and their signal transducers exceeds the scope of this chapter. Some sensing systems represent "generic" recognition strategies capable of sensing injuries caused by a range of insults, whereas others detect insults due to a specific mechanism. Sensor systems based on the ancient leucine-rich repeat (LRR) include the TLRs and the NACHT-LRRs (including the nucleotide-binding oligomerization domain [NOD] and NACCHT-, LRR-pyrin domain [PYD]-containing proteins [NALPs]). Other, C-type lectin receptors recognize different bacterial carbohydrate structures, as well as some gram-negative outer membrane proteins. Proteinase-activated receptors constitute a third family of receptors activated by cellular injury and tissue damage that may link the innate immune and nervous systems to the inflammatory response. Periodic publication of excellent reviews provides frequent updates on these and other mammalian sensing systems (2,8,30,36,54). Examples of mechanism-specific injury sensors include the family of prolyl hydroxylases that sense cellular hypoxia (57) and the retinoic acid inducible gene I (RIG-I) RNA helicase sensor of double-stranded viral RNA (59).

Toll-like Receptors as a Prototypical General Injury-sensing System

Despite their recent description, the TLRs, their intracellular signal transduction pathways, and the cellular responses their activation triggers have taken center stage in the attempts to understand innate immunity and the links between innate and adaptive immune responses. Many reasons underlie this intense interest, but a common thread to all is that TLRs represent a true sensing system capable of detecting a broad range of injuries, endogenous and exogenous. Conservation of elements of this system (LRRs, immunity-associated kinases, etc.) across kingdom—not just species—lines suggests that these motifs represent a common strategy for different hosts, one forged in the evolutionary crucible. The following text reviews core features of this system, discusses both the general principles

of sensing and response and the higher-order complexities of detecting and initiating cellular responses to injury, and ultimately highlights what remains unknown and challenges current investigators. Readers are referred to the several excellent review articles that are published each year on the growing understanding of TLR recognition and signaling (1,2,39).

TLR/IL-1R Superfamily. The first TLR discovered was the *Drosophila* protein Toll. Later, sequencing of RNA expressed in multiple mouse and human tissues, and public deposition of these sequences, led to the recognition of other receptors that resembled Toll (43). Humans express 11 TLR family members. Their basic structure consists of an ectodomain composed of LRRs that differ in number and organization. The structure of these ectodomains distinguishes one TLR from another and confers on each its recognition specificity. In the case of TLR4, the major endotoxin sensor, MD2, is also associated with the ectodomain and is required for endotoxin recognition. The intracellular domain, common to both TLR and the IL-1 receptor subfamilies, is composed of a Toll/IL-1R (TIR) domain. Across different receptors, amino acid identity ranges from 20% to 30%, but in conserved regions, the similarity is higher. This intracellular domain engages the intracellular signaling apparatus (1) (**Fig. 17.1**).

The activation of TLRs triggers intracellular signal transduction. As depicted in **Figure 17.2** (48), receptor engagement induces the assembly of a multiprotein receptor complex through protein domain interactions, phosphorylation, and the displacement of proteins from different subcellular compartments. Myeloid differentiation adapter protein (MyD88), a dual-domain adaptor protein, is recruited to the activated

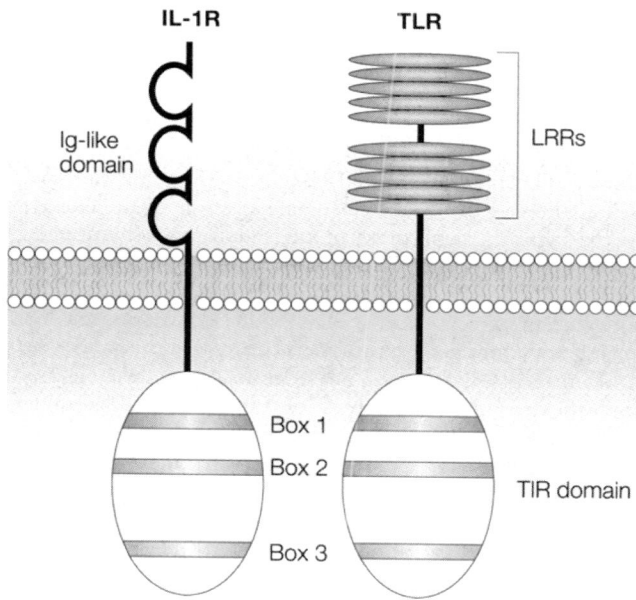

FIGURE 17.1. Humans express 11 Toll-like receptors (TLRs). Their basic structure consists of an ectodomain composed of leucine-rich repeats (LRRs) and an intracellular domain, common to both TLR and the IL-1 receptor subfamilies, containing a Toll/IL-1R (TIR) domain. The structure and organization of the LRRs within these ectodomains differ in number and organization for each TLR and confer recognition specificity on each.

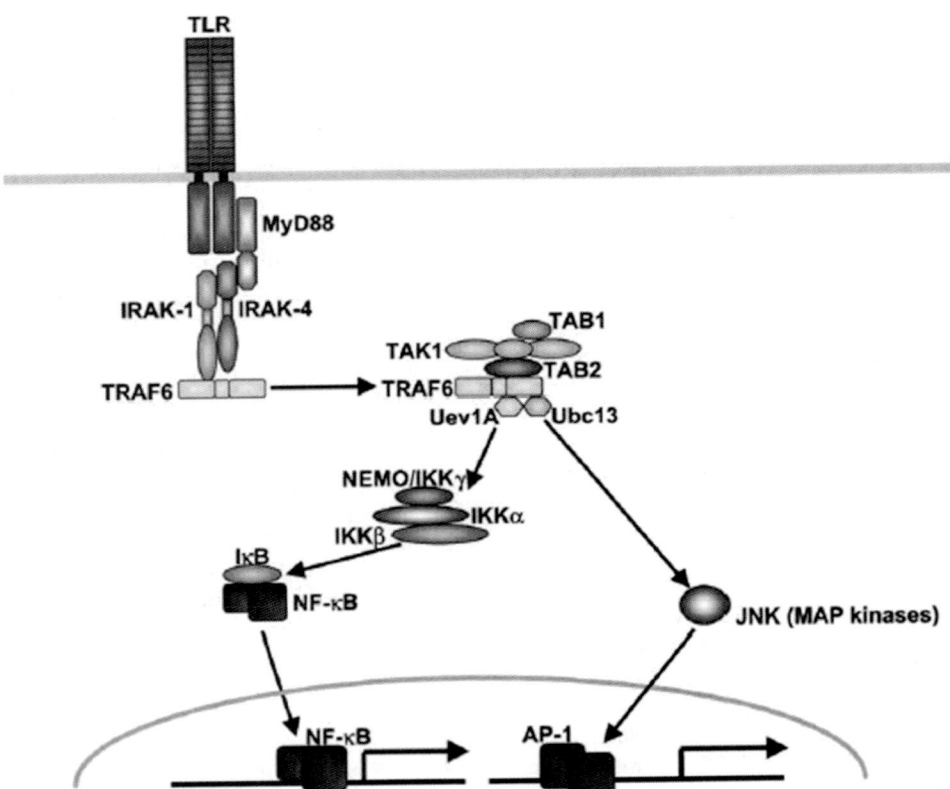

FIGURE 17.2. TLR-mediated My-D88-dependent signaling pathway. Upon receptor stimulation, MyD88, a dual-domain adaptor protein, migrates from the cytosol to the activated receptor complex through TIR:TIR domain interactions. IL-1 receptor-associated kinase (IRAK)-4, IRAK1, and TRAF6 are then recruited to the nascent complex, via death domain-mediated associations between IRAK family members and MyD88. IRAK4 phosphorylates IRAK1, which then undergoes extensive autophosphorylation and conformational changes. Hyperphosphorylated IRAK-1, together with the ubiquitin ligase TRAF6, dissociates from the receptor complex, and interacts with a complex containing the kinase TAK1 and the adapters TAB1 and TAB2 at the membrane (not shown). Phosphorylation of TAB2 and TAK1 leads to IRAK1 degradation at the membrane, translocation of the complex to the cytosol, recruitment of two additional ubiquitin ligases, ubiquitination of TRAF, and activation of TAK1, which triggers additional kinase cascades that lead to NFκB, stress-activated protein kinase (SAPK or JNK) activation, and new proinflammatory gene expression.

receptor complex through TIR:TIR domain interactions. The MyD88 death domain, in turn, provides a platform for IL-1 receptor-associated kinase (IRAK)-4 and IRAK1 recruitment to the receptor complex. IRAK4 phosphorylates IRAK1, which then undergoes extensive autophosphorylation and conformational changes, interacts with the ubiquitin ligase TNF receptor-associated factor 6 (TRAF6), dissociates from the receptor complex, and associates with a complex containing the TGF-β activated protein kinase (TAK1) and the adapters TAK1-binding proteins (TAB)-1 and -2 at the membrane (not shown). Phosphorylation of TAB2 and TAK1 leads to IRAK1 degradation at the membrane, translocation of the complex to the cytosol, recruitment of two additional ubiquitin ligases, ubiquitination of TRAF, and activation of TAK1, which triggers additional kinase cascades that lead to NFκB, stress-activated protein kinase (SAPK or JNK) activation, and new proinflammatory gene expression (1).

As reagents, techniques, and questions have become more sophisticated, the elucidation of this process has undergone refinement. TLRs, in fact, activate multiple intracellular pathways; which pathways are activated depends both on the adapters present and the receptors being activated. For example, TLR4 activates both MyD88-dependent and MyD88-independent cascades, the latter through other adapter proteins, TIR domain-containing adaptor protein inducing interferon beta (TRIF), TRIF-related adapter molecule (TRAM), and Rieske iron-sulfur protein (RIP1), which lead to the expression of IFN-β and other interferon-inducible genes. TLR3 does not activate the MyD88-dependent pathway. Moreover, some of the TLRs (e.g., 3, 7, 8, and 9) are not even expressed on the cell surface, but rather within the endosomal compartment (21). A schematic summary of TLR signaling cascades is

contained in **Figure 17.3.** For a more comprehensive map of the TLR signaling network, please consult the work of Oda and Kitano (39).

TLR signal transduction highlights two general signaling concepts about the cellular response to injury signals. The first is that signaling protein oligomerization begets activation. In the case of receptors, adapters, and kinases, the interaction of TIR domains in TLRs and MyD88 fosters death domain–mediated associations between MyD88 and IRAK4 and IRAK1, a prerequisite for IRAK1 phosphorylation and activation by IRAK4. An analogous cascade of associations leads to activation of the ubiquitin ligase activity of TRAF6. A second theme regarding intracellular signaling following TLR activation is that kinase activity subserves at least two critical functions in the response to injury signals. Phosphorylation activates proteins targeted by kinases. Thus, IRAK4 phosphorylates IRAK1, activating its own catalytic activity, both autocatalytic and that of interferon response factor (IRF)-7. Kinase activity also mediates signal propagation. Hyperphosphorylated IRAK1 is unstable in the receptor complex; it dissociates and moves, with TRAF6, to interact with the TAK1/TAB kinase complex. Catalytic activity of the TAK1 kinase activates two additional kinase complexes: IκB kinase and mitogen-activated protein kinase kinase (MKK6). Thus, the vectorial property of kinase function is responsible for the injury signal's arrival in the nucleus—in the forms of NFκB and cJun transcription factors—to effect changes in gene expression.

Cellular Responses

Cellular responses to injury signals fall into two broad categories: genomic and nongenomic. Genomic responses refer to those reactions that involve changes in gene expression. They

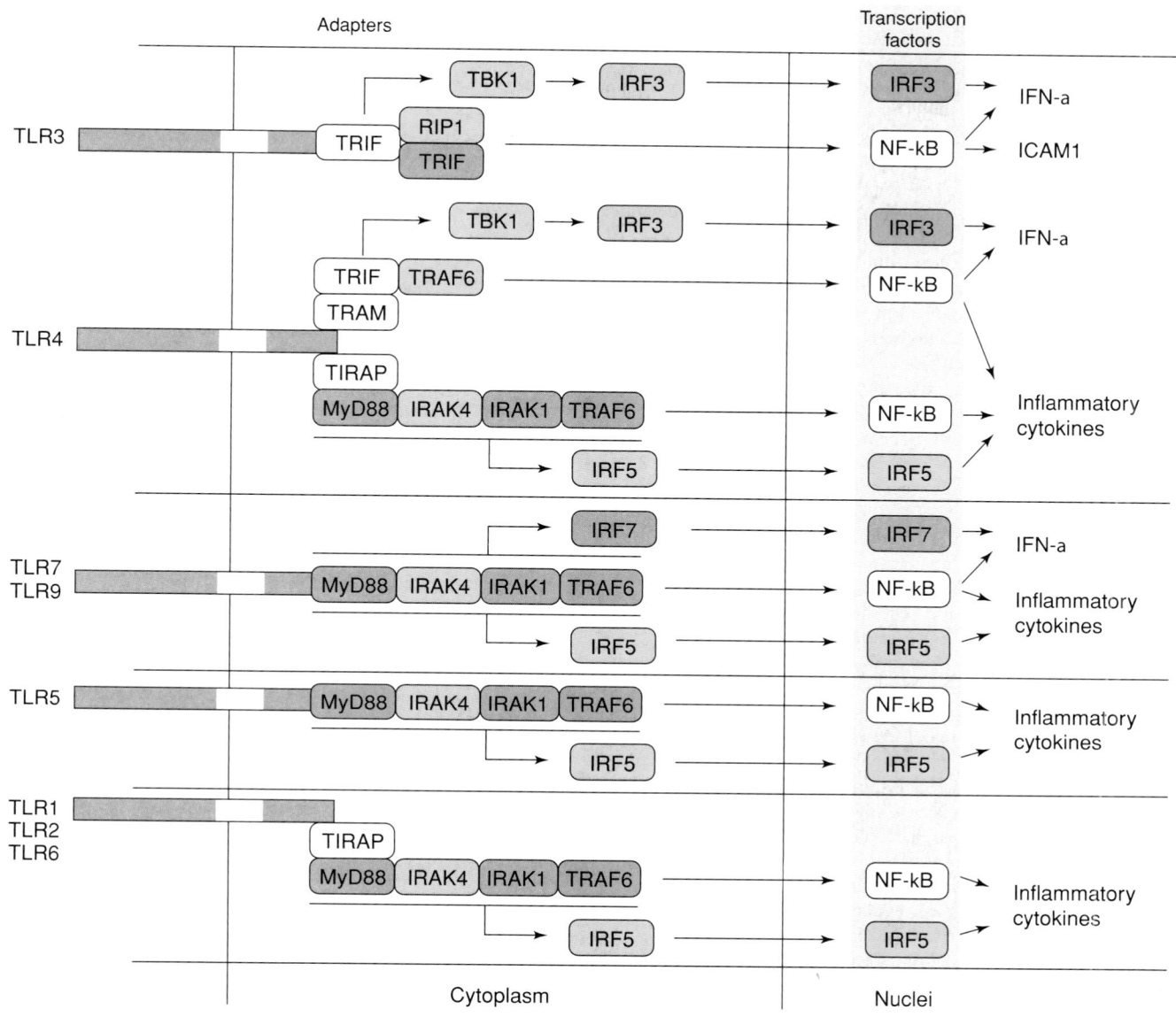

FIGURE 17.3. Schematic representation of TLR signaling pathways. Human TLRs and major intracellular pathways, including essential transcriptional activators, are depicted. All TLRs, except TLR3, signal to the nucleus via the MyD88-dependent pathway that activates NFκB and several interferon response factors (IRFs), which in turn induce genes essential to the inflammatory response. Several pathways and targets have been omitted, and many have yet to be described.

can either be upregulatory or suppressive, promoting gene transcription and translation or inhibiting them. Many signals, if not most, that indicate the presence of cellular injury involve activation of the transcription factor NFκB, making this molecule a central regulator of the inflammatory response. Nongenomic responses involve activation or release of preformed effector stores. Retrograde release of substance P from C fibers (afferent sensory nerves involved in nociception) constitutes an example of a nongenomic response.

Nuclear Factor-κB and Genomic Responses to Injury. Although originally identified in activated B cells and believed to be a regulator of immunoglobulin expression, NFκB orchestrates many aspects of the inflammatory response. NFκB actually consists of 10 related genes that encode transcription

factors or their inhibitors, constituting a system of proinflammatory responsiveness. The interaction of these dimers with the inhibitor proteins of the IκB family prevents DNA binding of the transcription factors with the promoter sequences of NFκB-responsive genes. Detection of an injury signal, either primary (via TLRs, NLRs, or other receptors) or secondary (through proinflammatory cytokine receptors), triggers degradation of the IκB proteins, freeing the transcription factors to interact with the promoters of responsive genes. In reality, two distinct NFκB pathways exist. The one just described, called the *canonical pathway*, is responsible for regulating the inflammatory response, including the proliferation and apoptosis of lymphoid cells involved in this response. The second, *noncanonical pathway* belongs more appropriately to the realm of adaptive immunity, because it is responsible for the development of those lymphoid organs that are necessary for appropriate antigen processing, presentation, and mounting of the adaptive immune response (15).

When activated, NFκB influences the expression of over 500 genes involved in the inflammatory response. An examination of these genes reveals a map of the inflammatory response to injury and infection (see http://people.bu.edu/gilmore/nf-kb/target/index.html for a recent tally of target genes). Genes regulated by NFκB belong to several categories that are essential to the initiation, regulation, or termination of the inflammatory response. Genes that promote the local inflammatory response include those specifying other transcription factors (interferon regulatory factors, Jun B, Bcl3, c-myb, c-myc, and glucocorticoid receptor); cytokines (IL-1, TNF-α, macrophage inflammatory protein [MIP]-1, IFN-γ, and IL-2); chemokines (IL-8, monocyte chemotactic protein [MCP]-1, RANTES); receptors for cytokines, chemokines, and membrane-bound ligands (TLR2, NOD2, TNF receptor, MHC II, CD40, and CD86); and cell adhesion molecules (intercellular adhesion molecule [ICAM]-1, vascular cell adhesion molecule [VCAM]-1, fibronectin, P-selectin, and DC-SIGN). Other genes include those involved in the acute phase (C-reactive protein, serum amyloid A, LPS binding protein, and β-defensins) and stress (superoxide dismutases, inducible nitric oxide synthase, cyclooxygenase [COX]-2, and several cytochrome p450 genes) responses. Yet, additional genes under the control of NFκB regulate apoptosis (*Bax, Fas, Bcl-2,* and *caspase-11*) and growth factors and their receptors (fibroblast growth factor [FGF]-8, insulin-like growth factor binding protein [IGFBP]-1, erythropoietin [Epo], granulocyte-colony stimulating factor [GCSF], vascular endothelial growth factor [VEGF]-C). The sheer range of genes influenced by NFκB hints at the complexity of mechanisms to achieve cell type-specific, context-specific, and stimulus-specific responses. Specificity mechanisms that affect NFκB activity, govern transcription on NFκB-regulated promoters, and radiate from NFκB dimer isoforms all point to the presence of an elaborate regulatory apparatus that is the current focus of research efforts (15).

The final steps in the cellular response to injury signals involve translation of RNA transcripts into effector proteins and the transport or release to their site of activity. The expression of many proinflammatory molecules, particularly cytokines, is under translational control, and many of these molecules possess a common mRNA sequence in the 3′-untranslated region (9) that is the target of multiple proteins that permit translation of the message (12,13,24). Secretion of proinflammatory cytokines and chemokines, release of soluble receptors, and induction of membrane-bound receptors and adhesion molecules mark the initiation of the efferent arm of the innate immune response, the subject of the next section.

Summary of Essential Characteristics of an Injury-Sensing Apparatus

Our understanding of how cells sense injury has progressed rapidly in the last decade. The TLRs and their intracellular signaling pathway constitute one type of global injury sensing system. The receptors are widely distributed, and their expression increases in response to threats to host integrity in tissues that do not normally express them. They are also sensitive,

becoming activated in the presence of low concentrations of agonist. Many of these receptors are promiscuous, capable of recognizing multiple signals, both exogenous and endogenous. Finally, in healthy states, the system is quiescent, with signal and sensor remaining apart from one another.

As in any surveillance system, the TLR-NFκB sensing module accomplishes several different functions in response to injury or infection. First, it translates the injury signal into a language intelligible to the cell interior (in the case of the TLR/IL-1R pathway, a common language used by 10 of 11 TLRs, the IL-1R, IL-18R, and three other IL1R family members). Proximal elements of the pathway process and distribute the signal to multiple downstream effectors, leading to genomic and nongenomic responses. Understanding how the signal is processed—that is, how adaptors, kinases, ligases, and transcription and translation factors integrate and parse information transferred from the cell surface, endosomal compartment, cytosol, and nucleus—in different cell types has received increased emphasis as the characterization of individual components approaches completion. Attempts to understand the processing of different and complex arrays of injury signals, as occurs during infection, are beginning to embrace complex systems-based concepts that describe cells' (and, indeed, entire organisms') responses by difficult-to-predict, emergent properties.

LOCAL RESPONSE AND ALERTING HOST DEFENSE

Once sentinel cells have detected injury or microbial invasion, they unleash a response with the goal of containing the insult and eliminating invading microbes and injured and dying cells. The host must engage both local tissue and systemic components to accomplish these dual objectives, the latter to muster distant resources (e.g., mobilize marginated neutrophils, produce acute-phase reactants, etc.) and support the local response. Through cytokine, chemokine, and antimicrobial peptide production and action, neuroendocrine system activation, localized endothelial cell changes, leukocyte influx into the injured tissue, and the acute-phase response, the host attempts to neutralize the threat to its integrity and restore homeostasis.

Because even the basic inflammatory response is so complex, the following summary includes only a few details—important ones, to be sure, but by no means comprehensive. The synopsis also outlines the acute local injury and neutrophil influx responses to bacterial tissue invasion or localized tissue necrosis (e.g., following ischemia). This reaction depicts the earliest activation of innate immunity. Chronic inflammatory responses, as occur with some pathogens or in chronic inflammatory states (e.g., autoimmunity), use analogous localization mechanisms but differ in the types of cells recruited and the involvement of adaptive immunity.

Requirements for Effective Injury Response

As indicated earlier, a suitable host defense system must marshal both local and distant resources to confront the threat. Tissue adjacent to the microbial invasion site should commence the containment and elimination of damaged tissue or invading microorganisms, while recruiting additional support to the site of injury from more remote sources. In the afferent arm, the host must translate the primary injury signal, detected by specialized sensor cells, into a language intelligible to all host cells. This translation function alerts uninjured but at-risk cells in the vicinity of injury and amplifies the original injury signal. Finally, communication networks must distribute the signal to more distant sites critical to supporting and coordinating the integrated inflammatory response (e.g., CNS, liver). The efferent arm first directs effectors to the site of injury. Neurogenic inflammation, cytokine production, altered local endothelium, and chemokine gradients promote leukocyte arrival at the injury site and prime them to enact their assigned inflammatory actions. This vectorial component is essential to proper localization of the injury response. Failure to localize or the indiscriminate activation of inflammatory functions away from infectious foci or injury sites may underlie certain parainfectious syndromes, such as ARDS, severe sepsis, or disseminated intravascular coagulation (DIC) (35). The efferent limb of a host defense system then concentrates the inflammatory response to a limited area, while ensuring containment of invading microorganisms and toxic inflammatory products to that site. A balance between potent local proinflammatory effectors and systemic anti-inflammatory mediators is essential to this circumscription function (34).

Local Response

An effective local response must accomplish four objectives. It must first ensure placement of effectors at the injury site. Because effectors range in size from small molecules to proteins to large leukocytes, the local response utilizes various mechanisms to achieve this first goal. The local reaction must also contain microbial invasion and limit the impact of necrotic cell death on both adjacent and distant tissues. Failure to do so would result in systemic spread of pathogens and toxic substances that could destabilize the host. As containment is accomplished, the local response must clean up the detritus of injury, including both contained microbes and dead and dying host cells. Finally, the local inflammatory response initiates the healing process. Depending on the affected tissue and the injury mechanism, healing may involve regeneration, scarring, or a combination of the two. Healing will not be discussed further.

Three general processes are critical during an acute inflammatory response. First, the initial injury signal must undergo local amplification, a process that involves spreading an intelligible alarm and generating injury location information. The second process involves alteration of the local vasculature to permit soluble and cellular effectors in the bloodstream to leave the vascular space and prevent microbes and toxins from entering the circulation. Last, leukocytes migrate from the vascular space to the injury site in a regulated process that destroys invaders and infected cells, scavenges injured and dying tissue, and promotes an adaptive immune response to infections. These processes are discussed in greater detail below.

Local Amplification of Injury Signal

Specialization poses interesting problems for the host. Tissues evolved to enact particular functions (e.g., gas exchange, blood circulation, or solute excretion) often lack other capacities. Many specialized cell types either lack or exhibit deficiencies in the ability to sense injury. TLR protein expression, both scattered and nonubiquitous, illustrates this point. When a tissue is threatened at one site, however, the host must have a means to alert surrounding cells and engage their participation in mounting a protective response. In mammals, at least two systems exist to perform this essential function. The first consists of different systems of soluble mediators collectively referred to as *cytokines*, whereas the second utilizes the peripheral nervous system.

Cytokines. Cytokines refer to soluble proteins or glycoproteins made by cells to affect the behavior of other cells (22). They are usually produced in response to a stimulus (as opposed to constitutively), act over a short distance, and are distinguished from hormones and growth factors based on arbitrary criteria, although properties and functions often overlap. Some cytokines are pleiotropic, and others exhibit a narrow spectra of targets and effects. Various schemata have been used to classify families of cytokines.

The Proinflammatory Cytokines: TNF-α and IL-1β. Shortly after local injury or microbial invasion, specialized injury-sensing cells produce and release both TNF-α and IL-1β. Although structurally unrelated and recognized by different receptors, the expression of these two cytokines is under similar control, and they elicit overlapping biologic effects. Transcription of both mRNAs is regulated by NFκB, and a shared AU-rich region in the 3' untranslated region, common to many proinflammatory molecules, controls mRNA stability and, thus, message translation. Secretion of these cytokines, however, follows distinct pathways. TNF-α is synthesized as a precursor, membrane-anchored secretory protein. A novel pathway targets trimeric pro–TNF-α to a recycling endosome and triggers its cleavage and extracellular release by its processing enzyme, TNF-α–converting enzyme (TACE), following membrane fusion. Following a nonclassical secretory route, pro–IL-1β and its processing protease, caspase 1, are both targeted to specialized secretory lysosomes. Extracellular ATP then provides a second stimulus that triggers cleavage of the procytokine to mature IL-1β and its secretion via exocytosis.

The mature cytokines bind to ubiquitous cognate receptors, triggering activation of NFκB and other key intracellular inflammatory mediators. These molecules lead, in turn, to the production and release of additional molecules that activate local endothelium, serve as chemoattractants, and begin to cycle off the acute proinflammatory response.

The net effect of TNF and IL-1 action is threefold:

■ These cytokines convert a cryptic injury signal into a language shared by most cells in an affected tissue, by virtue of near ubiquitous receptor distribution.
■ They spread the alarm to a greater number of cells in the area of injury. This propagation function amplifies the original injury signal by inducing more cells to contribute to the local inflammatory response.
■ This initial proinflammatory cytokine response provides the host with positional information about the site of injury. The intensity of the response is highest closest to the primary injury or invasion site. Chemokine concentrations are highest nearer the center of injury, diminishing in a radial fashion. Endothelial activation is also more intense in vessels closer to the infection or site of necrosis than in more distant vessels.

ELR+ CXC chemokines. Chemokines are cytokines that exert chemotactic functions. The approximately 50 chemokines belong to at least four families that are classified according to molecular structure, although the four families and individual molecules exhibit redundant functions (29). The CXC chemokines contain two cysteine residues separated by a variable residue at their amino terminus. These molecules are further subdivided according to the presence (ELR+) or absence (ELR−) tripeptide motif. The ELR+ CXC chemokines are considered the primary neutrophil chemoattractants, with IL-8 (or CXCL8, according to other nomenclature) representing the prototype. These molecules interact with two cognate receptors (CXCR1 and CXCR2) with similar biologic effects. Synthesis of the ELR+ CXC chemokines occurs in response to proinflammatory stimuli, either as a result of direct infection (e.g., LPS), injury (e.g., hypoxic–ischemic injury), or primary cytokine (TNF-α or IL-1β) stimulation.

Through an overlapping, multistep process, IL-8 and other ELR+ CXC chemokines enable the movement of neutrophils out of the vascular space to the site of inflammation. Initial interaction between IL-8 and CXCR1 and -2 may occur as neutrophils rolling along the endothelium arrest, allowing high-avidity interactions between ligand and receptor (5). IL-8 forms a gradient, mediated in part by immobilization on basement membrane proteins, with highest concentrations at the site of inflammation that decrease with distance from the primary focus. Neutrophils migrate down the chemokine gradient from lower to higher concentration, becoming more activated as they approach the site of infection or injury.

Thus, the CXC ELR+ chemokines, as well as other inducible chemokines, enact three essential functions for the acute local response: (a) They provide positional information to cellular effectors migrating to the inflammatory focus; (b) because the concentration gradient is continuous, these molecules also map out the route to the site; and (c) finally, they gradually arm the leukocyte, enhancing its level of activation as the effector cell approaches the center of maximal injury. The latter function maximizes destructive potential where appropriate and minimizes the chances of damage to uninjured tissue.

Neurogenic Inflammation. The term *neurogenic inflammation* refers to a specific reaction to infection or injury mediated by the peripheral nervous system. In this reaction, primary sensory nerve fibers actually carry out an efferent function (antidromic transmission) that promotes local inflammation. Following local injury, narrow-diameter, unmyelinated C-fibers in close proximity to, or membrane contact with, innate immune cells (especially mast cells) release neuropeptides, in particular substance P and calcitonin gene–related peptide. These neuropeptides, in turn, act on local immune cells, nerves, endothelium, and vascular smooth muscle to elicit many effects, including the cardinal signs of inflammation. Substance P, for example, promotes vasodilation, plasma extravasation, leukocyte activation, and adhesion molecule expression on endothelium (44) and leads to enhanced sensitization to painful stimuli (hyperalgesia). Most known inducers or enhancers of neurogenic inflammation are endogenous (bradykinin, glutamate, and acetylcholine), raising the question of whether the enhancement represents an amplification step only. However, heat, ATP, and hydrogen ions can also precipitate neurogenic inflammatory response, and other primary stimuli may yet be identified. Moreover, the sympathetic nervous system promotes neurogenic inflammation, as sympathectomy abrogates this reaction (as, for example, in the protective effect of prior brachial plexus injury [58]), and increased sympathetic activity in certain arthritis models is associated with more severe joint destruction (6).

Localized Vascular Response

The vasculature plays a critical role in the acute and subacute response to infection and injury. It routes both plasma, which contains potent antibacterial and proinflammatory proteins, and nonresident cells, principally different types of leukocytes, close to the site of insult. An effective inflammatory response, therefore, maximizes the delivery of these soluble and cellular components to the injury neighborhood, providing for both increased flux and correct localization, and it facilitates extravasation of these mediators, while at the same time preventing a systemic spread of toxins or microbes from the focus.

Vasodilation and Increased Permeability. Different types of injury (e.g., ingrown toenails, bacterial pharyngitis, blunt trauma) provoke similar initial responses. Whether sensed directly, by the presence of class-identifying molecules, or indirectly by the presence of tissue damage, the challenge provokes an initial response that involves the release of preformed mediators. Histamine, serotonin (from mast cells), and substance P (from sensory neurons) collaborate to induce local arteriolar vasodilatation, giving rise to hyperemia in the vicinity of the injury. These substances, together with others that potentiate further release of these primary mediators (e.g., bradykinin, tryptase, vasoactive intestinal peptide, and prostaglandin [PGE$_2$]), also trigger formation of reversible gaps between endothelial cells, leading to increased vascular permeability, transudation, and angiogenic edema. The wheal-flare reaction seen with urticaria or dermographism illustrates this early response even in the absence of any significant injury, but more damage is accompanied by a cellular infiltrate that develops later.

Vasodilation promotes the bulk movement of blood components to the region of injury or microbial invasion, while increased permeability permits translocation of soluble effectors out of the vascular space. The net effect of these combined processes is threefold: (a) targeting of antimicrobial and proinflammatory molecules to the site of injury or invasion; (b) increased bulk fluid delivery to the focus, which dilutes and neutralizes toxic mediators to help minimize secondary tissue damage; (c) increased interstitial fluide, which increases lymphatic flow, irrigates the focus, and facilitates development of the adaptive immune response to pathogens in the wound site by delivering antigens to draining lymph nodes.

Endothelial activation. The arteriovenous vasculature is not, as this discussion might imply, simply a conduit for blood components. It provides essential information about the location and intensity of an injury, serves as a portal for the cellular infiltrate of inflammation, and regulates its own role in this response. However, the endothelium, in concert with the peripheral nervous system, confers this important additional functionality on the blood vessels. Although the endothelium has multiple functions during the inflammatory response, two are discussed here.

The histologic hallmark of inflammation is the presence of leukocytes at the injury site or infection focus. Although most leukocytes traffic from the arteriovenous vasculature through the tissue to the lymphatic vascular system before returning to blood, carrying out continuous surveillance, a few, usually of monocytic lineage, take up residence in specific tissues. Following different acute insults, however, neutrophils rapidly congregate in large numbers at the site of injury, in a directed, nonrandom fashion. Activated endothelium in the vicinity of injured tissues furnishes both the information regarding the location of the inflammatory focus to leukocytes patrolling the vascular space and the means to initiate migration out of the vessel to the injury site.

After microbial invasion or other tissue damage, the postcapillary venules become the principal site of leukocyte extravasation. Two critical forces determine the efficiency with which this process occurs. The first is the relatively low shear stress (force exerted by flowing blood along the vessel wall that opposes the tendency to adhere to the vessel wall) in this part of the microcirculation. The second is the expression of molecules on the activated endothelial cell surface that promote leukocyte adherence and help these cells resist the shear stress of blood flow, help reduce their profile, and facilitate their migration out of the vessel.

Endothelial activation is a complex process. Multiple factors influence the degree of activation. The intensity of the injury itself or the pathogen load is a primary determinant of activation. More extensive local tissue damage, higher bacterial or viral load, and higher local primary cytokine concentration (particularly IL-1-β and TNF-α, but also IFN-γ) increase the intensity of the endothelial response in the region of injury. Localized shear stress, uninjured stromal cells (e.g., smooth muscle cells and fibroblasts), and even the extracellular matrix further modulate endothelial activation. One of the principal responses of activated endothelium is adhesion molecule and chemokine expression. Upregulation of selectins and vascular cell adhesion molecule (VCAM)-1 helps to halt rolling neutrophils (**Fig. 17.4**) and endothelial surface-associated chemokines, such as MCP-1, interact with the arrested leukocyte, triggering integrin signaling, subsequent flattening, and the transendothelial migration of the leukocytes out of the vascular space into the adjacent tissue (37). From there, they begin their migration down

changing chemokine gradients through the tissue to the injury site.

Thrombosis. Coagulation and inflammation are closely linked, although the detailed knowledge of this relationship is still emerging. In fact, the systems that protect against hemorrhage and microbial dissemination may have evolved from a common ancestral strategy that accomplished both. In the horseshoe crab, bacterial invasion precipitates a localized response that involves hemolymph coagulation and hemocyte agglutination, immobilizing the invader and preventing systemic spread prior to engulfment or killing (17). This limulus coagulation response forms the basis for current endotoxin detection tests. Both inflammation and coagulation influence each other. In general, local inflammation tends to downregulate natural anticoagulant systems, favoring thrombosis, whereas processes that skew the balance of procoagulation and anticoagulation forces toward antithrombosis and fibrinolysis have anti-inflammatory effects (10).

Coagulation is a surface-associated phenomenon. Under normal circumstances, the apical surface of the vascular endothelium possesses anticoagulant properties that discourage thrombus formation. However, tissue injury or infection can either disrupt endothelial continuity or induce changes in the endothelial surface that favor thrombus formation. Direct injury to the vessel exposes the soluble components of the extrinsic coagulation cascade to tissue factor expressed on monocytes, smooth muscle cells, and fibroblasts, thus triggering a proteolytic sequence that results in thrombin formation. Thrombin, in turn, exerts both procoagulant functions (fibrin formation, platelet shape change, activator release, and aggregation) and proinflammatory effects (vasoconstriction and cytokine production). Thrombosis can also occur within the vascular space with an intact endothelium. Although less well understood, intravascular coagulation can also occur in the setting of both localized and systemic inflammation. Factors that favor the occurrence of intravascular coagulation include an increase in negatively charged membrane surfaces (e.g., increased circulating microvesicles); the downregulation of the natural anticoagulant, activated protein C (through decreases in thrombomodulin and the endothelial cell protein C receptor); and

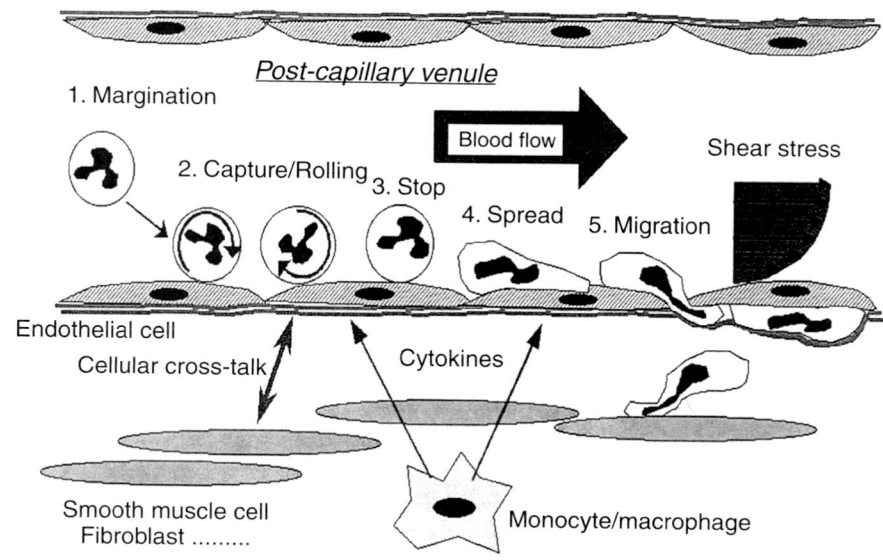

FIGURE 17.4. Leukocyte recruitment to inflamed tissue. Upregulation of selectins and VCAM-1 helps to halt rolling neutrophils; endothelial surface–associated chemokines, such as MCP-1, interact with the arrested leukocyte, triggering integrin signaling, subsequent flattening, and the transendothelial migration of the leukocyte out of the vascular space into the adjacent tissue. From there, they begin their migration down changing chemokine gradients through the tissue to the injury site.

neutrophil-mediated endothelial-cell damage (converting the endothelium into a procoagulant surface).

The net effect of thrombosis is threefold. First, as in the horseshoe crab, it isolates an area of injury, preventing blood flow into or out of the affected zone. This containment prevents nutrient delivery to the site. Oxygen deprivation seals the fate of most host cells in the immediate vicinity of injury or invasion, but it may prevent viral replication or intracellular bacterial survival (by killing the parasitized host cell) and even extracellular aerobic pathogen survival. Containment also protects against systemic microbial spread or dissemination of the toxic products of tissue damage. Second, thrombosis delimits a zone of nonviability. Other cells in the vicinity remain at risk, but those deprived of blood flow constitute the tissue lost to the primary injury. Third, thrombosis is also a signal of host injury. By altering local hemodynamics and amplifying proinflammatory stimuli both directly and indirectly, this process contributes additional information about the location, size, and severity of the threat to the host.

Leukocyte Effector Response

Leukocytes enact different effector programs, depending on their lineage and the insult to which they respond. Neutrophils perform distinct functions from T lymphocytes, and neutrophils will respond differently to tissue injured by hypoxic–ischemic injury or microbial invasion. The effector response involves arriving at the correct site, carrying out the appropriate host defense reactions, and providing for resolution of one phase of the response and initiating the subsequent phase. An overview of neutrophil function in acute inflammation follows. Macrophage and lymphocyte recruitment and activity are also essential to resolving an acute inflammatory response, but space precludes a discussion of their roles in this response.

Following transendothelial migration, neutrophils must traverse the tissue to the injury focus. They must first be able to sense chemoattractant concentration differences in the extracellular milieu. They must then use those gradients to orient (polarize) the cell to head toward higher concentrations. Finally, they must be able to physically displace themselves through the tissue.

Neutrophils actually sense at least two broad categories of chemoattractants: intermediary and end-target. Molecules such as the ELR+ CXC chemokines, produced as a result of the primary injury or infection or during the initial amplification phase, belong to the former class. Chemotactic bacterial products (such as formyl-Met-Leu-Phe) or the complement component C5a generated at the site of infection constitute end-target chemoattractants. Moreover, neutrophils exhibit a preferential response to the latter class of molecule; given a choice between the two classes of agents, regardless of the concentration of either, neutrophils will respond preferentially to those agents generated at the site of infection. This hierarchical responsiveness is attributable to the intracellular signaling pathway triggered by each, with intermediary chemokines acting through the phosphatidylinositol 3-kinase (PI3K) pathway and end-target molecules activating the p38 mitogen-activated protein kinase (MAPK) pathway (14).

How neutrophils become polarized in response to slight differences in chemokine concentration is still being elucidated. To date, evidence indicates that, despite a uniform distribution of chemokine receptors on the leukocyte surface, extracellular chemoattractant concentration differences translate into an asymmetric accumulation of lipid products of PI3K signaling at the edge of the leukocyte that faces the highest chemokine concentration. This distribution affects the intracellular distribution of cytoskeletal molecular motor components that will carry out leukocyte locomotion (27).

The movement of neutrophils through the tissues depends on transient adhesive interactions between integrin superfamily members and ligands that compose the extracellular matrix (ECM; e.g., collagen, laminin, fibronectin, tenascin). In this role, leukocyte integrins act as (a) anchoring proteins, providing physical interaction between ECM proteins (through binding of their ectodomains) and intracellular cytoskeletal molecules (via the cytoplasmic domains); and (b) signal transducers, communicating binding and release information, together with signals to enhance the neutrophil's activation state as it approaches the injury site. The $\beta1$ integrin family mediates these interactions and coordinates locomotion through the ECM, although the migration process requires more than integrin–ECM interactions (27).

As they approach the injured site, neutrophils undergo progressive activation, such that, by arrival, they are fully primed to perform the appropriate effector function. Actual effector responses are determined by what the neutrophils encounter at the site and involve a combination of release and activation of preformed mediators (e.g., granule proteins/peptides, reactive oxygen species [ROS]) with new gene expression.

The presence of bacteria at the injury site may or may not prompt phagocytosis. When bacteria cannot be phagocytosed, the neutrophil releases antimicrobial and proteolytic proteins and generates ROS, resulting in bacterial and tissue destruction. Microbial engulfment, in contrast, triggers granule content release into the phagosome and generation of ROS to destroy the ingested bacteria, as well as a two-stage genomic response that involves upregulation of 305 and downregulation of 297 genes. In the first wave, cytokines and chemokines that recruit and activate macrophages and lymphocytes and support wound healing are expressed. Following this first surge of new gene expression, a second response ensues, with upregulation of proapoptotic genes and downregulation of receptors for different inflammatory mediators and injury-sensing proteins (cytokines, chemokines, immunoglobulins, and TLRs). Neutrophils then undergo apoptosis and are ingested by macrophages, marking entrance into the resolution phase of the acute inflammatory response (51).

Neutrophils recruited to sterile injury sites exhibit a similar initial proinflammatory genomic response but, in the absence of phagocytosis, express antiapoptotic genes and prolong the period of neutrophil protection against infection (51). Less is known about the genomic response of neutrophils that respond to sites with significant necrotic tissue damage.

Alerting Host Defense

Although much of the local inflammatory response outlined in the preceding section is tissue autonomous (i.e., triggered by the involved tissues themselves), when the insult is significant enough, it triggers a supporting systemic response that overlaps with the host's reaction to environmental stress. Signs of systemic responses may include fever, activation of the hypothalamic-pituitary-adrenocortical axis and the hypothalamic-adrenomedullary-autonomic nervous system, and acute-phase protein production. Defining thresholds for the activation of these responses is difficult because they vary depending on the baseline state of the host at the time of injury or infection. However, two generalizations about the intact response bear mention. First, although this response supports the local inflammatory process, its net impact on the host appears to be anti-inflammatory, making the host temporarily less reactive to inflammatory and infectious stimuli (34). Second, proper activation and modulation requires coordination between both hard-wired and soluble components. Because space limitations preclude a complete discussion, the following paragraphs will focus on two critical intermediaries that alert the host to a localized threat to its integrity: the peripheral nervous system and the cytokine IL-6.

Peripheral Nervous System

The peripheral nervous system refers to the network of nerves that either resides entirely within non-CNS tissue or that originates or terminates in the CNS, but has the principal function of carrying signals to or from the visceral organs or somatic tissues. These nerves contain a variety of fibers. As alluded to earlier, they may be afferent or efferent and may subserve either somatic or autonomic functions. In alerting the host to local injury or infection, the afferent component of both somatic and autonomic nerves enact an essential function.

Infections or injuries to the viscera activate afferent neurons that form part of the vagus nerve. When stimulated, these afferent fibers signal to neurons with connections throughout the CNS, including the hypothalamus and cortex. The host responds by increasing its thermal balance point (fever), local cytokine production in the CNS, and secretion of pituitary hormones (adrenocorticotropic hormone [ACTH], α-melanocyte stimulating hormone [MSH]) that support the host's ability to handle the stress of visceral injury or infection, including behaviors such as the fight–flight response, and maintenance of an anti-inflammatory milieu. If the insult is noxious enough, the host may sense pain referred to the body wall, represented by the area of sensory cortex activated by the autonomic afferent signals (e.g., periumbilical region during appendicitis; left shoulder, neck, and jaw with myocardial ischemia). Acute vagotomy, in contrast, attenuates the ability of experimental animals to mount a fever when injected intraperitoneally with LPS, even though they produce higher TNF-α and IL-1β concentrations. Vagotomized humans, so treated because of severe peptic ulcer disease (believed to be precipitated by stress), do not, however, appear to have deficient responses to visceral infections or injuries, suggesting the existence of redundant sensing systems to alert the host to threats within body cavities.

Injuries to the limbs and body wall activate peripheral sensory fibers that transmit an array of complex information about the insult to the CNS and trigger efferent responses that further behaviors and physiologic responses to separate from noxious stimuli (withdrawal) and support the local inflammatory response to the injury or infection, including many of those referred to in the preceding paragraph.

Interleukin-6

IL-6 is the best-studied soluble activator of a systemic response to local injury or infection. It is synthesized in response to primary injury signals (e.g., LPS and other microbial products) and secondary amplifiers (TNF-α and IL-1β). Unlike these primary and secondary signals, which appear in the circulation only following massive or overwhelming insult, IL-6 represents a convenient, if nonspecific, marker of localized inflammation. Although this cytokine exhibits marked pleiotropy, only pyrogen and acute-phase response activator will be highlighted.

First, IL-6 links the inflammatory focus to the CNS, effecting changes in host physiology and behavior to confront the challenge posed by the insult. Clinically, the most notable effect of IL-6 on the CNS is its role in the febrile response, although it also modulates activation of the hypothalamic-pituitary-adrenal axis. In its function as a "pyrogenic cytokine," it enters the circulation via lymphatic and hematogenous routes following release from tissue-based and extravasated leukocytes and endothelium. As it circulates through the vasculature of the CNS, it interacts with specialized neurons (the circumventricular organ system) that sample the circulating milieu. Elevated serum IL-6 concentrations induce PGE_2 synthesis within these neurons and secretion in the hypothalamus, leading to the febrile response. This response in humans involves redistributing the circulation away from the periphery until the higher temperature is reached; in smaller species, it involves behavioral changes, such as huddling.

IL-6 serves as a critical bridge between the site of inflammation and the liver, the second major organ supporting the innate immune response to infection and injury, and it constitutes the most important soluble trigger of the acute-phase response—a complex stereotyped reprogramming of hepatic protein synthesis. Elevated IL-6 levels stimulate the synthesis of proteins to support the host response. C-reactive protein, a pentraxin with potent antimicrobial and anti-inflammatory properties, mannose-binding protein, and serum amyloid P are three acute-phase proteins whose expression is regulated by IL-6. IL-6 also suppresses the synthesis of other proteins, such as albumin and haptoglobin, as part of this hepatic genomic response.

REGULATION AND OUTCOME OF INFLAMMATION

Any system that detects and responds to injury to the host must be regulated. Failure to control and ultimately terminate an inflammatory reaction would result in a self-perpetuating, destructive spiral. Unfortunately, very little is known about higher-order regulation of the innate immune response at this writing. Three categories of controls can be envisioned. In the first, an effective host defense system must regulate the *type* of response. The mobilization of natural killer (NK) cells to eliminate a staphylococcal skin infection would be wasteful, but failure to do so in hepatitis C infection could be lethal to the host. Knowledge of how the host recruits the right kinds of cells to different injuries is fragmented and confusing, especially given the overlapping cellular and receptor targets for different cytokines (gp130-mediated signaling) and chemokines (e.g., CXCR1 and -2) and hierarchical relationships among different chemoattractant molecules.

The second type of control regulates the *intensity* of a response according to the threat imposed by the insult. The generation of an exuberant pyogenic reaction with extensive distal thrombosis that results in autoamputation would be excessive for a hangnail, but might be more appropriate in an ascending fasciitis. In the case of neutrophil recruitment, activation state increases with proximity to the inflammatory focus, stemming in part from increasing chemoattractant concentrations. However, less is known about how the host determines how many neutrophils are enough to accomplish the specific task (a form of polling) and regulates their arrival (an executive function).

Finally, the responses, regardless of type or intensity, should have a beginning, middle, and end. Therefore, the third type of control involves *phasing*. IL-6-*trans*-signaling, in which the balance between IL-6, its soluble receptor, and the receptor antagonist soluble gp130 determines the biologic response, exemplifies an elegant, self-regulating system that both promotes and suppresses IL-6 function at the inflammatory focus (20).

Systems biology approaches that account for multiple inputs and extreme complexity will ultimately shed more light on these regulatory issues than reductionist methods characteristic of the molecular biology era. Moreover, development of new therapies that target the inflammatory response will depend on a more complete understanding of its regulation.

Outcome of Inflammation: Demarcation of Three Domains

The injury itself and the host's response establish an ongoing dialectic. Until its resolution, this exchange defines three domains within any host that are both anatomic and functional. At the site of injury or microbial invasion, and radiating outward, some tissue and function are irretrievably lost (**Fig. 17.5,** Domain 1). The extent of this domain is determined solely by the magnitude of the primary injury. Factors that affect the magnitude of the initial insult include time (e.g., duration of ischemia), force (energy of impact, speed of body or projectile), and virulence or infectivity of microbe. Beyond this core of destruction lies a field of tissue at risk for loss (Domain 2). The loss of at-risk tissue (Domain 1-to-2 transition) is referred to clinically as "secondary injury." The concept of at-risk tissue is analogous to a "watershed area" or "penumbra" in ischemic or traumatic neurologic injuries. Similarly, the idea of a functional Domain 2 is encompassed by the notion of "stunned" or "hibernating" myocardium. Multiple factors determine the proportion of tissue or function that is ultimately lost or preserved, including the magnitude of primary injury, genetic background of host (which influences the injury response), nongenetic modifiers of the host response (e.g., nutrition, immunosuppression), and exogenous interventions. Most therapeutic interventions seek to prevent or minimize secondary injury (i.e., decrease the extent of Domain 2), and many aim to modulate the inflammatory response.

Outside the vulnerable area resides tissue unaffected by the injury (Domain 3). Although **Figure 17.5** depicts these domains graphically, it fails to capture the dynamic tension at the interfaces between them. Necrotizing pneumonia, characterized by the microbial invasion site and necrotic center surrounded by alveolar, airway, and supporting tissue vulnerable to progressive invasive disease and flanked by functionally normal lung, illustrates this concept clinically. The size or mass of each domain will be determined by the magnitude of the injury and the host's response to it, which can be either insufficient or excessive and lead, in either instance, to additional damage.

Organ function and host survival depend on sufficient Domain 3 mass to maintain homeostasis. In general, loss of between 75% and 90% of functional tissue (e.g., nephrons, cardiac myocytes) exceeds an organ's capacity to compensate and results in overt organ failure. Occasionally, this loss of function is transient, suggesting the existence of either poorly functioning at-risk tissue that recovers and restores organ function, rejoining Domain 3, or significant regenerative capacity. If, however, organ function fails to return, host survival is threatened. In this scenario, organ transplantation often constitutes the best, although still suboptimal, solution to restore the lost function of certain organs. Replacement therapy (e.g., insulin use for endocrine pancreatic failure) represents an alternative when the lost function is relatively simple to mimic.

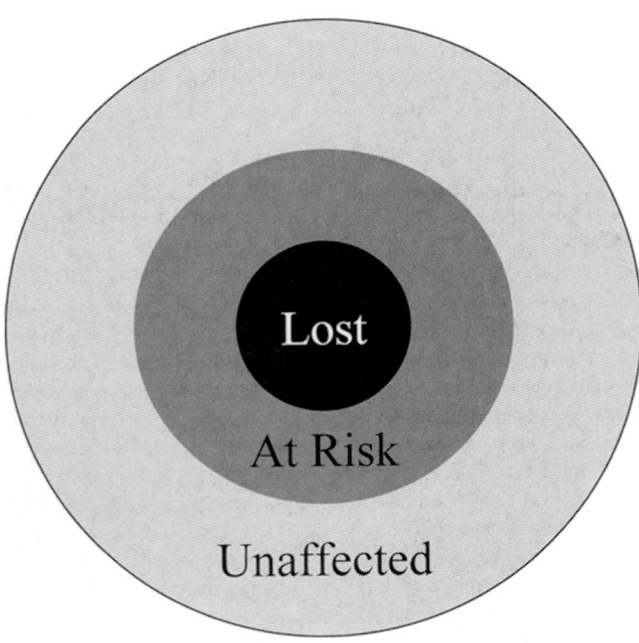

FIGURE 17.5. Outcome of inflammation: demarcation of three domains. The size or mass of each domain will be determined by the magnitude of the injury and the host's response to it. The response itself can be appropriate, insufficient, or excessive and lead, in the latter two circumstances, to additional tissue damage or loss of function.

CONCLUSIONS AND FUTURE DIRECTIONS

To conclude this introduction to innate immunity and inflammation, a few key points about this system should be highlighted. First, innate immunity is essential to survival; without it, the host would fall victim to even the commensal organisms that reside on mucosal surfaces or the skin. Second, although often characterized as "primitive," especially in comparison to adaptive immunity, innate immunity also exhibits tremendous complexity and is tightly integrated with multiple nonimmune systems (vascular, neuroendocrine) in the host. Despite its complexity, however, it really evolved to respond to small or moderate injuries. Severe insults, such as massive trauma or overwhelming septicemia—conditions treated in ICUs throughout the world—may trigger widespread activation of innate immunity, but rather than protecting the host, this activation usually worsens the host's condition, causing ARDS, shock, and DIC. Finally, therapeutic manipulation of this response will ultimately depend on much more detailed knowledge of the interactions between hosts and the insults that trigger innate immune responses in different tissues.

KEY POINTS

■ Innate immunity refers to the cells, subcellular elements, and molecules that protect the host from spread of infection and tissue damage.

■ Innate immune function is essential for host survival, and its sophistication acknowledges the complexity of diverse evolutionary pressures that face the mammalian genome.

■ The acute inflammatory response demonstrates innate immunity at work.

■ Microbial molecules that activate innate immunity are better understood than endogenous injury signals.

■ Current understanding of host injury-sensing mechanisms, while increasing, remains limited.

■ The ability to prevent or successfully manage devastating problems treated in the ICU, including severe sepsis, ARDS, DIC, and multiorgan dysfunction, will depend on successful decoding of the regulation of the innate immune response.

References

1. Akira S, Takeda K. Toll-like receptor signalling. *Nat Rev Immunol* 2004; 4:499–511.
2. Akira S, Uematsu S, Takeuchi O. Pathogen recognition and innate immunity. *Cell* 2006;124:783–801.
3. Beck G, Habicht G. Immunity and the invertebrates. *Sci Am* 1996;60–66.
4. Beutler B. Innate immunity: An overview. *Mol Immunol* 2004;40:845–59.
5. Bizzarri C, Beccari AR, Bertini R, et al. ELR(+) CXC chemokines and their receptors (CXC chemokine receptor 1 and CXC chemokine receptor 2) as new therapeutic targets. *Pharmacol Ther* 2006;112(1):139–49.
6. Black PH. Stress and the inflammatory response: A review of neurogenic inflammation. *Brain Behav Immun* 2002;16:622–53.
7. Burnet FM. *The Clonal Selection Theory of Acquired Immunity.* Cambridge: Cambridge University Press, 1959.
8. Cambi A, Figdor CG. Levels of complexity in pathogen recognition by C-type lectins. *Curr Opin Immunol* 2005;17:345–51.
9. Caput D, Beutler B, Hartog K, et al. Identification of a common nucleotide sequence in the 3'-untranslated region of mRNA molecules specifying inflammatory mediators. *Proc Natl Acad Sci USA* 1986;83:1670–4.
10. Esmon CT. Inflammation and the activated protein C anticoagulant pathway. *Semin Thromb Hemost* 2006;32(Suppl 1):49–60.
11. Gallucci S, Lolkema M, Matzinger P. Natural adjuvants: Endogenous activators of dendritic cells. *Nat Med* 1999;5:1249–55.
12. Gueydan C, Droogmans L, Chalon P, et al. Identification of TIAR as a protein binding to the translational regulatory AU-rich element of tumor necrosis factor alpha mRNA. *J Biol Chem* 1999;274:2322–6.
13. Gueydan C, Houzet L, Marchant A, et al. Engagement of tumor necrosis factor mRNA by an endotoxin-inducible cytoplasmic protein. *Mol Med* 1996;2:479–88.
14. Heit B, Tavener S, Raharjo E, et al. An intracellular signaling hierarchy determines direction of migration in opposing chemotactic gradients. *J Cell Biol* 2002;159:91–102.
15. Hoffmann A, Baltimore D. Circuitry of nuclear factor kappaB signaling. *Immunol Rev* 2006;210:171–86.
16. Hume DA. The mononuclear phagocyte system. *Curr Opin Immunol* 2006;18:49–53.
17. Iwanaga S. The molecular basis of innate immunity in the horseshoe crab. *Curr Opin Immunol* 2002;14:87–95.
18. Janeway CA Jr. Approaching the asymptote? Evolution and revolution in immunology. *Cold Spring Harb Symp Quant Biol* 1989;54(Pt 1):1–13.
19. Jiang D, Liang J, Fan J, et al. Regulation of lung injury and repair by Toll-like receptors and hyaluronan. *Nat Med* 2005;11:1173–9.
20. Jones SA. Directing transition from innate to acquired immunity: Defining a role for IL-6. *J Immunol* 2005;175:3463–8.
21. Kawai T, Akira S. Pathogen recognition with Toll-like receptors. *Curr Opin Immunol* 2005;17:338–44.
22. Klein J, Václav H. *Immunology,* 2nd ed. Malden, MA: Blackwell Science, Ltd.; 1997:722.
23. Lederberg J. Genes and antibodies: Do antigens bear instructions for antibody specificity or de they select cell lines that arise by mutation? *Science* 1959;129:1649–53.
24. Lewis T, Gueydan C, Huez G, et al. Mapping of a minimal AU-rich sequence required for lipopolysaccharide-induced binding of a 55-kDa protein on tumor necrosis factor-alpha mRNA. *J Biol Chem* 1998;273:13781–6.
25. Ley K. History of inflammation research. In: Ley K, ed. *Physiology of Inflammation,* 1st ed. New York: Oxford University Press; 2001:1–10.
26. Li M, Carpio DF, Zheng Y, et al. An essential role of the NF-kappa B/Toll-like receptor pathway in induction of inflammatory and tissue-repair gene expression by necrotic cells. *J Immunol* 2001;166:7128–35.
27. Lindbom L, Werr J. Integrin-dependent neutrophil migration in extravascular tissue. *Semin Immunol* 2002;14:115–21.
28. Lotze MT, Tracey KJ. High-mobility group box 1 protein (HMGB1): Nuclear weapon in the immune arsenal. *Nat Rev Immunol* 2005;5:331–42.
29. Mantovani A. The chemokine system: Redundancy for robust outputs. *Immunol Today* 1999;20:254–7.
30. Martinon F, Tschopp J. NLRs join TLRs as innate sensors of pathogens. *Trends Immunol* 2005;26:447–54.
31. Matzinger P. Tolerance, danger, and the extended family. *Annu Rev Immunol* 1994;12:991–1045.
32. Medzhitov R, Preston-Hurlburt P, Janeway CA Jr. A human homologue of the Drosophila Toll protein signals activation of adaptive immunity. *Nature* 1997;388:394–7.
33. Munford RS. Personal communication. 2006.
34. Munford RS, Pugin J. Normal responses to injury prevent systemic inflammation and can be immunosuppressive. *Am J Respir Crit Care Med* 2001;163:316–21.
35. Munford RS, Tracey KJ. Is severe sepsis a neuroendocrine disease? *Mol Med* 2002;8:437–42.
36. Murray PJ. NOD proteins: An intracellular pathogen-recognition system or signal transduction modifiers? *Curr Opin Immunol* 2005;17:352–8.
37. Nash GB, Buckley CD, Rainger G, eds. The local physicochemical environment conditions the proinflammatory response of endothelial cells and thus modulates leukocyte recruitment. *FEBS Lett* 2004;569:13–17.
38. Noble PW, McKee CM, Cowman M, et al. Hyaluronan fragments activate an NF-kappa B/I-kappa B alpha autoregulatory loop in murine macrophages. *J Exp Med* 1996;183:2373–8.
39. Oda K, Kitano H. A comprehensive map of the toll-like receptor signaling network. *Mol Syst Biol* 2006;2:2006.0015. Epub April 18, 2006.
40. Poltorak A, He X, Smirnova I, et al. Defective LPS signaling in C3H/HeJ and C57BL/10ScCr mice: Mutations in Tlr4 gene. *Science* 1998;282:2085–8.
41. Rietschel ET, Westphal O. Endotoxin: Historical perspectives. In: Brade H, Opal SM, Vogel SN, et al., eds. *Endotoxin in Health and Disease.* New York: Marcel Dekker, Inc.; 1999:1–30.
42. Rocha e Silva M. A brief survey of the history of inflammation. 1978. *Agents Actions* 1994;43:86–90.
43. Rock FL, Hardiman G, Timans JC, et al. A family of human receptors structurally related to Drosophila Toll. *Proc Natl Acad Sci USA* 1998;95:588–93.
44. Schaible HG, Del Rosso A, Matucci-Cerinic M. Neurogenic aspects of inflammation. *Rheum Dis Clin North Am* 2005;31:77–101, ix.
45. Seong SY, Matzinger P. Hydrophobicity: An ancient damage-associated molecular pattern that initiates innate immune responses. *Nat Rev Immunol* 2004;4:469–78.
46. Shi Y, Evans JE, Rock KL. Molecular identification of a danger signal that alerts the immune system to dying cells. *Nature* 2003;425:516–21.
47. Shi Y, Zheng W, Rock KL. Cell injury releases endogenous adjuvants that stimulate cytotoxic T cell responses. *Proc Natl Acad Sci USA* 2000;97:14590–5.
48. Takeda K, Akira S. TLR signaling pathways. *Semin Immunol* 2004;16:3–9.
49. Termeer C, Benedix F, Sleeman J, et al. Oligosaccharides of hyaluronan activate dendritic cells via toll-like receptor 4. *J Exp Med* 2002;195:99–111.
50. Termeer CC, Hennies J, Voith U, et al. Oligosaccharides of hyaluronan are potent activators of dendritic cells. *J Immunol* 2000;165:1863–70.
51. Theilgaard-Monch K, Porse BT, Borregaard N. Systems biology of neutrophil differentiation and immune response. *Curr Opin Immunol* 2006;18:54–60.
52. Thomas L. *The Lives of a Cell: Notes of a Biology Watcher.* New York: The Viking Press, 1974.
53. Vaara M. Lipopolysaccharide and the permeability of the bacterial outer membrane. In: Brade H, Opal SM, Vogel SN, et al., eds. *Endotoxin in Health and Disease.* New York: Marcel Dekker, Inc.; 1999:31–38.

54. Vergnolle N. The inflammatory response. *Drug Dev Res* 2003;59:375–81.
55. Wallin RP, Lundqvist A, More SH, et al. Heat-shock proteins as activators of the innate immune system. *Trends Immunol* 2002;23:130–5.
56. Wasserman SA. A conserved signal transduction pathway regulating the activity of the rel-like proteins dorsal and NF-kappa B. *Mol Biol Cell* 1993;4:767–71.
57. Wenger RH, Stiehl DP, Camenisch G. Integration of oxygen signaling at the consensus HRE. *Sci STKE* 2005;2005:re12.
58. Willis TM, Hopp RJ, Romero JR, et al. The protective effect of brachial plexus palsy in purpura fulminans. *Pediatr Neurol* 2001;24:379–81.
59. Yoneyama M, Kikuchi M, Natsukawa T, et al. The RNA helicase RIG-I has an essential function in double-stranded RNA-induced innate antiviral responses. *Nat Immunol* 2004;5:730–7.

CHAPTER 18 ■ CELLULAR ADAPTATIONS TO STRESS

DEREK S. WHEELER • HECTOR R. WONG

Adaptability is probably the most distinctive characteristic of life.
Hans Selye, The Story of the Adaptation Syndrome (1950)

Biologic stress is a common phenomenon in virtually all forms of critical illness and stems from either the disease process itself (e.g., hypoxia or ischemia) or from the therapies employed in the intensive care unit (e.g., oxidant stress from therapeutic oxygen or mechanical stress from positive pressure ventilation). Whereas some therapeutic strategies in the ICU are directly targeted at these stressors (e.g., antibiotics directed toward microbial stress or fluid replacement in the setting of hypovolemic stress), most therapeutic strategies are fundamentally supportive. As such, many forms of therapy in the ICU provide time and a platform to allow for endogenous cellular stress adaptations to take place. The success or failure of these cellular responses is critical to the eventual development of organ failure and, consequently, to patient outcome.

All cells respond to stress through the activation of primitive, evolutionarily conserved, genetic programs that maintain homeostasis and ensure cell survival (**Fig. 18.1**). *Stress adaptation*, which is known in the literature by a myriad of terms, including *tolerance, desensitization, conditioning,* and *reprogramming*, is a common paradigm found throughout nature, in which the primary exposure of a cell or organism to a stressful stimulus (e.g., heat, ischemia, hypoxia, endotoxin) results in an adaptive response, by which a subsequent second exposure to the same stimulus produces a minimal response. More interesting is the phenomenon of cross-tolerance, by which a primary exposure to a stressful stimulus results in an adaptive response, whereby the cell or organism is resistant to a subsequent stress that differs from the initial stress (i.e., exposure to heat stress that leads to resistance to hypoxia). Several examples of stress adaptation are well described and are discussed in greater detail in the next sections, including the heat shock response, ischemic preconditioning (IP), and endotoxin tolerance.

It is imperative that physicians who care for critically ill and injured children possess an understanding of these concepts, because an understanding of stress adaptation is necessary to recognize the current limits of supportive care and to move the field forward with respect to research endeavors and novel therapeutic strategies. Hence, the goal of this chapter is to introduce some fundamental concepts of how cells adapt to stress. Generalized adaptive responses to various cell stressors will be reviewed first, followed by a brief discussion of some of the more commonly implicated mediators of these responses.

THE HEAT SHOCK RESPONSE

The heat shock response was first described over four decades ago in common fruit flies exposed to increased environmental temperature. What was once an obscure observation of questionable biologic relevance has now evolved into a fundamental tenet of how cells adapt in response to, and survive, a broad variety of biologic stresses (23,24,36). The heat shock response is characterized by the rapid expression of a unique group of proteins, collectively known as *heat shock proteins* (Hsps) when a cell or organism is exposed to environmental stress. The structure, mode of regulation, and function of Hsps are highly conserved throughout the entire evolutionary tree, and Hsps have been identified in virtually all eukaryotic and prokaryotic species examined to date. Although classically described as a response to heat stress (hence the term *heat shock response*), Hsps can be induced by a wide variety of nonthermal stressors and pharmacologic agents (**Table 18.1**). For this reason, the terms "stress response" and "stress proteins" may be more appropriate. Many of these stimuli are relevant to the critically ill patient, and it is now well established that critically ill patients are capable of expressing Hsps (i.e., mounting a heat shock response) (14,17,28,37). Moreover, and particularly germane to a textbook on pediatric critical care medicine, the experimental literature suggests that younger animals have a greater capacity to express Hsps compared with older animals (15).

Hsps comprise a large family of proteins that are found in virtually every cellular compartment, including the nucleus, cytoplasm, and mitochondria (**Table 18.2**). In addition, recent evidence indicates that extracellular forms of Hsps also exist and are biologically functional. By convention, Hsps are classified according to their molecular mass (e.g., Hsp25 represents the 25-kDa family of Hsps) and range in molecular mass from 7 to 110 kDa (e.g., Hsp25, Hsp32, Hsp47, Hsp60, Hsp70, Hsp90, and Hsp110). Although the expression of Hsp was initially noted in cells following acute stress, several members of this family of proteins are constitutively expressed and play important roles in cellular homeostasis. Some Hsps have additional functions that are not related to heat shock, although they are still classified as Hsps. For example, the enzyme heme oxygenase is also known as Hsp32 (discussed in greater detail later). In addition, ubiquitin, inhibitor of κB (IκB), and endothelial nitric oxide synthase (eNOS) are occasionally listed as Hsps, in that they can be induced by classic heat shock. Many Hsps are constitutively expressed (Hsp90 is one of the most abundant proteins found inside the cell), whereas others are rapidly and highly expressed in response to cellular stress. Among the

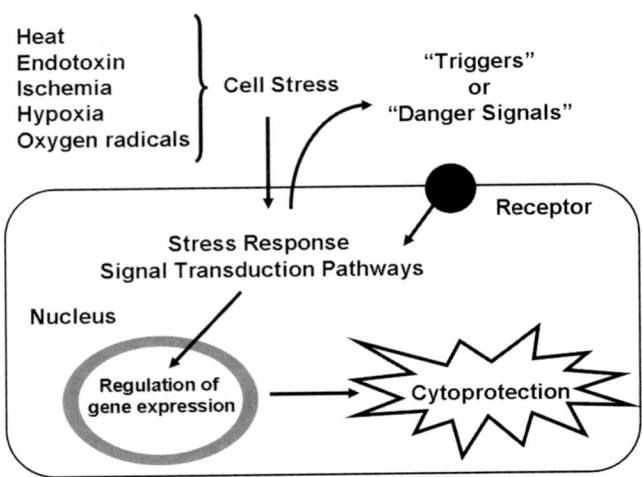

FIGURE 18.1. Simplified representation of the basic mechanisms of cellular adaptation. Exposure to stress (e.g., heat, endotoxin, ischemia, oxygen radicals, hypoxia, etc.) results in (1) the direct activation of stress response pathways and/or (2) the release of "triggers" or endogenous "danger signals" that activate stress response pathways (these "danger signals," therefore, serve both an autocrine and paracrine function). These stress response pathways converge upon various transcription factors, protein kinases, and ion channels to generate a stress response—a cytoprotective response characterized by the phenomenon of stress tolerance.

latter, Hsp72 is one of the more well-studied inducible Hsps in the context of cellular adaptations to stress and consequent protection against cellular injury (cytoprotection).

Regulation of the Heat Shock Response

Cells respond to stressful stimuli (e.g., heat shock) by increasing the gene expression of Hsps at a level proportional to the severity of the stress. For example, a temperature threshold of 4°C to 8°C above the normal growing temperature is required for induction of Hsp expression (23). Heat stress purportedly affects the tertiary and quaternary structure of intracellular proteins, and the intracellular accumulation of denatured proteins is believed to be the universal signal that results in the stress-induced gene expression of Hsps. Experimental support for this purported mechanism is shown by the fact that the microinjection of denatured proteins into cells results in up-regulation of Hsp expression.

A family of transcription factors, known as heat shock factors (Hsfs) controls the regulation of Hsp gene expression (23). To date, only three Hsfs have been identified in humans (Hsf1, Hsf2, and Hsf4), although Hsf1 appears to be the most important stress-responsive Hsf. The Hsfs are characterized by a highly conserved amino-terminal, helix-turn-helix, DNA-binding domain, as well as by a carboxy-terminal domain, which activates transcription of DNA into messenger RNA (i.e., a transactivating domain). Hsf1 is present as a constitutively phosphorylated monomer during the resting, unstressed

TABLE 18.1

INDUCERS OF THE STRESS RESPONSE

Type of stress	Agent	Comments
Environmental	Temperature	
	Heavy metals	Cadmium, zinc
	Ethanol	
	Oxygen radicals	
Metabolic	Hyperosmolality	
	Glucose starvation	
	Tunicamycin	
	Calcium ionophores	
	Amino acid analogs	
Clinical	Ischemia/reperfusion	Reperfusion seems to be the limiting factor
	Shock	
	Anoxia	
	Endotoxin	
Pharmacologic	Sodium arsenite	Used extensively in vitro and in vivo
	Herbimycin A	Tyrosine kinase inhibitor
	Geldanamycin	Tyrosine kinase inhibitor and Hsp90 inhibitor
	Prostaglandin A1	Other prostaglandins are also active
	Dexamethasone	
	Aspirin	Lowers temperature threshold for Hsp induction
	Non-steroidal anti-inflammatory drugs	Lowers temperature threshold for Hsp induction
	Pyrrolidine dithiocarbamate	Antioxidant; inhibitor of NFκB
	Diethyldithiocarbamate	
	Bimoclomol	Hydroxylamine derivative, nontoxic
	Serine protease inhibitors	Concomitant inhibition of NF-κB
	Curcumin	Major constituent of tumeric; anti-inflammatory
	Geranylgeranylacetone	Antiulcerative agent

TABLE 18.2

THE MAJOR FAMILIES OF HEAT SHOCK PROTEINS

Name	Size (kDa)	Localization	Bacterial homolog	Some known and possible functions
Ubiquitin	8	Cytosol/nucleus	—	Nonlysosomal degradation pathways
Hsp 27	27	Cytosol/nucleus	—	Regulator of actin cytoskeleton; molecular chaperone; cytoprotection
Heme oxygenase	32	Bound to ER, extends to cytoplasm	—	Degradation of heme to bilirubin; resistance to oxidant stress
Hsp 47	47	ER	—	Collagen chaperone
Hsp 60	60	Mitochondria	Gro EL	Molecular chaperone
Hsp 70	72	Cytosol/nucleus	Dna K	Highly stress inducible; involved in cytoprotection against diverse agents
	73	Cytosol/nucleus	—	Constitutively expressed chaperone
Hsp 90	90	Cytosol/nucleus	htpG	Regulation of steroid hormone activity
Hsp 110	110	Nucleolus/cytosol	Clp family	Protects nucleoli from stress

state. Hsp70, a product of Hsf1 activation, appears to associate with Hsf1 and retain it in its monomeric form and, therefore, may play an important role in downregulating Hsf1 activation. Following heat shock, Hsf1 undergoes trimerization and rapidly translocates into the nucleus. Although trimerization is sufficient for DNA binding, the stimulation of transcription by Hsf1 (i.e., transactivation) requires the phosphorylation of specific serine residues on Hsf1 itself, adding yet another layer of regulatory control. Once activated in this manner, Hsf1 binds to a specific sequence of DNA present in the promoter region of the Hsp gene, known as the heat shock element (HSE). The HSE is defined by a tandem repeat of the nucleotide pentamer nGAAn ("n" denoting less conserved nucleotides) arranged in an alternating orientation, either "head-to-head" (e.g., 5'-nGAAnnTTCn-3') or "tail-to-tail" (e.g., 5'-nTTCnnGAAn-3'). Binding of the HSE by Hsf1 leads to rapid transcription of Hsp mRNA and subsequent protein translation.

Heat Shock Proteins and Cytoprotection

The most well-known biologic function of Hsps is their ability to serve as molecular chaperones (24,36). In this role, Hsps serve to fold, transport, and stabilize intracellular proteins. Because many forms of cellular injury lead to misfolding of intracellular proteins and to defects in intracellular protein processing and trafficking, the molecular chaperone properties of Hsps are thought to play a major role in the mechanisms by which the heat shock response confers protection in such diverse forms of cellular injury. Experimentally, the heat shock response can be induced by either thermal stress or through pharmacologic induction (see **Table 18.1**). In either case, it is now well established that induction of the heat shock response confers protection in various animal models of critical illness, including septic shock, acute lung injury, oxidant stress, and ischemia–reperfusion injury (39). That Hsp72 plays a major role in cytoprotection is evident by studies in which Hsp72 is overexpressed genetically and the experimental animals are afforded similar protection to that seen by induction of Hsp72 through thermal stress or pharmacologic induction.

The Heat Shock Response and Inflammation

Another mechanism by which the heat shock response confers cytoprotection is through its ability to modulate cellular proinflammatory responses. Numerous studies have demonstrated, in both in vitro and in vivo experimental models, that induction of the heat shock response inhibits subsequent production of cytokines, chemokines, and nitric oxide when cells are exposed to proinflammatory stimuli. One major mechanism by which the heat shock response inhibits cellular proinflammatory responses is through inhibition of the nuclear factor (NF)-κB signal-transduction pathway (18). NF-κB is a transcription factor that regulates the expression of many genes involved in inflammation (see Chapter 17). The heat shock–mediated inhibition of the NF-κB pathway involves inhibition of IκB kinase and increased expression of the endogenous NF-κB inhibitory protein, IκBα. These inhibitory effects of heat shock on cellular proinflammatory responses and the NF-κB pathway appear to be relatively specific, rather than a global downregulation of cellular function and gene expression.

Extracellular Heat Shock Proteins

Until recently, Hsps have been regarded as exclusively *intracellular* proteins. Recent studies, however, clearly illustrate that Hsps can also exist in the *extracellular* compartment. For example, adult patients suffering from major trauma have increased serum levels of Hsp72 (28). Critically ill children with septic shock also have increased serum levels of Hsp72, and the absolute levels are much higher than those reported for critically ill adult patients following multisystem trauma (37). The latter may be reflective of an increased capacity of children to express Hsps compared with adults, consistent with the experimental literature previously mentioned. Research that characterizes the developmental time course for the expression and response of Hsps to critical illness in children has yet to be conducted.

Whether increased levels of extracellular Hsps represent the active release/secretion of Hsps or a nonspecific release of Hsps from dying cells remains to be determined. Current evidence indicates that both processes are operative (11). Regardless of how Hsps enter the extracellular compartment, emerging evidence indicates that extracellular Hsps are biologically active. For example, Hsp72 has been demonstrated to activate proinflammatory and antibacterial responses in macrophages (2,3,11). In this context, extracellular Hsps are said to serve as "danger signals" for the innate immune system.

The biologic role, if any, of extracellular Hsps in critical illness remains to be defined, and is currently an active area of investigation. It is possible that extracellular Hsps are simply an epiphenomenon of illness severity that reflects induction of the heat shock response in critically ill patients. The experimental data mentioned earlier, however, indicate that extracellular Hsps are capable of modulating the innate immune system, and, if so, this is likely to be of significance to the critically ill patient. The difficulty of elucidating this significance is highlighted by the observations that increased extracellular Hsps correlate with improved survival in adult patients with trauma (28) and that they correlate with illness severity and mortality in children with septic shock (37).

The Heat Shock Response as a Therapeutic Strategy

Recognition that induction of the heat shock response confers broad cytoprotection against diverse forms of cellular injury has generated interest in developing clinically feasible strategies to safely induce the heat shock response (36). Deliberate induction of hyperthermia is not likely to be feasible, given the metabolic consequences of severe hyperthermia in critically ill patients. A related concept is the controversial issue of not treating fever in critically ill patients (29), which may also not be feasible due to the metabolic and neurologic consequences of high fever in children, not to mention societal attitudes toward fever control in children. Pharmacologic strategies to induce the heat shock response are hampered by the relative toxicity of the currently available agents. One agent that shows promise

in critically ill patients, however, is the amino acid glutamine, which appears to have feasibility as a relatively safe and effective inducer of the heat shock response in humans (38,41).

ISCHEMIC PRECONDITIONING

The phenomenon of IP, in which multiple, brief ischemic episodes (i.e., preconditioning) protect the heart from a subsequent sustained ischemic insult, was first described in 1986, with use of a canine model of myocardial ischemia produced by coronary occlusion (26). Four cycles of brief (5-min) ischemia prior to a more prolonged period of ischemia (40 mins) reduced infarct size by nearly 75% (**Fig. 18.2**). Since that time, IP has been shown to reduce the infarct size in every other species tested, and both in vitro data involving cardiomyocytes and clinical data from small case series suggest that IP is cytoprotective in humans as well (7,31). IP is more readily recognized in the clinical setting in the context of the acute coronary syndrome, in which patients who have at least one episode of prodromal angina are somewhat protected from a subsequent, more severe episode of myocardial ischemia (i.e., "the cardiac warm-up phenomenon").

Although the mechanism(s) that underlie IP have not been fully elucidated, it appears that the cytoprotective response consists of an early ("classical" IP) and a late ("delayed" IP) phase (7,31). For example, cytoprotection appears within minutes of the preconditioning stimulus and lasts only 2 to 3 hrs (early phase, or first window of protection), although tissue protection later reappears 24 hrs after the preconditioning stimulus (late phase or second window of protection). Classic IP depends mainly on the activation of ion channels and/or post-translational modification of preexisting cellular proteins, which makes intuitive sense, given the rapidity with which this response occurs. On the other hand, delayed preconditioning involves the simultaneous activation of multiple stress-responsive genes and de novo synthesis of several proteins (including ion channel proteins, receptor proteins, enzymes, and molecular chaperones, such as the Hsps discussed earlier),

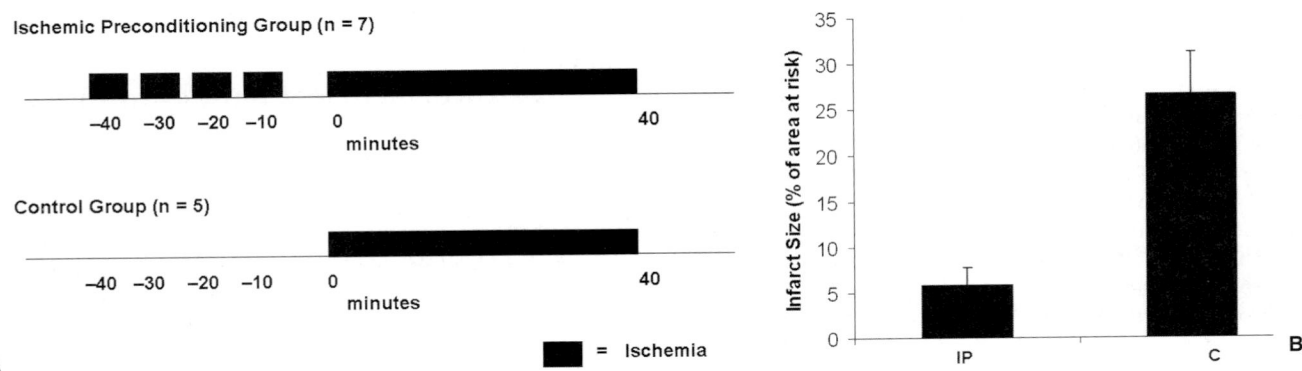

FIGURE 18.2. A: Experimental protocol used in the landmark study by Murry, Jennings, and Reimer (26). In the ischemic preconditioning (IP) group, dogs ($n = 7$) were exposed to four 5-min cycles of myocardial ischemia (produced by temporary coronary occlusion), followed by 5 mins of reperfusion prior to a sustained 40-min period of myocardial ischemia. Longer episodes of IP (i.e., 10-min cycles) were associated with excessive mortality. Animals in the control (C) group ($n = 5$) were exposed to the sustained 40-min period of myocardial ischemia alone. Animals were sacrificed at 4 days, and infarct size was measured. **B:** Infarct size (expressed as the percentage of the area at risk) was reduced by approximately 75% in the IP group compared with the C group, ($p < 0.05$).

which ultimately results in the development of a cytoprotective phenotype.

Although IP was first described in the heart, preconditioning has also been described in the liver, kidney, lung, and brain (10,34). At present, limited data suggest that IP occurs in the human intestine as well. Finally, preconditioning is not confined to one organ, but can also limit infarct size in remote, non-preconditioned organs (so-called *remote preconditioning*).

Classical Ischemic Preconditioning

Adenosine appears to play a major role as both a trigger and an effector of classic IP. As discussed in Chapter 19, ischemia leads to the rapid degradation of ATP to adenosine, which subsequently accumulates in the ischemic tissue. In addition to adenosine, several other potential mediators of classic IP are released by the ischemic myocardium, including bradykinin, norepinephrine, opioids, and reactive oxygen species (ROS). Adenosine appears to mediate classic IP via stimulation of adenosine receptor subtypes A_1 and A_3, thereby activating cytoprotective pathways that involve protein kinase C (PKC) (especially the isoforms PKC-δ and PKC-ϵ), phosphatidylinositol 3-kinase (PI3K), and several mitogen-activated protein kinases (MAPK), including extracellular receptor kinase (ERK), c-jun kinase (JNK), and p38 MAPK. The ATP-sensitive potassium (K_{ATP}) channel, especially the mitochondrial K_{ATP} channel, appears to play a crucial role in classic IP as well (and may involve Hsp27), although a detailed review of this subject is well beyond the intended scope of this chapter.

Delayed Ischemic Preconditioning

IP was previously thought to be a transient phenomenon, lasting for only a brief period after the initial preconditioning stress. Subsequent studies have shown, however, that the cytoprotective response reappears 24 hrs later (31). Although not as robust as the earlier phase of cytoprotection, this second window of protection lasts up to 72 hrs. This distinctive time course strongly suggests that delayed IP is mediated, at least in part, by upregulation of gene expression and the subsequent synthesis of new proteins. Although classic and delayed IP share several key features (especially the agents that trigger the cytoprotective response, e.g., adenosine, bradykinin, opioids, and norepinephrine), endogenous protection via nitric oxide (NO) appears to play an important role as a trigger of delayed IP. The activation of several stress responsive signal transduction pathways converge upon the transcription factor, NF-κB (see Chapter 17), resulting in upregulation of gene expression of various stress-responsive, cytoprotective proteins, including superoxide dismutase (SOD), inducible NOS (iNOS), cyclooxygenase (COX)-2, aldose reductase, and Hsp. K_{ATP} channels are also potentially involved in delayed IP, although the mechanisms are not well understood.

Ischemic Preconditioning as a Therapeutic Strategy

The clinical correlate of IP, the so-called "cardiac warm-up phenomenon," has been shown to have a protective effect in patients who progress to acute coronary syndrome (35). The cytoprotective effect appears to significantly diminish if more than 24 hrs lapse between prodromal angina and myocardial infarction. Similarly, patients who experience a transient ischemic attack during the week prior to a stroke have a more favorable recovery. These epidemiologic studies, especially when viewed in conjunction with the wealth of experimental and animal data currently available, clearly support the concept that IP is operative in the clinical setting. However, making the transition from the bench to the bedside has been slow and difficult. Pharmacologic preconditioning (e.g., targeting the adenosine receptor or K_{ATP} channel) in patients who undergo coronary angioplasty has produced encouraging results. Classic or pharmacologic preconditioning has been used in several small clinical trials in patients who undergo cardiothoracic surgery (e.g., coronary artery bypass grafting, cardiopulmonary bypass, lung resection surgery), hepatic surgery (especially liver resection and liver transplantation), and vascular surgery.

Two important caveats deserve mention. First, whereas IP may be less successful in older patients, especially the elderly, few experimental studies have examined the effect of IP in young, immature animals, and virtually no clinical studies have been performed in the pediatric population. Second, evidence suggests that IP may not be protective in patients with comorbid conditions, such as diabetes mellitus and hypercholesterolemia, in whom IP would potentially have the greatest benefit. Clearly, additional studies are necessary, both at the bench and the bedside, before strategies centered on IP are widely utilized in the clinical arena.

HYPOXIC PRECONDITIONING

Hypoxic preconditioning is very similar, both conceptually and mechanistically, to the two aforementioned stress responses—the heat shock response and IP. Hypoxic preconditioning has been described in the brain, heart, and other tissues, and refers to a period of hypoxia that confers tolerance to a subsequent and otherwise lethal period of hypoxia. Although the fundamental mechanisms intrinsic to hypoxic preconditioning remain to be elucidated, experimental studies suggest a central role for the transcription factor hypoxia inducible factor (HIF)-1 (32,33).

Hypoxia Inducible Factor

HIF-1 is composed of two basic helix-loop-helix (bHLH) proteins of the PAS family (named for Per, ARNT, and Sim, the first members identified), HIF-1α and HIF-1β. HIF-1α contains an N-terminal DNA-binding domain, two transcriptional activating domains (NAD and CAD, for N-terminal activation domain and C-terminal activation domain, respectively), and an oxygen-dependent degradation domain (ODD). HIF-1β (also called aryl hydrocarbon receptor nuclear translocator or ARNT) is expressed constitutively in all cells regardless of oxygen tension, but appears to be essential to the induction of HIF target genes. The list of HIF target genes includes genes for vascularization, energy metabolism, vascular tone, and erythropoiesis (**Table 18.3**). In addition, heme oxygenase (HO)-1 expression is, in part, dependent on HIF-1 activity.

TABLE 18.3

HIF TARGET GENES

Genes involved in vascularization
Vascular endothelial growth factor (VEGF)
VEGF receptor FLT-1

Genes involved in energy metabolism
Aldolase
Enolase I
Glucose transporter 1
Glucose transporter 3
Glyceraldehyde phosphate dehydrogenase
Hexokinase
Insulin-like growth factor
Lactate dehydrogenase
Phosphofructokinase
Phosphoglycerate kinase
Pyruvate kinase

Genes involved in regulation of vascular tone
α_{1B}-Adrenergic receptor
Endothelin-1
Nitric oxide synthase (NOS2; inducible isoform of NOS)

Genes involved in regulation of iron metabolism and
  erythropoiesis
Erythropoietin
Heme oxygenase-1
Transferrin
Transferrin receptor

Regulation of Hypoxia Inducible Factor

The regulation of HIF-1 is quite unique and deserves mention. HIF-1α gene transcription is highly inducible by hypoxia, although the exact mechanism is not well understood at present (32,33). The unique feature of HIF-1 gene regulation is that HIF-1α is continually synthesized in the cell, even under con-ditions of normoxia. Under conditions of normoxia, two proline residues are hydroxylated by one or several candidate prolyl hydroxylases, resulting in a change in conformation of the HIF-1α protein. The von Hippel-Landau protein (pVHL) binds to diproline-hydroxylated HIF-1α, leading to the recruitment of several other factors to this complex, including elongin C, elongin B, Rbx 1, and Cul-2 (22). This multimeric complex acts as an E_3 ubiquitin ligase, and HIF-1α (specifically, the ODD) is polyubiquitinated and subsequently degraded by the 26S proteasome complex. Thus, under conditions of normoxia, HIF-1α is continuously produced and degraded. Conversely, under conditions of hypoxia, pVHL dissociates from the HIF-1α protein, thereby interrupting the cycle that leads to polyubiquitination and continuous degradation of HIF-1, and thus leading to a rapid elevation of intracellular HIF-1α protein, which is then free to dimerize with HIF-1β, translocate to the nucleus, and bind to hypoxia response elements (HRE) to induce transcription of HIF target genes (**Fig. 18.3**). This unique aspect of HIF-1α regulation provides a mechanism for rapidly activating HIF-1 in the context of hypoxia. Importantly, Hsp90 may be critical to the stabilization of HIF-1α under conditions of hypoxia.

Hypoxia Inducible Factor and Cytoprotection

The biologic importance of HIF-1 has been established in transgenic mice with targeted deletions of either *HIF-1α* or *HIF-1β* (32,33). For example, mice homozygous for deletions of either subunit (*HIF-1$\alpha^{-/-}$* or *HIF-1$\beta^{-/-}$*) die during embryogenesis secondary to insufficient vascular development. In contrast, heterozygote mice (*HIF-1*) appear to develop normally. When exposed to hypoxia, however, these animals have an impairment of the classical responses and adaptations to hypoxia, as described later.

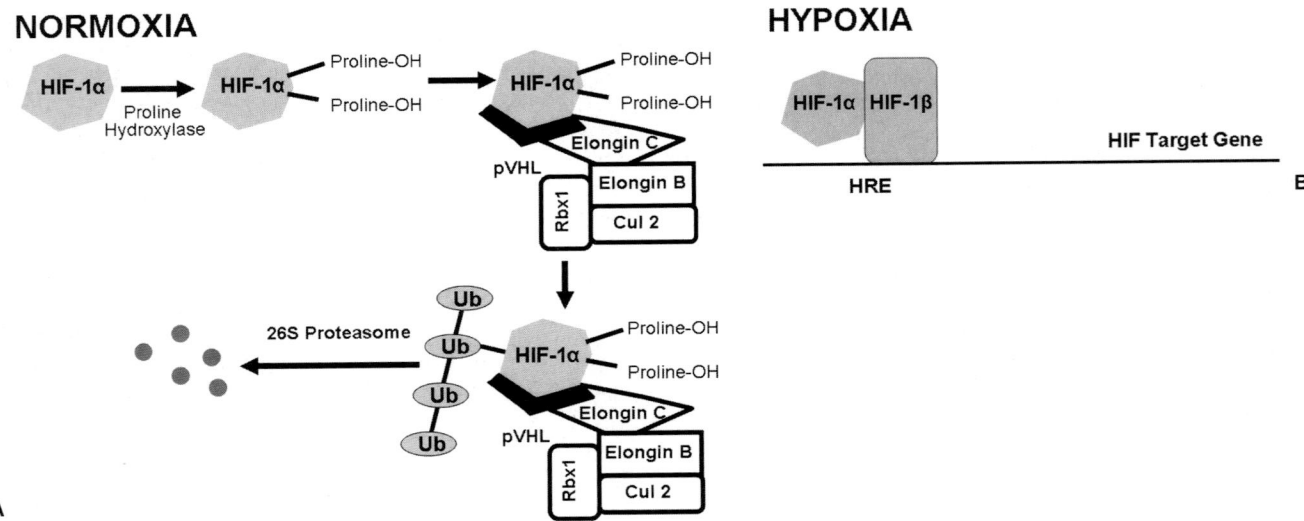

FIGURE 18.3. Regulation of HIF-1. **A:** Under conditions of normoxia, HIF-1α associates with the von Hippel-Lindau protein (pVHL) and forms a complex resulting in its polyubiquitination and continuous degradation by the 26S proteasome. **B:** Under conditions of hypoxia, HIF-1α dissociates from pVHL and combines with HIF-1β to translocate to the nucleus, where it upregulates HIF-target genes. HRE, hypoxia response elements.

The cytoprotective properties of HIF-1 relate primarily to the HIF-1–dependent target genes that allow for adaptation to hypoxia. For example, induction of the HIF-1–dependent gene *erythropoietin* leads to an increased production of red blood cells, thereby increasing the oxygen-carrying capacity of blood to compensate for hypoxia. This type of cytoprotective response is particularly important, for example, in children with cyanotic heart disease. Another example involves the HIF-1–dependent gene vascular endothelial growth factor (*VEGF*), which is a critical growth factor for the development of blood vessels. In tissues subjected to ischemia, such as the myocardium, expression of VEGF promotes the development of neovascularization as a potential means of increasing blood flow to the ischemic tissue. Yet another role for HIF-1 involves HIF-1–dependent expression of inducible nitric oxide synthase (discussed later) and IP of the myocardium.

Although the heat shock response and classic IP allow for more immediate forms of cytoprotection, the cytoprotective responses and adaptations associated with hypoxic preconditioning and HIF-1 activation are comparatively slower to develop and allow for longer-term adaptation. In addition, some of the responses induced by HIF-1 activation can be maladaptive/pathologic, depending on duration of activation. For example, HIF-1 activation is thought to play a role in the development of pulmonary vascular disease and pulmonary hypertension in the setting of chronic hypoxia. Thus, a greater understanding of HIF-1 regulation and activity will be necessary to manipulate HIF-1 activity as a therapeutic option.

ENDOTOXIN TOLERANCE

Lipopolysaccharide (LPS), or endotoxin, a membrane glycolipid of gram-negative bacteria, is a potent inducer of proinflammatory gene expression. In keeping with the concept of stress adaptation and the tolerance paradigm, primary exposure of a cell or organism to LPS (preconditioning) produces a change in phenotype, whereby a second exposure to LPS produces a minimal response (**Fig. 18.4**). For example, LPS

administration produces fever, tachycardia, tachypnea, and hemodynamic instability (i.e., the systemic inflammatory response syndrome, or SIRS) in laboratory animals, whereas a second dose of LPS produces a relatively minimal response. Similarly, LPS induces a dramatic increase in tumor necrosis factor (TNF)-α gene expression in human peripheral blood monocytes (PBMC), although a second exposure produces a markedly attenuated response, with decreased TNF-α gene expression.

Molecular Mechanisms of Endotoxin Tolerance

Although the basic concept has been known for decades, the fundamental mechanisms occurring at the molecular level that lead to endotoxin tolerance remain to be fully elucidated (5,9). Two distinct phases are historically described—early, or classic, endotoxin tolerance and late endotoxin tolerance (note the similarities to early or classic IP and delayed IP described earlier). Early (classic) endotoxin tolerance is transient (generally lasting <72 hrs following preconditioning) and is nonspecific, in that endotoxin derived from one bacterial species can induce tolerance to endotoxin derived from yet another bacterial species. Classic endotoxin tolerance occurs independently of antibody formation. Conversely, late tolerance (>72 hrs following preconditioning) is type specific (i.e., specific to endotoxin derived from a particular bacterial species) and antibody dependent. The remainder of this discussion will focus on classic endotoxin tolerance.

An in-depth, conceptual understanding of normal LPS signaling is essential before discussing the purported mechanistic basis of endotoxin tolerance. As discussed in Chapter 17, LPS binding to its receptor complex (Toll-like receptor (TLR)4/CD14/MD2) is facilitated by LPS-binding protein (LBP), triggering a cascade of events that culminates in the recruitment of the myeloid differentiation adapter protein (MyD88) and the interleukin (IL)-1 receptor-associated kinase (IRAK) to this complex. IRAK undergoes autophosphorylation and recruits the additional adapter protein, TNF receptor associated factor (TRAF)-6, which then phosphorylates and activates an upstream, heterotrimeric member of the NF-κB pathway, the IκB protein kinase complex (IκK-α, -β, and -γ, which is also called NEMO), resulting in the phosphorylation of IκBα. Once phosphorylated, IκBα is targeted for polyubiquitination and degradation by the 26S proteasome. Degradation of IκBα unmasks the nuclear localization sequence of the p50 subunit, and nuclear translocation of NF-κB occurs. NF-κB then binds to the NF-κB consensus sequence to initiate the transcription of a number of key proinflammatory-related genes.

One potentially attractive mechanism of endotoxin tolerance is the downregulation of cell surface expression of individual components of the LPS receptor complex (e.g., TLR4, CD14, MB-2). Based on conflicting data from both in vitro and in vivo studies, it appears that this mechanism is unlikely. Rather, alterations in the intracellular components of the LPS signal transduction appear more likely (**Fig. 18.5**), including decreased expression of IRAK-1 (perhaps with the concomitant upregulation of its inhibitor, IRAK-M), increased expression of IκBα, or alteration of the normal components of NF-κB (i.e., a shift from the p65/p50 heterodimer toward the transcriptionally inactive p50/p50 homodimer) (5,9). Additional

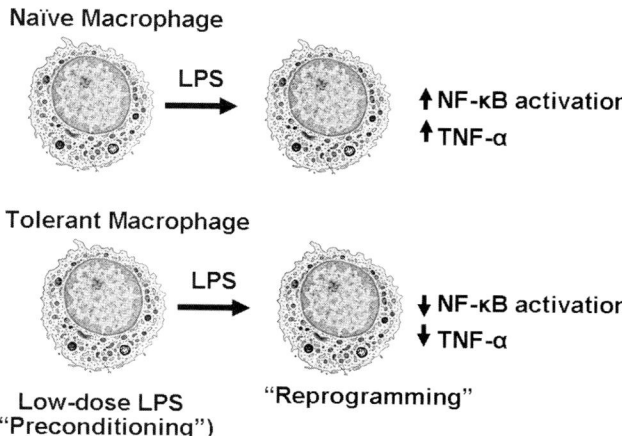

FIGURE 18.4. Classic endotoxin tolerance. Naïve macrophages respond to LPS with an increase in NF-κB–dependent, proinflammatory gene expression (e.g., TNF-α). Macrophages preconditioned with low-dose LPS are more resistant to a subsequent dose of LPS and show less NF-κB–dependent proinflammatory gene expression.

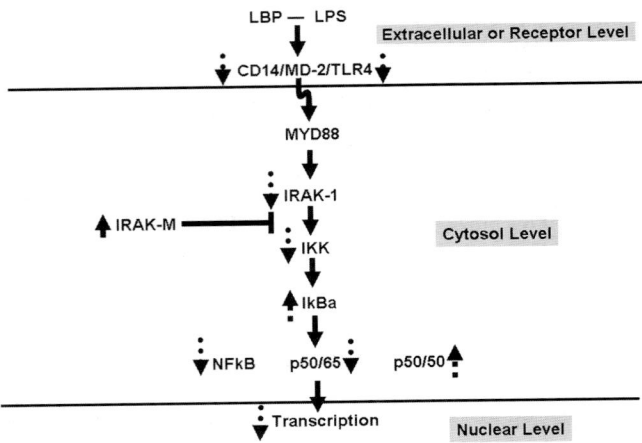

FIGURE 18.5. Potential mechanisms of endotoxin tolerance.

mechanisms are probably involved, and additional mechanistic insight is required.

Does Endotoxin Tolerance Have Clinical Relevance?

The common assertion that endotoxin tolerance represents a global downregulation of proinflammatory gene expression is perhaps incomplete and not entirely accurate. For example, although TNF-α production is significantly diminished in tolerant cells, as well as in tolerant animals, the production of other proinflammatory cytokines, such as IL-1β and IL-6, may be increased, decreased, or unchanged, depending on the experimental model. Several studies have noted that PBMC isolated from both children and adults with SIRS (secondary to surgery, trauma, cardiopulmonary bypass, or cardiac arrest and resuscitation, etc.) and septic shock show strikingly similar alterations in intracellular signal transduction pathways that are consistent with the endotoxin tolerance phenotype (5). For example, impaired ex vivo cytokine production following LPS stimulation has been demonstrated in leukocytes obtained from patients with sepsis and trauma. Furthermore, low levels of LPS-stimulated ex vivo cytokine production from these patients have been associated with poor clinical outcome, an anti-inflammatory response commonly referred to as "immunoparalysis." Children with evidence of immunoparalysis experience increased rates of sepsis and prolonged lengths of stay in the PICU after cardiac surgery (1). However, from a conceptual standpoint, immunoparalysis appears to be strikingly different from classic endotoxin tolerance in one regard. Early studies suggested that preconditioning macrophages and mononuclear cells with small doses of LPS (i.e., classic endotoxin tolerance) resulted in both (a) a diminished proinflammatory response to a subsequent dose of LPS and (b) *increased* phagocytosis and resistance to bacterial infection (the latter not being consistent with the concept of immunoparalysis). Endotoxin tolerance, therefore, may not necessarily equate with immunoparalysis. Additional studies are necessary to provide further insight into the potential clinical relevance of endotoxin tolerance.

HEME OXYGENASE

Heme Oxygenase Biochemistry

The visible transformation of a common bruise is a well-known colorimetric reaction that depends on the enzyme, heme oxygenase (HO). HO is the first and rate-limiting step in the degradation of heme (purple hue) to biliverdin (green hue), and finally to bilirubin (yellow hue) (**Fig. 18.6**). Three known isoforms of HO exist: HO-1, HO-2, and HO-3. In the context of cellular adaptation to stress, HO-1 appears to be the most relevant isoform. HO-1 is identical to Hsp32 and is highly inducible by a variety of cellular stressors and stimuli, including heme, nitric oxide, cytokines, heavy metals, hyperoxia, hypoxia, endotoxin, and heat shock (25).

HO-1 activity is present in virtually all organs. The importance of HO-1 in human health and disease was recently demonstrated by the first description of complete HO-1 deficiency in humans (40), in which a 6-year-old boy had complete HO-1 deficiency and a clinical condition characterized by severe growth retardation, hemolytic anemia, tissue iron deposits, widespread evidence of endothelial cell damage, and increased susceptibility to oxidant injury. These findings are remarkably similar to the phenotype commonly observed in *HO-1*–null mice.

Heme Oxygenase-1 and Cytoprotection

In vitro studies that involve gene transfection or gene transfer approaches have provided clear evidence that *HO-1* confers cytoprotection (25,27). For example, overexpression of *HO-1* conferred protection against oxygen toxicity, hemoglobin toxicity, TNFα-mediated apoptosis, and *Pseudomonas*-mediated cellular injury and apoptosis. Experiments in animal models, involving either pharmacologic induction of *HO-1* or genetic overexpression of *HO-1*, have confirmed that *HO-1* confers cytoprotection in vivo. Induction of *HO-1* by intravenous hemoglobin protected rats against the lethal effects of endotoxemia. Lung epithelial overexpression of *HO-1*, via an adenovirus vector, conferred protection in rats exposed to hyperoxia, and cardiac-specific overexpression conferred protection in a murine model of ischemia. In a cardiac xenograft transplantation model, increased expression of *HO-1* improved graft survival, further stirring interest in *HO-1*–mediated cytoprotection in the field of transplant biology.

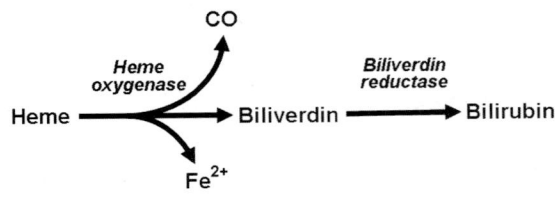

FIGURE 18.6. Heme oxygenase is the rate-limiting enzyme in the conversion of heme to bilirubin, generating ferritin and carbon monoxide as by-products.

Mechanisms of Heme Oxygenase-1 Cytoprotection

The byproducts of HO enzymatic activity include carbon monoxide (CO), bilirubin, and ferritin (see **Fig. 18.6**), and each of these by-products has been postulated to play a role in cytoprotection. Ferritin is known to protect against oxidant stress by regulating the otherwise corrosive reactions generated by the combination of oxygen and iron, and bilirubin can function as a potent antioxidant. The most recent work in the field, however, implicates CO-related cell signaling as the key component of HO-1–mediated cytoprotection (6,12,30). CO shares a variety of properties with NO, including neurotransmission, regulation of vascular tone, and activation of soluble guanylate cyclase. The reported biologic effects of CO include potent anti-inflammatory effects (via the MAPK pathway), antiapoptotic effects, and antioxidant effects. In vivo administration of low concentrations of inhaled CO protected rats against hyperoxia-mediated acute lung injury, and administration of exogenous CO to cardiac tissue protected the tissue against ischemia–reperfusion injury, following transplantation. These studies are particularly intriguing because the amount of CO administered is within the range administered to patients who undergo lung diffusion scans.

ANTIOXIDANT SYSTEMS

Oxidant Stress

Although the use of oxygen is requisite for aerobic organisms, this process inevitably leads to the production of ROS, including NO, hydrogen peroxide, superoxide anion, hydroxyl radicals, and peroxynitrite. When produced in large amounts, ROS can cause excessive oxidant stress, which leads to cellular and tissue injury. ROS-mediated cellular and tissue injury involves damage to genomic and mitochondrial DNA, lipid peroxidation, and protein modification. In addition, cell death secondary to oxidant stress can occur from either necrosis or apoptosis.

Potent antioxidant systems have evolved to counterbalance the normal production of ROS that occurs during many cellular processes, as well as the excessive amounts of ROS that can occur during pathologic states (19). Despite this elegant counter-regulatory system, ROS can lead to cellular injury when either a component of the antioxidant system is defective or when the high-level production of ROS overwhelms an otherwise intact antioxidant system. Recognition of this critical balance and the mechanisms involved in defending against ROS holds potential for the design of therapeutic strategies directed toward restoring the balance between ROS production and endogenous antioxidant systems.

Superoxide Dismutases

The SOD family includes Mn-SOD, Cu/Zn-SOD, and Fe-SOD; they exist within the mitochondrial and cytoplasmic cellular compartments and in the extracellular compartment. SOD is capable of efficiently converting two superoxide molecules to hydrogen peroxide and oxygen (**Fig. 18.7**). The impor-

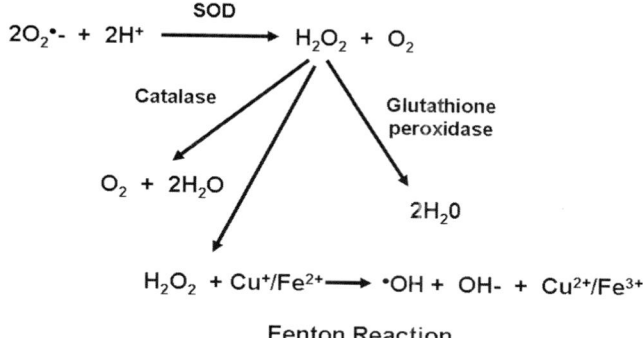

FIGURE 18.7. Schematic depicting the activities of superoxide dismutase (SOD), catalase, and glutathione peroxidase. SOD converts two molecules of superoxide anion to form hydrogen peroxide and water. The hydrogen peroxide produced from this reaction can be further reduced by either catalase or glutathione peroxidase. Catalase converts two molecules of hydrogen peroxide to oxygen and water. Glutathione peroxidase converts hydrogen peroxide to two molecules of water using glutathione as a substrate. In addition, the reduction of hydrogen peroxide by catalase and glutathione peroxidase decreases the participation of hydrogen peroxide in the Fenton reaction, which can lead to the formation of hydroxyl radicals.

tance of SOD in cellular adaptation to stress is illustrated by gene knockout studies and by numerous studies that demonstrate that genetic overexpression of SOD confers protection against oxidant stress (20). In addition, mutations of human Cu/Zn-SOD are strongly linked to development of amyotrophic lateral sclerosis and are likely to be operative in certain critically ill patients. Unfortunately, pharmacologic strategies to augment SOD activity have not been successful to date, despite its showing tremendous promise in the preclinical setting.

Catalase and Glutathione Peroxidase

Catalases are synergistic with SOD by converting hydrogen peroxide to water and oxygen (see **Fig. 18.7**). By lowering intracellular levels of hydrogen peroxide, catalases can also prevent the formation of hydroxyl radicals that could occur via the Fenton reaction (see **Fig. 18.7**). Glutathione (GSH) peroxidases consist of a least four isoforms in mammals, and are widely distributed in many tissues. Similar to catalases, all members of the GSH peroxidases can convert hydrogen peroxide to water by using glutathione as a substrate.

Thioredoxin

Thioredoxin and thioredoxin reductase serve as another major antioxidant mechanism in mammals (4). In conjunction with nicotinamide adenine dinucleotide phosphate (NADPH), thioredoxin reductase leads to the reduction of the active disulfide site of thioredoxin. Thioredoxin, in turn, can broadly function as a protein disulfide reductant. In addition, the thioredoxin system provides an efficient mechanism for the regeneration of various low molecular-weight antioxidants, such as vitamin E, vitamin C, selenium-related compounds, lipoic acid, and ubiquinones.

NITRIC OXIDE

Nitric Oxide Biochemistry

NO is well known to the pediatric intensivist as a therapeutic, inhaled gas used in the context of increased pulmonary vascular resistance or pulmonary hypertension. NO is also produced endogenously by the enzyme NOS, which converts L-arginine to citrulline and NO (8,16,21). NOS exists as three isoforms: eNOS, iNOS, and neuronal NOS (nNOS). The terms "eNOS" and "nNOS" are relative misnomers, because both isoforms are widely distributed beyond the endothelium and central nervous system. Both eNOS and nNOS are constitutively active, calcium dependent, and produce relatively small amounts of NO. iNOS derives its name from the observation that it requires new gene expression for maximal activity. iNOS is calcium independent and is responsible for the high-level production of NO following proinflammatory stimuli. It is now recognized, however, that the eNOS and nNOS genes can undergo regulation (i.e., induction) under certain conditions and that iNOS can be constitutively active. The human genes for the NOS isoforms are now categorized based on the order in which they were cloned: human nNOS is *NOS1*, human iNOS is *NOS2*, and human eNOS is *NOS3*.

One of the primary mechanisms by which NO affects cellular function is through the activation of soluble guanylate cyclase, which leads to increased intracellular levels of cyclic guanosine monophosphate (cGMP) (8,16,21). In that NO is a free radical gas, other important NO mechanisms that affect cellular function include reactions with metal complexes, nitrosation, nitration, and oxidation reactions. The degree to which any one of these mechanisms is operative in a given biologic process is, in turn, highly dependent on the amount of NO produced and the biologic milieu.

Nitric Oxide and Cytoprotection

Since the discovery that NO is produced endogenously, a large number of biologic and physiologic processes have been described as being regulated by NO. Thus, it is not surprising that NO can function as both a cytoprotective and a cytotoxic molecule (8,16,21). This section will focus on NO-dependent cytoprotection, but it should be remembered that, for virtually each example of cytoprotection, an example of NO functioning in an opposite manner can be found.

Apoptosis can be modulated by NO and is perhaps the most prominent and well-studied example of NO-mediated cytoprotection (13). The antiapoptotic effects of NO have been demonstrated in multiple cell types and in the context of multiple proapoptotic signals. The mechanisms by which NO inhibits apoptosis are quite diverse. These include induction of HO-1 and Hsp72, cGMP-mediated regulation of intracellular calcium, inhibition of caspase activity, inhibition of cytochrome C release, and preservation of the intracellular antiapoptotic protein, Bcl-2.

NO can also be protective in whole organs: liver, kidney, brain, heart, and intestine (16). The mechanisms by which NO protects these organs involves vascular dilation, prevention of platelet and neutrophil adherence, antioxidant effects, antiapoptotic effects, and induction of other such cytoprotec-

tive mechanisms as Hsp72 and HO-1. Thus, NO can protect organs during various forms of injury or stress by maintaining blood flow, preventing thrombosis, limiting inflammation, decreasing oxidant stress, and/or preventing apoptosis. Again, the degree to which any one of these mechanisms is operative, or predominant, depends on the type of injury/stress, the amount of NO produced, and the biologic context in which the NO is produced.

The cytoprotective properties of NO are indisputable, and many biologically plausible mechanisms account for the observed cytoprotective effects. The availability of commonly used NO-donors (e.g., sodium nitroprusside and nitroglycerin) and novel NO-donors potentially allows for the direct application of the cytoprotective properties in the clinical setting as a means of affording organ and tissue protection during a variety of disease states. Enthusiasm for this approach must be tempered, however, by the known dual nature of NO as both a cytoprotective and cytotoxic molecule.

CONCLUSIONS AND FUTURE DIRECTIONS

In this chapter, we have described a broad range of cellular adaptations to stress. The adaptations range from broad responses that confer generalized cytoprotection (e.g., the heat shock response) to responses limited to specific forms of cellular stress (e.g., antioxidant responses to oxidative stress). The importance of these adaptations in the clinical care of critically ill children cannot be overstated. Much of critical care–related intervention is directed at organ support, which, in effect, provides a platform for and timeframe in which to allow cellular stress adaptations to become operative. It is through these responses, then, that many critically ill children ultimately recover from a given illness or injury. Conversely, inadequate adaptations or failure to adapt can lead to organ failure and death, despite optimal organ support.

An important challenge in the field is to devise safe, therapeutic strategies to manipulate and/or enhance these adaptations for the benefit of our patients. By understanding the molecular mechanisms that allow for adaptations, the field will be better positioned to meet this challenge. The evolution and development of novel pharmacologic agents, molecular-based strategies, and even gene-based therapy collectively hold the potential to effectively manipulate and harness these forms of cellular adaptation to perform as a therapeutic strategy that goes well beyond organ support.

KEY POINTS

- The heat shock response and Hsps provide protection against a broad variety of cellular stresses and injuries.
- The heat shock response and Hsps are potent modulators of inflammation-associated signal transduction.
- Extracellular Hsps are emerging as important signaling molecules in innate immunity and other cellular processes.
- Ischemic preconditioning describes a specific form of cellular adaptation, whereby brief periods of nonlethal ischemia confer cellular resistance to subsequent and otherwise lethal periods of ischemia.

- Hypoxic preconditioning is a similar concept to that of IP, but it is specific to hypoxic conditions, rather than ischemia.
- HIF is a key molecule in cellular adaptations to hypoxia.
- Endotoxin tolerance describes an intriguing adaptation, whereby cellular exposure to low levels of endotoxin reprograms the cellular response to subsequent exposure to higher levels of endotoxin.
- The clinical significance of endotoxin tolerance to medicine and innate immunity remains unclear at the present time.
- HO performs a broad range of cytoprotective roles, and a large portion of this protective effect seems to be mediated by carbon monoxide, which is a primary end-product of HO-mediated degradation of heme.
- ROS are inevitably derived from the requisite use of oxygen by aerobic organisms, and excessive amounts of ROS can lead to oxidative cellular and tissue injury.
- The major antioxidant mechanisms that serve to protect against ROS include superoxide dismutase, catalase, glutathione peroxidase, thioredoxin, and thioredoxin reductase.
- NO is produced by NOS, which exists in three isoforms, all of which convert L-arginine to citrulline and NO.
- NO affects cellular function primarily through the activation of soluble guanylate cyclase, but it can also undergo reactions involving metal complexes, nitrosation, nitration, and oxidation reactions.
- NO has both cytotoxic (maladaptive) and cytoprotective (adaptive) properties, depending the amount of NO produced and the biologic context.

References

1. Allen ML, Peters MJ, Goldman A, et al. Early postoperative monocyte deactivation predicts systemic inflammation and prolonged stay in pediatric cardiac intensive care. *Crit Care Med* 2002;30:1140–5.
2. Asea A, Kraeft SK, Kurt-Jones EA, et al. HSP70 stimulates cytokine production through a CD14-dependant pathway, demonstrating its dual role as a chaperone and cytokine. *Nat Med* 2000;6:435–42.
3. Asea A, Rehli M, Kabingu E, et al. Novel signal transduction pathway utilized by extracellular HSP70: Role of toll-like receptor (TLR) 2 and TLR4. *J Biol Chem* 2002;277:15028–34.
4. Burke-Gaffney A, Callister ME, Nakamura H. Thioredoxin: Friend or foe in human disease? *Trends Pharmacol Sci* 2005;26:398–404.
5. Cavaillon JM, Adrie C, Fitting C, et al. Endotoxin tolerance: Is there a clinical relevance? *J Endotoxin Res* 2003;9:101–7.
6. Choi AM, Otterbein LE. Emerging role of carbon monoxide in physiologic and pathophysiologic states. *Antioxid Redox Signal* 2002;4:227–8.
7. Das DK, Maulik N. Cardiac genomic response following preconditioning stimulus. *Cardiovasc Res* 2006;70:254–63.
8. Dimmeler S, Zeiher AM. Nitric oxide and apoptosis: Another paradigm for the double-edged role of nitric oxide. *Nitric Oxide* 1997;1:275–81.
9. Fan H, Cook JA. Molecular mechanisms of endotoxin tolerance. *J Endotoxin Res* 2004;10:71–84.
10. Hausenloy DJ, Yellon DM. Survival kinases in ischemic preconditioning and postconditioning. *Cardiovasc Res* 2006;70:240–53.
11. Johnson JD, Fleshner M. Releasing signals, secretory pathways, and immune function of endogenous extracellular heat shock protein 72. *J Leukoc Biol* 2006;79:425–34.
12. Kim HP, Ryter SW, Choi AM. CO as a cellular signaling molecule. *Annu Rev Pharmacol Toxicol* 2006;46:411–49.
13. Kim YM, Bombeck CA, Billiar TR. Nitric oxide as a bifunctional regulator of apoptosis. *Circ Res* 1999;84:253–56.
14. Kindas-Mugge I, Hammerle AH, Frohlich I, et al. Granulocytes of critically ill patients spontaneously express the 72 kD heat shock protein. *Circ Shock* 1993;39:247–52.
15. Kregel KC. Heat shock proteins: Modifying factors in physiological stress responses and acquired thermotolerance. *J Appl Physiol* 2002;92:2177–86.
16. Kroncke KD, Fehsel K, Kolb-Bachofen V. Nitric oxide: Cytotoxicity versus cytoprotection – how, why, when, and where? *Nitric Oxide* 1997;1:107–20.
17. Lai Y, Kochanek PM, Adelson PD, et al. Induction of the stress response after inflicted and non-inflicted traumatic brain injury in infants and children. *J Neurotrauma* 2004;21:229–37.
18. Malhotra V, Wong HR. Interactions between the heat shock response and the nuclear factor-kappa B signaling pathway. *Crit Care Med* 2002;30:S89–95.
19. Mathers J, Fraser JA, McMahon M, et al. Antioxidant and cytoprotective responses to redox stress. *Biochem Soc Symp* 2004;157–76.
20. McCord JM. Superoxide dismutase in aging and disease: An overview. *Methods Enzymol* 2002;349:331–41.
21. Michel T, Feron O. Nitric oxide synthesis: Which, where, how, and why? *J Clin Invest* 1997;100:2146–52.
22. Mole DR, Maxwell PH, Pugh CW, et al. Regulation of HIF by the von Hippel-Lindau tumour suppressor: Implications for cellular oxygen sensing. *IUBMB Life* 2001;52:43–7.
23. Morimoto RI, Kline MP, Bimston DN, et al. The heat-shock response: Regulation and function of heat-shock proteins and molecular chaperones. *Essays Biochem* 1997;32:17–29.
24. Morimoto RI, Santoro MG. Stress-inducible responses and heat shock proteins: New pharmacologic targets for cytoprotection. *Nat Biotechnol* 1998;16:833–38.
25. Morse D, Choi AM. Heme oxygenase-1: From bench to bedside. *Am J Respir Crit Care Med* 2005;172:660–70.
26. Murry CE, Jennings RB, Reimer KA. Preconditioning with ischemia: A delay of lethal cell injury in ischemic myocardium. *Circulation* 1986;74:1124–36.
27. Otterbein LE, Choi AM. Heme oxygenase: Colors of defense against cellular stress. *Am J Physiol Lung Cell Mol Physiol* 2000;279:L1029–37.
28. Pittet JF, Lee H, Morabito D, et al. Serum levels of Hsp 72 measured early after trauma correlate with survival. *J Trauma* 2002;52:611–17; discussion 7.
29. Ryan M, Levy MM. Clinical review: Fever in intensive care unit patients. *Crit Care* 2003;7:221–25.
30. Ryter SW, Otterbein LE, Morse D, et al. Heme oxygenase/carbon monoxide signaling pathways: Regulation and functional significance. *Mol Cell Biochem* 2002;234–235:249–63.
31. Sanada S, Kitakaze M. Ischemic preconditioning: Emerging evidence, controversy, and translational trials. *Int J Cardiol* 2004;97:263–76.
32. Semenza GL. HIF-1: Mediator of physiological and pathophysiological responses to hypoxia. *J Appl Physiol* 2000;88:1474–80.
33. Semenza GL. Surviving ischemia: Adaptive responses mediated by hypoxia-inducible factor 1. *J Clin Invest* 2000;106:809–12.
34. Sharp FR, Ran R, Lu A, et al. Hypoxic preconditioning protects against ischemic brain injury. *J Am Soc Exp Neuro Therap* 2004;1:26–35.
35. Sitzer M, Foerch C, Neumann-Haefelin T, et al. Transient ischaemic attack preceding anterior circulation infarction is independently associated with favourable outcome. *J Neurol Neurosurg Psychiatry* 2004;75:659–60.
36. Westerheide SD, Morimoto RI. Heat shock response modulators as therapeutic tools for diseases of protein conformation. *J Biol Chem* 2005;280:33097–100.
37. Wheeler DS, Fisher LE Jr, Catravas JD, et al. Extracellular hsp70 levels in children with septic shock. *Pediatr Crit Care Med* 2005;6:308–11.
38. Wischmeyer PE. The glutamine story: Where are we now? *Curr Opin Crit Care* 2006;12:142–8.
39. Wong HR. Potential protective role of the heat shock response in sepsis. *New Horiz* 1998;6:194–200.
40. Yachie A, Niida Y, Wada T, et al. Oxidative stress causes enhanced endothelial cell injury in human heme oxygenase-1 deficiency. *J Clin Invest* 1999;103:129–35.
41. Ziegler TR, Ogden LG, Singleton KD, et al. Parenteral glutamine increases serum heat shock protein 70 in critically ill patients. *Intensive Care Med* 2005;31(8):1079–86.

CHAPTER 19 ■ SHOCK AND REPERFUSION INJURY

BASILIA ZINGARELLI

Ischemia and reperfusion injury is a critical pathophysiologic event common to several clinical conditions, including myocardial infarction, cerebral and intestinal ischemia, stroke, cardiopulmonary bypass, solid-organ transplantation, soft-tissue flaps, and extremity reimplantation. It can also occur as a consequence of collapse of systemic circulation, as in *cardiovascular shock* with low cardiac output, which results in inadequate tissue perfusion (ischemia) and typically requires cardiovascular resuscitation (reperfusion).

Ischemia usually results from a dramatic reduction of oxygen supply in the whole organism or in defined tissue territories, and rapidly results in cell metabolic derangement, molecular alterations, and dysfunction sequelae. Occasionally, ischemia may result from increased metabolic requirements or impaired oxygen utilization at the cellular level, despite adequate oxygen delivery. If not reversed within a short period, the altered cellular metabolism progresses to complete depletion of the energetic pools, accumulation of waste and toxic products, and eventually, to cell death.

The main therapeutic intervention in clinical conditions of ischemia requires the restoration of blood flow (reperfusion) and/or recovery of the normal oxygen levels (reoxygenation) by providing circulatory and respiratory support. Once perfusion is reestablished tissue ischemia is generally reversed. However, restoration of blood flow initiates a paradoxical injury process known as *reperfusion injury,* which is characterized by an exaggerated inflammatory response and may lead to cellular death and further organ dysfunction. The intense inflammation triggered by ischemia and reperfusion injury may also precipitate inflammatory damage in organs not involved in the initial ischemic insult. This condition is termed *multiple organ dysfunction syndrome* (MODS) (see Chapter 21) and is the leading cause of death in ICUs.

_____The biochemical and molecular changes of ischemia and reperfusion are complex; these include the formation of several toxic inflammatory mediators, reactive oxygen species (ROS), and reactive nitrogen species (RNS) by different inflammatory and parenchymal cells, the disturbances of the microcirculation and endothelium barrier, and the alteration of the coagulation and complement cascades. To counteract this deleterious inflammatory response, the tissues also attempt to adapt within the altered metabolic environment by deploying cellular mechanisms of defense (see Chapter 18).

OXYGEN DELIVERY AND ACUTE CELLULAR OXYGEN DEFICIENCY

According to the Fick equation, oxygen delivery (DO_2) depends on two variables: the arterial oxygen content (CaO_2) and the cardiac output (CO). In turn, CO depends on the heart rate and the stroke volume, which is determined by myocardial contractility and the ventricular preload and afterload (**Fig. 19.1**). In the pediatric patient, CO depends more on heart rate than on stroke volume because, at this stage, the development of the myocardial contractile mass is incomplete. In addition to adjusting CO, tissue perfusion and metabolic demands may also be maintained by modification of the systemic vascular resistance through compensatory changes in the local vasomotor tone (see Fig. 19.1).

Therefore, *acute cellular oxygen deficiency* may result as a consequence of a reduction of CaO_2, because it may occur in conditions of local tissue ischemia caused by arterial occlusion within the perfusion territory of an affected vessel (myocardial or splanchnic infarction, cerebral ischemia, solid-organ transplantation, soft-tissue and limb reimplantation). Limited pump flow due to decrease in CO is, instead, the cause of global ischemia observed in conditions of cardiovascular shock. However, in some clinical conditions, inadequate tissue energetic metabolism may derive from an increase of total body oxygen consumption (VO_2), despite a normal oxygen delivery. For example, during septic shock, tissue oxygenation may be inadequate even in the presence of normal blood flow due to a major increase in metabolic demand and impaired oxygen extraction.

DEFINITION AND CLASSIFICATION OF SHOCK

Shock is defined as a state of acute circulatory dysfunction that results in a failure to deliver sufficient oxygen and other nutrients to meet the metabolic demands of the tissues (2). Shock is a progressive process characterized by three stages, depending on the causative factors, the cellular compensatory responses, and the ischemia and reperfusion injury. In the early *compensated stage*, a number of neurohormonal compensatory physiologic mechanisms act to maintain blood pressure and preserve adequate tissue perfusion. At this stage, shock may be reversible, even without therapeutic intervention. However, when these compensatory mechanisms fail, shock may progress to an *uncompensated stage* that requires, and may still respond to, therapeutic interventions. Unfortunately, in the *irreversible stage*, shock progresses to a remarkable degree of organ and tissue injury, which is unresponsive to conventional therapy and leads to the death of the patient.

Five main types of shock are described (**Table 19.1**). *Hypovolemic shock* is the most common type of shock in children and is caused by a reduction in the volume of blood by hemorrhage, nonhemorrhagic volume depletion, or dehydration

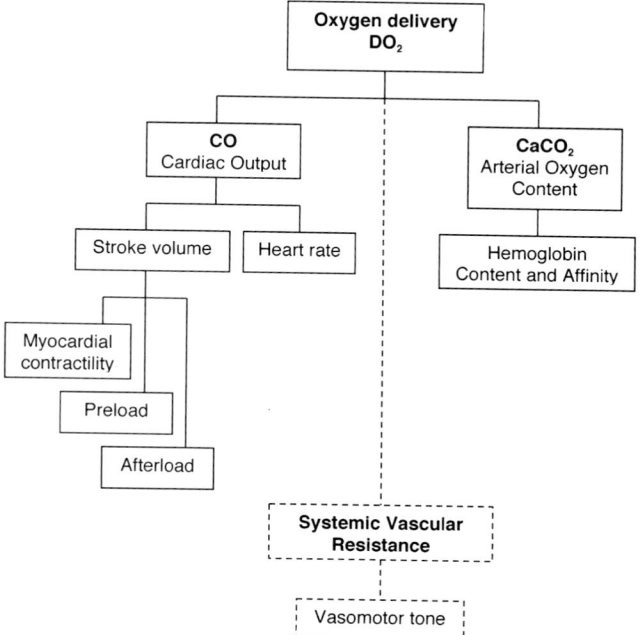

FIGURE 19.1. Variables of oxygen delivery. Oxygen delivery (DO_2) depends on cardiac output (CO) and arterial oxygen content (Cao_2). CO depends on heart rate and stroke volume, which is determined by myocardial contractility and the ventricular preload and afterload. Cao_2 depends on hemoglobin content, affinity, and saturation. Modification of the systemic vascular resistance contributes to maintenance of tissue perfusion through changes in the local vasomotor tone and affects CO by altering afterload.

TABLE 19.1

CLASSIFICATION OF SHOCK

Type	Clinical syndrome
Hypovolemic	Hemorrhage
	Nonhemorrhagic fluid depletion
	Vomit
	Diarrhea
	Severe burn
	Internal sequestration
	Diabetes
	Nephrotic syndrome
	Other form of dehydration
Cardiogenic	Myocardial infarction
	Sever congestive failure
	Cardiac surgery
	Dysrhythmias
	Myocarditis
	Cardiopulmonary bypass
	Septic shock
	Drug intoxication
Obstructive	Cardiac tamponade
	Pneumothorax
	Massive pulmonary embolus
Distributive	Septic shock
	Toxic shock syndrome
	Anaphylaxis
	Neurogenic shock
	Endocrinologic shock
	Drug intoxication
Dissociative	Methemoglobinemia
	Carbon monoxide poisoning

(especially in young children). *Cardiogenic shock* is caused by a decline in CO secondary to myocardial damage and/or dysfunction. This type of shock is less frequent in children, but may be seen in neonates with congenital heart disease, in older patients immediately after repair of congenital heart defects, and in patients with myocarditis, thyrotoxicosis, and pheochromocytoma. *Septic shock* may also be included in the category of cardiogenic shock because of the occurrence of myocardial depression induced by inflammatory mediators. *Distributive shock* results from abnormalities in flow distribution secondary to impaired vasomotor tone, despite a normal or high CO. The most common cause of distributive shock in children is sepsis, especially in the early stage. Other types of distributive shock are *anaphylactic shock* from systemic allergic reactions and *neurologic shock* from spinal cord injuries. Drug intoxication by barbiturates, phenothiazines, and antihypertensives may also cause maldistribution. *Obstructive shock* is uncommon in children and is caused by a mechanical obstruction that impairs an adequate CO. The most common causes are pericardial tamponade and congenital heart lesions characterized by left ventricular outflow obstruction (i.e., critical aortic stenosis). Other causes are tension pneumothorax and, less frequently, pulmonary embolism. *Dissociative shock* is also uncommon in children and results from clinical conditions associated with inadequate tissue oxygenation secondary to abnormal affinity of hemoglobin for oxygen, such as methemoglobinemia and carbon monoxide poisoning.

The specific pattern of response and related pathophysiology, clinical manifestations, and treatments vary with the eti-

ology of shock, and the reader is referred to the clinical section of this book for further discussion.

CELLULAR AND MOLECULAR MECHANISMS OF INJURY

Metabolic Derangement and Energy Failure During Ischemia

The cells of all tissues undergo metabolic changes when deprived of oxygen and other nutrients. The quantitative and kinetic features of these metabolic responses are different for each specialized cell type and depend on the function and structure of the cell. Brain and myocardium are the most sensitive tissues to acute deficiency in oxygen, and even a short period of ischemia can lead to deleterious and irreversible effects.

Furthermore, the etiologic factor of the clinical condition of shock or ischemia also has profound effects on many fundamental aspects of cell metabolism and function. The pathophysiologic effects of cardiogenic and hypovolemic shock are related predominantly to the acute deficiency of oxygen, whereas the pathophysiologic effects of septic shock result largely from the overwhelming production of inflammatory mediators. In shock associated with sepsis, in fact, bacterial products interact directly with several cell types, including macrophages, neutrophils, monocytes, endothelial cells, and myocytes, to activate the innate immune response and to stimulate the production of numerous inflammatory toxic mediators. The excessive inflammatory response is then responsible for hemodynamic compromise, widespread tissue ischemia, and reperfusion injury (**Fig. 19.2**).

Independent of the cause of ischemia and cell specificity, however, a time-dependent cascade of metabolic responses is shared among all cell types during ischemia (**Fig. 19.3**). After only a few seconds of ischemia, oxidative phosphorylation and mitochondrial ATP production are seriously compromised. Therefore, levels of ATP and other high-energy phosphates—mainly creatine phosphate—decline rapidly, and the breakdown products of adenine nucleotides, such as inorganic phosphate and adenosine, accumulate. The cell shifts from oxidative metabolism to an inefficient anaerobic glycolysis, producing only 2 moles of ATP per 1 mole of glucose, instead of the 38 moles of ATP normally produced during aerobic metabolism. This collapse of high-energy phosphate compounds impairs the energy-dependent cell processes, especially membrane ion pumps (Na^+/H^+ exchanger). DNA and protein synthesis are also suppressed, although some specific proteins, for example, heat shock protein 70 (Hsp70) and protein kinase C (PKC), may be induced in an attempt by the cell to adapt to the hypoxic environment (see Chapter 18).

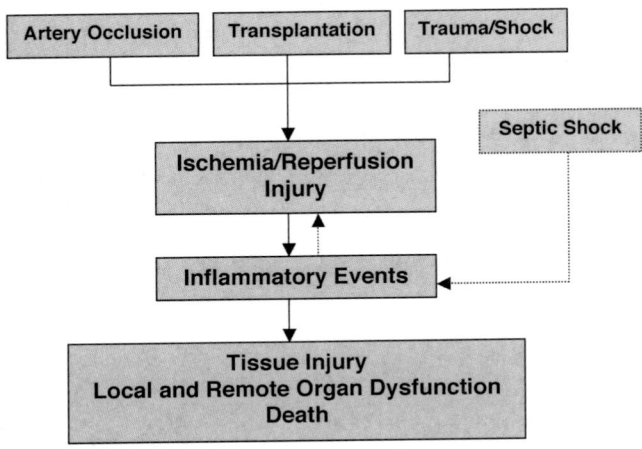

FIGURE 19.2. Kinetics of pathophysiologic events of shock and reperfusion. The pathophysiologic effects of acute local ischemia (after artery occlusion or organ transplantation) or acute global ischemia (after trauma and severe hemorrhage) are related predominantly to the acute deficiency of oxygen and the subsequent reperfusion injury at the time of reoxygenation. In septic shock, an overwhelming inflammatory response is first activated by bacterial products and precedes the hemodynamic compromise and widespread tissue ischemia and reperfusion injury.

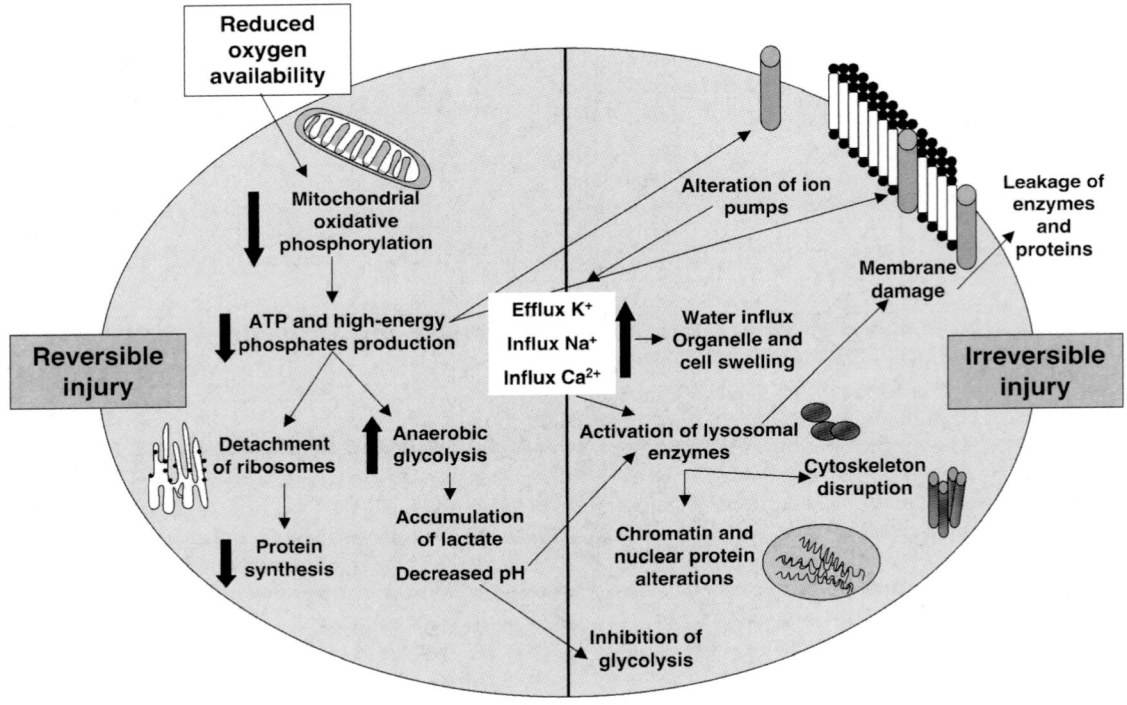

FIGURE 19.3. Metabolic and cellular derangement during ischemia. Reduction in oxygen availability compromises mitochondrial oxidative phosphorylation. Levels of ATP and other high-energy phosphates rapidly decline. The cell shifts from oxidative metabolism to an inefficient anaerobic glycolysis, producing less ATP. This energy failure slows the rate of protein synthesis and impairs the energy-dependent ion pumps, leading to an increase of intracellular levels of sodium (Na^+) and calcium (Ca^{2+}), an influx of water, and a decrease of intracellular levels of potassium (K^+). Water influx into the cell leads to swelling of the cytoplasm and organelles, such as mitochondria and endoplasmic reticulum, further impairing mitochondrial oxidative phosphorylation and protein synthesis. Accumulation of hydrogen ions and lactate results in intracellular acidosis and inhibition of glycolysis. At this time, if oxygen supply is not restored, cell injury becomes irreversible. Increase of intracellular Ca^{2+} causes activation of lysosomal enzymes and disrupts mitochondria, further uncoupling oxidative phosphorylation. Activated proteases also cleave cytoskeletal filaments and impair membrane permeability. Finally, physical disruption of the cell membrane occurs and is associated with leakage of cellular enzymes and proteins into the plasma.

Increased anaerobic glycolysis for ATP production leads to the accumulation of hydrogen ions and lactate, resulting in intracellular acidosis and the inhibition of glycolysis. Membrane depolarization and failure of ATP-dependent ion pumps lead to an efflux of potassium and influx of sodium and calcium. The increase of intracellular sodium concentration is accompanied by water influx into the cell, leading to swelling of the cytoplasm and organelles such as mitochondria and endoplasmic reticulum. Within seconds or minutes, these abnormalities become sufficiently severe to reduce cell function. In the heart, this metabolic derangement translates into a reduction of the contractile force generated by actin-myosin cross-bridge formation; in the gut, altered intestinal absorptive function is associated with translocation of bacteria from the intestine to the lymphatic vessels and blood stream. At this point, if oxygen supply is restored, cell injury is reversible.

However, if ischemia persists, cell injury may become irreversible. The cytosolic and mitochondrial concentration of calcium also increases due to changes in the cell calcium transport systems. Mitochondria show amorphous matrix densities and granular dense bodies of calcium phosphate, which are considered the earliest sign of irreversible ischemic cell injury. Mitochondria play an important role in ischemic damage. Indeed, the excessive energy demand is likely to represent a crucial factor in the ensuing irreversible damage of cells, especially in cardiomyocytes, where the cell volume occupied by mitochondria is the greatest among all the cell types. A major role in the progression toward cell death might be attributed to the opening of the *mitochondrial permeability transition pore*, a high-conductance channel whose opening leads to an increase of mitochondrial inner membrane permeability to solutes with molecular masses up to 1,500 Da. The opening of these pores releases stored calcium into the cytosol, and dissipation of the mitochondrial inner transmembrane potential uncouples the electron transport system from ATP hydrolysis. These events abolish mitochondrial ATP production, leading to energy failure, enhanced production of ROS, and the release of apoptotic factors, thus contributing to cell death (9).

This altered metabolic milieu, with a sustained increase in cytosolic and mitochondrial calcium, causes the activation of a number of enzymes (proteases, phospholipases, ATPases) and disrupts mitochondrial and lysosomal membranes, further uncoupling mitochondrial oxidative phosphorylation and promoting the release of other acid hydrolases. Activated proteases also cleave cytoskeletal filaments and impair their anchoring and stabilizing function. These changes collectively lead to a progressive increase in membrane permeability, severe derangements of intracellular electrolytes, and ATP exhaustion (50).

The terminal event after prolonged ischemia is cell death, which occurs mainly by necrosis and is associated with physical disruption of the cell membrane and, consequently, widespread leakage of cellular enzymes or proteins across the cell membrane and into the plasma. This latter phenomenon may provide important diagnostic tools of cell damage (such as the serum increase of creatine kinase and troponin levels for the diagnosis of myocardial infarction). However, apoptosis is also a major contributor of cell death and is activated by release of proapoptotic components from the altered mitochondria.

Reperfusion Injury

Rapid and sustained restoration of oxygen and nutrient supply to the ischemic tissue is the major goal in the treatment of patients with clinical conditions of global or local ischemia. This therapeutic intervention has the potential to relieve ischemia and can result in the recovery of cell function and prevention of cell death. Upon reperfusion, if the cell injury is still reversible, electron transfer and ATP synthesis restart, the internal ectoplasmatic pH is restored, and other metabolic processes are reestablished. The severity and duration of ischemia are the main factors that influence recovery: The earlier the reperfusion and/or reoxygenation is established, the more favorable the clinical outcome for the patient.

Paradoxically, however, reoxygenation initiates a cascade of events that may lead to additional cell injury, known as *reperfusion injury*, in tissues that previously had been ischemic but not necessarily irreversibly damaged. The underlying pathophysiologic mechanisms of this phenomenon are still not well understood. At least four major components contribute to reperfusion injury: oxidative and nitrosative stress, endothelial dysfunction and microvascular injury, neutrophil activation, and complement system activation.

Oxidative and Nitrosative Stress

The production of excessive quantities of ROS and RNS is an important mechanism of reperfusion injury. The reactive species include highly unstable oxygen and nitrogen molecules, such as superoxide (O_2^-), hydrogen peroxide (H_2O_2), oxidized lipoproteins, lipid peroxides, nitric oxide (NO), and peroxynitrite (ONOO) (18). ROS and RNS can be formed by several mechanisms; they can be produced by a reduction of molecular oxygen in altered mitochondria; by enzymes such as xanthine oxidase (XO), nicotinamide adenine dinucleotide phosphate (NADPH) oxidase, cytochrome P450, nitric oxide synthase (NOS) and cyclooxygenase (COX); and by auto-oxidation of catecholamines. The source of reactive species varies from cell to cell and from stage to stage during the ischemia and reperfusion event. For example, in myocytes, but to a much lesser extent than in other cell types, the production of oxyradicals starts early in the ischemic period in altered mitochondria and is further enhanced during reperfusion. At reperfusion, a massive activation of XO is a major source of ROS in endothelial cells, and COX may contribute to this oxidative stress. Cytochrome P450 accounts for the production of ROS in lung epithelial cells, and NADPH oxidase accounts for ROS production in infiltrated neutrophils. The production of potent RNS appears to be more ubiquitous, because a number of inflammatory mediators may lead to the induction of NOS in several cell types. In addition, the antioxidant mechanisms of the cell may be compromised and may further favor the accumulation of reactive species.

These reactive species mediate tissue injury by two main mechanisms: (a) directly, by inducing the damage of important cellular macromolecules and (b), indirectly, by activating signal transduction pathways that result in the production of inflammatory mediators and/or apoptotic mediators.

Sources of Reactive Oxygen and Nitrogen Species

Mitochondria

The generation of ROS starts during ischemia in the mitochondria. Although it might be expected that ischemia, caused by a low partial pressure of oxygen, would decrease oxyradical production, this paradoxic increase is secondary to the altered redox balance of the mitochondria. With ischemia, the metabolic reduction of the adenine nucleotide pool leaves the respiratory chain cytochromes in a more fully reduced state, allowing them to directly transfer (i.e., "leak") electrons to the residual molecular oxygen entrapped within the inner mitochondrial membrane. This electron leakage appears capable of producing large amounts of superoxide radical. Reintroduction of oxygen with reperfusion reenergizes the mitochondria, but electron leakage further increases because of low ADP content, thus enabling more reactions with molecular oxygen and yielding to the excessive "burst" of ROS.

Xanthine Oxidoreductase System

The xanthine oxidoreductase (XOR) enzyme system plays an important role in the catabolism of purines, catalyzing the oxidation of hypoxanthine to xanthine and the oxidation of xanthine to uric acid. Despite its wide tissue distribution, the enzyme is mostly localized in endothelial and epithelial cells, and exists in two interconvertible forms, XO and xanthine dehydrogenase (XDH) (37). During ischemia, XDH is converted to the oxidase form by a protease activated by the intracellular overload of calcium. At the same time, degradation of ATP leads to an accumulation of hypoxanthine in the ischemic tissue. During reperfusion, with the presence of large quantities of molecular oxygen and high concentrations of hypoxanthine, XO yields a burst of superoxide (**Fig. 19.4**). Recently, the XOR enzyme system has been shown to catalyze the reduction of nitrates and nitrites to nitrites and NO, respectively, thus also contributing to NO generation. This activity is more prominent under acidic conditions and may contribute to a pathophysiologic enhancement of NO production in ischemic or hypoxic tissues.

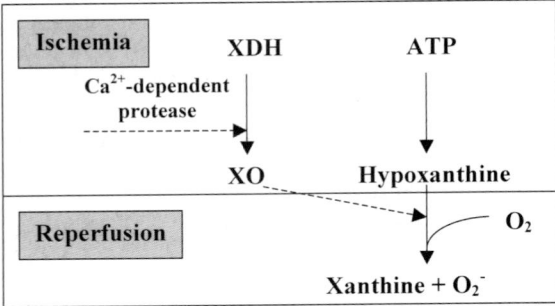

FIGURE 19.4. Superoxide production by the xanthine oxidase. During ischemia, xanthine dehydrogenase (XDH) is converted to xanthine oxidase (XO) by a protease activated by the intracellular overload of calcium. At the same time, degradation of ATP leads to accumulation of hypoxanthine in the ischemic tissue. At reperfusion, large quantities of molecular oxygen are reintroduced into the cell. Both molecular oxygen and hypoxanthine then serve as substrates for XO to produce superoxide.

The hypothesis that generation of superoxide by XO may play an important pathogenetic role in reperfusion injury has been supported by studies demonstrating that the inactivation of XO with allopurinol ameliorates reperfusion-induced tissue damage (14). However, the role of XO in reperfusion injury is not fully confirmed. For example, it appears that the conversion of XDH to XO is too slow to play a major role in the pathogenesis of ischemia and reperfusion injury in the liver (13). Furthermore, the distribution of the XO among tissues varies with very low activity detected in the human heart, where it is located in the endothelium only, but not in the myocytes.

Interestingly, it appears that ischemia and reperfusion in any tissue may lead to the release of XOR into the circulation. Elevated plasma levels of XOR have been reported in adult patients who were subjected to limb ischemia–reperfusion (20), liver transplantation (43), or small-intestine ischemia–reperfusion. In critically ill infants and children with shock subsequent to severe sepsis, trauma, or major surgery, high XO activity has been detected in urine. This elevation in XO activity index appears to correlate with high blood levels of oxidized glutathione (a marker of oxidative stress) and with the clinical symptoms of an excessive proinflammatory response (39). It has been suggested that, once in the circulation, XOR may contribute to the development of MODS. These circulating levels may, in fact, bind to the endothelial cells of distant sites and contribute to the initiation of oxidative damage in organs remote from the original ischemic tissue (37).

Nitric Oxide Synthase Pathway

NO is a highly reactive gas that is synthesized from L-arginine by a family of enzymes referred as to NO synthases (NOSs) (see Chapter 18). Three isoforms of NOS have been characterized: neuronal (nNOS, or type 1), inducible (iNOS, or type 2), and endothelial (eNOS, or type 3) (11). The eNOS and nNOS isoforms are constitutively expressed, calcium/calmodulin dependent, and produce low amounts of NO. The designation of these constitutive isoforms does not strictly reflect their tissue expression, because eNOS and nNOS are not only found in endothelial and neuronal cells but also in other cell types, including cardiomyocytes and muscle cells. The iNOS isoform is a calcium/calmodulin-independent enzyme that is responsible for the production of large amounts NO. Although not detected under normal conditions, the expression of the iNOS isoform is induced in response to microbial products, inflammatory cytokines, and growth factors in almost every cell type during diverse pathologic conditions, including sepsis, hemorrhagic shock, trauma, and ischemia.

Under normal conditions, the constitutive forms of NOS release low concentrations of NO, which are critical to normal physiology. For example, the nNOS-derived NO acts as a neurotransmitter and a second messenger. The eNOS-derived NO is the physiologic mediator of normal vascular tone. Once formed by vascular endothelial cells, NO diffuses to adjacent smooth muscle cells, activates soluble guanylate cyclase, produces cyclic guanosine monophosphate (cGMP), and reduces intracellular calcium concentration, thus resulting in vasodilatation. Apart from its direct vasodilatory effect, the endothelium-derived NO also maintains normal tissue perfusion and vascular permeability by inhibiting platelet aggregation, leukocyte adherence, and smooth muscle proliferation in the vascular system. In cardiomyocytes, under physiologic conditions, both constitutive forms of NOS (types 1 and 3) have

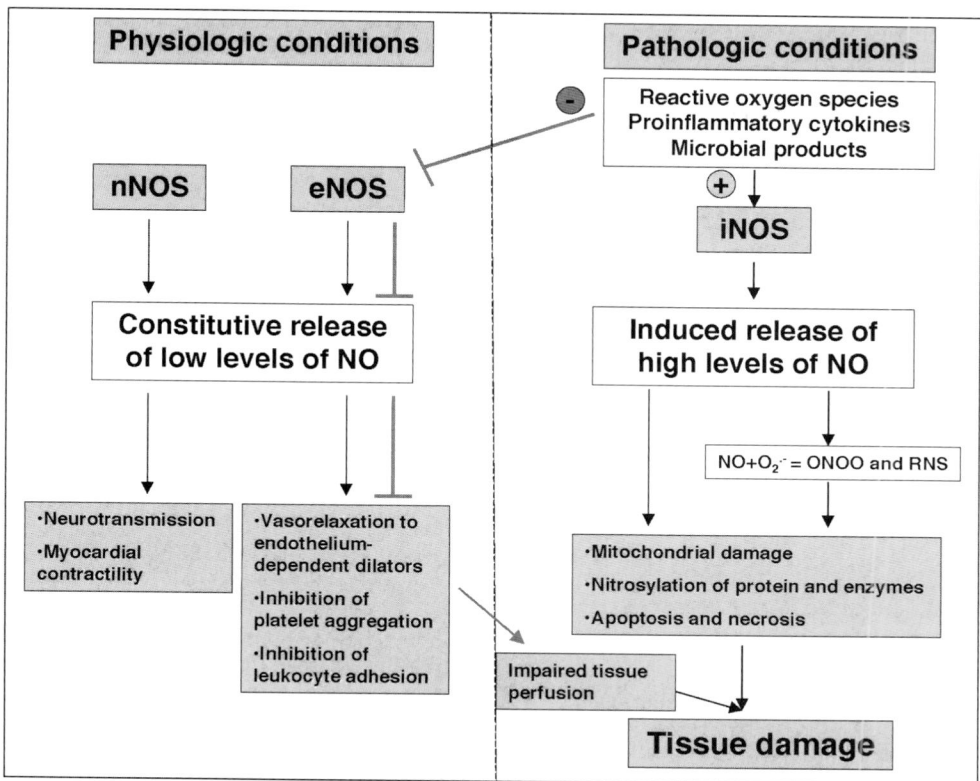

FIGURE 19.5. Activation of nitric oxide synthase (NOS) enzymes during physiologic conditions and during pathologic conditions after shock and reperfusion injury. Under normal conditions, the constitutive forms of NOS (nNOS and eNOS) release low concentrations of NO, which acts as a neurotransmitter, modulator of myocardial contractility, or modulator of vascular tone. The endothelium-derived NO also maintains normal tissue perfusion and vascular permeability by inhibiting platelet aggregation and leukocyte adherence. After prolonged ischemia and immediately at the onset of reperfusion, reactive oxygen species, several inflammatory mediators, and bacterial products may reduce NO production from the constitutive eNOS, impairing vascular relaxation to endothelium-dependent vasodilators and predisposing the endothelium to platelet aggregation and leukocyte adhesion. In prolonged shock and severe ischemia and reperfusion, an inducible form of NOS (iNOS) is activated and produces large amounts of NO. Cytotoxic effects may be mediated directly by high levels of NO and/or indirectly by other reactive nitrogen species (RNS) and peroxynitrite, which is formed from the reaction of NO with superoxide. NO and RNS may inhibit the mitochondrial respiratory chain, induce nitrosylation of proteins and enzymes, and cause cell apoptosis and necrosis.

been described to release NO, which regulates cardiac function through their direct effects on several aspects of cardiomyocyte contractility, from the fine regulation of excitation–contraction coupling (with positive inotropic and lusitropic effects) to modulation of autonomic signaling and mitochondrial respiration (11,36).

Changes in the activation of the NOS enzymes and in the production of NO occur during conditions of shock and reperfusion injury. The best-characterized events are the impairment of eNOS activity and induction of iNOS (**Fig. 19.5**). During sepsis or after prolonged ischemia, and immediately at the onset of reperfusion, the burst of oxidants scavenges NO, thus reducing its availability in the endothelium (33); the release of proinflammatory cytokines also cooperates to reduce NO production from the constitutive eNOS by reducing eNOS mRNA stability and expression (47). This reduced availability of NO is a major contributing factor in the development of endothelial dysfunction after ischemia and reperfusion in the heart and other vascular beds. In fact, the reduction of NO release from the endothelium impairs vascular relaxation to endothelium-

dependent vasodilators and predisposes the vascular endothelium to platelet aggregation and leukocyte adhesion. Because of the very important effects of NO on vascular tone and thrombogenicity, drugs that can modulate NO levels (e.g., nitroglycerin) have long been used as therapeutic agents for the various angina syndromes, and they are used in congestive heart failure and in patients with left ventricular dysfunction. Because the local vasodilatory effects of NO in the lung vascular bed appear to improve oxygenation, inhaled NO gas is currently used in sepsis associated with persistent pulmonary hypertension or in high-risk pediatric patients to manage lung failure secondary to acute respiratory distress syndrome (ARDS) (28).

In severe ischemia and reperfusion, high levels of NO are produced by iNOS and may be responsible for potentially noxious effects. Cytotoxic effects may be mediated directly by NO and/or indirectly by reactive NO-derived byproducts. As a highly unstable gas with an unpaired electron, NO can cause direct oxidation or S-nitrosylation of biomolecules. Moreover, the inherent radical nature of NO allows reactions with other free radicals or oxygen to yield other reactive intermediates, which then contribute to cell dysfunction and death. One of the most potent reactive intermediates is peroxynitrite, which is formed from the reaction of NO with superoxide. Peroxynitrite causes the oxidation of sulfhydryls, lipid peroxidation, and RNA and DNA breakage (1,24,58); it reacts with thiols and induces the nitration of tyrosine residues in proteins to form nitrotyrosine, thus altering protein structure and function. In the highly oxidative milieu of reperfused tissue, in addition to peroxynitrite, several other chemical reactions that involve nitrite, hypochlorous acid, and peroxidases can induce tyrosine nitration and contribute to tissue damage (24). The deleterious effects of RNS are mainly related to mitochondrial damage, collapse of the energetic capacity, and the induction of apoptosis by the release of proteins from the mitochondria, and necrosis by lysis of plasma membrane (24,27).

Nitrate and nitrite are stable end-products of NO and can be measured in plasma, serum, urine, and other biologic fluids. Although concentration of these metabolites may be influenced by liver and kidney function, dietary intake of nitrates, or pharmacologic intake of NO donors, the increase in nitrite/nitrate levels in biologic samples can be considered a marker of increased activation of NOS in septic patients, and it correlates with severity of illness and mortality scores (15). High levels of nitrites and nitrates can be also found in shock without sepsis and transplantation, and they are suggestive of an exaggerated proinflammatory response with poor outcome (52).

The role of NO in shock and ischemia and reperfusion injury is not completely known, because several experimental studies using inhibitors of NO synthesis have reported controversial data (18). In an effort to reverse the severe hypotension in septic patients, nonselective pharmacologic NOS inhibitors, which can repress NO production from both the constitutive and the inducible isoforms, have been developed and studied in clinical trials in adult patients. Although treatment with these NOS inhibitors is able to increase mean arterial blood pressure, mortality appears to be increased as well (31,51). Use of iNOS inhibitors has not been tested in the pediatric population.

Therefore, it appears that multiple factors, such as NO concentration, redox status of the cell, and the NO:superoxide radical ratio, determine whether NO serves as a cytoprotective or cytotoxic agent. Certainly, in acute conditions of ischemia, the physiologic release of endothelium-derived NO is important for the regulation of microvascular permeability and the maintenance of local perfusion. Conversely, in sepsis and severe prolonged ischemia and reperfusion, overproduction of NO may mediate deleterious effects.

Decreased Activity of Antioxidant Mechanisms

Under physiologic conditions, cells have a substantial ability to tolerate reactive species by safely metabolizing them to water and other stable molecules through enzymatic and nonenzymatic pathways (40) (see Chapter 18). The enzymatic pathways are catalase and glutathione peroxidase, which coordinate the catalysis of hydrogen peroxide to water, and superoxide dismutase, which facilitates the formation of H_2O_2 from superoxide. The nonenzymatic pathways include intracellular antioxidants, such as vitamins C, E, and β-carotene, ubiquinone, lipoic acid, urate, cysteine, and glutathione (GSH), which serves as a reducing substrate for the enzymatic activity of glutathione peroxidase. Thioredoxin and thioredoxin reductase form an additional redox regulatory system, because they catalyze the

regeneration of antioxidant molecules, such as ubiquinone (Q10), lipoic acid, and ascorbic acid.

However, this orchestrated homeostasis fails when the robust reperfusion-induced generation of reactive species exceeds the cellular antioxidant activity (40). In addition, intracellular levels of GSH decline with a concomitant accumulation of the oxidized and inactive form of glutathione (GSSG). Maladaptive decreases of other nonenzymatic antioxidants may also occur. For example, plasma levels of ascorbate and atrial levels of vitamin E are reduced in patients after cardiopulmonary bypass (6). In cerebrospinal fluid samples from infants and children with severe traumatic brain injury, a progressive compromise of antioxidant defenses has been characterized by ascorbate depletion and decreased glutathione levels, and has been associated with increased free radical–mediated lipid peroxidation (8).

However, oxidative stress and antioxidant capacity in the pediatric age group have not been adequately characterized, because the ability to directly measure oxidative stress within tissues is markedly limited. Furthermore, despite many studies in experimental models of reperfusion injury and the availability of a wide array of antioxidant agents, it is still undetermined whether antioxidant supplementation may have any clinical therapeutic application in ischemia and reperfusion (16,22).

Direct Cytotoxic Effects of Reactive Oxygen Species and Reactive Nitrogen Species

Damage of Macromolecules

ROS and RNS are extremely reactive, and cause direct structural damage of many enzymes, proteins, lipids, and DNA. The most common chemical reactions include the oxidation of sulfhydryl groups and thioethers, as well as the nitration and hydroxylation of aromatic compounds. Modification of these macromolecules can cause the inactivation of critical enzymes and can induce denaturation that renders proteins nonfunctional. For example, tyrosine nitration induced by peroxynitrite or nitrogen derivatives may lead to a dysfunction of superoxide dismutase and cytoskeletal actin (18,27,40). Lipid peroxidation results in the disruption of the cell membrane, as well as the membranes of cellular organelles, and causes the release of such highly cytotoxic products as malondialdehyde. Oxidation of sulfhydryl groups is responsible for the inhibition of critical mitochondrial enzymes of the respiratory chain (1) (Fig. 19.6).

DNA Damage and Activation of Poly(ADP-ribose) Polymerase-1

Another important interaction of ROS and RNS occurs with nucleic acids. Oxidative attack on the deoxyribose moiety will lead to the release of free bases from DNA, generating strand breaks with various sugar modifications and simple abasic sites at which DNA bases are lost. Nitrosative attack will lead to nitrated guanine nucleosides and nucleotides, which may further contribute to oxidative stress via the production of superoxide mediated by various reductases and may disturb or directly modulate various important enzymes, such as guanosine triphosphate (GTP)-binding proteins and cGMP-dependent

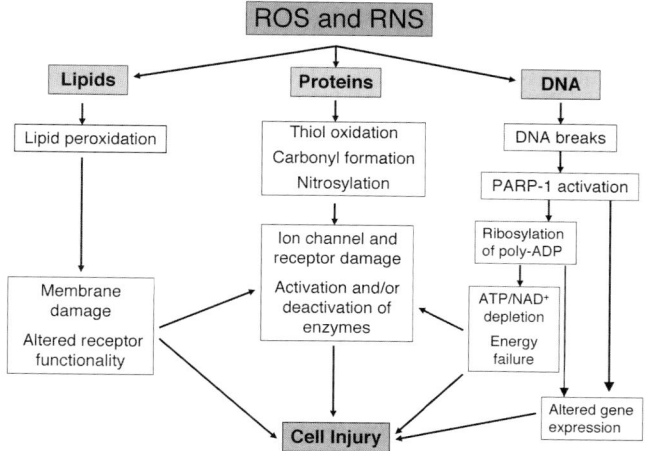

FIGURE 19.6. Direct cellular damage induced by ROS and RNS. ROS and RNS induce oxidation, carbonyl formation, and nitrosylation of lipids, proteins, and DNA. Modification of these macromolecules can cause disruption of the cell membrane, deactivation or activation of critical enzymes, and denaturation of ion pumps or membrane receptors. ROS and RNS also interact with DNA, generating strand breaks with various sugar modifications. In an attempt to repair DNA damage, poly(ADP-ribose) polymerase-1 (PARP-1) is activated. The process of poly(ADP-ribosyl)ation initiates an energy-consuming cycle, which rapidly depletes the intracellular NAD$^+$ and ATP energetic pools and alters gene expression, further enhancing cell injury.

enzymes. Alteration of the genetic material contributes then to the general decline in cellular functions and, ultimately, to death (24).

To maintain genomic stability, the cell employs many different repair pathways to remove DNA damage. Poly(ADP-ribose) polymerase (PARP)-1 is a chromatin-associated nuclear enzyme that recognizes DNA nicks and breaks and possesses DNA repair function. Once activated by the occurrence of DNA breakage, PARP-1 cleaves NAD$^+$ into ADP-ribose and nicotinamide, attaches ADP-ribose to various nuclear proteins and PARP-1 itself, and then extends the initial ADP-ribose group into a nucleic acid–like polymer, poly(ADP)ribose. Although poly(ADP-ribosyl)ation is an attempt by the cell to repair DNA, it appears that this process may be more harmful than beneficial and further amplifies tissue damage. PARP-1, in fact, initiates an energy-consuming cycle that rapidly depletes intracellular NAD$^+$ and ATP energetic pools, slows the rate of glycolysis and mitochondrial respiration, and progresses to a loss of cellular viability, postulated as a *suicide phenomenon* (16). Several experimental reports in rodents have demonstrated that the activation of PARP-1 is a major cytotoxic pathway of tissue injury in different pathologies associated with shock and reperfusion injury, including hemorrhagic shock, cardiopulmonary bypass, sepsis, and myocardial, cerebral, and splanchnic infarction (16,55,58). In addition to the energetic failure, PARP-1 activation and poly(ADP-ribosyl)ation may also cause tissue damage by playing a role in gene expression. Experimental reports have suggested that PARP-1 alters the function of a variety of transcription factors, including the proinflammatory factor nuclear factor (NF)-κB and the cytoprotective heat shock factor-1 (Hsf-1), thus modulating the gene expression of several inflammatory mediators (56,57).

Indirect Cytotoxic Effects of Reactive Oxygen Species and Reactive Nitrogen Species

Activation of Mitogen-Activated Protein Kinases and Phosphatase

In addition to directly injuring cells, ROS and RNS have the potential to induce tissue damage through the regulation of signal transduction pathways that modulate the proinflammatory phenotype of the cell. Because of their reactivity, ROS and RNS induce structural and functional changes within the critical thiol groups or amino acid residues of mitogen-activated protein kinases (MAPKs) and phosphatases, which are important components of an extensive network of signal transduction pathways (54). MAPKs mediate the transduction of extracellular signals from the receptor levels to the nuclear transcription factors (see Chapter 17). These kinases activate each other by sequential steps of phosphorylation, whereas their inactivation is mediated by phosphatases through dephosphorylation. Specifically, ROS and RNS activate cytosolic or membrane-bound enzymes, which then begin sequential phosphorylation and dephosphorylation events. Important oxidant-sensitive kinases in shock and reperfusion injury include the extracellular signal-regulated kinase 1 and 2 (ERK 1/2), c-Jun amino-terminal kinase (JNK), p38 MAPK, and inhibitor κB kinase (IκK). Phosphorylation of ERK, JNK, p38, and IκK activates nuclear proteins and transcription factors, and ultimately regulates the transcription of several genes of inflammatory mediators (54).

Activation of Nuclear Transcription Factors

At the nuclear level, NF-κB is important in the expression of many genes, the proteins of which are involved in the inflammatory response (see Chapter 17). NF-κB is ubiquitously found in all mammalian cells and is usually present in the cytoplasm of the cell in an inactive state bound to an inhibitory protein known as inhibitor κBα (IκBα). A common pathway for the activation of NF-κB occurs when its inhibitor protein IκBα is phosphorylated by the upstream kinase IκK. After IκBα is phosphorylated, a process of proteolytic digestion of this protein is activated. Degradation of IκBα allows NF-κB to migrate to the nucleus, where it activates the transcription of target genes (59).

Specific MAPKs, such as JNK, control the activation of *fos* and *jun* family protooncogenes and their protein products (c-jun, jun-B, jun-D, c-Fos, and others). These "early response protooncogene" products dimerize to form the activator protein (AP)-1, another nuclear transcription factor that is also purportedly regulated by ROS and RNS and involved in the expression of genes of inflammatory mediators (54).

These signaling cascades are rapid, enabling the cells to respond to environmental changes by inducing a prompt production of inflammatory mediators, thus determining the functional outcome in response to stress. Downstream products of NF-κB and AP-1 activation include cell adhesion molecules and inflammatory cytokines (messenger molecules) that are important for leukocyte activation and leukocyte recruitment, tumor necrosis factor (TNF)-α, and NOS (regulator of vascular tone). It is important to note that several of the inflammatory mediators that are regulated by NF-κB (e.g., TNF-α and

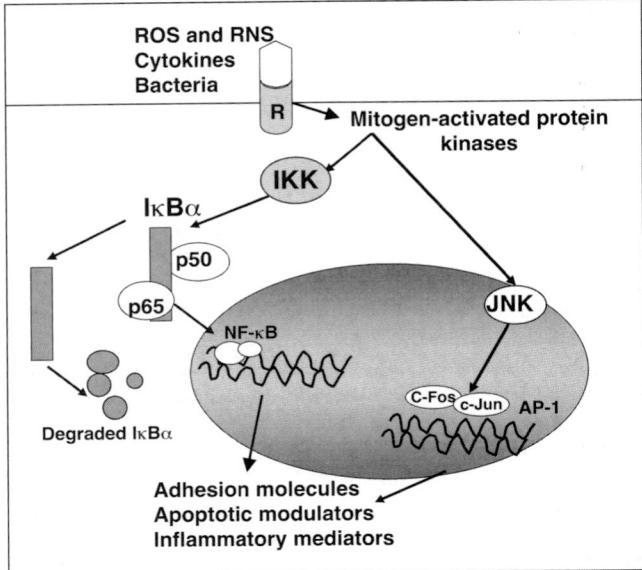

FIGURE 19.7. Activation of transcription by ROS and RNS. ROS, RNS, cytokines, and bacterial products are potent stimuli for the activation of a cascade of mitogen-activated protein kinases. At the downstream of this cascade, the inhibitor κB kinase (IκK) phosphorylates inhibitor κBα (IκBα), allowing its proteolytic degradation. This event unmasks the nuclear factor-κB (NF-κB), which is free to translocate into the nucleus to initiate gene transcription. Similarly, c-Jun aminoterminal kinase (JNK) phosphorylates c-Jun, allowing its dimerization with c-Fos, thus forming the transcription factor activator protein (AP)-1. Activation of both NF-κB and AP-1 induces production of adhesion molecules, apoptotic modulators, and inflammatory mediators, such as cytokines and enzymes.

interleukin [IL]-1) and/or AP-1 can, in turn, further activate these transcription factors, thus creating a self-maintaining inflammatory cycle that increases the severity and duration of the inflammatory response (54,59) (**Fig. 19.7**).

Clinical data suggest a pathologic role for NF-κB in reperfusion injury, sepsis, and multiple organ failure. NF-κB binding has been shown in peripheral leukocytes of septic patients. Increased NF-κB binding activity positively correlated with severity of illness, and it was significantly increased in nonsurvivors, compared with survivors, of septic shock (12,41). On the contrary, resolution of inflammation is associated with low DNA binding of the transcription factor. In patients with acute appendicitis, NF-κB DNA binding was elevated and correlated with the severity of symptoms. This increased activity returned to baseline values within 18 hrs after appendectomy (42). In patients who underwent major vascular surgery, activation of NF-κB in neutrophils was significantly elevated and correlated with a higher incidence of postoperative organ dysfunction in comparison with patients who did not exhibit a marked elevation of NF-κB activation (19). In children who underwent congenital heart surgery on cardiopulmonary bypass, NF-κB nuclear translocation was examined in myocardial tissue samples, and it was found that the myocardial activation of NF-κB and the subsequent inflammatory cascade may contribute to the pathophysiology of congenital heart disease in infants and children (38).

These clinical findings suggest that NF-κB may represent a therapeutic target during shock and reperfusion injury. Numer-

ous reports have demonstrated that pharmacologic inhibitors of NF-κB exert beneficial effects in models of myocardial ischemia and reperfusion injury, hemorrhagic shock, and sepsis (59). However, this potential therapeutic approach hypothesis remains to be investigated in human studies.

Complement System Activation

The complement system is an important pathway of innate immune defense and inflammation. The principal biologic functions include cell lysis of foreign organisms, phagocytic clearance of immune complexes, antigen presentation to lymphocyte, and recruitment of inflammatory cells to the site of injury. The complement system is composed of more than 30 plasma proteins, glycoproteins, and soluble or membrane-bound receptors. Most complement system proteins exist in plasma as inactive precursors that cleave and activate each other in a proteolytic cascade in response to different mechanisms. Three different pathways of activation have been described: *classical*, *alternative*, and *lectin-binding* (**Fig. 19.8**). The classical pathway is initiated by antigen–antibody complexes and/or inflammatory proteins, such as C-reactive protein and serum amyloid protein. The alternative pathway is initiated by surface molecules that contain carbohydrates and lipids, such as bacteria, fungal yeast cells, and some parasite surface molecules. The lectin-binding pathway is initiated by the binding of mannose-binding lectin protein (MBL), resulting in activation of MLB-associated serine-proteases (MASPs). Complement system components are numbered in the order in which they were discovered, which is almost the same as the order in which they function in the activation cascade. Although the stimulating factors for each pathway are distinct, each one has a similar terminal sequence that creates the active factors C5a and the complex C5b–C59, also known as the *membrane attack complex* (MAC), which is believed to mediate tissue injury. C5a is one of the most proinflammatory peptides with pleiotropic functions. Upon binding to high-affinity receptors, such as the C5aR receptor on neutrophils, monocytes, and macrophages, C5a serves as a powerful *chemoattractant* for these cells and promotes their activation, leading to the oxidative burst and release of lysosomal enzymes and proinflammatory cytokines (23). C5a can also bind to specific C5aR receptor in epithelial cells and activate the release of inflammatory mediators, such as cytokines. MAC is the *killer* molecule of the complement system. Its main function is to disrupt the phospholipid bilayer of target cells, leading to cell lysis and death by the formation of transmembrane channels. MAC also has other important functions, which it shares with C5a. They both activate the coagulation pathway, induce expression of adhesion molecules on endothelial cells, and decrease the release of NO (causing vasoconstriction), thus amplifying the loss of vascular homeostasis and endothelial dysfunction (23,25). In addition, the classical, alternative, and lectin-binding pathways have as their by-products a number of *anaphylatoxins* and *opsonins*. Anaphylatoxins cause increased vascular permeability, smooth muscle contraction, and mast cell degranulation. Complement system fragments called *opsonins* adhere to microorganisms and promote leukocyte chemoattraction, antigen binding, and phagocytosis, and the activation of macrophage and neutrophil-killing mechanisms. Under physiologic conditions, numerous inhibitory molecules are present in the plasma

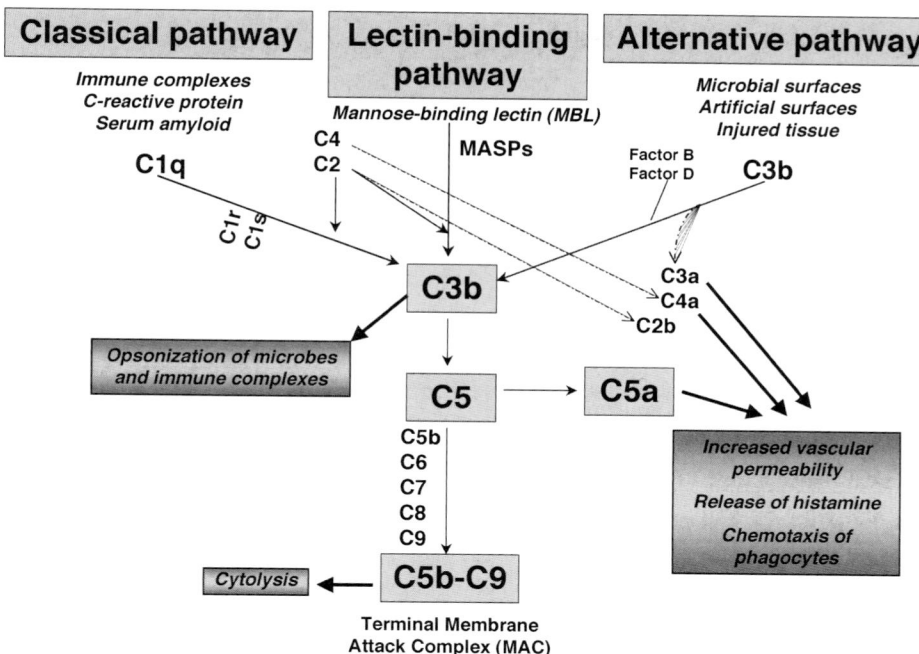

FIGURE 19.8. Activation of complement system. Three different pathways activate the complement system during shock and reperfusion: classical, lectin, and alternative pathway. The classical pathway is initiated by antigen–antibody complexes or inflammatory proteins, such as C-reactive protein and serum amyloid protein. The lectin pathway is initiated by the binding of mannose-binding lectin protein (MBL), resulting in activation of MLB-associated serine-proteases (MASPs). The alternative pathway is initiated by surface molecules that contain carbohydrates and lipids, such as bacterial, fungal yeast cell, and some parasite surface molecules. The terminal common step of these pathways is the activation of C5a and the complex C5b–C59, also known as the *membrane attack complex* (MAC), which mediates tissue injury. Other by-products of the complement cascade, *anaphylatoxins* and *opsonins*, contribute to tissue injury by facilitating phagocytosis and by increasing vascular permeability, smooth muscle contraction, and mast cell degranulation.

(serum proteases and complement system inhibitors) and on the endothelial surface (decay accelerating factor and membrane cofactor protein), which protect the host against complement system injury (23,25).

Data from numerous experimental animal studies of ischemia and reperfusion injury in different organ systems, as well as from clinical studies, support the concept that activation of the complement system is a crucial pathogenetic event of tissue injury (5,23). All three pathways are activated in ischemia and reperfusion injury and seem to be involved in an organ-dependent manner (25). Complement system activation has been demonstrated in myocardial infarction, and in ischemia of the intestine, hind limb, kidney, liver, hemorrhagic shock, and sepsis. During cardiopulmonary bypass procedure, the contact of blood with the artificial surfaces of the bypass equipment can also activate complement system proteins (25). In addition, endothelial dysfunction during reperfusion may alter the protective mechanism mediated by the complement system inhibitors, thus contributing to its exaggerated activation.

Numerous experimental studies have demonstrated beneficial effects of complement system inhibition in ischemia and reperfusion–induced injury (10). However, only a few clinical trials have been conducted thus far. Two recent human clinical studies tested a novel C5 complement system monoclonal antibody, pexelizumab, combined with thrombolytic therapy (34) or angioplasty (21) after myocardial infarction. No significant effects of the C5 antibody against preexisting myocardial infarcts were found in either trial. However, a 70% reduction in 90-day mortality was observed when patients were treated with a bolus and continued infusion of pexelizumab (21). Interestingly, clinical benefit was not related to infarct size, extent of ST elevation, or evidence of angiographic or electrocardiographic reperfusion (4). TP-10, a recombinant soluble complement receptor type 1 (sCR1), has been developed for the potential treatment of reperfusion injury (following surgery, ischemic disease, and organ transplantation), organ rejection,

acute inflammatory injury to the lungs, and autoimmune diseases (46). A phase I/II trial of TP-10 conducted in 15 children under 12 months of age who were undergoing cardiac surgery for congenital heart defects showed that TP10 administration was safe and appeared to decrease the complement system activation induced by cardiopulmonary bypass and to protect vascular function (29). Although unconfirmed, these clinical reports suggest that strategies to inhibit the complement system pathway may offer new therapeutic approaches to manage critically ill patients.

Endothelial Dysfunction

As a continuous monolayer on the luminal surfaces of both arteries and veins, the endothelium plays an essential role in the homeostasis of coagulation, fibrinolysis, angiogenesis, and vascular tone. In ischemia and reperfusion injury, the endothelium is one of the first organs to demonstrate signs of dysfunction and modification. As a result of oxidative stress and reduced bioavailability of the constitutive production of NO, vasodilation is impaired and vascular permeability increases, leading to edema formation and enhancement of interstitial pressure. When these detrimental changes occur in capillaries and arterioles, the local circulation of blood may be impaired, a phenomenon known as *no-reflow*. Changes in endothelial adhesiveness also occur, allowing the recruitment of circulating leukocytes from the bloodstream into the ischemic tissue. This event plays an important physiologic role in the resolution of the damage, as leukocytes participate in the destruction of foreign antigens and in the remodeling of injured tissue. However, the recruitment and transmigration of leukocytes may further compromise the integrity of the endothelial barrier and augment damage to parenchymal cells. Activated leukocytes, indeed, release proteolytic enzymes (e.g., elastase, collagenase, cathepepsin, hyaluronidase) and proinflammatory mediators and augment the oxidative burden by producing ROS and

RNS. Furthermore, leukocytes physically plug postcapillary venules and small arterioles, thereby contributing to the no-reflow phenomenon and exacerbating the ischemic damage. Additionally, alteration of the endothelial surface and aggregation and activation of platelets trigger dysregulation of the coagulation and fibrinolytic systems (48).

Recruitment and Transmigration of Leukocytes

____The emigration of circulating leukocytes from the blood into the inflamed tissue involves a sequence of three complex steps: rolling, firm adhesion, and transmigration of leukocytes. This multistep process is coordinated by endothelial adhesion molecules, which are expressed on the endothelial surface and recognized by specific receptors on the leukocyte membrane (**Fig. 19.9**). Three families of adhesion molecules have been identified: the selectins, the immunoglobulin gene superfamily, and the integrins (35).

The initial interaction between leukocytes and endothelium is transient, resulting in the *rolling* of leukocytes along the wall of postcapillary venules at a very slow velocity distinctly below that of flowing blood. The selectin family mediates this rolling process and is composed of three members named according to the cells in which they were originally discovered: P-selectin (platelets and endothelial cells), E-selectin (endothelial cells), and L-selectin (leukocytes). P-selectin is preformed and stored in α-granules of platelets and Weibel-Palade bod-

ies of endothelial cells. Therefore, it is rapidly translocated to the cell surface after exposure to ROS and RNS, thrombin, histamine, or complement. E-selectin is expressed on the endothelial cells after stimulation with proinflammatory cytokines (TNF-α and IL-1) several hours following ischemia and reperfusion injury. The corresponding ligands for selectins on the surface of the leukocyte are sialylated Lewis^x and A blood-group antigens. In addition to endothelial cells, leukocytes also express a selectin (L-selectin), which binds to a specific sulfated Lewis^x ligand on endothelial cells (35).

The rolling leukocytes then become activated by local factors generated by the endothelium, resulting in their arrest and *firm adhesion* to the vessel wall. The activating factors include cytokines, chemoattractants (e.g., leukotriene B4, C5a, platelet activating factor), and chemoattractive chemokines, which bind to and activate integrins on leukocytes. Finally, this firm attachment allows the *transmigration* or *diapedesis* of the leukocyte across the endothelial monolayer and basement membrane into the tissues (35).

Firm adhesion and transmigration are mediated by the interaction of β_2 integrins (also known as CD11/CD18) and β_1 integrins on the surface of leukocytes, with immunoglobulin gene superfamily members expressed by endothelium (35). The intercellular adhesion molecules (ICAMs), ICAM-1, ICAM-2, and ICAM-3; vascular cellular adhesion molecule (VCAM)-1 (VCAM-1); and platelet-endothelial cell adhesion molecule (PECAM) are members of the immunoglobulin superfamily. ICAM-1 is constitutively expressed at low levels on the endothelium and is responsible for the firm adhesion of

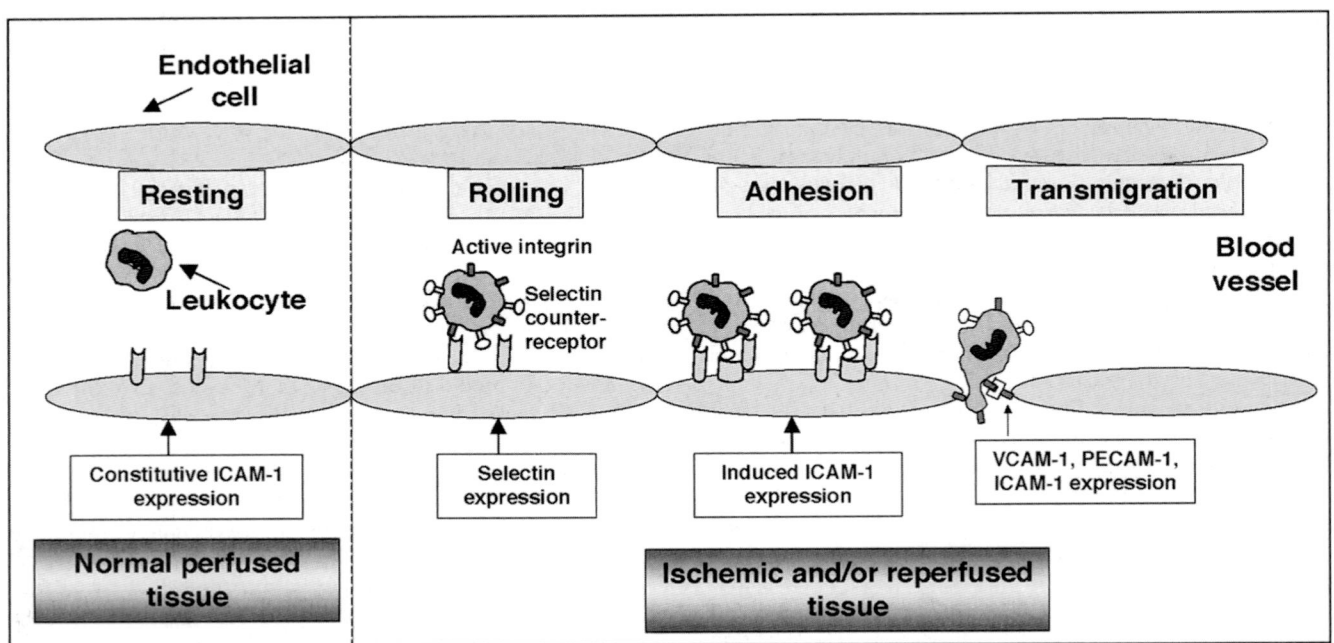

FIGURE 19.9. Leukocyte migration across the endothelial barrier. During the resting state, no interaction occurs between leukocytes and the endothelium, which expresses low levels of intercellular adhesion molecule (ICAM)-1. During ischemia and reperfusion, the mechanisms of transendothelial migration can be regarded as having three steps: rolling, adhesion, and transmigration. During the *rolling* phase, selectins are expressed on the surface of endothelial cells and corresponding ligands for selectins are expressed on leukocytes, leading to a slowing and attachment of circulating leukocytes to the vessel wall. During the *adhesion* and *transmigration* phases, the interaction of β_2 and β_1 integrins on the surface of leukocytes with immunoglobulin gene superfamily members, such as ICAM-1, VCAM-1, and PECAM-1, allows firm adhesion of leukocytes and their transmigration into the parenchyma.

neutrophils. Its surface expression is further enhanced during inflammation on endothelial cells after exposure to oxidants or cytokines (35). In addition to being present on endothelial cells, ICAM-1 is also present on leukocytes, epithelial cells, cardiomyocytes, and fibroblasts, thus contributing to the tissue margination of leukocytes (53). The CD11/CD18 family of integrins is the counter-receptor for ICAM-1 and ICAM-2. VCAM-1 is expressed only after exposure to inflammatory mediators or cytokines on endothelial cells, binds to the integrin very late activation antigen-4 (VLA4 group/β_1 integrin) that is found on leukocytes, and appears particularly important in wound healing (35).

As a consequence of the modification of endothelial adhesiveness, platelets also accumulate in the vessels, resulting in further impairment of microcirculation and contributing to the prothrombotic phenotype of the endothelium. Circulating platelets roll and adhere to the endothelium or subendothelial matrix using similar adhesion molecules and release substances that are able to cause further chemotaxis and migration of circulating leukocytes. This process is particularly relevant in the brain microvasculature, where shear forces are high and adhesion molecule expression is low, and platelets may play an important role as a bridge between the leukocytes and endothelium (30).

After being expressed on the cell surface, adhesion molecules are rapidly shed into the bloodstream. The detection of these circulating adhesion molecules has been employed as a sensitive marker of endothelium dysfunction, and has been widely reported in patients with sepsis or ischemic conditions. For example, increased blood levels of ICAM-1 in septic adults correlate well with the severity of inflammation and the course of sepsis (i.e., MODS and death) (44,49). In pediatric heart transplant recipients, systemic expression of adhesion molecules and plasma coagulation markers correlates with the occurrence of transplant coronary artery disease and/or rejection (26). Similarly, the upregulation and expression of soluble P-selectin indicates neutrophil activation in children who undergo cardiopulmonary bypass and correlates significantly with surgery time, aortic cross-clamping time, inotropic support, postoperative Pediatric Risk of Mortality score, hypotension, and tachycardia (32).

Because the abnormal sequestration of leukocytes is a central component in the development of reperfusion injury, therapeutic strategies that employ the use of antibodies raised against adhesion molecules have been attempted to inhibit the inflammatory response. Experimental studies in a number of animal models of myocardial, splanchnic, cerebral, and hepatic reperfusion damage after ischemia have largely been successful (3). In the clinical setting, however, the few studies that have been conducted to test the efficacy of these agents in organ transplantation, hemorrhagic shock, and myocardial infarction have produced unsatisfactory results (3,7,17,45,53).

CONCLUSIONS AND FUTURE DIRECTIONS

Several mechanisms cooperate in a complementary and synergistic manner in the pathophysiology of ischemia and reperfusion injury. The knowledge of the precise sequence of these biochemical and molecular events has enormous clinical rele-

vance, because it would imply the possibility of improving recovery using specific interventions that would target these cellular pathways. As described throughout the chapter, most basic science studies, which have been conducted in experimental animals, have reported that the use of antioxidants, antibodies against adhesion molecules, inhibition of complement factors, or inhibition of PARP-1 and NF-κB, may, indeed, prevent or delay cell death. Despite these many studies, as yet, no definitive clinical indications have been revealed for the application of these novel agents in shock and reperfusion injury in humans. Multiple clinical trials have attempted to alter the progression of the inflammatory response in adult patients. Although successful progress in some clinical trials has been reported, other novel strategies have failed. Reasons for these equivocal results may include individual injury patterns, inappropriate timing of drug administration, and suboptimal drug levels at the target site. In addition, the study protocols have focused on single mechanisms only, whereas the inflammatory network of reperfusion is more complex, including several concomitant and interconnected pathways. In the PICU, novel therapeutic drug protocols are further limited by the paucity of information related to these agents in the pediatric population. In the future, a better understanding of the pathologic mechanisms at the site of injury will identify exact primary targets for drug interventions. In addition, progress in diagnostic tools for the monitoring of inflammatory status may provide valuable information for the appropriate timing and management of critically ill patients.

KEY POINTS

- Ischemia results from a dramatic reduction of oxygen supply to tissues and/or organs and rapidly results in cell metabolic derangement, molecular alterations, and dysfunction sequelae.
- Timely reperfusion of the ischemic tissue is the mandatory treatment of patients with clinical conditions of ischemia. However, reperfusion initiates a cascade of events that causes additional cell injury, a phenomenon called *reperfusion injury.*
- The production of excessive quantities of ROS and RNS is an important mechanism of reperfusion injury. These reactive species mediate tissue injury by two main mechanisms: directly, by inducing damage of important cellular macromolecules and indirectly, by activating signal transduction pathways.
- As highly reactive species, ROS and RNS induce the alteration of the structure and function of many enzymes, proteins, lipids, and DNA.
- ROS and RNS initiate signaling cascades that result in a prompt production of inflammatory mediators, such as cytokines, adhesion molecules, chemokines, and metabolic enzymes, thus determining the functional outcome of the cell in response to ischemia.
- The complement system is activated in an attempt to induce lysis of foreign organisms and to promote phagocytic clearance of immune complexes and the recruitment of inflammatory cells at the site of injury. However, this system can amplify endothelial dysfunction and the parenchymal damage during reperfusion.

- Endothelial dysfunction is an early event of reperfusion and is triggered by the endothelial generation of ROS and RNS. Endothelial dysfunction is characterized by the development of a procoagulant phenotype, loss of vascular responsiveness to vasodilator and vasoconstrictor agents, increased vascular permeability, and adhesiveness to platelets and leukocytes.

- In the early phase of shock and reperfusion, leukocytes are present mainly in the intravascular space (attached to the endothelium), and they play an important role in endothelial injury. At later stages, leukocytes migrate into the tissues and exacerbate parenchymal damage.

- The production of ROS and RNS, endothelial injury, activation of the complement system, release of neutrophil-attractive factors, and leukocyte infiltration (leading to further production of reactive species and proteolytic enzymes) constitute a vicious cycle, which is ultimately responsible for parenchymal injury.

- Current experimental research has raised the exciting prospect that pharmacologic intervention aimed at interrupting the various levels of the ischemia–reperfusion injury cycle may ameliorate cell dysfunction and prevent death. However, large clinical trials are necessary to determine whether these novel therapeutic interventions may be beneficial to the patient.

References

1. Alvarez B, Radi R. Peroxynitrite reactivity with amino acids and proteins. *Amino Acids* 2003;25:295–311.
2. American Heart Association. 2005 American Heart Association guidelines for cardiopulmonary resuscitation and emergency cardiovascular care of pediatric and neonatal patients: Pediatric advanced life support. *Pediatrics* 2006;117:E1005–28.
3. Anaya-Prado R, Toledo-Pereyra LH, Lentsch AB, et al. Ischemia/reperfusion injury. *J Surg Res* 2002;105:248–58.
4. Armstrong PW, Mahaffey KW, Chang WC, et al. Concerning the mechanism of pexelizumab's benefit in acute myocardial infarction. *Am Heart J* 2006;151:787–90.
5. Arumugam TV, Shiels IA, Woodruff TM, et al. The role of the complement system in ischemia-reperfusion injury. *Shock* 2004;21:401–9.
6. Ballmer PE, Reinhart WH, Jordan P, et al. Depletion of plasma vitamin C but not of vitamin E in response to cardiac operations. *J Thorac Cardiovasc Surg* 1994;108:311–20.
7. Baran KW, Nguyen M, McKendall GR, et al. Double-blind, randomized trial of an anti-CD18 antibody in conjunction with recombinant tissue plasminogen activator for acute myocardial infarction: Limitation of myocardial infarction following thrombolysis in acute myocardial infarction (LIMIT AMI) study. *Circulation* 2001;104:2778–83.
8. Bayir H, Kagan VE, Tyurina YY, et al. Assessment of antioxidant reserves and oxidative stress in cerebrospinal fluid after severe traumatic brain injury in infants and children. *Pediatr Res* 2002;51:571–8.
9. Bernardi P, Krauskopf A, Basso E, et al. The mitochondrial permeability transition from in vitro artifact to disease target. *FEBS J* 2006;273: 2077–99.
10. Bhole D, Stahl GL. Therapeutic potential of targeting the complement cascade in critical care medicine. *Crit Care Med* 2003;31(Suppl 1):S97–104.
11. Bian K, Murad F. Nitric oxide: Biogeneration, regulation, and relevance to human diseases. *Front Biosci* 2003;8:D264–78.
12. Bohrer H, Qiu F, Zimmermann T, et al. Role of NF-κB in the mortality of sepsis. *J Clin Invest* 1997;100:972–85.
13. Brass CA. Xanthine oxidase and reperfusion injury: Major player or minor irritant? *Hepatology* 1995;21:1757–60.
14. Bulger EM, Maier RV. Antioxidants in critical illness. *Arch Surg* 2001;136: 1201–7.
15. Carcillo JA, Fields AI, American College of Critical Care Medicine Task Force Committee Members. Clinical practice parameters for hemodynamic support of pediatric and neonatal patients in septic shock. *Crit Care Med* 2002;30:1365–78.
16. Chiarugi A. Poly(ADP-ribose) polymerase: Killer or conspirator? The "suicide hypothesis" revisited. *Trends Pharmacol Sci* 2002;23:122–9.
17. Faxon DP, Gibbons RJ, Chronos NA, et al. The effect of blockade of the CD11/CD18 integrin receptor on infarct size in patients with acute myocardial infarction treated with direct angioplasty: The results of the HALT-MI study. *J Am Coll Cardiol* 2002;40:1199–204.
18. Ferdinandy P, Schulz R. Nitric oxide, superoxide, and peroxynitrite in myocardial ischaemia-reperfusion injury and preconditioning. *Br J Pharmacol* 2003;138:532–43.
19. Foulds S, Galustian C, Mansfield AO, et al. Transcription factor NF-κB expression and postsurgical organ dysfunction. *Ann Surg* 2001;233:70–8.
20. Friedl HP, Smith DJ, Till GO, et al. Ischemia-reperfusion in humans: Appearance of xanthine oxidase activity. *Am J Pathol* 1990;136:491–5.
21. Granger CB, Mahaffey KW, Weaver WD, et al. Pexelizumab, an anti-C5 complement antibody, as adjunctive therapy to primary percutaneous coronary intervention in acute myocardial infarction: The complement inhibition in myocardial infarction treated with angioplasty (COMMA) trial. *Circulation* 2003;108:1184–90.
22. Granot E, Kohen R. Oxidative stress in childhood – in health and disease states. *Clin Nutr* 2004;23:3–11.
23. Guo RF, Ward PA. Role of C5a in inflammatory responses. *Annu Rev Immunol* 2005;23:821–52.
24. Halliwell B. Free radicals, proteins and DNA: Oxidative damage versus redox regulation. *Biochem Soc Trans* 1996;24:1023–7.
25. Hart ML, Walsh MC, Stahl GL. Initiation of complement activation following oxidative stress: *In vitro* and *in vivo* observations. *Mol Immunol* 2004;41:165–71.
26. Hilgendorff A, Kraemer U, Afsharian M, et al. Value of soluble adhesion molecules and plasma coagulation markers in assessing transplant coronary artery disease in pediatric heart transplant recipients. *Pediatr Transplant* 2006;10:434–40.
27. Ischiropoulos H. Biological selectivity and functional aspects of protein tyrosine nitration. *Biochem Biophys Res Commun* 2003;305:776–83.
28. Kinsella JP, Abman SH. Inhaled nitric oxide therapy in children. *Paediatr Respir Rev* 2005;6:190–8.
29. Li JS, Sanders SP, Perry AE, et al. Pharmacokinetics and safety of TP10, soluble complement receptor 1, in infants undergoing cardiopulmonary bypass. *Am Heart J* 2004;147:173–80.
30. Liu L, Kubes P. Molecular mechanisms of leukocyte recruitment: Organ-specific mechanisms of action. *Thromb Haemost* 2003;89:213–20.
31. Lopez A, Lorente JA, Steingrub J, et al. Multiple-center, randomized, placebo-controlled, double-blind study of the nitric oxide synthase inhibitor 546C88: Effect on survival in patients with septic shock. *Crit Care Med* 2004;32:21–30.
32. Lotan D, Prince T, Dagan O, et al. Soluble P-selectin and the postoperative course following cardiopulmonary bypass in children. *Paediatr Anaesth* 2001;11:303–8.
33. Ma XL, Weyrich AS, Lefer DJ, et al. Diminished basal nitric oxide release after myocardial ischemia and reperfusion promotes neutrophil adherence to coronary endothelium. *Circ Res* 1993;72:403–12.
34. Mahaffey KW, Granger CB, Nicolau JC, et al. Effect of pexelizumab, an anti-C5 complement antibody, as adjunctive therapy to fibrinolysis in acute myocardial infarction: The COMPlement inhibition in myocardial infarction treated with thromboLYtics (COMPLY) trial. *Circulation* 2003;108: 1176–83.
35. Malik AB, Lo SK. Vascular endothelial adhesion molecules and tissue inflammation. *Pharmacol Rev* 1996;48:213–29.
36. Massion PB, Feron O, Dessy C, et al. Nitric oxide and cardiac function: Ten years after, and continuing. *Circ Res* 2003;93:388–98.
37. Meneshian A, Bulkley GB. The physiology of endothelial xanthine oxidase: From urate catabolism to reperfusion injury to inflammatory signal transduction. *Microcirculation* 2002;9:161–75.
38. Mou SS, Haudek SB, Lequier L, et al. Myocardial inflammatory activation in children with congenital heart disease. *Crit Care Med* 2002;30: 827–32.
39. Nemeth I, Boda D. Xanthine oxidase activity and blood glutathione redox ratio in infants and children with septic shock syndrome. *Intensive Care Med* 2001;27:216–21.
40. Nordberg J, Arner ES. Reactive oxygen species, antioxidants, and the mammalian thioredoxin system. *Free Radic Biol Med* 2001;31:1287–312.
41. Paterson RL, Galley HF, Dhillon JK, et al. Increased nuclear factor ?B activation in critically ill patients who die. *Crit Care Med* 2000;28:1047–51.
42. Pennington C, Dunn J, Li C, et al. Nuclear factor-κB activation in acute appendicitis: A molecular marker for extent of disease? *Am Surg* 2000;66: 914–8.
43. Pesonen EJ, Linder N, Raivio KO, et al. Circulating xanthine oxidase and neutrophil activation during human liver transplantation. *Gastroenterology* 1998;114:1009–15.
44. Reinhart K, Bayer O, Brunkhorst F, et al. Markers of endothelial damage in organ dysfunction and sepsis. *Crit Care Med* 2002;30:S302–12.
45. Rhee P, Morris J, Durham R, et al. Recombinant humanized monoclonal antibody against CD18 (rhuMAb CD18) in traumatic hemorrhagic shock: Results of a phase II clinical trial. Traumatic Shock Group. *J Trauma* 2000; 49:611–20.
46. Rioux P. TP-10 (AVANT Immunotherapeutics). *Curr Opin Investig Drugs* 2001;2:364–71.

47. Schulz R, Kelm M, Heusch G. Nitric oxide in myocardial ischemia/reperfusion injury. *Cardiovasc Res* 2004;61:402–13.
48. Seal JB, Gewertz BL. Vascular dysfunction in ischemia-reperfusion injury. *Ann Vasc Surg* 2005;19:572–84.
49. Sessler C, Windsor A, Schwartz M. Circulating ICAM-1 is increased in septic shock. *Am J Respir Crit Care Med* 1995;151:1420–7.
50. Taegtmeyer H, King LM, Jones BE. Energy substrate metabolism, myocardial ischemia, and targets for pharmacotherapy. *Am J Cardiol* 1998;82: K54–60.
51. Watson D, Grover R, Anzueto A, et al. Cardiovascular effects of the nitric oxide synthase inhibitor NG-methyl-L-arginine hydrochloride (546C88) in patients with septic shock: Results of a randomized, double-blind, placebo-controlled multicenter study (study no. 144–002). *Crit Care Med* 2004;32:13–20.
52. Wong HR, Carcillo JA, Burckart G, et al. Nitric oxide production in critically ill patients. *Arch Dis Child* 1996;74:482–9.
53. Yonekawa K, Harlan JM. Targeting leukocyte integrins in human diseases. *J Leukoc Biol* 2005;77:129–40.
54. Yoshizumi M, Tsuchiya K, Tamaki T. Signal transduction of reactive oxygen species and mitogen-activated protein kinases in cardiovascular disease. *J Med Invest* 2001;48:11–24.
55. Zingarelli B. Importance of poly (ADP-ribose) polymerase activation in myocardial reperfusion injury. In: Szabó C, ed. *Cell Death: The Role of Poly(ADP-ribose) Polymerase.* Boca Raton: CRC Press LLC; 2000: 41–60.
56. Zingarelli B, Hake PW, O'Connor M, et al. Absence of poly(ADP-ribose) polymerase-1 alters nuclear factor-κB activation and gene expression of apoptosis regulators after reperfusion injury. *Mol Med* 2003;9:143–53.
57. Zingarelli B, Hake PW, O'Connor M, et al. Differential regulation of activator protein-1 and heat shock factor-1 in myocardial ischemia and reperfusion injury: Role of poly(ADP-ribose) polymerase-1. *Am J Physiol Heart Circ Physiol* 2004;286:H1408–15.
58. Zingarelli B, O'Connor M, Wong H, et al. Peroxynitrite-mediated DNA strand breakage activates poly-adenosine diphosphate ribosyl synthetase and causes cellular energy depletion in macrophages stimulated with bacterial lipopolysaccharide. *J Immunol* 1996;156:350–8.
59. Zingarelli B, Sheehan M, Wong HR. Nuclear factor-κB as a therapeutic target in critical care medicine. *Crit Care Med* 2003;31:S105–11.

CHAPTER 20 ■ PHARMACOLOGY

ATHENA F. ZUPPA • JEFFREY S. BARRETT

The word *pharmacology* is derived from the Greek "pharmacon," or drug, and "logos," or science. It is more formally defined as the study of how chemical substances interact with living systems. If these substances have medicinal properties, they are typically referred to as *pharmaceuticals*. Pharmacology, then, encompasses drug composition, drug properties, interactions, toxicology, and desirable effects that can be used in therapy of diseases. Underlying the discipline of pharmacology are the fields of pharmacokinetics (PK) and pharmacodynamics (PD), which focus on the movement of the various molecular entities contained within a pharmaceutical as it traverses bodily space and the actions of the active moieties once they arrive at the intended physiologic site within the body. Each of these disciplines can be further defined by the underlying processes that dictate specific pathways (e.g., absorption, distribution, metabolism, elimination). Hence, pharmacology is essential to our understanding of how drugs work and how to guide their administration.

Pediatric pharmacotherapy can be challenging due to developmental changes that may alter drug kinetics, pathophysiologic differences that may alter pharmacodynamics, disease etiologies that may differ from those of adults, and other factors that may result in great variation in safety and efficacy outcomes. The situation becomes more convoluted when one considers critically ill children and the paucity of well-controlled pediatric clinical trials in this vulnerable population. Caregivers who prescribe medications to critically ill children must have some understanding of the basic processes that govern the current dosing recommendations for their patients. In many situations, understanding the source and nature of the data used to support such guidance is helpful from the standpoint of managing expectations of patient response to pharmacotherapy and considering whether dosing modifications should be made. Our comfort in using drugs in critically ill children is often based on the populations previously studied (adults, mainstream pediatric patients, etc.) and the knowledge gained from previous experience.

A review of the pharmacologic principles that generally guide pharmacotherapy is provided in this chapter, with a focus on specific topics relevant to the research and development of pharmaceuticals in critically ill children. In addition, the current knowledge on dosing medications commonly prescribed for critically ill children is reviewed.

SCIENTIFIC FOUNDATIONS

Pharmacokinetics

Absorption

Absorption is the process of drug transfer from its site of administration to the bloodstream. The rate and efficiency of absorption depend on the route of administration. For intravenous (IV) administration, absorption is complete; the total dose reaches the systemic circulation. Drugs administered enterally may be absorbed by either passive diffusion or active transport.

Bioavailability

The *bioavailability* (F) of a drug is defined by the fraction of the administered dose that reaches the systemic circulation. If a drug is administered intravenously, the bioavailability is 100% and F = 1.0. When drugs are administered by routes other than IV, the bioavailability is usually <100%. Bioavailability is reduced by incomplete absorption, first-pass metabolism, and distribution into other tissues.

Distribution

The volume of distribution (Vd) is a hypothetical volume of fluid through which a drug is dispersed. A drug rarely disperses solely into the water compartments of the body. Instead, most drugs disperse to several compartments, including adipose tissue, and bind to plasma proteins. The total volume into which a drug disperses is called the *apparent volume of distribution*. This volume is not a physiologic space, but rather a conceptual parameter. It relates the total amount of drug (Drug) in the body to the concentration of drug (C_p) in the blood or plasma:

$$Vd = Drug/C_p \qquad [20.1]$$

Figure 20.1 represents the fate of a hypothetical drug after IV administration. After administration, a maximal plasma concentration is achieved, and the drug is immediately distributed. The plasma concentration then decreases over time. This initial phase is called the *α-phase* of drug distribution, in which the decline in plasma concentration reflects the distribution of the drug. Once a drug is distributed, it undergoes metabolism and elimination. The second phase is called the *β-phase*, in which the decline in plasma concentration reflects drug metabolism and clearance. In equations, the terms A and B are intercepts with the Y axis. The extrapolation of the β-phase defines B. The dotted line is generated by subtracting the extrapolated line from the original concentration line. This second line defines α and A. The serum concentration (C) can be determined using the formula:

$$C = Ae^{-\alpha t} + Be^{-\beta t} \qquad [20.2]$$

The distribution and elimination half-lives can be determined by equations 20.3 and 20.4, respectively (10,11):

$$t_{1/2\alpha} = 0.693/\alpha \qquad [20.3]$$

and

$$t_{1/2\beta} = 0.693/\beta \qquad [20.4]$$

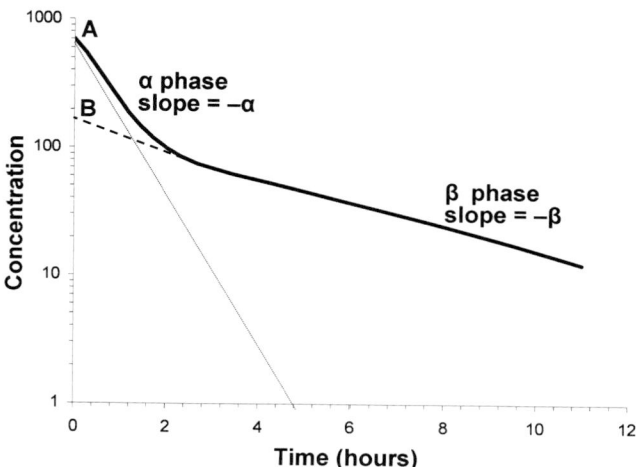

FIGURE 20.1. Semi-logarithmic plot of concentration versus time after an IV administration of a drug that follows two-compartment pharmacokinetics.

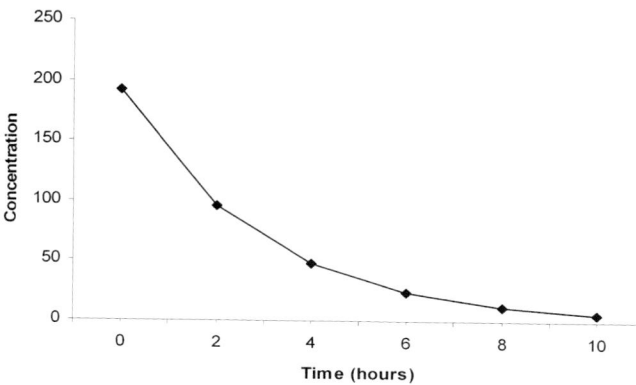

FIGURE 20.2. Concentration versus time profile of a drug demonstrating first-order elimination.

For drugs in which distribution is homogenous along the varied physiologic spaces, the distinction between the α and β phases may be subtle and, essentially, a single phase best describes the decline in drug concentration.

Metabolism

Overview. The metabolic transformation of drugs is catalyzed by enzymes, and most reactions follow Michaelis Menten kinetics:

$$V = [(V_{max})(C)/Km] + (C) \qquad [20.5]$$

where

V is the rate of drug metabolism
C is the drug concentration
Km is the Michaelis Menten constant.

In most situations, the drug concentration is much less than Km, and Equation 20.5 simplifies to

$$V = (V_{max})(C)/Km \qquad [20.6]$$

In this case, the rate of drug metabolism is directly proportional to the concentration of free drug, and follows first-order kinetics. A constant percentage of the drug is metabolized over time, and the rate of elimination is proportional to the amount of drug in the body. Most drugs used in the clinical setting are eliminated in this manner. The concentration time curve of drug that follows first-order elimination is represented in **Figure 20.2**. A semi-logarithmic plot results in a straight line (**Fig. 20.3**).

A few drugs, such as aspirin, ethanol, and phenytoin, are used at higher doses in certain clinical scenarios, resulting in higher plasma concentrations than would be seen at standard doses. In these situations, C is much greater than Km, and Equation 20.5 reduces to:

$$V = (V_{max})(C)/(C) + V_{max} \qquad [20.7]$$

The enzyme system becomes saturated by a high free-drug concentration, and the rate of metabolism is constant over time. This condition is called *zero-order kinetics*, and a constant amount of drug is metabolized per unit time. A large increase in serum concentration can result from a small increase in dose for drugs that follow zero-order elimination. A plot of concentration versus time will result in a straight line (**Fig. 20.4**). A semi-logarithmic plot of concentration versus time demonstrates a convex line (**Fig. 20.5**).

Phase I and Phase II Biotransformation

The liver is the principal organ of drug metabolism. Other tissues that display considerable drug metabolic activity include the gastrointestinal tract, lungs, skin, and kidneys. Following oral administration, many drugs are absorbed intact from the small intestine and transported to the liver via the portal system, where they are metabolized. This process is called *first-pass metabolism* and may greatly limit the bioavailability of orally administered drugs.

In general, all metabolic reactions can be classified as either phase I or phase II biotransformations. Phase I reactions usually convert the parent drug to a polar metabolite by introducing or unmasking a more polar site (e.g., –OH, –NH$_2$). If phase I metabolites are sufficiently polar, they may be readily excreted. However, many phase I metabolites undergo a subsequent reaction in which endogenous substances, such as glucuronic acid, sulfuric acid, or an amino acid, combine with the metabolite to form a highly polar conjugate. Many drugs undergo these

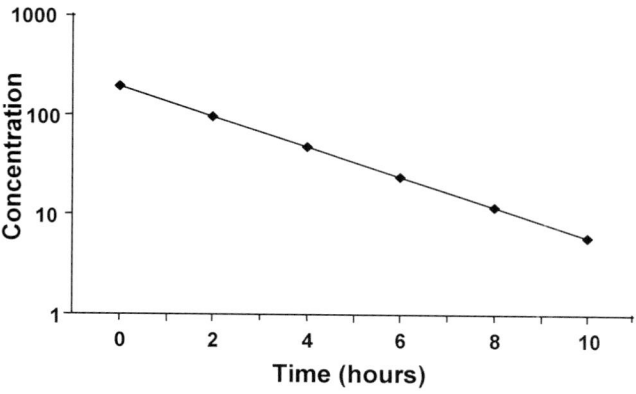

FIGURE 20.3. Semi-logarithmic plot of concentration versus time of a drug demonstrating first-order elimination.

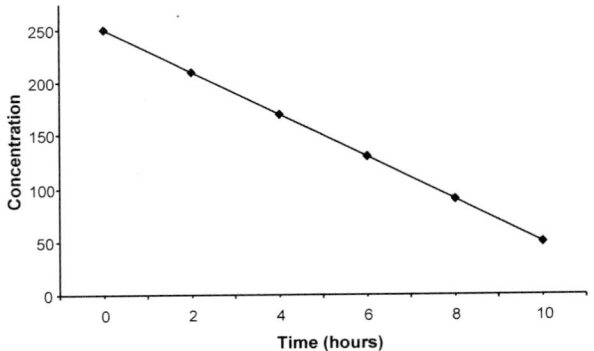

FIGURE 20.4. Concentration versus time of a drug demonstrating zero-order elimination.

sequential reactions. However, phase II reactions may precede phase I reactions, as in the case of isoniazid.

Phase I reactions are usually catalyzed by enzymes of the cytochrome P450 system. These drug-metabolizing enzymes are located in the lipophilic membranes of the endoplasmic reticulum of the liver and other tissues. Three families, CYP1, CYP2, and CYP3, are responsible for most drug biotransformations. The CYP3A subfamily accounts for >50% of phase I drug metabolism, predominantly by the CYP3A4 subtype. CYP3A4 is responsible for the metabolism of drugs commonly used in the intensive care setting, including acetaminophen, cyclosporine, diazepam, methadone, midazolam, spironolactone, and tacrolimus. Most other drug biotransformations are performed by CYP2D6 (e.g., clozapine, codeine, flecainide, haloperidol, oxycodone), CYP2C9 (e.g., phenytoin, S-warfarin), CYP2C19 (e.g., diazepam, omeprazole, propranolol), CYP2E1 (e.g., acetaminophen, enflurane, halothane), and CYP1A2 (e.g., acetaminophen, caffeine, theophylline, warfarin). Drug biotransformation reactions may be enhanced or impaired by multiple factors, including age, enzyme induction or inhibition, pharmacogenetics, and the effects of other disease states (35,41).

Elimination

Clearance (Renal, Hepatic, Other). Elimination is the process by which a drug is removed or "cleared" from the body.

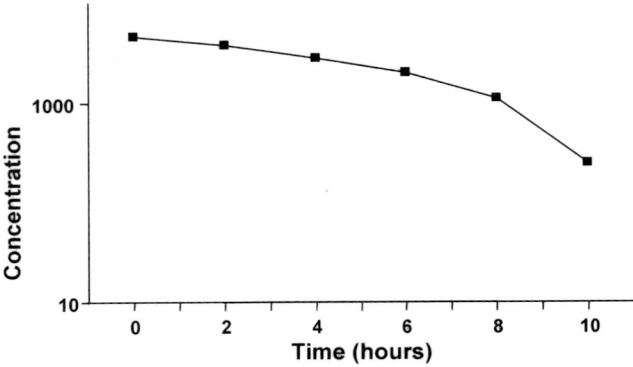

FIGURE 20.5. Semi-logarithmic plot of concentration versus time of a drug demonstrating zero-order elimination.

Clearance (CL) is usually considered to be the amount of blood from which all drug is removed per unit time (volume/time). The kidneys and liver are the main organs responsible for drug clearance. The total body clearance of a drug is equal to the sum of the clearances from all mechanisms, typically partitioned into renal and nonrenal clearance. Most elimination by the kidneys is accomplished through glomerular filtration. Glomerular integrity, the size and charge of the drug, water solubility, and the extent of protein binding determine the amount of drug filtered at the glomerulus. Highly protein-bound drugs are not readily filtered. Therefore, estimation of the glomerular filtration rate has traditionally served as an approximation of renal function.

In addition to glomerular filtration, drugs may be eliminated from the kidneys via active secretion. Secretion occurs predominantly at the proximal tubule, where active transport systems secrete primarily organic acids and bases. Organic acids include most cephalosporins, loop diuretics, methotrexate, nonsteroidal anti-inflammatories, penicillins, and thiazide diuretics. Organic bases include ranitidine and morphine. As drugs move toward the distal convoluting tubule, the concentration increases. High urine flow rates decrease the concentration of drug in the distal tubule, decreasing the likelihood that a drug will diffuse from the lumen. For both weak acids and bases, the nonionized form of the drug is reabsorbed more readily. Altering the pH (ion trapping) can minimize reabsorption by placing a charge on the drug and preventing its diffusion. For example, salicylate is a weak acid. In case of salicylate toxicity, urine alkalinization places a charge on the molecule and increases its elimination by reducing tubular reabsorption.

The liver also contributes to elimination through metabolism or excretion into the bile. After a drug is secreted in the bile, it may be either excreted into the feces or reabsorbed via enterohepatic recirculation (10,35,41).

The half-life of elimination is the time it takes to clear half of the drug from plasma. It is directly proportional to the Vd, and inversely proportional to CL (10):

$$t_{1/2\beta} = (0.693)(Vd)/CL \qquad [20.8]$$

Organ Dysfunction

Renal Dysfunction

Renal failure can impact drug pharmacokinetics through several mechanisms. The binding of acidic drugs to albumin is reduced because accumulated organic acids compete with albumin-binding sites and because uremia changes the structure of albumin. Altered albumin binding leads to altered Vd and, consequently, to altered elimination half-life (41). Renal insufficiency is likely to decrease the clearance of drugs that are normally >30% eliminated unchanged in the urine, which results in a prolonged $t_{1/2\beta}$ of drugs such as digoxin, aminoglycosides, insulin, and others (41).

Hepatic Dysfunction

Drugs that undergo extensive first-pass metabolism may have a significantly higher oral bioavailability in patients with liver failure than in normal subjects. Gut hypomotility may delay the peak response to enterally administered drugs in these patients. Hypoalbuminemia or altered glycoprotein levels may affect the fractional protein binding of acidic or basic drugs, respectively. Altered plasma protein concentrations may affect the extent of tissue distribution of drugs that are normally highly protein bound. The presence of significant edema and ascites may alter the Vd of highly water-soluble agents, such as aminoglycoside antibiotics. The capacity of the liver to metabolize drugs depends on hepatic blood flow and liver enzyme activity, both of which can be affected by liver disease. In addition, liver disease affects P450 isoforms in a variable manner; some P450 isoforms are more dysfunctional in the context of liver disease than others. This variability in susceptibility leads to heterogenous effects of liver disease on P450-dependent drug metabolism (41,55).

Cardiac Dysfunction

Circulatory failure, or shock, can alter the pharmacokinetics of drugs frequently used in the intensive care setting. Drug absorption may be impaired because of bowel wall edema. Passive hepatic congestion may impede first-pass metabolism, resulting in higher plasma concentrations. Peripheral edema inhibits absorption by intramuscular parenteral routes. The balance of tissue hypoperfusion versus increased total body water with edema may unpredictably alter Vd. In addition, liver hypoperfusion may alter drug-metabolizing enzyme function, especially flow-dependent drugs such as lidocaine (41).

Physiologic Differences in Children That Affect Drug Disposition

As children develop and grow, changes in body composition, development of metabolizing enzymes, and maturation of renal and liver function all have an impact on drug disposition (10,11).

Renal

Glomerular filtration and tubular secretion are significantly reduced in the premature and full-term neonate, as compared with older children. Maturation of renal function is a dynamic process that begins during fetal life and is complete by early childhood. Maturation of tubular function is slower than that of glomerular filtration. The glomerular filtration rate is approximately 2 to 4 mL/min/1.73 m^2 in term neonates, but it may be as low as 0.6 to 0.8 mL/min/1.73 m^2 in preterm neonates. The glomerular filtration rate increases rapidly during the first 2 weeks of life and continues to rise until adult values are reached at 8 to 12 months of age. For drugs that are dependent on renal elimination, impaired renal function decreases clearance and increases the half-life. Therefore, for drugs that are primarily eliminated by the kidney, dosing should be performed in an age-appropriate fashion that takes into account maturational changes in kidney function (10,11,38).

Hepatic

Hepatic biotransformation reactions are substantially reduced in the neonatal period. At birth, the cytochrome P450 system is 28% that of the adult (10,11). The expression of phase I enzymes, such as the P450 cytochromes, changes markedly during development. CYP3A7, the predominant CYP isoform expressed in fetal liver, peaks shortly after birth and then declines rapidly to levels that are undetectable in most

adults. Within hours after birth, CYP2E1 activity surges, and CYP2D6 becomes detectable soon thereafter. CYP3A4 and CYP2C (CYP2C9 and CYP2C19) appear during the first week of life, whereas CYP1A2 is the last hepatic CYP to appear, at 1 to 3 months of life (38). The ontogeny of phase II enzymes is less well established than the ontogeny of reactions that involve phase I enzymes. Available data indicate that the individual isoforms of glucuronosyltransferase (UGT) have unique maturational profiles with pharmacokinetic consequences. For example, the glucuronidation of acetaminophen (a substrate for UGT1A6 and, to a lesser extent, UGT1A9) is decreased in newborns and young children, as compared with adolescents and adults. Glucuronidation of morphine (a UGT2B7 substrate) can be detected in premature infants as young as 24 weeks of gestational age (38).

Gastrointestinal

Overall, the rate at which most drugs are absorbed from the gastrointestinal tract is slower in neonates and young infants than in older children. As a result, the time required to achieve maximal plasma levels of enterally administered drugs is longer in the very young (38). The effect of age on enteral absorption is not uniform, and it is difficult to predict (10,11). Gastric emptying and intestinal motility are the primary determinants of the rate at which drugs are presented to, and dispersed along, the mucosal surface of the small intestine. At birth, the coordination of antral contractions improves, resulting in a marked increase in gastric emptying during the first week of life. Similarly, intestinal motor activity matures throughout early infancy, with consequent increases in the frequency, amplitude, and duration of propagating contractions (38).

Changes in the intraluminal pH in different segments of the gastrointestinal tract can directly affect both the stability and the degree of ionization of a drug, thus influencing the relative amount of drug available for absorption. During the neonatal period, intragastric pH is relatively elevated (>4). Thus, oral administration of acid-labile compounds such as penicillin G produces greater bioavailability in neonates than in older infants and children (33). In contrast, drugs that are weak acids, such as phenobarbital, may require larger oral doses in the very young to achieve therapeutic plasma levels. Other factors that impact the rate of absorption include age-associated development of villi, splanchnic blood flow, changes in intestinal microflora, and intestinal surface area (38).

Body Composition

Age-dependent changes in body composition alter the physiologic spaces into which a drug may be distributed (38). The percent of total body water drops from approximately 85% in premature infants to 75% in full-term infants, to 60% in the adult. Extracellular water decreases from 45% in the infant to 25% in the adult. Total body fat in the premature infant can be as low as 1%, as compared to 15% in the normal, term infant. Many drugs are less bound to plasma proteins in the neonate and infant than in the older child (10,11).

Much of drug distribution is a result of simple passive diffusion along concentration gradients and subsequent binding of the drug to tissue components. However, tissue transporters capable of producing a biologic barrier also contribute to drug distribution. An example is P-glycoprotein, a member of the ATP-binding cassette family of transporters that functions as an efflux transporter capable of extruding selected substances from cells. The expression and localization of P-glycoprotein in specific tissues facilitates its ability to limit the cellular uptake of selected substrates to these sites (e.g., the blood–brain barrier [BBB], hepatocytes, renal tubular cells, and enterocytes). Limited data are available regarding the ontogeny of P-glycoprotein expression in humans. A single study of the expression of P-glycoprotein in the central nervous system (CNS) in tissue obtained postmortem from neonates born at 23 to 42 weeks of gestational age suggests a pattern of localization similar to that in adult mice late in gestation and at term. However, the level of P-glycoprotein expression appeared to be lower than that in adults (66). Limited data in neonates suggest that the passive diffusion of drugs into the CNS is age dependent, as reflected by the progressive increase in the ratios of brain phenobarbital to plasma phenobarbital from 28 to 39 weeks of gestational age, demonstrating the increased transport of phenobarbital into the brain (48).

Pharmacodynamics

Pharmacodynamics, in general terms, seeks to define what the drug does to the body (i.e., the effects or response to drug therapy). Pharmacodynamics modeling attempts to characterize measured, physiologic parameters before and after drug administration, with the effect defined as the change in a physiologic parameter relative to its pre-dose or baseline value. *Baseline* is defined as the physiologic parameter without drug dosing and may be complicated in certain situations due to diurnal variations. Efficacy can be defined numerically as the expected sum of all beneficial effects following treatment. Similarly, toxicity can be characterized either by the time course of a specific toxic event or the composite of toxic responses attributed to a common toxicity.

Overview

Pharmacodynamic response to drug therapy evolves only after active drug molecules reach their intended site(s) of action. Hence, the link between pharmacokinetic and pharmacodynamic processes is implicit. Differences in pharmacodynamic time course among drug entities can be broadly associated with

the nature of the concentration–effect relationship as being *direct* (effect is directly proportional to concentration at the site of measurement, usually the plasma) or *indirect* (effect exhibits some type of temporal delay with respect to drug concentration either because of differences between site of action and measurement or because the effect of interest results after other physiologic or pharmacologic conditions are satisfied).

Direct-effect relationships are easily observed with cardiovascular agents. Pharmacologic effects such as blood pressure, ACE-inhibition, and inhibition of platelet aggregation can be characterized by direct-response relationships. Such relationships can usually be defined by three typical patterns—linear, hyperbolic E_{max}, and sigmoid E_{max} functions (**Fig. 20.6**). In each case, the plasma concentration and drug concentration at the effect site are proportional. Likewise, the concentration–effect relationship is assumed to be independent of time.

Other drugs exhibit an indirect relationship between concentration and response. In this case, the concentration–effect relationship is time dependent. One explanation for such effects is hysteresis. *Hysteresis* refers to the phenomenon in which a time lapse exists between the cause and its effect. With respect to pharmacodynamics, this time lapse most often indicates a situation in which a delay exists in equilibrium between plasma drug concentration and the concentration of active substance at the effect site. Three broad conditions can account for this phenomenon: The active drug response site is not in the central compartment, the mechanism of drug action involves new protein synthesis, or the particular drug has active metabolites.

More complicated models (indirect-response models) have been used to express the same observations but typically necessitate a greater understanding of the underlying physiologic process (e.g., cell trafficking, enzyme recruitment, etc.). The salient point is that pharmacodynamic characterization and dosing guidance derived from such characterization stand to be more informative than drug concentrations alone.

Pharmacogenomics

Pharmacogenomics is the study of how an individual's genetic inheritance affects his response to drugs. Pharmacogenomics

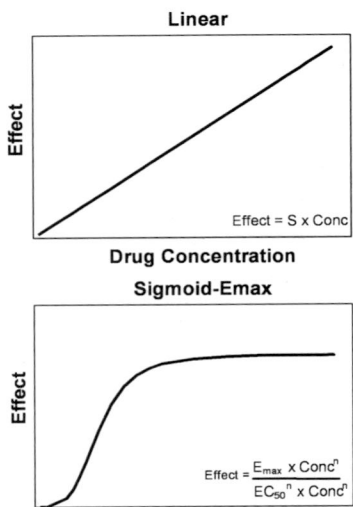

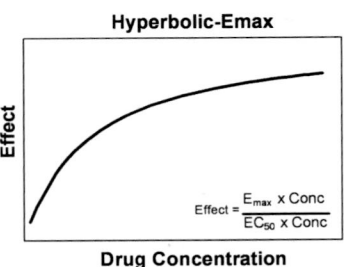

FIGURE 20.6. Representative pharmacodynamic relationships for drugs that exhibit direct responses: linear, hyperbolic, and sigmoid E_{max} relationships shown. S is the slope of the linear response; E_{max} refers to the maximum effect observed; EC_{50} refers to the concentration at which 50% of the maximal response is achieved, and n is the degree of sigmoidicity or shape factor (sometimes referred to as the Hill coefficient).

holds the promise that drugs might one day be tailored to individuals and adapted to each person's own genetic makeup. Environment, diet, age, lifestyle, and state of health all can influence a person's response to medicines, but understanding an individual's genetic composition is thought to be a key to creating personalized drugs with greater efficacy and safety. Pharmacogenomics combines traditional pharmaceutical sciences, such as biochemistry, with annotated knowledge of genes, proteins, and single nucleotide polymorphisms (see Chapter 16).

APPLICATION TO PEDIATRIC INTENSIVE CARE

Benzodiazepines

Benzodiazepines are often used to provide sedation and amnesia. Benzodiazepines exert their anxiolytic, amnestic, anticonvulsant, and muscle-relaxing effects through interaction at specific binding sites on neuronal γ-aminobutyric acid (GABA) receptors (46). Benzodiazepines facilitate the inhibitory action of GABA on neuronal impulse transmission. The potency of individual medications is determined by their receptor affinity. Benzodiazepines enhance inhibitory synaptic transmission by mimicking and increasing the actions of GABA-mediated chloride influx at the GABA receptor.

Chronic administration of benzodiazepines can lead to decreased receptor activity and drug tolerance. Tolerance is a common finding in ICU patients who receive benzodiazepines or other sedative agents for periods >24 hrs. Withdrawal syndromes have been reported with the cessation of midazolam and other benzodiazepine infusions. Risk factors for acute withdrawal include high infusion rates, prolonged duration, and abrupt cessation. For these reasons, gradual tapering of sedative infusions and substitution with longer-acting agents (e.g., diazepam) are suggested to reduce the chance of withdrawal reactions. Benzodiazepines also are noted for occasionally producing paradoxic reactions, including increased agitation and delirium (76).

Diazepam

Diazepam is highly lipid-soluble and highly protein-bound and distributes quickly into the brain. It is available in IV and oral preparations. Diazepam administration results in antegrade but not retrograde amnesia. It reduces the cerebral metabolic rate for oxygen consumption and thus decreases cerebral blood flow in a dose-dependent manner. As do other benzodiazepines, diazepam raises the seizure threshold (76). After enteral dosing, diazepam demonstrates a bioavailability of 100%. It has a Vd of 1.1 to 2.9 L/kg (29,76) and is 98% protein bound (29). Diazepam is metabolized by hepatic microsomal enzymes (CYP2C19) to active compounds such as desmethyldiazepam and oxazepam. Desmethyldiazepam has a long elimination half-life of 100 to 200 hrs and is eliminated by the kidneys. Oxazepam has an elimination half-life of 10 hrs. The elimination half-life of diazepam averages 72 hrs, varies widely, and is increased in the elderly, neonates, and patients with liver disease. Metabolism is also affected by genetics, gender, endocrine status, nutritional status, smoking, and concurrent drug therapy (76). The mean plasma clearance is 0.27 to 0.37 mL/kg/min and is independent of liver blood flow (50).

Diazepam alone has minimal cardiovascular depressant effects, although systemic vascular resistance is reduced slightly, producing a small decline in arterial blood pressure. Respiratory drive is minimally decreased by diazepam alone but is profoundly depressed when diazepam (or another benzodiazepine) is used in combination with opioids. Diazepam elimination is decreased by such drugs as cimetidine, fluconazole, and valproic acid (76).

Midazolam

Midazolam is three to four times more potent than diazepam (76). It is rapidly absorbed after administration of the oral syrup formulation, with adolescents absorbing the drug at approximately half the rate observed in younger children (ages 2 to <12 years). In children 6 months to 16 years, the absolute bioavailability of midazolam averaged 36%, with a very broad range (9%–71%). No relationship between midazolam bioavailability and age was observed (53). The pKa of midazolam (6.1) is especially important because it permits a conformational change in midazolam's structure, depending on pH. As currently marketed, midazolam is buffered to a pH of 3.5, opening its imidazole ring and increasing its water solubility. At physiologic pH, however, the diazepine ring closes rapidly and midazolam becomes lipid soluble. As a consequence, the effects of midazolam are rapid.

Midazolam is 95% protein bound, with a Vd of 1.9 L/kg (76). Midazolam undergoes extensive metabolism by the cytochrome P4503A subfamily (e.g., CYP3A4 and CYP3A5) to a major hydroxylated metabolite (1-OH-midazolam). 1-OH-midazolam is equipotent to midazolam and is subsequently metabolized to 1-OH-midazolam-glucuronide by uridine diphosphate-glucuronosyltransferases (UGTs). 1-OH-midazolam-glucuronide also appears to have sedative properties when concentrations are high, as has been observed in adult patients with renal failure (18).

The elimination half-life of midazolam is prolonged, and clearance is reduced in adolescents as compared with younger children. In healthy children 6 months to <2 yrs, 2 years to <12 years, and 12 years to <16 years, the clearance was 11.3, 10, and 9.3 mL/kg/min, respectively (53). Adult clearance is estimated at 6.6 mL/kg/min (29). CYP3A4/5 activity reaches adult levels at between 3 and 12 months of postnatal age (42). Developmental differences in CYP3A activity may therefore alter the pharmacokinetics of midazolam in pediatric intensive care patients of different ages. Similarly, the UGTs exhibit developmental changes in activity. However, because the specific UGTs involved in the conjugation of 1-OH-midazolam are not yet known, the impact of ontogeny on this reaction remains to be determined (18).

Less than 1% of midazolam is excreted unchanged in the urine. The elimination half-life of midazolam is 2 hrs in young, healthy adults but increases rapidly in the elderly and following major surgery (76). 1-OH-midazolam-glucuronide is renally excreted, with an elimination half-life of 1 hr with normal renal function (18). This results in high concentrations in the presence of renal failure and is responsible for prolonged sedation (50).

Midazolam is metabolized by hepatic microsomal oxidation. The oxidative pathway is susceptible to many factors, including hepatic disease, advanced age, and drug inhibition. The most dramatic changes in the pharmacokinetics of midazolam in the critically ill may result from altered hepatic metabolism.

Accumulation occurs in critically ill patients at the peak of their illness, with low or absent concentrations of 1-hydroxy midazolam, suggesting failure of liver metabolism (62). A number of drugs, including cimetidine, erythromycin, propofol, and diltiazem, have been reported to delay midazolam metabolism and therefore increase its duration of effect.

The accumulation of the active metabolite also may be important in some ICU patients. As with other benzodiazepines, midazolam causes dose-related respiratory depression and, in large doses, can cause vasodilation and hypotension (76). As with many highly lipid soluble drugs, drug accumulates in peripheral tissues and in the bloodstream rather than being metabolized after continuous infusion for extended time periods. When the infusion is discontinued, peripheral-tissue stores release midazolam back into the plasma, and the duration of clinical effect can be prolonged. Obese patients with larger volumes of distribution and elderly patients with decreased hepatic and renal function may be at higher risk for prolonged sedation from midazolam (23).

Lorazepam

Lorazepam is the least lipid soluble of the three benzodiazepines and traverses the BBB most slowly, resulting in delayed onset and prolonged duration of effect (76). Lorazepam is well absorbed orally and demonstrates a bioavailability of 93% after oral administration (29). It is absorbed rapidly after intramuscular injection, and plasma concentrations peak within 60 mins. It is approximately 90% protein bound and has a Vd of 2 L/kg. Lorazepam is metabolized to inactive products by hepatic glucuronidation. The pharmacokinetics of lorazepam do not change significantly in the elderly or in critically ill populations. The elimination half-life ranges from 10 to 20 hrs but is prolonged by liver and end-stage kidney disease (76). Clearance is estimated at 1.1 mL/kg/min (29). Because lorazepam is insoluble in water, it is manufactured with polyethylene glycol. This drug vehicle may be associated with lactic acidosis, hyperosmolar coma, and a reversible nephrotoxicity after high doses or prolonged infusions (76). At the time of this writing, the National Institutes of Health are sponsoring a multi-institution clinical trial designed to specifically address the pharmacokinetics and pharmacodynamics of lorazepam in critically ill children.

Flumazenil

Flumazenil acts at the benzodiazepine binding site on the GABA receptor to antagonize the effects of benzodiazepine agonists. Flumazenil is chemically and structurally similar to other benzodiazepine receptor agonists. Flumazenil produces a reversal of benzodiazepine-induced sedative and amnestic effects. Clinical effects are seen immediately after IV administration. Flumazenil does not reverse the effects of opioids, barbiturates, alcohol, or other GABA-mimetic agents (76). Flumazenil is short acting, and careful clinical observation is crucial if the therapeutic intent is to avoid the recurrence of benzodiazepine-induced sedation. Repeated administrations may be necessary to maintain its antagonistic action (39).

Flumazenil is 40% to 50% plasma protein bound, with a Vd of 0.6 to 1.6 L/kg (29,39). It is cleared rapidly from the plasma by hepatic metabolism (76). Less than 0.2% of an IV dose is recovered unchanged in the urine, and three metabolites of flumazenil have been identified (39). The elimination half-life of flumazenil is approximately 1 hr, which is significantly shorter than that of many of the benzodiazepine compounds used clinically (76). The clearance is estimated at 17 mL/kg/min (29). Flumazenil can precipitate withdrawal and/or seizures in patients with benzodiazepine dependence caused by chronic exposure (76).

Barbiturates

Barbiturates are weak acids that are absorbed and rapidly distributed to all tissues and fluids, with high concentrations in the brain, liver, and kidneys. High lipid solubility is the dominant factor in the distribution of barbiturates within the body. The more lipid-soluble the barbiturate, the more rapidly it penetrates all tissues of the body. Barbiturates are bound to plasma and tissue proteins to varying degrees, with the degree of binding increasing directly as a function of lipid solubility. Barbiturates are absorbed in varying degrees following oral, rectal, or parenteral administration.

Thiopental

Thiopental is an ultra–short-acting barbiturate, commonly administered for the induction of general anesthesia and treatment of intracranial hypertension. Another use of high-dose thiopental therapy is in the management of status epilepticus refractory to more conventional therapy. Following a single IV dose, unconsciousness occurs within 10 to 20 secs, the depth of anesthesia may increase for up to 40 secs, and then decrease as thiopental is redistributed out of the brain until consciousness returns in 5 to 10 mins (29,57).

Thiopental is 85% protein bound, with a Vd of 2.3 L/kg. Thiopental is almost completely metabolized in the body, with a very small percentage excreted unchanged in urine. Oxidation to the thiopental carboxylic acid is the major step of detoxification in humans, and the urinary excretion of this product accounts for approximately 10% to 25% of the administered doses. The elimination half-life is 9 hrs, and its CL is 3.9 mL/kg/min (29,57). Thiopental produces apnea and should be not administered unless the means for assisted ventilation are immediately available. It also decreases cardiac output somewhat. However, in the presence of hypovolemia, sepsis, or circulatory failure, therapeutic doses may result in circulatory collapse (29). Intramuscular injection or extravasation of thiopental produces severe tissue necrosis.

Pentobarbital

Pentobarbital is a major metabolite of thiopental. Pentobarbital has two enantiomeric forms: R- and S-pentobarbital. The S-enantiomer causes a longer duration of sedation than does the R-enantiomer in humans. High-dose pentobarbital infusions have been advocated as an effective adjunct in controlling persistent intracranial hypertension after severe head trauma in patients who are refractory to conventional therapy. Pentobarbital has a potent effect on GABA-sensitive chloride channels and is a potent CNS depressant. Following IV administration, the onset of action is almost immediate for pentobarbital. Pentobarbital enters the brain more rapidly than do phenobarbital or diazepam and is a very potent antiepileptic drug. Pentobarbital has also been recommended as a sedative agent for diagnostic imaging studies (25,34).

Pentobarbital is metabolized primarily by the hepatic microsomal enzyme system, and the metabolic products are excreted in the urine and, less commonly, in the feces (49). The CL of the S-enantiomer is less than that of the R-enantiomer (43 vs. 32 mL/min), and the Vd of the S-enantiomer is slightly less than the R-enantiomer (1.1 vs. 1.2 L/kg). The S-enantiomer is also more strongly protein bound in plasma (73.5% vs. 63.4% for the R-enantiomer) (12). In a study of seven healthy adult men and women, 100 mg of pentobarbital was administered as an IV bolus. A two-compartment model determined the central Vd to be 0.44 L/kg, with a peripheral Vd of 0.56 L/kg (Vd = 1 L/kg). The elimination half-life was 22.3 hrs (20). Pentobarbital pharmacokinetics were assessed in 10 adults with severe nonpenetrating head injury. An IV loading dose (10 mg/kg) was infused over 1 hr, followed by a continuous infusion at 0.5 to 3.0 mg/kg/hr. The mean $t_{1/2}$ and Vd were significantly less than values reported for the healthy control subjects (6). In another study of six adult patients with severe head injury, the mean CL was 0.7 mL/kg/min, with a Vd of 1 L/kg and an elimination half-life of 19.1 hr. Considerable variation in individual patient parameters was observed (73).

The pharmacokinetics of pentobarbital were examined in 11 children with Reye syndrome, hypoxic encephalopathy, or acute head injury. Nine of these patients were hypothermic (<32°C). The total CL and Vd were respectively 0.4 mL/kg/min and 0.8 L/kg—less than that reported in the normothermic adult volunteers following IV doses of pentobarbital. The elimination half-life of 25.5 hrs was not significantly different from previously reported values (59). Pentobarbital administration has potential respiratory-depressant and hypotensive side effects. Tolerance may develop with prolonged use.

Opioids

Opioids are endogenous or exogenous substances that bind to receptors found in the CNS and peripheral tissue. Three classes of opiate receptors have been characterized: $\mu 1$ and -2, $\kappa 1$ to -3, and $\delta 1$ and 2.

The $\mu 1$ (spinal) and $\mu 2$ (supraspinal) subtypes are present in the CNS. Stimulation of these receptors produces analgesia, respiratory depression, and miosis. The primary opioids stimulating the μ receptors include fentanyl, methadone, morphine, and sufentanil. $\kappa 1$ receptors elicit spinal analgesia when stimulated. The pharmacologic properties of $\kappa 2$ receptors remain unknown. The analgesic effects of $\kappa 3$ receptors are exerted through supraspinal mechanisms. Drugs with higher affinity for κ receptors include butorphanol, levorphanol, naloxone, and nalbuphine.

The primary activity of enkephalins, endogenous analgesic ligands in the brain and adrenal glands, is to trigger the activation of δ receptors. The stimulation of δ receptors induces spinal and supraspinal analgesia. Two subtypes of δ receptors are present: $\delta 1$ and $\delta 2$. Sufentanil is the only analgesic with known agonism for the δ receptor, although it has less affinity for δ and κ receptors than for μ receptors (28).

Opioids lead to a dose-dependent, centrally mediated respiratory depression, mediated by the $\mu 2$ receptors in the medulla. The carbon dioxide response curve is shifted to the right, and the ventilatory response to hypoxia is obliterated. Opioids have little hemodynamic effect on patients with euvolemia whose blood pressure is not sustained by the sympathetic nervous system, but may cause hypotension in the hypovolemic patient. Opiate side effects include nausea, vomiting, decreased gastrointestinal motility (constipation), urinary retention, and pruritus (23). A withdrawal syndrome characterized by irritability, agitation, hypertension, nausea, vomiting, diarrhea, or sweating will occur if opioid administration is weaned abruptly after prolonged usage.

Morphine

Morphine is a potent μ-receptor agonist with additional κ-receptor activity (28). Morphine's onset of action is relatively slow (5–10 min) because of low lipid solubility. The duration of action is dose-dependent, but is approximately 4 hrs after a single dose (23). Morphine has a bioavailability of 24%. It is 35% protein bound, with a Vd estimated at 3.3 L/kg (29). Metabolism primarily occurs through the liver by glucuronide conjugation, and excretion occurs through the kidney. Morphine's predominant metabolite, morphine-6-glucuronide, is an active analgesic and may accumulate in patients with renal failure. This active metabolite is several times more potent than morphine itself (28). The elimination half-life is 1.9 hrs, and CL is estimated at 24 mL/kg/min (29).

The pharmacologic effects of morphine include analgesia, respiratory depression, gastrointestinal effects (nausea and vomiting), orthostatic hypotension, sedation, and altered mentation (28). Morphine administration may cause histamine release (23).

Hydromorphone

Hydromorphone is a morphine-like agonist and a semisynthetic opioid analgesic with roughly three- to fourfold greater potency than morphine. Hydromorphone, like morphine, provides analgesic effects within 15 to 30 mins of administration (28). Its metabolism primarily occurs by the liver to hydromorphone-3-glucuronide. Although it has been recommended as an alternative to morphine for patients in renal failure (54), hydromorphone's metabolite may accumulate in renal failure, resulting in neuroexcitability and cognitive impairment (28).

Meperidine

Meperidine is primarily a μ-receptor agonist and has approximately one-tenth the potency of morphine. The analgesic effects of meperidine are detectable within 5 mins of IV administration and 10 mins after intramuscular or subcutaneous administration (28). Meperidine is useful for drug-induced rigors and pain symptoms, such as those that accompany administration of amphotericin B. Meperidine has a bioavailability of 52%. It is 58% protein bound, with a Vd of 4.4 L/kg (29). It is metabolized through the liver to an active metabolite, normeperidine, which has a half-life of 15 to 30 hrs (28). Meperidine has an elimination half-life of 3.2 hrs, with a CL of 17 mL/kg/min (29). Normeperidine accumulates in renal failure and produces neurotoxicity, which may result in tremors, myoclonic jerks, and seizures. Case reports of seizures with meperidine have been noted with administration by patient-controlled analgesia pumps (27). Risk for seizures is also reported in patients with renal insufficiency, with sickle-cell anemia, and in those receiving high-dose meperidine (28). Hence, meperidine is now used only rarely.

Fentanyl

Fentanyl is a synthetic opioid commonly used in anesthesia and in the ICU for pain management and sedation. Fentanyl is 50 to

100 times more potent than morphine and provides a relatively quick (almost immediate) onset of action and short duration (~0.5–1 hr). Fentanyl is more lipid soluble than morphine and has a more rapid onset of action due to quicker penetration of the CNS. Fentanyl may be administered by the IV, IM, epidural, transdermal, and intrathecal routes (28,70). Fentanyl has a very low bioavailability due to a high first-pass effect and, consequently, is not administered by the oral route. It is 84% protein bound, with a Vd of 4 L/kg (29).

Fentanyl is metabolized by the liver to inactive metabolites that are eliminated by the kidney. It has an elimination half-life of 3.7 hrs and a CL of 13 mL/kg/min. Metabolism is determined primarily by liver perfusion, and diseases that decrease liver blood flow, such as cardiac failure, may decrease the clearance of fentanyl. Although renal failure does not significantly alter the pharmacokinetics and pharmacodynamics of fentanyl in most patients, a few studies have demonstrated increases in the Vd and $t_{1/2}$ in critically ill patients with renal failure who are receiving continuous fentanyl infusions (29,70). Long-term, continuous infusions of fentanyl may result in a prolonged elimination half-life and duration of action as a result of drug accumulation in peripheral tissues. Unlike morphine, fentanyl is not associated with mast-cell histamine release and may be preferred in patients who are susceptible to the cardiovascular effects of morphine (70). Rapid administration has been associated with rigidity of the chest wall, which produces apnea and inability to apply assisted ventilation until the patient receives neuromuscular blockade.

Naloxone

Naloxone is an opiate antagonist. Small doses can result in the prompt reversal of opiate-induced respiratory depression, sedation, analgesia, and hypotension. Naloxone can be administered endotracheally. The duration of action is 1 to 4 hrs, and the Vd is 2.1 L/kg. Naloxone undergoes significant first-pass metabolism and is metabolized in the liver by conjugation with glucuronic acid. CL is estimated at 22 mL/kg/min, with an elimination half-life of 1.1 hrs (29). Caution must be used when treating opiate overdose in a patient with pain. Doses of 0.001 to 0.010 mg/kg should be titrated to achieve the desired clinical effect.

Ketamine

Ketamine is a racemic mixture consisting of two optical enantiomers, R(−) and S(+). Administration produces a dose-dependent CNS depression that leads to a dissociative state, characterized by profound analgesia and amnesia but not necessarily loss of consciousness. Ketamine is a bronchodilator that causes minimal respiratory depression, and protective airway reflexes are more likely to be preserved than with other anesthetics. However, increased oral secretions can occur with its use. It is used clinically for indications such as induction of anesthesia in hemodynamically compromised patients or active asthmatic disease; intramuscular sedation of uncooperative patients, particularly children; supplementation of incomplete regional or local anesthesia; sedation in the intensive care setting; and for short, painful procedures, such as dressing changes in burn patients.

Ketamine is structurally related to phencyclidine, binds to the phencyclidine receptor in the N-methyl-D-aspartate

(NMDA) channel, and inhibits glutamate activation of the channel in a noncompetitive manner (23,40). It is minimally protein bound and has a Vd of 1.8 L/kg. The $t_{1/2}$ is 2.3 hrs, and CL is 15 mL/kg/min. The compound is metabolized extensively by the hepatic cytochrome P450 system. The primary metabolite, norketamine, is only one-third to one-fifth as potent as the original compound but may be involved in the prolonged analgesic actions of ketamine. The metabolites of norketamine are excreted by the kidneys (29,40). Common side effects include emergence delirium and severe hallucinations. These effects can be reduced with concomitant administration of a benzodiazepine, such as midazolam. Although ketamine administration is generally associated with increases in heart rate, cardiac output, and blood pressure, hypotension from direct myocardial depression can occur (23).

Propofol

Propofol is an alkylphenol IV anesthetic. Its exact mechanism of action is unclear, but it is thought to act at the GABA receptor. It is an oil at room temperature and is prepared as a lipid emulsion. Propofol is highly lipid soluble and rapidly crosses the BBB. Onset of sedation is rapid (1–5 mins), and duration of action is dose dependent but usually very short (2–8 mins) because of rapid redistribution to peripheral tissues. When continuous infusions are used, the duration of action may be increased, but it is rare for the effect to last longer than 60 mins after the infusion is stopped (23). Propofol is a hypnotic agent that, like benzodiazepines, provides a dose-dependent suppression of awareness from mild depression of responsiveness to obtundation. It is a potent anxiolytic and a potent amnestic agent but does not possess analgesic properties (23).

The pharmacokinetics of propofol in healthy individuals who are undergoing surgery are characterized by a rapid distribution phase of 1.3 mins and a rapid redistribution phase of 30 mins (50). Propofol is metabolized primarily by conjugation in the liver to inactive glucuronide and sulfate metabolites, which are then cleared by the kidney. The elimination half-life is 4 to 7 hrs. Metabolism of propofol does not appear to be significantly altered by hepatic or renal disease. However, in critical care populations, clearance is generally slower than in the general population, probably secondary to decrease in hepatic blood flow (50).

Propofol pharmacokinetics are distinct and can be contrasted with the pharmacokinetics of other commonly used IV-administered sedatives. Propofol pharmacokinetics are best described by a three-compartment model: a central compartment (essentially blood volume), a rapidly equilibrating compartment, and a slowly equilibrating, or deep-tissue, compartment (60). Following an IV bolus dose, rapid equilibration occurs between blood and the highly perfused tissue of the brain, thus accounting for the rapid onset of anesthesia. Plasma levels initially decline rapidly as a result of both rapid distribution and metabolism. Distribution, however, is not complete, and a true steady-state is not rapidly achieved. Initiation of a continuous IV infusion can maintain a pseudo-steady-state plasma drug concentration. The deep-tissue compartment eventually is saturated, which results in an increase in plasma drug concentrations if infusions are maintained at a constant rate. The rate at which equilibration occurs is a function of the rate and duration of the infusion. Another important aspect of propofol pharmacokinetics is that the drug can limit its own clearance. Propofol is eliminated by hepatic conjugation to inactive metabolites, which are excreted by the kidney. Studies have indicated that after a 2 mg/kg bolus dose of propofol for induction of cardiac anesthesia, blood flow in the liver is reduced by 14%. Bolus doses of propofol may cause a small but persistent change in blood flow to the liver, which results in decreased clearance that leads to plasma concentrations that are higher than those predicted by an infusion. In addition to hepatic blood flow, other factors, such as age, lean body mass, and central blood volume, have been found to affect the induction dose of anesthesia. Younger children require larger doses for induction (37), and critically ill patients with low cardiac output usually require smaller doses (9). In addition, the presence of such opiates as fentanyl decreases the amount of propofol needed by 50% to 55% (36).

Apnea may occur after a loading dose. Administration can cause significant decreases in blood pressure, especially in hypovolemic patients, mainly as a result of preload reduction from the dilation of venous capacitance vessels. A lesser effect is mild myocardial depression. Because it is delivered in a lipid carrier, hypertriglyceridemia is a possible side effect of propofol (23). Lactic acidosis has been associated with its use in the pediatric population (14). Recent reports of dysrhythmia, heart failure, metabolic acidosis, hyperkalemia, and rhabdomyolysis have been described in adults treated with high doses of propofol (>80 mcg/kg/min) (15). Although propofol is highly effective for procedural sedation in the PICU, it is not approved for long-term continuous sedation because of the risk of rhabdomyolysis, acidosis, and death after prolonged administration in children.

Etomidate

Etomidate is an ultra–short-acting, nonbarbiturate, hypnotic agent without analgesic effects. IV administration of 0.3 mg/kg will induce sleep for approximately 5 mins. Cardiovascular and respiratory adverse events are minimal (29). Etomidate administration is associated with a transient 20% to 30% decrease in cerebral blood flow. Etomidate is rapidly metabolized in the liver to inactive metabolites, and approximately 75% of the administered dose is excreted in the urine during the first day after injection (35). Involuntary muscle movements are a frequent occurrence. Etomidate may inhibit adrenal steroidogenesis, causing a decrease in plasma cortisol concentrations (29). The effect of etomidate on steroidogenesis has recently led to controversy regarding its use in the care of critically ill patients (3). Although a single administration can be highly effective, we recommend avoiding repeated administration of etomidate in a critically ill patient.

Dexmedetomidine

Dexmedetomidine is a highly selective α_2 agonist, with hypnotic and anxiolytic properties attributed to the α_{2A} adrenoreceptors in the locus caeruleus. Analgesic properties are a result of the stimulation of α_2 adrenoreceptors in the brain, spinal cord, and peripheral sites (8). Dexmedetomidine is being increasingly used in the adult ICU setting because it allows postoperative patients to remain sedated but to be aroused easily with gentle stimulation (69). Furthermore, it produces sedation without respiratory depression or the risk of a withdrawal syndrome after prolonged infusion. Only limited pharmacokinetic data are currently available to help guide dosing in children.

Dexmedetomidine demonstrates a rapid distribution phase, with a distribution half-life of approximately 6 mins. The steady-state Vd of dexmedetomidine is 1.6 L/kg. Protein binding in healthy adult male and female volunteers was 94%. Dexmedetomidine undergoes almost complete biotransformation, with very little unchanged dexmedetomidine excreted in urine or feces. Biotransformation involves both direct glucuronidation and cytochrome P450-mediated metabolism. The major metabolic pathways of dexmedetomidine are: (a) direct N-glucuronidation to inactive metabolites; (b) aliphatic hydroxylation (mediated primarily by CYP2A6) of dexmedetomidine to generate 3-hydroxy dexmedetomidine, the glucuronide of 3-hydroxy dexmedetomidine, and 3-carboxy dexmedetomidine; and (c) N-methylation of dexmedetomidine to generate 3-hydroxy N-methyl dexmedetomidine, 3-carboxy N-methyl dexmedetomidine, and N-methyl O-glucuronide dexmedetomidine. The elimination half-life of dexmedetomidine is approximately 2 hrs, and CL is estimated to be 9 mL/kg/min. Approximately 95% of the administered dose is recovered as metabolites in the urine, and 4% in the feces. In clinical studies, hypotension and bradycardia were the significant treatment-emergent adverse events reported in dexmedetomidine patients compared with placebo patients (1).

Neuromuscular Blockers

During neurotransmission, the neurotransmitter acetylcholine is synthesized, stored in vesicles at the neuromuscular junction, released into the synapse, and bound to nicotinic receptors in the muscle endplate. Acetylcholine acts as an agonist at the neuromuscular junction. Muscle contraction occurs when the impulse generated in a neuron creates an action potential that is chemically transmitted across the synapse.

The postsynaptic nicotinic receptor at the neuromuscular junction is the major site of action of depolarizing and nondepolarizing neuromuscular blockers. Nondepolarizing neuromuscular blockers act as antagonists, combine with the nicotinic receptors, and block the action of acetylcholine. They also antagonize presynaptic nicotinic acetylcholine release, possibly contributing to blockade. Succinylcholine and depolarizing agents act by a different mechanism that is less well understood. Like acetylcholine, succinylcholine depolarizes the membrane and opens sodium channels. Because succinylcholine is fairly resistant to acetylcholinesterase and not metabolized locally at the neuromuscular junction, it persists longer than acetylcholine and results in longer depolarization and a brief initial period of fasciculation. This is followed by a block in neurotransmission and the onset of flaccid paralysis, both of which are secondary to the inability of acetylcholine to initiate a propagating action potential at an already depolarized endplate (45).

Succinylcholine

Succinylcholine is structurally similar to acetylcholine. It is used because of its favorable pharmacokinetic profile, with quick onset and short duration (45). Administration is followed by muscle fasciculations and subsequent neuromuscular blockade approximately 60 secs after IV dosing. The blockade remains for approximately 5 to 10 mins (11). Succinylcholine is eliminated by plasma cholinesterase, has a very short duration of action, and can be used independent of a patient's renal and hepatic status. Prolongation of blockade occurs in patients with conditions associated with plasma cholinesterase deficiency and with high doses (45). The elimination half-life is 3 hrs (11). Succinylcholine can cause severe, although uncommon, adverse drug reactions, such as malignant hyperthermia, increased intraocular pressure, masseter muscle rigidity, rhabdomyolysis, bradycardia, and hyperkalemia (11,45). It is contraindicated in patients with spinal cord injury, severe burns, neuromuscular disorders, or preexisting hyperkalemia.

Pancuronium

Pancuronium is a nondepolarizing neuromuscular blocking agent. Onset of action occurs 4 to 6 mins after administration and remains for 120 to 180 mins (29). Pancuronium is 7% protein bound, with a Vd of 0.26 L/kg. The CL is estimated at 1.8 mL/kg/min (29). Approximately 60% to 80% of pancuronium is eliminated by the kidney (11). In patients with renal failure, pancuronium CL is decreased significantly (45). Pancuronium is largely excreted unchanged in the urine, but a small percentage is metabolized to 3-desacetylpancuronium, which may accumulate after prolonged infusion. Although only 10% is eliminated by the liver, pancuronium also accumulates in fulminant hepatic failure (11,50). Its administration causes tachycardia, largely due to the blocking of cardiac muscarinic cholinergic receptors (11).

Vecuronium

Vecuronium, a steroid-based compound derived from pancuronium, is also a nondepolarizing neuromuscular blocker (50). Onset of action occurs 2 to 4 mins after administration and remains for 30 to 40 mins (29). The Vd is 0.2 L/kg (29). Vecuronium, like pancuronium, is deacetylated in the liver to produce 3-desacetyl, 17-desacetyl, and 3,17-desacetyl derivatives, which are respectively, two times, 17 times, and 35 times less potent than the parent vecuronium compound (50). Even though it is primarily metabolized, cumulative effects of vecuronium are evident in renal transplant recipients and patients with severe renal failure. This effect is attributable to its metabolite, 3-desacetyl vecuronium, which has 80% of the activity of the parent drug and reportedly accumulates to a greater degree in patients with renal failure. Vecuronium may also accumulate in patients with hepatic failure because of decreased biliary uptake (11). In the presence of normal hepatic and renal function, the elimination half-life of vecuronium is 1.33 to 1.8 hrs (50). Vecuronium's active metabolites are associated with prolonged effects lasting hours to days, which may be seen in patients with end-stage renal disease (45).

Atracurium and Cisatracurium

Atracurium is a nondepolarizing neuromuscular blocker of intermediate duration (50). Onset of action occurs 2 to 4 mins after administration and remains for 30 to 40 mins. Atracurium has a Vd of 0.16 L/kg, an elimination half-life of 0.3 hrs, and a CL of 6.2 mL/kg/min (29). Atracurium (and cisatracurium) are eliminated by Hofmann elimination, which is a spontaneous nonenzymatic degradation at physiologic pH and temperature. Because of these pharmacokinetic properties, atracurium is commonly regarded as an appropriate agent when neuro-

muscular blockade is necessary in patients with multiorgan dysfunction. In contrast to atracurium, cisatracurium is associated with less risk of dose-dependent histamine release and hence less risk of urticaria, bronchospasm, or hypotension.

Atracurium is metabolized to the inactive metabolites laudanosine and a monoquaternary acrylate, both of which may be toxic. Laudanosine may accumulate in patients with renal insufficiency and in those receiving long-term infusions. Rare instances have been reported of patients developing seizures while receiving prolonged infusions of atracurium, presumably because of laudanosine accumulation. However, at therapeutic doses of atracurium, laudanosine concentrations may not reach adequate levels to produce a neurotoxic effect. Laudanosine and the monoacrylate are further metabolized, conjugated, and excreted in the urine. The activity of these final metabolites is unknown (45). Hypothermia and acidosis decrease the clearance of atracurium, because Hofmann elimination is pH- and temperature-dependent (45).

Mivacurium

Mivacurium is a nondepolarizing neuromuscular blocker (50). Onset of action occurs 2 to 4 mins after administration and remains for 12 to 18 mins (29). Mivacurium is eliminated by plasma cholinesterase, has a very short duration of action, and can be used independent of a patient's renal and hepatic status (45). As with succinylcholine, plasma cholinesterase deficiency prolongs the action of mivacurium. Higher doses are associated with histamine release (29).

Sympathomimetics

Dopamine

Dopamine is the metabolic precursor of norepinephrine and epinephrine. It is a central neurotransmitter, also found in the sympathetic nervous system and in the adrenal medulla. Dopamine stimulates dopamine (D_1 and D_2) receptors in the brain and in the vascular beds of the kidneys, mesentery, and coronary arteries. By activating cyclic AMP, D_1-receptor activation leads to vasodilation. It also stimulates α and β receptors, although its affinity for these receptors is lower (47). Low infusion rates (1–5 mcg/kg/min) augment renal sodium excretion through dopamine receptor agonism. Intermediate dosing (5–10 mcg/kg/min) results in chronotropic and inotropic effects through β-receptor agonism. Administration of these doses usually results in an increase in systolic blood pressure, minimal change in diastolic pressure, and a subsequent increase in pulse pressure. Systemic vascular resistance is unchanged secondary to the balance of dopamine's ability to reduce regional arteriolar resistance in the mesentery and kidneys, with only a minor increase in other vasculature. Higher doses (10–20 mcg/kg/min) result in increased vascular resistance secondary to a predominant α effect (29).

Dopamine hydrochloride is used only intravenously (29). As for all sympathomimetics, the central venous route is preferred over a peripheral vein. In hemodynamically stable adult patients, the steady-state Vd and the elimination half-life increased with the dose. At a dose of 3 mcg/kg/min the Vd was 0.78 L/kg, and the elimination half-life was 22 min, increasing to 1.58 L/kg and 38 min, with a dose of 6 mcg/kg/min (43). Similar values (elimination half-life of 26 min) were reported in hemodynamically stable children, aged 3 months to 13 years, who were recovering from cardiac surgery or shock (21). In critically ill newborn infants with sepsis and hypotensive shock, the Vd averaged 1.8 L/kg, and total body clearance averaged 115 mL/kg/min (9). Dopamine is a substrate for monoamine oxidase (MAO) and catechol-O-methyltransferase (COMT) (29). In hemodynamically stable adult patients, dopamine CL ranged between 50 and 56 mL/kg/min and was independent of the dose (43). Plasma dopamine clearance ranges from 60 to 80 mL/kg/min in adults and is lower in patients with renal or hepatic disease. CL in children <2 years of age is approximately twice that in older children (82 vs. 46 mL/kg/min) (47).

A marked variation in CL was thought to explain the variation in dose amount required to achieve a desired clinical response in critically ill newborn infants (9). A study that evaluated the impact of hemodialysis on dopamine pharmacokinetics in seven adult patients reported that the fraction removed by dialysis was only 2.5% (2). Dopamine toxicity includes tachycardia, hypertension, and dysrhythmias, and an increase in myocardial oxygen consumption. Dopamine depresses the ventilatory response to hypoxemia by as much as 60%. It can decrease arterial Po_2 by interfering with hypoxic pulmonary vasoconstriction. Dopamine administration may suppress the release of thyrotropin (68).

Dobutamine

Dobutamine resembles dopamine structurally and is delivered as a racemate. The (+) isomer is a strong β agonist and α_1 antagonist, whereas the (−) dobutamine isomer is a weak β antagonist and a potent α_1 agonist. Dobutamine has somewhat greater selectivity for β_1 than β_2 receptors. As a result of opposing α_1 activities, dobutamine produces significant inotropic support, with less chronotropic and vasopressor activity (29). Doses of 5 to 20 mcg/kg/min are employed for inotropic support.

Dobutamine hydrochloride is used only intravenously. Dobutamine's Vd is 0.2 L/kg, with steady-state concentrations achieved within 10 mins of the initiation of the infusion (29). In 10 children who were post–cardiac surgery and in 17 with shock, who ranged in age from 0.13 to 16.6 years, the elimination half-life was 25.8 min (61). Dobutamine's major metabolites are conjugates of dobutamine and 3-O-methyl dobutamine (29). Typical clearance values in sick children are 70 to 100 mL/kg/min (26). In a study of 12 critically ill children aged 1 month to 17 years, dobutamine plasma clearance rates ranged from 40 to 130 mL/kg/min, and dobutamine pharmacokinetics followed a first-order kinetic model (26). Dobutamine increases myocardial oxygen demand and may predispose to arrhythmias (29). Acute high-dose dobutamine lowers thyroid-stimulating hormone by an unknown mechanism (44).

Epinephrine

Epinephrine is useful in treating shock associated with myocardial dysfunction and hypotension. Epinephrine activates α_1, β_1, and β_2 receptors. It is a principal hormone of stress, and produces widespread metabolic and hemodynamic effects. β_1 receptors are affected by very low plasma concentrations of epinephrine, seen at doses of 0.05 to 0.1 mcg/kg/min. The earliest effects of epinephrine are an increase in heart rate and inotropy. Myocardial oxygen utilization may increase out of proportion to the increase in force of contraction. At these doses, stimulation of β_2 receptors promotes relaxation of re-

sistance arterioles, promoting a decrease in systemic vascular resistance and diastolic blood pressure. Higher plasma concentrations result in activation of α_1 receptors, with a subsequent increase in systemic vascular resistance. At moderate doses (0.1–1 mcg/kg/min), the α stimulation is often balanced by the improved cardiac output and relaxation of the arteriolar beds. High-dose infusions (1–2 mcg/kg/min) are associated with significant vasoconstriction and possible compromise of blood flow to individual organs. The most predominant vascular effects are seen in the smaller arterioles, although veins and large arteries also have a response. The effect of epinephrine infusions on blood flow to hepatic, splanchnic, and renal vascular beds is variable and depends on baseline hemodynamics, disease state, and epinephrine dose. Even when epinephrine infusion leads to improved blood pressure and cardiac output, blood flow to abdominal viscera may decrease as flow is diverted to heart, brain, and skeletal muscle.

Epinephrine has many uses. It is commonly used in the treatment of respiratory diseases with elements of bronchospasm. It can also be used to treat the symptoms of hypersensitivity reactions to drugs and other allergens (29). In the pediatric critical care environment, the most frequent indications for IV epinephrine are cardiogenic shock and septic shock with reduced stroke volume. Patients with septic shock who do not improve after aggressive volume repletion and treatment with dopamine and/or dobutamine may benefit from epinephrine. Epinephrine is the principal drug used in CPR after cardiac arrest (see Chapter 23).

Epinephrine is not effective after oral administration because it is rapidly oxidized and conjugated in the gastrointestinal mucosa and liver. Absorption from subcutaneous tissues is slow because of vasoconstriction. When inhaled, the actions of the drug are largely restricted to the respiratory system; however, systemic tachycardia can occur (29). Enhanced automaticity and increased oxygen consumption are the major toxicities. A severe imbalance of myocardial oxygen delivery and consumption may produce electrocardiographic changes consistent with ischemia. Hypokalemia secondary to β_2-adrenergic stimulation and hyperglycemia secondary to α-adrenergic–mediated insulin suppression are associated with epinephrine administration.

Norepinephrine

Dopamine is carboxylated at the β carbon to produce norepinephrine. Norepinephrine differs from epinephrine in that it lacks the methyl substitution on the amino group. Norepinephrine has little β_2 activity but is a potent α_1 and β_1 agonist. Infusions in normal subjects result in elevations of systemic vascular resistance because the α_1 effects are not opposed by β_2 stimulation. Reflex vagal activity reduces the heart rate, blunting the expected chronotropic effect of β_1 stimulation. Stoke volume increases, but cardiac output changes minimally. Peripheral vascular resistance increases in most vascular beds, including the kidney, liver, and skeletal muscle. Glomerular filtration is maintained, unless the decrease in renal blood flow is very substantial. Mesenteric vessels are also constricted, decreasing splanchnic and hepatic blood flow. Coronary blood flow increases due to direct coronary dilation and increase in blood pressure (29).

Norepinephrine is administered intravenously (29). The elimination half-life of IV norepinephrine is 2 to 2.5 mins (64). Norepinephrine is metabolized by enzymatic degradation, either by COMT or MAO. It is also cleared from the plasma by neuronal and tissue uptake (64). The CL of norepinephrine in healthy adults is 24 to 40 mL/kg/min. Limited pediatric pharmacokinetic data are available (64). Norepinephrine administration may result in compromised organ blood flow. It may improve blood pressure without improving perfusion, most commonly seen with a low cardiac index and elevated capillary wedge pressure (19,22).

Isoproterenol

Isoproterenol, the synthetic N-isopropyl derivative of norepinephrine, is a potent, nonselective β-adrenergic agonist with very low affinity for α-adrenergic receptors. The principal cardiovascular effects relate to its inotropic, chronotropic, and peripheral vasodilator effects. Isoproterenol increases heart rate and enhances contractility. Peripheral vasodilatation produces a decrease in systemic vascular resistance. The increase in inotropy and chronotropy in the face of decreased systemic vascular resistance results in an increase of cardiac output. Isoproterenol relaxes almost all smooth muscle but has a significant impact on bronchial and gastrointestinal smooth muscle. Pulmonary bronchial and vascular bed β_2-adrenergic receptor agonism results in bronchodilation and pulmonary vasodilation. If normal prior to the isoproterenol infusion, mesenteric and renal perfusion decreases. However, if isoproterenol is administered in a shock state, the increase in cardiac output may result in increase in blood flow to these tissues (29).

Isoproterenol is readily absorbed when given parenterally or as an aerosol. Isoproterenol is metabolized predominantly by COMT (29). The pharmacokinetics of isoproterenol in infants and children was studied in pediatric patients who were either postoperative from cardiac surgery or being treated for reactive airway disease. The volume of distribution was 0.2 L/kg. The average CL was 42.5 mL/kg/min, and the average plasma half-life was 4.2 mins (54). Isoproterenol increases myocardial demand for oxygen and decreases supply by decreasing coronary filling. If the patient is intravascularly fluid depleted and not provided with fluid resuscitation, hypotension may occur with the institution of the drug (29).

Phenylephrine

Phenylephrine demonstrates predominantly α_1-adrenergic agonism. It causes marked vasoconstriction of the arterial and venous capacitance vessels, resulting in a rise in blood pressure and a sinus bradycardia due to vagal reflexes (13).

Vasodilators

Sodium Nitroprusside

Despite its widespread use, quality pharmacokinetic and pharmacodynamic data regarding the use of sodium nitroprusside (SNP) in children are limited. Experiences with sodium nitroprusside used to induce deliberate hypotension in small cohorts of children have been described (7,17). Investigators observed that younger subjects required more SNP than did older subjects to achieve comparable degrees of blood pressure control. In their small retrospective cohort, doses of 10 mcg/kg/min were necessary to achieve satisfactory blood pressure response. Three possible responses to nitroprusside administration in children were described: (a) a constant response to "conventional" doses <3 mcg/kg/min, (b) a tachyphylactic response characterized by continuously escalating dose requirement (>3 mcg/kg/min) to achieve a satisfactory blood pressure, and (c) resistance to the blood pressure–lowering effects of the drug. They cautioned against using total doses that exceeded 3 mcg/kg/min or continuing administration of nitroprusside in the latter two scenarios. Another group compared SNP to nitroglycerin for inducing hypotension in a group of 14 adolescents; they found that doses of SNP between 6 and 8 mcg/kg/min were superior to nitroglycerin at any dose in the reliable induction of hypotension for children and adolescents undergoing scoliosis, craniofacial, or hepatic surgery (75). In a randomized trial comparing nitroprusside to nicardipine in 20 healthy adolescents with idiopathic scoliosis undergoing spinal fusion, target blood pressures were easily obtainable in both groups, and operating conditions were comparable (30). The time to restoration of baseline blood pressure after termination of the infusion was significantly longer in the nicardipine group. Interestingly, blood loss was significantly greater in the SNP group. Details on nitroprusside dose requirements were not provided.

A well-described potential side effect of nitroprusside is cyanide and/or thiocyanate toxicity. IV SNP degradation results in the release of free cyanide. Cyanide accumulation can cause a metabolic acidosis, arrhythmia, excessive hypotension, and death. Cyanide can subsequently be converted to serum thiocyanate using thiosulfate. Thiocyanate is ultimately renally eliminated (35). SNP metabolism was described in 10 children who received SNP at doses up to 10 mcg/kg/min (mean infusion rate, 6 mcg/kg/min) while undergoing cardiopulmonary bypass for repair of complex congenital cardiac defects (51). Cyanide levels rose as a function of time while SNP was infused, and they rapidly fell when SNP was discontinued. Despite the fact that some children demonstrated plasma cyanide levels above the generally accepted threshold of 0.5 mcg/mL, no patients developed clinically apparent toxicity. Adverse effects include nausea, vomiting, agitation, and muscular twitching. Acute psychosis from thiocyanate intoxication can result from prolonged therapy, especially in patients with renal failure.

Hydralazine

Hydralazine causes the direct relaxation of arteriole smooth muscle. Venous capacitance vessels are not dilated, and postural hypotension is uncommon. IV hydralazine may be used for hypertensive emergencies but is rarely the sole agent with which to treat hypertension (29). It is well absorbed but undergoes significant first-pass metabolism, making the systemic bioavailability low. It is 87% protein bound, and has a Vd of 1.5 L/kg. The rate of acetylation is genetically determined, with approximately 50% of the US population being fast acetylators and the other 50%, slow. The elimination half-life is 1 hr, although the systemic effect may remain for up to 12 hrs. The CL is 50 mL/kg/min (29). Sympathetic stimulation can result in an increased heart rate, increased renin activity, and subsequent fluid retention. Side effects include headache, nausea, flushing, and palpitations. Administration can result in a syndrome that resembles systemic lupus and is characterized by serum sickness, hemolytic anemia, vasculitis, and glomerulonephritis (29).

Nicardipine

Nicardipine is a calcium-entry blocker (slow-channel blocker or calcium-ion antagonist) that inhibits the transmembrane influx of calcium ions into cardiac muscle and smooth muscle without changing serum calcium concentrations. The effects of nicardipine are more selective to vascular smooth muscle than to cardiac muscle. In animal models, nicardipine produces a relaxation of coronary vascular smooth muscle at drug levels that cause little or no negative inotropic effect. In humans, nicardipine produces a significant decrease in systemic vascular resistance. The degree of vasodilation and the resultant hypotensive effects are more prominent in hypertensive patients. In hypertensive patients, nicardipine reduces the blood pressure at rest and during exercise. In normotensive patients, a small decrease of approximately 9 mm Hg in systolic and 7 mm Hg in diastolic blood pressure may occur.

Nicardipine is completely absorbed following oral administration. The systemic bioavailability is approximately 35% following an oral dose. The pharmacokinetics of nicardipine are nonlinear due to a saturable hepatic first-pass metabolism. Following oral administration, plasma levels are detectable at as early as 20 mins, and maximal plasma levels are achieved generally at between 1 and 4 hrs. Following oral administration, increasing doses result in disproportionate increases in plasma levels. Increasing the dose twofold may increase maximum plasma levels four- to fivefold. Rapid dose-related increases in nicardipine plasma concentrations are seen during the first 2 hrs after initiation of an infusion, and concentrations reach a steady state at approximately 24 to 48 hrs. Upon termination of the infusion, plasma concentrations rapidly decline, with at least a 50% decrease during the first 2 hrs (74). The Vd is approximately 8.3 L/kg, and the elimination half-life in adults is 8.6 hrs (74).

Nicardipine undergoes extensive hepatic metabolism via the P450 pathway. Transformation of the N-benzyl side-chain position 3 is the primary site of breakdown. Oxidation to the pyridine analog is another source of metabolism (67). Virtually no unchanged drug is found in the urine. Although nicardipine is principally metabolized by the liver, lower clearance has been reported in patients with renal impairment (74). Cimetidine increases plasma levels. Patients receiving the two drugs concomitantly should be carefully monitored. Concomitant administration of nicardipine and cyclosporine results in elevated plasma cyclosporine levels. Plasma concentrations of cyclosporine should therefore be closely monitored, and its dosage reduced accordingly, in patients treated with nicardipine (74).

Miscellaneous

Nitric Oxide

Nitric oxide (NO) is produced by many cells of the body. It relaxes vascular smooth muscle by binding to the heme moiety of cytosolic guanylate cyclase, activating guanylate cyclase, and increasing intracellular levels of cyclic guanosine $3',5'$-monophosphate, which then leads to vasodilation. NO has a half-life of only a few seconds in vivo. However, because it is soluble in both aqueous and lipid media, it readily diffuses through the cytoplasm and plasma membranes. NO has effects on neuronal transmission and on synaptic plasticity in the CNS. When inhaled, NO produces pulmonary vasodilation and thus finds its principal use in the treatment of pulmonary hypertension.

Inhaled NO appears to increase the PaO_2 by dilating pulmonary vessels in better-ventilated areas of the lung, redis-tributing pulmonary blood flow away from lung regions with low ventilation:perfusion ratios toward regions with normal ratios. Although this therapy transiently improves oxygenation in patients with acute respiratory failure, it has not improved long-term outcomes.

In addition to its hemodynamic effects, inhaled NO may inhibit platelet aggregation. These effects are dose-dependent, in that both excesses and deficiencies of the gas have been implicated in the genesis and/or evolution of many significant diseases. At high concentrations (>80–100 ppm), inhaled NO has proinflammatory and prooxidant effects, increasing macrophage production of tumor necrosis factor (TNF)-α, interleukin (IL)-1, and reactive oxygen species (71,72). Concentrations up to 80 ppm appear to reduce the number and activity of pulmonary neutrophils. The dose of 50 ppm appears to reduce the migration of neutrophils from the vascular compartment to the airways and inhibits chemotaxis (58).

The pharmacokinetics of NO have been studied only in adults. NO is absorbed systemically after inhalation. Most of it traverses the pulmonary capillary bed, where it combines with hemoglobin that is 60% to 100% oxygen saturated. At this level of oxygen saturation, NO combines predominantly with oxyhemoglobin to produce methemoglobin and nitrate. At low oxygen saturation, NO can combine with deoxyhemoglobin to transiently form nitrosylhemoglobin, which is converted to nitrogen oxides and methemoglobin upon exposure to oxygen. Within the pulmonary system, NO can combine with oxygen and water to produce nitrogen dioxide (NO_2) and nitrite, respectively, which interact with oxyhemoglobin to produce methemoglobin and nitrate. Thus, the end products of NO that enter the systemic circulation are predominantly methemoglobin and nitrate. Nitrate has been identified as the predominant NO metabolite excreted in the urine, accounting for $>70\%$ of the NO dose inhaled. Nitrate is cleared from the plasma by the kidney at rates approaching the rate of glomerular filtration. No studies have been conducted to assess the interaction of inhaled NO with other drugs. Hence, clinical interactions with other medications used in the treatment of respiratory failure cannot be ruled out. Inhaled NO has been administered in combination with dopamine, dobutamine, corticosteroids, and surfactant without interactions being detected (24).

Both relative and absolute contraindications have been described for the use of NO. An absolute contraindication is warranted in the rare condition of methemoglobin reductase deficiency. The primary concerns related to the administration of inhaled NO are the formation of NO_2, methemoglobinemia, and the "rebound effect." The latter describes a phenomenon in which significant increases in pulmonary vascular resistance (rebound pulmonary hypertension) occur following termination of inhaled NO. NO_2 production is another potential concern with the use of inhaled NO. NO_2 is produced from NO and oxygen and can cause oxidative pulmonary damage, resulting in the generation of free radicals, which can oxidize amino acids and begin lipid peroxidation of the cellular membrane (24,65).

Milrinone

Milrinone has combined inotropic and vasodilating effects ("inodilator"), as well as lusitropic effects (63). It is a bipyridine derivative of amrinone, primarily used for the treatment of congestive heart failure and commonly used to support cardiac output after congenital heart surgery in neonates, infants, and children. The drug is primarily cleared through renal secretion (85%), with 15% undergoing glucuronidation, and is 70% protein bound (77). Pharmacokinetic studies suggest that the CL of milrinone is greater and its Vd is larger in children than in adults (31,52), but infants appear to have lower milrinone clearance than do children (52).

A recent study of pediatric patients <6 years of age who received milrinone as a slow-loading dose followed by a constant-rate infusion after cardiac surgery used population modeling to describe milrinone pharmacokinetics (4). The pharmacokinetics were best described by a weight-normalized, one-compartment model. The Vd of 482 mL/kg was independent of age, whereas CL increased linearly with age. A comparable two-compartment model had a central Vd of 66 mL/kg, peripheral Vd of 269 mL/kg, CL of 6.29 mL/kg/min, and an intercompartmental CL of 4.75 mL/kg/min. In pediatric patients who underwent biventricular cardiac surgery, the Vd and CL of milrinone were reported as 900 mL/kg and 3.8 mL/kg/min for infants and 700 mL/kg and 5.9 mL/kg/min for children, respectively (52). In a population of neonates who underwent Norwood Stage I single-ventricle palliation, a loading dose of 100 mcg/kg during cardiopulmonary bypass resulted in plasma peak and trough milrinone concentrations similar to those achieved with 50-mcg/kg loading doses in other clinical settings (5).

Due to impaired renal clearance during the immediate postoperative period, a standard infusion of 0.5 mcg/kg/min resulted in drug accumulation during the initial 12 hrs of drug administration. Immediately postoperatively, milrinone clearance was significantly impaired (0.4 mL/kg/min), improved by the twelfth postoperative hour, and approached steady-state clearance by postoperative day 4. The weight-normalized population estimate for steady-state clearance in this population was 2.6 mL/kg/min, which is less than that reported for older infants postoperative from cardiac surgery (78).

Vasopressin

Vasopressin is an exogenous, parenteral form of antidiuretic hormone. Antidiuretic hormone is produced in the parvocellular and magnocellular neurons within the supraoptic and paraventricular nuclei of the hypothalamus. It is stored and released by the posterior pituitary gland in response to increases in plasma osmolality or as a baroreflex response to decreases in blood pressure and/or blood volume.

The cellular effects of vasopressin are mediated by two major receptors, V_1 and V_2. V_1 receptors have been further subdivided as V_{1a} and V_{1b}. The V_{1a} receptor is the most widespread and is found in vascular smooth muscle, myometrium, the bladder, adipocytes, hepatocytes, platelets, renal medullary interstitial cells, vasa recta in the renal circulation, epithelial cells in the renal cortical collecting duct, spleen, testis, and many CNS structures. Only the adenohypophysis is known to contain V_{1b} receptors. V_2 receptors are predominantly found in the principal cells of the renal collecting duct system. V_2 receptors mediate the most predominant renal response to vasopressin, resulting in increased water permeability in the collecting duct. These V_2-mediated effects occur at much lower concentrations than are required to engage V_1-receptor–mediated actions. Other renal activities mediated by V_2 include increased urea and sodium (Na^+) transport, increasing the urine concentrating ability of the kidneys.

The cardiovascular effects of vasopressin are complex. Vasopressin administration results in significant vasoconstriction, mediated by V_1 receptors. Vascular smooth muscle in the skin, skeletal muscle, fat, pancreas, and thyroid gland appear to be most sensitive, with vasoconstriction also occurring in gastrointestinal tract, coronary vessels, and brain. Activation of V_2 receptors increases circulating concentrations of procoagulant factor VIII and von Willebrand factor, and vasopressin is presumed to stimulate the secretion of these factors from storage sites in the vascular endothelium (29). Diabetes insipidus is a disease of impaired renal conservation of water, either secondary to an inadequate secretion of vasopressin (central diabetes insipidus), as seen with many patients who have sustained traumatic brain injury, or an insufficient renal response to vasopressin (nephrogenic diabetes insipidus). Vasopressin is most commonly indicated in the treatment of patients with high urine flow due to central diabetes insipidus (16).

Due to its vasoactive effects, vasopressin therapy has been evaluated in the specific setting of cardiac arrest and refractory hypotension in septic shock (56). It was recently recommended by the American Heart Association as an alternative to epinephrine for adult patients in ventricular fibrillation, and it is used to control upper gastrointestinal hemorrhage given its ability to cause vasoconstriction of the mesenteric vasculature.

Vasopressin must be administered parenterally because it is degraded by trypsin in the gastrointestinal tract. The duration of antidiuretic effect following intramuscular or subcutaneous administration is approximately 2 to 8 hrs. The hormone distributes throughout the extracellular fluid but does not bind to plasma proteins. Vasopressin is degraded primarily in the liver and kidneys, and has a plasma half-life of 10 to 35 mins. Approximately 5% of a subcutaneously administered dose is excreted unchanged in the urine within 4 hrs (32). Large doses can result in cardiac complications, such as arrhythmias and decreased cardiac output.

CONCLUSIONS AND FUTURE DIRECTIONS

Pharmacology is an important discipline that underlies the management of pharmacotherapy, or the safe and effective administration of pharmaceuticals. Understanding pharmacologic principles is essential for the proper application of pharmacotherapeutic modalities in critically ill children. Although much of the pharmacologic knowledge used to derive dosing guidance for critically ill children is obtained from adult and other pediatric populations, research into understanding the dose requirements for critically ill children is more active than ever before.

Because children are typically not subject to dose-escalation studies similar to those conducted in the adult population, initial estimation of dose requirements in pediatrics is often based on various arbitrary descriptors of body size; the lack of well-conducted pharmacodynamic and pharmacokinetic studies is often replaced by extrapolation from adult or animal data. Likewise, the pediatric susceptibility to adverse drug reactions is often difficult to predict. Past therapeutic mishaps have clearly shown that dosing derived from adult studies cannot easily be extrapolated to infants and children. In addition, many adult dosage forms, such as tablets and capsules, are inappropriate for neonates, infants, and preschool children. Likewise, targeted investigations in critically ill pediatric populations are now occurring with greater frequency, as the scientific community has a greater appreciation of the risk of ignorance and the incredible burden placed on the caregivers of this population. As these data become available, it is likewise incumbent upon caregivers to educate themselves to this guidance and be able to apply such knowledge to their own practice.

KEY POINTS

- An understanding of pharmacokinetics and pharmacodynamics can allow for a rational approach toward prescribing medications for critically ill children.
- Drug absorption, distribution, metabolism, elimination, and the response to medications are impacted by age and disease state.
- Many medications are prescribed for children based on dosing guidance from adult studies.
- Care providers must be cautious of the high risk of drug interactions and adverse reactions in the intensive care setting.

References

1. Abbott. Precedex Product Label, 2003.
2. Allen E, Pettigrew A, Frank D, et al. Alterations in dopamine clearance and catechol-O-methyltransferase activity by dopamine infusions in children. *Crit Care Med* 1997;25:181–9.
3. Annane D. ICU physicians should abandon the use of etomidate! *Intensive Care Med* 2005;31:325–6.
4. Bailey JM, Hoffman TM, Wessel DL, et al. A population pharmacokinetic analysis of milrinone in pediatric patients after cardiac surgery. *J Pharmacokinet Pharmacodyn* 2004;31:43–9.
5. Bailey JM, Levy JH, Kikura M, et al. Pharmacokinetics of intravenous milrinone in patients undergoing cardiac surgery. *Anesthesiology* 1994;81:616–22.
6. Bayliff CD, Schwartz ML, Hardy BG, et al. Pharmacokinetics of high-dose pentobarbital in severe head trauma. *Clin Pharmacol Ther* 1985;38:457–61.
7. Bennett NR, Abbott TR. The use of sodium nitroprusside in children. *Anaesthesia* 1977;32:456–63.
8. Bhana N, Goa KL, McClellan KJ. Dexmedetomidine. *Drugs* 2000;59:263–8; discussion 9–70.
9. Bhatt-Mehta V, Nahata MC, McClead RE, et al. Dopamine pharmacokinetics in critically ill newborn infants. *Eur J Clin Pharmacol* 1991;40:593–7.
10. Carruthers SG, Hoffman BB, Melmon KL, eds. *Melmon and Morrelli's Clinical Pharmacology.* New York: McGraw-Hill, 2000.
11. Chernow B, ed. *The Pharmacologic Approach to the Critically Ill Patient.* Baltimore: Williams and Wilkins, 1994.
12. Cook CE, Seltzman TB, Tallent CR, et al. Pharmacokinetics of pentobarbital enantiomers as determined by enantioselective radioimmunoassay after administration of racemate to humans and rabbits. *J Pharmacol Exp Ther* 1987;241:779–85.
13. Cooper DW, Carpenter M, Mowbray P, et al. Fetal and maternal effects of phenylephrine and ephedrine during spinal anesthesia for cesarean delivery. *Anesthesiology* 2002;97:1582–90.
14. Cray SH, Robinson BH, Cox PN, et al. Lactic acidemia and bradyarrhythmia in a child sedated with propofol. *Crit Care Med* 1998;26:2087–92.
15. Cremer OL, Moons KG, Bouman EA, et al. Long-term propofol infusion and cardiac failure in adult head-injured patients. *Lancet* 2001;357:117–8.
16. David JL. Desmopressin and hemostasis. *Regul Pept* 1993;45:311–7.
17. Davies DW, Greiss L, Kadar D, et al. Sodium nitroprusside in children: Observations on metabolism during normal and abnormal responses. *Can Anaesth Soc J* 1975;22:553–60.
18. de Wildt SN, de Hoog M, Vinks AA, et al. Population pharmacokinetics and metabolism of midazolam in pediatric intensive care patients. *Crit Care Med* 2003;31:1952–8.
19. Desjars P, Pinaud M, Bugnon D, et al. Norepinephrine therapy has no deleterious renal effects in human septic shock. *Crit Care Med* 1989;17:426–9.
20. Ehrnebo M. Pharmacokinetics and distribution properties of pentobarbital in humans following oral and intravenous administration. *J Pharm Sci* 1974;63:1114–18.
21. Eldadah MK, Schwartz PH, Harrison R, et al. Pharmacokinetics of dopamine in infants and children. *Crit Care Med* 1991;19:1008–11.
22. Fukuoka T, Nishimura M, Imanaka H, et al. Effects of norepinephrine on renal function in septic patients with normal and elevated serum lactate levels. *Crit Care Med* 1989;17:1104–7.
23. Gehlbach BK, Kress JP. Sedation in the intensive care unit. *Curr Opin Crit Care* 2002;8:290–8.
24. Gianetti J, Bevilacqua S, De Caterina R, et al. Inhaled nitric oxide: More than a selective pulmonary vasodilator. *Eur J Clin Invest* 2002;32:628–35.
25. Greenberg SB, Adams RC, Aspinall CL, et al. Initial experience with intravenous pentobarbital sedation for children undergoing MRI at a tertiary care pediatric hospital: The learning curve. *Pediatr Radiol* 2000;30:689–91.
26. Habib DM, Padbury JF, Anas NG, et al. Dobutamine pharmacokinetics and pharmacodynamics in pediatric intensive care patients. *Crit Care Med* 1992;20:601–8.
27. Hagmeyer KO, Mauro LS, Mauro VF, et al. Meperidine-related seizures associated with patient-controlled analgesia pumps. *Ann Pharmacother* 1993;27:29–32.
28. Hall LG, Oyen LJ, Murray MJ, et al. Analgesic agents. Pharmacology and application in critical care. *Crit Care Clin* 2001;17:899–923, viii.
29. Hardman JG, Limbird LE, eds. *Goodman and Gilman's The Pharmacologic Basis of Therapeutics.* New York: McGraw-Hill, 1996.
30. Hersey SL, O'Dell NE, Lowe S, et al. Nicardipine versus nitroprusside for controlled hypotension during spinal surgery in adolescents. *Anesth Analg* 1997;84:1239–44.
31. Hoffman TM, Wernovsky G, Atz AM, et al. Efficacy and safety of milrinone in preventing low cardiac output syndrome in infants and children after corrective surgery for congenital heart disease. *Circulation* 2003;107:996–1002.
32. Holmes CL, Patel BM, Russell JA, et al. Physiology of vasopressin relevant to management of septic shock. *Chest* 2001;120:989–1002.
33. Huang NN, High RH. Comparison of serum levels following the administration of oral and parenteral preparations of penicillin to infants and children of various age groups. *J Pediatr* 1953;42:657–8.
34. Hubbard AM, Markowitz RI, Kimmel B, et al. Sedation for pediatric patients undergoing CT and MRI. *J Comput Assist Tomogr* 1992;16:3–6.
35. Katzung BG, ed. *Basic and Clinical Pharmacology.* New York: McGraw Hill, 2001.
36. Kazama T, Ikeda K, Morita K, et al. Reduction by fentanyl of the Cp50 values of propofol and hemodynamic responses to various noxious stimuli. *Anesthesiology* 1997;87:213–27.
37. Kazama T, Ikeda K, Morita K, et al. Relation between initial blood distribution volume and propofol induction dose requirement. *Anesthesiology* 2001;94:205–10.
38. Kearns GL, Abdel-Rahman SM, Alander SW, et al. Developmental pharmacology—drug disposition, action, and therapy in infants and children. *N Engl J Med* 2003;349:1157–67.
39. Klotz U, Kanto J. Pharmacokinetics and clinical use of flumazenil (Ro 15-1788). *Clin Pharmacokinet* 1988;14:1–12.
40. Kohrs R, Durieux ME. Ketamine: Teaching an old drug new tricks. *Anesth Analg* 1998;87:1186–93.
41. Krishnan V, Murray P. Pharmacologic issues in the critically ill. *Clin Chest Med* 2003;24:671–88.
42. Lacroix D, Sonnier M, Moncion A, et al. Expression of CYP3A in the human liver—evidence that the shift between CYP3A7 and CYP3A4 occurs immediately after birth. *Eur J Biochem* 1997;247:625–34.
43. Le Corre P, Malledant Y, Tanguy M, et al. Steady-state pharmacokinetics of dopamine in adult patients. *Crit Care Med* 1993;21:1652–7.
44. Lee E, Chen P, Rao H, et al. Effect of acute high dose dobutamine administration on serum thyrotrophin (TSH). *Clin Endocrinol (Oxf)* 1999;50:487–92.
45. McManus MC. Neuromuscular blockers in surgery and intensive care, Part 1. *Am J Health Syst Pharm* 2001;58:2287–99.
46. Mendelson WB. Neuropharmacology of sleep induction by benzodiazepines. *Crit Rev Neurobiol* 1992;6:221–32.
47. Notterman DA, Greenwald BM, Moran F, et al. Dopamine clearance in critically ill infants and children: Effect of age and organ system dysfunction. *Clin Pharmacol Ther* 1990;48:138–47.
48. Painter MJ, Pippenger C, Wasterlain C, et al. Phenobarbital and phenytoin in neonatal seizures: Metabolism and tissue distribution. *Neurology* 1981;31:1107–12.
49. *Physicians' Desk Reference.* Montvale, NJ: Thomson Healthcare, 2006.
50. Power BM, Forbes AM, van Heerden PV, et al. Pharmacokinetics of drugs used in critically ill adults. *Clin Pharmacokinet* 1998;34:25–56.
51. Przybylo HJ, Stevenson GW, Schanbacher P, et al. Sodium nitroprusside metabolism in children during hypothermic cardiopulmonary bypass. *Anesth Analg* 1995;81:952–6.
52. Ramamoorthy C, Anderson GD, Williams GD, et al. Pharmacokinetics and side effects of milrinone in infants and children after open heart surgery. *Anesth Analg* 1998;86:283–9.
53. Reed MD, Rodarte A, Blumer JL, et al. The single-dose pharmacokinetics of midazolam and its primary metabolite in pediatric patients after oral and intravenous administration. *J Clin Pharmacol* 2001;41:1359–69.
54. Reyes G, Schwartz PH, Newth CJ, et al. The pharmacokinetics of isoproterenol in critically ill pediatric patients. *J Clin Pharmacol* 1993;33:29–34.

55. Rodighiero V. Effects of liver disease on pharmacokinetics. An update. *Clin Pharmacokinet* 1999;37:399–431.

56. Rosenzweig EB, Starc TJ, Chen JM, et al. Intravenous arginine-vasopressin in children with vasodilatory shock after cardiac surgery. *Circulation* 1999;100:II182–II6.

57. Russo H, Bressolle F. Pharmacodynamics and pharmacokinetics of thiopental. *Clin Pharmacokinet* 1998;35:95–134.

58. Sato Y, Walley KR, Klut ME, et al. Nitric oxide reduces the sequestration of polymorphonuclear leukocytes in lung by changing deformability and CD18 expression. *Am J Respir Crit Care Med* 1999;159:1469–76.

59. Schaible DH, Cupit GC, Swedlow DB, et al. High-dose pentobarbital pharmacokinetics in hypothermic brain-injured children. *J Pediatr* 1982;100:655–60.

60. Schuttler J, Ihmsen H. Population pharmacokinetics of propofol: A multicenter study. *Anesthesiology* 2000;92:727–38.

61. Schwartz PH, Eldadah MK, Newth CJ, et al. The pharmacokinetics of dobutamine in pediatric intensive care unit patients. *Drug Metab Dispos* 1991;19:614–9.

62. Shelly MP, Mendel L, Park GR. Failure of critically ill patients to metabolise midazolam. *Anaesthesia* 1987;42:619–26.

63. Shipley JB, Tolman D, Hastillo A, et al. Milrinone: Basic and clinical pharmacology and acute and chronic management. *Am J Med Sci* 1996;311:286–91.

64. Steinberg C, Notterman DA. Pharmacokinetics of cardiovascular drugs in children. Inotropes and vasopressors. *Clin Pharmacokinet* 1994;27:345–67.

65. Troncy E, Collet JP, Shapiro S, et al. Inhaled nitric oxide in acute respiratory distress syndrome: A pilot randomized controlled study. *Am J Respir Crit Care Med* 1998;157:1483–88.

66. Tsai CE, Daood MJ, Lane RH, et al. P-glycoprotein expression in mouse brain increases with maturation. *Biol Neonate* 2002;81:58–64.

67. Urien S, Albengres E, Comte A, et al. Plasma protein binding and erythrocyte partitioning of nicardipine in vitro. *J Cardiovasc Pharmacol* 1985;7:891–8.

68. Van den Berghe G, de Zegher F, Lauwers P, et al. Dopamine suppresses pituitary function in infants and children. *Crit Care Med* 1994;22:1747–53.

69. Venn RM, Grounds RM. Comparison between dexmedetomidine and propofol for sedation in the intensive care unit: Patient and clinician perceptions. *Br J Anaesth* 2001;87:684–90.

70. Volles DF, McGory R. Pharmacokinetic considerations. *Crit Care Clin* 1999;15:55–75.

71. Wang YG, Rechenmacher CE, Lipsius SL. Nitric oxide signaling mediates stimulation of L-type Ca^{2+} current elicited by withdrawal of acetylcholine in cat atrial myocytes. *J Gen Physiol* 1998;111:113–25.

72. Weinberger B, Fakhrzadeh L, Heck DE, et al. Inhaled nitric oxide primes lung macrophages to produce reactive oxygen and nitrogen intermediates. *Am J Respir Crit Care Med* 1998;158:931–38.

73. Wermeling DP, Blouin RA, Porter WH, et al. Pentobarbital pharmacokinetics in patients with severe head injury. *Drug Intell Clin Pharm* 1987;21:459–63.

74. Wyeth Laboratories. Product Information: Cardene IV, nicardipine. Philadelphia, 1999.

75. Yaster M, Simmons RS, Tolo VT, et al. A comparison of nitroglycerin and nitroprusside for inducing hypotension in children: A double-blind study. *Anesthesiology* 1986;65:175–9.

76. Young CC, Prielipp RC. Benzodiazepines in the intensive care unit. *Crit Care Clin* 2001;17:843–62.

77. Young RA, Ward A. Milrinone. A preliminary review of its pharmacological properties and therapeutic use. *Drugs* 1988;36:158–92.

78. Zuppa AF, Nicolson SC, Adamson PC, et al. Population pharmacokinetics of milrinone in neonates with hypoplastic left heart syndrome undergoing stage I reconstruction. *Anesth Analg* 2006;102:1062–69.

CHAPTER 21 ▪ MULTIPLE ORGAN DYSFUNCTION SYNDROME

YONG Y. HAN • THOMAS P. SHANLEY

Perhaps no clinical entity epitomizes the discipline of critical care medicine as well as the condition known as multiple organ dysfunction syndrome (MODS). Numerous pharmacologic and technologic advances, reviewed in other chapters in this text, have led to substantial improvements in the stabilization and support of the acutely presenting, critically ill patient. The past decades have witnessed dramatic decreases in mortality rates from diseases that were once almost universally lethal. However, arising concomitantly with this ability to alter the natural course of acute illness are new clinical dilemmas, characterized by the evolution of these apparently "averted" fatalities into delayed, and often protracted, nebulous deaths marked by the progressive dysfunction of multiple organs. Almost irrespective of the initial, life-threatening primary insult—severe infection, extensive burns, massive trauma, significant hypoxic–ischemic events, refractory shock, cardiopulmonary arrest, or other serious injury—the progression of sequential organ dysfunction seen in MODS has emerged as a final common pathogenic pathway that constantly threatens the survival of critically ill children and challenges the clinical acumen of critical care physicians. Yet, almost ironically, despite gaining considerable ability to recognize the clinical manifestations of MODS and its associated epidemiologic and prognostic implications, our understanding of its underlying pathophysiologic mechanisms remains incomplete, and specifically targeted therapies remain limited. As a result, numerous theories, supported in part by both experimental and observational data, have been espoused in an attempt to define the mechanisms of this process and to identify novel means for treating this often fatal syndrome.

Although each of our subspecialty colleagues in cardiology, pulmonology, nephrology, neurology, or hematology can provide expert advice regarding how to best treat their specific organ system of interest, the optimal management of MODS often requires the careful balancing and orchestration of multiple therapeutic modalities, because treatment for one organ system may deleteriously hinder the recovery of another. This chapter attempts to provide a global overview of MODS through a review of the definition and epidemiology of pediatric MODS, a discussion of some of the prevailing and alternate mechanistic theories thought to contribute to the pathogenesis and pathophysiology of MODS, and a brief description of therapeutic interventions that may impact the clinical course of MODS.

RECOGNIZING AND DEFINING MULTIPLE ORGAN DYSFUNCTION SYNDROME

In many respects, the emergence of MODS as a clinical entity parallels the "birth" of Critical Care Medicine as a subspecialty discipline. Prior to the advent of modern ICUs in the mid-1950s and the successful development of contemporary life-support technologies, most patients afflicted with acute, life-threatening, critical illness died from overwhelming primary injury. However, as advances in surgery, anesthesiology, and medicine began to empower physicians with potentially life-saving interventions, early critical care pioneers began to recognize that their initial resuscitative efforts were often thwarted by the onset of a perplexing clinical entity characterized by the development of secondary physiologic derangements in organs previously "spared" from the primary insult. Initial reports of this phenomenon often focused on single-organ dysfunction, such as respiratory failure, as a complicating feature of the primary disease process or of the resuscitation itself. In 1950, one of the earliest pathologic descriptions was provided of what would later be recognized as acute respiratory distress syndrome (ARDS), which the authors proposed was a complication of fluid resuscitation for shock (21). The notion that this clinical entity could entail *multisystem* involvement was suggested as early as 1963, in a report that described "high-output respiratory failure" as an important cause of death from peritonitis or ileus (8). Although this study also focused primarily on respiratory derangements, the authors did acknowledge potential contributions from hematologic, renal, and cardiovascular system breakdowns that led to patient demise. The fundamental observation that overwhelming infections could lead to MODS dates back to the late 1960s. In 1967, the pattern of septic shock progression was reported in a large case series, and the sequential evolution of organ failure was detailed in many of the patients (33). Two years later, the clinical syndrome of serial respiratory, cardiovascular, and hepatic failure was described following hemorrhage from acute gastric stress ulcers complicated by gram-negative sepsis (45). However, noninfectious triggers for MODS were also observed and, in a related manner, in 1973, sequential failure of multiple organs was discussed in a seminal series of patients who underwent repair of ruptured aortic aneurysms (48). Shortly after these reports, Baue wrote a landmark editorial in 1975, proposing that this observed "multiple, progressive, or sequential systems failure" represented a distinct clinical entity that was, indeed, often more difficult to combat and more refractory to medical therapy than the triggering insult itself (3). Over the ensuing years, several additional terms or phrases were utilized to describe this clinical concept, including "multiple organ failure (MOF)," "remote organ failure," and "multiple system organ failure (MSOF)." Particularly relevant to our specific discipline of Pediatric Critical Care Medicine, in 1986, "multiple organ system failure (MOSF)" in children was first described, with consideration for age-adjusted criteria for organ failure (56).

In an attempt to bring consistency to the definition and characterization of MODS (as well as "sepsis"), a Consensus Conference was convened by the American College of Chest Physicians (ACCP) and the Society of Critical Care Medicine (SCCM) in 1991 (with conference proceedings published in 1992). The stated goals of the conference were "to provide a conceptual and a practical framework to define the systemic inflammatory response to infection, which is a progressive injurious process that falls under the generalized term 'sepsis' and includes sepsis-associated organ dysfunction" (2). At that time, an emphasis was placed on the understanding (a) that MODS reflected a *continuum of dysfunction,* rather than a *dichotomous state* of normal function versus failure, (b) that this condition was potentially *reversible,* and (c) that the degree of organ dysfunction could change over time. Additionally, in discussing the mechanism(s) responsible for the development of MODS, it was acknowledged that numerous host, pathogen, and treatment factors were likely to impact the course of MODS (2). To reflect consensus approval for these proposed concepts, conference delegates adopted to use "multiple organ dysfunction syndrome" as the preferred term to describe this now widely accepted clinical entity. Moreover, to reflect differences in the pathophysiologic triggers that lead to MODS, the concepts of *primary* versus *secondary* MODS were introduced. Thus, primary MODS developed from the direct result of a well-defined insult in which organ failure occurred early and could be directly attributed to the insult itself (e.g., meningococcemia). In contrast, following a latent period after the initial insult, secondary MODS emerged as a consequence of a maladaptive host response to the injury, most commonly an infectious complication. Interestingly, in differentiating between primary versus secondary MODS in children, Proulx et al. presented alternate, time-based definitions, defining primary MODS as the occurrence of MODS within the first week of PICU admission, without evidence of sequential organ dysfunction, and secondary MODS as the onset of MODS more than 7 days after PICU admission or sequential organ dysfunction to a maximal number of organ failures occurring more than 72 hrs after the initial diagnosis of MODS (38). At this time, it remains uncertain whether the etiology-based or time-based definition of primary versus secondary MODS will be adopted for pediatric MODS, and appropriate clarification should be noted when discussing these concepts.

Reaching consensus uniformity in concept, definition, and specific physiologic criteria for MODS marked an important hurdle in the adult healthcare areas, because clinicians and investigators could now speak a "common language" in describing MODS. However, despite the adage that "children are not little adults," remarkably, it was not until 2002 that a simi-

lar consensus expert panel in the area of pediatric critical care medicine met to address *pediatric-specific* definitions and criteria for sepsis and organ dysfunction (17). Hence, variability between pediatric studies to date has remained a significant obstacle to a more comprehensive clinical understanding of pediatric MODS.

Meanwhile, in 2001, a decade after the 1991 ACCP/SCCM conference, the definitions derived from that conference were revisited (results were published in 2003) during a joint consensus conference sponsored by the SCCM, the European Society of Intensive Care Medicine, the ACCP, the American Thoracic Society, and the Surgical Infection Society (30). The primary consensus point derived from the 2001 meeting was that, although the definitions from 1991 were generally robust enough for continued clinical application, they did not allow for a precise "staging" of the host response to an inflammatory trigger. To address this deficiency, a staging system, similar to that used for cancer biology and based on a PIRO system, was proposed (**Table 21.1**). The PIRO system involves characterization of the *p*redisposition of the host to be affected, the *i*nsult/*i*nfection that is triggering the response, the *r*esponse of the host (e.g., presence of the systemic inflammatory response syndrome [SIRS], biomarkers), and the degree of *o*rgan dysfunction (30). Thus, the quantification of organ dysfunction and improved mechanistic understanding of the pathophysiology of MODS remain essential goals of ongoing critical care research.

Scoring Systems

Derived from an assortment of clinical observations and definitions and markers of organ dysfunction, a number of proposed scoring systems have been developed, variably validated, and applied to multiple clinical series, with the goal of "quantifying" the severity of MODS. Unfortunately, the heterogeneity of these numerous scoring systems has complicated the consistency of objectively recording MODS severity for the purposes of study comparison and mortality prediction. In adults, the main scoring systems include Multiple Organ Dysfunction Score (MODS), the Logistic Organ Dysfunction Score (LODS), and the Sequential Organ Failure Assessment (SOFA) score, each of which has aimed to quantify the severity of MODS as a single score and correlate this score to outcome in adult patients.

During the early evolution of pediatric MODS quantification (that predated the 1991 ACCP/SCCM Consensus Conference), organ dysfunction was viewed dichotomously rather than in a continuum, and the total number of organs with dysfunction (0 to 5, 6, or 7, depending on the inclusion of the hepatic and gastrointestinal systems) was used to score the severity of MODS in children. As would have been predicted, this score (sometimes referred to as the Organ Failure Index score) correlated to mortality. The first series of age-specific criteria to reflect organ dysfunction in children from 1986 (56) were modestly refined to include criteria for hepatic and gastrointestinal failures (38,55). The adult definition that MODS required the simultaneous involvement of two or more organ systems was also adopted for pediatric MODS.

Although the initial age-adjusted criteria for organ *failure* provided a set of diagnostic criteria by which clinicians could identify MODS (**Table 21.2**), it was not until 1999 that a formal

TABLE 21.1

THE PIRO SYSTEM

Domain	Present	Future	Rationale
Predisposition	Premorbid illness, age, sex, cultural beliefs	Genetic polymorphisms in components of the inflammatory response; better understanding of host–pathogen interaction	Premorbid factors impact on the morbidity and morality of an acute trigger; consequences of insult are genetically influenced
Insult/Infection	Culture and sensitivity of pathogens, detection of diseases amenable to source control	Assay of microbial products (e.g., LPS, PCR for DNA); gene transcript profiles	Characterizing insult in order to target specific therapies against triggering insult/pathogen
Response	SIRS; other signs of sepsis (e.g., CRP)	Markers of inflammation (IL-6, PCT); impaired host response, detection of specific therapeutic targets (LPS, TNF)	Mortality and response to therapy vary with measures of disease severity; mediator-targeted therapy
Organ dysfunction	Measured as number of failing organs or score (MODS, SOFA, LODS, PEMOD, PELOD)	Dynamic measures of cellular response to insult: apoptosis, cell stress	Response to therapy not possible if damage present; identifying cellular injury to utilize therapies

LPS, lipopolysaccharide; PCR, polymerase chain reaction; CRP, c-reactive protein; PCT, procalcitonin; TNF, tumor necrosis factor; MODS, Multiple Organ Dysfunction Score; SOFA, Sequential Organ Failure Assessment; LODS, Logistic Organ Dysfunction Score; PEMOD, Pediatric Multiple Organ Dysfunction; PELOD, Pediatric Logistic Organ Dysfunction. From Levy MM, Fink MP, Marshall JC, et al. 2001 SCCM/ESICM/ACCP/ATS/SIS International Sepsis Definitions Conference. *Crit Care Med* 2003;31:1250–6, with permission.

attempt to develop and validate a pediatric organ *dysfunction* score was reported. The authors used two developmental methods: the PEdiatric Multiple Organ Dysfunction (PEMOD) system and the PEdiatric Logistic Organ Dysfunction (PELOD) score (28). The intended purpose for designing such a scoring system was not necessarily to predict mortality, because the mortality rate for pediatric MODS was substantially lower when compared with that of adults; rather, the purpose was to more accurately describe and quantify clinical complications among PICU patients using changes in the organ dysfunction score as a surrogate outcomes measure.

The creation of the PEMOD and PELOD scoring systems was carefully described in the initial report. Of note, age-dependent physiologic variables (e.g., heart rate) were stratified into four age groups: neonates (<1 month), infants (1–12 months), children (1–12 years), and adolescents (>12 years). The weight of each variable in predicting mortality was independently determined, and four levels of increasing severity were defined to which weighted "values" of 0, 1, 10, or 20 were assigned. In the final compilation, the weight of each organ dysfunction and severity was integrated into a score, with 12 variables retained (**Table 21.3**). Following its description, the PELOD score was subjected to a validation study that included over 1,800 children in seven PICUs across Europe and North America (29). The predictive value of the PELOD score for a mortality end-point was fairly accurate during the first 5 days of admission to the PICU (receiver operating characteristic curve area, 0.79–0.85). However, it is important to again highlight the difference in a scoring system such as PELOD (which was designed to serve as a surrogate measure of outcome) with that of actual prognosticating

scoring systems such as PRISM or PIM (which were designed specifically to maximize the ability to predict mortality outcome).

As mentioned earlier, most recently, first in 2002 (17) and then in 2004 (6), a consensus expert panel in Pediatric Critical Care Medicine met to review available scoring systems for pediatric MODS. The primary goal of this effort was to generate a reproducible assessment of organ dysfunction that would allow the tracking of functional improvement or decline, which could then serve as a meaningful end-point for clinical trials. The panel's review centered on those scores that had been derived during the preceding years. Although not advocating the use of any one particular scoring system, the panel did develop specific criteria for defining organ dysfunction based on these summary scoring systems (**Table 21.4**) (17). They advised that for study enrollment purposes, cardiovascular and respiratory organ dysfunction should be present, with subsequent monitoring of other organ system function. They also proposed using *organ dysfunction–free days* as a study end-point, as was designed into the Resolution of Organ Failure in Pediatric Patients with Severe Sepsis (RESOLVE) trial, which examined the efficacy of drotrecogin-α (i.e., recombinant activated protein C) to hasten the resolution of organ failure in pediatric severe sepsis (see the "Treatment of MODS" section later in this chapter). It remains uncertain how well this metric will perform over time. The ultimate goal is to assimilate scoring systems, such as the PELOD score, with additional biologic information (e.g., biomarkers, genetic predisposition, and pharmacogenomics) to more accurately determine the beneficial effects of newly developed therapeutic strategies for sepsis and MODS.

TABLE 21.2

CRITERIA FOR PEDIATRIC ORGAN SYSTEM FAILURE IN INFANTS AND CHILDREN

Cardiovascular system
1. Systolic blood pressure less than 40 mm Hg for patients <1 yr of age, or <50 mm Hg for patients >1 year of age
2. Heart rate <50 beats/min or >220 beats/min for patients <1 yr of age, or <40 beats/min or >200 beats/min for patients >1 yr of age
3. Cardiac arrest
4. Serum pH <7.2 with a normal $Paco_2$
5. Continuous IV infusion of inotropic or vasopressor agents to maintain blood pressure and/or cardiac output (excluding dopamine ≤5 mcg/kg/min)

Respiratory system
1. Respiratory rate >90 breaths/min for patients <1 yr of age, or >70 breaths/min for patients >1 yr of age
2. $Paco_2$ >65 torr
3. Pao_2 <40 torr in the absence of cyanotic congenital heart disease
4. Mechanical ventilation (>24 hrs in the postoperative period)
5. Pao_2/Fio_2 ratio <200 in the absence of cyanotic congenital heart disease

Central nervous system
1. Glasgow Coma Score <5
2. Fixed and dilated pupils in the absence of mydriatic medications

Hematologic system
1. Hemoglobin level <5 g/dL
2. White blood cell count <3,000 cells/mm^3
3. Platelet count <20,000 cells/mm^3
4. D-Dimer >0.5 mcg/mL with prothrombin time >20 sec and partial thromboplastin time >60 sec in the absence of antithrombotic medications and/or primary liver disease

Renal system
1. Serum urea nitrogen level >100 mg/dL
2. Serum creatinine level >2 mg/dL in the absence of preexisting renal disease
3. Need for acute dialysis

Hepatic system
Total serum bilirubin >3 mg/dL in the absence of hemolysis, hyperbilirubinemia of the newborn, breast-feeding–related hyperbilirubinemia, or primary liver disease

Gastrointestinal system
Gastroduodenal bleeding plus one of the following, thought to be directly the result of gastroduodenal bleeding:
1. Decrease of hemoglobin of >2 g/dL
2. Requirement for blood transfusion
3. Hypotension
4. Need for gastric or duodenal surgery
5. Death

MODS is defined as the simultaneous occurrence of at least two organ dysfunctions. Information in table is as derived by Wilkinson JD, Pollack MM, Glass NL, et al. Mortality associated with multiple organ system failure and sepsis in pediatric intensive care unit. *J Pediatr* 1987;111:324–8, and later modestly modified by Proulx F, Fayon M, Farrell CA, et al. Epidemiology of sepsis and multiple organ dysfunction syndrome in children. *Chest* 1996;109:1033–7.

EPIDEMIOLOGY OF MULTIPLE ORGAN DYSFUNCTION SYNDROME

Incidence

Until uniformly defined and scored, the incidence of MODS in both adult and pediatric populations was difficult to determine. While complicated by the development of varying criteria, definitions, and scores in adult ICU patients, the incidence of MODS has ranged broadly from 14% to 54%, depending on the specific patient population admitted to an adult ICU (34), with the highest rates consistently observed in those adult patients diagnosed with sepsis and/or postsurgical patients (20,34). In pediatric studies, the incidence of MODS among general PICU populations has ranged from 11% to 57% (**Table 21.5**) (16,27,29,38,39,47,55,56). Clearly, the incidence of MODS depends on a number of factors, including surgical/postoperative status (e.g., trauma vs. transplantation vs. congenital heart repair), premorbid conditions (e.g., cancer, immunodeficiency, stem cell transplant [up to 50% with MODS]), and the triggering insult (e.g., 95% of infants who present with postasphyxial injury have MODS) (44).

The most comprehensive evaluation of the incidence of MODS in hospitalized children (and encompassing non-PICU patients) was reported by investigators who utilized the Healthcare Cost and Utilization Project Kids' Inpatient Database (KID), which included discharge and billing/coding (i.e.,

TABLE 21.3

PEDIATRIC LOGISTIC ORGAN DYSFUNCTION (PELOD) SCORE

Organ system and variables	Points by level of severity for each system			
	0	1	10	20
Respiratory system				
PaO$_2$/FIO$_2$	>70 *and*		≤70 *or*	
PaCO$_2$	≤90 *and*		>90	
Mechanical ventilation	No ventilation	Ventilation		
Cardiovascular system				
Heart rate (beats/min)				
<12 yrs	≤195		>195	
≥12 yrs	≤150		>150	
Systolic BP	*and*		*or*	
<1 month	>65		35–65	<35
1 month–1 yr	>75		35–75	<35
1–12 yrs	>85		45–85	<45
>12 yrs	>95		55–95	<55
Neurologic system				
GCS	12–15 *and*	7–11	4–6 *or*	3
Pupillary reaction	Both reactive		Both fixed	
Hepatic system				
ALT	<950 *and*	≥950 *and*		
PT/INR	>60 *or* <1.4	≤60 *or* ≤1.4		
Renal system: Creatinine				
<7 days	<1.59		≥1.59	
7 days–1 yr	<0.62		≥0.62	
1–12 yrs	<1.13		≥1.13	
>12 yrs	<1.59		≥1.59	
Hematologic system				
White blood cell count	>4.5 *and*	1.5–4.4 *or*	<1.5	
Platelet count	≥35,000	<35,000		

GCS, Glasgow Coma Score; ALT, alanine aminotransferase; PT, prothrombin time; INR, International Normalized Ratio. From Leteurtre S, Martinot A, Duhamel A, et al. Development of a pediatric multiple organ dysfunction score: Use of two strategies. *Med Decis Making* 1999;19:399–410, and Leteurtre S, Martinot A, Duhamel A, et al. Validation of the paediatric logistic organ dysfunction (PELOD) score: Prospective, observational, multicentre study. *Lancet* 2003;362:192–7, with permission.

ICD-9-CM) data on over 1.1 million pediatric patients from 22 states to estimate the overall incidence of MODS in children (23). In this series, over 50,000 children (4.5%) were admitted with at least one organ system dysfunction and, depending on how MODS was defined from the coding system, the incidence of MODS was either 3.3% or 0.5% (23). Although this relatively low incidence of MODS among hospitalized children might have deceptively suggested that the overall health burden of MODS was minor, this study also highlighted the tremendous and disproportionate impact that MODS carried on length of stay, resource utilization, and mortality for the unfortunate minority of infants and children who had suffered organ dysfunction.

Specific Etiologies

As alluded to earlier, only a few studies of MODS in children have been conducted. As a result, description is incomplete of the various factors that contribute to both the initiation of and outcome from MODS in children, including age, triggering pathology, and premorbid conditions (i.e., chronic illness, immunosuppression, etc.). Despite this limitation, some clear patterns emerge from the reports to date. For example, it is clear that sepsis is a principal trigger of MODS, not only among adult ICU patients but also in the PICU population, in whom the incidence of MODS in children with sepsis ranges from 24% to 73% (see **Table 21.5**) (13,26,43). Other medical diagnoses reported to be associated with pediatric MODS include asphyxial insults, inborn errors of metabolism, hypoxemic respiratory failure (acute lung injury/ARDS), acute renal failure, pancreatitis, intracranial hemorrhage, and neurodegenerative diseases (39). Of course, MODS often presents in pediatric surgical patients, with the incidence varying by study population. In various epidemiologic studies, surgical diagnoses that have been associated with the development of MODS among children include post–cardiac surgery, multiple trauma, liver transplantation, and bowel obstruction (39). Less is known regarding the influence of chronic diseases and premorbid conditions on the incidence of MODS. Information on specific patient populations exists, such as for allogeneic bone-marrow transplantation (relative risk of MODS estimated to be 38.67; confidence interval [CI], 5.47–273.2) (12) or oncologic patients admitted to the PICU for complications that arise during the course of chemotherapy (MODS incidence on the order of 50%).

TABLE 21.4

PEDIATRIC ORGAN DYSFUNCTION CRITERIA: THE DIAGNOSTIC CRITERIA FOR PEDIATRIC MODS BASED ON 2002 INTERNATIONAL PEDIATRIC SEPSIS CONSENSUS CONFERENCE

Cardiovascular dysfunction
Despite administration of isotonic IV fluid bolus $\geq$40 mL/kg in 1 hr:
- Decrease in BP (hypotension) <5% percentile for age or systolic BP <2 SD below normal for age*
  OR
- Need for vasoactive drug to maintain BP in normal range (dopamine $\geq$5 mcg/kg/min or dobutamine, epinephrine, or norepinephrine at any dose
  OR
- Two of the following:
  Unexplained metabolic acidosis: base deficit >5.0 mEq/L
  Increased arterial lactate >2 times upper limit of normal
  Oliguria: urine output <0.5 mL/kg/hr
  Prolonged capillary refill: >5 sec
  Core to peripheral temperature gap >3°C

Respiratory system
- Pao_2/Fio_2 ratio <300 in the absence of cyanotic congenital heart disease or preexisting lung disease
  OR
- $Paco_2$ >65 torr or 20 mm Hg above baseline $Paco_2$
  OR
- Proven need or >50% Fio_2 to maintain saturation $\geq$92%
  OR
- Need for nonelective invasive or noninvasive mechanical ventilation

Central nervous system
- GCS $\leq$11
  OR
- Acute change in mental status with a decrease in GCS $\geq$3 points from abnormal baseline

Hematologic system
- Platelet count <80,000/mm^3 or a decline of 50% in platelet count from highest valued recorded over 3 days (for chronic heme-onc patients)
  OR
- INR >2

Renal system
- Serum creatinine level greater than twice the upper limit for age or twofold increase in baseline creatinine

Hepatic system
- Total serum bilirubin $\geq$4 mg/dL (in the absence of hemolysis, hyperbilirubinemia of the newborn, or primary liver disease)
  OR
- ALT twice upper limit of normal for age

BP, blood pressure; SD, standard deviations; GCS, Glasgow Coma Score; INR, International Normalized Ratio; ALT, alanine aminotransferase. From Goldstein B, Giroir B, Randolph A. International pediatric sepsis consensus conference: Definitions for sepsis and organ dysfunction in pediatrics. *Pediatr Crit Care Med* 2005;6:2–8, with permission.

Outcome

Due to variations in criteria that define organ dysfunction and other factors, the mortality rate for children who meet MODS criteria has ranged widely from 12% to 57% in a general PICU population (see **Table 21.5**). Additionally, the mortality rate for specific subpopulations grouped according to underlying disease, premorbidities, and surgical status invariably influences MODS outcomes. Of particular interest has been the subpopulation of patients with sepsis. Whereas adult studies have suggested that patients with sepsis-related MODS carry a higher mortality risk than do other etiologies, early pediatric studies did not corroborate adult observations (38,55). On the other hand, more recent pediatric studies have tended to agree with the adult observation that sepsis portends a negative survival

impact for patients with MODS (27,47). The reason for this apparent discrepancy between the earlier and later studies is unclear but can be attributed, in part, to methodologic differences. However, despite these variances, all studies examining patients with both MODS and sepsis have demonstrated a consistent pattern of increasing mortality risk with increasing sepsis severity.

Regardless of the triggering insult, every epidemiologic report has substantiated the observation that mortality risk correlates with the number of organs failing. Although not all children with MODS necessarily go on to die, it is rather astonishing to note that 90% to 100% of all deaths that occur in PICUs have been associated with MODS (see **Table 21.5**), suggesting that to impact outcome, an improved mechanistic understanding of the pathophysiology of MODS is necessary to either attenuate the progression of organ failure once

TABLE 21.5

SUMMARY OF EPIDEMIOLOGIC STUDIES EXAMINING PEDIATRIC MODS AND SEPSIS-RELATED MODS[a]

	MODS - PICU								MODS - Hospital	Sepsis - PICU		
	Wilkinson 1986 (56)	**Wilkinson 1987 (55)**	**Proulx 1994 (39)**	**Proulx 1996 (38)**	**Goh 1999 (16)**	**Leteurtre 2003 (30)**	**Tantalean 2003 (47)**	**Leclerc 2005 (28)**	**Johnston 2004 (41)**	**Saez-Llorens 1995 (43)**	**Duke 1997 (13)**	**Kurko 2003 (27)**
Setting	1 PICU - USA	5 PICUs - USA	1 PICU - France	1 PICU - France	1 PICU - Malaysia	7 PICUs - France/ Canada/ Switzerland	1 PICU - Peru	3 PICUs - France/ Canada	22 state database - USA	1 PICU - Panama	1 PICU - Australia	1 PICU - USA
Study Design	prospective	prospective	prospective	prospective	partly prospective	prospective	prospective	prospective	retrospective	retrospective	prospective	retrospective
Study Dates	1980–1982	1984–1985	1990–1991	1991–1992	1995–1996	1998–2000	1996–1997	1997	1997	1981–1992	?	1998–1999
Study Duration	13.5 months	7 months	9 months	13 months	19 months	18 months	6 months	5 months	12 months	12 years	?	2 years
Number of Admissions	831	726	777	1,058	495	1,806	276	593	1,152,854	4,529	?	2,346
MODS Definition/Critera	modified Wilkinson 1986 (56) study	modified Wilkinson 1986 (56)	modified Wilkinson 1986 (56)	modified Wilkinson 1987 (55)	Wilkinson 1987 (55)	Leteurtre 1999 [PELOD] (29)	study	Leteurtre 1999 [PELOD] (29)	ICD-9-CM coding study	study	modified Wilkinson 1987 (55)	modified Wilkinson 1987 (55)
Maximum MODS (i.e. OFI)	5	7	5	7	7	6	7	6	6	5	6	7
MODS Incidence	226/831 (27.2%) [b]	177/726 (24.4%)	85/777 (10.9%)	191/1058 (18.1%)	84/495 (17.0%)	965/1806 (53.4%)	156/276 (56.5%)	269/593 (45.4%)	6112/1152854 (0.5%) [d]; 37682/1152854 (3.3%) [e]			
Overall MODS Mortality	60/226 (26.5%) [b]	83/177 (46.9%)	43/85 (50.6%)	68/191 (35.6%)	48/84 (57.1%)	111/965 (11.5%)	65/156 (41.7%)	51/269 (19.0%)	1633/6112 (26.7%) [d]; 3684/37682 (9.8%) [e]			
1 OD Mortality	2/241 (0.8%)	25/97 (25.8%)				3/471 (0.6%)	6/85 (7.1%)	0/150 (0%)	1856/45274 (4.1%)			
2 OD Mortality	15/142 (10.6%)	30/48 (62.5%)	2/34 (5.9%)	?/86	20/45 (44.4%)	14/457 (3.1%)	23/78 (29.5%)	7/156 (4.5%)	1048/4854 (21.6%)			
3 OD Mortality	36/62 (58.1%)	28/32 (87.5%)	29/36 (80.6%)	?/59	16/26 (61.5%)	29/285 (10.2%)	21/54 (38.9%)	16/75 (21.3%)	441/1007 (43.8%)			
4 OD Mortality	9/12 (75.0%)	28/32 (87.5%)	7/9 (77.8%)	?/24	12/13 (92.3%)	24/125 (19.2%)	16/19 (84.2%)	19/27 (70.4%)	144/251 (57.4%)			
5 OD Mortality	no patients	included in 4 OD	5/6 (83.3%)	?/13	included in 4 OD	30/70 (42.9%)	4/4 (100%)	7/9 (77.8%)	included in 4 OD			
6 OD Mortality	xxxxx	included in 4 OD	xxxxx	?/6	included in 4 OD	14/28 (50%)	1/1 (100%)	2/2 (100%)	included in 4 OD			
7 OD Mortality	xxxxx	included in 4 OD	xxxxx	?/3	included in 4 OD	xxxxx	no patients	xxxxx	xxxxx			
Sepsis Definition	N/A study	N/A study	N/A	modified 1991 ACCP/ SCCM (2)	modified 1991 ACCP/ SCCM (2)	N/A	modified 1991 ACCP/ SCCM (2)	modified 1991 ACCP/ SCCM (2)	ICD-9-CM coding study	study	modified 1991 ACCP/ SCCM (2)	2002 ACCM Guidelines (9)
Sepsis Incidence		21%, 21%, 24% [c]		316/1058 (29.9%)			127/276 (46.0%)	138/593 (23.3%)		815/4529 (18.0%)		147/2346 (6.3%)
Sepsis Mortality				?/316	27/44 (61.4%)		47/127 (37.0%)	27/138 (19.6%)		319/815 (39.1%)	10/31 (32.2%)	18/143 (12.6%)

(continued)

289

TABLE 21.5
(CONTINUED)

	MODS - PICU								MODS - Hospital	Sepsis - PICU		
	Wilkinson 1986 (56)	Wilkinson 1987 (55)	Proulx 1994 (39)	Proulx 1996 (38)	Goh 1999 (16)	Leteurte 2003 (30)	Tantalean 2003 (47)	Leclerc 2005 (28)	Johnston 2004 (41)	Saez-Llorens 1995 (43)	Duke 1997 (13)	Kutko 2003 (27)
Sepsis Category Mortality												
Sepsis				?/245			16/76 (21.1%)	9/103 (8.7%)		27/171 (15.8%)		N/A
Severe Sepsis				?/46			17/30 (56.7%)	6/17 (35.3%)		201/497 (40.4%)		N/A
Septic Shock				?/25			14/21 (66.7%)	12/18 (66.7%)		91/147 (61.9%)		13/96 (13.5%)
Among MODS Patients												
Sepsis Incidence		84/177 (47.5%)	19/85 (22.4%)	72/191 (37.7%)	44/84 (52.4%)		87/156 (55.8%)	98/269 (36.4%)				
No Sepsis Mortality		44/93 (47.3%)		45/119 (37.8%)	21/40 (52.5%)		20/69 (29.0%)	24/171 (14.0%)				
Sepsis Mortality		39/84 (46.4%)		23/72 (31.9%)	27/44 (61.4%)		45/87 (51.7%)	27/98 (27.6%)				
Sepsis Catergory Mortality												
Sepsis				9/41 (22.0%)	2/9 (22.2%)			9/68 (13.2%)				
Severe Sepsis				2/8 (25.0%)	13/20 (65.0%)			6/13 (46.2%)				
Septic Shock				12/23 (52.2%)	12/15 (80.0%)			12/17 (70.6%)				
Among Sepsis Patients												
MODS Incidence								98/138 (71.0%)		197/815 (24.2%)	11/29 (37.9%)	70/96 (72.9%)
No MODS Mortality								0/40 (0%)		175/618 (28.3%)	3/20 (15.0%)	0/26 (0%)
MODS Mortality								27/98 (27.6%)		144/197 (73.1%)	7/11 (63.6%)	13/70 (18.6%)
Overall Mortality	62/831 (7.5%)	83/726 (11.4%)	43/777 (5.5%)	68/1058 (6.4%)	50/495 (10.1%)	115/1806 (6.4%)	71/276 (25.7%)	51/593 (8.6%)	4635/1152854 (0.4%)			
Mortality without MODS	2/62 (3.2%)	0/83 (0%)	0/43 (0%)	0/68 (0%)	2/50 (4%)	4/115 (3.5%)	6/71 (8.5%)	0/51 (0%)				
Mortality with MODS	60/62 (96.8%)	83/83 (100%)	43/43 (100%)	68/68 (100%)	48/50 (96%)	111/115 (96.5%)	65/71 (91.5%)	51/51 (100%)				

a Many of these data were not explicitly reported in the original studies and have been extracted from the text through interpolation and reverse calculations.
b The mortality rate was reported as 54% in the original paper.
c Incidence of sepsis reported from three of the five PICUs in the study.
d MODS defined by dysfunction of two or more organs.
e MODS defined by study.
MODS, multiple organ dysfunction syndrome; OD, organ dysfunction; OFI, organ failure index; PELOD, pediatric logistic organ dysfunction.

initiated or reverse the process once established. Thus, the following section addresses the numerous mechanistic theories ascribed to explain the development of MODS.

PATHOPHYSIOLOGY OF MULTIPLE ORGAN DYSFUNCTION SYNDROME

Although the definition proposed by the ACCP/SCCM Consensus Conference broadly describes MODS as the "presence of altered organ function in an acutely ill patient such that homeostasis cannot be maintained without intervention" (2), the dominant conceptual framework upon which the pathogenesis of MODS has traditionally been viewed has been within the context of dysregulated (immuno)inflammation. Early theories asserted that widespread organ dysfunction was a manifestation of unintended collateral damage stemming from an exaggerated or uncontrolled SIRS secondary to a severe inciting injury. However, mounting disappointment from the failures of numerous anti-inflammatory strategies to improve patient outcomes strongly suggested that this hyperinflammation model was incomplete. Additionally, the growing realization that an endogenous compensatory anti-inflammatory response syndrome (CARS) existed (5) and that this counter-regulatory process could, under certain conditions, also deleteriously modulate the host response to injury have led to more recent theories that promote the notion that MODS reflects an imbalance or *dissonance* between these pro- and anti-inflammatory forces.

Extensive experimental and clinical data continue to support the veracity of dysregulated inflammation as an important contributor to the pathogenesis of MODS. However, perhaps analogous to the proverbial blind men perceiving different "truths" through inspection of different parts of an elephant, it may be possible that our current perspective of MODS through this inflammatory model, although fundamentally sound, may represent only part of a larger network of interdependent processes that go awry in the setting of MODS. For example, the bioenergetic and metabolic derangements that are also clearly recognized as integral to the development of MODS have yet to be fully explained through inflammatory mechanisms. In this regard, it may be informative to briefly take a step back and attempt to examine "the whole elephant," so that a more comprehensive picture of MODS can be obtained before further focusing on the specific details of the prevailing dysregulated inflammation paradigm.

What Constitutes Normal Physiologic Homeostasis?

In attempting to construct a broader conceptual framework, we observe that, by its very definition, the concept of MODS is inherently tied to that of *homeostasis* (or more precisely, the *loss* of homeostasis). Hence, it appears that, to better understand MODS, we should first explore what constitutes normal physiologic homeostasis. As described in many introductory Biology courses, homeostasis can be considered a state of dynamic equilibrium in which the internal environment of a living entity is maintained in a relatively narrow physiologic range

while resisting perturbations that are caused by variations in its external environment. When applied to a single cell or simple organism, this concept is relatively easy to comprehend, because the internal and external environments are clearly demarcated by a cell wall or membrane. However, also inherent to its very definition, MODS is a clinical syndrome that can arise only in sophisticated, multiorgan, higher-order species; in this context, the concept of homeostasis encompasses additional complexity, because it must address spatial and hierarchical considerations related to the sheer increase in the size and specialization of physiologic functions that characterize the higher-order organism. In other words, the concept of homeostasis relevant to MODS carries both micro- and macroenvironmental meanings, because multiple dynamic equilibriums simultaneously maintained at the local (i.e., cellular) and regional (i.e., tissue or organ) levels collectively integrate in a highly organized, well-orchestrated, and hierarchical manner to support the global dynamic equilibrium of the whole organism. Although at first glance this latter, multidimensional notion of homeostasis might be confusingly complex, it is possible to systematically deconstruct and reconstruct its multiple layers to provide some clarity to this intricate picture.

Recall that all complex, multicellular, higher-order species, including human beings, start life as a single-cell entity and that subsequent embryologic development proceeds through a well-ordered sequence of steps that demonstrates remarkable similarities to the march of evolution from primordial single-cell organism to modern, complex, multiorgan life forms. Drawing from these parallels in embryonic and evolutionary development, we can begin to appreciate that the same types of physical, spatial, physiologic, and logistic obstacles to evolutionary progress must also be overcome to permit embryonic development from a single cell into a complex mature life form. In this regard, we recognize that vital prerequisite physiologic functions must be sequentially gained at each step of development and that any disruption of these basic functions at earlier stages prohibits the existence of later stages. Therefore, examining the obligatory shifts in homeostatic function through the progression of evolution may provide insight into our own biologic makeup and reveal potential areas of vulnerability with respect to the development of MODS.

Taking this approach, one might ask, "What are the necessary elements for a unicellular organism or single cell to maintain homeostasis and sustain life?" In very simplistic terms, they involve transport, (energy) metabolism, and communication/regulation. As alluded to earlier, at their most fundamental level, all living organisms are organic, water-filled biologic systems composed of proteins, carbohydrates, lipids, and nucleic acids enclosed by physical barriers that demarcate an internal milieu that is distinct from the external environment. The presence of this physical barrier immediately necessitates that cells must adapt some *transport* mechanism to import biomolecules and substrates essential for building and maintaining the cell's internal biologic system (and conversely, export undesired biologic "waste"). However, simply combining these bioelements does not itself constitute a living entity, and the "breath of life" is instilled only when this static picture is set into motion through active cellular *metabolism*. Metabolism entails both anabolic and catabolic activities and encompasses DNA replication, protein synthesis, maintenance of cell membrane integrity, and a host of other vital cellular functions. However, perhaps the most critical facet of cellular metabolism involves the generation of adequate *energy* or fuel to drive this cellular machinery. A more detailed discussion of energy metabolism is warranted and will be addressed shortly but, in the interim, it is imperative to recognize that, although cellular transport assembles the components of the life machine and energy metabolism sets this machine into motion, precise regulatory control of cellular activity is necessary to maintain the ongoing operation of the life machine. This need for regulatory control implies the presence of a sophisticated "communication network" that senses changes in both internal and external conditions to signal appropriate responses to regain equilibrium from any perturbation. This "network" must simultaneously adjust the flux of biomaterials and rate of energy production to meet specific demands that might be imposed on the cell at any particular moment. For example, the highly conserved heat shock response can be viewed as a series of regulatory communication switches that are triggered in response to high ambient temperature (as well as other stressors) and that mobilize factors to assist in proper protein folding to protect against protein degradation. As another example, a cell preparing for mitosis actively imports nucleic acids for DNA replication and escalates energy production (i.e., imports and consumes more glucose or lipid) to meet increased metabolic demands. Alternatively, it may sense that insufficient biomaterials are available and signal to abort mitosis altogether. Thus, at the cellular level, a series of regulatory controls and feedback mechanisms that are closely tied to continuous environmental monitoring are necessary to maintain homeostatic functions.

Before discussing how these concepts of transport, energy metabolism, and communication/regulation become modified as focus is shifted from a unicellular organism to a multicellular entity, a specific aspect of cellular energy metabolism deserves special attention. Although certain proto-eukaryotic cells and plant life are able to harness light energy directly from their environment, most other cell types extract their energy from the controlled breakage of high-energy carbon–carbon bonds in organic material (e.g., glucose), which is ultimately converted into the universal energy currency form of adenosine triphosphate (ATP). In the absence of oxygen, cellular capacity to generate ATP is severely restricted (two ATPs per glucose molecule consumed) and, although primitive life forms can still exist, advanced evolutionary progress through anaerobic energy metabolism alone is impossible. Hence, biologic transformation from anaerobic to aerobic metabolism, characterized by the emergence of mitochondria as subcellular organelles that utilize oxygen to perform oxidative phosphorylation (also known as *cellular respiration*), marks a critical leap in evolutionary development. This exponential increase in ATP-generating capacity per organic substrate consumed (theoretically up to 36–38 ATPs per glucose molecule) can fuel a vast array of previously unsupportable metabolic activities. At the same time, this functional transformation does not come without a price, because strict aerobic entities like mammalian cells are now vulnerable to periods of anoxia or hypoxia or to any impairment of mitochondrial function. Additionally, the inadvertent release of toxic oxygen moieties (i.e., reactive oxygen species, ROS) from occasional basal errors in oxidative phosphorylation can occur. Thus, the same oxidative properties of oxygen that afford more efficient ATP production can, in Janus-like fashion, also inflict "self-injury" by damaging sensitive parts of the cellular machinery. Ironically, the very mitochondria that unintentionally produce these toxic oxygen moi-

eties are probably most at risk for self-injury. A self-amplifying, vicious cycle can be set into motion by which mitochondrial oxidant injury can lead to increased errors in oxidative phosphorylation, which leads to increased production of ROS and, consequently, to more self-injury. This dangerous cycle, if left unchecked, can ultimately lead to a functional anaerobic state and bioenergetic failure despite adequate oxygen. Hence, an indispensable task that cells must perform in tandem with the transition from anaerobic to aerobic energy metabolism is the creation of a powerful cellular antioxidant defense system to prevent rampant proliferation of this autodestructive cycle (see Chapter 18). One popular theory of aging (which can be viewed in some respects as the development of MODS in *really slow motion*) proposes that incremental oxidative damage to mitochondrial DNA encoding components of the electron transport chain mount over time and lead to a progressive decline in cellular energy production capacity, limited compensatory reserves to tolerate stress, and, ultimately, to cellular demise.

In observing that cellular energy metabolism in higher-order organisms depends on a constant oxygen (and nutrient) supply, mitochondrial integrity, and robust antioxidant defense mechanisms, we can begin to appreciate how any disturbance to the delicate balance of these elements can set the stage for the development of the bioenergetic derangements observed in MODS; this becomes especially evident in our later discussion on bioenergetic failure and apoptosis.

Transport and Energy Metabolism

As described earlier, cellular transport at the single-cell level principally involves the import of biomaterial into the cell, most notably vital nutrients (e.g., carbohydrates or lipids) necessary for energy metabolism. Although gases such as oxygen and small lipophilic molecules can diffuse across cell membranes along a concentration gradient, cellular transport is often facilitated by specialized channels or transport proteins that can selectively recognize specific substrates to import. Unless a cell specifically possesses mobility function, it is important to remember that its nutrient supply is limited by what is available in its immediate surroundings and by any convective and diffusive forces. Although it is not usually considered in the single-cell setting, the most basic concept of *shock*, which is the state in which cellular metabolic demand cannot be met due to insufficient nutrient supply or mitochondrial dysfunction, can be applied to describe conditions of oxygen depletion (hypoxic shock) and glucose depletion (hypoglycemic shock). In the absence of limited exogenous nutrient supply, the flux of biomaterials is regulated by internal signals that control the activity of these channels or transport proteins. Although specific transport problems at the single-cell level are most often genetic in nature and are generally of little interest with respect to MODS, it is tempting to speculate whether the recent clinical observations of hyperglycemia and relative insulin resistance that occurs during critical illness might somehow reflect transient dysfunction of the glucose transport receptor from which paradoxic *intracellular hypoglycemia* (i.e., glycopenic shock) ensues despite the presence of abundant bloodstream glucose.

Evolution from a single cell into a simple, multicellular organism such as a flatworm (phylum Platyhelminthes) requires little change in transport function, because each individual cell is within proximity to the outside environment and can obtain sufficient nutrients for survival from diffusion. However, as the multicellular entity gains additional complexity and increases in size, its metabolic needs exceed what can be supported by diffusion alone. Thus, it must adapt a means to transport vital biomaterials across large spatial domains so that every cell receives a continuous nutrient supply irrespective of its location within the organism. We recognize this critical adaptation of transport function in the higher-order organism as the *circulatory system*—the intimate link between transport and energy metabolism. As a result, derangements in the physiologic components of this functional "pump" mechanism—preload, contractility, afterload—give rise to the more familiar classifications of shock states—hypovolemic, cardiogenic, and distributive—associated with global circulatory collapse. It is important to note that, although circulatory compromise certainly results in a state of energy deficit caused by an imbalance between energy production and energy expenditure that we call "shock," this state is not necessarily contingent on the presence of hypotension, because cellular energy deficits may continue to mount despite the return to normal blood pressures. Although our discipline has clearly understood for years the urgency to reverse shock and attempt to avert the fulminate development of MODS, we have only recently appreciated the implication that, despite restoration of global circulation, microcirculatory perfusion defects from evolving microvascular derangements may continue and lead to persistent *regional* shock that seems to herald progressive organ dysfunction.

Communication/Regulation

As described earlier, cell communication at the unicellular level is primarily *intra*cellular and directed solely for self-regulation of biologic activity in response to changes in internal and external signals. A host of both negative and positive feedback loops keeps the internal conditions of the cell within a narrow and optimal physiologic range that is necessary to maintain general cellular metabolism. External stimuli are sensed through specialized receptor complexes (typically located on the cell surface but possibly also present in the cell nucleus) that, upon binding by specific chemical signals (i.e., ligands), activate a conditioned response from the cell. For example, ligand binding of the tyrosine kinase family of receptors may, after signal transduction and a series of signal amplification and regulatory sequences, initiate important steps for cellular growth and differentiation. Although not a typical feature of unicellular communication, an example of *autocrine* communication has been described in the context of T cells and monocytes, in which they release chemical signals to stimulate their own proliferation.

As the organism becomes multicellular, communication expands to encompass *inter*cellular dimensions, to regulate cell–cell interactions and to coordinate cellular functions so that the composite organism behaves as a single unit or entity. Initially, intercellular communication may be little more than simply sustaining direct cell–cell contact, as in the example of the sponge colony (phylum Porifera), whose individual cells are capable of functioning completely independently of the other. However, even this seemingly simple task of initiating cell–cell contact still requires that the cells of the organism gain the ability to distinguish "self" from "nonself," it and is facilitated through mutual cell surface ligand–receptor bindings through the expression of specific adhesion molecules. This capacity to discriminate "friend" from "foe" becomes especially relevant as an array of Toll-like receptors evolve to help recognize foreign pathogens. These and other components of an *innate immune system* in primitive organisms (and conserved in later,

higher-order life forms) play a critical role in defending against unwelcome invaders and infection.

As the organism grows more complex through specialization of cellular function, with a concomitant differentiation into specific tissues and organs that necessitates obligate interdependence, a vast hierarchic intercellular communication network must evolve. Paradoxically, despite the profound intricacies of this network, the mode of intercellular communication remains remarkably similar to the single-cell paradigm, as effector cells release chemical signals that bind to specific receptors on recipient cells to elicit the desired responses. Cells in direct contact through specialized adhesion molecules or in close proximity to each other communicate via *paracrine* signals, whereas far-reaching communication (made feasible by the emergence of the circulatory system) is afforded by *endocrine* signals. Meanwhile, regulatory control for the entire organism is orchestrated through the evolution of specialized neuroendocrine cells that further differentiate into (a) neuronal cells that form the critical central and peripheral nervous systems, and (b) a variety of discrete endocrine cells that collectively form the endocrine system. Through mutual coordination, these specialized cells serve to regulate global physiologic functions via neurotransmitters, electrical signals, and specific hormonal signals. In this context, it is remarkable how a single cell can manage to integrate hundreds and perhaps thousands of different signals being transmitted at any given moment into an appropriate functional response. This amazing task is even more noteworthy when we consider that a large group of cells can coordinate their activities to collectively function in unison as a single entity (i.e., an organ). In this regard, it is easy to see how aberrant signals, disruption of signal processing, or inadequate or improper response to regulatory signals can have far-reaching consequences that may jeopardize the delicate homeostatic balance of the organism.

Linking Transport and Communication Functions with the Immune and Coagulation Systems

Earlier, we presented the case for how the development of the circulatory system stemmed from the evolutionary need to overcome diffusion limitations as organisms grew larger, more complex, and more metabolically active. This same evolutionary pressure most likely facilitated the development of specialized cells (e.g., erythrocytes) to enhance oxygen transport in the circulation to overcome the limited solubility of oxygen in the liquid phase. The concepts of hemorrhagic and anemic shock arise from our dependence on this specific oxygen transport system. However, it would be a gross oversimplification to suggest that energy metabolism has remained the sole function of the circulatory system, because this same system serves to facilitate remote cell-to-cell communication, not only through the endocrine means as mentioned earlier, but also through mobile cellular components. In this regard, it may be important to examine certain aspects of the cellular constituents of the circulatory system to provide a framework for a later discussion on the contribution of inflammation to MODS.

Circulatory systems have been classified into two distinct types, open and closed, with the former being the more primitive form. The open system can still be seen in insects and horseshoe crabs (phylum Arthropoda for both), whereas the closed system prevails in higher-order mammals, including human beings (phylum Chordata). In the setting of an open circulatory system, no real distinction exists between intravascular and interstitial space, and a simple breach of the outer body would allow loss of all extracellular fluid (hemolymph), as well as provide an opening for bacterial invasion and infection. Bacterial invasion is particularly troublesome; any infection has the potential to quickly become systemic, because bacteria can use the very convective flow of hemolymph to spread throughout the entire organism. Hence, evolutionary survival requires adaptive mechanisms to seal the tear in the body wall to prevent further loss of bodily fluid and to kill and eliminate the foreign invaders. This survival requirement is met through the development of a specialized cell known as a *hemocyte* or *amoebocyte*, which is believed to be the precursor to the pluripotent hematopoietic cell before it diverged into the three lines (leukocytes, megakaryocytes, and erythrocytes) associated with closed circulatory systems. In addition to its erythrocyte-like, oxygen-carrying function, the primitive hemocyte bears the earliest semblance of the cellular component of the innate immune system, possessing the critical ability to distinguish "self" from "nonself." As alluded to earlier, through specialized receptors on its surface, thought to be homologous precursors to our Toll-like receptors, the hemocyte recognizes unique bacterial components and becomes activated to mobilize cellular defenses. It releases chemokine-like signals to recruit other hemocytes to the site of injury; it also releases fibrin-like substances that can form a "clot." This clot formation seals the breach in the body wall to prevent further loss of hemolymph and, at the same time, immobilizes bacteria to facilitate hemocyte phagocytosis and bacterial killing. Thus, in the open circulatory system, combined *coagulation* and *inflammatory* responses beneficially serve to achieve the common goals of gaining *hemostasis* and preventing systemic spread of life-threatening infection. For organisms that retain tissue regenerative capabilities, this dual function can provide a considerable survival advantage. As an example, if a horseshoe crab's leg is seriously injured and infected, the entire appendage can be "clotted off," discarded, and a new limb can regrow in its place, thereby sacrificing a "nonessential" body part so that the organism itself can continue to live. (As an aside, the Limulus amoebocyte lysate assay utilized for detecting endotoxin is derived from the horseshoe crab and operates on this very clotting principle). However, for human beings and other higher-order organisms that have limited tissue-regeneration capacities, this early evolutionary survival benefit can become a potential liability, because the loss of limb becomes permanent. In observing the open circulatory system that precedes our closed system, we can appreciate how cells that are considered key to the modulation of inflammation were once closely tied to the functions of energy metabolism, as well as to clotting and coagulation.

Systemic Inflammatory Response and Immune Dysregulation

Keeping in mind the observation that sepsis-induced inflammation is one of the principal triggers for the development of MODS, and that MODS reflects the loss of homeostatic function, it may be reflective to consider the normal function of the inflammatory response before ascribing to dysregulated inflammation a role in MODS. Similar to the response to injury observed for open circulatory systems, inflammation that occurs in the setting of our closed circulatory system is, in many respects, also stereotyped (albeit more sophisticated). This conditioned reaction entails a series of communication cascades, triggered by cellular or tissue injury, that attempts to orches-

trate the mobilization of reparative mechanisms to restore function at the affected site of injury. For example, localized trauma to a limb that causes mechanical crush or sheer injury to soft tissue releases into the circulation chemical substances, including the well-known cytokines such as tumor necrosis factor (TNF)-α and interleukin (IL)-1β, that relax vascular smooth muscle cells (causing local vasodilatation of vessels), activate endothelial cells to increase capillary permeability, and attract circulating leukocytes to the site of injury. These events culminate in exudation of fluid and plasma proteins, leukocyte transmigration, and the classic findings of *rubor* (redness), *calor* (heat), *tumor* (swelling), and *dolor* (pain). The activation of several plasma protein cascades (all with phylogenetic-related homologs in the open circulatory system) involving complement, coagulation/fibrinolysis, and bradykinin occurs as part of this evolutionarily imprinted response to injury.

During this response, the first wave of leukocytes recruited to the site of injury is composed primarily of circulating neutrophils, which are "caught" at the affected vascular site by endothelial cell adhesion molecules (e.g., intercellular adhesion molecule [ICAM]-1) binding with neutrophil adhesion molecules (e.g., β_2 integrins), both of which are upregulated in response to early cytokine release (TNF-α and IL-1β). Adherent neutrophils within the vascular space are subsequently "lured" by chemotactic molecules, including chemokines (e.g., IL-8/CXCL8), complement products (e.g., C5a), and leukotrienes (e.g., LTB$_4$), into the extravascular space and site of injury. This well-characterized leukocyte–endothelial–cell-adhesion cascade has been one of the most important biologic discoveries in the past two decades with regard to advancing the understanding of inflammation-mediated tissue injury. The purpose of neutrophil recruitment is to scavenge cellular debris and concomitantly combat any foreign invaders through phagocytosis and the release of lysosomal enzymes, including proteases and myeloperoxidases, which help to fight infection and break down damaged scaffolding proteins in preparation for subsequent reparative processes. The next wave of cells is comprised of those from the monocyte/macrophage and fibroblast lineages, drawn in by a myriad of cytokines and chemokines. These cells are enlisted to repopulate the site, lay down fresh scaffolding proteins, and reestablish intercommunication pathways. Even as this local activity reaches a maximal level, additional signals from these immune cells begin the process of downregulating this proinflammatory cascade, referred to as CARS, which is the result of a coordinated action by a series of mediators (e.g., IL-10, TGF-β, IL-1 receptor antagonist protein [IL1Ra], among other cytokines) to reduce local leukocyte traffic, assist in reabsorbing extravascular fluid, and begin reparative processes so that normal functioning can be reestablished (5). Most commonly, the degree to which this inflammatory response is activated parallels the degree of tissue injury, such that small or trivial injuries remain completely localized.

In this light, it is easy to comprehend how either inadequate "containment" or overexuberance of the inflammatory signals for this normally beneficial response can result in the physiologic perturbation that leads to the clinical manifestation of MODS. In some cases, moderate injuries result in the modest systemic spillover of immune-mediated inflammatory communication into the general circulation, resulting in symptoms remote from the site of injury/invasion and eliciting the well-recognized SIRS. With devastating injuries, complete systemic spillover of all inflammatory processes may occur. Thus, what was intended to be a beneficial local response by the host becomes an overwhelming perturbation of systemic homeostasis, characterized by significant elevations in cytokines (TNF-α and IL-1β) and upregulation of the inducible form of nitric oxide synthase (iNOS), which, in concert with other mediators, causes loss of vasomotor tone, capillary leak, and myocardial depression, culminating in inadequate cardiac output and shock—that imbalance between substrate delivery-energy production and energy demands. Without aggressive fluid and inotropic/vasopressor resuscitation, persistent global shock leads to ongoing hypoxic–ischemic injury, eliciting even more inflammatory signals and creating a self-amplifying vicious cycle.

The inflammation-centered paradigm described here also supports an additional hypothesis regarding the cause of MODS: the so-called "gut hypothesis," which states, that during a period of hypotension or shock, hypoperfusion of the intestines compromises the integrity of immunologic barriers, allowing for *translocation* of endogenous gut flora or their bacterial products (e.g., endotoxin) into the systemic circulation, thereby similarly triggering, or perhaps amplifying, the SIRS response. In this manner, a localized injury that results in an inadequately regulated or "contained" inflammatory response results in splanchnic hypoperfusion and subsequent bacterial translocation and further systemic activation of the immune-inflammatory-coagulation systems (11). This so-called "gut hypothesis" has some attractive aspects, in that it could explain the high prevalence of bacteremia in the absence of an identifiable septic focus in MODS and that enteric organisms are most commonly cultured from this group of patients.

An overall appreciation of this reviewed pathobiology explains the early traditional paradigm, in which massive activation and dysregulation of proinflammation was believed to be the culprit for MODS development. As a result, it was believed that attenuating the magnitude of this hyperinflammatory response might allow the host to more effectively restore homeostasis. As mentioned earlier, although demonstrating some benefits in controlled experimental settings, numerous anti-inflammatory strategies failed to translate into clinical improvements. This realization occurred around the same time that clinicians began to recognize that many people who died from MODS had either persistent infection or were prone to acquire new (often nosocomial) infections. Additionally, translational investigators were providing a better understanding of the natural communication sequence of inflammation and the important contribution of endogenous counter-regulatory signals that comprise CARS. They hypothesized that this, too, might become dysregulated. Hence, a population of patients was identified who demonstrated an inability to mount an appropriate inflammatory response to typical triggers. Such patients were, in fact, characterized as functionally immunodeficient, immunocompromised, or, in some descriptions, "immunoparalyzed" (53). Such a state of immune *dissonance* placed them at risk of being unable to clear invading pathogens, which led to an alternative theory that a "second hit" (infectious or otherwise) caused the clinical progression to MODS. For this reason, it has been suggested that perhaps boosting the immune response (using, for example, interferon-γ or granulocyte-macrophage colony-stimulated factor, GM-CSF) may, in fact, help patients with MODS clear persistent infections or better withstand secondary infectious challenges (e.g.,

ventilator-associated pneumonia). Whether this approach will be successful remains to be determined.

In summary, working within the framework of normal immune responses, dysregulation of these evolutionary beneficial processes can explain a number of the theories that have been used to explain the pathophysiology of MODS.

Coagulation/Thrombosis and Microcirculatory Impairment

Given the early combined phylogenetic functions of the coagulation and innate immune systems, it should come as no surprise that both systems become activated when tissue injury or infection occurs. Pediatricians have clinically recognized for years the dreaded, limb-threatening thrombotic complications of *purpura fulminans* from disseminated meningococcemia. Yet almost inexplicably, the potential contribution of the coagulation system to the development and progression of MODS has long been overshadowed by the almost exclusive attention to dysregulated immunoinflammation. Rather than being considered an active "co-conspirator" with inflammation, the coagulation system has been mostly viewed as a "subordinate" system, the primary role of which has been to defend against life-threatening bleeding. When acknowledged as a potential pathologic process, concern about coagulation abnormalities has typically centered around excessive bleeding risks from impaired hemostatic function—similar to consumptive coagulopathy from disseminated intravascular coagulation—while often neglecting thromboembolic problems. However, with the recent finding of a survival benefit afforded by the use of recombinant activated protein C in adults with severe sepsis (4), renewed interest has arisen in more closely examining the intrinsic link between coagulation and inflammation, and their combined roles in the development of MODS. Hence, we now acknowledge that the same destructive injuries that launch the "cytokine storm" of inflammation and precipitate shock concomitantly activate the coagulation cascade and impair fibrinolysis, resulting in a functional hypercoagulable state that can lead to disseminated microvascular thrombosis. That inflammation and coagulation are intimately entwined in the development of microvascular thrombosis is further supported by autopsy findings that demonstrate neutrophils in addition to platelets and fibrin as comprising clots in the microcirculation. Clearly, the development of microthrombi throughout multiple organs in the body results in their dysfunction on the basis of local ischemia and inadequate substrate delivery. However, even with reestablishment of global circulation using early interventions, ongoing microvascular thrombosis (often manifest clinically as new-onset thrombocytopenia) can cause persistent microcirculatory ischemia and tissue injury that continue to fuel the vicious cycle of ischemia/shock–(re)injury–inflammation described earlier. In this regard, the idea that persistent *regional* shock contributes to the development of MODS is gaining broader appeal.

Along these lines, the concept of thrombocytopenia-associated multiple organ failure (TAMOF), which has been described as a thrombotic microangiopathic process akin to thrombotic thrombocytopenic purpura (TTP) and characterized by increased von Willebrand Factor (vWF) and/or decreased ADAMTS13 (a disintegrin and metalloprotease, with thrombospondin-1-like domains, member 13) activity has been recently proposed as a mechanism for the development of MODS (36). The function of vWF, a prothrombogenic protein produced by the vascular endothelium and platelets, is to assist in hemostatic function at a site of vascular/endothelial injury. vWF is normally released into the circulation as large multimeric complexes, the sizes of which correlate to their platelet thrombogenicity. However, the propensity of vWF to form a spontaneous clot is minimized in part by its circulating in a compact, less thrombogenic form and by circulating proteases, notably ADAMTS13, that degrade vWF into smaller multimers. After localized vascular injury, activation of the endothelium or increased shear stress at the site causes the large vWF multimers to unfold, which uncovers their full thrombogenic potential and causes the trapping of platelets and the formation of a platelet-vWF clot that serves to create a platelet plug to stop bleeding. Once hemostasis has been achieved, the balance between thrombosis/fibrinolysis shifts in favor of increased fibrinolytic activity and eventual restoration of normal microcirculatory flow and function. The hypothetical pathogenesis of TAMOF relates to the notion that severe injury triggers massive systemic endothelial (and platelet) activation, which heralds a thrombotic microangiopathic process throughout all vascular beds. Alternatively, it has also been suggested that systemic release of proinflammatory mediators (e.g., TNF-α) can similarly activate the formation of large vWF multimers, while reducing ADAMTS13 amount and/or activity, resulting in disseminated microvascular thrombosis and organ failure. This topic has been reviewed by Tsai HM (49). These hypotheses regarding the pathogenesis of TAMOF have also raised the intriguing possibility that plasma exchange, by clearing (unfolded) large vWF multimers while simultaneously replacing ADAMTS13 with fresh plasma, may improve MODS by diminishing circulating vWF multimers.

This "microcirculatory hypothesis" of MODS becomes even more complicated when the additional biologic complexity introduced by the reestablishment of adequate blood flow to organs is considered. The phenomenon of *reperfusion injury* that follows a period of thrombosis-mediated ischemia can result in substantial cellular and tissue injury due to oxygen radical generation, as reviewed in Chapter 19 and elsewhere (19). Thus, even when the primary insult of hypoperfusion is addressed with the reestablishment of oxygenated blood flow, a second wave of injurious mediators in the form of oxidant stresses may be encountered. The provision of antioxidant therapies has shown some clinical benefits in specific situations of reperfusion injury (41), although whether this effect can be achieved globally in the setting of resuscitation from hypoxic–ischemic insult to prevent MODS remains to be determined.

Mitochondrial Dysfunction, Bioenergetic Failure, and Apoptosis

Throughout the preceding discussion, we emphasized the strict dependence of higher-order organisms on maintaining aerobic energy metabolism for their survival. From this perspective, we presented the concept that the development of MODS may result from the accumulation of cellular energy deficits that arise from global and regional shock states related to severe injury or its accompanying immunoinflammatory-coagulation response. In this paradigm, any energy debt must be repaid quickly if cells, tissues, and organs are to regain function, homeostasis, and survive. In this regard, rapid reversal of shock through aggressive restoration of global and regional circulation to ensure adequate oxygen and nutrient delivery is paramount for the prevention of complete bioenergetic failure and necrotic cell

death. Yet, even after apparent patient stabilization through such interventions, a perplexing condition has been observed in which cells are unable to utilize oxygen, characterized clinically by increasing lactic acidosis in the face of diminished oxygen extraction and elevated mixed venous oxygen saturations. This condition has been referred to as "cytopathic hypoxia" (15) (a slight misnomer in our opinion, because there is no true hypoxia). The purported mechanism for impaired oxygen utilization stems from an acquired state of mitochondrial dysfunction (perhaps deserving of the term *mitochondrial shock*), a concept discussed earlier with respect to mitochondrial oxidant self-injury from the inadvertent release of free radicals from oxidative phosphorylation. Although previously the mitochondria was presented as an important source for ROS production, we acknowledge that, under pathologic conditions, an ample supply of ROS can also be generated elsewhere. For example, activated neutrophils that produce superoxide for bacterial killing have been implicated as one such source. Another source is through the upregulation of iNOS in endothelial cells during acute inflammation that results in the production of significant amounts of nitric oxide (NO), a "weak" free radical that can reversibly inhibit complex IV of the mitochondrial electron transport chain (ETC) (7). NO can also combine with superoxide to form peroxynitrite, a considerably stronger free radical capable of damaging a wide range of cellular components, including DNA, proteins, lipid membranes, and mitochondria.

Regardless of specific source, the onslaught of these additional reactive oxygen and nitrogen species (now commonly abbreviated as "RONS") can potentially overwhelm cellular antioxidant defenses that attempt to attenuate RONS-mediated damage. Thus, a relative overabundance of RONS can cause direct inhibition of the mitochondrial ETC. As mentioned before, any resultant mitochondrial damage can precipitate a self-destructive, vicious cycle, as well as impair the very energy production capacity necessary to escape energy debt. In addition, an overabundance of RONS can inhibit or decrease the expression of certain mitochondrial enzymes involved in energy metabolism (e.g., pyruvate dehydrogenase, *cis*-aconitase) upstream to the ETC, which effectively results in the degradation of the chemiosmotic gradient (i.e., mitochondrial membrane potential $[\Delta\Psi]$) driving oxidative phosphorylation. In either circumstance, the end result is cellular bioenergetic failure.

It has also been noted that, under certain situations, cells may continue to die after resuscitation. However, rather than classic necrotic cell death that typically characterizes complete energy depletion, these cells often quietly "disappear" by apoptosis, or programmed cell death. As a result, a fundamental question puzzling critical care physicians has been: Why would cells undergo apoptosis when global patient stabilization has been achieved? One possible explanation may be that these cells had reached the critical "point of no return," and committal signals for apoptosis had already been activated before patient resuscitation and stabilization. Alternatively, ongoing exogenous inflammatory signals (e.g., TNF-α, Fas) or other endogenous signals (e.g., DNA damage, p53) may push cells precariously on the edge of survival to choose apoptotic death. Here, the critical role of mitochondria in determining cellular fate becomes highlighted. Although previously regarded as an organelle simply responsible for energy metabolism, the mitochondrion has recently attained considerable stature through the discovery that it can trigger apoptosis (32). The fact that mitochondria would acquire this role makes intuitive sense because they are in the best position to gauge whether the energy costs associated with cellular repair might be too excessive, leaving apoptosis as the better option for the organism as a whole in the face of potentially limited resources. Intense research has been devoted to better understand the exact mechanisms involved in mitochondrial-mediated apoptosis; however, a comprehensive review is beyond the scope of this particular discussion, and we briefly present only a few important concepts and steps.

Although somewhat controversial, it has been proposed that a number of cellular stressors, such as oxidant stress or low ATP states, trigger the conformational alignment of various mitochondrial proteins integral to its inner and outer membranes, such that physical "pores" are formed, allowing free passage of molecules of <1.5 kDa (59). Creation of these pores effectively "short circuits" the mitochondrion, collapsing the $\Delta\Psi$ that drives oxidative phosphorylation and ATP production. In addition, the osmotic influx of water into the mitochondrial matrix leads to significant swelling and rupture of the outer membrane, which allows the release of cytochrome c, a non–membrane-bound component of the mitochondrial ETC, along with other proapoptotic proteins into the cytosol. In the cytosol, cytochrome c binds with Apaf-1 and, together in multimeric fashion, they form a structure called the *apoptosome*. The apoptosome recruits procaspase-9, which then becomes activated to caspase-9 and, in turn, cleaves and activates procaspase-3 to caspase-3, the key executioner of apoptosis (reviewed by Jin and El-Deiry [22]).

For the intensivist, a better understanding of the mechanistic regulation of apoptosis may seem irrelevant unless these processes can be therapeutically manipulated for patient benefit. In this regard, the development of target "therapies" to alter apoptotic signaling has been especially challenging because the tightly regulated process of apoptosis serves an important functional role in maintaining the overall homeostasis of the organism. Although our instinctive response is to view cell death negatively, the careful, controlled elimination of cells that have outlived their usefulness benefits the organism by creating room for new, more robust, and efficient cells. Clearly, any potential intervention must selectively target *pathologic* apoptosis while sparing *physiologic* apoptosis if it will have any chance for clinical relevance. Whether this is possible remains to be determined.

TREATMENT OF MULTIPLE ORGAN DYSFUNCTION SYNDROME

Perhaps the most disappointing realization regarding the epidemiology, pathophysiology, and outcome related to MODS has been the inability to significantly alter the course of this clinical challenge after it has developed. As a result, *prevention* has been espoused as the treatment of choice for addressing this difficult clinical entity. We have approached this problem from the viewpoint of MODS reflecting a loss of homeostasis due to a number of derangements in normal cellular function, and we would submit that the goal in approaching MODS is to prevent this loss of homeostasis. In reviewing those processes necessary for maintaining biologic homeostasis (the global goal of the host), it is intuitively obvious to acknowledge the fundamental

role of those therapies that fall under the rubric of "supportive care" and that are familiar to all practicing intensivists. These include several of the therapeutic principles outlined in accompanying chapters. Clearly, effective, early resuscitation in the form of restoration of ventilation and oxygenation, adequate intravascular volume resuscitation (including red blood cells in the setting of severe anemia), and maintenance of adequate organ perfusion pressure using lusitropic, inotropic, vasopressor, or afterload-reducing therapies as needed, are key mainstays of therapy (9). Although these are intuitively obvious goals, how they are achieved may impact the severity and outcome of MODS.

Without a doubt, the institution of mechanical ventilation can be a life-saving therapy when used to restore adequate oxygenation and ventilation in spontaneously breathing patients. However, as has been learned over the past 30 years, mechanical ventilation can also be associated with detrimental consequences. It has been well established that the use of high inspiratory pressures (plateau pressures >30 cm H_2O) (*barotrauma*), excessive tidal volumes ($\geq$12 mL/kg) (*volutrauma*), and inadequate positive end-expiratory pressure (PEEP) (*atelectatrauma*) can worsen lung injury (*ventilator-induced lung injury, VILI*) and, in some circumstances, result in the systemic release of inflammatory mediators from the lung—a pathophysiologic principle collectively termed *biotrauma* (37). Several lines of evidence support the notion that injurious ventilation causes inflammatory gene expression in lungs (57); this reaction is not always limited to the lung (40), and a protective ventilatory strategy diminishes systemic cytokine expression, in association with less MODS (1).

Other theories derived from additional experimental work include the hypotheses that VILI may promote bacterial translocation (31), release proapoptotic factors from the lung, and/or suppress peripheral immune responses related to counter-regulation of lung inflammation (54). Regardless of the precise cause(s), these observations have led to the therapeutic principle of a protective lung strategy achieved by limiting tidal volumes and/or plateau pressures and avoiding excessive lung collapse by utilizing sufficient PEEP. Nevertheless, it is sobering to concede that, despite the application of these principles to critically ill patients who require mechanical ventilatory support, many patients still succumb to MODS.

Equally as obvious to employ are the principles of hemodynamic support; however, this too does not always ensure a favorable outcome. Perhaps no better example of the potential beneficial effect of this approach exists than the observation that, when achieved, goal-directed therapy in adult sepsis may be able to ameliorate the severity of organ dysfunction (as estimated by surrogate Acute Physiology and Chronic Health Evaluation, APACHE, scores) (42). Whether achieving early, goal-directed targets, such as superior vena cava oxygen saturation levels >70%, is as effective at reducing organ failure and mortality in pediatric patients as has been shown in adults remains an intriguing question. Nevertheless, despite what otherwise appears to be adequate delivery of oxygen, as reflected by normal cardiac output and oxygen saturation levels, it is clear that, in many circumstances, this is insufficient to meet the patient's metabolic demands. This relative failure or inadequacy of typically "normal" oxygen delivery has been termed *pathologic supply-dependent oxygen consumption* by some, and implies that a critical imbalance between oxygen delivery and consumption has been reached. Unfortunately, the *supranormal* delivery of oxygen achieved by augmenting cardiac output, hemoglobin concentration, and/or hemoglobin oxygen saturation does not consistently reverse this physiologic state. Certain theories, backed by scant experimental evidence, have been proffered to explain this phenomenon, including maldistribution of perfusion at the microcirculatory level (10), initiation of a futile energy cycle of the cell mediated by inflammatory cytokines (46), and molecular alterations in cellular respiration that affect oxygen uptake by the cell (25). Regardless of the ultimate pathologic cause, it is humbling to note that strict adherence to our long-practiced principles of hemodynamic support will not always prevent the progression of MODS in our patients and keeps the pursuit of "insulin for oxygen" one of the "Holy Grails" in sepsis research. Thus, in the end, although guided by the principles of lung-protective mechanical ventilation and hemodynamic resuscitation and support, the clinician will inevitably continue to face challenges from MODS.

Other mainstays of therapy include immediate control of any source of "injury," earliest achievable institution of enteral feeding, and avoidance of excessive fluid overload. Whether the trigger is traumatic in nature or related to an identifiable nidus of infection, "source control" achieved in association with the institution of timely and accurate antibiotic coverage remains one of the most important predictors of outcome in critically ill patients. In studies of critically ill adults, the early initiation of enteral nutrition has been consistently demonstrated to improve ICU outcomes, including the degree of MODS. However, some studies have questioned whether the enteral route is indeed superior to parenteral nutrition and capable of preventing MODS if a positive nitrogen balance is maintained and adequate caloric delivery is achieved. Also, whether adding enteral bacterial decontamination or immunoactive nutritional supplements (e.g., glutamine) to the nutritional approach ultimately impacts the incidence and outcome of MODS remains incompletely studied. Finally, a clear association has been established between fluid overload and MODS in critically ill pediatric patients (18). It has been suggested that using continuous renal replacement therapy early in the course of illness to avoid excessive fluid overload (>15% above dry weight) may improve mortality rates in patients with established MODS (18). However, whether this approach translates broadly to the PICU population remains to be determined.

Finally, two recent therapeutic advances achieved in the critically ill adult population deserve comment. In light of the link between inflammation and coagulation with MODS, investigators hypothesized that pharmacologically targeting both systems may prove beneficial in patients with severe sepsis who were at substantial risk for developing MODS. Activated protein C (APC), or drotrecogin-α, has been shown to possess both anticoagulant and anti-inflammatory activity (24). A phase III trial involving administration of recombinant APC in adults with severe sepsis demonstrated an absolute reduction in mortality of 6.1% (4), although notably, this effect was most pronounced in the sickest (uppermost APACHE score quartile) and oldest patient groups. In one of the largest multicentered trials in pediatric critical care performed to date (resolution of organ failure in pediatric patients with severe sepsis, RESOLVE), investigators tested the efficacy of APC in decreasing the number and/or length of organ failure in children with severe sepsis using a surrogate of organ failure–free days. As is now well known, this study was terminated due to lack of efficacy (35),

suggesting that the pathobiology at play in critically ill adults may differ from that in children.

In a similar manner, adult intensivists around the world have become aware of the benefit of achieving tight glycemic control in their critically ill patients. The early study by van den Berghe et al. demonstrated that maintaining blood glucose at a level between 80 and 110 mg/dL reduced mortality in an adult surgical ICU from 8.0 to 4.6% ($p < 0.04$) with the greatest reduction in mortality involving deaths due to MODS with a proven septic focus (52). Since this report, a number of studies have attempted to corroborate the finding in broader patient populations. In general, it appears that this therapeutic approach may positively impact outcomes in critically ill adults; however, the impact appears to depend on both the patient population and the length of ICU stay (51). Furthermore, it appears that hyperglycemia may also be associated with increased mortality and organ failure in children (14), although hypoglycemia, which could result from overly aggressive correction of hyperglycemia may be equally detrimental (58). In fact, consistent with the hypothesis of dysregulated homeostasis presented earlier, the worst outcomes have been observed in those children who demonstrated the greatest degree of variability in serum glucose (i.e., from lowest to highest value), suggesting that tight physiologic regulation of this system had been lost (58). Whether the clinical benefits observed with tight glycemic control are derived from attenuating the effects of high glucose on impairing physiologic function (i.e., glucose toxicity) or they reflect insulin as being a beneficial, therapeutic modulator of critical illness remains incompletely known (reviewed by Van den Bergh [50]). Most importantly, whether the same approach of tight glucose control in critically ill children with severe sepsis and MODS has a favorable outcome remains to be studied. Unlike the developed adult, resultant hypoglycemia in the developing infant and child may have devastating consequences—a reality those involved in the design of such a future study must address. In summary, it remains to be seen whether the recent therapeutic successes enjoyed by adult intensive care physicians—lung-protective ventilation, drotrecogin-α therapy, and tight glucose control—ultimately translate to similar pediatric success stories. Clearly, an improved mechanistic understanding of the biologic processes that mediate the initiation, propagation, and resolution of organ dysfunction in critically ill children is needed before achieving similar improvements in our therapeutic armamentarium.

CONCLUSIONS AND FUTURE DIRECTIONS

Our clinical and epidemiologic understanding of pediatric MODS has expanded substantially since its initial recognition as a distinct clinical entity, although the interpretation of the cumulative data has been complicated by the methodologic heterogeneity between studies. However, with recent consensus agreements reached for *pediatric-specific* definitions and criteria for MODS, we are hopeful that greater clarity will emerge through more uniformity in future investigations. Yet, despite our increasing ability to recognize the clinical manifestations of MODS and its associated epidemiologic and prognostic implications, we remain frustrated by the current limitations of our therapeutic armamentarium. As a result, as with every challenging clinical syndrome that prematurely robs the precious lives of the children for whom we care, our discipline must remain committed to advancing our biologic and mechanistic understanding of this fatal syndrome so that future development of novel, viable therapies for MODS can be realized.

To assist with this endeavor, we have presented a conceptual paradigm to support the view that MODS reflects the ultimate loss of homeostasis at the cellular, tissue/organ, and whole-body levels. From this perspective, it is possible to make connections among many of the prevailing theories that have attempted to explain the pathogenesis of MODS. Despite the promise for improving patient outcomes held by our expanding scientific and medical knowledge base and the ever-advancing, life-sustaining technologies, the looming presence of potential death from MODS remains. We urge equipoise in this relatively young discipline as it considers new scientific discoveries and confronts the excitement they may generate. We predict that, in the near future, the impact of intensive glucose control, early goal-directed therapy (perhaps with novel, noninvasive measures of oxygen delivery), and the influence of lung-protective ventilatory strategy on organ failure and outcomes will be studied in a prospective manner in children. However, amid the struggle to achieve physiologic balance at the patient's beside, the physician must exhibit patience, perhaps above all other virtues. It may be as important to know what *not to do* as it is to know what to do, particularly as evidence of novel therapeutic advances are realized in adults that are not replicated or even studied in children. We must be cognizant that our ever-increasing ability to achieve perfect "numbers," although a source of great professional pride, may not necessarily serve the best interest of the patient.

As stated in the introduction to this chapter, MODS epitomizes the discipline of Critical Care Medicine. As such, we must continue to balance the concerns of each of our subspecialty colleagues regarding their particular organ system of interest, because it is our responsibility to orchestrate the multiple therapeutic modalities aimed at restoring global homeostasis. Finally, it is important not to lose sight of the humanistic side of our profession, because family members of those children for whom we care often place their faith in spiritual and religious "forces," even as they place their faith and trust in our clinical judgment.

KEY POINTS

■ MODS can be triggered by a number of pathologic insults (e.g., sepsis, multiple trauma, hypoxia–ischemia) and is among the most common causes of death in children in PICUs.

■ Consensus definitions for pediatric-specific, physiologic criteria for MODS have recently been proposed, so that clinicians and investigators can achieve greater uniformity in determining the epidemiology of, and outcomes from, pediatric MODS.

■ Living organisms achieve survival by maintaining precise physiologic homeostasis. Evolution to a multiorgan species creates an increasingly complex interplay among the systems (e.g., transport, [energy] metabolism, and communication/regulation) necessary for survival. Within this paradigm, perturbations that lead to a failure to maintain

normal function within these systems can result in physiologic derangement and organ dysfunction.

■ A number of theories are attributed to the development of MODS, including dysregulated immunoinflammation, bioenergetic failure/apoptosis, hypercoagulability with microvascular thrombosis, and intestinal barrier failure that results in bacterial translocation.

■ In pediatric critical care medicine, the mainstay of therapy for MODS remains general supportive care through careful orchestration and balancing of multiple therapeutic modalities.

■ Future studies must determine the impact of tight glucose control, lung-protective strategies of mechanical ventilation, anticoagulation therapy, and renal replacement therapy/plasmapheresis on the progression of, and outcome from, MODS.

References

1. Acute Respiratory Distress Syndrome Network. Ventilation with lower tidal volumes as compared with traditional tidal volumes for acute lung injury and the acute respiratory distress syndrome. *N Engl J Med* 2000;342:1301–8.
2. American College of Chest Physicians/Society of Critical Care Medicine Consensus Conference. Definitions for sepsis and organ failure and guidelines for the use of innovative therapies in sepsis. *Crit Care Med* 1992;20:864–74.
3. Baue AE. Multiple, progressive, or sequential systems failure. A syndrome of the 1970s. *Arch Surg* 1975;110:779–81.
4. Bernard GR, Vincent JL, Laterre PF, et al. Efficacy and safety of recombinant human activated protein C for severe sepsis. *N Engl J Med* 2001;344:699–709.
5. Bone RC. Sir Isaac Newton, sepsis, SIRS, and CARS. *Crit Care Med* 1996;24:1125–8.
6. Brilli RJ, Goldstein B. Pediatric sepsis definitions: Past, present, and future. *Pediatr Crit Care Med* 2005;6:S6–8.
7. Brown GC. Nitric oxide inhibition of cytochrome oxidase and mitochondrial respiration: Implications for inflammatory, neurodegenerative and ischaemic pathologies. *Mol Cell Biochem* 1997;174:189–92.
8. Burke JF, Pontoppidan H, Welch CE. High output respiratory failure: An important cause of death ascribed to peritonitis or ileus. *Ann Surg* 1963;158:581–95.
9. Carcillo JA, Fields AI. Clinical practice parameters for hemodynamic support of pediatric and neonatal patients in septic shock. *Crit Care Med* 2002;30:1365–78.
10. De Blasi RA, Palmisani S, Alampi D, et al. Microvascular dysfunction and skeletal muscle oxygenation assessed by phase-modulation near-infrared spectroscopy in patients with septic shock. *Intensive Care Med* 2005;31:1661–8.
11. Deitch EA, Morrison J, Berg R, et al. Effect of hemorrhagic shock on bacterial translocation, intestinal morphology, and intestinal permeability in conventional and antibiotic-decontaminated rats. *Crit Care Med* 1990;18:529–36.
12. Diaz MA, Vicent MG, Prudencio M, et al. Predicting factors for admission to an intensive care unit and clinical outcome in pediatric patients receiving hematopoietic stem cell transplantation. *Haematologica* 2002;87:292–8.
13. Duke TD, Butt W, South M. Predictors of mortality and multiple organ failure in children with sepsis. *Intensive Care Med* 1997;23:684–92.
14. Faustino EV, Apkon M. Persistent hyperglycemia in critically ill children. *J Pediatr* 2005;146:30–4.
15. Fink MP. Bench-to-bedside review: Cytopathic hypoxia. *Crit Care* 2002;6:491–9.
16. Goh A, Lum L. Sepsis, severe sepsis and septic shock in paediatric multiple organ dysfunction syndrome. *J Paediatr Child Health* 1999;35:488–92.
17. Goldstein B, Giroir B, Randolph A. International pediatric sepsis consensus conference: Definitions for sepsis and organ dysfunction in pediatrics. *Pediatr Crit Care Med* 2005;6:2–8.
18. Goldstein SL, Somers MJ, Baum MA, et al. Pediatric patients with multiorgan dysfunction syndrome receiving continuous renal replacement therapy. *Kidney Int* 2005;67:653–8.
19. Granger DN. Role of xanthine oxidase and granulocytes in ischemia-reperfusion injury. *Am J Physiol* 1988;255:H1269–75.
20. Guidet B, Aegerter P, Gauzit R, et al. Incidence and impact of organ dysfunctions associated with sepsis. *Chest* 2005;127:942–51.
21. Jenkins MT, Jones RF, Wilson B, et al. Congestive atelectasis/A complication of the intravenous infusion of fluids. *Ann Surg* 1950;132:327–47.

22. Jin Z, El-Deiry WS. Overview of cell death signaling pathways. *Cancer Biol Ther* 2005;4:139–63.

23. Johnston JA, Yi MS, Britto MT, et al. Importance of organ dysfunction in determining hospital outcomes in children. *J Pediatr* 2004;144: 595–601.

24. Joyce DE, Nelson DR, Grinnell BW. Leukocyte and endothelial cell interactions in sepsis: Relevance of the protein C pathway. *Crit Care Med* 2004;32:S280–6.

25. Kozlov AV, Staniek K, Haindl S, et al. Different effects of endotoxic shock on the respiratory function of liver and heart mitochondria in rats. *Am J Physiol Gastrointest Liver Physiol* 2006;290:G543–9.

26. Kutko MC, Calarco MP, Flaherty MB, et al. Mortality rates in pediatric septic shock with and without multiple organ system failure. *Pediatr Crit Care Med* 2003;4:333–7.

27. Leclerc F, Leteurtre S, Duhamel A, et al. Cumulative influence of organ dysfunctions and septic state on mortality of critically ill children. *Am J Respir Crit Care Med* 2005;171:348–53.

28. Leteurtre S, Martinot A, Duhamel A, et al. Development of a pediatric multiple organ dysfunction score: Use of two strategies. *Med Decis Making* 1999;19:399–410.

29. Leteurtre S, Martinot A, Duhamel A, et al. Validation of the paediatric logistic organ dysfunction (PELOD) score: Prospective, observational, multicentre study. *Lancet* 2003;362:192–7.

30. Levy MM, Fink MP, Marshall JC, et al. 2001 SCCM/ESICM/ACCP/ATS/SIS International Sepsis Definitions Conference. *Crit Care Med* 2003;31: 1250–6.

31. Lin CY, Zhang H, Cheng KC, et al. Mechanical ventilation may increase susceptibility to the development of bacteremia. *Crit Care Med* 2003;31:1429–34.

32. Liu X, Kim CN, Yang J, et al. Induction of apoptotic program in cell-free extracts: Requirement for dATP and cytochrome c. *Cell* 1996;86:147–57.

33. MacLean LD, Mulligan WG, McLean AP, et al. Patterns of septic shock in man – a detailed study of 56 patients. *Ann Surg* 1967;166:543–62.

34. Moreno R, Vincent JL, Matos R, et al. The use of maximum SOFA score to quantify organ dysfunction/failure in intensive care. Results of a prospective, multicentre study. Working Group on Sepsis related Problems of the ESICM. *Intensive Care Med* 1999;25:686–96.

35. Nadel S, Goldstein B, Williams MD, et al. Drotrecogin alfa (activated) in children with severe spesis: a multicentre phase III randomised controlled trial. *Lancet* 2007;369:836–43.

36. Nguyen T, Hall M, Han Y, et al. Microvascular thrombosis in pediatric multiple organ failure: Is it a therapeutic target? *Pediatr Crit Care Med* 2001;2:187–96.

37. Plotz FB, Slutsky AS, van Vught AJ, et al. Ventilator-induced lung injury and multiple system organ failure: a critical review of facts and hypotheses. *Intensive Care Med* 2004;30:1865–72.

38. Proulx F, Fayon M, Farrell CA, et al. Epidemiology of sepsis and multiple organ dysfunction syndrome in children. *Chest* 1996;109:1033–7.

39. Proulx F, Gauthier M, Nadeau D, et al. Timing and predictors of death in pediatric patients with multiple organ system failure. *Crit Care Med* 1994;22:1025–31.

40. Ranieri VM, Suter PM, Tortorella C, et al. Effect of mechanical ventilation on inflammatory mediators in patients with acute respiratory distress syndrome: A randomized controlled trial. *JAMA* 1999;282:54–61.

41. Rayner BS, Duong TT, Myers SJ, et al. Protective effect of a synthetic antioxidant on neuronal cell apoptosis resulting from experimental hypoxia reoxygenation injury. *J Neurochem* 2006;97:211–21.

42. Rivers E, Nguyen B, Havstad S, et al. Early goal-directed therapy in the treatment of severe sepsis and septic shock. *N Engl J Med* 2001;345:1368–77.

43. Saez-Llorens X, Vargas S, Guerra F, et al. Application of new sepsis definitions to evaluate septic pediatric patients with severe systemic infections. *Pediatr Infect Dis J* 1995;14:557–61.

44. Shah P, Riphagen S, Beyene J, et al. Multiorgan dysfunction in infants with post-asphyxial hypoxic-ischaemic encephalopathy. *Arch Dis Child Fetal Neonatal Ed* 2004;89:F152–5.

45. Skillman JJ, Bushnell LS, Goldman H, et al. Respiratory failure, hypotension, sepsis, and jaundice. A clinical syndrome associated with lethal hemorrhage from acute stress ulceration of the stomach. *Am J Surg* 1969;117:523–30.

46. Soriano FG, Liaudet L, Szabo E, et al. Resistance to acute septic peritonitis in poly(ADP-ribose) polymerase-1-deficient mice. *Shock* 2002;17:286–92.

47. Tantalean JA, Leon RJ, Santos AA, et al. Multiple organ dysfunction syndrome in children. *Pediatr Crit Care Med* 2003;4:181–5.

48. Tilney NL, Bailey GL, Morgan AP. Sequential system failure after rupture of abdominal aortic aneurysms: An unsolved problem in postoperative care. *Ann Surg* 1973;178:117–22.

49. Tsai HM. Current concepts in thrombotic thrombocytopenic purpura. *Annu Rev Med* 2006;57:419–36.

50. Van den Berghe G. How does blood glucose control with insulin save lives in intensive care? *J Clin Invest* 2004;114:1187–95.

51. Van den Berghe G, Wilmer A, Hermans G, et al. Intensive insulin therapy in the medical ICU. *N Engl J Med* 2006;354:449–61.

52. Van den Berghe G, Wouters P, Weekers F, et al. Intensive insulin therapy in the critically ill patients. *N Engl J Med* 2001;345:1359–67.

53. Volk HD, Reinke P, Docke WD. Clinical aspects: From systemic inflammation to "immunoparalysis." *Chem Immunol* 2000;74:162–77.

54. Vreugdenhil HA, Heijnen CJ, Plotz FB, et al. Mechanical ventilation of healthy rats suppresses peripheral immune function. *Eur Respir J* 2004;23:122–8.

55. Wilkinson JD, Pollack MM, Glass NL, et al. Mortality associated with multiple organ system failure and sepsis in pediatric intensive care unit. *J Pediatr* 1987;111:324–8.

56. Wilkinson JD, Pollack MM, Ruttimann UE, et al. Outcome of pediatric patients with multiple organ system failure. *Crit Care Med* 1986;14:271–4.

57. Wilson MR, Choudhury S, Goddard ME, et al. High tidal volume upregulates intrapulmonary cytokines in an in vivo mouse model of ventilator-induced lung injury. *J Appl Physiol* 2003;95:1385–93.

58. Wintergerst KA, Buckingham B, Gandrud L, et al. Association of hypoglycemia, hyperglycemia, and glucose variability with morbidity and death in the pediatric intensive care unit. *Pediatrics* 2006;118:173–9.

59. Zoratti M, Szabo I. The mitochondrial permeability transition. *Biochim Biophys Acta* 1995;1241:139–76.

CHAPTER 22 ■ AIRWAY MANAGEMENT

ALLAN de CAEN • JONATHAN DUFF • ASHRAF H. COOVADIA • ROBERT LUTEN • ANN E. THOMPSON • MARY FRAN HAZINSKI

The accurate assessment and safe management of the airway is fundamental to the care of critically ill or injured children. The anatomy, development, and evaluation of the pediatric airway, basic airway management, and management of the difficult airway are reviewed in this chapter, with emphasis on techniques for securing the airway.

THE ANATOMY OF THE AIRWAY

The larynx consists of nine cartilages, including the thyroid, cricoid, epiglottis, corniculate, cuneiform, and arytenoid cartilages. These cartilages are covered by folds of mucosa, connective tissue, and muscle; laryngeal tissue folds define the glottis. The superior, inferior, and recurrent laryngeal nerves innervate the larynx. Supraglottic sensation is mediated by the superior laryngeal nerve, and infraglottic sensation is mediated by the inferior laryngeal nerve. The recurrent laryngeal nerve provides most laryngeal motor innervation. Only the cricothyroid muscle is innervated by the superior laryngeal nerve. The airway is lined with ciliated and squamous epithelium that is highly vascular and overlies a rich network of lymphatic vessels.

DEVELOPMENTAL AIRWAY CONSIDERATIONS

The anatomy of the pediatric airway differs from the adult airway until it reaches mature position at approximately 8 to 14 years of age.

The major differences between the pediatric and the adult airway are size, shape, and position in the neck. Tracheal diameter and length increase with age. Tracheal dimensions reported from postmortem examinations have been verified using MRI (41) (Table 22.1). Because the diameter of the pediatric trachea is small, relatively small compromise in tracheal radius can significantly increase resistance to airflow and work of breathing. Resistance to airflow is inversely related to the *fourth* power of the radius during quiet breathing, when airflow is laminar, but is inversely related to the *fifth* power of the radius when airflow is turbulent. When respiratory distress is present, providers should attempt to keep the child as quiet as possible, minimizing agitation to reduce turbulent flow, airway resistance, and work of breathing.

The infant's tongue is large in proportion to the rest of the oral cavity and is closer to the palate; therefore, it can easily obstruct the airway. Laryngoscopic stabilization of the tongue is more difficult in the infant and child than in the adult.

The child's subglottic airway is smaller and more compliant, and the supporting cartilage is less well developed than in the adult. As a result, upper airway obstruction (e.g., caused by croup, epiglottitis, or extrathoracic foreign body) can produce tracheal collapse and stridor. The epiglottis is proportionally larger in the child than in the adult, and the ligamentous connection between the base of the tongue and the epiglottis (the hyoepiglottic ligament) is not as strong in the young child as in the adult. These differences can influence the selection of laryngoscope blade (straight versus curved) for the intubation of young children (see discussion in the section Endotracheal Intubation, Intubation Procedure). Although most of the child's laryngeal mucosa is loosely connected to the underlying tissues, it is tightly connected in the area of the vocal cords and at the laryngeal surface of the epiglottis. Subglottic inflammation is typically contained below this level; however, with little room to accommodate even modest inflammation at the level of the vocal cords or epiglottis, such inflammation can lead to a gross distortion of tissue planes and anatomic positions.

The glottic opening lies at approximately the cervical level of C2 or C3 in the infant or child and at the level of C3 or C4 in the adolescent or adult. This position places the pediatric glottic opening at the base of the proportionally larger and predominantly intraoral tongue (**Fig. 22.1**). This position of the pediatric airway has been described as "*anterior*" when compared to the mature airway, because the airway may become "hidden" behind the tongue on laryngoscopy. The pediatric airway is actually more *superior* (i.e., higher or more cephalad) *and* more *anterior* than the adult airway. MRI studies in children document anterior angulation (nearly 10 degrees from the vertical) at approximately the level of the sternal notch (41). Airway webcam videos are available at http://www.airwaycam.com/vol2.html.

On the basis of cadaver studies, it has long been accepted that the child's larynx is cylindrical from side to side but conical in the transverse or anterior-posterior dimension, with the tip of the cone at the level of the cricoid cartilage. Pediatric studies using MRI have confirmed this conical shape. In these studies of anesthetized, spontaneously breathing children, the smallest transverse diameter of the larynx was at and immediately below the level of the vocal cords, rather than at the cricoid cartilage (26). However, because the vocal cords and subglottic tissues can be distended, the rigid cricoid ring is still the smallest functional part of the infant airway (26). As the child grows to adulthood, the larynx becomes more cylindrical in shape, with the narrowest segment at the level of the vocal cords (see **Fig. 22.1, Table 22.2**). These anatomic variations make intubation of the child more difficult than intubation of

TABLE 22.1

TRACHEAL DIMENSIONS

Age (yrs)	Tracheal diameter (mm)	Superior tracheal limb length (mm)	Inferior tracheal limb length (mm)	Combined tracheal length (mm)
0–1	4.91 ± 0.88	27.94 ± 5.75	16.74 ± 7.78	44.68
1–2	6.68 ± 3.37	30.54 ± 5.74	20.11 ± 10.01	50.65
2–4	6.38 ± 1.86	31.87 ± 5.92	26.36 ± 5.91	58.23
4–6	8.4 ± 0.98	35.88 ± 14.03	27.84 ± 11.98	63.72
6–8	8.88 ± 1.51	35.45 ± 11.34	29.43 ± 10.80	64.88
8–10	9.35 ± 1.70	39.53 ± 6.95	35.48 ± 9.19	75.00
10–12	9.55 ± 1.14	38.53 ± 6.97	34.03 ± 7.31	72.56
12–14	10.46 ± 2.32	41.81 ± 9.28	40.19 ± 12.99	82.00
≥14	12.99 ± 1.35	47.21 ± 13.56	44.30 ± 17.14	91.51

Measurements are listed ± sample SD.
From Reed JM, O'Conner DM, Myer CM 3rd. Magnetic resonance imaging determination of tracheal orientation in normal children. Practical implications. *Arch Otolaryngol Head Neck Surg.* 1996;122(6):605–608, with permission.

the adult, requiring more expertise and more precise selection of endotracheal tube (ETT) size. If the child's ETT is too large, it can cause subglottic pressure ischemia and necrosis, leading to subglottic stenosis.

Oral intubation with direct laryngoscopy requires the establishment of a line of vision from the mouth and teeth to the vocal cords (i.e., the glottic opening). This line of vision requires the alignment of three axes: the oral, pharyngeal, and laryngeal. Normally, the laryngeal axis is perpendicular to the oral axis and forms a 45-degree angle with the pharyngeal axis. The provider must position the patient to align these axes for optimal airway patency and for successful intubation.

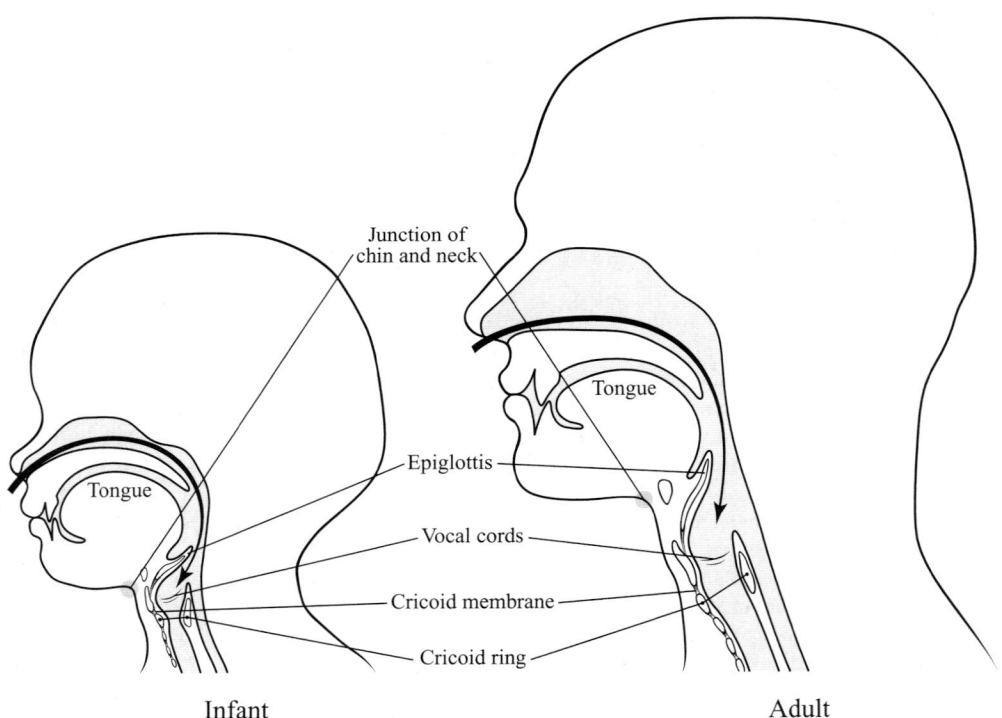

FIGURE 22.1. The anatomic differences particular to children are these: 1. Higher, more anterior position of the glottic opening. (Note the relationship of the vocal cords to the chin/neck junction.) 2. Relatively larger tongue in the infant, which lies between the mouth and glottic opening. 3. Relatively larger and more floppy epiglottis in the child. 4. The cricoid ring is the narrowest portion of the pediatric airway versus the vocal cords in the adult. 5. Position and size of the cricothyroid membrane in the infant. 6. Sharper, more difficult angle for blind nasotracheal intubation. 7. Larger relative size of the occiput in the infant. From Luten RC, Kissoon NJ. In: Wallis R, Luten LC, Murphy MF et al., eds. *Manual of Emergency Airway Management*, 2nd ed. Philadelphia: Lippincott Williams & Wilkins, 2004: 217, with permission.

TABLE 22.2

ANATOMIC DIFFERENCES BETWEEN ADULT AND PEDIATRIC AIRWAYS

Anatomy	Clinical significance
Tongue occupies relatively large portion of the oral cavity.	High anterior airway position of the glottic opening compared with that in adults
High tracheal opening (relative to cervical vertebrae): C1 in infancy C3 to C4 at 7 years of age C4 to C5 in the adult	Straight blade preferred over curved blade to push distensible anatomy out of the way to visualize the larynx
Large occiput may cause flexion of the airway, and large tongue can fall against the posterior pharynx when child is supine.	Sniffing position opens the airway. The larger occiput actually elevates the head toward the sniffing position in most infants and children (neck must be extended). A towel may be required under shoulders to elevate torso relative to head in small infants.
Cricoid ring is the narrowest portion of the child's trachea (vocal cords are the narrowest portion in the adult).	Uncuffed tubes may provide adequate seal, as they can fit snugly at the level of the cricoid ring. Selection of correct tube size is essential because use of excessively large tube may cause mucosal injury.
Consistent anatomic variations with age, with fewer anatomic abnormal variations related to body habitus, arthritis, and chronic disease.	Age-related variations: <2 years: High anterior airway 2–8 years: Transition >8 years: Small adult
Large tonsils and adenoids may bleed. More acute angle between epiglottis and laryngeal opening makes endotracheal intubation difficult.	Blind nasotracheal intubation not indicated in children. May cause failure of attempted nasotracheal intubation.
Small cricothyroid membrane.	Needle cricothyrotomy difficult; surgical cricothyrotomy is impossible in infants and small children.

Adapted from Luten RC, Kissoon NJ. Approach to the pediatric airway. In: Walls R, ed. *Manual of Emergency Airway Management,* 2nd ed. Philadelphia: Lippincott Williams & Wilkins, 2004.

The rescuer aligns the three axes in an older child or adult by placing a towel or other support beneath the occiput to tilt the neck forward (from the shoulders) and by lifting the chin to extend the neck. A technique to align the axes in younger children is placing them in the *sniffing position* (**Fig. 22.2**). Because children younger than ~2 years of age have a relatively large occiput, it is unnecessary to place a towel or other support under the occiput to tilt the neck. Such tilting naturally occurs when the child lies supine on a flat surface. The provider may only need to lift the chin to produce slight extension of the neck and align the axes. Providers should avoid hyperextension of the infant's neck because it can cause airway obstruction. In fact, for small infants it may be necessary to balance the disproportionate occipital size by placing a support under the shoulders. In all ages, the axes are correctly aligned for orotracheal intubation if the external auditory canal is anterior to the front edge of the patient's shoulders (see **Fig. 22.2**).

BASIC AIRWAY ASSESSMENT

Before performing any invasive airway procedure, the provider must assess the child to identify the potentially difficult airway. The three basic components of this assessment are the oropharyngeal examination, evaluation of atlanto-occipital joint extension, and measurement of the potential mandibular displacement area. Although the combination of these three assessments predicts the difficult adult airway, no comparative pediatric data exist.

The Oropharyngeal Examination

The degree of mouth opening is assessed by asking the cooperative patient to open the mouth to the widest extent possible and to protrude the tongue as far as possible, enabling assessment of the palate, the range of motion of the temporomandibular joint, and the size of the tongue relative to the oral cavity. The *Mallampati assessment* (**Fig. 22.3**) classifies the degree of airway difficulty based on the ability to visualize the faucial pillars, soft palate, and uvula with exposure of the glottis (28). With a Class 1 airway (i.e., all three pharyngeal structures can be visualized), laryngoscopy yields adequate "laryngeal exposure" in >99% of adult patients, whereas with a Class 3 airway (i.e., glottis cannot be exposed), laryngoscopy yields "adequate exposure" in only 7% of adult patients (28). Limited pediatric data suggest that this technique has a high (50%) false-positive rate for identifying difficult pediatric airways (16).

Evaluation of Atlanto-occipital Joint Extension

Reduced range of neck motion (reduced *atlanto-occipital joint extension*) will preclude successful alignment of the airway axes, making it difficult to visualize the glottic opening. An atlanto-occipital extension of 35 degrees is normal for adults, with no comparable pediatric data.

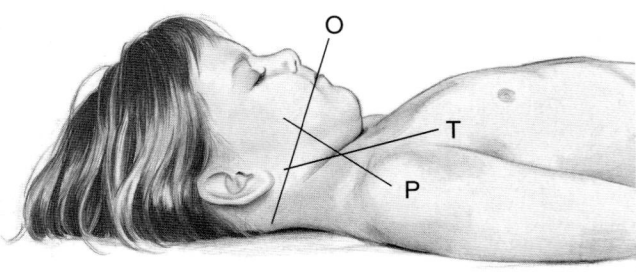

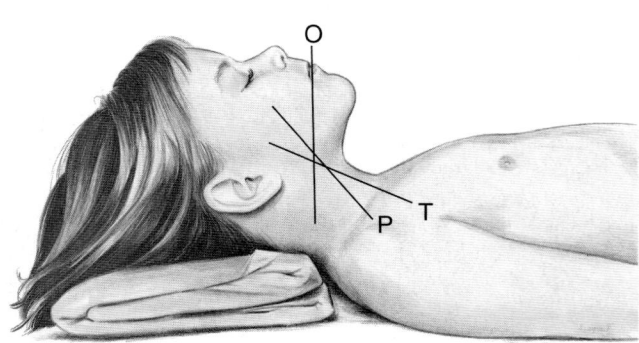

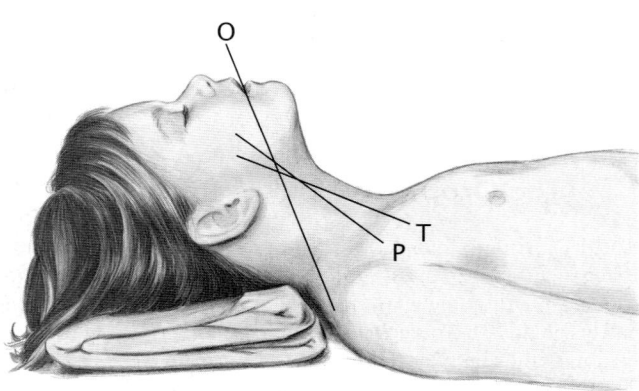

FIGURE 22.2. Correct positioning of the child over 2 years of age for ventilation and tracheal intubation. The oral (O), pharyngeal (P) and laryngeal/tracheal (T) axes are optimally aligned for intubation when the child is placed in the "sniffing" position. For infants and children younger than 2 years of age, the prominent occiput often provides the needed movement of the head forward of the shoulders. In the child over 2 years of age (shown here), a small towel is placed under the head (to lift the head forward) and the neck is slightly extended. The opening of the ear canal should be above or just anterior to the front of the child's shoulder. **A:** Resting position. **B:** Proper forward movement of head relative to shoulders. **C:** Proper positioning with both head position and neck extension for intubation: The oral, pharyngeal, and laryngeal/tracheal axes are aligned. From Pediatric Advanced Life Support. American Heart Association, Inc., 2002, with permission.

Evaluation of Potential Mandibular Displacement Area

To perform successful laryngoscopy, the intubator must be able to deflect supraglottic soft tissue structures such as the tongue into the pharyngeal space. This potential space is defined by the space from the lateral and anterior aspects of the mandible to the hyoid bone. Reduction in the volume of this potential space (e.g., due to mandibular hypoplasia or an increase in the volume of submandibular soft tissue) or an increase in the volume of soft tissue that must be displaced (e.g., enlarged tongue) will make it difficult to visualize the larynx. The size of this potential space can be estimated with the neck extended by evaluating the *thyromental distance*, the distance between the upper aspect of the thyroid cartilage/hyoid bone and the lower aspect of the mandible. When this distance is small, the angle between the pharyngeal and laryngeal axes will be more acute, making it difficult to align these axes to visualize the larynx. The potential mandibular displacement area is considered adequate for the adult and child if, with the head in neutral position, two fingers (3 cm) can be placed between the hyoid bone and the anterior ramus of the mandible. The minimum hyoid-to-mandible distance for an infant is 1.5 cm (3).

BASIC AIRWAY MANAGEMENT

Initial Maneuvers to Clear Airway

If the child is awake, with mild-to-moderate airway obstruction and no suspected cervical spine injury, she should be allowed to assume a position of comfort. The airway is suctioned as needed, and oxygen is administered. If the child is obtunded, the airway can become obstructed by a combination of neck flexion, jaw relaxation, displacement of the tongue against the posterior pharyngeal wall, and collapse of the hypopharynx. A simple jaw-thrust maneuver is the most effective method of opening the airway, although a head tilt-chin lift may also be successful. Providers should use the jaw thrust to open the airway if cervical spine injury is suspected, and they must perform the jaw thrust to provide effective bag-mask ventilation. If no cervical spine injury is suspected, or if the airway cannot be opened using the jaw thrust, the provider should open the airway using a head tilt-chin lift maneuver.

Oral and Nasal Airways

Oropharyngeal Airway

The *oropharyngeal airway* (OPA) consists of a flange, a short bite-block segment, and a curved plastic body that provides an airway and suction channel through the mouth to the pharynx. It is designed to relieve airway obstruction by fitting over the tongue to hold it and the soft hypopharyngeal structures away from the posterior wall of the pharynx. An OPA may be used in the *unconscious* child if manual attempts to open the airway (e.g., head tilt-chin lift or jaw thrust) fail to provide and maintain a clear, unobstructed airway. Use of an OPA in patients with intact cough or gag reflexes may stimulate gagging and vomiting; therefore; it is not recommended.

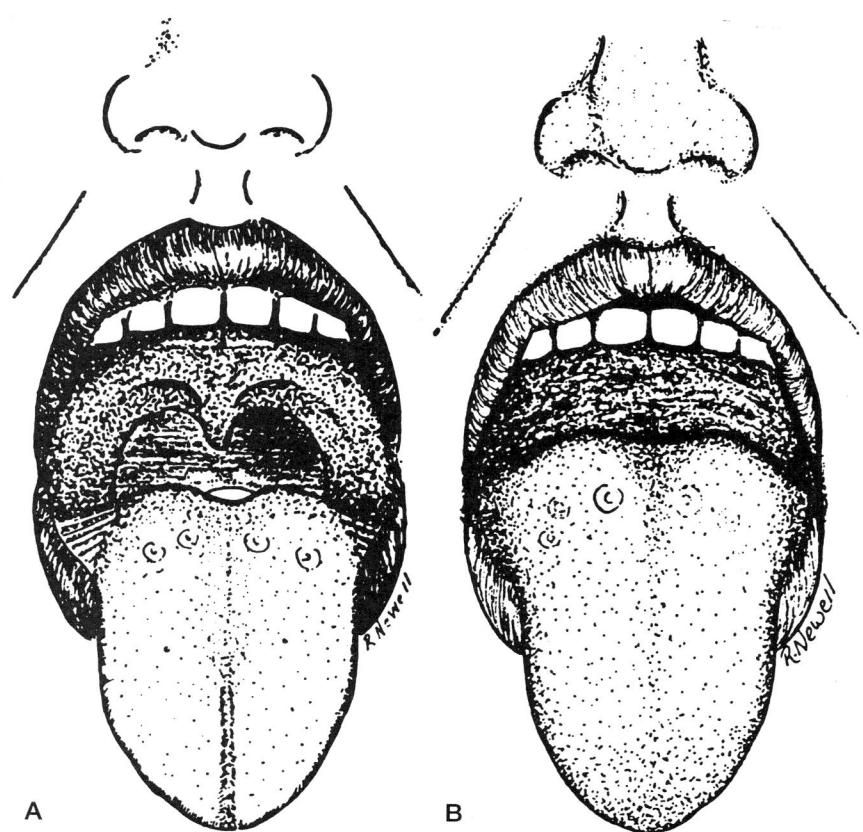

FIGURE 22.3. A: Tonsillar pillars, soft palate, and uvula are clearly visualized—a Class 1 airway. **B:** None of the pharyngeal structures are visualized—a Class IV airway. From Mallampati SR, Gatt SP, Gugino LD, et al. A clinical sign to predict difficult tracheal intubation: A prospective study. *Canadian Anaesth Soc J* 1985;32:429–34, with permission.

A correctly sized OPA will extend from the corner of the mouth to the angle of the jaw. If the OPA is too large, it may obstruct the pharynx; if it is too small, it may push the base of the tongue back against the posterior pharynx. A tongue depressor may be used to insert the OPA directly into place. The OPA may also be inserted sideways and then rotated (90 degrees) into position. Upside-down insertion with 180-degree rotation is not routinely recommended because it may injure tissues or push the tongue posteriorly.

Nasopharyngeal Airways

A *nasopharyngeal airway* (NPA) is a soft rubber or plastic tube (a shortened endotracheal tube can be used) that provides an airway and channel for suctioning between the nares and the pharynx. NPAs may be used in patients with or without an intact cough and gag reflex.

NPAs are available in sizes 12 to 36 French. A 12-French NPA (approximately the size of a 3-mm ETT) will generally fit the nasopharynx of a full-term infant. The NPA should be smaller than the inner aperture of the nares, and its proper length is approximately equal to the distance from the tip of the nose to the tragus of the ear. If the NPA is too long, it may cause vagal stimulation and bradycardia, or it may injure the epiglottis or vocal cords.

Once the airway is inserted, it should be reevaluated frequently. If the airway is too large, it will cause sustained blanching of the alae nasi (nostrils) after insertion. The airway can irritate the mucosa or lacerate adenoidal tissue and cause bleeding. These complications may aggravate airway obstruction and complicate airway management. Physical irritation of the larynx may stimulate coughing, vomiting, or laryngospasm.

Bag-Mask Ventilation

Bag-mask ventilation is an essential skill that requires adequate training and frequent use or periodic retraining. Providers must be proficient in selecting the correct mask size, opening the airway, making a tight seal between the mask and face, delivering effective ventilation, and monitoring the patient. In the out-of-hospital setting, bag-mask ventilation can be as effective as endotracheal intubation when the transport interval is short, particularly when providers have limited training or experience in pediatric intubation (15,47).

The most common technique for single-rescuer bag-mask ventilation involves the "E-C clamp" technique. The rescuer tilts the child's head and uses the last three fingers of one hand (forming a capital letter "E") to lift the jaw while pressing the mask against the face with the thumb and forefinger of the same hand (creating a "C"). The second hand squeezes the bag to deliver each breath over 1 sec to produce visible chest rise. It is important that the jaw is lifted to open the airway and the mask is simultaneously held tightly against the face. The rescuer should not simply press the mask down on the face, because this can close the airway and prevent effective ventilation.

For larger patients, those with a difficult airway, or those with reduced lung compliance, a two-person, bag-mask technique may be necessary. The first rescuer uses both hands to lift the jaw and open the airway while holding the mask to the face; the second rescuer squeezes the bag. Both rescuers should ensure that each breath produces visible chest rise.

Advanced Airways

Advanced airways should be placed within a healthcare system that has established processes for continuous quality improvement, including protocols (e.g., indications for intubation, device selection, medications, and technique for confirmation of tube placement), verification of healthcare provider training and experience, monitoring of complication rates, and a system for remedial training.

General Indications for an Advanced Airway

An unstable airway may result from an altered level of consciousness or compromised airway reflexes, from intrinsic airway or lung parenchymal disease, or from hemodynamic compromise. The general indications for advanced airway placement include actual or anticipated compromise in airway patency, ventilation, or oxygenation. Specific examples include loss of airway protection from impaired central nervous system function, need for hyperventilation to treat increased intracranial pressure (ICP), and inadequate ventilation or ventilatory drive despite oxygen administration. Advanced airway placement may be appropriate if deterioration of the patient's respiratory status is anticipated or if a "borderline" patient must be moved into a poorly monitored or poorly controlled environment (e.g., sedation of a patient in the CT scanner or the interhospital transport of a child).

Choice of Advanced Airway

The ETT has long been considered the optimal advanced airway. However, evidence in a prehospital setting documented that endotracheal intubation may offer no survival benefit over bag-mask ventilation when the transport interval is short. In addition, when personnel assigned to intubate the patient lack adequate training and experience, the incidence of complications, such as unrecognized esophageal intubation, is unacceptably high (15,47). Alternatives to the ETT that have been studied in children include the bag-and-mask and the laryngeal mask airway (LMA).

Data are inadequate to support the routine use of any single approach to airway management in pediatric critical care. The optimal technique for advanced airway insertion is affected by the clinical situation (patient condition and available resources) and the competence of the provider. The provider must weigh potential benefits of the advanced airway against potential risks of the procedure, and should verify correct advanced airway placement immediately after insertion, when the patient is moved, and with any clinical deterioration.

Placement of an advanced airway during attempted cardiopulmonary resuscitation (CPR) also requires the weighing of potential risks and benefits. During CPR, intubation requires interruption of life-saving interventions such as cardiac compressions, and it may cause hypoxemia, reflux, and aspiration. Unrecognized tube misplacement is likely to be fatal. The rescuer must weigh these risks against the potential benefit of establishing an advanced airway in a timely fashion. An advantage of advanced airway placement during CPR is that, after placement, compressions can be provided continuously, without pauses for ventilation.

The intubator should always have a second strategy to provide oxygenation and ventilation if the initial airway approach fails. Bag-mask ventilation may provide this second strategy.

Endotracheal Intubation

Endotracheal intubation (ETI) requires the preparation of equipment and personnel, patient assessment and positioning, and provision of adequate monitoring, oxygenation, and ventilation. Orotracheal intubation is usually performed initially because it is typically a faster route of insertion with fewer complications.

Preparation. Preparation for laryngoscopy and intubation is essential; many "difficult airways" are normal airways that have been inadequately supported. While providing effective oxygenation and ventilation using a bag and mask, the provider should quickly perform a basic airway assessment (see section on Basic Airway Assessment) before attempting intubation. After establishing that the airway can be intubated, the provider should assemble the necessary equipment and personnel and establish monitoring (**Table 22.3**).

Because infants and children vary widely in size, the use of a reference device, such as a length-based resuscitation tape, is helpful in guiding the selection of intubation equipment. Although the use of age-based formulas (**Table 22.4**) to estimate the initial choice of cuffed and uncuffed tracheal tubes is more reliable than estimates based on the size of the fifth finger, these formulas are not as accurate as length-based tapes in predicting appropriate ETT size (9).

It may be necessary to modify equipment selection based on the patient's condition. For example, providers generally use smaller-than-predicted ETTs in the setting of upper airway obstruction. As noted earlier, the intubator must always have an alternate approach in mind to manage the airway in the event that the initial approach fails.

Appropriate positioning of the patient prior to intubation is critical. To directly visualize the glottis, the intubator must position the child to align the axes of the mouth, pharynx, and trachea ("the sniffing position"; see discussion in the section Developmental Airway Considerations). Incomplete extension or hyperextension of the neck or failure to use appropriate age-related head positioning can convert a normal airway into a "difficult" one. The intubator should avoid manipulation of the neck if a risk exists of cervical spinal instability.

Intubation Procedure. Procedural monitoring is essential during ETI, including the monitoring of heart rate, blood pressure, oxygen saturation, and, when possible, end-tidal capnometry/capnography prior to and immediately following ETI. Children have higher oxygen consumption (per kilogram body weight) than do adults and may rapidly become hypoxemic during the procedure, so that the intubator must provide adequate oxygenation before the intubation attempt. The intubator should terminate ETI efforts and initiate bag-mask ventilation if the patient's heart rate, oxygenation, or clinical appearance deteriorates.

After pharmacologic preparation of the patient (if appropriate), bag-mask ventilation should be interrupted to insert the ETT under direct visualization. The laryngoscope blade is used to deflect the tongue and lift the supraglottic structures (or tent the epiglottis) to visualize the glottis. The ETT is inserted through the vocal cords.

TABLE 22.3

EQUIPMENT FOR ENDOTRACHEAL INTUBATION

Monitoring Equipment (apply before intubation if at all possible)
Cardiorespiratory monitor (including monitoring of blood pressure, if possible)
Pulse oximeter

Length-based Tape to Estimate Tube and Equipment Sizes

Suction Equipment
Tonsil-tipped suction device or large-bore suction to suction pharynx
Suction catheter of appropriate size to suction endotracheal tube
Suction canister and device capable of generating suction of −80 to −120 mm Hg (a wall-suction device capable of generating −300 mm Hg is preferred)

Bag and Mask
Check size and oxygen connections
Connected to high-flow oxygen source with reservoir (capable of providing ∼100% oxygen)

Medications
Anticholinergics (atropine)
Sedatives
Paralytics
Appropriate IV equipment and syringes for administration of medications

Intubation Equipment
Stylet
Cuffed and uncuffed tubes of estimated size and cuffed and uncuffed tubes that are 0.5 mm larger and smaller than estimated sizes
Laryngoscope blades (curved and straight) and handle with working light (keep extra batteries and bulb ready)
Water-soluble lubricant
Syringe to inflate tube cuff (if appropriate)
Towel or pad to place under patient (if appropriate)

Confirmation Device(s)
Exhaled CO_2 detector (pediatric size for patients <15 kg and adult size for patients >15 kg)
Esophageal detector device may be used for children who are >20 kg with a perfusing rhythm

Tape/device to Secure Tube
Tape and tincture of benzoin or
Commercial device

TABLE 22.4

FORMULAS FOR ESTIMATION OF ENDOTRACHEAL TUBE SIZE AND DEPTH OF INSERTION

Size

Uncuffed tubes for children >2 years:
Endotracheal tube (internal diameter in mm) $= \dfrac{\text{Age (y)}}{4} + 4$

Cuffed tubes for children >2 years
Endotracheal tube (internal diameter in mm) $= \dfrac{\text{Age (y)}}{4} + 3$

Depth of insertion
Depth of insertion (cm) = (age in years/2) + 12
Depth of insertion = (ETT internal diameter) × 3

---

successfully visualize the glottis. If the provider can only visualize the posterior aspects of the glottis, successful intubation may be possible by using a stylet to create a bend (a "hockey stick") in the end of the tracheal tube. Intubators must ensure that the tip of the stylet does not protrude beyond the end of the tracheal tube.

The tracheal tube should be positioned with the tube's marker line placed at or distal to the vocal cords. Cuffed tubes should be placed so that the cuff is positioned immediately below the level of the cords. Correct depth of insertion can be estimated from formulas using the child's age or the ETT size (**Table 22.4**).

Verification of Placement. Once the tube has been placed, it should be held firmly while correct placement is verified with clinical examination and a confirmation device. No single method for confirmation of tube placement is completely accurate and reliable; therefore, both clinical assessment and a confirmation device are necessary. To perform clinical confirmation, bag-tube ventilation is provided while the intubator observes for chest rise, auscultating bilaterally over the anterior chest, both axillae and the stomach, and observing for water vapor in the tracheal tube on exhalation. Either exhaled carbon dioxide (CO_2) detectors or an esophageal detector device may be used for device confirmation.

After confirmation of correct tube position, the tube should be taped in place and the depth of insertion should be recorded (in cm) at the lip. Hand ventilation is provided using a bag with attached manometer to assess for the presence of leak around the tracheal tube. Correct tube selection should permit an audible air leak around the tube when the inflation pressure exceeds 15 to 25 cm H_2O. Absence of a leak with this pressure suggests that the tube is too large or that the cuff inflation pressure is too high; either condition can cause tracheal mucosal injury. If a cuffed tube is used, the cuff should be deflated until an air leak is detectable at the appropriate pressures, and cuff pressure should be kept at <20 cm H_2O. If an uncuffed tube is in place, and no air leak is detected with the application of 15 to 25 cm H_2O pressure, it may be necessary to replace the tube with a smaller size when the patient is stable.

If a leak is present at inspiratory pressures of <15 to 25 cm H_2O, the tube may be too small or the cuff may be incompletely inflated. Such an air leak can prevent the creation of any positive end-expiratory pressure and may complicate mechanical ventilation. Although most ventilators can compensate for some air leak, excessive air leak is undesirable. Further inflation

---

A curved blade is often more effective for intubation of the older child (>2 years), whereas a straight blade is typically reserved for younger children and those with a "difficult airway." However, no real rule has been defined as to which blade should be used. Both curved and straight blades should be available.

If, despite appropriate head positioning, the intubator cannot see the glottis during the attempt, an assistant should perform external laryngeal manipulation (backward, upward, and rightward push—BURP) to attempt to bring the glottis into view. If the glottis is still difficult to visualize, bag-mask ventilation should be provided and the patient's head repositioned, with verification that the external auditory canal is anterior to the front edge of the patient's shoulder. It may be helpful to ask an assistant to place a finger in the right side of the patient's mouth and pull to the right, which may create more room to

of the cuff may help, provided the cuff inflation pressure remains at <20 cm H_2O. If an uncuffed tube is used, and it is impossible to provide adequate ventilation, replacement of the tube with a larger or cuffed tube should be considered.

Nasotracheal Intubation

Nasotracheal intubation is rarely performed as a primary intubation technique in the emergently ill or injured child. It is more commonly performed "electively" after primary oral intubation, with the hopes of improving patient comfort (e.g., reducing gagging) or increasing ease of tube stabilization (with reduced kinking or biting, when compared to oral tracheal tubes, and reduced secretion-induced tube slippage). Relative contraindications to nasotracheal intubation include coagulopathy, maxillofacial injury, or basilar skull fracture.

To perform nasotracheal intubation, the lubricated tube is passed through one of the nares and guided through the larynx with McGill forceps. Care is taken to avoid lacerating or rupturing the laryngeal tube balloon during manipulation of the tube with the forceps. Blind nasotracheal intubation, as taught for awake intubation of adults, is generally difficult to perform in children. Several anatomic characteristics of the pediatric airway and the need for a cooperative patient limit the feasibility of this procedure in children younger than 8 to 10 years of age.

Complications of nasotracheal intubation include nose bleed (especially problematic if no other airway is in place), pressure-induced ischemic injury to the rim of the nares, and nasal deformity due to nasal septal pressure necrosis (more likely when a tube is in place for long periods in premature infants). In older children, nasal intubation may be associated with a greater risk of sinusitis or otitis media than is oral intubation.

Rapid-sequence Intubation

General Principles. Rapid-sequence intubation (RSI) is a technique used to secure the airway in the patient who presents with a full (or presumed full) stomach, where even moderate preintubation gastric insufflation by bag-mask ventilation may cause gastric regurgitation and pulmonary aspiration. The steps of the classic RSI include (18):

- A basic airway assessment, including relevant patient history using the *SAMPLE* mnemonic (*s*igns and *s*ymptoms, *a*llergies, *m*edications, *p*ast history, *l*ast meal, *e*vents leading to intubation) to assess the risk/suitability for the use of anesthetics or paralytics.
- Preparation of personnel and equipment and establishment of monitoring.
- Preoxygenation (or more accurately, denitrogenation) for 2 to 3 mins with 100% O_2, delivered via a tight-fitting mask, which helps to maintain oxygenation during the period of apnea that follows.
- Administration of an IV anesthetic/sedative/analgesic and almost simultaneous delivery muscle relaxant.
- Application of cricoid pressure (once patient is deeply sedated).
- A period of apnea until the patient has full muscle relaxation.
- Tracheal intubation.
- Removal of cricoid pressure only after tube position is confirmed and the tube cuff (if present) is inflated.

RSI in children is particularly challenging for several reasons. As discussed earlier, the normal child can rapidly develop arterial oxygen desaturation after relatively short periods of apnea. The desaturation will be more rapid if the child is hypoxic prior to the procedure. Some patients who require emergent intubation (e.g., those with intracranial or pulmonary hypertension) will be intolerant of even brief periods of hypercapnia associated with apnea. For these reasons, a "modified RSI technique" is often used in the intubation of critically ill children. After establishment of monitoring, some degree of bag-mask ventilation is provided while cricoid pressure is applied to minimize gastric distention. This technique should prevent or delay the onset of hypoxia and hypercarbia and their sequelae.

Before initiating RSI, the provider must determine if the patient will tolerate the procedure. Some patients have tenuous airways that allow for some oxygenation during spontaneous ventilation. Administration of sedatives and paralytics will remove spontaneous respiratory effort. If the provider is unable to maintain the patient's airway (with or without intubation), hypoxia and hypercarbia can develop rapidly. Examples of scenarios in which RSI may lead to "losing the airway" include patients with significant airway obstruction, facial trauma, or congenital craniofacial anomalies.

Medications. Several types of medications are used during RSI (18,49) (**Table 22.5**). No perfect combination of drugs exists for all patients; providers should select drugs based on the patient's condition and the provider's expertise. Not every patient needs general anesthesia for intubation, but most children require some degree of sedation to facilitate intubation and to reduce their awareness of paralysis and intubation.

Bradycardia can develop during RSI as the result of airway manipulation and as a side effect of some RSI drugs. It can significantly reduce oxygen delivery, especially in patients with limited cardiac output. The American Heart Association Pediatric Advanced Life Support guidelines (18) and the American College of Emergency Physicians (49) recommend the use of atropine for children who undergo RSI who are <1 year of age, for children 1 to 5 years of age who are receiving succinylcholine, and for adolescents who are receiving a second dose of succinylcholine. However, atropine may not be effective in preventing bradycardia (13,32). Although atropine can reduce oral secretions (facilitating airway visualization), the time to the onset of this effect is longer (15–30 mins) than most practitioners are prepared to wait before instrumenting the airway.

A number of sedative, amnestic, and analgesic agents are used during RSI, often interchangeably. Although anesthesia can be achieved using high doses of *benzodiazepines* (e.g., midazolam, lorazepam, and diazepam), these agents are more commonly used to facilitate intubation in patients who require only sedation/amnesia or to supplement other sedative/anesthetic agents (e.g., ketamine or fentanyl). They provide no analgesic effect. Because they do blunt endogenous catecholamines, they can have negative hemodynamic effects and will produce respiratory depression, especially when combined with other agents, such as opioids.

Any of the *opioids* can provide anesthesia at high doses but usually at a hemodynamic (i.e., hypotensive) cost. Fentanyl (a synthetic opioid) is commonly used during RSI. Although it provides rapid onset of analgesia at relatively low doses (i.e., 2–4 mcg/kg IV), it must be given 5 mins prior to laryngoscopy to blunt the hemodynamic response to intubation (i.e., heart rate

TABLE 22.5

RAPID-SEQUENCE INTUBATION DRUGS AND DOSES

Drug	Dose/Route	Duration	Comments
Cardiovascular adjuncts			
Atropine	IV: 0.01–0.02 mg/kg (min: 0.1 mg max: 1 mg)	>30 min	• Inhibits bradycardic response to hypoxia; may cause tachycardia • May cause pupil dilation
Glycopyrrolate	IV: 0.005–0.01 mg/kg (max: 0.2 mg)	>30 min	• Inhibits bradycardic response to hypoxia; may cause tachycardia
Sedative hypnotic agents/analgesics			
Diazepam	IV: 0.1–0.2 mg/kg (max: 4 mg)	30–90 min	• May cause respiratory depression or potentiate depressant effects of narcotics and barbiturates
Lorazepam	IV: 0.05–0.1 mg/kg (max: 4 mg)	4–6 hr	• May cause hypotension
Midazolam	IV: 0.1–0.3 mg/kg (max: 4 mg)	1–2 hr	• Minimal cardiac depression • Occasional respiratory depression • No analgesic properties
Fentanyl citrate	IV, IM: 2–4 mcg/kg	IV: 30–60 min IM: 1–2 hrs	• May cause respiratory depression, hypotension, chest wall rigidity with high-dose (>5 mg/kg) infusions • May elevate ICP
Anesthetic agents (in doses indicated)			
Thiopental	IV: 2–5 mg/kg	5–10 min	• Negative inotropic effects and often causes hypotension • Decreases cerebral metabolic rate and ICP • Potentiates respiratory depressive effects of narcotics and benzodiazepines • No analgesic properties
Etomidate	IV: 0.2–0.4 mg/kg	5–15 min	• Decreases cerebral metabolic rate and ICP • May cause respiratory depression • Minimal cardiovascular effects • Causes myoclonic activity; may lower seizure threshold • Causes cortisol suppression; contraindicated in patients dependent on endogenous cortisol response • No analgesic properties
Lidocaine	IV: 1–2 mg/kg	~30 min	• Causes myocardial and CNS depression with high doses • May decrease ICP during RSI • Hypotension occurs infrequently
Ketamine	IV: 1–2 mg/kg IM: 3–5 mg/kg	30–60 min	• May increase blood pressure, heart rate, cardiac output • May cause increased secretions, laryngospasm • Causes limited respiratory depression • Bronchodilator • May cause hallucinations, emergence reactions
Propofol	IV: 2 mg/kg (up to 3 mg/kg in young children)	3–5 min	• May cause hypotension, especially in hypovolemic patients • May cause pain on injection • Highly lipid soluble • Causes less airway reactivity than barbiturates
Neuromuscular blocking agents			
Succinylcholine	Infant IV: 2 mg/kg Child IV: 1–1.5 mg/kg IM: Double the IV dose	3–5 min	• Depolarizing muscle relaxant; causes muscle fasciculation • May cause rise in ICP and intraocular and intragastric pressures • May cause rise in serum potassium • May cause hypertension • Avoid in renal failure, burns, crush injuries, or hyperkalemia
Atracurium	IV: 0.5 mg/kg	30–40 min	• Metabolized by plasma hydrolysis • May cause mild histamine release
cis-Atracurium	IV: 0.1 mg/kg, then 1–5 mg/kg/min	20–35 min	• Metabolized by plasma hydrolysis • May cause mild histamine release
Rocuronium	IV: 0.6–1.2 mg/kg	30–60 min	• Few cardiovascular effects
Vecuronium	IV: 0.1–0.2 mg/kg	30–60 min	• Few cardiovascular effects

Adapted from Hazinski M, Zaritsky A, Nadkarni V, et al. Rapid Sequence Intubation. In: *PALS Provider Manual*. Dallas: American Heart Association, 2002; and Venkataraman ST, Khan N, Brown A. Validation of predictors of extubation success and failure in mechanically ventilated infants and children. *Crit Care Med* 2000;28:2991–6.
ICP, intracranial pressure; RSI, rapid-sequence intubation

and blood pressure changes) (22). Because fentanyl has limited sedative/amnestic effects, it is frequently used with benzodiazepines. High bolus doses of fentanyl (≥ 5 mcg/kg) can cause acute onset of chest wall rigidity, which can be prevented by coadministration of a paralytic agent.

Anesthetic agents used during RSI include ketamine, propofol, thiopental, and etomidate. Ketamine is a dissociative anesthetic with analgesic and amnestic properties. It increases heart rate, systemic blood pressure, and cardiac output, making it a useful anesthetic for patients with acute hemodynamic instability. Although it theoretically may produce hypotension in catecholamine-depleted patients (e.g., chronic congestive heart failure), it is commonly used in children with myocardial depression or pulmonary hypertension. Its bronchodilator properties can be beneficial when patients with acute bronchospasm are intubated. Ketamine was long thought to increase intracranial blood flow and exacerbate intracranial hypertension. However, if effective ventilation is provided before intubation to avoid hypercapnia, ketamine is not associated with increased ICP and may actually decrease ICP (1). Emergence delirium and prolonged and recurrent hallucinations occur frequently (especially in adolescents) and may be prevented by co-dosing with a benzodiazepine. Because ketamine can increase airway secretions, pretreatment with atropine or glycopyrrolate should be considered if timing allows.

Propofol is a nonbarbiturate anesthetic with rapid onset and a short duration of action. It is an effective anesthetic, but side effects may include hypotension from negative inotropy and vasodilatation. It has no analgesic properties.

Thiopental is a short-acting barbiturate that leads to rapid onset of anesthesia and amnesia. Although it is very effective in reducing intracranial hypertension through its reduction of cerebral metabolism and cerebral blood flow, it may produce severe vasodilation, negative inotropy, and hypotension, thus limiting its use in critically ill children to those with adequate cardiovascular function.

Etomidate is a short-acting IV hypnotic agent that provides anesthesia while maintaining hemodynamics and cerebral perfusion without raising ICP. These features have made it desirable for use in the care of the patient with head injury. It is a respiratory depressant and lacks any analgesic properties. Limited retrospective adult data suggest that the use of etomidate for intubation might predispose the critically ill patient to acute adrenal insufficiency and worsened hemodynamics for as long 24 hrs after dosing (8,20). Etomidate may lower the seizure threshold and may cause myoclonus, coughing, or hiccupping.

Other potential RSI drugs include lidocaine and neuromuscular blockers. Although IV or endotracheal lidocaine is given to suppress reflex autonomic and airway responses to laryngoscopy (especially in the setting of increased ICP), the pediatric literature supporting lidocaine's efficacy is limited (see discussion in the section on Intracranial Hypertension below).

Neuromuscular blocking agents are used to facilitate the visualization and intubation of the airway. The use of these agents during RSI has been shown to increase the likelihood of successful intubation (44). Clinical indicators of adequate paralysis include lack of spontaneous movements, respiratory effort, and blink reflex, as well as jaw relaxation, manifested by the ability to fully open the patient's mouth without resistance.

The two broad groups of neuromuscular blocking agents are the depolarizing and nondepolarizing agents, distinguished by their action on receptors at the neuromuscular junction. *Depo-larizing neuromuscular blockers* bind the postsynaptic receptor of the neuromuscular junction, leading to unsynchronized depolarization of the postsynaptic membrane, which causes transient muscular fasciculation (seen less commonly in smaller infants) and then paralysis as the receptors remain occupied. Succinylcholine is the most commonly used agent in this group. The advantages of this drug include rapid onset and relatively short duration of action. Pharmacokinetics and dosing characteristics vary with patient age. Complications occur in 0.3% to 1% of children (31), including acute hyperkalemia, malignant hyperthermia, and masseter spasm with subsequent airway obstruction. This drug normally causes a modest rise in serum potassium (typically 0.5–1 mEq/L) but may produce significant hyperkalemia in specific at-risk patients (54); these include patients with burns (the response is proportional to the extent of the burn), peripheral nerve injury, renal failure, neuromuscular disease, or major trauma with rhabdomyolysis. The risk of acute hyperkalemia in the child with previously undiagnosed neuromuscular disease triggered a US Food and Drug Administration warning that succinylcholine is contraindicated in pediatric intubation "…except when used for emergency tracheal intubation or in instances where immediate securing of the airway is necessary." Although the risk of hyperkalemia may be reduced by the simultaneous use of defasciculating, nondepolarizing agents (48), such drugs will substantially increase succinylcholine dose requirements. Because nondepolarizing paralytics are available with rapid onset of action, succinylcholine's role in pediatric neuromuscular blockade may be extremely limited. Despite the theoretical contraindications to succinylcholine in the setting of ocular trauma and increased ICP, limited clinical literature documents these complications (50).

Nondepolarizing neuromuscular blockers (e.g., rocuronium and atracurium) bind the postsynaptic receptors of the neuromuscular junction, without causing postsynaptic depolarization and neuromuscular transmission. The literature shows that "high" doses of these agents can create adequate conditions for intubation in times to onset similar to those of succinylcholine. The onset of action is shortened if a "priming dose" is given 3 to 5 mins prior to the intubation, but this will prolong the period of muscle relaxation (7). The provider must be ready to assume control of the airway and ventilation when a priming dose is used in children, because some will develop profound muscle weakness with a priming dose.

Rocuronium, a derivative of vecuronium, has few cardiovascular side effects. A dose of 1 mg/kg of rocuronium can produce conditions for intubation comparable to succinylcholine within 1 min, but its duration is much longer than succinylcholine.

Other nondepolarizing neuromuscular blockers are available, each with its own pharmacologic profile and advantages and disadvantages. Atracurium and cis-atracurium are both eliminated by Hoffman elimination; thus, their clearance is independent of renal or hepatic function. They also have the potential for histamine release.

Cricoid Pressure. The "Sellick maneuver" puts direct pressure on the cricoid cartilage, compressing the upper esophageal sphincter, thus preventing reflux of gastric contents from the esophagus into the airway and preventing the insufflation of air into the stomach during positive-pressure ventilation (PPV). Care must be taken with its application. Cricoid pressure can distort the upper airway, preventing effective visualization of the airway and effective bag-mask ventilation. The use of cricoid pressure in patients with laryngeal or cervical spine pathology is controversial because it may cause cervical spine movement. It is contraindicated in patients with a cough or gag reflex.

Laryngeal Mask Airway

The LMA consists of a small mask with an inflatable cuff that is connected to a plastic tube with a universal adaptor. It is designed to be placed in the oropharynx with its tip in the hypopharynx and the base of the mask at the epiglottis. When the cuff of the mask is inflated, it creates a seal with the supraglottic area, allowing air flow between the tube and the trachea.

The LMA can be used with spontaneously breathing patients to deliver PPV or as a guide for insertion of another airway device, such as an ETT, airway-exchange catheter, lighted stylet, or flexible fiberoptic bronchoscope. The maximum seal pressure possible is ~25 cm H_2O, which may limit effective PPV in critically ill children. Use in conscious patients requires sedation to minimize airway protective reflexes, including laryngospasm and bronchospasm.

The ease of insertion and relatively low complication rate have made the LMA an important component of the management of patients with difficult airways. However, because it is a supraglottic device, it is less effective in patients with glottic or subglottic pathology. Complications due to malpositioning of the device (resulting in airway obstruction) or increased difficulty of insertion are more common in younger children (35), but the complication rate decreases with increased operator experience. As of 2006, no clinical reports of LMA use during pediatric cardiac arrest were available.

The original LMA, the LMA Classic, is a multiuse device with sizes for neonates through adults (**Table 22.6**). It is important to choose the correct size; if the LMA is too large, it will be difficult to place, and if it is too small, it will not maintain an adequate seal to deliver effective PPV. The combined widths of the patient's index, middle, and ring fingers can be used to estimate the size of the LMA (14).

TABLE 22.6

LMA AIRWAY SELECTION AND CUFF INFLATION VOLUMES

LMA airway size	Patient size	Maximum cuff inflation volumes (mL)
1	Neonates/infants up to 5 kg	4
1½	Infants 5–10 kg	7
2	Infants/children 10–20 kg	10
2½	Children 20–30 kg	14
3	Children 30–50 kg	20
4	Adults 50–70 kg	30
5	Adults 70–100 kg	40
6	Adults >100 kg	50

*These are maximum clinical volumes that should never be exceeded. It is recommended that the cuff be inflated to 60 cm H_2O intracuff pressures.
From LMA. Available at: http://www.lmana.com/faqs.php#faq03. Accessed March 26, 2007.

Several techniques have been described for inserting LMAs in children. Classically, the LMA is inserted with the patient positioned as for ETI. The LMA can be inserted with the cuff fully deflated and lubricated; it is advanced with the aperture of the mask facing toward the tongue until the rescuer feels resistance, and the cuff then is inflated. Cuff inflation may push the LMA slightly out of the mouth. The LMA may also be inserted with the cuff partially inflated (i.e., with half of the recommended volume) and the LMA mask inverted or turned to the side. Once the LMA is fully inserted, it is rotated to normal position and the cuff is fully inflated (23,34).

LMA insertion causes less airway trauma and hemodynamic changes than laryngoscopy. LMAs will not prevent aspiration of refluxed gastric contents.

Other Airway Devices

The Esophagotracheal Combitube. The Combitube is a dual-lumen, dual-cuff airway device. The tube is blindly placed; therefore, it is usually inserted with the distal tip in the esophagus. When the two cuffs are inflated (one distal in the esophagus and the second in the oropharynx), the larynx is trapped between them and ventilation can be provided through the first (pharyngeal) lumen. If the tip of the tube is placed in the trachea (<5% of insertions), the second lumen must be used for ventilation. The provider must accurately determine the location of the distal tip to ensure ventilation through the correct lumen. In that the smallest size is designed for patients over 4 feet in height, its use in children is limited.

Gum Elastic Bougie and Airway-exchange Catheter. The *gum elastic bougie* can be inserted blindly into the airway and used as a guide for insertion of an ETT. The *airway-exchange catheter* was designed to be placed through an existing ETT and used as a guide for exchanging that ETT for a new one. It can also be used to intubate the larynx directly if an ETT will not pass through the larynx; the ETT is then threaded over the airway-exchange catheter into the airway. Some airway-exchange catheters have a central lumen, allowing oxygenation or insertion over a guidewire.

Fiberoptic Intubation

Endotracheal intubation over a flexible fiberoptic bronchoscope has become an important method by which to secure the airway in patients when direct ETI is impossible. The bronchoscope can be inserted blindly or under direct visualization. Experienced operators have a very high success rate.

The bronchoscope has an operator-guided flexible port and a port that can be used for administering medications, providing suction, or passing a guidewire. Once the fiberoptic bronchoscope is inserted into the trachea, a guidewire can be passed through the suction port or a preloaded ETT can be passed over the scope into the trachea. The fiberoptic scope also allows direct visualization of the larynx to identify trauma or congenital anomalies of the larynx before intubation, and it can be used in intubated patients to assess persistent atelectasis, airway injury, or pulmonary hemorrhage, and to perform bronchial alveolar lavage.

Very small, ultra-thin bronchoscopes are available for tube sizes as small as 3.0 mm, although most of these scopes do not have a suction port, are very delicate, and are difficult to control. Cooperative older children may tolerate flexible laryngoscopy awake, but most patients will require sedation to minimize gagging and laryngospasm. Topical anesthesia can be given through the scope to attenuate airway protective reflexes. Ideally, the child will be breathing spontaneously, which allows dynamic visualization of the glottic structures to identify malacia or vocal cord paralysis and provides a margin of safety if ETI is unsuccessful. Fiberoptic intubation can injure airway structures.

Other inexpensive and easy-to-use fiberoptic devices are available to aid intubation. The *optical stylet* can be placed down even small ETTs to provide a fiberoptic view of the airway (46). Video intubation laryngoscopes, such as the GlideScope, have been used in neonates and children (53).

Confirmation of Advanced Airway Placement

Exhaled Carbon Dioxide. Both clinical assessment and a device should be used to confirm advanced airway placement immediately after insertion, when the patient is moved, and whenever the intubated patient deteriorates. Accuracy of exhaled CO_2 and esophageal detector devices have been reported following ETT placement in children, but their accuracy has not been reported with other advanced airways. Experience is limited in cardiac arrest.

In a child with a perfusing rhythm, the detection of exhaled CO_2 using a colorimetric detector or capnometer is both sensitive and specific for ETT placement. In cardiac arrest, or with a large pulmonary embolus, pulmonary blood flow may be extremely low; therefore inadequate CO_2 may be detected despite correct tracheal tube placement. Bolus IV epinephrine administration during resuscitation may transiently reduce pulmonary blood flow, reducing the exhaled CO_2 below the limits of detection. In experimental pediatric cardiac arrest, the sensitivity of CO_2 detection was 85% and the specificity was 100% (4) for tracheal tube placement. Both with a perfusing rhythm and in cardiac arrest, the detection of exhaled CO_2 after six initial breaths (to wash out any CO_2 that entered the stomach during bag-mask ventilation) reliably indicates placement of the tube in the trachea. If tube position is in doubt during CPR, the rescuer should confirm tube position with direct laryngoscopy.

Two sizes of colorimetric exhaled CO_2 devices are available: one for children who weigh <15 kg and the other for patients who weigh >15 kg. Use of the larger detector with a small child could result in failure to detect exhaled CO_2 despite correct tracheal tube placement. In addition, use of even the smaller detector in infants who weigh <2 kg will add substantial dead space to the ventilator circuit.

Severe airway obstruction (e.g., status asthmaticus) and pulmonary edema may impair CO_2 elimination sufficiently to cause failure to detect exhaled CO_2 in adults, but these problems have not been reported in children. If the detector is contaminated with acidic gastric contents or acidic drugs, such as tracheally administered epinephrine, the colorimetric detector may stop reacting. Despite these potential limitations, monitoring exhaled CO_2 is an important tool for confirming the initial placement and position of a tracheal tube. A fall in exhaled CO_2 (with capnography or capnometry) indicates tube displacement more rapidly and reliably than pulse oximetry.

When time permits, a chest radiograph should be obtained to confirm the proper depth of tube insertion. The tip of the tube should be in mid-trachea, at approximately the level of the third or fourth thoracic vertebra. Most commercially available ETTs have marks that indicate depth of insertion; the depth marker at the child's teeth or lips should be noted before the

tube is secured and throughout intubation. Position of the tip of the tube will move with changes in head position; the tube will move further into the trachea when the neck is flexed.

Esophageal Detector Device. The esophageal detector device is accurate when used to confirm ETT placement in children who have a perfusing rhythm and are >20 kg in weight (45). At this writing, no published evidence exists on the sensitivity or reliability of the device in children in cardiac arrest.

Lighted Intubation Stylet

The lighted intubation stylet, also known as the *light wand*, is essentially a rigid stylet with a fiberoptic light at the tip. Pediatric versions can be inserted through ETTs as small as 2.0 mm. The lighted stylet is portable, relatively inexpensive, and produces less laryngeal stimulation than laryngoscopy; airway injury is uncommon with this device.

The lighted stylet can be used as a traditional stylet, inserted with direct laryngoscopy or blindly if direct laryngoscopy is impossible. Blind placement of an ETT over the stylet can be very useful in cases of limited neck and/or jaw mobility because it does not require full mouth opening or neck extension. The lighted stylet can be used when large amounts of blood and secretions are present, unless they are sufficiently thick to disrupt transillumination. Failure of placement can be due to subglottic stenosis, vocal cord closure, or entrapment of the tip in the vallecula or the aryepiglottic folds.

The lighted stylet does take time to insert, and the hypoxemic patient may not tolerate the procedure. It is therefore relatively contraindicated in the "cannot intubate, cannot oxygenate" scenario. Because the procedure requires that the airway be midline, it is contraindicated in conditions where the glottis is deviated laterally or when laryngeal pathology is present. Any condition that limits transmission of light through the anterior neck (e.g., mass lesions, scarring, or massive edema or obesity) will also interfere with use of the stylet.

Percutaneous Needle Cricothyrotomy/Tracheostomy

Indications. Every publication or lecture on pediatric airway management refers to the technique of needle cricothyrotomy as the rescue procedure of last resort. Although limited literature and sparse clinical experience support its use, clinicians who manage pediatric emergencies must be familiar with the procedure and its equipment and indications.

Needle cricothyrotomy/tracheostomy is indicated as a lifesaving procedure in patients who present or progress to the "cannot intubate, cannot oxygenate" scenario, with obstruction proximal to the glottic opening, or in patients with abnormal anatomy that precludes laryngoscopic visualization of the glottic opening. The classic indication is the child with epiglottitis when bag-mask ventilation and intubation have failed. Other clinical indications include facial trauma and angioedema. The procedure is rarely helpful in foreign-body aspiration if the object cannot be visualized by direct laryngoscopy, because it is unlikely that the obstruction is located proximal to the level of the cricothyroid membrane. It also would be of questionable value in the patient with croup because a small ETT can usually bypass the subglottic obstruction.

Equipment. If the procedure is necessary, the use of familiar equipment such as an IV catheter with ventilation bag is recommended. Bag-catheter ventilation can provide effective oxygenation but not ventilation. The use of potentially harmful and rarely employed procedures, such as jet ventilation through a catheter, has high potential for complications. It is a good practice to preassemble a needle cricothyrotomy/tracheostomy kit (pre-made kits are available), seal it in a transparent bag, and tape it in an accessible place in the resuscitation area. Providers should practice with the equipment (especially manual ventilation through the catheter) prior to use. The simplest equipment, appropriate for use in infants, consists of a 14-gauge over-the-needle catheter, a 3.0-mm ETT adapter, and a 5-mL syringe.

Several alternatives to conventional catheters are available for needle cricothyrotomy. A short (6 cm), Cook 15-gauge, plastic-covered, wire mesh, transtracheal catheter is less likely to kink (obstruct) than a traditional catheter. Several commercially available cricothyrotomy devices are inserted using a modified Seldinger technique to place the airway. A jet-ventilation catheter (VBM Medical, Inc.) is simple, practical in design, and comes in three different sizes to accommodate all pediatric patients, but little published data supports its use.

Procedure. The child is placed in the supine position with a towel under the shoulders to produce exaggerated neck extension. Doing this forces the trachea anteriorly, so that it is easily palpable and can be stabilized with two fingers of one hand. Although it is ideal to puncture the cricothyroid membrane (the cricoid ring is less likely to narrow during healing), this membrane may be difficult to palpate in infants, and insertion of the catheter through adjacent structures is unlikely to cause life-threatening complications. The upper trachea should be considered functionally as a large palpable vein, which should be isolated and cannulated, with the catheter directed at the shallowest angle practical. For this reason, the procedure is probably better called *percutaneous needle tracheostomy*; the priority is to quickly establish adequate airway and oxygenation through a needle placed in the trachea. Once the catheter is in place, the 3.0-mm ETT adapter and a ventilation bag with oxygen are attached and bag-catheter ventilation is begun. Placement is confirmed by clinical examination (chest rise and breath sounds may be difficult to appreciate) and detection of exhaled CO_2. The small catheter radius will normally cause high resistance to ventilation that should not be mistaken for signs of a misplaced catheter, poor lung compliance, or a pneumothorax. The required inspiratory pressures are well above the limits of the pop-off valve for any ventilation bag; therefore, the valve must be occluded to provide gas flow through the catheter.

Jet ventilation through a cricothyrotomy should only be considered by those experienced in its use and preferably in children older than 5 or 6 years of age. If bag-catheter ventilation provides adequate oxygen saturation, it is preferable to jet ventilation. If jet ventilation is used, the provider should start with low psi (20 mm Hg) and titrate to adequate chest excursion and oxygen saturation. Extreme caution is required to avoid the complications of excessive flow and resultant barotrauma.

Support of Patient with Advanced Airway

Warmed and humidified oxygen should be provided to patients with advanced airways, because the airway bypasses the hu-

midification and warming functions of the upper airway. Sedation should be titrated to maintain patient comfort. Periodic suctioning of the airway is required because secretion clearance is impaired. Providers must frequently verify tube patency and proper tube position. Continuous monitoring of exhaled CO_2 is recommended during transport to enable the early detection of tube obstruction or displacement.

Complications of Endotracheal Intubation

Complications of ETI can be divided into immediate or procedure complications (associated with the placement of the artificial airway) and later complications. Later complications include those that occur while the artificial airway is in place and those that develop during and following extubation.

Procedure Complications. Any airway intervention may convert a *potentially* compromised airway to an *actually* compromised airway and may create hypoxia and hypercarbia. In addition, placement of an advanced airway often requires interruption or postponement of other interventions (e.g., chest compressions during CPR) that may have a greater impact on patient survival. In some settings (e.g., in the prehospital setting with short transport intervals or healthcare settings in which providers have limited opportunities for intubation), more emphasis should be placed on good basic airway management than on advanced airway placement.

Immediate complications of intubation can result from the medications required for intubation, from trauma to (e.g., laceration of) airway structures or injury to the cervical spine, and from the physiologic effects of laryngoscopy and PPV. Laryngoscopy can cause increased intracranial and intraocular pressures, coughing, regurgitation, aspiration, and laryngospasm, especially in the patient with inadequate sedation. The potential for airway injury increases with a difficult airway and with multiple intubation attempts. Dental injury is common in school-aged children with loose deciduous teeth. The risk of injury can be minimized by careful laryngoscopy (with appropriate patient sedation) and selection of appropriate tube size.

Accurate initial and ongoing assessment of ETT placement is essential. Esophageal intubation and gastric dilation will quickly result in hypoxia and increase the risk of aspiration. A misplaced tube should be detected with careful clinical assessment and evaluation of exhaled CO_2 immediately after tube placement. Mainstem bronchus intubation (more commonly right sided) can result in atelectasis, hypoxia, and pneumothorax.

Later Complications. While the tube is in place, providers should assess the nares, lip, and tongue for signs of pressure injury. Ulcers may develop on the arytenoids, posterior vocal cords, subglottic area, anterior tracheal wall, and epiglottis. Oropharyngeal aspiration has been documented in 28% of intubated pediatric patients, and it is more likely to occur with oral intubation and in patients with lower sedation scores (2). The use of cuffed ETTs may decrease this risk. Finally, ventilator-associated pneumonia and sinusitis can be sources of morbidity in intubated patients.

Unplanned extubation increases hospital and PICU lengths of stay and occurs in 5% to 14% of intubated patients (29,43). It appears to be more common in younger children, those intubated orally, those documented to be more agitated, and when greater than a 1:1 patient-to-nurse ratio is provided. Interestingly, less than half of patients reported to have unplanned extubation require reintubation, suggesting the need for more aggressive identification of patients who require extubation.

ETI results in hyperemia, edema, and mucosal hemorrhage, which can progress to ulceration, erosion, and eventual chronic fibrosis. Fibrosis typically develops in the subglottic region; it is circumferential but may be asymmetric and result in granuloma formation, especially posteriorly. Late complications can develop up to 6 weeks after extubation and include laryngeal and tracheal granulomas, vocal cord paralysis, and subglottic stenosis.

Subglottic stenosis following extubation is observed in fewer than 8% of intubated patients (52). The number of intubations appears to be independently associated with the development of airway injury (17). Duration of intubation is also associated with an increased risk of subglottic stenosis, although injuries have been reported even after short-term intubations (see discussion in the next section). In that no apparent "safe" duration of intubation has been defined, the decision to switch to tracheostomy should be patient specific and not related to an arbitrary time limit.

Planned Extubation and Postextubation Care

Weaning from the ventilator and extubation may be attempted after resolution of the conditions that necessitated intubation. The patient should have adequate airway protective reflexes, as demonstrated by an intact cough, gag, and swallow. Sedation should be weaned so that the patient has adequate airway reflexes and ventilatory drive. Neuromuscular blockade should be completely reversed and confirmed by train-of-four testing or evaluation of spontaneous movement.

Oxygenation and ventilation should be adequate with minimal ventilatory support (e.g., $\leq$4–6 cm H_2O positive end-expiratory pressure, enough pressure support to overcome ETT resistance, and minimal FIO_2). The patient should successfully complete a trial of spontaneous breathing with pressure support, volume support, or T-piece. Ideally the patient should have an air leak around the ETT with inflation pressures of >15–25 cm H_2O, although this test has poor sensitivity for predicting postextubation stridor, especially in younger children (33). Finally, cardiac function should be adequate to tolerate the increase in left ventricular afterload that develops with the withdrawal of PPV (39).

Once criteria for extubation are met, the ETT and oropharynx are suctioned to help to prevent aspiration and laryngospasm. Oral and gastric feeding is suspended for 4 to 6 hrs prior to extubation in case reintubation is required. If a cuffed tube is in place, the cuff is deflated prior to extubation. Oxygen (100%) is provided, and the lungs are fully inflated as the tube is withdrawn to provide a buffer for possible laryngospasm. For children with airway anomalies, extubation in the operating suite may be appropriate.

After extubation, humidified oxygen is provided, and the patient is monitored for signs of extubation failure. Extubation failure occurs in 4.1% to 29% of patients (depending on the definition of failure and the study population) and results in increased PICU and hospital lengths of stay and possibly in mortality (24). Upper airway obstruction, pulmonary dysfunction, and respiratory muscle weakness are the most common causes of failure (24). Patients who fail extubation tend to be

younger, intubated longer, and have chronic medical problems (11,24). Some bedside measurements of respiratory function, including spontaneous tidal volume indexed to body weight, FIO_2, mean airway pressure, oxygenation index, fraction of total minute ventilation provided by the ventilator, peak ventilation inspiratory pressure, dynamic compliance, and mean inspiratory flow, have been shown to predict the level of risk for extubation failure (51).

Noninvasive ventilation has been touted as a treatment for patients who develop postextubation respiratory failure. However, large adult trials failed to demonstrate benefit and documented some harm (12).

The complications of extubation include aspiration, laryngospasm, bronchospasm, and upper airway edema, causing stridor. Risk of aspiration can be reduced by ensuring that the stomach is empty, the patient is awake, and the oropharynx is clear of secretions before extubation. Laryngospasm results from stimulation of the larynx by secretions or by the ETT, especially in a patient who is not fully awake. Under most circumstances, it can be treated by the application of continuous positive airway pressure until the spasm resolves, although some patients require muscle relaxants and reintubation. Some experts recommend application of firm pressure just posterior to the mandibular ramus (medial to the earlobe) to break laryngospasm. Bronchospasm is common in asthmatic patients after extubation and can be treated with inhaled β-adrenergic agonists.

Postextubation stridor is more common in patients who are 1 to 4 years of age, those who have traumatic or multiple intubations, and those with airway abnormalities. Postextubation stridor has also been associated with excessive tube movement and use of a relatively large ETT. Hoarseness and croupy cough, with or without respiratory insufficiency, develop within the first 3 hrs after extubation, peak within 8 hrs, and usually resolve by 24 hrs, although residual hoarseness can persist for up to 72 hrs. The stridor is often caused by subglottic edema but may result from neurologic impairment, laryngomalacia, subglottic stenosis, or vocal cord paralysis. In an endoscopic survey of children with persistent postextubation stridor, most had laryngotracheitis with or without neurologic dysfunction. Only 20% of children had structural airway problems, such as stenosis or vocal cord paralysis (25).

The treatment of postextubation stridor includes administration of humidified air or oxygen, racemic epinephrine, and possible corticosteroids. Nebulized racemic epinephrine (0.5 mL of 2.25% solution in 2.5 mL of saline) produces vasoconstriction and reduces edema. The use of dexamethasone for the prevention and treatment of postextubation stridor remains controversial. A meta-analysis of trials of dexamethasone (0.25–0.5 mg/kg/dose) found that it reduced the incidence of postextubation stridor but did not significantly reduce the reintubation rate (30). However, other than hyperglycemia, dexamethasone produces no significant side effects. Oxygen in helium may be administered because this mixture is less dense than pure oxygen, allows higher inspiratory flow at lower resistance, and can improve comfort. However, patients who require a >40% inspired O_2 concentration may not receive enough helium to experience benefit.

Extubation failure may require reintubation until the reason for the failure can be treated or resolves. Persistent postextubation stridor is an indication for diagnostic bronchoscopy.

THE DIFFICULT AIRWAY: ASSESSMENT AND MANAGEMENT

Assessment and Physiology

A difficult airway is present if the intubator experiences difficulty in providing effective bag-mask ventilation or difficulty with tracheal intubation. The difficult pediatric airway is best managed not by heroic intervention and uncommonly used techniques but, instead, by anticipation and careful planning. Much of the information that will guide risk assessment and management decisions can be obtained from a careful patient history and a focused physical examination.

Caregivers should be questioned and old records obtained to determine if previous intubations have been difficult. A history of previous acute or chronic upper airway obstruction, including symptoms of stridor, snoring, or sleep apnea, suggests a potentially difficult airway. A history of obesity, limited jaw or neck movement, facial trauma, or laryngeal abnormalities can also suggest a difficult airway. Craniofacial anomalies can be associated with difficult airways and may be isolated or associated with syndromes or other organ system dysfunction that could complicate intubation. As noted earlier under Developmental Airway Considerations, any condition that interferes with alignment of the oral, pharyngeal, and laryngeal axes will complicate and may prevent intubation. Also as noted earlier, the child is positioned appropriately for orotracheal intubation if the external auditory canal is anterior to the front edge of the patient's shoulders. Assessment of the visibility of the uvula, tonsils, and posterior pharyngeal wall can help to predict a difficult airway. However, these techniques have not been validated in children and may be difficult to perform in an uncooperative, critically ill child.

General Management of the Difficult Airway

General Principles

The most critical aspects of difficult-airway management are the anticipation of difficulties and development of a suitable backup plan. Hypoxia and airway obstruction can develop very quickly in young children with airway compromise.

The American Society of Anesthesiologists has developed an algorithm for the approach to and management of the difficult airway. Often, the most difficult decision is whether to attempt conventional intubation or to proceed directly to more advanced techniques.

A kit with the equipment necessary to deal with the difficult airway should be readily available and should include different types and sizes of laryngoscope blades, ETTs and LMAs, forceps, stylets, a needle cricothyrotomy/tracheostomy kit, and an intubating bronchoscope. If a surgical airway is anticipated, notify personnel skilled at emergent cricothyrotomy and tracheostomy. If sedation is necessary for airway management, the use of short-acting and/or reversible agents is preferred, but the safety of the airway is the priority.

If initial tracheal intubation fails, changing laryngoscope blades should be considered, to improve visualization of glottic structures. The patient's position is manipulated as needed to improve alignment of the oral-pharyngeal-laryngeal axes and to provide external laryngeal manipulation (backward, upward, and rightward push—BURP). If the initial intubation attempt is unsuccessful, consider alternate airway strategies, rather than repeatedly attempting unsuccessful intubations and possibly causing further airway trauma. If the child was difficult to intubate, prepare carefully for extubation, because edema may make reintubation even more difficult. Consider extubating patients with an airway exchange catheter in place until successful extubation is confirmed.

Management of Specific Problems

Awake Intubation

Although awake intubation (i.e., intubation without sedation) is an important strategy for use in an adult patient with a difficult airway, it can be very difficult to perform in an uncooperative child. The risks of intubating an awake, struggling, frightened child must be weighed against the need for maintaining spontaneous breaths if intubation fails. Intubation without sedation is appropriate in cardiopulmonary arrest and may be appropriate for the child in severe shock.

Sedation may be titrated to minimize discomfort but avoid deep sedation. This approach allows intubation without severely compromising airway reflexes, respiratory drive, or hemodynamics. If available, a relatively short-acting inhalational anaesthetic such as sevoflurane can create appropriate conditions for intubation and maintain respiratory drive. Short-acting medications, such as propofol, ketamine, or benzodiazepines, may be titrated to balance patient cooperation and cardiopulmonary stability. However, this balance can be difficult to maintain, especially in younger children. Lidocaine spray may minimize gagging and laryngospasm.

Full Stomach

One of the risks associated with instrumenting the pediatric airway is the potential for reflux and aspiration of gastric contents. Airway reflexes that usually protect against aspiration may be suppressed by sedatives and anesthetics, neuromuscular blockers, or underlying disease or injury. Aspiration of as little as 0.4 mL/kg of gastric contents can cause significant acute lung injury (38). Acidic gastric fluid (especially when the pH is <2.5) is particularly injurious. Others factors that influence the severity of aspiration include the size of the particles involved, the bacterial content, and the patient's underlying cardiopulmonary status. Immediate sequelae of aspiration can include bronchospasm, acute pneumonitis, and acute respiratory distress syndrome (ARDS).

Providers should attempt to minimize the risk of aspiration by making the patient NPO as soon as the possibility of intubation arises. However, it may be impossible to delay intubation to await gastric emptying. Because time to gastric emptying can be increased by acute illness and some medications, even patients who have been NPO for ≥6 hrs may be at risk. Altered bowel motility and processes that increase intra-abdominal pressure (e.g., obesity, ascites, or abdominal masses) can also increase risk of gastric reflux and aspiration. Therapy to modify the pH (e.g., antacids or H_2 blockers) prior to intubation is thought to reduce lung injury from the aspiration of gastric contents, but little data support this claim. Although some drugs given 60 to 90 mins prior to intubation may reduce the volume and acidity of pediatric gastric secretions (27), this option is not practical if the airway must be secured emergently.

If the child with a potentially full stomach requires intubation, RSI is performed. The use of cricoid pressure during ventilation may reduce the risk of aspiration, especially if PPV (and potential gastric insufflation) is limited prior to intubation. Placing a nasogastric tube before intubation may not reliably empty the stomach and may increase the risk of aspiration by keeping the esophageal sphincter open.

Cervical Spine Abnormalities and Injuries

Cervical spine anomalies and conditions that limit neck movement interfere with visualization of the larynx. Cervical spine abnormalities may be associated with conditions such as Goldenhar and Klippel-Fiel syndromes, juvenile idiopathic arthritis, spondyloarthropathies, and neuromuscular scoliosis. Airway management in these patients is further complicated if the disease process affects the temporomandibular joint, limiting mouth opening.

In patients with an unstable cervical spine, movement of the neck required for direct laryngoscopy could result in subluxation of the spine and spinal cord injury. Atlanto-axial instability occurs in 10% to 30% of patients with Down syndrome. A history of neurologic symptoms and flexion/extension cervical spine radiographs can help to screen for these patients. In cases of uncertainty, it is prudent to treat all children with Trisomy 21 as if they have unstable cervical spines. In trauma patients, cervical spine instability is assumed to be present in all patients with a head or neck injury or a consistent mechanism of injury.

In patients with presumed or diagnosed cervical spine instability, one healthcare provider should be designated to be responsible for stabilizing the neck during airway manipulation until the airway is secured and immobilization devices can be applied. In these cases, a straight blade may provide a better view of the glottic structures, although more advanced airway techniques such as fiberoptic intubation are sometimes required. Establishment of an adequate airway is a priority.

Intracranial Hypertension

Successful airway management for a patient with increased ICP includes both advanced airway placement and prevention of secondary neurologic injury. Laryngoscopy and intubation trigger spikes in ICP. In addition, intubation may be complicated by the presence of facial trauma or a potentially unstable cervical spine.

For intubation of patients with isolated intracranial hypertension, anesthetic agents such as thiopental and propofol may be beneficial. Although fentanyl has been shown to raise ICP (10), literature suggests that ketamine might actually lower ICP (1). Lidocaine may have a neuroprotective role in preventing intracranial hypertension, especially when coupled with other anesthetic agents. Neuromuscular blockade is thought to allow for a safer intubation with smaller rises in ICP, but the effects on ICP probably result from the simultaneous use of anesthetic agents. Controversy still exists as to whether succinylcholine's rapid action offsets its potential side effects, including drug-induced fasciculation and consequent increases in ICP. Because patients with increased ICP do not tolerate the mild hypoxia and hypercapnia that can develop with a traditional RSI, a modified RSI is typically used. Unintentional hyperventilation that may reduce cerebral blood flow should be avoided.

When intubating the trachea of a patient with intracranial hypertension associated with multisystem disease, intubators should remember that what is theoretically good for the brain might not benefit the rest of the body. Many anesthetic agents produce vasodilation that may compound the abnormal hemodynamics seen with trauma and septic shock.

Shock

When intubating the trachea of a child in shock, the provider must be aware of normal cardiopulmonary interactions (see Chapter 64). The reduced left ventricular afterload that results from PPV may be beneficial when myocardial contractility is poor. However, securing the airway of these patients carries risk. PPV reduces preload, potentially reducing cardiac output (36). Small infants can have an augmented vagal response to PPV, leading to bradycardia and further reduction in cardiac output. These changes with PPV can be exacerbated by hypovolemia or reduced cardiac contractility.

The provider should assume that the child in shock has a full stomach and should use an RSI technique for placement of an advanced airway. It may be necessary to optimize hemodynamics by administering bolus IV fluids or inotropes before attempting the intubation. Potential bradycardia (as a result of vagal or drug-related effects) should be anticipated, and prophylactic use of atropine should be considered. Intubation sedatives/anesthetics should be selected with careful consideration of their associated hemodynamic effects; no anesthetic agent is risk-free. Drugs with potent vasodilatory effects, such as propofol and thiopental, should be used with extreme caution. Ketamine is a useful drug in the hemodynamically unstable patient, but even it has negative inotrope effects. Fentanyl at low doses is commonly used but also has some vasodilatory effects. Etomidate maintains blood pressure during intubation but has potential adrenal suppressive effects, especially in septic patients; these effects can worsen hemodynamic instability. Neuromuscular blockade (using rapid-onset agents such as rocuronium) should be considered to minimize the risk of aspiration.

Facial or Laryngotracheal Injury

Although trauma to the airway structures is relatively uncommon, it can significantly complicate airway management. Facial injuries may be associated with profuse bleeding, fractures, and aspiration of blood, gastric contents, or teeth. Concurrent orbital and intracranial injuries are common and can affect management (see section on Open Globe). A free-floating (fractured) maxilla can cause compression of the nasopharynx and airway obstruction.

If the patient is breathing spontaneously with no signs of obstruction, oxygen administration by mask may be adequate. However, ongoing hemorrhage and edema may create the need for an advanced airway. Orotracheal intubation with cricoid pressure and aggressive suctioning is often all that is required. If injury or uncontrollable bleeding obstructs the view of the larynx, fiberoptic or surgical techniques may be needed. Nasotracheal intubation is contraindicated until basal skull fracture can be ruled out because the tube can migrate intracranially.

Neck injuries can result in direct trauma to the larynx. Soft-tissue injury, including edema, hematoma, arytenoid dislocation, laryngotracheal separation, and vocal cord paralysis, can occur. Fractures are rare. Laryngeal injuries should be suspected in any patient with anterior neck trauma and hoarseness, stridor, subcutaneous emphysema, or pneumomediastinum/pneumothorax. Injuries to other structures in the neck such as the great vessels, esophagus, and cervical spine must be ruled out. When laryngeal injury is present, it is helpful to evaluate it endoscopically before intubation to exclude laryngotracheal separation that will increase the risk of soft-tissue intubation.

Many injuries and problems can cause progressive and potentially life-threatening laryngeal swelling. For these problems, early airway intervention is crucial before increasing edema makes intubation impossible. Inhalation injury should be anticipated in any burn patient with facial burns, singed nasal hairs, carbonaceous debris in the airway, or a history of closed-space exposure. Caustic ingestion can have a similar effect on airway structures. Anaphylaxis and hereditary angioedema are abrupt reactions that can result in severe airway edema, obstruction, and cardiovascular collapse. In these conditions, epinephrine and early airway management are keys to therapy.

Iatrogenic injuries can cause airway obstruction. Vocal cord paralysis results from damage to the recurrent laryngeal nerve and can result from central causes (head injury, hydrocephalus) or direct injury (e.g., difficult birth or mediastinal or neck surgery, such as coarctation repair). Stridor, aspiration, and a weak cry are common symptoms. Subglottic stenosis, congenital or secondary to ETI, may necessitate use of a smaller-than-predicted ETT size.

Open Globe

When a child has a penetrating eye injury, extrusion of vitreous contents can occur during intubation. Rises in ocular pressure, produced by any Valsalva maneuver (such as crying, coughing, gagging, or straining) will exacerbate this risk. The best combination of drugs to facilitate the intubation of such a patient is RSI with adequate amounts of analgesia and sedation. IV lidocaine may be helpful in preventing the rise in intraocular pressure. Succinylcholine and ketamine have historically been associated with vitreous extrusion in this setting, although adult data challenge this dogma. Once intubated, the patient requires ongoing sedation/analgesia to prevent straining against the tracheal tube or gagging, which could result in increased ocular pressure.

Mediastinal Mass

The anterior mediastinal space can occasionally be occupied by masses, most commonly neoplasms. Malignant lesions such as lymphoma (Hodgkins or non-Hodgkins) are common, but nonmalignant lesions can occur as well. The diagnosis may be made during preanesthesia respiratory function testing, with a finding of partial intrathoracic airway obstruction. The diagnosis may also be made through the use of chest radiographs, CT scans, echocardiography, or MRI.

Patients with mediastinal airway or cardiovascular compression can be relatively asymptomatic until anesthesia is initiated. Changes in airway tone or chest wall compliance that result from anesthesia or neuromuscular blockade can lead to collapse or compression of the airway and nearby vascular structures, with consequent cardiorespiratory collapse. Although the airway may be intubatable, the mass may compress the trachea distal to the end of the tracheal tube, precluding effective oxygenation and ventilation even after intubation.

Respiratory distress may result from a malignant pleural effusion or from partial intrathoracic airway obstruction. Compression of mediastinal vascular structures can lead to superior vena caval syndrome.

The basic principle of management of the patient with a mediastinal mass is to keep the patient breathing spontaneously. The lateral or even prone position may minimize airway compression. While the provider is preparing for intubation, the head of the bed should be elevated to help to maintain lung volumes. Anesthetic agents with minimal hemodynamic effects (e.g., ketamine) should be used. Preload should be optimized with IV fluids to counteract the mass compression of vascular structures. Acute airway obstruction may be successfully managed with the use of rigid bronchoscopy or median sternotomy and extracorporeal life support. These solutions will only be possible if this complication is anticipated and equipment and personnel are prepared in advance.

Craniofacial Abnormalities

Craniofacial anomalies such as Pierre Robin, Treacher-Collins, and Goldenhar syndromes can create a difficult airway. Visualization of the glottis by direct laryngoscopy can be difficult if not impossible in these conditions.

Micrognathia is common in these conditions, causing a cephalad positioning of the larynx, thus resulting in a more "anterior" airway with a smaller anterior mandibular space for displacement of the tongue during laryngoscopy. Glossoptosis, the downward and backward displacement of the tongue, will also interfere with visualization of the larynx. Other craniofacial anomalies that can complicate airway management include gross macrocephaly, midface hypoplasia, maxillary protrusion, facial asymmetry and a high arched palate, a small mouth, a short muscular or immobile neck, and facial clefts. Patients with cleft palate can develop obstruction of the oropharynx during sedation if the tongue falls into the cleft, although this can be prevented with the use of an oropharyngeal airway. The LMA can provide an effective airway for children with craniofacial anomalies (5).

Macroglossia

Macroglossia is an enlargement of the tongue, present in patients with Beckwith-Wiedemann syndrome and Trisomy 21. These syndromes are also characterized by hypotonia, and the combination can make bag-mask ventilation difficult. A curved blade may be preferable for visualization of the vocal cords in these patients (19).

Infiltration of the Soft Tissues

Infiltration of the soft tissues will result in a decreased area for displacement of upper airway structures during laryngoscopy, making it more difficult to view the glottis. In addition, the infiltration can distort the glottis. Hemangiomas grow rapidly during infancy and can cause airway compromise either from mass effect or acute airway hemorrhage. Subglottic hemangiomas can cause complete airway obstruction in infants. Venous lymphatic malformations (cystic hygromas) can continue to grow through childhood; they may grow rapidly due to infection or hemorrhage, and may compromise the airway. Management of these problems requires early detection and possible insertion of an advanced airway.

Obesity

The obese child can present challenges during basic (noninvasive) and advanced airway and ventilation support. Children with obesity have limited oxygen reserve. Increased chest wall and abdominal tissue and reduced chest compliance compromise diaphragm excursion and reduce functional residual capacity during both spontaneous and assisted ventilation. Oxygenation is often further compromised by ventilation–perfusion mismatch. Chronic airway obstruction and hypoventilation can produce alveolar hypoxia and pulmonary hypertension that may be detected during preanesthetic clinical exam, augmented by electrocardiogram and echocardiogram (revealing right ventricular strain).

Obese children often have relatively short necks with fatty infiltration of the upper airway structures, creating a relative macroglossia. Fatty infiltration may also distort the airway. When combined with commonly associated airway anomalies (e.g., tongue size and position in the child with Down syndrome), airway obstruction is likely. Superimposed infection, even from "benign" upper respiratory viral illnesses, or altered airway tone with sleep, anesthesia, or muscle relaxation, can further compromise the airway.

It is difficult for one person to hold the airway open and provide bag-mask ventilation for the very obese child because the child's jaw, head, and neck are very heavy. Two rescuers or the insertion of a nasal/oral airway may be required. Positioning of the obese child's airway may be complicated by the presence of fatty infiltration of the posterior thorax. Only limited additional padding under the torso may be necessary to place the child in the sniffing position; in fact, doing so may hyperextend the neck, partially obstructing the airway and compromising visualization during laryngoscopy.

Medication dosages and ETT size should be based on ideal body weight. However, the increased adipose tissue will increase the volume of distribution of some medications used in RSI (such as fentanyl, succinylcholine, and rocuronium), and these must be dosed based on actual body weight (6). The use of large laryngoscope blades and short laryngoscope handles (for age) may be necessary to adequately visualize the obese child's larynx. If intubation attempts fail, alternative airway devices such as LMAs can be used. As a final option, cricothyrotomy can be performed. If it is difficult to identify the traditional landmarks, the incision is made halfway between the hyoid bone and the sternal notch, because this approximates the position of the cricothyroid membrane (40).

Mucopolysaccharidosis and Musculoskeletal Syndromes

The deposition of mucopolysaccharides in the airway leads to macroglossia, tonsillar hypertrophy, thickening of the oral mucosa, and obstruction of nasal passages. A short neck is common. The temporo-mandibular joints and cervical spine may be involved, limiting jaw and neck mobility. Patients with Morquio syndrome are at risk for atlanto-axial subluxation. The airway infiltration worsens with age; therefore, intubation becomes more difficult (and sometimes impossible) as the child ages. This situation can occur with Hurler syndrome at as early as 2 years of age. The use of an LMA to aid fiberoptic intubation has been described in this population, although it is not always successful (21).

Foreign-body Aspiration

Foreign-body aspiration is a common cause of airway obstruction in children <2 years of age. Food, especially nuts and seeds, are the most commonly aspirated foreign objects. They can lodge in any part of the airway from the nasal passage to the lung parenchyma. The trachea and the mainstem bronchi are common sites of foreign body deposition. Because the left bronchus angles more acutely from the trachea in older children and adults, more right-bronchus foreign-body aspiration is observed in these older patients. Because the angle of the left bronchus is not as acute, left-bronchus foreign-body aspiration is more common in smaller children than in adults.

A high index of suspicion is necessary to diagnose foreign-body aspiration because many choking episodes are not witnessed, and findings in physical and radiographic examinations are nonspecific. Cervical and chest films should be obtained, especially in the case of a radio-opaque foreign body. If the inspiratory chest film is normal, an expiratory chest film can demonstrate air trapping due to endobronchial foreign bodies causing partial bronchial obstruction. If foreign-body aspiration is at all suspected, endoscopy is indicated. Any sharp object or any object causing acute upper airway obstruction with respiratory failure should be removed on an urgent basis. Back slaps/chest thrusts in responsive infants and abdominal thrusts in responsive older children can be attempted if endoscopy is not immediately available. Flexible bronchoscopy can be used for diagnosis, but a rigid scope is almost always required for removal.

Acute Infectious Airway Obstruction

Infections of the deep neck space, including parapharyngeal, retropharyngeal, and peritonsillar infections, can lead to airway compromise. A high index of suspicion is required for diagnosis, because these infections are relatively rare. Symptoms include fever, neck swelling, pain, torticollis, limited neck movement, drooling, and trismus (37). A protruding tongue can suggest infection in the submandibular or sublingual space (Ludwig angina). These conditions can rapidly progress to airway compromise. Therapy includes early antibiotics and surgical evaluation.

Laryngotracheobronchitis (croup) presents with hoarseness, barky cough, and stridor and is almost always viral in origin. Only the most severe cases that are not responsive to steroids and nebulized racemic epinephrine require intubation. Subglottic narrowing may necessitate use of a much smaller ETT than predicted.

Bacterial laryngotracheobronchitis (bacterial tracheitis) is most commonly caused by *Staphylococcus aureus*. It often begins with a viral prodrome similar to croup but progresses rapidly with high fever, severe stridor, and respiratory distress.

Acute epiglottis is an airway emergency characterized by acute inflammation of the supraglottic region. Fortunately, this problem has almost vanished with the introduction of the *Haemophilus influenzae* type B vaccine. Epiglottitis is marked by sudden onset of fever, dysphagia, drooling, a "hot-potato voice," and toxemia. Unlike croup and bacterial tracheitis, cough is rarely present. Older patients often present in the "tripod" position to maximize air entry. Antibiotic therapy should be instituted as soon as possible.

Patients with impending airway obstruction from upper airway infection or any other rapidly progressive process should be taken to the operating room or ICU immediately for assessment. Urgent consultation with pediatric anesthesia and otolaryngology specialists is required. Control of the airway is the priority. It is imperative to keep the child calm and allow the child to remain in the position of comfort; placing the child supine or performing unnecessary procedures such as blood sampling can trigger laryngospasm and irreversible airway obstruction. Examinations should be limited until all necessary equipment and personnel are available to treat airway collapse. Patients should always be accompanied by a physician skilled in airway procedures. The utility of a lateral neck radiograph in these patients is controversial and can agitate them, resulting in further airway compromise.

Intubation in the operating room using an inhalational anesthetic is preferred. Swelling and distortion of upper airway structures can be so extreme that intubation is impossible and a surgical airway is required. In the spontaneously breathing child, the visualization of air bubbles during exhalation can help to locate the glottic opening, and the ETT can be blindly placed in that area. The appropriate tube size will allow a small amount of air leak and is usually 0.5–1.0 mm smaller in diameter than the predicted ETT size. It is important to remember that smaller-diameter tubes may not be sufficiently long for larger patients. Muscle relaxants are contraindicated until the airway is secure. If the child collapses acutely and experienced personnel are not yet available, bag-mask ventilation should be attempted while personnel and equipment are assembled.

The resolution of acute airway obstruction can result in postobstructive pulmonary edema. It has been reported in 2% to 10% of all patients with upper airway obstruction and in a higher percentage of those patients who require intubation. Various etiologies of airway obstruction have been associated with the development of pulmonary edema, including foreign bodies, laryngospasm, obstructed ETT, and croup. It usually develops within a few minutes to a few hours following the onset of obstruction, and usually resolves in ≤72 hrs. Proposed mechanisms include negative intrapleural pressure transmitted to the alveoli, creating a hydrostatic gradient that favors extravascular fluid movement. Negative intrapleural pressure can increase venous return to the right heart with bowing of the interventricular septum (increasing left ventricular end-diastolic pressure and thus pulmonary venous pressure) and increased right ventricular output and pulmonary blood flow (42). The edema is often asymptomatic, and treatment is supportive; PPV with positive end-expiratory pressure is occasionally required.

CONCLUSIONS AND FUTURE DIRECTIONS

High-resolution visual imaging using cameras on the distal end of the tracheal tube, light wand stylets, and laryngoscopes are rapidly being developed. Realistic simulation mannequins can facilitate training and experience before a clinical need for airway intervention arises. In addition, the use of simulation programs can enhance the development of teamwork, practice, and evaluation of preparation and protocols. Intensive and continuous quality improvement using such tools as the National Emergency Airway Registry can provide feedback and data on the impact of these technologies on airway management (44).

More information is necessary, however, on the effectiveness of simulator mannequin training and the necessary intervals for retraining in airway techniques. Successful acute airway management requires adequate training, frequent experience, and a process of continuous quality improvement. However the need for provider experience must be weighed against the need of the child for an experienced provider to establish an airway under urgent conditions.

KEY POINTS

- An appreciation of the differences in anatomy, physiology, and changes with age of the child's airway is essential for successful and safe airway management.
- Children desaturate rapidly; hence, time for deliberation is limited when airway support is needed. Modification of the standard RSI technique may therefore be necessary.
- Attention to choice of equipment (type and size), appreciation of the pathology for which intubation is required, and presence of personnel with the requisite skills are necessary for successful airway support.
- Successful acute airway management requires that providers anticipate the development of a difficult airway and have a primary and secondary plan for management.
- The difficult pediatric airway is best managed not by heroic intervention and uncommonly used techniques but, rather, by anticipation and planning, careful patient positioning, effective bag-mask ventilation, and advanced airway insertion, as needed.

References

1. Albanese J, Arnaud S, Rey M, et al. Ketamine decreases intracranial pressure and electroencephalographic activity in traumatic brain injury patients during propofol sedation. *Anesthesiology* 1997;87:1328–34.
2. Amantea SL, Piva JP, Sanches PR, et al. Oropharyngeal aspiration in pediatric patients with endotracheal intubation. *Pediatr Crit Care Med* 2004;5:152–6.
3. Berry F. Anesthesia for the child with a difficult airway. In: Berry F, ed. *Anesthetic Management of Difficult and Routine Pediatric Patients.* New York: Churchill Livingstone; 1990: 167–98.
4. Bhende MS, Karasic DG, Karasic RB. End-tidal carbon dioxide changes during cardiopulmonary resuscitation after experimental asphyxial cardiac arrest. *Am J Emerg Med* 1996;14:349–50.
5. Brambrink AM, Braun U. Airway management in infants and children. *Best Pract Res Clin Anaesthesiol* 2005;19:675–97.
6. Brunette DD. Resuscitation of the morbidly obese patient. *Am J Emerg Med* 2004;22:40–7.
7. Cheng CA, Aun CS, Gin T. Comparison of rocuronium and suxamethonium for rapid tracheal intubation in children. *Paediatr Anaesth* 2002;12:140–5.
8. Cohan P, Wang C, McArthur DL, et al. Acute secondary adrenal insufficiency after traumatic brain injury: A prospective study. *Crit Care Med* 2005;33:2358–66.
9. Daugherty RJ, Nadkarni V, Brenn BR. Endotracheal tube size estimation for children with pathological short stature. *Pediatr Emerg Care* 2006;22: 710–7.
10. de Nadal M, Ausina A, Sahuquillo J, et al. Effects on intracranial pressure of fentanyl in severe head injured patients. *Acta Neurochir Suppl* 1998;71: 10–2.
11. Edmunds S, Weiss I, Harrison R. Extubation failure in a large pediatric ICU population. *Chest* 2001;119:897–900.
12. Esteban A, Frutos-Vivar F, Ferguson ND, et al. Noninvasive positive-pressure ventilation for respiratory failure after extubation. *N Engl J Med* 2004;350:2452–60.
13. Fastle RK, Roback MG. Pediatric rapid sequence intubation: Incidence of reflex bradycardia and effects of pretreatment with atropine. *Pediatr Emerg Care* 2004;20:651–5.
14. Gallart L, Mases A, Martinez J, et al. Simple method to determine the size of the laryngeal mask airway in children. *Eur J Anaesthesiol* 2003;20:570–4.
15. Gausche M, Lewis RJ. Out-of-hospital endotracheal intubation of children. *JAMA* 2000;283:2790–2.

16. George E, Haspel KL. The difficult airway. *Int Anesthesiol Clin* 2000;38:47–63.

17. Gomes Cordeiro AM, Fernandes JC, Troster EJ. Possible risk factors associated with moderate or severe airway injuries in children who underwent endotracheal intubation. *Pediatr Crit Care Med* 2004;5:364–8.

18. Hazinski M, Zaritsky A, Nadkarni V, et al. Rapid Sequence Intubation. In: *PALS Provider Manual*. Dallas: American Heart Association, 2002.

19. Infosino A. Pediatric upper airway and congenital anomalies. *Anesthesiol Clin North Am* 2002;20:747–66.

20. Jackson WL Jr. Should we use etomidate as an induction agent for endotracheal intubation in patients with septic shock?: A critical appraisal. *Chest* 2005;127:1031–8.

21. Khan FA, Khan FH. Use of the laryngeal mask airway in mucopolysaccharidoses. *Paediatr Anaesth* 2002;12:468.

22. Ko SH, Kim DC, Han YJ, et al. Small-dose fentanyl: Optimal time of injection for blunting the circulatory responses to tracheal intubation. *Anesth Analg* 1998;86:658–61.

23. Kundra P, Deepak R, Ravishankar M. Laryngeal mask insertion in children: A rational approach. *Paediatr Anaesth* 2003;13:685–90.

24. Kurachek SC, Newth CJ, Quasney MW, et al. Extubation failure in pediatric intensive care: A multiple-center study of risk factors and outcomes. *Crit Care Med* 2003;31:2657–64.

25. Lin CD, Cheng YK, Chang JS, et al. Endoscopic survey of post-extubation stridor in children. *Acta Paediatr Taiwan* 2002;43:91–5.

26. Litman RS, Weissend EE, Shibata D, et al. Developmental changes of laryngeal dimensions in unparalyzed, sedated children. *Anesthesiology* 2003;98:41–5.

27. Maekawa N, Nishina K, Mikawa K, et al. Comparison of pirenzepine, ranitidine, and pirenzepine-ranitidine combination for reducing preoperative gastric fluid acidity and volume in children. *Br J Anaesth* 1998;80:53–7.

28. Mallampati SR, Gatt SP, Gugino LD, et al. A clinical sign to predict difficult tracheal intubation: A prospective study. *Can Anaesth Soc J* 1985;32:429–34.

29. Marcin JP, Rutan E, Rapetti PM, et al. Nurse staffing and unplanned extubation in the pediatric intensive care unit. *Pediatr Crit Care Med* 2005;6:254–7.

30. Markovitz BP, Randolph AG. Corticosteroids for the prevention of reintubation and postextubation stridor in pediatric patients: A meta-analysis. *Pediatr Crit Care Med* 2002;3:223–6.

31. McAllister JD, Gnauck KA. Rapid sequence intubation of the pediatric patient. Fundamentals of practice. *Pediatr Clin North Am* 1999;46:1249–84.

32. McAuliffe G, Bissonnette B, Boutin C. Should the routine use of atropine before succinylcholine in children be reconsidered? *Can J Anaesth* 1995;42:724–9.

33. Mhanna MJ, Zamel YB, Tichy CM, et al. The "air leak" test around the endotracheal tube, as a predictor of postextubation stridor, is age dependent in children. *Crit Care Med* 2002;30:2639–43.

34. Nakayama S, Osaka Y, Yamashita M. The rotational technique with a partially inflated laryngeal mask airway improves the ease of insertion in children. *Paediatr Anaesth* 2002;12:416–9.

35. Park C, Bahk JH, Ahn WS, et al. The laryngeal mask airway in infants and children. *Can J Anaesth* 2001;48:413–7.

36. Pepe PE, Raedler C, Lurie KG, et al. Emergency ventilatory management in hemorrhagic states: Elemental or detrimental? *J Trauma* 2003;54:1048–55; discussion 1055–57.

37. Rafei K, Lichenstein R. Airway infectious disease emergencies. *Pediatr Clin North Am* 2006;53:215–42.

38. Raidoo DM, Rocke DA, Brock-Utne JG, et al. Critical volume for pulmonary acid aspiration: Reappraisal in a primate model. *Br J Anaesth* 1990;65:248–50.

39. Randolph AG, Wypij D, Venkataraman ST, et al. Effect of mechanical ventilator weaning protocols on respiratory outcomes in infants and children: A randomized controlled trial. *JAMA* 2002;288:2561–8.

40. Ray RM, Senders CW. Airway management in the obese child. *Pediatr Clin North Am* 2001;48:1055–63.

41. Reed JM, O'Conner DM, Myer CM 3rd. Magnetic resonance imaging determination of tracheal orientation in normal children. Practical implications. *Arch Otolaryngol Head Neck Surg* 1996;122:605–8.

42. Ringold S, Klein EJ, Del Beccaro MA. Postobstructive pulmonary edema in children. *Pediatr Emerg Care* 2004;20:391–5.

43. Sadowski R, Dechert RE, Bandy KP, et al. Continuous quality improvement: Reducing unplanned extubations in a pediatric intensive care unit. *Pediatrics* 2004;114:628–32.

44. Sagarin MJ, Chiang V, Sakles JC, et al. Rapid-sequence intubation for pediatric emergency airway management. *Pediatr Emerg Care* 2002;18:417–23.

45. Sharieff GQ, Rodarte A, Wilton N, et al. The self-inflating bulb as an airway adjunct: Is it reliable in children weighing less than 20 kilograms? *Acad Emerg Med* 2003;10:303–8.

46. Shukry M, Hanson RD, Koveleskie JR, et al. Management of the difficult pediatric airway with Shikani Optical Stylet. *Paediatr Anaesth* 2005;15:342–5.

47. Stockinger ZT, McSwain NE Jr. Prehospital endotracheal intubation for trauma does not improve survival over bag-valve-mask ventilation. *J Trauma* 2004;56:531–6.

48. Theroux MC, Rose JB, Iyengar S, et al. Succinylcholine pretreatment using gallamine or mivacurium during rapid sequence induction in children: A randomized, controlled study. *J Clin Anesth* 2001;13:287–92.

49. Thompson A. Pediatric airway management. In: Fuhrman B, Zimmerman J, eds. *Pediatric Critical Care*, 3rd ed. Philadelphia: Mosby, 2005.

50. Vachon CA, Warner DO, Bacon DR. Succinylcholine and the open globe. Tracing the teaching. *Anesthesiology* 2003;99:220–3.

51. Venkataraman ST, Khan N, Brown A. Validation of predictors of extubation success and failure in mechanically ventilated infants and children. *Crit Care Med* 2000;28:2991–6.

52. Walner DL, Loewen MS, Kimura RE. Neonatal subglottic stenosis–incidence and trends. *Laryngoscope* 2001;111:48–51.

53. Weiss M, Hartmann K, Fischer JE, et al. Use of angulated video-intubation laryngoscope in children undergoing manual in-line neck stabilization. *Br J Anaesth* 2001;87:453–8.

54. Zelicof-Paul A, Smith-Lockridge A, Schnadower D, et al. Controversies in rapid sequence intubation in children. *Curr Opin Pediatr* 2005;17:355–62.

CHAPTER 23 ■ CARDIOPULMONARY RESUSCITATION

ROBERT A. BERG • KATSUYUKI MIYASAKA • ANTONIO RODRIGUEZ-NUÑEZ • MARY FRAN HAZINSKI •
DAVID ZIDEMAN • VINAY M. NADKARNI

Pulseless cardiac arrest is typically defined as the cessation of cardiac mechanical activity, determined by the absence of a palpable central pulse, unresponsiveness, and apnea. Separating severe hypoxic-ischemic shock with poor perfusion from the nonpulsatile state of cardiac arrest can be challenging at any age. This critical assessment and definition can be especially difficult in infants because of their anatomic and physiologic characteristics. In adults, a rescuer's ability to make this determination by pulse check is neither sensitive nor specific (30,72). The pulse check is even more problematic in infants and children. In adults, pulses can typically be palpated until the systolic pressure is <50 mm Hg. Because the normal systolic blood pressure in neonates is generally in the 60s, a decrease in blood pressure to "nonpalpable pulse" may occur earlier in the continuum from hypoxic-ischemic shock to nonpulsatile cardiac standstill. Furthermore, the strongest accessible central arterial pulse to palpate in an adult is the carotid pulse; however, the short, fleshy neck of a baby, along with the potential to compress the airway and impede respiration, limits the appropriateness of using the carotid location to assess central pulse presence in infants. Early detection of impending cardiac arrest is essential because lack of prompt recognition and effective intervention results in certain death or profound neurologic devastation. Effective cardiopulmonary resuscitation (CPR) and advanced life support targeted to the etiology, timing, intensity, and duration of the cardiac arrest can optimize the potential to restore an apparently dead child back to life. Impressively, that once lifeless child has the potential for a full, vigorous, high-quality life.

MECHANISM OF DISEASE

Cardiac arrest is the end result of diverse etiologies and pathophysiologic mechanisms, ultimately leading to an electrical or mechanical cardiac arrest due to progressive hypoxic-ischemic events or metabolic disturbances.

Arrhythmogenic ("electrical") cardiac arrests are typically due to ventricular fibrillation (VF) or rapid ventricular tachycardia (VT). These arrhythmias can result from (a) *congenital cardiac abnormalities* associated with myocardial ischemia (e.g., coronary artery anomalies), genetic channelopathies associated with prolonged QT syndrome, familial cardiomyopathies (e.g., hypertrophic, dilated, arrhythmogenic right ventricular dysplasia), or mitochondrial diseases, or from (b) *acquired cardiomyopathies* from drugs/toxins (e.g., doxorubicin cardiomyopathy, drug-induced prolonged QT syndrome), a hypoxic-ischemic event with inadequate myocardial oxygen delivery, cardiac surgical injury, commotio cordis, mechanically induced VF, ischemia during CPR, and inappropriate unsynchronized cardioversion shock.

Mechanical ("pump") cardiomyopathic arrests are typically due to inadequate myocardial oxygen delivery from asphyxial, ischemic, metabolic (e.g., hypoglycemia, hypocalcemia, severe acidosis), or pharmacologic (e.g., β-blocker, calcium channel blocker, or barbiturate toxicity) problems. A myriad of etiologic events can result in severe asphyxia, severe hypoxia, severe ischemia, or a combination of all three, ultimately resulting in myocardial pump failure. These pump problems typically manifest as hypoxic-ischemic cardiac dysfunction and circulatory shock with a cardiogenic component before progressing to cardiac arrest. Therefore, the best outcomes from these processes occur with early recognition, monitoring, and aggressive intervention to treat the prearrest condition, thereby preventing progression to pulseless cardiac arrest.

PHASES OF CARDIAC ARREST AND CARDIOPULMONARY RESUSCITATION

Interventions to improve outcome from pediatric cardiac arrest should be targeted to optimize therapies according to the etiology, timing, duration, intensity, and "phase" of resuscitation, as suggested in **Table 23.1**. Cardiac arrest has at least four phases: prearrest, no-flow (untreated cardiac arrest), low-flow (CPR), and postresuscitation. The prearrest phase represents the greatest opportunity to impact patient survival by preventing pulseless cardiopulmonary arrest.

Interventions during the no-flow phase of untreated, pulseless cardiac arrest focus on early recognition of cardiac arrest and initiation of basic and advanced life support. When oxygen delivery to the brain or heart is insufficient, CPR should be started. The goal of effective CPR is to optimize coronary perfusion pressure and blood flow to critical organs during the low-flow phase. Basic life support using continuous, effective chest compressions (i.e., push hard, push fast, allow full chest recoil, minimize interruptions, and do not overventilate) is the emphasis in this phase.

The postresuscitation phase is a high-risk period for brain injury, ventricular arrhythmias, and other reperfusion injuries. Injured cells can hibernate, die, or partially or fully recover function. Overventilation (hyperventilation) is frequent, and can have adverse effects during and following CPR. Interventions such as systemic hypothermia during the immediate postresuscitation phase strive to minimize reperfusion injury

TABLE 23.1

PHASES OF CARDIAC ARREST AND RESUSCITATION

Phase	Interventions
Prearrest phase (protect)	Optimize community education regarding child safety Optimize patient monitoring and rapid emergency response Recognize and treat respiratory failure and/or shock to prevent cardiac arrest
Arrest (no-flow) phase (preserve)	Minimize interval to BLS and ALS (organized response) Minimize interval to defibrillation, when indicated
Low-flow (CPR) phase (resuscitate)	"Push hard, push fast" Allow full-chest recoil Minimize interruptions in compressions Avoid overventilation Titrate CPR to optimize myocardial blood flow (coronary perfusion pressures and exhaled CO_2) Consider adjuncts to improve vital organ perfusion during CPR Consider ECMO if standard CPR/ALS not promptly successful
Postresuscitation phase: Short-term rehabilitation	Optimize cardiac output and cerebral perfusion Treat arrhythmias, if indicated Avoid hyperglycemia, hyperthermia, hyperventilation Consider mild post-resuscitation systemic hypothermia Debrief to improve future responses to emergencies
Postresuscitation phase: Longer-term rehabilitation (regenerate)	Early intervention with occupational and physical therapy Bioengineering and technology interface Possible future role for stem cell transplantation

BLS, basic life support; ALS, advanced life support; ECMO extracorporeal membrane oxygenation; CPR, cardiopulmonary resuscitation

and support cellular recovery. The postarrest phase may have the most potential for innovative advances in the understanding of cell injury and death, inflammation, apoptosis, and hibernation, ultimately leading to novel interventions. Thoughtful attention to the management of temperature, glucose, blood pressures, coagulation, and optimal ventilation may be particularly important in this phase. The rehabilitation stage of postresuscitation concentrates on the salvage of injured cells, recruitment of hibernating cells, and reengineering of the reflex and voluntary communications of these cell and organ systems to improve functional outcome.

The specific phase of resuscitation should dictate the timing, intensity, duration, and focus of interventions. Emerging data suggest that interventions that can improve short-term outcome during one phase may be deleterious during another. For example, intense vasoconstriction during the low-flow phase of cardiac arrest may improve coronary perfusion pressure and probability of return of spontaneous circulation (ROSC). The same intense vasoconstriction during the postresuscitation phase may increase left ventricular afterload and worsen myocardial strain and dysfunction. Our current understanding of the physiology of cardiac arrest and recovery only enables the titration of blood pressure, global oxygen delivery and consumption, body temperature, inflammation, coagulation, and other physiologic parameters to attempt to optimize outcome. Future strategies will likely take advantage of emerging discoveries in cellular inflammation, thrombosis, reperfusion, mediator cascades, cellular markers of injury and recovery, and transplantation technology.

IS CARDIOPULMONARY RESUSCITATION EFFECTIVE FOR CHILDREN?

In a report of successful resuscitation using closed-chest cardiac massage, asphyxiated children in the operating room who received immediate, effective resuscitation attained excellent outcomes (58). When cardiac arrest is witnessed and of short duration, excellent outcomes *can* occur after various types of bystander CPR, including mouth-to-mouth rescue breathing alone, chest compressions alone, or standard chest compressions and mouth-to-mouth rescue breathing. Nevertheless, some reports question the effectiveness and advisability of prehospital pediatric CPR.

To further delineate these issues, prehospital pediatric asphyxial arrests were simulated in animal models. In the first study (11a), asphyxia was induced by clamping the tracheal tube of piglets until cardiac arrest occurred, defined by loss of aortic pulsation. The mean time until loss of aortic pulsations was 8.9 ± 0.4 mins. After loss of aortic pulsations, animals were randomized to simulated bystander CPR or no CPR until simulated emergency medical service (EMS) arrival 8 mins later. After a complete cardiac arrest, 24-hr survival was clearly superior in the group that received both chest compressions and rescue breathing, compared with either alone or no CPR. A similar study was performed using intervention at a slightly earlier point in the asphyxial process, when the pulse was "no longer palpable," as defined by a systolic pressure <50 mm Hg (i.e., after severe hypotension but before complete loss of aortic pulsation) (12). After this injury without complete cardiac arrest, 24-hr survival was best when both chest compressions and rescue breathing were provided, but rescue breathing alone and chest compressions alone were individually better than no CPR at all. Interestingly, most of the animals with 24-hr survival had ROSC before the simulated EMS arrival. CPR was clearly not futile in these models of prehospital pediatric cardiac arrest; excellent CPR was remarkably effective when provided early enough.

Such laboratory studies put clinical reports in context. In a large, prospective study in Houston, taking place over the course of 3.5 years, it was demonstrated that the outcomes from pediatric prehospital cardiac arrests were dismal: Only six of the 300 children (2%) survived to hospital discharge, and only one of the six survived without significant neurologic deficits (88). However, EMS providers determined the diagnosis of cardiac arrest when they arrived at the scene. As in most prehospital reports, children in cardiac arrest who attained ROSC after bystander CPR but before EMS arrival were excluded from analysis. Importantly, 41 children who had received bystander CPR were not in cardiac arrest at the time of EMS arrival; all 41 presumably had drowning-related cardiac arrests, and all survived with good neurologic outcomes. Most exhibited evidence of significant hypoxic-ischemic injury when they arrived at the hospital, suggesting "real" cardiac arrest at the scene. In contrast, none of the other 24 children with drowning-related cardiac arrests who were still in cardiac arrest when the EMS personnel arrived survived with a good neurologic outcome.

Prospective evaluation of a decade-long, population-based study of pediatric drowning-related events in Houston (77) demonstrated 421 children with drowning events in a population of approximately 2 million total, with approximately 400,000 children (annual incidence of 10.0 per 100,000 children); of these 421 children, 234 required resuscitation. Bystander CPR was administered to 193 resuscitated children (82%), and 72% of these children were long-term survivors. Ninety-nine percent of the long-term survivors were neurologically intact. However, if the child was still apneic and pulseless when EMS personnel arrived, <5% were revived, and none of these subsequent survivors were ultimately neurologically intact. These data and similar data from others (66, 88, 107) are consistent with the animal data, reported clinical experience, and in-hospital pediatric CPR data: CPR can be quite effective for asphyxial cardiac arrests, but the timing of interventions is critically important.

In summary, animal and human data both indicate that well-performed CPR for children is quite effective. In addition, these data support the notion that high-quality basic life support early is more important than advanced life support late. Prompt action by a citizen bystander in the prehospital setting or a provider in the in-hospital setting is generally more effective than late heroic efforts in the ICU.

EPIDEMIOLOGY

Pediatric In-hospital Arrests

The true incidence of pediatric pulseless arrest is difficult to estimate, complicated by inconsistent definitions and assessment of pulselessness in children. Cardiac arrests were reported in 1.8% of all children admitted to PICUs in the US (90) and in 6% of children admitted to one PICU in Finland (97).

Several well-designed in-hospital pediatric CPR investigations with long-term follow-up have established that pediatric CPR and advanced life support can be remarkably effective (**Table 23.2**). Almost two-thirds of these cardiac arrest patients were initially successfully resuscitated (i.e., attained sustained ROSC). Most of these arrests/events occurred in PICUs due to progressive life-threatening illnesses that had not responded to treatment despite critical care monitoring and supportive care. Almost three-quarters of survivors to discharge had good neurologic outcome. The 1-year survival rates of 10% to 44% are better than reported outcomes following out-of-hospital pediatric CPR.

Only a few studies have used the more rigorous Utstein-style reporting for in-hospital pediatric cardiac arrests and CPR. Two describe all CPR events at children's hospitals in Brazil (80) and Finland (97). The most common causes of the events were progressive respiratory failure and progressive shock. Approximately two-thirds of the children attained sustained ROSC, and 1-year survival was 15% and 18%, respectively.

Recently published Utstein-style reports of in-hospital pediatric cardiac arrests are derived from the multicentered National Registry of Cardiopulmonary Resuscitation (NRCPR) of the American Heart Association (73). The NRCPR is a prospective, multicentered observational registry of in-hospital cardiac arrests and resuscitations. The large size, scope, and quality of the NRCPR distinguish this North American data, which characterize the process and outcome of pediatric in-hospital CPR events. Summaries of these important characteristics are presented in **Tables 23.3** and **23.4**.

In these NRCPR reports, a cardiac arrest was explicitly defined as cessation of cardiac mechanical activity, determined by the absence of a reported palpable central pulse, unresponsiveness, and apnea. Events were excluded if the cardiac arrest began out-of-hospital, involved a newborn in a delivery room or NICU, or was limited to a shock by an implanted cardioverter-defibrillator. Most of these arrests occurred in children with progressive respiratory insufficiency and/or progressive circulatory shock. These children often had progressive underlying critical illnesses despite aggressive critical care monitoring and therapy. Therefore, 95% of these arrests were witnessed and/or monitored, and only 14% occurred on a general pediatric ward. Before the arrest, 57% of these children were mechanically ventilated, 38% had continuous vasopressor infusions, and 29% had continuous direct arterial blood pressure monitoring.

Despite the diverse and complex clinical circumstances that led to their arrests, 52% attained sustained ROSC, 36% survived for 24 hrs, and 27% survived to hospital discharge. Outcomes for these children were substantially better than reported outcomes for adults in this registry (adjusted Odds Ratio [OR], 2.3; 95% Confidence Interval [CI], 2.0–2.7). Importantly, 65% of these children had good neurologic outcome, defined as: (a) Pediatric Cerebral Performance Category of 1, 2, or 3, or (b) no change from baseline Pediatric Cerebral Performance Category.

Of importance, 200 children who received chest compressions without pulselessness during this same observation period were excluded from the NRCPR cardiac arrest analysis because they did not ever completely lose their pulse during the event. Similar to the two previous Utstein-style pediatric

TABLE 23.2

SUMMARY OF REPRESENTATIVE STUDIES OF OUTCOME FOLLOWING IN-HOSPITAL
PEDIATRIC CARDIAC ARREST

Author, year	Setting*	# of patients	ROSC	Survival to discharge	Good neurologic survival
Samson 2006 (83)	In-hospital Initial VF/VTCA	104	73 (70%)	36 (35%)	34 (33%)
Samson 2006 (83)	In-hospital subsequent VF/VTCA	149	52 (35%)	16 (11%)	12 (8%)
Nadkarni 2006 (73)	In hospital CA	880	459 (52%)	236 (27%)	154 (18%)
Reis 2002 (80)	In hospital CA	129	83 (64%)	21 (16%)	19 (15%)
Extracorporeal Life Support Organization, 2005 (45)	In hospital CA resuscitation by ECMO	232	N/A All needed ECMO	88 (38%)	Not reported
Suominen 2000 (97)	In-hospital CA	118	74 (63%)	1-year survival 21 (18%)	Not reported
Parra 2000 (76)	Pediatric CICU CA	32	24 (63%)	14 (44%)	8 (25%)
Chamnanvanakij 2000 (22)	In-hospital intubated NICU patients with chest compressions for bradycardia	39	33 (85%)	CPR 20 (51%) CA 10%	CPR 5 (13%) (6 lost to follow-up)
Slonim 1997 (90)	In-hospital PICU CA	205	Not reported	28 (14%)	not reported
Torres 1997 (100)	In-hospital CA	92	Not reported	1-year survival 9 (10%)	7 (8%)
Zaritsky A 1987 (108)	In hospital CA	53	Not reported	5 (9%)	Not reported
Young 1999 (107)	Meta-analysis in hospital CA	544	Not reported	129 (24%)	Not reported
Lopez-Herce 2005 (66)	Mixed in-hospital & out-of-hospital CA	213	110 (52%)	45 (21%)	34 (16%)
Tunstall-Pedoe 1992 (101)	Mixed in-hospital & out-of-hospital CA	3,765	1,411 (38%)	706 (19%)	Not reported

ROSC, return of spontaneous circulation; VF, ventricular fibrillation; VT, ventricular tachycardia; CA, cardiac arrest; ECMO, extracorporeal membrane oxygenation; CICU, cardiac ICU; CPR, cardiopulmonary resuscitation

in-hospital studies, only 82% of children who received chest compressions fit the definition of pulseless cardiac arrest. As expected, children who received chest compressions for bradycardia with pulses had a much higher survival-to-hospital discharge rate (60%) than those with pulseless cardiac arrest (27%, $p < 0.001$).

Pediatric Out-of-hospital Arrests

Outcomes following pediatric out-of-hospital arrests appear to be worse than those following in-hospital arrests (**Table 23.5**). These poor outcomes are in part due to prolonged periods of "no flow" and in part due to specific diseases with especially poor outcomes. Many pediatric out-of-hospital cardiac arrests are not witnessed, and only approximately one-third of children with an out-of-hospital cardiac arrest are provided with bystander CPR. Therefore, the no-flow period is typically quite prolonged before EMS personnel provide CPR, and neurologic outcomes are generally worse among children who are survivors of out-of-hospital arrest compared with those with in-hospital arrests.

Two common types of out-of-hospital cardiac arrests have especially poor outcomes: traumatic arrests and those associated with sudden infant death syndrome (SIDS). Traumatic cardiac arrests typically result either from airway compromise and severe, prolonged hypoxia or from exsanguination that results in profound circulatory shock; not surprisingly, chest compressions with an empty heart are not likely to provide adequate coronary and cerebral perfusion. Sudden infant death syndrome patients are typically discovered a long time after cardiac arrest, with understandably poor outcome. In most series of out-of-hospital pediatric cardiac arrests, more than one-third of the children have the diagnosis of SIDS.

PEDIATRIC VENTRICULAR FIBRILLATION

Ventricular fibrillation is an uncommon but not rare electrocardiographic rhythm during out-of-hospital pediatric cardiac arrests. Two studies reported VF as the initial rhythm in 19% to 24% of out-of-hospital pediatric cardiac arrests, but these

TABLE 23.3

CHARACTERISTICS OF PEDIATRIC IN-HOSPITAL CARDIAC ARRESTS FROM THE NATIONAL REGISTRY OF CARDIOPULMONARY RESUSCITATION OF THE AMERICAN HEART ASSOCIATION

Characteristic	Pediatric cardiac arrest ($n = 880$) (100%)
Age, years	
Mean (SD)	5.6 (6.4)
Median (range)	1.8 (0–17.0)
Sex	
Male	473 (54)
Female	407 (46)
Race/ethnicity	
White	447 (51)
Black	226 (26)
Hispanic	105 (12)
Other/unknown	102 (12)
Patient type	
Inpatient	750 (85)
Emergency department	121 (14)
Other (outpatient, visitor, or employee)	9 (1)
Illness Category	
Medical, cardiac	158 (18)
Medical, noncardiac	402 (46)
Surgical, cardiac	150 (17)
Surgical, noncardiac	62 (7)
Trauma	91 (10)
Other*	17 (2)
Preexisting Conditions	
Respiratory insufficiency	511 (58)
Hypotension/hypoperfusion	319 (36)
Congestive heart failure	273 (31)
Pneumonia/septicemia/other infection	259 (29)
Arrhythmia	182 (21)
Renal insufficiency	104 (12)
Diabetes mellitus	11 (1)
Metabolic/electrolyte abnormality	178 (20)
Baseline depression in CNS function	151 (17)
Metastatic or hematologic malignancy	43 (5)
Myocardial infarction	21 (2)
None†	69 (8)
Hepatic insufficiency	55 (6)
Acute CNS nonstroke event	94 (11)
Acute stroke	5 (1)
Major trauma	97 (11)
Toxicologic problem	12 (1)

Data are expressed as number (%) unless otherwise specified. Because of rounding, percentages may not all total 100. Preexisting conditions total more than the total number of patients due to patients having more than one preexisting condition present at the time of admission to hospital.
*All 17 were obstetrics.
†No documented preexisting conditions.
SD, standard deviation; CNS, central nervous system
Data from Nadkarni VM, Larkin GL, Peberdy MA, et al. First documented rhythm and clinical outcome from in-hospital cardiac arrest among children and adults. *JAMA.* 2006;295:50–57, with permission.

TABLE 23.4

EVENT CHARACTERISTICS OF PEDIATRIC IN-HOSPITAL CARDIAC ARRESTS FROM THE NATIONAL REGISTRY OF CARDIOPULMONARY RESUSCITATION OF THE AMERICAN HEART ASSOCIATION

Characteristic	Pediatric cardiac arrest ($n = 880$)
Event location	
Intensive care unit	570 (65%)
Emergency department	116 (13%)
General inpatient	123 (14%)
Diagnostic area	21 (2%)
Outpatient, other, or unknown	20 (2%)
Operating department or postanesthetic care	30 (3%)
First documented pulseless rhythm	
Asystole	350 (40%)
VF and pulseless VT	120 (14%)
VF	71 (8%)
Pulseless VT	49 (6%)
PEA	213 (24%)
Unknown by documentation	197 (22%)
Discovery status at time of event*	
Witnessed and/or monitored	834 (95%)
Witnessed and monitored	727 (83%)
Witnessed and not monitored	73 (8%)
Monitored and not witnessed	34 (4%)
Not monitored and not witnessed	46 (5%)
Immediate cause(s) of event	
Acute respiratory insufficiency	455 (57%)
Hypotension	483 (61%)
Acute myocardial infarction or ischemia	12 (2%)
Metabolic/electrolyte disturbance	95 (12%)
Acute pulmonary edema	33 (4%)
Acute pulmonary embolism	6 (1%)
Airway obstruction	41 (5%)
Toxicologic problem	9 (1%)

Data are expressed as number (%). Because of rounding, percentages may not total 100. Totals do not sum to total number of pediatric patients for discovery status at time of event and immediate cause(s) of event characteristics due to patients having more than one characteristic.
*The National Registry of Cardiopulmonary Resuscitation definition of monitored includes electrocardiogram, apnea/bradycardia, or pulse oximeter.
VF, ventricular fibrillation; VT, ventricular tachycardia; PEA, pulseless electrical activity.
Data from Nadkarni VM, Larkin GL, Peberdy MA, et al. First documented rhythm and clinical outcome from in-hospital cardiac arrest among children and adults. *JAMA.* 2006;295:50–57, with permission.

studies excluded SIDS deaths. In studies that include SIDS victims, the frequency drops to the range of 6%–10% (91). It is important to note that electrocardiographic rhythms are often not attained as promptly in children as in adults and that VF eventually converts into asystole over time. Therefore, the reported prevalence of VF depends on the aggressiveness and timing of monitoring and the inclusion criteria for the report.

The incidence of VF varies by setting and age. In special circumstances, such as tricyclic antidepressant overdose, cardiomyopathy, post–cardiac surgery, and prolonged QT

TABLE 23.5

SUMMARY OF REPRESENTATIVE STUDIES OF OUTCOME FOLLOWING OUT-OF-HOSPITAL PEDIATRIC CARDIAC ARREST

Author, year	Setting	# of patients	ROSC	Survival to discharge	Favorable neurologic survival
Gerein 2006 (37)	OOH CA Canada	503	Not reported	10 (2%)	Not reported
Donoghue 2005 (26)	OOH CA Systematic review	5,693	Not reported	689 (12%)	228 (4%)
Berg M 2005 (10)	OOH CA Shockable rhythm	13	13 (100%)	0 (0%)	0 (0%)
Young 1999 (107)	Meta-analysis OOH CA	1568	Not reported	132 (8%)	Not reported
Sirbaugh 1999 (88)	OOH CA	300	33 (11%)	6 (2%)	1 (<1%)
Suominen 1998 (98)	OOH CA After trauma	41	10 (24%)	3 (7%)	2 (5%)
Suominen 1997 (96)	OOH CA	50	13 (26%)	8 (16%)	6 (12%)
Schindler 1996 (85)	OOH CA	80	43 (54%)	6 (8%)	0 (0%)
Kuisma 1995 (60)	OOH CA	34	10 (29%)	5 (15%)	4 (12%)
Dieckmann 1995 (25)	OOH CA	65	3 (5%)	2 (3%)	1 (1.5%)
Lopez-Herce 2005 (66)	Mixed in-hospital & OOH CA	213	110 (52%)	45 (21%)	34 (16%)
Tunstall-Pedoe 1992 (101)	Mixed in-hospital & OOH CA	3765	1411 (38%)	706 (19%)	Not reported

ROSC, return of spontaneous circulation; OOH, out-of-hospital; CA, cardiac arrest

syndromes, VF is a more likely rhythm during cardiac arrest. Commotio cordis, or mechanically initiated VF due to relatively low-energy chest-wall impact during a narrow window of repolarization (10–30 msec before the T wave peak in swine models), is reported predominantly in children 4–16 years old. Out-of-hospital VF cardiac arrest, uncommon in infants, occurs more frequently in children and adolescents. The variance of VF by age was highlighted in a study that documented VF/VT in only 3% of children in cardiac arrest who were 0 to 8 years old versus 17% of children who were 8–19 years old (4). Although VF is often associated with underlying heart disease and generally considered the "immediate cause" of cardiac arrest, "subsequent" VF can also occur during resuscitation efforts. In studies of VF among asphyxiated piglets, the incidence of VF was 28%–33% during resuscitation. Asphyxia-associated VF is also well documented among pediatric near-drowning patients (39).

Recent studies indicate that VF and VT (shockable rhythms) occur in 27% of in-hospital cardiac arrests at some time during the arrest and resuscitation. Although the rhythms during most in-hospital cardiac arrests (both in children and adults) are asystole and pulseless electrical activity (PEA), in many arrests, the rhythms are VF or pulseless VT. Among the first 1,005 pediatric in-hospital cardiac arrests in the NRCPR (83), 10% had an initial rhythm of VF/VT, an additional 15% had subsequent VF/VT (i.e., some time later during the resuscitation efforts), and another 2% had VF/VT, but the timing of the arrhythmia was not clear.

Traditionally, VF and VT have been considered "good" cardiac arrest rhythms, resulting in better outcomes than asystole and PEA. Of note, survival to discharge was much more common among children with an initial shockable rhythm than among children with shockable rhythms that occurred later during the resuscitation. Even in the setting of progressive res-

piratory failure and shock with an initial electrocardiogram of asystole or PEA, a substantial number of these children developed subsequent shockable VF/VT during CPR. Surprisingly, the subsequent VF/VT group had worse outcomes than children with asystole/PEA who never developed VF/VT during the resuscitation: 11% with subsequent VF/VT during resuscitation from asystole/PEA versus 27% with asystole/PEA alone. These data suggest that outcomes after *initial* VF/VT are "good," but outcomes after *subsequent* VF/VT are substantially worse, even compared to asystole/PEA rhythms.

Why was the outcome so poor in the subsequent VF/VT group? Plausible explanations include: (a) a delay in the diagnosis of subsequent VF/VT during the resuscitative efforts, (b) adverse effects of resuscitative interventions (e.g., too much epinephrine), and (c) severity of underlying myocardial pathology.

Termination of Ventricular Fibrillation: Defibrillation

Defibrillation (defined as termination of VF) is necessary for the successful resuscitation from VF cardiac arrest. Note that termination of fibrillation can result in asystole, PEA, or a perfusing rhythm. The goal of defibrillation is the return of an organized electrical rhythm with pulse. When prompt defibrillation is provided soon after the induction of VF in a cardiac catheterization laboratory, the rates of successful defibrillation and survival approach 100%. When automated external defibrillators are used within 3 mins of adult-witnessed VF, long-term survival can occur in >70% (18,103). In general, the mortality increases by 7%–10% per minute of delay to defibrillation. Early and effective, near-continuous chest compressions can attenuate the incremental increase in mortality with delayed defibrillation. The provision of high-quality CPR can improve outcome and save lives. Because pediatric cardiac arrests are commonly due to progressive asphyxia and/or shock, the initial treatment of choice is prompt CPR. Therefore, rhythm recognition is relatively less emphasized compared with adult cardiac arrests. However, successful resuscitation from VF does require defibrillation. The earlier VF can be diagnosed, the more successfully it can be treated.

Determinants of Defibrillation (Termination of Ventricular Fibrillation)

Successful termination of VF (defibrillation) is achieved by attaining current flow adequate to depolarize a critical mass of myocardium. Current flow (amperes) is primarily determined by the shock energy (joules), which is selected by the operator, and the patient's transthoracic impedance (ohms).

During the 1970s, animal studies using monophasic shock waveforms established that adequate electrical current flow through the myocardium led to successful defibrillation, and too much current flow resulted in postresuscitation myocardial damage and necrosis. In addition, factors that affected transthoracic impedance were identified as paddle size, thoracic gas volume, electrode/paddle contact, and conducting paste. Small paddle size increases resistance and thereby decreases current through the myocardium. On the other hand, paddles/pads larger than the heart result in current flow through extramyocardial pathways and less current through the heart (consequently, less flow for effective defibrillation). Poor electrode paddle contact and larger lung volumes (gas) result in greater impedance, whereas conducting paste and increased pressure at the paddle-skin contact decrease impedance. Transthoracic impedance could be decreased with multiple "stacked" shocks, partly due to increased skin blood flow after electrical shocks. These studies established that current density (current flow through the myocardium) is the primary determinant of both the effectiveness of the shock and myocardial damage.

Pediatric Defibrillation Dose

Early recommendations (from the 1970s) for initial defibrillation doses as high as 200 J for all children were extrapolated from adult data. Despite clinical experience indicating that such doses were effective, providing these large energies to infants and children seemed potentially dangerous, with animal data (11) demonstrating histopathologic myocardial damage at doses >10 J/kg. Other animal data indicated that 0.5–10 J/kg was adequate for defibrillation in a variety of species.

In a retrospective study of the efficacy of the 2-J/kg pediatric defibrillation strategy, 71 transthoracic defibrillation attempts on 27 children were evaluated (41). These children were 3 days to 15 years old and weighed 2.1–50 kg. Fifty-seven of 71 shocks were within 10 J of the 2-J/kg pediatric doses, and 91% (52/57) of these shocks were effective at terminating VF. The authors did not report any other outcome measures (e.g., successful termination of fibrillation to a perfusing rhythm, 24-hr survival, survival to discharge). Subsequent clinical usage suggests that the 2-J/kg dose is effective for short-duration, in-hospital defibrillation, although this conclusion has not been rigorously evaluated.

As noted earlier, current density determines the effectiveness and harm of the shock. Moreover, differences in paddle size, defibrillation energy dose, and the individual's transthoracic

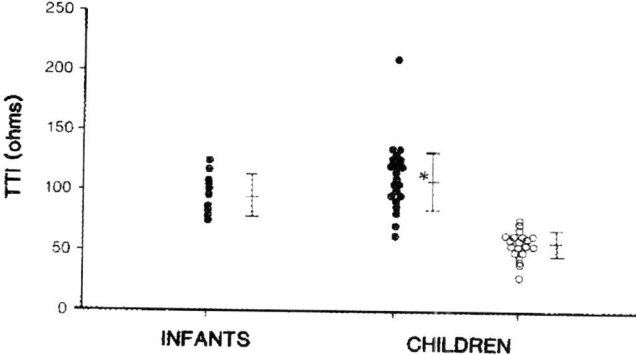

FIGURE 23.1. Effect of Paddle size and age on transthoracic impedance (TTI). ●, pediatric paddles; ○, adult paddles; *$p < 0.001$ vs. adult paddles; bar indicates standard deviation. From Atkins DL, Sirna S, Kieso R, et al. Pediatric defibrillation: importance of paddle size in determining transthoracic impedance. *Pediatrics.* 1988;82:914–918, with permission.

impedance are the main determinants of current density. Therefore, investigators explored the effects of paddle size, age, and weight on transthoracic impedance in children (5) (**Fig. 23.1**). As expected, transthoracic impedance increased substantially with pediatric paddles. Based on those data, the AHA recommends that "pediatric" or "small" paddles only be used in infants (1). More importantly, the authors of this study established that the relationship between transthoracic impedance and weight is not linear. The mean transthoracic impedance in their children was approximately 50 Ω with 83 cm² adult paddles and varied threefold among children. With pediatric or small pads (44 cm²), the mean impedance was approximately 70 Ω in 3.8–36-kg children. The impedances of their infants were slightly lower than that of their older children, but the range of each was wide, and the overlap substantial (5). Note that the mean transthoracic impedance in adults is typically approximately 60 to 80 Ω and that it also varies by more than threefold. These data suggest that the adjustment of pediatric energy dose to weight (2–4 J/kg) requires further study.

Pediatric Defibrillation Doses for Prolonged Ventricular Fibrillation

Of the approximately 16,000 children with cardiac arrest each year in North America, only 5%–20% present with an initial rhythm VF. Very little data have been published regarding pediatric defibrillation doses for prolonged VF. Therefore, the approach to pediatric prolonged VF is extrapolated from adult recommendations. For adults, the same defibrillation dose is recommended after brief-duration or prolonged-duration VF, even though the monophasic 200-J dose is often less effective at terminating prolonged VF (~60% termination of prolonged VF compared with >90% for short duration VF). Defibrillation is typically achieved using biphasic defibrillators, and the 150-J or 200-J biphasic adult automated external defibrillator (AED) dosage is nearly 90% successful at terminating prolonged VF (much better than the ~60% effectiveness with 200-J monophasic defibrillation). The presently recommended pediatric VF dose of 2 J/kg by monophasic waveform is safe, but data are limited regarding effectiveness for prolonged VF. A recently published animal study (11) regarding defibrillation after 7 mins of untreated VF in 4–24-kg piglets suggests that 2 J/kg may not be adequate. Twenty-four piglets were shocked with 2 J/kg, followed by 4 J/kg. The pediatric dose of 2 J/kg monophasic shocks was uniformly unsuccessful at terminating fibrillation in all 24 piglets. This should not be over-interpreted; interspecies differences could exist in defibrillation thresholds.

However, a small clinical study of pediatric defibrillation (10) attempts also confirms that a 2-J/kg defibrillation dose is often inadequate. Eleven children received 14 pediatric-dose shocks for VF in the Tucson EMS over a 5-year period, using the same definition as the earlier-mentioned pediatric in-hospital (i.e., brief duration) defibrillation study (2 J/kg ± 10 J) (41). Only 7 of 14 shocks (50%) terminated out-of-hospital (prolonged) VF, versus 52 of 57 shocks (91%) in their 27 in-hospital patients (p <0.01). This small series suggests that further evaluation of shock dose for prolonged VF is important.

Standard weight-based dosing strategy for pediatric defibrillation is not easily implemented in AEDs. Manufacturers have developed alternatives that attenuate the pediatric dose to 50–86 J biphasic. This dose is safe and effective in piglets after either brief or prolonged VF. In addition, the 50-J/75-J/86-J shocks were more effective than a weight-based 2-J/kg dose at initial termination of fibrillation after prolonged VF. In addition, in piglet studies that modeled prolonged out-of-hospital pediatric VF (7 mins of untreated VF), adult biphasic shocks of 200 J/300 J/360 J were compared with a "pediatric" biphasic AED dose of 50 J/75 J/86 J. Pediatric dosing resulted in fewer elevations of cardiac troponin T levels (14), less postresuscitation myocardial dysfunction (i.e., lesser decreases of left ventricular ejection fraction 1–4 hrs postresuscitation), and superior 24-hr survival with good neurologic outcome. These data support the use of attenuating electrodes with adult AEDs for pediatric defibrillation.

It is important to remember that the lack of shock delivery for pediatric VF is 100% lethal. Therefore, adult defibrillation doses are preferable to no defibrillation dose. A single-case report in the literature demonstrated that an adult AED dose could save the life of a 3-year-old child in VF. That child was defibrillated with a biphasic shock of 150 J (9 J/kg) (40). He survived without any apparent adverse effects. In particular, he had no elevations of serum creatine kinase or cardiac tro-ponin I and had normal postresuscitation ventricular function on echocardiogram.

Pediatric Automated External Defibrillators

Ventricular fibrillation is prolonged in nearly all children with out-of-hospital VF by the time EMS personnel and defibrilla-tors arrive. Automated external defibrillators have been rec-ommended for children <8 years old (2,81,82). Before such recommendations could be made, two issues were considered: (a) the safety and efficacy of the AED diagnostic rhythm anal-ysis program in children, and (b) the safety and efficacy of the AED shock dosage.

An important concern was that babies and small children with sinus tachycardia or supraventricular tachycardia can have very high heart rates that might be misinterpreted as "shockable" by AEDs with diagnostic programs developed for adult arrhythmias. Fortunately, published studies regarding the rhythm-analysis programs from several manufacturers have es-

tablished that they are quite sensitive and specific (6,20) in de-tecting the shockable rhythm of VF (6,20,82). Both algorithms were less sensitive at detecting the very uncommon shockable rhythm of VT, but were quite specific (i.e., the algorithm did not misinterpret other rhythms as VT and therefore did not recommend shocking a "nonshockable" rhythm). Ideally, the device should demonstrate high specificity for pediatric shock-able rhythms—that is, the device will not recommend a shock for nonshockable rhythms. At this writing, the evidence is in-sufficient to support a recommendation for or against the use of AEDs in children <1 year of age.

INTERVENTIONS DURING THE PREARREST PHASE

Interventions during the pre-arrest phase focus on prevention. For example, infant safety seats and safe driving to prevent traumatic arrests, water safety programs to prevent drown-ing arrests, medication safety caps to prevent drug poisoning arrests are all well-known, highly effective efforts to prevent cardiac arrests. Because early recognition, prevention, and an-ticipation of cardiac arrest is better than treatment, medical emergency teams (rapid response teams) are being trained to recognize and intervene when cardiac arrest is impending. Because many pediatric cardiac arrests are due to progres-sive respiratory failure and shock, the main focus of Pediatric Advanced Life Support (PALS) is the early recognition and treatment of respiratory failure and shock in children (i.e., prevention of cardiac arrest during the prearrest phase). Early warning systems, criteria of activation, and demonstrated ca-pability to decrease the incidence of and improve outcomes fol-lowing in-hospital pediatric arrest are developing (29,99,102).

INTERVENTIONS DURING THE CARDIAC ARREST (NO-FLOW) PHASE AND CARDIOPULMONARY (LOW-FLOW) PHASE: CARDIOPULMONARY RESUSCITATION

Airway and Breathing

One of the most common precipitating events for cardiac arrest in children is respiratory insufficiency. Adequate oxygen de-livery to meet metabolic demands and the removal of carbon dioxide are the goals of initial assisted ventilation. Effective bag-mask ventilation skills remain the cornerstone of provid-ing effective emergency ventilation. Effective ventilation does not necessarily require a tracheal tube. In one randomized, con-trolled study of children with out-of-hospital respiratory arrest (35), children who were treated with bag-mask ventilation did as well as children treated with prehospital endotracheal in-tubation. Emergency airway techniques such as transtracheal jet ventilation and emergency cricothyroidotomy are rarely, if ever, required during CPR. During CPR, cardiac output and pulmonary blood flow are approximately 10%–25% of that during normal sinus rhythm. Consequently, much less ventila-tion is necessary for adequate gas exchange from the blood traversing the pulmonary circulation during CPR. Animal and adult data indicate that overventilation during CPR is common and can substantially compromise venous return and cardiac output. Most concerning, these adverse hemodynamic effects during CPR, combined with the interruptions in chest compressions that are typically necessary to provide airway management and rescue breathing, can contribute to worse survival outcomes.

Although airway and breathing are prioritized in the ABC (airway, breathing, circulation) assessment approach, special circumstances may impact that priority order. In animal models of sudden VF cardiac arrest, acceptable PaO_2 and $PaCO_2$ persist for 4 to 8 mins during chest compressions without rescue breathing. Moreover, many animal studies indicate that outcomes from sudden, short-duration VF cardiac arrests are at least as good with chest compressions alone as with chest compressions plus rescue breathing. In addition, several retrospective studies of witnessed VF cardiac arrest in adults also suggest that outcomes are similar after bystander-initiated CPR with either chest compressions alone or chest compressions plus rescue breathing. A randomized, controlled study of dispatcher-assisted, bystander CPR in adults found a trend toward improved survival in those patients who received chest compressions alone compared to those who received dispatcher-instructed ventilation and chest compressions (42). In contrast, animal studies of asphyxia-precipitated cardiac arrests have established that rescue breathing is a critical component of successful CPR (12).

If adequate oxygenation and ventilation are important for survival from any cardiac arrest, why is rescue breathing not initially necessary for VF, yet quite important in asphyxia? Immediately after an acute fibrillatory cardiac arrest, aortic oxygen and carbon dioxide concentrations do not vary from the prearrest state because there is no blood flow, and aortic oxygen consumption is minimal. Therefore, when chest compressions are initiated, the blood flowing from the aorta to the coronary and cerebral circulations provides adequate oxygenation at an acceptable pH. At that time, myocardial oxygen delivery is limited more by blood flow than by oxygen content. Adequate oxygenation and ventilation can continue without rescue breathing because the lungs serve as a reservoir for oxygen during the low-flow state of CPR. In addition, ventilation can occur due to chest compression–induced gas exchange and spontaneous gasping during CPR in victims of sudden cardiac arrest. Therefore, arterial oxygenation and pH can often be adequate using chest compressions alone for VF arrests.

For the infant or child, foregoing ventilation may not be appropriate because respiratory arrest and asphyxia generally precede pediatric cardiac arrest. During asphyxia, blood continues to flow to tissues; therefore, arterial and venous oxygen saturations decrease while carbon dioxide and lactate increase. In addition, continued pulmonary blood flow before the cardiac arrest depletes the pulmonary oxygen reservoir. Therefore, asphyxia results in significant arterial hypoxemia and acidemia prior to resuscitation, in contrast to VF. In this circumstance, rescue breathing can be life saving.

Circulation

Providing basic life support with continuous effective chest compressions is generally the best way to provide circulation during cardiac arrest. Basic life support is often provided poorly or not provided at all. The most critical elements are to *push hard* and *push fast*. Because no flow occurs without chest compressions, it is important to minimize interruptions in chest compressions. To allow good venous return in the decompression phase of external cardiac massage, it is important to allow full-chest recoil and to avoid overventilation. The latter can prevent venous return because of increased intrathoracic pressure.

The use of closed-chest cardiac massage to provide adequate circulation during cardiac arrest was initially demonstrated in small dogs with compliant chest walls. Based on reasonable extrapolation, these investigators felt that closed-chest cardiac massage would be effective with children but might not be effective with adults. Therefore, the first patients successfully treated with closed-chest cardiac massage were children. The presumed mechanism of blood flow was direct compression of the heart between the sternum and the spine in these children with compliant chest walls. Later investigations indicated that blood could also be circulated during CPR by the thoracic pump mechanism. That is, chest compression–induced increases in intrathoracic pressure can generate a gradient for blood to flow from the pulmonary vasculature, through the heart, and into the peripheral circulation. Regardless of mechanism, cardiac output during CPR seems to be greater in children (and immature animals) with compliant chest walls than in adults with less-compliant chest walls. Interestingly, recent NRCPR data indicate that outcomes from in-hospital cardiac arrest are substantially better in infants than in older children (69), perhaps because of superior perfusion during CPR.

Circumferential Versus Focal Sternal Compressions

In adults and animal models of cardiac arrest, circumferential (Vest) CPR provides better CPR hemodynamics than point compressions. In smaller infants, it is often possible to encircle the chest with both hands and depress the sternum with the thumbs, while compressing the thorax circumferentially. In an infant model of CPR (48,70), this "two-thumb" method of compression resulted in higher systolic and diastolic blood pressures and a higher pulse pressure than did traditional two-finger compression of the sternum.

Duty Cycle

Duty cycle is the ratio of time of compression phase to the entire compression–relaxation cycle. In a model of human adult cardiac arrest (33,43), cardiac output and coronary blood flow are optimized when chest compressions last for 30% of the total cycle time. As the duration of CPR increases, the optimal duty cycle may increase to 50%. In a juvenile swine model, a relaxation period of 250–300 ms (a duty cycle of 40%–50% if 120 compressions are delivered per min) correlated with improved cerebral perfusion pressure when compared with shorter duty cycles of 30% (24).

Open-chest Cardiopulmonary Resuscitation

Excellent, standard closed-chest CPR generates approximately 10%–25% of baseline myocardial blood flow and a cerebral blood flow that is approximately 50% of normal. By contrast, open-chest CPR can generate a cerebral blood flow that approaches normal. Although open-chest massage improves coronary perfusion pressure and increases the chance of successful defibrillation in animals and humans, surgical thoracotomy is impractical in many situations. A retrospective review of 27 cases of CPR following pediatric blunt trauma (15 with open-chest CPR and 12 with closed-chest CPR) demonstrated that open-chest CPR increased hospital costs without altering rates of ROSC or survival to discharge (87). However, survival in both groups was 0%, indicating that the population may have been too severely injured or too late in the process to benefit from this aggressive therapy. Open-chest CPR is often provided to children after open-heart cardiac surgery and sternotomy. The earlier institution of open-chest CPR may warrant reconsideration in selected special resuscitation circumstances.

Ratio of Compressions to Ventilation

Compression:ventilation (C:V) ratios and tidal volumes recommended during CPR are based on rational conjecture and educational retention theory. Ideal C:V ratios for pediatric patients are unknown. Recent physiologic estimates suggest the amount of ventilation needed during CPR is much less than the amount needed during a normal perfusing rhythm because the cardiac output during CPR is only 10%–25% of that during normal sinus rhythm (51). The benefits of positive-pressure ventilation (increased arterial content of oxygen and carbon dioxide elimination) must be balanced against the adverse consequence of impeding circulation.

Maximizing systemic oxygen delivery during single-rescuer CPR requires a tradeoff between time spent doing chest compressions and time spent doing mouth-to-mouth ventilations. Theoretically, neither compression-only nor ventilation-only CPR can sustain systemic oxygen delivery. The best ratio depends on many factors, including the compression rate, tidal volume, blood flow generated by compressions, and the time that compressions are interrupted to perform ventilations. A chest C:V ratio of 15:2 delivered the same minute ventilation as CPR with a chest C:V ratio of 5:1 in a mannequin model of pediatric CPR, but the number of chest compressions delivered was 48% higher with the 15:2 ratio (57,92).

In adults, mathematical models (7) of oxygen delivery during CPR performed with variable ratios of healthcare-provider chest compressions to ventilations suggest that the optimal C:V ratio is approximately 30:2 and, for lay rescuers, closer to 50:2. Mathematical models of C:V ratios suggest that matching the amount of ventilation to the amount of reduced pulmonary blood flow during closed-chest cardiac compressions should favor very high compression-to-ventilation ratios. The effect of C:V ratio on oxygen delivery to peripheral tissues has been demonstrated (7). Ignoring the amount of ventilation provided by chest compressions alone, neither compression-only nor ventilation-only CPR can sustain oxygen delivery to the periphery for prolonged periods of CPR. As mentioned earlier, the best ratio depends on many factors (i.e., compression rate, tidal volume, blood flow generated by compressions, and time that compressions are interrupted to perform ventilations). These factors can be related in a mathematical formula based on physiology, because they change as a function of the size of the patient. Such considerations may help refine the amount of ventilation recommended for both adults and children. The ratio of chest compressions to ventilations during no-flow and low-flow phases of cardiopulmonary-cerebral resuscitation remains an area of high interest, controversy, and future research. These formulas, adjusted to the known physiologic variables in children, have suggested the potential to simplify the C:V

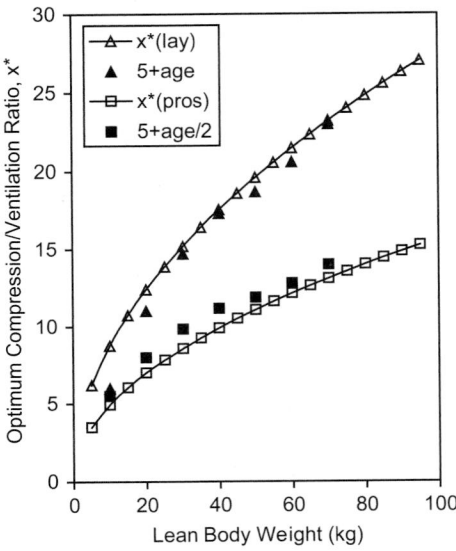

FIGURE 23.2. Scaling rules for optimum compression:ventilation (C:V) ratios in pediatric basic life support. Open symbols represent theoretical C:V ratios for optimal oxygen delivery, scaled for persons having a wide range of body weight. Lay rescuers (*lay*) are assumed to take 8 secs to deliver one rescue breath in an adult-sized individual, in keeping with the observations of Chamberlain and coworkers. Professional rescuers (*pros*) are assumed to take 2.5 secs to deliver one rescue breath. Solid symbols indicate approximations to the theoretical curves, based on average body weights of children ages 1 to 18 years, according to the rules "5 + patient age in years" for lay rescuers and "5 + one-half patient age in years" for professional rescuers. From Babbs CF, Nadkarni V. Optimizing chest compression to rescue ventilation ratios during one-rescuer CPR by professionals and lay persons: Children are not just little adults. *Resuscitation* 2004;61:173–81, with permission.

ratio of 15 chest compressions to two ventilations in children (8,92) (**Fig. 23.2, 23.3**).

Intraosseous Vascular Access

Intraosseous (IO) vascular access provides access to a noncollapsible marrow venous plexus, which serves as a rapid, safe, and reliable route for the administration of drugs, crystalloids, colloids, and blood during resuscitation. Intraosseous vascular access can often be achieved in 30–60 secs. A specially designed IO bone-marrow needle with a stylet is preferred to prevent obstruction of the needle with cortical bone. The IO needle is typically inserted into the anterior tibial bone marrow; alternative sites include the distal femur, medial malleolus or the anterior superior iliac spine, and the distal tibia. In adults and older children, the medial malleolus, distal radius, and distal ulna are optional locations.

Resuscitation drugs, fluids, continuous catecholamine infusions, and blood products can be safely administered through the IO route. The onset of action and drug levels following IO infusion during CPR are comparable to those achieved following vascular administration, including central venous administration. Intraosseous vascular access may also be used to obtain blood specimens for chemistry, blood gas analysis, and blood typing and cross-matching, (53) although administration of sodium bicarbonate through the IO cannula eliminates the close correlation with mixed venous blood gases.

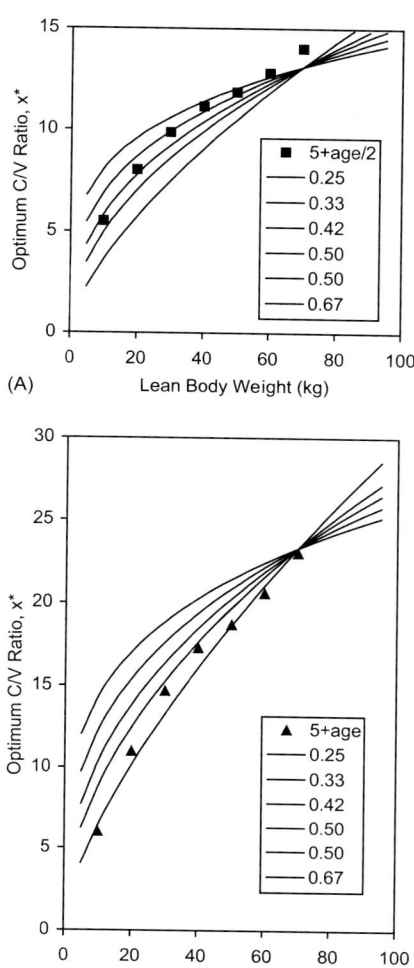

FIGURE 23.3. Sensitivity analysis for scaling rules for optimum compression:ventilation (C:V) ratios in pediatric basic life support. The general effect of body size upon the optimum C:V ratio is insensitive to changes in the exponent of body weight. **A:** Calculations for professional rescuers. **B:** Calculations for lay rescuers. From Babbs CF, Nadkarni V. Optimizing chest compression to rescue ventilation ratios during one-rescuer CPR by professionals and lay persons: Children are not just little adults. *Resuscitation* 2004;61:173–81, with permission.

Complications have been reported in <1% of patients following IO infusion; these include tibial fracture, lower extremity compartment syndrome, severe extravasation of drugs, and osteomyelitis. Most of these complications may be avoided by careful technique. Although microscopic pulmonary fat and bone marrow emboli have been demonstrated in animal models (75), they have never been reported clinically and appear to occur just as frequently during cardiac arrest without IO drug administration. Animal data and one human follow-up study indicate that the local effects of IO infusion on the bone marrow and bone growth are minimal.

Endotracheal Drug Administration

Intraosseous vascular access has largely replaced the need for endotracheal drug administration, although important drugs were commonly administered via the endotracheal tube before vascular access was achieved. In particular, epinephrine, atropine, naloxone, and lidocaine were commonly administered via the endotracheal route. Sodium bicarbonate and calcium may be very irritating to the airways and lung parenchyma and are not recommended for endotracheal administration.

Absorption of drugs into the circulation after endotracheal administration depends on dispersion over the respiratory mucosa, pulmonary blood flow, and the matching of the ventilation (drug dispersal) to perfusion. The small volumes of drug that remain as droplets in the tracheal tube are obviously not effective. Inadequate chest compressions that result in poor pulmonary blood flow will also limit absorption of the drug and prevent its delivery to the heart and systemic circulation. Preexisting pathophysiologic conditions such as pulmonary edema, pneumonitis, and airway disease also affect the pharmacokinetics of endotracheally administered drugs. Another confounding factor is that the vasoconstrictive effects of epinephrine may limit local pulmonary blood flow, thereby diminishing drug uptake and delivery. It is therefore not surprising that drug absorption varies greatly and that optimal drug doses have not been determined. Animal studies reveal a wide variability in plasma epinephrine levels and physiologic effects after endotracheal administration. On average, 10 times as much endotracheal epinephrine is required to attain peak plasma levels comparable to those of IV administration (47). Moreover, a prolonged depot effect typically occurs after endotracheal epinephrine administration, which can lead to postresuscitation hypertension, tachycardia, and ventricular arrhythmias.

Medication Use During Cardiac Arrest

Although animal studies indicate that epinephrine can improve initial resuscitation success after both asphyxial and VF cardiac arrests, no single medication has been shown to improve survival outcome from pediatric cardiac arrest.

Vasopressors

During CPR, epinephrine's α-adrenergic effect on vascular tone is most important. The α-adrenergic action increases systemic vascular resistance, increasing diastolic blood pressure, which in turn, increases coronary perfusion pressure and blood flow and increases the likelihood of ROSC. Epinephrine also increases cerebral blood flow during CPR because peripheral vasoconstriction directs a greater proportion of flow to the cerebral circulation. The β-adrenergic effect increases myocardial contractility and heart rate and relaxes smooth muscle in the skeletal muscle vascular bed and bronchi, although this effect is of less importance. Epinephrine also increases the vigor and intensity of ventricular fibrillation, increasing the likelihood of successful defibrillation.

High-dose epinephrine (0.05–0.2 mg/kg) improves myocardial and cerebral blood flow during CPR more than standard-dose epinephrine (0.01–0.02 mg/kg) and may increase the incidence of initial ROSC (17,65). The administration of high-dose epinephrine, however, can worsen a patient's postresuscitation hemodynamic condition by causing increased myocardial oxygen demand, ventricular ectopy, hypertension, and myocardial necrosis (13). Prospective and retrospective studies indicate that the use of high-dose epinephrine in adults or children does not improve survival and may be associated with a worse neurologic outcome (9,19).

A randomized, controlled trial of rescue high-dose epinephrine versus standard-dose epinephrine following failed initial standard-dose epinephrine for pediatric in-hospital cardiac arrest demonstrated a worse 24-hr survival in the high-dose epinephrine group (1/27 vs. 6/23, $p < 0.05$) (78). In particular, high-dose epinephrine seemed to worsen the outcome of patients with asphyxia-precipitated cardiac arrest. High-dose epinephrine cannot be recommended routinely for initial therapy or rescue therapy.

Wide variability in catecholamine pharmacokinetics and pharmacodynamics dictates individual titration. A life-saving dose during CPR for one patient may be life-threatening to another. High-dose epinephrine should be considered as an alternative to standard-dose epinephrine in special circumstances of refractory pediatric cardiac arrest (e.g., patient on high-dose epinephrine infusion prior to cardiac arrest) and/or when continuous direct arterial blood pressure monitoring allows titration of the epinephrine dosage to diastolic (decompression phase) arterial pressure during CPR. Nevertheless, high-dose epinephrine has not been demonstrated to improve outcome and should only be used with caution.

Vasopressin is a long-acting endogenous hormone that acts at specific receptors to mediate systemic vasoconstriction (V_1 receptor) and reabsorption of water in the renal tubule (V_2 receptor). In experimental models of cardiac arrest (104,105), vasopressin increases blood flow to the heart and brain and improves long-term survival when compared to epinephrine. Vasopressin may decrease splanchnic blood flow during and following CPR. In randomized, controlled trials of in-hospital and out-of-hospital arrests in adults (93,106), vasopressin had comparable efficacy to epinephrine. Vasopressin did not improve outcome compared with epinephrine.

In a piglet model of prolonged VF, the use of vasopressin and epinephrine in combination resulted in higher left ventricular blood flow than either pressor alone, and both vasopressin alone, and vasopressin plus epinephrine resulted in superior cerebral blood flow than did epinephrine alone (67,105). By contrast, in a piglet model of *asphyxial* cardiac arrest, return of spontaneous circulation was more likely in piglets treated with epinephrine than in those treated with vasopressin. A case series of four children who received vasopressin during six prolonged cardiac arrest events suggests that the use of bolus vasopressin may result in return of spontaneous circulation when standard medications have failed (68). Vasopressin has also been reported to be useful in low-cardiac-output states associated with sepsis syndrome and organ recovery in children. Although vasopressin will not likely replace epinephrine as a first-line agent in pediatric cardiac arrest, preliminary data suggest that its use in conjunction with epinephrine in pediatric cardiac arrest deserves further investigation.

Calcium

For in-hospital pediatric cardiac arrests, hypocalcemia is not uncommon. Although calcium administration is only recommended during cardiac arrest for hypocalcemia, hyperkalemia, hypermagnesemia, and calcium-channel-blocker overdose, it is commonly used for in-hospital pediatric cardiac arrests, especially those that occur post-cardiac surgery. The administration of calcium has not been demonstrated to improve outcome in cardiac arrest (94). Animal studies suggest that calcium administration may worsen reperfusion injury (55).

Buffer Solutions

Cardiac arrest results in lactic acidosis from inadequate organ blood flow and poor oxygenation. Acidosis depresses myocardial function, reduces systemic vascular resistance, and inhibits defibrillation. Nevertheless, the routine use of sodium bicarbonate for a child in cardiac arrest is not recommended. Clinical trials that involved critically ill adults with severe metabolic acidosis did not demonstrate a beneficial effect of sodium bicarbonate. However, because the presence of acidosis may depress the action of catecholamines, the use of sodium bicarbonate seems rational in an acidemic child who is refractory to catecholamine administration. The administration of sodium bicarbonate is more clearly indicated in the patient with a tricyclic antidepressant overdose, hyperkalemia, hypermagnesemia, or sodium-channel-blocker poisoning.

The buffering action of bicarbonate occurs when a hydrogen cation and a bicarbonate anion combine to form carbon dioxide and water. If carbon dioxide is not effectively cleared through ventilation, its build-up will counterbalance the buffering effect of bicarbonate. Other side effects with sodium bicarbonate include hypernatremia, hyperosmolarity, and metabolic alkalosis. THAM is a non-carbon-dioxide-generating buffer that can be used during cardiac arrest. Note that excessive alkalosis decreases calcium and potassium concentration and shifts the oxyhemoglobin dissociation curve to the left.

Antiarrhythmic Medications: Lidocaine and Amiodarone

The administration of antiarrhythmic medications should not delay the administration of a shock for a patient with VF. However, after unsuccessful attempts at electrical defibrillation, medications to increase the effectiveness of defibrillation should be considered. In both pediatric and adult patients, the first administered medication for ventricular fibrillation is epinephrine. If epinephrine with or without vasopressin and a subsequent repeat attempt to defibrillate are unsuccessful, the antiarrhythmic agents amiodarone or lidocaine should be considered.

Lidocaine has been recommended traditionally for shock-resistant VF in adults and children. However, amiodarone is the only antiarrhythmic agent that has been prospectively determined to improve survival to hospital admission in the setting of shock-resistant VF when compared to placebo (27,59). Furthermore, patients who received amiodarone for shock-resistant out-of-hospital ventricular fibrillation had a higher rate of survival to hospital admission than did patients who received lidocaine alone. Neither of these (27,59) randomized, controlled trials included children. Although no comparisons of antiarrhythmic medications for pediatric refractory VF have been published, extrapolation of the adult studies has led to the recommendation of amiodarone as the preferred antiarrhythmic agent for children.

POSTRESUSCITATION INTERVENTIONS

Temperature Management

Mild, induced hypothermia is a promising goal-directed, postresuscitation therapy for adults. Two seminal articles established that induced hypothermia (32°–34°C) could improve outcome for comatose adults after resuscitation from VF cardiac arrest (16,50). In both of these randomized, controlled trials, the inclusion criteria were patients >18 years who were persistently comatose after successful resuscitation from nontraumatic VF. The multicentered European study had a goal of 32°C–34°C for the first 24 hrs postarrest (50). The mean time until attainment of this temperature goal was 8 hrs. Six-month survival with good neurologic outcome was superior in the hypothermic group (75/136 vs. 54/137; RR, 1.40; CI, 1.08–1.81). Similarly, death at 6 months postevent occurred less often in the hypothermic group (56/137 vs. 76/138; RR, 0.74; CI, 0.58–0.95). The second study reported good outcomes in 21/43 (49%) of the hypothermic group versus 9/34 (26%) of the control group ($p = 0.046$, OR 5.25; CI, 1.47–18.76) (16). Importantly, hypotension occurred among over half of the patients in both groups and was aggressively treated with vasoactive infusion in the European study. Similarly, more than half of Bernard's patients received epinephrine infusions during the first 24 hrs postresuscitation.

Interpretation and extrapolation of these studies to children is difficult. Fever following cardiac arrest, brain trauma, stroke, and other ischemic conditions are associated with poor neurologic outcome. Hyperthermia following cardiac arrest is common in children (44). It is reasonable to believe that mild, induced, systemic hypothermia may benefit children who are resuscitated from cardiac arrest. However, benefit from this treatment deserves to be rigorously studied in children and in adult patients with non-VF arrests. At a minimum, it is advisable to avoid even mild hyperthermia in children following CPR. Scheduled administration of antipyretic medications *and* use of external cooling devices are often necessary to avoid hyperthermia in this population. Emerging neonatal trials of selective brain cooling and systemic cooling may show promise in neonatal hypoxic-ischemic encephalopathy, suggesting that induced hypothermia may improve outcomes (38,86).

Postresuscitation Myocardial Support

Postarrest myocardial stunning occurs commonly after successful resuscitation in animals, adults, and children. In addition, most adults who survive to hospital admission after an out-of-hospital cardiac arrest die in the postresuscitation phase, many due to progressive myocardial dysfunction. Animal studies demonstrate that postarrest myocardial stunning is characterized by a global biventricular systolic and diastolic dysfunction and typically resolves after 1 or 2 days (36,54). Postarrest myocardial stunning is pathophysiologically similar to sepsis-related myocardial dysfunction and postcardiopulmonary bypass myocardial dysfunction, including increases in inflammatory mediator and nitric oxide production. Postarrest myocardial stunning is worse after a more prolonged untreated cardiac arrest, after more prolonged CPR, after defibrillation with higher energy shocks, and after a greater number of shocks.

Optimal treatment of postarrest myocardial dysfunction has not been rigorously established. As noted earlier, this myocardial dysfunction has been treated with various continuous inotropic/vasoactive agents, including dopamine, dobutamine, and epinephrine, in both children and adults. In addition, milrinone improves the hemodynamic status of children with post-

cardiopulmonary bypass myocardial dysfunction and septic shock. Finally, the new inotropic agent levosimendan has also been effective in the treatment of animal models of postresuscitation myocardial dysfunction (49), treatment of myocardial stunning in adults (34), and pediatric low-cardiac output (32).

Although prospective, controlled trials in animals have demonstrated that the myocardial dysfunction can be effectively treated with vasoactive agents, no data demonstrate improvements in outcome. Nevertheless, because myocardial dysfunction is common and can lead to secondary ischemic injuries to other organ systems or even cardiovascular collapse, treatment with vasoactive medications is a rational therapeutic choice that may improve outcome. The hemodynamic benefits in animal studies of postarrest myocardial dysfunction, pediatric studies of post-cardiopulmonary bypass myocardial dysfunction, and pediatric sepsis-related myocardial dysfunction support the use of inotropic/vasoactive agents in this setting (3,21,46,52,61,62). In addition, adult studies document the common occurrence of postarrest hypotension and/or poor myocardial function "requiring" inotropic/vasoactive agents. In summary, because treatment of postarrest myocardial dysfunction with inotropic/vasoactive infusions can improve the patient's hemodynamic status, such treatment should be routinely considered and titrated to effect. Unfortunately, evidence-based therapeutic targets for goal-directed therapy are ill defined.

Blood Pressure Management

It has been demonstrated that 55% of adults who survived out-of-hospital cardiac arrests required in-hospital vasoactive infusions for hypotension unresponsive to volume boluses (64). Compared to healthy volunteers, adults resuscitated from cardiac arrest have impaired autoregulation of cerebral blood flow. Hence, they may not maintain cerebral perfusion pressure in the face of systemic hypotension and, likewise, may not be able to protect the brain from acutely increased blood flow in the face of systemic hypertension. It is rational to presume that blood pressure variability should be minimized as much as possible following resuscitation from cardiac arrest.

A brief period of hypertension following resuscitation from cardiac arrest may diminish the no-reflow phenomenon. In animal models, brief, induced hypertension following resuscitation results in improved neurologic outcome compared to normotension. In a retrospective human study, postresuscitative hypertension was associated with a better neurologic outcome after controlling for age, gender, duration of cardiac arrest, duration of CPR, and preexisting diseases (9). It seems reasonable to aggressively treat and prevent hypotension. Moreover, severe sustained hypertension is not desirable.

Glucose Control

Hyperglycemia following adult cardiac arrest is associated with worse neurologic outcome after controlling for duration of arrest and presence of cardiogenic shock (63). In animal models of asphyxial and ischemic cardiac arrest, the administration of insulin and glucose, but not the administration of glucose alone, improved neurologic outcome compared to administration of normal saline (15). Data for evidence-based titration of specific end-points is not available.

Extracorporeal Membrane Oxygenation—Cardiopulmonary Resuscitation

Perhaps the ultimate technology to control postresuscitation temperature and hemodynamic parameters is extracorporeal membrane oxygenation (ECMO). The concomitant administration of heparin may optimize microcirculatory flow. The use of veno-arterial ECMO to reestablish circulation and provide controlled reperfusion following cardiac arrest has been published, but prospective, controlled studies are lacking. Nevertheless, these series have reported extraordinary results with the use of ECMO as a rescue therapy for pediatric cardiac arrests, especially from potentially reversible acute postoperative myocardial dysfunction or arrhythmias. In one study, 11 children who suffered cardiac arrest in the PICU after cardiac surgery were placed on ECMO during CPR after 20–110 mins of CPR (28). Prolonged CPR was continued until ECMO cannulae, circuits, and personnel were available. Six of these 11 children were long-term survivors without apparent neurologic sequelae. More recently, two centers have reported an additional remarkable eight pediatric cardiac patients who were provided with mechanical cardiopulmonary support during CPR within 20 mins of the initiation of CPR. All eight survived to hospital discharge (71). Cardiopulmonary resuscitation and ECMO are not curative treatments. They are simply cardiopulmonary supportive measures that may allow tissue perfusion and viability until recovery from the precipitating disease process. As such, they can be powerful tools. Most remarkably, in a report of 66 children who were placed on ECMO during CPR over 7 years, the median duration of CPR prior to establishment of ECMO was 50 mins, and 35% (23/66) of these children survived to hospital discharge (71). Additional centers corroborate this finding (23). It is important to emphasize that these children had brief no flow periods, excellent CPR during the low-flow period, and a well-controlled postresuscitation phase.

The potential advantages of ECMO come from its ability to maintain a tight control of physiologic parameters after resuscitation: blood flow rates, oxygenation, ventilation, anticoagulation, and body temperature can be manipulated precisely through the ECMO circuit. As we learn more about the processes of secondary injury following cardiac arrest, ECMO might enable controlled perfusion and temperature management to minimize reperfusion injury and maximize cell recovery.

POSTRESUSCITATION OUTCOMES

The most important postresuscitation outcomes are survival with favorable neurologic outcome and acceptable quality of life. Many studies report end-points of return of sustained circulation or survival to hospital discharge. Information is limited about neurologic outcomes and predictors of neurologic outcome after both adult and pediatric cardiac arrests. Barriers to the assessment of neurologic outcomes of children after cardiac arrests include the constantly changing developmental context that occurs with brain maturation. Prediction or prognosis for future neuropsychologic status is a complex task, particularly after an acute neurologic insult. Little information is available regarding the predictive value of clinical neurologic examinations, neurophysiologic diagnostic studies

(e.g., electroencephalogram or somatosensory-evoked potentials), biomarkers, or imaging (CT, MRI, or positron-emission tomography) on eventual outcomes following cardiac arrest or other global hypoxic-ischemic insults in children. CT scans are not sensitive in detecting early neurologic injury. The value of MRI studies following pediatric cardiac arrest is not yet clear. However, MRI with diffusion weighting should provide valuable information about hypoxic-ischemic injury in the subacute and recovery phases. Emerging data suggest that burst-suppression pattern on postarrest electroencephalogram is sensitive and specific for poor neurologic outcome (74). One study showed somatosensory-evoked potential was highly sensitive and specific in pediatric patients after cardiac arrest (84). However, somatosensory-evoked potentials are not standardized in the pediatric population, and they are difficult to interpret. Many children who suffer a cardiac arrest have substantial preexisting neurologic problems. For example, 17% of the children with in-hospital cardiac arrests from the NRCPR were neurologically abnormal before the arrest (73). Thus, comparison to prearrest neurologic function of a child is difficult and adds another barrier to the assessment and prediction of postarrest neurologic status.

Biomarkers are emerging tools with which to predict neurologic outcome. In an adult study, the serum level of neuron-specific enolase and S100b protein showed prognostic value. Neuron-specific enolase of >33 mcg/L and S100b of >0.7 mcg/L were highly sensitive and specific for poor neurologic outcome (death or persisting unconsciousness) (79). The validation of those biomarkers in pediatric postarrest patients requires further study.

Most pediatric cardiac arrest outcome studies have not included neurologic outcomes. Investigations that include neurologic outcomes have generally used the Pediatric Cerebral Performance Category, a gross outcome scale. Many neuropsychologic tests can detect more subtle, clinically important neuropsychologic sequelae from neurologic insults. Neuropsychologic outcomes are important issues for future pediatric cardiac arrest outcome studies.

QUALITY OF CARDIOPULMONARY RESUSCITATION AND RESUSCITATION INTERVENTIONS

Despite evidence-based guidelines, extensive provider training, and provider credentialing in resuscitation medicine, the quality of CPR is typically poor. Slow compression rates, inadequate depth of compression, and substantial pauses are the norm. The mantra of "push hard, push fast, minimize interruptions, allow full-chest recoil, and don't overventilate" can markedly improve myocardial, cerebral, and systemic perfusion and improve outcomes (31). The quality of postresuscitative management has also been demonstrated to be critically important to improve resuscitation survival outcomes (95).

CONCLUSIONS AND FUTURE DIRECTIONS

Outcomes from pediatric cardiac arrest and CPR appear to be improving. An evolving understanding of the pathophysiology of events and titration of the interventions to the timing, etiology, duration, and intensity of the cardiac arrest event can improve resuscitation outcomes. Exciting discoveries in basic and applied science are on the immediate horizon for study in specific populations of cardiac arrest victims. By strategically focusing therapies to specific phases of cardiac arrest and resuscitation and to evolving pathophysiology, critical care interventions hold great promise to lead the way to more successful cardiopulmonary and cerebral resuscitation in children. In the future, the treatment of sudden death in children requires more evidence-based and less anecdotal interventions. Timing of therapeutic interventions to prevent arrest and to protect, preserve, and promote restoration of intact neurologic survival is of the highest priority. Emerging technology interfaced with evolving teams and systems of postresuscitative care will likely facilitate high-quality interventions and ensure optimal odds for survival.

Exciting new epidemiologic studies, such as the NRCPR for in-hospital cardiac arrests and the large-scale, multicentered Resuscitation Outcome Consortium funded by the National Heart, Lung, and Blood Institute, are providing new data to guide our resuscitation practices and generate hypotheses for new approaches to improve outcomes. It is increasingly clear that excellent basic life support is often not provided. Innovative technical advances, such as directive and corrective real-time feedback, can increase the likelihood of effective basic life support. In addition, team dynamic training and debriefing can substantially improve self-efficacy and operational performance.

Induced hypothermia is a promising neuroprotective and cardioprotective postarrest intervention. Experimental data suggest that it can and should be considered as an intra-arrest intervention, especially during prolonged CPR efforts. Chemical hibernation, controlled reanimation, and emergency preservation and resuscitation techniques are being considered.

Mechanical interventions such as ECMO or other cardiopulmonary bypass systems are already commonplace interventions during prolonged in-hospital cardiac arrests. Technical advances are likely to further improve our ability to provide such mechanical support.

In the past, the concept of evidence-based pediatric cardiac arrest recommendations seemed fanciful. Recommendations were based on extrapolated animal and adult data. These suboptimal approaches are no longer acceptable. Pediatric cardiac arrest clinical trials have started with the randomized controlled trial of high-dose epinephrine versus standard dose epinephrine as rescue therapy for in-hospital pediatric cardiac arrests. Clinical trials are necessary for appropriate evidence-based recommendations for treatment of pediatric cardiac arrests. It is likely that the evolution of systems such as "cardiac arrest centers," similar to trauma, stroke, and myocardial infarction centers, is likely to facilitate the appropriate intensive care to patients who require specialized postresuscitation care.

KEY POINTS

- Effective CPR and advanced life support targeted to the etiology, timing, intensity, and duration of the cardiac arrest can optimize the potential to restore an apparently dead child back to life.

- Sudden arrhythmogenic ("electrical") cardiac arrests are typically due to VF or rapid VT and respond to rapid electrical defibrillation.

- Mechanical ("pump") cardiomyopathic arrests are typically due to inadequate myocardial oxygen delivery from asphyxial, ischemic, metabolic, or pharmacologic problems and usually require mechanical support (CPR) to restore perfusion.

- Cardiac arrest has at least four phases: prearrest, no-flow (untreated cardiac arrest), low-flow (CPR), and postresuscitation. The interventions needed in each phase are specific to the phase of resuscitation.

- Animal and human data indicate that well-performed CPR for children is quite effective and support the notion that high-quality basic life support early is more important than advanced life support late.

- Outcomes following pediatric out-of-hospital arrests appear to be worse than those following in-hospital arrests. Two common types of out-of-hospital cardiac arrests have especially poor outcomes: traumatic arrests and those associated with SIDS.

- The incidence of VF varies by setting and age. In special circumstances, such as tricyclic antidepressant overdose, cardiomyopathy, post-cardiac surgery, and prolonged QT syndromes, VF is a more likely rhythm during cardiac arrest.

- Defibrillation (termination of VF) is necessary for successful resuscitation from VF cardiac arrest. Defibrillation can result in asystole, PEA, or a perfusing rhythm. Successful defibrillation is achieved by attaining current flow adequate to depolarize a critical mass of myocardium.

- One of the most common precipitating events for cardiac arrest in children is respiratory insufficiency. Adequate oxygen delivery to meet metabolic demands and removal of carbon dioxide are the goals of initial assisted ventilation.

- Providing basic life support with continuous effective chest compressions and minimal pauses and interruptions, is generally the best way to provide circulation during cardiac arrest.

- Mild induced hypothermia is a promising goal-directed, postresuscitation therapy for adults. However, benefit from this treatment deserves to be rigorously studied in children and in adult patients with non-VF arrests.

- Optimal treatment of postarrest myocardial dysfunction has not been rigorously established; it has been treated with various continuous inotropic/vasoactive agents in both children and adults.

- ECMO may provide the ultimate control of postresuscitation temperature and vital organ perfusion, and has been demonstrated with good outcomes in selected resuscitation circumstances. The concomitant administration of anticoagulants may optimize microcirculatory flow.

- Despite evidence-based guidelines, extensive provider training, and provider credentialing in resuscitation medicine, the quality of CPR is typically poor. Slow compression rates, inadequate depth of compression, and substantial pauses are the norm. A mantra of "push hard, push fast, minimize interruptions, allow full-chest recoil, and don't overventilate" can markedly improve myocardial, cerebral, and systemic perfusion and improve outcomes.

References

1. 2005 American Heart Association (AHA) guidelines for cardiopulmonary resuscitation (CPR) and emergency cardiovascular care (ECC) of pediatric and neonatal patients: Pediatric advanced life support. *Pediatrics* 2006;117:e1005–28.

2. 2005 American Heart Association (AHA) guidelines for cardiopulmonary resuscitation (CPR) and emergency cardiovascular care (ECC) of pediatric and neonatal patients: Pediatric basic life support. *Pediatrics* 2006;117:e989–1004.

3. Abdallah I, Shawky H. A randomised controlled trial comparing milrinone and epinephrine as inotropes in paediatric patients undergoing total correction of Tetralogy of Fallot. *Egyptian Journal of Anaesthesia* 2003;19:323–9.

4. Appleton GO, Cummins RO, Larson MP, et al. CPR and the single rescuer: At what age should you "call first" rather than "call fast"? *Ann Emerg Med* 1995;25:492–4.

5. Atkins DL, Sirna S, Kieso R, et al. Pediatric defibrillation: Importance of paddle size in determining transthoracic impedance. *Pediatrics* 1988;82:914–8.

6. Atkinson E, Mikysa B, Conway JA, et al. Specificity and sensitivity of automated external defibrillator rhythm analysis in infants and children. *Ann Emerg Med* 2003;42:185–96.

7. Babbs CF, Kern KB. Optimum compression to ventilation ratios in CPR under realistic, practical conditions: A physiological and mathematical analysis. *Resuscitation* 2002;54:147–57.

8. Babbs CF, Nadkarni V. Optimizing chest compression to rescue ventilation ratios during one-rescuer CPR by professionals and lay persons: Children are not just little adults. *Resuscitation* 2004;61:173–81.

9. Behringer W, Kittler H, Sterz F, et al. Cumulative epinephrine dose during cardiopulmonary resuscitation and neurologic outcome. *Ann Intern Med* 1998;129:450–6.

10. Berg MD, Samson RA, Meyer RJ, et al. Pediatric defibrillation doses often fail to terminate prolonged out-of-hospital ventricular fibrillation in children. *Resuscitation* 2005;67:63–7.

11. Berg RA, Chapman FW, Berg MD, et al. Attenuated adult biphasic shocks compared with weight-based monophasic shocks in a swine model of prolonged pediatric ventricular fibrillation. *Resuscitation* 2004;61:189–97.

11a. Berg RA, Hilwig RW, Kern KB, et al. Ewy GA. Simulated mouth-to-mouth ventilation and chest compressions (bystander cardiopulmonary resuscitation) improves outcome in a swine model of prehospital pediatric asphyxial cardiac arrest. *Crit Care Med* 1999;27(9):1893–9.

12. Berg RA, Hilwig RW, Kern KB, et al. "Bystander" chest compressions and assisted ventilation independently improve outcome from piglet asphyxial pulseless "cardiac arrest." *Circulation* 2000;101:1743–8.

13. Berg RA, Otto CW, Kern KB, et al. High-dose epinephrine results in greater early mortality after resuscitation from prolonged cardiac arrest in pigs: A prospective, randomized study. *Crit Care Med* 1994;22:282–90.

14. Berg RA, Samson RA, Berg MD, et al. Better outcome after pediatric defibrillation dosage than adult dosage in a swine model of pediatric ventricular fibrillation. *J Am Coll Cardiol* 2005;45:786–9.

15. Berger PB. A glucose-insulin-potassium infusion did not reduce mortality, cardiac arrest, or cardiogenic shock after acute MI. *ACP J Club* 2005;143:4–5.

16. Bernard SA, Gray TW, Buist MD, et al. Treatment of comatose survivors of out-of-hospital cardiac arrest with induced hypothermia. *N Engl J Med* 2002;346:557–63.

17. Brown CG, Martin DR, Pepe PE, et al. A comparison of standard-dose and high-dose epinephrine in cardiac arrest outside the hospital. The Multicenter High-Dose Epinephrine Study Group. *N Engl J Med* 1992;327:1051–5.

18. Caffrey SL, Willoughby PJ, Pepe PE, et al. Public use of automated external defibrillators. *N Engl J Med* 2002;347:1242–7.

19. Callaham M, Madsen C, Barton C, et al. A randomized clinical trial of high-dose epinephrine and norepinephrine versus standard-dose epinephrine in prehospital cardiac arrest. *JAMA* 1992;268:2667–72.

20. Cecchin F, Jorgenson DB, Berul CI, et al. Is arrhythmia detection by automatic external defibrillator accurate for children? Sensitivity and specificity of an automatic external defibrillator algorithm in 696 pediatric arrhythmias. *Circulation* 2001;103:2483–8.

21. Ceneviva G, Paschall JA, Maffei F, et al. Hemodynamic support in fluid-refractory pediatric septic shock. *Pediatrics* 1998;102:e19.

22. Chamnanvanakij S, Perlman JM. Outcome following cardiopulmonary resuscitation in the neonate requiring ventilatory assistance. *Resuscitation* 2000;45:173–80.

23. de Mos N, van Litsenburg RR, McCrindle B, et al. Pediatric in-intensive-care-unit cardiac arrest: Incidence, survival, and predictive factors. *Crit Care Med* 2006;34:1209–15.

24. Dean JM, Koehler RC, Schleien CL, et al. Age-related changes in chest geometry during cardiopulmonary resuscitation. *J Appl Physiol* 1987;62:2212–9.

25. Dieckmann RA, Vardis R. High-dose epinephrine in pediatric out-of-hospital cardiopulmonary arrest. *Pediatrics* 1995;95:901–13.

26. Donoghue AJ, Nadkarni V, Berg RA, et al. Out-of-hospital pediatric cardiac arrest: An epidemiologic review and assessment of current knowledge. *Ann Emerg Med* 2005;46:512–22.

27. Dorian P, Cass D, Schwartz B, et al. Amiodarone as compared with lidocaine for shock-resistant ventricular fibrillation. *N Engl J Med* 2002;346:884–90.

28. Duncan BW, Ibrahim AE, Hraska V, et al. Use of rapid-deployment extracorporeal membrane oxygenation for the resuscitation of pediatric patients with heart disease after cardiac arrest. *J Thorac Cardiovasc Surg* 1998;116:305–11.

29. Duncan H, Hutchison J, Parshuram CS. The Pediatric Early Warning System score: A severity of illness score to predict urgent medical need in hospitalized children. *J Crit Care* 2006;21(3):271–8.

30. Eberle B, Dick WF, Schneider T, et al. Checking the carotid pulse check: Diagnostic accuracy of first responders in patients with and without a pulse. *Resuscitation* 1996;33:107–16.

31. Edelson DP, Abella BS, Kramer-Johansen J, et al. Effects of compression depth and pre-shock pauses predict defibrillation failure during cardiac arrest. *Resuscitation* 2006;71:137–45.

32. Egan JR, Clarke AJ, Williams S, et al. Levosimendan for low cardiac output: A pediatric experience. *J Intensive Care Med* 2006;21:183–7.

33. Feneley MP, Maier GW, Kern KB, et al. Influence of compression rate on initial success of resuscitation and 24-hour survival after prolonged manual cardiopulmonary resuscitation in dogs. *Circulation* 1988;77:240–50.

34. Garcia Gonzalez MJ, Dominguez Rodriguez A. Pharmacologic treatment of heart failure due to ventricular dysfunction by myocardial stunning: Potential role of levosimendan. *Am J Cardiovasc Drugs* 2006;6:69–75.

35. Gausche M, Lewis RJ. Out-of-hospital endotracheal intubation of children. *JAMA* 2000;283:2790–2.

36. Gazmuri RJ, Weil MH, Bisera J, et al. Myocardial dysfunction after successful resuscitation from cardiac arrest. *Crit Care Med* 1996;24:992–1000.

37. Gerein RB, Osmond MH, Stiell IG, et al. What are the etiology and epidemiology of out-of-hospital pediatric cardiopulmonary arrest in Ontario, Canada? *Acad Emerg Med* 2006;13:653–8.

38. Gluckman PD, Wyatt JS, Azzopardi D, et al. Selective head cooling with mild systemic hypothermia after neonatal encephalopathy: Multicentre randomised trial. *Lancet* 2005;365:663–70.

39. Graf WD, Cummings P, Quan L, et al. Predicting outcome in pediatric submersion victims. *Ann Emerg Med* 1995;26:312–9.

40. Gurnett CA, Atkins DL. Successful use of a biphasic waveform automated external defibrillator in a high-risk child. *Am J Cardiol* 2000;86:1051–3.

41. Gutgesell HP, Tacker WA, Geddes LA, et al. Energy dose for ventricular defibrillation of children. *Pediatrics* 1976;58:898–901.

42. Hallstrom AP, Cobb LA, Johnson E, et al. Dispatcher-assisted CPR: Implementation and potential benefit. A 12-year study. *Resuscitation* 2003;57:123–9.

43. Halperin HR, Tsitlik JE, Guerci AD, et al. Determinants of blood flow to vital organs during cardiopulmonary resuscitation in dogs. *Circulation* 1986;73:539–50.

44. Hickey RW, Kochanek PM, Ferimer H, et al. Hypothermia and hyperthermia in children after resuscitation from cardiac arrest. *Pediatrics* 2000;106:118–22.

45. Hintz SR, Benitz WE, Colby CE, et al. Utilization and outcomes of neonatal cardiac extracorporeal life support: 1996–2000. *Pediatr Crit Care Med* 2005;6:33–8.

46. Hoffman TM, Wernovsky G, Atz AM, et al. Efficacy and safety of milrinone in preventing low cardiac output syndrome in infants and children after corrective surgery for congenital heart disease. *Circulation* 2003;107:996–1002.

47. Hornchen U, Schuttler J, Stoeckel H, et al. Endobronchial instillation of epinephrine during cardiopulmonary resuscitation. *Crit Care Med* 1987;15:1037–9.

48. Houri PK, Frank LR, Menegazzi JJ, et al. A randomized, controlled trial of two-thumb vs. two-finger chest compression in a swine infant model of cardiac arrest. *Prehosp Emerg Care* 1997;1:65–7.

49. Huang L, Weil MH, Sun S, et al. Levosimendan improves postresuscitation outcomes in a rat model of CPR. *J Lab Clin Med* 2005;146:256–61.

50. Hypothermia After Cardiac Arrest Study Group. Mild therapeutic hypothermia to improve the neurologic outcome after cardiac arrest. *N Engl J Med* 2002;346:549–56.

51. Idris AH, Staples ED, O'Brien DJ, et al. Effect of ventilation on acid-base balance and oxygenation in low blood-flow states. *Crit Care Med* 1994;22:1827–34.

52. Innes PA, Frazer RS, Booker PD, et al. Comparison of the haemodynamic effects of dobutamine with enoximone after open heart surgery in small children. *Br J Anaesth* 1994;72:77–81.

53. Johnson L, Kissoon N, Fiallos M, et al. Use of intraosseous blood to assess blood chemistries and hemoglobin during cardiopulmonary resuscitation with drug infusions. *Crit Care Med* 1999;27:1147–52.

54. Kamohara T, Weil MH, Tang W, et al. A comparison of myocardial function after primary cardiac and primary asphyxial cardiac arrest. *Am J Respir Crit Care Med* 2001;164:1221–4.

55. Katz AM, Reuter H. Cellular calcium and cardiac cell death. *Am J Cardiol* 1979;44:188–90.

56. Kern KB, Hilwig RW, Berg RA, et al. Efficacy of chest compression-only BLS CPR in the presence of an occluded airway. *Resuscitation* 1998;39:179–88.

57. Kinney SB, Tibballs J. An analysis of the efficacy of bag-valve-mask ventilation and chest compression during different compression-ventilation ratios in manikin-simulated paediatric resuscitation. *Resuscitation* 2000;43:115–20.

58. Kouwenhoven WB, Jude JR, Knickerbocker GG. Closed-chest cardiac massage. *JAMA* 1960;173:1064–7.

59. Kudenchuk PJ, Cobb LA, Copass MK, et al. Amiodarone for resuscitation after out-of-hospital cardiac arrest due to ventricular fibrillation. *N Engl J Med* 1999;341:871–8.

60. Kuisma M, Suominen P, Korpela R. Paediatric out-of-hospital cardiac arrests—epidemiology and outcome. *Resuscitation* 1995;30:141–50.

61. Laitinen P, Happonen JM, Sairanen H, et al. Amrinone versus dopamine-nitroglycerin after reconstructive surgery for complete atrioventricular septal defect. *J Cardiothorac Vasc Anesth* 1997;11:870–4.

62. Laitinen P, Happonen JM, Sairanen H, et al. Amrinone versus dopamine and nitroglycerin in neonates after arterial switch operation for transposition of the great arteries. *J Cardiothorac Vasc Anesth* 1999;13:186–90.

63. Langhelle A, Tyvold SS, Lexow K, et al. In-hospital factors associated with improved outcome after out-of-hospital cardiac arrest. A comparison between four regions in Norway. *Resuscitation* 2003;56:247–63.

64. Laurent I, Monchi M, Chiche JD, et al. Reversible myocardial dysfunction in survivors of out-of-hospital cardiac arrest. *J Am Coll Cardiol* 2002;40:2110–16.

65. Lindner KH, Ahnefeld FW, Bowdler IM. Comparison of different doses of epinephrine on myocardial perfusion and resuscitation success during cardiopulmonary resuscitation in a pig model. *Am J Emerg Med* 1991;9:27–31.

66. Lopez-Herce J, Garcia C, Dominguez P, et al. Outcome of out-of-hospital cardiorespiratory arrest in children. *Pediatr Emerg Care* 2005;21:807–15.

67. Lurie K, Voelckel W, Plaisance P, et al. Use of an inspiratory impedance threshold valve during cardiopulmonary resuscitation: A progress report. *Resuscitation* 2000;44:219–30.

68. Mann K, Berg RA, Nadkarni V. Beneficial effects of vasopressin in prolonged pediatric cardiac arrest: A case series. *Resuscitation* 2002;52:149–56.

69. Meaney PA, Nadkarni VM, Cook EF, et al. Higher survival rates among younger patients after pediatric intensive care unit cardiac arrests. *Pediatrics* 2006;118:2424–33.

70. Menegazzi JJ, Auble TE, Nicklas KA, et al. Two-thumb versus two-finger chest compression during CRP in a swine infant model of cardiac arrest. *Ann Emerg Med* 1993;22:240–1.

71. Morris MC, Wernovsky G, Nadkarni VM. Survival outcomes after extracorporeal cardiopulmonary resuscitation instituted during active chest compressions following refractory in-hospital pediatric cardiac arrest. *Pediatr Crit Care Med* 2004;5:440–6.

72. Moule P. Checking the carotid pulse: Diagnostic accuracy in students of the healthcare professions. *Resuscitation* 2000;44:195–201.

73. Nadkarni VM, Larkin GL, Peberdy MA, et al. First documented rhythm and clinical outcome from in-hospital cardiac arrest among children and adults. *JAMA* 2006;295:50–7.

74. Nishisaki A, Sullivan J, 3rd, Steger B, et al. Retrospective analysis of the prognostic value of electroencephalography patterns obtained in pediatric in-hospital cardiac arrest survivors during three years. *Pediatr Crit Care Med* 2007;8:10–7.

75. Orlowski JP, Julius CJ, Petras RE, et al. The safety of intraosseous infusions: Risks of fat and bone marrow emboli to the lungs. *Ann Emerg Med* 1989;18:1062–7.

76. Parra DA, Totapally BR, Zahn E, et al. Outcome of cardiopulmonary resuscitation in a pediatric cardiac intensive care unit. *Crit Care Med* 2000;28:3296–300.

77. Pepe PE, Wigginton JG, Mann DM, et al. Prospective, decade-long, population-based study of pediatric drowning-related incidents. *Acad Emerg Med* 2002;9:516–7.

78. Perondi MB, Reis AG, Paiva EF, et al. A comparison of high-dose and standard-dose epinephrine in children with cardiac arrest. *N Engl J Med* 2004;350:1722–30.

79. Piazza O, Cotena S, Esposito G, et al. S100B is a sensitive but not specific prognostic index in comatose patients after cardiac arrest. *Minerva Chir* 2005;60:477–80.

80. Reis AG, Nadkarni V, Perondi MB, et al. A prospective investigation into the epidemiology of in-hospital pediatric cardiopulmonary resuscitation using the international Utstein reporting style. *Pediatrics* 2002;109:200–9.

81. Samson RA, Berg RA, Bingham R. Use of automated external defibrillators for children: Sn update—an advisory statement from the Pediatric Advanced Life Support Task Force, International Liaison Committee on Resuscitation. *Pediatrics* 2003;112:163–8.

82. Samson RA, Berg RA, Bingham R, et al. Use of automated external defibrillators for children: An update: An advisory statement from the Pediatric Advanced Life Support Task Force, International Liaison Committee on Resuscitation. *Circulation* 2003;107:3250–5.

83. Samson RA, Nadkarni VM, Meaney PA, et al. Outcomes of in-hospital ventricular fibrillation in children. *N Engl J Med* 2006;354:2328–39.

84. Schellhammer F, Heindel W, Haupt WF, et al. Somatosensory evoked potentials: A simple neurophysiological monitoring technique in supra-aortal balloon test occlusions. *Eur Radiol* 1998;8:1586–9.

85. Schindler MB, Bohn D, Cox PN, et al. Outcome of out-of-hospital cardiac or respiratory arrest in children. *N Engl J Med* 1996;335:1473–9.

86. Shankaran S, Laptook A, Wright LL, et al. Whole-body hypothermia for neonatal encephalopathy: Animal observations as a basis for a randomized, controlled pilot study in term infants. *Pediatrics* 2002;110:377–85.

87. Sheikh A, Brogan T. Outcome and cost of open- and closed-chest cardiopulmonary resuscitation in pediatric cardiac arrests. *Pediatrics* 1994;93:392–8.

88. Sirbaugh PE, Pepe PE, Shook JE, et al. A prospective, population-based study of the demographics, epidemiology, management, and outcome of out-of-hospital pediatric cardiopulmonary arrest. *Ann Emerg Med* 1999;33:174–84.

89. Skrifvars MB, Saarinen K, Ikola K, et al. Improved survival after in-hospital cardiac arrest outside critical care areas. *Acta Anaesthesiol Scand* 2005;49:1534–9.

90. Slonim AD, Patel KM, Ruttimann UE, et al. Cardiopulmonary resuscitation in pediatric intensive care units. *Crit Care Med* 1997;25:1951–5.

91. Smith BT, Rea TD, Eisenberg MS. Ventricular fibrillation in pediatric cardiac arrest. *Acad Emerg Med* 2006;13:525–9.

92. Srikantan SK, Berg RA, Cox T, et al. Effect of one-rescuer compression/ventilation ratios on cardiopulmonary resuscitation in infant, pediatric, and adult manikins. *Pediatr Crit Care Med* 2005;6:293–7.

93. Stiell IG, Hebert PC, Wells GA, et al. Vasopressin versus epinephrine for inhospital cardiac arrest: A randomised controlled trial. *Lancet* 2001;358:105–9.

94. Stueven HA, Thompson B, Aprahamian C, et al. The effectiveness of calcium chloride in refractory electromechanical dissociation. *Ann Emerg Med* 1985;14:626–39.

95. Sunde K, Pytte M, Jacobsen D, et al. Implementation of a standardised treatment protocol for post resuscitation care after out-of-hospital cardiac arrest. *Resuscitation* 2007;73:29–39.

96. Suominen P, Korpela R, Kuisma M, et al. Paediatric cardiac arrest and resuscitation provided by physician-staffed emergency care units. *Acta Anaesthesiol Scand* 1997;41:260–5.

97. Suominen P, Olkkola KT, Voipio V, et al. Utstein style reporting of in-hospital paediatric cardiopulmonary resuscitation. *Resuscitation* 2000;45:17–25.

98. Suominen P, Rasanen J, Kivioja A. Efficacy of cardiopulmonary resuscitation in pulseless paediatric trauma patients. *Resuscitation* 1998;36:9–13.

99. Tibballs J, Kinney S, Duke T, et al. Reduction of paediatric in-patient cardiac arrest and death with a medical emergency team: Preliminary results. *Arch Dis Child* 2005;90(11):1148–52.

100. Torres A, Jr., Pickert CB, Firestone J, et al. Long-term functional outcome of inpatient pediatric cardiopulmonary resuscitation. *Pediatr Emerg Care* 1997;13:369–73.

101. Tunstall-Pedoe H, Bailey L, Chamberlain DA, et al. Survey of 3765 cardiopulmonary resuscitations in British hospitals (the BRESUS Study): Methods and overall results. *Br Med J* 1992;304:1347–51.

102. VandenBerg SD, Hutchison JS, Parshuram CS, et al. Paediatric Early Warning System Investigators. A cross-sectional survey of levels of care and response mechanisms for evolving critical illness in hospitalized children. *Pediatrics* 2007;119(4):e940–6.

103. Valenzuela TD, Roe DJ, Nichol G, et al. Outcomes of rapid defibrillation by security officers after cardiac arrest in casinos. *N Engl J Med* 2000;343:1206–9.

104. Voelckel WG, Lindner KH, Wenzel V, et al. Effects of vasopressin and epinephrine on splanchnic blood flow and renal function during and after cardiopulmonary resuscitation in pigs. *Crit Care Med* 2000;28:1083–8.

105. Voelckel WG, Lurie KG, Lindner KH, et al. Comparison of epinephrine and vasopressin in a pediatric porcine model of asphyxial cardiac arrest. *Circulation* 1999;36:1115–8.

106. Wenzel V, Krismer AC, Arntz HR, et al. A comparison of vasopressin and epinephrine for out-of-hospital cardiopulmonary resuscitation. *N Engl J Med* 2004;350:105–13.

107. Young KD, Seidel JS. Pediatric cardiopulmonary resuscitation: A collective review. *Ann Emerg Med* 1999;33:195–205.

108. Zaritsky A, Nadkarni V, Getson P, et al. CPR in children. *Ann Emerg Med* 1987;16:1107–11.

CHAPTER 24 ■ TRANSPORT

MONICA E. KLEINMAN • AARON J. DONOGHUE • RICHARD A. ORR • NIRANJAN "TEX" KISSOON

Pediatric critical care is delivered in dedicated specialty units within tertiary care centers. Critically ill or injured children who are admitted to a PICU have an improved outcome compared with children who are admitted to an adult ICU (61). Therefore, it is often necessary to transfer critically ill or injured children to the appropriate level of pediatric critical care services. Pediatric transport programs and teams permit hospitals to extend critical care services into the community so that patients can benefit from specialty care prior to and during interfacility transfer. Transport is a particularly high-risk phase of a child's care due to the need to travel in a mobile environment with limited space and resources. However, the patient's status may actually improve prior to arrival at the tertiary center due to the initiation of specific critical care therapies that would ordinarily not be available until after admission to the ICU.

HISTORIC DEVELOPMENT OF PEDIATRIC TRANSPORT PROGRAMS

Transport medicine is a relatively new specialty within pediatric critical care. The first formal guidelines for air and ground transport of pediatric patients were issued by the American Academy of Pediatrics (AAP) in 1986 (4). Shortly thereafter, the AAP granted task force status to interhospital transport, and the Section on Transport Medicine was officially established in 1995. More comprehensive guidelines were published in 1993 (32), with subsequent revisions in 1999 and 2006 (51,73).

TRANSPORT IN DEVELOPING COUNTRIES

Most of this chapter focuses on the development and attributes of highly sophisticated tertiary care transport systems in developed countries; however, many alternatives and ingenious systems have evolved in resource-limited settings or less-developed emergency medical and tertiary care networks. Transport is a neglected aspect of care in many areas of the world due to lack of resources (trained personnel, vehicles, resources to pay personnel, lack of roads, and attacks on transport vehicles during conflicts) (23). Under these circumstances, adverse events are high and improvement in outcomes is not demonstrated. Deciding whether developing and transitional countries should have PICU transport involves a balance of the overall health priorities of that community, and decisions can only be made locally with full knowledge of continuous quality improvement data. Sophisticated transport systems are unlikely to decrease overall mortality if resources are simply diverted from one entity to another. Sophisticated transport efforts may be of little benefit and may not lead to improved outcomes if pre-PICU practice (IV fluids, supplemental oxygen, bag-valve-mask ventilation and intubation equipment, proper monitoring and resuscitation protocols, etc.) and tertiary PICU facilities are not improved first (36). In resource-limited settings, therefore, the cost benefit of a retrieval team must be balanced against compelling and competing primary healthcare priorities such as nutrition, primary care, and immunizations (30). These competing interests and limitations aside, home-grown solutions include bicycles with trailers, tricycles with platforms, motor boats, and ox carts in Tanzania, and taxis and buses driven by drivers with prehospital training in emergency management in Ghana. In many other areas of the world, no transport options are available. Despite severely limited resources for such communities, from a patient perspective, the principles and considerations for sound transport medicine are the same in resource-rich and resource-poor settings.

ORGANIZATION OF PEDIATRIC TRANSPORT SYSTEMS

Pediatric critical care transport programs are part of the continuum of care of emergency medical services (EMS) for children and are intended to provide a safe environment during transport between healthcare institutions. In designing a pediatric transport program to meet the specific needs of the region served, considerations should include the resources of the referring and receiving hospitals, the characteristics of the patient population, and the area's geography and accessibility.

Most specialty pediatric transport services are hospital based. Several models exist, including the use of on-duty staff who are relieved of other duties to perform patient transport, "on-call" staff who respond from home, and dedicated pediatric transport team members who are on site and do not have other patient care responsibilities. Each program design has obvious advantages and disadvantages in terms of mobilization time, personnel utilization, and cost. No consensus exists concerning the volume of patient transfers required to justify a dedicated pediatric transport team, and each institution must consider the economic and staffing implications of the various program structures.

Established transport services have certain organizational features in common. In addition to trained and qualified staff, essential components include: (a) on-line medical control by qualified physicians, (b) ground and air ambulance capabilities, (c) a coordinated communications system, (d) written clinical and operational guidelines, (e) a comprehensive program for quality and performance improvement, (f) a database to track activity and permit patient follow-up, (g) medical and nursing leadership, (h) administrative resources, and (i) institutional endorsement and financial support (73).

PREHOSPITAL CARE VERSUS CRITICAL CARE TRANSPORT

Emergency medical service includes all aspects of basic life support, advanced life support, and critical care transport in which emergency care is provided at a scene and/or in a vehicle. Emergency medical service encompasses the prehospital and interfacility components of transport and includes hospital-based specialty teams. Most pediatric critical care transport programs provide interfacility transport but do not routinely respond to the scene of an accident or emergency, except if a crash is encountered during travel or if a multicasualty incident or disaster occurs.

Prehospital care providers have variable educational backgrounds and experience in the care of critically ill or injured children. Less than 10% of all ambulance calls nationwide are for infants and children; only a few involve advanced life support, and even less can be classified as critical care. Overall, this frequency translates into three pediatric patient encounters per month for approximately 60% of the nation's paramedics, with <3% of the nation's paramedics providing emergency care for ≥15 children per month (64). As a result, in the prehospital setting, an adult patient is more likely to receive appropriate intervention than a child who has a similar problem.

Limited provider exposure to critically ill children leads to a problem in maintaining pediatric assessment and treatment skills. It has been demonstrated that, in a program with 50 active advanced life support providers in the current EMS system, each provider is expected to have one pediatric bag-valve-mask case every 1.7 years, one pediatric intubation case every 3.3 years, and one intraosseous cannulation case every 6.7 years (11). It has also been demonstrated that the ability of a prehospital provider to intubate or provide bag-valve-mask ventilation for a child deteriorates significantly in the 6 months following initial training (37). These data should be considered when selecting the appropriate mode of interfacility transport for an ill or injured pediatric patient.

Currently, no federal regulations specifically address the emergency care of children. The federally funded EMS for Children (EMS-C, www.ems-c.org) program, founded in 1984, has as its mission to ensure that all children and adolescents receive state-of-the-art emergency care throughout the EMS system, from prevention through rehabilitation. The EMS-C program provides grants to states to improve existing EMS systems and to develop and evaluate protocols and procedures for treating children.

THE TRANSPORT ENVIRONMENT

Mobile Intensive Care

The care of critically ill or injured children during interfacility transport presents unique challenges for assessment, monitoring, diagnosis, and treatment. Thorough preparation and equipment are required to permit safe and effective manage-

ment during transport. The clinical assessment of patients, both by physical examination and through the use of monitoring equipment, is more difficult in a mobile environment as compared with the ICU. Both ground and air transport result in noise levels that can prohibit auscultation of lung and heart sounds. Vehicular motion and vibration can result in artifacts in pulse oximetry, electrocardiography, and oscillometric blood pressure monitoring. However, it is possible to perform advanced procedures in a mobile environment. Published reports have described successful endotracheal intubation, pleural decompression, and intraosseous access during both air and ground transports. In general, however, the risk of performing a procedure during transport is considered higher than in a stationary setting. As a result, the threshold for establishing a secure airway, for example, is lower when interfacility transport is required.

The capacity for laboratory analysis during transport has traditionally been limited, other than the use of reagent strips or glucometers for blood glucose measurement. Recent technologic advances have produced handheld and portable devices that enable point-of-care testing through the use of rapid assays, thus permitting the analysis of whole-blood chemistries and blood gases. A retrospective review of point-of-care testing use over 5 years by a single institution's critical care transport team showed that point-of-care testing led to significant management changes in 30% of patients, with bedside blood gas analysis having the highest impact on therapy (31). A similar prospective study was performed in which the transport team sampled arterial blood at the referring hospital and during transport; the results influenced management in 86.2% of the patients, with adjustment in mechanical ventilation being most common (68).

With advances in technology, most therapies available in the ICU can be employed during critical care transport; examples include mechanical ventilation (invasive and noninvasive), continuous infusions, administration of inhaled nitric oxide, and cardiac pacing. Limitations to the performance of specific therapies are largely due to the inability to safely secure equipment for travel. Despite this, several programs have invested in the necessary vehicle modifications to permit such advanced therapies as extracorporeal membrane oxygenation (ECMO) and high-frequency oscillatory ventilation (HFOV) during interfacility transport (28,50,72).

Ground Transport Considerations

Transport by ground is the most common modality of interfacility and prehospital transport. The advantages of ground transport include virtually ubiquitous access, low cost, and ability to respond in most weather conditions. Ambulances are more spacious than most aeromedical transport vehicles and provide the option to perform procedures or clinical interventions in a stationary setting when necessary. Specially equipped ambulances for pediatric patients have the capability to transport newborns and small infants in isolettes and can be modified to provide adequate infant and child restraint devices, even for critically ill patients.

The disadvantages of ground transport include severe winter weather, traffic congestion, and road and highway conditions. The use of sirens to facilitate the navigation of traffic, although helpful in expediting transport in urban areas, can impair the ability of the team to perform any clinical tasks dependent on auscultation. Teams that perform only ground transports should develop a strong working relationship with teams that provide rotor- and fixed-winged transports to allow for optimal coordination of efforts when transporting critically ill children is time sensitive or involves travel over long distances.

Aeromedical Transport

Aeromedical transport is widely available in the US and other developed countries. Both rotor-wing (helicopter) and fixed-wing (airplane) aircraft can be adapted for use as critical care transport vehicles. The use of aeromedical services requires an understanding of the unique physiologic stresses and logistic issues associated with rotor- and fixed-wing transport.

Altitude Physiology

Barometric pressure is defined as the sum of the partial pressures of each of the component gases in the atmosphere; it represents the force or weight exerted by the atmosphere at any given altitude. Barometric pressure at sea level is 760 mm Hg and decreases as altitude increases. At altitudes that are within the physiologic range, the component gases exist in constant proportions: nitrogen (78%), oxygen (21%), and minute percentages of other gases, such as carbon dioxide, helium, and hydrogen.

Dalton's Law states that the total pressure of a gas represents the sum of the partial pressures of the different gas components:

$$P_T = P_1 + P_2 + P_3 \ldots \qquad [24.1]$$

As total barometric pressure decreases with increasing altitude, the partial pressure of each gas is reduced. Likewise, the addition of another gas to the mixture decreases the partial pressure of all other gases.

The partial pressure of any inspired gas is determined by the barometric pressure (P_B) and the fraction of the atmospheric gas it represents. In the case of oxygen, for example, P_{IO_2} at sea level can be calculated as follows:

$$
\begin{aligned}
P_{IO_2} &= P_B \times F_{IO_2} \\
&= 760 \text{ mm Hg} \times 0.21 \\
&= 159 \text{ mm Hg} \qquad [24.2]
\end{aligned}
$$

At an altitude of 8,000 feet, the partial pressure of inspired oxygen is reduced as follows:

$$
\begin{aligned}
P_{IO_2} &= P_B \times F_{IO_2} \\
&= 565 \text{ mm Hg} \times 0.21 \\
&= 118 \text{ mm Hg} \qquad [24.3]
\end{aligned}
$$

Whereas P_{IO_2} represents the partial pressure of inspired oxygen, the actual partial pressure of oxygen at the alveolar level is affected by the presence of water vapor and carbon dioxide, both of which reduce the partial pressure of oxygen in accordance with Dalton's Law. The amount of carbon dioxide in the alveolar space is, in part, determined by the patient's metabolism—that is, *the respiratory quotient.*

The *alveolar gas equation* defines the relationship between the alveolar partial pressure of oxygen (P_{AO_2}), P_B, fraction of oxygen in inspired gas (F_{IO_2}), alveolar partial pressure of carbon dioxide (P_{aCO_2}), and the respiratory quotient (R), as

follows:

$$P_{AO_2} = (P_B - P_{H_2O}) \times F_{IO_2} - (P_{aCO_2}/R) \qquad [24.4]$$

Assuming that R is 0.8, P_{aCO_2} is normal (i.e., ~40 mm Hg), and the partial pressure of water vapor at body temperature (37°C) is 47 mm Hg, the P_{AO_2} while breathing room air at sea level is calculated as follows:

$$
\begin{aligned}
P_{AO_2} &= (760 \text{ mm Hg} - 47 \text{ mm Hg}) \times 0.21 - (40/0.8) \\
&= 99 \text{ mm Hg} \qquad [24.5]
\end{aligned}
$$

Thus, with increasing altitude and decreasing P_B, the resultant P_{AO_2} will decrease. P_{AO_2} can be restored to baseline values by increasing the F_{IO_2}. If other factors remain constant, the F_{IO_2} required to maintain the same P_{AO_2} at a lower barometric pressure can be calculated as follows:

$$F_{IO_{2(1)}} \times (P_{B(1)} = F_{IO_{2(2)}} \times (P_{B(2)} \qquad [24.6]$$

The maintenance of a specific barometric pressure in the cabin of an aircraft (i.e., cabin pressurization) ameliorates this effect to some extent, but this is possible only in fixed-wing aircraft and not in helicopters.

A decrease in the ambient barometric pressure has the potential to affect any gas-filled compartment in the body. *Boyle's Law* states that an inverse relationship exists between volume and pressure of a gas; therefore, a decrease in pressure results in an increase in volume. The formula for Boyle's Law is:

$$P_1 V_1 = P_2 V_2 \qquad [24.7]$$

where: P_1 = pressure at altitude 1
$\quad\quad\quad V_1$ = volume at altitude 1
$\quad\quad\quad P_2$ = pressure at altitude 2
$\quad\quad\quad V_2$ = volume at altitude 2

The significance of decreased barometric pressure is dependent on the altitude at which an unpressurized aircraft operates. Most medical helicopters travel at between 1500 and 5000 feet above ground level. If ground level represents sea level, then barometric pressure will decrease by 20% at 5000 feet, with a consequent 20% increase in gas volume. Most commercial aircraft will maintain a cabin pressure that is equivalent to approximately 8000 feet above sea level, corresponding to a 30% decrease in barometric pressure and a 30% increase in the volume of air-filled spaces.

Gas in normal anatomic compartments (e.g., bowel, middle ears) or in abnormal locations (e.g., pneumothorax) has the potential to undergo physical changes as a result of increased altitude, as does air in devices with gas-inflated medical components (e.g., compression stockings, endotracheal tube cuffs, etc.). In an in vivo study of intubated adults undergoing aeromedical transport, the tracheal cuff pressures increased by an average of 23 cm H_2O at an altitude of 3000 feet (39). It is essential to anticipate and address the potential for gas expansion by such interventions as gastric drainage, pleural decompression, and replacement of air in an endotracheal tube cuff (using saline) prior to transport.

Rotor-wing (Helicopter) Transport

Rotor-wing transport is much more common than fixed-wing and has a long history of use in prehospital and interfacility patient transport. The greatest advantage of helicopter transport is the speed with which a helicopter can be deployed and complete a trip. This advantage may be important in densely populated urban areas, where traffic can impede expeditious ground-based transport, but it is particularly significant for rural areas, where greater distances must be covered. Delays in helicopter response due to need for refueling, reconfiguration, or pilot duty time may reduce the impact of air transport on shortening the time to arrival at the receiving facility. Although significant variability is involved due to geography, staffing, helipad accessibility, and the need for refueling or reconfiguration, helicopter transport is faster than ground transport if the patient is more than 45 miles from the receiving facility (21).

The disadvantages of helicopter transport include a high level of noise, which impairs or sometimes totally eliminates the ability to use a stethoscope, and vibration, which can interfere with patient evaluation. Esophageal stethoscopes designed to fit under flight headphones may ameliorate the difficulty with auscultation, but they are in limited use. Hypothermia is a major risk for infants during helicopter transport if an isolette is not used. In the unpressurized cabin of a helicopter, ambient air has less moisture, which leads to increased risk of airway plugging from secretions. Humidified gases should be used as early as possible.

The use of transport helicopters also requires the presence of a helipad or a suitable landing zone; in the case of interfacility transport, it may be necessary for a helicopter to land at a local airport if the referring hospital has no on-site helipad. Time saved by air transport can be diminished by the need for ground ambulance transfer between the helicopter and the referring and/or receiving hospital. Weather has a more profound affect on helicopter transport than other vehicular modalities, and helicopter flights can be unavailable due to weather as frequently as 20% of the time, depending on the region.

Cost is another significant disadvantage of helicopter transport. The cost effectiveness of scene flights by prehospital aeromedical teams, primarily for trauma patients, has been called into question for both adults and children (14). Investigations into whether air transport has a significant impact on patient outcomes have yielded mixed results (see Outcomes section). Several studies have demonstrated that air transport is an overutilized resource for pediatric patients, most likely reflecting the discomfort of community providers with the management of children (57). In one retrospective review, 33% of pediatric trauma patients transported by helicopter were discharged home from the emergency department (ED); among the same population, only 4% were taken directly to the operating room (24).

Fixed-wing (Airplane) Transport

Fixed-wing transport is typically reserved for travel over long distances. It has the advantage of the fastest speed of the three commonly used transport modalities. Additional advantages include cabin pressurization, which minimizes the adverse physiologic effects of altitude, and the ability to fly in weather conditions that may not be favorable for helicopter transport. The disadvantages of fixed-wing transport include the same considerations with regard to noise and movement as encountered in a helicopter. Additionally, the available workspace in a fixed-wing vehicle is usually less than in either helicopters or ambulances. Use of fixed-wing transport also requires the presence of airports close to both referring and receiving hospitals, and such a transport necessarily entails ground transportation to and from the airports, with multiple patient transfers from ambulance to aircraft. Fixed-wing transport requires ad-

ditional time to mobilize due to the need to file a flight plan. Finally, very high cost remains a disadvantage.

Intrahospital Transport

The transport of a critically ill child outside of the PICU occurs commonly due to the need for diagnostic evaluation and procedures in areas such as the radiology suite and operating room. Intrahospital transport presents challenges that are similar to interfacility transport, namely, the need to provide critical care in a nonoptimal environment with limited resources.

For any given procedure or test that requires travel outside of the ICU, the clinician must weigh the risks and benefits to the patient. A patient whose condition has not been stabilized or who may deteriorate if specific therapies are interrupted should only be transported if the proposed study or intervention is essential to direct therapy or definitively manage a critical problem. The requirements for such a transport include adequate personnel, equipment, monitoring, and medications such that the level of care and monitoring provided during the time spent outside the ICU is similar to that in the ICU. Monitoring, at a minimum, must include electrocardiography, pulse oximetry, and noninvasive blood pressure. Most portable monitors are also equipped with the capability to measure arterial blood pressure, intracardiac or pulmonary artery pressure, central venous pressure, and intracranial pressure. Capnography during transport is essential for the intubated patient, both to provide a noninvasive measure of ventilation and to ensure early recognition of a displaced or obstructed endotracheal tube. Equipment and medications for emergent airway management should be available for all patients who have an artificial airway or who may require assisted ventilation. All monitors and equipment must be portable and capable of operation by battery power, with verification of a fully charged state prior to leaving the ICU. It is important not to rely on the presence or availability of such equipment in the other hospital areas to which the patient is being transported.

Respiratory support during intrahospital transport is commonly indicated; a respiratory therapist or other provider familiar with the devices being used for the patient in the ICU should be present on all such transports. A patient may either be ventilated using a manual resuscitation bag or a portable transport ventilator. In general, manual ventilation results in significantly increased variability in end-tidal carbon dioxide concentration as compared to transport ventilators (22). In a cohort of 12 children undergoing repeated $PaCO_2$ measurements during intrahospital transport, unintentional hyperventilation was very common, with resultant $PaCO_2$ levels of <25 mm Hg occurring in 62% of measurements taken (66). It is also essential to have access to an adequate supply of oxygen and/or compressed air during the anticipated travel time. Most patients can be safely ventilated with 100% oxygen during brief intrahospital transports.

The largest study to date to examine adverse occurrences during pediatric intrahospital transport found that, during 269 events, significant physiologic derangements, as evidenced by vital sign changes, occurred 72% of the time and that equipment-related problems occurred during 10% of the transports (70). A significant therapeutic intervention was necessary in 14% of patients. Adverse occurrences were more common in patients who received mechanical ventilation, and interventions were also more commonly necessary in this group (34%, as compared to 9% of nonventilated patients). Multivariate analysis demonstrated an association between length of transport and the likelihood of an adverse event, whereas no association was found with age of patient or number of team members accompanying the patient.

Safety Considerations

By its nature, interfacility transport carries additional potential risks for healthcare providers and other individuals (i.e., parents). Collisions during air and ground interfacility transport are uncommon but can result in injury to, and death of, patients, clinicians, and vehicle operators, as well as disruption of care delivery systems due to loss of work days and damage to vehicles and equipment. A survey of transport teams comprised of National Association of Children's Hospitals and Related Institutions (NACHRI) members found that a total of 66 collisions were reported over 5 years (46). No association between number of collisions and total number of transports by the team was apparent, and all fatalities occurred secondary to air transport crashes.

Despite the known advantages of appropriate child restraint devices, their use in ground ambulances is uncommon because of the perception that children cannot be adequately monitored and treated while restrained. In a recent survey of prehospital EMS providers, only half reported that they had adequate knowledge about securing a critically ill child for transport, and 23% indicated that they permitted children to travel while sitting on an adult's lap at least some of the time (40). In comparison, none of the specialty pediatric transport personnel surveyed permitted this practice. Ground transport providers should be familiar with state and local regulations regarding child restraint, which often do not exempt emergency vehicles.

PRINCIPLES OF TRANSPORT MEDICINE

The philosophy of pediatric transport advocates a seamless transition from the referring hospital to the receiving institution, with no decrement in the level of care or monitoring during travel. The initiation of specific critical care therapies prior to transport is indicated if they will improve the safety and outcome of the transport. Transferring a child prior to stabilization is associated with significant risk of deterioration en route and a delay in receiving appropriate care. For the few situations in which a time-sensitive intervention is needed that cannot be provided at the referring hospital, such as a craniotomy for an expanding epidural hematoma, one-way transfer using referring-hospital staff may be preferable.

RESUSCITATION AND STABILIZATION

It is the responsibility of the referring hospital to use its best available resources to stabilize a child prior to transport. In the interest of time, the referring physician may initiate the transport process during ongoing efforts at patient stabilization. It must be determined by the referring physician that the benefit of transferring a child to another center for further management outweighs the risk of the transport itself. It may be helpful for the referring physician to consult with the medical control physician at the receiving hospital regarding the advantages of transfer for a particular patient. Further interventions once the transport team arrives may be necessary; the goals of such additional measures are to ensure optimal patient care and safety during travel while minimizing additional time at the referring facility. These include ensuring the security and proper function of vascular lines, assessing endotracheal tube patency and position, evaluating oxygenation and ventilation, and administering additional medications such as sedatives or analgesics. Point-of-care laboratory testing may be applied when appropriate.

Not surprisingly, time spent by transport teams at referring institutions has been shown to be significantly increased when patients require advanced procedural interventions, such as endotracheal intubation, central venous or arterial access, or thoracostomy tube placement; by contrast, simpler procedures, such as IV placement, blood gas analysis, and nasogastric tube placement, have not been associated with such delays (18). The transport team and medical control physician must weigh the benefits of remaining at the referring hospital to perform procedures or to place catheters for invasive monitoring against the risk of further delays in patient transfer to the tertiary center.

Preparation for Transport

For the referring facility, preparation for the transport of pediatric patients begins with a baseline level of readiness for pediatric assessment, resuscitation, and treatment. Unfortunately, multiple studies have documented that many facilities have considerable deficiencies in the availability of specialized equipment and medications and inadequate training for hospital personnel for the care of the critically ill child (56). No uniform requirements exist for specific credentials or certifications for hospital ED personnel; these are determined by individual institutions. Facilities staffed by board-certified emergency medicine physicians may provide a higher level of pediatric emergency care; however, medical command physicians and transport teams from receiving hospitals should not make assumptions about any given level of knowledge or skill.

Community hospitals should maintain a current list of receiving hospitals and their contact numbers. Once the process of transporting a child is initiated, the referring hospital should be requested to prepare the appropriate documentation, which often includes chart duplication and copies or digital images of radiographs. When possible, it is preferable for the parent(s) or caretaker(s) to remain with the patient until the transport team arrives, to provide informed consent for the transport. All communications should be well documented, ideally through the use of continuously recorded telephone lines that can be used for all transport-related conversations.

Prior to their arrival, the transport team members should discuss and anticipate the patient's needs to ensure an appropriate level of continued care while in transit. Devices for respiratory support and vascular access should be carried by the team, and their function should be checked prior to departure. Medications in weight-appropriate doses and infusions (either in use at the time of transport or anticipated to become necessary) should be prepared in advance. Portable monitors should include the capability for invasive monitoring (arterial, intracranial, capnography) when such monitors are known to be in use or believed to be necessary for the patient's management during transport. The team should know the patient's ongoing medical issues to be able to devise a plan in case of deterioration or complications; in some instances, this may involve consultation with the medical command physician and/or relevant specialists by telephone during stabilization and transport. Additional assessment and stabilization should be thorough but efficient; the adequacy of the resuscitation and stabilization is more important that the amount of time spent on scene at the referring institution.

Communication

Initial communication should include a direct conversation between the referring physician and the receiving physician. Information provided by the referring facility should include the patient's history; the clinical status, including a complete set of vital signs; and an assessment of respiratory, cardiovascular, and neurologic function. The patient's management through the time of the call should be described completely.

The receiving physician may be asked for medical advice pertaining to the ongoing treatment of the patient. Such advice should be clearly documented. Giving medical advice to a referring facility, depending on the level of comfort and capability of the referring facility with respect to critically ill or injured children, can be fraught with potential difficulty. It is essential to provide such advice in a constructive and diplomatic way and not to convey any sense of criticism. Training for physicians who act as medical control for transported patients should include attention to the importance of effective communication.

Communication with family members prior to transport may be challenging.. Time constraints and the need for rapid interventions and evacuation very frequently result in conversations that are brief and hurried, despite an often increased level of concern and anxiety in family members. At a minimum, the risks and benefits of interfacility transfer must be explained and consent obtained, either in person or by phone. Studies have demonstrated that these brief encounters, while difficult, can be very effective at achieving levels of communication that parents view as satisfactory and that the cost incurred by delays on the order of minutes by longer family encounters is small (53). Training program educators should be mindful of these concerns and should include specific training directed toward optimizing such communication skills.

Family and Ethical Considerations

Do-Not-Attempt-Resuscitation Orders

The treatment of disorders that have previously been fatal in children continues to improve; consequently, many children are surviving with chronic conditions for longer periods of time. In some cases, these children may be at an ongoing risk of death or critical illness. With this trend, advanced directives and do-not-attempt-resuscitation (DNAR) orders are becoming more prevalent for pediatric patients. The expressed wishes of a patient and/or the family can vary considerably with respect to interventions and measures that are included in the advanced directives.

The existence of a DNAR order or advance directive does not imply that the child should not receive any treatment; in general, these orders address specific interventions at the time of a respiratory or cardiorespiratory arrest. Children for whom a DNAR order has been written may still present for emergency care due to issues with pain management, fear or uncertainty about the trajectory of deterioration, or unanticipated changes in condition. Existing data from pediatric EDs have demonstrated that patients with DNAR orders frequently present to these settings when acutely ill. Therefore, pediatric transport teams may be requested to transport a child with an existing DNAR order to a tertiary facility. The consent by a patient or parent to be transported is generally regarded as a request for a higher level of care when, in fact, many factors may lead to a request for transfer: desire for end-of-life care by familiar caretakers, uncertainty as to whether the patient is actually at end of life, or inability to control symptoms such as pain or anxiety. Nonetheless, the possibility still exists that patients or their caretakers may have preexisting preferences with respect to interventions or procedures that they would not want performed regardless of circumstances. A complete exploration of these preferences in the face of such an ambiguous situation, coupled with ongoing acute illness and the need for expedient care, can be extremely challenging. Although attempts to generate systems to track advanced directives in children in EDs are made, they are limited by design to individual hospitals and their referral areas.

Transport team members should inquire about the presence of advanced directives for patients in their care, and they should not assume that such inquiries will have been made by the providers at the referring facility. Transport team members should also obtain specific details about the terms of an advanced directive. When the patient's deterioration appears rapid, it is important to discuss the potential events during transport with family members who have decision-making capacity. When ambiguity exists or family members appear uncertain about their decisions, it is highly preferable for them to accompany the patient on the transport if possible (see Family Presence section). If family members are unavailable or unable to reach consensus, it may be appropriate to offer limited resuscitation measures in an effort to reach the receiving hospital, at which point life-sustaining care can be withdrawn if appropriate.

Death on Transport

It is unusual for children to die during interfacility transport. By policy, most critical care transport programs will not depart from the referring facility with active cardiopulmonary resuscitation in progress. Exceptions to this rule include situations such as accidental hypothermia, in which a prolonged period of cardiac arrest may be tolerated without severe neurologic injury. Pediatric transport services may respond to a referring facility to find that a patient has failed to respond to resuscitative measures but the resuscitation team chose to continue efforts until arrival of the team. Transport team members should review the patient's status for any potentially reversible causes of refractory arrest and, in consultation with the medical control physician, use usual and customary criteria to discontinue resuscitation. They may be called upon to provide emotional support for the family as well as the referring hospital staff.

Transport team members should be familiar with state regulations regarding notification of the regional organ procurement organization and medical examiner's office following the death of a pediatric patient. In most states in the US, it is illegal for anyone other than authorized funeral homes and the medical examiner's office staff to transport a patient who has been pronounced dead. Transporting a child's body to the referring facility for autopsy, for example, requires that the child be sent to the referring hospital's morgue and then transported by an authorized party. In general, if cardiac arrest occurs after the team departs from the referring facility, the team should continue resuscitative efforts until arrival at the receiving facility. Under certain circumstances and in consultation with the medical control physician, it may be appropriate to divert to a closer facility.

Family Presence

Permitting family members to remain physically present during acute medical care for their children is an issue that has been systematically evaluated with respect to CPR and invasive procedures in the ED (33,38). Policy statements that encourage family presence in these situations now exist, but to date, no such formal recommendations have been formulated with respect to family presence during critical care transport.

Special considerations related to the presence of a family member or caretaker during interfacility transport include the effect on care delivery, safety, and the emotional milieu for patients, parents, and staff. Additional seats for passengers are present in most ambulances and approximately one-half of helicopters used for transport in the United States, but opinions and policies regarding the presence of parents during critical care transport vary greatly. Possible advantages associated with parental presence include emotional benefit to the patient, decreased parental anxiety, caretaker availability for procedural consent when necessary, and improved public relations. Disadvantages include limitations of space, distraction or increased anxiety for the crew, and increased parental or patient anxiety.

Data on the effect of parental presence during transport is limited but, for the most part, report its safety without impedance of care. A national survey of pediatric transport programs showed that 63% of 103 responding programs permitted parents to travel with their children in the ambulance, but parents actually accompanied the team during only 28% of transports (75). Parents who accompanied their children during transport reported less anxiety in themselves and their children, compared with parents whose children were transported without parental accompaniment (74). Physicians and nurses experienced very little additional stress or difficulty performing interventions when necessary, and the majority of practitioners described the experience as beneficial (19). Adverse events occurred in only 11 of 279 (3%) transports, and most of the recorded adverse events were parent-related as opposed to patient-related. This study resulted in the adoption of parental presence as standard practice for the South Thames Retrieval Service, one of the largest pediatric transport services in the UK.

TRANSPORT CONSIDERATIONS FOR SPECIFIC POPULATIONS

Pediatric critical care transport team members must have a diverse set of skills and the flexibility to adapt to changing environments and situations—all perhaps within a single shift or day of the week. Familiarity with the special considerations for unique populations will contribute to the transport service's effectiveness and quality of care.

Pediatric Emergency Department Considerations

It is estimated that <10% of hospitals in the US have dedicated pediatric EDs. The majority of pediatric emergency care, therefore, is provided in EDs that serve both adults and children, whose resources for pediatric emergency care are variable. The AAP and American College of Emergency Physicians have jointly published guidelines for the care of children in the ED, addressing leadership, personnel, equipment, and policies and procedures (5). At present, no method is uniformly accepted for categorizing EDs based on their capabilities with regard to pediatric emergency care. The AAP has endorsed a statement by the Society for Academic Emergency Medicine that, whereas physically separate care areas for children are ideal, they are not mandatory for the provision of quality pediatric emergency care (7). Despite the existence of recommendations from national organizations, many EDs are underequipped for the treatment of critically ill or injured children.

Trauma Centers

Trauma is the leading cause of death for children between the ages of 6 months and 14 years; consequently, the interfacility transport of critically injured children is a frequent occurrence. It is essential that pediatric transport team members be familiar with the trauma capabilities of receiving institutions. The American College of Surgeons Committee on Trauma has developed a classification system for trauma center levels based on predefined criteria for staffing, facilities, and other resources; it designates an individual institution through a process called *verification* (http://www.amtrauma.org/tiep/reports/ACSClassification.html). Level 1 trauma centers may be classified as Level 1 pediatric and/or adult trauma centers. As expected, to be so designated, these facilities must meet additional requirements for specially trained pediatric medical and surgical specialists. Guidelines for prehospital transport destination based on trauma center level are typically determined by state or regional EMS protocols. Pediatric trauma patients may or may not be given special consideration within a state's trauma system, depending on the availability and accessibility of pediatric trauma centers in the region.

Most pediatric trauma patients suffer blunt injuries that are typically managed nonoperatively. Pediatric trauma resuscitation focuses on airway management, ventilatory support, and restoration of intravascular volume. Approximately 30% of pediatric trauma patients will require an operation at some point during their hospitalization. A retrospective review was performed of over 68,000 trauma patients under the age of 18 whose information was available through the National Trauma Data Bank (1). Excluding patients with isolated orthopedic injuries, 7.8% of patients with blunt trauma underwent emergent surgical procedures defined as surgery within 4 hrs following admission. The indications for surgery were general surgical (4.5%), neurosurgical (2.1%), or other (1.2%). When the patient population was limited to children ≤13 years of age, only 5.5% of patients underwent emergency operative procedures other than orthopedic surgery.

A small percentage of injured children (e.g., patients with expanding epidural hematomas) will require immediate surgery on arrival to the trauma center. In these cases, it is important that transport programs work with receiving hospitals to develop procedures for direct admission of selected patients to the operating room or other appropriate location. Components of a "direct-to-the-OR" protocol include a communication system to notify the appropriate surgical service(s) and other essential personnel (e.g., anesthesia, operating room nursing, blood bank, radiology). In most cases, eligible patients should already have a secure airway and any imaging that would be considered essential (e.g., CT scan) prior to surgery.

For most pediatric trauma patients, the most common complication during interfacility transport is airway compromise. As discussed earlier, despite the importance of pretransport stabilization, it is common for injured children to be rapidly transferred from community facilities due to their lack of comfort with pediatric patients. Children who were transported by helicopter were likely to be transferred significantly more quickly from referring hospitals than were adults with equal severity of injury (34).

Given the nonoperative nature of most pediatric trauma cases, trauma specialists and transport providers debate regarding whether direct transfer from the scene of the injury to a trauma center is preferable to secondary transfer after stabilization at a nontertiary hospital. Proponents of the former method cite rapid access to diagnostic and surgical services, whereas proponents of the latter emphasize the importance of early airway and shock management. Several studies have supported the position that early and ongoing resuscitation of the pediatric trauma patient improves outcome and should not be compromised in the interest of rapid transfer. The outcomes of injured children transported from the scene directly to a trauma center were compared with those of children who were first stabilized in a community hospital and later transferred by air (49). The patients were stratified by injury severity (minor = index injury severity score <15, major = index injury severity score >15). The overall mortality rate was lower for the group that underwent secondary interfacility transport (5.5% vs. 8.7%, p <0.05). The most severely injured patients were the most likely to benefit, with a mortality of 15.5% versus 26.7%. The authors concluded that stabilization at a community hospital prior to transfer to a trauma center may improve survival for injured children.

PICU Considerations

As with trauma centers and NICUs, PICUs may be classified by level based on their resources and capabilities. Guidelines for PICUs have been updated by the AAP and the Society of Critical Care Medicine (6). Level I facilities are those that provide a full range of pediatric subspecialty services and meet specific requirements for availability of personnel, equipment, and support services on a 24-hr basis. For Level II facilities, some of these resources are considered optional, with continued minimum requirements for staffing and other services. In most states, the classification of PICUs is an informal practice that has no bearing on patient triage or transfer or the type or complexity of care that is permitted at a particular institution. The availability of certain services, however, may be regulated by a state agency such as the Department of Public Health, which may have the authority to license ICU beds, approve expansion of services and physical facilities, and control expenditures for capital resources. Such regulations may impact hospital-based transport programs, which may be required to demonstrate sufficient need in the region or state to expand physical facilities or enact major purchases, such as aircraft.

Despite evidence that supports improved outcomes with admission to PICUs, a significant number of critically ill infants and children continue to be admitted to hospitals that lack pediatric specialty facilities or expertise (9). Nearly 10% of all US hospitals without PICU facilities admit critically ill and injured children, and 7% of these hospitals routinely admit these children to adult ICUs rather than transferring them to a pediatric facility. Of the hospitals that keep children, few have protocols for obtaining pediatric consultation for emergencies, and many do not have appropriately sized equipment for pediatric patients (9).

Burn Centers

The management of the pediatric burn patient may require specific resources because serious burns are both uncommon and highly complex. Although adult burn units are commonly found at major medical centers, specialized care for pediatric burn patients is concentrated among a small number of facilities, such as the nationwide Shriner's Hospital system. Transfer to a pediatric burn center is often a secondary or even tertiary transport following resuscitation and/or stabilization at a community hospital or trauma center without a burn unit.

Critical care transport programs should work with the closest regional pediatric burn center to develop procedures for the triage of seriously burned children either directly to the burn center or in secondary transfer following resuscitation and stabilization at another facility. The American Burn Association (www.ameriburn.org) has developed guidelines for the transfer of pediatric patients to a pediatric burn center (8) (**Table 24.1**). Burn patients are often transported by helicopter, but in many instances, air transport may be unnecessary due to an observed practice of "overtriage." Studies have shown that referring physicians regularly overestimate burn size, favoring the use of air transport and thus increasing the costs of acute burn care (63,65).

NICU Considerations

Unlike trauma centers or PICUs, NICUs are typically licensed by the individual state to provide a specific level of services for neonatal patients. The level of NICU care is usually designated by the state's hospital regulatory agency, such as the Department of Public Health, whose definitions may vary from state to state. The AAP recommends a uniform classification and subclassification of NICUs based on their capabilities (2) (**Table 24.2**).

TABLE 24.1

AMERICAN BURN ASSOCIATION BURN UNIT REFERRAL CRITERIA

1. Partial thickness burns >10% total body surface area
2. Burns that involve the face, hands, feet, genitalia, perineum, or major joints
3. Third-degree burns in any age group
4. Electrical burns, including lightning injuries
5. Chemical burns
6. Inhalation injury
7. Burn injury in patients with preexisting medical disorders that could complicate management, prolong recovery, or affect mortality.
8. Any patients with burns and concomitant trauma (e.g., fractures) in which the burn injury poses the greatest risk of morbidity or mortality. In such cases, the patient may be initially stabilized in a trauma center before being transferred to a burn unit. Physician judgment will be necessary in such situations and should be in concert with the regional medical control plan and triage protocols.
9. Burned children in hospitals without qualified personnel or equipment for the care of children.
10. Burn injury in patients who will require special social, emotional, or long-term rehabilitative intervention.

Extracorporeal Membrane Oxygenation and Inhaled Nitric Oxide

Extracorporeal membrane oxygenation, a form of extracorporeal life support, is provided at approximately 115 centers in the US, a number that has decreased over the past 10 years, reflecting the decreased demand for ECMO due to the use of therapies such as HFOV, inhaled nitric oxide (iNO), and surfactant replacement.

TABLE 24.2

LEVELS OF NEONATAL INTENSIVE CARE UNITS

Level I (Basic)
Neonatal resuscitation
Postnatal care of healthy newborns
Care of infants born at 35–37 weeks' gestation who are physiologically stable
Stabilization of sick newborns or those who are <35 weeks' gestational age prior to transfer to a higher-level facility

Level II (Specialty)
Neonatal resuscitation
Postnatal care of infants born at >32 weeks' gestation and birth weight >1,500 g, care of newborns who are moderately ill and do not require urgent subspecialty services
Care of premature infants who are convalescing after a course in a Level III nursery

Level III (Subspecialty)
Neonatal resuscitation
Postnatal care that includes advanced life support and/or comprehensive care for high-risk or critically ill newborns

In 1999, the Food and Drug Administration approved the use of iNO for the treatment of hypoxic respiratory failure in term and near-term neonates with clinical or echocardiographic evidence of pulmonary hypertension. As a result, many newborn ICUs, including facilities that do not have ECMO capabilities, began to provide iNO therapy. The initiation of iNO therapy in a non-ECMO center is controversial, because it may delay transfer to a facility with ECMO capability. This practice has major implications for critical care transport teams, who may be called upon to urgently transfer a critically ill newborn who is already receiving maximal medical therapy, including iNO, in a non-ECMO facility. Therefore, it is essential that non-ECMO centers that provide iNO therapy for neonatal respiratory failure work closely with an ECMO center to develop criteria for the transfer of these infants, with a goal of ensuring a "window of opportunity" during which the transport can be safely accomplished. These guidelines should be evaluated regularly by reviewing the outcome of infants transported for ECMO. A certain incidence of "unnecessary" transports (i.e., infants who are referred for, but ultimately do not require, ECMO) may be necessary if the transfer criteria are adequately conservative. Furthermore, any transport team that may be called upon to transport a newborn who is already receiving iNO therapy must have the capability of providing iNO during transport, because abrupt discontinuation may result in serious deleterious effects (3,71).

The decision to initiate iNO on transport should reflect a consideration of the potential risks and benefits of its use outside the ICU, including the severity of illness and distance or time to the receiving facility. The practice of empirically initiating iNO on transport to facilitate the transition from HFOV to conventional mechanical ventilation has been reported, but no evidence suggests that it improves patient safety or outcome (47).

Ideally, a newborn with hypoxic respiratory failure whose trajectory predicts the need for ECMO will be transferred to an ECMO center prior to meeting criteria for cannulation or becoming too unstable to transport. When this is not possible, a few select programs have the capability to respond to requests for transport by mobilizing an ECMO team that is capable of cannulating the patient at the referring facility, then transporting while on ECMO to the base institution (28,50,72). Although labor intensive, expensive, and associated with high risk, this practice has been carried out safely and successfully in both civilian and military programs.

In general, the Extracorporeal Life Support Organization recommends that a neonate whose condition is deteriorating be transferred at a time when the conversion to conventional ventilation can still be tolerated and suggests that an infant who has not improved after 6 hrs of HFOV be considered a candidate for expedient transfer (67). Individual institutions may use the alveolar-arterial oxygen difference, the oxygenation index, or the persistence of a PaO_2 of <50 torr as predictors of the need for ECMO. Unfortunately, published experience indicates that the transfer of newborns for ECMO often occurs after the patient has reached commonly agreed upon criteria for cannulation (58).

The staff at the ECMO center that accepts a newborn in transfer should clearly indicate to the referring physician that the patient is being transported as an ECMO candidate, without a guarantee that ECMO will be provided. This approach minimizes the possibility that the referring hospital or the family will question the decision to transport in the event that ECMO is not required. Furthermore, it communicates the fact that the ECMO center will be evaluating the patient and determining if the infant is an appropriate candidate for ECMO after arrival.

The decision to cannulate for ECMO may be facilitated by requesting that the referring facility perform certain diagnostic studies while the transport team is mobilizing and responding. These studies include an echocardiogram to evaluate for noncorrectable conditions or cyanotic heart disease that might have been misdiagnosed as pulmonary hypertension. In addition, a cranial ultrasound to assess for the presence of intracranial hemorrhage may be helpful. Because the receiving facility will need to type and cross-match the patient's blood, it is unnecessary to perform this at the referring hospital, unless a need for the transfusion of blood products during transport is anticipated.

ADMINISTRATIVE AND TRAINING ISSUES

Finances and Reimbursement

Emergency medical care for critically ill or injured children should be provided regardless of the patient's insurance status or ability to pay. Likewise, a transport team's response to a request for emergent interfacility transfer should not depend on financial considerations. However, it is important to recognize that transport services are resource intensive and, when considered in isolation, represent a source of revenue loss for an individual patient. Administrators must understand that transport teams facilitate patient entry into the hospital's system and cannot be expected to be independently profitable. On a less-measurable basis, the availability of high-quality transport services is expected to promote satisfaction and appreciation among referring physicians and families.

Most costs (e.g., equipment and personnel costs) associated with operating a transport service are fixed. Significant expenses include vehicle maintenance, insurance, and repairs; durable equipment; and disposable supplies. As in other areas of healthcare, personnel salaries and benefits compose most of a transport team's budget. In that transport team members are often more senior and experienced, their salaries may be accordingly higher.

Transfer Agreements and Marketing

It is important to cultivate relationships with referral facilities to improve both market share and the coordination of patient care. In the current financial climate, many smaller hospitals are reducing pediatric subspecialty services and referring sicker children to tertiary facilities. Transfer agreements establish policies that clearly define administrative procedures and the roles and responsibilities of the referring and receiving facilities. These agreements may include language that indicates acceptance of acutely ill patients by the receiving hospital, as well as an understanding that recuperating patients will be returned to the referring facility. Transfer agreements must comply with local, state, and federal mandates. The EMS-C program has

TABLE 24.3

REQUIREMENTS OF THE EMERGENCY MEDICAL TRANSPORTATION AND LABOR ACT

1. The transferring hospital provides medical treatment to the best of its ability, based on available resources.
2. The transferring physician contacts the receiving facility to determine that qualified personnel and space are available for treatment and to identify a receiving physician who will accept the patient.
3. The transferring hospital sends copies of all available medical records related to the patient's emergency medical condition.
4. The transfer is affected through qualified personnel and transportation equipment, including the use of advanced life support, if appropriate.

published sample pediatric transfer guidelines for adoption by different states or programs (www.ems-c.org).

Legal Considerations

The practice of interfacility patient transfer is regulated by federal laws that serve to protect patients who present to a hospital facility with an emergency condition. The Consolidated Omnibus Budget Reconciliation Act was first passed in 1986; one component of this legislation was the Emergency Medical Transportation and Labor Act (EMTALA). The EMTALA was created to prevent "patient dumping"; that is, the transfer to another facility of an individual who does not have the ability to pay for services, without assessment or stabilizing treatment (**Table 24.3**). The EMTALA was last revised in November 2003, and regular revisions can be expected in the future (www.cms.hhs.gov/EMTALA) (16). Although these laws pertain to the United States only, the general principle of providing the best care, including transport accessibility to all children regardless of ability to pay, should be supported by all clinicians. Physicians' awareness of the laws in their practice locale and their advocacy for what is best for children should be a priority and may lead to improvements, even in situations with limited resources (55).

Risk Management and Insurance

Because transport team members are exposed to activities that may place them at increased risk of injury and death, programs should consider requesting additional insurance coverage for staff while on transport. Unlike personnel who function solely within a hospital environment, transport team members are exposed to a higher risk of accidents and injuries during ground and air transports. Their job description may include lifting and carrying, and they may work in extreme weather conditions. Although it has been determined that collisions and crashes by pediatric and neonatal teams are uncommon, collective data suggest that one collision or crash occurs for every 1,000 patient transports. Collisions or crashes that involve death are less common and occur at a rate of 0.55 injuries or deaths per 1,000 transports (46). Although deaths occur (most frequently as the result of aircraft crashes), ground collisions account for most transport-related injuries. Injuries sustained during ground collisions tend to be moderate to severe. Because transport team members tend to be young, with many productive years ahead of them, disability coverage is important to provide financial security following an accident or work-related injury.

Quality Improvement

The construction of a well-functioning transport program begins with a strong foundation of personnel, training, equipment, communication system, and vehicles (ambulance, helicopter, or fixed-wing aircraft). Continued monitoring and evaluation of the transport program are critical to ensuring quality patient care and promoting the program's success.

Essential Elements of a Quality Improvement Plan

A written plan is essential for the development of a quality improvement (QI) program. The plan should begin with an explanation of the mission of the transport service and the goals for the QI program. It should delineate the lines of authority for performing quality measurement activities and should list how that authority interfaces with the governing body for the transport service. A QI program should establish criteria to ensure that the standards of care are practiced by individuals and groups, linking the transport team with the medical director, administrative team, risk management, and other pertinent disciplines to identify opportunities to improve care. Transport programs should analyze every component of the services that they provide to ensure effective, consistent, safe, and state-of-the-art care.

The Role of the Medical Director in the Quality Improvement Process

The medical director must actively participate in the QI process if it is to be a viable component of the transport program. The medical director serves in various capacities as a resource, supervisor, moderator, evaluator, and educator. Activities for the medical director related to QI include interviewing, hiring, educating personnel, developing treatment protocols, and directing the overall transport system. Supervision of patient care during transport (i.e., on-line medical control) via direct communication is another important component of ensuring quality of care. The medical director should oversee the post-transport case-review process, including audits of charts, recorded audiotapes, and morbidity and mortality conferences.

Quality Improvement and Accreditation

Within the transport arena, the Commission on Accreditation of Medical Transport Systems (CAMTS) is an organization that aims to improve the quality of patient care and safety of the transport environment through its voluntary accreditation process. Although originally focused on air transport services, CAMTS now surveys ground, rotor-wing, and fixed-wing programs. Accreditation consists of an application process, site survey, and program review to evaluate the program using measurable standards and objective criteria. Accreditation standards are revised every 2 to 3 years with input from representatives of the medical profession to reflect the dynamic nature of the critical care transport field. As of September 2006, 127 services in North America were accredited by CAMTS.

The most recent CAMTS standards for accreditation became effective on January 1, 2007 (www.camts.org).

Education, Certification, and Licensure

Transport team leadership (clinicians, administrators, and medical directors) should determine educational and certification requirements for their team members. Initial training includes core material that may be supplemented as needed to address specific educational needs. At present, no uniform national curriculum exists for transport clinicians, either adult or pediatric. Several organizations have nationally recognized certifications for certain types of transport team members, such as flight nurses and critical care paramedics. Although board certification or a certificate of special competency in transport medicine has not yet been established, most doctors who direct or provide care as pediatric transport physicians are board certified in emergency medicine, critical care, or neonatology. Attending physicians who provide medical control to the team must be licensed to practice medicine in the state in which the base hospital is located. If physicians in training (fellows or residents) are part of the transport team, requirements for participation and supervision must be developed. Compliance with training requirements and preparation for clinical transport experience should be documented by the fellowship training director.

Multiple, standardized life-support courses provide certification in specialty areas such as neonatal resuscitation, pediatric resuscitation, advanced trauma care, and disaster management. Teams that transfer only neonatal patients may require certifications specific to their patient population, whereas teams that transfer more than one age group or both children and adults will have additional requirements. Regarding procedural skills, skill acquisition is accomplished through initial training, and performance evaluation occurs in a precepted setting. Recommendations have been published for procedural training for pediatric and neonatal transport nurses, as well as guidelines for skill assessment and retention (44,45).

The term "scope of practice" describes the clinical abilities and skill set for each team member, and may vary depending on an individual's educational background or experience, even among staff with the same professional degree. Transport services or healthcare institutions should be familiar with the policies and procedures that govern scope of practice in their locality.

Healthcare providers are licensed by the state in which they practice, usually through the Department of Health or related state agency. Transport team members must be licensed for their professional practice according to the regulations of the state in which their service is based. Paramedics also have the option of national certification but still require state licensure. Many transport teams provide services in multiple states or even in multiple countries. It is not necessary for each transport team professional to be licensed in every jurisdiction in which they provide patient care; instead, they are considered to be practicing within their home state for purposes of licensure, regardless of the patient's location. Transport team members are typically credentialed by the institution where they are based or with which they are primarily affiliated. However, by the nature of their work, they regularly provide patient care in facilities in which they do not have clinical privileges. This situation is best addressed by the creation of preapproved inter-facility transfer agreements between the referring and receiving institutions.

Standard operating guidelines, protocols, and procedures should be established for transport team members by the team's leadership. Protocols define a team's usual approach to specific patient problems and, for nonphysician teams, provide standing orders for therapies that do not require contact with medical control. Protocols also allow the team to function in the event that a patient's condition changes and the medical control physician cannot be immediately contacted.

Resident Education in Transport Medicine

Transport represents an excellent educational opportunity for residents in training but may conflict with the efficiency and effectiveness of a dedicated transport team. Interfacility transport requires a unique set of skills, distinct from the traditional hospital-based training of most residency programs. It is essential that personnel utilized to provide care during interfacility transport be properly trained, familiar with the unique demands of providing care in a mobile environment, and prepared to handle the variety of patient contingencies that may arise during ground and air transport. The addition of a trainee to the transport team composition should only occur with adequate preparation and education so that patient and team safety are not jeopardized. Practically, space or weight considerations may be an issue, because vehicles used by transport teams have limited room and capacity. Further studies are warranted to determine if pediatric resident involvement in a transport medicine rotation improves the resident's level of skill and confidence or adds value to the service.

The Residency Review Committee of the Accreditation Council for Graduate Medical Education refers to pediatric resident involvement in critical care transport in its program requirements for residency education in pediatrics as follows: (a) participation in decision making in the admitting, discharging, and transferring of patients to the ICU; and (b) resuscitation, stabilization, and transportation of patients to the ICU and within the hospital (www.acgme.org). In a recent survey of 138 pediatric residency programs, 80% of base hospitals operated a pediatric critical care transport team (27). Team leadership was provided by nurses in 44% of pediatric transports. Of the remaining programs, 70% used residents as team leaders. The prerequisites for resident participation were variable, but most often included completion of a NICU or PICU rotation (85%) or certification in the Neonatal Resuscitation Program or Pediatric Advanced Life Support (94%). If a residency program elects to include transport medicine as a clinical rotation, a specific curriculum should be developed for resident physicians in training

OUTCOMES

It is difficult to measure the impact of interfacility transport care or events on the ultimate outcome of a critically ill patient. Most studies have used surrogate end-points rather than long-term clinical outcomes or mortality. In a systematic review of outcomes of interfacility transport for adult patients who were intubated and mechanically ventilated, data were insufficient to conclude risk factors for morbidity and mortality (26). Evidence for or against a particular practice or specific therapy is limited by the absence of randomized, controlled trials, especially in pediatric critical care transport. Two national leadership conferences have identified key questions in the field, most of which would require multicentered studies for answers (20,76).

Transport Scoring Systems

In contrast to transported neonates, the ability to predict which pediatric patients are at high risk for deterioration during interfacility transport has been elusive (15). Several scoring systems have been developed based on pretransport data, but their utility is limited by the subjective nature and variable accuracy of referring physicians' assessments. The association between pretransport variables and in-hospital mortality was studied, and factors identified at the time of referral for transport that were predictive of mortality were systolic blood pressure, respiratory rate, oxygen requirement, and altered mental status, similar to those variables that are used to evaluate risk of mortality at the time of admission to the ICU (59). Importantly, the risk of mortality correlated with the likelihood of deterioration and the need for major interventions or procedures during transport.

Team Composition

Pediatric critical care transport teams may be staffed with a variety of personnel combinations including registered nurses or nurse practitioners, physicians, respiratory therapists, and paramedics. A consensus does not exist among transport experts as to the ideal team composition, and optimal staffing may depend on the patient's condition, anticipated clinical needs, and available resources at the referring facility. In many European countries and Australia, it is commonplace for physicians to serve as team members for both prehospital and interhospital transports. Several adult studies have demonstrated improved survival for trauma patients when physicians are included in the team composition (29), whereas others have shown no benefit. To date, no studies have been conducted to evaluate the effect of physician-versus-nonphysician team composition on the outcome of transported pediatric patients.

With adequate pretransport stabilization, most pediatric transports occur without the need for advanced procedures (42). With regard to specific skills, nonphysician teams compare favorably with physician-staffed teams. A 95.1% success rate has been reported for endotracheal intubation in children <13 years of age by a single, nonspecialty, nurse-paramedic, critical care transport team (35). In contrast, other aeromedical transport programs have reported worse performance when comparing adult with pediatric intubations. It was concluded in all of these studies that additional training in airway management in children and the use of medications (e.g., neuromuscular blockade) to facilitate intubation would likely result in a greater success rate.

As might be expected, when cognitive skills are considered, a greater difference is observed between physicians and nonphysicians. The training and performance of pediatric transport nurses were compared with that of third-year pediatric residents with regard to radiographic interpretation (43). The transport nurses had <10 hrs of instruction, whereas the residents had an average of 133 hrs of formal training in radiology. The correlation with a radiologists' interpretation was approximately 66% for the house staff and 34% for the transport nurses. The transport nurses' training was apparently more focused, and they had higher scores on the assessment of radiographs with pneumothoraces.

Specialty Pediatric Teams Versus General Teams

Mortality was significantly reduced when a specialized team was employed for the transport of neonates who weighed <1.5 kg, compared with those transported by alternative means (17). Infants were warmer, less hypotensive, and less acidotic on admission to the NICU when they were transported by a physician and nurse who were trained in neonatal care.

Pediatric critical care transport exposes patients to risks that may be mitigated by the use of specially trained and equipped personnel. In a prospective study to evaluate the morbidity associated with interhospital transport by a nonspecialty team, the risk of adverse events was compared between patients who underwent interfacility transport and a control group of patients admitted to the PICU from within the receiving institution (41). Of 177 transported patients, significant adverse events occurred in 15.3%, whereas the incidence of adverse events was 3.6% in the 195 control patients. Although the severity of illness was slightly greater in the group of patients who required transport, the difference in adverse events persisted among the most severely ill patients when controlling for risk of mortality.

Inadequate stabilization and adverse events were reduced when transport team members received specialized pediatric training (52). In this study, 72% of all preventable insults on transport occurred with emergency medical attendants who had no formalized pediatric training; 20% occurred with emergency medical attendants who had received an intensive 18-month pediatric training module; and only 8% occurred when the patients were transported by a pediatric intensive care team. Similarly, it was demonstrated that pediatric patients who were transported by nonspecialized teams had a 10-fold increase in transport-related adverse events (e.g., inadvertent extubation) compared with patients who were transported by pediatric specialty teams, after adjusting for severity of illness and number of interventions (25).

A study from the Netherlands prospectively compared patient care during interhospital transport when children were accompanied either by the referring physicians or by specialty transport (retrieval) teams (69). Patients transported by referring physicians had a higher incidence of respiratory insufficiency (56.9% vs. 41.1%) and a lower incidence of circulatory insufficiency (27.0% vs. 41.1%) as their primary diagnosis. Despite this, fewer of the children transported by the referring physician received ventilatory support (47.4% vs. 72.3%). Notably, they also had a higher rate of significant complications and need for acute interventions immediately upon arrival at the receiving hospital's PICU.

In a prospective risk assessment of 1,085 children transported to a children's hospital, patients who were transported by nonspecialized transport teams were more likely to suffer from an unplanned event (odds ratio, 22.2) and in-hospital mortality (odds ratio, 2.4) when compared with children who were transported by specialized teams, after adjusting for severity of illness, age, and diagnosis (60). Mobilization time, scene time, and total transport time did not predict unplanned events or death.

A systematic review of the literature to evaluate the evidence that supported the use of specialist transport personnel for critically ill adult and pediatric patients included a total of 4,534 patients from six cohort studies (12). When adjusted for severity of illness, only one study demonstrated a clinically relevant improvement in outcome—survival to 6 hrs—when specialty personnel accompanied the patient.

In addition to outcome, transport by specialty teams has also been shown to impact costs. A case-controlled study of head-injured children was conducted, and costs associated with secondary adverse events during transport were calculated, with the Glasgow Coma Scale score used for case severity adjustment (54). Investigators found more preventable insults among those patients transported by untrained escorts than among those transported by trained escorts, with the majority of insults in the untrained escort group occurring due to hypoxia. It was determined that the additional cost of care resulting from secondary adverse events that occurred during transport by untrained escorts was $135,952.

Air Versus Ground Transport

The primary difference between transport by air and transport by ground is the reduction in time to arrival at the tertiary facility; the patients most likely to benefit are those with emergent conditions that require an intervention that is not available at the referring hospital or during transport. Examples include patients with neurosurgical conditions (shunt malfunction, intracranial hemorrhage) or those with airway obstruction that requires specialized management (e.g., foreign body aspiration, congenital anomalies). In a retrospective analysis of pediatric patients transported to an urban trauma center, it was found that patients transported by air had higher injury severity scores and were more likely to require ICU admission and rehabilitation services. After adjusting for injury severity, patients transported by air were found to have improved survival rates (57). It was estimated that approximately one patient was saved (i.e., an unexpected survivor) for every 100 helicopter transports.

The adult literature contains multiple studies that show improvement in mortality for severely injured patients transported by helicopter, while at the same time acknowledging that the majority of trauma patients have non–life-threatening injuries. A meta-analysis of adult trauma patients transported from the scene of injury to a trauma center analyzed 22 studies and 37,350 patients (13). A non–life-threatening injury was defined as one with a >90% survival based on trauma score–injury severity score methodology. Approximately 60% of patients had minor injuries based on their scores. A total of 25.8% of patients were discharged within 24 hours after arrival at the trauma center. The challenge for aeromedical transport teams, therefore, is to more accurately predict which patients are likely to benefit from scene transport by helicopter.

No studies have directly compared interfacility ground and air transport for pediatric patients. The decision to use a particular mode of transport must balance the anticipated benefits to the individual patient with the potential threats to patient and team safety.

Telemedicine

One obvious justification for the use of critical care transport services is the need for evaluation by experts who are located in another facility. New technology makes it possible for patient assessment or test interpretation to be performed remotely, potentially improving pretransport care or, at the other extreme, obviating the need for patient transfer. The feasibility of telemedicine use during pediatric critical care transport was demonstrated in a cohort of 15 patients between the ages of 3 months and 14 years (48). Patients who presented to the ED were simultaneously evaluated directly by a pediatric emergency medicine physician and remotely by a pediatric critical care physician via a broadband audiovisual link. With regard to important clinical findings, the telemedicine physician performed with a sensitivity of 87.5% for abnormal findings and a specificity of 93% for normal findings.

A specific area in which the benefits of telemedicine have been demonstrated is the use of remote echocardiography interpretation. *Tele-echocardiography* has been used successfully to evaluate newborns with suspected congenital heart disease, preventing unnecessary transport for diagnostic testing for those infants who are clinically well. The use of remote interpretation of neonatal echocardiograms was reported at two community hospitals in South Dakota. Of 72 patients, transport was deemed necessary for only 8 newborns (11%) with cardiac disease or persistent pulmonary hypertension (10). A study of a larger series of patients described the use of real-time echocardiogram interpretation by pediatric cardiologists using videoconferencing technology (62). Of the 500 studies performed, 266 revealed significant findings, including complex congenital heart disease and decreased cardiac function. The tele-echocardiography results had an immediate impact on patient management in 151 cases. Importantly, only 19 patients required emergency transport to the tertiary care center, and the average time interval between request for echocardiogram and the availability of results was reduced from over 12 hrs to 28 mins.

CONCLUSIONS AND FUTURE DIRECTIONS

Historically, the incorporation of new therapies and strategies into the transport environment has lagged behind their implementation in the ICU, largely due to cost and logistical issues (e.g., portability). Importantly, this delay provides the opportunity to evaluate whether the potential benefit of a specific treatment or technique merits its adaptation for use in a mobile setting. It is essential to remember that the most valuable resource is the trained and prepared transport team member who can anticipate the patient's trajectory of illness and respond to changes in the patient's condition. Ultimately, the safety of the journey and the outcome for the patient depend most on the expertise and skill of the healthcare providers and the strength of the system within which they practice.

KEY POINTS

- Pediatric critical care transport programs are designed to improve the safety and outcome for critically ill or injured children who require interfacility transfer for specialized care. Resuscitation and stabilization prior to transport are important principles to prevent patient deterioration between hospitals.

- Providing intensive care in a mobile environment is associated with unique challenges and risks in comparison to the inpatient setting. Aeromedical transport is associated with additional physiologic stresses that should be considered when preparing a patient for interfacility transport.

- Most critical care therapies can be provided during transport, although little evidence exists for specific treatments that improve patient outcome.

- Specialized pediatric transport teams appear to have advantages over general critical care teams in terms of appropriateness of therapy and adverse events and, in one study, reduced mortality. In most cases, pediatric patients are more likely to benefit from the expertise of the transport team members than from the speed of travel.

- Healthcare providers involved in interfacility transports should be familiar with the resources of receiving hospitals with regard to pediatric emergency, intensive care, and trauma services, as well as the responsibilities of referring physicians specified by federal regulations.

References

1. Acierno SP, Jurkovich GJ, Nathens AB. Is pediatric trauma still a surgical disease? Patterns of emergent operative intervention in the injured child. *J Trauma* 2004;56:960–4.
2. American Academy of Pediatrics, Committee on Fetus and Newborn. Levels of Neonatal Care. *Pediatrics* 2004;114:1341–7.
3. American Academy of Pediatrics, Committee on Fetus and Newborn. Use of Inhaled Nitric Oxide. *Pediatrics* 2000;106:344–5.
4. American Academy of Pediatrics, Committee on Hospital Care: Guidelines for Air and Ground Transportation of Pediatric Patients. *Pediatrics* 1986;78:943–50.
5. American Academy of Pediatrics, Committee on Pediatric Emergency Medicine, and American College of Emergency Physicians. Care of Children in the Emergency Department: Guidelines for Preparation. *Pediatrics* 2001;107:777–81.
6. American Academy of Pediatrics, Section on Critical Care and Committee on Hospital Care. Guidelines and Levels of Care for Pediatric Intensive Care Units. *Pediatrics* 2004;114:1114–25.
7. American Academy of Pediatrics, Statement of Endorsement. Pediatric Care in the Emergency Department. *Pediatrics* 2004;113:420.
8. American College of Surgeons Committee on Trauma. Resources for the optimal care of the injured patient: Guidelines for the operations of burn units, 1999.
9. Athey J, Dean JM, Ball J, et al. Ability of hospitals to care for pediatric emergency patients. *Pediatr Emerg Care* 2001;17:170–4.
10. Awadallah S, Halaweish I, Kutayli F. Tele-echocardiography in neonates: Utility and benefits in South Dakota primary care hospitals. *S D Med* 2006;59:97–100.
11. Babl FE, Vinci RJ, Bauchner H, et al. Pediatric prehospital advanced life support care in an urban setting. *Pediatr Emerg Care* 2001;17:36–7.
12. Belway D, Henderson W, Keenan SP, et al. Do specialist transport personnel improve hospital outcome in critically ill patients transferred to higher centers? A systematic review. *J Crit Care* 2006;21:8–17.
13. Bledsoe BE, Wesley AK, Eckstein M, et al. Helicopter scene transport of trauma patients with nonlife-threatening injuries: A meta-analysis. *J Trauma* 2006;60:1257–65.
14. Brathwaite CE, Rosko M, McDowell R, et al. A critical analysis of on-scene helicopter transport on survival in a statewide trauma system. *J Trauma* 1998;45:140–4.
15. Broughton SJ, Berry A, Jacobe S, et al, and the Neonatal Intensive Care Unit Study Group. The mortality index for neonatal transportation score: A new mortality prediction model for retrieved neonates. *Pediatrics* 2004;114:e424–8.
16. Centers for Medicare and Medicaid Services (CMS), HHS. Medicare program: Clarifying policies related to the responsibilities of Medicare-participating hospitals in treating individuals with emergency medical conditions. Final rule. *Federal Register* 2003;68:53222–64.
17. Chance GW, Matthew JD, Gash J, et al. Neonatal transport: A controlled study of skilled assistance. *J Pediatr* 1987;93:662–6.

18. Chen P, Macnab AJ, Sun C. Effect of transport team interventions on stabilization time in neonatal and pediatric interfacility transports. *Air Med J* 2005;24:244–7.

19. Davies J, Tibby SM, Murdoch IA. Should parents accompany critically ill children during inter-hospital transport? *Arch Dis Child* 2005;90:1270–3.

20. Day S, McCloskey K, Orr R, et al. Pediatric interhospital critical care transport: Consensus of a national leadership conference. *Pediatrics* 1991;88:696–704.

21. Diaz MA, Hendy GW, Bivins HG. When is the helicopter faster? A comparison of helicopter and ground ambulance transport times. *J Trauma* 2005;58:148–53.

22. Dockery WK, Futterman C, Keller SR, et al. A comparison of manual and mechanical ventilation during pediatric transport. *Crit Care Med* 1999;27:802–6.

23. Duke T Transport of seriously ill children: A neglected global issue. *Intensive Care Med* 2003;29:1414–6.

24. Eckstein M, Jantos T, Kelly N, et al. Helicopter transport of pediatric trauma patients in an urban emergency medical services system: A critical analysis. *J Trauma* 2002;53:340–4.

25. Edge WE, Kanter RK, Weigle CG, et al. Reduction of morbidity in interhospital transport by specialized pediatric staff. *Crit Care Med* 1994;22:1186–91.

26. Fan E, MacDonald RD, Adhikari NK, et al. Outcomes of interfacility critical care adult patient transport: A systematic review. *Crit Care* 2005;10(1):R6.

27. Fazio RF, Wheeler DS, Poss WB. Resident training in pediatric critical care transport medicine: A survey of pediatric residency programs. *Pediatr Emerg Care* 2002;16:166–9.

28. Foley DS et al. A review of 100 patients transported on extracorporeal life support. *ASAIO J* 2002;48:612–9.

29. Garner A, Rashford S, Lee A, et al. Addition of physicians to paramedic helicopter services decreases blunt trauma mortality. *Aust NZ J Surg* 1999;69:697–701.

30. Goh AYAbdel-Latif M, Lum LC. Outcome of children with different accessibility to tertiary pediatric intensive care in a developing country–a prospective cohort study. *Intensive Care Med* 2003;29(1):97–102.

31. Gruszecki AC, Hortin G, Lam J, et al. Utilization, reliability, and clinical impact of point-of-care testing during critical care transport: Six years of experience. *Clin Chem* 2003;1017–9.

32. *Guidelines for Air and Ground Transportation of Neonatal and Pediatric Patients* Elk Grove Village: American Academy of Pediatrics, 1993.

33. Guidelines for Cardiopulmonary Resuscitation and Emergency Cardiovascular Care, Part 2: Ethical issues. *Circulation* 2005;112:IV-6–11.

34. Harrison T, Thomas SH, Wedel SK. Interhospital aeromedical transports: Air medical activation intervals in adult and pediatric trauma patients. *Am J Emerg Med* 1997;15:122–4.

35. Harrison TH, Thomas SH, Wedel SK. Success rates of pediatric intubation by a non-physician staffed critical care transport service. *Pediatr Emerg Care* 2004;20(2):101–7.

36. Hatherill M, Waggie Z, Reynolds L. Transport of critically ill children in a resource-limited setting. *Intensive Care Med* 2003;29(9):1547–54.

37. Henderson DP. Education of paramedics in pediatric airway management effects of different retaining methods on self-efficacy and skill retention. *Acad Emerg Med* 1998;171:429 (abstract).

38. Henderson DP, Knapp JF. Report of the National Consensus Conference on Family Presence During Pediatric Cardiopulmonary Resuscitation and Procedures. *J Emerg Nurs* 2006;32:23–9.

39. Henning J, Sharley P, Young R. Pressures within air-filled tracheal cuffs at altitude—an in vivo study. *Anaesthesia* 2004;59:252–4.

40. Johnson TD, Lindholm D, Dowd D. Child and provider restraints in ambulances: Knowledge, opinions, and behaviors of emergency medical services providers. *Acad Emerg Med* 2006;13:886–92.

41. Kanter RK, Boeing NM, Hannan WP, et al. Excess morbidity associated with interhospital transport. *Pediatrics* 1992;90:893–8.

42. King BR, Foster RL, Woodward GA, et al. Procedures performed by pediatric transport nurses: How "advanced" is the practice? *Pediatr Emerg Care* 2001;17:410–3.

43. King BR, Wolfson BJ, Geller E. A comparison of the radiographic interpretation skills of pediatric transport nurses and pediatric residents. *Pediatr Emerg Care* 1999;15:373–5.

44. King BR, Woodward GA. Procedural training for pediatric and neonatal transport nurses: Part I—training methods and airway training. *Pediatr Emerg Care* 2001;17:461–4.

45. King BR, Woodward GA. Procedural training for pediatric and neonatal transport nurses: Part 2—procedures, skills assessment, and retention. *Pediatr Emerg Care* 2002;18:438–41.

46. King BR, Woodward GA. Pediatric critical care transport—the safety of the journey: A five-year review of vehicular collisions involving pediatric and neonatal transport teams. *Prehosp Emerg Care* 2002;6:449–54.

47. Kinsella JP, Griebel J, Schmidt JM, et al. Use of inhaled nitric oxide during interhospital transport of newborns with hypoxemic respiratory failure. *Pediatrics* 2002;109:158–61.

48. Kofos D, Pitetti R, Orr R, et al. Telemedicine in Pediatric Transport: A feasibility study. *Pediatrics* 1998;102:e58.

49. Larson JT, Dietrich AM, Abdessalam SF, et al. Effective use of the air ambulance for pediatric trauma. *J Trauma* 2004;56:89–93.

50. Linden V, Palmer K, Reinhard A, et al. Inter-hospital transportation of patients with severe acute respiratory failure on extracorporeal membrane oxygenation—national and international experience. *Intensive Care Med* 2001;27:1643–8.

51. MacDonald MG, Ginzburg HM, eds. *Guidelines for Air and Ground Transport of Neonatal and Pediatric Patients,* 2nd ed. Elk Grove Village: American Academy of Pediatrics, 1999.

52. Macnab AJ. Optimal escort for interhospital transport of pediatric emergencies. *J Trauma* 1991;31:205–9.

53. Macnab AJ, Gagnon F, George S, et al. The cost of family-oriented communication before air medical interfacility transport. *Air Med J* 2001;20:20–2.

54. Macnab AJ, Wensley DF, Sun C. Cost-benefit of trained transport teams: Estimates for head-injured children. *Prehosp Emerg Care* 2001;5:1–5.

55. McDonnell WM, Roosevelt GE, Bothner JP. Deficits in EMTALA knowledge among pediatric physicians. *Pediatr Emerg Care* 2006;22:555–61.

56. McGillivray D, Nijssen-Jordan C, Kramer MS, et al. Critical pediatric equipment availability in Canadian hospital emergency departments. *Ann Emerg Med* 2001;37:371–6.

57. Moront ML, Gotschall CS, Eichelberger MR. Helicopter transport of injured children: System effectiveness and triage criteria. *J Pediatr Surg* 1996;31:1183–6.

58. The Neonatal Inhaled Nitric Oxide Study Group. Inhaled nitric oxide in full-term and nearly full-term infants with hypoxic respiratory failure. *N Engl J Med* 1997;336:597–604.

59. Orr RA, Venkataraman ST, McCloskey KA, et al. Measurement of pediatric illness severity using simple pretransport variables. *Prehosp Emerg Care* 2001: 5;127–33.

60. Orr R, Venkataraman S, Seidberg N. Pediatric specialty care teams are associated with reduced morbidity during pediatric interfacility transport. *Crit Care Med* 1999;27:A30.

61. Pollack MM, Alexander SR, Clarke N, et al. Improved outcomes from tertiary center pediatric intensive care: A statewide comparison of tertiary and nontertiary intensive care facilities. *Crit Care Med* 1991;19:150–9.

62. Sable CA, Cummings SD, Pearson GD, et al. Impact of telemedicine on the practice of pediatric cardiology in community hospitals. *Pediatrics* 2002;109:e3.

63. Saffle JR, Edelman L, Morris SE. Regional air transport of burn patients: A case for telemedicine? *J Trauma* 2004;57:57–64.

64. Scribano PV, Baker MD, Holmes J, et al. Use of out-of-hospital interventions for the pediatric patient in an urban emergency medical services system. *Acad Emerg Med* 2000;7:745–50.

65. Slater H, O'Mara MS, Goldfarb IW. Helicopter transport of burn patients. *Burns* 2002;28:70–2.

66. Tobias JD, Lynch A, Garrett J. Alterations of end-tidal carbon dioxide during the intrahospital transport of children. *Pediatr Emerg Care* 1996;12:249–51.

67. Van Meurs K, Lally KP, Peek G, et al, eds. *ECMO: Extracorporeal cardiopulmonary support in critical care,* 3rd ed. Ann Arbor: Extracorporeal Life Support Organization, 2002.

68. Vos G, Engel M, Ramsay G, et al. Point-of-care blood analyzer during the interhospital transport of critically ill children. *Eur J Emerg Med* 2006;13:304–7.

69. Vos GD, Nissen AC, Nieman FH, et al. Comparison of interhospital pediatric intensive care transport accompanied by a referring specialist or a specialist retrieval team. *Intensive Care Med* 2004;30:302–8.

70. Wallen E, Venkataraman ST, Grosso MJ, et al. Intrahospital transport of critically ill pediatric patients. *Crit Care Med* 1996;23:1588–95.

71. Westrope C et. al. Experience with mobile inhaled nitric oxide during transport of neonates and children with respiratory insufficiency to an extracorporeal membrane oxygenation center. *Pediatr Crit Care Med* 2004: 5;542–6.

72. Wilson BJ, Jr., Heiman HS, Butler TJ, et al. A 16-year neonatal/pediatric extracorporeal membrane oxygenation transport experience. *Pediatrics* 2002;189–93.

73. Woodward GA, Insoft RM, and Kleinman ME, eds. *Guidelines for Air and Ground Transport of Neonatal and Pediatric Patients,* 3rd ed. Elk Grove Village: American Academy of Pediatrics, 2006.

74. Woodward GA, Insoft RM, Shaver AL, et al. The state of pediatric interfacility transport: Consensus of the Second National Pediatric and Neonatal Interfacility Transport Medicine Leadership Conference. *Pediatr Emerg Care* 2002;18:38–43.

75. Woodward GA, Fleegler EW. Should parents accompany pediatric interfacility ground ambulance transports? The parent's perspective. *Pediatr Emerg Care* 2000;16:383–90.

76. Woodward GA, Fleegler EW. Should parents accompany pediatric interfacility ground ambulance transports? Results of a national survey of pediatric transport team managers. *Pediatr Emerg Care* 2001;17:22–7.

CHAPTER 25 ■ INVASIVE PROCEDURES

STEPHEN M. SCHEXNAYDER • PRAVEEN KHILNANI • NAOKI SHIMIZU • ARNO L. ZARITSKY

Invasive procedures are required in the routine care of many critically ill children. Complications from these procedures can be life-threatening, necessitating careful assessment and informed consent of the risk versus benefit. Anatomically correct task trainers (e.g., mannequins) are not available for many procedures; therefore, procedures are frequently learned on real patients under the guidance of experienced clinicians. However, ongoing performance of procedures is important to assess and maintain competence and reduce the risk of complications.

CENTRAL VENOUS CATHETERIZATION

Central venous catheter (CVC) placement is frequently required in the care of critically ill and injured children. Common indications for placement include reliable venous access for medication administration, monitoring of central venous pressure and central venous oxygen saturation, parenteral nutrition, and frequent blood sampling. This constitutes increased use of CVCs and decreased use of pulmonary artery catheters for goal-directed therapies in the ICU. CVCs are also placed for hemodialysis, hemofiltration, and apheresis in the PICU.

Contraindications for the procedure are based on balancing the benefits and risks: bleeding, infection, thrombosis, air or clot embolus, vessel puncture or injury, nerve or lymphatic injury, catheter malfunction, wire-induced arrhythmia, or catheter displacement. Bleeding complications may be the most common adverse associated events, and subclavian catheters are frequently avoided in very young and coagulopathic patients due to inability to effectively compress the subclavian vessels. With appropriate training, vessel cannulation complications can be reduced using visualization techniques, such as bedside ultrasound. Recent advances demonstrate that catheter-related bloodstream infection, the most common complication of CVC, can be substantially reduced by using a "bundle" of practices advocated as part of the "Saving 100,000 Lives" campaign of the Institute of Health Care Improvement (4).

Three sites are commonly used for pediatric CVC placement: femoral, internal jugular, and subclavian. Increasingly, peripherally inserted central catheters are used from both upper and lower extremity sites, often by interventional radiologists in infants and children, but these techniques will not be described here. Although data from adults indicate a lower risk of infection from subclavian sites, conclusive data in children are lacking. Regardless of site, attention to detail in CVC placement can reduce CVC infections. Recommended insertion techniques for all sites include strict hand scrubbing prior to placement, skin antisepsis with chlorhexidine, and full barrier precautions (operator wearing hair covering, mask, sterile gown, and gloves, and use of a large sterile-field drape). Sedation and analgesia plus local anesthesia should be routinely used for pediatric CVC placement, both for patient comfort and to facilitate placement and reduce complications related to patient movement.

Most CVCs are placed using the wire-guided (Seldinger) technique, in which a needle or catheter-over-needle unit is introduced into the desired vein, blood is aspirated, and a guidewire is placed through the needle or catheter. Advancing the guidewire through the veins into the chambers of the heart, particularly into the ventricle, may cause cardiac arrhythmias. With multilumen catheters and soft single-lumen catheters, a dilation step is frequently required next and is performed by passing the dilator over the guidewire after the needle has been removed. Care must be taken to insert the dilator only to the estimated depth of the vessel, as the stiffness of the dilator may penetrate the posterior wall of the vessel. Catheters should be flushed with saline or diluted heparin flush solution prior to insertion, and their lumens should be occluded to reduce the chance of air embolism. In hypovolemic patients, volume resuscitation through a peripheral or intraosseous site prior to attempted CVC placement will facilitate successful cannulation for all central veins.

In children with severe hypoxemia or cyanotic congenital heart disease, recognition of inadvertent arterial placement can be difficult due to poorly saturated arterial blood. A sterile IV, saline-filled extension tubing set may be attached to the needle prior to dilation of the vessel. The distal end of the IV tubing should be opened, and the tubing should be raised to ~10 cm above the body surface. Arterial placement should result in pulsatile blood that pushes saline from the tubing at this level, while venous placement frequently results in oscillations of the fluid column with respiration. In patients with low venous pressures, the fluid will frequently flow into the patient at the 10-cm height, and care should be taken to avoid air embolism. In equivocal cases, a sterile pressure transducer set can be attached to the tubing to verify pressures and differentiate arterial and venous waveforms. The preferred location for the tip of the catheter is controversial and not supported by good data. Most authorities recommend placement at or above the junction of the superior vena cava and right atrium for upper body catheters (44).

Femoral Venous Catheterization

For femoral venous cannulation, the lower extremity should be positioned with slight external rotation at the hip and flexion at the knee (frog-leg appearance). A rolled towel under the buttock may facilitate successful venous access, particularly in smaller children. Restraining the leg in the desired position

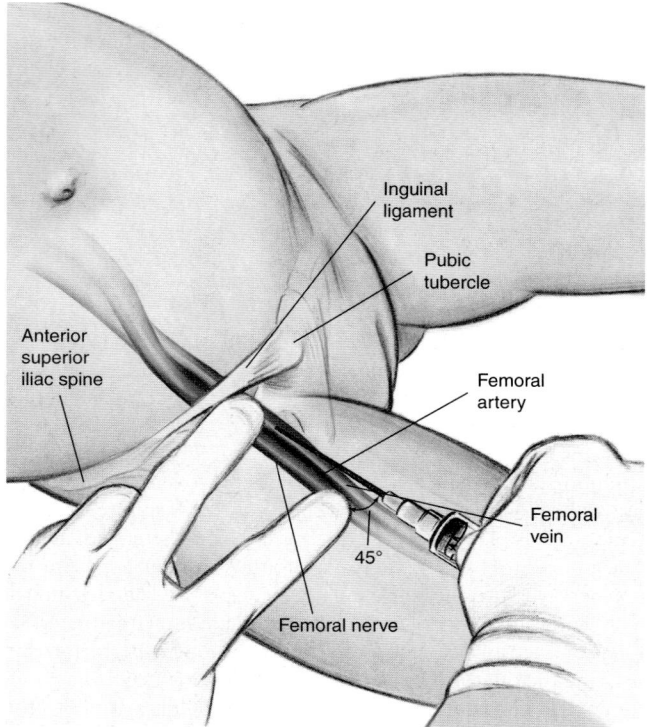

FIGURE 25.1. Femoral vein cannulation technique. From *Pediatric Advanced Life Support.* American Heart Association, Inc., 2002, with permission.

will help to maintain optimal conditions. The femoral artery should be located by palpation or ultrasound or, in the pulseless patient, assumed to be at the midpoint between the pubic symphysis and anterior superior iliac spine. The area over the intended puncture site should be infiltrated with local anesthetic. During cardiopulmonary resuscitation, pulsations may be felt in the femoral vein or artery; therefore if cannulation is not successful medial to the pulsations, one should aim for the pulsation during cardiopulmonary resuscitation. The needle should be inserted 1–2 cm below the inguinal ligament, just medial to the femoral artery, and slowly advanced while negative pressure is applied to a syringe attached to the introducer needle (**Fig. 25.1**). The needle should be directed at a 15–45-degree angle toward the umbilicus, depending on the size of the child, with a flatter approach used in infants than in older children. Once the free flow of venous blood is observed, the syringe should be removed while the needle is carefully stabilized and the guidewire is introduced gently. Some manufacturers include a specially designed syringe (Raulerson) that allows the guidewire to pass through the syringe without removing the needle when placing larger catheters. The guidewire should pass easily with minimal resistance; *force should not be applied* to overcome a great deal of resistance. Once the guidewire is in place, the Seldinger technique (as described earlier) should be employed. Some experts recommend a lateral abdominal x-ray when femoral venous catheters are placed to document that the catheter has not been placed in the lumbar venous placement (8). Lumbar venous placement occurs more commonly from the left versus the right femoral vein. The catheter should be secured with suture or a special sutureless catheter securement device (e.g., Stat-lock, Venetec International, San Diego, California).

Subclavian Venous Catheterization

For cannulation of the subclavian vein, positioning of the patient in a head-down position (Trendelenburg) of approximately 30 degrees increases upper body venous pressures, which causes distention of the central veins. This positioning also minimizes the risk of introduced air embolism traveling to the brain. The patient's neck should be extended and a rolled towel placed beneath the patient, along the axis of the thoracic spine. However, some authorities recommend keeping the head in a neutral (midline) position in children to optimize the diameter of the vein (36) or slightly flexing the neck and turning the head toward the puncture site when using the right side approach in infants (26). The shoulders should be maintained in neutral position with the arms at the patient's side (56).

In the smaller intubated patient, sedation, analgesia, and temporary neuromuscular blockade will facilitate proper patient positioning and reduce complications related to patient movement. In intubated patients, care should be taken to avoid kinking, disconnection, or dislodgement of the endotracheal tube. Bilateral breath sounds should be verified after proper patient positioning. Both the left and right sides have been advocated as preferable, although no clear-cut evidence exists for one side versus the other. The junction of the middle and proximal thirds of the clavicle should be located, and a small (25-gauge) needle should be used to infiltrate local anesthesia. The needle should be introduced just under the clavicle at the junction of the middle and medial thirds and slowly advanced while negative pressure is applied with an attached syringe (**Fig. 25.2**). The needle should be inserted parallel with the frontal plane and directed medially and slightly cephalad, under the clavicle toward the lower end of the fingertip in the sternal notch. When patients are mechanically ventilated, the needle is advanced while someone holds the ventilator in an expiratory hold position to minimize the risk of pneumothorax. When free flow of venous blood is obtained, the needle should be stabilized and the syringe removed while a fingertip is placed over the needle hub to prevent air entrainment. The guidewire should be introduced during inspiration in a patient on positive-pressure ventilation or during exhalation in a spontaneously breathing patient (to avoid air embolus). The Seldinger technique as described above should then be followed. Once the CVC is placed, the catheter should be secured with sutures and a chest x-ray should be obtained to verify catheter location prior to using the catheter and to rule out complications, such as pneumothorax or hemothorax.

Internal Jugular Catheterization

Internal jugular catheterization can be achieved via multiple approaches. Right-sided approaches are preferred due to potential injury to the thoracic duct on the left side. The carotid artery should be palpated, as it lies medial to the internal jugular vein within the carotid sheath. For all approaches, the patient should be positioned supine and in a slight (15–30 degree) Trendelenburg position, with a roll under the shoulders and with the head turned away from the puncture site.

In the anterior approach, the needle is introduced along the anterior margin of the sternocleidomastoid, halfway between the mastoid process and sternum and directed toward

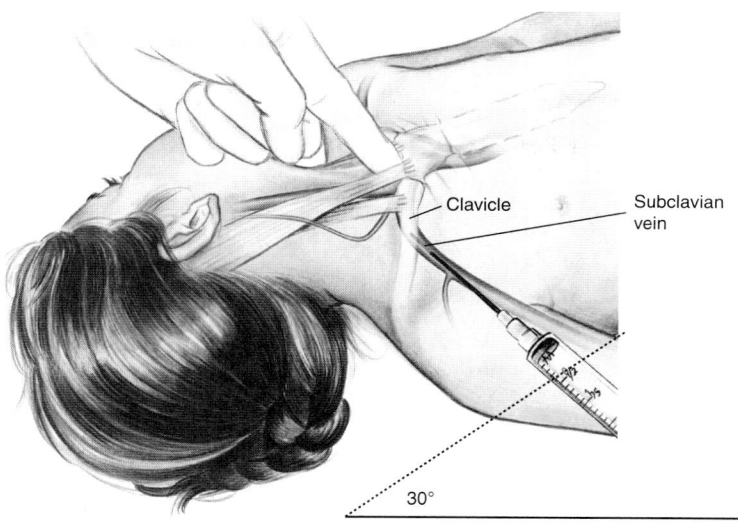

FIGURE 25.2. Cannulation of the subclavian vein. From *Pediatric Advanced Life Support*. American Heart Association, Inc., 2002, with permission.

the ipsilateral nipple (**Fig. 25.3A**). In the middle approach, the needle enters the apex of a triangle formed by the clavicle and the heads of the sternocleidomastoid muscle (**Fig. 25.3B**). The skin should be punctured with the needle at a 30-degree angle while the needle is directed toward the ipsilateral nipple. For the posterior approach, the needle should be introduced along the posterior border of the sternocleidomastoid cephalad to its bifurcation into the sternal and clavicular heads (**Fig. 25.3C**). The needle should be aimed toward the suprasternal notch. In all approaches, the needle should be advanced during exhalation to minimize the chance of pneumothorax, and the syringe should be aspirated as the needle is advanced. When the vein is entered and free flow of venous blood is established, the needle should be stabilized and the syringe removed while the hub of the needle is covered to prevent air entrainment. The guidewire should then be introduced and advanced a distance that approximates the distance to the junction of the superior vena cava and right atrium.

Complications

Early complications include early perforations (vessels and other structures) that may be related to the needle, guidewire, dilator, or catheter, or later perforations related to catheter-induced erosion. Hemothorax, hydrothorax, and pericardial tamponade may occur with upper body CVCs or long femoral CVCs. The risk of catheter-induced erosion increases with stiffer catheters and when the catheter tip abuts a vessel or cardiac wall. Pneumothoraces may occur using the subclavian and internal jugular approaches, whereas retroperitoneal hemorrhage may occur using femoral approaches. Hemorrhagic complications may be reduced through the correction of coagulopathies prior to CVC attempts. Catheter fracture may occur at any point, and may require retrieval under fluoroscopy.

Catheter-related bloodstream infection (CRBSI) is the most common complication of CVC and can be reduced by employing strict attention to the insertion technique. In addition to insertion technique, minimizing entry into the catheter, daily assessment of the continued need for the catheter, and employing chlorhexidine skin prep during dressing changes are recommended (40). A chlorhexidine-containing sponge at the insertion site may also reduce CRBSI (35). For longer-term catheters, a vancomycin-heparin lock solution reduces CRBSI when the catheters are not being used (18), although daily evaluation for the continued need for the catheter is considered an important part of CRBSI-reduction strategies. Both antibiotic-impregnated and antiseptic-impregnated catheters have been shown to reduce CRBSI; comparisons between the two products have demonstrated lower CRBSI rates, with rifampin/minocycline catheters compared to chlorhexidine/silver sulfadiazine-treated products (13). Deep venous thrombosis is associated with all catheters sites but is most frequently recognized with femoral venous catheters (57).

Ultrasound Assistance in Central Venous Catheter Placement

Ultrasonography is used increasingly at the bedside to assist in the placement of CVCs. While many of the reports describe the technique for adults, recent reports demonstrate the usefulness of ultrasound guidance to reduce complications in infants and children when the internal jugular vein is being cannulated (9,61). One small series reported the use of ultrasound in pediatric femoral vein catheterization (50). A number of commercial systems are available; most of these are designed for adults, but some manufacturers have modified their technology for use in pediatrics. A higher-frequency probe that provides good anatomic detail is necessary in children. The anatomy seen for internal jugular catheter placement is demonstrated in **Figure 25.4**.

Some operators use the technology to mark the vein prior to attempted puncture (static technique), while others use real-time imaging to guide the needle puncture and CVC placement (dynamic technique). In a study of adults at an academic medical center emergency department, the use of bedside ultrasound was demonstrated to decrease by more than fourfold the mean time from skin puncture to obtaining a blood return (38). A review of published trials demonstrated a significant reduction in failure rate, number of attempts, and arterial puncture when ultrasound was compared to conventional technique using anatomical landmarks, but the technique increased costs in adults (29). A meta-analysis of published pediatric trials

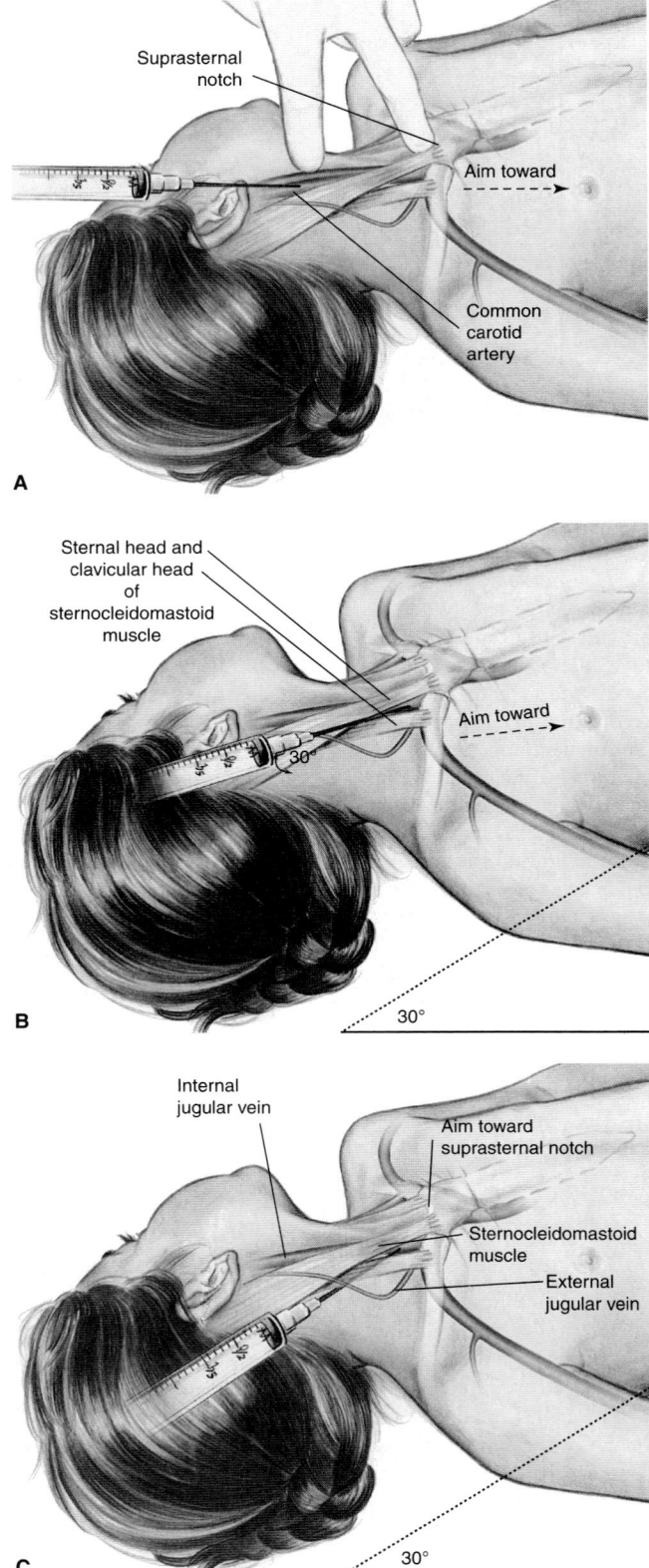

FIGURE 25.3. Technique for catheterization of the internal jugular vein. **A:** Anterior route. **B:** Middle route. **C:** Posterior route. From *Pediatric Advanced Life Support*. American Heart Association, Inc., 2002, with permission.

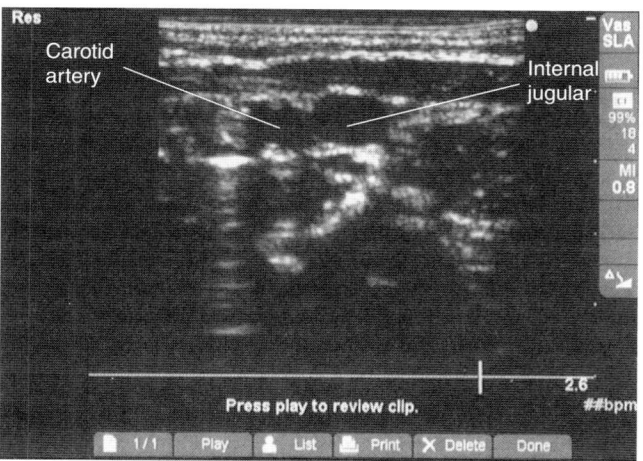

FIGURE 25.4. Anatomy seen during an ultrasound-assisted placement of a central venous line.

demonstrated an overall risk reduction of 85% for failed placement and a 73% risk reduction in complications when using ultrasound for internal jugular approaches (25).

Higher success rates are generally found when real-time images are obtained and used to guide needle and catheter insertion during the procedure. In children, an assistant can be very helpful to keep the transducer in the correct position. To maintain strict antisepsis, the assistant must utilize full-barrier precautions and use a long, sterile sheath to maintain the integrity of the sterile field. Ultrasonic gel is also required inside the sterile sheath.

To train providers on CVC placement, anatomic models are available (Blue Phantom, Kirkland, WA) that can be used to simulate ultrasound-guided CVC placement for adults. Other nonanatomically correct models allow practicing the use of ultrasound for the puncture of smaller vessels, and some centers use turkey thighs for practicing vessel cannulation using ultrasound guidance.

INTRAOSSEOUS INFUSION

Intraosseous (IO) needle placement and infusion are essential techniques for pediatric resuscitation. Recent guidelines recommend IO access for all ages and during cardiopulmonary arrest when no vascular access is present (1). IO infusions have drug delivery times equivalent to peripheral and central IVs and can be used to administer all medications that can be given IV. Blood can be drawn for laboratory analyses and culture, and this route can deliver continuous medication infusions. The IO route is preferred for drug delivery during cardiopulmonary resuscitation compared with endotracheal drug delivery.

The most common site for IO placement is the proximal tibia. The distal tibia, distal femur, calcaneus, and anterior superior iliac spine are alternate lower body sites (**Fig. 25.5**). For the upper body, use of the humerus and radius has been described (**Fig. 25.6**). A sternal IO catheter placement system is available for adults (FAST, Pyng Medical, Richmond, British Colombia). Spring-loaded needles (BIG, WaisMed, Houston, TX) are available in both adult and pediatric sizes. A drill for IO access (EZ-IO, Vidacare Corp., San Antonio, TX) has also been approved by the U.S. Food and Drug Administration for

use in the tibia and humerus of both children and adults. Because commercial products and their insertion techniques vary widely, practitioners should refer to manufacturers' direction for the use and insertion of these newer IO devices.

Although standard hypodermic needles and spinal needles have been used, success rates are lower with these than with the use of a bone marrow aspiration or biopsy needle with a stylet. Moreover, a needle with a stylet is recommended to limit the risk of obstructing the needle lumen with bone during insertion.

The desired placement site should be located; in all cases, placing an IO needle into a fractured bone should be avoided. The overlying skin should be prepared with chlorhexidine or povidone-iodine and the extremity supported on a firm surface; the physician's hand should not be placed behind the extremity. If the IO is being placed near a joint, the needle should be directed slightly away from the joint, although injury to the epiphysis is unlikely. The needle should be advanced through the skin, and when the needle reaches the periosteum, a firm twisting motion should be used to advance the needle through the cortical bone into the marrow cavity. It is important to twist, rather than push, the needle into the bone to minimize bending of the needle. Once a decrease in resistance is felt, the needle should be advanced no further. The cap should then be unscrewed and the stylet removed from the needle. Aspiration of bone marrow should be attempted; if no marrow can be aspirated, infusion of a small amount of saline should be attempted. Infusion with little or no resistance indicates successful placement. At this point, a reattempt at aspiration will yield pink-tinged saline in the syringe hub. The IO needle should be stabilized, and 10–20 mL of normal saline should be injected while signs of infiltration are noted (swelling or induration). If successful placement is confirmed, an infusion set should be connected to the needle for fluid and drug administration.

Multiple IO attempts should not be made in the same bone due to potential extravasation of medications and fluids from the site of a previous attempt. IO infusions are indicated only for short-term use (hours) until more reliable vascular access can be obtained. Complications of IO infusion include infection, compartment syndrome, and, potentially, growth failure if the IO is placed in the epiphysis. The area should be frequently observed during fluid administration in order to detect infiltration as early as possible. While fat emboli have been documented in the pulmonary circulation of animals that have an IO placed, no effects on gas exchange or pulmonary shunt were observed (41). The IO should be removed as soon as sufficient IV access has been established.

ARTERIAL CATHETERIZATION

Arterial access is frequently used in the care of critically ill infants and children for arterial blood gas and other blood sampling, as well as continuous blood pressure monitoring. Like central venous catheterization, sedation and analgesia plus local anesthesia facilitate the successful placement of arterial lines. To minimize infection risks, sterile technique should be employed in the placement of arterial catheters.

Radial artery catheterization is frequently performed in the PICU, although radial artery catheter placement can be difficult in patients with shock. Some authorities recommend

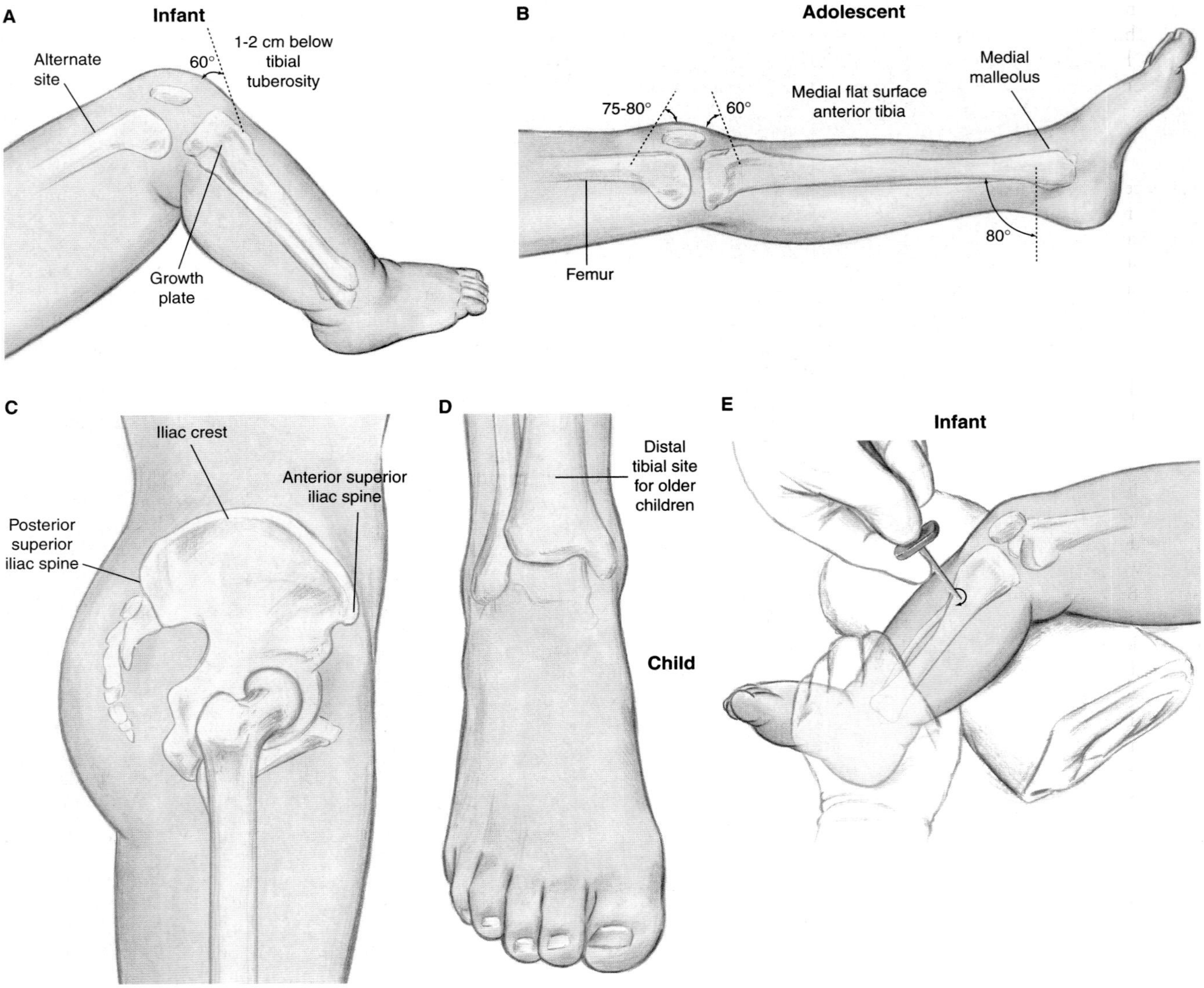

A **Infant**

Alternate site

60°

1-2 cm below tibial tuberosity

Growth plate

B **Adolescent**

75-80°

60°

Medial flat surface anterior tibia

Medial malleolus

80°

Femur

C

Iliac crest

Anterior superior iliac spine

Posterior superior iliac spine

D

Distal tibial site for older children

Child

E **Infant**

FIGURE 25.5. **A**: Locations for intraosseous infusion (IOI) in an infant. **B**: Locations for IOI in the distal tibia and the femur in older children. **C**: Location for IOI in the iliac crest. **D**: Location for IOI in the distal tibia. **E**: Technique for IOI infusion needle. From *Pediatric Advanced Life Support*. American Heart Association, Inc., 2002, with permission.

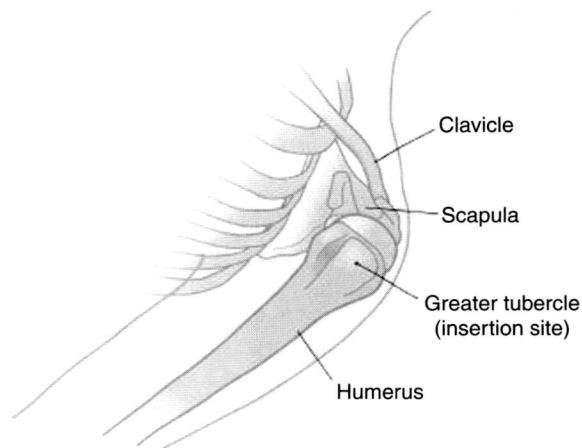

Clavicle

Scapula

Greater tubercle (insertion site)

Humerus

FIGURE 25.6. Placement of intraosseous needle in the humerus.

verifying and documenting collateral circulation through the palmar arch via the use of the modified Allen's test. In this bedside test, the blood is displaced from the hand while both the ulnar and radial arteries are occluded. After the hand becomes pale, the pressure on the ulnar artery is released. The hand should regain its well-perfused state quickly after release of the ulnar artery if collateral circulation is adequate.

For catheterization of the radial artery, the wrist should be placed on an appropriately sized arm board with a small roll under the dorsal surface of the wrist. In the responsive patient, local anesthesia should be infiltrated on the radial pulse after skin antisepsis with chlorhexidine. Some authors recommend puncture of the skin surface with a 20-gauge needle to reduce the chance of damaging the catheter as it passes through the skin.

Once the skin has been entered, several techniques can be used to pass the catheter. In all approaches, the catheter should be advanced over the needle assembly at a 30-degree angle to the skin. Some operators prefer to pass the needle completely through the artery in order to transfix the vessel. Once blood return has ceased, the needle is withdrawn slightly, and the catheter is advanced once blood flow returns. Other techniques include inserting a catheter over the needle through the skin until blood flow is noted. At that point, the catheter is slowly advanced while the needle is kept immobile. The catheter should advance easily. The third technique involves placement of the catheter using the Seldinger technique.

Once the catheter is in place, tubing connected to a pressure monitoring system should be attached. Attachment of the tubing should include a Luer-lock design to minimize the chance of exsanguination from a disconnected arterial catheter. For this reason, pressure monitoring should be instituted quickly so that a disconnection in the system will be rapidly recognized. The catheter should be secured in place using suture, tape, or a specially designed arterial access anchoring device.

The femoral artery is occasionally used in hemodynamically unstable patients when other access sites are difficult. The patient should be positioned in the same manner as described for femoral venous catheterization. The site of puncture should be directly over the point of maximal pulsation in the femoral triangle. Because of the relatively deeper location of the femoral artery, the Seldinger technique is recommended for this site. Complications are related to emboli and thrombosis of the artery. Emboli from the femoral artery may travel distally and cause foot or toe ischemia.

Both the dorsalis pedis and posterior tibial arteries can be cannulated in the foot. The posterior tibial artery is best approached with the foot dorsiflexed, while the dorsalis pedis artery is cannulated with the foot in mid-plantar flexion.

The axillary artery is rarely used in children but can occasionally be a useful location when other sites have been exhausted or the condition of overlying skin prohibits their use (22). The Seldinger technique is preferred for this site. When the axillary artery is used, great care should be taken to eliminate all bubbles from the tubing circuit, as flushing can introduce air bubbles in a retrograde fashion into the subclavian artery, and they potentially can move into the carotid and cerebral circulation. Due to the absence of collateral circulation, the brachial artery is not recommended for arterial access.

For radial (and presumably other peripheral) catheters, use of a papaverine-containing heparin saline solution has been demonstrated to prolong arterial catheter life (24).

THORACENTESIS/TUBE THORACOSTOMY

Tube thoracostomy or thoracentesis is sometimes required in the management of critically ill and injured infants and children. Both procedures may be rapidly required for patients in extremis, or they may be performed in a purely elective manner. Both procedures may be required to drain abnormal accumulations of matter within the chest, which may include air (pneumothorax), blood (hemothorax), fluids (hydrothorax), or pus (empyema). Any abnormal collection in the pleural space may interfere with respiratory function and, in severe cases, will impair cardiovascular function. In simple pneumothorax, air accumulates in the pleural space surrounding the lung, caus-

ing a collapse of a portion of the lung on the affected side. When the pressure rises and exceeds the pressure in the opposite side of the chest, the affected side shifts the mediastinum toward the unaffected side and further impairs gas exchange in the functioning lung (tension pneumothorax). In this condition, when the pressure rises to a level above central venous pressure, cardiac output is impaired through the inhibition of venous return and may result in cardiopulmonary arrest. When the pleural space has direct communication with the atmosphere in a spontaneously breathing patient, open pneumothorax ("sucking chest wound") is present.

Not all pneumothoraces require drainage. In small pneumothoraces in spontaneously breathing patients, observation alone may be sufficient, although data in children are lacking. Breathing 100% oxygen may be helpful in facilitating reabsorption of the pneumothorax.

Needle Thoracostomy

Emergent decompression is indicated when a tension pneumothorax is suspected in a deteriorating patient. In these circumstances, awaiting a confirmatory chest x-ray is unnecessary. A needle or catheter-over-needle unit (IV catheter) is inserted perpendicular to the chest wall and advanced along the superior border of the third rib (second intercostal space) in the midclavicular line until a rush of air is heard. A syringe may also be attached to the end of the needle-catheter unit and air aspirated as the procedure is completed. When a catheter-over-needle unit is used, the needle is removed and the catheter is left in place. When spontaneous respirations are present, a stopcock should be attached to prevent air entry into the chest. Repeated aspiration of air through a syringe attached to the stopcock may be required until a tube thoracostomy can be performed.

Thoracentesis

Thoracentesis may be used to symptomatically relieve respiratory distress in patients with large effusions (e.g., postoperative cardiac surgery patients) and capillary leak syndromes (e.g., sepsis) and to obtain pleural fluid for diagnostic studies.

Contraindications to thoracentesis are relative and must be weighed against the risks and benefits. If a small volume of fluid is present, the risks are substantially higher, as they are in patients who are coagulopathic or uncooperative or in patients who are being ventilated with positive pressure. Sedation and analgesia are generally required in pediatric patients and are discussed in Chapter 12. Topical anesthetics, such as lidocaine-prilocaine or liposomal lidocaine, applied at least 1 hr prior to the procedure may reduce the discomfort of the infiltration of local anesthetics.

When possible, patients are generally positioned in a seated, upright position to obtain pleural fluid. A young child may be held in an upright position by an assistant, or an older child may be positioned leaning over a padded tray table. In mechanically ventilated patients, using a partial lateral decubitus position, with the side containing the fluid in the dependent position (generally with the patient at a 30–45-degree angle to the bed), may facilitate obtaining fluid. For simple aspiration of air, the supine position can be used with the technique described under needle decompression.

The usual site for a thoracentesis to obtain fluid is the posterior axillary line near the tip of the scapula, which represents the seventh intercostal space during full inspiration. The area is cleaned with an antiseptic, such as chlorhexidine or povidone-iodine, and the area is infiltrated with local anesthetic using a fine (27–30-gauge) needle. A longer, 22–25-gauge needle is then used to infiltrate local anesthetic into the deeper soft tissue and to locate the superior border of the rib, to avoid the neurovascular bundle that runs under the inferior surface of the rib. The periosteum is infiltrated, and the needle is advanced into the pleural space until fluid is aspirated. The depth at which the fluid is obtained should be noted and can be marked by clamping a sterile hemostat to the needle at the skin when the proper insertion depth is noted. If a catheter-over-needle unit is used, the unit is advanced just past the point at which fluid is obtained; the plastic catheter is then advanced into the chest cavity. The needle is then removed, and a stopcock or extension tubing is attached. If the fluid is very viscous, a larger (14–16-gauge) needle or catheter will facilitate successful removal of the fluid, while a smaller gauge (20–22-gauge) may be sufficient for thin fluid. Aspiration should be continued until the desired volume for diagnostic studies is aspirated or until respiratory distress is relieved if the procedure is for symptom control.

Pneumothorax may occur after thoracentesis, and a chest x-ray is frequently obtained after the procedure. Pneumothorax is more common when patients are undergoing positive pressure ventilation. Hemothorax may also occur. Pulmonary edema from a large volume of fluid removal has not been described in children, although it has been noted in adults when over 1 L of fluid is removed.

Tube Thoracostomy

Tube thoracostomy is performed in the PICU setting for the ongoing drainage of air or pleural fluid. Tube thoracostomy may also be required in the care of postoperative cardiac patients for the management of pleural effusions and chylothoraces. As with thoracentesis, no definite contraindications are associated with tube thoracostomy, but coagulopathies should be corrected when feasible in non–life-threatening situations. In patients with hemothorax, the hemothorax may tamponade ongoing bleeding; therefore, adequate vascular access and volume resuscitation should precede drainage, and blood should be readily available to anticipate the need for rapid blood transfusion.

Sedation and analgesia are generally required in pediatric patients, as this procedure is quite painful. Generous local anesthesia will decrease sedation and analgesia requirements, although care must be taken with small children to avoid inadvertent administration of a toxic dose of local anesthesia (maximum dose of lidocaine without epinephrine, 5 mg/kg or 1 mL/kg of a 0.5% solution; lidocaine with epinephrine, 7 mg/kg or 1.4 mL/kg of a 0.5% solution). The usual site of entry is into the fourth or fifth intercostal space in the anterior or midaxillary line. In the prepubertal child, the nipple usually overlies the fourth intercostal space. After puberty, the fourth intercostal space is usually located at the inferior border of the breast. The skin entry site should be infiltrated one intercostal space inferior to the anticipated entry to the chest wall, continuing along the anticipated track of the catheter and between the intercostal spaces, as noted previously.

The skin should be prepared with an antiseptic solution, such as chlorhexidine or povidone-iodine. For classical chest tube placement, a skin incision in an axis parallel to the rib is made through the area and blunt dissection is performed using a curved hemostat or Kelly clamp through the incision site and directed up to the superior intercostal space that has been chosen for chest wall entry (**Fig. 25.7**). The clamp should be inserted with the tip closed; the tip is then spread to dissect the tissues. When the dissection has reached the area chosen for pleural penetration, the clamp should be pushed firmly through the pleura while control is maintained so that the chest wall is not penetrated too deeply. In larger children, a finger can be inserted through the tract to manually break up any adhesions that can be felt. The clamp can be placed through the most distal side hole of the tube and clamped at the end of the tube to facilitate guiding the tube. A second clamp placed near the distal end of the tube prevents the free flow of pleural fluid or blood once the tube is in place.

Once the tube tip is within the thorax, the clamp should be opened and the tube advanced sufficiently so that the most proximal hole of the tube is within the thoracic cavity. While the tube is held securely, the drainage system should be connected, and the distal clamp on the tube released to allow drainage. Several techniques for securing the tube have been described, including a purse-string suture and sutures on each side of the skin incision. Commercial devices for securing tubes without sutures are available. Tapes may also be applied to reinforce the stability of the tube.

A number of percutaneous chest drainage systems are available, including pigtail catheters and tube-over-obturator systems (ThalQuik, Cook Critical Care, Bloomington, IN). Most of these systems involve needle puncture into the thorax, followed by placement of a reinforced wire through the needle, dilation of the track, and finally, tube placement using an obturator introducer over the wire (**Fig. 25.8**). Care should be taken with these systems to avoid deeply inserting stiff dilators into the chest, with the subsequent risk of injury. The dilator should only be inserted to the depth needed to penetrate the chest wall and facilitate passage of the tube into the thorax.

Once the tube is in place, it should be observed for air leaks. If an air leak persists for more than a few minutes, all connections should be checked to ensure air is not being entrained through a loose connection. Once the tube is secured, an x-ray should be taken to verify the tube position and observe resolution of the pneumothorax or effusion. If pneumothorax is ongoing despite a working thoracostomy tube, an airway injury or bronchopleural fistula may be present.

In general, when tube drainage has fallen to <2–3 mL/kg over 24 hrs, the tube may be considered for removal. If the tube was placed for a pneumothorax and no active air leak is present, a several-hour trial of observation without suction (water seal) is recommended, obtaining another x-ray to assess reaccumulation of the pneumothorax prior to removing the tube. Most significant reaccumulations have been shown to be clinically evident using this method (42,43). When the decision is made to remove the tube, treatment with analgesics will reduce discomfort. Topically applied anesthetic creams have been shown to reduce pain and to be superior to IV morphine when left in place for 3 hrs (60). Intrapleural bupivacaine has

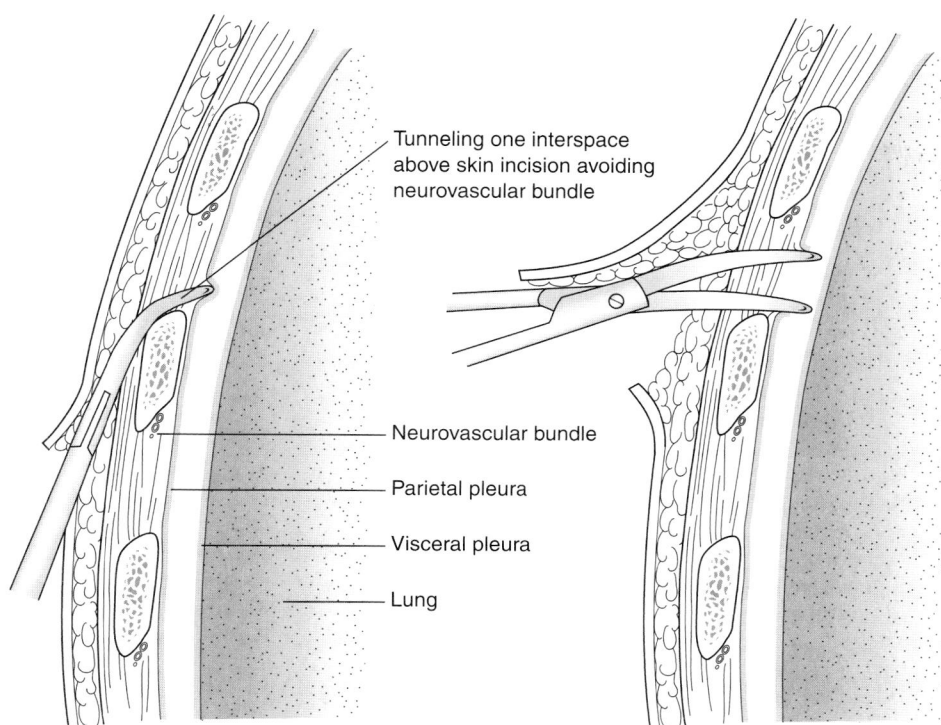

Tunneling one interspace
above skin incision avoiding
neurovascular bundle

Neurovascular bundle

Parietal pleura

Visceral pleura

Lung

FIGURE 25.7. Chest tube thoracostomy.

also been used but has not been demonstrated to be effective in adult trials (45).

PERICARDIOCENTESIS

Pericardiocentesis is required for life-threatening cardiac tamponade or for elective removal of fluid for diagnostic purposes. This procedure may be required after pediatric cardiovascular surgery or during the initial stabilization of pediatric trauma. When practical, pericardiocentesis may be performed in the cardiac catheterization laboratory with electrocardiographic and hemodynamic monitoring and fluoroscopic imaging or, alternatively, under real-time echocardiography guidance. If echocardiography is not available in the catheterization laboratory, prior echocardiographic imaging is recommended to localize and size the effusion. Because of the potentially life-threatening immediate complications associated with pericardiocentesis, surgical exploration is an alternative to an emergent procedure if time allows. Elective removal of pericardial fluid in the presence of a chronic or recurrent pericardial accumulation should be accomplished with echocardiography guidance or surgical exploration to enhance safety.

Although trauma is one of the major causes of cardiac tamponade, it is rarely associated with blunt trauma in children. It may result from stab wounds to the heart or from penetration of a fractured rib into the heart. Gunshot wounds usually result in fatal hemorrhage rather than pericardial tamponade. The classic clinical presentation of "paradoxical pulse" and severe hypotension with distended neck veins is seen in adults and children. The pathophysiology of cardiac tamponade results from reduced filling of the right heart during diastole because of the pressure of blood within the contained pericardium exceeds venous return pressures, causing a decrease in cardiac

output and, ultimately, hypotension. Any sick child with signs of elevated venous pressures (jugular venous distension, hepatomegaly, pulmonary edema), tachycardia, hypotension, and a prominent "paradoxical pulse" must be suspected of having pericardial tamponade. If the physical findings and signs suggest tamponade, confirmation of the diagnosis is ideally obtained by echocardiography, although in some cases immediate intervention without delay may be required.

Pericardiocentesis is indicated for the emergent correction of life-threatening cardiac tamponade. The mere presence of excessive pericardial fluid, however, is generally not an indication for an emergent procedure. Pericardiocentesis has several potentially severe complications and should only be performed emergently when evidence of life-threatening circulatory compromise is observed. Under these conditions, the benefits of the procedure outweigh its risks.

Immediate complications associated with this procedure include puncture and laceration of the ventricular epicardium or myocardium, laceration of a coronary artery or vein, and hemopericardium secondary to laceration of the ventricle, coronary vessels, or great vessels. Lethal arrhythmias such as ventricular fibrillation or ventricular tachycardia may also occur. Pneumothorax may also occur. Delayed complications include slowly developing pneumothorax and pneumopericardium, diaphragm perforation, peritoneal puncture with subsequent peritonitis or false-positive aspirate, esophageal puncture with subsequent mediastinitis, pericardial leakage and development of a cutaneous fistula, and local infection.

Recommended needle sizes are a 20-gauge needle (1 inch, or 2.5 cm) for infants, a 20-gauge needle (1.5–2 inches, or 3–5 cm) for children, and an 18- or 20-gauge needle (3 inches, or 7.5 cm) for adolescents. Some operators prefer an electrocardiogram (ECG) lead attached to the needle to detect epicardial contact of the needle. Over-the-needle IV catheters may also be used in

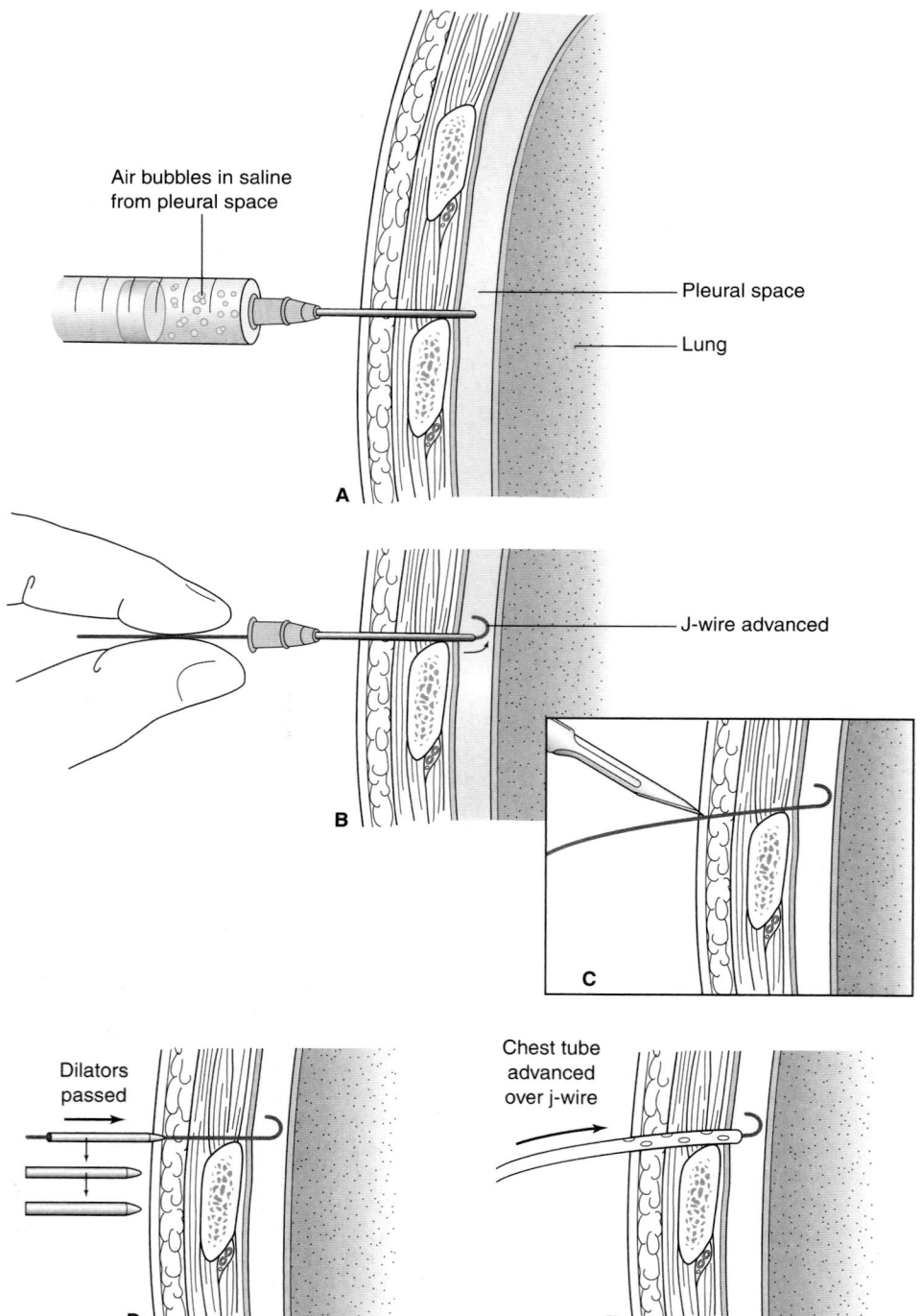

Air bubbles in saline from pleural space

Pleural space

Lung

A

J-wire advanced

B

C

Dilators passed

D

Chest tube advanced over j-wire

E

FIGURE 25.8. Wire-guided placement of chest-drainage system.

smaller children, but most do not allow attachment of an ECG lead.

The child's vital signs should be monitored during and after the procedure. If the patient is not intubated, airway management and resuscitation equipment, including a defibrillator, should be immediately available. If time allows, the xiphoid and subxiphoid areas and thorax should be disinfected. The child should be placed in a head-up position, if possible, to promote anterior pooling of the effusion.

The overlying skin should be infiltrated with lidocaine, and a small stab incision should be made with a blade just below and to the left of tip of the xiphoid process to facilitate easier passage of the needle. Some experts prefer to enter the chest just to the right of the xiphoid tip. An 18- or 20-gauge pericardiocentesis needle is ideal for percutaneous drainage. A small syringe containing 1% lidocaine without epinephrine is attached to the needle via a 3-way stopcock so that local anesthetics may be administered as the needle is advanced. The 3-way stopcock is also attached to tubing, which may be used to monitor intrapericardial pressure. Although many sources advocate the use of an ECG lead clipped to the pericardiocentesis needle with an alligator clamp, this feature may not be essential.

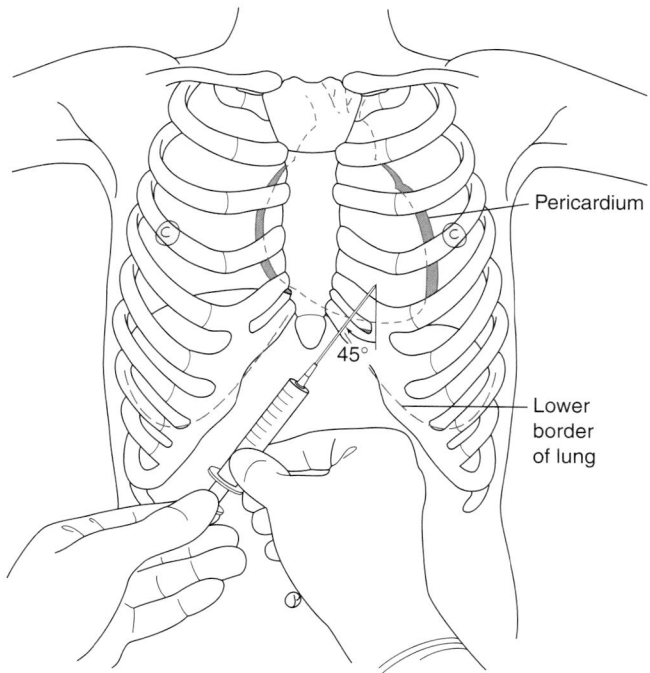

FIGURE 25.9. Needle placement for pericardiocentesis. The needle should be inserted into the skin incision site at a 45-degree angle to the skin and directed toward the left nipple or the tip of the left scapula.

The needle should be inserted into the skin incision site at a 45-degree angle to the skin and directed toward the left nipple or the tip of the left scapula (**Fig. 25.9**). The needle is advanced slowly, aspirating and injecting lidocaine until pericardial fluid is aspirated. Once pericardial fluid is obtained, the intrapericardial pressure is recorded if the system is being transduced. In the setting of pericardial tamponade, the intrapericardial pressure should be equal to the central venous pressure.

If an ECG lead is attached to the needle, contact with the ventricular wall is indicated by ECG changes. The most common manifestations are "current of injury" patterns (ST segment changes and T-wave inversion, QRS complex widening) or PVCs caused by ventricular irritation. If any of these ECG changes are seen, the needle should be withdrawn slightly until the ECG change disappears. If the ECG tracing does not normalize, the needle should be removed completely. In addition, a recording of the intrapericardial pressure could identify intraventricular placement if a ventricular waveform is documented.

Once the needle tip is in the correct position, the stopcock is disconnected and a J-tipped guidewire is introduced into the pericardial space. Often, a dilator is then inserted over the wire, a pigtail pericardial catheter is advanced over the guidewire, and then the guidewire is removed before evacuation of the pericardial fluid. If the needle tip enters a blood-filled pericardial sac, as much non-clotted blood as possible should be withdrawn. Some experts report that blood aspirated from the pericardial sac will not clot; blood aspirated from the heart chambers will clot within 4–6 mins, although this is not universally accepted. Whether the blood clots or not depends on its source of origin. For instance, if the cause of the pericardial tamponade is catheter perforation of a heart chamber, the pericardial blood will often clot even though it is not drawn directly from the heart chamber. Fluid aspirated at the time of pericardiocentesis should be sent for the laboratory examinations.

Even in an emergency setting, it is preferable to use a pericardiocentesis needle, guidewire, and catheter rather than a needle alone, although an 18- or 20-gauge catheter-over-needle system may be substituted if necessary. It is quite hazardous to attempt to drain a pericardial effusion with a needle alone because of the possibility of laceration of the myocardium or coronary vessels. As much fluid as possible should be aspirated, and the intrapericardial pressure following the procedure should be less than 3 mm Hg, with negative deflections during spontaneous inspiration.

The catheter may be withdrawn immediately after the procedure or left in place for up to 24–48 hrs if reaccumulation of fluid is of concern. Echocardiography should be performed following the procedure to document evacuation of the fluid and to determine catheter position. If echocardiography is immediately available, it can be used during the procedure to verify correct catheter placement and ensure adequate drainage during the procedure.

TRANSPYLORIC FEEDING TUBE PLACEMENT

Nutrition is an integral part of the management of critically ill and injured children. Either parenteral or enteral routes can provide nutritional support. Whenever possible, enteral nutrition is the method of choice, as it reduces complication rates and maintains gut integrity.

Nasogastric tube feeding is the first choice of enteral nutrition, but it may be poorly tolerated in critically ill children as a result of gastroparesis. In this setting, transpyloric placement of a feeding tube into the duodenum or jejunum is often recommended to support early feeding, improve tolerance of enteral nutrition, and decrease the risk of aspiration pneumonia. However, achieving small-bowel feeding tube placement can be difficult, time consuming, and costly, and it may delay the initiation of enteral nutrition. Transpyloric tube feeding is commonly indicated when children are unable to tolerate oral or gastric feeding but have adequate gastrointestinal function.

Blind insertion of a transpyloric tube is usually performed at bedside using a weighted or unweighted tube. Right lateral decubitus positioning and motility (prokinetic) agents, such as metoclopramide or erythromycin, are occasionally used. Even if post-pyloric position is not achieved soon after the insertion, the tube may migrate through the pylorus over time.

An immediate x-ray to confirm transpyloric placement may not always be necessary. Ultrasonography can also be used for placement confirmation (21). If a child is stable and requires early establishment of feeding, fluoroscopic-guided insertion may be considered, although if bedside fluoroscopy is not available, the risks of moving critically ill children to the radiology suite should be considered. Various alternative bedside techniques, including pH assisted, magnet/endoscope guided, and spontaneous passage with or without motility (prokinetic) agents have been suggested as alternative techniques to facilitate tube passage through the pylorus.

Complications during insertion include gastrointestinal tract perforation and tube misplacement. Similar to malplacement of a nasogastric tube, tracheal or bronchial intubation may occur during feeding tube placement, particularly in patients who are receiving sedation and neuromuscular blockade. Perforations of the gastrointestinal tract and formation of an enterocutaneous fistula are reported, particularly in infants. Development of pyloric stenosis during transpyloric tube feeding has also been reported in infants (34). Obstruction of a long, narrow transpyloric tube is one of the more common problems.

Gastric air insufflation may allow rapid placement of feeding tubes into the small bowel with fewer attempts, compared with a standard insertion technique in children (12,54). For this technique, an unweighted nasoenteric feeding tube attached to a 3-way stopcock and a 60-mL syringe is inserted through the nares into the stomach. After 10 mL/kg of air is injected, the tube is advanced a distance estimated to position the tip of the tube proximal to the pylorus. An additional 10 mL/kg of air is then injected, and the tube is advanced the distance necessary to place the tube in the fourth part of the duodenum. The success rate using this technique was reported in multiple pediatric studies as 86%–92%, compared to <50% in the control group (12).

Another placement technique uses a feeding tube with a pH sensor at the distal tip. pH-assisted transpyloric tube placement was reported as a safe, easy bedside alternative to other techniques in critically ill infants and small children. The success rate using this technique was reported in a pediatric study as 97%, compared with 53% in the control group (16).

Recently, the use of a magnet-tipped feeding tube, dragged into proper position with an external magnet, has been described (17). The feeding tube was manufactured to include a magnet and a magnet field sensor in the distal tip, connected by a thin insulated wire to a small light at the proximal end. A larger hand-held magnet was held over the epigastrium to magnetically capture the tube tip, indicated by the illumination of the proximal light. The tube tip was then maneuvered by the hand-held magnet along the lesser curvature of the stomach, through the pylorus, and into the duodenum. The success rate has been reported between 60%–95% inconsistently (5).

Endoscopic tube placement provides additional anatomic information and may allow for earlier initiation of enteral feedings. However, the efficacy and success rate is not uniform, and it requires the availability of an experienced pediatric endoscopist. Some studies demonstrate a failure to improve transpyloric intubation rates and tube dislodgement during endoscope removal.

The use of metoclopramide, a prokinetic agent, has been recommended to achieve transpyloric placement, but its efficacy is controversial. A Cochrane Database Systematic Review of four clinical studies reported no statistically significant difference between IV and intramuscular metoclopramide administered to promote tube migration (51). IV administration of 10 mg and 20 mg of metoclopramide was equally ineffective in facilitating transpyloric intubation.

Some studies reported that gastric feeding using erythromycin as a prokinetic is equivalent to transpyloric feeding in meeting the nutritional goals of the critically ill (19). Erythromycin has been tried as a prokinetic agent instead of metoclopramide, to enhance gastric motor activity and emptying; however, its efficacy is inconsistent. Some reports described that erythromycin infusion (3 mg/kg) and electromyogram signal guidance can facilitate rapid transpyloric feeding tube placement with an initial success rate of 80%.

ABDOMINAL PARACENTESIS

Abdominal paracentesis is a percutaneously performed procedure for sampling and drainage of the peritoneal cavity in patients with ascites, peritonitis, or blunt abdominal trauma. Therapeutic indications for this procedure include an increase in intra-abdominal pressure (IAP) that causes some combination of significant respiratory distress, cardiovascular compromise, oliguria, acidosis, or raised intracranial pressure. In the PICU, common etiologies of massive ascites include fluid resuscitation for treatment of shock (e.g., in meningococcemia), viral hemorrhagic shock (e.g., Dengue shock syndrome), trauma, severe burns, and multiorgan dysfunction with fluid overload from capillary leak syndromes.

Diagnostic indications include new onset ascites, chronic ascites with clinical deterioration and suspected peritonitis, pancreatitis, and intraperitoneal bleeding. Diagnostic peritoneal lavage is not routinely recommended in the evaluation of patients with blunt trauma due to high false-negative rates (23) and due to the widespread and rapid availability of CT scanning, which is noninvasive and provides more organ-specific information to guide potential surgical intervention. Various causes of ascites include portal hypertension, inferior vena cava obstruction, heart failure, nephrotic syndrome, lymphomas, leukemias or neoplasms that involve liver or mediastinum, chronic pancreatitis, or cirrhosis of the liver. The differential diagnosis of clinical symptomatology related to ascites is shown in **Table 25.1** (52).

No absolute contraindications are associated with abdominal paracentesis. It should be avoided in a patient with an acute abdomen who requires immediate surgery. Both coagulopathies and thrombocytopenia are considered as relative contraindications; however, prophylactic use of platelets or fresh frozen plasma for performing this procedure is not recommended. Special caution is necessary in patients with severe bowel distension, history of previous abdominal or pelvic surgery, or distended bladder not adequately drained by a Foley catheter. Insertion sites where abdominal scar or cellulitis is apparent should be avoided due to the possibility of adherent bowel with scars and introduction of infection with cellulitis. While abdominal paracentesis is a relatively safe procedure (47), perforation of bowel and bladder, persistent leakage of fluid, intra-abdominal bleeding, infection, and hypovolemic shock may occur.

Paracentesis kits are usually available. When they are not, the following supplies should be assembled: skin disinfectant, sterile gloves and mask, sterile drape, local anesthetic, 3–10-mL syringe with small (25-gauge) needle for anesthesia, 20–22 gauge over-the-needle catheter for smaller children, and a 16–20-gauge catheter for larger children. Large syringes and a 3-way stopcock should be available. When ongoing drainage is planned, a pigtail catheter kit should be available, along with a collection bag to drain the removed fluid.

The diagnosis of ascites should be clinically confirmed by shifting dullness, flank dullness, and fluid waves on abdominal examination (10). Clinical examination will usually identify patients with moderate to severe ascites, but some patients

TABLE 25.1

DIFFERENTIAL DIAGNOSES OF FLUID IN ABDOMEN

Ascites associated with abdominal tenderness
Peritonitis
Pancreatitis
Congestive heart failure
Constrictive pericarditis
Biliary peritonitis
Hepatitis
Hepatic venous obstruction (Budd-Chiari syndrome)
Intraperitoneal bleeding (trauma, ectopic pregnancy)
Hepatic abscess

Ascites associated with no abdominal tenderness and low serum albumin
Protein-losing enteropathy
Nephrotic syndrome
Malnutrition
Portal hypertension
Congenital syphilis
Cirrhosis

Ascites associated with no abdominal tenderness and normal serum albumin
Portal hypertension
Tuberculous peritonitis
Chylous ascites
Renal disease
Malignancy
Obstructive uropathy
Wilson disease
Hematocolpos

with mild to moderate ascites may be missed (20). Abdominal ultrasound can detect even small quantities of fluid (as low as 150 mL) and should be used to aid in diagnosis and to perform ultrasound-guided aspiration. Sedation is usually required and is discussed in Chapter 12.

In ascites, the bowel tends to float in the nondependent midline area. Therefore, the area of needle insertion should be dependent and lateral in children (58), although some authorities prefer the midline 2 cm below the umbilicus (46). The patient should be placed in a supine position, with head elevated and the bladder empty. Using sterile technique, the insertion site is prepared with chlorhexidine or povidone-iodine. The skin and subcutaneous tissue are infiltrated with a local anesthetic. Alternatively, lateral insertion can be accomplished, preferably in the left lower quadrant, a few centimeters above the inguinal ligament, lateral to the rectus abdominis muscle (37,48). A Z-track method minimizes the risk of fluid leak, compared with a direct linear-track insertion. The Z-track can be applied by placing caudal traction on the skin after the needle has been inserted perpendicular to the abdominal wall.

Once the initial needle insertion is made through the skin and subcutaneous tissues, negative pressure is maintained with the syringe, while the needle is advanced further until a pop is felt as the needle enters the peritoneal cavity and free fluid is aspirated. If a catheter-over-needle system is used, the catheter is advanced over the needle into the peritoneal cavity and the needle is removed. Approximately 20–30 mL of fluid is usually enough for diagnostic studies, but for therapeutic drainage, more fluid may be required until the abdomen is visibly lax and

the patient's respiratory distress improves. Ascitic fluid may be sent for cell count with differential count, specific gravity, glucose, total protein, alkaline phosphatase, albumin, amylase, LDH, ammonia, creatinine, potassium, bilirubin, triglycerides, cellular morphology, aerobic and anaerobic cultures, viral and fungal cultures, acid-fast bacilli stain and culture, and Gram stain, as clinically indicated. Corresponding serum chemistries should also be sent. A large volume drained quickly can result in shock and hypotension; therefore, no more than 15–20 mL/kg should be drained at one time (58). Positional change may be necessary to facilitate drainage of the ascitic fluid. A pigtail catheter may be used if drainage is required over the following 24–48 hrs, leaving the catheter in place. After the removal of the needle or the catheter, a sterile pressure dressing should be applied.

The rate of complications is reported as 1%–3% (10). Complications include bowel or bladder perforation, bleeding, subcutaneous hematoma, infection, persistent leak, scrotal edema, and hypotension. Perforation of the bladder can be prevented if care is taken to empty the bladder prior to the procedure (37). As the risk of bowel perforation is high in patients with a history of previous surgery and adhesions, it can be prevented by avoiding old scars at the insertion site, to prevent injury to an adherent bowel loop (53). Ultrasound-guided paracentesis will also reduce risk in this setting.

Bowel perforation will usually close quickly without leak unless intraluminal pressure is high. Blood vessel perforation may result in bleeding, which usually stops quickly unless portal hypertension or severe coagulopathy is present. Perforation of solid organs can occur, but usually bleeding will stop spontaneously. Introduction of infection into the peritoneal cavity is possible; therefore, strict aseptic technique should be used. Scrotal edema (or labial edema in females) has been reported in patients with massive ascites (presumably from the tracking of fluid along tissue planes), and the use of small needles may prevent this complication (5). The persistent leak of ascitic fluid is rare but usually responds to pressure and potentially may be prevented by use of the Z-track method. Hypotension from hypovolemia can occur if >20 mL/kg of fluid is aspirated from the peritoneal cavity.

The fluid is initially evaluated by visual inspection. The fluid is normally straw-colored but may be turbid in chemical or infectious peritonitis. Chylous ascites will yield milky or yellowish fluid (59). Bile-stained fluid may be associated with pancreatitis or gall bladder or common bile duct perforation (2). Blood-tinged fluid is seen with visceral disruption or traumatic paracentesis (10).

In peritonitis, >50% polymorphonuclear leukocytes will be seen. Lymphocytes will predominate with chylous ascites (usually >90% lymphocytes) or tuberculous peritonitis (10). If paracentesis is used to diagnose the need for surgery in necrotizing enterocolitis, brownish fluid indicates perforation or necrotic bowel. If Gram stain reveals bacteria, surgery or drainage procedures may be considered for necrotizing enterocolitis (31).

Low glucose is seen with bacterial or tuberculous peritonitis. An absolute glucose of <60 mg/dL is considered low, or if the ascitic fluid glucose is less than two thirds of the serum glucose level. Total protein of <2.5 g/dL, a fibrinogen level of 0.3% to 4% of total protein, a fluid-to-serum protein ratio of <0.5, and specific gravity of <1.015 are consistent with a transudate. Alkaline phosphatase is greater than twice the serum level in

TABLE 25.2

COMPARISON OF ASCITIC FLUID OF DIFFERENT ETIOLOGIES

Spontaneous bacterial peritonitis	>250 cells/mL Total protein is >1 g/dL LDH and glucose may be normal pH may be low or normal Culture and Gram stain may be negative Serum-ascitic albumin gradient is usually >1.1 g
Secondary bacterial peritonitis	Total protein is >3 g/dL LDH is >serum LDH Glucose is <50 mg/dL >500 cells/mL with polymorphonuclear predominance Gram stain is positive Serum-ascitic albumen gradient is <1.1 g/dL pH is not a reliable correlate of bacterial peritonitis
Chylous ascites	Milky or yellow fluid, but may be clear WBC = 1000–5000, with lymphocytic predominance (usually >90%) Triglyceride level >> serum triglycerides (>1500 g/dL) Total protein is <3 g/dL
Pancreatic ascites	Turbid, tea-colored, or bloody fluid Elevated total WBC count and protein Amylase and lipase are > serum levels; in patients <4–6 months of age, amylase may be low, but lipase is always higher
Tuberculous ascites	Bloody or yellow fluid, firm clots Total protein is >2.5 g/dL WBC >1000 with predominant lymphocytes Glucose is <30 mg/dL
Urine ascites	Protein is <1 g/dL Potassium and creatinine are >serum
Malignant ascites	Bloody fluid ⇑Protein and LDH ⇓Glucose Serum-ascitic albumen gradient is <1.1 g/dL
Nephrotic syndrome	Total protein is <2.5 g/dL
Biliary ascites	Bile-stained fluid Bilirubin >> serum bilirubin (100–400 mg/dL)

LDH, lactate dehydrogenase; WBC, white blood count

patients with perforated or necrotic viscus. The ammonia level is twice as high as serum ammonia in patients with strangulated bowel and duodenal perforation. Ascitic fluid amylase is greater than serum amylase in patients with pancreatitis, pancreatic pseudocyst, intestinal perforation, or strangulation. In urinary ascites, ammonia, creatinine, and potassium concentrations will be elevated (10). Serum-ascitic albumin gradient is defined as the difference between serum and ascitic fluid albumin concentrations. A gradient of ≥1.1 g correlates with portal hypertension (27). A comparison of ascitic fluid composition in different types of ascites is shown in **Table 25.2**.

TRANSURETHRAL BLADDER CATHETER PLACEMENT AND BLADDER PRESSURE MONITORING

Transurethral bladder catheter placement is commonly performed in the PICU as an integral part of strict intake and output monitoring of fluid balance, and has recently been used in certain specific situations for monitoring IAP. Contraindications to transurethral catheter placement include urethral trauma or blood at the tip of the meatus, prostatic displacement on rectal examination in males, obvious pelvic fracture, or perineal hematoma. Complications include trauma to the urethra and bladder, vaginal catheterization, urinary tract infection, intravesical knotting of the catheter, paraphimosis, and hematuria.

The measurement of bladder pressure as a surrogate for IAP is used to detect intra-abdominal hypertension (IAH), leading to abdominal compartment syndrome (ACS). A number of physiologic derangements have been described with IAH, including cardiovascular, pulmonary, and renal effects (11). Many pediatric reports suggest the importance of monitoring IAP in an attempt to detect IAH early, allowing early intervention and potentially preventing associated complications (15,28,39).

Among the common clinical situations in which IAP can increase is trauma that leads to accumulation of blood, fluid,

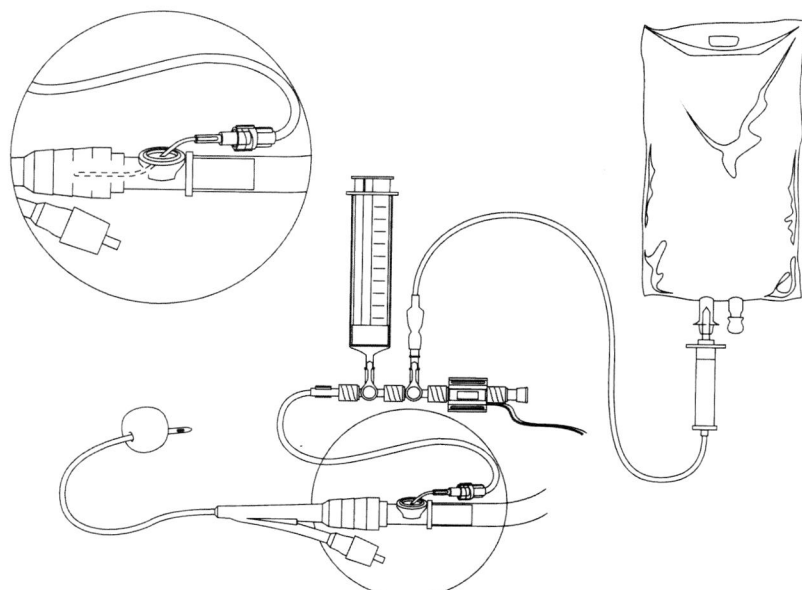

FIGURE 25.10. A closed, needle-free system for measurement of intravesicular pressure. Normal saline (1000 mL), a 60-mL Luer-lock syringe, and a segment of pressure tubing are attached to a disposable pressure transducer connected to two stopcocks. An 18-gauge angiocatheter is inserted into the culture aspiration port of the urinary drainage tubing, and the needle is removed, with the plastic infusion catheter left in place. The infusion catheter is connected to the pressure tubing, and the system is flushed with normal saline. The infusion catheter may be taped to the urinary drainage tubing for added security.

or edema; nontraumatic bowel ischemia, infarction, and gastrointestinal hemorrhage can also lead to increased IAP due to edema or fluid collection. IAP increases in the PICU are commonly seen in (a) children with septic shock with capillary leak, (b) children with multiorgan dysfunction syndrome (MODS), (c) severely burned or trauma patients with ischemia–reperfusion injury following fluid resuscitation, and (d) those who are post-liver transplantation or post-surgical closure of an abdominal wall defect. Although specific pediatric indications for IAP monitoring have not been established, patients at risk for significant increases in IAP include (a) those with blunt abdominal injury; (b) those with MODS, meningococcemia, dengue shock syndrome, severe burns, or high cumulative fluid balance who are mechanically ventilated; and (c) those who are postoperative with abdominal packing.

Increased IAP can lead to inferior vena cava compression with a reduction of venous return, which causes a low cardiac output with impaired renal perfusion and oliguria. In severe cases, raised IAP can lead to intra-abdominal arterial occlusion. It can also lead to respiratory compromise due to impaired diaphragmatic excursion, raised airway pressures, and reduction of pulmonary blood flow, with consequent hypoxemia and hypercarbia. Abdominal tamponade also leads to increased intracranial pressure and reduction in cerebral perfusion pressure. In summary, signs of ACS include abdominal distension, oliguria, hypoxia, hypotension, and acidosis. Early monitoring of IAP should be considered in situations in which the patient is already exhibiting signs of ACS or is at high risk of developing it.

Although various techniques of IAP monitoring, including intragastric pressure and intravesical pressure, have been described, measurement of intravesical pressure is considered a gold standard for IAP measurement (27). The technique for intravesical pressure measurement was first described by Kron (32) and later modified by Cheatham (7). Recent reports suggest the inaccuracy of clinical examination in detecting IAH (30) and a need for standardization and development of clinical practice guidelines for adults (55). Although measurement of IAP has been recommended in pediatric patients with abdomi-

nal wall defects (33) and in children with major burns, routine measurement of intra-abdominal bladder pressure is not yet a common practice in the PICU. In pediatric patients, various indirect methods of measuring intravesical pressure have been compared recently (14). The set-up is schematically shown in **Fig. 25.10.**

To monitor intravesical pressure, the urinary catheter must have a closed drainage system, and the patient must be in the supine position. The transducer system should be connected to the monitor, with connection to a bag of saline. A 30-mm or 60-mm pressure scale on the monitor is selected, a 60-mL syringe is attached to the distal stopcock, and the symphysis pubis is taken as the zero reference point. The bladder drainage system is clamped distal to the catheter and drainage bag connection. The sampling port of the catheter is cleaned with an antiseptic swab, and a large (18-gauge) needle is inserted into the sampling port. The stopcock attached to the syringe is turned off to the patient. The saline bag is then opened toward the syringe, and the syringe is filled with saline flush. The stopcock is turned off to the pressure bag, and 1 mL/kg of saline from the syringe is injected into the bladder. Any air seen between the clamp and the urinary catheter should be expelled by opening the clamp and allowing the saline to flow back past the clamp before reapplying the clamp. The pressure waveform typically shows a small variation between inspiration and expiration, with the end-expiratory pressure taken as the IAP. A printed strip facilitates measurement of the IAP. Once the pressure measurement is made, the needle is removed from the sampling port and catheter drainage tubing is unclamped. The amount of saline injected should be accounted for in the output charting.

When a transducer is not available, the catheter tubing is simply raised vertically above the symphysis pubis at a 90-degree angle to the patient's pelvis, and the tubing is unclamped. The distance in centimeters between the symphysis pubis zero point and the maximal height of the fluid column is recorded (7). This minimally invasive technique is popular in some institutions because it is quick and can be easily performed by the staff, without the need for a transducer set-up.

A closed commercial monitoring and drainage system that utilizes an inline valve allows monitoring without the need to use a needle to connect to the sampling port of the catheter (AbViser, Wolfe Tory Medical Inc., Salt Cake City, UT).

Normal pediatric values are not established for IAP. Based on adult data (6), normal range of IAP is considered to be 0–12 mm Hg. IAH is defined as an IAP of >12 mm Hg. ACS may occur with an IAP of >20 mm Hg. The severity of IAH has also been described as mild (10–20 mm Hg), moderate (>20–40 mm Hg), and severe (>40 mm Hg). The incidence of ACS is 15% in adult studies, much higher than the reported pediatric incidence of 0.7% (3), which may reflect a failure to recognize this condition in the pediatric population. A high index of suspicion in patients at risk for developing ACS and measurement of IAP early during the course of illness are required to recognize this condition.

Various interventions to reduce IAP include gastric suction, enemas, diuretics, muscle relaxants, paracentesis, and surgical decompression, as clinically indicated. Because the level of IAP at which ACS occurs in children is unknown, some have suggested that a distended abdomen, oliguria, and/or hypoxia and hypercarbia plus increased airway pressure justify abdominal decompression (28). Some authors recommend decompression at >25 mm Hg in patients who are treated by silo decompression (15). Paracentesis may provide an alternative to operative intervention in pediatric patients with severe traumatic liver injuries and ACS related to fluid and blood accumulation (49).

CONCLUSIONS AND FUTURE DIRECTIONS

Invasive procedures are a routine part of pediatric critical care. Complications can range from trivial to life-threatening, requiring an assessment of the risk and benefit for each procedure. Informed consent is appropriate in less urgent circumstances. Operator training, practice, and experience reduce risks. Future improvements in device technology may also reduce infectious and mechanical complications. Sedation and analgesia are often required when performing invasive procedures in children.

KEY POINTS

■ Central venous catheterization is frequently required in the PICU. Femoral, subclavian, and internal jugular site choices in children are largely a function of operator experience and local practice. Data from adults suggest subclavian CVCs are associated with the least risk for infectious complications, and these should be considered in adolescents in appropriate settings.

■ Intraosseous infusion is an emergency vascular access technique appropriate for children and adolescents of all ages.

■ Thoracostomy is frequently required in critical care, and newer wire-guided techniques are increasingly used.

■ Arterial catheterization remains the gold standard for arterial pressure monitoring and is necessary in some critically ill patients.

■ Pericardiocentesis may be required emergently for pericardial tamponade, but imaging modalities (ultrasound or fluoroscopy) may improve safety when time permits.

■ Transpyloric feeding tube placement may be performed blindly at the bedside with good success rates; magnet-tipped and pH-guided tubes may be useful in experienced hands.

■ Abdominal paracentesis is useful for both diagnostic and therapeutic purposes in the PICU.

■ Bladder pressure monitoring via a transurethral bladder catheter can allow monitoring of bladder pressure as a surrogate marker for intra-abdominal pressure. Pressures >12 mm Hg are considered high, and >25 mm Hg may require surgical intervention.

■ Infectious complications, one of the most frequent adverse events of invasive procedures, can be reduced by strict attention to full surgical barrier precautions, skin disinfection with chlorhexidine, and by removing invasive devices as quickly as possible. Antibiotic catheters may also reduce infectious complications as well.

■ Ultrasound is a promising bedside technology for the reduction of risks in many procedures. As clinicians gain experience with this technology, safety of the procedures will likely improve as well as the availability of higher-resolution devices.

References

1. American Heart Association Guidelines for Cardiopulmonary Resuscitation and Emergency Cardiovascular Care. *Circulation* 2005;112(24 Suppl):IV1–203.
2. Athow AC, Wilkins ML, Saunders AJ. Pancreatic ascites presenting in infancy, with review of literature. *Dig Dis Sci* 1991;36:245–7.
3. Beck R, Halberthal M, Zonis Z, et al. Abdominal compartment syndrome in children. *Pediatr Crit Care Med* 2001;2:51–6.
4. Berwick DM, Calkins DR, McCannon CJ, et al. The 100,000 lives campaign: Setting a goal and a deadline for improving health care quality. *JAMA* 2006;295:324–7.
5. Boivin M, Levy H, Hayes J. A multicenter, prospective study of the placement of transpyloric feeding tubes with assistance of a magnetic device. *The Magnet-Guided Enteral Feeding Tube Study Group. JPEN J Parenter Enteral Nutr* 2000;24:304–7.
6. Cheatham ML. Intraabdominal hypertension. *New Horiz* 1997;96–115.
7. Cheatham ML, Safcsak K. Intraabdominal pressure: A revised method for measurement. *J Am Coll Surg* 1998;186:594–5.
8. Chen CC, Tsao PN, Yau KI. Paraplegia: Complication of percutaneous central venous line malposition. *Pediatr Neurol* 2001;24:65–8.
9. Chuan WX, Wei W, Yu L. A randomized-controlled study of ultrasound prelocation vs anatomical landmark-guided cannulation of the internal jugular vein in infants and children. *Paediatr Anaesth* 2005;15:733–8.
10. Cochran WJ. Ascites. In: McMillan JA, De Angelis CD, Feigin RD, eds. *Oski's Pediatrics: Principles and Practice.* Philadelphia: Lippincott, 1994.
11. Cullen DJ, Coyle JP, Teplick R, et al. Cardiovascular, pulmonary, and renal effects of massively increased intra-abdominal pressure in critically ill patients. *Crit Care Med* 1989;17:118–21.
12. Da Silva PS, Paulo CS, de Oliveira ISB, et al. Bedside transpyloric tube placement in the pediatric intensive care unit: A modified insufflation air technique. *Intensive Care Med* 2002;28:943–6.
13. Darouiche RO, Raad, II, Heard SO, et al. A comparison of two antimicrobial-impregnated central venous catheters. *Catheter Study Group. N Engl J Med* 1999;340:1–8.
14. Davis PJ, Koottayi S, Taylor A, et al. Comparison of indirect methods of measuring intra-abdominal pressure in children. *Intensive Care Med* 2005;31:471–5.
15. DeCou JM, Abrams RS, Miller RS, et al. Abdominal compartment syndrome in children: Experience with three cases. *J Pediatr Surg* 2000;35:840–2.
16. Dimand RJ, Veereman-Wauters G, Braner DA. Bedside placement of pH-guided transpyloric small bowel feeding tubes in critically ill infants and small children. *JPEN J Parenter Enteral Nutr* 1997;21:112–4.
17. Gabriel SA, Ackermann RJ. Placement of nasoenteral feeding tubes using external magnetic guidance. *JPEN J Parenter Enteral Nutr* 2004;28:119–22.
18. Garland JS, Alex CP, Henrickson KJ, et al. A vancomycin-heparin lock solution for prevention of nosocomial bloodstream infection in critically ill neonates with peripherally inserted central venous catheters: A prospective, randomized trial. *Pediatrics* 2005;116:e198–205.

19. Gharpure V, Meert KL, Sarnaik AP. Efficacy of erythromycin for postpyloric placement of feeding tubes in critically ill children: A randomized, double-blind, placebo controlled study. *JPEN J Parenter Enteral Nutr* 2001;25: 160–5.

20. Glauser JM. Paracentesis. In: Roberts JR, Hedges JR, eds. *Clinical Procedures in Emergency Medicine*. Philadelphia: WB Saunders, 1991.

21. Greenberg M, Bejar R, Asser S. Confirmation of transpyloric feeding tube placement by ultrasonography. *J Pediatr* 1993;122:413–5.

22. Greenwald BM, Notterman DA, DeBruin WJ, et al. Percutaneous axillary artery catheterization in critically ill infants and children. *J Pediatr* 1990;117:442–4.

23. Heller M, Jehle D. *Ultrasound in Emergency Medicine*. Philadelphia: WB Saunders, 1995.

24. Heulitt MJ, Farrington EA, O'Shea TM, et al. Double-blind, randomized, controlled trial of papaverine-containing infusions to prevent failure of arterial catheters in pediatric patients. *Crit Care Med* 1993;21:825–9.

25. Hind D, Calvert N, McWilliams R, et al. Ultrasonic locating devices for central venous cannulation: Meta-analysis. *Br Med J.* 2003;327:361.

26. Jung CW, Bahk JH, Kim MW, et al. Head position for facilitating the superior vena caval placement of catheters during right subclavian approach in children. *Crit Care Med* 2002;30:297–9.

27. Kandel G, Diamant NE. A clinical view of recent advances in ascites. *J Clin Gastroenterol* 1986;8:85–99.

28. Kawar B, Siplovich L. Abdominal compartment syndrome in children: The dilemma of treatment. *Eur J Pediatr Surg* 2003;13:330–3.

29. Keenan SP. Use of ultrasound to place central lines. *J Crit Care* 2002;17:126–37.

30. Kirkpatrick AW, Brenneman FD, McLean RF, et al. Is clinical examination an accurate indicator of raised intra-abdominal pressure in critically injured patients? *Can J Surg* 2000;43:207–11.

31. Kosloske AM, Papile L, Burstein J. Indication for operation in acute necrotizing enterocolitis. *Surgery* 1980;87:502–6.

32. Kron IL, Harman PK, Nolan SP. The measurement of intra-abdominal pressure as a criterion for abdominal re-exploration. *Ann Surg* 1984;199:28–30.

33. Lacey SR, Bruce J, Brooks SP, et al. The relative merits of various methods of indirect measurement of intra-abdominal pressure as a guide to closure of abdominal wall defects. *J Pediatr Surg* 1987;22:1207–11.

34. Latchaw LA, Jacir NN, Harris BH. The development of pyloric stenosis during transpyloric feedings. *J Pediatr Surg* 1989;24:823–4.

35. Levy I, Katz J, Solter E, et al. Chlorhexidine-impregnated dressing for prevention of colonization of central venous catheters in infants and children: A randomized controlled study. *Pediatr Infect Dis J* 2005;24:676–9.

36. Lukish J, Valladares E, Rodriguez C, et al. Classical positioning decreases subclavian vein cross-sectional area in children. *J Trauma* 2002;53:272–5.

37. Mallory A, Schaefer JW. Complication of diagnostic paracentesis in patients with liver disease. *JAMA* 1978;239:628–30.

38. Miller AH, Roth BA, Mills TJ, et al. Ultrasound guidance versus the landmark technique for the placement of central venous catheters in the emergency department. *Acad Emerg Med* 2002;9:800–5.

39. Neville HL, Lally KP, Cox CS, Jr. Emergent abdominal decompression with patch abdominoplasty in the pediatric patient. *J Pediatr Surg* 2000;35:705–8.

40. O'Grady NP, Alexander M, Dellinger EP, et al. Guidelines for the prevention of intravascular catheter-related infections. *Centers for Disease Control and Prevention. MMWR Recomm Rep* 2002;51:1–29.

41. Orlowski JP, Julius CJ, Petras RE, et al. The safety of intraosseous infusions: Risks of fat and bone marrow emboli to the lungs. *Ann Emerg Med* 1989;18:1062–7.

42. Pacanowski JP, Waack ML, Daley BJ, et al. Is routine roentgenography needed after closed tube thoracostomy removal? *J Trauma* 2000;48:684–8.

43. Pacharn P, Heller DN, Kammen BF, et al. Are chest radiographs routinely necessary following thoracostomy tube removal? *Pediatr Radiol* 2002;32:138–42.

44. Polderman KH, Girbes AJ. Central venous catheter use. *Part 1: Mechanical complications. Intensive Care Med* 2002;28:1–17.

45. Puntillo KA. Effects of interpleural bupivacaine on pleural chest tube removal pain: A randomized controlled trial. *Am J Crit Care* 1996;5:102–8.

46. Ruddy RM. Section VII, Procedures: Peritoneal Tap. In: Fleisher GR, Ludwig S, Henretiz FM, et al., eds. *Textbook of Pediatric Emergency Medicine*. Baltimore: William and Wilkins, 2000.

47. Runyon BA. Paracentesis of ascitic fluid: A safe procedure. *Arch Intern Med* 1986;146:2259–61.

48. Runyon BA. Care of patients with ascites. *N Eng J Med* 1994;330:337–42.

49. Sharpe RD, Pryor JP, Gandhi RR, et al. Abdominal compartment syndrome in the pediatric blunt trauma patient treated with paracentesis: Report of two cases. *J Trauma* 2002;53:380–2.

50. Sheridan RL, Petras L, Lydon M. Ultrasonic imaging as an adjunct to femoral venous catheterization in children. *J Burn Care Rehabil* 1997;18:156–8.

51. Silva CC, Saconato H, Atallah AN. Metoclopramide for migration of naso-enteral tube. *Cochrane Database Syst Rev.* 2002;CD003353.

52. Simon JE. Abdominal distension. In: Fleisher GR, Ludwig S, Henretiz FM, et al., eds. *Textbook of Pediatric Emergency Medicine*, 4th ed. Baltimore: William and Wilkins, 2000.

53. Smith SD, Vasquez WD. Ascites. In: O'Neill JA, Rower MI, Grossfield JL, et al., eds. *Pediatric Surgery*. Baltimore: Mosby Year Book, 1998.

54. Spalding HK, Sullivan KJ, Soremi O, et al. Bedside placement of transpyloric feeding tubes in the pediatric intensive care unit using gastric insufflation. *Crit Care Med* 2000;28:2041–4.

55. Sugure M. Intraabdominal pressure time for clinical practice guidelines. *Intensive Care Med* 2002;28:389–91.

56. Tan BK, Hong SW, Huang MH, et al. Anatomic basis of safe percutaneous subclavian venous catheterization. *J Trauma* 2000;48:82–6.

57. Trottier SJ, Veremakis C, O'Brien J, et al. Femoral deep vein thrombosis associated with central venous catheterization: Results from a prospective, randomized trial. *Crit Care Med* 1995;23:52–9.

58. Tuggle DW. Abdominal paracentesis. In: Blumer JL, ed. *A Practical Guide to Pediatric Intensive Care*. St Louis: Mosby Year Book, 1990.

59. Unger SW, Chandler JG. Chylous ascites in infants and children. *Surgery* 1983;93:455–61.

60. Valenzuela RC, Rosen DA. Topical lidocaine-prilocaine cream (EMLA) for thoracostomy tube removal. *Anesth Analg* 1999;88:1107–8.

61. Verghese ST, McGill WA, Patel RI, et al. Ultrasound-guided internal jugular venous cannulation in infants: A prospective comparison with the traditional palpation method. *Anesthesiology* 1999;91:71–7.

CHAPTER 26 ■ RECOGNITION AND INITIAL MANAGEMENT OF SHOCK

SIMON NADEL • NIRANJAN "TEX" KISSOON • SUCHITRA RANJIT

Shock is a complex clinical syndrome in which the cardiovascular system fails in its primary function of substrate delivery and metabolite removal, resulting in anaerobic metabolism and tissue acidosis. If unchecked, irreversible cellular damage occurs. In general, all shock states eventually lead to decreased delivery or impaired utilization of essential cellular substrates and, finally, to eventual loss of normal cellular function. Because circulatory function is dependent on blood volume, vascular tone, and cardiac function, shock states may result from abnormalities in one or more of these factors or from cellular metabolic disturbances due to inability to utilize substrates delivered to the tissue by the circulation.

Shock is divided into three major categories: hypovolemic, cardiogenic, and distributive, with a degree of overlap. Hypovolemic shock is a result of inadequate circulating blood volume, owing to blood or fluid loss, or insufficient fluid intake. Cardiogenic shock occurs when cardiac compensatory mechanisms fail and may occur in infants and young children and in patients with preexisting myocardial disease or injury. Distributive shock, such as septic and anaphylactic shock, is associated with peripheral vasodilatation, arterial and capillary shunting past tissue beds with pooling of venous blood, and decreased venous return to the heart. This categorization is an oversimplification, as several mechanisms may be contributing in the same patient. The end result, however, is failure to provide energy substrates to meet the metabolic demand of the tissues.

Shock is a clinical diagnosis, but its recognition remains problematic in children. Shock may be present long before hypotension occurs. Children will often maintain their blood pressure until the late stages of shock; therefore, the presence of systemic hypotension is not required to make the diagnosis of shock in children, as it is in adults (53). For example, septic shock in pediatric patients has been defined as tachycardia (which may be absent in the hypothermic patient) with signs of decreased perfusion, including decreased peripheral pulses compared with central pulses, altered alertness, flash capillary refill or capillary refill of >2 secs, mottled or cool extremities, and decreased urine output (5). Hypotension is a sign of late and decompensated shock in children, if present in a child with these other features.

Although distinct clinical presentations and classifications of shock in children have been characterized (e.g., warm and cold shock, fluid-refractory shock, and catecholamine-resistant shock), these are not particularly helpful in diagnosis or management. Shock in children should be recognized by clinical and laboratory signs that include tachypnea and tachycardia, peripheral vasodilation (warm shock) or cool extremities (cold shock), altered mental status, hypothermia or hyperthermia, together with reduction of urine output, metabolic acidosis, or increased blood lactate. In addition to clinical and hemodynamic variables, shock can be defined in terms of its metabolic consequences, such as oxygen use variables or cellular variables.

CLASSIFICATION OF SHOCK

Quantitative Shock (Decreased Oxygen Delivery)

Decreased Flow (e.g., Hypovolemic, Cardiogenic Shock)

Decreased flow may be the consequence of either decreased circulating volume (absolute or relative hypovolemia) or failure of the cardiac pump. Hypovolemia is "absolute" due to dehydration from extracellular fluid, blood, or plasma loss and "relative" when fluid administration is inadequate to compensate for loss of vascular tone, as in sepsis or anaphylaxis, or due to vasodilating agents. In relative hypovolemia, a discrepancy exists between the circulating volume of blood and the vascular capacity. In addition, abnormal sympathetic tone is associated with altered capillary recruitment. Therefore, relative hypovolemia is associated with altered redistribution of flow among and within organs.

Cardiac failure resulting in shock can be due to myocardial injury (infectious or ischemic) or obstructive lesions [increased right ventricular afterload, increased pulmonary vascular resistance, increased left ventricular afterload, increased systemic vascular resistance (SVR)], and/or from lack of ventricular filling (decreased right ventricular or left ventricular preload, valvular lesions, decrease in filling time due to tachycardia).

Decreased Oxygen Content (CaO₂), (e.g., Hemorrhagic Shock, Acute Hypoxemic Respiratory Failure, Poisoning)

Hemorrhagic shock is usually a result of hypovolemia and anemia. However, anemia is not necessarily associated with hypovolemia (e.g., in hemolysis). When anemia is associated with hemorrhage (hypovolemia), the decrease in oxygen delivery (DO_2) is substantially greater than either insult alone. Decreased oxygen-carrying capacity of hemoglobin (Hb), and therefore inadequate DO_2, may also result in shock. For instance, with carbon monoxide poisoning, a decrease in DO_2 results from competitive binding of carbon monoxide in preference to O_2. This process is exacerbated by abnormal O_2 utilization, as carbon monoxide interferes with oxidative phosphorylation, resulting in a decreased oxygen extraction ratio (O_2ER). In this case, shock is both distributive and quantitative. In any respiratory cause of acute hypoxia, decreased arterial oxygen saturation (SaO_2) leads to a decrease in DO_2 as soon as cardiac output is unable to compensate for metabolic needs.

Distributive Shock (Decreased Oxygen Extraction)

Distributive shock often coexists with hypovolemic and/or cardiogenic shock. Distributive shock occurs when blood is redistributed among organs such as secondary to sepsis, anaphylaxis, or vasodilating agents. In addition, especially in sepsis, a decrease in capillary recruitment secondary to altered vascular reactivity, disseminated intravascular coagulation, endothelial cell dysfunction, or increased blood cell adhesiveness and abnormal mitochondrial function (mitochondrial injury or dysfunction) may be present. These changes contribute to the inability to fully utilize oxygen that is delivered. Spinal cord injury is a specific form of distributive shock that leads to profound hemodynamic changes. Sudden loss of sympathetic outflow from the spinal cord leads to a sudden decrease in total peripheral resistance and cardiac output, while central venous pressure (CVP) remains unchanged. The hypotension improves within days due to reasons that are not totally understood but may include synaptic reorganization or hyper-responsiveness of alpha receptors.

PATHOPHYSIOLOGY OF SHOCK

Oxygen Delivery (DO_2)

Circulatory failure results in a decrease in oxygen delivery (DO_2) to the tissues and is associated with a decrease in cellular partial pressure of oxygen (PO_2). When a critical PO_2 is reached, oxidative phosphorylation is limited by the lack of oxygen, leading to a shift from aerobic to anaerobic metabolism. The result is a rise in cellular and blood lactate concentration and a concomitant decrease in ATP synthesis. Because ATP provides the energy for cellular function, a decrease in or lack of ATP is the final common pathway of cellular insult in all forms of shock. ADP and hydrogen ion accumulate and, together with raised serum lactate, lead to metabolic and lactic acidosis.

Adequate tissue oxygenation is not an absolute number but relies on a DO_2 sufficient to meet tissue oxygen demand (47). Oxygen demand varies according to tissue type and according to time. Although oxygen demand cannot be measured or calculated, oxygen uptake or consumption (VO_2) and DO_2 can both be quantified and are linked by the relationship:

$$VO_2 = DO_2 \times O_2ER$$

where
O_2ER = oxygen extraction ratio (O_2ER in%, VO_2 and DO_2 in mLO_2/kg/min)
DO_2 = total flow of oxygen in arterial blood

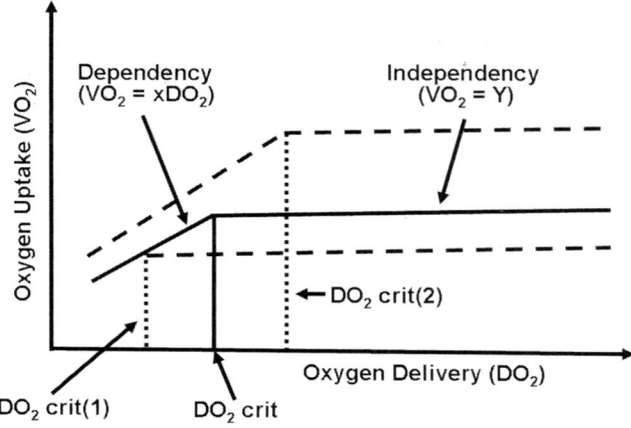

FIGURE 26.1. Relationship of oxygen uptake (VO_2) to oxygen delivery (DO_2): When VO_2 is supply independent (Independency), whole-body O_2 needs are met. When VO_2 becomes dependent on DO_2 (Dependency), VO_2 becomes linearly dependent on DO_2 at the critical DO_2 (DO_2crit), which corresponds to the definition of "dysoxia." DO_2crit is influenced by global oxygen requirements: When VO_2 is decreased (i.e., during sedation and hypothermia), the DO_2crit is also decreased [DO_2crit(1)]. When VO_2 is increased (i.e., agitation, hyperthermia, sepsis), DO_2crit is increased [DO_2crit(2)].

DO_2 is related to cardiac output (CO) and arterial oxygen content (CaO_2):

$$DO_2 = CO \times CaO_2$$

CaO_2 is the product of Hb (g/100 mL), arterial oxygen saturation (SaO_2,%), and Hb oxygen-carrying capacity (1.39 mL O_2/g Hb):

$$CaO_2 = Hb \times SaO_2 \times 1.39$$

Under normal conditions, oxygen demand equals VO_2 (roughly equivalent to 2.4 mL O_2/kg/min for a DO_2 of 12 mL O_2/kg/min, which corresponds to an O_2ER of 20%). The rate of oxygen delivered is physiologically larger than the rate of uptake or consumption; i.e., DO_2 is adapted to oxygen demand. When demand increases (e.g., during exercise), DO_2 must adapt and increase.

During circulatory shock or hypoxemia, as DO_2 declines, VO_2 is maintained by a compensatory increase in O_2ER; VO_2 and DO_2, therefore, remain independent. However, if DO_2 falls further, a critical point is reached (DO_2crit). O_2ER can no longer increase to compensate for the fall in DO_2, and at this point, VO_2 becomes dependent on DO_2. If VO_2 is higher, this DO_2crit is also higher (**Fig. 26.1**).

O_2ER increases because of redistribution of blood flow and capillary recruitment. Redistribution of blood flow occurs via an increase in sympathetic adrenergic tone and central vascular contraction in organs (e.g., the skin and gut), which have a low O_2ER. Blood is often preferentially shifted to maintain perfusion of critical organs (e.g., the brain and heart) that have a high O_2ER. Capillary recruitment is responsible for peripheral vasodilatation.

Mixed Venous Oxygen Saturation

In the clinical setting, mixed venous O_2 saturation (SvO_2) can be useful in assessing whole body VO_2-DO_2 relationships.

According to the Fick equation, tissue VO_2 is proportional to cardiac output:

$$VO_2 = cardiac\ output \times (CaO_2 - CvO_2)$$

where

$$CvO_2 = mixed\ venous\ blood\ oxygen\ content$$

To some extent, CaO_2 and CvO_2 are proportional to SaO_2 and SvO_2, respectively, by the relationship:

$$VO_2\ is\ proportional\ to\ CO \times (SaO_2 - SvO_2) \times Hb \times 1.39$$

Therefore, it becomes apparent that:

$$SvO_2\ is\ proportional\ to\ SaO_2 - VO_2/(CO \times Hb \times 1.39)$$

An examination of this relationship reveals that four conditions may cause SvO_2 to decrease: hypoxemia (decrease in SaO_2), increase in VO_2, reduction in CO, and decrease in Hb concentration. At DO_2crit, SvO_2 is approximately 40% (SvO_2crit), with an O_2ER of 60% and a SaO_2 of 100%. For the same decrease in CaO_2 (induced by either a decrease in Hb or SaO_2), the decrease in SvO_2 will be more pronounced if cardiac output cannot increase proportionately (43). Hence, SvO_2 represents adequacy of the response of global cardiac output to CaO_2 decrease.

A 40% SvO_2 can be taken as an imbalance between arterial blood O_2 supply and tissue O_2 demand, with evident risk of dysoxia. In the clinical setting, a decrease in SvO_2 of 5% from its normal value (65%–77%) represents a significant fall in DO_2 and/or an increase in O_2 demand. If treatment is instituted to restore SvO_2 to the normal range (such as fluid resuscitation, inotropic therapy, or red cell transfusion), the measurement of CO, as well as SaO_2 and Hb, should be instituted to choose and monitor response to therapy.

ASSESSMENT

Assessment of Global Blood Flow

Global blood flow is dependent on preload, myocardial function, afterload, and heart rate. Regional flow distribution is not homogeneous and is dependent on central and peripheral vascular tone, which ultimately results in the composite, SVR. As a gross simplification, mean arterial pressure (MAP) can be estimated as the product of flow by SVR, such that if flow decreases, MAP remains stable when SVR increases; this corresponds to an increase in sympathetic adrenergic tone and central volume contraction in low-O_2ER organs and preserved peripheral vasodilatation in high-O_2ER organs. Under these circumstances, overall O_2ER increases and SvO_2 decreases.

Good data are not available for the selection of threshold blood pressures that should be maintained in these situations, particularly in children. Arbitrary values of a systolic of 90 mm Hg or a MAP of 60 mm Hg in adults have been chosen, with population standards for age in children (18). During circulatory shock, when DO_2crit is breached, VO_2-DO_2 dependency, with a rise in blood lactate level, implies oxygen debt. In adults and children, hyperlactemia (and thus oxygen debt) is related to the likelihood of multiorgan failure and mortality (21,23).

The hemodynamic variables important in shock also relate to flow to vital organs. Flow (Q) varies directly with perfusion pressure (dP) and inversely with resistance (R), mathematically represented by:

$$Q = dP/R$$

For the whole body, this relationship is represented by:

$$CO = MAP - CVP/systemic\ vascular\ resistance$$

This relationship also holds for organ perfusion. In the kidney, for example:

$$Renal\ blood\ flow = mean\ renal\ arterial\ pressure - mean\ renal\ venous\ pressure/renal\ vascular\ resistance$$

Some organs, including the kidney and brain, have vasomotor autoregulation that maintains flow in low-pressure states. However, even in organs with autoregulation capabilities, at some critical point, perfusion pressure is reduced below the ability to maintain blood flow. The purpose of treatment of shock is to maintain perfusion pressure above the critical point below which blood flow cannot be effectively maintained in individual organs.

Because the kidney receives the second highest blood flow of any organ in the body, measurement of urine output can be used as an indicator of adequate perfusion pressure (with the exception of patients with hyperosmolar states leading to osmotic diuresis). In this regard, maintenance of MAP with norepinephrine has been shown to improve urine output and creatinine clearance in hyperdynamic sepsis. However, maintenance of supranormal MAP above this point is likely of no benefit (26).

Measurement of cardiac output and oxygen consumption, Cardiac Index (CI) × (arterial oxygen content − mixed venous oxygen), has been proposed as being of benefit in patients with persistent shock, because a CI between 3.3 and 6.0 L/min/m^2 and oxygen consumption of >200 mL/min/m^2 are associated with improved survival (36). Assuming a hemoglobin concentration of 10 g/dL and 100% arterial oxygen saturation, a CI of >3.3 L/min/m^2 would correlate to a mixed venous oxygen saturation of 70% in a patient with a normal oxygen consumption of 150 mL/min/m^2. Oxygen consumption is the product of CI, arterial oxygen content, and oxygen extraction. Therefore, an oxygen consumption of 150 mL/min/m^2 = 3.3 L/min/m^2 × [1.36 × 10 g/dL × 100 + PaO$_2$ × 0.003] × [100% − 70%].

To apply any therapeutic intervention, early recognition of shock is crucial. Previously well children with intact cardiovascular homeostatic mechanisms can compensate extremely well during hypoperfusion states. For this reason, it may be difficult to differentiate the early phases of compensated shock. Constant vigilance and repeated reevaluation is therefore required to recognize the early phases of shock.

Assessment of Regional Blood Flow

Skin Temperature Gradient

Body temperature gradients have long been used as a parameter of peripheral perfusion. In the presence of a constant environmental temperature, changes in skin temperature are the result of changes in skin blood flow (18). The temperature gradients, peripheral-to-ambient (dTp-a) and central-to-peripheral (dTc-p), can better reflect cutaneous blood flow than skin temperature itself. In the presence of constant environmental conditions, dTp-a decreases and dTc-p increases during vasoconstriction. A gradient of 3°–7°C occurs in patients who are hemodynamically stable (6). Moreover, an increase in dTp-a of >4°–6°C over 12 hrs was observed in survivors of hypovolemia and low cardiac output (22).

Optical Monitoring

Optical methods apply light with different wavelengths directly to tissue components, using the scattering characteristics of tissue to assess various states of these tissues. At physiologic concentrations, the molecules that absorb most light are hemoglobin, myoglobin, cytochrome, melanins, carotenes, and bilirubin. These substances can be quantified and measured in tissues using simple optical methods. The assessment of tissue oxygenation is based on the specific absorption spectrum of oxygenated Hb (HbO_2), deoxygenated Hb, and cytochrome aa3 (Cytaa3). Commonly used optical methods for peripheral monitoring are perfusion index, near-infrared spectroscopy, laser-Doppler flowmetry, and orthogonal polarization spectral.

Peripheral Perfusion Index. The peripheral perfusion (flow) index (PFI) is derived from the photoelectric plethysmographic signal of pulse oximetry and has been used as a noninvasive measure of peripheral perfusion in critically ill patients (28). The principle of pulse oximetry is based on two light sources with different wavelengths (660 nm and 940 nm) transmitted through the cutaneous vascular bed of a finger or earlobe. Deoxygenated Hb absorbs more light at 660 nm, and HbO_2 absorbs more light at 940 nm. A detector measures the intensity of the transmitted light at each wavelength, and the oxygen saturation is derived by the ratio between the red light (660 nm) and the infrared light (940 nm) absorbed. As other tissues, such as connective tissue, bone, and venous blood, also absorb light, pulse oximetry distinguishes the pulsatile component of arterial blood from the nonpulsatile component of other tissues. Using a two-wavelength system, the nonpulsatile component is then discarded, and the pulsatile component is used to calculate the arterial oxygen saturation. The overall hemoglobin concentration can be determined by a third wavelength at 800 nm, with a spectrum that resembles that of both Hb and HbO_2. The resulting variation in intensity of this light can be used to determine the variation in arterial blood volume (pulsatile component). The PFI is calculated as the ratio of the light that reaches the detector of the oximeter between the pulsatile component (arterial compartment) and the nonpulsatile component (other tissues) and is calculated independently of the patient's oxygen saturation. Alteration in peripheral perfusion is accompanied by variation in the pulsatile component, and because the nonpulsatile component does not change, the ratio changes. As a result, the value displayed on the monitor reflects changes in peripheral perfusion.

Near-infrared Spectroscopy. Near-infrared spectroscopy (NIRS) offers a technique for continuous, noninvasive, bedside monitoring of tissue oxygenation. As with pulse oximetry, NIRS uses the principles of light transmission and absorption to measure the concentrations of hemoglobin, oxygen saturation (StO_2), and Cytaa3 in tissues. NIRS has a greater tissue penetration than pulse oximetry and provides a global assessment of oxygenation in all vascular compartments (arterial, venous, and capillary). In addition to blood flow, evaluation of HbO_2 and Hb, NIRS can assess the Cytaa3 redox state. Cytaa3 is the end receptor in the oxygen transport chain that reacts with oxygen to form water, and most cellular energy is derived from this reaction. Cytaa3 remains in a reduced state during hypoxemia. The absorption spectrum of Cytaa3 in its reduced state shows a weak peak at 70 nm, whereas the oxygenated form does not. Therefore, monitoring changes in the Cytaa3 redox state can provide a measure of the adequacy of oxidative metabolism.

The use of NIRS in deltoid muscle during resuscitation of severe trauma patients has recently been reported (4,33). A strong association was found between elevated serum lactate levels and elevated Cytaa3 redox state during 12 hrs of shock resuscitation and the development of multiorgan failure (4). A good relationship was also shown between tissue O_2 (StO_2), systemic oxygen delivery, and lactate during and after resuscitation in severely injured patients over a period of 24 hrs (33). A study in septic and nonseptic adults used NIRS to measure both regional blood flow and oxygen consumption after venous occlusion (15). The potential to monitor regional perfusion and oxygenation noninvasively at the bedside makes clinical application of both PFI and NIRS technology of particular interest in intensive care.

Orthogonal Polarization Spectral. Orthogonal polarization spectral (OPS) is a noninvasive technique that uses reflected light to produce real-time images of the microcirculation. Light from a source passes through the first polarizer and is directed toward the tissue by a set of lenses. As the light reaches the tissue, the depolarized light is reflected back through the lenses to a second polarizer or analyzer and forms an image of the microcirculation, which can be recorded. The technology has been incorporated into a small hand-held video-microscope, which can be used in both research and clinical settings.

OPS can assess tissue perfusion using functional capillary density; i.e., the length of perfused capillaries per observation area (measured as cm/cm^2). Functional capillary density is a very sensitive parameter for determining the status of nutritive perfusion to the tissue, and it is an indirect measure of oxygen delivery.

One of the most easily accessible sites in humans for perfusion monitoring is the mouth. OPS produces clearly defined images of the sublingual microcirculation by placement of the probe under the tongue. The use of OPS to assess the sublingual tissues provides information about the dynamics of microcirculatory blood flow and, therefore, has been used to monitor the perfusion during clinical treatment of circulatory shock. It has shown the effects of improvements in microcirculatory blood flow with dobutamine and nitroglycerin in volume resuscitated septic patients (10,42). Limitations of the technique include movement artifacts, semiquantitative measures of perfusion, the presence saliva or blood, observer-related bias, and inadequacy of sedation to prevent patients from moving or damaging the device.

In septic patients, OPS has shown that microvascular alterations are more severe in patients with a worse outcome and that these microvascular alterations can be reversed using vasodilators (8).

In patients with cardiac failure and cardiogenic shock, the number of small vessels and the density of perfused vessels are lower than in controls, and the proportion of perfused vessels is higher in survivors than in nonsurvivors (9). Although alterations in the sublingual microcirculation may not be representative of other microvascular beds, changes in the sublingual circulation evaluated by capnometry during hemorrhagic shock have reflected changes in perfusion of splanchnic organs (24).

Transcutaneous Oxygen and Carbon Dioxide Measurements. The continuous noninvasive measurement of oxygen and carbon dioxide tension is possible because both gases can diffuse through the skin. At ambient temperature, the skin is not very permeable to gases, but at higher temperatures, the ability of the skin to transport gases is improved. Oxygen sensors for transcutaneous electrochemical measurements are based on polarography: an amperometric transducer in which the rate of a chemical reaction is detected by the current drained through an electrode. The sensor heats the skin to 43°–45°C, which causes dermal capillary hyperemia and increases local oxygen tension by shifting the oxygen dissociation curve in the heated dermal capillary blood. Transcutaneous sensors enable the estimation of arterial oxygen pressure (PaO_2) and arterial carbon dioxide pressure ($PaCO_2$) and have been successfully used for monitoring these values in both neonates and in adults.

The newborn infant is suitable for this method because of its thin epidermal layer. However, in older children and adults, the skin is thicker, causing the transcutaneous oxygen partial pressure ($PtcO_2$) to be lower than PaO_2. The correlation between $PtcO_2$ and PaO_2 also depends on the adequacy of blood flow. Low blood flow caused by vasoconstriction during shock overcomes the vasodilatory effect of the $PtcO_2$ sensor, resulting in tissue hypoxia beneath the $PtcO_2$ sensor. The fact that the $PtcO_2$ sensor does not accurately reflect the PaO_2 in low-flow states such as shock enables the estimation of cutaneous blood flow through the relationship between the two variables. Some have suggested the use of a transcutaneous oxygen index (tc-index), i.e., the changes in $PtcO_2$ relative to changes in PaO_2 (46).

When blood flow is adequate, $PtcO_2$ and PaO_2 values are almost equal and the tc-index is close to 1. During low flow states, such as shock, the $PtcO_2$ drops and becomes dependent on the PaO_2 value, and the tc-index decreases. A tc-index below 0.7 has been associated with hemodynamic instability. One group found a good correlation ($r = 0.86$) between tc-index and cardiac index in patients with shock (46). However, the relationship between tc-index and cardiac index appeared less reliable in hyperdynamic shock.

Transcutaneous carbon dioxide partial pressure ($PtcCO_2$) has been also used as an index of cutaneous blood flow. Differences between $PaCO_2$ and $PtcCO_2$ have been explained by local accumulation of CO_2 in the skin due to hypoperfusion. Because the diffusion constant of CO_2 through skin is approximately 20 times greater than O_2, $PtcCO_2$ is less sensitive to changes in hemodynamics than $PtcO_2$.

$PtcO_2$ and $PtcCO_2$ have also been used as early indicators of tissue hypoxia and subclinical hypovolemia in acutely ill patients in the emergency department (49) and operating room (44). Nonsurvivors had lower $PtcO_2$ values and higher $PtcCO_2$ values than did survivors. These differences were evident even shortly after the patient's arrival. The authors reported critical tissue perfusion threshold values of a $PtcO_2$ of 50 mm Hg for more than 60 mins and a $PtcCO_2$ of 60 mm Hg for more than 30 mins. Patients who failed to avoid these critical thresholds had 89%–100% mortality.

One of the main limitations of this technique is the necessity of blood gas analysis to obtain the tc-index and $PaCO_2$. In addition, the sensor position must be changed every 1–2 hrs to avoid burns. After each repositioning, a period of 15–20 min is required for stability, which limits its use in emergency situations. Also, the time required for calibration limits its early use in the emergency department, and critical $PtcO_2$ and $PtcCO_2$ values have not yet been established. Therefore, this technology therefore has not gained widespread acceptance in clinical practice.

Tissue Capnometry. Measurement of the tissue-arterial CO_2 tension gradient has been used to reflect the adequacy of tissue perfusion. Gastric and ileal mucosal CO_2 clearance has been the primary reference for measurements of regional PCO_2 gradient during circulatory shock (12). The regional PCO_2 gradient represents the balance between regional CO_2 production and clearance. In low flow states, tissue CO_2 increases as a result of a stagnation phenomenon (7). Comparable decreases in tissue blood flow during circulatory shock have also been demonstrated by measuring the sublingual tissue PCO_2 ($PslCO_2$) (38).

The currently available system for measuring $PslCO_2$ consists of a disposable PCO_2 sensor and a battery-powered, handheld instrument. Clinical studies have suggested that $PslCO_2$ is a reliable marker of tissue hypoperfusion. In one study of emergency department patients, patients with physical signs of circulatory shock and high blood lactate levels had higher $PslCO_2$ values, and a $PslCO_2$ threshold value of 70 mm Hg was predictive for the severity of circulatory failure (50).

As with PCO_2 in the gut mucosa, $PslCO_2$ is also influenced by $PaCO_2$. Hence, the gradient between $PslCO_2$ and $PaCO_2$ ($Psl-aCO_2$) may be more specific for tissue hypoperfusion. In one study, the $Psl-aCO_2$ gradient was a sensitive marker for tissue perfusion and a useful endpoint for the titration of goal-directed therapy (30). $Psl-aCO_2$ differentiated better than $PslCO_2$ alone between survivors and nonsurvivors, and a difference of >25 mm Hg indicated a poor prognosis. Limitations of this technique include the necessity of blood gas analysis to obtain $PaCO_2$. In addition, normal and pathologic $Psl-aCO_2$ values are not well defined.

In clinical practice, a more complete evaluation of tissue oxygenation can be achieved by adding noninvasive assessment of perfusion in peripheral tissues to global parameters. Noninvasive monitoring of peripheral perfusion can be applied early to patients in the emergency department, operating room, or on hospital wards. This approach can employ both simple physical examination and newer technologies just discussed. Although these methods may reflect variations in peripheral perfusion with certain accuracy, more studies are necessary to define the precise role of such methods in the evaluation of children in shock.

Clinical Assessment

History

In many cases, such as overt hemorrhage, the cause of shock is obvious. However, a detailed history in less obvious situations is vital to decisions regarding appropriate management. The early diagnosis of shock requires knowledge of the conditions that predispose children of different ages and comorbidities to shock. For instance, a history of congenital heart disease, immunodeficiency, trauma, surgery, toxin ingestion, or allergies is important.

Children who are febrile, who have an identifiable source of infection, or who are hypovolemic are at increased risk of developing shock. In neonates, the maternal and birth history is required, especially with regard to timing and duration of rupture of membranes, maternal fever, blood loss, fetal distress, and other obstetric information. In the case of trauma, history regarding the mechanism and timing of injury, whether excessive blood loss has occurred, and the level of consciousness before hospital arrival is vital. A history of immunodeficiency, use of immunosuppressive agents, duration and height of fever, and associated features, such as lethargy, vomiting, diarrhea, decreased oral intake, and decreased level of consciousness or awareness, may suggest infection and the possibility of septic shock or dehydration. Other details, such as environmental exposure, drug ingestion, previous medical history, and allergies, are also important.

Physical Examination

As children often will maintain their blood pressure until they are severely ill (53), the presence of systemic hypotension is not required to make the diagnosis of shock, as in adults. In guidelines published by the American College of Critical Care Medicine, Carcillo and colleagues defined shock in pediatric patients as tachycardia (which may be absent in the hypothermic patient), with signs of decreased organ or peripheral perfusion, including decreased peripheral pulses compared with central pulses, altered alertness, flash capillary refill or capillary refill >2 secs, mottled or cool extremities, or decreased urine output (5). Hypotension is a sign of late shock and should not be relied on to make the diagnosis. Moreover, the classifications of shock in children (e.g., warm and cold shock, fluid-refractory shock, or catecholamine-resistant shock) are not helpful for diagnosis but may dictate therapy.

Shock in children can be recognized before hypotension occurs by clinical and laboratory signs that include altered mental status, tachypnea and tachycardia, hypothermia or hyperthermia, and changes in peripheral perfusion [vasodilation (warm shock) or cool extremities (cold shock)], together with reduction of urine output, metabolic acidosis, or increased blood lactate.

In addition to these classifications of shock, it is also helpful to consider three stages in shock: compensated, decompensated, and irreversible. In the early, compensated stage, homeostatic mechanisms are functioning to maintain vital organ perfusion. Blood pressure, urine output, and cardiac function may all appear normal; however, early cellular metabolic alterations are taking place. In decompensated shock, circulatory compensation fails because of dysoxia, ischemia, endothelial cell injury and dysfunction, the upregulation and elaboration of inducible gene products, and the release of toxic materials from host cells and microorganisms (either invasive or from the patient's gut). Eventually, cellular function deteriorates and widespread abnormalities occur in all organ systems, eventually leading to multiorgan failure. When this process has caused such widespread organ dysfunction, death is inevitable despite temporary support, and the irreversible stage of shock is reached. The point at which irreversibility is reached is becoming more advanced as technology and supportive care improves.

The physical examination may reveal a decrease in tissue perfusion, which is identified by changes in body surface temperature, prolonged capillary refill time, and impaired organ function. Decreased skin perfusion and temperature reflects a predominance of the sympathetic neurohumoral response to hypovolemia (27). Skin temperature is measured using the dor-

sal surface of the examiner's hands or fingers because these areas are most sensitive to temperature perception. Patients are considered to have cool extremities (a) if all examined extremities are cool to the examiner or (b) if only the lower extremities are cool, despite warm upper extremities, in the absence of peripheral vascular disease. Clinical signs of poor peripheral perfusion consist of cold, pale, clammy, and mottled skin, associated with an increase in capillary refill time. In particular, skin temperature and capillary refill time have been advocated as an indicator of the adequacy of peripheral perfusion (25,32,41,43,45). In a study that related the measurement of distal extremity skin temperature (evaluated by subjective physical examination) as a marker of peripheral perfusion with biochemical and hemodynamic markers of hypoperfusion in adult patients in the ICU, an association was reported in patients with cold peripheries (including septic patients) between poor peripheral perfusion with lower cardiac output and higher blood lactate levels, indicating more severe tissue hypoxia (25).

Capillary refill time (CRT) has become widely accepted as a reflection of intravascular volume, especially in children and in the assessment of trauma. A value <2 secs at normal ambient temperature is considered adequate. CRT has been validated as a measure of peripheral perfusion, with significant variation in children and adults. A study on a normal population reported that CRT varied with age and sex (41). It was found that a CRT of <2 secs was a normal value for most young children and young adults, but that CRT varied with age, being substantially higher in healthy women (2.9s) and in the elderly (4.5s). A poor correlation may exist between CRT, heart rate, blood pressure, and cardiac output (41,45); however, prolonged CRT in pediatric patients has been found to be a good predictor of dehydration, reduced stroke volume, and increased blood lactate levels (32,43). The findings of these studies show that monitoring of skin temperature and CRT are valuable in hemodynamic monitoring during circulatory shock and should be the first approach to assess any critically ill patient. Less data is available regarding the clinical utility of these measures once the patient has been admitted to the ICU.

Laboratory Markers of Shock

Serial blood gas and arterial lactate evaluation are widely used to complement the clinical assessment of systemic perfusion by quantifying the extent of tissue hypoperfusion and providing useful trends with which to titrate therapy. Normalization of blood pressure may not indicate reversal of the shock state in a patient who has ongoing metabolic acidosis and/or elevated arterial lactate.

Mixed venous O_2 saturation (SvO_2) can be useful in assessing whole-body VO_2-DO_2 relationships. Recent studies have used central venous oxygen saturation ($ScvO_2$) to detect global O_2 deficiency (39). An important feature is that $ScvO_2$ can be monitored continuously with fiberoptic probes. Early identification of patients with severe sepsis and shock and rapid initiation of goal-directed therapy to achieve adequate tissue oxygenation by improving DO_2 ($ScvO_2$ monitoring) has been shown to significantly improve mortality (39).

In the clinical setting, a decrease in SvO_2 of 5% from its normal value (65%–77%) represents a significant fall in DO_2 and/or an increase in O_2 demand. If treatment is instituted to restore SvO_2 to the normal range (such as fluid resuscitation, inotropic therapy, or red cell transfusion), measurement of CO, as well as SaO_2 and Hb should be instituted to introduce the appropriate corrective therapy. The implication is that the strategy for managing shock relies on early and rapid estimation of O_2 deficit, rapidly followed by corrective therapy and ongoing monitoring, dependent on the most likely cause of dysoxia (39).

While lactate and base deficit estimations together with $ScvO_2$ measurement are invaluable for detection and monitoring of global O_2 deficiency, regional and tissue perfusion may not be accurately assessed using these indices. With increasing emphasis on the importance of optimizing regional perfusion, other measures to assist in the definition of shock states have come into clinical use in recent years. Some of these technologies will be mentioned briefly because they are not widely used in the initial stages of resuscitation from shock. Moreover, they may be more useful in monitoring the response to therapy in the PICU.

THERAPEUTIC PRINCIPLES

Monitoring

Apart from repeated clinical examinations, the minimal monitoring appropriate for patients who are either in incipient or actual shock includes continuous electrocardiography, pulse oximetry, continuous invasive or rapid and regular noninvasive blood pressure, and urine catheter for continuous measurement of urine output. A central venous catheter allows CVP monitoring, which may indicate the need for fluid if the CVP is <8 mm Hg. In addition, the catheter allows rapid infusion of drugs and fluids and monitoring of $ScvO_2$ (a surrogate for mixed SvO_2). However, a central venous catheter insertion for CVP monitoring is not essential in the early stages of management of a child in shock.

In the sedated, ventilated patient, recordings of systolic pressure variation and/or pulse pressure variation may be helpful. The heart remains preload dependent until systolic pressure variation is <10 mm Hg, and/or pulse pressure variation is <10% (34). Blood gas analysis, which examines metabolic acidosis and lactate concentration, gives an indication of global oxygenation, which reflects the adequacy of cardiac output and oxygen delivery.

A pulmonary artery catheter (ideally with continuous CO monitoring and with a fiberoptic SvO_2 device) and/or any noninvasive flow assessment (transesophageal Doppler or echocardiography) is recommended when cardiac output is difficult to assess according to the Frank-Starling curve. In this context, the effect of fluid administration on cardiac output and oxygen delivery/consumption should be assessed and titrated.

Symptomatic Treatment

General Supportive Measures

Emergency therapy should be given to all patients while the specific diagnosis is being established. Supplemental O_2 and respiratory support should be titrated in response to acute respiratory failure (whether primary respiratory failure, as in acute lung injury, or secondary, as a result of shock). Acute circulatory failure should be initially treated by fluid challenge. If intravascular volume is optimized and myocardial contractil-

ity remains reduced, support with vasoactive agents w with vasoactive agents ill be necessary. In the case of distributive shock (e.g., anaphylaxis or acute vasodilation), adrenaline or vasoconstrictors should be considered. Suggested protocols for management in the emergency department and shortly after transition to the ICU is outlined in **Figures 26.2** and **26.3**.

Fluid Infusion

Fluid challenge is the first step in therapy. The goal is to optimize left ventricular preload to improve DO_2 by increasing cardiac output as in the Frank-Starling curve. However, this increases the risk of pulmonary interstitial edema. It has been reported that up to 60 mL/kg fluid may be given in the first hour of therapy to children with septic shock, without increasing the risk of pulmonary edema, while resulting in a consequent improvement in outcome (19).

In septic shock it is widely accepted that maximal preload and, thus, cardiac output are obtained at a pulmonary artery occlusion pressure of 12–15 mm Hg. However, recent studies have revealed no clear evidence of benefit of pulmonary artery catheters (20) and their routine use in children is limited.

Clinical fluid requirement is usually determined in the emergency situation by clinical parameters, such as a combination of heart rate, blood pressure, peripheral perfusion, and urine output, and these are supplemented by invasive monitoring of CVP and arterial pressure, as well as biochemical parameters of global perfusion, such as venous oxygen saturation, serum lactate, strong ion gap, and base deficit.

The choice of fluid for resuscitation is also a subject of intense debate. Several studies have cast doubt on previously accepted theories that colloid solutions are better for fluid replacement in critical illness, as colloids were thought to be more likely to be retained intravascularly and thus less likely to exacerbate capillary leakage, especially in the lung. A meta-analysis by the Cochrane Albumin Reviewers suggested that 4.5% human albumin solution (HAS) may be associated with excess mortality when compared with saline for various indications, including hypovolemia (1). However, other investigators have suggested that the use of 4.5% HAS may be associated with improvements in morbidity (48). These meta-analyses prompted a large, randomized, controlled study in nearly 7000 critically ill adults that showed that use of either 4% HAS or normal saline for fluid resuscitation in patients in ICUs resulted in similar outcomes at 28 days (13). However, in subgroup analyses of patients included in this study, HAS seemed to have a protective effect in patients with septic shock, and normal saline seemed to have a protective effect in patients with traumatic brain injury. The reasons for these subgroup findings are unclear, but should be examined in future studies.

Few large, properly controlled studies of the differences between various fluids for resuscitation of pediatric shock have been conducted. In one analysis of children with dengue shock syndrome, no difference was seen between patients resuscitated with crystalloid or colloid solutions (52). However, this is a very specific form of septic shock in which, despite increased capillary permeability, patients become hemoconcentrated, a condition not seen in other forms of septic shock. In addition, few large, properly conducted studies of the use of artificial colloid solutions have been performed in children; therefore doubt remains regarding the short-term and long-term effects of the artificial colloid solutions. However, the use of normal

SUGGESTED EMERYGENCY DEPARTMENT SEPSIS PROTOCOL

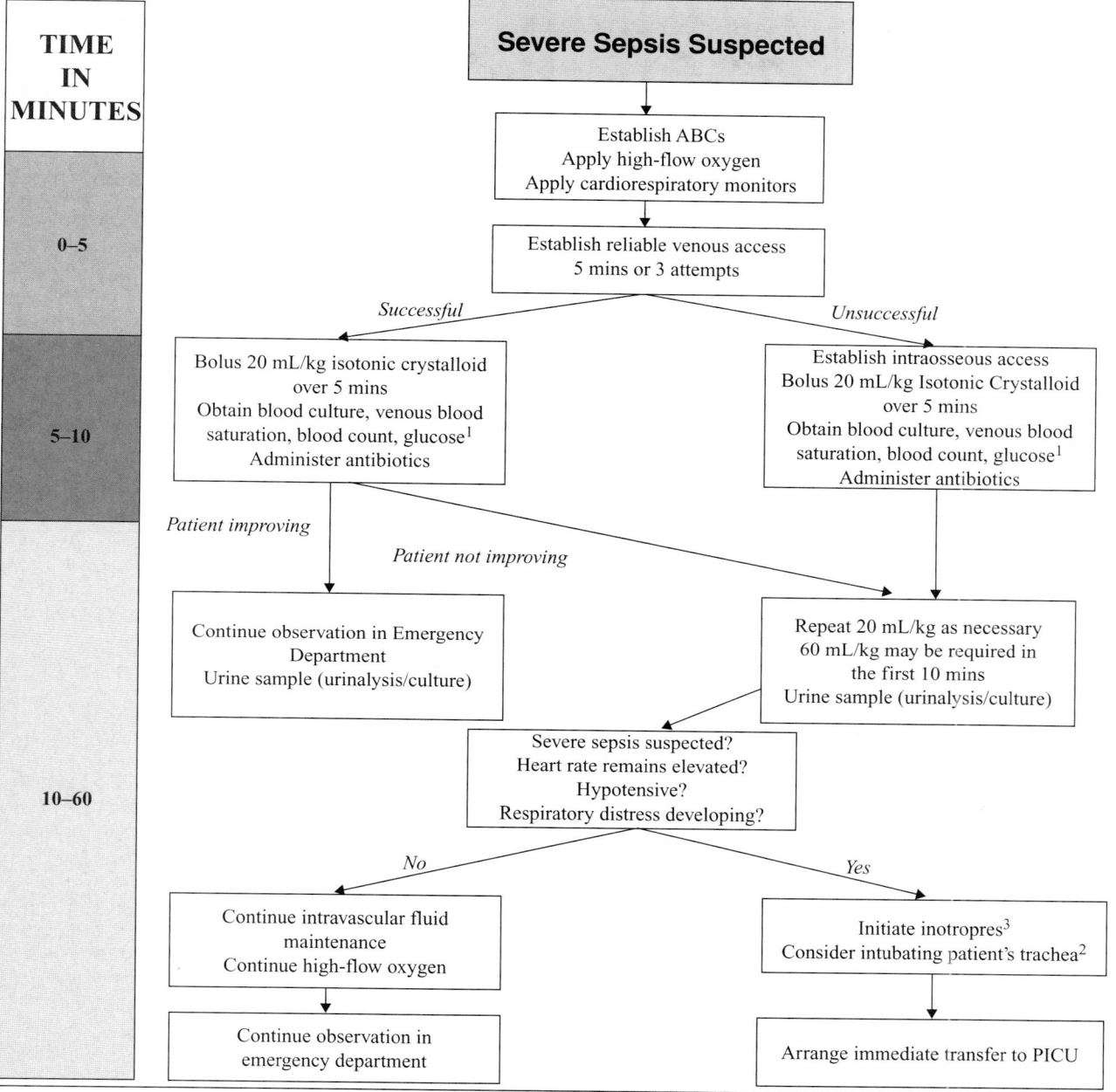

FIGURE 26.2. Suggested emergency department sepsis protocol.

1. Blood sample includes blood culture, complete blood count with differential, electrolytes, BUN, creatinine, venous blood saturation, lactate, ionized calcium, glucose.

2. Consider: Vagolytic (atropine 20 mcg/kg); Induction agent with minimal hypotensive effect (ketamine 1 mg/kg); Paralytic (rocuronium 1 mg/kg or succinylcholine 2 mg/kg).

3. Recommended inotropes if peripheral access only: dopamine 10 mcg/kg/min, epinephrine 0.1–0.2 mcg/kg/min. Recommended inotropes if central access: dopamine 10 mcg/kg/min, epinephrine 0.05–2 mcg/kg/min, norepinephrine (0.05–2 mcg/kg/min).

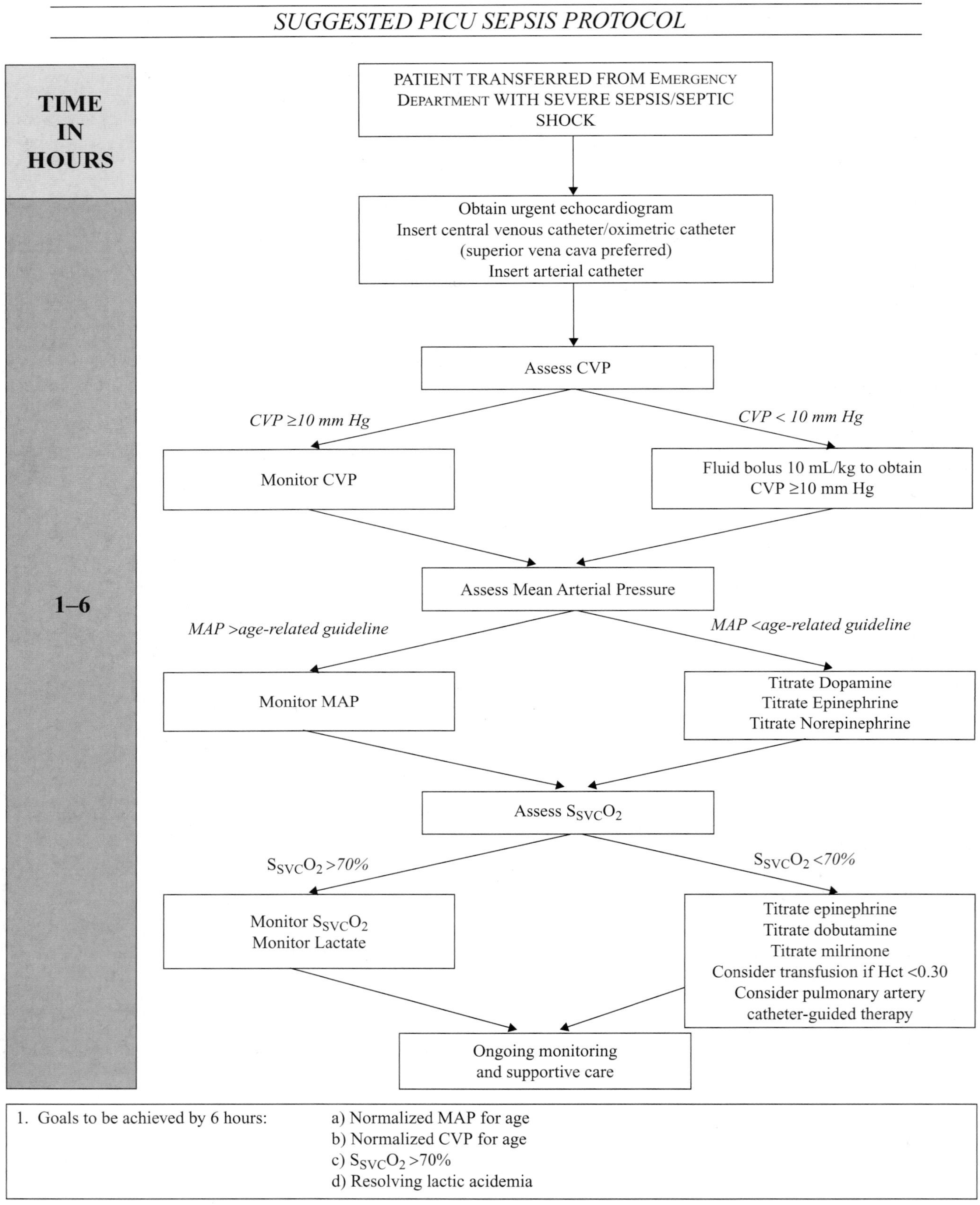

SUGGESTED PICU SEPSIS PROTOCOL

TIME IN HOURS

1–6

PATIENT TRANSFERRED FROM EMERGENCY DEPARTMENT WITH SEVERE SEPSIS/SEPTIC SHOCK

Obtain urgent echocardiogram
Insert central venous catheter/oximetric catheter
(superior vena cava preferred)
Insert arterial catheter

Assess CVP

CVP ≥10 mm Hg → Monitor CVP

CVP < 10 mm Hg → Fluid bolus 10 mL/kg to obtain CVP ≥10 mm Hg

Assess Mean Arterial Pressure

MAP >age-related guideline → Monitor MAP

MAP <age-related guideline → Titrate Dopamine / Titrate Epinephrine / Titrate Norepinephrine

Assess $S_{SVC}O_2$

$S_{SVC}O_2 >70\%$ → Monitor $S_{SVC}O_2$ / Monitor Lactate

$S_{SVC}O_2 <70\%$ → Titrate epinephrine / Titrate dobutamine / Titrate milrinone / Consider transfusion if Hct <0.30 / Consider pulmonary artery catheter-guided therapy

Ongoing monitoring and supportive care

1. Goals to be achieved by 6 hours:
   a) Normalized MAP for age
   b) Normalized CVP for age
   c) $S_{SVC}O_2 >70\%$
   d) Resolving lactic acidemia

FIGURE 26.3. Suggested PICU sepsis protocol. CVP, central venous pressure; MAP, mean arterial pressure.

saline as the initial fluid for shock resuscitation is reasonable (3).

Antibiotic Therapy

Ample evidence suggests that early administration of appropriate antibiotics reduces mortality in critically ill patients with bloodstream infections. The choice of antibiotics is vital and should be guided by the susceptibility of likely pathogens in the community and the hospital, as well as any specific knowledge about the patient, including underlying disease and the clinical syndrome. The regimen should cover all likely pathogens, as there is little margin for error in critically ill patients. A guide to aid in the selection of the most appropriate early antibiotic based on the suspected source can be found in **Table 26.1**. The eventual choice will also depend on prevalent pathogens and susceptibilities in the community and hospital.

Although restricting the use of antibiotics is important for decreasing the development of antibiotic-resistant pathogens, critically ill children with severe sepsis or septic shock warrant broad-spectrum therapy until the causative organism and its antibiotic susceptibilities are available. The antimicrobial regimen should always be reassessed after 48–72 hrs on the basis of microbiologic and clinical data, with the aim of narrowing the antibiotic spectrum to reduce (a) the risk of development of antimicrobial resistance, (b) toxicity, and (c) costs.

Blood Replacement

Usually, blood replacement is not required unless shock is due to acute hemorrhage or anemia. However, an Hb of >8–10 g/dL is thought to be useful in patients with severe sepsis and/or decreased cardiac contractility (11). In these patients, the decreased Hb concentration is not compensated by an increase in cardiac output, and DO_2crit is reached more rapidly.

Vasoactive Agents

Catecholamines help in restoration of perfusion pressure and augmentation of cardiac output to ensure sufficient DO_2, which should allow regional flow distribution and improved O_2ER. All catecholamines are inotropic agents and can be classified as (a) *inodilators* when they combine inotropic properties with vasodilation (e.g., dobutamine and milrinone; these agents increase flow), and (b) *inoconstrictors* when they combine inotropic properties with vasoconstricting effects (e.g., dopamine, adrenaline, noradrenaline; these agents increase perfusion pressure). Due to variations in individual sensitivities, dose titration of inotropes is mandatory.

More potent vasoactive agents, such as vasopressin and its derivatives, and inhibitors of nitric oxide synthase are now being used in children with shock (31). These agents cause a rise in blood pressure. However, just as a low blood pressure is not necessary to diagnose shock in children, restoration of blood pressure may not necessarily be a surrogate for clinical benefit in any patient. Indeed, in a large clinical trial of an antagonist of nitric oxide synthase that was used in an attempt to reverse sepsis-induced hypotension, the required rise in blood pressure was mirrored by a significant increase in mortality (29).

OTHER THERAPEUTIC PRINCIPLES

A number of treatments are clearly essential for the management of any patient in shock. Infectious source control and its eradication are vital. In addition, treatment of hypoxia and identification and treatment of ongoing fluid losses or occult hemorrhage are mandatory. If, despite these basic therapeutic principles shock continues, advanced supportive measures may be required.

The importance of correcting metabolic abnormalities has been emphasized in anecdotal guidelines in children with meningococcal shock (37). However, clinical studies of the use of bicarbonate therapy to correct shock-induced metabolic acidosis failed to show any improvement in cardiac output or reduction in inotrope requirement, regardless of the degree of acidemia (14). Treatment for adults has moved toward goal-directed therapies, with the targets for children in the process of being defined.

Replacement low-dose steroid therapy has been shown to be beneficial in patients with septic shock and evidence of adrenal hyporesponsiveness, especially in those with high or increasing requirements for inotropes (2). This benefit has not yet been demonstrated in pediatric patients. However, similar adrenal hyporesponsiveness has been shown in children (35), and stress doses of steroids are now commonly used in children who require high-dose inotropes.

CONCLUSIONS AND FUTURE DIRECTIONS

Shock is a clinical diagnosis. The mainstay of therapy is to recognize the seriously ill child before shock progresses to irreversibility. Once shock is present, attempts must be made to prevent its progression. Without a specific marker to determine the irreversible point in shock, heroic efforts to reverse shock, such as the use of extracorporeal devices for cardiac support, may be reasonable. However, regardless of the initial type of shock, by the time shock advances to gross abnormalities in volume status, vascular tone, cardiac function, cellular energetics, and multiorgan function, it is very likely that purely mechanical devices will not correct all of these existent abnormalities (51). Further definition of specific goal-directed therapies, with evidence-based targets for prevention or non-progression of shock is on the horizon.

KEY POINTS

- Clinical evaluation must include full assessment of respiratory and cardiovascular status, including oxygenation, respiratory rate and work of breathing, heart rate, blood pressure, peripheral perfusion, urine output, and level of consciousness.
- Laboratory evaluation should include markers of global oxygenation, including arterial blood gas and lactate measurement.
- Rapid assessment of global oxygen variables can be obtained by mixed venous or central venous oxygen saturation.
- Many methods of evaluation of regional tissue oxygenation and microvascular blood flow are being developed; the most useful include near infrared spectroscopy and orthogonal polarization spectral.

TABLE 26.1

	NEONATE (<1 mo)	INFANT (1–3 mos)	PEDIATRIC (>3 mos)
Sepsis Unknown Source	Ampicillin + [gentamicin or cefotaxime] Ampicillin 50 mg/kg/dose IV and q6h (q8h if <1 wk old) **plus** Gentamicin 2.5 mg/kg/dose IV q8 hrs (q12 hrs if <1 week old) and Acyclovir 20 mg/kg/dose IV q8 hrs **OR** Ampicillin 50 mg/kg/dose IV and q6h (q8 hrs if <1 wk old) **plus** Cefotaxime 50 mg/kg/dose IV and q8 hrs (q12 hrs if <1 wk old)	Ampicillin + cefotaxime Ampicillin 50 mg/kg/dose IV & q6 hrs **plus** Cefotaxime 50 mg/kg/dose & IV q6 hrs	Cloxacillin + Cefotaxime Cloxacillin 50 mg/kg/dose IV and q6 hrs (Max 2 g/dose) **plus** Cefotaxime 50 mg/kg/dose IV and q6 hrs (Max 2 g/dose)
CNS Suspected Source			Cefotaxime ± Vancomycin Cefotaxime 75 mg/kg/dose IV and q6 hrs (Max 2 g/dose) **plus** Vancomycin 20 mg/kg IV × 1 dose, then 15 mg/kg/dose IV q6 hrs
		Shunt/EVD Meropenem 40 mg/kg dose IV and q8 hrs (Max 2g/dose) plus Vancomycin 20 mg/kg IV × 1 dose, then 15 mg/kg/dose IV q6 hrs	
Pneumonia Suspected Source		Cloxacillin + Cefotaxime Cloxacillin 50 mg/kg/dose IV and q6 hrs (Max 2 g/dose) **plus** Cefotaxime 50 mg/kg/dose IV and q6 hrs (Max 2 g/dose)	Cloxacillin + Cefotaxime +/- azithromycin Cloxacillin 50 mg/kg/dose IV and q6 hrs (Max 2 g/dose) **plus** Cefotaxime 50 mg/kg/dose IV and q6 hrs (Max 2 g/dose) **plus** Azithromycin 10 mg/kg/dose PO/IV × 1 dose (Max 500 mg), then 5 mg/kg/dose PO/IV q24 hrs (max 250 mg/dose) × 5 days
GU Suspected Source	**No known anatomic abnormalities or first presentation:** Ampicillin + gentamicin Ampicillin 50 mg/kg/dose IV and q6 hrs (q8 hrs if <1 wk old) **plus** Gentamicin 2.5 mg/kg/dose IV NOW and q8 hrs (q12 hrs if <1 wk old) **Known abnormality of GU tract:** Piperacillin + gentamicin Piperacillin 75 mg/kg/dose IV q6 hrs (q8 hrs if <1 wk old) **plus** Gentamicin 2.5 mg/kg/dose IV q8 hrs (q12 hrs if <1 wk old)	> 1 mo old: **No known anatomic abnormalities or first presentation:** Ampicillin + gentamicin Ampicillin 50 mg/kg/dose IV and q6 hrs (Max 3g/dose) **plus** Gentamicin 7 mg/kg/dose IV and every q24 hrs **Known abnormality of GU tract:** Piperacillin/ tazobactam + gentamicin Piperacillin/tazobactam 75 mg/kg/dose piperacillin component IV q6 hrs (Max 4 g/dose) plus Gentamicin 7 mg/kg/dose IV **NOW** and every q24 hrs	
Skin/ Soft Tissue Suspected Source	Clindamycin + Penicillin + Gentamicin **OR** Clindamycin + Cefotaxime Clindamycin 5 mg/kg/dose IV and q6 hrs (q8 hrs if <1 wk old) **plus** Penicillin 50,000 units/kg/dose IV and q6 hrs (q8 hrs if <1wk old) **plus** Gentamicin 2.5 mg/kg/dose IV and q8 hrs (q12 hrs if <1wk old) **OR** Clindamycin 5 mg/kg/dose IV **NOW** and q6 hrs (q8 hrs if <1wk old) **plus** Cefotaxime 50 mg/kg/dose IV **NOW** and q8 hrs (q12 hrs if <1 wk old)	> 1 mo old: Clindamycin + Penicillin + Gentamicin **OR** Clindamycin + Cefotaxime Clindamycin 13 mg/kg/dose IV and q8 hrs (Max 900 mg/dose) **plus** Penicillin 65,000 units/kg/dose IV and q4 hrs (Max 4 million units/dose) **plus** Gentamicin 7 mg/kg/dose IV and q24 hrs **OR** Clindamycin 13 mg/kg/dose IV and q8 hrs (Max 900 mg/dose) **plus** Cefotaxime 50 mg/kg/dose IV and q6 hrs (Max 2 g/dose) **if Group A Strep suspected** **Add IV immunoglobulin (IVIG) 1 g/kg/dose IV q24 hrs × 2 doses** ****ordered from blood bank**	
Immunocompromised/Febrile Neutropenic Patient	> 1 mo old: Piperacillin/tazobactam + gentamicin Piperacillin/tazobactam 75 mg/kg/dose piperacillin component IV NOW and q6 hrs (Max 4 g/dose) **plus** Gentamicin 7 mg/kg/dose IV and q24 hrs		

- The "Holy Grail" of shock management would be a rapid, noninvasive, reliable method of assessing deficits in both regional and local oxygenation.
- Management is dependent on understanding causes of shock and giving both cause-directed and early goal-directed therapies.
- Well-controlled, randomized trials for children with shock states are urgently required to evaluate the most appropriate and effective aspects of therapy.

References

1. Alderson P, Bunn F, Lefebvre C, et al. Human albumin solution for resuscitation and volume expansion in critically ill patients. *Cochrane Database Syst Rev* 2004;4:CD001208.
2. Annane D, Sebille V, Charpentier C, et al. Effect of treatment with low doses of hydrocortisone and fludrocortisone on mortality in patients with septic shock. *JAMA* 2002;288:862–71.
3. Boluyt N, Bollen CW, Bos AP, et al. Fluid resuscitation in neonatal and pediatric hypovolemic shock: a Dutch Pediatric Society evidence-based clinical practice guideline. *Intensive Care Med* 2006;32(7):995–1003.
4. Cairns CB, Moore FA, Haenel JB, et al. Evidence for early supply independent mitochondrial dysfunction in patients developing multiple organ failure after trauma. *J Trauma* 1997;42:532–6.
5. Carcillo JA, Fields AI, Task Force Committee Members: Clinical practice variables for hemodynamic support of pediatric and neonatal patients in septic shock. *Crit Care Med* 2002;30:1365–1378.
6. Curley FJ, Smyrnios NA. Routine monitoring of critically ill patients. In: Irwin RS, Cerra FB, Rippe JM, eds. *Intensive Care Medicine*. New York: Lippincott. Williams & Wilkins. 2003;250–70.
7. De Backer D, Creteur J, Preiser JC, et al. Microvascular blood flow is altered in patients with sepsis. *Am J Respir Crit Care Med* 2002;166:98–104.
8. De Backer D, Creteur J. Regional hypoxia and partial pressure of carbon dioxide gradients: what is the link? *Intensive Care Med* 2003;29:2116–2118.
9. De Backer D, Creteur J, Dubois MJ, et al. Microvascular alterations in patients with acute severe heart failure and cardiogenic shock. *Am Heart J* 2004;147:91–99.
10. De Backer D, Creteur J, Dubois MJ, et al. The effects of dobutamine on microcirculatory alterations in patients with septic shock are independent of its systemic effects. *Crit Care Med* 2006;34:403–8.
11. Dellinger RP, Carlet JM, Masur H, et al. Surviving sepsis campaign guidelines for management of severe sepsis and septic shock. *Crit Care Med* 2004;32:858–73.
12. Fiddian-Green RG, Baker S. Predictive value of the stomach wall Ph for complications after cardiac operations: comparison with other monitoring. *Crit Care Med* 1987;15:153–156.
13. Finfer S, Bellomo R, Boyce N, et al. A comparison of albumin and saline for fluid resuscitation in the intensive care unit. *N Engl J Med* 2004;350:2247–56.
14. Forsythe SM, Schmidt GA. Sodium bicarbonate for the treatment of lactic acidosis. *Chest* 2000;117:260–7.
15. Girardis M, Rinaldi L, Busani S, et al. Muscle perfusion and oxygen consumption by near-infrared spectroscopy in septic shock and non-septic-shock patients. *Intensive Care Med* 2003;29:1173–1176.
16. Goldman AP, Kerr SJ, Butt W, et al. Extracorporeal support for intractable cardiorespiratory failure due to meningococcal disease. *Lancet* 1997;349:466–9.
17. Goldstein B, Giroir B, Randolph A. International Consensus Conference on Pediatric Sepsis. International pediatric sepsis consensus conference: Definitions for sepsis and organ dysfunction in pediatrics. *Pediatr Crit Care Med* 2005;6:2–8.
18. Guyton AC. Body temperature, temperature regulation, and fever. In: Guyton AC, Hall JE, eds. *Textbook of Medical Physiology*. Philadelphia: Saunders, 1996:911–22.
19. Han YY, Carcillo JA, Dragotta MA, et al. Early reversal of pediatric-neonatal septic shock by community physicians is associated with improved outcome. *Pediatrics* 2003;112:793–9
20. Harvey S, Harrison DA, Singer M, et al. Assessment of the clinical effectiveness of pulmonary artery catheters in management of patients in intensive care (PAC-Man): A randomised controlled trial. *Lancet* 2005;366:472–7.
21. Hatherill M, Waggie Z, Purves L, et al. Mortality and the nature of metabolic acidosis in children with shock. *Intensive Care Med.* 2003;29:286–91.

22. Henning RJ, Wiener F, Valdes S, Weil MH. Measurement of toe temperature for assessing the severity of acute circulatory failure. *Surg Gynecol Obstet* 1979;149:1–7.
23. Husain FA, Martin MJ, et al. Serum lactate and base deficit as predictors of mortality and morbidity. *Am J Surg* 2003;185:485–91.
24. Jin X, Weil MH, Sun S, et al. Decreases in organ blood flows associated with increases in sublingual PCO_2 during hemorrhagic shock. *J Appl Physiol* 1998;85:2360–4.
25. Kaplan LJ, McPartland K, Santora TA, et al. Start with a subjective assessment of skin temperature to identify hypoperfusion in intensive care unit patients. *J Trauma* 2001;50:620–7.
26. LeDoux D, Astiz ME, Carpati CM, et al. Effects of perfusion pressure on tissue perfusion in septic shock. *Crit Care Med* 2000;28:2729–2732.
27. Lima AP, Beelen P, Bakker J. Use of a peripheral perfusion index derived from the pulse oximetry signal as a noninvasive indicator of perfusion. *Crit Care Med* 2002;30:1210–1213.
28. Lima A, Bakker J. Noninvasive monitoring of peripheral perfusion. *Intensive Care Med* 2005;31:1316–26.
29. Lopez A, Lorente JA, Steingrub J, et al. Multiple-center, randomized, placebo-controlled, double-blind study of the nitric oxide synthase inhibitor 546C88: Effect on survival in patients with septic shock. *Crit Care Med* 2004;32:21–30.
30. Marik PE, Bankov A. Sublingual capnometry versus traditional markers of tissue oxygenation in critically ill patients. *Crit Care Med* 2003;31:818–22.
31. Matok I, Vard A, Efrati O, et al. Terlipressin as rescue therapy for intractable hypotension due to septic shock in children. *Shock* 2005;23:305–10.
32. McGee S, Abernethy WB, III, Simel DL. Is this patient hypovolemic? *JAMA* 1999;281:1022–9.
33. McKinley BA, Marvin RG, Cocanour CS, et al. Tissue hemoglobin O_2 saturation during resuscitation of traumatic shock monitored using near infrared spectrometry. *J Trauma* 2000;48:637–42.
34. Michard F, Boussat S, Chemla D, et al. Relation between respiratory changes in arterial pulse pressure and fluid responsiveness in septic patients with acute circulatory failure. *Am J Respir Crit Care Med* 2000;162:134–8.
35. Pizarro CF, Troster EJ, Damiani D, et al. Absolute and relative adrenal insufficiency in children with septic shock. *Crit Care Med* 2005;33:855–9.
36. Pollack MM, Fields AI, Ruttimann UE. Distributions of cardiopulmonary variables in pediatric survivors and nonsurvivors of septic shock. *Crit Care Med* 1985;13:454–459.
37. Pollard AJ, Britto J, Nadel S, et al. Emergency management of meningococcal disease. *Arch Dis Child* 1999;80:290–6.
38. Povoas HP, Weil MH, Tang W, et al. Comparisons between sublingual and gastric tonometry during hemorrhagic shock. *Chest* 2000;118:1127–32.
39. Rivers E, Nguyen B, Havstad S, et al. Early goal-directed therapy in the treatment of severe sepsis and septic shock. *N Engl J Med* 2001;345:1368–77.
40. Ronco JJ, Fenwick JC, Tweeddale MG, et al. Identification of the critical oxygen delivery for anaerobic metabolism in critically ill septic and nonseptic humans. *JAMA* 1993;270:1724–30.
41. Schriger DL, Baraff L. Defining normal capillary refill: Variation with age, sex, and temperature. *Ann Emerg Med* 1988;17:932–5.
42. Spronk PE, Ince C, Gardien MJ, et al. Nitroglycerin in septic shock after intravascular volume resuscitation. *Lancet* 2002;360:1395–6.
43. Steiner MJ, DeWalt DA, Byerley JS. Is this child dehydrated? *JAMA* 2004;291:2746–54.
44. Tatevossian RG, Wo CC, Velmahos GC, et al. Transcutaneous oxygen and CO_2 as early warning of tissue hypoxia and hemodynamic shock in critically ill emergency patients. *Crit Care Med* 2000;28:2248–53.
45. Tibby SM, Hatherill M, Murdoch IA. Capillary refill and core-peripheral temperature gap as indicators of haemodynamic status in paediatric intensive care patients. *Arch Dis Child* 1999;80:163–6.
46. Tremper KK, Shoemaker WC. Transcutaneous oxygen monitoring of critically ill adults, with and without low flow shock. *Crit Care Med* 1981;9:706–9.
47. Vallet B, Tavernier B, Lund N. Assessment of tissue oxygenation in the critically ill. *Eur J Anaesthesiol* 2000;17:221–9.
48. Vincent JL, Navickis RJ, Wilkes MM. Morbidity in hospitalized patients receiving human albumin: a meta-analysis of randomized, controlled trials. *Crit Care Med* 2004;32:2029–38.
49. Waxman K, Sadler R, Eisner ME, et al. Transcutaneous oxygen monitoring of emergency department patients. *Am J Surg* 1983;146:35–8.
50. Weil MH, Nakagawa Y, Tang W, et al. Sublingual capnometry: a new noninvasive measurement for diagnosis and quantitation of severity of circulatory shock. *Crit Care Med* 1999;27:1225–9.
51. Werns SW. Percutaneous extracorporeal life support: reserve for patients with reversible causes of shock and cardiac arrest. *Crit Care Med* 2003;31:978–80.
52. Wills BA, Nguyen MD, Ha TL, et al. Comparison of three fluid solutions for resuscitation in dengue shock syndrome. *N Engl J Med* 2005;353:877–89.
53. Zaritsky AL, Nadkarni VM, Hickey RW, et al., eds. *Pediatric Advanced Life Support Provider Manual*. Dallas: American Heart Association, 2002.

CHAPTER 27 ■ MULTIPLE TRAUMA

JOHN SCOTT BAIRD • ARTHUR COOPER

EPIDEMIOLOGY OF PEDIATRIC TRAUMA

Trauma is the forceful disruption of bodily homeostasis, and it remains the leading cause of death in children and young adults in the US and other developed countries (**Fig. 27.1**). It comprises injuries described as unintentional, as well as those that are intentional, including child abuse. Approximately half of all injuries to children involve multiple organs or body regions, and these injuries are associated with a higher case-based fatality rate. Blunt injury is far more common than penetrating injury in children, although the latter is more deadly (**Table 27.1**). During the last 25 years in the US, the population-based mortality rate for unintentional pediatric injury has fallen by more than 50% (28), although it remains the commonest cause of death for all pediatric patients in the most recent year for which statistics are available (2003), followed in older adolescents by homicide and suicide. Indeed, although mortality rates for the leading causes of pediatric death have declined over the last several decades in all developed countries, they have declined least for trauma (**Fig. 27.2**). Most pediatric deaths from trauma are associated with motor vehicles, and most occur prior to hospital admission. The morbidity of pediatric trauma increases with increasing severity of injury and is manifested frequently by functional limitations following major injury; the overall cost is difficult to estimate, although it is likely enormous.

If economics is the dreary science, then the epidemiology of trauma is the desperate science, particularly regarding children: Trauma remains the "neglected disease of modern society," as it was originally described in a monograph by the National Academy of Sciences over 40 years ago (1). Organizing a community for pediatric trauma care requires not only specialized knowledge of the evaluation and management of childhood injury, but also the ability to ensure that the special needs of children are met throughout the entire continuum of trauma care—from prevention, through prehospital care, transport, emergency care, operative and intensive care, recovery, and rehabilitation. Reductions in the rates of pediatric trauma morbidity and mortality are the result of concerted efforts during the last few decades, which have involved research, education, legislation, and an investment in medical services at all levels. Further declines in pediatric trauma morbidity and mortality in the US will require an even broader and more vigorous public health approach, probably modeled after some of the more successful European countries (Sweden, Italy, the UK, and the Netherlands).

Injuries are, for the most part, not true "accidents," but predictable events rooted in a complex web of social, cultural, and economic factors that impact upon the host, agent, and environment. They have been shown to respond to established harm-reduction strategies based within the community. The National Safe Kids Campaign (www.safekids.org) and the Injury Free Coalition for Kids (www.injuryfree.org) have both proven effective in reducing the burden of childhood injury (15). Comorbidities common to many injured children and adolescents include limited access to healthcare, altered family dynamics (including child abuse), increased risk-taking behavior (including substance abuse and intoxications), and suicidal intent, among others. Strategies to limit such comorbidities are likely to prove useful in reducing childhood injuries.

PEDIATRIC INJURY: MECHANISMS AND PATTERNS

Intracranial injuries are the cause of most pediatric trauma deaths (due at least in part to the untoward effects of traumatic coma on airway patency, breathing control, cerebral perfusion, and the anatomic features unique to children). The evaluation and management of neurologic injuries will be reviewed elsewhere in the text. Most blunt trauma in childhood is unintentional, but 7% of serious injuries are due to intentional physical assault (of which nearly half, or 3%, are due to child abuse) (20). Blunt injuries outnumber penetrating injuries in children by a ratio of 12:1, a ratio that has decreased in recent years. While blunt injuries are more common, penetrating injuries are more lethal. The automobile is responsible for approximately 75% of all childhood deaths, which are split between those that result from pedestrian trauma and those that result from occupant injuries (20). Although younger children are more likely to die as a result of injuries sustained while they are passengers in automobile accidents, older children and adolescents are more likely to die due to injuries sustained as bicycle riders or pedestrians. In general, children are more likely than adults to die from injuries sustained in an automobile crash (35), suggesting a greater susceptibility.

Injury mechanism is the main predictor of injury pattern (**Table 27.2**). Pedestrian motor vehicle trauma may result in the Waddell triad of injuries to the head, torso, and lower extremities, while occupant injuries include head, face, and neck trauma in unrestrained passengers, and cervical spine injuries, bowel disruption or hematoma, and Chance fractures of the spine in restrained passengers. Bicycle trauma results in head injury in unhelmeted riders and upper extremity and upper abdominal injuries, the latter as the result of contact with the handlebar. Low falls, the most common cause of childhood

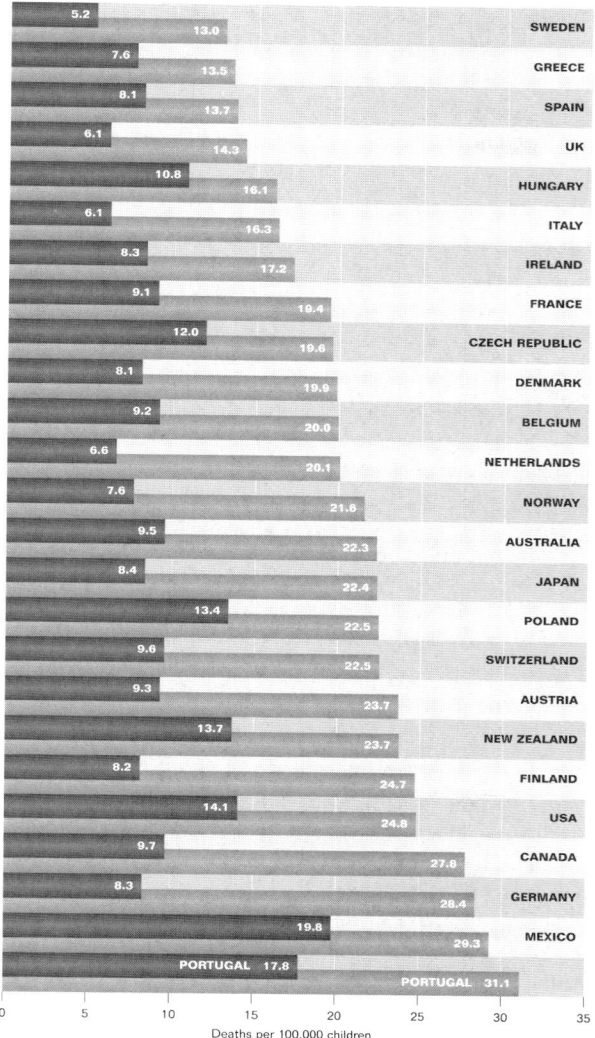

FIGURE 27.1. Annual deaths due to injury in children during the 1970s (light bars) and 1990s (dark bars). From UNICEF. A league table of child deaths by injury in rich nations. *Innocenti Report Card* No. 2, February 2001. UNICEF Innocenti Research Centre, Florence. © The United Nations Children's Fund, 2001.

injury, rarely produce significant trauma, but high falls (from the second story or higher) are associated with serious head injuries, with the addition of long-bone fractures (at the third story), and intrathoracic and intra-abdominal injuries (at the fifth story, the height from which 50% of children can be expected to die following a high fall) (7). With the growing popularity of extreme sports (including extreme skiing and surfing, in-line skating, mountain bicycling, rock climbing, skateboarding, snowboarding, and ultra-endurance racing) in which risk may be underappreciated, patterns of adolescent traumatic injury are likely to change.

This chapter includes a review of the pathophysiology associated with trauma and a discussion of a management scheme for the multiple-injured pediatric patient. Because multiple trauma potentially impacts all other organ systems, the reader is referred to other chapters in this text that discuss specific organ injuries in greater detail. Yet while it is important to realize that the involvement of multiple organ systems is the rule fol-

TABLE 27.1

INCIDENCE AND MORTALITY OF PEDIATRIC TRAUMA

Injury mechanism	Incidence (%)	Mortality (%)
Blunt	92	3
Fall	27	<1
Motor vehicle injury—occupant	21	4
Motor vehicle injury—pedestrian	12	5
Bicycle	9	2
Penetrating	8	5
Gunshot wound	2	10
Stabbing	3	3
Crush	<1	3

Adapted from Cooper A. Early assessment and management of trauma. In: Ashcroft KW, Holcomb GW, Murphy JP, eds. *Pediatric Surgery.* Philadelphia: Elsevier, 2005:168–84.

lowing major trauma in children, due chiefly to their small size, the proportionately larger size of the head, and the proportionately smaller size of the torso, major pediatric blunt trauma is more a disease of airway and breathing than of bleeding and shock.

PATHOPHYSIOLOGY

The effects of injury on a child are related to the amount of kinetic energy transferred: half of the mass of the impacting object times its velocity squared. Because the child's body is smaller, this energy is compacted into a smaller space. As a result, involvement of many organ systems is common with significant pediatric trauma. In addition, the increased elasticity of immature bone results in increased soft-tissue injury when the impact is confined to a smaller space. In blunt trauma, the forces of impact are dependent upon such factors as the size and speed of the vehicle or the vertical displacement following a fall. In penetrating trauma, the forces of violation are dependent upon the weapon used (e.g., the size of the missile it discharges and the velocity with which it is delivered).

Irrespective of the exact mechanism of injury, the body's physiologic responses to trauma tend to be similar and essential for survival: reflexive increases in vasomotor tone in response to hemorrhage help to maintain effective circulating blood volume and vital organ perfusion, as do catecholamine-mediated increases in cardiac output. Organs involved in these and related reflex arcs following acute traumatic injury include the central and peripheral nervous systems, the cardiovascular system, the adrenal glands, the kidneys, and the liver. The resultant collection of reflex responses mediated by these organ systems helps to define the stress response following injury. Because cardiac output is dependent on preload, afterload, and myocardial contractility, changes in intravascular volume and systemic vascular resistance following major trauma may compromise oxygen delivery.

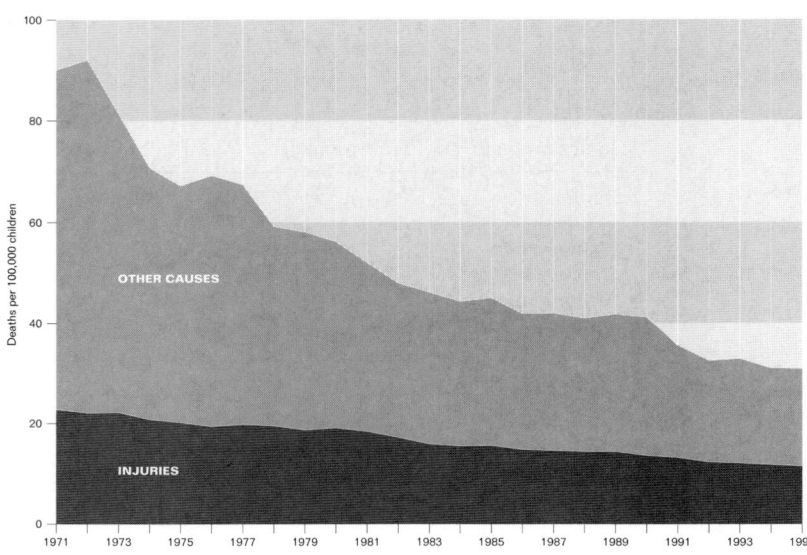

FIGURE 27.2. Death rates from injuries versus all other causes in children (up to 14 years old) of developed countries, 1971–1995. From UNICEF. A league table of child deaths by injury in rich nations. *Innocenti Report Card* No. 2, February 2001. UNICEF Innocenti Research Centre, Florence. © The United Nations Children's Fund, 2001.

TABLE 27.2

COMMON INJURY MECHANISMS AND CORRESPONDING INJURY PATTERNS IN CHILDHOOD TRAUMA

Injury mechanism	Details	Injury pattern
Motor vehicle injury—occupant	Unrestrained	Head/neck injuries Scalp/facial lacerations
	Restrained	Abdomen injuries Lower spine fractures
Motor vehicle injury—pedestrian	Single injury	Lower extremity fractures
	Multiple injuries	Head/neck injuries Chest/abdomen injuries Lower extremity fractures
Fall from height	Low	Upper extremity fractures
	Medium	Head/neck injuries Scalp/facial lacerations Upper extremity fractures
	High	Head/neck injuries Scalp/facial lacerations Chest/abdomen injuries Extremity fractures
Fall from bicycle	Unhelmeted	Head/neck injuries Scalp/facial lacerations Upper extremity fractures
	Helmeted	Upper extremity fractures
	Handlebar impact	Abdomen injuries

Adapted from Cooper A. Early assessment and management of trauma. In: Ashcroft KW, Holcomb GW, Murphy JP, eds. *Pediatric Surgery*. Philadelphia: Elsevier, 2005:168–84.

Baroreceptors located in the walls of large arteries in the thorax and neck respond to changes in blood pressure by exciting or inhibiting the medullary vasoconstrictor and vagal parasympathetic centers, with resultant changes in vasomotor tone, chronotropy, and inotropy. Maximum sympathetic vasoconstriction following trauma that results in global brain ischemia may occur, at least for the first few minutes following injury. Other responses to the stress of trauma include the release of angiotensin by the kidneys, cortisol and aldosterone by the adrenal glands, and vasopressin by the posterior pituitary gland, as well as various local compensatory mechanisms, which, in the presence of diminished blood volume, help to contract circulation or shift fluid into the intravascular compartment. Tissue injury may also activate cascades that contribute to the stress response, involving complement, cytokines, eicosanoids, histamine, kinins, nitric oxide, and serotonin, as well as a variety of hormonal mediators, among others.

The stress response is usually self-limited and adaptive, but when severe injury occurs, the response may be profound and result in a hypermetabolic state, defined as an increase in substrate consumption, which may be pathologic when persistent. Persistent unopposed hypermetabolic state may occur in severely injured children and is characterized by prolonged catabolism, with resultant impaired healing and immunodeficiency. A shift in protein production to acute-phase proteins, including α1-antitrypsin, C-reactive protein, complement components, fibrinogen, and haptoglobin, among others, is common and appears to be mediated by cytokines, such as interleukin (IL)-1, IL-6, and IL-8 (38). Inflammation remote to the site of injury may occur and manifest as systemic inflammatory response syndrome and/or multiple organ dysfunction syndrome, although the incidence of these entities following trauma appears to be lower in children, compared with adults (19).

Recently, attention has been focused on the contribution of genotype to trauma outcome. Many different genes are likely to be important in modulating the stress response, improving healing, and avoiding complications. Therefore, an understanding of the genetic contribution to posttraumatic inflammation does not easily lend itself to routine clinical investigations. Among the different defense mechanisms utilized by cells in animal models, innate (as opposed to adaptive) immune components appear to exert a powerful effect on outcome following inflammation and/or injury. Innate responses to inflammation and injury include many of the mediators and/or cascades noted previously, as well as toll-like receptors and the transcription factor known as nuclear factor (NF)-κB. Activation of both has been described in animal models following trauma, and evidence has been shown of NFκB activation in adults with severe trauma (40). Activation of NFκB results in the expression of hundreds of genes, including those responsible for the production of adhesion molecules, cytokines, immune recognition receptors, neutrophil adhesion receptors, and proteins involved in antigen presentation. These mediators (cytokines in particular) appear to be responsible for remote inflammation in the setting of major trauma and sepsis.

The production of various acute-phase proteins in the liver appears to be mediated by specific cytokines after activation and translocation of NFκB to the nucleus (**Fig. 27.3**): IL-1–like cytokines [IL-1α, IL-1β, tumor necrosis factor (TNF)-α, and TNF-β] are associated with the production of C-reactive protein and complement C3, whereas IL-6–like cytokines (IL-6,

leukemia inhibitory factor, IL-11, and others) are associated with the production of fibrinogen, haptoglobin, α1-antitrypsin, etc. The various functions of these acute-phase proteins include bacterial killing and phagocytosis, thrombosis and fibrinolysis, control of proteolysis, and various repair processes; these proteins thus work to restore homeostasis following inflammation or injury and are part of a carefully orchestrated response.

Roger Bone hypothesized that trauma is, in part, an inflammatory critical illness, much like sepsis, and both may be characterized by a vigorous cytokine response (11). As trauma victims often have diminished cellular and humoral immunity, an increased risk of multiple organ dysfunction (even in organ systems remote from the site of injury), and other evidence of systemic inflammation, investigators have searched for a common cause. Cytokines participate in immunity, multiple organ dysfunction, and systemic inflammation: These low-molecular-weight proteins are extraordinarily potent and influence a broad range of cellular functions. The increase in cytokines following major trauma occurs locally at the site of injury (and perhaps in sites remote from injury) and occasionally spills out in high enough plasma concentrations to produce systemic inflammation. Recent evidence suggests that severity of injury (29,45,51,59), progression to multiorgan system failure (41), and mortality (59) are all associated with increasing plasma concentrations of IL-2, IL-6, and/or IL-8 sampled within a few hours of multiple trauma. Marked elevations in IL-6 have been noted in hemorrhage following trauma (39). As similar traumatic insults may be associated with different outcomes, it is likely that genetic polymorphisms at multiple alleles, including those involved in cytokine production, contribute to the variability in outcome, though evidence remains insufficient to date. In addition, developmental aspects that involve differences in these responses have not yet been explored. Moreover, the hypothesis that excessive cytokine release following trauma may be maladaptive and contribute to worsening injury is still an hypothesis, and further investigation is required.

The trauma-associated hypermetabolic state in children also involves a shift in the hormonal milieu from anabolic to catabolic mediators, including an increase in cortisol, epinephrine, and glucagon concentrations, concurrently with a decrease in activity of insulin and the somatotropic axis hormones (growth hormone and insulin-like growth factors [IGFs]). Both insulin and growth hormone resistance occur in critically ill children, including those with major trauma, and contribute to the trauma-associated hypermetabolic state. Antagonism against IGFs may be partially responsible for decreased levels and activity of insulin and IGFs, leading to insulin resistance. Additionally, cytokines, such as TNF-α, may further inhibit the somatotropic axis.

Stress hyperglycemia (serum glucose of >200 mg/dL) is common following pediatric trauma (54) and is related to insulin and growth hormone resistance in the presence of enhanced gluconeogenesis. An association appears to exist between hyperglycemia and poor outcome in adults with traumatic injury (33,60). Mechanisms that underlie the association between hyperglycemia and poor outcome are not fully understood, although a shift to anaerobic metabolism with increased lactate production and brain tissue acidosis, impaired neutrophil activation due to impaired superoxide production, and increased oxidant stress from the generation of advanced glycation end-products have all been implicated. The association

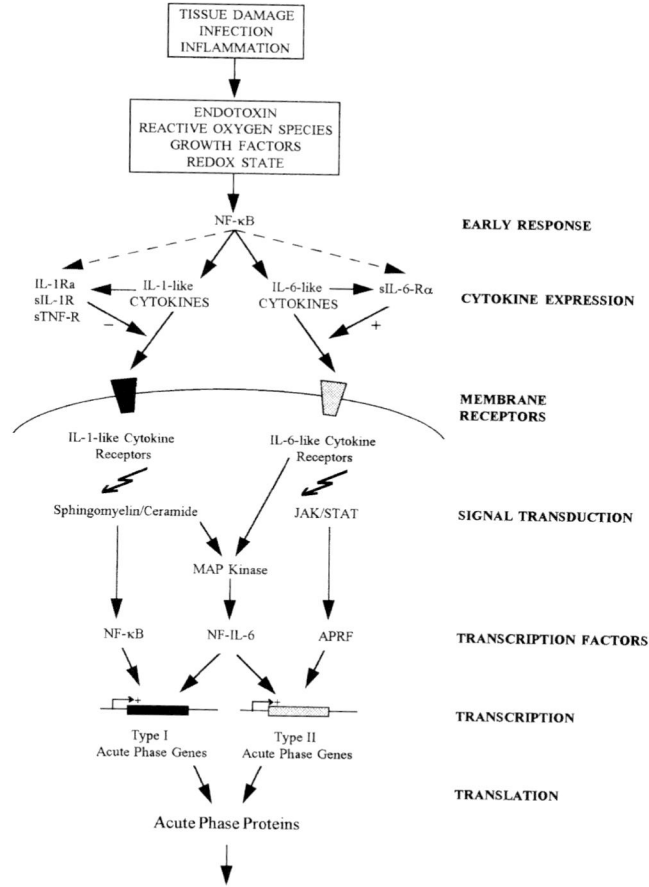

FIGURE 27.3. Main events leading to the acute phase response in trauma, infection, or inflammation, including the role of NFκB and cytokines in the induction of protein translation From Moshage H. Cytokines and the hepatic acute phase response. *J Pathol.* 1997;181:257–66.

between hyperglycemia and poor outcome has been noted with both early and persistent hyperglycemia, and control of hyperglycemia was associated with an improved outcome in critically ill adults, including some with multiple trauma (55). In an animal model, insulin attenuated the production of cytokines associated with the acute stress response following thermal injury (30). Children with hyperglycemia and traumatic brain injury or burn injury (26) also appear to have a poorer outcome, and insulin reduced both IL-1β and TNF-α 15 days after injury and increased IL-10 30 days after injury in children with severe burn injury (31). The change in cytokine response appeared to be unrelated to glycemia. However, the effect of insulin therapy on mortality in pediatric trauma is still unknown.

Hormonal components of the stress response also include arginine vasopressin (AVP). The release of AVP from the posterior pituitary is stimulated by increasing plasma osmolality or declining extracellular fluid volume, the latter mediated via stretch receptors in the atria and the baroreceptor reflex arc. AVP release is more sensitive to small increases in plasma osmolality, but large declines in extracellular fluid volume mandate rapid increases in AVP, regardless of plasma osmolality. AVP release is also stimulated by some of the factors associated with the stress response, including dopamine, hypoxemia, and hypocapnia, as well as certain cytokines. Once released, AVP activates specific renal tubular receptors that are responsible for controlling how the kidneys handle free water, and it activates receptors in vessel walls responsible for regulation of vasomotor tone. AVP release may be stimulated following pediatric trauma, particularly head trauma (25), resulting in water retention with hyponatremia in the absence of hypovolemia—the syndrome of inappropriate antidiuretic hormone secretion. Alternatively, AVP release may be deficient following pediatric head trauma, resulting in a dilute diuresis with hypernatremia-diabetes insipidus.

INITIAL ASSESSMENT

Emergency Medical Services

Pediatric trauma resuscitation should begin as soon as possible after the injury, ideally through pediatric-capable emergency medical dispatchers who provide instructions to lay rescuers at the scene. It continues upon the arrival of prehospital professionals, including first responders, emergency medical technicians, and paramedics. The emphasis in pediatric prehospital trauma care is on aggressive support of vital functions during what has been called the "platinum half hour" of early pediatric trauma care.

The transport of critically injured children requires special expertise: Paramedics who routinely perform these tasks receive extra pediatric training, as well as support from experienced physicians, nurses, and other healthcare professionals. Additional support, which is essential for this type of service, includes an ongoing review of adverse events, equipment and personnel needs, and policies and procedures. Prehospital transport of critically injured children frequently presents a critical choice to emergency medical personnel—"scoop and run or stay and play." Although a universal answer to this dilemma is not possible, it is clear that as time is spent at the trauma site, the "platinum half hour" ticks away, and de-

lay should be avoided whenever possible. Transport between healthcare facilities is often appropriate for injured children who require special medical expertise available at another hospital, or as a component of regionalization of pediatric critical care. Some pediatric hospitals have established specialized teams for this type of interhospital transport of critically ill and injured patients. Private ambulance services with pediatric expertise, either in the prehospital or interhospital setting, provide an additional choice in many communities. Yet, transport of critically injured children is not risk-free, because adverse events (including obstructed endotracheal tubes and loss of vascular access) occur at nearly twice the rate during interhospital transport as in the PICU and 10 times more frequently with nonspecialized teams than with specialized teams. At a minimum, transport providers must be capable of critical pediatric assessment and monitoring, and they must be highly skilled in the techniques of pediatric endotracheal intubation and vascular access, as well as in fluid and drug administration in critically ill and injured children. Whenever possible, interhospital transport of such patients should be conducted by specialized pediatric transport teams staffed by physicians and nurses with special training.

Trauma centers are hospitals with special expertise in trauma care, and centers verified by the American College of Surgeons are classified as Level One (with the most comprehensive array of specialists and services, often located in large academic medical centers), Level Two (with most but not all of the specialists and services available in Level One), and Level Three (only core specialists and services are available; usually located in smaller community hospitals). In some states, pediatric trauma centers have also been designated; these are now similarly classified, except that Level Three centers cannot be separately verified for pediatric trauma. Hospitals and clinics without trauma center designation (nontrauma centers) are still part of the regional trauma system and should be capable of routine resuscitation and stabilization of injured patients.

Severely injured children in the US who are cared for in hospitals with a PICU or in pediatric trauma centers have an improved outcome (22,43). The common denominator for these sites is accumulated expertise caring for critically ill children, and this expertise is both essential and difficult to quantify. However, as few institutions possess the resources to provide such a level of care, the number of qualified centers is limited, even in larger metropolitan areas, where a full range of pediatric specialty services may be available at more than one institution. Referral of critically ill and injured children to qualified centers (i.e., regionalization) is a well-established practice, and critically injured children should undergo primary transport to these institutions wherever possible. Nevertheless, every receiving hospital must be capable of initiating resuscitation and stabilizing critically injured children, and have transfer agreements in place with hospitals that have full pediatric capabilities.

Scoring

A global assessment represented by a single number that is capable of stratifying risk and survival following traumatic injury has long been a goal among trauma researchers. Scores developed to help in this regard include the Injury Severity Score and the Revised Trauma Score (**Tables 27.3** and **27.4**), although neither specifically addresses the pediatric population. The

TABLE 27.3

TRAUMA SCORES COMMONLY USED IN CHILDREN: PEDIATRIC TRAUMA SCORE

Points	+2	+1	−1
Size (kg)	>20	10–20	<10
Airway	Normal	Maintained	Unmaintained
Systolic blood pressure (mm Hg)	>90	50–90	<50
CNS	Awake	Obtunded	Coma
Open wound	None	Minor	Major
Skeletal trauma	None	Closed	Open-Multiple

Glasgow Coma Scale (GCS) is used to assess gross neurologic status following injury (and requires modification for infants and small children), while the Pediatric Risk of Mortality III and Pediatric Index of Mortality II are focused on the outcome of all patients admitted to a PICU.

Among the scores utilized to assess and predict outcome in critically injured children, the Pediatric Trauma Score (**Table 27.3**) is acceptable for outcome assessment and for field use and is recognized by the American College of Surgeons Committee on Trauma and the American Pediatric Surgical Association Trauma Committee. A Pediatric Trauma Score of <9 is consistent with significant risk of mortality, and identifies patients with an Injury Severity Score of >9. However, the Pediatric Trauma Score has not consistently proven superior to other scores, particularly the Revised Trauma Score. At present, reliance on anatomic, physiologic, and mechanistic criteria for primary transport to a trauma center with pediatric expertise appears to be equally useful, and this is the approach currently preferred for field triage of injured adults and children by the American College of Surgeons Committee on Trauma.

Primary Survey

The body regions most frequently injured in major childhood trauma are the head and neck, abdomen, and lower extremities, while in minor childhood injury, soft tissue and upper extremity injuries predominate. Because most pediatric trauma is blunt trauma that involves the head, it is primarily a disease of airway and breathing, rather than circulation, bleeding, and shock. Even so, while neuroventilatory derangements (in effect, abnormalities in GCS and respiratory rate) are five times more common than hemodynamic derangements (abnormalities in blood pressure) in the children with significant mortality risk in the National Pediatric Trauma Registry, the latter are twice as lethal as the former. The primary survey—the ABCs:

airway, breathing, and circulation (D may be added for disability or gross neurologic impairment, and E for exposure and environment as noted below)—is thus vitally important in the evaluation and treatment of pediatric victims of multiple or severe trauma, and repeated evaluation is necessary. Resuscitation of the child trauma victim is conducted concurrently with the primary survey, in a continuous cycle of assessment, intervention, and reassessment.

The primary survey is completed by fully exposing, i.e., undressing, the injured child to more fully assess injury. In an environment at room temperature, children rapidly lose heat due to their large body surface area relative to their body mass and due to their increased minute ventilation and its accompanying heat of vaporization. Additionally, the younger the child, the less subcutaneous tissue is available for heat insulation. It is incumbent on the clinical team to prevent hypothermia in this setting, as it may further compromise control of hemorrhage and cardiorespiratory function.

Airway (and Cervical Spine Stabilization)

All else will be futile if the first step of trauma management, airway control, is ineffective. As a corollary, consideration of cervical spine stabilization is mandatory with this first step, and the best approach is a plan formulated well in advance. When endotracheal intubation is required for respiratory failure, rapid-sequence (oral) intubation is reasonable following appropriate cervical spine protection, working under the warranted assumption that each patient has a full stomach. Intubation will be additionally necessary for the child in decompensated shock. Exceptions to this approach will be reviewed.

All patients undergoing a primary survey should receive supplemental oxygen with an FiO2 of 1. An airway obstructed by soft tissues and secretions is opened (utilizing the modified jaw thrust maneuver with or without an oropharyngeal airway to displace the mandible) while proper cervical spine precautions

TABLE 27.4

TRAUMA SCORES COMMONLY USED IN CHILDREN: REVISED TRAUMA SCORE

Glasgow Coma Scale	Systolic blood pressure (mm Hg)	Respiratory rate (breaths/min)	Points
13–15	>89	10–29	4
9–12	76–89	>29	3
6–8	50–75	6–9	2
4–5	1–49	1–5	1
3	0	0	0

are taken (maintaining the cervical spine in a neutral position with bimanual cervical spine stabilization, followed by application of a semirigid cervical extrication collar and long backboard). The airway is then cleared utilizing a large-bore, Yankauer-type suction device, and assessment can proceed to the next step. A head tilt is avoided in patients with possible cervical spine injury. The larynx is more superior and anterior in children (see Chapter 22), and oral intubation is difficult for those without pediatric experience.

Important considerations regarding pediatric endotracheal intubation include: (a) nasal intubation is contraindicated in patients with severe facial or head trauma, including, in particular, those with cerebrospinal fluid leak, and blind intubation is discouraged; (b) trauma patients should be considered to have a full stomach, independent of their last documented meal, as gastric emptying time may be delayed in this setting; (c) children are more likely to develop respiratory failure than are adults with equivalent injury; (d) the patient's hemodynamic status will help to determine the most appropriate therapeutic approach; and (e) while an uncuffed endotracheal tube may be utilized in the field or the emergency department, a cuffed endotracheal tube may be indicated in the PICU, particularly if respiratory compliance appears to be diminished during bag valve mask ventilation. The routine use of noninvasive ventilation in injured children, particularly those with head, face, or neck injury, is contraindicated. Finally, children are much less tolerant of prolonged hypoxia than are adults; with full denitrogenation, the typical adult can sustain approximately 4 mins of apnea without hypoxia. However, infants may only tolerate 30 seconds of apnea, even if fully preoxygenated, because the infant's functional residual capacity is relatively smaller, while oxygen consumption is greater than that of the adult. Denitrogenation is thus essential in children and accomplished by 3–5 minutes of tidal breathing at an FiO_2 of 1.

The details of pediatric rapid-sequence intubation, including appropriate medications and algorithms, are reviewed in Chapter 22. In most pediatric victims of multiple trauma, the indications, practice, and complications of endotracheal intubation are clear and easily understood. When endotracheal intubation is unsuccessful, or in patients with significant facial, head, neck and/or airway injury, the laryngeal mask airway is of limited use, as it is inserted blindly; in addition, it may not completely seal the airway, so that aspiration remains a distinct possibility. Fiberoptic-assisted intubation may be helpful in patients with injury to the upper airway; indeed, endoscopy is mandatory for suspected injury to the larynx, trachea, or bronchi.

Surgical approaches to establish an airway for trauma patients include needle and surgical cricothyroidotomy. A needle cricothyroidotomy is appropriate for trauma patients with upper airway obstruction (above the larynx) after failed orotracheal intubation or because significant upper airway injury renders an attempt at intubation futile, but it is contraindicated in the presence of laryngotracheal injury, as it may exacerbate the injury. A needle cricothyroidotomy is merely a temporary expedient, and plans for the next step should be made concurrently. An emergent surgical cricothyroidotomy is indicated for trauma patients with significant laryngeal injury or following failed procedures to secure an airway; some practitioners also perform an urgent tracheostomy for acute, posttraumatic asphyxia. Adequate support for both procedures in a setting outside the operating room is essential, as it is very easy to lose the airway due to hemorrhage, edema, subcutaneous air, or relaxation of muscle tone following anesthesia.

Breathing

As soon as a patent airway is assured, the patient should continue to receive an FiO_2 of 1. If ventilation is inadequate, positive pressure ventilatory (PPV) assistance should be offered. Inadequate ventilation is characterized by decreased breath sounds, an abnormal respiratory pattern, and clinical evidence of hypercarbia (including an increase in sympathetic tone, which may be unappreciated in the setting of major trauma); hypoxia occurs late in the course. Hypercarbia may rise rapidly without obvious signs, although decreased responsiveness is the rule. The FiO_2 can then be titrated to maintain an oxygen saturation of approximately 95%.

Laboratory examinations, often helpful in this setting, should not be relied upon to determine therapy; a chest radiograph or even an arterial blood gas level generally confirms what has been clinically obvious for some time. Waiting for the chest radiograph to drain a tension pneumothorax (indicated by decreased breath sounds, deviated trachea, progressive respiratory distress, and hemodynamic compromise) in a patient with multiple trauma is not helpful. Nor is it helpful to rely on the arterial blood gas level to decide whether to intubate a patient; that decision is a clinical one, equally dependent on the patient's ability to adequately exchange gas and on the need to maintain and protect the airway.

Ensuring adequate minute ventilation and oxygenation during PPV for each age range involves making appropriate choices in a stressful situation; in addition, technology continues to change rapidly. It is essential that pediatric intensivists be involved in the prescription for mechanical ventilation early in the course. Age-appropriate initial settings are reviewed in Chapter 34.

Circulation

Attention devoted to the maintenance of adequate circulation will help attenuate the stress response and may prevent delayed inflammatory complications of major trauma. The basic steps in the management of hemorrhagic shock are control of active hemorrhage, placement of IV lines, and volume replacement or resuscitation, as necessary.

Control of Active Hemorrhage. Most children in hypotensive shock following traumatic injury are victims of uncontrolled hemorrhage, which can be reversed only if promptly recognized and appropriately treated. Potential sites of unrecognized hemorrhage include those body cavities large enough to sequester significant volumes of blood (hemithorax, retroperitoneum, pelvis, thigh compartments). Control of active hemorrhage involves the principles of hemostasis, which have not changed in several decades and include as the first and most important step direct pressure over all actively bleeding wounds. Tourniquet techniques have rarely been advocated or used in civilian practice in recent years, although current military experience suggests a possible role in control of exsanguinating hemorrhage from a traumatic amputation. Military antishock trousers (MAST) may also be helpful in selected patients with decompensated shock due to poorly controlled hemorrhage from a lower extremity fracture or an unstable pelvis. When confronted with a MAST-suited patient, careful attention is mandatory; deflation should not be attempted until the primary survey is complete and a plan for possible surgical intervention is formulated. In addition, deflation should be conducted sequentially: The abdominal portion is deflated first, followed by each of the lower extremity compartments, and blood pressure and perfusion must be stabilized following each deflation.

Coagulopathies in injured children typically are related to dilution of platelet and plasma coagulation factors during extensive resuscitation and transfusion, although hypothermia may also contribute. The appropriate platelet count "trigger" for transfusion is debated, although better indicators may be platelet function, as well as the rate of decline. Nevertheless, when platelets fall below 50,000/mm^3, with clinical evidence of bleeding, it is appropriate to begin a platelet transfusion. A general guideline is to administer 6 units to an adult or 0.1–0.2 units/kg to a child. Empiric platelet and fresh frozen plasma transfusions should be considered when more than two blood volumes (or 80 mL/kg of packed red blood cells in a child) have been transfused during resuscitation. Laboratory tests of the coagulation system are used to guide specific replacement; the prothrombin time, partial thromboplastin time, and platelet count are routinely monitored. Mixing studies may be appropriate for the evaluation of abnormal results. If fibrinolysis is suspected, an appropriate laboratory assessment is also indicated (D-dimer, fibrinogen). Efficacious therapies for hemorrhage with coagulopathy include the replacement of specific coagulation components, avoiding inhibition of coagulation factors, and consideration of aprotinin and aminocaproic acid if excessive fibrinolysis is contributing to hemorrhage. In addition, as activated factor VII is sufficient to initiate the activation of thrombin from prothrombin and thus initiate coagulation, therapy with recombinant activated factor VII offers another potential treatment for severe, unresponsive hemorrhage. A large, randomized, placebo-controlled trial of activated recombinant factor VII in adults with severe traumatic hemorrhage showed a significant reduction in red blood cell transfusions in patients with severe blunt trauma and a trend to transfusion reduction in penetrating trauma (10). No equivalent trials in children are currently available.

Placement of Intravenous Lines. The child who presents with major trauma with signs of hypovolemic shock (rapid, thready pulse, cool, mottled skin, prolonged capillary refill, decreased pulse pressure, altered sensorium) will require volume resuscitation. However, shock is less obvious in children for a variety of reasons: The mobile mediastinum may shift under tension and more easily compensate for obstructive lesions, the pediatric vasculature is better able to constrict in response to hypovolemia, and the cardiovascular system is healthier than it is in adults. In general, children can maintain systemic vascular resistance (and thus afterload and systemic blood pressure) far longer than adults can with similar injuries. Finally, frank hypotension is a late sign of pediatric shock and may not develop until 30%–35% of circulating blood volume is lost, leading to a "deceptive" presentation of shock in children.

Vascular access should be rapidly obtained in children with major trauma; a delay may be catastrophic. Even in the absence of signs of (hypovolemic) shock, vascular access should be immediately available. Resuscitation is best carried out by means of large bore peripheral catheters placed percutaneously in median antecubital veins at the elbow or in the saphenous veins at the ankle. In the event that access cannot be established rapidly in younger children, intraosseous access may be utilized. Access by central venous catheter in the femoral, internal jugular, or subclavian veins or by cutdown in the ankle or groin is helpful during resuscitation if experienced operators are immediately available and other means of vascular access are inadequate. Following acute resuscitation, arterial and central venous catheterization is indicated for children with ongoing cardiorespiratory compromise.

Volume Replacement. Simple hypovolemia usually responds to 20–40 mL/kg of warmed isotonic solution, but frank hypotension (clinically diagnosed by a systolic blood pressure <70 mm Hg plus twice the age in years) typically requires 10–20 mL/kg warmed packed red blood cells in addition. Any injured child who cannot be stabilized using this regimen likely has internal bleeding and requires emergency operation for control of hemorrhage. If a child presents in shock and has no signs of intrathoracic, intra-abdominal, or intrapelvic bleeding, but fails to improve despite seemingly adequate volume resuscitation, other forms of shock (obstructive, cardiogenic, neurogenic) should be considered, and the following questions asked: (a) Has tension pneumothorax or cardiac tamponade developed? (b) Is there an unrecognized myocardial contusion? (c) Was a spinal cord injury missed on physical examination?

Over-resuscitation that contributes to hemorrhage or edema in injured children is not so much a problem as insufficient or delayed resuscitation. Edema following over-resuscitation is generally clinically relevant only in the presence of neurologic injury and can be avoided by titrating volume resuscitation to measures of tissue perfusion. However, close attention to the estimated blood volume as a function of size is essential, and may help to provide valuable estimates of the severity of hemorrhage (**Table 27.5**).

A classification of hypovolemia based on clinical findings suggests that most injured children will not become hypotensive until more than 30% of their estimated blood volume is lost. With blood loss of 10%–15% of the total blood volume (mild blood volume loss, or Class I hemorrhage in older patients), clinical symptoms most often include only mild tachycardia in children. As more blood loss occurs—up to 30% of the total blood volume (Class II in older patients)—a further increase in tachycardia occurs, with diminished peripheral pulses. With a loss of 30%–45% of the circulating blood volume (moderate blood volume loss, or Class III in older patients), a marked decrease in urinary output occurs, central pulses are thready and peripheral pulses are lost, pulse pressure narrows, and mental confusion is evident; the blood pressure may be only mildly decreased. With loss of more than 45% of the circulating blood volume (Class IV in older patients), the clinical findings include coma and frank hypotension.

The ongoing controversy regarding colloid versus crystalloid resuscitation fluids has abated somewhat in the last few years. Meta-analyses of trials in critically ill (mostly adult) patients (4,44) suggest that outcome following resuscitation with albumin or other colloid solutions is no different when compared to crystalloid solutions. In addition, studies in young trauma patients treated with colloids or crystalloids showed no differences in the development of pulmonary edema or in pulmonary dysfunction. Crystalloid solutions, generally cheaper than colloids and immediately available to the clinician, are thus quite popular for the initial resuscitation of injured children. However, an animal model of hemorrhagic shock suggests that resuscitation with albumin is associated with lower

TABLE 27.5

CLASSIFICATION OF ESTIMATED BLOOD VOLUME LOSS BY CLINICAL SIGNS

System	Mild[a] 15%–30% total blood volume loss	Moderate[b] 30%–45% total blood volume loss	Severe[c] >45% total blood volume loss
Cardiovascular	Tachycardia with weak, thready pulses	Tachycardia with absent peripheral pulses and weak, thready central pulses; mild hypotension with narrow pulse pressure	Tachycardia followed by bradycardia; hypotension
CNS	Anxious, irritable, confused	Lethargic, dulled response to pain	Comatose
Skin	Cool, mottled; prolonged capillary refill	Cyanotic unless anemic; markedly prolonged capillary refill	Pale, cold
Urine output	Minimally decreased	Minimal	None

[a]Corresponds to Class I/II blood loss in adults.
[b]Corresponds approximately to Class III blood loss in adults.
[c]Corresponds approximately to Class IV blood loss in adults.
Adapted from *Advanced Trauma Life Support*, 7th ed. Chicago: American College of Surgeons, 2004.

levels of inflammatory cytokines in the lungs and the circulation (61), as well as a decrease in lung apoptosis (17), compared to resuscitation with Ringer lactate. In addition, the possibility that infusion of a colloid solution could more rapidly restore the adequacy of circulation—perhaps in specific subgroups with shock—remains a tantalizing prospect, and the use of colloid solutions in trauma resuscitation is not likely to disappear soon.

Resuscitation with hypotonic solution is contraindicated for several reasons: (a) excess free water will exacerbate edema formation, particularly in the central nervous system (CNS); (b) subsequent changes in osmolality are poorly tolerated in critically ill patients; and (c) blood products and other parenteral medications may not be compatible with these solutions.

Isotonic crystalloid solutions commonly utilized for resuscitations (often while blood products are being prepared) include normal saline and Ringer lactate. The excessive use of normal saline may lead to a hyperchloremic metabolic acidosis, which can obscure underlying metabolic acidosis secondary to hypoperfusion. The lactate in Ringer lactate is metabolized by the liver to bicarbonate; therefore, this solution provides a buffer, so long as hepatic function remains intact. In patients with severe hepatic injury, it may be reasonable to limit lactate intake. Plasmalyte is another isotonic solution that provides buffer as acetate and gluconate, although it may not be available at some sites.

Hypertonic saline may offer some benefits in hemorrhagic shock, including a redistribution of extracellular water due to tonicity changes; as hypertonic saline increases extracellular fluid osmolality, a tonicity gradient helps to pull water from the intracellular compartment. In animal models, hemodynamic effects include an improvement in inotropy (46,57), as well as less neutrophil activation and less gut and lung injury compared to that with Ringer lactate (18,48). Even small volumes of hypertonic saline may be helpful in this regard, and the concept of small-volume hyperosmolar resuscitation may have utility in pediatric trauma. In some patients with multiple trauma, including neurologic injury, the judicious use of hypertonic (3%) saline may therefore be appropriate, although data from large clinical trials are not yet available, nor are ex-

tensive clinical data in children without neurologic injury, and appropriate limits for extracellular osmolality are still controversial. It is also likely that an equivalent amount of chloride from 3% saline contributes equally to the development of hyperchloremic metabolic acidosis, similar to that occurring with normal saline. Reliance on hypertonic saline to the exclusion of isotonic resuscitation fluids is not supported at this time.

Albumin (molecular weight: 69 kDa) is a naturally occurring plasma protein that provides approximately 80% of the intravascular colloid oncotic pressure. It is a human blood product, although heat treated; therefore, it is not associated with infectious disease risks. Both 5% and 25% (or "salt-poor") albumin have been used in the resuscitation of pediatric trauma patients; 5% is preferred for acute resuscitation. Other colloid solutions include 6% hydroxyethyl starch and low-molecular-weight dextran; the latter agent is seldom used in the trauma setting, because it induces platelet dysfunction, interferes with cross-matching of blood, and may be filtered by the renal tubules, leading to renal failure. Hydroxyethyl starch is a synthetic colloid that consists of a hydroxyethyl-substituted, branched-chain amylopectin with a molecular weight of 69 kDa. Although its elimination half-time is 17 days, in clinical practice, it expands the plasma volume for only 24–36 hrs. Adverse effects include an inhibition of platelet aggregation following the administration of more than 15–20 mL/kg.

The treatment of hemorrhagic shock must include transfusion of blood products, particularly in patients with moderate to severe blood volume loss (i.e., Class III and Class IV in older patients). The hematocrit of a unit of packed red blood cells will depend on the anticoagulant used. With citrate phosphate dextrose, the average hematocrit is 65%–75%, whereas the more commonly used adenine anticoagulants are associated with hematocrits of 50%–60%. In the emergent resuscitative phase of therapy in Class III and Class IV patients, time may not allow a full type and cross-match to be accomplished before transfusion. When using uncross-matched blood, it is best to obtain at least an ABO and Rh type and partial cross-match. If time does not permit even a preliminary screen, ABO and Rh type-specific, uncross-matched blood is still preferable (and more abundant) to type O-negative, Rh-negative, uncross-matched blood. In the absence of type-specific blood, the latter can be used, although cross-matching may still be helpful to ensure the absence of A and/or B antibodies. Blood warmers should be used whenever possible, especially if the volumes delivered are great or if the patient is small. Several types are available, and they are often found in the operating room. The use of blood replacement products, such as stroma-free hemoglobin and human polymerized hemoglobin, holds great promise and possible benefit in adult hemorrhagic shock; however, their use in children is still investigational.

Although the majority of patients will respond to timely intravascular repletion of volume and hemoglobin, some severely injured patients in Class III and/or Class IV have persistent perfusion defects that will not correct without immediate surgical intervention. Rarely, infusion of vasoactive medications like epinephrine or the use of a MAST suit may help to bridge the time from primary resuscitation to operating room.

Disability (Abbreviated Neurologic Exam)

Assessment of disability and the neurologic status completes the primary survey ("ABCD") and relies on the use of the GCS (to assess level of consciousness), an evaluation of papillary responses (to exclude mass lesions), and other evidence of an altered mental status. Traumatic coma (GCS ≤8) and pupillary asymmetry mandate immediate involvement of neurosurgical consultants. It is important to make at least a preliminary assessment of the neurologic status while the severely injured patient is being prepared for endotracheal intubation, although this exercise should not divert the clinician; rather, a few seconds should be sufficient to make a mental note of the pupillary responses and GCS. Documentation can wait, but cannot be ignored, since serial measurements of GCS are no less valuable than the initial measurement.

Monitoring Resuscitation

Resuscitation proceeds concurrently with continuous reevaluation at this stage, and the most sensitive monitors of adequate circulation in children include the vital signs and evidence of perfusion, filling pressures, and urinary output. Although noninvasive monitoring (e.g., SpO_2, $ETCO_2$) will suffice for many patients, the use of invasive monitoring may be warranted in selected patients, if potential benefits outweigh known risks. However, continuous reassessment by a knowledgeable and observant bedside physician will still be needed to guide resuscitation.

The most sensitive monitor of cardiac output and volume status in a child is the heart rate. The adequacy of circulation is assessed by noting the quality, rate, and regularity of the pulse and secondarily by obtaining the blood pressure. Progressively weakening central pulses, particularly with other signs of poor perfusion, suggest an impending cardiac arrest. On the other hand, bounding peripheral pulses with an active precordium do not guarantee that all will be well in patients with a stress response following severe trauma. Respiratory rates in children generally require careful assessment, as a cursory examination over a few seconds is likely to miss periods of apnea, intermittent distress, or progressive deterioration. A respiratory rate of 25/min is inappropriately low in the injured infant, while a respiratory rate of 50/min is inappropriately

high in the injured adolescent. Blood pressure may be normal despite a 25% to 30% loss of total blood volume. Nevertheless, beat-to-beat monitoring of blood pressure via an intra-arterial catheter is an important component of pediatric intensive care, and such catheters provide ready access for blood sampling.

The perfusion of distal extremities is monitored by assessing capillary refill and skin turgor and by looking for cyanosis or other signs of circulatory embarrassment. A capillary refill greater than 2 seconds suggests poor distal perfusion. Adequate lighting is essential to detect such findings, as is maintenance of normal body temperature.

The central venous pressure may be a helpful marker of intravascular volume, particularly in patients with extensive fluid resuscitation. It is measured from a catheter within the vena cava, as near to the right atrium as possible and, when measured at end-expiration/end-diastole, offers a good estimate of right atrial and right ventricular pressure (in the absence of pericardial or other cardiovascular disease). Although a single determination of central venous pressure may not accurately reflect effective circulating blood volume, repeated determinations, particularly following carefully monitored fluid boluses, may more accurately reflect filling pressure and blood volume. The Weil criteria for central venous pressure change with hypovolemia following intravascular fluid bolus therapy, also known as the "2–5 rule," may be helpful in deciding when to offer further volume resuscitation: If the response to a fluid bolus within 10 mins of starting the bolus is an increase in central venous pressure of <2 mm Hg or >5 mm Hg, it is continued or discontinued, respectively (56). A flow-directed, balloon-tipped pulmonary artery catheter to measure pulmonary capillary wedge pressure (potentially a good estimate of left atrial pressure) may offer a survival benefit in the most severely injured adult trauma patients (24).

Urinary output should be measured in all seriously injured children as an indicator of renal perfusion, because this may be a surrogate for tissue perfusion of other vital organs. As such, urinary output provides a valuable marker for the adequacy of fluid resuscitation. Hourly trends are more important and clinically relevant than average daily results and should be at least 1–2 mL/kg/hr in older children and adolescents and at least 0.5–1 mL/kg/hr in infants and younger children. Hourly output may vary due to technologic issues, and attention must be paid to ensure accuracy. Leaking around catheters is common, and measurement of fluid losses in wet clothing and sheets improves accuracy. Occasionally, sediment occludes the small catheters utilized in infants and children, and catheter flushes with small amounts of sterile saline may be helpful. Placement of a urinary catheter via the transurethral route should be deferred in patients with urethral injury, including those with pelvic fractures and/or gross hematuria.

Urinary output and other clinical markers, including the vital signs, may not always permit discrimination between those with compensated and uncompensated shock, or allow recognition of adequate volume resuscitation. Additional helpful markers of adequate resuscitation include mixed venous oxygen saturation, arterial lactic acid concentration, and the base deficit. These should be measured serially and trended to provide the most information. Lack of improvement in arterial lactic acid concentration and/or base deficit despite appropriate volume resuscitation may indicate ongoing hemorrhage and increased risk of mortality.

Secondary Survey

Complete History and Physical Examination

Once the primary survey is complete, resuscitation is ongoing, and shock is being effectively treated, a secondary survey is undertaken for the definitive evaluation of the injured child. The primary survey and associated resuscitation efforts should be well advanced within 15 minutes of arrival in the trauma resuscitation area. The secondary survey consists of a "SAMPLE" history (*s*ymptoms, *a*llergies, *m*edications, *p*ast illnesses, *l*ast meal, *e*vents and environment) and a complete head-to-toe examination that addresses all body regions and organ systems, along with a complete history of the injury. Continued reassessment and resuscitation must proceed with the secondary survey. The examination should be targeted to the head and neck (for any history of blunt injury above the clavicles, alteration in level of consciousness, or neck pain or swelling), to the chest (for any history of chest pain, noisy or rapid breathing, respiratory insufficiency, or hemoptysis), and to the abdomen (for any history of abdominal pain, bruising or tenderness, distention, pelvic instability, or vomiting, especially if the emesis is stained with blood or bile). In examining the child, the physician's first responsibility is to identify life-threatening injuries that may have been overlooked during the primary survey, such as tension pneumothorax, massive hemothorax (unilaterally decreased breath sounds with dullness to percussion and a displaced trachea), and gastric dilatation (upper abdominal distention with hyperresonance to percussion).

A head that demonstrates any sign of drainage from the nose or ears or any evidence of mid-face instability, suggests the presence of a basilar skull fracture (which precludes the passage of a nasogastric tube) or an oromaxillofacial fracture (which may compromise the airway). Hemotympanum and Battle sign point toward a basilar skull fracture. A neurologic examination as complete as circumstances allow should be performed. Following the lateral cervical spine radiograph (omitted acutely if it distracts from ongoing resuscitation, so long as the cervical spine is protected), the neck is examined for tenderness, swelling, torticollis, or spasm, suggesting the presence of a cervical spine fracture (which may not be detected on lateral cervical spine films; i.e., spinal cord injury without radiologic abnormality, or SCIWORA). The trachea should be midline, and the large vessels of the neck examined. A chest that discloses (a) point tenderness, palpable bony deformity, crepitus, or subcutaneous emphysema on inspection or palpation; (b) inadequate chest rise or air entry on auscultation or percussion; or (c) asymmetry in excursion suggests the presence of a rib fracture or air or blood in the thorax (mandating a search for a pneumothorax or hemothorax). Muffled or distant heart sounds with jugular venous distention may suggest cardiac tamponade (although the latter may be difficult to detect if the child has a short, fat neck; it may also be absent with concurrent hypovolemia). An abdomen that remains distended following gastric decompression suggests the presence of intra-abdominal bleeding (most often from the spleen or liver) or a disrupted hollow viscus (especially if fever, tenderness, or guarding are found together with abdominal distention or nasogastric aspirate stained with blood or bile).

All skeletal components should be palpated for evidence of instability or discontinuity, especially bony prominences, such as the anterior superior iliac spines, which commonly are in-jured in major blunt trauma. In the absence of obvious deformities, fractures should be suspected if bony point tenderness (or hematoma or spasm of overlying muscles), an unstable pelvic girdle, or perineal swelling or discoloration is appreciated. Most long-bone fractures will be self-evident, but such injuries are occasionally missed during the secondary survey, emphasizing the need to assume that a fracture is present on the basis of history alone (even if no deformity is obvious) until proven otherwise; in addition, frequent reexamination is necessary of all injured extremities for evidence of pain, pallor, pulselessness, paresthesias, and paralysis (the classic signs of associated vascular trauma, or, when advanced, compartmental hypertension). The back should be completely examined. Appropriate components of the secondary survey should be repeated at intervals.

Laboratory Examinations

Although screening laboratory examinations may be of limited value in injured children generally, they are an integral part of the secondary survey, and their utility increases with severity of injury. Selected laboratory examinations may serve to provide early warning to the treating physician of impending deterioration, especially when physical findings are minor or questionable. Arterial blood gases are of paramount importance in determining the adequacy of ventilation (P_aCO_2), oxygenation (P_aO_2), and perfusion (base deficit), although the critically important determinant of blood oxygen content and, hence, tissue oxygen delivery (assuming the P_aO_2 exceeds 60 mm Hg) is the blood hemoglobin concentration. Serial hematocrits (obtained at regular intervals until the patient is stable) are essential to the management of severely injured children, as is a type and cross-match sent as early as possible from the emergency department. In the presence of abdominal injury or occult hemorrhage, elevations in serum transaminases or amylase and lipase suggest injury to the liver or pancreas; the infrequency of pancreatic injury makes the latter far less cost effective than the former. Coagulopathy is more common in children with extensive resuscitation or traumatic brain injury, and a screen that includes the prothrombin time and partial thromboplastin time should be performed in these patients. Urinalysis should be performed on children with suspected abdominal injury; urine that is grossly bloody or is positive for blood by dipstick (of note, myoglobin may yield false positive results) or microscopy (which shows 20 or more red blood cells per high-power field) suggests renal trauma and, therefore, damage to adjacent organs (due to the high incidence of associated injuries). A pregnancy test is advisable for injured adolescent females. Point-of-care laboratory examinations may be particularly helpful, because results are immediately available and, when appropriately chosen, likely to be clinically relevant.

Radiologic examinations are an integral part of the secondary survey. Arrangements should be made, before plain films are ordered, to obtain CT scans, as indicated. Once these are completed, whatever plain films are required may be obtained. However, at no time should imaging studies take precedence over resuscitation from life-threatening injuries, nor should an unstable patient be taken to the radiology department, nor should the physician and nurse fail to accompany and continuously monitor a critically injured child. CT scans of the head should be obtained whenever the patient has suffered a loss of consciousness or neurologic injury is suspected. To the extent that hemodynamic stability permits, CT scans of the abdomen should be obtained in the presence of signs of internal bleeding (abdominal tenderness, distention, bruising, or gross hematuria), a history of hypotensive shock (which has responded to volume resuscitation), penetrating injury, or major trauma. Generally, patients with severe, multiple trauma that prevents a complete physical examination benefit from routine CT of the head, thorax, abdomen, and pelvis, although normal results do not exclude injury; spiral or helical CT scanners in this setting may allow for optimal use of IV contrast, given the increased rapidity and resolution of such scans.

Angiography, often following preliminary identification of such injury by CT, is appropriate for further study of injuries to large vessels in selected patients. Interventional radiologists may then be able to offer an alternative to surgical intervention, including embolization and stenting. When interventional radiology procedures are not advisable, such information obtained by angiography may still prove helpful for vascular surgical intervention.

Although the incidence of SCIWORA (almost exclusively a pediatric diagnosis and uncommon even when originally described several decades ago) is low, it is a frequent cause of spinal cord injury in children. SCIWORA is a result of high-energy injuries, usually associated with automobile accidents, and is characterized by normal radiographic studies (either plain films or CT scans) with demonstrable defects on MRI. In some children with SCIWORA, a delayed clinical presentation of neurologic injury occurs, and the optimal time for MRI following such injury is still unknown.

Focused assessment by sonography in trauma (FAST) may be useful in detecting intra-abdominal blood, with the additional advantage that assessments can be performed serially at the patient's bedside; however, FAST is not yet sufficiently reliable to exclude abdominal injury. Nevertheless, the role of FAST in the diagnosis of abdominal injury is likely to increase, while the role of diagnostic peritoneal lavage decreases. A detailed sonographic examination may be useful for those cases in which intra-abdominal injury is suspected and CT cannot be obtained, either due to lack of equipment, a history of allergy to iodinated contrast agents, or pregnancy. Echocardiography is often helpful in the evaluation of thoracic injury, because it may reveal anatomic or functional cardiovascular injury or injury adjacent to cardiovascular structures.

Management

The management of pediatric trauma is the responsibility not of a single individual or specialty, but of a multidisciplinary team of pediatric-capable health professionals. It continues with the secondary survey and frequent reevaluation of vital functions and concludes with rehabilitation, and it encompasses the operative, critical, acute, and convalescent phases of care. Avoidance of secondary injury (injury due to persistent or recurrent hypoxia or hypoperfusion) is a major goal and mandates reliance on continuous monitoring.

Any child who requires resuscitation should initially receive no oral intake because of the temporary paralytic ileus that often accompanies major blunt abdominal trauma, and because general anesthesia may later be required. However, isotonic IV fluid should be administered at a maintenance rate, presuming both normal hydration at the time of the injury and normalization of both vital signs and perfusion status following resuscitation. Gastric tube decompression and a urinary catheter

should be placed unless proscribed by signs of a craniofacial or pelvic fracture, respectively.

With few exceptions, hypotensive pediatric trauma patients require immediate operation, while nonoperative management of blunt visceral trauma is most often successful. Penetrating injuries of the head, neck, and abdomen also require surgical intervention, but most intrathoracic injuries, whether blunt or penetrating, require only tube thoracostomy. Resuscitative emergency department thoracotomy has a dismal outcome in children, and is no longer routinely performed. Survival approaches zero following blunt traumatic cardiac arrest at any point during resuscitation, and following penetrating traumatic cardiac arrest absent signs of life in the field or in the emergency department. Emergency thoracotomy in the operating room is also rarely performed in children, except for massive hemothorax (20 mL/kg), ongoing hemorrhage (2–4 mL/kg/hr) from the chest tube, or persistent massive air leak or food or salivary drainage from the chest tube. Laparotomy is always required for gunshot wounds to the abdomen, as well as for penetrating abdominal injury associated with hemorrhagic shock, peritonitis, or evisceration. Thoracoabdominal injury should be suspected (a) whenever the torso is penetrated between the nipple line and the umbilicus (anteriorly) or the costal margin (posteriorly), (b) if peritoneal irritation develops following thoracic penetration, (c) if food or chyme is recovered from the chest tube, or (d) if injury trajectory imaging studies suggest the possibility of diaphragmatic penetration. If one or more of these signs is present, tube thoracostomy should be performed expeditiously, followed by laparotomy or laparoscopy for repair of the diaphragm and damaged organs. Skeletal injuries constitute the majority of cases in which surgical intervention is necessary. All penetrating wounds are contaminated and must be treated as infected, while accessible missile fragments should be removed (once swelling has subsided) to prevent the development of lead poisoning (especially those in contact with bone or joint fluid).

Analgesia appropriate for the injury is essential and may require frequent titration by experienced nursing staff. Most children with multiple trauma benefit from parenteral opiate therapy. Age-appropriate rating devices to assess for pain are available and should be monitored frequently during the first few days following injury. Physician staff should be notified when increasing needs for analgesia are noted. Patient-controlled analgesia (also with parenteral opiate) is indicated for capable older children and adolescents with significant injury-associated pain. Alternative methods of analgesia that may be valuable for some patients include local anesthesia, epidural analgesia, and nonopioid analgesia; adjunctive use of sedative-hypnotic agents may also be helpful in some injured children.

Glucose supplementation is unnecessary in most noninfant trauma victims, at least during the first day of therapy following major trauma, unless hypoglycemia or underlying disease is noted. Patients who receive supplemental glucose and those with an increased risk for hyperglycemia (i.e., a history of diabetes) should be closely monitored. Although the appropriate threshold for intervention in hyperglycemia associated with pediatric trauma is unknown, it is common practice to treat patients with glycosuria. When an insulin infusion is used to treat hyperglycemia, close attention to avoid hypoglycemia is essential. Following the acute injury and recovery, euglycemia is a reasonable goal, with maximized caloric intake.

Early involvement of social services, psychiatric support, pastoral care, and responsible law enforcement and child protective agencies is mandatory, especially in cases of intentional injury. Efforts must be made to attend to the emotional needs of the child and family, especially for those families who are forced to suffer the death of a child or a sibling. In addition to loss of control over their child's destiny, parents of seriously injured children may also feel enormous guilt, whether or not these feelings are warranted. The responsible physician should attempt to create as normal an environment as possible for the child and to allow parents to participate meaningfully in postinjury care. In so doing, treatment interventions will be facilitated, as the child perceives that parents and staff are working together to ensure an optimal recovery.

The care of children with major traumatic injury also involves nutritional support of nitrogen (even more than energy) and, in patients who are not eating, prophylactic therapy to prevent gastric stress ulcer bleeding. Tetanus-prone wounds require tetanus toxoid, with or without tetanus immune globulin, depending on immunization status and degree of contamination.

A critical result of the secondary survey in severe pediatric trauma is the answer to an urgent question regarding disposition: the radiology department, the operating room, or the PICU? The subsequent intrahospital transport of severely injured children requires planning, equipment, and professional support. Both the nurse responsible for the patient and the primary resuscitating physician should accompany a critically injured child, allowing for the transfer of important data and a plan of management.

Definitive Management of Non-neurologic Injuries

The definitive management of childhood trauma begins once sustentative care (the primary survey and resuscitation phases) has concluded. Definitive management of childhood trauma depends on the type, extent, and severity of the injuries sustained. Injuries to the torso (chest and abdomen) and skeleton are reviewed in this section. In patients treated with or without acute surgical intervention, it is important to note that later surgical interventions may be required, particularly in patients with persistent or worsening organ dysfunction.

Chest Trauma

Intrathoracic injuries occur in 6% of pediatric trauma victims (14), with the majority (86%) due to blunt injury, mostly (74%) automobile related. Most of these injuries will be manifest during the primary survey, although occasionally (with pulmonary contusions or lacerations, tracheobronchial injuries, etc.), identification will be delayed for several hours following injury. About 50% of children with thoracic injury require a thoracostomy. The thoracic injury pattern includes lung contusion and laceration (48%), pneumothorax and hemothorax (41%), and rib and sternal fractures (32%). Thus, a routine portable chest radiograph (anterior-posterior) will be helpful in most patients. Injuries to the heart, diaphragm, great vessels, bronchi, and esophagus occur less frequently. A chest CT scan is often helpful in patients with severe thoracic injuries, and may help to grade the severity of other lung injury, including contusion.

Because blunt trauma is nearly 10 times more deadly when associated with major intrathoracic injury, this condition serves as a marker of injury severity, even though it is the proximate cause of death in <1% of all pediatric blunt trauma.

The child compensates poorly for respiratory derangements associated with serious thoracic injury, due to (a) larger oxygen consumption (as noted previously); (b) a smaller functional residual capacity compared to closing capacity, with a resultant tendency to atelectasis; (c) lesser pulmonary compliance, yet greater chest wall compliance (which dictate chiefly a tachypneic response to hypoxia); and (d) horizontally aligned ribs and rudimentary intercostal musculature (which make the small child a diaphragmatic breather). The chest wall of the child often escapes major harm because the pliable nature of the cartilaginous ribs permits compression without radiographic fracturing. Pulmonary contusions are the typical result, and they are seldom life-threatening. Pneumothorax and hemothorax, due to lacerations of the lung parenchyma and intercostal vessels, are less common results but place the child in grave danger of sudden, marked ventilatory and circulatory compromise as the mediastinum shifts. A flail chest is unlikely until ribs are more completely ossified. Traumatic asphyxia secondary to blunt thoracic trauma with a closed glottis results in petechial hemorrhages in the upper portion of the body but may require only a few days of mechanical ventilatory support.

Critical care of the respiratory insufficiency that accompanies severe thoracic injury emphasizes the avoidance of further injury related to atelectrauma, barotrauma, biotrauma, and volutrauma, using the least amount of oxygen and respiratory support necessary to maintain the P_aO_2 at 70–80 mm Hg (hence, an S_pO_2 of 90%–100%). In the absence of acute lung injury (P_aO_2/FiO_2: 200–300), normocarbia is recommended. If acute lung injury is present or likely to develop, volutrauma should be avoided by using tidal volumes of 6–8 mL/kg and permissive hypercapnia, so long as head injury is not present, to attenuate further lung injury and lessen progression to acute respiratory distress syndrome (ARDS). Positive end-expiratory pressure sufficient to prevent end-expiratory collapse of small airways should be used to minimize atelectrauma. If peak inspiratory pressure cannot be maintained below 30 cm H_2O with minimal attendant barotraumas (less in the presence of air leak syndromes or fresh bronchial or pulmonary suture lines), alternative strategies should be considered, including high-frequency oscillatory ventilation, pronation, and lung surfactant. The role of extracorporeal membrane oxygenation (ECMO) for trauma patients remains uncertain due to the possibility of further hemorrhage during mandatory anticoagulation, although a recent case series included five children with respiratory failure and abdominal and/or thoracic injury treated successfully with venovenous ECMO. Median mechanical ventilation prior to ECMO was 6 days. Hemorrhage occurred frequently during ECMO, but it was manageable (23).

Pulmonary Contusion, Laceration, and Hematoma. Pulmonary parenchymal injury due to blunt trauma is characterized by alveolar hemorrhage, consolidation, and edema, leading to decreased gas exchange and pulmonary compliance. It may manifest as hemoptysis, subcutaneous emphysema, and respiratory distress, and occurs commonly in children with thoracic injury. Laboratory examinations may reveal hypoxemia on an arterial blood gas and a density in the lung fields on chest radiograph. A laceration in the pulmonary parenchyma may result from blunt or penetrating thoracic trauma and manifest as hemoptysis or hemothorax, often with an associated pneumothorax. Most pulmonary lacerations are minor and do not require specific therapy. Persistent hemorrhage from a laceration or contusion may result in a pulmonary hematoma; distinction of this entity from a simple contusion is not clearly defined.

Secondary complications of pulmonary contusion are not uncommon and include aspiration and infection; ARDS develops in up to one-fifth of children with pulmonary contusion (5). Careful attention to fluid intake is essential in patients with pulmonary contusion. The management of respiratory insufficiency in patients with these complex injuries was reviewed earlier. Pulmonary contusions uncomplicated by aspiration, overhydration, or infection can be expected to resolve in 7–10 days, mandating the judicious use of pulmonary toilet, crystalloid fluid (i.e., avoiding overhydration), loop diuretics, and selective antibiotic therapy to preclude the development of ARDS. Fluid and blood in lung parenchyma provide an excellent "culture medium" for bacterial infection, and care must be taken to recognize early signs of superinfection of a pulmonary contusion.

Hemopneumothorax. Blunt or penetrating trauma that leads to a communication between the pleural space and the atmosphere results in an immediate accumulation of air (and possibly blood) into the pleural space, with contralateral mediastinal shift. Often, these injuries are associated with rib fractures. Penetrating trauma is associated with a higher incidence of hemopneumothorax than is blunt trauma. Air passes freely in and out of a large chest wall defect, but if the opening is small, ingress may occur during inspiration and obstruction may occur during expiration, leading to further shift of the mediastinum (i.e., a tension pneumothorax). As more air and/or blood collects in the thorax with worsening mediastinal shift, obstruction to venous return and cardiac output lead to shock. However, some patients may be minimally symptomatic, and a screening chest radiograph is appropriate in children with thoracic trauma. In any case, collections of blood and/or air in the pleural space of an injured child should be expeditiously drained.

Initial therapy of hemopneumothorax in this setting includes a sterile, occlusive dressing to convert the open chest wall injury to a closed injury. A tube thoracostomy inserted via the fifth intercostal space in the mid-axillary line via open or Seldinger technique is then connected to a collection chamber with an applied pressure of −20 cm H_2O; a water-seal chamber connected in series will facilitate the identification of air leaks in the system. In young children with thin chest walls, a short subcutaneous tunnel created between the skin incision and the entry point into the pleural space helps prevent air leaks around the tube. The management of a tube thoracostomy requires significant nursing skills, including knowledge of appropriate dressings, the ability to troubleshoot the system (including both air leak and obstruction scenarios), and an understanding of the patient's tolerance and analgesia requirements. The water-seal chamber should be frequently checked to assess for air leaks, while the collection chamber may reveal blood, serosanguineous, or other exudative fluid. Video-assisted thoracoscopy (VATS) may be helpful when residual collections of blood persist. Definitive management of an open chest wound requires surgical intervention in the controlled environment of the operating room following stabilization.

Rib Fractures and Flail Chest. Rib fractures occur in approximately one-third of children with blunt thoracic trauma (14), and their occurrence suggests a mechanism of injury characterized by significant energy transfer. The presence of rib fractures in an injured child appears to be a marker of more severe injury and increased risk of mortality. Rib fractures in infants and young children are frequently associated with child abuse, particularly in the absence of a history of major blunt trauma. Cardiopulmonary resuscitation is rarely associated with anterior rib fractures. Fracture of a first rib may be a marker of major vascular injury in children. Treatment of isolated rib fractures includes adequate analgesia and chest physiotherapy to prevent atelectasis and pneumonia. Older children may be able to use incentive spirometry and deep-breathing exercises.

A flail chest is rare in children and is characterized by a chest wall segment that has lost continuity with the thorax and moves paradoxically with changes in intrathoracic pressure: *in* with inspiration and *out* with expiration. This injury is the result of major thoracic blunt trauma and is usually associated with multiple rib fractures, such that contiguous ribs have two or more fractures, as well as a pulmonary contusion. Diagnosis is made by the visual inspection of paradoxical movement of the chest wall, although it may be less obvious or absent in young children with small flail segments. Definitive management includes controlled mechanical ventilation; the inflated lung acts as a splint, stabilizes the rib fractures, and decreases pain associated with the chest wall injury. Continued therapy is mainly directed at the underlying pulmonary contusion. Intercostal or epidural analgesia may be helpful. Prolonged mechanical ventilatory support and surgical fixation may be necessary in rare cases.

Myocardial Contusion. Although myocardial contusion may occur in adults with significant thoracic trauma, mostly in automobile drivers whose chests are crushed against the steering column, similar injuries are rare in children. Symptoms include chest pain, dysrhythmias, and myocardial dysfunction. Signs on physical examination include tachycardia or dysrhythmia, a gallop rhythm, and findings consistent with cardiogenic pulmonary edema. Laboratory examinations may reveal the presence of cardiomegaly, as well as myocardial dysfunction on electrocardiography and/or echocardiography, and elevated myocardial enzymes. Treatment is primarily supportive. Because children with myocardial contusion are at risk for sudden and lethal dysrhythmias, even if the initial electrocardiogram is unremarkable, they require admission to a PICU and continuous cardiac monitoring.

Sudden death that occurs with a relatively minor blunt injury to the chest is known as *commotio cordis* and is seen principally in male adolescents in association with athletic events. The mechanism of injury appears to be ventricular dysrhythmia, and because the energy of impact is often low, associated injury is not generally present. Survival is low but would likely improve with more widespread community access to defibrillation.

Cardiac Tamponade. Pericardial contusions and lacerations may lead to hemopericardium and subsequent cardiac tamponade, although this appears to be an uncommon complication in children. Rising pericardial pressure obstructs both venous return and cardiac output, leading to Beck's triad (pulsus paradoxus, a quiet precordium, and distended neck veins), at least in some affected adolescents and adults; shock is the result. In younger victims of major thoracic trauma, unexplained tachycardia may be an early sign of tamponade, and examination of neck veins may be less revealing. Additional data that may be helpful include a jugular venous pressure tracing with absent Y descent—at least in older patients with a central venous catheter—and, occasionally, the presence of *pulsus alternans*. Treatment in severely injured patients with a suggestive history and physical examination should not be delayed. FAST examination in selected patients may be quite helpful, and may be available expeditiously. A CT scan without a large pericardial effusion is useful for patients at increased risk in whom the clinical suspicion is lower. Other helpful laboratory tests include a chest radiograph, electrocardiography, and echocardiography (in particular, the presence of right atrial diastolic collapse in patients with a pericardial effusion). Expansion of intravascular volume is a helpful temporizing measure as the patient is prepared for a pericardiocentesis or operative placement of a pericardial window. Because most anesthetic agents are associated with a decrease in systemic vascular resistance and a subsequent fall in preload, local anesthesia may be a good choice for emergency pericardiocentesis. Positive-pressure ventilation, with or without intubation, is not well tolerated in these patients either, until at least partial decompression has occurred. Sedation with agents that permit spontaneous ventilation without significant decreases in myocardial contractility and systemic vascular resistance are helpful in patients who are unable to tolerate the procedure; ketamine and etomidate have been used. Bedside pericardiocentesis with contemporaneous placement of a drainage catheter via Seldinger technique may help temporize unstable patients until definitive repair in the operating room can be undertaken.

Rupture of the Diaphragm. Traumatic rupture of the diaphragm results from severe compression forces over the lower chest and upper abdomen, and patients generally have severe associated injuries. This injury has been recognized with increased frequency in the pediatric trauma patient following blunt trauma or with lap-belt injuries. Rupture is far more common on the left side, almost certainly because the right diaphragm is buttressed, and partially occluded, by the liver. A small tear in the diaphragm may not cause immediate symptoms, but eventually results in progressive herniation of abdominal contents through the diaphragmatic defect, as negative intrathoracic pressure gradually sucks abdominal viscera through the defect. The diagnosis should be suspected when the left diaphragm is not clearly visualized or is abnormally elevated or shaped, when abdominal visceral shadows are abnormally located on the initial chest radiograph, or when a nasogastric tube terminates in the hemithorax. Radiographic evaluation may be unreliable in the setting of penetrating injury. Treatment is operative repair. Unfortunately, significant delays in diagnosis are not uncommon.

Aortic Disruption. Although injury to the aorta is uncommon in children, it may occur following severe deceleration injuries and/or a fall from extreme heights. It is associated with a high mortality rate and other significant thoracic injuries, and most children with this injury die at the scene. Among the rare survivors, clinical symptoms and signs include back pain, a machinery-type heart murmur that classically radiates to the back, and hemorrhagic shock. A widened mediastinum, loss of the aortic knob, deviation of the trachea to the right, fracture of the first or second ribs, and apical capping may also suggest its presence in this setting. Arch aortography, a chest CT or MRI, and transesophageal echocardiography are frequently needed to adequately delineate the injury. Preoperative β-blockade may be appropriate in selected patients. Treatment is emergent thoracotomy and surgical repair, most often under cardiopulmonary bypass.

Tracheobronchial Tears. Rupture of the tracheobronchial tree due to blunt or penetrating thoracic trauma is often difficult to diagnose; most patients with major tracheobronchial tears die at the scene. Survivors may include some children suffering "clothesline" injuries to the neck, in whom an airway can be established distal to the injury. Affected patients often have symptoms and signs of airway obstruction (dyspnea and stridor), as well as pneumothorax, pneumomediastinum, and subcutaneous emphysema. A persistent—and often large—air leak following tube thoracostomy also suggests the possibility of a tracheobronchial tear, usually located near the carina in children with severe thoracic trauma. Blind airway suctioning is contraindicated when tracheobronchial tears are suspected, and bronchoscopy may be diagnostic. Because PPV may exacerbate the leak, careful management of airway pressures and fluid intake is essential. High-frequency oscillatory ventilation and other therapeutic modalities may be helpful and should be considered early in the course of injury. Some patients require multiple tube thoracostomies or emergent operative intervention to repair the leak. Isolation of the affected airway with one-lung ventilation, if possible, or even ECMO, may be life saving.

Abdominal Trauma

The abdomen of the child is vulnerable to injury for several reasons. Flexible ribs cover only the uppermost portion of the abdomen; thin layers of muscle, fat, and fascia provide little protection to the large solid viscera; the pelvis is shallow, lifting the bladder into the abdomen. Moreover, the overall small size of the abdomen predisposes the child to multiple rather than single injuries. Finally, gastric dilatation due to air (which often confounds abdominal examination by simulating peritonitis) leads to ventilatory and circulatory compromise by limiting diaphragmatic motion, increasing risk of aspiration, and causing vagally mediated dampening of the normal tachycardic response to hypovolemia.

Serious intra-abdominal injuries occur in 8% of pediatric trauma victims (14) and include injuries to the liver (27%), spleen (27%), kidneys (25%), and gastrointestinal tract (21%). Injuries to the genitourinary tract, pancreas, abdominal blood vessels, and pelvis are infrequent (5% or less) and, with the exception of injuries to abdominal blood vessels, account for few of the deaths that result from intra-abdominal injury. Penetrating abdominal injury is much less common than blunt trauma in children, and most of these patients will need surgical exploration following resuscitation and stabilization.

Physical signs of significant abdominal injury in children include diminished bowel sounds, tenderness to palpation, guarding, rebound tenderness, and other signs of peritoneal irritation. Depending on the mechanism of injury, some children may develop an abdominal wall hematoma (i.e., the "seatbelt sign" due to a restraint). Although the physical examination usually is abnormal in children with significant intra-abdominal injury, the findings may not be specific. Frequent reexamination is essential, because the possible need for intervention does not abate immediately following the injury.

Laboratory examinations that should be reviewed in the child with abdominal injury (as noted previously) include serial hematocrits, a type and cross-match, a complete blood count, serum transaminases, a coagulation screen (prothrombin time and partial thromboplastin time), urinalysis, and amylase and lipase in patients at increased risk. Abdominal radiographs should be assessed for evidence of free air. Following plain abdominal radiographs in children with suspected abdominal injury, CT scanning is the imaging study of choice; it is readily available, noninvasive, and has helped reduce the need for acute surgical interventions. It is recommended for both blunt and penetrating injury. Because the extent of abdominal injury may be more difficult to appreciate from the pediatric physical examination than is the extent of thoracic injury, imaging results often help guide resuscitation.

Although intravenous contrast is essential (in the absence of renal failure or allergy) to optimize the information from an abdominal CT scan, some controversy exists about the role of intraluminal contrast: Time spent preparing the patient for the scan is increased, there may be an increased risk of aspiration, and the contrast may traverse the alimentary canal slowly in patients with major trauma; in addition, common abdominal injury patterns in children typically involve solid rather than hollow viscera, potentially limiting the utility of intraluminal contrast. Nevertheless, double (intraluminal and intravenous) contrast CT scans of the abdomen are quite helpful in many injured children, and are preferred in many trauma centers.

Key findings on abdominal CT scans include vascular blush and other signs of contrast extravasation, although evidence of extravasation does not mandate emergency laparotomy, as is true for adults. A FAST examination may be useful to confirm abnormalities in children who are too unstable to undergo a CT scan but is less helpful when negative. Subsequent imaging procedures that may prove useful include radionuclide scans and an intravenous urogram for renal trauma in selected patients.

Most solid visceral injuries are successfully treated nonoperatively, especially those involving kidneys (98%), spleen (95%), and liver (90%) (50). Acute management should follow consensus guidelines. The extent of intra-abdominal injury in a child may be difficult to determine because of an inadequate history, a presumed inconsequential injury, or the frequent absence of external clinical signs of internal injury. Bleeding from renal, splenic, and hepatic injuries is mostly self-limited and resolves spontaneously in nearly 100%, 95%, and 90% of such cases, respectively, unless the patient presents in hypotensive shock or the transfusion requirement exceeds 40 mL/kg of body weight (half of the circulating blood volume) within 24 hours of injury. Although uncommon, vascular injury (excluding solid organ injuries) in children, whether in the thorax or abdomen, is associated with high mortality. The role of peritoneal lavage to diagnose intra-abdominal hemorrhage in children has markedly declined, with an increased reliance on radiologic imaging and nonoperative management. The indications for immediate abdominal surgery in pediatric trauma patients include evidence of ongoing intra-abdominal hemorrhage (shock), evidence of hollow viscus perforation (peritonitis), and evisceration. Some experts would add major renal and collecting system disruption as well as major pancreatic ductal disruption to this list,

although nonoperative management has also been advocated for these injuries. When hemorrhage is ongoing, the transfusion of blood products requires careful attention; rapid transfusions may be best accomplished using specific devices and catheters, warming of blood products is essential, and close monitoring of blood chemistry will help to prevent or treat resultant electrolyte problems and metabolic acidosis. Laparotomy for the management of renal, pancreatic, gastrointestinal, and genitourinary injuries is performed utilizing damage control methods for patients in extremis and staged closure for patients with abdominal compartment syndrome. Resuscitation in the PICU of patients treated with a damage-control approach may permit a more controlled reoperation, with an improved outcome as observed in adult patients, but data in children are lacking. In any case, an open abdomen following either damage control or decompressive laparotomy mandates adequate protection of the viscera from microbial contamination, evaporative water and heat loss, and desiccation.

Appreciation of the likelihood of multiple injuries in children mandates prioritization; for example, "uncontrolled intra-abdominal hemorrhage takes precedence over a stable thoracic aorta tear" (9). Angiographic interventional radiology may be useful in selected cases, particularly where bleeding is severe and easily accessible.

Liver and Spleen. The spleen and liver are the most commonly injured organs in blunt abdominal trauma, and each accounts for approximately one-fourth of all intra-abdominal injuries. Diagnosis is made by abdominal CT in hemodynamically stable patients. A grading system for anatomic findings in splenic and hepatic injury has been developed by the American Association for the Surgery of Trauma (36) (**Table 27.6**); this system may also prove helpful in predicting outcome. In hemodynamically unstable patients, diagnosis is based on operative findings. However, conservative management is the rule, because the majority of patients are not hemodynamically unstable and most do not progress to frank, uncontrolled intra-abdominal hemorrhage. Nevertheless, operative intervention must be readily available if nonoperative management is contemplated. Complications specific to conservative management have not yet been completely characterized.

Of particular importance in the evaluation of patients for potential surgical intervention is hemodynamic stability: Is the hematocrit stable, even if low? If so, hemorrhage may have stopped; continuing hemorrhage is indicated by a falling hematocrit. An ongoing requirement for transfusion in the first few hours of resuscitation may also indicate an increased risk for vascular injury that requires surgery. Is evidence of continued intra-abdominal hemorrhage seen on imaging procedures, or are the base deficit and serum lactate concentrations continuing to worsen? If so, a laparotomy may be indicated.

An evidence-based guideline utilizing CT scan findings for the treatment of children with liver and spleen injuries below grade V has been proposed and includes ICU admission for patients with grade IV injury, several weeks of activity restriction depending on grade of injury, and no need for routine follow-up imaging (50). However, the relatively small study size, given the infrequency of late solid-organ hemorrhage, suggests that continued outcomes research is needed.

Kidneys and Urinary Tract. Children are more susceptible to renal trauma than adults are due to the reasons cited earlier;

TABLE 27.6

GRADING SYSTEM[a] FOR HEPATIC AND SPLENIC INJURIES

Injury	Grade I	Grade II	Grade III	Grade IV	Grade V	Grade VI
Hematoma: liver, spleen	Subcapsular, <10% surface area	Subcapsular, 10%–50% surface area; intraparenchymal diameter <10 cm (liver) vs. <5 cm (spleen)	Subcapsular, >50% surface area or expanding; ruptured subcapsular or parenchymal hematoma; intraparenchymal hematoma >10 cm (liver) vs. >5 cm (spleen) or expanding			
Laceration: liver	Capsular tear <1 cm parenchymal depth	1–3 cm parenchymal depth, <10 cm in length (liver) vs. not involving a trabecular vessel (spleen)	>3 cm parenchymal depth or involving trabecular vessels (spleen)	Parenchymal disruption of 25%–75% of hepatic lobe, or 1–3 segments within a lobe	Parenchymal disruption >75% of hepatic lobe, or >3 segments within a lobe	
Laceration: spleen					Shattered spleen	
Vascular injury: liver				Involvement of hilar vessels with >25% devascularization	Juxtahepatic venous injuries	Hepatic avulsion
Vascular injury: spleen					Hilar injury with devascularization	

[a]Advance one grade for multiple injuries, up to grade III.
Adapted from Moore EE, Cogbill TH, Jurkovich GJ, et al. Organ injury scaling: spleen and liver (1994 revision). *J Trauma.* 1995;38:323–4.

TABLE 27.7

GRADING SYSTEM[a] FOR RENAL INJURY

Injury	Grade I	Grade II	Grade III	Grade IV	Grade V
Contusion	Microscopic or gross hematuria, normal urologic studies				
Hematoma	Subcapsular, nonexpanding	Nonexpanding perirenal hematoma confined to renal retroperitoneum			
Laceration		<1 cm parenchymal depth (renal cortex) without urinary extravasation	>1 cm parenchymal depth (renal cortex) without urinary extravasation	Extending through renal cortex, medulla and collecting system	Shattered kidney
Vascular injury				Main renal artery or vein injury with contained hemorrhage	Avulsion of renal hilum

[a]Advance one grade for multiple injuries to the same organ.
Adapted from Moore EE, Shackford SR, Pachter HL, et al. Organ injury scaling: Spleen, liver, and kidney. *J Trauma*. 1989;29:1664–6.

in addition, the child's kidney occupies a proportionally larger retroperitoneal space. Blunt trauma is more frequent than penetrating trauma, usually leading to a hematoma. However, lacerations of the kidney are not uncommon and result mostly from crush injuries against the ribs or spine.

Gross hematuria remains the most reliable indicator of serious urologic injury and mandates radiographic examination. Microscopic hematuria is less sensitive in this regard, although the degree of hematuria does not necessarily correlate with severity of urologic injury. Because insertion of a urethral catheter itself can cause hematuria, the urine that is examined should ideally be a spontaneously voided specimen. Because rhabdomyolysis following crush injury may present with pigmented urine and a urinalysis positive for heme, it is important to distinguish this entity: Red blood cells on microscopic analysis of urine suggest urologic hemorrhage rather than myoglobinuria. An abdominal CT scan with intravenous contrast is the most appropriate initial test for hemodynamically stable children with suspected renal trauma. The American Association for the Surgery of Trauma developed a grading system (Table 27.7) for renal injury utilizing CT scan results, which has been used in management (37). A "one-shot" trauma intravenous urogram, which may be performed in the operating room for patients who require emergent surgical exploration, provides some gross information about renal function.

The conservative management of renal injury in grades I to III is routine. In children with grades IV and V renal injury, indications for surgical exploration include persistent hemorrhage, expanding or uncontained retroperitoneal hematoma, or suspected renal pedicle avulsion. In addition, those with substantial devitalized renal parenchyma and/or urinary extravasation may also be candidates. Occasionally angiographic control of renal hemorrhage is feasible.

The ureters are protected by muscle and soft tissue and are rarely injured, although ureteropelvic junction disruption may occur following severe abdominal trauma; delayed radiographic imaging may be helpful in this setting. Surgical repair of these injuries may include multiple reconstruction proce-

dures following acute recovery. The bladder is less protected in children due to its position. Rupture of the bladder dome—the weakest area—leads to an intraperitoneal leak, whereas pelvic fractures associated with rupture of the bladder wall or base give rise to an extraperitoneal leak. If the bladder is not filled with contrast for a CT scan, diagnosis may be delayed. The approach for surgical repair of a ruptured bladder depends on the site of the leak; a cystostomy is often helpful. Pelvic fractures are also associated with urethral injury, particularly in males, and blood is generally present at the urethral meatus of affected patients. Diagnosis mandates retrograde urethrography. Management depends on the severity and site of urethral injury and may include multiple reconstruction procedures and cystostomy.

Rhabdomyolysis secondary to crush injuries may be associated with renal dysfunction and failure; serum muscle enzymes are dramatically elevated, and early treatment with hydration (and possibly urinary alkalinization) is helpful. Renal replacement therapy is appropriate for patients with trauma-associated renal failure, whether or not rhabdomyolysis is present. This therapy may permit optimization of nutritional support, especially when meticulous fluid balance is essential. The threshold for initiation of renal replacement therapy in trauma-associated renal insufficiency, particularly in children, remains controversial.

Gastrointestinal Tract. The esophagus is a thoracic organ, although rarely injured by blunt thoracic trauma. Blunt injuries to the remainder of the gastrointestinal tract may follow several patterns, including crush injury (the organ is compressed against the spine), burst injury (the filled, distended viscus is compressed rapidly), and shear injury (tethers, including neurovascular structures, of an organ are damaged by rapid acceleration/deceleration). Subsequent damage may include hematoma, laceration, perforation, or transection of the gastrointestinal tract, and symptomatology may change over hours or days. Blunt stomach injury is more frequent in children than in adults and usually results in a perforation or "blowout" injury along the greater curvature. Nasogastric drainage may be bloody, and radiographic studies are generally positive for free air. Duodenal injuries are less frequent than other injuries of the gastrointestinal tract due in part to a retroperitoneal—and somewhat protected—location. Because this location may also serve to hide clinical signs of injury, it is reassuring to note that CT scans (preferably with double contrast) appear to differentiate well between duodenal hematoma and perforation in children. Hematomas and/or perforations that involve the remainder of the small bowel may be difficult to diagnose early, because peritoneal signs may take several hours to develop fully. Significant blunt injuries to the large bowel generally lead to the rapid development of symptoms and an abnormal physical examination. Diagnosis of gastrointestinal tract perforation following trauma in children is mostly the result of careful, repeated physical examination, although CT scans and other laboratory examinations are helpful, particularly in patients who are unable to respond appropriately or comply with the examination.

The management of gastrointestinal tract perforation in children is surgical; nonoperative management of duodenal hematomas has also been used successfully and is indicated as initial treatment. Because adults with a hematoma in the colonic wall may develop delayed perforation, the appropriate management strategy for this entity in children is debated. A colostomy may also be necessary for extensive large bowel injury with perforation and significant fecal contamination, although in its absence, primary repair is often feasible in an otherwise healthy child without shock or the need for multiple blood transfusions.

Pancreas. Although infrequently injured in children due in part to its retroperitoneal location, the pancreas may be injured with severe blunt abdominal trauma; a delay in diagnosis may occur, and affected children generally have multiple associated injuries. Diagnosis depends mainly on CT scan results, although clinical and laboratory data may also be useful. Endoscopic retrograde cholangiopancreatography (ERCP) with possible stenting, may be helpful for selected patients with duct disruption. Routine surgical intervention is not recommended, but distal pancreatectomy may have a role in selected patients. Pseudocyst formation related to duct disruption has been reported in approximately one-third of children with pancreatic injuries (49); nonoperative management with parenteral nutrition, gut rest, and drainage procedures, when appropriate, are recommended.

Abdominal Compartment Syndrome. Trauma-associated abdominal compartment syndrome is not common in children but may occur following blunt trauma or burn injury. Massive fluid resuscitation may be associated with the development of this syndrome. The syndrome is recognized by increasing intra-abdominal pressure, and the pathophysiology involves decreased abdominal organ perfusion with decreased venous return from the lower half of the body. Hypoperfusion injury leads to further tissue edema and progressive hypoperfusion, and abdominal distention with organ dysfunction occurs. Oliguria and respiratory insufficiency are common clinical findings in children.

Diagnosis involves instilling 1 mL/kg of sterile saline via the bladder catheter and measuring the pressure; pressure greater than 25 mm Hg (or ~18 cm H_2O) is diagnostic (the refer-

ence point is the symphysis pubis). A lower pressure threshold (16 mm Hg, or ~12 cm H_2O) for the diagnosis of abdominal compartment syndrome in children with organ dysfunction has been suggested (8) and may prove more clinically relevant. The mortality rate associated with this complication is high, but the condition itself is easily treated by decompressive laparotomy, often with temporary patch abdominoplasty.

Skeletal Trauma

The porous nature of immature cortical bone may lead to an increased incidence of fractures in children compared to adults. As immature bone is also more elastic, fractures in children are often incomplete or nondisplaced. Fractures in childhood are also unique as a result of the presence of growth plates, the rapid rate of healing, a tendency to remodel in the plane of the fracture, and a high incidence of ischemic vascular injuries. In addition, long-term growth disturbances may complicate childhood fractures. Diaphyseal fractures of the long bones cause significant overgrowth, while physeal (growth plate) fractures, particularly if severe (Salter-Harris types 3 and 4), cause significant undergrowth. Joint dislocations and ligamentous injury are less common in children. The periosteum is also thicker in children and may assist in stabilization of underlying fractures.

Fractures are rarely an immediate cause of death in blunt trauma, although they are the leading cause of disability; they are present in 26% of serious blunt injury cases and constitute the principal anatomic diagnosis in 22%. Upper extremity fractures outnumber lower extremity fractures by 7:1, although in serious blunt trauma, this ratio is 2:3. The most common long-bone fractures sustained during childhood pedestrian motor vehicle crashes are fractures of the femur and tibia, whereas falls typically are associated with both upper and lower extremity fractures if fall height is significant (from the top of a bunk bed or the window of a high-rise dwelling, not from falls from standard-height beds or down the stairs). The delayed diagnosis of fractures in multiply injured children may occur; the frequency depends on age and diagnostic method.

Because isolated long-bone and pelvic fractures are rarely associated with significant hemorrhage, a diligent search must be made for another source of bleeding if signs of hypotensive shock are observed. This search frequently leads to the abdomen, although infants and children may also lose substantial amounts of blood in the thorax or head. For a more detailed discussion of open fractures, amputations, and other forms of severe skeletal trauma, the reader is referred to orthopedic texts.

Fractures. Because long-bone fractures are rarely life threatening unless associated with major bleeding (bilateral femur fractures or unstable pelvic fractures), the general care of the injured patient takes precedence over orthopedic care, but early stabilization will serve both to decrease patient discomfort and limit the amount of blood loss. Closed treatment predominates for fractures of the clavicle, upper extremity, and tibia, while fractures of the femur increasingly involve the use of internal fixation. Careful inspection of all wounds is necessary, as an open fracture may be associated with an innocuous-appearing puncture wound. If an open fracture is suspected, do not reexamine it repeatedly; a simple dressing with immobilization of the extremity is appropriate. It is worth noting that open fractures significantly increase the risk of developing a compartment syndrome. Operative treatment is required for complex open fractures (for debridement and irrigation), displaced supracondylar fractures (due to their association with ischemic vascular injury), and major or displaced physeal fractures (which must be reduced anatomically). Owing to the ability of most long-bone fractures to remodel, reductions need not be perfectly anatomic, but remodeling is limited in torus and greenstick fractures, as the hyperemia typical of complete fractures is unlikely to occur.

The critical care of skeletal injuries consists of careful immobilization as appropriate, with emphasis on the prevention of immobilization-related complications (such as friction burns and decubitus ulcers) through the use of supportive and assistive devices (such as egg-crate or similar mattresses and a trapeze to permit limited freedom of movement). Prolonged skeletal traction in children with fractures may be associated with hypertension and hypercalcemia, although a direct relationship appears unlikely; both respond to mobilization. Frequent neurovascular checks are essential to assess for the development of arterial insufficiency, a hallmark of the compartment syndrome.

The care of open fractures includes antibiotics, generally a first-generation cephalosporin unless significant comminuted bone from a high-energy injury is present (in which case, addition of an aminoglycoside is reasonable). Complications, including traumatic fat embolism following long-bone fracture and rhabdomyolysis following severe crush injury are rare, but require aggressive care when present. The former may be associated with ARDS and/or emboli to other organs, and early stabilization of long-bone fractures is helpful, while the latter is treated as previously noted. Early rehabilitation is vital to optimal recovery and mandates routine physiatric consultation on admission to the PICU.

Compartment Syndrome. Fracture-associated arterial insufficiency is recognized by the presence of a pulse deficit on serial examination, but detection of the compartment syndrome usually requires the measurement of compartment pressures; elevated compartment pressures impair capillary perfusion, and ischemia develops rapidly. This syndrome can develop occasionally, even in the absence of trauma, with extravasation of IV fluid. Symptoms include the 5 Ps: pallor, pulselessness, paresthesia, paralysis, and pain. The last, pain, is the earliest sign of the syndrome, is often out of proportion to the injury, and may be difficult to treat, even with opiates. Frequent, repeated neurovascular checks of multiply traumatized children are essential to detect this devastating complication early.

Fasciotomy is indicated when the compartment pressure is greater than 40 cm H_2O, although lower pressures may mandate treatment if the child is symptomatic or if the capillary perfusion pressure is reduced. The utility of an absolute pressure limit for children of different ages is controversial, and the diagnosis remains, in part, a clinical one. Fasciotomy in the lower extremities is often performed simultaneously for all adjacent compartments and, following fasciotomy, the skin wounds are left open to heal by delayed primary closure or skin grafting.

CHILD ABUSE

When the history of injury in a child is inconsistent with the severity of injury, child abuse must be considered. Child abuse is the presumed underlying cause of 3% of major traumatic injuries in children, although the actual incidence is difficult to determine. A detailed review of the mechanisms, patterns, presentation, and findings of physical abuse is beyond the scope of this chapter, but child abuse may be suspected whenever a delay in obtaining treatment is unexplained; when the history is vague or otherwise incompatible with the observed physical findings; when the caretaker blames siblings, playmates, or other third parties; or when the caretaker protects other adults rather than the child. Although the recognition and sociomedicolegal management of suspected cases of child abuse require a team approach, assessment and medical treatment of physical injuries is no different than for any other mechanism of injury. Confrontation and accusation hinder treatment and rehabilitation and have no place in the management of any injured child, regardless of the nature of the injury (although reports of suspected child abuse must be filed with local child protective services in every state and territory in the US).

Victims of child abuse are younger, more severely injured, and more likely to die from their injuries than are other pediatric trauma patients. More importantly, morbidity in this group is worse. These patients are more likely to require custodial care and have more significant functional limitations (21). The "shaken baby syndrome" comprises a unique set of symptoms and signs peculiar to nonaccidental trauma; this entity is also known as the "whiplash shaken infant syndrome" (12). These patients have intracranial and intraocular hemorrhages in the absence of external trauma to the head or fracture of the calvaria, and the "shaking" injuries are the result of bleeding from the easily torn bridging veins of the infant's meninges during rapidly applied forces of acceleration-deceleration, forces which are dramatically increased if concomitant impact is also present. Ophthalmologic examination often reveals retinal hemorrhages of varying severity, occasionally with retinal detachment. The prognosis is poor for many affected infants. Additional patterns of injury secondary to physical abuse include burns and contusions, particularly in patterns suggesting a mechanism, such as cigarette or hot iron burns, or fingerprint contusions, as well as asphyxiation, blunt abdominal injury, multiple fractures of various ages, and sexual abuse.

The physical examination is often normal in abused infants and children; it may also be normal initially and change over several hours, mandating frequent reexamination. Findings on physical examination may include signs of general neglect, such as poor skin hygiene, malnutrition, failure to thrive, hematomas, and petechiae of various ages and distribution (although the color of cutaneous contusions is not generally a sensitive and specific indicator of contusion age), bite marks, burn injuries, abrasions, strap or belt injuries, and soft-tissue swelling (**Fig. 27.4**). An ophthalmologic examination is mandatory in infants who are possible abuse victims; pupillary dilatation should be performed sequentially, using shorter-acting agents to avoid prolonged, bilateral mydriasis. Particular attention should also be directed at evidence of sexual abuse, such as condylomata, perianal and genital hematoma, other venereal disease (oral and genital), and pain in the anogenital area.

In addition to routine laboratory examinations for childhood trauma, infant victims of abuse require an examination for skeletal injury; either a skeletal survey with chest

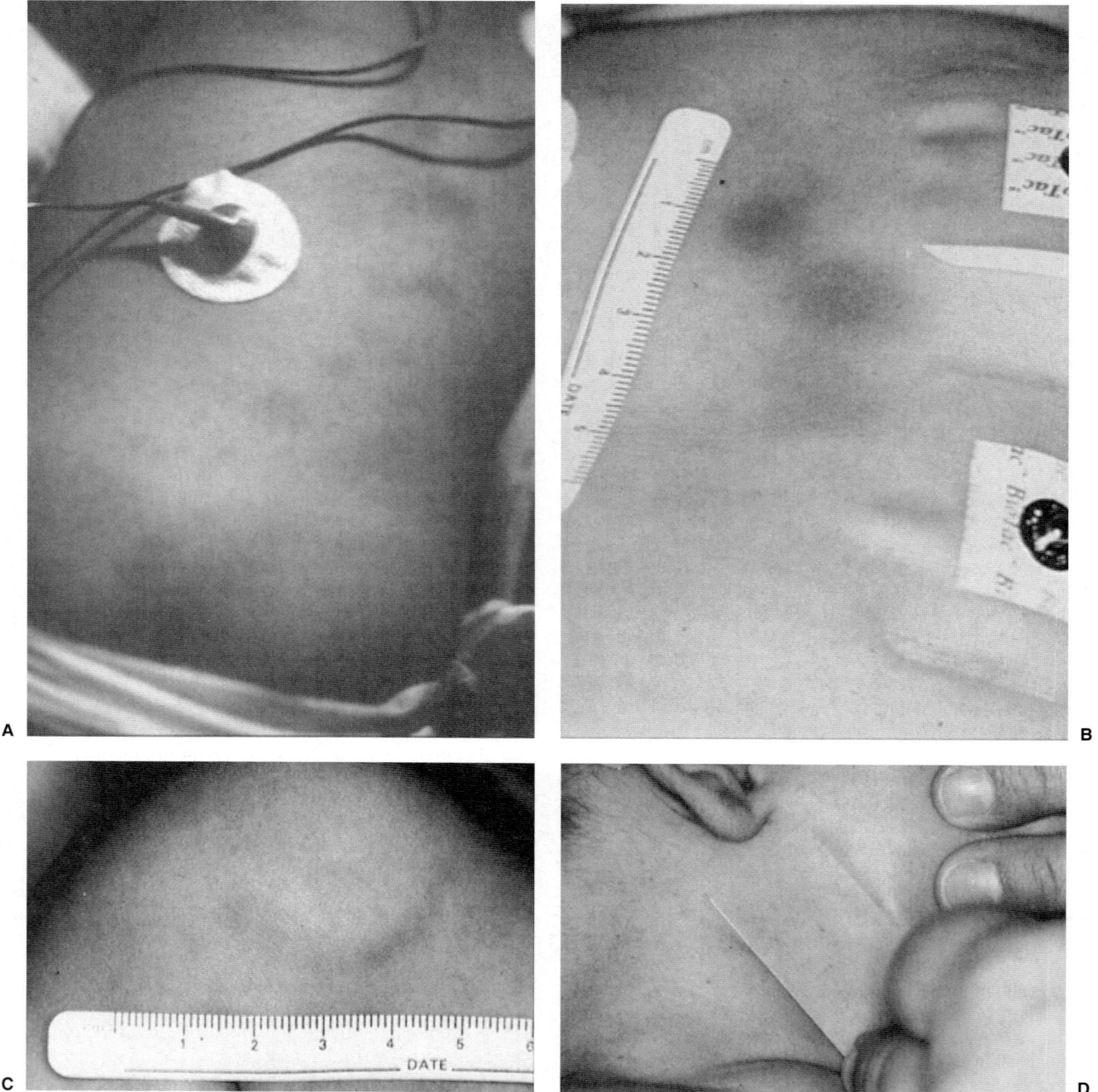

FIGURE 27.4. Cutaneous findings in child abuse. **A, B:** Fingerprint contusions of various ages on back of one baby and chest wall of another. **C:** Bite mark on knee. **D:** Petechiae on neck of asphyxiated baby.

radiograph (possibly including oblique rib films) or a bone scan are commonly used. Further testing, including radiographic imaging, will depend on the presentation and differential diagnosis. Radiographic manifestations of child abuse include new and old injuries, subperiosteal hemorrhages, epiphyseal separations, periosteal shearings, metaphyseal fragmentations, previously healed periosteal calcifications, and shearing of the metaphysis.

The diagnosis of child abuse is uncomfortable, even for experienced physicians; it is frequently a diagnosis of exclu-sion, considered only after more "acceptable" diagnoses are ruled out. However, the diagnosis of child abuse is rarely made with absolute certainty on the initial presentation, and the physician's role is to serve as an advocate for children. The possibility of abuse should therefore be investigated expeditiously, because it is equally important to protect siblings still in the home. The prompt involvement of social services and responsible child protective services allows the intensive care unit staff to attend to the child's medical problems.

COMPLICATIONS

The case fatality rate following pediatric trauma is approximately 2.5% overall, but the morbidity associated with pediatric trauma is much greater and increases with increasing severity of injury. Mild-to-moderate functional limitations were present at discharge in one-fourth of injured children without traumatic neurologic injury (3). The incidence is much higher in children with traumatic neurologic injury, and severe functional limitations, including cognitive impairment, behavioral disturbances, and a decline in academic performance, are all generally associated with these injuries. Severe functional limitations are present in most children following major trauma and may persist for months or longer. The direct cost of pediatric trauma care in the US is enormous, but the burden, including direct and indirect costs, related to pediatric trauma morbidity is unknown, although likely just as significant. Rehabilitation and physical therapy appear to be underutilized in some injured children, and more appropriate use of these services could help reduce this burden. Referrals for these services should be made early in the hospital course. Of note, socially disadvantaged families may experience barriers to long-term follow-up services for their injured children (32). Vigilance to ensure appropriate follow-up in all injured children should be the goal.

Primary and secondary injury, including complications, contribute to morbidity and mortality; of note, injury-related complications appear to be more frequent than treatment-related complications. Functional limitations, troublesome episodes of anxiety and stress, and infection (often treatment related) are all common complications of pediatric trauma. Thromboembolic events and ventilator-associated pneumonia appear to occur less frequently than in injured adults.

Acute Stress and Posttraumatic Stress Disorder

The anxiety and stress associated with pediatric traumatic injury impact the patient, the family, and, often, the community. It would not be surprising if these symptoms persisted for some time, although the time course and incidence is not yet well described. Symptoms of stress immediately following childhood injuries associated with automobiles were reported in 88% and 83% of pediatric patients and their parents, respectively (58). In addition, 40% of these families (patients and/or parents) experienced "broad distress" or significant symptoms across multiple symptom categories. These families benefit from referral to behavioral health specialists with expertise in treating families after traumatic events.

When symptoms are present more than a month following a traumatic event, posttraumatic stress disorder (PTSD) may be diagnosed; this diagnosis is suggested by avoidance of reminders of the event, persistent hyperarousal symptoms, and unwanted recollections of the event. The occurrence of PTSD in children appears to be high, irrespective of the severity of injury. Between one-fourth and one-third of all children are affected up to 18 months following injury (16,34,47). Not surprisingly, it is also high in the parents and family members of victims. Although research on treatment methods is scanty currently, referral for psychologic care should be considered for all patients and families with suggestive symptoms. Therapeutic options include pharmacotherapy, behavioral therapy, and various educational initiatives, among others.

Infection

Because fever, leukocytosis, and other signs of inflammation are commonly observed in injured children during the acute-phase response, they are neither sensitive nor specific to infection. Resorption of large hematomas, atelectasis, long-bone fractures, and retained necrotic tissue all may contribute to or suggest an inflammatory response. Continued vigilance is necessary to ensure that occult infection does not complicate the care of injured children.

Approximately 10% of severely injured children develop infection, and the majority of these are nosocomial (42), including catheter-related sepsis, urinary tract infection in patients with indwelling urinary catheters, and ventilator-associated pneumonia. Trauma-related infections are much less common and typically involve the wound, abdomen, or CNS. Broad-spectrum IV antibiotics are often prescribed following significant penetrating trauma and/or open fractures, but not following blunt trauma. Routine antibiotic therapy following trauma, including burn injury, is not indicated, because it may lead to the selection of resistant organisms and does not seem to prevent infection.

Injured children who develop an infection have a longer hospital stay, but mortality is generally unaffected (42), in part because significant clinical deterioration during hospitalization usually mandates empiric, broad-spectrum antibiotic therapy. Antibiotic therapy is also begun for severely injured children with wound infection, cellulitis, or thoracostomy tube. A urinary tract infection in a child with an indwelling catheter usually mandates catheter removal or at least catheter exchange, whereas venous catheter–related sepsis mandates a new venous catheter and empiric antibiotic therapy.

Thromboembolic Events

The incidence of thromboembolic events appears to be very low in injured children compared with adults, although epidemiologic data is lacking. Significant deep venous thromboses and/or pulmonary emboli have been noted in less than 0.1% of children who are hospitalized for traumatic injury (6,52). As a result, routine prophylaxis is not indicated for infants and children who are hospitalized with traumatic injury. While it is possible that adolescents have a gradually increasing risk of thrombotic events after acute traumatic injury, to date, little evidence supports this. Compression stockings and pneumatic sequential decompression devices are appropriate in older adolescents who are likely to require prolonged bed rest or in the presence of other risk factors in those able to tolerate these devices. Assuming that hemorrhage has been controlled, further therapy to prevent thrombotic complications should be considered for those adolescents with a history of venous stasis and/or injury or prothrombotic conditions. Individualized therapy that involves the trauma surgeon and a pediatric hematologist is most helpful in this setting, at least until the promulgation of well-supported clinical guidelines.

In the presence of deep venous thrombosis and/or pulmonary embolism in injured children, the decision to employ therapeutic anticoagulation must be carefully evaluated by the entire trauma team. Both therapeutic anticoagulation and vena cava filters have been used successfully in injured pediatric patients (27), although the evidence is limited. Even less evidence supports the role for thrombolysis, surgical thrombectomy, or other vascular procedures (i.e., stenting) in injured children with thrombotic complications that involve large veins. The management of arterial injuries, including surgical (for threatened limbs) and conservative approaches ("watch and wait" with anticoagulation for nonthreatened but mildly ischemic limbs), has been successful in children.

CONCLUSIONS AND FUTURE DIRECTIONS

Among the areas of basic science research, the effect of genotype—in particular the contribution of factors such as NFκB—is a target of vigorous current research. Improvements in clinical care, including analgesia, particularly of younger patients, optimal control of glucose in critically injured children, the early institution of rehabilitative services, and improvement in our ability to address the emotional needs of injured children and their parents also deserve further investigation. Continued improvements in monitoring equipment, including the development of bioimpedance technology and pulse wave form analysis, may offer early evidence of clinically significant physiologic derangements without the problems associated with invasive devices. Epidemiologic investigations in risk and the prevention of injury are likely to identify important targets for intervention. However, it is worth reemphasizing that further declines in morbidity and mortality associated with pediatric trauma are most likely to come from a concerted social, cultural, and economic approach involving prevention and including education, legislation, and the expansion of pediatric emergency medical services at every level. Pediatric critical care practitioners should play an important role in this effort.

KEY POINTS

■ Trauma is the leading cause of pediatric deaths in developed countries; most children suffer significant morbidity following major trauma. Further reductions in morbidity and mortality related to pediatric trauma are possible but will require a multidisciplinary approach.

■ Blunt trauma is more frequent than penetrating trauma, although the latter is more deadly. The mechanism of injury often predicts the pattern of injuries and suggests a management strategy.

■ The ABCDs (airway, breathing, circulation, and disability) are the focus of the primary survey and mandate appropriate interventions and continued reassessment during the "golden hour" (or "platinum half-hour") following injury. Respiratory failure is a frequent complication of major pediatric trauma, whereas hypotension is less common and a late finding.

■ The goal of the secondary survey is to definitively evaluate the injured child, and it should proceed concurrently with

ongoing resuscitation efforts by a multidisciplinary team. Laboratory examinations are an important component.

■ Common visceral injuries in children include contusions, hematomas, and lacerations of the lungs, liver, spleen, or kidneys, as well as pneumothorax, hemothorax, rib fractures, and gastrointestinal tract injury. Important aspects of these injuries in children include the role of nonoperative management and the provision of meticulous intensive care.

■ Common complications of major pediatric trauma include functional limitations, troublesome anxiety and stress, and infection (often related to treatment). The optimal recognition and management of each of these problems remains to be determined.

References

1. Accidental Death and Disability: The Neglected Disease of Modern Society. In: Committee on Trauma and Committee on Shock DoMS, National Research Council, National Academy of Sciences, ed. Washington: National Academy of Sciences, 1966.
2. *Advanced Trauma Life Support, 7th edition.* Chicago: American College of Surgeons, 2004.
3. Aitken ME, Jaffe KM, DiScala C, et al. Functional outcome in children with multiple trauma without significant head injury. *Arch Phys Med Rehabil* 1999;80:889–95.
4. Alderson P, Bunn F, Lefebvre C, et al. Human albumin solution for resuscitation and volume expansion in critically ill patients. *Cochrane Database Syst Rev* 2004:CD001208.
5. Allen GS, Cox CS, Jr. Pulmonary contusion in children: Diagnosis and management. *South Med J* 1998;91:1099–106.
6. Azu MC, McCormack JE, Scriven RJ, et al. Venous thromboembolic events in pediatric trauma patients: Is prophylaxis necessary? *J Trauma* 2005;59:1345–9.
7. Barlow B, Niemirska M, Gandhi RP, et al. Ten years of experience with falls from a height in children. *J Pediatr Surg* 1983;18:509–11.
8. Beck R, Halberthal M, Zonis Z, et al. Abdominal compartment syndrome in children. *Pediatr Crit Care Med* 2001;2:51–6.
9. Bliss D, Silen M. Pediatric thoracic trauma. *Crit Care Med* 2002;30: S409–15.
10. Boffard KD, Riou B, Warren B, et al. Recombinant factor VIIa as adjunctive therapy for bleeding control in severely injured trauma patients: Two parallel randomized, placebo-controlled, double-blind clinical trials. *J Trauma* 2005;59:8–15; discussion, 8.
11. Bone RC. Toward a theory regarding the pathogenesis of the systemic inflammatory response syndrome: What we do and do not know about cytokine regulation. *Crit Care Med* 1996;24:163–72.
12. Caffey J. The whiplash shaken infant syndrome: Manual shaking by the extremities with whiplash-induced intracranial and intraocular bleedings, linked with residual permanent brain damage and mental retardation. *Pediatrics* 1974;54:396–403.
13. Cooper A. Early Assessment and Management of Trauma. In: Ashcroft KW, Holcomb GW, Murphy JP, eds. *Pediatric Surgery.* Philadelphia: Elsevier, 2005:168–84.
14. Cooper A, Barlow B, DiScala C, et al. Mortality and truncal injury: The pediatric perspective. *J Pediatr Surg* 1994;29:33–8.
15. Davidson LL, Durkin MS, Kuhn L, et al. The impact of the Safe Kids/Healthy Neighborhoods Injury Prevention Program in Harlem, 1988 through 1991. *Am J Public Health* 1994;84:580–6.
16. de Vries AP, Kassam-Adams N, Cnaan A, et al. Looking beyond the physical injury: posttraumatic stress disorder in children and parents after pediatric traffic injury. *Pediatrics* 1999;104:1293–9.
17. Deb S, Sun L, Martin B, et al. Lactated Ringer's solution and hetastarch but not plasma resuscitation after rat hemorrhagic shock is associated with immediate lung apoptosis by the up-regulation of the Bax protein. *J Trauma* 2000;49:47–53; discussion, 5.
18. Deitch EA, Shi HP, Feketeova E, et al. Hypertonic saline resuscitation limits neutrophil activation after trauma-hemorrhagic shock. *Shock* 2003;19:328–33.
19. Dilley A, Wesson DE. Pediatric Organ Failure. In: Wesson DE, ed. *Pediatric Trauma.* New York: Taylor & Francis Group, 2006;197–209.
20. DiScala C. *National Pediatric Trauma Registry Annual Report.* Boston: Tufts University Rehabilitation and Childhood Trauma Research and Training Center, 2002.
21. DiScala C, Sege R, Li G, et al. Child abuse and unintentional injuries: A 10-year retrospective. *Arch Pediatr Adolesc Med* 2000;154:16–22.

22. Farrell LS, Hannan EL, Cooper A. Severity of injury and mortality associated with pediatric blunt injuries: Hospitals with pediatric intensive care units versus other hospitals. *Pediatr Crit Care Med* 2004;5:5–9.

23. Fortenberry JD, Meier AH, Pettignano R, et al. Extracorporeal life support for posttraumatic acute respiratory distress syndrome at a children's medical center. *J Pediatr Surg* 2003;38:1221–6.

24. Friese RS, Shafi S, Gentilello LM. Pulmonary artery catheter use is associated with reduced mortality in severely injured patients: A National Trauma Data Bank analysis of 53,312 patients. *Crit Care Med* 2006;34:1597–601.

25. Gionis D, Ilias I, Moustaki M, et al. Hypothalamic-pituitary-adrenal axis and interleukin-6 activity in children with head trauma and syndrome of inappropriate secretion of antidiuretic hormone. *J Pediatr Endocrinol Metab* 2003;16:49–54.

26. Gore DC, Chinkes D, Heggers J, et al. Association of hyperglycemia with increased mortality after severe burn injury. *J Trauma* 2001;51:540–4.

27. Grandas OH, Klar M, Goldman MH, et al. Deep venous thrombosis in the pediatric trauma population: An unusual event: Report of three cases. *Am Surg* 2000;66:273–6.

28. Guyer B, MacDorman MF, Martin JA, et al. Annual summary of vital statistics-1997. *Pediatrics* 1998;102:1333–49.

29. Hoch RC, Rodriguez R, Manning T, et al. Effects of accidental trauma on cytokine and endotoxin production. *Crit Care Med* 1993;21:839–45.

30. Jeschke MG, Einspanier R, Klein D, et al. Insulin attenuates the systemic inflammatory response to thermal trauma. *Mol Med* 2002;8:443–50.

31. Jeschke MG, Klein D, Herndon DN. Insulin treatment improves the systemic inflammatory reaction to severe trauma. *Ann Surg* 2004;239:553–60.

32. Keenan HT, Runyan DK, Nocera M. Child outcomes and family characteristics 1 year after severe inflicted or noninflicted traumatic brain injury. *Pediatrics* 2006;117:317–24.

33. Laird AM, Miller PR, Kilgo PD, et al. Relationship of early hyperglycemia to mortality in trauma patients. *J Trauma* 2004;56:1058–62.

34. Landolt MA, Vollrath M, Ribi K, et al. Incidence and associations of parental and child posttraumatic stress symptoms in pediatric patients. *J Child Psychol Psychiatry* 2003;44:1199–207.

35. Meier R, Krettek C, Grimme K, et al. The multiply injured child. *Clin Orthop Relat Res* 2005;432:127–31.

36. Moore EE, Cogbill TH, Jurkovich GJ, et al. Organ injury scaling: spleen and liver (1994 revision). *J Trauma* 1995;38:323–4.

37. Moore EE, Shackford SR, Pachter HL, et al. Organ injury scaling: Spleen, liver, and kidney. *J Trauma* 1989;29:1664–6.

38. Moshage H. Cytokines and the hepatic acute phase response. *J Pathol* 1997;181:257–66.

39. Murata A, Ogawa M, Yasuda T, et al. Serum interleukin 6, C-reactive protein and pancreatic secretory trypsin inhibitor (PSTI) as acute phase reactants after major thoraco-abdominal surgery. *Immunol Invest* 1990;19:271–8.

40. Nakamori Y, Ogura H, Koh T, et al. The balance between expression of intranuclear NF-kappaB and glucocorticoid receptor in polymorphonuclear leukocytes in SIRS patients. *J Trauma* 2005;59:308–14; discussion 14–5.

41. Partrick DA, Moore FA, Moore EE, et al. Jack A. Barney Resident Research Award winner. The inflammatory profile of interleukin-6, interleukin-8, and soluble intercellular adhesion molecule-1 in postinjury multiple organ failure. *Am J Surg* 1996;172:425–9; discussed 9–31.

42. Patel JC, Mollitt DL, Tepas JJ, 3rd. Infectious complications in critically injured children. *J Pediatr Surg* 2000;35:1174–8.

43. Potoka DA, Schall LC, Gardner MJ, et al. Impact of pediatric trauma centers on mortality in a statewide system. *J Trauma* 2000;49:237–45.

44. Roberts I, Alderson P, Bunn F, et al. Colloids versus crystalloids for fluid resuscitation in critically ill patients. *Cochrane Database Syst Rev* 2004: CD000567.

45. Roumen RM, Hendriks T, van der Ven-Jongekrijg J, et al. Cytokine patterns in patients after major vascular surgery, hemorrhagic shock, and severe blunt trauma. Relation with subsequent adult respiratory distress syndrome and multiple organ failure. *Ann Surg* 1993;218:769–76.

46. Rowe GG, McKenna DH, Corliss RJ, et al. Hemodynamic effects of hypertonic sodium chloride. *J Appl Physiol* 1972;32:182–4.

47. Schreier H, Ladakakos C, Morabito D, et al. Posttraumatic stress symptoms in children after mild to moderate pediatric trauma: A longitudinal examination of symptom prevalence, correlates, and parent-child symptom reporting. *J Trauma* 2005;58:353–63.

48. Shi HP, Deitch EA, Da Xu Z, et al. Hypertonic saline improves intestinal mucosa barrier function and lung injury after trauma-hemorrhagic shock. *Shock* 2002;17:496–501.

49. Shilyansky J, Sena LM, Kreller M, et al. Nonoperative management of pancreatic injuries in children. *J Pediatr Surg* 1998;33:343–9.

50. Stylianos S. Evidence-based guidelines for resource utilization in children with isolated spleen or liver injury. The APSA Trauma Committee. *J Pediatr Surg* 2000;35:164–7; discussion 7–9.

51. Svoboda P, Kantorova I, Ochmann J. Dynamics of interleukin 1, 2, and 6 and tumor necrosis factor alpha in multiple trauma patients. *J Trauma* 1994;36:336–40.

52. Truitt AK, Sorrells DL, Halvorson E, et al. Pulmonary embolism: Which pediatric trauma patients are at risk? *J Pediatr Surg* 2005;40:124–7; discussion 7.

53. UNICEF. A league table of child deaths by injury in rich nations. Innocenti Report Card No 2 2001. http://www.unicef-icdc.org/publications/pdf/repcard2e.pdf. Accessed on Nov 15, 2006.

54. Valerio G, Franzese A, Carlin E, et al. High prevalence of stress hyperglycaemia in children with febrile seizures and traumatic injuries. *Acta Paediatr* 2001;90:618–22.

55. van den Berghe G, Wouters P, Weekers F, et al. Intensive insulin therapy in the critically ill patients. *N Engl J Med* 2001;345:1359–67.

56. Weil MH, Henning RJ. New concepts in the diagnosis and fluid treatment of circulatory shock. Thirteenth annual Becton, Dickinson and Company Oscar Schwidetsky Memorial Lecture. *Anesth Analg* 1979;58:124–32.

57. Wildenthal K, Mierzwiak DS, Mitchell JH. Acute effects of increased serum osmolality on left ventricular performance. *Am J Physiol* 1969;216:898–904.

58. Winston FK, Kassam-Adams N, Vivarelli-O'Neill C, et al. Acute stress disorder symptoms in children and their parents after pediatric traffic injury. *Pediatrics* 2002;109:E90.

59. Yagmur Y, Ozturk H, Unaldi M, et al. Relation between severity of injury and the early activation of interleukins in multiple-injured patients. *Eur Surg Res* 2005;37:360–4.

60. Yendamuri S, Fulda GJ, Tinkoff GH. Admission hyperglycemia as a prognostic indicator in trauma. *J Trauma* 2003;55:33–8.

61. Zhang H, Voglis S, Kim CH, et al. Effects of albumin and Ringer's lactate on production of lung cytokines and hydrogen peroxide after resuscitated hemorrhage and endotoxemia in rats. *Crit Care Med* 2003;31:1515–22.

CHAPTER 28 ■ DROWNING AND NEAR DROWNING: SUBMERSION INJURIES

KATHERINE BIAGAS

Submersion injuries are the second leading cause of accidental death in children. A drowning event is a fatal submersion injury; a near-drowning event is one in which the victim survives, albeit possibly with important disabilities. In the US, submersion events account for approximately 1000 deaths and more than 3000 emergency department visits annually for children <19 years of age (1,35). Despite advances in medical care and efforts to prevent such events, outcomes from all but brief submersion events remain, in many cases, quite poor.

EPIDEMIOLOGY

Most submersions occur in fresh water, with a large proportion of these occurring in natural bodies of water—rivers, creeks, lakes, and ponds. Submersions also occur frequently in domestic sites—home pools, spas, or bathtubs—and recreational community pools, water parks, schools, etc. (19). An investigation of specific drowning sites in the US demonstrated that, for the country as a whole, as few as 4% of events occur in salt water, although this incidence is higher in coastal communities (8).

Three groups of children are at particular risk for submersion injuries: the very young, adolescent males, and nonwhites. Submersion events that involve infants and toddlers commonly occur in sources of water in the home (8). Infants who are 6–11 months of age largely drown in bathtubs, and the use of infant bathtub seats does not prevent such events (9). Older infants and toddlers may drown as the result of a fall into a shallow body of water such as a wading pool, spa, or bathtub (3,8,38). Moreover, infants and toddlers are the group least likely to have a witnessed drowning event (38), a condition associated with longer submersion time and poorer outcomes. In this age group, males and females drown with equal frequency; in all other age groups, submersion event rates are higher in males than in females (8,38).

Boys who are 15–19 years of age have the second highest drowning rate. Events in this age group are generally related to recreational water activities. This population has the highest rate of drowning while swimming, boating, or driving a car, even when compared with adults who, over a lifetime, engage in such activities to a greater extent (38). African American boys have a higher drowning incidence with such events usually recreation related. A fourfold increased incidence in 5–9-year-old and a >10-fold increased incidence in 15–19-year-old African American males have been demonstrated, as compared with their Caucasian counterparts (8). Moreover, fatal submersion injuries are higher in African Americans and Hispanics than the general pediatric population (25).

Certain medical conditions may predispose children to submersion (Table 28.1). Drowning risk is elevated in children with epilepsy, with the highest number of events occurring in bathtubs and pools (15). Epilepsy, excluding other neurologic disabilities, results in a 10-fold increased risk of submersion events (15). In one report, 7% of pediatric drowning victims had a prior history of seizure (38). Hyperventilation with swimming exertion may even predispose a child with epilepsy to have a seizure, thus precipitating the drowning event.

Patients with long QT syndrome (LQTS) or other cardiac "channelopathies" are at increased risk for drowning events (2,7,11). Ventricular tachyarrhythmias in such patients may be exacerbated by swimming. In one report, 91% of patients who presented for evaluation of possible LQTS and had personal or family history of swimming-related syncope had mutations in the LQTS1 gene (11). Swimming is an arrhythmogenic trigger because the action activates the "diving reflex," which alters autonomic stability. This diving reflex is elicited in mammals by contact of the face with cold water and consists of breath-holding, bradycardia, and intense peripheral vasoconstriction. Swimming also involves physical exertion, which may be a syncopal trigger in some (11). Screening of relatives is recommended for anyone suspected of having a swimming-related arrhythmia syndrome. Counseling regarding safe water-related activities and β-blockade therapy are recommended for affected individuals.

The use of alcohol or other intoxicating substances is associated with submersions in older adolescents. Alcohol usage is found in 20% of all submersion injuries in adolescents 15 years and older (38) and in 25%–50% of recreational water deaths in adolescents and adults (31,35). Moreover, the intoxicated victim may vomit, with aspiration of gastric contents. Other medical conditions that less frequently predispose to drowning include depression, coronary artery disease, cardiomyopathy, hypoglycemia, and hypothermia.

Submersion injuries in older children and adolescents may be associated with cervical spine injury. The incidence of such injury is low, estimated at 0.5%–5.0% of submersions (24,46). The mechanism of injury is diving or falling into a body of water with a blow that hyperextends the cervical spine. A history of diving is usually elicited (46). When evaluating victims of unwitnessed events, the possibility of associated cervical spine injury should be considered. Immobilization of the cervical spine at the scene is imperative. As with other injuries of the spine, the diagnosis of injury is a clinical one and is based on suspicion about the mechanism of injury and the patient's neurologic condition. Radiographs of the cervical spine may be normal despite debilitating cord injury (41), and MR imaging may be necessary to confirm the clinical suspicion.

TABLE 28.1

MEDICAL CONDITIONS THAT PREDISPOSE CHILDREN TO SUBMERSION EVENTS

Seizure disorder
Long QT syndrome or other "channelopathies"
Use of alcohol or other illicit substances
Other conditions that less frequently predispose to drowning:
   Depression
   Coronary artery disease
   Cardiomyopathy
   Hypoglycemia
   Hypothermia

PATHOPHYSIOLOGY

The initial sequence of events in drowning was studied during the 1930s, using animals, and consists of the following: initial struggle sometimes with a surprise inhalation, suspension of movement and exhalation of a little air, frequently followed by swallowing, violent struggle, convulsions with spasmodic respiratory efforts through an open mouth, loss of reflexes, and death. This sequence has been confirmed in many cases by bystanders who witness the struggle and subsequent motionlessness. During the initial seconds of submersion, small amounts of fluid are aspirated, often causing laryngospasm. Victims who are resuscitated at this phase will have little water aspiration, but ventilation by rescue breathing may be difficult because of glottic closure. If the victim loses muscle tone, larger quantities of fluid may be aspirated. In addition, a victim may swallow a large amount of fluid and may vomit, aspirating gastric contents.

The development of hypothermia is extremely common with submersion. The presence of hypothermia, in most cases, should not be interpreted as a "cold-water drowning," a particular situation that will be discussed later. Rather, hypothermia is usually secondary to rapid radiant heat losses in tepid water. As core temperature drops below the mid-30s°C, the victim may develop muscular weakness, and aspiration is facilitated. At lower core temperatures, unconsciousness ensues. Atrial fibrillation occurs with core temperatures in the low 30s°C and ventricular fibrillation or asystole with severe hypothermia (core temperature <28°C) (25,35). Coagulopathy, platelet dysfunction, and immunologic dysfunction also may occur with severe hypothermia.

Fluid and Electrolyte Disturbances

Much has been made of possible fluid shifts and electrolyte disturbances occurring during submersions. Postmortem examination has demonstrated mild-to-moderate hyponatremia of victims who drowned in fresh water and moderate hypernatremia and hyperchloremia in those who drown in salt water. However, clinically important abnormalities in serum electrolyte concentrations usually are not found in patients who survive the event. Exceptions to this generality are found in near-drownings that occur in high-salinity water such as found in the Dead Sea. In addition, hypermagnesemia has been described in seawater drowning, probably a result of both aspiration and ingestion (13). Similarly, important disorders of vascular volume are not often found after drowning. Fresh-water-associated hemodilution and hypervolemia are generally mild. Hypovolemia after saltwater drowning may be seen in severe cases, usually in victims who do not survive.

Respiratory and Cardiovascular Dysfunction

Submersion victims experience some period of hypoxia. For those with brief episodes, hypoxemia is limited to the duration of hypopnea or apnea and may resolve with rescue or initial resuscitation efforts. However, many patients, even those with relatively short-duration hypoxia, may develop increased permeability of pulmonary capillaries, with alveolar fluid leak and dysfunction of surfactant. In patients with longer hypoxic episodes or alveolar aspiration, these processes are more aggressive, with resultant lung collapse, alveolar derecruitment, intrapulmonary shunting, raised pulmonary vascular resistance, and ventilation-perfusion mismatching. Additional cardiac dysfunction may lead to left atrial hypertension and pulmonary-capillary engorgement, furthering pulmonary capillary leak. Large and small airway dysfunction may occur, exacerbating gas exchange problems by trapping gas (29). In combination, these processes create the clinical syndromes of acute lung injury and, later, acute respiratory distress syndrome (ARDS) (26). Aspiration of gastric contents may add caustic injury to airways and alveoli, worsening gas trapping and hypoxemia. Neurogenic pulmonary edema may contribute to deficits in gas exchange and lung function.

The hallmark of cardiovascular dysfunction with submersion injury is shock (33). Systemic and pulmonary vascular resistances are raised with hypothermia and sympathetic activity associated with the diving reflex. With these processes, ventricular end-diastolic pressures are raised, as are atrial pressures, with resultant congestion of central and pulmonary veins. Myocardial contractility is diminished with hypoxemia. Poor myocardial contractility, in combination with raised systemic vascular resistance, results in lower cardiac output. The clinical examination is one of "cold" shock, with poor perfusion and end-organ dysfunction. The degree to which such derangements are reversible with resuscitation efforts is related to the duration of hypoxemia and low-flow states. Important end-organ (kidneys, liver, etc.) dysfunctions may be demonstrable during the patient's hospitalization but usually fully recover with supportive care.

Hypoxic-Ischemic Brain Injury

The most important sequela of submersion injuries is global hypoxic-ischemic brain injury. The combination of hypoxemia and low-flow states results in a host of pathologic processes, including energy failure, lipid peroxidation, production of free radicals, inflammatory responses, and release of excitotoxic neurotransmitters. Disruption of neuronal and glial functions and architecture occurs. Neuronal losses occur with activation of immediate early genes (40) and initial neuronal death, followed days later by so-called "delayed neuronal drop out." The vascular end zones are particularly vulnerable, and "watershed" infarctions may be appreciated on CT scans. With a more extensive hypoxic-ischemic insult, a CT scan of the brain may show a "reversal sign" or global "ground glass" appearance, with attenuation of signal in the supratentorial intracranial contents or entire brain, respectively.

Submersion in Ice-Cold Water

While the functional outcome after submersion injury is usually related to the duration and depth of the hypoxic-ischemic insult, brain function may be preserved in cold-water drowning, with good and even normal neurologic outcomes observed despite extensive submersions. Numerous reports have documented dramatic cases of intact neurologic functioning in children who drowned in icy water (6,14,23,44). The term "cold-water drowning" is a misnomer, in that the submersion must occur in ice-cold water and, with very rare exceptions (34), is a phenomenon restricted to northern climates (5). Patients who have drowned in more temperate water but who have become hypothermic should be considered to have hypothermia from prolonged submersion. Such secondary hypothermia is often a poor prognostic sign.

Young children are particularly susceptible to rapid cooling of the brain in icy water because of little subcutaneous fat insulation and a large head-to-body ratio. Moreover, activation of the diving reflex slows metabolism and preserves some perfusion to the heart and brain. Additionally, neurologic preservation can be seen when the lower body is submersed in ice water and the head remains above water, allowing the victim to continue to breathe. The result is rapid brain cooling in the face of residual perfusion and provision of brain substrates.

MANAGEMENT

Management at the scene should focus on rapid restoration of oxygenation and spontaneous circulation with basic cardiopulmonary resuscitation. Emergency medicine services should be summoned as quickly as possible. No attempts should be made to drain water from the lungs before initiation of rescue breathing. Bystanders should perform mouth-to-mouth breathing even before the victim is removed from the water. Trained rescuers, equipped with a buoyant rescue aid, should attempt in-water rescue breathing of the victim found in deep water (37). Once on solid ground, chest compressions should be performed unless the presence of a pulse is established. As previously discussed, cervical spine immobilization should be performed in cases with a history of diving, or when the cause of drowning is not known. Spinal immobilization is otherwise unnecessary and should not interfere with resuscitative efforts. Advanced life support should be initiated by paramedics for victims who do not regain spontaneous breathing and consciousness with rescue breaths. Bag-valve-mask ventilation with supplemental oxygen is sufficient to restore circulation in some victims. Endotracheal intubation with manual ventilation, administration of fluid boluses, defibrillation, and administration of bolus vasoactive medications (32) may be required in others; however, these efforts should not be pursued to the extent that transportation of the victim to a hospital is delayed.

Management in the Emergency Department

Definitive management of submersion injuries begins in the emergency department. Advanced life support should focus on establishment of adequate oxygenation and ventilation, adequate circulation, and determination of neurologic functioning (Table 28.2). Initial neurologic status is approximated using the Glasgow Coma Scale, a 3–15-point combination score reflecting best verbal, motor, and eye-opening functions in response to graded stimuli. A more thorough neurologic examination is performed later. Repeated Glasgow Coma Scale determinations during the first 12 hrs of treatment and repeated neurologic examinations throughout hospitalization are necessary to document improvement in function. More importantly, frequently repeated examinations may detect deterioration in neurologic condition (e.g., deterioration in neurologic function with the onset of subclinical seizures), which must be evaluated for possible treatable causes.

In the emergency department, definitive warming should be initiated for all but mild hypothermia (35–36°C) and performed in concert with resuscitation efforts. The simplest warming techniques include the use of warmed IV fluids, external radiant heat, ventilation with heated gas, and immersion in a warm bath. More aggressive efforts are necessary for moderate hypothermia: warmed peritoneal lavage or dialysis fluids and/or bladder washes with warm fluids. For severe hypothermia, passive rewarming can induce "rewarming shock," with peripheral vasodilatation and impaired cardiac output. The use of cardiopulmonary bypass has been advocated for core rewarming in severe hypothermia (44,49). Failure to restore circulation after 30 mins of rewarming to ≥32°C suggests that further resuscitation efforts will not be successful. However, rewarming efforts should not be overly aggressive. Studies of hypothermic treatment in adults with cardiac arrest demonstrate that brain cooling is neuroprotective and that better-than-expected neurologic outcomes are possible (4,21,50). Given this encouraging data, consideration should be given to maintaining mild hypothermia (core temperature of 32–35°C) in children who remain comatose after submersion (47). Certainly, overwarming should be avoided.

Management in the PICU

Children who do not regain full consciousness in the emergency department should be transferred to a pediatric intensive care facility. There, ongoing efforts should be to aggressively treat any cardiorespiratory dysfunction. An "open lung" strategy should be employed for patients with acute lung injury or ARDS. Usual ventilator settings include limiting ventilator peak pressures to 25 torr, tidal volumes to 6–8 mL/kg, and fraction of inspired oxygen to <0.60. Liberal use of positive end-expiratory pressure may improve oxygenation dramatically. Permissive hypercapnia, a commonly used lung-protective strategy, is contraindicated if intracranial hypertension is suspected. Administration of exogenous surfactant was used successfully to treat severe ARDS following submersion injury when surfactant wash out/dysfunction was suspected (36). Extracorporeal membrane oxygenation was used successfully in similar circumstances (17). Continuous vasoactive

TABLE 28.2

IMPORTANT PRINCIPLES FOR THE MANAGEMENT OF CHILDREN WITH SUBMERSION INJURY

IN THE EMERGENCY DEPARTMENT	
Establish adequate oxygenation and ventilation	Intubate airway of unconscious or hypoventilating children
	Provide supplemental oxygen
Establish normal circulation	Bolus IV fluids (NS) for hypotension
	Initiate use of vasopressor infusions (epinephrine, consider addition of vasopressin) for continued hypotension
Neurologic examination	Determine Glasgow Coma Scale score
	Control seizures with bolus administration of anticonvulsants (lorazepam, phenobarbital, or fosphenytoin)
Rewarming of hypothermia, unless mild (35–36°C)	Use warmed fluids and ventilation with heated gas
	Consider bladder washes with warmed fluids
	Consider cardiopulmonary bypass
Transfer patient for definitive care	Transfer to inpatient unit for observation if full neurologic and cardiovascular function are rapidly restored
	Transfer to a PICU if full function not restored
IN THE PICU	
Employ ventilator strategies for ALI/ARDS	Limit ventilator peak pressures to <25 torr
	Limit tidal volumes to 6–8 mL/kg
	Limit fraction of inspired oxygen to <0.60
	Liberal use of PEEP
	Consider the use of exogenous surfactant or ECMO for continued hypoxemia
Treat myocardial dysfunction	Titrate vasoactive infusions to normal cardiac output and adequate end-organ perfusion
Employ brain-protective strategies	Avoid hyperthermia
	Treat clinical and subclinical seizures
	Use mild systemic cooling (35–36°C) for 24–48 hrs
	Frequent neurologic reassessments and adjunct studies of function as indicated
Refer to a rehabilitation facility for persistent neurologic injury upon recovery	

NS, normal saline; ALI, acute lung injury; ARDS, acute respiratory distress syndrome; PEEP, positive end-expiratory pressure; ECMO, extracorporeal membrane oxygenation

infusions may be required to treat myocardial dysfunction and correct abnormal peripheral vascular resistance. Treatment should concentrate on normalizing blood pressure, organ perfusion, and gas exchange as quickly as possible, and frequent repeated examinations are necessary to detect deterioration in cardiorespiratory function.

The other focus of ICU care is restoration of cerebral function, although no definitive treatment exists to reverse the neuronal injury processes previously discussed. Instead, care of the brain is supportive. Normal cardiorespiratory function should be maintained. Hypermetabolic states, such as seizures and fevers, should be aggressively treated. Routine electroencephalography (EEG) should be used to detect subclinical seizures and to titrate antiepileptic therapy. In cases of severe global brain injury, consideration should be given to maintaining mild hypothermia for 24–48 hrs, as previously discussed. To maintain a hypothermic state, patients may require the use of neuromuscular blocking agents, which will interfere with performance of the neurologic examination. In addition, intracranial hypertension may be found in cases of severe brain injury. Despite previous enthusiasm for monitor-

ing and treatment of intracranial pressure, no evidence suggests that such management affects ultimate outcome. Rather, raised intracranial pressure is a marker of poor neurologic prognosis.

PREVENTION

The outcome of a drowning event is determined in the first few minutes of submersion. As options are available in terms of primary therapy for these injuries, an emphasis on prevention is necessary. Prevention strategies have focused on calling attention to the common causes of childhood drowning, specifically bathtub drowning and recreation-related incidents (48). Slogans such as, "Don't Turn Your Back On Me" alert parents to the proper supervision of infants and toddlers. Other alerts focus on specific events; e.g., the installation of a home pool. Most pool-related submersions occur within the first 6 months of pool exposure (45). The absence of proper pool fencing may increase the odds of pool-related drowning by as much as three- to five-fold (45). Written alerts about drowning risks are generally distributed to customers upon purchase of a new pool.

Additional prevention campaigns have focused on the family pediatrician. The American Academy of Pediatrics issued a policy statement in 2003 to guide pediatricians in incorporating regular, age-appropriate teaching about water safety in their anticipatory guidance to families. Their recommendations can be found at The Injury Prevention Program website, www.aap.org/family/tippmain.htm. Additional prevention tips are available at the Consumer Product Safety Commission website, http://www.cpsc.gov/. Such strategies have met with some success. Reduction in some types of submersions was noted in the UK perhaps due to initiatives on children's safety in water (42).

OUTCOMES

Outcome from drowning is related to the extent of cerebral injury. However, this outcome is difficult to predict. Poor prognostic signs include an unwitnessed event, prolonged time to resuscitation, the need for cardiopulmonary resuscitation at the scene and in the emergency department (22), and prolonged coma. The best independent predictor of survival is submersion time (39,43); however, in many patients, these data are not known. In Toronto, investigators found the presence of a detectable heartbeat and hypothermia at the initial examination in the emergency department to be discriminate predictors of good outcome versus death or persistent vegetative state (5). However, these findings may not be generalizable; rather, they may reflect the somewhat unique occurrence in Ontario of submersion in frigid water. In the emergency department, a physical examination remarkable for nonreactive pupils or a Glasgow Coma Scale score of ≤5 predict poor neurologic outcome (30); but, these are not absolute predictors.

Specific prognostic scales are similarly less satisfactory in discriminatory function. The Pediatric Risk of Mortality Score (PRISM), a predictor of mortality in critical illness, discriminates between death and the presence or absence of poor outcome, but it is unable to distinguish between different degrees of neurologic dysfunction (20). Other clinical classification systems developed specifically for drowning events have been similarly inadequate (12). A reasonable approach, therefore, is to avoid determining which patients should receive initial treatment based on prognostic factors. Rather, the "treat-them-all approach" applies, with aggressive efforts despite initial lack of heartbeat (30). The adage, "you're not dead until you're warm and dead," applies with vigorous resuscitative efforts, including rewarming, as needed. Prognosis is deferred until circulation is restored and perfusion optimized. At that time, the patient can be more completely examined.

In those who remain with coma or altered mental status upon restoration of normal circulation, prognosis is usually determined using interim assessments. Repeated clinical neurologic examinations are perhaps the most reliable basis for estimate of outcome. Adjunct studies are often necessary. CT is used in the initial assessment of patients, especially in patients with a history of possible associated traumatic injury. Repeated brain CT scans often add little more information. MRI and MR spectroscopy can detect more subtle injury (16,27). Serial MR scans obtained 3 to 4 days after injury in a series of near-drowning victims admitted to a PICU provided excellent predictive values (16); however, ultimate brain dysfunction has been reported despite normal MR scans (23). Electrophysiologic studies may provide additional information. The early use of electroencephalography may be limited by the need for sedatives in the initial recovery phase, but persistent low attenuation of the electroencephalogram is a poor prognostic sign (28). Brainstem auditory-evoked responses have been used to evaluate function in prolonged outcome with some success (18). Use of a series of electrophysiologic modalities, including sleep recordings, brainstem auditory-evoked responses, somatosensory-evoked potentials, and polysomnography to generate a more complete picture of functioning in 5 comatose children after near-drowning events suggested that better prediction could be attained using all of these modalities over the use of EEG alone (10). No single prognostic test or assessment can reliably discriminate good from poor functional outcomes in all victims of submersion injury; moreover, no indicator is sufficiently reliable to be the sole determinant of whether to withdraw or withhold therapy in a victim of submersion injury.

CONCLUSIONS AND FUTURE DIRECTIONS

Submersion injury is one of the leading causes of accident-related mortality and morbidity in childhood. The pathophysiologic processes of such injury are those of hypoxia-ischemia. At present, therapy is focused on restoration of oxygenation and circulation at the scene, with rapid transfer to an emergency department and pediatric intensive care facility when the patient does not experience rapid, full recovery. At present, therapy for brain injury is largely limited to good supportive care and avoidance of secondary insults. The impact of advancements in critical care in the last decade, such as the use of surfactant or inhaled nitric oxide for submersion-related ARDS has not been studied. However, such therapies remain promising and should be considered. Similarly, the use of mild hypothermia early in the PICU course should be considered for submersion victims with neurologic deficits. However, as the central nervous system suffers the most enduring damage in these patients, substantial improvements in outcomes will not be realized until more effective primary therapies for hypoxic-ischemic brain injury are found.

KEY POINTS

- Submersion injury is the leading cause of accident related death and disability.
- Two age groups are primarily affected: infants and toddlers, and adolescents.
- Therapy consists of rapid restoration of respiration and circulation.
- Therapy for brain injury includes supportive care and, possibly, mild hypothermia.
- No specific prognostic tests or examinations exist.
- Prevention of submersion injuries is an important public health goal.

References

1. Water-related injuries: Fact Sheet, in *National Center for Injury Prevention and Control*. Atlanta, Center for Disease Control and Prevention, 2004.

2. Ackerman MJ, Tester DJ, Porter CJ, et al. Molecular diagnosis of the inherited long-QT syndrome in a woman who died after near-drowning. *N Engl J Med* 1999;341:1121–5.

3. Agran PF, Anderson C, Winn D, et al. Rates of pediatric injuries by 3-month intervals for children 0 to 3 years of age. *Pediatrics* 2003;111:e683–92.

4. Bernard SA, Gray TW, Buist MD, et al. Treatment of comatose survivors of out-of-hospital cardiac arrest with induced hypothermia. *N Engl J Med* 2002;346:557–63.

5. Biggart MJ, Bohn DJ. Effect of hypothermia and cardiac arrest on outcome of near-drowning accidents in children. *J Pediatr* 1990;117:179–83.

6. Bolte RG, Black PG, Bowers RS, et al. The use of extracorporeal rewarming in a child submerged for 66 minutes. *JAMA* 1988;260:377–9.

7. Bradley T, Dixon J, Easthope R. Unexplained fainting, near drowning and unusual seizures in childhood: Screening for long QT syndrome in New Zealand families. *N Z Med J* 1999;112:299–302.

8. Brenner RA, Trumble AC, Smith GS, et al. Where children drown, United States, 1995. *Pediatrics* 2001;108:85–9.

9. Byard RW, Donald T. Infant bath seats, drowning and near-drowning. *J Paediatr Child Health* 2004;40:305–7.

10. Cheliout-Heraut F, Rubinsztajn R, Ioos C, et al. Prognostic value of evoked potentials and sleep recordings in the prolonged comatose state of children. Preliminary data. *Neurophysiol Clin* 2001;31:283–92.

11. Choi G, Kopplin LJ, Tester DJ, et al. Spectrum and frequency of cardiac channel defects in swimming-triggered arrhythmia syndromes. *Circulation* 2004;110:2119–24.

12. Christensen DW, Jansen P, Perkin RM. Outcome and acute care hospital costs after warm water near drowning in children. *Pediatrics* 1997;99:715–21.

13. Cohen DS, Matthay MA, Cogan MG, et al. Pulmonary edema associated with salt water near-drowning: New insights. *Am Rev Respir Dis* 1992;146:794–6.

14. Corneli HM. Accidental hypothermia. *J Pediatr* 1992;120:671–9.

15. Diekema DS, Quan L, Holt VL. Epilepsy as a risk factor for submersion injury in children. *Pediatrics* 1993;91:612–6.

16. Dubowitz DJ, Bluml S, Arcinue E, et al. MR of hypoxic encephalopathy in children after near drowning: Correlation with quantitative proton MR spectroscopy and clinical outcome. *AJNR Am J Neuroradiol* 1998;19:1617–27.

17. Eich C, Brauer A, Kettler D. Recovery of a hypothermic drowned child after resuscitation with cardiopulmonary bypass followed by prolonged extracorporeal membrane oxygenation. *Resuscitation* 2005;67:145–8.

18. Fisher B, Peterson B, Hicks G. Use of brainstem auditory-evoked response testing to assess neurologic outcome following near drowning in children. *Crit Care Med* 1992;20:578–85.

19. Gilchrist J, Gotsch K, Ryan G. Non-fatal and fatal drownings in recreational water settings- United States, 2001–2002. *MMWR Morb Mortal Wkly Rep* 2004;53:447–52.

20. Gonzalez-Luis G, Pons M, Cambra FJ, et al. Use of the Pediatric Risk of Mortality Score as predictor of death and serious neurological damage in children after submersion. *Pediatr Emerg Care* 2001;17:405–9.

21. Holzer M, Bernard SA, Hachimi-Idrissi S, et al. Hypothermia for neuroprotection after cardiac arrest: Systematic review and individual patient data meta-analysis. *Crit Care Med* 2005;33:414–8.

22. Horisberger T, Fischer E, Fanconi S. One-year survival and neurological outcome after pediatric cardiopulmonary resuscitation. *Intensive Care Med* 2002;28:365–8.

23. Hughes SK, Nilsson DE, Boyer RS, et al. Neurodevelopmental outcome for extended cold water drowning: A longitudinal case study. *J Int Neuropsychol Soc* 2002;8:588–95.

24. Hwang V, Shofer FS, Durbin DR, et al. Prevalence of traumatic injuries in drowning and near drowning in children and adolescents. *Arch Pediatr Adolesc Med* 2003;157:50–3.

25. Ibsen LM, Koch T. Submersion and asphyxial injury. *Crit Care Med* 2002;30:S402–8.

26. Kim KI, Lee KN, Tomiyama N, et al. Near drowning: Thin-section CT findings in six patients. *J Comput Assist Tomogr* 2000;24:562–6.

27. Kreis R, Arcinue E, Ernst T, et al. Hypoxic encephalopathy after near-drowning studied by quantitative 1H-magnetic resonance spectroscopy. *J Clin Invest* 1996;97:1142–54.

28. Kruus S, Bergstrom L, Suutarinen T, et al. The prognosis of near-drowned children. *Acta Paediatr Scand* 1979;68:315–22.

29. Laughlin JJ, Eigen H. Pulmonary function abnormalities in survivors of near drowning. *J Pediatr* 1982;100:26–30.

30. Lavelle JM, Shaw KN. Near drowning: Is emergency department cardiopulmonary resuscitation or intensive care unit cerebral resuscitation indicated? *Crit Care Med* 1993;21:368–73.

31. Levy DT, Mallonee S, Miller TR, et al. Alcohol involvement in burn, submersion, spinal cord, and brain injuries. *Med Sci Monit* 2004;10:CR17–24.

32. Lienhart HG, John W, Wenzel V. Cardiopulmonary resuscitation of a near-drowned child with a combination of epinephrine and vasopressin. *Pediatr Crit Care Med* 2005;6:486–8.

33. Lucking SE, Pollack MM, Fields AI. Shock following generalized hypoxic-ischemic injury in previously healthy infants and children. *J Pediatr* 1986;108:359–64.

34. Modell JH, Idris AH, Pineda JA, et al. Survival after prolonged submersion in freshwater in Florida. *Chest* 2004;125:1948–51.

35. Moon RE, Long RJ. Drowning and near-drowning. *Emerg Med (Fremantle)* 2002;14:377–86.

36. Onarheim H, Vik V. Porcine surfactant (Curosurf) for acute respiratory failure after near-drowning in 12-year-old. *Acta Anaesthesiol Scand* 2004;48:778–81.

37. Perkins GD. In-water resuscitation: A pilot evaluation. *Resuscitation* 2005;65:321–4.

38. Quan L, Cummings P. Characteristics of drowning by different age groups. *Inj Prev* 2003;9:163–8.

39. Quan L, Wentz KR, Gore EJ, et al. Outcome and predictors of outcome in pediatric submersion victims receiving prehospital care in King County, Washington. *Pediatrics* 1990;86:586–93.

40. Robinson DA, O'Brien PK, Gheewala RM, et al. Differential expression of neuronal fos protein after cold water drowning and controlled rewarming. *J Am Coll Surg* 2004;198:404–9.

41. Robles LA, Curiel A. Posttraumatic cervical disc herniation: An unusual cause of near drowning. *Am J Emerg Med* 2005;23:905–7.

42. Sibert JR, Lyons RA, Smith BA, et al. Preventing deaths by drowning in children in the United Kingdom: Have we made progress in 10 years? Population-based incidence study. *BMJ* 2002;324:1070–1.

43. Suominen P, Baillie C, Korpela R, et al. Impact of age, submersion time and water temperature on outcome in near-drowning. *Resuscitation* 2002;52:247–54.

44. Thalmann M, Trampitsch E, Haberfellner N, et al. Resuscitation in near drowning with extracorporeal membrane oxygenation. *Ann Thorac Surg* 2001;72:607–8.

45. Thompson DC, Rivara FP. Pool fencing for preventing drowning in children. *Cochrane Database Syst Rev* 2005;CD001047.

46. Watson RS, Cummings P, Quan L, et al. Cervical spine injuries among submersion victims. *J Trauma* 2001;51:658–62.

47. Williamson JP, Illing R, Gertler P, et al. Near-drowning treated with therapeutic hypothermia. *Med J Aust* 2004;181:500–1.

48. Wintemute GJ. Childhood drowning and near-drowning in the United States. *Am J Dis Child* 1990;144:663–9.

49. Wollenek G, Honarwar N, Golej J, et al. Cold water submersion and cardiac arrest in treatment of severe hypothermia with cardiopulmonary bypass. *Resuscitation* 2002;52:255–63.

50. Zeiner A, Holzer M, Sterz F, et al. Mild resuscitative hypothermia to improve neurological outcome after cardiac arrest. *A clinical feasibility trial. Hypothermia After Cardiac Arrest (HACA) Study Group. Stroke* 2000;31:86–94.

CHAPTER 29 ■ BURNS, ELECTRICAL INJURIES, AND SMOKE INHALATION

ROGER W. YURT • JOY D. HOWELL • BRUCE M. GREENWALD

The derangements of physiology that occur after major burn injury in a child are among the most challenging problems in modern medical care. The loss of skin integrity exposes the child to the exterior environment of bacterial, fungal, and viral pathogens. At the same time, the wounds provide a portal for loss of fluid and body heat. Beyond these local changes are the systemic responses that further stress the homeostatic mechanisms that usually maintain a stable internal environment for the patient. This chapter addresses the evaluation and care of the child with a major burn, electrical injury, and/or smoke inhalation injury. However, information will be provided regarding lesser wounds as well, as it is not uncommon for patients to present with multisystem injury in addition to a burn injury.

EVALUATION OF THE PATIENT

The distraction created by the appearance of large areas of blistering, tissue loss, and disfigurement associated with a burn injury can lead to a fixation on that injury and a lack of recognition that burn-injured patients are trauma patients. In that regard, initial evaluation should be the same as for any patient who has sustained injury. Thus, the basic ABCs of ensuring adequacy of an airway, that the patient is ventilating, and that circulation is intact must be addressed. A rapid overall evaluation of the patient is performed as resuscitation is initiated. The specific details of evaluating a child with burn injury will be addressed here. The aspects of evaluation of additional traumatic injury are addressed in Chapter 27.

Extent of Burn Injury

The extent of tissue injury caused by a burn is quantified by the surface area and the depth of injury. Determination of the extent of injury provides a basis for estimation of fluid requirements for resuscitation and for determining an overall care plan. In addition, in that a positive correlation exists between extent of injury and mortality, this determination provides information on prognosis. For estimation of the extent of surface area involved, a Lund & Browder chart or Berkow's formula should be used. The "rule of nines" cannot be used in children <15 years. The distribution of surface area by age is shown in the chart that is in use at the William Randolph Hearst Burn Center (Table 29.1).

Evaluation of depth of injury is readily determined at the extremes of depth, such that partial-thickness injury is easy to differentiate from full-thickness injury. A first-degree burn is characterized as erythematous, painful, and dry, while a third-degree burn, also known as a full-thickness burn, is leathery, dry, and insensate. Burn injuries at an intermediate depth of partial thickness are more difficult to assess. They are divided into superficial and deep partial thickness wounds. Whether superficial or deep, these wounds appear very similar on physical examination. They are erythematous, moist, and sensate. Evaluation of these wounds is complicated by the fact that they evolve over time, are frequently not homogenous with regard to depth, and are dynamic over the first days after injury. Attempts to use advanced instrumentation, such as laser Doppler and infrared sensing devices, have not yet proved to be of value in routine evaluation of this depth of injury. A more recent report suggests that laser Doppler imaging may be of value in estimating depth of injury in children (19). The importance of differentiating these depths of injury relates to the fact that a superficial partial-thickness burn will re-epithelialize in 2 weeks, whereas a deep partial-thickness wound heals by epithelialization and contraction. To avoid scarring, the deeper wound must be treated by skin grafting. Except for small surface area wounds, full-thickness wounds should be either excised and closed primarily or grafted with the patient's skin. A cross-section of skin with indication of the various depths of injury is depicted in **Figure 29.1**.

Types of Injury

The depth of the injury in burns that are caused by scalding, flame, or contact with a hot object is directly related to the temperature, duration of exposure, and thickness of the tissue. Three zones of injury have been identified in burn-injured skin. The outer zone of coagulative necrosis includes necrotic tissue that is irreversibly damaged by heat or chemical. Below that is the zone of stasis in which some viable tissue remains. This dynamic region is subject to further necrosis if it is not protected from further physical damage. Care must be taken to avoid aggressive methods of debridement and harsh cleansing agents. In addition, delivery of nutrient blood flow and oxygen is important in this region, and compromised cardiac output due to inadequate resuscitation can increase the depth of injury. The zone adjacent to the zone of stasis has been termed the zone of hyperemia, given the increased blood flow and local inflammatory response to the injury.

Chemical burns cause denaturation of protein and disruption of cellular integrity. The degree of injury is dependent on the time of exposure, the strength of the agent, and the solubility of the agent in tissue. Alkaline agents tend to penetrate deeper into tissues than do acids, with an exception

TABLE 29.1

DISTRIBUTION OF BODY SURFACE AREA BY AGE AS PERCENTAGE OF TOTAL
BODY SURFACE AREA

Area	Age in years				
	0–1	1–4	5–9	10–14	15
Head	19	17	13	11	9
Neck	2	2	2	2	2
Anterior trunk	13	13	13	13	13
Posterior trunk	13	13	13	13	13
Each buttock	2.5	2.5	2.5	2.5	2.5
Genitalia	1	1	1	1	1
Each upper arm	4	4	4	4	4
Each lower arm	3	3	3	3	3
Each hand	2.5	2.5	2.5	2.5	2.5
Each thigh	5.5	6.5	8	8.5	9
Each leg	5	5	5.5	6	6.5
Each foot	3.5	3.5	3.5	3.5	3.5

being hydrofluoric acid, which penetrates lipid membranes very readily.

The major concern in evaluating patients who sustain electrical injuries is that the surface injury, which may appear similar to other burn injuries, is often not indicative of the extent of injury. In the local area of injury, subcutaneous tissue, muscle, and bone may be injured. Electrical current follows the path of least resistance and will pass through nerve and blood vessels preferentially and cause injury to these tissues. If the current passes through the torso, organ injury may result. Injury of the heart is primarily associated with arrhythmia. Injuries of other viscera, including the pancreas and gastrointestinal tract, have been reported. Practice guidelines for the management of electrical injury suggest that patients who contact a low voltage (<1000 volts) source can be cared for as outpatients if they have no electrocardiographic abnormalities, no history of loss of consciousness, and no other reason for admission (2). Patients who contact high-voltage sources are usually admitted and placed on cardiac monitoring. Creatine kinase levels, including the MB subunit, do not reliably indicate the extent of myocardial injury, and the published guidelines indicate that data are insufficient to determine if troponin levels give an accurate index of the extent of injury. The physician should always have a high index of suspicion that deep injury has oc-

curred and that exploration of extremities will be necessary if compartment pressures rise, perfusion is compromised, or neurologic changes occur. Late sequelae of electrical injury, which may occur months or even years after injury, include the development of cataracts and transverse myelitis of the spinal cord.

Injury caused by exposure to ionizing radiation may be limited to the skin but is often deeper. Because these wounds do not heal well, care must be taken to avoid additional damage of the tissue. The vasculitis that is associated with these injuries is usually a life-long problem.

Neglect and Abuse

As the incidence of child abuse has been reported to be as high as 16% of children admitted to burn centers in the US (17), the index of suspicion should be high when a child is injured by burning. Most of these injuries occur in children between 2 and 4 years of age. The determination of whether abuse or neglect has occurred is based on the characteristics of the wounds and the history provided. A history that is inconsistent with the findings on physical exam is sufficient reason to launch a deeper investigation into the injury. Conflicting histories should also lead to a search for additional information about the incident.

Well-defined lines of demarcation between burned and unburned skin in a scald burn and the absence of splash burns are suggestive of intentional injury. However, splash burns can also be seen in intentional scald-burning cases. In addition, sparing of areas of skin may be suggestive of an intentional injury, particularly seen when the extremity is held in flexion and the area around the joint is protected and spared. Contact burns also present with well-defined margins; the object that caused the injury can often be determined by the outline of the wound.

A recent study reported that 69.6% of children admitted to the burn center were victims of neglect, and indicated that the incidence was highest in 3–6-year-olds, those with low socioeconomic status, and those with a family size of 6 or more (44). All states in the US require the reporting of suspected neglect and/or abuse of children.

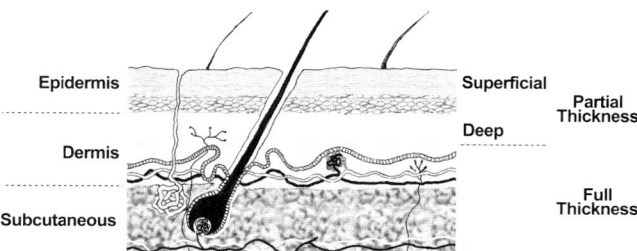

FIGURE 29.1. Schematic depiction of a cross-section through skin. The epidermis, dermis, and subcutaneous layers are shown. The levels of burn injury are divided into partial thickness, which may be superficial or deep, and full thickness.

Inhalation Injury

Although it is commonly thought that inhalation injury to the upper airway and parenchyma of the lung is due to thermal injury to the airway, this is almost never the case. The upper airway can dissipate heat effectively, and only occasionally has direct inhalation of superheated steam been found to cause inhalation injury. Inhalation of products of combustion causes inhalation injury. Upper airway injury edema associated with aspiration of hot liquid at the time of a scald injury is a rare injury seen in children. Signs of upper airway obstruction will often lead to intubation of the airway in this group of patients.

Providing care for a child with an inhalation injury is dependent on an understanding of the pathophysiology that is associated with the damage caused by the injury. The majority of injuries to the lung are caused by inhalation of toxic chemical products of combustion, in particular, aldehydes. Carbon monoxide and cyanide poisoning may occur as well. These toxins cause erythema and edema of the airway and lead to blistering, ulceration, erosions, and sloughing of the mucosa of the airway. The local edema, infiltration of the tissue with polymorphonuclear leukocytes, and sloughing of bronchial mucosa can lead to the formation of an endobronchial cast and obstruction of terminal bronchioles. Pulmonary edema occurs from increases in pulmonary lymph flow and microvascular permeability. The debris in the airway cannot be cleared because of the injury to the mucosa and disruption of the mucociliary transport mechanism. The obstruction of the small airways and the accumulation of carbonaceous material and necrotic debris provide a fertile ground for the development of infection. Some authors have reported that the incidence of pneumonia in patients with inhalation injury is as high as 70% within a week of injury (34).

In the management of burn and trauma patients, airway evaluation and management are of paramount importance and begin with an assessment of airway patency and quality of respirations. Chest x-ray, arterial blood gas determination, and pulmonary function testing are usually normal during the first 3 days following injury. Patients, who sustain injury in a closed space, have burns above the clavicle, singeing of facial hair, hoarseness, or carbonaceous sputum should be assumed to have sustained an inhalation injury. Elevated carboxyhemoglobin levels will confirm exposure to carbon monoxide but are not diagnostic for injury to the lung. Because the primary concern early after inhalation injury is obstruction of the airway, the upper airway should be evaluated immediately, usually in the emergency department. Flexible bronchoscopy provides the opportunity to confirm the diagnosis. Xenon ventilation/perfusion scans show air trapping when parenchymal injury is present; however, this test does not provide quantitative information on the extent of injury.

Decision to Transfer to Specialized Care

The resources required to care for patients with significant burn injury are not available at many medical centers. For this reason, a regionalized system for care of the burn-injured patient has been developed. Although travel time and distance to a burn center are of concern, transfer of burn-injured patients

TABLE 29.2

CRITERIA FOR REFERRAL FOR CARE OF A PATIENT WITH A BURN INJURY TO A REGIONAL BURN CENTER

For adults and pediatric patients with second- and third-degree cutaneous burns, burn center candidates are identified according to the following:

1. Partial thickness burns greater than 10% total body surface area
2. Burns that involve the face, hands, feet, genitalia, perineum, or major joints
3. Third-degree burns in any age group
4. Electrical burns, including lightning injury
5. Chemical burns
6. Inhalation injury
7. Burn injury in patients with preexisting medical disorders that could complicate management, prolong recovery, or affect mortality
8. Any patients with burns and concomitant trauma (such as fractures) in which the burn injury poses the greatest risk of morbidity or mortality. In such cases, if the trauma poses the greater immediate risk, the patient may be initially stabilized in a trauma center before being transferred to a burn unit. Physician judgment will be necessary in such situations, and should be in concert with the regional medical control plan and triage protocols.
9. Burned children in hospitals without qualified personnel or equipment for the care of children
10. Burn injury in patients who will require special social, emotional, or long-term rehabilitative intervention

From *Guidelines for the Operations of Burn Units* (pp. 55–62), Resources for Optimal Care of the Injured Patient: 1999, Committee on Trauma, American College of Surgeons.

after initial evaluation has been shown to be safe, especially if initiated early after injury. Patients with burns over >30% of their body surface area (BSA); children with injury of critical body parts, such as genitalia; and those with significant preexisting disease should be cared for in a burn center. Specific guidelines have been published by the American Burn Association (8) (**Table 29.2**).

RESUSCITATION

General Principles

Peripheral venous cannulation is preferred over central venous access and may be performed through burn-injured tissue if access through noninjured sites is not available. Children with >10% total BSA injury require IV fluid resuscitation and should have a urinary catheter. In addition, patients who have sustained a major injury should have a nasogastric tube placed to decompress the stomach. During transport and resuscitation, every effort should be made to maintain body temperature. Patients should be wrapped in clean sheets or blankets and, in the initial phase in the emergency care area, the room should be warmed. Resuscitation fluids should be warmed.

Fluid Resuscitation

Burn injury leads to intravascular volume depletion because fluid is lost into burn-injured tissue, through the wound, and into noninjured tissue. The major losses occur during the first 24 hrs following the injury, and it is generally agreed that during this period, crystalloid solutions should be used. As fluid shifts from the vascular space are massive in major injuries, formulae have been developed to provide an estimate of the fluid requirements. In addition to intravascular volume loss, myocardial depression occurs in the first 24–36 hrs after injury. Every guideline that has been developed carries with it the mandate that the patient's response to resuscitation—not the formula—be used as the actual determinant of fluid administration. The goal of resuscitation is to maintain adequate intravascular volume to support tissue perfusion and thereby preserve organ function. The adequacy of resuscitation in burn injury is based on observation of blood pressure, heart rate, and urine output. The patient is "titrated" with fluid to maintain normal blood pressure, heart rate, and hourly urine output of 1 mL/kg/hr in the infant and young child and 0.5 mL/kg/hr in the child >12 years of age or >50 kg in weight.

The Parkland formula is a crystalloid-based formula that provides the foundation for current methods of resuscitation (6). This formula calls for the initiation of resuscitation with lactated Ringer solution at a rate based on the BSA of burn injury and the patient's body weight. The calculated resuscitation volume for the first 24 hrs is:

$$(4 \text{ mL/kg} \times \% \text{BSA burn}) + \text{maintenance fluids} \qquad [29.1]$$

Maintenance fluids (5% dextrose in lactated Ringer solution) should be estimated (100 mL/kg for the first 10 kg, 50 mL/kg for the second 10 kg, and 20 mL/kg above 20 kg body weight) for children who weigh <40 kg. For adults and children who weigh >40 kg, maintenance fluids are not included in the estimate of fluid requirements. Half of this volume is given in the first 8 hrs after injury, and the other half is given in the following 16 hrs. To minimize the volume of fluid during resuscitation, some investigators have recommended the use of higher concentrations of sodium in the resuscitation fluid. Others have not had success with hypertonic saline resuscitation regimens; moreover, some have reported higher complication and mortality rates compared to historic controls in whom lactated Ringer was the resuscitation solution (18).

At the Shriners Burn Center in Galveston, Texas, an alternative formula used for calculating resuscitation fluid for the first 24 hrs after injury calls for lactated Ringer solution based upon surface area of injury in square meters (SA) with maintenance fluid (5% dextrose in lactated Ringer's) based on total BSA in square meters:

$$(5000 \text{ mL} \times \text{SA burn}) + (2000 \text{ mL} \times \text{total BSA}) \qquad [29.2]$$

The current evidence continues to support a crystalloid-based regimen in the range of 2–4 mL/kg/% BSA burn in the first 24 hrs. However, more recent data indicate that patients who have sustained inhalation injury—and all patients in general—are receiving more than estimated needs. This change, which Pruitt reviewed and called "fluid creep" (27), may be due in part to a much more aggressive use of analgesics in recent years, which appears to cause vasodilatation and exacerbation of the discrepancy between intravascular volume and the capacity of the intravascular space (37). Of concern are the complications associated with excessive volume resuscitations, which include pulmonary edema and increased subeschar pressures in the extremities and the abdomen, leading to compartment syndrome.

After the first 24 hrs, fluids are given to meet maintenance requirements and to replace ongoing losses. The hourly evaporative fluid loss from the patient's wounds can be estimated as:

$$(25 + \% \text{ BSA burn}) \times \text{total BSA} \qquad [29.3]$$

The evaporative losses are primarily free water. However, to avoid rapid changes in sodium concentration in children, this loss is replaced with a salt-containing solution, such as 5% dextrose in 0.2% normal saline. The loss of serum protein is clinically significant when the burn injury exceeds 40% BSA. When the injury is this size or larger, the loss is replaced in the second 24 hrs after injury with 5% albumin solution. The volume required can be estimated as:

$$0.3\text{–}0.4 \text{ mL/kg} \times \% \text{ BSA burn} \qquad [29.4]$$

The ultimate goal in the postresuscitation period is to maintain normal blood pressure, heart rate, urine output, and serum sodium.

Hypoalbuminemia

In burn patients, hypoalbuminemia is a frequent finding, and the etiology is multifactorial. Increased losses of albumin occur directly via drainage from burn wounds, as well as diffusely, as a consequence of profound capillary leakage ignited by the cascade of inflammatory mediators triggered by the burn injury. Albumin production is also reduced in critical illness, likely due to an increase in the production of acute phase proteins. Additionally, in the immediate postresuscitation phase, a dilutional contribution to hypoalbuminemia may occur if intravascular volume is increased. Chronic illness and malnutrition are other potential causes of nonacute hypoalbuminemia.

Albumin contributes 80% of the normal colloid oncotic pressure (13); therefore, hypoalbuminemia is associated with edema, particularly of the pulmonary interstitium and bowel wall. Albumin is often administered in an effort to avoid exacerbating acute lung injury, diarrhea, feeding intolerance, impaired wound healing, and the resultant complications.

The use of albumin in burn patients and in those with critical illness has been extensively studied, with great variability in results. Although some studies have suggested an increased risk of mortality associated with hypoalbuminemia, when the data from these studies are carefully analyzed, increased mortality is primarily seen in patients whose serum albumin was low at the time of presentation and in patients with extensive burns, infectious complications, chronic illness, and malnutrition (13). The extent of burn injury and incidence of sepsis appear to be the true risk factors for mortality. Studies that suggest an increased mortality associated with the administration of albumin have been refuted by a recent multi-institutional, randomized, double-blinded study that showed no difference in mortality in adult ICU patients resuscitated with saline vs. albumin (10).

The precise threshold at which hypoalbuminemia actually becomes clinically significant has only been investigated in animal studies. In humans, the preponderance of evidence from randomized, controlled trials that evaluate feeding intolerance, diarrhea, pulmonary dysfunction, and mortality as end points demonstrated that mild-to-moderate hypoalbuminemia is well tolerated in previously healthy patients (31). Among burn patients with hypoalbuminemia, serum albumin gradually normalizes, especially in the context of aggressive nutritional support, and higher serum albumin concentration is seen in patients who receive enteral, as compared to parenteral, nutrition. Therefore, routine albumin repletion may not be warranted, but more rigorously conducted studies are necessary to clarify the issue. The present practice in the William Randolph Hearst Burn Center is to ensure appropriate caloric delivery, preferably by the enteral route, as quickly as possible and—in critically ill pediatric patients—25% albumin should be added if the serum level is below 3 mg/dL.

Management of Inhalation Injury

Therapy consists of aggressive pulmonary toilet, use of mucolytics, and early identification and treatment of infection and supportive care. Administration of nebulized heparin is associated with reduced atelectasis and improved pulmonary function, compared to historic controls (9). Prophylaxis with antibiotics is not used; corticosteroids are of no benefit and are potentially harmful (20).

The level of support that is required may range from supplemental oxygen to advanced modes of assisted ventilation and hyperbaric oxygen therapy. For patients with evidence of inhalation injury, supplemental oxygen should be provided via nasal cannula or simple facemask, both of which will add additional humidification. If stridor due to upper airway inflammation and edema is present, racemic epinephrine may be employed to transiently relieve the obstruction to airflow. Helium/oxygen admixtures (Heliox) reduce resistance to turbulent airflow and, in turn, improve the work of breathing in situations of upper airway obstruction. Heliox is most frequently used to treat upper airway obstruction following extubation. When the airway is compromised, these patients should be intubated to permit definitive assessment and airway control. Based on a recent survey of pediatric burn centers, approximately 12% of pediatric burn victims require intubation, with approximately 70% of those intubated having sustained inhalation injury (35).

Until quite recently, Pediatric Advanced Life Support guidelines called for the use of uncuffed endotracheal tubes in children under 8 years of age (25). This practice has not been universally adhered to, especially by physicians inexperienced in the care of patients with severe restrictive and obstructive lung disease in whom the presence of a leak around the endotracheal tube would impair oxygenation and ventilation. However, ample evidence suggests that cuffed endotracheal tubes can be safely and effectively used in critically ill and burned pediatric patients. The size of the endotracheal tube when using a cuffed tube should be at least 0.5 cm smaller than an uncuffed tube. The current Pediatric Advanced Life Support guidelines recommend use of the formulas: (age/4) + 3 for cuffed endotracheal tubes and (age/4) + 4 for uncuffed tubes (25).

The prevalence of acute respiratory distress syndrome (ARDS) in mechanically ventilated adults with major burns has been estimated to be as high as 54% (7). Although the prevalence in pediatric burn patients is likely lower, acute lung injury and ARDS represent significant clinical challenges, especially in very young patients. Ventilator modes employed in the management of children with respiratory failure vary at both small and large pediatric burn centers. Pressure control ventilation and synchronized intermittent mandatory ventilation are the most frequently used modes, while more advanced modes are reserved for patients with severe restrictive lung disease. The use of lung protective strategies, as applied to all children with acute lung injury, is appropriate. These strategies include low tidal volume/high positive end-expiratory pressure (PEEP), airway pressure release ventilation (APRV) and high frequency oscillatory ventilation (HFOV) (14). Early excision and closure of the burn wound, as well as lung protective ventilation strategies, are the two main priorities in the management of burn patients with ARDS.

HFOV has been used as a rescue therapy in burn patients with ARDS who fail conventional mechanical ventilation. One center has reported the use of HFOV not only as rescue therapy, but also as a modality employed in the operating room for treating patients who require surgical intervention. As the timing of burn excision has a significant impact on survival following burn injury, the use of HFOV in the operating room has been considered by these authors to be important in maximizing survival. In addition, these authors reported much poorer outcomes in burn patients with smoke inhalation on HFOV compared to those without smoke inhalation (7). High-frequency percussive ventilation has been used in adult burn patients with ARDS, but its use has not been reported in pediatric burn victims.

The mode of mechanical ventilation employed in the care of the pediatric burn patient should ultimately be governed by the level of pulmonary dysfunction with synchronized intermittent mandatory ventilation plus pressure support being a reasonable default mode for the patient with little-to-no lung disease. Pressure-control ventilation and pressure-regulated volume control are alternatives, especially in patients who demonstrate high peak pressures. Cuffed endotracheal tubes and lung protective ventilator strategies should be employed in patients at risk for acute lung injury. Low tidal volume/high PEEP is used initially and progresses to HFOV or APRV in patients who require PEEP in excess of 10 cm of H_2O. It should be noted that the practice guidelines for burn care, developed by the American Burn Association, indicate that insufficient data exist to support a standard treatment guideline (1).

Timing of Tracheostomy in Pediatric Burn Victims

Tracheostomy is classically utilized in patients following a prolonged course of endotracheal intubation. However, early tracheostomy has also been used safely in a cohort of pediatric burn patients. A retrospective review of 38 children with burn injury who underwent early tracheostomy over a 2 1/2-year period reported no cases of tracheal stenosis, tracheomalacia, or acute airway emergencies in 38 children with burn injury in whom early tracheostomy was performed 2–4 days after the initiation of assisted ventilation (23). The patient population consisted mainly of children with burns of the face and head, and approximately 67% had inhalation injury. Thirteen percent had ARDS, and the mean $PaO_2 : FiO_2$ ratio prior to tracheostomy was 300. The average time to decannulation was 6 weeks. The authors concluded, based on the lack of complications and modest (15%) improvement in PaO$_2$: FiO$_2$ ratio, that tracheostomy should be considered in all children with severe burns in whom a prolonged course of mechanical ventilation is anticipated (23). Further study is warranted to precisely define the appropriate patient population and appropriate timing of tracheostomy in pediatric burn victims. Currently, tracheostomy is generally reserved for patients who have failed extubation or for those projected to require chronic mechanical ventilation, i.e., neurologically devastated patients.

WOUND CARE

General Principles

The objective of wound care is to avoid infection and protect the wound from further injury. Small (<2 cm) blisters are often left intact, whereas larger blisters and full-thickness wounds should be débrided and covered with a topical agent. Debridement is often very painful and is therefore carried out under general anesthesia or deep sedation. Ketamine is the anesthetic agent of choice because of its profound cutaneous analgesia. Propofol is an alternative, although the risk of hypotension and/or hypoventilation is greater than with ketamine. Even in the absence of debridement, burns are painful, and patients usually require opioid analgesia. Pain management is discussed in detail in Chapter 12.

Inpatient wound care is provided in a warm environment in an area reserved for wound care in a burn center. Agents that may cause additional tissue damage are avoided, and the circulation of the wound is protected by avoiding hypotension, hypoxemia, and hypothermia and by excluding the use of α-adrenergic agents, which are likely to lead to additional tissue ischemia. Sterile gloves should be worn at all times when a wound is manipulated. Chemical injury of tissue is treated with irrigation with copious amounts of either normal saline or tap water for as long as 6 hrs. Neutralizing agents are not used because they can lead to additional tissue damage caused by heat generated in an exothermic reaction between the chemicals. Hydrofluoric acid injuries can lead to systemic hypocalcemia; therefore, brief irrigation should be followed by topical application of calcium gluconate gel. If pain persists, clysis of the wound with calcium gluconate is used, except in digits. For injury to distal extremities, intra-arterial infusion of calcium gluconate has been recommended.

Prophylaxis Against Wound Infection

Systemic antimicrobial prophylaxis is not used in patients who are admitted to the hospital. The wounds are closely observed for infection, and treatment is initiated if infection occurs. Opinions vary regarding the use of antibiotics in the outpatient setting. If it is anticipated that compliance with a topical therapy regimen will be poor, systemic prophylaxis should be provided.

The advent of effective topical antimicrobial agents has substantially reduced the mortality associated with burn wound infection. The commonly used agents and their advantages and disadvantages are listed in **Table 29.3**. The ideal topical regimen rests on the use of an agent with good prophylactic antimicrobial activity that also provides an opportunity to easily evaluate the wound and to perform regular physical therapy. According to a recent international survey (16), silver sulfadiazine is the topical agent most commonly used for partial-thickness (32% of centers), mixed partial- and full-thickness (34% of centers), and full-thickness (30% of centers) burn wounds. An aqueous solution of silver nitrate (0.5%) has been used for years for its topical antimicrobial activity; however, only 4% of

TABLE 29.3

TOPICAL ANTIMICROBIAL AGENTS FOR TREATMENT OF BURN INJURY BY TYPE

	Application	Advantages	Disadvantages
OINTMENT			
Bacitracin	2nd degree burns, small areas	Not water soluble, good on face	Not indicated for large surface area
CREAM			
Silver sulfadiazine	2nd and 3rd degree burns	Soothing, good for range of motion	Possible neutropenia; little penetration
Mafenide acetate	2nd and 3rd degree burns	Penetrates eschar	Painful, metabolic acidosis
SOLUTION			
Aqueous silver nitrate (0.5%)	2nd and 3rd degree burns	Good antimicrobial	Hyponatremia, stains wound, little penetration
Mafenide acetate (5%)	Graft dressing, open wound soak	Broad activity, moist dressing	Not used for unexcised wound
IMPREGNATED DRESSINGS			
Acticoat	2nd degree burns	Dressing change every 3 days	Only 2nd degree
Aquacel Ag	2nd degree burns	Leave on for 21 days	Less flexibility and ease of motion; only 2nd degree burns

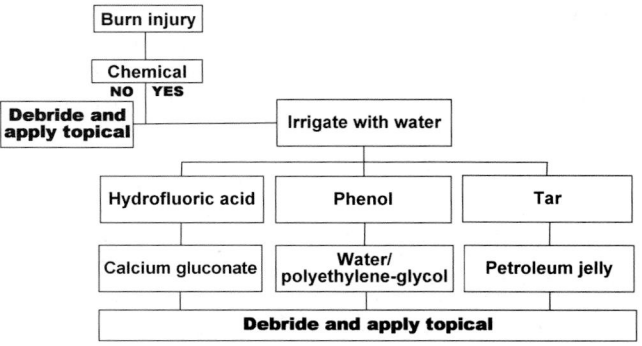

FIGURE 29.2. An algorithm for burn wound care. Chemical injuries require irrigation and, in some cases, additional treatment prior to debridement and application of topical antimicrobials.

centers currently use this agent as a primary topical. Because these agents do not penetrate burn wounds well, they are indicated for prophylaxis against infection, but not for therapy. Mafenide acetate does penetrate the wound and is the agent used for therapy of burn wound infection. More recent approaches include the use of silver as an antimicrobial; preliminary reports suggest that Acticoat, a silver-coated synthetic mesh dressing, provides antimicrobial activity in a dressing that may be left on a partial-thickness wound for 2 to 3 days. A more recent product, Acticoat 7, is reported to have antimicrobial activity that is sufficient to allow it to protect wounds for 7 days. Aquacel Ag Hydrofiber has been used with success on partial-thickness burn wounds. The advantages of this product are that the dressing does not have to be changed, and antimicrobial activity is equivalent to silver sulfadiazine. Ease of movement and flexibility was decreased with this product, compared to silver sulfadiazine. Silver sulfadiazine is not used in infants <2 months of age or in patients who are near-term pregnant due to concern that kernicterus is associated with exposure to sulfonamides. An algorithm for wound care is shown in **Figure 29.2.**

Surgical Care

Excision and closure of wounds have the advantage of reducing the extent of injury and eliminating the risk of wound infection. Tangential excision, which is the sequential removal of layers of necrotic tissue until viable tissue is identified, is the most commonly used method of excision of burn-injured tissue. The advantage of this method is that it yields the best cosmetic and functional result; however, it is also associated with considerable blood loss. Tourniquets, applied during excision of extremity wounds, have been shown to minimize blood loss. This approach presents a challenge to even the experienced burn surgeon because identification of the depth to excise to viable tissue is difficult to ascertain in the absence of capillary bleeding. Alternatively, deep excision of the wound to the level of the fascia is associated with minimal blood loss and is used when wounds are deep, full thickness, and infected, or when large areas are excised. The cosmetic results are poor, and lymphatic drainage is impaired after this type of excision.

One of the major advances in burn care has been the recognition that patients in whom the wounds are excised early after injury have fewer complications. The usual approach is to be-

gin excision within the first 3–4 days after injury (39). Although no randomized, prospective study has indicated that outcome is affected by early intervention, it is widely held that the overall improved outcome in burn-injured patients over the past 20 years is in large part due to this approach. Excision has been initiated by some within the first 24 hrs after injury (36); however, most authors suggest that this is too early, and excision is better performed when the patient with a large burn has been stabilized. In addition to the stability of the patient, other factors, such as coexistent injuries and inhalation injury, affect the timing of operative intervention. In the patient with wounds that will require grafting (i.e., deep partial and full thickness over >40% of the body surface area, a strategy for surgical intervention must be developed that accounts for available donor sites, with a goal of reducing the amount of open wound as quickly as possible. In such cases, closure of the wound takes precedence over cosmetic and functional considerations.

At the present time, the ultimate closure of the excised wound requires the use of autograft. If sufficient donor sites are available, the preferred skin graft in children is a split-thickness autograft (0.15–0.20 mm in thickness). A thicker, full-thickness graft is preferred for cosmetic reconstruction and in areas where scarring would lead to functional compromise. However, this thickness of donor skin requires that the donor site be grafted. When donor sites are limited, autograft can be expanded by passing it through a mechanical meshing device that allows it to be enlarged up to six times the surface area of the original donor skin. For practical purposes, the skin is not usually meshed to a size greater than four times the initial area.

Closure of the excised wound may be staged by temporarily covering it with biologic or manufactured dressings. Allograft provides for closure of the wound and may also be used as a test graft in areas where infection is of concern or when the adequacy of the excised wound bed is suspect. If an allograft is left in place for longer than 10 to 14 days, it becomes incorporated into the wound, and the wound must be excised to remove it. In recent years, a number of skin substitutes have been developed that replace the function of some or all layers of the skin. Integra Life Sciences Corporation provides a temporary epidermis as an outer layer of silastic and an inner layer matrix for the growth of a neodermis. Success with use of this product has been reported by a number of authors, all of whom noted an improved result in cosmesis and function but increased rates of infection when the wound bed was contaminated. A thin layer of epidermis must ultimately be grafted onto the neodermis. *AlloDerm* is human dermis that has been processed to extract cells and their components. This nonantigenic matrix provides a scaffold for a new dermis upon which a thin epidermal graft may be placed. This product has been used to improve cosmetic outcome and because a thin epidermal graft can be placed upon it. The advantage that these products offer for patients with large surface areas of injury is that donor sites are available in shorter time frames for recropping of epidermis for further grafting.

Immediate application of other products, such as pigskin or *Biobrane* (a synthetic membrane composed of silastic and a chondroitin sulfate–coated surface), on partial-thickness wounds moderates pain and eliminates the need to change dressings, but these slough off when applied to deep partial-thickness wounds.

Circumferential Burns

Circumferential burn wounds present unique problems associated with compromise of the tissue underneath the wound. In the extremities, the combination of increased extravascular fluid in the wound and underlying tissues and the lack of elasticity of the burn wound can lead to subeschar pressures that compromise blood flow to viable tissue. All extremities with circumferential full-thickness burns should be elevated to minimize edema formation and should be evaluated hourly for the classic signs of vascular compromise: pallor, pain, paresthesia, paralysis, and poikilothermia. Because these signs are often difficult to evaluate in a burn-injured extremity, additional assessment of Doppler-measured blood flow in the distal extremity should also be performed. Loss of Doppler signals may not be seen until after damage has occurred; therefore, the threshold for performing an escharotomy to release subeschar pressure should be low. An escharotomy is performed by making an incision through the eschar on the lateral surface of the extremity. An additional escharotomy may be required on the medial surface as well. The preferred sites for escharotomy are indicated in **Figure 29.3**. A multicentered study has suggested that delay in decompression of extremities may be associated with occult intracompartmental infection (32). Decompression of the hand should be performed when full-thickness burn injury leads to compromise of blood flow and function. Escharotomies are performed in fingers in the mid axial line on the ulnar side and on the radial side of the thumb, so as to preserve tactile sensation of the surfaces of opposition of the fingers and thumb.

In a similar way, a "compartment syndrome" can occur in the chest or abdomen in patients with circumferential full-thickness burn injury in these areas. A decrease in pulmonary compliance in these patients may indicate that decompression is necessary. Escharotomy of the chest in the anterior axillary line will often decrease the inspiratory pressures required to maintain tidal volume. If circumferential full-thickness burns of the abdomen and back are present, an escharotomy following the costal margin may be necessary. Incision of the eschar may be performed with a scalpel, but is often done with electrocautery so that minor bleeding can be controlled. Because full-thickness wounds are insensate and avascular, anesthesia is not necessary, and these procedures may be performed under sterile conditions at the bedside. Circumferential full-thickness burns on the abdominal wall can contribute to the development of increased intra-abdominal pressure during resuscitation. If an abdominal compartment syndrome develops, it may be relieved by escharotomy, drainage of peritoneal fluid, or decompressive laparotomy.

INFECTION

General Aspects in Burn Injury

The systemic inflammatory response that is associated with a major burn ignites a cascade of events that presents as a clinical syndrome that is difficult to distinguish from infection. Virtually all children that sustain burn injury have fever; severely burn-injured patients often have core body temperatures of 39–39.5°C, and they frequently develop an intestinal ileus, become disoriented, develop hyperglycemia, and sustain changes in fluid balance. The burn wound has been described as a "black box" in which a local inflammatory process occurs that leads to introduction of mediators of inflammation into the systemic circulation and causes activation of cells as they pass through the milieu of the wound. These events compound the responses to injury and are described here to point out that they distinguish the burn-injured patient from patients with other injuries. It appears that the incidence of infection is higher in burn-injured children compared to other critically ill children. Reported nosocomial infection rates in burn-injured children are high in all cases, with a central catheter infection rate of 4.9/1000 catheter days, a burn-wound infection rate of 5.6/1000 burn unit days, a ventilator-associated pneumonia rate of 11.4/1000 ventilator days, and a urinary catheter-related urinary tract infection rate of 13.2/1000 urinary catheter days (43).

An increased susceptibility to infection related to the extent of burn injury has also been suggested experimentally in animal models that demonstrate the activation of polymorphonuclear leukocytes (PMNs). Serum cytokine levels are elevated within the first week following a burn injury in children. Both proinflammatory [IL-6, IL-8, IL-1β, monocyte chemoattractant protein (MCP)-1, macrophage inflammatory protein (MIP)-1β, IL-13, IL5, and IL-7] and anti-inflammatory [IL-10, granulocyte colony-stimulation factor (G-CSF), IL-17, interferon (IFN)-γ, IL-12, p70, and IL-4] serum cytokine levels have been found in significantly higher amounts in burn-injured children compared to normal controls (11). The net result of the activation of these cells and mediator pathways appears to be indiscriminant recruitment of the normal pathways that maintain homeostasis, which leads to susceptibility to infection, further local tissue injury, and distant organ dysfunction.

BURN–WOUND INFECTION

In an attempt to standardize the evaluation and classification of infection in the wounds of the burn-injured patient, a subcommittee of the American Burn Association has provided a proposal for categorization of these infections (24). Although these guidelines are open for comment at this time, they provide

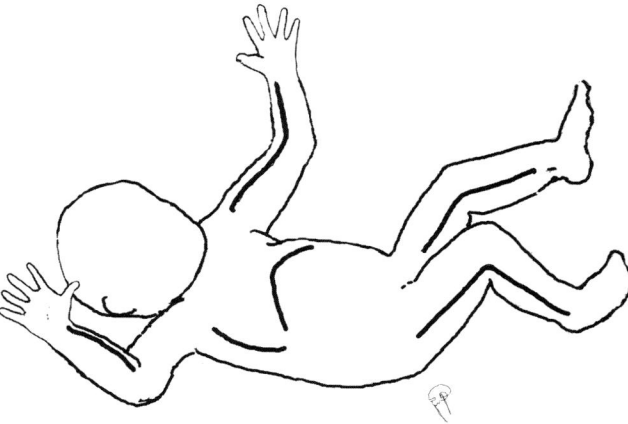

FIGURE 29.3. This diagram shows where surgical incisions (escharotomy) are performed in patients who have compromised blood flow due to circumferential full-thickness burns. The incisions are made laterally and/or medially with the patient in the true anatomic position, as shown.

a foundation for describing the four categories of wound-related infection and are used here as a basis for describing the infections that occur in the patient with burn injury.

Impetigo

This infection "involves the loss of epithelium from a previously reepithelialized surface such as a grafted burn, a partial-thickness burn allowed to heal by secondary intention, or a healed donor site" (28). This definition assumes that no other cause for epithelial loss is present such as mechanical damage, hematoma formation, or ischemia of the tissue. This infection, which has also been termed *melting graft syndrome*, is not necessarily associated with systemic signs of infection, fever, or an elevated white blood cell count. Although it is often caused by streptococcal or staphylococcal species, it may be caused by other organisms as well. Burn-wound surface cultures, which give no insight into what is occurring within the wound, are helpful in determining the inciting organism in these infections. Treatment consists of local care of the wound and systemic antibiotics.

Open Surgical Wound Infection

These infections are associated with a surgical intervention that has not healed. As defined by the subcommittee, they may occur in an ungrafted, excised burn or at unhealed donor sites and are associated with culture-positive purulent exudates. In addition, at least one of the following conditions is present: (a) loss of synthetic or biologic covering of the wound; (b) changes in wound appearance, such as hyperemia; (c) erythema in the uninjured skin surrounding the wound; or (d) systemic signs, such as fever or leukocytosis.

These infections require a change in local wound care, usually the addition of a topical antimicrobial, more frequent dressing changes, and the administration of systemic antibiotics.

Cellulitis

Burn-associated cellulitis must be differentiated from the normal local inflammatory response to a burn injury that is manifest as erythema at the margin of the wound. This finding differs from cellulitis by its localized nature (usually <1–2 cm from the margin of the wound) and by the lack of extension beyond that zone. The guidelines suggest that, in addition to a requirement for antibiotic treatment, the definition of cellulitis requires at least one of the following: (a) localized pain, tenderness, swelling, or heat at the affected site; (b) systemic signs of infection, such as hyperemia, leukocytosis, or septicemia; (c) progression of erythema and swelling; or (d) signs of lymphangitis, lymphadenitis, or both.

Invasive Infection

The diagnosis of invasive burn-wound infection rests on the recognition of changes in the wound, which include black, purple, or reddish discoloration; maceration; or early separation of eschar and systemic manifestations of infection. In addition to the clinical assessment of the wound, biopsy may be performed for quantitative culture or histologic evaluation. A tissue culture with >100,000 organisms is cultured from a gram of tissue. However, considerable variability in results with this technique and the lack of correlation with histologic findings have limited its application to use for identification of organisms in wounds. Histologic evaluation, although not readily available at most institutions, is diagnostic for invasive infection when organisms are identified in viable tissue. Invasive wound infection requires surgical excision of the wound to the level of viable tissue and administration of systemic antibiotics. The topical antimicrobials, with the exception of mafenide acetate, which may be used in preparation for excision, are not used for therapy for invasive burn-wound infection because they do not penetrate eschar.

The criteria for diagnosis of invasive infection, as outlined in the American Burn Association guidelines, include the following:

- Inflammation of the surrounding uninjured skin
- Histologic examination that shows invasion by the infectious organism into adjacent viable tissue
- Isolation of an organism from the blood in the absence of other infection
- Signs of the systemic inflammatory response syndrome (such as hyperthermia, hypothermia, leukocytosis, tachypnea, hypotension, oliguria, or hyperglycemia at a previously tolerated level of carbohydrate intake) and mental status changes

Pneumonia

The use of effective topical antimicrobials for prevention and therapy of wound infection, along with earlier surgical intervention in wound care, has led to a decrease in the incidence of wound infection, and respiratory failure is now the leading cause of death in the patient with thermal injury. Although inhalation injury is a prominent cause of respiratory complications in these patients, the incidence of pneumonia and ARDS is high, even when direct lung injury is not present. A review of autopsies on burn-injured children revealed that 44% had pneumonia at the time of death (3). Standard care includes early detection of pulmonary infection by Gram stain of sputum and culture of secretions, with respiratory support with assisted ventilation when pulmonary failure develops. The issue of how to make the diagnosis of pneumonia in a burn-injured patient has not been resolved. Pneumonia was diagnosed clinically in only 28% of children who were proven to have it at autopsy (3). This same study showed a very poor correlation with bronchoalveolar lavage (BAL) and protected bronchial brush (PBB) results. Additional studies suggest that BAL, with a positive result defined as >1000 colony forming units (CFU) per milliliter, and PBB are not sensitive enough in children to make the diagnosis of pneumonia but are helpful in detecting tracheobronchitis after inhalation injury (33). BAL has been reported to be useful in diagnosis and directing therapy in adult burn-injured patients with ventilator-associated pneumonia (42). In those studies, a positive BAL was considered to be at least 10,000 CFU/mL. The presence of white blood cells and bacteria in the sputum associated with other signs of infection should prompt the initiation of systemic antimicrobials that target the organisms that predominate in the flora of the unit at the time. Specific antimicrobials are then selected when culture results are available.

Suppurative Thrombophlebitis

Bacterial colonization of venous catheters in patients in ICUs, and in particular of central catheters in burn-injured patients, has been reported to be as high as 25%. No general consensus exists regarding how to minimize catheter-related infections. Some centers require that all peripheral, central venous, and arterial catheters be changed over a guidewire on day 3 and that a new site be used on day 6. Others have suggested that once-a-week catheter replacement is sufficient to maintain an acceptable rate of catheter-related bloodstream infection in children (33). The reason for concern, especially in burn-injured individuals, is that suppurative thrombophlebitis can be an insidious and life-threatening infection. The only findings may be persistent fever and a bacteremia that continues despite appropriate antibiotic treatment. The classic findings (edema, erythema, pain, and a palpable cord at an IV site) that are associated with phlebitis may not be identifiable. Diagnosis is confirmed by aspiration of purulent material from the affected vein, and treatment consists of excision of the involved vein to the point at which bleeding is encountered and the vessel is normal.

Suppurative Chondritis

The cartilage of the ear has minimal protection and blood supply and is highly susceptible to infection when the overlying tissue is damaged. Dressings should not be applied to the ear, and pillows should not be used. Auricular burns should be treated with twice-daily open wound care and gently débrided. The topical agent of choice is mafenide acetate because it penetrates eschar and avascular cartilage. When suppurative chondritis occurs, systemic antibiotics are of little value due to the avascular nature of the tissue, and the ear must be surgically drained under anesthesia by bivalving of the ear, with excision of infected and necrotic tissue.

Bacteremia Associated with Wound Manipulation

It is anticipated that debridement and surgical excision of burn wounds will lead to bacteremia; however, the data to support this are variable. Sasaki et al. observed transient bacteremia in 21% of burn care procedures (30), while others have reported that more than 40% of burn patients had positive blood cultures following burn excision. It appears that the incidence of bacteremia following wound manipulation is related to the extent of injury. This finding is supported by the 8% incidence of bacteremia in patients with 31%–60% total body surface area (TBSA) burns, compared to a 75% incidence in those with >60% TBSA burns. More recent studies have suggested that the incidence of bacteremia associated with wound manipulation is low in the early period after injury. Nevertheless, bacteremia related to burn care, especially in patients with a large burn injury, may seed distant sites, such as cardiac valves or the brain, and it is likely that, in this population of patients, perioperative administration of antibiotics that are active against the flora of the wound is of benefit.

Other Infections

As in any seriously injured patient, the associated immunocompromise may set the stage for infection at any site. Burn-injured patients have a high incidence of urinary tract infections and pneumonia. They may also develop other infections, such as appendicitis, but often do not present with classic features due to a suppressed inflammatory response. A high index of suspicion is necessary to detect these infections. Additional infections of concern in the burn-injured patient are listed below.

Sinusitis

One source of sepsis that is frequently overlooked in the burn patient is nosocomial sinusitis. Factors that predispose to sinusitis are indwelling catheters for nasogastric or nasoduodenal feeding and nasotracheal intubation, especially in patients with inhalation injury. The clinical diagnosis of nosocomial sinusitis is difficult because purulent nasal discharge is absent in 73%, a majority of cases. The diagnosis is made by culture of drainage fluid and by CT scan of the sinuses. Once the diagnosis is made, treatment consists of removal of all tubes and catheters, initiation of appropriate antibiotic therapy, and drainage. If a nasotracheal tube is present, it should be changed to the orotracheal route. In some cases, it may be necessary to perform a tracheostomy to adequately control the infectious process.

Bacterial Endocarditis

Immune compromise, recurrent bacteremia, and the frequent use of central venous catheters in the patient with burn injury are risk factors for the development of endocarditis. The association of central venous and pulmonary artery catheters with the development of bacterial endocarditis in burn-injured patients is well documented. Similar to suppurative thrombophlebitis, bacterial endocarditis is insidious and should be suspected when blood cultures are positive without an obvious source and with a fever of unknown origin—particularly in burn-injured patients, as the incidence of bacterial endocarditis has been reported to be as much as 14–70 times higher than in other ICU patients. The presence of a new cardiac murmur supports the diagnosis, which should be confirmed by echocardiography. In the past, bacterial endocarditis was associated with nearly 100% mortality in the patient with burn injury, but early diagnosis with surgical intervention has led to improved survival in recent years. Antibiotic therapy is based upon blood culture results and should continue for 4–6 weeks.

HYPERMETABOLISM AND NUTRITION

The classic description of the metabolic response to injury includes an early ebb phase that is characterized by low cardiac output and a decreased metabolic rate followed by a hypermetabolic phase that starts at 24–36 hrs after injury. An approximate 50% increase in protein metabolism and energy expenditure occurs due to hypermetabolism, fluid losses,

TABLE 29.4

FORMULA FOR NUTRITIONAL SUPPORT IN THE BURN PATIENT

Infants (0–12 months)	2100 kcal/m^2 plus 1000 kcal/m^2 burn
Children 1–11 years	1800 kcal/m^2 plus 1300 kcal/m^2 burn
Children 12 years and older	1500 kcal/m^2 plus 1500 kcal/m^2 burn

sepsis, and inflammation in children following a large burn injury, and this catabolic state can persist for 9–12 months. The stress hormones (cortisol, epinephrine, and glucagon) all increase, mediating increased gluconeogenesis, glycogenolysis, muscle breakdown, and bone loss. Furthermore, the anabolic effects of insulin and growth hormone are antagonized in patients with burns. Early and aggressive nutritional support has been shown to reduce the elevated resting energy expenditure (REE) in burn victims. Most investigations have led to the conclusion that measurement of REE by indirect calorimetry is the best way to estimate caloric needs in children during the hypermetabolic phase. The use of the Harris Benedict formula, the World Health Organization formula, or the Schofield-HW equation showed poor correlation with REE in children after major burn injury (38). It has been shown that male children have a higher metabolic rate than females after injury and that children who are <3 years of age have only a slight increase in metabolic rate (22). Furthermore, studies confirm that hypermetabolism persists for over 12 months following injury. Nutritional support in the burn patient is usually guided by a formula, such as that used at the Shriners Burn Center, especially when indirect calorimetry is not available (Table 29.4).

The enteral route is the preferred route for administration of nutrition. A nasogastric or nasoduodenal tube should be placed as soon as the initial evaluation and burn resuscitation are complete and, in the absence of contraindications, enteral feeds should be initiated within 24 hrs of injury. However, feeding intolerance, as evidenced by significant gastric residual volume and diarrhea, may limit use of the gastrointestinal tract for caloric delivery. Diarrhea is a commonly encountered problem in the burn population. The etiology is likely multifactorial, and commonly postulated sources include antibiotic use, nosocomial infection, bowel wall edema, hyperosmolarity and insufficient fiber content of enteral formulas, and compromised mucosal integrity. However, diarrhea is usually noninfectious and, despite physiologic plausibility, is not worsened by hypoalbuminemia. Factors associated with a decreased incidence of diarrhea in burn victims include fat intake <20% of overall caloric intake, vitamin A intake >10,000 IU/day in adults, and early implementation of enteral feeds (<48 hrs post-burn) (12).

In addition to vitamin A, other vitamins, minerals, and trace elements may be required in excess of recommended daily allowances, including calcium, magnesium, vitamin D, zinc, copper, and other micronutrients. It is believed that upregulation of the parathyroid gland calcium-sensing receptor contributes to hypocalcemia and hypomagnesemia. The current standard is to supplement calcium and magnesium until serum levels are within the normal range. Zinc and copper levels are also diminished following thermal injury. These micronutrients have important roles in bone matrix formation, linear growth, wound healing, and immunity (41). Levels are thought to be low because of wound losses, increased urinary excretion, and the activity of IL-1 and other cytokines produced during the acute phase response. Calcium supplementation can impair zinc absorption and decrease copper retention. No clear consensus exists regarding appropriate zinc and copper supplementation in burn-injured patients.

In addition to early and aggressive nutritional support, attempts have been made to pharmacologically mitigate the hypermetabolic state that persists following burn injury. The hypermetabolism, which can be blunted to some extent by β-blockade, has led some to recommend the use of propranolol in children. A recent randomized, prospective, placebo-controlled study showed that propranolol given via nasogastric tube in doses of 0.3–1.0 mg/kg body weight every 4–6 hrs decreases heart rate by 11% (5). These studies also showed that the hepatomegaly that routinely occurs in severely burn-injured children was virtually eliminated. Although side effects of β-blockade (e.g., hypotension and bronchospasm) may occur, none were noted in this fully monitored group of critically ill children.

Muscle wasting, decreased bone mineralization, and retarded linear growth can be quite profound. In the early 1990s, recombinant human growth hormone was evaluated, initially in adults and later in children. Safety concerns surrounding its use were noted in several European studies. Although, pediatric patients did not appear to have the same issues, daily subcutaneous injections limited patient compliance. In the mid-1990s, testosterone was shown to improve protein synthesis; however, hepatotoxicity, acne, hirsutism, and virilization in females limit its utility. In the late 1990s, a synthetic testosterone analog, oxandrolone, was studied in adult and pediatric burn patients. In a 12-month randomized, placebo-controlled, double-blinded study in pediatric patients with burns of 40% BSA or greater, it was found to produce an earlier normalization of serum albumin, prealbumin, and retinol-binding protein and to improve lean body mass and bone mineral content. In treated patients, as compared to controls, this study reported no acne, facial hair, hirsutism, or hepatotoxicity (15). Despite these results, oxandrolone is not yet considered to be standard care following burn injury in children.

Glycemic Control

As noted previously, protein metabolism and energy expenditure increase by approximately 50% in children following a large burn injury. The etiology of this catabolic state is multifactorial but favorably impacted by insulin administration. Hyperglycemia in burn patients is associated with increased morbidity and mortality. Additionally, maintenance of normoglycemia has recently been shown to reduce mortality in critically ill medical and surgical patients (40). Administration of exogenous insulin can overcome insulin resistance, retard protein catabolism, and promote normoglycemia. Analysis of the benefit of insulin administration appears to favor maintenance of normoglycemia over insulin dosage as the true source of improved outcomes (40). Emerging evidence demonstrates that intensive insulin therapy can be safely and effectively implemented in the pediatric population, and its use in the pediatric burn population may lower infection rates and improve survival (26). Additionally, the combined benefits of glycemic control in the critically ill patient and the favorable effects of insulin in promoting protein synthesis and preventing protein catabolism support the use of insulin administration to achieve glycemic control in the burn patient. No blood glucose goal has been established for the critically ill pediatric patient; however, a reasonable target for blood glucose should be levels that range between 90 and 120 mg/dL. Careful attention must be paid to avoiding hypoglycemia, however. Members of the healthcare team participating in the care of pediatric burn patients should be sensitized to the importance of glucose monitoring and the recognition of hypoglycemia, especially in very young or nonverbal children. Standing insulin orders should only be written for patients who demonstrate persistent hyperglycemia while they receive constant glucose delivery in the form of enteral tube feedings or parenteral nutrition.

OUTCOME

Survival after burn injury has improved significantly during the past 20 years and appears to have reached a plateau over the past 10 years (29). Because mortality rates have changed, the suggestion of two decades ago that mortality could be estimated as the sum of age and percent of the body surface area that sustained thermal injury no longer holds true. However, multiple studies have confirmed that patient age and extent of injury are the two most powerful predictors of outcome. Review of the records of more than 187,000 victims of burn injury indicates than mortality has decreased from 6.2% in 1995 to 4.7% in 2005 (21). These data also demonstrate the significant contribution of age to mortality risk in children. The mortality for a burn injury of 60%–69.9% TBSA was 50% in the newborn to 1.9-year-old group, 22.6% in those between 2 and 4.9 years of age, and 18.3% in those between 5 and 19.9 years of age. Although it has been suggested that the rate of survival in girls is greater than in boys, this was unconfirmed by a 2005 study (4).

An increased mortality rate when thermal injury is associated with inhalation injury is well recognized, with reported increases in mortality as high as 20% with inhalation injury. A comparative study of patients matched for burn size and age reported a mortality rate of 9.6% in patients without inhalation injury, compared to 46.6% in those with inhalation injury (34). To specifically prognosticate the outcome for the thermally injured patient, most authors have suggested that multivariate statistical techniques, such as probit or regression analysis, be applied.

REHABILITATION

Advances in medical care leading to increased survival from thermal injury have led to a renewed emphasis on quality of life after these injuries. Rehabilitation of the patient with a burn injury begins from the time of initial medical care, requires intense care in the first year after injury, and often, continued life-long care. Splinting of injured extremities begins as soon as the patient is stabilized, and range-of-motion exercises begin within the first 24 hrs. The team approach is important to coordinate therapy, surgical intervention, and medical care.

As soon as wounds have a stable epidermal closure, usually within 2 weeks after grafting or primary healing has occurred, attention is turned to wound and scar management. Garments that apply pressure to the wounds are tailor-made for the patient and worn 24 hrs per day. The opportunity to modulate the development of cicatrix is restricted to the time when the wound is immature and actively remodeling. This period may extend up to a year post injury, but mechanical intervention is of little benefit beyond that time. Surgical intervention for cosmetic deformity is usually delayed until the wound is mature, as is intervention for functional restriction, unless a surgical procedure is necessary to allow for physical therapy.

CONCLUSIONS AND FUTURE DIRECTIONS

Advances in the care of the burn-injured child have paralleled progress in critical care, with additional improvements in resuscitation and wound care leading to a decrease in mortality from burn injury. The current challenge is to improve the quality of life after major injury, and future directions include advances to improve texture, color, and elasticity of grafted areas. Microvascular techniques for reconstruction will become increasingly important to replace major tissue loss and improve cosmetic outcomes.

KEY POINTS

- Initial evaluation of the patient includes determination of depth of injury and extent of surface area involved. These are trauma patients and may have other injuries in addition to the burn.
- Fluid resuscitation in the first 24 hrs is based on a formula to calculate the amount of lactated Ringer solution to infuse. The formula is only a guide; adjustments are made based on vital signs and urine output.
- Silver sulfadiazine is the topical agent most commonly used for burn wounds. Early excision of the wound is now standard of care in the burn-injured patient.
- Hypermetabolism is very prominent in the burn-injured child. Proteins and calories must be provided to address these needs, beginning on the day of injury. Hypermetabolism persists for 9–12 months post-injury.
- Outcomes have improved to the extent that all children should be resuscitated regardless of extent of injury.

References

1. Arenholz DH, Cope N, Dimick AR, et al. Inhalation injury: Initial management. *J Burn Care Rehabil* 2001;(Suppl):23S–6S.
2. Arnoldo B, Klein M, Gibran NS. Practice guidelines for the management of electrical injuries. *J Burn Care Research* 2006;27:439–47.
3. Barret JP, Ramzy PI, Wolf SE, et al. Sensitivity and specificity of bronchoalveolar lavage and protected bronchial brush in the diagnosis of pneumonia in pediatric burn patients. *Arch Surg* 1999;134:1243–6.
4. Barrow RE, Przkora R, Hawkins HK, et al. Mortality related to gender, age, sepsis, and ethnicity in severely burned children. *Shock* 2005;23:485–7.
5. Barrow RE, Wolfe RR, Dasu MR, et al. The use of beta-adrenergic blockade in preventing trauma-induced hepatomegaly. *Ann Surg* 2006;243:115–20.
6. Baxter CR, Shires T. Physiologic response to crystalloid resuscitation of severe burns. *Ann NY Acad Sci* 1968;150:874–94.
7. Cartotto R, Ellis S, Smith T. Use of high-frequency oscillatory ventilation in burn patients. *Crit Care Med* 2005;33(3):S175–81.

8. Committee on Trauma. Guidelines for the operations of burn units in resources for optimal care of the injured patient. *Bull Am Coll Surg* 1999;55–62.

9. Desai MH, Mlcak R, Richardson J, et al. Reduction in mortality in pediatric patients with inhalation injury with aerosolized heparin/N-acetylcystine therapy. *J Burn Care Rehabil* 1998;19:210–2.

10. Finfer S, Norton R, Bellomo R, et al. The SAFE study: Saline vs. *albumin for fluid resuscitation in the critically ill*. *Vax Sanguinis* 2004;87(Suppl 2):S123–31.

11. Finnerty CC, Herndon DN, Przkora R, et al. Cytokine expression profile over time in severely burned pediatric patients. *Shock* 2006;26:13–9.

12. Gottschlich MM, Warden GD, Havens MM, et al. Diarrhea in tube-fed burn patients: Incidence, etiology, nutritional impact, and prevention. *J Parenter Enteral Nutr* 1988;12(4):338–45.

13. Greenhalgh DG, Housinger TA, Kagan RJ, et al. Maintenance of serum albumin levels in pediatric burn patients: A prospective, randomized trial. *J Trauma* 1995;39(1):67–74

14. Habashi NM. Other approaches to open-lung ventilation: Airway pressure release ventilation *Crit Care Med* 2005;33(3):Suppl 228–40.

15. Hart DW, Wolf SE, Ramzy PI, et al. Anabolic effects of oxandrolone after severe burn. *Ann Surg* 2001;233(4):556–64.

16. Hermans MHE. Results of a survey on the use of different treatment options for partial and full-thickness burns. *Burns* 1998;24:539–51.

17. Hight DW, Bakalar HR, Lloyd JR. Inflicted burns in children. *JAMA* 1979;242:517–20.

18. Huang PP, Stucky FS, Dimick AR. Hypertonic sodium resuscitation is associated with renal failure and death. *Ann Surg* 1995;221:543–57.

19. La Hei ER, Holland AJA, Martin HCO. Laser Doppler imaging of pediatric burns: Burn wound outcome can be predicted independent of clinical examination. *Burns* 2006;32:550–3.

20. Levine BA, Petroff PA, Slade CL, et al. Prospective trials of dexamethasone and aerosolized gentamicin in the treatment of inhalation injury in the burned patient. *J Trauma* 1978;18:188–93.

21. Miller SF, Bessey PQ, Schurr MJ, et al. National burn repository 2005: A ten-year review. *J Burn Care Res* 2006;27:411–3.

22. Mlcak RP, Jeschke MG, Barrow RE, et al. The influence of age and gender on resting energy expenditure in severely burned children. *Ann Surg* 2006;244:121–30.

23. Palmieri TL, Jackson W, Greenhalgh DG. The benefits of early tracheostomy in severely burned children. *Crit Care Med* 2002;30(4):922–4.

24. Peck MD, Weber J, McManus A, et al. Surveillance of burn wound infections: a proposal for definitions. *J Burn Care Rehabil* 1998;19:386–9.

25. Pediatric Advanced Life Support *Circulation* 2005;112:[Suppl I]:IV 167–187.

26. Pham TN, Warren AJ, Phan HH, et al. Impact of tight glycemic control in severely burned children. *J Trauma*. 2005;59:1148–54.

27. Pruitt BA, Jr. Protection from excessive resuscitation "pushing the pendulum back." *J Trauma* 2000;49:567–8.

28. Ramzy PI, Jeschke MG, Wolf SE. Correlation of bronchoalveolar lavage with radiographic evidence of pneumonia in thermally injured children. *J Burn Care Rehabil* 2003;24:382–5.

29. Ryan CM, Schoenfeld DA, Thorpe WP, et al. Objective estimates of the probability of death from burn injuries. *N Engl J Med* 1998;338:362–6.

30. Sasaki TM, Welch GW, Herndon DN, et al. Burn wound manipulation-induced bacteremia. *J Trauma* 1979;19(1):46–8.

31. Sheridan RL, Prelack K, Cunningham JJ. Physiologic hypoalbuminemia is well tolerated by severely burned children. *J Trauma* 1997;43(3):448–52.

32. Sheridan RL, Tompkins RG, McManus WF, et al. Intercompartmental sepsis in burn patients. *J Trauma* 1994;36:301–5.

33. Sheridan RL, Weber JM. Mechanical and infectious complications of central venous cannulation in children: Lessons learned from a 10-year experience placing more than 1000 catheters. *J Burn Care Research* 2006;27:713–8.

34. Shirani KZ, Pruitt BA Jr, Mason AD. The influence of inhalation injury and pneumonia on burn mortality. *Ann Surg* 1986;205:82–7.

35. Silver GM, Freiburg C, Halerz M, et al. A survey of airway and ventilator management strategies in North American pediatric burn units. *J Burn Care Rehabil* 2004;25:435–40.

36. Still JM, Law EJ, Craft-Coffman B. An evaluation of excision with application of autografts or porcine xenografts within 24 hours of injury. *Ann Plast Surg* 1996;36:176–9.

37. Sullivan SR, Friedrich JB, Engrav LH, et al. "Opioid creep" is real and may be the cause of "fluid creep." *Burns* 2004;30:583–90.

38. Suman OE, Mlcak RP, Chinkes DL, et al. Resting energy expenditure in severely burned children: Analysis of agreement between indirect calorimetry and prediction equations using the Bland-Altman method. *Burns* 2006;32:335–42.

39. Tompkins RG, Remensnyder JP, Burke JF, et al. Significant reductions in mortality for children with burn injuries through the use of prompt eschar excision. *Ann Surg* 1988;208:577–85.

40. Van den Berghe G, Wouters PJ, Bouillon R, et al. Outcome benefit of intensive insulin therapy in the critically ill: Insulin dose versus glycemic control. *Crit Care Med* 2003;31(2):359–66.

41. Voruganti VS, Klein GL, Lu H, et al. *Impaired zinc and copper status in children with burn injuries: Need to reassess nutritional requirements*. *Burns* 2005;31:711–6.

42. Wahl WL, Ahrns KS, Brandt MM, et al. Bronchoalveolar lavage in diagnosis of ventilator-associated pneumonia in patients with burns. *J Burn Care Rehabil* 2005;26:57–61.

43. Weber JM, Sheridan RL, Pasternak MS, et al. Nosocomial infections in pediatric patients. *Am J Infect Control* 1997;25:195–201.

44. Yasti AC, Tumer AR, Atli M, et al. A clinical forensic scientist in the burns unit: Necessity or not? A prospective clinical trial. *Burns* 2006;32:77–82.

CHAPTER 30 ■ TERRORISM AND MASS CASUALTY EVENTS

PHILIP L. GRAHAM, III • GEORGE L. FOLTIN • F. MERIDITH SONNETT

Over the last decade significant concerns about the risks of mass casualty events that involve explosives, chemical, biological, radiological, and nuclear weapons have become increasingly widespread. These concerns intensified substantially subsequent to September 11, 2001, when the magnitude of US vulnerability to terrorism-related mass casualty incidents became incontrovertible. New editions of many standard medical texts now include a full chapter dedicated to disaster preparedness, underscoring the grim realization that physicians and other healthcare workers must be prepared for an event that results in mass causalities. "Front-line" healthcare workers (first responders and emergency department staff) require education and training in early recognition and initial management of the injuries and conditions associated with weapons of mass destruction. Similar education and training is needed for those healthcare workers who will be responsible for the on-going management of these victims. Pediatric critical care physicians and their counterparts in adult healthcare will be expected to be familiar with the myriad of distinct injuries and illnesses associated with exposure to agents used in terrorist attacks, as well as the appropriate treatment and management strategies.

PEDIATRIC-SPECIFIC DISASTER PREPAREDNESS

Traditionally, the vast majority of disaster preparedness efforts have focused on the needs of adults, even though children represent the most vulnerable proportion of victims (32). Past experience with natural mass casualty and terrorism-related events (e.g., Oklahoma bombing, Tokyo subway Sarin attack, Hurricane Katrina, and on-going terror-related attacks in the Middle East) highlight the fact that the worldwide medical community is not sufficiently prepared to manage victims of such events and that it is the least well prepared for pediatric casualties (9,15,25). The unique needs of children must be explicitly defined as they relate to the anatomic, physiologic, and psychologic differences between children and adults. Evidence-based guidelines and recommendations for the development of comprehensive, pediatric-focused, disaster preparedness programs, published in 2004, underscored the crucial need for pediatric-specific medical expertise to optimize the care and outcomes of pediatric victims of disasters and terrorism-related events. This important document represents one of the first and most extensive publications to address the large gaps in current pediatric disaster preparedness (27). The vulnerabilities that are unique to pediatric disaster victims are highlighted in **Table 30.1**.

Children are disproportionately affected by terrorism-related events and require prolonged and extensive medical care that substantially exceeds the needs of adult victims. The anatomy and physiology of children differs from adults, and it is, therefore, important to anticipate the different patterns of illness and injury that pediatric victims of a mass casualty terrorist attack would sustain. Gaining an understanding of the properties and characteristics of agents that might be employed in terrorist attacks and of the epidemiology and patterns of injury will help to better prepare medical centers and healthcare workers. Literature and past experience with terrorist attacks highlight the enormous burden mass casualty events would have on hospital ICUs (3,37).

This chapter will prepare the pediatric critical care clinician to care for victims of terror-related incidents and will focus on:

■ PICU response to mass casualty events, including surge capacity
■ Recommendations for critical care treatment and management of pediatric victims of terrorism who survive initial prehospital or emergency department resuscitation
■ The presentation, characteristics, treatment options, and on-going critical care management of specific agents: blast/explosive, biological, chemical, and radiological and nuclear

PREPARING FOR SURGE IN THE PICU

The unique physiology of children dictates that they will be overly represented among the victims of a chemical or biological incident (9). Advance planning for a mass-casualty event must include comprehensive evaluation and preparation for implementation of systems to support communication, staffing, supplies, capacity, infection control, availability of durable equipment, assessment of current patient status, and clinical standards. Best practice dictates that a PICU representative should be designated to critically evaluate the unit's emergency preparedness status.

Disaster Notification System

All hospitals have a disaster notification system; often, however, pediatric interests are not adequately or appropriately represented. Every PICU should have a well-defined plan for clinician recall in the event of a mass-casualty event. Specific clinicians who live close to the hospital and who have

TABLE 30.1

PEDIATRIC-SPECIFIC VULNERABILITIES FROM EXPOSURE TO TERRORISM-RELATED AGENTS

Increased respiratory exposure (higher minute ventilation, live "closer to the ground")

Increased dermal exposure (less fat, thinner, more permeable skin; larger body surface area/mass ratio)

Increased risk of dehydration due to toxin-induced vomiting and diarrhea (decreased intravascular volume, larger body surface area/mass ratio)

Increased risk of hypothermia during decontamination procedures (larger body surface area/mass ratio)

Immunologic immaturity, resulting in more virulent disease manifestations; greater permeability of blood–brain barrier

Developmentally less capable of escaping attack and taking appropriate protective actions (developmental immaturity, dependence on adult caregivers who may be severely injured or dead)

Increased incidence of multiple-organ injury (thoracic cage not as well developed, less protection of visceral organs)

Increased incidence of head injury (head is larger proportionally; calvarium is thinner and offers less protection of brain matter, more susceptible to penetrating and blunt trauma)

Adapted from Henretig FM, Ciesiak TJ, Eitzen EM Jr. Biologic and chemical terrorism. J Pediatr 2002;141:311–26.

family situations that allow them to report to the hospital on short notice should be predesignated as "first responders." The healthcare workers who support the "first responder" pool are expected to perform their function when communication systems may be inoperable. A disaster plan should specify the location where staff will report upon notification of a disaster. The plan should make provisions for at least two shifts of healthcare workers. It is critical to hold a second wave of responders "on reserve," with a plan to have them report later (e.g., 12 hrs) after the start of the incident. Periodic disaster drills must be conducted so that these systems can be tested and adjustments in the execution can be made, as necessary.

Pre-event Planning

Pre-event planning for increased supply needs is an important element of a comprehensive emergency preparedness plan. Developing an inventory of critical supplies and determining current stocks is a first step. Every hospital and ICU must decide how many days of "stand-alone" supplies should be stockpiled for a mass-casualty event, when normal delivery routes are apt to be disrupted. The Joint Commission of Accreditation of Health Care Organizations currently recommends 48–72 hrs of supplies (24), but this may be expanded in the future.

Critical care bed capacity may be expanded by using stretchers, cots, or additional beds in existing PICU locations. Additionally, critical care may be provided in alternative locations, such as postoperative holding areas, catheterization laboratories, procedure rooms, the NICU, and the emergency depart-

ment. Plans for such expansions must be made in concert with the hospital staff members who understand the electric and medical gas systems that supply these areas.

Institutions with established PICUs have a role in supporting surrounding facilities that do not have PICU resources. A strategy to integrate this potentiality must be included in pre-event planning. An effective plan must be developed and coordinated between the disaster preparedness teams from lead institutions and local facilities that lack PICU capability.

Infection Control Measures

Infection control during a mass-casualty incident of any type will be challenging and, during a biological event, may be critically important to avoid propagation of the pathogen. Infection control precautions can be divided into a two-tiered approach, with *standard precautions* as the first tier, or foundation, for the prevention of transmission of infectious pathogens. Standard precautions include hand hygiene, which is the single most effective tool for minimizing disease transmission, and use of personal protective equipment (PPE) for all contacts with blood, body fluids, nonintact skin, and mucous membranes. The second tier of precautions is termed *extended precautions,* the use of which is recommended when specific pathogens are known or suspected, and includes *contact precautions*, *droplet precautions*, and *airborne infection isolation precautions* (18). In a biological event, standard precautions will continue to be critically important, but expanded precautions may also be necessary. Ensuring a supply of PPE requires planning because the demand will be great when multiple victims of a biological attack require care. The provision of multiple *airborne infection isolation environments* (i.e., negative pressure rooms) is beyond the capability of most hospitals. Alternative processes, such as portable high-efficiency particulate air filtration and isolation tents, may mitigate risk.

Equipment Needs

Durable medical equipment, such as ventilators, monitoring systems, and IV administration systems, may be limited in mass-casualty situations. Stockpiling, cooperative vendor and mutual aid agreements, government assistance, and altered standards of care may all play roles in the provision of care.

In-Patient Disposition in Surge Capacity Plans

Most ICUs in the US operate at close to capacity (19). In the event of increased demand for critical care, the needs of existing patients must be determined. It will be possible to transfer some patients out of the PICU to general medical or surgical units; a few may be stable enough to be discharged home. Transferring patients to other facilities is also an option to help increase ICU capacity; however, in a mass-casualty event, most healthcare facilities will be equally overwhelmed. In general, these strategies only have the ability to increase capacity by 20–50%.

Emergency Mass Critical Care

Emergency mass critical care is a term used to define the level of care that would be required in the event of a mass casualty that results in enormous numbers of people needing medical and surgical treatment. The vast number of victims who require critical care would overwhelm existing medical delivery systems, which would not be able to maintain traditional standards of care (34). A plan for *emergency mass critical care* must be developed and should include the following strategies:

a. Provide only the most basic critical care interventions.
b. Expand the scope of noncritical care-trained providers.
c. Provide critical care in noncritical care settings.
d. Alter triage decision making, including withholding of care.

This approach to mass-casualty events is in the process of being developed, and the directives are less well articulated for pediatric patients than for adults. Hospital ethics committees may find it beneficial to begin these considerations in the pre-event period.

TERRORIST-RELATED EVENTS

Blasts and Explosives

Epidemiology

Although theoretical concern is increasing that terrorists will deploy chemical, biological, radiological, and nuclear agents, to date, explosive devices have been utilized most commonly. The effects of blast trauma have similarities to those of conventional trauma, in that victims can sustain blunt, penetrating, burn, crush, and inhalational injuries. Blast injuries, however, do not occur in isolation and display unique injury patterns. Victims usually sustain simultaneous injuries with multisystem effects, rendering the medical management of those who survive exceedingly complex (7,15,26).

Children who are exposed to explosive/blast attacks are particularly vulnerable to multiple organ injury for the following reasons:

- Their smaller mass results in greater force applied per unit of body surface area. Because they have less fat and elastic connective tissue, the chest, abdominal, and pelvic organs are relatively less protected and, therefore, susceptible to greater injury (15).
- Children are more susceptible to fractures at the incompletely calcified growth plates of bones.
- The pediatric chest wall is more pliable, placing children at greater risk for significant cardiac and pulmonary injury (15,20).

Information compiled following the 1995 Oklahoma City bombing provided important data about the injuries that were sustained by the pediatric victims (33). Of the 816 casualties, 66 were children, 19 of whom died. Of the children who died, 16 (84%) were seated next to windows. The pattern of injury in the 19 children who died was: 100%, soft tissue injures; 37%, abdominal or thoracic injuries; 31%, amputations; 47%, arm fractures; 29%, leg fractures; 21%, burns. Ninety percent sustained skull fractures, 88% of those with cerebral evisceration ("skull capping").

TABLE 30.2				

COMPARISON OF RESOURCE UTILIZATION BETWEEN CHILDREN INJURED IN TERROR-RELATED AND CHILDREN INJURED IN NON–TERROR-RELATED TRAUMA

	Terror[a]		Non-terror[a]	
	n	%	n	%
Total	138	100	8363	100
OPERATIONS/PROCEDURES				
Yes	77	55.8	1908	22.8
No	61	44.2	6455	77.2
ICU STAY				
Yes	45	32.6	633	7.6
No	93	67.4	7726	92.4
TOTAL LENGTH OF HOSPITAL STAY				
<7 days	83	61.5	7466	89.7
≥8 days	52	38.5	861	10.3
DESTINATION AT DISCHARGE				
Home	89	65.0	8036	96.1
Rehabilitation	23	16.7	80	1.0
Death	7	5.1	57	0.7
Transfer	9	6.5	112	1.3
Other	10	6.7	78	0.9

[a]Significant (p <0.0001) difference between the 2 groups was found for all variables.
Adapted from Aharonson-Daniel L, Waisman Y, Dannon Y. Epidemiology of terror-related versus non-terror related traumatic injury in children. Pediatrics. 2003;112:280e–284e.

Injury characteristics of the 47 children who sustained non-fatal injuries included: 2 open, depressed skull fractures with extrusion of brain matter, 2 closed-head injuries, 3 arm fractures, 1 leg fracture, 1 arterial injury, 1 splenic injury, 5 tympanic membrane (TM) perforations, 3 corneal abrasions, and 4 burns. Fifteen percent required hospitalization.

A comprehensive analysis of the epidemiology of blast and explosive events in children published in 2003 highlights the pattern of blast specific injures and resource utilization in pediatric victims of terrorist acts in Israel (3,37). These data were compared with non–terror-related pediatric injuries. The majority of children injured in blast attacks sustained multiple injuries, had a higher percentage of neurologic injury and medical instability, and had a greater need for both immediate acute care and prolonged pediatric intensive care. The differences in medical resource utilization between the 2 groups are outlined in **Table 30.2**. These data underscore the fact that hospital and healthcare resources have been significantly affected by mass casualty events and that such events would likely overwhelm current medical systems.

Blast Properties

Explosives can be categorized according to speed, size, weight, TNT equivalents, source, original purpose, and adulterant components ("dirty bomb," bolts, nails). Typically, explosives

TABLE 30.3

OVERVIEW OF MECHANISM OF BLAST INJURY

Classification	Characteristics	Anatomic area affected	Types of injuries
Primary	Unique to high-order explosives, results from the impact of the overpressurization wave	Gas-filled structures: lungs, gastrointestinal tract, auditory system	Blast lung or pulmonary barotrauma, bowel rupture, tympanic membrane rupture, traumatic brain injury
Secondary	Results from shrapnel and flying debris	Can cause injury to any anatomic area	Penetrating foreign body to globe, chest, abdomen
Tertiary	Results from acceleration-deceleration forces from blast that propels victims	Can cause injury to any anatomic area	Traumatic amputation, fractures to face, pelvis, ribs, spine
Quaternary	Results from exposure to blast-related events, such as fire and collapsed building structures	Can cause injury to any anatomic area	Crush injuries, first- and second-degree burns, exacerbation of underlying disease states

Adapted from: CDC Mass Trauma Preparedness and Response website at http://www.bt.cdc.gov/masscasualties/explosions.asp#classification. Accessed September 2006.

are categorized as high-order explosives (HE) and low-order explosives (LE). HE create supersonic overpressurization shock waves and require detonation. Examples of HE are all military bombs, TNT, ammonium nitrate fuel oil, and C-4 "plastic" explosives. HE explosions result in primary blast injury (PBI) (26,39).

LEs produce subsonic explosions and do not create the shock wave characterized by HE. They are composed of propellants and undergo deflagration rather than the detonation caused by HE. In comparison to HE, the release of energy from LE is slower. Although LE explosions are associated with significant mortality and morbidity, they rarely result in the characteristic pulmonary and central nervous system (CNS) injuries unique to PBI from HE. primarily result in penetrating injuries from shrapnel and flying debris, crush, blunt, and burn injuries, and they include pipe bombs, gunpowder, and pure petroleum-based bombs (Molotov cocktails) (26,39).

Environmental Factors

The severity of blast-related injury depends upon the environment in which the blast occurs. Mortality and morbidity are significantly greater when the blast occurs in a confined space or is associated with a collapsed building or other enclosed space (17). Open spaces (e.g., street corner, open market) are associated with a 10% fatality rate, confined spaces (e.g., bus) are associated with a 20% fatality rate (70% of fatalities die at the scene), and enclosed spaces (within a structure, e.g., building) are associated with a 20% fatality rate (90% of fatalities die at the scene).

Mechanism of Injury

The severity of injury from blast trauma is related almost exclusively to three main factors: the distance of the victim from the site of explosion (32), the environment in which the explosion occurs (open versus confined space) (25), and the proximity to solid surfaces (blast waves are reflected off of solid surfaces and increase the victim's level of exposure). PBIs occur exclusively from exposure to HE and result in specific injury patterns (13,26). The mechanisms of injury from blast exposures can be divided into four relatively distinct categories: primary, secondary, tertiary, and quaternary. Secondary, tertiary, and quaternary injuries often occur simultaneously and can result from either LE or HE. Penetrating and blunt trauma are the predominant types of injuries in post-explosion survivors. Blast lung injury (BLI) (described below) is the most common injury causing death in those victims initially surviving an explosion. An overview of the mechanisms of blast injury is provided in **Table 30.3**.

Clinical Sequelae of Blast Injuries

Primary Blast Injury

The injuries of PBI are directly related to the effects on air filled organs. The organ systems most commonly affected are pulmonary, GI, and auditory. Brain, cardiothoracic, and ocular structures are affected as well. These injuries are described in the following sections.

Blast Lung Injury

Pulmonary barotrauma that results in pulmonary contusion and air embolism represents the most common cause of death from PBI.

Pathophysiology. Macro and micro tears in pulmonary tissue that result in pulmonary hemorrhage, edema, and loss of structural integrity are the major causes of damage in PBI. On a cellular level, shock waves produce an inflammatory response; IL-8 is released, causing mobilization of polymorphonuclear leukocytes (PMLs) into the systemic circulation (36). The release of proinflammatory cytokines promotes the expression of the CD11b receptor complex on the PML surface, leading to adhesion at the site of injury. This "reaction" impairs gas exchange at the level of the alveoli. Air emboli result when the integrity of the blood vessels is interrupted and interface between blood vessels and air spaces occurs, allowing air bubbles to escape into the circulation (22,28,36).

Clinical Findings. The clinical triad of apnea, bradycardia, and hypotension is usually evident immediately post-explosion.

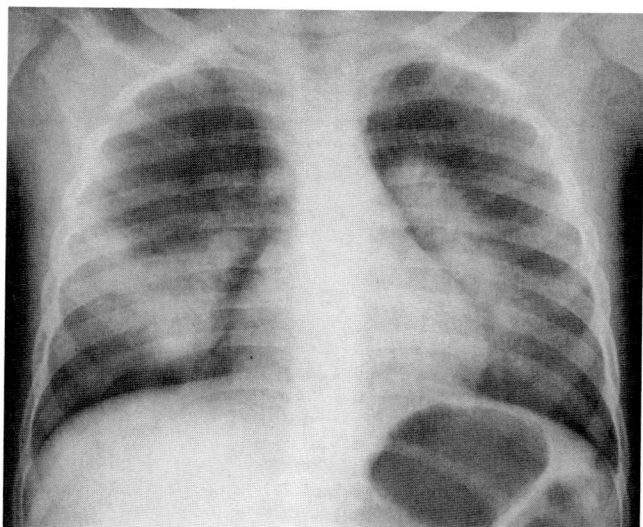

FIGURE 30.1. Typical "butterfly" pattern" blast lung injury. From Sosna J, Sella T, Shaham D, et al. Facing the new threats of terrorism: Radiologists' perspectives based on experience in Israel. *Radiology.* 2005;237(1):28–36, with permission.

Symptoms may, however, present and/or progress for up to 48 hrs post-explosion. Deterioration results in acute respiratory failure and/or acute respiratory distress syndrome (ARDS). Chest x-ray reveals a classic white butterfly pattern (35) (**Fig. 30.1**).

The diagnosis of BLI should be considered in any victim with dyspnea, cough, chest pain, or hemoptysis following exposure to a blast. The pulmonary injuries evident on a microscopic level range from petechiae to massive hemorrhage. The signs and symptoms associated with BLI are listed in **Table 30.4**.

The development of air emboli, a specific and particularly ominous complication of BLI, is directly related to the degree of injury sustained. The risk of mortality is high, given that emboli can occlude coronary and cerebral vessels, as well as cardiac outflow tracts, resulting in myocardial ischemia, stroke, and shock. Additional significant morbidity is related to ocular vessel occlusion, causing blindness, and vital end-organ ischemia (38).

It is crucial that those clinicians who care for patients with blast exposure be cognizant of the early manifestations of air embolization. It may be difficult to diagnose because other serious clinical conditions have similar presenting signs and symptoms. A heightened sense of suspicion in these select cases is paramount to optimizing the patient's outcome.

Treatment and Management. By definition, patients in the ICU have survived the initial resuscitation phase of their treatment. If BLI is aggressively treated initially, the potential for survival is greater. Initial treatment consists of administration of 100% oxygen therapy and maintaining a patent airway. Most victims will require mechanical ventilation. The risk of pneumothoraces (simple and tension) is high. Prophylactic chest tube placement is recommended prior to induction of anesthesia and/or interinstitutional transport. Massive hemoptysis is managed with endotracheal intubation and selective ventilation of the uninvolved lung, although this technique may be difficult in small children. Determining the source of bleeding is

TABLE 30.4

OVERVIEW OF BLAST-RELATED INJURY

System	Injury or condition
Auditory	Traumatic tympanic membrane rupture, disruption of middle and inner ear structures (ossicles and cochlea)
Respiratory	Blast lung, pulmonary barotrauma, hemothorax, pneumothorax, pulmonary hemorrhage, arteriovenovenous fistula from air embolism, aspiration pneumonitis
Gastrointestinal	Bowel perforation, organ rupture, mesenteric ischemia from air embolism
Cardiovascular/ circulatory	Cardiac contusion; air embolism, which causes myocardial infarction, cardiogenic shock, peripheral vascular injury
Ocular	Globe rupture, foreign bodies, orbital fractures, air embolism
Neurologic	Closed brain injury, concussion, cerebral and spinal cord infarcts from air embolism
Renal/genitalia	Renal contusion, laceration, fracture, testicular rupture
Musculoskeletal	Bony fractures, traumatic amputations, crush injuries, compartment syndrome, burns, lacerations

Adapted from: CDC Mass Trauma Preparedness and Response website at http://www.bt.cdc.gov/masscasualties/explosions.asp#classification. Accessed on September 2006.

often a great challenge. In some cases, both lungs are involved, also rendering selective ventilation unrealistic (4,39).

Diagnostic imaging or medical interventions may aid in confirming the diagnosis of air embolism. Echocardiography, CT scan, and bronchoscopy can provide direct visualization of air bubbles. Transesophageal echocardiography allows visualization of air particles as small as 2 μm. Suspicion of coronary artery air emboli must be managed aggressively with oxygen and attempts to stop the further passage of air. A tight-fitting mask with 100% oxygen must be applied immediately. Rapid and aggressive treatment to stop air entry into the circulation system is indicated. The approach used to treat air emboli in the blast trauma patient is extrapolated from the standard treatment recommended for massive air embolization caused by nonexplosion-related blunt or penetrating trauma. Thoracotomy on the affected side is usually recommended; however, blast injuries may be associated with multiple sites of injury, and selective thoracotomy may not be effective (4). The safest management strategy is to place the patient in either a modified left lateral decubitus/prone position or injured-lung side down position to increase venous pressure on that side and reduce/minimize embolization. Placing affected patients in these positions makes the most anatomic and physiologic sense, though data is not adequate to support this management strategy as improving overall outcomes. An additional mode of therapy that has theoretic potential for treating air emboli is hyperbaric oxygen therapy. Although experience is scant with this approach in the setting of blast injuries, it has been successful in treating cerebral emboli that develop from diving decompression injuries, by reducing air bubble volume (4,39).

The use of positive pressure ventilation (PPV) has been recommended but is controversial and should only be considered in circumstances of severe respiratory failure or massive hemoptysis. Documented reports of sudden cardiovascular, respiratory, and neurologic collapse with the initiation of PPV make it difficult to recommend. The risk of pulmonary alveolar rupture from PPV is significant, resulting in additional formation of air emboli that might enter the circulation, resulting in fatal coronary artery emboli (4).

Mechanical ventilation for patients with BLI who require intubation presents a similar challenge as does the use of PPV. Treatment recommendations for the ARDS and pulmonary contusions that result from conventional trauma and disease provide guidelines for the clinical manifestations of BLI. General principles include maintaining low tidal volumes and peak inspiratory pressures and high peak end-expiratory pressures. Extracorporeal oxygenation may be considered as a last resort. Specifics of management are discussed in detail in Chapters 36 and 37.

Much of the data on BLI survival and outcomes come from the experience and retrospective review of victims of terrorist blast attacks in Israel. Most BLI survivors require mechanical ventilation. Severe BLI is, not surprisingly, associated with the highest mortality rates and includes profound hypoxemia (PaO_2/FIO_2 <60 mm Hg), bilateral pneumothoraces, and bilateral lung infiltrates on x-ray. Those victims of moderate and mild BLI have better potential to recover fully if treated aggressively with the supportive measures just described (26).

Gastrointestinal Blast Injury

Injury to the GI tract is the second most common lethal injury from exposure to a blast. As with other air-filled organs, the overpressurization wave from a blast attack causes extensive compression and distortion of the GI tract. The manifestations of "blast-abdomen" are generally delayed, presenting from 8–36 hrs postexposure. These are patients who will have survived to inpatient admission, most likely, to the ICU.

Pathophysiology. The terminal ileum and colon are especially vulnerable to blast effects. These areas are at significant risk for perforation. The small intestine, which has less air than the terminal ileum and large colon, is not as dramatically affected. Solid-organ rupture is a lethal effect of blast injury. Fractures of the liver and spleen, ruptured testicle, and subcapsular and retroperitoneal hematomas represent high-morbidity injuries following blast trauma. These injuries may be difficult to diagnose for a variety of reasons. Onset of symptoms is often delayed; other more immediately obvious injuries may distract the physician from the often subtle initial findings that would suggest significant abdominal trauma (12,38).

Clinical Findings. The signs and symptoms associated with intra-abdominal injury are listed in **Table 30.5**. These findings are often subtle and may be overshadowed, clinically, by other critical injuries. Recognizing that evidence of abdominal injury

TABLE 30.5

SIGNS AND SYMPTOMS ASSOCIATED WITH BLAST ABDOMINAL INJURY

Absence of bowel sounds
Abdominal pain
Abdominal distension
Hematochezia
Hypotension
Involuntary guarding
Rebound tenderness
Nausea and vomiting
Orthostasis/syncope
Testicular pain
Tenesmus

Adapted from Foltin GL, Schoenfeld D, Shannon M. *Pediatric Terrorism and Disaster Preparedness A Resource for Pediatricians.* AHRQ Publication Nos. 06(07)-0056 and 06(07)-0056-1, October 2006. Agency for Healthcare Research and Quality, Rockville, MD. http://www.ahrq.gov/research/pedprep/resource.htm. Accessed May 2007.

may develop slowly and insidiously is crucial in preventing unnecessary morbidity and mortality.

Management. The initial management of these patients in the emergency department includes meticulous attention to the ABCs of Advanced Trauma Life Support protocols (airway with C-spine control, breathing, and circulation). Once a patient has arrived in the ICU, the diagnosis of abdominal blast injury may already have been addressed. The critical care physician must know, however, that abdominal injuries in these circumstances are a significant cause of delayed mortality. CT scan, ultrasonography, and diagnostic peritoneal lavage are the most reliable methods used to detect intra-abdominal injury. CT scan provides excellent data on intra-abdominal hemorrhage, organ injury, free intraperitoneal air, and intramural hematomas, but CT is not reliable for detecting hollow viscus perforation in early stages.

For patients who may be compromised from other significant injuries, it is reasonable to begin prophylactic antibiotics until such time that a definitive intervention/procedure can confirm an intact bowel and GI tract. Exploratory laparotomy may be required to identify a peritoneal source of bleeding in the hemodynamically unstable patient. Any surgical intervention for these patients carries an enormous risk given the other severe injuries likely sustained as a result of the blast. In general, patients who require surgery under these circumstances do poorly (7).

Blast Auditory Injury

The auditory system is extremely susceptible to injury from blast explosions. Given this vulnerability, the ear is the organ most frequently injured in a blast event. Auditory injuries are frequently overlooked, however, because victims of blast attacks will likely have distracting life-threatening injuries. Fortunately, following damage from blast injuries, the external ear heals well. Healing of the middle and inner ear occurs less reliably. Permanent sensorineural hearing loss occurs in approximately 30% of victims as a result of profound irreversible injury to the sensory epithelial tissue located in the inner ear (hair cells of the organ of Corti). Typically, however, hearing loss and tinnitus are temporary and resolve within hours to days after exposure to a blast (12,16). The TM is often perforated as a result of exposure to a blast overpressurization wave. In the setting of blast injury, TM rupture may be a marker for more significant organ injury.

Pathophysiology. Sound waves travel through the ear canal, interface with the TM, and are then transmitted via the ossicles through the air-filled middle ear. These sound waves are then converted to nerve impulses when they reach the cochlea of the inner ear. The organ of Corti, located on the cochlea, is comprised of specialized sensory epithelia (hair cells). These specialized sensory epithelial cells transmit sound wave information to the vestibulocochlear nerve (cranial nerve VIII). This delicate, intertwined system is severely disrupted from exposure to the overpressure wave created by blast attack (12).

Clinical Findings. The clinical findings expected from blast injury to the auditory canal are highlighted in **Table 30.6**. Damage to the auditory canal may be overlooked because of the severity of associated injuries. It is important to remain cognizant of the signs and symptoms of auditory damage. A thorough evaluation of the auditory canal and hearing function should be conducted when the patient is stabilized and awake. If damage has been identified, measures must be taken to promote healing and prevent further structural and functional damage (12).

Management. In cases in which a blast injury results in disfiguring injuries that include exposed cartilage, management may require the skills of a plastic or ear, nose, throat (ENT) surgeon. Evaluation of the middle ear must be achieved to determine if the TM is ruptured. The ear canal may be obstructed by blood or other debris and must be carefully cleaned in order to obtain visualization of the TM. In the setting of TM disruption, antibiotics are recommended only in the case of infection. The vast majority of TM ruptures heal spontaneously. However, a small proportion do not heal and require surgical grafting. It is therefore imperative that an ENT surgeon follow-up to

TABLE 30.6

SIGNS AND SYMPTOMS ASSOCIATED WITH BLAST AUDITORY INJURY

Tinnitus
Otalgia
Otorrhea
Tympanic rupture
Ossicular chain disruption and fracture
Perilymphatic fistula
Conductive and sensory hearing loss
Basilar membrane rupture

Adapted from Foltin GL, Schoenfeld D, Shannon M. Pediatric Terrorism and Disaster Preparedness A Resource for Pediatricians. AHRQ Publication Nos. 06(07)-0056 and 06(07)-0056-1, October 2006. Agency for Healthcare Research and Quality, Rockville, MD. http://www.ahrq.gov/research/pedprep/resource.htm. Accessed May 2007.

confirm adequate healing or referral for longer-term follow-up. Cholesteatoma is a complication associated with blast TM perforations. These infections result in significant bony destruction and have the potential to invade the intracranial space. Long-term follow-up should be arranged for these patients to help prevent this infrequent but debilitating complication (12).

No reliably proven treatment including corticosteroids, vasodilators, and vitamin supplements exists for blast-induced sensorineural hearing loss. While little, if any, data support reversal of symptoms or improved outcomes with these therapies, some investigators suggest using the strategies aggressively in cases in which the alternative may be total permanent deafness. Environmental factors that include noise restraint may play a role in healing. In the ICU setting, this may be challenging. However, reasonable attempts should be made to control excessive and extraneous noise in the surrounding environment (16).

Effects of Blast Explosives on Other Organ Systems

Cardiovascular Effects

Victims of blast exposure may suffer profound cardiovascular injury, causing mortality without significant signs of external trauma (23). Researchers have studied the effects of blast attacks on the cardiovascular system in survivors and in animal models. The clinical triad of bradycardia, hypotension, and apnea results from a vagally mediated reflex response to exposure to a blast attack (30). The cardiovascular system normally responds to decreases in heart rate, stroke volume, and cardiac index by increasing systemic vascular resistance, thereby increasing or maintaining blood pressure to maintain cardiac output and brain perfusion. In victims of blast injury, this normal reflex increase in systemic vascular resistance does not occur, resulting in a dramatic fall in blood pressure. If the initial insult from the blast is not lethal, return of normal cardiovascular function may occur within several hours.

It is important to recognize that hypotension may also be a result of significant volume loss from internal hemorrhage or major musculoskeletal injury. Direct injury to the heart and blood vessels often occurs as a result of exposure to a blast wave. Victims suffer from coronary vessel embolization and cardiovascular ischemia (7).

Clinical Signs and Symptoms. Myocardial damage or ischemia may result in the characteristic signs and symptoms associated with acute myocardial infarction: chest pain, shortness of breath, nausea, and diaphoresis. Hypotension, tachycardia, and poor perfusion, as previously mentioned, may be the result of volume loss from internal injuries.

Management. Supportive therapy represents the most reasonable approach to victims who suffer from cardiovascular injury. Maintaining euvolemia should be the goal of fluid therapy. Aggressive volume replacement typically utilized for routine trauma patients is not the best approach for victims of blast attacks. In these cases, impaired pulmonary function is likely, given the mechanism of injury, and increased fluids may further compromise lung function.

Ophthalmologic Injuries

Serious ophthalmologic injury occurs in 10%–28% of survivors of PBI. Injuries are overwhelmingly a result of secondary blast injury, from flying debris inflicting a wide range of penetrating eye trauma. Globe rupture represents the most significant of these injuries, which also include orbital fractures, hyphema, corneoscleral and lid lacerations, traumatic cataracts, optic nerve damage, and retinitis (13,26).

Management. As with auditory injuries, eye trauma will generally be addressed after life-threatening conditions are treated and stabilized in the emergency department setting. However, blast-related eye injuries often require relatively immediate intervention to optimize outcome. Best outcomes are associated with interventions that occur within 12 hrs of injury (8).

Neurologic Injury

PBI can cause significant injury to the brain, which results from rapid shifts in air pressure caused by the blast wave. High incidence of cranial injury is seen in children exposed to primary blast attacks. Of those who survive, injuries include concussion, barotrauma from acute gas embolization, and coup and contrecoup injuries. Air emboli can cause cerebral infarcts and occlude spinal cord vessels. The resulting neurologic deficits are due to mild to severe traumatic brain injury. It has been estimated that the mortality rate of victims who sustain neurologic injury is 8–25% (7).

Pathophysiology. Many of the pathophysiologic factors that cause brain damage following traumatic brain injury play a role in PBI. These include increased levels of inducible nitric oxide synthase, injury due to excitotoxicity, and oxidative stress. Patterns of disease include diffuse axonal injury (26). Direct effects of cerebral hemorrhage that results in increased intracranial pressure (ICP) also contribute significantly to the severity of traumatic brain injury. Open and closed brain injury may be caused by tertiary blast effects, which are characterized by victims being thrown from the intensity of the "blast-wind" (26).

Clinical Signs and Symptoms. Signs and symptoms of neurologic injury may vary from mild to severe and can include headache, vertigo, altered mental status, focal neurologic deficits, seizures, paresthesias, and coma.

Management. The severity of the injury will dictate the level of management. Standard measures to reduce increased ICP should be employed as needed. Expertise of a neurosurgeon will be necessary to implement invasive techniques, such as intraventricular drain insertion, craniectomy, surgical removal of foreign body imbedded in brain tissue, and control of intracranial hemorrhage, to treat and manage brain injury. Those children who survive and have sustained any level of traumatic brain injury should be closely monitored after discharge and should undergo formal neurologic evaluation to determine the need for rehabilitation.

NONCONVENTIONAL WEAPONS

The acronym CBRN is commonly used for nonconventional terror weapons: chemical-biological-radiological-nuclear.

Chemical

Chemical agents include nerve, asphyxiant, choking/pulmonary, and blistering/vesicant. The agents of chemical terrorism may originate from military, industrial, medical, or other sources. In the event of chemical agent attack, the prehospital system will likely be overwhelmed with victims seeking care. As with any terror event, in addition to those actually harmed, many more "worried well" may present for care, further stressing the healthcare system.

Initial Approach to Chemical Attack

The single most important first step for treating all chemical exposures is the initial decontamination strategy. Immediate removal of patient clothing can eliminate approximately 90% of contaminants. After the clothing is removed, the patient's skin and eyes may require decontamination. In most cases, decontamination of skin can be accomplished by gentle and thorough washing with water and soap, if available. Thorough decontamination should occur before a patient enters the hospital. Special challenges are encountered in decontaminating pediatric patients, including susceptibility to hypothermia, behavioral regression, and the need to decontaminate caretakers. Further details of decontamination and PPE will not be addressed here, as patients should have been completely decontaminated before any interaction with a pediatric intensive care physician.

Nerve Agents

Pathophysiology. Nerve agents are similar to organophosphate insecticides and include cholinesterase inhibitors, such as Sarin, Soman, and VX. Nerve agents inhibit the action of acetylcholinesterase at cholinergic neural synapses, where acetylcholine then accumulates. These agents are generally colorless, odorless, tasteless, and nonirritating to the skin. Nerve agent vapors are denser than air and tend to accumulate in low-lying areas, putting children at risk for higher exposure. The agents used in terrorist attacks are inhaled and absorbed through skin and mucous membranes.

Clinical Signs and Symptoms. Symptoms are characteristic of muscarinic excess (rhinorrhea, bronchorrhea, bronchospasm, vomiting, diarrhea) as well as nicotinic excess (respiratory muscle paralysis and peripheral muscle fasciculation, followed by paralysis). Ocular symptoms include miosis, eye pain, vision changes, and tearing. Tachycardia or bradycardia may be present. CNS toxicity includes headache, agitation, and seizures (2).

Management. Emergent treatment of nerve agent toxicity is described in **Table 30.1**. Initial treatment includes administration of atropine followed by pralidoxime, with liberal use of benzodiazepines. Autoinjector kits ("Mark 1" kits contain a 2-mg dose of atropine and a 600-mg dose of pralidoxime) have become increasingly available in prehospital settings; however, dosing for small children and infants is not well established. The Food and Drug Administration recently approved a pediatric-sized atropine autoinjector ("AtroPen" is produced in three sizes: 0.25 mg, 0.5 mg, and 1 mg of atropine), but corresponding pralidoxime autoinjectors are not available. If pediatric patients survive a nerve agent attack and arrive at a critical care environment, they will likely need atropine and benzodiazepines for several days. Adult survivors of nerve agent exposure have required up to 20 mg of atropine over the first 24 hrs and have received pralidoxime doses repeated hourly or by infusion (500 mg/hr). Topical cycloplegics may reduce nerve agent-induced ocular pain.

Asphyxiants

Pathophysiology. Asphyxiants are toxic compounds that inhibit cytochrome oxidase, causing cellular anoxia and lactic acidosis (high anion gap). Hydrogen cyanide, the most commonly known toxicant in this class, is a colorless liquid or gas that smells like bitter almonds and has a strong affinity for the heme ring. Cyanide is also believed to be a direct neurotoxin that contributes to an excitatory injury in the brain, probably mediated by glutamate stimulation of NMDA receptors.

Clinical Signs and Symptoms. Exposure to hydrogen cyanide produces rapid onset of tachypnea, tachycardia, and flushed skin, followed by nausea, vomiting, confusion, weakness, trembling, seizures, and death. Death may occur as quickly as 8 mins after exposure. "Classic" signs of cyanide poisoning include severe dyspnea without cyanosis. The symptoms of cyanide toxicity and nerve agents may be difficult to distinguish. Cyanide exposure results in seizure activity that begins within seconds of inhalation, and death occurs within minutes, generally with little cyanosis or other findings. Nerve agent toxicity has a more

protracted course and includes symptoms described in the previous section; cyanosis will occur at a late stage, if at all.

Management. Initial management includes early administration of 100% oxygen, correction of acidosis, and seizure control. Patients who have few symptoms at presentation do not need antidotes. After decontamination, victims of cyanide poisoning may require specific therapy (**Table 30.7**). Sodium thiosulfate or amyl nitrate transform hemoglobin into methemoglobin, which combines with cyanide (removed from cytochrome oxidase) to form cyanomethemoglobin, allowing for the resumption of cellular respiration. The administration of sodium thiosulfate accelerates the normal enzymatic conversion of cyanide to thiocyanate complex, which can then be eliminated. Initial nitrate treatment may result in profound hypotension. Patients who survive the initial exposure and receive specific treatment will likely require intensive care to manage respiratory failure, ARDS, acidosis, shock, and seizures.

Choking/Pulmonary Agents

Pathophysiology. Choking agents include chlorine and phosgene, which are in the gaseous form at room temperature. Phosgene smells like "freshly mown hay." Chlorine has a strong, characteristic odor. When inhaled, these agents produce massive mucosal irritation and edema, as well as significant damage to lung parenchyma. Chlorine acts primarily on the tracheobronchial tree at the level of the respiratory epithelium of the

---

TABLE 30.7

CENTERS FOR DISEASE CONTROL CATEGORY A CHEMICAL AGENTS

Agent	Findings	Treatment
Nerve agents: Sarin, Soman, VX	Rhinorrhea, bronchorrhea, bronchospasm, respiratory muscle paralysis, eye pain	Airway, breathing, circulation support, 100% oxygen Atropine: 0.05–0.1 mg/kg (0.1–5 mg) IM, IV, ETT, IO q2–5 mins for secretions and respiratory symptoms *THEN* Pralidoxime (2-PAM): 25–50 mg/kg IM or IV (max 1 g IV, 2 g IM) repeat in 30 mins, then every 60 mins for weakness and/or high atropine requirement Diazepam: 0.3 mg/kg (max 10 mg) IV OR equivalent benzodiazepine IM, IV, IO[a]
Asphyxiants: Cyanide	"Cherry red skin," tachypnea, seizures	Airway, breathing, circulation support, 100% oxygen If conscious: No antidote If unconscious: Sodium nitrate 3%: 0.12–0.33 mL/kg (max 10 mL) slowly IV (minimum 5 mins). Often causes orthostatic hypotension. Sodium thiosulfate: 25%: 1.65 mL/kg over 10–20 mins (max 50 mL) Sodium bicarbonate for acidosis after above if unresponsive
Choking agents: Chlorine, phosgene	Eye, nose, throat irritation (especially chlorine); bronchospasm, pulmonary edema (especially phosgene)	Symptomatic care, possible bronchoscopy, aggressive management of pulmonary edema
Blistering/vesicant: "Mustard" Lewisite	Skin erythema; vesicle and ocular inflammation; respiratory tract inflammation	Symptomatic care, "burn" care, possible use of hematopoietic growth factors British Anti-Lewisite (BAL) (if available) 3 mg/kg IM q4–6 hrs for systemic effects in severe cases

[a] Some authorities recommend seizure prophylaxis with benzodiazepines, others suggest use for treatment. IM, intramuscularly; ETT, endotracheal tube; IO, intraosseous

bronchi and larger bronchioles. The resultant effects include necrosis and denudation, often with the formation of pseudomembranes. Phosgene tends to harm the gas-exchange regions of the respiratory system (respiratory bronchioles, alveolar ducts, and alveoli), causing pulmonary edema (15).

Clinical Signs and Symptoms. Chlorine and phosgene gas have both immediate and delayed effects depending on the level of exposure. Symptoms that occur soon after exposure portend a poor prognosis, indicating exposure to a massive dose (5). Chlorine victims tend to have coughing, stridor, and bronchospasm, while those exposed to phosgene typically have progressive dyspnea.

Management. After initial decontamination, management follows the standard recommendations for acute lung injury, including administration of oxygen and bronchodilators. Corticosteroids are often added to the treatment regimen. Pseudomembrane formation may lead to airway obstruction and may require bronchoscopic intervention. Bacterial superinfections are commonly seen several days after exposure and require culture-directed, aggressive antimicrobial therapy. For patients with pulmonary edema, adequate oxygenation, generous use of positive end-expiratory pressure, and careful attention to fluid balance are critical.

Blistering/Vesicant Agents

Pathophysiology. Blistering agents include sulfur mustard and Lewisite. Both were employed during World War I as maiming agents. Mustard is an alkylating compound associated with a low death rate but a high complication rate in exposed victims. Sulfur mustard is an alkylating agent that is highly toxic to rapidly reproducing and poorly differentiated cells; skin, pulmonary parenchyma, and bone marrow are frequently damaged. Although mortality is considerably lower than that caused by other chemical weapons such as nerve agents, sulfur mustard results in levels of morbidity that would overwhelm the healthcare system if large numbers of victims were exposed. Lewisite is an arsenical compound that affects skin and eyes immediately upon exposure (15).

Clinical Signs and Symptoms. Symptoms generally begin 12 hrs postexposure and include eye, skin, and pulmonary irritation, as well as blister formation. Proximal airway involvement includes rhinorrhea, hoarseness, and cough. Bacterial superinfection is common. All cellular elements of the bone marrow can be affected; megakaryocytes and granulocyte precursors are more susceptible than those of the erythropoietic system. Injury to the GI mucosa from mustard can lead to a delayed onset of more severe vomiting, diarrhea, abdominal pain, and prostration.

Management. The treatment and management for mustard exposure is primarily supportive but may include hematopoietic growth factors, such as granulocyte colony-stimulating factor and granulocyte-macrophage colony-stimulating factor. Typically, treatment will entail those interventions required to support damage to lung, skin, and soft tissue. Skin lesions are treated similarly to those of burn victims; fluid losses in these cases tend to be less than those that occur in "traditional" burn victims. Treatment for Lewisite is also primarily support-

ive; however, a specific antidote exists (British Anti-Lewisite) but is unlikely to be commonly available.

Biological Agents

The Centers for Disease Control has categorized potential agents of bioterror into 3 groups based on their potential threat. Category A agents, which constitute the highest threat, include anthrax, plague, tularemia, smallpox, the viral hemorrhagic fevers, and botulism. These agents vary widely in their infectivity, lethality, and availability of treatments. Smallpox and anthrax are particularly concerning; both of these agents can potentially be grown easily in large quantities and be disbursed by aerosol, exposing large numbers of people. As evidenced by the 2001 anthrax attacks in the US, even a small number of clinical cases of a bioterror-induced illness can panic a population and result in enormous resource utilization. Critical care physicians may be the first to recognize that such an attack has occurred. Clusters of patients with acute respiratory distress with fever (signs and symptoms consistent with anthrax, plague, tularemia), similar characteristic rash with fever (signs and symptoms consistent with smallpox and viral hemorrhagic fevers), or neurologic syndromes (botulism) should prompt immediate notification of hospital infection control teams and public heath authorities (15).

Anthrax

Pathophysiology. Anthrax disease is caused by the spore-forming, gram-positive bacterium *Bacillus anthracis*. Three types of anthrax affect humans: cutaneous anthrax, which is acquired when a spore enters the skin through a cut or an abrasion; GI tract anthrax, contracted from eating contaminated food, primarily meat from an animal that died of the disease; and pulmonary, or inhalation anthrax, which results from breathing in airborne anthrax spores. Cutaneous anthrax accounts for 95% of anthrax disease in this country. In cutaneous and GI anthrax, low-level infection occurs, leading to local edema and necrosis. Spores are phagocytosed by macrophages and germinate. In inhalational disease and in some cases of cutaneous and GI diseases, macrophages that contain bacilli detach and migrate to the regional lymph nodes and cause regional hemorrhagic lymphadenitis. Bacteria spread through the blood and lymph, resulting in septicemia. Anthrax bacilli secrete two exotoxins (edema toxin and lethal toxin) that are active in host cells. Edema toxin results in massive edema via a cyclic-AMP pathway, and lethal toxin causes an inflammatory activation of macrophages, leading to a cytokine storm state (14).

Clinical Signs and Symptoms. Cutaneous lesions in the form of papules appear 1–7 days after exposure. Papules progress to form vesicles and then ulcerate, resulting in a black eschar which covers the lesion. The incubation time of inhalational anthrax is most commonly thought to be 1–7 days, but periods of up to 2 months have been described. Inhalational illness is biphasic; 1–6 days after exposure, victims develop nonspecific upper respiratory infection-type symptoms; they then appear to recover. Later-appearing symptoms include high fever, respiratory distress, shock, and death (75% fatality rate if untreated). The chest x-ray may be notable for mediastinal widening and

TABLE 30.8

CENTERS FOR DISEASE CONTROL CATEGORY A BIOLOGICAL AGENTS

Agent	Findings	Treatment
Inhalational: Anthrax	Febrile, widened mediastinum, effusions, sepsis	Ciprofloxacin: (10 mg/kg/dose) IV (max 400 mg) q12 hrs OR doxycycline: 2.2 mg/kg/dose IV (max 100 mg) q12 hrs AND 1–2 other drugs[a]
Plague	Pneumonia, sepsis	Gentamicin: 2.5 mg/kg/dose IV q8 hrs OR doxycycline: 2.2 mg/kg/dose IV (max 100 mg) q12 hrs OR ciprofloxacin: (10 mg/kg/dose) IV (max 400 mg) q12 hrs OR chloramphenicol 25 mg/kg q6 hrs IV (max 4 g/ day)[b]
Tularemia	Pneumonia, hilar adenopathy	Gentamicin: 2.5 mg/kg/dose IV q8 hrs OR doxycycline: 2.2 mg/kg/dose IV (max 100 mg) q12 hrs OR ciprofloxacin: (10 mg/kg/dose) IV (max 400 mg) q12 hrs
Smallpox	Multiple firm pustules all in the same stage of evolution, fever	Vaccination for exposure within 96 hrs Potential use of cidofovir or analogs
Viral hemorrhagic fevers	Fever, bleeding, shock	Supportive, ribavirin for some etiologies (Lassa)
Botulism	Flaccid afebrile descending paralysis	Antitoxin, supportive care

[a]Penicillin, amoxicillin, clindamycin. Most authorities would treat with three to four drugs for 2 weeks, then switch to monotherapy or dual therapy to complete in 60 days when sensitivities are known. Anthrax may have either natural or engineered resistance elements.
[b]Recommended for plague meningitis. Serum levels and hematologic adverse events must be monitored.

may lack infiltrates. Blood cultures may be positive, and meningitis often occurs in more than 50% of victims (31).

Management. Specific multiagent antimicrobial therapy is required, as well as aggressive ventilatory and intravascular support for the multiorgan system failure that occurs in severely affected patients. Antimicrobial treatment is detailed in **Table 30.8**. A monoclonal antibody against one of the anthrax toxins was approved for prevention and treatment of anthrax in 2006, but its efficacy has been demonstrated in animal models only. Person-to-person transmission of anthrax is not possible; therefore, standard precautions are the only required infection control measures.

Yersinia pestis

Pathophysiology. *Yersinia pestis* causes plague, which can naturally occur in septicemic, bubonic, or pneumonic forms. Like anthrax, a bioterrorist incident that involves plague would likely occur through aerosolization and result in pneumonic involvement. Direct inhalation of the bacillus results in pneumonic plague and subsequent bacteremia and septicemia. The bacillus causes a multilobar hemorrhagic and necrotizing bronchopneumonia.

Clinical Signs and Symptoms. After an incubation period of 2–8 days (less for aerosolized exposure), rapidly progressive pulmonary disease with hemoptysis and cyanosis develops. Cough with purulent sputum (gram-negative rods may be seen) may be present. Pneumonia is evident on chest x-ray. Untreated pneumonic plague progresses to respiratory failure and shock, resulting in death in nearly 100% of victims.

Management. Immediate early treatment (**Table 30.8**) with an aminoglycoside or doxycycline is critical. Chloramphenicol is the recommended treatment regimen when plague-induced

meningitis occurs. Patients with pneumonic plague should be cared for using droplet precautions until they have received 72 hrs of antibiotic therapy (21).

Francisella tularensis

Pathophysiology. *Francisella tularensis* is a highly virulent, small, nonmotile, aerobic, gram-negative, coccobacillus that causes tularemia after host contact with infected animal carcasses or fluids, in glandular, oculoglandular, oropharyngeal, septicemic, typhoidal, and pneumonic forms. A bioterror aerosol release of *F. tularensis* primarily causes pulmonary disease, although other forms are possible. *F. tularensis* is a facultative intracellular bacterium that multiplies within macrophages, allowing it to invade the lymph nodes, lungs, pleura, spleen, and liver.

Clinical Signs and Symptoms. After 1–14 days postexposure, victims develop an influenza-like illness and atypical pneumonia; chest x-ray may show hilar adenopathy. After inhalational exposure, hemorrhagic inflammation of the airways develops and progresses to necrotizing pneumonia. Pleural disease is common. Bacteremia may be common in early stages.

Management. Treatment (**Table 30.8**) with gentamicin or doxycycline reduces mortality from 30% to 10% (31). Person-to-person spread of tularemia is not possible; therefore, standard precautions are the only infection control measure required (21).

Terror-related Viral Agents

Variola Virus—Smallpox

Pathophysiology. Since naturally occurring smallpox disease no longer exists, a single case of smallpox (Variola virus) anywhere in the world would be considered evidence that a bioterror attack has occurred. Much of the population does not have immunity to this disease, and children have not been vaccinated in the US since 1971. It is not known if the smallpox virus exists outside of official stores in the US and Russia, but some fear that it does. Variola infection follows the transmission of infective aerosolized droplets to the oropharyngeal or respiratory mucosa. The infective dose is believed to be only a few virions. Macrophages are the first cells infected; the virus then migrates along the lymphatics and multiplies in regional lymph nodes. Infected macrophages migrate from these vessels into the epidermis, and necrosis and edema follow. Polymorphonuclear leukocytes then migrate into these areas, forming pustules.

Clinical Signs and Symptoms. Individuals infected with smallpox present clinically with a general viral prodrome that is characterized by high fever and constitutional symptoms. The characteristic rash of smallpox begins on the face and rapidly spreads centrifugally. The patient's fever decreases with the onset of rash and infectivity begins. Lesions progress as a group through stages of being macular, papular, vesicular, and finally as deep, hard, large pustules that crust after 8–10 days. These crusts eventually separate (2–4 weeks), leaving scars. Once the crusts are separated, the patient is no longer infectious. Historic mortality rates in unimmunized populations were approximately 30% and were higher in children <1 year of age. Death most often occurred in the second week of illness from multiorgan failure secondary to overwhelming viremia.

Management. Treatment is primarily supportive. Appropriate antibiotic coverage for bacterial superinfections will likely be required. Cidofovir has been shown to have a beneficial effect in animal models, but its efficacy in humans is unknown (6). If smallpox occurs, mass vaccination campaigns must take place; vaccination within 72–96 hrs after exposure provides good protection against disease and excellent protection against fatal disease (6). Vaccinia immune globulin has no clinical benefit for patients who are infected with smallpox. Persons hospitalized with smallpox should be cared for in a negative-pressure environment, with staff using both airborne and contact precautions. Ideally, only staff previously vaccinated for smallpox should care for victims.

Viral Hemorrhagic Fevers

Pathophysiology. The viral hemorrhagic fevers are a group of infections caused by a variety of agents (e.g., Ebola and Lassa). The clinical manifestations are similar, and include rash and fever. Bleeding diathesis which can progress into severe hemorrhagic disease can occur, manifested as bleeding from internal organs and mucous membranes.

Clinical Signs and Symptoms. After an incubation period ranging from 2–28 days, victims of the viral hemorrhagic fevers develop rash and fever, variable bleeding diatheses, petechiae, mucosal hemorrhages, hematuria, and GI bleeding. Diagnosis of the specific agents is made epidemiologically or by acute and convalescent titers.

Management. Treatment advice must be obtained from public health authorities; ribavirin might be effective for several of the viruses. Florid cases will require extensive amounts of blood products to support victims. Empiric isolation should include airborne and contact precautions, unless the exact nature of the virus is known.

Terror-related Preformed Toxins

Pathophysiology. *Clostridium botulinum* is a spore-forming anaerobe that produces the most lethal toxin that exists, with an LD50 in humans estimated at 0.000001 mg/kg (1). Botulism occurs naturally in three main forms: food-borne botulism, wound botulism, and infant botulism. An intentional release of botulism toxin would result in cases of inhalational disease. The seven known serotypes of botulism toxin act by inhibiting acetylcholine release, thereby decoupling the nervous system from skeletal muscle, causing death from aspiration and respiratory arrest. Each serologic type of toxin acts on one or more proteins of the soluble N-ethylmaleimide-sensitive factor-attachment protein receptor (SNARE) complex, which mediates exocytosis of acetylcholine. Recovery from botulism occurs in part by recovery of function in poisoned presynaptic terminals. Axonal sprouting, with creation of new presynaptic terminals, is of equal or greater importance in recovery. Both processes occur over weeks to months.

Clinical Signs and Symptoms. The epidemiology of a botulism terror attack would likely include multiple victims presenting for care from between hours to 3 days after exposure. Lack of acetylcholine release at the neuromuscular junction produces weakness of skeletal muscles, initially causing an acute, afebrile, descending paralysis, with cranial nerve palsies and progressive respiratory failure. Inhibition of acetylcholine release also occurs at the parasympathetic terminals, leading to autonomic signs and symptoms. No change in sensation or level of consciousness occurs.

Management. Close monitoring of the respiratory effort of botulism victims is critical; bedside pulmonary function testing allows for the decision of ventilatory support to be made efficiently. Treatment is supportive; without treatment, patients may need ventilatory support for weeks. Even a small attack could overwhelm a municipality's supplies of ventilators. The CDC has stocks of a bivalent (A and B) equine antiserum that can considerably reduce the amount of time that victims require ICU care. An investigational equine serotype E antitoxin has also been developed, and the US military holds an investigational heptavalent (A-G) antitoxin. As with any equine product, skin testing and possible desensitization are necessary; serum sickness is likely. Human-to-human spread of botulism does not occur; therefore, standard precautions are the only infection control measures required.

Radiological/Nuclear

Radiological and nuclear terrorism have a wide spectrum of possible effects. Regardless of the magnitude of the damage or contamination, widespread panic will occur within the affected geographic area. Radiological terror involves exposing portions of the population to radioactive materials, most likely with a radiological dispersal device (or "dirty bomb"). Such devices use conventional explosives to disperse radioactive materials that have potential to contaminate limited geographic areas. The ensuing panic may lead to injuries during unplanned evacuations.

A nuclear attack involves fission; immediate morbidity and mortality result from the explosive force of the detonation. Acute radiation syndrome (or "radiation sickness") can occur in the survivors of a nuclear attack. Despite widespread concerns over potential attacks on nuclear power plants, such an attack would likely cause radiological exposure, as opposed to a full blown nuclear event. Nuclear experts believe that a nuclear reactor "meltdown" would be prevented by the multitude of safety devices that nuclear power plants have in place (15,29).

Decontamination

Unlike some of the biological and chemical scenarios described previously, decontamination of radiological victims is less time sensitive. Critical and life-threatening conditions should be treated before decontamination occurs. As with chemical exposures, removal of clothing will eliminate 90% of contamination. If a patient is exposed to radioactive material and is alive upon arrival at a hospital, he is very unlikely to be sufficiently contaminated to cause harm to healthcare workers. After stabilization of conventional injuries, the patient can be disrobed and washed with soap and water (run-off should be contained). The eyes may then be flushed. Standard precautions are the only measures required for healthcare workers who do not come into direct contact with radioactive dust or debris.

Pathophysiology. For both radiological and nuclear victims, a dose- and time-dependent illness occurs at predictable intervals after exposure. Acute radiation syndrome is most likely to occur in those who are exposed to a nuclear detonation but who were far enough away not to die from the blast effects. A radiological dispersal device is significantly less likely to cause acute radiation syndrome. Military, industrial, and medical exposures can also lead to acute radiation syndrome. Progenitor and rapidly dividing cells are the most significantly affected by radiation exposure; the hematopoietic, reproductive, and GI systems are the most severely affected.

Clinical Signs and Symptoms. Victims of radiation exposure are likely to initially have a nonspecific prodrome (hours to days of nausea, vomiting, and fatigue), followed by a latent period, culminating in illness that can occur from days to weeks after exposure. All cell lines of the hematopoietic system are the first to be affected. Severely affected patients have total loss of their hematopoietic system, much like a bone marrow transplant patient who has had a fully ablative preparative regimen. Hemorrhage and sepsis are common. The GI system is affected, causing mucosal sloughing, hemorrhage, obstruction, and sepsis. Radiation pneumonitis can occur and requires aggressive ventilatory support. High doses of radiation cause acute microvascular injury to the CNS. Intractable seizures and elevated ICP are associated with high morbidity.

Management. Treatment is supportive (fluids, nutrition, antimicrobials, skin care, hematopoietic growth factors). The possibility of rescue hematopoietic stem cell transplantation exists for a select group of victims—those who have received a dose of radiation that is lethal to the bone marrow but not other body systems (10). The full spectrum of assessment and treatment of radiation sickness is beyond the scope of this text, but several important points to consider include:

- Health physicists and/or nuclear medicine physicians will help to determine the specific exposure and prognosis.
- Life-threatening injuries should be treated before decontamination.
- Specific antidotes are unlikely to be helpful in the critical care environment (it is possible that some victims will have been given potassium iodide in an attempt to avoid the carcinogenic effects of radioactive iodine, which could be released in a nuclear power plant incident), but some chelating agents may have efficacy.

While all PICUs will be able to treat one or more victims of severe radiation exposure, these patients will require tremendous resource utilization, and surge capacity may be quickly overwhelmed. Expert nuclear medicine and health physicist advice and guidance will be critical in determining which victims are most likely to benefit from critical care interventions. This expertise will help to determine if exposure-specific treatments are available.

CONCLUSIONS AND FUTURE DIRECTIONS

Emergency preparedness has become a high priority endeavor for governmental and healthcare institutions and a critical necessity. Plans that appropriately and adequately include the treatment and management of children lag behind the developed strategies that address adult mass casualty victims. Improving the systems of emergency care, in general, requires coordination between federal, state, regional, and municipal agencies (11). Advocating for the needs of children as an integral component of these efforts is crucial. Developing best practice models that can be widely adopted should be based on evidence-based standards. A 2004 consensus report meticulously describes important first steps in accomplishing these necessary goals (27). An important stated objective is expanding and refining our current knowledge base as it relates to the needs of pediatric victims of terrorism. The report underscores the need for strong advocacy to ensure the implementation of the proposed recommendations and guidelines.

KEY POINTS

- Terrorism and mass casualty events affect a disproportionate number of children.
- Children have unique anatomic, physiologic, developmental, and psychologic needs, compared to adult victims of terrorism.
- Historically, the needs of pediatric victims of terrorist attacks have not been sufficiently addressed in formal disaster preparedness strategies.
- In pediatric survivors of blast injuries, it is crucial to be familiar with delayed-onset signs and symptoms associated with high morbidity.
- The single most important first step in responding to a chemical, biological or radiological event is rapid and thorough decontamination of victims by healthcare workers wearing adequate PPE.

■ Organ systems (e.g., auditory, ophthalmic) overlooked during resuscitative efforts must be comprehensively evaluated.

■ Supportive measures are the mainstay of treatment and management for survivors of terror attacks; however, specific pharmacologic and medical interventions may mitigate mortality and morbidity.

■ All physicians should be cognizant of the status of surge equipment, supplies, and availability of personnel at their institutions.

■ Physicians should educate themselves on evacuation plans: What if a Hurricane Katrina-like event were to happen at your location?

■ Hospital preparedness should be coordinated with regional, municipal, and public health entities.

■ Facilities that have PICUs have a role to support surrounding facilities that do not have PICU resources. Strategies for coordination should be established and regularly practiced.

References

1. Abramowicz M, ed. Drugs and vaccines against biological weapons. *The Medical Letter on Drugs and Therapeutics* 2001;43:87–9.
2. Abramowicz M, ed. Prevention and treatment of injury from chemical warfare agents. *The Medical Letter on Drugs and Therapeutics* 2002;44:1–4.
3. Aharonson-Daniel L, Waisman Y, Dannon YL, et al. Epidemiology of terror-related versus non-terror-related traumatic injury in children. *Pediatrics* 2003;112:e280–4.
4. Argyros, GJ. Management of primary blast injury. *Toxicology* 1997;121:105–15.
5. Beary JF, Aronstein WS, Chines AA. Chemical terrorism: Diagnosis and treatment of exposure to chemical weapons. UpToDate Patient Information website http://patients.uptodate.com/topic.asp?file=dis-med/4586; 2005:version 14.1. Accessed December 14, 2006.
6. Breman JG, Henderson DA. Diagnosis and Management of Smallpox. *N Engl J Med* 2002;346:1300–8.
7. Centers for Disease Control. Explosions and blast injuries: A primer for clinicians. CDC Mass Trauma Preparedness and Response webpage at http://www.bt.cdc.gov/masscasualties/explosions.asp#classification. Accessed September 17, 2006.
8. Chisholm P. Mobile ophthalmic surgical teams. Military Medical Technology Online Archives 2005; Vol. 9, Issue 4, at http://www.military-medical-technology.com/article.cfm?DocID=1021 Accessed September 11, 2006.
9. Committee on Environmental Health and Committee on Infectious Diseases. Chemical-biological terrorism and its impact on children: A subject review. *Pediatrics* 2000;105:662–8.
10. Committee on Environmental Health. Radiation Disasters and Children. *Pediatrics*. 2003;111:1455–66.
11. Committee on the Future of Emergency Care in the United States Health System Board on Health Care Services. *Hospital-based emergency care: At the breaking point*. Washington, DC: Institute of Medicine of the National Academies; National Academy of Sciences, 2006.
12. Cripps NP, Glover MA, Guy RJ. The pathophysiology of primary blast injury and its implications for treatment. Part II: The auditory structures and abdomen. *J R Nav Med Serv* 1999;85:13–24.
13. DePalma RG, Burris DG, Champion HR. Current Concepts Blast Injuries. *N Engl J Med* 2005;352:1335–42.
14. Dixon TC, Meselson M, Guillemin J. Anthrax. *N Engl J Med*. 1999;341:815–26.
15. Foltin GL, Schoenfeld D, Shannon M. Pediatric Terrorism and Disaster Preparedness A Resource for Pediatricians. AHRQ Publication Nos. 06(07)-0056 and 06(07)-0056-1, October 2006. Agency for Healthcare Research and Quality, Rockville, MD. http://www.ahrq.gov/research/pedprep/resource.htm. Accessed May 2007.
16. Garth RJN. Blast injury of the ear: An overview and guide to management. *Injury* 1995;26:363–6.
17. GNYHA Briefing on Blast Injury and Mass Casualty Events (October 17, 2005). Asymmetric War (Terrorism) and the Epidemiology of Blast Trauma at http://www.gnyha.org/45/Default.aspx. Accessed September 17, 2006.
18. Graham PL. Healthcare-associated infections. In: Burg F, Ingelfinger JR, Polin RA, Gerson AA, eds. *Current Pediatric Therapy*, 18th ed. Philadelphia: Saunders Elsevier, 2006;692–7.
19. Halpern NA, Pastores SM, Greenstein RJ. Critical Care Medicine in the United States 1985–2000: An analysis of bed numbers, use, and cost. *Crit Care Med* 2004;32:1254–9.
20. Henretig FM, Cieslak TJ, Eitzen EM. Biologic and chemical terrorism. *J Pediatr* 2002;141:311–26.
21. Henretig FM, Cieslak TJ, Madsen JM, et al. Emergency Department awareness and response to incidents of biological and chemical terrorism. In: Fleisher G, Ludwig S. *Textbook of Pediatric Emergency Medicine*, 5th ed. Philadelphia: Lippincott Williams & Wilkins, 2006:135–61.
22. Horrocks CL. Blast Injuries: Biophysics, pathophysiology, and management principles. *J R Army Med Corps* 2001;147:28–40.
23. Irwin RJ, Lerner MR, Bealer JF, et al. Cardiopulmonary physiology of primer blast injury. *J Trauma* 1997;43:650–5.
24. Joint Commission of Accreditation of Health Care Organizations http://www.jointcommission.org/NR/rdonlyres/9C8DE572-5D7A-4F28-AB84-3741EC82AF98/0/emergency-preparedness.pdf Accessed September 11, 2006.
25. Keim ME, Pesik N, Twum-Danso NA. Lack of hospital preparedness for chemical terrorism in a major US city: 1996–2000. *Prehosp Disast Med* 2003; 18:193–9.
26. Lavonis E. Blast injuries. Emedicine website. Available at: http://www.emedicine.com/emerg/topic63.htm. Accessed September 4, 2006.
27. Markenson D, Redlener I. Pediatric terrorism preparedness national guidelines and recommendations: Findings of an evidence-based consensus process. *Biosecur Bioterror* 2004;2:301–19.
28. Mayorga MA. The pathology of primary blast overpressure injury. *Toxicology* 1997;121:17–28.
29. Mettler FA, Voelz GL. Major radiation exposure—what to expect and how to respond. *N Engl J Med* 2002;346:1554–61.
30. Ohnishi M, Kirkman RJ, Watkins PE. Reflex nature of the cardiorespiratory response to primary thoracic blast injury in the anaesthetized rat. *Exp Physiol* 2001;86:357–64.
31. Patt HA, Feigin RD. Diagnosis and management of suspected cases of bioterrorism: A pediatric perspective. *Pediatrics* 2002;109:685–92.
32. Peam J. Children and war. *J Paediatr Child Health* 2003;39:166–72.
33. Quintana DA, Jordan FB, Tuggle DW, et al. The spectrum of pediatric injuries after a bomb blast. *J Pediatr Surg* 1997 Feb;32:307–10.
34. Rubinson L, Nuzzo SM, Talmor DS, et al. Augmentation of hospital critical care capacity after bioterrorist attacks or epidemics: Recommendation of the Working Group on Emergency Mass Critical Care. *Crit Care Med* 2005;3:2393–2403.
35. Sosna J, Sella T, Shaham D, et al. Facing the new threat of terrorism: Radiologists' perspectives based on experience in Israel. *Radiology* 2005;237:28–36.
36. Tsokos M, Paulsen F, Petri S, et al. Histological, immunohistochemical, and ultra-structural findings in human blast lung injury. *Am J Respir Crit Care Med* 2003;168:549–55.
37. Wasiman Y, Aharonson-Daniel L, Mor M. The impact of terrorism on children: A two-year experience. *Prehospital and Disaster Medicine* 2003;18:242–8.
38. Wightman JM, Gladish SL. Explosions and blast injuries. *Ann Emerg Med* 2001;37:664–78.
39. Wightman JM, Gladish SL. Explosions and blast injuries: A primer for clinicians. Atlanta: Centers for Disease Control and Prevention at http://www.cdc.gov/masstrauma/preparedness/primer.pdf. Accessed September 17, 2006.

CHAPTER 31 ■ POISONING

G. PATRICIA CANTWELL • RICHARD S. WEISMAN

Childhood poisoning remains a common occurrence despite widespread educational efforts by healthcare providers and the utilization of childproof medication dispensers. The challenge to the pediatric intensivist can be daunting in determining which ingestions are potentially high risk and which are inconsequential. Yearly data collection reveals that more than 2 million exposures to toxic substances are reported to poison centers throughout the US. The overwhelming majority of toxic exposures cause minimal to no effect; morbidity and mortality associated with these exposures are extremely uncommon (40). Poisoning that occurs in children less than 5 years of age is generally accidental and accounts for approximately 85%–90% of pediatric poisoning. Poisoning in a child older than 5 years is generally considered intentional and comprises the remaining 10%–15% of childhood poisonings (28). Unintentional overdoses may occasionally occur in teenagers who take alcohol and street drugs. Teenagers are also subject to hospitalization following suicide attempts or suicide gestures. The Toxic Exposure Surveillance System of the American Association of Poison Control Centers reports ingestion to be the primary route of exposure to toxic substances (40). Risk factors for childhood exposure include exploratory behavior, child abuse, the possibility of environmental exposures, suicide attempts in children, and neonates exposed to toxins in utero.

EPIDEMIOLOGY

Poisoning may occur with differing modes of exposure. Exposures may occur via ingestion, ocular exposure, topical exposure, envenomation, inhalation, and transplacental exposure. The ingestion of poisonous plants is common in children and may account for approximately 5%–10% of calls to poison control centers. It is difficult to establish a clear-cut list of problem plants, as many plants have both edible and toxic parts, are difficult for non-botanists to identify accurately, and have variable plant names, and for many plants, the quantity necessary to produce toxicity is unclear.

Management of childhood poisoning is challenging due to the existence of hundreds of prescription medications, household chemicals, stings and envenomations, illicit and designer drugs, and increased use of nonprescription and herbal medications. Pediatric fatalities are most often associated with the following agents: analgesics, hydrocarbons, antidepressants, gases and fumes, stimulants and street drugs, cardiovascular drugs, anticonvulsants, sedatives/hypnotics/antipsychotics, and chemicals. The agents that most frequently prompt calls to poison control centers are cosmetics and personal care products, cleaning substances, analgesics, foreign bodies, topical agents, and plants.

CLINICAL APPROACH TO THE POISONED CHILD

The acute management of the poisoned child generally begins in the emergency department. Recommendations for the management of the poisoned child have been challenging due to limited research based upon small-case series, animal studies, and case reports. Initial evaluation involves the process of triage and the determination of appropriate decontamination and treatment regimens. The intensivist may be immediately involved, as aggressive interventions are often required before it is possible to determine a comprehensive history, physical examination, and diagnostic testing. Urgent priorities include the focus on a primary survey that involves attention to the patient's airway, breathing, and circulation (ABCs). Following the establishment of life-saving supportive care, a detailed evaluation can be meticulously performed. Toxins may cause respiratory failure by depression of the respiratory drive, hypoperfusion of the central nervous system (CNS), coma with impaired/absent protective airway reflexes, or direct toxic effects on the pulmonary system. Airway management mandates a low threshold for rapid-sequence intubation due to the potential for loss of protective airway reflexes and expectation of a full stomach, with risk for aspiration. Many toxins may cause extreme hemodynamic instability due to dysrhythmias and/or hypotension. Comprehensive stabilization involves attention to respiratory, cardiovascular, neurologic, and metabolic aberrancies. It is critical for healthcare providers to ensure safety of personnel in initiating treatment; decontamination and proper personal protective equipment may be required prior to proceeding with management. Optimal clinical management of the critically ill, poisoned patient mandates a seamless transfer of information and patient care from the emergency department to the ICU. The mainstay of intensive care management is meticulous supportive care with attention to emergent airway management (Chapter 22), respiratory failure (Chapters 46 and 47), hemodynamic collapse (Chapter 26), and management of the comatose patient (Chapter 53). These entities are discussed in detail in respective chapters, while specifics related to particular poisons are highlighted below.

PATIENT HISTORY

A comprehensive history for the potential of toxic exposure may be obtained from witnesses, family members, friends, and emergency medical services personnel. It is important to obtain a list of all available toxins within the household, including over-the-counter medications and nonpharmaceutical agents (e.g., plants, cleaning agents). A comprehensive history

TABLE 31.1

TOXICITY LEVELS OF SELECTED MEDICATIONS AND MEDICATION CLASSES

Agents	Minimum potential lethal dose	Maximum dose available	Potentially fatal units in a 10-kg child
Antimalarials			
Chloroquine	20 mg/kg	500 mg	1
Hydroxychloroquine	20 mg/kg	200 mg	1
Camphor	100 mg/kg	200 mg/mL	5 mL
Imidazolines			
Clonidine	0.01 mg/kg	0.3 mg; 7.5 mg/patch	1
Tetrahydrozoline	2.5 to 5 mL	0.1%	2.5 to 5 mL
Methyl Salicylates	150 to 200 mg/kg	1400 mg/mL	1.1 to 1.4 mL
Sulfonylureas			
Glipizide	0.1 mg/kg	5 mg	1
Glyburide	0.1 mg/kg	10 mg	1

From Matteucci MJ. One pill can kill: Assessing the potential for fatal poisonings in children. *Pediatr Ann* 2005;34:964–968, with permission.

must also include focused information about the environment, circumstances preceding and surrounding a toxic exposure, smells or unusual items, the occupation of those in the home, and queries regarding the presence of a suicide note. Obtaining an accurate history in adolescent poisonings is especially challenging due to the potential use of multiple substances, possible drugs of abuse, prolonged time between ingestion and presentation, and attempts at concealing accurate information. Additional information includes the maximum amount of toxin available and the minimum amount per kilogram that produces symptoms. It is helpful to estimate the quantity of liquid toxins by quantifying a swallow: 5–10 mL in a young child and 10–15 mL in an adolescent. A useful mnemonic to recall is the "over-the-counter" or "OTC" designation for medications, which can also mean "oblivious to toxic contents" (13). The history must include potential illnesses of family members, which can serve to identify possible culprit medications. It is vital to obtain product containers or medication labels to identify specific toxic contents. Extremely dangerous single agents are camphor, chloroquine, hydroxychloroquine, imipramine, desipramine, quinine, methyl salicylate, theophylline, thioridazine, and chlorpromazine. A number of medications have been determined to be potentially lethal to a child who weighs 10 kg and ingests of just one tablet, capsule, or teaspoonful (23) (**Table 31.1**).

A comprehensive history must include evaluation for indoor air pollutants, which may include carbon monoxide, cyanide, ozone, smoke, volatile hydrocarbons, and mercury vapor.

After obtaining the history, early contact with the *regional poison control center (1-800-222-1222)* provides rapid access to a toxicology consult. Specific signs and symptoms can serve to focus a differential diagnosis. Prompt assimilation of metabolic and kinetic information allows the determination of a potential clinical course. The clinician may be caught off-guard in cases of delays between the onset of ingestion and development of symptoms. It is especially helpful to obtain assistance in identifying and managing odd drugs and chemicals. Centralized databases provide information about possible public health threats in the event of multiple poisonings.

PHYSICAL EXAMINATION

General

A comprehensive physical examination can be crucial in determining which agents are involved in causing toxic symptoms. Careful assessment of vital signs combined with a thorough physical examination serves to narrow a broad array of differential diagnoses and allows for specific initial treatment interventions. The intent of this chapter is not to review every possible poisoning, but rather to provide a methodical approach to organizing physical findings that can focus therapy and guide specific diagnostic evaluations. The signs and symptoms that suggest specific classes of poisoning are generally grouped into syndromes and referred to as toxidromes. These groupings are essential for the successful recognition of poisoning patterns. Herbal poisoning and dietary supplements have also been implicated with a host of typical symptomatologies (42) (**Tables 31.2 and 31.3**). An approach to the classic toxidromes can be misleading, depending on the amount of toxic exposure, competing toxins or medications, and patient comorbidities. The classic toxidromes may be grouped into four categories: sympathomimetic, cholinergic, anticholinergic, and opiate-sedative-ethanol syndromes.

Many nonspecific findings are related to the gastrointestinal (GI) system and include nausea, vomiting, abdominal pain, and loose stools. Elevated body temperature serves to identify specific toxic agents. Careful physical examination elucidates findings of significant concern that can serve to identify the heralding features of a particular toxidrome.

Cardiopulmonary

As noted in the primary survey, the priority exam is geared at recognition of life-threatening compromise of airway, breathing, and circulation. Toxins may cause an array of aberrations of the cardiovascular system, including hypertension/

TABLE 31.2

EXAMPLES OF KNOWN HERBAL PRODUCTS AND THEIR ASSOCIATED
TOXIC EFFECTS

Herbal product	Toxic chemicals	Effect or target organ
Monkshood (*Aconitum* sp.)	Aconite	Cardiac arrhythmias, shock, weakness, seizures, coma, paresthesias, nausea, emesis
Wormwood (*Artemisia absinthium*)	Thujone	Seizures, dementia, tremors, headache, ataxia
Chaparral (*Larrea divericata*)	Nordihydroguaiaretic acid	Nausea, emesis, hepatitis
Cinnamon oil (*Cinnamomum* sp.)	Cinnamaldehyde	Dermatitis, abuse syndrome
Comfrey (*Symphytum officinale*)	Pyrrolizidines	Hepatic veno-occlusive disease
Crotalaria sp.	Pyrrolizidines	Hepatic veno-occlusive disease
Eucalyptus (*Eucalyptus globulus*)	1,8 cineol	Drowsiness, ataxia, seizures, nausea, vomiting, coma
Garlic (*Allium sativum*)	Allicin	Nausea, emesis, anorexia, weight loss, bleeding, platelet dysfunction
Heliotropium sp.	Pyrrolizidines	Hepatic veno-occlusive disease
Jin bu huan	Tetrahydropalmatine	Hepatitis
Kava (*Piper methysticum*)	Kavapyrones	Hepatitis, cirrhosis
Laetrile	Cyanide	Coma, seizures, death, respiratory failure
Licorice (*Glycyrrhiza glabra*)	Glycyrrhetic acid	Hypertension, hypokalemia, dysrhythmias
Ma Huang (*Ephedra sinica*)	Ephedrine	Hypertension, dysrhythmias, stroke, seizures
Nutmeg (*Myristica fragrans*)	Myristicin, eugenol	Hallucinations, emesis, headache
Strychnos nux-vomica	Strychnine	Seizures, abdominal pain, respiratory failure
Pennyroyal (*Mentha pulegium; Hedeoma* sp.)	Pulegone	Centrilobular liver necrosis, fetotoxicity, abortion
Senecio sp.	Pyrrolizidines	Hepatic veno-occlusive disease

From Woolf AD. Herbal remedies and children: Do they work? Are they harmful? *Pediatrics* 2003;112:
240–246, with permission.

hypotension due to direct action of the toxin on vascular smooth muscle, neurogenic effects on autonomic nervous centers, and direct cardiogenic or renal effects. These specific physical findings are best expressed in tabular form (12) (Table 31.4).

Neurologic

The neurologic examination is especially important, as many toxins can be expected to depress the level of consciousness by directly interfering with respiratory drive or hypoxia from loss of protective airway reflexes. Neurologic deterioration can be catastrophic; therefore, frequent exams must be documented. One must anticipate the potential for manifestation of seizure activity. The pupillary exam is an extremely useful neurologic finding. Various toxins interfere with the autonomic innervation of the pupil and may manifest as miosis or mydriasis. Symmetrical pupillary changes are typical of toxic exposures, with asymmetry most commonly evidencing a structural or focal neurologic abnormality. It is essential to recognize that polydrug toxicity may involve agents with competing actions on the

pupillary response. Management based on the isolated evaluation of pupil size may lead to misdiagnosis. Further confounding the exam may be the possibility of traumatic brain injury or intracranial hemorrhage that stems from the toxic exposure. An extensive list of toxins that includes over-the-counter medications, common household products and drugs of abuse is associated with an altered sensorium. Additionally, one must be cognizant of potential abstinence syndromes in patients suffering from chronic substance abuse. Drug withdrawal may be heralded by agitation, abnormal vital signs, irritability, and an altered sensorium. Nystagmus, tinnitus, and visual disturbances are commonly observed neurologic findings in selected intoxications.

Dermatologic Manifestations and Telltale Odors

Dermatologic examination may yield the identification of varied toxins. Inhalant abuse may lead to skin rashes around the nose and mouth. Needle tracks or characteristic tattooing are

TABLE 31.3

TWELVE MOST DANGEROUS DIETARY SUPPLEMENTS

Name (also known as)	Dangers
DEFINITELY HAZARDOUS *Documented organ failure and known carcinogenic properties*	
ARISTOLOCHIC ACID *Aristolochia* sp. (birthwort, snakeroot, snakeweed, sangree root, sangrel, serpentary, serpentaria); *Asarun canadens* (wild ginger)	Potent human carcinogen; can cause kidney failure and death
VERY LIKELY HAZARDOUS *Banned in some countries, FDA warning, or adverse effects in studies*	
COMFREY *Symphytun officinale* (ass ear, black root, blackwort, bruisewort, consolidate radix, consound, gum plant, healing herb, knitback, knitbone, salsify, slippery root, symphytum radix, wallwort)	Abnormal liver function or irreversible damage; deaths reported
ANDROSTENEDIONE *4-androstene-3* (17-dione, andro, androstene)	Increased cancer risk; decrease in HDL cholesterol
CHAPARRAL *Larrea divaricate* (creosote bush, greasewood, hediondilla, jarilla, larreastat)	Abnormal liver function or irreversible damage; deaths reported
GERMANDER *Teucrium chamaedrys* (wall germander, wild germander)	Abnormal liver function or irreversible damage; deaths reported
KAVA *Piper methysticum* (ava, awa, gea, gi, intoxicating pepper, kao, kavain, kawa-pfeffer, kew, long pepper, malohu, maluk, meruk, milik, rauschpfeffer, sakau, tonga, wurzelstock, yagona, yangona)	Abnormal liver function or irreversible damage; deaths reported
LIKELY HAZARDOUS *Adverse events reported, theoretical risks*	
BITTER ORANGE *Citrus aurantium* (green orange, kijitsu, neroli oil, Seville orange, and shangzhou zhiqiao, sour orange, zhi oiao, zhi xhi)	High blood pressure; risk of arrhythmias, heart attack, and stroke
LOBELIA *Lobelia inflata* (asthma weed, bladderpod, emetic herb, gagroot, lobelie, indian tobacco, pukeweed, vomit wort, wild tobacco)	Breathing difficulty, rapid heartbeat, low blood pressure, diarrhea, dizziness; possible related deaths reported
ORGAN/GLANDULAR EXTRACTS Brain, adrenal, pituitary, placenta, other gland "substance" or "concentrate"	Theoretical risk of mad cow disease, especially from brain extracts
PENNYROYAL OIL *Hedeoma pulegioides* (lurk-in-the-ditch, mosquito plant, piliolerial, pudding grass, pulegium, run-by-the-ground, squaw balm, squawmint, stinking balm, tickweed)	Liver and kidney failure, nerve damage, convulsions, abdominal tenderness, burning of the throat; deaths reported
SCULLCAP *Scutellaria lateriflora* (blue pimpernel, helmet flower, hoodwort, mad weed, mad-dog herb, mad-dog weed, quaker bonnet, scutelluria, skullcap)	Abnormal liver function or damage
YOHIMBE *Pausinystalia yobimbe* (johimbi, yohimbehe, yohimbine)	Changes in blood pressure, arrhythmias, respiratory depression, myocardial infarction; deaths reported

From Natural Medicines Comprehensive Database 2004 and Consumers Union's medical and research consultants. Data extracted from *Consumer Reports,* May 2004.

TABLE 31.4

CLINICAL MANIFESTATIONS OF POISONING

SKIN

Cyanosis (unresponsive to oxygen-methemoglobinemia)	Nitrates, nitrites, phenacetin, benzocaine
Red flush	Carbon monoxide, cyanide, boric acid, anticholinergics
Sweating	Amphetamines, LSD, organophosphates, cocaine, barbiturates
Dry	Anticholinergics
Bullae	Barbiturates, carbon monoxide
Jaundice	Acetaminophen, mushrooms, carbon tetrachloride, iron, phosphorus
Purpura	Aspirin, warfarin, snakebite

TEMPERATURE

Hypothermia	Sedative hypnotics, ethanol, carbon monoxide, phenothiazines, TCAs, clonidine
Hyperthermia	Anticholinergics, salicylates, phenothiazines, TCAs, cocaine, amphetamines, theophylline

BLOOD PRESSURE

Hypertension	Sympathomimetics (especially phenylpropanolamine in over-the-counter cold remedies) organophosphates, amphetamines, PCP
Hypotension	Narcotics, sedative hypnotics, TCAs, phenothiazines, clonidine, β-blockers, calcium channel blockers

PULSE RATE

Bradycardia	Digitalis, sedative hypnotics, β-blockers, ethchlorvynol, calcium channel blockers
Tachycardia	Anticholinergics, sympathomimetics, amphetamines, alcohol, aspirin, theophylline, cocaine, TCAs
Arrhythmias	Anticholinergics, TCAs, organophosphates, phenothiazines, digoxin, β-blockers, carbon monoxide, cyanide, theophylline

MUCOUS MEMBRANES

Dry	Anticholinergics
Salivation	Organophosphates, carbamates
Oral lesions	Corrosives, paraquat
Lacrimation	Caustics, organophosphates, irritant gases

RESPIRATION

Depressed	Alcohol, narcotics, barbiturates, sedative/hypnotics
Tachypnea	Salicylates, amphetamines, carbon monoxide
Kussmaul	Methanol, ethylene glycol, salicylates
Wheezing	Organophosphates
Pneumonia	Hydrocarbons
Pulmonary edema	Aspiration, salicylates, narcotics, sympathomimetics

CENTRAL NERVOUS SYSTEM

Seizures	TCAs, cocaine, phenothiazines, amphetamines, camphor, lead, salicylates, isoniazid, organophosphates, antihistamines, propoxyphene, strychnine
Pupils, miosis	Narcotics (except Demerol and Lomotil), phenothiazines, organophosphates, diazepam, barbiturates, mushrooms (muscarine types)
Mydriasis	Anticholinergics, sympathomimetics, cocaine, TCAs, methanol, glutethimide, LSD
Blindness, optic atrophy	Methanol
Fasciculation	Organophosphates
Nystagmus	Diphenylhydantoin, barbiturates, carbamazepine, PCP, carbon monoxide, glutethimide, ethanol
Hypertonus	Anticholinergics, strychnine, phenothiazines
Myoclonus, rigidity	Anticholinergics, phenothiazines, haloperidol
Delirium/psychosis	Anticholinergics, sympathomimetics, alcohol, phenothiazines, PCP, LSD, marijuana, cocaine, heroin, methaqualone, heavy metals
Coma	Alcohols, anticholinergics, sedative hypnotics, narcotics, carbon monoxide, tricyclic antidepressants, salicylates, organophosphates, barbiturates
Weakness, paralysis	Organophosphates, carbamates, heavy metals

GASTROINTESTINAL SYSTEM

Vomiting, diarrhea, abdominal pain	Iron, phosphorus, heavy metals, lithium, mushrooms, fluoride, organophosphates, arsenic

Adapted from Guzzardi L, Bayer MJ. Emergency management of the poisoned patient. In: Bayer M, Rumack BH, Wanke LA, eds. *Toxicologic emergencies.* Bowie, MD: Robert J. Brady, 1984.

TABLE 31.5

TOXINS ASSOCIATED WITH CHARACTERISTIC BREATH ODORS

Toxin	Characteristic odor
Acetone	Acetone
Arsenic	Garlic
Camphor	Mothballs
Chloroform	Sweet
Cyanide	Bitter almond
Ethanol	Ethanol
Hydrogen sulfide	Rotten eggs
Isopropanol	Acetone
Methyl salicylate	Wintergreen
Nicotine	Stale tobacco
Organophosphates	Garlic
N-Pyridylmethylnitrophenylurea (Vacor rat poison)	Peanuts
Paraldehyde, chloral hydrate	Pears (urine)
Phenol, cresol	Phenolic
Phosphorus	Garlic
Salicylates	Acetone
Thallium	Garlic
Turpentine	Violets

From Woolf AD. Principles of toxin assessment and screening. In: Fuhrman BP, Zimmerman J, eds. *Pediatric Critical Care*, 3rd ed. Philadelphia: Mosby, Elsevier, 2006:1511–31, with permission.

suggestive of IV drug use. Meticulous skin examination must focus upon commonly employed intravascular access sites, including the groin, neck, supraclavicular areas, dorsum of the feet, and tongue. Adverse drug reactions and allergic dermatitis may occur from exposure to drugs, plants, or chemicals. Alopecia can lead to the identification of long-term exposure to a variety of toxic chemicals. Jaundice is yet another dermatologic finding of significance that should suggest consideration of specific toxic exposures in the differential diagnosis. Telltale odors are another means of compartmentalizing a variety of toxins (**Table 31.5**). Agents may have saturated the clothing or skin, or may be emanated via the breath.

LABORATORY EVALUATION

Basic Principles

The laboratory evaluation generally confirms a diagnosis that has already been established based on the history and physical examination. In some circumstances, important decisions about therapy will be made based upon quantitative drug or toxin levels in blood specimens. These include acetaminophen, ethanol, methanol, ethylene glycol, lithium, salicylates, iron, lead, mercury, arsenic, phenobarbital, carbon monoxide, methemoglobin, and theophylline. It is extremely important to be aware of the spectrum of toxins screened by individual hospital laboratories. Most laboratories routinely screen for acetaminophen, ethanol, barbiturates, opiates, anticonvulsants, benzodiazepines, phenothiazines, and salicylates. A number of drugs of abuse may be included, specifically, am-

phetamines, cocaine, and tetrahydrocannabinol. A "negative" toxicology screen by no means excludes the possibility of a toxic exposure. Opioids, such as hydrocodone, oxycodone, methadone, fentanyl, meperidine, and propoxyphene, may not be detected by some opiate screening methodology, such as the immunoassay. It is extremely helpful to be specific about identifying toxins of interest, so that the laboratory personnel have input into the ideal screening evaluation. In certain instances, toxins may be better detected in urine than in blood. Analysis of gastric contents may be helpful in elucidating a particular toxin if they are collected before absorption is likely. Comprehensive drug screens and drug levels are often obtained to glean positive toxin identification and quantification; however, the results are generally not available in time to affect any initial interventions. Many physicians do not fully understand the limitations of toxicology screens or the implications of positive versus negative results. For example, a urine drug screen is devised to detect the parent drug or metabolites up to a number of days following the use of a drug. It follows that a positive urine drug screen may not necessarily confirm that symptoms are due to the agent identified by the test. A number of immunoassays are poorly sensitive and specific, which can lead to false-positive and false-negative results. Consultation with a toxicologist at the regional poison control center (800-222-1222) is helpful in selecting and interpreting test results. The National Institute for Drug Abuse has established the commonly employed "drug of abuse screen" (NIDA-5), which utilizes immunoassay for amphetamines, marijuana, cocaine, opiates, and phencyclidine.

Prioritization of laboratory analysis is directed at the identification of immediately life-threatening situations. It is essential to obtain acetaminophen levels in virtually all poisoned patients to ensure that urgent management can be addressed, if necessary. Prompt determination of blood glucose level should be accomplished in any patient with an altered sensorium.

Anion Gap

Electrolytes and blood urea nitrogen (BUN)/creatinine levels allow for the determination of an anion gap acidosis, basic electrolytes, and the assessment of renal function. The anion gap calculation is:

$$Na\,(mEq/L) - [Cl\,(mEq/L) + HCO_3\,(mEq/L)]$$

The normal anion gap is generally 3–16 mEq/L. Agents that cause an elevated anion gap metabolic acidosis are listed in Table 31.6.

TABLE 31.6

METABOLIC ACIDOSIS [NA − (Cl + HCO$_3$)]: MUDPILES

Methanol
Uremia
Diabetic ketoacidosis
Paraldehyde and phenformin
Isoniazid and iron
Lactic acidosis
Ethanol and ethylene glycol
Salicylates

TABLE 31.7

CHARACTERISTIC URINE COLOR CHANGES

Orange to red-orange
Rifampin, deferoxamine, mercury, phenazopyridine, chronic lead poisoning

Pink
Cephalosporins or ampicillin

Brown
Chloroquine or carbon tetrachloride

Green to blue
Amitriptyline

Electrocardiogram

The 12-lead electrocardiogram is an invaluable tool in the evaluation of potential intoxication, particularly in detecting dysrhythmias and conduction abnormalities, such as widening of the QRS complex or prolongation of the QT interval. Cardiovascular toxicity is a common cause of death that results from antidepressant overdose and can manifest as myocardial depression, ventricular fibrillation, and ventricular tachycardia. The electrocardiogram is useful both in diagnosis and in management.

Urinalysis

Urine color may be helpful in the identification of a number of toxins (**Table 31.7**). It is important to obtain urine pregnancy tests on any patient of child-bearing age.

Urinalysis may reveal specific crystals (calcium oxalate crystals in ethylene glycol poisoning) or myoglobinuria. The presence of myoglobinuria is suggestive of rhabdomyolysis, which is followed by determination of serum creatinine phosphokinase. A positive urine ferric chloride test (phenylpyruvic acid) is indicative of a phenothiazine or salicylate overdose.

Blood Gas Analysis

Arterial blood gas analysis is useful for the evaluation of acid-base status, and the addition of co-oximetry can target carboxyhemoglobin, methemoglobinemia, and sulfhemoglobin.

Osmolality

Intoxication with methanol, ethanol, ethylene glycol, acetone, and isopropanol can be recognized due to their propensity to increase serum osmolality. Calculated serum osmolality is determined by the following:

$$2 \times Na\ (mEq/L) + blood\ urea\ nitrogen\ (g/L)/2.8$$
$$+ glucose\ (mg/dL)/18$$

The osmolar gap is evaluated by subtracting the calculated osmolality from the measured osmolality. Normal osmolar gap is 3–10 mOsm/kg H_2O. Conversion factors may be utilized to determine an estimated serum concentration of alcohols and glycols (43). Calculation of the osmolar gap may be con-founded by the presence of lipemia or other osmotically active agents often used in the ICU, such as mannitol or contrast for diagnostic imaging procedures.

Ancillary Testing

Additional baseline laboratory evaluation may be particularly prudent in the evaluation of the patient. Complete blood cell count with platelets and leukocyte differential, blood clotting parameters (prothrombin time and partial thromboplastin time), liver function tests, and possible electroencephalogram may prove useful.

Radiologic Imaging

Radiographic evaluation is particularly useful in ingestion of certain foreign bodies, as well as in the instance of a number of radiopaque drugs, metals, and chemicals. In the event of the ingestion of disc batteries, it is warranted to obtain serial chest/abdominal x-rays to document the movement of the foreign body through the GI tract. Radiographic evaluation has identified efforts at drug smuggling via body packing with cocaine-filled containers. Chest and abdominal x-rays are extremely helpful in locating a number of radiopaque pills or tablets and in elucidating aspiration or pulmonary edema. Pill bezoars may be identified when contrast is utilized for the study. Radiopaque compounds may be grouped by the mnemonic "COINS": chloral hydrate and cocaine packets, opiate packets, iron and heavy metals (lead, arsenic, mercury), neuroleptics, and sustained–release or enteric coated tablets.

MANAGEMENT

Toxicology Resources

It is absolutely essential to employ all available resources when dealing with a patient exposed to an unintentional or intentional toxic exposure. Numerous resources enable the practitioner to have rapid access to a wealth of information regarding drug identification, pharmacokinetics, drug interactions, and precautions. It is especially important to have a link to resource information for patterns of drug toxicity and current therapies for exposure in the event of chemical terrorism. The regional poison control hotline is a mainstay for reference. Additional helpful resources are the Poisindex computer database (Micromedex Corporation, Greenwood Village, CO) and Drug Information Centers located in most large medical centers.

Toxicokinetics

Toxicokinetics, or pharmacokinetics in the poisoned patient, can provide important conceptual information to the healthcare provider. It is vital to consider the differences between adult and pediatric patients to make appropriate modifications to poisoning treatment recommendations that may have been developed for adult patients. Principles of toxicokinetics focus on the dynamics of the processes of absorption, distribution, metabolism, and elimination of drugs or toxins.

Prevention of absorption is a mainstay of toxicology. Washing a toxin from the skin or removing a victim from an environment with a toxic gas may dramatically reduce toxicity. Preventing absorption from the GI tract is more complex, as the drug or toxin must dissolve in aqueous gastric fluids and traverse several lipophilic membranes prior to reaching the vascular compartment. Consequently, factors such as pH and pKa of the toxin and lipid solubility of the drug may alter absorption. Timely administration of activated charcoal may allow the drug or toxin an opportunity to be adsorbed to activated charcoal within the GI lumen. Enteric-coated tablets and sustained-release formulations have been designed to delay and sustain the absorption process. Kinetically, this delayed absorption results in a lengthier time to achieve peak serum concentrations, which prolongs the duration of action of the drug. Whole-bowel irrigation may allow enteric-coated tablets or sustained-release formulations to transit the GI tract before absorption begins. Drugs with complex or slow dissolution or absorption are most amenable to activated charcoal.

Distribution is the process of the drug or toxin moving from the intravascular compartment into tissue. This process is impacted by protein binding, pH, and lipophilicity of the drug or toxin. The volume of distribution (Vd) is equal to the amount of drug in the body divided by the peak concentration of the drug in the blood compartment.

$$Vd = \text{concentration in body}/[\text{plasma}]$$

Age-specific volume of distribution for drugs and toxins can be found in the medical literature. The larger the volume of distribution, the more likely the drug will transit from the intravascular compartment into the tissue. Toxins with large volumes of distribution include camphor, antidepressants, digoxin, opioids, phenothiazines, and phencyclidine. Drugs with small volumes of distribution include ethanol, methanol, salicylate, lithium, valproic acid, and phenobarbital. In the event that Vd is <1, the drug or toxin may usually be removed by hemodialysis. The volume of distribution formula can also be useful in predicting peak drug or toxin levels when the amount ingested is known.

Protein binding plays an important role in the distribution process. Drugs and toxins that are highly bound to plasma proteins will exist in the intravascular compartment in both the bound and unbound form. The unbound form of a drug is always the pharmacologically active component. Albumin and α_1 acid glycoprotein are two of the most common plasma proteins that bind drugs. Highly protein-bound drugs include carbamazepine, phenytoin, valproic acid, warfarin, and salicylate. If a patient has reduced levels of plasma proteins, a proportional increase in the unbound, active form of the drug must be used. For example, phenytoin has a therapeutic range of 10–20 mcg/mL in a patient with normal albumin levels. In a patient with a 20% reduction in albumin level, the therapeutic range must be adjusted to 8–16 mcg/mL. Consequently, this may necessitate a dose reduction and may explain why toxicity (nystagmus, ataxia, CNS depression) may be seen in patients within the normally reported therapeutic range. Alternatively, many centers now measure the free fraction of phenytoin to determine the effects of protein binding on activity. A level of 1–2 mcg/mL generally is considered therapeutic. Protein binding is

also known to be pH dependent, a principle that is extremely important in the management of tricyclic antidepressant poisoning, as discussed later in this chapter.

Metabolism is an important route of elimination and involves a complex array of enzymes that are designed to generally improve the water solubility of drugs and their metabolic breakdown products. Among the enzyme systems frequently involved in this process are the cytochrome P450 monooxygenase enzymes. Many of these enzymes have specific isoenzymes that can be induced (cigarette smoke, omeprazole, rifampin) or inhibited (amiodarone, cimetidine, erythromycin, grapefruit juice, ketoconazole), resulting in toxicity or subtherapeutic levels. Patients with hepatotoxicity or poor hepatic perfusion may exhibit increased drug levels and decreased drug clearance if they are receiving a drug with a high hepatic extraction ratio.

Renal elimination is the most common route of elimination. Many drugs are metabolized in the liver to water-soluble metabolites so that they may be renally cleared. Renal elimination or glomerular filtration rate parallels, but does not equal, the creatinine clearance. As the creatinine clearance decreases and serum creatinine increases, it is likely that the drug and toxin clearance is being proportionally reduced. Clearance is a valuable tool in predicting and projecting drug half-life and rates of elimination. Clearance (Cl) is equal to the volume cleared of drug/toxin per unit of time, expressed as mL/min or L/hr.

$$Cl = \text{dose rate}/\text{steady state plasma concentration}$$

The clearance calculation is beneficial to determine how quickly a drug is being removed from the body and if hemodialysis with a known clearance can prove useful in altering the elimination profile.

Decontamination Principles

Decontamination may be individualized, depending upon the type and route of exposure and the amount of time that elapses from ingestion. The approach to the poisoned patient has evolved significantly over the years. Aggressive gastric decontamination was once the rule of thumb for the management of every child, and syrup of ipecac was routinely prescribed by the general pediatrician as a component of anticipatory guidance.

Syrup of Ipecac

Syrup of ipecac is a derivative of the ipecacuanha plant, the active components of which are emetine and cephaeline. These substances lead to vomiting by means of central chemotactic stimulation and local effects on the gastric mucosa (10). Research has shown that this agent is useful if given within minutes of ingestion but that the benefit is extremely time limited. Most importantly, clinical evidence has not revealed that syrup of ipecac resulted in improved patient outcomes, even with early administration. Pitfalls in the utilization of syrup of ipecac include its contraindicated use in the event of airway compromise, caustic ingestion, or hydrocarbon ingestion, and adverse reactions of lethargy, drowsiness, and prolonged vomiting. The American Academy of Clinical Toxicology (AACT) and the European Association of Poisons Centres and Clinical

Toxicologists (EAPCCT) issued a firm position statement that "syrup of ipecac should not be administered routinely in the management of poisoned patients ... its routine administration in the emergency department should be abandoned" (16). Literature exists regarding inappropriate utilization of ipecac and lack of efficacy when administered in the home setting (6). Recent data reveal that documented use of ipecac has been scant, a finding that is further supported by the position statement of the American Academy of Pediatrics, which followed the aforementioned AACT policy (1), and is outlined in current guidelines published by the American Association of Poison Control Centers (22).

Gastric Lavage

A mainstay of gastric decontamination has been the utilization of gastric lavage (38). The proper technique of gastric lavage involves the insertion of a large-bore orogastric tube into the stomach, followed by administration and aspiration of fluid, with the intent of recovering newly ingested toxins. This technique can be particularly traumatizing to a young child and is truly associated with risk in a patient with any degree of impaired airway protection. Contraindications to gastric lavage include compromised upper airway protection, ingestion of corrosive substances or hydrocarbons, and patients at risk for GI perforation or hemorrhage.

Complications associated with this technique have been pulmonary aspiration, respiratory compromise, mechanical injury/perforation, and electrolyte imbalances (38,39). A position statement from the AACT/EAPCCT stipulates that gastric lavage

> should not be employed routinely in the management of poisoned patients. No evidence suggests that its use improves clinical outcome, and it may cause significant morbidity. [Gastric lavage] should not be considered unless a patient has ingested a potentially life-threatening amount of a poison and the procedure can be undertaken within 60 mins of ingestion. Even then, clinical benefit has not been confirmed in controlled studies (39).

Incorrectly performed, gastric lavage places a patient at significant risk for complications and unlikely clinical benefit. It is no wonder that the documented utilization of gastric lavage has declined over the years (40).

Activated Charcoal

Activated charcoal is a particularly efficacious therapy in the management of most poisonings, as it can potentially decrease the absorption of a broad array of toxins and is only ineffective in a small number of cases (**Table 31.8**). Activated charcoal adsorbs drugs and chemicals by weak Van der Waals forces that prevent absorption. Activated charcoal is prepared by superheating highly carbonaceous materials with activating agents (e.g., steam or carbon dioxide) to form a substance with a significant surface area, which provides the basis for its high adsorptive capacity (14). Numerous studies have shown that activated charcoal is quite efficacious as a single agent in achieving gastric decontamination. The adsorptive utility of activated charcoal does depend upon how quickly it can be administered after the toxic ingestion. Activated charcoal was found to reduce the mean bioavailability of drugs by 69.1% when

TABLE 31.8	
AGENTS NOT ADSORBED BY CHARCOAL	

Common electrolytes
Iron
Mineral acids or bases
Alcohols
Cyanide
Most solvents
Most water insoluble compounds (hydrocarbons)
Pesticides
Lithium

administered within 30 mins after ingestion. The most recent AACT/EAPCCT policy statement stipulates that,

> activated charcoal should not be routinely administered in the management of poisoned patients ... the greatest benefit is within one hour of ingestion ... there are insufficient data to support or exclude its use after one hour of ingestion. There is no evidence that the administration of activated charcoal improves clinical outcome (11).

Even so, widespread practice has followed the convincing indirect evidence that efforts at early administration of activated charcoal are useful in reducing absorption of drugs and toxins (35). It is important to note that the inability of existing studies to show benefit after 1 hr does not exclude a potential benefit of activated charcoal administered 2–3 hrs post-ingestion. Additional studies with larger populations, greater sensitivities, and better-defined end points are needed. The generally accepted dose of activated charcoal is based upon in vitro studies, which support a charcoal-to-drug ratio of 10:1. It follows that the usual dosage for unquantified ingestions is 1 g/kg. Activated charcoal is contraindicated in the event of an inadequately protected airway, heralded by absent gag reflex or extreme somnolence. If the administration of activated charcoal is deemed to be ideal, the patient may undergo rapid-sequence intubation to attain a protected airway. Extreme caution must be utilized when the toxic agent is known to slow GI motility (e.g., tricyclic antidepressants, calcium channel blockers, and opiates).

Activated charcoal may be found in preparation with sorbitol, a common cathartic. Data are conflicting regarding the administration of the combination of a charcoal-cathartic, and improvement in patient outcomes has not been documented (30). The consensus is that the isolated use of cathartics has no role in the management of the poisoned patient, and a sound recommendation is lacking regarding the routine use of a cathartic in combination with activated charcoal (30).

Activated charcoal has additional utility when given in multiple doses for substances with prolonged half-lives and small volumes of distribution. Agents amenable to the use of multidose activated charcoal are carbamazepine, dapsone, phenytoin, phenobarbital, quinine, salicylates, and theophylline. The mechanism of action appears to be via the interruption of enterohepatic and enteroenteric recirculation of drugs by sequestration of the drug in the gut lumen due to its concentration gradient. Clinical judgment must be utilized, as the clinical benefits of this therapy have not been proven with firm controlled studies, and the therapy is contraindicated in the presence of decreased peristalsis or bowel obstruction.

Whole-Bowel Irrigation

The technique of whole-bowel irrigation utilizing osmotically balanced polyethylene glycol electrolyte solutions (PEG-ES) appears attractive in that it can enhance the elimination of toxins prior to their absorption. A definite theoretical benefit can be gained in aiding elimination following ingestions of heavy metals, iron, sustained-release or enteric-coated tablets, and illegal drug packets. However, definitive clinical recommendations regarding this practice have not been established (31). Recommendations regarding dosing of PEG-ES have proposed target goals of 1500–2000 mL/hr in adults, 1000 mL/hr in children ages 6–12 years, and 500 mL/hr in children 9 months to 6 years of age. Utilization of this technique has absolutely no role in the management of patients with an unprotected airway, hemodynamic compromise, intractable vomiting, and GI hemorrhage, ileus, perforation, or obstruction (31).

Surgical Decontamination

Emergent surgical GI decontamination may prove useful in rare cases. For example, surgical intervention would be indicated in the event of mechanical bowel obstruction or bowel ischemia due to heroin or cocaine drug packets. Surgical intervention may be an option in the event of massive iron ingestion with failure to evacuate the GI tract.

Antidotes

Antidotal therapy is a vital component of management, as it may prove useful in initiating therapy and in definitively identifying a particular toxin (**Tables 31.9, 31.10**). However, antidotes are only available for a limited number of toxins and it is crucial to be aware of potential adverse reactions. It is essential to be familiar with specific antidotes that must be readily available in both the emergency department and ICU. The crux of management truly centers upon aggressive supportive care rather than administration of an antidote. Specific toxins and their antidotes as well as modes of enhancing elimination are listed in Table 31.9.

Flumazenil is an extremely useful benzodiazepine antagonist that can result in dramatic improvement in a depressed sensorium due to a benzodiazepine overdose. Flumazenil is a 1,4-imidazobenzodiazepine that competes with the benzodiazepines for receptor sites in the CNS that bind γ-aminobutyric acid (GABA), a primary inhibitory neurotransmitter; hence, it is classified as a benzodiazepine receptor antagonist. Flumazenil has a shorter duration of action than most benzodiazepines. The sedative and respiratory depression effects of the benzodiazepine may outlast the effects of flumazenil reversal. The major adverse reactions reported with flumazenil use are seizures and dysrhythmias. Seizures induced by flumazenil are difficult to manage because the benzodiazepine (GABA) receptors are blocked. The association of seizures has occurred in patients who were physically dependent upon benzodiazepines, those utilizing benzodiazepines for control of seizures, those with an underlying seizure disorder, and individuals treated for a combined ingestion of benzodiazepines and tricyclic antidepressants. Flumazenil may be especially helpful in managing a pure benzodiazepine overdose but should be avoided in unknown overdoses or in mixed ingestions.

The intensivist must be extremely familiar with the utilization of naloxone, an opiate-receptor antagonist that proves particularly useful in effecting rapid reversal of narcotic toxicity. Administration and dosing are discussed in the opioid toxidrome section of this chapter.

Extracorporeal Elimination

Aggressive supportive therapies to enhance toxin elimination have included hemoperfusion and hemodialysis (7). Randomized, prospective, controlled studies have not established solid guidelines for the utilization of such therapies. General guidelines have been suggested for circumstances that may warrant such techniques, including progressive clinical deterioration refractory to aggressive supportive care, ingestion and/or absorption of a potentially lethal dose of toxin, blood concentrations that indicate serious intoxication, and impaired organ function that limits the normal route of toxin elimination. Hemodialysis is effective for the removal of small compounds that are concentrated in the intravascular compartment and are loosely protein bound. Charcoal hemoperfusion is preferred in the instance of toxicity with larger, lipid-soluble compounds with greater affinity for plasma proteins.

Hemodialysis is indicated for the management of severe salicylate and lithium exposures, following toxic exposures to methanol and ethylene glycol, and occasionally when hydrophilic drugs with low volumes of distribution and low protein binding result in severe or life-threatening clinical effects and other, less-invasive therapeutic options are not available. Successful hemodialysis is dependent upon membrane permeability, correlation between the plasma drug concentration and drug toxicity, plasma levels in a potentially fatal range or the presence of a substance with high likelihood to be metabolized to a toxic substance, and ability to significantly enhance clearance. Consultation with the Poison Control Center and a nephrologist is often helpful in determining if hemodialysis is indicated. Although distinct theoretical benefits support utilization of extracorporeal therapies in the management of acute intoxications, few intoxicants require these techniques.

Hemoperfusion involves the passage of blood through an extracorporeal circuit and cartridge that contains an adsorbent and return of the detoxified blood to the patient. Using hemoperfusion is advantageous over using hemodialysis for a few drugs (e.g., theophylline); however, overdoses of theophylline have become extremely rare. For this reason, few institutions have experience with this technique; cartridges have become difficult to obtain and may not be available in many areas. Cartridges may become saturated with the toxin following 2 or more hours of use, which limits efficacious removal. Generous amounts of heparin are required to prevent the cartridges from clotting due to the adsorption of heparin by the charcoal. One must weigh the risk-benefit ratio of these therapies when considering their use.

Diuresis

Drug elimination may be facilitated by ensuring adequate renal flow 2–5 mL/kg/hr. This brisk diuresis will reduce drug

TABLE 31.9

SELECTED ANTIDOTES AND METHODS OF ENHANCING TOXIN ELIMINATION

Antidote	Toxin
Antivenoms	
Crotalidae	North American Pit Viper envenomation
Polyvalent (ACP)	
Polyvalent immune Fab	
Micruris sp.	Eastern or Texas coral snake envenomations
Latrodectus mactans	Black widow spider envenomation
Atropine	Organophosphate (OP), carbamate poisoning, bradydysrhythmias, Centruroides envenomation
Calcium (chloride or gluconate)	Calcium-channel blocker overdose, hydrofluoric acid ingestion/exposure
Cyanide antidote package	Cyanide, acetonitrile (artificial nail remover), amygdalin (peach, apricot pits), nitroprusside (thiosulfate only)
Amyl nitrite	
Sodium nitrite	
Sodium thiosulfate	
Deferoxamine	Iron
Digoxin-specific antibody fragments	Digoxin, digitoxin, natural cardiac glycosides (e.g., oleander, red squill, Bufo toad venom)
Flumazenil	Benzodiazepines
Fomepizole	Toxic alcohols (ethylene glycol, methanol)
Glucagon	Calcium-channel blocker, β-blocker toxicity
Glucose (dextrose)	Sulfonylureas, insulin, hypoglycemia (multiple toxins)
Hydroxocobalamin (vitamin B_{12})[a]	Cyanide, acetonitrile, amygdalin, nitroprusside
Insulin (high dose)/euglycemia[b]	Calcium-channel blocker, β-blocker toxicity
Methylene blue	Methemoglobinemia
N-acetylcysteine	Acetaminophen, pennyroyal oil, carbon tetrachloride
Naloxone	Opioid toxicity
Octreotide	Sulfonylurea toxicity
Physostigmine	Antimuscarinic delirium (as a diagnostic tool only)
Pralidoxime	OP poisoning (insecticides, nerve agents)
Protamine sulfate	Heparins
Pyridoxine	Isoniazid, monomethylhydrazine (rocket fuel), Gyromitra mushrooms
Thiamine	Deficiency states (e.g., alcoholism, anorexia nervosa)
Sodium bicarbonate	Sodium channel blocking cardiotoxins, salicylates

Method of removal	Indication
Dialysis	Toxic alcohols, salicylates, lithium, theophylline, valproic acid, atenolol, sotalol, others
Urinary alkalinization with sodium bicarbonate	Salicylates, phenobarbital, chlorpropamide, chlorophenoxy herbicides, methotrexate

[a] Not FDA approved for this use.
[b] Anecdotal experience.
From Barry JD. Diagnosis and management of the poisoned child. *Pediatr Ann* 2005;34:937–46, with permission.

concentration in the distal tubules and effectively decrease a concentration gradient, which reduces the chance of reabsorption and enhances elimination. Diuresis is occasionally combined with techniques to alter the urinary pH, a principle that is based upon the premise that reabsorption across the renal tubular epithelium occurs only when a compound is nonionized and lipid soluble. The ionized versus nonionized portion of a drug depends upon the pKa of the drug and the pH of the urine or plasma. It is possible to alter the pH of the urine and enhance the proportion of ionized drug, which essentially traps the drug in the tubular lumen, thereby reducing reabsorption and enhancing excretion. Elimination of drugs with pKa values in the range of 3.0–7.2 may be enhanced by alkalinizing the urine. Drugs and toxins with which

alkalinization of the urine has shown to be effective in enhancing elimination include salicylate, phenobarbital, chlorpropamide, and the chlorophenoxy herbicides. Alkalinization of the urine may be achieved by adding sodium bicarbonate (50–75 mEq/L) to the IV fluids. It is imperative to ensure vigilance in following serum potassium and sodium levels as alkalinization is accomplished. Although in theory, acidification of the urine may enhance elimination of a weak base, there is virtually no indication for acid diuresis in management of the poisoned patient. The utilization of aggressive diuresis poses a risk for fluid overload, with cerebral edema, pulmonary edema, and hyponatremia. It is essential to monitor urinary pH, serum sodium, and potassium and acid-base balance.

TABLE 31.10

USEFUL DIAGNOSTIC TRIALS

Agent suspected	Agent administered	Dose	Positive results
Benzodiazepines	Flumazenil	0.2–0.3 mg/kg IV (maximum 3 mg)	Improved consciousness
Iron	Deferoxamine	40 mg/kg IM (maximum 2 g)	"Vin rosé" urine color
Opiates	Naloxone hydrochloride	0.03 mg/kg (up to 4 mg)	Improved consciousness
Organophosphate	Atropine	0.1 mg/kg	Mydriasis, less secretions
Phenothiazine (dystonia)	Diphenhydramine	1–2 mg/kg IV (maximum 25 mg)	Resolution
Phenothiazine (neuroleptic malignant syndrome)	Dantrolene	1–3 mg/kg IV	Resolution
Insulin reaction	Dextrose	1 g/kg IV	Improved consciousness
Isoniazid	Pyridoxine	5 g IV	Seizures abate; improved consciousness

From Woolf AD. Principles of toxin assessment and screening. In: Fuhrman BP, Zimmerman J, eds. *Pediatric Critical Care*. 3rd ed. Philadelphia, PA: Mosby Elsevier, 2006:1511–31, with permission.

Several agents are particularly useful to employ as diagnostic trials in elucidating the presence of a particular toxin (**Table 31.10**). Utilization of specific antibodies has been extremely efficacious in binding to offending drugs, reversing their toxicity, and enhancing elimination. This therapy has shown dramatic results in severe digoxin intoxication, as discussed later. Specific antibodies are also commonly used for the treatment of crotalid and elapid envenomations.

TOXIDROMES

The physical examination may lend itself to the association of a constellation of signs associated with particular substances or groups of substances, most commonly referred to as toxidromes. Elucidation of toxidromes is dependent upon careful review of vital signs, mental status, pupillary size and reactivity, skin characteristics (moisture, temperature, and color), bowel sounds, muscle tone, respiratory effort, and the presence of tremors. The following review of toxidromes is meant to provide a descriptive overview, with tables for rapid ref-

erence. Further in-depth discussion may be sought in medical toxicology references.

Sympathomimetic/Adrenergic Agents

Common sympathomimetic adrenergic agents are listed in **Table 31.11**. Signs and symptoms of sympathomimetic toxicity (**Table 31.12**) are dependent upon the target receptor sites. It is common to witness tachycardia and hypotension due to the stimulatory and vasodilatory effects of β-agonists. α-Agonists are associated with severe hypertension and reflex bradycardia. Sympathetic effects may be rendered by direct adrenergic stimulation or via indirect action through release of norepinephrine. Hyperthermia, rhabdomyolysis, and myoglobinuria are attributed to increased metabolic activity. Myocardial ischemia may occur, as well as ischemic or hemorrhagic stroke. This classification generally includes the amphetamines, cocaine, ephedrine, pseudoephedrine, phenylpropanolamine, and other adrenergic stimulants. The methylxanthines caffeine and theophylline are not sympathomimetics, but they may result in similar symptomatology.

Benzodiazepines are useful in reducing CNS catecholamine release and thereby are effective in controlling severe hypertension, tachycardia, agitation, and extreme muscle activity. It is essential to recognize that use of a β-blocking agent to control tachycardia and hypertension may result in unopposed

TABLE 31.11

SYMPATHOMIMETIC AGENTS

Albuterol
Amphetamines
Caffeine
Catecholamines
Cocaine
Ephedrine
Ketamine
Lysergic acid diethylamide (LSD)
Methamphetamine
Phencyclidine (PCP)
Phenylephrine
Phenylpropanolamine
Pseudoephedrine
Terbutaline
Theophylline

TABLE 31.12

SYMPATHOMIMETIC TOXIDROME

Agitation
Seizures
Mydriasis
Tachycardia
Hypertension
Diaphoresis
Pallor
Cool Skin
Fever

α-receptor stimulation. For this reason, β-blockers are best avoided, and a benzodiazepine alone or with nitroprusside or phentolamine should be used when control of hypertension and tachycardia becomes necessary. Cocaine toxicity can result in depletion of catecholamines, which may cause late cardiovascular collapse. It follows that short-acting antihypertensive agents are preferred for treating these overdoses.

The sympathomimetic toxidrome is not seen with toxicity due to such centrally acting α-agonists as clonidine. These agents result in decreased sympathetic outflow and cause reflex bradycardia, hypotension, and CNS and respiratory depression.

Cholinergic Agents

Toxins and poisons that increase the effect of the cholinergic nervous system are classified as cholinergic agonists. These substances include muscarinic agents, nicotinic agents, and cholinesterase inhibitors (Table 31.13). Muscarinic agents act at postganglionic, parasympathetic nerve endings and in sweat glands. The direct acting muscarinic agonists result in excessive parasympathetic activity. Nicotinic agents act at sympathetic and parasympathetic autonomic ganglia. Cholinesterase inhibitors result in an accumulation of acetylcholine at the cholinergic synapse.

This toxidrome is effectively managed with atropine. Nicotine is known to cause salivation, nausea, and vomiting. Tachycardia, hypertension, and tachypnea are generally followed by bradycardia, hypotension, and respiratory failure. Central effects include initial agitation, followed by seizures, lethargy, coma, and possible neuromuscular blockade. Management of nicotine poisoning is accomplished with aggressive supportive care.

Organophosphate pesticides and nerve agents are examples of cholinesterase inhibitors. It is possible to have a mixed tox-

TABLE 31.13

CHOLINERGIC TOXIDROME FEATURES

Muscarinic effects (DUMBBELS)
Diarrhea
Urinary incontinence
Miosis
Bradycardia
Bronchorrhea
Emesis
Lacrimation
Salivation
Nicotinic effects
Fasciculations
Weakness
Paralysis
Tachycardia
Hypertension
Agitation
Central effects
Lethargy
Coma
Agitation
Seizures

icity, but parasympathetic toxicity is most commonly seen. The mechanism of action of organophosphate toxicity occurs by the binding and inactivation of acetylcholinesterase, with a subsequent excess of nicotinic and muscarinic activity in the peripheral and central nervous systems. The preponderance of acetylcholine results in depolarization of the neuromuscular junction. The enzyme is eventually phosphorylated, and cholinesterase activity resumes following synthesis of a new enzyme. Carbamates, which are also used as pesticides, reversibly bind to acetylcholinesterase and ultimately undergo spontaneous hydrolysis, which results in a restoration of cholinesterase activity within hours. The central manifestations of carbamate toxicity are less severe, as they do not easily penetrate the CNS. The symptoms of organophosphate toxicity depend upon the route, duration of exposure, and the absorbed dose. Dermal exposure results in local hyperhidrosis, which is followed by systemic involvement as the drug is absorbed.

Topical decontamination with utilization of personal protective equipment is essential. Inhalational exposure is marked by upper airway involvement and subsequent respiratory distress. Vomiting and drooling are most commonly seen following ingestion. Fatality is usually attributed to respiratory failure that results from bronchorrhea, bronchospasm, diminished respiratory drive, and neuromuscular blockade. Seizures and severe CNS toxicity occur following large exposures to household products or small exposures to industrial pesticides and "nerve agents."

Management of organophosphate toxicity involves expeditious administration of atropine to reverse the muscarinic effects, an oxime (Pralidoxime) to facilitate reactivation of acetylcholinesterase, which reverses the neuromuscular blockade, and benzodiazepines to control seizures. Atropine administration is guided by the effect of drying secretions rather than by heart rate or pupil size. Pralidoxime is not generally administered in the case of carbamate toxicity, because the carbamates bind to acetylcholinesterase; consequently, the effects are self-limited.

A caveat of rapid sequence intubation in the management of organophosphate poisoning involves the potential for prolonged paralysis. The production of acetylcholinesterase and plasma cholinesterase is inhibited, which prolongs the half-life of succinylcholine.

Anticholinergic Agents

Agents that produce antimuscarinic properties result in a constellation of symptoms and signs referred to as the anticholinergic toxidrome (Tables 31.14, 31.15). These agents act at muscarinic receptors of the CNS, targeting organs of the parasympathetic nervous system and the sympathetic nervous system (the sweat glands). This toxidrome is extremely similar to the sympathomimetic toxidrome but may be distinguished by examination of the mucous membranes and skin and by auscultation for bowel sounds. Sympathomimetic toxicity results in diaphoresis and cool skin, while anticholinergic toxicity is notoriously marked by impaired sweating and warm, dry skin. Sympathomimetics result in hyperactive bowel sounds, while anticholinergics cause diminished bowel sounds and even ileus. Tachycardia, mydriasis, urinary retention, flushing, and hyperthermia are found with both sympathomimetic and

TABLE 31.14

ANTICHOLINERGIC AGENTS

Antihistamines—diphenhydramine, hydroxyzine
Atropine
Benztropine mesylate
Carbamazepine
Cyclic antidepressants
Cyclobenzaprine
Hyoscyamine
Jimsonweed
Oxybutynin
Phenothiazines
Scopolamine
Trihexyphenidyl

anticholinergic toxicity. Hypertension also occurs with both sympathomimetic and anticholinergic exposures; however, it is generally less severe with anticholinergic toxicity than with sympathomimetic toxicity.

Management must focus on controlling agitation to minimize hyperthermia in the face of impaired sweating mechanisms. Benzodiazepines may be extremely helpful in managing symptoms. Physostigmine, a cholinesterase inhibitor, may be employed with the intent of reversing central and peripheral manifestations of the anticholinergic toxidrome; however, it is not recommended for management of tricyclic antidepressant toxicity because of reported convulsions and asystole.

Opioid Agents

Agents that result in the opioid toxidrome are classified as opiates (substances derived from opium) and opioids (substances derived from opium and synthetically derived agents with similar properties). These terms are used interchangeably, as the pharmacologic effects are similar. Most opioids and opi-

TABLE 31.15

ANTICHOLINERGIC TOXIDROME

Agitation
Delirium
Coma
Mydriasis
Dry mouth
Warm, dry, flushed skin
Tachycardia
Hypertension
Fever
Urinary retention
Decreased bowel sounds
Associated expressions
"Mad as a Hatter"
"Blind as a Bat"
"Red as a Beet"
"Hot as a Hare"
"Dry as a Bone"

ates cause a triad of respiratory depression, coma, and miosis. An exception is meperidine, with which toxicity is manifested by respiratory depression, coma, and mydriasis; additionally, seizures are reported to occur with meperidine toxicity. Physical findings often include bradycardia, hypotension, and decreased GI motility. Diphenoxylate and methadone present a particular hazard to toddlers due to low-dose ingestions (27).

Management involves administration of naloxone, an opiate-receptor antagonist that results in rapid reversal of toxicity. Naloxone is generally initiated at 0.1 mg/kg/dose IV in children and 1–2 mg/dose in adolescents and adults to achieve reversal of respiratory depression. If a partial response is observed, up to 10 mg may be necessary. Alternate administration can be accomplished by a variety of routes: subcutaneous, intramuscular, and endotracheal. It is critical to note that administration of naloxone may precipitate an acute withdrawal syndrome in opiate-dependent patients. If opiate dependency is suspected, it is prudent to initiate therapy with lower doses. The duration of action of naloxone is shorter than the action of many opiates; therefore, it is essential to strongly consider subsequent dosing or even administration of continuous infusion. Naloxone has been associated with the development of pulmonary edema, although this condition may occur as a result of opiate toxicity (36). Nalmefene is a longer-acting opiate-receptor antagonist; it administration should be preceded by a test dose of naloxone to rule out the possibility of acute withdrawal. Nalmefene is not thought to carry significant advantages, as compared to a continuous naloxone infusion.

Clonidine is a centrally acting α-agonist that is often included in the opiate toxidrome due to the diminished sympathetic tone, its ability to cause miosis and CNS and respiratory depression in overdose, and its occasional reversal with naloxone. Controversy exists regarding the utilization of naloxone in clonidine toxicity. In the event of respiratory failure, aggressive supportive care mandates initiation of airway management prior to the administration of naloxone.

Many opiates (e.g., codeine, hydrocodone, oxycodone, and propoxyphene) are formulated in combination with acetaminophen or aspirin. Therefore, it is extremely important to maintain a high index of suspicion for toxicity from such compounds. Fentanyl patches contain a high concentration of drug per patch; significant toxicity can result from ingestion as well as inhalation.

FOCUSED REVIEW OF COMMON TOXINS

It is beyond the scope of a textbook of pediatric critical care medicine to do justice to the field of toxicology in attempting to review specific pharmacology, pathophysiology, clinical manifestations, and management for each toxin. The earlier discussion was designed to provide a succinct, common sense approach to dealing with a poisoned child or adolescent. Such tools will guide the practitioner to locate appropriate resources and adeptly stabilize the patient. The following section will review a number of the most commonly seen toxins in the emergency department that require subsequent care in the ICU.

Acetaminophen

Acetaminophen is by far the most commonly ingested drug in the case of intentional overdoses. It presents a significant concern due to its toxicity, which can result in fulminant hepatic failure. An understanding of the pharmacokinetics of acetaminophen metabolism is essential to developing a management plan. Acetaminophen is metabolized in the liver by glucuronidation and sulfation-forming nontoxic metabolites that are renally excreted. In event of an overdose, metabolism via the CYP2E1, CYP1A2, and CYP3A4 subfamilies of the cytochrome P-450 pathway produces N-acetyl-p-benzoquinoneimine (NAPQI), which conjugates with reduced glutathione (2). Glutathione is depleted in the case of a significant overdose, which allows the toxic intermediate NAPQI to bind to the hepatocytes and result in cell death. This metabolite is detoxified by reduced glutathione when acetaminophen is taken in appropriate doses. Excessive doses of acetaminophen completely overwhelm the liver's ability to detoxify NAPQI, which results in hepatic necrosis (**Fig. 31.1**). The clinical manifestations of acetaminophen intoxication are commonly described in four stages.

The initial presentation of an acetaminophen overdose is usually heralded by nausea and vomiting within 12–24 hrs, although some patients may be completely asymptomatic (Stage I). This is clearly a reason to screen for acetaminophen levels in all ingestions. Acidosis may be present in extreme overdoses. The liver transaminases usually are noted to be elevated by 24 hrs following ingestion (Stage II), at which time clinical symptoms often abate. Liver function abnormalities peak at 48–72 hrs following ingestion, and symptomatology returns with nausea, vomiting, and anorexia (Stage III). The clinical course may result in complete recovery or fulminant hepatic failure. The recovery phase (Stage IV) generally lasts approximately 7–8 days. It is important to know that cases of fulminant hepatic failure with jaundice, encephalopathy, and bleeding occur infrequently. The most efficacious therapy involves the administration of N-acetylcysteine (NAC), which serves as a precursor

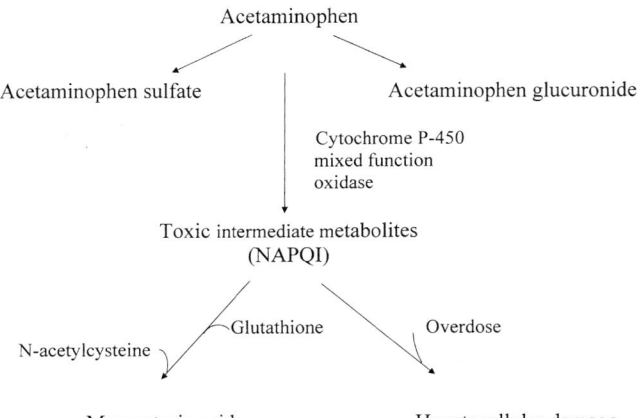

FIGURE 31.1. The intermediate metabolite NAPQI is responsible for hepatic injury associated with acetaminophen toxicity; it is ordinarily detoxified by the addition of sulfhydryl groups. Glutathione acts as a sulfhydryl group donor but, in massive overdose, it is not present in sufficient quantity to protect the liver. N-acetylcysteine acts as a sulfhydryl group donor to detoxify NAPQI when glutathione is depleted.

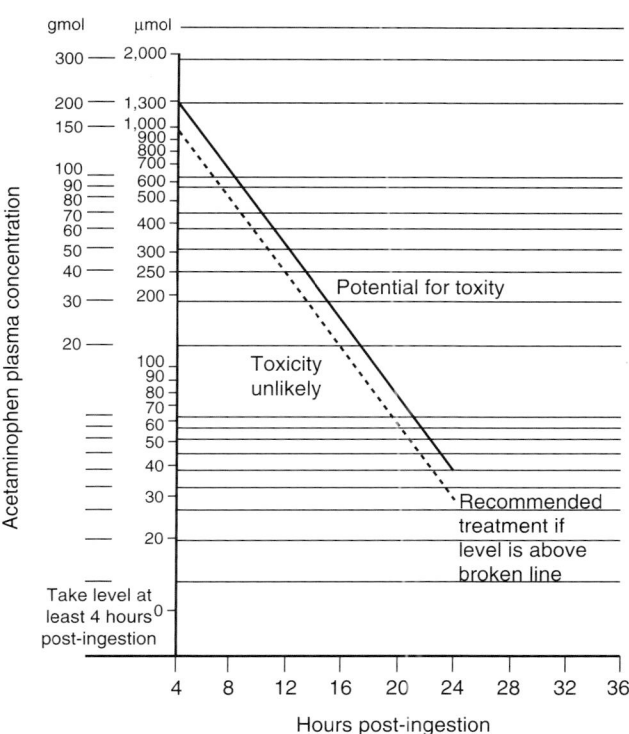

FIGURE 31.2. Use of nomogram in management of acute acetaminophen overdose. From Joshi P, Toxidromes and their treatment. Acetaminophen level is obtained at ≥4 hrs after ingestion. Level is then plotted on nomogram. Above the broken line = administer full course of acetylcysteine. Below the broken line = acetylcysteine not necessary. From Fuhrman BP, Zimmerman JJ, eds. *Pediatric Critical Care, 3rd ed.* Philadelphia: Mosby, Elsevier, 2006:1521–31, with permission.

to facilitate the synthesis of glutathione (**Fig. 31.1**). Initiation of NAC is usually recommended within 10 hrs following ingestion; however, it has been beneficial when administered up to 24 hrs following ingestion. Timely utilization of NAC has been proven to reduce the incidence of hepatotoxicity. A decision to employ this therapy is based upon application of the Rumack-Matthew nomogram (15) (**Fig. 31.2**) in plotting a serum level of acetaminophen drawn at least 4 hrs following ingestion. In the event that blood levels are not immediately available, treatment decisions should be based upon a suggestive history. The therapy can be stopped if a nontoxic level is eventually obtained. Oral dosing of NAC begins with a loading dose of 140 mg/kg, followed by maintenance therapy of 70 mg/kg every 4 hrs for 17 doses. Therapy should continue until all doses are administered, even though the acetaminophen plasma level drops below the toxic range. NAC can also be administered IV in a 20-hr protocol. Initially, the patient receives a 150-mg/kg loading dose over 15 mins, followed by 50 mg/kg over 4 hrs, and then 100 mg/kg over the final 16 hrs. Care must be taken to ensure that the NAC is appropriately diluted and that the patient will not become fluid overloaded.

Salicylates

It is essential that physicians in the PICU are aware of the many forms of salicylates. Acetylsalicylic acid (ASA), or aspirin, is the most commonly encountered form, but bismuth subsalicylate, sodium salicylate, and magnesium salicylate are often encountered in various drugs. Aspirin is contained in a wide variety of medications, including antihistamines, sympathomimetics, anticholinergics, opiates, and acetaminophen. Oil of wintergreen, comprised of 98% methyl salicylate, is a particularly dangerous compound. Another less commonly considered mode of intoxication occurs via exposure to topical aspirin-containing compounds that are ingested or absorbed cutaneously. In general, doses of <100 mg/kg produce minimal toxicity; however, doses that exceed 300 mg/kg can yield catastrophic clinical symptoms and often prove deadly. Aspirin with a pKa of 3.5 exists largely in the non-ionized, insoluble form in the stomach. A low gastric pH causes most of the aspirin to remain in the non-ionized form; hence, it dissolves inefficiently. If a patient has been taking an H_2 antagonist, a proton-pump inhibitor, or antacids, the pH of the stomach will become less acidotic, rendering the aspirin to have improved solubility and more rapid absorption.

Respiratory alkalosis is often the first feature of salicylate intoxication; it results from increased minute ventilation. Nausea, vomiting, dehydration, and tinnitus are commonly seen. CNS manifestations include lethargy, coma, and seizures. The mechanism of action involves the uncoupling of oxidative phosphorylation, resulting in hyperpyrexia and acidosis. The severity of acidosis is also contributed to by an inhibition of the tricarboxylic acid cycle. It is not unusual to have a mixed acid-base status manifested by either respiratory alkalosis, metabolic acidosis, or a mixed respiratory alkalosis-metabolic acidosis. The concomitant ingestion of CNS depressants can blunt the respiratory drive and result in a more profound metabolic acidosis. Salicylate intoxication may mimic the presentation of diabetes mellitus due to its effects on carbohydrate metabolism, with resultant hyperglycemia and glycosuria. Chronic salicylate toxicity has been associated with fatal complications of pulmonary and cerebral edema. Diagnosis of chronic salicylate intoxication requires a high index of suspicion, as the presentation may appear as an altered sensorium, sepsis, diabetic ketoacidosis, respiratory failure, or cardiopulmonary disease.

Salicylate intoxication is quickly diagnosed by assessing the plasma salicylate concentration, thereby measuring the concentration of salicylic acid and its metabolites. Preliminary diagnosis may be rapidly made by utilizing the ferric chloride or Phenistix test. Ferric chloride added to a urine sample that contains salicylate will turn the specimen purple. Blood or urine that contains salicylate will turn the Phenistix brown. Determination of serum salicylate levels should be made 2 and 6 hrs following ingestion of immediate-release preparations. In the event of a significant overdose or ingestion of enteric-coated tablets, it is important to monitor levels every 2–4 hrs to establish a peak level. Levels should be monitored for at least 24 hrs in the event of an ingestion of sustained-release or enteric-coated capsules due to their very erratic absorption.

Targeted therapy in salicylate ingestion is directed at prevention of absorption early on with activated charcoal and alkalinization of the urine to enhance the elimination as described earlier. Meticulous monitoring of urine pH is necessary to avoid significant alkalemia. Acetazolamide is not utilized to achieve an alkaline diuresis, as it results in a systemic metabolic acidosis. Hemodialysis is quite efficacious, and is recommended for extremely elevated serum salicylate levels (>100 mg/dL), presence of renal insufficiency, significant volume overload, and pulmonary edema or severe electrolyte aberrations. The benefit of hemodialysis is the ability to achieve rapid correction of fluid and electrolyte abnormalities, correct acid-base disturbances, and enhance salicylate clearance.

ALCOHOLS

Ethanol

Ethanol is reported to be the most commonly ingested alcohol and poses a hazard not only in beverage form, but is contained in a variety of other products, such as mouthwash, perfume and cologne, and topical antiseptics. Children may present with nausea, vomiting, stupor, and ataxia. Infants and toddlers may dramatically develop coma, hypothermia, and hypoglycemia when ethanol levels exceed 50–100 mg/dL. Metabolic acidosis is typically found. Adolescents tend to have more typical signs of intoxication with levels of 100–150 mg/dL. Deaths directly attributed to alcohol ingestion are usually associated with alcohol concentrations >500 mg/dL. It is critical to have a concept of the concentration of alcohol when considering the potential toxicities. An ingestion of approximately 1 g/kg of ethanol will raise the blood alcohol level to 100 mg/dL. The following estimates of toxicity may be extrapolated: beer (5% alcohol), 10–15 mL/kg; wine (14% alcohol), 4–6 mL/kg; and 80-proof liquor (40% alcohol), 1–2 mL/kg. Binge drinking has been a catastrophic activity of adolescents and college students.

Emergent assessment and management of potential respiratory compromise is a priority, as is rapid blood glucose determination. Ethanol is rapidly absorbed from the GI tract, so that GI decontamination is rarely necessary. However, in adolescents, activated charcoal is useful due to a significant risk of co-ingestions.

The metabolism of alcohol by the hepatic enzyme alcohol dehydrogenase is dose dependent. In general, the rate of reduction is reported to range from 10–25 mg/dL/hr. Hemodialysis may increase the rate of elimination significantly, but it is rarely necessary. Patients with impaired liver function or significant toxicity (levels >450–500 mg/dL) may be candidates for hemodialysis.

Isopropyl Alcohol

Isopropyl alcohol is a component of many home products, including rubbing alcohol, aftershave lotions, perfumes, skin lotions, and antifreeze compounds. Young children are at risk for accidental ingestion, while adolescents may utilize the products as an ethanol substitute. Ingestion is typically the most common route, but infants may be poisoned via inhalation of isopropyl vapors during sponging for a fever. The toxic dose is reported to be 1 mL/kg of 70% isopropyl alcohol; ingestion of more than a swallow is potentially toxic in children. Toxicity is manifested by vomiting, abdominal pain, and often, hematemesis due to gastritis. Neurologic manifestations include lethargy, dizziness, ataxia, and possible coma. In patients who have ingested isopropyl alcohol, the unusual finding of ketosis and ketonemia without an acidemia may be seen. Isopropyl alcohol is metabolized to acetone. Children are at extreme risk for hypoglycemia. Ethanol, fomepizole, and hemodialysis are usually not indicated in the management of isopropyl alcohol intoxication.

Methanol and Ethylene Glycol

Methanol and ethylene glycol are toxic alcohols most commonly found in antifreeze compounds, and both are known to cause CNS depression. The substances are metabolized by alcohol dehydrogenase, which results in extremely toxic metabolites. Methanol is metabolized to formic acid, which causes severe metabolic acidosis and retinal toxicity. Ethylene glycol is ultimately metabolized to oxalate, which results in severe metabolic acidosis, hypocalcemia, and renal failure.

Ingestions that exceed 0.5 mL/kg may result in significant toxicity, and ingestions >1 mL/kg may prove to be fatal. Determination of an elevated osmolal gap is helpful, as these compounds are osmotically active and may raise the measured serum osmolality. It must be recognized that the presence of a normal osmolal gap (−8 to +12) does not exclude significant levels of toxic alcohols. Toxicity may be documented with serum levels of the parent compounds; however, in the event of a late presentation, levels may be undetectable following complete metabolism. The laboratory hallmarks of ethylene glycol and methanol poisoning are a high anion gap metabolic acidosis and an elevated osmolal gap.

The cornerstone of management has been aimed at blocking alcohol dehydrogenase to negate the formation of the toxic metabolites. Although ethanol has been utilized, it is fraught with difficulties in titration, as well as side effects of inebriation, CNS depression, hypoglycemia, and hypotension. Fomepizole has become the accepted drug of choice in blocking alcohol dehydrogenase. Following the administration of fomepizole, the parent alcohol compounds are renally excreted: methanol with a half-life of 54 hrs and ethylene glycol with a half-life of 19.7 hrs. Thiamine and pyridoxine should be administered IV every 6 hrs to patients who have ingested ethylene glycol. Thiamine has been shown to stimulate the conversion of glyoxylate to α-hydroxy-β-ketoadipate, and pyridoxine stimulates the conversion of glyoxylate to nontoxic glycine. Both of these may theoretically reduce metabolism to oxalic acid and calcium oxalate; however, evidence based benefits have not been established. Folic acid should be given to patients who have ingested methanol, as it has been shown in animals to speed the metabolism of formic acid to carbon dioxide and water. Hemodialysis is recommended in the instance of high levels of methanol or ethylene glycol, especially with concomitant metabolic acidosis, electrolyte abnormalities, and renal impairment of visual disturbance.

CAUSTICS

The ingestion of caustic compounds requires an understanding of the differing pathophysiology between alkaline and acid products. Alkaline injury results from a liquefaction necrosis caused by saponification of cellular fats and protein degradation. This process quickly results in very deep injury, mostly involving the oropharynx and proximal esophagus. Affected tissue often turns a white-gray color

(saponification necrosis) and becomes friable and structurally unstable. Perforation is common with severe exposures. Automatic dishwasher detergents possess extremely high alkalinity and are thought to be the most dangerous detergent in most households (21).

Acid ingestion results in a superficial coagulation necrosis, with marked heat production and eschar formation. Ingested acid is often absorbed, resulting in metabolic acidosis, hemolysis, and renal failure. The coagulative necrosis seen with acid ingestions often involves the length of the esophagus, extending into the stomach. Injury potential is dependent upon the type of chemicals involved, the quantity and concentration, duration of contact, liquid versus solid, diluents present and the vulnerability of the tissues affected.

Caustic ingestions pose risk to the GI tract and may result in respiratory damage. Significant caustic ingestions are marked by nausea, vomiting, oropharyngeal plaques, burns and tissue edema, dysphagia, drooling, and refusal to eat or drink. The clinical presentation may involve generalized systemic signs, including hyperpyrexia, respiratory distress, hemodynamic instability, hypocalcemia (with hydrofluoric acid ingestion), and metabolic acidosis (with acidic ingestion). Perforation may be marked by abdominal pain, subcutaneous emphysema, pneumothorax, pneumomediastinum, or peritonitis.

Management of the caustic toxin involves aggressive decontamination, with washing and diluting of dermal or ocular exposures, fresh air and oxygen for inhalational injury, and removal of as much substance from the mouth as possible in the ingestion of a caustic solid. The pH of the ocular fluids should be determined following irrigation to ensure neutralization of caustics; normal pH of tears is 7. Alkali eye exposures mandate an urgent ophthalmologic consult. Serial radiographs are utilized to track swallowed button batteries. Button batteries lodged in the esophagus must be expeditiously removed; those in the stomach or intestines generally pass intact.

If the patient can immediately drink a small amount of water or milk, it may help to reduce esophageal injury by washing the caustic into the stomach. Damage following the ingestion of a liquid occurs within seconds to minutes, offering little opportunity to dilute the toxin. After the immediate phase, when tissue damage is occurring, dilution of the ingested caustic is not recommended because of the limited possibility for benefit and the greater potential for harm due to perforation or even pulmonary aspiration. Tissue damage may continue for a slightly longer period when a solid caustic agent has been ingested. Additionally, with the anticipation of sedation for diagnostic endoscopy, the patient must remain with an empty stomach. Neutralization of a caustic substance is contraindicated, as the resultant exothermic reaction can yield more extensive tissue destruction. Ipecac, gastric lavage, and activated charcoal are not indicated. Endoscopy is recommended within the first 24 hrs following ingestion to quantify actual tissue damage. Risk for perforation is significant if endoscopy is delayed over 48 hrs due to loss of tissue integrity. The role of steroids has been controversial in reducing inflammation, granulation, and stricture formation. Steroids may be indicated in the event of laryngeal edema and bronchospasm. Antibiotics have no role in the absence of documented bacterial involvement or an existing secondary infection. Patients must be monitored for complications of mediastinitis, pneumonitis, and peritonitis.

Carbon Monoxide

Carbon monoxide poisoning is a major factor in deaths related to fire, but exposure may occur due to the incomplete combustion of any carbon-containing fuel (e.g., natural gas, fuel oil, gasoline, propane, charcoal). Such poisonings are often reported with improperly vented wood- or coal-burning stoves and from an inadequately ventilated automobile exhaust pipe. Carbon monoxide exposure results in significant tissue hypoxia due to the extremely high binding affinity with hemoglobin (200–300 times that of oxygen) and a leftward shift and change in shape (hyperbolic configuration) of the oxyhemoglobin dissociation curve. Carbon monoxide also binds to cytochrome oxidase and interferes with electron transport and adenosine triphosphate production. Definitive diagnosis is made by cooximetry and determination of the carboxyhemoglobin level. Frequently reported signs and symptoms are associated with a specific level of carboxyhemoglobin (**Table 31.16**); however, exact correlation between carboxyhemoglobin levels and symptomatology is often lacking. It is important to recognize that the blood carboxyhemoglobin levels will fall rapidly and may not truly reflect the degree of cellular dysfunction. Transcutaneous measurement of oxygen saturation by pulse oximetry will be falsely normal, as pulse oximetry cannot differentiate oxyhemoglobin from carboxyhemoglobin.

The mainstay of therapy is directed at removing the patient from the source of contamination and expeditious delivery of 100% oxygen. The half-life of carboxyhemoglobin is dependent upon the mode of delivery of varying oxygen concentrations (**Table 31.17**). Hyperbaric oxygen therapy is particularly useful in extreme cases, because it both dramatically decreases the concentration of carboxyhemoglobin and accelerates the

TABLE 31.16

CARBON MONOXIDE INHALATION

Carboxy-hemoglobin level	Intoxication classification	Symptoms
5%		*Impaired judgment* *Altered fine motor skills*
20%	Mild	*Headache* *Dyspnea* *Visual changes* *Confusion*
30%	Moderate	*Drowsiness, dulled sensorium* *Faintness* *Nausea/vomiting* *Tachycardia*
40%–60%	Moderate – Severe	*Weakness* *Poor coordination* *Loss of recent memory* *Impending cardiovascular and neurologic collapse*
>60%	Severe	*Coma* *Convulsion* *Death*

TABLE 31.17

HALF-LIFE OF CARBOXYHEMOGLOBIN

Oxygen concentration	t 1/2
21%	5 hrs
100% (mask, ET)	90 min
Hyperbaric oxygen, 2–3 atmospheres	30 min

ET, endotracheal

removal of carbon monoxide from cytochrome oxidase. A caveat in consideration of hyperbaric oxygen therapy is the lack of pediatric clinical trials; it follows that utilization of hyperbaric oxygenation is controversial. However, strong consideration should be given to early consultation with a hyperbaric oxygen therapy facility for patients who have experienced loss of consciousness or syncope or who continue to exhibit neurologic symptoms while receiving oxygen therapy. Hyperbaric therapy has no role if such a transfer would compromise patient stabilization and the accessibility/capability for providing intensive care management. Complications associated with hyperbaric therapy include barotraumas (pneumomediastinum, pneumothorax, tympanic membrane rupture), oxygen toxicity (seizures), and claustrophobic reactions in a small chamber. It is disheartening that carbon monoxide poisoning that presents with loss of consciousness or syncope, even with initially low carboxyhemoglobin levels, may ultimately result in delayed or persistent neurologic sequelae.

Cyanide

Cyanide toxicity may result from a number of differing exposures. Often used as an industrial reagent, it is also found as a component of smoke in household fires that involve plastics and other synthetic materials. Hydrogen cyanide is generated by the combustion of plastics in home and industrial fires. The seeds of a number of edible fruits (apples, cherries, peaches, and pears) contain cyanogenic glycosides that are converted to cyanide in the GI tract. Nitroprusside is metabolized to cyanide; therefore, close monitoring for toxicity is necessary when utilized in the ICU, especially with existing renal failure.

The ingestion of cyanide salts (sodium cyanide, potassium cyanide) results in their conversion to hydrogen cyanide by the presence of gastric acids. This compound is then absorbed. Cyanide quickly causes toxicity via the inhalational route by binding to cytochrome A3, preventing the uptake of oxygen by cytochrome oxidase and the electron transport chain. Tissue hypoxia results due to a complete lack of oxygen utilization, with failure to produce ATP.

Management is especially challenging, as the signs and symptoms are nonspecific but reflect profound hypoxia. Death often occurs within minutes of exposure. Patients do not present with cyanosis; venous oxygen saturation is elevated, which reflects the inability of the cells to utilize oxygen. Successful treatment requires rapid diagnosis and administration of the antidote (**Fig. 31.3**). The antidote kit contains amyl nitrite ampules and IV sodium nitrite to produce methemoglobinemia. The amyl nitrite is administered by inhalation while IV access

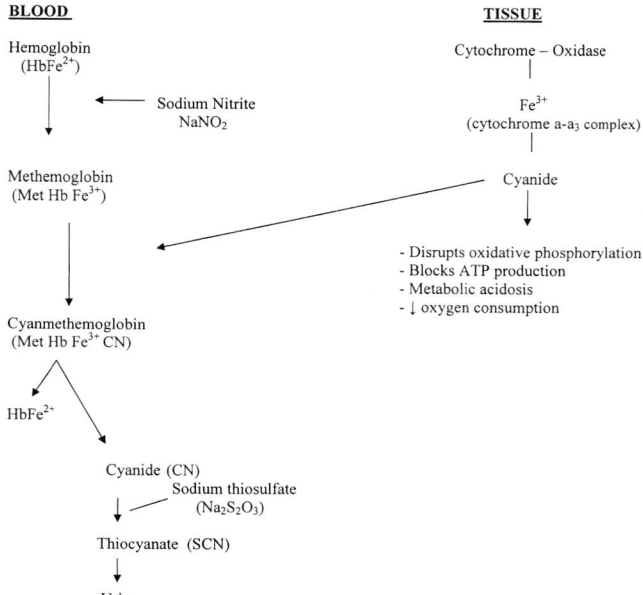

BLOOD   TISSUE

Hemoglobin (HbFe^{2+})

Cytochrome – Oxidase

Sodium Nitrite NaNO$_2$

Fe^{3+} (cytochrome a-a$_3$ complex)

Methemoglobin (Met Hb Fe^{3+})

Cyanide

- Disrupts oxidative phosphorylation
- Blocks ATP production
- Metabolic acidosis
- ↓ oxygen consumption

Cyanmethemoglobin (Met Hb Fe^{3+} CN)

HbFe^{2+}

Cyanide (CN)

Sodium thiosulfate (Na$_2$S$_2$O$_3$)

Thiocyanate (SCN)

Urine

FIGURE 31.3. Sodium nitrite (NaNO$_2$) causes an oxidant stress, which results in the formation of methemoglobin. The ferric ion of methemoglobin competes with cytochrome oxidase for cyanide, dissociates cyanide from the tissue, and forms cyanmethemoglobin. Sodium thiosulfate (Na$_2$S$_2$O$_3$) facilitates the conversion of the cyanide (CN) contained in cyanmethemoglobin to thiocyanate (SCN).

is obtained. Once an IV site is available, the sodium nitrite is given to produce an approximate 20% methemoglobinemia. The utility of methemoglobin is that it has an even higher binding affinity for cyanide than cytochrome A3 and will remove the cyanide-forming cyanmethemoglobin. Sodium thiosulfate is then administered as a substrate for the enzyme rhodanase, which will form sodium thiocyanate and regenerate the methemoglobin to scavenge another molecule of cyanide from the cytochrome oxidase chain. The sodium thiocyanate will then be cleared by the kidneys and eliminated in the urine. It is important to judiciously administer the initial nitrites to minimize the risk of hypotension, as both are potent vasodilators. Although cyanide toxicity may be present in fire victims, nitrite administration is particularly risky because the resultant methemoglobin formation would exacerbate the already diminished oxygen-carrying capacity due to carbon monoxide exposure.

Iron

Iron toxicity poses extreme detriment in the case of a significant ingestion. Iron exists in a variety of salts that contain differing proportions of elemental iron. Doses of elemental iron that exceed 20 mg/kg generally cause GI irritation. Systemic toxicity usually does not occur unless the elemental iron dose exceeds 60 mg/kg. The first phase of iron intoxication usually occurs within 30 mins of ingestion and is marked by vomiting, diarrhea, and possible hematemesis or hematochezia. This stage may require aggressive fluid resuscitation due to profound fluid and electrolyte losses. The latent period, or second phase, is heralded by a resolution of the GI manifestations, but the patient continues to have a nonspecific malaise. Tachycardia may be present following the previous fluid derangements,

and metabolic acidosis may be developing. The third phase occurs 12 hrs following ingestion and is manifested by profound hemodynamic instability and shock. The fourth phase is depicted by liver failure. Scarring or strictures of the GI tract may occur due to the corrosive effect of the iron. It is highly unusual to be faced with systemic iron toxicity without the prodromal GI symptoms.

Iron toxicity warrants serious consideration of GI lavage or whole-bowel irrigation because it is not effectively adsorbed by charcoal. Whole bowel irrigation is effective in decreasing iron absorption and is helpful in breaking up pill concretions that can result in direct mucosal injury. The coalescence of iron tablets in the stomach or duodenum has resulted in hemorrhagic infarction, with subsequent perforation, peritonitis, and death. A reasonable risk of pyloric stenosis or bowel stenosis may present at 4–6 weeks following ingestion.

Serum iron levels should be determined within 6 hrs of ingestion. If patients remain asymptomatic by 6 hrs following ingestion, it is highly unlikely that systemic illness will develop. Metabolic acidosis or acidemia correlates with toxicity. A white blood cell count >15,000/mm^3 with a serum glucose level >150 mg/dL may sometimes be found and may have some predictive value of elevated serum iron levels. Deferoxamine chelation (gradually increasing to 15 mg/kg/hr IV) is indicated for serum iron levels >500 mcg/dL or in the event of hemodynamic collapse. Deferoxamine must be administered with caution for multiple reasons. It is derived from *Streptomyces pilosus*, and a percentage of patients will probably have allergic reactions. If deferoxamine is administered too rapidly, it causes hypotension and in adults; if greater than 6–8 g is administered in 24 hrs, pulmonary fibrosis can occur. If symptoms appear refractory to management following 24 hrs of chelation therapy, it is recommended to decrease the deferoxamine infusion due to its association with development of acute respiratory distress syndrome. Chelation therapy is continued until the serum iron level returns to normal, the metabolic acidosis resolves, the patient clinically improves, and the urine color returns to normal. Determination of total iron-binding capacity is not useful in acute management, as the presence of free iron interferes with the assay, which results in a falsely elevated reading of total iron-binding capacity.

Critical care management must focus upon the potential for cardiopulmonary failure with profound hypotension, extreme metabolic acidosis, hypo- or hyperglycemia, anemia and colloid losses due to GI hemorrhage, renal failure secondary to shock, and hepatic failure, which exacerbates the bleeding diathesis. Brisk urine output is essential for the excretion of the iron-deferoxamine complex.

CALCIUM CHANNEL BLOCKERS

Various calcium channel antagonists (e.g., nifedipine, amlodipine, felodipine, nicardipine, verapamil, diltiazem) are used in the management of cardiovascular and renal diseases. Calcium channel blockers are used for their action on L-type calcium channels in the heart and vascular smooth muscle. The blockade of cardiac calcium channels causes negative inotropic, chronotropic, and dromotropic effects. Vasodilation results from the blockade of calcium channels in arteriolar smooth muscle. The dihydropyridine calcium channel antagonists (nifedipine, amlodipine, felodipine, nicardipine) may result in hypotension and reflex tachycardia. The life-threatening consequences of blocked calcium channels include bradydysrhythmias [pacemaker cell inhibition and atrioventricular (AV) block] and profound hypotension (vasodilatation and impaired contractility) (25). Electrocardiographic changes include prolonged PR interval, inverted P waves, AV dissociation, AV block, ST-segment changes, sinus arrest, and asystole. Cerebral hypoperfusion may present as altered mental status, seizures, and coma. Management considerations include reports of noncardiogenic pulmonary edema, which necessitates judicious fluid resuscitation and ventilatory support. GI hypomotility, ileus, and constipation may occur due to inhibition of GI motility hormone release (32). Fluid resuscitation is generally successful in symptomatic management. IV calcium and vasopressors may be employed in the instance of refractory hypotension (5). Activated charcoal should be administered and repeated if the calcium channel blocker is in a sustained-release formulation. Whole-bowel irrigation should also be considered for patients with ingestions of sustained-release calcium channel blockers.

Overdosage of verapamil and diltiazem is complicated by their propensity to cause cardiogenic shock/pump failure. Management in this case may be enhanced by the utilization of dobutamine or phosphodiesterase inhibitors (milrinone, amrinone). Glucagon has been considered a specific therapy for refractory hypotension due to its effect in increasing cyclic adenosine monophosphate (cAMP), activating cAMP-dependent protein kinase, and effecting transient release of intracellular calcium (29). Recommended dosing advises an IV bolus 0.15 mg/kg, followed by an infusion of 0.05–0.1 mg/kg/hr (3). The utilization of high dose insulin has been proposed to offset the hyperglycemia caused by impaired insulin release from the calcium channel blocker toxicity (9). Hyperinsulinemia/euglycemia therapy has been reported to reverse cardiogenic shock in the instance of calcium channel blocker toxicity (8). In severe cases that are refractory to medical management, alternative therapies may include use of transvenous pacing, a ventricular assist device, or extracorporeal life support.

β-BLOCKERS

β-Adrenergic antagonists are classified according to their site of receptor activity. β_1 receptors are located in cardiac, renal, and adipose tissue. β_1 receptor agonists result in positive inotropic and chronotropic effects, renin release, and lipolysis. β_1-selective agents include atenolol, metoprolol, esmolol, and acebutolol. Propranolol, nadolol, and pindolol have activity at β_1 and β_2 receptors. β_2 receptors are located in the liver and smooth muscle of blood vessels, trachea, bronchi, and GI tract. Catecholamine stimulation that targets β_2 receptors results in increased glycogenolysis or gluconeogenesis, vasodilatation, bronchial relaxation, and decreased GI motility. β-Adrenergic antagonists competitively inhibit the effects of the sympathetic neurotransmitters at the respective receptor sites. Some β-blocking agents have additional actions, such as propranolol, which causes sodium channel blocking activity, and labetalol, which has α-receptor blocking activity.

β-Blocker toxicity results in bradycardia, hypotension, and conduction delay. Severe toxicity may result in arrhythmias, including torsades de pointes, ventricular fibrillation, and asystole. Patients may occasionally present with bronchospasm. Hypoglycemia is frequently seen in β-blocker toxicity. Propranolol not only causes hemodynamic compromise, but due to its lipid solubility, it has the potential to cross the blood-brain barrier and result in coma and seizures. Labetalol can have conflicting actions and may cause vasodilation and β-receptor blockade. Sotalol, a β-blocker with type III antiarrhythmic activity, may cause dose-dependent prolongation of the QT interval and subsequent torsades de pointes. Acebutolol toxicity is one of the most severe, in that it predisposes to ventricular repolarization abnormalities, resulting in ventricular arrhythmias (20).

Management may merely require hemodynamic monitoring if the patient presents with asymptomatic bradycardia. Atropine is often helpful to reverse bradycardia and hypotension. It is important to consider that therapy with mixed β agonists may result in an exacerbation of hypotension due to β_2 receptor-mediated vasodilatation. Epinephrine infusions have been reported to be efficacious in overcoming the β-adrenergic blockade. The phosphodiesterase inhibitors amrinone and milrinone are thought to carry the benefit of blocking the breakdown of cAMP, thereby enhancing cardiac contractility. Contractility may also be enhanced by the action of glucagon, which increases intracellular cAMP. Severe toxicity may be managed with similar therapies in calcium channel blocker overdose, including transvenous pacing and extracorporeal life support. Benzodiazepines are helpful to manage seizures. Bronchospasm that is not abated with inhaled β_2 agonists might respond to anticholinergic agents.

Digoxin

Digoxin and digitalis glycosides are commonly utilized to manage cardiac failure and tachydysrhythmias. Digoxin improves cardiac contractility by increasing intracellular calcium concentration due to blockade of Na/K-ATPase. It enhances vagal tone and causes sinoatrial and AV nodal depression. Digoxin toxicity is marked by an increase in sympathetic tone and likelihood of increased automaticity.

Clinical manifestations of digoxin overdose include nausea, vomiting, altered sensorium, and cardiac dysrhythmias. The most typical dysrhythmias of digoxin toxicity are bidirectional ventricular tachycardia and atrial tachycardia with AV block. Hyperkalemia results from the blockade of Na/K-ATPase. The diagnosis of acute digoxin toxicity can be documented with a serum digoxin level.

Heart block or sinus bradycardia may be managed with atropine. In the event of serious cardiac dysrhythmias, therapy should commence with digoxin-specific Fab fragments (Digibind, DigiFab). It is absolutely essential to avoid any drugs whose action is to depress activity of the sinoatrial or atrioventricular nodes. Fab therapy restores the activity of the Na^+-K^+ pump and consequently results in resolution of hyperkalemia. Although calcium is employed in treating significant hyperkalemia, it should be avoided due to the action of digoxin, which causes an increase in intracellular calcium. Indications for utilization of Fab therapy in children include (a) a known ingestion of at least 0.1 mg/kg, (b) a digoxin level of >5 ng/mL and signs and symptoms of digoxin toxicity, (c) the occurrence of life-threatening arrhythmias, or (d) a serum potassium level of >6 mEq/L. The ingestion of the oleander plant, which contains cardiac glycoside, may present as digoxin toxicity and may respond to Fab therapy.

TRICYCLIC ANTIDEPRESSANTS

The tricyclic antidepressants are utilized for a variety of disorders, such as enuresis, pain syndromes, and psychiatric disorders, consequently posing a risk for accidental and intentional ingestions. This class of medication carries the potential for serious toxicity and may result in a broad array of clinical manifestations. The tricyclic compounds have anticholinergic properties that result in the anticholinergic toxidrome. Their inhibition of α-adrenergic receptors can result in sedation and hypotension. They cause blockade of cardiac sodium channels, which results in decreased myocardial contractility and delayed conduction, manifested by widening of the QRS complex. Clinical symptoms have been related to the degree of QRS widening: seizures (QRS >100 ms) and arrhythmias (QRS >160 ms). Some investigators have reported the presence of an R wave in lead aVR $\geq$3 mm or an R wave : S wave ratio in lead aVR $\geq$0.7 to be a superior predictor of severe toxicity (19). Blockade of the potassium channel results in prolongation of the QT interval. Seizures have been attributed to effects of the tricyclics on GABA and on the reuptake of biogenic amines in the CNS. Consequently, it is possible to have a strong clinical impression of tricyclic toxicity in the presence of the anticholinergic syndrome, hypotension, widening of the QRS complex, and seizures. In general, severe toxicity is expressed very early in the course of management. Patients initially require meticulous monitoring, although in the absence of QRS widening, cardiac conduction anomalies, hypotension, altered sensorium, and seizures within the initial 6 hrs, it is unlikely that the patient will deteriorate. Supportive management is indicated for the control of anticholinergic symptoms. Seizure management is generally accomplished with benzodiazepines. It is extremely important to avoid the use of flumazenil as reversal if a possibility of co-ingestion of benzodiazepines exists, as this may precipitate tricyclic-induced seizure activity. Sodium bicarbonate is utilized to achieve serum alkalinization (pH >7.4 and <7.55) when the QRS is widened or in the face of ventricular arrhythmias (18). Alkalinization significantly increases the protein binding of free drug to α_1 acid glycoprotein, resulting in rapid restoration of normal cardiac conduction. The administration of sodium bicarbonate is targeted at narrowing of the QRS and is titrated accordingly, by bolus dosing or continuous infusion. It is fairly standard practice to monitor the electrocardiogram for approximately 6 hrs following the discontinuation of a continuous bicarbonate infusion. Patients who receive sodium bicarbonate often become hypokalemic, requiring careful monitoring and replacement therapy. Tricyclic antidepressants block the reuptake of norepinephrine at the neuromuscular junction, leading to catecholamine depletion. For this reason, vasopressors (e.g., norepinephrine and epinephrine) may be needed to maintain adequate vascular tone and blood pressure. Catecholamine depletion renders a poor response to dopamine, the effectiveness of which is dependent upon releasable stores of norepinephrine (44). In the case of hypotension refractory to vasopressor therapy, extracorporeal membrane oxygenation may be effective.

Carbamazepine toxicity may mirror the above constellation of symptoms and signs, as it is a benzodiazepine derivative structurally related to the tricyclic antidepressants. Toxicity has manifested following drug interactions with erythromycin, isoniazid, cimetidine, and propoxyphene. Management principles are directed at supportive care, with a high index of suspicion for respiratory failure, seizures, and hemodynamic instability. Charcoal may be utilized to prevent absorption. Vasopressors and anticonvulsant therapies may be necessary.

HERBAL TOXICITY/NUTRITIONAL SUPPLEMENT TOXICITY

Nutritional supplements have risen to the forefront as a potential for significant toxicity. These agents have not been regularly monitored by laws or mandatory safety guidelines, and their ready availability renders the feeling that they are safe to use. The 12 most dangerous supplements with alternate names and associated clinical manifestations are listed in **Table 31.3**. This information can be reviewed on the Consumer Reports website (www.consumerreports.org). A number of herbal remedies have been reported to carry significant toxicity and are listed in **Table 31.2**. Management of these poisonings can be summarized by aggressive supportive care and therapies directed at control of specific symptoms.

CLUB DRUGS

The increased popularity of club drugs emerged with the rave scene—all-night, semi-private parties characterized by techno music, dancing, visual effects with strobe lighting and lasers, and illicit use of drugs and alcohol. Substance abuse at these events most commonly includes the utilization of ecstasy and amphetamines, as well as marijuana, cocaine, inhalants, ketamine, and γ-hydroxybutyrate (GHB). It is important to recognize that these agents often find themselves in the hands of adolescents. The practitioner must remain cognizant of an array of common drugs of abuse, along with their respective street names (**Table 31.18**).

A number of substances are abused via inhalation (**Table 31.19**). The inhalants are categorized by hydrocarbons (aliphatic and halogenated hydrocarbons and solvents), nitrous oxide, and nitrites. These agents are typically abused by techniques commonly referred to as sniffing, bagging, or huffing. Sniffing involves inhalation of the vapor from an open container or surface containing the volatile agent. Bagging refers to the user placing the compound into a large bag and inhaling directly from the bag. With huffing, the user places the inhalant into a rag or handkerchief, which is held under the nose, and inhales deeply. The rapid absorption from the lungs and the high lipid solubility of these agents results in rapid entry to the brain. Clinical effects usually occur within seconds to minutes. It is essential to recognize that these compounds can cause significant organ damage (26) (**Table 31.20**). Inhalation of volatile compounds may result in chemical pneumonitis. CNS depression may result in depression of airway reflexes, which may lead to catastrophic aspiration and respiratory arrest.

Ecstasy (X, E, XTC, Adam)

Ecstasy, 3,4-methylenedioxymethylamphetamine (MDMA), is a selective serotoninergic neurotoxin that is utilized to foster

TABLE 31.18

COMMON DRUGS OF ABUSE AND THEIR STREET NAMES

Category substance name	Street names
Marijuana	Dope, ganja, joint, Mary Jane, pot, weed
Tobacco	Smoke, chew, beedi, snuff, cigar
Alcohol	Booze
Cocaine	Crack, candy, rock, Charlie, toot, snow
Methamphetamine	Crystal, meth, ice, speed, fire
Ritalin (Methylphenidate)	MPH, Vitamin R, skippy
MDMA (methylenedioxy-methamphetamine)	Adam, clarity, ecstasy, XTC
GHB (γ-hydroxybutyrate)	Georgia home boy, G, liquid ecstasy
Ketamine	Special K, K, Vitamin K
PCP (phencyclidine)	Angel dust
LSD (lysergic acid diethylamide)	Acid, Big D, blotters, cube
Heroin (diacetylmorphine)	Brown sugar, H, horse
OxyContin (oxycodone HCL)	Oxy, OC, killer
Vicodin (hydrocodone bitartrate with acetaminophen)	Vike, Watson-387
Benzodiazepines	Downers, sleeping pills
Rohypnol (flunitrazepam)	Roofies, roofinol, rope, R2
Anabolic steroids	Roids, juice
Inhalants	Poppers, snappers, whippets

From Nanda S, Konur N. Adolescent drug and alcohol use in the 21st century. *Pediatr Ann* 2006;35:193–9, with permission.

a sense of enhanced empathy, relaxation, and closeness. A significant danger associated with obtaining ecstasy pills is the risk of contaminants. Contaminants such as aspirin or caffeine may exacerbate fluid losses. Other commonly found contaminants include methylenedioxyamphetamine (MDA), paramethoxyamphetamine, phencyclidine (PCP), and heroin, all of which can cause serious toxicity. Some deaths reported from ecstasy were actually felt to be secondary to high concentrations of the contaminant paramethoxyamphetamine (37). Dehydration is a frequent manifestation of ecstasy toxicity. Mild cases may present with anxiety attacks, muscle cramping, severe trismus, or urinary retention due to spasm of the urethral sphincter. Acute intoxication with MDMA is heralded by hyperthermia, malignant hyperthermia, rhabdomyolysis, disseminated intravascular coagulation, acute renal failure, seizures, cardiac arrhythmias, intracranial hemorrhage, brain infarction, or death (33). Hyperpyrexia results from a recalibration of the thermoregulatory center by MDMA and other amphetamine derivatives. Significant hyponatremia is commonly found and has been attributed to the consumption of large amounts of water to counteract the increased insensible fluid losses from hyperpyrexia.

γ-Hydroxy Butyrate (G, Liquid Ecstasy, Liquid E)

γ-Hydroxyl butyrate (GHB) is a CNS depressant that results in a state of euphoria, disinhibition, and heightened sexuality, making it a "date-rape drug." GHB had been sold in health food stores as a sleeping aid and a stimulant of muscle growth and human growth hormone. It was declared illegal for use in the US in 1991, followed by the illegalization of GHB precursors in 2000 (34). Dose-dependent side effects include drowsiness, dizziness, nausea, vomiting, amnesia, hallucinations,

TABLE 31.19

COMMONLY ABUSED INHALANTS

Solvents	Commercial products	Medical gases	Aliphatic nitrites
Paint thinners	Butane lighters	Chloroform	Cyclohexyl nitrite
Gasoline	Whipping cream aerosols	Ether	Amyl nitrite
Glue	Spray paint	Halothane	Butyl nitrite
Felt-tip marker fluid	Hair and deodorant sprays	Nitrous oxide	
	Shoe polish		

Data from *Monitoring the Future National Results on Adolescent Drug Use: Overview of Key Findings.* Bethesda, MD: National Institute on Drug Abuse. 2004 NIH Publication No. 05-5726.

TABLE 31.20

EFFECTS OF INHALANTS

Effect	Inhalant
Hearing loss	Trichloroethylene, toluene
Peripheral neuropathies or limb spasms	Hexane, nitrous oxide
CNS or brain damage	Toluene
Bone marrow damage	Benzene
Liver and kidney damage	Toluene, chlorinated hydrocarbons
Blood oxygen depletion	Organic nitrates, methylene chloride

Data from *Monitoring the Future National Results on Adolescent Drug Use: Overview of Key Findings.* Bethesda, MD: National Institute on Drug Abuse. 2004 NIH Publication No. 05-5726.

convulsions, respiratory failure, coma, and death. Aggressive supportive care is the mainstay of management. Intubation is generally unnecessary, as patients tend to have a sudden reversal of loss of consciousness. Emergence may be marked by myoclonic jerking, confusion, or combativeness. If trismus is present, the accompanying ingestion of ecstasy or other stimulants should be suspected. Deaths reported from GHB intoxication usually emanate from the concomitant use of other respiratory depressants, such as alcohol or ketamine (37).

Methamphetamines (Tina, Ice, Crystal Meth, Tweak, Crank, Glass)

Methamphetamine may be taken orally, rectally, intravenously, or smoked; it is most commonly snorted intranasally. This agent is extremely physically addictive. Symptomatology follows the pattern of the sympathomimetic toxidrome. The clinical presentation may include headaches, pallor, tachycardia, hypertension, chest pain, palpitations, arrhythmias, hyperthermia, rhabdomyolysis, convulsions, and death (24). Patients will often be extremely agitated and anxious, flushed, and diaphoretic and have mydriasis. Management of these patients includes fluid and electrolyte replacement, as well as utilization of benzodiazepines that are effective in controlling agitation, hypertension, and seizures. Most patients do well with aggressive supportive care.

Cocaine

Cocaine toxicity is incorporated within the sympathomimetic toxidrome but deserves mention with the specific club drugs. It may be used by inhalation (cocaine alkaloid, or "crack"), nasal insufflation, or the IV or GI route. It is absorbed in the hydrochloride or base form. Crack cocaine is considered the most potent and addictive form; it is also the most common form that is unintentionally ingested by small children. Infants may be exposed to cocaine in breast milk or via passive inhalation of vapors from crack cocaine (41). Cocaine results in an adrenergic storm by blocking reuptake of catecholamines at adrenergic nerve endings. Clinical manifestations include extreme

CNS stimulation, along with cardiovascular and respiratory effects. Seizures, hypertension, and hyperthermia may lead to cardiac ischemia, CNS bleeding and infarction; end-organ failure may progress to hemodynamic collapse, coma, and death. An acute coronary syndrome results from the combined effects of cocaine: stimulation of β-adrenergic myocardial receptors increases myocardial oxygen demand, while the α-adrenergic and 5-hydroxytryptamine agonist effects cause coronary artery constriction. Cocaine results in a variety of dysrhythmias (wide complex tachycardia and ventricular fibrillation) due to adrenergic stimulation and sodium channel blockade. It is difficult to accurately identify a cocaine-related myocardial infarction, because the electrocardiogram may by abnormal even in the absence of myocardial infarction. Furthermore, serum creatine kinase concentrations are typically elevated without an accompanying myocardial infarction. This elevation is attributed to rhabdomyolysis, which mandates a need for aggressive diuresis. Serum troponin levels are helpful in the evaluation for cocaine related myocardial infarction (17).

Myocardial ischemia due to cocaine-induced vasoconstriction usually appears within 1 hr after exposure, corresponding with the time frame for peak concentration. It is important to realize that, as concentrations of cocaine's major metabolites (benzoylecgonine and ecgonine methyl ester) rise, there may be an associated delayed vasoconstriction. This pattern of metabolism explains the clinical delay often seen with myocardial ischemia or infarction.

Management commonly includes the liberal use of benzodiazepines, which control seizure activity and have also been reported to be efficacious in reducing heart rate and systemic arterial pressure (17). Hypertensive crisis must be controlled to minimize cerebrovascular or myocardial injury. Management of pediatric acute coronary syndrome may be represented by the mnemonic MONA (morphine, oxygen, nitroglycerin, aspirin). Recommended dosing of nitroglycerine in children is by IV infusion: initial dose of 0.25–0.5 mcg/kg/min, titrated by 0.5–1 mcg/kg/min every 3–5 mins as needed; in general, the dose range is 1–3 mcg/kg/min. Cocaine-induced vasoconstriction of the coronary arteries may be reversed with phentolamine, an α-adrenergic antagonist. β-Adrenergic blockers are contraindicated in the management of cocaine-induced acute coronary syndrome.

CONCLUSIONS AND FUTURE DIRECTIONS

Management of the poisoned child is often accomplished by pediatricians and emergency medicine physicians. The intensivist becomes involved in cases of significant cardiopulmonary instability or those that require for meticulous monitoring due to the distinct potential for an ingested agent to result in clinical deterioration. Vigilant supportive care remains the hallmark of management and is important in asymptomatic poisonings and in life-threatening toxicity. Toxicology literature contains an abundance of research targeted at antidotes and decontamination strategies. The reality remains that pediatric ingestions are ideally managed by prevention, and it is essential to recognize that the only way to decrease morbidity and mortality from poisoning is to focus efforts at prevention. Parents must receive diligent anticipatory guidance about the variety of common household substances that contain often-overlooked, potentially lethal ingredients. The universal poison control number should be posted in all homes, clinics, schools, and hospitals. Diligence in advancing public health education and garnering increased funding for research will ideally serve to combat morbidities associated with pediatric poisoning.

KEY POINTS

- Childhood poisoning remains a common occurrence, making it imperative for continuum of care, from the prehospital environment to the emergency department and the ICU. It is mandatory to quickly establish ingestions that pose significant risk versus those that are inconsequential.

- A comprehensive history, focused physical examination, and thoughtful laboratory evaluation provide an excellent template for assessing risk of toxicity and enabling the practitioner to avail the use of a multitude of poison resources.

- Identification of toxidromes requires meticulous attention to clinical signs and symptoms. The toxidromes are grouped as sympathomimetic/adrenergic, cholinergic, anticholinergic, and opioid.

- The laboratory evaluation generally serves to confirm a diagnosis that has been made based upon the history and physical examination. The negative toxicology screen does not exclude the possibility of a toxic exposure. Targeted determination of electrolytes, osmolality, glucose, electrocardiogram, urinalysis, and radiographic imaging may be particularly helpful in eliciting the etiology of a suspected toxin.

- Familiarity with specific toxins and their antidotes enables immediate initiation of therapy, as well as the ability to definitively identify certain toxins.

- Toxicokinetic principles focus upon the processes of absorption, distribution, metabolism, and elimination of drugs or toxins. Knowledge and application of these processes provides the mainstay of specific management of the poisoned child.

- Supportive care remains the crux of therapy for *all* poisonings. Aggressive airway management with attention to airway reflexes is by far the most important management principle. Careful evaluation and maintenance of ventilation is critical. Hemodynamic compromise must be expeditiously recognized and corrected. It is possible to anticipate many aberrations in the cardiopulmonary and neurologic systems with knowledge of the adverse effects of different drug classes.

- Prevention strategies are key in decreasing morbidity and mortality. All healthcare providers in the US must be familiar with the Universal Poison Control number—1–800-222–1222.

References

1. Poison treatment in the home. American Academy of Pediatrics Committee on Injury, Violence, and Poison Prevention. *Pediatrics.* 2003;112:1182–85.
2. Alander SW, Dowd D, Bratton SL, et al. Pediatric acetaminophen overdose: risk factors associated with hepatocellular injury. *Arch Pediatr Adolesc Med* 2000;154:346–50.
3. Bailey B. Glucagon in beta-blocker and calcium channel blocker overdoses: A systematic review. *J Toxicol Clin Toxicol* 2003;41:595–602.
4. Barry JD. Diagnosis and management of the poisoned child. *Pediatr Ann* 2005;34:937–46.
5. Belson MG, Gorman SE, Sullivan K. Calcium channel blocker ingestion in children. *Am J Emerg Med* 2000;18:581–6.
6. Bond GR. Home syrup of ipecac use does not reduce emergency department use or improve outcome. *Pediatrics* 2003;112:1061–4.
7. Borkan SC. Extracorporeal therapies for acute intoxications. *Crit Care Clin* 2002;18:393–420.
8. Boyer EQ, Duic PA, Evans A. Hyperinsulinemia/euglycemia therapy for calcium channel blocker poisoning. *Pediatr Emerg Care* 2002;18:36–7.
9. Boyer EW, Shannon M. Treatment of calcium-channel-blocker intoxication with insulin infusion. *N Engl J Med* 2001;344:1721–2.
10. Chomchai CG. Ipecac syrup. In: Olson KR, ed. *Poisoning & Drug Overdose*, 4th ed. New York, NY: Lange Medical Books/McGraw-Hill 2004:228–9.
11. Chyka PA, Seger D, American Academy of Clinical Toxicology; European Association of Poisons Centres and Clinical Toxicologists. Position statement: Single-dose activated charcoal. *J Toxicol Clin Toxicol* 1997;35:721–41.
12. Guzzardi L, Bayer MJ. Emergency management of the poisoned patient. In: Bayer M, Rumack BH, Wanke LA, ed. *Toxicologic Emergencies.* Bowie, MD: Brady RJ, 1984.
13. Hochman J, Tunnessen WW Jr. Pediatric puzzler. *Contemporary Pediatr* 1995;12:121–31.
14. Howland MA. Antidotes in depth: Activated charcoal. In: Goldfrank LR, Flomenbaum NE, Lewin NA, et al. eds. *Goldfrank's Toxicologic Emergencies,* 7th ed. New York: McGraw-Hill 2002:469–74.
15. Joshi P. Toxidromes and their treatment. In: Fuhrman BP, Zimmerman JJ, eds. *Pediatric Critical Care,* 3rd ed. Philadelphia: Mosby, Elsevier, 2006: 1521–31.
16. Krenzelok EP, McGuigan M, Lheur P, American Academy of Clinical Toxicology; European Association of Poisons Centres and Clinical Toxicologists. Position statement: Ipecac syrup. *J Toxicol Clin Toxicol* 1997;37:699–709.
17. Lange RA, Hillis LD. Cardiovascular complications of cocaine use. *N Engl J Med* 2001;345:351–8.
18. Liebelt EL. Targeted management strategies for cardiovascular toxicity from tricyclic antidepressant overdose: The pivotal role for alkalinization and sodium loading. *Pediatr Emerg Care* 1998;14:293–98.
19. Liebelt EL, Francis PD, Woolf AD. ECG lead aVR versus QRS interval in predicting seizures and arrhythmias in acute tricyclic antidepressant toxicity. *Ann Emerg Med* 1995;26:195–201.
20. Love JN. Acebutolol overdose resulting in fatalities. *J Emerg Med.* 2000;18:341–344.
21. Mack RB. Dishwasher detergent toxicity—Here's looking at you, kid. *Contemp Pediatr* 1993;49–58.
22. Manoguerra AS, Cobaugh DJ. Guidelines for the Management of Poisonings Consensus Panel. Guideline on the use of ipecac syrup in the out-of-hospital management of ingested poisons. American Association of Poison Control Centers, 2004; *Clin Tox* 2005;1:1–10.
23. Matteucci MJ. One pill can kill: Assessing the potential for fatal poisonings in children. *Pediatr Ann* 2005;34:964–8.
24. McEvoy AW, Kitchen ND, Thomas DG. Lesson of the week: Intracerebral haemorrhage in young adults: The emerging importance of drug misuse. *Br Med J* 2000;320:1322–24.
25. Moser LR, Smythe MA, Tisdale JE. The use of calcium salts in the prevention and management of verapamil-induced hypotension. *Ann Pharmacother* 2000;34:622–29.
26. Nanda S, Konnur N. Adolescent drug and alcohol use in the 21st century. *Pediatr Ann* 2006;35:193–99.
27. Osterhoudt KC. The toxic toddler: Drugs that can kill in small doses. *Contemp Peds* 2000;17(3):73–85.
28. Osterhoudt KC, Shannon M, Henretig FM. Toxicologic emergencies. In: Fleisher GR, Ludwig S, eds. *Textbook of Pediatric Emergency Medicine,* 4th ed. Philadelphia: Lippincott Williams and Wilkins, 2000:887–942.
29. Papadopoulos J, O'Neil MG. Utilization of a glucagon infusion in the management of a massive nifedipine overdose. *J Emerg Med* 2000;18:453–5.
30. Position paper: Cathartics. *J Toxicol Clin Toxicol* 2004;42:243–53.
31. Position paper: Whole bowel irrigation. *J Toxicol Clin Toxicol* 2004;42:843–54.
32. Ray JM, Squires PE, Meloche RM. L-type calcium channels regulate gastrin release from human antral G cells. *Am J Physiol* 1997;273:G281–G8.
33. Shannon M. Methylenedioxymethamphetamine (MDMA, "Ecstasy"). *Pediatr Emerg Care* 2000;16:377–80.
34. Shannon M, Quang LS. Gamma-hydroxy-butyrate, gamma-butylolactone, and 1,4,-butanediol: a case report and review of the literature. *Pediatr Emerg Care* 2000;6:435–40.
35. Smilkstein MJ. Techniques used to prevent gastrointestinal absorption of toxic compounds. In: Goldfrank LR, Flomenbaum NE, Lewin NA, et al., eds. *Goldfrank's Toxicologic Emergencies,* 7th ed. New York: McGraw-Hill 2002:44–57.
36. Sterrent C, Brownfield J, Korn CS, et al. Patterns of presentation in heroin overdose resulting in pulmonary edema. *Am J Emerg Med* 2003;21:32–34.
37. Tellier PP. Club Drugs: Is it all ecstasy? *Pediatr Ann* 2002;31:550–6.
38. Tucker JR. Indications for, techniques of, complications of, and efficacy of gastric lavage in the treatment of the poisoned child. *Curr Opin Pediatr* 2000;12:163–5.

39. Vale JA, American Academy of Clinical Toxicology; European Association of Poisons Centres and Clinical Toxicologists. Position statement: Gastric lavage. *J Toxicol Clin Toxicol* 1997;35:711–9.

40. Watson WA, Litovitz TL, Lein-Schwartz W, et al. 2003 Annual Report of the American Association of Poison Control Centers Toxic Exposure Surveillance System. *Am J Emerg Med* 2004;22:335–404.

41. Winecker RE, Goldberger BA, Tebbett IR. Detection of cocaine and its metabolites in breast milk. *J Forensic Sci* 2001;46:1221–3.

42. Woolf AD. Herbal remedies and children: Do they work? Are they harmful? *Pediatrics.* 2003;112:240–6.

43. Woolf AD. Principles of toxin assessment and screening. In: Fuhrman BP, Zimmerman JJ, eds. *Pediatric Critical Care,* 3rd ed. Philadelphia: Mosby, Elsevier, 2006:1511–1531.

44. Zaritsky AL. Catecholamines, inotropic medications, and vasopressor agents. In: Chernow B, ed. *The Pharmacologic Approach to the Critically Ill Patient,* 3rd ed. Baltimore: Williams & Wilkins 1994:387–404.

CHAPTER 32 ■ THERMOREGULATION

PAMELA FEUER • THYYAR M. RAVINDRANATH • DAVID G. NICHOLS

PHYSIOLOGY OF THERMOREGULATION

Normal body temperature is maintained constant by a balance of heat loss and heat gain with the assistance of an efficient thermoregulatory mechanism. Extreme environmental temperature variations, however, can overcome this effective thermoregulatory function and lead to heat- or cold-related illnesses.

Body temperature consists of core and shell temperatures. Rectal, esophageal, and oral temperatures represent core temperature, while axillary and skin temperatures are examples of shell temperature. Core temperature determines the risk of injury to various organs in the body. Air temperature, air movement, thermal radiation, sweating, skin blood flow, and temperature of underlying tissue all influence shell temperature (21). Thermoreceptors for the shell reside in the skin. Core thermoreceptors exist in the cortex, hypothalamus, midbrain, medulla, spinal cord, and deep abdominal structures in addition to the skin (2,43). Upon sensing temperature change, these receptors transmit afferent impulses via the lateral spinothalamic tract to the central thermostat located in the preoptic/anterior hypothalamus, which maintains the temperature set point (39). Thermoregulation is initiated when sensed temperature is different from the set point. The conditions associated with failed thermoregulatory mechanisms that lead to hyperthermia or hypothermia will be discussed in this chapter.

Heat Gain

Warm-blooded animals have the capacity to raise body temperature above their environmental temperature, which occurs when endogenous or exogenous heat gain exceeds heat loss. Heat is generated in the human body from basal metabolism, physical activity, food consumption, metabolic activity, emotional modification, hormonal effects, and medications. The body may also acquire heat passively when the environmental temperature exceeds body temperature.

Heat Loss

Heat is lost from the body via conduction, convection, radiation, and evaporation. In most situations humans produce more heat than necessary and dissipate the excess heat into the environment.

Conduction is heat loss by the transfer of heat from a warmer to a cooler object when the two objects are in direct contact. The amount of heat loss depends on the contact area and the temperature difference between the body and the other surface. Usually, only 3% of body heat is lost by conduction. However, conduction may be a major source of heat loss in wet clothing or immersion incidents, because of the excellent conductive properties of water.

Convection is heat loss by the movement of air or fluid that circulates around the skin. More heat is carried away from the body in windy conditions, as the movement of air rapidly removes the insulating layer of warmer air normally around the body surface. Approximately 12%–15% of body heat is lost by convection.

Radiation is heat loss due to infrared heat emission to surrounding air. Heat loss occurs primarily from the head and noninsulated areas of the body and can occur rapidly. Radiation can account for 55%–65% of heat loss.

Evaporation is heat loss by the change of water from a liquid to gas state via the skin or respiration. Evaporation normally accounts for 25% of heat loss, but can depend on surface area, temperature difference, and humidity. Evaporative heat loss is greatest in cold, dry, and windy conditions (34).

HYPERTHERMIA

Definitions

Hyperthermia refers to body temperature elevation beyond the hypothalamic set point because of inadequate heat loss and/or excessive heat gain. Cytokines do not mediate this temperature elevation, in contrast to fever (see below), as the hypothalamic set point itself has not changed. Hence, antipyretics (aspirin, acetaminophen, nonsteroidal anti-inflammatories), which lower the set point, have no effect. Extreme temperature elevations (>41°C) are common in the hyperthermic patient.

Fever is a regulated temperature elevation (>38.5°C) to a new higher set point in the hypothalamus. It is caused by the release of pyrogens from macrophages/monocytes, typically cytokines IL-1, tumor necrosis factor (TNF), interferon (IFN)-γ, and IL-6, in response to inflammatory stimuli such as infection, malignancy, autoimmune disease, etc. Cytokine-induced fever rarely exceeds 41°C, with the exception of some cases of encephalitis and meningitis.

Classification of Hyperthermia Syndromes

Hyperthermia syndromes maybe be classified as environmental (or exertional), drug (or toxin)- induced, or of genetic/unknown origin. Considerable overlap exists among these groups, as patients with a genetic predisposition may be more susceptible to environmental/exertional or drug-induced hyperthermia.

The patient presentation among these syndromes has many features in common that are related to the temperature elevation. However, certain aspects of the presentation may be unique or exaggerated, depending on the specific entity. In humans, hyperthermia may induce euphoria instead of discomfort, resulting in failure to seek prompt medical attention. Even in the severest form of heat illness, early clinical signs are nonspecific. The severity of heat-related injury depends on the degree of core temperature elevation and its duration. Therefore, preventive measures, early diagnosis, and aggressive treatment are essential components of a good outcome.

Heat Stroke (Environmental/Exertional Heat-related Illness)

Heat-related illnesses constitute a spectrum of diseases that ranges from heat stress—a benign condition—to heat stroke—a potentially fatal condition. The milder conditions (variously termed heat rash, heat cramps, heat edema, and heat exhaustion) generally do not require PICU management.

Heat stroke is characterized by an elevation of core temperature above 40°C. It is subdivided into classic or environmental and exertional heat stroke. The mechanism of classic heat stroke that follows high environmental temperature is not known. However, exertional heat stroke may be linked to a genetic predisposition. Individuals with a predominance of type II muscle fibers are more susceptible to exertional heat stroke. These individuals have lower exercise capacity and accumulate more lactate, which, in turn, directly activates the cell membrane sodium/potassium pump (Na/K-ATPase). Activation of Na/K-ATPase affects intracellular sodium/calcium and depletes the energy stores of the cells (19). The loss of mitochondrial function and disturbed calcium (Ca^{2+}) homeostasis activate phospholipase A_2, resulting in the production of free radicals, prostaglandins, leukotrienes, and calcium-dependent proteases and eventual development of rhabdomyolysis (33). Rhabdomyolysis results from free radical-induced lipid peroxidation and overload of cellular and mitochondrial calcium, which lead to muscle necrosis.

Prevention

With knowledge of the risk factors for heat stroke, effective preventive methods can be applied successfully. For example, children are not as well adapted as adults are to extreme heat. As a result, children tend to become hyperthermic during physical activity in hot environments, for some of the reasons that follow (14). The ratio of surface area to body mass is larger in children; hence, they gain greater heat from the environment on a hot day. The ratio of metabolic heat produced per mass unit is greater in children during physical exertion. Children have lower sweating capacity when compared to adults, resulting in their inability to loose heat by evaporation, although children can effectively eliminate heat in a mildly warm climate or in a neutral thermal environment, they are unable to eliminate heat when air temperature exceeds 35°C. Humidity is a major component of heat stress in children. Physical activity in a warm environment without acclimatization leads to heat-related illnesses. The process of acclimatization to hot surroundings is slower in children when compared to adults. Approximately

8–10 exposures of 30–45 mins each are necessary to attain sufficient acclimatization in children. The rate of exposure is at a rate of one per day or one every other day. Children frequently do not consume enough water to replenish fluid lost during physical activity. Dehydration is a risk factor for heat-related illness. Additionally, children generate an increase in core body temperature, when compared to adults, for a given level of dehydration. Hence, children should be encouraged to drink adequate quantities of fluids before and during physical activity. The risk factors are listed in Table 32.1 (14,22).

Identifying high-risk groups can prevent heat-related illness. Heat-related mortality and morbidity is reduced when safe havens are established that provide air conditioning, hydration, and medical equipment for those in need. The news media can play a key role in educating the public in the prevention of heat-related illnesses. Administration of 5 oz of fluid (e.g., cold tap water) for a 40-kg child and 9 oz for an adolescent is adequate to ensure hydration and is recommended even when the children are not thirsty (14). The addition of salt to induce thirst would increase fluid consumption and prevent heat-related illness. A gradual acclimatization process should be encouraged, with the duration of intense physical activity reduced when air temperature and relative humidity are elevated.

TABLE 32.1

RISK FACTORS FOR HEAT-RELATED ILLNESS

Factors	Description
Age	Elderly, children
Sex	Male due to increase in muscle mass and strenuous activity
Socioeconomic factors	Lack of access to air conditioners; individuals living in upper floors of apartment buildings especially with flat roof tops; social isolation; closed doors and windows during hot weather conditions
Weather conditions	Factors that prevent heat loss from the body: reduced wind, elevated barometric pressure, high humidity, high environmental temperature at or above body temperature for prolonged periods of time
Drugs	Alcohol, anticholinergics, amphetamines, anti-Parkinson medications, β-blockers, cocaine, diuretics, ecstasy, ephedra-containing diet supplements, neuroleptics, phenothiazines, tricyclic antidepressants
Body habitus	Obesity
Clothing	Thick, nonabsorbable clothing
Illnesses	Mental handicap; febrile illnesses; dehydrating illnesses such as diabetes insipidus, diabetes mellitus, diarrhea and vomiting; skin diseases such as anhidrosis; heat-producing illnesses such as thyrotoxicosis; lack of sleep, food, or water; diminished sweating as in cystic fibrosis; lack of acclimatization; previous heat stroke
Exertional heat illness	Athletes, military personnel, manual laborers

Measurement of environmental stress can be used to prevent heat-related injuries associated with activity in hot environments. The wet-bulb globe temperature (WBGT) index is widely used to measure environmental stress as an index of heat stress. The WBGT index consists of three metrics weighted as follows:

$$WBGT = (0.7\ Twb) + (0.2\ Tg) + (0.1\ Tab) \qquad [32.1]$$

The first metric, Twb, refers to wet-bulb temperature. It is obtained by covering a dry-bulb thermometer that is not immersed in water with a water-saturated cloth and placing it in direct sunlight. The second metric, Tg, refers to black-globe temperature and is obtained by placing, in direct sunlight, a dry bulb in a metal globe. Lastly, Tab refers to a measurement of air temperature without direct sunlight using a dry bulb thermometer. A portable monitor is used to measure the WBGT index, with temperature values reported in Celsius or Fahrenheit, and risk categories can be stratified based on it. "Very high risk" is associated with values over 28°C, "high risk" is placed in the range of 23–28°C, "moderate risk" falls in the range of 18–23°C, and temperatures below 18°C fall into the "low risk" category. The activities should be modified accordingly (7).

Core Pathophysiology

Compensated Response

Thermoregulation. A major portion of heat is lost from the body via the skin, and perspiration-induced evaporation is responsible for most heat loss. The skin's blood flow enhances heat loss through conduction and convection. Cutaneous vasodilatation that results from increased skin blood flow brings skin temperature nearer to core temperature. The increase in cutaneous blood flow that results from an elevated core temperature is ninefold greater than the increase that results from an elevation in the skin temperature (43).

The sympathetic nervous system controls blood flow through the skin by modulating adrenergic vasoconstrictor and vasodilator fibers. During heat stress, tonic cutaneous vasoconstriction is inhibited and vasodilatation is induced, resulting in an increase in skin blood flow. An elevation in skin temperature results from convection of heat from striated muscles and internal organs to the surface (48). Cutaneous blood flow at rest constitutes 5%–10% of total cardiac output (200–500 mL/min). Heat stress-induced vasodilatation increases cutaneous blood flow to 60% of cardiac output (8 L/min).

Acclimatization. Acclimatization is an adaptation response that can take up to several weeks following exposure to a hot environment. Adaptation responses include an increase in plasma volume, enhanced cardiovascular performance, activation of renin-angiotensin-aldosterone axis, an ability to increase sweating, salt retention by sweat glands and kidneys, an enhancement of glomerular filtration rate, and inhibition of rhabdomyolysis (31).

Systemic Inflammatory Response: Cytokine Release. Serum of TNF-α, IL-1, IL-6 and endotoxin levels are increased following elevation in body temperature. The ensuing systemic inflammatory response involves epithelial cells, endothelial cells, and leukocytes. These cells modulate cytokine response to heat injury, resulting in healing and repair, thereby preventing multiorgan dysfunction (26).

Cell-survival Response: Heat Shock Proteins. Heat stress induces heat shock elements, which leads to an accelerated transcription of heat shock proteins (Hsps). These proteins bestow cells with the ability to survive injury. The mechanism of resisting injury involves Hsps acting as molecular chaperones, i.e., proteins that assist other proteins in achieving proper folding, thus preventing further protein denaturation. It has been observed that Hsps modulate baroreceptor reflex response following heat stress and blunt bradycardia and hypotension (35).

Decompensated Response

Temperature. The height of temperature elevation and its duration determine organ injury. Body temperatures in the 41–42°C range lead to tissue injury within 1–8 hrs. Temperatures that exceed 49°C induce tissue injury in 5 mins. Hypovolemia follows excessive dehydration, lowering preload and therefore cardiac output, with a resultant decrease in skin blood flow. Loss of heat by conduction and convection is limited, and thermoregulation is compromised. Decreased blood volume from hypovolemia decreases sweating, thereby reducing heat loss by evaporation. Reflexes that help to maintain central blood volume and blood pressure override thermoregulatory signals for cutaneous vasodilatation, resulting in an inability to lose heat by evaporation (17).

Exaggerated Systemic Inflammatory Response. The balance between proinflammatory mediators such as TNF-α, IL-1β, IFN-γ, and anti-inflammatory mediators, such as soluble TNF-α (sTNF-α) and IL-10, determines the extent of tissue injury. The predominance of proinflammatory mediators leads to systemic inflammation with subsequent multiorgan dysfunction (13).

Gastrointestinal Ischemia. Vasodilatation-induced shift of blood flow from the core to the peripheral circulation results in reduced blood flow to the gastrointestinal tract, with subsequent gut ischemia. Gut ischemia disrupts immunologic and gut mucosal barrier function, and the ensuing translocation of endotoxin and release of proinflammatory cytokines. Proinflammatory cytokines promote endothelial activation and release of endothelin and nitric oxide. Specific to this discussion, the cytokine mediators cause thermoregulatory failure and alter hemodynamic function, resulting in the progression of heat-related illness (10,24,25).

Activation of Coagulation Cascade. The activation of coagulation cascade as a result of heat injury is supported by the presence of the thrombin-antithrombin complex and decreased levels of naturally synthesized anticoagulation proteins such as protein C, protein S, and antithrombin III. The activation of fibrinolysis is indicated by the appearance of D-dimer, decreased levels of plasminogen, and the presence of the plasmin-antiplasmin complex (11). Heat injury induces a prothrombotic state by enhancing the expression of adhesion molecules.

Inadequate Heat Shock Protein Response. Progression of heat-related illness is associated with attenuated release of Hsps. Advanced age, failure to acclimatize, and genetic factors are associated with inadequate Hsp release (41).

CLINICAL FEATURES

Heat stroke affects multiple organs and results in their dysfunction. The clinical effects seen in various organs are discussed below.

Central Nervous System

Individuals who suffer from heat exposure can present with delirium, seizures, lethargy, and coma due to metabolic disturbances, cerebral edema, or ischemia. The cerebellum is particularly sensitive to high temperatures (3). Neurologic complications include intracranial bleed, cerebral infarct, cerebral edema, central pontine myelinolysis, and Guillain-Barré syndrome. Intracranial bleed occurs acutely and is related to the disseminated intravascular coagulation (DIC) that accompanies heat stroke. Cerebral infarct results from cerebral thrombosis secondary to hemoconcentration. Cerebral pontine myelinolysis may be related to rapid changes in serum osmolality with little alteration in serum sodium. Immune system activation by cytokines following heat stroke disrupts the blood-brain barrier and exposes peripheral nerves to antigen, resulting in the Guillain-Barré syndrome, usually seen 7–10 days after heat stroke.

Cardiovascular System

Heat elimination by evaporation involves translocation of blood from central circulation to the periphery, which can lead to hypotension, especially in the presence of hypovolemia. Hypotension may also be due to the production of nitric oxide that results from heat-related illnesses (6). Patients with heat stroke may present with either hyperdynamic or hypodynamic circulation, with elevated systemic vascular resistance, low cardiac output, and variable pulmonary vascular resistance.

Electrocardiographic Changes

Victims of heat stroke show electrocardiographic changes that include rhythm disturbances, conduction defects, and changes in the QT interval and the ST segment. Rhythm disturbances such as sinus tachycardia, supraventricular tachycardia, and atrial fibrillation are observed. Conduction defects such as right bundle branch block and intraventricular conduction defects have been noted. Prolonged QT may be due to hypomagnesemia, hypocalcemia, or hypokalemia, which result from heat-related injuries. The presence of ST segment changes indicates myocardial ischemia, which can lead to myocardial infarction. The predisposing factors for myocardial ischemia include tachycardia and increased oxygen demand from hyperthermia, combined with hypotension from hypovolemia.

Respiratory System

Heat stroke may result in respiratory failure secondary to acute respiratory distress syndrome (ARDS) (see Chapter 46). The exact time of onset of ARDS following heat stroke is unpredictable. DIC that accompanies heat injury may trigger the onset of ARDS.

Acid-Base, Electrolyte, and Renal Disorders

Renal System

Acute renal failure is attributed to hypovolemia, rhabdomyolysis, DIC, and direct effects of thermal injury. A variety of acid-base and electrolyte derangements follow from the primary heat-related illness, compounded by rhabdomyolysis and renal insufficiency.

Lactic acidosis with compensatory respiratory alkalosis occurs in exertional heat stroke. *Hyponatremia* is seen following sweat losses of >5 L/day and upon rehydration. It also occurs during the early stages of acclimatization to heat, during vigorous exercise (e.g., marathon or triathlon), and during prolonged and repeated exercise in the heat. *Hypokalemia* is seen initially as a consequence of respiratory alkalosis that is induced by hyperventilation secondary to hyperthermia, catecholamine secretion, sweat losses, and renal losses from hyperaldosteronism due to physical activity in a hot environment. Persistent high temperature, perfusion failure, and hypoxemia all lead to magnesium-dependent Na/K-ATPase pump malfunction. The resultant potassium seepage from cells may cause *hyperkalemia*, which is exacerbated by renal failure. Although hyperkalemia and hypokalemia occur in heat-related injury, hypokalemia is the predominant effect observed. Acute *hypophosphatemia* occurs from the increase in glucose phosphorylation as a result of alkalosis. Later in the course, sustained tissue injury leads to leakage of phosphate from the cells, which complexes with extracellular calcium and results in *hypocalcemia*. Hypocalcemia and hypophosphatemia also can be secondary to hypomagnesemia, lack of bone responsiveness to parathyroid hormone or deficient parathyroid hormone secretion. *Hyperuricemia* occurs due to augmented release and diminished excretion of uric acid secondary to rhabdomyolysis and renal failure, respectively. The mechanisms involve release of purine from injured muscle and inhibition of uric acid excretion in the urine due to metabolic acidosis. *Hypomagnesemia* follows excessive sweating. However, a rapid decline in urinary magnesium excretion results in normal serum magnesium levels. Prolonged intense exercise can induce the uptake of magnesium by erythrocytes, mononuclear cells, and muscle, leading to clinically significant hypomagnesemia. *Hypoglycemia* occurs due to rapid depletion of glycogen, rapid utilization of glucose, and liver dysfunction from splanchnic ischemia, which results in failure to convert lactate to glucose.

Gastrointestinal Tract

Gut ischemia results in liver dysfunction with elevated alanine transaminase, aspartate transaminase, bilirubin, γ-glutamyl transpeptidase, and lactic dehydrogenase. Peak elevation in liver enzymes occurs 72 hrs following heat injury. Liver damage may be due to either direct heat injury or hypoxemia secondary to splanchnic ischemia. Fulminant liver failure is very uncommon following heat injury.

Hematology and Immunology

DIC occurs and is worsened by liver dysfunction. Splanchnic ischemia leads to translocation of endotoxin, with subsequent release of proinflammatory mediators, including TNF-α, IL-1, IL-2, IL-6, IL-8, platelet activating factor, arachidonic acid, and vasoactive amines, and resultant multisystem organ dysfunction.

Musculoskeletal System

Elevated serum creatine phosphokinase (CPK) indicates rhabdomyolysis. It occurs in most cases of exertional heat stroke and less frequently in classical heat stroke. The consequences of rhabdomyolysis include hyperkalemia leading to cardiotoxicity, myoglobinuria resulting in renal failure, shock from sequestration of fluid into injured muscle, and muscle necrosis of the diaphragm leading to respiratory failure. Compartment syndrome can result from severe edema of the muscles of the extremities. Hence, it is important to monitor arterial pulsation, perfusion, and sensation of the swollen extremities and to measure direct tissue pressure in suspected cases of compartment syndrome.

DIFFERENTIAL DIAGNOSIS

Diagnosis of heat stroke should be suspected in anyone who presents with a core temperature of >40.6°C, hot, dry skin, and changes in mental status that include delirium, and seizures. The differential diagnoses are listed in **Table 32.2**. Septic shock closely mimics heat-related illness. A good history and physical examination can exclude many diagnostic entities such as complications related to thyroid disease, drug toxicities, and malignant hyperthermia.

LABORATORY EVALUATION

Laboratory tests are performed to evaluate target organ injury and confirm the diagnosis by ruling out other disease entities.

Urine

Urine analysis may show elevated specific gravity with low urine output from dehydration and hypovolemia. Protein in the urine indicates muscle breakdown. The presence of red blood cells, myoglobin, and tubular casts denotes acute tubular necro-

sis as a consequence of hypovolemia and rhabdomyolysis. The finding of myoglobinuria is especially important, as it is diagnostic of rhabdomyolysis in this setting, for which specific emergency therapy is necessary (see below). Urine drug screen is performed when drug ingestion is suspected.

Complete Blood Count

Leukocytosis on a complete blood count may be due to systemic inflammation from heat-related illness or sepsis. Elevated hemoglobin and hematocrit indicates hemoconcentration due to dehydration. Thrombocytopenia, elevation in hypersegmented neutrophils, and atypical lymphocytosis are also features of heat injury. At times, spherocytes and, less commonly, schistocytes, ovalocytes, and stomatocytes are observed on the blood smear. These changes are reversed within 4–7 days following effective treatment of heat injury.

Serum Chemistry

Serum chemistry typically reveals hyponatremia, hypokalemia followed by hyperkalemia, hyperphosphatemia, and hypocalcemia. Hypoglycemia is also noted in victims of heat stroke. Elevated blood urea nitrogen and creatinine levels can be observed as a consequence of dehydration and ensuing prerenal azotemia or renal failure. Increase in CPK follows rhabdomyolysis.

Liver Function Test

Elevation in aspartate aminotransferase (AST) and alanine aminotransferase (ALT) are noted due to liver dysfunction, an attribute of multiorgan failure from heat stroke.

Coagulation Profile

Activation of the extrinsic pathway of coagulation following heat stroke promotes coagulopathy (DIC). Elevation in prothrombin time, partial thromboplastin time, and D-dimer and decrease in platelets are seen as a consequence of coagulopathy.

Arterial Blood Gas

Evaluation of arterial blood gases reveals respiratory alkalosis in cases of classic heat stroke and metabolic acidosis in cases of exertional heat strokes. Hypoxemia with low Pao_2/Fio_2 ratio occurs as a result of heat stroke complicated by ARDS.

Imaging

A chest x-ray is useful in confirming the presence of ARDS and in detecting the presence of infective or aspiration pneumonia. CT imaging of the brain is performed to diagnose central nervous system (CNS) complications of heat stroke victims such

TABLE 32.2

DIFFERENTIAL DIAGNOSES OF HEAT STROKE

Entities	Etiologies
Central nervous system	Meningitis, encephalitis, and hypothalamic infarction
Thyroid	Graves disease, thyroid storm
Infection	Sepsis
Drugs	Toxicity from anticholinergic, antidepressants, amphetamines, hallucinogens, cocaine, PCP, monoamine oxidase inhibitors, neuroleptics, and salicylates
Drug withdrawal	Narcotics, benzodiazepines
Metabolic	Diabetic ketoacidosis
Miscellaneous	Malignant hyperthermia

as cerebral infarction or edema. Patients with heat-related illnesses suffer from cardiac arrhythmias, which can be confirmed with a 12-lead electrocardiogram. An echocardiogram is indicated in patients who present with clinical suspicion of myocardial dysfunction.

Spinal Tap

A spinal tap is useful in suspected cases of meningitis or encephalitis, both of which can closely mimic the encephalopathy that accompanies heat stroke. The clinician should be cognizant of raised intracranial pressure due to associated CNS complications, as well as DIC, which accompanies heat stroke, both of which are relative contraindications for a spinal tap.

COMPLICATIONS

Complications following heat-related illness are enumerated in **Table 32.3.**

TREATMENT

Heat Stroke

Heat stroke is a medical emergency that requires prompt and aggressive treatment to prevent mortality. Prompt attention to the ABCs of resuscitation is required here and in every other form of hyperthermia.

Therapy at the Scene
Emergency cooling should be undertaken without delay (4). The victim should be moved to a shaded area, tight clothing should be removed, and the victim should be sprinkled with water from any source and fanned constantly. Cooling victims below 39°C within 30 mins greatly improves the outcome from heat-related injury. The core temperature is measured during the application of the cooling process, and various methods of cooling are available. Currently, no prospective study recommends one method over another (45). Various methods of cooling and their advantages and disadvantages are listed in **Table 32.4.**

TABLE 32.3

COMPLICATIONS OF HEAT-RELATED ILLNESS

Organs system	Complications
Central nervous system	Encephalopathy, coma, seizures, hemiplegia, cerebellar injury
Cardiovascular	Myocardial injury
Pulmonary	Acute respiratory distress syndrome
Gastrointestinal	Ischemia or infarction
Renal	Acute renal failure
Muscular	Rhabdomyolysis
Hematology	Disseminated intravascular coagulation, thrombocytopenia
Metabolic	Lactic acidosis

Supplemental oxygen should be provided to hypoxic individuals, and the airway should be secured with an endotracheal tube in comatose patients with loss of protective airway reflexes. Shivering and consequent increase in body temperature can be prevented by the administration of diazepam. Vital signs, including core temperature via rectal or esophageal route are monitored continuously. Vascular access is established with a wide bore catheter. Ringer's lactate or normal saline is used for hydration. Hydration status should be assessed by physical examination of skin perfusion and urine output monitoring by means of a Foley catheter. Overhydration should be avoided to minimize the development of pulmonary edema and cerebral edema that can follow heat stroke. Seizures from heat stroke can effectively be treated with diazepam. The victim should be moved to a tertiary care medical center as soon as possible.

Therapy at the Tertiary Center
Those victims who had their airway controlled are placed on positive-pressure ventilation with supplemental oxygen to correct hypoxemia. Positive end-expiratory pressure should be titrated to treat hypoxemia and to keep FIO_2 below the toxic level of 0.5. Body cooling (see **Table 32.4**) should be continued until core temperature is below 39°C with core temperature monitored every 5 mins by one of the methods mentioned above. IV fluids should be given via a wide bore catheter, and a central venous line should be placed for central venous pressure measurement. Fluids are given based on physical examination of perfusion status, status of the pulse, and measurement of urine output via a Foley catheter. Overhydration must be avoided for the reasons stated earlier. Low cardiac index, elevated central venous pressure, mild right-heart failure, and low systemic vascular resistance are seen in most victims of heat stroke. However, effective cooling results in vasoconstriction and increased blood pressure. Victims of heat stroke need careful titration of fluids, as they develop noncardiogenic pulmonary edema and cerebral edema. Some victims may present with low cardiac index, elevated central venous pressure, and hypotension, which necessitate inotropic support. Low cardiac index, low central venous pressure, and hypotension may be seen in other victims and necessitate liberal fluids. It is important to avoid α-adrenergic agents if at all possible, as the associated vasoconstriction prevents heat loss from the skin. It is also prudent to avoid the administration of anticholinergic agents, as they prevent sweating and increase body temperature.

Blood glucose and serum electrolytes are measured frequently and corrected appropriately. Hypocalcemia is corrected cautiously due to the risk of deposition of calcium carbonate and calcium phosphate in injured skeletal muscles.

Rhabdomyolysis, identified by elevated creatine kinase and myoglobinuria, requires aggressive hydration to increase urine output to >3 mL/kg/hr. The addition of sodium bicarbonate to the IV fluids prevents tubular precipitation of myoglobin if the urine pH is raised to >6.5. In addition to volume expansion, mannitol 0.25 g/kg IV may be used as an osmotic diuretic to increase urine flow.

Once rhabdomyolysis has been diagnosed, the patient may face several additional life-threatening problems, including renal failure, pulmonary edema, worsening electrolyte derangements, and compartment syndrome. Oliguric renal failure secondary to acute tubular necrosis (see Chapter 96) may

TABLE 32.4

METHODS OF COOLING

Cooling methods	Description	Advantages	Disadvantages
EXTERNAL COOLING			
Immersion	Immersion of body in ice water	Faster cooling, greater temperature gradient between core and periphery	Vasoconstriction; interferes with heat loss; shivering; interferes with resuscitative measures
Body-cooling unit	Spraying finely atomized water mixed with warm air to keep body temperature above 32°C–33°C	Faster cooling (mean cooling rate of 0.31°C/min or 32.6°F/min); comfortable to the patient; heat is lost by evaporation and convection	Sophisticated unit that requires maintenance and storage
Wet sheet and fan	Patients are covered with a sheet, water is sprayed over the sheet, and fans are used to blow over the wet sheet	Heat lost by evaporation; heat loss is comparable to body-cooling unit; easy maintenance	
Ice packs	Ice packs are placed over the groin, axillae, and neck	Simple and readily available; inexpensive; shorter cooling time when combined with evaporative technique	Longer cooling time compared to evaporative technique
CORE COOLING			
Cold-water irrigation	Gastric, bladder, peritoneal lavage, extracorporeal technique	Not well studied	Invasive, especially peritoneal and extracorporeal techniques
IV fluids	Cold IV fluid administration	Not studied	Noninvasive

lead pulmonary edema, unless the fluid administration rate is decreased. Hemofiltration or dialysis may be necessary to remove excess fluid volume and treat electrolyte abnormalities in the patient with heat stroke, rhabdomyolysis, and acute tubular necrosis.

Extreme hyperkalemia, hyperphosphatemia, and hyperuricemia may occur. Although standard measures to treat hyperkalemia (bicarbonate, calcium chloride, insulin, and glucose administration) apply in this setting, it is likely that the patient will have already been alkalinized. In addition, the benefits of calcium administration in preventing dysrhythmias must be balanced against the risk of precipitation of calcium phosphate crystals in injured muscle. If meticulous monitoring of the electrocardiographic pattern shows signs of hyperkalemia (tall T waves, prolonged P-R interval, widened QRS, any dysrhythmia), the risk-benefit ratio argues for calcium administration. Aggressive lowering of the serum potassium level is paramount with: (a) glucose 1 g/kg and insulin 0.1 unit/kg IV; (b) sodium polystyrene sulfonate (Kayexalate) 1 g/kg via nasogatric tube every 2–6 hrs, and/or (c) dialysis. Hyperphosphatemia is managed with phosphate binders (sevelamer) and dialysis. Hyperuricemia is managed with hydration, alkalinization, and drug therapy, including allopurinol and recombinant uricase (rasburicase).

Acute renal failure is seen in 30% of patients with exertional heat stroke and in 5% following classic heat stroke. The most important aspect in the prevention of renal failure is to adequately hydrate patients. If oliguria persists despite adequate hydration and in the presence of normal blood pressure, patients who are at high risk for pulmonary edema may need invasive monitoring (e.g., central venous pressure) to titrate fluid therapy. A trial dose of furosemide and mannitol is given to induce diuresis. Early dialysis should be considered in those who have renal failure.

Shock can follow rhabdomyolysis from sequestration of large quantities of fluid into the injured muscles in the first 24 hrs following heat injury. The administered fluid may contribute to edema in injured muscles, which can lead to compartment syndrome in the extremities. Compartment syndrome generally occurs on the third or fourth day following injury and results in a secondary elevation of creatine kinase due to muscle necrosis from compression by trapped fluid. Fasciotomy is recommended if an increase in compartment pressures is documented, or if clinical signs such as pulselessness, paresthesias, pain, or paralysis of the extremity are present.

Coagulation abnormalities peak at ~24–36 hrs; hence, prothrombin time, partial thromboplastin time, platelet count, and fibrin split products are obtained at admission and at intervals thereafter. DIC is treated with blood products. The use of ε-aminocaproic acid for fibrinolysis is extremely dangerous and provides no long-term benefit; it has also been shown to cause rhabdomyolysis. The other contributing factor for coagulopathy is liver dysfunction, which is treated with supportive care. Liver transplantation is seldom needed for liver dysfunction following heat stroke.

Intracranial pressure monitoring has not been reported in heat stroke victims; however, it is individualized based on bedside clinical evaluation and should be considered if DIC has been excluded or corrected in a comatose patient with suspected cerebral edema documented by CT scan.

Outcomes

A total of 4780 deaths from heat stroke was reported between the years 1979 and 2002 in the US. In children who are <15 years of age, mortality was as high as 6% (24).

HYPERTHERMIA SYNDROMES

Malignant Hyperthermia

Malignant hyperthermia (MH) is a genetic syndrome that requires exposure to certain potent inhaled general anesthetics (halothane, isoflurane, sevoflurane) and/or the depolarizing muscle relaxant succinylcholine. The inheritance pattern in 50% of patients is autosomal dominant, caused by a point mutation in the gene encoding the ryanodine receptor RYR1 (the Ca^{2+} release channel of the sarcoplasmic reticulum). This mutation leads to sustained Ca^{2+} release from the sarcoplasmic reticulum upon exposure to a triggering agent. Patients without a family history may have other spontaneous mutations that produce the MH phenotype. Because of the variable genotype, the diagnosis is still usually made with the halothane (or caffeine) contracture test on skeletal muscle obtained during biopsy. Patients who are suspected to have MH should undergo testing at an MH testing center, wear a "Medic Alert" bracelet, and obtain up-to-date information from the Malignant Hyperthermia Association of the United States at www.mhaus.org.

The incidence of MH is 1 in 4000 for mild presentations and 1 in 250,000 for the fulminant form. Patients with certain neuromuscular disorders such as muscular dystrophy, myotonia, and central core disease are at increased risk.

The cardinal features of MH include muscle rigidity (sustained contracture), which is often first detected when masseter spasm prevents opening of the mouth for intubation. The sustained muscle contracture generates heat and greatly increased muscle metabolism, which in turn, lead to increased carbon dioxide production (increased end-tidal carbon dioxide [E_TCO_2] concentration), acidosis, tachypnea, and tachycardia (including ventricular tachycardia). The body temperature often exceeds $41°C$. In the absence of prompt medical intervention, rhabdomyolysis supervenes, with the risk of hyperkalemia, ventricular tachycardia, myoglobinuric renal failure, and cardiac arrest.

Although MH presents most commonly in the operating room, the pediatric intensivist must be thoroughly familiar with the course and management because of the possibility of recrudescence of MH in the ICU. Also, the increasing use of inhaled anesthetics in the ICU to treat refractory asthma or provide sedation increases the risk of MH occurring initially in the PICU. All patients who develop intraoperative MH must be admitted to an ICU because recrudescence of MH occurs in 20% of patients, especially in those with a muscular body type. (12). The time between the initial onset of MH and recrudescence averages 13 hrs.

Therapy for MH consists of immediate discontinuation of inhaled anesthesia and/or succinylcholine. The inspired gas is converted to 100% oxygen at high flow rates to wash out residual anesthetic as rapidly as possible. The muscle relaxant dantrolene, 2.5 mg/kg IV, is given as rapidly as possi-

ble. The dose may be repeated to control signs of hypermetabolism. Cold normal saline, 15 mL/kg, is administered rapidly if temperature is >39°C. Emergency laboratory testing involves serum potassium, creatine kinase, arterial blood gas, and coagulation tests to evaluate hyperkalemia, rhabdomyolysis, metabolic acidosis, and DIC, respectively. The complications should be treated rapidly. Hyperkalemia is the presumed cause of any ventricular dysrhythmia during MH until proven otherwise, such that glucose, insulin, bicarbonate, and calcium are added to primary antidysrhythmia therapy (e.g., amiodarone or cardioversion).

Malignant Hyperthermia-like Syndrome

In 2003, a new syndrome resembling MH was described. (27). However, in contrast to classic MH, these patients had not been exposed to anesthetics or succinylcholine; rather they presented with type II diabetic coma and a hyperglycemic, hyperosmolar nonketotic state. Hyperthermia occurred typically after administration of insulin, although exceptions have been described. The patients were usually obese African American males with acanthosis nigrans. Rhabdomyolysis, hemodynamic instability, and organ failure punctuate the course of this condition, which has been termed *malignant hyperthermia-like syndrome* (MHLS). The mortality rate is high (>50%).

The etiology of MHLS is unknown. The insulin preservative, m-creosol, underlying fatty acid oxidation defects (e.g., short-chain acyl-CoA dehydrogenase deficiency), and infection have all been proposed as contributing to the cause of MHLS. It is likely that multiple factors contribute to MHLS, and each case requires a careful workup for enzyme defects, infection, and toxins.

Therapy for MHLS should include the immediate administration of dantrolene, based on limited case reports to date (30). Because dantrolene must be diluted in sterile water, a calculated dose of hypertonic saline can be administered concurrently to prevent a rapid decline in serum osmolality, which may precipitate cerebral edema. Cooling methods outlined in **Table 32.4** are indicated until temperature is <39°C.

The correct management of IV fluids, glucose, and electrolytes is critical. After a sufficient volume of normal saline has been administered rapidly to restore blood pressure and perfusion, the remaining volume deficit and ongoing losses are replaced more slowly over 72 hrs. Hydration alone often lowers serum glucose such that a lower dose of insulin can be used (0.05 units/kg/hr) to correct hyperglycemia without precipitating rapid osmotic shifts.

Neurolept Malignant Syndrome

Neurolept malignant syndrome (NMS) is a rare clinical syndrome associated with the use of antipsychotic drugs and characterized classically by four cardinal signs: muscle rigidity, mental status changes (confusion, agitation, catatonia, encephalopathy, coma), hyperthermia, and autonomic instability (tachycardia, labile hypertension, diaphoresis). Atypical presentations may occur where only two or three of the cardinal signs are present.

Every type of neurolept agent that antagonizes D_2 dopamine receptors has been associated with NMS, including haloperidol, chlorpromazine, fluphenazine, risperidone, cloza-pine, and olanzapine. The anti-emetic and gastric motility agents promethazine and metoclopramide have also been implicated in NMS. Risk factors for NMS appear to correlate with potent antipsychotics (e.g., haloperidol), rapid dose escalation, concomitant use of lithium, and comorbid diseases such as acute infection. Although no controlled trials have been reported to support specific medical therapy, dantrolene, bromocriptine, and amantadine have been tried. We favor the use of dantrolene. All antipsychotic drugs known to trigger NMS must be discontinued emergently. Monitoring, laboratory testing, and supportive care follow the approach described for other hyperthermia syndromes. Benzodiazepines may be used to control agitation. Psychosis or catatonia may require electroconvulsive therapy. Once NMS has resolved, antipsychotic medications, preferably of lower potency and without the concomitant use of lithium, can be reintroduced gradually and titrated to effect.

Serotonin Syndrome

Serotonin syndrome (SS) is a clinical syndrome that exhibits signs of excess postsynaptic serotonergic neurotransmission, which may include hyperthermia. The classic triad of SS signs includes abnormalities of mental status (agitation, delirium), neuromuscular function, (hyperreflexia, clonus, hypertonicity, tremor), and autonomic function (hyperthermia, tachycardia, hypertension, diaphoresis, vomiting, diarrhea). Clonus may be spontaneous, inducible, or ocular. SS is often confused with NMS, but clonus is not a prominent finding in NMS. Furthermore, NMS develops over days and weeks, whereas SS usually develops within 24 hrs. Given the multiplicity of potential signs and symptoms, patients will present with variations of the classic triad, and a high index of suspicion is needed in any patient who is receiving medications that increase serotonergic activity (**Table 32.5**).

Overall, hyperthermia occurs in 50% of patients with SS but is universal among the sickest SS patients in the PICU. The Hunter Serotonin Toxicity Criteria incorporate the most important findings (clonus, agitation, diaphoresis, tremor, hyperreflexia, hypertonicity, hyperthermia) into a decision-making rule set that is sensitive (84%) and very specific (97%) for SS (18).

The management of SS relies upon supportive care, as outlined for other hyperthermia syndromes. The serotonergic drug is discontinued immediately. Agitated patients should receive benzodiazepine sedation. If the triggering agent is a monoamine oxidase inhibitor (MAOI), which has caused hypotension, then it is prudent to avoid inotropes (e.g., dopamine) that are metabolized by monoamine oxidase inhibitors. After fluid volume resuscitation, a direct-acting vasoconstrictor such as phenylephrine is preferred to treat hypotension. The cause of hyperthermia in SS is related to muscle activity. Therefore, severely hyperthermic patients should undergo rapid-sequence induction of anesthesia, endotracheal intubation, and neuromuscular blockade to eliminate motor activity until hyperthermia resolves. The antidote for SS is cyproheptadine, a histamine-1 (H_1) receptor antagonist with nonspecific serotonergic (5-HT1A and 5-HT2A) antagonistic properties. Because cyproheptadine is only available as an oral formulation (tablet or syrup), it should be given via nasogastric tube at a total daily dose of 0.25 mg/kg divided every 6 hrs. The maximum daily dose is 12 mg for children 2–6 years and 16 mg for children 7–14 years old. After discontinuation of the triggering agent and institution of supportive care plus cyproheptadine, most patients will show marked improvement within 24 hrs.

Sympathomimetic and Anticholinergic-induced Hyperthermia Syndromes

Drug-induced hyperthermia from sympathomimetic or anticholinergic poisoning is discussed in Chapter 31.

HYPOTHERMIA

Hypothermia and cold-induced injuries include a spectrum of conditions that range from frostnip and frostbite to severe hypothermia, all of which may cause minor-to-significant morbidity and mortality. Although hypothermia is most common during exposure to cold environments, it can also develop secondary to other causes, such as toxin exposures, metabolic derangements, infections, and CNS or endocrine system dysfunction. Environmental cold injury may be most obvious in cold climates but can also occur in warmer climates that have rapid temperature changes or with the use of indoor cooling methods such as air conditioning.

Definitions

Frostnip is a mild form of cold injury. It is a nonfreezing injury of skin tissues, usually of the face, fingertips, or toes of patients who are exposed to cold temperatures of ~15°C. Ice-crystals form in the tissues, but no tissue destruction occurs. Frostnip is associated with pallor and numbness or tingling of the affected skin until warming occurs. A more significant nonfreezing injury is termed *chilblains*, which can occur as tissue temperature drops below 15°C. The walls of small vessels break and tissues swell. Treatment of frostnip and chilblains usually involves simple rewarming. Dressing warmly, covering ears, keeping hands and feet dry, and seeking a warmer environment when hands and feet feel cold can prevent frostnip and chilblains.

Frostbite is the destruction of skin or other tissues caused by freezing between 6.1°C and –15°C. It is classified as superficial—affecting skin and subcutaneous tissues—or deep—affecting bones, joints, and tendons (9,42). Intracellular and extracellular ice crystals form in the tissues during freezing; vascular stasis and tissue ischemia follow. Below-freezing temperatures, low windchill, high humidity, and prolonged exposure to cold are risk factors. Superficial frostbite leads to pallor, edema, blistering, and desquamation. Deep frostbite can lead to hemorrhagic blisters, anesthesia, hyperesthesia, ulceration, and gangrene. Treatment involves removal of nonadherent wet clothing, rapid rewarming, and avoidance of rubbing damaged tissue. Preparation and protection from the effects of cold weather is the best prevention for frostbite.

Hypothermia is defined as a core body temperature of <35°C (95°F). Humans can only adapt to their environment and maintain core temperature within a narrow range. When this adaptive thermoregulation is overwhelmed, the body

TABLE 32.5

DRUGS THAT INCREASE SEROTONIN LEVELS AND MAY PRECIPITATE SEROTONIN SYNDROME

Class	Mechanism	Examples
Dietary supplement	Increases serotonin formation	L-tryptophan
Illicit drug	Increases release of serotonin	Amphetamines, ecstasy, cocaine
Weight loss drug (amphetamine derivatives)	Increases release of serotonin	Phentermine, fenfluramine, dexfenfluramine
Herbal medication	Prevents reuptake of serotonin into the presynaptic neuron	St. John's wort
Antidepressant: Selective serotonin reuptake inhibitor	Prevents reuptake of serotonin into the presynaptic neuron	Citalopram, escitalopram, fluoxetine, paroxetine, sertraline
Antidepressant: Tricyclic antidepressant	Prevents reuptake of serotonin into the presynaptic neuron	Amitriptyline, amoxapine, desipramine, doxepin, imipramine, maprotiline, nortriptyline, protriptyline, trimipramine
Antidepressant: Selective serotonin/norepinephrine reuptake inhibitor	Prevents reuptake of serotonin and norepinephrine into the presynaptic neuron	Bupropion, trazodone, nefazodone, venlafaxine
Antidepressant: Monoamine oxidase inhibitor	Inhibits metabolism of serotonin	Phenelzine, tranylcypromine, isocarboxazid
Antibiotic: Monoamine oxidase inhibitor (MAOI)	Inhibits metabolism of serotonin	Linezolid
Migraine drug	Activates serotonin 5-HT1 receptors	Almotriptan (Axert), naratriptan (Amerge), sumatriptan (Imitrex), zolmitriptan (Zomig)
Anti-emetics	Prevents reuptake of serotonin into the presynaptic neuron	Ondansetron, granisetron
Anti-tussive	Prevents reuptake of serotonin into the presynaptic neuron	Dextromethorphan
Analgesic	Activates serotonin 5-HT1 receptors	Fentanyl

cannot generate sufficient heat to continue natural function and hypothermia occurs. Hypothermia is classified as mild (35–32°C), moderate (<32–28°C), or severe (<28°C) based on core body temperature (47). Determining the severity of hypothermia is sometimes difficult because standard clinical thermometers measure only as low as 34.4°C. Therefore, when hypothermia is suspected, it is important to record core body temperature using low-reading rectal thermometers or electronic rectal, esophageal, or bladder thermistor probes. All organ systems are affected by hypothermia, but the CNS and the cardiovascular system are the most sensitive. The degree of hypothermia has implications regarding expected pathophysiologic changes and appropriate therapeutic modalities.

Mechanisms of Disease

The pathophysiology of hypothermia is related to mechanisms of heat loss (see earlier sections), temperature homeostasis, cellular effects, and organ system response.

Temperature Homeostasis

Thermoregulation. Thermoregulatory response to cold requires input from peripheral skin receptors and core thermoreceptors along the distribution of the internal carotid arteries and the posterior hypothalamus. The cutaneous nerve-ending cold receptors are located more superficially and in greater numbers than warm receptors. Afferent impulses are transmitted via the spinothalamic tracts and relayed to the hypothalamus. Core thermoreceptors are less well understood, but the response of the peripheral vasculature to sympathetic input appears to be modulated by the temperature of circulating blood. Thermosensitive neurons are located throughout the CNS in close proximity to arteries, so that blood and brain temperature are closely coupled.

Thermogenesis. Thermogenesis, or heat production, normally occurs in obligatory ways, such as that due to basal metabolism and exercise. When cooling occurs despite this heat generation, facultative thermogenesis occurs via voluntary physical activity, shivering, or humoral response. Shivering is the production of heat by muscle tremor and produces a fivefold increase in metabolic rate. Humoral thermogenesis involves sympathetic release of norepinephrine and subsequent expression of mitochondrial uncoupling proteins, which then leads to the production of heat by uncoupling of the metabolic chain from oxidative phosphorylation in the inner membranes of mitochondria. Norepinephrine and epinephrine are also released from the adrenal medulla, inducing glycogenolysis in muscle and liver cells (48).

Heat Conservation. The conservation of heat occurs in response to cold stress. The response by the cutaneous circulation is a locally initiated and mediated vasoconstrictor response via the release of norepinephrine from sympathetic nerve endings acting on peripheral α_2-receptors and a reflex response initiated by skin cooling over the general body surface. Skin blood flow can be downregulated to nearly zero in extreme cold. Local sensory blockade can interfere with the adrenergic response, allowing for reversal to vasodilation (e.g., in the hands, during local cooling). As whole-body cooling proceeds, the prevailing vasoconstrictor mechanisms are nonadrenergic (5). Heat may be conserved with insulation secondary to subcutaneous fat and by normal behavioral responses to cold exposure, both of which may be less effective at the extremes of age.

Cellular and Tissue Effects

Cold exposure and freezing of tissue can cause direct cellular injury by the formation of extracellular ice crystals, which in turn, produces intracellular dehydration, elevation of intracellular electrolytes, and temperature-induced protein changes. Further temperature reduction leads to intracellular crystallization and mechanical destruction of cells (42). A shift in the oxyhemoglobin dissociation curve to the left leads to further tissue hypoxia. Vasoconstriction contributes to hypoperfusion and stasis, and endothelial injury causes thromboembolism. During cooling, cyclic freezing and thawing can occur in extremities, resulting in the release of prostaglandin F2 and thromboxane A2, which potentiates vasoconstriction, platelet aggregation, and thrombosis. In mice, moderate systemic hypothermia causes accelerated microvascular arteriole and venule thrombus formation by activation of the GPIIb-IIIa fibrinogen receptor (36). Cold-induced inhibition of coagulation-cascade enzymes and platelet dysfunction also occurs, which can lead to bleeding. Thawing of frozen tissue results in marked edema that is secondary to melting of ice crystals, cell damage, lack of endothelial integrity, and thrombosis.

Organ System Response to Hypothermia

All organ systems are affected by significant hypothermia. The responses at different degrees of hypothermia are summarized in Table 32.6. The most significant of these effects occur in the central nervous, cardiovascular, and renal systems. Even with mild systemic hypothermia, the CNS responses are slowed, and severe mental status changes and unconsciousness occur below 32°C. Myocardial irritability develops and frequently leads to arrhythmias, initially atrial and then ventricular, including ventricular fibrillation below 28°C. Below 32°C, a J (Osborn) wave may be seen on electrocardiogram, represented by a hump at the QRS-ST junction in the inferior and lateral precordial leads (38).

A cold-induced diuresis occurs with mild hypothermia. Initially, increased renal blood flow occurs after peripheral vasoconstriction. However, with falling temperature, loss of distal tubular reabsorption of water and sodium and a resistance to the action of antidiuretic hormones occur, which can result in significant intravascular volume depletion in the hypothermic patient.

Cold-water Immersion. The organ system response to immersion in cold water versus exposure to cold air can be dramatically different at the onset of the insult. An initial "cold shock" results in uncontrolled respiratory gasping and hyperventilation, tachycardia, and hypertension. Respiratory alkalosis and cerebral vasoconstriction occur. However, the heat loss by conduction in cold water is approximately 20 times greater than in air, leading to very rapid cooling and decrease in organ blood flow. Conditions that involve total immersion, including the head, initiate a "diving reflex" that consists of apnea, marked bradycardia, increased peripheral vascular resistance, and increased blood supply to the brain and heart due to parasympathetic neural output in addition to the sympathetic activity from cold exposure (29). The early shunting of oxygen to essential vascular beds and the subsequent overall decrease in

---

TABLE 32.6

ORGAN SYSTEM RESPONSES TO HYPOTHERMIA

Severity of hypothermia	Central nervous system	Cardiovascular	Respiratory	Metabolic, renal, endocrine	Neuromuscular
Mild (35–32°C)	Depressed cerebral metabolism; confusion; amnesia; ataxia	Vasoconstriction; tachycardia followed by bradycardia; increased cardiac output; hypertension	Tachypnea followed by progressive decrease in minute ventilation; bronchospasm; impaired mucosal function	Increased metabolism; increased oxygen consumption; cold diuresis; impairment of renal-concentrating ability; hypovolemia	Increased tone with shivering, followed by muscle fatigue
Moderate (<32–28°C)	Unconsciousness; papillary dilatation; diminished gag reflex	Bradycardia; decreased contractility; slowed cardiac conduction; J waves on ECG; arrhythmias	Hypoventilation with acidosis despite decrease in CO_2 production; V/Q mismatch; decreased oxygen consumption	Decreased renal blood flow; no insulin activity	Extinction of shivering; hyporeflexia; muscle rigidity
Severe (<28°C)	Decreased or no EEG activity; nonreactive pupils; loss of ocular reflexes	Progressive decrease in BP, cardiac output, and heart rate; ventricular arrhythmias (fibrillation); asystole	Lung capillary damage; pulmonary edema; further decreased oxygen consumption; apnea	Decrease in basal metabolism; acidosis; renal failure	Areflexia; rhabdomyolysis

ECG, electrocardiogram; EEG, electroencephalogram; BP, blood pressure.

metabolic rate due to rapid cooling may provide an explanation for the very prolonged submersion survival times seen in children.

Etiology of Hypothermia

Common Causes

Hypothermia may occur due to a variety of causes and can be accidental or nonaccidental and environmental or nonenvironmental. The majority of cases of hypothermia are caused by environmental exposure. The diagnosis of environmental hypothermia can be obvious in patients found in cold outdoor environments, but may be overlooked in patients found indoors. Etiologies of hypothermia include conditions that cause increased heat loss, decreased heat production, impaired thermoregulation, and other miscellaneous clinical conditions (Table 32.7).

Predisposing Factors

Preexisting and concomitant factors can increase the susceptibility to hypothermia. Infants and children have a high ratio of body surface area to mass and, therefore, faster cooling rates. Adolescents and those with relative linearity also cool more quickly. In addition, low body fat decreases tissue insulation, and small muscle mass results in lower absolute metabolic heat production (46). Neonates and the elderly can be dysthermic at seasonal temperature extremes. Minimal differences in thermoregulation exist between eumenorrheic females and males of similar body type and fitness. However, during cold exposure, females in the luteal and follicular phase of menstruation have greater decreases in temperature than males (23).

Alcohol and sedative drugs cause cutaneous vasodilation and inhibit the shivering response to cold exposure. In addition, these substances lead to impairment in awareness of the cold and in the necessary judgment to seek shelter and warm clothing.

Clinical Presentation and Diagnosis

In that hypothermia can occur without exposure to a cold environment, the diagnosis must be considered in those patients who present with the recognized clinical features and with an accurately measured core body temperature. The cardiovascular examination in patients with hypothermia is often difficult. Pulses are difficult to appreciate due to profound bradycardia and frozen extremities. Many hypothermic changes may be seen on electrocardiogram. The clinical features noted in mild, moderate, and severe hypothermia are listed in **Table 32.8.**

Laboratory Data

Hypothermia leads to acidosis, altered blood clotting, and decreased kidney and renal function. Hypokalemia and hyperkalemia occur, and hyperkalemia becomes prominent with increased severity of hypothermia. Liver function tests are abnormal secondary to reduced cardiac output. Hyperglycemia occurs in acute hypothermia, but hypoglycemia may be seen in subacute or chronic hypothermic conditions. Previously, blood gas temperature correction was thought to be necessary for correct interpretation of acid-base and respiratory status. However, current data support the use of only uncorrected blood gas values to guide therapy (44). Hypothermia results in prolongation of prothrombin and partial thromboplastin times secondary to the inhibition of the enzymatic reactions of the coagulation cascade. Thrombocytopenia can occur due to bone marrow suppression and splenic sequestration.

Clinical Management

Hypothermia is a medical emergency that requires prehospital care, which may include a need for basic life support and advanced cardiac life support, depending on the severity. All patients should be removed from the cold environment, and wet clothing must be removed. Patients must be rewarmed. The method of rewarming is determined by the severity of

TABLE 32.7

ETIOLOGIES OF HYPOTHERMIA

Increased heat loss	Decreased heat production	Impaired thermoregulation	Other clinical states
Environmental	**Neuromuscular insufficiency**	**Central nervous system failure or abnormalities**	Multisystem trauma
Immersion	Age extremes	Hemorrhage/infarction	Sepsis
Nonimmersion	Impaired shivering	Trauma	Shock
Iatrogenic	Lack of adaptation	Birth asphyxia	Systemic acidoses
Exposure	**Insufficient fuel**	Tumors	Pancreatitis
Cold IV infusions	Hypoglycemia	Malformations	Uremia
Emergency deliveries	Malnutrition	Metabolic causes	Familial dysautonomia
Heat stroke treatment	Extreme physical exertion	Ethanol	Water intoxication
Dermatologic	Impaired mobility	Pharmacologic: barbiturates, narcotics, phenothiazines, lithium	Episodic spontaneous hypothermia with hyperhidrosis
Burns	**Endocrinologic failure**	**Peripheral nervous system failure**	
Exfoliative dermatitis	Hypothyroidism	Neuropathies	
Induced vasodilation or impaired peripheral vasoconstriction	Hypopituitarism	Diabetes	
Ethanol	Hypoadrenalism	Acute spinal cord transection	
Pharmacologic: phenothiazines, α-blockers			

TABLE 32.8

CLINICAL FEATURES OF HYPOTHERMIA

	Mild hypothermia (35°C–32°C)	Moderate hypothermia (<32°C–28°C)	Severe hypothermia (<28°C)
Thermoregulatory	Shivering	Extinction of shivering	No shivering
Respiratory	Tachypnea	Hypoventilation, respiratory acidosis, hypoxemia, aspiration pneumonia, atelectasis	Apnea, pulmonary edema, acute respiratory distress syndrome
Cardiovascular	Tachycardia, hypertension	Bradycardia, hypotension, prolonged QT interval, J wave, atrial arrhythmias	Pulseless electrical activity, atrial and ventricular fibrillation, asystole
Gastrointestinal	Ileus, nausea, vomiting	Pancreatitis, gastric erosions	Pancreatitis, gastric erosions
Renal/fluid/electrolyte	Cold diuresis, hypokalemia, alkalosis	Hyperkalemia, hyperglycemia, lactic acidosis	Hyperkalemia, hyperglycemia, lactic acidosis
Muscular	Hypertonia	Rigidity	Rhabdomyolysis
Hematologic		Hemoconcentration, hypercoagulability	Thrombocytopenia, disseminated intravascular coagulation, bleeding
Neurologic	Disorientation, impaired judgment, dysarthria, ataxia, hyperreflexia	Agitation, hallucination, unconsciousness, dilated pupils, diminished gag reflex, hyporeflexia	Coma, nonreactive pupils, areflexia, brain-dead-like state

hypothermia and other clinical parameters. Little evidence supports the benefit of one method of rewarming over another. However, anecdotal evidence suggests that, unless the patient has full monitoring and critical care support systems, slow rewarming is safer than rapid rewarming (8).

Passive External Rewarming

Passive rewarming—the use of blankets to cover the head, neck, and body—reduces evaporative heat loss and can rewarm at a rate of 0.5–4°C per hour. This method will be unsuccessful if shivering or other thermoregulatory mechanisms are absent. Passive external rewarming is usually an adequate treatment modality for patients with mild hypothermia.

Active External Rewarming

Active external warming—the application of heat directly to the skin—is only effective if the patient has an intact circulation that can return peripherally rewarmed blood to the core. Hot water bottles may cause burns to cold and vasoconstricted skin. Warm blankets and heating blankets rewarm at variable rates and may also produce burns to the skin. Radiant warmers can also produce skin burns if patients are not covered with blankets. Forced-heated-air devices such as the Bair Hugger device can rewarm at a rate of 1–2.5°C per hour by heat transfer via convection. Warm water immersion is not recommended because the patient cannot be monitored. External methods of rewarming are usually effective for mild-to-moderate hypothermia. Complications of active external warming are core temperature "after-drop" secondary to the rapid return of cold peripheral blood to the heart, acidosis due to return of pooled lactic acid to the central circulation, and hypotension secondary to venous pooling.

Active Internal Rewarming

The modalities for active internal rewarming have a spectrum of invasiveness and potential complications. These methods are necessary for treating patients with severe hypothermia. The rewarming method should be chosen based on available resources, monitoring, and support systems and on the presence of cardiac arrest or fibrillation.

Active internal warming methods include heated (42°C), humidified air via an endotracheal tube and heated (42°C) IV fluids via rapid infusion. Together, these methods can warm at a rate of 1–2°C per hour. More invasive techniques include body cavity lavage (gastric, bladder, colon, pleural, peritoneal) with warmed saline, which can warm at a rate of 1–4°C per hour. The most invasive methods of active internal rewarming are extracorporeal and include continuous arteriovenous or venovenous warming, hemodialysis and cardiopulmonary bypass. The first three require the presence of a pulse and adequate blood pressure. Cardiopulmonary bypass is highly effective and can increase core temperature by 1–2°C every 3–5 mins. In addition, it provides the benefit of full circulatory support. Cardiopulmonary bypass is the method indicated for severe hypothermia associated with either the failure of less-invasive, active rewarming techniques, or severe hypothermia accompanied by cardiac arrest, or a nonperfusing cardiac rhythm. In a series of young, healthy patients (including 7 children) with accidental deep hypothermia, survival with good neurologic outcome was reported in the 15 of 32 patients who received cardiopulmonary bypass (49). An algorithm for the rewarming approach to the hypothermic patient is shown in **Figure 32.1**.

Management of Patients with Arrhythmias and Cardiac Arrest

Patients with hypothermia develop dysrhythmias. Most dysrhythmias correct with rewarming alone. Initial rewarming procedures, endotracheal intubation, vascular access, and patient transport should be performed gently, as these patients are prone to develop ventricular fibrillation. Hypothermic patients with cardiac arrest or nonperfusing rhythms require modification of conventional advanced life support protocols, as their

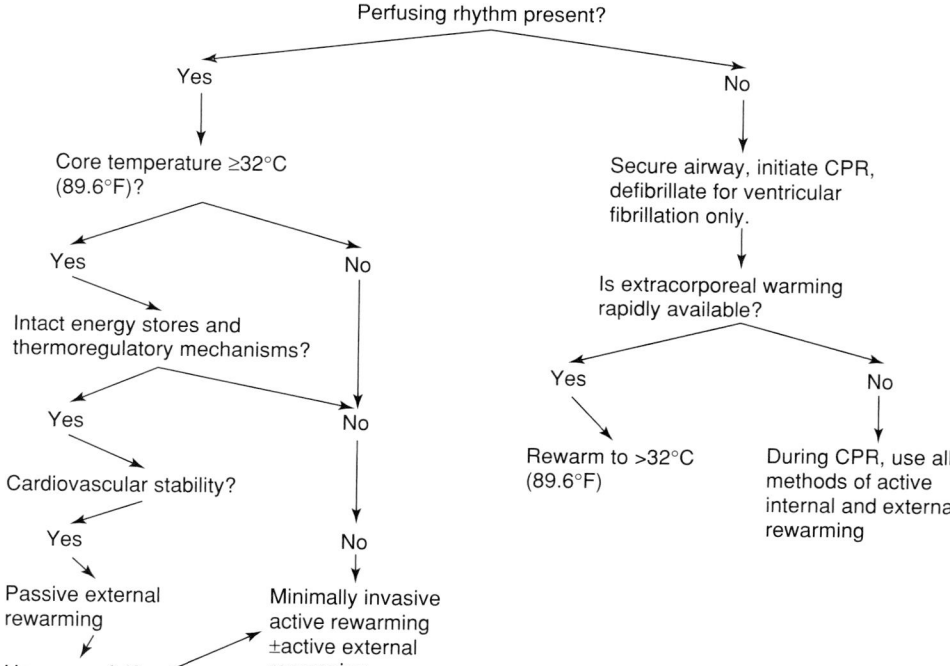

FIGURE 32.1. Rewarming approach for hypothermia.

hearts may be unresponsive to cardiovascular drugs, defibrillation, and pacemaker stimulation. For those with moderate hypothermia, cardiopulmonary resuscitation should be initiated and if indicated, defibrillation should be attempted. However, IV resuscitative medications should be spaced at longer intervals secondary to reduced drug metabolism and potential for toxic accumulation of these medications in the peripheral circulation. In the patient with severe hypothermia and cardiac arrest, cardiopulmonary resuscitation should be initiated, but attempts at ventricular fibrillation and administration of resuscitative medications should be withheld until the patient is rewarmed above 30°C with active internal rewarming methods. Resuscitative efforts in the severely hypothermic patient may be very prolonged, especially if extracorporeal warming is unavailable. Although a patient may appear clinically dead, resuscitative efforts should continue at least until the patient has been rewarmed to near normal core temperature (1).

Other Management Considerations

Laboratory evaluation of the hypothermic patient may demonstrate numerous abnormalities to consider in the context of current acute and chronic conditions. Evaluation should include serum electrolytes, blood glucose, renal function tests, arterial blood gases and pH, complete blood cell count, and coagulation studies. Drug toxicology screens and blood alcohol level should be obtained when appropriate. The patient's hematocrit may be elevated as a result of decreased plasma volume due to a decrease in core temperature. In the patient who is moderately to severely hypothermic, a normal hematocrit may indicate acute blood loss or preexisting anemia. Hyperglycemia is often present in acute hypothermia; however, hypoglycemia may be seen in the setting of subacute or chronic hypothermia or alcohol intoxication and should be treated. Hypokalemia is commonly seen in mild hypothermia, but hyperkalemia—common with moderate and severe hypothermia—is a marker

of acidosis, cell death, and renal failure. Lower temperatures also enhance the cardiac toxicity of hyperkalemia (37). Hypothermic coagulopathies commonly occur, especially in association with major trauma.

Aggressive volume resuscitation is warranted in hypothermic patients secondary to the dehydration caused by cold diuresis and the vascular expansion with vasodilatation upon rewarming. No evidence exists for the empiric administration of steroids or antibiotics. However, stress-dose steroids should be administered in patients with a known history of adrenal insufficiency and should be considered if body temperature fails to normalize despite the use of appropriate warming techniques. Antibiotics should be administered to patients in whom it is suspected that infection is the etiology of the hypothermic presentation (40).

Outcomes

Averages of 689 deaths per year between the years 1979 and 2002 were attributed to hypothermia in the US. The annual death rates are now 0.2 per 100,000 population but were higher prior to 1990. The majority of deaths in 2002 were in males and those older than 65 years of age. However, adolescent boys aged 15–19 had a death rate of 0.5 per 100,000 population (28).

The outcome of hypothermia depends on the cause and comorbid conditions that precipitated the hypothermia. The abnormal physiologic conditions that occur with hypothermia are generally reversible with rewarming. Overall patient mortality is reported as 12%. However, with moderate-to-severe hypothermia, overall mortality approaches 40%. The lowest initial temperatures recorded in those who survived from hypothermia were 14.2°C in a child (16) and 13.7°C in an adult (20); both had good neurologic recovery after rescue and rewarming with cardiopulmonary bypass. The presence of asphyxia or hypoxic brain damage prior to the development of hypothermia increases the risk of mortality, as does serious underlying disease. In patients with multisystem trauma, hypothermia below 32°C is associated with 100% mortality.

"Rewarming shock," multisystem organ dysfunction, sepsis, and tissue injury remain frequent morbidities and can contribute to mortality. Psychological and neurodevelopmental disturbances have been reported in infant and newborn survivors of accidental hypothermia (15).

Prevention

Hypothermia and frostbite are devastating and potentially avoidable conditions, and education and preparation are essential toward achieving prevention. Urban poverty, socioeconomic conditions, and extremes of age are major factors in the incidence of accidental hypothermia in urban areas. Those who participate in winter sports and wilderness enthusiasts also fall into high-risk groups. Alcohol use can contribute to the potential for hypothermia in all risk groups due to behavioral and physiologic alterations. Strategies for the prevention of hypothermia include being educated on signs and symptoms and creating a winter survival kit with blankets, nonperishable food, water, first aid, and medications. Public health strategies that can target high-risk groups include resources to provide frequent checks on those at risk, improved insulation, adequate heating, and shelters to minimize cold exposure.

Warm, layered clothing worn during outdoor activities minimizes convective heat loss. Covering the head with a hat or a scarf minimizes heat loss from radiation. As a rule, infants and young children should be dressed in one additional layer of clothing more than an adult would wear in similar cold conditions. In addition, children's outdoor play time should be limited and include periods of time indoors to warm-up. If signs and symptoms of mild hypothermia are present, returning to an indoor environment can prevent progression to a life-threatening condition. Caretakers of children or adults who have an underlying condition that predisposes to hypothermia need anticipatory guidance on risks and prevention. Education of public safety personnel and healthcare workers to recognize hypothermia and to know effective treatment strategies can also help to prevent hypothermia-related morbidity and mortality.

CONCLUSIONS AND FUTURE DIRECTIONS

Heat-related illnesses consist of a group of disorders that range from benign heat cramps to devastating heat strokes. Early diagnosis and rapid treatment prevent the high mortality and morbidity associated with heat stroke. A preventive strategy is an important part of the overall therapeutic approach that can be effectively implemented to thwart a poor outcome.

Heat-induced inflammatory cascade cannot be interrupted once it is initiated. Corticosteroids, anti-endotoxin antibodies, interleukin receptor antagonists, and nuclear factor (NF)-κβ blockers have been used in experimental settings. The interruption of activated coagulation cascade by replacing deficient levels of naturally occurring anticoagulant factors, such as activated protein C and tissue factor pathway inhibitor may modulate the inflammatory cascade, which may ameliorate systemic inflammation and the subsequent multiorgan dysfunction. Upregulation of Hsps to protect cells from heat-related illnesses is another logical therapeutic choice aimed at preventing irreversible cell damage.

Cold-induced injuries and hypothermia are a group of disorders that range from frostnip and frostbite to devastating profound hypothermia. Early recognition of localized cold injury and rapid rewarming prevent limb-threatening conditions. Although hypothermia typically occurs after exposure to low ambient temperature, numerous other conditions may precipitate a fall in core body temperature. Early recognition and rapid treatment can limit the morbidity and mortality in less severe cases of hypothermia. Severe hypothermia requires the rapid initiation of complex and invasive modalities in centers that can provide tertiary and quaternary care. Despite a very high expected mortality, a good outcome is possible for patients who present clinically dead when they are treated with extracorporeal life support for rewarming and prolonged resuscitation. Preventive strategies are necessary to reduce the incidence of accidental hypothermia.

To date, no validated prognostic indicators have been identified that determine potential recovery from severe accidental hypothermia. Further study might improve treatment and rewarming algorithms. Understanding the mechanisms of circulatory dysfunction during rewarming of hypothermic patients may result in management strategies to optimize tissue oxygen delivery and vascular bed reperfusion (32). Ongoing study of organ system response to hypothermia and its treatment may also elucidate mechanisms by which hypothermia provides protective effects during its therapeutic use for conditions such as cardiac arrest.

KEY POINTS

- Extreme variations in environmental temperature disrupt thermoregulatory function and lead to heat-related illness.
- Children are more prone to develop heat-related illness due to their inability to adapt to extreme heat; prevention is essential in avoiding these complications.
- Modulation of the systemic inflammatory response is an important determinant of compensated versus decompensated response to heat-related injury.
- Heat stroke is a medical emergency. Prompt and aggressive cooling to below 39°C within 30 mins of onset of illness prevents a high mortality rate.
- Efficacy of one method of cooling over another has not been proven.
- Hypothermia can occur due to exposure to cold and many other etiologies when thermoregulation is overwhelmed or dysfunctional.
- Children are at increased risk for hypothermia due to their body morphology and faster cooling rates.
- The choice of rewarming method for hypothermia is dependent upon the degree of hypothermia and the presence or absence of cardiac arrest.
- Resuscitation of the hypothermic patient with cardiac arrest should be continued until rewarming has occurred.
- Prevention and early recognition can limit the incidence, morbidity, and mortality of accidental hypothermia.

References

1. 2005 American Heart Association Guidelines for Cardiopulmonary Resuscitation and Emergency Cardiovascular Care, Part 10.4: Hypothermia. *Circulation* 2005;112:136–8.
2. Adair ER, Black DR. Thermoregulatory response to RF energy absorption. *Bioelectricmagnetics* 2003;Suppl 6:S17–38.
3. Albukrek D, Bakon M, Moran DS, et al. Heat stroke-induced cerebellar atrophy: Clinical course, CT and MRI findings. *Neuroradiology* 1997;39:195–7.
4. Al-Harthi SS, Yaqub BA, Al-Nozha MM, et al. Management of heat stroke patients by rapid cooling at Mecca pilgrimage. *Saudi Med J* 1986;7:369.
5. Alverez, GE, Zhao, K, Kosiba, WA, et al. Relative roles of local and reflex components in cutaneous vasoconstriction during skin cooling. *J Appl Physiol* 2006;100:2083–8.
6. Alzeer AH, Al-Arifi A, Warsy AS, et al. Nitric oxide production is enhanced in patients with heat stroke. *Intensive Care Med* 1999;25:58–62.
7. Armstrong LE, Epstein Y, Greenleaf JE, et al. Heat and cold illnesses during distance running. *Medicine and science in sports medicine* 1996;28:i–x.
8. Aslam, AF, Aslam, AK, Vasavad, BC, et al. Hypothermia: Evaluation, electrocardiographic manifestations, and management. *Am J Med* 2006;119, 297–301.
9. Biem J, Koehncke N, Classen D. Out of the cold: Management of hypothermia and frostbite. *Can Med Assoc J* 2003;168: 305–11.
10. Bosenberg AT, Brock-Utne JG, Gaffin SL, et al. Strenuous exercise causes systemic endotoxemia. *J App Physiol* 1988;65:106–8.
11. Bouchama A, Bridey F, Hammami MM, et al. Activation of coagulation and fibrinolysis in heat stroke. *Thromb Hemost* 1996;76:909–15.
12. Burkman JM, Posner KL, Domino KB. Analysis of the clinical variables associated with recrudescence after malignant hyperthermia reactions. *Anesthesiology* 2007;106(5):901–6.
13. Chang DM. The role of cytokines in heat stroke. *Immunol Invest* 1993;22: 553–61.
14. Committee on Sports Medicine and Fitness, AAP. Climatic heat stress and the exercising child and adolescent. *Pediatrics* 2000;106:158–9.
15. Culic S. Cold injury syndrome and neurodevelopmental changes in survivors. *Arch Med Res* 2005;36:532–8.
16. Dobson JA, Burgess. Resuscitation of severe hypothermia by extracorporeal rewarming in a child. *J Trauma* 1996;40:483–5.
17. Donaldson GC, Keatinge WR, Saunders RD. Cardiovascular response to heat stress and their adverse consequences in healthy and vulnerable human population. *Int J Hyperthermia* 2003;9:225–35.
18. Dunkley EJ, Isbister GK, Sibbritt D, et al. The Hunter Serotonin Toxicity Criteria: Simple and accurate diagnostic decision rules for serotonin toxicity. *QJM* 2003;96(9):635–42.
19. Epstein Y. Predominance of type II fibers in exertional heat stroke. *Lancet* 1997;350:83–4.
20. Gilbert M, Busund, R, Skagseth A, et al. Resuscitation from accidental hypothermia of 13.7°C with circulatory arrest. *Lancet* 2000;355:375–6.
21. Gilbert SS, Van den Heuvel CJ, Ferguson SA, et al. Thermoregulation as a signaling system. *Sleep Med Rev* 2004;8:81–93.
22. Grogan H, Hopkins PM. Heat stroke: Implications for critical care and anaesthesia. *Br J Anaesth* 2000;88:700–7.
23. Grucza R, Pekkarinen H, Hanninen O. Different thermal sensitivity to exercise and cold in men and women. *J Ther Bio* 1999;24:397–401.
24. Hall DM, Baumgardner AR, Oberley TD, et al. Splanchnic tissues undergo hypoxic stress during whole-body hyperthermia. *Am J Physiol* 1999;276: G1195–203.
25. Hall DM, Buettner GR, Oberley LW, et al. Mechanism of circulatory and intestinal barrier dysfunction during whole body hyperthermia. *Am J Physiol Heart Circ Physiol* 2001;280:H509–21.
26. Hietala J, Nurmi T, Danarinen A, et al. Acute-phase proteins, humoral and cell-mediated immunity in environmentally induced hyperthermia in man. *Eur J Appl Physiol Occup Physiol* 1982;49:271–6.
27. Hollander AS, Olney RC, Blackett PR, et al. Fatal malignant hyperthermia-like syndrome with rhabdomyolysis complicating the presentation of diabetes mellitus in adolescent males. *Pediatrics* 2003;111(6 Pt 1):1447–52.
28. Hypothermia-Related Deaths-United States, 2003–2004. *Morb Mortal Wkly Rep* 2004;54:173–5.
29. Kawakami Y, Natelson BH, DuBois AB, Cardiovascular effects of face immersion and factors affecting diving reflex in man. *J App Physiol* 1967;23: 964–70.
30. Kilbane BJ, Mehta S, Backeljauw PF, et al. Approach to management of malignant hyperthermia-like syndrome in pediatric diabetes mellitus. *Pediatr Crit Care Med* 2006;7(2):169–73.
31. Knochel JP. Catastrophic medical events with exhaustive exercise "white collar rhabdomyolysis." *Kidney Int* 1990;38:709–19.
32. Kondratiev TV, Flemming K, Myhre ESP, et al. Is oxygen supply a limiting factor for survival during rewarming from profound hypothermia. *Am J Physiol Heart Circ Physiol* 2006;291:H441–50.
33. Larner AJ. Dantrolene for exertional heat stroke. *Lancet* 1992;339:182.
34. Lee-Choing TL, Stiff JT. Disorder of temperature regulation. *Compr Ther* 1995;21:697–704.
35. Li PL, Chao YM, Chan SH, et al. Potentiation of baroreceptor reflex response by heat shock protein 70 in nucleus tractus solitarii confers cardiovascular protection during heat stroke. *Circulation* 2001;103:2114–9.
36. Lindenblatt, N, Menger, MD, Klar, E, et al. Sustained hypothermia accelerates microvascular thrombus formation in mice. *Am J Physiol Heart Circ Physiol* 2005;289:2680–7.
37. Mallet, ML. Pathophysiology of accidental hypothermia. *Q J Med* 2002; 95:775–85.
38. Mattu A, Brady WJ, Perron AD. Electrocardiographic manifestations of hypothermia. *Am J Emerg Med* 2002;20:314–26.
39. McAllen RM. Preoptic thermoregulatory mechanism in detail. *Am J Physiol Regul Integr Comp Physiol* 2004;287:R272–3.
40. McCullough L, Arora S. Diagnosis and treatment of hypothermia. *Amer Fam Phys* 2004;70:2325–32.
41. Moseley PL. Heat shock proteins and heat adaptation of the whole organism. *J Appl Physiol* 1997;83:1413–17.
42. Murphy JV, Banwell PE, Roberts AHN, et al. Frostbite: Pathogenesis and treatment. *J Trauma* 2000;48:171–8.
43. Passlick-Deetjen J, Bender-Stoll E. Why thermosensing? A primer on thermoregulation. *Nephrology Dialysis Transplantation* 2005;20:1784–9.
44. Shapiro BA. Temperature correction of blood gas values. *Respir Care Clin N Am* 1995;1:69–76.
45. Smith JE. Cooling methods used in the treatment of exertional heat illness *BJSM* 2005;39:503–7.
46. Stocks JM, Taylor NAS, Tipton MJ, et al. Human physiological responses to cold exposure. *Aviat Space Environ Med* 2004;75:444–57.
47. Ulrich AS, Rathlev NK. Hypothermia and localized cold injuries. *Emerg Med Clin N Am* 2004;22:281–98.
48. Van Someren EJ, Raymann RJ, Scherder EJ, et al. Circadian and age related modulation of thermoreception and temperature regulation: Mechanism and functional implications. *Aging Res Rev* 2002;1:771–8.
49. Walpoth BH, Walpoth-Aslan BN, Mattle HP, et al. Outcome of survivors of accidental deep hypothermia and circulatory arrest treated with extracorporeal blood warming. *N Engl J Med* 1997;337:1500–5.

CHAPTER 33 ■ ENVENOMATION SYNDROMES

JAMES TIBBALLS • KENNETH D. WINKEL

Numerous terrestrial and marine animals envenomate, or poison, human victims around the world, causing characteristic syndromes. Children are over-represented among the victims. Many envenomation syndromes threaten life and cause serious illness. Treatment in some syndromes is the application of mechanical ventilation and intensive cardiovascular support but also include the application of specific therapies and, in some syndromes, the administration of antivenom. Included in this chapter is a description of the animals, their toxins or poisons, the syndromes that they cause, and the appropriate treatment for each. Sites of actions of some toxins and poisons on neuromuscular function are shown in **Figure 33.1**.

SNAKEBITE

Venomous Snakes and Snakebite

Snakebite occurs on all continents except Antarctica, with the highest incidence in the developing countries of the tropics. The true incidence of snakebite is unknown, but it has been estimated that up to 2 million bites occur throughout the world annually, with 100,000–200,000 deaths (8). The greatest number of bites occurs in the highly populated, rural areas in Asia, with children being frequent victims.

Medically significant venomous snakes can be classified into 2 major families: the *Elapidae* and the *Viperidae*. The elapids are front-fanged, terrestrial snakes and include the most dangerous Australian snakes (such as the taipan, brown, death adder, tiger, and black snakes); the cobras, mambas and kraits of Asia and Africa; and the coral snakes of the Americas. The venoms of elapid species are highly neurotoxic, with an additional effect of cytotoxicity in some species (e.g., spitting cobras). Vipers have characteristically large, front, foldable fangs and venom that is less toxic but notable for inducing bite-site swelling and tissue destruction. These snakes include the rattlesnakes of the Americas and the old- and new-world vipers. A small number of venomous colubrids, a family of back-fanged snakes, such as the African boomslang, are also medically important. A fourth family is the *Hydrophiidae*, or sea snakes, which are found along much of the IndoPacific coastline, predominantly in the tropics.

Venom

Snake venom is a complex mixture of toxic and nontoxic substances—mostly proteins—that display neurotoxic, myotoxic, procoagulant and anticoagulant, and cytotoxic and hemolytic properties. The composition of venoms influences the clinical presentation of snakebites (**Table 33.1**).

Diagnosis of Envenomation

A high index of suspicion should be maintained in children who suddenly become ill while unsupervised outside, particularly in rural areas and in the summer months.

Signs of Snakebite

Signs of snakebite, but not necessarily envenomation, may include puncture marks (usually on limbs) that (a) may be difficult to see, (b) may consist of single, double or multiple puncture marks or scratch marks, and (c) may be bleeding or oozing; multiple punctures suggest severe envenomation. Another sign of snakebite is regional tender lymphadenopathy, which may also be present after bites from nonvenomous snakes and is thus not by itself an indication for antivenom.

Symptoms of Envenomation

The symptoms of envenomation may include local effects and specific and non-specific features. Local effects are swelling, bleeding/oozing, and pain. Specific features include painful, tender muscles (myolysis); blurred vision, diplopia, difficulty swallowing or breathing, slurred speech, weakness, paraesthesia (neurotoxicity); and spontaneous bleeding from mucosal surfaces, and continual bleeding from the bite site or venipunctures (coagulopathy). Nonspecific features include headache, nausea, vomiting, abdominal pain, collapse, and unconsciousness (may be transient).

Signs of Envenomation

Signs of envenomation include (a) progressive limb swelling, blistering and discoloration; (b) irritability, confusion, coma; (c) bleeding from bite, venipuncture, or other sites (care should be taken with puncture of arterial or central venous sites in the presence of potential coagulopathy, and intramuscular injections should be avoided); (d) dark urine (myoglobinuria, hematuria); and (e) ptosis, dysarthria, weakness/paralysis, dyspnea, respiratory failure (neurotoxicity).

Laboratory Investigations

Laboratory investigations should include the following:

- Snake venom detection kit (SVDK)—Preferably bite site, but secondarily urine or blood—only in Australia and Papua New Guinea

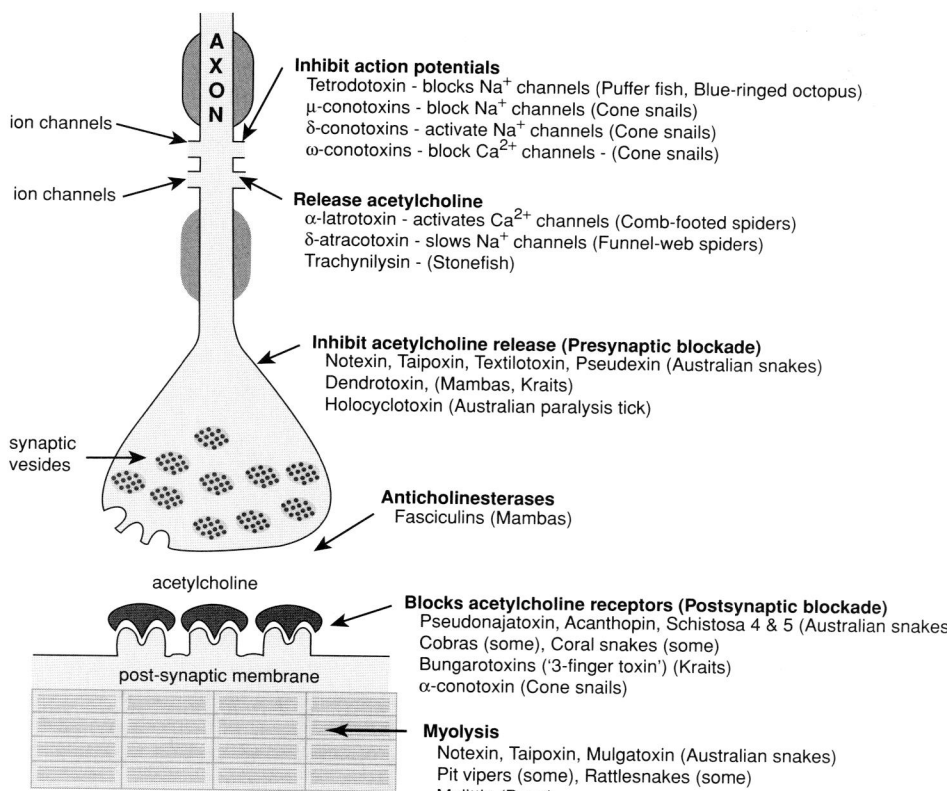

FIGURE 33.1. Sites of action of some major toxins and poisons on nerve, neuromuscular junction, and muscle.

- Coagulation studies—Prothrombin time (INR/PT), activated partial thromboplastin time (aPTT), activated clotting time (ACT), D-dimer, fibrogen degradation products (X-FDP), and fibrinogen levels. In remote areas where sophisticated clotting tests are unavailable, a simple test of coagulation may be performed by placing a sample of the patient's blood in a plain glass tube. It should clot within 10 mins in the absence of coagulopathy. If it remains unclotted at 20 mins (the "20-min whole-blood clotting test"), it is a highly sensitive and specific test of coagulopathy.
- Creatine kinase for myolysis
- Urinalysis for hemoglobin, myoglobin
- Renal function testing—Renal function may be impaired secondary to myoglobinuria or other mechanisms.
- Electrolytes—Particularly potassium (K$^+$), which may be elevated with rhabdomyolysis
- Full blood count—The white cell count is usually only mildly elevated; significant leukocytosis may indicate other pathology. Thrombocytopenia may occur with some snakebites both in isolation and as part of disseminated intravascular coagulopathy (DIC) or microangiopathic hemolytic anemia.

Differential Diagnosis of Venomous Snakebite

On occasion, the diagnosis of snakebite may be unclear; this is more likely in young children or others unable to give a clear history (e.g., found unconscious), in patients bitten at night, in dense scrub where snakes may not be seen, or occasionally in persons engaged in catching or keeping snakes. Differential diagnosis of venomous snakebite includes nonvenomous snakebite; bite or sting by other venomous creature (e.g., hymenoptera, spider, octopus, jellyfish); cerebrovascular accident; ascending neuropathy, e.g., Guillain-Barré Syndrome; acute myocardial infarction; allergic reaction (note that some patients, particularly snake handlers, may have allergic reactions to snake venoms and to antivenoms); hypoglycemia/hyperglycemia; drug overdose; closed head injury.

The symptoms and signs of envenomation and the time course follow a predictable sequence (Table 33.2), but the time course may vary enormously between individual patients, as they are influenced by such factors as amount of venom injected; body weight, age, and state of health of the patient; and time elapsed since the bite and site of the bite. Variation between snake species and between snakes of the same species is also important; for example, the size and maturity of the snake and the time since it last injected venom may influence the severity of the envenomation.

Effects of envenomation are genera and species specific. Bite site swelling and tissue necrosis may be severe after Asian cobra and pit viper bites, may lead to a compartment syndrome, and may even require limb amputation. Myolysis is particularly prominent in envenomations from South American pit vipers, sea snakes, and black snakes. Death adder and king cobra envenomations are specifically neurotoxic. Myolysis may lead to renal failure, a complication that is particularly severe in cases of Russell's viper envenomation. Some snake venoms, including those from many elapid species, contain both postsynaptic and presynaptic neurotoxins, the latter being difficult to reverse if

TABLE 33.1

THE CLINICAL FEATURES OF VARIOUS MEDICALLY SIGNIFICANT VENOMOUS SNAKES OF THE WORLD

Region and species	Clinical features				
	Neurotoxic	Coagulopathic	Local cytotoxic	Myotoxic	Other
South America					
Bothrops spp (lance-headed vipers)	–	++	++	+	Shock, renal failure
Crotalus durrissus terrificus (pit vipers)	++	++	–	+++	Renal failure
North America					
Crotalus spp. (pit vipers)	+	++	++	+	Shock, renal failure
Micrurus spp. (coral snakes)	++			++	
Australia-Papua New Guinea					
Oxyuranus spp. (taipan)	+++	+++		+	Renal failure
Acanthophis spp. (death adder)	+++				
Notechis spp. (tiger)	+++	+++		++	Renal failure
Pseudechis spp. (black)	+	++	–	+++	Renal failure
Pseudonaja spp. (brown)	++	+++			Renal failure
Asia					
Daboia russelii (Russell's viper)	–/+	+++	++	+++	Shock, renal failure
Naja spp. (cobras)	+++		+++		Shock
Naja philippinensis (Philippines cobra)	+++	–	+	–	Shock
Ophiophagus hannah (King cobra)	+++				
Echis carinatus (saw-scaled viper)	–	++	+++	–	Shock, renal failure
Bungaris spp. (kraits)	++		–	–	
Calloselasma rhodostoma (Malayan pit viper)		+++	+++		Shock, renal failure
Europe					
Vipera spp. (European adders)	+/–	+	+		Shock, renal failure
Africa					
Cerastes cerastes (Saharan horned viper)		+++	++		Shock
Echis ocellatus (carpet viper)		+++	++		Shock, renal failure
Naja spp. (African spitting cobras)			+++		
Bitis gabonica (gaboon viper)	+	+++	+++		Cardiotoxic
Bitis arietans (puff adder)		++	+++		Cardiotoxic
Dendroaspis spp. (mambas)	+++		+/++		
IndoPacific					
Hydrophids (sea snakes)	+++		+	++/+++	Renal failure

The symbols represent subjective degrees of severity: –, little clinical effect; +, mild effect of envenomation; ++, moderate effect; +++, severe effect. This is only an approximate guide as the extent of the envenomation syndrome varies with the species or subspecies.
Adapted from Cheng AC, Currie BJ. *J Intensive Care Med.* 2004;19:259–69 and Meier J, White J. *Clinical toxicity of animal venoms and poisons.* Florida: CRC Press, 1995.

the patient is not treated promptly. Coagulation disturbances, frequently secondary to DIC or defibrination, are common after many elapid and viper bites, although severe hemorrhage is infrequent.

Treatment of Venomous Snakebite

First Aid

The role of first aid is important in the prehospital setting and may be important in the hospital as well. A significant number of snakebites, perhaps the majority, do not result in systemic envenomation. Many snakes are not venomous or mildly venomous; further, with many bites by venomous snakes, only a small amount of venom, or no venom, may be injected. However, these situations cannot often be readily determined, and it is thus prudent to treat all snakebites as potentially serious envenomations and to give first aid. At least 95% of bites occur on the limbs; approximately 60% involve a lower limb.

Many first aid practices are useless with snake envenomation. Venom may be injected quite deeply; consequently, little venom is removed by incision or excision (cutting or sucking). These practices are not recommended and may be dangerous, particularly in the coagulopathic patient. The use of arterial tourniquets, especially for prolonged periods, may also be dangerous and is no longer recommended for any type of venomous bite or sting. Suction devices are ineffective and may even worsen local tissue damage.

TABLE 33.2

EXPECTED SEQUENCE OF MAJOR SYSTEMIC SYMPTOMS AND SIGNS AFTER ENVENOMATION BY ELAPID SNAKE SPECIES

<1 hr after bite
Headache
Nausea, vomiting, abdominal pain
Transient hypotension associated with confusion or loss of consciousness
Coagulopathy (laboratory testing or whole-blood clotting time)
Regional lymphadenitis

1–3 hr after bite
Paresis/paralysis of cranial nerves, e.g., ptosis, double vision, external ophthalmoplegia, dysphonia, dysphagia, myopathic facies
Hemorrhage from mucosal surfaces and needle punctures secondary to DIC
Tachycardia, hypotension
Tachypnea, shallow tidal volume

>3 hr after bite
Paresis/paralysis of truncal and limb muscles
Paresis/paralysis of respiratory muscles (respiratory failure)
Peripheral circulatory failure (shock), hypoxemia, cyanosis
Rhabdomyolysis
Dark urine (due to myoglobinuria or hemoglobin)
Renal failure secondary to combinations of shock, hypoxemia, DIC, rhabdomyolysis and hemolysis
Coma secondary to cerebral hypoxemia or ischemia, occasionally due to hemorrhage

A more rapid illness may develop after multiple bites or in small child.
DIC, disseminated intravascular coagulation.

Pressure-immobilization First Aid

Pressure-immobilization first aid for venomous bites and stings was developed experimentally in the 1970s by Struan Sutherland for Australian elapid envenomation (40). In this technique (Fig. 33.2), a continuous bandage is applied, as tightly as binding a sprained ankle, to the whole limb; and a splint is then applied to prevent movement. For example, for a bite on the ankle, the bandage is applied continuously from the toes upward to include the bite site and is extended above the knee, and a splint applied to prevent use and movement of the limb. The rationale is compression of lymphatic channels and inactivation of the "muscle pump" by which lymph flows and by which venom reaches the circulation. Experimental studies suggest that compression without immobilization is ineffective. Retarding the movement of venom from the bite site into the circulation "buys time" for the patient to reach medical care.

Pressure immobilization is recommended for use in bites by all Australian venomous snakes and other purely neurotoxic elapids, such as kraits, mambas, and coral snakes. While clinical trials are lacking, case reports suggest that pressure-immobilization is safe and probably effective in delaying the movement of venom into the circulation (32). If applied correctly, pressure-immobilization first aid may be safely left in situ for several hours, unlike arterial tourniquets which may cause ischemic and/or nerve damage. Additional studies support the efficacy of this technique to retard the movement of venom from the eastern diamond-back rattlesnake (39) and Indian cobra (41). A variant of the technique, featuring a "pressure pad" applied to the bite site, has been trialed with modest success in Burma (31,46).

The timing of removal of a pressure-immobilization bandage is important. Once an asymptomatic patient has reached a hospital that has appropriate antivenom, first aid measures may be removed. Bandages and splints should not be left in place for prolonged periods in this circumstance. If, on removal of first aid measures, the patient's condition deteriorates, the bandages can be re-applied while antivenom is administered. If a patient arrives at the hospital with obvious envenomation but without pressure-immobilization, it should be applied. Pressure bandages may be cut away locally from a bite site to allow swabs to be taken for venom detection, and new bandages can be quickly applied.

Resistance to a universal recommendation for use of pressure-immobilization for snakebite has centered on concerns about potentiating local tissue damage by trapping venom locally. The rationale for this concern appears sound when the significant local toxicity of species such as North American crotalids and Asian pit vipers is compared with the limited local effects of most Australian elapids. Therefore, immobilization without pressure remains a routine first aid recommendation for crotalid and viper bites (28).

Medical Treatment of Envenomation

The principles of treatment are resuscitation, antivenom administration and treatment of specific effects of venom. A careful history and examination should be undertaken, with reference to the features of envenomation described above as well as previous envenomations and allergies to antivenom or to horse serum. A thorough history will assist in diagnosis and aid in decision making with respect to definitive treatment. Samples for venom detection (if relevant) and for pathology should be obtained, and an attempt made to identify the genus of snake, if possible (see later section). The key question is whether or not to give antivenom, an issue that should be regularly reassessed,

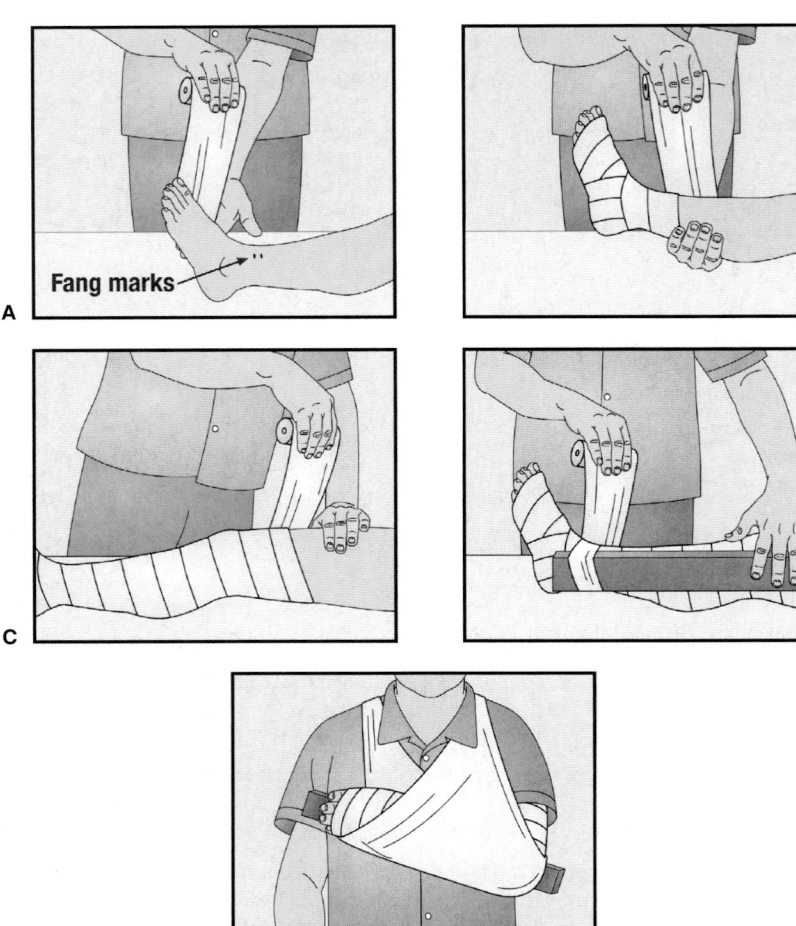

A

B

C

D

E

FIGURE 33.2. Pressure-immobilization first aid. A–C: Commencing distal to bite, apply bandage as tightly as binding a sprained ankle, enveloping the bite site, and extending above major joint. D,E: Apply splint to prevent use of limb, thereby preventing muscle use and lymph flow. From Tibballs J. Envenomation in Australia. In: Wheeler DS, Wong HR, Shanley TP, eds. *Pediatric Critical Care Medicine.* Heidelberg: Springer-Verlag, 2007.

as snakebite is a highly dynamic situation that reflects ongoing absorption of venom.

If the patient has not developed any symptoms or signs of envenomation, nor any indication of coagulopathy or myolysis on blood taken 4–6 hrs after the removal of first aid (or after the bite if no first aid was used), then the patient has probably not sustained a significant envenomation, although delayed onset of symptoms up to 24 hrs after bites have been described. Particular care is required if a neurotoxic elapid bite is suspected, as few signs may be present apart from late-onset neurotoxicity. Overnight observation is desirable, especially if the patient is a young child or comes from a remote area. Ideally, envenomated patients should be admitted to the ICU and observed for a period of at least 24 hrs, depending on the clinical circumstances. Frequent neurologic observations should be performed, and pathology studies should be repeated regularly to monitor progression of the illness.

Local Effects. Vipers cause troublesome local complications such as skin blistering, limb swelling, and tissue necrosis. Although progressive limb swelling is an indication for antivenom use, its effectiveness at reducing local venom effects remains controversial, as does fasciotomy. As compartment syndrome is an infrequent complication of even locally necrosing snakebites, intracompartment pressures should be carefully monitored before consideration of surgical intervention (47).

Local blistering may progress to full-thickness skin necrosis over 3–7 days; such sites are particularly prone to infection.

Coagulopathy. Uncorrected or worsening coagulopathy after initial antivenom treatment is an indication that circulating procoagulants or anticoagulants remain unneutralized and that further antivenom is required. The frequency at which clotting studies should be repeated is controversial. After circulating antivenom has been neutralized, it may be 4–6 hrs or longer before reconstitution of plasma clotting factors has occurred sufficiently to normalize coagulation tests. A lack of improvement in clotting times on retesting may therefore represent insufficient antivenom or insufficient time for regeneration of clotting factors, while improvement in coagulation may represent the efficacy of antivenom or the natural recovery from the disease. Active bleeding, despite adequate quantities of antivenom, is an indication for factor replacement. Whole blood should only be reserved for significant anemia and volume loss. Although the management of asymptomatic but coagulopathic patients is controversial, extrapolation from other hematologic conditions suggests that coagulopathy with parameters exceeding critical thresholds (INR >3, aPTT >50 sec, platelets <50,000/mm^3, and fibrinogen <75 mg/dL) is associated with a major bleeding risk of 1% over a few days (10) and thus warrants specific coagulation factor replacement.

Neurotoxicity. Descending paralysis, starting with ptosis and external ophthalmoplegia and progressing to respiratory failure, is typical of bites by Elapidae (including sea snakes) and a few species of Viperidae (47). In severe envenomations that result in respiratory failure, supplemental oxygen and endotracheal intubation with mechanical ventilation are indicated. If antivenom is delayed or inadequate doses are given, recovery may be prolonged (days to weeks).

Rhabdomyolysis and Renal Failure. Many factors may contribute to renal failure, including shock, a direct toxic effect of venom, rhabdomyolysis, and DIC (7). Although various measures (such as alkalinization of the urine with sodium bicarbonate ($NaHCO_3$) and mannitol to create a forced diuresis) have been advocated, these practices remain controversial, with poor evidence (7). Hyperkalemia secondary to rhabdomyolysis may be treated with the usual medications, including calcium (Ca), insulin, and glucose. Hemodialysis may occasionally be required, particularly in cases in which treatment has been delayed.

Shock and Cardiotoxicity. Monitoring of central venous pressure may be useful in the titration of IV fluid in patients who have not responded to fluid challenge for hypotension. The etiology of shock may vary with the snake species and includes fluid sequestration into necrotic tissue, altered vascular permeability, acute reactions to venom or antivenom, and either direct or secondary cardiotoxicity due to hypoxemia or hypotension. Shock occurs, for example, with *Echis* and *Bitis* species envenomation in which electrocardiographic abnormalities, such as septal T-wave inversion, sinus bradycardia, atrioventricular block, and other conduction defects, are observed, but their clinical significance has not been well defined (47). Disseminated intravascular coagulation may be associated with myocardial ischemia and pulmonary hypertension.

Other. Spitting cobras and the South African rinkhals spray venom from the tips of their fangs into a victim's eyes, causing painful chemical conjunctivitis with the risk of corneal ulceration, anterior uveitis, and secondary infection. The eyes should be irrigated immediately with generous volumes of water (47).

All patients should receive appropriate tetanus and antibiotic prophylaxis if the bite wound is contaminated (but not otherwise). Rarely, the snake's fangs may break and become embedded in the wound, acting as a foreign body and a nidus for infection. Other treatments include analgesia (avoid sedating or narcotic agents such as morphine if possible). Prolonged bed rest may cause contractures, which may be prevented by splinting, and rehabilitation physiotherapy should be started as early as possible (47).

Antivenom

Antivenom is the only specific treatment for bites by venomous snakes. The type of antivenom is determined by the genus of species of snake and by geographic factors. Anticholinesterase inhibitors such as neostigmine may assist in the emergency management of predominantly post-junctional neurotoxic envenomations, such as by the Philippine cobra (48) and Papuan death adder (7), due to the curare-like actions of their neurotoxins.

Indications for Antivenom

Antivenom is indicated if evidence is observed of systemic envenomation or progressive limb swelling or necrosis. If pressure-immobilization first aid is in place, symptoms or signs of envenomation, including laboratory signs, may only become apparent when first aid measures are removed. Such evidence includes physical symptoms or signs such as headache, nausea or vomiting, irritability, confusion or collapse, hypotension, neurologic impairment, abnormal bleeding, hematuria, or myoglobinuria. Laboratory investigations consistent with systemic envenomation include a disordered coagulation profile (or noncoagulable blood in whole-blood clotting test), low or undetectable levels of fibrinogen or raised levels of FDPs, elevated serum creatine kinase level, hemoglobinuria or myoglobinuria. Puncture marks and lymphadenopathy are not indications, per se, for antivenom, as these can occur in bites from nonvenomous snakes or when little or no venom is injected. Similarly, a positive SVDK result at the bite site is not in itself an indication for antivenom, as venom may be present on the skin or clothing but not in sufficient quantity in the circulation to cause systemic envenomation.

Choice of Antivenom

The correct choice of antivenom is crucial. Antivenoms only neutralize the venoms used in their production. Generally they provide little or no neutralization of other snake venoms, although some neutralization of other species, particularly within the same genus, may be expected. The correct antivenom may be selected on the basis of positive morphologic identification of the snake or by use of a SVDK.

Identification of the offending snake aids the choice of the appropriate antivenom and alerts clinicians to particular features characteristic of envenomation by that type of snake. In cases of snakebite that involves zoo staff, herpetologists, or other experienced snake handlers, the snake's identity may be known (although this cannot always be relied upon, particularly in the case of amateur collectors). Identification of snakes by the general public or by hospital staff, even when the offending snake accompanies the patient to hospital, is frequently unreliable. Formal identification by a herpetologist is ideal. Sometimes the snake is not seen or is only glimpsed in retreat, rendering identification impossible or unreliable. In the case of snakebite that involves small children, a history may be vague or entirely lacking. In all of these circumstances a contingency plan for choice of antivenom should be based on knowledge of local species. The occurrence of bites by exotic snakes, i.e., snakes from other countries kept in zoos or private collections, is very problematic. Local poison information centers may be able to locate an appropriate antivenom.

Australia and Papua New Guinea are the only countries that have a commercially available SVDK. This test is a rapid, two-step, enzyme immunoassay in which reactions occur with antibodies to the venoms of major Australian snake genera. Venom from a bite-site swab or a blood or urine sample reacts with specific antibodies in different reaction wells, resulting in a color change that indicates the snake group involved and the type of snake antivenom that may be required.

Bite-site swabs are considered the most reliable sample for use in a SVDK, provided the bite site has not been washed. Blood and urine samples (or other biologic sample) may also be used but are less reliable. Urine in particular may be used if presentation has been delayed or if the bite site (unusually) cannot be identified. The kit has "built-in" positive and negative controls that must be checked to validate the test results. The test is regarded as highly reliable, but like all tests, it must have a rate of false negatives and false positives, although these rates are as yet undefined.

Although a positive SVDK test of blood or urine confirms that envenomation has occurred, it is not *per se* an indication to give antivenom. Conversely, a negative SVDK result does not mean that envenomation has not occurred, as venom may be present in a concentration below the detection limit or may not yet have reached the blood or have been excreted in the urine. The information should be used in conjunction with other information (such as clinical presentation, knowledge of snakes in the geographic area, identification of snakes brought to hospital with the patient) to determine which antivenom to use if the patient is significantly envenomated.

If a reliable identification of the snake cannot be made, polyvalent antivenom or a selection of monovalent that covers likely species should be used. For example, in Australia a combination of brown and tiger snake antivenoms is satisfactory for all snake envenomation (by indigenous species) in the state of Victoria, and tiger snake antivenom alone is satisfactory for the state of Tasmania; however, elsewhere, polyvalent antivenom that contains aliquots of tiger, brown, black, death adder, and taipan antivenoms is required.

Administration of Antivenom

Snake antivenoms are given by the IV route. Skin testing for allergy to antivenom is not recommended, as it is unreliable and may delay urgent therapy. Antivenoms should be diluted in at least 100 mL of normal saline, 5% dextrose, or Hartmann's solution immediately prior to administration. Initial administration should be slow, while the patient is observed for signs of allergic reaction. If no reaction is observed, the infusion may be run over 15–30 mins. If the patient reacts to the antivenom, the rate may be slowed or the infusion ceased temporarily. If reaction is severe, treatment with adrenaline, antihistamines, corticosteroids, or plasma volume expanders should be undertaken as required. The decision to recommence antivenom should be based on the clinical state of the patient. In the case of the patient with a known allergy to antivenom or to horse serum, the decision to withhold antivenom should be based on the severity of envenomation and availability of resuscitation facilities and skills.

The neutralization efficacy of antivenoms and doses are variable. The initial doses recommended for particular envenomations are provided by product information and are based on the *average* venom yields from the snake concerned and the severity of the presenting signs and symptoms. The amount of venom injected is quite variable. Few rigorous clinical trials have been undertaken on the efficacy of antivenoms internationally. Further, antivenoms are often used for their "paraspecific" efficacy, in that the identity of the snake is unknown and venom from only a few species is used to manufacture polyvalent antivenoms. However, in Australia, evidence exists that manufacturer-recommended doses may be insufficient to reverse coagulopathy associated with the bites of several Australian venomous snakes, notably the brown snake (38,45). Larger initial doses should also be considered in the presence of evidence of severe envenomation (multiple bites, rapidly progressive symptoms, large snakes). The dose of antivenom for children should not be reduced according to their weight because the amount of venom injected by the snake is independent of the victim's size.

Thus, the dose of antivenom cannot be specified with absolute reliability. Antivenom requirements of individual patients will vary considerably. Some patients with minimal envenomation may not require antivenom, whereas severely envenomated patients may require multiple doses. Recurrence of coagulopathy may occur, particularly with the use of newer Fab-type antivenoms, leading to the need for further doses of antivenom (10). Advice may be available from local poison information (control) centers.

Adverse Reactions to Antivenom

As snake antivenoms are biologic protein products manufactured by a variety of techniques from animal sources, the rate of adverse reaction varies considerably in frequency and severity. Overall, adverse reactions are common and may be divided into early hypersensitivity reactions (true anaphylactic reactions are probably less common compared with anaphylactoid reactions), pyrogenic reactions, and late allergic reactions (serum sickness). Limited data are available to estimate the incidence of each type of reaction. In general, the highest rates of acute reaction, up to 80%, occur in unfractionated equine antivenoms (e.g., Haffkine Institute polyvalent snake antivenom in India) (14), whereas the lowest rates are observed with Fab-type ovine antivenoms (e.g., Crofab polyvalent crotalid antivenom in the US) (10).

Facilities and skills should be readily available for dealing with such complications as anaphylaxis before the administration of antivenoms. In particular, prior to the administration of antivenom, epinephrine (10 mcg/kg) should be prepared for use in the event of hypotension or bronchospasm. Epinephrine is the treatment of choice in conjunction with bronchodilators, H_1 receptor blockers, fluid replacement, and corticosteroids.

Premedication for Antivenom

Premedication to reduce adverse antivenom reactions has been controversial, and evidence for its efficacy had been lacking. However, a randomized, double-blinded, placebo-controlled trial of the efficacy of low-dose subcutaneous epinephrine to prevent acute adverse reactions to snake antivenom in Sri Lanka in 1999 demonstrated a fourfold reduction in such reactions (33). In addition, no adverse reactions (such as intracranial hemorrhages) were observed in the premedicated patients, supporting the safety of this recommendation. Although this study has been criticized for lacking statistical power and its relevance to antivenoms with much lower reaction rates (7), premedication with subcutaneous adrenaline is particularly recommended for polyvalent antivenom in a low-resource setting. Adults should receive 0.25 mg of epinephrine by the subcutaneous route (0.005 mg/kg for children). To avoid hypertension in a coagulopathic patient with the potential for bleeding, epinephrine as a premedicant should not be given IV. Similarly, epinephrine should not be administered intramuscularly, as this may also lead to hypertension and to hematoma formation in the presence of coagulopathy. Although traditionally used, antihistamines are not recommended on the basis of findings of a randomized, placebo-controlled trial in Brazil (14) and because they confound the effects of venom by sedative and hypotensive actions.

Serum Sickness

Serum sickness due to the deposition of immune complexes is a recognized complication of the administration of foreign protein solutions such as antivenoms. Symptoms include fever, rash, arthralgia, lymphadenopathy, and a flu-like illness. It usually occurs 7–10 days after antivenom administration. The possibility of serum sickness and its usual symptoms and signs should be discussed with the patient prior to discharge so that it may be recognized and treated early. Corticosteroids should be considered if a large volume of antivenom, such as polyvalent antivenom or multiple ampules of monovalent antivenom, have been administered or if the patient has a history of exposure to equine protein. Both the incidence and severity of delayed serum sickness may be reduced by the administration of prednisolone, 1–2 mg/kg daily for 5 days after the administration of antivenoms.

SPIDER BITE

Spiders have a truly global distribution in nearly all environments, with thousands of species described. Consequently, spider bite is one of the most common problems in toxicology. Fortunately, in most cases only transient local or radiating pain, bite-site redness, swelling, and itchiness occur. In that virtually nothing is known about the venom of most spiders, the most appropriate approach is general treatment based on presenting symptoms. Spiders with the greatest potential for harm include funnel-web spiders (*Atrax* or *Hadronyche* spp.), comb-footed spiders (*Latrodectus* spp.), and the necrotizing species, the most important of which are the recluse or violin spiders (*Loxosceles* spp.), each of which require specific treatment.

Funnel-web Spiders

More than 30 species of highly dangerous funnel-web spiders are found mainly on the eastern seaboard of Australia. While many remain unnamed and their venoms unstudied, all funnel-web spiders belong either to the genus *Atrax* or *Hadronyche*. Funnel-web spiders are the most dangerous spiders in the world, as they have caused death within 2 hrs. Fortunately, severe envenomation is uncommon and no fatalities have occurred since the introduction of an antivenom in 1980 (26). Identification and classification of funnel-webs is often difficult, and some resemble the less dangerous trapdoor spiders. Any dark-colored or brown spider that is 2–3 cm in body size on the eastern seaboard of Australia should be regarded, from a medical perspective, as if it were a funnel-web. Capture and formal identification of the spider is helpful.

Venom

Unlike most spiders, the venom of the male Sydney funnel-web spider is more toxic than that of the female. While the venoms have many components, the key polypeptide neurotoxins of approximately 42 amino acids are the γ-atracotoxins (γ-ACTXs), which act by slowing sodium current inactivation, resulting in spontaneous repetitive generation of action potentials. This process triggers the release of excessive catecholamines and eventual exhaustion of predominantly sympathetic neurotransmitters, leading to a characteristic biphasic clinical syndrome. Acetylcholine is also released at neuromuscular junctions and in the autonomic nervous system.

Envenomation

The syndrome is generally characterized by two phases; the first begins within minutes of the bite, and the second occurs when the secretions subside, typically many hours later. Historically, deaths have occurred in either phase of the envenomation. The characterization of phases 1 and 2 of envenomation by the funnel-web spider, as well as its treatment, are listed in **Table 33.3.** However, it should be noted that most definite bites by funnel-web spiders are asymptomatic.

If no symptoms or signs of envenomation have begun 4 hrs after the removal of first aid measures or post-bite, the patient may be discharged. (Most patients who present to the hospital will not have been envenomated.) Tetanus status should be assessed and prophylaxis provided if indicated. Follow-up is necessary for potential secondary infection. Wound cultures and appropriate antibiotic therapy may be needed.

Comb-footed (Widow) Spiders

The "comb-footed" spiders of the family *Theridiidae* are ubiquitous throughout the world, with more than 100 species described within one genus alone. The *Latrodectus* species, including the widow, button, koppie, or redback spiders, are the most medically significant. Globally, this genus is probably the most important cause of spider bite, with *Latrodectus* antivenom producers on every continent. In Australia, more redback spider (*L. hasselti*) antivenom is reported used than any other antivenom. Mortality from this envenomation is rare (25).

Venom

The exact mechanism(s) by which *Latrodectus* sp. toxins produce the clinical effects are poorly understood, as is the precise cause of death in the rare fatalities. The key toxin, α-Latrotoxin, a high-molecular-weight protein of ~100–120 kDa, appears to be relatively invariant between *Latrodectus* species. It is a presynaptic neurotoxin that stimulates the release of catecholamines from sympathetic nerves and acetylcholine from motor nerve endings. This action has both receptor-mediated and receptor-independent phases. In a remarkable contrast to most envenomation syndromes, widow spider envenomation may progress and persist for days to months.

Envenomation

Bites by widow spiders produce a recognizable syndrome—"latrodectism"—that may necessitate antivenom administration. Usually the bite is painful, but it may be relatively painless and, unless the spider is seen, may initially go unnoticed. Puncture marks and swelling are uncommon. The onset of symptoms and signs is highly variable, but progression of the illness is generally slow. Effects may persist for weeks after an untreated bite and have been successfully treated with black widow or redback spider antivenom weeks or even months after the bite.

Signs and symptoms include (a) local pain that radiates from the bite site and involves the entire limb, which increases over the first hour and typically persists for greater than 24 hrs; (b) localized redness, piloerection, painful regional

TABLE 33.3

EFFECTS AND TREATMENT OF ENVENOMATION BY FUNNEL-WEB SPIDERS

Phase 1
Local Effects
- Bite site may be painful for days to weeks because of direct trauma and acidity of venom, but no local necrosis has been recorded.
- Local swelling and erythema

General Effects
- Numbness around the mouth, and spasms or fasciculation of the tongue
- Nausea and vomiting, abdominal pain, and acute gastric dilatation
- Profuse sweating, salivation, lacrimation, piloerection, and severe dyspnea
- Confusion progressing to coma
- Hypertension, tachycardia, and vasoconstriction (hypotension may occur later)
- Local and generalized muscle fasciculation and spasm, which may be prolonged and violent (facial, tongue, or intercostal muscles and including trismus)

Phase 2
- Hypotension
- Hypoventilation and apnea
- Acute noncardiogenic pulmonary edema
- Coma and, finally, irreversible cardiac arrest

Treatment
- Maintenance of airway, breathing and circulation
- Prompt application of a PIB to affected limb, as for neurotoxic elapid snake bite. The PIB should only be removed once the patient has reached a location where appropriate resuscitation can be given and antivenom is available.
- If the PIB is removed and the patient deteriorates, it should be reapplied.
- If antivenom is not available, the PIB should be kept in place, because evidence from animal experiments suggests that venom may be inactivated at the bite site
- Administration of IV antivenom
- Intubation and ventilation for respiratory failure and to reduce intracranial pressure (note: endotracheal intubation may be hindered by excessive salivary secretions and violent fasciculations)
- Supportive care (additional) may include:
  - Atropine in doses sufficient (20 mcg/kg initial dose) to reduce salivation and bronchorrhea
  - Nasogastric aspiration to relieve gastric dilatation
  - Muscle relaxants and sedatives to facilitate mechanical ventilation
  - Sympathetic blockade for hypertension and severe tachycardia
  - Fluid resuscitation in the event of hypotension, but with caution because of risk of noncardiogenic pulmonary edema

PIB, pressure-immobilization bandage

lymphadenopathy, and sweating (sometimes affecting only the bitten limb but sometimes occuring in a distribution unrelated to the bite site); (c) systemic features, including fever, hypertension, tachycardia, nausea and vomiting, abdominal pain, headache, lethargy and insomnia; (d) migratory arthralgia and paraesthesias. Children generally present with irritability and local pain, erythema, and nonspecific maculopapular rashes. Myalgia/neck spasms in children >4 years of age seem to be a prominent feature.

Rare complications include neurologic symptoms associated with the neuromuscular blockade and possibly excessive catecholamine release, e.g., muscle weakness or twitching, myocarditis, rhabdomyolysis, paralysis, and death.

Treatment

Antivenom should be administered for pain that is unrelieved by simple analgesia (e.g., local application of ice or oral analgesics) and/or with systemic symptoms or signs of envenomation such as vomiting, severe headache, abdominal pain and collapse, hypertension, arthralgia, or myalgia. When the clinical findings are atypical but the history is suggestive, a trial of antivenom may be helpful both diagnostically and therapeutically. The usual dose is a single vial, but occasionally several

vials may be required, especially in the setting of more than one bite and in those presenting late. Typically, antivenom is effective within the first 2 hrs after injection, but occasionally symptoms can reappear, necessitating a further dose. The dose should not be reduced for children, whose lower body weight renders them theoretically more susceptible to severe envenomation.

The reaction rate to redback antivenom (manufactured by CSL, Ltd.) is low, observed in one series as 0.5%; therefore, premedication is usually not recommended, but patients with a history of horse allergy or prior exposure to equine immunoglobulin may be at higher risk for acute or delayed allergic reactions. The incidence of serum sickness is unclear but is certainly low; therefore, corticosteroids are not recommended routinely. Use of redback antivenom at different stages of pregnancy without problems and without increase in the frequency of malformation or other direct or indirect harmful effects on the human fetus has been reported. Unlike most other antivenoms, administration of widow or redback spider antivenom may be effective even several weeks after a bite.

Unlike snake antivenoms, redback and widow antivenom may be administered by the intramuscular route. However, if envenomation is severe, or if response to intramuscular injection is poor, the IV route can be used. If given IV, the antivenom should be diluted in 100–500 mL of crystalloid solution (normal saline, Hartmann solution, or dextrose) and run over 15–30 mins.

The redback antivenom is also effective against other widow spiders that cause "latrodectism-like" symptoms. However, more research is required before the full range of indications is established. For example, envenomation by the brown house, cupboard, or "false-widow" spiders (*Steatoda* spp.), although they belong to a separate genus within the same family as redback spiders (Theridiidae), is effectively treated with redback antivenom. Like the redback-type spiders, they are found throughout the world, but bites have been poorly documented. Physically, they are slightly smaller in size, with a similar body shape to the redback, but they lack the distinctive red coloration on the ventral abdominal surface. Instead, they may have a yellow or cream stripe or spots. With all *Steatoda* and *Latrodectus* spp., the female is the larger and more dangerous (but male and juveniles may still bite and envenomate). The envenomation syndrome is similar to that caused by the redback spider but less severe: bite-site pain and redness, swelling, sweating, piloerection, pain radiating to involve the limb, chest pain, nausea and vomiting, shivering, lethargy, tachycardia, and hypertension have all been observed after these spider bites. It therefore seems prudent to treat these bites in the same manner as a *Latrodectus* envenomation.

Recluse or Violin Spiders

Loxosceles spiders are another group with a wide distribution, with more than 50 species described from equatorial to subtemperate regions, but only a few species have been implicated in human envenomation—loxoscelism—and are capable of causing necrotizing skin lesions (17). The important species in South America are *L. gaucho, L. intermedia,* and *L. laeta,* while in North America, they are *L. deserta* and *L. reclusa* (17).

Venom

The venom from *Loxosceles* species has variable toxicity. For instance, *L. deserta, L. rufescens,* and *L. arizonica* are thought to cause relatively mild lesions. In general, the *Loxosceles* species in South America cause a higher incidence of the systemic illness in humans than do those from elsewhere. The venoms contain proteases, hydrolases, lipases, hyaluronidase, alkaline phosphatase, and collagenase, among other enzymes. Sphingomyelinase D is one of the most important components of the venom responsible for development of dermonecrosis, myolysis, and hemolysis. The mechanism of action is a very complex and multifactorial process. The characteristic dermonecrotic lesion results from the venom's direct effect on the cellular and basal membrane components and on the extracellular matrix. The initial interaction between the venom and tissues causes complement activation; migration of polymorphonuclear lymphocytes; liberation of proteolytic enzymes, cytokines, and chemokines; platelet aggregation; and blood flow alterations that result in edema and ischemia, with development of necrosis.

Envenomation

The diagnosis of *Loxosceles* envenomation is usually based on the clinical examination findings and patient history, as the spider is seldom identified. For that reason, the real incidence of envenomation is unknown and misdiagnosis frequent. Envenomation causes two syndromes: cutaneous loxoscelism and viscerocutaneous loxoscelism.

Cutaneous Loxoscelism. Cutaneous loxoscelism is characterized by a dermonecrotic lesion at the bite site that can take weeks to heal. Most *Loxosceles* envenomations result in little more than a mild inflammatory reaction, but in a small subset of victims bitten, a necrotic skin ulcer develops within 2 to 6 hrs after the bite, with the site developing severe burning pain accompanied by localized intradermal hemorrhage, erythema, pruritus, and swelling. It is often surrounded by a perimeter of blanched skin that results from venom-induced vasoconstriction. A larger area of erythema may also evolve in reaction to the chemical mediators that leach into the surrounding tissue. A fine, macular eruption over the entire body has occasionally been noted. By day 3 or 4, the initial hemorrhagic areas degrade into a central area of blue necrosis, which eventually forms an eschar that sinks below the surface of the skin. This common pattern is referred to as the "red, white, and blue sign." This appearance of the wound differentiates this bite from non-necrotic ulcers, which tend to maintain a red lesion that remains raised above the surrounding skin.

Eschars eventually dehisce, leaving a necrotic center that heals by secondary intention, usually with scar formation. Plastic surgery is sometimes required to repair the affected area. The average time from treatment to healing of a suspected bite averages 15 days, with a range from 0 to 78 days. If ulceration has not developed by 2–3 days after the bite, necrosis will not usually develop. Secondary infection at a *Loxosceles* envenomation site is rare, although a more generalized rash can simulate cellulitis. Venom-induced lymphangitis can also be confused with a secondary infection. Transient and mild constitutional signs and symptoms (e.g., myalgia, malaise, fever, chills, nausea, vomiting, generalized rashes, and headache) may occur that are not as severe as the systemic illness, although the early stages of systemic illness may be similar.

Viscerocutaneous Loxoscelism. Viscerocutaneous loxoscelism is a severe systemic illness that sometimes occurs after *Loxosceles* envenomation in addition to the local damage. It consists of a low grade fever, arthralgia, diarrhea, vomiting, coagulopathy, DIC, hemolysis, petechia, thrombocytopenia, urticaria, and sometimes rhabdomyolysis. Hemolysis and rhabdomyolysis can cause acute renal failure. Although viscerocutaneous loxoscelism occurs 48–72 hrs after envenomation, it has occurred at as early as 24 hrs (17). It has a higher incidence in the pediatric population.

The prevalence of viscerocutaneous loxoscelism ranges from 0.7% to 27% and varies geographically, perhaps because *L. reclusa,* the predominant species in the US, seldom causes the systemic illness caused by *L. laeta,* the predominant South American species. Deaths due to these bites usually occur in children <7 years of age, presumably because the ratio of venom quantity to body weight in small children is higher than in other age groups. Necrosis at the envenomation site occurs in up to half of all patients. Despite extensive research, no cost-effective or time-effective diagnostic test to confirm envenomation is commercially available.

Treatment of Cutaneous Loxoscelism

Despite the fact that loxoscelism is a leading cause of spider-bite morbidity in some regions, a definitive therapy is not established. Various interventions have been proposed: dapsone, surgical excision, steroids, hyperbaric oxygen therapy, and antivenom therapy (17).

Polymorphonuclear-cell Inhibitors. Sulfones (i.e., dapsone) inhibit polymorphonuclear lymphocyte degranulation, reducing local tissue inflammation and subsequent destruction caused by these cells. These inhibitors antagonize the intracellular calcium release that results in the expression of granule markers that occur with venom-induced endothelial cell activation. Dapsone has been investigated for loxoscelism in multiple animal and human studies, with inconclusive results. Because of its side effects (including cholestatic jaundice, hepatitis, leukopenia, methemoglobinemia, hemolytic anemia, and rarely, peripheral neuropathy) and limited supporting data, the benefit-to-risk ratio of dapsone has been questioned. Nonetheless, its use is advocated in the US and Brazil.

Surgical Excision. Surgical debridement and skin grafting was one of the first interventions used for cutaneous loxoscelism, and it has been explored as treatment both alone and in conjunction with dapsone. Although preliminary results found improved outcome when the two were used together, early surgical management in general has been found to be ineffective and sometimes harmful as an initial management technique. The poor cosmetic results that occurred in early interventions were due to increased levels of acute-phase reactants, secondary to surgery, that exacerbate venom effects and prolong tissue injury.

A wound may take several days to reach maximum size (which is predictive of healing time). Surgical excision only after a delay of 2–8 weeks allows dissipation of venom and the subsequent acute-phase reactants. Ultimately, 3% of all cutaneous loxoscelism patients require skin grafting once the acute phase of envenomation has passed and either the size of the lesion (>2 cm) or comorbidities such as peripheral vascular disease or diabetes mellitus make primary healing less likely. A delay of weeks is required for the wound to "declare itself" by stability of the area of necrosis or shrinkage. Prior to this, frequent evaluation is necessary to assess the wound, and delayed surgical treatment should only be considered when a lesion fails to heal or complications occur.

Wound Care. Many topical wound treatments have been proposed. Although no prospective studies have been published on decontamination, the most important intervention might be wound irrigation. Venom can remain in a wound for up to 5 days before elimination. A direct correlation between diffusion of venom from the wound and the degree of dermal inflammation has been described.

Corticosteroids. The controversy over systemic corticosteroids for both systemic and cutaneous loxoscelism started relatively early in the development of treatment modalities. Clinical studies are small and limited, hindered by lack of confirmation that lesions were actually *Loxosceles* envenomations. Various reviews indicate that, while systemic corticosteroids are not recommended for the cutaneous form of loxoscelism, they might have a role for viscerocutaneous loxoscelism. Although corticosteroids are advocated in Brazil for systemic illness but not simple necrotic ulcers, data are insufficient to merit steroid use in either the cutaneous or the viscerocutaneous forms of *Loxosceles* envenomation. Nonetheless, the immunosuppression of corticosteroids early in the course of a systemic reaction might ameliorate immune-mediated morbidity.

Antibiotics. In the US, necrotic lesions of any cause are usually treated with oral antibiotics to prevent infection, although this may be unnecessary if necrotic ulceration is highly likely to be due to envenomation. As early envenomation can appear to be caused by infection, this might account for the high incidence of antibiotic use. Indeed, early *Loxosceles* bites are often misdiagnosed as infections until the characteristic necrotic lesion ensues. In a classical envenomation lesion, antibiotics are not indicated in the absence of evidence of infection.

Hyperbaric Oxygenation. Hyperbaric oxygenation therapy has been used for cutaneous loxoscelism. Its proposed efficacy is promotion of neovascularization with increased oxygen availability to ischemic tissue. However, no conclusive evidence supports its use.

Antivenom Therapy. At this writing, commercial *Loxosceles* antivenoms are available through four sources (Institute Butantan in São Paulo and Centro de Produção e Pesquisa em Imunobiológicos in Paraná, both in Brazil; The Institutos Nacionales de Salud in Lima, Peru; and Instituto Bioclon in Mexico), but none are available in the US. The Brazilian Ministry of Health has the most extensive use of antibody treatment and has developed guidelines for its use in large cutaneous lesions and extensive necrosis or systemic illness (17). Antivenom is also used to decrease the severity of reaction and shorten healing time, depending on how early after the bite it is administered. However, no large-scale, prospective studies have been undertaken, and administration is not without risk of allergic reactions.

In most clinical investigations, a significant delay usually occurs between the actual bite and presentation for treatment. This delay previously had been considered to render antiserum administration ineffective, as the most damaging effects occur in the first 3–6 hrs of the bite in animal studies and in vitro. However, work using a rabbit model suggests that IV equine anti-*Loxosceles* serum reduces the size of venom-induced lesions if used up to 12 hrs after intradermal injection of venom. Taken together, all these studies suggest potential value of delayed use of antivenom to decrease lesion size and/or limit systemic illness, but more clinical trials are needed. In countries where antivenom is used, the usual indication is systemic loxoscelism, although clinical trial data are lacking.

Treatment of Viscerocutaneous Loxoscelism

Loxosceles species venoms vary in strength and are highly potent, with an LD_{50} in the milligram-per-kilogram range in mice. A full envenomation can deliver up to 0.07 mg of venom. Rare deaths from loxoscelism may be secondary to renal failure, and hemolysis as suggested by pediatric case reports. Renal failure results from hemolysis and from direct nephrotoxic effect, which may be more pronounced in children. Children, particularly those <7 years of age, are often more susceptible to the viscerocutaneous form of loxoscelism. Although relatively rare, once the systemic form of loxoscelism is fully manifested, it carries significant morbidity and mortality. A critically ill child without an obvious cause of illness should prompt consideration of *Loxosceles* envenomation, particularly in an endemic area. A bite mark may be overlooked on physical exam. Measures such as fluid administration and vasopressor support to maintain renal perfusion and augment clearance of hemoglobin and myoglobin secondary to hemolysis and rhabdomyolysis can reduce the severity of renal damage.

The degree of hemolysis can be profound and may necessitate blood transfusion. Although the use of corticosteroids for viscerocutaneous loxoscelism is universally accepted as a means to help protect reticulocytes from the venom effect, data to support this practice are limited. Hemolysis may occur in delayed onset of a systemic reaction after development of a dermonecrotic lesion. A patient with an isolated dermal lesion discharged home should be instructed to watch carefully for a change in urine color, which is indicative of this complication.

SCORPION STINGS

Of the 800 known species of scorpions, many cause serious and life-threatening illness (2). These nocturnally active creatures inhabit areas with warm or hot dry climates within a 45° latitude of either side of the Equator.

Venom

Scorpion venom is a complex mixture of mucopolysaccharides, hyaluronidase, serotonin, histamine, protease inhibitors, histamine releasers, and protein neurotoxins that inhibits inactivation of voltage-gated sodium channels (20), resulting in release of transmitters at sympathetic, parasympathetic, and neuromuscular receptors.

Envenomation

Distinctive syndromes of envenomation are caused by members of a limited number of scorpion families in Mexico and Central America, southern American States (Texas, Arizona, New Mexico), South America (Brazil, Venezuela, Colombia, Argentina), India and Nepal, Middle East, North Africa, and Central and South Africa (**Table 33.4**). Children are more susceptible than adults, possibly because scorpion venom targets the brain and heart more in younger animals (29).

Life-threatening cardiovascular and neurotoxic effects are caused by most species, except *Centruroides sculpturatus*, whose effects are essentially confined to neurotoxicity. A systemic inflammatory response with cytokine release, kinin release, and complement activation may lead to multiorgan failure. Mortality is variable, reported in Tunisia as 7.6% of 951 victims over a 13-year period up to 2002 (5) but as only 0.2% of 825 victims patients in 1994–1995 (1). Elsewhere, mortality was recorded in Morocco as 1.3% of 1212 cases (37), and in Egypt as 12.5% of 41 children (22).

Neurologic Effects

Although pain is the universal feature of envenomation by scorpions, a wide variety of other neurologic symptoms and signs may constitute a syndrome, as determined by the specific species. Generally, envenomation may cause the following: coma, convulsions, cerebral edema, external ophthalmoplegia, mydriasis, meiosis, agitation, rigidity, tremor, twitching, tongue and muscle fasciculation, respiratory failure, gastric and pancreatic hypersecretion, bradycardia, tachycardia, salivation, sweating, abdominal pain, vomiting, and priapism.

TABLE 33.4

SPECIES, DISTRIBUTION, AND EFFECTS OF SCORPIONS

Geographic region	Species	Cardiotoxic	Neurotoxic
India	*Buthus tamulus* *Mesobuthus tamulus* (Indian red scorpion)	+++	++
Middle East and North Africa	*Leiurus quinquestriatus* *Androctonus crassicauda*	+++	++
Brazil	*Tityus serrulatus*	+++	++
Mexico	*Centruroides suffusus*	+	++
Southern states of the US	*Centruroides sculpturatus* (*exilicauda*)	−	++
Central and South Africa	*Parabuthus transvaalicus* *Parabuthus granulatus*	+	++

The symbols represent subjective degrees of severity: −, little clinical effect; +, mild effect of envenomation; ++, moderate effect; +++, severe effect. This is only an approximate guide as the extent of the envenomation syndrome varies with the species or subspecies.
Adapted from Amitai Y. Scorpions. In: Brent J, Wallace KL, Burkhart KK, et al., eds. *Critical Care Toxicology*. Philadelphia: Mosby, Elsevier 2005:1213–20.

Cardiovascular Effects

Multiple mechanisms lead to cardiovascular failure. Myocardial ischemia or myocarditis with raised CPK-MB isoenzymes and cardiac troponin I levels may occur in children (22). Experimentally, direct cardiotoxicity and release of endogenous catecholamines are responsible for high vascular resistance in both systemic and pulmonary circulations, low cardiac output, and elevated left atrial pressure.

Treatment

Antivenom Therapy

The efficacy of scorpion antivenoms, derived from various animals, has been debated. Numerous case series and retrospective reviews have cited beneficial effects and improvement in outcome. For example, coincident with introduction of antivenom and adjunctive therapy, the mortality among 24,000 patients in 18 health regions in Saudi Arabia was reduced from 4%–6.8% to <0.05%. However, only one randomized, controlled trial has been performed (1), which in 825 victims older than 10 years of age, found no benefit, irrespective of the clinical severity on presentation. Although there is little doubt that antivenom reduces serum concentration of venom, the clinical relevance of this effect is questionable. In animal experiments, simultaneous administration of antivenom with venom is protective, but antivenom delayed even by 10 mins fails to alter hemodynamic effects. Moreover, the incidence of acute and delayed adverse reactions to antivenom may not be inconsequential and must be weighed against the degree of envenomation, local knowledge of species and their effects, and duration since envenomation.

Physicians experienced in treating scorpion envenomation suggest reserving antivenom therapy for patients with significant systemic toxicity, which includes arrhythmia, hypertension, hypotension, seizures, coma, or pulmonary edema. Lesser manifestations warrant at least admission to the ICU. Antivenom should only be administered intravenously, with preparedness to treat an acute adverse reaction and followed-up to treat possible serum sickness. If indicated, the dose should not be reduced because of child status (2).

Supportive Therapy

Supportive cardiovascular therapy is important in severe envenomation. Intensive monitoring and titration of vasodilator and inotropic agents is required, along with judicious mechanical ventilation. In early envenomation, catecholamine release causes hypertension, but this may later culminate in cardiac failure and hypotension. Hydralazine, nifedipine, and oral prazosin have been used successfully clinically, while phentolamine has been used experimentally. In 19 patients with pulmonary edema of whom 11 required mechanical ventilation and 10 had peripheral circulatory failure, infusion of dobutamine markedly improved cardiac output, systemic arterial pressure, and right ventricular ejection fraction, while it decreased pulmonary artery occlusion pressure (13). A titratable vasodilator would be beneficial at least in the hypertensive phase of the syndrome and, possibly, later in conjunction with an inotropic agent. The use of hydrocortisone has not influenced outcome.

BEE, WASP, AND ANT (HYMENOPTERA) STINGS

While reactions to most stings by Hymenoptera are mild and self-limiting, a life-threatening, immediate, hypersensitivity reaction (anaphylaxis) may occur for which the same treatment protocol should be adopted regardless of the responsible creature. Although anaphylaxis is more common in children, morbidity is greater in the elderly due to greater comorbidities such as coronary atherosclerosis and medications such as β-antagonists and ACE inhibitors. Most bee and wasp species are solitary, and they only sting in self-defense, but social bees and wasps use their sting to defend their nests, resulting in multiple stings and, occasionally, massive envenomation.

Bee Stings

Within the superfamily *Apoidea*, subfamilies include the social bumble bees (*Bombinae*) and honey bees (*Apinae*). The common honeybee (*Apis mellifera ligustica*) is well established throughout the world and is an important cause of Hymenopteran stings. It does not tend to attack in a swarm, unlike the aggressive "Africanized" honey bee (*Apis mellifera scutellata*) that is responsible for mass envenomations in the Americas. Cases of massive bee envenomation (venom toxicity) are rare outside of those areas in which the Africanized strain is endemic. While most bee stings are trivial, rapid death may follow either mass stings or anaphylactic reactions in hypersensitive individuals (even after a single sting). Most bee sting-related deaths are among outdoor workers, especially farmers, truck drivers, and beekeepers (and their families, including children).

Wasp Stings

Most social wasps belong to one of the two subfamilies of Vespidae: Vespinae and Polistinae. The subfamily Vespinae includes four genera: *Dolichovespula* "yellow jackets" (18 species), *Vespula* "common social wasps," with some species also called "yellow jackets" (~25 species), *Vespa* "hornets" (20 species; these large, potentially very dangerous wasps inject more toxic venom, in larger quantities, than bees and smaller wasps), and *Provespa* (3 species). Within the subfamily Polistinae, some species of the paper wasps, genus *Polistes* (*P. annularis, P. exclamans, P. fuscatus, P. metricus*), are of medical importance. Vespinae are found in Eurasia, North America, and North Africa. The US is home to 17 native species of yellow jacket, the exotic European hornet (*Vespa crabro*), and the European wasp (*Vespula germanica*). *Vespula* yellow jackets have spread and become well established in non-native regions such as Australia, New Zealand, South American, and South Africa. In northern Australia, serious wasp stings are generally due to native paper wasps. In Asia, deaths frequently occur in children and young adults from stings of oriental and tropical *Vespa* wasps, which pose a particular hazard to those who climb coconut palms, gather fruit, work in coffee or rubber plantations, and cut trees or bamboo.

Like bees, wasps are colony insects that construct large nests, often among the lower tree branches, where they can be accidentally disturbed, provoking an aggressive swarm attack. A wasp nest near a home or school should be destroyed, preferably at night when the wasps are less likely to attack, by experienced personnel wearing protective clothing,

Ant Stings

Ants (family Formicidae) are widespread, with approximately 8800 species worldwide. However, relatively few species are medically important, and these can be divided into two major groups, distinguished by the development of a venom injection apparatus. The first group gives an irritating bite that they then spray with secretions from their abdominal glands. The second group causes painful true stings, injecting allergenic venom. These are typified by the *Myrmecia* ants in Australia and the fire ants (*Solenopsis* spp.) in the Americas. Other groups also cause occasional allergic reactions.

The red imported fire ant, *Solenopsis invicta*, is of particular clinical significance. It forms super colonies and is an aggressive, territorial species that swarms onto an intruder before stinging. Stings are multiple, usually in the tens or hundreds. Approximately one-quarter of patients stung will develop some degree of allergy. Numerous fatalities, but rarely among children, have occurred in the US, where the fire ant has become widespread since its introduction in the 1930s. It has recently become established in Australia (36). Fire ant venom contains alkaloids known as *piperidines*, which produce a very painful, burning sensation, unlike that of other hymenoptera, and cause a characteristic urticarious pustule at the sting site.

Venoms

In a typical wasp sting, 2–20 mcg of venom is injected. It consists of active amines (serotonin, histamine, tyramine, catecholamines), histamine-releasing peptides or mastoparans, wasp kinins (which are pain-inducing molecules), and antigen 5 (the most active allergen). In addition, venoms contain several enzymes, including phospholipases, hyaluronidases, and cholinesterases which contribute to the allergic response. The venom of some wasp species contains neurotoxins and acetylcholine. Despite some common components, wasp venom components vary greatly among species, with variable lethal doses. Hornets (*Vespa*) have potent venom (LD_{50} ranging from 1.6 to 4.1 mg/kg in four *Vespa* spp.) that can deliver lethal doses in as few as 50–200 stings. Social wasps (*Vespula* and *Dolichovespula*) have less potent venom (LD_{50} ranging from 3.5 to 15 mg/kg) and also deliver smaller quantities of venom per sting.

In contrast, a single bee sting typically contains ~50 mcg of venom that consists of enzymes, small proteins and peptides, and amines. Melittin, which hydrolyzes cell membranes, thereby changing cell permeability and inducing pain, is the primary component of bee venom, making up 50% of the venom dry weight. Another component, phospholipase A_2, is a major allergen that also causes pain and hemolysis. Additional components are hyaluronidase ("spreading factor" that allows venom components to permeate tissue), amines (histamine, dopamine, norepinephrine), and peptide 401 (mast cell degranulating peptide that triggers the inflammatory cascade). Honey bee venom has a median lethal dose in mice of 3 mg/kg

body weight. In humans, the LD_{50} is estimated at 19 stings/kg, translating into roughly 500–1500 stings to deliver a lethal dose. Africanized honeybees deliver slightly less (but equally toxic) venom than European honeybees.

Deaths due to venom toxicity have occurred within 4 hrs but may be delayed until 7–9 days after stinging. Secondary infection is a greater risk after wasp stings compared with bee stings, as the former are predators on insects and scavengers of sugar sources rather than being pure pollen and nectar feeders. Wasps also reuse their stings and may break the skin with their mandibles.

Envenomation by Bee, Wasp, and Ant Stings

Simple Stings

Bee, wasp, and ant stings in nonallergic individuals produce immediate burning pain, redness, and swelling at the sting site. Pain usually subsides over some hours, while redness and swelling resolve more slowly.

Multiple Stings

The effects of multiple stings are dramatically amplified, and systemic effects include headache, vomiting, thirst, pain, edema, discolored urine (hematuria and/or myoglobinuria), jaundice, and confusion. Rhabdomyolysis with resultant acute renal failure may occur. Intravascular hemolysis, coagulopathy, thrombocytopenia, metabolic disturbances, encephalopathy, liver dysfunction, and myocardial damage have also been reported (18). Death from venom toxicity has been recorded in many countries, generally when a patient has more than 200, and usually 500, bee stings but may also occur after as few as 25–30 wasp or hornet stings. Hospitalization is mandatory for anyone who receives more than 10 stings.

Systemic Allergy

Hypersensitive patients may develop rapid, catastrophic anaphylaxis that causes death in minutes. Severe systemic reactions are less common in children than in adults, but the risk of recurrence can persist for decades, with a 30% chance of a similar reaction even 20 years after sting (15). In some patients, venom allergy may cause large local reactions that may involve the swelling of the whole limb within 24 hrs.

Treatment for Bee, Wasp, and Ant Stings

Simple Stings

The stinger should be removed as soon as possible (the method is unimportant) to limit the amount of venom injected. The majority of single bee stings do not require treatment, although cold packs and oral analgesia are valuable. Wasps and ants do not leave their sting behind; therefore each individual may sting multiple times. Large, local reactions usually respond well to symptomatic treatment with nonsteroidal anti-inflammatory agents and topical steroid creams. Oral steroids and antihistamines are often used.

Anaphylaxis

Treatment for anaphylaxis is based on administration of epinephrine as definitive therapy, supported by oxygen, β agonists for bronchoconstriction, steroids, and IV fluid (for hypotension). Individuals at risk for anaphylaxis from insect stings must carry, and be taught to use, injectable adrenaline (such as EpiPen, an automated device for prehospital intramuscular injection of epinephrine) immediately after a sting. Two dosages are available (child, 150 mcg; adult, 300 mcg). An Australian study of Hymenoptera sting mortality (21) revealed that most patients who died from anaphylaxis had a known insect sting allergy. Patients with a history of anaphylaxis to bee or wasp venom and a positive skin test should also have maintenance immunotherapy (injection of small quantities of pure bee or wasp venom) for at least 3–5 years. This protocol provides 80% protection from further episodes of bee sting anaphylaxis and 98% protection against wasp-sting anaphylaxis. Long-term immune tolerance induced by venom immunotherapy is greater in children than in adults (15).

Multiple Stings

Patients with serious systemic effects due to envenomation may require resuscitation. Renal function should be closely monitored. Prolonged hemofiltration or dialysis may be required. Permanent renal damage may necessitate long-term dialysis. Tetanus status should be checked and, in cases of multiple wasp stings, septicemia should be anticipated and antibiotic prophylaxis considered. Children are at greater risk of toxicity due to the higher dose of venom per unit of body mass.

TICK BITE

Ticks are arthropod ectoparasites that feed on blood, piercing the skin of a host with a hypostome. A complex mixture of chemicals is secreted to enable long-term attachment to, and maintain blood flow from, the host. Such substances inhibit hemostasis, augment local blood flow, and suppress the inflammatory and immune responses of the host. Ticks cause a number of different problems, including allergy, transmission of infection (zoonoses), secondary infection, foreign-body granuloma if not removed in entirety, and paralysis.

Tick paralysis occurs in several parts of the world. In Australia, paralysis is caused by the female *Ixodes holocyclus* (Australian paralysis tick) and, to a lesser extent, by *I. cornuatus* (42). At least 20 deaths occurred in New South Wales alone between 1900 and 1945 before the availability of an antitoxin. *I. holocyclus* is restricted to scrub and brush country in coastal regions from Cairns on the eastern coast of Queensland through New South Wales to the southeastern parts of Victoria, where its range overlaps with *I. cornuatus*.

In North America, 40 species of indigenous soft ticks (*Argasidae*) and hard ticks (*Ixodidae*) parasitize humans, but many foreign ticks are also discovered attached to victims who return from abroad (23). In the southern and Atlantic states, the soft tick *Amblyomma americanum* (Lone Star tick) predominates; in the eastern states, *Dermacentor variabilis* (American dog tick) and *Ixodes scapularis* (blacklegged tick) predominate; and in the Rocky Mountains and certain western states, *Dermacentor andersoni* (Rocky Mountain wood tick) is common.

In far western states, *I. pacificus* (western blacklegged tick) is found. Parasitism by the soft ticks, *Ornithodoros* spp., occurs in western states. Paralysis and occasional death usually occur among children who are <8 years of age and *Dermacentor andersoni* is often the cause (11). In South Africa, a number of species are considered potentially dangerous, especially *Argas walkerae*. Mild cases have been reported in Europe and the UK.

Ticks are vectors of rickettsial diseases, symptoms of which essentially consist of fever, rash, and myalgia. In Australia, ticks are vectors of *Coxiella burnetii*, which causes Q fever, and of *Rickettsia australis*, which causes North Queensland tick typhus and rickettsial spotted fevers in Victoria. In America, *Dermacentor andersoni* is the vector for *Rickettsia rickettsii* and *R. peacockii*, the causative agents of Rocky Mountain spotted fever and other spotted fevers.

Lyme disease, named after Lyme, Connecticut, in the US, where it was first described, is caused by tick bite. It is a multisystem, infectious disease caused by a spirochete, *Borrelia burgdorferi*, which is carried by ixodid ticks. The principle features of the syndrome are a rash, arthritis, various neurologic manifestations, and myocarditis. The disease is widespread in North America and Europe, where *I. dammini*, *I. pacificus*, and *I. ricinus* are responsible. In Australia, sporadic cases occur and are probably transmitted by *I. holocyclus*.

In Europe, severe viral encephalitis and hemorrhagic fevers are caused by viruses of the genera *Flavivirus*, *Nairovirus*, and *Coltivirus*, which are transmitted by tick bite. The ticks mainly responsible are of the genera *Ixodes* (*ricinus*, *persulcatus*), *Haemaphysalis*, and *Dermacentor* (*reticulates*, *pictus*). Diseases such as tick-borne encephalitis, Omsk hemorrhagic fever, louping ill and Crimean-Congo hemorrhagic fever have very low mortality.

Envenomation

Human victims and their clinicians may be unaware of the presence of a tick until progressive muscle weakness and ataxia develops; even then, unless a thorough search for an engorged tick is conducted, it may not be noticed. The tick may be above the hairline, in a skin fold, or in any body orifice. Local edema and inflammation may signal its presence, but it may also make it difficult to see and extract. Regional lymphadenopathy may be present. If a hypersensitivity to tick secretions has developed, local changes may be dramatic.

Several protein neurotoxins of ~5 kDa molecular weight that cause ascending paralysis in experimental animals have been identified in *I. holocyclus* saliva (43). They probably inhibit release of neurotransmitters. Intoxication occurs after the tick has been feeding for 3 or more days. By this time, its weight will have increased from a mere 1 mg to ~450 mg. Significant illness is more common in children, and the first obvious evidence of poisoning may be unsteadiness in walking or lethargy. Usually, the child becomes subdued and sleepy and refuses food. The paralysis commences as ascending symmetrical weakness that progresses to involve the upper limbs and, terminally, the muscles involved with swallowing and breathing. Neurologic examination will reveal a paralysis of a lower motor neuron type. The deep tendon reflexes are diminished or absent, and the plantar response generally remains flexor in type. Early cranial nerve involvement, particularly both internal and external ophthalmoplegia, may occur. In older children and adults, the presenting complaint may be difficulty in reading. Double vision, photophobia, nystagmus, or pupillary dilation may be present.

Nerve paralysis may be limited to the vicinity of the engorging tick, as in, for example, unilateral facial nerve palsy caused by a tick embedded behind the ear; however, in most cases, it is general. Neurophysiologic studies reveal general, low-amplitude, compound muscle action potentials with normal conduction velocities, normal sensory studies, and normal response to repetitive stimulation (16). Occasionally, cardiac failure due to toxic myocarditis may occur in humans.

Differential Diagnosis

The diagnosis may be difficult if the victim has traveled with the tick in situ to a different part of the country, from a rural to an urban environment, or to another country where tick paralysis is unknown. Once the possibility of tick paralysis is considered, a careful search for the culprit(s) may confirm the diagnosis. General flaccidity or paralysis may be mistaken for poliomyelitis and vice versa, as they share some clinical similarities. Other diagnoses to be considered are diphtheria, myasthenia, Guillain-Barré syndrome, botulism, myopathies, and a variety of inflammatory and toxic neuropathies. A facial nerve palsy may be mistaken for a viral infection.

Laboratory Investigations

Hematologic investigations and lumbar puncture performed in several cases have not been helpful. Eosinophilia does not occur. However, plasma creatine kinase and troponin determinations should be made.

Treatment

Prompt and careful removal of the offending tick(s) is essential. The sprayed application of a personal insect repellent that contains pyrethrins or synthetic pyrethroid rapidly kills the tick and causes the hypostome and chelicerae (mouth parts) to lose turgidity and shrink away from the host tissue. Extrication is then easily effected by use of curved forceps, the points of which are pressed into position on either side of the tick's mouth parts, pressing well down into the skin, avoiding any pressure on the tick's body, and closing firmly on the hypostome before attempting to lift the tick out. The engorged body of the tick should not be grasped by the fingers or forceps, as this may result in incomplete removal and the expression of toxin. An alternative method of extraction is by gentle upward traction of a thread encircling the mouth parts. Surgical excision of the tick is not necessary, nor is application of a pressure-immobilization bandage after removal of the tick(s), as the onset of paralysis is slow.

If paralysis has occurred, mechanical ventilation may be required for several days. Due to delay in the onset of the effects of the toxin, the onset of paralysis may be delayed until after removal of a tick(s) in an asymptomatic victim, and the effects

may worsen after the removal of the tick in an already poisoned victim. Adequate observation after tick removal is necessary, even if the victim, particularly a child, is well at the time of its discovery and removal. Failure to recover should prompt a further search for additional ticks.

In Australia, the production of a tick antitoxin derived from infested dogs has been recently discontinued.

Apart from neurotoxic effects, the likelihood of zoonosis and secondary infection must be considered, and tetanus prophylaxis brought up-to-date. The possibility of renal damage should be considered if rhabdomyolysis occurs.

JELLYFISH STINGS

All four classes of the phylum Cnidaria (Hydrozoa, Scyphozoa, Cubozoa, Anthozoa), are characterized by possession of nematocysts (stinging cells) and cause human envenomation. Three of the classes are described as "jellyfish" because of their gelatinous, free-floating medusal life-cycle stage. Of these, Scyphozoa are true jellyfish, Cubozoa are "Box jellyfish," whereas Hydrozoa are hydroids. Large chirodropid (multi-tentacled) cubozoan jellyfish have killed or seriously injured numerous victims, while small carybdeid (single-tentacled) cubozoan jellyfish and some species of hydroids have occasionally caused deaths (44).

Chirodropidae

Chirodropids are large jellyfish with a box-shaped bell from whose four corners arise numerous long tentacles. The most important chirodropid is *Chironex fleckeri* (Australian box jellyfish). *C. fleckeri* inhabit waters of northern Australia and the IndoPacific region, including Vietnam, the Philippines, Malaysia, Thailand, and probably Indonesia. It has caused approximately 70 deaths in Australia. Chirodropid deaths in nearby countries may have been due to *C. fleckeri* or another closely related species, *C. quadrigatus* (49). *C. fleckeri* and similar chirodropids have a white or translucent cubic or box-shaped bell as large as a 2-gallon bucket (i.e., 20 × 30 cm) and weighing >6 kg. Four bundles of up to 15 translucent extensile tentacles stream out from 4 pedalia (fleshy arms) under the bell. Tentacles of mature specimens stretch 3 meters. The wide, ribbon-like tentacles are covered with millions of nematocysts (spring-loaded syringes), which discharge toxins via a penetrating everting thread or tube upon contact. The threads have little denticles that enable them to drill 1 mm into the dermis of human skin. As the tube everts and penetrates skin, it releases venom directly into any transfixed capillaries, ensuring rapid toxicity.

Venom

Animals injected with a lethal venom dose die within 15 mins from cardiorespiratory arrest. Toxic components include an ~70-kDa hemolytic component (hemolysin), a dermatonecrotic factor, and a lethal protein component with probable direct cardiotoxicity induced by calcium influx as the result of membrane pore formation (6).

Envenomation

C. fleckeri is rarely noticed by a victim until contact with tentacles occurs, usually while wading or swimming in shallow water. The tentacles are easily torn from the jellyfish by the encounter and, in adhering to the victim's skin, resemble earthworms of a pink, grey, or bluish hue. During the first 15 mins, pain increases in mounting waves despite removal of the tentacles. The victim may scream and become irrational. The lesions are distinctive and resemble marks made by a whip that is 8–10 mm wide with a "frosted ladder pattern" that matches the bands of nematocysts on the tentacles. Whealing is prompt and massive. Edema, erythema, and vesiculation soon follow, and when these subside (after some 10 days), patches of full-thickness necrosis leave permanent scars. Severity of injury is related to size of the jellyfish and the extent of tentacle contact. Most stings are quite minor. The mechanism of death in humans is not known with certainty, but case reports suggest a consequence of combined cardiovascular and respiratory failure.

Antivenom

C. fleckeri antivenom is the only jellyfish antivenom manufactured worldwide and has been in use since 1970. It is concentrated immunoglobulin derived from the serum of sheep injected with *C. fleckeri* venom. Each vial contains sufficient activity to neutralize 20,000 IV LD_{50} mouse doses. Antivenom is used in ~10% of envenomations. It is not effective against Australian *Chiropsalmus sp.* venom.

Treatment of Envenomation

The severity and rapidity of envenomation necessitate decisive action, the mainstays of which include first aid, cardiopulmonary resuscitation, and antivenom administration. First aid measures include retrieval of the victim from the water to avoid further contact with the creature(s) and to prevent drowning; basic life support; inactivation of undischarged nematocysts by pouring vinegar (4%–6% acetic acid) over adhering tentacles for at least 30 secs to prevent further envenomation. (Alcohol in any form must *not* be used for this purpose.) Vinegar-treated tentacles are harmless, but if vinegar is not available, tentacles may nonetheless be picked off safely by rescuers, as only a harmless prickling of the fingers may occur. Advanced cardiopulmonary resuscitation should be performed on the beach (if possible), during transportation, and in the hospital. Three vials of antivenom should be administered.

Calcium Channel Blockade. The use of verapamil, although theoretically appealing, is probably harmful due to its hypotensive effects and therefore is contraindicated. It has not been used successfully in humans or animals (34). *C. fleckeri* venom causes a large elevation of cytosolic calcium (Ca^{2+}) in rat myocytes not prevented by verapamil (6).

Magnesium. Magnesium may prove to be an important adjunctive therapy in envenomation. Prophylactic administration did not prevent cardiovascular collapse induced by venom in rats but improved the effectiveness of antivenom from 40% to 100% (34).

Ice Packs. Mildly painful stings respond well to application of ice packs after they have been doused with vinegar.

Indications for Antivenom

Antivenom should be administered as soon as possible in the following circumstances: (a) unconsciousness, cardiorespiratory arrest, hypotension, dysrhythmia, or hypoventilation; (b) difficulty with breathing, swallowing, or speaking; (c) severe pain (parenteral analgesia is also usually required); or (d) possibility of significant skin scarring. The initial dose is three ampules infused IV, diluted 1:10 with a crystalloid solution.

Laboratory Diagnosis

The simplest and quickest way to confirm *Chironex* envenomation is detection of characteristic nematocysts on microscopic examination of a 4–8-cm-long piece of ordinary transparent sticky tape that has been applied to the sting site. The tape is applied to a lesion, stroked several times, removed, and with its sticky side up, affixed onto a glass slide. Microscopic examination of skin scrapings is an alternative. Nematocysts of *C. fleckeri* and *Chiropsalmus* sp. are difficult to distinguish.

Prevention

People should never swim, wade, or paddle in the subtropical waters of Australia (beaches, estuaries) when a "jellyfish alert" has been issued. Swimming should be restricted to the safe months of the year and to beaches enclosed by jellyfish-resistant nets ("stinger enclosures"). If water must be entered because of a person's occupation or hobby, protective clothing should be worn.

Other Chirodropids

Lesions produced by another highly dangerous Australian chirodropid jellyfish, *Chiropsalmus* sp., are narrower and milder, and the tentacular contact is far less than that of *Chironex fleckeri*. Lethal chirodropids are found elsewhere in the world, including in the Gulf of Mexico, where a fatality was attributed to *C. quadrumanus*. Another, *C. quadrigatus* (Habu-kurage), inhabits Japanese waters.

Carybdeids

Carybdeids (order Carybdeidae, class Cubozoa) are also box jellyfish: the bell is cubic but from each corner arises an arm (pedalium) that usually bears only a single tentacle in contrast to those of chirodropids, which bear many tentacles. Although many exist in all except colder oceans, species of medical importance are *Carybdea rastoni* (the jimble), *Carukia barnesi* (irukandji), and *Carybdea alata* (Hawaiian box jellyfish).

Carybdea rastoni

C. rastoni is a four-tentacled small jellyfish often found in swarms, with a very wide distribution in the Western Pacific Ocean and most Australian and Japanese waters. The bell is translucent and usually not much larger than 2 cm across. Its tentacles stretch ~5 cm to perhaps 30 cm.

Venom and Envenomation. Purified protein toxins cause vasoconstriction (perhaps by release of catecholamines), release of prostaglandins, and contraction of smooth muscle (44). Tentacles bear ovoid nematocysts. Stings are usually immediately painful, with linear lesions frequently four in number, ranging from 10 to 20 cm in length, and may blister. No specific management is recommended.

Carukia barnesi, The Irukandji

Morphologic differentiation of *Carukia barnesi* and *Carybdea rastoni* may be difficult; both are small carybdeids with a box-shaped bell and four tentacles. *C. barnesi* is found from Exmouth in Western Australia, across northern Australia, and down the Queensland coast as far south as Mackay. Its squarish bell is barely 12 mm wide, and its four tentacles vary in length up to 35 cm. Clumps of nematocysts (mammilations) appear as tiny red dots over the bell whereas, on the tentacles, they are in tightly packed "collars" and in ring formations. The body and tentacles are almost completely transparent in water.

Venom and Envenomation. The venom contains a potent neuronal sodium channel modulator that releases high levels of catecholamines, with resultant tachycardia, increased cardiac output, and systemic and pulmonary hypertension (50). This hyperadrenergic state may partially explain the clinical features of the "Irukandji syndrome." The victim rarely sees the offending jellyfish but is often aware of a sting, usually slight, to the upper body while swimming in deep water. Sometimes the sting is unnoticed, and it is the onset of symptoms that forces the victim to leave the water. The sting area contains no banding or puncture marks, just an oval area of barely perceptible erythema that measures approximately 5 cm by 7 cm. Irregularly spaced papules ("goose pimples") up to 2 mm in diameter develop within 20 mins of the sting and then fade, but erythema may last several days.

From 5 mins to as late as 2 hrs after the sting, but usually after ~30 mins, a distinctive severe syndrome develops. Severe low back pain, cramping muscle pains, nausea, vomiting, profuse sweating, headache, restlessness, and agitation almost invariably occur, sometimes with hypertension. Abdominal pain is associated with spasm of the muscles of the abdominal wall, and cramps occur in the muscles of the limbs. Occasionally, loss of consciousness occurs due to cerebral edema. Also occasionally, acute cardiac failure occurs and manifests as pulmonary edema, poor contractility, low cardiac output, and raised cardiac enzymes (19). The onset of pulmonary edema is delayed, occurring several to many hours after the sting. The mechanism of cardiac failure is speculative but appears to be secondary to hypertension or direct myocardial depression. It seems unlikely that the relatively brief period of only mild-to-moderate hypertension before the onset of cardiac failure is the sole cause.

Most stings have been mild, although 2 fatalities in northern Australia have been attributed to unseen jellyfish causing the Irukandji syndrome. In these fatalities, intracerebral hemorrhage was associated with severe hypertension. Irukandji syndrome is not confined to Australian water and has been reported in Papua New Guinea, Hawaii, Japan, China, southern US (Florida), Qatar, and Thailand, possibly due to other carybdeids (44).

Treatment. Pain relief is the most important feature of management in mild-to-moderate cases. Repeated doses of IV or intramuscular opiates may be required, with care not to cause

hypotension. In a series of 10 victims with Irukandji syndrome, IV magnesium salts provided pain relief and a reduction in blood pressure (9). Otherwise, treatment includes oxygen therapy, diuretics, vasodilators, inotropic support, and mechanical ventilation or application of continuous positive airway pressure. Antihypertensive therapy may be required in the initial phase of management. Infusions of phentolamine have been used successively for this purpose, although a "titratable" nitrate (nitroprusside) is preferred.

Carybdea alata (Hawaiian Box Jellyfish)

The *Carybdea alata* species has a bell approximately 8 cm in height and 5 cm in width, with tentacles approximately 0.5 m in length. Its sting causes moderate pain and may be responsible for an Irukandji syndrome (51). Immersion of the sting in hot water gives pain relief (27).

Physalia physalis (Portuguese Man-of-War); Physalia utriculus (Bluebottle)

These jellyfish are the most frequent cause of significantly painful stings. Three deaths have been attributed to the Atlantic *P. physalis* on the southeast coast of the US, but no fatalities have been attributed to *P. utriculus* in Australia.

Species of *Physalia* are found in all hot and temperate waters of the world. Each jellyfish is a colony of hydrozoans grouped into four specific roles. One group (the "sail") forms a gas-filled float that keeps the colony on the surface and enables wind-assisted travel. The float of *P. physalis*, the multi-tentacled species, measures from 2–25 cm in length, while in *P. utriculus* is smaller—up to 10 cm in length. Another group involves reproduction, while another has polyps and tentacles with nematocysts, acting as a "keel" or "sea anchor" and is responsible for the collection of food. A fourth group performs digestion. The long fishing tentacle of a large multi-tentacled species may be 30 m long, while that of a single-tentacled species is 2–3 m. Being a creature floating on the surface in armadas, *Physalia* presents a significant hazard to swimmers. *Physalia* stranded on a beach may cause stings if handled.

Envenomation and Venom. The main lethal toxin, physalitoxin, is a glycoprotein with cardiovascular toxicity that results from formation of nonselective channels or pores in membranes (12). Upon contact, contracted tentacles produce a lesion, usually linear, like a row of beans or buttons, while uncontracted tentacles may give fine linear stings. The offending creature is usually easily identified. Undischarged nematocysts are spherical.

Treatment. Most stings are quite minor. In the few reported deaths, victims were in cardiac arrest within minutes of contact with tentacles. Death in one case was attributed primarily to respiratory arrest. No specific antivenom is available.

FISH STINGS

Numerous fish have dorsal or pectoral spines that may inflict a traumatic wound made worse by deposition of venom (42).

Stonefish

Species of the stonefish genus *Synanceia* (*Synanceja*) are found throughout the entire IndoPacific region and, in Australia, from Brisbane to 500 km north of Perth. Stonefish are easily mistaken for a piece of rock or dead coral that has become encrusted with marine growth. The venom apparatus is purely defensive and plays no role in the capture of prey. Stonefish have 13 dorsal spines, each of which carries two basal venom glands. When disturbed, the spines become erect. When trodden upon, venom is forced out of the tips of the spines into the victim's foot.

Venom

Venoms of all three species (*S. verrucosa, S. horrida, S. trachynis*) depress the cardiovascular and neuromuscular systems and have a direct effect on muscle. Less dangerous effects are hemolysis, an increase in vascular permeability, and effects due to a host of enzymes that include hyaluronidase. Experimentally, venom injected intravenously causes hypotension, respiratory distress, and paralysis by direct myotoxicity. Various protein toxins have been isolated that are cytotoxins, release acetylcholine and other transmitters, cause myolysis, and cause cardiovascular collapse by negative inotropic actions and vasodilation.

Envenomation

Stings are extremely painful. The victim may become irrational. The severity of the signs and symptoms is usually in direct proportion to the depth of penetration of the spine(s) and the number of spines involved. In addition to local swelling and pain, muscle weakness and paralysis may develop in the affected limb, and shock may occur. Fatalities have occurred in IndoPacific regions, and one has been reported in Australia.

Antivenom

Stonefish antivenom, a pure equine F(ab)$_2$ preparation, is manufactured by Commonwealth Serum Laboratories (Pty) in Australia. It neutralizes the venoms of *S. trachynis, S. verrucosa,* and *S. horrida.* Vials contain approximately 2 mL, which in vitro will neutralize 20 mg of venom.

Treatment

The initial priority is pain relief. No attempt should be made to retard the movement of venom from the stung area, as this will only enhance local pain and tissue damage. Relief in minor cases may be achieved by bathing or immersing the sting with warm-to-hot water. In severe cases, pain relief may only be obtained by the combined use of antivenom and opiate drugs. A local anesthetic may be injected into the track of the sting and the surrounding area. A regional nerve block should be considered.

Antivenom is recommended for all cases, except in those that involve only a single puncture wound with moderate discomfort. The initial dose of antivenom is determined by the number of spines and depth of penetration. One vial (2000 units of antivenom in 2 mL) is sufficient for every one to two spine punctures. Antivenom is usually given intramuscularly. In very severe cases, three or more vials may be required and the use of the IV route should be considered, particularly if the pain is widespread or the patient is in shock. Antivenom should not be injected in or around the area of the sting.

The injured limb should be comfortably immobilized. Administration of an antibiotic (e.g., trimethoprim-sulfamethoxazole, third-generation cephalosporins, or imipenem) active against pathogens found in salt or brackish water (*Vibrio* spp., *Aeromonas* spp., *Plesiomonas* spp.) is recommended. Tetanus prophylaxis should be given according to the victim's immune status. Severe injuries may require early surgical debridement of dead tissue and drainage. Skin grafting may be necessary when antivenom has been delayed and considerable ulceration exists. Sometimes a sting remains painful for months, or recurrent inflammation or discharge occurs, usually due to a spine fragment, which being semitransparent and deeply embedded, may be undetectable except by surgical exploration or ultrasound examination.

Other Stinging Fish

Numerous other fish with stinging spines of the families Scorpaenidae (scorpion fish), Synanceiidae, and Trachinidae are to be found in the world's oceans and fresh waters. Examples are the butterfly cod (*Pterois volitans*), waspfish (*Apistops caloundra*), scorpion cods (*Scorpaena cardinalis*), South Australian cobbler (*Gymnapistes marmoratus*), fortescue (*Centropogon australis*), bullrout (*Notesthes robusta*), gurnard perch (*Neosebastes pandus*), goblinfish (*Glyptauchen panduratus*), ghoul (*Inimicus caledonicus*), and numerous catfish, weeverfish, rabbitfish, and spinefeet (*Siganus lineatus* and *spinus*). Many envenomations occur among amateur collectors of *Pterois volitans*. The mechanical penetration or laceration by spines is painful enough, but many also envenomate.

Treatment

Little is known about the nature of the venoms associated with the dorsal spines of the many stinging fish. There are no antivenoms. Otherwise, the management of a wound is as for stonefish.

Stingrays

Stingrays have barbed tails that may inflict serious leg, abdominal, or chest wounds. Direct damage by penetration of the stinging barb is usually of greater importance than the introduction of the venom or a marine pathogen. A swimmer cruising the ocean floor is at risk of a serious chest wound when disturbing settled rays, as is the occupant of an open small boat when a ray leaps from the water surface.

Significant wounds require exploratory surgery because the wound track may contain a trail of glandular and integumentary sheath material as well as necrotic tissue. Penetrating wounds to the chest or abdomen must be explored because of likely internal damage. Tetanus and introduction of marine bacterial infection are possible.

OCTOPUS BITE

At least six species of *Hapalochlaena*, the blue-ringed or blue-lined octopuses, are found around the coast of Australia.

Species also exist in the IndoPacific waters, including those surrounding Papua New Guinea, New Zealand, and southern Japan. These small creatures, rarely larger than 20 cm from the tip of one arm to the tip of another, have characteristic dark brown or ochre bands over the body and arms with irregularly shaped blue circles, lines, and figures-of-eight superimposed. When the animal is disturbed, these markings become brilliant, iridescent, peacock blue. The saliva of three species—*H. lunulata*, *H. fasciata*, and *H. maculosa*—is highly venomous and is delivered when the octopus bites. Although the active toxin in saliva was originally named *maculotoxin*, it is in fact, *tetrodotoxin* (TTX) (35). It produces flaccid paralysis by reversibly blocking neuronal sodium channels. Other components in the saliva are phenolic amines and a hyaluronidase.

Envenomation

Most bites occur when an octopus is brought into contact with human skin. Fatalities and near- fatalities follow a fairly similar pattern: the octopus, having been found in a rock pool, is caught and placed usually on the back of the hand or arm of a victim while being shown to interested parties. The victim is generally unaware of any actual bite, but symptoms of envenomation occur within 5 or 10 mins and commence with weakness and numbness about the face and neck, combined with difficulty in breathing and nausea. Vomiting often occurs. In severe cases, a state of complete flaccid paralysis and apnea may progress rapidly. Cardiac function remains unaltered until hypoxemia occurs.

Treatment

No specific therapy is available. The pressure-immobilization method of first aid should be applied immediately to the bitten area, if accessible. Rescue breathing followed by mechanical ventilation must be instituted and continued until recovery, usually after several hours. From a clinical viewpoint, the syndrome of envenomation differs from tetrodotoxic fish poisoning only because of the route of absorption of the toxin: after an effective bite by *Hapalochlaena* spp., death could occur within 30 mins due to the sudden onset of a flaccid paralysis, but ingestion of tetrodotoxic fish flesh may lead to vomiting, severe abdominal pain, and the onset of paralysis over several hours.

CONE SNAIL STING

Cone snails are mollusks that inhabit conical-shaped shells, prized by collectors. They fire a venom-laden miniature harpoon to rapidly paralyze prey such as fish. They inhabit the floor of tropical and subtropical seas. Venoms contain numerous small proteins that target voltage-sensitive sodium, calcium, potassium, N-methyl-D-aspartate (NMDA)-glutamate, and nicotinic acetylcholine receptor channels. These conotoxins cause rapid disruption of neuronal transmission, neurotransmitter release (particularly acetylcholine), and neuroreceptor activation. Several ω-conotoxins, including MVIIA and CVID, which are selective N-type calcium channel inhibitors, are antinociceptive, and at least one is commercially available for the treatment of chronic pain.

Treatment

The unwary human who handles a live cone shell is at risk of serious illness or death, although deaths have been few. A sharp, stinging pain is followed by local numbness or paresthesia. In serious envenomation, weakness and incoordination of voluntary muscles occurs rapidly and is accompanied by vision, swallowing, and speech disturbances. Respiratory failure due to paresis or paralysis may eventuate. The only specific management is mechanical ventilation. Spontaneous recovery of full neuromuscular function may take days to weeks.

FISH THAT ARE POISONOUS TO EAT

Fish that are poisonous to eat contain a variety of toxins, including TTX, ciguatoxin (CTX), maitotoxin, and histamine, among others. The toxins, produced by bacteria or *dinoflagellates*, accumulate in the flesh or contaminate the flesh in fish being prepared for consumption. Filter-feeding shellfish also accumulate toxins produced by dinoflagellates, namely saxitoxins, okadaic acid, domoic acid, and brevetoxins.

Tetrodotoxin Poisoning

Hundreds of species of tetrodotoxic fish exist in sea waters. Characteristic features are absence of scales, large eyes, and teeth arranged as four plates (tetraodontiformes). Many have spikes, and most, when threatened, inflate themselves into spheres, using either air or water, and thus have common names such as puffer fish, toad fish, globe fish, toado, swell fish, and balloon fish. TTX is concentrated in the fish liver, ovaries, intestine, and skin but easily contaminates flesh being prepared for consumption. In Japan, the flesh of selected toad fish, fugu, is a culinary delight, as traces of TTX produce a pleasant tingling gustatory sensation.

Tetrodotoxin

TTX, one of the most potent toxins known, was originally extracted from the eggs of puffer fish. The most important effects are upon nerve fibers, where blockage of excitability occurs and causes flaccid paralysis. Because of the unique action of TTX as a sodium channel blockade, it has been extensively studied by neurophysiologists. Passage of action potentials along nerves is prevented by selective inhibition of the sodium-carrying mechanism, while the movement of potassium is not disturbed. The effect is selective for some sodium channels, not sodium ion. This nerve-blocking potential is greatest in peripheral nerves, affecting sensory and autonomic nerve fibers. Skeletal and smooth muscle and, to a lesser extent, cardiac muscle have their excitability reduced by TTX. The central effects are depression of spinal reflex pathways, induction of vomiting, and hypothermia. Hypoventilation is due to paralysis of peripheral nerves, while hypotension is due to blockade of vasomotor nerves and direct suppression of vascular smooth muscle, causing vasodilation. The medullary vasomotor and respiratory centers are not affected. Myocardial cells are relatively insensitive to TTX.

TTX has been isolated from the skin of Central American frogs of the genus *Atelopus*, from skin glands of the Californian newt of the genus *Taricha*, from the posterior salivary glands of the blue-ringed octopus, *Hapalochlaena maculosa*, from the Pacific goby fish, from certain flatworms, and from a variety of other creatures, including starfish and crabs. This widespread distribution has yet to be satisfactorily explained, but the toxin may be produced by bacteria present in these species (42).

Poisoning

Signs and symptoms of poisoning develop within 10–45 mins of consumption. Most victims have some nausea, but vomiting is uncommon. Mildly poisoned victims usually experience only "tingling" sensations, but the severely poisoned rapidly develop serious illness. Consciousness may remain unimpaired until near death; those who survive a near-fatal episode may recall careless comments made by relatives or hospital staff. Poisoning is classified into four grades:

- Grade 1: Perioral numbness with or without gastrointestinal symptoms
- Grade 2: Numbness of tongue, face, and other areas of skin; early motor paralysis and incoordination; slurred speech and ataxia, but peripheral reflexes intact
- Grade 3: Widespread paralysis, dyspnea, dysphonia, and hypotension, but consciousness retained
- Grade 4: Severe hypoxia, near-complete paralysis, and hypotension; death due to rapid respiratory failure

Differential Diagnosis

The diagnosis is usually straightforward, especially when a number of individuals have shared a meal. Although puffer fish are not ciguatoxic fish, the illness ciguatera may present in a similar fashion but later, usually 2–12 hrs after consumption of fish easily identified as not puffer fish. The ciguatera sufferer usually has reversed sensations; in particular, hot objects feel cold and vice versa, whereas this phenomenon is absent in tetrodotoxic poisoning.

Treatment

Apart from gastric lavage, TTX poisoning has no antidote or specific treatment; treatment is supportive. Vomiting should be induced, provided that the victim has no difficulty in swallowing or protection of the airway. If aspiration is possible, gastric lavage should be performed after endotracheal intubation. If symptoms are confined to paresthesias and mild weakness without hypoventilation, light sedation with a benzodiazepine or other sedative for anxious patients may be desirable, and close observation must be maintained until symptoms recede. If dysphagia is present, oral intake must be suspended and IV infusion started to maintain hydration and prevent hypotension.

Any difficulty in dealing with saliva or respiratory secretions is an indication for endotracheal intubation, as is increasing dyspnea, rising respiratory rate, or progressive hypercapnia. The short, natural course of intoxication makes tracheostomy unnecessary. As these patients are conscious (unless acutely hypoxic), adequate sedation is required, with full anesthesia for intubation.

Fluid administration should be regulated according to hemodynamic parameters. As TTX causes vasodilatation and cardiac depression in severe toxicity, plasma volume replacement is necessary, along with an inotropic agent. Atropine may be ineffective in preventing bradycardia, which may respond to isoproterenol or epinephrine. Complete atrioventricular dissociation may require temporary pacemaker insertion.

Anticholinesterases. Although anticholinesterases have been administered many times to victims of poisoning with varied responses, neither theoretical grounds nor convincing experimental evidence explain why such drugs should be beneficial, as the toxin causes paralysis not by an action at the neuromuscular junctions but on motor axons and on muscle membranes. Anticholinesterases are not recommended but, if administered, should be given in conjunction with an antimuscarinic agent to prevent bradycardia.

Laboratory Investigations

Although Japanese scientists have used mouse bioassay and various gas and liquid chromatography techniques to analyze gastric and intestinal contents of victims, these are not generally available.

Ciguatera

Ciguatera is a polymorphic illness contracted from consumption of fish that are contaminated with CTXs. Gastrointestinal and neurologic effects predominate. The name ciguatera is derived from "cigua," Spanish for a small Caribbean snail that is poisonous to eat.

Toxin is passed up the food chain, reaching high concentration in the flesh of the larger carnivorous fish, such as Spanish mackerel (*Scomberomorus commersoni*). The toxin is generated in a dinoflagellate, *Gambierdiscus toxicus*, present in the benthic biodendritus and named after the Gambier Islands in French Polynesia, where it was discovered. It is tasteless and is not destroyed by cooking. Some evidence suggests that certain cyanobacteria produce toxins with effects similar to those of ciguateric fish, with the implication that such bacteria are the origin of CTXs (42). CTXs are potent ichthyotoxins, which may explain why human fatality is low; i.e., only mildly affected fish survive to be caught and consumed.

Ciguatera occurs in all tropical and subtropical sea waters up to 30° latitude. However, because of international and interstate commerce and tourism, the illness may occur virtually anywhere outside endemic areas. At least 400 species of tropical shore fish have been known to produce ciguatera. The numbers of the dinoflagellate increase dramatically after damage to coral reefs, either by natural phenomena or activities by man, such as jetty construction.

Ciguatoxins

CTXs are a group of lipophilic polycyclic ethers (24) that bind to site 5 of the voltage-sensitive sodium channel, thereby increasing sodium permeability and triggering acetylcholine and norepinephrine release, increased excitability in sensory neurons, and potentiation of effects of norepinephrine on smooth muscle. Neuronal excitability is also increased by blockage of voltage-gated potassium channels. Nerve excitability in many parts of the autonomic nervous system alters visceral and thermoregulatory responses and causes smooth muscle contraction.

Experimentally, CTXs cause diarrhea, increased peristalsis (treated with atropine), and increased mucus secretion. Also experimentally, CTXs in low concentrations cause transient positive inotropy, which can be blocked with atropine and α- and β-adrenergic antagonists. In high concentrations, CTXs cause negative inotropy, which can be reversed with lidocaine. Repeated doses of CTXs cause cardiac necrosis, interstitial fibrosis, and bilateral ventricular hypertrophy. Arrhythmias, including bradycardia, atrioventricular conduction disturbances, and transient hypertension, precedes terminal hypotension and cardiac failure. Death in unventilated experimental animals is due to respiratory depression and arrest.

Poisoning

Although this polymorphic illness has many variations, a typical case involves gastroenteritic symptoms for 1 or 2 days, weakness, myalgia and arthralgia for several days to a week, and paresthesias for several days to several weeks.

The most common symptoms among 20,000 cases in French Polynesia (3) were grouped into four main categories: neurologic, digestive, cardiovascular, and generalized. From these, paresthesia, arthralgia, myalgia, vertigo, ataxia, diarrhea, vomiting, nausea, bradycardia, hypotension, pruritus, and asthenia account for the most frequent or typical signs and symptoms, with an incidence of 15% to 90% in victims. Approximately 77% of patients developed symptoms within 12 hrs of ingestion of fish. The recovery period varied from several days to months. The fatality rate was <1%, with death occurring from cardiac rather than respiratory failure, but the latter has occurred secondary to prolonged central neurologic depression. The paresthesias, numbness, and tingling are more often circumoral but may also involve the extremities. Other symptoms described include lacrimation, salivation, metallic taste, sweating, headache, neck stiffness, chills, shaking, dysuria, dyspnea, and abdominal pain.

Usually, the victim has no fever but shuns food and finds drinking water to be painful; indeed, some 25% of affected patients complain of painful or loose teeth in their sockets. An erythematous rash is common, and sometimes general desquamation occurs. By 10 hrs after the meal, the acute symptoms have subsided. The patient is left weak and exhausted and still suffering from tingling and numbness, which may last for 7 days or longer.

Some of the features of ciguatera poisoning are quite characteristic. Inability to discriminate temperatures and reversal of temperature perception (dysesthesia) are diagnostic. Victims often notice burning or pain on their skin when exposed to cold water. Often, hot objects feel cold and vice versa. Such persons must take great care not to scald themselves when bathing. The paradoxical reversal of temperature sensation, commonly described in ciguatera poisoning, is considered to be the result of an exaggerated and intense nerve depolarization in peripheral small A-delta myelinated and in C-polymodal nociceptor fibers. Ciguatoxin-1 depolarizes and contracts arterial smooth muscle. In New Caledonia, the illness is called "*la gratte*" or "the itch." Pruritus and paresthesia may involve the soles of the feet and palms of the hands.

Recovery occurs within 48 hrs to 7 days in mild cases but takes several weeks for severe cases. Sometimes, sensitivity to any kind of fish develops, and in other cases, vague tingling sensations, pruritus, and even ataxia may persist for years. In cases of death, these symptoms may occur after 10 mins, but they usually occur after several days. Should the patient survive a very severe poisoning, it may be a year or more before full recovery.

Differential Diagnosis. Sometimes the toxic fish is transported and eaten far from its place of origin and poses a diagnostic challenge for clinicians unless they make a connection with fish consumption. TTX poisoning is easily distinguished from ciguatera, and bacterial contamination of seafood will produce a very rapid onset of gastrointestinal symptoms without peripheral neurologic effects.

Treatment

This poison has no specific treatment or antidote. Patients with marked gastrointestinal fluid loss will require parenteral fluid and electrolyte replacement. Patients with severe cases may need endotracheal intubation and mechanical ventilation. Generally, patients with milder cases need no special treatment other than attentive nursing. Sedation is usually required, and opiates may be necessary.

Numerous drugs have been tried with limited success in the treatment of ciguatera poisoning. Among these are mannitol (*vide infra*), corticosteroids, analgesics, tricyclic antidepressants, antihistamines, calcium gluconate, atropine, phentolamine, pralidoxime, nifedipine, tiapride, and vitamins B_6 and B_{12}. No blinded controlled study of any drug, including mannitol, has been published. Gastric lavage would not be helpful (and possibly dangerous) unless the victim presented with severe signs soon (within 1 hr) after poisoning. The efficacy of activated charcoal is unknown, but in that appearance of symptoms is usually delayed at least several hours, it is unlikely to be helpful.

Mannitol. IV mannitol has been extolled as an effective treatment, but convincing clinical evidence of its efficacy has yet to be provided. Improvement in 24 patients was reported within minutes of treatment (30). The most notable improvements were in neurologic symptoms and muscular dysfunction, whereas gastrointestinal symptoms disappeared more slowly. Recovery of 2 patients in coma was described: "One patient stood up and asked for orientation within 10 mins after mannitol therapy was started; the other patient, though confused, sat up after 5 mins." Numerous other reports of case series have been published (42); although all are suggestive of benefit, none are definitely conclusive. A randomized, unblinded trial compared mannitol to the standard treatment, which included calcium with vitamins and glucose, in selected patients (4). In that study, the mannitol group had significant reductions of paresthesia and gastrointestinal effects after 1 hr but no further improvement after 24 hrs. No improvements occurred in the other effects of ciguatoxicity in the mannitol-treated group. The efficacy of mannitol has been investigated in laboratory studies, with mixed results (42).

Laboratory Investigations

Numerous methods of detecting CTX have been developed but none are readily available and all involve specialized laboratories in regional centers. The mouse bioassay is the most widely used.

Maitotoxin Poisoning

Maitotoxins are water-soluble polyether toxins that are distinct from CTXs but also associated with the marine unicellular dinoflagellate *Gambierdiscus toxicus*. First recognized in the gut of the "maito," the surgeonfish *Ctenochaetus striatus*, they probably contribute to the constellation of symptoms, particularly gastrointestinal, in ciguatera. Many of the in vitro effects of maitotoxin are prevented by calcium channel blockers such as verapamil.

Treatment

No specific treatment exists. In that maitotoxicity is a possible contributory component of ciguatera, the same treatment may be appropriate, with the possible consideration of calcium channel blockade.

Scombroid Poisoning

Scombroid poisoning occurs worldwide when scombroid fish, such as tuna or mackerel or other large oceanic fish, become contaminated with enteric bacteria. The toxin responsible is histamine converted from histidine in the flesh by bacteria. Large amounts of histamine may develop in dead fish if they are not promptly frozen or if they are allowed to thaw too long before they are cooked, as cooking does not destroy histamine. The illness may also be contracted from canned or smoked fish.

The contaminated fish is not putrefied and looks and smells normal, but a sharp or peppery taste is sometimes noted. *Proteus morgani* is the only bacterial species able to produce histamine in high enough concentrations to cause human poisoning. Other substances present in spoiled fish may enhance the activity of histamine, facilitate its absorption, or inhibit its inactivation, as histamine is degraded in human intestines and the illness cannot be mimicked by ingestion of histamine.

Scombroid poisoning should be differentiated from "seafood allergy" and bacterial food poisoning by careful history elucidation. Typical symptoms in order of frequency are diarrhea, hot flushing or sweating, bright erythematous rash, nausea and vomiting, headache, abdominal pain, palpitations, burning in the mouth, fever, and dizziness. Facial edema is sometimes present and respiratory distress may occur. Occasionally, cardiac arrhythmias or hypotension occur. Onset of illness is usually within 30 mins of fish ingestion and lasts only 8–12 hrs but is sometimes prolonged. The illness occurs worldwide and has been stated as the most significant cause of illness associated with seafood in the US and the most frequent in Canada.

Treatment

Mild poisoning, restricted to rash, flushing, sweating, tachycardia, palpitations, and headache, may require a parenteral antihistamine (H_1 and H_2 antagonists). Moderate poisoning with gastrointestinal symptoms may require IV fluid replacement. Severe poisoning with bronchospasm, hypotension, or airway obstruction may require epinephrine (parenteral or inhaled), bronchodilator, and airway protection. No deaths have been reported.

Laboratory Investigations

Contaminated fish contain large amounts of histamine, while histamine and its metabolite N-methylhistamine, are excreted in the urine in high concentrations for approximately 24 hrs after poisoning.

Shellfish Poisoning

Certain species of dinoflagellates (microalgae, plankton) produce toxins that are ingested by filter feeding bivalve mollusks (e.g., mussels, clams, oysters, scallops, and cockles) that, in turn, may be ingested by crabs and lobsters. Life-threatening illnesses may result from ingesting the mollusks or other creatures that ingest them, with the most serious being paralytic shellfish poisoning and diarrhetic shellfish poisoning. The toxins are not destroyed by cooking.

Paralytic Shellfish (Saxitoxin) Poisoning

Toxins. A group of toxins, paralytic shellfish poisons, or saxitoxins, named after the butter clam *Saxidomus gigantea* from which the first saxitoxin was isolated, block sodium channels in a manner similar to, but not identical to, structurally unrelated TTX. Tissues that are affected are neural, cardiac, skeletal muscle, and vascular smooth muscle. Human poisoning has been caused by a few species of the dinoflagellates that are members of the plankton genera *Alexandrium*, *Pyrodinium* and *Prorocentrum*. Members of these genera bloom sporadically, creating "red tides" in sea or fresh waters. At such times, mollusks become heavily contaminated. Outbreaks of shellfish poisoning have occurred in many parts of the world. The toxins are also produced by organisms other than dinoflagellates, including numerous cyanobacteria (blue-green) algae which injure animals when overgrowth (a bloom) occurs.

Poisoning. Neurologic, respiratory, and cardiovascular symptoms usually develop within 30 mins. Experimentally, saxitoxin causes a rapid onset of respiratory and cardiovascular failure. The toxin is excreted by glomerular filtration.

Treatment. Only supportive treatment is available, including airway protection, mechanical ventilation, and inotropic support. From animal studies of saxitoxin poisoning and its treatment, 4-aminopyridine holds promise. This drug selectively blocks potassium channels in excitable membranes, facilitates neurotransmitter release at synapses, and has reversed saxitoxin-induced cardiorespiratory collapse.

Laboratory Investigations. Although numerous assays for saxitoxin and its derivatives have been devised, none may be performed rapidly or easily.

Diarrhetic Shellfish (Okadaic Acid) Poisoning

Diarrhetic shellfish poisoning is characterized by gastroenteritis after ingestion of shellfish, in particular mussels that have fed on marine dinoflagellates (plankton) of the genera *Dinophysis* and *Prorocentrum*, which manufacture the polyether okadaic acid and its numerous derivatives. Symptoms of nausea, vomiting, diarrhea, abdominal pain, and fever occur within 30 mins and last more than 8 hrs. This poisoning has is no specific treatment.

Amnestic Shellfish (Domoic Acid) Poisoning

Amnestic shellfish poisoning is characterized by acute gastrointestinal symptoms and unusual neurologic abnormalities in people who have eaten mussels. Severely poisoned patients have experienced hemiparesis, seizures, hypotension, ophthalmoplegia, abnormalities of arousal ranging from agitation to coma, and residual severe anterograde memory deficits. The agent responsible is domoic acid, an analog of the neuroexcitatory transmitter glutamic acid, which is produced by blooms of species of the diatom genus *Pseudo-nitzschia* and in clams and crabs. No specific treatment is available.

Brevetoxin Poisoning

Brevetoxins are a family of polyethers that is similar to CTXs is associated with "red tide" algal blooms, particularly with the dinoflagellate *Ptychodiscus brevis*. They accumulate in filter-feeding shellfish such as oysters. Like CTXs, they bind to site 5 of voltage-sensitive sodium channels.

Brevetoxins induce release of acetylcholine and catecholamines from central and peripheral neuronal sites and possible acetylcholine from neuromuscular junctions. Experimentally, initial effects include bradycardia, hypotension, and bradypnea, followed by hypertension, tachycardia, cardiac arrhythmias, and respiratory arrest. Ventilated animals succumb to cardiovascular collapse. Interestingly, neurotoxicity is prevented by co-application of NMDA receptor antagonists, such as ketamine, dextromethorphan, and dextrorphan. No specific treatment is available.

CONCLUSIONS AND FUTURE DIRECTIONS

Syndromes that result from envenomation by terrestrial and marine creatures often necessitate invasive treatment and monitoring, particularly of cardiac and respiratory function. Although the toxins of some creatures and features of their envenomation syndromes are relatively well known (e.g., of some snake and spider bites), the nature of the toxins and envenomation syndromes that result, for example, from scorpion and jellyfish envenomation remain obscure. Many of these areas deserve basic scientific and clinical research.

In addition to general therapy, numerous syndromes require specific therapy that can only be anticipated from knowledge of the effects of the toxins and poisons involved. Effective first aid also constitutes an important part of the management of some envenomations, such as those from elapid snake and funnel-web spider bites; in these instances, first aid should not be neglected when the victim arrives in hospital, as it serves to limit the amount of venom that reaches the circulation of a victim. In several syndromes, antivenom therapy is the key to successful treatment and good outcome. Unfortunately, antivenoms for the toxins of many creatures do not exist, while some manufacturers of snake antivenoms around the world are ceasing or scaling back production because of lack of profitability.

KEY POINTS

- Snakebite causes most mortality attributed to envenomation, particularly in developing countries. The main snake species belong to families of Elapidae and Viperidae. Snake venoms cause neurotoxic, myotoxic, procoagulopathic and anticoagulopathic, cytotoxic, and hemolytic effects.

- Snakebite is not always accompanied by envenomation, but its management includes first aid that consists of pressure-immobilization bandaging of the bitten limb (for neurotoxic elapid bites), resuscitation, appropriate antivenom therapy, and treatment of systemic effects of venom. Hypoxemia, hypotension, rhabdomyolysis, and DIC may combine to cause renal failure, for which support may be needed. Antivenom administration should be preceded by the administration of subcutaneous adrenaline to prevent and ameliorate adverse reactions.

- Bites by spiders are very common, but only a few species of spider threaten life. These include bites by Australian funnel-web spiders; they cause muscle fasciculation followed by weakness and respiratory failure, which along with bronchorrhea, is due to acetylcholine release. Hypertension and coma occur secondary to catecholamine release, which later culminates in heart failure, hypotension, and pulmonary edema. An antivenom is available and pressure-immobilization bandaging of the bite site is an effective first aid technique.

- Globally, bites by comb-footed spiders, such as the Australian red-back spider and the North American widow spider (genus *Latrodectus*), are the most important. They cause severe pain, inflammatory signs, and hypertension. Antivenoms are available in several countries.

- Bites by some North and South American recluse spiders may cause dermatonecrotic lesions alone or in combination with gastrointestinal illness, coagulopathy, hemolysis, and sometimes rhabdomyolysis, with subsequent renal failure. Antivenoms are available.

- Scorpion stings may threaten life in India, Africa, Brazil, Mexico, and the southern American states. All cause severe pain and, depending on the species, life-threatening cardiovascular effects and a wide range of neurotoxicity. The efficacy of antivenoms is debatable, but judicious vasodilator and inotropic therapy, along with mechanical ventilation, may be required.

- Bee and wasp stings worldwide and some ant stings may cause life-threatening anaphylaxis. Envenomation syndromes may occasionally be encountered with multiple stings. Prominent bee species are the common honeybee (*Apis mellifera*) and wasps of the genera *Vespa, Vespula, Provespa,* and *Polistes*. Prominent ants are the Australian *Myrmecia* species (jumping jack and bull-ants) and the American *Solenopsis* spp. (fire ants). Treatment is as for anaphylaxis.

- Tick bite may cause allergy and zoonosis, especially rickettsial diseases, Lyme disease, viral encephalitis, and hemorrhagic fever. Species that cause paralysis in North America are of the genera *Dermacentor, Amblyomma,* and *Ixodes*; in South Africa, *Argas*; and in Australia, *Ixodes*. The onset of flaccid paralysis is slow. Mechanical ventilation may be required until spontaneous recovery after tick removal.

- Although many species of jellyfish cause painful stings, few threaten life. Most deaths from jellyfish stings have been due to the chirodropid (jellyfish with many tentacles arising from corners of a bell) Australian box jellyfish (*Chironex fleckeri*), whose stings cause rapid cardiorespiratory failure by unknown mechanisms. An antivenom is available.

■ Similar chirodropid jellyfish inhabit the IndoPacific region. Of the carybdeid jellyfish (single tentacles arising from corners of a bell), the Hawaiian box jellyfish (*Carybdea alata*), Australian jimble (*Carybdeid rastoni*), and irukandji (*Carukia barnesi*) cause significant pain, and stings by the latter may be accompanied by hypertension and late cardiac failure. Treatment includes pain relief, oxygen therapy, diuretics, vasodilators, inotropic support, mechanical ventilation or application of continuous positive airway pressure, and possible antihypertensive therapy.

■ Although stings by *Physalia* spp. (Portuguese man-of-war, bluebottle) are the most frequent worldwide, few deaths have been recorded.

■ Numerous fish have spines that inject venom when they are handled or trodden upon, causing very painful lesions. The most prominent are species of the genus *Synanceia* (stonefish), which inhabit the IndoPacific region. An antivenom is available. Occasionally, the barbs of stingrays cause severe penetrating chest trauma.

■ Several species of Australian *Hapalochlaena* (blue-ringed) octopuses inject TTX, which causes the rapid onset of flaccid paralysis, necessitating mechanical ventilation for several hours.

■ Some mollusc cone snails fire a venom-laden mini-harpoon, which bears protein toxins that cause rapid paralysis.

■ Some fish are poisonous to eat, including numerous worldwide tetrodotoxic species (order Tetraodontiformes) that cause paralysis. Tropical and subtropical species cause ciguatera, an acute gastrointestinal illness that is accompanied by a polymorphic long-lasting neurologic illness for which mannitol may be effective. Scombroid poisoning is due to consumption of fish that are contaminated by bacteria that manufacture histamine, which causes flushing, tachycardia, hypotension, and bronchospasm. Consumption of some shellfish may cause toxin-related paralysis or gastrointestinal illness.

References

1. Abroug F, El Atrous S, Nouira S, et al. Serotherapy in scorpion envenomation: A randomised controlled trial. *Lancet* 1999;354:906–9.
2. Amitai Y. Scorpions, In: Brent J, Wallace KL, Burkhart KK, et al., eds. *Critical Care Toxicology.* Philadelphia: Elsevier Mosby; 2005:1213–20.
3. Bagnis RA. Clinical features on 19,890 cases of ciguatera (fish poisoning) in French Polynesia. *Toxicon.* 1987;26:16.
4. Bagnis R, Spiegel A, Boutin JP, et al. Evaluation of the efficacy of mannitol in the treatment of ciguatera in French Polynesia. *Medicale Tropicale.* 1992;52:67–73.
5. Bahloul M, Chaari A, Khlaf-Bouaziz N, et al. Gastrointestinal manifestations in severe scorpion envenomation. *Gastroenterol Clin Biol.* 2005;29:1001–5.
6. Bailey PM, Bakker AJ, Seymour JE, et al. A functional comparison of the venom of three Australian jellyfish—*Chironex fleckeri, Chiropsalmus* sp., and *Carybdea xaymacana*— on cytosolic Ca^{2+}, haemolysis and *Artemia* sp. lethality. *Toxicon* 2005;45:233–42.
7. Cheng AC, Currie BJ. Venomous snakebites worldwide with a focus on the Australia-Pacific region: Current management and controversies. *J Intensive Care Med.* 2004;19:259–69.
8. Chippaux JP. Snake-bites: Appraisal of the global situation. *Bull World Health Organ.* 1998;76:515–24.
9. Corkeron M, Pereira P, Makrocanis C. Early experience with magnesium administration in Irukandji syndrome. *Anaesth Intens Care.* 2004;32, 666–9.
10. Dart RC, McNally J. Efficacy, safety, and use of snake antivenoms in the United States. *Ann Emerg Med.* 2001;37:181–8.
11. Dworkin MS, Shoemaker PC, Anderson DE. Tick paralysis: 33 human cases in Washington State. *Clin Infect Dis.* 1999;29:1435–9.
12. Edwards L, Luo E, Hall R, et al. The effect of Portuguese man-of-war (*Physalia physalis*) venom on calcium, sodium and potassium fluxes of cultured embryonic chick heart cells. *Toxicon* 2000;38:323–35.
13. Elatrous S, Nouira S, Besbes-Ouanes L, et al. Dobutamine in severe scorpion envenomation: Effects on standard hemodynamics, right ventricular performance, and tissue oxygenation. *Chest* 1999;116:748–53.
14. Fan HW, Marcopito LF, Cardoso JL, et al. Sequential randomized and double-blind trial of promethazine prophylaxis against early anaphylactic reactions to antivenom for Bothrops snake bites. *BMJ.* 1999;318:1451–2.
15. Golden DB. Insect allergy in children. *Curr Opin Allergy Clin Immunol* 2006;6:289–93.
16. Grattan-Smith PJ, Morris JG, Johnston HM, et al. Clinical and neurophysiological features of tick paralysis. *Brain* 1997;120:1975–87.
17. Hogan C, Barbaro KC, Winkel KD. Loxoscelism: Old obstacles, new directions. *Ann Emerg Med* 2004;44:608–624.
18. Levick NR, Schmidt JO, Harrison J, et al. Bee and wasp sting injuries in Australia and the USA: Is it a bee or is it a wasp and why should we care? In: Austin AD, Dowton M, eds. *The Hymenoptera: Evolution, Biodiversity and Biological Control.* Canberra: CSIRO Publishing, 2000.
19. Little M, Pereira P, Mulcahy R, et al. Severe cardiac failure associated with presumed jellyfish sting. Irukandji syndrome? *Anaesth Intens Care.* 2003;31:642–7.
20. M'barak S, Fajloun Z, Cestele S, et al. First chemical synthesis of a scorpion alpha-toxin affecting sodium channels: The Aah I toxin of *Androctonus australis hector. J Pept Sc.* 2004;10:666–77.
21. McGain F, Winkel KD. Ant sting mortality in Australia. *Toxicon* 2002;40:1095–100.
22. Meki AR, Mohamed ZM, Mohey El-deen HM. Significance of assessment of serum cardiac troponin I and interleukin-8 in scorpion envenomed children. *Toxicon* 2003;41:129–37.
23. Merten HA, Durden LA. A state-by-state survey of ticks recorded from humans in the United States. *J Vector Ecol* 2000;25:102–13.
24. Murata M, Legrand AM, Ishibashi Y, et al. Structures and configurations of ciguatoxin from moray eel *Gymnothorax javanicus* and its likely precursor from the dinoflagellate *Gambierdiscus toxicus. J Am Chem Soc.* 1990;112:4380–4386.
25. Nimorakiotakis B, Winkel KD. Spider bite. Part 1: Spider bite: The redback spider and its relatives. *Aust Fam Physician.* 2004;33:153–7.
26. Nimorakiotakis B, Winkel KD. Spider bite. Part 2: Funnel web and common spider bites. *Aust Fam Physician.* 2004;33:244–51.
27. Nomura JT, Sato RL, Ahern RM, et al. A randomised paired comparison trial of cutaneous treatments for acute jellyfish (*Carybdea alata*) stings. *Am J Emerg Med.* 2002;20:624–6.
28. Norris RL, Bush SP. North American venomous reptile bites. In: Auerbach PS, ed. *Wilderness Medicine,* 4th ed. St. Louis: Mosby, 2001:896–926.
29. Nunan EA, Moraes MF, Cardoso VN, et al. Effect of age on body distribution of tityustoxin from *Tityus serrulatus* scorpion venom in rats. *Life Sci.* 2003;73:319–25.
30. Palafox NA, Jain LG, Pinano AZ, et al. Successful treatment of ciguatera fish poisoning with intravenous mannitol. *JAMA.* 1988;259:2740–2.
31. Pe T, Mya S, Myint AA, et al. T. Field trial of efficacy of local compression immobilization first-aid technique in Russell's viper (*Daboia russelii siamensis*) bite patients. *Southeast Asian J Trop Med Public Health.* 2000;31:346–8.
32. Pearn J, Morrison J, Charles N, et al. First-aid for snakebite: Efficacy of a constrictive bandage with limb immobilization in the management of human envenomation. *Med J Aust.* 1981;2:293–5.
33. Premawardhena AP, de Silva CE, Fonseka MM, et al. Low-dose subcutaneous adrenaline to prevent acute adverse reactions to antivenom serum in people bitten by snakes: Randomised, placebo controlled trial. *BMJ* 1999;318:1041–3.
34. Ramasamy S, Isbister GK, Seymour JE, et al. The in vivo cardiovascular effects of box jellyfish *Chironex fleckeri* venom in rats: Efficacy of pretreatment with antivenom, verapamil and magnesium sulphate. *Toxicon* 2004;43:685–90.
35. Sheumack DD, Howden MEH, Spence I, et al. Maculotoxin: A neurotoxin from the venom glands of the octopus *Hapalochlaena maculosa* identified as tetrodotoxin. *Science* 1978;199:188–9.
36. Solley GO, Vanderwoude C, Knight GK. Anaphylaxis due to red imported fire ant. *Med J Aust* 2002;176:518–9.
37. Soulaymani-Bencheikh R, Soulaymani A, Semlali I, et al. Scorpion poisonous stings in the population of Khouribga. *Bull Soc Path Exot* 2005;98:36–40.
38. Sprivulis P, Jelinek GA, Marshall L. Efficacy and potency of antivenoms in neutralizing the procoagulant effects of Australian snake in dog and human plasma. *Anaesth Intens Care.* 1996;24:379–81.
39. Sutherland SK, Coulter AR. Early management of bites by the eastern diamond-back rattlesnake (*Crotalus adamanteus*): Studies in monkeys (*Macaca fascicularis*). *Am J Trop Med Hyg.* 1981;30:497–500.
40. Sutherland SK, Coulter AR, Harris RD. Rationalisation of first aid measures for elapid snakebite. *Lancet.* 1979;1:183–6.
41. Sutherland SK, Harris RD, Coulter AR, et al. First aid for cobra (*Naja naja*) bites. *Indian J Med Res.* 1981;73:266–8.
42. Sutherland SK, Tibballs J. *Australian Animal Toxins.* Melbourne: Oxford University Press, 2001.

43. Thurn M. *Tick toxinology: Isolation and characterisation of the toxin from the Australian Paralysis tick, Ixodes holocyclus.* PhD thesis, University of Technology, Sydney, 1994.
44. Tibballs J. Australian venomous jellyfish, envenomation syndromes, toxins and therapy. *Toxicon* 2006;48:830–859.
45. Tibballs J, Sutherland SK. The efficacy of antivenom in prevention of cardiovascular depression and coagulopathy induced by brown snake (*Pseudonaja*) species venom. *Anaesth Intens Care.* 1991;19:530–4.
46. Tun-Pe, Aye-Aye-Myint,Khin-Ei-Han, et al. Local compression pads as a first-aid measure for victims of bites by Russell's viper (*Daboia russelii siamensis*) in Myanmar. *Trans R Soc Trop Med Hyg.* 1995;89:293–5.
47. Warrell D. Treatment of bites by adders and exotic venomous snakes. *Br Med J.* 2006;331:1244–7.
48. Watt G, Theakston RD, Hayes CG, et al. Positive response to edrophonium in patients with neurotoxic envenoming by cobras (*Naja naja philippinensis*): A placebo-controlled study. *N Engl J Med.* 1986;315:1444–8.
49. Williamson JA, Fenner PJ, Burnett JW, et al. *Venomous & Poisonous Marine Animals: A Medical and Biological Handbook.* Sydney: New South Wales University Press, 1996.
50. Winkel KD, Tibballs J, Molenaar P, et al. The cardiovascular actions of the venom from the Irukandji (*Carukia barnesi*) jellyfish: Effects in human, rat and guinea pig tissues in vitro, and in pigs in vivo. *Clin Exp Pharmacol Physiol.* 2005;32:777–8.
51. Yoshimoto CM, Yanagihara AA. Cnidarian (coelenterate) envenomations in Hawai'i improve following heat application. *Trans Roy Soc Trop Med & Hyg.* 2002;96:300–3.

CHAPTER 34 ■ MECHANICAL VENTILATION

MARK J. HEULITT • GERHARD K. WOLF • JOHN H. ARNOLD

In simple terms, the lung-ventilator unit can be thought of as a tube with a balloon network on the end, with the tube representing the ventilator tubing, endotracheal tube (ETT), and airways and the balloon network representing the alveoli. During mechanical ventilation, the forces generated are a combination of effort provided by the patient's muscles during spontaneous breathing attempts and support derived from the ventilator. The movement of gas is determined by forces, displacements, and the rate of change of component displacements, which are distensible. To generate a volume displacement, the total forces have to overcome both the elastic and resistive elements of the lung and airway/chest wall. To generate gas flow, the total forces must overcome the resistive forces of the airway, the ventilator tubing, and the ETT to allow gas to flow into or out of the lung, depending on driving pressure gradients.

This discussion of mechanical ventilation will first focus on an understanding of how the patient's physiologic changes occur to generate these forces, both by intrinsic patient effort and from forces generated by ventilator output. How the ventilator controls the variables of flow, volume, and pressure to generate these forces and how these controllers interface with the patient will then be examined. Finally, the indications, settings, and modes of ventilatory support available to clinicians who care for infants and children will be discussed.

PHYSIOLOGY OF MECHANICAL VENTILATION

In physiology, force is measured as pressure $\left(pressure = \frac{force}{area}\right)$, displacement is measured as volume (volume = area × displacement), and the relevant rate of change is measured as flow (e.g., average flow $= \frac{\Delta volume}{\Delta time}$; instantaneous flow $= \frac{dv}{dt}$; where d represents the derivative of volume with respect to time). The key components in positive-pressure mechanical ventilation are the pressure necessary to cause a flow of gas to enter the airway and increase the volume of gas in the lungs. The volume of gas (ΔV) going to any lung unit (the balloons in our simplified example) and the gas flow ($\dot{V}$) may be related to the applied pressure (ΔP) by

$$\Delta P = \Delta V/C + \dot{V} \cdot R + k$$

where R is the airway resistance, C is the lung compliance and k is a constant that defines end-expiratory pressure.

The above equation is known as the *equation of motion* for the respiratory system. The sum of the muscle pressures and the ventilator pressure is the applied pressure to the respiratory system. The muscle pressure represents the pressure generated by the patient to expand the thoracic cage and lungs. Unfortunately, this force is not able to be measured directly. In contrast, the ventilator pressure is the transrespiratory pressure (from the mouth to the alveolar space) generated by the ventilator during inspiration. Combinations of these pressures are generated when a patient is breathing on a positive-pressure ventilator. For example, when respiratory muscles are at complete rest, the muscle pressure is zero; thus, the ventilator must generate all of the pressure necessary to deliver the tidal volume (VT) and inspiratory flow. The reverse is also true—when the patient is making some respiratory effort and generating muscle pressure, the degree of support that must be supplied by the ventilator is less. Multiple modes of ventilator support can be used to assist the patient in this circumstance. With the basic principle behind the equation of motion defined, it must be applied to the forces that must be overcome to generate gas flow. The total pressure applied to the respiratory system (P_{RS}) of a ventilated patient is the sum of the pressure generated by the ventilator (measured at the airway, P_{AO}) and the pressure developed by the respiratory muscles (P_{MUS}).

$$P_{RS} = P_{AO} + P_{MUS} = \frac{V}{C} + \dot{V} \times R + k$$

where:

$\dot{V} =$ flow
$R =$ airway resistance
$\frac{V}{C} =$ respiratory system compliance
$k =$ the constant that represents the measured alveolar end-expiratory pressure.

P_{AO} and $\dot{V}$ can be measured by the pressure and flow transducers in the ventilator. Volume is derived mathematically from the integration of the flow waveform.

To generate a volume displacement, the total forces have to overcome elastic and resistive elements of the lung and airway/chest wall, represented by V/C and $\dot{V} \times R$, respectively. V/C depends on both the volume insufflated in excess of resting volume and on respiratory system compliance. To generate a flow of gas, the total forces must overcome the resistive forces of the airway and the ETT against the driving pressure gradients. Given the physics principle that any action has an opposing reaction, at any moment during inspiration, a balance is maintained of forces attempting to expand the lung and the chest wall and those opposing lung and chest wall expansion. We commonly measure the result of these forces as the airway pressure (P_{AWO}). Opposing pressures to lung and chest wall expansion are the sum of elastic recoil pressure ($P_{elastic}$), flow resistive pressure ($P_{resistive}$), and inertance pressure ($P_{inertance}$) within the respiratory system. Thus:

$$P_{AWO} = P_{elastic} + P_{resistive} + P_{inertance}$$

Inertial forces relate to the energy required for initiation of gas movement and are usually negligible during conventional ventilation; thus, this component is commonly ignored. For conventional ventilation, the forces exemplified in the equation of motion can be expressed as:

$$P_{AWO} = P_{elastic} + P_{resistive}$$

If the elastic forces are the product of elastance and volume ($P_{elastic} = E \times V$), and resistive forces are the product of flow and resistance ($Resistive = \dot{V} \times R$), the formula can be written as:

$$P_{AWO} = (Elastance \times Volume) + (Resistance \times Flow)$$

Elastance is the inverse of compliance. If compliance is substituted for elastance in the equation, the equation of motion results:

$$P_{AWO} = \frac{Volume}{Compliance} + Resistance \times Flow$$

It is important to note that the quotient of volume displacement over compliance of the respiratory system represents the pressure necessary to overcome the elastic forces above the resting lung volume (known as the functional residual capacity, FRC). The FRC represents the quantity of air remaining in the lungs at the end of a spontaneous expiration. Pressure, volume, and flow are all measured relative to their baseline values. Thus, for a patient on a ventilator, the pressure necessary to cause inspiration is measured as the change in airway pressure above positive end-expiratory pressure (PEEP), representing the change from baseline pressure to peak inspiratory pressure. For example, in a patient breathing spontaneously on continuous positive-airway pressure (CPAP), the ventilator pressure is zero; thus, the patient must utilize respiratory muscles to generate all of the work of breathing (WOB) and the force necessary to expand the lungs and chest, to enable forward gas flow into the alveoli. The same principle can be applied to the volume generated during inspiration (known as the tidal volume), which is the change in volume in the lung during inspiration above FRC. The pressure necessary to overcome the resistive forces of the respiratory tract is the product of the maximum airway resistance (R_{max}) and the inspiratory flow. Flow is measured relative to its end-expiratory value and is usually zero at the beginning of an inspiratory effort, unless an intrinsic PEEP ($PEEP_i$) is present. In this circumstance, flow may still be occurring within the lung as alveoli attempt to achieve their baseline state—that is, due to time-constant differences, overfilled alveoli may be emptying into underfilled alveoli to help both to achieve their "best" resting volume. This effect is known as *pendelluft*. When $PEEP_i$ is present, it will take more "effort" from the patient and the ventilator to generate enough flow to move gas into the lung.

At this point in the discussion of mechanical ventilators, those factors that are directly clinician-controlled must be differentiated from those that occur indirectly. For example, pressure, volume, and flow are directly controlled variables, while other important factors such as resistance and compliance are dependent upon the resistive and elastic properties of the respiratory system and cannot be directly controlled.

VENTILATOR CONTROLLERS

Each ventilator is essentially a controller of pressure, volume, or flow in the equation of motion. The manner in which each variable is controlled, described as the *mode of ventilation*, determines how the ventilator delivers the mechanical breath. In the equation of motion, the form of any of the variables (pressure, volume, and flow are expressed as functions of time) can be predetermined. This principle serves as the theoretical basis for classifying ventilators as *pressure, volume,* or *flow* controllers (**Fig. 34.1**). The necessary and sufficient criteria for determining which variable is controlled are listed in **Table 34.1**. It is important to recognize that any ventilator can only directly control one variable—pressure, volume, or flow—at a time. Thus, a ventilator is simply a technology that controls the airway pressure waveform, the inspired volume waveform, or the inspiratory flow waveform, and pressure, volume, and flow are referred to in this context as *control variables*.

Most clinicians think of ventilators in terms of modes of ventilation. However, the mode of ventilation is meant to be a description of the way in which a mechanical breath is delivered. The determinants of how a mechanical breath is delivered are summarized not only in the control variables, but also in the phase and conditional variables (**Fig. 34.1**). Again, control variables are the independent variables that are either pressure, volume, or flow. *Conditional* variables are determinants of a response to a preset threshold, which are both clinician set and influenced by dependent and independent variables. Phase variables are those that are used to start, sustain, and end the

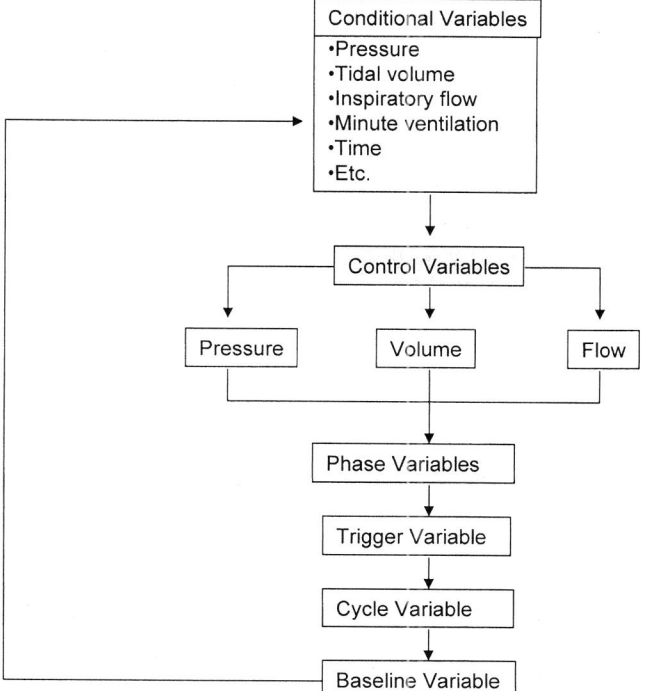

FIGURE 34.1. Flow chart to emphasize that each breath may have a different set of control and phase variables, depending upon the mode of ventilation. From Chatburn RL. Classification of mechanical ventilators. *Respir Care.* 1992;37:1009–25, with permission.

TABLE 34.1

VENTILATOR CONTROLLERS

Flow controller (constant flow controller)	Pressure controller (constant pressure controller)	Volume controller (variable flow controller)
Modes VC, SIMV-VC **Equation** $$Flow = \frac{Pressure}{Resistance}$$	**Modes** PC, SIMV-PC, PRVC **Equation** $$Flow = \frac{Volume}{Compliance}$$ $Pressure = Resistance \times Flow$	**Modes** VC **Equation** $Flow = Pressure \times Compliance$
Independent variables Flow *Dependent variables* Pressure	*Independent variables* Pressure *Dependent variables* Volume Flow	*Independent variables* Volume *Dependent variables* Pressure
Limiting variables Volume *Trigger variables* Time Pressure Flow	*Limiting variables* Pressure *Trigger variables* Time Pressure Flow	*Limiting variables* Volume *Trigger variables* Time Pressure Flow

VC, volume control; SIMV-VC, synchronized, intermittent mandatory ventilation-volume control; PC, pressure control; SIMV-PC, synchronized, intermittent mandatory ventilation-pressure control; PRVC, pressure regulated volume control.

phase. During inspiration, the phase variables include the trigger variable (determines the start of inspiration), limit variable (determines what sustains inspiration), and cycle variable (determines the end of inspiration).

Control Variables

Control variables relate to the elastic and resistive forces that must be overcome to allow gas delivery to the patient. An initial discussion of the elastic components of the equation of motion as it relates to pressure will help to simplify the explanation. It is known that compliance relates to the change in volume in the lung as a result of a change in pressure. Thus, pressure is related to volume and to the patient's compliance.

$$Pressure = \frac{Volume}{Compliance}$$

If the clinician sets pressure as the control variable, volume varies directly with the compliance of the respiratory system. Thus, pressure is the independent variable set by the clinician, and volume is the dependent variable determined by the level of pressure. When the pressure pattern is preset by the clinician, the ventilator operates as a pressure controller. The volume becomes a function of compliance, so that a decrease in compliance allows less volume to be delivered for the same pressure. During expiration, the elastic and resistive elements of the respiratory system are passive, and expiratory waveforms are not directly affected by the modes of ventilation or the controller. However, as the respiratory cycle is a set period of time, any change in the inspiratory time can influence expiratory time and, to a certain extent, the expiratory profile.

For the resistive components of the equation of motion:

$$Pressure = Resistance \times Flow$$

When a ventilator operates as a constant-pressure controller—for example, in pressure-control (PC) mode, pressure-regulated volume control (PRVC) mode, and synchronized, intermittent mandatory ventilation-pressure control (SIMV-PC) mode—pressure is an independent, or controlled, variable (**Table 34.1**). The set pressure will be delivered and maintained constant throughout inspiration, independent of what resistive or elastic forces of the respiratory system might be. Even though pressure is constant, the delivered VT will vary as a function of compliance and resistance, and the flow will also vary exponentially with time.

A waveform from a ventilator operating as a pressure controller is displayed in **Figure 34.2**. Under this condition, volume and flow become the dependent variables, and their patterns will depend upon compliance and resistance. When a pressure pattern is preset (constant in a PC mode), flow-time and volume-time waveforms vary exponentially with time and are a function of compliance and resistance.

It is now clear that flow and resistance are associated only with the resistive components of the equation of motion. The elastic component refers to volume and compliance. Considering the resistive components of the equation of motion:

$$Pressure = Resistance \times Flow \quad OR \quad Flow = \frac{Pressure}{Resistance}$$

Thus, if the clinician sets flow as function of time, pressure then varies with resistance. Flow is the independent variable, and pressure is the dependent variable. When a flow pattern is preset, the ventilator operates as a flow controller; pressure is a function of resistance, and the inspiratory pressure-time waveform varies linearly with time. Volume increases linearly

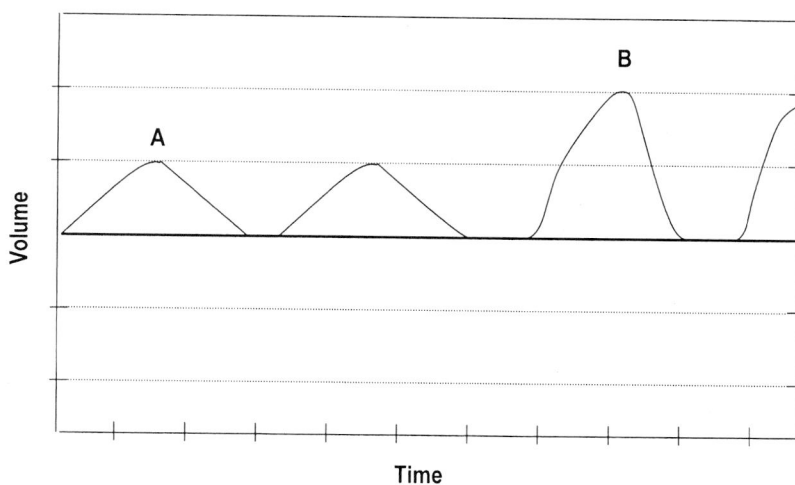

Time

FIGURE 34.2. Volume-time wave form from a constant pressure mode of ventilation. **A:** Increased resistance. With inspiration, an abnormal increase in tidal volume and decrease in inspired tidal volume occur, as compared to tracing B (normal resistance). Expiration has an abnormal linear decay to baseline. **B:** Normal resistance. During inspiration, a normal exponential increase in tidal volume occurs. Expiration has a normal exponential decay to baseline.

with time, although it does not have a direct relation to flow. Based on the equation of motion, volume does have an indirect relationship to flow, as volume is the integral of flow and flow is the derivative of volume. Again, expiration is passive, and the expiratory profile is not directly affected by mode of ventilation, but rather by compliance and resistance, even though the set inspiratory time can influence the expiratory time and, to a certain extent, the expiratory profile.

When a ventilator operates as a constant-flow controller (volume-controlled, VC, and SIMV-VC modes), flow is the independent variable. Regardless of the resistive or elastic forces of the respiratory system, the set flow will be delivered and maintained constant throughout inspiration. Pressure and VT will vary with time, depending on the compliance and resistance.

Waveforms from a ventilator operating as a flow controller are illustrated in **Figure 34.3.** Flow is the independent variable (controlled variable); pressure and volume are dependent variables. When a flow pattern is preset (constant in this case), pressure and volume are the dependent variables; they vary linearly with time and are functions of compliance and resistance. The modern ventilator can operate as a *flow controller* or as a *pressure controller.* As a flow controller, the most common

pattern is *constant flow,* also referred to as a *square-wave flow* pattern. In this mode, the flow increases to a set level that is maintained for the duration of the inspiratory time. The pressure and volume that the patient receives are a function of compliance and resistance. When a ventilator is set as a pressure controller, the observed pressure pattern is constant and results in a square-wave pressure pattern.

From the equation of motion, it can be stipulated that, with the ventilator operating as a constant-flow controller, the pressure and volume are linear functions of time. The various ventilators are able to deliver various flow patterns. To have flow patterns different from the most common types, which are constant and exponentially decelerating, the ventilator must be controlled by a microprocessor, which performs a series of sequential adjustments dictated by an algorithm to produce various flow patterns, including decelerating ramp, ascending ramp, and sinusoidal. These flow patterns are used in various volume-cycled modes. Again, volume-cycled ventilation is still controlled by flow, and the independent variable set is flow. It is important to note that the decelerating rate of flow is controlled by an algorithm that does not reflect the elastic and resistive elements of the respiratory system. Abnormalities in these elements may result in flow-starvation asynchrony, as the flow

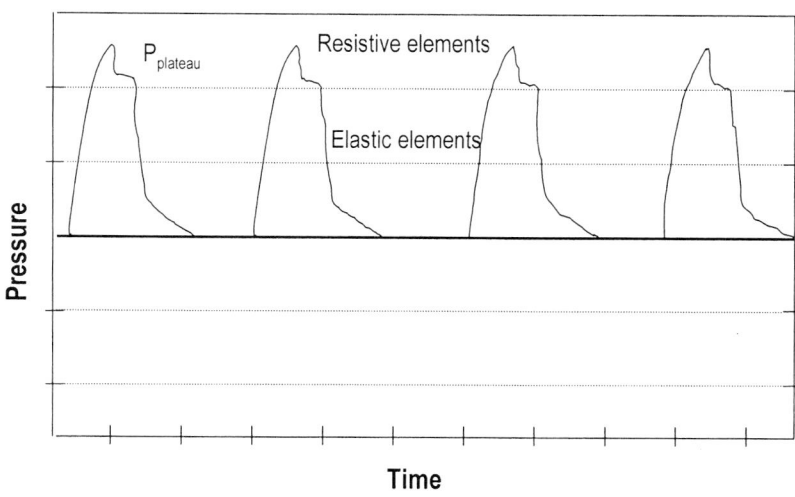

Time

FIGURE 34.3. Pressure-time waveform from a constant flow mode illustrating resistive and elastic elements of the respiratory system.

from the ventilator may be inadequate to meet patient needs. Not all ventilators can provide novel flow patterns.

Describing the flow and pressure patterns observed in different modes of ventilation is often confusing jargon. To expand further, in PC ventilation, the pressure pattern is "square," but flow increases rapidly at the beginning of the inspiratory phase to generate the set pressure limit, then decays exponentially over the inspiratory time. This flow pattern is described as *decelerating flow*. It is said that the major difference between volume and pressure ventilation is based on the square-wave and the decelerating flow patterns observed. In PC mode, the initial "snap" of high flow to reach the set pressure limit has been thought to be potentially beneficial in opening stiff alveoli in conditions such as acute respiratory distress syndrome (ARDS) or surfactant deficiency. It has been proposed that a decelerating flow favors better gas exchange and improves distribution of ventilation among lung units with heterogeneous time constants. For this reason, clinicians often choose PC ventilation in patients with poor compliance, although the true benefit of PC versus other modes has not been well established in animal or clinical studies.

Volume is most closely associated with the elastic component of the equation of motion. The resistive component of the equation is most dependent on resistance and flow. The elastic components can be rearranged to display how volume is determined:

Volume = Pressure × Compliance

If the clinician sets volume as a function of time, pressure then varies with compliance. Volume is the independent variable, and pressure is the dependent variable.

Theoretically, when a ventilator sets a volume pattern, it operates as a volume controller. However, to be a true volume controller, the ventilator must measure volume directly in order to set the volume pattern. Most ventilators cannot directly measure volume; rather, they calculate volume delivered from flow that occurs over a period of time. Most ventilators use volume as a limiting variable, meaning that inspiration stops when the preselected volume is reached. When inspiration stops at the preset volume value, the ventilator is referred to as *volume cycled*, but it is really acting as a flow controller. That is, the ventilator is set to deliver a set VT at a certain number of breaths per minute and a specified inspiratory time, which determines the patient's minute ventilation. The ventilator gives a certain flow to meet the set requirements.

Understanding the delivery of a positive-pressure breath to a patient requires an understanding of the relationship of gas delivery to overcoming the resistive and elastic elements of the patient and the ventilator system.

Volume Measurement

The goals of modern mechanical ventilation in infants and children have focused on preventing overdistension of alveoli by limiting VT, thus reducing volutrauma (25,42,43). Exact knowledge of both inspired and expired gas volumes with a sufficient level of precision is essential to optimize ventilator settings using lung-protective techniques. During the inflation phase of mechanical ventilation, pressure rises within the ventilator circuit, causing elongation and distension of the gas within the circuit. This gas becomes compressed within the ventilator tubing and never reaches the patient. The volume associated is termed the *compressible volume of the circuit*. While in most circumstances, this volume is standard within different sizes of circuits, variation can occur. Knowing the compressible volume within the ventilator circuit is important in determining the actual VT being delivered to the patient's lungs. When compression volume is accounted for in determining patient VT, the resultant volume is termed the *effective tidal volume*, which means that this is the tidal volume that reaches the patient's lungs. Effective tidal volume (eVT) can be calculated thusly:

$$eVT = (VT_E) - [\text{circuit compensation} \times (PI_{max} - PEEP)]$$

where:

VT_E = expired tidal volume
PI_{max} = maximal inspiratory pressure.

The optimal site for monitoring volumes in infants and children is unclear. The inability to accurately measure VT in a conventional ventilator is caused by several factors, including (a) difficulty of compensating for volume loss in the ventilator circuit or in the humidifier and (b) changes in temperature, humidification, and secretions, which may also influence the amount of gas that gets delivered from the ventilator to the actual patient. Air leaks around the ETT itself, especially in small patients with uncuffed tubes, are another source of volume measurement error. Measuring VT at the proximal airway eliminates most circuit compliance and other dead-space factors. Therefore, it has been recommended that the proximal airway be the only site at which to obtain accurate volume measurements in infants and children (44). To measure volumes at the proximal airway, a pneumotachograph must be positioned at the patient's airway opening or at the ETT. Unfortunately, this technique has disadvantages that are especially apparent in infants and children. A pneumotachograph placed at the proximal ETT opening creates dead space of its own, which can be detrimental in infants who already have small VTs (37). In addition, the proximally placed pneumotachograph may impair admittance to the ETT and airways and make suctioning more difficult. Secretions can also result in contamination of the pneumotachograph and distort observed measurements. Finally, the weight of the pneumotachograph at the proximal end of the ETT increases its overall weight and may result in an increased risk of extubation.

Given the importance of knowing the true VT delivered to a patient, it is essential to determine which is the most accurate, safe, and efficient site to monitor. It is also important to understand the reliability of conventional displays of VT generated by most ventilators. Three clinical studies have compared the ventilator-displayed VT (measured at the exhalation valve for exhaled VT displays) with the VT measured at the ETT. One group studied 98 ventilated infants and children using the Servo 300™ ventilator; 70 patients were ventilated with an infant circuit (compliance: 0.61 mL/cm H_2O), and 28 patients were ventilated with a pediatric circuit (compliance: 1.0 mL/cm H_2O) (15). In the patients with the infant circuit, poor correlation was noted between the expiratory VT measured with the pneumotachometer and the ventilator-displayed VT ($R^2 = 0.54$). Poor correlation ($R^2 = 0.58$) was also noted between the expiratory VT measured with the pneumotachometer and the calculated effective VT. In pediatric circuits, greater correlation occurred between the pneumotachometer-measured expiratory

VT, the ventilator-displayed VT, and the calculated effective VT ($R^2 = 0.84$ and $R^2 = 0.85$, respectively).

A second group studied 54 ventilated infants and children using the Servo 300™ ventilator with the pediatric circuit (compliance: 1.35 mL/cm H_2O) and adult circuit (compliance: 2.4 mL/cm H_2O) [17]. The VT measured at the ETT was significantly less than the ventilator-measured tidal VT and varied between 2% and 91%, with a mean (standard deviation) error of 32% (20%) in 40 children with the pediatric circuit and 18% (6%) in 16 children with the adult circuit. The VTs displayed by the ventilator were also significantly different from the calculated effective VT (−63.3% to +29.1%), with substantial underestimation of VT from the VT displayed or the effective VT in many patients with small VTs. The third group studied 30 ventilated infants, 1–23 months old, on Servo 300™ ventilators with neonatal (compliance: 0.63: mL/cm H_2O) and pediatric (compliance: 1.13: mL/cm H_2O) circuits [59]. This study demonstrated that the expiratory VT measured at the ETT was less than the expiratory VT displayed by the ventilator. When the ventilator was in the VC mode, the median difference was −36% (range: −5% to −2%), while the median was −35% (range: −6% to −60%) in the PC mode. The calculated effective VT was not statistically different from the ventilator-measured VT in PC mode; however, individual differences were large (range: −26% to +52%). The calculated effective VT was less than the VT measured at the ETT in the VC mode, with large individual differences (median: −23%, range: −48% to +21%). All of these clinical studies have recommended that the VT should be measured at the ETT in infants and small children. As stated previously, the effective VT can be calculated as the ventilator-measured expired VT. However, this method fails to take into account volume lost internally in the ventilator. Manufacturers have attempted to compensate for these volume losses by measuring compression volume loss in the system. The compliance factor can be calculated as

$$K_c = \frac{d_v}{(P_1 - P_0)}\ mL/cmH_2O$$

where:

  K_c = the compliance factor
  d_v = the total integrated volume
  P_0 and P_1 = start and target pressures.

Data demonstrate good agreement in volume measured at the ventilator when compensation adjustment is on, as compared to volume measured at the proximal airway [44]. The use of circuit-compliance compensation improved the agreement between the volume measured by the ventilator in an animal trial; pediatric pigs had improved agreement between the two volume methods attributable to circuit-compliance compensation (with circuit-compliance compensation "on," 0.97; with circuit-compliance compensation "off," 0.88; $p = 0.027$). It is essential for the clinician to understand the accuracy of the delivery of VT to their patients, especially in patients with small volumes, such as infants.

In a clinical study of 68 ventilated pediatric patients aged between 2 days and 18 years of age, the principal observation was that, when compression volume was compensated for by a computer algorithm, a negative bias occurred. Displayed volume was lower than that set by the clinician, but agreement was good when using compensation, with a concordance correlation between 0.90 and 0.98. Accuracy, expressed as percent difference, improved only in older patients [5]. A limitation of this study, as well as previous studies that utilized an airway sensor or pneumotachograph as the reference value of volume is the short time frame in which volumes were measured. A potential limitation of the airway sensor is the increased opportunity for the sensor to be contaminated by airway secretions and foreign substances, as compared to a pneumotachograph located within the ventilator. The potential for contamination, and thus degradation of the accuracy of the signal, of an airway sensor increases with increased length of time that the sensor is in place. In all of these studies, the airway sensor was only in place for a limited period. Caution must be used in extrapolating measurements from previously cited studies when the airway sensor is not left in place over a prolonged period.

Collectively, studies have shown that the ventilator-displayed VT, without software compensation for circuit compliance, generally overestimates the true delivered VT. Conversely, when the circuit-compliance compensation feature is on, the ventilator-displayed VT generally underestimates the true delivered VT.

Phase Variables

Discussion to this point has focused on the control variable required for a mechanical ventilator to deliver a breath to the patient and the interactions that occur with the delivery of that breath. The following discussion focuses on what have been described as *phase variables* [20]. Phase variables control the ventilator during the period of time between the beginning of one breath and the initial phase of the next breath. In other words, phase variables are important in determining how a ventilator initiates, sustains, and ends inspiration and what it does between inspirations. Expiration, being passive, is not described in this terminology. In each phase, a particular variable is measured and used to initiate, sustain, and end the phase. The phase variables include the trigger variable (determines the initiation of inspiration), limit variable (determines what sustains inspiration), and cycle variable (determines the termination of inspiration).

Trigger Variables

Patient ventilator system interactions can be initiated under two settings: The ventilator can deliver a controlled breath independent of the patient's desire, or it can be coordinated with the patient's effort. Ventilators will measure one or more of the variables associated with the equation of motion (e.g., pressure, volume, flow, or time). Inspiration is initiated when one of these variables reaches a preset variable. A patient-triggered breath, sometimes known as *interactive ventilation*, provides patients with some autonomy to alter breathing patterns in response to their ventilatory demand. Such systems necessitate an interface between the ventilator and the patient to allow for rapid, measured responses from the ventilator to meet patient needs. For such systems to operate, they must sense a signal from the patient and recognize the beginning of inspiration. Second, they must pressurize the system to allow for delivery of the breath to the patient. Finally, the system must recognize the end of inspiration and thus termination of the breath. Ideally, if this interaction could be facilitated by direct interaction between the patient and mechanical ventilator, delays and patient discomfort created by the temporary or relative unavailability of the caregiver at the patient's bedside could be eliminated.

Initial recognition of the signal from the patient to begin inspiration is commonly referred to as *triggering*. Triggering can be subdivided into pretrigger and trigger phases (70). The pretrigger phase has been defined as the time from the onset of inspiration until triggering occurs. The trigger phase is the time from triggering until the maximum flow of gas occurs. The most common trigger variables are time and flow.

In *time triggering*, the ventilator initiates a breath according to a set frequency independent of the patient's spontaneous efforts. In flow triggering, the ventilator senses the patient's inspiratory effort as a change in flow from the baseline flow and begins inspiration independent of the set breath frequency. Ventilator features that affect the trigger phase include the response time of the ventilator and the presence of bias flow. *Bias flow* is a continuous delivery of fresh gas circulating through the inspiratory and expiratory limbs of the circuit. Theoretically, bias flow reduces the WOB by making flow available to satisfy the earliest demand of the patient during inspiration, before the flow is initiated during the pretrigger phase. Increased patient effort to trigger the ventilator and delayed response of the ventilator to the patient's effort can be translated directly into increased WOB.

Current ventilator designs have improved patient-ventilator interactions by improving both the signal sensed by the ventilator and the response time of the ventilator. Today, all ventilators have the capability to utilize a flow signal as the trigger signal from the patient to the ventilator. Flow triggering has the advantage of allowing the patient to trigger the ventilator with less effort, and it has a faster response time (45). The process of creating somewhat seemingly small amounts of negative pressure in pressure-triggered breaths is made increasingly more difficult when the patient has a smaller ETT and/or in the presence of $PEEP_i$.

Theoretically, patient-triggered ventilation could be improved if a signal could be acquired from the patient that represented the earliest attempt by the patient to acquire a breath and if that signal could represent the amount of effort or drive from the patient for that breath. This approach is represented in what has been termed *neurally adjusted ventilatory assist*, or NAVA (4). The NAVA approach to mechanical ventilation is based on the acquisition of the patient's neural respiratory output as it is transmitted through the phrenic nerve to the diaphragm. This signal is acquired via an esophageal catheter with an imbedded series of electrodes that capture the electrical activity signal of the diaphragm, known as E_{di}. NAVA responds by providing the requested level of ventilatory support to the patient from the E_{di}. The advantage of this system is the ability to acquire the patient's desire to trigger the ventilator quickly and to offer feedback between patient effort and ventilator output. At this writing, NAVA is being investigated in clinical trials in Europe in neonatal, pediatric, and adult patients.

Work of Breathing

Work is equal to the force applied to an object multiplied by the distance the object travels. That is, work = force × distance or $W = F \times D$. If work is applied into the three dimensions of the respiratory system, work becomes the pressure applied to yield a change in the volume of the system and can be expressed as:

$$W = P \times V \quad \text{or} \quad W = \int_0^v P \times dv$$

where $\int_0^v P$ is the integral of the pressure across the respiratory system as a function of volume, and dv is the change in the volume of the respiratory system.

The concept of work associated with the functioning of the respiratory system has been known since the seminal analysis of Otis et al. (62). They elucidated that several forces were encountered while breathing, including the elastic forces of the chest wall and lungs, viscous and turbulent resistance of air, nonelastic tissue impedance, and inertia. Basically, motion requires work. Work is performed when pressure changes the volume of the respiratory system and is the product of pressure and volume integrated over time with respect to volume. Work is performed on the respiratory system by externally applied pressures from the ventilator via positive pressure, respiratory muscles, or both, as the lungs expand and contract. To achieve normal ventilation, the body performs work (WOB) to overcome the elastic and frictional resistance of the lungs and chest wall. Total work of breathing (WOB_T) is the sum of elastic work (WOB_E) and resistive work (WOB_R). Elastic WOB represents physiologic work to expand the lungs and chest wall. Resistive WOB is considered a measure of imposed WOB and includes work caused by the breathing apparatus, such as the ETT, breathing circuit, and ventilator demand-flow system. Artificial airways and physiologic resistive work on the airways are responsible for a large part of the imposed resistive work, with the mechanical ventilator also contributing some portion of resistive work (12).

Clinicians have long recognized that increased WOB occurs in patients being weaned from prolonged mechanical ventilation, when the patient begins to breathe spontaneously and take on more of the WOB. Patient-related factors, equipment factors, and decision-making affect weaning of patients from mechanical ventilation and, thus, WOB. Equipment factors relate to the ability of the mechanical ventilator to meet the needs of the patient. It has been demonstrated in a lung model that the amount of WOB varies according to the device utilized (9). These equipment factors have an increased significance in patients with poor pulmonary reserve or high airway resistance, where the WOB associated with the equipment is increased (61,69). These factors also have an increased significance in pediatric patients, in whom equipment is often associated with increased WOB (16).

Limit Variable

The limit variable is the modality that sustains inspiration. Inspiration time is defined as the time interval from the beginning of inspiratory flow to the beginning of expiratory flow. During inspiration, pressure, volume, and flow increase above their end-expiratory values.

If one or more of these variables increases only as high as a preset value, this variable will be referred to as the *limit variable*. It is important to recognize that the limit variable determines what *sustains* inspiration but differs from the *cycle variable*, which determines the *end* of inspiration. Therefore, a limit value does not terminate inspiration but increases to a preset value.

Cycle Variable

The cycle variable is the modality that terminates inspiration once a preset value is obtained, and this variable must be measured. The cycle variable also differs according to the mode of ventilation used. In PSV, the termination of the breath traditionally is triggered when either an absolute level of flow or a fixed percentage of peak inspiratory flow is reached. Until recently, this gave the clinician little control over the ventilator cycling off as it relates to the patient's pathology. For example, in a patient with increased airway resistance and dynamic hyperinflation, it may be desirable to shorten the inspiratory phase and prolong the expiratory phase. By changing the cycle-off variable, the patient's inspiratory phase can be shortened, allowing the patient a longer expiratory phase. The opposite is also true for patients with decreased pulmonary compliance. In this circumstance, the clinician might want to prolong the inspiratory phase and provide a shorter expiratory phase. Thus, termination of the breath can be extended by delaying the beginning of expiration.

PATIENT-VENTILATOR ASYNCHRONY

Patient-ventilator asynchrony is failure of two controllers to act in harmony (52). A patient on mechanical ventilation has the clinician-controlled mechanical pump of the ventilator and the patient's own respiratory muscle pump. Factors that affect patient-ventilator synchrony are listed in **Table 34.2** and can be subdivided into equipment factors, patient factors, and decision-making factors. Evaluation of patient-ventilator synchrony can also be subdivided into four phases that consist of issues of triggering, adequacy of flow delivery, adequate breath termination, and effects of PEEP and/or $PEEP_i$ (60).

Trigger Asynchrony

Trigger asynchrony is defined as the presence of muscular effort that results in a ventilator trigger (19). The incidence of patient-ventilator asynchrony is not well studied in pediatric patients. Clinical studies in adults have demonstrated trigger asynchrony in all of the common ventilator modes. Asynchrony occurs because of failure of the patient's drive to breathe, observed when additional support is provided by the base mode of the ventilator and the patient's drive to breathe decreases. Trigger asynchrony is also associated with the development of auto-PEEP.

To trigger the ventilator, mechanically ventilated patients with obstructive lung disease who develop $PEEP_i$ must generate a negative intrapleural pressure to match the value of $PEEP_i$ plus the sensitivity threshold. When inspiratory effort by the patient is less than that threshold value, the ventilator will not deliver a breath, which causes effort by the patient without a response being generated from the ventilator. Thus, dynamic hyperinflation ($PEEP_i$) leads to frequent nontriggering of breaths in patients with obstructive lung disease. Such non-

TABLE 34.2

VENTILATOR–PATIENT SYNCHRONY

Equipment factors
Trigger variables
Sensitivity settings
Response time of the ventilator
Inspiratory flow characteristics
Mode of ventilation
Expiratory valve design
Design of positive end-expiratory pressure valve and operation
External factors and equipment to the ventilator

Patient factors
Sedation and pain control
Patient's inspiratory effort and drive
Patient's disease process
Intrinsic positive end-expiratory pressure
Size of the airway
Presence of airway leak
Nutritional status
Patient homeostasis

Decision-making factors
Deleterious effects of patient-ventilator asynchrony
Patient fights the ventilator
Increased level of sedation
Higher work of breathing
Muscle damage
Ventilation-perfusion mismatch
Dynamic hyperinflation
Delayed or prolonged weaning
Prolonged intensive care or hospital stay
Higher costs

triggered breaths represent wasted breathing effort on the part of the patient and lead to patient-ventilator asynchrony, as the patient becomes distressed from the lack of ventilator response to their attempts to initiate a breath. In assist-control modes, the ventilator must be set to respond to the patient's breathing effort for the patient to receive any breathing assistance. In patients with obstructive lung disease or those in whom $PEEP_i$ is present, application of external PEEP may reduce nontriggered breaths by narrowing the difference between mouth pressure and alveolar pressure at end expiration. Similarly, in patients with high resistance to airflow from airway edema or constriction (such as asthma) who often also have air trapping and high levels on $PEEP_i$, application of external PEEP can help to "stent open" airways and improve flow during tidal expiration. Both of these conditions may have the elastic threshold load and WOB reduced by the use of extrinsic PEEP.

Flow Asynchrony

Flow asynchrony occurs whenever the ventilator flow does not match the patient's flow need. Flow delivered from the ventilator can be in either a fixed (such as in VC ventilation) or variable flow pattern (PC or PRVC). In VC mode, flow is fixed so that a set level of flow is delivered with each breath. As WOB is the sum of the work performed by the ventilator and the work performed by the patient, reduction in ventilator support or patient work will reduce the level of support. During ventilation with variable flow, the peak flow depends on a number of factors: set target pressure, patient effort, and the compliance and resistance of the respiratory system. In PC mode, the clinician can set the target pressure and the rate of flow acceleration or rise time. The control flow of acceleration varies according to the manufacturer, but the principles remain the same. A slower rise time may limit the ability of the ventilator to meet the patient's inspiratory demand. Studies of flow asynchrony during PC ventilation or PSV have implied that many patients require a rapid rise time to match increased ventilatory demand (55).

In a study that assessed whether adjustments in the initial flow or breath termination criteria affected patient–ventilator synchrony, the ventilator pattern response to PSV of 33 adult patients was studied under conditions with two parameters: seven different levels of delivered initial PSV flow, and during PSV termination that occurred when peak flow fell to 50% and 25%. It was found that an optimal initial flow could be defined for a given level of PSV, which resulted in the patient gaining a maximal pressure and volume from the ventilator. When the initial PSV flows were above and below this optimal flow, faster breathing rate, shorter inspiratory times, smaller VTs, and a tendency for airway pressure to fall short of the preset value occurred. Although increasing the inspiratory flow in PSV in adults may thus be useful, recommending the same maneuver in pediatric patients may be deleterious. Because pediatric patients have smaller ETTs, increased flow may lead to increased turbulence of gas and possible increased patient-ventilator asynchrony.

Termination Asynchrony

Termination asynchrony occurs when neural inspiratory time and ventilator inspiratory time do not coincide. The ability of the ventilator mode to terminate a breath when the patient desires constitutes an important factor in reducing the incidence of dyssynchrony. When the patient experiences high airway resistance, such as in bronchopulmonary dysplasia or chronic obstructive pulmonary disease, the inspiratory phase of a ventilator breath may be prolonged when a mode is selected that allows the patient to trigger spontaneous breaths. This situation can occur in PSV, resulting in early activation of expiratory muscles with premature termination of the ventilator breath.

Termination asynchrony can be caused by delayed termination or premature termination, with the most common being delayed termination. Generally, delayed termination results in dynamic hyperinflation, which then may result in missed trigger attempts as the patient is not able to overcome the effects of PEEP$_i$ and trigger the ventilator. Premature termination of a breath can also have deleterious effects with resultant asynchrony. In a 2001 study, premature termination led to substantially reduced V$_T$, increased respiratory rate, decreased inspiratory time, and increased WOB (76). A solution to help alleviate termination asynchrony has been incorporated into later-generation ventilators. This additional control allows for adjusting flow that causes the ventilator to cycle from the inspiratory phase to the expiratory phase (cycle-off) and allows for exhalation to be active. The effects of changing cycle-off when the ventilator begins exhalation as a function of peak inspiratory flow, in a ventilator with an active exhalation system, show that at a cycle-off set at 1%, the breath is terminated earlier than with the cycle-off set at 40%. In one study, WOB was not different between the two settings for cycle-off. How-

ever, considerable differences in the areas under both the time/flow and pressure/flow curves can be expected (46).

Expiratory Asynchrony

Expiratory asynchrony occurs due to a shortened or prolonged expiratory time, as well as patient efforts during expiration, when the ventilator is unresponsive. Shortened expiratory time creates the potential for hyperinflation secondary to air trapping and thus induces PEEP$_i$.

Historically, when patient effort signaled the ventilator to open the expiratory valve, the ventilator was no longer responsive to the patient's demands. Recently, manufacturers have introduced active exhalation valves that continue to sense patient effort during exhalation and respond to the patient effort. If the patient generates an effort during exhalation, the ventilator can terminate exhalation and respond to the patient effort. This mechanism is in contrast with systems that only allow the patient to attempt to pull flow from the bias flow in the system but require the patient to wait for expiration to terminate before another ventilator breath could be generated or triggered.

WHY ARE CHILDREN DIFFERENT?

Infants and children are both anatomically and physiologically different from adults, which limits the application of adult studies to the care of young children on mechanical ventilation. These differences decrease with the growth of the child. In a study of infants and children intubated for elective surgery, it was found that resistance of the respiratory system (R$_{rs}$) and airway resistance (R$_{aw}$) decreased as height increased (53). A comparison of this relationship with the reported power function of lung volume changes suggests that R_{rs} is actually lower, relative to lung size, in infants than in older children. That is, increases in lung volumes are greater than decreasing resistance; therefore, specific resistance (*resistance × volume*) would increase with decreasing height. Thus, it is speculated that the airways do not grow at the same rate as the increase in lung tissue. In infants, lung volume may increase at a greater rate than the increase in airway diameter, which may be one reason why infants are especially prone to air trapping and hyperinflation in circumstances of airway narrowing or elevated resistance, such as in bronchiolitis.

It also appears that mechanical ventilation has detrimental effects on the airways of infants that include changes in the dimensions and mechanical properties of the airways. The extent of ventilation-induced deformation appears to be directly related to the compliance of the airway and inversely related to age. Anatomically, it has been demonstrated that the airways after mechanical ventilation have an increase in tracheal diameter, thinning of cartilage and muscle, disruption of the muscle-cartilage junction, and focal abrasions of the epithelium (24). In comparison to airways that have never been exposed to mechanical ventilation, airways that have been exposed are difficult to expand but easy to collapse (63). Also, these airways show greater resistance to airflow. These findings result clinically in patients with flow limitation, gas trapping, and increased dead space, airway resistance, and WOB (79).

Infants and young children also are at a mechanical disadvantage because of the high compliance and low elastic recoil of the infant and young child's chest wall. The child must perform more work to move the same VT than a more mature person, as part of the WOB is lost in distortion of the rib cage. The low elastic recoil of the chest wall places infants and young children at greater risk of lung collapse, as most tidal breathing takes place in the range of the closing capacity of the lung. Also, infants have a reduced ability to generate muscle force due to the shape of their rib cage, location of the insertion of their diaphragm, reduced muscle mass, and lower oxidative capacity (11).

INDICATIONS FOR MECHANICAL VENTILATION

No controlled studies have elucidated or evaluated the indications for the use of mechanical ventilation in pediatric patients. The use of mechanical ventilation in this population has evolved over the past 10 years as we have expanded our knowledge of lung injury caused by it (42,43). Also, the use of noninvasive intermittent mandatory ventilation (IMV) has increased, and the need for every patient to be intubated to offer positive-pressure mechanical ventilation is no longer absolutely necessary. The indications for the use of mechanical ventilation are diverse and include both primary respiratory and nonrespiratory causes. The decision to place a patient on positive-pressure mechanical ventilation is a combination of clinical judgment, assessing symptoms and signs of the need for mechanical ventilation, and laboratory tests. In essence, the decision to place a patient on either invasive or noninvasive positive-pressure mechanical ventilation represents the patient's inability to deal with increased inspiratory loads and maintenance of airway patency or inability to maintain gas exchange. Inspiratory loads consist of inertial (obesity, chest wall density), threshold (artificial loads placed on airway), resistive (upper airway obstruction, asthma, artificial airway), and elastic (kyphoscoliosis, pulmonary restriction, chest wall trauma, pleural effusions, pneumonia, pulmonary edema, pulmonary fibrosis, hyperinflation) loads.

DETERMINING INITIAL SETTINGS FOR MECHANICAL VENTILATION

After the decision is made to place the patient on mechanical ventilatory support, it is essential that the settings of the mechanical ventilator be directed toward the indications for ventilatory support. Essentially, mechanical ventilatory support can be subdivided into three phases: acute, maintenance, and weaning. The acute phase of mechanical ventilation is the initial phase when the clinician matches the patient's disease process with the ventilatory mode and level of support. It is during the acute phase that the clinician must optimize mechanical ventilator support while minimizing potential deleterious effects. The initial settings of mechanical ventilatory support are dependent upon the patient's age and mode of support and can be subdivided into volume-targeted and pressure-targeted modes. The selection of ventilator settings is also directed by the clinician's desire to eliminate ventilator-induced lung injury. It is essential for the clinician to recognize that the goal of mechanical ventilatory support is not to normalize the patient's blood gases at the cost of ventilator-induced lung injury. For patients

with obstructive lung disease, such as asthma, this lung protection strategy would include the prevention of high airway pressures and hyperinflation-associated complications. Initial settings would include a lower VT and prolonged exhalation times. Allowing such patients to breathe spontaneously in a support mode is ideal, as it allows the patient more control over the exhalation time. However, as some intubated asthmatics have elevated levels of $PaCO_2$, this strategy may result in agitation in the patient and, therefore, an increase in sedation. The level of PEEP in patients with obstructive disease has traditionally been set at minimal levels, secondary to the development of auto-PEEP, due to the patient's increased airway resistance with inadequate lung emptying during exhalation. However, some patients may require levels of PEEP to match the level of auto-PEEP to splint airways open, ensuring adequate oxygenation and improving exhalation.

Patients with decreased thoracic compliance must have ventilatory settings directed toward lung recruitment to reduce the severity of ventilator-induced lung injury. As discussed in previous sections, this lung protection strategy is primarily accomplished by limiting distending volume, the change in pressure to distend the alveoli, and the level of end-expiratory pressure. This strategy is directed toward reducing the cyclic collapse and re-expansion of the alveoli due to inadequate levels of PEEP and thus the inability to maintain the alveoli open throughout the respiratory cycle.

LUNG RECRUITMENT

Lung recruitment is a strategy aimed at re-expanding collapsed lung tissue and maintaining high PEEP to prevent subsequent "derecruitment." The benefits of optimal lung recruitment and prevention of derecruitment involves (a) a reduction in the intrapulmonary shunt fraction with an improvement in arterial oxygenation, (b) an improvement in pulmonary compliance by shifting the compliance curve to the point where less pressure is required for the same change in volume, and (c) prevention of a cyclic opening, collapse, and reopening of alveolar units with each breath associated with ventilator-induced lung injury. To recruit collapsed lung tissue, sufficient pressure must be imposed to exceed the critical opening pressure of the affected lung. Lung recruitment has gained widespread interest as a tool for opening closed lung units. The widespread use of low VTs may increase the risk of reabsorption atelectasis in the basal parts of the lung, which eventually may lead to consolidation of the affected areas. This atelectatic effect is further enhanced by high-inhaled O_2 concentrations. In certain patients, the use of a recruitment maneuver may provide a long-term improvement in oxygenation. If a proper PEEP level can be determined and set, the effect will stabilize and further protect the lung by avoiding cyclical opening and closing of lung units.

Ideal patients for recruitment maneuvers are those with putative ARDS in the early phase of the disease (before the onset of fibroproliferation). These patients will continue to be poorly oxygenated in spite of a high FIO_2. Preexisting focal lung disease that may predispose to barotrauma should be regarded as a relative contraindication to the maneuver (e.g., extensive apical bullous lung disease). Patients with "secondary" ARDS (e.g., following abdominal sepsis) are thought to be more likely to respond favorably to the maneuver than patients with "primary" lung disease and acute lung injury.

Several methods are used clinically to accomplish an opening of collapsed alveoli. The common denominator for most of these methods is to intermittently apply an increased positive pressure in the lung for a limited time. One method utilizes the graphical display of dynamic inspiratory compliance (C_{dyni}), which indicates the response of the patient's lung mechanics to each change in applied airway pressure and inspiratory VT (VT_i). For example, during a stepwise increase of the end inspiratory pressure (EIP), a corresponding increase in VT will occur. C_{dyni} is defined as:

$$Cdyni = \frac{VTi}{EIP - PEEP}$$

As long as the relative increase in EIP and VT are linear, the C_{dyni} will appear constant, reflecting the pressure–volume relation in the lung over time. With a continued stepwise increase in EIP, eventually less increase will occur in the corresponding VT, which is indicated by a slight decrease in C_{dyni}. Additional increase in EIP at this point may result in a gradually smaller increase in VT, accompanied by a decrease in C_{dyni}. This pattern may illustrate that the frequency of opening of collapsed alveoli is reduced relative to increase in pressure and that further increase in EIP may result in overdistension of already opened alveoli.

PEEP Titration

C_{dyni} may also be a useful parameter by which to find the appropriate level of PEEP that may prevent alveolar collapse during expiration, thereby helping to guide the titration of effective PEEP. This assessment may be performed by a stepwise decrease of the initial PEEP level and should be completed before the recruitment maneuver is performed. As PEEP is carefully decreased, the C_{dyni} will initially increase with each decrease of PEEP, indicating a relief of overdistended areas in the lung. Subsequently, the C_{dyni} will reach a plateau at which C_{dyni} no longer increases when the PEEP level is decreased. After further decrease in the PEEP level, the C_{dyni} will begin decreasing, indicating initial collapse of alveoli that can no longer be kept open at the current PEEP level. Effective PEEP should be set at 2–3 cm H_2O above the indicated collapse pressure as a safety margin after a preceding recruitment maneuver.

Another method is to identify the critical opening pressure of the airways by utilizing a static pressure-volume loop to generate the lower inflection point (**Fig. 34.4**). As the lung is inflated from zero end-expiratory pressure, the clinician attempts to identify the point at which the volume abruptly changes, termed the *lower inflection point*. As the lung is further inflated, the pressure-volume slope increases to the point at which the volume no longer changes with each change in pressure. This flattening of the pressure-volume loop is referred to as *beaking* (as in a bird's beak, referring to the pattern of the graphed pressure-volume loop) and represents overdistension of the lung. The next phase of the pressure-volume loop occurs when expiration begins and the lung begins to deflate; the pressure point at which rapid loss of volume begins to occur has been termed the *deflection point*. Ideally, the clinician utilizes the identification of the inflection and defection points to select the PEEP level necessary to maintain the lung open throughout inspiration and expiration, without allowing for overdistension. This technique is difficult to accurately deter-

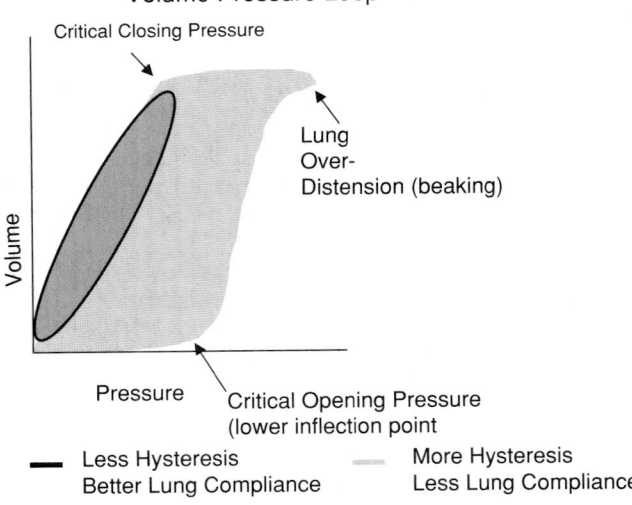

Volume Pressure Loop

FIGURE 34.4. Two pressure volume loops superimposed on the same graph. The dark gray loop represents a lung with normal pulmonary compliance. The light gray loop demonstrates a lung with decreased pulmonary compliance. Illustrated on this loop is the critical opening pressure or point when volume increases once critical pressure is reached, point of lung over distention where there is pressure change without volume and the critical closing pressure.

mine at the bedside, especially in children. Because an accurate static pressure-volume loop also requires that the patient not generate spontaneous breaths, neuromuscular blockade is often required.

Measures of Lung Recruitment

C_{dyni} can be used as a measure of improvement in lung compliance during lung recruitment; however, other measures should be utilized to ensure recruitment without overdistension of the recruited alveoli. If the lung is recruited, oxygenation, pulmonary compliance, and ventilation should improve. It is important not to be misled by an improvement of oxygenation alone as a measure of lung recruitment. An increase in PEEP can reduce cardiac output and increase PaO_2 despite a decrease in O_2 delivery. The CO_2 concentration in expired air depends on alveolar ventilation, cardiac output, and the metabolic state. The elimination of CO_2 via expired gas during normal conditions can be calculated using the Brody formula, which predicts CO_2 production during resting conditions:

$$\dot{V}CO_2\,(elimination/minute) = V/Q \times 10 \times BW^{0.75}$$

A measure of CO_2 at the airway is $VTCO_2$, which can be calculated by dividing $\dot{V}CO_2$ by the respiratory rate. When a stepwise increase of EIP is applied to a collapsed lung, $VTCO_2$ will increase with each pressure step due to increased ventilation of already opened alveoli and recruitment of collapsed areas, allowing for additional diffusion of CO_2 from the blood into the alveolar space.

With a continued stepwise increase of EIP, $VTCO_2$ will continue to increase to a point at which no additional alveoli can be recruited without impeding alveolar blood supply. Alveoli already opened could also be overdistended, thus decreasing the diffusion of the CO_2 into the alveoli. Both circumstances will correspond to a drop in $VTCO_2$.

POSITIVE END-EXPIRATORY PRESSURE

PEEP can be added to any mode of mechanical ventilation and is produced by a number of devices that regulate the pressure in the expiratory limb of the ventilator circuit. The effect of PEEP is as a distending pressure to increase the FRC (volume of gas at the end of exhalation in the lung). By maintaining this pressure above the pressure in which the lungs collapse (closing pressure), atelectasis or alveolar collapse is minimized. The ultimate effect is decreased intrapulmonary shunting of blood and improved arterial oxygenation.

PEEP increases intrathoracic pressure and causes potential hemodynamic consequences by transmitting the applied PEEP to transmural capillary pressure, which affects the right and left heart. The most dramatic effect of increased PEEP is decreased venous return to the right heart. In children with normal cardiac function, compensation for this effect can easily be made by increasing intravascular volume with administration of isotonic crystalloids or colloids.

MODES OF VENTILATION

Intermittent Mandatory Ventilation

IMV is a mode of mechanical ventilation that allows the patient to breathe spontaneously between machine-cycled or clinician-controlled mandatory breaths. During IMV, a preset number of positive-pressure (mandatory) breaths is delivered between which the patient can breathe spontaneously. The mandatory breaths can control variables of volume (clinician-preset volume with flow limit, volume, or time cycled) or pressure (pressure limited, time cycled). IMV can be contrasted with single-control modes (assist control, PC, VC) because the patient is allowed to breath spontaneously between mandatory breaths. The most common mode of IMV is SIMV, in which mandatory, or machine, breaths are synchronized via a timing window to the patient effort at the patient's intrinsic respiratory rate rather than the breaths being evenly spaced over each minute (**Fig. 34.5**). Commonly, this mode is combined with pressure support, which provides support to nonmandatory breaths. The

main disadvantage of SIMV, as compared to assist-control, is that the clinician may overestimate the amount of support, which leads to patient fatigue, as the WOB is increased (54). Another disadvantage in infants and children is that the support modes used during SIMV are not volume targeted but are usually limited by pressure. Thus, small changes in airway resistance or pulmonary compliance may lead to a decrease in VT obtained with the supported breaths, resulting in inadequate gas exchange and patient distress, especially if the mandatory breath rate is low.

Pressure-Controlled Ventilation

During PC ventilation, a pressure-limited breath is delivered during a preset inspiratory time at the preset respiratory rate (**Fig. 34.6**). The VT is determined by the preset pressure limit and the compliance and resistance of the respiratory system. The flow waveform is always decelerating in PC. Gas flows into the chest along the pressure gradient. As the alveolar pressure rises with increasing alveolar volume, the rate of flow drops off (as the pressure gradient between the airway opening and the alveolar space narrows). The set pressure is maintained for the duration of inspiration.

PC ventilation has several advantages. The higher initial flow associated with PC ventilation more easily meets the patient's flow demands, especially in patients with "stiff" lungs. The peak inspiratory pressure during PC ventilation is usually less compared to VC ventilation for the same obtained VT. During PC breaths, the distribution of ventilation may be more even in a lung with heterogeneous mechanical properties. That is, the initial high flow opens alveoli, and the constant pressure maintained during inspiration may allow gas to flow from more well-distended alveoli to more collapsed areas and thus distribute gas more efficiently throughout the lung. PC is also useful in the patient with an air leak. Although volume is lost through the leak, the ventilator will continue to attempt to compensate by maintaining the airway pressure for the duration of the inspiratory phase.

PC ventilation also has several disadvantages. It does not guarantee minute ventilation, and therefore, requires closer observation by the healthcare provider. The delivered VT will change as the patient's lung mechanics or effort changes.

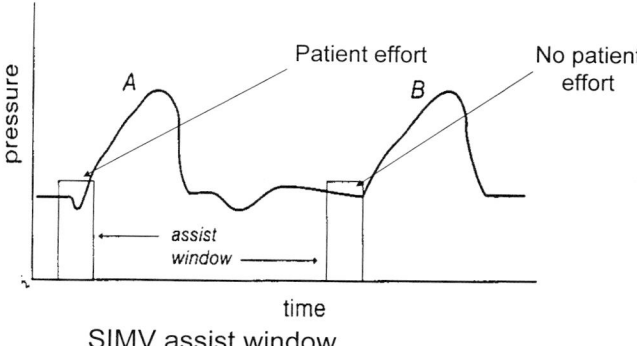

FIGURE 34.5. Two SIMV breaths. The first is patient triggered and the second is machine triggered. If the patient does not trigger a breath in the assist window the ventilator will deliver a machine breath at the start of the next window.

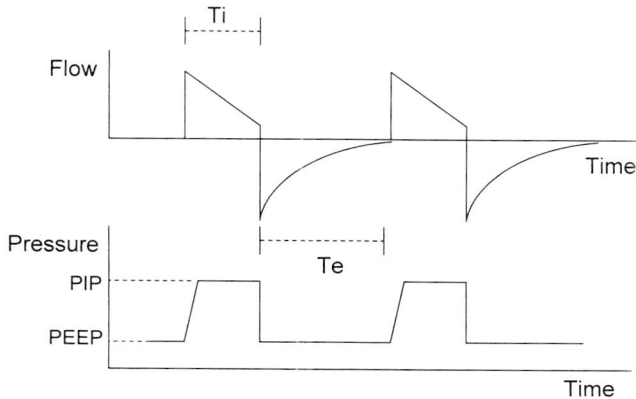

FIGURE 34.6. Pressure-controlled breath. Note the flow pattern is rapidly decelerating from high initial flow to baseline.

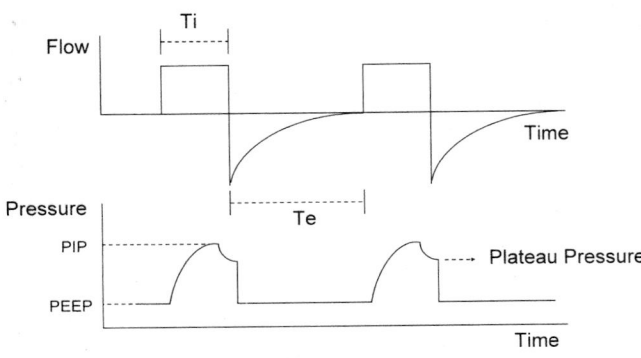

FIGURE 34.7. Volume-controlled breath. Note the flow pattern is square with an initial high flow that is maintained during inspiration and then quickly terminated at expiration.

Worsening of the patient's compliance or resistance results in decreased VT delivered and may result in hypoventilation and hypoxia. Conversely, an improvement in patient compliance or increasing patient effort can lead to a higher VT with alveolar overdistension (volutrauma).

Volume-controlled Ventilation

In the VC ventilation mode, the ventilator delivers a preset VT with a constant flow during a preset inspiratory time at the preset respiratory rate (**Fig. 34.7**). Airway and alveolar pressures are dependent variables and will rise or fall depending upon changes in lung mechanics or patient effort. VC ventilation has some advantages. By setting the volume to be delivered and the breath rate, the clinician has control over the patient's minute ventilation and CO_2 clearance, provided only a small leak is present around the ETT. Ventilator-induced lung injury due to alveolar overdistension (volutrauma) can also be less in volume-control mode.

VC ventilation also has disadvantages. The constant-flow type of breath delivery in VC ventilation may not meet patient demands, especially if the patient has poorly compliant lungs that may benefit from the initial accelerated flow that occurs with PC ventilation, resulting in asynchrony between the patient's breathing efforts and the ventilator; this disadvantage leads to distress and often an increase in sedation requirements. The peak inspiratory pressure is higher in VC ventilation compared to PC ventilation for the same obtained VT.

Proportional-assist Ventilation

Proportional-assist ventilation (PAV) is designed so that, theoretically, the level of ventilatory support is proportional to patient effort. This mode was designed to increase or decrease airway pressure by amplifying airway pressure proportional to inspiratory flow and volume. Unlike other modes in which a preset volume or pressure determines the level of support, in PAV, the level of support is determined in an interaction between the patient and the ventilator.

Most of the studies that utilized PAV have been observational, with limited reports in children. In patients sup-

ported with PAV, a greater variability was seen in VT than in PSV. However, PAV appears to be associated with better comfort. The current technology is associated with concerns regarding the interface with accurate measurements of elastance and resistance and regarding the issue of "runaway control" with changes in ETT resistance, presence of auto-PEEP, and a nonlinear relationship elastance and resistance. Despite some potential advantages, no studies have demonstrated outcome benefits. PAV is currently not available in the US.

Airway-pressure-release Ventilation

Airway-pressure-release ventilation (APRV) is essentially a high-level CPAP mode that is terminated for a very brief period. The elevated baseline helps oxygenation, and the timed releases assist CO_2 removal. This mode allows the patient to spontaneously breathe during all phases of the cycle (**Fig. 34.8**). APRV is different from other modes of ventilation in that it is based on an intermittent decrease in airway pressure, rather than an increase. APRV has been successfully used in various forms of respiratory failure and acute lung injury in both adults and children.

In addition to FiO_2, the operator-controlled parameters in APRV mode are: P_{high}, T_{high}, P_{low}, and T_{low}, where P and T equate to pressure and time. P_{high} should be set at a level equivalent to the plateau pressure being used in a conventional mode when transitioning to APRV. If APRV is the first mode to be used, P_{high} is set at ~20–30 cm H_2O, P_{low} at zero, T_{high} at ~4–6 sec, and T_{low} initially at ~0.2–0.6 sec. T_{low} should then be adjusted based on the expiratory gas flow waveform so that the expiratory flow falls to ~25%–75% of peak expiratory flow. Generally, T_{low} will be shortened in restrictive disease and lengthened in obstructive disease.

The P_{high} and T_{high} regulate end-inspiratory lung volume and provide a significant contribution to the mean airway pressure (MAP). MAP correlates to mean alveolar volume and is critical for maintaining an increased surface area of open air spaces for diffusive gas movement. As a result, these parameters control oxygenation and alveolar ventilation. Counterintuitive to conventional concepts of ventilation, the extension of T_{high} can be associated with a decrease in $PaCO_2$ as machine frequency decreases. P_{low} and T_{low} regulate end-expiratory lung volume and should be optimized to reduce airway closure/derecruitment and not as a primary ventilation adjustment. Generally, to maintain maximal recruitment T_{high} should occur at the optimal P_{high} or CPAP level. To minimize derecruitment, the time (T_{low}) at P_{low} is brief. Partial assistance (pressure support or automatic-tube compensation) can also be added to the spontaneous breaths. When the patient's underlying condition improves, APRV can gradually be weaned by lowering the P_{high} and extending the T_{high}. The goal is to arrive at straight CPAP.

APRV has several advantages. Clinical studies have shown that oxygenation and ventilation can be maintained at lower pressures with APRV when compared with conventional ventilatory management. Additionally, improvements in hemodynamic parameters and splanchnic perfusion have been reported. As the patient is able to breathe spontaneously throughout the entire respiratory cycle with this mode of

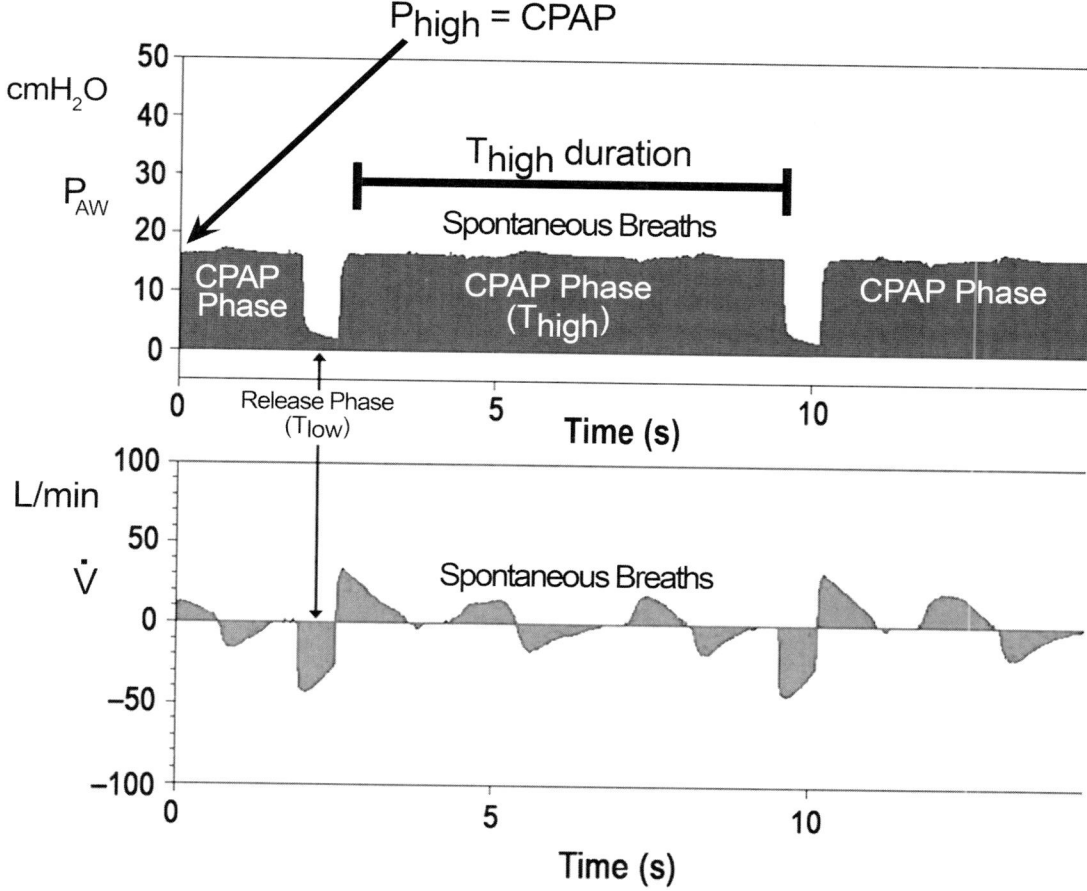

FIGURE 34.8. Patient breathing on APRV. The CPAP phase (P_{high}) is intermittently released to a P_{low} for a brief duration (T_{low}) reestablishing the CPAP level on the subsequent breath. Spontaneous breathing may be superimposed at both pressure levels and is independent of time-cycling. Adapted from Habashi N. Other approaches to open-lung ventilation: Airway pressure release ventilation. *Crit Care Med* 2005;33(3) Suppl:S228–S240.

ventilation, the need for heavy sedation and neuromuscular blockade is much less than with other modes of ventilation.

APRV, like all other modes, also has some disadvantages. APRV is a form of PC ventilation; therefore, mechanical VT varies according to lung mechanics. Also, the spontaneous breaths during the long inflation period can further increase end-inspiratory lung volume beyond that set by the inflation pressure; therefore, APRV may be less effective as a strategy to limit alveolar overdistension. APRV has not been well compared to other forms of conventional ventilation in a controlled fashion.

Hybrid Techniques

Hybrid techniques, also described as dual-controlled ventilation, are modes that allow the clinician to set a volume target while the ventilator delivers a PC breath. Dual control of the breath in these hybrid modes is designed to be either intrabreath (within a breath) or interbreath (breath to breath). Examples of dual control *intrabreath* modes are volume-assured pressure support and pressure augmentation. In these modes, the venti-

lator switches from PC to VC during a single breath. Examples of dual-control *interbreath* modes are PRVC, adaptive pressure ventilation, variable PC, and Autoflow™. In these modes, the pressure limit is increased or decreased automatically to maintain a clinician-selected target volume. Frequently used hybrid modes are discussed in the following sections.

Pressure-regulated Volume Control

PRVC (or adaptive pressure ventilation, variable PC, Autoflow™, or Volume Control Plus™) is a dual-control, breath-to-breath mode. PRVC has a variable decelerating flow pattern, with breaths time cycled. During PRVC, the pressure and volume are regulated. Thus, all breaths are volume targeted, with pressure adjusted to reach that volume target. PRVC often incorporates a "compliance curve" that is developed within the ventilator computer, as it gives several initial breaths at varying VTs that increase incrementally up to the set value. From this information, the ventilator computes the pressure target required to deliver the desired VT. Depending on the respiratory system compliance, the pressure associated with the tidal breath can vary over time. If the patient's compliance decreases, the pressure required to ensure the volume breath can be increased up to within 5 mm Hg of the set pressure-alarm limit. If the patient's compliance improves, the pressure required to deliver the volume breath will be reduced. Thus, a specific VT and minute ventilation is assured, while pressure-induced lung damage is minimized. The proposed advantage of this mode is a constant $\dot{V}_E$ and VT with automatic weaning of the pressure limit as the patient's compliance improves.

Volume-assured Pressure Support

Volume-assured pressure support and pressure augmentation are described as a dual control within a breath mode, where the ventilator switches from PC to VC within the breath. In this mode, the clinician chooses a volume target and the breath begins as a pressure-limited, flow-cycled breath, either spontaneously (pressure support) or mechanically. When inspiratory flow has decelerated to the minimum set level, delivered volume is measured. If the target volume has been met or exceeded, the breath ends. If the delivered volume has not met the target, the breath is transitioned to a volume-targeted breath by prolonging inspiration at the minimum flow and increasing the inspiratory pressure until the delivered volume has been obtained. The theoretical advantages of these modes are the ability to maintain constant VT and minute volume with a resultant lower WOB. Little evidence is available on its use in infants and children, and no recent studies have been conducted to demonstrate its use. Concerns exist that severe patient-ventilator asynchrony can be observed with pressure- and volume-assured ventilation if the patient is breathing spontaneously and inspiration is prolonged.

Support Modes of Ventilation

Pressure-support Ventilation

PSV is a form of mechanical ventilatory support that delivers a clinician-selected amount of positive airway pressure to assist an intubated patient's spontaneous inspiratory effort. PSV is used either as low-level PSV to overcome the patient's work associated with the ETT or as high-level PSV as a stand-alone ventilatory support mode. The rationale for the use of low-level PSV is that an airflow resistance associated with an ETT produces an undesirable high pressure-volume workload that may compromise comfort and ventilatory function with spontaneous breathing during IMV breaths. Higher levels of PSV can be used as a stand-alone mode by applying whatever level of inspiratory pressure is necessary for a desired VT and minute ventilation. However, it should be noted that if changes occur in the patient's resistance and/or compliance, the VT delivered may vary greatly and potentially under- or overventilate the patient.

Volume-support Ventilation

Volume-support ventilation is a volume-targeted mode of ventilation that is essentially pressure support with VT as a feedback. In this mode, the level of inspiratory pressure is adjusted with each breath to reach a targeted clinician-selected volume. All breaths are patient triggered, pressure limited, and flow cycled.

As outlined in the weaning section, volume-support ventilation is utilized in patients once they demonstrate that they are ready to be weaned, which is best demonstrated when the patient begins to trigger the ventilator above the set rate. When the patient triggers the ventilator, the patient's set VT is reduced by 15%, and the pressure associated with maintaining adequate minute ventilation and gas exchange is followed over time. As the patient's compliance improves, the required pressure to deliver the VT will be diminished. Patients may be extubated from volume support once the required peak inspiratory pressure is ≤20 cm H_2O, PEEP is ≤6 cm H_2O, and standard extubation criteria are met (resolution of cause for intubation, ability to protect the airway, hemodynamic stability, etc.). By using the peak inspiratory pressure as a guide for extubation, the clinician is utilizing an indirect measure of improvement of pulmonary compliance to guide clinical improvement. Hybrid modes such as ventilator-support ventilation have an advantage in pediatric patients by maintaining a clinician-targeted volume even if changes occur in the patient's airway resistance (e.g., increased secretions) and/or pulmonary compliance. As the patient initiates all ventilator breaths, however, most hybrid modes will automatically alarm and switch to an assist-control or SIMV mode if the patient becomes apneic or breaths are inadequate to meet VT goals to prevent deleterious patient events.

Closed-loop Methods

An important factor in successful weaning of mechanical ventilation is the ability of the clinician to manipulate the ventilator so that it responds to the patient's physiologic respiratory demands by providing more or less support, as needed. If the ventilator itself could make these adjustments, based upon the patient's physiologic needs and ventilatory pattern, it would provide optimal weaning (66).

Automode

Automode is a patient-interactive mode that uses a computer-directed algorithm to direct both control and support modes depending on the patient's needs (47). When Automode is enabled, it allows the ventilator to switch between volume control/volume support (VC/VS), pressure control/pressure support (PC/PS), and pressure regulated volume control/volume support (PRVC/VS), with spontaneously triggered breaths. When Automode is activated, the ventilator will switch to the corresponding support mode when the patient triggers two consecutive breaths. The ventilator remains in the support mode as long as the patient continues to breathe spontaneously. If the patient stops triggering, the ventilator automatically switches back to the clinician-selected control mode.

Volume-assured Pressure Support/ Pressure Augmentation

Volume-assured pressure support and pressure augmentation are described as dual-control-within-a-breath modes in which the ventilator switches from PC to VC within the breath. The theoretical advantage of these modes is their ability to maintain constant VT and minute volume, with a resultant lower WOB. Little evidence is available on their use in infants and children, and no recent studies demonstrate its use.

Automatic Tube Compensation

Automatic tube compensation (ATC) utilizes calculated tracheal pressure to compensate for ETT resistance via a closed loop control (40). The calculation for determining tracheal pressure is:

$$\text{Tracheal pressure} = \text{proximal airway pressure} - (\text{tube coefficient} \times \text{flow}^2)$$

Thus, the known resistive coefficients of the ETT and measurement of instantaneous flow are used to apply pressure proportional to the resistance of the entire respiratory cycle. Theoretically, the interest in ATC has been in eliminating the imposed WOB during inspiration. As discussed in the description of PRVC and volume support, the use of ATC has theoretical advantages in pediatric patients with small ETTs, and it has an increased potential for large swings in airway resistance due to secretions that may limit the amount of support for the patient. The theoretical advantages are (a) compensation for the WOB imposed by the artificial airway, (b) adjustment of the level of inspiratory flow to meet the patient's demand (similar to PAV), and (c) compensation for imposed expiratory resistance to reduce air trapping. However, the advantages are not always realized at the bedside. During expiration, the calculated tracheal pressure is greater than the airway pressure, and under those conditions, negative airway pressure could reduce expiratory resistance. However, as ATC cannot reduce PEEP to <0 cm H_2O during exhalation, expiratory resistance may not have complete compensation. Also, kinks, bends, or secretions in the ETT may lead to changes in airflow resistance, again causing incomplete compensation. The evidence for the advantages of ATC is strictly anecdotal, and its role in pediatric patients is yet to be determined.

HIGH-FREQUENCY VENTILATION

High-frequency ventilation (HFV) delivers minimal tidal volumes that approximate the anatomic dead space at rates exceeding the normal respiratory rate. Tidal volumes of 1–3 mL/kg are delivered at rates from 3–20 Hz (180–1200 breaths/min). The limitation of delivered tidal volumes and optimization of alveolar recruitment, which minimizes atelectrauma (21) and volutrauma (41), has become one of the main strategies of mechanical ventilation in patients with ARDS (1). At least theoretically, HFV provides lung-protective ventilation by applying maximal MAP and recruitment while delivering minimal tidal volumes.

Classification of Devices

During HFV, an oscillating waveform is generated by rapidly altering gas flow. While inspiration during HFV is always active, depending on the device, expiration can be either active or passive. During passive expiration, the elastic recoil of the lungs generates a positive transpleural pressure and expiration. During active expiration, the air is actively withdrawn out of the lungs as the diaphragm or piston of an oscillator travels away from the airway opening in the ventilator circuit. The devices described differ by the technical modalities through which HFV is achieved. The nomenclature of devices is not en-

tirely straightforward, and hybrid devices exist that combine HFV with conventional ventilation.

High-frequency Oscillation Ventilation

A nearly square waveform is generated either by a diaphragm or by a piston (64). Inspiration and expiration are active. Gas is forced into the lungs and actively withdrawn from the airways, as the diaphragm or piston travels forward and backward. Fresh gas flow pressurizes the system to the required MAP. The magnitude of the oscillations (often referred to as ΔP) is controlled by the distance traveled by the piston or the diaphragm. The inspiratory time is set as a percentage of the respiratory cycle and determines the ratio of inspiratory-to-expiratory (I:E) time. An inspiratory time of 33% or 50%, resulting in an I:E ratio of 1:2 or 1:1, is frequently used in the clinical setting.

High-frequency Jet Ventilation

During high-frequency jet ventilation, a jet ventilator is combined with a conventional ventilator. The gas flows from two sources: The jet ventilator is the source of the small delivered tidal volumes, whereas the conventional ventilator is the source of the bias flow. Inspiration is active, whereas expiration is passive and driven by elastic recoil of the lungs and chest wall. Jet ventilation can be delivered during CPAP or conventional ventilation. The resulting tidal volume of the jet ventilator is a result of the driving pressure of the jet, resistance of the ETT, and the set inspiratory time. Inspiratory and expiratory times are variable in most devices. High-frequency jet ventilation has been evaluated in a number of neonatal trials (30,50).

High-frequency Flow Interrupters

With the use of high-frequency flow interrupters, a valve mechanism in the expiratory limb of the ventilator rapidly alters flow, causing a pulsating gas flow. Some conventional ventilators provide this mode as a back-up mode to transition to high-frequency flow interrupters without switching the ventilator. Due to their limited bias flow, high-frequency flow interruption devices are usually used in the neonatal setting.

Examples of Commercially Available Devices

Neonatal Devices

The Life Pulse High-Frequency Ventilator (Bunnell, Salt Lake City, UT) is a jet-ventilator used in neonates. The ventilator is connected to a conventional ventilator at the patient's ETT with a special adapter. The jet ventilations are added to the conventional ventilation that the patient is receiving. The respiratory rate varies between 4 and 11 Hz (240–660 breaths/min), with airway pressure monitored at the ETT.

The Babylog 8000 plus (Draeger Medical, Telford, PA) is a conventional ventilator with the option to ventilate in a high-frequency mode (high-frequency flow interruption). Small delivered tidal volumes are generated by rapidly switching the expiratory valve. The bias flow is up to 30 L/min. The ventilator can oscillate between 5 and 20 Hz (300–1,200 breaths/min). HFV can be applied during CPAP or SIMV.

Pediatric and Adult Devices

The Sensormedics 3100 A/B (Viasys, Yorba Linda, CA) is a device used for high-frequency oscillation ventilation (HFOV). Oscillations are generated with a diaphragm. Fresh gas is provided by a bias flow system, with frequencies ranging from 3 to 15 Hz (180–900 breaths/min). The Sensormedics 3100 A is used for neonates and infants, with bias flow ranging from 0 to 40 L/min and MAPs ranging from 3 to 45 cm H_2O. The Sensormedics 3100 B is approved for adults and larger children who weigh >35 kg. In comparison to the 3100A, the 3100B has a more powerful diaphragm, can provide a larger bias flow (0–60 L/min), and can apply higher MAPs of up to 55 cm H_2O. The Sensormedics 3100 A/B generates effective gas exchange in neonates, infants, and adults. Such devices have been evaluated in large, multicentered trials (8,22,23).

Mechanisms of Gas Exchange

The mechanisms of gas exchange during HFV are different from conventional ventilation. While HFV is frequently used in the clinical setting, it seems counterintuitive that this modality of ventilation produces adequate oxygenation and removal of CO_2. Of interest, species such as dogs are capable of spontaneous respiratory rates of 5–6 Hz (240–300 breaths/min) while they are panting. Despite the fact that tidal volumes approach the anatomic dead space, adequate gas exchange is still maintained (58). During HFV, gas exchange is achieved by a number of different mechanisms (**Fig. 34.9**). Although described as distinct modes in this chapter, all modes of gas exchange interact with each other during HFV of the architecturally unique human lung.

Ventilation of Alveolar Units with Short Path Lengths: Bulk Ventilation

When a small tidal volume is delivered, it may reach the proximal alveolar units with short path lengths by bulk ventilation, resulting in direct ventilation of this fraction of lung units. This mode of gas exchange closely resembles conventional ventilation, but only the most proximal and most compliant alveoli are ventilated directly in this fashion during HFV.

Ventilation in the Conducting Airways: Taylor Dispersion and Convective Dispersion

In 1953, Taylor first described the dispersion of particles in the presence of laminar flow (74). When the velocity of gas flow increases, the initial planar surface of a gas column transforms into a parabolic surface, allowing a greater deal of longitudinal mixing and dispersion. The center of the gas column is believed to travel faster than the outer areas, allowing further diffusion and mixing downstream. Turbulence that occurs when this gas column reaches a bifurcation will partly replace laminar mixing, resulting in dispersion of gas molecules and further contributing to gas exchange. Convective dispersion occurs when a uniform column of air is transformed into a parabolic shape. Air molecules undergo mixing as molecules in the center of the gas column move to the tip of the parabolic shape and the molecules near the wall stay behind.

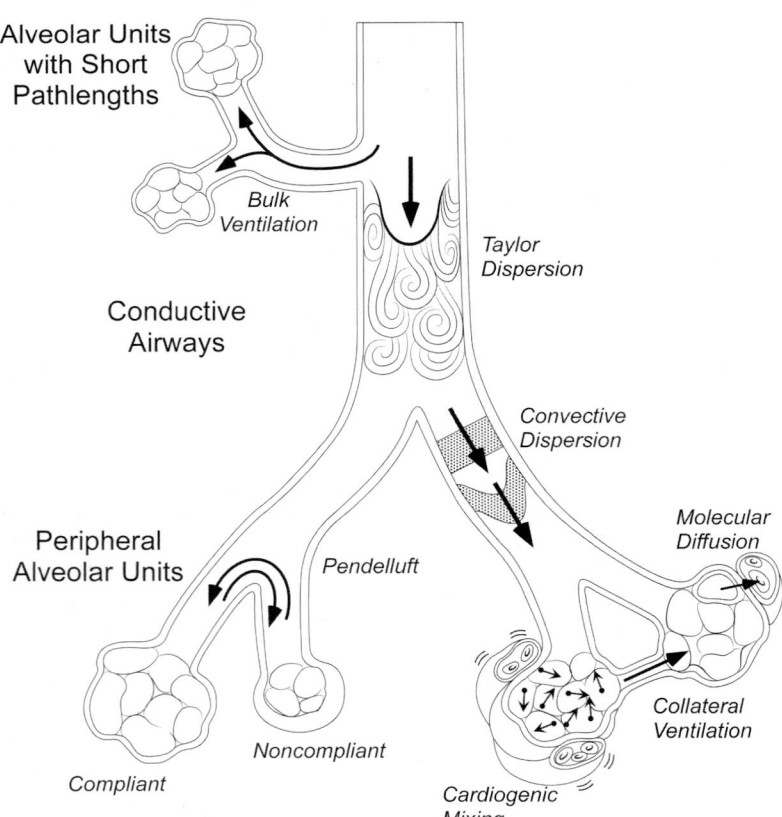

FIGURE 34.9. Mechanisms of gas exchange during high-frequency ventilation.

Ventilation of Peripheral Alveolar Units: Pendelluft and Collateral Ventilation

The heterogeneous nature of ARDS results in significant regional heterogeneity of lung mechanical properties: noncompliant, atelectatic areas are adjacent to compliant, overinflated areas. The regional time constant (τ = resistance × compliance) describes the rate of filling and emptying of a lung unit. Noncompliant areas fill and empty at a faster rate than compliant areas. Pendelluft (from the German: *pendel*, pendulum and *luft*, air) means that gas equilibrates between compliant and noncompliant lung units, resulting in regional mixing of gas. Pendelluft is an inspiratory and an expiratory phenomenon. At end expiration, air moves from the compliant to the noncompliant area, as the compliant area is still emptying when the noncompliant area is already empty. At end inspiration, air moves from the noncompliant area, which is already filled, to the compliant area, which is still filling (18). During HFV, this concept is believed to contribute to gas exchange, potentially ventilating areas otherwise not penetrated directly by HFV.

Collateral ventilation occurs between neighboring alveoli through collateral channels such as the interalveolar pores of Kohn. Collateral ventilation has been suggested as a mechanism of gas transport during HFV, although the high resistance of the collateral channels may limit the overall contribution to gas exchange during HFV (7).

Ventilation near the Alveolocapillary Membrane: Molecular Diffusion and Cardiogenic Mixing

Passive diffusion of gas molecules through the alveolocapillary membrane is the predominant form of gas transport during HFV and conventional ventilation in the peripheral lung units. Cardiac-induced pressure changes in the vascular bed add to gas mixing on the alveolar level. These mechanisms of gas exchange are not unique to HFV, as they also occur during conventional ventilation.

In summary, gas exchange during HFV is a function of several different mechanisms of gas transport in the conducting airways and alveolar units, which interact in a complex fashion. The various modes have a regional distribution: in the more proximal alveoli, direct ventilation of alveoli by bulk flow is predominant. In large airways such as the trachea and the left and right main stem, Taylor-type dispersion and convective dispersion take place. In the small peripheral airways and the alveoli, Pendelluft, collateral ventilation, molecular diffusion, and cardiogenic mixing play the main role (18).

Technical Description of High-frequency Ventilation

Alveolar Recruitment

Mean Airway Pressure. Alveolar recruitment is associated with improving gas exchange (56,67). Optimal lung volume during HFV has been described as the lowest MAP that achieves oxygenating efficiency and maintains lung volume (14). An increase in MAP during HFV is achieved by narrowing the orifice of the expiratory valve or by increasing the bias gas flow. MAP and pressure amplitude are significantly altered by the ETT (39). Decreasing the size of the ETT leads to a decrease of the

peak-to-trough pressure amplitude. The diameter and length of the ETT also affect MAP.

Distal airway pressures vary in response to changes in the I:E ratio during HFV. Data from animal models using alveolar capsules indicate that MAP is nonhomogeneously distributed throughout the lung. Air trapping occurs if the inspiratory time is increased at the expense of the expiratory time. Data from animal models further suggest that distal alveolar pressures can exceed proximal MAPs during I:E ratios >1:2 (2,3,39). This phenomenon has led to the recommendation that I:E ratios be limited to 1:2 in the clinical setting.

Carbon Dioxide Elimination

Alveolar Ventilation. Several investigators have shown that alveolar ventilation is a function of the rate of oscillations and the squared tidal volume ($V_{CO_2} = f \times V_T^2$) (13,49). Tidal volume contributes more to CO_2 elimination than frequency does, as tidal volume is squared in the formula. The relation between alveolar ventilation and tidal volume is further complicated by the branching generations of the tracheobronchial tree. In experimental studies using fluid models of branching tubes, the oscillatory diffusivity has been described as (18,38):

$$D_{osc} = f^{0.9} \times V_T^{2.2} \text{ and } D_{osc} = f^{1.4} \times V_T^{1.8}$$

In the clinical setting, it is appropriate to estimate alveolar ventilation as a product of the device frequency and the square of the delivered tidal volume.

Any maneuver that alters tidal volume will alter CO_2 removal. Increasing the amplitude leads to increasing tidal volumes and improves CO_2 elimination. Conversely, decreasing the amplitude decreases CO_2 elimination by directly decreasing delivered tidal volume.

Respiratory Frequency. During HFOV, the device frequency has a significant effect on delivered tidal volume. With an increasing respiratory rate, the inspiratory time is decreased and the oscillations of the diaphragm become less efficient, resulting in decreased delivered tidal volumes. As tidal volumes are more important than rate for CO_2 elimination, increasing the respiratory rate during HFV paradoxically diminishes CO_2 clearance. Conversely, decreasing the rate results in more efficient oscillations, larger tidal volumes, and improved CO_2 clearance.

The following clinical example illustrates the described relationship. During HFOV with the Sensormedics 3100, the inspiratory time is set as a percentage of the total respiratory cycle. If the inspiratory time is set at 33% and the rate is decreased from 10 Hz to 8 Hz, the inspiratory time increases from 33 msecs to 42 msecs. The increased inspiratory time at lower device frequency will lead to more efficient oscillations, increased delivered tidal volumes (**Fig. 34.10**), and increased CO_2 elimination.

Effect of an Endotracheal Tube Leak. Creating an ETT cuff leak has been suggested as an alternative way to enhance CO_2 clearance in the setting of hypercarbia despite a maximized amplitude and a low rate. The clearance enhancement will occur by promoting a path of CO_2 egress via a path outside of the ETT. After the ETT cuff has been deflated to produce a cuff leak, the proximal MAP will decrease. The expiratory valve or bias flow should be adjusted to maintain the same MAP for this maneuver to be effective (78).

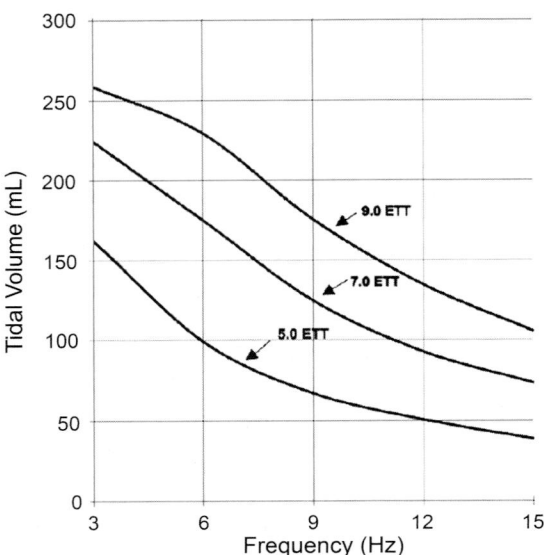

FIGURE 34.10. Tidal volumes (mL) and respiratory rate (Hz) during high-frequency oscillation ventilation with the Sensormedics 3100B (Viasys, Yorba Linda, CA). Increasing the rate leads to lower tidal volumes. Note the effect of the endotracheal tube size on tidal volumes. ETT, endotracheal tube. From the Sensormedics 3100B user manual, with permission.

WEANING FROM MECHANICAL VENTILATORY SUPPORT

Weaning of mechanical ventilatory support has traditionally been a mix of science and art. Although a relative consensus exists as to when mechanical ventilation should be initiated in the presence of respiratory insufficiency, the management of pediatric patients during recovery from respiratory failure remains largely subjective and is predominately determined by institutional or individual practices or preferences.

The median age of pediatric patients who receive mechanical ventilatory support is 1 year (36,65). The percentage of pediatric patients on mechanical ventilation for >12 hrs was 35% in one study (36), while only 17% required ventilation for >24 hrs in another report (65). The median duration of mechanical ventilation in these studies was 6–7 days. Of the patients who required mechanical ventilation, pneumonia (15%) and neurologic problems (14%) were reported as the underlying reason for initiation of mechanical ventilation.

As discussed earlier, mechanical ventilation in children can be subdivided into three phases: acute, maintenance, and weaning phases. The acute phase of mechanical ventilatory support includes primary lung recruitment. Once the lung is recruited and the patient's ventilatory support is decreased to levels that do not expose the patient to detrimental levels of inspired O_2 and distending volume ($FIO_2 \leq 0.6$; VT, 4–6 mL/kg; peak inspiratory pressure <35 cm H_2O), the patient goes into the maintenance phase. The maintenance phase refers to that period spent waiting for improvement in the disease process that led to the need for intubation. Usually, only FIO_2 and PEEP are actively adjusted during this period. The patient moves from the maintenance phase to the weaning phase when the patient

sends a signal (e.g., triggering the ventilator with spontaneous breathing efforts) to the clinician that weaning will be tolerated. Once weaning begins, the clinician must identify when the patient will tolerate removal of the ETT. The following discussion will review how weaning principles are applied to children.

The physiology of the WOB was discussed previously. To be successfully weaned off of the ventilator, the patient must be able to perform the WOB and have adequate neural control of airway reflexes.

Predictive Indices for Discontinuation from Mechanical Ventilatory Support

Mechanical ventilation is required for as long as the load on the respiratory pump exceeds its capacity. Predicting the success of weaning of pediatric patients from mechanical ventilation has been defined by using clinical signs and symptoms. Although an astute clinician might be able to predict the time that a patient is ready to start weaning, extubation failure still occurs in up to 24% of cases. Attempts have been made to devise some objective predictive indices that might help to identify the optimal time for extubation. These indices or parameters assess different physiologic functions of the respiratory system, including the differentiation between the elastic and resistive components of pulmonary dysfunction; defining alteration or limitation in inspiratory/expiratory airflow; determining the magnitude of driving pressure, work, and effort to maintain VT; and defining sequential changes to monitor the progression and resolution of the underlying disease process.

It is also likely that individual pulmonary mechanics or function-testing criteria per se might not have the same discriminatory power as composite parameters due to the multiple factors that influence successful withdrawal of mechanical ventilation. For this reason, it has been proposed that integrated indices that are a composite of two or more measurements may be more predictive of success. However, despite the inclusion of a variety of respiratory functions with good predictive value in adults, these integrated indices do not seem to be reliable predictors of success or failure in infants and children (28,51).

Clinical Trials of Weaning

A limited number of clinical trials of weaning from mechanical ventilation have been conducted in children. In adult patients, numerous studies, such as spontaneous breathing trials and respiratory therapist-driven protocols, have demonstrated the advantage of weaning strategies.

One trial studied 257 consecutive infants and children who received mechanical ventilation for at least 48 hrs and were deemed ready to undergo a breathing trial by their primary physician (35). Patients were randomly assigned to undergo a trial of breathing with either pressure support of 10 cm H_2O or a T piece. Bedside measurements of respiratory function were obtained immediately before discontinuation of mechanical ventilation and within the first 5 min of breathing through a T piece. The decision to extubate a patient at the end of the breathing trial was made by the primary clinician, who was unaware of the results of respiratory function measurements. Of 125 patients in the pressure-support group, 99 (79.2%) completed the breathing trial and were extubated, and 15.1% required reintubation within 48 hrs. Of the 132 patients in the T-piece group, 102 (77.5%) completed the breathing trial and were extubated, with 13 of them (12.7%) requiring reintubation within 48 hrs. The percentage of patients who remained extubated for 48 hrs after the breathing trial did not differ between groups (67.2% pressure support vs. 67.4% T piece, $p = 0.97$).

Process of Weaning

Weaning is a dynamic process that usually begins during patient recovery at some undefined point that is determined by the bedside physician. This subjective bias inevitably decreases the reproducibility of any study and makes results difficult to extrapolate to clinical practice. Standard indices for assessing patient weaning ability include (a) resolution of the etiology of respiratory failure and stable respiratory status; (b) decreased FIO_2 (usually to <50%) and decreased PEEP to 5 cm H_2O; (c) respiratory rate to <60 for infants <12 months of age, to <40 for preschool and school-aged children, and to <30 for adolescents; (d) no acidosis (pH <7.35) or hypercapnia (PCO_2 >60 torr). Other parameters that indirectly assess oxygenation and compliance include a P:F ratio of >267 (PaO_2 >80 torr on FIO_2 of 0.3), SpO_2 >94% on FIO_2 $\leq$0.5, peak inspiratory pressure <20 cm H_2O, PEEP $\leq$5 cm H_2O, combined with adequate respiratory muscle function, and hemodynamic stability without evidence of shock. These criteria include good perfusion (e.g., capillary refill <3 secs), age-appropriate blood pressure (above −2 SD cut-off for age), and good cardiac function (e.g., no requirement of infusions of vasoactive and/or inotropic medications, with the exception of dopamine $\leq$5 mcg/kg^{-1}/min^{-1}). Patients must be easily arousable to verbal or physical stimulation (e.g., pediatric Glasgow Coma Scale score of $\geq$11) and must be capable of moving an uninjured upper and lower extremity against gravity. Patients must also have acceptable serum potassium, magnesium, and phosphorous concentrations.

The individual who makes the decision to wean the patient may also have an impact on the length of mechanical ventilation. Decision making by respiratory care practitioners (RCPs) has long been felt to have the potential to reduce the length of mechanical ventilation because the respiratory therapist is more available to be at the bedside and perform frequent patient assessments. Respiratory therapist-driven weaning protocols are being examined as an alternative to current standard practices of weaning, which are physician-driven (29,48). RCPs classically perform diagnostic functions, such as blood gases, pulse oximetry, end-tidal CO_2 measurements, and airway function screenings; they also have the expertise to interpret these data. In a controlled trial of 300 adult patients who were randomized to daily screening and spontaneous breathing trials by RCPs, the intervention group had a 25% reduction in the median number of days of mechanical ventilation (29). A study of 223 pediatric patients demonstrated a decrease in total length of ventilation, weaning time, and time to extubation in patients weaned by an RCP-driven protocol versus physician-directed weaning (71).

Adjuncts to Weaning

Pharmacologic Agents

Routine administration of corticosteroids is a frequent adjunct for extubation. The anti-inflammatory effects of steroids form the basis of this approach. Two well-designed trials of dexamethasone therapy prior to extubation in children have unequivocally demonstrated that steroids reduce postextubation stridor (6,75). The inferences from these trials are strengthened because they were truly blinded studies. In contrast to the demonstrated effect on stridor, the effect of corticosteroids on reintubation is unclear. In one of the two studies, 7 of 32 patients who did not receive steroids required reintubation in contrast to 0 of 31 patients who received steroids. The trend in the second study was in the opposite direction, with 4 of 77 children who did not receive steroids and 9 of 76 who did receive steroids requiring reintubation. It is unclear why these studies demonstrated opposite results. Thus, while dexamethasone therapy may reduce stridor, no definitive evidence suggests that it reduces reintubation. Both of these trials found reintubation rates of >10% (6,75).

Heliox

After endotracheal extubation, upper and total airway resistances may frequently be increased, resulting in high inspiratory effort to breathe. A few patients, ranging from 5% to 16%, develop postextubation airway obstruction and frank respiratory distress (6). In addition, a substantial number of patients develop inspiratory distress after extubation, leading to reintubation (31,32). In these patients, an increase in upper airway and total inspiratory resistance may contribute to this respiratory distress. As discussed earlier, infants and children have both anatomic and physiologic differences from adults that predispose them to airway edema and dysfunction.

Helium-oxygen (HeO_2) mixture (heliox) has a low density and a high kinematic viscosity, allowing for a reduction in airway resistance. Some studies showed that it could have beneficial effects in the treatment of upper airway obstruction (57). The use of HeO_2 mixture in adults (10) and in children (26) with upper airway obstruction has been reported in several anecdotal series and a few studies, and it has become one of the more accepted indications for HeO_2 use (57). Although the effects of heliox have been shown predominantly by observational studies, the fact that the immediate improvement obtained with HeO_2 breathing was reversed when it was discontinued even briefly suggested an independent beneficial effect of the gas related to its physical properties.

Noninvasive Mechanical Ventilatory Support

The process of discontinuing mechanical ventilation must balance the risk of complications due to unnecessary delays in extubation with the risk of complications due to premature discontinuation and the need for reintubation. The use of noninvasive positive-pressure ventilation is a promising therapy after failure of extubation but has not yet been shown to reduce the need for reintubation or reduce post-intubation mortality

(33). In principle, as most pediatric patients require reintubation due to poor or excessive effort (68), noninvasive support may allow the patient to bridge to extubation.

While noninvasive ventilation is a valuable technique for ventilatory support in pediatric patients, is has limitations that can cause it to fail. For noninvasive ventilatory support to function properly, the mask or nasal prongs must adequately seal to the patient. The varying physical sizes and the lack of tolerance of masks, or even prongs, can limit the utility of noninvasive ventilation in children. The variety of devices that are available for noninvasive support seems to be addressing some of these issues. Success with noninvasive techniques has been reported to avoid the need for tracheal intubation in some groups, such as immunosuppressed patients with asthma or respiratory insufficiency. However, no study to date has proven that noninvasive ventilation is superior to tracheal intubation and conventional mechanical ventilation. Some clinicians assert that use of noninvasive ventilation in acute respiratory failure merely prolongs the time to tracheal intubation and thus may be of little benefit; these claims have also not been demonstrated. One form of noninvasive ventilation that seems to be increasing in popularity is the use of high-flow nasal cannula therapy. In studies of premature infants, use of support devices, such as Vapotherm, has shown equivalent changes in WOB and lower-airway pressure measurements as those provided by continuous positive-pressure ventilation using nasal prongs.

Recognition of Weaning Failure

Failure of weaning can be categorized by increased respiratory load or decreased respiratory capacity. Increased respiratory load is represented by increased elastic load (unresolved lung disease, secondary pneumonia, abdominal distension, and hyperinflated lungs), increased resistive load (thickened airway secretions, partially occluded ETT, upper airway obstruction), or increased minute ventilation (pain and irritability, sepsis/hyperthermia, metabolic acidosis). Decreased respiratory capacity is represented by decreased respiratory drive (sedation, central nervous system infection, traumatic brain injury, hypocapnia/alkalosis), muscular dysfunction [muscular catabolism and weakness (malnutrition), severe electrolyte disturbances], and neuromuscular disorder (diaphragmatic dysfunction, prolonged neuromuscular blockade, cervical spinal injury).

Extubation failure with subsequent reintubation in pediatric patients ranges between 14% and 24% (34–36,68). In a study of 632 pediatric patients, the failure rate of planned extubation was 4.9%. The rate of failure increased with the length of time patients received mechanical ventilation, with patients ventilated for >24 hrs having a failure rate of 6.0% and those ventilated for >48 hrs having a failure rate of 7.9% (27). Predicting extubation outcome in patients is usually based upon clinical judgment. However, attempts have been made to identify specific predictors of extubation failure. The success of these predictors has been mixed. Investigators adapted adult integrated indices to pediatric patients by normalizing the VT and dynamic compliance to body weight (11). Extubation failure was defined as reintubation within 24 hrs; the failure rate was 19%.

A study of 208 pediatric patients who were ventilated for at least 24 hrs identified criteria for low risk (<10%) and high risk (25%) of extubation failure on the basis of direct measurements of pulmonary function (51). For this study, the rate of patients who required reintubation within 48 hrs (excluding those who failed secondary to upper-airway obstruction) was 16.3%. Thirty-four of the 208 patients studied were reintubated, for an overall failure rate of 16.3%. Of the patients who failed extubation, 65% required reintubation secondary to poor or excessive effort. Extubation failure increased significantly with decreasing VT indexed to body weight of a spontaneous breath, increasing FIO_2, increasing MAP, increasing oxygenation index, increasing fraction of total minute ventilation provided by the ventilator, increasing peak ventilatory inspiratory pressure, or decreasing mean inspiratory flow.

Advances in Weaning

To wean patients optimally and ensure patient comfort, ventilator adjustments must be made moment to moment in response to the patient's immediate physiologic needs. It is, of course, unrealistic for any member of the medical, nursing, or respiratory care staffs to perform in this manner. In response to this need for improved patient-ventilator interactions, some researchers have experimented, with promising results, with an interactive, computer-directed, closed-loop weaning system (72,73,77).

Weaning from mechanical ventilation remains a complex and poorly standardized area of respiratory care. Technical advancements in integration of patient effort and mechanical response have great potential to revolutionize this field to the benefit of patients.

CONCLUSIONS AND FUTURE DIRECTIONS

Mechanical ventilation can be considered as it relates to the issues of (a) equipment utilized to support the patient, (b) our understanding of what reduces potential iatrogenic lung injury and maintenance of the patients normal physiology, and (c) how best to make decisions concerning the initiation, level of support, and removal of mechanical ventilatory support. The equipment used for mechanical ventilation continues to evolve, including new modes and interfaces between the patient and the ventilator. Traditionally, the site of the signal from the patient to the ventilator has been at either the patient's airway or at the ventilator. New technologies are being evaluated that would allow the signal to be acquired as it moves from the patient's brain to the diaphragm. This technique will allow for a quantification of the patient's respiratory effort and thus regulate the level of support delivered by the ventilator to the patient's effort.

Further research is required to better understand the complex issues concerning how the lung is injured during positive-pressure mechanical ventilation. We have finally begun to understand what injures the lung, but it is still not clear how best to apply this knowledge to ventilation of critically ill patients to help prevent ongoing injury. The development of databases and collaborative groups such as the ARDSnet, the PALISI network, and the Pediatric Critical Care Research Network have great potential to enlist large groups of patients toward answering these many questions. Technically improved monitoring devices to study lung mechanics and the effects of treatment are also becoming available. Reliability and acceptance of research efforts will have an important impact on the use of mechanical ventilation in the future. Efforts at reducing or eliminating secondary lung damage from infection and other inciting causes may also change the landscape of the types of patients who require mechanical ventilation.

Before weaning from the ventilator can become more of a science and less of an art, more knowledge is required to define the optimal method of separating the patient from mechanical ventilation once their disease process improves.

KEY POINTS

- The lung-ventilator unit can be thought of as a tube with a balloon network on the end, with the tube representing the ventilator tubing, ETT, and airways and the balloon network representing the alveoli.
- To generate gas flow, the total forces must overcome the resistive forces of the airway, the ventilator tubing, and the ETT to allow gas to flow into or out of the lung, depending on driving pressure gradients
- The *equation of motion* for the respiratory system relates how volume (ΔV), pressure (ΔP), and flow ($\dot{V}$) interact to move gas into and out of the lung:

$$\Delta P = \Delta V/C + \dot{V} \cdot R + k$$

where R is the airway resistance, C is the lung compliance, and k is a constant that defines end-expiratory pressure.
- The manner in which each variable (pressure, volume, or flow) is controlled, described as the *mode of ventilation*, determines how the ventilator delivers the mechanical breath.
- Compliance relates to the ease of inflation of lung units and is determined by:

$$\text{Compliance} = \Delta\text{ Volume } / \Delta\text{ Pressure}$$

- In PC ventilation, the pressure pattern is "square," but flow increases rapidly at the beginning of the inspiratory phase to generate the set pressure limit and then decays exponentially over the inspiratory time. This flow pattern is described as *decelerating flow*.
- Clinicians often choose PC ventilation in patients with poor compliance, although the true benefit of PC versus other modes has not been well established in animal or clinical studies.
- If the clinician sets volume as a function of time, pressure then varies with compliance. Volume is the independent variable, and pressure is the dependent variable.
- Understanding the factors involved in tidal volume measurement and how they are determined in different ventilators and techniques is important in patient management.
- The volume of gas that becomes compressed within the ventilator tubing and never reaches the patient is termed the *compressible volume of the circuit*.
- When compression volume is accounted for in determination of patient VT, the resultant volume is termed the *effective tidal volume*, which means that this is the tidal volume that reaches the patient's lungs.
- Effective tidal volume (eVT) can be calculated as:

$$\text{eVT} = (\text{VT}_E) - [\text{circuit compensation} \times (\text{PI}_{max}) - \text{PEEP}]$$

- While measuring tidal volume at the airway opening may give the best estimate of tidal volume in the lungs, this

can be associated with problems such as losing air around uncuffed ETTs, unreliable measuring sensors, and potential extubation from the weight of the measuring device.
- The manner in which each variable (pressure, volume, or flow) is controlled, described as the *mode of ventilation*, determines how the ventilator delivers the mechanical breath.
- *Control* variables are the independent variables that are either pressure, volume, or flow. *Conditional* variables are determinants of a response to a preset threshold which are both clinician-set and influenced by dependent and independent variables. *Phase* variables are those that are used to start, sustain, and end the phase.
- Most ventilators cannot directly measure volume; rather, they calculate volume delivered from flow that occurs over a period of time.
- Studies have shown that the ventilator-displayed VT, without software compensation for circuit compliance, generally overestimates the true delivered VT. Conversely, when the circuit-compliance compensation feature is on, the ventilator-displayed VT generally underestimates the true delivered VT.
- The NAVA approach to mechanical ventilation is based on the acquisition of the patient's neural respiratory output as it is transmitted through the phrenic nerve to the diaphragm.
- In infants, the fact that lung volume may increase at a greater rate than airway diameter may be one reason why infants are especially prone to air trapping and hyperinflation.
- The high compliance and low elastic recoil of the infant/young child's chest wall results in increased WOB to move the same tidal volume as an adult.
- Patient-ventilator asynchrony is a result of factors related to ventilator triggering, adequacy of flow delivery, adequate breath termination, and effects of PEEP and/or PEEP$_i$.
- The goal of mechanical ventilatory support is not to normalize the patient's blood gases at the cost of ventilator-induced lung injury.
- For patients with obstructive lung disease, lung protection may include a lower tidal volume and prolonged exhalation times. A support mode with spontaneous breathing may also be useful.
- In patients with poor compliance, maintaining lung recruitment without excessive distending volume changes in pressure to distend the alveoli and end-expiratory pressure may limit ventilator-induced lung injury.
- Lung injury prevention is directed toward reducing cyclic collapse and re-expansion of alveoli due to inadequate PEEP.
- Widespread use of low tidal volumes may result in reabsorption atelectasis in basal lung areas. This effect can be enhanced by the use of high inhaled O_2 concentrations. PEEP may be protective in these circumstances.
- It is important not to be misled by an improvement of oxygenation alone as a measure of lung recruitment. An increase in PEEP can reduce cardiac output and increase PaO_2 despite a decrease in O_2 delivery.
- The effect of PEEP is as a distending pressure to increase the FRC (volume of gas at the end of exhalation in the lung).
- The peak inspiratory pressure in PC ventilation is usually lower than in VC ventilation.

- PC ventilation does not guarantee minute ventilation. Worsened compliance or resistance in the patient will result in decreased VT.

- Tidal volume is assured in VC ventilation.

- The constant flow pattern in VC may not meet patient demands, especially in patients with poorly compliant lungs.

- APRV is a high-level CPAP mode that is terminated for brief periods.

- Dexamethasone, heliox, and noninvasive ventilation may be helpful in preventing intubation or reintubation in patients with respiratory illness.

- Bulk convection, pendelluft, Taylor dispersion, convective dispersion, cardiogenic mixing, collateral ventilation, and molecular diffusion are distinct modes of gas exchange that interact with each other during HFOV.

- Increasing the MAP increases alveolar recruitment and oxygenation during HFOV.

- Alveolar ventilation is a function of the rate of oscillations and the squared tidal volume ($V_{CO2} = f \times VT^2$).

- Tidal volume delivery and CO_2 elimination are directly related to the peak-to-trough pressure amplitude, and negatively correlated with device frequency.

- The presence of an ETT cuff leak may further contribute to CO_2 clearance.

References

1. Acute Respiratory Distress Syndrome Network. Ventilation with lower tidal volumes as compared with traditional tidal volumes for acute lung injury and the acute respiratory distress syndrome. N Engl J Med 2000;342:1301–8.
2. Allen JL, Frantz ID, 3rd, Fredberg JJ. Heterogeneity of mean alveolar pressure during high-frequency oscillations. J Appl Physiol 1987;62:223–8.
3. Allen JL, Fredberg JJ, Keefe DH, et al. Alveolar pressure magnitude and asynchrony during high-frequency oscillations of excised rabbit lungs. Am Rev Respir Dis 1985;132:343–9.
4. Allo JC, Beck JC, Brander L, et al. Influence of neurally adjusted ventilatory assist and positive end-expiratory pressure on breathing pattern in rabbits with acute lung injury. Crit Care Med 2006;34(12):2997–3004.
5. Alsaati BZ, Thurman TL, Holt S, et al. Reliability of measured tidal volume in mechanically ventilated pediatric patient in the PICU (abstract). PAS 2005;57:2421.
6. Anene O, Meert KL, Uy H, et al. Dexamethasone for the prevention of postextubation airway obstruction: A prospective, randomized, double-blind, placebo-controlled trial. Crit Care Med 1996;24:1666–9.
7. Armengol J, Jones RL, King EG. Collateral ventilation during high-frequency oscillation in dogs. J Appl Physiol 1985;58:173–9.
8. Arnold JH, Hanson JH, Toro-Figuero LO, et al. Prospective, randomized comparison of high-frequency oscillatory ventilation and conventional mechanical ventilation in pediatric respiratory failure. Crit Care Med 1994;22:1530–9.
9. Banner MJ, Downs JB, Kirby RR, et al. Effects of expiratory flow resistance on inspiratory work of breathing. Chest 1988;93:795–9.
10. Barach A. The use of helium in the treatment of asthma and obstructive lesions in the larynx and trachea. Ann Intern Med 1935;9:739–65.
11. Baumeister BL, el-Khatib M, Smith PG, et al. Evaluation of predictors of weaning from mechanical ventilation in pediatric patients. Pediatr Pulmonol 1997;24:344–52.
12. Beydon L, Chasse M, Harf A, et al. Inspiratory work of breathing during spontaneous ventilation using demand valves and continuous flow systems. Am Rev Respir Dis 1988;138:300–4.
13. Boynton BR, Hammond MD, Fredberg JJ, et al. Gas exchange in healthy rabbits during high-frequency oscillatory ventilation. J Appl Physiol 1989;66:1343–51.
14. Brazelton TB, 3rd, Watson KF, Murphy M, et al. Identification of optimal lung volume during high-frequency oscillatory ventilation using respiratory inductive plethysmography. Crit Care Med 2001;29:2349–59.
15. Cannon ML, Cornell J, Tripp-Hamel DS, et al. Tidal volumes for ventilated infants should be determined with a pneumotachometer placed at the endotracheal tube. Am J Respir Crit Care Med 2000;162:2109–12.
16. Carmack J, Torres A, Anders M, et al. Comparison of inspiratory work of breathing in young lambs during flow triggered and pressure triggered ventilation. Respir Care 1995;40:28–34.
17. Castle RA, Dunne CJ, Mok Q, et al. Accuracy of displayed values of tidal volume in the pediatric intensive care unit. Crit Care Med 2002;30:2566–74.
18. Chang HK. Mechanisms of gas transport during ventilation by high-frequency oscillation. J Appl Physiol 1984;56:553–63.
19. Chao DC, Scheinhorn DJ, Stearn-Hassenpflug M. Patient-ventilator trigger asynchrony in prolonged mechanical ventilation. Chest 1997;112:1592–9.
20. Chatburn RL. Classification of mechanical ventilators. Respir Care 1992;37:1009–25.
21. Chu EK, Whitehead T, Slutsky AS. Effects of cyclic opening and closing at low- and high-volume ventilation on bronchoalveolar lavage cytokines. Crit Care Med 2004;32:168–74.
22. Courtney SE, Durand DJ, Asselin JM, et al. High-frequency oscillatory ventilation versus conventional mechanical ventilation for very-low-birth-weight infants. N Engl J Med 2002;347:643–52.
23. Derdak S, Mehta S, Stewart TE, et al. High-frequency oscillatory ventilation for acute respiratory distress syndrome in adults: A randomized, controlled trial. Am J Respir Crit Care Med 2002;166:801–8.
24. Deoras KS, Wolfson MR, Bhutani VK, et al. Structural changes in the trachea of preterm lambs induced by ventilation. Pediatr Res 1989;26:434–7.
25. Dreyfuss D, Saumon G. Barotrauma is volutrauma, but which volume is the one responsible? Intensive Care Med 1992;18:139–41.
26. Duncan P. Efficacy of helium-oxygen mixtures in the management of severe viral and post-intubation croup. Can Anaesth Soc J 1979;26:206–12.
27. Edmunds S, Weiss I, Harrison R. Extubation failure in a large pediatric ICU population. Chest 2001;119(3):897–900.
28. El-Khatib M, Jamaleddine G, Soubra R, et al. Pattern of spontaneous breathing: Potential marker for weaning outcome. Spontaneous breathing pattern and weaning from mechanical ventilation. Intensive Care Med 2001;27(1):52–8.
29. Ely EW, Baker AM, Dunagan DP, et al. Effects on the duration of mechanical ventilation of identifying patients capable of breathing spontaneously. N Engl J Med 1996;335(25):1864–9.
30. Engle WA, Yoder MC, Andreoli SP, et al. Controlled, prospective, randomized comparison of high-frequency jet ventilation and conventional ventilation in neonates with respiratory failure and persistent pulmonary hypertension. J Perinatol 1997;17:3–9.
31. Epstein SK, Ciubotaru RL, Wong JB. Effect of failed extubation on the outcome of mechanical ventilation. Chest 1997;112:186–92.
32. Epstein SK, Ciubotaru RL. Independent effects of etiology of failure and time to reintubation on outcome for patients failing extubation. Am J Respir Crit Care Med 1998;158:489–93.
33. Esteban A, Frutos-Vivar F, Ferguson ND, et al. Noninvasive positive-pressure ventilation for respiratory failure after extubation. New Engl J Med 2004;350(24):2452–60.
34. Farias JA, Alia I, Retta A, et al. An evaluation of extubation failure predictors in mechanically ventilated infants and children. Intensive Care Med 2002;28(6):752–7.
35. Farias JA, Retta A, Alía I, et al. A comparison of two methods to perform a breathing trial before extubation in pediatric intensive care patients. Intensive Care Med 2001;27(10):1649–54.
36. Farias JA, Frutos F, Esteban A, et al. What is the daily practice of mechanical ventilation in pediatric intensive care units? For the International Group of Mechanical Ventilation in Children. Intensive Care Med 2004;30:918–25.
37. Figueras J, Rodriguez-Miguelez JM, Botet F, et al. Changes in TcPCO2 regarding pulmonary mechanics due to pneumotachometer dead space in ventilated newborns. J Perinat Med 1997;25:333–9.
38. Fletcher PR, Epstein RA. Constancy of physiological dead space during high-frequency ventilation. Respir Physiol 1982;47:39–49.
39. Gerstmann DR, Fouke JM, Winter DC, et al. Proximal, tracheal, and alveolar pressures during high-frequency oscillatory ventilation in a normal rabbit model. Pediatr Res 1990;28:367–73.
40. Guttmann J, Haberthur C, Mols G. Automatic tube compensation. Respir Care Clin N Am 2001;7:475–501, x.
41. Hernandez LA, Peevy KJ, Moise AA, et al. Chest wall restriction limits high airway pressure-induced lung injury in young rabbits. J Appl Physiol 1989;66:2364–8.
42. Heulitt MJ, Anders M, Benham D. Acute respiratory distress syndrome in pediatric patients: Redirecting therapy to reduce iatrogenic lung injury. Respir Care 1995;40:74–85.
43. Heulitt MJ, Bohn D. Lung-protective strategy in pediatric patients with acute respiratory distress syndrome. Respir Care 1998;43:952–60.
44. Heulitt MJ, Holt SJ, Thurman TL, et al. Reliability of measured tidal volume in mechanically ventilated young pigs with normal lungs. Intensive Care Med 2005;31:1255–61.
45. Heulitt MJ, Torres A, Anders M, et al. Comparison of total resistive work of breathing in two generations of ventilators in an animal model. Pediatr Pulmonol 1996;22:58–66.
46. Heulitt MJ, Wankum P, Holt S, et al. Evaluation of the effects of an active exhalation valve and changing cycle offtime during pressure support ventilation in a neonatal animal model (abstract). Pediatric Research 2003;53:2711.
47. Holt SJ, Sanders RC, Thurman TL, et al. An evaluation of Automode, a computer-controlled ventilator mode, with the Siemens Servo 300A ventilator, using a porcine model. Respir Care 2001;46:26–36.
48. Horst HM, Mouro, D, Hall-Jenssens, RA, Pamukov, N. Decrease in ventilation time with a standardized weaning process. Arch Surg 1998;133:483–9.

49. Kamitsuka MD, Boynton BR, Villanueva D, et al. Frequency, tidal volume, and mean airway pressure combinations that provide adequate gas exchange and low alveolar pressure during high frequency oscillatory ventilation in rabbits. *Pediatr Res* 1990;27:64–9.
50. Keszler M, Donn SM, Bucciarelli RL, et al. Multicenter controlled trial comparing high-frequency jet ventilation and conventional mechanical ventilation in newborn infants with pulmonary interstitial emphysema. *J Pediatr* 1991;119:85–93.
51. Khan N, Brown A, Venkataraman ST. Predictors of extubation success and failure in mechanically ventilated infants and children. *Crit Care Med* 1996;24(9):1568–79.
52. Kondili E, Prinianakis G, Georgopoulos D. Patient-ventilator interaction. *Br J Anaesth* 2003;91:106–19.
53. Lanteri CJ, Sly PD. Changes in respiratory mechanics with age. *J Appl Physiol* 1993;74:369–78.
54. Leung P, Jubran A, Tobin MJ. Comparison of assisted ventilator modes on triggering, patient effort, and dyspnea. *Am J Respir Crit Care Med* 1997; 155:1940–8.
55. MacIntyre NR, Ho LI. Effects of initial flow rate and breath termination criteria on pressure support ventilation. *Chest* 1991;99:134–8.
56. Maggiore SM, Jonson B, Richard JC, et al. Alveolar derecruitment at decremental positive end-expiratory pressure levels in acute lung injury: Comparison with the lower inflection point, oxygenation, and compliance. *Am J Respir Crit Care Med* 2001;164:795–801.
57. Manthous CA, Morgan S, Pohlman A, Hall JB. Heliox in the treatment of airflow obstruction: A critical review of the literature. *Respir Care* 1997; 42:1034–42.
58. Meyer M, Hahn G, Buess C, et al. Pulmonary gas exchange in panting dogs. *J Appl Physiol* 1989;66:1258–63.
59. Neve V, Leclerc F, Noizet O, et al. Influence of respiratory system impedance on volume and pressure delivered at the Y piece in ventilated infants. *Pediatr Crit Care Med* 2003;4:418–25.
60. Nilsestuen JO, Hargett KD. Using ventilator graphics to identify patient-ventilator asynchrony. *Respir Care* 2005;50:202–34; discussion 32–4.
61. Nishimura M, Hess D, Kacmarek RM. The response of flow-triggered infant ventilators. *Am J Respir Crit Care Med* 1995;152:1901–9.
62. Otis AB, Fenn WO, Rahn H. Mechanics of breathing in man. *J Appl Physiol* 1950;2:592–607.
63. Penn RB, Wolfson MR, Shaffer TH. Effect of ventilation on mechanical properties and pressure-flow relationships of immature airways. *Pediatr Res* 1988;23:519–24.
64. Pillow JJ. High-frequency oscillatory ventilation: Mechanisms of gas exchange and lung mechanics. *Crit Care Med* 2005;33:S135–41.
65. Randolph AG, Meert KL, O'Neil ME, et al. Pediatric Acute Lung Injury and Sepsis Investigators Network. The feasibility of conducting clinical trials in infants and children with acute respiratory failure. *Am J Respir Crit Care Med* 2003;167:1334–40.
66. Ranieri VM. Optimization of patient-ventilator interactions: Closed-loop technology to turn the century. *Intensive Care Med* 1997;23:936–9.
67. Ranieri VM, Eissa NT, Corbeil C, et al. Effects of positive end-expiratory pressure on alveolar recruitment and gas exchange in patients with the adult respiratory distress syndrome. *Am Rev Respir Dis* 1991;144:544–51.
68. Randolph AG, Wypij D, Venkataraman ST, et al. Pediatric Acute Lung Injury and Sepsis Investigators (PALISI) Network. Effect of mechanical ventilator weaning protocols on respiratory outcomes in infants and children: A randomized controlled trial. *JAMA* 2002;288(20):2561–8.
69. Sanders RC, Jr. , Thurman TL, Holt SJ, et al. Work of breathing associated with pressure support ventilation in two different ventilators. *Pediatr Pulmonol* 2001;32:62–70.
70. Sassoon CS. Mechanical ventilator design and function: The trigger variable. *Respir Care* 1992;37:1056–69.
71. Schultz TR, Lin RJ, Watzman M, et al. Weaning children from mechanical ventilation: A prospective randomized trial of protocol directed versus physician directed weaning. *Respiratory Care* 2001;46(8):772–82.
72. Strickland JH Jr, Hasson JH. A computer-controlled ventilator weaning system. *Chest* 1991;100:1096–9.
73. Strickland JH Jr, Hasson JH. A computer-controlled ventilator weaning system. A clinical trial. *Chest* 1993;103:1220–6.
74. Taylor GI. The dispersion of soluble matter in solvent flowing slowly through a tube. *Proc R Soc London* 1953;223:446–68.
75. Tellez, DW, Galvis, AG, Storgion, SA, et al. Dexamethasone in the prevention of postextubation stridor in children. *J Pediatr* 1991;118:289–94.
76. Tokioka H, Tanaka T, Ishizu T, et al. The effect of breath termination criterion on breathing patterns and the work of breathing during pressure support ventilation. *Anesth Analg* 2001;92:161–5.
77. Tong DA. Weaning patients from mechanical ventilation. A knowledge-based system approach. *Comput Methods Programs Biomed* 1991;35(4):267–78.
78. Van de Kieft M, Dorsey D, Morison D, et al. High-frequency oscillatory ventilation: Lessons learned from mechanical test lung models. *Crit Care Med* 2005;33:S142–7.
79. Wolfson MR, Bhutani VK, Shaffer TH, et al. Mechanics and energetics of breathing helium in infants with bronchopulmonary dysplasia. *J Pediatr* 1984;104:752–7.

CHAPTER 35 ■ INHALED GASES

ANGELA T. WRATNEY • DONNA S. HAMEL • IRA M. CHEIFETZ

The provision of inhaled gases provides a therapeutic resource fundamental to the management of respiratory disease in critical care medicine. The clinical and pathophysiologic processes associated with respiratory failure are directly targeted by medical gases used in the PICU. Therefore, critical care personnel must be familiar with the following inhaled medical gases and medications: (a) O_2, (b) inhaled nitric oxide (iNO), (c) helium-oxygen mixtures (heliox), (d) inhaled bronchodilators, (e) hypoxic gas mixtures, (f) exogenous CO_2 administration, and (g) inhalational anesthetics. This chapter includes a discussion of the pharmacologic and therapeutic mechanisms, the appropriate delivery system technology, and important considerations for each of the inhaled therapies used in the PICU.

The nasal passages and upper airway warm, humidify, and filter air for the respiratory system. Thus, in the provision of inhaled gas therapies that bypass the upper airway or are administered with high pressure or flow, careful attention to temperature control, humidification, and infection control is warranted. Failure to do so may result in hypothermia, inspissated secretions, and airway injury and potentially contribute to the development of ventilator-associated pneumonia (8).

Administration of inhaled medical gases also requires environmental safeguards. For some gases (iNO and inhalational anesthetics), specialized gas-scavenging equipment is required to prevent contamination of the ambient air, while other gas therapies, due to their ability to support combustion, must be delivered in a well-ventilated area with frequent turnover of the ambient air. The risk of fire, although rare, may be increased in underventilated areas, such as under occlusive drapes (i.e., during sterile procedures), or during procedures that utilize electrical devices (e.g., electrocautery units). As with any medical therapy, administration of inhaled gas therapies requires staff education, safety training, and compliance with local and governmental regulations.

OXYGEN

The percent fraction of inspired oxygen (FIO_2) in ambient air is 21%. For medical use, 100% oxygen is mass produced from fractional distillation of atmospheric air. O_2 is provided to patients with impaired respiratory function to improve arterial saturation, to vasodilate the pulmonary capillary bed, and to enhance systemic oxygen delivery.

Oxygen Metabolism

O_2 is essential for cellular aerobic metabolism. Oxidative phosphorylation of NADH within the mitochondria generates 36 moles of ATP for every mole of glucose consumed. Under anaerobic conditions, glycolysis consumes energy stores and results in the production of lactic acid.

During the process of normal cellular metabolism, reactive oxygen species (ROS), such as the superoxide anion (O_2^-), O_2 radical ($O_2\bullet$), hydroxyl radical (OH^-), and hydrogen peroxide (H_2O_2), are produced. ROS cause oxidative injury to proteins, DNA, and lipids. Organs rich in lipids and proteins, such as the pulmonary and central nervous system, are especially at risk. Endogenous antioxidant enzyme systems, such as superoxide dismutase (SOD), glutathione peroxidase, and catalase, attempt to clear ROS to limit cellular injury (**Table 35.1**). SOD converts superoxide and hydrogen to O_2 and H_2O_2, while catalase detoxifies this product into H_2O and O_2. Glutathione peroxidase binds oxygen radicals with lipids to produce lipid hydroxides and water. Additional endogenous scavengers include cholesterol, α-tocopherol (vitamin E), ascorbic acid (vitamin C), selenium, and bilirubin.

Antioxidant defense systems may be overwhelmed when exposed to high FIO_2 or during prolonged O_2 exposure. Individual patient susceptibility to O_2 toxicity may derive from variations in the duration and fractional percent of O_2 exposure, the underlying disease state, antioxidant availability, and individual genetic variations (27).

Oxygen Delivery Systems

Dependent on the desired FIO_2, a variety of devices exist for administering supplemental O_2 (**Table 35.2**). The flow provided by the O_2 delivery system will either be sufficient to meet the inspiratory flow needs of the patient (high-flow systems), or it will be insufficient (low-flow systems), causing the patient to entrain additional room air flow. High-flow delivery systems provide a more stable, measurable delivery of the FIO_2 independent of patient respiratory effort. High-flow delivery devices can be used with masks, tracheostomy collars, nebulizers, and O_2 tents or hoods. Low-flow systems include nasal cannulae, simple face masks, or face masks with a reservoir (non-rebreather or partial rebreather).

Nasal Cannulae

The nasal cannulae provide a comfortable, lightweight, and inexpensive method for low-flow O_2 delivery (0.1–6 L/min). FIO_2 delivery ranges between 24% and 50%. Although variable in the actual FIO_2 delivered, a general "rule of thumb" states that for each liter of supplemental O_2 provided, the inspired O_2 concentration increases by ~4% (5). Rapid respiratory rates, higher tidal volumes, and shorter inspiratory times cause increased air dilution and reduce the actual inspired FIO_2. Two caveats bear mentioning for use of nasal cannulae in the infant: (a) when administering low flow (e.g., flow <1 L), the actual

TABLE 35.1

REACTIVE OXYGEN SPECIES AND THE ENDOGENOUS ANTIOXIDANT
DEFENSE SYSTEMS

Reactive oxygen species	Chemical symbol	Antioxidant defense(s)
Superoxide anion	O_2^-	Superoxide dismutase
Hydrogen peroxide	H_2O_2	Glutathione peroxidase and catalase
Hydroxyl radical	$OH \cdot$	Nonenzymatic mechanisms (e.g., vitamin C)

flow and FIO_2 provided may be highly inaccurate due to the frequent occurrence of system leaks, displaced nasal prongs, and the limitations in flow meter calibration; and (b) when administering higher flow (e.g., >2 L), the infant may receive a significant degree of support from the high-inspired FIO_2 and/or the positive end-expiratory pressure (PEEP) produced (36).

Face Masks

Simple face masks fit over the patient's nose and mouth, providing an FIO_2 delivery of between 35% and 55% O_2. A nonrebreathing face mask consists of a simple face mask adapted with a reservoir bag and an inflow system for fresh gas infusion to increase FIO_2 delivery to close to 100% O_2. Two one-way valves, located between the mask and the reservoir and at one of the side exhalation ports, ensure that each inspiratory breath consists of fresh gas and that exhaled gas is eliminated without entrainment of room air. As a safety mechanism, the other side exhalation port is kept open to allow the entrainment of room air in the event that gas flow to the mask system is interrupted. Similarly, a partial rebreathing mask consists of a mask with an attached reservoir bag and an inflow gas source. However, the system lacks the unidirectional valve between the face mask and the reservoir. Thus, it allows the mixing of the exhaled CO_2 gas from the patient with the O_2 in the reservoir bag. To avoid rebreathing exhaled CO_2, the inspired gas flow rate should be maintained at or above 6 L/min.

Venturi masks are high-flow systems that provide fixed concentrations of 24%, 28%, 31%, 35%, 40%, or 50% O_2. These concentrations are obtained by delivering manufacturer-recommended flow rates necessary to generate specific oxygen-to-air entrainment ratios. The flow velocity of O_2 entering the mask causes the entrainment of air through side ports in the device. Dependable O_2 concentrations are administered as long as total gas flow exceeds the patient's peak inspiratory flow.

TABLE 35.2

FRACTION OF INSPIRED OXYGEN PROVIDED BY
VARIOUS DELIVERY SYSTEMS

	FIO_2 delivery	Flow required
Nasal cannula	24%–50%	<6 L
Face mask	<60%	6–10 L
Venturi mask	<60%	Variable
Partial rebreather	<60%	15 L
Nonrebreather	~100%	15 L

Oxygen Hood and Tent

O_2 hoods are transparent enclosures designed to surround the head of a neonate or small infant. O_2 tents are available to allow the patient to move freely within a larger O_2-rich environment. These devices may be used to provide a continuous flow of humidified O_2 in a temperature-controlled environment for the infant or toddler who is agitated by a nasal cannula. These devices are generally small enough to recover the FIO_2 quickly when the seal is disturbed. However, an O_2 analyzer must be used to analyze the O_2 concentration close to the patient, as the O_2 can form layers, creating a gradient up to 20% (29).

Important Considerations

The administration of O_2 is a universal practice in the PICU but is not without risks. O_2-mediated pulmonary toxicity is pathologically very similar to acute respiratory distress syndrome (ARDS) (10). Clinically, the patient may complain of chest pain, cough, and tracheal inflammation. Physiologically, decreased pulmonary compliance and abnormal gas exchange result from impaired surfactant activity. Pathologically, inflammatory cell infiltrates contribute to proteolytic damage, loss of the alveolar-capillary membrane integrity, and pulmonary edema. Although an FIO_2 of 0.50 is commonly regarded as safe, the literature reports that toxicity may be seen with even brief periods of exposure to low levels of O_2 (17). A safe level or duration of FIO_2 exposure has not been established. Reviewing the ongoing need for O_2 therapy for every patient is a good practice guideline.

When supplemental O_2 fails to improve the hypoxemia, one of several pathophysiologic states [including hypoventilation, airway obstruction, diffusion abnormalities, ventilation-perfusion (V/Q) mismatch, and hemoglobinopathies], which disturb alveolar gas exchange or O_2 binding in the capillary, may be present. An extreme form of V/Q mismatch is known as a *physiologic* or *anatomic shunt*. Physiologic right-to-left shunts occur when pulmonary blood passes from systemic veins to systemic arteries without first exchanging gas with the alveoli. Patients with intrapulmonary shunts may benefit from invasive or noninvasive positive pressure ventilation to improve lung volume and V/Q matching. Patients with an anatomic right-to-left intracardiac shunt (i.e., cyanotic congenital heart disease) are hypoxemic and cannot increase their arterial O_2 content in response to supplemental O_2.

Administering oxygen to patients with a chronically compensated respiratory acidosis will induce a mild increase in measured blood $PaCO_2$. Hypercarbia is hypothesized to occur secondary to (a) loss of hypoxic pulmonary vasoconstriction,

(b) decreased stimulation of peripheral chemoreceptors to the central respiratory center, and (c) the decreased CO_2-binding affinity of oxyhemoglobin (i.e., the Haldane effect) (34).

INHALED NITRIC OXIDE

Named "Molecule of the Year" by *Science* magazine in 1992, endogenous nitric oxide (NO) is an essential gaseous cell mediator in neurotransmission, inflammatory cell activation, and vascular smooth muscle relaxation. Therapeutically, iNO is used as a selective pulmonary vasodilator to enhance V/Q matching, to treat pulmonary arteriolar hypertension, and to reduce pulmonary vascular resistance and right ventricular cardiac work.

Pharmacology

Endogenous NO is synthesized within most cells of the human body from arginine and O_2 by one of three isoforms of NO synthase (NOS): neural, inducible, and endothelial. Constitutive production is found in the vascular endothelium, neurons, platelets, adrenal medulla, and macula densa of the kidney. NO is also produced under pathologic conditions by the inducible NOS found within macrophages, hepatocytes, and airway epithelial and smooth muscle cells.

NO induces upregulation of cytosolic guanylyl cyclase, triggering the activation of cyclic guanosine 3′,5′-monophosphate (cGMP)-dependent protein kinases (**Fig. 35.1**). Ultimately, this cascade results in smooth muscle cell relaxation and pulmonary arteriolar vasodilation due to decreased intracellular calcium

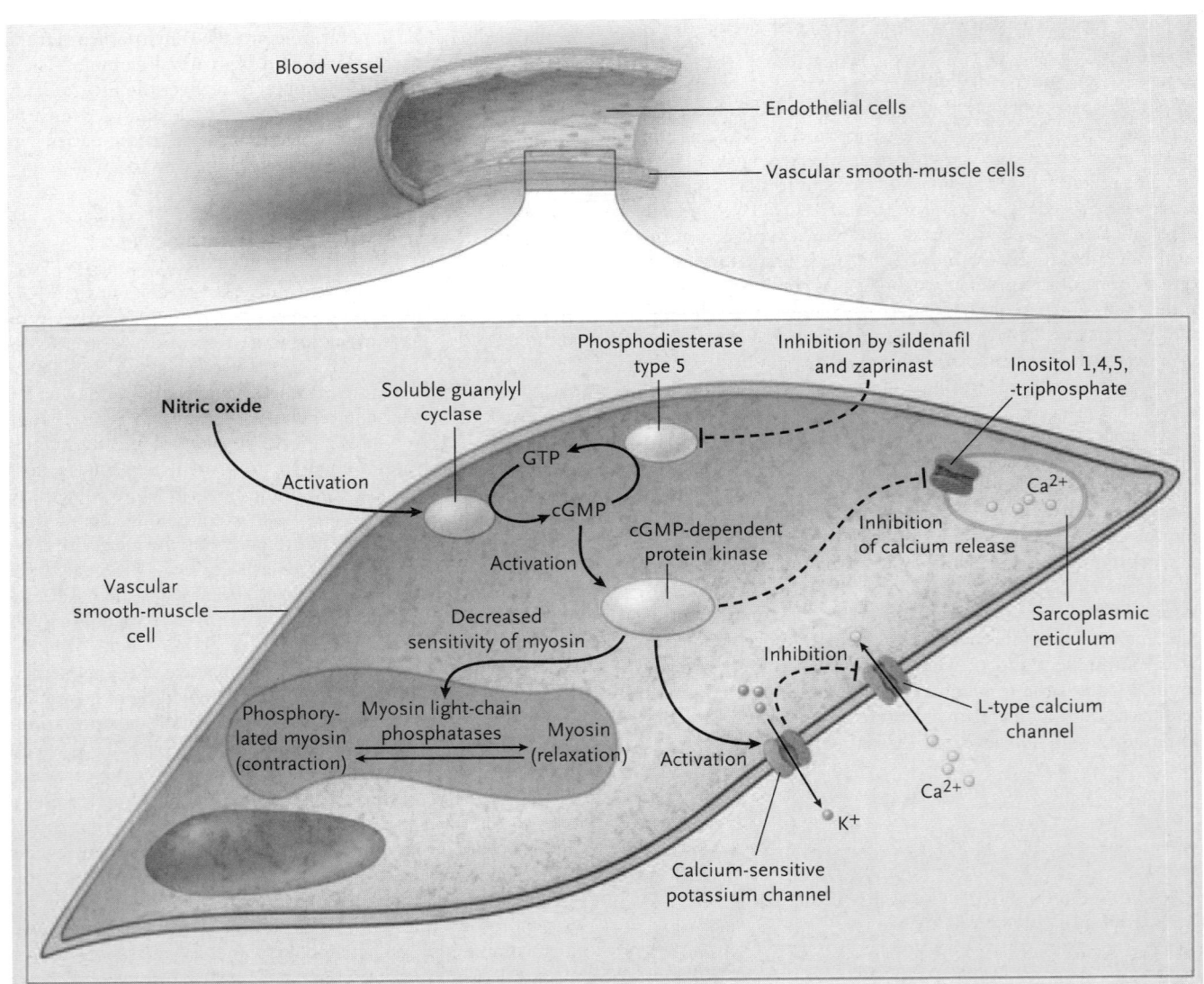

FIGURE 35.1. iNO causes pulmonary vascular endothelial smooth muscle cell relaxation, induces pulmonary capillary smooth muscle cell relaxation, and induces upregulation of guanylyl cyclase, resulting in cytosolic increase of cyclic guanosine 3′,5′-monophosphate (cGMP). cGMP-dependent protein kinase (cGKI) ultimately lowers the intracellular calcium concentration and decreases the sensitivity of myosin to calcium-induced contraction. From Griffiths MJD, TW Evans. Drug therapy: Inhaled nitric oxide therapy in adults. *N Engl J Med* 2005;353:2683–95.

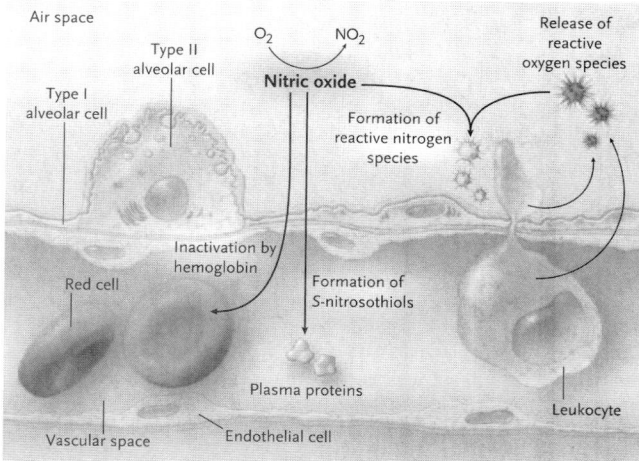

FIGURE 35.2. The biochemical fates of inhaled nitric oxide. Systemic uptake of iNO is limited by nitric oxide-binding to oxyhemoglobin, heme-iron, and plasma proteins. Depending upon the relative concentration of O_2 and free radicals (reactive oxygen species), nitrogen dioxide (NO_2) and reactive nitrogen species (i.e., peroxynitrite) may be produced. From Griffiths MJD, TW Evans. Drug therapy: Inhaled nitric oxide therapy in adults. *N Engl J Med* 2005;353:2683–95.

levels. Phosphodiesterase enzymes cause cGMP levels within the smooth muscle cell to fall. Phosphodiesterase enzyme inhibitors (e.g., sildenafil, zaprinast, and dipyridamole) preserve the cGMP-dependent cascade and may provide a synergistic increase in the vasodilatory effects of iNO.

iNO provides a therapeutic, selective pulmonary vasodilator. This selectivity results from NO reactions which limit movement and activity of iNO to the pulmonary vascular bed (37). Systemic uptake of NO is limited by three scavenging mechanisms: (a) NO-oxyhemoglobin binding (forming methemoglobin and nitrate), (b) NO-binding to plasma proteins (forming nitrosothiols, which potentially store NO activity and inhibit platelet aggregation), and (c) NO-heme iron binding to form nitrosylhemoglobin. NO can also react with free radicals when available (**Fig. 35.2**) to form nitrogen dioxide (NO_2) or peroxynitrite ($ONOO^-$). Protein nitration and oxidative lung injury can result from these toxic reactions and may underlie the pathologic mechanism for hyperoxic or ischemia-reperfusion injury. The biochemical fate of NO may depend upon the relative concentrations of the various blood components (oxyhemoglobin, iron, plasma proteins), ROS, and antioxidants.

Nitric Oxide Delivery Systems

NO gas is produced at high temperatures by a catalyst-induced oxidation of ammonia and is then stored with nitrogen as the balancing gas. iNO is generally delivered during mechanical ventilation but can also be delivered to nonintubated patients via a tight-fitting face mask, transtracheal O_2 catheter, or nasal cannula. iNO should not be administered via an O_2 hood due to the potential for accumulation of toxic nitrogen dioxide byproducts within the hood.

During mechanical ventilation, a constant desired concentration of NO is delivered to the patient, independent of ven-

tilator mode or flow rate. An integrated NO delivery unit and nitrogen dioxide monitoring system, such as the Ohmeda INOvent Nitric Oxide delivery system (Datex-Ohmeda, Madison, WI) is generally used. With this system, the minimum delivered concentration of iNO is 0.1 ppm, at a flow rate between 4 and 120 L/min. iNO is injected directly into the inspiratory limb of the ventilator circuit in synchrony with each inspiratory breath. iNO has an effective half-life of 15–30 sec. Therefore, to ensure that the iNO flow is not interrupted in the event the patient must be disconnected from the ventilator, a separate connector is used to facilitate iNO delivery via a manual bag system. iNO delivery with the Bunnell Life Pulse High-Frequency Jet ventilator has been used in the clinical setting for premature infants with respiratory distress syndrome and has been tested with infant lung models (40).

For delivery via nasal cannula to the nonventilated patient, effective NO delivery has been validated for flow rates as low as 1 L/min. Accurate delivery below 5 ppm is not possible with the current technology.

Important Considerations

During iNO administration, the appropriate monitoring and measurement of NO_2 and methemoglobin levels is necessary to prevent potential NO-induced toxicity. NO_2 forms from the reaction of NO with O_2, and its level is continuously measured using electrochemical sensors. When administering iNO at doses <40 ppm, toxic levels of NO_2 (<2 ppm) rarely occur (13,18). Methemoglobin is produced from NO reaction with oxyhemoglobin, which converts the iron to the ferric or oxidized state ($Fe3^+$). Normally, methemoglobin is converted within the red cell by NADH-cytochrome b5 reductase to restore ferrous hemoglobin ($Fe2^+$). Methemoglobinemia may result in patients with inefficient methemoglobin reductase activity or in those who are exposed to high concentrations of iNO or O_2. Blood methemoglobin levels should be monitored within 4 hrs of initiating iNO and after every 24 hrs of continued treatment.

Patients should be monitored for rebound pulmonary hypertension and hypoxemia when iNO therapy is being weaned. Nitration produced during exogenous iNO leads to impaired endothelial NOS activity (33). Therefore, abrupt discontinuation of iNO may precipitate V/Q mismatch, pulmonary hypertension, and hemodynamic compromise. iNO must be steadily tapered, with concurrent clinical and hemodynamic evaluation, to safely identify the patient's response to weaning of iNO therapy.

Dosing and duration of iNO therapy may depend on the therapeutic target defined for each patient (i.e., improved V/Q matching versus decreased pulmonary arterial pressure). The effective dose of iNO may depend on the degree of reversible pulmonary arterial hypertension, the extent of V/Q mismatching, and the concurrent level of alveolar recruitment. iNO doses between 5 and 20 ppm should produce a clinically apparent response in oxygenation and/or pulmonary vascular resistance. Continuous iNO of >40 ppm does not produce greater benefit; rather, it can produce increased measured levels of methemoglobin and nitrogen dioxide. In patients with hypoxemic respiratory failure, alveolar derecruitment has been associated with a poor response to iNO therapy at recommended doses. In patients with pulmonary hypertension, a decrease in pulmonary vascular resistance by 30% during a trial of 10 ppm iNO for 10 mins has been predictive of those likely to derive a clinical response to oral agents (35). Although commonly used to improve hypoxemia in patients with ARDS, a growing body of literature fails to support the benefit of iNO on important clinical outcomes, such as number of ventilator-free days or survival. The effect of iNO administration on pain crises and acute chest syndrome in patients with sickle cell anemia is the subject of current clinical trials.

HELIUM-OXYGEN MIXTURES (HELIOX)

Helium is administered clinically as a helium-oxygen mixture, referred to as *heliox*. Although helium is biologically inert and provides no direct pharmacologic or biologic effects, heliox provides a medical gas therapy with unique therapeutic application to respiratory processes associated with high airways resistance or obstructive pathology (19). Due to its low density, heliox can significantly decrease respiratory distress and work of breathing, and may improve the deposition of bronchodilator therapy to obstructed lower airways. Heliox provides a rapidly acting inhaled therapy that may afford the patient greater comfort and improved gas exchange while he awaits the therapeutic onset of slower, definitive medical therapies (i.e., corticosteroids).

Pharmacology

Helium is an odorless, tasteless, noncombustible gas. It is commercially produced from natural gas by liquefaction or by thermal release of helium from uranium ore. Helium (0.179 micropoise) is approximately one-seventh the density of air (1.293 micropoise) and O_2 (1.429 micropoise). The density of heliox is dependent on the relative percentage of helium compared to O_2. The higher the concentration of helium, the lower the concentration of O_2 and the lower the total density of the inhaled gas (**Fig. 35.3**). Premixed heliox provide 20% O_2 (80:20 mixture), 30% O_2 (70:30 mixture), or 40% O_2 (60:40 mixture).

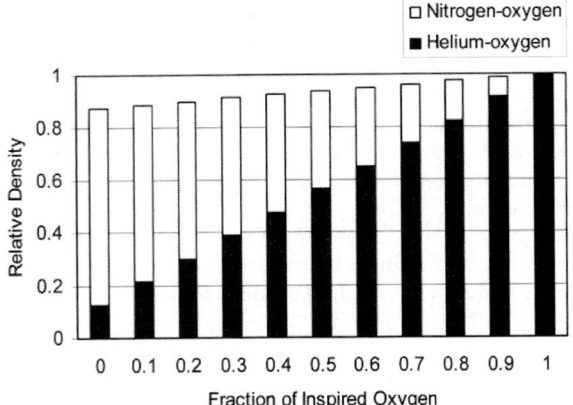

FIGURE 35.3. Helium-oxygen mixtures provide a low-density inhaled gas. The greater the fractional percentage of helium administered, the lower the density of the helium-oxygen mixture.

Gas flow at high velocity through a relatively small cross-sectional area (e.g., gas flow within the upper airway or through partially obstructed air passages) is typically turbulent, whereas gas flow across a large cross-sectional area (e.g., in the lung periphery) is typically laminar. The lower density of heliox, as compared to O_2-enriched air, improves gas flow through high-resistance airways with turbulent gas flow. Turbulent gas flow is mathematically defined by the Bernoulli principle as:

$$Q = (2 \Delta P / \rho)^{1/2}$$

where Q = turbulent gas flow rate, ΔP = airway driving pressure, and ρ = gas density.

As gas flow becomes less turbulent in the affected airways, flow velocity is reduced and the flow pattern may transition from turbulent to more laminar. This transitional zone is represented by the Reynolds number (Re). A lower Re indicates gas flow with greater laminar flow characteristics.

$$Re = 2Vr\rho/\eta$$

where V = gas velocity, r = airway radius, ρ = gas density, and η = gas viscosity.

The low density of heliox allows greater gas flow through airways with high resistance and decreases the Re in airways with transitional gas flow pattern to generate more laminar flow of gas delivery to the distal airways. Furthermore, CO_2 diffuses four times as rapidly in heliox mixtures than in air or O_2 gas alone, which may contribute to the tendency for heliox to rapidly improve ventilation and to reduce the patient's work of breathing (16). Conflicting results from clinical and laboratory trials may suggest the effectiveness of heliox to improve deposition of inhaled bronchodilator in the distal airways and to improve gas movement, as measured by spirometry (1).

Heliox Delivery Systems

Heliox is normally administered to nonventilated patients in respiratory distress via a face mask with a reservoir bag or nonrebreather mask. To retain the low density and therapeutic properties of heliox, any delivery system must minimize entrainment of room air. Therefore, administration with a tight-fitting mask is appropriate, while administration via nasal cannula or a loose-fitting mask is ineffective. Additionally, administering heliox via a tent is impractical, as the helium portion of the gas mixture layers at the top of the tent. The delivery device may include a Y-piece attachment, placed between the mask and the reservoir bag, to add a nebulizer for concurrent bronchodilator administration. Due to the production of less turbulent air flow, a minimum flow rate of 12 L/min is required to aerosolize the treatment (22). An O_2 analyzer should be placed in-line with the patient inspiratory limb when administering heliox to ensure that a known fractional percent of O_2 is being supplied to the patient.

Heliox delivery through mechanical ventilators may also be effective to reduce air trapping and airways resistance in partially obstructed airways (4). Most mechanical ventilators can be adapted to administer heliox, but calibration is required. Ventilators are designed and calibrated for a mixture of O_2 and air; thus, adding heliox gas, which is of a different density, viscosity, and thermal conductivity, can affect both the delivered and measured tidal volumes (31). Some ventilators and in-line respiratory mechanic monitors have calibration settings for heliox. Otherwise, suggested correction factors are available for most ventilators in the US and Europe (39). Heliox has only been thoroughly studied and clinically used when administered through a conventional mechanical ventilator. The use of heliox in conjunction with "nonconventional" ventilation, such as high-frequency oscillatory ventilation (HFOV) and high-frequency jet ventilation (HFJV), is based on laboratory evaluations and sporadic case reports (23). Routine use of heliox with nonconventional ventilation cannot be recommended at the current time.

Heliox administration can also alter the function of respiratory diagnostic and monitoring equipment. Unless appropriately calibrated for heliox use, diagnostic equipment, flow meters, gas blenders, and monitoring devices will erroneously report low flow and tidal volume readings. The delivered flow rate of an 80:20 heliox mixture is 1.8 times greater than the set flow rate, and the flow rate of a 70:30 heliox mixture is 1.6 times greater. Thus, for every 10 L/min flow of an 80:20 heliox mixture that is set, 18 L/min is actually delivered. One must account for the greater flow rate delivery when heliox is used.

Important Considerations

Helium must always be administered with O_2. Although tanks of 100% helium are available, an interruption in O_2 delivery could result in the accidental administration of pure helium, which could be fatal. Continuous in-line monitoring of inspired O_2 concentration is essential to ensure adequate O_2 delivery to the patient.

Consideration must be given to the patient's O_2 requirement. The higher the fraction of inspired O_2 required, the lower the helium concentration and the lower the therapeutic benefit derived. However, even those patients with high O_2 requirements ($FIO_2 \geq 0.80$) may have improved gas exchange with the administration of heliox, allowing for reduced O_2 therapy.

The effects of heliox and improvement in the work of breathing are typically apparent within several minutes. A brief therapeutic trial can quickly assess for a clinical response, either by the patient's subjective report or based upon serial examination of respiratory effort, quality of air entry, and gas exchange. Devices that measure indices of pulmonary status, such as peak flow and FEV_1, must be calibrated for heliox.

Clinically, it is appropriate to forewarn the patient that, during heliox use, their voice may become high-pitched and their ability to generate an effective cough will be reduced. Coughing typically produces a high-velocity burst of turbulent expiratory air flow to expel upper airway irritants. When heliox is in use, air flow turbulence is minimized and coughing efficacy may be reduced. The patient may be instructed to remove the mask briefly to wash out the heliox gas effects in order to generate an effective cough.

INHALED BRONCHODILATOR THERAPY

Lower airway respiratory disease is often accompanied by bronchoconstriction, inflammatory cell activation, mucosal edema formation, and inspissated secretions. Inhaled bronchodilator therapy is provided to relieve lower airway bronchoconstriction, reduce airway resistance, and improve V/Q matching. Inhaled bronchodilators are often given in combination with other pharmacologic agents, including anti-inflammatory agents, decongestants, mucolytic agents, and pulmonary vasodilators, to reverse multiple processes that limit effective gas exchange.

Pharmacology

Inhaled bronchodilator therapy may include the use of β-adrenergic receptor agonists and/or anticholinergic receptor blockade. The inhaled β-agonists (e.g., albuterol, metaproterenol, pirbuterol, levalbuterol, fenoterol, and salbutamol) interact with type 2 β-receptors (β_2) on the luminal surface of bronchial smooth muscle cells. β-agonists can also bind β_2 receptors found on a variety of other cell types to decrease mast-cell mediator release, increase mucociliary transport, alter vascular tone, limit edema formation, and inhibit neutrophil, eosinophil, and lymphocyte functional responses (14). The inhaled anticholinergic agent ipratropium bromide competitively inhibits acetylcholine binding at the M_3 muscarinic receptor located on bronchial smooth muscle cells to decrease intracellular cyclic AMP (cAMP) and cause bronchodilation.

Although systemic uptake of inhaled agents is negligible, clinically notable side effects may result due to receptor binding at nonpulmonary sites and nonselective receptor binding. β_2 receptors on arteriolar smooth muscle cells in skeletal muscles and the liver lead to vasodilation, decreased systemic vascular resistance, tremors, and decreased insulin release, which may become clinically evident with a widened pulse pressure, hyperglycemia, and hypokalemia. Rarely, prolonged administration of β-agonists can elevate creatine phosphokinase and lactate dehydrogenase. β-adrenergic type 1 receptor binding causes tachycardia, palpitations, and/or arrhythmias. Nonselective binding by ipratropium at M_2 receptor sites located on sympathetic nerve terminals could theoretically provoke bronchoconstriction, but this effect is limited by the very poor systemic absorption of the inhaled drug.

Albuterol is a 1:1 racemic mixture of the R- and S-isomers. The R-isomer, levalbuterol, is responsible for the drug's bronchodilating activity, while the S-isomer has been proposed to contribute to a higher incidence of side effects, toxicity, and tolerance, which have been observed following chronic β-agonist use (15). Although often purported to decrease side effects, levalbuterol has not been shown to provide a significant advantage over albuterol in bronchodilator effect, side-effect profile, or in preventing hospital admission (6). Levalbuterol use should be reserved for those patients who have a known history of adverse effects to albuterol.

Aerosol Delivery Systems

Three principal types of devices are used to generate therapeutic aerosols: nebulizers, metered-dose inhalers (MDIs), and dry-powder inhalers (DPIs). All three types of devices may be equally effective for aerosol administration to the spontaneously breathing patient, but the DPIs are ineffective devices for use in mechanically ventilated patients.

Nebulizers

Nebulizers physically "shatter" liquid into small particles to create an aerosol that can be effectively inhaled. Drug delivery to the distal airways is achieved by creating particle sizes between 1 and 5 μm. Particles that are too large (<10 μm) are deposited primarily in the oropharynx, and particles that are too small (<1 μm) are not effectively inhaled (1). To create the aerosol, a pressurized gas jet (air, O_2, or heliox) is forced through a small orifice above the medication reservoir, breaking the surface tension of the liquid to form large droplets. Typically, a baffle within the reservoir recycles larger droplets into the liquid reservoir to enable the formation of smaller particles, which can be entrained into the inspiratory gas stream that is inhaled by the patient. In place of a baffle, some nebulizers contain a vibrating mesh or plate with multiple apertures to produce a very fine-particle fraction. Alternatively, ultrasonic nebulizers create an aerosol by transmitting ultrasonic waves to the surface of the solution to create an aerosol. The aerosol is delivered to the patient during an inspiratory breath or by a fan operated within the nebulizer. Small-volume ultrasonic nebulizers are commercially available for delivery of inhaled bronchodilators; large-volume ultrasonic nebulizers are available for sputum induction in adult patients. Lastly, specialized small-volume nebulizers are equipped with filters, a scavenging system, and one-way valves and should be used for inhaled medications (e.g., pentamidine, ribavirin, rhDNase, and tobramycin) when it is necessary to prevent contamination of the ambient environment.

Three variables affect nebulizer output: initial fill volume (volume of medication and sterile diluent), nebulization time, and gas flow rate. An increase in any one of these variables increases the effective delivery of inhaled medication. During nebulization, water vapor evaporates and the aerosol becomes more concentrated, thus delivering a greater fraction of medication with each inspiratory cycle. A minimum driving gas flow rate of 8 L/min is required when using air or O_2; due to the lower density of heliox and less turbulent gas flow properties, a gas flow rate >12 L/min is required to aerosolize the treatment when heliox is used as the driving gas (22).

Newer breath-actuated nebulizers significantly increase drug delivery by releasing aerosol only upon inhalation, rather than throughout the respiratory cycle. Inhaled aerosols can be effectively administered to the infant and pediatric patient using a face mask or a mouthpiece. A mouthpiece may be preferred, as it can be used to direct aerosol therapy to the mouth of the younger patient. The mask may not be well tolerated in the younger patient, and an improper fit can cause significant deposition of aerosol to the eyes, resulting in papillary dilation.

Metered-Dose Inhaler

An MDI consists of drug suspended in a mixture of propellants, surfactants, preservatives, flavoring agents, and dispersal agents within a pressurized canister. The mixture is released from the MDI canister through a metering valve and stem into an actuator boot. To improve effective delivery for the pediatric patient, a spacer or valved holding chamber is commonly used. The MDI is actuated once every 15–20 sec into the accessory device, to reduce the need to coordinate with inspiration. A spacer device is an open-ended tube or bag that allows the MDI plume to expand and the propellant to evaporate. A

valved holding chamber incorporates a one-way valve to release aerosol from the chamber only during inspiration. Drug particle deposition on the inner surfaces of these devices can occur, resulting in less effective drug delivery. To avoid this particle deposition, the device must be washed prior to use to remove static charges on the plastic material of the chambers.

Dry-Powder Inhalers

A DPI creates aerosol by drawing air through a dose of powdered medication. The advantage of the DPI is that it is breath-actuated, thus delivering medication only upon inhalation, reducing the problem of coordinating inspiration with actuation. However, release of the drug requires high-inspiratory flow rates <50 L/min, which limit the use of the DPI in patients <6 years of age and in the neuromuscularly weak patient. The DPI is not effective for aerosol delivery during mechanical ventilation, as the high ambient humidity causes the dry powder to clump and create larger particles that do not aerosolize well.

Mechanically Ventilated Patients

Inhaled bronchodilators may be effectively administered and equally therapeutic in the mechanically ventilated patient using a nebulizer or MDI (11). To increase the effective drug delivery during mechanical ventilation, attention to several aspects of delivery is required: (a) location of delivery within the ventilator circuit, (b) humidity within the circuit, and (c) ventilator flow (Table 35.3). In terms of location of delivery, the

---

TABLE 35.3

RECOMMENDED TECHNIQUES FOR METERED-DOSE INHALER AND NEBULIZER USE DURING MECHANICAL VENTILATION

Metered-
  dose inhaler
Agitate MDI and warm to hand temperature
Place MDI adaptor into inspiratory limb of circuit (18–30 cm
  from the Y-piece connector)
Attach MDI to adaptor in ventilator circuit (chamber-style is
  best)
Actuate ≥6 puffs at beginning of inspiratory cycle
Cycle each actuation with a spontaneous or ventilator
  inspiratory cycle
Wait ≥5 sec between actuations
Assess patient response

Nebulizer
Establish dose to be administered
Place drug in nebulizer reservoir; fill with sterile water to
  ≥4 mL
Place nebulizer in inspiratory circuit ≥18–30 cm from the
  patient Y-piece connector
Initiate driving gas flow of oxygen ≥6 L/min; ≥12 L/min
  when heliox used
Turn off flow by or continuous flow during nebulization
Continue nebulization treatment until sputtering occurs
  indicating end of treatment
Remove nebulizer and return ventilator to previous settings
Assure no leak in circuit
Assess patient response

Adapted with permission from James B. Fink, MS, RRT.

nebulizer device or MDI (fitted with a chamber) provides optimum medication delivery when placed in the inspiratory limb of the ventilator circuit ~18–30 cm from the endotracheal tube Y-piece connector. Furthermore, the ventilator circuit distal to the device should have no kinks, elbow connectors, or other obstructions to gas flow. This location allows the circuit to act as a spacer reservoir and limits medication entrainment along plastic surfaces. Regarding humidity within the circuit, it significantly decreases aerosol deposition. Positioning the delivery device so that it bypasses the humidifier increases medication delivery by a factor of nearly 4 (30). Due to the high humidity, increased dosage of medication is often required to achieve a therapeutic effect in mechanically ventilated patients (12). Required MDI actuations may range from 6–40 puffs (depending on patient age and size) to produce a therapeutic effect. In the neonatal and pediatric population, the required doses of specific aerosolized medications are not known. Attention to ventilator gas flow is important to affect drug delivery. Greater aerosol delivery occurs when MDI actuation is synchronized with a delivered inspired breath, a larger tidal volume, or the use of an end-inspiratory pause. For all of the previously mentioned reasons, direct application of medication into the endotracheal tube is not recommended.

Using an MDI versus continuous nebulizer treatment for the intubated patient is associated with the relative advantages of decreased personnel time required for administration, no requirement to disconnect ventilator circuit (when an in-line MDI chamber is used), and no requirement to alter ventilator settings during administration. Additionally, the disadvantages with an in-line nebulizer treatment include alteration of inspiratory flows, additional bias flow in the ventilator circuit that may interfere with patient-triggered modes of ventilation, and the possibility for aerosol particles to deposit and crystallize on the expiratory mechanisms, creating inadvertent expiratory resistance or intrinsic PEEP (20,21).

Important Considerations

Effective administration of inhaled aerosol therapy in the pediatric patient depends on the delivery system used, optimizing delivery technique with the use of an appropriate accessory device (e.g., spacer or aerosol chamber), and optimizing the technical aspects of drug delivery during mechanical ventilation.

NITROGEN (HYPOXIC GAS) AND CARBON DIOXIDE ADMINISTRATION

PICUs that manage patients with single ventricle congenital heart disease may at times use supplemental nitrogen gas (forming a hypoxic gas mixture) or exogenous CO_2 administration to increase pulmonary vascular resistance (PVR) in an effort to control the ratio of pulmonary (Q_p) to systemic (Q_s) blood flow. A patent ductus arteriosus in these patients is vital to either systemic or pulmonary blood flow based on the underlying structural cardiac defect. In the care of some patients with ductal-dependent, single-ventricle, congenital heart disease, excessive pulmonary blood flow may lead to clinically significant systemic hypoperfusion. With single-ventricle physiology, cardiac output is distributed based on the relative vascular resistances between the pulmonary and systemic circulation. The ideal balance of these two circulations is reflected by an oxygenation saturation of ~80%. No controlled studies have determined if maintaining the systemic saturation near 75% with the use of supplemental nitrogen decreases morbidity and mortality in the preoperative period (38).

As centers gain more experience with this complex population of cardiac patients, treatment strategies are placing significantly more focus on maintaining adequate total cardiac output (systemic O_2 delivery) and less emphasis on inhaled gas therapies to alter the pulmonary-systemic blood flow ratio. Therefore, the administration of nitrogen or CO_2 to these patients has recently decreased, as improved preoperative care for the single-ventricle patient has allowed better systemic O_2 delivery without the exogenous administration of these gases.

Hypoxic Gas Mixtures

The addition of nitrogen gas to inspired room air via an endotracheal tube or hood results in a hypoxic or subambient O_2 mixture (i.e., FIO_2 <21%), referred to as *hypoxic gas* or *subambient O_2 therapy*. The fraction of inspired O_2 content in these gas mixtures ranges from 15% to 20%.

Hypoxic Gas Delivery Systems

Caution must be advised when delivering hypoxic gas mixtures to mechanically ventilated patients. Hypoxic gas mixtures are obtained by nitrogen dilution—the addition of low-flow nitrogen into the ventilator circuit. Administration of nitrogen and compressed air through a mechanical ventilator overrides important safety features. The FIO_2 control knob is no longer a control of administered O_2 but, rather, a control of either air or nitrogen. Therefore, if this knob is inadvertently turned (in either direction), the delivered concentration of hypoxic gas mixture may be significantly altered. It is impossible to deliver a hypoxic gas mixture via a ventilator and not defeat a safety mechanism. The O_2 analyzer alarm limits must be reset or turned off during hypoxic gas administration. Furthermore, commercially available O_2 analyzers do not accurately monitor these lower O_2 concentrations (32). Thus, the technical delivery of a hypoxic gas mixture requires expertise and vigilance to these considerations. For patient safety, clinical examination must be augmented by continuous monitoring of the delivered FIO_2 and the measured O_2 saturation in addition to frequent arterial blood gas sampling.

Carbon Dioxide

PVR is affected by alveolar O_2 tension, capillary CO_2 tension, and blood pH. Exogenous CO_2 may provide a dose-dependent increase in PVR. Some patients may respond to an elevated $PaCO_2$ of 45–50 mm Hg, whereas in other patients, levels as high as 80–95 mm Hg $PaCO_2$ may be required. As the $PaCO_2$ tension increases, the resultant blood pH may fall and acidemia may occur. Although the impact of acidemia on cardiac function has been studied extensively, great debate continues on its overall hemodynamic effects. Nonetheless, treatment of acidemia with buffering agents, such as bicarbonate or tromethamine (THAM), especially in patients with underlying cardiac dysfunction, seems commonplace in many ICUs.

Carbon Dioxide Delivery Systems

Exogenous CO_2 may be administered into the ventilator outflow port and measured by a capnometer in the inspiratory limb of the ventilator circuit. Increased $PaCO_2$ and acidemic pH are potent stimulators of respiration. Therefore, during exogenous CO_2 administration, minute ventilation must be maintained constant with the administration of sufficient sedation and, if necessary, neuromuscular blockade. Decreases in the ventilator set tidal volume and respiratory rate to achieve hypoventilation may have similar results as exogenous CO_2 administration, but if ventilator settings are decreased significantly, arterial desaturation may result secondary to the loss of lung volume. The therapeutic range of exogenous CO_2 is 1%–4% (8–30 mm Hg). The quantity of CO_2 in room air is 0.03% (0.22 mm Hg). Published nomograms aid in selecting the blender settings required to deliver precise concentrations of O_2 and CO_2 through a double-blender system (7).

Important Considerations

For some centers, hypoxic gas and/or exogenous CO_2 mixtures allow extra time to undertake an elective surgical repair. In other centers, the need for administration of these gas mixtures itself suggests that the operation is no longer elective and urgent operative repair is required. Regardless of the selected therapy, the goal of preoperative stabilization/management emphasizes adequate systemic O_2 delivery. Caution must always be advised with any inhaled medical therapy that requires the alteration of, or impairs, safety features. Although hypoxic gas mixtures and CO_2 administration may achieve a similar degree of balance between the pulmonary and system blood flow, exogenous CO_2 gas therapy may do so without the need to defeat important safety controls. These therapies require technical skill and a thorough understanding of the underlying physiology to ensure appropriate use and patient safety.

INHALATIONAL ANESTHETICS

Inhalational anesthetics have been administered in the critical care unit to aid in the treatment of medically refractory bron-

chospasm (isoflurane, desflurane), for refractory pain (isoflurane, N_2O), and for sedation (isoflurane, desflurane). The published literature suggests that few centers within the US routinely use volatile anesthetic agents within the ICU; whereas, internationally, the use and broader clinical applications for these agents are more common (9). These agents provide an appealing alternative to more traditional intravenous therapies provided in the ICU because they provide (a) the rapid onset and titration of therapeutic effects, (b) a low side-effect profile, (c) limited metabolism that is independent of renal or hepatic function, (d) the relief of bronchospasm, and (e) the potential to provide adequate sedation yet preserve spontaneous respiratory effort.

General Principles of Inhalation Anesthetics

To reach peak sedative effect, the inspired concentration must first reach equilibrium within the pulmonary alveolar capillary and subsequently reach equilibrium within the brain tissue. A low blood solubility (i.e., low blood:gas partition coefficient) establishes rapid equilibrium between the partial pressures of inspired gas within the alveolus, pulmonary capillary, and brain tissue (Table 35.4). Clinically, this allows for rapid and easily titratable effects on the respiratory and central nervous systems.

The end-tidal alveolar gas concentration is continuously monitored to determine the mean alveolar concentration (MAC) of the volatile agent administered to the patient. For each inhaled anesthetic agent, 1 MAC refers to the concentration required to prevent movement in 50% of patients in response to surgical stimuli. *MAC-hours* references the patient's level of anesthetic exposure in hours. For example, the MAC-hours for isoflurane is derived by dividing the end-tidal concentration by 1.15 (26). Notably, these references have not been established in ICU patients with multiple organ dysfunction or for long-term sedation.

Isoflurane

Isoflurane (1-chloro-2,2,2-trifluoroethyl difluoromethyl ether) is a fluorinated, nonflammable ether that is volatile at room temperature. It induces rapid anesthetic induction and

TABLE 35.4

COMPARISON OF ANESTHETIC POTENCY FOR INHALATIONAL ANESTHETICS USED IN THE PICU

		Partition coefficient at 37°C	
Anesthetic agent	MAC (%)*	Alveolar gas: blood	Blood: brain
Isoflurane	1.2	1.40	2.6
Desflurane	6.0	0.45	1.3
N_2O	105.0#	0.47	1.1

*MAC, minimum alveolar concentration; MAC%, concentration of inhaled agent required to prevent movement in response to surgical stimuli in 50% of patients.
#Hyperbaric conditions are required to reach 1 MAC.

recovery due to a low blood:gas partition coefficient. In the ICU, isoflurane has been used to treat pain, sedation, and severe bronchospasm in cases refractory to conventional medical therapies. Published case reports suggest that administration produces therapeutic benefit within 1 hr and is associated with an improvement in intrinsic PEEP, obstructive physiology, and inspiratory and expiratory resistive indices (28).

Pharmacology

The mechanism of action for isoflurane's bronchodilatory properties is not well established. Isoflurane may affect multiple pathways involved in the relief of bronchospasm, although no direct effect on histamine levels or smooth muscle contraction is measurable. It is postulated that isoflurane activates the sympathetic system to cause elevated endogenous catecholamine levels, leading to bronchodilation. Isoflurane is eliminated almost completely from the lungs, with only 0.2% undergoing oxidative metabolism via cytochrome P450 2E1. Thus, elimination is dependent on exposure duration (MAC-hours), minute ventilation, and cardiac output.

Isoflurane dosing in the ICU setting is initiated at 0.5% and titrated to clinical effect up to 2% (25). When used for anesthesia, induction is achieved with 3% isoflurane in O_2 and maintained with 1.5%–2.5%. If oversedation occurs, the effects may be quickly reversed by temporarily discontinuing therapy and administering 100% FIO_2. Dose-dependent side effects include systemic vasodilation and increased sympathetic stimuli, which result in increased cardiac output, skin flushing, and tachycardia. Isoflurane increases cerebral blood flow and may raise intracranial pressure, but it reduces cerebral O_2 consumption. Isoflurane is also a potent coronary vasodilator, the use of which results in improved coronary blood flow and decreased myocardial O_2 consumption.

Isoflurane Delivery Systems

Use of inhalation anesthetics within the ICU requires proper facilities, personnel training, and equipment to ensure a safe environment for patients and staff. To safely administer isoflurane outside of the operative setting, specialized equipment for monitoring and scavenging the volatile anesthetic are needed. An anesthesia machine or adaptation of the ICU ventilator is required for delivery. For the mechanically ventilated ICU patient, the anesthesia machine has the disadvantage of offering limited ventilatory modalities, flow patterns, and inspiratory-to-expiratory ratios. The ICU ventilator most commonly adapted for use with inhaled anesthetics is the Servo 900C anesthesia system (Siemens, Solna, Sweden), which includes a calibrated liquid injection vaporizer (Siemens vaporizer 925) and an active scavenging system (Servo Evac 180). Caution must be advised in administering an inhaled anesthetic with nontraditional equipment. Active scavenging systems and appropriate turnover of ambient air is required to protect patients and staff from inadvertent exposure. The scavenging system should collect all exhaled gases, including ventilator exhaust, gas emitted around an endotracheal tube leak, gases emitted when the ventilator circuit is disconnected, and any gas collected within the anesthesia bag during manual ventilation (9).

Continuous infrared monitoring equipment for both the inspired and expired concentrations of the inhalational agent is necessary. The high- and low-concentration alarms are set within a narrow range to immediately detect variations from desired settings.

Important Considerations

The safety of prolonged administration, particularly in the critically ill patient, has not been established. Case reports suggest that prolonged administration can be associated with an abstinence syndrome (2). Symptoms, which are reversible, include agitation, choreoathetoid movements, hypertension, tachycardia, diaphoresis, and diarrhea. These symptoms have been reported in patients who received >70 MAC-hours of isoflurane. The abstinence syndrome may be prevented or treated with the gradual withdrawal of the inhalation agent or use of IV sedation as the agent is withdrawn.

Fluoride ion nephrotoxicity is also associated with prolonged isoflurane exposure (24). Nephrotoxicity has been reported with serum fluoride levels $\geq$50 μM. A peak serum fluoride level of 26.1 μM was noted in 10 pediatric patients after 441 MAC-hours of isoflurane sedation (2). Periodic monitoring of renal function and ability to concentrate is warranted. Continuous temperature monitoring is necessary to detect the rare but treatable onset of malignant hyperthermia. Dantrolene sodium should be readily available at the bedside for any patient receiving inhaled isoflurane.

Nitrous Oxide

Nitrous oxide, or dinitrogen monoxide (N_2O), may be administered as an inhaled analgesic agent for patients in the PICU. N_2O is a relatively weak anesthetic agent, producing analgesia at low concentrations (20%) and requiring near-toxic concentrations to produce deep sedation. For this reason, N_2O is commonly administered in the operating room in combination with other inhalational agents.

Pharmacology

N_2O is produced from thermal decomposition of ammonium nitrate. Concentrations between 20% and 80% produce analgesia and dose-dependent levels of sedation. N_2O must always be administered with O_2, and cannot be administered above concentrations of 80% due to the limitation imposed on fractional percentage of O_2 supplied.

N_2O is eliminated via the lungs with metabolism that is independent of renal or hepatic function. A small fraction is eliminated via diffusion through the skin. Dose-dependent side effects include increased respiratory rate and depressed tidal volume, generally with minimal resultant effects on minute ventilation and CO_2 tension. NO increases cerebral blood flow and intracranial pressure, but these effects may be abolished when coadministered with IV sedation or narcotics.

Nitrous Oxide Delivery Systems

N_2O can be effectively delivered via nasal cannula, face mask, or non-rebreather mask. Concurrent administration with O_2 is required to ensure a fresh flow of O_2 to the patient. Safe-handling practices must be followed when using N_2O, as both it and O_2 gases support combustion. Flow meters that are ordinarily calibrated for the administration of O_2 and nitrogen require calibration for the delivery of N_2O.

Important Considerations

N_2O is contraindicated for any patient with pathologic air-filled cavities and with an increased risk of or prior history of pulmonary hypertension. Air-filled cavities contain nitrogen, which is highly insoluble. N_2O displaces nitrogen within any air-containing body cavity. N_2O will enter the cavity faster than nitrogen can escape, thus increasing the volume and pressure within the cavity. Therefore, N_2O administration may result in expansion of an existing pneumothorax, pulmonary bullae, intracranial air, vascular air embolus, bowel obstruction, or intraocular air bubble. N_2O also increases systemic and pulmonary venous tone, a response that may be exaggerated in patients with preexisting pulmonary hypertension.

Although a weak sedative, increased concentrations of N_2O can markedly depress ventilatory response to hypoxia. Thus, N_2O should always be administered with O_2, and O_2 saturation monitoring is mandatory. N_2O administration may cause megaloblastic anemia and a peripheral neuropathy secondary to vitamin B_{12} deficiency (3). Despite the potential complications of N_2O, it is overall a safe and effective inhalational agent when titrated to provide therapeutic pain relief.

CONCLUSIONS AND FUTURE DIRECTIONS

Inhaled medical gas therapies and medications provide a powerful therapeutic modality to improve systemic O_2 delivery in patients with cardiorespiratory disease. Critical care personnel should understand the therapeutic potential and appropriate delivery and safe-handling practices of commonly used inhaled gas therapies. This chapter has emphasized the following commonly used gas therapies and medications: (a) O_2, (b) iNO, (c) heliox, (d) inhaled bronchodilators, (e) hypoxic gas mixtures, (f) exogenous CO_2 administration, and (g) inhalational anesthetics. In the future, the spectrum of pharmacologic agents that may be delivered via aerosol or inhalational gas will increase to directly target pulmonary processes or as a vehicle for systemic bioavailability.

KEY POINTS

- Inhaled medical gas therapies are commonly used within the PICU to improve patient comfort, pulmonary gas exchange, and systemic O_2 delivery.
- All personnel who administer inhaled gas therapies should be aware of the common therapeutic indications, pharmacologic properties, technical delivery systems, and the safe-handling practices for each agent.
- Depending on the etiology of the ventilation-perfusion mismatch, restoring optimal alveolar gas exchange may involve supplemental O_2 administration to raise the alveolar O_2 tension, inhaled NO to vasodilate the pulmonary vascular bed in patients with increased pulmonary vascular resistance, heliox therapy to support alveolar gas exchange in obstructive disease processes, hypoxic gas mixtures or supplemental CO_2 therapy to balance systemic-to-pulmonary blood flow in patients with single ventricle physiology, or the provision of bronchodilator aerosols or inhalation anesthetic agents to relieve severe airway bronchospasm.

References

1. Anderson M, Svartengren M, Bylin G, et al. Deposition in asthmatics of particles inhaled in air or in helium-oxygen. *Am Rev Respir Dis* 1993;147(3): 524–8.
2. Arnold JH, Truog RD, Rice SA. Prolonged administration of isoflurane to pediatric patients during mechanical ventilation. *Anesth Analg* 1993;76:520–6.
3. Berger JJ, Modell JH, Sypert GW. Megaloblastic anemia and brief exposure to nitrous oxide: A causal relationship. *Anesth Analg* 1988;67:197–8.
4. Berkenbosch JW, Grueber RE, Dabbagh O, et al. Effect of helium-oxygen (heliox) gas mixtures on the function of four pediatric ventilators. *Crit Care Med* 2003;31(7):2052–8.
5. Branson RD. The nuts and bolts of increasing arterial oxygenation: Devices and techniques. *Respir Care* 1993;38:672–86.
6. Carl JC, Myers TR, Kirchner HL, et al. Comparison of racemic albuterol and levalbuterol for treatment of acute asthma. *J Pediatr* 2003 Dec;143(6): 731–6.
7. Chatburn RL, Anderson SM. Controlling carbon dioxide delivery during mechanical ventilation. *Respir Care* 1994;39:1039–1046.
8. Cook D, De Jonghe B, Brochard L, et al. Influence of airway management on ventilator-associated pneumonia: Evidence from randomized trials. *JAMA* 1998;279(10):781–787. Erratum in: *JAMA* 1999;281(22):2089.
9. Curley MA, Molengraft JA. Providing Comfort to Critically Ill Pediatric Patients: Isoflurane. *Crit Care Nurs Clin North Am* 1995;7:267–74.
10. Deneke SM, Fanburg BL. Normobaric oxygen toxicity of the lung. *N Engl J Med* 1980;303:76.
11. Duarte AG, Momii K, Bidani A. Bronchodilator therapy with metered-dose inhaler and spacer versus nebulizer in mechanically ventilated patients: Comparison of magnitude and duration of response. *Respir Care* 2000;45: 817–23.
12. Georgopoulos D, Mouloudi E, Kondili E, et al. Bronchodilator delivery with metered-dose inhaler during mechanical ventilation. *Crit Care* 2000; 4(4):227–34.
13. Gerlach H, Keh D, Semmerow A, et al. Dose-response characteristics during long-term inhalation of nitric oxide in patients with severe acute respiratory distress syndrome: A prospective, randomized, controlled study. *Am J Respir Crit Care Med* 2003;167:1008–15.
14. Gern JE, Lemanske RF, Jr. Beta-adrenergic agonist therapy. *Immunol Allergy Clin North Am* 1993;13:839.
15. Gibson P, Powell H, Ducharme F, et al. Long-acting beta2-agonists as an inhaled corticosteroid-sparing agent for chronic asthma in adults and children. *Cochrane Database Syst Rev* 2005:CD005076.
16. Gluck EH, Onorato DJ, Castriotta R. Helium-oxygen mixtures in intubated patients with status asthmaticus and respiratory acidosis. *Chest* 1990;98:693–8.
17. Griffith DE, Holden WE, Morris JF, et al. Effects of common therapeutic concentrations of oxygen on lung clearance of 99m Tc DTPA and bronchoalveolar lavage albumin concentrations. *Am Rev Respir Dis* 1986;134:233–7.
18. Griffiths MJD, TW Evans. Drug therapy: Inhaled nitric oxide therapy in adults. *N Engl J Med* 2005;353:2683–95.
19. Gupta VK, Cheifetz IM. Heliox administration in the pediatric intensive care unit: An evidence-based review. *Ped Crit Care Med* 2005;6:204–11.
20. Hanhan U, Kissoon N, Payne M, et al. Effects of in-line nebulization on preset ventilatory variables. *Respir Care* 1993;38:474–8.
21. Hess D. Inhaled bronchodilators during mechanical ventilation: Delivery techniques, evaluation of response, and cost effectiveness. *Respir Care* 1994;39:105–22.
22. Hess DR, Acosta FL, Ritz RH, et al. The effect of heliox on nebulizer function using a heliox-driven nebulizer albuterol bronchodilator. *Chest* 1999;115:184–9.
23. Katz AL, Gentile MA, Craig DM, et al. Heliox does not affect gas exchange during high-frequency oscillatory ventilation if tidal volume is held constant. *Crit Care Med* 2003;31(7):2006–9.
24. Kong KL. Isoflurane sedation for patients undergoing mechanical ventilation: Metabolism to inorganic fluoride and renal effects. *Br J Anaesth* 1990;64:159–62.
25. Kong KL. Inhalational anesthetics in the intensive care unit. *Crit Care Clin* 1995;11:887–902.
26. Kong KL, Willats SM, Prys-Roberts C. Isoflurane compared with midazolam for sedation in the intensive care unit. *BMJ* 1989;298:1277–80.
27. Lodato RF. Oxygen toxicity. *Critical Care Clinics* 1990;6:749–65.
28. Maltais F, Sovilj, Goldberg P, et al. Respiratory mechanics in status asthmaticus. Effects of inhalational anesthesia. *Chest* 1994;106:1401–6.
29. McPherson SP. Gas regulation, administration and controlling devices. In: McPherson SP, ed. *Respiratory Therapy Equipment*, 4th ed. St. Louis: CV Mosby, 1990;50–78.
30. Miller DD, Amin MM, Palmer LB, et al. Aerosol delivery and modern mechanical ventilation: In vitro/in vivo evaluation. *Am J Respir Crit Care Med* 2003;168:1205–9.
31. Myers TR. Therapeutic gases for neonatal and pediatric respiratory care. *Respir Care* 2003;48:399–422.
32. Myers TR, Chatburn RL. Accuracy of oxygen analyzers at sub atmospheric concentrations used in treatment of hypoplastic left heart syndrome. *Respiratory Care* 2002;47:1168–72.

33. Pearl JM, Nelson DP, Raake JL, et al. Inhaled nitric oxide increases endothelin-1 levels: A potential cause of rebound pulmonary hypertension. *Crit Care Med* 2002;30:89–93.

34. Sassoon CS, Hassell KT, Mahutte CK. Hyperoxic-induced hypercapnia in stable chronic obstructive pulmonary disease. *Am Rev Respir Dis* 1987; 135:907–11.

35. Sitbon, O, Brenot, F, Denjean, A, et al. Inhaled nitric oxide as a screening vasodilator agent in primary pulmonary hypertension. *Am J Respir Crit Care Med* 1995;151:384–9.

36. Sreenan C, Lemke RP, Hudson-Mason A, et al. High-flow nasal cannula in the management of apnea of prematurity: a comparison with conventional nasal continuous positive airway pressure. *Pediatrics* 2001;107:1081–83.

37. Stamler JS, Jaraki O, Osborne J, et al. Nitric oxide circulates in mammalian plasma primarily as an S-nitroso adduct of serum albumin. *Proc Natl Acad Sci USA* 1992;89:7674–7.

38. Tabbut S, Ramamurthy C, Montenegro LM, et al. Impact of inspired gas mixtures on preoperative infants with HLHS during controlled ventilation. *Circulation* 2001;104:1159–64.

39. Tassaux D, Jolliet P, Thouret JM, et al. Calibration of seven ICU ventilators for mechanical ventilation with helium-oxygen mixtures. *Am J Respir Crit Care Med* 1999;27:1603–7.

40. Platt DR, Swanton D, Blackney D. Inhaled nitric oxide (iNO) delivery with high-frequency jet ventilation (HFJV). *J Perinatol* 2003;23: 387–91.

CHAPTER 36 ■ EXTRACORPOREAL LIFE SUPPORT

STEVEN A. CONRAD • HEIDI J. DALTON

Severe cardiopulmonary failure is one of the more challenging disorders to manage in the ICU, and conventional means of support are frequently inadequate. Conventional support, which seeks to augment the function of the natural heart and lungs through mechanical ventilation and pharmacologic support, is limited in its effectiveness when organ dysfunction is severe. Furthermore, ventilator-induced lung injury and myocardial dysfunction are recognized complications of aggressive application of these therapies, leading to a poor outcome (20,33).

Extracorporeal life support (ECLS) is the application of extracorporeal circulation for the support of patients with severe cardiopulmonary failure. ECLS has its origins in cardiopulmonary bypass for cardiac surgery, a technology pioneered in the 1950s to permit intracardiac surgery. Development of improved bypass technologies ensued, to the extent that cardiopulmonary bypass is now a routine procedure in cardiac surgery. The transition of extracorporeal technologies from the operating room to the bedside in the ICU has a tumultuous yet interesting history. Today the application of ECLS has almost universal acceptance during the neonatal period and widespread acceptance in the pediatric age group.

RATIONALE

It is widely recognized that patients with severe respiratory failure succumb with multiple organ dysfunction despite the ability of mechanical ventilation to maintain blood gas levels at survivable levels. Attention has turned to the concept of *ventilator-induced lung injury*, in which the excessive levels of applied ventilatory support required for the lungs to maintain gas transfer can result in mechanical injury to the lungs and induction of local and systemic inflammation through mechanotransduction pathways (13,19,33). These effects are compounded by cardiovascular impairment induced by mechanical ventilation, as well as by myocardial depression associated with systemic inflammation and multiorgan dysfunction.

Evidence for this concept in humans is only indirect, however. Reduction in the level of tidal volume (i.e., lung distension) has been shown in a large adult trial to improve survival in acute respiratory distress syndrome (ARDS) (1). Two randomized trials of ECLS in adult patients did not show a survival benefit for ECLS, but these trials did not utilize the concept of lung rest. A recent randomized trial of ECLS in adult patient using lung-protective ventilator strategies found a significant survival benefit in patients receiving ECLS.

In pediatric patients, evaluation of the concept of ventilator-induced lung injury has taken an approach different from that in adults. A comparative trial of conventional mechanical ventilation with high-frequency oscillation (HFOV) revealed a lower frequency of barotrauma and improved outcome in the HFOV group. High-frequency oscillation maintains alveolar distension with much lower cyclic tidal stresses on the lung parenchyma and represents a lung-protective strategy (24). In addition to parenchymal injury, mechanical ventilation can also induce injury to the distal airways (18). Known as *ventilator-induced airway injury*, it can contribute to both acute and chronic lung dysfunction in infants. Lung-protective ventilatory strategies should therefore include attention to dynamic ventilatory patterns and to the degree of static inflation.

DOCUMENTING THE EXTRACORPOREAL LIFE SUPPORT EXPERIENCE

The Extracorporeal Life Support Organization (ELSO, Ann Arbor, MI) is a consortium of healthcare centers that use extracorporeal circulation for support of severe cardiopulmonary failure. These centers contribute detailed data to a registry on each ECLS case performed. The registry currently has data on over 32,000 cases performed at 145 centers since the first neonatal case in 1976. The vast majority of ECLS cases in the US and a growing number of international cases are reported to ELSO. Thus, the registry data is highly representative of ECLS over the past three decades.

CIRCUIT COMPONENTS

The components of an ECLS circuit, although based on the traditional cardiopulmonary bypass circuit, have been developed or adapted for long-term support (**Fig. 36.1**). Vascular cannulas are placed for blood drainage and reinfusion. A small drainage reservoir (bladder) helps to ensure continuous availability of blood for the pump. A roller-head or centrifugal pump provides the blood flow through the circuit. An artificial lung (membrane oxygenator) provides gas exchange, and a heat exchanger maintains a controlled temperature of reinfused blood. Other circuit components allow for infusion of medications, incorporation of a hemofilter for fluid control, and monitoring systems for blood gas, flow, and pressure.

Vascular Cannulas

Extracorporeal support requires blood flows equal to the cardiac output [for venoarterial (VA) support] and sometimes

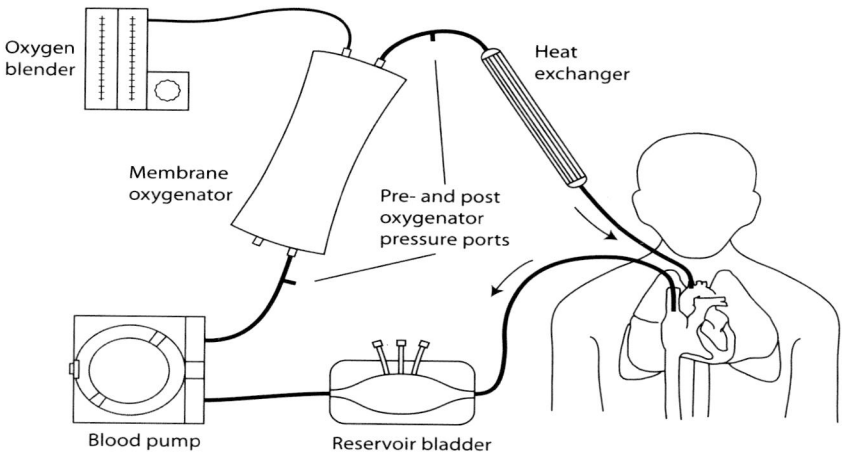

FIGURE 36.1. Components of a typical extracorporeal circuit. The circuit consists of a drainage reservoir (bladder), blood pump, membrane lung, heat exchanger, and connecting tubing.

higher [100–120 mL/kg/min for venovenous (VV) or hybrid support]. Cannulas of sufficient sizes to support this level of flow are necessary. The single-lumen cannulas used for vascular access are not unique to ECLS, having been developed for cardiovascular surgery. Most cannulas are constructed of polyurethane and may include wire reinforcement to prevent kinking. Cannulas that are placed percutaneously require appropriately sized tissue dilators.

Traditional cannulation employs two single-lumen cannulas, one for venous drainage and a second for return to the venous or arterial circulation. Single-lumen cannulas are used in all modes of support. The cannula size chosen is dictated by the size and flow requirements of the patient and the size of the vessel(s) available for cannulation. Neonates have vessels that range from ~8–10 French (fr) (carotid artery) to 12–15 fr (internal jugular vein), whereas adolescents can accommodate up to 20 fr arterial and 24 fr venous (and larger).

Double-lumen cannulas have been developed specifically for VV ECLS (Origen Biomedical, Austin TX) (**Fig. 36.2**). Placed through the internal jugular, these cannulas have two drainage ports located at both atriocaval junctions and a reinfusion port located between these two and directed toward the tricuspid valve. Unlike single-lumen cannulation approaches, the double-lumen cannula is designed to reduce recirculation by capturing blood that returns via both venae cava.

Blood flow through a vascular cannula is complex and nonlinearly dependent on pressure, and thus, not generally predictable from traditional hydraulic equations. The relationship between the pressure gradient applied to a cannula and the resultant flow is characterized and published as pressure-flow curves (**Fig. 36.3**). The M-number system was developed to characterize flow through ECLS cannulas and represents a single index of resistance based on a correlation between Reynolds numbers and friction factor. The number is experimentally determined for each catheter and allows comparison of expected flows among different cannulas. A higher M-number represents a higher resistance and thus a lower flow at a given driving pressure.

Blood Pumps

Two types of blood pumps are currently used for extracorporeal membrane oxygenation (ECMO), and they are the same pumps used for cardiopulmonary bypass. The most popular is the *roller pump*, a positive-displacement pump in which a rotating roller head squeezes a length of blood tubing against a backing plate as the roller head rotates (**Fig. 36.4**). This pump is used with gravity drainage; therefore, an assist reservoir (bladder) is required at the pump inlet to maintain a continuous supply of blood to the pump, as inlet occlusion can result in large negative pressures (−500 mm Hg or more). In the event of outlet tubing obstruction, the pump can generate pressures high enough to cause tubing rupture, requiring continuous monitoring of circuit pressures. When properly used and monitored, this type of pump has a low incidence of complications.

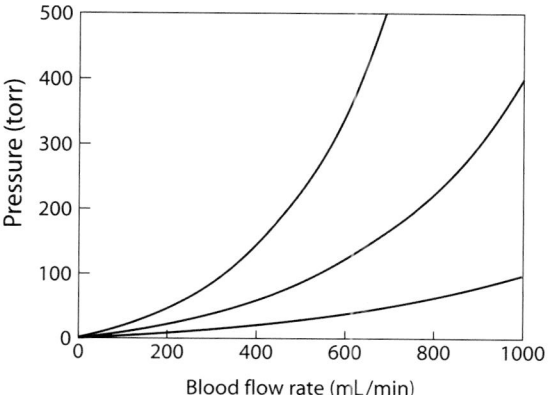

FIGURE 36.3. Pressure-flow curve for three different vascular access cannulas. The relationship between pressure and flow is nonlinear due to presence of side-holes, tapering, and development of turbulence.

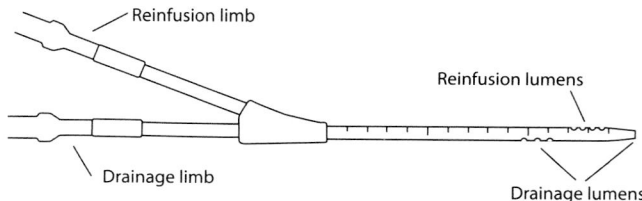

FIGURE 36.2. Double-lumen cannula for single-vessel (right internal jugular) access for venovenous extracorporeal life support.

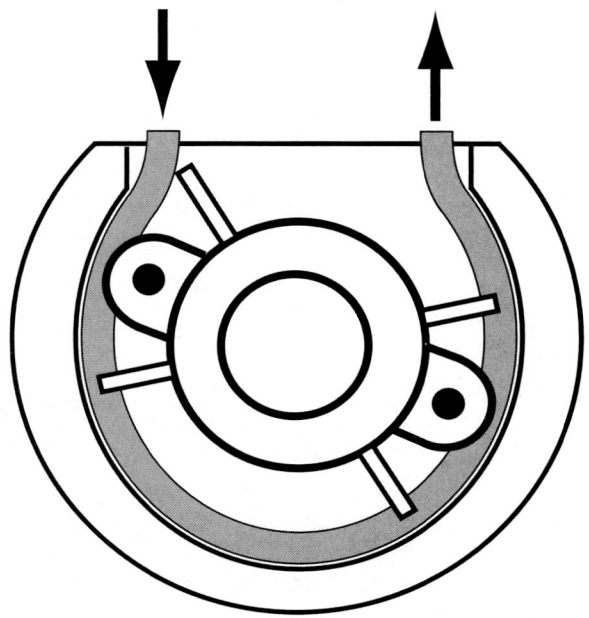

FIGURE 36.4. Roller pump used in extracorporeal circulation. The pump functions by having the rotor pinch and nearly occlude the raceway tubing against a backing plate, and the rotation forces blood through the tubing. The blood flow rate is linearly related to the size of the tubing and the rotational speed of the rotor.

The *centrifugal pump* is a nonocclusive pump that generates flow via a spinning rotor with vanes (**Fig. 36.5**). The device generates an active suction at the pump inlet. Occlusion of the inlet or outlet will result in only modest negative inlet or positive outlet pressures. Although this pump is safer from mechanical complications, hemolysis can develop rapidly in the case of tubing obstruction and is the most common complica-

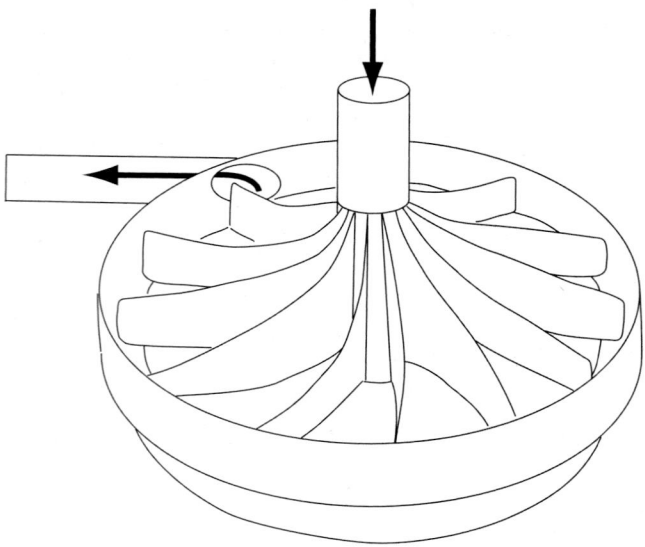

FIGURE 36.5. Centrifugal pump used in extracorporeal circulation. The tapered vanes on the roto create a centrifugal effect that forces blood from the central inlet port to the outer circumference, where it exits.

tion of the use of a centrifugal pump. Maintaining an adequate venous drainage and using a low-resistance oxygenator and a sufficiently large return cannula are effective strategies in preventing hemolysis.

Venous Assist Reservoir (Bladder)

Roller-pump systems require a continuous availability of blood at the inlet to avoid development of large negative pressures and hemolysis, which is ensured by placing a small assist reservoir, or bladder, just before the pump inlet. Gravity-assist is achieved by placing the reservoir and pump ~100 cm below the level of the cannula, providing a hydrostatic siphon for drainage and maintaining a positive pressure at the pump inlet. The reservoir also buffers against fluctuations in drainage. If drainage decreases, for example, due to hypovolemia, the reservoir will begin to empty, signaling the need for correction of the cause for poor drainage. Most roller-pump systems have the capability of servoregulation. A switch situated in the reservoir holder opens when the bladder empties, turning off the pump and allowing time for filling of the reservoir. With the pump off, the bladder refills and the pump resumes operation.

Membrane Lung

The membrane lung, commonly called a *membrane oxygenator*, provides gas exchange between the blood and the atmosphere. Although called an oxygenator, it is more appropriately called an artificial lung, as it transports CO_2 as well as O_2. The need to provide support for days to weeks imposes challenging requirements on oxygenator design. The two designs discussed here have traditionally been used for ECMO, and new designs are emerging.

Silicone Membrane Devices

The spiral-wound solid silicone sheet membrane lung (**Fig. 36.6**) has been used in the majority of ECMO cases since its inception. It consists of two long sheets of silicone sealed at the edges and wound on a polycarbonate support. Gas manifolds are attached at the ends, and other manifolds provide blood distribution between the rolls. Sizes range from 0.6–4.5 m^2. The larger devices have integrated heat exchangers.

Microporous, Hollow-fiber Devices

Microporous, hollow-fiber devices, most commonly used for cardiopulmonary bypass, are increasing in popularity for ECMO because of their improved gas-exchange performance and low resistance to blood flow. The hollow-fiber membranes are constructed of hydrophobic polymers with pores that range in size from 0.2–0.7 μm. These pores remain occupied with gas and present a gas-liquid interface for gas exchange. When in contact with water, or in short-term contact with plasma, the stability of these interfaces is maintained. After several hours of contact with plasma, however, leakage of plasma ensues and gas exchange is impaired, the cause of which is most likely the adherence of bipolar phospholipids creating a hydrophilic surface.

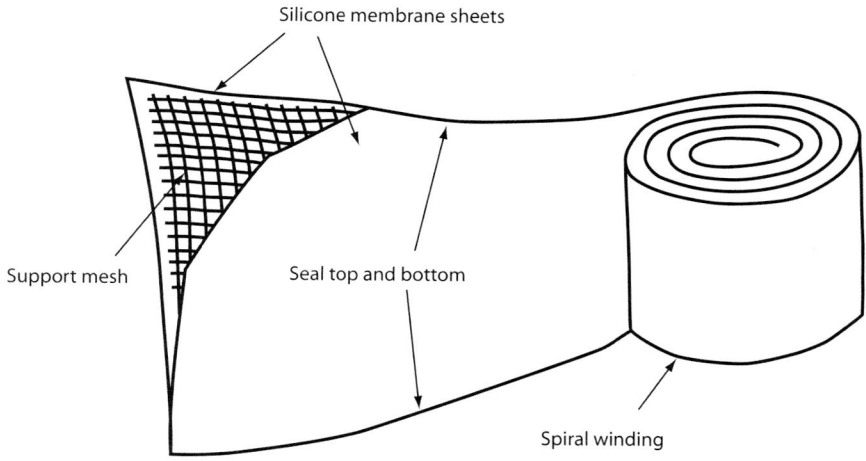

FIGURE 36.6. Solid silicone membrane lung used for ECLS. The silicone sheets are sealed at the edges and wound into a cylinder. The blood path is on the interior of the sheets, with the sweep gas on the exterior.

Monitoring Systems

An ECMO circuit is integrated with monitoring systems to ensure safe operation and effective gas transfer. Pressure monitors are used to monitor the development of excessive pressures across the device, providing an indication of the development of clotting and impairment of blood flow. In-line monitors in the drainage and postoxygenator circuit provide real-time information on venous and arterial saturation, pH, and hemoglobin concentration. Temperature monitors are used to monitor circuit and patient temperatures.

SUPPORT MODES

As ECMO has evolved from cardiopulmonary bypass (e.g., VA bypass with intrathoracic vascular cannulation), the initial application mode of ECMO was also venoarterial. While VA sup-

port remains important, especially with cardiac dysfunction, VV support has begun to supplant the traditional VA mode, primarily for respiratory failure. A hybrid support mode that combines features of VA and VV has been described. More recently, pumpless arteriovenous (AV) support has been shown to be clinically feasible for management of hypercarbic states. Each of these modes has particular advantages and disadvantages for different clinical situations (**Table 36.1**).

Venoarterial

VA support is based on cardiopulmonary bypass, in which blood is drained from the right atrium via the central venous system and returned to the proximal arterial system (**Fig. 36.7**). Both ventricles and the intervening pulmonary system are bypassed. In most cases partial support is achieved, with some residual pulmonary blood flow present. Cardiac and pulmonary support is provided with this mode. Cannulation

TABLE 36.1

COMPARISON OF CARDIOPULMONARY BYPASS AND DIFFERENT MODES OF ECLS

	CPB	VA ECMO	VV ECMO	VVA ECMO	AVCO$_2$R
Setting	Cardiac surgery	Prolonged support	Prolonged support	Prolonged support	ED or ICU support
Support	Total cardiac and pulmonary	Cardiac and pulmonary	Pulmonary	Cardiac and pulmonary	Pulmonary
Cannulation	Intrathoracic (surgical)	Extrathoracic (surgical)	Extrathoracic (percutaneous)	Extrathoracic (percutaneous)	Extrathoracic (percutaneous)
Blood pump	Roller or centrifugal	Roller or centrifugal	Roller or centrifugal	Roller or centrifugal	None (pumpless)
ECMO blood flow (fraction of CO)	Total (100%)	Subtotal (70%–90%)	Subtotal	Subtotal (1/3 arterial, 2/3 venous)	Low (10%–20%)
Pulmonary flow	None	Low	Unchanged	Moderate decrease	Unchanged
Length of support	Hours	Days to weeks	Days to weeks	Days to weeks	Days
Anticoagulation	ACT >400	ACT 180–200	ACT 180–200	ACT 180–200	ACT 200–220
Reservoir	Large	Small or none[a]	Small or none[a]	Small or none[a]	None

[a]Reservoir used for roller pump, optional for centrifugal pump.
CPB, cardiopulmonary bypass; VA, venoarterial; ECMO, extracorporeal membrane oxygenation; VV, venovenous; VVA, venovenoarterial; AVCO$_2$R, arteriovenous carbon dioxide removal; ED, emergency department; CO, cardiac output; ACT, activated coagulation time

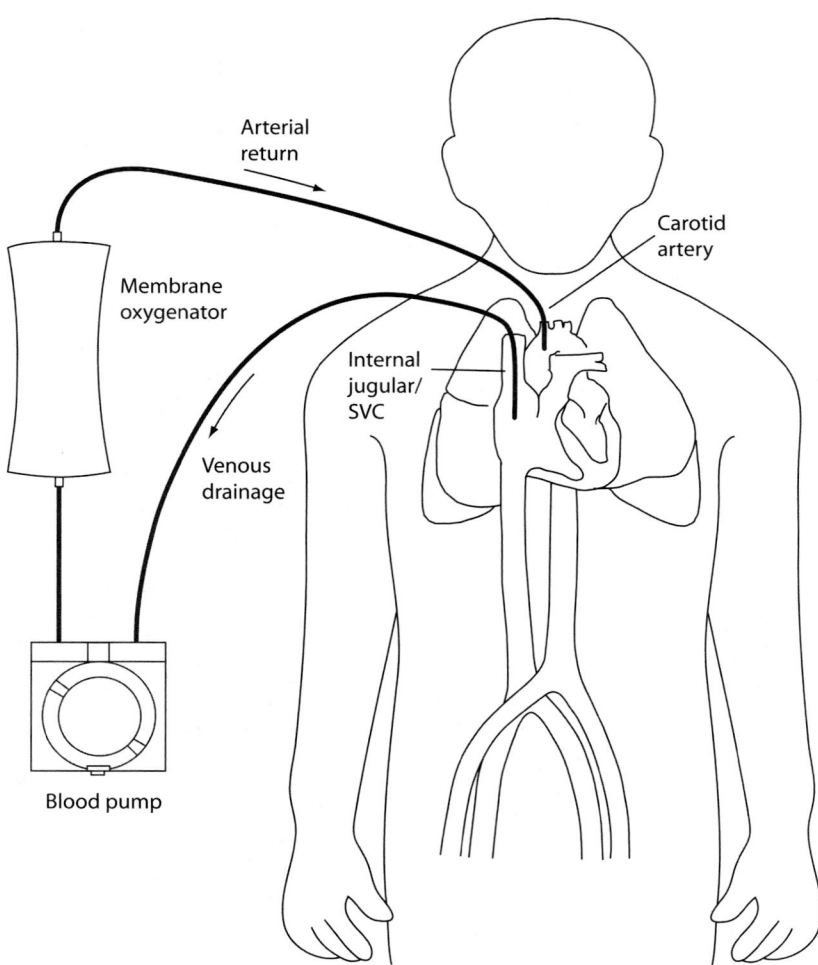

FIGURE 36.7. Venoarterial mode of extracorporeal life support via the cervical approach. Blood is drained from the right atrium and returned to the arterial system via the carotid artery into the proximal aorta. SVC, superior vena cava.

is usually performed by surgical access to the right internal jugular vein for right atrial drainage and to the right carotid artery for return to the aortic root. This mode provides the highest levels of systemic arterial saturation but may be associated with lower coronary O_2 saturation when bypass is partial in patients with severe respiratory failure, as poorly saturated native cardiac output may be directed toward the coronary ostia. The gas-exchange advantages of VA support are offset by a higher potential for complications, such as cerebral embolism, the reduction in pulmonary blood flow, and the loss of the right carotid circulation from ligation.

In place of the cervical approach, cannulation may be made through the femoral vessels (**Fig. 36.8**). This approach lends itself to percutaneous cannulation. Flow returning to the femoral artery will predominantly perfuse the lower half of the body, although retrograde flow up the aortic arch will also occur. The extent of retrograde flow is often dependent on the adequacy of native cardiac output, with more flow reaching the upper aorta under conditions of poor intrinsic cardiac function. With good cardiac function, the heart and brain predominantly receive blood from the native cardiopulmonary system. Thus, in patients with severe pulmonary failure and good cardiac function, desaturated blood may perfuse the brain and heart. Monitoring adequate cerebral oxygenation is important with this mode and can be performed by using cerebral near-infrared spectroscopy (NIRS) monitors, placing pulse oximetry devices on the ear or nose, and following mental status. Venous saturation entering

the right heart is often elevated in this mode by the mixing of the lower-body arterialized blood returned from the ECLS circuit with intrinsic venous blood; thus, adequate oxygenation to the native cardiopulmonary circuit can be obtained. While this mode has been used successfully, a recently introduced hybrid venovenoarterial mode overcomes limitations and may be even more efficient (see page 549).

Venovenous

VV ECLS can effectively support pediatric patients with respiratory failure (31) and is rapidly becoming the preferred mode for management of severe respiratory failure in children. VV support is a more recent development than VA support, having its origins in extracorporeal CO_2 removal (ECCO$_2$R). ECCO$_2$R was conceived as a low-flow VV mode that focused on CO_2 removal to support reduced levels of mechanical ventilation as part of a lung-protective ventilation strategy. Extension of this concept to higher blood flows and cannulation to minimize recirculation have allowed support for severe oxygenation failure. This mode provides prepulmonary oxygenation by draining blood from the central venous circulation and returning it back into the venous circulation (**Fig. 36.9**). The reinfused blood elevates mixed venous saturation, diminishes the effect of intrapulmonary shunt, and delivers blood with a higher saturation to the coronary arteries. No direct cardiac

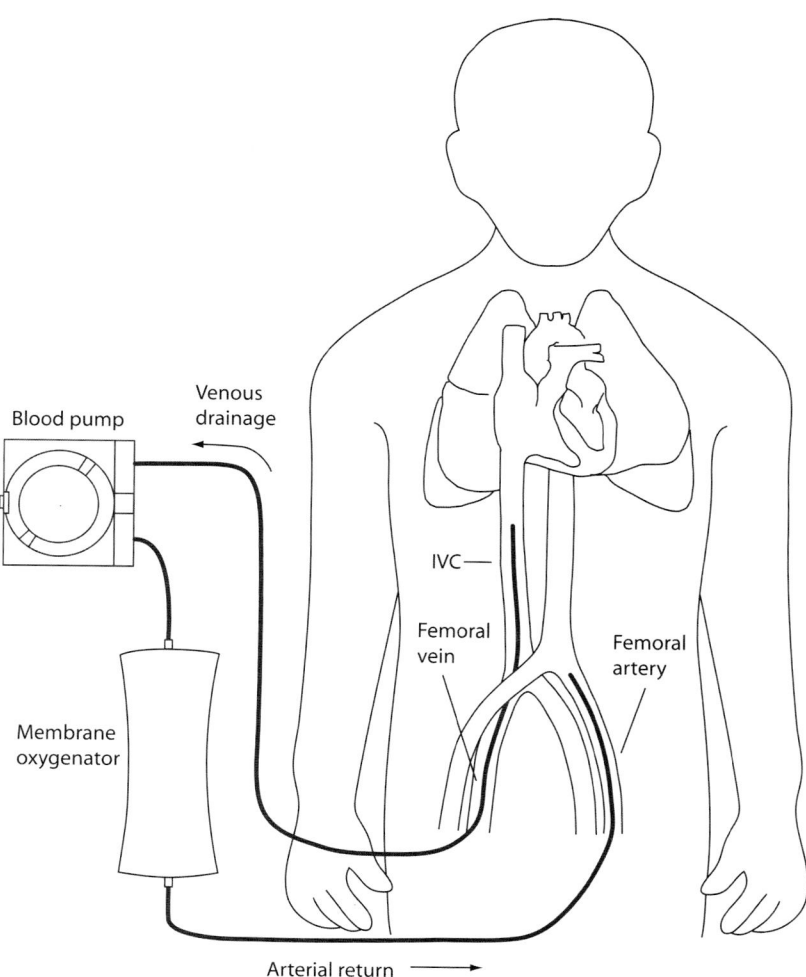

Blood pump

Venous drainage

Membrane oxygenator

IVC

Femoral vein

Femoral artery

Arterial return

FIGURE 36.8. Venoarterial mode of extracorporeal life support via the femoral approach. Blood is drained from inferior vena cava and returned to the arterial system via the femoral artery into the distal aorta. IVC, inferior vena cava.

support is delivered, although myocardial function commonly improves, often considerably, by elevation of myocardial oxygenation and reduction in intrathoracic pressures. VV support may be successfully applied even in the presence of inotrope dependence (38).

An attractive aspect of VV support is the ability to cannulate the veins percutaneously, avoiding surgical vascular access and largely eliminating bleeding from the vascular access site. The carotid artery and jugular are spared from ligation, and venous return through the jugular can be maintained. Central nervous system (CNS) complications are potentially lower with VV support (6), perhaps due to the less invasive nature of the vascular access technique. Cannulation is typically performed through the right internal jugular vein and the right common femoral vein. The more recent development of double-lumen cannula for patients who weigh up to 10 kg has allowed even simpler access, requiring only a single cannulation through the internal jugular vein (35). Recirculation, in which some of the return flow into the venous system is directed back into the drainage cannula, is present to a variable degree and reduces overall gas transfer. Venous drainage may be obtained from the internal jugular and returned to the femoral sites, or the direction of flow may be reversed (drainage from femoral with return to the jugular). Draining from the femoral veins has the advantage of reduced recirculation;

however, usually less venous flow can be obtained than if drainage is via the jugular cannula. (37). A three-cannula approach can be used to minimize recirculation even further (23) (**Fig. 36.10**).

Venovenoarterial

The venovenoarterial (VVA) mode is a recently introduced hybrid mode that combines VV support for pulmonary failure and partial VA support, with the advantage of percutaneous cannulation. The typical circuit consists of a drainage cannula in the right femoral vein and two return cannulae connected via a Y-connection, one in the right internal jugular vein and the second in a femoral artery (**Fig. 36.11**). Blood flow between the two return limbs is controlled to achieve approximately ~30% flow into the arterial system by restricting the flow (often with a simple screw clamp) to the venous cannula. VVA support is ideally suited for larger pediatric patients who require partial cardiac support in addition to pulmonary support.

Arteriovenous

The concept of pumpless AV support of gas exchange was described over 40 years ago, but has not been feasible until

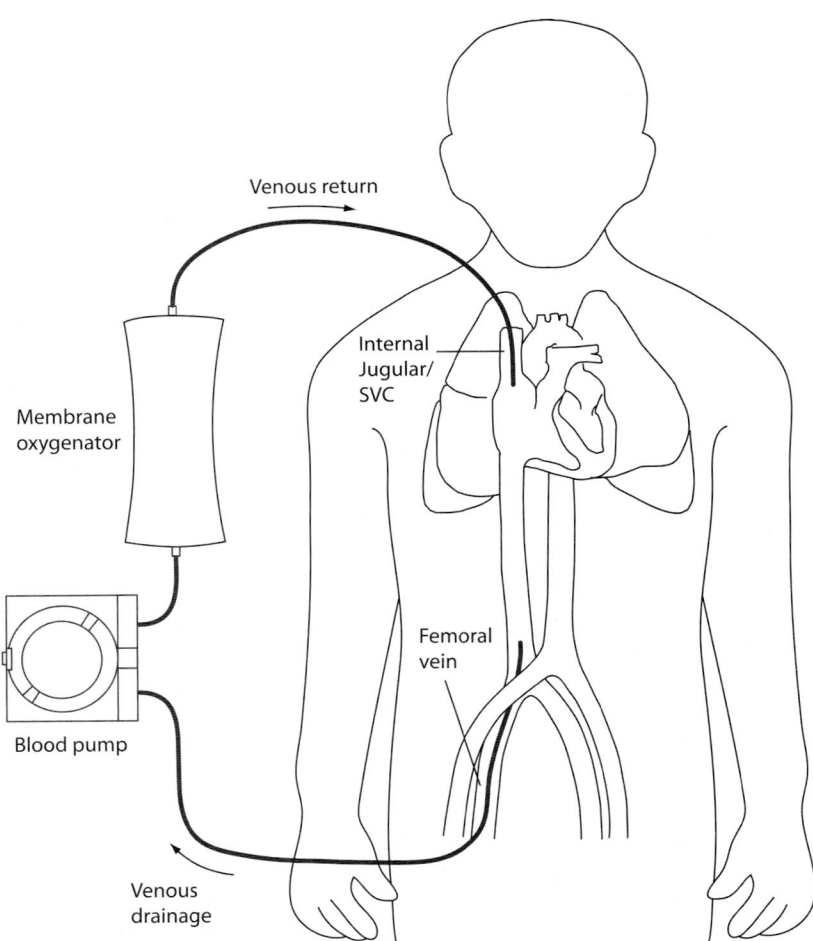

Venous return

Internal Jugular/SVC

Membrane oxygenator

Femoral vein

Blood pump

Venous drainage

FIGURE 36.9. Venovenous mode of extracorporeal life support. Blood is drained from the inferior vena cava and returned to the proximal superior vena cava (SVC) or right atrium.

the recent development of low-resistance, high-efficiency membrane lungs. The arterial-venous pressure gradient drives flow through a membrane lung without the need for a pump. Because arterial blood is usually well-oxygenated, oxygen transfer is limited, but CO_2 is readily removed. The applications of AV CO_2 removal ($AVCO_2R$) are identical to those of $ECCO_2R$, without the need for an extracorporeal pump, i.e., reduction in mechanical ventilatory support and control of hypercapnia.

Clinical trials in the US and Europe in adults have established the ability of AV support to safely remove CO_2 and allow for reduced ventilatory support (10,26). A blood flow of 15%–20% of cardiac output is required and is well tolerated in the absence of significant cardiac depression.

Application in pediatric patients for acute hypercapnia has been limited but successful, with a patient as young as 4 years of age successfully supported for 5 days (Louisiana State University Hospital, unpublished data). The advantages of this approach are the use of a very simplified circuit and elimination of the problems associated with pumped systems, such as tubing rupture, hemolysis, and platelet destruction.

CANNULATION TECHNIQUES

Vascular cannulation is perhaps the most challenging aspect of ECLS, and is the most limiting factor with respect to the

ability to provide an adequate level of support. The traditional approach has been an open surgical approach with vessel ligation. Percutaneous approaches are replacing surgical approaches where feasible.

Percutaneous Cannulation

The trend in vascular cannulation is toward percutaneous or modified percutaneous techniques, as this approach is more rapid and is associated with less bleeding complications and simplified decannulation. VV support is now almost exclusively approached percutaneously. The dual-lumen catheter by Origen Biomedical is available in 12-, 15-, and 18-fr sizes and is suitable for neonates and infants up to 10–12 kg. Larger sizes are under development and may prove suitable for larger patients. This cannula has both drainage and reinfusion lumens. The catheter is placed by percutaneous puncture of the right internal jugular, optionally under ultrasound guidance, using the well-described Seldinger technique. A guidewire exchange system is available, in which the initial puncture is made with a small needle and guidewire (0.018 inch), followed by an exchange for a larger wire (0.035 inch) that is suitable for dilation and advancement of the cannula.

VV cannulation in children who weigh >10–12 kg is accomplished by use of single-lumen cannulas in the femoral and right

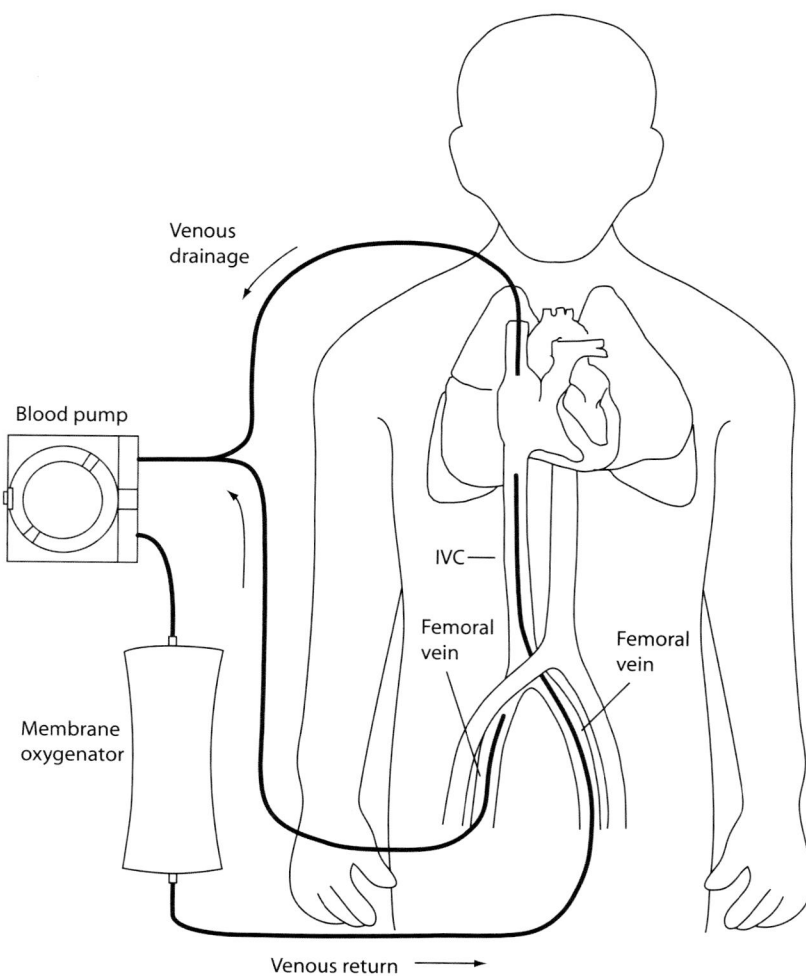

FIGURE 36.10. Venovenous support using three cannulas. This approach drains from the inferior (IVC) and superior vena cava, with return near the right atrium, minimizing recirculation.

internal jugular veins. The internal jugular is large enough to accommodate a single-reinfusion cannula (18–24-fr, depending on size). In larger children, a single femoral drainage cannula is usually suitable. The femoral veins in smaller children are smaller in relation to body size, and two drainage cannulas may be employed if drainage from a single site is inadequate. Choice of cannula size is dictated by the required flow (50–100 mL/kg). Ultrasound measurement is helpful in determination of vessel size and selection of an appropriately sized cannula.

A modified percutaneous technique for cannulation of the internal jugular vein in neonates has been described that uses a limited surgical exposure of the internal jugular with percutaneous cannulation under direct visualization of the vein (30). The correct cannula size can then be determined.

Percutaneous arterial cannulation is limited to the femoral artery in larger children. As this vessel is usually too small to accommodate full VA support, this approach is limited to the provision of partial support. In the presence of respiratory failure, hybrid VVA support may be a suitable option.

AV support for AVCO$_2$R requires a lower blood flow than that required for oxygenation support, on the order of 15%–20% of the cardiac output. Percutaneous cannulation of the femoral vessels with a 10–12-fr arterial cannula and 14–16-fr

venous cannula provides adequate flow (500–1000 mL/min) for complete CO$_2$ removal in hypercapnic states (10).

Peripheral Surgical Cannulation

The open surgical technique is the original method of cannulation for ECLS and remains the approach of choice today for VA support through the common carotid artery and internal jugular vein. A transverse incision is made above the right clavicle over the vessels, and dissection is performed to expose the carotid sheath (**Fig. 36.12**). The sheath is opened, and the vessels and vagus nerve identified. The vein is usually exposed first, with ligatures placed proximally and distally. The carotid is similarly exposed and prepared. An arteriotomy is made following distal ligation, and the arterial cannula is placed. Venotomy and venous cannulation follow next. The wound is closed and cannulas are secured in place.

Surgical placement of a dual-lumen venous cannula for VV bypass is performed in a similar manner, although without the need for carotid ligation and arteriotomy. Inability to percutaneously insert a dual-lumen cannula or development of complications during insertion are usually managed by conversion to an open surgical approach.

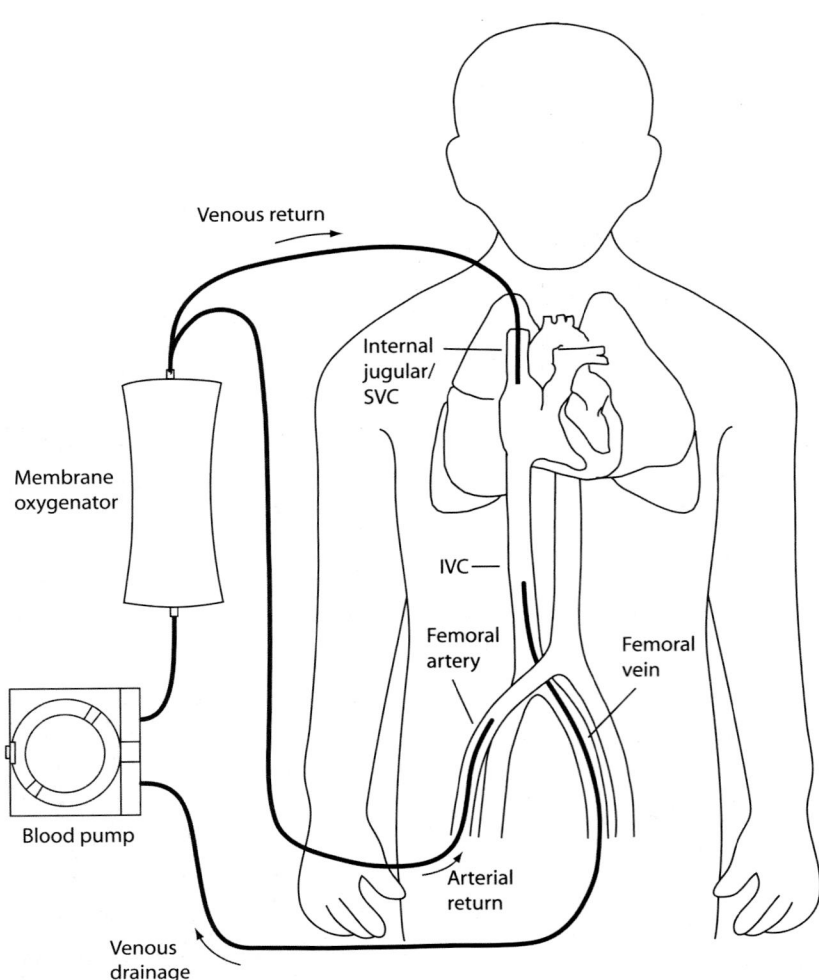

FIGURE 36.11. Hybrid venovenoarterial mode of extracorporeal life support. Blood is drained from the inferior vena cava (IVC) and returned to the right atrium, as in venovenous support. In addition, some of the returning blood is diverted to the femoral artery.

Transthoracic Cannulation

ECLS following failure to wean from cardiopulmonary bypass or sternotomy for resuscitation can be managed using the same cannulas placed for intraoperative support. These cannulas are placed into the right atrium and ascending aorta and are secured with purse-string sutures. The chest is incompletely closed (allowing the cannula to exit the wound) and dressed. If hemodynamic function improves in a short period of time, the patient can be weaned from support, and decannulated in the operating room. If long-term support is deemed necessary, the patient can be converted to peripherally placed cannulas, as bleeding is less with this approach.

Decannulation

Termination of ECLS is followed by decannulation. If cardiopulmonary function is marginal after cessation of support, the decision may be made to maintain the cannulas in place for several hours or more. Provisions for maintaining anticoagulation and continuous flushing of the cannulas must be made.

Surgically placed cannulas are removed by opening the surgical site, partially withdrawing the cannulas, proximally ligating the vessels, and removing the cannula. The wound is irrigated and closed. Percutaneous cannulas are removed by withdrawal, followed by pressure over the site. At the venous site, a suture may be placed to close the tract just proximal to the insertion site. Removal of percutaneous arterial cannulas up to ~16 fr can usually be managed nonoperatively, but larger cannulas may require arterial repair.

DETERMINANTS OF ECLS CIRCUIT PERFORMANCE

Delivery of sufficient O_2 and removal of CO_2 to support the patient with severe cardiopulmonary failure depends upon an adequate extracorporeal blood flow, efficient transfer of O_2 and CO_2 in the membrane oxygenator, and minimization of recirculation.

Blood Flow

The blood path in the extracorporeal circuit includes the vascular cannulas, circuit tubing, oxygenator, and heat exchanger. The point of greatest impedance to blood flow is in the vascular cannulas, in particular the venous drainage cannula, as it depends upon gravity drainage (roller pump) or a low level of

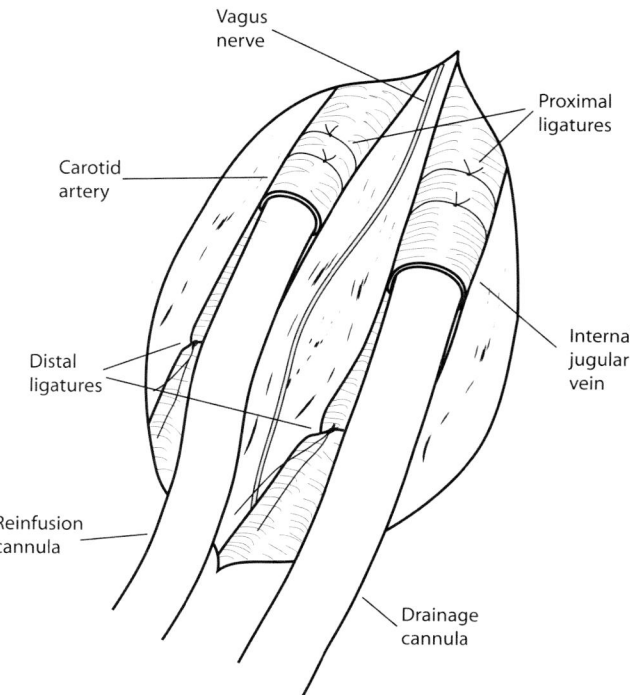

FIGURE 36.12. Open surgical approach to cervical cannulation. The carotid sheath is opened, the vessels are exposed, and ligatures are placed. An arteriotomy and venotomy provide access to the lumen for cannula insertion.

suction (centrifugal pump). Optimization of conditions for venous drainage, including selection of cannula size, is essential. The relationship between pressure and flow is nonlinear (**Fig. 36.3**). At lower blood flows, laminar flow predominates and is approximately described by the Hagen-Poiseuille equation, with flow (Q) directly related to pressure gradient (ΔP) and inversely related to catheter length (L):

$$\dot{Q} = \left(\frac{\pi r^4}{8\eta}\right)\frac{\Delta P}{L}$$

At higher flows, and as a result of catheter design (e.g., side holes), flow becomes nonlinearly related to pressure, and use of experimentally determined pressure-flow curves that are provided by manufacturers can be used. An alternative to published flow curves is the use of the M-number system, which seeks to ascribe a single number that defines flow impedance of a catheter or length of tubing (28).

The catheter dimension that has greatest influence on blood flow is the diameter; thus, the goal is to place the catheter with the largest diameter and shortest length as allowed by the venous anatomy. As gravity-assisted drainage can yield up to ~100 cm H_2O, this pressure can be used to estimate maximal blood flow for a given catheter. Actual flow depends on adequate venous return as well as proper depth and intravascular positioning of the venous cannula.

Membrane Oxygenator Gas Transfer

Blood delivered by the extracorporeal circuit must be fully saturated with O_2 by the membrane oxygenator to have maximal achievable O_2 delivery. A membrane oxygenator can fully saturate blood only up to a certain flow, above which saturation falls off and total O_2 delivery reaches a plateau. The rated flow of an oxygenator is the flow at which blood entering under standardized inlet conditions that simulate normal venous O_2 saturation (75%) is raised to 95%, and represents the maximal efficient flow for the device. Above the rated flow, O_2 transfer becomes diffusion limited, and O_2 saturation diminishes.

Gas transfer by the membrane oxygenator is determined by several factors. The membrane surface area, membrane diffusion coefficient, and thickness of the blood film in the oxygenator are determined by the manufacturer. The partial pressure gradient between the blood and gas phases is in part governed by blood and sweep gas flows. The choice of the membrane oxygenator is usually made on selecting a sufficiently large surface area device to accommodate the calculated blood flow (50–100 mL/kg/min).

Recirculation

Recirculation, in which some of the blood reinfused into the patient from the circuit is diverted back into the drainage cannula, rather than continue into the pulmonary circulation, is unavoidable in VV ECLS. The efficiency of extracorporeal support is reduced in proportion to the recirculation fraction (R), which can be theoretically calculated through the measurement of O_2 saturations in a fashion analogous to calculation of transpulmonary shunt fraction:

$$R = \frac{C_{pre}O_2 - C_{\bar{V}}O_2}{C_{post}O_2 - C_{\bar{V}}O_2}$$

where $C_{pre}O_2$ and $C_{post}O_2$ are the O_2 content of pre- and post-oxygenator blood. $C_{\bar{V}}O_2$ represents the true mixed venous blood O_2 content leaving the tissues and cannot be measured in the pulmonary artery (which on ECLS, is influenced by the blood returned by the circuit). This value can be estimated by sampling venous blood proximal to the drainage cannula and out of the recirculation path. Alternative methods for measuring recirculation include ultrasound dilution (49) and thermodilution (44), but these have not been widely adopted.

The amount of recirculation is influenced by cannula placement and can sometimes be increased by attempts to compensate by increasing the flow. The dual-lumen cannula attempts to minimize recirculation by draining from both the superior and inferior aspects of the right atrium (34). With two-cannula support, drainage from the inferior vena cava via the femoral vein and reinfusion into the superior vena cava via the internal jugular usually results in less recirculation than flow in the reverse direction (36). A three-cannula technique (two short drainage and one long reinfusion) has been shown to improve extracorporeal blood flow and reduce recirculation (23).

CLINICAL APPLICATIONS AND SELECTION OF PATIENTS

Hypoxemic Respiratory Failure

The pediatric patient beyond the first 2 weeks of life differs from the neonate in both physiology and spectrum of causes of acute respiratory failure. The features of fetal physiology,

TABLE 36.2

CRITERIA USED IN SELECTION OF PATIENTS FOR ECLS FOR PULMONARY SUPPORT IN HYPOXEMIC RESPIRATORY FAILURE

Severe, potentially reversible acute respiratory failure
Lack of response to conventional support measures[a]
Severe hypoxemia, e.g.,: $\quad$ Pao$_2$/Fio$_2$ <100 $\quad$ Oxygenation Index (OI) >40 $\quad$ Qs/Qt >0.5
Elevated inflation pressures, e.g.,: $\quad$ MAP >20 on conventional ventilation, >25 on HFOV $\quad$ Persistent air leak or interstitial air $\quad$ Cardiovascular depression with shock (pH <7.25)
Lack of irreversible ventilator-induced lung injury, e.g.,: $\quad$ Duration of mechanical ventilation <7 days

[a]Conventional support may include measures such as high frequency oscillation (HFOV), inhaled nitric oxide, prone positioning, surfactant, or others.
Qs/Qt, intrapulmonary shunt; MAP, mean airway pressure; HFOV, high frequency oscillatory ventilation

including fetal right-to-left shunts, have largely disappeared by the end of this period. Respiratory failure in the newborn due to persistent pulmonary hypertension and meconium aspiration is replaced by pulmonary infection, pulmonary aspiration, systemic sepsis and other conditions. These illnesses often trigger ARDS and are frequently accompanied by extrapulmonary organ system involvement. The most common cause of hypoxemic respiratory failure in the pediatric age group that leads to support with ECLS is viral pneumonia (26%), followed by ARDS (13%), bacterial pneumonia (10%), and aspiration pneumonitis (6%) (9). The remaining fraction comprises respiratory failure due to a number of other etiologies.

The selection of patients for ECLS is founded in a set of criteria that have evolved over time and have historically predicted high mortality (**Table 36.2**). The essential element of these criteria is to select patients with severe oxygenation impairment, risk of ventilator-induced pulmonary injury, and the capacity for pulmonary recovery. Measures of oxygenation impairment include the oxygenation index (OI), Pao$_2$/Fio$_2$ ratio (P/F ratio), or intrapulmonary shunt fraction. The OI takes into account the inflation pressures associated with the oxygenation variables and has been the traditional index used in neonates and younger children. The P/F ratio and intrapulmonary shunt are two interrelated measures that do not include an inflation pressure component, but they have been most commonly applied in older children and adults.

The avoidance of ventilator-induced lung injury is a major goal of ECLS; thus, patients who require excessive inflation pressures, even in the absence of life-threatening hypoxemia, should be considered for extracorporeal support. This is particularly important if lactic acidosis and shock result from high levels of ventilatory support. The presence of barotrauma (radiographic evidence of pneumomediastinum or pulmonary interstitial air, or persistent air leak) should lead to consideration of ECLS, especially if it is progressive and uncontrollable.

Even with these guidelines, the decision of whether to place a patient on extracorporeal support requires consideration of other factors, including comorbid conditions, contraindications to anticoagulation, duration of pre-ECLS cardiac arrest and quality of resuscitation and duration of mechanical ventilation prior to ECLS. The former contraindications to ECLS have given way to individualized decisions of risk assessment and potential benefit. It may be prudent to undertake high-risk or uncertain cases (e.g., uncertain neurologic status following cardiac arrest) with the provision that ECLS will be withdrawn if clinical information is discovered that would suggest futility.

VV support is the preferred ECLS mode for hypoxemic respiratory failure. The presence of inotropes, once used as an indication to proceed to VA support, is not a contraindication to VV support (38). In most cases, inotrope requirements are reduced, as the myocardium recovers from hypoxemia. The presence of shock despite inotropes, however, would be best supported with the VA approach.

Hypercapnic Respiratory Failure

Severe hypercapnia with respiratory acidosis, in particular severe asthma, is effectively managed by VV extracorporeal support. As CO$_2$ is more effectively exchanged in the membrane lung than is O$_2$, blood flows lower than that required for oxygenation are effective in control of hypercapnia. The concept of low-flow ECCO$_2$R was first described as an adjunct to enable lung-protective ventilation in adult ARDS. An extracorporeal blood flow of ≤20% of the cardiac output is sufficient for control of hypercapnia, although higher flows may be required if hypoxemia is present. Another advantage of extracorporeal support of severe asthma is the ability to perform bronchoscopy to remove secretions and debris.

An alternative to VV ECCO$_2$R is pumpless AVCO$_2$R. Percutaneous cannulation of the femoral artery and vein can be rapidly performed, and crystalloid priming of the circuit is simple. AVCO$_2$R can normalize pH and Pco$_2$, even in severe asthma. Decannulation is simple, as the small size of the arterial cannula permits hemostasis through direct pressure alone.

Acute Myocardial Dysfunction

ECLS has been a primary mode of support for pediatric patients with circulatory failure from acute myocardial dysfunction and accounts for the indication for support in over half of all pediatric ECLS cases beyond the neonatal period (9). The majority of cases have involved postoperative support following cardiac surgery, but cardiomyopathy and myocarditis are frequent reasons for cardiac support with ECLS. Familiarity with ECLS for pulmonary failure and the lack of availability of suitable pediatric ventricular assist devices are reasons for the use of ECLS, although small trials suggest that ECLS is of comparable efficacy to ventricular assist devices (15) and may be advantageous following cardiac transplantation (46).

Early initiation of support following recognition of circulatory failure is essential. Patients who are placed on ECLS in the operating room (rather than being delayed to the ICU) following open heart surgery have a better survival (2,7), most likely due to prevention of shock, acidosis, and cardiac arrest.

Prolonged low cardiac output and shock in the face of appropriate fluid management and pharmacologic support can result in neurologic injury and other organ dysfunction and should be avoided by early consideration of ECLS.

VA support is the mode of choice, as it provides cardiopulmonary bypass and maintains systemic circulatory flow at normal levels. Patients placed on ECLS in the operating room may be centrally cannulated, but the cervical approach with carotid and internal jugular cannulation is commonly practiced. Recent experience with the percutaneous femoral approach suggests that this cannulation route may be easy and successful. In the face of severe myocardial dysfunction in which the ventricle cannot empty against the afterload associated with ECLS-maintained arterial pressure, persistent elevation of end-diastolic pressure can result in pulmonary hypertension, pulmonary edema, pulmonary hemorrhage, and impairment of myocardial recovery. When required, the left heart can be decompressed via atrial septostomy (41), which can be performed in the cardiac catheterization suite or at the bedside. A recent report of percutaneous insertion of a miniature axial-flow rotary pump under bedside echocardiographic guidance suggests that this device may provide an alternative, less invasive approach that avoids the need for transport to the cardiac catheterization suite (50).

Nonsurgical causes of severe myocardial dysfunction are also supported with ECLS. Cardiomyopathies unrelated to cardiac surgery differ from the postoperative causes of myocardial dysfunction, in that recovery may take place after prolonged support. Acute myocarditis can follow a rapidly progressive course and result in death in a majority of cases. In a series of 15 patients with viral myocarditis and acute deterioration who were managed with mechanical support (12 with ECLS), survival was 80% (14). Support ranged in duration from 48–400 hrs, with a median of 140 hrs. Ventricular function in those recovering without transplantation was normal at follow-up periods up to 5.3 years. In another series of 14 patients with fulminant myocarditis managed with percutaneous femorofemoral VA ECLS, 10 patients (71%) survived. A smaller series reported survival in 4 of 5 patients with acute myocarditis, all but one of whom were managed with percutaneous femorofemoral bypass (8).

VA ECLS can be used to bridge to transplantation. Patients with cardiomyopathy have a better prognosis than those with congenital heart disease when bridged to transplantation. Acute viral myocarditis carries a good prognosis (17).

Weaning from VA ECLS is initiated when signs of ventricular recovery are noted. An early manifestation of recovery is improvement in pulsatility, as evidenced by an increase in pulse pressure. Echocardiography permits serial noninvasive assessment of ventricular contractility and can assess the response to changes in ventricular loading that are associated with reduction in flow. Once ventricular recovery begins, the extracorporeal flow is gradually reduced, and the patient is assessed clinically for adequacy of perfusion. Measurements of blood gases, mixed venous O_2 saturation, and cardiac function by echocardiography ensure that native cardiac function is adequate. When the patient can tolerate a low extracorporeal flow and maintain good perfusion, the ECLS circuit is discontinued and the cannulas are removed. Predictors of nonsurvival include persistent elevation of lactate (4,43), prolonged duration of support (2,4,43), progressive multiple organ dysfunction and nosocomial pneumonia (27).

Extracorporeal Cardiopulmonary Resuscitation

Recognition of the poor rate of recovery from cardiac arrest following external chest compression, particularly after prolonged efforts, has led to the expanded use of rapid-deployment ECLS. Also termed extracorporeal cardiopulmonary resuscitation (ECPR) or resuscitation extracorporeal membrane oxygenation (R-ECMO), this technique involves the rapid institution of ECLS during cardiac arrest via percutaneous cannulation of the femoral vessels or through a reopened sternotomy and mediastinal cannulation and a pre-primed or rapidly primed ECLS circuit.

A multi-institutional report of ECLS for a variety of emergent conditions (including cardiac arrest) in a general hospital population demonstrated feasibility and a survival of 20% (22). No patients with unwitnessed arrest survived. In pediatric patients who are post-cardiac surgery, survivals of 60% with rapid ECLS, even after average resuscitation times of 1 hr, have been reported (11,15).

ECPR is the most rapidly growing application for ECLS and has been used more frequently in pediatrics than in neonates and adults. In a single-center report of resuscitation ECLS following cardiac arrest in cardiac surgery patients, 73% survived (47).

Age-specific Considerations

The basic principles of ECLS are applicable across all age groups, from neonatal to adult. The primary differences with respect to age include cannulation approach and circuit specifications.

Cannulation approaches differ as a result of both differences in vascular anatomy and availability of various types of vascular cannulas. In infants, the femoral veins are small relative to the internal jugular and are generally not large enough to support adequate flow. The internal jugular is the vein of choice in infants. For respiratory support with VV ECLS, the dual-lumen cannula is preferred, placed either by the percutaneous or modified-percutaneous approach. Currently, the cannula is manufactured up to 18 fr in size, capable of supporting an infant who weighs up to 10–12 kg. For cardiac support with VA ECLS, surgical access to the internal jugular and the carotid with single-lumen cannula is the method of choice. In children larger than 10–12 kg (for which a dual-lumen cannula is not available), the femoral and internal jugular vessels can be used for the two- or three-cannula method for VV ECLS. Representative cannula sizes for children of different ages are given in **Table 36.3**. The circuit used for infants who weigh up to 10–12 kg employs 1/4-inch (6-mm) tubing, with 3/8- (10-mm) to 1/2-inch (13-mm) tubing used for larger children. The size of the membrane lung is also dependent on patient size. Representative circuit components for different sizes are also listed in **Table 36.3**.

PHYSIOLOGY OF EXTRACORPOREAL CIRCULATION

Extracorporeal circulation induces profound influences on human physiology, both desirable, as in the form of enhanced O_2

TABLE 36.3

REPRESENTATIVE CIRCUIT COMPONENTS FOR ECLS BASED ON PATIENT WEIGHT

	Weight (kg)					
	3–6	6–12	12–25	25–40	40–70	>70
Tubing size (inches)	¼	¼	⅜	⅜	⅜	⅜
Raceway size (inches)	¼–⅜	⅜	⅜–½	½	½	½
Centrifugal pump size[a]	Pediatric	Pediatric	Adult	Adult	Adult	Adult
Solid membrane lung size (m²)	0.8	1.5	2.5	3.5	4.5	4.5 × 2
Hollow fiber lung size (m²)	0.33–0.6	0.4–0.9	0.8–2.0	2.0–2.5	2.0–2.5	2.0–2.5
Venous cannula size (fr)[b]	12–15	14–18	15–19	19–21	21–23	23–25
Arterial cannula size (fr)[b]	10–12	12–15	14–17	16–19[c]	17–21[c]	19–23[c]
Dual-lumen venous cannula	12–15	15–18	n/a	n/a	n/a	n/a

[a]Centrifugal pump size is determined by tubing size.
[b]Individual considerations may require the use of other sizes.
[c]Smaller size is applicable to percutaneous. Hybrid support may involve sizes smaller than those listed.
fr, French; n/a, not available as of this publication

delivery, and undesirable, such as from the adverse effects on blood coagulation.

Perfusion

Systemic blood flow during VA ECLS is the sum of native cardiac output and blood flow through the circuit. As circuit blood flow is raised, less venous return is available to the native heart. As the proportion of systemic flow provided by the nonpulsatile blood pump increases, stroke volume diminishes and is recognized as a diminishing pulse pressure on the arterial waveform. In severe cardiac dysfunction, systemic blood flow may be provided totally by the extracorporeal circuit.

During total bypass, the left ventricle continues to receive some blood flow, mostly from the Thebesian veins (in the myocardial wall) and deep bronchial veins, and possibly intermittent flow across the pulmonary circulation. It slowly distends, so that intermittent pulsatile waveforms may appear. When cardiac contractility is sufficiently impaired and unable to eject blood against the afterload provided by the circuit, no pulsatile blood flow is noted. Distension of the left ventricle may lead to left atrial hypertension, pulmonary venous congestion, and pulmonary hemorrhage. Further, a distended left ventricle may impair myocardial blood flow and oxygenation. The role of left-heart decompression in this circumstance has already been discussed.

Nonpulsatile flow has potentially deleterious effects, including increased peripheral vascular resistance through higher levels of catecholamines (42) and reduced NO production (29), reduced renal and cerebral (48) perfusion, and impaired release of cortisol. The clinical relevance of these effects has been debated, but nonpulsatile flow does not appear to be detrimental during long-term ECLS if adequate total systemic perfusion is maintained. During VV ECLS, systemic blood flow is provided solely by the native heart and, therefore, remains pulsatile.

AV support represents an AV vascular shunt, reducing systemic blood flow by the blood flow through the circuit. Introducing such a shunt decreases afterload, and the heart will normally increase total cardiac output such that systemic blood flow to tissues is maintained. This compensatory increase may not occur if myocardial dysfunction is present. The use of this mode of support must be made cautiously in the presence of myocardial dysfunction, and monitoring for inadequate perfusion should be performed.

Oxygen Delivery

Systemic O_2 delivery during ECLS is dependent on the mode of support and the degree of native lung function. During VA ECLS, in which native pulmonary blood flow is parallel to the circuit flow, O_2 delivery is the total of that provided by fully saturated blood from the extracorporeal circuit mixed with that provided by the native lungs. With total bypass, systemic O_2 delivery is provided totally by the circuit and is equal to the product of the pump flow and the O_2 content of fully saturated blood:

$$DO_2 = \dot{Q}_{pump} \cdot C_{pump}O_2$$

With partial bypass, blood from the lungs is often poorly saturated due to pulmonary dysfunction, and therefore functions as a shunt, decreasing the total O_2 content relative to the amount of native pulmonary blood flow:

$$DO_2 = \dot{Q}_{pump} \cdot C_{pump}O_2 + \dot{Q}_{pul} \cdot C_{pul}O_2$$
$$= \dot{Q}_{total} \cdot \left[\frac{\dot{Q}_{pump}}{\dot{Q}_{total}} \cdot C_{pump}O_2 + \frac{\dot{Q}_{pul}}{\dot{Q}_{total}} \cdot C_{pul}O_2 \right]$$

In VV support, the circuit and the native pulmonary circulation are in series, and the effects of O_2 content provided by the pump and that provided by the native lungs is additive. The resulting O_2 delivery is the incremental O_2 content added to the true mixed venous O_2 saturation by the circuit and the lungs:

$$DO_2 = \dot{Q}_{total} \cdot \left[C_{\bar{V}}O_2 + \Delta C_{pump}O_2 + \Delta C_{pul}O_2 \right]$$

Due to incomplete drainage and recirculation, the amount added by the extracorporeal circuit will not result in fully saturated blood in the pulmonary artery, usually reaching

85%–90%. If pulmonary dysfunction is severe, no additional O_2 will be added by the lungs and systemic O_2 delivery will be based on the saturation provided to the pulmonary artery (usually 85%–90% but sometimes lower). If native lung function is present, additional O_2 will be transferred, and arterial saturation will be higher. When the lungs undergo recovery, the arterial blood may become fully saturated.

AV ECLS does not provide any significant degree of O_2 delivery, as the blood provided to the membrane already contains arterial levels of O_2. Even under profound hypoxemic conditions, the small fraction of blood through the circuit ($\leq 20\%$ of cardiac output) would not contribute substantially to overall O_2 delivery. It is therefore most applicable to hypercapnic states without significant hypoxemia. Removal of CO_2 by this route can reduce alveolar partial pressure of CO_2 and improve the gradient for pulmonary O_2 transfer; however, under conditions of increased inspired O_2 fraction, this effect is not clinically significant.

Blood Component Damage

The mechanical pumping of blood and resulting high flow through a system that is recognized to produce high shear rates results in injury to erythrocytes, platelets, and plasma proteins. Shear force represents a deforming force applied to blood components and is defined as the velocity gradient applied to the component. High shear rates can occur throughout the circuit, such as rapid directional changes at catheter side holes and edges, cavitation in the blood pump, and turbulence. The raceway of roller pumps and the rotating vanes of centrifugal pumps where they contact the blood are a known source of shear forces. High shear rates applied to erythrocytes induce membrane changes (altered deformability) or disruption (hemolysis). Roller pumps cause more hemolysis than centrifugal under proper operating conditions, but the rate of hemolysis is usually not clinically significant. Under improper operating conditions, however, both are capable of significant hemolysis. Elevated shear forces cause hemolysis, platelet deposition, and denaturation of plasma proteins and lipoproteins. Injury to plasma proteins, platelets, and white blood cells contributes to activation of coagulation and inflammation.

Activation of Coagulation

The extracorporeal circuit represents a large, nonendothelial contact surface that is known to induce profound effects on the coagulation system. The response is initiated during short-term support (e.g., during operating room cardiopulmonary bypass) and during long-term support with ECLS, with activation of the contact, intrinsic, extrinsic, and common pathways. The result is conversion of prothrombin to thrombin and of fibrinogen to fibrin. Fibrin polymers link to form a fibrin mesh and then cross-linked.

Several serine protease inhibitors of coagulation [e.g., antithrombin III (ATIII)] are activated, along with procoagulant proteins, but this physiologic system is overwhelmed by the degree of activation of coagulation by the circuit. Systemic anticoagulation, such as with heparin, is thus required. Heparin accelerates the action of ATIII but does not inhibit thrombin formation. As a result, it is not an ideal anticoagulant but remains a drug of choice for numerous reasons, including the great degree of experience with its use.

Systemic Inflammation

In addition to activation of coagulation, the extracorporeal circuit induces a systemic inflammatory response. Mediated by humoral and cellular components of the immune system, this response is complex, variable, and not completely understood. Activation of macrophages and other immune system-related cells results in the production of proximal proinflammatory mediators, including tumor necrosis factor (TNF), IL-1 and IL-6. Proinflammatory cytokines have numerous actions that result in systemic inflammation, including increases in neutrophil adhesion and migration, stimulation of neutrophil phagocytosis, and degranulation and release of reactive O_2 species. Eicosanoids (e.g., the thromboxanes) are more distal mediators of inflammation, particularly in the lungs, and are increased in extracorporeal circulation.

Neutrophils are activated by the introduction of extracorporeal circulation and are likely to be activated by the underlying disease state before initiation of ECLS. Hypoxemia, ischemia, and reperfusion contribute to pre-ECLS neutrophil priming. Neutrophils are not only activated by cytokine and bioactive lipids, but once activated can themselves produce proinflammatory cytokines and additional arachidonic acid products that mediate inflammation. Neutrophil degranulation results in release of proteolytic and cytotoxic enzymes. Formation of reactive O_2 species ensues, which is important for normal microbial killing. When released systemically, however, reactive O_2 species can damage endothelial and other cells, resulting in endothelial activation, microvascular coagulation, organ dysfunction, and capillary leak syndrome.

PATIENT MANAGEMENT

Circuit Priming

The extracorporeal circuit volume is large relative to the patient's blood volume, mandating that the circuit be primed with a solution that contains normal electrolyte concentration and acceptable acid-base status, oncotic pressure, and hemoglobin concentration. Priming begins with balanced electrolyte solution (such as Normosol or PlasmaLyte). Packed red blood cells and concentrated albumin or fresh frozen plasma. ECPR circuits often have priming volumes that are small enough to allow initiation with a bloodless prime. As citrated blood is acidic and depleted in calcium, bicarbonate (or THAM) and calcium chloride (after heparin) are included. Electrolytes, in particular potassium and ionized calcium, and pH are measured. Additional calcium and/or bicarbonate is added as needed. High potassium levels, especially in smaller patients, require gradual initiation of support. An alternative is to use hemofiltration to normalize electrolytes and pH.

Initiation of Support

Preparation of the patient prior to cannulation includes adequate sedation and analgesia. Activated clotting time

(ACT) is measured prior to heparin administration to obtain a baseline. If percutaneous cannulation is chosen, ultrasonographic measurement of vessel size and patency may be performed and may be used to guide needle insertion. Neuromuscular blockers are administered just prior to cannulation to prevent inspiratory efforts during cannula insertion that can result in a large air embolism.

Cannulation takes place at the bedside under local anesthesia or in a nearby procedure suite if fluoroscopy is used. An initial bolus of heparin (50–100 U/kg) is administered just prior to cannulation. After vascular access is achieved, the primed circuit is connected and flow is initiated at a low-flow rate, increased incrementally to the target rate over several minutes. Rapid initiation of flow may result in sudden acid-base and electrolyte shifts, with resultant hypotension or arrhythmia.

The target flow rate depends on patient size. Infants require 100–200 mL/kg/min. VV support targets the higher end of the range due to recirculation. Pediatric patients require ~100 mL/kg/min, and adolescents require 50–100 mL/kg/min.

Ventilator Management

Although the goal for ventilator management is to provide a protective ventilation strategy, no single strategy is universally practiced. The goal is to maintain alveolar distention, avoid overdistension and atelectasis, minimize cyclic shear stress associated with tidal ventilation, and reduce exposure to elevated concentrations of O_2. High-frequency oscillation with a mean airway pressure sufficient to minimize atelectasis may be used, although pulmonary toilet restrictions and need for sedation often negate any benefit. Use of pressure-limited ventilation, elevated levels of positive end-expiratory pressure (PEEP) (10–20 cm H_2O), low respiratory rate (6–10 per min), and small tidal volumes (4–6 mL/kg) will meet these goals. An appropriate level of PEEP can be obtained by recording a bedside slow dynamic pressure-volume curve and examining the inflection points on the inspiratory and expiratory curves. Recognition that patients on ECLS may be better served with less sedation and more interaction has led many centers to adopt pressure-support ventilation with elevated levels of PEEP (12–20 cm H_2O). Spontaneous breathing with coughing better clears lower airway secretions. Adjuncts to mechanical ventilation include bronchoscopy to facilitate removal of airway secretions and prone positioning.

Hemodynamic Management

The requirement for vasoactive agents is almost universal in patients about to undergo extracorporeal support. Patients with severe acute respiratory failure also have some degree of myocardial dysfunction. Right ventricular dysfunction due to acute pulmonary hypertension, myocardial depression from systemic inflammation, and altered ventricular filling due to high ventilation requirements are major contributors to myocardial dysfunction. Inotropic and vasopressor agents are weaned after initiation of support. Even patients on VV support can usually be weaned from high levels of pharmacologic support as a result of improved myocardial oxygenation and decreased right ventricular afterload. Most patients require some

vasoactive agents initially while on ECLS, albeit at lower levels. After the initial period of support, vasoactive agents can often be weaned off completely.

Sedation and Analgesia

Provision of sedation and analgesia is part of the management of all critically ill children, and ECLS is no exception. The same medications used for routine ICU sedation are also used in ECLS, usually consisting of a benzodiazepine (midazolam or lorazepam) and an opioid analgesic (morphine or fentanyl). Dosing requirements may be elevated, as drugs may be adsorbed by the circuit, tolerance can develop, and hemofiltration can remove administered drugs.

A major trend in extracorporeal support is to minimize sedation and allow spontaneous breathing, and even interaction with staff and family. Use of minimal doses of benzodiazepines and narcotics can be supplemented by other agents. Atypical antipsychotic agents are effective in reducing agitation and delirium without sedation, and dexmedetomidine provides sedation from which the patient can be easily aroused. Propofol is a short-acting agent that is easily titratable; however, it cannot be used with microporous, hollow-fiber oxygenators. The lipid component can decrease surface tension at the pores of the membrane, leading to plasma leakage.

Assessment of Adequacy of Support

A goal of extracorporeal support is to provide sufficient blood flow to meet metabolic demands and avoid tissue hypoxia, while not providing excessive flow. Flow in excess of demand increases the risk of adverse effects without conferring any benefit. Extracorporeal flow requirements differ among the various modes of support.

Cardiac support with VA ECLS provides the fraction of total cardiac output that cannot be provided by the native heart. In many cases, especially early during support before myocardial recovery takes place, total cardiac output must be provided by the extracorporeal circuit. Normal regulatory mechanisms for adjusting cardiac output are not present, and circuit flow must be adjusted to meet metabolic demands. Mixed venous O_2 saturation (Svo_2) in the normal range of 70%–75% is the usual goal, and flow is adjusted accordingly. In VA mode, blood in the drainage limb of the circuit represents true Svo_2, allowing for continuous monitoring during support. Arterial blood during VA support should have normal O_2 saturation (>95%) and CO_2 tension, and it reflects the mixing of blood that results from native cardiac output and that due to extracorporeal support. During full support, these values are close to those of blood leaving the oxygenator, such that reduction in the sweep gas flow and the Fio_2 in the sweep gas may be necessary to avoid hyperoxia and hypocapnia.

Assessment is more difficult during VV support. Measurement of true Svo_2 is precluded during this mode, as blood in the pulmonary artery is a mixture of blood returning from the tissues and the oxygenated blood provided by the circuit. Arterial saturation is then the result of O_2 transfer through the native lungs added to pulmonary artery saturation. In severe lung dysfunction, not uncommon during the initial phase of

ECLS, the lungs may not transfer O_2, and arterial saturation equals that of the pulmonary artery. VV support cannot provide full saturation of the venous blood as a result of incomplete drainage and recirculation, thus arterial saturation during this mode of support is typically 80%–85%. These levels are well tolerated if cardiac output is maintained. Assessing adequacy of support, therefore, depends on other assessments, such as resolution of lactic acidosis and clinical indices of perfusion. Thermodilution cardiac output measurements are not reliable during VV support, as the thermal indicator will be lost to the circuit and falsely high cardiac output measurements will be recorded.

A technique to estimate true Svo_2 if a pulmonary artery catheter is in place during VV support is to temporarily interrupt support. Within a few seconds, the blood supplied by the circuit will have passed the pulmonary artery, and Svo_2 measured at this time will be close to true Svo_2. This procedure is not commonly practiced, as it entails some degree of risk, and many patients will not be able to tolerate any cessation of support, however brief.

Fluids and Renal Replacement Therapy

Maintenance of normal intravascular volume is critical during ECLS, as adequate venous return is necessary to maintain pump flow. Insufficient volume can be detected by poor filling of the bladder and downregulation of the pump. In centrifugal pump systems without a bladder, blood flow variation at a constant pump speed heralds inadequate venous return and mandates prompt correction to avoid hemolysis. Volume can be replaced with crystalloid, colloid, or blood products. If blood products are required, they are the first choice. Because patients on ECLS have a capillary leak syndrome, use of colloids, maintenance of colloid oncotic pressure (e.g., total protein >5.5), and minimization of crystalloid administration is commonly practiced.

Excess interstitial edema leads to organ dysfunction, contributing to worsening pulmonary, cardiac, gastrointestinal, and renal function. Diuretics (intermittent or continuous infusion) are the first choice in reducing interstitial edema, but if response to diuretics is inadequate, hemofiltration can be easily incorporated into the ECLS circuit. Hemofiltration is used in approximately one-third of ECLS runs—for renal failure and for fluid management in the absence of renal failure. Low oncotic pressure (total protein <5.5 g/dL) is corrected with fresh frozen plasma (if also indicated for coagulation management) or concentrated albumin infusion (1–2 g/kg).

Hemofiltration can be performed by inserting a hemofilter between high-pressure and low-pressure points in the circuit, such as preoxygenator and into the bladder, respectively. This configuration acts as a shunt, reducing blood flow to the patient; therefore, circuit flow must be monitored beyond the insertion point and compensated for the loss to the hemofilter. Many centers insert a pumped hemofiltration system in series with the drainage limb of the ECLS circuit, allowing for more precise control of blood flow, replacement fluid volume, and ultrafiltration rate.

Plasmapheresis for plasma exchange in the management of sepsis syndrome or immunologic disorders and extracorporeal liver support for hepatic failure can also be performed through the ECLS circuit without the need for additional vascular access.

Anticoagulation and Hematologic Management

The ECLS circuit is procoagulant, requiring continuous administration of a systemic anticoagulant. Inadequate anticoagulation leads to clot formation in the circuit, which can affect circuit performance, accelerate platelet deposition, and induce systemic fibrinolysis. By far, most experience has been with heparin, and it remains the initial drug of choice. The level of anticoagulation is measured with a bedside assessment of ACT. Maintaining the ACT between 180 and 200 secs seems to best balance the risk of bleeding complications and circuit clotting.

Platelet consumption is ongoing during ECLS support, and daily transfusions are not uncommon during the early phase of support. A platelet count of 80,000–100,000 is maintained during the initial phase of support and during management of bleeding complications, but lower values may be accepted once transfusion requirements have stabilized and bleeding is not problematic. Red blood cell transfusions are often required, especially in the presence of overt bleeding. Even in the absence of bleeding, transfusion requirements are above normal, as red blood cell life span is shortened and erythropoietin deficiency and resistance are present in critical illness. The target hemoglobin is 11–13 g/dL, which provides sufficient O_2-carrying capacity. Blood with a short storage life is preferred.

Nutritional Support

It is well established that enteral nutrition has substantial benefits over IV nutrition in critically ill patients and is the preferred route of administration. Parenteral nutrition has given way to enteral nutrition as the route of choice, which is well tolerated in adults (39) and neonates (32) on ECLS. Initiation of enteral nutritional support should begin after resuscitation is complete and perfusion is restored, usually within 12–24 hrs. The absence of bowel sounds does not predict intolerance and should not be used as a reason to withhold feeding. Postpyloric feeding may be better tolerated than gastric, but the addition of promotility agents, such as erythromycin, allows successful gastric feeding in most patients.

Contraindications to the enteral route include mechanical obstruction, ischemic bowel, and recent bowel resection. IV nutritional support is used when the enteral route is contraindicated, or to supplement it when full support cannot be achieved by the enteral route alone. IV lipids administered to patients supported with a microporous, hollow-fiber oxygenator can result in plasma leakage. Newer hollow-fiber devices that have solid membranes or siloxane coating of the fibers are resistant to leakage.

Weaning from Support

Following sufficient recovery of organ function to enable termination of extracorporeal support, the transition from ECLS (weaning) is initiated. In VA support, the extracorporeal flow rate can be gradually reduced at intervals, with serial assessment of perfusion, myocardial function, and blood gases until a terminal flow of 5–10 mL/kg, or about 10% of full support. The response to cardiac loading is assessed with serial echocardiography. Ventilator settings are increased to compensate but only to levels considered safe (e.g., PIP $\leq$30 cm H_2O, FIO_2 $\leq$40%, PEEP $\leq$10 cm H_2O, and rate <30). In circuits with a bridge between the drainage and reinfusion lines, the bridge can be opened to maintain flow in the circuit while the patient cannulas are clamped and flushed. If successful, the patient is decannulated. The use of a bridge is decreasing, as it requires constant attention and can contribute to the formation of clots. In this case, patients are decannulated after the terminal flow is reached.

In VV support, weaning is simpler, as no cardiac support is provided. Flow is decreased to reduce the amount of extracorporeal O_2 delivery as ventilator settings are increased. Once a low flow is reached, the sweep gas to the oxygenator is turned off, eliminating all gas exchange support. If tolerated at acceptable ventilator settings, the circuit is discontinued and the patient is decannulated.

The duration of support required for cardiac or pulmonary recovery is variable. The average duration of support for postoperative cardiac dysfunction is 5–7 days, and it is slightly longer at 7–9 days for myocarditis and nonoperative cardiomyopathy. Support duration is longer for pulmonary dysfunction, averaging 11–13 days, depending on the diagnosis. It had once been common practice to terminate support in apparently refractory cases if organ function had not returned after a period of time (perhaps 2–3 weeks) under the assumption that organ damage was irreversible by this time. Recent experience, however, indicates that organ function can recover after extended periods of time, and support for 2–3 months or more with recovery is no longer uncommon. The decision to withdraw support is, therefore, an individualized one that includes underlying diagnosis, extent of organ dysfunction, complications, and perhaps further diagnostic tests to establish irreversibility.

COMPLICATIONS

Vascular Injury

The procedure of cannulation entails placement of a large vascular cannula, imposing the risk of injury to the vessel or failure to complete cannulation. These complications may be more common in percutaneous cannulation, as the vessels are not directly visualized, but they can occur during surgical approaches as well. Vascular injury can present as posterior perforation with extravascular placement, subintimal placement, or vessel transection. Failure to complete cannulation may result from an attempt to place a cannula larger than the vein can accommodate or from placement of the guidewire in a tributary rather than in the major vessel. These will usually require surgical exploration and management.

Ultrasonography can be used to measure vessel size prior to percutaneous cannulation to aid in selecting appropriately sized cannulas and in identifying abnormal venous anatomy prior to insertion. Ultrasonography is also helpful in guiding needle entry during vessel puncture, enhancing the chance of successful cannulation. Use of fluoroscopy during percutaneous catheter insertion can help to identify aberrant guidewire placement and reduce the chance of vascular injury.

Bleeding

Bleeding complications are among the most common problems associated with ECLS. Bleeding can occur at surgical (including cannulation) sites but can also be unrelated to procedures or trauma. Bleeding can be life threatening, such as with intracranial hemorrhage. The initial approach to bleeding management is to identify causes that are surgically correctable (e.g., as a bleeding vessel at a cannulation site). If no such treatable cause is found, the platelet count is increased and the level of anticoagulation is decreased. An ACT of 160–180 secs, and perhaps 140–160 secs may be required for a period of time. If bleeding continues despite these efforts, pharmacologic agents may be helpful. Aminocaproic acid has historically been the predominant pharmacologic agent that helps to control bleeding on ECLS. Aminocaproic acid binds reversibly to plasminogen, blocking the binding of plasminogen to fibrin and its activation to plasmin, thus inhibiting thrombolysis. A loading dose of 100 mg/kg is administered, followed by a continuous infusion of 25–50 mg/kg. Due to its tendency to induce thrombosis and cause clotting in circuits, aminocaproic acid has been replaced in some centers by aprotinin. Aprotinin is a serine protease inhibitor that inhibits the intrinsic pathway of coagulation and fibrinolysis, attenuates the release of proinflammatory cytokines, reduces vascular permeability, and enhances platelet function. It is administered in a loading dose of 10,000 KIU/kg, followed by a continuous infusion of 2500 KIU/kg/hr. The loading dose can be added to the circuit prime in patients with bleeding complications prior to initiation of ECLS or in those with a high risk of bleeding. Recent reports of the use of recombinant factor VII have also shown promise (12) for the control of bleeding on ECLS. Life-threatening or uncontrollable bleeding may require the discontinuation of ECLS.

Heparin-induced thrombocytopenia due to heparin-associated antibodies (Type II HIT) is an uncommon but potentially life-threatening complication of heparin use. A precipitous fall in platelet count 5 days or more after initiation of heparin in the presence of thrombotic complications mandates discontinuation of heparin and substitution of an alternative anticoagulant. Argatroban is a direct thrombin inhibitor that is gaining acceptance as the alternative to heparin (40,51), and can be titrated with the ACT. Type I HIT may occur during ECLS but is unlikely to be distinguished from circuit-related thrombocytopenia.

Infection

Infections related to ECLS are uncommon but represent an additional morbidity that can impact outcome. Infection related to vascular cannulation is greater for open surgical than for percutaneous cannulation. The greatest infection risk is in transthoracic, centrally cannulated patients. Strict aseptic technique during placement and ongoing catheter care are essential. Limitation of other, non-ECLS vascular catheters is also important in reducing infection risk. Routine ICU guidelines for reducing pulmonary infection risk also apply to patients on ECLS.

Sepsis was once considered a contraindication to ECLS, but it is now not uncommon to support patients with sepsis-induced cardiopulmonary dysfunction. Hemodynamic support guidelines for pediatric septic shock include ECLS as a modality that may improve outcome (5).

OUTCOME FROM ECLS

Approximately 33,000 patients from all age groups who have undergone extracorporeal support have been reported to the ELSO registry as of June 2006 (16). Most were in the neonatal age group, but 7241 were from the pediatric age group (**Table 36.4**). Almost half of these were cardiac support cases, and most of the remaining were respiratory support cases. A small but growing experience with extracorporeal cardiopulmonary resuscitation (ECPR, 470 patients) was also reported.

Survival in pediatric ECLS for respiratory failure is 64%, with 56% surviving to hospital discharge. The survival in cardiac support is lower, with 60% surviving ECLS and 44% surviving to discharge. ECPR has the lowest survival (39% to discharge), but considering the moribund condition of these children, this level of survival is nothing short of remarkable.

Several single-center series of pediatric cases have been published. A series from the UK in pediatric respiratory failure patients who had a $Pao_2:Fio_2$ ratio of 61 reported a 71% survival. A series of 128 pediatric patients with severe respiratory failure was reported at the University of Michigan, with 77% recovering pulmonary function and 71% surviving to hospital discharge (45). Approximately half of these were initiated on VV support, and 11% required switching to VA support. In the 121 patients supported for oxygenation failure, the mean $Pao_2:Fio_2$ ratio was 58, and in the seven supported for hypercapnia, the mean $Paco_2$ was 128 torr. A series of 82 patients with severe respiratory failure managed with VV support was recently reported, with a survival of 77% (31).

Long-term Outcomes

One of the most devastating sequelae associated with ECLS is neurologic impairment. Unlike the neonatal experience, no large-scale outcome studies that focus on the pediatric age group have been reported. The ELSO registry reports complication rates, but with respect to neurologic complications, these largely represent short-term complications. Clinically diagnosed brain death was reported in 5.8% of pediatric patients who were supported for respiratory failure and in 4.5% of those supported for cardiac failure. Seizures, either clinically or electroencephalographically determined, were reported in 8.1% of respiratory support cases and 13.5% of cardiac support cases. CNS infarction or hemorrhage was reported in 3.5%–5% of cases. Survival in the non-brain death cases with neurologic complications was lower, at ~50% of overall survival rate. Although these short-term complications are not accurate representations of long-term problems, they identify a cohort of patients with a higher risk.

Several small studies have reviewed neurologic outcome of pediatric patients following ECLS for cardiac failure. In a series of 64 children following cardiac surgery reported by the University of Michigan, 44% had neurologic impairment at time of discharge (25). Most of these children had hemodynamic compromise prior to initiation of ECLS. More recently, a report from the University of California, San Francisco, on 53 infants supported with ECLS following cardiac surgery demonstrated a 28% incidence of motor dysfunction and 50% cognitive dysfunction (21).

Less data is available following support for respiratory failure. One study prospectively evaluated 9 children at yearly intervals out to 3 years after ECLS (3). Evaluation consisted of neurodevelopmental testing, electroencephalogram, auditory and visual-evoked potentials, and brain imaging. One third of surviving children demonstrated impairment at 1 year following ECLS, which persisted to the 3-year evaluation session. Physiologic variables before and during ECLS, such as oxygenation index and blood gases, did not correlate with outcome.

TABLE 36.4

OVERALL OUTCOMES IN ECLS AS REPORTED TO THE EXTRACORPOREAL LIFE SUPPORT ORGANIZATION, ANN ARBOR, MI, AS OF JUNE 2006

	Total	Survived ECLS		Survived to discharge	
Neonatal					
Respiratory	20,631	17,582	85%	15,748	76%
Cardiac	2,734	1,588	58%	1,034	38%
ECPR	255	165	65%	101	40%
Pediatric					
Respiratory	3,271	2,105	64%	1,835	56%
Cardiac	3,500	2,091	60%	1,537	44%
ECPR	470	238	51%	185	39%
Adult					
Respiratory	1,209	716	59%	627	52%
Cardiac	652	285	44%	204	31%
ECPR	183	79	43%	58	32%

ECPR, Extracorporeal cardiopulmonary resuscitation

CONCLUSIONS AND FUTURE DIRECTIONS

Technical advances in ECLS have contributed to improvements in outcome and a reduction in complications. Further technical improvements have the potential to make ECLS safer and perhaps more effective. The availability of dual-lumen cannulas for infants has reduced the complexity of support. Development of similar catheters for larger pediatric patients is under way and will enable single-cannula extracorporeal support for pediatric respiratory failure in all age groups. Newer membrane oxygenators that offer the performance of hollow-fiber devices with the low failure rate and longevity of solid silicone oxygenators are under development. Advances in centrifugal pump design have resulted in an increased use of these devices over traditional roller pumps for ECLS. Newer pump and oxygenator configurations that are more compact, safe, and efficient may widen the use of these techniques in patients of all ages. Finally, research and development of implantable cardiac or pulmonary support devices in small patients may one day obviate the need for ECMO as we know it today.

KEY POINTS

- ECLS is the application of extracorporeal circulation and gas exchange, including ECMO and related techniques.
- ECLS has the potential to improve outcome in patients with severe, potentially reversible, cardiac or pulmonary failure with a high risk of mortality, at least in large part through its ability to provide circulatory support during cardiac recovery and to reduce the risk of ventilator-induced lung injury.
- Most support for respiratory failure is achieved with VV ECLS that provides prepulmonary oxygenation. Cardiac support is achieved with VA ECLS, which provides partial cardiopulmonary bypass. Hybrid VVA and AV are newer modes that have been introduced for selected cases.
- Percutaneous cannulation has largely replaced surgical cannulation for VV pulmonary support. Surgical cannulation is still required for most cardiac support, but percutaneous cannulation for partial support is used in selected cases.
- ECPR is the emergent application of ECLS to support patients who are sustaining refractory or recurrent cardiopulmonary arrest.
- ECLS induces profound changes in cardiopulmonary physiology, coagulation, and inflammation, which require management in addition to that of the underlying disease.
- The most common complication of ECLS is bleeding, requiring anticoagulation management, blood component or factor replacement, and, possibly, surgical intervention.
- Survival following ECLS for pulmonary support in severe pediatric respiratory failure is ~65%, with ~60% surviving following cardiac support and 50% following ECPR.

References

1. Acute Respiratory Distress Syndrome Network. Ventilation with lower tidal volumes as compared with traditional tidal volumes for acute lung injury and the acute respiratory distress syndrome. *N Engl J Med* 2000;342:1301–8.
2. Aharon AS, Drinkwater DC, Jr., Churchwell KB, et al. Extracorporeal membrane oxygenation in children after repair of congenital cardiac lesions. *Ann Thorac Surg* 2001;72:2095–101.
3. Amigoni A, Pettenazzo A, Biban P, et al. Neurologic outcome in children after extracorporeal membrane oxygenation: Prognostic value of diagnostic tests. *Pediatr Neurol* 2005;32:173–9.
4. Baslaim G, Bashore J, Al-Malki F, et al. Can the outcome of pediatric extracorporeal membrane oxygenation after cardiac surgery be predicted? *Ann Thorac Cardiovasc Surg* 2006;12:21–7.
5. Carcillo JA, Fields AI. Clinical practice parameters for hemodynamic support of pediatric and neonatal patients in septic shock. *Crit Care Med* 2002;30:1365–78.
6. Cengiz P, Seidel K, Rycus PT, et al. Central nervous system complications during pediatric extracorporeal life support: Incidence and risk factors. *Crit Care Med* 2005;33:2817–24.
7. Chaturvedi RR, Macrae D, Brown KL, et al. Cardiac ECMO for biventricular hearts after paediatric open heart surgery. *Heart* 2004;90:545–51.
8. Chen YS, Wang MJ, Chou NK, et al. Rescue for acute myocarditis with shock by extracorporeal membrane oxygenation. *Ann Thorac Surg* 1999;68:2220–4.
9. Conrad SA, Rycus PT, Dalton HJ. Extracorporeal Life Support Registry Report 2004. *ASAIO J* 2005;51:4–10.
10. Conrad SA, Zwischenberger JB, Grier LR, et al. Total extracorporeal arteriovenous carbon dioxide removal in acute respiratory failure: A phase I clinical study. *Intensive Care Med* 2001;27:1340–51.
11. Del Nido PJ, Dalton HJ, Thompson AE, et al. Extracorporeal membrane oxygenator rescue in children during cardiac arrest after cardiac surgery. *Circulation* 1992;86:II300–4.
12. Dominguez TE, Mitchell M, Friess SH, et al. Use of recombinant factor VIIa for refractory hemorrhage during extracorporeal membrane oxygenation. *Pediatr Crit Care Med* 2005;6:348–51.
13. Dos Santos CC, Slutsky AS. Mechanotransduction, ventilator-induced lung injury and multiple organ dysfunction syndrome. *Intensive Care Med* 2000;26:638–42.
14. Duncan BW, Bohn DJ, Atz AM, et al. Mechanical circulatory support for the treatment of children with acute fulminant myocarditis. *J Thorac Cardiovasc Surg* 2001;122:440–8.
15. Duncan BW, Hraska V, Jonas RA, et al. Mechanical circulatory support in children with cardiac disease. *J Thorac Cardiovasc Surg* 1999;117:529–42.
16. Extracorporeal Life Support Organization. International Summary. Ann Arbor: Extracorporeal Life Support Organization, 2006.
17. Fiser WP, Yetman AT, Gunselman RJ, et al. Pediatric arteriovenous extracorporeal membrane oxygenation (ECMO) as a bridge to cardiac transplantation. *J Heart Lung Transplant* 2003;22:770–7.
18. Greenspan JS, Shaffer TH. Ventilator-induced airway injury: A critical consideration during mechanical ventilation of the infant. *Neonatal Netw* 2006;25:159–66.
19. Halbertsma FJ, Vaneker M, Scheffer GJ, et al. Cytokines and biotrauma in ventilator-induced lung injury: A critical review of the literature. *Neth J Med* 2005;63:382–92.
20. Halbertsma FJ, Vaneker M, Scheffer GJ, et al. Cytokines and biotrauma in ventilator-induced lung injury: A critical review of the literature. *Neth J Med* 2005;63:382–92.
21. Hamrick SE, Gremmels DB, Keet CA, et al. Neurodevelopmental outcome of infants supported with extracorporeal membrane oxygenation after cardiac surgery. *Pediatrics* 2003;111:e671–5.
22. Hill JG, Bruhn PS, Cohen SE, et al. Emergent applications of cardiopulmonary support: A multiinstitutional experience. *Ann Thorac Surg* 1992;54:699–704.
23. Ichiba S, Peek GJ, Sosnowski AW, et al. Modifying a venovenous extracorporeal membrane oxygenation circuit to reduce recirculation. *Ann Thorac Surg* 2000;69:298–9.
24. Imai Y, Slutsky AS. High-frequency oscillatory ventilation and ventilator-induced lung injury. *Crit Care Med* 2005;33:S129–34.
25. Kulik TJ, Moler FW, Palmisano JM, et al. Outcome-associated factors in pediatric patients treated with extracorporeal membrane oxygenator after cardiac surgery. *Circulation* 1996;94:II63–8.
26. Moller JC, Schaible TF, Ahrens W, et al. Pumpless extracorporeal lung assist. *Lancet* 2000;356:1112.
27. Montgomery VL, Strotman JM, Ross MP. Impact of multiple organ system dysfunction and nosocomial infections on survival of children treated with extracorporeal membrane oxygenation after heart surgery. *Crit Care Med* 2000;28:526–31.
28. Montoya JP, Merz SI, Bartlett RH. A standardized system for describing flow/pressure relationships in vascular access devices. *ASAIO Trans* 1991;37:4–8.
29. Nakano T, Tominaga R, Nagano I, et al. Pulsatile flow enhances endothelium-derived nitric oxide release in the peripheral vasculature. *Am J Physiol Heart Circ Physiol* 2000;278:H1098–104.
30. Peek GJ, Firmin RK, Moore HM, et al. Cannulation of neonates for venovenous extracorporeal life support. *Ann Thorac Surg* 1996;61:1851–2.
31. Pettignano R, Fortenberry JD, Heard ML, et al. Primary use of the venovenous approach for extracorporeal membrane oxygenation in pediatric acute respiratory failure. *Pediatr Crit Care Med* 2003;4:291–8.

32. Piena M, Albers MJ, Van Haard PM, et al. Introduction of enteral feeding in neonates on extracorporeal membrane oxygenation after evaluation of intestinal permeability changes. *J Pediatr Surg* 1998;33:30–4.

33. Plotz FB, Slutsky AS, van Vught AJ, et al. Ventilator-induced lung injury and multiple system organ failure: a critical review of facts and hypotheses. *Intensive Care Med* 2004;30:1865–72.

34. Rais-Bahrami K, Walton DM, Sell JE, et al. Improved oxygenation with reduced recirculation during venovenous ECMO: Comparison of two catheters. *Perfusion* 2002;17:415–9.

35. Reickert CA, Schreiner RJ, Bartlett RH, et al. Percutaneous access for venovenous extracorporeal life support in neonates. *J Pediatr Surg* 1998;33:365–9.

36. Rich PB, Awad SS, Crotti S, et al. A prospective comparison of atrio-femoral and femoro-atrial flow in adult venovenous extracorporeal life support. *J Thorac Cardiovasc Surg* 1998;116:628–32.

37. Rich PB, Awad SS, Kolla S, et al. An approach to the treatment of severe adult respiratory failure. *J Crit Care* 1998;13:26–36.

38. Roberts N, Westrope C, Pooboni SK, et al. Venovenous extracorporeal membrane oxygenation for respiratory failure in inotrope dependent neonates. *ASAIO J* 2003;49:568–71.

39. Scott LK, Boudreaux K, Thaljeh F, et al. Early enteral feedings in adults receiving venovenous extracorporeal membrane oxygenation. *JPEN J Parenter Enteral Nutr* 2004;28:295–300.

40. Scott LK, Grier LR, Conrad SA. Heparin-induced thrombocytopenia in a pediatric patient receiving extracorporeal membrane oxygenation managed with argatroban. *Pediatr Crit Care Med* 2006;7:473–5.

41. Seib PM, Faulkner SC, Erickson CC, et al. Blade and balloon atrial septostomy for left heart decompression in patients with severe ventricular dysfunction on extracorporeal membrane oxygenation. *Catheter Cardiovasc Interv* 1999;46:179–86.

42. Sezai A, Shiono M, Nakata Ki, et al. Effects of pulsatile CPB on interleukin-8 and endothelin-1 levels. *Artificial Organs* 2005;29:708–13.

43. Shah SA, Shankar V, Churchwell KB, et al. Clinical outcomes of 84 children with congenital heart disease managed with extracorporeal membrane oxygenation after cardiac surgery. *ASAIO J* 2005;51:504–7.

44. Sreenan C, Osiovich H, Cheung PY, et al. Quantification of recirculation by thermodilution during venovenous extracorporeal membrane oxygenation. *J Pediatr Surg* 2000;35:1411–4.

45. Swaniker F, Kolla S, Moler F, et al. Extracorporeal life support outcome for 128 pediatric patients with respiratory failure. *J Pediatr Surg* 2000;35:197–202.

46. Taghavi S, Zuckermann A, Ankersmit J, et al. Extracorporeal membrane oxygenation is superior to right ventricular assist device for acute right ventricular failure after heart transplantation. *Ann Thorac Surg* 2004;78:1644–9.

47. Thourani VH, Kirshbom PM, Kanter KR, et al. Venoarterial extracorporeal membrane oxygenation (VA-ECMO) in pediatric cardiac support. *Ann Thorac Surg* 2006;82:138–44.

48. Undar A, Masai T, Yang SQ, et al. Effects of perfusion mode on regional and global organ blood flow in a neonatal piglet model. *Ann Thorac Surg* 1999;68:1336–42.

49. van Heijst AF, van der Staak FH, de Haan AF, et al. Recirculation in double-lumen catheter veno-venous extracorporeal membrane oxygenation measured by an ultrasound dilution technique. *ASAIO J* 2001;47:372–6.

50. Vlasselaers D, Desmet M, Desmet L, et al. Ventricular unloading with a miniature axial flow pump in combination with extracorporeal membrane oxygenation. *Intensive Care Med* 2006;32:329–33.

51. Young G, Yonekawa KE, Nakagawa P, et al. Argatroban as an alternative to heparin in extracorporeal membrane oxygenation circuits. *Perfusion* 2004;19:283–8.

CHAPTER 37 ■ RENAL REPLACEMENT THERAPIES

WARWICK W. BUTT • PETER W. SKIPPEN • PHILLIPPE JOUVET

Over the last 20 years, renal replacement therapy (RRT) has become a standard therapy in children in the PICU. RRT is used to remove exogenous or endogenous toxins and to restore water, acid-base, or electrolyte balance. In children, RRT requires specific expertise due to (a) the wide variation in the sizes of children who are treated (from 2–100 kg); (b) the variety of diseases associated with ARF and their specific indications, such as inborn errors of metabolism, cardiac failure, and sepsis; and (c) the variety of available techniques: peritoneal dialysis (PD), intermittent hemodialysis, and continuous renal replacement therapies [such as continuous venovenous hemofiltration (CVVH), continuous venovenous hemodialysis (CVVHD), and continuous venovenous hemodiafiltration (CVVHDF)]. The diseases that cause acute renal failure (ARF) and that require RRT have been described in several recent large reviews (9,17,55,65). The frequency of use of RRT in the PICU is between 2% and 7% of all patients admitted in some series (9,19,32,65). In general, the survival rate of children in the PICU who require RRT is worse than that of children who do not receive it. The overall mortality rate in children who receive RRT at the Royal Children's Hospital, Melbourne, in 2005, increased from 4% to 17% (cardiac, 3.3%–12.7%; noncardiac, 4.4%–50%), and the average length of stay increased from 4.5 days to 12.7 days (cardiac) and from 3.5 days to 15.4 days (noncardiac).

This chapter includes a review of the technical aspects of the commonly performed RRTs in the PICU, the respective renal and nonrenal indications for each type of therapy (which are relatively standard and are shown in **Table 37.1**), and a guide to aid the determination of which type of RRT is most appropriate for the individual patient (**Table 37.2**) (5,50,56).

BASIC PHYSIOLOGY

Developmental Changes in Renal Function

The term newborn infant has a renal blood flow of ~20% that of an adult. Consequently, the glomerular filtration rate is also markedly reduced, as is tubular excretion and reabsorption. The normal age-related changes in glomerular filtration rate and renal blood flow are shown in **Table 37.3**.

Clearance

Renal clearance is a quantitative measure of the rate of removal of a substance by the kidneys from the blood. It is expressed in terms of the volume of blood that could be completely cleared

of a substance in 1 min and is expressed as mL/min. Clearance is often standardized by adjusting for body surface area, and the units are described as mL/min/m^2.

Dialysis

Dialysis represents the process of exchange between two fluids (water and solute) across a semipermeable membrane. Usually, the fluids are representing by blood and dialysis fluid. Two main mechanisms are involved in the exchange of water, and two are involved in the exchange of solute.

   Osmosis—The movement of fluid along a concentration gradient (from low to high concentration).
   Hydrostatic Pressure—The force a fluid under pressure exerts against the walls or edges of the area in which it is contained. This pressure tends to force fluid from an area of high pressure to an area of low pressure across a semipermeable membrane.
   Diffusion—The movement of solute across a semipermeable from a high- to a low-concentration area.
   Convection (Bulk Flow, Solvent Drag)—The movement of solute that occurs in conjunction with, and linked to, fluid movement.

PERITONEAL DIALYSIS

PD is the oldest, simplest, and still the most commonly used form of RRT in children. PD is the bidirectional exchange of fluid and solute between dialysis fluid and blood in the peritoneal cavity across the peritoneal membrane, which covers all loops of bowel and reflects to cover the anterior and posterior surfaces of the abdomen to form a cavity. The membrane is constituted of fenestrated capillaries, interstitial connective tissue, and a thin layer of mesothelial cells. Solute and fluid move between gaps in the cells and between pores or channels in the interstitium. The other major mechanism involved in fluid and solute clearance is peritoneal lymph drainage. Up to 50% of capillary ultrafiltrate can be reabsorbed via the lymphatics, which can further affect negative fluid balance. The lymphatics can also absorb large molecules from the peritoneum that can enter the vascular system via the thoracic duct, limiting the type and strength of osmotic substances used in PD. PD is performed simply by allowing dialysis solution to run into the peritoneum, remain in situ ("dwell") for a time, and then drain for a period of time. This process completes one cycle, which can be repeated as desired. Similar to hemodialysis, PD corrects fluid and electrolyte abnormalities, metabolic acidosis,

TABLE 37.1

INDICATIONS FOR RENAL REPLACEMENT THERAPY

Renal
Oliguria (unresponsive to diuretics and/or fluid challenge)
Anuria (nonobstructive)
Metabolic acidosis
Hyperkalemia
Azotemia
Uremia symptoms (encephalopathy, myopathy, pericarditis, bleeding)
Hyperphosphatemia

Nonrenal
Fluid overload
Anticipated large transfusion in trauma or coagulopathy
Inborn errors of metabolism
Sepsis
Post-cardiopulmonary bypass systemic inflammatory response syndrome
Pancreatitis
Drug overdose

TABLE 37.3

NORMAL RENAL FUNCTION AT DIFFERENT AGES

Age	GFR mL</min/m^2	RBF mL/min/m^2
Preterm	15	40
Term	20	90
1–2 wks	50	220
6 mo–1 yr	80	350
1–3 yrs	100	540
Adult	120	620

GFR, glomerular filtration rate; RBF, renal blood flow

and azotemia through the processes of osmosis, diffusion, and filtration.

Physiology of Peritoneal Dialysis

The surface area of the peritoneal cavity is directly proportional to the patient's body surface area (~0.6 m^2/m^2 of body surface area), and peritoneal permeability is similar in all patients from 2 years to adulthood (6,14,38). Infants and small children have a large surface area to body weight ratio, which may explain the better efficiency of PD in small children when compared to adults (**Fig. 37.1**). Both molecular size (weight and three-dimensional shape) and amount of charge affect passage through the peritoneal membrane: The larger the molecule, the lower the permeability; the more highly charged the molecule, the lower the permeability. Fluid removal follows an osmotic gradient and is, therefore, more dependent on the concentration of the dialysis solution itself than on the peritoneal membrane. The peritoneal membrane is relatively impermeable to protein, unless diseases, such as sepsis, systemic inflammatory response syndrome, cardiopulmonary bypass (CPB), pancreatitis, or shock, have caused a marked increase in capillary permeability. Clearance achieved by PD depends on the size of the molecule (smaller molecules are cleared more quickly) (**Fig. 37.2**), the dialysis fluid osmolality (the higher the glucose concentration, the more rapid the fluid removal) (**Fig. 37.3**), the dwell time (most fluid removal occurs within the first 60 mins, because the concentration gradients change the most during this period) (**Fig. 37.4**), and the volume of dialysis fluid (the larger the volume, the greater the clearance because more fluid is in contact with the peritoneal membrane and its large surface area) (**Fig. 37.5**) (29). Fluid removal also depends on the retention effect of lymphatic drainage on fluid being removed from the peritoneum and returned to the vascular compartment. Although this process occurs slowly, it becomes important over time (65) (**Fig. 37.6**).

TABLE 37.2

SPECIFICS OF THE THREE TECHNIQUES OF RRT IN THE PICU

	PD	HDi	CRRT
METHOD SPECIFICITIES			
Vascular access (ECC)	No	Yes	Yes
Complex method with specific expertise	Low	High	Moderate
Systemic anticoagulation	No	Frequent	Frequent
DIALYSIS DOSE			
Efficacy to remove a toxin	Moderate	High	High
Efficacy to remove fluid	Moderate	Moderate	High
CLINICAL SITUATION INDICATION			
Hemodynamic instability	Yes	No	Yes
Intracranial hypertension	Yes	±	Yes
ARDS	±	Yes	Yes
Abdominal surgery	±	Yes	Yes

PD, peritoneal dialysis; HDi, intermittent hemodialysis; CRRT, continuous renal replacement therapies; ECC, extracorporeal circulation; ARDS, acute respiratory distress syndrome

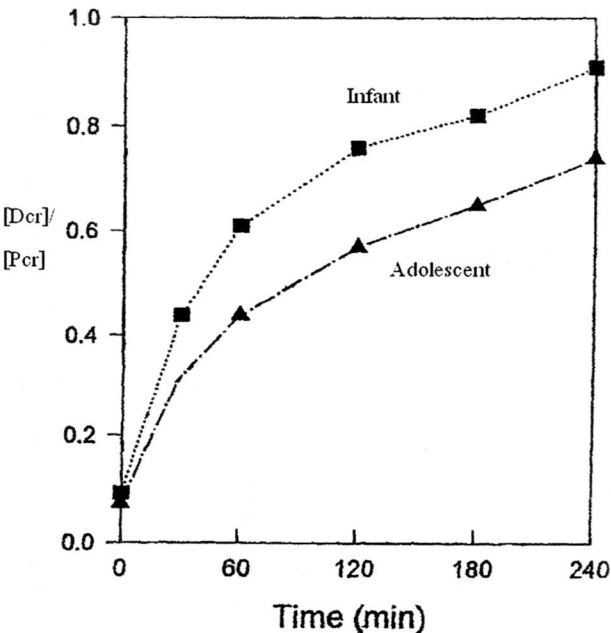

FIGURE 37.1. Clearance achieved by peritoneal dialysis over time. Dcr:Pcr ratio of dialysis creatinine to plasma creatinine against duration of dwell time. From Warady BA, *J Am Soc Nephrol* 1996;14:236–9, with permission.

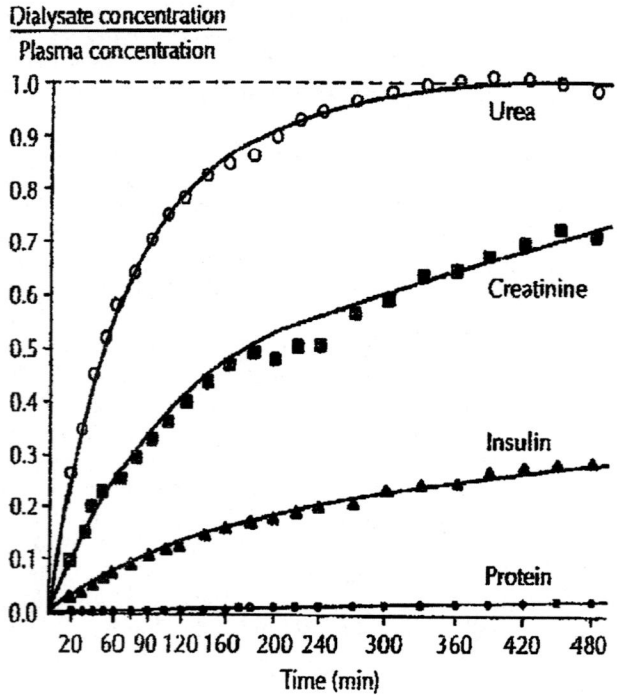

FIGURE 37.2. Variation of solute clearance as determined by molecular size. From Krediet RT, Peritoneal anatomy and physiology during peritoneal dialysis. In Horl WH et al., *Replacement of Renal Function by Dialysis,* 5e. Kluwer Academic Publishers, 2004, with permission.

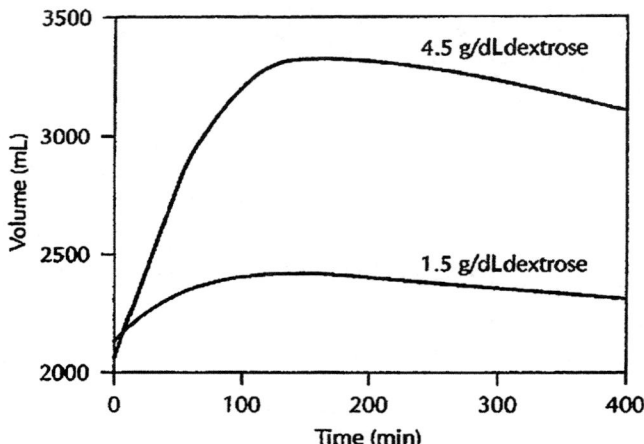

FIGURE 37.3. Dialysis fluid tonicity and effect on water removal. From Mujias S, *Kidney Intl* 2002;62 (S81):S17–22, with permission.

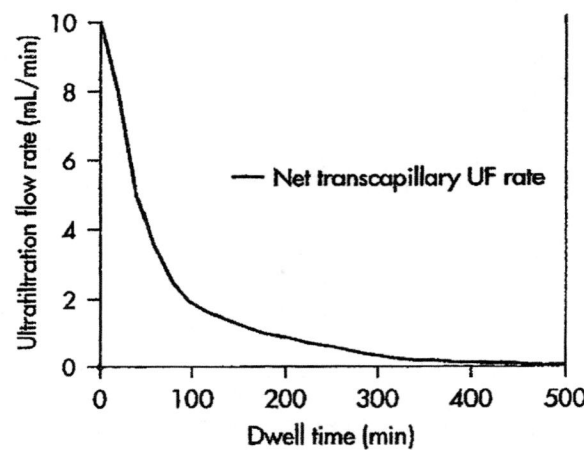

FIGURE 37.4. Effect of dwell time on fluid removal. From Nolph KD, *Kidney Intl* 1981;20:543–8, with permission.

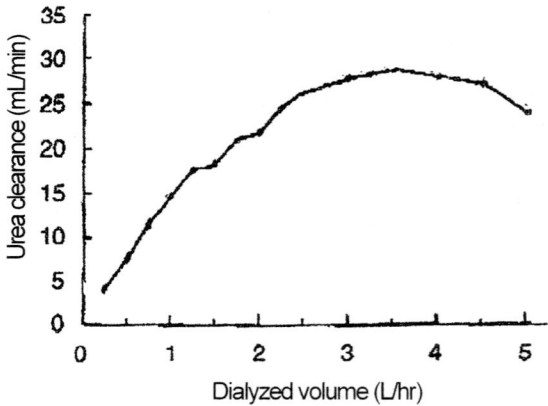

FIGURE 37.5. Volume of peritoneal dialysis fluid and urea clearance in adults. From Keshaviah P, *J Am Soc Nephrol* 1994;4:1820–6, with permission.

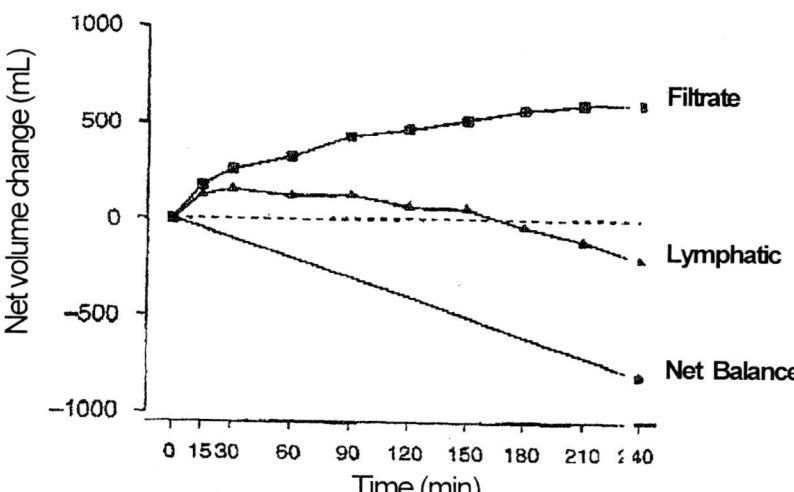

FIGURE 37.6. Change in fluid removal and net fluid balance over time in adults with 3-liter volume of peritoneal dialysis fluid. From Mactier RA, *J Clin Invest* 1987;80:1311–16, with permission.

Indications for Peritoneal Dialysis

- Standard indications for RRT are shown in **Table 37.1**
- Neonates/small infants
- Following CPB in infants who weigh <10 kg
- Difficult vascular access

Contraindications

- Defect in peritoneal membrane or cavity, such as diaphragmatic hernia, gastroschisis, omphalocele, postsurgical thoracoabdominal communication
- Abdominal sepsis with adhesions
- Necrotizing enterocolitis
- Ventriculoperitoneal shunt (relative)
- Profound shock or cardiac failure (relative)
- Massive rapid clearance required (relative)

Catheters Used for Peritoneal Dialysis

The Tenckhoff catheter is most commonly used for PD; it is available as either a straight or curled catheter. It can be inserted by a surgeon in the operating theater (after CPB) or in the PICU. The catheters range in size and diameter. Larger patients require longer lengths and larger-diameter tubing. Typical sizes for infants and small children are 10-, 12-, and 14-French (fr), with 45 cm length for acute PD. Infection is minimized by use of correct aseptic technique at the time of insertion, correct technique when dealing with the circuit or dialysis fluids, and a soft silicon catheter with a Dacron cuff near the skin entry site. At some centers, the catheter is inserted with a long, subcutaneous tunnel in both acute and chronic PD. Administration of a single dose of prophylactic antibiotics has also been recommended (41).

Manual versus Automated Peritoneal Dialysis

PD is a simple treatment to perform, and the process is easily automated. However, because automation involves substantial cost in establishing and training staff to be familiar with the technology and alarms, many ICUs use manual, nonmechanical therapy, which is managed by the bedside nurse.

Continuous-flow Peritoneal Dialysis

When a higher clearance is required, the use of continuous-flow PD has been used successfully. Urea clearances of 30–50 mL/min have been achieved with this technique (1). However, it is not routinely used because it necessitates the insertion of two catheters (one for fluid administration and one for removal) in the abdomen.

Complications

Similar to other methods of RRT, PD can be associated with *fluid and electrolyte abnormalities*, in particular, potassium, sodium and, in small infants, lactate. Significant potential also exists for fluid imbalance, with too much or too little fluid being removed. Overall fluid balance, central filling pressures, and electrolyte balance of patients who receive PD must be closely monitored to avoid complications.

Peritonitis is an uncommon complication that is mainly related to poor aseptic insertion or poor aseptic handling of the circuit and stopcocks. Close monitoring for symptoms (cloudy dialysis effluent, abdominal pain, fever, poor function) and signs (abdominal tenderness, fever, elevated white cell count) of peritonitis is essential to proper care. In some PICUs, a daily sample of PD fluid is drawn for microbiological microscopy and culture. Diagnosis of peritonitis is confirmed if the dialysate is cloudy, if the white blood cell count is >100/mm^3, and if >50% of the cells are polymorphonuclear cells. Early empiric therapy with intraperitoneal cefazolin and gentamicin is commenced. A single IV dose of vancomycin may also be given if the patient is clinically unstable.

Evidence of a pneumoperitoneum is also found in some patients with PD. Pneumoperitoneum usually results from air entrainment in the dialysis fluid, rather than from bowel perforation, although making the distinction between the two is

TABLE 37.4

VARIOUS PERITONEAL DIALYSIS SOLUTIONS USED IN THE PICU

	I	II	III	IV
Glucose (mg/dL)	1.5	1.5	4.25	4.25
Sodium (mm/L)	156	132	152	132
Chloride (mm/L)	105	95	110	96
Magnesium (mm/L)	0.28	0.25	0.29	0.25
Calcium (mm/L)	2.0	1.25	2.1	1.8
Lactate (mm/L)	0	40	0	40
Bicarbonate (mm/L)	34	0	35	0
Acetate (mm/L)	11.4	0	12	0

I, Isotonic, lactate free; II, isotonic; III, hypertonic, lactate free; IV, hypertonic

obviously important. Bowel perforation at the time of insertion is rare but is always a potential concern.

Catheter-related problems with PD can occur frequently. Poor flow into the peritoneum can occur from kinking of the catheter, crystallization around the catheter instillation/drainage holes, or infection. Poor drainage can occur with kinking, malposition of the catheter or from omentum that becomes wrapped around catheter drainage holes. Leakage at the site of entry can also occur from local irritation or infection of the site of entry or initial poor surgical technique. PD catheters placed in patients postoperative from cardiovascular surgery may also leak fluid into the thoracic cavity, especially if the catheter has been placed from the open thoracic cavity through the diaphragm into the abdomen (which should be avoided). In this circumstance, instilled PD fluid frequently leaks out of the chest tubes, without spending enough time in the abdominal cavity to exchange solute and fluids.

Hernias (inguinal) due to increased intra-abdominal pressure can occur, and the development of scrotal fluid (hydrocele) is common in the neonate. *Peritoneal fluid eosinophilia* may occur due to a reaction to the plastic tubing and may also be seen in fungal infection. *Peritoneal sclerosis*, in which thick, fibrinous tissue forms over the bowel and abdominal wall, occurs in rare circumstances and is often associated with repetitive episodes of prior peritonitis.

Dialysis Fluid Composition

In deciding to commence dialysis, what is to be removed and how much to be removed must be clearly defined, thereby determining the nature of the type of RRT applied.

The choice of PD solution depends on the amount of fluid to be removed, the age of the patient, and whether metabolic acidosis is present. Increased fluid removal usually involves the use of more hypertonic solutions. In the presence of metabolic acidosis, using a dialysis solution that does not contain lactate may be beneficial. Various solutions are shown in Table 37.4.

A decision must also be made regarding choice of volume of PD. Instillation of 10–20 mL/kg normally provides good clearance and minimal risk of intra-abdominal hypertension. Increased volume of dialysate to 30–40 mL/kg gives a better clearance of solutes but an increased likelihood of intra-abdominal hypertension or respiratory embarrassment.

Choice of additives to PD solution: Potassium can be either added or removed, heparin (institutional preference is usually 500 U/L) is often included, and antibiotics may be added depending on institutional preference.

Cycle time: Usually a total time of 30–240 mins (depending on diagnosis and clearance required) is provided for instillation, dwell time, and drainage, with dwell time providing 66%–85% of the total cycle time.

Cardiopulmonary Interactions

PD is the most common form of RRT in neonates and small children after bypass (64). PD continues to be effective even in low-cardiac output states, in hypotension conditions, and in infants with vasoconstrictors. However, as PD volumes increase or muscle relaxants are ceased and abdominal muscle tone increases, the potential increases for impairment of ventilation, gas exchange, and decreased cardiac performance. In a small study, it was found that dialysis volumes of up to 30 mL/kg did not result in intra-abdominal hypertension and had no negative effects on cardiac output, oxygen delivery, or respiratory function (39). In this study, cardiac index was highest with 10 mL/kg, rather than with 0 or 20 mL/kg. Intra-abdominal pressure may be easily and accurately measured using a bladder catheter with a balloon filled to a volume of 1 mL/kg (13) and connected to a pressure-monitoring column or device. Debate exists over the exact pressures that constitute intra-abdominal hypertension and the "best" way to monitor intra-abdominal pressure. A recent review of intra-abdominal hypertension and abdominal compartment syndrome discusses potential problems that can arise (7).

CONTINUOUS RENAL REPLACEMENT THERAPY

Continuous renal replacement therapy (CRRT) is perceived to be a "gentler" form of removal of fluid and solute. It can, over time, be equivalent in efficiency to intermittent hemodialysis and has the benefit of more hemodynamic stability. The initial

TABLE 37.5

FILTRATION IN 58 CHILDREN AT ROYAL CHILDREN'S HOSPITAL, MELBOURNE (1986–1989)

	AV ($n = 17$)	VV ($n = 41$)
Duration (hrs)	40 (14–142)	49 (3–220)
Filter life (hrs)	27 (4–47)	53 (3–126)
Ultrafiltration rate (mL/min/m²)	6 (17–18)	19 (5–43)
Blood flow (mL/min)	30 (15–30)	65 (25–100)
Filtration fraction%	17 (10–25)	13 (5–30)

AV, Arteriovenous; VV, Venovenous; n, number of patients. Data expressed as median (range).

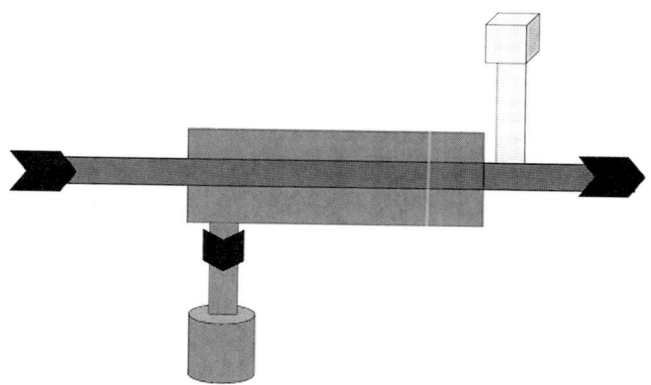

FIGURE 37.7. Continuous arteriovenous hemofiltration.

description of arteriovenous filtration was in adults and was subsequently described in children in 1986 (50). An abstract presented at the Pediatric Critical Care Colloquium in October 1989 described 58 children with a mixture of arteriovenous and venovenous filtration; these children ranged from 2 days to 16 years of age and weighed 2.4–86 kg. The authors reported improved filtration rate and filter life with venovenous compared to arteriovenous filtration (26) (**Table 37.5**). The initial experience with CRRT was very encouraging, particularly in newborns with inborn errors of metabolism in whom very large volumes of ultrafiltrate and solute removal could be achieved (58). Scattered case reports followed, including small series about the safety of the use of CRRT in 13 seriously ill infants who weighed <5 kg (48) and as an adjunctive therapy in 27 children with sepsis (46). In the last decade, several large series have reported the safety, efficacy, and outcome of children who were treated with CRRT. A study of 122 children with ARF found a higher mortality in those patients who received vasopressor therapy (35). Similar findings were noted in a series of 98 children (54). In a series that was corrected for patient severity of illness, it was noted that the amount of fluid overload present at the time of starting CRRT was related to outcome (18), suggesting that earlier use of CRRT to control fluid balance may improve outcome. Other authors have noted that outcome was related more to the underlying disease than to the treatment applied (57).

Goals of Pediatric Continuous Renal Replacement Therapy

The goals of CRRT for the intensivist include restoring fluid and electrolyte balance, improving lung function by decreasing lung water and capillary permeability, improving hemodynamics by removing inflammatory mediators or bacterial toxins, managing ARF by removing nitrogenous waste products and restoring acid-base balance, maintaining fluid balance while allowing nutrition or blood products to be given safely, purifying blood in conditions such as sepsis or metabolic disorders (e.g., hyperammonemia), and clearing ingested drugs or toxins. While many of these functions are still theoretical, the surge in use of CRRT in the ICU may provide data to further elucidate which indications are truly effective and beneficial.

Types of Continuous Renal Replacement Therapy

Continuous Arteriovenous Hemofiltration

In continuous arteriovenous hemofiltration (CAVH) mode, the drainage catheter is placed in an artery and the return catheter is placed in a vein (either peripheral or central). CAVH is simple to operate but has low ultrafiltrate production, especially in small patients or those with hypotension. It also provides a potential volume load to the heart in small infants that may not be well tolerated. In this mode, blood flows from artery to vein and filtrate production depends on the patient's blood pressure, the filter surface area, and the height of the collecting system below the filter. Although useful in adults, CAVH has been shown to be very inefficient in children (**Fig. 37.7**).

Continuous Venovenous Hemofiltration

Continuous venovenous hemofiltration (CVVH) may be performed with a double-lumen catheter, which contains both a drainage and return lumen that is placed in a central vein. CVVH may also be performed with separate catheters placed into two different peripheral or central veins. Clearance and fluid balance goals are chosen by the staff, and the parameters are set on the dialysis machine as shown in **Figure 37.8**):

Choose filtrate rate: $F = UFR = GFR$ (clearance of solute)

Choose fluid removal rate: $F - RF$
If no dialysis to be done concurrently: $D = 0$
Where:

$$F = \text{filtration rate}$$
$$UFR = \text{ultrafiltration rate}$$
$$GFR = \text{glomerular filtration rate}$$
$$RF = \text{replacement fluid}$$
$$D = \text{dialysate flow rate}$$

Slow Continuous Ultrafiltration

Slow continuous ultrafiltration (SCUF) uses a low volume of filtrate with no replacement solution and is useful in removing small amounts of fluid (**Fig. 37.9**). Ideally, this can be done by using arterial drainage and venous return, which can eliminate the need for a pump.

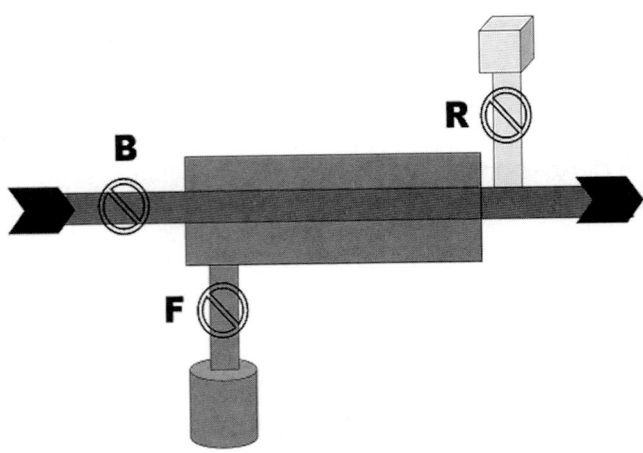

FIGURE 37.8. Continuous venovenous hemofiltration (postfilter replacement). B, blood flow; R, replacement fluid rate; F, filtration rate.

Continuous Venovenous Hemodialysis

In continuous venovenous hemodialysis (CVVHD), solute clearance and fluid balance are chosen by the staff and set on the dialysis machine (**Fig. 37.10**):

D:	dialysate flow rate (clearance)
Choose fluid removal rate:	F − D
No replacement fluid:	RF = 0

Continuous Venovenous Hemodiafiltration

In continuous venovenous hemodiafiltration (CVVHDF), both solute clearance and fluid balance goals are chosen by staff and then set on dialysis machine (**Fig. 37.10**):

Determine replacement fluid rate, then

$$F − D − RF = fluid\ balance$$

Where:

D = dialysate flow (clearance)
F − D = filtration rate (clearance)
RF = replacement fluid

Physiology of Continuous Renal Replacement Therapy

The filtration of blood during CRRT is analogous to native glomerular filtration and is determined by fluid movement across a semipermeable membrane down a pressure gradient.

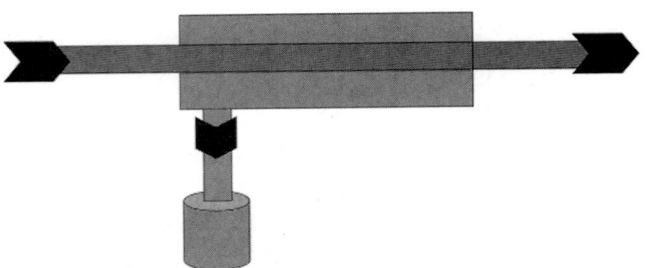

FIGURE 37.9. Slow continuous ultrafiltration (SCUF).

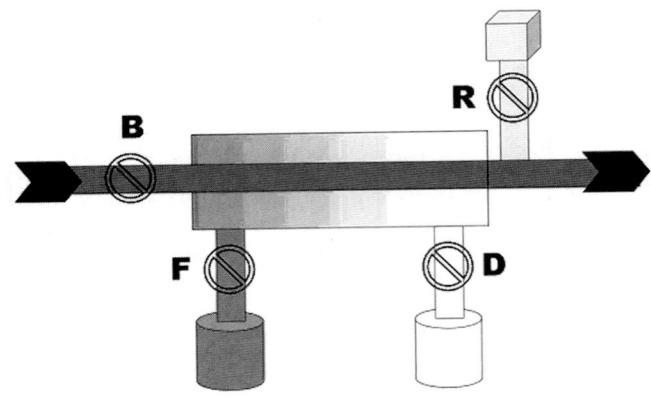

FIGURE 37.10. CVVHDF (postfilter replacement). B, blood flow; R, replacement fluid rate; F, filtration rate; D, dialysate flow rate.

Bulk flow of solute (convection) also occurs concurrently. Simply stated, the dialysis filter acts as a sieve, allowing molecules dissolved in water to be carried along to the other side. Each filter is composed of many microtubules that act independently of each other but function with the same principles. The process of convective ultrafiltration is driven by three key factors: filter blood flow, transmembrane pressure, and filtration fraction.

Filter Blood Flow

Poiseuille's Law governs laminar flow through a tube and is defined by the following parameters:

$$Qb = \Delta p − \pi r4/8l\mu$$

Where:

Qb = blood flow
Δp = change in pressure across the tube
r = radius of the tube
l = length of the tube
μ = viscosity of the blood

In CAVH, Δp is the difference between the filter inlet and filter outlet pressure. In CVVH, desired blood flow is set on the dialysis machine (**Fig. 37.11**). Lower blood flow across the filter can result in a higher tendency for clotting to occur. As the filter clots, resistance to flow will increase and filter pressure will increase as well. These parameters are monitored on the device.

Transmembrane Pressure

Transmembrane pressure (TMP) is the major force that acts on water and solute clearance outside the microtubule. Fluid moves through the microtubule into the external chamber of the filter, where it is removed as ultrafiltrate. The relationship between ultrafiltrate production and TMP is shown in **Figure 37.11**. The amount of ultrafiltrate obtained varies with the surface area, length and type of material from which the filter is made, and the patient's blood viscosity.

$$TMP = (Pi + Po)/2 − Pn$$

HF 400 ULTRAFILTRATION RATE

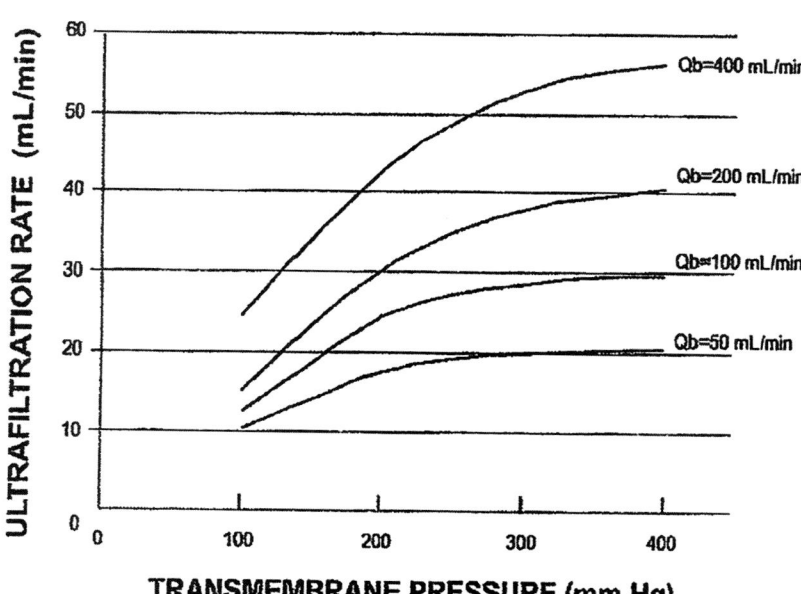

FIGURE 37.11. Relationship between ultrafiltration rate and transmembrane pressure: effect of blood flow. From *Technical Specifications Manual*, Renal Systems Minneapolis, MN, with permission.

Where:

Pi = filter inlet pressure
Po = filter outlet pressure
Pn = absolute value of the hydrostatic pressure
    on the filtrate side of the membrane (which is
    usually negative)

In CAVH, the transmembrane pressure is usually determined by the height difference between the filter and the continuous column of filtrate as it enters the collecting bag. In CVVH, the transmembrane pressure can be altered by the amount of suction applied to the filtrate line by the dialysis pump.

Filtration Fraction

Filtration fraction represents the efficiency of filtration, is determined by the rate of production of ultrafiltrate/rate of filter blood flow (UFR/BF), and depends on:

- TMP
- Surface area of the filter (**Fig. 37.12**)
- Permeability of the membrane
- Plasma oncotic pressure (**Fig. 37.13**)
- Hematocrit

The clearance of a substance in CRRT modes that involve hemodialysis depends on the dialysis flow rate, blood flow rate, the surface area of the filter, and the dialysis fluid composition. When using CRRT primarily for filtration, UFR/m² gives the approximate effective clearance that can be achieved. Clearance can be increased with higher blood flow, higher transmembrane pressures, and higher filtration fractions. Thus, larger surface area and increased filter permeability will increase the efficiency of filtration, whereas higher hematocrits and high plasma protein concentration will decrease efficiency of filtration (**Figs. 37.12** and **37.13**). It is important to note that use of fluid replacement solutions, either in the pre- or postfilter

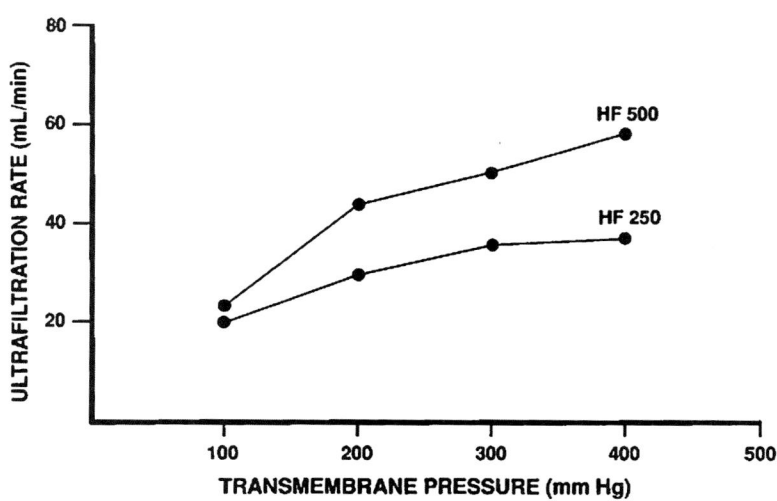

FIGURE 37.12. Relationship between ultrafiltration rate and transmembrane pressure: effect of filter surface area. From *Technical Specifications Manual*, Renal Systems Minneapolis, MN, with permission.

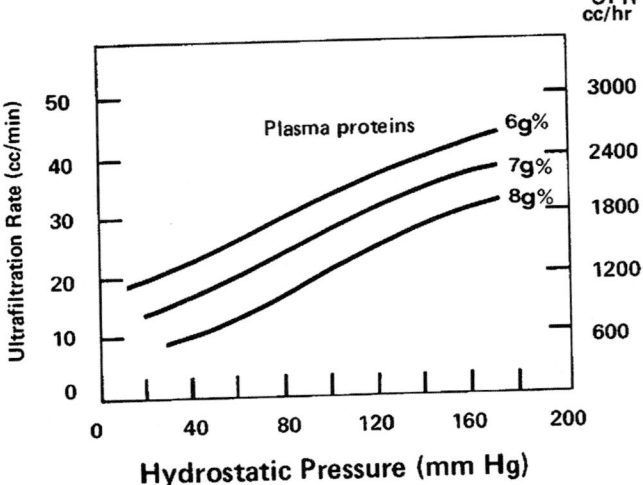

FIGURE 37.13. Effect of plasma protein concentration on ultrafiltration rate. From *Technical Specifications Manual*, Renal Systems Minneapolis, MN, with permission.

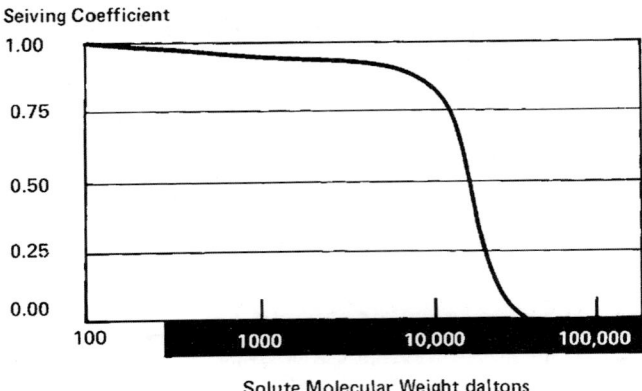

FIGURE 37.14. Filter solute removal: relationship of sieving coefficient and molecular weight. From *Technical Specifications Manual*, Renal Systems Minneapolis, MN, with permission.

positions, can also affect the duration of filtration that occurs over a 24-hr period and the adsorption and solute clearance of a substance.

Substances are removed from the blood via two mechanisms: the passing of *solute* through the filter or *adsorption* to the surface of the plastic tubing and the filter itself.

Solute Removal

The substances that are removed by the filter vary, depending on the type of filter used and the modality of filtration. Examples of solutes removed are shown in **Table 37.6** and **Figure 37.14**. The *sieving coefficient* is the concentration of a substance in the filtrate divided by the concentration of the same substance in the plasma. Many small molecules have a sieving coefficient of ~1. Given that the solute clearance equals

the filtrate flow times the sieving coefficient, it follows that the clearance of many solutes is determined by the filtrate flow rate. For example, creatinine clearance (Ccr, sieving coefficient of 1) is the same as the ultrafiltration rate (Ccr = UFR).

The concept of the sieving coefficient and filtrate flow works well to determine the plasma clearance of many substances, especially when simple methods, such as SCUF are used. However, at higher flow rates that may be used with CVVH, large amounts of replacement solutions may be used, which can also dramatically change plasma levels of solutes. Many commercial replacement solutions exist.

Significant convective clearance occurs of "middle" molecules, including cytokines, complement, tumor necrosis factor (TNF), IL-1, IL-6, and IL-8, prostaglandin, myocardial depressant factor, interferon, and even Gram-positive bacterial exotoxins. These substances have molecular weights of up to 17–28 kDa. In addition to molecular weight, clearance of a substance depends on its charge and three-dimensional arrangement. Clearance can also be affected by the type of material used in the filter membrane (polysulfone or polyacrylonitrile).

Differences in solute clearance between CVVH, CVVHD, and CVVHDF from a study in small piglets using a polysulphone membrane are shown in **Table 37.7**. Differences between type of dialysis and clearance were greater with larger molecules (47). In another study that compared CVVH and CVVHD in 10 patients, little difference for urea and creatinine clearance was noted, a slight (4%) increase in uric acid clearance occurred with CVVH, and a significant (19%) increase in vancomycin clearance with CVVH occurred, suggesting that CVVH offers some potential for the removal of middle molecules (21). This finding was confirmed in another study that showed that larger molecules, such as insulin, myoglobin, heparin, and vancomycin, are cleared well by CVVH (16). Other recent reviews of CVVH in the PICU environment have also supported these findings (4,28). A very interesting comparison of CVVHD and CVVH (with pre- and postmembrane dilution) found that CVVHD and postdilution CVVH gave similar urea and creatinine clearances that were 15% better than those achieved with predilution CVVH. Postdilution clearances were only measured at low-flow rates, however, because of concern regarding filter hemoconcentration and clotting. This study concluded that CVVHD was the optimal modality for small-molecule clearance during CRRT (40).

TABLE 37.6

SIEVING COEFFICIENTS FOR CLEARANCE OF VARIOUS SOLUTES

Solute	Sieving coefficient
CO_2	1.124
Blood urea nitrogen	1.048
Chloride	1.046
Phosphorus	1.044
Glucose	1.043
Creatinine	1.020
Uric acid	1.016
Sodium	0.993
Potassium	0.985
Magnesium	0.879
Creatine phosphokinase	0.676
Calcium	0.637
Total bilirubin	0.030
Direct bilirubin	0.030
Total proteins	0.021
Albumin	0.008

TABLE 37.7

MEAN SOLUTE EFFLUENT:PLASMA RATIO (SD) FOR EACH TECHNIQUE

Solute	CVVH	CVVHD	CVVHDF	ANOVA
Urea	0.957 (0.038)	0.876 (0.109)	0.754 (0.123)	$p = 0.002$
Creatinine	0.942 (0.050)	0.934 (0.056)	0.814 (0.057)	$p = 0.002$
All amino acids	0.996 (0.344)	0.904 (0.196)	0.778 (0.180)	$p < 0.001$
Vancomycin	0.739 (0.082)	0.643 (0.063)	0.509 (0.081)	$p < 0.001$
Phenytoin	0.302 (0.028)	0.297 (0.036)	0.265 (0.035)	$p = 0.067$

SD, standard deviation; CVVH, continuous venovenous hemofiltration; CVVHD, continuous venovenous hemodialysis; CVVHDF, continuous venovenous hemofiltration; ANOVA, analysis of variance

Adsorption

It is clear that proteins (especially fibrinogen and albumin) and cytokines (such as TNF and IL) are adsorbed to the plastic surface of the circuit. It is also clear that this adsorption is probably small in amount, and unless circuits are changed frequently (every few hours), the adsorption effect is probably of minimal significance (20,63).

Indications for Continuous Renal Replacement Therapy

The indications for CRRT can be renal (such as ARF) or nonrenal. Intensive care indications are shown in **Table 37.1**. The types and frequencies of conditions treated with extracorporeal RRT are shown in **Table 37.8**.

Contraindications to Continuous Renal Replacement Therapy

Very few absolute contraindications to CVVH exist. Even in the presence of intracranial hemorrhage or systemic bleeding, CVVH can be safely performed by using no anticoagulation, using small doses of heparin with close serial monitoring of anticoagulation by activated clotting time (ACT), or using regional anticoagulation provided by heparin/protamine or

citrate/calcium. Although some centers consider an intracerebral hemorrhage an absolute contraindication to CRRT, others would use a regional circuit anticoagulation technique or citrate/calcium.

Circuit Components

Catheters

A large range of double-lumen, variable-length catheters is available. These catheters contain a proximal withdrawal lumen that has multiple side holes and a distal, single-end lumen for reinfusion to the patient. They are firm so that they will not collapse with suction applied by the system. Recommended CVVH catheters for children of different sizes and ages are listed in **Table 37.9**.

Much debate surrounds the best vascular site for catheter placement, especially in small infants. The largest accessible percutaneous vessel is the subclavian vein, followed by the internal jugular and femoral veins. More serious insertion complications occur with subclavian vein cannulation, followed by internal jugular vein cannulation and femoral vein cannulation. Ultrasound localization of vessels during placement may limit complications and improve success of catheter insertion. The closer the tip of the vascular filtration catheter is to the right atrium, the better the flow obtained, although placing the catheter deep in the right atrium is associated with a greater risk

TABLE 37.8

SPECTRUM OF DISEASES/INDICATIONS FOR HEMOFILTRATION IN ICU

	Patients (277)	Filters (1003)
Sepsis (infection)	120 (43%)	443 (44.0%)
Acute renal failure	46 (16.6%)	206 (20.5%)
Systemic inflammatory response syndrome	35 (12.6%)	133 (13.2%)
Fluid and electrolyte	32 (11.5%)	76 (7.6%)
Inborn errors of metabolism	19 (6.8%)	44 (4.4%)
Liver failure	12 (4.3%)	38 (3.2%)
Oncology (sepsis, bone marrow transplant)	9 (3%)	36 (3.6%)
Other	4 (1.4%)	27 (2.7%)

No patients treated with plasmapheresis or hepatic support, such as molecular absorbent regeneration (MARS), are included in table.
From Butt, Royal Childrens Hospital Melbourne, unpublished data.

TABLE 37.9

SUGGESTED SIZES OF CATHETERS FOR USE IN CVVH

Patient size	Catheter size (manufacturer)
Neonate	Single-lumen 5 fr (Cook) Dual-lumen 7.0 fr (Cook/MedComp)
3–6 kg	Dual-lumen 7.0 fr (Cook/MedComp) Triple-lumen 7.0 fr (MedComp)
6–30 kg	Dual-lumen 8.0 fr (Arrow, Kendall)
>15 kg	Dual-lumen 9.0 fr (Arrow, Kendall)
>30 kg	Dual-lumen 10.0 fr (Arrow, Kendall) Triple-lumen 12.5 fr (Arrow, Kendall)

fr, French

of perforation. At high blood flow rates, maximum drainage capacity may be reached for the cannula and negative pressure can be generated in the dialysis circuit. Both blood drainage and blood return can be impaired. Alterations in circuit pressure (either too negative or too positive) outside the set alarm limits will cause constant cessation of filtration. In situations in which drainage is inadequate, the filter connections can be reversed so that the inflow (blood drainage) cannula is the single end hole and the blood-return lumen is the side hole. Although this may increase recirculation of blood back into the dialysis circuit, the improved blood flow obtained may allow adequate filtration to continue.

Filters

The key elements to the filter used for dialysis are:

Size—The larger the surface area, the higher the filtration fraction and the less the hemoconcentration that occurs within the filter. Larger filters, however, have larger priming volumes and slower blood flow within the filter.

The type of membrane—Filters may be composed of microtubules or a plate membrane, and the material may be either polysulphone or polyacrylonitrile nitrate. The minor differences in filtration fraction and sieving coefficients that exist between membranes are, for practical purposes, not relevant.

The filters used for CRRT vary around the world. In principle, large filters can be used even in small infants when venovenous circuits are used. The authors commonly use either 0.25 m^2 or 0.5 m^2 surface area filters, which allow for improved filter performance at lower blood flows and less hemoconcentration but require more anticoagulation because of the slower blood flow (**Table 37.10**).

Heater

The use of extracorporeal circulation and the infusion of solute with high flow create a substantial heat loss. Continuous monitoring of core temperature is necessary, and the use of heating systems is recommended. Newborns and small infants are kept warm with radiant incubators, and older children are warmed with warming blankets. Blood circuit and dialysate warmers are often used. Occasionally, a heat exchanger is added to the circuit. For older children, the circuit may also be covered with aluminium foil (space blanket material) to minimize heat loss. If these procedures are unsuccessful, a heat exchanger can be added to the circuit.

TABLE 37.10

HEMOFILTERS COMMERCIALLY AVAILABLE FOR CRRT IN CHILDREN IN 2005

Company	Name of hemofilter	Membrane structure type	Membrane type	Membrane surface (m²)	Priming volume (mL)
Amicon	Minimiser Plus	MT	PS	0.08	15
	Diafilter 10S	MT	PS	0.20	15
	Diafilter 20S	MT	PS	0.25	38
	Diafilter 30S	MT	PS	0.60	58
Baxter	PHSF 400 gold	MT	PS	0.30	28
	PHSF 700 gold	MT	PS	0.71	53
	PHSF 700 gold	MT	PS	1.25	83
Fresenuis	F-5	MT	PS	1.00	63
	F-6	MT	PS	1.3	82
Gambro	FH 22	MT	C	0.16	11
	FH 66	MT	P	0.60	43
Hospal	Multiflow 60	MT	AN69	0.60	92
	Multiflow 100	MT	AN69	0.90	130
	HF 1000	MT	PAE	1.15	128
	HF 1400	MT	PAE	1.40	186
Renaflo	HF 250	MT	PS	0.25	27
	HF 400	MT	PS	0.30	28
	HF 500	MT	PS	0.50	39

MT, microtubule; PS, polysulfone; AN69, polyacrylonitrile; P, polyamine; PAE, polyarylethersulfone; C, cuprophane

TABLE 37.11

HEMOFILTRATION REPLACEMENT SOLUTION

	mmol/L
Sodium	140
Calcium	2
Magnesium	1
Chlorine	100
Acetate	23
Bicarbonate	25
Potassium	3
Phosphate	1
Dextrose	0.18%

TABLE 37.12

CONTINUOUS RENAL REPLACEMENT THERAPY: ANTICOAGULATION STRATEGIES

Prefilter heparin 10 U/kg/hr
Heparin 10–20 U/kg/hr with monitoring of activated clotting time
Regional anticoagulation (prefilter heparin and postfilter protamine usually at a ratio of 100 U of heparin per 1 mg of protamine)
Regional citrate anticoagulation (prefilter citrate and postfilter calcium; special calcium-free dialysate needed)
Low-molecular-weight heparin
Prostacyclin (5 mcg/kg/hr)

Replacement Solution

The same solutions are used for dialysate and replacement fluids in CRRT. Commercial solutions usually include sodium, buffer, calcium, and magnesium, with concentrations similar to plasma. When prolonged CRRT is required, glucose and phosphorus should be present in the solution to limit depletion in the patient (Table 37.11). Many commercial solutions are available, many of which contain lactate. In children with impaired lactate metabolism due to liver failure, critical illness, circulatory failure, or inborn errors of metabolism, significant lactic acidosis may occur with use of these solutions. This problem can be rectified by using a solution that contains a bicarbonate buffer rather than lactate.

Pre- or Postfilter Replacement

Views vary regarding location of replacement fluid within the CRRT circuit. The advantages of replacement fluid placement prior to the filter (predilution) are (a) increased urea clearance as diffusion of red cell urea into the plasma occurs, and (b) a slight increase in filter survival due to hemodilution of blood and clotting factors. Thus, predilution placement is preferred in some PICUs. However, predilution placement decreases the sieving coefficient of most solutes by lowering the filter inlet concentration of these substances. A study in adults that compared pre- and postfilter replacement showed increased filter survival with predilution from 13–18 hrs (61). As most pediatric filter survival is >48 hrs, either with pre- or postfilter replacement, factors other than placement of replacement fluid within the circuit may be important in determining filter life between pediatric and adult patients.

Anticoagulation

Many strategies are used to prevent clotting in the extracorporeal circuits of RRT. Examples are listed in Table 37.12. It is vital to remember that many factors lead to clotting within the circuit. They include kinking of catheters; high circuit resistance; obstruction to inflow (blood drainage from patient) of catheter (often by side-hole occlusion by the vessel wall); slow blood flow or stasis; high blood viscosity due to high hematocrit, high plasma proteins, or from hemoconcentration due to excess fluid filtration; fibrin-strand formation from binding to

the plastic surface of tubing or the filter; circulating procoagulants (particularly in sepsis or systemic inflammatory response syndrome); and inadequate anticoagulation. While one study in adults showed minimal difference in CRRT efficiency between use of no anticoagulation, heparin, or regional anticoagulation, blood flows used in adult patients are much higher than those used in children and whether these same effects would be obtained in children is questionable (60). The majority of pediatric CRRT is performed with anticoagulation of some type. Examples of a CVVHDF circuit with various anticoagulation options are shown in Figure 37.15. While a wide variety of anticoagulants has been used in children (8), most PICUs follow one of the following schemes:

- Infusion of 10–20 U/kg heparin pre-filter and maintenance of measured at ACT 1.5 times normal.
- Regional anticoagulation with citrate infused prefilter at 1 mL/30 mL blood flow rate, with a goal of a prefilter ionized Ca^{2+} of <0.4 and a postfilter calcium infusion to maintain a circuit ionized Ca^{2+} of >1. Patients with cardiovascular compromise may require higher levels of ionized calcium (>1.2).
- Infusion of 10–20 U/kg heparin prefilter and 1–2 U/kg heparin postfilter and maintenance of ACT at 1.5 times normal

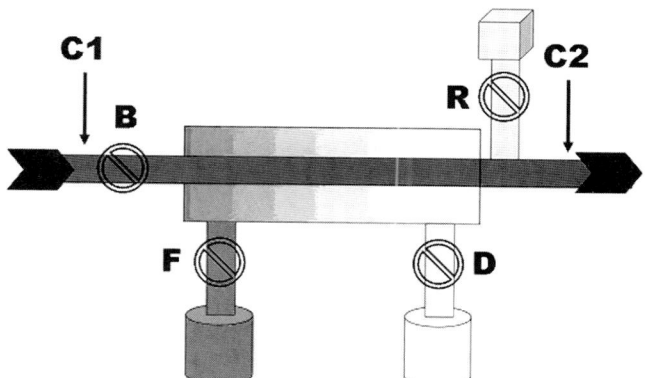

FIGURE 37.15. Continuous venovenous hemodiafiltration (CVVHDF) (postfilter replacement) with different anticoagulation options: C1 options—heparin, citrate, prostacyclin. C2 options—heparin, Ca^{2+}, protamine, nothing. B, blood flow; R, replacement fluid rate; F, filtration rate; D, dialysate rate.

(to limit clots on the return line and tip of vascular access catheter).

■ Regional anticoagulation with heparin infused prefilter with 10–20 U/kg/hr and reversed postfilter with protamine (1 mg for every 100 U of heparin given prefilter).

The easiest form of anticoagulation is a simple heparin infusion with regular monitoring of bedside ACTs and daily laboratory coagulation tests. In situations of marked coagulopathy, such as sepsis, severe brain injury, trauma, liver failure, or active bleeding, it is logical to use regional anticoagulation, whereby the circuit is anticoagulated but the effect is reversed prior to blood return to the patient. Using some form of anticoagulation with these types of clinical situations is imperative because circulating procoagulants will often cause filter clotting if no anticoagulation is used. The most common method of regional anticoagulation used in the PICU is citrate/calcium, while the use of heparin and protamine predominates in adult patients. Some favor citrate/calcium in the PICU because the heparin/protamine complex itself is an anticoagulant that prolongs the ACT and the exact dose of protamine is not certain in pediatrics.

Circuit Priming

With many modern CVVH systems, circuit priming is automatic. In children who weigh >15 kg, circuit priming is often performed with the use of 0.9% saline with 5 U/mL heparin. In smaller infants, however, a blood prime or albumin of 4%–5% is recommended to avoid hemodilution at the session start (25). Small infants are also prone to hypotension when CVVH is started, and ionized calcium and hemodynamics should be carefully monitored. Some centers have vasoactive medications (e.g., epinephrine) ready for administration to counteract hypotension during initiation of CVVH.

Calculation of Machine Settings

The first decision to be made is the mode of CRRT to be used. Most centers usually have a single type of CRRT.

For Continuous Venovenous Hemofiltration

A determination must be made regarding the type of clearance required, remembering that solute clearance with CVVH is equivalent to the filtration rate:

F = UFR = GFR, which usually means an ultrafiltration flow rate of 10–20 mL/min/1.73m^2, or alternatively 10–50 mL/kg/hr.

Once the UFR is chosen, blood flow is usually maintained at at least three times that of the UFR. Fluid balance with CVVH is calculated simply as UFR minus the replacement fluid and any other fluid administered to patient.

Frequent monitoring of clearance of substances such as water, urea, lactate, etc., may result in alterations of filtrate flow and, depending on the filtration fraction, a change in blood flow may also be required

For Continuous Venovenous Hemodialysis

D: dialysate flow rate (clearance)
Choose fluid removal rate: F − D
No replacement fluid: RF = 0

A decision is made about the clearance requirements, and a dialysate flow is calculated and set, as are the fluid removal goals. Fluid balance is merely

Filtrate flow − (dialysate flow + IV fluids).

Frequent monitoring of urea, creatinine, and electrolytes determines the adequacy of clearance. If clearance is inadequate, more flow or a larger membrane filter will improve clearance. This modality is usually used for ARF.

For Continuous Venovenous Hemodiafiltration

Usually, clearance is determined with 50% as dialysis and 50% as filtration. Fluid balance is:

Filtrate flow − (dialysis flow + replacement fluid + IV fluids).

Frequent monitoring of urea, electrolytes, and fluid balance is essential. Adjustment to increase clearance of small molecules is obtained by increasing dialysis flow (and filtrate flow in an equal amount). Clearance of middle molecules requires an increase in the percentage of filtrate flow as filtration.

Complications

Extracorporeal Therapy

■ *Access*—To avoid limb ischemia and arterial bleeding complications, arterial access is not commonly used.
■ *Infection*—Infection is usually related to catheter insertion sites.
■ *Technical*—Equipment may malfunction.
■ *Clotting of blood vessel or membrane filter*—Clotting is often related to the size of the catheter in relation to the size of the vessel. Clotting may also be increased in instances of infection. Despite the use of heparin, clots in the blood vessel used for cannulation can occur in 30%–50% of patients with large filtration catheters. Clotting of the filter is increased if there is a high filtration fraction, which caused hemoconcentration, in instances of slow blood flow in large surface area filters, or if long microtubules with high resistance are used. Clotting is also increased with frequent interruption of flow (3), poor anticoagulation, or in conditions with circulating procoagulants (e.g., sepsis or diffuse intravascular coagulopathy).
■ *Bleeding*—Patient bleeding may occur, but the degree of anticoagulation used for the dialysis circuit is fairly low or regional to minimize bleeding risk.
■ *Embolism*—Although uncommon, embolization of air clots or debris returning from the circuit can occur.

Continuous Renal Replacement Therapy

■ *Fluid imbalance*—Hypovolemia or fluid overload may occur from imbalances in fluid intake and filtration flow. In small infants, large volume changes may develop quickly and lead to hemodynamic compromise. Continuous monitoring of central venous filling pressures, blood pressure, and heart rate and use of venous saturation and lactate are helpful in monitoring patient status.

- *Electrolyte abnormalities*—Changes in electrolytes may occur if nonstandard solutions are used or if large volume changes go undetected.
- *Metabolic acidosis or alkalosis*—Either abnormality can occur. Alkalosis is more common with citrate anticoagulation, while use of dialysis or replacement solutions that contain lactate can lead to metabolic acidosis from hyperlactatemia.
- *Unwanted clearance*—CVVH leads to clearance of water-soluble vitamins and amino acids that must be replaced in long-term use.
- *Hypothermia*—Hypothermia occurs often from extracorporeal blood cooling. Temperature monitoring should be maintained. When routine measures are not sufficient, an in-line heater or tube-warming device should be used.
- *Thrombocytopenia*—It is not uncommon to see a decrement in platelet count of up to 50% of baseline values every time a patient is placed on a new filter. The exposure to a new filter does not seem to affect white blood cell count or to cause a rise in cytokines or inflammatory mediators.
- *Hypotension on connection of circuit and patient*—In patients with circulatory shock on vasopressors, hypotension and circulatory collapse can occur. It is believed that this is not due to volume shifts, but due to binding of catecholamines to the plastic of the circuit. Thus, in patients on large doses of vasoconstrictors and inotropic drugs, an effective strategy may be to double drug infusion rates before starting CVVH and then beginning with a slow blood flow that is gradually increased over 5–10 mins to the desired rate. Once initiation of CVVH has safely occurred, filtration can begin. Some centers use either rapid infusion of volume or a vasoconstrictor, such as metaraminol (Aramine), phenylephrine or norepinephrine, to treat the hypotension that often accompanies initiation of CVVH in patients on large amounts of vasoactive medications.
- *Hypoxia*—In neonates with severe lung disease (not those on extracorporeal membrane oxygenation, ECMO), hypoxemia from initial exposure to blood used in a "blood-primed" circuit may be avoided by an elevation in F_{IO_2} up to 100% in the ventilator.

HEMODIALYSIS

Hemodialysis (HD) is the extracorporeal exchange of fluid and solute that occurs across an artificial semipermeable membrane between blood and dialysis fluid that are moving in opposite (countercurrent) directions. HD uses dialyzers with larger surface area, higher blood flow rates, and higher dialysis flow rates than CRRT. Thus, HD is much more efficient at removing solute than CRRT. However, the intermittent nature of the technique (sessions usually last 4–6 hrs and are often repeated three times per week) lends itself to being used in stable children with chronic renal failure or ARF due to renal disease (such as hemolytic-uremic syndrome or glomerulonephritis). HD can be used in children in the PICU for indications of both renal failure and nonrenal failure. It can also be used in hemodynamically stable children with hyperammonemia (44), inborn errors of metabolism (36), and drug overdoses in which rapid substance removal may be desirable. Recent modifications and technical advances have allowed some critically ill children to receive daily HD or sustained, low-efficiency dialysis.

Physiology of Dialysis

Fluid Removal

Fluid removal is accomplished via the process of ultrafiltration along a hydrostatic pressure gradient called the *TMP gradient*, which is determined by the pressure difference across the semipermeable membrane minus the plasma oncotic pressure (which tends to retain fluid in the blood) and is of the order of 20–30 mm Hg.

$$TMP = (Pb - Pd) - Po$$

Where:

- Pb = pressure on the blood side of the membrane.
- Pd = pressure on the dialysis side of the membrane (often negative).
- Po = plasma oncotic pressure due to plasma protein concentration.

High-flux dialyzers are extremely permeable to water, while standard (low-flux) dialyzers are less permeable. The permeability of a membrane is defined as Kuf, which is the amount of ultrafiltrate at a particular TMP, and is measured as mL/hr × mm Hg. High-flux membranes permit high ultrafiltration rates, thereby allowing bulk flow (also known as solute drag) to occur and larger middle molecules to be removed (**Fig. 37.16**). Low-flux membranes remove less water and produce lower amounts of solute drag.

Solute Removal

Solute removal occurs by diffusive transport along a concentration gradient. The larger the concentration gradient, the faster the removal of solute or waste products.

$$Cl = Qb \times (Ci - Co)/Ci$$

Where:

- Cl = clearance.
- Qb = blood flow mL/min.
- Ci = concentration of solute at inlet.
- Co = concentration of solute at outlet.

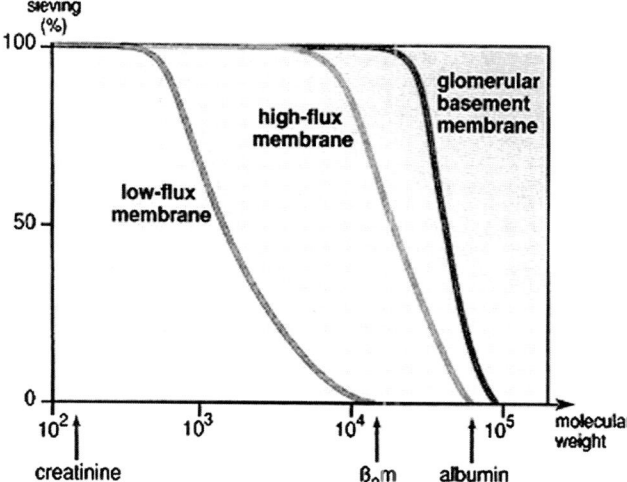

FIGURE 37.16. Sieving curves for different membranes showing which solutes can be convectively transported. From *Technical Specifications Manual*, Fresenius Medical Care, Germany.

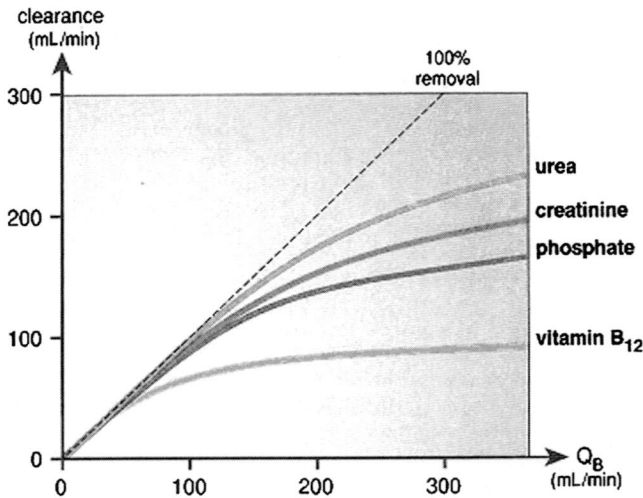

FIGURE 37.17. Clearance of small- and medium-sized molecules in relation to blood flow rate, (Q_B), for a low-flux, synthetic dialyzer. At low Q_B, clearance equals Q_B, i.e., the removal is 100%. From *Technical Specifications Manual,* Fresenius Medical Care, Germany.

Solute removal also depends on the time allowed for dialysis, as well as the volume of distribution for the particular solute; their relationship to clearance is:

$$Ci/Co = e^{-(KT/V)}$$

Where:

  e = base of natural logarithm
  K = clearance at a given blood flow
  T = time of dialysis
  V = volume of distribution for the solute.

Countercurrent flow is very important to improving the efficiency of solute removal because it maintains a continuous concentration gradient along the entire length of the dialyzer fibers.

Small molecules below 300 Da move easily across the membrane (**Fig. 37.17**). Increasing flow rates will increase solute transfer (increased blood flow brings more concentrated solute, while increased dialysate flow maintains low solute levels, thereby maintaining the concentration gradient); thus, small-molecule clearance is flow dependent. Large molecules do not diffuse as easily and, therefore, are not flow dependent, but

they are dependent on physical characteristics (thickness, surface area, and type) of the plastic that constitutes the membrane dialyzer.

Circuit

Catheters

In general similar catheters are used in acute HD and in CRRT. A large range of catheters for acute HD are commercially available; from 6.5–7 French in the newborn, to 14 French in the large adolescent. Currently most centers use double-lumen catheters for acute HD. These are inserted in the usual way into the femoral, internal jugular, or subclavian vein and must be large enough to obtain blood flow rates of 3–5 mL/kg/min to achieve adequate solute clearance. Some of the larger catheters also have an extra infusion lumen that can be used as a central venous access port.

Dialyzer

A large range of commercially available dialyzer membranes is used, and they have a number of features in common: small priming volume, biocompatibility (with minimal cytokine release), known sieving and filtration coefficients, known and consistent relationships between solute clearance and blood and dialysate flows, and low pressure drop across the membrane. Some centers use the Fresenius polysulfone dialyzers, the characteristics of which are listed in **Table 37.13**. Two types of dialyzers are available: *hollow-fiber* (capillary), which is used in most major centers, and *plate dialyzers*. Plate dialyzers are more complex than hollow-fiber types. They contain 40–70 pairs of membrane sheets layered in a stack. Blood flows between each pair of membrane sheets, while dialysis occurs in the middle of each pair of sheets. The flow in plate dialyzers is nonlaminar, but some evidence suggests that reduced clotting occurs, especially at low flows.

Modern membrane materials, such as polysulfone, polyamide, and polyacrylonitrile, are more biocompatible than the cellulose membranes of the past. Modern membranes have slightly different sieving coefficients, but the choice of membrane used is often a matter of personal preference. Membrane permeability may be divided into *diffusive* (related to thickness, charge, and type of plastic) and *hydraulic* (related to Kuf) (**Fig. 37.17**). It is prudent to choose a membrane size that has a surface area that is less than the surface area of the patient

TABLE 37.13

PERFORMANCE CHARACTERISTICS OF A FRESENIUS POLYSULFONE DIALYZER

	Surface area m^2			
	0.4	0.8	1.3	1.6
Clearance urea mL/min	125	170	243	247
UF-coefficient (mL/hr)/mm Hg	1.7	8.0	13.0	16.0
V Priming volume	28	42	82	102
ΔP blood (300 mL/min)	–	142	91	71
ΔO dialysate (500 mL/min)	–	23	19	16
Blood flow mL/min	200	200	300	300

UF, ultrafiltration; mm Hg, millimeters mercury (the higher the number the greater the UF coefficient)

and a priming volume that is less than 10% of the patient's circulating blood volume.

Priming the Circuit

In older children, the circuit is usually primed with saline or albumin. In children who weigh <10 kg, in children in whom the priming volume is <10%–15% of estimated patient blood volume, or in patients who are hemodynamically compromised, it is common practice to use a blood prime similar that often used with CRRT. Hematocrit of the priming fluid should be >40%. The amount of albumin and packed red blood cells to be added to the circuit and tubing can be calculated as:

$$(V_{prbc} \times Hct_{prbc}/P_{hct}) - V_{prbc} = V_{alb}$$

Where:

V_{prbc} = the volume of packed red blood cells for the prime

Hct_{prbc} = the hematocrit of the prime red blood cells

P_{hct} = the desired hematocrit of the prime

V_{alb} = the volume of 5% albumin to be added to the prime solution.

Anticoagulation

Heparin is the main method of anticoagulation. Other types of anticoagulation include enoxaparin, prostacyclin infusion, or regional anticoagulation with heparin/protamine or citrate/calcium. Each center will have its own protocol, for example, initial heparin dose for infants 5–15 kg is 10–16 U/kg, for children 15–25 kg, it is 16–20 U/kg, and for children >25 kg, it is 25–65 U/kg. Maintenance heparin for children <25 kg is 10–20 U/kg/hr, and for children >25 kg, it is 20–30 U/kg/hr.

Monitoring anticoagulation levels using bedside testing of ACT is essential, with a goal level 1.5–2 times normal, depending on the patient's diagnosis, clinical condition, and risk for bleeding. Enoxaparin (Clexane, Lovenox) offers the advantage of a single dose, less fibrin and platelet deposition and, in the long term, less osteoporosis and abnormal lipid levels (12). This medication is currently not available for anticoagulation in the US.

When bleeding is a concern, regional anticoagulation with citrate can be given as in CRRT, with a target ionized calcium of 0.3 predialyzer. To prevent systemic hypocalcemia, a calcium infusion is administered to maintain the patient's ionized calcium level at >0.9–1.2 (30). Heparin/protamine as a combination for regional anticoagulation is popular in adult ICUs but is uncommonly used in the PICU.

Choice of Dialysis Solution

It is important to remember that solute exchange in HD is a two-way process, so that the goals are removal of waste, normalization of electrolytes, addition of buffer, and maintenance of solute. In an excellent review article, the authors discuss the concept of "designer dialysate," in which dialysis fluid can be ordered to suit individual patient needs, and they discuss the components to be provided in the dialysate fluid (53).

Removal of waste implies no urea, no creatinine, and minimal phosphate in the dialysis fluid. Normalization of elec-

trolytes in particular focuses on key electrolytes of plasma including sodium, potassium, calcium, magnesium, and chlorine. Also, blood glucose should be maintained at a normal level. Finally, it is important to add buffer to prevent deal the metabolic acidosis that can be induced with dialysis. Buffering is usually accomplished by the addition of bicarbonate in concentrations of 30–35 mmol/L to the dialysis fluid.

Complications

Extracorporeal Therapy

Vascular access risks in extracorporeal therapy are similar to those in CRRT; namely, those associated with insertion of large catheters into central veins. Risks from problems related to insertion, infection, thrombosis, embolism, and hemorrhage. Longer-term complications include vascular stenosis and vessel occlusion with clot. Catheter clots are fairly common and may be treated with clot lysis techniques using tissue plasminogen activator or urokinase, although the risk of bleeding with these medications must be recognized. Technical malfunction of equipment is always a potential risk, but proper care, training of staff, and troubleshooting algorithms can limit the effects of technical failure to the patient.

Hemodialysis

Disequilibrium syndrome occurs when the patients' plasma becomes hypotonic relative to their brain cells and water enters the brain. Initial symptoms include nausea, headache, dizziness, and vomiting but can rapidly progress to seizures or coma. Children most at risk are those with high serum sodium or urea and those in whom very rapid HD is performed. When disequilibrium syndrome is recognized or in high-risk patients, an attempt should be made to have slow changes of solute occur by using low blood flow rates to decrease the rate of clearance. Mannitol at doses of 0.5–1.0 g/kg may also be helpful.

Hemolysis can occur during dialysis from use of dialysate solution that is hypotonic, hyperthermic, hyponatremic, or contaminated with formaldehyde, bleach, copper, or nitrates. Other causes of hemolysis include use of faulty blood pumps, which causes trauma to blood cells; inadequate anticoagulation leading to clot formation; and excess suction in the venous drainage line due to hypovolemia or kinking/obstruction of the dialysis catheter. The main danger that results from hemolysis is acute hyperkalemia that can cause arrhythmia and high plasma-free hemoglobin.

Anaphylaxis reactions still occur, albeit much less frequently than with the older styles of cellulose/cuprophane membranes. *Bacteremia/infection* can occur with poor aseptic technique. *Air embolus* is also possible, as is a blood or dialysate leak. *Hypothermia/hyperthermia* can occur if heaters or temperature baths malfunction. Dosage adjustment of drugs, both due to renal failure and removal of drug by HD, is essential (62). These events are all potentially dangerous and require constant supervision of the procedure by vigilant, well-trained, specialist staff.

Recirculation can occur because of high blood flows and, in small children especially, the proximity of the two ends (the drainage and reinfusion holes) of the catheters. The percentage of recirculation can be calculated as:

$$\% \text{ recirculation} = 100 \times U_{systemic} - U_{arterial}/U_{systemic} - U_{venous}$$

No recirculation is occurring when $U_{arterial} = U_{systemic}$.
Some recirculation is occurring if $U_{arterial} < U_{systemic}$.
Where U = urea concentration.

If recirculation is greater than 20%, the efficiency of HD is diminished and should be corrected.

Patient Monitoring During Dialysis

Blood pressure, heart rate, respiratory rate, SaO_2, electrocardiogram, and temperature should be continuously monitored. Parameters, such as blood glucose, ACT, hematocrit, and blood viscosity, should be serially monitored. Technical parameters of the dialysis machine, such as arterial and venous pressures, TMP, and ultrafiltrate rate, must also be carefully watched. Clinical symptoms of headaches, nausea, dizziness, and muscle cramps should be assessed. Neurologic observations of mental status and Glasgow Coma Scale score should be included as part of routine clinical assessment during dialysis.

Modifications to Standard Intermittent Hemodialysis

Daily HD was compared to intermittent hemodialysis (HDi) in a randomized, prospective, controlled trial and, not surprisingly, the daily HD group had improved outcome in terms of uremia and blood pressure control and shorter total time for dialysis. Most importantly, lower mortality was seen in patients who received daily dialysis (28% vs. 46%, $p = 0.01$) (19,53). This more frequent and potentially less destabilizing treatment may mean that HDi has a new role in PICU patients with sepsis or multiorgan failure.

Sustained low-efficiency daily diafiltration (SLEDD-f) for critically ill patients who require RRT is a combination of HDi and hemofiltration (not dissimilar to CVVHDF) that shows promise and may be a useful form of RRT in ICU (34,38).

HOW TO CHOOSE THE RIGHT TYPE OF RENAL REPLACEMENT THERAPY

Three main types of RRT—PD, HDi, and CRRT—are available at most modern PICUs in large pediatric hospitals and, for various reasons, the staffs will have made decisions regarding which type of RRT will be used in which clinical situation. In general, PD is used in small infants (<10 kg) after cardiac surgery and in those patients with early-onset chronic renal failure. The choice between HDi and the various modes of CRRT is more difficult and will often depend on personal preference. However, in general, CRRT tends to be used in the very sick or unstable patient with multiorgan failure, while HDi tends to be used in patients with ARF due to renal disease. Some units will use only CRRT in the PICU to avoid confusion among staff members and to maintain their skills for a particular type of CRRT. Thus, the type of CRRT present in a particular PICU may vary from center to center. Some units use mainly CVVHF in the PICU, while others use primarily CVVHDF.

A number of meta-analyses have been performed to identify if one form of CRRT is better than another. One analysis showed a benefit to treatment with CRRT compared to HDi (relative risk, 0.72; $p < 0.01$) (27), while an analysis of 6 trials showed no difference in mortality or outcome of renal failure when either dialytic mode was used (59). Clearly, intensivists and nephrologists should work together to provide effective RRT, irrespective of which mode is chosen.

PROGNOSIS IN ACUTE RENAL FAILURE

Over the last 20 years, CRRT has become a standard treatment in the PICU (43). Although some technical limitations have had to be overcome and randomized, controlled trials are lacking, increasing animal and human experience continues to document the efficacy of the technique. The first multicentered outcome of children who received CRRT in multiorgan dysfunction syndrome reported lower central venous pressure and less fluid overload in survivors, as compared to nonsurvivors. The investigators hypothesized that early use of CRRT might be expected to improve survival (18). Similar findings confirmed that less fluid overload occurred in survivors, especially with three or more organ system failures (15). Both of these studies help to confirm the role of CRRT in critically ill children, although controversy remains regarding when and how it should be implemented.

SPECIAL SITUATIONS

Newborn Babies

A large review of the causes of renal failure in newborn infants and available RRT for these babies was published in 2004 (2). The type of RRT offered to newborn infants depends on two key factors: local preference and the disease that is causing the need for RRT. After cardiac surgery, many centers would prefer PD. Catheters can be placed in the operating theater in a sterile and safe manner. PD enables controlled hypothermia for arrhythmia management, and RRT is likely to be needed for a relatively brief duration. PD avoids the need for anticoagulation and does not require specialized vascular-access catheters, with their attendant risks of infection, emboli, and vascular thrombosis, which can be a very important factor for future management of the patient with heart disease who may need further surgery or cardiac catheterizations.

In neonates and small infants with inborn errors of metabolism, all forms of extracorporeal RRT (CVVH, CVVHD, and CVVHDF) have been used, with rapid decrease in branched chain amino acids, keto-acids, lactate, and ammonia, resulting in minimizing cerebral injury (23,42). In newborns with sepsis, CVVH has been used alone or in combination with ECMO with encouraging results; the reasons quoted have included cytokine clearance and maintenance of fluid balance and renal support during ARF. In infants with chronic renal failure, nephrologists must determine the long-term plan, and a combination of modalities may be required.

Extracorporeal Membrane Oxygenation

Patients with sepsis or cardiogenic shock who receive ECMO for hemodynamic support often (43%) develop acute fluid overload or ARF. Given that these patients have all of the risks of extracorporeal therapy and are anticoagulated, it appears that minimal disadvantage is associated with adding CVVH, CVVHDF, or CVVHD. In 35 patients who received both therapies, 43% survived to hospital discharge, and renal function returned to normal in 93% (37). Usually, the CVVH circuit runs from the higher-pressure to the lower-pressure end of the oxygenator, representing a small shunt; it can also be run separately from the ECMO circuit in the usual fashion by using a CRRT machine. HD can also be performed while patients are on ECMO by means of connecting to the ECMO circuitry.

Sepsis

During the 1990s, CVVH was shown to improve gas exchange, hemodynamics, and survival in many different animal models of sepsis (10). Safety of filtration in critically ill infants and as adjunctive therapy was reported in 1994 and 1995 (25). A number of papers report cytokine removal in septic adults (11,20,51), while a randomized, controlled trial showed decreased mortality in critically ill adults with high-volume filtration (>35 mL/kg). In this study, <15% had a diagnosis of sepsis (49). Mechanisms of benefit appear to be related to "dampening the immune mediator response" and limiting peak levels of cytokines and other mediators of sepsis by both adsorption and filtration (45,52,63). Many emerging case series show improvements in hemodynamics and oxygenation and decreases in vasoactive drug requirements; however, to date, the numbers of patients are small and no true survival benefit has been established. It may be likely that early use of CVVH will improve fluid balance, cardiac performance, and oxygenation in children; indeed, many PICUs currently use CVVH as standard-of-care treatment. Unfortunately, no randomized, controlled trial has confirmed benefit of CRRT in critically ill children. Other therapies, such as plasmapheresis, adsorption with polymyxin, and coupled plasma adsorption, are being used in different parts of the world for similar reasons, but they also lack good evidence of benefit.

Cardiopulmonary Bypass

Cardiopulmonary bypass (CPB) presents a unique situation in which it is known beforehand that a patient will suffer a significant insult that leads to a systemic inflammatory response with a marked cytokine response. Much effort is directed toward limiting this response with the use of pre-insult corticosteroids, heparin-bonded circuits, albumin-priming of circuits, and modified ultrafiltration at the end of CPB. A preliminary study from Vienna in 1984 showed improvement in postoperative ventricular function in 27 adults who received hemofiltration at the end of surgery. An unpublished, randomized, controlled trial of prophylactic PD for 24 hrs in 160 children who weighed <10 kg after cardiac surgery, conducted in 1986–1987 (Tables 37.14 and 37.15) showed a nonsignificant trend to improvement with the dialysis group. A 1996 study, in which PICU staff members were blinded, examined the effect of high-volume (5 L/m²), zero-balanced hemofiltration in 20 children who underwent CPB (22). Significant differences were noted in postoperative bleeding, decreased time to extubations, and improved oxygenation in patients who received hemofiltration. Decreased TNF, IL-10, C3a, and myeloperoxidase were noted after filtration, while 24 hrs later, IL-1, IL-6, IL-8, and myeloperoxidase were decreased. A 1997 report on the use of PD in 32 children with ARF after cardiac surgery

TABLE 37.14

RANDOMIZED TRIAL OF PERITONEAL DIALYSIS IN INFANTS AFTER CARDIOPULMONARY BYPASS

	PD (n = 82)	No routine PD (n = 78)
Weight (kg)	4.3 ± 1.6	4.2 ± 1.8
Cardiopulmonary bypass (mins)	56 ± 27	54 ± 30
F$_{IO_2}$ >0.5 (hrs)	21 ± 27	40 ± 100
ICU duration (hrs)	85 ± 138	105 ± 160

PD, peritoneal dialysis
From Butt et al., unpublished data.

noted improved fluid removal along with improved cardiac and pulmonary function (65). Only minor complications were encountered and reported, reflecting on the overall safety of the technique. In 2001, a prospective randomized, controlled trial of modified ultrafiltration after CPB was conducted in 573 adults. Patients who received modified ultrafiltration had a slightly lower mortality, significantly lowered postoperative morbidity, and a decreased need for blood transfusion (33). It appears that the common use of modified ultrafiltration and early use of PD in many pediatric cardiac surgical programs, although unproven, may well be justified.

Liver Failure

For discussion of extracorporeal therapies in hepatic failure, see Chapter 88.

TRAINING OF HEALTHCARE PROVIDERS IN THE PICU

The incidence of RRT in the PICU varies according to the specific case-mix of the hospital—from 0.7–7% (9,19,32). In the PICU, all modes of RRT (PD, HDi, CRRT) are used, with increased use of CRRT in >50% of patients (64). Despite increased use, the multiple techniques available may make it

TABLE 37.15

RANDOMIZED TRIAL OF PERITONEAL DIALYSIS IN INFANTS AFTER CARDIOPULMONARY BYPASS

	PD (n = 82)	No PD (n = 78)
Serum potassium >6 (mmol/L)	4	7
Serum potassium <3 (mmol/L)	10	16
Se sodium (mmol/L)	140	137
Glucose 2–4 (mmol/L)	2	5
Glucose >28 (mmol/L)	4	6
Serum protein (g/L)	57	50
Serum urea (mmol/L)	7.2	6.1
Serum creatinine (mmol/L)	0.03	0.03
Fluid–mL/kg/hr	–4.1	–1.2

From Butt et al., unpublished data.

difficult to maintain staff competency and expertise in all aspects of RRT with the same degree of proficiency. Attempts to address this dilemma have led to several options. It simplicity allows the training of all nurses in manual PD. The specific nature of the skills required and the low frequency of use of HDi in the PICU necessitate special training, and nephrology staff should be included in the care of patients while they are on HDi in the PICU. For CRRT, three main methods of patient support are currently in use in various PICUs (24):

- *CRRT is exclusively performed by the nephrology staff.* This strategy has the advantage of specific and well-trained personnel. On the other hand, it limits the use of the technique to hours when these personnel are in-house and can slow the use of CRRT in an emergency.
- *CRRT is exclusively managed by PICU nurses.* The advantage of this approach is that the patient is entirely managed by the PICU staff. The difficulty is to maintain the nurses' skills and expertise at the appropriate levels, which may be facilitated by limiting the number of nurses and support staff who are involved in CRRT to a core group of individuals.
- *CRRT is managed both by the nephrology staff and PICU staff, with a pool of nurses on call.* This structure combines the expertise of both specialities and is promoted in many centers in North America.

CONCLUSIONS AND FUTURE DIRECTIONS

The ultrafiltration and solute clearance obtained during PD is dependent on the volume and osmolality of the dialysis fluid, the dwell time, and the permeability of the child's peritoneal membrane to a particular substance. Fluid is removed due to an osmotic gradient which diminishes over time. Shortening the total cycle time or increasing the dialysate glucose concentration usually improves fluid removal by maintaining the osmotic gradient at a higher degree. Solute clearance is diffusion related, thus, the larger the volume of dialysis fluid instilled, the greater the available surface area covered and the higher the efficiency of PD. Although efficiency for solute removal can also be increased with longer dwell times, for smaller molecules, short dwell times of 20 mins are adequate. Since the effectiveness of PD is not hampered by low cardiac output or shock states, it can be used even in small infants with hemodynamic instability. The safety of PD is well known with minimal complexity and minimal effects on cardiorespiratory function. Complications with PD are usually minor and often involve difficulty with catheter placement or function (64). As children grow, the effectiveness of PD in critically ill children diminishes.

The use of RRT is increasing in the PICU, as is the use of similar therapies, such as plasmapheresis. These therapies are being applied to children with a wider range of nonrenal indications, as well as earlier in the course of renal insufficiency. The use of CRRT to diminish fluid overload and maintain fluid balance is an area of much investigation. All three modalities (CVVH, CVVHD, and CVVHDF) should be available for optimal patient care. The structure of RRT support services varies among centers to utilize local knowledge and expertise; clearly, cooperation between all concerned, including nephrologists and intensivists, is key.

KEY POINTS

- RRT is an integral part of the patient care provided within the PICU.
- PD is best for neonates and in infants who weigh <10 kg after cardiac surgery.
- HDi is best for acute or chronic renal failure and in hemodynamically stable infants with acute renal failure.
- CRRT is best for children who are hemodynamically unstable with renal and nonrenal reasons for treatment.
- CRRT in unstable children can be initiated safely using a protocol of doubling doses of inotropic and vasoconstrictor drugs and then gradually increasing blood flow through the circuit for 5 mins, followed by commencement of filtration.
- Anticoagulation is essential, and either systemic heparin (controlled by ACT) or a regional citrate/calcium technique is generally best.
- The type of CRRT varies by institutional preference and local expertise rather than by proven medical superiority.
- Protocols of care differ but are essential in making these treatments safe.

References

1. Amerling R, Glezerman I, Savransky E, et al. Continuous flow peritoneal dialysis: Principles and applications. *Semin Dial* 2003;16:335–40.
2. Andreoli SP. Acute renal failure in the newborn. *Semin Perinatol* 2004;28(2):112–23.
3. Baldwin I, Bellomo R, Koch B. Blood flow reductions during continuous renal replacement therapy and circuit life. *Intensive Care Med* 2004;30(11):2074–9.
4. Bellomo R. Continuous hemofiltration as blood purification in sepsis. *New Horiz* 1995;3:732–7.
5. Bock KR. Renal replacement therapy in pediatric critical care medicine. *Curr Opin Ped* 2005;17:368–74.
6. Bouts AH, Davin JC, Groothoff JW, et al. Standard peritoneal permeability analysis in children. *J Am Soc Nephrol* 2000;11:943–50.
7. Bradley-Stevenson C, Harish V. Intra-abdominal hypertension and the abdominal compartment syndrome. *Curr Paediatrics* 2004;14:191–6.
8. Brophy PD, Somers MJ, Baum MA, et al. Multi-centre evaluation of anticoagulation in patients receiving continuous renal replacement therapy (CRRT). *Nephrol Dial Transplant* 2005;20(7):1416–21.
9. Bunchman TE, McBryde KD, Mottes TE, et al. Pediatric acute renal failure: Outcome by modality and disease. *Ped Nephrol* 2001;16:1067–71.
10. Butt, W. Septic Shock. *Pediatr Clin North Am* 2001;48(3):601.
11. Cole L, Bellomo R, Hart G, et al. A phase II randomized, controlled trial of continuous hemofiltration in sepsis. *Crit Care Med* 2002;30:100–6.
12. Davenport A. Anticoagulation options for pediatric hemodialysis. *Minerva Urol Nefrol* 2006;58(2):171–80).
13. Davis PJ, Koottayi S, Taylor A, Butt W. Comparison of indirect methods of measuring intra-abdominal pressure in children. *Intensive Care Med* 2005;31:471–5.
14. Esperanca M, Collins D. Peritoneal dialysis efficiency in relation to body weight. *J Pediatr Surgery* 1996;1:162–9.
15. Foland JA, Fortenberry JD, Warshaw BL, et al. Fluid overload before continuous hemofiltration and survival in critically ill children: A retrospective analysis. *Crit Care Med* 2004;32:1771–6.
16. Forni LG and Hilton PJ. Current Concepts: Continuous hemofiltration in the treatment of acute renal failure. *New Engl J Med* 1997;336:1303–9.
17. Goldstein SL, Currier H, Graf C, et al. Outcome in children receiving continuous venovenous hemofiltration. *Pediatrics* 2001;107:1309–12.
18. Goldstein SL, Somers MJ, Baum MA, et al. Pediatric patients with multiorgan dysfunction syndrome receiving continuous renal replacement therapy. *Kidney Int* 2005;67:653–8.
19. Gong WK, Tan TH, Foong PP, et al. Eighteen years experience in pediatric acute dialysis: Analysis of predictors of outcome. *Pediatr Nephrol* 2001;16:212–5.
20. Heering P, Grabensee B, Brause M. Cytokine removal in septic patients with continuous venovenous hemofiltration. *Kidney Blood Press Res* 2003;26(2):128–34.
21. Jeffrey RF, Khan AA, Prabhu P, et al. A comparison of molecular clearance rates during continuous hemofiltration and hemodialysis with a novel

volumetric continuous renal replacement system. *J Artif Organs* 1994;18(6): 425–8.

22. Journois D, Israel-Biet D, Pouard P, et al. High volume, zero-balanced hemofiltration to reduce delayed inflammatory response to cardiopulmonary bypass in children. *Anesthesiology* 1996;85(5):957–60.
23. Jouvet P, Jugie M, Rabier D, et al. Combined nutritional support and continuous extracorporeal removal therapy in severe acute phase of maple syrup urine disease. *Intensive Care Med* 2001;27:1798–1806.
24. Jouvet P, Litalien C, Phan V, et al. Epuration extra-renale chez l'enfant. In: Bastien O, Honnore P, Robert R, eds. *Circulations extra-corporelles en reanimation.* Paris: Elsevier, 2006;193–210.
25. Jouvet P, Poggi F, Rabier JL, et al. Continuous venovenous hemodiafiltration in the acute phase of neonatal maple syrup urine disease. *J Inherit Metab Dis* 1997;20:463–72.
26. Keeley S, Butt W. Continuous filtration techniques in children: A description. Pediatric Critical Care Colloquium, Santa Monica, California, Oct 1989.
27. Kellum JA, Angus DC, Johnson JP, et al. Continuous versus intermittent renal replacement therapy: A meta-analysis. *Intensive Care Med* 2002;28:29–37.
28. Kellum JA, Cellomo R, Mehta R, et al. Blood purification in non-renal critical illness. *Blood Purif* 2003;21:6–13.
29. Kohaut EC. The effect of dialysate volume on ultrafiltration in young patients treated with CAPD. *Int J Pediatr Nephrol* 1986;7(4):13–19.
30. Kreuzer M, Vester U, Homing A, et al. Regional anticoagulation with sodium citrate in pediatric patients on intermittent hemodialysis therapy with bleeding risks. *Hemodial Int* 2004;8(1):108.
31. Litalien C, Merouani A, Phan et al. Thérapies Vasculaires D'épuration Extrarénale. In J Lacroix J, Gauthier M, Leclerc F, Hubert P, eds. *Urgences et soins intensifs pédiatriques.* 2nd ed. Montreal and Paris: Éditions de l'Hôpital Sainte-Justine and Elsevier-Masson, 2007.
32. Lowrie LH. Renal replacement therapies in pediatric multiorgan dysfunction syndrome. *Pediatr Nephrol* 2000;14:6–12.
33. Luciani GB, Menon T, Vecchi B, et al. Modified ultrafiltration reduces morbidity after adult cardiac operations: A prospective, randomized clinical trial. *Circulation* 2001;104(Suppl 1):1253–9.
34. Marshall MR, Ma T, Galler D, et al. Sustained low-efficiency daily diafiltration (SLEDD-f) for critically ill patients requiring renal replacement therapy: Towards an adequate therapy. *Nephrol Dial Transplant* 2004;19:877–94.
35. Maxvold NJ, Smoyer WE, Gardner JJ, et al. Management of acute renal failure in the pediatric patient: Hemofiltration versus hemodialysis. *Am J Kidney Dis* 1997;30:S84–8.
36. McBryde KD, Kudelka TL, Kershaw DB, et al. Clearance of amino acids by hemodialysis in arginosuccinate synthetase deficiency. *J Pediatr* 2004;144(4):536–40.
37. Meyer RJ, Brophy PD, Bunchman TE, et al. Survival and renal function in pediatric patients following extracorporeal life support with hemofiltration. *Pediatr Crit Care Med* 2001;2:238.
38. Morgenstern BZ. Equilibration testing: Close, but note quite right. *Pediatr Nephrol* 1993;7:290–1.
39. Morris, KP, Butt, W, Karl, TR. Effect of peritoneal dialysis on intra-abdominal pressure and cardio-respiratory function in infants following cardiac surgery. *Cardiol Young* 2004;14(3):293–8.
40. Parakininkas D, Greenbaum LA. Comparison of solute clearance in three modes of continuous renal replacement therapy. *Pediatr Crit Care Med* 2004;5(3):269–74.
41. Peritoneal dialysis associated peritonitis in children. *Nephrology* 2004;9: S45–51.
42. Puliyanda DP, Harmon WE, Peterschmitt MJ, et al. Utility of hemodialysis in maple syrup urine disease. *Pediatr Nephrol* 2002;17:239–42.
43. Quan A, Quigley R. Renal replacement therapy and acute renal failure. *Curr Opin Pediatr* 2005;17:205–9.

44. Rajpoot DK, Gargus JJ. Acute hemodialysis for hyperammonemia in small neonates. *Pediatr Nephrol* 2004;19(4):390–5.
45. Ratanarat R, Brendolan A, Ricci Z, et al. Pulse high-volume hemofiltration in critically ill patients: A new approach for patients with septic shock. *Semin Dial* 2006;19(1):69–74.
46. Reeves JH, Butt W. Blood filtration in children with severe sepsis: Safe adjunctive therapy. *Intensive Care Med* 1995;21(6):500–4.
47. Reeves JH, Butt WA. Comparison of solute clearance during continuous hemofiltration, hemodiafiltration, and hemodialysis using a polysulfone hemofilter. *ASAIO J* 1995;40(1):100–4.
48. Reeves JH, Butt W, Sathe AS. A review of venovenous haemofiltration in seriously ill infants. *J Paediatr Child Health* 1994;30(1):50–4.
49. Ronco C, Bellomo R, Homel P, et al. Effects of different doses in continuous veno-venous haemofiltration on outcomes of acute renal failure: A prospective randomised trail. *Lancet* 2000;356(9223):26–30.
50. Ronco C, Brendolan A, Bragantini L, et al. Treatment of acute renal failure in newborns by continuous arterio-venous hemofiltration. *Kidney International* 1986;29(4):908–15.
51. Ronco C, Ricci Z, Bellomo R. Importance of increased ultrafiltration volume and impact on mortality: Sepsis and cytokine story and the role of continuous veno-venous haemofiltration. *Nephrol Hypertens* 2001;10(6): 755–61.
52. Ronco C, Tetta C, Mariano F, et al. Interpreting the mechanisms of continuous renal replacement therapy in sepsis: The peak concentration hypothesis. *Artif Organs* 2003;27(9):792–801.
53. Sam R, Vaseemuddin M, Leong WH, et al. Composition and clinical use of hemodialysis. *Hemodial Int* 2006;10:15–28.
54. Smoyer WE, McAdams C, Kaplan BS, et al. Determinants of survival in pediatric continuous hemofiltration. *J Am Soc Nephrol* 1995;6:1401–9.
55. Stickle S, Brewer ED, Goldstein SL. Pediatric (PED) acute renal failure (ARF) update: Epidemiology and outcome from a three and one-half year experience (Abstract). *J Am Soc Nephrol* 2002;13:649.
56. Strazdins V, Watson AR, Harvey B. Renal replacement therapy for acute renal failure in children: European guidelines. *Pediatr Nephrol* 2004;19: 199–207.
57. Symons JM, Brophy PD, Gregory MJ, et al. Continuous renal replacement therapy in children up to 10 kg. *Am J Kidney Dis* 2003;41:984–9.
58. Thompson GN, Butt W, Shann FA, et al. Continuous venovenous hemofiltration in the management of acute decompensation in inborn errors of metabolism. *J Pediatr* 1991;118:879–84.
59. Tonelli M, Manns B, Feller-Kopman D. Acute renal failure in the intensive care unit: A systemative review of the impact of dialytic modality, mortality, and renal recovery. *Am J Kidney Dis* 2002;40:875–85.
60. Uchino S, Fealy N, Baldwin I, et al. Continuous venovenous hemofiltration without anticoagulation. *ASAIO J* 2004;50(1):76–80.
61. Uchino S, Fealy N, Morimatsu H, et al. Pre-dilution vs. post-dilution during continuous veno-venous hemofiltration: Impact on filter life and azotemic control. *Nephron* 2003;94(4):c94–8.
62. Veltri MA, Neu AM, Fivush BA, et al. Drug dosing during intermittent hemodialysis and continuous renal replacement therapy: Special considerations in pediatric patients. *Pediatr Drugs* 2004;1:45–65.
63. Venkataraman R, Subramanian S, Kellum J. Clinical review: Extracorporeal blood purification in severe sepsis. *Critical Care* 2003;7:139–45.
64. Warady BA, Bunchman T. Dialysis therapy for children with acute renal failure: Survey results. *Pediatr Nephrol* 2000;11–13.
65. Werner HS, Wensley DF, Lirenman DS, et al. Peritoneal dialysis in children after cardiopulmonary bypass. *J Thorac Cardiovasc Surg* 1997;113(1): 64–8.
66. Williams DM, Sreedhar SS, Mickell JJ, et al. Acute kidney failure: A pediatric experience over 20 years. *Arch Pediatr Adolesc Med* 2002;156:893–900.

CHAPTER 38 ■ BLOOD PRODUCTS IN THE PICU

JACQUES LACROIX • NAOMI L.C. LUBAN • EDWARD C.C. WONG

The ICU is a major consumer of blood and blood products; it is estimated that ~8% of blood at a regional center is used in the ICU (55). The rationale for the use of labile blood products—red blood cells (RBCs), plasma, platelets, and granulocyte concentrates—in the PICU is reviewed in this chapter.

RED BLOOD CELL TRANSFUSION

Transfusion of packed RBCs or whole blood is a common supportive measure in the PICU; up to 50% of critically ill children receive an RBC transfusion during their stay (38). RBCs contain hemoglobin (Hb), which transports vital O_2 to cells to enable them to survive. Thus, at first glance, it would seem sensible to maintain the Hb concentration and hematocrit of critically ill patients within an age-appropriate normal range. However, the concept of "permissive anemia" has become more popular because the safety of RBC transfusion has been questioned, at least in part due to the increased awareness among the general public regarding the risk of contracting viral diseases, especially human immunodeficiency virus (HIV) and hepatitis. Less well recognized is the fact that transfusion of RBCs can modulate the inflammatory process, which may increase the risk or extent of multiple organ dysfunction syndrome (MODS). Thus, an important yet unanswered question is: What are the risk-benefit and cost-benefit ratios of RBC transfusion in critically ill children?

In this section, O_2 delivery (Do_2) and other issues in the critically ill child will be discussed, evidence on the effectiveness and usefulness of RBC transfusion in the intensive care setting will be reviewed, and the published recommendations for RBC transfusions to critically ill infants and children will be examined.

Scientific Foundation of Red Blood Cell Transfusion

Oxygen Transport in Critically Ill Children

Adaptation to Anemia. Tissue hypoxia from low Do_2 may be due to a low Hb concentration (anemic hypoxia), cardiac output (stagnant hypoxia), or Hb saturation (hypoxic hypoxia). Anemia is defined as Hb concentrations below the "normal" range for age and occurs in ~40% of critically ill children treated in typical North American PICUs (10). Causes include repetitive phlebotomy losses, hemorrhage, intraoperative blood loss, chronic anemia (frequent in patients with cancer), and congenital anemia (e.g., sickle cell disease and thalassemia).

The major physiologic consequence of anemia is a reduction in the Do_2 capacity of blood. O_2 consumption (Vo_2) depends on substrate availability and on metabolic demands. When the metabolic rate of a critically ill patient is increased, more nutrients and O_2 are needed to meet his energy requirements, and a higher Do_2 may be required. Under a "critical threshold," Vo_2 diminishes if Do_2 decreases. Over this threshold, a fall in Do_2 does not cause a drop in Vo_2 because an increase in cellular O_2 extraction or in cardiac output can compensate for the Vo_2. These mechanisms are limited; therefore, a critical threshold of Do_2 exists under which Do_2 and Vo_2 fall simultaneously (Vo_2/Do_2 dependency).

In critically ill patients, two phenomena may be present. First, the stress encountered by patients due to their disease frequently increases Vo_2; this can upregulate the Do_2/Vo_2 curve. Second, the critical threshold may be increased, which may explain why pathologic O_2 supply dependence is reported in selected patients, especially those with severe sepsis and septic shock. When the metabolic rate of a critically ill patient is increased, more nutrients and O_2 are necessary to meet energy requirements, and a higher Do_2 may be required.

The formula used to calculate Do_2 is:

$$Cardiac\ Output \times Pao_2$$

The formula for Cao_2 (arterial O_2 content) is:

$$(Sao_2 \times Hb \times 1.34) + (0.003 \times Pao_2)$$

where:

Hb concentration is expressed in grams per deciliter
Cao_2 is expressed in millimeters of mercury (mm Hg).

Thus, anemia can significantly decrease O_2 carrying capacity. However, in the normal host, the amount of O_2 delivered to the tissue exceeds resting O_2 requirements by two- to fourfold. When the Hb concentration falls below 10 g/dL, several adaptive processes ensure a physiologic reserve to maintain Do_2. Theses processes include increased extraction of available O_2, increased heart rate and stroke volume (i.e., cardiac output), redistribution of blood flow from nonvital organs toward the heart and brain at the expense of the splanchnic vascular bed, and a shift to the left in the oxyhemoglobin-dissociation curve (i.e., a decrease in O_2 affinity).

Impairment in Adaptive Mechanisms. A number of diseases and host characteristics may impair the adaptive mechanisms to anemia in critically ill patients. The metabolic rate is increased in systemic inflammatory response syndrome (SIRS), sepsis, and MODS; consequently, a limited reserve is available if the patient has additional metabolic stresses. Patients with sepsis and MODS may also have impaired left ventricular function and poor regulation of vascular tone, restricting Do_2 and redistribution of blood flow, respectively.

A number of host characteristics specific to children and infants may impair their adaptive mechanisms. The energy requirements of young infants are much higher than those in adults. This difference is mostly attributable to growth, and it means that they need more substrates, including O_2 and nutrients. For instance, the basic nutritional requirement given by the enteral route is 110–140 CAL/kg/day (460–590 kJ/kg/day) for a child <1 year of age, while it is 50 CAL/kg/day (210 kJ/kg/day) for an adult. In addition to increased metabolic demands, major differences in O_2 transport also exist between adults and children in the first year of life. Fetal Hb has a left-shifted O_2 equilibrium curve, and the proportion of fetal Hb is significant during the first months of life. Physiologic anemia is expected during this period, partially explaining why the Hb concentration varies so much in the newborn and the infant. During the first weeks of life, myocardial compliance is decreased, significantly impairing diastolic filling, which limits increases in stroke volume. Moreover, the heart rate is already high, even at rest, in newborns (~140 ± 20/min) and infants (~130 ± 20/min), which also limits the ability to increase cardiac output. Heart failure, which directly impairs Do_2, is in many instances a direct consequence of congenital cardiac defects or surgical repair, a frequent occurrence in the PICU. Children with cyanotic congenital heart disease have Hb concentrations as high as 20 g/dL, which is a rare occurrence in adults. Moreover, the health status of children prior to entry to the PICU is usually better than that of adults, which might explain lower mortality rates in children as compared to adults (4%–5% versus >20%). Therefore, many characteristics specific to critically ill children alter their ability to physiologically adapt to low Hb concentrations.

Oxygen Kinetics. In healthy patients, Do_2 exceeds resting O_2 requirements, but despite significant reserves, safety margins may rapidly disappear during critical illness. Some investigators have shown that patients with sepsis do indeed have some Do_2/Vo_2 dependence, which has led some to hypothesize that disease processes, such as sepsis, induce tissue hypoxia by producing an abnormally elevated anaerobic threshold. The resultant tissue hypoxia eventually contributes to the evolution of irreversible and often fatal MODS.

Interventions that affect blood flow include mechanical ventilation, inotropic agents, vasodilators, and fluid loading; they have been employed to investigate and potentially treat pathologic supply dependence. Because Hb is the principal O_2 carrier in blood, a transfusion threshold of at least 10 g/dL in critically ill patients has often been advocated; nevertheless, few studies have examined the role of Hb and RBC transfusions as a means of alleviating supply dependence. In short, it seems that pathologic supply dependence exists in some critically ill patients. However, it remains uncertain if RBC transfusion is the most useful method to achieve the "optimal Do_2."

Microcirculatory Effects of Native and Transfused Red Blood Cells

The effect of transfused RBCs on systemic Do_2 has been the subject of many studies. A number of studies also describe the effect of transfused RBCs on the distribution of systemic blood flow to specific organs. For example, RBC transfusion may cause gut ischemia among septic adults, even if it increases Do_2 (10). However, it remains unclear how transfused RBCs influence Do_2 in the microcirculation due to the difficulty in obtaining in situ measurements of blood viscosity, microcirculatory flow, and Vo_2.

In theory, too low or too high viscosity is associated with a risk of decreasing blood flow through small vessels. Capillaries collapse if the hematocrit is too low, and RBC transfusion may be viewed "as a means of restoring blood viscosity" (52). On the other hand, capillary resistance to blood flow increases rapidly if the hematocrit level increases over 0.45, which may result in microcirculatory stasis and impaired Do_2 to the tissues. Other authors have suggested that hematocrit has limited effects on microcirculatory flow. The microcirculatory effects of transfused RBCs may also be related to the generation of inflammatory mediators: Some cytokines may mediate vasoconstriction or thrombosis of small vessels, causing local ischemia.

Transfused RBCs may also possess properties that differ from their in vivo counterparts. Several age-related changes occur during storage of RBC. Characteristically, older RBC units have lower levels of 2,3-DPG, which alters Hb's affinity for O_2. Low levels of 2,3-DPG produce a left shift in the oxyhemoglobin-dissociation curve that may impede O_2 availability to the tissues, even if the Do_2 is increased. In addition, storage decreases RBC membrane deformability through alterations in cell membrane characteristics, which may influence end-capillary oxygen diffusion. Hemolysis does occur in packed RBC units over time; the amount of free Hb may increase from 0.5 mg/dL in a 1-day-old RBC unit to 250 mg/dL in a 25-day-old unit (40). Intravascular free Hb may cause vasoconstriction, probably by binding nitric oxide (NO). In summary, RBC transfusions increase global Do_2 but may decrease microcirculatory flow and O_2 availability in some tissues.

Immunologic Effects of Allogenic Red Blood Cell Transfusions

Transfused RBCs may adversely affect the immunologic responses. Limited evidence suggests that transfused RBCs may result in clinically important immune suppression in the recipient. For example, transfusions of packed RBCs decrease the number of rejection episodes and improve renal and cardiac allograft survival, which may be related to the alterations in lymphocyte reactivity observed after blood transfusions.

Evidence also suggests that transfused RBCs may have inflammatory effects. Many proinflammatory molecules are detected in RBC units, including cytokines, complement activators, O_2 free radicals, histamine, lysophosphatidylcholine species, and other bioreactive substances that may initiate, maintain, or enhance an inflammatory process. The white blood cells (WBC) and the cytokines in unfiltered packed RBCs may trigger or maintain a SIRS in the RBC recipients. Giving an RBC transfusion to a critically ill patient with SIRS may stimulate their inflammatory syndrome, which may result in the development of MODS (second-hit theory of MODS). Not surprisingly, some data suggest that transfused critically ill patients are more vulnerable than other patients to contract nosocomial infections and MODS, which may ultimately result in higher mortality rates (26). Some data suggest that the inflammatory risks of RBC transfusion decrease significantly if the packed RBC units are prestorage-leukocyte depleted. The clinical effects of RBC transfusion on the immunologic responses of critically ill children remain to be determined. In summary, some evidence suggests that transfusion may cause immunosuppression, thereby increasing the risk of acquiring nosocomial infections. RBC transfusion can also reinforce SIRS, which can progress to MODS.

Complications of Red Blood Cell Transfusion

Even though blood products are safer than in the past, RBC transfusion can cause many adverse events (**Tables 38.1, 38.2, and 38.3**), which can be classified as early adverse reactions and delayed complications.

Early Reactions to Red Blood Cell Transfusion

Acute Reactions to Red Blood Cell Units. Any unexpected or unexplained change in the clinical condition of a patient during a transfusion or in the 24 hrs following an RBC transfusion should be considered (and evaluated) as an acute transfusion reaction and should be reported to the blood bank and/or the transfusion service.

The most serious noninfectious complications of blood product transfusions are listed in **Table 38.1**; some are defined in **Table 38.2**. Specific comments may be useful for some of these complications.

By definition, transfusion-related acute lung injury (TRALI) is pulmonary edema occurring during or within 6 hrs after the end of a transfusion. The European Haemovigilance Network has identified the diagnostic criteria of this condition as (a) acute onset of respiratory distress during or within 6 hrs after the end of a transfusion, (b) no sign of circulatory overload, and (c) radiographic evidence of bilateral pulmonary infiltrates. A Canadian Consensus Conference held in 2004 added two criteria: (a) evidence of acute lung injury as defined by intensivists, (b) no preexisting acute lung injury or presence of risk factors for same (37). The latter criterion is a problem in critically ill recipients of blood products because TRALI, a transfusion-associated circulatory overload, and an acute lung injury may coexist in the same patient. TRALI can be life-threatening, but mortality is low (5%–10%) (41). Most episodes of TRALI resolve within 48 hrs, which contrasts with cases of acute lung injury that are not transfusion related. The pathophysiology of TRALI is still a matter of debate, but passive infusion of human leukocyte antigens (HLA), antileukocyte antibodies, and/or blood storage-related biologically active lipids from the donor may be involved (37). Antileukocyte antibodies are found in some cases (8).

Acute hemolysis is another important acute reaction. Non-immunologic hemolysis can be caused by mechanical trauma to RBCs, excessive warming, or a bacterial contamination. Some cases of hemolysis are related to acute or delayed immunologic reaction that is caused by Rh or ABO incompatibility, or they are related to antibodies to other erythrocyte antigens (Kidd, Kell, etc.).

More than 25% of deaths attributable to RBC transfusion are caused by blood-group incompatibility. The most significant risk of death from blood transfusion is from ABO mismatch, resulting in hemolysis (1/60,000) and death (1/600,000). In most instances, mismatch occurs when a patient receives blood prepared for another patient. Such errors

TABLE 38.1

INCIDENCE OF BLOOD PRODUCT TRANSFUSION-RELATED ADVERSE EVENTS

Serious adverse events	
Respiratory system	
Transfusion-related acute lung injury	1:20,000–1:5000 (5%–10% fatal)
Cardiovascular system	
Fluid overload	1:700–1:15,000
Hypotension[a]	1/102,000
Hematologic system	
ABO-incompatible transfusion	1:38,000
Death due to ABO-incompatible transfusion	1:1.8 million
Acute hemolytic transfusion reaction	1:12,000
Delayed hemolytic transfusion reaction	1:4000–1:12,000
Posttransfusion purpura	1:143,000–1:294,000
Mistransfusion	1:14,000–1:19,000
Other	
Anaphylaxis	1:1600 (platelets)
	1:23,000 (red blood cells)
Graft-versus-host disease	1:1 million (Canada)
Less Serious Adverse Events	
Febrile nonhemolytic transfusion reaction	1:500
Allergic (urticaria)	1:250

[a]Hypotension can be caused by allergic or hemolytic reactions, septicemia, citrate toxicity, reaction to leukocyte reduction filters, etc. Such reactions have been reported with packed RBC units, plasma, platelets, and albumin (18).

TABLE 38.2

DEFINITION OF SOME TRANSFUSION-RELATED ADVERSE EVENTS

Febrile nonhemolytic transfusion reaction. A rise in temperature ≥1°C that cannot be explained by the patient's clinical condition (i.e., other causes of fever must be excluded). A febrile nonhemolytic transfusion reaction may be accompanied by dyspnea and/or anxiety. Some of the following symptoms can also be present: rigors, dyspnea, tachycardia, or headache.
Hemolytic transfusion reaction (manifestations may range from mild to fatal). Hemoglobinuria or hemoglobinemia (measured as plasma free hemoglobin above the normal range) with at least one of the following symptoms/signs: fever, dyspnea, hypotension and/or tachycardia, anxiety/agitation, pain.
Major allergic and anaphylactic reaction (may be fatal). At least one of the following symptoms/signs must be present: cardiac arrest; generalized allergic reaction or anaphylactic reaction; angio-edema (facial and/or laryngeal); upper airway obstruction; dyspnea, wheezing; hypotension, shock; precordial pain or chest tightness; cardiac arrhythmia; loss of consciousness.
Circulatory overload (transfusion-related cardiac overload, TACO). Fluid overload with at least one of the following criteria: dyspnea or cyanosis; pulmonary edema de novo, tachycardia de novo, or hypertension.
Coagulopathy. At least one of the following criteria: INR >2.0; aPTT >60 secs; positive assay for fibrin-split products; D-dimers >0.5 mg/mL.

INR, international normalized ratio; aPTT, activated partial thromboplastin time.

occur more often in an emergency setting and can be avoided with careful identification of patient and donor unit.

Some acute transfusion reactions are related to the speed of administration of the unit and to the volume administered. Citrate anticoagulant can cause acidemia; however, if the liver is able to metabolize the citrate, a metabolic alkalosis develops. Citrate toxicity results if the capacity of the liver to metabolize citrate is overwhelmed, which occurs when >3 mL/kg/min of packed RBC or >1 mL/kg/min of whole blood or plasma are administered; severe hypocalcemia can ensue.

The risk of hyperkalemia is significant, especially if a transfusion is given rapidly. All RBC units contain potassium, which increases during refrigerated storage: Potassium levels of 5 mmol/L after 1 day of storage, 22 mmol/L after 15 days, and >35 mmol/L after 25 days have been reported (40). Red cells stored in additive solutions have less potassium than those stored in citrate-monobasic sodium phosphate-dextrose (CPD) or CPD-adenine (CPDA-1). Irradiation further increases the concentration of potassium in the unit. To avoid hyperkalemia, transfusing at a rate of <0.3 mL/kg/min of RBCs is advised.

TABLE 38.3

ESTIMATED RISK OF INFECTIONS FROM BLOOD PRODUCTS TRANSFUSION[a]

Infectious agent	United States	Other countries
HIV (with NAT)	1:2.1 million (repeat donors) 1:1 million (first-time donors)	1:4.7 million (Canada)[a]
HCV (with NAT) 1000	1:1.9 million (repeat donors) 1:791,000 (first-time donors)	1:2.8 million (Canada)[a]
HTLV	1:641,000	1:1.9 million (Canada)
Hepatitis B virus	1:30,000–250,000	1:82,000 (Canada)[a] 1:470,000 (France)
Hepatitis A virus	1:10 million	
Malaria	1:4 million	
Chagas disease	Extremely low	
Cytomegalovirus[b]	Unknown	
West Nile virus	Unknown	
Bacterial contamination		
Platelets[c]	1:1000–1:3000	1:14,000–1:38,000 (France)
Platelet fatality[c]	1:140,000	1:172,000 (France)
RBCs	1:500,000	1:66,000 (New Zealand)
RBC fatality	1:8 million	1:1 million (France)

[a]Based on residual risk calculations published by Canadian Blood Bank Services and Héma-Québec (27).
[b]The risk to contract CMV from manufactured plasma derived products is theoretical if blood product is heat inactivated.
[c]Without pretransfusion culture of component.
HIV, human immunodeficiency virus; NAT, nucleic acid test; HCV, hepatitis C virus; HTLV, human T-lymphocyte viruses; RBC, red blood cell

Acute Reactions to Massive Transfusion. Massive transfusion is defined as the administration of >1 blood volume within a 24-hr period. Serious acute complications of massive transfusion include fluid overload, coagulopathy, thrombocytopenia, acidosis, hyperkalemia, and hypocalcemia.

The coagulopathy and thrombocytopenia observed after massive transfusion are attributed to hemodilution, hypothermia, administration of blood products with a prolonged duration of storage, and disseminated intravascular coagulation. Transfusion-related coagulopathy can be diagnosed if at least one of the following criteria is observed during or shortly after a massive transfusion: international normalized ratio (INR) of >2.0, activated partial thromboplastin time of >60 secs, positive assay for fibrin-split products, or D-dimers of >0.5 mg/mL (41).

Delayed Complications to Red Blood Cell Transfusion

Delayed complications to RBC transfusion may occur weeks or even years after the transfusion. Most are infectious. The most frequent or the most important infections attributable to blood and blood product transfusions are listed in **Table 38.3**. Although transfusion-transmitted hepatitis C virus and HIV have become exceedingly rare, the risk of transfusion-transmitted infectious diseases, including hepatitis B, parvovirus B19, bacterial contamination, cytomegalovirus (CMV), and viruses for which testing is not currently performed (e.g., transfusion-transmitted virus, human herpes virus-8, hepatitis G virus) continue to be major concerns. Transmission of insect-borne zoonoses (malaria, Babesia, *Bartonella quintana*) is now well recognized (27). Three cases of variant Creutzfeldt-Jakob disease transmitted by transfusion have been reported (62).

Erythrocyte alloimmunization, a particular concern in chronically transfused patients and young women, occurs in 8% of recipients (13), with higher rates in patients with sickle cell disease and thalassemia. The incidence rate of late hemolysis (delayed hemolytic transfusion reaction) is 1/255,000 (27) and is likely due to low titer alloimmunization. Delayed hemolytic transfusion reaction is also more common in patients with sickle cell disease.

Posttransfusion purpura is rare but severe. Occurring 5–10 days after transfusion in patients sensitized by prior transfusion or pregnancy, posttransfusion purpura results in platelet counts often below 10×10^9/L. The pathogenesis is unclear and is presumably related to the development of platelet-specific antibody following transfusion.

Graft-versus-host disease (GVHD) is another rare but significant adverse event. Posttransfusion GVHD (PT-GVHD) occurs 10–28 days following transfusion. The risk of PT-GVHD is significantly higher in patients with congenital or acquired immunodeficiency. PT-GVHD also occurs in immunosufficient patients who receive nonirradiated RBC units from an HLA-related identical family member or community donor. DiGeorge syndrome is not uncommon among children who require corrective cardiovascular surgery; such patients should receive irradiated units to prevent PT-GVHD. Oncology patients and those undergoing hematopoietic stem cell or solid-organ transplantation and who are on immunosuppressive therapy are also at risk and should receive irradiated blood.

Transfusion of Red Blood Cells: Application to the PICU

Practice Pattern

The most frequent justification for prescribing an RBC transfusion is a low Hb concentration. However, two surveys based on questionnaires and three observational studies demonstrated large variability in practice pattern with respect to an "acceptable" threshold Hb concentration.

In a survey of pediatric critical care practitioners designed to investigate RBC transfusion practices and clinical determinants that might alter transfusion thresholds in critically ill children, investigators reported a threshold Hb range from <7 g/dL to >13 g/dL (32). A survey of European pediatric intensivists reported similar results (39).

Two bedside observational cohort studies were undertaken to characterize the actual practice pattern of pediatric intensivists with respect to RBC transfusions (2,16) and confirmed variability among PICUs in different countries, ranging from 7 g/dL to 11 g/dL for patients with similar diagnoses. In a third study completed in 2005 by the PALISI Network, the average Hb concentration before RBC transfusion given in 30 North American PICUs was >9 g/dL in children <5 years of age (range: 4.7–17.8 g/dL).

A retrospective study of 240 critically ill children with an Hb concentration of ≤9 g/dL from five PICUs in the US showed that pediatric intensivists transfused all patients with an Hb concentration of ≤5.3 g/dL and 38 out of 41 with a concentration of ≤6.4 g/dL, while only 33 of the 105 patients with an Hb concentration of ≥8 g/dL were transfused. More variation in practice patterns was observed if the Hb concentration was above this value (20).

A lack of outcome data probably explains the striking variation in stated and observed practice patterns among pediatric critical care practitioners.

Current Evidence

Evidence That Anemia May Be Detrimental. Some data suggest that severe anemia may increase the risk of mortality in critically ill mammals and human beings. In healthy animals undergoing acute hemodilution, evidence of heart dysfunction appears once the Hb concentration drops below 3.3–4 g/dL. However, animals with 50%–80% coronary artery stenosis can show evidence of ischemic insult to the heart with an Hb concentration as high as 7–10 g/dL (46).

Two studies undertaken in patients who refused blood products for religious reasons suggest that very low Hb levels may increase mortality (4,5). These studies reported the incidence of death after bloodless surgery; the risk of death increased steadily once the postoperative Hb concentration dropped below 4 g/dL in healthy patients (5). A higher mortality risk was involved if heart disease was present, and the odds of mortality increased when Hb concentration dropped below 10 g/dL (4).

Few studies assess the relationship between anemia and mortality in acutely ill children. One group followed 2433 anemic African children <12 years of age who were hospitalized; 20% received an RBC transfusion (29). Mortality was lower in children who received a transfusion if the Hb level was below 4.7 g/dL and they presented with some respiratory distress. In 1997, the same group of investigators reported an improved survival in hospitalized Kenyan children who received transfusion, with Hb levels <5 g/dL associated with respiratory distress (30). Another prospective cohort study of 1269 Kenyan children hospitalized for malaria showed that RBC transfusion decreased mortality if anemia was severe (Hb level <4 g/dL) or if dyspnea was associated with an Hb level of <5 g/dL (11). These studies suggest that some benefit may be associated with keeping the Hb concentration of hospitalized children above 5 g/dL; this should also be true for critically ill children.

Evidence That Red Blood Cell Transfusion May Be Useful. In critically ill adults, Hb concentration under 10 g/dL can be well tolerated in high-risk surgical patients and in critically ill patients who are stabilized and volume resuscitated. No clinical studies that documented the safety of maintaining low Hb concentrations in critically ill patients existed until the landmark article by Hébert et al., which showed that in euvolemic critically ill patients, a conservative strategy (RBC transfusions with non-leukocyte depleted units given only if the Hb concentration dropped under 7 g/dL and maintained at 7–9 g/dL) was safer than a liberal strategy (RBC transfusions given if the Hb concentration dropped under 10 g/dL and maintained at 10–12 g/dL) (26). An adjusted multiple organ dysfunction score and the hospital mortality rate were statistically lower in the former group.

An extensive review of the published pediatric literature yielded three randomized clinical trials that evaluated RBC transfusion strategies in children. Two studies that were published more than 20 years ago did not involve critically ill children: Both evaluated the usefulness of hypertransfusion as a treatment of malignant disease. One international, randomized clinical trial evaluated RBC transfusion strategies in 116 African children hospitalized for malarial crises who had no congenital hemolytic anemia. In these patients with hematocrit levels that ranged from 0.12 to 0.17, RBC transfusion did not improve the mortality rate (1/53 vs. 2/53) in patients without respiratory or cardiovascular compromise, but the study was clearly underpowered (25).

Four case series are published on the effect of RBC transfusion on O_2 delivery and O_2 consumption in critically ill children: 2 involved children in septic shock (33,36), one involved the postoperative care of cardiac surgery (45), and the last evaluated children with cyanotic congenital cardiomyopathy undergoing elective catheterization (3). Hemodynamic parameters were compared before and after RBC transfusions. In each study, transfusing 10 mL/kg of packed RBCs significantly increased the Hb level and Do_2, but Vo_2 increased in only one study (33). These small studies do not support the hypothesis that RBC transfusion is useful in increasing Vo_2.

Red Blood Cell Transfusion: Current Guidelines

In most instances, RBC transfusions are given to critically ill children because their Hb concentrations are considered to be "too low." However, the decision to give an RBC transfusion should not be based solely on Hb concentration. According to a mailed survey, pediatric intensivists' decisions to transfuse were not based solely on Hb but also on many other determinants: low Sao_2, low Cao_2, or low cardiac output (poor Do_2); high blood lactate level, low central venous ($Scvo_2$) or mixed venous saturation of O_2 (Svo_2), poor Vo_2; high severity of illness, as measured, for example, by the pediatric risk of mortality (PRISM) score; active bleeding; emergency surgery (32). In spite

of this, pediatric intensivists stated that a low Hb concentration is a crucial part of their decision making in prescribing RBC transfusions to a nonbleeding patient.

An observational cohort study of 303 children consecutively admitted over 3 months to a university-affiliated PICU reported that 45 children (15%) received between one and 33 RBC transfusions, for a total of 103 transfusions. The justifications provided by the attending physicians for administering RBC transfusions included anemia (103/103, 100%), respiratory failure (84%), active bleeding (67%), hemodynamic instability (50%), blood lactate level of >2 mmol/L (10%), or suboptimal Do_2 (6%). In many cases, more than one reason was specified, but in 7 cases, no specific reason was given (16).

In a prospective cohort study of 985 consecutive PICU admissions at Sainte-Justine Hospital, the most significant determinants of an initial RBC transfusion were the presence of anemia (defined by an Hb level of <9.5 g/dL) during PICU stay [odds ratio (OR), 13.26; 95% confidence interval (CI), 8.04–21.88; p <0.001], an admission diagnosis of cardiac disease (OR, 8.07; 95% CI, 5.14–14.65; p <0.001), an admission PRISM score of >10 (OR, 4.83; 95% CI, 2.33–10.04; p <0.001), and the presence of MODS during PICU stay (OR, 2.06; 95% CI, 1.18–3.57; p = 0.01) (2).

In a prospective cohort study of 548 children undergoing cardiac surgery, determinants of perioperative transfusion of blood products—not only RBC—included younger age, higher preoperative hematocrit, complex surgery, low platelet count, and longer duration of hypothermia (58).

Cumulatively, these studies show that many host-related and disease-related characteristics, as well as the Hb concentration, account for the practice patterns of PICUs with respect to RBC transfusion. In practice, most pediatric intensivists think that a higher Hb concentration may be required for more severe illness. However, this does not imply that predictive scores, such as PRISM III or Pediatric Index of Mortality 2, or descriptive scores, such as the Pediatric Logistic Organ Dysfunction score, can be used to make decisions about RBC transfusion in a given patient. These scores were created and validated to assess groups of children, and it would be inappropriate to include them in a decision process for individual patients. Instinctively, RBC transfusions will increase Do_2 in more critically ill patients. The problem is that what constitutes severe anemia, how one defines severity of illness, and what Hb concentration directs transfusion therapy are unknown. Further, the severity of illness and specific disease confounds any global recommendations to direct either when a transfusion is indicated or the posttransfusion Hb concentration.

While RBC transfusion does not increase Sao_2 or Cao_2, it does increase the Hb concentration, which should improve arterial O_2 content. For example, doubling the Hb concentration from 6 g/dL to 12 g/dL will double the Cao_2. Thus, the efficacy of RBC transfusion to improve Do_2 is clear, but its usefulness is questionable.

In 1941, 2 anesthesiologists, Drs. Adams and Lundy, wrote: "When concentration of Hb is <8–10 g per 100 cubic centimeters of whole blood, it is wise to give a blood transfusion before operation." Thereafter, the "10/30" rule (Hb of 10 g/dL or hematocrit of 30%) was standard practice for more than 50 years. Concerns over the past 15 years regarding transfusion-related complications have prompted a critical review of transfusion practices. In 1995, the Blood Management Practice Guidelines Conference (50) recommended a threshold of 7 g/dL if no cardiopulmonary disease is present; it also recommended a transfusion threshold of 10 g/dL in the perioperative period. The guidelines emphasized that the decision to administer RBC should be based on sound clinical judgment rather than on a Hb value.

Current pediatric guidelines are based on "expert" opinion, common practice, and the adult literature, rather than on evidence-based pediatric data. Following review of the available evidence, panels of Canadian (13) and British experts (19) did not recommend transfusion at a predetermined Hb level, but rather advocated an individualized approach to RBC transfusion decisions even for the critically ill patient. The same panel of British experts also suggested that an Hb level as low as 7 g/dL might be an acceptable threshold in stable children (19).

Even though the optimal Hb concentration or transfusion threshold above which the benefits outweigh the risks and costs remains to be determined, the 3 observational studies described earlier suggest that an Hb concentration <5 g/dL may be detrimental to severely ill children (11,29,30). In practice, the consensus is that an RBC transfusion must be given to critically ill children if their Hb concentration drops below 5 g/dL (32,39).

Data show that stable critically ill children are able to support Hb concentrations as low as 7 g/dL. A large, international, randomized clinical trial, the Transfusion Requirements in PICU (TRIPICU) study, showed equivalence in 637 stable critically ill children who were allocated either to receive an RBC transfusion when the Hb concentration dropped below 7 g/dL (restrictive group) or when it dropped below 9.5 g/dL (31). The number of patients who developed new or progressive MODS (primary outcome) was similar in both groups: 38 (11.9%) in the restrictive versus 39 (12.3%) in the liberal group. No differences were reported in other major outcomes, including all-cause mortality (14 deaths after 28 days in both groups), nosocomial infection, and length of stay. This noninferiority trial suggests that most stable critically ill children can support an Hb concentration >7 g/dL.

It is probably appropriate to use a higher threshold and to increase the Hb through transfusion in those children who are unstable; however, no consensus defines the threshold. A randomized clinical trial was conducted in the emergency room of a university-affiliated American hospital in which a rapid (<6 hrs) and aggressive therapy-driven protocol had the specific goal of decreasing mortality in adults with severe sepsis and septic shock (44). RBC transfusions to maintain the hematocrit over 30% were given to patients in the experimental group if the O_2 saturation in the central cava vein was lower than 70% after fluid challenge, vasopressors, and inotropes. Mortality was 46.5% in the standard treatment group (133 patients) versus 30.5% in the "early goal-directed therapy" group (130 patients, $p = 0.009$). The applicability of this trial to children can be debated, but it suggests that the outcome of children with severe sepsis may be better if the Hb concentration is kept over 10 g/dL, at least during the first hours following diagnosis.

Some data suggest that critically ill children with severe congenital cardiovascular disease may benefit from a higher Hb concentration intraoperatively and immediately postoperative. Evidence suggests that a low hematocrit can be detrimental for brain development. In piglets, a lower hematocrit (20% vs. 30%) was associated with worse cerebrovascular injury after deep hypothermic circulatory arrest (47). Hemodilution is frequently used in the course of cardiopulmonary bypass, and decrease in cerebral blood flow may increase the risk of brain injury. A randomized clinical trial reported that the neurodevelopmental index of 73 children assigned to hemodilution with a higher hematocrit (27.8%) during the cardiopulmonary bypass was better than the index of 74 subjects assigned to a lower hematocrit (21.5%) (28). A higher Hb concentration may also be useful in the postoperative setting. Another group showed that the administration of 11 mL/kg of packed RBC units to 15 children postoperatively increased their Hb concentration from 8.4 to 9.9 g/dL, and increased their Do_2 from 20.5 to 26.2 mL/kg/min, but the Vo_2 did not change at all (4.5 mL/kg/min before and 4.4 mL/kg/min after the transfusion) (45). Presently, a consensus does not exist in terms of keeping the Hb concentration over 10, and even over 12 g/dL, or to permitting a hematocrit of 20%–25% (Hb, 7–8 g/dL) (19). It is possible that stable critically ill children with severe congenital cardiovascular disease need a higher Hb concentration than those without such disease, but this remains to be proven.

The optimal Hb concentration may be even higher in cases of cyanotic congenital cardiomyopathy than in other kinds of congenital heart disease: Thresholds as high as 13 g/dL and even 16 g/dL are recommended in some textbooks. However, no clinical studies have addressed the specifics of transfusion therapy in cyanotic heart diseases. A case series of 7 children reported that increasing Hb concentration from 13.7 g/dL to 16.4 g/dL was associated with decreased right-to-left shunt (3). However, experience with bloodless cardiac operation for congenital heart disease in children of Jehovah's Witnesses suggests that lower levels of Hb may be well tolerated, even in children with cyanotic cardiomyopathy (1). Thus, the statement that "the optimal Hb concentration for children with cyanotic heart disease has yet to be determined" remains as true today as it was in 1985 (3).

Maintenance of a higher Hb concentration may be an advantage in traumatic brain injury. A cohort of patients who were monitored after subarachnoid hemorrhage suggests that RBC transfusion may increase the risk of vasospasm and poor outcome (48). RBC transfusion increases brain tissue O_2 partial pressure ($Pbto_2$) (49), but whether this improves the outcome of patients with severe brain injury is unclear. The most appropriate Hb concentration in critically ill patients with traumatic, hypoxic, or blood vessel-related brain injury remains to be determined.

Debate also continues regarding the usefulness of blood transfusion as a preventive measure. Some evidence suggests that transfusion is appropriate for critically ill children with congenital anemia (e.g., sickle cell disease), with acute chest syndrome, or in advance of an operative procedure.

Administration of Blood Components

It is necessary to have a well-grounded understanding of the biology and physiology of the individual cellular and liquid components of whole blood in order to prescribe the proper component for patients. Transfusion should be undertaken only if the anticipated benefit outweighs the potential risk. Sound decision by the physician as to whether to transfuse a particular product can only be made with thorough knowledge of the many blood components now available.

The physician must explain the benefits and risks of transfusion to the patient (or the patient's family) and obtain informed consent in accordance with institutional guidelines. The transfusion process is initiated when a physician writes an order specifying the component and the volume to be given. In addition, pretransfusion medication (if indicated), rate and duration of administration, and use of a blood warmer or electromechanical device should be specified. The identity of the blood unit and the recipient must be verified at each step, starting from the collection of the sample for group, type, and cross-match, and continuing through release from the blood bank to the final infusion of the component. Verification may use a bar code or other identifier system. The patient's pretransfusion and posttransfusion vital signs must be recorded. All blood components must be administered through a macroaggregate particulate filter (170–260 μm), and the transfusion must be completed within 4 hrs of the time of release from the blood bank.

Special infusion sets for high flow typically have large filter surface areas and large-bore tubing. For massive transfusion, as in cases of trauma, rapid infuser/blood warmers are available. Other special sets include mechanical infusers, gravity drip sets, and, for transfusion of small volumes of blood products, syringe sets. Microaggregate filters can be used for RBCs to screen out microaggregates, which typically consist of degenerating platelets, leukocytes, and fibrin strands. "Third-generation" leukoreduction filters are used for the WBC reduction of both RBC and platelet products. Benefits include reduced risk of CMV transmission, human leukocyte antigen (HLA) alloimmunization, and febrile nonhemolytic transfusion reactions. These filters may be used prior to storage of blood products immediately before transfusion or at the bedside.

Solutions that can be coadministered with RBCs include normal saline (0.9% USP) and, under rare circumstances, 5% albumin, ABO-compatible plasma, or plasma protein fraction. Hypotonic or hypertonic saline, lactated Ringer solution, 5% dextrose, and medications must not be administered with blood or blood components, to avoid hemolysis and loss of anticoagulation and to distinguish transfusion-mediated reactions from reactions mediated by other causes. RBCs and whole blood can be safely warmed to 37°C, but not more than 42°C, using specifically designed devices. These devices are indicated for adults receiving rapid and multiple transfusions of RBCs or whole blood at a rate of >50 mL/kg/hr, infants receiving rapid transfusions of >15 mL/kg/hr, adults or infants receiving exchange transfusions, and patients with cold agglutinin disease.

Blood or blood components can be modified in several ways to accommodate the patient's clinical situation. RBC and platelet products can be issued in smaller amounts to either reduce donor exposure or decrease the probability of volume overload. Washing of RBCs or platelets may be necessary to reduce anaphylactoid reactions from foreign plasma protein exposure. For those patients who have a history of anaphylactic reaction to blood or blood components and who have demonstrable anti-IgA antibodies, IgA-deficient blood or blood components can be obtained. Similarly, those patients with antibodies to RBC antigens must receive RBC units negative for the antigens to which the patient has developed antibodies. Consultation with a transfusion medicine physician may be necessary in these cases.

Red Blood Cell Products

Whole Blood. Allogeneic whole-blood units are rarely used in the US because they lack the advantages offered by com-

ponent therapy. More frequently, whole-blood units are collected for autologous transfusion. The standard single unit of whole blood contains 450 mL of collected blood into 63 mL of anticoagulant-preservative solution. The hematocrit is usually between 36% and 44%, and the whole-blood unit must be stored at 1°C–6°C. Depending on the anticoagulant-preservative solution, the shelf life will range between 21 and 35 days. However, after 24 hrs of storage, few functional platelets or granulocytes remain, and amounts of factors V and VIII are significantly decreased.

Whole blood units, when available, may be used in patients who are actively bleeding, with massive volume loss (>25%), and who need both O_2-carrying capacity and blood volume expansion. However, these units should not be used for normovolemic patients because RBCs are preferred in this setting. In an average-sized adult, 1 unit of whole blood should increase the hematocrit concentration by 1 g/dL and the hematocrit by 3%–4%.

Other uses of whole-blood units include blood prime for therapeutic procedures in patients with small blood volumes, neonatal exchange transfusions, and primes for devices such as selected cardiac bypass procedures and continuous hemoperfusion. However, whole-blood units are often not available or are unsuitable because of the decreased coagulation factor concentrations, especially of factors V and VIII. In these cases, reconstitution using RBC units and plasma-compatible fresh frozen plasma (FFP) or 5% albumin often suffices.

Red Blood Cells. RBCs are prepared by removal of 200–250 mL of plasma from 1 unit of whole blood. Various anticoagulant-preservative solutions are used that influence the shelf life and hematocrit of the final product. Units prepared in CPD are ~250 mL in volume, with a hematocrit of 70%–80% and a 21-day shelf when they are stored at 1°C–6°C. Units prepared in CPDA-1 have a 35-day shelf life, with a similar volume and hematocrit as CPD-prepared units. More commonly in the US and Canada, additive RBC units are prepared. Additive solutions, such as AS-1 (Adsol: dextrose, adenine, mannitol, sodium chloride), AS-3 (Nutricel: dextrose, adenine, monobasic sodium phosphate, sodium chloride), and AS-5 (Optisol: dextrose, adenine, mannitol, sodium chloride), are available to extend the shelf life further—up to 42 days at 1°C–6°C. After hard packing of a whole-blood unit, the additives are added using sterile technique. Units prepared with 100 mL of additive solution are ~350 mL in volume, with a hematocrit of 50%–60%. They have essentially no plasma, and they flow rapidly.

RBCs are indicated for patients with anemia who require an increase in O_2-carrying capacity and RBC mass. As with whole blood, 1 unit of RBCs in an average-sized adult will usually raise the Hb concentration by 1 g/dL and the hematocrit by 3%–4%. In pediatric patients, a volume of 10 mL/kg (with an adjusted hematocrit of 80%) can be anticipated to raise the Hb concentration by 3 g/dL. For additive units (which have an adjusted hematocrit of 65%), a volume of 10 mL/kg can be expected to result in less than a 3-g/dL increment.

Leukocyte-reduced Red Blood Cells. One unit of RBCs contains ~10^8 WBC, which is approximately a log less than that contained in whole-blood units. Current prestorage, third-generation leukocyte reduction filters can provide a 3-log, or 99.9%, reduction of WBC content to <5 × 10^6 WBC and, with some filters, <1 × 10^6 per product. This leukocyte reduction step preferably occurs after collection at the blood center, where problem units and filter failure can be identified.

Leukocyte-reduced RBCs are indicated (a) for patients with repeated febrile, nonhemolytic transfusion reactions to cellular blood components, or (b) to minimize alloimmunization to foreign HLA antigens. Febrile, nonhemolytic transfusion reactions are typically caused by reactions to donor WBC or to cytokines present in the product. Patients who have persistent febrile, nonhemolytic transfusion reactions to bedside leukocyte-reduced products may benefit from the lower levels of cytokines present in prestorage leukocyte-reduced products. Alloimmunization to foreign HLA class I antigens is of significant concern for patients who may require repeated platelet transfusions. Because platelets also possess HLA class I antigens, patients sensitized to such antigens can become refractory to platelet transfusions. If the decision is made to use leukocyte-reduced RBCs to prevent alloimmunization, it should be made before the first transfusion, and leukocyte-reduced platelets should also be used.

Controversial and unproven indications for leukocyte-reduced RBCs include reduction of immunomodulation that may lead to an increased risk of cancer recurrence or bacterial infections, reduction in prion-transmitted disease, and reduction in *Yersinia enterocolitica* contamination of RBCs. Canada, many countries in Europe, and many blood centers in the US have already initiated universal prestorage leukocyte reduction.

Washed Red Blood Cells. RBC washing involves the use of sterile saline to remove the plasma that remains in an RBC unit. The procedure removes >98% of the plasma, including plasma proteins, microaggregates, and cytokines, as well as up to 20% of the RBCs. The procedure takes 1–2 hrs with an automated cell washer, and resultant product (~180 mL) is suspended in sterile saline to a hematocrit of 70%–80%. This product is indicated for severe, recurrent allergic reaction to blood components not prevented by premedication with one or more antihistamines. Typically, such reactions are caused by allergy to plasma proteins. Patients known to be severely IgA-deficient with a circulatory anti-IgA antibody may have anaphylactic reactions to the IgA present in blood components and should receive either RBCs from IgA-deficient donors (ordered well in advance) or washed RBCs. Because the washing process creates an open system, this component has a shelf life of only 24 hrs at 1°C–6°C. Washed RBCs are not a substitute for leukocyte reduction because washing reduces the WBC content by only 1 log.

Frozen Deglycerolized Red Blood Cells. A freezing process that involves a high glycerol concentration is used by blood centers for long-term storage (up to 10 years at −65°C or colder temperatures) of RBC units with rare phenotypes. Preparation requires thawing and deglycerolization using serial saline-glucose solutions. The final hematocrit is between 55% and 70%, with a 94%–99% reduction of WBC content and at least 80% of the original red cell mass remaining. Using a closed system, the shelf life of a thawed product is 2 weeks; units thawed using an open system mandate a shelf life of 24 hrs at 1°C–6°C.

Prescription of Red Blood Cell Transfusion

Proper selection of RBCs and platelets by group and type of the donor and recipient is detailed in **Table 38.4.**

Two formulas are helpful in determining transfusion volumes:

$$\text{Volume (mL)} = [(\text{Hb}_{\text{targeted}} - \text{Hb}_{\text{observed}}) \times \text{blood volume}]/\text{Hb}_{\text{RBC unit}}$$

where:

$\text{Hb}_{\text{targeted}}$ is the Hb concentration targeted posttransfusion (for example, 10 g/dL)

$\text{Hb}_{\text{observed}}$ is the most recently measured Hb concentration of the patient (g/dL)

Blood volume is expressed in milliliters

$\text{Hb}_{\text{RBC unit}}$ is the average Hb concentration in the packed RBC units (g/dL) prepared by the transfusion service.

The other formula is:

$$\text{Total body blood volume} = \text{weight} \times \text{blood volume}$$

where:

weight is expressed in kilograms

blood volume is expressed in liters per kilogram (0.08 L/kg if child is <2 years old and 0.07 L/kg if child is 2–14 years old).

For example, if the $\text{Hb}_{\text{observed}}$ in a 2-week-old baby weighing 3 kg is 6.5 g/dL, her blood volume is 240 mL (0.08 L/kg × 3 kg), and the $\text{Hb}_{\text{RBC unit}}$ is 19.5 g/dL (AS-3). If the attending intensivist wants to increase the Hb concentration of the baby ($\text{Hb}_{\text{targeted}}$) to 10 g/dL, the volume of the RBC unit to be transfused would be determined by the following formula:

$$\text{Volume} = [(10.0 - 6.5 \text{ g/dL}) \times 240 \text{ mL}]/19.5 \text{ g/dL} = 43 \text{ mL}$$

Older children of specific weight who are healthy can give their own blood, called *autologous donation.* Lay people and caregivers believe that such transfusion is without risk. If these units have been collected far in advance of the procedures, they may contain more inflammatory mediators, free Hb, and potassium. Moreover, these units are not leukocyte depleted, at least in Canada. The risk-benefit ratio of autologous RBC transfusion remains to be determined.

RBC substitutes would be useful if available and effective. Many artificial O_2 carriers have been studied, including various Hb solutions and perfluorocarbon derivatives (21). The safety of these products is of concern, and their usefulness is not proven. None can be recommended presently.

Conclusions

An RBC transfusion is the only effective way to rapidly increase the Hb level of critically ill patients because their response to iron and erythropoietin is too slow. The risk–benefit ratio must be taken into account when transfusion is being considered. While data exist regarding the risks attributable to RBC transfusion, the risks of anemia are poorly understood, making it difficult to communicate these risks to critically ill patients and their families. Some evidence suggests that severe anemia increases morbidity and mortality in critically ill children, and some reports improved outcome following transfusion in some patients. The unanswered issues are how to correctly identify those patients who will benefit from RBC transfusion and how to use markers that will help physicians determine whether RBC transfusion is truly beneficial for a given patient.

TABLE 38.4

COMPATIBILITY OF BLOOD PRODUCTS

If patient's blood type is:	O positive 37.4%[a]	O negative 6.6%	A positive 35.7%	A negative 6.3%	B positive 8.5%	B negative 1.5%	AB positive 3.4%	AB negative 0.6
These blood types will be compatible as packed red blood cells								
O positive	X	X						
O negative		X						
A positive	X	X	X	X				
A negative		X		X				
B positive	X	X			X	X		
B negative		X				X		
AB positive	X	X	X	X	X	X	X	X
AB negative		X		X		X		X
These blood types will be compatible as whole blood								
O positive	X	X						
O negative		X						
A positive			X	X				
A negative				X				
B positive					X	X		
B negative						X		
AB positive							X	X
AB negative								X
These blood types will be compatible as fresh frozen plasma								
O positive	X	X	X	X	X	X	X	X
O negative	X	X	X	X	X	X	X	X
A positive			X	X			X	X
A negative			X	X			X	X
B positive					X	X	X	X
B negative					X	X	X	X
AB positive							X	X
AB negative							X	X
These blood types are the first choice as platelets[b]								
O positive	X	X	X	X	X	X	X	X
O negative		X		X		X		X
A positive			X	X			X	X
A negative				X				X
B positive					X	X	X	X
B negative						X		X
AB positive							X	X
AB negative								X

[a]Proportion (%) of general population with this blood type.

[b]If the first choice is unavailable, other blood types may be used after volume reduction. Rh-negative patients may receive Rh-positive platelets in special situations with approval of the medical director.

Some argue that transfusion thresholds should be abandoned in favor of RBC transfusion to address specific physiologic needs. Such determinants as markers of Do_2, Vo_2, and Vo_2/Do_2 dependence (Vo_2/Do_2 ratio, blood lactate, O_2 extraction, central-venous or mixed-venous O_2 saturation) may modulate the decision of pediatric intensivists to prescribe an RBC transfusion, but the indications for transfusion are still not well characterized for these different determinants (53). In practice, the decision to prescribe an RBC transfusion is still based on Hb concentration.

In practice, the available data suggest that all critically ill children should receive an RBC transfusion if their Hb concentration drops below 5 g/dL; on the other hand, an RBC transfusion is probably not required if the Hb concentration remains above 7 g/dL. Practitioners must take into account determinants other than the Hb concentration, such as age, the severity of illness, and the observation of signs of organ dysfunction (e.g., high blood lactate level or low central venous O_2 saturation). For example, it seems appropriate to consider a higher threshold and a more aggressive RBC transfusion strategy in critically ill children who are hemodynamically unstable or who have significant cardiovascular disease. These recommendations must also be adapted to specific diseases (e.g., sickle cell disease, thalassemia, hemolytic uremic syndrome, cyanotic heart disease); further research is necessary to better characterize the appropriate threshold for these specific diseases.

Ex vivo production of erythrocytes and bloodless medicine, discussed later, may be other means by which to decrease the requirements of allogenous RBC transfusion.

PLASMA

Constitution of Plasma

One unit of plasma is the quantity of plasma obtained from 1 unit of whole blood; plasmapheresis of a single donor can yield 500–800 mL. A typical whole-blood unit contains between 180 and 300 mL of anticoagulated plasma. Solvent/detergent plasma (plasma SD) consists of a pool of 2500 plasma units that have been further processed to remove viral contaminants in a volume of 200 mL. Plasma SD is not a licensed product in the US. Source plasma or single-donor plasma is stored at −20°C after collection. FFP is separated from whole blood within 6 hrs of collection; it can be stored.

Scientific Foundation of Transfusion of Plasma

One milliliter of plasma contains ~1 unit of each of the coagulation factors, as well as a concentration of complement, trace elements, and other plasma proteins. Labile coagulation factors, such as factors V and VIII, are unstable in plasma stored for prolonged periods at 1°–6°C, which explains why plasma is usually stored frozen at or below −18°C. At collection, FFP must contain at least 87% of normal concentration of factor VIII, and the concentration of Factor VIII must remain over 0.70 IU/mL, according to standards in many countries. FFP also contains significant amounts of glucose (535 mg/dL), sodium (172 mEq/L), potassium (15 mEq/L), and proteins (5.5 g/dL with 60% albumin) (12).

Transfusion of Plasma: Application to PICU

In most instances, plasma is used in the PICU to treat disseminated intravascular coagulation, to restore the blood concentration of deficient coagulation factors associated with massive transfusion or some diseases, or for rapid reversal of the warfarin effect. The efficacy and usefulness of FFP to correct the INR has been challenged recently (15). FFP is sometimes used for isolated congenital coagulation factor deficiencies; recombinant or plasma-derived, pooled and virally inactivated factor concentrates are preferred when clinically indicated.

Plasma can be required in patients who received massive transfusion of packed RBC units or whole blood. However, dilution of coagulation factors rarely appears before the patient receives >1.5 times his/her blood volume. Some surgeons request that plasma be administered once the patient receives 100% of his/her blood volume replaced by RBCs and if clinical evidence of oozing or microvascular bleeding is present (13). Plasma is used as a treatment measure of symptomatic thrombotic thrombocytopenic purpura and its related clinical entities, hemolytic uremic syndrome, and HELLP syndrome (*h*emolysis, *e*levated *l*iver *e*nzymes, and *l*ow *p*latelets). Plasma is also used as replacement fluid in some plasma exchanges performed by apheresis. The use of plasmapheresis is still under investigation as a treatment measure of sepsis and MODS.

Historically, plasma transfusion was used to increase the blood pressure of patients in shock. However, the adminis-tration of FFP to 115 nonbleeding critically ill adults was associated with an increased risk of new-onset acute lung injury, while no difference was observed in the incidence of new bleeding episodes (9). Plasma is not recommended as a volume expander; crystalloids, synthetic colloids, or purified human albumin solutions are preferred.

Transfusion of Plasma: How

Compatibility testing is not required before plasma transfusion, unless large volumes are given. FFP must be ABO compatible with the recipient's RBCs; AB plasma can be administered in severe and acute situations. Plasma dosing is calculated at 10–20 mL/kg, followed by repeat laboratory evaluation using a coagulation profile. In some cases, multiple repeat doses are necessary.

FFP can be warmed in 7 mins using a microwave oven; however, only ovens specifically constructed for this task can be used, as standard microwaves will destroy the function of several coagulation factors. Thawed plasma must be used within 4 hrs of release to be used as FFP. A macroaggregate filter must be used.

The effectiveness of FFP is often judged by cessation of bleeding, as the normalization of a coagulation profile may not always be seen. An activated coagulation time, prothrombin time, activated partial thromboplastin time, and INR may not correct. Additional plasma may be administered if the INR is higher than 2.5; the blood level of coagulation factors V, VIII, or IX is lower than 0.2–0.3 U/mL; or the fibrinogen level is <75 mg/dL (0.75 g/L). Although coagulation tests are poor predictors of bleeding (15), additional transfusions may be helpful when abnormal laboratory tests are associated with active hemorrhage.

PLATELETS

Constitution of Platelets

A platelet concentrate can be prepared from a single donor (apheresis procedure) or from a single whole-blood collection. Platelet concentrates derived from whole-blood donors are pooled as necessary prior to issue. In contrast, a platelet concentrate from a single-donor apheresis procedure is the equivalent of 6–10 platelets derived from whole-blood donations. In the US and Canada, platelets derived from whole-blood donations are prepared using a platelet-rich plasma method, whereas in Europe, platelets are derived from whole-blood–derived platelets using a buffy-coat method. Nonleukoreduced platelets have ~10^6–10^8 leukocytes per unit. However, once leukoreduced, using current leukoreduction filters, <5×10^6 leukocytes (and often <1×10^6 leukocytes) per unit are present. Both apheresis and whole-blood–derived platelets contain substantial amounts of plasma, requiring the use of ABO-compatible platelets unless the plasma is substantially removed. However, platelet plasma is not an adequate source of coagulation factors, as factors such as factors V and VIII markedly decrease during platelet storage. Typical red cell content is substantially less with apheresis platelets (typically much less than 0.005 mL of RBCs per unit) than with whole-blood–derived platelet concentrates, which can contain on average

~0.5 mL of RBCs (6). In Europe and Canada, all platelet products undergo leukoreduction, while leukoreduction is largely practiced in most transfusion services and blood centers in the US. Leukoreduction has several uses, including significantly decreasing the risk of HLA alloimmunization, nonhemolytic febrile reactions, and transmission of CMV. The volume of a whole-blood–derived platelet concentrate is 50–70 mL while that of an apheresis platelet concentrate ranges from 200 to 300 mL. There are ~5.5 × 10^10 platelets per whole-blood–derived unit (also called an *equivalent unit*, or EU).

Platelets are stored at 20°–24°C and, after completion of infectious disease testing, can be used up to 5 days after collection. A Federal Drug Administration-approved post-marketing study (Post-Approval Surveillance Study of Platelet Outcomes, Release Tested; PASSPORT) in the use of 6- and 7-day-old platelets is underway. It has been shown that 1–4-hr corrected count increments (CCIs) using these platelets is equivalent to CCIs of platelets ≤5 days old in PICU patients (60). Platelets undergo irreversible activation when stored between 1° and 8°C; therefore, optimal storage temperature is between 20°C and 24°C. Future research using cold storage and special preservative solution may be possible and allow prolonged storage of platelet concentrates (24).

Scientific Foundation of Transfusion of Platelets

Thrombocytopenia and/or qualitative platelet defects increase the risk of bleeding, due to impairment in the ability to form a platelet plug. Platelet concentrates are given to patients at risk of bleeding in order to increase their platelet count or to supply them with more functional platelets.

Thrombocytopenia is defined by a platelet count of <150,000/mm^3 (150 × 10^9/L). The prevalence of ICU-acquired thrombocytopenia is 44% in critically ill adults (51) and is thought to be similar in the PICU. Thrombocytopenia is observed when increased platelet consumption or decreased platelet production occurs. High platelet consumption is frequently caused in the PICU by nonimmune-mediated mechanisms, such as disseminated intravascular coagulation, splenomegaly, and sepsis, and by immune-mediated mechanisms, as seen with alloimmunization in patients undergoing chemotherapy who have received numerous blood products, patients with autoimmune thrombocytopenia purpura, and patients who develop heparin-induced thrombocytopenia or other drug-induced antiplatelet antibodies. Heparin-induced thrombocytopenia has an incidence rate of ~1% among patients who have undergone cardiovascular surgery for congenital heart disease. Decreased bone marrow platelet production can result from medications (most notably chemotherapy), sepsis, and viral infections, the latter of which can result in bone marrow histiocytic hyperplasia with hemophagocytosis (acquired hemophagocytosis syndrome) (17).

Qualitative platelet function defects commonly occur in the ICU. It is most frequently caused by toxins, drugs (for example, salicylate, nitric oxide), exposure to extracorporeal circulation, and renal failure (uremia). Treatment of qualitative platelet function defects requires platelet transfusion in addition to the administration of certain drugs, such as antifibrinolytic agents (e.g., ε-aminocaproic acid), and the use of cryoprecipitate to treat the platelet function defect associated with uremia. Certain rare, inherited macrothrombocytopathies or other inherited qualitative platelet defects, such as Bernard-Soulier disease and Glanzmann thrombasthenia, may require the use of recombinant factor VIIa, which avoids the potential alloimmunization of foreign platelet glycoproteins Ib/IX and IIb/IIIa, respectively, which these patients lack.

Transfusion of Platelets: Application to the PICU

The purpose of platelet therapy is to stop an ongoing hemorrhage or to prevent bleeding. It has been reported that correction of thrombocytopenia reduces mortality of critically ill patients (51). The risk of pulmonary hemorrhage is significant in mechanically ventilated patients if the platelet count is <50,000/mm^3, and most intensivists will prescribe a platelet transfusion in such an instance. A platelet transfusion must also be considered if the platelet count of a patient with an active hemorrhage is <50,000–100,000/mm^3. Transfusion to keep the platelet level above a threshold of 100,000/mm^3 is recommended in the presence of an active intracranial hemorrhage or if extracorporeal membrane oxygenation (ECMO) is underway. It is also appropriate to consider a platelet transfusion even when the platelet count is higher than 100,000/mm^3 if bleeding is active and severe, or if bleeding is associated with a qualitative platelet defect.

In patients with thrombocytopenia due to decreased platelet production (such as seen in patients who have received chemotherapy), prophylactic platelet transfusion should be considered if the platelet count is <5,000–10,000/mm^3 or if the patient has additional risk factors for bleeding.

The administration of a large amount of crystalloids, packed RBCs, and/or whole blood (more than 1 blood volume), such as seen in surgical patients or in massive transfusion for trauma patients, can dilute the platelet count. In such instances, the platelet count and the coagulation status must be monitored closely.

Platelet transfusion should not be used for the treatment of idiopathic thrombocytopenic purpura, except in the presence of intracerebral or life-threatening bleeding. Platelets are contraindicated in cases of thrombotic thrombocytopenic purpura and heparin-induced thrombocytopenia because of increased thrombotic risk. Alternatives to platelet transfusion, such as 1-deamino(8-D-arginine) vasopressin (DDAVP) or antifibrinolytic agents, the use of steroids, plasmapheresis, and avoidance of heparin, when relevant, should be considered as first-line therapies.

Platelet dysfunction is usually associated with some thrombocytopenia in critically ill patients. When a platelet dysfunction is suspected, platelet transfusion can be considered only if the patient is bleeding. However, it is suggested by some experts to keep the platelet count over 100,000/mm^3 during the postoperative care of pediatric cardiac surgery patients because some platelet dysfunction is frequently observed up to 4–6 hrs after a cardiopulmonary bypass.

Transfusion of Platelets: How

It is prudent to use ABO-matched platelets. The use of ABO-incompatible platelets requires that the transfusion service remove a substantial amount of incompatible plasma. This additional procedure decreases the platelet content by 15%–20%, shortens the storage time to 4 hrs, and delays platelet release by ~1 hr. Administering 5–10 mL/kg of platelet concentrate (either whole-blood–derived or apheresis platelets) to infants who weigh <10 kg and administering 1 whole-blood–derived unit per 10 kg of weight (i.e., 1 unit for an 11–20-kg child, 2 units for a 21–30-kg child, etc.), or ~5 mL/kg if using apheresis or prepooled platelets, in older children who weigh >10 kg, should increase the platelet count by 50,000/mm^3. Such an increase is not always observed, usually because platelet consumption is high, a frequent occurrence with disseminated intravascular coagulation or with the use of techniques like ECMO and cardiopulmonary bypass. Assessment of an adequate platelet count increment requires calculating a CCI at 1 hr post-platelet transfusion, which should be >7500, using the formula below.

$$CCI = \frac{\text{platelet count increment per mm}^3 \times \text{body surface area per m}^2 \times 10^{11}}{\text{Total number of platelets transfused}}$$

For example, a 1-hr posttransfusion platelet count increment of 40,000/mm^3 in a patient with a body surface area of 0.9 m^2 who received 3 equivalent units ($3 \times 5.5 \times 10^{10}$) of platelets would produce a CCI of 21,818. CCIs <7,500 may be suggestive of platelet refractoriness and require the use of crossmatched or HLA-matched platelets. For these specialized products, it is necessary to consult the transfusion medicine service. Under certain circumstances, patients with renal failure may require volume-reduced platelets. Preparation of these platelets, much like ABO-incompatible platelets, also results in decreased storage life of platelets, decreases platelet content, delays release, and requires contacting the transfusion medicine service. From a regulatory perspective, platelet concentrates must be used within 4 hrs after release by the blood bank. Platelets should be transfused using a standard blood filter (pore size, 170–260 mcm). If a single, whole-blood–derived platelet concentrate is given, an 80-mcm filter may be used to avoid wastage. An anti-D immunoglobin preparation (WinRho SDR) may be given to avoid the development of anti-D if the patient is Rh$^-$ and the donor is Rh$^+$. However, this practice is largely defined by the patient's underlying immunosuppression, gender, and age, and the institution's defined clinical practice.

Despite leukoreduction, which reduces the leukocyte count by ~1000-fold, some leukocytes are always found in platelet concentrates. Thus, leukoreduction cannot substitute for irradiation to eliminate the risk of transfusion-associated GVHD, which is associated with 90% mortality despite treatment. Patients most at risk for transfusion associated GVHD include patients with congenital cellular immunodeficiency, patients undergoing stem cell or solid-organ transplantation or chemotherapy, and patients receiving HLA matched products or directed donations from blood relatives (61).

GRANULOCYTES

Constitution of Granulocyte Concentrates

Granulocyte concentrates are collected from donors who have undergone either steroid and/or growth factor (most commonly granulocyte colony-stimulating factor, GCSF) stimu-

lation. Donors typically undergo 7–10-L apheresis collection using a cell separator. Steroid-only-stimulated granulocyte collections result in only 1–2 × 10^{10} granulocytes per unit, whereas steroid- and growth factor-stimulated collections can yield 4–8 × 10^{10} granulocytes per unit. Because the density of granulocytes is near that of RBCs, a sedimentation agent, such as hetastarch, is given as a continuous IV solution to the donor during apheresis collection. The volume of a granulocyte product is typically between 250 and 300 mL.

Scientific Foundation of Transfusion of Granulocyte: Why

The degree of neutropenia as the result of chemotherapy correlates with the risk of infection. As a result, it has been hypothesized that the transfusion of granulocytes would benefit patients who are neutropenic for a protracted period. In fact, several studies have shown that transfused granulocytes have the ability to migrate to areas of infection, as shown by nuclear medicine imaging studies using ^{111}Indium radiolabeled granulocytes (34) and skin-window methodology (35). However, 7 randomized and nonrandomized studies published between 1972 and 1980 demonstrated lack of consistent efficacy of granulocyte transfusions in septic patients. Factors related to benefit included those patients who received at least 3–4 granulocyte transfusions, those who had prolonged neutropenia, and those who received larger granulocyte doses. In another study, patients who received >2 × 10^{10} granulocytes could demonstrate a >2,000/mm^3 increment in the absolute neutrophil count of the next morning (42). Based on several randomized, controlled clinical trials, however, its use as a prophylactic measure in neutropenic patients in the setting of bone marrow transplantation or remission/induction chemotherapy for acute myelogenous leukemia is not recommended, as no survival advantage over conventional therapy is achieved despite decreased infection or sepsis in the transfused patients. However, meta-analysis of these studies revealed granulocyte dose, leukocyte compatibility, and shorter duration of neutropenia to be major determinants for prevention of bacterial infection (54). Thus, the need for randomized clinical trials to definitively determine the efficacy and adverse side effects of steroid and GCSF-stimulated granulocyte products is clear. The future use of granulocytes will also depend on pharmacologic advances in antimicrobial and antifungal therapy—particularly antifungal therapy, as a number of new antifungal agents are currently under investigation.

Transfusion of Granulocyte: Application to PICU

Granulocyte transfusions should be considered in severely neutropenic patients with bacterial sepsis or fungal infections when antimicrobial or antifungal therapy appears to be ineffective and bone marrow recovery is expected to be delayed as long as 2–3 weeks. Granulocyte transfusions should also be considered in patients with granulocyte dysfunction with bacterial sepsis or fungal infection and lack of responsiveness to standard therapy. It is important that an infectious disease consult be obtained to ensure that optimal antimicrobial or antifungal therapy has been achieved prior to initialization of granulocyte transfusions. Because it is recommended that granulocyte transfusions of at least 1×10^{10} be transfused daily until clinical improvement, it is important to coordinate requests with the transfusion medicine service, as granulocyte collection requires prior stimulation of donors who must undergo apheresis.

Transfusion of Granulocyte: How

Because of the extremely high granulocyte count within a granulocyte product, granulocyte metabolic activity can rapidly deplete glucose, produce lactic acid, and increase cell death. This fact is accentuated because of the requirement to store granulocytes at room temperature, as cold storage inactivates neutrophils. From a regulatory standpoint, granulocytes must be transfused within 24 hrs; some even recommend transfusion as soon as possible. Because of this requirement, infectious disease testing cannot be completed prior to release; thus, a small but not insignificant risk of viral disease transmission exists. Consequently, donors who have been frequent platelet apheresis donors are chosen to minimize this risk. Often, CMV-seronegative or CMV "safe" products are required. Because granulocytes cannot be leukoreduced, the risk of CMV transmission is significant if CMV-seropositive granulocytes are given. This can be a significant problem because donors who volunteer to donate granulocytes have to endure the side effects of both steroids and GCSF. Because granulocytes have significant RBC and plasma content, granulocytes must be ABO compatible and crossmatched prior to release. HLA matching and/or leukocyte crossmatching may be considered; however, this is not always attainable. A relative contraindication to granulocyte transfusions is if the recipient has anti-HLA or anti-granulocyte antibodies because of the possibility of developing transfusion-associated acute lung injury. Granulocyte irradiation is recommended, given the immunocompromised state of the recipient and because of the possibility of HLA- or leukocyte-crossmatch compatibility or related family member donations. Granulocytes should be transfused over 1–2 hrs via a standard blood (150–200 mcm) filter, with intermittent agitation of the unit to avoid settling of the granulocytes. Transfusion of granulocytes is frequently accompanied by fever, chills, and allergic reactions and should be discontinued in the case of severe pulmonary reaction. Granulocyte transfusion should be separated by as much time as possible from amphotericin transfusion, as severe pulmonary reactions have been associated with the simultaneous infusion of both products. Overall efficacy of granulocyte transfusion can be ascertained either by clinical improvement or assessment of absolute neutrophil counts.

LIMITING BLOOD PRODUCT UTILIZATION

"*Primum non nocere*" ("First, do no harm") holds true with blood products as with any other medical technology. Therefore, all possible steps must be taken to use blood products only when necessary and to limit blood losses. The concept of bloodless medicine refers to all of the strategies that can be used to provide medical care without allogeneic blood transfusion, including blood conservation. Bloodless medicine strategy often begins before surgery by collecting autologous donation. Pre-

scribing erythropoietin and iron supplements before a surgery can help to optimize the preoperative Hb level (23). Where possible, all drugs that can increase the risk of bleeding (e.g., anticoagulants and drugs that inhibit platelet function) must be avoided.

Many strategies are advocated during surgery (56). Hemostasis must be optimized, and all bleeding must be controlled rapidly. The use of fibrin sealants and antifibrinolytic agents, such as aprotinin or tranexamic acid, can be useful (22). Technology like acute normovolemic hemodilution, autologous blood cell salvage, intraoperative autotransfusion, and deliberate hypotension, can also be considered, but their applicability to young children is questionable, with very few randomized clinical trials (56,59).

Management of anemia and bleeding from coagulopathy in the ICU is still a matter of debate. "Permissive anemia" is advocated by some experts (19). Prevention of bleeding episodes is another option, but how it should be accomplished is still a matter of debate. Phlebotomy remains a significant cause of blood loss, which can be decreased by limiting the number of blood tests and the volume of blood required. For example, closed-blood sampling, use of pediatric blood collection tubes, microanalysis techniques that require small sample volumes, and in-line measurement of blood gas can all be effective ways to minimize blood loss (14,43,57).

Days to weeks of therapy are necessary for erythropoietin and iron to effectively increase the Hb concentration in healthy patients; the response of critically ill patients to erythropoietin is blunted. Erythropoietin does not appear to be an efficient use of a costly and limited resource in the ICU, even though it is effective in critically ill adults (7). Its usefulness in the PICU remains to be determined.

CONCLUSIONS AND FUTURE DIRECTIONS

Transfusion of one or more blood products to critically ill children may be life saving, but can also cause clinically significant adverse events. The decision to proceed with transfusion of any blood product must be based on individualized indications. More randomized clinical trials are required to improve the use of blood products in the PICU. In critically ill children, adverse events related to the immunomodulatory effects of blood products on the inflammatory and the allergic systems are more frequent than transfusion-related infectious diseases. More clinical research is required to better describe the cost and benefits of transfusion of blood products and to improve the use of blood products in the PICU.

KEY POINTS

Red Blood Cell Transfusion

■ RBC transfusion is required in most critically ill children if their Hb level is <5 g/dL; evidence supporting this recommendation: 3 large observational studies in children (11,29,30) and 1 observational study in adult Jehovah Witnesses (5).

■ RBC transfusion is probably useful if the Hb level is between 5 and 7 g/dL; evidence supporting this recommendation: none.

■ The risk/benefit ratio of giving or not giving an RBC transfusion is similar in stable critically ill children if their Hb level is between 7 and 9.5 g/dL, and we recommend not transfusing in such an instance unless another determinant suggests that it may be useful for a specific patient; evidence supporting this recommendation: 1 large, randomized clinical trial (31).

■ No RBC transfusion is required if the Hb level is >9.5 g/dL; evidence supporting this recommendation: none, but no hard data support the decision to give a transfusion in such an instance.

■ It may be useful, at least during the first 6 hrs of treatment, to keep the Hb concentration over 10 g/dL (hematocrit >30%) in patients with severe sepsis or septic shock; evidence supporting this recommendation is related to 1 large, randomized clinical trial in adults (44).

■ The appropriate Hb concentration in critically ill children with heart disease is unknown.

Fresh Frozen Plasma

■ Most clinical uses of FFP are not supported by evidence from randomized clinical trials.

■ Active bleeding attributable to coagulation factor deficiency is usually considered an absolute indication for the use of FFP; prophylactic use of FFP is controversial.

■ Plasma should not be used as a volume expander.

Platelets

■ Platelets can be useful to treat bleeding caused by low platelet counts and/or dysfunctional platelets.

■ Calculation of the 1-hr posttransfusion CCI can help to assess efficacy of platelet transfusion.

■ A variety of specialized platelet products can be requested from the transfusion medicine service to avoid or minimize transfusion-associated GVHD, volume overload, and platelet refractoriness.

Granulocytes

■ Granulocyte transfusion should be considered in the treatment of bacterial sepsis or fungal infections in neutropenic patients or in patients with dysfunctional neutrophils who may have protracted periods of neutropenia and who appear to have no response to antimicrobial or antifungal therapy.

■ Further use of granulocyte transfusions will be defined by future randomized clinical trials and advancements in antimicrobial and antifungal therapy.

ACKNOWLEDGMENTS

The research program of our group on RBC transfusion is supported by the Canadian Institutes of Health Research, the Canadian Blood Bank Services, the Fonds de la Recherche en Santé du Québec and Héma-Québec. Jacques Lacroix had a consultant agreement with Johnson & Johnson. We thank the members of the Canadian Critical Care Trials Group and the Pediatric Acute Lung Injury and Sepsis Investigators (PALISI) Network for their support.

References

1. Alexi-Meskishvili V, Stiller B, Böttcher W, et al. Correction of congenital heart defects in Jehovah's Witness children. *Thorac Cardiov Surg* 2004;52:141–6.
2. Armano R, Gauvin F, Ducruet T, et al. Determinants of red blood cell transfusions in a pediatric critical care unit: A prospective descriptive epidemiological study. *Crit Care Med* 2005;33:2637–44.
3. Beekman RH, Tuuri DT. Acute hemodynamic effects of increasing hemoglobin concentration in children with a right to left ventricular shunt and relative anemia. *J Am Coll Cardiol* 1985;5:357–62.
4. Carson JL, Duff A, Poses RM, et al. Effect of anaemia and cardiovascular disease on surgical mortality and morbidity. *Lancet* 1996;348:1055–60.
5. Carson JL, Noveck H, Berlin JA, et al. Mortality and morbidity in patients with very low postoperative Hb levels who decline blood transfusion. *Transfusion* 2002;42:812–8.
6. Cid J, Lozano M. Risk of Rh(D) alloimmunization after transfusion of platelets from D+ donors to D− recipients. *Transfusion* 2005;45:453–4.
7. Corwin HL, Gettinger A, Pearl RG, et al. Efficacy of recombinant human erythropoietin in critically ill patients. *JAMA* 2002;288:2827–35.
8. Curtis BR, McFarland JG. Mechanisms of transfusion-related acute lung injury (TRALI): Anti-leukocyte antibodies. *Crit Care Med* 2006;34:S118–23.
9. Dara SI, Rana R, Afessa B, et al. Fresh frozen plasma transfusion in critically ill medical patients with coagulopathy. *Crit Care Med* 2005;33:2667–71.
10. Desmet L, Lacroix J. Transfusion in pediatrics. *Crit Care Clin* 2004;20:299–311.
11. English M, Ahmed M, Ngando C, et al. Blood transfusion for severe anaemia in children in a Kenyan hospital. *Lancet* 2002;359:494–5.
12. Ewalenko P, Deloof T, Peeters J. Composition of fresh frozen plasma. *Crit Care Med* 1986;14:145–6.
13. Experts Working Group. Guidelines for red blood cell and plasma transfusions for adults and children. *Can Med Assoc J* 1997;156:S1–24.
14. Fowler RA, Rizoli SB, Levin PD, et al. Blood conservation for critically ill patients. *Crit Care Clin* 2004;20:313–24.
15. Gajic O, Dzik WH, Toy P. Fresh frozen plasma and platelet transfusion for nonbleeding patients in the intensive care unit: Benefit or harm? *Crit Care Med* 2006;34:S170–3.
16. Gauvin F, Chaïbou M, Leteurtre S, et al. Pratique de transfusion de concentré globulaire en réanimation pédiatrique: Une étude descriptive prospective. *Réanimation Urgences* 2000;9:339–44.
17. Gauvin F, Toledano B, Champagne J, et al. Reactive hemophagocytic syndrome presenting as a component of multiple organ system failure. *Crit Care Med* 2000;28:3341–5.
18. Gauvin F, Toledano B, Hume HA, et al. Hypotensive reactions associated with platelet transfusion through leucocyte reduction filters. *J Intensive Care Med* 2000;14:329–32.
19. Gibson BE, Todd A, Roberts I, et al. Transfusion guidelines for neonates and older children. *Br J Haematol* 2004;124:433–53.
20. Goodman A, M, Pollack MM, Patel KM, et al. Pediatric red blood cell transfusions increase resource use. *J Pediatr* 2003;142:123–7.
21. Goodnough LT, Shander A, Brecher ME. Transfusion medicine: Looking to the future. *Lancet* 2003;361:161–9.
22. Goodnough LT, Shander A, Spence R. Bloodless medicine: Clinical care without allogeneic blood transfusion. *Transfusion* 2003;43:668–76.
23. Goudnough LT, Brecher ME, Kanter MH, et al. Transfusion medicine: Blood conservation. *N Engl J Med* 1999;340:525–33.
24. Hoffmeister KM, Josefsson EC, Isaac NA, et al. Glycosylation restores survival of chilled blood platelets. *Science* 2003;301:1531–4.
25. Holzer BR, Egger M, Teuscher R, et al. Childhood anemia in Africa: To transfuse or not transfuse? *Acta Trop* 1993;55:47–51.
26. Hébert PC, Wells G, Blajchman MA, et al. A multicenter, randomized, controlled clinical trial of transfusion requirements in critical care. *N Engl J Med* 1999;340:409–17.
27. Infectious Diseases and Immunization Committee, Canadian Paediatric Society. Transfusion and risk of infection in Canada: Update 2006. *Paediatr Child Health* 2006;11:158–62.
28. Jonas RA, Wypij D, Roth SJ, et al. The influence of hemodilution on outcome after hypothermic cardiopulmonary bypass: Results of a randomized trial in infants. *J Thorac Cardiovasc Surg* 2003;126:1765–74.
29. Lackritz EM, Campbell CC, Ruebush TK, et al. Effect of blood transfusion on survival among children in a Kenyan hospital. *Lancet* 1992;340:524–8.

30. Lackritz EM, Hightower AW, Zucker JR, et al. Longitudinal evaluation of severely anemic children in Kenya: The effect of transfusion on mortality and hematologic recovery. *AIDS* 1997;11:1487–94.
31. Lacroix J, Hébert PC, Hutchison JS, et al. Transfusion strategies for patients in pediatric intensive care units. *N Engl J Med* 2007;356:1609–19.
32. Laverdière C, Gauvin F, Hébert PC, et al. Survey of transfusion practices in pediatric intensive care units. *Pediatr Crit Care Med* 2002;3:335–40.
33. Lucking SE, Williams TM, Chaten FC, et al. Dependence of oxygen consumption on oxygen delivery in children with hyperdynamic septic shock and low oxygen extraction. *Crit Care Med* 1990;18:1316–9.
34. McCullough J, Clay M, Hurd D, et al. Effect of leukocyte antibodies and HLA matching on the intravascular recovery, survival, and tissue localization of 111-indium granulocytes. *Blood* 1986;67:522–8.
35. McCullough J, Clay M, Loken M, et al. Effect of ABO incompatibility on the fate in vivo of 111Indium granulocytes. *Transfusion* 1988;28:358–61.
36. Mink RB, Pollack MM. Effect of blood transfusion on oxygen consumption in pediatric septic shock. *Crit Care Med* 1990;18:1087–91.
37. Moore SB. Transfusion-related acute lung injury (TRALI): Clinical presentation, treatment, and prognosis. *Crit Care Med* 2006;34:S114–7.
38. Morris KP, Naqvi N, Davies P, et al. A new formula for blood transfusion volume in the critically ill. *Arch Dis Child* 2005;90:724–8.
39. Nahum E, Ben-Ari J, Schonfeld T. Blood transfusion policy among European pediatric intensive care physicians. *J Intensive Care Med* 2004;19:38–43.
40. Nishiyama T, Hanaoka K. Hemolysis in stored red blood cell concentrates: Modulation by haptoglobin or ulinastatin, a protease inhibitor. *Crit Care Med* 2001;29:1979–82.
41. Popovsky MA. *Transfusion Reactions, 2nd ed.* Bethesda: AABB Press, 2001;468.
42. Price TH, Bowden RA, Boeckh M, et al. Phase I/II trial of neutrophil transfusions from donors stimulated with G-CSF and dexamethasone for treatment of patients with infections in hematopoietic stem cell transplantation. *Blood* 2000;95:3302–9.
43. Rickard CM, Couchman BA, Schmidt SJ, et al. A discard volume of twice the deadspace ensures clinically accurate arterial blood gases and electrolytes and prevents unnecessary blood loss. *Crit Care Med* 2003;31:1654–8.
44. Rivers E, Nguyen B, Havstad S, et al. Early goal-directed therapy in the treatment of severe sepsis and septic shock. *N Engl J Med* 2001;345:1368–77.
45. Seear M, Wensley D, MacNab A. Oxygen consumption-oxygen delivery relationship in children. *J Pediatr* 1993;123:208–14.
46. Shander A. Anemia in the critically ill. *Crit Care Clin* 2004;20:159–78.
47. Shum-Tim D, MacDonald D, Takayuki S, et al. Low postoperative hematocrit increases cerebrovascular damage after hypothermic circulatory arrest. *Pediatr Crit Care Med* 2005;6:319–26.
48. Smith MJ, Le Roux PD, Elliott JP, et al. Blood transfusion and increased risk for vasospasm and poor outcome after subarachnoid hemorrhage. *J Neurosurg* 2004;101:1–7.
49. Smith MJ, Stiefel MF, Magge S, et al. Packed red blood cell transfusion increases local cerebral oxygenation. *Crit Care Med* 2005;33:1104–8.
50. Spence RK, for the Blood Management Practice Guidelines Conference. Surgical red blood cell transfusion practice policies. *Am J Surg* 1995;170:S3–15.
51. Strauss R, Wehler M, Mehler K, et al. Thrombocytopenia in patients in the medical intensive care unit: Bleeding prevalence, transfusion requirements, and outcome. *Crit Care Med* 2002;30:1765–71.
52. Tsai AG, Cabrales P, Intaglietta M. Blood viscosity: A factor in tissue survival? *Crit Care Med* 2005;33:1662–3.
53. Tucci M, Lacroix J. Goal-directed Blood Transfusion Therapies. In: Nadkarni VM, ed. *Current Concepts in Pediatric Critical Care Course.* Des Plaines: Society of Critical Care Medicine, 2006:103–20.
54. Vamvakas EC, Pineda AA. Determinants of the efficacy of prophylactic granulocyte transfusions: A meta-analysis. *J Clin Apheresis* 1997;12:74–81.
55. Walsh TS. Is stored blood good enough for critically ill patients? *Crit Care Med* 2005;33:238–9.
56. Weldon BC. Blood conservation in pediatric anesthesia. *Anesthesiology Clin N Am* 2005;23:347–61.
57. Widness JA, Madan A, Grindeanu LA, et al. Reduction in red blood cell transfusions among preterm infants: Results of a randomized trial with an in-line blood gas and chemistry monitor. *Pediatrics* 2005;115:1299–306.
58. Williams GD, Bratton SL, Ramamoorthy C. Factors associated with blood loss and blood product transfusions: A multivariate analysis in children after open-heart surgery. *Anesth Analg* 1999;89:57–64.
59. Wong EC. Acute normovolemic hemodilution: A critical evaluation of its safety and utility in pediatric patients. *Transfusion Alternatives Transfusion Med* 2004;6:10–21.
60. Wong EC, Criss VR, Bhatia T, et al. Clinical experience on the use of 6- and 7-day platelets in pediatric patients. *Transfusion* 2006;46:10A.
61. Wong ECC. Irradiated product. In: Hillyer C, Strauss R, Luban NLC, eds. *Handbook of Pediatric Transfusion Medicine, 1st ed.* Amsterdam: Elsevier, 2004;101–12.
62. Wroe SJ, Pal S, Siddique D, et al. Clinical presentation and pre-mortem diagnosis of variant Creutzfeldt-Jakob disease associated with blood transfusion: A case report. *Lancet* 2006;368:2061–7.

CHAPTER 39 ■ PLASMAPHERESIS AND TRANSFUSION THERAPY

PETER W. SKIPPEN • NIRANJAN "TEX" KISSOON • CARON STRAHLENDORF • WARWICK W. BUTT

Apheresis (from the Greek, "to take away") involves the withdrawal of whole blood that is then processed to separate and remove particular constituents before being returned to the donor. Different techniques of pheresis are used, depending on the substance to be removed. Centrifugation, which can be applied with or without adsorption, is the technique that has the broadest application. In the critical care setting, the most commonly used method of apheresis is plasma exchange using membrane filtration.

Apheresis in children is challenging due to technical difficulties (especially in younger ages and smaller sizes), a lack of generally accepted indications and treatment schedules, and unclear end points of therapy. These factors contribute to the lack of strict inclusion/exclusion criteria and rigorous protocols under which apheresis is applied. Without such protocols and criteria, it is difficult to evaluate the effectiveness of apheresis in the many conditions in which it is employed (38).

One use of apheresis is to remove substances that are supposedly responsible for causing disease. However, uncertainty remains as to whether targeted substances are the causative agents of illness or merely markers of the disease state. In addition, many of the diseases treated are uncommon and subject to spontaneous relapses and remissions. The benefit of apheresis in these illnesses is thus difficult to judge. In addition, patients often receive multiple treatments for disease at the same time that they receive apheresis, so that any observed clinical changes are confounded as to which therapy provides exact benefit. For example, increase in muscle strength in Guillain-Barré syndrome or polyneuropathy is considered a positive response to therapy. However, changes in strength may be subjective findings and may be influenced by simultaneous treatments with steroids and immunoglobulins, which these patients are often receiving.

Despite these limitations, it is evident that apheresis techniques are used with some frequency in the ICU. This chapter focuses on the most common indications for apheresis in the PICU and discusses the evidence that supports its effectiveness. Discussion is limited to its use emergently in critically ill patients rather than its elective use in stable, chronic patients outside of the ICU. Areas of future investigation will also be discussed.

APHERESIS PROCEDURES

Apheresis techniques involve an extracorporeal circuit whereby blood is removed from the patient, separated into its various components that are then modified by interaction with either a centrifuge or a filter, and then returned to the patient. The technique used in individual patients depends on the particular blood element targeted for removal and/or replacement—either plasma or cellular (**Fig. 39.1**). The terms *plasmapheresis* and *therapeutic plasma exchange techniques* are used interchangeably and have the same meaning. These procedures remove large particles (up to 3,000,000 Daltons), as compared with hemofiltration (up to 50,000 Daltons).

Apheresis by centrifugation employs a blood cell separator that separates the blood components on the basis of differences in density or specific gravity. Whole blood from the patient enters the instrument and is driven through a separation channel (a semirigid, rectangular, plastic tube shaped into a ring) that rotates, generating a centrifugal force (**Fig. 39.2**). The centrifugal force separates the blood into a packed red blood cell (RBC) layer, a plasma layer, and a buffy coat in between, according to their specific gravity (**Fig. 39.3**). The heavier red cells move to the outer wall, while the lighter plasma moves to the inside wall of the separation chamber. Selective collection or removal of cellular components, such as white blood cells in cases of hyperleukocytosis, can be targeted according to the goal of therapy. Therapeutic exchanges of cellular components or plasma involve both removal of the targeted component and replacement with donor cells, plasma, or albumin. For example, RBCs are exchanged with those removed from patients in sickle cell crisis, while plasma is used to replace that taken off when autoimmune immunoglobulins are targeted during conditions such as myasthenia gravis.

Apheresis using a semipermeable filter membrane separates plasma from the whole blood based upon differences in solute size. The filter membrane is composed of porous, hollow fibers that are encased in a plastic cylinder (**Fig. 39.4**). The pores are large enough to allow passage of all blood elements, except the cellular components (**Fig. 39.5**). The principal mechanisms that determine clearance are filter surface area, filter flow, transmembrane pressure, and the sieving coefficients of molecules cleared. Disadvantages of membrane separation techniques over centrifugation are the need for central venous access to generate adequate blood flow and the fact that membrane separation is limited to removal and replacement of the plasma component only. An advantage of membrane filtration is that it can be performed at the bedside using special filters and the same machines that are used for renal replacement therapy (**Fig. 39.6**). It can also be combined with renal replacement therapy as an adjunct technique.

In this age of improved automation, manual exchange transfusion is rarely performed, but it remains the preferred method in the neonatal period. Access is obtained via the umbilical vessels. Observed fluid shifts are often easier to monitor using the manual technique of exchange transfusion.

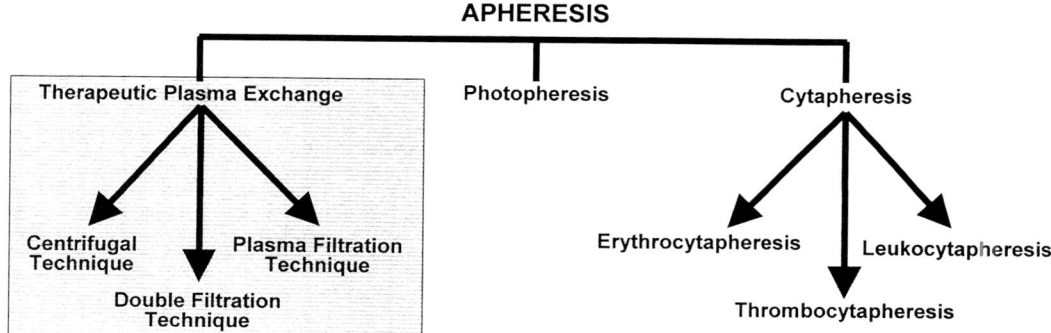

FIGURE 39.1. Apheresis refers to procedures that involve removing whole blood and separating it into its various components. Different techniques of apheresis exist. Blood components can be separated into various subunits based on therapeutic indications, and the remaining blood components are returned to the patient's bloodstream. Reproduced with permission from Gambro Canada.

PHYSIOLOGIC PRINCIPLES

Apheresis involves (a) the removal of substances that are implicated in causing some or all of the deleterious effects of a disease, or (b) the replacement of deficient substances from the plasma. For example, in diseases such as acute inflammatory demyelinating polyradiculopathy (AIDP) or myasthenia gravis, apheresis is used for the removal of autoimmune immunoglobulins. It can also be used to replace a plasma deficiency, such as in thrombotic thrombocytopenia purpura or help to modify the balance of proinflammatory and anti-inflammatory mediators in conditions such as sepsis.

While the exact mechanism of benefit of apheresis remains unclear for most therapeutic indications, the basic concepts are relatively simple. Apheresis techniques remove intravascular molecules more effectively than macromolecules that distribute widely in extravascular tissues. Extravascular molecules stored in the tissue may thus serve as a reservoir to replenish the bloodstream after circulating molecules have been removed by apheresis. The efficacy of an apheresis technique on removal of a molecule, therefore, depends on the molecule's distribution and the kinetics of production and catabolism. For most molecules, the rate of removal through apheresis far exceeds the rate of synthesis.

Molecular size is a more important factor affecting removal rates, as it determines access of the molecule to the intravascular space for removal by apheresis. For example, albumin, immunoglobulin G (IgG), IgA, and C3 complement are distributed similarly between the intravascular and extravascular space, whereas more than 75% of IgM and fibrinogen are retained within the intravascular space. As a result of these distributions, the proportion of these molecules removed from the intravascular compartment may be substantially different from that of the total body. Based on one-compartment modeling, a single-volume plasma exchange (approximately 40 mL/kg) using a continuous pheresis method will remove approximately 63% of the IgM and IgG from the intravascular compartment. The whole-body IgM and IgG levels, however, will only be reduced by 47% and 28%, respectively. If the exchange volume is increased to 1.5 times the estimated plasma volume, the IgM and IgG levels in plasma will fall even more (by 78%), while the whole-body IgM and IgG levels will fall by 59% and 35%, respectively (22).

The effects of repeated procedures on serum and total-body levels of targeted substances can be predicted based on an approximate 48-hr period for complete equilibration to occur between the intravascular and extravascular spaces. For example, a goal of reduction in whole-body immunoglobulins by 85%–90% would require four single-volume plasma exchanges to deplete whole-body IgM and six to seven exchanges to reduce IgG by a similar percentage. Increasing the exchange volume to 1.5 volume exchanges would reduce the number of total procedures required to only three to five to obtain similar removal of IgM and IgG.

In contrast to solute removal, removal of cells with apheresis is less efficient because of sequestration, which occurs in the liver and spleen, and adherence of cells to the vascular endothelium. Total circulating blood volume, rates of cell production, and release from extravascular sites also affect the amount of cellular depletion that can be obtained with apheresis. Because of these considerations, somewhat larger exchange volumes may be required to achieve clinically significant reductions in cell components. Modern cell separators are efficient in cellular depletions but require at least two times total blood volume exchanges for significant reductions to occur.

TREATMENT CONSIDERATIONS

Prior to considering apheresis therapy for a clinical condition in the PICU, one or more of the following considerations should be met:

- The target substance must be toxic to the patient or resistant to conventional therapy, or conventional therapy must have failed.
- The target substance must be accessible to apheresis; i.e., distributed primarily in the intravascular space.
- The target substance has a long half-life such that an extracorporeal clearance technique becomes more efficient than endogenous clearance.
- The target substance cannot be removed by simpler techniques, such as hemodialysis.

Successful apheresis requires meticulous attention to issues pertaining to vascular access, anticoagulation, and maintenance of intravascular volumes (18,22).

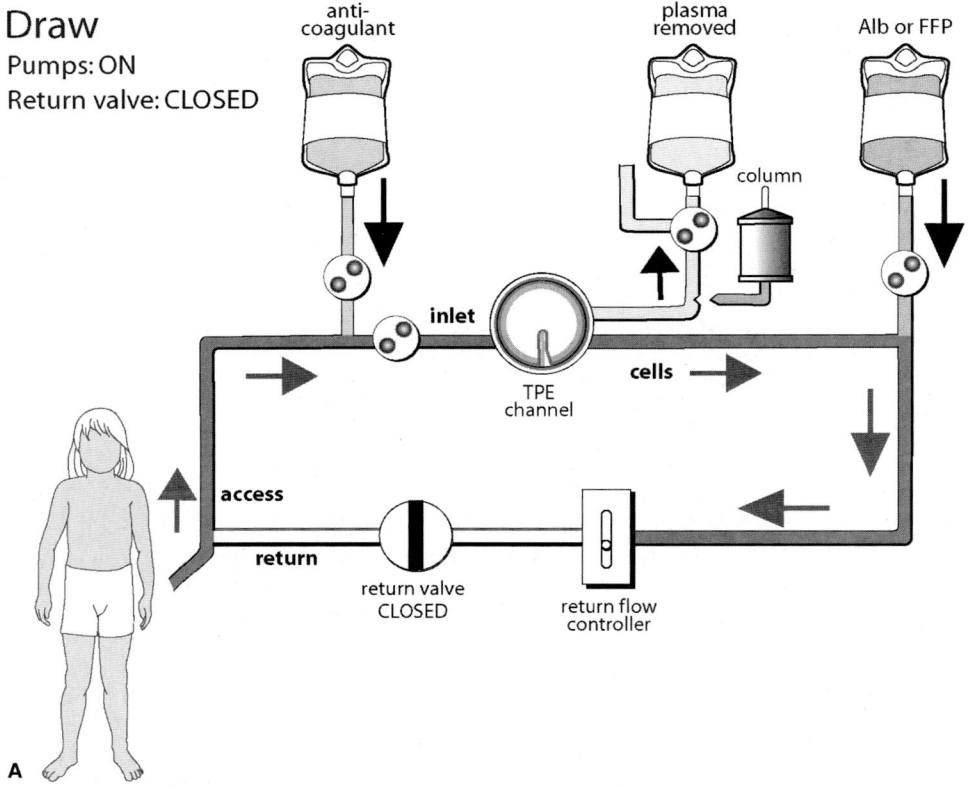

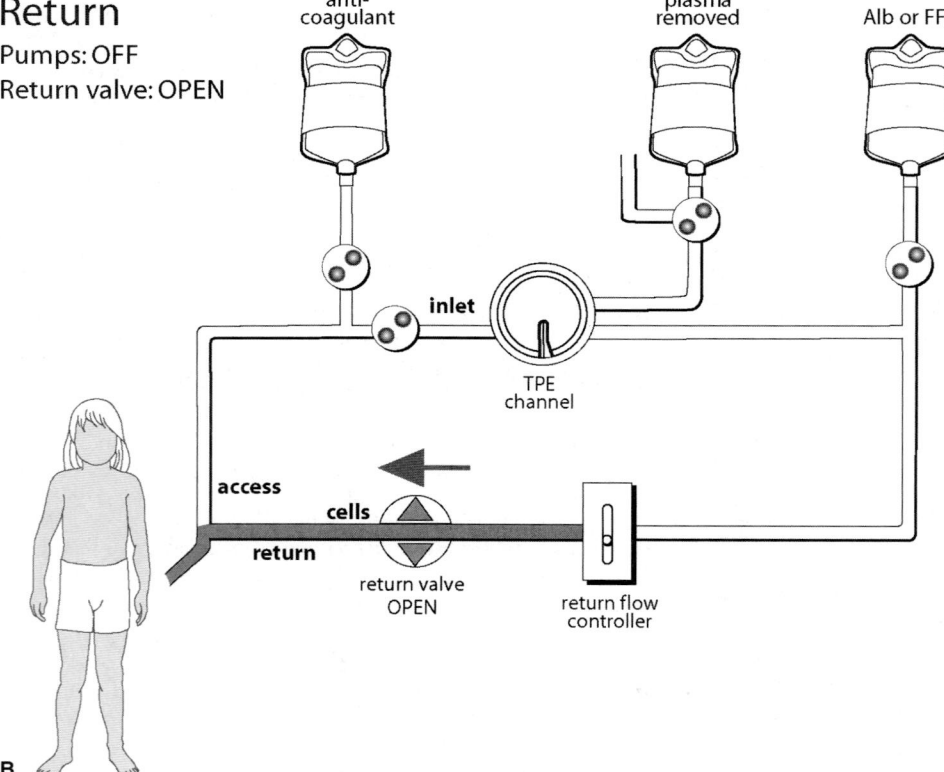

FIGURE 39.2. A: Schematic representation of centrifugal pump technique. In this figure, blood is withdrawn from the patient and separated into the various components. **B:** Blood is returned to the patient after separation and removal of the presumed noxious fraction of blood component. Reproduced with permission from Gambro Canada.

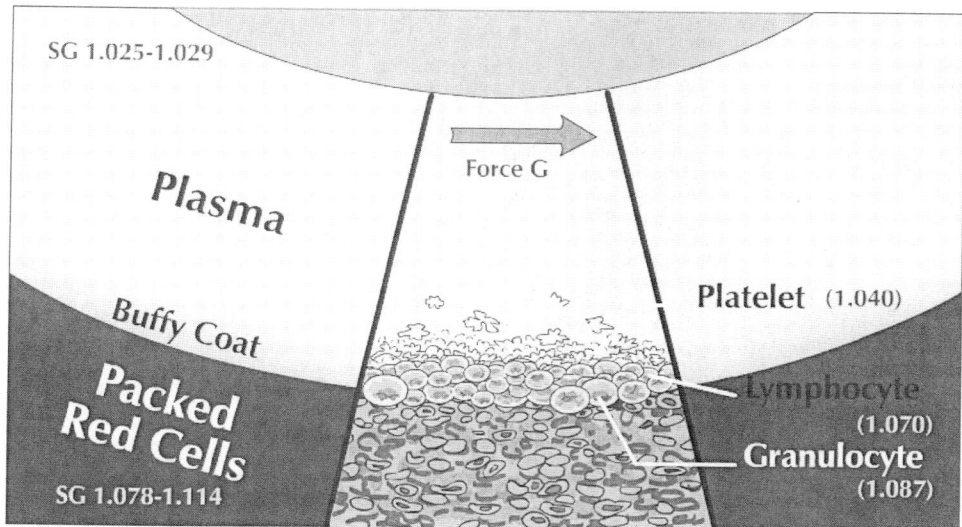

FIGURE 39.3. The mechanism of separation of blood components by centrifugal force based on specific gravity of the different blood elements in the separation chamber. The heaviest blood components are separated along the outside wall of the spinning channel. Plasma is the lightest component, and locates along the inside wall of the separation channel. Reproduced with permission from Gambro Canada.

Vascular Access

Like other hemofiltration procedures, adequate vascular access is a prerequisite to accommodate the high flow rates required to process between one and two blood volumes over the course of a few hours. Access flows of only 35–50 mL/min are required for centrifugal exchange, allowing the use of large-bore peripheral catheters, while membrane techniques require blood flow rates >100 mL/min, which necessitates central venous access. The size of the patient and technique used determine the actual access requirements. For example, depending on the size of the patient and the desired total filtration volume, a double-volume plasma exchange could be performed over 5–6 hrs with flows of only 25–60 mL/hr, using a large surface area filter, such as the Gambro PF 1000 or PF 2000. Intermittent apheresis techniques require cannulation of a single large vein. Continuous-flow procedures require cannulation of two vessels. In larger patients, this might be achieved through two large peripheral catheters: one for withdrawal and one for return of blood. In smaller children, peripheral veins are not adequate and central venous access using noncollapsible double-lumen hemodialysis

catheters is necessary. The catheter requirements are similar to those required for renal replacement procedures (see Chapter 37). A 6.5–7 French (fr) double-lumen catheter is usually suitable for patients who weigh up to 10–15 kg. Where available, an 8 fr catheter can be used in children up to 25 kg. A 10–11.5 fr catheter is suitable for adolescents.

For patients who require hemapoietic progenitor stem cell collection, a temporary dialysis catheter must often be inserted in the PICU. A cell separator is used to collect the desired number of CD34[+] cells. Although the collection is often not performed in the PICU, assistance may be requested from the PICU team for sedation and insertion of the catheter.

Anticoagulation

To maintain patency of the extracorporeal circuit, some form of anticoagulation must be used. As apheresis in the ICU patient is often used in the sickest patients with the highest bleeding risk, anticoagulation techniques that are regional in the apheresis circuit or that do not exert systemic anticoagulation are desired. A buffered citrate solution added to the patient's

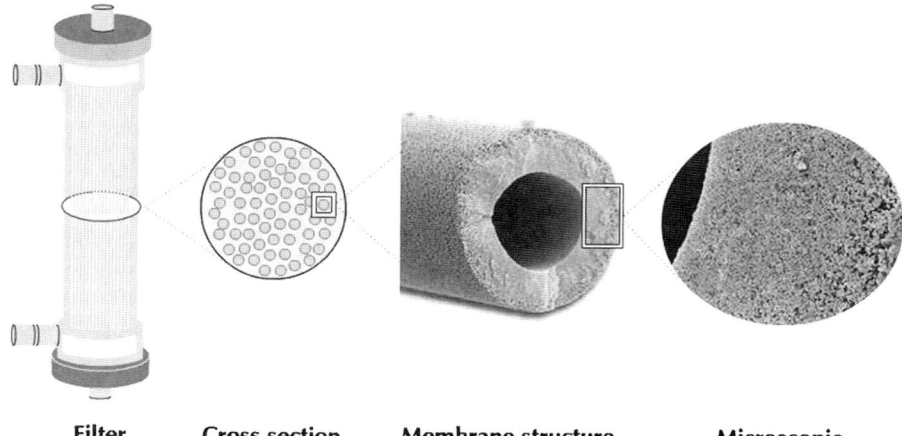

Filter   Cross section   Membrane structure   Microscopic membrane structure

FIGURE 39.4. Cross-section of a plasma membrane filter, demonstrating hollow-fiber technology. Whole blood is pumped through the plasma filter, generating a transmembrane pressure across the filter membrane. The pore sizes are large enough to allow passage of all plasma constituents except the cellular elements. The plasma-free blood is returned to the patient. Reproduced with permission from Gambro Canada.

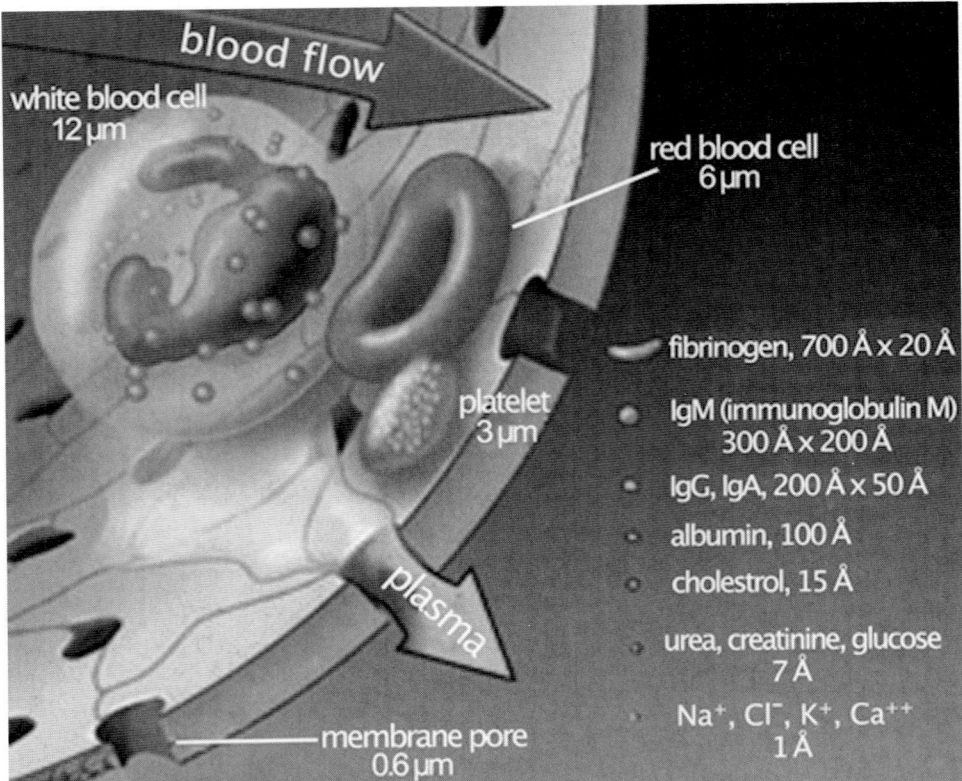

FIGURE 39.5. Cross-section of a single hollow fiber of a plasma membrane filter, demonstrating the pore sizes large enough to allow passage of all plasma constituents except the cellular elements. Reproduced with permission from Gambro Canada.

blood as it is withdrawn has become a common anticoagulant used for centrifugation apheresis procedures (**Fig. 39.1**). Citrate acts by chelating the ionized calcium in the extracorporeal circuit without inducing a systemic anticoagulant effect in the patient. Higher blood flows require higher citrate flows. Modern apheresis instruments automatically adjust citrate flow rates depending upon the blood flow rate into the extracorporeal circuit. Regional anticoagulation is achieved with circuit intracellular calcium (iCa^{2+}) levels between 0.3–0.4 mmol/L. Citrate has a half-life of 30 mins and is readily metabolized. A calcium bolus may be required to prevent or treat the clinical signs of hypocalcemia due to citrate toxicity. Alkalosis may also be encountered, depending on the duration of the exchange and the total volume of citrate solution infused.

Membrane separation techniques used in the PICU are often applied to the sickest patients who have high risk of bleeding as a consequence of their underlying disease. The risk of bleeding from anticoagulation must be balanced against the risk of clotting in the extracorporeal circuit. Unfractionated heparin is more commonly used for membrane separation techniques and is typically administered prefilter. When heparin is used as the anticoagulant of choice, circuit and patient activated clotting time (ACT) levels are monitored, with circuit ACTs ideally maintained around 1.5 times normal in an attempt to minimize patient bleeding complications. The membrane removes most of the heparin (free and protein bound). In some centers, unfractionated heparin is used concurrently with citrate, reducing the amount of both heparin and citrate required to prevent plasma filter clotting.

Large-volume exchanges deplete the patient's native circulating coagulation factors. Periodic monitoring of these factors is required, especially if products other than plasma are used for repletion and maintenance of intravascular volume.

Maintenance of Intravascular Volume

An important aspect of apheresis is maintaining constant intravascular volume during the procedure while removing the desired plasma or cellular components. The patient's fluid status may be altered through volume loss, overload, and/or hemodilution. The extent of initial volume loss depends on the comparative size of the extracorporeal circuit volume to the patient's blood volume, the hemodilution associated with the technique, the volume removed by the apheresis, and the replacement solution used. The ability of the critically ill child to compensate for acute volume or hemodilution changes depends upon the patient's cardiac, pulmonary, and renal functions. Any combination of crystalloid, albumin, fresh frozen plasma or IV immunoglobulin (IVIG) can be prescribed as replacement solutions to replace the plasma that is removed and discarded with the procedure, tailored to a specific child's other clinical issues (e.g., liver failure or severe sepsis). More commonly, dilution of plasma constituents may require replacement with blood component factors, depending upon the extent of the coagulation abnormality, risk factors for bleeding, the size of the exchange performed, and the replacement solution used.

The extracorporeal volume is dependent on the type of equipment and the technique (intermittent vs. continuous), and the type of procedure (e.g., leukapheresis vs. plasmapheresis). In smaller patients, extracorporeal volume depletion has a

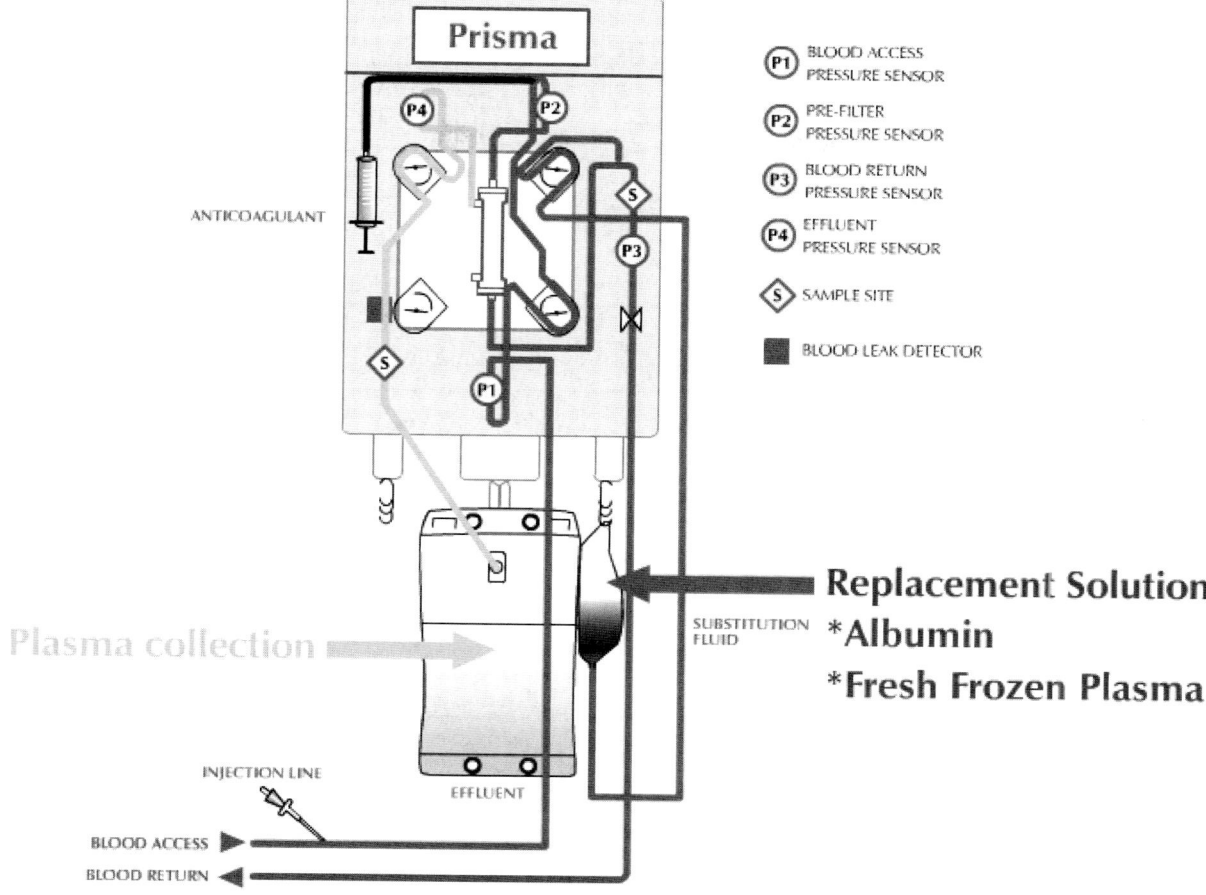

FIGURE 39.6. Schematic representation of Prisma membrane separation circuitry. Numerous manufacturers produce this technology, but the circuitry and separation principles are similar among manufacturers.

greater effect on hemodynamic parameters. A maximum extracorporeal volume to be removed should be established for each patient. Continuous techniques require lower priming volumes and are therefore the preferred choice for hemodynamically unstable or small children. Limits should be set on the volume shifts that occur during apheresis in unstable patients. It is generally recommended that volume shifts be <15% of the total blood volume during and after the procedure. Close monitoring of hemodynamic variables is required to ensure isovolemia and hemodynamic stability.

Maintenance of Red Cell Volume

The separation chambers in centrifugal apheresis instruments vary widely in their requirement for specific volumes of packed cells to establish and maintain separation gradients. A red cell deficit occurs (dependent upon the equipment chosen and procedure performed) as the centrifuge chamber is filled at the start of the apheresis procedure (**Table 39.1**). Volumes up to 1000 mL may be required to fill the chambers at initiation. A patient's age, weight, hematocrit, and clinical cardiorespiratory status determine tolerance of hemodilution and ability to maintain adequate oxygen delivery. Therefore, like volume

shifts, the safe minimum hematocrit should be established before the procedure.

Total blood volume and red cell volume must be calculated according to the patient age, sex, and body habitus. If the extracorporeal volume is >15% of the patient's total estimated blood volume, priming of the apheresis machine with packed red cells should be considered. In practice, to minimize the impact of the circuit extracorporeal volume on patients who weigh <25 kg, an allogeneic blood prime that is discarded at the end of the procedure is usually performed. An alternate technique involves using a blood prime when the desired RBC depletion exceeds 30% of the original circulating red cell volume. In larger patients or in those in whom some degree of hemodilution is likely to be well tolerated, isotonic crystalloid or colloid can be infused during the initiation of the procedure to maintain cardiovascular stability until the separation chamber is filled. Anemia may develop with repeated chronic apheresis, as small amounts of red cells are left in the disposable sets at the end of each procedure. During red cell exchanges or depletions, careful attention must be paid to the desired red cell volume and hematocrit to be maintained in the patient. The cell separator can be programmed to calculate and maintain the desired patient parameters.

TABLE 39.1

EXTRACORPOREAL VOLUMES OF VARIOUS SETS ON THE COBE SPECTRA SYSTEM

	Disposable tubing set volume	Total equivalent whole blood volume[a]	Total RBC volume[a]	Residual RBC volume[a]	Amount of blood diverted to tubing set from patient at start of procedure
Dual-needle TPE	285 mL	170 mL	68 mL	15 mL	150 mL
Dual-needle RBCX	285 mL	170 mL	68 mL	15 mL	100 mL
WBC procedures	285 mL	285 mL	114 mL	24 mL	150 mL

[a]The volumes are calculated based on a hematocrit of 40%.
RBC, red blood cell; TPE, therapeutic plasma exchange; RBCX, red blood cell exchange; WBC, white blood cell

Potential Complications of Apheresis Procedures

Complications related to apheresis are most commonly due to difficulties with vascular access or related to the procedure itself. Vascular access-related problems are discussed in Chapter 25. Procedure-related considerations include intravascular fluid, red cell volume shifts, and citrate toxicity. In addition, with erythrocytapheresis and leukapheresis procedures, reduction of platelets may occur. With any of the exchange procedures, it may be necessary to replace clotting factors and immunoglobulins.

Protein-bound drugs, such as acetylsalicylic acid, tobramycin, phenytoin, and β-blockers, may also be removed. These problems may be more clinically significant in small patients or in those who are critically ill and receiving apheresis techniques.

INDICATIONS

Most indications for apheresis fall within four main categories of disease: neurologic, hematologic/oncologic, autoimmune/rheumatic, and renal/metabolic. An additional ill-defined group includes sepsis syndrome and multiorgan failure with thrombocytopenia. Most apheresis is performed outside the realm of the PICU. Common conditions are listed in Table 39.2.

Evidence-based indications and guidelines for apheresis have been published by the American Society for Apheresis and endorsed by the American Association of Blood Banks (38). Current recommendations reveal few well-established indications and few with category I evidence (Tables 39.3, 39.4, and 39.5). Many of the indications for apheresis occur in patients with chronic disease, and these cases do not require the expertise of the intensive care team. On rare occasions, however, deranged physiology or complicating factors in these patients necessitates PICU admission. A few randomized, controlled trials of apheresis have been conducted in children, but most recommendations are derived from adult studies, anecdotal reports, or single-centered case series. The resulting evidence for the use of apheresis is often of lesser quality than for most other acute and critical illnesses. In addition to questions regarding the effectiveness of apheresis as a therapy in critically ill patients, other questions that remain unanswered include the frequency of therapy to be given, the total number of therapies applied, the replacement fluids that should be used, and the volume of exchange required. Despite all of these limitations, it would appear that the use of apheresis techniques in the PICU is rising at this writing. Further study should

TABLE 39.2

COMMON CONDITIONS TREATED WITH APHERESIS

Diagnosis	# of Patients	# of Filters	Average length (hrs)	Length range (hrs)	Average age (yrs)	Age range (yrs)
Sepsis	107	152	18.4	0–184	5.8	0–17
Autoimmune	53	290	6.7	1–184	8.6	0.1–15.5
Transplant	10	25	14.7	2–120	12.5	1.2–17.6
Oncology	6	8	10.6	4–44	9.5	1.8–15.7
Inborn error of metabolism	4	6	11	4–24	7	3–12.9
Liver	9	44	8.4	3–29	5.7	1.3–14.4
Hemophilia	1	1	4	4	1.40	1.4
Other	1	1	–	–	3.00	3
Pancreatitis	1	2	–	–	15.5	15.5
Pertussis	1	1	24	24	0.8	0.8
Poisoning/drug overdose	4	6	4.7	4	7.9	1.2–16.6

TABLE 39.3

GUIDELINES FOR APHERESIS—CATEGORY I

Disease	Procedure
Antiglomerular basement membrane antibody disease	Plasmapheresis
Thrombotic thrombocytopenic purpura	Plasmapheresis
Hyperleukocytosis	Leukapheresis
Sickle cell disease	Erythrocytapheresis
Thrombocytosis	Plateletpheresis
Posttransfusion purpura	Plasmapheresis
Guillain-Barré syndrome	Plasmapheresis
Chronic inflammatory demyelinating polyradiculoneuropathy	Plasmapheresis
Myasthenia crisis	Plasmapheresis
Demyelinating polyneuropathy with IgG and IgA	Plasmapheresis

Category I: Apheresis is standard and acceptable either as primary treatment or primary line adjunctive based on randomized, controlled trials or broad noncontroversial evidence.
Adapted from criteria endorsed by the American Association of Blood Banks. Smith JW, Weinstein R, Hillyer KL for the AABB Hemapheresis Committee. Therapeutic apheresis: A summary of current indication categories endorsed by the AABB and the American Society of Apheresis. *Transfusion* 2003;43:820–2.

TABLE 39.4

GUIDELINES FOR APHERESIS—CATEGORY II

Disease	Procedure
Rapidly progressive glomerulonephritis	Plasmapheresis
Acute renal failure post transplant	Plasmapheresis
Cryoglobulinemia (adults)	Plasmapheresis
Idiopathic thrombocytopenic purpura (refractory)	Immunoabsorption
Polycythemia vera or erythrocytosis	Erythrocytapheresis
Hyperviscosity (monoclonal IgM, IgA, IgG)	Erythrocytapheresis
Coagulation factor inhibitors	Plasmapheresis
Demyelinating polyneuropathy with IgM	Plasmapheresis/ immunoabsorption
Lambert-Eaton myasthenia syndrome	Plasmapheresis
Inflammatory bowel disease[a]	Plasmapheresis
Hypercholesterolemia[b]	Leukocyte pheresis Low-density lipoprotein apheresis

Category II: Evidence is generally supportive or adjunctive based on randomized, controlled trials or case studies.
[a]Data from Sawada K, Kusugami K, Suzuki Y. Leukocytapheresis in ulcerative colitis: Results of a multicentre double-blind prospective case-control study with sham apheresis as a placebo treatment. *Am J Gastroenterol* 2005;100:1362–69.
[b]Data from Ziajka P. Role of low-density lipoprotein apheresis. *Am J Cardiol* 2005;96(4):67–9.
Adapted from criteria endorsed by the American Association of Blood Banks. Smith JW, Weinstein R, Hillyer KL for the AABB Hemapheresis Committee. Therapeutic apheresis: A summary of current indication categories endorsed by the AABB and the American Society of Apheresis. *Transfusion* 2003;43:820–2.

TABLE 39.5

GUIDELINES FOR APHERESIS—CATEGORY III

Disease	Procedure
Hemolytic uremic syndrome	Plasmapheresis
Systemic lupus erythematosus	Plasmapheresis
Vasculitis	Erythrocytapheresis
Malaria or babesiosis	Plasmapheresis
Multiple sclerosis (acute, fulminant) (adults)	Plasmapheresis
Drug overdose and poisoning	Plasmapheresis
Acute hepatic failure	Plasmapheresis
Acute disseminated encephalomyelitis[a]	Plasmapheresis

Category III: Apheresis not indicated but reasonable as salvage therapy after failure of conventional therapy and lack of other options.
[a]Data from Khurana DS, Melvin JJ, Kothore SV. Acute disseminate encephalomyelitis in children: Discordant neurologic and neuroimaging abnormalities and response to plasmapheresis. *Pediatrics* 2005;116:431–6.
Adapted from criteria endorsed by the American Association of Blood Banks. Smith JW, Weinstein R, Hillyer KL for the AABB Hemapheresis Committee. Therapeutic apheresis: A summary of current indication categories endorsed by the AABB and the American Society of Apheresis. *Transfusion* 2003;43:820–2.

clarify some of the issues surrounding its efficacy and technical considerations.

AIDP, commonly referred to as Guillain-Barre syndrome, is the best-studied condition for which plasmapheresis is recommended. For all other category I indications, including thrombotic thrombocytopenic purpura (TTP), studies have been nonrandomized or case series. Despite this limitation, some disease states have demonstrated a remarkable reduction in mortality over time since the introduction of plasmapheresis. For example, the treatment of TTP with plasma exchanges has resulted in a markedly decreased mortality rate from 90% to 10% (29).

Emergency indications for apheresis relevant to the PICU include posttransfusion purpura and bleeding, TTP, red cell exchange for acute chest syndrome in sickle cell anemia, and pulmonary or central nervous system complications of hyperleukocytosis associated with acute leukemia (23). Even when indicated, the duration of therapy and number of treatments are unclear and will vary between conditions treated. For example, the treatment for Goodpasture syndrome, myasthenia gravis, and TTP is prolonged over weeks to months and is often associated with multiple other therapeutic interventions.

Most centers usually treat a small number of patients with varying diagnoses; hence, it is difficult to judge the effectiveness of apheresis for these conditions. The difficulty in judging clinical response to apheresis is exemplified by the following cases in which apheresis was used.

Neurologic Disease

A 14-year-old girl with AIDP secondary to mycoplasma was admitted to the PICU intubated and ventilated for progressive weakness and respiratory failure. She did not respond to the initial course of IVIG (2 g/kg) and was treated with four plasma exchanges (1.5× plasma volume exchanges on alternate days), commencing 4 days after admission. She was able to be extubated after the third course. This patient demonstrates a clear temporal relationship with clinical improvement and the initiation of plasmapheresis.

Another 15-year-old patient with AIDP secondary to systemic lupus erythematosus had a prolonged PICU course because of respiratory failure. She required several courses of plasma exchanges but was also treated with methylprednisone, cyclophosphamide, and IVIG. Although she improved over 3 weeks, it is difficult to judge the influence of plasma exchange on the clinical course of this patient in light of the other therapies that were offered.

In the 1980s, 2 large studies confirmed the effectiveness of plasmapheresis in Guillain-Barre syndrome (11,13). More recently, one group was able to stratify severity of illness and randomized each of these groups to a different number of exchanges (12). Based on this study, the Cochrane Group reviewed the effect of plasmapheresis session frequency and found no difference in response to four or six plasma exchanges in severe AIDP. No difference in efficacy of plasmapheresis over IVIG was noted (15).

Rheumatic/Autoimmune Disease

A 14-year-old girl presented to the pediatric intensive care unit with pulmonary hemorrhage and acute respiratory failure due to Wegener granulomatosis. Despite aggressive intensive care that included broad-spectrum antibiotics, RBC transfusions, and high-frequency oscillatory ventilation, she required extracorporeal life support 2 days after intubation for progressive hypoxemic respiratory failure. Following the diagnosis, she was started on cyclophosphamide and methylprednisolone and was given three plasma exchanges. She was weaned off of extracorporeal support 4 days after cannulation and extubated 10 days after admission. The confounding therapies are amply evident; hence, it is difficult to tease out the contribution of apheresis. Although vasculitis is only a category III indication, the additional risks associated with apheresis in a child already on extracorporeal life support were felt to be minimal and potentially beneficial.

Autoimmune Disease

A 9-year-old boy with neurologic cysticercosis developed toxic epidermal necrolysis after being administered carbamazepine for a seizure disorder. He required intubation 2 days after admission to the PICU for stridor, after which he received four daily doses of IVIG (1 g/kg/dose) without apparent response. Two days after intubation, he received daily plasmapheresis (1.5× volume exchanges with albumin replacement) for 5 days. Significant clinical improvement in the rash was seen within 48 hrs of initiating plasmapheresis, and he was extubated 6 days after commencing plasmapheresis. It was decided to treat this child based on a case series that showed some benefit in disease progression (rash and mucositis as seen in this child) despite IgG treatment. However, the role of plasmapheresis in the resolution of this patient's illness remains speculative.

HEMATOLOGIC/THROMBOTIC CONDITIONS

Hyperviscosity Syndromes

Hyperviscosity syndromes are characterized by sludging and decreased perfusion of the microvasculature due to increased blood viscosity. Hyperviscosity syndromes are classified on the basis of blood components (1) as (a) pleocytosis syndromes (increase in blood cells—red, white, or platelets), (b) sclerocitic syndromes (sickle cell, malaria), or (c) seiric syndromes (cryoglobulins, paraproteins). Only those conditions of relevance to pediatric practice are discussed here.

Pleocytosis Syndromes

Hyperleukocytosis. Leukapheresis, or therapeutic depletion of leukocytes, is used for hyperleukocytosis associated with leukemia. Extreme leukocytosis can cause sludging in the small vessels in the brain, leading to cerebral vascular hemorrhage. More commonly, pulmonary leukocytosis can result in respiratory compromise (34). Moreover, hyperleukocytosis is associated with early morbidity and mortality. Decreasing white blood cell loads to safe levels can be achieved easily with plasma exchange, evidenced by the effect of two leukapheretic exchanges (Table 39.6) in a 5-month-old with hyperleukocytosis due to acute leukemia. This child presented with a bulging fontanelle and acute respiratory failure and required intubation and mechanical ventilation shortly after admission to the PICU. The child was extubated 9 days after leukapheresis.

Neonatal Polycythemia. Exchange transfusion or erythrocytapheresis has been recommended for neonatal polycythemia because it may decrease blood viscosity and, hence, improve tissue perfusion and decrease hypoxemia and organ dysfunction. However, little documentation is available of long-term outcomes in neonates treated with exchange transfusion. Moreover, basic criteria as to whom should be treated are lacking. This is of importance because only 24% of neonates with cord hyperviscosity had polycythemia, and only 48% of polycythemic infants had hyperviscosity (10,36). Therefore, the traditional use of hematocrit as a clinical criterion for judging hyperviscosity is dubious. A recent systematic review found no

TABLE 39.6

RESULTS OF LEUKAPHERETIC EXCHANGES IN HYPERLEUKOCYTOSIS

	Initial parameters	Post 1st run	Post 2nd run
WBC × 10⁹/L	972	521	198
HgB g/L	52	66	64
Plt × 10⁹/L	18	76	42
Hct	0.16	0.20	0.20
Ca²⁺ mmol/L		0.94	0.99
WBC in effluent		406,000	440,650

WBC, white blood cell; HgB, hemoglobin; Plt, platelet; Hct, hematocrit long-term neurodevelopmental benefit from partial exchange in polycythemic infants and suggested that the long-term outcome is more likely related to the underlying cause of the polycythemia. Of concern was a relative risk of development of necrotizing enterocolitis of 8.68 in patients who received partial exchange (95% confidence interval, 1.06–71.1) (9).

Thrombocytosis. Uncontrolled thrombocytosis associated with myeloproliferative disorders may result in either severe thrombosis or hemorrhage. However, these conditions are rare in children. Platelet depletion (plateletpheresis) aims to reduce the platelet count to the near normal range (<600,000/mcL).

Sclerocytic Syndromes

Sickle Cell Disease. Exchange transfusion has been used in sickle cell disease for the treatment of stroke (8), severe intrahepatic cholestasis (7), prevention of sickling (2,19), and in bilateral retinal artery occlusion (41). However, most of these are anecdotal reports or small series that lacked controls. Of relevance to critical care practitioners is the unresolved debate over whether red cell transfusion is as effective as exchange transfusion and whether plasma exchange should be performed prior to patients undergoing cardiopulmonary bypass (14,26). However, the role of exchange transfusion in sickle cell crisis and in acute chest syndrome is well established. Evidence has shown that double-volume exchange transfusion lowers blood viscosity, relieves vaso-occlusion, and improves tissue oxygen delivery (40). The pre- and post-HbS quantification is helpful and may be a useful end-point to determine transfusion requirements. Improvement in tissue oxygen delivery could also be used as a reasonable end-point for titrating exchange transfusion in sickle cell disease. Other possible end-points, such as lowering of white blood count, platelets, or vascular cell adhesion molecule (VCAM)-1 levels, are short-lived and inconsistent, whereas no consistent pattern is seen in tumor necrosis factor (TNF)-α or IL1-α levels following exchange transfusion for sickle cell disease (21).

Malaria. The Centers for Disease Control recommends plasma exchange for *Plasmodium falciparum* infection when parasitemia is $\geq 10\%$, although exchange transfusion in malaria has yielded mixed results (31). The intent of transfusion in malaria is to reduce parasitic load and inflammatory mediators, such as TNF-α. A pediatric case series of 3 patients with renal and central nervous system involvement demonstrated good response and 100% survival using a single-volume RBC exchange transfusion (4). However, a meta-analysis of randomized clinical trials that evaluated chemotherapy-only versus exchange transfusion as adjunctive therapy reported that exchange transfusion failed to increase survival (33). Clinical experience suggests that patients with large parasitic loads may benefit from decreasing these levels and that doing so results in chemotherapy being more effective.

Miscellaneous Hematologic Disorders

Plasma therapies are also being applied to thrombotic disorders, the best known of which is TTP, which involves an acquired autoantibody-mediated severe deficiency of ADAMTS 13 (A disintegrin and metalloprotease with thrombospondin type 1 motif), a plasma metalloprotease that is responsible for

cleaving large von Willebrand factor multimers (24). Plasma exchange allows replacement of the deficient factor with fresh frozen plasma. Mortality for this condition has decreased from 90% to <10% following the introduction of plasma exchange as a therapy.

Posttransfusion purpura is a rare bleeding disorder of platelet alloimmunization. It appears with sudden onset of severe thrombocytopenia and purpura, and is often associated with life-threatening hemorrhage. No single modality has proven effective alone, but plasmapheresis has been effective after failure of corticosteroids and IVIG.

Other

Plasmapheresis in Sepsis

Sepsis is one of the leading causes of death in children. Clinical derangements are thought to be due to the action of inflammatory and anti-inflammatory mediators. The inhibition or removal of these mediators by plasmapheresis is thought to be of possible benefit (6). However, results have been mixed. The postulated benefits of plasmapheresis include modulation or removal of contributing or causal factors, such as endotoxin from bacteria, antigens, antibodies, cell debris, activating enzymes, coagulation activating factors, cytokines, compliment factors, removal of inhibitory factors, or a combination of these (25,39).

Although animal studies using plasma exchange have generally produced unfavorable results, several clinical studies have shown benefits, depending on the stated treatment effects. A small study of 30 patients (adults and children) with sepsis syndrome demonstrated the removal of a wide variety of acute-phase proteins and complement fragments, but did not influence IL-6 concentrations, thromboxane B_2, total white cell count, or platelet count. This study failed to show a difference in mortality or number of organs failing (32). A study of 106 consecutive adult patients with severe sepsis or septic shock randomized to either standard therapy or add-on plasmapheresis therapy reported a 28-day all-cause mortality of 33.3% (18/54) in the plasmapheresis group and 53.8% (28/52) in the control group (6). The number needed to treat was 4.9 for benefit of plasmapheresis over control. However, comparability of treatment groups was problematic.

Small pediatric studies have attempted to demonstrate an amelioration of the hemodynamic effects of sepsis, but lack of control of the volume and type of replacement solution given is a confounding variable (3). In another small study, some children with sepsis-induced multiorgan failure and thrombocytopenia were shown to have reduced or absent von Willebrand factor cleaving protease activity and increased tissue plasminogen activator type-1. Prolonged therapy with plasma exchange (up to 11 days) reversed the deficiency and was associated with an improvement in the multiorgan failure (28).

Apheresis in sepsis fails to demonstrate an improvement in outcome because many studies have small numbers of patients and historical controls. The low mortality rate in pediatric sepsis (10%–15%) requires the recruitment of large patient numbers to demonstrate a survival benefit in children. As a result, other outcome measures are being employed in pediatric studies, such as the pediatric logistic organ dysfunction (PELOD) score (20).

Plasma Exchange in Drug Toxicity

Plasma exchange may be of benefit for poisoning with drugs with high protein binding and low volume of distribution. It has been used effectively in vancomycin toxicity (5), theophylline poisoning (30,37), neonatal lead poisoning in combination with chelation (27), and isobutyl nitrate-induced methemoglobinemia (16). All are case reports that have shown relevant decreases in drug levels and good clinical outcomes. However, the lack of controls makes it difficult to ascertain the contribution of plasma exchange to outcomes.

CONCLUSIONS AND FUTURE DIRECTIONS

Future studies are necessary to define when apheresis should be used and specific outcome measures with which to determine its effectiveness. For instance, in sepsis, specific goals ultimately must be tied to a decrease in death and disability. For hyperviscosity syndromes such as polycythemia, measurement of viscosity may be an important surrogate end-point; however, long-term studies should be designed to determine the outcome of these patients. In sickle cell disease, goals such as improved tissue oxygenation or reducing hyperviscosity are favorable physiologic variables, provided they can be tied to relevant clinical end-points such as morbidity and mortality. The rationale for use of apheresis in immunologic conditions will rely on studies that address the influence of confounding therapies, long time lines, and the use of objective measurements to determine response. These studies are difficult to undertake and apheresis will continue to be one of several therapies offered in selected patients who suffer from these conditions.

KEY POINTS

- Apheresis refers to several techniques for the removal or modification of blood components.
- Technical difficulties in younger patients and the need for meticulous attention to vascular access, anticoagulation, and volume removed render apheresis challenging in the critically ill, unstable patient.
- Indications for apheresis fall into four main categories: neurologic, hematologic/oncologic, autoimmune/rheumatic, and renal/metabolic. Indications relevant to the PICU include posttransfusion purpura and bleeding, TTP, red cell removal in the acute chest syndrome of sickle cell disease, and hyperleukocytosis with pulmonary and central nervous system complications.
- The PICU indications may be associated with clear-cut end-points and outcomes, such as decreased levels of sickle cells or leukocytes; however, in diseases requiring chronic treatment, such as autoimmune and rheumatic diseases, the tendency for spontaneous relapse and remission and confounding therapies renders an evaluation of the effect of apheresis difficult.

ACKNOWLEDGMENT

The authors thank Gambro Canada for the use of Figures 39.1, 39.2, 39.3, 39.4, and 39.5.

References

1. Accorsi P, Passeri D, Onofrillo D, et al. Hyperviscosity syndrome in hematologic diseases and therapeutic apheresis. *Int J Artif Organs* 2005;28:1032–8.
2. Alvari JB. Sickle cell anemia: Pathophysiology and treatment. *Med Clin North Am* 1984;3:545–56.
3. Berlot G, Gullo A, Fasiolo S, et al. Hemodynamic effects of plasma exchange in septic patients: Preliminary report. *Blood Purif* 1997;15(1):45–53.
4. Boctor F. Red blood cell exchange transfusion as an adjunct treatment for severe plasma falciparum malaria, using automated or manual procedures. *Pediatrics* 2005;116(e592):e595.
5. Burkhart KK, Metcalf S, Shurnas E, et al. Exchange transfusion and multidose activated charcoal following vancomycin overdose. *J Toxicol Clin Toxicol* 1992;30(2):285–94.
6. Busund R, Kouklime V, Utrobin U. Plasmapheresis in severe sepsis and septic shock: A prospective randomized controlled trial. *Intensive Care Med* 2002;28:1434–9.
7. Chitturi S, George J, Ranjitkumar S, et al. Exchange transfusion for severe intrahepatic cholestasis associated with sickle cell disease? *J Clin Gastroenterol* 2002;35(4):362–3.
8. Cohen AR, Martin MB, Silber JH, et al. A modified transfusion program for prevention of stroke in sickle cell disease. *Blood* 1992;79(7):1657–61.
9. Dempsey EM, Barrington K. Short- and long-term outcomes following partial exchange transfusion in the polycythemic newborn: A systematic review. *Arch Dis Child Fetal Neonatal Ed* 2006;91:F2–F6.
10. Drew JH, Guaran RL, Cichello M, et al. Neonatal whole blood hyperviscosity: The important factor influencing later neurologic function is the viscosity and not the polycythemia. *Clin Hemorheol Microcirc* 1997;17(1):67–72.
11. French Cooperative Group on Plasma exchange in Guillain-Barre Syndrome. Efficiency of plasma exchange in Guillain-Barre Syndrome: Role of replacement fluids. *Ann Neurol* 1987;22:753–61.
12. French Cooperative Group on Plasma exchange in Guillain-Barre Syndrome. Appropriate number of plasma exchanges in Guillain-Barre Syndrome. *Ann Neurol* 1997;41:298–306.
13. Guillain-Barre Syndrome study group. Plasmapheresis and acute Guillain-Barre Syndrome. *Neurology* 1985;35:1096–104.
14. Hemming AE. Pro: Exchange Transfusion is required for sickle cell trait patients undergoing cardiopulmonary bypass. *J Cardiothorac Vasc Anesth* 2004;18(5):663–5.
15. Hughes RA, Raphael JC, Swan AV, et al. Intravenous immunoglobulin for Guillain-Barre Syndrome. *Cochrane database of systematic reviews* 2004;CD002063.
16. Jansen T, Barnung S, Mortensen CR, et al. Isobutyl-nitrite-induced methemoglobinemia; treatment with an exchange blood transfusion during hyperbaric oxygenation. *Acta Anaesthesiol Scand* 2003;47:1300–1.
17. Khurana DS, Melvin JJ, Kothore SV. Acute disseminate encephalomyelitis in children: Discordant neurologic and neuroimaging abnormalities and response to plasmapheresis. *Pediatrics* 2005;116:431–6.
18. Kim HC. Therapeutic pediatric apheresis. *J Clin Apher* 2000;15:129–57.
19. Kleinman SH, Hurvitz CG, Goldfinger D. Use of erythrocytapheresis in the treatment of patients with sickle cell anemia. *J Clin Apher* 1984;2(2):170–6.
20. Letreutre S, Martinot A, Duhamel A, et al. Validation of the pediatric logistic organ dysfunction (PELOD) score: Prospective multinational, multicentre study. *Lancet* 2000;362:192–7.
21. Liem RI, O'Gorman MR, Brown DL. Effect of red cell exchange transfusion on plasma levels of inflammatory mediators in sickle cell patients with acute chest syndrome. *Am J Hematol* 2004;76(1):19–25.
22. Linenberger ML, Price TH. Use of cellular and plasma apheresis in the critically ill patient: Part I: Technical and physiological considerations. *J Intensive Care Med* 2005;20:18–27.
23. Linenberger ML, Price TH. Use of cellular and plasma apheresis in the critically ill patient: Part II: Clinical indications and applications. *J Intensive Care Med* 2005;20:88–103.
24. McCarthy LJ, Dlott JS, Orazi A, et al. Thrombotic thrombocytopenia purpura: Yesterday, today and tomorrow. *Ther Apher Dial* 2004;8(2):80.
25. McMaster P, Shann F. The use of extracorporeal techniques to remove humoral factors in sepsis. *Pediatr Crit Care Med* 2003;4:2–7.
26. Messent M. Con: Exchange transfusion is not required for sickle cell trait patients undergoing cardiopulmonary bypass. *J Cardiothorac Vasc Anesth* 2004;18(5):666–7.
27. Mycyk MB, Leikin JB. Combined exchange transfusion and chelation therapy for neonatal lead poisoning. *Ann Pharmacother* 2004;38:821–4.
28. Nguyen TC, Han YY, Seidberg N, et al. Randomized controlled trial of plasma exchange for thrombocytopenia associated multiorgan failure in children. *Pediatr Res* 2001;49:42A.
29. Nguyen TC, Stegmayr B, Busund R. Plasma therapies in thrombotic syndromes. *Int J Artif Organs* 2005;28(5):459–65.
30. Osborn HH, Henry G, Wax P, et al. Theophylline toxicity in a premature neonate-elimination of kinetics of exchange transfusion. *J Toxicol Clin Toxicol* 1993;31(4):639–44.

31. Powell VI, Grima K. Exchange transfusion for malaria and babesia infection. *Transfus Med Rev* 2002;16(3):239–50.

32. Reeves JH, Butt W, Shann F. Continuous plasmafiltration in sepsis syndrome. *Crit Care Med* 1999;27:2096–104.

33. Riddle MS, Jackson JL, Sanders JW, et al. Exchange transfusion as an adjunct therapy in severe plasmodium falciparum malaria: A meta-analysis. *Clin Infect Dis* 2002;34(9):1192–8.

34. Rowe J, Lichtman M. Hyperleukocytosis and leukostasis: Common features of childhood Leukaemia. *Blood* 1984;63:1230–4.

35. Sawada K, Kusugami K, Suzuki Y. Leukocytapheresis in ulcerative colitis: Results of a multicentre double-blind prospective case-control study with sham apheresis as a placebo treatment. *Am J Gastroenterol* 2005;100: 1362–9.

36. Schimmel MS, Bromiker R, Soll RF. Neonatal polycythemia: Is partial exchange transfusion justified? *Clin Perinatol* 2004;31(3):545–53.

37. Shannon M, Wernovsky G, Morris C. Exchange transfusion in the treatment of severe theophylline poisoning. *Pediatrics* 1992;89(1):145–7.

38. Smith JW, Weinstein R, Hillyer KL for the AABB Hemapheresis Committee. Therapeutic apheresis: A summary of current indication categories endorsed by the AABB and the American Society of Apheresis. *Transfusion* 2003;43:820–2.

39. Vankataraman R, Subramanian S, Kellum JA. Clinical review: Extracorporeal blood purification in severe sepsis. *Critical Care* 2003;7:139–45.

40. Wayne AS, Kevy SV, Nathan DG. Transfusion management of sickle cell disease. *Blood* 1993;81(5):1109–23.

41. Weissman H, Nadel AJ, Dunn M. Simultaneous bilateral retinal arterial occlusions treated by exchange transfusion. *Arch Opthalmol* 1979;97: 2151–3.

42. Ziajka P. Role of low-density lipoprotein apheresis. *Am J Cardiol* 2005; 96(4):67–9.

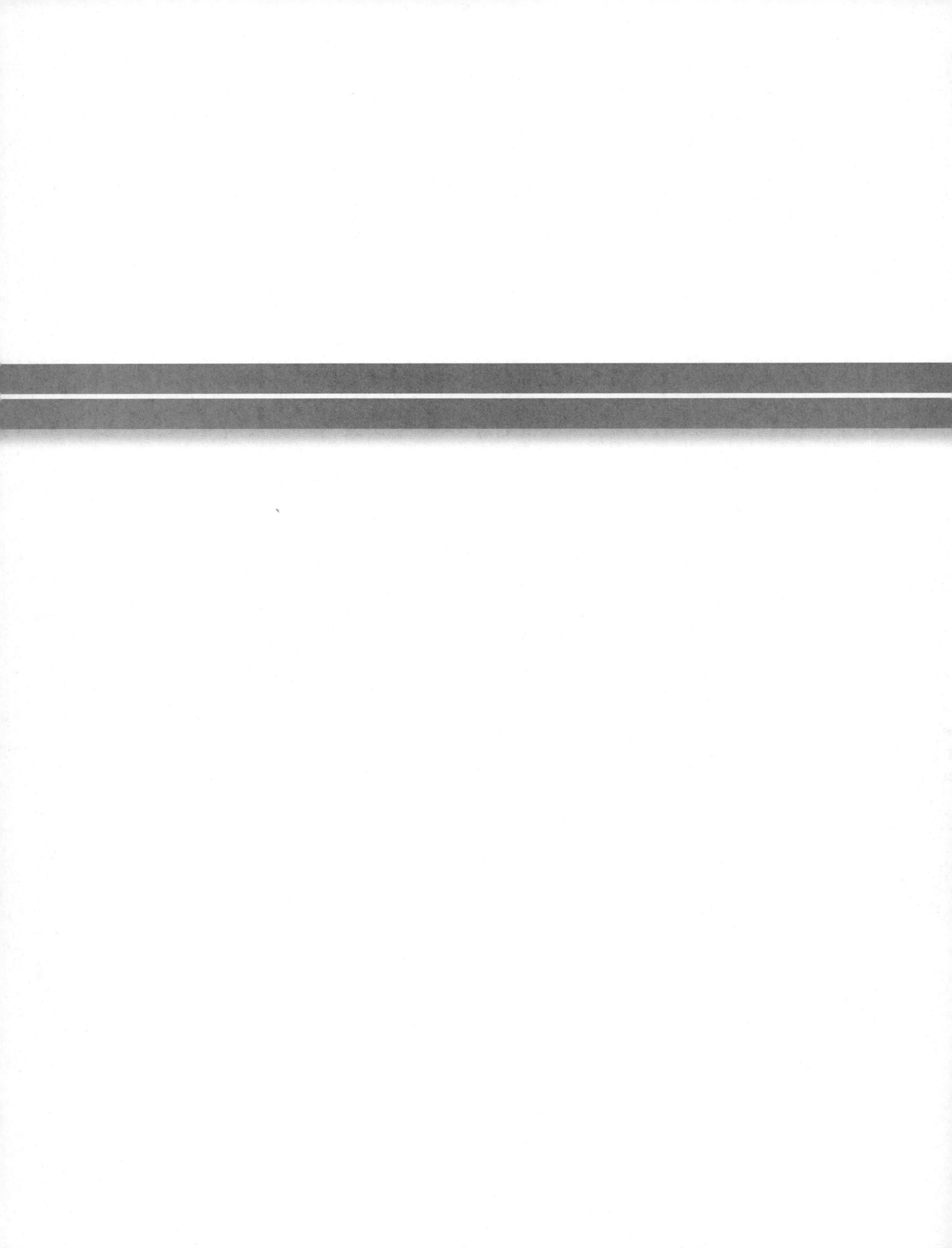

PART THREE ■ CRITICAL CARE ORGAN SYSTEMS

CHAPTER 40 ■ THE MOLECULAR BIOLOGY OF ACUTE LUNG INJURY

TODD CARPENTER • R. BLAINE EASLEY • KURT R. STENMARK

Acute lung injury (ALI) is an illness of great interest and importance in pediatric critical care. Children who suffer from ALI are often among the sickest and most challenging patients in the PICU. In addition, an even greater proportion of the patients in pediatric critical care present with respiratory illnesses that likely have substantial mechanistic overlap with ALI, even without cleanly fitting the clinical case definition of that condition. Understanding the cellular and molecular mechanisms that underlie ALI is important for understanding current and future approaches to treatment of many illnesses in the PICU.

The central derangement in ALI is the disruption of the alveolar-capillary barrier, which allows protein-rich plasma components to cross into the airspaces. Once alveoli are flooded, surfactant is inactivated and a cycle of inflammation and local hypoxia leads to injury progression, perhaps augmented by mechanical forces from the use of artificial mechanical ventilation and oxidant stress from high inspired O_2 concentrations. These changes comprise the early, acute phase of ALI, characterized by pulmonary edema, hypoxemic respiratory failure, poor lung compliance, and, often, some degree of pulmonary hypertension (**Fig. 40.1**). As the illness progresses, the disease enters a fibroproliferative phase, in which lung compliance improves but lung function remains poor as a result of progressive scarring and thickening of the lung interstitium. Ultimately, many patients recover lung function completely or nearly so, but substantial numbers of survivors have long-lasting pulmonary function deficits. While careful studies at bedside have led to improvements in outcome for this illness in the last decade, further progress will require a more detailed understanding of the molecular mechanisms of lung injury.

EDEMA FORMATION AND ACUTE LUNG INJURY

The movement of fluid out of the capillaries and into the alveolar airspace has several components. First, the endothelial barrier must be disrupted, allowing fluid out of the capillaries and into the interstitium. Next, the epithelial barrier must also be disrupted, allowing edema fluid into the airspaces. Finally, edema fluid must enter the alveoli at a rate that exceeds the capacity of alveolar liquid clearance mechanisms. An additional contributing factor is pulmonary microvascular pressure. For a given degree of capillary permeability, higher microvascular pressures drive more fluid across the endothelial barriers and, at high enough pressures, epithelial barriers.

Mechanisms of Increased Endothelial Permeability

The movement of fluid across the injured pulmonary vascular endothelium is thought to occur primarily via paracellular channels between the cells. The permeability of endothelial cell layers is largely determined by the state of intercellular junctions between endothelial cells and by the cytoskeleton of the individual endothelial cells (**Fig. 40.2**). Loosening of the intercellular junctions and/or contraction of the actin-myosin cytoskeleton allows the cells to pull apart, opening paracellular gaps for fluid movement across the barrier. Several types of junctions contribute to regulation of the lung endothelial barrier: tight junctions, adherens junctions, and focal adhesions. Tight junctions, comprised of a number of proteins, including occludens, claudins, and ZO proteins, are thought to be the major permeability-regulating element of the blood-brain barrier. Although some studies have implicated alterations in tight junction proteins in the control of lung vascular permeability, the role of tight junctions in this regard remains uncertain and is an area of active investigation. Recent literature suggests that adherens junctions may be more important than tight junctions in controlling lung permeability. In the pulmonary endothelium, adherens junctions are principally composed of vascular/endothelial-cadherin (VE-cadherin) and members of the catenin family of proteins, which then connect the extracellular side of the membrane to neighboring cells and intracellularly to the actin cytoskeleton. The breakdown of adherens junctions has been observed in cultured lung microvascular endothelial cells in response to permeability-increasing stimuli (e.g., thrombin and oxidant stress), and VE-cadherin function-blocking antibodies have been demonstrated to disrupt the alveolar-capillary barrier in vivo (4,12). A third type of intercellular junction, focal adhesions, connects the endothelial cell to the extracellular matrix via integrin receptors and a number of cytoplasmic focal adhesion proteins. The precise role of these junctions in ALI also remains uncertain, but accumulating evidence suggests that they, too, may be quite important. For example, rearrangement of focal adhesion complexes from the periphery of the cell to the ends of actin stress fibers has been observed in association with increases in endothelial permeability due to both cyclic stretch and vasoactive agonists such as thrombin (7).

Connected to these junctional complexes is the endothelial cytoskeleton, which has three principal components: actin fibers, microtubules, and intermediate filaments. Of these three

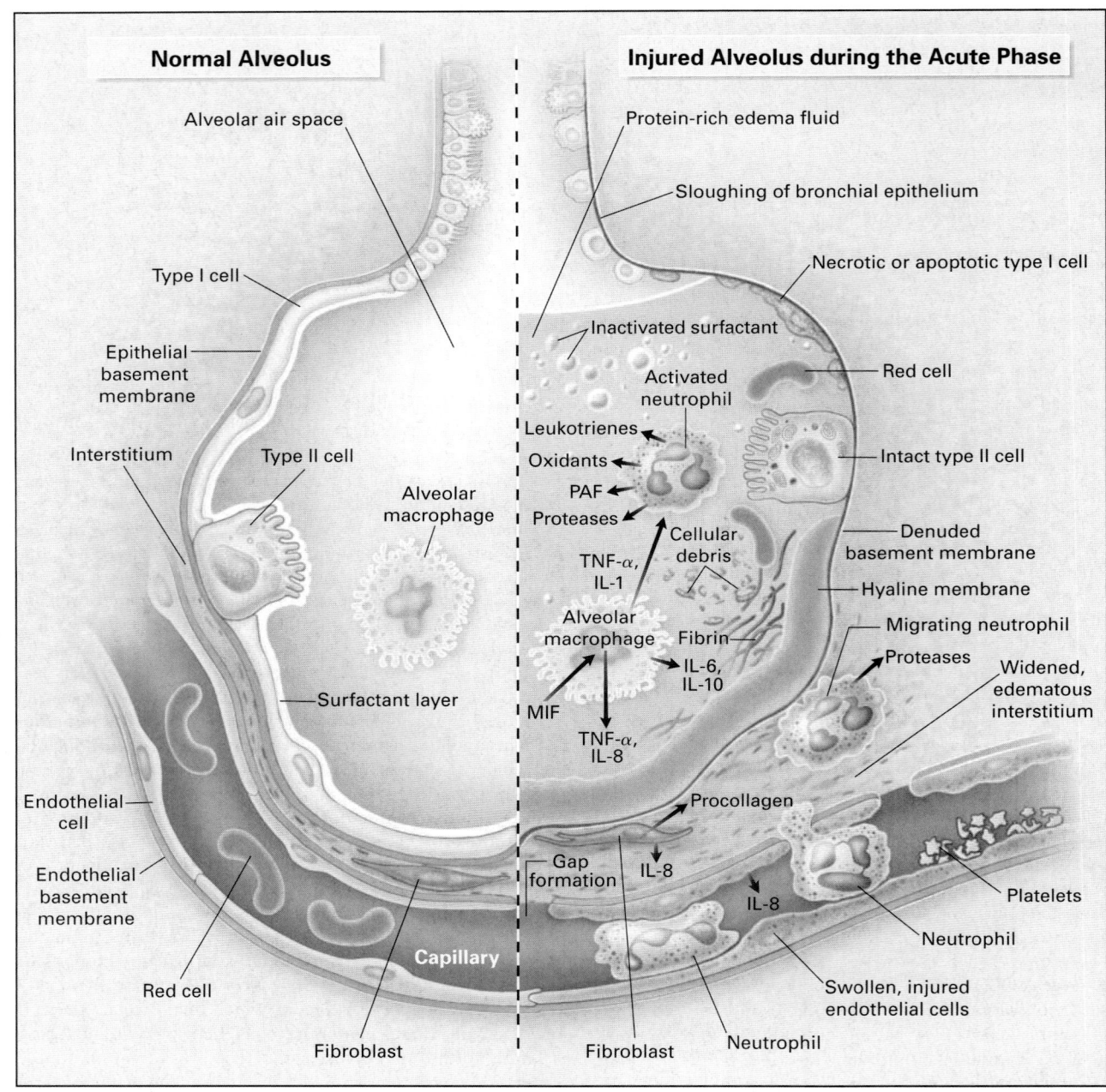

FIGURE 40.1. Cellular and molecular mechanisms of acute lung injury. Changes that occur as part of the early acute phase of lung injury are visible on the right half of the diagram in comparison to the left, including disruption of the endothelial and epithelial barriers, alveolar flooding, and influx of activated inflammatory cells into the alveolus and interstitium of the lung. From Ware LB, Matthay MA. The acute respiratory distress syndrome. *N Engl J Med* 2000;342:1334–49, with permission.

types of fibers, the actin cytoskeleton is the best studied and appears to be the most important in controlling lung endothelial barrier function (18). Actin fibers in unstimulated endothelial cells assume a "cortical" pattern, lined up around the periphery of the cell. Agonists that increase endothelial permeability cause actin fibers to rearrange into a more linear pattern ("stress fiber formation") and to interact with nonmuscle myosin, allowing the cell to contract away from its neighbors and create intercellular gaps in the monolayer. Stress fiber formation and actin-myosin interactions occur principally as a result of phosphorylation of the myosin light-chain (MLC) molecule. The extent of MLC phosphorylation, in turn, is regulated by a balance between the activity of two enzymes—myosin light-chain kinase (MLCK) and myosin phosphatase target subunit (MYPT). Many mediators with effects on endothelial barrier function exert their effects by modulating the activities of one or both of these enzymes.

Calcium handling is a key element in the control of the endothelial cytoskeleton. MLCK activation is generally a calcium-dependent process, and increased intracellular calcium

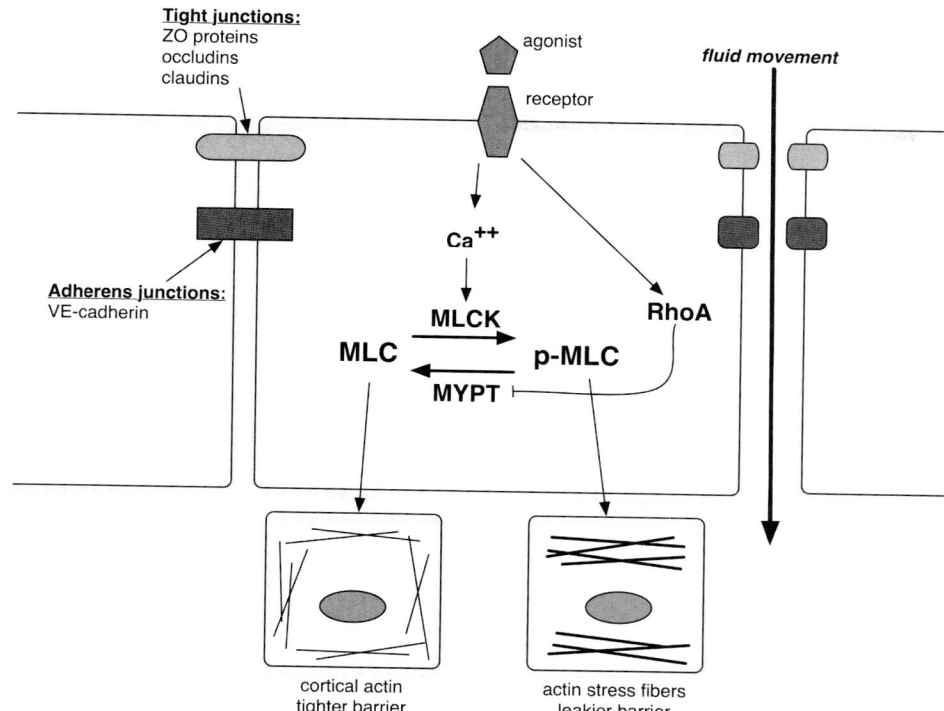

FIGURE 40.2. Molecular mechanisms that control endothelial permeability. Intact tight junctions and adherens junctions provide a barrier to paracellular fluid movement in unperturbed monolayers (*left side of figure*). Agonist stimulation leads to activation of MLCK via calcium influx and to suppression of myosin phosphatase activity via RhoA activation, with the net result of rearrangement of the actin cytoskeleton and increased actin-myosin interactions, leading to endothelial cell contraction. Combined with additional mechanisms that lead to the breakdown of intercellular junctions (tight junctions, adherens junctions), these changes cause endothelial cells to contract away from each other, allowing paracellular fluid flux (*right side of figure*). ZO, zonula occludens; VE-cadherin, vascular/endothelial-cadherin; MLCK, myosin light-chain kinase; MLC, myosin light chain; p-MLC, phosphorylated myosin light-chain; MYPT, myosin phosphatase target subunit

generally leads to increased endothelial permeability. In nonexcitable cells, such as endothelial cells, calcium entry is mediated primarily by a class of channels known as store-operated calcium (SOC) channels. This mechanism is activated by binding an agonist to its receptor on the endothelial cell surface, leading to generation of phospholipase C and release of calcium from sequestered intracellular stores. Depletion of the intracellular calcium stores triggers the opening of cell surface SOC channels, which further increases intracellular calcium, allowing calcium binding to calmodulin; calmodulin mediates activation of MLCK and a pathway involving RhoGTPases, which act on MYPT activity. The molecular identity of the endothelial cell SOC channels is not entirely determined, although the family of transient receptor potential channels (TRPC) has been identified as one form of SOC channel (20). Evidence that links TRPC channels to lung injury includes the finding that lung microvessels from TRPC-4 knockout mice show markedly reduced responses to permeability-increasing agonists such as thrombin. The precise role of SOC calcium entry in acute lung injury remains uncertain, however, because other studies have suggested that, while SOC channels regulate permeability in endothelial cells from larger conduit vessels, these channels are less important in controlling microvascular permeability and other mechanisms must provide the necessary intracellular calcium for microvascular permeability changes.

Due to its effects on MLC phosphorylation, the Rho family of GTPases has emerged as another key regulator of the actin cytoskeleton and of endothelial permeability (18,61). Rho family molecules function as molecular switches, cycling between an active guanosine triphosphate (GTP)-bound form and an inactive guanosine diphosphate (GDP)-bound form. The best studied of these proteins, RhoA, when activated, moves to the cell membrane and stimulates the activity of its downstream effectors, the Rho kinases, which then leads to phosphoryla-

tion of MYPT-1, reducing its activity and thus increasing MLC phosphorylation. The net effect of RhoA activation, then, is increased MLC phosphorylation, increased actin-myosin interaction, and increased endothelial cell gap formation. This mechanism of endothelial gap formation has been demonstrated to be important in endothelial permeability changes induced by mediators, including thrombin, tumor necrosis factor (TNF)-α, lysophosphatidic acid, and lipopolysaccharide. Interestingly, another member of the same Rho family of GTPases, Rac-1, appears to have opposite effects on permeability to those of RhoA, promoting a peripheral, cortical actin fiber pattern and increased barrier integrity. The downstream mediators that are responsible for these effects of Rac-1 are still uncertain.

While both calcium-dependent MLCK activation and Rho-mediated MYPT inactivation are clearly important in endothelial barrier regulation, the relative contributions of these two mechanisms remain incompletely understood. Nonetheless, most mediators implicated in ALI appear to act at least in part via these mechanisms.

Control of Pulmonary Vascular Tone

The regulation of pulmonary vascular tone is also important to the pathophysiology and treatment of ALI. Normal mechanisms of ventilation and perfusion matching are impaired in ALI, and the resultant maldistribution in pulmonary blood flow and increase in intrapulmonary shunting contributes to the severe systemic hypoxemia in these patients. Increased pulmonary arterial pressure is a common feature of ALI and correlates with worse outcome. The movement of fluid out of the vasculature and into the airspaces depends both on the permeability of the endothelial barrier and on the hydrostatic forces that drive fluid movement. Increased microvascular pressure can occur as a result of increased blood flow through a given vascular segment due to uneven arterial vasoconstriction or as a result of elevated pulmonary venous resistance. Both circumstances have been described in ALI (21,47). Increased microvascular pressure, in turn, can lead to microfractures of the capillary endothelium and even of the epithelium, which cause increased permeability. Newborn animals seem especially susceptible to this type of injury. These capillary "stress fractures" have been described with elevated left atrial pressure, high cardiac output states, and ventilator-induced lung injury (39,65). In addition, increased microvascular pressure alone has also been demonstrated to cause upregulation of adhesion molecule expression and increased intracellular calcium in endothelial cells, demonstrating a linkage between hydrostatic forces and inflammation in the lung microvasculature (37). Thus, while elevated pulmonary vascular pressures are severe enough to cause overt right heart failure in only a minority of patients with ALI, changes in vascular tone may contribute substantially to edema formation in many such patients and provide attractive targets for therapeutic intervention.

At the molecular level, increased vascular tone relies on mechanisms very similar to those involved in endothelial barrier function, although the target cell in this case is primarily the vascular smooth muscle cell. Most vasoconstrictive agonists, such as angiotensin II and endothelin (ET), bind G-protein–coupled receptors on the smooth muscle cell surface, stimulating phospholipase C, triggering diacylglycerol and inositol 1,4,5-triphosphate (IP3) formation, and leading to release of intracellular calcium stores and a rise in intracellular calcium concentration. In contrast to endothelial cells, however, smooth muscle cells also express voltage-gated ion channels, and when the intracellular calcium concentration reaches a threshold level, the cell depolarizes and opens voltage-gated calcium channels, flooding the cell with calcium. Calmodulin is then activated and, in turn, activates MLCK, which phosphorylates the MLC, enabling the interaction of myosin with actin and cell contraction. Some agonists also stimulate Rho/Rho kinase signaling, which reduces myosin phosphatase activity, leading to "calcium sensitization," in which contractile tone is increased independently of increased intracellular calcium. Molecules that affect vascular tone in the lung can be released by the vascular endothelium and by adventitial cells in the vascular wall, interstitial cells in the lung parenchyma, and circulating or inflammatory cells transiting the vascular bed. Recent work has increasingly focused on the role of those cells that surround the vessel as being key early mediators of many pulmonary vascular responses, in contrast to the previous concept of the endothelium as the primary controller of vascular tone.

Pulmonary vascular tone is the result of a balance between endogenous vasoconstrictors and vasodilators. ET is one of the most important endogenous vasoconstrictors. It is a 21-amino acid peptide expressed at high levels by many cells in the lung; it acts via two G-protein–coupled receptors, ET_A and ET_B. Binding of ET to the ET_A receptor on smooth muscle cells leads to intense constriction of either the airway or blood vessel involved. Activation of the ET_B receptor leads to various consequences, depending on the cell type that expresses it. In vascular smooth muscle, ET_B receptor stimulation generally acts similarly to ET_A receptor stimulation. The stimulation of endothelial ET_B receptors, however, triggers the release of nitric oxide

(NO) and causes vasodilation. On the endothelium, the ET_B receptor acts as a clearance receptor, internalizing and degrading circulating ET peptide from the bloodstream. In addition to its vascular effects, ET is a potent cytokine and contributes to both inflammatory responses and fibrosis. ET upregulates vascular endothelial growth factor (VEGF) in the lung, and angiopoietin-1 (Ang1) has been shown to downregulate ET. ET expression is also upregulated by hypoxia and a host of inflammatory cytokines, including transforming growth factor (TGF)-β.

The ET system has been clearly implicated in both human and experimental ALI. In humans, circulating ET levels are elevated and correlate with severity of illness in both adults and children. Lung ET content is also increased in experimental lung injuries. Endothelin antagonists given via either the parenteral or inhaled routes ameliorate lung injury in experimental settings as diverse as endotoxin-mediated injury, acid injury, surfactant depletion, and viral infection coupled with hypoxia. Whether the beneficial effects of ET antagonism in these settings are primarily due to improved pulmonary hemodynamics and reduced microvascular pressures, or to reduced inflammation and improved endothelial barrier function remains uncertain. Both mechanisms likely contribute.

NO, the most widely studied endogenous vasodilator, is also a signaling molecule with profound multitudinous effects in the lung. Its best-known function is as a vasodilator, although it has also been implicated in immune modulation, epithelial function, and control of endothelial permeability. While the precise mechanisms that underlie its vascular effects are still under investigation, NO acts in vascular smooth muscle by stimulating soluble guanylate cyclase to produce cyclic guanosine monophosphate (cGMP). cGMP activates a family of cGMP-dependent protein kinases that reduce intracellular calcium levels via an effect on calcium flux out of the sarcoplasmic reticulum and reduces calcium sensitization by activating myosin phosphatase. The net effect of these events is to reduce MLC phosphorylation and reduce vascular smooth muscle contraction. In addition to these effects on vascular tone, NO also appears to regulate endothelial permeability, although it has been reported to both increase and decrease lung microvascular permeability depending on the experimental setting studied (11,53).

NO is produced by a family of NO synthases (NOS). Endothelial NOS (eNOS) is constitutively expressed by endothelial cells, and neuronal NOS (nNOS) is expressed in neurons. Inducible NOS (iNOS) can be expressed by most mammalian cells as a response to inflammation or injury, in particular by lung macrophages and neutrophils in the setting of lung injury. Despite its widespread clinical use as an inhaled vasodilator to improve ventilation-perfusion matching in ALI, the literature regarding the physiologic and molecular roles of NO in the injured lung remains a confusing field. For example, while much available evidence suggests that lung injury is accompanied by increased NO in the lung, studies of nonselective NOS inhibitors in ALI have shown both improvement and worsening of edema formation. Similarly, the observed increase in local NO generation during lung injury would be expected to reduce vascular resistance; yet, the opposite is generally true in patients with acute respiratory distress syndrome (ARDS). The mechanisms that underlie this apparent insensitivity of the injured lung to NO remain uncertain.

The role of hypoxia in the control of pulmonary vascular tone is also pertinent to a discussion of ALI. Regional hypoxia is a characteristic of injured tissues and may be particularly evident in areas of dependent collapse in the injured lung, in which blood flow is reduced. Hypoxia can upregulate many of the transcriptional and signaling mechanisms that are active in the injured lung and may contribute to lung injury. Interestingly, while impaired ventilation-perfusion matching in the injured lung is a prominent mechanism of hypoxemia in ALI, hypoxic pulmonary vasoconstriction is generally blunted in patients with ARDS, and high O_2 concentrations do little to improve pulmonary hemodynamics. Thus, the elevation in pulmonary vascular resistance seen in ALI appears to be predominantly attributable to the effects of vasoactive mediators rather than to O_2 tension per se.

Epithelial Barrier Integrity and Function in Acute Lung Injury

Once plasma fluids have breached the endothelial barrier, they must cross the epithelial barrier to reach the alveolar airspace. By most estimates, the permeability of the epithelial barrier is approximately tenfold lower than that of the endothelial barrier, suggesting that the epithelium is the greater barrier to edema formation. Despite this fact, much more research has been directed at understanding endothelial permeability than epithelial permeability, perhaps because of the relative difficulty until recently of studying alveolar epithelial cells in vitro. In general, epithelial cells appear to form their barrier via intracellular junctions similar to those observed in the endothelium. Tight junctions exist in the alveolar epithelium and are comprised of claudins, occludens, and ZO proteins, as in other cell types. The particular claudin isoforms expressed appear to vary substantially from those in the endothelium and change with different stimuli, leading to the suggestion that alterations in claudin expression pattern provide a level of regulation of epithelial barrier function. Adherens junctions are also important in the epithelial barrier, although the predominant cadherin protein expressed is E-cadherin, rather than VE-cadherin as in the endothelium. In addition, changes in epithelial permeability are sometimes associated with actin cytoskeleton rearrangements, although evidence that implicates MLCK and Rho kinase activity in those events is lacking.

Despite the paucity of molecular detail about control of epithelial barrier permeability, many mediators capable of altering epithelial permeability have been described. Certainly, direct epithelial cell death, as a result of bacterial or viral infection or direct injury by inhaled toxins, can alter permeability, as can mechanical injury to the epithelium from ventilator-induced lung injury. Airway lipopolysaccharide, presumably acting via Toll-like receptors, increases epithelial permeability via a mechanism that involves neutrophil influx, and it can be partially blocked by NO. Other secondary mediators can also contribute. For example, TGF-β1 has been shown to increase epithelial cell monolayer permeability in vitro via a mechanism that is dependent on oxidant stress but not on MLCK. Hypoxia leads to increased epithelial permeability and breakdown of epithelial tight junctions. Cytokines, including TNF-α, IL-8, and epidermal growth factor (EGF) can also increase epithelial permeability.

A key advance in understanding pulmonary edema formation has been the description of the molecular mechanisms responsible for clearing alveolar edema fluid (42). For edema fluid to result in alveolar flooding, the movement of fluid into the airspaces must overwhelm these innate alveolar fluid clearance mechanisms (**Fig. 40.3**). Alveolar liquid clearance is largely the result of active sodium transport. Both type 1 and type 2 alveolar epithelial cells express Na/K-ATPases on their basolateral membranes. These enzymes, comprised of α and β subunits, actively pump sodium out of the epithelial cell and into the lung interstitium, exchanging three sodium molecules for two potassium molecules in the process. The epithelial cell also expresses epithelial sodium channels, or ENaCs, on its apical (luminal) surface. Three distinct ENaC subunits exist in mammals: ENaC-α, ENaC-β, and ENaC-γ. The functional channel is comprised of multimers of these subunits in a stoichiometry that remains unclear. ENaC channels allow sodium to move passively down the concentration gradient created by the basolateral pumps, out of the airspaces, and into the epithelial cell. The combined effect of the ENaC and Na/K-ATPases is to actively clear sodium from the airspaces across the epithelial barrier and into the interstitium, creating an osmotic gradient for water to follow. Water moves out of the alveolus along this osmotic gradient, both via specific water channels known as *aquaporins* and via paracellular routes.

A number of factors modulate the expression and activity of these molecules and may contribute to ALI. Interestingly, loss of specific aquaporins appears to do little to increase edema

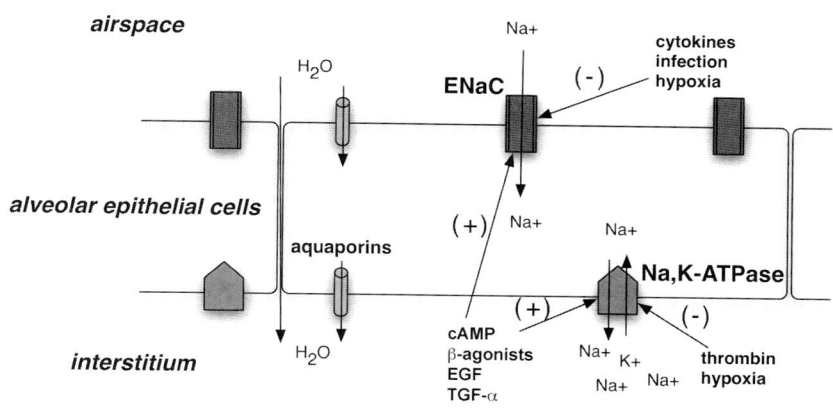

FIGURE 40.3. Molecular mechanisms regulating alveolar liquid clearance. Basolateral Na/K-ATPases (*pentagons*) pump sodium out the epithelial cell and into the interstitium, creating a gradient for sodium movement out of the airspaces via apical ENaC sodium channels (*rectangles*). Water follows this gradient out of the airspaces via aquaporin channels (*cylinders*) and paracellular routes (*arrow*). Stimuli, including cytokines, thrombin, hypoxia, and β-agonists, can increase or decrease ENaC and Na/K-ATPase function. ENaC, epithelial sodium channels; cAMP, cyclic adenosine monophosphate; EGF, epidermal growth factor; TGF-α, transforming growth factor alpha

accumulation, while changes in sodium channels or pumps have much greater effects, suggesting that water transport pathways other than aquaporins are the most important clearance routes in the intact lung. Relevant to lung injury, both inflammation and infection have been demonstrated to impair alveolar liquid clearance via alterations in sodium channel expression or activity. ENaC subunit expression is downregulated by cytokines, such as TNF-α and IL-1β, and by infection with *Pseudomonas aeruginosa* bacteria (13,55). Influenza virus and respiratory syncytial virus (RSV), in contrast, impair ENaC function without altering channel expression. In the case of RSV, this effect is mediated by uridine triphosphate release from the epithelium and stimulation of purinergic receptors. Hypoxia also impairs epithelial sodium transport by reducing both ENaC and Na/K-ATPase activity. Thrombin reduces lung liquid clearance by promoting endocytosis of Na/K-ATPases (60). Mediators that can increase alveolar liquid clearance have also been described. β-adrenergic agents, such as isoproterenol and dopamine, act via cyclic adenosine monophosphate (cAMP) to promote alveolar liquid clearance by increasing Na/K-ATPase activity and upregulating ENaC expression. Corticosteroids and aldosterone also increase ENaC expression.

The physiologic importance of these sodium and water transport mechanisms is apparent from both animal and human studies. Targeted deletion of the EnaC α-subunit in mice leads to respiratory distress and death shortly after birth from inability to clear fluid from the airspaces, whereas overexpression of the Na/K-ATPase β-subunit leads to increased alveolar liquid clearance in rats that are subjected to high tidal volume ventilation. In adult patients with ALI, alveolar fluid clearance rates are clearly impaired and clinical outcome correlates inversely with the degree of impairment, suggesting that those patients whose alveolar epithelial liquid clearance mechanisms sustain the greatest damage do worse clinically.

SURFACTANT BIOCHEMISTRY IN ACUTE LUNG INJURY

The loss of surfactant activity from epithelial cell death or dysfunction and direct surfactant inactivation by plasma proteins flooding the alveolus are prime characteristics of ALI. Pulmonary surfactant reduces surface tension in the air-liquid interface, facilitates the stability of the expanded alveolus, and is essential for normal lung function. In addition to its biomechanical properties, surfactant has been shown to contribute to the host's innate defense system and possess anti-inflammatory properties. The composition of surfactant is similar among various species and consists of ~90% lipids and 10% surfactant-related proteins. The lipid portion of surfactant contains 90% phospholipid, 75% of which is phosphatidylcholine (PC). Approximately 40% of the PC exists in desaturated form as dipalmitoylphosphatidylcholine (DPPC), which is believed to be the main surface-tension–reducing component at the air-liquid interface. Other lipid components, including phosphatidylglycerol (10% of total phospholipid), a few minor phospholipid species, and neutral lipids, such as cholesterol, assist in forming the surface-tension–lowering film that is associated with the air-liquid interface in the alveolus.

Surfactant proteins (SP-A, SP-B, SP-C, and SP-D) also play an important role in these processes, especially the small, hydrophobic proteins SP-B and SP-C. SP-B, present in the lung as a 16-kDa dimer, enhances the adsorption of surfactant lipids to the interface and promotes the transformation of this lipid layer into a DPPC-rich surface film able to reduce the surface tension to very low values during exhalation. SP-C, with a molecular mass of 4 kDa, is the most hydrophobic of the surfactant-associated proteins. SP-C is more intimately associated with the surfactant film than is SP-B, although the exact role of SP-C is less defined than that of SP-B. The two other proteins associated with surfactant are designated SP-A (32 kDa) and SP-D (43 kDa). These proteins are hydrophilic and belong to the collectin family. As collectins, their role appears predominantly related to host defense rather than to biophysical properties, although SP-A may contribute to surface tension reduction under stress conditions such as ALI.

Surfactant is synthesized in alveolar type II cells and secreted into the airspace via exocytosis. Within the airspace, alveolar surfactant exists as two structural forms (based on their buoyant density, composition, and function), designated as "large aggregates" and "small aggregates." Large aggregates are the heavier, surface-active components and contain the surfactant-associated proteins SP-A, SP-B, and SP-C. Small aggregates are lighter, vesicular forms that are not surface active and are the metabolic products of large aggregates with low amounts of surfactant protein. In normal lungs, both large and small aggregates are present in a consistent ratio, which is maintained through a dynamic process that involves the formation and secretion of large aggregates, subsequent conversion into small aggregates, and the clearance of small aggregates from the airspace.

Deficiencies of either surfactant phospholipids or surfactant proteins are associated with impaired lung function, including poor compliance, atelectasis, inflammation, infection, and hypoxemia. Analysis of bronchoalveolar lavage fluid (BALF) obtained from patients with ALI and from various animal models of ALI has confirmed that alterations of the endogenous surfactant system contribute to the lung dysfunction associated with ALI. These alterations include changes in the lipid profile, altered concentrations of surfactant-associated proteins, and shifts in the relative amounts of surfactant aggregate forms within the airspace. The specific lipid changes in ARDS include an overall decrease in the total amount of PCs and in the DPPC fraction, a decrease in phosphatidylglycerol, and an increase in other minor phospholipids. Changes to neutral lipids have not been studied extensively. The mechanisms that are responsible for these changes in lipid profile are related to altered synthetic and/or secretory pathways within the type II cell, as well as degradation of lipids within the airspace via phospholipase activity. In general, surfactant-associated protein concentrations are also decreased in BALF samples obtained from patients with ARDS, compared with samples from control subjects. This decrease in protein concentration, like that in lipids, may be because of alterations in type II cell metabolism and/or increased proteolytic activity within the airspace. Associated with these changes were increased levels of surfactant proteins in the serum of patients with ARDS. This finding likely reflects leakage of these proteins from the alveoli into the blood. Of potential clinical importance, serum levels of SP-A and SP-B were inversely related to oxygenation values, and serum levels of SP-D correlated with patient survival. The potential use of these measurements as markers of disease severity is currently being investigated.

provide opportunities for the future development of more specific interventions.

MEDIATORS OF ACUTE LUNG INJURY

Within this framework of basic mechanisms that underlie the formation of pulmonary edema, many additional mediators have been identified that amplify or extend injury. These mediators provide crucial links to the immune system and coagulation system and to the process of angiogenesis. While only a sampling of the mediators involved is discussed below (and summarized in **Table 40.1**), the important concept is that these multiple layers of mediators explain much of the difficulty encountered in devising effective targeted therapies for ALI and

Signaling and Transcriptional Mediators

Intracellular signaling pathways are an area of molecular medicine about which information has increased dramatically. These pathways both lead directly from cell-surface receptors to intracellular targets and cross-talk with each other, modulating and fine-tuning responses in complex networks. While a number of intracellular signaling pathways have been implicated in the development of ALI, one of the best described is the protein kinase C (PKC) family of serine/threonine kinases. These molecules have been implicated in signal transduction pathways important to many cellular functions, including the control of endothelial permeability in the injured lung. Direct

TABLE 40.1

KEY MOLECULAR MEDIATORS IMPLICATED IN ACUTE LUNG INJURY

Mediator	Source	Effects in ALI
SIGNALING MOLECULES		
Protein kinase C (PKC)	Intracellular	Increases microvascular permeability
TRANSCRIPTION FACTORS		
HIF-1	Intracellular	Upregulates hypoxia-responsive genes
NFκB	Intracellular	Regulates genes that control inflammatory responses
SMADs	Intracellular	Downstream of TGF-β; regulate genes that control endothelial and epithelial permeability, fibrosis
CYTOKINES		
TGF-β	Secreted by many cells	Increases endothelial and epithelial permeability; stimulates extracellular matrix production and fibrosis
TNF-α	Activated macrophages	Increases endothelial permeability
IL-1β	Activated macrophages	Increases endothelial permeability; amplifies immune responses; promotes epithelial repair
IL-6	Macrophages, endothelial cells, fibroblasts	Activates PKC, increases endothelial permeability
IL-10	Macrophages, lymphocytes	Inhibits cytokine production
HMGB1	Injured cells	Increases cytokine production
MIF-1	Macrophages, epithelial cells	Increases TNF-α, TLR-4 expression
CHEMOKINES		
IL-8	Alveolar macrophages	Neutrophil recruitment
GRO	Alveolar macrophages	Neutrophil recruitment
ENA-78	Alveolar macrophages	Neutrophil recruitment
ANGIOGENIC MEDIATORS		
VEGF	Epithelial cells, macrophages, smooth muscle	Increases endothelial permeability; involved in airway and vascular development and repair
Ang1	Vascular smooth muscle, endothelial cells	Reduces vascular permeability, decreases IL-8 expression
Ang2	Endothelial cells	Increases vascular permeability
OTHER MEDIATORS		
Thrombin	Cleavage of prothrombin	Increases endothelial permeability; activates TGF-β
S1P	Platelets	Reduces endothelial permeability
TGF-α		Promotes epithelial repair
KGF	Fibroblasts	Promotes alveolar epithelial proliferation
HGF	Fibroblasts	Promotes alveolar epithelial proliferation

stimulation of PKC activity with diacylglycerol increases microvascular permeability, and PKC inhibitors reduce the increased lung vascular permeability caused by thrombin, VEGF, O_2 free radicals, TNF-α, and polymorphonuclear neutrophils (PMNs). While the specific signaling networks responsible for the effect of PKC are still under investigation, PKC activation has been implicated in MLC phosphorylation in response to some agonists and in loosening of adherens junctions and focal adhesions in endothelial cells (58) (**Fig. 40.2**).

As with signaling, our understanding of transcriptional regulation of protein expression becomes more complex almost weekly. Among the many transcription factors currently thought to be involved in ALI, hypoxia-inducible factor (HIF)-1, nuclear factor κB (NFκB), and SMAD transcription factors figure prominently. HIF-1 is a ubiquitously expressed protein the accumulation and activity of which in the nucleus are critical in cellular responses to hypoxia. The expression of many of the mediators involved in ALI (including VEGF and ET-1, among others) is controlled, at least in part, by HIF-1. NFκB is the most prominent transcriptional regulator of inflammatory responses and cytokine production and, thus, may control the amplifying effects of those mediators in ALI. In animal studies, NFκB inhibition or antagonism ameliorates experimental lung injury (27). SMAD transcription factors are a family of molecules that act downstream of TGF-β and are implicated in control of endothelial and epithelial permeability, as well as in fibrotic responses. While increasing evidence links the SMADs with these processes, the downstream targets of SMAD activation in the setting of lung injury remain uncertain.

Cytokine Mediators

Many cytokines and proteins are implicated in the progression of ALI and affect multiple levels in the lung-injury process. Cytokines may directly affect lung cells, promoting endothelial or epithelial injury, or leading to fibroblast activation. They may also indirectly affect the injury process by recruiting circulating inflammatory or reparative cells.

One of the most important cytokines in the lung is TGF-β, a well-described mediator of ALI. Three isoforms of this cytokine have been identified, of which TGF-β1 is produced by endothelial cells. TGF-β is secreted by cells and stored in a latent form in the extracellular matrix. When enzymatically released from the latent form, active TGF-β binds to its receptors on the cell surface, phosphorylating and activating SMAD-family transcription factors, which then move into the nucleus and regulate the transcription of many other genes. TGF-β is nearly ubiquitously expressed and causes a plethora of conflicting effects. In the setting of ALI, however, TGF-β1 directly increases the permeability of cultured endothelial monolayers through mechanisms that appear to involve SMAD phosphorylation, activation of RhoA and p38 mitogen-activated protein kinase (MAPK), and the disruption of adherens junctions. TGF-β activation increases both endothelial and epithelial permeability. Findings demonstrate elevated lung TGF-β levels in both human ARDS and in animal models of lung injury, and TGF-β inhibition protects from experimental lung injury in animals. Recent evidence links the coagulation system (in the form of thrombin) with TGF-β activation and lung injury in the setting of both high tidal volume ventilation and bleomycin-induced

lung injury (29). These findings suggest that TGF-β activation is one of the pivotal steps in the initiation and propagation of ALI.

One of the key physiologic triggers of ALI is sepsis, and many of the cytokines involved in systemic inflammatory responses to sepsis have also been implicated in ALI. For example, TNF-α and IL-1β are cytokines predominantly produced by activated macrophages, and both are key elements of the systemic response to sepsis. TNF-α stimulation triggers the upregulation of adhesion molecules in human lung microvascular endothelial cells, which may lead to greater PMN attachment, cytoskeletal changes, and endothelial gap formation, which are mediated by activation of p38 MAPK, PKC isoforms, and RhoA. TNF-α has also been shown to induce the nitration of actin in endothelial cells, which may also cause endothelial barrier dysfunction in ALI. TNF-α levels have been measured in the BALF of ARDS patients and are often elevated, although, interestingly, levels have not correlated well with outcomes.

IL-1β has also been identified as a primary cytokine involved in the acute-phase inflammatory cascade in ALI. IL-1β has been shown to increase the permeability of cultured endothelial cell layers and can stimulate the production of a variety of chemotactic cytokines, such as IL-8, epithelial cell PMN activator (ENA-78), monocyte chemotactic peptide (MCP-1), and macrophage inflammatory peptide-1. Multiple investigators have identified this proinflammatory cytokine in BALF from patients with ARDS, along with its antagonist, IL-1 receptor antagonist (IL-1ra). IL-1ra completely inhibits binding of IL-1 to its primary cell-surface signaling receptor, IL-1R1. Strong correlations exist between measures of IL-1β activity and clinical lung injury severity and outcome in patients with ARDS. For example, investigators have used the ratio of IL-1:IL-1ra concentrations as a marker of the severity of lung injury. Studies of normal volunteers demonstrated a ratio of 1:1; however, patients with prolonged ARDS BALF demonstrated a ratio of 10:1, suggesting a role for IL-1 in maintaining the inflammatory state in ARDS. Signal transduction by the IL-1β ligand-receptor complex requires binding to a third protein, the soluble IL-1 receptor accessory protein (sIL-1RAcP). Because of the dynamic expression of anti-inflammatory ligands and the fact that soluble IL-1R1 competes with IL-1β activity, measurements of biologic activity in BALF are important to estimate proinflammatory activity. Supporting these observations, several investigators have characterized the biologic activity of IL-1β in ARDS edema fluids using microarray analysis and in an in vitro epithelial cell model of wound repair. These studies suggest a role for IL-1β in both fibroproliferation and epithelial repair.

Additional cytokines have been implicated in lung injury. IL-6 is consistently elevated in BALF and plasma from patients with ALI, and it increases endothelial permeability through activation of PKC. IL-10 is a potent anti-inflammatory cytokine identified in ARDS, and higher levels in BALF are associated with improved survival. IL-10 inhibits cytokine production by macrophages and is closely related to TNF-α expression. IL-10 also downregulates human leukocyte antigen HLA-DR expression on monocytes from patients with septic shock and may play a role in modulating the host response to infections. The ratio of concentrations of TNF-α to IL-10 was elevated in a group of 10 ARDS patients; however, a larger group of 46 patients with ARDS demonstrated a peak of IL-10 on day 1, falling to undetectable levels over 3 weeks, suggesting that in ARDS patients who survive up to 3 weeks, the TNF-α:IL-10 ratio favors a net anti-inflammatory condition over time.

A unique protein apparently involved in ALI is high-mobility group box 1 (HMGB1), which is a nuclear DNA-binding protein that is released from injured or necrotic cells and is a proinflammatory cytokine. It has been identified in the BALF and plasma of ARDS patients and has been implicated in both sepsis and ALI in animal models. HMGB1 is a late mediator of endotoxin lethality by activating downstream cytokine release. When given intratracheally in animals, HMGB1 induces acute inflammatory lung injury, characterized by PMN influx, lung edema, and local production of IL-1β, TNF-α, and the chemokine macrophage-inflammatory protein 2. Both ventilator-induced and endotoxin-induced lung injury can be ameliorated using anti-HMGB1 antibodies.

Macrophage migration inhibitory factor (MIF) is another cytokine that has been identified in BALF in ARDS. MIF is produced by alveolar macrophages and bronchial epithelial cells, and MIF and TNF-α each promote and reinforce the other's production. MIF potentiates the effects of endotoxin and Gram-positive bacterial products; it also regulates macrophage responses to endotoxin through its regulatory effect on Toll-like receptor-4 expression.

Inflammatory Cells and Chemokines

Several studies of serial BALF in ARDS have identified the importance of the acute inflammatory cell populations, their evolution over time, and their impact on clinical outcomes. For example, PMNs are abundant in BALF from patients with ARDS, and PMN products in BALF correlate with the physiologic abnormalities that occur. High numbers of PMNs in BALF, as well as their persistence after the first week of ARDS, are associated with increased mortality, particularly in sepsis. Despite these associations, the role of the PMN in lung injury remains a subject of some debate. PMNs and PMN products are clearly present in the injured lung, and in several experimental models, depletion of PMNs or blockade of their recruitment attenuated lung injury from clinically relevant insults. On the other hand, when PMNs are recruited into the normal human lung simply by instilling the chemoattractant LTB4, they can migrate without causing injury to the endothelial or epithelial barriers of the lung. In addition, although it is clear that lung cellular injury and clinical ARDS can occur in neutropenic patients, it is also true that after the initial lung injury, lung dysfunction can acutely worsen during the resolution of neutropenia, as PMNs are recruited to the injured lungs. These observations suggest that, although PMNs are neither necessary nor sufficient to cause lung injury in humans, activated PMNs can clearly contribute to the pathogenesis of the condition. Migrating PMNs, proinflammatory cytokines in the microvascular and tissue environments, and activated or damaged endothelial and/or epithelial cells act in concert to produce the lung dysfunction in ALI.

PMNs must be recruited from the bloodstream to gain access to the alveolar space and airways. Several of the most potent PMN chemoattractants have been identified in BALF from patients with ARDS. Early studies to identify the specific mediators that are responsible for PMN recruitment in the lungs of ARDS patients excluded some potential candidate molecules.

For example, Parsons et al. demonstrated the presence of PMN chemotactic activity in ARDS BALF and showed that it was *not* attributable to the components of the complement cascade (52). Similarly, the chemotactically active cleavage product of platelet basic protein, neutrophil activating peptide (NAP)-2 is *not* present in ARDS BALF. Over the last 15 years, however, a family of cytokines that are chemotactic for PMN, known as the CXC chemokines, has been described and characterized. An important subclass known as the ELR+ CXC chemokines contain a glutamyl-leucyl-arginine (ELR) motif that is critical to their neutrophil binding and chemotactic functions. The ELR+ CXC chemokines IL-8, ENA-78, growth-related oncogene (GRO), and granulocyte chemotactic peptide (GCP)-2 are all produced by human alveolar macrophages. IL-8, ENA-78, and GRO are present in biologically significant concentrations in BALF in ARDS, and their concentrations correlate with PMN concentrations. In general, as long as patients are ill enough to require continued mechanical ventilation, the concentrations of these CXC chemokines tend to remain logarithmically elevated above normal. Although GRO and ENA-78 concentrations are higher than IL-8 concentrations, IL-8 appears to be responsible for the majority of the PMN chemoattractant activity in human ARDS BALF. Several animal models of lung inflammation and injury also support the concept of IL-8 as the dominant PMN chemoattractant. For example, monoclonal antibodies to IL-8 significantly reduce lung injury and PMN migration in endotoxemia and acid-aspiration models (44).

Adding another level of complexity, two CXC chemokine receptors are found on human PMNs—CXCR1 and CXCR2. IL-8 can bind to either receptor with high affinity, whereas ENA-78 and GRO bind with high affinity only to CXCR2. On ligand stimulation, both chemokine receptors are rapidly internalized. CXCR1, however, is rapidly re-expressed (within minutes), whereas the re-expression of CXCR2 is considerably slower. In the presence of a systemic inflammatory process, such as severe sepsis, CXCR2 is tonically downregulated, and the function of CXCR1 predominates. Thus, among the multiple PMN chemotactic factors produced in humans, a small group appears to be particularly relevant to ARDS, with IL-8 and its cognate receptor, CXCR1, being the dominant receptor-ligand pair.

Thrombin

An interesting area of research has been the link between the coagulation system and lung injury (56,63). The close linkage between coagulation and inflammation, particularly in the setting of sepsis, has recently become clear. Proinflammatory cytokines activate the coagulation system, primarily via the upregulation of tissue factor expression on endothelial and inflammatory cells and subsequent activation of the extrinsic clotting cascade. The generation of thrombin via this mechanism leads to increased inflammation and cytokine release. Similar mechanisms are active in the alveoli in ALI or pneumonia, and these could contribute to the pathogenesis of lung injury. One likely mechanism for this effect is through the generation of thrombin in the lung. As has been described previously, thrombin has potent permeability-inducing effects that have led to its use as a common experimental stimulus for studying mechanisms of endothelial barrier control. Thrombin exerts its effects on endothelial cells by binding to its receptor, protease-activated receptor (PAR)-1, activating signaling cascades that lead to calcium release and the activation of RhoA, and then to cytoskeletal rearrangements and endothelial gap formation. In addition, thrombin stimulation can lead to the disruption of adherens junctions via signaling that is dependent on PKC. Thrombin stimulation of PAR-1 has also been linked experimentally to integrin-mediated TGF-β activation and consequent lung injury.

Angiogenic Mediators

An evolving paradigm in vascular biology is that injuries to a tissue may trigger gene expression of proangiogenic pathways. Many of the mediators involved in the formation of new blood vessels (angiogenesis) are activated by injury, and many of those mediators increase vascular permeability both in the lung and in other vascular beds. Three major families of molecules have been implicated in angiogenesis: the VEGFs, the angiopoietins, and the ephrins. While a role for the ephrins in regulating postnatal pulmonary vascular permeability remains speculative, solid evidence implicates both VEGF and angiopoietin family members in that process.

The VEGF family of receptors and ligands not only mediate blood vessel formation and increase vascular permeability. VEGF is produced and secreted by many cell types in the lung, including alveolar epithelial cells, vascular smooth muscle cells, microvascular endothelial cells, and lung fibroblasts. Inflammatory cells, such as neutrophils and monocytes, can also produce VEGF, as can stimulated alveolar macrophages. VEGF in the normal lung is highly compartmentalized, with alveolar levels far exceeding plasma levels. This alveolar reservoir of VEGF may play a role in promoting epithelial integrity under normal conditions and may affect endothelial permeability if the epithelium is damaged, allowing the highly concentrated alveolar VEGF to reach the endothelial layer. VEGF expression in the lung is strongly upregulated by hypoxia and by numerous cytokines and inflammatory mediators associated with ALI, including TNF-α, TGF-β, IL-6, and ET. VEGF exerts its effects via several receptors, the two best characterized of which are VEGFR1 (also known as flt-1) and VEGFR2 (also known as flk-1). These receptors are tyrosine kinases, able to initiate downstream phosphorylation cascades that activate numerous intracellular signaling molecules. Both VEGFR1 and VEGFR2 are expressed on pulmonary vascular endothelial cells and on airway and alveolar epithelial cells.

VEGF was originally described as "vascular permeability factor" due to its ability to dramatically increase endothelial permeability throughout the body. The effects of VEGF on vascular permeability in some vascular beds appear to involve the phosphorylation and activation of the intracellular signaling molecule Akt, which then causes the phosphorylation of eNOS, leading to increased NO production and increased cellular cGMP. The mechanism that connects NO and cGMP to increased permeability remains obscure, although recent evidence has linked it to activation of RhoA and MLC phosphorylation.

A growing body of evidence implicates VEGF in the pathogenesis of ALI, although considerable uncertainty remains regarding its exact roles. Overexpression of VEGF in the lungs of experimental animals leads to florid pulmonary edema, and VEGF antagonists reduce lung injury and edema formation in many lung-injury models, including viral infection, high tidal volume ventilation, and lipopolysaccharide. Studies of ARDS patients generally show increased plasma levels of VEGF early in the course of the disease. Airway levels of VEGF, in contrast, appear to decrease during the early phases of human ARDS and increase during recovery, a finding that has led to speculation that VEGF is required for healing of epithelial injury. VEGF may play different roles at different times in the course of ARDS and in different anatomic compartments of the lung, promoting edema formation initially but promoting epithelial repair in the later phase of the illness.

The angiopoietin family consists of several known ligands, the most important of which appear to be angiopoietin-1 (Ang1) and angiopoietin-2 (Ang2), and two receptors, TIE-1 and TIE-2. Both receptors are expressed in endothelial cells during development, but only TIE-2 is expressed at high levels in the lung in adult animals. During development, Ang1 binding to endothelial TIE-2 receptors leads to maturation of the developing vessel and stabilization of cell-cell contacts. Ang2 also binds to TIE-2 but acts as an antagonist to the effects of Ang1, causing vessel destabilization and loosened cell-cell contacts. Postnatally, Ang1 stimulation reduces vascular permeability and improves integrity of the vascular barrier, reduces PMN adhesion to the endothelium, and reduces endothelial IL-8 production. Mice exposed to lipopolysaccharide at doses sufficient to cause lung injury develop increased lung VEGF expression and reduced Ang1 expression, and Ang1 overexpression in those animals leads to reduced mortality and less lung injury (32). In contrast, circulating Ang2 levels are high in patients with sepsis and evidence of lung injury, and plasma from those patients leads to gaps in cultured endothelial cell monolayers (51). In addition, administration of Ang2 to healthy mice leads to pulmonary edema formation via increased capillary permeability, and Ang2 release from endothelial cells is stimulated by TNF-α and other cytokines. These findings suggest that the balance between Ang1 and Ang2 expression is an important mediator of endothelial barrier properties in the lung. The precise signaling mechanisms that underlie these effects of Ang1 and Ang2 are still under investigation, but they may involve Rho-family GTPases, as Ang1 has been reported to block RhoA activation, and the effects of Ang2 on the endothelium appear to be mediated by activation of Rho kinase and MLC phosphatase.

Mediators That Reduce Permeability

Sphingosine-1-phosphate (S1P) is a lipid mediator released from activated platelets that, in contrast to the mediators discussed previously, exerts a protective effect on the lung endothelial barrier (43). S1P binds to a class of G-protein–coupled receptors known as Edg receptors. The net effect of activation of Edg receptors in the endothelium is to activate Rac-1, leading to the rearrangement of actin into a cortical pattern, which results in reduced permeability and to the assembly of focal adhesions and cadherins junctions. Studies in experimental animals demonstrate a protective effect of S1P infusion on several forms of lung injury, including those associated with lipopolysaccharide and with high tidal volume ventilation. Interestingly, S1P has effects on barrier function in vivo that far exceed its molecular half-life, suggesting that it may alter the expression of some cytokines and adhesion molecules, thus modulating the immune response to lung injury (43). S1P may also have effects on other cell types in ALI. S1P leads to vasoconstriction in systemic and perhaps pulmonary vascular beds, and the administration of S1P into the airways leads to pulmonary edema via disruption of epithelial adherens and tight junctions (8). These cell type-specific differences in S1P effect likely relate to the specific Edg receptors and to different downstream signaling mechanisms from those receptors.

FIBROPROLIFERATIVE PHASE OF ACUTE RESPIRATORY DISTRESS SYNDROME

The pathophysiology of ARDS consists of overlapping acute inflammatory and delayed "repair/fibrotic" phases (64). Loss of alveolar capillary barrier function occurs early in ARDS and allows influx of proteinaceous fluid, blood, and inflammatory cells into the alveoli. Activation of the coagulation system and complement and the release of cytokines amplify the inflammatory response and contribute to further injury. It is now appreciated that overlapping with this acute exudative phase (rather than following it, as was previously thought) is a process of repair, markers of which have been identified as early as a few hours into the course of disease (41). This phase or process is characterized by the presence of intra-alveolar mesenchymal cells/fibroblasts, type II cell hyperproliferation, and extracellular matrix turnover. In many cases of ALI, the process of repair proceeds normally, with complete resolution of inflammation and fibrosis and a reestablishment of normal alveolar architecture.

In some instances, however, the resolution phase of ALI results in disordered repair of the alveolus, a process characterized by impaired fibrinolysis of the inflammatory coagulum, fibrocellular proliferation, architectural distortion of the lung parenchyma, and impaired angiogenesis. Clinically, the result of this fibroproliferative phase of ALI is a restrictive ventilatory defect and evidence of impaired alveolar membrane function, characterized by a prolonged reduction in the diffusing capacity for carbon monoxide (46).

Alveolar Epithelial Repair Following Acute Lung Injury

Restoration of the normal air space architecture requires reconstitution of the denuded type I alveolar epithelial cells that have undergone apoptotic and necrotic death during the exudative phase of ALI. Regeneration of type II epithelial cells, in coordination with extracellular matrix turnover, is important in reestablishing surfactant production and ion transport, functions essential for maintaining open and dry alveoli. It is apparent that orderly re-epithelialization suppresses fibroblast proliferation and matrix deposition after ALI (3,64). Thus, efficient restoration of the alveolar epithelium in the early phase of ALI/ARDS may speed recovery by enhancing alveolar liquid clearance and preventing the development of pulmonary fibrosis (6). In addition, the endothelium plays a critical role in the repair and remodeling of the alveolar capillary membrane (50).

Several mechanisms have major roles in alveolar epithelial repair in vivo and in vitro. Proliferation of alveolar type II cells is the most obvious and easily measurable event in epithelial repair in vivo, but 1–2 days transpire before it becomes significant (6). It is clear that other mechanisms probably contribute to early alveolar epithelial wound repair, especially in those situations in which progression to severe fibroproliferative changes does not occur. Recent studies have raised interesting possibilities. In vitro studies in an alveolar/epithelial wound repair model using primary alveolar type II epithelial cells isolated from rat lungs showed that cell spreading and migration are primarily responsible for efficient epithelial wound repair (25). Importantly, evidence derived from human BALF studies demonstrates that pulmonary edema fluid from patients with ALI/ARDS stimulates repair of epithelial monolayers that have been injured. One of the factors present in this edema fluid that helps support alveolar epithelial repair is IL-1β (23,24).

Evidence exists that epidermal growth factor (EGF), TGF-α, and their common receptor, epidermal growth factor receptor (EGFR), may also participate in epithelial repair following injury. TGF-α is elevated in edema fluid from patients with ALI/ARDS and induces alveolar/epithelial repair in vitro (34). Indeed, neutralizing antibodies to EGF and TGF-α decreased IL-1β–induced alveolar/epithelial repair. Further, blocking EGFR or its intracellular signaling through MAPK specifically inhibits the reparative effects of IL-1β in ALI (25). IL-1β appears to act in part by activating the EGF/TGF-α pathway in an autocrine/paracrine fashion. The potential value of using TGF-α or EGF to treat patients with ALI has not yet been evaluated.

Animal studies suggest that keratinocyte growth factor (KGF) and hepatocyte growth factor (HGF) may play a role in lung repair. KGF is produced primarily by fibroblasts and induces alveolar type II proliferation in vivo and in vitro (59). KGF has a protective effect against lung injury when administered before the injury (15). Further, elevated levels of KGF correlate with alveolar/epithelial cell proliferation following bleomycin injury, again supporting a role for KGF in epithelial repair (2,5). Experiments using specific inhibitors of the EGF/TGF-α pathway suggest that the effects of KGF are mediated again through the EGFR pathway. These findings, coupled with the previously-mentioned role of IL-1β and TGF-α, suggest that EGFR serves as a final common pathway in stimulating alveolar epithelial repair, at least in vitro (23). HGF is another potent mitogen for alveolar type II cells and is upregulated in fibroblasts following inflammatory cytokine stimulation (48). HGF is elevated in pulmonary edema in ALI/ARDS, supporting a role for HGF in epithelial repair (62).

In summary, alveolar/epithelial repair is extremely complicated and modulated by numerous growth factors and cytokines. These factors are secreted both from local cells, such as fibroblasts, and from inflammatory cells that accumulate in the alveolar space during lung injury. It is clear that proper communication must occur between the renewing epithelial cell populations, the underlying extracellular matrix, and the endothelial cells, which are undergoing constant changes in the setting of ALI. Much work is needed to establish how the alveolar/epithelial surface is repaired following ALI and how this repair process can ultimately be manipulated with therapeutic strategies to heal the injured lung.

Potential Mechanisms Involved in Fibroproliferative Phase of Acute Respiratory Distress Syndrome

Either during or following the acute inflammatory response to injury, interstitial fibroblasts migrate into the alveolar clot/coagulum, characterizing the beginning of the fibroproliferative phase of ALI (**Fig. 40.4**). The interstitial fibroblasts, either during or following migration, differentiate into myofibroblasts, which contain abundant α-smooth muscle actin and vinculin. This much more "metabolically active" fibroblast proliferates in its new location and exhibits upregulated expression of important integrin receptors, including the fibronectin receptor α5β1, CD44, and the receptor for hyaluronic acid–mediated motility (RHAMM), probably allowing for increased motility and specific interactions with the newly evolving microenvironment (40,70). Fibroproliferation is also seen in the microcirculation of the lung. In the airspace, fibroproliferation leads to shunt; in the microcirculation, it contributes to narrowing of the cross-sectional area, which contributes to pulmonary hypertension.

Transforming Growth Factor-β in the Fibroproliferative Phase

In addition to its likely roles in the acute phase of ALI, TGF-β also has an important role in the fibroproliferative responses observed in ALI (16,19,22). TGF-β is a major regulator of gene expression, particularly of extracellular matrix molecules, in mesenchymal cells and lung fibroblasts. It is a potent inducer of collagen synthesis, has the ability to directly cause differentiation of fibroblasts into myofibroblasts, and inhibits collagenase production (9,22,31). It is also clear that TGF-β induces

proliferation of same fibroblast populations, most probably through the induction of other growth factors, such as platelet-derived growth factor. TGF-β can establish an apparent state of autocrine stimulation in structural cells, including fibroblasts, resulting in chronic activation and possible differentiation to a more aggressive phenotype, a cell that would be consistent with nonresolving or severe disease. Indeed, investigators have described a population of alveolar mesenchymal cells isolated from patients with nonresolving ARDS that exhibited constitutive activation of prosurvival signaling pathways (28). These observations are important because they support the theory that, during the resolution of the fibrotic phase of lung injury, apoptosis of mesenchymal cells may be an essential component of normal repair and resolution. Conversely, they suggest that dysregulation of this process and appearance of cells that are resistant to apoptosis may lead to persistent or nonresolving ARDS.

Additional support for the role of TGF-β in the fibroproliferative responses can be detected in lungs of animal models of alveolar injury that leads to pulmonary fibrosis, as well as in human idiopathic pulmonary fibrosis during the active phase of ALI. The steady-state expression of TGF-β transcripts increases at ~1 week after intratracheal installation of bleomycin (66). These, as well as in vitro experiments, show that increased expression of TGF-β precedes the increased matrix deposition, supporting the involvement of this cytokine in the fibrotic process. Further support for the role of TGF-β comes from a bleomycin model in which a significant reduction in lung collagen accumulation and myeloperoxidase activity is noted when a concomitant IV administration of anti–TGF-β1 and –TGF-β2 antibodies is given to mice (26). The same inhibitory effect was reported in a mouse model of immune-induced lung fibrosis (14). An important source of TGF-β is the alveolar macrophage, because corticosteroids may modulate the late fibroproliferative stage of lung injury. It has been demonstrated that dexamethasone can inhibit macrophage secretion of

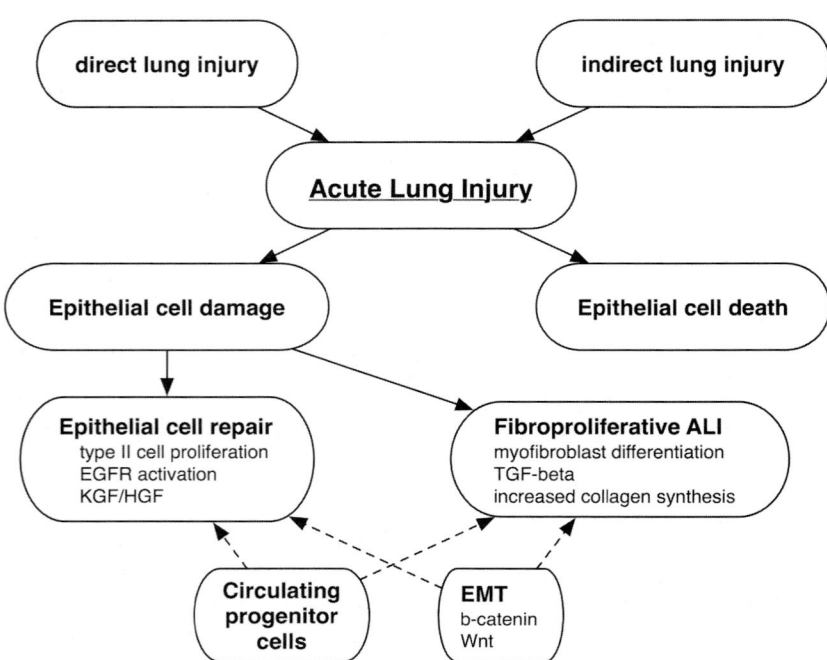

FIGURE 40.4. Fibroproliferation in lung injury. Direct and indirect triggers of ALI lead to epithelial cell damage and death. Recovery from epithelial damage can proceed to normal regulated repair mechanisms or to dysregulated mechanisms of fibroproliferation. Circulating progenitor cells and epithelial-mesenchymal transitions (EMT) may contribute to both repair and fibroproliferation. EGFR, epidermal growth factor receptor; TGF-β, transforming growth factor-β; KGF, keratinocyte growth factor; HGF, hepatocyte growth factor

IL-1 but, in fact, has very little effect on TGF-β1 secretion (33). Thus, it is possible that the variable efficacy of corticosteroid therapy in patients in the late stages of ALI is attributable to this divergence of effects, with corticosteroids causing a reduction in cytokine release but having little effect on TGF-β production by alveolar macrophages.

Epithelial-Mesenchymal Transdifferentiation in Fibroproliferative Acute Lung Injury

As accumulation of fibroblast or myofibroblast-like cells is critical in the fibroproliferative state of ALI, investigators have evaluated several pathways through which accumulation of these cells might occur. Work in other organ systems, especially the kidney, has suggested that transdifferentiation of epithelial cells into matrix-producing mesenchymal cells (fibroblasts and myofibroblasts) might be involved. Indeed, recent studies have suggested that transdifferentiation of epithelial cells into matrix-producing fibroblasts is a potential mechanism by which disordered epithelial repair promotes progression to the fibroproliferative stage of ALI (67). Several pathways regulate this process of epithelial-mesenchymal transdifferentiation (EMT). TGF-β again seems especially important (30,49). Another important pathway in the EMT process is the Wnt signaling pathway, which is interesting because several lines of investigation suggest that the mechanisms of resolution of ALI repair in adults are controlled, in part, by regulatory pathways that are important in lung morphogenesis and development (10,67). The Wnt pathway is one of numerous signaling pathways critical for precise temporal and spatial control of lung morphogenesis (57). Within this Wnt signaling pathway, β-catenin is a key regulatory protein. For instance, targeted deletion of β-catenin from the alveolar epithelium of developing mouse embryos results in complete disruption of the peripheral terminal alveolar saccule formation and in disturbances of pulmonary vasculogenesis (45). Interestingly, β-catenin expression is induced in type II epithelial cells in hyperoxia-exposed animals. It has been demonstrated that β-catenin signaling is upregulated in the reparative remodeling response to ALI (17). These studies suggest a strong association between enhanced expression of the cadherin/catenin axis with epithelial regeneration and EMT. Thus, EMT could contribute to myofibroblast proliferation and collagen deposition in ALI. Its role in lung fibrotic conditions deserves future attention.

Progenitor Cells in Acute Lung Injury

Evidence in a number of experimental systems suggests that mobilization of progenitor cells from the injured tissue or from the bone marrow may repair damage caused by a variety of insults (35,36). Numerous groups are exploring the possibilities that progenitor-type cells are involved in the injury process and/or potentially could be manipulated to ameliorate the disease process. Several experimental protocols have been developed to examine the effect of whole bone marrow transplantation, mesenchymal stem cell transplantation, and parabiosis on repair processes following injury. These models confirm that after lung damage, either with chemical agents or radiation,

injured recipient lungs can become repopulated with cells of donor origins, including type I and II epithelial cells, endothelial cells, and fibroblast and interstitial monocytes. These studies demonstrate that engraftment of stem cells into the lung is most robust following injury. Engraftment of donor cells in organs is minimal in control animals not subjected to chemical or radiation damage (1,54,69). It is also interesting to note that intact, noninjured bone marrow may be integral to protective responses. In one study, bone marrow ablation without transplantation caused changes in the lung reminiscent of emphysema in the absence of direct lung injury (54). Collectively, research suggests that when the lung is damaged by a variety of causes (chemicals, infection, radiation), progenitor cells are released from the bone marrow and attracted by as yet unidentified factors to the damaged lung. These cells act in a beneficial manner to repair the lung. For example, experiments in patients with ALI demonstrated that they have an increased number of circulating endothelial progenitor cells compared to healthy controls. Further, a greater number of circulating endothelial progenitor cells is associated with improved outcomes in a multivariable analysis that corrected for the effects for age, gender, and severity of illness scores. It should be noted, however, that progenitor cells could also, under certain circumstances, contribute to ongoing fibroproliferative responses, as has been demonstrated following bleomycin injury, in which a subset of circulating mesenchymal progenitor cells, termed *fibrocytes*, is recruited to the lung and contributes significantly to the fibroproliferative changes (38). Future studies will have to determine in more detail the role that these cells play in repair of the lung following injury.

CONCLUSIONS AND FUTURE DIRECTIONS

The large and evolving body of knowledge of the molecular biology of lung injury is highly complex and incomplete. Nonetheless, these complex molecular interactions and signaling networks both form the basis for current treatment strategies and suggest possible avenues for developing new therapies. Current approaches to ALI attempt to control edema formation primarily by reducing inflammation, by treating the underlying or exacerbating conditions, and by limiting ventilator-induced damage to the alveolar-capillary barrier. Observed reductions in circulating cytokines in patients who were ventilated with "lung protective" strategies confirm the validity of this approach. Otherwise, very little modern medicine is directed specifically at reducing lung microvascular permeability in the injured lung. Therapy directed at reducing microvascular pressures is generally reserved for patients in overt right heart failure, with the exception of inhaled NO, which is sometimes used to improve ventilation-perfusion matching in the injured lung. While inhaled NO has gained much attention for its ability to improve oxygenation in some patients with ALI, the effect is transient, and inhaled NO has not been demonstrated to alter the outcome of the illness, perhaps due to the multiple conflicting roles of NO in the injured lung. Efforts to reduce fluid intake and improve overall fluid balance have also been suggested as a means of reducing microvascular pressures favoring edema formation, although this strategy remains under study. While corticosteroids are under study for the prevention of late fibroproliferative changes in ALI, data in children do not yet exist and adult data demonstrate modest efficacy at best.

In terms of modulating epithelial function, the well-described surfactant lipid and protein changes in ALI have led to several trials of surfactant replacement as treatment for this condition. These trials have been generally disappointing. Whether the lack of efficacy in most studies results from ineffective delivery methods or insufficient replacement of surfactant proteins (as opposed to surfactant lipids) remains to be determined, but positive results from a recent trial of surfactant replacement in children seem certain to spur renewed interest in this approach (68).

Novel therapies directed at specific molecular mediators of lung injury have the potential to substantially improve the care of patients with ALI. In terms of the control of endothelial permeability, treatments directed more specifically at the preservation of endothelial barrier integrity hold promise. Rho kinase inhibitors appear effective in experimental animals, and several compounds are being tested in human clinical trials for other indications. Similarly, S1P analogs and HMG-CoA-reductase inhibitors (statins) both act via Rac activation to improve endothelial-barrier integrity and appear effective in ameliorating lung injury in animal models. Statins also prevent the posttranslational modifications necessary for RhoA activation and may prove helpful in both improving endothelial-barrier function and controlling vascular tone.

Therapies directed at mediators of the endothelial cytoskeleton may also prove viable. Current investigation of the utility of anticoagulant therapies, such as activated protein C, for ALI hope to exploit the linkage between coagulation and inflammation to ameliorate lung injury. Antiangiogenic therapies provide another possible avenue of investigation. VEGF antagonism may reduce endothelial permeability and edema formation, although this approach potentially could have detrimental effects on pulmonary vascular pressure and on epithelial regeneration. Available anti-VEGF agents are well tolerated as antineoplastic agents but have not yet been investigated for use in human ALI. Endothelin receptor antagonists are also well tolerated when used for pulmonary hypertension and may have beneficial effects in ALI, both by reducing vascular pressures and by reducing the generation of excessive amounts of other mediators, such as VEGF, although they remain unstudied for this indication in humans. Some investigators have suggested targeting transcriptional mediators, such as HIF-1 or NFκB, to reduce inflammation and injury in ALI. Additional novel therapies may be directed at the preservation or restoration of alveolar liquid clearance mechanisms. Studies of inhaled β-agonist to improve edema clearance in ALI are ongoing at present, as are preclinical studies of gene transfer therapies to increase the expression of sodium-transporting proteins. Finally, as our understanding of the reparative processes in the lung improves, therapies targeted at improving epithelial cell regeneration and reducing fibroproliferation may ultimately reduce the long-term consequences of ALI on lung function.

Clearly, many of the possible new approaches to interrupting the mechanisms that underlie lung injury are complicated by the multiple roles that many of these important mediators appear to play in the processes of both lung injury and repair. VEGF is one example of such a molecule, and many transcriptional regulators, including NFκB also contribute to the process of repair after injury. Enthusiasm over the possibility that antagonizing these mediators early in the course of ALI could alter its course and improve outcome is tempered by the possibility that such approaches could have deleterious effects on the recovery phase of lung injury. Devising strategies that reduce injury without reducing repair mechanisms remains a challenge and will require continued careful investigation of the molecular mechanisms that underlie both processes.

A final additional caveat in this discussion is the role of development. Most lung injury research has focused on adult animal models and adult patients, but some recent data suggest that the developing lung may be more susceptible to some injuries and less susceptible to others as compared to the adult lung. The molecular mechanisms that underlie these differences remain largely unexplored and may have profound implications for the development of future treatments for ALI in the PICU.

KEY POINTS

- Understanding the molecular mechanisms responsible for ALI is crucial to understanding both current and future treatments of ALI and other lung illnesses in the ICU.
- Pulmonary edema formation in early ALI requires disruption of the endothelial barrier via alterations in endothelial cell-cell and cell-matrix junctions, as well as rearrangement of the endothelial cell cytoskeleton.
- Pulmonary vascular tone may contribute to edema formation in early ALI, and many regulators of vascular tone in the injured lung, such as ET and NO, also act as signaling and cytokine mediators that participate in regulating inflammatory responses.
- Impairment of innate alveolar liquid clearance mechanisms involving ENaC and Na/K-ATPases contributes to pulmonary edema accumulation in ALI.
- Surfactant dysfunction and loss of surfactant proteins are critical features of lung injury.
- Many mediators, including transcription factors, signaling molecules, cytokines, chemokines, coagulation system proteins, and angiogenic mediators, amplify and extend the injury process in the lung.
- Repair of the injured lung involves both epithelial and mesenchymal cell proliferation, and may involve circulating progenitor cells and EMT.

ACKNOWLEDGMENTS

This work was supported by NIH SCOR Grant HL57144-10 and Program Project Grant HL14985-34 (KRS), and NIH Grant HL07743 (TC).

References

1. Abe S, Boyer C, Liu X, et al. Cells derived from the circulation contribute to the repair of lung injury. *Am J Respir Crit Care Med* 2004;170:1158–63.
2. Adamson IY, Bakowska J. Relationship of keratinocyte growth factor and hepatocyte growth factor levels in rat lung lavage fluid to epithelial cell regeneration after bleomycin. *Am J Pathol* 1999;155:949–54.
3. Adamson IY, Young L, Bowden DH. Relationship of alveolar epithelial injury and repair to the induction of pulmonary fibrosis. *Am J Pathol* 1988;130:377–83.
4. Angelini DJ, Hyun SW, Grigoryev DN, et al. TNF{alpha} Increases Tyrosine Phosphorylation of Vascular Endothelial-Cadherin and Opens the

Paracellular Pathway Through Fyn Activation in Human Lung Endothelia. *Am J Physiol Lung Cell Mol Physiol* 2006.

5. Atabai K, Ishigaki M, Geiser T, et al. Keratinocyte growth factor can enhance alveolar epithelial repair by nonmitogenic mechanisms. *Am J Physiol Lung Cell Mol Physiol* 2002;283:L163–9.

6. Berthiaume Y, Lesur O, Dagenais A. Treatment of adult respiratory distress syndrome: Plea for rescue therapy of the alveolar epithelium. *Thorax* 1999; 54:150–60.

7. Birukova AA, Chatchavalvanich S, Rios A, et al. Differential regulation of pulmonary endothelial monolayer integrity by varying degrees of cyclic stretch. *Am J Pathol* 2006;168:1749–61.

8. Brinkmann V, Baumruker T. Pulmonary and vascular pharmacology of sphingosine 1-phosphate. *Curr Opin Pharmacol* 2006;6(3):244–50.

9. Broekelmann TJ, Limper AH, Colby TV, et al. Transforming growth factor beta 1 is present at sites of extracellular matrix gene expression in human pulmonary fibrosis. *Proc Natl Acad Sci U S A* 1991;88:6642–6.

10. Chilosi M, Poletti V, Zamo A, et al. Aberrant Wnt/beta-catenin pathway activation in idiopathic pulmonary fibrosis. *Am J Pathol* 2003;162:1495–502.

11. Choi WI, Quinn DA, Park KM, et al. Systemic microvascular leak in an in vivo rat model of ventilator-induced lung injury. *Am J Respir Crit Care Med* 2003;167:1627–32.

12. Corada M, Mariotti M, Thurston G, et al. Vascular endothelial-cadherin is an important determinant of microvascular integrity in vivo. *Proc Natl Acad Sci U S A* 1999;96:9815–20.

13. Dagenais A, Gosselin D, Guilbault C, et al. Modulation of epithelial sodium channel (ENaC) expression in mouse lung infected with Pseudomonas aeruginosa. *Respir Res* 2005;6:2.

14. Denis M. Neutralization of transforming growth factor-beta 1 in a mouse model of immune-induced lung fibrosis. *Immunology* 1994;82:584–90.

15. Deterding RR, Havill AM, Yano T, et al. Prevention of bleomycin-induced lung injury in rats by keratinocyte growth factor. *Proc Assoc Am Physicians* 1997;109:254–68.

16. Dhainaut JF, Charpentier J, Chiche JD. Transforming growth factor-beta: A mediator of cell regulation in acute respiratory distress syndrome. *Crit Care Med* 2003;31:S258–64.

17. Douglas IS, Del Valle FD, Winn RA, et al. beta-Catenin in the Fibroproliferative Response to Acute Lung Injury. *Am J Respir Cell Mol Biol* 2006;34:274–85.

18. Dudek SM, Garcia JG. Cytoskeletal regulation of pulmonary vascular permeability. *J Appl Physiol* 2001;91:1487–500.

19. Fahy RJ, Lichtenberger F, McKeegan CB, et al. The acute respiratory distress syndrome: A role for transforming growth factor-beta 1. *Am J Respir Cell Mol Biol* 2003;28:499–503.

20. Freichel M, Vennekens R, Olausson J, et al. Functional role of TRPC proteins in native systems: Implications from knockout and knock-down studies. *J Physiol* 2005;567:59–66.

21. Ganter BG, Jakob SM, Takala J. Pulmonary capillary pressure. A review. *Minerva Anestesiol* 2006;72:21–36.

22. Gauldie J, Jordana M, Cox G. Cytokines and pulmonary fibrosis. *Thorax* 1993;48:931–5.

23. Geiser T. Mechanisms of alveolar epithelial repair in acute lung injury—a translational approach. *Swiss Med Wkly* 2003;133:586–90.

24. Geiser T, Atabai K, Jarreau PH, et al. Pulmonary edema fluid from patients with acute lung injury augments in vitro alveolar epithelial repair by an IL-1beta-dependent mechanism. *Am J Respir Crit Care Med* 2001;163: 1384–8.

25. Geiser T, Jarreau PH, Atabai K, et al. Interleukin-1beta augments in vitro alveolar epithelial repair. *Am J Physiol Lung Cell Mol Physiol* 2000;279: L1184–90.

26. Giri SN, Hyde DM, Hollinger MA. Effect of antibody to transforming growth factor beta on bleomycin induced accumulation of lung collagen in mice. *Thorax* 1993;48:959–66.

27. Haddad JJ. Science review: Redox and oxygen-sensitive transcription factors in the regulation of oxidant-mediated lung injury: Role for hypoxia-inducible factor-1alpha. *Crit Care* 2003;7:47–54.

28. Horowitz JC, Cui Z, Moore TA, et al. Constitutive activation of prosurvival signaling in alveolar mesenchymal cells isolated from patients with nonresolving acute respiratory distress syndrome. *Am J Physiol Lung Cell Mol Physiol* 2006;290:L415–25.

29. Jenkins RG, Su X, Su G, et al. Ligation of protease-activated receptor 1 enhances alphavbeta6 integrin-dependent TGF-beta activation and promotes acute lung injury. *J Clin Invest* 2006;116(6):1606–14.

30. Kalluri R, Neilson EG. Epithelial-mesenchymal transition and its implications for fibrosis. *J Clin Invest* 2003;112:1776–84.

31. Kaminski N, Allard JD, Pittet JF, et al. Global analysis of gene expression in pulmonary fibrosis reveals distinct programs regulating lung inflammation and fibrosis. *Proc Natl Acad Sci U S A* 2000;97:1778–83.

32. Karmpaliotis D, Kosmidou I, Ingenito EP, et al. Angiogenic growth factors in the pathophysiology of a murine model of acute lung injury. *Am J Physiol Lung Cell Mol Physiol* 2002;283:L585–95.

33. Khalil N, Whitman C, Zuo L, et al. Regulation of alveolar macrophage transforming growth factor-beta secretion by corticosteroids in bleomycin-induced pulmonary inflammation in the rat. *J Clin Invest* 1993;92:1812–8.

34. Kheradmand F, Folkesson HG, Shum L, et al. Transforming growth factor-

35. Korbling M, Estrov Z. Adult stem cells for tissue repair: A new therapeutic concept? *N Engl J Med* 2003;349:570–82.

36. Kotton DN, Summer R, Fine A. Lung stem cells: New paradigms. *Exp Hematol* 2004;32:340–3.

37. Kuebler WM, Ying X, Singh B, et al. Pressure is proinflammatory in lung venular capillaries. *J Clin Invest* 1999;104:495–502.

38. Lama VN, Phan SH. The extrapulmonary origin of fibroblasts: Stem/progenitor cells and beyond. *Proc Am Thorac Soc* 2006;3:373–6.

39. Lopez-Aguilar J, Piacentini E, Villagra A, et al. Contributions of vascular flow and pulmonary capillary pressure to ventilator-induced lung injury. *Crit Care Med* 2006;34:1106–12.

40. Lovvorn HN, 3rd, Cass DL, Sylvester KG, et al. Hyaluronan receptor expression increases in fetal excisional skin wounds and correlates with fibroplasia. *J Pediatr Surg* 1998;33:1062–9; discussion 9–70.

41. Marshall RP, Bellingan G, Webb S, et al. Fibroproliferation occurs early in the acute respiratory distress syndrome and impacts on outcome. *Am J Respir Crit Care Med* 2000;162:1783–8.

42. Matthay MA, Robriquet L, Fang X. Alveolar epithelium: Role in lung fluid balance and acute lung injury. *Proc Am Thorac Soc* 2005;2:206–13.

43. McVerry BJ, Garcia JG. In vitro and in vivo modulation of vascular barrier integrity by sphingosine 1-phosphate: Mechanistic insights. *Cell Signal* 2005;17:131–9.

44. Modelska K, Pittet JF, Folkesson HG, et al. Acid-induced lung injury. Protective effect of anti-interleukin-8 pretreatment on alveolar epithelial barrier function in rabbits. *Am J Respir Crit Care Med* 1999;160:1450–6.

45. Mucenski ML, Wert SE, Nation JM, et al. beta-Catenin is required for specification of proximal/distal cell fate during lung morphogenesis. *J Biol Chem* 2003;278:40231–8.

46. Neff TA, Stocker R, Frey HR, et al. Long-term assessment of lung function in survivors of severe ARDS. *Chest* 2003;123:845–53.

47. Nunes S, Ruokonen E, Takala J. Pulmonary capillary pressures during the acute respiratory distress syndrome. *Intensive Care Med* 2003;29:2174–9.

48. Ohmichi H, Matsumoto K, Nakamura T. In vivo mitogenic action of HGF on lung epithelial cells: Pulmotrophic role in lung regeneration. *Am J Physiol* 1996;270:L1031–9.

49. Okada H, Kalluri R. Cellular and molecular pathways that lead to progression and regression of renal fibrogenesis. *Curr Mol Med* 2005;5:467–74.

50. Orfanos SE, Mavrommati I, Korovesi I, et al. Pulmonary endothelium in acute lung injury: From basic science to the critically ill. *Intensive Care Med* 2004;30:1702–14.

51. Parikh SM, Mammoto T, Schultz A, et al. Excess Circulating Angiopoietin-2 May Contribute to Pulmonary Vascular Leak in Sepsis in Humans. *PLoS Med* 2006;3:e46.

52. Parsons PE, Fowler AA, Hyers TM, et al. Chemotactic activity in bronchoalveolar lavage fluid from patients with adult respiratory distress syndrome. *Am Rev Respir Dis* 1985;132:490–3.

53. Predescu D, Predescu S, Shimizu J, et al. Constitutive eNOS-derived nitric oxide is a determinant of endothelial junctional integrity. *Am J Physiol Lung Cell Mol Physiol* 2005;289:L371–81.

54. Rojas M, Xu J, Woods CR, et al. Bone marrow-derived mesenchymal stem cells in repair of the injured lung. *Am J Respir Cell Mol Biol* 2005;33:145–52.

55. Roux J, Kawakatsu H, Gartland B, et al. Interleukin-1beta decreases expression of the epithelial sodium channel alpha-subunit in alveolar epithelial cells via a p38 MAPK-dependent signaling pathway. *J Biol Chem* 2005;280: 18579–89.

56. Schultz MJ, Haitsma JJ, Zhang H, et al. Pulmonary coagulopathy as a new target in therapeutic studies of acute lung injury or pneumonia–A review. *Crit Care Med* 2006;34:871–7.

57. Shannon JM, Hyatt BA. Epithelial-mesenchymal interactions in the developing lung. *Annu Rev Physiol* 2004;66:625–45.

58. Siflinger-Birnboim A, Johnson A. Protein kinase C modulates pulmonary endothelial permeability: A paradigm for acute lung injury. *Am J Physiol Lung Cell Mol Physiol* 2003;284:L435–51.

59. Ulich TR, Yi ES, Longmuir K, et al. Keratinocyte growth factor is a growth factor for type II pneumocytes in vivo. *J Clin Invest* 1994;93:1298–306.

60. Vadasz I, Morty RE, Olschewski A, et al. Thrombin impairs alveolar fluid clearance by promoting endocytosis of Na+,K+-ATPase. *Am J Respir Cell Mol Biol* 2005;33:343–54.

61. van Nieuw Amerongen GP, van Delft S, Vermeer MA, et al. Activation of RhoA by thrombin in endothelial hyperpermeability: Role of Rho kinase and protein tyrosine kinases. *Circ Res* 2000;87:335–40.

62. Verghese GM, McCormick-Shannon K, Mason RJ, et al. Hepatocyte growth factor and keratinocyte growth factor in the pulmonary edema fluid of patients with acute lung injury. Biologic and clinical significance. *Am J Respir Crit Care Med* 1998;158:386–94.

63. Ware LB, Camerer E, Welty-Wolf K, et al. Bench to bedside: Targeting coagulation and fibrinolysis in acute lung injury. *Am J Physiol Lung Cell Mol Physiol* 2006;291:L307–11.

64. Ware LB, Matthay MA. The acute respiratory distress syndrome. *N Engl J Med* 2000;342:1334–49.

65. West JB. Invited review: Pulmonary capillary stress failure. *J Appl Physiol* 2000;89:2483–9; discussion 97.

66. Westergren-Thorsson G, Hernnas J, Sarnstrand B, et al. Altered expression

of small proteoglycans, collagen, and transforming growth factor-beta 1 in developing bleomycin-induced pulmonary fibrosis in rats. *J Clin Invest* 1993;92:632–7.

67. Willis BC, Liebler JM, Luby-Phelps K, et al. Induction of epithelial-mesenchymal transition in alveolar epithelial cells by transforming growth factor-beta1: Potential role in idiopathic pulmonary fibrosis. *Am J Pathol* 2005;166:1321–32.

68. Willson DF, Thomas NJ, Markovitz BP, et al. Effect of exogenous surfactant (calfactant) in pediatric acute lung injury: A randomized controlled trial. *JAMA* 2005;293:470–6.

69. Yamada M, Kubo H, Kobayashi S, et al. Bone marrow-derived progenitor cells are important for lung repair after lipopolysaccharide-induced lung injury. *J Immunol* 2004;172:1266–72.

70. Zaman A, Cui Z, Foley JP, et al. Expression and role of the hyaluronan receptor RHAMM in inflammation after bleomycin injury. *Am J Respir Cell Mol Biol* 2005;33:447–54.

CHAPTER 41 ■ RESPIRATORY PHYSIOLOGY

FRANK L. POWELL • GREGORY P. HELDT • GABRIEL G. HADDAD

PULMONARY GAS EXCHANGE

Pulmonary gas exchange describes the process of O_2 uptake and CO_2 elimination by the lungs to supply the metabolic demands of the body. This section of the chapter focuses on pulmonary gas exchange and how the lungs load adequate O_2 into the blood to meet tissue O_2 demand. It also covers the physiology of O_2 and CO_2 transport by the cardiovascular system and tissue gas exchange. Understanding pulmonary and tissue gas exchange also requires understanding O_2 and CO_2 blood dissociation curves, which are also discussed.

Normal O_2 values are shown in **Figure 41.1** as partial pressures (Po_2) that can be measured in gas, blood, and tissue samples from a resting adult at sea level. Partial pressure is calculated as the fraction of the total barometric pressure occupied by a given gas species:

$$P_x = F_x (P_{bar})$$

where F_x is the fractional concentration of gas "x" in a *dry* gas sample. Partial pressure is expressed in units of torr (1 torr = 1 mm Hg) or SI units of kilo Pascals (1 kPa = 7.5 mm Hg) in physiology.

The Po_2 decreases at every step, and this is called the O_2 *cascade*. The Po_2 drop between dry room air and inspired gas in the trachea (Pio_2) is due to humidification. Gas in the airways is saturated with water vapor at body temperature so that the total gas pressure available for O_2 and CO_2 inside the body is reduced. The water vapor pressure is 47 mm Hg at 37°C and 100% saturation. For a normal barometric pressure of 760 mm Hg at sea level:

Po_2 in dry ambient air = 0.21 × 760 mm Hg
= 160 mm Hg

Pio_2 in the airways = 0.21 × (760 − 47) mm Hg
= 150 mm Hg

Further decreases in Po_2 along the O_2 cascade are explained by the physiology of gas exchange. The large drop in Po_2 between inspired and alveolar gas is a function of ventilation. Diffusion across the blood-gas barrier and other factors, such as shunts and the mismatching of ventilation and pulmonary blood flow, explain the relatively small decrease in Po_2 between alveolar gas and arterial blood. The circulation and O_2 diffusion from capillaries to tissues cause the large decreases in Po_2 between arterial and venous blood, and between blood and mitochondria in the tissues

Gas exchange models are useful for quantifying respiratory function and diagnosing pulmonary disease. These models use a standard set of symbols developed for quantitative descriptions of respiratory physiology (**Table 41.1**). Generally, these models are based on the principle of conservation of mass, or *mass balance*, and they assume a steady state. *Steady state* means an equal and constant rate of gas transport at each step in the O_2 cascade, but it does not necessarily imply resting conditions. O_2 transport can be elevated but still equal at every step in the O_2 cascade (e.g., during steady-state exercise). However, non–steady-state conditions occur frequently (e.g., at the onset of exercise or in acute respiratory distress).

In an "ideal" model of alveolar gas exchange, arterial blood equilibrates with alveolar gas; therefore, the ideal alveolar-arterial Po_2 difference equals zero. In reality, the alveolar-arterial Po_2 difference exceeds zero, even in health (**Fig. 41.1**). Several factors, called *gas exchange limitations*, increase the alveolar-arterial Po_2 difference. Gas exchange limitations do not necessarily affect O_2 consumption at rest, but they can lower maximal O_2 consumption and decrease Po_2 values along the O_2 cascade in a steady state. The alveolar-arterial Po_2 difference is useful for diagnosing O_2 exchange limitations because different limitations respond differently to simple tests such as O_2 breathing.

The Blood-Oxygen Equilibrium Curve

The blood-O_2 equilibrium curves (O_2 dissociation curves) quantify O_2 carriage in blood as graphs of concentration versus partial pressure. It is necessary to consider both partial pressure and concentration because partial pressure gradients drive diffusive gas transport in lungs and tissues, but concentration differences determine convective gas transport rates in lungs and the circulation (see the section, Cardiovascular and Tissue Oxygen Transport).

This topic would be much simpler to explain and understand if O_2 was physiologically inert and occurred in blood only as physically dissolved gas. The concentration of a dissolved gas in a liquid is directly and linearly proportional to its partial pressure according to Henry's law ($C = \alpha P$, where α = solubility). However, O_2 also enters into chemical reactions with blood that (a) increase O_2 concentration in blood, and (b) allow physiologic modulation of O_2 transport by blood.

Normal O_2 concentration in arterial blood (Cao_2) is ~20 mL/dL. (The usual units for O_2 and CO_2 concentration in blood are mL/dL, also called volume %; 1 mL/dL $\approx$ 0.45 mmol/L.) However, only 0.3 mL/dL is physically dissolved gas; normal arterial Po_2 (Pao_2) is 100 mm Hg, and the physical solubility of O_2 in blood is 0.003 mL/(dL × mm Hg) at 37°C. If arterial blood contained only dissolved O_2, cardiac output would have to be 100 L/min to deliver enough O_2 to the tissues for a normal adult metabolic rate of 300 mL O_2/min!

Hemoglobin

Hemoglobin (Hb) is responsible for this dramatic increase in blood's O_2-carrying capacity. Hb consists of four polypeptide

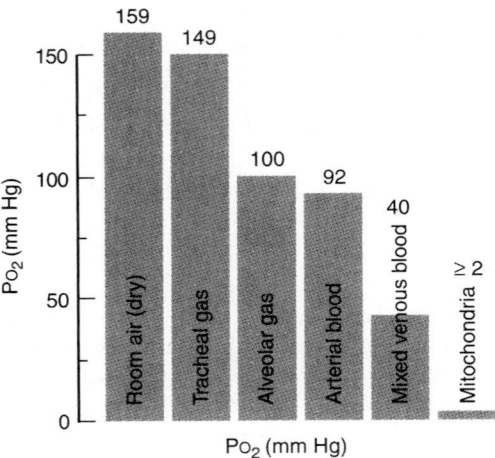

FIGURE 41.1. The "oxygen cascade" in a healthy subject breathing room air at sea level shows the pattern of Po_2 decrease between the different steps of O_2 transport. The difference between alveolar and arterial Po_2 occurs because of pulmonary gas exchange limitations. From Powell FL. Pulmonary gas exchange. In: Johnson LR, ed. *Essential Medical Physiology*, 3rd ed. Boston: Elsevier/Academic Press, 2003, with permission.

chains, each with a heme (iron-containing) protein that can bind O_2 with iron in the ferrous (Fe^{2+}) form. Methemoglobin results when iron is in the ferric form (Fe^{3+}) and cannot bind O_2. Small amounts of methemoglobin normally occur in blood and slightly reduce the amount of O_2 that can be bound to Hb. One gram of pure adult Hb can bind 1.39 mL of O_2 when fully saturated, but methemoglobin reduces this value to 1.34–1.36. The cellular packaging of Hb is important for the biophysics of the microcirculation, and it provides physiologic control of O_2 binding through cellular changes in the Hb microenvironment.

The four subunits of Hb include two α- and two β-chains, and variations in the amino acid sequence of these polypeptides explain the differences in Hb-O_2 affinity between species and at different stages of development. The three-dimensional shape of an Hb molecule, which is determined by the allosteric interactions of its four subunits, causes the O_2-equilibrium curve to be S-shaped, or sigmoidal (**Fig. 41.2**). O_2-equilibrium curves for individual α- and β-chains are not sigmoidal but simple convex curves similar to the O_2-equilibrium curve for myoglobin. Myoglobin occurs in muscle and has only a single polypeptide chain with one heme group. The sigmoidal shape of the O_2-Hb equilibrium curve facilitates O_2 loading into blood in the lungs and O_2 unloading from blood in the tissues.

Blood-Oxygen Equilibrium Curves

The two forms of the O_2-equilibrium curve are shown in **Figure 41.2**: (a) saturation of Hb with O_2 (So_2) versus Po_2, and (b) O_2 concentration in blood (Co_2) versus Po_2. Saturation quantifies the amount of O_2 in blood as the percentage of the total Hb sites available for binding O_2 that actually bind O_2 at a given Po_2. Therefore, saturation equilibrium curves are independent of Hb concentration in blood. In contrast, concentration curves quantify the absolute amount of O_2 in a volume of blood with a given Po_2, and they depend on the amount of Hb available.

O_2 capacity (O_{2cap}) is defined as the O_2 concentration in blood when Hb is 100% saturated with O_2. Pure Hb binds

TABLE 41.1

SYMBOLS IN RESPIRATORY PHYSIOLOGY

Primary variables (and units)	
C	Concentration or content (mL/dL or mmol/L)
D	Diffusing capacity [mLO_2 /(min × mm Hg)]
F	Fractional concentration in dry gas (dimensionless)
P	Gas pressure or partial pressure (mm Hg or cm H_2O)
$\dot{Q}$	Blood flow or perfusion (L/min)
R	Respiratory exchange ratio (dimensionless)
RQ	Respiratory quotient (dimensionless)
T	Temperature (°C)
V	Gas volume (L or mL)
$\dot{V}$	Ventilation (L/min)

Modifying symbols	
A	Alveolar gas
B	Barometric
D	Dead space gas
E	Expired gas
$\overline{E}$	Mixed-expired gas
I	Inspired gas
L	Lung or transpulmonary
T	Tidal gas
aw	Airway
w	Chest wall
es	Esophageal
pl	Intrapleural
rs	Transrespiratory system (total system)
a	Arterial blood
b	Blood (general)
c	Capillary blood
c'	End-capillary blood
T	Tissue
V	Venous blood
$\overline{v}$	Mixed-venous blood

Examples	
PAo_2 = Partial pressure of O_2 in alveolar gas
Pao_2 = Partial pressure of O_2 in arterial blood
$F\overline{E}co_2$ = Fraction of CO_2 in dry mixed, expired gas
$\dot{V}o_2$ = O_2 consumption per unit time
$\dot{V}A$ = Ventilation of the alveoli per unit time

1.39 mL O_2/g Hb, and **Figure 41.2** illustrates that the O_{2cap} for normal blood with a Hb concentration of 15 g/dL is 20.85 mL/dL (1.39 × 15). Physically dissolved also contributes a small amount to O_2 concentration. Therefore, total O_2 concentration in blood (in mL O_2/dL blood) is calculated as:

$$Co_2 = (O_{2cap} [So_2/100]) + (0.003 \, Po_2)$$

where:

$O_{2cap} = O_2$ capacity
$So_2 =$ saturation
$0.003 =$ physical solubility for O_2 in blood.

This equation and **Figure 41.2** show that dissolved O_2 is not a large component of O_2 concentration at Po_2 levels in arterial or venous blood (i.e., 100–40 mm Hg). The shape of the O_2-Hb equilibrium curves is complex and can be generated only experimentally or by sophisticated mathematical

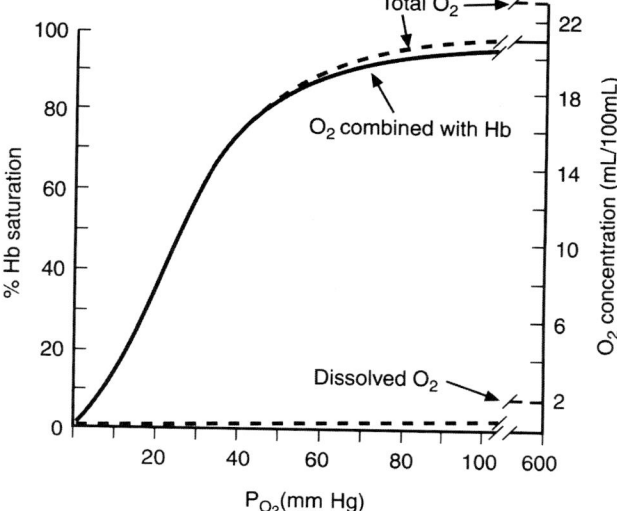

FIGURE 41.2. Standard human O_2-blood equilibrium (or dissociation) curve at pH = 7.4, Pco_2 = 40 mm Hg, and 37°C. Left ordinate shows O_2 saturation of hemoglobin (Hb) available for O_2 binding; right ordinate shows absolute O_2 concentration in blood. Most O_2 is bound to hemoglobin, and dissolved O_2 contributes very little to total O_2 concentration. From Powell FL. Oxygen and CO_2 transport in the blood. In: Johnson LR, ed. *Essential Medical Physiology*, 3rd ed. Boston: Elsevier/Academic Press, 2003, with permission.

algorithms. However, remembering only four points on the normal adult curve allows one to solve many common problems of O_2 transport:

(a) Po_2 = 0 mm Hg, So_2 = 0% (the origin of the curve)
(b) Po_2 = 100 mm Hg, So_2 = 98% (normal arterial blood, which is almost fully saturated)
(c) Po_2 = 40 mm Hg, So_2 = 75% (normal mixed venous blood)
(d) Po_2 = 26 mm Hg, So_2 = 50% (P_{50}, defined as the Po_2 at 50% saturation)

The P_{50} quantifies the affinity of Hb for O_2. For example, a decrease in P_{50} indicates an increase in O_2 affinity because O_2 saturation or concentration is greater for a given Po_2. In adult human blood, P_{50} = 26 mm Hg under standard conditions of partial pressure of CO_2 (Pco_2) = 40 mm Hg, pH = 7.4, and 37°C.

Modulation of Blood-Oxygen Equilibrium Curves

The O_2-equilibrium curve can be physiologically modulated in three ways: (a) the vertical height of the concentration curve (but not the saturation curve) can change, indicating a change in O_{2cap}, (b) the horizontal position of saturation and concentration curves can change, indicating a change in Hb-O_2 affinity, and (c) the shape of saturation and concentration curves can change, indicating a change in the chemical reaction between O_2 and Hb. The maximum height of the saturation curve cannot change by definition; the maximum is always 100% when O_2 is bound to all available Hb sites. However, changes in Hb concentration [Hb] will change the maximum height of the concentration curve, according to the relationship between O_{2cap} and [Hb] as described previously. Mean corpuscular Hb concentration (MCHC) quantifies [Hb] in red blood cells and hematocrit (Hct) quantifies the percentage of blood volume

that is red blood cells. Therefore [Hb], in g/dL of blood, depends on both of these factors:

$$[Hb] = MCHC\ Hct$$

Typical adult values of MCHC = 0.33, Hct = 45%, and [Hb] = 15 g/dL are used in **Figure 41.2**, which shows normal Cao_2 = 20 mL/dL and that Cao_2 = 15 mL/dL in mixed venous blood ($C\overline{v}_{oxygen}$). If [Hb] decreases, for example with decreased hematocrit in anemia, O_{2cap} and concentration decrease at any given Po_2. The O_{2cap} increases when [Hb] increases, for example, by the stimulation of red blood cell production in bone marrow by the hormone erythropoietin or by transfusion. Erythropoietin transcription is regulated by hypoxia-inducible factor (HIF)-1α that is released from cells in the kidneys in response to decreases in arterial O_2 levels. Polycythemia, or increased hematocrit, occurs with chronic hypoxemia in healthy people (e.g., during acclimatization to altitude) and with disease.

The horizontal position of the Hb-O_2 equilibrium curves reflects the affinity of Hb for O_2, and changes in horizontal position are quantified as changes in P_{50}. A decrease in P_{50} is referred to as a *left shift* of the equilibrium curve and indicates increased Hb-O_2 affinity; O_2 saturation or concentration is increased for a given Po_2. Similarly, increased P_{50}, or a *right shift*, reflects decreased Hb-O_2 affinity. The three most important physiologic variables that can modulate P_{50}—pH, Pco_2, and temperature—are shown in **Figure 41.3**.

The *Bohr effect* describes changes in P_{50} with changes in blood Pco_2 and pH. Decreased Pco_2 causes Hb-O_2 affinity to increase (decreased P_{50}), and increased Pco_2 causes Hb-O_2 affinity to decrease (increased P_{50}). As described later, pH decreases when Pco_2 increases and vice versa, and pH changes explain most of the Bohr effect with Pco_2 changes in blood. Hydrogen (H$^+$) binds to histidine residues in Hb molecules, thereby changing the conformation of Hb and the ability of heme sites to bind O_2. However, CO_2 also has a small, independent effect on Hb-O_2 affinity if pH is held constant. The physiologic advantage of the Bohr effect is that it facilitates loading in the lungs, where CO_2 is low and pH is high. In the tissues, the opposite occurs, and increased CO_2 causes pH to decrease and facilitates O_2 unloading from Hb to the tissues.

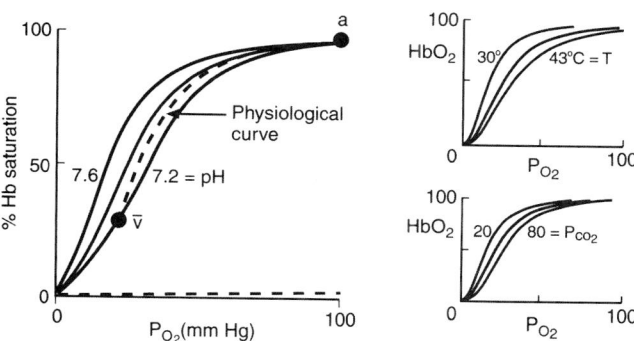

FIGURE 41.3. Effects of pH and Pco_2 (i.e., Bohr effect) and temperature on the position of the O_2-hemoglobin (HbO$_2$) equilibrium curve. The "physiological" curve connects the arterial (a) and mixed-venous points ($\overline{v}$), so that the in vivo curve is steeper than the standard curve at pH = 7.4. From Powell FL. Oxygen and CO_2 transport in the blood. In: Johnson LR, ed. *Essential Medical Physiology*, 3rd ed. Boston: Elsevier/Academic Press, 2003, with permission.

The affect of temperature on Hb-O_2 affinity also has physiologic advantages. Warm temperatures in intensely exercising muscles will increase P_{50} and decrease Hb-O_2 affinity to facilitate O_2 unloading to tissues.

A physiologic O_2-blood equilibrium curve can be defined as the curve that shows the change in blood O_2 concentration when Po_2 decreases from arterial to venous levels in the tissues or increases in the opposite direction in the lungs. The increase in Pco_2, decrease in pH, and potential increase in temperature between arterial and venous points make the physiologic curve steeper than individual curves (**Fig. 41.3**). This is an advantage for gas exchange because it increases the change in O_2 concentration for a given change in Po_2, thereby increasing O_2 uptake or delivery (see the section Cardiovascular and Tissue Oxygen Transport).

Hb-O_2 affinity is also affected by organic phosphates, with 2,3-diphosphoglycerate (2,3-DPG) being most important in humans. 2,3-Diphosphoglycerate is produced during glycolysis in red blood cells and increases P_{50} by interacting with hemoglobin β-chains to decrease their O_2-binding affinity. Physiologic stimuli that lead to enhanced O_2 delivery (e.g., chronic decreases in blood Po_2 levels) typically increase the concentration of 2,3-DPG and promote O_2 delivery to tissues. In blood stored in blood banks, 2,3-DPG is generally decreased, and the increased Hb-O_2 affinity can lead to problems in O_2 delivery after blood transfusion.

Carbon monoxide (CO) is a deadly gas that also modulates the Hb-O_2 dissociation curve by changing the shape and position of concentration or saturation curves. The affinity of Hb for CO is 240 times greater than it is for O_2, so even very small amounts of CO greatly reduce the capacity for Hb to bind O_2—that is, the O_{2cap}. However, CO also decreases the P_{50} and makes the Hb-O_2 curve less sigmoidal. CO causes a left shift of the curve by altering the ability of the Hb molecule to bind O_2; therefore, blood O_2 concentration remains high until Po_2 decreases to very low levels, which impairs O_2 unloading from blood to tissues. CO poisoning also has direct effects on cellular cytochromes, which contribute to its deadliness. CO is particularly dangerous because it is colorless and odorless, and the decrease it causes in arterial O_2 concentration is not sensed by respiratory control systems, which respond only to O_2 partial pressure, as explained in the Respiratory Control section. Hyperbaric O_2 exposure is used to treat CO poisoning because only very high Po_2 levels are effective at competing with CO for Hb-binding sites and driving CO out of the blood.

Oxygen Transport in Fetal Blood

The normal human fetus is exposed to a level of O_2 that would be considered severe hypoxia in adults, similar to the levels experienced on the summit of Mt. Everest! This is possible not only because the fetus is less sensitive to hypoxia than adults, but also because of fetal hemoglobin. Fetal Hb has a P_{50} of 20 torr, compared to 26 torr for adults, thus facilitating O_2 transfer to the fetus in the placenta (**Fig. 41.4**). Fetal Hb (HbF) is gradually replaced by adult hemoglobin in the first year. O_2 delivery across the placenta is ~8 mL O_2/min/kg of fetal mass, which is approximately twice the rate for an adult, but blood O_2 stores in the fetus are sufficient for only a few minutes of metabolism. O_2 delivery across the placenta is limited by blood flow and Po_2 levels in the mother and fetus, but not by diffusion. For example, decreasing maternal Pa_{O2} below 70 torr can reduce placental O_2 transfer. Increasing maternal Pa_{O2} to 600 torr, with O_2 breathing, can increase fetal umbilical O_2 tensions by 3–5 torr, which can be important if the fetus is suffering any hypoxic stress. Both the left shift of fetal versus adult O_2-Hb equilibrium curves and the high fetal O_2 capacity facilitate O_2 unloading from the mother to the fetus (**Fig. 41.4**). It is also significant that O_2 capacity is decreased in the mother near

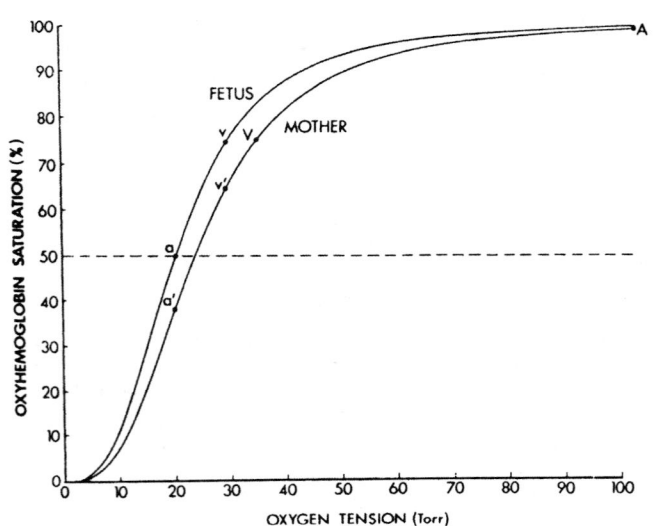
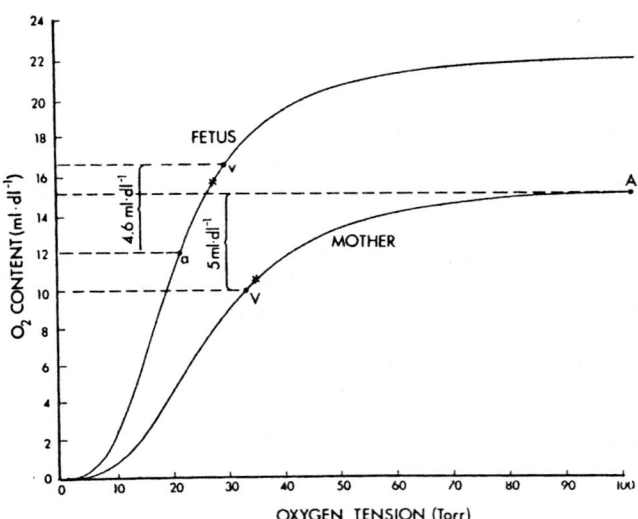

FIGURE 41.4. Oxygen-hemoglobin equilibrium curves for maternal and fetal hemoglobin. **A:** When Po_2 equilibrates between the fetal and maternal circulations, O_2 saturation is increased by 10% or more because of the lower P_{50} in fetal hemoglobin. **B:** Higher O_2 capacity of fetal compared to maternal blood further increases the amount of O_2 in blood for a given Po_2 and saturation. A = maternal arterial, V, maternal venous; a', umbilical (maternal) arterial; v', umbilical (maternal) venous; a, fetal arterial; v, fetal venous. From Powell FL. Pulmonary Gas Exchange. In: Johnson LR, ed. *Essential Medical Physiology*, 3rd ed. Boston: Elsevier Academic Press, 2003, with permission.

term (11.5 vs. 14 g/dL Hb). The Bohr effect also contributes to placental O_2 transport, as pH decreases from 7.42 in the maternal artery to 7.35 in the maternal vein.

Carbon Dioxide in Blood

The general principles of CO_2 transport by blood are similar to those for O_2, i.e., blood carries much more CO_2 than would be possible if it was only physically dissolved, and the CO_2-blood equilibrium curve is modulated by physiologic factors. In addition, CO_2 carriage by blood has important effects on acid-base balance.

CO_2-blood equilibrium (or dissociation) curves are nonlinear, but they have a different shape and position than O_2-blood equilibrium curves. Blood holds more CO_2 than O_2, in part because CO_2 is carried by blood in three forms (**Fig. 41.5**). Also, the CO_2-blood equilibrium curve is steeper than the O_2 curve, resulting in a smaller range of P_{CO_2} values in the body, compared with the range of P_{O_2} values, although the differences between arterial and venous concentrations are similar for CO_2 and O_2 (~5 mL/dL of blood). The resulting physiologic CO_2 dissociation curve between the arterial and venous points is much more linear than the physiologic O_2 dissociation curve (**Fig. 41.5**).

Forms of Carbon Dioxide in Blood

Physically dissolved CO_2 is a function of CO_2 solubility in plasma, which is 0.067 mL/(dL mm Hg) and 20 times more soluble than O_2. Still, dissolved CO_2 contributes only ~5% of total CO_2 concentration in arterial blood.

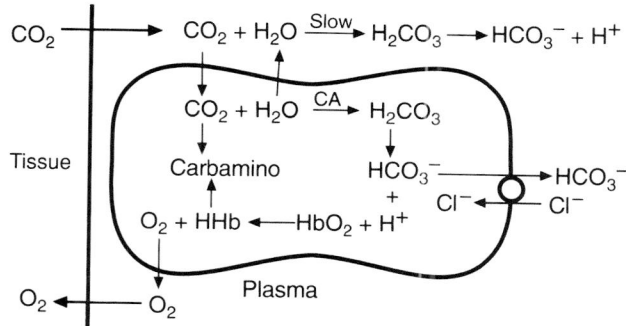

FIGURE 41.6. CO_2 and O_2 reactions in blood and tissues; the opposite reactions occur in the lungs. CA, carbonic anhydrase; HHb, protonated hemoglobin. From Powell FL. Oxygen and CO_2 transport in the blood. In: Johnson LR, ed. *Essential Medical Physiology*, 3rd ed. Boston: Elsevier/Academic Press, 2003, with permission.

Carbamino compounds comprise the second form of blood CO_2. These compounds occur when CO_2 combines with amine groups in blood proteins, especially with the globin of hemoglobin. However, this chemical combination between CO_2 and Hb is much less important than Hb-O_2 binding; therefore carbamino compounds comprise only 5% of the total CO_2 in arterial blood.

Bicarbonate ion (HCO_3^-) is the most important form of CO_2 carriage in blood. CO_2 combines with water to form carbonic acid, and this dissociates to HCO_3^- and H^+:

$$CO_2 + H_2O \leftrightarrow H_2CO_3 \leftrightarrow HCO_3^- + H^+$$

Carbonic anhydrase is the enzyme that catalyzes this reaction, making it almost instantaneous. Carbonic anhydrase occurs mainly in red blood cells, but it also occurs on pulmonary capillary endothelial cells and accelerates the reaction in plasma in the lungs. The uncatalyzed reaction will occur in any aqueous medium, but at a much slower rate, requiring >4 min for equilibrium. The rapid conversion of CO_2 to bicarbonate results in ~90% of the CO_2 in arterial blood that is carried in that form and has important implications for acid-base balance.

Figure 41.6 shows the carbonic acid reactions in plasma and red blood cells and illustrates important ion fluxes that occur with CO_2 transport in blood. CO_2 rapidly enters red blood cells from the plasma because it is soluble in cell membranes. Carbonic anhydrase catalyzes the rapid formation of HCO_3^- and H^+ in the cells, and some of this HCO_3^- is transported out by an electrically neutral bicarbonate-chloride exchanger. The chloride shift (*Hamburger shift*) is an increased intracellular chloride level with increased CO_2, or vice versa. The H^+ produced from CO_2 reacts with Hb and affects both the O_2 equilibrium curve (Bohr effect) and CO_2 equilibrium curve, as described next.

Modulation of Blood-Carbon Dioxide Equilibrium Curves

Hb-O_2 saturation is the major factor affecting the position of the CO_2 equilibrium curve. The *Haldane effect* increases CO_2 concentration when blood is deoxygenated or decreases CO_2 concentration when blood is oxygenated at any given P_{CO_2} (**Fig. 41.5**). The Haldane effect is actually another view of the same molecular mechanism that causes the Bohr effect on the

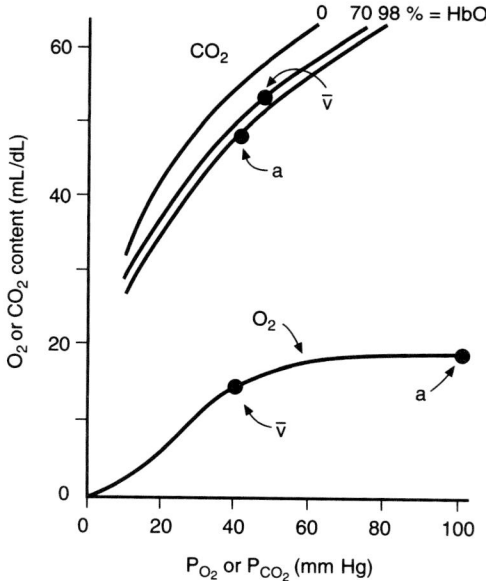

FIGURE 41.5. CO_2-blood equilibrium curve shown on same graph with O_2 equilibrium curve. Differences between the curves result in higher CO_2 concentrations in the blood and smaller P_{CO_2} differences between arterial (a) and venous ($\bar{v}$) blood. Hemoglobin-O_2 saturation affects the position of the CO_2 equilibrium curve (i.e., Haldane effect). From Powell FL. Oxygen and CO_2 transport in the blood. In: Johnson LR, ed. *Essential Medical Physiology*, 3rd ed. Boston: Elsevier/Academic Press, 2003, with permission.

O_2 equilibrium curve (described previously). H^+ ions from CO_2 can be thought of as competing with O_2 for Hb binding. Hence, increasing O_2 decreases the affinity of Hb for H^+ and blood CO_2 concentration (Haldane effect), and increased $[H^+]$ decreases the affinity of Hb for O_2 (Bohr effect). These interactions are summarized in **Figure 41.6.**

The Haldane effect promotes unloading of CO_2 in the lungs when blood is oxygenated and CO_2 loading in the blood when O_2 is released to tissues. The Haldane effect also results in a steeper physiologic CO_2-blood equilibrium curve (see **Fig. 41.5**), which has the physiologic advantage of increasing CO_2 concentration differences for a given PCO_2 difference.

Alveolar Ventilation and Alveolar PO_2

Ventilation is the first step in the O_2 cascade, and the level of alveolar ventilation ($\dot{V}_A$) is the most important factor determining arterial PO_2 for any given PIO_2 and level of O_2 demand ($\dot{V}O_2$) in healthy lungs. Total expired ventilation can be measured with a pneumotachometer or spirometer as the product of the volume of each breath, or tidal volume (V_T), and respiratory frequency (f_R):

$$\dot{V}_E = f_R\, V_T$$

However, all the tidal volume is not effective for gas exchange because the lung consists of a conducting zone, which does not exchange gas, and a respiratory zone, in which all gas exchange occurs. The conducting zone includes the conducting airways from the trachea to the terminal bronchioles, which occur at the 16th order of bronchial branching. The gas volume of the conducting zone equals the *anatomic dead space*. The respiratory zone comprises the rest of the lung from the 17th to 23rd orders of bronchial branching (i.e., respiratory bronchioles to alveolar sacs), and all gas exchange occurs there. With 23 orders of bronchial branching, total cross-sectional area of the airways in distal parts of the lung is greatly increased; therefore, the respiratory zone comprises most of the lung volume. For example, a normal adult will have a total lung capacity (TLC) of 6 L but an anatomic dead space of only 175 mL (~1 mL per pound of body weight).

$\dot{V}_A$ is the difference between total ventilation and dead space ventilation, and it is the effective conductance for pulmonary gas exchange. Total ventilation is not effective for gas exchange because part of the inspired tidal volume remains in the anatomic dead space (V_D). $\dot{V}_A$ can be determined using the *Fick principle*, which is a physiologic version of the principle of conservation of mass that describes gas transport by convection or bulk flow of air or blood. The Fick principle states that the amount of gas consumed or produced by an organ is the difference between the amount of the substance that enters the organ and the amount that leaves the organ. The formula for CO_2 elimination from the lungs ($\dot{V}CO_2$) is:

$$(\dot{V}CO_2) = (\dot{V}_A\, F_ACO_2) - (\dot{V}_I\, F_ICO_2)$$

where $\dot{V}CO_2$ is the difference between the CO_2 expired from the alveoli, and the amount of CO_2 inspired to the alveoli. F_ICO_2 is essentially zero; therefore, the equation can be simplified and rearranged to the *alveolar ventilation equation*:

$$\dot{V}_A = (\dot{V}CO_2/P_ACO_2)K$$

where:

$\dot{V}_A$ is expressed at body temperature and pressure saturated (i.e., L_{BTPS}/min)

$\dot{V}CO_2$ is expressed at standard temperature and pressure dry (i.e., mL_{STPD}/min)

P_ACO_2 is substituted for F_ACO_2

K is a constant (0.863).

In practice, arterial PCO_2 ($PaCO_2$) is substituted for alveolar PCO_2 (P_ACO_2) because the two values are equal in normal lungs, and an arterial blood sample is usually taken to evaluate gas exchange.

Alveolar Ventilation Equation Predicts Alveolar PCO_2

Rearranging the alveolar ventilation equation shows how $\dot{V}_A$ and P_ACO_2 (or $PaCO_2$) are inversely related for any given metabolic rate:

$$P_ACO_2 = (\dot{V}CO_2/\dot{V}_A)K$$

Hence, if $\dot{V}_A$ is doubled, P_ACO_2 is halved, regardless of the exact values for either variable. *Hyperventilation* is defined by a decrease in $PaCO_2$ from the normal value, implying excess $\dot{V}_A$ for a given $\dot{V}CO_2$. *Hypoventilation* is defined by an increase in $PaCO_2$, and this occurs when $\dot{V}_A$ is lower than normal for a given $\dot{V}CO_2$.

As explained previously, $\dot{V}_A$ is reduced from total ventilation by the amount of the dead space:

$$\dot{V}_A = f_R\, (V_T - V_D)$$

Although anatomic dead space can be measured with gas analyzers and flow meters, it is more clinically relevant to estimate physiologic dead space, which is also called *Bohr dead space*. Physiologic dead space includes all "wasted ventilation" and can exceed anatomic dead space, as described next. Physiologic dead space can be calculated from another rearrangement of the Fick principle applied to CO_2 elimination by the lungs as:

$$V_D/V_T = (P_ACO_2 - P_{\overline{E}}CO_2)/P_ACO_2$$

where $P_{\overline{E}}CO_2$ = *mixed-expired* PCO_2 that is measured by collecting all expired gas in a bag or a spirometer and includes gas exhaled from the alveoli *and* dead space. In practice, arterial PCO_2 is substituted for alveolar PCO_2 because it is easily measured.

Alveolar Gas Equation Predicts Alveolar PO_2

Alveolar PO_2 (P_AO_2) can be predicted from the *alveolar gas equation* that models an "ideal lung" with only physiologic dead space:

$$P_AO_2 = P_IO_2 - (P_ACO_2/R) + F$$

where:

P_IO_2 is inspired PO_2

P_ACO_2 is alveolar PCO_2

R is the respiratory exchange ratio

F is a constant that can be ignored under normal conditions (F = $P_ACO_2 \times F_IO_2$ [1 − R]/R and increases P_AO_2 only 2 mm Hg at normal O_2 and CO_2 levels).

In practice, arterial PCO_2 is substituted for alveolar PCO_2 because $PaCO_2 = P_ACO_2$ in normal lungs and arterial samples are easily obtained. The alveolar gas equation is only valid if inspired $PCO_2 = 0$, which is a reasonable assumption for room air breathing.

The *respiratory exchange ratio* (R) is the ratio of uptake to CO_2 elimination by the lungs:

$$R = \dot{V}_{CO_2}/\dot{V}_{O_2}$$

Under steady-state conditions, R equals the *respiratory quotient* (RQ), which is the ratio of CO_2 production to O_2 consumption in metabolizing tissues. RQ averages 0.8 on a normal, mixed, adult diet, but it can range from 0.67 to 1, depending on the relative amounts of fat, protein, and carbohydrate being metabolized. R can exceed this range in non-steady states, for example, when R exceeds 1 during hyperventilation. CO_2 stores in the body are much greater than O_2 stores because of bicarbonate in blood and tissues. R can increase because it takes longer to wash out the CO_2 stores than it does to charge up the much smaller O_2 stores in the body.

Substituting normal adult values in the alveolar gas equation predicts that $P_{AO_2} = 100$ mm Hg in breathing room air ($P_{AO_2} = 150 - 40/0.8$). Increases in $\dot{V}_A$ (hyperventilation) increases P_{AO_2} by decreasing P_{ACO_2}, whereas decreases in $\dot{V}_A$ (hypoventilation) decreases P_{AO_2}. Why ideal alveolar P_{O_2} is greater than measured arterial P_{O_2} is explained in the next section.

Diffusion

Diffusion of O_2 from alveoli to pulmonary capillary blood is the next step in the O_2 cascade after alveolar ventilation. It is important to note that blood leaving the pulmonary capillaries is in equilibrium with alveolar gas in healthy lungs under normal resting conditions. Hence, the small decreases between P_{AO_2} and P_{aO_2} shown in **Figure 41.1** are not caused by diffusion but by ventilation-perfusion mismatching in healthy lungs under normal conditions, as described in the next section.

O_2 moves from the alveoli to pulmonary capillary blood barrier according to Fick's first law of diffusion:

$$\dot{V}_{O_2} = \Delta P_{O_2} \times D_{O_2}$$

where:

ΔP_{O_2} is the average P_{O_2} gradient across the blood-gas barrier

D_{O_2} is a "diffusing capacity" for O_2 across the barrier.

Diffusion of a gas always occurs down a partial-pressure gradient, for example, from alveolar gas to pulmonary blood. Some readers may find it helpful to note the analogy between Fick's law for O_2 flux and Ohm's law for the flow of electrons (current = voltage/resistance). $\dot{V}_{O_2}$ is analogous to current, and ΔP_{O_2} is analogous to the potential energy difference of voltage. However, D_{O_2} is analogous to a *conductance*, which is the inverse of resistance (current = voltage × conductance). Flux can be increased either by increasing the P_{O_2} gradient or increasing the conductance (D_{O_2}).

D_{O_2} depends on both the molecular properties of the gas and the geometric properties of that membrane:

$$D_{O_2} = (\text{solubility}/MW)_{O_2} \cdot (\text{area}/\text{thickness})_{\text{membrane}}$$

Solubility is important because gas molecules must "dissolve" in a membrane before they can diffuse across it, and once dissolved, low-molecular-weight (MW) molecules move more quickly by the random motions of diffusion. Large surface areas increase the probability that an O_2 molecule will come into contact with the membrane through random motion, but

membrane thickness increases the distance that O_2 molecules must travel.

Pathway for Oxygen

The pathway of an O_2 molecule diffusing from alveolar gas to Hb inside an erythrocyte (red blood cell) in an adult lung (**Fig. 41.7**) is the anatomic basis for D_{O_2}. The total area of the blood-gas barrier is nearly 100 m^2 in adult lungs; it is extremely thin but variable in thickness and consists of several different layers. The "thin" side of a pulmonary capillary (0.3 μm) separates gas from plasma with (a) thin cytoplasmic extensions from type I alveolar epithelial cells, (b) a thin basement membrane, and (c) thin cytoplasmic extensions from capillary endothelial cells. The thicker side of a capillary has collagen in the interstitial space to provide mechanical strength in the alveoli. Epithelial and endothelial cell bodies are in alveolar corners between capillaries to further minimize the thickness of the gas exchange barrier. Finally, O_2 must diffuse through plasma and across the red blood cell membrane before it can combine with hemoglobin. The diffusing capacity for O_2 between the alveolar gas and hemoglobin is called the *membrane diffusing capacity for O_2*, or D_{MO_2}.

After O_2 diffuses into red blood cells, the finite *rate of reaction between O_2 and Hb* (abbreviated with the symbol θ) offers an additional "resistance" to O_2 uptake. The magnitude of this chemical resistance depends on θ and the total amount of Hb, which is a physiologic function of pulmonary capillary volume (V_C). This chemical resistance is in series with the membrane resistance, so that the total resistance to O_2 diffusion in the lung can be defined as:

$$1/D_{LO_2} = 1/D_{MO_2} + 1/(\theta V_C)$$

where D_{LO_2} *is the lung diffusing capacity for O_2.* (D_{LO_2} is a conductance; recall that conductance is the inverse of resistance, and resistors in series are additive.)

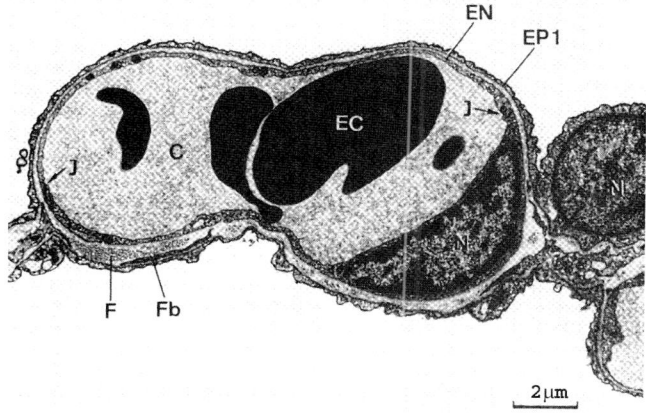

FIGURE 41.7. Electron micrograph of a pulmonary capillary showing the pathway for O_2 diffusion in the lung. O_2 diffuses from the alveolar space (open areas above and below capillary, C) through epithelial cell (*EP1*), interstitial space, endothelial cell (*EN*), and plasma before combining with hemoglobin in the erythrocyte (*EC*). Collagen fibers (*F*) and fibroblasts (*Fb*) thicken the interstitial space on one side of the capillary. N, nucleus; J, endothelial cell junctions. Scale marker = 2 μm. From Weibel ER. Design and morphometry of the pulmonary gas exchanger. In: Crystal RG, West JB, Barnes PJ, et al., eds. *The Lung: Scientific Foundations,* 2nd ed. Philadelphia: Lippincott Williams & Wilkins, 1997, with permission.

It is estimated that membrane and chemical reaction resistances to O_2 diffusion are approximately equal in normal lungs. Both Dm_{O_2} and V_C are under physiologic control through pulmonary capillary recruitment and distension. Therefore, $D_{L_{O_2}}$ increases with exercise by recruitment of Dm_{O_2} and θV_C. Methods for measuring $D_{L_{O_2}}$ are described below.

Po₂ Changes Along the Pulmonary Capillary

The normal time course of P_{O_2} changes along the capillary in adult lungs at normal P_{O_2} levels, and the P_{O_2} in capillary blood increases from mixed-venous levels at the beginning to arterial levels at the end of the capillary (**Fig. 41.8**). Alveolar P_{O_2} is constant everywhere outside the capillary because diffusion is rapid in the gas phase. Any O_2 moving into the blood is instantly replaced by diffusive mixing in the small alveolar spaces. Hence, the gradient for O_2 diffusion changes along the length of the capillary, and the ΔP_{O_2} value used in Fick's law is an average value, corresponding to the mean partial pressure gradient operating over the entire length of the pulmonary capillary.

The average capillary transit time of 0.75 seconds for adults (**Fig. 41.8**) is calculated from a cardiac output of 6 L/min and capillary volume of 75 mL (time = volume/flow rate). Note that diffusion equilibrium normally occurs between blood and gas in only 0.25 sec, providing a threefold safety factor. However, if $D_{L_{O_2}}$ is decreased sufficiently with lung disease, capillary P_{O_2} may not equilibrate with PA_{O_2} during the transit time (see **Fig. 41.8**, abnormal O_2 curve). In the abnormal case, $Pc'_{O_2} < PA_{O_2}$, which is defined as a *diffusion limitation for O_2*, where Pc' is used to designate end-capillary partial pressure.

Only two conditions lead to diffusion limitation for O_2 in healthy adults. First, elite athletes at maximal exercise, with very high O_2 consumption and cardiac outputs, can have transit

times that are too short for O_2 diffusion equilibrium. Capillary volume increases by recruitment and distension with elevated cardiac output, but this is not sufficient to balance the huge increase in flow rate that occurs in elite athletes. Second, normal adults exercising at altitude may not achieve diffusion equilibrium because transit time *and* PA_{O_2} decrease. Transit time will decrease with elevated cardiac output during exercise, but capillary volume recruitment and distension can preserve enough time for O_2 diffusion equilibrium to occur *if* PA_{O_2} is normal. However, PA_{O_2} is decreased at altitude, and this slows O_2 diffusion in two ways.

First, decreased PA_{O_2} slows O_2 diffusion by decreasing the P_{O_2} gradient that is driving diffusion. For example, at an altitude of 3,050 m (10,000 feet), the barometric pressure is only 523 mm Hg and PI_{O_2} is 100 mm Hg [0.21 (523−47) mm Hg]. In a normal individual doing mild exercise at this altitude, PA_{O_2} is measured to be ∼55 mm Hg. $P\bar{v}_{O_2}$ decreases much less than this because of the shape of the O_2-blood equilibrium curve (see the section, Cardiovascular and Tissue Oxygen Transport). Measurements show that $P\bar{v}_{O_2}$ is 24 mm Hg at altitude, compared with 30 mm Hg at sea level, with this amount of exercise. Therefore, the P_{O_2} gradient at the beginning of the capillary decreases from 70 mm Hg with mild exercise at sea level (100−30 mm Hg) to 31 mm Hg (55−24 mm Hg) at altitude. The exact values in this example are not as important as the general concepts that the shape of the O_2-blood equilibrium curve maintains $P\bar{v}_{O_2}$ in exercise at altitude (see Cardiovascular and Tissue Oxygen Transport), and this decreases the P_{O_2} gradient for diffusion in the lung.

Decreasing PA_{O_2} also slows the rate of rise in P_{O_2} because gas exchange is occurring on the steep portion of the O_2-blood equilibrium curve. This means that a given increase in O_2 concentration is not effective at increasing P_{O_2} toward the alveolar equilibrium value. In contrast, the flat shape of the O_2-blood equilibrium curve around normal PA_{O_2} levels promotes diffusion equilibrium. Small amounts of O_2 diffusing from alveolar gas into capillary blood cause large increases in P_{O_2}; therefore capillary P_{O_2} rapidly approaches equilibrium with PA_{O_2} in normoxia.

Note that both of these types of diffusion limitation in normal lungs are different than hypoxemia typically encountered in the ICU. In patients, metabolic rates and cardiac outputs may be depressed. Hypoxemia from a decrease in lung diffusing capacity (e.g., thickening of the blood-gas barrier from edema) may be corrected by increasing inspired O_2 levels.

Diffusion-limited and Perfusion-limited Gases

Dramatic differences in the time course of diffusion equilibrium for different gases in the lung are also shown in **Figure 41.8**. The anesthetic gas nitrous oxide (N_2O) achieves equilibrium rapidly, whereas CO never comes close to diffusion equilibrium. Understanding the differences between these gases is not only important for anesthesiology and emergency medicine, but it also helps in understanding the physiologic mechanisms for O_2 diffusion limitations.

The uptake of a gas that achieves diffusion equilibrium depends on the magnitude of pulmonary blood flow. For example, N_2O diffuses rapidly from the alveoli to capillary blood (**Fig. 41.8**); therefore, the only way to increase its uptake is to increase the amount of blood flowing through the alveolar capillaries. N_2O is an example of a *perfusion-limited gas*. Changes in the diffusing capacity have no effect on the uptake

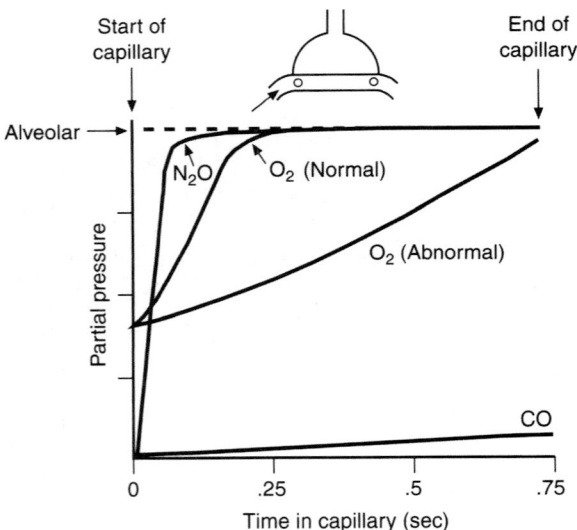

FIGURE 41.8. The time course of the increase in partial pressure for different gases diffusing from alveolar gas into pulmonary capillary blood. Nitrous oxide and O_2 under normal conditions equilibrate very quickly, but CO or O_2 under abnormal conditions do not equilibrate in the time it takes blood to flow through the capillary in adults (0.75 sec). From Powell FL. Pulmonary gas exchange. In: Johnson LR, ed. *Essential Medical Physiology*, 3rd ed. London: Elsevier Academic Press, 2003, with permission.

of a perfusion-limited gas or its partial pressure in the blood and body. All anesthetic and "inert" gases that do not react chemically with blood are perfusion-limited. Under normal resting conditions, O_2 is also a perfusion-limited gas.

The uptake of a gas that does not achieve diffusion equilibrium could obviously increase if the diffusing capacity increased. CO is an example of such a *diffusion-limited gas* (**Fig. 41.8**). As Hb has a very high affinity for CO, the effective solubility of CO in blood is large. Therefore, increases in the CO concentration in blood are not effective at increasing partial pressure of carbon monoxide (P_{CO}), which keeps blood P_{CO} lower than alveolar P_{CO} and results in a large disequilibrium and diffusion limitation. Under abnormal conditions, O_2 may become a diffusion-limited gas (**Fig. 41.8**).

In practice, the only diffusion-limited gases are CO and O_2 under hypoxic conditions. All other gases are perfusion-limited, including O_2 under normoxic conditions in healthy lungs. CO is diffusion-limited because it is always much more soluble in blood than in the blood-gas barrier. The same applies for O_2 in hypoxia, when the slope of the O_2-blood equilibrium curve is much steeper than the slope for physically dissolved O_2 in plasma (see **Fig. 41.5**). However, at high P_{O_2} levels, the slope of the blood-O_2 equilibrium curve equals the slope of the solubility curve in plasma and O_2 behaves like inert gases.

Measuring Diffusing Capacity

The diffusing capacity of the lung can be measured from the uptake of a diffusion-limited gas such as CO. If very low levels of CO are inspired (~0.1%), Hb saturation with CO is very low, arterial oxygenation is not disturbed, and no toxic effects occur. Also, the amount of CO entering the capillary blood does not increase blood P_{CO} significantly because CO is so soluble in blood. Therefore, the lung-diffusing capacity for CO (D_{LCO}) can be defined by Fick's first law of diffusion as:

$$D_{LCO} = \dot{V}_{CO}/P_{ACO}$$

where $\dot{V}_{CO}$ = CO uptake by the lung and the gradient driving CO diffusion equals P_{ACO} because average capillary $P_{CO} = 0$. In theory, although D_{LCO} could be used to calculate the D_L for O_2 by correcting for physical factors that determine diffusing capacity (MW and solubility), only D_{LCO} is reported clinically.

In the *steady-state D_{LCO} method*, the individual breathes a low level of CO for a couple of minutes. CO uptake is then calculated from the Fick principle using measurements of ventilation and inspired and expired P_{CO}. Alveolar P_{CO} can be estimated from expired P_{CO}. In the *single breath D_{LCO} method*, an individual takes a breath with a low concentration of CO and holds the breath for 10 sec. This method also requires a simultaneous measurement of lung volume (e.g., by helium dilution) to calculate $\dot{V}_{CO}$ from P_{CO} changes in the lung. Alveolar P_{CO} is estimated from expired P_{CO} and corrected for the change that occurs during the breath hold.

D_{LCO} in healthy adults is ~25 mL/(min × mm Hg) and can increase twofold to threefold with exercise, as expected for capillary recruitment and distension. D_{LCO} also changes with O_2 level because the rate of chemical reaction between CO and Hb is deceased by Hb oxygenation, and D_{LCO} has a chemical reaction rate component (θ V_C) similar to D_{LO_2}. In lung disease, D_{LCO} may be affected by other factors, such as unequal distributions of alveolar volume, pulmonary blood flow, and

diffusing properties. Such factors explain why morphometric estimates of diffusing capacity, based on anatomic measurements of the blood-gas barrier surface area, thickness, etc., are approximately twice as large as functional measurements of diffusing capacity. Because other factors can affect D_{LCO} measurement, it is sometimes referred to as a *transfer factor* instead of the diffusing capacity.

Limitations of Pulmonary Gas Exchange

Gas exchange limitations in the lungs can reduce P_{O_2} throughout the O_2 cascade. Such limitations do not decrease resting $\dot{V}_{O_2}$, although they may limit maximal O_2 consumption during exercise. Hypoxemia is defined as a decrease in blood P_{O_2}, and arterial hypoxemia, or decreased P_{aO_2}, indicates a limitation of pulmonary gas exchange. Gas exchange limitation does not imply a decrease in resting O_2 consumption, because P_{O_2} will adjust throughout the O_2 cascade to maintain O_2 consumption in a steady state. For example, $P_{\bar{v}O_2}$ (and cardiac output, $\dot{Q}$) will change as necessary to satisfy the cardiovascular Fick equation when O_2 consumption increases.

Gas exchange limitations not only decrease P_{aO_2}, but some also increase the alveolar-arterial P_{O_2} difference. The concept of an "ideal" lung without limitations was introduced previously and, under such ideal conditions, $P_{AO_2} - P_{aO_2} = 0$ mm Hg. However, in reality, P_{AO_2} calculated from the alveolar gas equation is greater than P_{aO_2} measured from an arterial blood sample, and the alveolar-arterial P_{O_2} difference increases with *most* (but not all) gas exchange limitations.

The four kinds of pulmonary gas exchange limitations are: (a) hypoventilation, (b) diffusion limitations, (c) pulmonary blood-flow shunts, and (d) mismatching of ventilation and blood flow in different parts of the lung. The following sections explain how each of these limitations decreases P_{aO_2}, and how the alveolar-arterial P_{O_2} difference is useful for diagnosing the causes of hypoxemia in a patient.

Hypoventilation

By definition, hypoventilation occurs if arterial P_{CO_2} is greater than normal. Hypoventilation is the only pulmonary gas exchange limitation that does not increase the alveolar-arterial P_{O_2} difference. Therefore, pure hypoventilation causes hypoxemia and increases arterial P_{CO_2}, but the alveolar-arterial P_{O_2} difference is normal. The magnitude of hypoxemia caused by hypoventilation is predicted by the alveolar gas equation:

$$P_{AO_2} = P_{IO_2} - (P_{ACO_2}/R)$$

Hypoventilation increases P_{ACO_2}, according to the inverse relationship between $\dot{V}_A$ and P_{ACO_2} described by the alveolar ventilation equation, which is easiest to understand when R = 1 and P_{AO_2} decreases 1 mm Hg for every 1 mm Hg increase in P_{ACO_2}. Conceptually, P_{IO_2} represents the total amount of gas inspired, and gas exchange replaces each molecule of O_2 consumed with one molecule of CO_2. Hence, P_{AO_2} is simply the difference between P_{IO_2} and P_{ACO_2} when R = 1. However, a normal value for R is 0.8, and this magnifies the effects of hypoventilation and increased P_{ACO_2} on hypoxemia.

Two primary classes of problems cause hypoventilation are (a) mechanical limitations and (b) ventilatory control abnormalities. Abnormal respiratory mechanics, such as increased airway resistance or decreased compliance with lung disease, may limit the effectiveness of the respiratory muscles in generating $\dot{V}A$. Also, the respiratory muscles themselves may be damaged and ineffective at generating the pressures necessary for normal ventilation. In all of these cases, the ventilatory control system may be normal in terms of sensing PaO_2 and $PaCO_2$ changes and sending neural signals to the respiratory muscles to increase ventilation. However, abnormal control of ventilation can also occur.

Diffusion Limitations

Pulmonary diffusion limitation is defined as disequilibrium between the partial pressure of a gas in the alveoli and pulmonary capillaries. Therefore, diffusion limitations decrease PaO_2 by increasing the alveolar-arterial PO_2 difference, which occurs when (a) the pressure head driving O_2 diffusion across the blood-gas barrier (PaO_2) is too low, or (b) the lung's diffusing capacity for O_2 (DL) is not sufficient for the O_2 demands of the body.

As described previously, diffusion limitations can occur in normal adults when PaO_2 is decreased at high altitude and O_2 demand is increased during hard exercise. Increased O_2 demand alone can increase the alveolar-arterial PO_2 difference and cause arterial hypoxemia in some elite athletes during maximal exercise at sea level. In lung disease, the measured $DLCO$ can decrease with destruction of surface area and capillary volume (e.g., emphysema) or thickening of the blood-gas barrier (e.g., edema), but $DLCO$ must decrease to <50% of normal before arterial hypoxemia is observed in resting patients. Hypoventilation and ventilation-perfusion mismatch can also lower PaO_2 and decrease the pressure gradient driving diffusion. Arterial hypoxemia caused by a diffusion limitation can be relieved rapidly by increasing inspired O_2 (within several breaths), which increases the driving pressure for O_2 from the alveoli into the blood.

Shunts

The ideal models used to analyze alveolar ventilation and diffusion have considered gas exchange as occurring in a single compartment so that arterial PO_2 equals PO_2 in the blood leaving the pulmonary capillaries ($PaO_2 = Pc'O_2$). In reality, arterial blood is not pure pulmonary capillary blood; it also includes shunt flow. *Shunt* is defined as deoxygenated venous blood flow that enters the arterial circulation without going through ventilated alveoli in the pulmonary circulation. This kind of shunt is also called *right-to-left shunt*, to distinguish it from left-to-right shunt, which shunts systemic arterial blood into pulmonary artery flow with some congenital heart defects. Right-to-left shunt decreases PaO_2 by diluting end-capillary blood with deoxygenated venous blood.

Shunt is calculated by applying the principle of mass balance to a two-compartment model, which splits total cardiac output ($\dot{Q}t$) between a shunt flow to an unventilated compartment ($\dot{Q}s$) and flow to a normally ventilated alveolar compartment (**Fig. 41.8**) and defines shunt flow as a fraction of total cardiac output:

$$\dot{Q}s/\dot{Q}t = (Cc'O_2 - CaO_2)/(Cc'O_2 - C\bar{v}O_2)$$

$\dot{Q}s/\dot{Q}t$ is calculated in practice by measuring arterial and mixed-venous blood samples in an individual during 100% O_2 breathing, which removes any diffusion limitation in ventilated alveoli; therefore, $Pc'O_2 = PaO_2 - CaO_2$ and CvO_2 are measured directly. $Cc'O_2$ is estimated from PaO_2 using an O_2-blood equi-

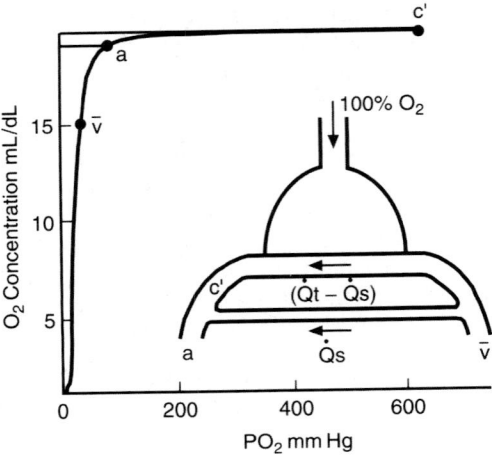

FIGURE 41.9. Two-compartment model for shunt flow ($\dot{Q}$ s) and effective pulmonary blood flow ($\dot{Q}t - \dot{Q}s$). Oxygen-blood equilibrium curve illustrates how small shunt flows of mixed-venous blood ($\bar{v}$) significantly decrease PO_2 in arterial blood (a) relative to PO_2 in end-capillary blood leaving the alveoli (c'). From Powell FL. Pulmonary gas exchange. In: Johnson LR, ed. *Essential Medical Physiology*, 3rd ed. London: Elsevier/Academic Press, 2003, with permission.

librium curve, where PaO_2 is calculated from the alveolar gas equation. (It should be noted, however, that FIO_2 appears in the constant "F" in the alveolar gas equation, and this constant should not be neglected when $FIO_2 = 1.0$.)

The effect of shunt on PaO_2 is illustrated in **Figure 41.9**. Alveolar and end-capillary PaO_2 are predicted to be more than 600 mm Hg during pure O_2 breathing. However, shunt significantly decreases PaO_2 because of the shape of the O_2-blood equilibrium curve. The large increase in PO_2 with O_2 breathing does not increase $Cc'O_2$ enough to offset the low level of $C\bar{v}O_2$. Therefore, persistent hypoxemia during 100% O_2 breathing indicates a shunt if all the alveoli are effectively ventilated with 100% O_2. (Exceptions to this condition may occur with ventilation-perfusion mismatching in lung disease, as described later.) If PaO_2 can be increased above 150 mm Hg during O_2 breathing, and cardiac output is normal, then 1% shunt increases the alveolar-arterial PO_2 difference by about 20 mm Hg.

In healthy adults, shunt during O_2 breathing averages <5% of cardiac output, including (a) venous blood from the bronchial circulation that drains directly into the pulmonary veins, and (b) venous blood from the coronary circulation that enters the left ventricle through the Thebesian veins. If shunt is calculated during room air breathing, it is called *venous admixture*. Venous admixture is larger than the shunt during O_2 breathing because it is an "as if" shunt, which includes the effects of low PO_2 from poorly ventilated alveoli. Venous admixture occurs even in healthy lungs with ventilation-perfusion mismatching, as described in the next section.

Ventilation-Perfusion Mismatching

Mismatching of ventilation and blood flow in different parts of the lung is the most common cause of alveolar-arterial PO_2 differences in health and disease. It is also the most complicated mechanism of hypoxemia and will be approached in two steps. First, the effect of the alveolar ventilation-perfusion ratio ($\dot{V}_A/\dot{Q}$) on P_{AO_2} is described for an ideal lung. Second, the mechanisms that result in heterogeneity between $\dot{V}_A/\dot{Q}$ ratios in different parts of lungs and the effect of this on P_{AO_2} are considered. It is important to understand that only this second factor increases the alveolar-arterial P_{O_2} difference ($P_{AO_2} - P_{aO_2}$).

The $\dot{V}_A/\dot{Q}$ Ratio

The effects of changing $\dot{V}_A/\dot{Q}$ were introduced previously in the section on Alveolar Ventilation and P_{AO_2}. P_{AO_2} increases with $\dot{V}_A$ according to the alveolar ventilation and alveolar gas equations. $\dot{V}_A/\dot{Q}$ adds the concept of blood flow. The effect of $\dot{V}_A/\dot{Q}$ on P_{AO_2} can be understood by thinking of $\dot{V}_A$ as bringing O_2 into the alveoli and thinking of $\dot{Q}$ as taking it away. If $\dot{Q}$ suddenly increases and removes more O_2 from the alveoli (recall that O_2 is normally a perfusion-limited gas), then P_{AO_2} will decrease. However, if $\dot{V}_A$ increases O_2 delivery to match increased O_2 removal (returning the $\dot{V}_A/\dot{Q}$ ratio to normal), then P_{AO_2} will return to normal. Decreasing $\dot{V}_A/\dot{Q}$ has the opposite effect and decreases P_{AO_2}.

The O_2- CO_2 diagram shows the effects of changing $\dot{V}_A/\dot{Q}$ in an ideal lung, modeled as a single alveolus in a steady state, with no shunts or diffusion limitations (**Fig. 41.10**). As $\dot{V}_A/\dot{Q}$ is the alveolar ventilation-perfusion ratio, dead space is not a factor. The "$\dot{V}_A/\dot{Q}$ line" on the CO_2- O_2 diagram shows all of the possible P_{CO_2}-P_{O_2} combinations that could occur in this ideal lung, with $\dot{V}_A/\dot{Q}$ ratios ranging from 0 to infinity. When $\dot{V}_A/\dot{Q} = 0$, a shunt is indicated. Because the shunt alveolus is not ventilated, it will equilibrate with mixed-venous blood, and the $\dot{V}_A/\dot{Q} = 0$ point corresponds to $P_{\bar{v}O_2}$ and $P_{\bar{v}CO_2}$. Dead space is indicated when $\dot{V}_A/\dot{Q}$ is infinite. As dead space receives no blood flow, this alveolus equilibrates with inspired gas, and the infinite $\dot{V}_A/\dot{Q}$ point corresponds to P_{IO_2}. Normal P_{ACO_2} and P_{AO_2} values are shown for a normal $\dot{V}_A/\dot{Q}$ of 0.8.

The important point to notice about the $\dot{V}_A/\dot{Q}$ line is that changes in $\dot{V}_A/\dot{Q}$ around the normal value affect P_{AO_2} more than they do P_{ACO_2} (note the different CO_2 and O_2 scales in **Fig. 41.9**). This generalization holds even if the $\dot{V}_A/\dot{Q}$ line is altered by changing mixed-venous or inspired gas (which changes the

endpoints), or by physiologic changes in the O_2-blood or CO_2-blood equilibrium curves (which determine the exact shape of the $\dot{V}_A/\dot{Q}$ line).

$\dot{V}_A/\dot{Q}$ Mismatching Between Different Alveoli

In real lungs, total alveolar ventilation and cardiac output must be distributed between some 300 million alveoli. This distribution is not perfectly uniform. This results in $\dot{V}_A/\dot{Q}$ heterogeneity, or different $\dot{V}_A/\dot{Q}$ ratios in different parts of the lung; $\dot{V}_A/\dot{Q}$ *mismatching* refers to spatial $\dot{V}_A/\dot{Q}$ heterogeneity between functional units of gas exchange in real lungs—not a mismatch between total $\dot{V}_A$ and $\dot{Q}$ or a deviation of the overall $\dot{V}_A/\dot{Q}$ from 1. Changes in the $\dot{V}_A/\dot{Q}$ ratio in an ideal lung or in a single alveolus change P_{AO_2}, as described previously (**Fig. 41.10**), but this does not change the alveolar-arterial P_{O_2} difference from the ideal value of zero. In contrast, $\dot{V}_A/\dot{Q}$ heterogeneity between lung units does decrease P_{aO_2} and increases the alveolar-arterial P_{O_2} difference.

Regional differences in alveolar ventilation occur because of the mechanical properties of the lung. In upright adults, gravity tends to distort the lung, and alveoli in the apex are more expanded than those in the base of the lung, resulting in basal alveoli operating on a steeper part of the lung's compliance curve, so that $\dot{V}_A$ is greater at the bottom than at the top of the lung. $\dot{V}_A$ per unit lung volume differs by a factor of 2.5 between the top and bottom of the upright adult lung (**Fig. 41.11**).

Regional differences in blood flow occur because of the effects of gravity on the pulmonary circulation, as described previously. Briefly, capillary pressure is greater at the bottom than at the top of the upright lung, which reduces local vascular resistance at the bottom of the lungs and increases regional blood flow. **Figure 41.10** illustrates that $\dot{Q}$ per unit lung volume changes by a factor of 6 between the top and bottom of the upright adult lung, or relatively more than $\dot{V}_A$. The net result is a large decrease in $\dot{V}_A/\dot{Q}$ between the top and bottom of upright adult lungs (**Fig. 41.11**).

This $\dot{V}_A/\dot{Q}$ heterogeneity between different regions of the lung leads to regional differences in P_{AO_2} and P_{ACO_2}, corresponding to differences predicted by the $\dot{V}_A/\dot{Q}$ line on the CO_2-O_2 diagram (**Fig. 41.10**). For example, $\dot{V}_A/\dot{Q}$ in the upright adult lung at rest ranges from 3.3 at the top of the lung to

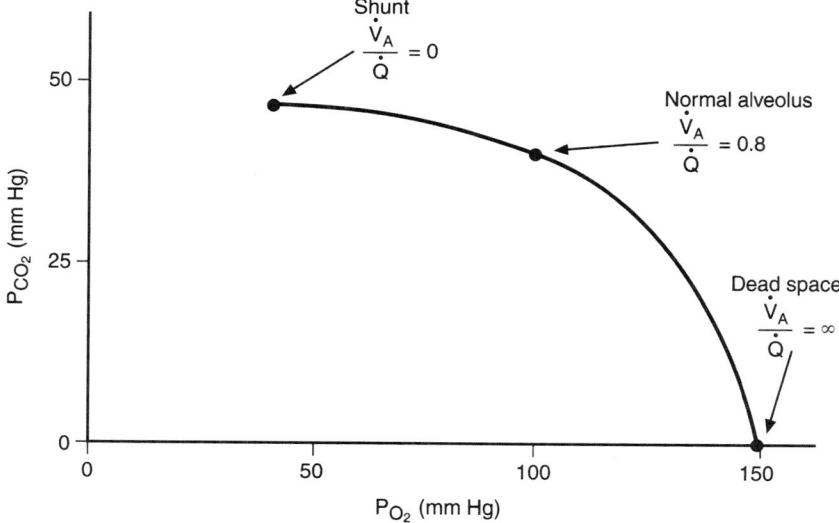

FIGURE 41.10. O_2-CO_2 diagram. The ventilation-perfusion curve describes all possible P_{O_2}-P_{CO_2} combinations in the alveoli [in an ideal lung ($P_{AO_2} = P_{aO_2}$)]. Mixed-venous values occur in alveoli with no ventilation (shunt) and inspired values occur in alveoli with no perfusion (dead space). From Powell FL. Pulmonary gas exchange. In: Johnson LR, ed. *Essential Medical Physiology*, 3rd ed. London: Elsevier/Academic Press, 2003, with permission.

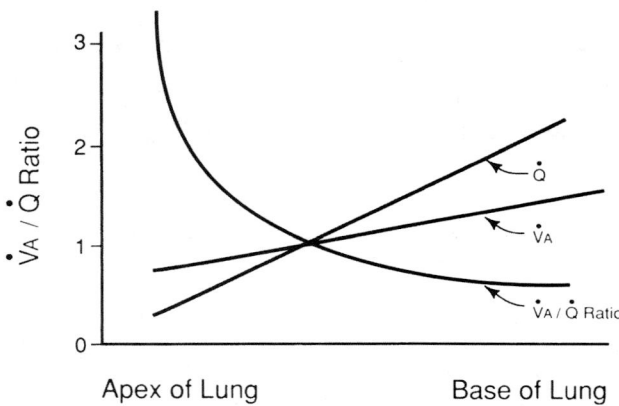

FIGURE 41.11. Gravity results in regional differences in alveolar ventilation ($\dot{V}A$) and blood flow between the apex and base of adult lungs, which causes the $\dot{V}A/\dot{Q}$ ratio to decrease ~2.5-fold from the top to the bottom of the lung. From Powell FL. Pulmonary Gas Exchange. In: Johnson LR, ed. *Essential Medical Physiology*, 3rd ed. Boston: Elsevier Academic Press, 2003, with permission.

0.6 at the bottom, decreasing P_{AO_2} from 132 mm Hg at the top of the lung to 89 mm Hg at the bottom. $P_A CO_2$ increases from 28 mm Hg at the top of the lung to 42 mm Hg at the bottom. These regional differences in alveolar gas cause O_2 uptake and CO_2 elimination to decrease from the top to the bottom of the lung. However, O_2 uptake decreases more than CO_2 elimination, corresponding to the larger decrease in P_{AO_2}, and this decreases R (the respiratory exchange ratio) between the top and the bottom of the lung. Exercise reduces regional heterogeneity of $\dot{V}A/\dot{Q}$, alveolar gases, and gas exchange by increasing blood flow at the top of the lung.

$\dot{V}A/\dot{Q}$ heterogeneity also causes heterogeneity in the P_{O_2} of the end-capillary blood ($P_{c'O_2}$) because alveolar-arterial P_{O_2} equilibrium occurs in any region with a normal diffusing capacity. The mechanism by which $\dot{V}A/\dot{Q}$ heterogeneity leads to hypoxemia is illustrated in **Figure 41.12**. Diffusing capacity is assumed normal; therefore, $P_{c'O_2}$ equals P_{AO_2} in each functional unit of gas exchange with a different $\dot{V}A/\dot{Q}$. In that arterial blood is a mixture of blood draining each unit, O_2 concentration in the "mixed" arterial blood is a flow-weighted average of blood from individual units. The "high" $\dot{V}A/\dot{Q}$ unit contributes relatively little to total blood flow, and $C_{c'O_2}$ is not increased significantly by the high P_{AO_2} because the blood-O_2 equilibrium curve is flat at high P_{O_2}. The "low" $\dot{V}A/\dot{Q}$ unit contributes relatively more to total blood flow, and $C_{c'O_2}$ is decreased significantly because the blood-O_2 equilibrium curve is steep at low P_{O_2}. Consequently, C_{aO_2} is weighted toward the level in the low $\dot{V}A/\dot{Q}$ units, and P_{AO_2} is lower than the numerical average of P_{AO_2} from all three alveoli.

$\dot{V}A/\dot{Q}$ heterogeneity increases the measured alveolar-arterial P_{O_2} difference without increasing alveolar-arterial P_{O_2} difference in any single gas exchange unit (**Fig. 41.12**). P_{O_2} in the mixed alveolar gas can be calculated as a flow-weighted mixture of the gas expired from all of the units. Increases in P_{O_2} can effectively balance decreases in P_{O_2} in the gas phase because partial pressure and concentration (or fraction, F) are linearly related for O_2 in the gas phase, unlike O_2 in blood. However, mixed P_{AO_2} exceeds the numerical average of P_{O_2} from the three units because the high $\dot{V}A/\dot{Q}$ unit contributes more volume to mixed alveolar gas.

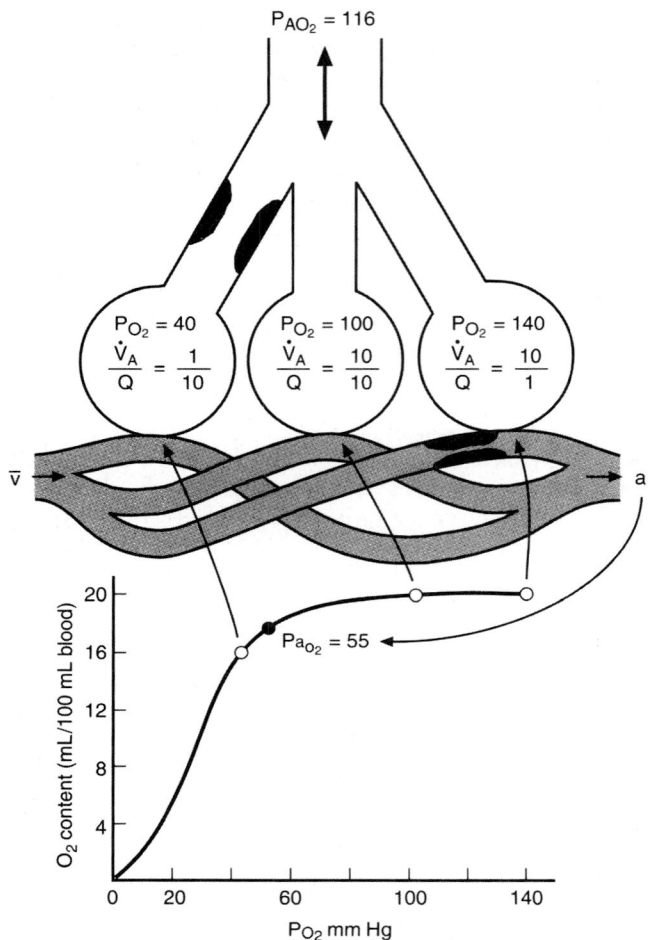

FIGURE 41.12. A three-compartment model showing how $\dot{V}A/\dot{Q}$ differences between lung units can increase the difference between mixed-alveolar P_{O_2} (P_{AO_2} = 116 mm Hg) and mixed-arterial P_{O_2} (P_{aO_2} = 55 mm Hg). Inspired P_{O_2} is assumed normal (150 mm Hg). Alveolar P_{O_2} in any individual unit is assumed equal to the P_{O_2} in end-capillary blood from that unit (*open circles on O_2 dissociation curve in lower panel*). However, P_{O_2} in mixed arterial blood is weighted toward P_{O_2} in the low $\dot{V}A/\dot{Q}$ units, and P_{O_2} in mixed alveolar gas is weighted toward P_{O_2} in the high $\dot{V}A/\dot{Q}$ units. The shape of the O_2 dissociation curve also contributes to the large alveolar-arterial P_{O_2} difference. From Powell FL. Pulmonary Gas Exchange. In: Johnson LR, ed. *Essential Medical Physiology*, 3rd ed. Boston: Elsevier Academic Press, 2003, with permission.

Therefore, $\dot{V}A/\dot{Q}$ heterogeneity decreases P_{aO_2} *and* increases P_{AO_2} from ideal values, and the alveolar-arterial P_{O_2} is increased. This mechanism increases the alveolar-arterial partial pressure difference for any gas, including CO_2 and anesthetic gases. However, $\dot{V}A/\dot{Q}$ affects O_2 more than other gases because the shape of the blood-O_2 equilibrium curve depresses P_{aO_2}. High and low $\dot{V}A/\dot{Q}$ regions can offset the effects of each other more effectively for CO_2 and anesthetic gases because the blood-equilibrium curves are relatively linear for these gases. Consequently, increasing overall ventilation is effective at overcoming P_{aCO_2} increases from $\dot{V}A/\dot{Q}$ heterogeneity, and the ventilatory control reflexes are quite effective at maintaining normal P_{aCO_2} by this mechanism.

$\dot{V}A/\dot{Q}$ heterogeneity occurs in normal lungs and explains the normal alveolar-arterial P_{O_2} in healthy young adults.

However, only half of the $\dot{V}A/\dot{Q}$ heterogeneity necessary to explain the normal alveolar-arterial PO_2 difference is caused by gravitational-dependent differences in $\dot{V}A$ and $\dot{Q}$ at different heights in the lung. Significant intraregional $\dot{V}A/\dot{Q}$ heterogeneity occurs between functional units of gas exchange (acini) at any given height in the lung. $\dot{V}A/\dot{Q}$ heterogeneity is also the most common cause of hypoxemia in lung disease.

The exact nature of $\dot{V}A/\dot{Q}$ heterogeneity can be measured by several methods, but they are generally restricted to the research laboratory and not useful clinically. $\dot{V}A/\dot{Q}$ heterogeneity can be diagnosed clinically by eliminating other causes of hypoxemia. Hypoventilation can be ruled out if arterial PCO_2 is normal. Diffusion limitation can be ruled out if the measured $DLCO$ is at least 50% of normal or if breathing high inspired O_2 relieves hypoxemia and decreases the alveolar-arterial PO_2 difference. However, 100% O_2 breathing will also eliminate hypoxemia from $\dot{V}A/\dot{Q}$ heterogeneity if all of the alveoli equilibrate with inspired PO_2. With pure O_2 breathing, only O_2 and CO_2 (plus water vapor) are in the alveolar gas, and PAO_2 is at least 600 mm Hg in all alveoli. In practice, $\dot{V}A/\dot{Q}$ heterogeneity includes poorly ventilated lung units; it may take up to 30 min to wash nitrogen out of all the alveoli during O_2 breathing. Consequently, O_2 breathing improves hypoxemia from $\dot{V}A/\dot{Q}$ heterogeneity but not nearly as quickly as it does with a pure diffusion limitation (which requires <1 min). If shunt is present, 100% O_2 breathing will never resolve the hypoxemia or decrease the alveolar-arterial PO_2 difference.

Other clinical measures of $\dot{V}A/\dot{Q}$ heterogeneity include physiologic shunt and dead space. Low $\dot{V}A/\dot{Q}$ gas exchange units and shunt have similar effects on PaO_2. Therefore, physiologic shunt (or venous admixture) can be used to quantify $\dot{V}A/\dot{Q}$ heterogeneity. Physiologic shunt is measured with the Berggren shunt equation (described previously) in an individual breathing less than 100% O_2 and usually room air (see the section, Shunts). $\dot{V}A/\dot{Q}$ heterogeneity causes hypoxemia "as if" there were an increase in shunt, thereby increasing physiologic shunt. Similarly, the effects of high $\dot{V}A/\dot{Q}$ units on PaO_2 resemble the effects of dead space. Therefore, physiologic dead space (see previous discussion) can be used to quantify the effects of $\dot{V}A/\dot{Q}$ heterogeneity on PaO_2 and $PaCO_2$ "as if" there were an increase in anatomic dead space. Note that both physiologic shunt and dead space will be less than the actual amounts of blood flow or ventilation going to abnormal $\dot{V}A/\dot{Q}$ units because shunt and dead space represent the extremes of the $\dot{V}A/\dot{Q}$ ratio, and actual $\dot{V}A/\dot{Q}$ ratios between 0 and infinity will have smaller effects on alveolar and arterial PO_2 and PCO_2 (**Fig. 41.10**).

It is important to note that the alveolar ventilation equation introduced previously does not accurately quantify $\dot{V}A$ when arterial PCO_2 is substituted for alveolar PCO_2 if significant $\dot{V}A/\dot{Q}$ heterogeneity is present. $\dot{V}A/\dot{Q}$ heterogeneity causes alveolar PCO_2 to be less than arterial PCO_2. Hence, the total ventilation to all alveoli is underestimated if arterial PCO_2 is used in the alveolar ventilation equation. Because it is difficult to measure mixed alveolar PCO_2, the alveolar ventilation equation is not used on people with lung disease.

Ventilation-perfusion inhomogeneities are common in clinical practice. The use of even small doses of supplemental O_2 is effective because the alveolar PO_2 is increased substantially by even small amounts of O_2. For example, the PAO_2 is raised by ~5–6 torr per percent supplemental O_2. In lung regions with low $\dot{V}A/\dot{Q}$, supplemental O_2 dramatically reduces the venous admixture due to the shape of the oxyhemoglobin-dissociation curve. Even an FIO_2 of 0.25 will produce an alveolar PO_2 that will saturate the blood in regions of the lung with a $\dot{V}A/\dot{Q}$ ratio as low as 0.2. At an FIO_2 of 0.4, virtually all venous admixture due to ventilation-perfusion mismatch is eliminated, and the remainder of the alveolar-arterial gradient is due to pure shunt.

Carbon Dioxide Exchange

Physiologic CO_2 transport follows the same general principles described for O_2 in the previous sections. For example, the Fick principle was used previously to calculate $PaCO_2$; the Fick principle can also be used to calculate the normal arterial-venous CO_2 concentration difference:

$$\dot{V}CO_2 = \dot{Q}(CaCO_2 - C\bar{v}CO_2)$$

For normal values of $\dot{V}CO_2 = 240$ mL of CO_2/min and $\dot{Q} = 6$ L/min, the arterial-venous CO_2 concentration difference is 4 mL/dL, which differs from the normal value for O_2 only by the difference in $\dot{V}CO_2$ and $\dot{V}CO_2$ (or by their ratio, which equals R).

Differences between CO_2 and O_2 exchange result mainly from (a) differences in the O_2 and CO_2 dissociation curves, and (b) differences in the effects of CO_2 and O_2 on ventilatory control reflexes. PCO_2 differences are much smaller than PO_2 differences between arterial and venous blood, although the concentrations are similar, because CO_2 is more soluble in blood. As explained previously, $PaCO_2$ is the most important value in determining the resting level of ventilation, and ventilatory reflexes tend to increase $\dot{V}A$ as much as necessary to restore normal $PaCO_2$ when gas exchange is altered.

Hypoventilation has almost the same effect on both O_2 and CO_2. Differences between decreases in PaO_2 and increases in $PaCO_2$ with hypoventilation are explained by the effect of the normal respiratory exchange ratio (R) in the alveolar gas equation. A normal R = 0.8 magnifies PaO_2 changes for a given $PaCO_2$ change.

Diffusion limitation affects CO_2 and O_2 similarly, but normal ventilatory control reflexes will increase $\dot{V}A$ and return $PaCO_2$ to normal. Calculating a diffusing capacity for CO_2 is less certain than for O_2 because resistances from the chemical reactions of CO_2 in the blood are more uncertain. Membrane-diffusing capacity for CO_2 is greater than DMO_2 because CO_2 solubility is much greater than O_2 solubility, but other factors are similar or identical. (Recall that D = [solubility/MW]$_{gas}$ × [area/thickness]$_{membrane}$). However, under normal circumstances, the rate of equilibration between alveolar gas and capillary blood is estimated to be similar for v and O_2, requiring ~0.25 sec for equilibrium. CO_2 equilibrium is slower than expected with its large membrane-diffusing capacity, in part because chemical reactions for CO_2 in blood are slow. Also, both membrane and blood solubility are high for CO_2, and the membrane:blood solubility ratio determines the rate of diffusion equilibrium, as described previously.

The effects of shunts and ventilation-perfusion mismatching on $PaCO_2$ are similar and relatively small for two reasons: (a) $PaCO_2$ changes little when shunt or low $\dot{V}A/\dot{Q}$ units increase CO_2 concentration because the CO_2-blood equilibrium curve is so steep, and (b) the linearity of the physiologic CO_2 dissociation curve means that increases in CO_2 concentration are offset by increasing $\dot{V}A$, which decreases $PaCO_2$. Normal ventilatory control will increase the overall $\dot{V}$ as necessary to restore $Paco_2$ toward normal. In fact, some patients with shunts and low $\dot{V}A/\dot{Q}$ units may actually have decreased $Paco_2$ if hypoxemia is severe enough to override the normal control of $Paco$. The extra ventilation necessary to compensate for shunt and low $\dot{V}A/\dot{Q}$ units contributes to physiologic dead space calculated by the Bohr method. The difference between physiologic and anatomic dead space is sometimes called *alveolar dead space*, which represents an "as if" amount of wasted ventilation that could explain measured CO_2 exchange if no shunt or $\dot{V}A/\dot{Q}$ mismatching were present in the lung.

Cardiovascular and Tissue Oxygen Transport

The mitochondria are the ultimate site of O_2 consumption and CO_2 production. Hence, gas exchange also occurs in the tissues as O_2 diffuses out of the circulation to meet metabolic demands. O_2 diffuses from the alveoli into pulmonary capillary blood; it is then pumped to the tissues in arterial blood by the heart and finally diffuses back out of the systemic capillaries to mitochondria in the tissues. The heart also pumps O_2-poor venous blood back to the lungs, where it is reoxygenated. The magnitude of the Po_2 decrease between arterial and venous blood (**Fig. 41.1**) depends on both the cardiovascular O_2 delivery and tissue O_2 demand.

O_2 delivery is the product of cardiac output and arterial O_2 concentration ($\dot{Q}$ Cao_2). The tissues will extract enough O_2 to meet their needs as long as O_2 supply is sufficient. Hence, O_2 supply and demand determine venous O_2 levels. These factors are related by the Fick principle, which describes O_2 transport by the cardiovascular system as:

$$\dot{V}o_2 = \dot{Q}(Cao_2 - C\overline{v}o_2)$$

where $\dot{V}o_2$ is O_2 consumption, $\dot{Q}$ is cardiac output, and the last term is the arterial-venous O_2 concentration difference. This equation can be used to calculate cardiac output from measurements of $\dot{V}o_2$ and blood O_2 concentrations.

The Fick principle can predict the arterial-venous O_2 concentration difference from adult resting values for O_2 consumption ($\dot{V}o_2 = 300$ mL/min) and cardiac output ($\dot{Q} = 6$ L/min): (300 mL of O_2/min)/(6,000 mL of blood/min) $= 5$ mL O_2/dL blood. If the normal value for $Cao_2 = 20$ mL of O_2/dL of blood, $C\overline{v}o_2 = 15$ mL/dL. Notice that the venous O_2 level is determined by (a) the ratio of metabolism to blood flow, and (b) arterial O_2 concentration, which is determined by alveolar Po_2 and the O_2-blood equilibrium curve. The O_2-blood equilibrium curve (see the previous section, Oxygen in Blood) is used to convert $C\overline{v}o_2$ (15 mL/dL) to mixed-venous O_2 saturation (75%) and $P\overline{v}o_2$ (40 mm Hg).

The cardiovascular Fick principle is graphically presented in **Figure 41.13** to illustrate the importance of the shape of the O_2-blood equilibrium curve. In the right panel, the height of the shaded rectangle represents the arterial-venous O_2 concentration difference, and its width represents cardiac output (normalized to 100 g of body mass). The area of the rectangle is the product of these two factors, and represents $\dot{V}o_2$.

Changes in $\dot{V}o_2$ can be achieved by increasing cardiac output ("flow reserve") and/or increasing the arterial-venous O_2 difference. The dashed lines in **Figure 41.13** show the consequences of increasing $\dot{V}o_2$ by increasing venous O_2 extraction

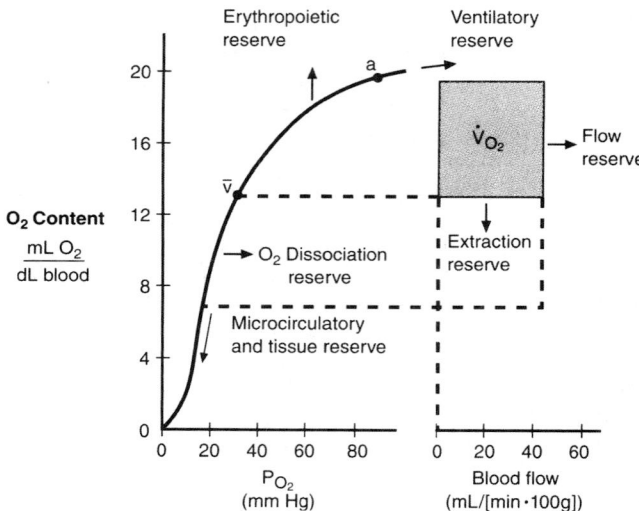

FIGURE 41.13. Graphic representation of O_2 transport by the cardiovascular system. (*Left*) O_2-blood equilibrium curve showing arterial (a) and mixed-venous ($\overline{v}$) points. (*Right*) Graphic representation of the Fick principle for cardiovascular O_2 transport. Horizontal axis is blood flow normalized to body mass; vertical axis is O_2 concentration from the left panel; shaded area is O_2 consumption. "Reserves," which can increase $\dot{V}o_2$, are described in the text. From Powell FL. Pulmonary gas exchange. In: Johnson LR, ed. *Essential Medical Physiology*, 3rd ed. London: Elsevier/Academic Press, 2003, with permission.

("extraction reserve"). Changes in $P\overline{v}o_2$ are minimized with large decreases in venous O_2 concentration by the shape of the O_2-blood equilibrium curve. A right shift of the curve can increase $P\overline{v}o_2$ for a given $C\overline{v}o_2$ ("O_2-dissociation reserve"). Maintaining a high $P\overline{v}o_2$ is important for tissue gas exchange and the "microcirculatory and tissue reserve," as discussed later. All these reserves are important mechanisms for meeting increased O_2 demands during exercise.

Increases in O_2 delivery are achieved primarily through increases in cardiac output in normoxic conditions. Increasing alveolar and arterial Po_2 is not effective at increasing Cao_2 in normoxic conditions because the slope of the O_2-blood equilibrium curve is flat at normal Pao_2 values ("ventilatory reserve"; **Fig. 41.13**). However, changes in Pao_2 are much more effective at changing O_2 delivery when Po_2 is low (e.g., at altitude, when exchange occurs on a steeper part of the O_2-blood equilibrium curve). Changes in hematocrit and hemoglobin concentration, which occur with chronic hypoxia, can increase O_2 delivery by increasing total O_2 concentration for any given Po_2 ("erythropoietic reserve"). The erythropoietic reserve is the physiologic basis for the questionable practice of "blood doping," which uses blood transfusions or artificial erythropoietin in attempts to increase maximal O_2 consumption and athletic performance.

Tissue Gas Exchange

Tissue gas exchange describes the process of O_2 moving out of systemic capillaries to the mitochondria in cells by diffusion. Therefore, O_2 consistency that is required for transport in tissues is described by Fick's first law of diffusion, similar to diffusion across the blood-gas barrier in the lung:

$$\overline{V}o_2 = \Delta Po_2 \times Dto_2$$

where ΔP_{O_2} is the average P_{O_2} gradient between capillary blood and the mitochondria, and $D_{t_{O_2}}$ is a tissue-diffusing capacity for O_2. Interestingly, anatomic estimates of $D_{t_{O_2}}$ for the whole body are similar to anatomic estimates of $D_{m_{O_2}}$ in the lung.

The main difference between O_2 diffusion in tissue and in the lung is that diffusion pathways are much longer in tissue. Tissue capillaries may be 50 μm apart, so that the distance from the capillary to mitochondria can be 50 times longer than the thickness of the blood-gas barrier (<0.5 μm). Long diffusion distances can lead to significant P_{O_2} gradients in tissues. Also, the P_{O_2} gradient varies along the length of a capillary as O_2 leaves the blood, and capillary P_{O_2} decreases from arterial to venous levels. A mathematical model called the *Krogh cylinder* can be used to predict P_{O_2} profiles in metabolizing tissue. This model predicts that P_{O_2} in cells farthest away from a capillary, or at the venous end of the capillary, may be zero when O_2 demand is increased. However, as mitochondria function normally until P_{O_2} decreases below a few millimeters of mercury, so metabolism will continue under all but these most extreme conditions.

During increased O_2 demand (e.g., exercise in skeletal muscle, absorption in the gut, nervous activity in the brain), additional capillaries may be recruited, which helps to maintain adequate O_2 supply by decreasing diffusion distances. Factors that increase or maintain $P_{\bar{v}_{O_2}}$ also help tissue O_2 diffusion by enhancing the P_{O_2} gradient. These factors include the steep shape of the O_2-blood equilibrium curve in the venous range and right shifts of the curve by temperature, P_{CO_2}, and pH changes such as in exercising muscle. $P_{\bar{v}_{O_2}}$ is sometimes used as an index of tissue O_2 exchange because it represents the minimum pressure head driving O_2 diffusion in the body.

Myoglobin may facilitate O_2 diffusion in muscle by shuttling O_2 to sites far away from a capillary. Measurements show that P_{O_2} in skeletal muscle is much more uniform than predicted by the Krogh cylinder model and that myoglobin may shuttle O_2 to the venous end. The implications of this finding for differences in O_2 transport between muscle (e.g., during myocardial ischemia) and brain (e.g., during a stroke) remain to be determined.

LUNG MECHANICS, RESPIRATORY, AND AIRWAY MUSCLES

The primary functions of the respiratory system are to transport O_2 from the environment to metabolizing cells and to remove CO_2 from the body. The first step in O_2 transport is ventilation of the lungs, which is a function of lung mechanics and the functioning of respiratory and airway muscles, as discussed in this section.

Pressure-Flow Relationships in the Respiratory System

The mammalian lung has a natural tendency to collapse. The respiratory muscles and the chest wall oppose this tendency and apply a continuous tension to the structure of the lungs to maintain lung volume at end-expiration. The tension within the

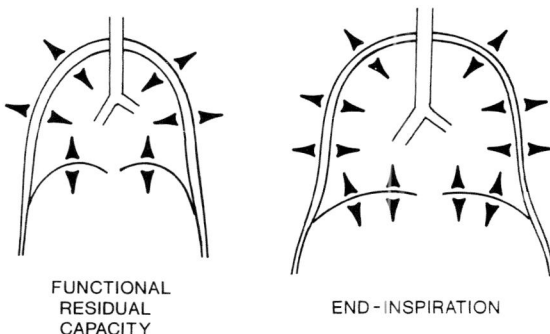

FUNCTIONAL RESIDUAL CAPACITY   END-INSPIRATION

FIGURE 41.14. Elastic recoil, represented by the arrows, increases with increasing lung volume. It produces the negative pleural pressure at end expiration. From Heldt GP. The mechanics of breathing: developmental aspects and practical applications. In: Boynton BR, Carlo WA, Jobe AH, eds. *New Therapies for Neonatal Respiratory Failure.* Cambridge: Cambridge University Press, 1994, with permission.

lung is generated by its fibrous structure and by the gas-liquid interface in the distal airways and alveoli. The sum of the forces that make the lungs collapse is referred to as the *elastic recoil* (**Fig. 41.14**) and is reflected in the amount of pressure that must be applied across the lungs to produce both the end-expiratory lung volume and changes in the lung volume with breathing. During mechanical ventilation, this pressure is predominantly the pressure applied to the endotracheal tube.

The basic relationships of pressures and flow in the respiratory system for a patient on a mechanical ventilator are shown in **Figure 41.15**. In panel A, the patient breathes spontaneously without positive end-expiratory pressure (PEEP). The respiratory muscles contract, and the pleural pressure (P_{pl}) decreases during inspiration from a negative value at end-expiration, which reflects the elastic recoil of the lungs. The transpulmonary pressure (P_{tp}), or the difference between the airway pressure (P_{aw}) and P_{pl}, also decreases, which produces the inspiratory flow (shown negative in the figure by convention). The elastic recoil of the lungs increases linearly with lung volume. The dashed lines on the P_{pl} record indicate the recoil pressure. The decrease in the transpulmonary pressure leads the elastic recoil pressure. This difference is the pressure that is needed to overcome the pulmonary resistance (P_{rs}) shown in the panel. The small decrease in P_{aw} reflects the resistance of the airway circuit. During expiration, the P_{pl} increases, and the elastic recoil of the lungs raises the alveolar pressure (P_A) to produce expiratory flow. The pressure change again leads that of the elastic recoil pressure to overcome the expiratory resistance.

Panel B shows one respiratory cycle when 5 cm H_2O of PEEP is added. A small increase in the end-expiratory P_{pl} is seen, and the P_{tp} is more negative due to an increased lung volume with the addition of PEEP. Inspiratory and expiratory flows are generated by the same mechanism as the situation without PEEP. Panel C shows one respiratory cycle when a synchronized breath is given by the ventilator. The change in P_{tp} is greater, as the ventilator pressure is added to the P_{pl}, which produces a larger breath. The flow rates are higher, and P_{rs} is greater. Note that in these three breaths, the conventions for the pressures are equivalent.

The inset shows the flow-volume loops for breath A on no PEEP, B on PEEP, and on C that produced with the ventilator.

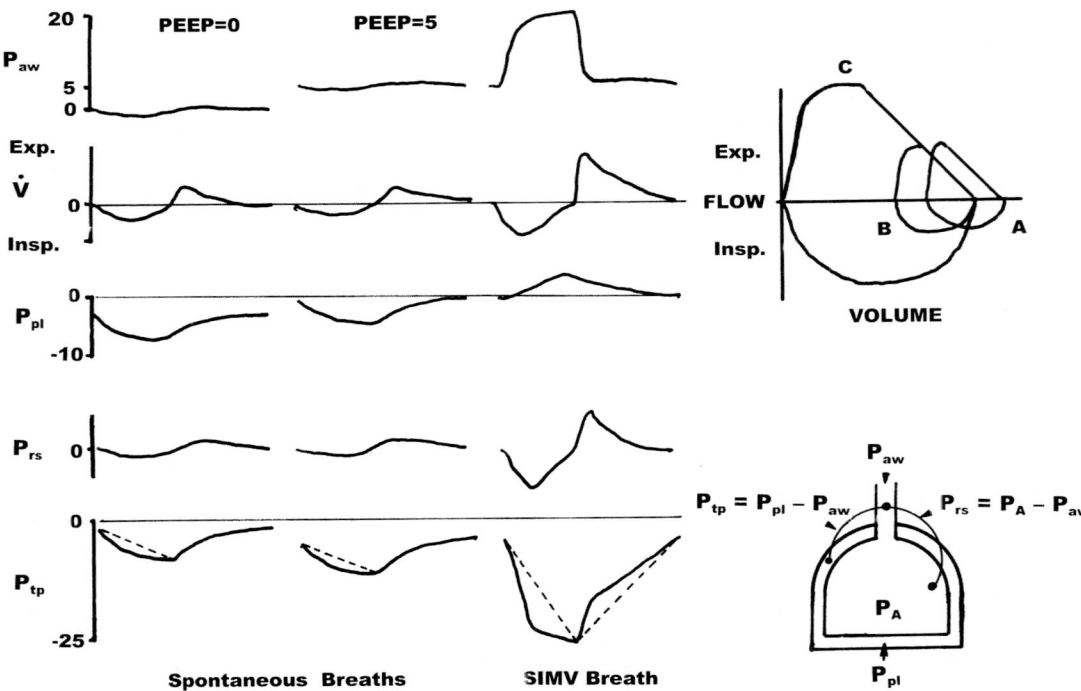

FIGURE 41.15. Recording of the airway pressure (P_{aw}), flow ($\overline{V}$), pleural pressure (P_{pl}), resistive pressure (P_{rs}), and transpulmonary pressure (P_{tp}) as defined in the diagram in the lower right corner. Three breaths are represented: two during spontaneous breathing with and without PEEP and one synchronized, intermittent, mandatory ventilator (SIMV) breath. Note that the P_{pl} is higher at end expiration while on PEEP and that the P_{tp} is more negative. The elastic line (*dashed*) has been added to the P_{tp} and represents the pressure needed to overcome the elastic recoil. The fall in P_{tp} leads the elastic line during inspiration and lags during expiration. The difference is P_{rs}, or the pressure needed to overcome the resistance of the airways and the lung tissue. The flow-volume loops of the three breaths are shown in the upper right corner. Note that the end-expiratory volume is larger in breaths B and C and that the expiratory flow-volume relationship is parallel in all three breaths. This represents the intrinsic flow limitation of the lungs that is independent of effort and only dependent on elastic recoil.

The end-expiratory volumes are greater for B and C than for A. The slope of the expiratory flow-volume curves are the same, even though shifted in volume. As discussed later, the expiratory flow limitation is independent of the effort made by either the patient or the ventilator.

In the clinical setting, measurements of pulmonary mechanics at the bedside in even the smallest infants can be made. Flow is measured with a pneumotachograph, which is a linear resistor of very low resistance that is placed on the endotracheal tube or on a face mask or nasal prongs. The P_{pl} is estimated by placing an esophageal pressure catheter in the lower thoracic esophagus. Proper measurement of esophageal pressure takes some experience, and the position of the pressure catheter is tested by performing an airway occlusion at end-expiration. The change in the airway occlusion pressure should be equal to the change in the esophageal pressure when the catheter is in proper position because, during occlusion, no resistive or elastic losses occur between the P_{pl} and the airway. Since the chest wall in infants is very compliant, it takes very little pressure to inflate it. Therefore, the airway pressure is used as the transpulmonary pressure for most clinical measurements. This must be remembered when results of the monitor on the ventilator in older children are interpreted or when the chest wall compliance is significant, for example, in a very edematous patient.

Developmental Aspects of the Lung as They Affect Elastic Recoil

From a mechanical viewpoint, the embryology of the lung determines much of the nonsurfactant properties of the lung. Two major systems of elastic fibers distribute the stress on the lung that is induced by decreases in intrapleural pressure so as to evenly inflate the lung. The first system is that of the airways, and the second originates from the pleural surface that grows toward the hilum. The airway system provides the even distribution of gas to the alveolar ducts, and the second system provides the matrix to evenly distribute the tension from the pleural surface to the alveolar ducts. These two systems develop simultaneously as the lung bud grows centripetally into the pleural space.

Lung development begins with the formation of the respiratory diverticulum at 4 weeks from the ventral wall of the foregut. The location of the bud on the gut tube is determined by the transcription factor TBX4, and the epithelium of the lungs, larynx, and bronchi are of endodermal origin. The cartilaginous, muscular, and connective tissues are derived from the splanchnic mesoderm that surrounds the foregut. The respiratory diverticulum expands caudally, and the tracheoesophageal ridges grow to separate it from the foregut. The ridges close to form the tracheoesophageal septum. The lung bud then expands into the mesoderm, forming the pleural space.

The lung bud forms the tracheal and two lateral outpouchings—the bronchial buds that become the main stem bronchi by the fifth week of gestation. Subsequent growth of the lung buds extend into the body cavity, forming the pericardioperitoneal canals, which ultimately are separated from the peritoneal and pericardial cavities by the pleuroperitoneal and pleuropericardial folds. The mesoderm, which covers the outside of the lungs, develops into the visceral pleura. The somatic mesoderm layer, covering the body wall in the inside, becomes the parietal pleura. The secondary bronchi divide repeatedly in a dichotomous fashion, forming the 10 segmental bronchi on the right and left, which are completed by the 17th week of gestation.

Differentiation of the lungs is under the control of the extracellular matrix that is laid down in the mesenchyme, into which the developing lung bud grows. During the pseudoglandular stage (5–16 weeks), airway branching is complete to the level of primitive respiratory bronchioles. Each terminal bronchiole divides into two or more respiratory bronchioles, which in turn, divide into three to six alveolar ducts by the end of the canalicular stage (16–24 weeks). The saccular stage then continues until birth, during which time the distal airways are differentiated until near term. Alveolarization occurs for many months after birth.

Much of the early branching is controlled by the presence of the proteoglycan syndecan, a molecule that is abundant in the mesenchyme and is critical to the formation of epithelial tubes. Epidermal growth factor supports the branching of the growing epithelium during the first 25 weeks of gestation. Fibronectin, a glycoprotein, directs the growth of the basement membrane and the formation of the collagen matrix. It ties the growth of the cells and the basement membrane via fibril formation, and it has three domains that bind to the collagen, heparin sulfate proteoglycans, and cells. The growth and branching of the epithelium into the airway structure are also under control of laminin, a large glycoprotein that is part of the basement membrane. Cellular interactions with laminin are mediated primarily through several molecules that bind to it: entactin for cell adherence; dystroglycan, which directs differentiation; and perlecan, which transduces stretching and is a signaling molecule for the action of dystroglycan. Cadherins are calcium-dependent molecules that direct the adherence of cells to each other, helping to form the cellular sheets and tubes of the alveolar ducts that will act as a vestibule for several additional generations of alveoli.

The terminal saccular stage, beginning at 25 weeks of gestation, is characterized by further widening of the airspaces and rearrangement of capillaries to form a more intimate air-blood interface. Thinning of the alveolar membrane and reduction in the mesenchymal mass also occur. The process of thinning of the alveolar septae is associated with a highly organized deposition of elastin fibrils in the transitory alveolar ducts. Elastin is later deposited maximally in secondary crests, which protrude into future airspaces that form the foundation of future alveolation. Lung volume grows by protrusion and lengthening of these secondary crests that are made of three layers. The central layer consists of fibroblastic cells and is associated with connective tissue that has developing capillaries on both sides. Fibroblast proliferation causes the crests to develop into alveolar duct septae and produce elastin, collagen, and proteoglycans.

As the septae are lengthening, type II cells proliferate. The extracellular matrix induces production of surfactant-associated proteins A, B, and C. As the septae thin out, the capillaries remodel to form a single capillary network. This fusion forms the central lamina densa of the basement membrane, which contains type IV collagen, which is extremely strong.

The main elastic elements of the lung are collagen and elastin. Collagen fibers are formed by binding fibrils together in a gel-like matrix with proteoglycans. Collagen is not very distensible but, when combined with elastin, forms interwoven strands similar to that of rubber and cotton, which are elastic with limited distensibility.

The central airways have two such collagen/elastin layers; one longitudinal and one circumferential, which grow out past the respiratory and terminal bronchioles and become thin fibers that spiral into the alveolar ducts. This network of fibers strengthens the mouth of the alveolar ducts and extends to several distal generations of alveoli. These fibers are continuous with the fibers of the blood vessels, airways, and the pleura.

Simultaneous with the development of the airways, the thick primary layer of the visceral pleura forms a system of fiber bags that grow toward the hilum from the pleural surface. These bags hold the developing subunits of the developing airways, of which the bottoms equally divide the pleural surface. The sides of each bag interdigitate with the fibers of the interlobular septae. The interlobular septae are fused with the alveolar septae they enclose. Tension developed at the pleural surfaces is thereby transmitted tangentially to the pleural surface and toward the hilum through the interlobular septae. This arrangement gives the lung isotropy, which makes each alveolar unit mechanically interdependent with its neighbors, so that the entire network is homogeneously self-inflating. In addition, spiral fibers at the level of the alveolar ducts maintain their patency when stretched during inspiration to enhance even entry of gas into each vestibule. The alveolar duct structure is especially important for maintaining alveolar expansion at low lung volumes. It is estimated that this system of fiber bags that originate from the pleura contributes 30% to the overall elastic recoil of the lung.

The airway and pleural systems may complement each other in distributing mechanical stress. They also form the continuous interstitial matrix, from the alveolar septae to both of the perivascular and pleural lymphatics, for transport of lymph to keep the air-blood interface from flooding. Although collagen and elastin are virtually always found together throughout the lung, they have independent mechanical effects that depend on lung volume. Destruction of elastic experimentally causes increased lung compliance at low and middle volume ranges (25%–40% of TLC). Experimental destruction by collagenase results in an increase in compliance at high lung volumes. Together, they contribute to a smooth pressure-volume curve, with stabilization of stress from the pleural surface, down to the smallest unit of gas exchange, and centrally to the hilum.

Surface Tension and Elastic Recoil

The elastic skeleton of the lung predicts a simple, linear relationship between the volume of the lung and the pressure applied across it. It has long been observed that pulmonary surfactant contributes greatly to the pressure-volume (PV) characteristics of the lungs. The observations just noted also

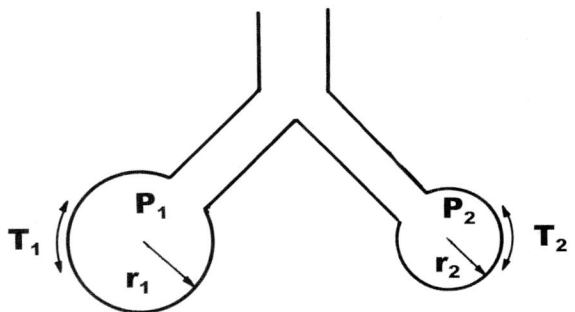

FIGURE 41.16. The distension pressure of two theoretical alveoli connected by a single airway is related by the law of La Place. In the larger alveolus, $P_1 = 2 \times$ tension$_1$/r$_1$, and in the smaller alveo, $P_2 = 2 \times$ tension$_2$/r$_2$. If tension$_1$ = tension$_2$, the distending pressure of the smaller alveolus will be greater and will collapse into the larger alveolus. Alternatively, a greater pressure will be required to recruit the smaller alveolus, leading to overdistension and barotrauma to the larger alveolus.

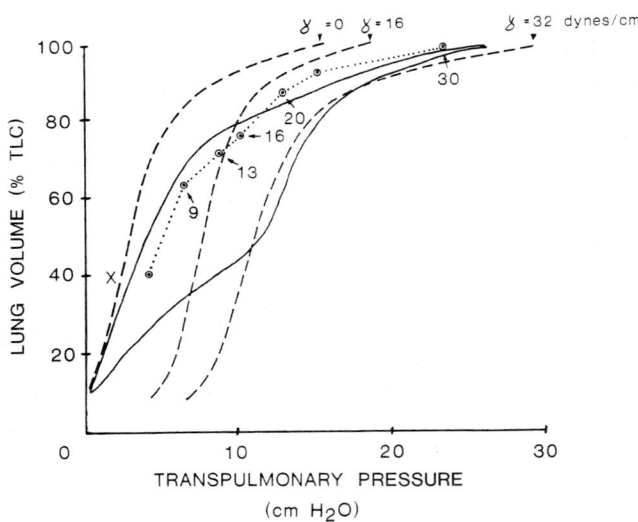

FIGURE 41.17. Summary of surface-tension effects on elastic recoil based on several types of experimental data. The solid curve shows the air inflation, with hysteresis. Dashed curves are deflation pressure-volume curves for lungs filled with perfluorocarbon liquids with fixed surface tensions of 0, 16, and 32 dyne/cm. Data points from direct alveolar surface-tension estimates using a micropuncture technique are shown joined by the dotted line. The **X** represents alveolar-wash surface tension in rat lungs. These four different techniques confirm the significant decrease in surface tension in vivo with lung inflation, which maintains lung stability at low lung volumes. TLC, total lung capacity. From Heldt GP. The mechanics of breathing: developmental aspects and practical applications. In: Boynton BR, Carlo WA, Jobe AH, eds. *New Therapies for Neonatal Respiratory Failure.* Cambridge: Cambridge University Press, 1994, with permission.

demonstrate that the surfactant system of the lung contributes to this hysteresis in the PV curves.

In the first approximation, the PV relationship of an air-liquid interface can be modeled with a bubble on the end of a blow-tube, by the law of La Place (**Fig. 41.16**):

$$P = 2 \times \text{surface tension}/r$$

where:

P = the pressure applied, is the surface tension of the air-liquid interface

r = the radius of the bubble.

The two theoretical alveoli presented in **Figure 41.16** have unequal radii. If the surface tension were the same in both alveoli, the alveolus with the smaller diameter would collapse into the larger one, as the pressure exerted by the surface-tension forces would be greater by this law. The fact that the pulmonary surfactant decreases on compression overcomes this problem and makes lung inflation more homogeneous.

Measurements of the alveolar sepal stretch provide an estimate of the radius of the alveoli and the surface-area changes of the lung during inflation. The relationship of surface tension to area has been studied by three approaches in an effort to understand the in vivo behavior of the PV curve. The first was the study of surface-tension measurements in vitro on a Langmuir-Wilhelmy balance during compression of surface-active film from lung extracts. The second approach was to construct PV curves in air-filled lungs and compare them to curves obtained from lungs filled with liquids (perfluorocarbons and kerosene) with fixed interfacial surface tension. The third approach was by direct estimate of alveolar surface tension using a microdroplet, wherein a micropipette (diameter $\sim$2 μm) was used to place a drop of fluorocarbon directly onto the alveolar surface through a micropuncture in the pleural surface. The fluorocarbon has a fixed low surface tension and spreads into a lens the diameter of which reflects the surface tension of the alveolar film.

Data from these three approaches are summarized in a plot of lung volume versus P$_{tp}$ in **Fig 41.17**. Even though less hysteresis was seen in the PV curve in lungs inflated with liquids of fixed surface tension, it still represented several centimeters of H$_2$O, which may represent tissue "creep," as described in

solid mechanics, or tissue remodeling. Inflation with liquids of increasing surface tension requires more pressure to open the lung, but lung inflation proceeds with equal ease until 80% of TLC is reached, when the compliance is markedly decreased. The equilibrium surface tension value of 25 dynes/cm, derived from the Langmuir-Wilhelmy balance data, has been added to the data interpolated from both the liquid-filled lung and micropipette measurements. The inflections in the PV curves for gas-filled lungs near 16 and 20 dynes/cm, by direct micropuncture measurements, coincide with this equilibrium value of the surface tension. At lung volumes above this point, the film spreads and tissue forces become dominant due to the collagen in the elastic skeleton. The value of surface tension, measured at TLC (30 dynes/cm) is less than that of the fixed fluorocarbon (32 dynes/cm), corresponding to a considerably decreased transpulmonary pressure at TLC. At lung volumes below this point, film compression leads to marked lowering of the surface tension and collapse of the film. At 40% of TLC, values as low as 0.5 dynes/cm have been measured in cats.

The currently accepted model for the dynamics of the surfactant effect can be summarized as follows. Assuming that a sufficient amount of surfactant exists, surface-active material (SAM) is actively adsorbed to the surface film during lung inflation. Relatively bare areas of the air-liquid interface are filled from the subphase from the previously compressed packed film. During lung deflation, differential desorption of the SAM occurs. Areas with little SAM are squeezed out of the film by SAM-rich areas. At low lung volumes, the film is compressed far from the equilibrium state, becomes unstable, and is desorbed from the monolayer film. Saturated lipid, di-palmitoylphosphatidylcholine (DPPC), produces the most stable interfacial film, especially on compression. As the lipid is compressed, non-DPPC elements are squeezed out of the monolayer. Surfactant-associated proteins smooth out the process of adsorption-desorption from inspiration to expiration and stabilize the film under compression. This process can explain much of the hysteresis of the PV curve.

The alveolar duct is pivotal to this process and is the point at which the interplay between the elastic skeleton and surfactant is most important. When lungs are washed of surfactant, the alveolar ducts increase in size, which suggests that alveolar collapse redistributes the stress to the more proximal airway. At 23–30 weeks gestation, the time when many infants are born prematurely, the elastic fibers are not yet developed and cannot bear the additional stress imposed by alveolar collapse. This effect is even greater during mechanical ventilation. Rupture of both the airways and the capillaries at this point causes the formation of edema and hyaline membranes, which are the primary pathologic precursor of bronchopulmonary dysplasia.

Surfactant replacement therapy is a well-established therapy for premature infants with respiratory distress syndrome. The surfactant is manufactured from the washings or homogenates of animal lungs and processed for separation of surfactant lipids and surfactant-associated proteins. The primary synthetic surfactant, Exosurf, is not as effective as natural surfactants and has fallen out of common clinical usage. Therapy is most effective if given either prophylactically at birth or within the first 2 hrs after birth. Infants treated with surfactant have rapidly decreased O_2 and ventilatory requirements and can be weaned from mechanical ventilation more quickly. Surfactant therapy is most effective for infants of 26–32 weeks' gestation, probably because their primitive alveoli are smaller than the nonalveolated saccules of younger infants and because of unavoidable complications of extreme prematurity. The use of prenatal steroids accelerates the appearance of endogenous surfactant and makes extremely premature infants more responsive to replacement therapy. A number of surfactants are commercially available, and despite manufacturers' claims or individual preferences, they have not been shown to have different effects in clinical trials. Surfactant therapy has also been used in treatment of neonatal pneumonia and congenital diaphragmatic hernia in small studies that have demonstrated positive effects.

Flow Limitation

The second element in the mechanics of breathing concerns where and how airflow limitation occurs. In purely elastic systems, the energy put into the system that causes deformation is released back to the system when the deformation is relieved. In purely resistive systems, the energy put into the system during deformation is lost, usually in the form of heat. This dissipation of energy in the lungs occurs both in the airways and tissue. The pulmonary resistance is usually thought to be that of the airways during spontaneous breathing, as most pathological states involve bronchoconstriction. Nevertheless, tissue resistive forces can more than equal those of the airways under certain pathologic states.

Airway resistance is usually modeled by the aerodynamics of flow through tubes. Flow through the airways is driven by

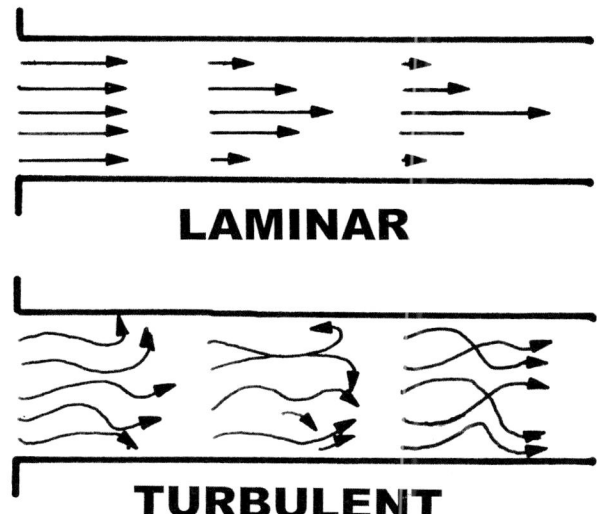

FIGURE 41.18. Flow velocity profiles for laminar and turbulent flow represented by velocity vectors during entry flow into a long, straight tube. In laminar flow, the profile is flat across the diameter of the tube but quickly attains a predictable parabolic profile. A balance is maintained between the convective force on the gas down the tube (related to density and velocity) and the viscous resistive forces developing the profile. In turbulent flow, random axial movement of the gas dissipates energy at a greater rate than during laminar flow, which is dependent on the density of the gas rather than on its viscosity. A very thin boundary layer forms next to the wall of the tube. Turbulent flow develops only at the peripheral airways, and laminar flow is characteristic of the larger airways.

a pressure drop between the alveoli and the atmosphere—or the endotracheal tube in the case of ventilated patients. The decrease in the pressure in the direction of the gas flow represents a dissipation of the kinetic energy of the gas. The rate of this dissipation depends on the conditions of flow. In laminar flow, the gas has a precisely ordered velocity profile, with the flow in the center being the greatest, decreasing to zero at the walls (**Fig. 41.18**). A boundary layer of very low flow forms at the walls. Laminar flow was first described by Poiseuille and theoretically has the least possible pressure drop or energy dissipation for a given flow and tube diameter:

$$\text{Resistance} = 8 \times \text{viscosity} \times \text{length}/\pi * \text{radius}^4$$

The resistance is dependent on the viscosity of the gas and is inversely proportional to the fourth power of the radius. This is an important consideration when endotracheal tubes of very small radius, as in the premature infant (<3.5 mm internal diameter).

A balance exists between the inertia of the gas and the viscous drag, which is expressed by the Reynolds number. This dimensionless number is proportional to the product of the gas density, the flow rate, and the diameter of the tube. When the Reynolds number is greater than ~2300, the inertial forces are greater than the viscous forces, and laminar flow cannot be established. Rather than moving in smooth lines straight down the tube, the gas is turbulent. The axial movement of the gas increases the pressure against the walls, and energy is dissipated at a greater rate than during laminar flow. During laminar flow, the pressure drop is proportional to the flow rate.

During turbulent flow, the pressure drop is proportional to the square of the flow rate.

A third type of flow regime is that of unsteady flow. If the gas in a long, straight tube is moved in a laminar fashion by a sinusoidal pressure generator, the flow profile has to reverse with each cycle. The gas in the center of the tube must reverse velocity greater than that close to the wall, and the flow lags behind that of the gas close to the wall (asymmetric gas flow profiles), causing an underestimation of the pressure drop at points of maximal flow acceleration. This type of flow regime is most applicable during high-frequency oscillatory ventilation. It is also relevant in small endotracheal tubes for newborns during conventional ventilation of >60 breaths/min, when the inertia of the gas can cause an underestimation of airway pressure of several cm H_2O.

These simplified theoretical models can help to explain the pressure drop in the airways. The airways are not long, straight tubes, but branches. From estimates of the Reynolds number and the dimensions of the airways obtained from anatomic casts, flow in the large airways is turbulent. Laminar flow becomes established between the 4th and the 15th generation of airways, depending on the flow rate of the gas.

The airways are also flexible tubes. The airway will collapse if the transmural pressure becomes negative. The peribronchial pressure is approximately equal to the P_{pl}. Flow is limited by the local wave speed of the gas it contains. The wave speed is the maximum speed with which a pressure drop at the thoracic outlet can be transmitted to the distal gas. Applying additional pressure upstream, such as during active expiration, does not allow transmission of the pressure or flow downstream because the transmural pressure in the large airways becomes negative. During inspiration (**Fig. 41.19A,B,C**), P_{pl} becomes more negative, the elastic recoil pressure increases, and the airways are supported by the negative pressure. During forced expiration,

the P_{pl} adds to the elastic recoil pressure, producing the positive alveolar pressure to generate expiratory flow. When gas moves from the distal airways to the central airways, it is accelerated, as the cross-sectional area of the airways decreases rapidly. This acceleration requires a pressure drop down the airway in addition to viscous losses. At the point at which the expiratory flow equals that of the wave speed, the transmural pressure becomes negative, and a choke point is established, called the *equal pressure point* (**Fig. 41.19D**). Flow is then limited by the downstream segment and is independent of the expiratory effort. The higher the flow, the greater the pressure required. Therefore, the transmural pressure primarily reflects the elastic recoil pressure of the lung, because the lung parenchyma is closely linked mechanically to the peribronchiolar space. Thus, at high lung volume, when recoil pressure is greatest, the flow limitation is in the second and third generation of bronchi. At lower lung volumes, flow decreases and the sites of flow limitation move peripherally. This phenomenon explains the linear shape of the expiratory flow-volume curve that is the basis of spirometric pulmonary function testing. Many measures applied to this curve, such as the fraction of the expired volume at one second, mid-expiratory flow, etc., are used to detect flow limitation at various points in the airways.

The P_{rs} is a mixture of laminar and turbulent flow. Flow in the large airways is turbulent, and the resistance in this flow regime is density dependent. In cases of extreme large-airway obstruction, the resistance can be reduced by reducing the density of the gas with the use of a mixture of helium and O_2 (Heliox). This reduction may help to relieve obstruction such that intubation of the patient is avoided. The primary limitation is the O_2 requirement of the patient that dilutes the helium in the mixture.

A Consolidated Model of the Dynamics of Breathing

The respiratory system has been classically modeled as a three-element physical system, consisting of an elastance, a resistance, and an inertial element (**Fig. 41.20**). The equation of motion for this system is as follows:

$$P_{tp} = [(1/C) \times V] + (R \times \dot{V}) + (I \times \dot{V})$$

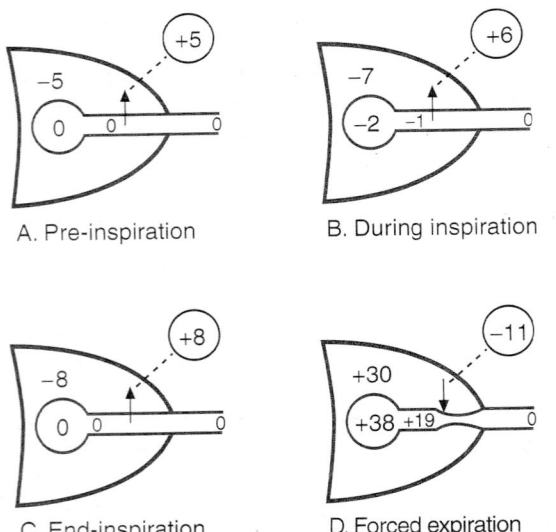

A. Pre-inspiration

B. During inspiration

C. End-inspiration

D. Forced expiration

FIGURE 41.19. Dynamic compression of the airways during forced expiration, caused by negative transmural airway pressure (**D**) beyond the equal pressure point. From Powell FL. Mechanics of breathing. In: Johnson LR, ed. *Essential Medical Physiology*, 3rd ed. London: Elsevier/Academic Press, 2003, with permission.

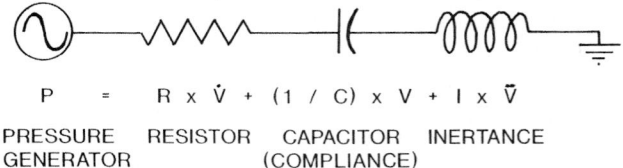

P   =   R x $\dot{V}$ +   (1 / C) x V   +   I x $\tilde{V}$

PRESSURE   RESISTOR   CAPACITOR   INERTANCE
GENERATOR   (COMPLIANCE)

FIGURE 41.20. Model of the respiratory system consisting of a pressure generator (the transpulmonary pressure) and a resistor, capacitor, and inertance connected in series. The values of the individual components are computed from the measurements of the pressure and flow into and out of the system, using the equation of motion to fit the experimental data. From Heldt GP. The mechanics of breathing: developmental aspects and practical applications. In: Boynton BR, Carlo WA, Jobe AH, eds. *New Therapies for Neonatal Respiratory Failure*. Cambridge: Cambridge University Press, 1994, with permission.

where:

Ptp is the pressure inflating the lungs (transpulmonary pressure)

C = the compliance, or 1/elastance

R = resistance

I = the inertance.

The compliance represents the elastic recoil of the lung, determined by the tissue elastic and surface tension forces. The resistance consists of the dissipative forces of the airways and tissue. As described previously, the airway component is both laminar and turbulent, or transitional, as described by Röhrer's equation:

$$P \text{ resistive} = K1 \times (\dot{V} + K2) \times \dot{V}^2$$

where K1 and K2 are coefficients that represent the relative proportions of laminar and turbulent resistive drops.

Clinical Implications

For most purposes, these parameters can be calculated by fitting these equations to the measured transpulmonary pressure and the resultant flow. These parameters are often displayed on ventilators and ventilator monitors and are of clinical usefulness in understanding and directing ventilator management. Infants who are treated with surfactant, for example, have increases in compliance, as would be expected from recruitment of alveoli. Infants who develop bronchopulmonary dysplasia have higher resistances in the first week of life and lower compliances. The use of steroids in bronchopulmonary dysplasia has been shown to yield improved gas exchange, reduced mechanical ventilatory requirements, and improvements in compliance. Bronchodilator therapy in infants with bronchopulmonary dysplasia results in statistically significant reductions in pulmonary resistance. Theophylline has been reported to reduce pulmonary and airway resistances in infants with bronchopulmonary dysplasia and, when used in conjunction with diuretics, appears to have a synergistic effect. The response to acute and chronic administration of furosemide has mixed results.

This classical model has limitations, which may explain why bedside measurement of mechanics tend to be nonspecific as a diagnostic test and why the parameters have a large coefficient of variation even within a diagnostic category. No standards have been established for the method of measurement, nor do age- or weight-related standard curves exist, as in spirometry. Ideally, both the compliance and resistance should be normalized for lung volume; however, lung volume is difficult or impossible to measure in mechanically ventilated infants or children due to leaks around the endotracheal tube. Finally, during mechanical ventilation, significant gas trapping occurs when either the resistance or compliance is high. The lung does not have adequate time to empty during the relatively short expiratory times. As mentioned previously, certain ventilator paradigms also lead to an underestimation of the airway pressure that is seen at the alveolar level due to turbulent flow in the proximal airway where the airway pressure is measured. Thus, these parameters can change due to changes in the pattern of mechanical ventilation and not due to changes in the mechanics of the lung.

Another limitation of the classical method of calculating mechanics is due to nonlinearities of both elastance and resistance.

The elastic and resistive properties of the lung are coupled: At lung volumes above 50% TLC, elastic recoil increases with a decrease in the resistance because airway diameters are larger at higher lung volumes. This phenomenon explains why the flow-volume curves are straight over a large range of lung volumes during forced expiration in normal lungs and even in disease states. The time constant of the lungs, or the product of the compliance and resistance, remains constant even though both the compliance and resistance are changing in a complementary fashion.

The apparent complementary coupling between elastance and resistance has been studied by several methods in an effort to interpret these measurements. Several mechanisms are proposed, including interactions of the fiber network of the pleura and terminal airways; tissue "creep," or dissipative changes in lung tissue with large inflations; the cross-bridge dynamics of smooth airway muscle; and surface active forces. The latter appears to be plausible, especially in young children. The alveolar duct is the site of the interaction of the elastic skeleton and the surface-active material. Although the alveolar duct does not impose a great contribution to total pulmonary resistance, it does interact with the process of alveolar recruitment. The act of cyclic recruitment (popping open) and de-recruitment represents a resistive loss. By the same mechanism, recruitment and de-recruitment would involve changes in the elastance. Both the patency of the alveolar ducts and stability of the alveoli are greatly under the influence of surfactant. Thus, this could be a single mechanism to explain this coupling.

The Forced Oscillation Technique

Another approach toward understanding the coupling of elastance and resistance is to measure the input impedance of the respiratory system with the forced oscillation technique (FOT). The measurement is made by applying a pressure signal comprised of a range of frequencies using a loudspeaker at the airway opening. This method has the advantage that it does not involve the performance of any maneuver on the part of the patient and, in infants, takes advantage of the Hering-Breuer reflex. Impedance is a complex description of the resistance, elastance, and inertance of a system. It consists of resistive and reactive components when changes in pressure and flow are in phase or out of phase, respectively. The airway and tissue elastances and the inertia of the accelerated air in the airways determine the reactive components. The resistance and reactance is computed as a function of the frequency as shown in **Fig. 41.21**. The resulting spectra demonstrate different and separate mechanical properties of the airways and acinar tissues. At low frequencies, tissue resistance and reactance change in a curvilinear fashion with frequency. At higher frequencies, the tissue properties become less pronounced and the spectrum reveals the reactance and inertance primarily of the airways. The resonant frequency is where the reactance is zero, which represents the frequency at which the tissue reactive and inertial components are equal. The parameters derived from fitting a model to these spectra include the airway resistance and inertance (R_{aw} and I_{aw}, respectively) and the tissue damping (G) and elastance (H). The coupling of the elastance and resistance of the tissues is the *hysteresity*, or the ratio of G to H. The use of these parameters gives a more complete description of the

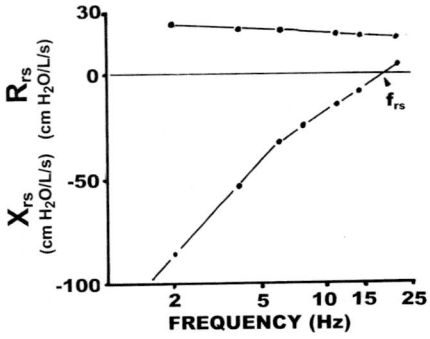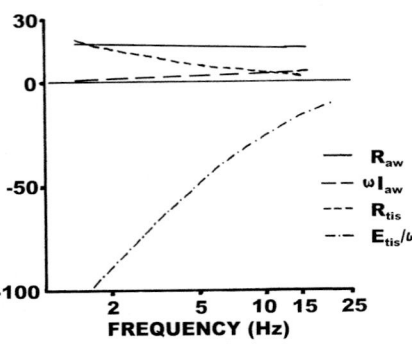

FIGURE 41.21. Impedance spectra measured by forced oscillation technique. **A:** The system resistance and reactance (X_{rs}) are plotted against frequency content of the forced pressure waveform. The point at which X_{rs} is zero is the resonant frequency (f_{rs}) of the system. **B:** The data are fit to a model that separates the contributions of the airway (R_{aw}) and tissue (R_{tis}) resistances, reactive elastance (E_{tis}/ω), and reactive inertance (ωI_{aw}) from the spectra in the left panel. Adapted from Gappa M, Pillow JJ, Allen J, et al., Lung function tests in neonates and infants with chronic lung disease: lung and chest-wall mechanics. Pediatr Pulm. 2006;41:291–317.

visco-elastic properties of the lung, as their coupling is significant and their separation is difficult.

Clinical Relevance of Forced Oscillation Technique

The FOT has provided unique insight into the pathophysiology of infants that has not been provided by classical calculation methods. The contribution of tissue viscoelasticity to total respiratory system impedance is significant, as demonstrated by studies both on surfactant-deficient lambs and human infants. The separation of the airway and tissue components using FOT is implied by the hysteresity, which is decreased after antenatal steroids, antenatal endotoxin exposure, postnatal surfactant treatment, and increasing postnatal size. The dependence of mechanics on the volume of the lungs is more dependent on the mechanical properties of the tissues, and the airway resistance measured by this method is relatively unchanged by increases in lung volume.

In older children, standards are available for some of these parameters based on height. The resistance at 10 Hz is concordant with spirometry obtained in most asthmatic children. The resistance at 5 or 8 Hz is significantly increased in children after maximal bronchodilation and is correlated with the clinical asthma score during acute asthmatic attacks. At age 8, significant increases in the resistance at 5 Hz and the decreases in the resonant frequency were found in children with bronchopulmonary dysplasia over a population of normal controls. Good agreement is also seen between the resistance at 5 Hz and airway resistance measured by body plethysmograph. Bronchodilator responsiveness can be demonstrated in children <7 years, with a cutoff value of an increase of 41% in the baseline resistance at 5 Hz. These changes appear to be longer-lasting with the FOT method than with spirometry after the administration of short-acting bronchodilators. In methacholine bronchoprovocation testing, the reactance at 5 Hz is more sensitive than the FEV_1 or the specific airway conductance, especially in children aged 4–6 years.

The FOT is, in theory, easily applied to young children. It requires the patient to simply breathe quietly on the measurement system. The resistance and reactance at frequencies below 10 Hz correspond well with spirometric values for bronchodilation and bronchial challenge testing. In a recent study of asthmatics aged 2–4 years at high risk of developing asthma, it was possible to train them to perform both spirometry and the FOT with >80% success with one training session. The application of the method to intubated infants and children is surprisingly more difficult because the endotracheal tube imposes a very large resistance that masks the changes in the calculated parameters. The method, with more standardization, will be a valuable tool in the future for assessing the effects of therapies on mechanically ventilated patients.

PULMONARY CIRCULATION

Although the systemic and pulmonary circulations share many common features, they also exhibit important differences in structure and function, and further differences occur in the pulmonary circulation with developmental changes between the fetus, newborn, and adult.

A general principle for adult pulmonary circulation is that the lung is the only organ to receive the entire cardiac output. Because the amount of blood pumped by the right and left ventricles is equal and because the pulmonary and systemic circulations are in series, adult lungs receive the same amount of blood flow as the rest of the body, placing the lung in a unique position to process blood. Many of the structure-function relationships in the pulmonary circulation are explained by the fact that the lungs must handle high rates of blood flow.

Pulmonary Vascular Pressures

The pressures in the adult pulmonary circulation are generally lower than in the systemic circulation. For example, pulmonary artery pressure (systolic/diastolic) averages 25/8 mm Hg versus 120/80 mm Hg for the systemic arteries. Pressures at the end of the systemic circulation in the right atrium average 2 mm Hg, compared to 5 mm Hg in the left atrium, which collects pulmonary venous return. The pulmonary circulation is "pressure passive," i.e., it can accommodate large changes in flow with little changes in pressure. This is important, as the pulmonary circulation must receive the entire cardiac output (under normal circumstances), and minimizing the work of perfusing the lungs and allowing systemic venous return to pass to the systemic ventricle at low pressure decreases the overall circulatory work. These differences between pulmonary and systemic circulations occur for two main reasons. First, the pulmonary circulation supplies only a single organ; therefore, a large pressure head is not necessary to distribute blood flow to multiple organs at different distances from the heart. The right ventricle only needs to generate sufficient pulmonary artery pressure to lift blood to the top of the lung. Low pressures mean that the pulmonary artery and its branches can have relatively thin walls, and they have much less connective tissue and smooth muscle compared with systemic arteries and arterioles. Pulmonary vascular pressures are so low that they are often measured in units of cm H_2O, rather than mm Hg (1.3 cm H_2O = 1 mm Hg). Second, pulmonary capillaries are not supported on the outside by tissue. As pulmonary capillaries are exposed to open gas spaces in the alveoli, they are more susceptible than systemic capillaries to *stress failure,* or bursting open, if their internal hydrostatic pressure is too high. All capillaries must be extremely thin to allow effective diffusion of gases.

The pressure drop from artery to vein is more uniform in the adult pulmonary circulation than in the systemic circulation, and this is the same for the circulation in newborns. Direct and indirect measurements indicate that pulmonary capillary pressure is near the mean of the average pulmonary arterial and venous pressures. Pulmonary capillaries contribute to more of the total pressure drop from artery to vein than do systemic capillaries. Therefore, capillaries are more important determinants of total resistance in the pulmonary circulation, compared with the systemic circulation.

Pulmonary vascular pressures can be altered by a variety of physiologic and pathologic conditions in adults. For example, mean pulmonary artery pressure can increase to more than 35 mm Hg during exercise, and pulmonary venous pressure can exceed 25 mm Hg in patients with congestive heart failure. Pressures in the pulmonary circulation also vary with normal breathing and especially with artificial ventilation because the heart is surrounded by the intrapleural space, in which pressure decreases during normal inspiration and increases during normal expiration (see the previous section on Lung Mechanics). During positive-pressure artificial ventilation, alveolar and intrapleural pressures may increase considerably during inflation, leading to large increases in pulmonary circulatory pressures. When alveolar and arterial pressures both increase, pulmonary vascular resistance may increase. Similarly, PEEP during artificial ventilation may increase pulmonary circulatory pressures and resistance in some circumstances, but not all, depending on the initial lung volume. The changes in pulmonary pressures and resistance between the fetal and adult states are described in the section Perinatal Pulmonary Circulation.

Pulmonary Vascular Resistance

The hydraulic analogy of Ohm's law can be used to define the relationship between pulmonary vascular pressure, flow, and resistance:

$$\Delta P = \dot{Q} \times PVR$$

where:

ΔP is the pressure gradient between the inlet and outlet of a vessel (in mm Hg or cm H_2O)
$\dot{Q}$ is blood flow (L/min)
PVR is pulmonary vascular resistance.

PVR is by definition the resistance for both lungs; in adults, it is ~1.7 (mm Hg × min)/L for a normal cardiac output of 6 L/min, with an average pressure drop of 10 mm Hg from the pulmonary artery to left atrium.

The resistance to flow through a vessel obviously depends on its dimensions. The dimensions of pulmonary vessels are

strongly influenced by several external forces, unlike the situation for rigid pipes in a plumbing system, or even in systemic arteries. The fundamental geometry of the pulmonary capillary network is also different from pipes or systemic capillaries. The numerous capillaries in the alveolar wall constitute an almost continuous sheet for blood flow between two flat membranes held together by numerous posts—called *sheet flow*; the resistance to sheet flow can be less than the resistance to flow through a network of tubes. Therefore, Poiseuille's law, which describes the resistance to laminar flow through a tube (resistance = 8 viscosity length/π radius^4), is not strictly correct for predicting the effects of pulmonary capillary dimensions on resistance. Still, PVR increases with length and decreases by a power function of the radius of pulmonary capillaries. Because the pulmonary capillaries are surrounded by the open air spaces of the alveoli, rather than solid tissue as in other organs, the primary determinant of vessel size in the lungs is the *transmural pressure*, which is the pressure difference between inside and outside the vessel:

$$P_{transmural} = P_{inside} - P_{outside}$$

Therefore, increasing pulmonary arterial pressure will increase flow by two mechanisms: (a) the pressure gradient for Ohm's law is increased, and (b) the transmural pressure is increased, which increases vessel size and decreases PVR (**Fig. 41.22**). Increasing pulmonary venous pressure also decreases PVR, because some of this pressure increase is transmitted to the capillaries and dilates them. As discussed previously, capillary dimensions significantly affect PVR. Hence, pressure affects resistance and vice versa in the pulmonary circulation, in contrast to the systemic circulation, in which resistance primarily affects pressure.

Alveolar pressure is the outside pressure for calculating transmural pressure in most pulmonary vessels. Alveolar pressure varies with the ventilatory cycle, but it is generally near

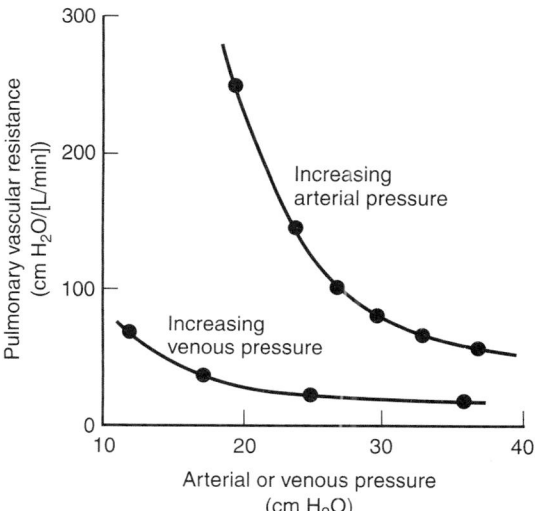

FIGURE 41.22. Pulmonary vascular resistance decreases with increasing pulmonary arterial or pulmonary venous pressure, while the other pressure is held constant. This is because increasing either pressure increases capillary pressure and causes recruitment and distention of pulmonary capillaries. From Powell FL. Structure and function of the respiratory system. In: Johnson LR, ed. *Essential Medical Physiology,* 3rd ed. London: Elsevier/Academic Press, 2003, with permission.

zero (i.e., atmospheric pressure). Therefore, vascular pressure is the primary determinant of transmural pressure in pulmonary vessels. However, large positive alveolar pressures can occur with some forms of artificial ventilation, as well as with PEEP and this will tend to collapse pulmonary capillaries. In other words, increased pulmonary arterial or venous pressures do not necessarily decrease vascular resistance unless they result in an increased transmural pressure, which dilates the capillaries.

Increasing transmural pressure can affect capillary dimensions by two mechanisms: recruitment and distention. At very low pressures, some capillaries may be closed, and increasing pressure will open them by recruitment. At higher pressures, capillaries are already open, but they may be distended or stretched by increased transmural pressure. Together, recruitment and distention increase the effective size of the pulmonary capillaries and reduce PVR.

Another important determinant of pulmonary vessel size is lung volume, but this effect differs for different types of vessels. Extra-alveolar vessels are surrounded by lung parenchyma, which acts as a tether or support structure to hold the vessels open. Therefore, lung volume is more important than alveolar pressure for determining the dimensions of extra-alveolar vessels. At high lung volumes, above functional residual capacity (FRC), the extra-alveolar vessels are pulled open by tissues outside the vessels. At low lung volumes, below FRC, this tethering effect is reduced and the extra-alveolar vessels narrow. Also, extra-alveolar vessels have smooth muscle and elastic tissue that tend to collapse the vessels at low lung volumes. The effects of lung volume on alveolar vessels are generally opposite those on extra-alveolar vessels. At high lung volumes, the alveolar wall is stretched and becomes thinner, reducing the size of pulmonary capillaries and alveolar vessels. At low lung volumes, the alveolar wall is not stretched and the capillaries relax open to a wider dimension. These factors account for why PVR is at its lowest at FRC—the lung volume at which normal tidal ventilation occurs. When end-expiratory lung volume (EELV) is greater or less than physiologic FRC, PVR is increased. In addition, compliance is optimal at FRC and decreased with EELV above or below FRC. In a similar fashion, lung resistance is also minimized at FRC and increased at EELV either above or below it.

It is important to note that circulation in the fetal and neonatal lung is *not* as pliable because all of the capillaries are apparently fully recruited, even under resting conditions. Experiments on newborn lambs show no increase in pulmonary diffusing capacity with increased left atrial pressure, in contrast to the increase observed in adult sheep (and humans), as capillary recruitment and distention increase the surface area available for diffusion.

Fetal and Perinatal Pulmonary Circulation

The anatomy of the pulmonary circulation in the fetus differs from the adult because the placenta is the primary gas-exchange organ in utero (**Fig. 41.23**). Fetal blood flows into the placenta through the umbilical arteries. O_2 diffuses from the maternal circulation into the fetus. Diffusion is relatively inefficient in the placenta compared to the lungs, but O_2 transfer is enhanced by the high O_2 affinity of fetal, compared to adult, hemoglobin (see the section Oxygen in Blood). The end result is a maximum Po_2 of 30 torr in the fetal circulation in blood leaving the placenta

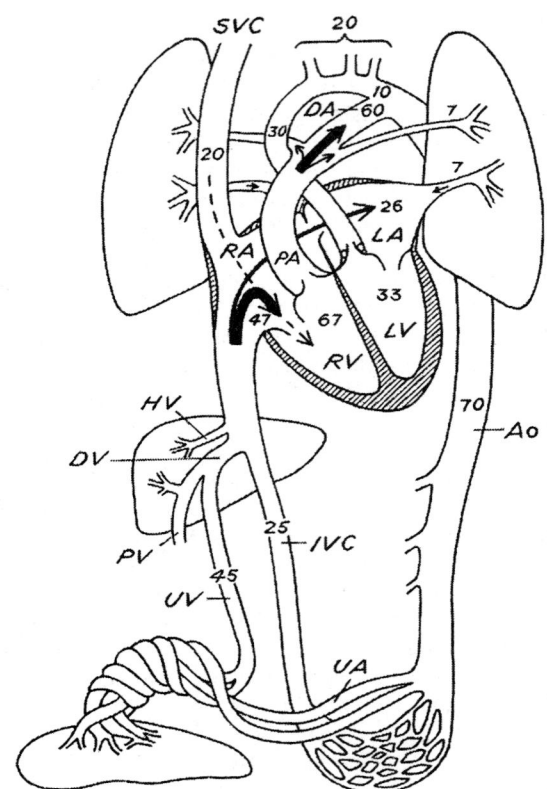

FIGURE 41.23. Schematic representation of human fetal circulation. Numbers refer to blood flow in mL/min through the main vascular channels. Numbers refer to blood flow in milliliters per minute through the main vascular channels. SVC, superior vena cava; DA, ductus arteriosus; RA, right atrium; PA, pulmonary artery; LA, left atrium; RV, right ventricle, LV, left ventricle; Ao, aorta; HV, hepatic vein; DV, ductus venosus; PV, portal vein; UV, umbilical vein; IVC, inferior vena cava; UA, umbilical artery. Adapted from Comroe, JH. *Physiology of Respiration*, Chicago: Year Book Medical Publishers, 1965.

and entering the inferior vena cava. Some of the oxygenated blood in the inferior vena cava flows directly from the right into the left atrium via the foramen ovale, which is a normal connection between the right and left atria in the fetus. Hence, blood leaving the left ventricle in the aorta has a relatively high Po_2, diluted only by other systemic venous blood in the inferior vena cava to ~25 torr. The rest of the blood returning from the inferior vena cava mixes with blood returning from the superior vena cava in the right atrium, reducing the Po_2 to 19 torr in the right ventricle.

Blood is pumped from the right ventricle into the pulmonary artery, but only 10% flows into the lungs; the remainder goes into the aorta via the ductus arteriosis, which is a shunt vessel normally present in the fetus. The small pulmonary blood flow is important for the normal development of the lungs and the surfactant system (see the previous section, Pulmonary Vascular Pressures). The ductus arteriosis joins the aorta distal to the carotid and coronary arteries. This anatomy maximizes the Po_2 in blood that perfuses the brain and heart because Po_2 is greater in the left ventricle than in the right ventricle (**Fig. 41.23**). It is important to note that the output of the left ventricle is only approximately half that of the right ventricle in the fetus, in contrast to being equal in adults, because the ductus arteriosis shunts blood from the pulmonary to systemic circulations.

The pressures in the fetal pulmonary circulation are high relative to adults because of the connection between the pulmonary arteries and the ductus arteriosis, which comes from the left ventricle, as well as high pulmonary vascular resistance in the fetal lung. Hypoxic pulmonary vasoconstriction helps to keep the pulmonary vascular resistance high in the fetus. The high pressures, and perhaps hypoxia, produce a well-developed smooth muscle layer in the pulmonary circulation of the fetus, especially compared to the adult.

At birth at term, the first few breaths expand the lungs, filling them with a relatively high O_2 tension, which makes several dramatic changes in the physiology. Hypoxic pulmonary vasoconstriction is reduced, and the pulmonary capillaries are stretched, opening them so that pulmonary blood flow greatly increases. The infant breathes deeply and rapidly, lowering the Pco_2 and raising the pH, which enhances the effects of decreased hypoxic pulmonary vasoconstriction (**Fig. 41.24**).

With the increase in pulmonary blood flow upon air breathing at birth, left atrial pressure increases, thus closing the flap-like foramen ovale. This closure is also aided by the decrease in right atrial pressure as the umbilical blood flow decreases. Flow through the ductus arteriosis decreases as resistance to pulmonary blood flow decreases and the ductus constricts in response to increased Po_2 and circulating prostaglandin (PGE_2).

This transition takes place in three stages. The first, which reduces the PVR to ~50% of the fetal level, occurs with the first few effective breaths. The second stage can take up to ~1 hr, during which time the ductus arteriosus constricts, and relief of the hypoxic pulmonary vasoconstriction is stabilized. During this stage, the systemic circulation is influenced by right-to-left shunting at the level of both the ductus arteriosus and the foramen ovale; the peripheral circulation can be sluggish and some degree of peripheral cyanosis can occur. During this stage, the PVR is reduced by ~75% of the fetal level. This third stage

takes several hours to several days, during which complete relaxation of the hypoxic vasoconstriction and remodeling of the vascular smooth muscle occur.

Distribution of Pulmonary Blood Flow

The distribution of pulmonary blood flow throughout the pulmonary vascular tree and to different parts of the lung is not uniform. This finding was first demonstrated in measurements of pulmonary blood flow at different heights in the lungs of erect adults. Relative blood flow increased progressively from top to bottom of the lung.

The effect of gravity on pulmonary vascular pressures is a major factor determining the regional differences in blood flow in the upright human lung. The pulmonary vasculature can be considered a continuous hydrostatic column that is ~30 cm tall in the upright human lung, meaning that a hydrostatic pressure difference of 30 cm H_2O (or 23 mm Hg) exists between vessels at the top and bottom of the lung. As this pressure difference is nearly as large as the pulmonary artery pressure, it has profound effects on regional distribution of blood flow. Evidence for a gravitational mechanism includes (a) a reduction in the gradient for blood flow when in the erect posture and during exercise, when pulmonary arterial pressure increases, and (b) a reduction in the gradient of blood flow when in the supine posture. A dorsal-ventral gradient can be measured when the subject is supine, and the vertical gradient is reversed in those suspended upside down.

These effects using the zone model for pulmonary blood flow developed by West are illustrated in **Figure 41.25**. This model conceptually divides the lung into three zones to explain how gravity affects blood flow up the lung through alveolar vessels at different heights. Zone 1 occurs at the top of the lung, where the pulmonary arterial pressure is not sufficient to pump blood to the top. In this case, pulmonary arterial pressure is less than the hydrostatic pressure column between the heart and the top of the lung. Alveolar pressure, even if zero, is greater than arterial pressure; thus, the capillaries collapse. Zone 1 does not

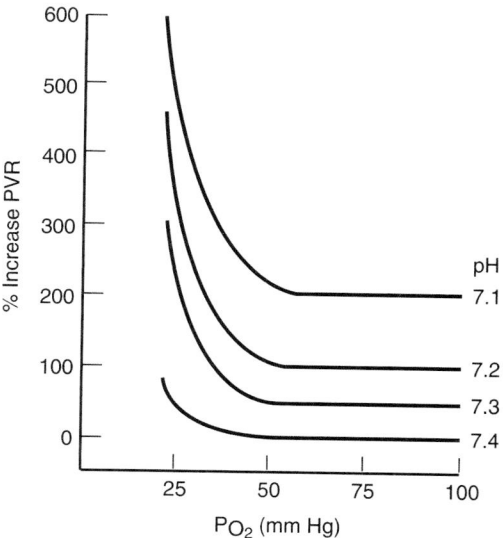

FIGURE 41.24. Deceasing O_2 in inspired gas (Po_2) causes hypoxic vasoconstriction and increases pulmonary vascular resistance (PVR). Arterial acidosis exaggerates this effect in newborns and may be important in helping to establish the adult pattern of circulation. From Powell FL. Pulmonary Gas Exchange. In: Johnson LR, ed. *Essential Medical Physiology*, 3rd ed. Boston: Elsevier Academic Press, 2003, with permission.

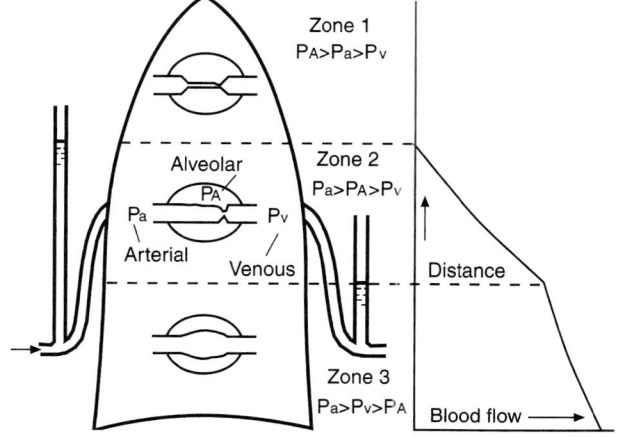

FIGURE 41.25. West's zone model for pulmonary blood flow predicts increasing blood flow down the lung because of the effects of gravity on pressures. Pa, arterial pressure; PA, alveolar pressure; Pv, venous pressure. From Powell FL. Structure and function of the respiratory system. In: Johnson LR, ed. *Essential Medical Physiology*, 3rd ed. London: Elsevier/Academic Press, 2003, with permission.

occur in the normal adult lung because the normal pulmonary arterial pressure (30 cm H_2O) is greater than the height of a water column between the heart and top of the lung ($\sim$15 cm).

Zone 2 describes the flow in most of the lung, where pulmonary arterial pressure is increased by the hydrostatic column and blood flow occurs. Venous pressure is less than alveolar pressure because these veins may be below the level of the heart. Intravascular pressure decreases from the arterial to venous level along the capillary, and at some point the alveolar pressure exceeds capillary pressure, which tends to collapse the capillary and reduce flow. If flow actually stops, pressure in the capillary rises toward the arterial level until the capillary is reopened and flow resumes. In zone 2, the relevant pressure gradient driving blood flow is the arterial-alveolar difference, and venous pressure is not important in determining zone 2 flow. Systems with flow determined by upstream and outside (instead of downstream) pressures are called *Starling resistors*. **Figure 41.25** shows flow progressively increasing down zone 2 because the hydrostatic column increases arterial pressure while alveolar pressure is constant. Both capillary recruitment and distention can contribute to increased flow in zone 2.

Zone 3 occurs near the bottom of the lung, where venous pressure is increased sufficiently by the hydrostatic column to exceed alveolar pressure. Therefore, the arterial-venous pressure difference determines blood flow in zone 3. **Figure 41.25** shows flow increasing down zone 3 because the hydrostatic column distends the capillaries.

Despite the success of the zone model at predicting regional differences in blood flow based on gravity, additional differences in blood flow occur, for example, between the center and the periphery of the lung at a given height up the lung. Local stresses and the anatomic details of vascular branching may contribute to such intraregional heterogeneity of blood flow. Local stresses may result from differences in vasoconstrictor influences (see next section) as well as bronchoconstriction, which affect pulmonary capillary dimensions through traction. Intraregional heterogeneity may explain up to half of the total heterogeneity of blood flow in the lungs.

The effect of mechanical ventilation on lung zones should also be considered. Clearly, elevating alveolar pressure will convert some zone 2 lung to zone 1 and some zone 3 lung to zone 2. Thus, the effect of mechanical ventilation could be to create more alveolar dead space (zone 1) and improve V/Q matching in zone 2.

Hypoxic Pulmonary Vasoconstriction

Hypoxic pulmonary vasoconstriction is an important physiologic mechanism that actively controls blood flow in adult lungs. Hypoxic pulmonary vasoconstriction is a direct response of vascular smooth muscle in pulmonary arterioles to decreased alveolar P_{O_2}. The cellular mechanism involves potassium channels in the pulmonary artery endothelium that are sensitive to O_2 levels. Hypoxic pulmonary vasoconstriction can be reduced by low concentrations of inhaled nitric oxide (NO) (20 ppm NO) in humans. Nitric oxide also relaxes systemic vessels through a cyclic guanosine monophosphate (cGMP) pathway. Hypoxic pulmonary vasoconstriction is not a reflex response, and it can even be induced in rings of pulmonary arterioles in vitro. This is opposite the vasodilatory effect of hypoxia in systemic arterioles.

A direct vasoconstrictor response to local alveolar P_{O_2} allows blood flow to be selectively diverted away from poorly ventilated regions of the lung. Hence, hypoxic pulmonary vasoconstriction is important for matching unequal distributions of ventilation and blood flow throughout the lungs. This response might be more important during the transition in the circulatory pattern at birth (see the previous section, Fetal and Perinatal Pulmonary Circulation). Hypoxic pulmonary vasoconstriction reduces blood flow through the fetal lung when it is not ventilated. This response is greatest in the fetus and serves an essential function in utero, where its absence leads to hydrops, hypoxia, and fetal demise.

Figure 41.24 shows the effect of P_{O_2} on pulmonary vascular resistance in a neonatal animal; the main effect of P_{O_2} occurs at very low levels, which are found in the fetus. However, blood pH has an effect even at high P_{O_2}; therefore, the increase in pH with the onset of air breathing will also reduce pulmonary vascular resistance as P_{O_2} increases with air breathing in the newborn. Other physiologic factors capable of influencing the adult pulmonary circulation include a weak vasoconstrictor effect from the sympathetic nervous system and potent vasoconstriction by endothelins, which are peptides released by pulmonary epithelial and endothelial cells (e.g., endothelin-1). The fetal and neonatal pulmonary circulations are also exquisitely sensitive to vasoconstrictors such as serotonin and vasodilators such as acetylcholine because the smooth muscle is more developed to support the higher pressures compared to adults.

Some of the most fascinating discoveries in the past decade have been in the area of smooth muscle contraction and the ionic basis for blood flow changes in the pulmonary circulation. Potassium (K^+) channels play a major role in smooth muscle cells and their contractility in response to hypoxia. For example, hypoxia, through a decrease in K^+ channel activity, depolarizes the cell membrane of smooth muscle cells in the wall of arterioles and thus activates voltage-dependent calcium (Ca^{2+}) channels, which open, and consequently Ca^{2+} ions enter into these cells following the concentration gradient. This increase in Ca^{2+} ions will activate contraction, inducing a constriction of such vessels. This could happen during hypoxic breathing, in local hypoxia such as in sickle cell disease, or during sleep-induced hypoventilation and obstructive sleep apnea.

How does the patent ductus close when the vessels are bathed in higher local O_2 levels at the time of birth as compared with fetal P_{O_2}? It is very interesting to note that the same response in K^+ channel activity occurs in these vessels in response to normoxia, as a result of the activation of a mitochondrial O_2 sensor in these cells that generates a diffusible redox mediator, hydrogen peroxide (H_2O_2). This, in turn, inhibits certain K^+ channels and leads to constriction in Pa_{O_2}, which is rather normal and not low.

Bronchial Circulation

The bronchial circulation is part of the systemic circulation and serves the metabolic needs of the large airways and blood vessels. The bronchial circulation does not extend to the gas-exchange zone, which is served by the pulmonary circulation. Bronchial arteries arise from the aorta and intercostal arteries, and the bronchial circulation returns blood to the heart by two pathways. Bronchial veins from large airways return approximately half of the bronchial blood flow to the right heart via the azygos vein. The other half of the bronchial circulation drains directly into the pulmonary circulation, which adds deoxygenated blood to the oxygenated blood returning to the left heart and constitutes an anatomic shunt. As blood flow through the bronchial circulation is only 1%–2% of cardiac output in normal adults, this anatomic shunt has a small affect on arterial O_2 levels. However, the anatomic shunt can increase with inflammatory airway disease and cause significant reductions in arterial O_2 levels.

Lung Fluid Balance

The pulmonary capillaries are extremely thin and contain pores that allow fluid to move across their walls. Starling's law describes the forces that govern fluid flux across capillary walls, and an understanding of these forces is necessary to understand both normal and pathologic lung fluid balance. Starling's law states that the net fluid flux across the capillary depends on a balance of hydrostatic forces (P) and colloid osmotic (or oncotic) forces (π):

$$\text{Net fluid flux} = K_{fc}\,[(Pc - Pi) - \sigma(\pi c - \pi i)]$$

where K_{fc} is a filtration coefficient that depends on the total surface area of the capillary and the number and size of pores in the capillary. Hydrostatic pressure in the capillary (Pc) tends to move fluid out, and interstitial pressure (Pi) tends to move fluid into the capillary. Conversely, capillary osmotic pressure (πc) tends to hold fluid in the capillary, and interstitial osmotic pressure (πi) tends to draw fluid out of the capillary. The osmotic reflection coefficient (σ) describes the effectiveness of osmotic pressure at moving fluids and can range from 0 to 1. Conceptually, σ compares the size of the pore to the osmotically active solute: $\sigma = 0$ if the solute can move freely through the pore, and $\sigma = 1$ if the solute cannot move through the pore.

Normally, the balance of forces results in net filtration, or the movement of a few milliliters per hour of fluid out of the capillaries in adults. Normal Pc $\approx$ 10 mm Hg, and normal Pi in the lungs is subatmospheric, so that a positive hydrostatic force moves fluid out of the capillaries. The interstitial space around alveolar capillaries is not compliant, and filtration in this region tends to increase local interstitial pressure. This local pressure increase is thought to provide a gradient moving filtrate toward the interstitium around the extra-alveolar vessels. Filtrate in this extra-alveolar region can be reabsorbed by the bronchial circulation or collected by lymphatics, which also return the fluid to the vascular system.

Normal plasma protein concentration is ~7.5 g/dL (mainly albumin); this exerts an osmotic pressure of ~28 mm Hg. The interstitium contains only ~5 g/dL of protein with an osmotic pressure of 15–20 mm Hg. Therefore, the osmotic forces promote absorption. Also, osmotic forces provide a natural feedback system in which increased filtration dilutes the interstitial space, thus reducing the osmotic gradient pulling fluid out of the capillaries. The osmotic pressure depends on the number of molecules in solution.

When this normal balance of forces is disturbed, filtration can exceed the capacity of reabsorption and lymphatic drainage, and fluid accumulates in the interstitium. Edema is the accumulation of excess filtrate outside the capillaries. Pulmonary edema fluid accumulates first in the peribronchiolar and perivascular spaces; this is called *interstitial edema*. In-

terstitial edema can alter local ventilation and perfusion and make gas exchange inefficient by decreasing compliance, increasing the work of breathing, and ultimately leading to loss of lung volume. As interstitial fluid accumulates, it can enter into the alveolus causing alveolar edema. Only in severe pathologic states does fluid cross directly from the capillary lumen into the alveolus because the intact fused basement membrane between the endothelial and epithelial cells is quite impervious to water. When damaged, however, water (and, when damage is severe, protein and red blood cells) can flood the alveolus directly from the capillaries. Alveolar edema, or flooding of excess filtrate into the alveolar spaces, is more serious because it can totally block ventilation and cause blood flow shunts in affected lung regions. The exact mechanisms that result in alveolar edema are not known, but they involve exceeding the lung's capacity for lymphatic drainage and changes in solute and fluid transport across airway epithelial cells. Alveolar type II epithelial cells normally transport sodium chloride to the basolateral surface, and water follows, keeping the alveoli dry.

Edema fluid can have low or high protein concentration. Hydrostatic edema, which may occur with elevated pulmonary capillary pressures in congestive heart failure, results in filtrate with low protein concentrations. Other lung injuries, such as acute respiratory distress syndrome, may alter the permeability of the capillary endothelium (i.e., changes) and produce a protein-rich edema fluid.

RESPIRATORY CONTROL

General Concepts

In the past century, especially in the past two or three decades, we have learned a great deal about respiratory control. Using a series of "concepts" the following sections will detail our current understanding of respiratory control and explore some ideas related to it in early life and during human development, providing examples of aberrant or abnormal respiratory control conditions and consequences in terms of tissue hypoxia.

Respiratory Control Concept 1

Respiration is controlled via a negative feedback system, using a controller in the central nervous system (CNS). The overall aim of the respiratory feedback loop is to keep blood gases in a normal range with the least possible energy expenditure and O_2 consumption. The afferent limb consists of receptors that send information to a central controller. For example, the carotid bodies inform the central controller of the O_2 level. Both airway and carotid body sensors compare actual and baseline (or programmed) "set" signals to generate error signals. The carotid sinus nerve fibers, which carry impulses generated by the carotid glomus cells, synapse in the medulla oblongata. The efferent limb is that part of the feedback loop that is responsible for the execution of the decision made centrally (i.e., the respiratory muscles and their innervation) after integrating afferent signals. Among many muscles of respiration, the external intercostal and diaphragm muscles are the major muscles. Activity and timing of the airway muscles are very critical in determining airway resistance and patency.

Negative feedback resists change and occurs because the controller attempts to rectify deviations from normal. For example, if CO_2 increases because of lack of ability to remove CO_2 adequately (e.g., airway obstruction), the output of the controller is increased to increase alveolar ventilation and decrease CO_2. If O_2 is reduced in the blood (observed Po_2 is very different from a "programmed or set" Po_2 that carotid glomus cells detect as abnormal), these cells will fire to stimulate phrenic nerve activity via the CNS.

Respiratory Control Concept 2

Central neuronal processing and integration in the brainstem is hierarchical. Respiratory muscles are recruited to perform different tasks at different times, such as for respiration, jumping, splinting the abdomen, and doing Valsalva maneuvers. In other conditions, respiratory muscles can be totally inhibited; e.g. while one is delivering a speech, CO_2 responsiveness is decreased substantially because respiratory muscles are recruited mostly for speech at the expense of respiration. Another example relevant to infants is bottle- or breast-feeding, which is sometimes associated with a reduction in ventilation and Po_2 because respiratory muscles and breathing efforts are inhibited. If presented with a number of neurophysiologic signals (representing options about various needs), the central controller can enhance or reduce the response to certain stimuli at the expense of others. Therefore, a hierarchy is used by brainstem networks in determining the response of the respiratory system at any one time. Temporal and spatial summation of excitatory and inhibitory postsynaptic potentials will be critical in deciding the behavior of these neurons. In addition, their cellular and membrane properties will indeed affect their output. Furthermore, changes in the state of consciousness modulate the ability of the brainstem to respond to afferent stimuli. Age is very important, as the response of the brainstem to stimuli varies with maturation and cortical input to brainstem structures.

A clinical correlation is the mechanical feedback that controls respiration in newborns. In addition to chemoreceptors, powerful mechanoreceptors in the lungs and chest wall function to preserve lung volume. Nowhere is this more evident than in the newborn, in whom the respiratory muscles are weak, whose lung mechanics are deranged, and whose oxygenation depends on maintenance of the FRC. The mechanoreceptors function to prolong inspiratory effort, shorten the expiratory time, and cause dynamic gas trapping. This tachypnea is commonly seen even in infants with normal gas exchange on mechanical ventilation. The mechanoreceptors are incorporated in the control of the airway muscles as well. Infants have expiratory grunting that can augment the expiratory transpulmonary pressure by several centimeters of H_2O to significantly increase their FRC.

Respiratory Control Concept 3

Brainstem neurons have cellular and membrane properties that allow them to beat (cycle) spontaneously. These properties play a role in generating rhythmic respiratory neuronal behavior. The central controller has two basic functions that are inherently linked: (a) integration of afferent information, and (b) generation and maintenance of respiration. These tasks are believed to be performed by different neuronal groups, but it is not known in precise mechanistic terms how each function takes place. The respiratory controller is probably a group of neurons that form a network. Respiratory neurons most likely do not have special inherent membrane properties (e.g., bursting, spontaneous depolarization properties) that would make

their membrane potential spontaneously oscillate. Rather, the output of the network that they form oscillates because of the special interconnections and synaptic interactions among these respiratory neurons.

Data have suggested that the respiratory rhythm is generated by an oscillating neuronal network in the ventrolateral formation of the medulla. The region that seems to be essential for the rhythm is the pre-Botzinger Complex (PBC), as all cranial nerve activity ceases after this region is separated from the lower brainstem. The properties of individual neurons in this area, how interconnected they are, and the nature of their synapses with neurons in the brainstem and other more rostral regions remain to be elucidated. Although the PBC is certainly a possible site for respiratory rhythm generation, the argument that this is the main site is unproven. Several experiments argue that the PBC is the rhythm generator: (a) drugs injected in the PBC alter breathing frequency, (b) lesions in the PBC do the same, and (c) respiratory afferents synapse in the PBC. However, it has not been shown that these types of experiments done in other areas have been negative. Data have delineated other sites that may control expiratory rhythms rather than inspiratory rhythms, as hypothesized for the PBC.

Respiratory Control Concept 4

Respiratory rhythm generation in central neurons is most likely a result of integration between network, synaptic, cellular, and molecular characteristics. Rhythmic movements, such as locomotion or heart beat, are generally based either on the action of endogenous "burster" neurons (or conditional bursters) or on a network of neurons, which by virtue of their connections, oscillate. In the case of networks, previous literature has suggested that central neurons can no longer be considered as just "followers." A very clear example of such an oscillating network is a set of neurons that have been well studied in *Tritonia diomedea*. In this animal, the central pattern generator responsible for escape swimming has been extensively studied and its properties well appreciated. The functional interaction of one set of synapses, for example, between C2 and ventral swim interneurons (VSIs) neurons is based on the fact that VSI-B neurons possess membrane properties that allow the excitation from C2 to be delayed, which is an important mechanism in the overall function of the *Tritonia* motor program. This current turns on with membrane depolarization but then quickly inactivates; hyperpolarization of the membrane potential removes this inactivation.

For dorsal and ventral medullary respiratory neurons, investigators have discovered a number of impressive membrane currents that can shape their repetitive firing. These include not only the classic sodium and K^+ currents responsible for the action potential, but also an A-current, two types of Ca^{2+} currents, Ca^{2+}-activated K^+ currents, inward-rectifier currents, ATP-sensitive K^+ currents, and others.

Data from studies of the cellular and membrane properties and synaptic efficiency of newborn neurons reveal differences in the integrated output from adult neural networks. For example, both active and passive cellular properties in newborn dorsal respiratory group cells are different from those in adults. Newborn brainstem neurons have less spike-frequency adaptation, less inward-rectifier currents, different after-hyperpolarization, a wider action-potential waveform, and no delayed excitation. Such electrophysiologic maturational changes are related to changes in a number of variables that pertain to cytosolic and membrane structure and function. For example, the distribution of ion channels and receptors on cell membranes, as well as the structural and functional nature and the regulation of ion channels, change with age in early life.

Respiratory Control Concept 5

Afferent information is not essential for generation of breathing, but modulates respiration. A multitude of afferent messages converge on the brainstem. Chemoreceptors and mechanoreceptors in the larynx and upper airways sense stretch, temperature, and chemical changes over the mucosa and relay this information to the brainstem. Afferent impulses from these areas travel through the superior laryngeal nerve and vagus. Changes in O_2 or CO_2 tensions are sensed at the carotid and aortic bodies, and afferent impulses travel through the carotid and aortic sinus nerves. Thermal or metabolic changes are sensed by skin or mucosal receptors or by hypothalamic neurons and are carried through spinal tracts to the brainstem. Afferent information is not a prerequisite for the generation and maintenance of respiration. When the brainstem and spinal cord are removed from the body and maintained in vitro, rhythmic phrenic activity can be detected for hours. Other in vivo experiments in chronically instrumented dogs in whom several sensory systems are simultaneously blocked indicate that afferent information is not necessary to stimulate the inherent respiratory rhythm in brainstem respiratory networks. However, both in vitro and in vivo studies demonstrate that, in the absence of afferent information, the inherent rhythm of the central generator (indexed by respiratory frequency) is slowed, and therefore, chemoreceptor afferents can play a role in modulating respiration and rhythmic behavior.

Among the many types of afferent information that affect the respiratory output of the CNS, CO_2 and O_2 are some of the most potent. If "afferent" is considered to be any information that converges on the brainstem respiratory network, CO_2 is certainly an important and powerful stimulus to respiration, even though it is sensed mostly in the CNS itself. Almost any change in CO_2 induces a change in ventilation and vice versa (for any given metabolic rate). A nearly normal ventilatory response to increased CO_2 can be observed in experimental animals that have no afferent input to the CNS from peripheral sensory nerves; e.g., removing the carotid bodies reduces the ventilatory response to CO_2 by a modest 20%. Chemoreceptors, in several specialized regions in the medulla, are particularly sensitive to changes in CO_2 and pH, although the exact mechanisms for responding to CO_2 and pH in these regions may not be understood. Furthermore, it is important to realize that nerve cells in the CNS, whether in these specialized regions or not, are responsive to CO_2 and pH as they do have either exchangers (e.g., Na/H exchanger) or ion channels (e.g., Na^+ channels) that are responsive to CO_2 and/or pH, and hence modulate cell excitability and neuronal output.

Developmental Aspects of Respiratory Control

Developmental studies have spanned a range of questions regarding such issues as the development of brainstem neurons, respiratory muscles, afferent receptors and systems (including the carotid bodies), and the end organs (lungs). These various aspects of respiratory control are not mature at birth.

Central Aspects of Respiratory Control

In vitro studies in the neonatal rat (whole brainstem preparation) have shed light on fundamental newborn issues. We know now that the young rat brainstem in vitro (which is very immature in the first week of postnatal life) does not require any peripheral drive for central oscillator discharge. The inherent respiratory rate is markedly reduced, however, and it is clear from these studies that peripheral and possibly central (rostral to the medulla and pons) input is necessary to maintain the respiratory output at a much higher frequency.

In that (a) the discharge of central neurons in the adult or neonate is affected by peripheral input, including input from the vagus nerve, and (b) the respiratory feedback system can operate on a breath-by-breath basis, the question has arisen as to whether the lack of myelination in the neonatal nerve fibers that subserve feedback affects function. Indeed, this is the case not only because of lack of myelination and potential delays in signaling, but also because inspiratory and expiratory discharges are so fast that they preclude the effect of peripheral input on the CNS *within* the same breath. Clearly, peripheral afferent may have effects on subsequent breaths. Therefore, whether breath-by-breath feedback is as effective in the young as in the adult remains an open question.

Differences between neonates and adults are also observed in response to endogenous stimuli such as responses to neurotransmitters or modulators. Young and immature animals respond differently to neurotransmitters, as documented by work in opossum. Glutamate injected in various locations in the brainstem, even in large doses, induces respiratory pauses, while it is clearly stimulatory in the older mature animal. Such inhibitory neurotransmitters as γ-aminobutyric acid (GABA) have also been used, and they have age-dependent effects in the opossum. Indeed, a chloride (Cl^-)-mediated inhibition is noted in the adult but not in the neonate in the isolated brainstem.

Peripheral Sensory Aspects

The primary O_2 sensors in the body, the carotids, show major differences between the newborn and the adult. Recordings from both single-fiber afferents and sinus nerves show major differences between the fetus and newborn and between newborn and adult. For example, it has been demonstrated that fetal chemoreceptor activity is present in the normal fetus and that a large increase in activity may be evoked by decreasing Po_2 in the ewe. As would be predicted, the large increase in Pao_2 at the time of birth virtually shuts off chemoreceptor activity in the newborn. However, this decreased sensitivity does not last long, and a normal adult-like sensitivity takes place by 1–2 weeks after birth.

A number of factors, both external and endogenous, play a role in this process. For example, arterial chemoreceptors are subject to external and hormonal influences, which may affect the sensor or alter tissue Po_2 within the organ. Neurochemicals may also play a major role as modulators of chemosensitivity. For example, endorphins are documented to decrease in the newborn period, and the effect of exogenous endorphin is inhibition of chemoreceptor hypoxia sensitivity. However, it has been shown that, even in the absence of external modulatory factors (hormonal or neural), chemosensitivity of the newborn chemoreceptor is less than in the adult. Nerve activity of rat carotid bodies in vitro following transition from normoxia to hypoxia is approximately fourfold greater in carotid bodies harvested from 20-day-old rats compared to 1- or 2-day-old rats. This finding corresponds well with the maturational pattern of the respiratory response to hypoxia in intact animals and suggests that major maturational changes occur within the carotid body itself. Histologic, biophysical, and neurochemical changes occur with development, but the significance of these changes is dependent on assumptions of how the organ senses Po_2. For example, the maturational increase in chemosensitivity may be attributed to a maturational change in the biophysical properties of glomus cells. In one model, hypoxia inhibits a membrane-localized K^+ channel that is active at rest, and the resulting depolarization leads to calcium influx and increased neural activity in adult carotid cells. Support for this mechanism has been obtained from cultured, adult rabbit glomus cells, the outward (or K^+) current of which is apparently inhibited by hypoxia. In comparison, glomus cells harvested from immature animals (e.g., rats) show a decrease in whole-cell K^+ current during hypoxia, but the decrease in K^+ current is attributed to a decreased activation of a Ca^{+2}-dependent K^+ current and not to a specialized K^+ channel sensitive to Po_2.

The ventilatory response to CO_2 also shows developmental changes. For example, premature infants and full-term newborns have a reduced response to CO_2 for several days (or weeks) in early life, which has been shown by studies to result from a complex integration of changes in neural control (maturation of the CNS or peripheral nerves) and respiratory mechanics (chest-wall mechanics and/or respiratory muscles).

In comparison to the adult, peripheral chemoreceptors assume a greater role in the newborn period. Although not essential for initiation of fetal respiratory movements, peripheral chemoreceptor denervation in the newborn results in severe respiratory impairment and high probability of sudden death. Lambs, following denervation, fail to develop a mature respiratory pattern and, more importantly, suffer a 30% mortality rate weeks or months following surgery. In other species, denervation leads to lethal respiratory disturbances. Denervated rats suffer from severe desaturation during REM sleep, and piglets suffer periodic breathing with profound apneas during quiet sleep. Of particular interest is the observation that these lethal impairments only occur during a fairly narrow developmental window, and denervation before or after this period results in minor alterations in respiratory function. This window of vulnerability, which is unmasked by denervation in the newborn period, supports the speculation that the sudden infant death syndrome (SIDS) may be due to immaturity or malfunction of peripheral chemoreceptors.

Oxygen Deprivation, Oxygen-sensing and Cell Injury

Pathologic conditions cause respiratory failure. All cardiorespiratory diseases can potentially produce respiratory failure, and this may be deleterious to other organs because of the ensuing acidosis and hypoxia. It is the hypoxia that should be avoided at all cost, as human tissues, especially the CNS, have low tolerance to a microenvironment devoid of O_2.

A great deal is known about the effect of the lack of O_2 on tissues at various ages, including fetal, postnatal, and adult. The carotid bodies discharge and have an effect on ventilation when the Pao_2 reaches below 55–60 torr. In general, other tissues react to such levels of Pao_2 but in very different ways. For example, tissue growth may be affected if Pao_2 is at the level when carotids start discharging. The effect on most tissues, however, is that they develop remarkable dysfunction when Pao_2 is below 35–40 torr. For example, the brain, which is among the most sensitive to the lack of O_2, has a resting (no hypoxia-induced) interstitial O_2 tension in the range of 20–35 torr, depending on age, region (white vs. gray matter), neuronal metabolism, temperature, proximity to blood vessels, etc.

Major questions remain about the mechanisms that lead to injury or that protect tissues from it. In the case of the nervous system, a number of mechanisms are activated during O_2 deprivation. Some events that take place during lack of O_2 are membrane biophysical events (e.g., those pertaining to Na^+ and K^+ channels); increased anaerobic metabolism; increased intracellular levels of H^+ and Ca^{2+}; increased concentrations in extracellular neurotransmitters (e.g., glutamate and aspartate); radical production; activation of kinases, protease, and lipase; injury and destruction of important cytoskeletal proteins; and gene regulation of a number of proteins (e.g., c-fos, NGF, HSP-70).

CONCLUSIONS AND FUTURE DIRECTIONS

From the point of view of the intensivist, the respiratory system is much more than the lung per se. It is the lung, the respiratory muscles, the chest cage, the blood and cardiovascular system, the brain (especially the brainstem), the endocrine system and, often, the gastrointestinal tract. The respiratory system indeed is a reflection of the health and integrity of a number of systems in the body. Although many of the physiologic principles have been long described, a number of new ideas and discoveries presented in this chapter will no doubt affect our future thinking and allow us to better care for children. Some of these new ideas have been described: aquaporins and gas channels, the effect of CO_2 on lung development, the ion channels that control the smooth muscle contraction in the pulmonary vasculature and patent ductus arteriosus, and the ion channels that are important for ion flux in the absence of adequate oxygenation.

KEY POINTS

- Oxygen diffusion from alveolar gas to pulmonary capillary blood is effective at equilibrating alveolar and arterial Po_2 ($Pao_2 = Pao_2$) under most conditions.
- Most of the O_2 transported in blood is bound to hemoglobin, and this combination is sensitive to CO_2, pH, temperature, and phosphates. Developmental differences in O_2-hemoglobin binding are explained by differences between adult and fetal hemoglobin.
- The pulmonary circulation has lower pressures and thinner vessel walls than the systemic circulation. Pulmonary vascular resistance is highly dependent on mechanical forces in the lungs and, in contrast to the systemic circulation, is increased by hypoxia.
- The four major causes of arterial hypoxemia are hypoventilation, shunt, diffusion limitation, and

ventilation-perfusion mismatch, which can be diagnosed by relatively simple tests and the alveolar-arterial P_{O_2} difference ($PA_{O_2} - Pa_{O_2}$).

■ Pulmonary mechanics is classically modeled as a capacitor (the elastance), a resistor (the airway and tissue resistance), and an inductor (primarily the inertia of the gas in the large airways) as a series circuit.

■ The elastic mechanical structure of the lungs, in conjunction with the surfactant system, makes the lung inflate uniformly and retain its end-expiratory volume to promote a good match of ventilation to perfusion. Mechanical ventilation of the immature lungs has special considerations, including surfactant replacement therapy.

■ Airflow limitation is a prominent feature of diseased lungs and is usually inferred from spirometric pulmonary function testing. Airflow limitation during mechanical ventilation may depend on the degree of inflation of the lungs, the resistance of the artificial airway, and the pattern of ventilation.

■ Recent developments of the forced oscillation technique have provided a deeper insight into the various mechanical components of the lung and may be applied clinically.

■ The first step in O_2 transport is alveolar ventilation ($\dot{V}_A$), which is a function of respiratory rate, tidal volume, and dead space volume.

■ Breathing is controlled by a negative feedback from chemoreceptors sensing arterial blood gas levels and mechanoreceptors from the lungs, airways, and chest wall acting on a respiratory rhythm generator in the brainstem.

■ The respiratory rhythm is generated by the integration of network, synaptic, and cellular properties of central neurons but it can be changed voluntarily, as well as being modulated by reflexes and being sensitive to the state of consciousness.

■ Developmental changes in respiratory control, and sensitivity to hypoxia, are explained by maturation of the CNS, peripheral sensory processes, the lung, and respiratory muscles.

ACKNOWLEDGMENTS

This work was supported by grants HL081823 (FLP) and 5 P01 HD 32573–11 (GGH).

References

Pulmonary Gas Exchange

1. Bauer C. Structural biology of hemoglobin. In: Crystal RG, West JB, Weibel ER, et al., eds. *The Lung: Scientific Foundations, Vol1, 2nd ed.* Philadelphia: Lippincott-Raven, 1997:1615–24.
2. Farhi LE, Tenney SM, eds. Gas Exchange. In: Geiger SR, ed. *Handbook of Physiology, Sec. 3, The Respiratory System.* Bethesda: American Physiologic Society, 1987.
3. Longo LD, Nystrom GA. Fetal and Newborn Respiratory Gas Exchange. In: Crystal RG, West JB, Weibel WR, et al., eds. *The Lung: Scientific Foundations, Vol. 2,* 2nd ed. Philadelphia: Lippincott-Raven, 1997:2141–49.
4. Roughton FJW. Transport of Oxygen and Carbon Dioxide. In: Fenn WO, Rahn H, eds. *Handbook of Physiology, Sec. 3, Respiration.* Bethesda: American Physiological Society, 1964:767–826.
5. Wagner PD. Diffusion and chemical reaction in pulmonary gas exchange. *Physiol Rev* 1997;57:257–312.
6. West JB, Wagner PD. Ventilation-perfusion Relationships. In: Crystal RG, West JB, Weibel WR, et al., eds. *The Lung: Scientific Foundations, 2nd ed.* Philadelphia: Lippincott-Raven, 1997:1693–710.

Lung Mechanics, Respiratory and Airway Muscles

7. Boynton BR, Carlo WA, Jobe AH, eds. *New Therapies for Neonatal Respiratory Failure. A Physiological Approach.* New York: Cambridge University Press, 1994.
8. Comroe JH. Retrospectroscope: Premature science and immature lungs. I. Some premature discoveries. *Am Rev Respir Dis* 1977;166:127–135.
9. Fredberg JJ, Stamenovic D. On the imperfect elasticity of lung tissue. *J Appl Physiol* 1989;67:2408–19.
10. Gappa M, Pillow JJ, Allen J, Mayer O, et al. Lung function tests in neonates and infants with chronic lung disease:Lung and chest-wall mechanics. *Pediatr Pulmonol* 2006; 41:291–317.
11. Oostveen E, MacLeod D, Lorino H, et al. The forced oscillation technique in clinical practice: Methodology, recommendations, and future developments. *Eur Respir J* 2003;22:1026–41.

Pulmonary Circulation

12. Fishman AP, ed. Circulation and non-respiratory functions, Vol. I. In: Geiger SR, *Handbook of Physiology, Sec. 3, The Respiratory System.* Bethesda: American Physiological Society, 1985.
13. Tod ML, Cassin S. Fetal and Neonatal Pulmonary Circulation. In: Crystal RG, West JB, Weibel WR, et al., eds. *The Lung: Scientific Foundations, Vol 2,* 2nd ed. Philadelphia: Lippincott-Raven, 1997;2129–39.

Respiratory Control

14. Dekin MS, Haddad GG. Membrane and cellular properties in oscillating networks: Implications for respiration. *J Appl Physiol* 1990;69(3):809–21.
15. Donnelly DF, Haddad GG. Respiratory changes induced by prolonged laryngeal stimulation in awake piglets. *J Appl Physiol* 1986;61:1018–24.
16. Donnelly DF, Haddad GG. Prolonged apnea and impaired survival in piglets after sinus and aortic nerve section. *J Appl Physiol* 1990;68(3):1048–52.
17. Haddad GG, Donnelly DF. O_2 Deprivation induces a major depolarization in brainstem neurons in the adult but not in the neonatal rat. *J Physiol (London)* 1990;429:411–28.
18. Haddad GG, Donnelly DF, Getting PA. Biophysical properties of hypoglossal neurons in-vitro: Intracellular studies in adult and neonatal rats. *J Appl Physiol* 1990;69:1509–17.

CHAPTER 42 ■ RESPIRATORY MONITORING

IRA M. CHEIFETZ • SHEKHAR T. VENKATARAMAN • DONNA S. HAMEL

WHY MONITOR?

Monitoring respiratory function is crucial to the management of critically ill children to (a) aid with diagnosis, (b) understand the pathophysiology of a disease, (c) assess the status and progress of the disease, and (d) provide guidelines for management.

In mechanically ventilated children, respiratory monitoring can also assist in understanding and optimizing patient-ventilator interactions, provide alerts and alarms, and aid in weaning.

Monitoring, which was once dependent solely on physical assessment and direct clinical observation, now includes elaborate automated surveillance of a tremendous number of cardiorespiratory physiologic and ventilator performance variables. Noninvasive monitoring techniques assess gas exchange and pulmonary mechanics, supplement physical assessment, and provide a continuous data stream, with alarms to identify changes in the child's status and to alert caregivers when necessary. Although physical examination remains clinically relevant, the role of the clinician has evolved and now must include the incorporation of all aspects of cardiorespiratory monitoring into a comprehensive, responsive assessment system. The appropriate integration and interpretation of all data are essential for efficient, high-quality, cost-effective, pediatric critical care.

In that the respiratory system removes carbon dioxide (CO_2) and facilitates oxygen (O_2) transport, quantifying and evaluating these two primary functions will be the focus of this chapter. The continuum of respiratory monitoring from basic physical assessment to complex, automated monitoring systems is addressed, and clinical indications, principles of operation, and functional limitations are discussed.

PHYSICAL ASSESSMENT

It is a concerning phenomenon of modern intensive care that physical examination, and especially the stethoscope, are used with decreasing frequency. Clinical scoring systems have been developed to evaluate the clinical parameters of skin color, nasal flaring, retractions, accessory muscle use, and the presence and severity of an abnormal sound (e.g., rales, wheeze, or stridor). Scoring systems generally demonstrate that the more pronounced the abnormality, the worse the prognosis (37). As these parameters can only be discerned by visual and auditory assessments, physical examination and assessment should never be replaced by technology. Technology should be used to augment physical assessment. Physical examination is, in fact, often the deciding factor between monitor error and a true change in a child's status.

Respiratory Rate and Pattern

Respiratory rate was one of the earliest parameters monitored. Historically, physical examination was the primary method by which to measure respiratory rate but, through the evolution of technology, several techniques are now used for measuring respiratory movements. Impedance pneumography is the method used most often for spontaneously breathing children. This method requires the placement of at least three leads over the chest: one over the heart and one each on the opposite sides of the lower lateral thorax. A small current is passed through one electrode, and the amount of current that passes through the chest is measured by the other electrode pair. The impedance to current flow varies with the fluid content of the chest, which in turn varies with the respiratory cycle. These differences can be converted by a microprocessor into a waveform and visually displayed on a monitor. Like many other physiologic parameters, respiratory rate and pattern vary, and each child should be evaluated with reference to the age-adjusted norms and pathophysiologic state.

The respiratory pattern in children has generated debate, particularly in the definitions of respiratory pauses, periodic breathing, and apnea. In general, respiratory pauses last <5 secs and occur in children who are <3 months of age. Pauses occur in groups of three or more, are separated by <20 secs, and generally resolve by 6 months of age without medical intervention. The definition of apnea is even more troublesome because of the role of sudden infant death syndrome (SIDS) in infant mortality and the substantial effort underway to prevent this tragic occurrence. A National Institutes of Health Conference consensus statement on infantile apnea defined apnea as cessation of breathing for >20 secs or any respiratory pause associated with bradycardia, pallor, or cyanosis. The relationship between infantile apnea and SIDS remains controversial (1).

GUIDELINES AND PRINCIPLES

Technologic advances of monitoring systems provide clinicians with reliable information regarding important physiologic variables and alert the patient care team to changes in these parameters, especially as they violate preset alarm limits. These monitors and systems generate trends so that changes in clinical condition can be more readily recognized.

Important management decisions are based on information provided by the monitor. The monitoring system must provide information pertinent to patient management and answers that will directly guide clinical interventions. All data provided by the monitoring system must be easily and quickly interpretable

TABLE 42.1

FUNDAMENTAL QUESTIONS REGARDING MONITORING

1. What should be monitored?
   a. What physiologic parameters do we want to monitor?
   b. Why should these parameters be monitored?
2. What is actually being measured?
   a. Are the parameters actually measured directly?
   b. Or, are inferences being made about the parameters based on measuring other variables?
3. If inferences are made, how do the monitors work?
   a. What are the assumptions behind the measurements, if any?
   b. Are assumptions being violated?
   c. How precise and accurate are the measurements?
4. What are the goals of monitoring?
   a. Diagnostic
      i. Type of physiologic impairment
      ii. Severity of physiologic impairment
   b. Therapeutic
      i. Selection of appropriate treatment
      ii. Measure effect of intervention(s)
   c. Prognostic
      i. Mortality
      ii. Morbidity
   d. Warning/alarms
      i. To alert about a change in patient status
      ii. To prevent catastrophic events

at the bedside and remotely. Additionally, the data must be accurate, and the technology must be sensitive enough to detect absolute values and changes. The technology must be practical, easily attached to the patient, dependable, and space efficient. Patient safety must always be the primary goal.

The primary monitoring question is often, "What should be monitored?" (**Table 42.1**). Technology enables the monitoring of multiple parameters continuously or at various intervals. However, the fact that every cardiorespiratory parameter can

be monitored does not mean that it should be monitored. Clinicians must address what is practical and clinically relevant to the management of each child, given the pathophysiology and the individual clinical scenario and keeping in mind that the answer is likely to change over time. Physical assessment and observation should always be used to complement electronic surveillance.

Assessment of Gas Exchange

The primary functions of the cardiorespiratory system are to provide adequate oxygen to the tissues and to eliminate CO_2 (**Fig. 42.1**). Cardiorespiratory distress in infants and children is often associated with abnormalities in oxygenation and ventilation and, thus, requires diligent monitoring. Monitoring of oxygenation includes an assessment of oxygen transfer in the lungs, oxygen transport to the tissues and organs by the circulatory system (O_2 delivery, Do_2), and oxygen transfer to and utilization by the tissues (**Fig. 42.2**). Elimination of CO_2 similarly involves CO_2 production by the tissues, transfer of CO_2 from the tissues to venous blood, transport of CO_2 by the circulatory system to the lungs, and elimination of CO_2 by alveolar ventilation in the exhaled gas (**Fig. 42.2**).

Assessment of the Lung as an Oxygenator

Indices used to assess the lung as an oxygenator are: (a) arterial oxygen tension (Pao_2), (b) arterial blood oxygen saturation (Sao_2), (c) intrapulmonary shunt fraction (Qs/Qt), (d) alveolar-to-arterial oxygen tension difference ($PA-ao_2$), (e) arterial-to-alveolar oxygen tension ratio (Pao_2/PAo_2), and (f) arterial-to-fraction of inspired oxygen ratio (Pao_2/Fio_2). Pao_2, represents the net effect of oxygen exchange in the lung. At sea level, the normal Pao_2 in a newborn infant is between 40 and 70 mm Hg when breathing room air. With increasing age, the Pao_2 increases until it reaches an adult value of 90–120 mm Hg. Hypoxemia is defined as a Pao_2 lower than the acceptable range for age, whereas hypoxia is inadequate tissue oxygenation. For a child, a Pao_2 of <60 mm Hg is defined as hypoxemia,

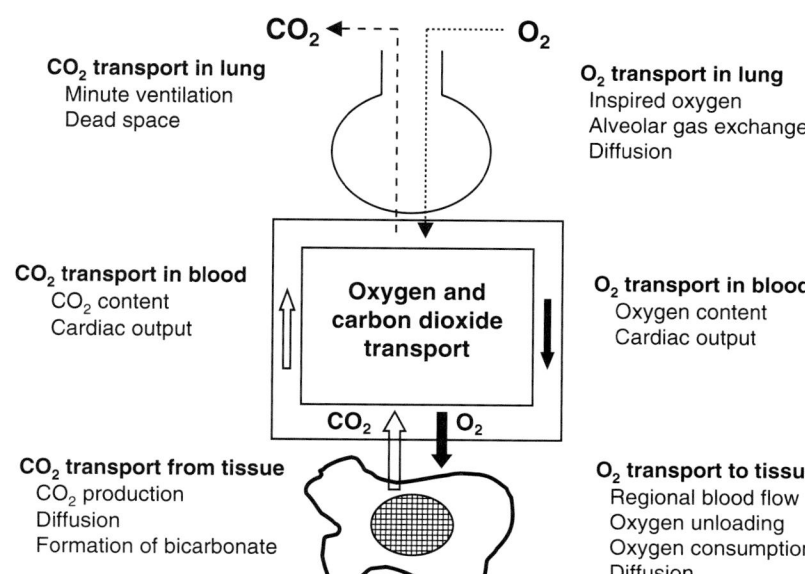

CO₂ transport in lung
Minute ventilation
Dead space

CO₂ transport in blood
CO₂ content
Cardiac output

CO₂ transport from tissue
CO₂ production
Diffusion
Formation of bicarbonate

O₂ transport in lung
Inspired oxygen
Alveolar gas exchange
Diffusion

O₂ transport in blood
Oxygen content
Cardiac output

O₂ transport to tissue
Regional blood flow
Oxygen unloading
Oxygen consumption
Diffusion

FIGURE 42.1. Physiology of oxygenation and ventilation. The primary functions of the cardiorespiratory system are to provide adequate O_2 to the tissues and to eliminate CO_2 via the lungs. This gas transfer process involves an elaborate interaction between the lungs, circulatory system, and the tissues throughout the body.

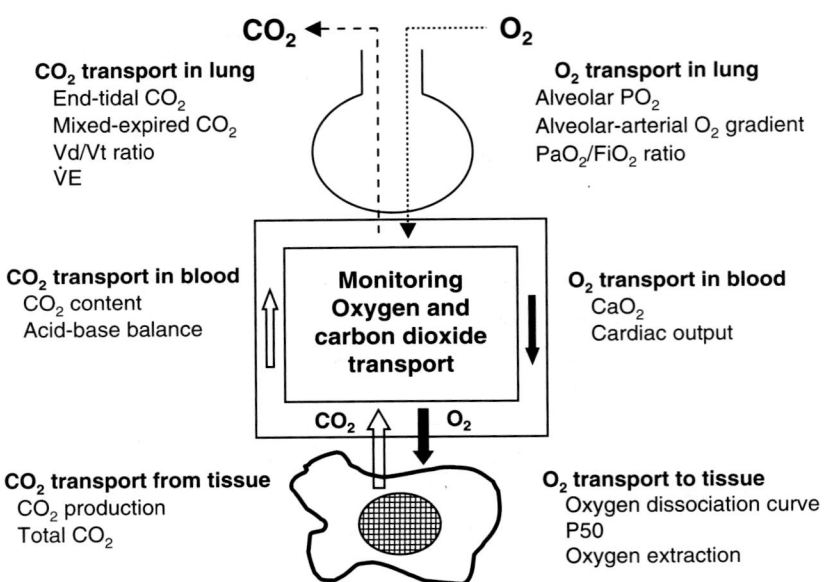

FIGURE 42.2. Variables associated with cardiorespiratory monitoring at each point in the transport of O_2 and CO_2. Monitoring of oxygenation includes an assessment of O_2 transfer in the lungs, O_2 transport to the tissues and organs by the circulatory system (i.e., O_2 delivery), and O_2 transfer to and utilization by the tissues. Elimination of CO_2 similarly involves CO_2 production by the tissues, transfer of CO_2 from the tissues to venous blood, transport of CO_2 by the circulatory system to the lungs, and elimination of CO_2 by alveolar ventilation in the exhaled gas. CO_2, carbon dioxide; E_TCO_2, end-tidal CO_2; Vd/VT ratio, dead space-to-tidal volume ratio; $\dot{V}_E$, expired minute volume; HCO_3, bicarbonate; Hb, hemoglobin; PA_O2, alveolar partial pressure of O_2; $PA_{-a}O_2$, alveolar-to-arterial O_2 tension difference; Pa_O2, arterial partial pressure of O_2; FI_O2, fraction of inspired O_2; Ca_O2, arterial O_2 content; Sa_O2, arterial O_2 saturation.

although that may be an acceptable level for a newborn. Pa_O2 is measured by obtaining an arterial blood sample. Alternatively, it can be estimated by measurement of the transcutaneous oxygen tension, as discussed later in this chapter.

Qs/Qt is defined as the fraction of right ventricular output that enters the left ventricle without oxygen transfer. In the absence of intracardiac shunts, Qs/Qt is calculated by the formula:

$$Qs/Qt = (Cc'_{O_2} - Ca_{O_2})/(Cc'_{O_2} - Cv_{O_2})$$

where:

Cc'_{O_2} = oxygen content of the pulmonary venous blood, assuming the lung to be a perfect oxygenator
Ca_{O_2} = arterial oxygen content
Cv_{O_2} = the mixed venous oxygen content.

Oxygen content is the amount of O_2 carried by a unit volume of blood and is equal to the amount bound to hemoglobin (Hb) and dissolved in plasma. One gram per deciliter of Hb will carry 1.34 mL of O_2 when it is fully saturated. The amount dissolved in plasma depends on the solubility coefficient of O_2. For every millimeter of mercury increase in partial pressure of oxygen (P_{O_2}), the amount of dissolved O_2 increases by 0.003 mL. Therefore, the oxygen content of whole blood is calculated as $(Hb \times 1.34 \times S_{O_2}/100) + (0.003 \times P_{O_2})$. Intrapulmonary shunt may consist of one or more of three components: anatomic shunt, capillary shunt, and venous admixture. Cc'_{O_2} is most affected by FI_{O_2}, Ca_{O_2} is affected mostly by intrapulmonary shunting, and Cv_{O_2} is affected mostly by cardiac output and O_2 consumption. Calculation of intrapulmonary shunt requires the sampling of mixed venous blood using a pulmonary artery catheter. This calculation is cumbersome and assumes that all alveolar spaces behave equally. When a pulmonary artery catheter is not available (as is usually the case), one of the indices described below may be used as an index of shunting.

$PA_{-a}O_2$, Pa_{O2}/PA_{O2}, and Pa_{O2}/FI_{O2}

If the lung were a perfect oxygenator, pulmonary venous O_2 would be identical to the alveolar P_{O_2} (PA_{O2}), and if the right

ventricular output traverses the ideal lung, Pa_{O2} would be the same as pulmonary venous O_2. PA_{O2} is calculated from the simplified alveolar gas equation,

$$PA_{O2} = (P_B - P_{H_2O}) \times FI_{O2} - Pa_{CO2}/RQ$$

where:

P_B = barometric pressure
P_{H_2O} = partial pressure of water vapor (47 mm Hg when fully saturated with H_2O)
RQ = respiratory quotient (CO_2 production/O_2 consumption).

With intrapulmonary shunting, Pa_{O2} is less than PA_{O2}. $PA_{-a}O_2$, Pa_{O2}/PA_{O2}, and Pa_{O2}/FI_{O2} are indices that reflect the extent to which the Pa_{O2} deviates from PA_{O2} as a measure of intrapulmonary shunting. The normal $PA_{-a}O_2$ is usually <20 mm Hg in a child and <50 mm Hg in a newborn. A large $PA_{-a}O_2$ represents intrapulmonary shunting or venous admixture. $PA_{-a}O_2$ is affected not only by intrapulmonary shunting, but also by mixed venous oxygen saturation. A major limitation of this index is that it changes unpredictably with increasing FI_{O2}. To compare gradients over time, FI_{O2} must remain constant. To be reliable, the arterial-to-mixed venous P_{O_2} difference must also be constant. Unlike $PA_{-a}O_2$, Pa_{O2}/PA_{O2} changes much more predictably with increasing FI_{O2}. Thus, it is preferred over $PA_{-a}O_2$ as an index of oxygen transfer in the lung and can be used to predict changes in Pa_{O2} when FI_{O2} is altered. Pa_{O2}/FI_{O2} ratio is the easiest index to calculate and does not require calculation of PA_{O2}. The disadvantage is that it does not adjust for alveolar CO_2. At high FI_{O2}, this error becomes quite small. The normal Pa_{O2}/FI_{O2} in a child is >400 mm Hg breathing room air at sea level.

Oxygen Delivery

Oxygen delivery (D_{O2}) is the amount of O_2 delivered by the cardiovascular system to the tissues every minute. It is calculated as

$$D_{O2} = Ca_{O2} \times CI$$

where CI = the cardiac index in mL/min/m^2.

A normal Do_2 in a child is ~650–750 mL/min/m^2. The major determinants of Do_2 are Hb and CI. Mild hypoxemia can be compensated by increasing either Hb or CI or both. If Do_2 is adequate to meet the tissue O_2 demands, the absolute Pao_2 is not critical.

Assessment of Oxygen Utilization

Oxygen consumption ($\dot{V}o_2$) is the amount of O_2 utilized by the body in a minute, and it can be measured by analyzing the inspired and expired gases using a Douglas bag or calculated using the Fick equation, where $\dot{V}o_2 = CI(Cao_2 - Cvo_2)$. Fever, thyrotoxicosis, and increased catecholamine release or administration increase the metabolic rate and increase $\dot{V}o_2$. Hypothermia and hypothyroidism tend to decrease $\dot{V}o_2$. Measurement of $\dot{V}o_2$ may be important in critically ill patients, especially those with moderately severe cardiorespiratory dysfunction. Under normal conditions, $\dot{V}o_2$ is independent of Do_2. In some critically ill patients, $\dot{V}o_2$ becomes Do_2 dependent. If clinically possible, Do_2 should be increased until $\dot{V}o_2$ is no longer Do_{2-} dependent.

Mixed Venous Oxygen Saturation

Mixed venous oxygen saturation (Svo_2) is commonly used as a measure of the balance between O_2 demand and supply. A low Svo_2 usually signifies that Do_2 is significantly decreased and the body is extracting more O_2 from the blood. This commonly occurs with hypovolemic and cardiogenic shock. In sepsis (where maldistribution of peripheral blood flow is present) and in inborn errors of metabolism (where O_2 utilization can be abnormal), Svo_2 may be normal or high despite O_2 deficits in the tissues. A high Svo_2 is usually seen in hypothermia because of decreased O_2 demand and in brain death, as the brain usually constitutes a major site of the total body O_2 consumption.

The O_2 saturation of Hb reaches stability in the right ventricular outflow tract after the differences in saturation from the various venous sources that comprise the venous return (i.e., inferior vena cava, superior vena cava, coronary sinus, and Thebesian veins) equilibrate. The normal saturation of the Hb in the pulmonary artery is ~78% in the normal person (range 73%–85%).

Rearrangement of the terms of the Fick equation indicates that Cvo_2 and, hence, Svo_2 are related to $\dot{V}o_2$ and cardiac output (Q_T) such that increases in $\dot{V}o_2$ or decreases in Q_T result in a reduction of Svo_2:

$$Svo_2 = Cvo_2 - \text{dissolved } O_2/(Hb \times 1.34)$$
$$Cvo_2 = Cao_2 - (\dot{V}o_2/Q_T)$$

where Hb equals the hemoglobin concentration.

Additional causes of changes in Svo_2 are listed in **Table 42.2**.

Although continuous monitoring of mixed venous O_2 saturation is interesting, clear-cut clinical indications for this technique remain to be demonstrated in children. As most children in the intensive care setting do not have pulmonary artery catheters, pediatric intensivists usually use superior vena cava saturations as a surrogate for true mixed venous O_2 saturations. It has been demonstrated that exact numerical values of mixed venous and central O_2 saturations are not equivalent in varying hemodynamic conditions; however, for clinical

purposes, the trends between these values were found to be reliable and presumably clinically valuable (14). It should be further noted, though, that investigators have reported no clear relationship between central and mixed venous O_2 saturations (19).

TABLE 42.2

COMMON CLINICAL CONDITIONS ASSOCIATED WITH CHANGES IN MIXED VENOUS O_2 SATURATION

Reduction in Svo_2
  ↓ O_2 delivery
    ↓ cardiac output
    ↓ arterial O_2 saturation
    ↓ hemoglobin concentration
  ↑ O_2 consumption

Increase in Svo_2
  ↑ O_2 delivery
  ↓ O_2 consumption
    ↓ O_2 extraction
Left-to-right intracardiac shunt
Sepsis

Svo_2, venous oxygen saturation

PULSE OXIMETRY

One of the most important advances in respiratory monitoring was the development of pulse oximetry (Spo_2), which provides a continuous, noninvasive measure of the percent O_2 saturation of arterial hemoglobin. Although pulse oximetry technology existed in the 1930s, the original hardware was bulky and required heating of the tissue bed. Thus, pulse oximetry did not become widely available until the 1980s with the development of advanced microprocessor technology. Additional advances included light-emitting diodes, plethysmography, and spectrophotometry. These technologic accomplishments made pulse oximetry relatively inexpensive, very safe, reasonably accurate, and portable.

Oxygen-dissociation Curve

The arterial O_2 saturation of Hb (Sao_2) is the percent oxyhemoglobin in the arterial blood. The O_2-dissociation curve describes the avidity with which O_2 binds to Hb. Acidemia, hypercarbia, increased temperature, and increased red-cell 2,3-diphosphoglycerate (2,3-DPG) level shift the curve to the right.

Beer-Lambert Law

A discussion of the physics of pulse oximetry requires understanding of the Beer-Lambert Law, which states that the concentration of a solute in a solvent can be determined by light absorption. The logarithmic relationship that exists between the transmission of light through a solution and the concentration

HEMOGLOBIN EXTINCTION CURVES

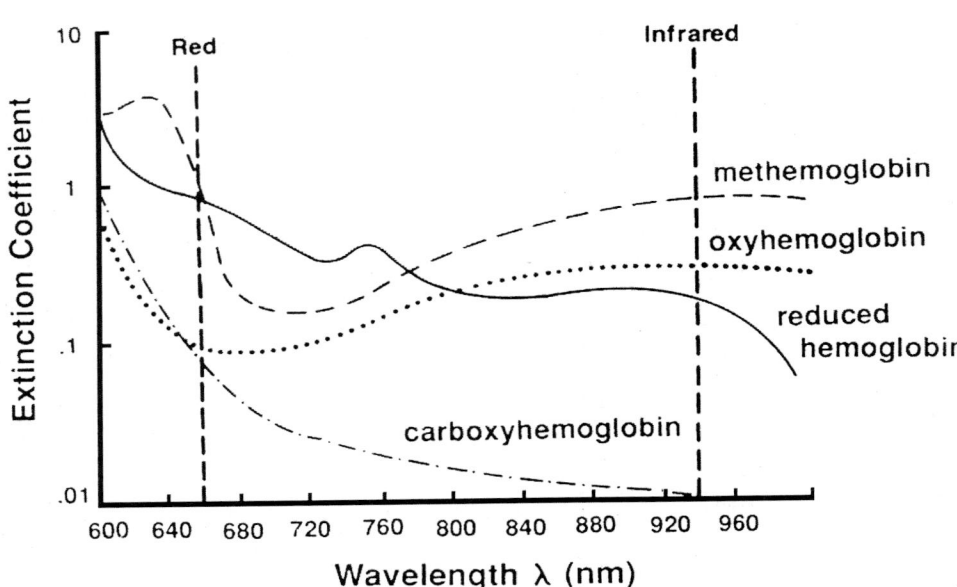

FIGURE 42.3. Hemoglobin extinction curves. The extinction curves of four hemoglobin species (oxyhemoglobin, reduced hemoglobin, methemoglobin, and carboxyhemoglobin) are displayed from red (660 nm) to infrared (940 nm). Tremper KK, Barker SJ. Pulse oximetry. *Anesthesiology* 1989;70:98–108, with permission.

of a given solute is expressed as:

$$C = \frac{\log_{10}(I \text{ out}/I \text{ in})}{\alpha d}$$

where:

- C = concentration
- I = intensity of the light
- d = distance the light travels through a solution
- α = absorption coefficient of the solute and is wave-length dependent.

Pulse oximetry estimates arterial O_2 saturation by measuring the absorption of light in tissues. As pulse oximetry assesses whether or not O_2 is attached to Hb, the relevant solutes are reduced Hb and oxyhemoglobin and their respective absorption characteristics. Wavelengths of 660 nm (red) and 940 nm (infrared) are used because the absorption characteristics of these two hemoglobins are significantly different at these two wavelengths (Fig. 42.3).

Beer's spectrophotometric principle is applied using a light-emitting diode and optical plethysmography. A miniaturized light source is applied to an area of the body that is narrow enough to allow light to traverse a pulsating capillary bed and be sensed by a photo detector (optical plethysmography). When light passes through a pulsating vascular bed, the transmitted light has nonpulsatile and pulsatile components (Fig. 42.4). The nonpulsatile component is assumed to represent light transmitted through the tissues, capillaries, and veins. The pulsatile component is assumed to represent light transmitted through the arterial bed.

As each heartbeat physiologically produces arterial (i.e., O_2-saturated) blood, the increase in O_2 saturation of the Hb results in an increased absorption of light. The pulse oximeter is empirically calibrated by comparing these ratios to direct arterial blood saturations obtained in healthy human volunteers. The O_2 saturation is calculated by comparing absorbencies at baseline (BA) and during the peak (PA) of a transmitted pulse at

660 nm (red) and 940 nm (infrared):

Red absorbance (R)/infrared absorbance (IR)
$$= (PA_{660}/BA_{660})/(PA_{940}/BA_{940})$$

The oximetry-determined plethysmographic signal amplitudes at various saturations and the algorithm used by the microprocessor to determine the Spo_2 by the R/IR ratio are shown in **Figures 42.5** and **42.6**. By using the two wavelengths of light, the pulse oximeter determines "functional saturation."

$$\text{Functional } Spo_2 = Hbo_2/(Hbo_2 + Hb)$$

where:

Hbo_2 = oxygenated Hb
Hb = nonoxygenated Hb.

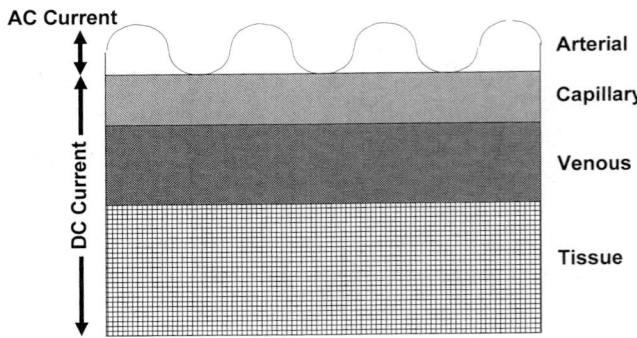

FIGURE 42.4. Spectrophotometric profile of transmitted light across a vascular bed. Pulse oximetry is characterized by a miniaturized light source applied to an area of the body that is narrow enough to allow light to traverse a pulsating capillary bed and be sensed by a photo detector. When light passes through a pulsating vascular bed, the transmitted light has nonpulsatile and pulsatile components. The pulsatile component is assumed to be due to arterial pulsations, while the nonpulsatile component represents light transmitted through the tissues, veins, and capillaries.

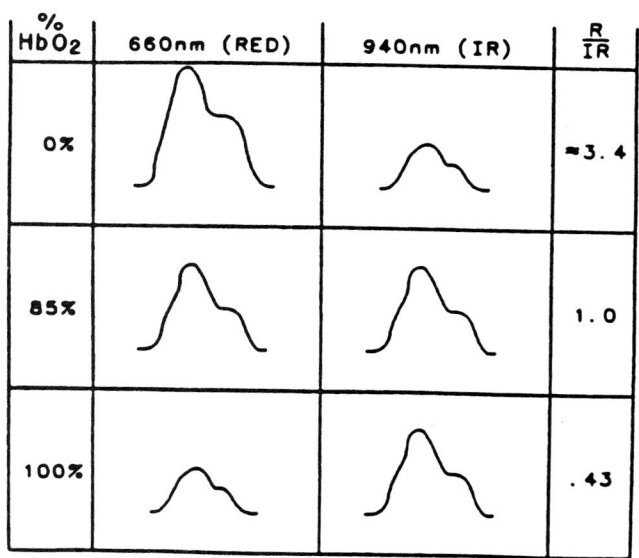

FIGURE 42.5. Relative plethysmographic (pulse-added) signal amplitudes, assuming the transmission intensities are similar. From Eisenkraft J. Pulse oximetry desaturation due to methemoglobinemia. *Anesthesiology.* 1988;68:279–82, with permission.

Functional Spo_2 is contrasted with the fractional Spo_2 measured by co-oximetry on most blood gas analyzers, which provides the ratio of oxygenated Hb to the sum of *all hemoglobin types*, including carboxyhemoglobin (COHb) and methemoglobin (MetHb), which do not carry O_2:

$$Fractional\ Spo_2 = O_2Hb/(Hbo_2 + Hb + COHb + MetHb)$$

The disadvantage of determining functional saturation is that other, possibly clinically significant Hb species, such as carboxyhemoglobin and methemoglobin, will be missed. This shortcoming can be overcome in ambiguous clinical situations by using periodic co-oximetry that uses four to six wavelengths to determine the fractional saturation.

It has been determined conclusively that the O_2 saturation of normal Hb determined by pulse oximetry correlates very closely with the O_2 saturation determined by the co-oximeter (correlation coefficient of 0.98) when the saturation is between 70% and 100% in the well-perfused, normothermic person (8,26,39), without significant quantities of other Hb moieties.

Many of the differences that have been reported in the accuracy of pulse oximeters are a result of the differences in the signal processing software and calibration curves for various brands of devices. Most manufacturers claim confidence limits of $\pm 2\%–4\%$ for readings >70%. During periods of desaturation <70%, the bias and precision are substantially worse and with greater variability, as a limited amount of calibration data exists for these low saturations. This issue primarily applies to children with cyanotic heart disease. For children expected to have normal saturations, the same clinical response should be prompted by any saturation <70%, regardless of the exact number.

Overall, pulse oximetry is based on three major assumptions: (a) only two forms of hemoglobin are present: oxyhemoglobin and deoxyhemoglobin; (b) the pulsatile component of the spectrophotometric absorbance is due only to the arterial blood; and (c) the algorithms derived from human volunteers apply to all patients. If any of these three assumptions are violated, then the pulse oximeter will not reflect the correct arterial O_2 saturation.

Factors That Affect the Performance of Pulse Oximeters

The technology of pulse oximetry has clear limitations, most of which are predictable from the basic physics of this technology (26) (**Table 42.3**). They affect the bias, precision, and applicability of the instrument and, in turn, can affect clinician confidence in the oximeter and its readings. As with all monitoring systems, pulse oximetry should never replace physical

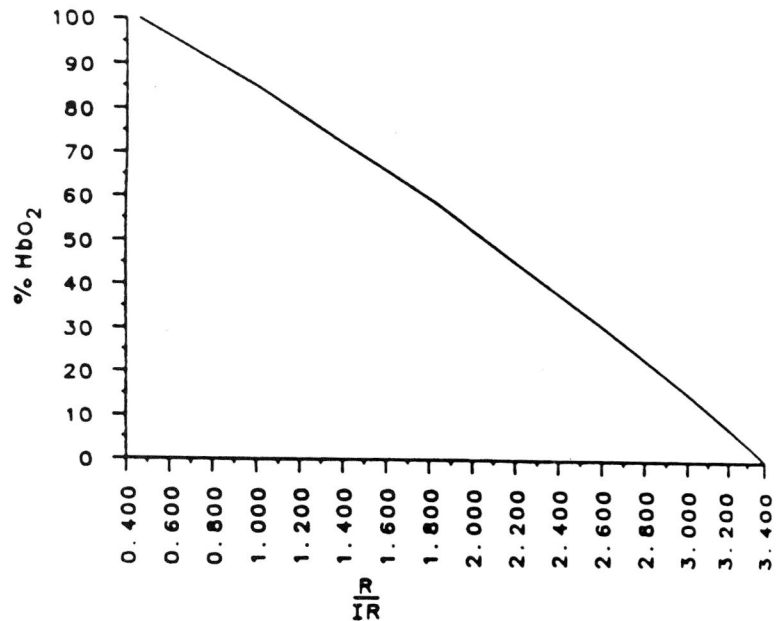

FIGURE 42.6. Algorithm relating % HbO_2 as *ordinate* to the ratio of the plethysmographic signal amplitudes and R/IR (or 660/940 nm) as *abscissa.* From Eisenkraft J. Pulse oximetry desaturation due to methemoglobinemia. *Anesthesiology* 1988;68:279–82, with permission. R, red absorbance; IR, infrared absorbance.

TABLE 42.3

FACTORS THAT CONTRIBUTE TO POTENTIAL
INACCURACY OF PULSE OXIMETRY

Poor cardiac output/low perfusion states
Motion artifact
Increased venous pulsations
Optical interference from environment
Dyshemoglobinemias: carbon monoxide, methemoglobinemia,
    fetal hemoglobin
Dyes and pigments: methylene blue, indocyanine green

examination and overall clinical assessment of a patient's respiratory status. Factors that affect the performance of pulse oximeters include artifacts introduced by patient motion, poor peripheral perfusion, and false alarms. Newer pulse oximeters have additional technology (generally advanced software algorithms) to improve performance during low-perfusion states and patient motion, as described later. Whether these newer technologies are superior is not clear (3,6,20).

Dyshemoglobinemia

The term *dyshemoglobinemia* refers to an abnormal species of Hb that results in the reduced ability of the Hb molecule to carry O_2 to the tissues because of combination with substances other than O_2 (e.g., carbon monoxide) or molecular alterations that do not allow O_2 to combine with the Hb molecule in an efficient manner (e.g., methemoglobin and fetal Hb). The absorption spectra for the dyshemoglobins are shown in **Figure 42.3.**

Carboxyhemoglobin

Carboxyhemoglobin is interpreted as oxyhemoglobin by the photo detector of the two-light-source photo oximeter. Thus, functional SpO_2 overestimates the true HbO_2, but fractional SpO_2 decreases dramatically (26). Data and clinical experience make it imperative that co-oximetry be used to determine O_2 saturation in the suspected presence of carboxyhemoglobin, such as in the patient with known smoke inhalation or with coma of uncertain cause (i.e., potential carbon monoxide poisoning). Note that carboxyhemoglobin and oxyhemoglobin have very similar absorbencies at 660 nm.

Methemoglobin

Methemoglobin absorbs light significantly at both the 660-nm and the 940-nm wavelengths, thereby confusing the oximeter photo detector into believing that both oxyhemoglobin and reduced Hb are increased. The microprocessor-driven algorithm results in the R/IR approaching unity and an SpO_2 of ~85% on the calibration curve (**Fig. 42.6**).

Methylene Blue

Methylene blue has a maximum absorbance at 668 nm. The oximeter interprets this extra absorbance as reduced Hb and, therefore, a lower SpO_2. Clinically, this is seen as a sudden (<30 secs) drop in saturation when methylene blue is injected for therapeutic or diagnostic purposes, such as testing urinary tract patency or treating methemoglobinemia. This effect generally is limited to ~2 mins.

Optical Interference

As pulse oximeters use optical devices, their performance may be affected by external light sources. Light from surgical lamps, bilirubin lights, fluorescent lights, infrared heating lamps, and direct sunlight can result in inaccurate but apparently normal values. Pulse oximeter probes are designed with wraps or shields to help to minimize this interference from external light. This has become less of a concern with recent improvements in pulse oximetry algorithms.

Low Perfusion States

Pulse oximetry depends on optical plethysmography (i.e., a pulsatile change in arterial blood). Thus, abnormalities in propagation of the pulse result in clinically significant inaccuracies of pulse oximetry. Traditionally, shock states, high vasopressor doses, severe edema, and peripheral vascular disease made it difficult for the pulse oximeter sensor to distinguish true signal from background; however, improvements have enabled saturation monitoring despite decreased perfusion (15).

Motion Artifact

Excessive motion of the photosensor causes intermittent contact with the skin and mechanically modulates the path length of the transmitted light and the amplitude and intensity of the received light. This variance in light transmission and reception through the monitoring site can produce false arterial pulse waveforms that the oximeter may not be able to differentiate from the true arterial waveforms, thus, producing spurious saturation values. Clinicians should verify pulse-rate accuracy in the assessment of pulse oximetry values to avoid misinterpretation in the face of motion artifact. New-generation oximeters incorporate software algorithms to better minimize motion artifact (3,6).

Clinical Applications

Over the past decade, pulse oximetry has become an integral part of all ICU monitoring (2). A key premise of this use is that pulse oximeters identify early changes in a child's cardiorespiratory status, allowing for a rapid response. However, few reports have supported this generally accepted assumption. Several clinical studies demonstrate that a fall in SpO_2 often precedes any change in other vital signs (21,31). A concern with pulse oximetry is the high occurrence rate of false alarms and clinically insignificant true alarms (32). Recent advances in the software algorithms have helped to decrease this concern to some degree; however, physical assessment remains the definitive evaluation tool.

The principal use of pulse oximetry is in the detection of hypoxemia, which is generally defined as an SpO_2 reading of <90%. It has been shown that, with the introduction of pulse oximetry into the operating room, the rate of unanticipated admissions to the ICU decreased from 64 per 10,000 patients to 25 per 10,000 patients (12). In 20,802 surgical patients, a 19-fold increase in the detection of hypoxemia (SpO_2 <90%) was demonstrated, compared to the control (nonmonitored) group (30). Other uses of oximetry include (a) titration of FIO_2, (b) as a screening test for cardiopulmonary disease, and (c) as a method for reducing unnecessary arterial blood gases in select patient populations.

TRANSCUTANEOUS MEASUREMENT OF GAS TENSION

In the late 1970s and early 1980s, professionals in neonatal critical care became highly enthusiastic about transcutaneous blood gas determination (transcutaneous O_2 tension, $P_{Tc}O_2$, and transcutaneous CO_2 tension, $P_{Tc}CO_2$) using miniaturized Clark Po_2 and Severinghaus Pco_2 electrodes. With transcutaneous technology, the skin is warmed to facilitate hyperperfusion and allow diffusion of gases through the dermal and epidermal layers. Monitors measure the Po_2 and CO_2 electrochemically. Electrodes are attached to the skin by adhesive patches to well-perfused, non-bony surfaces. The abdomen, inner thigh, lower back, and chest are desirable sites in neonates, as are the chest, abdomen, and lower back in larger children and adults. Perhaps the greatest benefit of this technology is continuous monitoring and trending that reduce the frequency of blood gas measurement and, hence, potentially decrease blood transfusions in neonates and infants.

Transcutaneous monitoring has been limited by the need for frequent calibration of electrodes, cost of supplies, occasional burns induced by the warming component, inaccuracy when the skin is not well perfused, reported inaccuracies in older patients, and the development of more advanced pulse oximetry technology. Accurate estimation of $Paco_2$ with transcutaneous technology over a wide range of CO_2 values has been reported in children with respiratory failure, including those who require high-frequency oscillatory ventilation (4,5). Furthermore, one report indicated that transcutaneous O_2 and CO_2 monitoring can be used to continuously evaluate tissue perfusion and serve as an early warning in critically ill children during resuscitation (34).

Physiologic Basis for Transcutaneous Monitoring

To measure O_2 tension across the skin, O_2 must be able to diffuse from the capillaries to the skin surface. In 1851, Gerlach was able to demonstrate that O_2 and CO_2 could diffuse through the skin of animals and humans. The O_2 tension measured on the surface of unheated skin is ~0–5 mm Hg in adults, ~0–10 mm Hg in term infants, ~10–15 mm Hg in larger premature infants (birth weight, 1.5–2 kg), and ~15–25 mm Hg in smaller premature infants (birth weight, <1.5 kg). In 1951, Baumberger and Goodfriend reported that when a finger was immersed in a phosphate buffer solution heated to ~45°C, the partial pressure of the solution approached Pao_2 in adults. Subsequently, it was shown that Pao_2 can be measured through the skin in newborns and adults by vasodilating the skin blood vessels with drugs or heat. To determine the conditions under which $P_{Tc}O_2$ approximates Pao_2, an understanding of the structure and blood flow through the skin is essential.

Structure and Blood Supply of the Skin

The skin consists of the dermis and epidermis (**Fig. 42.7**). The dermis is supplied through a rich network of arteriovenous anastomoses in the subcutaneous tissue and through U-shaped capillary loops that arise from the arteriovenous plexus. The

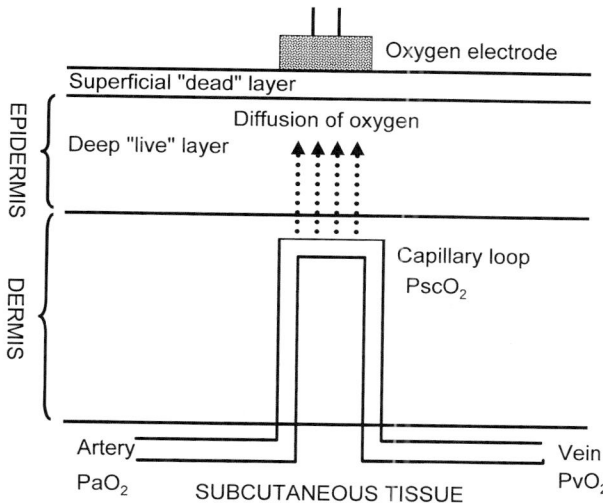

FIGURE 42.7. Schematic cross-section of the skin. The structure and blood supply of the skin, which consists of the dermis and epidermis, is displayed. O_2 diffuses out of the capillary into the tissues and can be measured by an electrode placed on the surface of the skin. $Psco_2$, skin capillary O_2 tension; Pao_2, arterial partial pressure of O_2; $P\bar{v}o_2$, partial O_2 pressure in venous blood.

epidermis consists of a deep, "viable" layer that utilizes O_2 and a superficial, "dead" part that does not consume O_2. O_2 supply to the dermis occurs by diffusion of O_2 from the capillary to the tissues as blood traverses from the arterial to the venous side of the capillaries by diffusion. The epidermis is supplied with O_2 by diffusion from the dome of the capillary to the deep layers of the epidermis.

Gas Exchange in the Skin

O_2 tension decreases linearly along the skin capillaries due to O_2 consumption in the dermis, which results in an arteriovenous difference in Po_2, with the Po_2 in the capillary dome being intermediate. O_2 diffuses from the capillary dome to the deep part of the epidermis due the differences in Po_2 across the layer. O_2 consumption results in a further drop in O_2 tension across this layer (**Fig. 42.8**). As the superficial, "dead part" of the epidermis does not consume O_2, the Po_2 at the interface of the superficial and deep layers of the epidermis would be measured on the skin surface as transcutaneous O_2 tension.

Assuming that no change occurs in O_2 consumption as blood flow to the dermis increases, the difference between arterial and venous O_2 content decreases. As the flow becomes excessive, this difference becomes exceedingly small. The effect of increasing blood flow on $P_{Tc}O_2$ in the normal newborn infant is shown in **Figure 42.9**. As Hb concentration remains the same, the difference in the O_2 partial pressures between arterial and venous blood becomes negligible, and capillary dome Po_2, being intermediate between arterial and venous Po_2, reflects arterial O_2.

Principle of Operation

In early studies with $P_{Tc}O_2$ monitoring, blood flow was increased using vasodilators such as nicotinic acid. Currently,

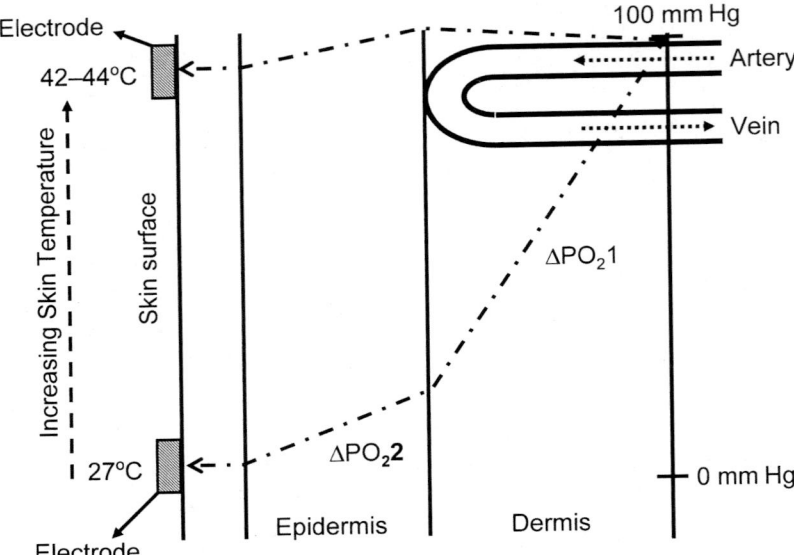

FIGURE 42.8. Schematic drawing of the O_2 profile in the skin. O_2 tension decreases along the skin capillaries due to O_2 consumption, predominantly in the dermis. Po_2, partial pressure of O_2. $\Delta Po_2 1$ represents the O_2 pressure drop in the dermis and $\Delta Po_2 2$ represents the drop in O_2 tension in the epidermis. When the skin is not heated, the surface O_2 is about 0–8 mm Hg in an infant. When the skin is heated to 42–44°C, the blood flow to the skin increases such that the supply of O_2 is in excess of the O_2 consumption of the underlying tissue. Then, the surface O_2 tension approximates arterial Po_2. Adapted from Venkataraman SP. Assessment of oxygenation and ventilation. In: Singh NC, ed. *Manual of Pediatric Critical Care*. Philadelphia: WB Saunders, 1997, with permission.

most transcutaneous monitors incorporate a heating element maintained at 42–44°C. Raising the temperature of blood has two opposing effects: (a) increased temperature shifts the O_2-dissociation curve to the right, causing the O_2 tension in the tissues to rise due to unloading of O_2, and (b) increased temperature raises O_2 consumption of the skin. As these effects act in opposite directions, they tend to offset each other, and the degree to which they offset each other determines any inaccuracy in $P_{Tc}O_2$.

The modern transcutaneous O_2 sensor consists of an electrode that has a platinum cathode and a silver reference anode encased in an electrolyte solution and separated from the skin by a membrane permeable to O_2. The electrode is heated (usually 42–44°C). The heating of the skin increases blood flow and arterializes the blood in the capillaries underneath the electrode, as described previously. O_2 diffuses from the arterialized capillary bed through the epidermis and the membrane into the electrode, where it is reduced at the cathode, thereby generating an electric current that is converted into the partial pressure measurements displayed by the monitor.

Clinical Applications

Transcutaneous O_2 monitoring has been used extensively in newborn infants with cardiorespiratory distress to estimate arterial O_2 tensions. The correlation between $P_{Tc}O_2$ and Pao_2 is excellent only when the blood pressure is within normal limits and peripheral circulation is normal. In circumstances where peripheral circulation is affected by hypotension, acidosis, or drugs, the correlation becomes poor (**Table 42.4**).

$PTcO_2$ monitoring in newborn infants has been primarily used to closely follow Pao_2 to maintain normoxemia (defined as a Po_2 of 50–100 mm Hg). In this range, the correlation between $P_{Tc}O_2$ and Pao_2 is excellent. To provide clinically useful information, it is important that not only normoxemia is detected, but also hypoxemia (Pao_2 <50 mm Hg) and hyperoxemia (Pao_2 >100 mm Hg). $P_{Tc}O_2$ has been found to correlate with Pao_2 in the range between 30 and 200 mm Hg. $P_{Tc}O_2$ tends to underestimate O_2 tensions >200 mm Hg and to overestimate Po_2 <30 mm Hg.

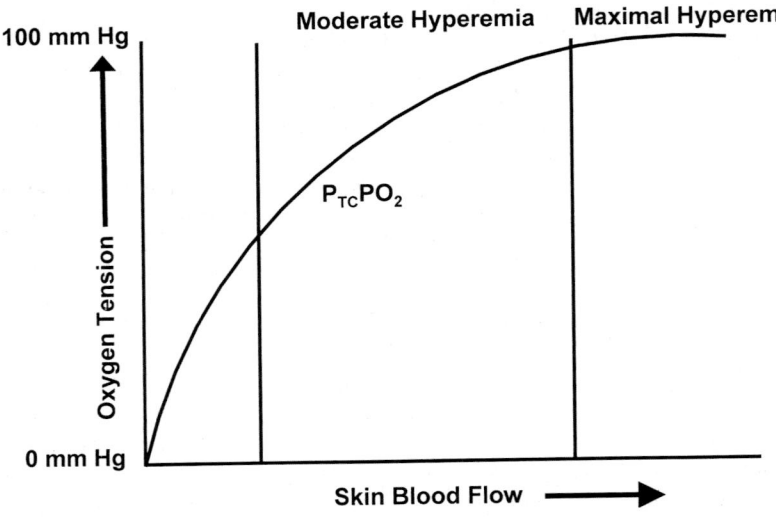

FIGURE 42.9. Influence of flow on the $P_{Tc}O_2$ with constant tissue respiration. The effect of increasing blood flow on $P_{Tc}O_2$ in the normal, newborn infant by hyperemia is displayed. If hemoglobin concentration remains the same, the difference in the O_2 partial pressures between arterial and venous blood becomes negligible, and capillary dome Po_2 reflects arterial O_2 as measured by transcutaneous technology. $P_{Tc}O_2$, transcutaneous partial pressure of O_2.

TABLE 42.4

CONDITIONS ASSOCIATED WITH POOR CORRELATION BETWEEN $P_{Tc}O_2$ AND PaO_2

1. Shock	<2 Standard deviations below mean for age
2. Acidosis	pH <7.1
3. Hypothermia	Temperature <35°C
4. Following cardiac surgery	Probably due to 1, 2, and 3
5. Skin edema	Severe
6. Cyanotic heart disease	PaO_2 <30 mm Hg
7. Tolazoline infusion	Probably related to shunting in the skin blood vessels

$P_{Tc}O_2$, transcutaneous partial pressure of CO_2; PaO_2, arterial oxygen tension

TABLE 42.5

ADVANTAGES AND DISADVANTAGES OF $P_{Tc}O_2$ MONITORING

Advantages

Provides a reliably accurate measure of PaO_2 continuously and noninvasively

Accurate over a wide range of PaO_2 values

Very useful in neonates to maintain PaO_2 within a narrow range

Provides a trend of PaO_2 over time

Can detect variability and large changes in PaO_2 when SaO_2 is >95%

Provides a measure of circulatory dysfunction when $P_{Tc}O_2$ is <PaO_2

Disadvantages

Requires frequent calibration

Requires frequent site changes due to the possibility of local burns on the skin

Requires a warm-up time of 10 mins

Underestimates PaO_2 in hyperoxic range (>150 mm Hg)

Overestimates PaO_2 in hypoxic range (<50 mm Hg)

Less useful with increasing age

$P_{Tc}O_2$, transcutaneous partial pressure of CO_2; PaO_2, arterial oxygen tension; SaO_2, arterial blood oxygen saturation

In critically ill newborns with mild circulatory failure, $P_{Tc}O_2$ can still reflect PaO_2, provided maximal hyperemia can be achieved. With moderate to severe circulatory failure, $P_{Tc}O_2$ no longer correlates with PaO_2. In these patients, $P_{Tc}O_2$ reflects skin perfusion more than PaO_2. The efficacy of various therapeutic maneuvers can be evaluated by their ability to restore the relationship between $P_{Tc}O_2$ and PaO_2.

In adults with peripheral vascular disease, $P_{Tc}O_2$ measurements have proven valuable in assessing adequacy of perfusion and in monitoring the effects of medical or surgical treatment. Transcutaneous O_2 monitoring is a form of surface oximetry of tissues. If O_2 could diffuse across the skin, it could theoretically diffuse through other tissues. In fact, studies have shown that O_2 diffuses across the intestines, liver, kidneys, and testicles. In several animal studies, O_2 monitoring on the surface of these organs has been used to assess the viability of these tissues. The hyperoxia test used to diagnose cyanotic heart disease has been extended to assess the viability of tissues. Viable tissues respond to increased inspired O_2 concentration by a rise in O_2 tension on the surface of the organ, and nonviable tissues have no response to increased O_2 concentration. The advantages and disadvantages of $P_{Tc}O_2$ monitoring are summarized in **Table 42.5**.

CAPNOGRAPHY

Capnography is the graphic waveform produced by variations in CO_2 concentration through the respiratory cycle as a function of time. Capnography can be either time- or volume-based (i.e., volumetric). Both time- and volume-based capnography respond to changes in ventilatory strategies and cardiac function. Time-based capnography is best known as end-tidal CO_2 (E_TCO_2) monitoring. In addition to the E_TCO_2 measurements provided by time-based capnography, volumetric capnography has been used to measure anatomic dead space, pulmonary capillary perfusion, and effective ventilation.

Sampling Techniques

Various capnography monitoring devices are available. In clinical practice, capnometers use two sampling techniques: sidestream and mainstream. The sidestream sampler aspirates a small quantity of gas continuously from the ventilator circuit, or at the nares in spontaneously breathing patients (i.e., via a nasal cannula). This sampling method allows for the monitoring of respiratory gases without the additional dead space and weight associated with the more common mainstream adapters. However, several disadvantages exist, including (a) the aspiration of mucous and water condensation into the sampling tubing, which can block the flow of gas, and (b) excessive scavenging of the gas flow, which may decrease minute ventilation in small children and infants. Slow aspiration rates can result in a significant time delay, and rapid aspiration rates can result in aspiration of fresh gas and an artifactual lowering of the end-tidal CO_2 value.

Mainstream capnography incorporates a light-emitting source and detector on separate sides of an airway adaptor. This equipment does not aspirate gas but is occasionally susceptible to secretions and humidity that cover the light source or detector. Recent technologic advances have greatly reduced the weight of these connectors, which decreases traction and tension on the endotracheal tube (ETT), as had been reported with earlier generations of this technology. Dead space has been reduced to 1 mL in the neonatal sensor and no longer poses a rebreathing problem in infants and children.

The two main techniques of capnography measurement are infrared spectroscopy and mass spectroscopy. Infrared spectroscopy requires three components: an infrared light source, a gas chamber, and a detector. Its success depends on the fact that each gas has unique absorption characteristics that can be used to quantify the amount (partial pressure) of a particular gas by application of the Beer-Lambert principle.

E_TCO_2 is defined as the peak CO_2 value during expiration and is dependent on adequate pulmonary capillary blood flow of CO_2-rich blood to alveoli, which in turn depends on adequate right and left heart function. The normal E_TCO_2 in healthy subjects is a <5 mm Hg different than the $PaCO_2$,

TABLE 42.6

CLINICAL CONDITIONS ASSOCIATED WITH ALTERATIONS IN E_TCO_2

Increases in E_TCO_2
Increased pulmonary capillary blood flow
Increased cardiac output
Hypoventilation
Increased CO_2 production
Sudden release of a tourniquet
Sodium bicarbonate administration

Decreases in E_TCO_2
Decreased pulmonary capillary blood flow
  Pulmonary hypertension
  Pulmonary embolus (thrombus or air)
Decreased cardiac output
Hyperventilation
Ventilator circuit leak
Obstructed endotracheal tube
Hyperventilation
Decreased CO_2 production

Absent E_TCO_2
Esophageal intubation
Ventilator disconnect

representing normal anatomic dead space of the upper airway. Clinical conditions associated with alterations in E_TCO_2 are shown in **Table 42.6.**

Evaluation of Respiratory Pattern

The phasic changes in CO_2 concentration that occur during the respiratory cycle are demonstrated in **Figure 42.10.** Evaluation of the respiratory pattern is aided by noting the near-zero end-inspiratory CO_2 value in the normal capnogram, the plateau at end expiration, and the highest CO_2 recorded (E_TCO_2). The capnogram converts these phasic values of CO_2 into electrical signals and displays them as respiratory rate, inspiratory CO_2, and E_TCO_2, as a waveform and/or digitally, allowing analysis of changes that take place breath-to-breath and over longer periods of time.

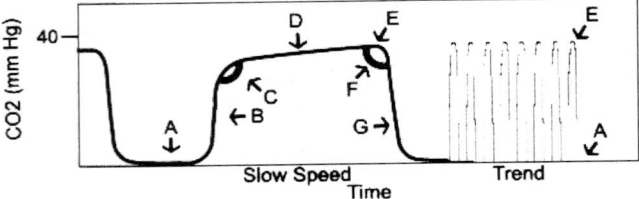

FIGURE 42.10. Normal features of a capnogram. *A*, baseline, represents the beginning of expiration and should start at zero. *B* is the transitional part of the curve represents mixing of dead space and alveolar gas. *C* is the α angle represents the change to alveolar gas. *D* is the alveolar part of the curve represents the plateau average alveolar gas concentration. *E* is the end-tidal CO_2 value. *F* is the β angle represents the change to the inspiratory part of the cycle. *G* is the inspiration part of the curve shows a rapid decrease in CO_2 concentration. From Thompson JE, Jaffe MB. Capnographic waveforms in the mechanically ventilated patient. *Respir Care* 2005;50(1):100–9, with permission.

Clinical Applications

Practical uses of E_TCO_2 monitoring in the ICU include adequacy of alveolar ventilation during mechanical ventilation, respiratory-rate monitoring, patient-ventilator system function, and ETT patency and positioning. Many institutions use capnography at intubation for a rapid assessment of ETT placement by confirming the presence of CO_2 in the exhaled gas, and some centers use it for the duration of mechanical ventilation to monitor for inadvertent dislodgement of the ETT.

Inadvertent placement of the ETT into the esophagus is one of the most serious complications of attempted endotracheal intubation (23). Esophageal intubation is not a rare occurrence, and early detection can be life saving. Assessment of four different methods of ETT placement verification found capnography to be the most rapid and reliable method for evaluation when compared to auscultation and transillumination (23).

While the validation of ETT placement in the trachea is improved with E_TCO_2 monitoring (23), limitations do exist (27). False-positive readings (i.e., the monitor displays an end-tidal CO_2 value when the ETT is not in the trachea) may occur following prolonged bag-valve-mask ventilation prior to intubation, following ingestion of antacids or carbonated beverages, or when the tip of the ETT is in the pharynx. False-negative readings (i.e., no end-tidal CO_2 value is displayed when, in fact, the ETT is in trachea) may occur if the patient has severe airway obstruction, poor cardiac output, pulmonary emboli, or pulmonary hypertension. When discrepancies appear between the capnometer reading and the physical assessment, further investigation is necessary.

Capnography can be used to great advantage in mechanically ventilated patients if the waveform is displayed and analyzed along with the numeric data. Mechanical failures can be detected, the adequacy of respiratory support can be analyzed, and changes can be made in the mode of ventilation to maximize the efficiency of ventilation, decrease the patient's work of breathing (WOB), and improve patient ventilator synchrony (**Figs. 42.11** through **42.13**).

Time-based versus Volumetric Capnography

While both time-based and volumetric capnography provide the measurement and display of end-tidal CO_2, many differences exist between the techniques. It is important to determine (a) which values are pertinent to the specific patient population being monitored, and (b) the primary clinical objectives.

Time-based capnography is limited to the measurement and display of the respiratory waveform and the E_TCO_2 value. The E_TCO_2 value displayed represents the partial pressure of CO_2 present at the end of exhalation (**Fig. 42.10**). The E_TCO_2 measurement can also be used to trend changes in $PaCO_2$ for patients in whom physiologic dead space is not significantly elevated or changing. However, this ability is weakened when significant physiologic dead space exists and impaired cardiac output is present. Impaired cardiac output can be caused by excessive positive end-expiratory pressure (PEEP). Optimization of mechanical ventilation may be better achieved with volumetric capnography than with time-based capnography, as mean airway pressure (i.e., PEEP) can be titrated based on changes in CO_2 elimination (19).

Advances in technology allow the integration of flow and volume to be graphically displayed (**Fig. 42.14**), which is the

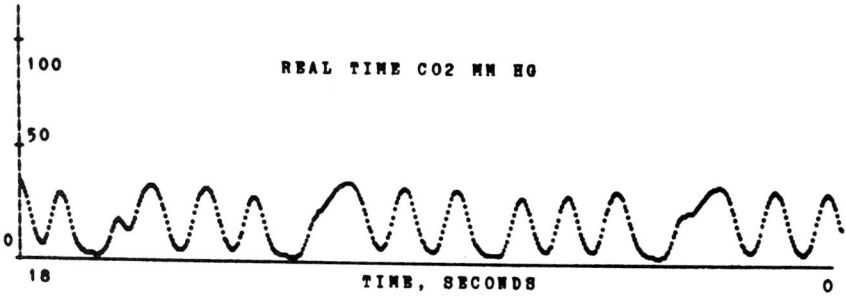

FIGURE 42.11. Chaotic respiratory pattern in a patient unable to tolerate spontaneous ventilation. From Carlon GC, Ray C, Miodownik S, et al. Capnography in mechanically ventilated patients. *Crit Care Med.* 1988;16:550–556, with permission.

basis of volumetric capnography. The display of measurements throughout the entire respiratory cycle is achieved providing a myriad of valuable information. Volumetric capnography provides a measurement of CO_2 production (Vco_2) and enables calculation of alveolar minute ventilation and the ratio of volume of dead space (Vd) and tidal volume (VT), Vd/VT. As many important management decisions are based on determination of VT and the resultant changes in gas exchange, accuracy of these values is essential (17,33).

The net volume of CO_2 eliminated through the lungs each minute (Vco_2) varies depending on CO_2 production, ventilation, circulation/perfusion and, to a lesser degree, diffusion. Vco_2 signals future changes in $Paco_2$, thus making Vco_2 a valuable marker for changes in the cardiorespiratory status of the ventilated patient (28). As CO_2 production varies between patients and within a patient over time, absolute values are not as significant as trends. As with O_2 consumption, CO_2 production and elimination comprise a continuous process. Therefore, Vco_2 rapidly reflects changes in ventilation and perfusion, regardless of the etiology. Vco_2 reflects the body's physiologic response to changes in mechanical ventilation. Capnography is a very useful and sensitive clinical tool that reflects the cardiorespiratory status and metabolic state of the patient.

The single-breath CO_2 waveform consists of three phases (**Fig. 42.14**). Phase 1 represents gas exhaled from the upper airways (i.e., gas exhaled from anatomic dead space), which generally is devoid of CO_2 (19). Therefore, a prolongation of phase 1 indicates an increase in anatomic dead space ventilation (Vd_{ana}). Phase 2 is the transitional phase from upper to lower airway ventilation. Changes in phase 2 reflect changes in perfusion. Phase 3 is the area of alveolar gas exchange, and represents changes in gas distribution. For example, when a maldistribution of gas exists, the slope of phase 3 will increase.

When weaning from mechanical ventilation, it is important to ensure that the volume of gas delivered actually participates in gas exchange (i.e., effective ventilation). Volumetric capnography provides clinicians with a continuous numerical representation of effective ventilation. While no definitive studies have been conducted to prove the value of monitoring volumetric capnography on patient outcomes, monitoring the effective gas exchange effects of each ventilator parameter adjustment seems intuitive.

Responses to changes in ventilatory strategies and cardiac function can be detected with both time-based and volume-based (i.e., volumetric) capnography. Many conditions, such as pulmonary embolism, pulmonary hypertension, air embolism, and severe cardiac dysfunction increase dead-space ventilation, impair gas exchange, and cause a significant decrease in the expired CO_2 concentration. Therefore, continuous capnographic monitoring can alert clinicians to potentially detrimental changes in a child's cardiorespiratory condition. Changes in capnography tend to occur more rapidly than changes in pulse oximetry.

MONITORING RESPIRATORY MECHANICS

Respiratory Inductive Plethysmography

Respiratory inductive plethysmography (**Fig. 42.15**) consists of two coils of insulated wires sewn in a sinusoidal pattern in elastic-fabricated bands. One band encircles the chest, with the upper level of the band just under the axillae, and the other encircles the abdomen, with the band located midway between the lower ribs and the upper edge of the iliac crests and care taken to avoid the lower ribs. If prolonged monitoring is planned, the bands can be taped to the skin. Movement generates voltage changes by generating magnetic fields in the rib cage and abdominal bands that are proportional to cross-sectional area changes and can be interpolated to indicate changes in thoracic volume. Before obtaining measurements on a patient, a reference volume signal from a spirometer must be fed into the calibration unit.

Following calibration, the sum signal from the rib cage and abdominal sensors must be validated against a simultaneous spirometer (or an integrated pneumotachometer) during tidal breathing. To verify the accuracy of the measurements, a repeat validation procedure must be performed after recording for a significant period of time. If the measurements are being made without any change in posture, either the isovolume or multiple linear-regressions technique may be used for calibration without substantial loss of accuracy. If a change in posture is planned, only the least-squares method is likely to retain its accuracy over time.

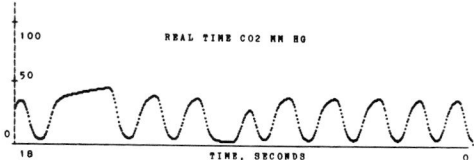

FIGURE 42.12. Intermittent mandatory ventilation without pressure support. Note irregular respiratory pattern, tachypnea, absence of alveolar plateau, low E_TCO_2, and high baseline CO_2. From Carlon GC, Ray C, Miodownik S, et al. Capnography in mechanically ventilated patients. *Crit Care Med* 1988;16:550–6, with permission.

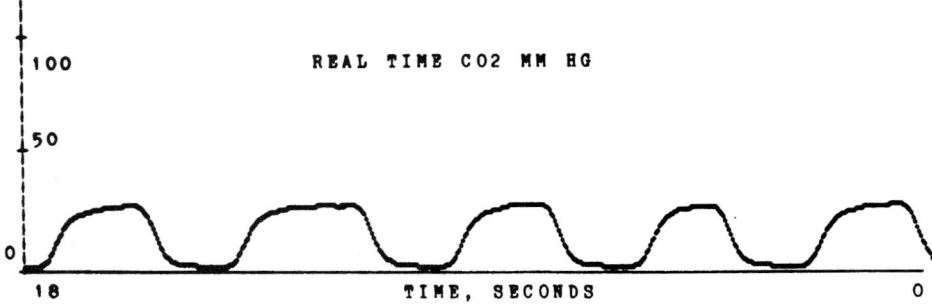

REAL TIME CO2 MM HG

100

50

0

18   TIME, SECONDS   0

FIGURE 42.13. Same patient as in Figure 42.12, 15 mins after addition of 20 cm H_2O pressure support. A normal capnogram and respiratory rate can now be observed. From Carlon GC, Ray C, Miodownik S, et al. Capnography in mechanically ventilated patients. *Crit Care Med* 1988;16:550–6, with permission.

Application in Critically Ill Patients

Minute ventilation is the product of VT and respiratory frequency (f):

$$V = VT/T_i \times T_i/T_{tot} \times 60$$

where:

V = minute ventilation (L/min)
T_i = inspiratory time (sec)
T_{tot} = total respiratory cycle (sec).

The parameter VT/T_i is the mean inspiratory flow, and T_i/T_{tot} is the fractional inspiratory time.

VT/T_i is a measure of respiratory drive and correlates well with other indices of respiratory drive such as $P_{0.1}$ and the ventilatory response to hypercapnia. $P_{0.1}$ is the pressure generated in the first 100 msec after the onset of inspiratory effort against an occluded airway and provides a measure of respiratory drive, as described later in this chapter.

Few pediatric studies have examined the utility of respiratory inductive plethysmograph in critical illness. Use of this technique to diagnose bilateral diaphragmatic paralysis has been reported (38). In adults, an index of rapid, shallow breathing (f/VT) >100 has been associated with a higher weaning

failure. In children, f/VT ratio does not predict extubation failure (36).

Monitoring of Respiratory Muscle Function

Maximal inspiratory pressure (P_{Imax}), often called negative inspiratory force, is defined as the maximal static pressure that can be generated with forceful efforts against an occluded airway. P_{Imax} may provide a noninvasive index of global muscle strength (13). P_{Imax} is usually measured after expiration to residual volume. In nonintubated patients, P_{Imax} is measured as the largest pressure sustained for at least 1 sec. On the other hand, P_{Imax} in intubated patients is the peak pressure that can be generated. In intubated patients, a one-way valve and manometer are attached to the airway, which permits exhalation but not inspiration. As the patient breathes spontaneously through the one-way valve, the pressures become more and more negative. The period of occlusion is maintained for at least 10–20 secs.

In normal infants, P_{Imax} during crying has been reported to be -118 ± 21 cm H_2O. In children 6–17 years of age, the P_{Imax} has been reported to be -70 to -110 cm H_2O, and pubertal children are capable of generating P_{Imax} of -80 to -120 cm H_2O (25,29). In adults, a P_{Imax} more negative than -30 cm H_2O has been reported to be associated with extubation success in adults, and a value less negative than -20 cm H_2O has been associated with extubation failure. In children, P_{Imax} has poor discriminative capacity between extubation success and failure (16). Despite the published utility of P_{Imax}, it is common practice to measure P_{Imax} prior to extubation in children, especially those with neuromuscular weakness (e.g., Guillain-Barré syndrome, weakness from prolonged neuromuscular blockade, etc.) and to defer extubation unless the P_{Imax} is more negative than -20 cm H_2O.

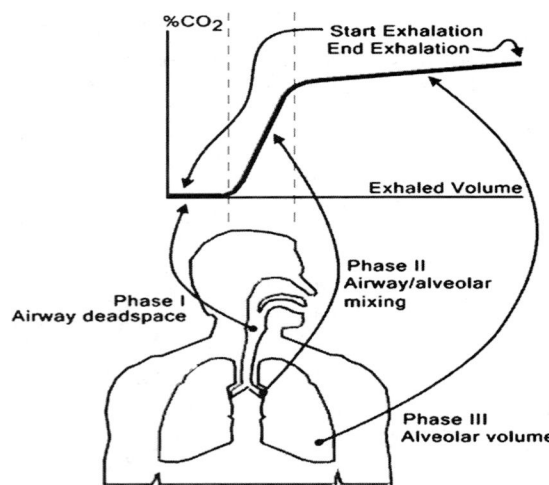

%CO2

Start Exhalation
End Exhalation

Exhaled Volume

Phase I
Airway deadspace

Phase II
Airway/alveolar
mixing

Phase III
Alveolar volume

FIGURE 42.14. Volumetric capnogram. The initial portion of the volumetric capnogram (phase 1) represents the quantity of CO_2 eliminated from the large airways. Phase 2 is the transitional zone, which represents ventilation from both small and large airways. The third phase of the capnogram represents CO_2 elimination from the alveoli and, thus, the quantity of gas involved with alveolar ventilation. Figure Courtesy of Respironics, Inc., and its affiliates, Wallingford, Connecticut.

Monitoring Respiratory Mechanics in Ventilated Patients

In a relaxed patient during mechanical ventilation, measurements of respiratory mechanics can be obtained by rapid airway occlusion during constant-flow inflation, when the proximal airway pressure increases as the lung is inflated to a maximal pressure (P_{max}). Rapid airway occlusion at end-inspiration results in an immediate drop in both airway pressure and transpulmonary pressure (P_{tp}) from P_{max}, followed

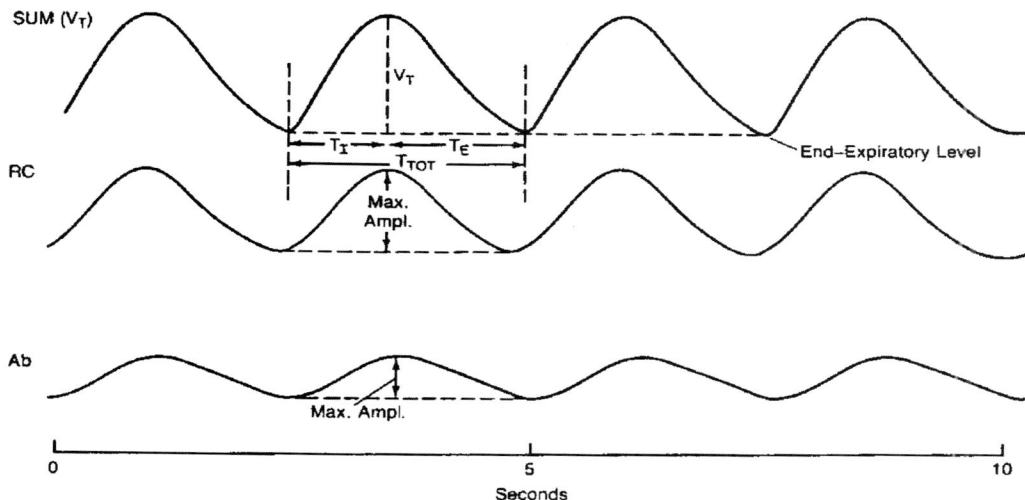

FIGURE 42.15. Schematic recording of the respiratory cycle obtained through a respiratory inductive plethysmograph. The algebraic sum of the ribcage (*RC*) and the abdominal (*Ab*) excursions equals VT. T_I is the inspiratory time (sec), T_E is the expiratory time, and T_{TOT} is the total respiratory cycle (sec). From Tobin MJ. Respiratory monitoring in the intensive care unit. *Am Review of Respir Dis* (*Am J Resp Crit Care Med*) 1988;138:1625–42, with permission.

by a gradual decrease until a plateau (P_{plat}) is achieved after 3–5 secs (**Fig. 42.16**). The pressure drop from P_{max} can be partitioned into an initial almost linear drop followed by a slower, multi-exponential decrease to P_{plat}. P_{plat}, P_{tp}, and esophageal pressure (P_{es}) represent the static recoil pressure of the total respiratory system, lung, and chest wall, respectively.

Compliance and Elastance

Compliance is defined as a change in volume divided by a change in transmural pressure. *Elastance* is the reciprocal of compliance. Lung compliance is defined as the change in lung volume divided by the transalveolar pressure, which is equal to the difference between the alveolar pressure (P_{alv}) at the end of inflation and the pleural pressure (P_{pl} or P_{es}). At the bedside, the P_{plat} can be substituted for P_{alv} and tidal volume can be substituted for a change in lung volume (C_{lung}):

$$C_{lung} = VT/(P_{plat} - P_{es})$$

C_{lung} is also called *static lung compliance* (C_{stat}). Since esophageal pressure is often not measured in children, C_{lung} can be calculated by:

$$C_{lung} = VT_{(effective)}/(P_{plat} - PEEP)$$

where $VT_{(effective)}$ is the tidal volume delivered to the patient (usually measured at the hub of the ETT or estimated by subtracting the compressible volume lost in the circuit from the ventilator-delivered tidal volume).

Chest-wall compliance is defined as the change in thoracic volume divided by the transthoracic pressure [atmospheric pressure (P_{atm}) – P_{es}]. To compare among patients, compliance values should be indexed to body weight.

Dynamic Compliance

Dynamic compliance (C_{dyn}) is defined as the change in volume divided by the change in airway pressure from end-expiration to end-inspiration during a mechanical breath. It is commonly calculated by dividing the VT by the difference between P_{max}

and end-expiratory pressure.

$$C_{dyn} = VT/(P_{max} - PEEP)$$

In patients without intrinsic PEEP ($PEEP_i$), the end-expiratory pressure to be used is the set PEEP. In patients with $PEEP_i$, the end-expiratory pressure to be used for the calculation of C_{dyn} is $PEEP_i$.

Tidal Volume Measurement

In adults, the inspiratory VT displayed by the ventilator can generally be used for compliance calculations and for most aspects of mechanical ventilation. However, it must be noted that the delivered tidal volume (VT_{del}) is distributed between the ventilator circuit and the patient. For infants and children, an accurate measurement of VT is essential. Thus, the issue is determining the ideal location at which VT measurements should be obtained, as VT can be measured at the ETT or at the ventilator.

In infants and children, the fraction of the VT_{del} that is distributed to the ventilator circuit is substantially higher than in adults and can be as much as 70% in critically ill infants (7). Measuring delivered VT at the ventilator does not compensate for the compliance of the ventilator circuit, for uncontrolled variations in the circuit setup, or for changes over time. A VT measured with a pneumotachometer positioned between the ETT and the ventilator circuit more reliably measures the VT actually delivered to neonatal and pediatric patients (7,9,11). To determine the actual VT delivered to the lungs without requiring additional equipment (i.e., a pneumotachometer), a mathematical formula can be used to correct for the compliance of the ventilator circuit:

$$VT_{eff} = VT_{del} - C_{vent}(PIP - PEEP)$$

where:

VT_{eff} = effective tidal volume that reaches the ETT
PIP = peak inspiratory pressure
C_{vent} = compliance of the ventilator circuit.

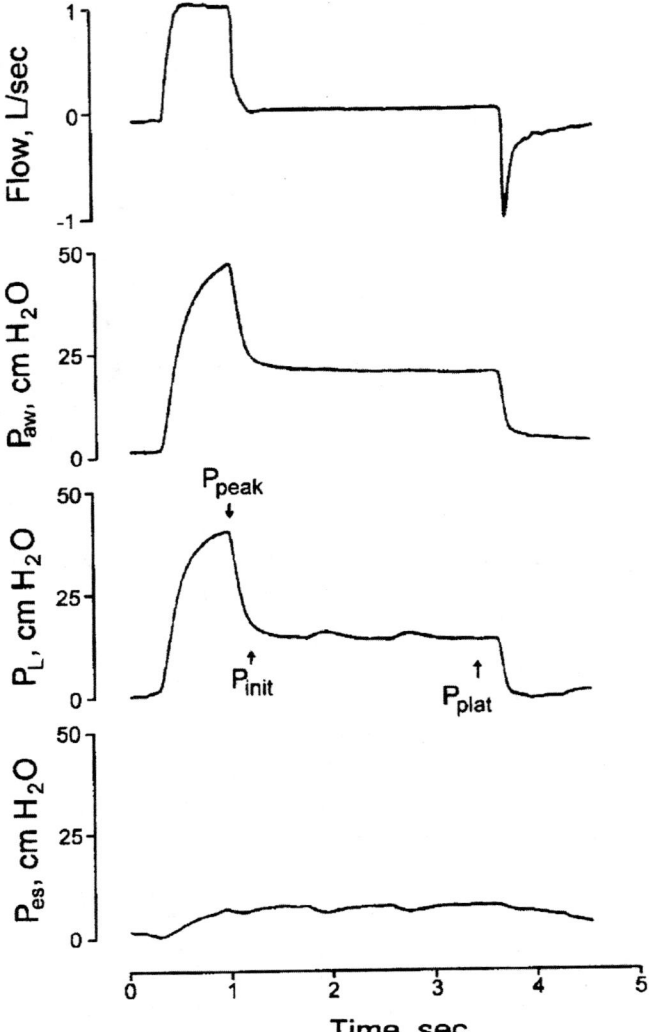

FIGURE 42.16. Flow (inspiration upward), airway pressure (P_aw), transpulmonary pressure (P_L), and esophageal pressure (P_es) tracings in a representative patient during passive ventilation. An end-inspiratory occlusion produced a rapid decline in both P_aw and P_tp from a peak value to a lower initial value, followed by gradual decrease until a plateau is achieved. From Jubran A, Tobin MJ. Passive mechanics of lung and chest wall in patients who failed and succeeded in trials of weaning. *Am J Resp Crit Care Med* 1997;155:916–21, with permission.

This calculated VT represents the ventilator-determined VT minus the volume "lost" due to the distensibility (compliance) of the ventilator circuit. It should be noted that the calculated values can differ from those measured at the ETT (7,9,11). Additionally, it is preferable to index tidal volumes to body weight to be able to compare across patient populations. When calculating compliances as described here, the VT_eff should be used instead of the ventilator VT.

Intrinsic PEEP

The static recoil pressure of the respiratory system at end expiration may be elevated in patients who receive mechanical ventilation, especially in those who have lower-airway disease and obstruction. With lower-airway obstruction, inspiration may begin before exhalation is complete, thus, resulting in an end-expiratory alveolar pressure that remains elevated above the proximal airway pressure. This positive recoil pressure, or static PEEP_i, can be quantified in relaxed patients by using an end-expiratory hold maneuver on a mechanical ventilator immediately before the onset of the next breath. Patients who are spontaneously breathing may need to overcome PEEP_i to trigger a ventilator. Thus, PEEP_i increases the WOB and can contribute to muscle fatigue. Excessive PEEP_i may also result in poor triggering because the patient is unable to generate the necessary negative pressure in the central airway. This problem can be largely overcome by flow triggering.

Static Pressure-Volume Curves

A static pressure-volume curve of the respiratory system can be constructed in a paralyzed patient by measuring airway pressure as the lungs are progressively inflated and deflated with a graduated volumetric syringe, the "super-syringe technique." In small children, the aliquots of volume should be 1–2 mL/kg. The pressure-volume (PV) curve has both inflation and deflation portions. It should be noted that this technique is rarely used in clinical practice.

The inspiratory phase of the PV curve consists of three sections. As the lung is inflated from low lung volumes, the initial lung compliance is low. Then, as airway pressure is increased, lung compliance improves, which continues until the lung is fully inflated. Inflating the lung further results in a reduction in the lung compliance at the end of inflation (**Fig. 42.17**). The junction between the first and second portion of the curve is called the *lower inflection point* (LIP). The LIP can be discerned by visual inspection of the PV curve. More accurately, the LIP can be calculated by intersecting the lines from the first and second portions of the curve. Alternatively, the LIP can be calculated by measuring the steepest point of the second section and marking the LIP as the point of a 20% decrease in slope from this steepest point. The junction of the second and third portions of the curve is called the *upper inflection point* (UIP). The UIP can be measured in the same way as the LIP, except the UIP would represent a 20% increase from the point of the greatest slope. The LIP is thought to represent the point of alveolar recruitment, and the UIP is thought to represent

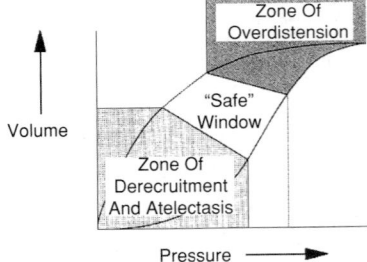

FIGURE 42.17. Pressure-volume curve. The inspiratory phase of the pressure-volume curve consists of three sections. As the lung is inflated from an initial low lung volume, the lung compliance is low. As airway pressure is increased, lung compliance improves, which continues until the lung is fully inflated. Inflating the lung further results in a reduction in the lung compliance at the end of inflation as the lung overdistends. The goal is to ventilate in the "safe window." From Froese AB. High-frequency oscillatory ventilation for adult respiratory distress syndrome: Let's get it right this time! *Crit Care Med.* 1997;25(6):906–8, with permission.

overdistension of the lung. In patients with acute lung injury, some investigators have recommended that PEEP should be set at a pressure slightly above the lower inflection point on a static PV curve.

Work of Breathing and Pressure-Time Product

WOB can be measured using esophageal manometry and measurement of tidal volume during spontaneous breathing. *Work* is defined as *force multiplied by displacement*. WOB can be estimated by integrating pressure and volume of a spontaneous breath.

A significant limitation of the measurement of WOB is that it may underestimate the total energy expenditure and O_2 consumption of the respiratory muscles. To overcome this problem, many have suggested the use of the pressure-time product for respiratory muscles. This also requires esophageal manometry but does not require simultaneous measurement of tidal volume. The pressure-time product is calculated as the time integral of the difference between P_{es} measured during assisted ventilation and the recoil pressure of the chest wall (35). The method of measuring the recoil pressure of the chest wall has been described previously.

Mechanical Ventilators and Airway Graphics Monitoring

Mechanical ventilators deliver gas at a pressure, generating flow and resulting in a change in patient lung volume. Most mechanical ventilators in the PICU permit continuous monitoring of respiratory mechanics and include graphic display of VT, gas flow (V), and airway pressure (P_{aw}).

Output waveforms are useful tools with which to study ventilator operation and provide a graphic display of the various modes of ventilation. Waveform analysis can be used to optimize mechanical ventilatory support and to analyze ventilator incidents and alarm conditions. Using this technology, it is possible to shape the form of ventilatory support to improve patient-ventilator synchrony, reduce WOB, and calculate a variety of physiologic parameters related to respiratory mechanics (35). The goal of this section is to provide clinicians with a clinical tool that can optimize their mechanical ventilation strategies through the application of airway graphic analysis.

A primary goal of graphic analysis is to quantitate respiratory pathophysiology by evaluating tidal volume, airway pressures, compliance, airway resistance, and pressure-volume and flow-volume relationships. Airway graphic analysis can help to determine the effectiveness of various interventions. Additionally, adverse effects, including alveolar overdistension, air leak, dynamic hyperexpansion ("gas trapping"), and patient-ventilator asynchrony, can be diagnosed and corrected.

Airway Scalars

Airway scalars are the most commonly reported waveforms. Scalars are comprised of three distinct waveforms: flow, pressure, and volume (y-axis) plotted against time (x-axis). Convention dictates that, in these waveforms, positive values correspond to inspiration events and negative values correspond to expiration. A simultaneous comparison of all three waveforms facilitates analysis of the patient-ventilator interface. Patient-ventilator asynchrony becomes evident when the timing and magnitude of flow, pressure, and volume are disproportionate or delayed. Additionally, each of these parameters (flow, pressure, and volume) can be plotted against each other. PV and flow-volume loops can be particularly helpful in assessing alterations in resistance, compliance, WOB, pulmonary overdistension, and premature termination of exhalation.

Optimal measurements are obtained when the pressure- and flow-monitoring device (pneumotachometer) is positioned between the ETT and ventilator circuit. Although resistance of the ETT is a component of the pressure graphic, pressures reported are generally considered to reflect proximal airway pressures. Volume is generally measured by integrating the flow signal over time. The upward deflection of the graphic represents the volume delivered to the patient, while the downward deflection represents the total expiratory volume. Inspiratory and expiratory volumes should be equal. However, it is not uncommon in patients with uncuffed ETTs or with cuffed ETTs that have inadequate cuff inflation for the expiratory volume to be less than the inspiratory volume. Percentage leak can be calculated and may aid in the decision to change the ETT size or to evaluate the adequacy of the cuff.

Scalar Display of Volume-limited Ventilation

A typical airway graphic during time-cycled, volume-limited ventilation is displayed in **Figure 42.18.** The top graphic

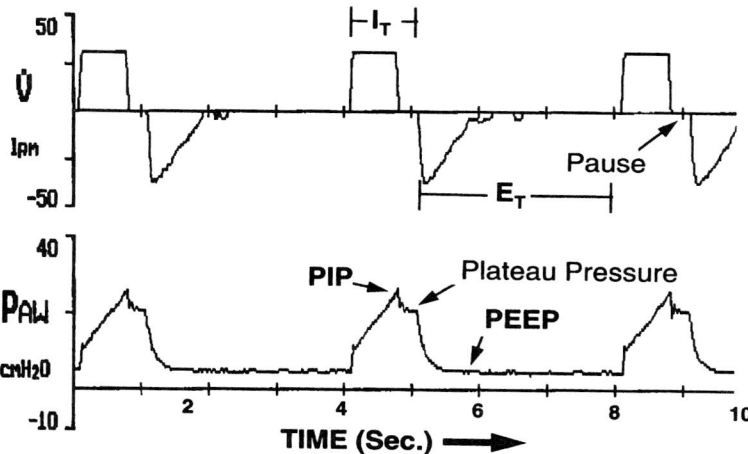

FIGURE 42.18. Normal scalar display of flow versus time and airway pressure versus time for volume-limited ventilation. P_{aw}, airway pressure; PIP, peak inspiratory pressure; PEEP, positive end-expiratory pressure. Figure courtesy of VIASYS Healthcare Inc., Yorba Linda, California.

displays flow on the vertical axis and time on the horizontal axis. The bottom graphic displays airway pressure versus time. During volume-limited ventilation, the VT is set, and the PIP is determined by lung compliance, airway resistance, inspiratory time (T_i), and flow characteristics.

Traditionally, this mode of ventilation is characterized by a square-wave, constant-flow inspiratory flow pattern. Constant-inspiratory flow corresponds to a linear increase in airway pressure until the preset VT is reached. When an unacceptable PIP occurs during volume-limited ventilation with a square-wave, constant-inspiratory flow pattern, consideration of increasing T_i, decreasing VT (allowing permissive hypercapnia) (18), or changing the ventilation mode to a variable, decelerating inspiratory flow pattern (24) will decrease the PIP. It should be noted that many newer-generation ventilators offer volume-limited ventilation with a variable, decelerating inspiratory flow pattern (i.e., pressure-regulated volume control).

In **Figure 42.18**, an inspiratory pause has been set and is represented by the lengthened T_i and the period of zero flow prior to exhalation. The plateau pressure corresponds to this zero-flow period during inspiration. The flow returns to zero during expiration, indicating the completion of exhalation.

Scalar Display of Pressure-limited Ventilation

A typical airway graphic during pressure-limited ventilation with a variable, decelerating inspiratory flow pattern (i.e., pressure control) is displayed in **Figure 42.19**. During pressure-limited ventilation, the PIP is set, and the VT is determined by lung compliance, airway resistance, and delivered flow rate. In the following discussions, PIP refers to the total peak inspiratory pressure above zero and not a set inspiratory pressure above PEEP. This characteristic flow pattern results in a curvilinear increase in airway pressure until the PIP is reached. Note the more rapid increase in pressure during the initial phase of a pressure-limited breath versus the linear increase in airway pressure that occurs with a volume-limited breath (**Fig. 42.18**). Due to Because of the length of the T_i, flow returns to zero while airway pressure is maintained. During pressure-limited

ventilation, if VT decreases, increasing the PIP limit, increasing the T_i, or optimizing the PEEP should be considered. At a similar VT, the decelerating flow pattern of pressure-limited ventilation results in a decrease in PIP (24) and an increase in pulmonary compliance when compared to volume-limited ventilation with a square-wave, constant-inspiratory flow pattern.

During acute respiratory distress syndrome (ARDS), pulmonary compliance is decreased. If PIP is held constant when compliance decreases, VT will be reduced and gas exchange will be impaired. This decrease in VT may result in respiratory acidosis. The approach to the loss of VT consists of allowing this to occur (i.e., permissive hypercapnia) (18) or increasing airway pressures (PIP and/or PEEP) to recruit lung volume.

Pressure-Volume and Flow-Volume Loops

PV and flow-volume loops provide insight into the patient's pathophysiology and the response to therapeutic interventions. PV loops depict pressure on the horizontal axis and volume on the vertical axis. The first portion of inspiratory curve in **Figure 42.17** shows a significant increase in pressure with little increase in volume (low compliance). The following portion shows a rapid up-sloping, depicting an increase in volume per pressure delivered (high compliance). This point is termed the *lower inflection point* and is created by a sudden opening of the alveoli. A sharp intersection is seen at the end of inspiration and the start of expiration. At the onset of expiration, a significant reduction in pressure with a smaller reduction in volume is seen. It should be noted that accurate inflection and deflection points can only be discerned with a static lung-inflation technique, using very low inspiratory flow, as previously described. The dynamic curves displayed on standard airway graphics monitors do not accurately detect inflection and deflection points, as gas flow is a significant variable.

The flow-volume loop depicts flow on the vertical axis and volume on the horizontal axis. Inspiration is seen on the upper portion of the loop, with exhalation depicted on the lower portion. Inspiratory volume is increased with increases in inspiratory flow. When flow terminates, expiration begins. Peak

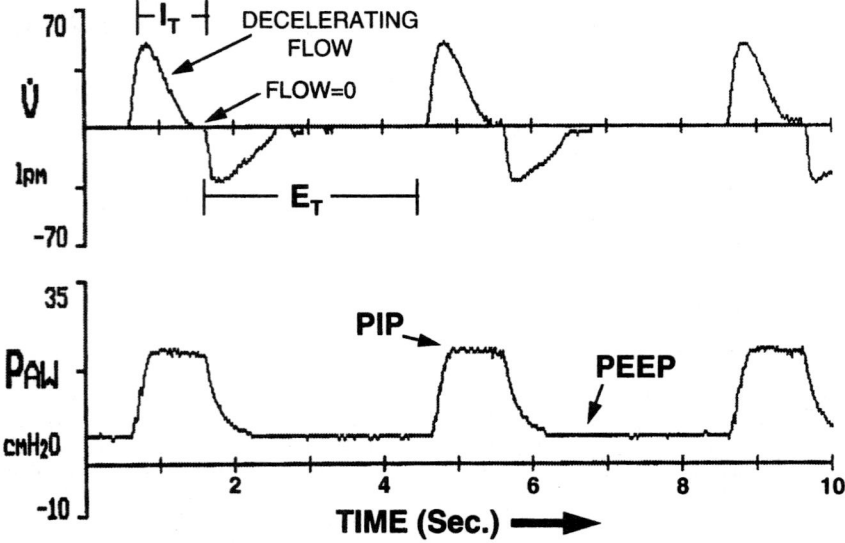

FIGURE 42.19. Normal scalar display of flow versus time and airway pressure versus time for pressure-limited ventilation. Figure courtesy of VIASYS Healthcare, Inc., Yorba Linda, California.

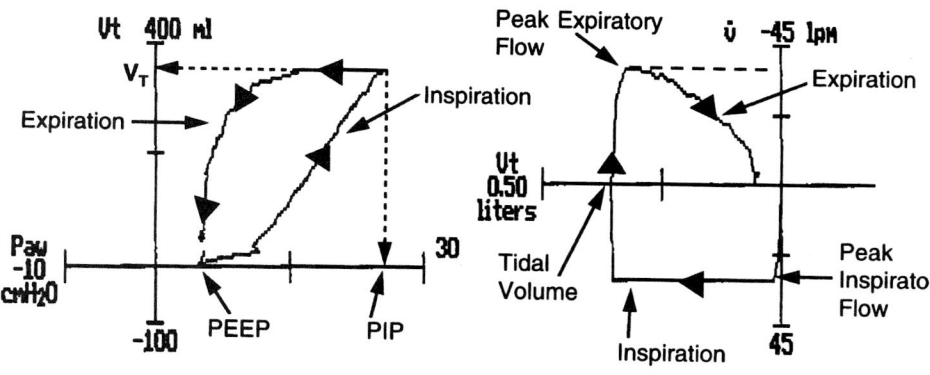

FIGURE 42.20. The pressure-volume graphic displays tidal volume on the vertical axis and airway pressure on the horizontal axis. The flow-volume graphic displays flow on the vertical axis and tidal volume on the horizontal axis. Note that in this flow-volume loop, the delivered inspiratory flow is represented during traditional volume-limited ventilation below the baseline as a square wave. Figure courtesy of VIASYS Healthcare, Inc., Yorba Linda, California.

expiratory flow rate is reached when the expiratory flow rate begins to decay.

Pressure-Volume and Flow-Volume Loops in Volume-limited Ventilation

The typical PV and flow-volume loops during volume-limited ventilation are displayed in **Figure 42.20.** As the ventilator delivers gas to the patient, airway pressure increases from the set PEEP level until the set VT is reached and inspiration is terminated. During exhalation, both volume and pressure are reduced in the airways until exhaled flow reaches zero, signifying the termination of the breath. Alterations in the shape of the inspiratory limb of the PV loop provide insight into the compliance of the lung and the presence of various abnormalities, including alveolar atelectasis and overdistension. Dynamic compliance, which is the slope of the line connecting the PEEP with the PIP, is calculated as

$$VT_{del}/(PIP - PEEP)$$

Note in **Figures 42.20** and **42.21** that only a small amount of volume is delivered during the initial phase of inspiration. As the inspiratory pressure increases, the critical opening pressure is achieved, and the tidal volume is delivered. Hysteresis, which is a nonlinear change in the PV relationship over time, is present during both inspiration and expiration. ARDS reduces pulmonary compliance (compare **Fig. 42.20** with **Fig. 42.21**). A decrease in compliance results in higher airway pressures being required to achieve a similar VT. As a result, the PV loop flattens, and the curvature of the inspiratory and expiratory limbs

decreases (decreased hysteresis). Note that, during the initial phase of inspiration, airway pressure increases, with little gas being delivered to the patient, due to alveolar collapse and a decrease in lung volume during the expiratory phase. To reexpand the collapsed alveoli, the initial phase of inspiration requires an elevation of airway pressure prior to delivering a significant volume of gas. Therefore, the initial phase of the inspiratory limb (re-expansion interval) is less sloped than the later phase of inspiration. Subsequently, the PIP may be increased. Increasing the PEEP may maintain alveolar patency during the expiratory phase and minimize this re-expansion interval (**Fig. 42.22**).

The evaluation of inspiratory and expiratory flow patterns can provide important information as to the presence of increased inspiratory or expiratory resistance (**Fig. 42.23**). In patients with elevated resistance, the response of these abnormalities to various interventions, including suctioning, altering the inspiratory time, and/or bronchodilator therapy, can then be assessed.

Pressure-Volume and Flow-Volume Loops in Pressure-limited Ventilation

The decelerating flow pattern of pressure-control ventilation results in a more rapid rise in airway pressure during the initial phase of inspiration, versus a traditional, volume-limited breath. The corresponding PV loop is demonstrated in **Figure 42.24.** During the initial phase of inspiration, the airway pressures are higher for a given VT, and the PV loop demonstrates an initial "scooping." Although the initial airway pressures are

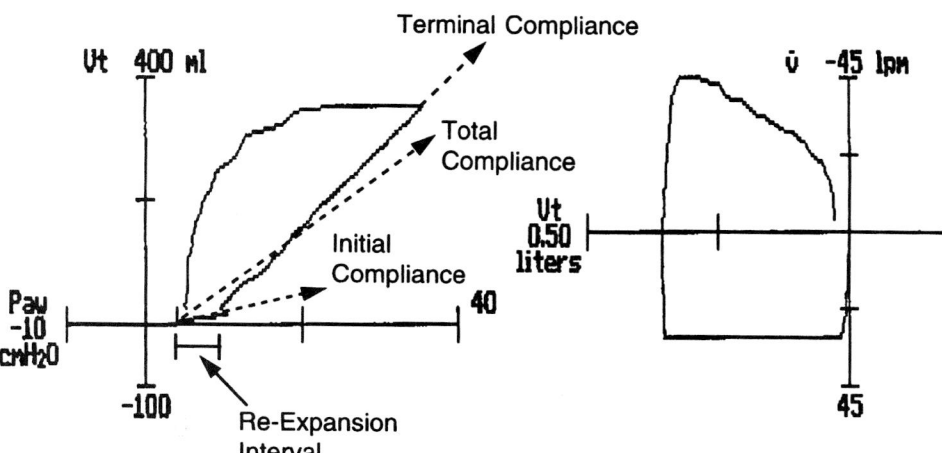

FIGURE 42.21. Pressure-volume and flow-volume loops for volume-limited ventilation during adult respiratory distress syndrome. Figure courtesy of VIASYS Healthcare, Inc., Yorba Linda, California.

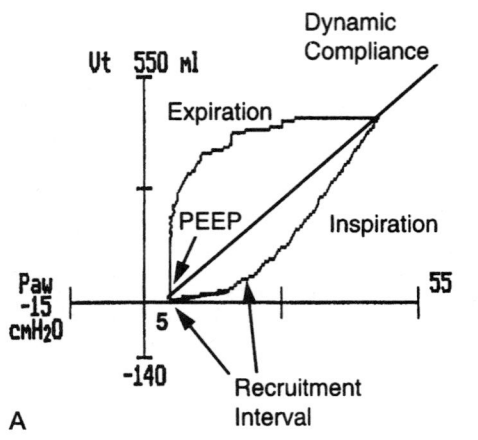

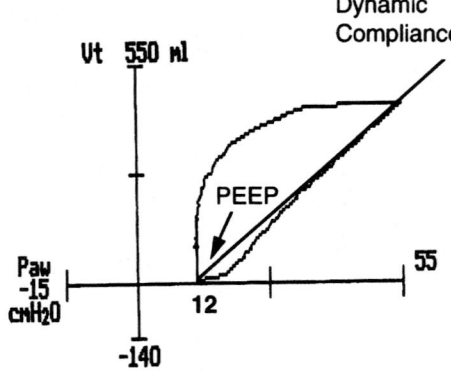

A

B

FIGURE 42.22. Pressure-volume loops indicating the optimization of PEEP during adult respiratory distress syndrome. **A:** Compliance at PEEP +5 cm H_2O. **B:** Compliance at PEEP +12 cm H_2O. Figure courtesy of VIASYS Healthcare, Inc., Yorba Linda, California.

higher for a given VT, the VT is delivered at a lower PIP, and dynamic compliance improves in this setting. This increase in dynamic compliance is demonstrated by the increased slope of the inspiratory loop (line connecting PEEP with PIP). The decelerating, variable inspiratory flow of pressure-control ventilation is higher than the fixed, constant flow of volume-limited ventilation. Thus, the peak inspiratory flow generated may better match the inspiratory demands of the patient.

Detection of Overdistension Using Pressure-Volume Loops

Pulmonary overdistension is defined as an abrupt decrease in compliance at the termination of a breath, demonstrated in the PV loop depicted in **Figure 42.25**. Overdistension occurs when the volume limit of some components of the lung is approached. As the ventilator attempts to provide gas to the patient, airway pressures increase, with little volume being deliv-

ered. Dynamic compliance is decreased, with the inspiratory loop having a reduced slope and terminal "beaking." Overdistension is clinically significant, as it can increase dead space, lead to volutrauma, and increase pulmonary vascular resistance. To eliminate overdistension, the set PIP or VT should be decreased. Additionally, optimization of PEEP may be beneficial. Excessively high PEEP can lead to overdistension of the more compliant regions of lung. PEEP, therefore, should be titrated carefully, as outlined here.

Flow-Volume Loops Demonstrating Airway Obstruction

In **Figure 42.26A**, the delivered inspiratory flow is represented below the baseline as a decelerating wave. During early exhalation, near-complete obstruction to flow results in a high expiratory resistance. In **Figure 42.26B**, the airway obstruction is more severe, and both the inspiratory and expiratory phases are involved. In the inspiratory phase, the decelerating wave form is blunted and approaches a square wave, while in the expiratory phase, the peak flow is limited. Despite an increase in PIP, the VT is reduced as a result of the severity of the obstruction. Both inspiratory resistance and expiratory resistance are elevated, indicating a fixed airway obstruction. Abnormalities of inspiratory and expiratory flow patterns can provide important information as to the presence of airway obstruction and the response of the obstruction to various interventions. Flow abnormalities may be associated with a variety of conditions, including a kinked or blocked ETT (ETT size, position, and need for suctioning should be evaluated), airway obstruction from anatomic causes, and bronchoconstriction (bronchodilators and/or steroids should be considered).

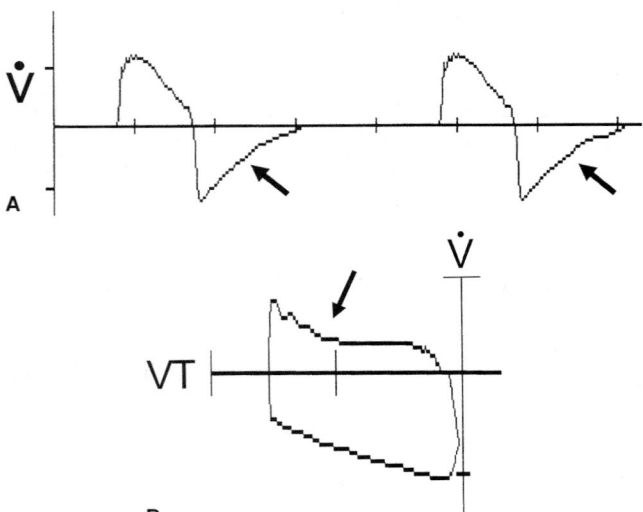

FIGURE 42.23. Increased expiratory resistance. **A:** Airway flow (*V*) is displayed over time. As noted by the arrows, exhalation is significantly prolonged, representing an increased expiratory resistance. **B:** Airway flow is graphed on the vertical axis and tidal volume (*VT*) on the horizontal axis. The arrow again indicates that expiratory flow increases as the expiratory flow rate is greatly reduced early in exhalation.

Optimizing Positive End-expiratory Pressure During Acute Respiratory Distress Syndrome

The decreased slope of a PV loop indicates decreased compliance; ARDS causes a loss of alveolar stability and the development of diffuse atelectasis. Alveolar collapse and a decreased end-expiratory lung volume may occur during the expiratory phase if the airway pressures are not adequate to maintain alveolar patency and opening volume. In **Figure 42.22A**, the PEEP is set at 5 cm H_2O, a setting that is inadequate to maintain alveolar patency and at which a significant amount of alveolar

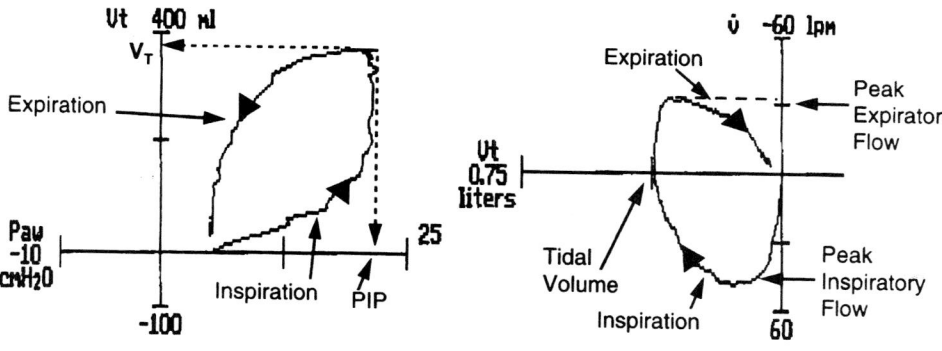

FIGURE 42.24. Normal pressure-volume and flow-volume loops for pressure-limited ventilation. VT, tidal volume. Figure courtesy of VIASYS Healthcare, Inc., Yorba Linda, California.

atelectasis and decreased lung volume occurs during the expiratory phase. During the initial phase of inspiration, re-expansion of the collapsed alveoli is necessary, and the airway pressures increase before a volume of gas is delivered to the patient. Once the opening pressure is reached, the VT is delivered.

The pressure cost of re-expansion is the amount of inspiratory airway pressure that is necessary to initiate the delivery of gas volume. The VT can be delivered only after the critical opening pressure is reached. The development of a significant amount of alveolar atelectasis results in a high pressure cost of re-expansion, which elevates the opening pressure and the PIP that are required to deliver the same VT.

Optimizing PEEP is an essential management strategy in patients with lung injury. By increasing the PEEP from 5 to 12 cm H_2O (**Fig. 42.22B**), a greater number of alveoli are maintained patent during the expiratory phase, and lung volume increases toward normal functional residual capacity. During the initial phase of inspiration, lower airway pressures are required to achieve lung opening, and the pressure cost of re-expansion is less than in **Figure 42.22A**. As lung volume is restored toward functional residual capacity by optimizing PEEP, the PIP required to deliver the VT may decrease over time. As a result, the lung is more compliant, and the VT can be delivered with a smaller change in airway pressure. These effects may

be more dramatic over time, as collapsed alveoli continue to be recruited. Additionally, the risk for ventilator-induced lung injury may decrease as PIP decreases.

Excessive levels of PEEP cause detrimental effects on cardiorespiratory function. These effects include (a) a reduction of venous return and cardiac output secondary to increased intrathoracic pressure, and (b) overdistension of compliant lung units with redistribution of blood flow to the less compliant lung units. To optimize PEEP using graphics, the level of PEEP is increased gradually until the best balance is achieved in the following variables: the lowest PIP to deliver the desired VT, the highest compliance, and the best O_2 delivery (requires a determination/estimate of cardiac output and a measurement of arterial oxygenation).

Dynamic Hyperexpansion/Intrinsic Positive End-expiratory Pressure

The square-wave, constant-flow pattern during inspiration is demonstrated in **Figure 42.27**, as in **Figure 42.18**. The respiratory rate and T_i have been increased, resulting in a dramatic increase in mean airway pressure. With inadequate time to complete exhalation before the next breath is initiated, dynamic hyperexpansion or "gas trapping" occurs. Dynamic hyperexpansion occurs with premature termination of exhalation. Prolongation of the T_i may be beneficial in certain clinical conditions (i.e., ARDS) by decreasing PIP and increasing mean airway pressure, which would be expected to improve oxygenation.

Dynamic hyperexpansion may result in $PEEP_i$, which elevates the baseline airway pressure (externally applied PEEP + $PEEP_i$). However, $PEEP_i$ is relatively uncontrolled compared to set PEEP, which can be more reliably titrated to achieve the desired oxygenation and ventilation end points. The increase in the baseline airway pressure secondary to $PEEP_i$ results in an increase in PIP that is required to maintain the set VT during volume-limited ventilation, or it results in a decrease in VT during pressure-limited ventilation (i.e., set total PIP).

The combination of an increased PIP and development of $PEEP_i$ will cause the mean airway pressure to rise. $PEEP_i$ may be desirable in the management of ARDS, as it results in improved oxygenation. However, careful monitoring of the amount of $PEEP_i$ is required to limit the development of secondary lung injury and hemodynamic compromise due to the increased mean intrathoracic pressure. While prolongation of the T_i may be beneficial, the resulting increase in intrathoracic pressure may compromise cardiac output by limiting venous return. Volume

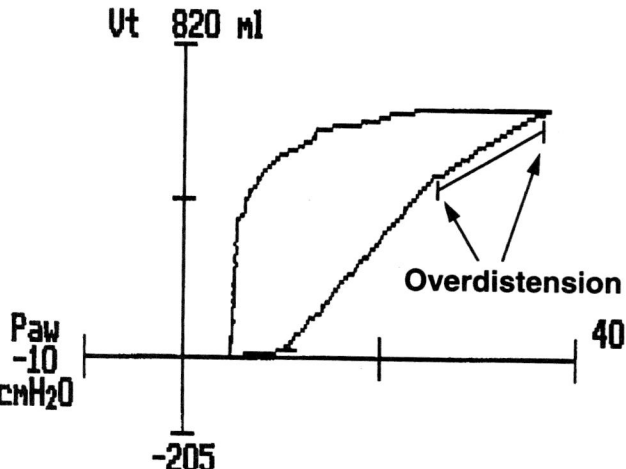

FIGURE 42.25. Pressure-volume loop demonstrating overdistension. Figure courtesy of VIASYS Healthcare, Inc., Yorba Linda, California.

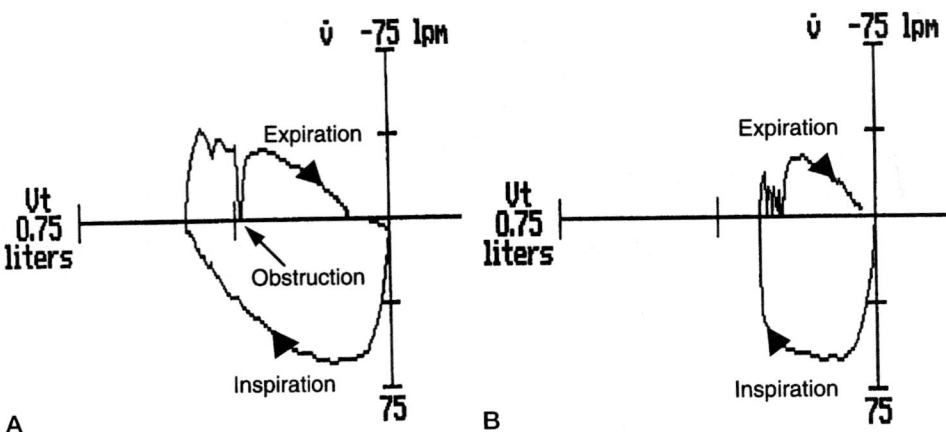

FIGURE 42.26. Flow-volume loops demonstrating airway obstruction. **A:** Mild airway obstruction, resulting in a high expiratory resistance. **B:** Severe airway obstruction that involves increased inspiratory and expiratory resistance. Figure courtesy of VIASYS Healthcare, Inc., Yorba Linda, California.

loading and/or the institution of inotropes may limit the effects of dynamic hyperexpansion/PEEP$_i$ on cardiovascular performance.

Patient Ventilator Asynchrony: Inaccurate Sensing of Patient Effort

Patient effort decreases airway pressure (arrows 1–3 in **Fig. 42.28**) and/or flow from baseline. Decreased airway pressure or flow (depending on the ventilator settings chosen) should result in an assisted mechanical breath in supported ventilation modes. However, with inadequate trigger sensitivity (**Fig. 42.28**), the ventilator is unable to determine that a patient effort has occurred (**Fig. 42.28**, patient breaths 1–3). During patient breath 4, the ventilator delivers the preset VT at the preset rate without regard to patient effort. Inadequate sensing of patient effort leads to tachypnea, increased WOB, patient-ventilator asynchrony, and patient discomfort ("fighting the ventilator"). To improve patient-ventilator synchrony in conditions when the patient effort is not appropriately sensed, trigger sensitivity must be improved. Flow triggering is generally more sensitive

than pressure triggering, as a small change in flow requires less inspiratory effort than a change in pressure.

Asynchrony may also occur when an air leak leads to the loss of PEEP, resulting in excessive ventilator triggering. This reduction in airway pressure or flow may be misinterpreted by the ventilator as a patient effort and result in a mechanical breath being triggered. This abnormality, commonly referred to as *autocycling*, may lead to frequent ventilator triggering without patient effort. In this case, the trigger sensitivity setting and/or the ETT air leak must be assessed.

Patient-Ventilator Asynchrony: Inadequate Ventilatory Support

Figure 42.29 reveals a patient effort that results in a decrease in airway pressure (arrows 1 and 2) and triggering of a mechanical breath. However, the constant inspiratory flow of the delivered mechanical breath is inadequate to meet the patient's inspiratory demands. The patient is not satiated by the constant inspiratory flow of the mechanical breath and, as a result, attempts to initiate a spontaneous breath during the mechanical breath (arrow 3), causing a transient reduction of airway

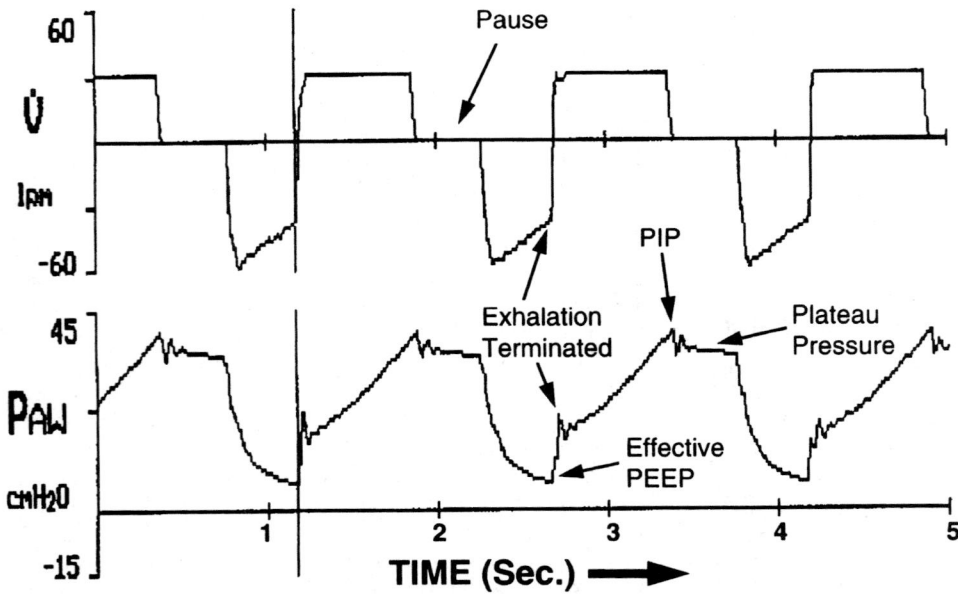

FIGURE 42.27. Scalar display of flow versus time and airway pressure versus time for volume-limited ventilation during adult respiratory distress syndrome. Premature termination of exhalation, which results in dynamic hyperexpansion (gas trapping), is shown. Figure courtesy of VIASYS Healthcare, Inc., Yorba Linda, California.

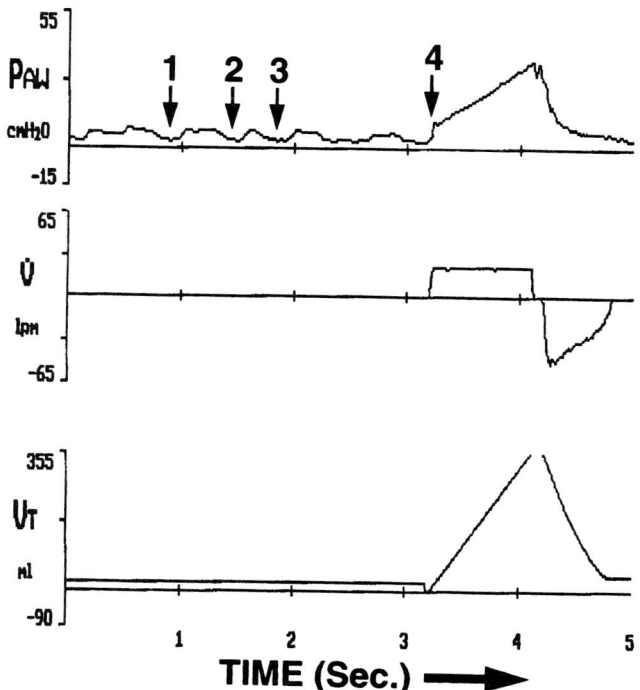

FIGURE 42.28. Scalar display of flow versus time, airway pressure versus time, and tidal volume versus time, representing patient-ventilator asynchrony to inadequate sensing of the patient effort. Figure courtesy of VIASYS Healthcare, Inc., Yorba Linda, California.

pressure, which is signified by a decrease in the airway pressure tracing during inspiration (flow asynchrony). Inadequate ventilatory support to meet the patient's inspiratory needs leads to tachypnea, increased WOB, and patient discomfort ("fighting the ventilator").

In volume-limited ventilation, a reduction of the inspiratory airway pressure as a result of a patient effort (arrow 3) during the mechanical breath may result in an increase in peak inspiratory pressure (arrow 4) being required to achieve the set VT. Increasing the flow rate during patient-assisted, volume-limited ventilation (i.e., constant, square-wave inspira-

tory flow) may eliminate flow asynchrony. The clinician should titrate the flow rate to reduce the drop in airway pressure (arrow 3) and return the airway pressure tracing to a more normal configuration. Additionally, decreasing the T_i or changing to another mode of ventilation with a variable, decelerating inspiratory flow is often beneficial. A variable flow mode may better meet the inspiratory demands of the patient. Such modes include pressure-support ventilation, pressure-assist/control ventilation, and pressure-regulated volume control. When increasing the flow rate or changing the inspiratory flow pattern is unsuccessful, inadequate ventilatory support should be considered as the cause of the patient-ventilator asynchrony.

Airway Graphics—Summary

With the technical advances that have occurred in providing mechanical ventilation for children, multiple modes of ventilation and parameters must be set and monitored by the clinician. The use of airway graphics and continuous capnography provide invaluable tools to help to design the most appropriate strategy for each child and to assess the efficacy of these management strategies (35). Airway graphics provide rapid assessment of the various respiratory parameters, help to generate and test hypotheses of patient management, and monitor for the presence of adverse effects of mechanical ventilation.

Esophageal and Gastric Manometry

Esophageal and gastric manometry are invasive methods by which to assess pressures generated during breathing. Esophageal manometry requires placement of an air-filled balloon attached to a catheter or a fluid-filled catheter in the lower third of the esophagus. In adults, polyethylene catheters with an internal diameter of 1.4 mm and a length of ~100 cm are commonly used. In children, fluid-filled catheters may be preferable, as their frequency response is high due to the noncompressibility of the fluid column in the catheter. The distal end of both systems should have multiple holes. Fluid-filled catheters must be constantly flushed to keep the catheter free of gas bubbles. Ideally, the tip of the catheter should be placed at the junction of the middle and lower third of the esophagus. To validate the position and measurement in spontaneously breathing patients, a dynamic occlusion test is employed. This

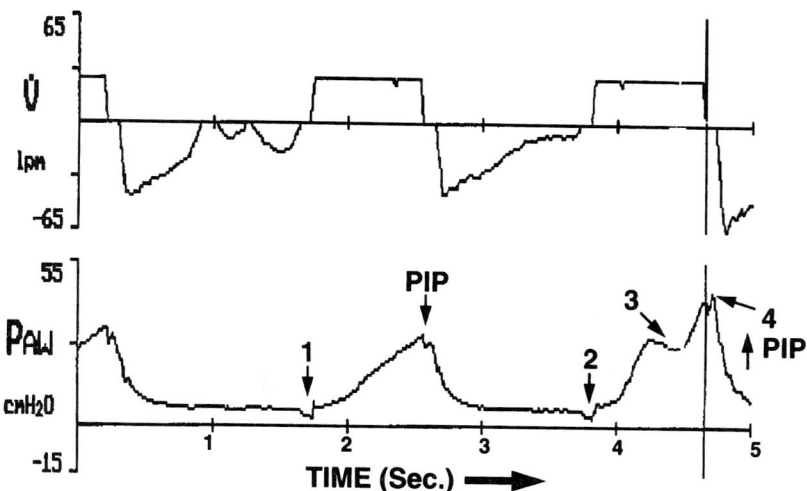

FIGURE 42.29. Scalar display of flow versus time and airway pressure versus time, representing patient-ventilatory asynchrony secondary to inadequate ventilatory support. Figure courtesy of VIASYS Healthcare, Inc., Yorba Linda, California.

requires breathing through an occluded airway, similar to the measurement for P_{Imax}. The change in proximal airway pressure should be the same as the change in the esophageal pressure. To validate the measurements in paralyzed patients, external pressure using a cuirass or a body plethysmograph can be used.

Constraints in measuring esophageal pressure include distortion of the esophagus, esophageal contraction, and uneven distribution of pleural pressures. When combined with measurement of flow and volume at the airway, esophageal manometry can be used to measure WOB, as described later. It has been shown that esophageal pressure monitoring complements readiness testing when patients are being weaned from mechanical ventilation (22).

Measurements of Diaphragmatic Function

Transdiaphragmatic Pressure

Transdiaphragmatic pressure (P_{di}) is defined as the difference between intrathoracic and abdominal pressures. It is usually calculated as the difference between P_{es} and gastric pressure (P_{ga}). Measurement of P_{di} is useful in the diagnosis of diaphragmatic strength, weakness, and fatigability, although few studies have been conducted in critically ill children.

Diaphragmatic Ultrasonography and Fluoroscopy

Diaphragmatic ultrasonography and fluoroscopy can be useful tools in detecting and diagnosing diaphragmatic paresis and paralysis. Diaphragmatic paresis and paralysis can occur from injury to the phrenic nerve or diaphragmatic muscle weakness. Diaphragmatic paresis is diagnosed by the reduction in diaphragm excursion during spontaneous breathing. Unilateral diaphragmatic paralysis can result in paradoxic movement of the diaphragm, when during inspiration, the normal diaphragm moves downward and the paralyzed diaphragm moves upward. It is important that testing be performed without positive pressure applied to the airway.

Measures of Inspiratory Drive

The pressure generated after the onset of inspiratory effort against an occluded airway in the first 100 msec ($P_{0.1}$) provides a measure of respiratory drive. In adults, $P_{0.1}$ can be used to predict weaning outcome. For extubated children, $P_{0.1}$ can be measured by placing a tight-fitting mask over the face and attaching a one-way valve that allows exhalation but not inspiration. When the valve is activated, the patient makes an inspiratory effort against an occluded airway and the pressure can be recorded through a side port in the system. In children who are mechanically ventilated, $P_{0.1}$ can be measured using either a one-way valve attached to the ETT, similar to that used to measure P_{Imax}, and the pressure can be recorded through a side port. Alternatively, with ventilators that allow an expiratory hold maneuver, holding the expiratory "pause/hold" button causes the inspiratory valve to remain closed at expiration. When the patient initiates a spontaneous breath, the inspiratory effort occurs with the airway occluded, and the pressure generated can be recorded to measure $P_{0.1}$. It is important that there be no leak in the system. This maneuver cannot be performed with an uncuffed ETT.

Factors that influence the measurement of $P_{0.1}$ include chest-wall distortion (a problem in young children with compliant chest walls), alteration in expiratory lung volume, time constant of the respiratory system, expiratory muscle activity (such as in lower airway obstruction), shape of the driving pressure wave, and pressure-flow phase lags.

An easier index to measure is the mean inspiratory flow (derived by dividing the VT by the T_i), which can be determined in intubated patients by measuring spontaneous VT and T_i using a pneumotachometer attached to the ETT without applying positive pressure to the airway. It can also be measured using respiratory inductive plethysmography, as previously described.

CONCLUSIONS AND FUTURE DIRECTIONS

As deterioration in respiratory status, including the need for mechanical ventilation, is the most common indication for admission to the PICU, monitoring of the respiratory system is of utmost importance to the pediatric intensivist. Respiratory monitoring is crucial to the optimal management of a critically ill infant or child to aid with diagnosis, to augment understanding of the child's pathophysiology, to assess the status and progress of a disease, and to provide data for management. Methods of monitoring the respiratory system have improved immensely in recent years, including advances in the areas of pulse oximetry, transcutaneous monitoring, and capnography. While physical examination continues to have significant clinical relevance, the incorporation of all aspects of cardiorespiratory monitoring into a comprehensive, responsive assessment system is essential to the management of critically ill infants and children.

The future of respiratory monitoring will clearly include continued hardware and software advances. More importantly, the future will likely bring an improved assessment of the available data, including smart prompts to help guide complex clinical decisions and closed feedback loops, in which the monitored data will be incorporated into management devices (i.e., ventilators) to affect routine patient care without the direct intervention of a clinician.

KEY POINTS

- Technology augments physical examination. A physical exam is often the deciding factor between monitor error and a true change in a child's status.
- Cardiorespiratory distress in infants and children is often associated with abnormalities in oxygenation and ventilation and thus requires diligent monitoring.
- Pulse oximetry is an integral part of all PICU monitoring systems. A key premise of pulse oximeters is that they are capable of early identification of changes in a patient's cardiorespiratory status, allowing for a rapid response. Recent software advances have helped to improve the clinical usefulness of this monitoring tool.
- Significant advances have occurred in transcutaneous monitor technology. The continuous monitoring and trending of CO_2 and O_2 can be useful in critically ill patients, especially in neonates and infants.
- Capnography (both time- and volume-based) is playing an increasingly important role in the management of critically

ill infants and children. Responses to changes in ventilatory strategies and cardiac function can be detected and trended with capnography.

■ Waveform analysis can be used to optimize mechanical ventilation and to analyze ventilator incidents and alarm conditions. Using this technology, it is possible to shape the form of ventilatory support to improve patient-ventilator synchrony, reduce WOB, and calculate physiologic parameters related to respiratory mechanics.

References

1. Anonymous. VIII ESPID Conference (European Society for the Study and Prevention of Infant Death), the International Conference on Prevention of Infantile Apnea and Sudden Infant Death on the Verge of the Millennium. *Pediatr Res* 1999;45(5):1A–52A.
2. Aoyagi T, Miyasaka K. Pulse oximetry: Its invention, contribution to medicine and future tasks. *Anesth Analg* 2002;94(1):S1–S3.
3. Barker SJ. "Motion-resistant" pulse oximetry: A comparison of new and old models. *Anesth Analg* 2002;95(4):967–72.
4. Berkenbosch JW, Lam J, Burd RS, et al. Noninvasive monitoring of carbon dioxide during mechanical ventilation in older children: End-tidal versus transcutaneous techniques. *Anesth Analg* 2001;92:1427–31.
5. Berkenbosch JW, Tobias JD. Transcutaneous carbon dioxide monitoring during high-frequency oscillatory ventilation in infants and children. *Crit Care Med* 2002;30(5):1024–7.
6. Bohnhorst B, Peter CS, Poets CF. Pulse oximeters' reliability in detecting hypoxemia and bradycardia: Comparison between a conventional and 2 new generation oximeters. *Crit Care Med* 2002;28(5):1565–8.
7. Cannon ML, Cornell J, Tripp-Hamel DS, et al. Tidal volume measurements in infants should be obtained with a pneumotachometer located at the endotracheal tube. *Am J Resp Crit Care Med* 2000;162(6):2109–12.
8. Carter BG, Wiwczaruk D, Hochmann M, et al. Performance of transcutaneous PCO$_2$ and pulse oximetry monitors in newborns and infants after cardiac surgery. *Anaesth Intensive Care* 2001;29(3):260–5.
9. Castle RA, Dunne CJ, Mok Q, et al. Accuracy of displayed tidal volume in the pediatric intensive care unit. *Crit Care Med* 2002;39(11):2566–74.
10. Chawla LS, Zia H, Gutierrez G, et al. Lack of equivalence between central and mixed venous oxygen saturation. *Chest* 2004;126(6):1891–6.
11. Chow LC, Vanderhal A, Raber J, et al. Are tidal volume measurements in neonatal pressure-controlled ventilation accurate? *Pediatr Pulmonol* 2002; 34:196–202.
12. Cullen DJ, Nemeskal AR, Cooper JB, et al. Effect of pulse oximetry, age, and ASA physical status on the frequency of patients admitted unexpectedly to a postoperative intensive care unit and the severity of their anesthesia-related complications. *Anesth Analg.* 1992;74(2):181–8.
13. Dimitriou G, Greenough A, Raffert GF, et al. Effect of maturity on maximal transdiaphragmatic pressure in infants during crying. *Am J Respir Crit Care Med* 2001;164:433–6.
14. Dueck MH, Klimek M, Appenrodt S, et al. Trends but not individual values of central venous oxygen saturation agree with mixed venous oxygen saturation during varying hemodynamic conditions. *Anesthesiology* 2005;103(2):249–57.
15. Durbin CG Jr, Rostow SK. More reliable oximetry reduces the frequency of arterial blood gas analyses and hastens oxygen weaning after cardiac surgery:
a prospective, randomized trial of the clinical impact of a new technology. *Crit Care Med* 2002;30(8):1735–40.
16. Farias JA, Alia I, Retta A, et al. An evaluation of extubation failure predictors in mechanically ventilated infants and children. *Intensive Care Med* 2002;28:752–7.
17. Hatzakis GE, Davis GM. Fuzzy logic controller for weaning neonates from mechanical ventilation. Proceedings/AMIA. *Annual Symposium*, 2002:315–9.
18. Hemmila MR, Napolitano LM. Severe respiratory failure: Advanced treatment options. *Crit Care Med* 2006;34(9):S278–S290.
19. Johnson JL, Breen PH. How does positive end-expiratory pressure decrease pulmonary CO$_2$ elimination in anesthetized patients? *Respiratory Physiology,* 1999;118(2–3):227–36.
20. Jopling MW, Mannheimer PD, Bebout DE. Issues in the laboratory evaluation of pulse oximeter performance. *Anesth Analg* 2002;94:S62–8.
21. Jubran A. Pulse oximetry. *Intensive Care Med* 2004;30(11):2017–20.
22. Jubran A, Grant BJ, Laghi F, et al. Weaning prediction: Esophageal pressure monitoring complements readiness testing. *Am J Resp Crit Care Med* 2005; 171(11):1252–9.
23. Knapp S, Kofler J, Stoiser B, et al. The assessment of 4 different methods to verify tracheal tube placement in the critical care setting. *Anesthesia Analg* 1999;88(4):766–70.
24. Kocis KC, Dekeon MK, Rosen HK, et al. Pressure-regulated volume control vs. volume control ventilation in infants after surgery for congenital heart disease. *Pediatr Cardiol* 2001;22(3):233–7.
25. Koechlin C, Matecki S, Jaber S, et al. Changes in respiratory muscle endurance during puberty. *Pediatr Pulmonol* 2005;40:197–204.
26. Lee WW, Mayberry K, Crapo R, et al. The accuracy of pulse oximetry in the emergency department. *Am J Emerg Med* 2000;18(4):427–31.
27. Li J. Capnography alone is imperfect for endotracheal tube placement confirmation during emergency intubation. *J Emerg Med* 2001;20(3):223–9.
28. Manthous CA. The anarchy of weaning techniques. *Chest* 2002;121(6): 1738–40.
29. Matecki S, Prioux J, Jaber S, et al. Respiratory pressures in boys from 11–17 years old: A semi-longitudinal study. *Pediatr Pulmonol* 2003;35(5):368–74.
30. Moller JT, Johannessen NW, Espersen K, et al. Randomized evaluation of pulse oximetry in 20,802 patients: II. Perioperative events and postoperative complications. *Anesthesiology* 1993;78(3):445–53.
31. Ochroch EA, Russell MW, Hanson WC, et al. The impact of continuous pulse oximetry monitoring on intensive care unit admissions from a post-surgical care floor. *Anesth Analg* 2006;102(3):868–75.
32. Poets CF, Urschitz MS, Bohnhorst B. Pulse oximetry in the neonatal intensive care unit (NICU): Detection of hyperoxemia and false alarm rates. *Anesth Analg* 2002;94(1):S41–3.
33. Soo Hoo GW, Park L. Variations in the measurement of weaning parameters: A survey of respiratory therapists. *Chest* 2002;121(6):1947–55.
34. Tatevossian RG, Wo CCJ, Velmahos GC, et al. Transcutaneous oxygen and CO$_2$ as early warning of tissue hypoxia and hemodynamic shock in critically ill emergency patients. *Crit Care Med* 2000;28(7):2248–53.
35. Tobin MJ, Jubran A, Laghi F. Patient-ventilator interaction. *Am J Resp Crit Care Med* 2001;163(5):1059–63.
36. Venkataraman ST, Khan N, Brown A. Validation of predictors of extubation success and failure in mechanically ventilated infants and children. *Crit Care Med* 2000;28:2991–6.
37. Wallach PM, Roscoe L, Bowden R. The profession of medicine: An integrated approach to basic principles. *Acad Med* 2002;77(11):1168–9.
38. Willis BC, Graham AS, Wetzel R, et al. Respiratory inductance plethysmography used to diagnose bilateral diaphragmatic paralysis: A case report. *Pediatr Crit Care Med* 2004;5(4):399–402.
39. Wouters PF, Gehring H, Meyfroidt G, et al. Accuracy of pulse oximeters: The European multi-center trial. *Anesth Analg* 2002;94(1):S13–S110.

CHAPTER 43 ■ STATUS ASTHMATICUS

MICHAEL T. BIGHAM • RICHARD J. BRILLI

Asthma is the most common chronic disease of childhood and accounts for a growing number of pediatric hospitalizations each year (9,22). Although the prevalence of asthma has reached a plateau, asthma-related mortality continues to be high (3,27). Consequently, national organizations continue to provide guidelines that describe optimal treatment for this common childhood illness (37). A clinical description of the pathophysiology, clinical presentation, and current treatment for children hospitalized in the PICU with status asthmaticus is the focus of this chapter.

DEFINITION

The word "asthma" is derived from the Greek verb "aazein," meaning to exhale with open mouth, to pant. The first recorded use of this word was 2700 years ago in Homer's *Iliad*, where it was used to describe hard breathing or short-drawn breaths. Homer described a warrior who died after a furious battle with "asthma and perspiration." Asthma was first used in a clinical context by Hippocrates (circa 460–360 BC). Asthma was mixed into his descriptions of respiratory findings, such as dyspnea, tachypnea, and orthopnea. The best clinical description of asthma in antiquity was by the Greek physician Aretaeus, approximately 500 years after Hippocrates. He devoted an entire chapter of his writings to detailed descriptions of asthma, suggesting that the cause of asthma was "a coldness and humidity of pneuma but the result was a thick viscid humor." Today, discussion does not include pneuma or viscid humor; rather, asthma is defined as "a chronic inflammatory disorder... causing recurrent episodes ... of wheezing, breathlessness, chest tightness, (and) coughing .... associated with airflow obstruction that is often reversible" (37). Status asthmaticus is a condition of progressively worsening bronchospasm and respiratory dysfunction due to asthma, which is unresponsive to standard conventional therapy and may progress to respiratory failure and the need for mechanical ventilation (2). For this review, status asthmaticus is defined as severe asthma that fails to respond to inhaled β agonists, oral or IV steroids, and O_2, and that requires admission to the hospital for treatment.

EPIDEMIOLOGY

Worldwide, an estimated 300 million people suffer from asthma. In children, the prevalence of asthma varies significantly by country, with the highest rates in the UK, Australia, and New Zealand, and the lowest in Eastern Europe, China, and Indonesia. Asthma prevalence is increasing in children <12 years of age and in regions with progressive urbanization. In the US, asthma affects 6 million children <18 years of age and is the leading cause of chronic illness in children. The economic burden of asthma is substantial, with ~10 million missed school days and $US726 million lost because of missed work. Asthma accounts for 470,000 (adults and children) annual hospital admissions across the US and is the leading cause of hospital admission for children <18 years of age (23). It is estimated that 13%–55% of all dollars spent on asthma care are hospital related, and status asthmaticus remains a leading cause of PICU admission (30).

Asthma-related death rates in American children nearly doubled between 1980 and 1995, but recently have stabilized (9). The number of asthma deaths in all age groups in the US is ~5000 per year, with 150–200 of those occurring in children <15 years of age (22). Most asthma-related deaths in children occur as a result of respiratory failure or cardiopulmonary arrest that occurs prior to obtaining medical care. Models that seek to predict fatal asthma focus upon identifying clinical, psychosocial, and ethnic risk factors (39). Clinical risks include a past history of ICU admission, respiratory failure, or rapid, sudden, severe deterioration (31,36). Psychosocial and ethnic risk factors include poor compliance with outpatient medical treatment, failure to perceive the severity of asthma attack, inner-city residence, denial of disease severity, and nonwhite race. African American children are four to six times more likely to die from asthma than are white children. Despite the aforementioned risk factors, nearly half of fatal asthma exacerbations occur in children with mild asthma. It is suggested that some of these deaths occur in a subpopulation of patients with decreased sensitivity to dyspnea or another group with "sudden asphyxial asthma" (19,34). This latter entity is characterized by rapid, sudden, severe airway obstruction that progresses to hypoxemic respiratory arrest over a short period, usually before presentation to medical care.

MECHANISM OF DISEASE: CORE PATHOPHYSIOLOGY

Genetics

No single asthma gene has been identified. It is likely that the disease is both polygenetic and environmentally influenced. More than 20 chromosomal regions have been linked to asthma. The most consistently linked regions have been on chromosomes 2q, 5q, 6p, 12q, and 13q (24). It is known that asthma inheritance is likely related to the inheritance of atopy. Studies in twins with asthma reveal significant genetic similarities but not identical phenotypic manifestations of asthma. This variation in disease severity may occur because airway hyperresponsiveness may be genetically distinct from atopy and is further confounded by gene-gene and gene-environmental interactions. The gene polymorphisms of the β_2 adrenergic receptors Arg16Gly and Gln27Glu have been examined in depth in an effort to clarify the phenotypic variability of airway hyperresponsiveness. A recent metaanalysis showed that the Arg16Gly allele of the β_2 adrenergic receptor gene predisposes to nocturnal asthma, but neither polymorphism modulates the risk for bronchial hyperresponsiveness (13). The clinical application of specific genetic profiles to both asthma prevention and treatment remains in the future.

Inflammation and Immunobiology

Asthma is an inflammatory disease characterized by air-flow obstruction due to airway hyperresponsiveness and bronchospasm and airway inflammation with mucosal edema and mucous plugging of the small airways. Airway inflammation is characterized by the submucosal cellular infiltrate of eosinophils, mast cells, and CD4 lymphocytes. The presence of these cells correlates with disease severity. The cascade of inflammation begins with degranulation of mast cells, usually in response to allergen exposure. Activated mast cells release histamine and leukotrienes, both activators of early airway smooth muscle spasm. The activated mast cells further activate T lymphocytes, which produce inflammatory cytokines (TH2) and IL-4, -5, and -13 (8). In addition, chemokines (leukotriene B4) are released, which attract neutrophils and promote further activation of the proinflammatory cascade. Submucosal infiltration by eosinophils, neutrophils, and activated lymphocytes, is responsible for late or delayed bronchospasm. The differentiation between "early" and "delayed" bronchospasm is important because early bronchospasm may be more sensitive to bronchodilating agents, while late bronchospasm is refractory to bronchodilation and more sensitive to anti-inflammatory therapy. This inflammatory environment results in overproduction of mucus; injury to airway epithelium that exposes nerve endings, which augments airway irritability; hyperresponsiveness; and mucosal edema. The final common pathway for the inflammatory cascade is bronchoconstriction and mechanical airway obstruction by edema and mucus.

The autonomic nervous system also contributes to bronchoconstriction through parasympathetic activation of M_3 receptors by acetylcholine and excitatory nonadrenergic, noncholinergic pathways mediated by tachykinins. Similar parasympathetic pathways stimulate mucous production and concomitant airway obstruction.

Pulmonary Mechanics and Gas Exchange Abnormalities

Pulmonary mechanical dysfunction occurs as a result of pathologic changes in bronchial smooth muscle contraction, mucosal edema, and increased mucous production, which cause decreased airway diameter and increased airflow resistance. During inspiration, negative pleural pressure causes physiologic intrathoracic airway dilation; however, during expiration, pleural pressure approaches zero, causing physiologic intrathoracic airway narrowing. In status asthmaticus, with pathologically narrowed and obstructed airways, these physiologic differences in airway diameter result in easier air entry

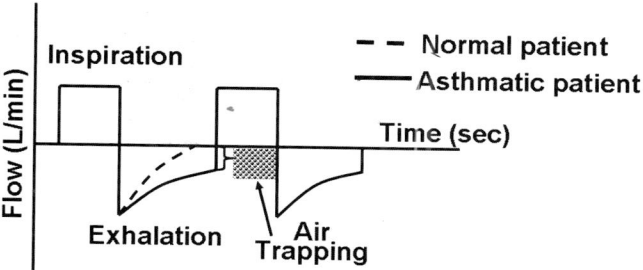

FIGURE 43.1. Flow-time waveform showing persistence of air flow at end expiration and resultant air trapping.

during inspiration but airflow obstruction during expiration, causing air trapping with each breath and lung hyperinflation (**Fig. 43.1**). With higher end-expiratory lung volumes, coupled with the fact that bronchospasm leads to increased airway resistance and reduced expiratory flow, expiration becomes an active, rather than passive, process that results in high energy expenditure and substantial increased work of breathing (WOB). Diaphragmatic flattening from hyperinflation causes additional mechanical disadvantages for the muscles of expiration and additional energy expenditure. Both forced expiratory volume and forced vital capacity are decreased in status asthmaticus as a result of high airway resistance. Total lung volumes are increased because of increased functional residual capacity.

Gas exchange abnormalities in status asthmaticus are due to ventilation-perfusion ($\dot{V}/\dot{Q}$) mismatch, including increased intrapulmonary shunt (atelectasis) and increased dead space (airway overdistension) that result from small airway obstruction due to mucous plugging, edema, and bronchoconstriction. Typically, these gas exchange abnormalities initially manifest as hypoxemia and hypocarbia. Atelectasis from small-airway obstruction causes areas of decreased ventilation but adequate pulmonary blood flow, and the resultant shunt leads to arterial hypoxemia. As disease severity worsens, greater distal airway obstruction causes alveolar distention and increased pulmonary dead space. To compensate for this worsening $\dot{V}/\dot{Q}$ mismatch, tachypnea occurs. Despite increasing dead space to tidal volume ratio (V_d/V_t), hypocarbia persists because minute ventilation increases. Finally, intercostal and diaphragmatic muscles fatigue. Increased minute ventilation is unable to compensate for the greatly increased V_d/V_t ratio, and hypercarbia results. As fatigue worsens, progressive hypoxemia and hypercarbia ensue and result in respiratory failure.

Cardiopulmonary Interactions in Asthma

Dynamic hyperinflation in severe asthma can have significant cardiopulmonary consequences. First, high lung volumes stretch the pulmonary vasculature, increasing pulmonary vascular resistance and increasing right ventricular afterload, which may compromise right ventricular function. In addition, fluctuations in pleural pressures produce significant effects on the intrathoracic vessels and right atrial venous return. During the large, negative intrathoracic pressure observed during inspiration, left ventricular afterload is increased and systolic blood pressure is decreased. Exaggerated variation in systolic blood pressure associated with intrathoracic pressure variation

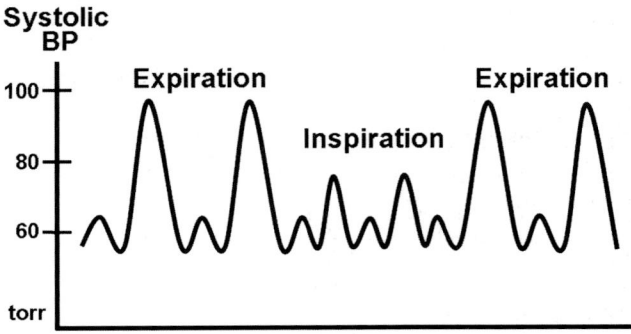

FIGURE 43.2. Pulsus paradoxus in status asthmaticus.

during inspiration is termed *pulsus paradoxus* (17) (**Fig. 43.2**). Systolic blood pressure decreases of >10–15 torr are associated with declining respiratory function in children with status asthmaticus (17).

CLINICAL PRESENTATION AND DIFFERENTIAL DIAGNOSIS

Differential Diagnosis

Children with moderate-to-severe status asthmaticus have varying degrees of respiratory distress and gas exchange abnormalities. Wheezing is the clinical hallmark of asthma; however, it is critical to consider the broad differential of the wheezing child prior to embarking on a diagnostic and therapeutic course to treat status asthmaticus. The differential diagnosis of wheezing is large, but the possibilities can be grouped into diagnoses that require differentiation at the time of first evaluation and those that may allow a more deliberative evaluation. Four disparate clinical entities must be distinguished when the patient is first evaluated because each of these entities results in different diagnostic and therapeutic approaches. These entities are asthma, pneumonia, foreign-body aspiration, and congestive heart failure (**Fig. 43.3**).

Other diagnostic considerations in the differential diagnosis of wheezing can be divided into upper and lower airway diseases. These clinical entities are more likely to present with chronic or recurrent symptoms, and, as such, a more contemplative evaluation may take place. Upper airway obstruction, while usually presenting with stridor, can also present with wheezing. Diagnostic considerations include fixed anatomic lesions, such as vocal cord paralysis, anatomic webs, and airway hemangiomas, or dynamic airway obstruction, such as laryngeal malacia, tracheal malacia, or bronchomalacia. Congenital anomalies, such as complete tracheal rings and bronchial slings, may also present with wheezing. Lower airway diseases that should be considered in addition to infection and congestive heart failure include cystic fibrosis and α_1 antitrypsin deficiency.

History

Children with status asthmaticus typically present with respiratory distress, cough, and wheezing that has progressed over

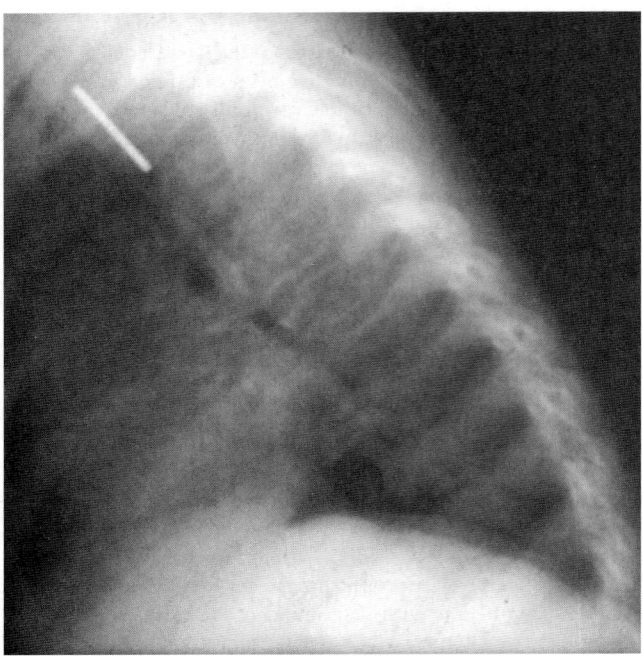

FIGURE 43.3. Chest radiograph of patient who presented with diffuse wheezing, revealing a coin in the esophagus.

1–2 days. Allergen exposure or upper respiratory tract infection are often triggers for the onset of illness and are frequently identified by the child or family as inciting events. In contrast, foreign-body aspiration will usually present with an abrupt onset of clinical symptoms. Assessing the time course of a wheezing episode is important to help distinguish diagnostic considerations and to determine the urgency of required therapeutic interventions. The presence of fever suggests lower respiratory infection, though asthma and pneumonia can both be present at the same time. When time permits, it is important to determine the presence of high-risk factors for asthma severity and fatality, including previous severe sudden deterioration, past PICU admissions, and previous respiratory failure with the need for mechanical ventilation.

Physical Exam

The rapid assessment of a child with status asthmaticus should focus upon determining the severity of airway obstruction. The use of the "rapid 30-sec cardiopulmonary assessment," as described by the American Heart Association, will allow quick determination of general appearance, airway patency, effectiveness of respiratory effort, and adequacy of circulation (4). Children with severe status asthmaticus often appear lethargic and diaphoretic, are unable to phonate, and have severe retractions with paradoxic thoracoabdominal breathing. Poor air movement found on chest auscultation is an ominous sign of impending respiratory or cardiopulmonary failure.

Wheezing, which reflects turbulent air flow in obstructed airways, is usually equally audible on both hemithoraces. Asymmetric wheezing may imply unilateral atelectasis, pneumothorax, or foreign body. Expiratory wheezing alone is found

TABLE 43.1

BECKER PULMONARY INDEX SCORE FOR ASTHMA

Score	Respiratory rate	Wheezing	Inspiratory/ expiratory ratio	Accessory muscle use
0	<30	None	1:1.5	None
1	30–40	Terminal expiration	1:2.0	1 site
2	41–50	Entire expiration	1:3.0	2 sites
3	>50	Inspiration and entire expiration	>1:3.0	3 sites or neck strap muscle use

in mild-to-moderate illness, whereas expiratory plus inspiratory wheezing is present in moderate-to-severe status asthmaticus. The "silent chest" is an ominous sign and may indicate either pneumothorax or the complete absence of air flow due to severe airway obstruction and imminent respiratory failure. Hypoxemia, as estimated by measured pulse oximetry, is another sign of asthma severity. Several clinical asthma scores have been used to objectively assess the severity of status asthmaticus (41). The Becker asthma score (Table 43.1), modified by DiGiulio, determines severity by rating the acuity of four clinical characteristics—respiratory rate, wheezing, inspiratory:expiratory ratio, and accessory muscle use—and has the advantage of not requiring a PaO_2 measurement, which is used in the Wood/Downes score (15). A Becker score >4 is considered moderate status asthmaticus and has been used as entry criteria for several inpatient asthma treatment trials. Children with scores ≥7 should be admitted to the ICU. While such scores are valuable in clinical studies, they are not effective in predicting progression of clinical illness. Serial measurements allow an objective determination of disease progression, though significant interobserver variability is often associated with assigning clinical scores, which limits the usefulness of scoring systems in the active clinical environment.

Laboratory Evaluation

Laboratory tests commonly obtained in children with status asthmaticus include arterial or venous blood gas determination, complete blood count, and a basic metabolic panel. For spontaneously breathing children with status asthmaticus, clinical interventions should be primarily based upon the physical examination and not upon blood gas determinations. Typically, early in the course of severe asthma, arterial hypoxemia and hypocarbia are found as a result of $\dot{V}/\dot{Q}$ mismatch and hyperventilation. As the air trapping worsens and V_d/V_t increase, hypocarbia may be replaced by normal or elevated $PaCO_2$. Normal $PaCO_2$ in a tachypneic, hyperventilating child with status asthmaticus warrants close clinical observation and may be a sign of early respiratory muscle fatigue. Lactic acidosis is often present in status asthmaticus and usually reflects a combination of dehydration and excess lactate production from overuse of the respiratory musculature. Rarely, it can suggest poor perfusion from impaired cardiac function that is associated with the increased ventricular afterload caused by negative intrathoracic pressures (up to minus 60 to 100 cmH_2O). The presence of leukocytosis on complete blood count may suggest respiratory

infection as the source of wheezing, though it can also represent a stress response to steroid administration or a response to β-agonist therapy. The white blood cell count in conjunction with chest x-ray and the presence or absence of fever will help to determine the need for antibiotic therapy. A basic metabolic panel may be useful to assess the degree of dehydration and the level of electrolyte disturbance. Hypokalemia may result from intracellular potassium shifts from exposure to β-agonist therapy in children with status asthmaticus. Determining serum magnesium values may be important because the correction of relative hypomagnesemia in status asthmaticus may improve outcome.

Radiographic Evaluation

A chest x-ray is not required at the time of hospital admission for all spontaneously breathing children with status asthmaticus; however, all children with first-time wheezing or patients who require PICU admission should receive a chest x-ray. Clinically relevant findings, such as evidence of an infectious infiltrate, pneumothorax, cardiomegaly, pulmonary edema, or even unsuspected chest masses, may be identified.

CLINICAL MANAGEMENT

Emergency Management in Anticipation of PICU Admission

Most children with asthma who are seen in the emergency department do not require hospital admission. Others with mild-to-moderate status asthmaticus require inpatient care and are usually treated with O_2, inhaled bronchodilators, and systemic corticosteroids. A small percentage of children require PICU admission. Clinical parameters that suggest the need for PICU admission are ill defined; however, children with past PICU admissions or a history of rapid clinical deterioration, children with severe distress (inspiratory and expiratory wheezing, limited air entry, air hunger, and inability to phonate) despite initial bronchodilator therapy, or those with a Becker asthma score ≥7 should be considered for PICU admission. Other indications for PICU admission include the child's sense of impending clinical doom, altered mental status, respiratory arrest, and a rising $PaCO_2$ coupled with clinical signs of fatigue (26). Recognizing the severely ill child with status asthmaticus and providing rapid aggressive care in the emergency department can interrupt a cycle of progressive air trapping, air hunger, and respiratory fatigue, and potentially prevent the onset of respiratory failure that may require mechanical ventilation.

Emergency-department management of a child with severe status asthmaticus should focus upon the assessment of impending respiratory failure, followed by therapeutic interventions, including, but not limited to, obtaining IV access, providing supplemental O_2 and continuous inhaled β-agonists, and administering IV methylprednisolone. Some suggest that IV magnesium and/or IV β-agonists should be administered in the emergency department to aggressively treat severe status asthmaticus and prevent progression to the need for mechanical ventilation.

PICU Management

General Care Issues

Children admitted to the PICU require IV access, continuous cardiorespiratory monitoring, and continuous pulse oximetry. For spontaneously breathing children in the PICU, frequent blood gas monitoring is not required. Such children can usually be managed with close clinical observation without indwelling arterial or central venous catheters. For children who require mechanical ventilation, a Foley catheter and arterial and central venous access are required.

Fluids

Critically ill children with status asthmaticus are often dehydrated as a result of decreased oral intake prior to admission and increased insensible fluid losses from increased minute ventilation. Providing appropriate fluid resuscitation and ongoing maintenance fluid is essential; however, overhydration should be avoided because these children are at risk for pulmonary edema due to microvascular permeability, increased left ventricular afterload, and alveolar fluid migration associated with the inflammatory lung process in asthma.

Oxygen

Most children with severe status asthmaticus will have some degree of mucous plugging, atelectasis, $\dot{V}/\dot{Q}$ mismatch, and hypoxemia. In those lung segments with atelectasis, compensatory hypoxic pulmonary vasoconstriction is often present. Treatment with inhaled β-agonists may induce generalized pulmonary vasodilatation and, as a result, exacerbate $\dot{V}/\dot{Q}$ mismatch and worsen hypoxemia. O_2 should be a part of the management for *all* children with status asthmaticus.

Corticosteroids

The overriding physiologic derangement in asthma is airway inflammation, and corticosteroids are a mainstay in the management of both acute and chronic asthma. Among their many actions, glucocorticosteroids suppress cytokine production, granulocyte-macrophage colony-stimulating factor, and inducible nitric oxide synthase activation, which are all important components of the inflammatory processes involved in the pathophysiology of asthma. As a result of their immunosuppressive activity, corticosteroids impede recruitment and activation of inflammatory cells, decrease airway mucous production, and attenuate microvascular permeability.

Systemically administered corticosteroids reduce asthma hospitalization rates and hospital length of stay (28). Inhaled corticosteroids are of no clinical benefit in the treatment of status asthmaticus. While some emergency-department data suggest that enteral and parenteral administration of corticosteroids are of equal efficacy, the child in the PICU is less likely to tolerate oral medications, and therefore, oral steroid administration is of limited value in these cases (5). Methylprednisolone is the most common agent used in the PICU and is preferred because of its limited mineralocorticoid effects. The initial dose is 2 mg/kg, followed by 0.5–1 mg/kg/dose administered IV every 6 hrs. Other agents that are sometimes used include dexamethasone and hydrocortisone. Systemic corticosteroids begin to exert their effect in 1–3 hrs and reach maximal effect in 4–8 hrs (12). Treatment duration depends upon the severity of illness but generally continues until the asthma exacerbation is resolved. Short courses of steroid treatment are generally well tolerated. Side effects often observed in the critically ill child include hyperglycemia, hypertension, and occasionally, agitation related to steroid-induced psychosis. These symptoms may be difficult to separate from those induced by β-agonist therapy. Prolonged steroid use may cause hypothalamic-pituitary-adrenal axis suppression, osteoporosis, myopathy, and weakness. The incidence of myopathy and weakness is increased when neuromuscular blocking agents are concomitantly administered in the mechanically ventilated asthmatic patient (21).

Inhaled β-Agonists

β-agonists, as sympathomimetic agents, cause direct bronchial smooth muscle relaxation and are key components of acute and chronic asthma therapy. Bronchial smooth muscles express β_2 adrenergic receptors, which are activated by binding with β-agonists. Activation of the receptor, which is G-protein–coupled, results in activation of adenylate cyclase and increased cyclic AMP (cAMP) and cAMP-dependent protein kinase (protein kinase A, PKA). PKA promotes calcium (Ca^+) efflux and inhibits Ca^+ influx in the sarcolemma, while enhancing Ca^+ uptake in the sarcoplasmic reticulum. This PKA-dependent Ca^+ regulation results in decreased actin-myosin interactions and smooth muscle relaxation. In the treatment of status asthmaticus, inhaled β-agonists are a bridge to support ventilation and oxygenation until the anti-inflammatory effects of corticosteroids take effect.

In the US, albuterol and terbutaline are commonly available, short-acting, selective β_2 agonists used for inhalation therapy. Terbutaline is less β_2 selective, compared to albuterol and, therefore, used less often for inhalation therapy than albuterol. Albuterol for inhalation is available in two forms: albuterol (salbutamol) and levalbuterol. Albuterol is a racemic mixture of two equal parts of mirror image forms: R-enantiomers and S-enantiomers. The R-enantiomer is the pharmacologically active enantiomer. The S-enantiomer is considered pharmacologically inactive, has a longer elimination half-life, and may contribute to airway irritation as a spasmogen. Levalbuterol consists solely of the R-enantiomer of albuterol, and some have suggested that levalbuterol has improved efficacy with fewer adverse effects when compared to racemic albuterol. In comparison trials, the use of levalbuterol has not proved superior to racemic albuterol (25). Currently, racemic albuterol remains the mainstay of inhaled β-agonist therapy in the ICU.

The delivery of albuterol in both acute and nonacute asthma has been studied extensively. The two primary delivery mechanisms are via small-volume nebulizer and metered-dose inhaler (MDI), usually with a vehicle-delivery device (i.e., spacer). Breath-actuated, inhaled β-agonist delivery devices are another relatively new delivery method; however, little data are available regarding the use of these devices in children with status asthmaticus. Intermittent MDI dosing is infrequently used in the critically ill child with status asthmaticus. Continuous albuterol nebulization is superior to intermittent dosing and is the primary delivery format for inhaled β-agonist therapy. With continuous inhalation, patients have more rapid clinical improvement than with intermittent administration. The usual dose of continuous albuterol nebulization is 0.15–0.5 mg/kg/hr, or 10–20 mg/hr. During weaning from continuous albuterol inhalation, some practitioners transition children to intermittent albuterol MDI treatments—usually four to eight puffs per dose, with each puff delivering 90 mcg.

Untoward side effects of continuous albuterol nebulization are common but relatively minor in severity. Sinus tachycardia is most common but rarely problematic. Other cardiovascular-related effects include palpitations, hypertension, diastolic hypotension, and, rarely, ventricular cardiac dysrhythmias. Excessive central nervous system (CNS) stimulation, including hyperactivity, tremors, and nausea with vomiting, are not uncommon. Hypokalemia and hyperglycemia are the most common metabolic derangements associated with albuterol use. Neither usually requires treatment, though supplemental potassium beyond maintenance amounts is sometimes necessary. Periodic serum potassium levels should be monitored during inhaled β-agonist treatment.

Intravenous and Subcutaneous β-Agonists

IV and subcutaneous administration of β-agonists is most beneficial in children with severe status asthmaticus and limited respiratory air flow, when distribution of inhaled medications may be significantly reduced. Nonselective β-agonists, such as ephedrine, epinephrine, and isoproterenol, are rarely used because of their high side-effect profile and the availability of more selective IV or subcutaneous agents.

Terbutaline, a relatively selective β_2 agonist, is available in the US for IV or subcutaneous administration. Because of its greater selectivity, terbutaline has largely supplanted the use of epinephrine for subcutaneous administration. Subcutaneous administration of β-agonists is primarily used for children with no IV access and as a rapidly available adjunct to inhaled β-agonists. Subcutaneous dosing for terbutaline is 0.01 mg/kg/dose, with a maximum dose of 0.3 mg. The dose may be repeated every 15–20 mins for up to three doses. IV terbutaline therapy starts with a loading dose of 10 mcg/kg over 10 mins, followed by continuous infusion at 0.1–10 mcg/kg/min. In the authors' experience, the usual range for effective IV terbutaline dosing is 1–8 mcg/kg/min.

The side effects of subcutaneous- or IV-administered terbutaline are similar to those of inhaled β-agonists. Some have suggested that the risk of myocardial ischemia is increased with the administration of relatively selective IV β-agonists. To date, this concern remains small, though data are limited. The authors believe that it is valuable to prospectively monitor cardiac-specific enzymes (creatine phosphokinase or troponin) in children who are receiving IV β-agonists, including terbutaline (11).

Methylxanthines

The role of methylxanthine therapy for critically ill children with status asthmaticus has changed as more selective β-agonists have become available. Methylxanthines promote relaxation of the bronchial smooth muscles; however, the exact mechanism of action remains controversial. Suggested mechanisms include increase of intracellular cAMP levels by blocking phosphodiesterase 4, control of intracellular calcium flux, inhibition of endogenous catecholamine release, and prostaglandin antagonism. In the 1970s, methylxanthines were a mainstay in the treatment of severe status asthmaticus, but recent data have made their use in the ICU controversial. For children with status asthmaticus who are hospitalized on the general-care ward, theophylline adds little to O_2, intermittent inhaled β-agonist bronchodilators, and corticosteroids (6). Theophylline added to a regimen that includes inhaled and/or IV β-agonists, inhaled ipratropium bromide, and corticosteroids significantly improved clinical asthma score over time but did not reduce PICU length of stay in critically ill asthmatic children (29). In another randomized trial, no difference was observed in the rate of clinical asthma score improvement between 3 treatment groups—theophylline alone, terbutaline alone, or terbutaline plus theophylline—when these regimens were added to standard therapy with inhaled β-agonists, corticosteroids, and O_2 (40). Theophylline therapy may be helpful in those critically ill children who are not responsive to steroids, inhaled and IV β-agonists, and O_2.

Theophylline is administered by continuous IV infusion following a loading dose of 5–7 mg/kg infused over 20 min. In general, a loading dose of 1 mg/kg will raise the serum theophylline level by 2 mcg/mL. For maximum therapeutic benefit, the goal serum theophylline level is 10–20 mcg/mL. Serum theophylline levels should be measured 1–2 hrs after the loading dose is completed. The continuous infusion should begin immediately after the bolus at a rate of 0.5–0.9 mg/kg/hr. The infusion should be adjusted to maintain levels, as noted previously. Theophylline clearance is reduced in infants and adolescents. In these age groups, the usual dose for continuous infusion is closer to 0.5 mg/kg/hr. Serum levels >20 mcg/mL are associated with adverse effects that include nausea, jitters or restlessness, tachycardia (racing heart), and overall irritability. Serum levels >35 mcg/mL have been associated with seizures and cardiac dysrhythmias. Careful attention to serum drug level measurements is required to minimize the risk of untoward side effects.

Anticholinergics

Ipratropium bromide is the most frequently used agent to provide anticholinergic effects in the treatment of status asthmaticus. Ipratropium promotes bronchodilation without inhibiting mucociliary clearance, as occurs with atropine. Acting as a parasympatholytic, aerosolized ipratropium antagonizes acetylcholine effects by blocking acetylcholine interactions with the muscarinic receptor on bronchial smooth muscle cells. By this mechanism, intracellular cyclic guanosine monophosphate levels are reduced and bronchial smooth muscle contraction is impaired.

When administered in the emergency department, ipratropium bromide reduced both hospital admission rates and clinical asthma scores. For children hospitalized with mild-to-moderate status asthmaticus, ipratropium has no additional clinical benefit over inhaled β-agonists and corticosteroids alone (14). Inhaled ipratropium has not been evaluated in critically ill children with status asthmaticus. While ipratropium therapy has no proven benefit in moderately ill children with asthma, the authors believe that it is prudent to add inhaled ipratropium therapy to the management of critically ill children who are not responding to other aggressive measures.

Ipratropium bromide can be delivered either by aerosol or MDI. Initial dose range is 125–500 mcg (if nebulized) or four to eight puffs (if via MDI) administered every 20 mins for up to three doses. The subsequent recommended dosing interval is every 4–6 hrs. Ipratropium has few adverse effects because it has poor systemic absorption. The most common untoward effects are dry mouth, bitter taste, flushing, tachycardia, and dizziness.

Magnesium Sulfate

Magnesium acts as a bronchodilator primarily through its activity as a calcium channel blocker and its role in activation of adenylate cyclase in smooth muscle cells. As result of these mechanisms, magnesium inhibits calcium-mediated smooth muscle contraction and facilitates bronchodilation.

The value of magnesium administration in the treatment of status asthmaticus remains controversial. Some studies, completed in the emergency department setting, demonstrate that magnesium administered either IV or by aerosol, can reduce hospitalization rates, improve short-term pulmonary function testing, and improve clinical asthma scores over time (7,10). Other studies have shown no benefit with magnesium treatment (33). No data are available regarding the efficacy of magnesium therapy in the ICU setting.

The usual dose of magnesium is 25–50 mg/kg/dose over 30 min, administered every 4 hrs. Magnesium can also be given by continuous infusion at a rate of 10–20 mg/kg/hr. With either dosing regimen, some have suggested a target magnesium level of 4 mg/dL to achieve maximal effect.

Side effects of magnesium administration include hypotension, CNS depression, muscle weakness, and flushing, though in the studies previously mentioned, no significant untoward effects were reported. Severe complications, such as cardiac arrhythmia including complete heart block, respiratory failure due to severe muscle weakness, and sudden cardiopulmonary arrest, may occur in the setting of very high serum magnesium levels (usually >10–12 mg/dL). Serum magnesium levels should be regularly monitored.

To date, magnesium therapy remains an unproven therapy in critically ill children with status asthmaticus. Nevertheless, given its low risk profile and its demonstrated benefit in the emergency department setting, it is appropriate to consider adding magnesium therapy to the treatment regimen of children in the PICU who are not responding to more conventional treatment measures.

Helium-Oxygen

Helium is a biologically inert, low-density gas that, when administered by inhalation in a mixture with O_2, reduces air flow resistance in small airways by reducing turbulent flow and enhancing laminar gas flow. These characteristics may also enhance particle deposition of aerosolized medications in distal lung segments. In aggregate, these characteristics make administration of a mixture of helium and O_2 (80% helium/20% oxygen—heliox) an attractive therapeutic option in the man-

agement of status asthmaticus, in which turbulent air flow and high airway resistance are common.

Clinical studies that examined the efficacy of helium/oxygen administration in status asthmaticus have yielded conflicting results. A recent Cochrane review concluded that heliox was not beneficial in asthma, though most of the studies cited were in adults. In contrast, some small studies in nonintubated children with moderately severe asthma have shown improvement in lung function and clinical asthma score with heliox therapy. Most recently, Kim et al. demonstrated that the use of heliox to drive continuous albuterol nebulization treatments for children in the emergency department with moderately severe status asthmaticus was associated with significantly improved clinical asthma scores (20). In the PICU, the use of heliox in mechanically ventilated children reduces peak airway pressure by lowering airway resistance, and it may enhance weaning from mechanical ventilation (1). The use of heliox is sometimes limited by the degree of hypoxemia in the patient. If substantial supplemental O_2 is added to the two available mixtures of helium/oxygen (80/20 and 70/30), the salutary effect of low-density gas administration on reducing turbulent gas flow is lost.

Heliox remains unproven therapy in critically ill children with status asthmaticus. For children who are not improving with conventional therapy or children who are receiving high-pressure mechanical ventilatory support, heliox may be a reasonable adjunct therapy.

Noninvasive Mechanical Ventilation

Mortality rates in mechanically ventilated children with status asthmaticus increase compared to those children who do not require mechanical ventilation. Noninvasive positive-pressure ventilation (NIPPV) is an alternative to conventional mechanical ventilation in these patients. A systematic review that examined data in these patients concluded that insufficient quality data are available to make recommendations about the use of NIPPV in patients with asthma. Other reports in small groups of adults suggest that NIPPV can prevent tracheal intubation. In one study, children were subjected to a crossover trial between NIPPV and standard therapy. The NIPPV group showed reduced WOB and dyspnea, compared to the standard therapy group (35). At this writing, noninvasive ventilation remains an unproven therapy for children with status asthmaticus; however, it is relatively easy to institute and a trial may be warranted prior to the institution of conventional mechanical ventilation.

Mechanical Ventilation

In status asthmaticus, tracheal intubation is indicated for children following cardiorespiratory arrest, those with refractory hypoxemia, or those with significant respiratory acidosis unresponsive to pharmacotherapy. Mechanical ventilation is intended to provide support while the underlying pathology resolves. Currently, <1% of children with status asthmaticus require mechanical ventilation. Of the children admitted to the PICU, only 5%–10% require mechanical ventilation, and many of those patients are intubated prior to arrival in the PICU (39). Children who require mechanical ventilation are at increased risk for pulmonary barotrauma, nosocomial infection, pulmonary edema, circulatory dysfunction, steroid/muscle relaxant-associated myopathy, and death (**Fig. 43.4**).

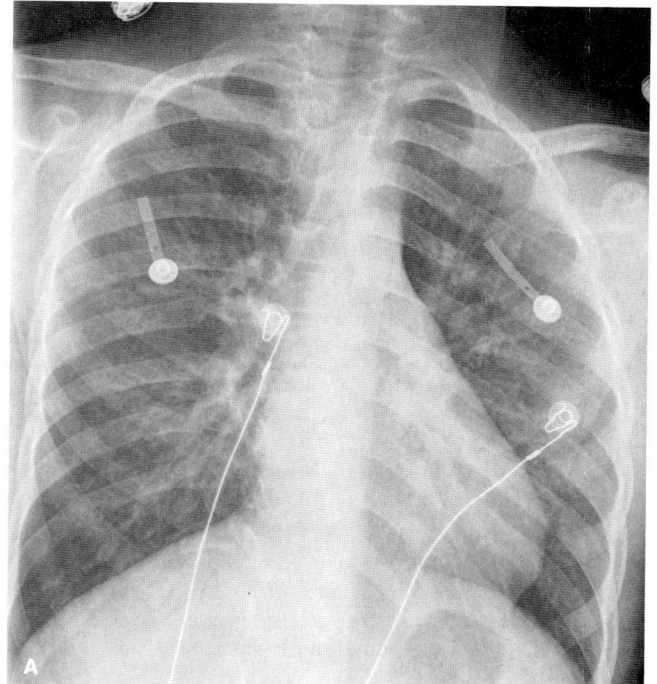

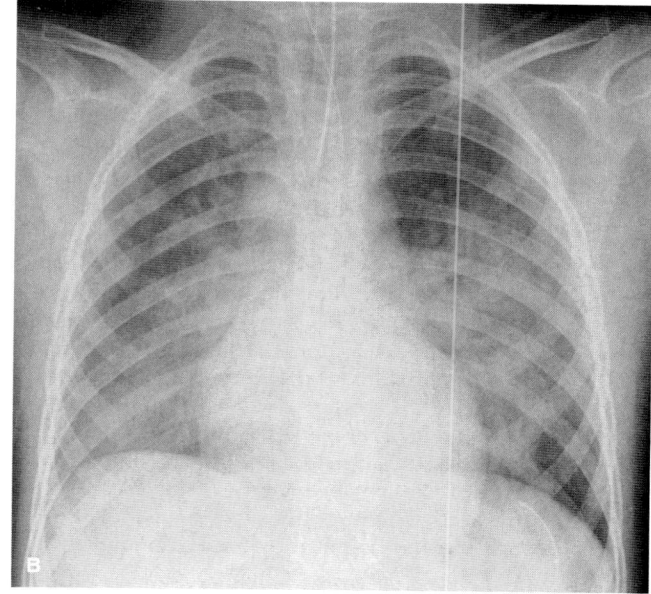

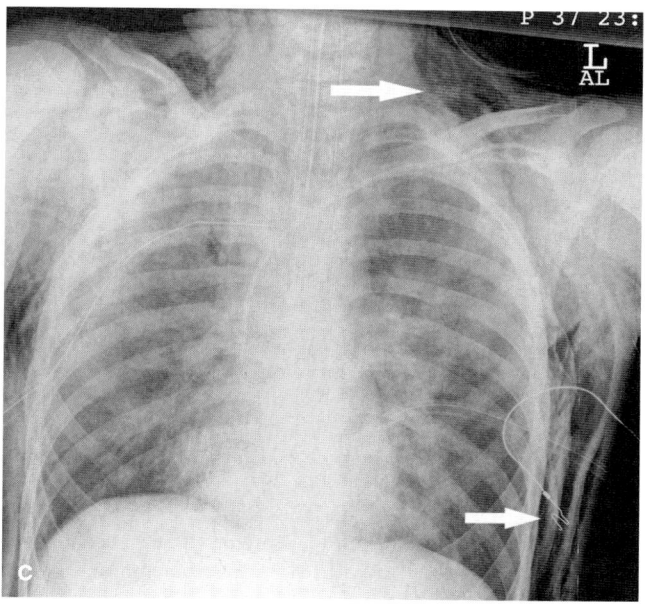

FIGURE 43.4. Pulmonary complications. **A:** Hyperinflation and air trapping. **B:** Pulmonary edema in patient receiving mechanical ventilation; note bilateral airspace disease. **C:** Significant barotrauma with bilateral pneumothoraces, requiring chest tubes and large amount of subcutaneous air (*arrows*).

Tracheal intubation of the asthmatic child with respiratory failure requires preparation and anticipation of patient deterioration. It should be performed by the most skilled individual available. Hypotension should be anticipated because many patients have relative hypovolemia that may be exacerbated by reduced preload as positive-pressure ventilation is initiated and by reduced vascular tone induced by anesthetic agents used for tracheal intubation. Histamine-producing agents, such as morphine or atracurium, must be avoided. Ketamine is an excellent anesthetic agent for induction because of its relatively long half-life, bronchodilating properties, and relative preservation of hemodynamic stability. A cuffed endotracheal tube with the largest diameter appropriate for the age of the child

should be used, as high ventilatory pressures are typical when treating mechanically ventilated children in status asthmaticus.

Ventilatory support in status asthmaticus should maintain adequate oxygenation, allow for permissive hypercarbia (moderate respiratory acidosis), and adjust minute ventilation (peak pressure, tidal volume, and rate) to maintain an arterial pH of >7.2. Ventilator management strategies should attempt to minimize dynamic hyperinflation and air trapping (**Fig. 43.1**), which can usually be accomplished by employing slow ventilator rates with prolonged expiratory phase, minimal end-expiratory pressure, and short inspiratory time.

The ideal mode of mechanical ventilation has not been established for asthmatic children with respiratory failure. Most of these children will display disparate time-constant physiology, though slow time constants will predominate. Volume-control ventilation with constant or accelerating flow wave forms will provide stable tidal volumes from breath to breath but, in the setting of dynamic airway resistance, may result in high peak airway pressures, uneven distribution of tidal breaths, and increased risk for pulmonary barotrauma. Pressure-control ventilation with decelerating flow pattern results in lower peak pressure, higher mean airway pressure, and better distribution of gas into high-resistance, long time-constant airways (32). In pressure-control mode with preset peak inspiratory pressure, rapidly changing airway resistance can result in (a) significant variation in delivered tidal volume and (b) increased risk of pulmonary barotrauma if airway resistance changes abruptly. Pressure-regulated volume control is a relatively new mode of mechanical ventilation. Although experience is limited with this mode of ventilation in patients with asthma, the decelerating flow pattern combined with the option to independently adjust pressure with a preset tidal volume is appealing to enhance gas distribution and minimize risk of barotrauma.

The use of positive end-expiratory pressure (PEEP) is controversial. Most authors suggest minimal PEEP because most patients with status asthmaticus already have increased functional residual capacity. High PEEP is likely to further increase functional residual capacity and exacerbate hyperinflation. Others argue that these patients have dynamic collapse of small airways during forced exhalation, and PEEP may stent small airways open at the end of expiration and facilitate full expiration. Review of graphically displayed flow-time curves will demonstrate whether expiratory flow is completed prior to the next breath (**Fig. 43.1**). Adjustments can then be made to the ventilator rate, inspiratory time, expiratory time, or PEEP to facilitate full expiration between breaths.

Other less conventional strategies have been used when standard mechanical ventilation approaches fail. The use of high-frequency ventilation has been described in a few case reports, though this mode of ventilation requires careful attention to the amplitude settings of the oscillator to avoid further hyperinflation. Some authors suggest using pressure-support ventilation without any preset rate and allowing the patient to breathe spontaneously. This strategy avoids complications associated with continuous or frequent use of muscle relaxants and has the further advantage of allowing the child to maintain forced exhalation while receiving support for inspiration. Tracheal gas insufflation has also been used to facilitate expiratory gas flow and reduce severe hypercarbia. Careful attention to secretion accumulation around the insufflation tube is necessary to avoid the development of tracheal tube mucous plugging.

Tracheal extubation should occur as soon as possible. Rapid weaning from the ventilator should take place—"declare them well and pull the tube." The presence of the breathing tube, especially in awake children, may irritate the airway and stimulate further bronchospasm. Decreasing peak inspiratory pressure, adequate air movement by auscultation, and graphic evidence of full expiration of inspired tidal volume are sufficient criteria for tracheal extubation, even if expiratory wheezing is still present on clinical exam.

Chest Physiotherapy

Chest physiotherapy (CPT) may augment airway clearance and encourage resolution of mucous plugging; however, it should only be considered in children with clear segmental or lobar atelectasis. In all other populations of children with status asthmaticus, CPT has no therapeutic benefit. Some suggest that CPT is irritating to the severe asthmatic and may actually worsen clinical symptoms. CPT is not recommended as part of routine management in the critically ill patient with status asthmaticus.

Antibiotics

Most asthma exacerbations are associated with, or triggered by, viral infections and not bacterial infections. For this reason, empiric antibiotic treatment for children with status asthmaticus is not indicated. Lower respiratory tract bacterial infections do occur in children with status asthmaticus. The most commonly identified organisms are *Mycoplasma pneumoniae* and *Chlamydia*. When findings on chest x-ray, leukocytosis, and fever suggest pneumonia, appropriate antibiotics should be administered, especially targeted at the organisms previously noted. Sinusitis is a common nonpulmonary infection found in children with status asthmaticus. When evidence of bacterial pneumonia is absent, and high fever and peripheral blood leukocytosis are present, the diagnosis of sinusitis should be considered, and, if found, antibacterial therapy should be instituted.

Sedation, Analgesia, Muscle Relaxants, Inhalational Anesthetics

Sedation of the unintubated asthmatic is generally not indicated. Some children who are excessively anxious and who are not hypoxemic or hypercarbic as a cause for their anxiety may benefit from sedation. Sedation should occur only in the closely monitored setting of the PICU. Ketamine is an excellent choice because it provides excellent sedation and bronchodilation with minimal risk of respiratory depression.

Mechanically ventilated children require sedation and, often, muscle relaxants to prevent ventilator-patient asynchrony and to reduce the risk of sudden cough-induced pulmonary barotrauma. Ketamine by continuous infusion is the first choice for sedation, usually combined with intermittent or continuous administration of benzodiazepines. Usual ketamine dosing is 1 mg/kg/hr and is adjusted to achieve sufficient sedation. Increased respiratory secretions occur with ketamine administration; however, these side effects are usually manageable. When opiates are used, fentanyl is preferred because morphine causes histamine release, which may exacerbate bronchospasm. Neuromuscular blocking agents are frequently required to facilitate mechanical ventilatory support. Vecuronium is a commonly used agent. The starting dose is 0.1 mg/kg/hr, which should be titrated to train-of-four monitoring—usually one to two twitches. Drug holidays can be used to reduce the risk of overdose, prolonged paresis, and myopathy that are sometimes observed in children who receive continuous infusions of the nondepolarizing neuromuscular blocking agents.

Inhaled general anesthetics have been used when all other measures are failing, and their bronchodilating properties have proven beneficial in the management of the intubated asthmatic (18). These agents should be administered in conjunction with anesthesia services. Hypotension and cardiac dysrhythmias are associated with their use and are more likely to occur in hypoxemic children.

Extracorporeal Membrane Oxygenation Support

When maximal medical therapy is failing, extracorporeal membrane oxygenation (ECMO) should be considered. Numerous case reports demonstrate high survival rates, even in a gravely ill patient population. The survival for children with refractory status asthmaticus who are placed on ECMO is ~90%.

OUTCOMES

Mortality rates for children with severe status asthmaticus who arrive at the hospital intact are nearly zero. Sophisticated ventilatory strategies, the availability of more selective, less toxic bronchodilating agents, and the selective use of ECMO has contributed to this good prognosis. Nearly all asthma deaths occur in those children who suffer a cardiopulmonary arrest prior to arrival for emergency hospital care. Improved outpatient management strategies are necessary to eliminate these deaths.

CONCLUSIONS AND FUTURE DIRECTIONS

Asthma is a disease that is increasing in worldwide prevalence and continues to have substantial clinical and financial impact on children and their families. Severe status asthmaticus is a life-threatening disorder that, if recognized and treated aggressively, has an extremely low mortality rate. It is incumbent upon the pediatric intensivist to rapidly diagnose and initiate therapy in these children. More work is required to recognize and provide earlier intervention options to those few asthmatics who suffer rapid-onset illness and resultant morbidity and mortality before they can receive emergent medical care.

Novel future therapies will likely involve modifying the inflammatory processes involved in the pathophysiology of asthma. Leukotriene modifiers and cytokine modulators may revolutionize asthma therapy, primarily in the outpatient arena, though these agents may also significantly impact ICU care as well. Other therapies on the horizon include phosphodiesterase inhibitors that are more specific than theophylline and anti-IgE monoclonal antibodies that reduce free IgE. Of these new asthma therapies, cytokine modulators and IgE inhibitors are receiving the most active research (38). Our understanding of viral-induced asthma is growing. Some suggest that an "asthma vaccine" to reduce viral-induced disease is at hand. Most experts are more realistic, suggesting that the multiple polymorphisms and interactions with environmental influences will preclude identification of an asthma cure.

KEY POINTS

- Asthma is the most common chronic disease of childhood and accounts for a growing number of pediatric hospitalizations each year.
- Status asthmaticus is a condition of progressively worsening bronchospasm and respiratory dysfunction caused by asthma; it is unresponsive to standard conventional therapy and may progress to respiratory failure and the need for mechanical ventilation.
- Asthma is an inflammatory disease that is characterized by air-flow obstruction due to airway hyperresponsiveness and bronchospasm and airway inflammation with mucosal edema and mucous plugging.
- Gas-exchange abnormalities in status asthmaticus are primarily due to V/Q mismatch, resulting from distal airway obstruction due to mucous plugging, edema, and bronchoconstriction.
- For patients who first present for evaluation of new-onset wheezing, four disparate clinical entities—asthma, pneumonia, foreign-body aspiration, and congestive heart failure—must be distinguished, because each of them requires different diagnostic and therapeutic approaches.
- For spontaneously breathing children with status asthmaticus, clinical interventions should be primarily based on the physical examination and not on blood gas determinations.
- The overriding physiologic derangement in asthma is airway inflammation, and corticosteroids are a mainstay in the management of both acute and chronic asthma. β-agonists, as sympathomimetic agents, cause direct bronchial smooth muscle relaxation and are key components in asthma therapy.
- IV and subcutaneous administration of β-agonists is most beneficial for patients with severe status asthmaticus and limited respiratory air flow, in whom distribution of inhaled medications may be significantly reduced.
- In status asthmaticus, tracheal intubation is indicated for patients who are post-cardiorespiratory arrest, those with refractory hypoxemia, or those with significant respiratory acidosis unresponsive to pharmacotherapy.
- When maximal medical therapy is failing, ECMO should be considered. The survival for patients with refractory status asthmaticus who are placed on ECMO is ~90%.

References

1. Abd-Allah SA, Rogers MS, Terry M, et al. Helium-oxygen therapy for pediatric acute severe asthma requiring mechanical ventilation. *Pediatr Crit Care Med* 2003;4:353–7.
2. Afzal M, Tharratt RS. Mechanical ventilation in severe asthma. *Clin Rev Allergy Immunol* 2001;20:385–97.
3. Akinbami LJ, Schoendorf KC. Trends in childhood asthma: Prevalence, health care utilization, and mortality. *Pediatrics* 2002;110:315–22.
4. American Heart Association. Recognition of respiratory failure and shock. In: Pediatric Advanced Life Support Provider Manual. Dallas: American Heart Association; 2002;23–42.
5. Becker JM, Arora A, Scarfone RJ, et al. Oral versus intravenous corticosteroids in children hospitalized with asthma. *J Allergy Clin Immunol* 1999; 103:586.
6. Bien JP, Bloom MD, Evans RL, et al. Intravenous theophylline in pediatric status asthmaticus: A prospective, randomized, double-blind, placebo-controlled trial. *Clin Pediatr* 1995;34:475–81.
7. Blitz, M. Aerosolized magnesium sulfate for acute asthma: A systematic review. *Chest* 2005;128:337–44.
8. Brightling CE, Symon FA, Birring SS, et al. TH2 cytokine expression in bronchoalveolar lavage fluid T lymphocytes and bronchial submucosal is a feature of asthma and eosinophilic bronchitis. *J Allergy Clin Immunol* 2002; 110:899–905.
9. Centers for Disease Control and Prevention. Asthma mortality and hospitalization among children and young adults-United States, 1980–1993. *MMWR Morb Mortal Wkly Rep* 1996;45(17):350–3.
10. Cheuk DK, Chau TC, Lee SL. A meta-analysis on intravenous magnesium sulphate for treating acute asthma. *Arch Dis Child* 2005;90:74–7.
11. Chiang VW, Burns JP, Rifai N, et al. Cardiac toxicity of intravenous terbutaline for the treatment of severe asthma in children: A prospective assessment. *J Pediatr* 2000;137:73–7.
12. Chipps BE. Assessment and treatment of acute asthma in children. *J Pediatr* 2005;147:288–94.

13. Contopoulos-Ioannidis DG. Meta-analysis of the association of beta 2-adrenergic receptor polymorphisms with asthma phenotypes. *J Allergy Clin Immunol* 2005;115:963–72.

14. Crave D, Kercsmar CM, Myers TR, et al. Ipratropium bromide plus nebulized albuterol for the treatment of hospitalized children with acute asthma. *J Pediatr* 2001;138:51–8.

15. DiGiulio GA, Kercmar CM, Krug SE, et al. Hospital treatment of asthma: Lack of benefit from theophylline given in addition to nebulized albuterol and intravenously administered corticosteroid. *J Pediatr* 1993;122:464–9.

16. Goldman MD, Mathieu M, Montely JM, et al. Inspiratory fall in systolic pressure in normal and asthmatic subjects. *Am J Respir Crit Care Med* 1995;151:743–50.

17. Jardin F, Farcot JC, Boisante L, et al. Mechanism of paradoxic pulse in bronchial asthma. *Circulation* 1982;66:887–94.

18. Johnston RG, Noseworthy TW, Friesen EG, et al. Isoflurane therapy for status asthmaticus in children and adults. *Chest* 1990;97:698–701.

19. Kikuchi Y, Okabe S, Tamura G, et al. Chemosensitivity and perception of dyspnea in patient with a history of near-fatal asthma. *N Engl J Med* 1994;330:1329–34.

20. Kim IK, Phrampus E, Venkataraman S, et al. Helium/oxygen-driven albuterol nebulization in the treatment of children with moderate to severe asthma exacerbations: A randomized, controlled trial. *Pediatrics* 2005;116:1127–33.

21. Leatherman JW, Fluegel WL, David WS, et al. Muscle weakness in mechanically ventilated patients with severe asthma. *Am J Respir Crit Care Med* 1996;153:1686–90.

22. Mannino DM, Homa DM, Akinbami LJ, et al. Surveillance for asthma: United States, 1980–1999. *MMWR Surveill Summ* 2002;51:1–13.

23. McCormick MS, Kass B, Elixhauser A, et al. Annual report on access to and utilization of health care for children and youth in the United States: 1999. *Pediatrics* 2000;105:219–30.

24. McCunney RJ. Asthma, genes, and air pollution. *J Occup Environ Med* 2005;47:1285–91.

25. Milgrom H, Skoner DP, Bensch G, et al. Low-dose levalbuterol in children with asthma: Safety and efficacy in comparison with placebo and racemic albuterol. *J Allergy Clin Immunol* 2001;108:938–45.

26. National Asthma Education and Prevention Program. Expert panel report 2: Guidelines for the diagnosis and management of asthma. NIH Publication No. 55-4051, 1997.

27. Pirie J, Cox P, Johnson D, et al. Changes in treatment and outcomes of children receiving care in the intensive care unit for severe acute asthma. *Pediatr Emerg Care* 1998;14:104–8.

28. Rachelefsky G. Treating exacerbations of asthma in children: The role of systemic corticosteroids. *Pediatrics* 2003;112:382.

29. Ream RS, Loftis LL, Albers GM, et al. Efficacy of IV theophylline in children with severe status asthmaticus. *Chest* 2001;119:1480–88.

30. Roberts JS, Bratton SL, Brogan TV. Acute severe asthma: Differences in therapies and outcomes among pediatric intensive care units. *Crit Care Med* 2002;30:581–5.

31. Robertson CF, Rubinfeld AR, Bowes G. Pediatric asthma deaths in Victoria: The mild are at risk. *Pediatr Pulmonol* 1992;13:95–100.

32. Sarnaik AP, Daphtary KM, Meert KL, et al. Pressure-controlled ventilation in children with severe status asthmaticus. *Pediatr Crit Care Med* 2004;5:133–8.

33. Scarfone RJ, Loiselle JM, Joffe MD, et al. A randomized trial of magnesium in the emergency department treatment of children with asthma. *Ann Emerg Med* 2000;36:572–8.

34. Sur S, Crotty TB, Kephart GM, et al. Sudden-onset fatal asthma. A distinct entity with few eosinophils and relatively more neutrophils in the airway submucosa? *Am Rev Repir Dis* 1993;148:713–9.

35. Thill PJ, McGuire JK, Baden HP, et al. Noninvasive positive-pressure ventilation in children with lower airway obstruction. *Pediatr Crit Care Med* 2004;5:408–9.

36. Turner MO, Noertjojo K, Vedal S, et al. Risk factors for near-fatal asthma. A case-control study in hospitalized patients with asthma. *Am J Respir Crit Care Med* 1998;157:1804–9.

37. US Department of Health and Human Services, Public Health Service, National Institutes of Health (NIH), et al. Guidelines for the diagnosis and management of asthma. Bethesda, MD: NIH Pub No 08-5846, 2007.

38. Weinberger M. Innovative therapies for asthma—Where we've been and where we're going: Innovative approaches of the past, present, and the future. *Paediatr Respir Rev* 2004;5:S113–4.

39. Werner, HA. Status asthmaticus in children. *Chest* 2001;119:1913–29.

40. Wheeler DS, Jacobs B, Kenreigh C, et al. Theophylline versus terbutaline in treating critically ill children with status asthmaticus: A prospective, randomized, controlled trial. *Pediatr Crit Care Med* 2005;6:142–7.

41. Wood DW, Downes JJ, Lecks HI. A clinical scoring system for the diagnosis of respiratory failure. *Preliminary report on childhood status asthmaticus. Am J Dis Child* 1972;123:227–8.

CHAPTER 44 ■ NEONATAL RESPIRATORY FAILURE

ELISABETH L. RAAB • LISA K. KELLY • PHILIPPE S. FRIEDLICH • RANGASAMY RAMANATHAN • ISTVAN SERI

Respiratory disease accounts for a major portion of admissions to the NICU. Respiratory symptoms in the neonate, such as tachypnea, cyanosis, grunting, flaring, and retractions, may be due to a primary pulmonary or intrathoracic process or may be the initial clinical manifestation of a wide range of non-respiratory processes, such as polycythemia, congenital heart disease, and bacteremia. Respiratory failure, due primarily to respiratory distress syndrome (RDS) in the preterm neonate and to infection, meconium aspiration syndrome, and congenital anomalies in the term infant, is a major cause of morbidity and mortality in the neonatal period and often has long-term implications for the future health of the child.

DEVELOPMENTALLY REGULATED DISEASE

Respiratory Distress Syndrome

RDS due to surfactant deficiency is a significant life-threatening condition that is seen primarily in preterm infants. The incidence of RDS is inversely proportional to gestational age: RDS occurs in ~50% of infants born before 29 weeks of gestational age and in 25% of infants born after 29 weeks. Despite significant improvements in perinatal care practices, the incidence of prematurity has not decreased over recent years. In fact, the incidence of prematurity is increasing in the US. One out of 8 babies is born preterm, which translates into ~480,000 preterm births each year in the US. Fortunately, with the use of maternal prenatal steroids to accelerate fetal organ development in general and lung maturity and surfactant release in particular, the incidence and severity of RDS have decreased by nearly 50%. Prenatal steroid exposure followed by postnatal surfactant therapy has been shown to have a synergistic effect in reducing the mortality and morbidity in preterm infants with RDS (39).

The newborn lung provides an extensive surface area for gas exchange, ~1 m²/kg body weight. Pulmonary surfactant coats the alveolar surface at the air-liquid interphase and maintains low surface tension, thus preventing collapse of the lung, especially at the end of expiration. Surfactant is composed of phospholipids (80–90%) and surfactant proteins (SP)-A, SP-B, SP-C, and SP-D. Disaturated phosphatidylcholine constitutes the major phospholipid. Surfactant is synthesized by the type II pneumocytes that line the alveoli and is stored as lamellar bodies. Lamellar bodies enter the alveoli by exocytosis and there transform into tubular myelin. Under the influence of SP-A, which is cosecreted along with the lamellar bodies from type II pneumocytes, tubular myelin unravels to form mono- and multilayers of phospholipids rich in SP-B and SP-C. Spreading and adsorption of phospholipids at the air-liquid interphase is dependent on SP-B, and to a lesser extent, on SP-C. Catabolism of secreted surfactant is primarily regulated by lung macrophages and SP-A. Remnants of SP-A, SP-B, and SP-C are taken up and recycled or degraded by type II pneumocytes. The composition of surfactant across different mammalian species is fairly constant, making it possible to modify surfactant from one species and use it in another species.

Surfactant therapy has decreased the mortality and incidence of pneumothorax in infants with RDS. However, short- and long-term morbidity continues to be a major problem, particularly among extremely low-birth-weight (ELBW, <1000 g) infants. Bronchopulmonary dysplasia (BPD), defined clinically as the need for supplemental O_2 at 36 weeks postmenstrual age, occurs in 30%–50% of ELBW infants. BPD is associated with poor lung function and repeated hospitalization for respiratory failure among survivors. BPD is a multifactorial disease, the origins of which include barotrauma that results from mechanical ventilation, volutrauma from using large tidal volumes, and "biotrauma" from the release of proinflammatory cytokines (e.g., IL-1, IL-8) and tumor necrosis factor (TNF). Preterm infants have a decreased capacity to produce anti-inflammatory cytokines (e.g., IL-10), which results in a persistent proinflammatory state. This condition leads to aberrant repair of the developing lungs following injury, resulting in alveolar and vascular hypoplasia. Preterm infants are born during the canalicular and saccular stages of lung development, which is the period of rapid growth of the lung parenchyma and pulmonary vasculature. Thus, injury at this stage can have a profound effect on the architecture and function of the lung. Preterm infants with RDS have decreased lung compliance due to high surface tension secondary to surfactant deficiency, which results in alveolar collapse and ventilation-perfusion (V̇/Q̇) mismatch. Exogenous surfactant therapy has significantly improved the outcome of preterm infants with RDS.

Delivery Room Management of Preterm Infants

Preterm infants with RDS have high surface tension and decreased lung compliance. Therefore, appropriate intervention in the delivery room is to provide continuous positive airway pressure (CPAP) to prevent alveolar collapse and to establish functional residual capacity. Even brief periods of large tidal volume breaths soon after birth have been shown to initiate lung injury and inactivate surfactant. CPAP stabilizes the alveoli, decreases the upper airway resistance, and promotes the release of preformed surfactant from type II pneumocytes. The care provided in the delivery room and over the course of the

697

first 12–24 postnatal hours is believed to have a larger cumulative impact on the outcome of the ELBW neonate than all of the other therapeutic interventions that the patient receives later during the hospitalization.

Surfactant Therapy for Respiratory Distress Syndrome

Surfactant therapy has been extensively evaluated in randomized, controlled trials in neonatal medicine and has become the standard of care for preterm infants with RDS. Surfactant therapy has been used *prophylactically* in preterm infants to optimize the distribution of the exogenously instilled surfactant by administering it while the lung is still fluid-filled. However, this approach has not been shown to be superior to postventilatory surfactant therapy, i.e., after the initial resuscitation and stabilization of the preterm infants. Nevertheless, *early rescue surfactant therapy* given within 30–120 mins of age has been shown to be better than *delayed rescue therapy* by decreasing the need for additional doses of surfactant and allowing faster weaning of supplemental O_2. Different surfactant preparations—synthetic, natural, and modified surfactants derived from animal sources—are available.

Synthetic surfactants include colfosceril palmitate (Exosurf), Pumactant (ALEC), Turfsurf, and lucinactant (Surfaxin). Of these four synthetic surfactants, the first three are no longer available for clinical use, and lucinactant has not yet been approved for clinical use by the US Food and Drug Administration. Seven different natural, modified surfactant preparations have been studied, including beractant (Survanta), calfactant (Infasurf), SF-RI 1 (Alveofact), and poractant alfa (Curosurf). They differ in composition, onset of response, duration of action, dosing volume, and the need for additional doses (**Table 44.1**). Preterm infants with RDS are typically given 100 mg/kg of phospholipids initially and subsequently at 6–12-hr intervals if the patient remains intubated and is receiving ≥30% O_2. Curosurf, one of the most concentrated surfactants available, is given at an initial dose of 200 mg/kg, but requires only the relatively low volume of 2.5 mL/kg intratracheally.

To date, 14 trials that compared natural versus synthetic surfactants (1,2,14, 20–22,30,34,36,41,45,47,50,61) (**Table 44.2**) and eight studies that compared different natural surfactants (6,7,8,33,44,51) (**Table 44.3**) have been published. A comparison of beractant and calfactant in the prophylactic treatment of RDS in preterm infants <1250 g showed no difference in mortality or BPD (8). However, mortality in a subgroup of infants <600 g was significantly lower in the beractant-treated group (26%), compared to 63% with calfactant. When these two surfactants were compared in the rescue treatment of RDS in 608 preterm infants, infants in the group treated with calfactant demonstrated lower F_{IO_2} and mean airway pressure at 72 hrs of age than those in the group treated with beractant. No significant differences in death or BPD were observed between infants in the two groups.

In a pilot trial that compared beractant and poractant alfa, investigators observed significant improvement in oxygenation, decreased peak inspiratory pressure, and decreased mean airway pressure, which persisted up to 24 hrs after administration of poractant alfa (51). No significant differences in mortality or BPD were noted between these two surfactants. In another study that compared alveofact, beractant, and poractant alfa, treatment with poractant alfa resulted in less days on mechanical ventilation and supplemental O_2 and shorter length of hospital stay (6). In a multicentered, randomized, controlled trial that compared poractant alfa and beractant, treatment with poractant alfa was associated with faster weaning of O_2, fewer additional doses of surfactant, and decreased mortality in preterm infants at <32 weeks' gestation when compared with beractant (44). Cumulatively, 36% of infants randomized to poractant alfa received ≥2 doses versus 68% in the beractant-treated group ($p < 0.05$). In a meta-analysis of the two studies that compared beractant and poractant alfa, neonatal mortality was significantly lower with poractant alfa (odds ratio, 0.35, 95% confidence interval, 0.13–0.92). A recent study that compared these two surfactants expanded on the observations of the previous trials and showed a more sustained improvement in oxygenation with poractant alfa than with beractant and a

---

TABLE 44.1

COMPOSITION AND DOSING OF NATURAL SURFACTANT PREPARATIONS COMMONLY USED IN PRETERM INFANTS WITH RESPIRATORY DISTRESS SYNDROME

Surfactant	Preparation, composition	Phospholipids (%)	Plasmalogen (mol%)	SP-B (mg/mmol PL)	SP-C	DPPC (mg/mL)	Dose (mL/kg)
Survanta	Minced Bovine Lung Extract/DPPC + Palmitic Acid + Tripalmitin added	84	1.5	0–1.3	1–20	25	4
Infasurf	Bovine Lung Lavage/DPPC, Cholesterol	95	NA	5.4	8.1	35	3
Curosurf	Minced Porcine Lung Extract/DPPC, Polar Lipids	99	3.8	2–3.7	5–11.6	80	1.25[a]

[a]Initial dose, 2.5 mL/kg.
PL, phospholipid; SP-B, surfactant protein B; SP-C, surfactant protein C; DPPC, dipalmitoyl phosphatidylcholine

TABLE 44.2

TRIALS COMPARING NATURAL VERSUS SYNTHETIC SURFACTANTS FOR THE PREVENTION OR TREATMENT OF RESPIRATORY DISTRESS SYNDROME IN PRETERM INFANTS

Trials (14)	Surfactant	N	P or Tx	Patients	Results
Horbar, 1993	Survanta vs. Exosurf	617	Tx	500–1500 g	Survanta: Lower 0–72-hr F_{IO_2} and MAP
Sehgal, 1994	Survanta vs. Exosurf	41	Tx	600–1750 g	No differences in any variables
Vermont-Oxford Network, 1996	Survanta vs. Exosurf	1296	Tx	501–1500 g	Survanta: Lower F_{IO_2} at 72 hrs, lower 0–72 hrs MAP; fewer air leaks
Hudak, 1996	Infasurf vs. Exosurf	1126	Tx	All with RDS	Infasurf: Lower 0–72 hrs F_{IO_2} and MAP; fewer air leaks
Hudak, 1997	Infasurf vs. Exosurf	846	P	<29 wks	Infasurf: Less RDS; lower 0–72-hr F_{IO_2} and MAP; fewer air leaks; more cystic PVL
Rollins, 1993	Curosurf vs. Exosurf	66	Tx	All with RDS	Curosurf: Lower F_{IO_2} and improved a/A P_{O_2} ratio
Alvarado, 1993	Survanta vs. Exosurf	66	Tx	<1500 g	Survanta: Decreased duration of PPV, O_2, and LOS
Pearlman, 1993	Survanta vs. Exosurf	121	Tx	All with RDS	No differences in any variables
Modanlou, 1997	Survanta vs. Exosurf	122	Tx	<1500 g	Survanta: Lower F_{IO_2}, MAP, and oxygenation index
da Costa, 1999	Survanta vs. Exosurf	89	Tx	<37 wks >1000 g	No difference
Kukkonen, 2000	Curosurf vs. Exosurf	228	Tx	All with RDS	Curosurf: Lower F_{IO_2} and MAP
Ainsworth, 2000	Curosurf vs. Pumactant	212	Tx	<30 wks	Curosurf: Decreased mortality (Trial stopped after interim analysis)
Sinha, 2005	Curosurf vs. Surfaxin	252 of 496	P	600–1250 g	No difference; 252 out of 496 original sample size enrolled
Moya, 2005	Exosurf vs. Surfaxin vs. Survanta	1294	P	600–1250 g	More effective than Exosurf; similar to Survanta

P, prophylaxis; Tx, rescue; MAP, mean airway pressure; RDS, respiratory distress syndrome; a/A P_{O_2}, arterial-to-alveolar oxygen tension; PVL, periventricular leukomalacia; PPV, positive-pressure ventilation; LOS, length of stay

TABLE 44.3

TRIALS COMPARING NATURAL SURFACTANTS FOR THE PREVENTION OR TREATMENT OF RESPIRATORY DISTRESS SYNDROME IN PRETERM INFANTS

Trials (8)	Surfactant	n	P or Tx	Patients	Results
Bloom, 1997	Survanta vs. Infasurf	374	P	<1250 g	No difference in any variables; Infasurf increased mortality in infants <600 g
Bloom,	Survanta vs. Infasurf	608	Tx	<2000 g	Infasurf: Lower average 0–72 hrs F_{IO_2} and MAP
Speer, 1995	Survanta vs. Curosurf	73	Tx	700–1500 g	Curosurf: Lower F_{IO_2}, PIP, MAP at 12–24 hrs
Baroutis, 2003	Alveofact vs. Survanta vs. Curosurf	80	Tx	<2000 g	Curosurf: Fewer days on O_2 and mechanical ventilation; decreased LOS
Ramanathan, 2004	Survanta vs. Curosurf	293	Tx	759–1750 g	Curosurf: Faster weaning, fewer doses, decreased mortality, cost effective
Malloy, 2005	Survanta vs. Curosurf	58	Tx	<37 weeks with RDS	Curosurf: Lower F_{IO_2} up to 48 hrs; fewer doses
Bloom, 2005	Survanta vs. Infasurf	749	P	23–29 weeks	Trial stopped early; original sample size 2,000; alive with BPD 34% vs. 33%; no differences in any outcomes
Bloom, 2005	Survanta vs. Infasurf	1361	Tx	401–2000 g	Trial stopped early; original sample size 2,080; alive with BPD 31% vs. 31%; no differences in any outcomes

P, prophylaxis; Tx, rescue; F_{IO_2}, fraction of inspired oxygen; MAP, mean airway pressure; PIP, peak inspiratory pressure; LOS, length of stay; RDS, respiratory distress syndrome; BPD, bronchopulmonary dysplasia significantly lower need for additional doses of poractant alfa compared to beractant (33). Surfactant trials and clinical outcomes from published studies are summarized in **Table 44.4**. Most, but not all, multiple, controlled trials have demonstrated better clinical outcomes and improved survival with natural surfactants than with synthetic surfactants. Among natural surfactants, poractant alfa may be associated with better clinical outcomes in preterm infants with RDS.

Oxygen Saturation Targeting and Permissive Hypercapnia

Despite the advances attributed to prenatal steroids, surfactant, and newer modes of ventilation, RDS continues to carry significant morbidity, including the risk of BPD. New strategies have evolved to improve outcomes. An aggressive approach to limiting exposure to O_2 is one of these widely adopted novel strategies. O_2 has numerous toxic effects, and of particular concern is the potential for O_2 to cause cellular injury—to the brain in particular—via production of O_2-derived free radicals. O_2 upregulates transcription factors, such as nuclear factor (NF) κB, and promotes release of proinflammatory cytokines, thus leading to persistent inflammation. Many centers now aim to keep the percent of O_2 saturation in the 80s or low 90s for preterm babies to decrease the chances of hyperoxygenation and free radical production. Although the data are scant and not well controlled, no evidence currently suggests adverse neurologic effects of the lower saturations. However, it is recommended that saturations be kept in the high 90s once an infant's corrected gestational age reaches the late preterm range.

Another recent change in neonatal practice is the adoption of permissive hypercapnia. Permissive hypercapnia involves allowing CO_2 levels in the blood to rise above 40 mm Hg to minimize the pressures (and volumes) required for ventilation and thereby potentially reduce the lung injury. This practice also allows for infants, who might have been reintubated in the past because of CO_2 retention, to remain extubated. Although procedures differ, CO_2 levels of 45–55 mm Hg are generally accepted, with some centers allowing higher CO_2 levels without changing ventilatory management. The side effects of this approach are unknown, but hypercapnia may decrease the autoregulatory capacity of cerebral vessels, potentially resulting in pressure-passive cerebral circulation (26). This is primarily of concern in the ELBW neonate during the immediate postnatal period. Therefore, the potential long-term neurodevelopmental effects of the hypercapnia-associated, pressure-passive cerebral circulation should be investigated.

Encouraged by data from nonrandomized studies at Columbia University in New York, many neonatologists are now attempting to avoid intubation and mechanical ventilation altogether, even in the tiniest babies. Using CPAP delivered via nasal prongs for newborns with respiratory distress soon after birth and a strategy of permissive hypercapnia, investigators at Columbia reported a low incidence of BPD, compared to other tertiary care centers, without a significant increase in mortality. As these findings must be confirmed in appropriately designed randomized clinical trials, some centers have chosen an intermediate approach, i.e., preterm infants less than an arbitrarily chosen gestational age (typically <28–30 weeks) with respiratory distress at birth are intubated for surfactant administration but extubated shortly thereafter. Although approaches differ, early extubation is now a widely shared goal among neonatologists. However, evidence that this approach is more effective in

reducing the incidence of medium- and long-term pulmonary and neurodevelopmental sequelae is not yet available.

Bronchopulmonary Dysplasia

Definitions and Epidemiology

BPD, often referred to as chronic lung disease of prematurity, is the most common chronic lung disease of childhood. The classic severe form of BPD as first reported in the late 1960s (40) (and discussed in detail later in this section) was described as a disease that affected infants born at 30–35 weeks of gestation with a history of hyaline membrane disease, significant ventilatory support, and prolonged O_2 exposure. Premature neonates born today are more likely to be more immature and to have received antenatal steroids, postnatal surfactant, and a shorter period of mechanical ventilation than those born during the 1960s. In addition, with advances in neonatal care and technology, infants born at earlier and earlier gestational ages are surviving. Consequently, the chronic lung disease of prematurity has changed and the classic severe form of BPD is seen less frequently, if at all. An increasing number of small, preterm infants are now surviving with a milder form of chronic lung damage, which has been described as "the new BPD." In addition to the changing pathophysiology of BPD, the definition of BPD has also recently changed. The initial definition of BPD was a requirement for O_2 at 28 days after birth. The definition has been revised to include the requirement for O_2 or ventilatory support at 36 weeks of corrected postnatal age (24). In addition to this "clinical" definition of BPD, it has been suggested that O_2 requirement at 36 weeks postmenstrual age should be challenged in every neonate, and only infants who fail to sustain O_2 saturations in the 90% range should be diagnosed with BPD (physiologic definition).

Infants commonly affected with this newer form of BPD are those of extremely low birth weight, usually born at less than 28 weeks of gestation. These infants typically receive antenatal corticosteroids and postnatal surfactant and initially do remarkably well, requiring low concentrations of supplemental O_2 and, often, only minimal ventilatory support for their initial RDS. However, subsequent complications, thought to be due at least in part to the dysregulated production of inflammatory cytokines, shift the balance from developmentally regulated, appropriate alveolar and vascular development to a process of premature maturation. This premature maturation of the lung is associated with an arrest in alveolar development and a loss of surface area for functional gas exchange. Scientific evidence suggests that this disordered development of the lung parenchyma may lead to important abnormalities in lung function, which may persist throughout the first decade of life and beyond (23).

Although severe BPD is now rare in infants born after 32 weeks of gestation, there is good evidence to suggest that the incidence of BPD may be increasing in infants who are born at <28 weeks of gestation or weigh <1000 g. Factors that contribute to this increase include more live births at this level of immaturity, more very low-birth-weight (VLBW) infants born in the US, and the improved neonatal survival for ELBW and VLBW infants. In the National Institute of Child Health & Development network, the incidence of BPD at 36 weeks postmenstrual age in infants between 500–1500 g has increased from

TABLE 44.4

OVERVIEW OF SURFACTANT TRIALS AND OUTCOME

Outcome variable	Survanta vs. exosurf	Infasurf* vs. exosurf	Infasurf* vs. survanta	Curosurf vs. exosurf**	Curosurf*** vs. ALEC	Curosurf*** vs. survanta	Alveofact vs. curosurf*** vs. survanta	Lucinactant vs. exosurf vs. survanta vs. curosurf
BPD	NIL	NIL	NIL	NIL	NIL	NIL	NIL	Less BPD[†]
IVH	NIL	Increased*,[‡]	NIL	Increased**	NIL	NIL	NIL	NIL
Mortality	NIL	NIL	Increased*	NIL	Decreased***	Decreased***	NIL	NIL
Doses	NIL	NIL	NIL	NIL	NIL	Fewer doses***	NIL	NIL
PPV days	NIL	NIL	NIL	NIL	NIL	NIL	Fewer days***	NIL
O₂ days	NIL	NIL	NIL	NIL	NIL	NIL	Fewer days***	NIL
LOS	NIL	NIL	NIL	NIL	NIL	NIL	Fewer days***	NIL

[‡]Prophylaxis trial; * observed with Infasurf; * observed with Infasurf in infants weighing <600 g in the prophylaxis trial; **observed with Exosurf; ***observed with Curosurf; † observed in arm of trial that compared Lucinactant with Exosurf (40.2% incidence of BPD in patients who received Lucinactant vs. 45% incidence of BPD in patients who received Exosurf, p = 0.045).
BPD, bronchopulmonary dysplasia; IVH, intraventricular hemorrhage; LOS, length of stay; NIL, no difference

19% in 1990 to 23% by the late 1990s. Furthermore, 60% of ventilated VLBW infants are at risk of O_2 dependency at 28 days of life, and 30% will still require O_2 at 36 weeks postnatal age (15). For the ELBW neonates, the incidence of BPD is estimated at 40%. Evidence shows that the need for mechanical ventilation increases the incidence of BPD to as high as 75%. Data from the Vermont Oxford Network database shows that the incidence of BPD has not decreased in the last 5 years. Furthermore, the relative risk of developing BPD increases by nearly twofold for each week of decrease in gestational age at birth.

The pathologic description of bronchopulmonary dysplasia by Northway divides the process into four distinct stages. Stage 1 describes the early findings of hyaline membrane disease, today referred to as RDS. Stage 2, occurs between days 4 and 10 of progression of the disease and is characterized by atelectasis, alternating with areas of emphysema, and increasing opacifications with air bronchograms on chest x-ray. In stage 3, typically present on days 11–30, permanent features of the disease appear, including bronchial and bronchiolar hyperplasia and cystic changes that were visible radiographically. The final stage (stage 4), presenting after the first postnatal month, is characterized by the pathologic findings of extensive fibrosis and destruction of the airways and alveoli. At this last stage, radiographic findings consist of fibrosis and areas of both consolidation and overinflation.

In comparison to this "classic" form of BPD, the "new BPD" shows more uniform lung inflation and only minimal fibrosis. In ELBW infants, the lung is completing the canalicular phase of lung development at the time of birth. It is believed that interference with the progress of alveolar development results in alveolar hypoplasia, the major abnormality described in the BPD of the premature infant seen today. In comparison to the classic form of BPD, characteristic features of the new BPD include formation of alveoli that are larger, more simplified, and fewer in number, and the presence of variable airway smooth muscle hyperplasia, with a significant decrease in airway lesions and interstitial fibroproliferation.

Etiology and Prevention

Identification of the risk factors for BPD and effective intervention strategies has been difficult due to significant differences among the studies in the time of disease assessment (28 days vs. 36 weeks of postnatal age). Nevertheless, the current understanding of BPD indicates a multifactorial etiology. By far, the most important factor is prematurity. In addition, intrauterine growth retardation places neonates at increased risk. While we still know little about the genetic contribution to the occurrence of BPD, a family history of lung disease, such as reactive airway disease, has been described as an additional risk factor.

Accumulating evidence suggests that inflammation plays a pivotal role in the pathogenesis of BPD. The inflammatory response can be triggered by a number of factors, including mechanical ventilation-associated barotrauma and volutrauma, free O_2 radicals, increased pulmonary blood flow [usually a result of a patent ductus arteriosus (PDA) with left-to-right shunting] and systemic or pulmonary infection acquired prenatally. The possible role of prenatal infection is supported by the increased incidence of BPD in infants born to mothers with chorioamnionitis. In addition, postnatal bacterial infection has clearly been shown to increase risk. Finally, infants whose airways are colonized with *Ureaplasma urealyticum* at birth ap-

pear to be at higher risk for BPD, although such an association has not been consistently demonstrated.

Among the markers of inflammation present in high concentrations in the tracheal aspirates of infants in whom BPD developed are interleukins IL-6, IL-8, IL-11, TNF-α, and tumor growth factor-β. Evidence exists of pulmonary alveolar macrophage activation in infants who subsequently develop BPD. These activated macrophages, especially when exposed to hyperoxia, are the likely sources of neutrophil chemotactant.

As mentioned previously, a significant association has been characterized between PDA and BPD. However, more recently, the relationship between ductal patency and the risk of developing BPD has been questioned. Although the human data are not definitive, animal data have demonstrated that prolonged left-to-right shunting through the PDA contributes to the development of BPD most likely via the shunt-induced increases in pulmonary blood flow, capillary pressure, and lung fluid secretion, and the compromised lung fluid clearance.

The association between O_2 toxicity and BPD has been known since the late 60s. Since that time, reports have continued to show an association between high supplemental O_2 exposure and lung damage in preterm infants who receive mechanical ventilation. The damage to the lung caused by O_2 toxicity appears to be mediated by reactive O_2 species, such as superoxide anion, hydrogen peroxide, and hydroxyl radicals, which are produced as molecular O_2 is reduced. The concept of oxidant and antioxidant imbalance in the preterm infant's lung has been supported in animal and human observational studies. Supplementation of the newborn preterm infant with retinoic acid derivatives has been shown to suppress formation of both superoxide and hydrogen peroxide (48). More recent evidence has shown that treatment of animals with antioxidants can protect against the formation of O_2 toxicity by-products involved in the pathogenesis of lung injury (9).

The association between mechanical ventilation of the preterm lung and the development of BPD has also been studied. Overdistension of the lung due to mechanical injury can cause leakage of fluid into the alveolar space and the release of proinflammatory cytokines. Animal studies have shown that prevention of overdistension lessens the degree of microvascular permeability abnormalities. Clinically, hyperventilation, hypocarbia, and the presence of an air leak, such as a pneumothorax and/or pulmonary interstitial emphysema, have all been linked to a higher relative risk of BPD.

In the past decade, significant improvements have been made in the mechanical ventilation strategies for preterm infants at risk of BPD. However, randomized clinical trials have not yet identified the mechanical ventilation mode associated with the lowest incidence of BPD. Theoretically, high-frequency oscillatory ventilation (HFOV), compared to conventional ventilation, offers greater prospects for more uniform lung inflation, with fewer areas of lung overdistension and reduced atelectasis. Nevertheless, a reduction in BPD has not been universally found in randomized clinical trials that compared HFOV to conventional ventilation. This may be, at least in part, due to differences in HFOV strategy and the baseline incidence of BPD among the different trials (13,25,35,56,60).

Accumulating evidence from animal and human studies demonstrates that end-expiratory lung volumes less than functional residual capacity and the resulting atelectasis are major contributors to the pathogenesis of BPD. In this paradigm, infants ventilated below functional residual capacity undergo repetitive overdistension of lung units. There is increasing evidence that optimal use of recruiting distending pressures, i.e., positive end-expiratory pressure (PEEP), may be associated with a lower risk of BPD. Indeed, it is now believed, although not yet proven, that appropriate use of PEEP or CPAP may be the most protective intervention in the prevention of BPD.

In addition to mechanical ventilatory strategies aimed at minimizing overdistension of the developing lung, many neonatologists, encouraged by data from nonrandomized, widely publicized studies from Columbia University, are now attempting to avoid intubation and/or mechanical ventilation in even the tiniest babies. As mentioned previously, using CPAP with nasal prongs in newborns with respiratory distress immediately after birth (regardless of gestational age or birth weight), combined with the strategy of permissive hypercapnia, physicians at Columbia University have reported a low incidence of BPD compared to other tertiary care centers, without any significant increase in mortality. The use of nasal CPAP immediately after birth appears to be associated with a lower incidence of BPD in other centers as well. Indeed, the best predictor of subsequent BPD is the need for endotracheal mechanical ventilation on the day of birth. Although as of yet, no large, randomized trials of this approach have been published, the use of nasal CPAP has been found to be effective in preventing failure of extubation in preterm infants following endotracheal intubation. In addition, the use of intermittent mandatory positive-pressure ventilation in nonintubated patients with BPD results in a decreased need for reintubation (18). Although approaches differ, early extubation is now a widely shared goal among neonatologists. Some centers continue to intubate VLBW infants after birth for surfactant administration, but the endotracheal tube is removed shortly after the surfactant has been given, resulting in a shorter duration of mechanical ventilation. However, no evidence suggests a significant decrease in the incidence of BPD in survivors who have received surfactant.

The issue of the optimal $PaCO_2$ level in the preterm infant has also been debated in recent years. Permissive hypercapnia, i.e., allowing CO_2 levels in the blood to rise above the normal value of 40 mm Hg to minimize the barotrauma and volutrauma required for ventilation, has been widely adopted. It is not unusual for neonatologists to allow $PaCO_2$ levels to be as high as 55–70 torr, especially in high-risk, ventilated, preterm neonates beyond the first postnatal week. Although no evidence has demonstrated an acute detrimental affect of permissive hypercapnia in the short-term, the long-term safety of permissive hypercapnia has not been studied. In addition, as mentioned previously, because hypercapnia may decrease the autoregulatory capacity of the cerebral vessels, the potential short- and long-term neurodevelopmental effects of the hypercapnia-associated, pressure-passive, cerebral circulation should be investigated, especially if permissive hypercapnia is used during the first postnatal days.

The role of inhaled nitric oxide (iNO) in the prevention of BPD has also generated much interest. The rationale for the use of iNO in preterm infants with RDS is based on its potential to reverse pulmonary hypertension, improve $\dot{V}/\dot{Q}$ matching, and decrease the inflammatory response. The first trial to demonstrate a significant decrease in the incidence of BPD or death in preterm infants treated with iNO was published in 2003 (46). In this single-centered trial, infants who were born before 34 weeks' gestation with RDS and who received mechanical ventilation and surfactant therapy were assigned to receive ei-

ther iNO or placebo. A significant decrease in the incidence of BPD was seen in the iNO cohort compared to controls (48.6% vs. 63.7%; relative risk, 0.76; 95% confidence interval, 0.6–0.97). Four other earlier trials that investigated the use of iNO in premature infants did not demonstrate a significant decrease in the incidence of BPD, although a trend toward a decreased incidence of BPD was seen in one study (29). Interestingly, the findings of 2 recent large, randomized, controlled trials appear to be encouraging for the use of low-dose iNO in the prevention of BPD in preterm infants (4,27). One trial found that iNO improves the pulmonary outcome for preterm infants at risk for BPD, without apparent short-term adverse effects, when started at 20 ppm between 7 and 21 postnatal days of age and administered at decreasing concentrations for a minimum of 24 days (4). The findings of the other trial indicate an iNO-associated improvement in the combined end-point of intracranial hemorrhage, periventricular leukomalacia, or ventriculomegaly when 5 ppm of iNO is started shortly after birth and given for 21 days or until extubation. However, in that the subpopulations of patients most likely to benefit from low-dose iNO treatment, the most appropriate timing, duration and dose of iNO administration and the long-term neurodevelopmental outcomes of iNO-exposed, high-risk preterm neonates are not known, the routine use of iNO for the prevention of BPD in preterm infants cannot yet be recommended, and iNO administration for the prevention of BPD should still be restricted to well-designed study protocols.

Steroids for the Prevention of Bronchopulmonary Dysplasia

Dexamethasone was a key part of efforts to prevent and/or treat BPD for many years. Indeed, premature infants who receive postnatal corticosteroids demonstrate decreased levels of inflammatory markers, and clinicians have used corticosteroids in hopes of decreasing the symptoms of BPD in high-risk populations. Although clinical trials have demonstrated short-term benefits, especially with respect to improving dynamic compliance and decreasing pulmonary resistance following treatment with corticosteroids, the overall impact of corticosteroids on BPD remains controversial. Significant adverse effects of dexamethasone administration, especially when high cumulative doses are given to preterm neonates, include hypertension, hyperglycemia, adrenal suppression, decreased growth, and abnormal neurodevelopment. In addition, the concomitant use of dexamethasone and a prostaglandin synthesis inhibitor, such as indomethacin, has been associated with an increased risk of spontaneous intestinal perforation during the first 2 postnatal weeks. As for the effect of postnatal administration of dexamethasone on neurodevelopmental outcome, follow-up data from randomized trials provide clear evidence that the administration of dexamethasone, in particular when given early and/or as a prolonged course, is associated with an increased incidence of adverse neurodevelopmental outcome (49). Therefore, dexamethasone is now reserved for patients with the most severe lung disease with respiratory failure, although, in general, no data support a better long-term pulmonary outcome with its use. Dexamethasone, if used at all, is now also given in lower doses and shorter courses than in the past. The American Academy of Pediatrics currently recommends that neonatologists counsel parents about the risks and benefits of dexamethasone prior to initiating treatment.

Some centers use low-to-medium doses of hydrocortisone to prevent and/or treat BPD in an uncontrolled manner. Therefore, very little data are available from appropriately designed randomized clinical trials regarding the efficacy or safety of the use of hydrocortisone compared to dexamethasone. As for the side effects (similar to those of dexamethasone), the concomitant administration of hydrocortisone and indomethacin has been associated with an increased risk of spontaneous intestinal perforation during the first 2 postnatal weeks (63). However, findings of observational studies using MRI and neurodevelopmental and intelligence testing suggest that, contrary to dexamethasone, hydrocortisone given over a period of 3 weeks in a cumulative dose of 50 mg/kg after the first postnatal week for the prevention and/or treatment of BPD in VLBW infants has no discernible effect at 7–8 years of age on cortical gray matter, white matter, and hippocampal volumes; motor and sensorineural development; or intelligence and memory (32,43).

In summary, no evidence suggests that dexamethasone (or hydrocortisone) administration to prevent or treat BPD in VLBW neonates improves pulmonary outcomes, and corticosteroid administration in general has significant side effects, including the occurrence of spontaneous intestinal perforation and poor neurodevelopmental outcome. Furthermore, despite the lack of evidence of untoward long-term central nervous system (CNS) effects of hydrocortisone, routine use of either medication must be discouraged, and their use should be restricted to brief administration of lower doses in patients with life-threatening respiratory failure despite optimum ventilatory and critical care support.

Management

The management and treatment of infants at risk of developing BPD should be directed toward (a) minimizing ventilatory support and alveolar overdistension, (b) supporting and maintaining functional residual capacity with optimal PEEP, (c) optimizing growth, and (d) judiciously using diuretics and bronchodilators. These goals can be achieved in part by employing optimal alveolar recruitment strategies to prevent atelectasis and sustain functional residual capacity, allowing as much as possible for synchrony between the infant and ventilation, and by embracing moderate permissive hypercapnia. In addition to carefully applying ventilation strategies, it is important to determine an appropriate target for the O_2 saturation in preterm infants. It should be emphasized that, in utero, the fetus is exposed to a Po_2 in the range of 25–30 mm Hg and an O_2 saturation of between 60%–80%. A large clinical trial that examined the care and treatment of retinopathy of prematurity revealed that infants maintained at O_2 saturations between 89–94% during the trial had a lower incidence of BPD than infants whose saturations were maintained over 96% (52). Based on these and other findings, significant changes in the targeted saturation range for premature infants have been instituted in many NICUs over the past 5 years. As mentioned previously, many centers now aim to keep the O_2 saturation percent for preterm neonates in the range of 80% to low 90's in the first postnatal weeks. Although the studies that have been done have typically been poorly controlled, no evidence currently suggests an adverse long-term neurodevelopmental impact of the presently targeted lower O_2 saturations. However, future studies must be designed to examine the potential side effects of lower O_2 saturations, including neurodevelopmental outcome and the potential for the development of pulmonary hyper-

tension and subsequent cor pulmonale during infancy or early childhood.

The optimization of growth and nutrition is essential to achieve early successful extubation. Careful attention to the infant's nutritional status is important for the promotion of lung growth. For example, vitamin A has been shown to decrease the incidence of BPD in clinical trials.

Diuretics have been used extensively to minimize pulmonary edema in the early stages of BPD. It has been reported that the use of loop diuretics, such as furosemide, improves lung mechanics and gas exchange in infants with established BPD. The use of thiazide diuretics, either alone or in combination with spironolactone (Aldactone), has been shown to improve lung function and mortality in clinical studies and in a meta-analysis of these clinical studies, respectively. The major drawbacks to the long-term use of diuretics are the metabolic complications, including a diuretic-induced hypochloremic and hypokalemic metabolic alkalosis. The hypochloremic alkalosis induced by diuretics can be detected by evaluating the electrolytes and blood gases in chronic BPD patients. Over time, these infants develop a compensatory respiratory acidosis in the presence of elevated serum bicarbonate. Therefore, ensuring adequate chloride and potassium intake is important when infants are receiving diuretics for the treatment of BPD. In addition, the long-term use of furosemide is associated with ototoxicity and significant hypercalciuria and nephrocalcinosis. Consequently, the routine, prolonged, and indiscriminate use of diuretic treatment in infants with BPD cannot be recommended.

By the time BPD is established, airway resistance is increased with clinical evidence of intermittent or persistent wheezing. The judicious use of inhaled β_2-adrenergic agonists is associated with improvement in ventilation. A common drug regimen includes inhaled albuterol therapy. Some neonatologists also use inhaled corticosteroids to minimize the inflammatory process that contributes to, and often causes, exacerbations of BPD. However, no evidence suggests that the use of inhaled corticosteroids improves pulmonary outcome.

Implications for Long-term Outcome

Fortunately, the mortality associated with BPD is significantly lower today than it was in the past (24). Nevertheless, it is estimated that the mortality rates associated with the most severe form of BPD and cor pulmonale can be as high as 40%, and the morbidities are significant. BPD is a multisystem disorder that affects more than just the lungs and is likely to remain, for those infants afflicted, a life-long condition.

Long-term morbidities associated with BPD include airway damage and cardiovascular complications, such as pulmonary hypertension and cor pulmonale. Some patients with BPD require tracheostomy for long-term mechanical ventilation. In the long-term follow-up of preterm infants, BPD is associated with poor neurodevelopmental outcome. However, it is not easy to separate the effects of BPD from the effects of immaturity and other complications of prematurity. Recurrent episodes of hypoxia with significant respiratory disease and the effects of the dysregulated inflammatory cytokines on both the lungs and the brain may explain, at least in part, the association between BPD and poor neurodevelopmental outcome. On the other hand, prolonged exposure to high concentrations of O_2 can lead to reactive O_2 species that may cause injury to the CNS—again, via a dysregulated inflammatory response. Furthermore, infants with BPD are often exposed to several pharmacologic agents, the effect of which on the developing CNS is not well established. Lastly, poor nutrition may play a role in the poor developmental outcome of children with BPD; they are often challenging to feed, and their supraphysiologic caloric requirements are often difficult to consistently achieve.

DISORDERS OF TRANSITION

Transient Tachypnea of the Newborn

Transient tachypnea of the newborn (TTN) was described in 1966 in a series of 8 term infants with early-onset respiratory distress, x-rays findings of increased pulmonary vascular markings, pulmonary edema, mild hyperexpansion, and mild cardiomegaly, and symptoms that resolved within 2–5 days. TTN has been shown to be due to a delay in the cessation of production and ensuing clearance of fetal lung fluid. The pathophysiology of TTN is dependent on an understanding of fetal lung fluid mechanics during gestation and early neonatal transition.

In fetal life, the lung epithelium actively secretes fluid into the intra-alveolar space at a rate of ~4–6 mL/kg/hr by late preterm gestation due to the upregulated activity of the 2-Cl^- K^+ Na^+ cotransporter pumping chloride, sodium, and potassium from the interstitium to the airspaces. This rate of fluid secretion slows in the 1–2 days preceding labor due to increased fetal catecholamine levels and β-receptor–mediated inhibition of the cotransporter in the lungs. The change in the hormonal milieu coincident with parturition changes the activity of other ion channels in the epithelium to actively absorb, rather than secrete, fluid primarily through activation of the Na/K-ATPase. Therefore, infants born by elective cesarean section (i.e., cesarean section without labor) are at higher risk for developing TTN and for overall pulmonary morbidity, most likely because they do not undergo the normal hormonal changes essential to the natural transition to extrauterine life, including a surge in epinephrine, norepinephrine, thyroid hormones, cortisol, etc.

Clinically, TTN presents with increased work of breathing, respiratory distress, hypoxemia, and CO_2 retention. The differential diagnosis includes sepsis, pneumonia, RDS, pulmonary hypertension, congenital lung malformation, and congenital heart disease. The diagnosis of TTN is one of exclusion. Early treatment is focused on supportive care with careful O_2 administration and positive pressure as needed, radiographs to rule out lung malformations, antibiotics while the infant is evaluated for sepsis, and an echocardiogram if indicated. TTN is by definition a transient disease, and although the infants may appear clinically sick with moderate respiratory failure initially, they typically improve significantly within 8–24 hrs. The initial chest x-ray findings of pulmonary edema, air bronchograms, and hyperexpansion also resolve within the same time frame, making x-rays an effective way to differentiate TTN from neonatal pneumonia, as the x-ray findings in pneumonia will persist beyond the first 24–48 hrs.

Persistent Pulmonary Hypertension of the Newborn

Persistent pulmonary hypertension of the newborn (PPHN) is a clinical syndrome of failure of pulmonary vascular transition to extrauterine life that results in increased pulmonary pressures, hypoxemia, and respiratory distress. Although the incidence is not precisely known, it is ~1–2 per 1000 live-born births and continues to account for significant neonatal morbidity and mortality despite recent advances in available therapies.

In utero, the placenta, not the lungs, serves as the organ of gas exchange, and pulmonary resistance is maintained at or above systemic levels to maintain low pulmonary blood flow (estimated at 10% of combined ventricular output around midgestation, increasing to 20–25% by term). Pulmonary vascular resistance is actively maintained, despite a rapidly growing vascular surface area, through constriction of the pulmonary vascular smooth muscle cells by a variety of pathways, including hypoxia, endothelin-1, and thromboxane. As the fetus approaches term gestation, vasodilatory pathways are upregulated and become increasingly dominant. The most well-studied and understood of these vasodilating pathways are the nitric oxide (NO) and prostacyclin pathways. Increases in cyclic guanosine monophosphate (cGMP) levels lead to vasorelaxation via a decrease in intracellular calcium. cGMP is inactivated by the phosphodiesterase (PDE) enzymes, specifically PDE5. Prostacyclin exerts its physiologic effect through an analogous pathway. As an arachidonic acid metabolite, prostacyclin's rate-limiting step involves the cyclooxygenase enzymes COX-1 and COX-2; however, the rate-determining step involves the enzyme prostacyclin synthase (PGIS). Prostacyclin activates adenylate cyclase to increase the production of cAMP from ATP, leading to decreased intracellular calcium concentration and, thus, vasorelaxation (**Fig. 44.1**). Endothelial nitric oxide synthase (eNOS), PGIS, and COX-1 expression are increased in the pulmonary endothelium as term gestation approaches, priming the vasculature to respond to vasodilatory stimuli.

At birth, multiple factors interact to regulate these pathways and dilate the pulmonary vasculature during the first few breaths, leading to an approximate 50% reduction in pulmonary resistance and a five- to tenfold increase in pulmonary blood flow. Critical signals for this transition are mechanical distension of the lung, falling CO_2 tension, and rising O_2 tension. Specifically, O_2 stimulates the activity of both eNOS and COX-1, leading to increased levels of NO and prostacyclin. Furthermore, increased O_2 tension increases ATP release from red blood cells, which also activates COX-1 and eNOS. Significant derangements in metabolic homeostasis, i.e., acidosis, hypoxemia, and hypercarbia, prevent the coordinated transition from vasoconstricting to vasodilating predominance, leading to the clinical syndrome of PPHN.

The most common precipitating diseases, most of which are described in greater detail elsewhere in this chapter, are meconium aspiration syndrome, sepsis/pneumonia, perinatal depression/acidosis, abnormal pulmonary vascular development, pulmonary hypoplasia, and idiopathic "black lung" PPHN. In patients with these diseases, it is essential to have an understanding of the different etiologies of PPHN to tailor therapy. However, regardless of the etiology, hypoxemic respiratory failure in these infants is evident from birth or shortly thereafter, often with progressive cardiovascular compromise. The differential diagnosis includes congenital heart disease (most commonly, obstructed total anomalous pulmonary venous return), sepsis/pneumonia, polycythemia, perinatal depression, and metabolic disease.

Initial treatment of PPHN includes correction of metabolic derangements, such as hypothermia, hypoglycemia, hypocalcemia, anemia, polycythemia, and hypovolemia. The use of

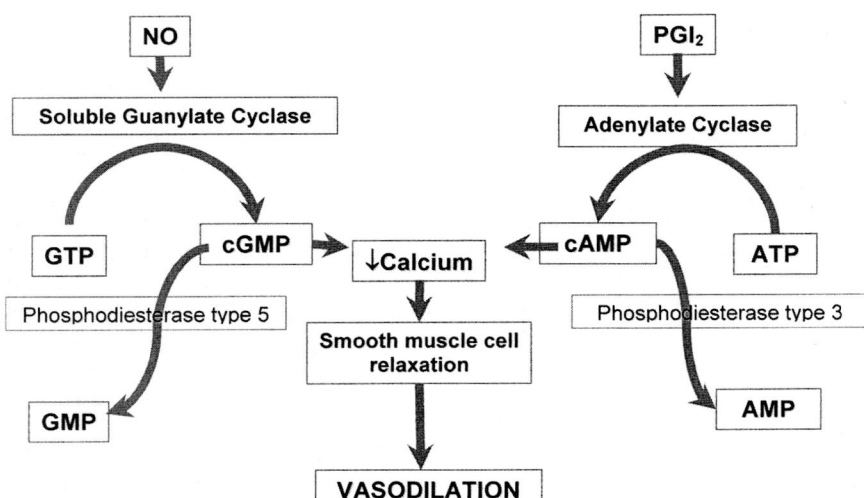

FIGURE 44.1. The parallel mechanisms of action of nitric oxide and prostacyclin working through the cyclic GMP and AMP systems via soluble guanylate cyclases and adenylate cyclase.

alkalinizing agents is controversial, and induced alkalosis has been linked with adverse outcomes; however, correction of metabolic acidosis to physiologic pH is standard therapy. The appropriate use of vasopressor/inotropes (dopamine or epinephrine), inotropes (dobutamine), and lusitropes (milrinone) to support systemic perfusion (cardiac output) and myocardial function without inducing unwanted increases in the pulmonary vascular resistance (PVR) is important. The historic practice of using vasopressors/inotropes to drive the blood pressure to supraphysiologic levels to "force" blood through the lungs cannot be recommended, as increased PVR may occur. Monitoring of the preductal (right arm or right side of the face) and postductal (lower extremity) saturations can provide a reasonable estimation of ductal-level shunting and severity of PPHN, assuming the ductus arteriosus is patent.

The goal of mechanical ventilation is to achieve "optimal" lung volume and recruitment (9–10 ribs) through the use of conventional or HFOV and to establish normal $Paco_2$ levels and normal oxygenation. Failure to achieve lung recruitment at or above functional residual capacity contributes to hypoxemia and high PVR. Conversely, hyperexpansion, particularly with the constant distending pressure of HFOV, may also worsen pulmonary hypertension by causing the compression of capillaries and small arterioles and decreased cardiac output by interfering with venous return to the heart. Some evidence suggests that HFOV will improve lung recruitment in homogenous lung disease and may improve delivery of NO to the alveolar surface (28). iNO has been shown in 2 large, multicentered, randomized, controlled trials to improve oxygenation and decrease the need for extracorporeal membrane oxygenation (ECMO) in term infants with hypoxemic respiratory failure and an oxygenation index of >25 when started at 20 ppm (37,11). Recent studies have looked at starting iNO therapy earlier or at lower doses and have not shown any improvement in patient outcome when compared to this standard regimen. Surfactant is beneficial in improving compliance and oxygenation in infants with specific diseases and is described in further detail in other sections of this chapter.

ECMO remains the final rescue therapy for infants with PPHN. The ECMO trial conducted in the UK and published in 1996 was a randomized, controlled trial of conventional therapy with or without ECMO as rescue therapy. This trial was largely completed before the widespread use of iNO and showed a clear survival benefit with ECMO versus conventional therapy (relative risk of death, 0.51; 95% confidence interval, 0.36–0.73) (57). More recent trials have studied the long-term effects of the newer, aggressive pre-ECMO therapy and not shown any changes in long-term outcome or time to discharge, at least as can be determined using the Extracorporeal Life Support Organization registry data (16).

The underlying principle in the treatment of PPHN is that, in the vast majority of cases, it is a reversible disease, and if one can avoid overt toxicity of the therapy and support the infant during the acute phase of the disease, the pulmonary vasculature will remodel and/or dilate and the long-term outcome will be excellent. The exception is when the process is not reversible, as when the vasculature is hypoplastic [hypoplastic lungs, congenital diaphragmatic hernia (CDH)] or malformed (alveolar capillary dysplasia). The pulmonary vascular transition after birth and the development of treatments to minimize or avoid the toxicities of current therapies remain active areas of research, especially because a large number of infants still require rescue therapy with ECMO.

Meconium Aspiration Syndrome

Approximately 13%–15% of all births in the US are complicated by meconium-stained amniotic fluid (MSAF), with 3%–6% subsequently developing meconium aspiration syndrome (MAS) (~25,000–30,000 cases per year), making MAS the most common cause of PPHN. Infants pass meconium in utero in response to stressful stimuli. A small subset of these infants who develop severe hypoxemia and acidosis and start gasping (second phase of apnea) will then aspirate the MSAF into their airway, creating the scenario that can lead to MAS. MAS occurs when an infant born through MSAF develops a subsequent pneumonitis, leading to respiratory distress and PPHN. In infants who have significant MAS, it is important to consider the cause of the passage of meconium and to be alert to signs of perinatal depression.

The management of the delivery of infants born through MSAF has evolved. The guidelines of the Neonatal Resuscitation Program no longer recommend the routine suctioning of the oropharynx of infants born through MSAF at the perineum (prior to delivery of the infant's body). However, the Neonatal Resuscitation Program does continue to recommend that non-vigorous infants born through MSAF be intubated and undergo tracheal suctioning by the neonatal team. In addition, it is no longer recommended to intubate and suction vigorous infants. This recommendation is largely based on a study that showed no improvement in outcome for the vigorous infants who had tracheal suctioning, compared with those who did not; it also showed increased complications in those who underwent routine intubation and intratracheal suctioning (64).

Meconium exerts its toxic effect primarily through activation of the inflammatory cascade, resulting in the development of chemical pneumonitis. Meconium aspiration leads to the release of cytokines, such as TNF-α, IL-1β, and IL-8, and activates the alternative complement pathway, which directly injures the lung parenchyma, leading to vascular leak, pneumonitis, and pulmonary edema. Evidence suggests that meconium pneumonitis triggers increased postnatal release of the potent vasoconstrictors endothelin-1 and thromboxane A2, worsening the pulmonary hypertension. Additionally, the meconium itself can cause intermittent airway obstruction with a "ball-valve" effect. The inflammatory response, the increase in vasoconstrictors, and the mechanical effect of meconium combine to make infants with meconium aspiration extremely sick, with poorly compliant lungs, a tendency toward air trapping, and a high risk of pneumothoraces. The ensuing respiratory failure and the dysregulated production of vasoconstrictors prevent the normal drop in PVR that is required for the transition to extrauterine life and may result in severe pulmonary hypertension and hypoxia. The typical x-ray findings include patchy infiltrates with patchy areas of atelectasis and hyperinflation.

Initial management of MAS includes supportive therapy, including intubation, cardiovascular support, analgesia, and antibiotics. Corticosteroids have been studied extensively in these infants and, although it remains controversial, the evidence at this time does not support the routine use of steroids in MAS. Meconium has been shown in laboratory settings to inactivate surfactant and to displace it from the alveolar surface. Indeed, surfactant replacement therapy improves lung compliance and oxygenation in infants with MAS and decreases the need for ECMO. iNO, a selective pulmonary vasodilator, is recommended for infants who do not respond to the previous therapies; iNO is further discussed in the section on PPHN.

CONGENITAL LUNG ANOMALIES

Congenital Diaphragmatic Hernia

CDH occurs in 1 per 2000–4000 live births and accounts for 1%–2% of infant mortality in the US. The mortality for infants with CDH remains ~30%, although this number is changing, as antenatal diagnosis has increased and certain centers are currently reporting significant increases in survival. However, increased antenatal diagnosis is uncovering what Harrison refers to as the "hidden mortality" of CDH, i.e., a previously underappreciated rate of intrauterine fetal demise with CDH and an increasing rate of elective termination. CDH occurs due to a failure of closure of the pleuroperitoneal folds at around ges-

tational week 5, resulting in a posterolateral diaphragmatic defect (Bochdalek hernia). The defect is most often on the left side, although ~10% will be on the right side and 2% will be bilateral. CDH is almost universally associated with lung hypoplasia primarily on the ipsilateral side; however, the contralateral side is typically hypoplastic as well.

CDH can occur as an isolated defect or, in ~40% of cases, in association with another major anomaly. CDH occurs as a feature of a number of syndromes (Denys-Drash, neonatal Marfan syndrome, Simpson-Golabi-Behmell, Beckwith-Wiedemann, Pallister-Killean, Fryns syndrome, etc.) with a variety of gene mutations, both known and unknown, and diverse inheritance patterns. Animal models exist, but none completely mimic the human disease. The most studied animal model is the nitrofen-induced diaphragmatic hernia rodent model. Nitrofen, a pesticide, causes CDH in roughly 50% of the litter after exposing the pregnant mouse or rat to the toxin on embryonic days 8–11. The phenotype of this model includes CDH, pulmonary hypoplasia, conotruncal cardiac defects, and intestinal malrotation. Interestingly, some of the defects (pulmonary hypoplasia in particular) are seen in littermates who do not develop the diaphragmatic defects. The nitrofen model has been studied extensively to determine the genetics of the disease. Although the etiology remains unknown, interesting findings include increased expression of vascular cell adhesion molecule (58), decreased expression of vascular endothelial growth factor (10), and downregulation of fibroblast growth factors 7 and 10 (55).

Antenatal screening is useful to begin to stratify patients based on risk. Important risk factors are associated anomalies and the degree of pulmonary hypoplasia. In one series of 174 infants with CDH, 31 had major cardiac anomalies (including ventricular septal defect, arch obstruction, tetralogy of Fallot, and transposition of the great arteries), and only 4 of the 31 survived (12). Currently, the best predictors of pulmonary hypoplasia are the lung:head ratio (LHR) and the presence or absence of liver herniated into the chest. The LHR compares the right lung volume at the level of the four-chamber view of the heart to the head circumference at 24–26 weeks of gestation, with LHR of <0.6 predicting a 0% survival, LHR of 0.6–1.35 predicting 57% survival, and LHR of >1.35 predicting 100% survival (31). Subsequent studies have confirmed a nearly universally fatal prognosis with an LHR of <1 and a good outcome with an LHR of >1.4. This stratification of risk groups was developed for studies of fetal intervention, the majority of which investigated permanent fetal tracheal occlusion. It is known that if the trachea is occluded in utero, the lungs become hyperplastic due to the blockage of fluid egress from the lung, and the in utero intrapulmonary dynamics are altered. It has been demonstrated in separate studies using animal models of CDH that tracheal occlusion could lead to improved lung growth. Unfortunately, human studies using the permanent fetal tracheal occlusion strategy have failed to show any benefit and have been complicated by an increased rate of premature deliveries. Currently, fetal intervention for CDH has no role outside of randomized, controlled trials at experienced centers that are assessing novel fetal treatment strategies, such as endoscopic intermittent tracheal obstruction.

When the presence of a CDH is known antenatally, the delivery room management focuses on immediate intubation, as bag-and-mask ventilation should be avoided to minimize distension of the stomach and the proximal intestine that would result in further compromise in lung expansion and cardiac filling. The stomach should immediately be decompressed with a sump tube. Many centers will routinely paralyze and sedate the infants to prevent them from swallowing air and to limit activity during the initial stabilization. However, no evidence suggests that the use of neuromuscular blockade in the delivery room (or later in the course) improves outcomes, while it carries several risks, among them, sensorineural hearing loss.

Even today, not all cases of CDH are diagnosed antenatally. A number of features should raise suspicion about the possibility of CDH in the newborn with early hypoxemic respiratory distress. On physical exam, breath sounds may be absent on the left side of the chest, the heart sounds may be shifted to the right, and the abdomen tends to be scaphoid due to some of the abdominal organs shifting to the thorax. It may be difficult to effectively ventilate and resuscitate the patient. A chest x-ray confirms the diagnosis: bowel loops are seen in the chest.

Historically, the infant with CDH constituted a surgical emergency, and the diaphragmatic defect was repaired as soon as possible. This practice led to high operative mortality, and over time, the focus changed to allowing time for the infant to be stabilized and the pulmonary vascular pressures to fall prior to surgery, also providing time to assess for the presence of associated defects or syndromes that are important in determining outcome, even if surgery is indicated. The shift toward delayed surgery has occurred with little evidence other than the findings of 2 small studies that showed no change in outcome from surgery in the first 24 hrs versus after the first 24 hrs. However, in current practice, surgery is often delayed for weeks, not 1 or 2 days.

Ventilator management of CDH has also evolved based on experimental data but with little evidence from randomized, controlled trials. One of the major problems in CDH is pulmonary hypoplasia; therefore, it makes physiologic sense to avoid barotrauma, limit peak inspiratory pressures to 24–26 cm H_2O, allow spontaneous ventilation, and adopt the strategy of permissive hypercarbia. It is well known that infants with CDH have a high incidence of pulmonary hypertension; however, it is important to remember that the pulmonary vasculature in these patients is developmentally abnormal and hypoplastic; therefore, aggressive ventilator goals are likely to increase ventilator-induced injury rather than acutely lower the pulmonary pressures. Many studies in animal models of CDH have shown a relative surfactant insufficiency. Human studies of surfactant replacement have demonstrated variable results, and data from the CDH registry do not support the use of surfactant in the term or near-term CDH infant (59).

As discussed previously, selective pulmonary vasodilation with iNO is effective in infants with hypoxemic respiratory failure without CDH; however, its role in CDH is less clear. The largest study of CDH patients with iNO was in a subpopulation of the Neonatal Inhaled Nitric Oxide Study (NINOS) randomized, controlled trial of iNO. In that trial, no change was observed in the combined outcome of death or need for ECMO with the use of iNO, but a trend toward an increase in ECMO utilization was seen (38). These data have been interpreted in several ways, with some advocating that iNO stabilizes patients enough to allow for ECMO cannulation. Nevertheless, survival was unchanged between the control and treated groups. Others question why patients with CDH did not have a sustained response and whether iNO actually

made the infants less stable and, thus, more likely to require rescue therapy with ECMO. The answer remains unknown. Currently, iNO is widely used in the CDH population, and recent evidence from the Extracorporeal Life Support Organization registry supports the observation that pre-ECMO use of iNO does not worsen outcome (16). Given the lack of evidence of a sustained response, it is reasonable to restrict the use of iNO in the CDH patient to ECMO centers or to the stabilization of a patient for transport to the regional ECMO center. Late pulmonary hypertension remains a significant problem in the CDH population. Researchers are investigating the role of pulmonary vasodilators such as sildenafil, inhaled prostacyclin, and chronic iNO therapy. At this writing, data are insufficient to recommend their routine use.

Congenital Cystic Adenomatoid Malformation and Bronchopulmonary Sequestration

Congenital Cystic Adenomatoid Malformation

Congenital cystic adenomatoid malformation (CCAM) of the lung is a rare developmental abnormality believed to occur due to a failure of the normal bronchoalveolar development between weeks 5 and 7 of gestation. The lesions are typically unilateral and isolated to one lobe, but can be bilateral in <10% of cases. Several classification systems exist for CCAM, but the most commonly used is the classification by Stocker:

- Type 1: 50% of lesions; contains between one and four large cysts, typically >3 cm in diameter
- Type 2: 40% of cases; multiple smaller (<1 cm diameter) cysts
- Type 3: 10% of cases; lesions appear solid due to multiple very small cysts

CCAM is often diagnosed antenatally and the information obtained from antenatal surveillance has helped to understand the natural progression of these lesions. They typically grow significantly between 20 and 26 weeks of gestation and can lead to mediastinal shift and hydrops fetalis, most commonly seen with type 3 or with a single dominant cyst. The development of hydrops is an extremely poor prognostic sign. Occasionally, the lesions can regress as pregnancy develops. Routine ultrasound surveillance approximately weekly during the period of active growth is recommended for all types of CCAM.

Clinically, infants with CCAM present with a spectrum of illness, from severe respiratory failure to asymptomatic. The severity of respiratory compromise cannot always be predicted. Initial management focuses on stabilizing the infant and confirming the diagnosis with a chest CT or MRI, if possible. Surgical resection is recommended after stabilization. Timing of the surgery depends on the severity of the symptoms and ranges from 1–2 days to 4–6 months of age; asymptomatic cases are typically delayed. However, resection is recommended in all cases due to the high likelihood of chronic infections in the lesion and the possibility of malignant transformation, which has been reported to occur at as early as 13 months of age.

Pulmonary Sequestration

Pulmonary sequestration is another cystic lesion of the lung, differentiated from CCAM by the origin of its blood supply, which is systemic rather than pulmonary. In 15%–20% of cases, multiple feeding vessels are involved. Sequestrations can be intrapulmonary or extrapulmonary and are believed to occur due to development of an accessory lung bud. However, the exact etiology and timing is not known. Males are four times more likely to have sequestrations, which are typically unilateral and more commonly on the left. Many infants with sequestration are asymptomatic at birth, although sequestrations may be diagnosed early as part of an evaluation that is triggered by the presence of other congenital anomalies. Rarely, patients may be symptomatic due to enlargement of the lesion. Sequestrations present a risk for recurrent infections—historically, this was the typical way sequestrations came to medical attention prior to routine prenatal ultrasonography. Resection of the lesion is recommended in the first year of life, although timing depends on the case. Very rarely, a mixed lesion of CCAM and sequestration may present. The outcome and treatment of afflicted neonates usually do not differ from those seen with CCAM or sequestration alone.

Pulmonary Hypoplasia

Pulmonary hypoplasia represents a broad spectrum of anatomic malformations, ranging from total bronchial agenesis to mild parenchymal hypoplasia, and may be either primary or secondary to other lesions. Primary pulmonary hypoplasia is typically unilateral and not associated with other malformations. Secondary pulmonary hypoplasia is by definition associated with other malformations, such as CDH (as discussed previously), skeletal or neuromuscular disease (in which the lack of fetal movement, an important stimulus to lung growth, does not occur), and oligohydramnios sequence. The latter will be the focus of this section.

Oligohydramnios is associated with either renal disease in the neonate or chronic amniotic fluid leak. Fetal urine output becomes the primary source of amniotic fluid after 20–22 weeks of gestation; before then, amniotic fluid is primarily produced by the placenta. Infants with bilateral renal agenesis, bilateral dysplastic kidneys, or obstructive uropathies have severe oligohydramnios due to the lack of fetal urine output. These infants, who have characteristic facial features and limb contractures that were described in 1946 by Potter, represent the most severely affected neonates and often have fatal lung hypoplasia, which is frequently complicated by multiple pneumothoraces after birth. Fetal intervention has been attempted in infants with obstructive uropathy; a stent may be placed in the bladder to drain the urine into the amniotic cavity, thereby restoring the amniotic fluid in the uterus and removing pressure from the kidneys. Results to date have been mixed; however, this method remains an active area of investigation.

Oligohydramnios related to amniotic fluid leak appears to have a slightly different pathophysiology, and the degree of pulmonary hypoplasia is very difficult to assess antenatally. Although the difference in pathophysiology remains incompletely understood, it is postulated that because the infants are still creating urine, the amniotic fluid volume is variable and therefore, the effects on lung growth are also variable. In these infants, the degree of pulmonary hypoplasia must be assessed postnatally by the ability to oxygenate and ventilate the infant. Management is focused on limiting barotrauma while assessing the degree of lung hypoplasia and associated anomalies.

ACQUIRED DISEASE

Air-leak Syndrome

Air-leak syndromes represent one of the most serious complications of assisted ventilation in the neonate. Air leaks begin with rupture of alveoli or distal airways and are associated with high ventilator pressures and severe lung disease. They can occur suddenly, often complicate the treatment of RDS, and may be life threatening if not rapidly identified and addressed.

Pulmonary Interstitial Emphysema

Pulmonary interstitial emphysema (PIE) results from overdistension of distal airways and usually occurs in the tiniest, most immature babies. The distribution of inspiratory gas is not uniform in infants with severe parenchymal lung disease, with the majority of the volume of each breath distributed to the more compliant lung units. As a consequence of this maldistribution, the more compliant lung units become overdistended and rupture. The ruptured airways provide a pathway for leakage of air into the connective tissues that leads to the clinically observed findings of PIE on x-ray (discussed later). As air moves within the connective tissues, it can further track toward the hilum of the lung. PIE increases the volume of gas within the lung parenchyma, thereby decreasing lung compliance and increasing airway resistance. An increased need for ventilation typically occurs as the result of increased respiratory dead space and reduced minute ventilation. Hypoxemia results from the reduction in alveolar ventilation and from intrapulmonary shunting. Death may occur due to inadequate ventilation and oxygenation.

PIE is diagnosed radiographically based on the characteristic linear and cyst-like radiolucencies that reflect the accumulation of interstitial air. PIE may involve a single lobe, one lung, or both lungs. The linear radiolucencies are coarse and rarely appear to branch. They must be differentiated from the smooth, branching, perihilar air bronchograms often seen with RDS. The cyst-like radiolucencies of PIE take the appearance of small bubbles, typically vary in size from 0.5 to 4 mm in diameter, and are often present in large numbers.

No precise treatment for PIE exists. Given the pathophysiology of the air leak, it is not surprising that neonatologists have used ventilatory techniques to minimize alveolar and airway distention to prevent PIE. When PIE is unilateral, it is often suggested that the infant be positioned with the affected side down. When PIE is bilateral or extensive, an attempt can be made to decompress the air leaks by using a short inspiratory time, low inflation pressures, and small tidal volumes. With the use of these techniques over time, the lungs will slowly deflate and areas of overdistension should improve. One drawback to this approach is that it is often difficult to achieve optimal or even adequate oxygenation and ventilation while allowing for the collapse of the PIE-affected areas of lung. HFOV may allow for adequate ventilation and oxygenation in infants with PIE at lower peak and mean airway pressures than with conventional ventilation.

Pneumomediastinum and Pneumothorax

Although tightly associated with assisted ventilation and RDS, as is PIE, pneumothorax and pneumomediastinum may occur spontaneously. Interestingly, 3%–5% of normal term newborns present with asymptomatic, spontaneous, non-tension pneumothoraces during the first few postnatal hours. These pneumothoraces are thought to be a consequence of the large negative intrapleural pressure that is generated by the newborn at the first few breaths that are required to inflate the lungs immediately after delivery. As for the neonatal population with lung disease, it is believed that up to 10% may develop airleak syndrome as a result of poor lung compliance and the need for mechanical ventilation. Pneumomediastinum usually occurs when air tracks through the peribronchial interstitium to the hilum, at which point air ruptures into the mediastinum. The accumulation of air through the mediastinum into the pleural space can produce a tension pneumothorax. When the collection of air is constrained to the mediastinum, it is unusual for the volume of air to cause circulatory compromise, due in part to the fact that the air can dissect from the mediastinum into the soft tissue, typically of the neck, producing subcutaneous emphysema. In contrast, tension pneumothorax can result in exceedingly high intrapleural pressures, collapsing the ipsilateral lung and causing mediastinal shift with concomitant hypoxia and hypercapnia. The resulting mediastinal shift can impede cardiac output and lead to cardiovascular collapse. In the preterm neonate, the development of a tension pneumothorax is also associated with an increased incidence of periventricular/intraventricular hemorrhage.

The diagnosis of pneumothorax and/or pneumomediastinum is easily confirmed by clinical examination and chest x-ray. Isolated pneumomediastinum is often asymptomatic or associated with mild respiratory symptoms. With a pneumothorax, infants are usually symptomatic with signs of respiratory distress (tachypnea, retractions, grunting, flaring), cyanosis, and poor perfusion. Bedside evaluation may reveal tachycardia with a narrow pulse pressure. It is important to note that differential breath sounds are an unreliable marker for the diagnosis of pneumothorax in infants. An acute clinical deterioration in a mechanically ventilated infant should prompt an urgent search for the possibility of an air leak.

Transillumination of the chest can sometimes be used to make the diagnosis of an air leak, but if time allows, the diagnosis should be confirmed by chest x-ray. Nitrogen washout is a therapy used for stable, minimally symptomatic non-mechanically ventilated neonates with air leak. The infant is placed on 100% inspired O_2, typically delivered via an Oxy-Hood, and monitored closely for resolution of the air leak. However, due to the toxicity associated with the use of 100% O_2, the risks of using the nitrogen washout technique may outweigh the risks associated with chest tube placement, especially in the unstable preterm infant, in whom recurrence of the pneumothorax is likely. Tube thoracostomy is indicated in neonates with cardiorespiratory compromise or those receiving mechanical ventilation. Needle aspiration may be useful for acute relief of a tension pneumothorax but should usually be followed by chest tube placement to allow for continued evacuation of the air leak while the lung tissue is healing. The chest tube is typically connected to 10–20 cm of negative water pressure, and drainage and radiographs are monitored to determine the timing of resolution of the air leak and readiness for removal of the tube.

Pulmonary Hemorrhage

Pulmonary hemorrhage has been associated with a wide range of predisposing conditions, including prematurity, mechanical ventilation, sepsis, PDA, and asphyxia. Pulmonary hemorrhage reflects hemorrhagic pulmonary edema in most cases. Studies done over 30 years ago compared the hematocrit and protein composition of the hemorrhagic fluid obtained from the lungs with arterial and venous samples of blood from infants with pulmonary hemorrhage and concluded that the lung effluent was usually hemorrhagic edema rather than whole blood. The pathophysiology may involve acute injury to the left ventricle, resulting in left ventricular failure, increased filtration pressure, and subsequent injury to the walls of capillaries in the lung, with resulting marked capillary leak. Pulmonary hemorrhage in sepsis is likely related to endotoxin release and consequent increased pulmonary microvascular permeability. An association exists between pulmonary hemorrhage and surfactant administration, especially in the presence of a PDA. It is thought that the increased risk of developing hemorrhagic pulmonary edema after surfactant results from the rapid and significant decline in PVR that is associated with surfactant administration and the subsequent increase in the left-to-right shunting through the PDA, resulting in severe pulmonary overcirculation.

The earliest clinical sign of pulmonary hemorrhage is usually the detection of blood-tinged secretions from the endotracheal tube. The amount of bloody fluid seen may be minimal or copious. On occasion, pulmonary hemorrhage can be dramatic, and fluid that resembles whole blood may egress in large volumes from the trachea. Chest x-ray may reveal fluffy infiltrates consistent with pulmonary edema, and the infant's respiratory status often deteriorates.

Treatment of pulmonary hemorrhage involves clearing the airway to prevent frank obstruction from the hemorrhagic fluid and adjusting support to provide adequate oxygenation and ventilation. However, every effort should be made to avoid unnecessary suctioning of the trachea, which may only exacerbate the bleeding. Increasing the mean airway pressure, typically achieved by increasing PEEP, helps to prevent the continued flow of blood into the trachea. Blood tests for the presence of coagulopathy or new-onset infection, as well as to monitor the hematocrit, are indicated. In most cases, packed red blood cell transfusion is unnecessary, and the additional volume only worsens the pulmonary edema. Therefore, volume administration in hypotensive neonates with pulmonary hemorrhage must be avoided, at least in the period immediately following the development of the hemorrhage. Despite the association between surfactant replacement for RDS and pulmonary hemorrhage, some evidence suggests that pulmonary hemorrhage causes increased surface tension and surfactant dysfunction and that some benefit may be derived from administration of surfactant once the patient has been stabilized.

Pulmonary Edema

Pulmonary edema describes the abnormal accumulation of fluid in the pulmonary interstitium and alveolar spaces that can compromise oxygenation and ventilation. Fluid in the lungs normally flows from capillaries that run from the alveolar septae into the pulmonary interstitium as a result of the gradient between the hydrostatic and oncotic pressures of the microvasculature and interstitium. The fluid is drained from the interstitium by lymphatic channels and thus returns to the intravascular space. Under normal conditions, fluid does not accumulate within the interstitium. However, if lymphatic drainage does not keep pace with filtration or if the alveolar membrane is injured, pulmonary edema can occur.

Pulmonary edema occurs in neonates in association with a variety of pathologic processes. Increased hydrostatic filtration pressure due to increased left atrial pressure is a common cause. Left atrial pressure may be elevated as a result of volume overload, presence of a PDA with left-to-right shunting, or obstruction to outflow due to congenital heart disease and abnormal anatomy. Some evidence suggests that increased filtration pressure from heart failure is the cause of the pulmonary edema seen with perinatal hypoxic ischemic injury. Pulmonary edema associated with sepsis likely results from increased capillary endothelial permeability that is caused by activated neutrophils and other inflammatory mediators.

Pulmonary edema is a common complication during both the acute and chronic periods of a preterm infant's NICU course. During the early postnatal period, pulmonary edema is associated with both PDA and RDS. With the significant decreases in PVR following delivery, a left-to-right shunting of blood takes place at the level of the ductus; the frequently significant increased pulmonary blood flow causes an increase in fluid filtration, leading to edema. Studies have shown an association (but not causation) between persistent ductal patency and BPD. In addition, altered epithelial permeability plays a role in the pathogenesis of pulmonary edema in neonates with RDS.

Pulmonary edema also complicates the management of patients with BPD and may occur for a number of reasons. A diminished pulmonary capillary bed or hypoxia, both seen in patients with BPD, may cause increased PVR. In addition, patients with BPD have abnormal plasma oncotic pressure, perhaps due to inappropriate control of vasopressin secretion or related to poor nutritional status. Capillary permeability may also be increased as a consequence of damage to the endothelium from the dysregulated release of proinflammatory cytokines and chemokines, infection, barotrauma and volutrauma, or O_2 toxicity. Long-term cardiac complications of BPD, i.e., cor pulmonale and left ventricular dysfunction, may contribute as well, increasing lymphatic and left atrial pressures, respectively.

Pulmonary edema complicates the respiratory management of the neonate. Every effort should be made to optimize nutrition and minimize barotrauma and excessive supplemental O_2 exposure during the patient's course. One must maintain a high degree of suspicion for persistent patency or reopening of the ductus arteriosus in VLBW neonates during the first days and weeks after delivery. Diuretics are frequently used as therapy for pulmonary edema to improve oxygenation and ventilation. Furosemide is typically used as the first-line agent of choice, but as discussed previously, chlorothiazide (Diuril) and spirolactone (Aldactone) are frequently preferred for the management of the chronic phase of BPD, especially in the outpatient setting, to minimize the requirement for potassium and chloride supplementation, reduce the need for outpatient blood work to monitor electrolyte values, and decrease the risk of sensorineural hearing loss associated with chronic furosemide administration.

Airway Injury

Despite the current trend toward early extubation and aggressive use of noninvasive mechanical ventilation in even the smallest neonates, a prolonged need for mechanical ventilation is often necessary for many of the sickest preterm infants. Prolonged intubation carries the risk for significant upper airway complications. For instance, marked stridor following extubation or a history of repeated failure to successfully extubate an infant may be due to airway injury secondary to long-term intubation. Injury can occur as a result of irritation from the endotracheal tube over time or from focal damage at the time of intubation and can range from edema, ulcerations, and granulations to vocal cord paralysis or subglottic stenosis. Studies have reported ulceration and granulation in 44%–47% of infants who survive prolonged intubation (19). A risk of necrotic damage to the trachea or bronchi with high-frequency jet ventilation also exists, especially if humidification of the inspired gas is inadequate.

Clinical subglottic stenosis was once reported to occur in as many as 9% of intubated neonates, but recent reports estimate the incidence at <2% (62). Stenosis occurs as a result of trauma to the subglottis from tube motion over time. The injury begins where the tube causes ischemia of the airway mucosa. Eventually, areas of ischemia ulcerate, exposing cartilage, which can become infected, and scarring and stenosis may result. The posterior subglottis is the region most commonly affected in neonates.

Every effort must be made to minimize trauma to the airway during hospitalization, particularly during intubation attempts. In addition, endotracheal tubes should be upsized only if a leak around the endotracheal tube is compromising adequate ventilation and if the larger tube passes easily through the subglottis. A brief course of periextubation dexamethasone may decrease postextubation stridor in preterm neonates who are at high-risk for subglottic edema. Nebulized racemic epinephrine may also help reduce stridor in the acute setting after extubations, although it carries the risk of rebound edema formation once the medication is discontinued. However, in some cases, these interventions are not enough to allow for safe, adequate gas exchange and reintubation may be necessary. In such circumstances, the airway should be evaluated. Typically, the initial evaluation is at the bedside by flexible bronchoscopy, but rigid laryngoscopy in the operating room is often indicated to more completely visualize the extent and location of injury to the airway. Even when numerous extubation attempts have failed, extubation is sometimes successful when reattempted, after allowing time for growth and healing, and if CPAP, nasal, or nasopharyngeal intermittent assisted ventilation is used after extubation. However, surgical intervention may be necessary when the laryngotracheal injury continues to impair oxygenation and/or ventilation. Surgical options include an anterior cricoid split or tracheostomy.

Infection

Neonatal sepsis occurs in 1 in 1000 term infants and in 1 in 4 preterm infants. Pneumonia, both congenital and acquired, frequently coexists with sepsis in the newborn period. The immature immune system puts the neonate at increased risk of infection, and pneumonia, in particular, is a significant cause of morbidity and mortality in the newborn. The preterm infant, whose immune system is markedly immature and who has diminished levels of serum immunoglobulin concentrations compared to the term newborn, is at particularly high risk. Risk factors for early-onset sepsis include premature delivery, multiple pregnancy, prolonged rupture of amniotic membranes (>18 hrs), maternal fever, maternal group B *Streptococcus* (GBS) colonization, and chorioamnionitis. Nosocomial pneumonia, unfortunately a relatively common complication, is associated with mechanical ventilation and prolonged hospital stays. Both congenitally acquired and nosocomial pneumonias may have long-term ramifications for survivors. A growing body of evidence points to the connection between infection and the development of BPD.

Congenital Pneumonia

Congenital pneumonia frequently coexists with sepsis and is a significant source of morbidity and mortality in neonates. Infection is typically acquired when organisms ascend into the uterine cavity, either during or prior to labor, and come into contact with the fetus. Consequently, prolonged rupture of membranes is a significant risk factor for neonatal sepsis. The lungs may become infected when the fetus swallows infected amniotic fluid. Infection can occur even when membranes are intact until just prior to delivery. Transmission of bacteria can occur hematogenously, from the mother's blood via the placenta, or via aspiration of organisms at the time of delivery as the newborn passes through the birth canal.

Group B *Streptococcus* is the most common pathogen that causes early-onset neonatal pneumonia in the US. Premature infants are at increased risk of infection, and the mortality rate is higher than in term infants. In 1996, the Centers for Disease Control and Prevention (CDC) developed guidelines for screening pregnant women for GBS colonization at 35–37 weeks' gestation. The rate of GBS colonization is estimated to be 20–30% for American women. It is currently recommended that colonized women and those with other risk factors for neonatal sepsis be given intrapartum antibiotic therapy beginning at least 4 hrs prior to delivery. The incidence of early-onset GBS infection has been reduced by 65% in communities that have adopted the CDC GBS-prevention guidelines and is now reported to be as low as 0.37 per 1000 live births. The majority of cases of early-onset GBS infection in the era of intrapartum GBS prophylaxis occur in mothers who tested negative for GBS at the time of screening (42). Other organisms that may cause pneumonia in the neonate include Gram-negative organisms, particularly *Escherichia coli*, group D *Streptococcus*, *Listeria*, pneumococci, *Staphylococcus* species, and fungus. *Chlamydia*, although acquired congenitally, typically presents as pneumonia at several weeks of age rather than in the immediate postnatal period. Interest has been renewed in the possibility that peripartum transmission of *Ureaplasma urealyticum* to the respiratory tract of the preterm neonate may contribute to the development of severe respiratory failure and/or BPD. Although more typically a cause of late-onset pneumonia in neonates, viruses (herpes simplex virus, enterovirus, and adenovirus, in particular) can also cause congenital pneumonia and may have a severe and sometimes fatal course.

It can be difficult to make a definitive diagnosis of pneumonia in the neonate. Neonates may present with respiratory distress at birth (or shortly after birth) for a wide range of reasons unrelated to infection. Tachypnea, retractions, grunting, and cyanosis can all result from processes as varied as transient tachypnea of the newborn, respiratory distress syndrome, CDH, pneumothorax, and polycythemia. In addition, neonates with pneumonia can present without focal respiratory signs, demonstrating only temperature instability (typically hy-

pothermia), glucose instability, or jaundice. Fever and cough, frequent findings in older patients, are uncommon in newborns with bacterial pneumonia.

It is often difficult to obtain bacterial confirmation of pneumonia in the neonate. Tracheal culture may not isolate the pathogen. However, numerous white blood cells on the aspirate may signal the presence of infection, and growth of an isolated organism, when present, can guide therapy. Blood cultures should be sent to evaluate for bacteremia and can help determine appropriate coverage when culture growth is observed. A chest x-ray is indicated to evaluate for infiltrates, although it is often difficult to differentiate an infiltrate from atelectasis, RDS, retained lung fluid, and the edema seen with certain cardiac anomalies; serial radiograms may be useful in differentiating the various processes. Appearance of an infiltrate may lag behind the onset of clinical symptoms by 24–48 hrs. *Staphylococcus aureus* pneumonia is classically associated with empyema and pneumatocele formation. A decreased or elevated white blood cell count and/or a predominance of immature white blood cell forms are suggestive of infection. Although nonspecific, an elevated c-reactive protein indicates the presence of an infectious or inflammatory process.

It is standard for antibiotic therapy to be started prior to the determination of a definitive diagnosis of pneumonia in the neonate. Treatment is usually begun as soon as respiratory symptoms develop or troubling lab findings are identified in an infant at risk for sepsis. Typical treatment pending identification of the pathogen is broad spectrum, consisting of a penicillin in addition to an aminoglycoside. Coverage should be narrowed if the causative organism is identified. The appropriate duration of antibiotic therapy for neonatal pneumonia has not been clearly established. Ten days of IV ampicillin and gentamicin is probably the most widely accepted treatment, but treatment duration varies. Given the high incidence of coexisting bacteremia, many neonatologists would treat a documented Gram-negative pneumonia for a minimum of 14 days and rule out the possibility of meningitic involvement. Supportive care is also critical; IV nutrition, mechanical or assisted ventilation, and hemodynamic support are often required during the acute phase of the illness. Pneumonia may be complicated by PPHN, and patients should be monitored closely to ensure adequate oxygenation and ventilation.

Nosocomial Pneumonia

Nosocomial infection, including pneumonia, is rare in healthy newborns admitted to well-baby nurseries, but is a serious and frequent complication of prolonged NICU admissions. Although not uniformly accepted, the CDC defines an infection as nosocomial if it occurs after admission to the NICU and was not vertically acquired from the mother. Nosocomial pneumonia is defined by the CDC in patients who are <1 year of age as the appearance of a new or progressive infiltrate on chest x-ray, increased respiratory secretions or a change in sputum character, and isolation of the pathogen from a tracheal aspirate, bronchial washing, or biopsy specimen.

The risk of nosocomial infection during a NICU stay is inversely proportional to the patient's gestational age and birth weight. Data published in 2001 reported ventilator-associated pneumonia per 1000 ventilator days stratified by birth weight to be 3.5 at <1000 g birth weight, 4.9 at 1001–1500 g, 1.1 at 1501–2500 g, and 0.9 at >2500 g birth weight (53). A 2003 prospective, single-centered study showed a ventilator-associated pneumonia rate of 28.3% in patients with birth weights of ≤2000 g who were admitted to the NICU for >48 hrs. The same study showed that ventilator-associated pneumonia is an independent predictor of both mortality and prolonged length of hospital stay (3).

A prior bloodstream infection and the prolonged need for mechanical ventilation have both been shown to predict a neonate's risk of a nosocomial pneumonia (3,54). Mechanical ventilation presents a risk because the respiratory tract, given time, will become colonized with bacteria, typically Gram-negative bacilli (*Pseudomonas aeruginosa, Klebsiella pneumoniae, E. coli*) or *Staphylococcus* species. Data that support a correlation between time of intubation and colonization have been published (17). Bacterial colonization of the respiratory tract can occur as a result of contaminated respiratory equipment, the presence of bacteria in oral secretions that pool around the endotracheal tube, or via transmission of bacteria during labor and delivery. Fungus, typically *Candida*, can also colonize the neonatal respiratory tract and potentially cause pneumonia and/or systemic disease. Viruses, particularly respiratory syncytial virus, may also cause nosocomial pneumonia in NICU patients.

Like congenital pneumonia, nosocomial pneumonia in the neonate can be difficult to diagnose. Nosocomial pneumonia should, in most cases, manifest itself with a clinical deterioration in the patient's respiratory status. The chest x-ray may show a focal infiltrate, but it is often difficult to clearly detect an infiltrate, as many preterm infants have significant radiographic findings of lung disease at baseline and frequently develop areas of atelectasis. A tracheal aspirate should be sent for Gram stain and culture, but it is important to realize that the most ventilated patients will have colonization of the respiratory tract with bacteria and will subsequently have growth of bacteria when tracheal aspirate cultures are sent. It is important to critically analyze tracheal aspirate results in an attempt to differentiate colonization from infection and determine the need for antibiotic therapy. The presence of many or a moderate amount of white blood cells has been used as an indicator of the presence of infection. In addition, growth of a single or predominant organism that is a known pathogen may be helpful. Growth of mixed flora and the presence of only a few white blood cells are more consistent with colonization. Respiratory secretions can be sent for viral testing when a viral etiology is suspected. It is rare in infants to have additional samples, such as bronchoalveolar lavage fluid or lung biopsy specimens, to send for culture.

Given that the pathogens responsible for nosocomial infections differ somewhat from those responsible for early-onset infections, the antibiotics administered for nosocomial pneumonia prior to identification of the responsible organism vary from those used for early-onset infection. Vancomycin is often used in combination with an aminoglycoside as the regimen of choice for a suspected nosocomial infection in the NICU. Vancomycin is used to optimally cover *Staphylococcus* species, particularly *S. epidermidis*, which is frequently oxacillin resistant and a common cause of infection in NICU patients. Some centers choose to treat neonates who develop nosocomial infections with double Gram-negative antibiotic coverage while awaiting culture results, the theory being that Gram-negative organisms typically cause more aggressive disease and vancomycin can always be added if clinical deterioration continues or significant growth of *S. epidermidis* from the cultures is seen.

Sometimes, antibiotic therapy is directed at the bacteria that are known colonizers in the infant based on growth seen on prior bacterial cultures and/or based on the pattern of unit-specific cultures and resistance panels.

CONCLUSION AND FUTURE DIRECTIONS

Although NICU survival has improved markedly over the years, particularly impacted by advances in knowledge and technology (e.g., surfactant, iNO, and ECMO), many survivors have long-term sequelae from their neonatal illnesses that will result in further illness and hospital admissions during childhood and potentially beyond. The burden of neonatal respiratory failure on society will be reduced as we make strides toward the following goals:

- Prevention or reduction of premature delivery (although currently, the incidence of premature delivery has been increasing).
- Development of well-informed guidelines for target parameters for O_2 saturations and CO_2 levels in the preterm neonate.
- A better understanding of developmental hemodynamics and effective treatment of cardiovascular compromise in the preterm and term neonate.
- A greater understanding of the optimal disease-specific approach to ventilator management in the neonate.
- Development of safe and effective in utero interventions to improve outcomes of CDH, CCAM, and congenital heart disease.
- Future technologic advances in ECMO that may reduce the need for anticoagulation and the chance of brain injury from hemorrhage.
- Interventions that may decrease the risk of perinatal transmission of infection and reduce the incidence of hospital-acquired infection in the neonate.

KEY POINTS

- Prematurity continues to be a significant source of neonatal mortality and long-term pediatric morbidity.
- Prenatal steroids, surfactant, and improvements in neonatal nutrition are the advances that have had the most important impact on improving neonatal survival.
- Increasingly sophisticated, disease-specific ventilator management should decrease long-term morbidity for critically ill neonates.
- Research must now focus on determining the impact of our physiologic interventions, such as the management of hypotension, oxygenation, and ventilation, on long-term neurodevelopmental outcome.

References

1. Ainsworth SB, Beresford MW, Millligan DWA, et al. Pumactant and poractant alfa for treatment of respiratory distress syndrome in neonates born at 25–29 weeks' gestation: A randomized trial. *Lancet* 2000;355:1387–92.
2. Alvarado M, Hingre R, Hakason D, et al. Clinical trial of Survanta versus Exosurf in infants <1500 g with respiratory distress syndrome. *Pediatr Res* 1993;33:A314.

3. Apisarnthanarak A, Holzmann-Pazgal G, Hamvas A, et al. Ventilator-associated pneumonia in extremely preterm neonates in a neonatal intensive care unit: Characteristics, risk factors, and outcomes. *Pediatrics* 2003;112:1283–9.

4. Ballard RA, Truog WE, Cnaan A, et al. for the NO CLD Study Group. Inhaled nitric oxide in preterm infants undergoing mechanical ventilation. *N Engl J Med* 2006;355:343–53.

5. Banks BA. Postnatal dexamethasone for bronchopulmonary dysplasia: A systematic review and meta-analysis of 20 years of clinical trials. *Neoreviews* 2002;3:E24–34.

6. Baroutis G, Kaleyias J, Liarou T, et al. Comparison of three treatment regimens of natural surfactant preparations in neonatal respiratory distress syndrome. *Eur J Pediatr* 2003;162:476–80.

7. Bloom BT, Clark RH. Infasurf-Survanta Clinical Trial Group. Comparison of Infasurf and Survanta in the prevention and treatment of respiratory distress syndrome. *Pediatrics* 2005;116(2):392–9.

8. Bloom BT, Kattwinkel J, Hall RT, et al. Comparison of Infasurf (calf lung surfactant extract) to Survanta in the treatment and prevention of respiratory distress syndrome. *Pediatrics* 1997;100(1):31–8.

9. Chang LL, Subramanian M, Yoder BA, et al. A catalytic antioxidant attenuates alveolar structural remodeling in BPD. *Am J Respir Crit Care Med* 2003;167:57–64.

10. Chang R, Andreoli S, Ng US, et al. VEGF expression is downregulated in nitrofen-induced congenital diaphragmatic hernia in rats. *J Pediatr Surg* 2004;30:1457–62.

11. Clark RH, Kueser TJ, Walker MW, et al. Low-dose nitric oxide therapy for persistent pulmonary hypertension of the newborn. *N Engl J Med* 2000;342:469–75.

12. Cohen MS, Rychik J, Bush DM, et al. Influence of congenital heart disease on survival in children with congenital diaphragmatic hernia. *J Pediatr* 2002;141:25–30.

13. Courtney SE, Durand DJ, for the Neonatal Ventilation Study Group. High-frequency oscillatory ventilation vs. conventional mechanical ventilation for very low birth weight infants. *N Engl J Med* 2002;347:643–52.

14. da Costa DE, Pai MG, Al Khusaiby SM. Comparative trial of artificial and natural surfactants in the treatment of respiratory distress syndrome of prematurity: Experience in a developing country. *Pediatr Pulmonol* 1999;27(5):303–4.

15. Ehrenkranz RA, Walsh-Sukys MC, for the NICHD Neonatal Research Network. New consensus definition of bronchopulmonary dysplasia (BPD-DEF) predicts pulmonary and neurodevelopmental outcomes in early infancy. *Pediatr Res* 2001;49:A276, #1579.

16. Fliman PJ, DeRegnier RO, Kinsella JP, et al. Neonatal extracorporeal life support: Impact of new therapies on survival. *J Pediatr* 2006;148:595–9.

17. Friedland DR, Rothschild MA, Delgado M, et al. Bacterial colonization of endotracheal tubes in intubated neonates. *Arch Otolaryngol Head Neck Surg* 2001;127(5):525–8.

18. Ho JJ, Subramaniam P, Henderson-Smart DJ, et al. Continuous distending pressure for respiratory distress syndrome in preterm infants. *The Cochrane Library*, Issue 2, Oxford: Update Software, Ltd., 2002.

19. Hoeve LJ, Eskici O, Verwoerd CD. Therapeutic for reintubation for post-intubation laryngotracheal injury in preterm infants. *Int J Pediatr Otorhinolaryngol* 1995;31(1):7–13.

20. Horbar JD, Wright LL, Soll RF, et al. A multicenter randomized trial comparing two surfactants for the treatment of neonatal respiratory distress syndrome. National Institute of Child Health and Human Development Neonatal Research Network. *J Pediatr* 1993;123:757–66.

21. Hudak ML, Farrell EE, Rosenberg AA, et al. A multicenter randomized masked comparison trial of natural versus synthetic surfactant for the treatment of respiratory distress syndrome. *J Pediatr* 1996;128:396–406.

22. Hudak ML, Martin DJ, Egan EA, et al. A multicenter randomized masked comparison trial of synthetic surfactant versus calf lung surfactant extract in the prevention of neonatal respiratory distress syndrome. *Pediatrics* 1997;100:39–50.

23. Jobe AH. An unknown: Lung growth and development after very preterm birth. *Am J Respir Crit Care Med* 2002;15(166):1529–30.

24. Jobe AH, Bancalari E. Bronchopulmonary dysplasia. *Am J Respir Crit Care Med* 2001;163:1723–9.

25. Johnson AH, Peacock JL, for the UK Oscillation Study Group. High-frequency oscillatory for the prevention of chronic lung disease of prematurity. *N Engl J Med* 2002;347:633–42.

26. Kaiser JR, Gauss CH, Williams DK. The effects of hypercapnia on cerebral autoregulation in ventilated very low birth weight infants. *Pediatr Res* 2005;58(5):931–5.

27. Kinsella JP, Cutter GR, Walsh WF, et al. Early inhaled nitric oxide therapy in premature newborns with respiratory failure. *N Engl J Med* 2006;355(4):354–64.

28. Kinsella JP, Troug WE, Walsh WF, et al. Randomized multicenter trial of inhaled nitric oxide and high frequency ventilation in severe, persistent pulmonary hypertension of the newborn. *J Pediatr* 1997;131:55–62.

29. Kinsella JP, Walsh WF, Bose CL, et al. Inhaled nitric oxide in premature neonates with severe hypoxaemic respiratory failure: A randomized controlled trial. *Lancet* 1999;354:1061–5.

30. Kukkonen AK, Virtanen M, Jarvenpaa AL, et al. Randomized trial comparing natural and synthetic surfactant: Increased infection rate after natural surfactant? *Acta Pediatr* 2000;89(5):556–61.

31. Laudy JA, Van Gucht M, Van Dooren MF, et al. Congenital diaphragmatic hernia: An evaluation of the prognostic value of the lung to head ratio and other prenatal parameters. *Prenat Diagn* 2003;23:634–9.

32. Lodygensky GA, Rademaker K, Zimine S, et al. Structural and functional brain development after hydrocortisone treatment for neonatal chronic lung disease. *Pediatrics* 2005;116(1):1–7.

33. Malloy CA, Nicoski P, Muraskas JM. A randomized trial comparing beractant and poractant treatment in neonatal respiratory distress syndrome. *Acta Paediatr* 2005;94(6):779–84.

34. Modanlou H, Beharry K, Padilla G, et al. Comparative efficacy of Exosurf and Survanta surfactants on early clinical course of respiratory distress syndrome and complications of prematurity. *J Perinatol* 1997;17:455–60.

35. Moriette G, Paris-Llado J, Walti H, et al. Prospective randomized multicenter comparison of high-frequency oscillatory ventilation and conventional ventilation in preterm infants of less than 30 weeks with respiratory distress syndrome. *Pediatrics* 2001;107:363–72.

36. Moya FR, Gadzinowski J, Bancalari E, et al. A multicenter, randomized, masked, comparison trial of Lucinactant, Colfosceril Palmitate, and Beractant for the prevention of respiratory distress syndrome among very preterm infants. *Pediatrics* 2005;115(4):1018–29.

37. Neonatal Inhaled Nitric Oxide Study Group. Inhaled nitric oxide in full-term and near-term infants with hypoxemic respiratory failure. *N Engl J Med* 1997;342:597–604.

38. Neonatal Inhaled Nitric Oxide Study Group. Inhaled nitric oxide and hypoxic respiratory failure in infants with congenital diaphragmatic hernia. *Pediatrics* 1997;99:838–45.

39. NIH Consensus Development Panel. Effect of Corticosteroids for fetal maturation on perinatal outcomes. *JAMA* 1995;273(1):413–8.

40. Northway WH Jr. , Rosan RC, Porter DY. Pulmonary disease following respirator therapy of hyaline-membrane disease: Bronchopulmonary dysplasia. *N Engl J Med* 1967;16(276):357–68.

41. Pearlman SA, Leef KH, Stefano JL, et al. A randomized trial comparing Exosurf versus Survanta in the treatment of neonatal RDS. *Pediatr Res* 1993;33:A340.

42. Puopolo KM, Madoff LC, Eichenwald EC. Early-onset group B streptococcal disease in the era of maternal screening. *Pediatrics* 2005;115(5):1240–6.

43. Rademaker KJ, Rijpert M, Uiterwaal CS, et al. Neonatal hydrocortisone treatment related to 1H-MRS of the hippocampus and short-term memory at school age in preterm born children. *Pediatr Res* 2006;59(2):309–13.

44. Ramanathan R, Rasmussen MR, Gerstmann DR, et al. North American Study Group. A randomized, multicenter masked comparison trial of poractant alfa (Curosurf) versus beractant (Survanta) in the treatment of respiratory distress syndrome in preterm infants. *Am J Perinatol* 2004;21(3):109–19.

45. Rollins M, Jenkins J, Tubman R, et al. Comparison of clinical responses to natural and synthetic surfactants. *J Perinatol Med* 1993;21:341–7.

46. Schreiber MD, Gin-Mestan K, Marks JD, et al. Inhaled nitric oxide in premature infants with respiratory distress syndrome. *N Engl J Med* 2003;349:2099–2107.

47. Sehgal SS, Ewing CK, Richards T, et al. Modified bovine surfactant (Survanta) versus a protein free surfactant (Exosurf) in the treatment of respiratory distress syndrome in preterm infants: a pilot study. *J Natl Med Assoc* 1994;86:46–52.

48. Shenai JMP, Mellen BG, Chytil F. Vitamin A status and postnatal dexamethasone treatment in BPD. *Pediatrics* 2000;106:547–53.

49. Shinwell ES, Karplus M, Reich D, et al. Early postnatal dexamethasone treatment and increased incidence of cerebral palsy. *Arch Dis Child Fetal Neonatal Ed* 2000;83:F177–81.

50. Sinha SK, Lacaze-Masmonteil T, Soler A, et al. A multicenter, randomized, controlled trial of Lucinactant versus Poractant alfa among very premature infants at high risk for respiratory distress syndrome. *Pediatrics* 2005;115:1030–8.

51. Speer CP, Gefeller O, Groneck P, et al. Randomised clinical trial of two treatment regimens of natural surfactant preparations in neonatal respiratory distress syndrome. *Arch Dis Child Fetal Neonatal Ed* 1995;72(1):F8–13.

52. STOP-ROP (Supplemental Therapeutic Oxygen for Prethreshold Retinopathy of Prematurity). A randomized controlled trial. *Pediatrics* 2000;105:295–310.

53. Stover BH, Shulman ST, Bratcher DF, et al. Nosocomial infection rates in US children's hospitals' neonatal and pediatric intensive care units. *Am J Infect Control* 2001;29:152–7.

54. Suara RO, Young M, Reeves I. Risk factors for nosocomial infection in a high-risk nursery. *Infect Control Hosp Epidemiol* 2000;21(4):250–1.

55. Teremoto H, Yoneda A, Puri P. Gene expression of fibroblast growth factors 7 and 10 is downregulated in the lung of nitrofen-induced diaphragmatic hernia in rats. *J Pediatr Surg* 2003;38:1021–4.

56. Thome U, Kossel H, Lipowsky G. Randomized comparison of high-frequency oscillatory ventilation with high-rate intermittent positive pressure ventilation in preterm infants with respiratory failure. *J Pediatr* 1999;135:39–46.

57. UK ECMO Collaborative Group. UK collaborative randomized trial of neonatal extracorporeal membrane oxygenation. *Lancet* 1996;348:75–82.

58. Unemoto K, Sakai M, Shima H, et al. Increased expression of ICAM-1 and VCAM-1 in the lung of nitrofen-induced congenital diaphragmatic hernia. *Pediatr Surg Int* 2003;19:365–70.

59. Van Meurs K, Congenital Diaphragmatic Hernia Study Group. Is surfactant therapy beneficial in the treatment of the term newborn infant with congenital diaphragmatic hernia? *J Pediatr* 2004;145:312–6.

60. Van Reempts P, Borstlap C, Laroche S, et al. Early use of high-frequency ventilation in the premature neonate. *Eur J Pediatr* 2003;162:219–26.

61. Vermont Oxford Neonatal Network. A multicenter randomized trial comparing synthetic surfactant with modified bovine surfactant extract in the treatment of neonatal respiratory distress syndrome. *Pediatrics* 1996;97:1–6.

62. Walner DL, Loewen MS, Kimura RE. Neonatal subglottic stenosis-incidence and trends. *Laryngoscope* 2001;111(1):48–51.

63. Watterberg KL, Gerdes JS, Cole CH, et al. Prophylaxis of early adrenal insufficiency to prevent bronchopulmonary dysplasia: A multicenter trial. *Pediatrics* 2004;114:1649–57.

64. Wiswell TE, Gannon CM, Jaco J, et al. Delivery room management of the apparently vigorous meconium-stained neonate: Results of the multicenter, international collaborative trial. *Pediatrics* 2000;105:1–7.

CHAPTER 45 ■ BRONCHIOLITIS AND PNEUMONIA

WERTHER BRUNOW DE CARVALHO • CíNTIA JOHNSTON • MARCELO CUNIO MACHADO FONSECA

BRONCHIOLITIS

Acute bronchiolitis (AB) is the most frequent and severe respiratory system syndrome involving children <2 years of age, with the peak incidence occurring at <12 months of age. AB has an epidemic pattern, with increases in prevalence during the fall and winter. In winter, AB is one of the most frequent causes of infant hospitalization. In the US, 2 out of 100,000 live-birth children die as a result of AB-associated complications (29).

AB is generally self-limited, with a low mortality rate (<1%). In high-risk children (those who are premature or immunocompromised or those who suffer from bronchopulmonary dysplasia or congenital heart disease), AB can be associated with prolonged disease and a mortality rate as high 30%. In developed countries, while the mortality rate among previously healthy children is low, AB is associated with high morbidity. More than half of AB patients have recurring episodes of wheezing and asthma until 7–11 years of age. Pharmacologic treatment of children with AB is a frequent practice, although no universal consensus as to efficacy or standard treatment exists.

Definition

AB is a lower respiratory tract syndrome with acute onset, predominantly involving infants <1 year old; however, it may occur in children up to 2–3 years of age. Typically, it begins with initial symptoms of an upper airway viral infection, such as fever and coryza. Within 4–6 days, the lower respiratory tract is involved, with clinical signs of cough, tachypnea, hyperinflation, chest retractions, widespread crackles, and wheezing.

Epidemiology and Etiology

Children <6 months old are at increased risk for developing severe AB disease. It is a seasonal disease that coincides with the viral agent epidemics of respiratory infection. Every year, more than 700,000 children in the US are seen in emergency rooms due to AB/respiratory syncytial virus (RSV), and approximately one-third of these infants are admitted for inpatient treatment (37). Most common in the winter season, AB now occurs year-round in areas with large contingents of international travelers who may bring the disease with them from the "winter" in their original country to a site in another season.

AB is an acute respiratory disease with bronchioli inflammation and obstruction. A wide range of agents (parainfluenza, adenovirus, influenza, *Mycoplasma pneumoniae*, rhinovirus,

Chlamydia pneumoniae, human metapneumovirus, and coronavirus) may cause AB; however, RSV (with its A and B subtypes) is by far the most frequently involved agent.

Environmental and genetic factors contribute to disease severity. Passive tobacco exposure increases hospitalization risk in AB (**Table 45.1**). Hospitalization due to AB has increased in the last 20 years, perhaps reflecting the increased survival of infants with comorbid conditions that may predispose them to contracting AB and the expanded use of pulse oximetry to identify hypoxemia and severity of illness.

Pathogens

The most frequently identified agents in lower respiratory tract infections in infants and young children are described in the next sections.

Influenza Virus

The child hospitalization rate associated with influenza virus is similar to that in the adult population (14). Clinical diagnosis has low sensitivity, mainly in children <3 years of age (53). In 2003–2004, an epidemic linked to the variant strain A/Fujian/411/2002 was predominant, increasing influenza infection complications as well as the mortality rate (6). In this study, the most frequent diagnosis before death was pneumonia (49%), followed by sepsis or shock (34%), laryngotracheobronchitis or croup (20%), disseminated intravascular coagulation (12%), AB (8%), and encephalopathy (6%). Studies conducted in Japan showed that ceasing influenza virus vaccination was associated with increased child mortality in those between 1 and 4 years of age (61).

Although influenza infection is self-limited, it may cause complications, such as pneumonia, Reye syndrome, myositis, febrile convulsion, and acute encephalopathy. Hospitalization, increased disease severity, and complications are more frequent in children <2 years old and in those with risk factors (asthma or other chronic pulmonary disease, severe heart disease, immunocompromise, hemoglobinopathies, and diabetes mellitus) (27).

Human Metapneumovirus

Human metapneumovirus (hMPV) was first described in 2001 in 28 Dutch children with RSV-like disease (64). A paramyxovirus was isolated in these children and identified as a new metapneumovirus family member based on viral data, gene sequence, and constellation. This serologic study showed that all children >5 years old had anti-hMPV antibody, suggesting a

TABLE 45.1

RISK FACTORS FOR CLINICAL WORSENING OF ACUTE BRONCHIOLITIS

Initial presentation	Tachypnea (RR >60–80 bpm or retractions)
	Hypoxia (SaO$_2$ 90%–95%)
	Feeding difficulty or dehydration
Age	Age <12 months (the younger the child, larger the risk)
Comorbidities	Bronchopulmonary dysplasia
	Congenital heart disease
	Cystic fibrosis
	Immunodeficiency
Prematurity	Gestation age <36 weeks
Other	Malnutrition
	Poverty
	Overcrowding
	Parents and/or family members who smoke
	Genetic RSV infection predisposition

RR, respiratory rate; SaO$_2$, arterial oxygen saturation; RSV, respiratory syncytial virus

high transmission level. This virus has probably been circulating in humans for the last 50 years.

The hMPV virus has universal distribution, especially during fall and winter seasons in temperate climates (52). It is associated with several clinical presentations, such as cold, AB, asthma exacerbation and airway obstructive disease, pneumonia, and occasionally, severe infections in immunocompromised patients (64). Severe AB can be caused by combined infection with hMPV and RSV (59).

Of the new metapneumovirus types, hMPV is the first known to infect humans (Paramyxoviridae family) (63). RSV belongs to a separate genus in the same family. hMPV has been identified in the nasopharynx aspirate of children and adults with respiratory system infection in several countries. The clinical syndrome of infected children ranges from mild respiratory symptoms to AB and pneumonia (32). The signs and symptoms of hMPV are fever (67%), cough (100%), rhinorrhea (92%), retractions (92%), wheezing (83%), vomiting (25%), and diarrhea (8%).

A hMPV infection causes AB (67%), pneumonia (17%), and acute otitis (50%). Average hospitalization time is 4.5 days, and one-third of the patients were in the hospital for >7 days. When reverse polymerase chain reaction (PCR) is performed, hMPV is found in 1.5–10% of children who had previously unexplained infection in the respiratory system (49).

hMPV mostly affects children <2 years of age, predominantly among those between 3 and 5 months. hMPV epidemics occur at different times than do those of other viruses. Due to its heterogeneity, multiple reinfections of hMPV may occur in the same patient, particularly in the aged and immunocompromised (52).

In a prospective study that evaluated 208 children <3 years old, hMPV was identified in 12 (6%) who were hospitalized due to acute respiratory system infection; RSV was found in 118 (57%), and influenza A was found in 49 (24%) (9). AB was diagnosed in 8 (68%), and pneumonia was diagnosed in 2

(17%) of the hMPV-infected children. Of the RSV-infected children, AB was diagnosed in 99 (84%), and pneumonia was diagnosed in 30 (25%). None of the children with hMPV needed to be treated in a PICU; however, 15% of those with RSV and influenza A did. hMPV is an important cause of disease in young infants, with similar but less severe clinical manifestations as RSV.

In another prospective study (20), hMPV was found in 14% of a sample of 749 children <2 years of age and was second only to RSV (76%) in frequency. The hMPV infection occurs more frequently in infants. Recurrent wheezing was noted in 49.3% of children, followed by AB (46.4%). O$_2$ therapy was necessary in 58% of the patients, although mechanical ventilation was required for only one child. Mean hospital length of stay was 5 ± 3 days.

Rhinovirus

Although the diseases caused by rhinovirus are not completely defined, its infection is the leading cause of asthma crisis in children and adults (33). During the first year of life, a twofold greater RSV infection rate is associated with wheezing when compared to infections caused by rhinovirus. In the third year of life, rhinovirus was found in 42% of 180 wheezing episodes, as compared to 16% for RSV, 8% for parainfluenza, and 4% for other viruses. The incidence of hMPV was not investigated. Risk factors for wheezing when evaluated in children at age 3 included passive smoke exposure [odds ratio (OR), 2.1], older siblings (OR, 2.5), allergic sensitization to foods at 1 year of age (OR, 2.0), any moderate to severe respiratory illness without wheezing during infancy (OR, 3.6), and at least 1 wheezing illness with RSV (OR, 3.0), rhinovirus (OR, 10) and/or non-rhinovirus/RSV pathogens (OR, 3.9) during infancy. Infection with rhinovirus was also the strongest viral predictor of subsequent wheezing at age 3 years (OR, 6.6; p <0.0001). In addition, 63% of infants who wheezed during rhinovirus seasons continued to wheeze in the third year of life, as compared to 20% of all other infants (OR, 6.6; p <0.0001) (35). It is still undetermined whether host factors such as innate immunologic response predispose to more severe disease and wheezing or if repeated viral respiratory diseases cause wheezing due to airway and pulmonary lesions.

Coronavirus

A causal relationship between febrile respiratory disease and a new coronavirus (other than human coronavirus) was initially shown in China in 2003 (34); this disease was named *acute respiratory syndrome*. Infants and young children were not detected as a risk group, and only a few cases were found in children <15 years old.

In young children, signs of upper airway infection are present; symptoms such as tremors, stiffness, and myalgia are usually not seen. Clinical manifestations are mild in young children when compared to adolescents and adults (30). Incubation time ranges from 2 to 7 days but may be >10 days, with fever higher than 38°C (100.4°F), dry cough, and dyspnea progressing to hypoxemia. Chest x-ray demonstrates early focal infiltration, progressing to generalization with interstitial infiltration in the majority of patients. Radiologic features are not distinct from bronchopneumonia caused by other pathogens. Laboratory changes include leukopenia or moderate lymphopenia with liver enzyme elevation.

TABLE 45.2

ADENOVIRUS CLINICAL SYNDROMES

System	Clinical manifestations
Respiratory	*Upper respiratory tract*
	Pharyngitis
	Coryza
	Lower respiratory tract
	Laryngotracheobronchitis
	Cough
	Acute bronchiolitis
	Pneumonia
Ocular	Conjunctivitis with respiratory disease
	Acute follicular conjunctivitis
	Epidemic keratoconjunctivitis
	Pharyngoconjunctival fever
Gastrointestinal	Diarrhea
	Immunocompromised host hepatitis
Urinary	Hemorrhagic cystitis
Nervous	Aseptic meningitis
	Meningoencephalitis, encephalitis
	Myelitis, acute flaccid palsy
	Myositis
Skin	Rash
Disseminated infections (immunocompromised newborns)	Multiple-organ failure

Adenovirus

Adenovirus is so named because it is frequently isolated from adenoid and other lymphatic tissues; 51 serotypes are currently identified. Adenovirus, a DNA virus, has no lipid viral envelope, is highly stable out of host cells, and may remain infectious at room temperature for 2 weeks. It is destroyed by heat (54°C, 129.2°F, for 30 mins), usual disinfectant and detergents, and by hand-cleaning agents. It is one of the most frequent causes of acute respiratory infection and conjunctivitis, and may be latent and cause later relapse. Adenovirus is transmittable between individuals by respiratory and eye drops and, in case of enteric adenovirus, by stools. The incubation time ranges from 5 to 10 days. It is not common in the first 6 months of life, suggesting protection by maternal antibodies. By 5 years, 75% of children have positive serology for adenoviruses. Serotypes 1–7 are responsible for acute respiratory diseases. Approximately 2%–3% of acute respiratory infections are caused by adenovirus, with >8% caused in children <2 years old (36). Lower respiratory system infections include pneumonia, AB, laryngotracheobronchitis, or a pertussis-like cough (**Table 45.2**).

Parainfluenza

The seasonal pattern of types 1, 2, and 3 parainfluenza viruses is curiously interactive. Every second year, type-1 parainfluenza virus causes a defined epidemic, with a larger number of croup cases than AB. Type-2 parainfluenza virus epidemic is erratic and comes just after a type-1 epidemic; a type-3 parainfluenza virus epidemic occurs yearly (mostly in spring and summer) and has prolonged duration in relation to types 1 and 2 (22). Parainfluenza viruses cause a disease similar to RSV with a lower hospitalization rate. Generally, these infections involve upper airways, and 30% to 50% of cases are complicated with acute otitis. Type-3 parainfluenza virus pneumonia and AB occur mainly in the first 6 months of life, with a lower incidence when compared to RSV.

Respiratory Syncytial Virus

Mostly based on the surface of G glucoproteins, RSV is divided into 2 large groups: A (dominant strain) and B. This virus grows optimally in a pH of 7.5; although sensitive to temperature, in gloves contaminated with RSV-infected nasal secretions it is recovered >1 hr later. Due to this stability, in a hospital setting, RSV may be considered a nosocomial agent. One is exposed to RSV after contact with ocular or nasal secretion. Serum antibodies appear to offer some protection against RSV infection. High maternal antibody levels are associated with lower infection rates in infants. Prophylactic administration of antibodies has been effective in reducing, but not eliminating, severe RSV disease. In humans and animals with deficient T cells, the infection is more severe, and RSV replication is longer (43).

Pathogenesis

AB caused by RSV results from infection and inflammation of the respiratory mucosa. Symptoms of lower respiratory tract obstruction are a consequence of the partial obstruction of the distal airways. Histologic examination frequently shows respiratory epithelium necrosis, monocytic inflammation with peribronchial edema, and distal airway obstruction with mucus and fibrin plugs. Infants are predisposed to AB due to the smaller distal airways and the absence of active immunity against RSV as well as to other respiratory viruses. Viral replication induces the production of inflammatory mediators by epithelial respiratory cells, contributing to the disease. Respiratory epithelial cell desquamation, mucosal edema, and increased airway smooth muscle reactivity cause AB respiratory symptoms. Inflammatory mediators produced by infected epithelial cells respond according to the involved viral agent. The relationship between disease severity and multiple-virus coinfection is not clear.

Differential Diagnosis

The absence of previous upper respiratory tract symptoms in a child who acutely begins to wheeze is suggestive of AB. In newborns with congenital heart disease, AB should be considered. Gastroesophageal reflux, aspiration pneumonia, and foreign-body aspiration may mimic AB symptoms.

Clinical Manifestations

AB usually occurs in winter but can be observed in any season. Parents usually report that affected children attend daycare centers or had contact with people with cold symptoms. In the beginning of the disease, children have abundant rhinorrhea and typically a "tight" cough, along with poor food intake (4–6 days after symptoms start). The degree of fever in infants depends on the infecting organism. Children experiencing AB

TABLE 45.3

WOOD-DOWNES SCORE

Score	Wheezing	Retraction	Respiratory rate	Heart rate	Ventilation	Cyanosis
0	No	No	<30	<120	Good Symmetrical	No
1	End expiratory	Subcostal/intercostal	31–45	>120	Regular Symmetrical	Yes
2	All expiration	Supraclavicular + nasal flaring	40–60		Very reduced	
3	inspiration and expiration	+ intercostal + suprasternal			Silent thorax	

The highest scores from each column are summed to attain the total severity score: 1–3, mild; 4–7, moderate; 8–14, severe. Adapted from Wood DW, Downes JJ, Lecks HI, et al. A clinical scoring system for the diagnosis of respiratory failure. Preliminary report on childhood status asthmaticus. *Am J Dis Child* 1972;123(3):227–8, with permission.

caused by RSV are frequently febrile by the time of consultation ($\geq$38.5°C, 101.3°F, in ~50% of patients), and those with influenza or parainfluenza usually have a fever >39°C (102.2°F).

Infants with AB often have significant tachypnea, mild-to-moderate hypoxia, and signs of respiratory distress, such as nasal flaring and respiratory accessory muscle use. Physical examination frequently demonstrates audible wheezing, crackles, or rhonchi (apical ventilatory pattern), and a prolonged expiratory phase. Other common findings are conjunctivitis, acute otitis, and rhinitis. Many infants have a distended abdomen due to pulmonary hyperinflation.

A mild leukocytosis with a normal differential is frequently found in infants experiencing AB. Hypoxia is detected by pulse oximetry or arterial blood gases. CO_2 retention may be seen in severe cases. Viruses may be detected from nasal samples by indirect fluorescence antibody detection, PCR, radioimmunoassay, or direct culture. Virus-diagnosing test results may be used to limit inappropriate use of antibiotics. Chest x-rays often show nonspecific findings, including hyperinflation, gross infiltrates that are typically migratory and attributable to postobstructive atelectasis, and peribronchial filling. AB is not an alveolar space disease and, when a true alveolar infiltrate is seen, secondary bacterial pneumonia should be suspected. Wood-Downes score may be used to evaluate and grade AB severity (68) (**Table 45.3**).

Treatment

Clinical judgment remains the gold-standard criterion for hospital admission and cannot be replaced by objective criterion. Arterial O_2 saturation (SaO_2) is the most consistent clinical predictor of a worsening clinical condition (the cut-off point ranging from 90% to 95%); however, most children in this SaO_2 range have good clinical outcomes in prospective cohort studies (38).

Factors such as age <3 months, past medical history, SaO_2, respiratory rate (RR), and cardiorespiratory effort should be observed. SaO_2 <95%, prematurity (<34 weeks of gestational age), congenital heart disease, neurologic disease, RR >70 bpm, pulmonary atelectasis, sick or toxic appearance, and age <3 months are associated with most severe disease (defined as inability to keep active and alert or well hydrated). An arterial saturation of <95% on pulse oximetry was the single best

predictor of a more severe total disease course (60). Generally, RR >80 bpm and hypoxia with SaO_2 <85% are predictors of the need for intensive care, but they have low sensitivity (30%) and specificity (97%) for predicting a worsening clinical picture (10). Admission to the PICU is appropriate if clinical (progressive respiratory distress leading to respiratory fatigue, apnea episodes) and/or diagnostic signs (PO_2 <60 mm Hg; PCO_2 >50 mm Hg) of respiratory failure are noted despite administration of supplemental O_2 (40%–50% FIO_2).

Treatment of children with AB has changed over the years and remains controversial. With no effective proven treatment, any therapeutic strategy has little definitive evidence.

Hydration and Oxygenation

Adequate hydration and oxygenation are the backbone of AB treatment. Offering oral/enteral fluids or, when feeding is not tolerated, IV fluids and O_2 support is essential. Although hydration greatly varies among institutions, approximately half of uncomplicated bronchiolitis patients may require IV fluids. Supplemental O_2, usually delivered via nasal prongs, is the single most useful therapy. SaO_2 should be kept above 92% (7). Careful monitoring, mainly among the more sick and high-risk children, is important, as more aggressive ventilatory support may be required (mask, nasopharyngeal continuous positive airway pressure ventilation, or even endotracheal ventilation), and the timely introduction of ventilatory support is important to prevent further complications. These measures, along with suitable monitoring, are universally accepted supportive treatment.

β_2 Agonists

The use of β_2 agonists still has no scientifically defined recommendation; however, in the clinical setting, it remains an almost universal practice to administer these agents to children with AB, at least on a trial basis. If clinical improvement does not immediately occur or if worsening is observed after 60 mins of inhalation, β_2 agonists should be discontinued. Airway diameter reduction and wheezing result from at least four causes in RSV infection: increased secretion production, sloughing of injured airway epithelium to lumen, mucosal and interstitial edema, and bronchoconstriction mediated by possible humoral and neurogenic mechanisms. The contribution of each factor varies among children, and the degree of bronchoconstriction varies considerably among patients. As β_2 agonists help to relieve bronchoconstriction, the degree of their effectiveness is directly related to the contribution of bronchoconstriction to wheezing (i.e., the greater the contribution, the more effective the agonists).

Bronchodilator treatment is more effective when administered early, presumably when the small airways are not obstructed by secretions and cellular debris. One study evaluated the response to β-agonists that were given by metered dose inhaler or nebulized treatment in children with severe disease who required intubation and mechanical ventilation (62). It was concluded that pulmonary compliance and resistance improved with both methods of treatment, and no complications were observed.

Results obtained with anticholinergics use (ipratropium bromide) are very limited. They were not superior to β_2 agonists alone and did not improve the results when used in combination. Theophylline appears to be indicated for clinical apnea, but no studies have been conducted to evaluate this indication.

Racemic Epinephrine

When compared to inhaled albuterol/fenoterol, epinephrine is more effective. A recent Cochrane review showed that epinephrine leads to small improvement on the clinical score but no change in the hospitalization rate (25). Racemic epinephrine 2.25% and L-epinephrine 0.1% are used at 0.1 mg/kg and 0.05 mg/kg, respectively, every 4 hrs. This treatment should only be used in the hospital setting with clinical, heart rate, and electrocardiographic monitoring. As a rebound effect may occur, the child should be observed for at least 1–2 hrs following cessation of treatment and a decision to discharge prematurely should be avoided.

When RSV infection pathogenesis is known, the response difference among epinephrine and albuterol is better understood. Due to α-adrenergic agonist activity, epinephrine is more effective at reducing interstitial mucosa edema and may be more effective than β-adrenergic bronchodilator therapy in opening small airways. β-agonists increase mucosal blood flow and thickness with edema and can exacerbate wheezing and respiratory distress. In addition, excessive use may increase O_2 consumption and therefore respiratory demand, further exacerbating respiratory failure.

Inhaled and Systemic Steroids

The use of inhaled and systemic steroids is also a controversial therapy, as these agents may produce little or no response at all. They are generally indicated for mild or moderate AB treatment. A Cochrane systematic review showed no benefit of systemic steroid use in the management of AB (51). Severely ill children who are receiving mechanical ventilation may benefit from steroid use; however, steroids do not prevent bronchospasm in patients following AB. The anti-inflammatory action of steroids may be effective, according to the pathophysiology of the infection caused by RSV; however, studies conducted to date do not justify the use of this treatment based on improvement of clinical findings, reduction in hospital admission, and hospital length of stay.

Aerosolized Recombinant Human DNAse

Studies have evaluated the effects of aerosolized recombinant human DNAse used for treatment of children with RSV in-

fection (45,47). In the first, a randomized, placebo-controlled study, the chest x-ray score significantly improved after DNAse administration, while no improvement or a worsening score was noted in the control group (47). However, other measurement differences, such as RR, wheezing, and retractions, were not significant between groups. Mucus in patients with cystic fibrosis, bronchiectasias, and RSV AB was shown to contain significant extracellular DNA from degenerated leukocytes and epithelial debris (47). DNA increased pulmonary secretion viscosity and adhesiveness. DNAse may also be effective in infections complicated by atelectasis, bronchial secretions, and mucous plugs that have high DNA concentration. Another group used DNAse, aerosolized or by cannula, twice daily until clinical improvement, for children without cystic fibrosis and with atelectasis; they found quick clinical improvement after 2 hrs and radiologic improvement after 24 hrs for most of the children (26).

Ribavirin

Ribavirin is an antiviral drug that inhibits the structural protein synthesis of the virus, reducing viral replication and immunoglobulin (Ig) E response. Following the initial excitement regarding this drug, problematic issues arose related to its high cost, logistic issues, possible teratogenesis, and low clinical efficacy. A Cochrane review found no conclusive evidence that ribavirin use is beneficial for AB due to RSV (65).

Antibiotics

Antibiotics have no benefit in treating RSV but are important in treating secondary bacterial infection, such as *Streptococcus* and *Staphylococcus*, which can occur following initial RSV infection.

Other Measures

Although limited evidence regarding the efficacy of adjunct therapies for AB exists, many treatments are used. These are discussed in brief here. Many have never been subjected to randomized, controlled trials.

Heliox

The helium-oxygen mixture (heliox) reduces the work of breathing and expiratory wheezing in children with obstructive disease. Studies that evaluated heliox effects on RSV-infected children demonstrated that this mixture can be useful as a supportive therapy that avoids respiratory failure and intubation, but that it has no benefit for patients who are receiving invasive mechanical ventilation (11,41). It is recommended that its use should be restricted to the intensive care setting.

Respiratory Physiotherapy

Although only 3 randomized, controlled clinical trials involving AB children and respiratory physiotherapy are available, this therapy is routine in some PICUs (8,48,66). In a systematic review, the recommended techniques for children with AB are based on positioning therapy, alveolar recruitment, expiratory airflow increase using hand vibration, and airway aspiration (54). Due to copious airway secretions in RSV, airway suctioning is an effective measure for tracheobronchial hygiene. Approximately 60% of respiratory resistance is in the upper airways, and as infants predominantly breathe through the nose, the clearance of these secretions may have a positive impact on work of breathing and relieve symptoms.

Extracorporeal Membrane Oxygenation

Extracorporeal membrane oxygenation (ECMO) is an option for severely ill children who cannot be supported by conventional mechanical ventilation due to their ventilation and cardiocirculatory condition. While use of ECMO for RSV is infrequent, good survival has been obtained, even with prolonged durations of this support while the patient is awaiting lung recovery (46).

Inhaled Nitric Oxide

Nitric oxide used in the treatment of children severely infected with RSV improved oxygenation (28) and respiratory system resistance. One study showed that some children benefit and others worsen or have no therapeutic benefit, concluding that inhaled nitric oxide does not improve pulmonary mechanics (50). The use of this therapy should be reserved for patients with severe hypoxemia, refractory to ventilatory support.

Exogenous Surfactant

Children with AB infected by RSV have surfactant deficiency in both quantity and ability to decrease alveoli superficial tension. The use of exogenous surfactant as potential treatment for AB patients was evaluated, and the results suggest that surfactant has an important role on small-airway patency as well as on pulmonary compliance; however, its use is restricted to patients in the ICU (15). Despite the positive response observed in some studies with surfactant, its clinical use remains infrequent. A new study evaluating its use in patients specifically with RSV is under way at this writing.

Conventional Mechanical Pulmonary Ventilation

Conventional mechanical ventilation, using control-pressure ventilation mode, is indicated in those children with either obstructive or restrictive hypoxemic disease; however, a mixed mode (pressure regulated, volume controlled) can also be chosen. Due to the possibility of intrinsic positive end-expiratory pressure (PEEP), efforts should be focused on maintaining a low RR (20 bpm) and an inspiratory:expiratory ratio of 1:3. Additionally, the initial PEEP should be ~5 cm H_2O, with adjustments being made according to the degree of alveolar recruitment and clinical response.

High-frequency Oscillation Ventilation

High-frequency oscillation ventilation is indicated for those patients whose condition continues to worsen despite conventional mechanical ventilation or for those with significant air leak (pneumothorax, interstitial emphysema, pneumopericardium). It is also indicated for patients with restrictive disease, with an oxygenation index > 13 at some centers. The main advantage of this therapy is the possibility of optimizing ventilation and oxygenation with a lower risk of pulmonary injury induced by mechanical ventilation.

Noninvasive Positive-pressure Ventilation

Noninvasive positive-pressure ventilation use in AB children keeps airways open, improves respiratory flow, maintains functional residual capacity, improves pulmonary compliance, facilitates secretion mobilization, reduces work of breathing, improves gas exchange, and preserves surfactant synthesis and release. This therapy is indicated as first-choice ventilatory support in children who are experiencing apnea episodes and for preventing the use of invasive mechanical ventilation. This noninvasive support can be performed using continuous positive airway pressure (CPAP) or bilevel positive airway pressure (BiPAP) ventilatory mode. New modes of high-flow nasal cannula therapy with devices such as Vapotherm may also be advantageous in some patients. When CPAP is chosen, it is recommended to start with 4–6 cm H_2O; if BiPAP is chosen, it is recommended to begin with an inspiratory pressure of 8 cm H_2O and expiratory positive airway pressure of 4 cm H_2O. Noninvasive positive-pressure ventilation parameter changes should be titrated to the child's clinical response.

Prophylaxis

Preventing RSV infection in young infants, mostly in those at high risk, is clearly the best strategy. Two measures are available for preventing RSV infection: use of vaccines (active immunization) and parenteral immunoglobulins. Efforts to obtaining an effective vaccine persist without positive results. Passive immunization against RSV may be made with monoclonal antibodies (palivizumab, approved by the US Food and Drug Administration in 1998). Once per month during the epidemic months, an intramuscular dose of 15 mg/kg should be administered. The efficacy of passive immunization is 1/200, and immunization reduces RSV hospitalization rates by 55%. Premature infants without chronic pulmonary disease benefit more from palivizumab. Updated directions for palivizumab use were published by the American Academy of Pediatrics in 2005 (2); its use is indicated in children with congenital heart disease and significant hemodynamic impairment.

Prognosis

Most children with AB, regardless of severity, recover without sequelae. The natural course of the disease usually ranges from 7 to 10 days; however, some children remain ill for weeks. Children predisposed to asthma may wheeze more when infected by RSV or another allergic stimulus. Debate remains concerning the exact mechanism of post-AB wheezing and if viral infection is the underlying cause or if wheezing is the consequence of airway disease (13).

PNEUMONIA

Pneumonia is an inflammation of the lung parenchyma. The etiology may be infectious or not, as in food, gastric juice, or foreign aspirations; hypersensitivity to inhaled materials (hydrocarbon and lipoid pneumonia); and drug- or radiation-induced pneumonitis. Pneumonia usually presents with clinical signs of alveolar alteration and radiologic signs of opacity, without lung volume loss. The term *bronchopneumonia* refers to characteristic clinical findings with multiple opacities on radiologic exam, generally poorly defined, without clear segmental limits, and associated with a more serious clinical presentation.

Pneumonia is one of the most frequent infections in children and one of the main causes that lead to hospitalization. More than 95% of the episodes of pneumonia in the world occur in developing countries. It is estimated that 150 million cases occur annually in children who are <5 years old (57).

Pneumonia can be classified according to the anatomic location (lobar, lobular, alveolar, or interstitial), the location where it was acquired (community or nosocomial), or the causative organism. Nosocomial pneumonia can be acquired during mechanical ventilation or not. Although universal definition is lacking, community-acquired pneumonia is usually defined as a lung infection with acute symptoms (fever, cough, dyspnea), associated with altered pulmonary auscultation (crackles) or with the presence of an acute infiltrate in chest x-ray in a not previously hospitalized or institutionalized child for at least 14 days before the first symptoms (5).

Pneumonia is a frequent nosocomial infection. According to the National Nosocomial Infections Surveillance System, pneumonia associated with mechanical ventilation is the second leading cause of nosocomial infection (20%), occurring more frequently in children between 2 and 12 months of age, and the most frequent microorganism is *Pseudomonas aeruginosa* (22%) (56). The European multicentered study group found a nosocomial infection rate of 23.6% in children, and the most frequent infection was pneumonia (53%), with *P. aeruginosa* (44%) being the most frequent pathogen (55). Another study in PICU patients found a nosocomial infection prevalence of 12% and, in this group, pneumonia was associated with mechanical ventilation in 22.7% (21).

When a child presents with recurrent pneumonia, the possibility of an underlying disease (e.g., acquired or congenital lung anatomical abnormalities, immunodeficiency, prematurity, lung sequestration, tracheoesophageal fistula, foreign body, cystic fibrosis, heart failure, palatine cleft, bronchiectasis, ciliary dyskinesia, neutropenia, and increased pulmonary blood flow) should be considered. Other predisposing factors are low socioeconomic level, parents who smoke, and PICU patients (mainly those who are intubated and require prolonged mechanical ventilation), prolonged postoperative period, supine position, use of nasogastric tubes, use of muscle-relaxing drugs, use of antacids and H_2 blockers (gastric colonization), coma, shock, and inadequate use of humidifiers.

Epidemiology

Community-acquired Pneumonia

In children who are <1 year of age, viruses are the main pneumonia-causative pathogens (44). In the neonatal period, the most frequent pathogens are herpes simplex and cytomegalovirus. In children >6 months of age, RSV, influenza, parainfluenza, adenovirus, rhinovirus, coronavirus, measles, rubella, chickenpox, cytomegalovirus, and herpes are more frequent.

In newborns and in infants <2 months old, the bacterial etiologies are more frequent: Group B Streptococci, gram-negative bacilli (maternal genital tract or hospital flora), *Staphylococcus aureus*, *Chlamydia trachomatis*, and congenital syphilis (less frequently). From 2 months to 5 years of age, *Streptococcus pneumoniae*, type B *Haemophilus influenzae*, and *S. aureus* are frequently found. The prevalence of *Mycoplasma pneumoniae* increases in children >3 years, and

the prevalence of *S. pneumoniae*, *M. pneumoniae*, type B Haemophilus influenza, and *Chlamydophila pneumoniae* increases in children ≥5 years of age.

Other pathogens, such as helminths (*Ascaris lumbricoides*, *Strongyloides stercoralis*, *Toxocara kennels*), hMPV (*Bordetella pertussis*, *Mycobacterium tuberculosis*, *Listeria monocytogenes*, *Legionella pneumophila*), Hantavirus (*Coxiella burnetii*), protozoa (*Toxoplasma gondii*, *Pneumocystis carinii*), fungi, and physical and chemical agents, can also be found.

Nosocomial Pneumonias

Pneumonias acquired after 48–72 hrs of hospitalization are considered nosocomial. The incidence of pneumonia occurring in ventilated patients after 48–72 hrs is termed *ventilator-associated pneumonia*. Identification and reduction of ventilator-associated pneumonia in the PICU is a current focus of infection-control efforts at many centers. The airways may be colonized by pathogens coming from pharyngeal, intestinal, and/or hospital flora. The main agents are gram-negative: *P. aeruginosa*, *Klebsiella* spp., *Escherichia coli*, *Enterobacter* spp., *Serratia marcescens*, and *Acinetobacter* spp. The gram-positive agents are *S. aureus* and *S. pneumoniae*. The fungi are *Candida albicans* and, in the patients with leukemia, lymphoma, or acquired immunodeficiency syndrome (AIDS) and in those who are post-organ transplant, the possibility of viral infections and *Pneumocystis carinii* should be considered.

Aspiration Pneumonia

Children with obstructive lesions of the gastrointestinal tract, diseases with hypotonia, dysautonomia, compromised consciousness, or gastroesophageal reflux and/or swallowing incoordination can aspirate or regurgitate, which can cause chemical pneumonitis. Often, there is a time lapse between the aspiration and the signs and symptoms of pneumonia. Previously healthy, nonhospitalized, patients can be infected with agents of their own oral flora (predominantly anaerobes), and hospitalized patients can be colonized by gram-negative bacteria.

Pathogenesis

Pneumonia may occur either by direct tracheal colonization or by direct invasion of the pulmonary parenchyma. The first-line protection against respiratory pathogens is the airway defense barriers, mainly the mucous membrane and the mucociliary layer, which are responsible for the clearance of foreign material or microorganisms. Once bacteria inoculate the respiratory tract, a normal inflammatory response (including antibodies, complement, phagocytes, and cytokines) begins and causes injury to the functioning pulmonary tissue (67).

The bacteria that cause pneumonia also have specific virulent factors that increase their survival and reproduction, resulting in more extensive lesions of the lung. Pneumonia can also be caused by a direct lung invasion; this is an important infective mechanism for *S. pneumoniae* and *S. aureus*.

Clinical Manifestations

Bacterial pneumonia in previously healthy children is not frequent, usually occurring after a viral infection or in the presence of an underlying chronic disease. The clinical features vary

TABLE 45.4

PNEUMONIA CLINICAL MANIFESTATIONS AND ETIOLOGIC AGENTS

Clinical manifestations	Etiologic agent
Fever	Virus, *Chlamydia*, *Mycoplasma pneumoniae*
Wheezing	Virus (+ respiratory syncytial virus)
Myalgia	Virus (+ influenza), *M. pneumoniae*
Upper airway distress	Virus (+ parainfluenza)
Conjunctivitis	*Chlamydia*, adenovirus
Cutaneous abscesses	*Staphylococcus aureus*
Purpuric cutaneous injuries	*Pseudomonas aeruginosa*
Paroxysmal cough	*Chlamydia*
Acute otitis	*Streptococcus pneumoniae*/type B *Haemophilus influenzae*
Effusion/empyema	*S. pneumoniae*/*S. aureus*
Sudden onset	*S. aureus*

according to the etiologic agent (**Table 45.4**), nutritional status, immunologic condition, and underlying disease.

The usual signs and symptoms are fever, lethargy, poor appetite, pallor or cyanosis, toxemia, agitation, vomiting, and abdominal distension. Signs and symptoms of lung compromise are respiratory distress (nasal flaring, intercostal and subcostal retractions, thoracic pain). The pulmonary signs vary, and alterations of the breath sounds, such bronchophony, crackles, reduction of the thoracic expansion on the compromised side, hemorrhage signs/empyema, or bronchial murmur may be present.

Tachypnea is the most sensitive parameter in children with pneumonia. Its precise predictive value depends on the underlying disease (39), but diagnosis should not be based solely on the presence of the tachypnea, which is present in other diseases, such as AB and asthma. Fever and cough are also frequent symptoms, and clinical signs of accessory ventilatory muscle retractions and altered pulmonary auscultation tend to be the most specific indicators of lower airway compromise (18). Other less-specific indicators include physical indisposition, vomiting, abdominal pain, and thoracic pain (suggestive of bacterial pneumonia). Wheezing can be observed in children with bacterial pneumonia, but it is more common in children with AB or with other viral lower airway infection.

Diagnosis

A diagnosis of pneumonia is possible in children who present with fever, cough, and tachypnea and have an infiltration on chest x-ray. However, several other diseases can have these signs and symptoms, such as AB, upper airway infection, congestive heart failure, pulmonary embolism, thoracic tumors, or inflammatory diseases (systemic vasculitis).

The diagnosis is essentially clinical, based on history, physical examination, and epidemiologic data. Chest x-rays are of great value, despite their not being specific. The radiologic pattern may suggest the disease etiology (**Table 45.5**). However, interobserver agreement on the infiltrate pattern (alveolar versus interstitial) or the presence of air bronchograms is poor (1). Chest ultrasonography may be useful to demonstrate and char-

acterize pleural effusions, septations, and collections. Chest CT may be necessary for further delineation. When the child develops persistent or progressive symptoms despite therapy, contrast CT can be useful to evaluate suppurative complications such as empyema or lung necrosis.

When the symptoms persist despite empiric therapy, fiberoptic bronchoscopy with bronchoalveolar lavage is a diagnostic option. In immunocompromised children in whom the selection of antibiotics is difficult, early bronchoscopy may be indicated.

Laboratory Studies

In the presence of pneumonia, the white blood cell count can be >25,000/mm^3 or even >35,000/mm^3 (42). Other inflammatory markers, such as C reactive protein, procalcitonin, and erythrocyte sedimentation rate, are usually elevated (**Table 45.6**). Bacterial blood cultures for the diagnosis and management of pneumonia, particularly when a bacterial etiology is suspected, are recommended (40). Bacterial isolation in blood cultures varies from 3% to 11%, but this rarely modifies the patient's management (12). Although uncommon, the identification of a specific organism (*S. pneumoniae* or *S. aureus*), along with the antimicrobial activity, can be especially useful in more serious cases or when pleural effusions are present. Viral diagnosis (culture or antigen detection using direct fluorescence) is not usually necessary, but in certain circumstances such as in immunocompromised children or to guide infection control precautions, it may be useful.

Polymerase chain reaction has high sensitivity and specificity for *Mycoplasma* infections, which can also be identified using serology (positive IgM indicates an acute infection). When *Legionella* infection is suspected, the pathogen urinary antigen is the diagnostic test of choice. The test remains positive for weeks after acute infection. When chest x-ray suggests a mycobacterium disease (mediastinal enlargement) or when epidemiologic risk factors increase the probability of tuberculosis infection, purified protein derivative of tuberculin (PPD) should be performed.

Treatment

Hospitalization Criteria

No scoring system, validated in children, exists that can be used to identify patients with specific risks and to guide hospitalization in pneumonia (58). Several admission criteria are used, including septic appearance, hypoxia that requires O$_2$ therapy, severe or moderate respiratory distress, difficulty in taking fluids or oral medications, and socioeconomic factors. Newborns with fever and pneumonia should be hospitalized, as well as those who had previous diseases complicated by pneumonia (**Table 45.7**).

Supportive Therapy

Supportive therapy includes maintenance of nutritional state, fluid, electrolyte, and acid-base balance, and temperature; 30-degree head elevations, heated and humidified O$_2$ therapy, thinning of secretions, and physiotherapy have all been suggested. Tracheal intubation and mechanical ventilation should

TABLE 45.5

PNEUMONIAS ETIOLOGY AND MOST FREQUENT RADIOLOGIC PATTERNS

Etiology	Radiologic pattern
Viral pneumonia	Diffuse interstitial infiltration Hyperinflation
S. pneumoniae pneumonia	Clinical findings do not always correspond to the radiologic findings. Lobar consolidation is frequent in older children (homogeneous condensation/presence of air bronchogram). Pleural reaction and effusion are not rare. The radiologic resolution can be completed after several weeks of the clinical resolution.
Streptococcal pneumonia	Diffuse bronchopneumonia Pleural effusion may occur. Radiologic resolution may last for weeks.
Staphylococcal pneumonia	At first, an unspecific bronchopneumonia image may be seen. Soon, the infiltration becomes more homogeneous and involves a lobe or hemithorax. In secondary film, forms may appear as not well delimited bronchopneumonia-associated nodular images. During evolution, pleural effusion/empyema may be seen. Pyopneumothorax and pneumatoceles of variable sizes are frequent.
Pneumonia due to type B H. influenzae	Usually lobar or segmental distribution Right-side predominant Pleural effusion is more frequent than in pneumococcal pneumonia. Pneumatoceles may be present.
Mycoplasma pneumoniae pneumonia	Bronchopneumonic or interstitial pattern Dense unilateral infiltration in ~75% of the cases, more frequently involving inferior lobes Lobar pneumonia is not frequent. Hilar lymphadenopathy in approximately one-third of cases Pleural involvement may occur.
Chlamydia trachomatis pneumonia	Hyperinsufflation Interstitial or diffuse alveolar infiltrate

be considered in the most severe cases of acute respiratory failure.

Age-related Antibiotic Therapy

Group B Streptococci and gram-negative bacteria prevail among newborns until the age of 3 weeks, and in most of the cases, IV ampicillin and gentamicin should be used. In severe disease, third-generation cephalosporin (cefotaxime) should be administered, along with ampicillin, to provide coverage for potential *L. monocytogenes*. In children between 3 weeks and 3 months, if the child is febrile, erythromycin 40 mg/kg/day should be prescribed every 6 hrs to treat *C. trachomatis*; if the child has a fever and toxic appearance, ceftriaxone 50 mg/kg/day every 24 hrs should be administered. If bacterial pneumonia is suspected in children between 4 months and 4 years, ampicillin 200 mg/kg/day every 6 hrs should be administered. In severe cases, ceftriaxone should be used.

In children >5 years old, azithromycin 10 mg/kg, followed by 5 mg/kg/day, can be used for routine treatment of atypical bacteria, particularly *M. pneumoniae* (58). Ceftriaxone, with or without macrolides, may be used in sicker children. In all ages, if the clinical manifestations suggest the presence of *S. aureus*, oxacillin or vancomycin should be used, depending on the prevalence of methicillin-resistant *Staphylococcus* in the community (Table 45.8).

Empiric Treatment of Nosocomial Pneumonias

Initial treatment should cover gram-negative and gram-positive pathogens, using semisynthetic penicillin (oxacillin/cloxacillin) with third- or fourth-generation cephalosporins (ceftriaxone/ceftazidime or cefepime). In the presence of a high incidence of methicillin-resistant *S. aureus*, vancomycin, teicoplanin, or clindamycin should be administered with third- or fourth-generation cephalosporin. An optional treatment would be vancomycin with imipenem or meropenem. If risk factors exist for fungal infection, amphotericin B or fluconazole should be administered. If the patient has received a bone marrow graft or has lymphoma, leukemia, or AIDS, it is necessary to enhance the antibiotic spectrum for *Pneumocystis carinii*, adding trimethoprim-sulfamethoxazole or pentamidine.

Specific Pneumonia Treatment

For the treatment of infections caused by *C. trachomatis* and *M. pneumoniae*, a macrolide is the drug of choice. For patients with suspicion of *S. pneumoniae* pneumonia, therapy is driven by the local antimicrobial susceptibility pattern, and ampicillin or ceftriaxone, in the cases of nonsusceptible pathogens, could be used. Vancomycin is rarely necessary for the treatment of *S. pneumoniae* pneumonia, even if the strain is not susceptible to penicillin. When infection due to type B *H. influenzae* is

TABLE 45.6

LABORATORY TESTS FEATURES

Diagnostic test	Characteristics
Blood count	Leukocytosis
	Leukopenia suggests a worse prognosis.
	Varied degrees of anemia
Erythrocyte sedimentation rate and reactive C protein	Nonspecific, used for follow-up control
Blood cultures	May be suggestive of bacterial etiology when very elevated.
	The ideal is to collect three samples before the beginning of the antibiotic therapy
	High specificity
	Variable sensibility depending on agent
Pleural fluid culture	Etiologic agent can be found in up to 60% of cases.
Tracheal aspirate culture	Intubated patients
	Growth $>10^5$–10^6 CFU/mL suggests infection.
Bronchoalveolar lavage culture (bronchoscopy)	High sensibility and specificity
	Growth $>10^4$ CFU/mL indicates infection.
Culture of material obtained from aspirative puncture	Growth $>10^3$ CFU/mL indicates infection.
Biopsies	Invasive method and therefore with restricted indications
Virus isolation and fibroblasts, HeLa, HEP2, and kidney monkey cells culture	Special restricted indications
	Good positivity/high cost
	Used mainly during epidemic offspring investigations
Respiratory virus serologies	Blood samples in acute and convalescent phases
	Investigation of antibody elevation against a specific virus—useful as an epidemiologic instrument.
	Has no diagnostic usefulness in the acute phase because the serologic result will confirm the etiology only after the end of the acute phase.
Detection of bacterial antigens in corporal fluids	Urine and pleural fluid
	Reactions occur against *S. pneumoniae*, *H. influenzae*, group B streptococcus, and *N. meningitidis* serotypes A, B, C, Y, and W135
	In ~90% of the pneumonias due to *H. influenzae* with bacteremia blood or urine, samples are positive for group B streptococci; 5–30% of the infections are due to *S. pneumoniae*.
Nasopharynx secretion sample Immunofluorescence	Detection of viral antigens
	Positivity up to 85% for RSV
Fast detection cryoagglutinins	The test is positive if defined micronodular agglutination occurs
ELISA	For virus and bacteria
Complement fixation reaction	Performed for virus and *Mycoplasma pneumoniae*
	Retrospective diagnosis

CFU, colony-forming units; ELISA, enzyme-linked immunoabsorbent assay

TABLE 45.7

HOSPITAL ADMISSION CRITERIA

<3--6 months
Acute respiratory failure (dyspnea, sustained tachypnea)
Toxemia/sepsis
Hemodynamic instability
Necessity for oxygen therapy
Domiciliary treatment failure
Extensive lung compromise
Immunosuppression, heart disease or other serious underlying disease
Socioeconomic factors
Pneumonia complications

suspected, ceftriaxone or ampicillin-sulbactam should be used because of the presence of β-lactamase–mediated resistance to ampicillin in several type B *H. influenzae* strains. For the majority of pathogens, the optimal duration of the antimicrobial therapy for complicated or uncomplicated pneumonia is not established. Data suggest the use of azithromycin for 5 days for the treatment of *C. pneumoniae* pneumonia (24).

The treatment of the *S. pneumoniae* pneumonia should be maintained until the child has no fever for at least 72 hrs, and the total duration of the therapy should not be <10–14 days. Fever can persist for several days after the beginning of appropriate therapy, reflecting the inflammatory cascade and tissue injury. Initial empiric therapy can be modified after the identification of the etiologic agent (**Table 45.9**).

TABLE 45.8

EMPIRIC TREATMENT OF COMMUNITY-ACQUIRED PNEUMONIAS ACCORDING TO AGE

Age	Treatment
Newborns up to 2 months	Possible infection due to Group B Streptococcus or gram-negative bacilli: Ampicillin plus Gentamicin or ampicillin plus Amikacin
	If *Chlamydia trachomatis* infection is suspected: Erythromycin
	Suspicion of Herpes: Acyclovir
	Suspicion of CMV: Ganciclovir
Nonfebrile pneumonia up to 3 months	Probable infection due to *Chlamydia trachomatis*: Erythromycin
Nonfebrile pneumonia 3–4 months to 5 years	Most frequent viral infections: Antivirals in special situations
2 months to 5 years	Possible agents: *Streptococcus pneumoniae*, *Haemophilus influenzae*, and *Staphylococcus aureus*
	Noncomplicated cases: oral amoxicillin, amoxicillin-clavulanate acid or cefuroxime
	Moderate to serious infection: IV amoxicillin-clavulanate, cefuroxime, or oxacillin plus chloramphenicol or third-generation cephalosporin
>5 years	*Mycoplasma pneumoniae* (frequent): macrolides (erythromycin, clarithromycin, azithromycin)
	Viral pneumonia is also possible
	Pneumonia and *H. influenzae*: noncomplicated cases: amoxicillin-clavulanate or cefuroxime (orally)
	Complicated cases: erythromycin plus cefuroxime (IV) or third-generation cephalosporin

Complications

Pneumonia complications include pleural effusions, empyema, extrapulmonary infection and sepsis, acute respiratory distress syndrome, shock, lung abscess, pneumothorax, atelectasis, and multiple organ system dysfunction. Pleural effusion and empyema are the most frequent complications.

Pleural Effusion

Pneumonia with pleural effusion is defined by the presence of fluids in the pleural cavity; it is termed *empyema* when this fluid contains pus (31). Pleural effusions can occur associated with many etiologic agents. *S. pneumoniae* is responsible for most of the cases, although *S. aureus* and *S. pyogenes* are also associated with high incidence of pleural effusion and empyema (23). Tuberculosis is also a frequent cause of pleural effusion, and it should be considered in the differential diagnosis of certain patients. Pleural effusions are classified as transudates and empyema, according to the laboratory analysis of the pleural fluid (**Table 45.10**). Additional data include a positive microbiologic study (Gram test, culture, or other diagnostic tests, such as PCR).

As in noncomplicated pneumonia, complementary tests have a limited value. Chest x-ray is indispensable for the correct diagnosis and follow-up of pleural effusion, demonstrating the magnitude and the evolution of this complication. Chest ultrasonography is also useful in the diagnosis and follow-up. CT findings have not been reliable in predicting which effusion will fulfill empyema criteria (16).

All children with a diagnosis of pleural effusion should have a diagnostic and sometimes therapeutic thoracentesis performed. Conservative treatment of pleural infection consists of isolated antibiotic therapy or antibiotic therapy and simple drainage (4). Most of the small parapneumonic effusions respond to antibiotic therapy without any additional intervention. However, the pleural effusions that increase volume and/or compromise breathing in an ill, feverish child must be drained. If the child has a significant pleural infection, a thoracostomy tube should be inserted. Repeated thoracentesis punctures are not recommended.

The initial empiric IV antibiotic therapy should cover *S. pneumoniae*. Broad-spectrum antibiotics are necessary for nosocomial infections, as well as those secondary to surgery, trauma, and aspiration. The antibiotic choice should be guided by the microbiologic results.

Intrapleural fibrinolytics may shorten hospital length of stay and are recommended by some for complicated parapneumonic effusions (loculated thick fluid) or empyema; however, only urokinase was analyzed in randomized, controlled trials involving children (3). Urokinase should be administered twice per day for 3 consecutive days: 10,000 units in 10 mL of normal saline for children <1 year of age and 40,000 units in 40 mL of normal saline in those ≥1 year old. Surgical treatment should be considered in patients who remain septic due to persistent pleural collection despite chest thoracostomy and antibiotic therapy. The three main surgical options are (a) video-assisted thoracic surgery; (b) minithoracotomy, which is similar to video-assisted thoracic surgery but is an open procedure; and (c) decortication, a more prolonged and complicated procedure. An organized empyema in a symptomatic child may require a thoracotomy and decortication.

TABLE 45.9

IDENTIFICATION OF THE ETIOLOGIC AGENT AND ANTIMICROBIALS

Agent	Antimicrobials
Chlamydia trachomatis	Erythromycin (40 mg/kg/day)
Chlamydia pneumoniae	Erythromycin (40 mg/kg/day)
Mycoplasma pneumoniae	Erythromycin (40 mg/kg/day)
Group B β-hemolytic streptococcus	Ampicillin (100 mg/kg/day)
	plus gentamicin (5 mg/kg/day)
	OR
	plus amikacin (15 mg/kg/day)
Streptococcus pneumoniae	
Sensitive to penicillin	Crystalline penicillin (100,000–250,000 U/kg/day)
Intermediate sensitivity	Penicillin (200,000–250,000 U/kg/day)
Resistant to the penicillin	Cefotaxime (200 mg/kg/day) or Ceftriaxone (100 mg/kg/day)
Resistant to penicillin and cephalosporins	Vancomycin (40–60 mg/kg/day)+ clindamycin (30–45 mg/kg/day)–erythromycin (40 mg/kg/day) (follow antibiogram orientation)
Haemophilus influenzae	
β-lactamase negative	Ampicillin (100 mg/kg/day)
β-lactamase positive	Cefotaxime (200 mg/kg/day) or ceftriaxone (100 mg/kg/day)
Staphylococcus aureus	
Methicillin sensitive	Oxacillin (200 mg/kg/day)
Methicillin resistant	Vancomycin (40–60 mg/kg/day) or teicoplanin (10 mg/kg/day) plus clindamycin (30–35 mg/kg/day).
Simian retrovirus, influenza b, parainfluenza	Ribavirin (15–20 mg/kg/day) (orally or IV) for immunocompromised patients, premature babies, those with chronic pulmonary diseases, congenital heart disease, or pulmonary hypertension, or critically ill patients
Influenza a and b	Amantadine 5 mg/kg/day (max. 150 mg/day)–from 1 year to 9 years of age (PO)
	Amantadine 100 mg every 12 hrs–>9 years of age (PO)
	Zanamivir 10 mg every 12 hrs–>12 years of age (inhaled)
Herpes simplex or zoster	Acyclovir (250 mg/m^2/8 hrs) (IV) (25–50 mg/kg/8 hrs) OR
	Foscarnet (60 mg/kg/8 hrs) (IV)
Cytomegalovirus	Ganciclovir 2,5 mg/kg/8 hrs initial (IV) 5 mg/kg/12 hrs (2–3 weeks) or foscarnet
Fungi	Amphotericin B (1 mg/kg/day)
	Liposomal amphotericin B (3 mg/kg/day) or fluconazole 6 mg/kg/day

Prognosis

Although hospitalization rates in children with pneumonia are increasing, in the US, a 97% reduction in the death rate was seen between 1939 and 1996 (17). Between 1995 and 1997, the estimated death rates (not adjusted for comorbidities) were 4% for children <2 years and 2% for those between 2 and 17 years (19). Improvements in intensive care treatment contributed to reduced mortality, which was higher in children with underlying diseases. Most children who develop pneumonia do not have long-term sequelae. Children who have noncomplicated parapneumonic effusions respond well to conservative treatment, without any residual lung lesion. Usually, the pleural disease due to virus or *Mycoplasma* resolves spontaneously. In contrast to adult patients, infants and children have a better ability to resolve pleural thickness without any subsequent detrimental effect in lung growth and function. The increased

incidence of methicillin-resistant *S. aureus* and organisms with increasing virulence factors may result in an increase in the occurrence of pneumonia and septic shock precipitated by these infections.

CONCLUSIONS AND FUTURE DIRECTIONS

Although AB is a frequent cause of consultation and hospitalization among young children only a small number—those with underlying diseases—have a high risk of developing a more severe disease. Treatment is limited to supportive care, including fluid replacement and O_2 therapy. Other therapeutic modalities are all controversial and the subject of additional studies. Future studies are necessary to further investigate the therapies that show early promise and to continue to search for more

TABLE 45.10

PLEURAL FLUID CHARACTERISTICS

	Transudate	Exudate
pH	>7.20	<7.20
Proteins (pleural fluid/ serum level rate)	<0.5	≥0.5
LDH (pleural fluid/ serum level rate)	<0.6	≥0.6
LDH (UI)	<200	≥200
Glucose (mg/dL)	>40	<40
Red cells (mm³)	<5000	>5000
Leukocytes (mm³)	<10,000 (PMN)	>10,000 (PMN)

LDH, lactate dehydrogenase; PMN, polymorphonuclear neutrophil

effective acute therapies. A genetic modification to alter the RSV genome, modifying the nonstructural protein NS1, is being developed to produce new vaccines. Novel antiviral treatments and vaccines are the main innovations to be achieved in terms of treatment and prophylaxis.

The incidence of nosocomial and community-acquired pneumonia and their complications remains elevated, with a high morbidity mainly in developing countries. However, clear evidence does not exist regarding how to best manage these patients. More adequate and accurate diagnostic methods are necessary to guide antimicrobial therapy, and new molecular diagnostic techniques will be useful. The emergence of resistant microorganisms perpetuates the need for continuous research for new antimicrobials. Strict control of nosocomial infections is of utmost importance, along with the use of vaccines and immunobiologic products.

KEY POINTS

Acute Bronchiolitis

■ AB can be caused by several pathogens, such as parainfluenza, adenovirus, influenza, M. pneumoniae, rhinovirus, C. pneumoniae, human metapneumovirus, and coronavirus.

■ Symptoms of lower respiratory tract obstruction are a consequence of the partial obstruction of the distal airways due to respiratory epithelial cell desquamation, mucosa surface edema, and increased airway smooth cells reactivity.

■ Gastroesophageal reflux, aspiration pneumonia, and foreign-body aspiration, may mimic AB symptoms.

■ Children who experience AB, mainly due to RSV, influenza, or parainfluenza, are frequently febrile (50% of the patients).

■ Significant tachypnea, mild to moderate hypoxia, and signs of respiratory distress, such as nasal flaring and respiratory accessory muscle use, are frequent findings on physical examination. Pulmonary auscultation with audible wheezing, crackles or rhonchi, and prolonged expiratory phase are also frequent findings.

■ Chest x-rays often show nonspecific findings, including hyperinflation and gross infiltrates that are typically migratory.

■ As AB is not an alveolar space disease, in the case of real alveolar infiltrate, secondary bacterial pneumonia should be suspected.

■ As an objective criterion for hospital admission of AB children does not exist, clinical judgment remains the gold-standard criterion.

■ The most consistent clinical predictor of clinical worsening is arterial O₂ saturation.

■ Disease severity is associated to SaO₂ <95%, prematurity <34 weeks of gestational age, congenital heart disease, neurologic diseases, RR >70 bpm, pulmonary atelectasis, and age <3 months.

■ If clinical and/or diagnostic signs of impending respiratory failure are present despite adequate supplemental O₂ therapy, admission to the PICU would be appropriate.

■ AB treatment still remains a polemic issue, as no effective proven treatment exists and, in most cases, the therapeutic strategy has no definitive evidence of efficacy.

■ Adequate hydration and oxygenation remain the backbone of AB treatment.

■ Although scientifically defined recommendations are lacking, use of β_2 agonists remains an almost universal practice.

■ When compared to albuterol/fenoterol, epinephrine is more effective. However, although inhaled epinephrine leads to clinical improvement, hospitalization rate remains unchanged.

■ The use of inhaled and systemic steroids produces scarce or no response; it, therefore, remains a controversial therapy.

■ As DNA increases pulmonary secretion viscosity and adhesiveness, DNAse, either aerosolized or by cannula, may be useful in AB patients.

■ At this writing, no conclusive evidence suggests that ribavirin use is beneficial for AB due to RSV.

■ Antibiotics have an important role in AB that is complicated by secondary bacterial infection.

■ The use of heliox has some evidence for clinical efficacy. However, therapies such as respiratory physiotherapy, exogenous surfactant, high-frequency oscillation ventilation, positive-pressure noninvasive ventilation, inhaled nitric oxide, and ECMO have limited evidence levels and have not been (and likely never will be) subjected to randomized, controlled trials for evaluation in AB. Such therapies may be appropriate in individual patients with severe disease.

■ According to the American Academy of Pediatrics, palivizumab should be used in children with congenital heart disease and significant hemodynamic impairment.

Pneumonia

■ Pneumonia associated with mechanical ventilation is the second highest cause of nosocomial infections.

■ The pathogenesis of pneumonia is dependent on host defense and microorganism virulence balance.

■ Bacterial pneumonia is not common in previously healthy children; it usually occurs after a viral infection or in the presence of an underlying chronic disease.

- Tachypnea is the most sensitive parameter in children with pneumonia.
- Diagnosis is essentially clinical, based on anamnesis, physical examination, and epidemiologic data.
- Although not specific, chest x-rays are of great value in diagnosing pneumonia.
- Chest sonography is useful in demonstrating and characterizing pleural effusions, septations, and collections.
- Blood cultures are recommended for the diagnosis and management of bacterial pneumonia.
- A pediatric-validated scoring system to guide hospitalization in pneumonia cases does not exist.
- Maintenance of the nutritional state, fluids, electrolyte and acid-base balance, and corporeal temperature; elevated decubitus; heated and humidified O_2 therapy; thinning of secretions; and physiotherapy are the backbone of pneumonia therapy.
- Antimicrobial therapy is guided according to epidemiologic and clinical data, the patient's age, the infective microorganism, and antimicrobial resistance.
- Consensus exists regarding the management of children with pleural effusion and empyema, the most frequent pneumonia complications, but it has little evidence of efficacy evidence.
- Most children who develop pneumonia have no long-term sequelae.

References

1. Albaum MN, Hill LC, Murphy M, et al. Interobserver reliability of the chest radiograph in community-acquired pneumonia. *PORT Investigators*. *Chest* 1996;110(2):343–50.
2. American Academy of Pediatrics. Revised indications for the use of palivizumab and respiratory syncytial virus immune globulin intravenous for the prevention of the respiratory syncytial infections (2003). http://aappolicy.aappublications.org/cgi/reprint/pediatrics; 112/6/1447.pdf (Accessed 2006).
3. Balfour-Lynn IM, Abrahamson E, Cohen G, et al. BTS guidelines for the management of pleural infection in children. *Thorax* 2005;60(1):i1–21.
4. Balfour-Lynn IM; Paediatric Pleural Diseases Subcommittee of British Thoracic Society Standards of Care Committee. Some consensus but little evidence: guidelines on management of pleural infection in children. *Thorax* 2005;60(2):94–6.
5. Bartlett JG, Dowell SF, Mandell LA, et al. Practice guidelines for the management of community-acquired pneumonia in adults. Infectious Diseases Society of America. *Clin Infect Dis* 2000;31(2):347–82.
6. Bhat N, Wright JG, Broder KR, et al. Influenza-associated deaths among children in the United States, 2003–2004. *N Engl J Med* 2005;353:2559–67.
7. Black CP. Systematic review of the biology and medical management of respiratory syncytial virus infection. *Respir Care* 2003;48(3):209–31.
8. Bohe L, Ferrero ME, Cuestas E, et al. Indications of conventional chest physiotherapy in acute bronchiolitis. Medicina (Buenos Aires) 2004;64:198–200.
9. Boivin G, De Serres G, Côtê S, et al. Human metapneumovirus infections in hospitalized children. *Emerg Infect Dis* 2003;9:634–40.
10. Brooks AM, McBride JT, McConnochie KM, et al. Predicting deterioration in previously healthy infants hospitalized with respiratory syncytial virus infection. *Pediatrics*. 1999;104(3 Pt 1):463–7.
11. Cambonie G, Milesi C, Fournier-Favre S, et al. Clinical effects of heliox administration for acute bronchiolitis in young infants. *Chest* 2006;129(3):676–82.
12. Campbell SG, Marrie TJ, Anstey R, et al. The contribution of blood cultures to the clinical management of adult patients admitted to the hospital with community-acquired pneumonia: a prospective observational study. *Chest* 2003;123(4):1142–50.
13. Carbonell-Estrany X, Kimpen JL. Introduction. RSV and RAD: possibilities for prevention? The link between respiratory syncytial virus and reactive airway disease. *Respir Res* 2002;3(1):S1–2.
14. Centers for Diseases Control. Prevention and control of influenza. *MMWR* 2005;54:1–40.
15. Davison C, Ventre KM, Luchetti M, et al. Efficacy of interventions for bronchiolitis in critically ill infants: a systematic review and meta-analysis. *Pediatr Crit Care Med* 2004;5(5):482–9.
16. Donnelly LF, Klosterman LA. CT appearance of parapneumonic effusions in children: findings are not specific for empyema. *AJR Am J Roentgenol* 1997; 169(1):179–82.
17. Dowell SF, Kupronis BA, Zell ER, et al. Mortality from pneumonia in children in the United States, 1939 through 1996. *N Engl J Med* 2000;342(19):1399–407.
18. Esposito S, Bosis S, Cavagna R, et al. Characteristics of Streptococcus pneumoniae and atypical bacterial infections in children 2–5 years of age with community-acquired pneumonia. *Clin Infect Dis* 2002;35(11):1345–52.
19. Feikin DR, Schuchat A, Kolczak M, et al. Mortality from invasive pneumococcal pneumonia in the era of antibiotic resistance, 1995–1997. *Am J Public Health* 2000;90(2):223–9.
20. García-Garcia ML, Calvo C, Martín F, et al. Human metapneumovirus infections in hospitalized infants in Spain. *Arch Dis Child* 2006;91:290–5.
21. Garrett DA, McKibben P, Levine G,, et al. Prevalence of nosocomial infections in pediatric intensive care unit patients at US children's hospitals. 4th Decennial International Conference on Nosocomial and Healthcare-Associated Infections. March 5–9, 2000; Atlanta, Georgia.
22. Hall CB. Respiratory syncytial virus and parainfluenza virus. *N Engl J Med* 2001;344(25):1917–28.
23. Hardie WD, Roberts NE, Reising SF, et al. Complicated parapneumonic effusions in children caused by penicillin-nonsusceptible Streptococcus pneumoniae. *Pediatrics* 1998;101(3):388–92.
24. Harris JA, Kolokathis A, Campbell M, et al. Safety and efficacy of azithromycin in the treatment of community-acquired pneumonia in children. *Pediatr Infect Dis J* 1998;17(10):865–71.
25. Hartling L, Wiebe N, Russell K, Patel H, Klassen TP. Epinephrine for bronchiolitis. *Cochrane Database Syst Rev* 2004; (1):CD003123.
26. Hendriks T, de Hoog M, Lequin MH, et al. DNase and atelectasis in noncystic fibrosis pediatric patients. *Crit Care* 2005;9(4):R351–6.
27. Hillenbrand K. Ativiral therapy for influenza infections. *Ped Rev* 2005; 26(11):427–8.
28. Hoehn T, Krause M, Krueger M, et al. Treatment of respiratory failure with inhaled nitric oxide and high-frequency ventilation in an infant with respiratory syncytial virus pneumonia and bronchopulmonary dysplasia. *Respiration* 1998;65(6):477–80.
29. Holman RC, Shay DK, Curns AT, et al. Risk factors for bronchiolitis-associated deaths among infants in the United States. *Pediatr Infect Dis J* 2003;22:483–90.
30. Hon KL, Leung CW, Cheng WT, et al. Clinical presentations and outcome of severe acute respiratory syndrome in children. *Lancet* 2003;361 (9370):1701–3.
31. Jaffe A, Balfour-Lynn IM. Management of empyema in children. *Pediatr Pulmonol* 2005;40(2):148–56.
32. Jartti T, van den Hoogen B, Garofalo RP, et al. Metapneumovirus and acute wheezing in children. *Lancet* 2002;360(9343):1393–4.
33. Kling S, Donniger H, Williams Z, et al. Persistence of rhinovirus RNA after asthma exacerbation in children. *Clin Exp Allergy* 2005;35:672–78.
34. Ksiazek TG, Erdman D, Goldsmith CS, et al. A novel coronavirus associated with severe acute respiratory syndrome. *N Engl J Med* 2003;348(20):1953–66.
35. Lemanske RF, Jackson DJ, Gangnon RE, et al. Rhinovirus illnesses during infancy predict subsequent childhood wheezing. *J Allergy Clin Immunol* 2005;116:571–77.
36. Langley JM. Adenoviruses. *Ped Rev* 2005;26(7):244–9.
37. Leader S, Kohlhase K. Recent trends in severe respiratory syncytial virus (RSV) among US infants, 1997 to 2000. *J Pediatr* 2003;143(5):S127–S32.
38. Lind I, Gill JH, Calabretta NC. What are hospital admission criteria for infants with bronchiolitis? *Clin Inquiries* 2006;55(1):67–69.
39. Lucero MG, Tupasi TE, Gomez ML, et al. Respiratory rate greater than 50 per minute as a clinical indicator of pneumonia in Filipino children with cough. *Rev Infect Dis* 1990;12(8):S1081–3.
40. Mandell LA, Bartlett JG, Dowell SF, et al. Update of practice guidelines for the management of community-acquired pneumonia in immunocompetent adults. *Clin Infect Dis* 2003;37(11):1405–33.
41. Martinon-Torres F, Rodriguez-Nunez A, Martinon-Sanchez JM. Heliox therapy in infants with acute bronchiolitis. *Pediatrics* 2002;109(1):68–73.
42. Mazur LJ, Kline MW, Lorin MI. Extreme leukocytosis in patients presenting to a pediatric emergency department. *Pediatr Emerg Care* 1991;7(4):215–8.
43. McCarthy CA, Hall CB. Respiratory syncytial virus: concerns and control. *Ped Rev* 2003;24:301–9.
44. McIntosh K. Community-acquired pneumonia in children. *N Engl J Med* 2002;346(6):429–37.
45. Merkus PJ, de Hoog M, van Gent R. DNase treatment for atelectasis in infants with severe respiratory syncytial virus bronchiolitis. *Eur Respir J* 2001;18(4):734–7.
46. Meyer TA, Warner BW. Extracorporeal life support for the treatment of viral pneumonia: Collective experience from the ELSO registry. Extracorporeal Life Support Organization. *J Pediatr Surg* 1997;32(2):232–6.
47. Nasr SZ, Strouse PJ, Soskolne E, et al. Efficacy of recombinant human deoxyribonuclease I in the hospital management of respiratory syncytial virus bronchiolitis. *Chest* 2001;120(1):203–8.

48. Nicholas KJ, Dhouieb MO, Marshal TG, et al. An evaluation of chest physiotherapy in the management of acute bronchiolitis. Changing clinical practice. *Physiotherapy* 1999;85 (12):669–74.

49. Nissen MD, Siebert DJ, Mackay IM, et al. Evidence of human metapneumovirus in Australian children. *Med J Aust* 2002;176(4):188.

50. Patel NR, Hammer J, Nichani S, et al. Effect of inhaled nitric oxide on respiratory mechanics in ventilated infants with RSV bronchiolitis. *Intensive Care Med* 1999;25(1):81–7.

51. Patel H, Platt R, Lozano JM, et al. Glucocorticoids for acute viral bronchiolitis in infants and young children. *Cochrane Database Syst Rev* 2004;(3):CD004878.

52. Pelletier G, Dery P, Abed Y, et al. Respiratory tract reinfections by the new human Metapneumovirus in an immunocompromised child. *Emerg Infect Dis* 2002;8(9):976–8.

53. Peltola V, Reunanen T, Ziegler T, et al. Accuracy of clinical diagnosis of influenza in outpatient children. *Clin Infect Dis* 2005;41(8):1198–200.

54. Perrotta C, Ortiz Z, Roque M. Chest physiotherapy for acute bronchiolitis in paediatric patients between 0 and 24 months old. *Cochrane Database Syst Rev.* 2005;(2):CD004873.

55. Raymond J, Aujard Y. Nosocomial infections in pediatric patients: a European, multicenter prospective study. European Study Group. *Infect Control Hosp Epidemiol* 2000;21(4):260–3.

56. Richards MJ, Edwards JR, Culver DH, et al. Nosocomial infections in pediatric intensive care units in the United States. National Nosocomial Infections Surveillance System. *Pediatrics* 1999;103(4):e39.

57. Rudan I, Tomaskovic L, Boschi-Pinto C, et al. Global estimate of the incidence of clinical pneumonia among children under five years of age. *Bull World Health Organ* 2004;82(12):895–903.

58. Sandora TJ, Harper MB. Pneumonia in hospitalized children. *Pediatr Clin North Am* 2005;52(4):1059–81.

59. Semple MG, Cowell A, Dove W, et al. Dual infection of infants by human metapneumovirus and human respiratory syncytial virus is strongly associated with severe bronchiolitis. *J Infect Dis* 2005;191:382–86.

60. Shaw KN, Bell LM, Sherman NH. Outpatient assessment of infants with bronchiolitis. *Am J Dis Child* 1991;145(2):151–5.

61. Sugaya N, Takeuchi Y. Mass vaccination of schoolchildren against influenza and its impact on the influenza-associated mortality rate among children in Japan. *Clin Infect Dis* 2005;41:939–47.

62. Torres A Jr, Anders M, Anderson P, et al. Efficacy of metered-dose inhaler administration of albuterol in intubated infants. *Chest* 1997;112(2):484–90.

63. van den Hoogen BG, Bestebroer TM, Osterhaus AD, et al. Analysis of the genomic sequence of a human metapneumovirus. *Virology* 2002;295(1):119–32.

64. van den Hoogen BG, De Jong JC, Groen J, et al. A newly discovered human pneumovirus isolated from Young children with respiratory tract disease. *Nat Med* 2001;7:719–24.

65. Ventre K, Randolph A. Ribavirin for respiratory syncytial virus infection of the lower respiratory tract in infants and young children. *Cochrane Database Syst Rev* 2004;(4):CD000181.

66. Webb MSC, Martin JA, Cartlidge PHT. Chest physiotherapy in acute bronchiolitis. *Arch Dis Childhood* 1985;60:1078–9.

67. Wijnands GJ. Diagnosis and interventions in lower respiratory tract infections. *Am J Med* 1992;92:9IS–97S.

68. Wood DW, Downes JJ, Lecks HI. A clinical scoring system for the diagnosis of respiratory failure. Preliminary report on childhood status asthmaticus. *Am J Dis Child* 1972;123(3):227–8.

CHAPTER 46 ■ ACUTE LUNG INJURY AND ACUTE RESPIRATORY DISTRESS SYNDROME

KATHLEEN M. VENTRE • JOHN H. ARNOLD

In 1967, Ashbaugh and colleagues described a syndrome of tachypnea, hypoxia, and decreased pulmonary compliance in a series of 11 adults and one child with respiratory failure. The pathologic features included interstitial and intra-alveolar edema and hemorrhage, as well as hyaline membrane formation. Overall, this condition seemed to have many features in common with the previously described infant respiratory distress syndrome. Although the syndrome had been widely recognized and reported for years, it was not until 1994 that a consensus definition entered the scientific literature (6). The American-European Consensus Conference suggested that the "adult" respiratory distress syndrome be renamed the "acute" respiratory distress syndrome (ARDS) to acknowledge the existence of this condition in children. The consensus document also established definitive criteria for the diagnosis of ARDS and a milder form of the syndrome, which the panel called "acute lung injury" (ALI). The panel defined ARDS as acute, noncardiogenic pulmonary edema with bilateral pulmonary infiltrates on chest x-ray and a ratio of PaO_2 to FIO_2 of ≤ 200. Acute lung injury was defined similarly, but with a ratio of PaO_2 to FIO_2 of 200–300 (**Table 46.1**). This consensus statement set the stage for a new era in clinical research in which the application of consistent diagnostic criteria gave way to higher-quality reviews, prospective cohort studies, and clinical trials that have shed considerable light on the epidemiology, pathophysiology, and factors that influence outcome of ARDS in children.

According to contemporary diagnostic criteria, ARDS and ALI account for a sizable share of the PICU caseload. Recent data indicate that ARDS occurs in 1%–4% of PICU admissions and that as many as 10% of PICU patients who receive mechanical ventilation meet diagnostic criteria for ARDS (26,61). Reported mortality varies between 20% and 75%, depending on the criteria used to identify cases, coexisting risk factors such as immunocompromise, and the presence of nonpulmonary organ failure (26). The highest mortality rates are reported in small, single-centered, retrospective studies from the 1980s and early 1990s, before consensus diagnostic criteria were developed. Since that time, the trend has been toward decreased mortality in pediatric ARDS, which likely reflects the use of more consistent diagnostic criteria, as well as genuine improvements in supportive care. A 6-month survey of nine North American PICUs reported in 2003 that mortality among ARDS patients who required mechanical ventilation at the time of screening was 4.3% (bone marrow transplant recipients were excluded from this cohort) (61). This figure is consistent with mortality reported in the control arm of a recent multicentered, randomized, controlled trial (RCT), from which bone marrow transplant patients were also excluded (16). By comparison, another recent clinical trial that did include bone marrow transplant

recipients and other immunocompromised patients reported a markedly higher control group mortality rate of 36%; mortality among the immunocompromised control children was 60% (88). In a recent multicentered, prospective cohort study that described the epidemiology of pediatric ALI and ARDS, Flori et al. found that overall hospital mortality was 22% among children with a PaO_2:FIO_2 ratio <300. The group that met criteria for ARDS (PaO_2: FIO_2 <200) had a mortality of 26% (26). These mortality figures are higher than those reported in recent pediatric trials and are more in line with those reported in contemporary adult ARDS trials. The most common diagnosis associated with the development of ALI and ARDS among the entire study cohort was pneumonia (35%). Sepsis was considerably less common; the prevalence of 13% in the study cohort contrasts with data generated several years earlier that suggested that sepsis was the most common cause of ARDS in both adults and children (26,42). Taken together, these studies report clearly different mortality data for pediatric ALI and ARDS. The study by Flori et al. is worthy of mention because its prospective design allowed for identification of cases early in the disease process. In fact, 28% of the cases were identified before mechanical ventilation was required (26). Thus, the advent of high-quality clinical research has greatly influenced our understanding of epidemiology and outcomes in pediatric ALI and ARDS over the past decade and promises to create opportunities to improve outcomes further, as innovative therapies can be tested at the onset of disease.

MECHANISM OF DISEASE: CORE PATHOPHYSIOLOGY

Host Genetic Factors

Our present understanding of the pathophysiology of ALI and ARDS comes from careful study of its clinical course in animal models and affected humans, as well as postmortem histopathologic data. More recently, some effort has been extended to apply techniques from molecular genetics to understanding the role of host factors by linking the presence of specific genetic polymorphisms to the development and/or severity of ARDS. In particular, specific polymorphisms in the genes that govern surfactant protein B production, host immune response, and hormonal pathways have all been associated with the development of ARDS (35,51,93), but the strength of the inferences drawn from such studies may be limited by the difficulty of accounting for posttranslational modifications and other interactions that could alter the relationship

TABLE 46.1

AMERICAN-EUROPEAN CONSENSUS CRITERIA FOR
ACUTE LUNG INJURY (ALI) AND THE ACUTE
RESPIRATORY DISTRESS SYNDROME (ARDS)

Acute onset
Bilateral pulmonary infiltrates on chest radiography
Pulmonary artery occlusion pressure ≤ 18 mm Hg or no
   clinical evidence of left atrial hypertension
$Pao_2:Fio_2$ ratio $\leq 300 = $ ALI
$Pao_2:Fio_2$ ratio $\leq 200 = $ ARDS

Adapted from Bernard GR, Artigas A, Brigham KL, et al. The
American-European Consensus Conference on ARDS. Definitions,
mechanisms, relevant outcomes, and clinical trial coordination. *Am J
Respir Crit Care Med* 1994;149:818–24.

between genotype and disease phenotype in the affected host
(55). Moreover, when interpreting such studies, careful attention must be given to details in their design, because erroneous
associations between the candidate gene and the phenotype of
interest can result if the study is not adequately powered to
detect a true positive association, if cases and controls are not
adequately matched, or if the finding is not replicated in an independent population of cases and controls (83). Although the
field of molecular genetics promises to aid in clarifying the interaction between host response and initiating factors in ARDS,
much more study should be accomplished in this area.

Initiating Factors

ARDS develops following either "direct" or "indirect" lung
injury. Pneumonia and pulmonary aspiration are among the
most common conditions with the potential to inflict direct
lung injury and ARDS, but traumatic pulmonary contusion,
fat embolism, submersion injury, and inhalational injury are
relatively common causes as well. The most common forms of
indirect lung injury include systemic conditions, such as sepsis,
shock, cardiopulmonary bypass, and transfusion-related lung
injury. One of the more important reasons for attempting to
distinguish between direct and indirect injury is that each of
these pathways is associated with distinct pathologic changes
in respiratory system mechanics that may be associated with
distinctly different clinical outcomes (32,62). For example, direct injury is suspected of causing regional consolidation from
destruction of the alveolar architecture, while indirect injury is
believed to be associated with pulmonary vascular congestion,
interstitial edema, and less severe alveolar involvement (32).
Patients with direct forms of lung injury tend to dominate enrollment in current clinical studies, in keeping with the current
predominance of pneumonia as the inciting factor for ARDS.
However, careful appraisal of study outcomes in other subgroups may reveal differences in the response to therapy. For
example, subgroup analysis from two recent RCTs that evaluated surfactant for treatment of ALI and ARDS has shown
an outcome benefit associated with the use of surfactant in patients with direct forms of lung injury and not in those with
indirect forms (73,88). Thus, defining the relative contribution
of direct versus indirect lung injury to the development of ALI

and ARDS with more precision will be an important step in allowing future clinical trials to test novel therapies among similar groups of patients and will likely depend on incorporating
uniform diagnostic criteria into well-designed epidemiologic
studies.

Phases of Disease

Regardless of the inciting factors, ARDS commonly progresses
through stages defined by their associated clinical, radiographic, and histopathologic features. The first, or exudative
phase, is characterized by the acute development of decreased
pulmonary compliance and arterial hypoxemia. The alteration
in pulmonary mechanics leads to tachypnea. Arterial blood
gas analysis typically reveals hypocarbia at this stage. The
chest x-ray usually reveals diffuse alveolar infiltrates from pulmonary edema. The proinflammatory events that occur during the exudative phase tend to create the setting for transition into the fibroproliferative stage of ARDS, during which
increased alveolar dead space and refractory pulmonary hypertension may develop as a result of chronic inflammation
and scarring of the alveolar-capillary unit. The fibroproliferative phase then gives way to a recovery phase, with restoration of the alveolar epithelial barrier, gradual improvement in
pulmonary compliance and resolution of arterial hypoxemia,
and eventual return to premorbid pulmonary function in many
patients (85).

Alveolar-Capillary Barrier Dysfunction and Edema Formation

By definition, the edema in ARDS is not caused by cardiac failure but results from disruption of the structural components
that regulate alveolar fluid balance under normal conditions.
Normally, the pulmonary capillary endothelial cells are connected by tight junctions that allow some movement of fluid,
but no movement of proteins or other solutes, into the interstitial space. The alveolar epithelium, on the other hand, normally is not permeable to fluid, proteins, or other solutes. The
rate of fluid movement into the interstitium is governed by the
net difference between hydrostatic pressure and osmotic pressure in the pulmonary capillaries, relative to the pulmonary
interstitium. Generally, fluid movement across a semipermeable membrane, such as the pulmonary capillary endothelial
layer, is characterized by the well-known Starling formula:

$$\dot{Q} = K_f [(P_c - P_{is}) - \sigma (\pi_{pl} - \pi_{is})]$$

where:

$\dot{Q}$ = filtration rate across the semipermeable membrane
K_f = membrane filtration coefficient
P_c = capillary hydrostatic pressure
P_{is} = interstitial hydrostatic pressure
σ = membrane reflection coefficient
π_{pl} = plasma oncotic pressure
π_{is} = interstitial oncotic pressure.

The small amount of fluid that accumulates in the interstitial space is usually cleared by the pulmonary lymphatic system.
The key pathophysiologic event that distinguishes the orderly
regulation of alveolar fluid balance in the normal state from

the dysfunction typified by ALI and ARDS is injury to the alveolar epithelium and/or pulmonary capillary endothelium. This injury can occur directly as the result of parenchymal injury or following a distant or systemic disease process that provokes the host immune response, causing neutrophil activation and elaboration of proinflammatory cytokines. Either pathway results in the opening of tight junctions and unregulated leakage of fluid, protein, and other solutes into the interstitium and, subsequently, into the alveolar space, which creates multiple mechanisms for impairment of gas exchange.

Surfactant Dysfunction and Alteration of Pulmonary Mechanics

Injury to the pulmonary surfactant system is one of the more serious manifestations of damage to the alveolar epithelium and subsequent alveolar flooding. Surfactant is produced mainly by alveolar epithelial type II cells and contains phospholipid and protein components. Its major function is to promote alveolar and small-airway stability by lowering surface tension, although its principal protein constituents also have an important role in facilitating clearance of infectious organisms (89,90). The Laplace equation illustrates the relationship between surface tension (T), cavity radius (r), and the pressure (P) required to maintain the patency of a spherical structure:

$$P = 2T/r$$

In reality, alveoli are polygonal rather than spherical, and their patency is facilitated by outward traction forces that are generated by the pulmonary interstitial matrix (60). Notwithstanding the inherent assumptions, application of Laplace's formula to explain alveolar inflation makes it easy to see that an increase in surface tension in a small cavity, such as an alveolus, will require elevated transalveolar pressures to achieve and maintain patency.

Following lung injury, surfactant production declines because of damage to alveolar epithelial cells, and the surface activity of any surfactant remaining in the alveolar space is impaired because of alterations in its phospholipid constituents, as well as from inactivation by alveolar exudates (38). It is important to appreciate how the loss of surfactant integrity dramatically alters the mechanical properties of the entire lung. In the nondiseased state, the interaction of surfactant with the elastic properties of the lung and chest wall produces *pulmonary hysteresis*, which allows for the maintenance of lung volume at lower transpulmonary pressures ($P_{transpulmonary} = P_{airway} - P_{pleural}$) during expiration than are required during inspiration. One way to demonstrate the volume-pressure relationships throughout the respiratory cycle is to perform a static inflation maneuver, in which discrete gas volumes are introduced into the lung up to total lung capacity, using a calibrated syringe ("super syringe"). Carefully measured volumes are similarly withdrawn from the lung to plot the volume-pressure relationships during lung emptying (**Fig. 46.1**). During inspiration, increasing transpulmonary pressure produces little change in lung volume until the patient reaches a lower inflection point on the inspiratory limb of the curve (lower P_{flex}) (**Fig. 46.2**). At that point, the change in lung volume produced by each upward increment of pressure (i.e., compliance) increases quickly, and then more slowly, until reaching an upper inflection point (upper P_{flex}) (Fig. 46.2) where compliance

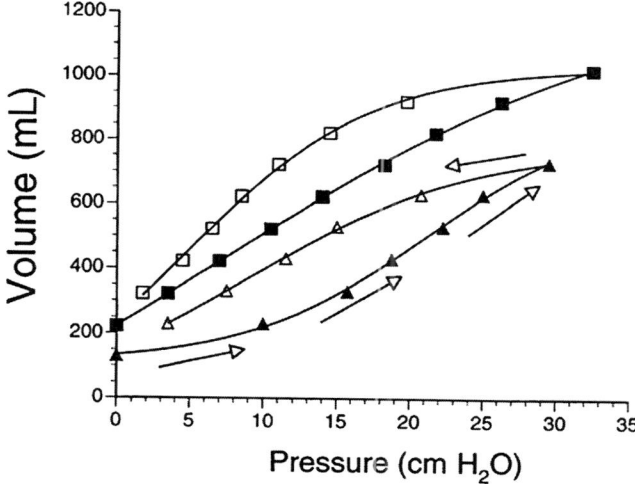

FIGURE 46.1. Pulmonary hysteresis. Volume–pressure relationships before and after lung injury. Inflation (*solid symbols*) and deflation (*open symbols*) volume–pressure data in a canine model before (*squares*) and 60 mins after (*triangles*) oleic acid–induced acute lung injury. During deflation (expiration), higher lung volumes are maintained at lower transpulmonary pressures. Original experimental data are fitted with a sigmoidal equation to construct the curves ($R^2 > 0.9997$). From Venegas JG, Harris RS, Simon BA. A comprehensive equation for the pulmonary pressure-volume curve. *J Appl Physiol* 1998;84:389–95, with permission.

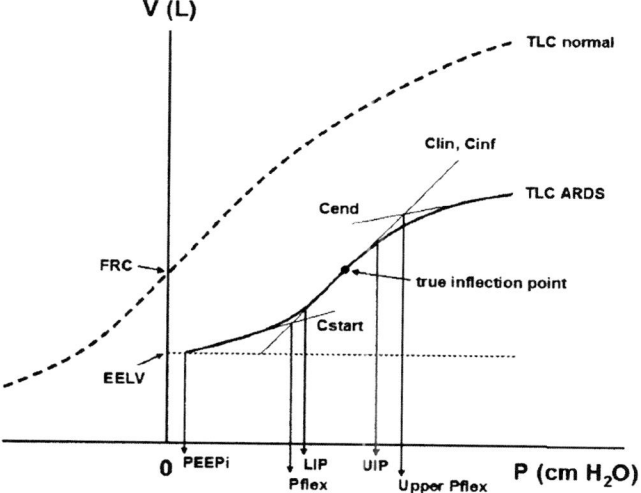

FIGURE 46.2. Volume–pressure curve in absence of disease (*dashed lines*) and in ARDS (*solid line*). Inspiratory curves are shown. Important transitions during lung inflation are indicated on the ARDS curve. Note that in ARDS, total lung capacity (TLC) is reduced, compared to TLC in the normal lung. In this example, a small amount of positive end-expiratory pressure (intrinsic PEEP, or $PEEP_i$) is present at EELV in the ARDS lung. EELV in the ARDS lung is below FRC. Compliance is indicated at various points as the slope of the volume-pressure curve. P_{flex} is indicated on the curve as the intersection of the low-compliance portion of the curve obtained at low lung volume (C_{start}). Upper P_{flex} is indicated at the transition between the nearly linear zone of maximal compliance (C_{lin}) and the zone of low compliance at high lung volume (C_{end}). The lower inflection point (LIP) and upper inflection point (UIP) are points at which the volume–pressure curve begins to depart from C_{lin} at the extremes of lung volume. The "true inflection point" marks the actual change in concavity of the volume–pressure curve. From Harris RS. Pressure-volume curves of the respiratory system. *Respir Care* 2005;50:78–98, with permission.

again decreases. The upward displacement of the expiratory limb relative to the inspiratory limb (Fig. 46.1) illustrates the difference in the transpulmonary pressures needed to maintain lung volume as the lung recoils and empties. This difference is potentiated by the properties of surfactant. In the injured lung, hysteresis is less pronounced, and the entire curve is displaced downward and to the right, reflecting the higher pressures required to achieve and maintain lung recruitment and an overall decrease in lung compliance that is evident throughout the respiratory cycle (Figs. 46.1 and 46.2).

The effect of alveolar and small-airways collapse on overall airway resistance can be explained by the Hagen-Poiseuille equation describing laminar flow in straight circular tubes:

$$R = (8\eta l)/\pi r^4$$

where:

R = resistance to flow
η = gas viscosity
l = tube length
r = airway radius.

From this equation, it follows that a reduction in airway caliber, from peribronchiolar edema or outright airway collapse, produces a marked increase in airways resistance. Respiratory system resistance can be studied in vivo by plotting the decline in tracheal pressure following end-inspiratory airway occlusion until flow ceases and a plateau pressure is reached. Such techniques have suggested that increased total respiratory system resistance is observed in patients with ARDS compared to controls, largely because of "mechanical unevenness" or instability of the respiratory system in this disease.

To create a more complete picture of pulmonary mechanics in ALI and ARDS, it is important to consider the properties of the abdomen and chest wall. It was first demonstrated in a swine model that increasing abdominal pressure results in a decrease in total lung capacity and lung volumes, leading to alterations in the volume-pressure relationship in the nondiseased lung that resemble what occurs in ALI and ARDS (56). Subsequently, the contribution of abdominal distension to the alteration of respiratory system mechanics in patients with ALI and ARDS was evaluated (62). Comparing patients with ARDS after major abdominal surgery to those with nonsurgical ARDS, the investigators plotted static volume-pressure curves of the respiratory system, chest wall, and lung by relating calibrated changes in lung volume to end-inspiratory plateau pressures obtained at the airway opening and in the esophagus. Static abdominal pressure was obtained by relating end-inspiratory gastric plateau pressure to gastric plateau pressure measured at end-expiratory lung volume (EELV). This study was able to identify clear differences in the shape of the volume-pressure curves obtained from patients with ARDS related to abdominal pathology in the postoperative setting versus "medical" ARDS. Specifically, the volume-pressure relationship of the chest wall among surgical ARDS patients was shifted downward and to the right relative to curves obtained from nonsurgical ARDS patients (**Fig. 46.3**). The differences in curve morphology between these 2 groups correlated with differences in static abdominal pressures, indicating a decrease in chest wall compliance in surgical ARDS that is attributable to increases in intra-abdominal pressure. In comparison, the nonsurgical ARDS group demonstrated chest wall compliance curves that resembled those produced by the preoperative sur-

gical controls (62). These observations suggest that ARDS impairs respiratory system mechanics in different ways, depending on the underlying etiology, a finding that has significant implications for understanding clinical outcomes in ALI and ARDS and for defining subgroups within a large and heterogeneous disease population that would most likely benefit from specific therapies or alternative management strategies.

Mechanisms of Alveolar Fluid Clearance

Once fluid accumulates in the alveolar space, its clearance is regulated by ion channels in distal airway Clara cells and in alveolar epithelial type I and type II cells. Alveolar type II cells can be isolated under experimental conditions and, thus, have been studied in great detail. Besides producing pulmonary surfactant, type II cells are also responsible for transepithelial ion transport (27). Sodium is taken up by channels on the apical surface of type II cells. This function can be suppressed by administration of the diuretic amiloride. Subsequently, Na/K-ATPases located on the basolateral cell membrane actively transport sodium back into the interstitial space, which creates the gradient for passive movement of water across the alveolar epithelium and back into the interstitium (86). (**Fig. 46.4**). The alveolar epithelial damage that occurs in ALI creates conditions that compromise the capacity of membrane proteins to regulate alveolar fluid balance. Moreover, in vitro and in vivo experimental models have shown that exposure of alveolar epithelium to hypoxia inhibits transepithelial sodium transport and decreases overall alveolar fluid clearance (84). The permeability edema that is the defining feature of early ARDS sets the stage for reduced compliance and an EELV that decreases below functional residual capacity (FRC) to a point approaching closing capacity, creating conditions that favor the development of regional atelectasis, intrapulmonary shunt, and alveolar hypoxia.

Alteration of Gas Exchange in Disease

At this point, it is clear that many potential sources of hypoxia exist in ALI and ARDS. It is easy to understand that edema in the interstitial compartment or in the alveolar space will inhibit gas exchange and that pulmonary blood flowing past compromised or collapsed lung units will be poorly oxygenated, thus lowering the O_2 content of pulmonary venous blood and reducing systemic O_2 content. The fraction of pulmonary blood flow that ultimately enters the systemic circulation without being oxygenated (the "shunt fraction," or venous admixture) can be approximated using the equation:

$$\dot{Q}_S/\dot{Q}_T = (C_{c'}o_2 - C_ao_2)/(C_{c'}o_2 - C_Vo_2)$$

where $\dot{Q}_S/\dot{Q}_T$ is the shunt fraction, $\dot{Q}_S$ is the amount of shunt flow, $\dot{Q}_T$ the total flow, $C_{c'}o_2$ is the end-pulmonary capillary O_2 content, Cao_2 is the arterial O_2 content, and C_Vo_2 is the mixed venous O_2 content.

Shunted blood is low in O_2 and high in carbon dioxide, but intrapulmonary shunt does not tend to elevate systemic $Paco_2$ because chemoreceptors sensitive to acute increases in $Paco_2$ stimulate respiratory drive, eliminating carbon dioxide before an increase would be detectable by blood gas analysis. Therefore, the arteriovenous carbon dioxide gradient

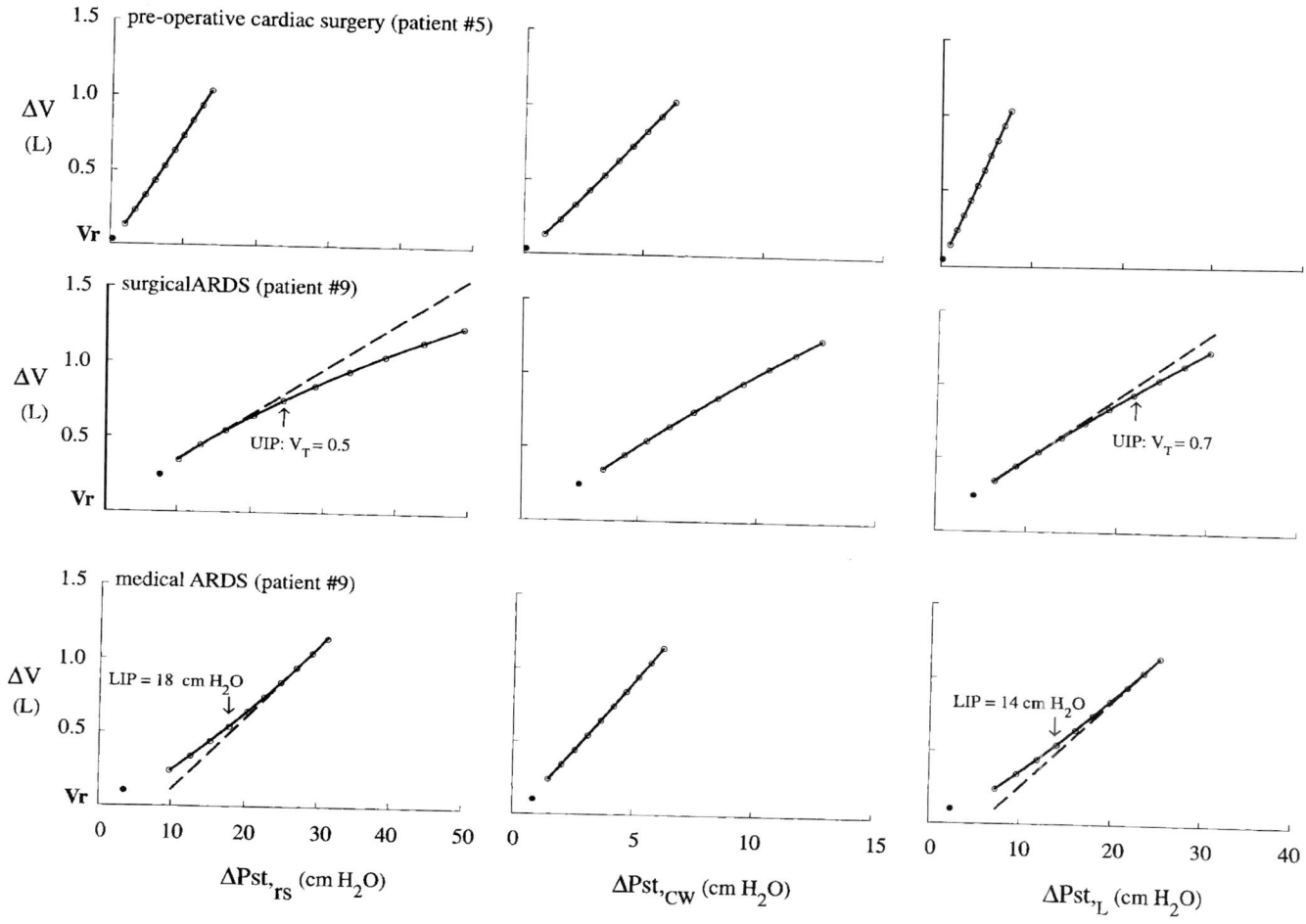

FIGURE 46.3. Static inflation volume–pressure curves of the respiratory system (rs), chest wall (cw), and lung (L) in one preoperative cardiac surgery (*top*), one surgical ARDS patient (*middle*), and one medical ARDS patient (*bottom*). Closed symbols indicate intrinsic PEEP (PEEP$_i$), with the corresponding increase in EELV. Dashed lines indicate zone of lowest elastance (highest compliance), as determined by regression analysis. Note that, in the nonsurgical ARDS patient, the chest wall compliance curve resembles the corresponding curve in the preoperative surgical control patient. The chest wall compliance curve in the surgical ARDS patient is shifted downward and to the right by comparison. ΔPst, changes in end-inspiratory static pressure; ΔV, changes in lung volume relative to equilibrium volume; UIP, upper inflection point; LIP, lower inflection point. From Ranieri VM, Brienza N, Santostasi S, Puntillo F, Mascia L, Vitale N, Giuliani R, Memeo V, Bruno F, Fiore T et al. Impairment of lung and chest wall mechanics in patients with acute respiratory distress syndrome: Role of abdominal distension. *Am J Respir Crit Care Med* 1997;156:1082–91.

under normal conditions is ~4–6 mm Hg. The phenomenon of "right-to-left" intrapulmonary shunt is ameliorated to some degree by pulmonary vasoconstriction, which redirects blood toward better-ventilated lung units. The pulmonary vascular bed uniquely contains smooth muscle that contracts in response to hypoxemia.

Clearly the relationship of alveolar ventilation ($\dot{V}$) to perfusion ($\dot{Q}$) is not anatomically fixed. Even in the absence of disease, the distribution of inspired gas is subject to gravitational forces acting on the lung (57). In the upright human lung, spontaneous breathing creates a decreasing gradient of transpulmonary pressure from lung apex to lung base. In other words, the driving pressure for alveolar filling is greater in the (nondependent) apex than it is at the (dependent) lung base. Consequently, the less distended, dependent alveoli are positioned on a more compliant portion of the volume-pressure curve, compared to the more distended nondependent alveoli

(**Fig. 46.5**). Therefore, dependent alveoli collectively account for a greater portion of alveolar ventilation than do nondependent alveoli (**Fig. 46.6**). The effects of gravity on the distribution of pulmonary blood flow are perhaps less straightforward. In the upright, isolated, and perfused canine lung, detection of blood flow using simple radiolabeled gas techniques has indicated that blood flow is greater in dependent regions as compared to nondependent regions. On a global level, gravity does have a role in creating higher pulmonary vascular hydrostatic pressure in dependent lung regions, which should theoretically produce a favorable matching of ventilation to perfusion, at least in the upright, nondiseased lung. However, high-resolution experimental techniques have demonstrated that local variability in pulmonary blood flow distribution cannot be completely explained by gravity and is more likely related to the pulmonary vascular architecture. Studying anesthetized dogs in the prone and supine position, investigators

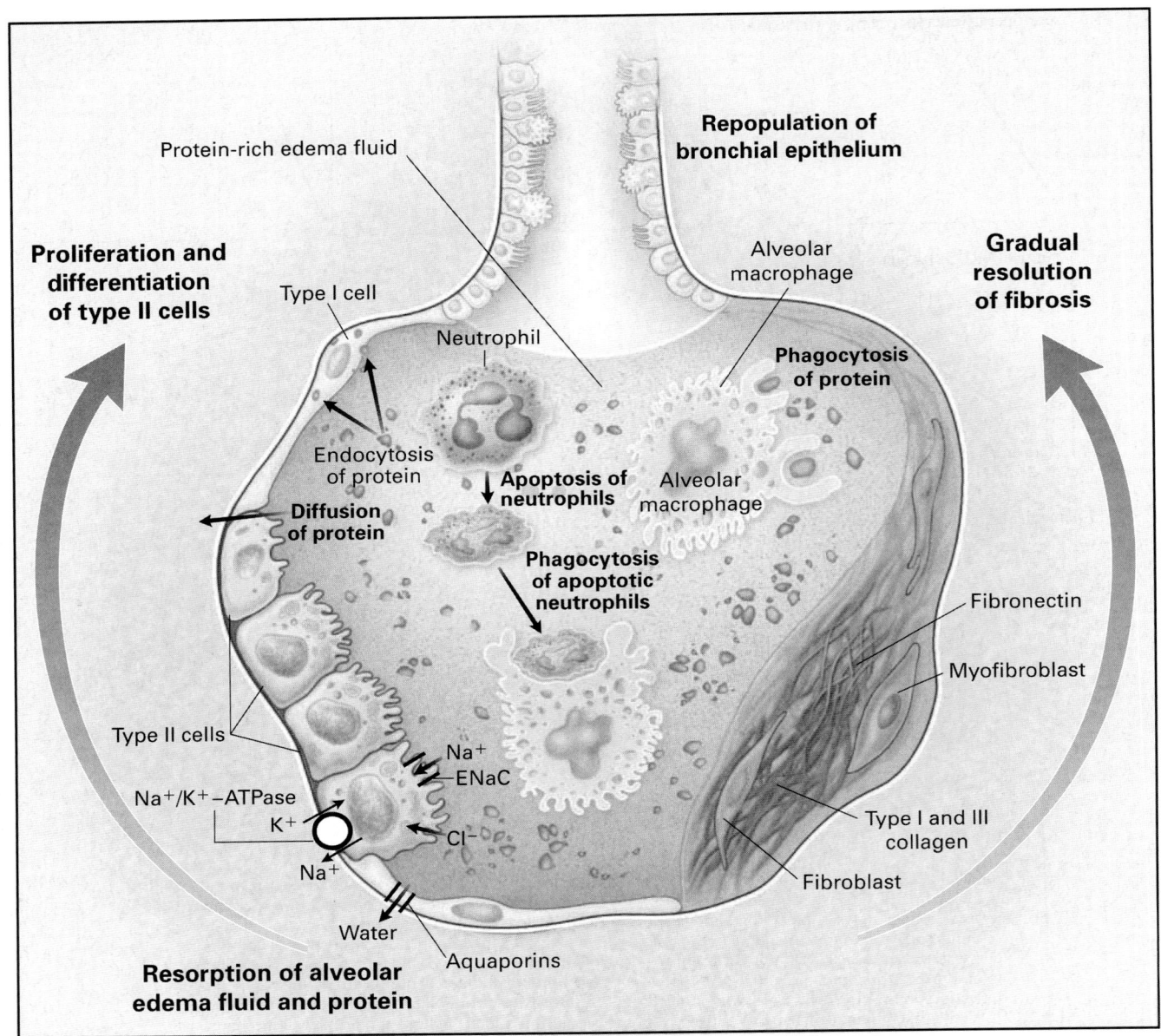

FIGURE 46.4. Cellular mechanisms of ARDS resolution. Repopulation of the alveolar epithelial barrier is evident on the left side of the figure and, within the alveolus, neutrophils are undergoing apoptosis and phagocytosis by alveolar macrophages. Structural elements governing fluid transport across the alveolar epithelium are illustrated. EnaC, epithelial sodium channel. From Ware LB, Matthay MA. The acute respiratory distress syndrome. *N Engl J Med* 2000;342(18):1334–49, with permission.

were able to characterize pulmonary blood flow distribution using inert, radiolabeled microspheres injected under low lung volume conditions (34). After injection, microspheres embolize within pulmonary capillaries, and sectioning of the lung into small segments reveals the spatial distribution of pulmonary blood flow. In the supine position, pulmonary blood flow was distributed preferentially to the dorsal (dependent) region, but marked heterogeneity of perfusion existed within tissue planes that were subject to identical gravitational forces (41). In the prone position, pulmonary blood flow was also preferentially distributed to the dorsal (now nondependent) region, and flow within isogravitational planes was more uniform (34,41).

Imbalances in the distribution of ventilation and perfusion create alveolar-capillary units that vary in their gas-exchanging efficiency according to the local distribution of alveolar gas flow relative to pulmonary blood flow. In healthy patients, ~10% of cardiac output does not come into contact with alveolar gas. This "physiologic shunt" fraction includes baseline $\dot{V}/\dot{Q}$ inequality, as well as blood from the bronchial, pleural, and thebesian veins, which returns to the systemic circulation without passing through the pulmonary vascular bed. The influence of $\dot{V}/\dot{Q}$ imbalance on blood gas tensions is magnified in ALI and ARDS, in which consolidation and collapse of lung units are widespread and fluid-filled alveoli act as low $\dot{V}/\dot{Q}$ lung units with the potential to create detectable elevations

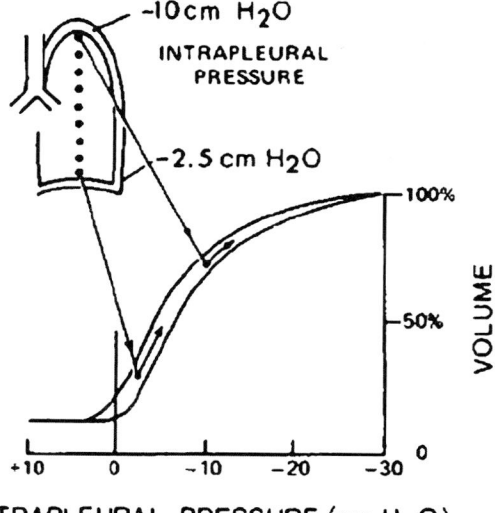

FIGURE 46.5. Regional differences in ventilation in the upright lung. The weight of the lung creates less negative intrapleural pressure at the lung base, while more negative intrapleural pressure is created at the apex. These differences translate into a decreasing transpulmonary pressure gradient from apical to dependent lung regions. From West JB. Mechanics of breathing. In: *Respiratory Physiology: The Essentials,* 4th ed. Baltimore: Williams and Wilkins, 1990;87–113, with permission.

in P_aCO_2 and decreases in P_aO_2. Consolidation of diseased alveoli creates radial traction on neighboring lung units that results in alveolar overdistension and pulmonary capillary narrowing, creating high $\dot{V}/\dot{Q}$ areas and adding to alveolar dead space. The addition of positive-pressure ventilation (PPV) adds to distension of nondependent alveoli and can displace local pulmonary blood flow, creating even more pronounced $\dot{V}/\dot{Q}$ inequality, particularly in supine patients in whom positive alveolar pressure enhances the gradient between gas distribution and pulmonary blood flow distribution. Use of the multiple inert gas elimination technique in experimental animals and human subjects has confirmed that, although both intrapulmonary shunt and $\dot{V}/\dot{Q}$ inequality contribute to impairment of gas exchange in ALI and ARDS, intrapulmonary shunt is the dominant cause of arterial hypoxemia in these conditions.

Host Immune Response: Role of Cytokines and Alteration of Hemostasis

The host immune response plays an important role in the pathogenesis of ALI and ARDS. Although injury begins with exposure to one or more inciting factors, the lung injury sequence is potentiated by inflammatory mediators that interact with the coagulation cascade to upset the usual balance between proinflammation and anti-inflammation, and procoagulation and anticoagulation. Following lung injury, activated macrophages located in the alveolar space secrete tumor necrosis factor (TNF-α) and IL-1β, two early-response agents of the innate immune system. These two early mediators subsequently stimulate the production of other proinflammatory interleukins, such as IL-6, and potentiate the interaction between β_2 integrins on neutrophils and intercellular adhesion molecule (ICAM-1) on vascular endothelial cells. This interaction attaches the neutrophil to the endothelium. Subsequently, IL-8 works together with the complement system (factors 3a and 5a), leukotriene B$_4$, and platelet-activating factor (PAF) to establish a chemotactic gradient that recruits neutrophils from their endothelial attachments into the alveolar space, where they are capable of elaborating O_2 and nitrogen free radical species (85) (**Fig. 46.7**). Release of reactive O_2 species potentiates additional damage to alveolar epithelial cells, leading to their dysfunction and apoptosis. In addition, reactive O_2 species upregulate expression of nuclear factor (NF-κB), a transcription factor that controls the expression of proinflammatory mediators and inhibits neutrophil apoptosis (68).

IL-6 stimulates the extrinsic coagulation pathway through interaction with tissue factor that is expressed on the surface of activated macrophages and the capillary endothelium and is bound to factor VIIa. The tissue factor VIIa complex activates prothrombin, resulting in the production of thrombin, which in turn converts fibrinogen to fibrin. The coagulation cascade also contains several negative feedback loops that are governed by substances such as antithrombin and activated protein C (APC), which serve to control the extent of thrombosis once it is triggered. Therefore, in the individual patient, it is possible to see evidence of vascular thrombosis and a local or systemic coagulopathy as a result of coagulation factor consumption and increased fibrin degradation from the interaction between TNF and platelet activator inhibitor (66). Recent

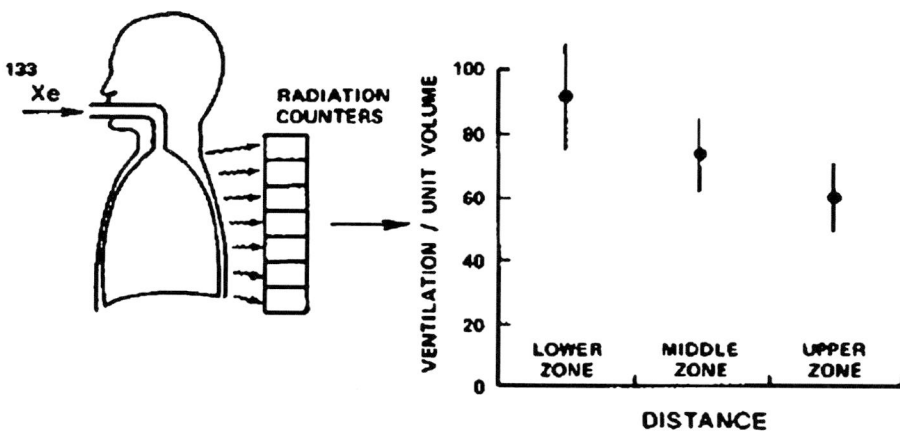

FIGURE 46.6. Regional differences in lung ventilation. Distribution of inhaled radiolabeled xenon gas is recorded by external radiation counters in a series of normal subjects. The ventilation per unit lung volume is greatest near the lung base ("lower zone") and is smallest toward the lung apex ("upper zone"). From West JB. Ventilation. In: *Respiratory Physiology: The Essentials,* 4th ed. Baltimore: Williams and Wilkins, 1990;11–20, with permission.

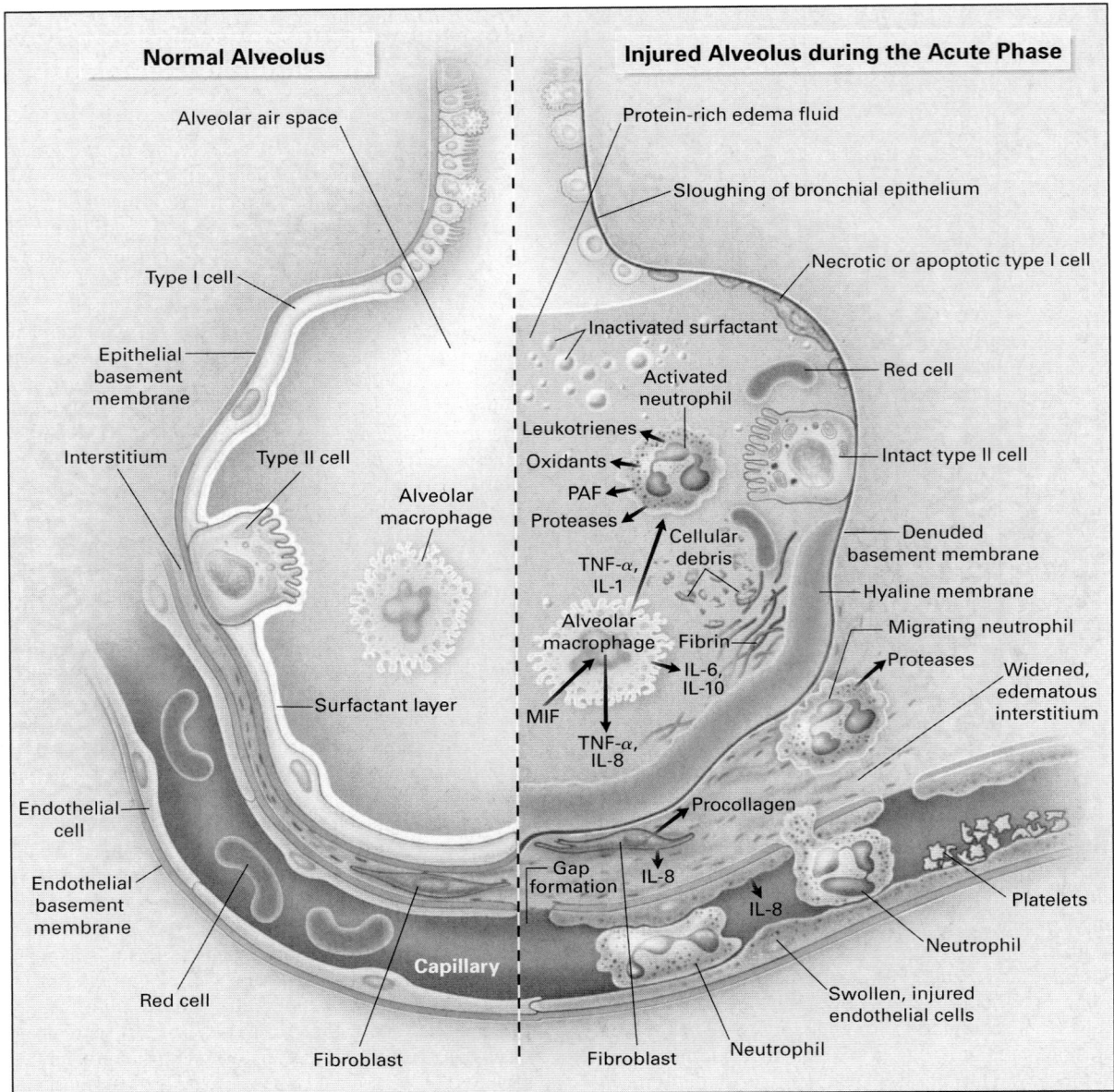

FIGURE 46.7. Cellular and molecular mechanisms of inflammation and alteration of hemostasis in ALI and ARDS. The normal alveolus is shown on the left, and the injured alveolus is shown on the right. From Ware LB, Matthay MA: The acute respiratory distress syndrome. *N Engl J Med* 2000;342(18):1334–49, with permission.

investigations have indicated that bronchoalveolar lavage (BAL) specimens from patients with lower respiratory tract inflammation contain elevated levels of soluble tissue factor and factor VII; APC has been identified in alveolar fluid, as well (67). Moreover, in small-animal models, the administration of high-dose antithrombin has been shown to prevent alveolar fibrin deposition and the development of lung injury in the context of endotoxemia (91).

Whether the individual patient with ALI and/or ARDS expresses, on balance, a predominantly procoagulant or anticoagulant phenotype seems likely to be a function of the interaction between host genetics and the specific inciting factors that lead to disease development. However, some experimental data now indicate that the supportive strategy selected by

the clinician can modify this process. For example, mechanical ventilation using large tidal volumes seems to be associated with release of platelet activator inhibitor-1 and reduced fibrinolytic activity in a small-animal model of lung injury (17). Another group of investigators recently reported that patients who were ventilated for 5 hrs with high (12 mL/kg) tidal volumes and zero positive end-expiratory pressure (PEEP) following elective surgery demonstrated significant elevation in levels of thrombin-antithrombin complexes, tissue factor, and factor VIIa in BAL fluid, as compared to those who were ventilated over the same period of time with small tidal volumes and PEEP equal to 10 cm H_2O (14). These findings indicate that the inflammatory response in ALI and ARDS alters the hemostatic balance in ways that might suggest novel targets for therapeutic intervention. They may also explain some of the hemodynamic consequences of the disease.

Amplification of the immune response to lung injury is thus a product of redundancies and interactions among components of the innate immune system (cytokines), the complement system (C3a, C5a), products of membrane phospholipid metabolism (leukotrienes, PAF), and the coagulation cascade. This process eventually transitions to a more specific immune response in which activated lymphocytes and monocytes produce anti-inflammatory cytokines, such as tumor growth factor-β, which have a role in downregulating the effects of proinflammatory cytokines on neutrophils and endothelial cells and elaboration of extracellular matrix, giving way to the fibroproliferative stage of disease. Resolution of inflammation in ARDS is also mediated by IL-10, an anti-inflammatory cytokine that attenuates fibrosis and the activity of NF-κB, inducing neutrophil apoptosis and allowing for repopulation of bronchial and alveolar epithelium (68).

Alteration of Cardiovascular Function: Effects on Pulmonary Hemodynamics

Overall, the elaboration of proinflammatory cytokines in ALI and ARDS initiates or potentiates the development of permeability edema, leading to alveolar hypoxia, thrombotic obstruction of the pulmonary microvasculature, and eventual interstitial fibrosis. Each of these pathophysiologic elements has the potential to increase pulmonary vascular resistance (PVR), adding to right ventricular afterload and potentially compromising cardiac output. Studies in open-chested and excised canine lung models established many years ago that PVR is dramatically affected by changes in lung volume. These experiments demonstrated that PVR is minimal (or "optimal") at the lung volume that corresponds to FRC, or normal EELV. As EELV increases toward total lung capacity, extra-alveolar vascular resistance drops as these vessels become less tortuous. However, intra-alveolar vascular resistance escalates very

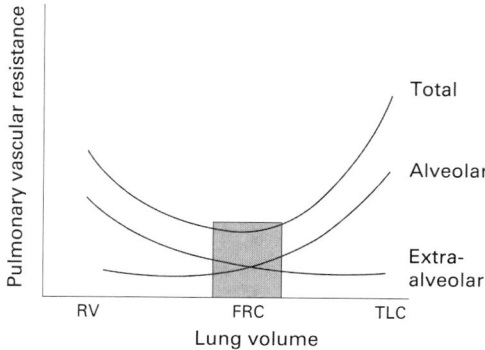

FIGURE 46.8. Effect of lung volume on pulmonary vascular resistance. "Optimal," or nadir PVR occurs at FRC. As lung volume increases toward total lung capacity (TLC), extra-alveolar resistance drops, while intra-alveolar vascular resistance escalates. As lung volume drops toward residual volume (RV), extra-alveolar vascular resistance increases as these vessels become tortuous, while alveolar hypoxia results in intra-alveolar vasoconstriction. The "Total," or net effect of these findings on overall PVR is represented by the uppermost curve. From Shekerdemian L, Bohn D. Cardiovascular effects of mechanical ventilation. *Arch Dis Child* 1999;80(5):475–80, with permission.

rapidly as alveolar distension begins to compress these vessels. The net effect of increasing lung volume on these two components of the pulmonary vascular bed is an exponential increase in PVR. As EELV drops toward residual volume, resistance of the extra-alveolar vessels increases as they become more tortuous. In addition, collapse of small airways as lung compliance falls results in alveolar hypoxia and reflex pulmonary vasoconstriction. Collectively, the effects of lung volume on PVR produce a parabolic curve whose nadir occurs at FRC (**Fig. 46.8**). Increases in PVR and right ventricular afterload at the extremes of lung volume can ultimately reduce systemic cardiac output, as increased end-diastolic volume in the highly compliant right ventricle (RV) shifts the interventricular septum toward the left, resulting in decreased left ventricular (LV) compliance and poor LV filling. These cardiopulmonary interactions suggest that strategies that emphasize the maintenance of alveolar volume while avoiding alveolar overdistension are not only necessary to improve gas exchange, but they are also likely to have a favorable effect on cardiovascular performance in ALI and ARDS.

CLINICAL PRESENTATION

Diffuse alveolar disease that meets criteria for ALI and ARDS produces a predictable sequence of clinical changes. When fluid accumulation in the interstitial space exceeds the absorptive capacity of the pulmonary lymphatics, lung compliance declines and tachypnea ensues as the patient attempts to generate adequate minute ventilation in the face of lower tidal volumes. The eventual leakage of proteinaceous fluid into the alveolar spaces interferes with native surfactant function, creating conditions that favor regional atelectasis and small-airways closure, as well as a decrease in EELV to a point near or below closing capacity, especially in small infants and those with highly compliant chest walls (e.g., patients with neuromuscular disease). At this point, hypoxia rapidly worsens and breathing becomes more labored in an effort to generate transpulmonary pressures sufficient to maintain alveolar patency. Hypocarbia is often present early in the disease process, when the patient first manifests tachypnea. However, as the work of breathing escalates, the $PaCO_2$ will further rise as respiratory muscle fatigue ensues. At this stage, positive pressure ventilation is required to open a sufficient number of atelectatic lung units for adequate gas exchange. On auscultation, the patient will typically demonstrate rales over areas of atelectasis or alveolar congestion and decreased air entry over areas that are largely consolidated. Occasionally, it is possible to appreciate wheezes over areas in which intermittent small-airways closure is occurring.

Imaging Studies

Clinical changes of early ALI and ARDS manifest on chest x-rays as diffuse alveolar infiltrates and air bronchograms that may be accompanied by pleural effusion and widespread atelectasis (**Fig. 46.9**). Areas of lung injury that are evolving into fibrosis may appear as prominent reticular opacities. Studies that have evaluated patients with ALI and ARDS using CT have facilitated an understanding that lung consolidation occurs along a gradient corresponding to the gravitational axis. Between these two regions lies a zone of airspace opacification

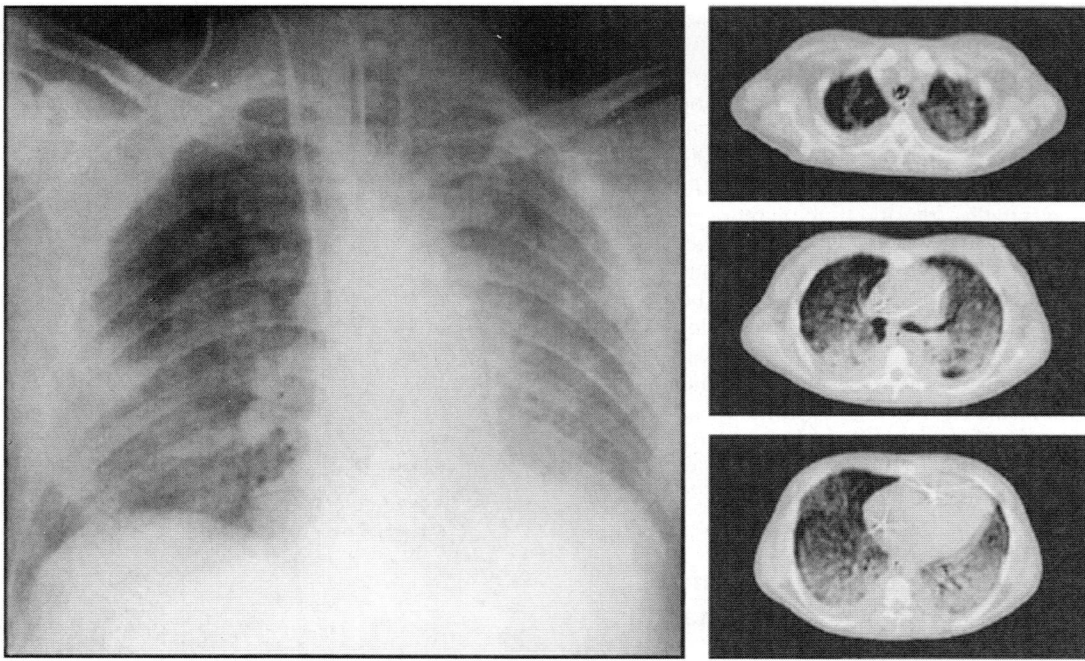

FIGURE 46.9. Nonuniform parenchymal involvement in acute respiratory distress syndrome (ARDS). Anterior-posterior (AP) chest x-ray and CT scans corresponding to lung apex, hilum, and base from a patient with sepsis and ARDS. Images are taken with the patient in supine position, at a PEEP of 5 cm H_2O. The CT scans illustrate the influence of the gravitational axis on the pattern of alveolar consolidation in ARDS: Nondependent regions are aerated, while dependent regions remain consolidated. From Gattinoni L, Caironi P, Pelosi P, et al. What has computed tomography taught us about the acute respiratory distress syndrome? *Am J Respir Crit Care Med* 2001;164:1701–11, with permission.

without consolidation (**Figs. 46.9** and **46.10**). The spatial distribution of ALI has been demonstrated in anesthetized and paralyzed dogs that were rotated while being injected with oleic acid in divided doses to encourage a diffuse pattern of lung injury (13). The animals were then exposed to high tidal volume ventilation while they were in either the supine or prone position. At the end of the experiment, all animals developed lung edema distributed, for the most part, to dependent areas. However, regardless of body position, histologic abnormalities were more severe in dorsal lung regions, in a pattern reflecting the preferential distribution of pulmonary blood flow, the pathway by which lung injury was initiated in this model.

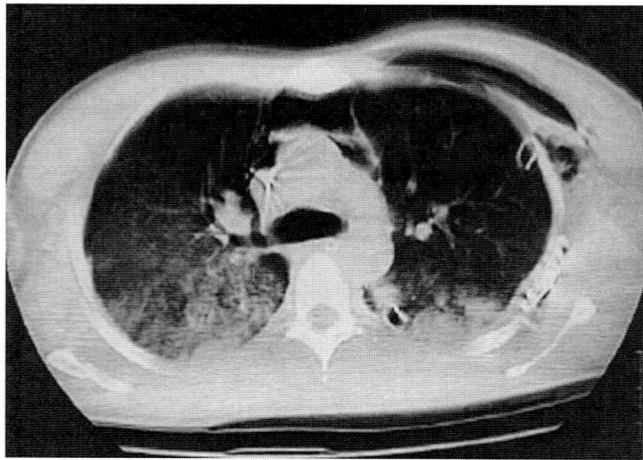

FIGURE 46.10. CT scan of a patient with ARDS, 5 days after multiple trauma. A view at the level of the carina shows diffuse alveolar opacification, with areas of consolidation located in dependent regions. From Gattinoni L, Caironi P, Pelosi P, et al. What has computed tomography taught us about the acute respiratory distress syndrome? *Am J Respir Crit Care Med* 2001;164:1701–11, with permission.

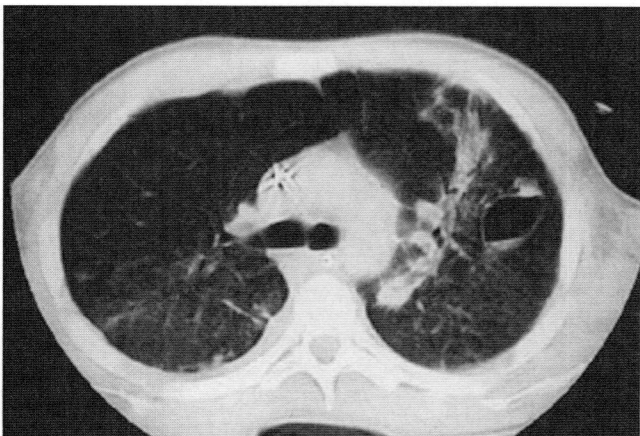

FIGURE 46.11. ARDS: CT changes 12 days later. The same patient seen in Figure 46.10 undergoes CT imaging 12 days after onset of ARDS. Alveolar opacities have largely cleared, giving way to reticular infiltrates. A pneumatocele is evident on the left, and an area of atelectasis is seen medial to it. From Gattinoni L, Caironi P, Pelosi P, et al. What has computed tomography taught us about the acute respiratory distress syndrome? *Am J Respir Crit Care Med* 2001;164:1701–11, with permission.

Development of dependent atelectasis in any patient oriented horizontally is not a new concept; CT images obtained in supine, anesthetized patients without lung disease who were administered neuromuscular blockade have identified the same phenomenon. However, serial CT imaging in patients with ALI and ARDS has revealed that, in later stages of the disease, fibrosis begins to be identifiable in nondependent areas that seemed to be relatively free of disease earlier in the course (**Figs. 44.10 and 44.11**). The reticular pattern of infiltration that appears in these areas seems to be associated with lengthy and aggressive strategies of mechanical ventilation (21), suggesting that the "natural history" of ALI and ARDS actually represents the combined effects of an initial biological insult and ventilator-associated injury (**Figs. 46.10 and 46.11**). Although CT images of the lung in diseases now categorized as ALI and ARDS have been available for study for nearly 20 years, it is not until recently that their implications began to be incorporated into management strategies that seek to limit lung injury by respecting the underlying pathophysiology of the disease.

PRINCIPLES OF CLINICAL MANAGEMENT

As more of the pathophysiologic elements involved in ALI and ARDS have been elucidated in the laboratory, considerable ef-

fort has been given toward translating them into innovative targets for therapeutic intervention. At the moment, therapeutic drug trials in this area have not identified an agent that improves clinically important outcome measures in a way that warrants its routine use in the management of all patients with ALI and ARDS (**Table 46.2**). The mainstay of therapy remains supportive care, of which a critically important component is the application of PPV (**Table 46.3**).

Positive-pressure Ventilation

Hypoxia is an essential feature of ALI and ARDS; the basis for its development is the breakdown of the alveolar-capillary barrier. Once this occurs, pulmonary compliance and EELV tend to decline dramatically and $\dot{V}/\dot{Q}$ imbalance ensues, which explains why hypoxia in ALI and ARDS is typically refractory to the provision of supplementary O_2 alone. Moreover, ongoing exposure to high concentrations of supplemental O_2 in the absence of effective reversal of atelectasis is associated with the development of lung injury that is remarkably similar to ALI and ARDS. Humans begin to consistently manifest this type of lung injury when they are exposed to an FIO_2 of >0.5. To stabilize consolidated or collapsed alveoli to a degree that is sufficient to provide oxygenation without the use of high FIO_2, PPV is necessary. In Ashbaugh's original description of ARDS, he reported that the hypoxemia associated with this disease could be

---

TABLE 46.2

RESULTS OF SELECTED CLINICAL TRIALS EVALUATING VENTILATION STRATEGIES OR PHARMACOLOGIC THERAPIES FOR ACUTE LUNG INJURY AND THE ACUTE RESPIRATORY DISTRESS SYNDROME

Intervention	Year	Number of patients	Findings	Study
Low tidal volume mechanical ventilation	2000	861	*22% relative mortality benefit*	NIH Acute Respiratory Distress Syndrome Network (2)
Prone positioning	2001	304	No mortality benefit	Gattinoni, et al. (33)
	2005[a]	102	No mortality benefit	Curley, et al. (16)
	2006	136	No mortality benefit[b]	Mancebo, et al. (49)
Conservative vs. liberal fluid administration strategy	2006	1000	No mortality benefit	NIH Acute Respiratory Distress Syndrome Network (87)
Surfactant	1996	725	No mortality benefit	Anzueto, et al. (4)
	2004	448	No mortality benefit	Spragg, et al. (73)
	2005[a]	152	Mortality benefit seen in surfactant group[c]	Willson, et al. (88)
Corticosteroids	1998	24	Mortality benefit[d]	Meduri, et al. (54)
	2006	180	No mortality benefit	NIH Acute Respiratory Distress Syndrome Network (75)
Inhaled nitric oxide	1998	177	No mortality benefit	Dellinger, et al. (20)
	1999[a]	108	No mortality benefit[e]	Dobyns, et al. (23)
	2004	385	No mortality benefit	Taylor, et al. (76)

[a]Pediatric Study.
[b]58% ICU mortality in control arm; study ultimately underpowered (see text).
[c]Study ultimately underpowered (see text). [d]Small study (see text).
[d]Crossover design (see text).
[e]Adapted from Ware LB, Matthay MA. The acute respiratory distress syndrome. *N Engl J Med* 2000;342:1334–49.

TABLE 46.3

SUGGESTED THERAPY GUIDELINES FOR ALI/ARDS

	Pulmonary	Cardiovascular	Other
Resuscitation	Supplemental O_2 Early arterial access for disease identification (PaO_2/FIO_2, OI) and early implementation of therapy Consider early NPPV for alveolar recruitment in alert, cooperative patient[a] Endotracheal intubation and PPV for respiratory failure failing noninvasive therapy Titrate PEEP to achieve $FIO_2 \leq 05.-0.6/SpO_2$ 88–95%. Limit tidal volume (6 mL/kg *ideal* body weight) and alveolar plateau pressure (≤ 30 cm H_2O)[b] Permissive hypercapnia unless contraindicated (coexistent increased intracranial pressure, etc.)	Crystalloid, colloid, or blood to optimize intravascular volume and support hemodynamics[c] Anticipate potentially adverse hemodynamic consequences of transition to PPV in setting of intravascular volume depletion Titrate supportive therapy to correct perfusion abnormalities and optimize urine output	Cultures Broad-spectrum antimicrobial agents Consider antifungal, antiviral, atypical agent coverage in immunocompromised population Consider early bronchoalveolar lavage in immunocompromised population
Escalation	Titrate PEEP upward if ongoing hypoxemia in setting of alveolar derecruitment. Early transition to HFOV if high inflation pressures are necessary Consider prone positioning in selected cases	Titrate fluid and vasoactive infusions to achieve age-appropriate blood pressure parameters and adequate end-organ function	Sedation/analgesia Neuromuscular blockade if necessary
Maintenance	Follow OI to track response to therapy Wean ventilator as allowable	Monitoring: CVP, serial clinical examination and review of organ function[d] Maintain euvolemia Diuretics	Nutrition: Implement enteral nutrition as early as feasible. Avoid excess glucose administration. Careful attention to nitrogen balance. Neuromuscular blockade: Daily infusion interruption and discontinue as soon as feasible Sedation and analgesia: Daily infusion interruption and wean during plateau phase of illness
Advanced therapy	OI not improving on optimal ventilator strategy/HFOV: Consider ECMO	Consider early renal replacement therapy for persistent hypervolemia and oliguria despite diuretics	

[a]Early NPPV may avert need for intubation in certain immunocompromised patients (40).
[b]Optimal tidal volume and plateau pressure are not known, but use of 6 cc/kg has been associated with a 22% relative mortality benefit compared to 12 mL/kg (2). High tidal volumes are also associated with proinflammatory cytokine release (2,3,63).
[c]Optimal hemoglobin concentration is not known. In absence of cardiovascular disease, hemoglobin of 7–9 g/dL is probably adequate and may avert adverse effects of red cell transfusion (39).
[d]Current data suggest pulmonary artery catheter use in ALI/ARDS is not associated with improved outcomes and may be associated with increased incidence of catheter-related complications (77). CVP must be interpreted in context of surrounding compartment pressure (e.g., intrathoracic pressure for superior vena cava lines) and/or myocardial compliance. In absence of coexisting intracardiac shunt, mixed venous O_2 saturation may clarify adequacy of cardiac output.
OI, oxygenation index ($100 \times$ mean airway pressure $\times$ FIO_2)/PaO_2; NPPV, noninvasive positive-pressure ventilation; PEEP, positive end-expiratory pressure; HFOV, high frequency oscillatory ventilation; CVP, central venous pressure; ECMO, extracorporeal membrane oxygenation
Adapted from Fackler JC, Arnold JH, Nichols DG, et al. Acute Respiratory Distress Syndrome. In: Rogers M, ed. *Textbook of Pediatric Intensive Care*, 3rd ed. Baltimore: Williams and Wilkins, 1996;197–233.

reversed with PEEP. In the decade that followed publication of this initial case series, a study conducted in a small number of patients with severe hypoxic respiratory failure demonstrated that upward titration of PEEP from 0 to 15 cm H_2O resulted in similar linear increases in EELV, PaO_2, and static compliance (25). A few years later, the effects of PEEP were evaluated in an oleic acid model of canine lung injury. In that study, increasing PEEP from 3 to 13 cm H_2O decreased intrapulmonary shunt fraction without altering pulmonary blood flow; alveolar septa were thicker and a greater portion of alveoli were flooded in the lungs ventilated without PEEP, as compared to those that were ventilated with PEEP. In lungs ventilated with PEEP, edema was confined to the perivascular space (48). It is tempting to conclude from these observations that PEEP reverses hypoxemia in ALI and ARDS by simply redistributing extravascular lung water and restoring EELV toward FRC. However, it is useful to look at these results in light of Webb and Tierney's study from the mid 1970s, in which they demonstrated that a pattern of injury resembling ARDS could be created in healthy lungs by mechanically ventilating with high peak inflation pressures, and applying PEEP in this context similarly limited edema formation. Taken together, these studies shed light on the possibility that besides restoring an interface for adequate gas exchange, stabilizing alveolar volume through the application of PEEP might also limit the development of ventilator-associated injury. While the salutary effects of PEEP have been well established, it is important to recognize the potential for PEEP to augment anatomical dead space by distending large airways, and potentially adding to alveolar dead space (see below).

When managing a patient with hypoxic respiratory failure, it is important to appreciate the effects of PPV on cardiovascular function. During normal breathing, negative intrathoracic pressure lowers intracavitary pressure in the right atrium and, together with positive intra-abdominal pressure, creates a gradient that promotes right atrial filling. Lung inflation toward FRC is associated with a decrease in PVR, which lowers right ventricular afterload, and pulmonary venous return proceeds unimpeded to the left heart and systemic circulation. Although PPV is required to restore lung volume toward FRC and achieve adequate gas exchange in hypoxic respiratory failure, it also increases right atrial pressure, diminishing the pressure gradient for systemic venous return and lowering right ventricular stroke volume. On the other hand, PPV tends to enhance LV function because of its favorable effects on LV afterload, as determined by transmural pressure (P_{tm}). P_{tm} is defined as the intracavitary pressure (P_{ic}) minus the surrounding, or pleural pressure (P_{pl}):

$$P_{tm} = P_{ic} - P_{pl}$$

This formula illustrates that LV transmural pressure (or afterload) is reduced in the setting of PPV and increased in the setting of negative-pressure ventilation. Although the gradient for cardiac filling can be manipulated by intravascular volume loading and the use of vasoactive infusions, the effects of PPV on overall cardiac output have much to do with the relationship between alveolar volume and pulmonary blood flow. It has been known for many years that the sensitivity of RV contractile function to RV afterload is such that acute changes in lung volume can produce increases in PVR capable of precipitating RV failure. The effects of this phenomenon on systemic cardiac output may outweigh any reduction in LV afterload

that occurs with the transition to PPV. Moreover, because gas distribution in mechanically ventilated patients is preferentially distributed to nondependent, high $\dot{V}/\dot{Q}$ areas, PEEP can exacerbate the tendency toward alveolar overinflation, adding to alveolar dead space and possibly escalating PVR. In summary, a sound physiologic basis supports the expectation that titrating positive pressure (or PEEP) in a way that achieves alveolar recruitment, avoids alveolar overdistension, and optimizes the relationship of ventilation to perfusion will provide adequate gas exchange while limiting the possibility for exposure to additional lung injury and potentially adverse cardiovascular effects.

Therapeutic goals for the use of positive pressure in the management of ALI and ARDS have evolved considerably over the past several decades. "Adequate gas exchange" was once defined as normal blood gas tensions, without regard for the level of mechanical support that was required to produce them. For the many reasons outlined previously, mechanical ventilation has come to be regarded as a legitimate source of injury important enough to impact survival in patients with ALI and ARDS. Comparison of CT images of the lung in mechanically ventilated patients during inspiration and expiration illustrates that gravitational forces likely create zones of differential susceptibility to mechanical injury, because tidal volumes are preferentially delivered to unconsolidated, nondependent lung units (31). In heterogeneous conditions, such as ALI and ARDS, it is difficult to know what level of PEEP will open enough alveoli to produce adequate oxygenation without creating conditions for ongoing stress-induced lung injury. Expert opinion has always varied when it comes to specifying precise algorithms for achieving adequate oxygenation. Recognizing the prudence of limiting a patient's exposure to high concentrations of supplementary O_2 and high transpulmonary pressures, a logical strategy suggests stepwise escalation of PEEP in 3–5-cm H_2O increments, until arriving at the minimum PEEP that allows for a PaO_2 in the range of 55–80 mm Hg, with peripheral O_2 saturation (SpO_2) of 88%–95%, using an FIO_2 of 0.5–0.6 (2).

The tidal volume selected by the clinician also deserves careful consideration, because multiple lines of evidence indicate that limiting phasic changes in lung volume and preventing alveolar overdistension at end-inspiration will reduce the risk of ventilator-associated lung injury (15,63,72). Large tidal-volume ventilation strategies have been associated with the development of ALI in patients with normal pulmonary function before intubation (30), and high-volume/low PEEP strategies have been associated with enhanced inflammatory cytokine expression in serum and BAL fluid samples in adults with ARDS (63). In 2000, the ARDS network demonstrated conclusively in a landmark multicentered RCT that limiting tidal volumes could result in significantly decreased mortality in ARDS. The trial was stopped early, after investigators found that patients randomized to receive tidal volumes of 6 mL/kg ideal body weight had a 22% relative reduction in mortality, compared to those randomized to receive tidal volumes of 12 mL/kg ideal body weight (2). The experimental arm of the study called for limitation of plateau pressures to $\leq$30 cm H_2O, while the control arm had plateau pressure limited to $\leq$50 cm H_2O. Management in both study arms also allowed for development of a modest respiratory acidosis, with pH >7.30. Remarkably, the investigators were also able to demonstrate a significant reduction in plasma levels of the proinflammatory cytokine IL-6 among patients in the low tidal volume group.

Ongoing interest in the lung-protective merits of low tidal volume ventilation has led to the expectation that high-frequency oscillatory ventilation (HFOV) would have an important role in the management of patients with ALI and ARDS. HFOV is an attractive mode of ventilation because of its unique ability to provide adequate gas exchange using tidal volumes below dead-space volume in the setting of continuous alveolar recruitment. Theoretically, high-frequency ventilation should provide the ultimate "open-lung" strategy of ventilation, with preservation of EELV, minimization of cyclic stretch, and avoidance of parenchymal overdistension at end-inspiration, amounting to ventilation on the most compliant portion of the volume-pressure curve while avoiding extremes of lung volume (Fig. 46.1). The first and largest multicentered, randomized trial to evaluate the effect of HFOV versus conventional ventilation in children was a crossover design that enrolled children with diffuse alveolar disease and/or air leak (5). The investigators randomized 70 patients to receive (a) conventional ventilation with limitation of peak inspiratory pressure, or (b) HFOV using a strategy that targeted a lung volume at which optimal oxygenation occurred (Sao$_2$ ≥90% and Fio$_2$ <0.6). For patients with air leak, airway pressure was further limited, while Fio$_2$ was preferentially increased to achieve saturations of ≥85% and pH ≥7.25 until the air leak resolved. The study found no difference in survival or duration of mechanical ventilation between the 2 groups, but significantly fewer children randomized to receive HFOV remained dependent on supplemental O$_2$ at 30 days. Post hoc analysis revealed that outcome benefits were not as great in those that crossed over to the HFOV arm, supporting the suggestion by numerous studies that use of HFOV will be more successful if employed early in the course of disease, using a strategy that emphasizes alveolar recruitment.

Fluid Management

Clinicians often face a dilemma when managing ALI and ARDS regarding how best to support hemodynamics without increasing alveolar fluid accumulation and ongoing pulmonary dysfunction. Decades ago, evidence from large-animal models of ALI indicated that lower cardiac filling pressures and intravascular pressures could limit extravascular lung water accumulation without impairing tissue oxygenation. Case series from the 1970s through the early 1990s also identified a relationship between fluid-restrictive management strategies and improved pulmonary compliance, as well as actual improvements in survival. However, contemporary lung-protective strategies of mechanical ventilation that have recently proven to reduce mortality in ALI and ARDS (2) often call for high levels of PEEP to stabilize alveolar volume, and intravascular volume supplementation may be necessary in this context to optimize $\dot{V}/\dot{Q}$ relations and improve overall cardiac output. With this in mind, the Acute Respiratory Distress Syndrome Clinical Trials Network (ARDSNet) designed a multicentered RCT to evaluate the effects of various fluid-management protocols on outcomes in ALI and ARDS using a contemporary "open lung," low tidal volume strategy. This trial randomized 1,000 intubated adults with evidence of ALI or ARDS for less than 48 hrs to receive either conservative or liberal administration of IV fluids (crystalloid, colloid, or

blood), with hemodynamic monitoring by pulmonary artery catheter or central venous catheter, according to a two-by-two factorial design (87). The protocol called for frequent hemodynamic assessment, with administration of a specified amount of fluid, furosemide, dobutamine, or a vasopressor, according to cardiac filling pressures, urine output, mean arterial blood pressure, and cardiac index or clinical perfusion. Patients in the liberal treatment arm received therapies targeting higher filling pressures (central venous pressure, CVP, of 10–14 mm Hg or pulmonary artery occlusion pressure of 14–18 mm Hg). Those in the conservative arm were assigned to receive therapies targeting lower filling pressures (CVP <4 mm Hg or pulmonary artery occlusion pressure of <8 mm Hg). In the final analysis, the investigators reported no interaction between the assigned fluid strategy and the assigned catheter. Mortality (the primary outcome) was similar between the conservative group (25.5%) and the liberal group (28.4%; $p = 0.30$). However, review of the secondary outcome measures revealed that the conservative strategy was associated with an improvement in oxygenation index ([100 × mean airway pressure × Fio$_2$]/P$_a$O$_2$) and a significant increase in ventilator-free days during the first 28 days of therapy (14.6 ± 0.5 vs. 12.1 ± 0.5; p <0.001), while it did not seem to increase the incidence of renal failure or need for dialysis (87). Interestingly, the "liberal" fluid management strategy produced cumulative fluid balances in study subjects that are comparable to both pre-study baseline cardiac filling pressures and published data reflecting "best practice" almost 20 years earlier (87). It is important to emphasize that the results of this study are relevant to patient management during the "maintenance" phase of therapy—after adequate initial resuscitation. Patients entered this study after hemodynamic variables were "optimized" (CVP 11.9 ± 0.3 and cardiac index 4.2 ± 0.1 L/min/m^2 in the conservative group; CVP 12.2 ± 0.3 and cardiac index 4.3 ± 0.1 L/min/m^2 in the liberal group), and patients with renal failure were excluded. Overall, this study is a good example of how individual components of supportive-care protocols for ALI and ARDS must be reevaluated in the context of the most current clinical evidence base, such as the benefits of "open-lung" low tidal volume ventilation, to achieve a more comprehensive understanding of how to optimize patient outcomes in these conditions.

Adjuvant Therapies in ALI and ARDS

Prone Positioning

Because alveolar consolidation occurs along the gravitational axis in ALI and ARDS, and because pulmonary blood flow is distributed preferentially to dorsal lung regions, it is logical to speculate that ventilation-perfusion relationships in the mechanically ventilated injured lung can be improved by manipulating body position. Animal models that demonstrated attenuation of lung injury by prone positioning offer support for this expectation (12,13). Specifically, one could also imagine that placing a patient prone might reduce chest wall compliance, thus transmitting airway pressure to the alveoli more efficiently and stabilizing alveolar volume over a larger portion of previously nonaerated lung units. Large-animal experiments have confirmed that prone positioning improves oxygenation and $\dot{V}/\dot{Q}$ matching, allows for the generation of transpulmonary pressure sufficient to open previously consolidated areas, and actually attenuates ventilator-associated lung injury (12,13,45). Prone positioning was first applied as part of a multicentered RCT in 2001 (33). In this study, patients randomized to the intervention arm received an average of 7 hrs of prone positioning per day. The majority showed an increase in PaO_2/FiO_2 of at least 10, with greatest effect occurring during the first hour prone. Interestingly, responders also manifested a favorable change in $PacO_2$. Nonetheless, mortality at the end of the 10-day period was comparable [prone, 21.1%, vs. supine, 25%; relative risk, 0.84; 95% confidence interval (CI), 0.56–1.27] (33). In 2004, another group evaluated prone positioning for a median of 8 hrs per day (interquartile range, 7.7–9.8) in a less-select group of adult patients with ALI and ARDS and documented similar improvements in oxygenation without a 28-day mortality benefit, as well as an increased incidence of adverse events referable to use of the prone position (37). The study reported in 2006 is also noteworthy for its efforts to identify a subgroup of ARDS patients who might benefit the most from prone positioning (49). These investigators randomized 136 adults with ARDS to supine or prone (a mean of 17 hrs/day for a mean of 10 days) within 48 hrs of meeting inclusion criteria. Many of their patients had significant comorbidities, including immunocompromise and nonpulmonary organ failures, and tidal volumes up to 10 mL/kg with peak inspiratory pressure up to 40 cm H_2O were allowed. The overall mortality in the control arm was 58%. These features make this study difficult to compare with others. This study was stopped short of its 200-patient goal because of a declining rate of enrollment. In the end, the authors were unable to demonstrate a significant mortality benefit, which was the primary outcome measure. However, they performed an interesting post hoc analysis among 103 patients with a simplified acute physiology II (SAPS II) score of <50 and among 33 patients with a SAPS II score of >50. In the group with lower SAPS scores, a statistically significant ICU mortality benefit from prone positioning (33% vs. 53%; $p = 0.049$) was reported.

The first group to systematically evaluate prone positioning in infants and children with ALI and ARDS conducted a multicentered trial that randomized patients to receive 20 hrs of prone positioning each day during the acute phase of illness for a maximum of 7 days (16). Customized cushions were used to stabilize the most compliant portion of the chest wall during prone positioning. Remarkably, the study protocolized almost every aspect of supportive care, including delivery of lung-protective mechanical ventilation, as well as explicit algorithms to guide sedation, hemodynamic management, nutrition, and skin care. The vast majority (>80%) of the patients enrolled in each study arm had direct pulmonary injury as the etiology of ALI or ARDS. In the end, this trial was stopped according to predetermined futility criteria, after enrolling 102 of an expected 180 patients. The investigators reported a very low mortality rate of 8% in each arm of the study. Despite favorable changes in PaO_2/FiO_2 and oxygenation index among patients who were randomized to use of the prone position, no difference in the number of ventilator-free days between the prone group and the supine group was observed (mean difference, −0.2 days; 95% CI, −3.6 to 3.2 days; $p = 0.91$) (16).

In the interest of future clinical trial development, perhaps it is useful to speculate about why such a thoughtfully designed clinical trial was unable to demonstrate an outcome benefit

associated with prone positioning, given the weight of the experimental evidence. First, the low mortality rate suggests that the protocols guiding supportive care were highly efficacious and may be worthy of incorporation into "standard care" algorithms. Reducing mortality in ALI and ARDS even further may require implementation of such treatment protocols earlier in the disease process. A second issue to consider is that prone positioning may still be useful for specific subpopulations that have not been exclusively studied in large trials, such as patients with increased chest wall compliance from baseline neuromuscular weakness or patients in whom chest wall compliance is increased as a result of pharmacologic neuromuscular blockade. Although existing data do not support routine use of prone positioning for patients with ALI and ARDS, the strong scientific basis for this intervention may prompt clinicians to use it in individual patients whose specific underlying physiology suggests that their gas exchange efficiency may improve as a result. Occasionally, in such cases, improvements in gas exchange may be substantial enough to allow the patient to wean from potentially injurious inflation pressures and/or fractional inspired O_2 concentrations.

Surfactant

Ten years after ARDS was first described, dysfunction of the surfactant system was identified in this disease, which helped to explain why its histopathologic features seem so similar to the respiratory distress syndrome associated with neonatal surfactant deficiency. Analysis of BAL fluid from postmortem lung specimens and from adult patients with respiratory failure demonstrated alterations in the lipid-to-protein ratio of endogenous surfactant and an overall increase in surface tension in ARDS, compared to healthy controls (38). Surfactant was thereafter identified as a potential therapy in ARDS, and the first multicentered RCT to evaluate its use in ARDS was published in 1996 (4). The investigators randomized patients with ALI or ARDS (PaO_2/FiO_2 <250), including only those with *indirect* lung injury referable to sepsis. In all, 725 adults received (a) synthetic surfactant (Exosurf, Glaxo-Wellcome), aerosolized for delivery into the inspiratory limb of the ventilator circuit, or (b) 0.45% aerosolized saline placebo for a maximum of 5 days. Both groups showed similar changes in the alveolararterial O_2 gradient and PaO_2/FiO_2 throughout the study period, and no difference in mortality (the primary outcome measure) was noted between the two groups; 30-day survival in each group was ~60%. A potential explanation for the lack of benefit in this study was the difficulty of delivering aerosolized surfactant to the lower airways in the intubated patient. Subsequent trials evaluating the use of surfactant replacement in ALI and ARDS delivered the drug by intratracheal instillation. One small, open-label study used semisynthetic bovine surfactant (Survanta), and the other larger multicentered trial used recombinant surfactant (Venticute) (36,73). Both studies demonstrated the safety and feasibility of administering intratracheal surfactant in the adult ALI and ARDS population, and both demonstrated some short-term improvement in oxygenation in patients in the intervention arm. However, neither study demonstrated a survival benefit.

Evidence on the use of surfactant in children comes in large part from a recent multicentered RCT that compared administration of modified bovine surfactant (Calfactant) with air placebo in 152 infants and children with ALI and ARDS (88).

The study was notable for attempting to blind study personnel and clinicians to the treatment and for its inclusion of immunocompromised patients, who are traditionally excluded from such studies. Aspects of patient care apart from the study intervention were not protocolized. The original power calculations called for recruiting 300 patients, but the pace of enrollment was slower than expected and the study closed after enrollment of 152 patients. Despite this, the authors reported a significant reduction in mortality in the surfactant patients, compared to the placebo patients (19% vs. 36%; $p = 0.03$), as well as significant improvements in oxygenation index. However, it should be emphasized that post hoc adjustment for immunocompromised status using logistic regression techniques eliminated the statistically significant mortality benefit from surfactant (adjusted odds ratio of mortality for placebo compared to surfactant, 2.11; 95% CI, 0.93–4.79; $p = 0.07$). The results suggest a possible benefit of surfactant in this population, but it is not clear if this finding is due to the intrinsic superiority of Calfactant compared to other preparations, or to other issues with the study design.

It is difficult to draw meaningful conclusions from this collection of trials because they differ so greatly with respect to the study population, surfactant composition, and surfactant dosing regimen. Each of the surfactant preparations studied differs in its protein and phospholipid ingredients, and these differences may translate into distinct clinical effects. It is also important to acknowledge the differences in mechanical ventilation strategy among these studies because both animal and human data indicate that response to exogenous surfactant seems to be diminished in the setting of mechanical ventilation using large tidal volumes, while surfactant function seems to be enhanced when strategies are used that promote alveolar stability throughout the respiratory cycle (81). Despite the evidence for surfactant dysfunction in ALI and ARDS, outcome benefits associated with the use of surfactant in this relatively heterogeneous patient cohort have not come close to those reported in association with its use in surfactant-deficient neonates with the neonatal respiratory distress syndrome. It is logical to speculate that the mechanical ventilation strategy used for ALI and ARDS may confound the effects of exogenous surfactant in these diseases, because such patients generally require mechanical ventilatory support for a longer period of time than do newborn infants with neonatal respiratory distress syndrome. Although the data have yet to identify a clear indication for the use of surfactant in ALI and ARDS, arriving at the "ideal" surfactant dose and composition, as well as the timing of its administration, will ultimately depend on understanding its interaction with the chosen mechanical ventilation strategy.

Corticosteroids

Numerous clinical trials have attempted to establish a role for corticosteroids in modulating the role of the immune response to improve clinical outcomes in patients with ALI and ARDS. Use of corticosteroids has inherent appeal because these agents are understood to limit transudation of plasma across the capillary endothelium and exert anti-inflammatory effects by downregulating expression of steroid-responsive genes coding for proinflammatory cytokines while upregulating those encoding for anti-inflammatory agents, such as IL-10 (64). Studies that evaluated short courses of high-dose corticosteroids administered early in ARDS were not able to demonstrate an outcome benefit, although the data on the use of corticosteroids in persistent ARDS are thought to be more encouraging. In actuality, the evidence cited by many clinicians to support administration of corticosteroids to patients with persistent ARDS is based on one single-centered trial that included only 24 patients, of whom 16 received methylprednisolone for ARDS with a lung injury score that failed to improve by day 7 of illness (54). The study found that patients in the methylprednisolone group had improved oxygenation and other indices of lung injury and reduced mortality (12% vs. 62%; $p = 0.03$).

More recently, the ARDSNet investigators have published a multicentered RCT that evaluated the use of methylprednisolone versus placebo in 180 patients who continued to meet consensus criteria for ARDS 7–28 days after onset of disease (6). As in the prior study, the methylprednisolone was administered and tapered over several weeks. The mechanical ventilation strategy varied according to year of enrollment, with tidal volumes decreasing over time, in accordance with evidence favoring the use of low tidal volume ventilation that emerged during the 7-year span of the study. Explicit criteria were used to govern ventilator weaning and subsequent extubation. Overall, the investigators did not find an interaction between time of enrollment, tidal volumes, and outcomes with regard to methylprednisolone administration. Mortality at 60 days (the primary outcome) did not differ between the placebo group (28.6%) and the methylprednisolone group (29.2%; $p = 1.0$), despite the fact that corticosteroids were associated with an improvement in short-term measures, such as oxygenation and respiratory system compliance, and shorter duration of vasoactive infusions. Finally, methylprednisolone was not associated with an increase in infectious complications, but the investigators did identify a higher incidence of neuromuscular weakness in the treatment group (75). However, it is important to note that, among patients who entered the study on or after day 14 of ARDS, methylprednisolone was associated with a significant increase in both 60- and 120-day mortality.

Although a much stronger study than its predecessors in many respects, this most recent corticosteroid trial leaves open a number of questions, including how best to address hyperglycemia and other collateral effects of corticosteroid administration in critically ill patients. The intuitive appeal of leveraging the host immune response to improve outcomes in inflammatory conditions such as ALI and ARDS is likely to endure, although the redundancy and complexity of the immune response will make it challenging to develop more precise immunomodulatory interventions. Prospects of future studies to translate corticosteroids or other anti-inflammatory therapies into an outcome benefit in ALI and ARDS will likely depend on developing additional insights into the role of inflammation and anti-inflammation in the pathogenesis and resolution of lung injury. Moreover, future studies must incorporate the evolving evidence base of "best practices" with regard to mechanical ventilation strategy and metabolic, hemodynamic, and sedation management.

Inhaled Nitric Oxide

Nitric oxide (NO) has been known for some time as the endogenous "endothelium-derived relaxing factor" that couples with the cyclic 3,5′-monophosphate (cGMP) system to mediate vasodilation by local smooth muscle relaxation and to modify immune function and platelet aggregation. In the lung, NO is produced by the endothelium, airway smooth muscle cells, inflammatory cells, platelets, epithelial cells, and fibroblasts as a product of the conversion of L-arginine to citrulline by the enzyme NO synthase. NO binds readily with hemoglobin, resulting in its own inactivation and the production of nitrosyl-hemoglobin and methemoglobin. NO can also interact with O_2 to form nitrogen dioxide (NO_2), which has been associated with provoking the host inflammatory response in laboratory animals exposed to ambient concentrations as low as 1.5 parts per million (ppm).

Considering that its exceedingly short half-life limits its effects to the immediate local environment, it follows that NO could serve as a selective pulmonary vasodilator if administered exogenously. Clinical trials of inhaled NO (iNO) in persistent pulmonary hypertension of the newborn demonstrated significant improvement in oxygenation and a decrease in the need for extracorporeal membrane oxygenation (ECMO) (65). Subsequently, iNO was investigated for its therapeutic potential in ALI and ARDS, with the idea of reversing pulmonary vasoconstriction, relieving microvascular obstruction by reducing platelet aggregation, improving gas exchange by improving the ratio of ventilation to perfusion in diseased lung units, and potentially reducing neutrophil adhesion and local inflammation. Results were promising in experimental animal models of ARDS (28), but in the clinical arena it has been difficult to demonstrate a benefit from iNO with respect to clinically relevant outcomes in ALI and ARDS.

In 1998, the multicentered Inhaled Nitric Oxide in ARDS Study Group published the results of a prospective RCT to evaluate safety and dose-response relationships in a total of 177 adults with ARDS from causes other than sepsis (20). The study found that iNO delivered in concentrations ranging from 1.25 to 40 ppm was well tolerated. Administration of iNO was associated with early but nonsustained increases in PaO_2 and transient decreases in oxygenation index. These short-term physiologic improvements did not translate to a measurable difference in mortality between the 2 groups. A few years later, the same group of investigators published a follow-up multicentered, blinded RCT that evaluated the use of low-dose iNO (5 ppm) in nonseptic adults with ALI and ARDS (PaO_2/FIO_2 ≤250) (76). Subgroup analysis in the former study had indicated that this dose was associated with an increase in ventilator-free days and decreased short-term mortality. As in their prior study, the investigators suggested guidelines for mechanical ventilation that emphasized titrating PEEP to optimize pulmonary compliance and reduce FIO_2, as well as limiting peak inspiratory pressures, but no specific treatment protocols were included. The study found that, despite association with transient increases in PaO_2, iNO at 5 ppm did not increase the number of days during which patients were alive and free of mechanical ventilation (mean difference, –0.1 day; 95% CI, –2.0 to 1.9 days; $p = 0.97$).

Data on the use of iNO in pediatric ALI/ARDS is for the most part limited to one multicentered RCT that randomized 108 children (mean PaO_2/FIO_2 84 ± 33 in control arm; 78 ± 30 in intervention arm) to treatment with mechanical ventilation alone or in combination with iNO at 10 ppm over at least 72 hrs (23). An "open-lung" strategy of mechanical ventilation was used, and the study protocol allowed for permissive hypercapnia. Patients were allowed to exit the study if they met

predetermined treatment failure criteria. This feature did not allow the study to identify a mortality benefit from iNO therapy. This study also showed acute but nonsustained improvements in oxygenation associated with iNO, and the number of treatment failures did not differ between study groups. Improvement in oxygenation was more prevalent and more sustained in children with an oxygenation index >25 at enrollment.

In summary, the data do not support routinely offering iNO to nonseptic patients with ALI and ARDS, but of course, some individuals suspected of having particularly reactive pulmonary vasculature may yet benefit from this therapy. In cases in which the clinician elects to use iNO as adjuvant therapy in ALI and ARDS, it seems logical to incorporate strategies for optimizing its delivery to the lower airways and alveoli. Because existing clinical trials do not incorporate specific protocols for mechanical ventilation, one can speculate that the collective results cannot control for a potential interaction between the effect of iNO and the ventilation strategy. Post hoc analysis of the original iNO study data (discussed previously) reported that delivering iNO in combination with HFO appeared to produce greater improvement in oxygenation than either therapy alone (22). These findings suggest that ventilation strategies that incorporate sustained alveolar recruitment may be more likely to potentiate any favorable effect of iNO.

Activated Protein C

Much data has accumulated over the past decade that has helped to elucidate the complex relationship between the inflammatory response and the coagulation system. We now know that the two systems interact to alter the hemostatic balance in inflammatory states. APC is a naturally occurring anticoagulant that reduces the tendency toward thrombosis by inhibiting coagulation factors Va and VIIIa (66). APC was once believed to be principally synthesized in the liver, but it has also been isolated from renal tissue, neural tissue, lung tissue, and even BAL fluid (66,91). A large, multicentered RCT was recently able to show a significant mortality benefit from the administration of APC to adults with severe sepsis, a portion of whom also met criteria for ARDS (8). This study outcome suggested a therapeutic potential in manipulating the hemostatic balance in the context of systemic inflammatory disease. However, investigators have not been able to replicate these results in children. The multicentered trial to evaluate the use of APC in infants and children with sepsis was closed early for low likelihood of achieving a favorable risk-to-benefit ratio. At interim analysis, the data monitoring committee for the trial identified an increase in central nervous system bleeding events among children in the APC arm, although mortality was not significantly different between the 2 study groups.

Some experimental evidence supports consideration of a future prospective clinical trial of APC in ALI and ARDS. For example, systemic levels of APC are reduced in patients with ALI and ARDS, even if sepsis is not present, and APC seems to reverse endotoxin-related coagulation and downregulate activity of platelet activator inhibitor-1 activity in the human lung (80). Moreover, intratracheal APC administration has been demonstrated to inhibit the development of pulmonary fibrosis in an experimental animal model of lung injury (92). Finally, systemic administration of APC in an ovine model of inhalational lung injury has been found to produce significant improvements in shunt fraction and pulmonary mechanics without provoking hemorrhagic complications (53). Interpreting the adult APC trial in light of this information raises the possibility that APC exerts key local effects, rather than generalized systemic effects, in patients with severe sepsis, and one such benefit may be the modulation of fibrin turnover in the lung (66). At present, a National Institutes of Health (NIH)-sponsored, phase II RCT of APC in adults with ALI and ARDS is under way. Given the previous experience with APC in children, it does not seem likely that a similar trial will take place in children. It should be emphasized that extrapolating the encouraging results that are obtained with APC therapy in adults to children requires extreme caution, as well as an appreciation of the low mortality rate in pediatric ALI and ARDS and the potential for serious hemorrhagic complications in infants and children.

Modifying Alveolar Fluid Clearance

Laboratory and clinical evidence has demonstrated at least short-term benefits from limiting fluid replacement and accumulation to improve pulmonary compliance in ALI and ARDS (46,87). Studies that related impairment of alveolar fluid clearance to increased mortality in ALI and ARDS suggest that attention to this aspect of care in these conditions should, in theory, offer the promise of reduced mortality. However, the potential for restrictive fluid strategies to translate into an overall clinical outcome benefit may be limited by the possibility of contributing to the development of hypoperfusion and organ dysfunction. Since the local cellular mechanisms of alveolar fluid accumulation and clearance in lung injury have been elucidated, these pathways have attracted interest as potential therapeutic targets with less apparent risk of provoking unwanted systemic effects. As described previously, airway epithelial ion and fluid transport is reduced by alveolar hypoxia, and recent data indicate that this phenomenon can be reversed by reoxygenation, as well as through stimulation of β_1 and β_2 receptors found on alveolar epithelial cells (84). For instance, alveolar fluid clearance appears to be stimulated by β-receptor agonists administered IV or instilled directly into the alveolar space (27). The β-agonist-mediated increase in alveolar fluid clearance is reversible by amiloride, suggesting that β-agonists are specifically upregulating transepithelial sodium transport (27). In fact, it has been demonstrated in a small-animal model of lung injury that exposing the alveoli of hypoxic animals to terbutaline at a dose previously demonstrated to provide therapeutic alveolar fluid concentrations in critically ill humans quickly reversed the hypoxia-related decrease in alveolar fluid clearance (84). In addition, β-agonists are suspected of having other potentially favorable effects, such as inhibiting endotoxin-induced proinflammatory cytokine release, endotoxin-related coagulation, and proinflammatory neutrophil activity (50,94). Attempts to use β-agonists in patients with ALI have so far been limited to small preclinical experiments and a single placebo-controlled trial (52,59). These studies demonstrated a decrease in extravascular lung water in the intervention group, including upregulation of alveolar fluid clearance. At the moment, a large, NIH-sponsored, multicentered RCT of aerosolized albuterol in ALI and ARDS, powered to detect a difference in ventilator-free days, is scheduled to begin.

Nutritional Support

Much attention has been given to the ideal method of delivering nutrition to critically ill patients and, over the past several years, a number of reports support the concept that enteral, rather than parenteral, nutrition can preserve functional integrity of the gastrointestinal mucosal barrier and decrease the potential for intestinal bacterial translocation and systemic infection. Moreover, at least one study has shown that providing enteral nutrition early in the ICU course can potentially reduce mortality and duration of hospital stay in patients with ARDS (74). Nonetheless, a substantial amount of practice variation exists with regard to timing, volume, and composition of enteral feeding in critically ill patients, and no clear consensus guidelines exist to guide clinician practice in this area.

One body of evidence does support the critical role of fatty acid metabolism in the inflammatory cascade. Specifically, linoleic and α-linolenic acid are essential fatty acids that are converted after ingestion to cell membrane-associated lipids, such as arachidonic acid, eicosapentaenoic acid (EPA), and docosahexaenoic acid (DHA), which possess a central role in host immunity. In inflammation, the activity of phospholipases release membrane lipid and the breakdown products of these compounds participate in the potentiation of the host immune response (**Fig. 44.12**). For example, lipoxygenases and cyclooxygenases acting on the arachidonic acid pathway release leukotrienes, prostaglandins, and thromboxanes, while metabolism of other membrane lipids, such as EPA and DHA, release far less active compounds, and the metabolic pathways that lead to their release seem to be inhibited by downregulation of required enzyme systems (44). The central role of the arachidonic acid pathway in inflammation results from the ubiquity of its parent compound, linoleic acid, in the human diet, leading to its over-representation as a cell membrane constituent relative to compounds in the α-linolenic acid family (69). Not surprisingly, increases in arachidonic acid metabolites have been documented in ALI and ARDS; leukotrienes, prostaglandins, and thromboxanes have been identified in plasma, urine, and BAL fluid and are believed to be accountable for many undesired collateral effects of the host immune response, such as vasoconstriction, platelet aggregation, and increased airway resistance. Administration of arachidonic acid precursors to patients with ALI and ARDS seems to increase thromboxane A_2 production, while inhibiting cyclooxygenase activity seems to improve gas exchange, relieve vasoconstriction, and decrease airways resistance (1,9). Thus, the ultimate constituents of cell membranes reflect the balance of ingested fatty acids, and dietary manipulations can influence the characteristics of the host inflammatory response.

Experience with providing alternative ratios of fatty acids in an attempt to repopulate host cell membranes has demonstrated that feedings enriched with ω-3 fatty acids, such as EPA and DHA, decrease proinflammatory cytokine concentrations in plasma and BAL fluid in animal models of ALI and ARDS (24). Apart from 2 clinical trials in ALI (29,71), data in humans is, for the most part, limited to populations with chronic inflammatory conditions (47,70). However, early results do indicate that such dietary manipulations are well tolerated, result

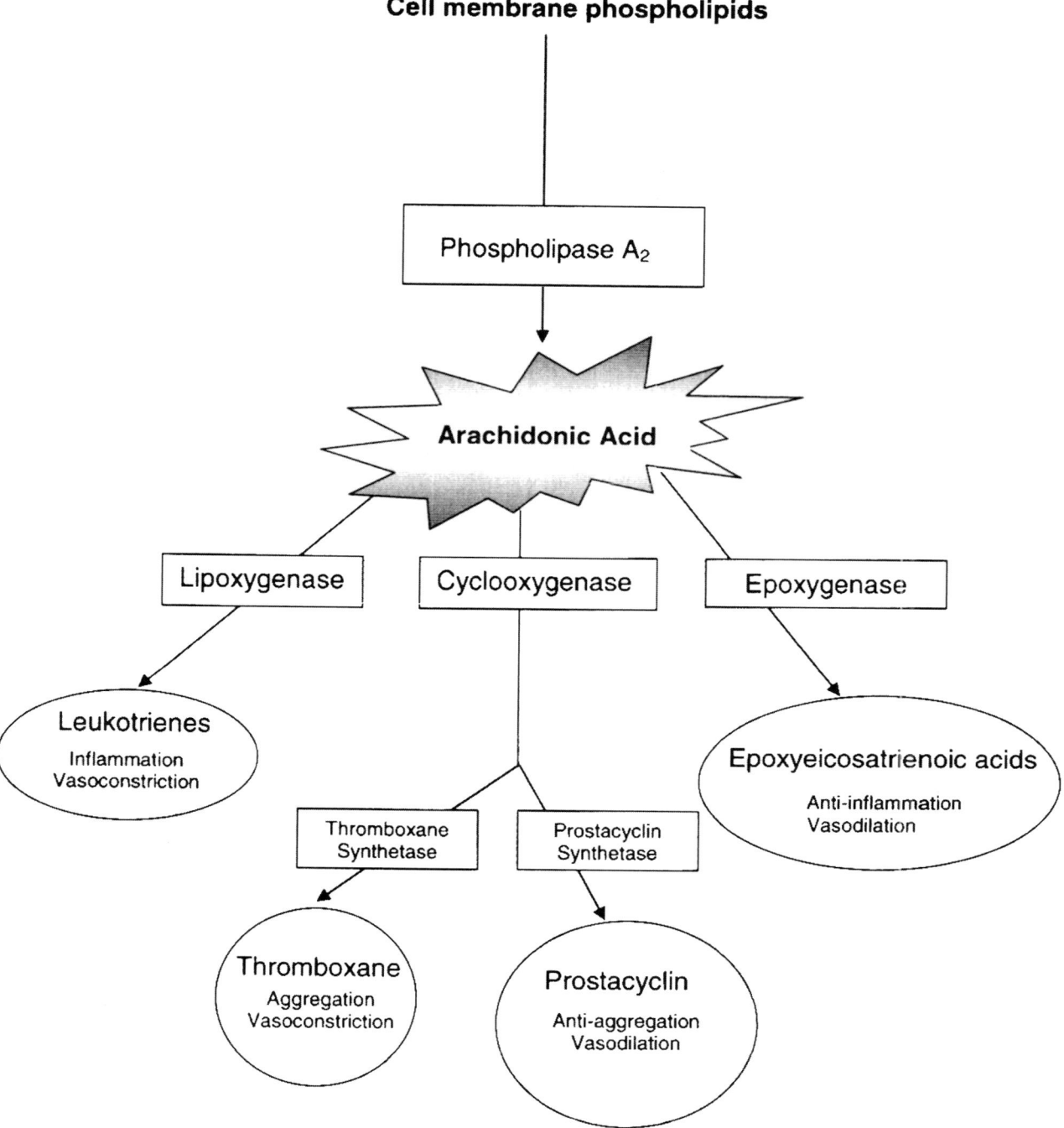

FIGURE 46.12. Cell membrane phospholipid metabolism.

in favorable global physiologic changes within days of their administration and, in some cases, have been associated with measurable clinical benefits. An NIH-sponsored, multicentered RCT is underway to address (a) whether rapidly advancing enteral feedings versus prolonged trophic enteral feedings is preferable in ALI and ARDS and (b) whether supplementation of enteral feedings with ω-3 fatty acids and antioxidant compounds can translate into an outcome benefit.

Role of Extracorporeal Membrane Oxygenation in Pediatric Acute Lung Injury and Acute Respiratory Distress Syndrome

Existing data indicate that ECMO is an effective therapy for hypoxemia associated with pulmonary hypertension in newborns. In the 30-year history of using ECMO for this purpose, nearly 20,000 neonates with respiratory failure have been supported with this technology, and data from the Extracorporeal Life Support Organization (ELSO) registry indicate an overall survival to discharge of 77% in this cohort (82). Highest survival rates occur among infants with the meconium aspiration syndrome (94%), and lowest survival is found among infants with congenital diaphragmatic hernia (52%) (82). These figures are impressive, considering that inclusion criteria for ECMO in most institutions involve selection of patients whose disease severity is estimated to correlate with a mortality of ~80%.

Use of ECMO for pediatric respiratory failure has not met with similar success. Current ELSO registry data indicate that overall survival in this cohort is ~40%–50%, although particularly experienced institutions are reporting survival rates of up to 70%–80% (10,82). These figures are lower than those reported in the neonatal population, perhaps because children who fail "conventional therapy" for ALI and ARDS represent a much more clinically heterogeneous group, with more protracted clinical courses and a higher likelihood of having coexisting nonpulmonary organ dysfunction. Increasingly, pediatric critical care specialists have come to recognize the potential for lung-protective ventilation strategies to limit the development of excess lung injury and cytokine-mediated dysfunction of distant organs. As protective ventilation protocols are more commonly implemented in clinical practice, "conventional therapy" is expected to produce an increasing number of survivors of more and more complex varieties of critical illness, and identifying a role for ECMO in this population is likely to become more difficult. In any case, the best outcomes can be expected from patients with reversible lung injury who are identified as failing conventional therapy before they begin to develop nonpulmonary organ failures. Early recognition of the patient with hypoxic respiratory failure who is destined to fail even the most strategic mode of mechanical ventilation is difficult but necessary to maximize the patient's prospects for survival. A growing amount of data indicate that the trend in oxygenation index, a measurement that characterizes oxygenation as a function of the intensity of ventilatory support, is a reliable indicator of a patient's prospects for responding to a course of mechanical ventilation for severe ALI and ARDS, and serial measures may assist the clinician in identifying patients who may benefit from ECMO, before they transition into a syndrome of irreversible multiorgan dysfunction (5,79).

OUTCOMES IN PEDIATRIC ACUTE LUNG INJURY AND ACUTE RESPIRATORY DISTRESS SYNDROME

Recent data indicate that mortality in pediatric ALI and ARDS seems to be decreasing. Retrospective case series published 10–15 years ago documented mortality rates of 50–75% (18,19,78), while mortality for pediatric ALI and ARDS in the setting of carefully designed prospective clinical trials is now reported as <10% (16,61). Recent prospective observational studies that include more heterogeneous patient cohorts report mortality rates of 22–27% (26,79), but overall mortality among children with ALI and ARDS remains less than the 30–40% mortality rates reported in contemporary adult

trials (2). Highest mortality rates have been traditionally associated with immunocompromised children who develop ALI and ARDS, although current data indicate that survival trends even among this vulnerable subgroup may be increasing in the era of lung-protective ventilation. For example, a recent case series (11) and a subgroup analysis of a larger observational study (79) report up to 40% survival among pediatric bone marrow transplant recipients who require mechanical ventilatory support for respiratory failure, a figure that is higher than those reported during the previous decade (43,58).

It has long been suspected that death from ALI and ARDS rarely occurs as a result of refractory impairment of gas exchange but that it more often occurs in association with the development of multiorgan dysfunction. In fact, current outcomes data support the fact that the presence of one or more nonpulmonary organ failures correlates with a six- to eightfold increase in the likelihood of mortality (26,79), which may explain why ECMO has been used as rescue therapy with only limited success in this population. Several potential mechanisms have been proposed by which multiorgan system failure could follow from single organ failure, including disordered systemic thrombosis and elaboration of proinflammatory cytokines as a result of ALI. Although the impact of anticoagulants, such as APC, on the incidence of nonpulmonary organ dysfunction in ALI has yet to be evaluated in a clinical trial, investigators have been able to demonstrate a decrease in the release of proinflammatory cytokines in patients who receive low-tidal-volume ventilation, compared to high-tidal-volume ventilation (2,63). In summary, a growing amount of data allows us to speculate that the mechanical ventilation strategy may impact outcome by interfering with the development of nonpulmonary organ dysfunction.

CONCLUSION AND FUTURE DIRECTIONS

ALI and ARDS can be conceptualized as the ultimate inflammatory consequences of a variety of potential insults to the lung. Rapid translation of core physiologic principles and laboratory observations to the clinical arena over the past decade has produced a number of high-quality trials in which the benefits of targeted therapies and supportive care strategies have been rigorously evaluated. The pediatric intensivist is faced with the challenge of providing supportive therapies that are carefully titrated to limit their potential for inflicting additional injury and exacerbating the host inflammatory response. Although mortality rates in pediatric ALI/ARDS seem to be decreasing, it is not clear which specific "advances" are responsible for this finding. Despite significant progress in understanding the pathophysiology of these diseases, attempts to translate novel therapies into clinically meaningful outcome benefits have been unsuccessful (Table 46.2). The only intervention that has proven to result in a significant mortality benefit in patients with ARDS is a simple variation on a form of therapy required by all patients with this disease, regardless of etiology; namely, low tidal volume ventilation (2). In any case, the low mortality now reported in pediatric ALI/ARDS trials may indicate the benefits of strictly protocolized, high-quality supportive care, but it also points out the challenges faced by clinical investigators when it comes to designing future trials with sufficient power to provide a reliable estimate of the effects of novel therapies in these diseases. Identifying additional opportunities to further improve outcomes in pediatric ALI/ARDS will likely depend on applying proven or promising therapies and care strategies at the earliest possible time in the disease process and clarifying which subgroups of ALI/ARDS patients stand to benefit from specific interventions.

KEY POINTS

- ALI and ARDS have multiple causes. The host inflammatory response is a key feature in the pathogenesis of these diseases.

- Recent RCTs using explicit supportive care protocols indicate that mortality in pediatric ALI/ARDS is decreasing.

- The mainstay of therapy in pediatric ALI/ARDS is supportive care. Low-tidal-volume mechanical ventilation is the one component of supportive therapy that is associated with a significant mortality benefit in ALI/ARDS.

- Steroids, fluid restriction, surfactant, prone positioning, and inhaled NO, although theoretically beneficial, will not benefit all children with ALI/ARDS when applied indiscriminately.

- Introducing therapy at the earliest possible time in the disease process will be an important goal in future pediatric ALI/ARDS trials.

References

1. Ketoconazole for early treatment of acute lung injury and acute respiratory distress syndrome: a randomized controlled trial. The ARDS Network. *JAMA* 2000;283:1995–2002.
2. Ventilation with lower tidal volumes as compared with traditional tidal volumes for acute lung injury and the acute respiratory distress syndrome. The Acute Respiratory Distress Syndrome Network. *N Engl J Med* 2000;342:1301–8.
3. Altemeier WA, Matute-Bello G, Frevert CW, et al. Mechanical ventilation with moderate tidal volumes synergistically increases lung cytokine response to systemic endotoxin. *Am J Physiol Lung Cell Mol Physiol* 2004;287:L533–42.
4. Anzueto A, Baughman RP, Guntupalli KK, et al. Aerosolized surfactant in adults with sepsis-induced acute respiratory distress syndrome. Exosurf Acute Respiratory Distress Syndrome Sepsis Study Group. *N Engl J Med* 1996;334:1417–21.
5. Arnold JH, Hanson JH, Toro-Figuero LO, et al. Prospective, randomized comparison of high-frequency oscillatory ventilation and conventional mechanical ventilation in pediatric respiratory failure. *Crit Care Med* 1994;22:1530–9.
6. Bernard GR, Artigas A, Brigham KL, et al. The American-European Consensus Conference on ARDS. Definitions, mechanisms, relevant outcomes, and clinical trial coordination. *Am J Respir Crit Care Med* 1994;149:818–24.
7. Bernard GR, Korley V, Chee P, et al. Persistent generation of peptido leukotrienes in patients with the adult respiratory distress syndrome. *Am Rev Respir Dis* 1991;144:263–7.
8. Bernard GR, Vincent JL, Laterre PF, et al. Efficacy and safety of recombinant human activated protein C for severe sepsis. *N Engl J Med* 2001;344:699–709.
9. Bernard GR, Wheeler AP, Russell JA, et al. The effects of ibuprofen on the physiology and survival of patients with sepsis. The Ibuprofen in Sepsis Study Group. *N Engl J Med* 1997;336:912–8.
10. Bohn D. Acute hypoxic respiratory failure in children. In: Van Meurs K LK, Peek G, Zwischenberger J (ed), ECMO: Extracorporeal cardiopulmonary support in critical care, 3rd edition. Ann Arbor: Extracorporeal Life Support Organization, 2006;329–61.
11. Bojko T, Notterman DA, Greenwald BM, et al. Acute hypoxemic respiratory failure in children following bone marrow transplantation: an outcome and pathologic study. *Crit Care Med* 1995;23:755–9.
12. Broccard A, Shapiro RS, Schmitz LL, et al. Prone positioning attenuates and redistributes ventilator-induced lung injury in dogs. *Crit Care Med* 2000;28:295–303.
13. Broccard AF, Shapiro RS, Schmitz LL, et al. Influence of prone position on the extent and distribution of lung injury in a high tidal volume oleic acid model of acute respiratory distress syndrome. *Crit Care Med* 1997;25:16–27.
14. Choi G WE, Bresser P, et al. Lung-protective mechanical ventilation attenuates fibrin generation in non-injured lungs (Abstract). *Am J Respir Crit Care Med* 2005;171:A244.
15. Chu EK, Whitehead T, Slutsky AS. Effects of cyclic opening and closing at low- and high-volume ventilation on bronchoalveolar lavage cytokines. *Crit Care Med* 2004;32:168–74.
16. Curley MA, Hibberd PL, Fineman LD, et al. Effect of prone positioning on clinical outcomes in children with acute lung injury: a randomized controlled trial. *JAMA* 2005;294:229–37.
17. Dahlem P, Bos AP, Haitsma JJ, et al. Alveolar fibrinolytic capacity suppressed by injurious mechanical ventilation. *Intensive Care Med* 2005;31:724–32.
18. Davis SL, Furman DP, Costarino AT, Jr. Adult respiratory distress syndrome in children: associated disease, clinical course, and predictors of death. *J Pediatr* 1993;123:35–45.
19. DeBruin W, Notterman DA, Magid M, et al. Acute hypoxemic respiratory failure in infants and children: clinical and pathologic characteristics. *Crit Care Med* 1992;20:1223–34.
20. Dellinger RP, Zimmerman JL, Taylor RW, et al. Effects of inhaled nitric oxide in patients with acute respiratory distress syndrome: results of a randomized phase II trial. Inhaled Nitric Oxide in ARDS Study Group.[comment]. *Critical Care Medicine* 1998;26:15–23.
21. Desai SR, Wells AU, Rubens MB, et al. Acute respiratory distress syndrome: CT abnormalities at long-term follow-up. *Radiology* 1999;210:29–35.
22. Dobyns EL, Anas NG, Fortenberry JD, et al. Interactive effects of high-frequency oscillatory ventilation and inhaled nitric oxide in acute hypoxemic respiratory failure in pediatrics. *Crit Care Med* 2002;30:2425–9.
23. Dobyns EL, Cornfield DN, Anas NG, et al. Multicenter randomized controlled trial of the effects of inhaled nitric oxide therapy on gas exchange in children with acute hypoxemic respiratory failure. *J Pediatr* 1999;134:406–12.
24. Endres S, Ghorbani R, Kelley VE, et al. The effect of dietary supplementation with n-3 polyunsaturated fatty acids on the synthesis of interleukin-1 and tumor necrosis factor by mononuclear cells. *N Engl J Med* 1989;320:265–71.
25. Falke KJ, Pontoppidan H, Kumar A, et al. Ventilation with end-expiratory pressure in acute lung disease. *J Clin Invest* 1972;51:2315–23.
26. Flori HR, Glidden DV, Rutherford GW, et al. Pediatric acute lung injury: prospective evaluation of risk factors associated with mortality. *Am J Respir Crit Care Med* 2005;171:995–1001.
27. Folkesson HG, Matthay M. Alveolar epithelial ion and fluid transport: Recent progress. *Am J Respir Cell Mol Biol* 2006;35(1):10–9.
28. Fratacci MD, Frostell CG, Chen TY, et al. Inhaled nitric oxide. A selective pulmonary vasodilator of heparin-protamine vasoconstriction in sheep. *Anesthesiology* 1991;75:990–9.
29. Gadek JE, DeMichele SJ, Karlstad MD, et al. Effect of enteral feeding with eicosapentaenoic acid, gamma-linolenic acid, and antioxidants in patients with acute respiratory distress syndrome. Enteral Nutrition in ARDS Study Group. *Crit Care Med* 1999;27:1409–20.
30. Gajic O, Dara SI, Mendez JL, et al. Ventilator-associated lung injury in patients without acute lung injury at the onset of mechanical ventilation. *Crit Care Med* 2004;32:1817–24.
31. Gattinoni L, Caironi P, Pelosi P, et al. What has computed tomography taught us about the acute respiratory distress syndrome? *Am J Respir Crit Care Med* 2001;164:1701–11.
32. Gattinoni L, Pelosi P, Suter PM, et al. Acute respiratory distress syndrome caused by pulmonary and extrapulmonary disease. Different syndromes? *Am J Respir Crit Care Med* 1998;158:3–11.
33. Gattinoni L, Tognoni G, Pesenti A, et al. Effect of prone positioning on the survival of patients with acute respiratory failure. *N Engl J Med* 2001;345:568–73.
34. Glenny RW, Lamm WJ, Albert RK, et al. Gravity is a minor determinant of pulmonary blood flow distribution. *J Appl Physiol* 1991;71:620–9.
35. Gong MN, Wei Z, Xu LL, et al. Polymorphism in the surfactant protein-B gene, gender, and the risk of direct pulmonary injury and ARDS. *Chest* 2004;125:203–11.
36. Gregory TJ, Steinberg KP, Spragg R, et al. Bovine surfactant therapy for patients with acute respiratory distress syndrome. *Am J Respir Crit Care Med* 1997;155:1309–15.
37. Guerin C, Gaillard S, Lemasson S, et al. Effects of systematic prone positioning in hypoxemic acute respiratory failure: a randomized controlled trial. *JAMA* 2004;292:2379–87.
38. Hallman M, Spragg R, Harrell JH, et al. Evidence of lung surfactant abnormality in respiratory failure. Study of bronchoalveolar lavage phospholipids, surface activity, phospholipase activity, and plasma myoinositol. *J Clin Invest* 1982;70:673–83.
39. Hebert PC, Wells G, Blajchman MA, et al. A multicenter, randomized, controlled clinical trial of transfusion requirements in critical care. Transfusion Requirements in Critical Care Investigators, Canadian Critical Care Trials Group. *N Engl J Med* 1999;340:409–17.
40. Hilbert G, Gruson D, Vargas F, et al. Noninvasive ventilation in immunosuppressed patients with pulmonary infiltrates, fever, and acute respiratory failure. *N Engl J Med* 2001;344:481–7.
41. Hlastala MP, Glenny RW. Vascular structure determines pulmonary blood flow distribution. *News Physiol Sci* 1999;14:182–6.

42. Hudson LD, Milberg JA, Anardi D, et al. Clinical risks for development of the acute respiratory distress syndrome. *Am J Respir Crit Care Med* 1995;151:293–301.

43. Keenan HT, Bratton SL, Martin LD, et al. Outcome of children who require mechanical ventilatory support after bone marrow transplantation. *Crit Care Med* 2000;28:830–5.

44. Kumar KV, Rao SM, Gayani R, et al. Oxidant stress and essential fatty acids in patients with risk and established ARDS. *Clin Chim Acta* 2000;298:111–20.

45. Lamm WJ, Graham MM, Albert RK. Mechanism by which the prone position improves oxygenation in acute lung injury. *Am J Respir Crit Care Med* 1994;150:184–93.

46. Long R, Breen PH, Mayers I, et al. Treatment of canine aspiration pneumonitis: fluid volume reduction vs. fluid volume expansion. *J Appl Physiol* 1988;65:1736–44.

47. MacLean CH, Mojica WA, Newberry SJ, et al. Systematic review of the effects of n-3 fatty acids in inflammatory bowel disease. *Am J Clin Nutr* 2005;82:611–9.

48. Malo J, Ali J, Wood LD. How does positive end-expiratory pressure reduce intrapulmonary shunt in canine pulmonary edema? *J Appl Physiol* 1984;57:1002–10.

49. Mancebo J, Fernandez R, Blanch L, et al. Multicenter Trial of Prolonged Prone Ventilation in Severe Acute Respiratory Distress Syndrome. *Am J Respir Crit Care Med* 2006.

50. Maris NA, de Vos AF, Dessing MC, et al. Antiinflammatory effects of salmeterol after inhalation of lipopolysaccharide by healthy volunteers. *Am J Respir Crit Care Med* 2005;172:878–84.

51. Marshall RP, Webb S, Bellingan GJ, et al. Angiotensin converting enzyme insertion/deletion polymorphism is associated with susceptibility and outcome in acute respiratory distress syndrome. *Am J Respir Crit Care Med* 2002;166:646–50.

52. Matthay MA, Abraham E. Beta-adrenergic agonist therapy as a potential treatment for acute lung injury. *Am J Respir Crit Care Med* 2006;173:254–5.

53. Maybauer M, Maybauer D, Fraser JT, et al. Recombinant human activated protein C improves pulmonary function in ovine acute lung injury resulting from smoke inhalation and sepsis. *Critical Care Medicine* 2006;34.

54. Meduri GU, Headley AS, Golden E, et al. Effect of prolonged methylprednisolone therapy in unresolving acute respiratory distress syndrome: a randomized controlled trial. *JAMA* 1998;280:159–65.

55. Mehta NM, Arnold JH. Genetic polymorphisms in acute respiratory distress syndrome: new approach to an old problem. *Crit Care Med* 2005;33:2443–5.

56. Mutoh T, Lamm WJ, Embree LJ, et al. Abdominal distension alters regional pleural pressures and chest wall mechanics in pigs in vivo. *J Appl Physiol* 1991;70:2611–8.

57. Newman JH. Pulmonary hypertension. *Am J Respir Crit Care Med* 2005;172:1072–7.

58. Nichols DG, Walker LK, Wingard JR, et al. Predictors of acute respiratory failure after bone marrow transplantation in children. *Crit Care Med* 1994;22:1485–91.

59. Perkins GD, McAuley DF, Thickett DR, et al. The beta-agonist lung injury trial (BALTI): a randomized placebo-controlled clinical trial. *Am J Respir Crit Care Med* 2006;173:281–7.

60. Prange HD. Laplace's law and the alveolus: a misconception of anatomy and a misapplication of physics. *Adv Physiol Educ* 2003;27:34–40.

61. Randolph AG, Meert KL, O'Neil ME, et al. The feasibility of conducting clinical trials in infants and children with acute respiratory failure. *Am J Respir Crit Care Med* 2003;167:1334–40.

62. Ranieri VM, Brienza N, Santostasi S, et al. Impairment of lung and chest wall mechanics in patients with acute respiratory distress syndrome: role of abdominal distension. *Am J Respir Crit Care Med* 1997;156:1082–91.

63. Ranieri VM, Suter PM, Tortorella C, et al. Effect of mechanical ventilation on inflammatory mediators in patients with acute respiratory distress syndrome: a randomized controlled trial. *JAMA* 1999;282:54–61.

64. Rhen T, Cidlowski JA. Antiinflammatory action of glucocorticoids–new mechanisms for old drugs. *N Engl J Med* 2005;353:1711–23.

65. Roberts JD, Jr. , Fineman JR, Morin FC, 3rd, et al. Inhaled nitric oxide and persistent pulmonary hypertension of the newborn. The Inhaled Nitric Oxide Study Group. *N Engl J Med* 1997;336:605–10.

66. Schultz MJ, Haitsma JJ, Zhang H, et al. Pulmonary coagulopathy as a new target in therapeutic studies of acute lung injury or pneumonia–a review. *Crit Care Med* 2006;34:871–7.

67. Schultz MJ, Millo J, Levi M, et al. Local activation of coagulation and inhibition of fibrinolysis in the lung during ventilator associated pneumonia. *Thorax* 2004;59:130–5.

68. Shimabukuro DW, Sawa T, Gropper MA. Injury and repair in lung and airways. *Crit Care Med* 2003;31:S524–31.

69. Simopoulos AP. Omega-3 fatty acids in health and disease and in growth and development. *Am J Clin Nutr* 1991;54:438–63.

70. Simopoulos AP. Omega-3 fatty acids in inflammation and autoimmune diseases. *J Am Coll Nutr* 2002;21:495–505.

71. Singer P, Theilla M, Fisher H, et al. Benefit of an enteral diet enriched with eicosapentaenoic acid and gamma-linolenic acid in ventilated patients with acute lung injury. *Crit Care Med* 2006;34:1033–8.

72. Slutsky AS, Tremblay LN. Multiple system organ failure. Is mechanical ventilation a contributing factor? *Am J Respir Crit Care Med* 1998;157:1721–5.

73. Spragg RG, Lewis JF, Walmrath HD, et al. Effect of recombinant surfactant protein C-based surfactant on the acute respiratory distress syndrome. *N Engl J Med* 2004;351:884–92.

74. Stapleton R, Stainberg D, Rubenfenld G, et al. Early versus delayed enteral feeding in medical ICU patients with acute lung injury. *Proc Amer Thor Soc* 2005;2:A36.

75. Steinberg KP, Hudson LD, Goodman RB, et al. Efficacy and safety of corticosteroids for persistent acute respiratory distress syndrome. *N Engl J Med* 2006;354:1671–84.

76. Taylor RW, Zimmerman JL, Dellinger RP, et al. Low-dose inhaled nitric oxide in patients with acute lung injury: a randomized controlled trial. *JAMA* 2004;291:1603–9.

77. The National Heart L, and Blood Institute Acute Respiratory Distress Syndrome (ARDS) Clinical Trials Network. Pulmonary-artery versus central venous catheter to guide treatment of acute lung injury. *New Engl J Med* 2006;354:2213–24.

78. Timmons OD, Dean JM, Vernon DD. Mortality rates and prognostic variables in children with adult respiratory distress syndrome. *J Pediatr* 1991;119:896–9.

79. Trachsel D, McCrindle BW, Nakagawa S, et al. Oxygenation index predicts outcome in children with acute hypoxemic respiratory failure. *Am J Respir Crit Care Med* 2005;172:206–11.

80. van der Poll T, Levi M, Nick JA, et al. Activated protein C inhibits local coagulation after intrapulmonary delivery of endotoxin in humans. *Am J Respir Crit Care Med* 2005;171:1125–8.

81. van Kaam AH, Haitsma JJ, Dik WA, et al. Response to exogenous surfactant is different during open lung and conventional ventilation. *Crit Care Med* 2004;32:774–80.

82. Van Meurs K, Hintz S, Sheehan A. ECMO for Neonatal Respiratory Failure. In: Van Meurs K, Lally K, Peek G, et al., eds. *ECMO: Extracorporeal Cardiopulmonary Support in Critical Care, 3rd ed.* Ann Arbor: Extracorporeal Life Support Organization 2006:273–306.

83. Vitali SH, Randolph AG. Assessing the quality of case-control association studies on the genetic basis of sepsis. *Pediatr Crit Care Med* 2005;6:S74–7.

84. Vivona ML, Matthay M, Chabaud MB, et al. Hypoxia reduces alveolar epithelial sodium and fluid transport in rats: reversal by beta-adrenergic agonist treatment. *Am J Respir Cell Mol Biol* 2001;25:554–61.

85. Ware LB, Matthay MA. The acute respiratory distress syndrome. *N Engl J Med* 2000;342:1334–49.

86. Ware LB, Matthay MA. Clinical practice. Acute pulmonary edema. *N Engl J Med* 2005;353:2788–96.

87. Wiedemann HP, Wheeler AP, Bernard GR, et al. Comparison of two fluid-management strategies in acute lung injury. *N Engl J Med* 2006;354:2564–75.

88. Willson DF, Thomas NJ, Markovitz BP, et al. Effect of exogenous surfactant (calfactant) in pediatric acute lung injury: a randomized controlled trial. *JAMA* 2005;293:470–6.

89. Wright JR. Pulmonary surfactant: a front line of lung host defense. *J Clin Invest* 2003;111:1453–5.

90. Wu H, Kuzmenko A, Wan S, et al. Surfactant proteins A and D inhibit the growth of Gram-negative bacteria by increasing membrane permeability. *J Clin Invest* 2003;111:1589–602.

91. Yamamoto K, Loskutoff DJ. Extrahepatic expression and regulation of protein C in the mouse. *Am J Pathol* 1998;153:547–55.

92. Yasui H, Gabazza EC, Tamaki S, et al. Intratracheal administration of activated protein C inhibits bleomycin-induced lung fibrosis in the mouse. *Am J Respir Crit Care Med* 2001;163:1660–8.

93. Ye SQ, Simon BA, Maloney JP, et al. Pre-B-cell colony-enhancing factor as a potential novel biomarker in acute lung injury. *Am J Respir Crit Care Med* 2005;171:361–70.

94. Zhang H, Kim YK, Govindarajan A, et al. Effect of adrenoreceptors on endotoxin-induced cytokines and lipid peroxidation in lung explants. *Am J Respir Crit Care Med* 1999;160:1703–10.

CHAPTER 47 ■ CHRONIC RESPIRATORY FAILURE

THOMAS G. KEENS • SHEILA S. KUN • SALLY L. DAVIDSON WARD

Advances in pediatric critical care medicine have increased survival from catastrophic childhood illnesses and injuries. However, this improved survival has come at a price. Sometimes, children who would otherwise have died survive with chronic illnesses (3,4,43,48). Children treated in the PICU for acute respiratory failure (ARF) may emerge with chronic lung disease. A smaller proportion of survivors develops chronic respiratory failure (CRF), and may require long-term ventilatory support (4,34,38,47). Many PICU children already had significant chronic disease when they were admitted (34). Thus, their reserve was likely already decreased, making it more likely that these patients may develop CRF (34). Rather than being maintained as long-term residents in the PICU, most of these children can now be cared for in the home, even if ventilatory support is required. Mechanical ventilation can now be performed in the home, providing a relatively good quality of life for many children (2,10,20,21,36). This chapter reviews CRF, what can be done to attempt to wean patients from long-term assisted ventilation in the PICU, and how to care for the child who requires home mechanical ventilation.

The ability to sustain spontaneous ventilation requires adequate function of the mechanisms that control ventilation, ventilatory muscle function, and lung mechanics. Significant dysfunction of any of these three components of the respiratory system may impair a child's ability to breathe spontaneously. Respiratory failure occurs when central respiratory drive and/or ventilatory muscle power are inadequate to overcome the respiratory load (Fig. 47.1). Chronic respiratory failure occurs if the cause of this imbalance is not reversible, and chronic ventilatory support will be required. Once the decision has been made to institute long−term mechanical ventilation in an infant or child with a stable or progressive disorder, the child cannot reside indefinitely in a PICU (1,2,10,20,21,36). Thus, children with CRF must be cared for in the home or in chronic care facilities. Chronic ventilatory support in the home is, for many patients, a safe and relatively inexpensive alternative.

The goals of home ventilatory support for children with CRF are quite different from the goals of assisted ventilation for children with ARF in the PICU (11,24,28,49). The former include (a) ensuring the medical safety of the child, (b) preventing or minimizing complications, (c) optimizing the child's quality of life, (d) maximizing rehabilitative potential, and (e) reintegrating the child with his family. Medical safety is ensured by attempting to normalize respiratory function. The child's quality of life is optimized by rehabilitation to as normal a lifestyle as possible and by reintegration into the family. To achieve these goals, it is necessary to adopt a different approach from that employed in the care of children with ARF.

RESPIRATORY SYSTEM IN CHILDREN

Neurologic control of breathing must ensure adequate ventilation to meet the metabolic needs of the body during sleep, rest, and exercise. Ventilation varies with the state of the individual. It becomes less adequate during sleep, and it is less responsive to modulation by chemoreceptor input during rapid eye movement (REM) or active sleep. It is not surprising that sleep is the most vulnerable period for the development of inadequate ventilation in disorders of respiratory control (5,24,49). Immaturity of the respiratory control systems in the infant and young child predispose to apnea and hypoventilation. Further, the infant spends ∼50% of sleep time in REM sleep (in contrast to 15–20% spent by the adult), and an infant sleeps for a longer portion of the day. Active sleep is associated with greater variation in respiratory timing and amplitude, resulting in periods of inadequate gas exchange. Thus, CRF always includes inadequate gas exchange during sleep.

The diaphragm must perform the work of breathing. Ventilatory muscles of normal strength and endurance may fatigue in the face of increased respiratory loads (31,35). On the other hand, weak ventilatory muscles may successfully perform the work of breathing when pulmonary mechanics are optimal, yet fail when pulmonary mechanics worsen, as during respiratory infections (17). The factors that predispose to ventilatory muscle fatigue include hypoxia, hypercapnia, acidosis, malnutrition, hyperinflation, changes in pulmonary mechanics that cause increased work of breathing, and disuse. The infant diaphragm has a significantly smaller proportion of fatigue−resistant muscle fibers and is weaker than the diaphragm of older children and adults (22). Thus, the infant is predisposed to ventilatory muscle fatigue. Underlying muscle pathology will further limit ventilatory muscle endurance. Therefore, infants and children are predisposed to respiratory failure compared to adults, because of differences in the control of sleep and breathing and decreased ventilatory muscle strength and endurance.

ACUTE RESPIRATORY FAILURE

The clinical picture, etiology, pathophysiology, medical management, and ventilator management of ARF are discussed in detail in other chapters of this text. For purposes of providing a better understanding of CRF, however, we can contrast it with aspects of ARF. Acute respiratory failure is most

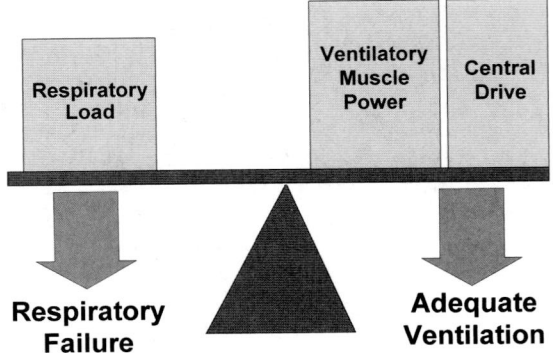

FIGURE 47.1. The respiratory balance. In normal individuals, ventilatory muscle power and central drive are more than adequate to overcome the respiratory load, tipping the balance to the right, which results in adequate ventilation. However, when ventilatory muscle power and/or central drive are sufficiently decreased and/or the respiratory load is sufficiently increased, or some combination thereof, ventilatory muscle power and central drive may not be sufficient to overcome the respiratory load. The balance will tip to the left, and respiratory failure will result.

commonly seen in children who experience the abrupt onset of a severe respiratory disorder, such as severe pneumonia or acute respiratory distress syndrome. This is accompanied by an increase in the respiratory load that exceeds the ability of the child's physiology to continue performing that level of work. The ventilatory muscles fatigue while attempting to exert increased effort for breathing (31,35). Thus, the child breathes inadequately, which results in hypoxia, hypercapnia, and acidosis. If the work of breathing is plotted on the ordinate, the fatigue threshold indicates the highest level of work that a subject can sustain indefinitely without fatigue (**Fig. 47.2**). If the work of breathing associated with a respiratory illness remains below the fatigue threshold, a child can continue to breathe spontaneously, and ARF may not occur. In a typical episode of

ARF, the work of breathing rapidly exceeds the child's fatigue threshold.

Most children with ARF can be weaned from mechanically assisted ventilation when the work of breathing decreases with recovery from the lung disease. Usually, in the PICU, ventilator settings for children with ARF are adjusted to provide the minimal level of support necessary to achieve adequate gas exchange. Weaning is performed in such a way that the patient assumes increasing proportions of the work of breathing. As the primary task of a child with ARF is to wean from assisted ventilation, settings are adjusted so that the child expends all available energy for the work of breathing, leaving little or no reserve for other activities. However, this strategy is only successful if the underlying cause of respiratory failure is subsiding.

CHRONIC RESPIRATORY FAILURE

Chronic respiratory failure implies that a chronic, perhaps irreversible, underlying respiratory disorder is causing respiratory insufficiency that results in inadequate ventilation or hypoxia (28). The diagnosis of CRF is usually made once repeated attempts to wean from assisted ventilation have failed for at least 1 month in a child without superimposed acute respiratory disease or a patient who has a diagnosis with no prospect of being weaned from the ventilator (such as high spinal cord injury) (**Fig. 47.3**). For purposes of this discussion, the term "prolonged respiratory failure" will be used for children who are difficult to wean from mechanically assisted ventilation but have not yet satisfied the time criteria for the diagnosis of CRF, defined as at least one month of ventilator dependence. Some children with prolonged respiratory failure will develop CRF if appropriate therapeutic interventions fail, but others will be able to be weaned from mechanically assisted ventilation. The proper approach to a patient with prolonged respiratory failure must include addressing all barriers to weaning. Keeping the

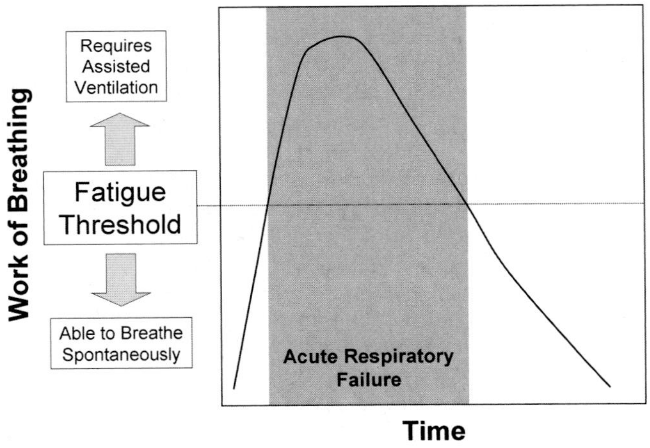

FIGURE 47.2. Acute respiratory failure. Work of breathing (*Y axis*) increases with worsening lung disease until it exceeds the fatigue threshold, at which point, mechanically assisted ventilation is required until the lung disease improves to the point at which work of breathing falls below the fatigue threshold (*shaded area*). Then, the child is able to perform the work of breathing required to breathe spontaneously and he can be weaned from mechanical ventilation.

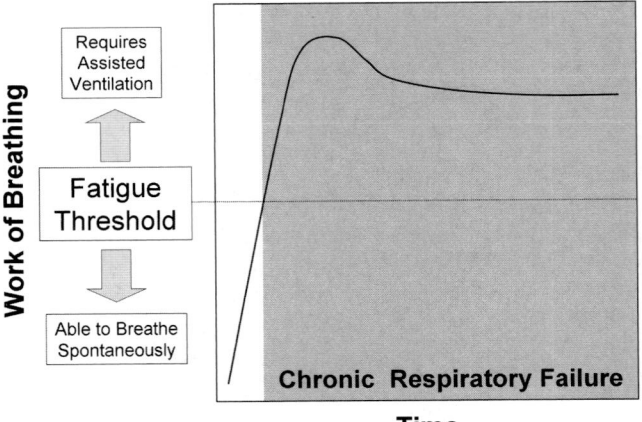

FIGURE 47.3. Chronic respiratory failure. Work of breathing (*Y axis*) increases with worsening lung disease until it exceeds the fatigue threshold. Mechanically assisted ventilation is required at this point (*shaded area*). However, the lung disease does not improve to the point that work of breathing falls below the fatigue threshold. Thus, the child is not able to perform the work of breathing required to breathe spontaneously and remains ventilator-dependent.

respiratory system balance in mind (Fig. 47.1), therapy should be directed toward reducing the respiratory load, improving ventilatory muscle power, and increasing central respiratory drive as much as possible.

Reduce the Respiratory Load

Reducing the respiratory load requires that pulmonary mechanics be optimized (26). Infection should be treated vigorously with appropriate antibiotics. Aggressive chest physiotherapy, with inhaled bronchodilators and anti-inflammatory agents, reduces atelectasis and pulmonary resistance by enhancing mucociliary activity and clearing secretions. In infants and young children, respiratory failure is often complicated by increased lung fluid, either interstitial or alveolar edema. Thus, diuretics may be helpful. Careful attention to electrolyte balance is required whenever diuretics are used.

Increase Ventilatory Muscle Power

Ventilatory muscle power is adversely affected by many conditions commonly present in children with chronic lung disease. The work output of the ventilatory muscles is measured as the generated pleural, airway, or transdiaphragmatic pressures (17). Fatigue of the ventilatory muscles occurs when muscle energy production is hindered (22,23,31,35). Ventilatory muscles cannot perform work if they cannot produce energy. Hypoxia, hypercapnia, and acidosis all decrease the efficiency of muscle energy production, predisposing the muscle to fatigue. Malnutrition decreases oxidative energy-producing enzymes in muscle. Hyperinflation places the diaphragm at a mechanical disadvantage, so that the same amount of muscle tension develops less pressure. Infants have decreased strength and endurance of the ventilatory muscles compared to adults or older children (22). If the child has received assisted ventilation for some time, muscle changes may occur from disuse (23). Thus, even a child who does not have a diagnosis of a neuromuscular disorder may have ventilatory muscle dysfunction or fatigue, contributing to respiratory failure. Bronchopulmonary dysplasia, for example, is a primary lung disease associated with hypoxia, hypercapnia, hyperinflation, malnutrition, and infancy, all of which decrease ventilatory muscle endurance. Thus, therapy should be directed toward adequate oxygenation and ventilation, removal of airway obstruction and hyperinflation, adequate nutrition, and ventilatory muscle training (23). Pharmacologic neuromuscular blockade, sedation, and pain medications may also decrease ventilatory muscle function. When possible, these medications should be weaned as tolerated. Attention to the optimization of ventilatory muscle function is an important adjunct to the treatment of any child with prolonged respiratory failure.

Ventilator weaning techniques should be designed to improve ventilatory muscle power in an attempt to raise the child's fatigue threshold (**Fig. 47.4**). The desired approach is similar to athletic training of any other skeletal muscle (23). Athletes train for performance by bursts of muscle activity (training stress) followed by rest periods. Sprint weaning is analogous to this form of athletic training, and ventilatory muscle training may result. Intermittent mandatory ventilation weaning imposes a

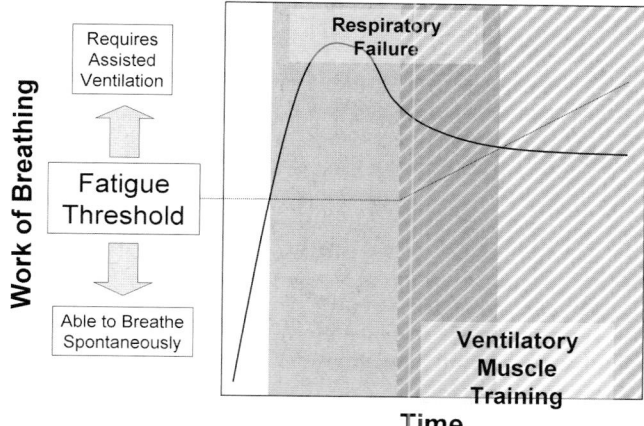

FIGURE 47.4. Ventilatory muscle training. Work of breathing (*Y axis*) increases with worsening lung disease until it exceeds the fatigue threshold. Mechanically assisted ventilation is required at this point (*shaded area*). The lung disease does not improve to the point that work of breathing falls below the fatigue threshold. However, ventilatory muscle training increases the work of breathing that the patient can perform (*hatched area*), thus raising the fatigue threshold until it exceeds the work of breathing. Respiratory failure overlaps ventilatory muscle training until the fatigue threshold exceeds the required work of breathing. Then, the child is able to perform the work of breathing required to breathe spontaneously and can be weaned.

gradually increasing functional demand on the ventilatory muscles, but it does not provide the alternating stress ("sprints") and rest training pattern. In our experience, some children who have not been weaned from mechanically assisted ventilation by traditional intermittent mandatory ventilation weaning approaches were able to be weaned by sprint weaning, though this may take several weeks.

In a child with prolonged respiratory failure, sprint weaning, or sprinting, is instituted in the following way. Ventilator settings are adjusted to completely meet the child's ventilatory demands by the use of a physiologic ventilator rate for age and the attainment of normal noninvasive monitoring of gas exchange (SpO$_2$ $\geq$95% and end-tidal PCO$_2$ [P$_{ET}$CO$_2$] of 30–35 torr). The goal is to provide total ventilatory muscle rest. The patient is then removed from the ventilator for short periods of time during wakefulness, approximately four times per day. In some cases, these initial sprints may last only 1–2 mins. The child is carefully monitored noninvasively during sprints to prevent hypoxia or hypercapnia, using pulse oximetry and P$_{ET}$CO$_2$ monitoring. Increased supplemental O$_2$ may be required during sprinting. Guidelines for terminating sprints, such as a SpO$_2$ of <95% or a P$_{ET}$CO$_2$ of >45–50 torr, should be provided as written orders. In addition, if the child develops signs of distress, tachypnea, retractions, diaphoresis, tachycardia, hypoxia, or hypercapnia, the sprint should be stopped. Note that the child with a respiratory control disorder may not exhibit these signs of distress. If the child develops signs of distress, tachypnea, retractions, hypoxia, or hypercapnia, the sprint is stopped. The length of each sprint is increased daily as tolerated. The physician should avoid the temptation to increase the sprint length too rapidly, as this often hinders the progress of weaning. Initially, sprinting should be performed only during wakefulness, as ventilatory muscle function and central respiratory drive are more intact during wakefulness than during sleep. Usually a

APPROACHES TO WEANING CHILDREN WITH PROLONGED RESPIRATORY FAILURE

Reduce the respiratory load	
Relieve bronchospasm	Aerosolized bronchodilator
	Aerosolized corticosteroids or other anti-inflammatory agents
Remove excessive pulmonary secretions	Chest physiotherapy
	If ventilatory muscle weakness, consider cough assist device
Reduce lung fluid and pulmonary edema	Diuretics with careful attention to electrolyte balance
Treat pulmonary infections	Antibiotics
	Consider aerosolized antibiotics for chronically colonized patients

Increase ventilatory muscle power	
Increase ventilatory muscle strength	Eliminate or reduce hyperinflation
Increase ventilatory muscle endurance	Adequate oxygenation
	Avoid hypercapnia
	Avoid acidosis
	Achieve optimal nutrition
	Reduce respiratory load (as above)
Train ventilatory muscles to improve strength and endurance	Sprint weaning

Improve central respiratory drive	
Avoid hypochloremic alkalosis	Maintain serum Cl^- $\geq$95 mEq/dL
	Avoid chronic alkalosis
Reset chemoreceptors	Ventilate to adequate oxygenation (Spo_2 $\geq$95%) and ventilation ($P_{ET}co_2$ $\leq$40 torr)
Avoid respiratory depression	Reduce or avoid central nervous system-depressant medications

child is weaned off the ventilator completely during wakefulness, before attempting to reduce sleeping ventilatory support. It is important to remember that sprint weaning requires that the child receive complete ventilatory support during rests (16). Because sprint weaning simulates athletic training, better success has been observed with this form of ventilator weaning in prolonged respiratory failure if ventilatory muscle fatigue is thought to be a component. In effect, this technique raises the fatigue threshold, so that a child can perform an increased level of work of breathing and sustain adequate spontaneous ventilation (23) (Fig. 47.4).

Improve Central Respiratory Drive

Central respiratory drive can be impaired by metabolic imbalance (5,24,46,49). Chronic metabolic alkalosis, for example, decreases central respiratory drive. Thus, electrolyte balance should be maintained, with careful attention to maintaining serum chloride concentrations of >95 mEq/dL and avoiding alkalosis. Chronic hypoxia and/or hypercapnia may cause habituation of chemoreceptors, leading to a decrease in central respiratory center stimulation and decreased central respiratory drive. Although methylxanthines have been used to stimulate central respiratory drive by some clinicians, Swaminathan demonstrated no effect of theophylline on ventilatory responses to hypercapnia or hypoxia in normal subjects (41). Further, children with central hypoventilation syndrome have chemoreceptor dysfunction, which does not respond to pharmacologic

stimulation (5,24,46,49). In general, pharmacologic respiratory stimulants are probably ineffective in the treatment of prolonged respiratory failure.

This three-pronged approach to children with prolonged respiratory failure may result in successful weaning from mechanically assisted ventilation (summarized in **Table 47.1**). However, when children remain ventilator-dependent for at least 1 month despite appropriate use of the techniques just described, and the respiratory load has been reduced, ventilatory muscle power has been improved, and central respiratory drive has been increased as much as possible, the cause of respiratory failure may be irreversible, or weaning the child from assisted ventilation may take several months to years. In either case, the diagnosis of CRF is made, and chronic ventilatory support will be required (28).

DECISION TO INITIATE CHRONIC VENTILATORY SUPPORT

Ideally, the decision to initiate chronic ventilatory support in a child may be made electively or nonelectively (15,40). In the past, most decisions to begin chronic ventilatory support were made nonelectively. Typically, a child develops ARF from a respiratory infection or pneumonia. The child is intubated, and mechanically assisted ventilation is initiated as a life-saving measure. Subsequently, it is not possible to wean the child from mechanical ventilation. Because it is often emotionally difficult to abruptly stop this therapy in an alert child who might experience severe distress without it, the transition to chronic ventilatory support is made. In this setting, the child and family often do not have the opportunity to discuss this therapeutic option in advance. Thus, the child and family are not really given a choice about whether or not to initiate chronic ventilatory support (40).

Increasingly, the decision to initiate chronic ventilatory support is being made electively to preserve physiologic function and improve the quality of life. Using this decision-making approach, the healthcare team begins the discussion of options for long-term care, including tracheostomy and chronic ventilatory support, in patients who can be expected to develop CRF (15,40). The most obvious example is the child with a progressive neuromuscular disorder, such as spinal muscular atrophy or muscular dystrophy (27). Discussion begins long enough before the anticipated need to allow the child and family to thoroughly evaluate the options, discuss their feelings, and reach a decision. If the family opts for chronic ventilatory support, then noninvasive ventilatory support is usually initiated first, or a tracheostomy is performed and positive-pressure ventilation (PPV) is started electively before the patient develops major complications of CRF (11,12,13,27). Since hypoventilation is more severe during sleep than during wakefulness, nocturnal assisted ventilation often prevents the development of pulmonary hypertension and other complications of chronic intermittent hypoxia (12). Nocturnal ventilation allows ventilatory muscle rest and improves endurance for spontaneous breathing while awake; therefore, it is actually associated with an enhanced quality of life (12,13). Further, with this approach, the child and family do have the opportunity to make a truly informed decision about whether or not to initiate chronic ventilatory support (40).

Consensus has not been reached regarding the length of time that a child can remain intubated before airway damage from prolonged intubation occurs. Therefore, an "outside limit" has not been reached on the length of time intubation is permitted before performing a tracheostomy. In practice, if a child requires PPV via tracheostomy, a tracheostomy should be surgically placed when the diagnosis of CRF is made.

CANDIDATES FOR HOME MECHANICAL VENTILATION

Children with CRF and relatively stable ventilator settings are candidates for home mechanical ventilation (19,24,28,49). The pulmonary component of the disorder is usually the most likely to provide instability. Therefore, the pulmonary disease must be such that the child does not require frequent adjustments in ventilator settings to maintain adequate gas exchange. Generally, the F_{IO_2} should be 40% or less. The requirement for peak inspiratory pressure (PIP) should be less than 40 cm H_2O. Although higher F_{IO_2} and PIP can be delivered by portable ventilators, patients requiring these settings may be too unstable to be successfully ventilated at home. Portable ventilators can now provide positive end-expiratory pressure and pressure support. Children with CRF fall into three basic diagnostic categories: ventilatory muscle weakness and neuromuscular diseases, central hypoventilation syndromes, and chronic pulmonary disease.

Ventilatory Muscle Weakness and Neuromuscular Diseases

Ventilatory muscle weakness has three physiologic consequences. Inspiratory muscle weakness prevents children from inspiring deeply, resulting in atelectasis. Expiratory muscle weakness prevents effective coughing, resulting in decreased removal of pulmonary secretions and foreign material from the lungs, both of which increase the incidence and severity of pneumonia, which is the leading cause of morbidity and mortality in children with neuromuscular disease. Frequent or severe pneumonias in a child with neuromuscular disease indicate that ventilatory muscle weakness is significant. Once weakness of the ventilatory muscles progresses sufficiently, hypoventilation and inadequate gas exchange result (31,35). Two basic types of ventilatory muscle weakness are seen in neuromuscular disease: progressive and nonprogressive. In progressive neuromuscular disease, such as spinal muscular atrophy or muscular dystrophy, muscle weakness worsens with time, resulting in an inevitable and predictable development of CRF (11,12,13,27,37,40). In nonprogressive neuromuscular diseases, such as congenital myopathies, the muscle weakness per se does not progress. However, a relative progression of impairment may occur, because muscle strength cannot increase to overcome the increasing functional demands as the body grows. Many children with static neuromuscular disorders become nonambulatory and ventilator-dependent at or near puberty, because of the marked increase in body mass associated with the pubertal growth spurt.

Often, children with chronically elevated P_{CO_2} of >55–60 torr, due to ventilatory muscle weakness, will develop progressive pulmonary hypertension. Although O_2 administration improves the Pa_{O_2} and relieves hypoxia, this treatment alone is inadequate, as hypoventilation persists with resulting pulmonary hypertension. Thus, these children require home mechanical ventilation (11,12,13,27).

Children with ventilatory muscle weakness make good candidates for home mechanical ventilation. Because the cause of their respiratory failure is primary muscle weakness, these patients usually do not have significant lung disease, which would require the need for frequent changes in ventilator settings. These children usually are much more stable on home mechanical ventilation and have less frequent pneumonias and hospital admissions than they did before the institution of home mechanical ventilation (11,12,13,27,37,40). Some children will require full-time ventilatory support, while others may require only nocturnal ventilatory support.

Central Hypoventilation Syndromes

The cause of CRF in children with central hypoventilation syndrome is inadequate central respiratory drive (5,24,25,29,30,44,46,49), and the cause can be congenital or acquired. The congenital form may be idiopathic (congenital central hypoventilation syndrome or Ondine curse) or due to an identifiable brainstem lesion (Arnold Chiari malformation in myelomeningocele). Acquired forms of central hypoventilation syndrome may be due to brainstem trauma, tumor, hemorrhage, stroke, infection, etc. In children with respiratory control disorders, usually little can be done to augment central respiratory drive (5,46). However, central respiratory drive can be further inhibited by metabolic imbalance, such as chronic metabolic alkalosis. Thus, serum chloride concentrations should be maintained at >95 mEq/dL, and alkalosis should be avoided. Pharmacologic respiratory stimulants are not helpful (41). Sedative medications and central nervous system depressants should be avoided, as these may cause apnea or hypoventilation. Children with respiratory control disorders are generally good candidates for chronic home mechanical ventilation (5,24,25,29,30,44,46,49). The same caveats for treating underlying pulmonary infections apply.

While central respiratory drive is impaired, the lungs and ventilatory muscles may be nearly normal, permitting reasonably stable ventilator settings to achieve adequate gas exchange. Some of these children will require full-time ventilatory support, while others will require ventilatory support only while sleeping (5,24,29,46,49). Because the ventilatory muscles are normal and the respiratory load is not substantially increased, this group of patients can be offered a variety of modalities for ventilatory support, including PPV, noninvasive ventilatory support, negative-pressure ventilators (NPV), and diaphragm pacing (5,6,24,25,29,42,45,46,49). In general, children with central hypoventilation syndrome make good candidates for home mechanical ventilation. Nevertheless, some children may have neurologic problems due to the underlying disorder, which may affect the long-term prognosis. Home mechanical ventilation is not a cure for the underlying neurologic disorder.

Chronic Pulmonary Disease

Chronic pulmonary disease may increase the work of breathing to a level higher than can be sustained by the child. Often, the underlying lung disease is intrinsically unstable, requiring frequent adjustments in ventilator settings, but some children with chronic pulmonary disease will stabilize to the point where home mechanical ventilation is possible (2,10,18,20,21,28). No consensus has been reached on the PCO_2 level at which a child with chronic lung disease is considered to be in chronic respiratory failure, and to require chronic ventilatory support. However, in our experience, children with a PCO_2 of ≥60 torr have a better clinical outcome if they receive chronic ventilatory support to keep the PCO_2 level at ≤45 torr than they do if they remain with elevated PCO_2. The improvement is seen primarily in improved growth, decreased hospitalization time, and avoidance of pulmonary hypertension. Many of these children will be able to wean from chronic ventilatory support with time. Bronchopulmonary dysplasia is a common chronic lung disease for which home ventilation has been used in children. Newer, continuous-flow home ventilators have permitted successful home mechanical ventilation in children with restrictive lung disease, such as hypoplastic lungs from thoracic restriction (skeletal dysplasias) or interstitial lung diseases. Home mechanical ventilation has also been used in children with advanced obstructive lung disease, such as cystic fibrosis, as a bridge to lung transplantation (18). It is important to note that children with unstable lung disease, requirements for high O_2 and peak inspiratory pressures, or the need for frequent changes in ventilator settings are poor candidates for home mechanical ventilation.

PHILOSOPHY OF CHRONIC VENTILATORY SUPPORT

For most children on home mechanical ventilation, weaning is not a realistic goal in the short term. To optimize quality of life, these children must have energy available for other physical activities. Thus, ventilators are adjusted to completely meet their ventilatory demands, leaving much of their energy available for other activities. For children without significant lung disease, ventilators are adjusted to provide a $P_{ET}CO_2$ of 30–35 torr and a SpO_2 of ≥95%. For children who do not require assisted ventilation while awake, ventilating to PCO_2 ≤35 torr during sleep is associated with better spontaneous ventilation while awake (16). Optimal ventilation also avoids atelectasis and the development of coexisting lung disease. It has also been our experience that children who receive chronic ventilatory support actually have fewer complications and generally do better clinically, with some degree of hyperventilation during assisted ventilation (5,12,16,24,28,30,49).

For the child who requires home mechanical ventilation, mobility and quality of life are maximized if the child can breathe unassisted for portions of the day. Even if a child cannot be weaned completely from assisted ventilation, nocturnal ventilation preserves waking quality of life and allows the ventilatory muscles a recovery period during the time when the patient is at highest risk for hypoventilation. In our experience, the weaning of daytime assisted ventilation is best accomplished by sprint weaning. From the perspectives of the patient, parent, and caretaker, it is preferable to have a child who can be away from a ventilator for several hours a day than to have a child who must remain on the ventilator at all times, even if the ventilator rate or settings are lower.

MODALITIES OF HOME MECHANICAL VENTILATION

The ideal ventilators for home use are different from those used in hospitals for the treatment of ARF (7,19). Because many children who require home mechanical ventilation do not have severe lung disease, a number of different techniques are available for providing chronic ventilatory support at home, including portable PPV via tracheostomy; bi-level positive airway pressure ventilation via a mask or other interface; negative-pressure chest shell (cuirass), wrap, or portable tank ventilator; or diaphragm pacing.

Portable Positive-Pressure Ventilator via Tracheostomy

Portable PPV via tracheostomy is the most common method of providing assisted ventilation for infants and children in the home (2,5,7,8,12,13,20,21,24,28,30,36,49). Commercially available electronic PPVs are battery-powered, are relatively portable, and maximize mobility. Portable PPVs are not as powerful, technologically sophisticated, or as versatile as hospital ventilators. Consequently, when infants and children acquire a superimposed respiratory infection, portable ventilators may not be capable of adequately ventilating the child, and hospitalization may be required. Most ventilator-assisted infants and small children are subject to frequent respiratory infections, which often require hospitalization and assisted ventilation with higher settings. A tracheostomy offers the advantage of providing ready access to the airway for hospital ventilators without the need for endotracheal intubation.

For home mechanical ventilation, small, uncuffed tracheostomy tubes are preferred, as the work of breathing required to overcome the increased resistance is performed by the ventilator, not the child. The rationale for the small uncuffed tracheostomy tube is to (a) minimize the risk of tracheomalacia or tracheal mucosal damage, (b) allow a large expiratory leak so that the child may speak, and (c) provide a margin of safety because the child may still be able to ventilate around the tracheostomy tube. Further, the use of a one-way, positive-closure speaking valve enables the child to phonate from early childhood and thus to speak relatively normally in childhood and adolescence (28).

Small, uncuffed tracheostomy tubes are associated with leaks, which can be large and variable, especially in small children. If the same peak inspiratory pressure is achieved on each breath, the lungs are inflated to the same tidal volume, dependent on pulmonary mechanics, regardless of the amount of leak around the tracheostomy. Because of this, pressure ventilation is preferred, and it can be easily utilized on newer portable home ventilators with continuous flow (14). Portable ventilators without continuous flow are volume-preset ventilators. A significant and, importantly, potentially variable portion of the ventilator-delivered breath escapes in the leak around the uncuffed tracheostomy. In some older children and adolescents, this leak is relatively constant, and a higher tidal volume setting can be used to compensate for the leak and achieve adequate ventilation at home. However, this tidal volume setting must be derived empirically, as it is not possible to predict the portion of a ventilator-delivered breath that escapes through the tracheostomy leak. In infants and smaller children, the tracheostomy leak is large and variable and can rarely be compensated for by a single tidal volume setting. In this situation, the tracheostomy leak can be compensated for by using the ventilator in a pressure-limited modality (also known as pressure plateau ventilation). Some commercially available, portable PPV have a high-pressure limit adjustment (pressure pop-off valve), which is separate from the high-pressure alarm, while others must use an external pressure-limit valve. The pressure limit is adjusted to the desired PIP. A high tidal volume setting is then chosen that is sufficient to inflate the lungs, compensate for tubing compliance, and accommodate the leak. The ventilator now functions as a pressure-preset ventilator (14). When the pressure limit is reached, the pressure will "plateau" at that level (**Fig. 47.5**). The remainder of the ventilator tidal volume is not delivered to the patient. For a small tracheostomy leak, the desired pressure limit will be achieved quickly, and a relatively large portion of the breath escapes through the ventilator. For a large tracheostomy leak, it will take longer to achieve the desired pressure limit, but the lungs will still be inflated to the same peak inspiratory pressure. In either case, the lungs will be inflated to the desired PIP, corresponding to a constant tidal volume. It is important to note that the ventilator's high-pressure alarm, useful in detecting an occluded tracheostomy tube, will not function when a pressure plateau is used. Thus, another alarm, such as a pulse oximeter, is required. Pressure-plateau ventilation is very successful in the home ventilation of infants

Pressure Plateau Ventilation

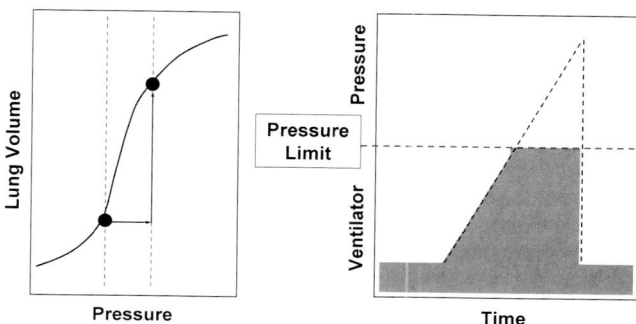

FIGURE 47.5. Pressure-plateau ventilation. If the lungs are inflated to the same pressure on every breath, the same tidal volume will be achieved, according to the pressure–volume characteristics of the lungs (*left panel*). To establish pressure plateau ventilation on a volume preset ventilator without continuous flow (*right panel*), the pressure limit is set with a pressure pop-off valve to the desired peak inspiratory pressure. The ventilator-delivered tidal volume is set high to inflate the lungs and to compensate for the tracheostomy leak and compliance factors of the ventilator circuit. Even though the tracheostomy leak is variable, the lungs will be inflated to the same inspiratory pressure on each breath, ensuring a predictable tidal volume.

and small children, and it has allowed us to ventilate these patients without the use of cuffed tracheostomy tubes or cumbersome continuous-flow devices. It is also useful in older children or adolescents who have large or variable tracheostomy leaks (14).

The development of newer portable ventilators with continuous flow has allowed more sophisticated adjustments of ventilation settings to minimize patient asynchrony and has allowed more medically complicated patients to be ventilated at home. For children and families who require home ventilation, a second ventilator is necessary if they require ventilatory support ≥20 hrs/day or if they live a long distance from respiratory home care vendors who can provide emergency service in the event of malfunction (28).

Tracheostomy

A tracheostomy is performed when CRF is evident. As previously discussed, a small size, uncuffed tracheostomy tube is preferred. After a tracheostomy is performed, it usually takes 7 days for the track to establish and mature. The first tracheostomy tube change is performed by an otolaryngologist to ensure that no complications arise with granulation tissue or a false track and to document easy reinsertion.

One of the most common complications for a child with a tracheostomy is mucous plugging. Mucous can obstruct the airway within minutes after being suctioned. No standard scheduled time for suctioning is defined, as each child is different, and tracheal suctioning needs vary. Hence, vigilance for airway obstruction must be keen and constant. Ventilator alarms and backup monitoring devices are not optimally designed to respond to mucous plugs, nor are they sensitive enough to signal airway obstruction quickly. Therefore, caregivers should be taught not to rely on alarms alone as an indication for the need to suction. Rather, they should be trained to observe early signs of airway obstruction. For a child who is ventilator-dependent, the tubing and the noise from the ventilator may make it difficult to discern the problem. Mucous plugging is reportedly more prevalent at nighttime, when bedside observation is less rigorous. As the consequence of mucous plugging can be serious, caregivers should be trained to routinely triage "a breathing problem" by inspecting the airway for its patency. When in doubt, caregivers should suction and then change the entire tracheostomy tube.

The weight of ventilator tubing pulling on the tracheostomy can cause erosion, laceration of the skin, and an exacerbation of granulation tissue growth. Bleeding from aggressive suctioning is another common problem, which uncommonly can lead to potential life-threatening bleeding in extreme situations. Granulation tissue forms from persistent irritation from suctioning and can obstruct the airway and compromise ventilation. Granulation tissue is an indication for bronchoscopy and possible laser removal. Tracheitis is a common complaint and requires medical attention. When systemic signs and symptoms of infection are not present, inhaled antibiotics are helpful to reduce upper respiratory infection and prevent pneumonia.

If a tracheostomy tube is dislodged accidentally, an immediate replacement is recommended to ensure adequate ventilation and airway access. Tracheostomy stomas can shrink down and close in a very short time. A spare tracheostomy tube is necessary as a backup at all times.

While we advocate a small, uncuffed tracheostomy tube, some patients require a customized length or an extension from the stoma site. Newly developed types allow choices. A few children, especially older ones, might need cuffed tubes to decrease the leak and allow better ventilation during sleep, when upper airway resistance decreases. Cuffed tubes, which are inflated during sleep, can almost always be deflated during wakefulness, permitting speech. Sometimes, cuffed tubes do not even require inflation to decrease the air leak and to improve ventilation. Choice of cuffed tubes should be made according to the needs of the child. Recommended cuffs can be tight to the shaft or with light, soft sleeves. In summary, the type, length, and size of the tracheostomy tube may have to be individualized to the patient, as these can influence ventilator parameters. As the patients grow, the tracheostomy tube must be upsized to provide adequate ventilation.

Ventilator Circuits

A circuit is required to deliver air from a PPV to the patient. Gas from the ventilator goes through a heated humidification system. Ventilator gas must be humidified for infants and children. The desired temperature range is 26–29°C (80–85°F). Condenser humidifiers are not as effective for infants and small children as are heated humidifiers, but they can be used for travel or for short periods. The circuit is usually connected to the tracheostomy with a swivel adapter. Dead space between the tracheostomy and exhalation valve should be minimized to avoid elevated PCO_2. Two to three circuits are generally provided for home care, and they are changed each day. The circuit (tubing, valve, and humidifier) not in use should be cleaned with mild soap and water, then rinsed in a disinfectant (such as 10% alkyl dimethylbenzyl ammonium chloride), and dried (28).

Monitoring and Alarm Systems

Infants and children who require home mechanical ventilation have very little respiratory reserve. These children may have rapid changes in their clinical condition, which affects the adequacy of both spontaneous and assisted ventilation. These rapid changes require constant awareness of the child's respiratory status. Caregivers should be trained to assess color change, chest excursion, respiratory distress, tachycardia, tachypnea, diaphoresis, edema, lethargy, and tolerance for spontaneous ventilation off the ventilator (28). Changes in these parameters may be clinical signs that ventilation is inadequate. These children can be checked by noninvasive blood gas monitoring, if available. In some cases, when in-home nursing care is used, nursing personnel can assist in the continual evaluation of the child's clinical condition. Alarm systems are crucial, but they do not take the place of a trained and attentive caregiver.

All PPV have a low-pressure alarm, which sounds in the event that a minimal pressure level is not achieved. These alarms are important to detect a sudden disconnect of the ventilator from the tracheostomy or other very large leak in the circuit, and they are usually set to sound if the maximal airway pressure achieved on a breath is less than the desired PIP minus 10 cm H_2O. However, if an infant or small child with a small tracheostomy is decannulated with the small tracheostomy still connected to the ventilator, sufficient resistance from the tracheostomy tube alone may keep the low-pressure alarm from sounding (26). Ventilators also have high-pressure alarms, which sound if the pressure required to deliver a breath is too high. Very useful in detecting a plug or occlusion of the tracheostomy tube, these alarms are usually set to sound if the maximal airway pressure achieved on a breath is greater than 10 cm H_2O above the desired PIP. As mentioned previously, high-pressure alarms will not sound if a ventilator is being used in a pressure-plateau or pressure-controlled mode. Therefore, an additional monitoring system external to the ventilator and monitoring the child directly is required. Currently, a pulse oximeter, which can alarm for low SpO_2 or low heart rate, is the recommended patient monitor. Alarms are usually set to sound for a SpO_2 of <85% or a heart rate below 60 bpm for ages 1–12 months and 50 bpm for those >1 year of age. High-heart rate alarms are not used. The pulse oximeter alarm should be used at all times during sleep and when a ventilator-dependent patient is not being observed.

More sophisticated home ventilators have low- and high-minute ventilation alarms. For those ventilators, which monitor inspired minute ventilation (V_I), low-minute ventilation alarms will sound for airway occlusion, and they should be set to sound for a V_I below the measured V_I. High-minute ventilation alarms will sound an alarm for a disconnect, and they should be set for a V_I above the measured V_I, assuming the alarm will sound if the ventilator is completely disconnected. High- and low-minute ventilation alarms, which monitor exhaled minute ventilation, are not useful with uncuffed tracheostomy tubes and variable leaks. Although these alarms may improve patient safety, they are not a substitute for the use of pulse oximetry as an additional alarm system.

Bi-level Positive Airway Pressure Ventilation by Mask or Nasal Prongs

Noninvasive intermittent PPV is delivered via a nasal mask, nasal prongs, or face mask using a bi-level positive airway pressure ventilator (5,9,18,25,29,33,37,42,44). This technique is commonly used in older children, but has also been used successfully in infants and small children. Bi-level ventilation can be used in children who require ventilatory support only during sleep and who have relatively mild intrinsic lung disease. Thus, bi-level ventilation is most frequently used in children with neuromuscular disorders and central hypoventilation syndromes (11,25,27,29,33,42,44). Bi-level ventilation has also been used for children with chronic lung disease who require ventilatory muscle rest (18). Bi-level ventilators are smaller, less expensive, and generally easier to use than conventional ventilators. Newer models have pressure and apnea alarms and adjustable rise times. Bi-level ventilators can provide variable continuous flow via a blower (fan), have a fixed leak (which prevents CO_2 retention), and can compensate for leaks around the mask. Inspiratory positive airway pressure (IPAP) and expiratory positive airway pressure (EPAP) can be adjusted independently. The IPAP-to-EPAP difference is proportional to tidal volume. When bi-level ventilators are used for ventilatory assistance rather than for obstructive sleep apnea, a large IPAP-to-EPAP difference is desirable. Tidal volume increases linearly, with an IPAP-to-EPAP difference of up to ~14 cm H_2O (29). Higher differences may increase tidal volume with stiff lungs. The lowest EPAP that can be used without CO_2 accumulation at the interface is 4 cm H_2O. The highest IPAP that can be used is generally 20 cm H_2O. However, most children need to begin with lower IPAP in the range of 10–14 cm H_2O and increase slowly as tolerated and as necessary (29). Humidification and supplemental O_2 can be added to the circuit, though they are not always necessary.

Four modes of bilevel ventilation can be used: continuous positive airway pressure; spontaneous mode, which assists patient-initiated breaths; timed mode, which controls ventilation at a set rate; and spontaneous/timed mode, which assists generated breaths as long as the patient breathes in accord with at least the set backup rate and adds control breaths if the patient does not breathe at the minimum backup rate. Only the spontaneous/timed and timed modes guarantee breath delivery and should be used in children with respiratory control disorders because these patients cannot be trusted to generate their own adequate respirations. Bi-level ventilation is not usually used 24 hrs/day, because the mask interferes with daily activities and social interaction, and the risk of skin breakdown increases significantly. Because of the risk of aspiration, children who are unable to remove their own masks should not have full-face masks unless they are closely observed. Most side effects related to bi-level ventilation are minimal, such as rhinitis, aerophagia, conjunctival injection, and skin breakdown, most of which can be avoided by proper fitting of the mask. Mask ventilation has been associated with some mid-face hypoplasia, although it is not clear if the mask was causative.

Noninvasive bi-level ventilation is not as powerful as PPV via tracheostomy. Thus, children may require intubation and more sophisticated ventilatory support during acute exacerbations, such as respiratory syncytial virus infections, the risk of which is higher in young children. The major benefit of bi-level ventilation is that a tracheostomy is not required. In general, children successfully managed with bi-level ventilation have less severe respiratory failure than those who require PPV via tracheostomy. Therefore, nonadherence with prescribed bi-level ventilation is more common than with PPV via tracheostomy.

Negative-Pressure Ventilation

Negative-pressure ventilators apply a negative pressure outside the chest and abdomen to generate inspiration (5,7,24,28,49).

A chest shell ventilator uses a dome-shaped shell that is fitted over the anterior chest and abdomen. The negative-pressure wrap ventilator is a "jump suit" that fits snugly around the neck, wrists, and ankles to minimize leaks. A metal "cage" inside the jump suit creates a space where negative pressure can be generated during inspiration. A portable tank is a NPV into which the child's torso is placed, with the head outside. Negative inspiratory pressure is generated inside the chest shell, wrap, or portable tank, which expands the chest and upper abdomen. The ventilator rate and the negative pressure to be developed inside the chest shell, wrap, or portable tank can be controlled. The negative pressure is proportional to the tidal volume, but may be limited by leaks around the chest shell or wrap. These ventilators can provide effective ventilation in children and adolescents, sometimes without a tracheostomy. However, with NPV, synchronous activation of the upper airway muscles does not occur as with spontaneous breathing. Thus, airway occlusion can occur when breaths are generated by a NPV during sleep. Therefore, infants and young children may require a tracheostomy. In that the major potential benefit of NPVs is that a tracheostomy may not be needed in older children, this technique may offer little advantage over PPV in the infant or young child.

For the negative-pressure chest shell ventilators to provide adequate ventilation, the chest shell must be closely fitted to the chest to avoid large leaks. Further, chest shells must be changed and refitted as the child grows. The adequacy of gas exchange produced by negative-pressure chest shell ventilation must be checked frequently to ensure that the chest shell fit and ventilator settings are optimal. Negative-pressure wrap ventilators or portable tanks need not conform exactly to the chest configuration. Thus, they are better suited for small children or some children with scoliosis or chest wall deformities. However, the effectiveness of NPV depends on the ability to move the chest wall. Thus, children with marked scoliosis or chest wall deformities that restrict chest wall motion are not good candidates for NPV.

Negative pressure ventilators are not as portable as electronic PPVs, nor are they battery-operated. Some patients have difficulty sleeping in the supine position necessitated by the chest shell or wrap. The portable tank does permit sleeping on the back or side. Skin irritation may occur when the chest shell rubs the skin, although this can usually be avoided by having the child sleep with a T–shirt under the chest shell and with the use of baby powder or corn starch on the skin. In general, children complain that NPVs are quite cool, because of the continuous movement of air. Thus, wearing a warm shirt is sometimes necessary for comfort, even during warm weather.

Negative pressure ventilation may permit decannulation of a tracheostomy. Children with congenital central hypoventilation syndrome have been successfully transitioned from PPV via tracheostomy to NPV to be rid of the tracheostomy after 5–6 years of age. Upper airway obstruction can be minimized by tonsillectomy and adenoidectomy. Reducing the inspiratory negative pressure and/or increasing the inspiratory time may also reduce obstructive apneas.

Negative pressure ventilation is not as powerful as PPV via tracheostomy. Thus, children may require intubation and more sophisticated ventilatory support during acute exacerbations (e.g., respiratory syncytial virus infections), the risk of which is higher in young children. The major benefit of NPV is that a tracheostomy may not be required. However, many of our patients who used NPV have changed to bi-level ventilation because it is more portable, generally easier to use, and a tracheostomy is not required.

Diaphragm Pacing

Diaphragm pacing generates breathing using the child's own diaphragm as the respiratory pump (5,6,45,46,49). Commercially available diaphragm pacing systems have battery-operated external transmitters. An antenna is taped on the skin over subcutaneously implanted receivers. The transmitter generates a train of pulses for each breath, which is transmitted through the antenna to the receiver under the skin, similar to radio transmission. The receiver converts this energy to standard electrical current, which is directed to a phrenic nerve electrode by lead wires. The electrical stimulation of the phrenic nerve causes a diaphragmatic contraction, which generates the breath. The amount of electrical voltage is proportional to the diaphragmatic contraction, which generates tidal volume. In children, simultaneous bilateral diaphragm pacing is generally required to achieve optimal ventilation. In older children or adolescents who have stable chest walls, adequate ventilation may be achieved by pacing only one side. In general, bilateral implantation of diaphragm pacer electrodes and receivers is recommended. But, if one side fails, adequate ventilation can often be achieved using only unilateral pacing (6).

Use of pacers requires that the phrenic nerves and the diaphragm function appropriately to enable effective ventilation. Therefore, ventilatory muscle myopathy and phrenic neuropathy are contraindications to pacer use. Obstructive apnea can be a complication of diaphragm pacing during sleep, because synchronous upper airway skeletal muscle contraction does not occur with inspiration. However, this can often be overcome by adjusting settings on the pacers to lengthen inspiratory time and/or decrease the force of inspiration. In general, diaphragm pacers can only be used up to ~14 hrs a day, and they cannot be used for 24 hrs continuously. Thus, patients who require ventilatory support 24 hrs a day should have an alternate form of ventilation for part of the day if pacers are used. Pacers can be used for daytime support of ambulatory children who require full-time ventilatory support, in combination with PPV at night (6,45).

Diaphragm pacing has the advantage that the diaphragm pacer system is small, light, battery-operated, and easily portable (6,45). Some adolescents believe diaphragm pacing is a "more natural way to breathe" than a ventilator and thus derive psychologic benefit. However, the surgical technique is tricky, and use of the pacers once implanted requires a fair amount of experience. Therefore, diaphragm pacing should generally be performed in centers with experience in the technique. This technique may provide benefit to select groups of children with central hypoventilation syndrome or high cervical spinal cord injury (5,6,45,46).

HOSPITAL MANAGEMENT PRIOR TO DISCHARGE

The underlying conditions that result in the need for home mechanical ventilation are not reversible with specific treatment (24,28,49). However, improvement in pulmonary mechanics will reduce the work of breathing, substantially increase the patient's ability to breathe spontaneously, and may allow weaning from assisted ventilation for some portion of the day, thus significantly improving mobility and quality of life.

Nearly all children who receive home mechanical ventilation develop chronic lung disease with elements of bronchoconstriction, chronic inflammation of the airway, and impaired mucociliary clearance. Therapy should be directed toward relief of bronchospasm, clearance of pulmonary secretions, reduction in lung water, treatment of pulmonary infections, and prevention of aspiration. These children usually benefit from aerosolized bronchodilators followed by intensive pulmonary physiotherapy on a routine basis. Patients should receive the routine immunizations and annual split virion influenza vaccine.

The patient's respiratory status must be stable on the home ventilator for at least 1–2 weeks prior to discharge (**Table 47.2**). It is important to emphasize that settings on a home ventilator do not provide the same ventilation as do the same settings on a hospital ventilator. Therefore, the child must be tested on home equipment before discharge (28). Invariably, ventilator settings must be increased on the home ventilator to achieve the same level of gas exchange achieved on a hospital ventilator. In the hospital, it is important to use the actual ventilator and circuits that the child will use in the home (19,28).

Patients tolerate a $Paco_2$ slightly lower than physiologic, 30–35 torr, which provides a margin of safety and eliminates any subjective feeling of dyspnea. In the home, ventilator settings cannot be changed frequently to maintain perfect blood gas values. Thus, settings should not be changed in response to minor variations in blood gas values, but only to correct persistent trends or major abnormalities (1,7,8,19,24,28,32).

TABLE 47.2

NEEDS OF THE VENTILATOR-ASSISTED CHILD PRIOR TO HOSPITAL DISCHARGE

1. Medical stability of the child's condition, permitting relatively constant ventilator settings
2. Family commitment to care for the ventilator-assisted child at home
3. Realistic assessment of the medical care requirements and arrangement for the family's ability to meet them, including in-home nursing assistance, if necessary
4. Thorough education of the family and other caregivers in technical aspects of medical care and equipment operation
5. Selection of a respiratory equipment vendor able to supply and service the desired equipment, with 24-hr emergency availability
6. Selection of a local primary pediatrician to provide well-child care, emergency care, and liaison with community resources
7. Informing of community emergency medical systems of the ventilator-assisted child and her needs
8. Notification of telephone and power companies to provide priority service in the event of interruption of service
9. Arrangement for routine and emergency transport from home to the medical center responsible for medical care
10. Arrangement for other medical, psychosocial, and developmental support, such as physical and occupational therapy, respite care, and school

TABLE 47.3

HOME RESPIRATORY EQUIPMENT FOR HOME MECHANICAL VENTILATION
(PPV VIA TRACHEOSTOMY)

1. Electronic portable PPV with:
   1 humidifier with humidifier jar
   1 heater and thermometer, water trap
   2 circuits with bleed-in adapter/connector
   Flex tubing
   Automobile cigarette lighter adaptor for car use, if available
2. Backup ventilator: Absolutely essential for patients who require ≥20 hrs/day of assisted ventilation or who are living long distances from medical and technical support
3. Deep-cycle marine gel battery with case and cables for operation of the ventilator and battery charger (unless built into the ventilator)
4. E-cylinder of oxygen with stand and regulator for emergency use
   Supplemental oxygen system, if necessary
5. Aerosol delivery system with:
   2 aerosol set-ups
   2 trach adapters
   2 22/15-cm connector/adapters
6. Portable suction machine with battery pack, connecting tubing, appropriately sized tracheal suction catheters, and tonsil fine-tip catheters
7. Resuscitation bag with appropriate size mask
8. Pulse oximeter as an alarm system (alarm settings: SpO_2 <85%; low–heart rate <60 bpm age 1–12 months, <50 bpm age ≥1 year; high–heart rate off)
9. Other essential accessories are:
   Tracheostomy tube holder
   Artificial nose (HMV = head moisture exchanger)
   In-line speaking valve
   Bacterial filter

The equipment essential for home care of the ventilator-assisted child is listed in **Table 47.3** (19,28). Service contracts for the maintenance of the ventilator and other respiratory equipment must be arranged. The respiratory equipment vendor should make home visits every month to verify proper operation of equipment, troubleshoot problems, and provide preventive maintenance. Prompt 24-hr emergency vendor support is essential in the event of equipment malfunction. A backup ventilator and other essential equipment should be provided to all families, but *must* be provided for children who are ventilator dependent ≥20 hrs/day or when they live long distances from medical or technical assistance (7,19,28). A resuscitation bag is necessary for resuscitation and to permit manual ventilation in the event of power failure or ventilator malfunction. The physical environment of the home should be evaluated for adequacy of space, grounded electrical outlets, and wiring (8,19,28,32).

Prior to discharge from the hospital, the family must become familiar with all aspects of their child's care. They must demonstrate competency in equipment operation, tracheostomy care, pulmonary physiotherapy, administration of medications (including aerosols), and cardiopulmonary resuscitation. Families must become adept at recognizing signs of respiratory compromise. Although most families become skilled in these tasks, it is not always realistic to expect that they can continuously care for their child unassisted in the home. Nurses with pediatric critical care expertise are helpful in assisting families for 8–24 hrs/day in the home care of their child, especially infants and young children. Before a child is discharged from the hospital, each nurse who will care for the child at home should receive in-service training on the child's care, preferably from the child's primary nurse (8,19,28,32).

Children who are ventilator-assisted in the home must be closely linked to a medical center capable of providing the subspecialty care required. Prior to home care, arrangements should be made for transportation to the hospital from the home or local emergency room in the event of an emergency. Currently available portable ventilators usually permit the families to transport their ventilator-assisted child for routine visits. When possible, a local primary pediatrician should be recruited to provide routine pediatric care. The local emergency room or paramedics should be familiar with the child and be able to provide emergency care or transport to the medical center when necessary. The local telephone and utility companies must be notified in writing of the patient's location and condition. In the event of a power outage or other interruption of service, the home ventilator patient should be given priority for restoration of service (19,28).

HOME MANAGEMENT OF THE VENTILATOR-ASSISTED CHILD

Routine evaluation of ventilator settings should be performed on a regular basis so that ventilation meets the changing requirements of the growing child. Although no consensus is available on the minimum frequency of evaluations, such evaluations are generally required more frequently in the first year of life (24,28). Older children who are medically stable probably only need such evaluations yearly. Following any change in the respiratory system (severe infection, hospitalization, etc.), settings should also be checked and readjusted. These evaluations are usually performed by polysomnography, and it is important to monitor $P_{ET}CO_2$ as an indication of the adequacy of ventilation. Sleep studies during daytime naps may also be adequate for the evaluation of ventilator settings if the child's clinical course is reasonably stable. Sleep studies may also be used to predict the success of sprint weaning during sleep when sprinting schedules are advancing in the home. In the absence of the availability of a sleep laboratory, an overnight hospital admission with continuous recording of SpO_2 and $P_{ET}CO_2$ may be sufficient to assess the adequacy of ventilator settings.

Some ventilator-assisted children will also require supplemental O_2. Supplemental O_2 may be required during spontaneous breathing and/or during mechanically assisted ventilation. O_2 requirements must be assessed at regular intervals using noninvasive monitoring of oxygenation. Supplemental O_2 is not a replacement for home ventilation in those patients with chronic hypoventilation.

Because home mechanical ventilation may not completely meet the ventilatory requirements at all times, even the most successfully managed patients may be exposed to periods of alveolar hypoxia and hypoventilation (**Table 47.4**). Thus, all ventilator-assisted children are at risk for development of pulmonary hypertension and cor pulmonale. The usual clinical findings of right heart failure may not be present until late in the course. Echocardiography may be a more sensitive method for following right heart function. Echocardiography to measure right ventricular dimensions, pulmonic valve systolic time intervals, septal morphology, pulmonic valve "a dip," pulmonic valve early systolic closure, and acceleration time of pulmonary artery flow (Doppler) should be obtained annually and more often if clinically indicated. When signs of pulmonary hypertension are discovered, it should be assumed that the level of mechanical ventilation is inadequate until proven otherwise. The patient should be hospitalized for continuous noninvasive monitoring of gas exchange and ventilator adjustments. Some patients who require assisted ventilation only while sleeping may hypoventilate intermittently while breathing spontaneously during wakefulness. If this occurs frequently, pulmonary hypertension may result, even if mechanical ventilation at night is adequate.

Common childhood illnesses pose a unique threat to the ventilator-assisted child. A number of normal host defenses against disease are either lost or impaired in these patients. For example, breathing via tracheostomy bypasses the normal humidifying and filtering functions of the upper airway, predisposing to inspissated secretions and tracheobronchitis. Ineffective cough leads to impaction and decreased clearance of pulmonary secretions. An inability to increase respiratory rate in response to fever may lead to dyspnea and hypoxia. Despite the use of preventive and therapeutic measures directed at these problems, even a relatively trivial upper respiratory infection may compromise the ventilator-assisted child. Ventilator adjustments, with an increased level of support, are usually needed. Patients ordinarily requiring ventilation only during sleep often need 24 hrs/day support during illnesses. Because of these changes in the ventilatory requirements, these patients may require hospitalization for blood gas monitoring and frequent ventilator changes. Hospital ventilators with greater flex-

TABLE 47.4

MANAGEMENT OF COMPLICATIONS OF HOME MECHANICAL VENTILATION

Medical problem	Management
Hypoxia	Evaluate oxygenation by noninvasive monitoring. If SpO_2 is <95%, add supplemental O_2 or increase ventilatory support.
Hypoventilation	Evaluate ventilator settings by noninvasive monitoring. If $P_{ET}CO_2$ is >35 torr, increase ventilatory support.
Chronic lung disease	Have a high index of suspicion. The diagnosis of chronic lung disease is often missed in ventilator-assisted children. Treatment includes bronchodilators (aerosolized and/or systemic), pulmonary physiotherapy, and diuretics.
Pulmonary hypertension	Ensure adequate oxygenation and ventilation. Periodically monitor electrocardiogram and echocardiogram for signs of pulmonary hypertension.
Pulmonary infections	Complete immunizations, including influenza A/B split virion vaccine. Treat respiratory infections aggressively with antibiotics and chest physiotherapy.
Growth delay	Ensure adequate caloric quantity and quality. Growth delay is a complication of chronic hypoxia or hypercapnia. Assess oxygenation and ventilation.

ibility than portable electronic ventilators are usually required to ensure adequate ventilation during these hospitalizations. After recovery, patients should demonstrate adequate ventilation on their home ventilator for at least a few days prior to discharge.

Placement of a ventilator-assisted child in the school system poses unique challenges to the teachers and the school district. Yet, many ventilator-assisted children can attend regular school, especially if they require assisted ventilation only during sleep. Whenever possible, it is desirable to educate a ventilator-assisted child in as normal a school setting as possible. When the discharge team works closely with school district personnel, the optimal educational setting for the child can often be arranged. Educating school officials about the true nature of the child's disorder often eases fear and facilitates school placement and acceptance. Obviously, some children are better served in special schools, but this is usually dependent on disease involvement in bodily systems other than the respiratory system (19,24,28).

Even with sophisticated management at home, ventilator-assisted children may succumb to a catastrophe stemming from a simple problem, such as a disconnected ventilator or plugged tracheostomy, emphasizing the need for compulsive care (39). However, home ventilator equipment failure is uncommon, occurring only approximately once every 1.3 patient-years, and Srinivasan found no serious sequelae to equipment failure in a home care program with attention to detail (39).

CONCLUSIONS AND FUTURE DIRECTIONS

Successful care of the ventilator-assisted child at home demands compulsive attention to detail on the part of medical personnel, the child, and the family. However, the potential rewards are great. Many ventilator-assisted children do quite well at home, and home care of these patients is a safe and relatively inexpensive management technique. The high motivation of parents for the care of their children in the home often results in a high quality of care. After the transition from hospital to home, parent-child relationships and child development are enhanced. Potential for rehabilitation in all aspects of daily living is increased, and many children will experience a near-normal lifestyle. Future technologic improvements are likely improve portability, effectiveness of ventilation, versatility of ventilation modalities and, potentially, the ability to care for more severely affected children at home.

KEY POINTS

- The respiratory system in children is vulnerable to CRF. With respiratory disorders, ventilatory muscle power and/or central respiratory drive may not be adequate to overcome the respiratory load, resulting in respiratory failure.

- CRF requires a different philosophy and strategy than ARF to treat it optimally. As these children will not wean quickly from mechanically assisted ventilation, their ventilatory needs should be fully supported by the ventilator, and weaning (if possible) requires optimizing the function of the lungs, ventilatory muscles, and central drive.

- Children with CRF can often be cared for at home. Candidates for home mechanical ventilation must have a stable respiratory disorder that does not require frequent changes in ventilator settings.

- Home mechanical ventilation is most commonly provided using PPV via tracheostomy. However, some children are able to use noninvasive techniques (bi-level positive airway pressure ventilation via mask, NPV, or diaphragm pacing), which may permit removal of their tracheostomies.

- Prior to hospital discharge, children using home mechanical ventilation and their families require thorough education, complete equipment testing including safety monitors, and arrangements for ancillary healthcare needs and community resources (school).

- Once at home, children using home mechanical ventilation require ongoing medical care from an interdisciplinary team who can address medical, developmental, psychosocial, and equipment needs.

References

1. Ambrosio IU, Woo MS, Jansen MT, et al. Safety of hospitalized ventilator-dependent children outside of the intensive care unit. *Pediatrics* 1998;101:257–9.
2. Appierto L, Cori M, Bianchi R, et al. Home care for chronic respiratory failure in children. *Paediatr Anaesthesia* 2002;12:345–50.
3. Ben Abraham R, Efrati O, Mishali D, et al. Predictors of mortality after prolonged mechanical ventilation after cardiac surgery in children. *J Crit Care* 2002;17:235–9.
4. Ben-Abraham R, Weinbroum AA, Roizin H, et al. Long-term assessment of pulmonary function tests in pediatric survivors of acute respiratory distress syndrome. *Med Sci Monit* 2002;8:153–7.
5. Chen ML, Keens TG. Congenital central hypoventilation syndrome: Not just another rare disorder. *Paediatr Respir Rev* 2004;5:182–9.
6. Chen ML, Tablizo MA, Kun S, et al. Diaphragm pacers as a treatment for congenital central hypoventilation syndrome. *Exp Rev Med Dev* 2005; 2:577–85.
7. Davidson Ward SL, Keens TG. Home mechanical ventilators and equipment. In McConnell MS, ed. *Guidelines for Pediatric Home Health Care.* Evanston, Illinois: American Academy of Pediatrics, 2002:177–86.
8. DeWitt PK, Jansen MT, Davidson Ward SL et al. Obstacles to discharge of ventilator assisted children from the hospital to home. *Chest* 1993;103: 1560–5.
9. Fauroux B, Boffa C, Desguerre I, et al. Long-term noninvasive mechanical ventilation for children at home: A national survey. *Pediatr Pulmonol* 2003;35:119–25.
10. Fauroux B, Sardet A, Foret D. Home treatment for chronic respiratory failure in children: A prospective study. *Eur Respir J* 1995;8:2062–6.
11. Finder JD, Birnkrant D, Carl J, et al. American Thoracic Society: Respiratory care of the patient with Duchenne muscular dystrophy. ATS Consensus Statement. *Amer J Respir Crit Care Med* 2004;170:456–65.
12. Gilgoff IS, Kahlstrom E, MacLaughlin E, et al. Long-term ventilatory support in spinal muscular atrophy. *J Pediatr* 1989;115:904–9.
13. Gilgoff RL, Gilgoff IS. Long-term follow-up of home mechanical ventilation in young children with spinal cord injury and neuromuscular conditions. *J Pediatr* 2003;142:476–80.
14. Gilgoff IS, Peng R-C, Keens TG. Hypoventilation and apnea in children during mechanical assisted ventilation. *Chest* 1992;101:1500–6.
15. Gilgoff IS, Prentice W, Baydur A. Patient and family participation in the management of respiratory failure in Duchenne's muscular dystrophy. *Chest* 1989;95:519–24.
16. Gozal D, Keens TG. Passive nighttime hypocapnic hyperventilation improves daytime eucapnia in mechanically ventilated children. *Amer J Respir Crit Care Med* 1989;157(3):A779.
17. Gozal D, Shoseyov D, Keens TG. Inspiratory pressures with CO_2 stimulation and weaning from mechanical ventilation in children. *Amer Rev Respir Dis* 1993;147:256–61.
18. Hodson ME, Madden BP, Steven MH, et al. Non-invasive mechanical ventilation for cystic fibrosis patients—a potential bridge to transplantation. *Eur Respir J* 1991;4:524–7.
19. Holecek MS, Nixon M, Keens TG. Discharge of the technology dependent child. In: Levine DL, Morriss FC, eds. *Essentials of Pediatric Intensive Care,* 2nd ed. New York: Churchill Livingston, 1997:1537–48.
20. Jardin E, O'Toole M, Paton JY, et al. Current status of long-term ventilation of children in the United Kingdom. *Brit Med J* 1999;318:295–9.
21. Kamm M, Burger R, Rimensberger P, et al. Survey of children supported by long-term mechanical ventilation in Switzerland. *Swiss Med Weekly* 2001;131:261–6.
22. Keens TG, Bryan AC, Levison H, et al. Developmental pattern of muscle fiber types in human ventilatory muscles. *J Appl Physiol: Respir, Environ, Exercise Physiol* 1978;44:909–13.
23. Keens TG, Chen V, Patel P, et al. Cellular adaptations of the ventilatory muscles to a chronic increased respiratory load. *J Appl Physiol: Respir Environ Exercise Physiol* 1978;44:905–8.
24. Keens TG, Davidson Ward SL. Syndromes affecting respiratory control during sleep. In: Loughlin GM, Marcus CL, Carroll JL, eds. *Sleep and Breathing in Children: A Developmental Approach.* Lung Biology in Health and Disease series. New York: Marcel Dekker, Inc., 2000:525–53.
25. Kerbl R, Litscher H, Grubbauer HM, et al. Congenital central hypoventilation syndrome (Ondine's curse syndrome) in two siblings: Delayed diagnosis and successful noninvasive treatment. *Eur J Pediatr* 1996;155:1059–64.
26. Kun S, Nakamura CT, Ripka JF, et al. Home ventilator low pressure alarms fail to detect accidental decannulation with pediatric tracheostomy tubes. *Chest* 2001;119:562–4.
27. Lyager S, Steffensen B, Juhl B. Indicators of need for mechanical ventilation in Duchenne muscular dystrophy and spinal muscular atrophy. *Chest* 1995;108:779–85.
28. Make BJ, Hill NS, Goldberg AI, et al. Mechanical ventilation beyond the intensive care unit: Report of a consensus conference of the American College of Chest Physicians. *Chest* 1998;113:289S–344S.

29. Marcus CL. Ventilator management of abnormal breathing during sleep: Continuous positive airway pressure and nocturnal noninvasive intermittent positive pressure ventilation. In: Loughlin GM, Marcus CL, Carroll JL, eds. *Sleep and Breathing in Children: A Developmental Approach.* Lung Biology in Health and Disease series. New York: Marcel Dekker, Inc., 2000:797–811.

30. Marcus CL, Jansen MT, Poulsen MK, et al. Medical and psychosocial outcome of children with congenital central hypoventilation syndrome. *J Pediatr* 1991;119:888–95.

31. Nickerson BG, Keens TG. Measuring ventilatory muscle endurance in humans as sustainable inspiratory pressure. *J Appl Physiol: Respir Environ Exercise Physiol* 1982;52:768–72.

32. Noyes J. Barriers that delay children and young people who are dependent on mechanical ventilators from being discharged from the hospital. *J Clin Nurs* 2002;11:2–11.

33. Paditz E. Nocturnal nasal mask ventilation in childhood. *Pneumologie* 1994;48:744–9.

34. Randolph AG, Meert KL, O'Neil ME, et al. The feasibility of conducting clinical trials in infants and children with acute respiratory failure. *Am J Respir Crit Care Med* 2003;167:1334–40.

35. Roussos C. S, Macklem PT. Diaphragmatic fatigue in man. *J Appl Physiol: Respirat Environ Exercise Physiol* 1977;43:189–97.

36. Sasaki M, Sugai K, Fukumizu M, et al. Mechanical ventilation care in severe childhood neurological disorders. *Brain Dev* 2001;23:796–800.

37. Simonds AK, Ward S, Heather S, et al. Outcome of paediatric domiciliary mask ventilation in neuromuscular and skeletal disease. *Eur Respir J* 2000;16:476–81.

38. Slater A, Shann F, Pearson G. PIM2: A revised version of the Pediatric Index of Mortality. *Intensive Care Med* 2003;29:278–85.

39. Srinivasan S, Doty SM, White TR, et al. Frequency, causes, and outcome of home ventilator failure. *Chest* 1998;114:1363–7.

40. Sritippayawan S, Kun SS, Keens TG, et al. Initiation of home mechanical ventilation in children with neuromuscular diseases. *J Pediatr* 2003;142:481–5.

41. Swaminathan S, Paton JY, Davidson Ward SL, et al. Theophylline does not increase ventilatory responses to hypercapnia or hypoxia. *Amer Rev Respir Dis* 1992;146:1398–1401.

42. Teague WG. Non-invasive positive pressure ventilation: Current status in paediatric patients. *Paed Resp Rev* 2005;6:52–60.

43. Tibby SM, Taylor D, Festa M, et al. A comparison of three scoring systems for mortality risk among retrieved intensive acre patients. *Arch Dis Child* 2002;87:4215.

44. Villa MP, Dotta A, Castello D, et al. Bi-level positive airway pressure (BiPAP) ventilation in an infant with central hypoventilation syndrome. *Pediatr Pulmonol* 1997;24:66–9.

45. Weese-Mayer DE. Diaphragm pacing in infancy and childhood. In: Loughlin GM, Marcus CL, Carroll JL, eds. *Sleep and Breathing in Children: A Developmental Approach.* Lung Biology in Health and Disease series. New York: Marcel Dekker, Inc., 2000: 813–24.

46. Weese-Mayer DE, Shannon DC, Keens TG, et al. Idiopathic congenital central hypoventilation syndrome: Diagnosis and management. *Amer J Respir Crit Care Med* 1999;160:368–73.

47. Weiss I, Ushay HM, DeBruin W, et al. Notterman. Respiratory and cardiac function in children after acute hypoxic respiratory failure. *Crit Care Med* 1996;24:148–54.

48. Welton JM, Meyer AA, Mandelkehr L, et al. Outcomes of and resource consumption by high-cost patients in the intensive care unit. *Am J Crit Care* 2002;11:467–73.

49. Witmans MB, Chen ML, Davidson Ward SL, et al. Congenital syndromes affecting respiratory control during sleep. In: Lee-Chiong T, ed. *Sleep: A Comprehensive Handbook.* Hoboken: John Wiley and Sons, 2006:517–27.

CHAPTER 48 ■ SLEEP AND BREATHING

SALLY L. DAVIDSON WARD • THOMAS G. KEENS

Sleep-related breathing disorders (SRBD) may be severe enough to warrant admission to the PICU for management, or these patients may require PICU monitoring following surgical therapy. In addition, previously unrecognized SRBD may complicate the course of PICU patients admitted for other reasons. This chapter contains a summary of the reasons why sleep represents a period of vulnerability for the respiratory system, how this results in an array of breathing disorders unique to sleep, and the common forms of SRBD that may be found in a PICU setting. Also included is an outline of the postoperative challenges encountered in caring for patients affected by SRBD, documentation of the presentation and differential diagnosis of infants with apparent life-threatening events, and a review of the impact of poor sleep quality on patients cared for in the PICU.

that is characteristic of this state affects all of the muscles of the upper airway and all of those involved in performing the work of breathing, with the only exception being the diaphragm. Loss of muscle tone leads to increased collapsibility of the upper airway and a decrease in functional residual capacity of the lungs, predisposing to upper airway obstruction or obstructive sleep apnea and impaired gas exchange (31,58). REM accounts for approximately 20% of normal sleep time in adults and children and 50% of sleep time in newborn infants; thus, the importance of REM sleep is not trivial in infants and children. In addition, important maturational differences in infancy predispose to respiratory instability, and these will be discussed in this chapter within the context of apparent life-threatening events and apnea of infancy.

RESPIRATORY CONTROL AND SLEEP

Breathing is under both voluntary and involuntary control during wakefulness. Chemoreceptor activity ensures that minute ventilation is appropriately matched to metabolic needs, whereas voluntary control of ventilation allows the integrated performance of complex behavioral activities. Because both voluntary and metabolic controls of breathing are active during wakefulness, even an anatomically small upper airway usually remains sufficiently patent for uncompromised breathing. However, respiratory control and upper airway muscle tone are state-specific, and, importantly, they are entirely different during sleep, predisposing to instability and upper airway obstruction. As normal individuals fall asleep, the arterial P_{CO_2} rises several torr. The proposed mechanism is "withdrawal of the wakefulness stimulus," suggesting that the sum total of the sensory input of wakefulness is a nonspecific stimulus to the neurologic centers of respiratory control (31). This sensory input is lost with sleep onset. Similarly, the wakefulness stimulus has an influence on the resting muscle tone of the upper airway, which, when withdrawn at the onset of sleep, may favor airway obstruction. Behavioral control of ventilation is absent during non-rapid eye movement (REM) sleep. Thus, adequate ventilation is critically dependent on chemical control. However, the ventilatory responses to hypoxemia and hypercapnia, both potent stimuli of chemoreceptor activity during wakefulness, are blunted during sleep. Important respiratory reflexes, such as coughing and swallowing, are also inhibited by sleep. The changes in lung volume that occur with moving from the upright to supine position reduce the caudal traction on the upper airway, thus increasing airway collapsibility (58). The respiratory pattern becomes irregular during REM sleep, with a variable rate and tidal volume and frequent respiratory pauses. Finally, during REM sleep, the skeletal muscle atonia

OBSTRUCTIVE SLEEP APNEA SYNDROME

The most common form of sleep-disordered breathing in childhood is obstructive sleep apnea syndrome (OSAS). Obstructive sleep apnea (OSA) is defined as an absence of airflow at the nose and mouth despite continued respiratory efforts. Discrete events that are partial in nature, i.e., reduced but not absent airflow, are termed *obstructive hypopneas* and are often accompanied by hypoxemia, hypercapnia, and sleep disruption, as shown in **Figure 48.1**. Continuous partial airway obstruction can result in obstructive hypoventilation. Children with OSAS present with snoring and difficulty breathing during sleep. Parents may describe gasping, choking, or observed apneas during their child's sleep. Because OSAS and snoring are often worse in the supine position, parents may move their children several times during the night. Nocturnal symptoms may be accompanied by behavioral or neurocognitive impairment during the day (22).

The patency of the upper airway during sleep is determined by the bony and soft tissue anatomy of the airway and the upper airway muscle tone. The latter is influenced both by state (wakefulness vs sleep; and REM vs. non-REM sleep) and by neural and chemical controls. The pharyngeal airway serves multiple purposes. To propel boluses of food, forceful constriction of the pharyngeal muscles is required, whereas speech requires dynamic changes in the structure and rigidity of the pharynx and larynx. Although respiration is best served by a rigid airway, these other functions require the pharynx to be collapsible. Thus, the neuromuscular function of the upper airway is critical to maintaining airway patency. If neural inputs that maintain airway patency during sleep are inadequate and/or if the airway is anatomically narrowed, OSAS may result. Findings on physical exam during wakefulness do not accurately predict the presence of OSAS during sleep, nor

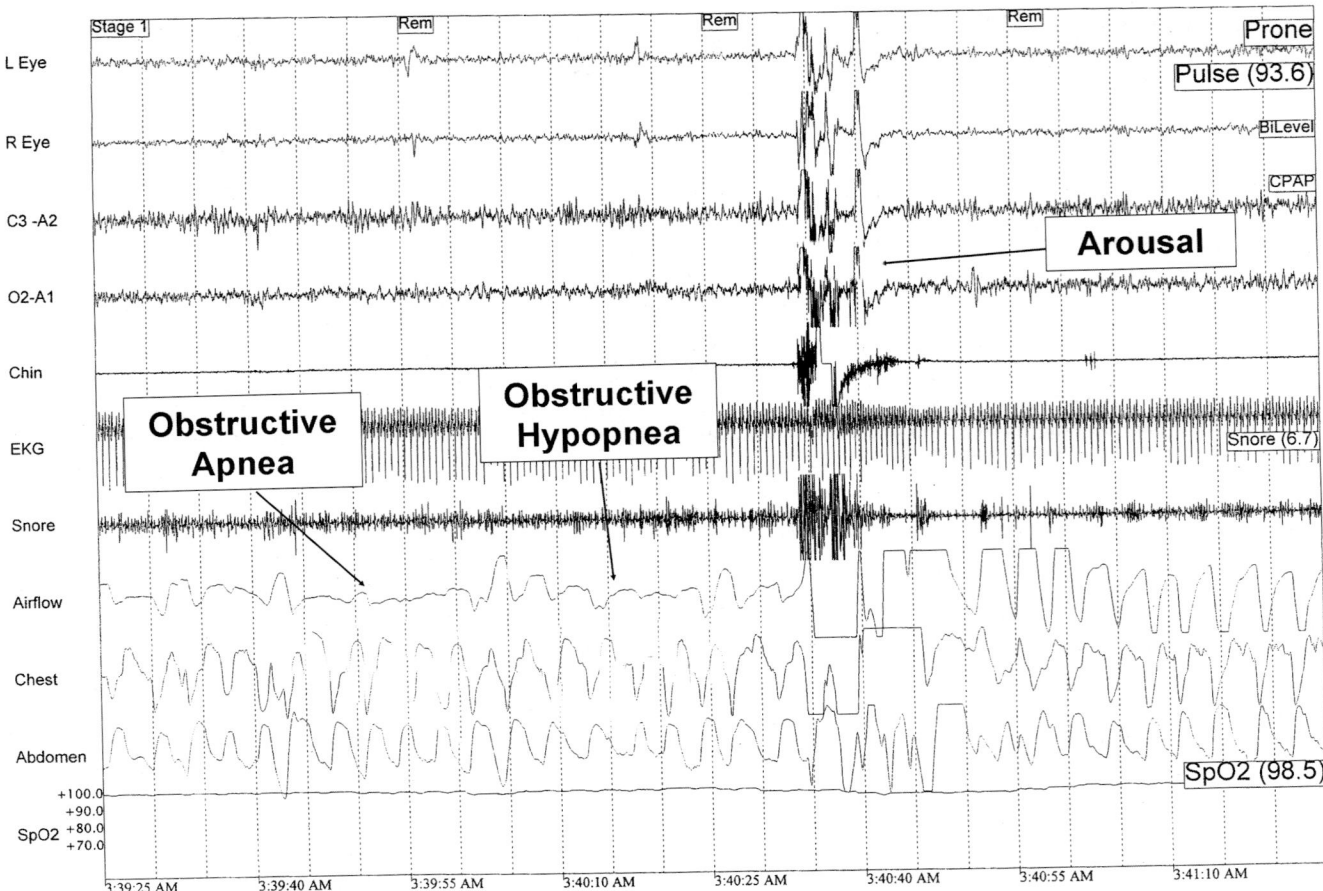

FIGURE 48.1. Obstructive events on polysomnogram. Two obstructive events are shown on this 2-min epoch recorded from a 4-year-old child with nightly snoring. The first event is an obstructive apnea, characterized by an absence of airflow despite continued respiratory effort. The second event is an obstructive hypopnea with reduced, but not absent, airflow. The events result in a mild desaturation and are terminated by an arousal from sleep, with restoration of airflow.

does correction of the anatomic defect by surgery invariably relieve all of the symptoms. The significant familial pattern to the risk of OSAS is likely related to both heritable anatomic and central nervous system factors (22,58).

A number of conditions predispose to OSAS; the most common are listed in **Table 48.1**. These etiologies have anatomically or functionally narrowed upper airways in common. With the onset of the obesity epidemic in children, the landscape of sleep-disordered breathing has changed dramatically. Many children and adolescents are now at risk for severe obesity-related OSAS. Obstructive apneas and hypopneas can result in continuous or episodic hypoxemia and/or hypoventilation during sleep, as well as repetitive arousals from sleep. These stimuli alter the function of the autonomic nervous system. Both systemic and pulmonary hypertension are recognized complications of OSAS. Because the protective response to OSA includes arousal, sleep can be fragmented. In the most severe cases, repeated arousal results in excessive daytime sleepiness, which is the most common presenting feature in adults with OSAS. However, this is not nearly as common in children, perhaps because they are less likely to arouse following each obstructive event. An exception to this is the morbidly obese child in whom excessive daytime sleepiness is often severe. Although children with OSAS may not have daytime sleepiness, they may suffer from other neurobehavioral complications, including school failure, hyperactivity, and mood or conduct disorders. It is plausible that the sleep disruption and hypoxemia of OSAS are responsible for the neurologic and behavioral complications, and one large population-based study found a correlation between the severity of OSAS and the extent of these complications (25). However, primary snoring (snoring without findings of OSAS on PSG) has been found by others to result in neurobehavioral difficulties (43). Further study is required to explore these relationships. Other complications of OSAS include failure to thrive, nocturnal enuresis, and worsening of parasomnias, such as sleepwalking (26).

TABLE 48.1

CONDITIONS THAT PREDISPOSE TO OBSTRUCTIVE SLEEP APNEA SYNDROME IN CHILDREN

Adenotonsillar hypertrophy
Obesity
Craniofacial abnormalities
Down syndrome
Sickle cell disease
Cerebral palsy

TABLE 48.2

NORMAL VALUES FOR PEDIATRIC
POLYSOMNOGRAPHY

	Normal	Abnormal
Apnea hypopnea index (events/hr)	<1	>1
Maximal end-tidal P_{CO_2} ($P_{ET}CO_2$; torr)	≤53	>54
Duration of hypoventilation ($P_{ET}CO_2$ >45 torr; % of total sleep time)	≤45%	>46%
Minimal SpO_2 (%)	92%	<91%
Fall in SpO_2 (%)	≤8%	>9%

Data from Marcus CL, Omlin KJ, Basinki DJ, et al. Normal polysomnographic values for children and adolescents. *Am Rev Respir Dis* 1992;146:1235–9.

TABLE 48.3

CONDITIONS WITH A HIGHER RISK OF
COMPLICATIONS FOLLOWING
ADENOTONSILLECTOMY

Age <3 years
Severe OSAS (profound hypoxemia, AHI >10, significant
   hypoventilation)
Morbid obesity
Neuromuscular disease
Pulmonary hypertension
Down syndrome
Craniofacial anomalies

OSAS, obstructive sleep apnea syndrome; AHI, apnea hypopnea index

Because neither history nor physical exam is sufficient to firmly establish the diagnosis of OSAS, a polysomnogram (PSG; sleep study) is required to reliably make the diagnosis (34). Normative PSG values have been established for children and are quite different from those used in adults, as shown in **Table 48.2** (34,57). The importance of using age-appropriate normative values is illustrated by the fact that normal children have only one or two obstructive apneas or hypopneas per hour of sleep, whereas adults may have as many as five obstructive events per hour of sleep and still be considered normal (31,34).

The first approach to therapy for OSAS is generally adenotonsillectomy (T&A), which should be performed following documentation of the syndrome by PSG. Surgical therapy is often completed in the ambulatory surgery center or with one night of inpatient postoperative observation (19,36). At least one study has demonstrated that children with mild OSAS will do well postoperatively from a respiratory standpoint, irrespective of the use of opiates for analgesia. Polysomnography was performed on the first postoperative night, revealing decreased obstructive events and oxygenation, as compared to the preoperative PSG, although sleep efficiency was decreased (18). However, some groups of patients are at higher risk for postoperative complications and will require a higher level of care. Complications of T&A include postoperative bleeding, upper airway obstruction secondary to airway edema, pulmonary edema, and respiratory failure (19,44,47,49). Diagnostic groups at the highest risk for postoperative complications are listed in **Table 48.3**(37,47).

Children at higher risk for postoperative complications should be admitted for overnight observation, and they may benefit from the intensive cardiorespiratory monitoring afforded by a PICU (19,54). In a retrospective series of 69 children who were observed postoperatively in the PICU following T&A, 23% had respiratory compromise, defined as an O_2 saturation less than 70% and/or hypercapnia. The patients with respiratory compromise were younger (3.4 vs. 6.1 years), had higher numbers of obstructive events per hour on preoperative PSG (49 vs. 19), and were more likely to have failure to thrive, abnormalities of cardiac function, or craniofacial abnormalities. Multiple regression analysis revealed that an age of <3 years and more than 10 obstructive events per hour of sleep were the most significant risk factors for postoperative respiratory compromise (37). Therefore, a preoperative review of the history and the PSG can identify which patients can

be scheduled for same-day surgery and those who will require postoperative care in the PICU. Omitting the PSG and performing T&A simply on the basis of a history of snoring and the presence of adenotonsillar hypertrophy puts children at risk for unexpected postoperative complications (36,37).

Increasingly, children with morbid obesity are presenting with OSAS, and OSAS is often severe in this group with very frequent obstructive events, profound hypoxemia, and significant hypoventilation. Similar to adults with OSAS, both systemic and pulmonary hypertension may be present (30). Unlike the majority of children with OSAS, respiratory control can be altered with re-setting of chemoreceptor function, resulting in daytime hypoventilation. In this instance, ventilation may be dependent on hypoxic drive, requiring that O_2 be used judiciously and necessitating close monitoring both preoperatively and postoperatively. In one retrospective review of 957 children who underwent T&A, of the 543 admitted to the hospital after surgery, 14 were identified as morbidly obese and were admitted to the PICU for observation. Three required assisted ventilation in the postoperative period (50).

Infants and children with craniofacial abnormalities characterized by micrognathia or midfacial hypoplasia can have severe OSAS. It has been reported that surgery for OSAS in patients with craniofacial malformations is less likely to succeed in infants <12 months of age and results in long hospital stays and difficulty with extubation, as compared to older infants and children who undergo similar procedures. Although older children with craniofacial abnormalities are more likely to improve with surgical intervention, they are still at risk for postoperative complications, such as lower respiratory tract infections or the need for a nasopharyngeal airway (24). Children with Down syndrome have multiple reasons for OSAS, including midfacial hypoplasia, relative macroglossia, hypotonia, obesity, and, occasionally, hypothyroidism. In a series of 16 children with Down syndrome, 25% required PICU care postoperatively and persistent symptomatic apnea and hypoxemia were common following T&A (8).

Therapy to support children with respiratory compromise following T&A or other airway surgery can include prolonged intubation or a nasopharyngeal airway. The use of noninvasive ventilation, either continuous or bilevel positive airway pressure (CPAP or BPAP), is attractive, as it avoids intubation and can often be performed on a pediatric unit after the patient is stable. However, some practitioners have questioned the safety of positive airway pressure in the immediate postoperative period, with concerns regarding subcutaneous emphysema, bleeding, or uncomfortable drying of the upper airway by positive pressure airflow. A study of 1321 patients following T&A described 9 patients managed postoperatively with positive airway pressure. Four patients were obese, 4 had underlying neurologic disease, 3 were asthmatic, and 3 were younger than 3 years of age. All tolerated positive-pressure therapy without complications. Two of the obese patients were eventually discharged home with positive airway pressure. Thus, noninvasive ventilation may have a role in the management of complicated patients immediately following adenotonsillectomy. Careful attention to the selection of the mask interface to avoid skin breakdown and the provision of adequate humidification are critical (16).

Most children with OSAS will be treated with T&A as first-line therapy, even if other anatomic or functional abnormalities are likely contributing to the upper airway obstruction. However, some will undergo a more extensive procedure, uvulopalatopharyngoplasty, which includes not only removal of the tonsils, but the tonsillar pillars and uvula as well. This procedure is most often reserved for patients with cerebral palsy or Down syndrome, who have a high probability for residual obstruction following T&A alone (8,29,33,51). Mandibular distraction osteogenesis is being used with increasing frequency for infants and children with syndromes that include micrognathia. Among them are Pierre Robin syndrome, Treacher-Collins syndrome, and conditions that include hemifacial microsomia (10,23). This procedure represents a considerable therapeutic advance, as previously many of these patients would have required a tracheostomy. A recent study of 15 infants with upper airway obstruction treated by internal mandibular distraction osteogenesis documented success and avoidance of tracheostomy in all but one infant. The infants in this series were kept intubated for 3–4 days postoperatively. This treatment approach also improved oral feeding ability, and no patients required placement of a feeding tube (23). Treatment of OSAS in patients with Beckwith-Wiedemann (and occasionally Down syndrome) may require tongue reduction surgery (29). As a whole, the group of children who require complex surgical treatment for OSAS tend to have more severe sleep-disordered breathing and other risk factors for postoperative difficulties. Thus, they should be observed for a period of time in the PICU, and may require several days of intubation following surgery. Despite surgical therapy, some will have only minimal improvement in OSAS, and they will need transition to long-term positive-pressure therapy (CPAP or BPAP), or they will require tracheostomy placement.

Occasionally, patients with OSAS will initially present with acute respiratory failure. This is less common in the current era, when the recognition of sleep-disordered breathing has increased, and the literature contains little evidence to guide treatment. These patients may be otherwise normal or have one of the risk factors listed in Table 48.3. Unlike the majority of children with OSAS, they may have experienced long-term hypercapnia with resulting blunting of their respiratory drive, necessitating extreme caution in the use of supplemental O_2. Injudicious application of high-flow O_2 in this situation can precipitate a respiratory arrest (35). Intubation and ventilation or continuous noninvasive ventilation to correct respiratory acidosis may be indicated. Less severe patients may be managed with placement of a nasopharyngeal tube, though

intubation may be technically difficult (40). Pulmonary hypertension with right heart failure and pulmonary edema is often present, which will require treatment with diuretics and cardiology evaluation. Longstanding upper airway obstruction may have prevented adequate clearance of pulmonary secretions, and treatment with antibiotics may be indicated. Systemic steroids can be administered to acutely decrease the size of adenoidal and tonsillar tissue. The patient should be stabilized before definitive surgical therapy is considered. In this instance, PSG documentation of OSAS is not required preoperatively, but it is necessary following therapy, as residual breathing difficulties during sleep are common following this presentation (36).

The preoperative history should include questions concerning potential sleep apnea because OSAS is estimated to affect ~3% of all children, and unrecognized sleep apnea can adversely affect surgical outcome (52). Further, changes in respiratory control following anesthesia can worsen symptoms of OSAS. Patients with OSAS are likely to have a greater degree of respiratory depression (lower minute ventilation, hypercapnia, and central apnea) with anesthesia that is further worsened by opiates, as compared to children without sleep-disordered breathing (53). The stress of surgery has important effects on sleep architecture that can result in sleep fragmentation and deprivation and REM sleep reduction. Studies in adults have revealed that, although REM sleep may be inhibited on the first postoperative night, REM sleep rebounds on the second or third night. While potentially important for all postoperative patients, in the presence of OSAS, this can result in more opportunity for REM-related hypoxemia or obstructive apneas, at a time when the intensity of monitoring may have been relaxed. In addition, the sleep fragmentation inherent in hospitalization may change upper airway neuromuscular function, favoring airway obstruction and apnea. Studies of adults with OSAS who underwent orthopedic procedures document cardiorespiratory complications in one-third of patients, including unplanned ICU transfers and reintubation (28). Therefore, careful screening of surgical patients for OSAS and recognition of OSAS in postoperative patients is warranted.

The adult OSAS literature contains evidence that stabilization by positive airway pressure (CPAP or BPAP) therapy prior to elective surgery significantly reduces the operative risk and improves the postoperative course as compared to untreated OSAS (28,46). Positive-pressure therapy can be administered continuously postoperatively, with a gradual wean to nighttime use only, allowing the use of adequate sedation and analgesia with less concern regarding respiratory depression. With the increased incidences of pediatric obesity, undoubtedly, more patients who have coexisting OSAS will require intensive care for various reasons. Some will suffer from the metabolic syndrome with insulin resistance and systemic hypertension. A significant number will have OSAS that may not be recognized until extubation, which will require transition to positive-pressure therapy and long-term follow-up by a pulmonary or sleep medicine specialist.

As discussed previously, the perioperative use of positive airway pressure therapy has been reported to reduce complications in adults with OSAS. Certainly, if this therapy has been used at home, arrangements must be made to continue it after surgery. Although patients with untreated OSAS may benefit from positive-pressure support after surgery, pressure titration and adaptation of the patient to the mask may be difficult when the child is recovering from surgery. Judicious use of narcotics in pain management, avoiding or minimizing sedation, and careful respiratory monitoring with frequent assessment of airway status are required with OSAS (28,40).

SUDDEN INFANT DEATH SYNDROME

Sudden infant death syndrome (SIDS) is defined as the sudden, unexpected death (apparently occurring during sleep) of an infant <1 year of age that remains unexplained after a thorough investigation, including performance of a complete autopsy and review of the circumstances of death and the clinical history (32,56). SIDS is the most common cause of nontraumatic death in infants between the ages of 1 month and 1 year, yet its cause remains unknown (4,21). The typical clinical scenario is that parents or caregivers place their apparently healthy baby down to sleep for an overnight sleeping period or a daytime nap. They return some time later to find that their baby has died. In some cases, the parents or caregivers have been within hearing distance of the baby, and they have returned within 30 mins of putting their baby down, to find that the baby has died during that short period of time. Yet, no sounds suggested that struggling occurred. Thus, SIDS appears to occur swiftly and silently.

Most SIDS infants are obviously dead when found. However, some receive cardiopulmonary resuscitation by emergency responders, and these infants are often transported from the place of death to a nearby hospital by emergency medical personnel. Most SIDS infants are not able to be resuscitated in the emergency department. However, in a very small percentage of babies, resuscitation successfully retrieves a heartbeat, though spontaneous ventilation does not return, and the infant is transported to a PICU on life support. Thus, pediatric intensivists care for "SIDS" infants in these situations.

For those babies who present with a sudden severe cardiorespiratory arrest and who are only resuscitated to the point that a heartbeat returns, the outlook is poor. These babies usually deteriorate and develop brain death within 24–48 hrs. Presumably, the initial event was so severe that neurologic damage occurred despite the brief success at regaining a heartbeat. However, these babies should be evaluated for disorders that can cause rapid death, including sepsis, trauma (particularly head trauma), cardiac lesions (serious arrhythmias or anomalous coronary arteries), metabolic disorders, respiratory disorders, (pneumonia or craniofacial abnormalities predisposing to obstructive sleep apnea syndrome). If child abuse or neglect is suspected, referral to professionals who specialize in evaluation for child abuse is indicated (2).

All states in the US and most Western countries require a thorough postmortem investigation, including an autopsy, to determine the cause of death of babies who die suddenly outside of a hospital. By definition, the autopsy does not reveal an identifiable cause of death in SIDS babies (21,32). In most jurisdictions, babies treated in the PICU still fall under the legal mandate for the coroner or medical examiner to determine the cause of death. In these cases, the death should most appropriately be viewed as having occurred where the baby was discovered in cardiopulmonary arrest, rather than in the hospital.

Thus, an examination of the death scene by trained coroner's investigators and a complete autopsy by a skilled pathologist should be performed.

Usually, the SIDS event is accompanied by such severe hypoxemia that internal organs are not useful for transplantation. Infrequently, however, a baby who is diagnosed with brain death but has a heartbeat on life support may be a suitable organ donor. If the intensivist believes that organs may be suitable for transplantation, permission of the medical examiner is usually required before organs can be harvested. A potential conflict exists between examination of vital organs by the medical examiner to determine the cause of death and using these organs for transplantation to save the life of other infants. If some organs do seem potentially useful for transplantation, most coroners and medical examiners will permit the transplant after discussion.

The most important aspect of the care of such SIDS infants is to provide the surviving family members with information about SIDS and resources for support. If the infant does not have evidence of trauma or another cause of death, SIDS is most likely to emerge as the cause of death after the postmortem evaluation. When speaking with the parents, the intensivist can indicate that it appears to have been a SIDS death, although further investigation and autopsy are necessary for confirmation. Parental grief following a SIDS death is complicated by the fact that no one can tell parents why their baby died. They tend to blame themselves, and their guilt tends to be even greater than that of parents whose babies died from known causes. As an authority in healthcare, the intensivist can emphasize to parents that SIDS is a natural cause of death. Based on our current knowledge, SIDS parents do nothing to cause the death, and they could not have done anything to prevent it. SIDS parent support groups are the single best resource for SIDS parents; group participants are available 24 hrs per day to speak with newly bereaved SIDS parents and to provide comfort and support. In the US, the national SIDS parent support organization is First Candle/SIDS Alliance. In the UK, the support organization is called the Foundation for the Study of Infant Deaths; in Canada, it is the Canadian Foundation for the Study of Infant Deaths; in New Zealand, it is the Cot Death Association; and in Australia, the organization is called SIDS and Kids.

By definition, SIDS occurs in the first year of life. It is most common between 2 and 4 months of age. It is less common in the first month of life, and ~95% of SIDS deaths have occurred when the victims were less than 6 months of age (4,21). SIDS is slightly more common in males. The risk of SIDS is higher in infants born prematurely or with low birth weight. Babies born to mothers who smoked cigarettes or used illicit drugs during pregnancy also face an increased risk. African-American and Native American babies are at increased risk. We now know that the sleeping environment plays an important role in SIDS (4). Sleeping in the prone position, on soft bedding, with soft items in the bed, overheating, and possibly bed sharing are all associated with an increased risk for SIDS. In 2004, the most recent year for which complete data are available, the incidence of SIDS in the US was 0.51 SIDS deaths per 1,000 live births, or ~1 in every 2000 babies born. The SIDS rate has fallen dramatically since 1992 due to the "Back to Sleep" campaign, which seeks to educate parents regarding safe infant sleep practices (4). However, some babies, whose parents follow these recommendations, still died from SIDS.

APPARENT LIFE-THREATENING EVENTS

An apparent life-threatening event (ALTE) is defined as an event that is frightening to the observer, in which the infant is observed to have color change (cyanosis or pallor), tone change (limpness, rarely stiffness), apnea, and in which vigorous stimulation, mouth-to-mouth breathing, or resuscitation are required to revive the infant (3,27,41). In most cases, observers feared that the infant was in the process of dying. Sometimes, infants appear to respond quickly, and they may appear entirely normal when medically examined at a later time. Other infants require intensive intervention or resuscitation, and they may still exhibit signs of a serious hypoxic event several minutes later (27). It is this latter group, with persistent cardiorespiratory instability, who will usually be admitted to a PICU for observation and treatment.

Initial Evaluation

ALTE is a clinical diagnosis based on an accurate history of the event by a witness (3,27,41). No diagnostic tests can be used to determine if a child experienced an ALTE. However, the presence of laboratory evidence for severe hypoxia (acidosis or elevated lactate, liver enzymes, or urinary hypoxanthines) can contribute to the assessment of the severity of the event. For a diagnosis of ALTE to be made, most clinicians require that significant intervention was necessary to revive the baby (41). For those infants with signs and/or persistent symptoms that suggest a major hypoxic episode, there is little doubt that something serious has occurred. These infants will require a diagnostic evaluation to discover the etiology of the event, which is necessary both to properly treat the underlying etiology and to reduce the chance for recurrent events.

Relationship Between an Apparent Life-threatening Event and Sudden Infant Death Syndrome

Clinically, infants who present with an ALTE are of concern because it has been believed that ALTEs are associated with an increased risk for SIDS. However, no scientific evidence supports this belief (3,27,45). The Collaborative Home Infant Monitoring Evaluation (CHIME) study monitored over 1,000 babies during sleep in their homes for 6 months (45). They did not find that ALTE babies had a higher risk of recurrent apneic events as compared to healthy term control infants (45). Further, the peak incidence of prolonged apnea in infants occurred at a much younger age than when SIDS occurs, suggesting that these prolonged apneas are not related to SIDS (13,45). Therefore, it is likely that most ALTE infants would not die from SIDS or another sudden cause, even if untreated. In addition, relatively few SIDS parents report that their babies had any serious apneas prior to death (20). The most important difference between ALTE and SIDS is that ALTE babies survive their episodes, while SIDS babies die. Babies with SIDS usually die from only one event. Babies with ALTE often have survived one or more events, even before treatment. Thus, the vast majority of ALTE babies do not die from SIDS, and the two conditions should not be equated (3,4,27,45).

The explanation for ALTE being a phenomenon of infancy lies in the fact that the cardiorespiratory physiology of infants is rapidly undergoing change and thus is intrinsically unstable. For example, central control of breathing is immature and all infants are predisposed to breathing pauses during sleep (45). Infants are exquisitely sensitive to hypoxic depression of ventilation. Thus, hypoxia that results from an apnea will exacerbate the apnea, rather than serve as a stimulus to resolve it. The infant diaphragm has both decreased strength and decreased endurance compared to older children or adults. Thus, the diaphragm is more susceptible to fatigue, especially in the face of increased respiratory loads such as may be caused by lung disease or obstructive apnea. Finally, newborn infants are born with only 10% of the alveoli they will have as adults. Thus, elastic support of alveoli, airways, blood vessels, and lymphatics is decreased, and these structures tend to collapse or be narrower in the face of any lung disease. All components of the respiratory system are immature and have decreased reserve. They can more readily go into respiratory failure, and apnea is a common response to a variety of stresses. Therefore, a number of diseases and stresses can cause cardiorespiratory compromise, and ALTE can be a result of many disorders that stress this system. Consequently, ALTE infants often have an identifiable cause for their events, and they deserve a careful diagnostic evaluation and appropriate treatment.

Diagnostic Evaluation

Infants who experienced an ALTE and are admitted to a PICU have evidence of ongoing cardiorespiratory instability, metabolic acidosis (presumably from a prolonged hypoxic event), or evidence of some other potentially life-threatening condition. They must first be evaluated for adequate cardiorespiratory status. An arterial blood gas, blood sugar, and chest x-ray are first-line diagnostic procedures. If the infant appears to be septic, a diagnostic evaluation for sepsis will be necessary, including a lumbar puncture. Other diagnostic evaluations should be performed as indicated by the clinical history of the event and physical examination (26). No cookbook series of diagnostic tests exists for all infants with ALTE. Testing should be guided by the specific circumstances of the ALTE infant and the event (27). A list of possible etiologies for ALTE and appropriate diagnostic testing is shown in **Table 48.4**. It should be emphasized that not all of these diagnostic studies are required for evaluating an ALTE; only those indicated by the history and physical examination.

Sleep studies are frequently used to evaluate infants with ALTE. Generally, these are not useful in predicting the recurrence risk for subsequent events (27). Therefore, they should not be used to decide if an infant will or will not have subsequent ALTEs. However, they are extremely useful in diagnosing sleep-disordered breathing, which may have contributed to or caused an ALTE, such as OSAS, hypoxia due to chronic lung disease, or central hypoventilation syndromes.

Etiology

As many as 50%–70% of ALTEs can be explained by an identified diagnosis (12,27). The most common causes of ALTE are shown in **Figure 48.2**. In some series, as many as 50% of ALTEs

TABLE 48.4

DIAGNOSTIC EVALUATION FOR APPARENT
LIFE-THREATENING EVENT INFANTS

Potential diagnosis/etiology	Diagnostic tests
Infection Sepsis Asphyxia	Complete blood count Arterial blood gas (pH)
Hypocalcemia Electrolyte Imbalance Dehydration	Serum electrolytes Serum calcium BUN, creatinine
Hypoglycemia	Blood sugar
Sepsis	Blood, urine, cerebrospinal fluid cultures
Pneumonia Chronic lung disease Congenital heart disease Cardiomyopathy	Chest x-ray Electrocardiogram Echocardiogram
Cardiac arrhythmia Prolonged QT interval syndrome	Electrocardiogram 24-hr Holter monitoring
Trauma Child abuse	Skeletal series Skull x-ray Head CT scan Retinoscopy
Seizures	Electroencephalogram
Gastroesophageal reflux disease	Barium swallow Gastric scintiscan, esophageal pH monitoring
Sleep-disordered breathing Obstructive sleep apnea Central hypoventilation syndrome	Overnight polysomnography
Upper airway obstruction Craniofacial abnormality Congenital airway anomaly	Laryngoscopy Bronchoscopy
Inborn errors of metabolism	Serum ammonia level Urine organic acids Plasma amino acids
Drug ingestion Toxic exposure	Serum and urine toxicology

are caused by gastrointestinal disorders (27). Although gastroesophageal reflux disease is frequently found on diagnostic testing for ALTE, it should not be assumed too quickly that this completely explains the event (5,27). Apneas have not temporally correlated with gastroesophageal reflux events on PSG (26). ALTEs of gastrointestinal origin usually occur during or shortly after feeding, they are more likely to occur during wakefulness, and they may be accompanied by choking, vomiting, or coughing. Neurologic problems account for up to 30% of ALTE in some series (27). Seizures are the most common neurologic etiology of ALTE. Electroencephalograms should be performed when seizures are suspected, but they may not be diagnostic. The diagnosis of seizures is based on a typical history. Congenital brainstem anomalies, especially Arnold Chiari type I or II, may cause apnea. When neurologic causes of ALTE are suspected, a brainstem MRI may be helpful in diagnosing brainstem anomalies.

Approximately 20% of ALTE may be due to respiratory disorders (27). Obstructive sleep apnea can occur with viral infections, such as respiratory syncytial virus, cytomegalovirus, or influenza. Craniofacial anomalies predispose to obstructive apnea in infants (17,38). Central nervous system depressant medications enhance susceptibility to OSAS. OSAS can be idiopathic in infants, especially if they are premature; and it is exacerbated by anemia. A history of noisy breathing, snoring, or excessive sweating during sleep should prompt a further evaluation for OSAS (26). Cardiovascular problems account for only ~5% of ALTEs (11,27).

It has been estimated that inborn errors of metabolism account for 2%–5% of ALTEs (6,27). ALTEs due to inborn errors of metabolism are often associated with fasting, fever, or vomiting. Inborn errors of β-oxidation of fatty acids have been described in ALTE babies with severe recurrent events, events that persist beyond a year of age, and in babies with a family history of previous infant deaths and/or severe apneas (6).

Less than 3% of ALTEs appear to be due to child abuse (27,48). The diagnosis of child abuse is clear when signs of trauma, previous fractures, or neglect (failure to thrive) are observed (2,52). A family history of previous SIDS, infant deaths, or ALTE, especially if associated with unusual circumstances, may increase suspicion for child abuse. However, it is not the primary role of the intensivist to rule in or out the diagnosis of child abuse. Rather, one should refer suspicious cases to experts in the field (2).

Management

The medical management of the ALTE infant in the PICU is directed toward stabilizing the cardiorespiratory status of the infant. Once this is achieved, a diagnostic evaluation, directed by the history and physical examination, is performed. If an identifiable cause explains the ALTE, the treatment should be directed toward that diagnosis. However, in as many as 30%–50% of ALTE infants, a specific etiology will not be determined, and these infants are said to have idiopathic ALTE or apnea of infancy (3,27,41). The appropriate post-PICU treatment of these infants is controversial.

Respiratory stimulants, such as methylxanthines, have not been shown to prevent subsequent ALTEs (27,41). They may not stimulate central control of breathing. They are associated with side effects, including gastroesophageal reflux, impaired arousal, depressed ventilatory responses, and an increased propensity for seizures (27,41). Therefore, methylxanthines are not useful in the long-term management of infants who experience an ALTE.

If a treatable cause for the ALTE cannot be found, and if the original event was of sufficient severity to be of concern about the sequelae of subsequent events, most clinicians will manage these patients with home apnea-bradycardia monitoring (3,27,41). While it is recognized that randomized, controlled trials have not been conducted to test the efficacy of home apnea-bradycardia monitoring in saving lives, this technique remains the most frequently chosen one for these infants. The most commonly used home monitors detect chest wall movement by transthoracic impedance, and they detect heart rate by electrocardiogram. These monitors can detect central apneas but not obstructive apneas. Chest wall movement may occur during obstructed breaths (Fig. 48.3), and the monitor will interpret that as uninterrupted breathing (45). Home apnea-bradycardia monitors alert parents and caregivers to

Most Common Causes of ALTE

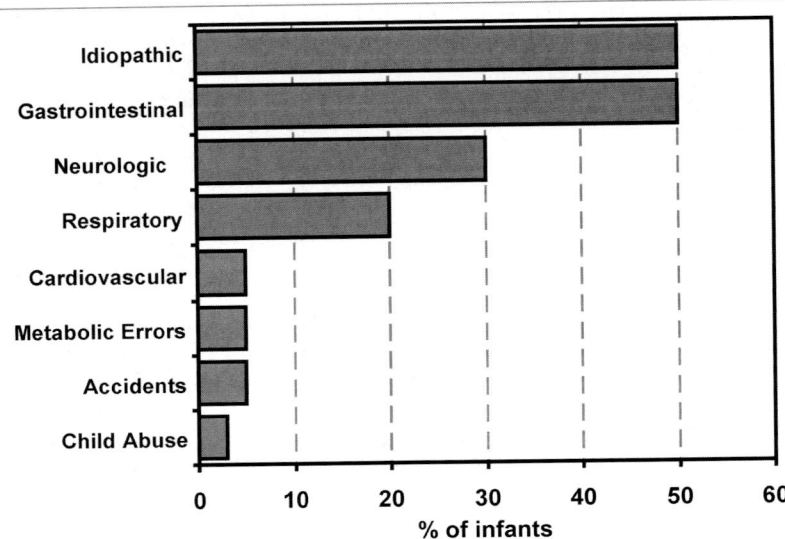

FIGURE 48.2. The most common causes of ALTE. The approximate proportion of infants (*X-axis*) who have ALTE that is attributed to one or more of the listed categories. Modified from the data summary in Kahn A. Recommended clinical evaluation of infants with an apparent life-threatening event. Consensus document of the European Society for the Study and Prevention of Infant Death, 2003. *Eur J Pediatr* 2004;163:108–15.

prolonged central apneic pauses and/or bradycardias by sounding an alarm (usually 90 decibels). Then, trained caregivers must respond to evaluate the event and revive the infant if necessary. Recommended alarm settings are listed in **Table 48.5**. The caregiver's progressive response to a home monitor alarm is shown in **Table 48.6**. Home monitors should have a memory that records what the monitor detects during and before an alarm sounds. Many home monitor alarms are actually caused by artifact due to poor signal. The recorded alarms, downloaded from the monitor memory, can be used to decide if monitor alarms in the home are detecting pathologic apneas or bradycardias.

Pulse oximetry, by measuring oxygenation, may sound the alarm for a more relevant physiologic event than will traditional home monitors. However, pulse oximeters may have excessive false alarms due to motion artifact. As technology improves, pulse oximeters may be useful as home monitors in the future.

The CHIME study found that if infants did not have a significant apnea or bradycardia within 2 months of the original event, they did not have one subsequently (45). Therefore, it appears to be safe to discontinue home apnea-bradycardia monitoring once an infant has gone 2 months without a significant event (3,45).

SLEEP IN THE PEDIATRIC INTENSIVE CARE UNIT

The purpose of sleep is not fully understood, but the consequences of sleep deprivation are well described. Addressing the impact of sleep deprivation on healthcare providers is one of the most important aims of improving healthcare safety. However, sleep deprivation also affects patients, particularly in the PICU. Inadequate sleep can cause neurocognitive and

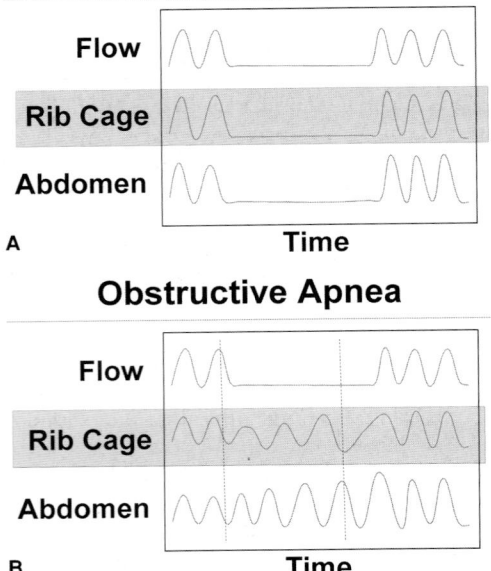

FIGURE 48.3. Home monitor detection of central and obstructive apnea. Home monitors detect breathing by chest wall motion (transthoracic impedance). They can detect central apneas (**A**), characterized by no chest wall movement (*gray area*). However, they cannot detect obstructive apneas (**B**), because chest wall movement continues during the obstructive event (*gray area*).

TABLE 48.5

RECOMMENDED ALARM SETTINGS FOR HOME APNEA-BRADYCARDIA MONITORS

Infant age (months post-term)	Apnea (seconds)	Low heart rate (beats/min)	High heart rate
0–1	20	80	Off
1–2	20	70	Off
3–12	20	60	Off
>12	25	50	Off

TABLE 48.6

CAREGIVER RESPONSES TO HOME APNEA-BRADYCARDIA ALARMS

Time (secs)	Action by caregiver
0–20	Time from the start of a central apnea until the home monitor sounds an alarm.
20–30	Caregivers reach the infant's location and observe the infant's color, tone, and breathing. Is this a real alarm?
30–40	Apply gentle stimulation (call the name, stroke the back, shake an extremity).
40–50	Apply vigorous stimulation (turn the baby face up if not supine), lift the baby, support the head, and move the baby.
>50	Begin cardiopulmonary resuscitation.

psychological deficits. Sleep deprivation is a physiologic stressor and can affect autonomic, immunologic, metabolic, and hormonal function. Finally, adults have identified poor sleep as one of the greatest hardships endured during their ICU stays (55).

Sleep in critically ill patients is characterized by an abnormal distribution, with sleep times scattered throughout a 24-hr period rather than consolidated at night. Thus total sleep time may not be affected but, because sleep is fragmented, its restorative properties may be lacking. The arrangement of sleep stages is also affected, with an increase in "light sleep" (stage 1) and decreased time in deeper sleep (stages 2, 3, 4, and REM). Sleep in the ICU is disrupted by frequent arousals and awakenings. Over one-third of adult patients recall poor sleep during their ICU stay, and the vast majority rate poor sleep as being moderately or extremely bothersome. In one study, only an inability to communicate by ventilated patients was rated as more stressful than the inability to sleep (42).

All hospitalized children are at risk for poor sleep from illness, pain, medications, therapies, and an unfamiliar sleep environment. However, the PICU environment is perhaps the most important factor in sleep disruption for the critically ill child. Noise and light levels are high in the PICU and are not conducive to sleep (1). Although monitors, alarms, ventilators, pagers, and other devices contribute to the ambient noise, talking appears to be the biggest culprit. Mechanical ventilation poses an additional challenge to a good night's sleep. Poor synchrony between the patient and the ventilator, intubation, the ventilator mode, intermittent suctioning, and an inability to communicate all may contribute to sleep disruption. The need for assisted ventilation may also be a marker for greater disease severity, with inherently poor sleep. The presence of sepsis alters sleep architecture and interferes with the normal circadian pattern of melatonin secretion (39,55).

The medications used in the PICU often affect sleep, both during and after use. Benzodiazepines and opioids cause REM suppression; consequently, a REM rebound effect follows discontinuation, which can result in nightmares or disturbing dreams. Sedation has some of the properties of natural sleep (decreased awareness of surroundings, decreased motor activ-

ity), but it is not known if or how well sedation mimics the proposed function and purpose of natural sleep, which likely includes restoration and maintenance of neural and somatic function. One study followed 2 children who received continuous sedation and neuromuscular blockade following laryngotracheoplasty by continuous polysomnography for 96 hrs. The PSG records revealed that sleep did occur under these conditions, but it was fragmented and occurred both during the day and the night (9). Another study of ventilated children who received continuous sedation and opiate analgesia found that sleep was severely fragmented and that REM sleep accounted for only 3% of total sleep time (1). A recent study of fentanyl withdrawal in neonates revealed that a reduction in sleep time was the most frequent troublesome sign (14). The use or discontinuation of many other classes of medications can also affect sleep. For example, an abrupt discontinuation of a β-blocker can fragment sleep dramatically. Therefore, a review of all medications, both current and recent, should be performed whenever sleep disturbance or deprivation affects children in the PICU (55).

Sleep deprivation results in a number of neurologic and behavioral complications. Reduced vigilance and reaction time are the impairments most relevant for sleep deprivation in healthcare providers. For patients, mood alterations (irritability) and organic brain dysfunction (delusions and hallucinations) are probably more important. Delirium can occur in the PICU setting and has serious negative prognostic implications. Although no link has been proven between sleep disturbance and delirium, this is clearly an important area for future research (15).

Sleep deprivation in critically ill patients may impair immunologic function. Animal studies have identified decreased cellular immunity with sleep deprivation. While it is true that the clinical significance of these findings is unknown, when a patient's survival may depend on their ability to mount an adequate immune response to multiple challenges, it seems prudent to enhance sleep quality whenever possible. Sleep loss affects the secretion of hormones that can play a role in the body's response to stress, including increases in cortisol, norepinephrine, and thyroid hormone. Critical illness can also alter these same hormones. Both sleep deprivation and critical illness cause insulin resistance that can be clinically significant. As the presence of sleep deprivation is potentially more amenable to change than the severity of the underlying illness, adopting strategies to enhance sleep in the PICU is a worthwhile endeavor (55).

Monsen et al. reported their efforts to reduce noise and sleep disturbance in a neurointensive care unit. Sleep disturbances were documented in subsets of patients in a total of fourteen 24-hr periods before the intervention in order to target efforts, and again after the intervention to evaluate effectiveness. Investigators found that routine nursing care activities were the most disturbing. Also implicated were inhalational treatments, CPAP, and ambient noise. A behavioral modification program was introduced for the staff, which included education about the concept of healthy sleep, or sleep hygiene, and how to structure activities to minimize sleep disruption. The findings of the study emphasized the need to limit care activities between the hours of midnight and 0500 to provide time for consolidated sleep, as well as the importance of engaging the ICU staff in continuous efforts to reduce noise levels (39). Controlling light exposure with open blinds during the day and decreased light at night has also been recommended.

CONCLUSIONS AND FUTURE DIRECTIONS

Sleep is a period of vulnerability for the respiratory system. Obstructive sleep apnea syndrome, ALTEs, and SIDS are manifestations of this vulnerability. The perturbations of physiology inherent in critical illness do not spare the process of sleep, and the environment of the PICU generally adds to sleep abnormalities rather than promoting healthy sleep. Goals for the future include identifying more exact methods of predicting which infants and children are at highest risk for severe OSAS and its attendant complications, understanding the etiologies of ALTE and SIDS and establishing strategies to prevent them from occurring, and developing approaches to minimize the effects of sleep disruption in the PICU setting.

KEY POINTS

- Obstructive sleep apnea occurs when the upper airway is functionally or anatomically narrowed. Sleep predisposes to airway instability and obstruction.

- Most children with OSAS can be treated with T&A in the ambulatory surgery center. However, those who are at risk for severe OSAS and for postoperative complications will need PICU care.

- In addition to adenotonsillectomy, OSAS can be successfully treated with other surgical approaches and by the use of positive airway pressure. Children with obesity-related OSAS will often require CPAP or BPAP to control OSAS.

- Children who present to the PICU for other reasons may have unrecognized OSAS. Screening for sleep-related breathing disorders should be part of the preoperative evaluation of all children who are to undergo elective surgical procedures. Continuous positive airway pressure can be used both before and after surgery for stabilization.

- The respiratory system in infancy is immature and intrinsically unstable. Infants may suffer an ALTE due to a number of etiologies that perturb the respiratory system. A targeted diagnostic evaluation and therapy directed at the underlying cause is indicated. Home monitoring is needed for infants at risk for subsequent events.

- SIDS is the most common cause of death for infants between the ages of 1 month and 1 year. The etiology of SIDS remains unknown, but the risk has been significantly reduced by the promotion of safe infant sleep practices. The parents of SIDS babies suffer overwhelming grief and need education and emotional support, which are best provided by SIDS parent organizations.

- Sleep fragmentation and deprivation occur in the PICU setting, and they may interfere with physiologic responses to stress and add to the discomfort of being a patient in the PICU. Many medications, therapies, and the PICU environment negatively impact sleep. A consideration of the importance of sleep in the PICU may enhance patient outcomes.

References

1. Al-samson RH, Cullen P. Sleep and adverse environmental factors in sedated mechanically ventilated patients. *Pediatr Crit Care Med* 2005;6:562–7.

2. American Academy of Pediatrics. Distinguishing sudden infant death syndrome from child abuse fatalities. *Pediatrics* 2001;107:437–41.

3. American Academy of Pediatrics Policy Statement. Apnea, sudden infant death syndrome, and home monitoring. *Pediatrics* 2003;111:914–7.

4. American Academy of Pediatrics Policy Statement. The changing concept of sudden infant death syndrome: Diagnostic coding shifts, controversies regarding the sleeping environment, and new variables to consider in reducing the risk. *Pediatrics* 2005;116, 1245–55.

5. Arad-Cohen N, Cohen A, Tirosh E. The relationship between gastroesophageal reflux and apnea in infants. *J Pediatr* 2000;137:321–6.

6. Arens R, Gozal D, Williams JC, et al. Recurrent apparent life-threatening events during infancy: A manifestation of inborn errors of metabolism. *J Pediatr* 1993;123:415–8.

7. Balbani APS, Weber Silke AT, Montovani JC. Update in obstructive sleep apnea syndrome in children. *Rev Bras Otorrinolaringol* 2005;71:74–80.

8. Bower CM, Richmond D. Tonsillectomy and adenoidectomy in patients with Down syndrome. *Int J Pediatr Otorhinolaryngol* 1995;33:141–8.

9. Carno MA, Hoffman LA, Henker R, et al. Sleep monitoring in children during neuromuscular blockade in the pediatric intensive care unit. *Pediatr Crit Care Med* 2004;5:224–9.

10. Chigurupati R, Massie J, Dargaville P, et al. Internal mandibular distraction to relieve airway obstruction in infants and young children with micrognathia. *Pediatr Pulmonol* 2004;37:230–5.

11. Dancea A, Cote A, Rohlicel C, et al. Cardiac pathology in sudden unexpected infant deaths. *J Pediatr* 2002;141:336–42.

12. Daniels H, Naulaers G, Deroost F, et al. Polysomnography and home-documented monitoring of cardiorespiratory pattern. *Arch Dis Child* 1999;81:434–6.

13. Davidson Ward SL, Keens TG, Chan LS, et al. Sudden infant death syndrome in infants evaluated by apnea programs in California. *Pediatrics* 1986;77:451–5.

14. Dominguez KD, Lomako DM, Katz RW, et al. Opioid withdrawal in critically ill neonates. *Ann Pharmacother* 2003;37:473–7.

15. Ely EW, Shitani A, Truman B, et al. Delirium as a predictor mortality in mechanically ventilated patients in the intensive care unit. *J Am Med Assoc* 2004;291:1753–62.

16. Friedman O, Chidekel A, Lawless SL, et al. Postoperative bilevel positive airway pressure ventilation after tonsillectomy and adenoidectomy in children: A preliminary report. *Int J Pediatr Otorhinolaryngol* 1999;51:177–80.

17. Guilleminault C, Pelayo R, Leger D, et al. Apparent life-threatening events, facial dysmorphia and sleep-disordered breathing. *Eur J Pediatr* 2000;159:444–9.

18. Helfaer MA, McColley SA, Pyzik PL, et al. Polysomnography after adenotonsillectomy in mild pediatric obstructive sleep apnea. *Crit Care Med* 1996;24:1323–7.

19. Halfaer MA, Wilson MD. Obstructive sleep apnea, control of ventilation, and anesthesia in children. *Pediatr Clin North Am* 1991;41:131–51.

20. Hoffman HJ, Damas K, Hillman L, et al. Risk factors for SIDS: Results of the National Institute of Child Health and Human Development SIDS Cooperative Epidemiological Study. *NY Acad Sci* 1988;533:13–30.

21. Hunt CE, Hauck FR. Sudden infant death syndrome. *Can Med Assoc J* 2006;174:1861–9.

22. Isono S. Upper airway muscle function during sleep. In: Loughlin GM, Carroll JL, Marcus CL, eds., *Sleep and Breathing in Children: A Developmental Approach.* New York: Marcel Dekker, Inc., 2000:261–92.

23. Izadi K, Yellon R, Mandell DL, et al. Correction of upper airway obstruction in the newborn internal mandibular distraction osteogenesis. *J Craniofacial Surg* 2003;14:493–9.

24. Januszkiewicz JS, Cohen SR, Burstein FD, et al. Age-related outcomes of sleep apnea surgery in infants and children. *Ann Plast Surg* 1997;38:465–77.

25. Kaemingk KL, Pasvogel AE, Goodwin JL, et al. Learning in children and sleep-disordered breathing: Findings of the Tucson Children's Assessment of Sleep Apnea (TuCASA) prospective cohort study. *J Int Neuropsychol Soc* 2003;9:1016–26.

26. Kahn A, Rebuffat E, Sottiaux M, et al. Arousals induced by proximal esophageal reflux in infants. *Sleep* 1991;14:39–42.

27. Kahn A. Recommended clinical evaluation of infants with an apparent life-threatening event. Consensus document of the European Society for the Study and Prevention of Infant Death, 2003. *Eur J Pediatr* 2004;163:108–15.

28. Kaw R, Michota F, Jaffer A. Unrecognized sleep apnea in the surgical patient: Implications for the perioperative setting. *Chest* 2006;129:198–205.

29. Kennedy DJ, Waters KA. Investigation and treatment of upper-airway obstruction: Childhood sleep disorders I. Obstructive sleep apnea syndrome is common and is associated with significant childhood morbidities. *MJA Practice Essentials* 2005;182:419–23.

30. Kessler R, Chaouat A, Schinkewitch P, et al. The obesity-hypoventilation syndrome revisited: A prospective study of 34 consecutive cases. *Chest* 2001;120:369–76.

31. Krimsky WR, Leiter JC. Respiratory control during sleep. In: Lee-Chiong T, ed., *Sleep: A Comprehensive Handbook.* Hoboken, NJ: John Wiley and Sons, Inc., 2006: 663–7.

32. Krous HF, Beckwith JB, Byard RW, et al. Sudden infant death syndrome (SIDS) and unclassified sudden infant deaths (USID): A definitional and diagnostic approach. *Pediatrics* 2004;114:234–8.

33. Magardino TM, Tom LW. Surgical management of obstructive sleep apnea in children with cerebral palsy. *Laryngoscope* 1999;109:1611–5.

34. Marcus CL, Omlin KJ, Basinki DJ, et al. Normal polysomnographic values for children and adolescents. *Am Rev Respir Dis* 1992;146:1235–9.

35. Marcus CL. Sleep-disordered breathing in children. *Am J Resp Crit Care Med* 2001;164:16–30.

36. Marcus C, Chapman D, Davidson Ward SL, et al. Clinical practice guideline: Diagnosis and management of childhood of obstructive sleep apnea syndrome. *Pediatrics* 2002;109:704–12.

37. McMolley SA, April MM, Carroll JL, et al. Respiratory compromise after adenotonsillectomy in children with obstructive sleep apnea. *Arch Otolaryngol Head Neck Surg* 1992;118:940–3.

38. McNamara F, Sullivan CE. Obstructive sleep apnea in infants: Relation to family history of sudden infant death syndrome, apparent life-threatening events, and obstructive sleep apnea. *J Pediatr* 2000;136:318–23.

39. Monson MG, Edell-Gustafsson UM. Noise and sleep disturbance factors before and after implementation of a behavioral modification programme. *Intens Crit Care Nurs* 2005;21:208–19.

40. Moos D, Cuddeford J. Implications of obstructive sleep apnea syndrome for the perianesthesia nurse. *J Perianesth Nurs* 2006;21:103–18.

41. National Institutes of Health Consensus Development Conference on Infantile Apnea and Home Monitoring. *Pediatrics* 1987;79:292–9.

42. Nelson JE, Meier DE, Oei EJ, et al. Self-reported symptom experience of critically ill cancer patients receiving intensive care. *Crit Care Med* 2001;29:277–82.

43. O'Brien LM, Mervis CB, Holbrook CR, et al. Neurobehavioral implications of habitual snoring in children. *Pediatrics* 2004;114:44–9.

44. Paradise JL, Bluestone CD, Colborn DK, et al. Tonsillectomy and adenoidectomy for recurrent throat infections in moderately affected children. *Pediatrics* 2002;110:7–15.

45. Ramanathan R, Corwin MJ, Hunt CE, et al. Cardiorespiratory events recorded on home monitors: Comparison of healthy infants with those at increased risk for SIDS. *J Amer Med Assoc* 2001;285:2199–207.

46. Rennotte MT, Baele P, Aubert G, Rodenstein DO. Nasal continuous positive airway pressure in the perioperative management of patients with obstructive sleep apnea submitted to surgery. *Chest* 1995;107:367–74.

47. Rosen GM, Muckle RP, Mahowald MW, et al. Postoperative respiratory compromise in children with obstructive sleep apnea syndrome: Can it be anticipated? *Pediatrics* 1994;93:784–8.

48. Samuels MP, Southall DP. Alarms during apparent life-threatening events. *Am J Respir Crit Care Med* 2003;167:A677.

49. Sher AE. Upper airway surgery for obstructive sleep apnea. In: Lee-Chiong T, ed., *Sleep: A Comprehensive Handbook*. Hoboken, NJ: John Wiley and Sons, Inc., 2006: 211–22.

50. Spector A, Scheid S, Hassink S, et al. Adenotonsillectomy in the morbidly obese child. *Int J Pediatr Otorhinolaryngol* 2003;67:359–64.

51. Thomas MM, Lawrence WC. Surgical management of obstructive sleep apnea in children with cerebral palsy. *Laryngoscope.* 1999;109:1611–5.

52. Warwick JP and Mason DG. Obstructive sleep apnoea syndrome in children. *Anaesthesia* 1998;53:571–579.

53. Waters KA, McBrien F, Stewart P, Hinde et al. Effects of OSA, inhalational anesthesia, and fentanyl on the airway and ventilation of children. *J Appl Physiol* 2002;92:1987–94.

54. Walker P, Whitehead B, Rowley M. Criteria for elective admission to the paediatric intensive care unit following adenotonsillectomy for severe obstructive sleep apnoea. *Anaesth Intensive Care* 2004;32:43–6.

55. Weinhouse GL and Schwab MD. Sleep in the critically ill patient. *Sleep* 2006;29:707–16.

56. Willinger M, James LS, Catz C. Defining the sudden infant death syndrome (SIDS): Deliberations of an expert panel convened by the National Institute of Child Health and Human Development. *Pediatr Pathol* 1991;11:677–84.

57. Witmans MB, Keens TG, Davidson Ward SL, et al. Obstructive hypopneas in children and adolescents: Normal values. *Am J Respir Crit Care Med* 2003;168:1540.

58. Woodson BT. Physiology of sleep-disordered breathing. In: Lee-Chiong T, ed., *Sleep: A Comprehensive Handbook*. Hoboken, NJ: John Wiley and Sons, Inc., 2006, 211–22.

CHAPTER 49 ■ ACUTE NEUROMUSCULAR DISEASE

SUNIT SINGHI • ALKA KHADWAL • ARUN BANSAL

A child with an acute neuromuscular disorder (NMD) requires critical care for respiratory assistance, including intubation of the trachea, mechanical ventilation, or both. The common scenarios that require critical monitoring or care involve the need for airway protection, assistance with oxygenation and/or ventilation, or intensive pulmonary toilet. Intubation of the trachea may be necessary for airway protection if bulbar muscle dysfunction is present. Mechanical ventilation, either noninvasively or with intubation, may be necessary if respiratory failure develops. Occasionally, children with acute NMDs will require airway management solely to facilitate pulmonary toilet. Typically, more than one of these three needs is present when a child with an acute NMD requires respiratory assistance.

Acute NMDs can be the primary reason for admission to the ICU. However, they may also develop de novo during the ICU stay and result in an increase in morbidity and mortality, in the length of hospital stay, and in healthcare costs. So-called "ICU-acquired neuromuscular weakness," comprising critical illness polyneuropathy (CIP) and critical illness myopathy (CIM) may occur more often in adults than primary NMDs such as Guillain-Barré syndrome (GBS), motor neuron disease, or myopathies (40). The incidence of these secondary illnesses (CIP/CIM) in children is less common than in adults, which may be due to under-recognition and under-reporting for children (62).

REGULATION OF RESPIRATION

Respiration is regulated by both voluntary and involuntary neural mechanisms. The cerebral cortex is responsible for voluntary control of breathing, whereas the brainstem, mainly the medulla oblongata with additional inputs from pons and vagus, provides involuntary control. Spontaneous breathing is produced by rhythmic discharge of motor neurons innervating the respiratory muscles under the control of brainstem and is regulated by alterations in arterial PaO_2, $PaCO_2$, and pH. The afferent limb of the respiratory feedback system is composed of input from the tissues and airways with receptor endings and chemoreceptors in the carotid bodies, which send information to the central nervous system (CNS). The efferent limb involves signals sent from the CNS via cranial and peripheral nerves to the respiratory muscles, which produce an increase or decrease in respiratory activity. This feedback system optimizes airway patency, work of breathing, and gas exchange.

NMDs can be classified according to the site of primary pathology: brain, spinal cord, peripheral nerve, neuromuscular junction, or the skeletal muscle (**Table 49.1**). In primary NMDs, ineffective motor nerve input to muscles may originate in diseases of the brain (central hypoventilation), spinal cord (trauma), anterior horn cells (poliomyelitis, spinal muscular atrophy), peripheral nerve (GBS), neuromuscular junction (botulism, myasthenia gravis), or skeletal muscle system (muscular dystrophy).

RESPIRATORY MECHANICS

The lungs and surrounding chest-wall muscles form the ventilatory apparatus, which is similar in function to a pump. The integrity of this "respiratory pump" and the central control from brain and nerves is essential for maintaining normal breathing. The primary muscle of breathing is the diaphragm. The accessory muscles of breathing are located in the neck and the upper chest wall and include the sternocleidomastoid, trapezius, intercostal, and rhomboid muscles. Inspiration is an active process during which an increase in intrathoracic volume is produced by chest and lung expansion, resulting from contraction that causes a downward movement of the diaphragm. The intercostal muscles stabilize the chest wall during changes in intrathoracic pressure. Expiration is a passive process during quiet breathing that results from elastic recoil of the lungs as the diaphragm relaxes to resume its resting configuration. The alternating inspiratory and expiratory activity moves gases in and out of the lung for gaseous exchange. As breathing becomes vigorous with increased activity (exercise) or in the presence of an airway obstruction, the accessory muscles of breathing augment ventilation.

Brain and brainstem diseases cause respiratory depression, characterized by central patterns of respiration, including hyperventilation; irregular, ataxic (or cluster) breathing; hiccups; hypopnea; and apnea. Bulbar involvement may cause impaired clearing of secretions and aspiration. Children unable to clear secretions are more prone to pulmonary infection, which can lead to further deterioration of the clinical condition. Malfunction of a motor nerve unit (i.e., anterior horn cell, axon of anterior horn cell with its myelin covering, neuromuscular junction, and the muscle innervated by the anterior horn cell) may result in an inability to protect the airway, dysfunction of respiratory muscles, or both. Impairment of breathing may occur as a

TABLE 49.1

ANATOMIC CLASSIFICATION AND EXAMPLES OF CONDITIONS WITH NEUROMUSCULAR WEAKNESS THAT REQUIRE PEDIATRIC INTENSIVE CARE

Brain
Intracranial hemorrhage
Hypoxic ischemic encephalopathy
Meningoencephalitis
Acute demyelinating encephalomyelitis

Spinal cord
Trauma
Epidural abscess
Myelitis
Acute poliomyelitis
Spinal muscular atrophy

Peripheral nerve
Guillain-Barré syndrome
Critical illness polyneuropathy
Toxic (lead, arsenic) neuropathy
Drug-induced neuropathy, e.g., vincristine
Diphtheric polyneuropathy
Acute porphyria
Phrenic nerve injury—diaphragmatic paralysis

Neuromuscular junction
Myasthenia gravis and congenital myasthenic syndromes
Prolonged neuromuscular blockade
Antibiotic (aminoglycoside, d-penicillamine) therapy
Snake bite and scorpion sting
Organophosphorus poisoning
Botulism
Tick paralysis
Hypermagnesemia

Muscle
Critical illness myopathy
Hypokalemia
Muscular dystrophies
Congenital myopathies
Acute rhabdomyolysis
Inflammatory myopathies, e.g., dermatomyositis

result of ineffective motor nerve stimulation or intrinsic muscle disease.

In neuromuscular weakness, a combination of abnormalities often contributes to ineffective gas exchange (**Fig. 49.1**). Unable to generate normal inspiratory effort, these patients take breaths of decreased tidal volume and increase their respiratory rate to maintain adequate alveolar ventilation. This pattern of rapid, shallow breathing can lead to a decrease in lung compliance, an increase in work of breathing, and a decrease in respiratory reserve. The decrease in tidal volume and minute ventilation contributes to hypoxemia and hypercapnia. An ineffective cough results in retention and aspiration of secretions and microatelectasis. Lack of muscle tone also leaves the recoil pressure of the lung relatively unopposed, resulting in decreased functional residual capacity and impairment in gas exchange. The development of respiratory symptoms may be relatively insidious or sudden. Most of these patients are not very active and may not complain of shortness of breath, but a minor respiratory infection can precipitate sudden respiratory collapse.

EVALUATION OF RESPIRATORY DYSFUNCTION IN A PATIENT WITH A NEUROMUSCULAR DISORDER

Respiratory muscle weakness and fatigue frequently contribute to ventilatory failure in the patient with an NMD. Monitoring of clinical parameters that indicate the severity and progression of weakness from the onset is very important (**Table 49.2**). Nocturnal respiratory dysfunction, increased chest infections, and the need to provide respiratory support have all been correlated with significant reductions in clinical parameters.

History

Patients with significant weakness of the oropharyngeal muscle may complain of intermittent choking, slurred speech, dysphonia, and difficulty in clearing secretions, or they may present with aspiration pneumonia. Patients may complain of shortness of breath at rest or on exertion, or they may have nonspecific symptoms such as restlessness, difficulty sleeping, or fatigue. Early morning headache, day-time somnolence, and poor school performance are suggestive of nocturnal hypoventilation, which causes hypoxemia and hypercapnia. Weakness of the diaphragm, to a greater extent than weakness of the intercostals, can result in daytime dependency on accessory muscles and can lead to nighttime hypoventilation, as the intercostal muscles can become hypotonic during sleep. Positional symptoms may be described by patients with acute NMDs. Patients with diaphragmatic weakness commonly use accessory muscles of breathing and report becoming distressed when supine. Patients with an intact diaphragm but weak intercostals and abdominal muscles may report respiratory distress in the upright position.

Examination

Speech may be slurred, or nasal escape of air due to oropharyngeal muscle weakness may occur. Laryngeal muscles involvement will result in dysphonia. Difficulty in initiating an explosive cough suggests glottic weakness. A weak cough should alert the examiner that the patient is at high risk of decompensation from retained secretions. Respiration may be rapid and shallow and fail to increase in response to the patient's activity. Patients may present in respiratory failure with a normal or decreased respiratory rate, a late and ominous sign for exhaustion and decompensation. A scaphoid appearance in the abdomen may relate to an isolated diaphragm weakness, with the diaphragm drawn up into the chest during inspiration.

In many neuromuscular syndromes, patients demonstrate a sign called *paradoxical breathing*. Early in the disease, weakness of the intercostal muscles is relatively greater than weakness of the diaphragm. The intercostal muscles usually stabilize the chest wall during inspiration. Paradoxical breathing occurs when, during inspiration, the chest wall is pulled inward due to weak intercostal muscles while the abdomen expands outward as the diaphragm contracts downward; this appears as a rocking motion of chest and abdomen. This pattern differs from normal inspiration in which diaphragm contraction

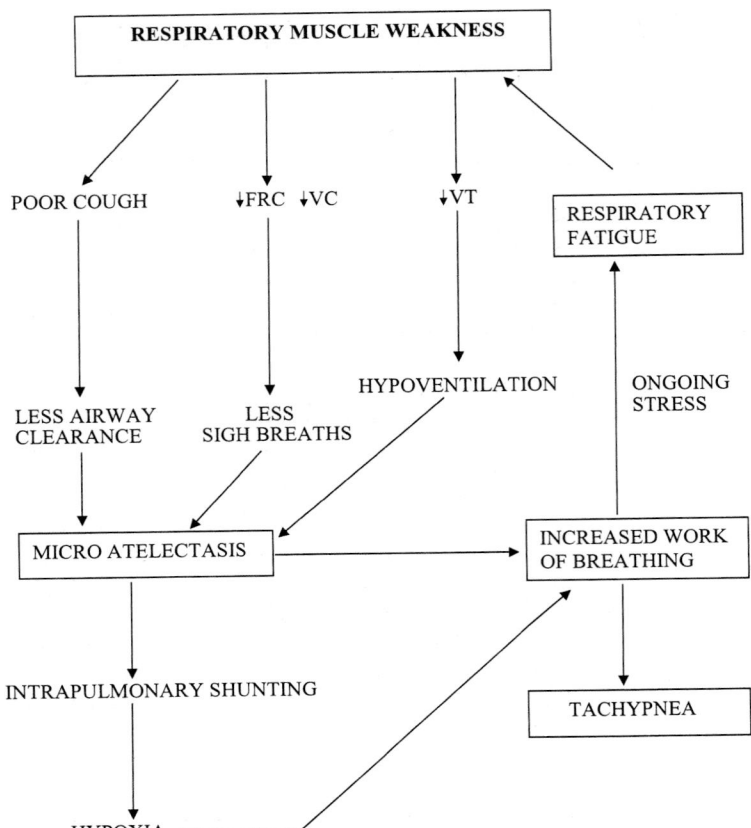

FIGURE 49.1. Pathophysiology of respiratory failure in neuromuscular disorders. FRC, functional residual capacity; VC, vital capacity; VT, tidal volume.

results in abdominal expansion and intercostal contraction causes chest expansion (i.e., synchronized motion of the abdomen and chest).

Abnormalities of, or progression of, blood gas values can be monitored as an indication of respiratory failure. Arterial blood gas monitoring may not be optimal, as changes in blood gases and oxygen saturation tend to occur late after patients can no longer compensate for increasing weakness.

Spirometry

A simple, single-breath counting test may be used at the bedside in older children and adolescents to assess severity and follow progression of weakness due to acute NMD. If the patient can count up to 10 in one breath, the forced vital capacity is likely to be at least 15–20 mL/kg. If they can count up to 25, the vital capacity is ~30–40 mL/kg. Monitoring the trend in single-breath counting may help to predict progression and the need for mechanical ventilation before actual respiratory failure.

A spirometric assessment can also be performed at the bedside in children >5 years to monitor both the severity of weakness and the progression of weakness using a measurement of vital capacity and two clinically helpful respiratory pressures. A normal vital capacity is measured from maximum inspiration to maximum expiration (normal values range from 55–80 mL/kg). Maximum static respiratory pressures are measured: maximum inspiratory pressure (measured at residual volume; normal values are −100 to −120 cm H_2O for adult males and

−80 to −100 cm H_2O for adult females) and maximum expiratory pressure (measured at total lung capacity, normal values 150–240 cm H_2O for adult males and 108–160 cm H_2O for adult females). These are considered sensitive indicators of respiratory muscle strength. Both minimal values and changes in values have been associated with clinically significant deterioration, including an inability to cough and clear secretions, increased incidence of pulmonary infections, increased nighttime ventilatory insufficiency, hypercarbia, and need for ventilatory assistance. Exact minimal measurements that require intervention are not available because of variations in respiratory impairment among disorders or among patients and the lack of data in children. A 20/30/40 rule has been suggested for adult patients for minimal values that raise concern for respiratory failure. A vital capacity of ~20 mL/kg, a maximum inspiratory pressure less negative than −30 cm H_2O, or a maximum expiratory pressure of <40 cm H_2O are minimal values that raise concern for respiratory problems in adults with acute NMD. Also reported as concerning are values that fall by 50% from baseline or >30% in a 24-hr period. It has been observed that life-threatening respiratory failure occurs when vital capacity drops below 20 mL/kg or 30% of predicted values (35).

Radiologic Studies

Radiographic findings are often late or nonspecific. Some helpful findings may include the following. On chest x-ray, an elevated hemidiaphragm, in fixed position during inspiration and

TABLE 49.2

CLINICAL AND LABORATORY PARAMETERS THAT ARE USEFUL IN ASSESSMENT OF ADEQUATE RESPIRATORY FUNCTION IN PATIENTS WITH NEUROMUSCULAR WEAKNESS

Clinical
Respiratory rate—Good index of response to hypoventilation caused by muscular weakness; tachypnea is the earliest response
Swallowing and handling of secretions
Quality of cough
Volume of speech
Single-breath count
Chest expansion
Presence of tachycardia/diaphoresis (nonspecific)
Use of accessory muscles
Orthopnea
Inward movement of abdomen during inspiration.
Breathing pattern alternates between accessory and major respiratory muscles, signifying weakness of major respiratory muscles
Change in status when sleeping—accessory muscle tone decreases
Rate of progression of generalized weakness

Laboratory
Vital capacity
Maximum inspiratory pressure
Maximum expiratory pressure
Sao_2, Pao_2, $Paco_2$, pH
Chest radiograph

expiration, suggests hemidiaphragm weakness or paralysis. A bell-shaped thoracic cage is indicative of intercostal muscle weakness or hypotonia. Nonspecific findings include patchy atelectasis or areas of consolidation in patients with aspiration or infection of the respiratory tract.

MANAGEMENT

Nonspecific or supportive management for respiratory failure and to avoid problems that result from generalized weakness will be discussed in this section. Specific management for disorders will be discussed later, with the discussion of the disorder. Respiratory management is one of the most critical aspects common to all of these disorders and includes airway protection and supportive ventilation, which should take priority over the investigation of the underlying cause and precipitating factors.

Respiratory Monitoring and Care

Ventilatory muscle insufficiency and diaphragmatic weakness may not correlate with general neuromuscular weakness. Respiratory function may be compromised even before clinical signs of ventilatory insufficiency are obvious. The onset of respiratory failure may be more rapid than the underlying neuropathy because of concomitant pulmonary infection. Because of these issues, respiratory status must be closely and carefully monitored.

The patient's ability to protect his airway should be assessed. Nasal speech, difficulty in swallowing, or protrusion

of the tongue indicate significant bulbar muscle involvement and imminent airway obstruction and ventilatory failure. Clinical manifestations of ventilatory muscle weakness include increased respiratory rate, decreased tidal volume, paradoxic inward chest movement during inspiration, and frequent change in breathing pattern. Active use of accessory muscles of respiration, acidosis, mechanical airway obstruction, and pneumonitis indicate weakness of major muscles of respiration. Hypercapnia is a late finding. Whenever possible, bedside spirometry should be performed. A forced vital capacity that falls below 15–20 mL/kg indicates increased risk of ventilatory failure. Patients unable to generate −20 to −30 cm H_2O of inspiratory force are also at higher risk for respiratory insufficiency. These assessments should be conducted every 2–4 hrs. Once admitted to the ICU, these patients should be monitored closely and oral fluids and feeds should be discontinued. Declining respiratory function is usually associated with a low threshold for intubation and ventilation.

Endotracheal Intubation

Intubation is considered (a) to protect the airway from severe aspiration because of oropharyngeal weakness; (b) to prevent respiratory failure from declining tidal volumes, hypoxemia despite supplemental oxygen, and hypercapnia; and, if necessary (c), to optimize pulmonary toilet.

Mechanical Ventilation

If in doubt, early assisted ventilation should be the preferred treatment so as to ensure adequate minute ventilation. In severe cases, intubation and controlled mechanical ventilatory support are required. If the patient is able to generate some effort, synchronized intermittent mechanical ventilation, pressure-support ventilation, or a combination of both are appropriate modes for ventilation. With synchronized intermittent mechanical ventilation, unassisted, spontaneous breathing may burden the accessory ventilatory muscles, but in pressure-support ventilation, inability to trigger breaths or unanticipated changes in lung compliance can result in insufficient ventilation. If fatigue, hypoxemia, or hypercapnia is encountered, the ventilatory support from either mode must be increased. Available data are limited regarding the use of noninvasive ventilation for children with acute NMDs. In a pilot study, 10 children with NMDs (2 with myasthenia gravis) who met criteria for intubation and ventilation were able to be managed with noninvasive ventilation (44).

Weaning. Weaning from mechanical ventilation should be started when ventilatory muscle strength begins to return, provided the *chest x-ray does not show* atelectasis or infiltrates and the oxygenation is good. A vital capacity >10 mL/kg and a maximum inspiratory force of at least −20 cm H_2O are useful indicators of ability to wean. Weaning from synchronized intermittent mechanical ventilation can be accomplished by gradual reducing ventilation breaths or by increasing the duration of spontaneous breathing and *time off of the ventilator*. Weaning from pressure-support ventilation can be accomplished by gradually decreasing the inspiratory pressure support. During weaning, the patient should not be allowed to become significantly tachypneic and end-tidal CO_2 should be monitored to confirm that Pco_2 is maintained within the normal range. Ventilatory support may be maintained at preweaning levels at night to provide rest. During sleep, some level of pressure support is usually required to prevent loss of lung volume and hypoxemia.

Generally, if a pressure support of 5 cm H_2O is well tolerated or the patient is maintaining minute ventilation without intermittent mechanical ventilation breaths, ventilation can be discontinued. A high-flow T-piece system with an end-expiratory pressure of 2.5–7.5 cm H_2O can be added to the endotracheal tube to prevent atelectasis during nonventilated periods. With increasing muscle strength, patients can be kept off of the ventilator for increasing periods using either continuous positive airway pressure or a T-piece circuit. Before considering endotracheal tube extubation, clinical assessment of bulbar muscle weakness is very important, as upper airway difficulties may compromise breathing after extubation.

Complications of Mechanical Ventilation. Complications of mechanical ventilation depend on the duration therapy. Nosocomial pneumonia and atelectasis are the most common complications. Long-term, invasive ventilation may result in tracheomalacia, tracheoesophageal fistula formation, or tracheal stenosis. Practicing sterile techniques during suctioning of the airway (no more often than necessary to minimize introduction of pathogens) may decrease the incidence of nosocomial pneumonia.

Tracheostomy

Advantages of early tracheostomy include increased comfort, airway safety, and help in weaning from ventilation. No guidelines exist for tracheostomy in children with these disorders. Some disease-specific data suggest that children are less likely to require tracheostomy than are adults.

General Supportive Care

General care is directed toward preventing complications that arise as a result of prolonged immobilization. Patients on ventilators require special attention in preventing pressure sores and nerve compression by frequent and gentle posture changes, padding, and the use of air or water mattresses. General care should include regular physiotherapy, with provision of splints to prevent joint contractures, prevention of deep vein thrombosis, keeping a conscious patient comfortable by careful positioning and repositioning, and early enteral nutrition to prevent gastric mucosal atrophy and to reduce the incidence of nosocomial infection. Inadequate intake of calories and protein may result in ventilator dependence. Parenteral nutrition should be reserved for patients with ileus. Handwashing, strict policies regarding IV and urinary catheter asepsis and antimicrobial procedures, avoidance of gastric alkalization, and infection surveillance can prevent nosocomial sepsis, which is a leading cause of mortality in the ICU.

Physiotherapy. Chest physiotherapy is believed to prevent mucus retention and segmental pulmonary collapse. To maintain joint mobility and prevent deep vein thrombosis in the limbs, early institution of occupational and physical therapy and use of heparin and support stockings are recommended for nonambulatory adult patients, but no specific recommendations exist for children.

Frequent Changes in Position. The use of water or air mattresses to prevent pressure sores and positioning and padding of limbs to prevent secondary nerve damage are advised. In-

flamed nerves appear to be more susceptible to pressure injury. A trochanteric roll may help to prevent peroneal nerve compression and footdrop. Frog positioning (i.e., knees flexed and apart, elbows partially flexed, and shoulders extended) may prevent pressure injury. In patients with facial nerve palsy, eye care is imperative to prevent eye desiccation and corneal injury.

Bowel Care. The risk of constipation is increased by prolonged immobilization and use of opiates for analgesia. Daily monitoring of bowel sounds by auscultation for early detection of ileus is recommended.

Bladder Care. Bladder catheterization is performed as a part of general nursing care, to maintain body hygiene and prevent distension. Whenever urinary retention is encountered, a sterile, closed, urinary drainage system should be used or manual decompression should be performed with close monitoring for the development and treatment of urinary tract infections (28). The risk of infection should be balanced against the benefit of catheterization.

Nutrition. Critical illness is a hypercatabolic state. To meet the patient's need for increased energy, enteral feeding should be started as soon as possible. Full-strength formula should be used to meet high-protein and high-caloric need.

Pain Relief. Pain relief may initially be achieved with paracetamol or nonsteroidal analgesics. Narcotic analgesics may also be necessary additionally. Carbamazepine or gabapentin may be used in case of neurogenic pain.

Psychological and Emotional Support. Psychological and emotional disturbances may require attention. In patients with quadriparesis or cranial nerve dysfunction who require mechanical ventilation, continuous psychological support and psychopharmacologic measures may be useful.

GUILLAIN-BARRÉ SYNDROME

Acute inflammatory demyelinating polyneuropathy, or GBS, is an acute, autoimmune (often postinfectious), usually demyelinating disorder of the peripheral nervous system characterized by areflexic weakness of limbs. The disease derives its name from two French neurologists Georges Guillain and Jean Alexandre Barré who, in association with Andre Strohl, an electrophysiologist, described the clinical, electrophysiologic, and cerebrospinal fluid (CSF) characteristics of the syndrome. The first modern description of an illness similar to GBS is credited to Jean Landry in 1859. The diagnostic criteria for GBS were reported by the National Institute of Neurological and Communicative Disorders and Stroke in 1978 and revised by Asbury and Cornblath in 1990 (4).

Epidemiology

With the prevention of paralytic poliomyelitis, GBS has become the most common cause of acquired, nontraumatic, generalized motor paralysis. The median annual incidence of GBS is ~1.3 (range 0.5–4.0) per 100,000 population (33) with a lower risk (0.5–1.5 per 100,000) in those under 18 years of age (55). The disease can occur at any age, in any race, and in all climates (seasonal variation from China). The average age of presentation in children ranges between 4 and 8 years, though children as young as 1 year may be affected. Males have a slight predilection for GBS (male:female ratio, 1.2:1).

Etiology and Pathogenesis

As many as 70% of patients experience an infectious illness in the 28 days preceding the onset of neurologic symptoms. Minor respiratory infections account for ~60% of these infections, followed by gastrointestinal ailments and nonspecific febrile illnesses. Various infections and other events implicated in the development of GBS are listed in **Table 49.3**.

The neurophysiologic and pathologic processes that underlie GBS are classified as acute inflammatory demyelinating polyradiculopathy (AIDP), acute motor axonal neuropathy (AMAN), or acute motor and sensory axonal neuropathy (AMSAN) (see the following pathology section for descriptions of these classifications). The Miller Fisher syndrome, a variant of GBS, is characterized by a triad of ophthalmoplegia, ataxia, and areflexia. AIDP is the most prevalent form of GBS and accounts for 85%–90% of cases in the West, while AMAN, originally described in a summer epidemic in rural in China, is seen in 60%–80% of patients with GBS from China and in 40% from Japan (33).

Cumulated evidence supports the observation that the peripheral nerve injury in GBS involves both humoral and cell-mediated immune responses that cause inflammatory cell infiltration and myelin destruction. An abnormal T-cell response, precipitated by preceding infection, results in abnormal immune stimulation. Molecular similarity of certain endogenous myelin and ganglioside antigens to constituents of the infecting organism results in hyperimmune responses being mounted by T-cell lymphocytes and macrophages directed against pe-

ripheral nerve fibers. It would appear that GBS results from a primary antibody response against a protein from an infecting organism that cross-reacts with patients' gangliosides (41). Activated T cells may stimulate B-cell proliferation, which produces antibodies to myelin, causes macrophage activation and recruitment, activates the complement system, or causes direct cytotoxic damage to myelin or Schwann cells. The activated macrophage and T cells gain access to peripheral nerves using two adhesion molecules: E-selectin (ELAM-1) and intracellular adhesion molecule (ICAM)-1.

Antibodies against anti-peripheral nerve neutral glycolipids have been found in patients with GBS. Significantly increased levels of antibodies to gangliosides GD1a, GD1b, GT1b, and other glycolipids have been detected in serum of GBS patients. Antibodies to GQ1b, a minor glycoside in peripheral nerves, were detected in 90% of patients with Miller Fisher syndrome (41). AMAN is frequently associated with antiganglioside antibodies (e.g., GM1, GM1b, GD1a), and evidence of preceding *Campylobacter jejuni* infection. Both IgG and IgM antibodies to ganglioside are present, but the early presence of IgG or IgA antibodies to GM1 is associated with a protracted illness and poor recovery.

Pathology

Demyelinating lesions are seen along the entire length of the peripheral nerve in GBS, including the nerve roots. All nerve types may be involved, including those serving autonomic, motor, and sensory systems. Generally, the motor nerve involvement is more than the sensory nerve involvement. AIDP typically shows segmental demyelination along with perivenular mononuclear cell infiltrate. At an early stage, the infiltrate is composed of small- and medium-sized lymphocytes that are subsequently replaced by macrophages involved in active phagocytosis of myelin. The immune target in AIDP appears to be within the Schwann-cell surface membrane or myelin.

The cytoplasmic projection of macrophages that penetrate through myelin gaps insinuate themselves between myelin lamellae and peel away layers of myelin from the axon (41). Macrophages have also been observed within axonal cylinders; this may explain some cases of GBS with axonal degeneration in the absence of severe demyelination. During the recovery phase, Schwann-cell proliferation with imperfect remyelination is seen. AMAN typically shows axonal degeneration of motor fibers with little or no demyelination. The immune response here seems to be directed primarily against the axonal membrane.

TABLE 49.3

INFECTIONS AND EVENTS REPORTED TO PRECEDE GUILLAIN-BARRÉ SYNDROME

Infections
Common cold
Gastrointestinal illness
Epstein-Barr virus
Cytomegalovirus
Viral hepatitis
Varicella (in 3%–4% children)
Campylobacter jejuni infection
Human immunodeficiency virus infection
Mycoplasma pneumoniae (in 1%–5%)
Japanese encephalitis virus
Falciparum malaria
Haemophilus influenzae

Immunization
Rabies vaccine (sample rabbit brain, suckling mouse)
Influenza vaccination
Hepatitis B
? Typhoid, tetanus

Minor surgery

Clinical Features

A common initial symptom of GBS is paresthesia of the toes and fingers, followed by progressive weakness of the lower limbs and/or unsteadiness in gait. As the disease progresses over a period of a few hours to days and weeks, weakness of the upper limbs occurs and cranial nerve palsies develop. This ascending weakness or paralysis is usually symmetrical. In half of the children, pain may be the initial complaint, resulting in the diagnosis being missed or delayed. Ataxia, limb pain, and back pain are more frequent in children than in adults. Urinary retention is seen in 10%–15% of children. Dysautonomia that presents as dizziness, sweating, and tachycardia may also occur.

The hallmark of GBS on physical examination is ascending motor weakness, along with areflexia. Lower-limb, deep-tendon reflexes are usually absent at presentation, but the upper limb reflexes may still be elicited, although with difficulty. Motor weakness may ascend up the body to involve respiratory muscles. The progression may occur slowly or rapidly, or in "fits and starts." Cranial nerve involvement (35%–50%), autonomic instability (26%), ataxia (23%), or dysesthesia (20%) may occur. The most common signs of autonomic dysfunction are either sinus tachycardia or bradycardia and hypertension. In ~20% of patients, arrhythmias and changes in peripheral vasomotor tone are seen, manifesting as hypotension and lability of blood pressure. Loss of normal vasoregulation has been associated with exaggerated hemodynamic responses to drugs and anesthetic agents. Loss of autonomic control of either systemic blood flow distribution or renin-aldosterone release and fluid loss from sweat glands commonly result in volume and electrolyte disturbances. Hyponatremia is common in GBS and has often been attributed to syndrome of inappropriate antidiuretic hormone, but excess antidiuretic hormone in these patients may also be caused by hypovolemia, hypotension, or positive-pressure ventilation.

Variant clinical features include fever at onset of neurologic symptoms, severe sensory loss with pain (myalgias and arthralgias, meningismus, radicular and back pain), sphincteric dysfunction (urinary retention), ileus, CNS involvement (cerebellar ataxia, extensor planter response, absent pupillary response, and rarely, loss of all brainstem reflexes), and papilledema. Studies show that adults with GBS may experience abnormal mental state, as evidenced by vivid dreams, hallucinations, delusions, and psychosis. Autonomic dysfunction, mechanical ventilation, and increased CSF proteins are risk factors for developing an abnormal mental state (10).

Variants of GBS are encountered, though less often, by an intensivist. These include descending GBS (facial or bulbar muscles are first to be involved), Miller Fischer syndrome variant (characterized by ophthalmoplegia, ataxia, and areflexia with relatively little weakness), and less common variants that include polyneuritis cranialis, pharyngocervicobrachial syndrome, acute sensory neuropathy of childhood, and acute pandysautonomia.

Diagnosis and Differential Diagnosis

The diagnosis of GBS may be difficult because of variable symptomatology and often unclear etiology of the disease. The possibility of GBS as a diagnosis should be considered in any patient with rapid onset of acute neuromuscular weakness. In its evolving phase, GBS must be differentiated from other conditions that cause progressive symmetric weakness, including transverse myelitis, acute polyneuropathies caused by toxins/heavy metals, organophosphorus poisoning, tick paralysis, acute porphyria, diphtheria polyneuropathy, myelopathies (poliomyelitis and other enteroviral infections of anterior horn cell), myasthenia gravis, and electrolyte disturbances (especially hypokalemia). Asymmetric involvement, preserved or brisk reflexes, and extensor planter response should suggest a diagnosis other than GBS. Myasthenia gravis (MG) presents with intact tendon reflexes, no dysautonomia, and a normal

CSF examination. Enteroviral infections usually cause CSF pleocytosis, and motor neuronal injury is found on electromyogram. Transverse myelitis causes a sensory-deficit level, urinary incontinence, and CSF pleocytosis. Botulism may mimic GBS but these patients have ophthalmoplegia with pupillary involvement, dry mouth, and ileus. Tick paralysis can cause an acute ascending paralysis with areflexia and is seen in North America and Australia. These patients have complete ophthalmoplegia but preserved sensation. A tick is usually found on the scalp or behind the ear. Certain laboratory tests seem particularly valuable in differentiating GBS from other conditions.

Lumbar Puncture

If lumbar puncture is performed a week after onset of weakness, the CSF findings typically suggest demyelination, e.g., elevated protein (>45 mg/dL) without CSF pleocytosis (<10 cells/mm^3) (often referred to as albuminocytologic dissociation). Serial spinal taps may be required if the initial findings are normal. Occasionally, the protein level may not rise throughout the illness, and a mildly elevated cell count (10–50 cells/mm^3) is all that is seen. More than 50 cells/mm^3 should prompt a reconsideration of the diagnosis of GBS.

Imaging

Two weeks after of onset of symptoms, lumbosacral MRI with gadolinium contrast may reveal enhancement of the cauda equina nerve roots. This finding has a diagnostic sensitivity for GBS of 83% and is present in 95% of typical cases (23).

Electrodiagnostic Studies

Peripheral neurophysiology within the first week of symptom onset shows characteristic features of peripheral demyelination, including abnormal temporal dispersion of compound muscle action potentials (CMAP); impersistence, prolonged, or absent F or H response; increased distal latencies and conduction block; and reduced conduction velocities of motor and sensory nerves. Features of axonal forms of GBS include lack of neurophysiologic evidence of demyelination and loss of amplitude of CMAP or sensory nerve action potentials to <80% of the lower limit of normal age-appropriate values. By the second week of illness, most patients show reduced CMAP, prolonged distal latencies, and reduced motor conduction velocities.

Management

Children with GBS are at risk for life-threatening respiratory complications and autonomic disturbance. Indications for PICU admission include rapid progression of motor weakness involving respiratory muscles, ventilatory insufficiency, pneumonia, severe bulbar weakness, autonomic instability, arrhythmia, or bradycardia. Complications related to therapy that require intensive care include fluid overload or anaphylaxis from IV immunoglobulin (IVIG) administration or hemodynamic instability related to plasmapheresis. These factors may exist alone or in combination.

Respiratory Monitoring and Care

It is reported that 15% of children with GBS develop respiratory failure that requires supportive mechanical ventilation (55). As impending respiratory failure for children with GBS has no clear indicators, close observation with serial assessment of ventilatory parameters (as described previously) is essential.

Endotracheal Intubation

Endotracheal intubation may be required in children with GBS to protect the airway from aspiration, overcome obstruction from loss of airway tone, or facilitate supportive mechanical ventilation. In GBS, rapid disease progression, presence of bilateral facial nerve palsy, and autonomic dysfunction have been associated with increased likelihood of intubation (35). Planning for early intubation to minimize pulmonary complications has been encouraged to prevent inherent risks of emergency intubation.

Dysautonomia and potential for succinylcholine-induced hyperkalemia may increase the risks of endotracheal intubation in patients with GBS. Dysautonomia may exaggerate the hemodynamic responses to the drugs used to induce anesthesia during intubation. Patients without full stomachs or ileus may benefit from topical/local anesthetic administration to blunt airway response, and short-acting benzodiazepine sedation and atropine decrease sudden hypotension and arrhythmia induced by airway manipulation. For patients who require emergency intubation (with full stomachs or ileus), a classic or modified rapid-sequence technique, including preoxygenation, cricoid pressure, atropine, lidocaine, a titrated (when possible) or reduced dose of a sedative, and short-acting nondepolarizing muscle relaxants (use of muscle relaxant must be weighed against the risk of a difficult airway) should be used. When feasible, careful titration of drugs with monitoring of heart rate, oxygen saturation, blood pressure, and electrocardiogram during intubation is preferred to prevent catastrophic responses.

Mechanical Ventilation

Independent predictors of the need for ventilation in adults with GBS were interval between the onset of symptoms to admission of <7 days, inability to cough, inability to stand, inability to flex arms or head, increasing liver enzymes, and vital capacity <60% of predicted (52). Clinical signs that indicate the need for mechanical ventilation include ventilatory muscle insufficiency, an increasing oxygen requirement to maintain SpO_2 >92%, or signs of alveolar hypoventilation (e.g., PCO_2 >50 torr). Other indications for initiating mechanical ventilation in GBS are forced vital capacity <15 mL/kg, rapid decline in vital capacity by 50% from baseline, and inability to generate a maximum negative inspiratory pressure of −20 cm H_2O. In GBS, recovery from respiratory failure is to be expected, even though some residual motor weakness may remain in the recovering phase.

Tracheostomy

No definitive guidelines exist for tracheostomy in children with GBS. Early tracheostomy may benefit patients who have severe GBS with clinical and electrophysiologic evidence of axonal involvement together with respiratory failure and autonomic dysfunction. With studies that report mean duration of ventilation ranging between 15 and 43 days, some patients can be spared tracheostomy. Tracheostomy in adult patients with GBS may be deferred until the end of the second week of illness, when definitive treatment is completed and potential for recovery can be predicted (28).

Autonomic Dysfunction

Autonomic failure has become a major factor in mortality from GBS. Fatal cardiovascular collapse due to autonomic dysfunction occurs in 2%–10% of seriously ill patients. Risk of dysautonomia is high in patients with respiratory failure, quadriplegia, or bulbar involvement. Heart rate, blood pressure, and electrocardiographic monitoring should be continued until patients are off of respiratory support. A reduction or absence of normal "beat to beat" variation in the heart rate suggests vagal involvement and may be an indicator for risk of arrhythmia in patients with GBS. Transcutaneous cardiac pacing may be used for symptomatic bradycardia. Hypotension may be treated with volume repletion, or if refractory to fluids, a pure α-agonist such as phenylephrine may be used to avoid potential arrhythmogenic effects from combined α- and β-agonists. When hemodynamic instability is severe, continuous arterial blood pressure recording should be performed to guide volume therapy. Hypertension may occur but, generally does not need specific treatment unless associated with signs of end-organ damage (i.e., pulmonary edema, encephalopathy, or subarachnoid bleed). A high index of suspicion for other medical complications (e.g., pulmonary embolism, pneumothorax, sepsis) should be considered before attributing cardiovascular complications to dysautonomia alone.

General Supportive Care

The patient with GBS who requires intensive care usually has a lengthy stay; hence, the general care in the ICU is as important as mechanical ventilation and specific therapy. Constipation is seen in more than 50% of patients with GBS as a result of adynamic ileus with or without other features of autonomic instability. Promotility drugs are contraindicated in patients with dysautonomia. Pain relief may be necessary, with acetaminophen usually the first choice. Opioids may be needed in addition, and carbamazepine or gabapentin may be used in case of neurogenic pain.

Specific Therapy—Immunomodulation

Various immunomodulatory therapies have been attempted in GBS. The Cochrane Neuromuscular Group has reviewed evidence regarding the use of steroids, plasma exchange, and IVIG in children and adults (26,27,46).

Corticosteroids

Current evidence does not support the use of corticosteroids in the treatment of GBS. A Cochrane review of 6 eligible trials that included a total of 195 corticosteroid-treated and 187 control subjects did not find significant difference in any disability-related outcome between the two groups. Hypertension only developed less often in the IV methylprednisolone group than in the control group. The reviewers concluded that corticosteroids should not be used in the treatment of GBS. A combination of methylprednisolone and IVIG does not offer additional advantage (27).

Plasma Exchange (Plasmapheresis)

Plasma exchange is believed to remove or dilute the humoral antibodies implicated in the pathogenesis of GBS. During each exchange, 40–50 mL/kg of plasma is replaced with a mixture of normal saline and albumin. The value of plasma exchange in younger children (<12 years old) is not clear, but in adults, it is beneficial. A review of 6 randomized trials that comprised 649 patients found plasma exchange to be beneficial (46). The plasma-exchange group showed reduced time to recover to walking, reduced need for artificial ventilation, decreased duration of ventilation, and lower rate of severe sequelae at 1 year. These advantages are best obtained if the plasma exchange is performed within 2 weeks of onset of illness. At least four exchanges have been found to be optimal for moderate to severely affected patients (i.e., unable to walk unsupported or worse), and two exchanges are sufficient for mildly affected patients (46). Relapses are seen in ~10% of patients within 3 weeks of plasmapheresis.

Plasmapheresis should be performed in centers with the expertise to perform the procedure in critically sick patients. Complications associated with the procedure include hematoma at vascular puncture site, pneumothorax following central venous catheterization, and sepsis. Mild hypotension that is responsive to fluid administration is common in children who undergo plasma exchange. Plasmapheresis is contraindicated in patients with severe hemodynamic instability, bleeding diathesis, and septicemia. Plasma exchange has been compared to CSF filtration, another new treatment, in a small trial. CSF filtration involves five or six cycles of daily filtration of 30–50 mL of CSF. No significant difference in outcome was noted between the two procedures (63).

Intravenous Immunoglobulin

IVIG has been shown to be equally beneficial to plasma exchange in GBS. IVIG is given as daily infusion (0.4 g/kg/day) for 5 days in the first 2 weeks of illness. Systematic data are inadequate to support the use of 1 g/kg/day for 2 days. IVIG has become the preferred treatment in GBS because of the ease of administration, especially in infants and children in whom central-venous access may be difficult.

Minor side effects of IVIG include headache, myalgia, and arthralgia; flu-like symptoms; fever; and vasomotor reactions. IgA-deficient patients may develop anaphylaxis after the first course of IgA-containing IVIG. Rarely, aseptic meningitis, congestive heart failure, vascular complications, and renal failure have been reported; therefore, IVIG should not be used in patients with congenital IgA deficiency, hyperviscosity syndromes, and congestive heart failure. In all of these conditions plasma exchange is the treatment of choice. A meta-analysis of 5 randomized trials that compared IVIG with plasma exchange (involving 536 patients, mostly adults, who were unable to walk and had been ill for <2 weeks) revealed that IVIG hastened recovery as much as plasma exchange (26). IVIG is also effective in children (32). In patients with severe GBS (i.e., unable to stand), IVIG reduced the need for mechanical ventilation and reduced the average length of PICU stay by 50%. Early recovery from muscle weakness and decreased length of intubation and ventilation contribute to reducing the incidence of pulmonary complications such as pneumonia and atelectasis (54).

The mechanism of action of IVIG is likely multifactorial and is believed to involve modulation of complement activation, binding and neutralization of idiotypic antibodies, saturation of Fc receptors on macrophages, and suppression of various inflammatory mediators, such as cytokines, chemokines, etc.

(11). Preliminary studies suggest that IVIG may be more efficacious than plasma exchange in patients with AMAN.

Outcome

The outcome of GBS is more favorable in children than in adults, and recovery, although it can be partial, is usually complete. The estimated mortality in childhood GBS is <5%; higher rates are seen in medically disadvantaged areas. Causes of death due to GBS include respiratory failure and cardiac arrest secondary to dysautonomia. Death may occur because of complications associated with immobility and mechanical ventilation, such as pneumonia, sepsis, acute respiratory distress syndrome, and thromboembolic events. Recovery usually begins 2–4 weeks after plateau of symptom progression. The median time from the onset of symptoms to full recovery was 66 days, with 90%–95% of full recoveries in children by 3–12 months. In a pediatric multicenter study (175 patients aged 11 months to 17.7 years), 74% could not walk at the peak of illness and 17% required mechanical ventilation for respiratory failure. On long-term follow-up, 92% were free of symptoms and the remainder could walk without support (31). Recurrence of symptoms, though less common in children, can be encountered in 6% of cases. One study reported that 12% of cases had recurrent symptoms within the first 2–3 weeks after IVIG therapy. Literature regarding the long-term outcome of children with GBS is limited; 75%–80% of children recover fully (41). Two studies, one before the use of IVIG and the other after its use, have shown no significant difference (23% vs. 24%) in long-term deficits (58). Younger age group (<9 years), rapid progression to maximal weakness (within 10 days), and need for mechanical ventilation emerged as important prognostic factors for long-term deficits (58). Predominantly axonal involvement and absence or severe reduction of the CMAP (<10% lower limit of normal) on electrophysiologic studies have been recognized as strong predictors of a longer time to becoming ambulatory. Early presence of IgG or IgA anti-GM1 antibodies, and serologic evidence of *C. jejuni* infection are laboratory features predictive of severe disease and poor outcome.

MYASTHENIA GRAVIS

Myasthenia gravis, literally, *grave muscle weakness*, is a disorder of the neuromuscular junction characterized by fluctuating weakness and fatigability of the voluntary skeletal muscles that result from autoimmune destruction of acetylcholine receptors (AchR). Its onset in childhood was first reported by Erb in 1879. In childhood, MG is categorized by age or immune-system involvement as (a) autoimmune MG or juvenile MG (JMG), (b) congenital MG or genetic MG, or (c) transient neonatal MG (TMG).

Epidemiology

The incidence of MG is estimated to be 4–6 per million per year, with a prevalence of 40–80 per million (39). MG is rare during childhood, and no epidemiologic data exist regarding children who have AchR autoantibodies, muscle-specific kinase antibodies, or the genetic form of the disease without antibody involvement. Approximately 10%–15% of all patients have onset before 20 years of age, with an estimated annual incidence of 1.1 per million total population. Some demographic differences are seen in the epidemiology of MG in children. The incidence is higher in African American than in Caucasian patients. In general, female preponderance is seen, but before puberty, both sexes are equally affected in the Caucasian population. This demographic difference may be the result of genetic differences or different predisposing environmental triggering factors (3).

Pathogenesis

The pathogenesis usually involves polyclonal IgG autoantibodies that are directed against AchR. Autoantibodies against nicotinic AchR are detectable in 85%–90% of cases of MG, and the remaining cases include either antibodies against other targets (e.g., muscle-specific kinase) or a genetic basis for abnormal neuromuscular transmission at the neuromuscular junction. The antibodies are produced by B cells, but autoreactive T cells are necessary for disease to occur. The cause of failure of T-cell tolerance and subsequent failure of B-cell tolerance is not yet fully understood. The autoantibodies cause disease at the neuromuscular junction by blocking the Ach binding sites on the receptors and inducing local deposition of complement. This results in a reduction in the number of functional AchRs with disruption of normal neuromuscular transmission, which manifests as weakness of skeletal muscles. Severity of weakness is proportional to the reduction in functional AchRs.

Patients with increased levels of autoantibodies against AchRs are termed *seropositive*. *Seronegative* (no AchR antibodies) patients may have autoantibodies against other antigens, such as muscle-specific kinase, acetylcholine premembrane receptor (PremRab), or other neighboring postsynaptic proteins. Alternatively, seronegative patients may have some genetic mutation of AchRs, or its associated protein, or a congenital absence of acetylcholine esterase. Many (40%–50%) seronegative MG patients with generalized weakness have antibodies against muscle-specific kinase. These patients have atypical illness characterized by involvement of facial, bulbar, neck, shoulder, and respiratory muscles, with less involvement of ocular muscles. They have variable response to first-line treatment, i.e., cholinesterase inhibitors (49).

The mechanism that triggers autoimmune destruction of AchRs is still unclear. Microbial infections have been implicated. Strong evidence suggests that the thymus gland plays a central pathophysiologic role as thymic hyperplasia is found in ~70% of cases. Thymomas and myasthenic thymus contain abundant AchR-reactive T cells.

Clinical Features

Juvenile Myasthenia Gravis

Juvenile MG (autoimmune MG of childhood) has an age of onset between 3 months and 16 years, mostly before 3 years (64), and a clinical picture that is similar to MG in adults. Symptoms are least apparent on awakening, and they become more evident later in the day. Weakness may remain localized to the eye muscles or it may progress to be generalized. Ocular involvement is present in most children with JMG, taking the form of intermittent drooping of eyelids with a persistent upward gaze or double vision, especially while reading. This weakness is variable and often asymmetric. In 10%–15% of children, weakness may be limited to the extraocular muscles, a condition known as *ocular MG*. Seventy-five percent of children who present initially with ocular symptoms develop progressive disease that results, within 4 years, in bulbar weakness or generalized weakness.

Almost 75% of patients have bulbar weakness at the time of initial presentation; for example, weakness of tongue and soft palate that results in nasal or slurred speech, especially after prolonged talking, or difficulty in chewing during meals due to weakness of muscles of mastication. Pharyngeal and laryngeal muscle weakness leads to dysphonia and choking on food and secretions. Facial muscle weakness results in a flattened, expressionless face and in drooling. Diminished strength of neck muscles may cause the tendency of the head to fall forward or backward, requiring manual assistance for holding up the head. Involvement of muscles of the legs results in fatigability and weakness while climbing stairs or running. This weakness tends to be symmetric and proximal; distal weakness is an atypical presentation of MG.

Systemic weakness that involves diaphragm and muscles of respiration may also occur and may be so severe as to cause respiratory failure. *Weakness of respiratory muscles in combination with bulbar weakness warrants hospitalization for immediate evaluation and management.*

On physical examination, findings are confined to the motor system, with no loss of sensation or coordination. Ptosis may be asymmetric, but extraocular muscle weakness is symmetric and fluctuating. Pupillary responses are not affected. Various maneuvers can be performed to unmask the underlying fatigability, including repetitive trips up and down the staircase, repetitive fun exercises in young children, having the patient count to 100 or chew for 30 seconds, and may provide a rough assessment of fatigable weakness. An adaptation of a scale devised by Osserman is used commonly to grade strength and fatigability (3):

- Grade I: Weakness restricted to extraocular muscles
- Grade IIa: Generalized mild weakness
- Grade IIb: Generalized moderate weakness
- Grade III: Generalized severe weakness
- Grade IV: Life-threatening weakness of respiratory muscles

The clinical state of the patient during the examination may not show correlation with the level of antibodies (64).

Transient Neonatal Myasthenia Gravis

Transient neonatal MS presents shortly after birth, occurring in 10%–20% of babies born to mothers with autoimmune MG. Passive transplacental transfer of circulating AchR antibodies is the cause. Correlation exists between the occurrence and severity of neonatal MG and AchR antibody titers in the mother and newborn. However, the condition may occur in babies of mothers in clinical remission or without elevated AchR titers. A high ratio of anti-embryonic muscle AchR antibodies to anti-adult muscle AchR antibodies correlates very well with the occurrence of neonatal MG.

The features of transient neonatal MG may develop within a few hours of birth. Infants may show a range of symptoms from mild hypotonia to a generalized weakness, feeble cry, difficult feeding, ptosis, facial weakness, or life-threatening respiratory distress. The syndrome usually resolves within 3 weeks but will occasionally persist for months. Every newborn of myasthenic mothers should be observed during the neonatal period for signs of muscle weakness, respiratory failure, and any impairment of bulbar muscles. Treatment includes anticholinesterase and, if indicated, ventilatory support. Very severe cases may require plasmapheresis (9).

Congenital Myasthenia Gravis

Congenital myasthenic syndromes are genetic disorders of neuromuscular transmission produced by mutations that alter the expression and function of ion channels, receptors, enzymes, or other accessory molecules necessary to maintain safe neuromuscular transmission. Most cases present at birth, but some may present later in childhood or adolescence. Severe cases present in infancy or early childhood. The presenting features include any combination of ptosis, ophthalmoparesis, dysphagia, dysarthria, poor feeding, weak cry, hypotonia, motor delay, respiratory distress, chronic respiratory and limb weakness, and arthrogryposis multiplex. Congenital MG must be differentiated from myopathies, muscular dystrophies, and JMG. Depending upon the defect, various treatment options are available, including pyridostigmine, 3,4-diaminopyridine, quinidine, and fluoxetine; however, immunotherapy has no role. Some disorders (slow-channel congenital MG, congenital acetylcholinesterase deficiency) progressively worsen over years due to progression of end-plate myopathy and degeneration of the postsynaptic region because of cationic overload. If patients with other abnormalities (AchR deficiency, fast-channel congenital MG, congenital choline acetyltransferase deficiency) survive infancy and childhood, they may show some improvement with age or develop static or slowly progressive weakness.

Emergencies in Myasthenia Gravis

Myasthenic crisis and cholinergic crisis are two emergencies in MG associated with acute, life-threatening respiratory failure. Myasthenic crisis is an acute exacerbation of the disease process that results in severe weakness from dysfunction of the neuromuscular junctions. Myasthenic crisis is characterized by respiratory failure due to weakness of either the upper airway muscles or of the diaphragm and other respiratory muscles. This condition can be precipitated by respiratory infection, sepsis, aspiration, surgical procedures, rapid tapering of corticosteroid or immunotherapeutic drugs, initiation of corticosteroid therapy, and exposure to drugs. Myasthenic crisis may be the initial presentation of undiagnosed MG. Twenty percent of patients with MG suffer from myasthenic crisis within the first year of illness, and approximately one-third of them experience another episode.

Cholinergic crisis is severe weakness usually caused by an overtreatment with cholinergic medication, resulting in overstimulation and blockade of the already functionally compromised neuromuscular junction by acetylcholine. The weakness due to cholinergic crisis may be indistinguishable from myasthenic crisis. The muscarinic effects of cholinesterase in-

hibitors (CEIs) increase bronchopulmonary secretions, which can obstruct the airway and cause aspiration. Patients show features of cholinergic excess, including excessive salivation, excessive lacrimation, diarrhea, sweating, pupillary constriction, and possibly, muscle fasciculation. Patients with compromised renal function are more susceptible to cholinergic crisis. Patients in crisis should be observed and monitored in an intensive care setting.

Cholinergic crisis and myasthenic crisis may be difficult to distinguish. CEI treatment should be withheld initially to avoid contributing to cholinergic overload in cholinergic crisis. CEI treatment is potentially harmful in patients with myasthenic crisis if they have significant weakness, as it may cause increased secretions and thus hasten respiratory failure. Supportive care is generally required for both crises. CEI is withheld and atropine is used to treat cholinergic crisis. Removal of triggers and institution of plasmapheresis or administration of IVIG may be necessary to treat myasthenic crisis. Steroids, immunotherapy, and thymectomy are not immediately useful for myasthenic crisis, as they may take weeks to be effective.

Diagnosis

The diagnosis of MG is based on clinical history, neurologic examination, and pharmacologic, electrophysiologic, and serologic testing.

Pharmacologic Testing

Edrophonium Chloride (Tensilon) Test. Tensilon is an IV cholinesterase-inhibiting agent with a rapid onset (30 secs) and a short duration (15 mins) of action. It acts by inhibiting the enzyme acetylcholinesterase, thereby allowing acetylcholine to diffuse widely throughout the synaptic cleft and to interact with AchRs, resulting in a larger and longer end-plate potential. The dose that produces improvement cannot be predicted, as the response is variable. Edrophonium is administered intravenously in incremental doses, beginning with 0.01 mg/kg up to maximum of 0.1 mg/kg and observing for improvement in function. Bradycardia can be a significant side effect; therefore, patients should be on a cardiac monitor, and atropine should be available. Relative contraindications to this test are a history of bronchial asthma or cardiac dysrhythmias. Any group of muscles can be tested, but it is considered more sensitive and useful when improvement in ptosis and double vision are used as the diagnostic end-points. The key is to identify precisely which muscle or muscle group is to be tested. Objective improvement in muscular strength is more important than the perception of improvement. The result of the test is influenced by the patient's maximal exertional effort prior to and after administration of the drug. The test is reasonably sensitive but not specific for MG. False-positive results can occur in other neuromuscular conditions (e.g., botulism, GBS, motor neuron disease, and lesions of brainstem). A video of the test is often helpful in recording, and later comparing, before and after drug effects.

Other Cholinesterase Inhibitors. Some patients may not show a response to edrophonium, but they may show improvement to neostigmine or pyridostigmine. These agents have an onset of action 5–15 mins after intramuscular administration, and their effect may last for up to 4 hrs. This longer duration of action (compared to edrophonium) may make neostigmine and pyridostigmine more useful in the evaluation of children. A therapeutic trial of oral pyridostigmine may have a subjective benefit on strength and fatigability that is not apparent after a single dose of edrophonium.

Electrophysiologic Testing

Repetitive Nerve Stimulation. A peripheral nerve is stimulated supramaximally and the CMAP is recorded with a surface electrode placed over the motor point of the muscle, along with a reference electrode placed distally over a tendon or bony prominence. Initial motor amplitudes are generally normal, but if any decrement in the motor response exceeds 10% with repeated nerve stimulation, the test is considered positive. The yield from the test is higher in the severe form of the disease and when muscle groups that have clinically significant weakness are tested.

Single-muscle-fiber Electromyography. Single-muscle-fiber electromyography is a highly specialized test. A fine-needle electrode is placed between two muscle fibers innervated by a single nerve. Variation in the action potentials of two muscle fibers is referred to as a "jitter." If >10% of muscle-fiber pairs have jitter exceeding the upper limit of normal jitter in that muscle, the test is considered positive. The test has a sensitivity of ~90%, but it is not very specific; it may be positive in other NMDs. Single-muscle-fiber electromyography examination may demonstrate fibrillation, which may indicate functional denervation of the muscle fibers and is generally a marker of more severe disease.

Serologic (Immunologic) Test

Measurement of antibodies to AchR by radio-immuno-precipitation assay is one of the most specific diagnostic tests for MG. These antibodies are present in 85% of patients with MG. As seronegative patients can become positive, monitoring of serology is helpful. The levels vary widely among patients with similar severity of weakness, and normal levels do not exclude the diagnosis. The level may be raised in other conditions, such as autoimmune liver disease, systemic lupus erythematosus, inflammatory myopathies, and first-degree relatives of patients with acquired MG. Other antibodies that are useful in the diagnosis of MG include AchR-modulating antibody, antibody to striated muscle, and antibody directed against skeletal muscle intracellular proteins. CD-cell examination may be abnormal in 85% of cases, mostly because of reduced levels of CD4+ or CD3+ and CD8+ (64).

Management

MG is no longer the uniformly fatal illness that it was in the past. It can now be managed with safe and effective therapies. Management in a PICU is indicated in patients with respiratory compromise or bulbar weakness and in those at risk for deterioration during initiation of therapy, myasthenic or cholinergic crisis, or perioperative management, including thymectomy.

Patients in myasthenic crisis have intact respiratory drive; hence, the reduction in tidal volume in evolving ventilatory failure is initially countered by increasing respiratory rate. Diaphragmatic weakness and excessive use of accessory muscles of respiration becomes evident. A weak cough or low, single-breath counting performance, denoting significant expiratory muscle weakness, also occurs. Respiratory compromise due to oropharyngeal and laryngeal muscle weakness may have normal tidal volume and vital capacity. With diaphragm and accessory muscle weakness, vital capacity will be reduced, as will maximum inspiratory pressure measurements. An inability to produce a maximal inspiratory pressure more negative than -20 mm Hg suggests the need for urgent intubation. Vocal cord weakness may be demonstrated by direct laryngoscopy.

Endotracheal Intubation

At the time of intubation, careful consideration should be given to the use of neuromuscular blocking agents because of prolonged and unpredictable duration of action. Resistance to the effects of succinylcholine is possible due to relative deficiency of AchRs, and higher doses may be needed to induce paralysis. Once the patient is paralyzed with succinylcholine, prolonged paralysis is highly likely, as is increased sensitivity to nondepolarizing neuromuscular blocking agents, which causes marked and prolonged paralysis. Short-acting, nondepolarizing agents may be less likely to result in unwanted prolonged paralysis, but unexpected prolongation of any paralytic should be anticipated.

Mechanical Ventilation

Initially, patients may be too weak to trigger the ventilator and will require controlled ventilation. Administration of pyridostigmine can be discontinued to facilitate mechanical ventilation and improve airway toilet and suctioning. No particular mode of mechanical ventilation is superior. If P_{CO_2} is not >50 mm Hg, noninvasive ventilation with bilevel positive-pressure ventilation may bypass the need for intubation in acute respiratory failure due to myasthenic crisis (45). In adults, proactive and thorough respiratory care reduces the risk of prolonged respiratory complications and the length of ventilation and ICU stay (61).

General ICU Care

Some medications exacerbate muscle weakness, and these should be avoided or stopped (**Table 49.4**).

Specific Therapies

The management of MG involves a graded approach in which the choice of treatment depends on the patient's age, severity, and rate of disease progression.

Cholinesterase Inhibitors. In patients with moderately severe muscle weakness but no evidence of respiratory failure, it is reasonable to increase the dose of pyridostigmine every few days until a satisfactory response is apparent. In patients in acute respiratory failure, one approach is to gradually increase the dose of pyridostigmine while undertaking a course of plasma exchange. These drugs cross the blood-brain barrier poorly and, therefore, no CNS side effects are seen. Rather, side effects are related to increased peripheral cholinergic activity and include bronchospasm, excessive salivation, bradycardia, nausea, diarrhea, and miosis.

Ach Release Promoters. Guanidine and 4-aminopyridine have been reported to improve ocular muscle and limb muscle strength in some patients, without any benefit for respiratory paralysis. These two drugs enhance the release of Ach from nerve terminals.

TABLE 49.4

PHARMACEUTICAL AGENTS WITH THE POTENTIAL TO AGGRAVATE MYASTHENIA GRAVIS

Antibiotics
Ampicillin, aminoglycosides (gentamicin, kanamycin, streptomycin, tobramycin), clindamycin, colistin, erythromycin, fluoroquinolones (e.g., ciprofloxacin, norfloxacin), lincomycin, neomycin, penicillin, polymyxin B, sulfonamides, tetracycline, trimethoprim-sulfamethoxazole, vancomycin

Anticonvulsants
Barbiturates, carbamazepine, gabapentin, phenytoin, trimethadione (no longer available in US)

Antirheumatic drugs
Chloroquine, penicillamine (could cause myasthenia gravis or elevation of antibodies)

Cardiovascular drugs
Bretylium, calcium-channel blockers (nifedipine, verapamil), lidocaine, oxprenolol, procainamide, propranolol and other β-blockers, quinidine

Psychotropic agents
Chlorpromazine, diazepam, lithium, promazine

Replacement hormones
Adrenocorticotropic hormone, corticosteroids, estrogens, oral contraceptives, thyroid hormones

Other drugs
Diuretics (lower serum potassium), interferon-α, iodinated radiographic contrast agents, muscle relaxants, magnesium, opioids, neuromuscular-blocking agents, quinine

Immunosuppressive Therapy

If no improvement in weakness is seen despite adequate CEI therapy, immunosuppressive drugs can be added. These include corticosteroids, azathioprine, cyclophosphamide, cyclosporine, and methotrexate. These drugs suppress the immune system by inhibiting both cellular and humoral mechanisms and reducing the damage due to autoimmunity. Limited evidence from randomized, controlled trials suggests that corticosteroid treatment offers short-term benefit in MG. However, corticosteroids are not better than azathioprine or IVIG (50). Pulsed, high-dose methylprednisolone has been used, with sustained response lasting for months.

Prednisolone, the most commonly used immunosuppressive agent, is added at a once-daily dose of 1.5–2 mg/kg in patients with moderate-to-severe disease that is refractory to CEIs. Improvement can occur within 2–3 weeks, but transient paradoxic deterioration in weakness may occur in ~50% of cases, and 10% may need mechanical ventilation (48). After maximum improvement is achieved, slow tapering of steroids is required. Some patients will need a maintenance of low-dose steroid (5–10 mg every other day) for years or for life.

Other agents are used in individuals who relapse on corticosteroids or in those with disabling steroid side effects (e.g., osteoporosis, psychosis, hypertension, myopathy, glaucoma, and infection). In adults, oral prednisolone combined with azathioprine results in fewer relapses, more remission, and less steroid usage. Other, newer immunosuppressants used in MG are mycophenolate mofetil and tacrolimus (48). Patients with disabling but stable symptoms with concerns about high-dose

steroids may receive mycophenolate mofetil. If these fail, azathioprine or cyclosporine is the next option.

Plasmapheresis

Plasmapheresis removes AchR antibodies from the circulation and has been advocated as an effective treatment for MG because it brings about improvement within a few days that lasts for several weeks (6). However, to date, only case series of plasma exchange in myasthenic crisis are available. Guidelines have not been established regarding number, volume, or frequency of exchanges. Five or six single-volume exchanges are performed on alternate days until an adequate response is obtained, which is usually seen after two to five exchanges. Plasmapheresis is used to prevent crises prior to thymectomy or any surgery. It is also used in very weak patients who are admitted for initiation of corticosteroid therapy and in cases that are refractory to CEIs and other immunomodulatory therapies. Two controlled trials that included a small number of patients failed to demonstrate a cumulative long-term effect of plasma exchange (19).

Intravenous Immunoglobulin

IVIG is considered to be as effective as plasmapheresis. In one randomized trial that compared IVIG to plasmapheresis, both were found to be equally effective (18). A systemic review of available randomized studies did not find any evidence that IVIG improves long-term functional outcome in moderate or severe MG or that it had a steroid-sparing effect (20). With 2 g/kg given over 5 days (0.4 g/kg/day), 60%–70% of patients are expected to show response within days to weeks, and the response lasts up to 60 days. In patients with acute respiratory failure or who are in myasthenic crisis, IVIG is used if plasmapheresis is not available or cannot be done (e.g., in young children with difficult venous access, in those in whom sepsis is the trigger for myasthenic crisis). IVIG may also be useful in patients who are refractory to other immunosuppressants.

Thymectomy

In a recent series of chest CT scanning in childhood MG, thymic proliferation and thymoma were found in approximately half of the cases (64). Some studies suggest that early removal of the thymus may adversely affect the immune status. However, the benefit of thymectomy for MG has not yet been established (48). Usually, thymectomy is recommended in moderate and severe MG that is inadequately controlled on CEIs. Studies show that the subgroup of MG that most benefits from thymectomy includes those with early onset, AchR antibody-positive MG. A consensus group concluded that the benefit of thymectomy in nonthymomatous autoimmune MG has not been established. They were unable to determine from the available studies whether the observed association between thymectomy and improved outcome was a result of thymectomy or because of differences in severity at baseline before therapy. Thus, for patients with nonthymomatous autoimmune MG, thymectomy should only be considered as an option to increase the probability of remission or improvement (25).

Perioperative Management of Patients with Thymectomy. Patients selected for thymectomy should have pulmonary function testing, including vital capacity and maximum expiratory force, both before and after cholinergic inhibition. If the patient is already on CEIs and can tolerate withdrawal of drug for 6–8 hrs, preoperative low maximum expiratory force off of CEIs indicates the risk of postoperative respiratory complications. In such cases, plasmapheresis for 5 days or IVIG is recommended. If the maximum expiratory force off of CEIs is satisfactory, early postoperative extubation is expected. CEIs are discontinued on the morning of surgery to avoid interactions and side effects in the operating room. Atropine is recommended to reduce secretions, and in patients on corticosteroids, preoperative, stress-dose, hydrocortisone is used for 3 days postoperatively.

Natural Course and Outcome of Myasthenia Gravis

The natural history of MG is highly variable. Weakness tends to be limited to ocular muscles in 10%–15% of patients. Approximately 50% of those who present with ocular features progress to develop systemic or bulbar weakness within the first 2 years of onset, with 75% progressing within 4 years (24). Spontaneous remission can occur, especially in younger children. In a large pediatric series, collected over 44 years, spontaneous remission was found in 7.6% within 3 years of onset of the disease and in 30.1% within 15 years (47). Seventy-five percent of children and adolescents with JMG who undergo thymectomy have complete remission, with improvement in up to 95% of cases (51). The course of congenital MG is more static or slowly progressive. A subset of congenital MG patients who do not respond to CEIs worsen over years with a progressive motor end-plate myopathy.

ACUTE INTERMITTENT PORPHYRIA

The word *porphyria* is derived from the Greek *porphuros*, which means red or purple. The porphyrias are a group of disorders caused by an enzymatic defect in many of the enzymes involved in heme biosynthesis. Four of these defects may present as acute porphyria, which is characterized by acute, life-threatening attack of neurovisceral symptoms (2). Acute intermittent porphyria (AIP) is the most common among all acute porphyrias; the average worldwide prevalence is 1 per 20,000, with an incidence of 1 new case per 100,000 per year. AIP has its highest incidence in people of Swedish descent. The incidence is reportedly 1.5 per 100,000 in the US Swedish population and 1 per 1000 in Lapland, Sweden (14). Other acute porphyrias are hereditary coproporphyria, variegate porphyria, and 5-aminolevulinic acid (ALA) dehydratase-deficient porphyria. These conditions are either acquired or inherited as autosomal dominant (except AIP, which is autosomal recessive) with weak penetrance.

Pathophysiology

The porphyrias are classified as hepatic or erythroid types, based on the site of expression of the enzyme defect, from which most of the heme biosynthetic inhibitors arise and where most of them accumulate, i.e., liver or erythrocytes. They are also classified as either acute or cutaneous, based of the predominant clinical presentation. The enzyme defect associated with each type of porphyria and the metabolic by-products that are likely to accumulate are shown in **Figure 49.2**. The abnormal functioning of enzymes may occur because of a defective gene or a toxin, which results in overproduction and accumulation of intermediates that are known as *porphyrins* or *porphyrin precursors*. Common to all acute porphyrias is overproduction and accumulation of ALA and porphobilinogen (PBG). AIP is due to reduced activity of PBG deaminase, the enzyme that catalyzes the conversion of PBG to hydroxymethylbilane. The neurovisceral symptoms are due to the neurotoxic effect of PBG and ALA and interaction of ALA with γ-aminobutyric acid (GABA) receptors (14).

Clinical Features

The classic features of acute porphyrias are abdominal pain, altered mental state, and peripheral neuropathy. Abdominal pain is present in most patients (14). Clinical presentation without abdominal pain is unusual. Pain in the limbs, back, neck, and chest occur in up to 70% of cases. A similar proportion have weakness and paresis (2). Patients may have different types of episodes because of a varied response to precipitating factors.

Abdominal pain is likely to be due to visceral neuropathy. It is usually diffuse but can be continuous or paroxysmal, and it can radiate to the legs. Typically, no rebound tenderness or guarding is found on examination. Nausea, vomiting, and constipation accompany the pain, but occasionally, diarrhea occurs. Radiologic examination of the abdomen does not show any abnormality.

Neurologic symptoms may involve both the central and peripheral nervous systems and include paresthesias, myalgias, paresis, neuropathy, seizures, and coma. Motor neuropathy of acute, severe attacks usually presents with paresis and muscle weakness at an early stage. The weakness begins proximally, in the arms rather than the legs. It is usually symmetric, resembling GBS, and can progress to quadriparesis and bulbar and respiratory muscle weakness. The deep tendon reflexes may be lost. Respiratory failure may occur in up to 20% patients (2). Neurologic symptoms are generally triggered or worsened by inadequate therapy and lack of diagnosis. Improvement may take a long time, but it is usually complete. Signs of autonomic nervous system involvement (e.g., tachycardia, hypertension, sweating) are common (2).

Psychiatric symptoms include insomnia (usually an early symptom), restlessness, anxiety, depression, confusion, hallucinations, delirium, disorientation, and confusion. These are usually associated with abdominal symptoms.

Hyponatremia frequently complicates the acute porphyrias and may precipitate seizures. Other electrolyte disturbances (e.g., hypokalemia, hypomagnesemia, hypochloremia) may also occur (14).

Precipitating Factors

Four main categories of factors can either induce or worsen an attack of acute porphyria: medications, starvation, hormonal factors, and infection. The medications include anticonvulsants (i.e., barbiturates, phenytoin, carbamazepine, diazepam) and antibacterials (i.e., chloramphenicol, erythromycin, metronidazole, sulfonamides) (**Table 49.5**). The mechanism by which medications cause an attack is induction or upregulation of

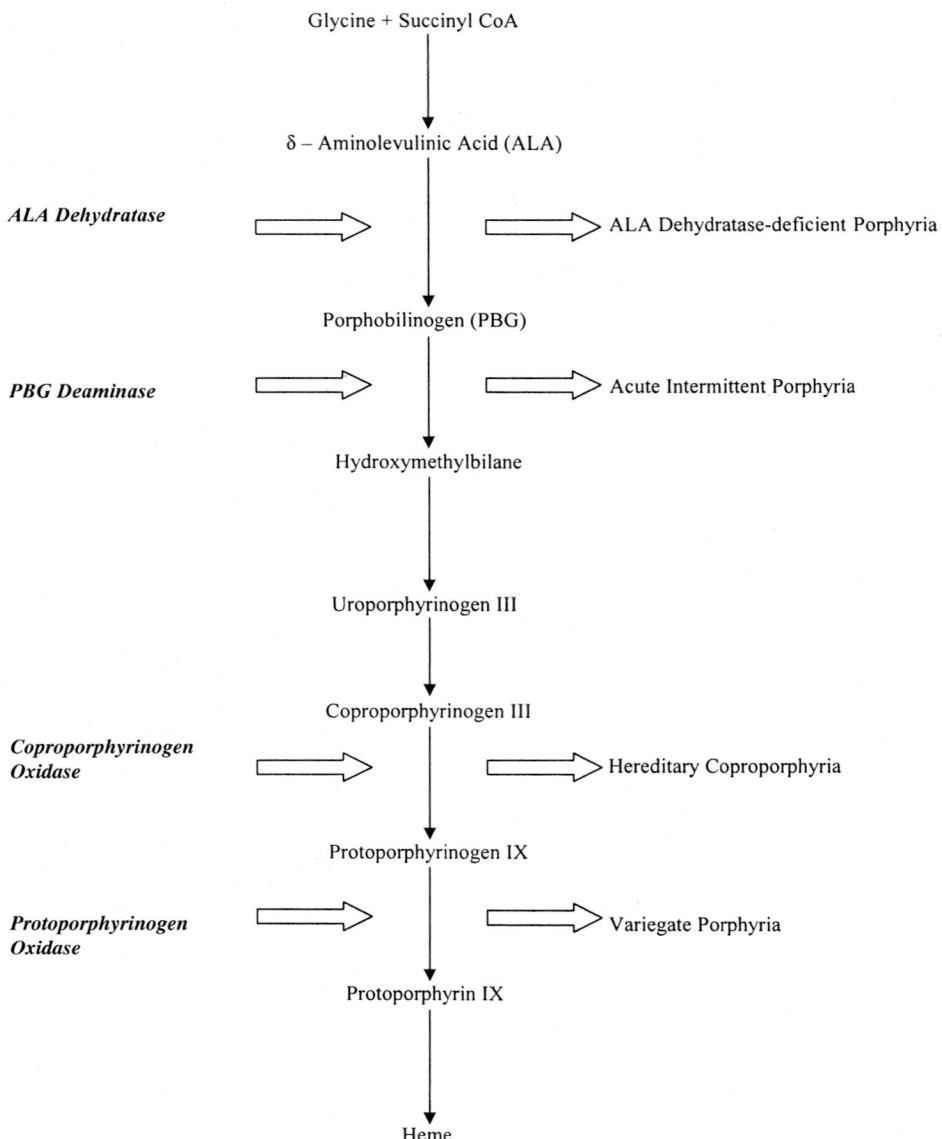

FIGURE 49.2. Heme biosynthetic pathway showing the enzyme defect causing acute hepatic porphyrias.

the cytochromes, which leads to depletion of heme stores, and induction of ALA synthesis. Starvation and dieting can precipitate an acute attack through the induction of ALA synthetase. Use of hormonal agents, estrogen, and oral contraceptives or endogenous excess of estrogen during pregnancy can also precipitate AIP. Both bacterial and viral infections induce an acute attack by catabolizing heme, which in turn, induces ALA synthetase and the accumulation of porphyrin precursors.

Diagnosis

Misdiagnosis or delayed diagnosis of porphyria is common. Therefore, acute porphyria should be considered in all patients who present with unexplained abdominal pain and neurovisceral symptoms and in any adolescent or female with acute onset of muscle weakness or respiratory paralysis. In a patient with abdominal pain, presence of hypertension, dark urine, muscle weakness, and pain should heighten the suspicion of an

acute porphyria. Whenever the diagnosis is suspected, a rapid test for increased urine PBG levels should be undertaken. The commonly used screening tests are the Watson-Schwartz test or the Hoesch test; these are qualitative in nature and have a low sensitivity of 40%–69%. Quantitative methods are more reliable and measure total 24-hr excretion of PBG and ALA during an acute attack.

Measurement of enzyme activity and DNA testing can determine the type of acute porphyria, and may be helpful in early identification of asymptomatic relatives. Half-normal activity of erythrocyte PBG deaminase confirms a diagnosis of AIP in patients with increased PBG. However, normal erythrocyte PBG deaminase activity does not exclude AIP because some mutations in the PBG deaminase gene lead to enzyme deficiency in the liver and other organs but not in erythrocytes (8). DNA studies can be conducted for genetic localization once the biochemical and enzymatic studies have confirmed the type of porphyria. Genetic counseling should be offered to these patients (8).

TABLE 49.5

COMMONLY USED DRUGS THAT ARE UNSAFE IN PORPHYRIA

Analgesics	Diclofenac and other nonsteroidal anti-inflammatories, pentazocine
Antihypertensives	α-methyl dopa, captopril, diltiazem, hydralazine, nifedipine
Antiepileptics	Phenytoin, barbiturates, carbamazepine, clonazepam (high dose), primidone, succinimides
Antibiotics and antibacterials	Sulfonamides, griseofulvin, chloramphenicol, doxycycline, erythromycin, ciprofloxacin, pyrazinamide, rifampicin
Diuretics	Furosemide, hydrochlorothiazide
Hormones and Endocrine agents	Estrogens (oral contraceptives), progesterone and synthetic progestins, sulfonylureas
Miscellaneous	Ergot compounds, imipramine, lidocaine, metoclopramide, cimetidine

Treatment of Acute Attack

The goals of treatment are to identify the triggering event, alleviate symptoms, and reverse ALA synthetase activity with medication. If an obvious trigger is identified, such as a drug, it should be stopped. Dehydration, malnutrition, or infection should be managed. Morphine or other opiate analgesics can be used to control pain. Propranolol can be used for hypertension, and diazepam can be used to acutely treat seizures. Long-term seizure control can be achieved with valproate or clonazepam. Hyponatremia and hypomagnesemia should be corrected. Gastrointestinal symptoms can be treated with chlorpromazine or phenothiazine.

Enzyme activity is reversed by administering 10% glucose and hemin infusion. These act by directly suppressing ALA synthetase activity (8). Hemin infusion is given in a dose of 3–4 mg/kg once daily for 4 days. Excessive production of porphyrin precursors is decreased within hours of hemin infusion and clinical improvement is seen within 2–4 days. Many studies, mostly uncontrolled, have shown that early initiation of hemin is associated with improved outcome. Use of the tin protoporphyrin has been shown to prolong remission induced by heme arginate. Hemin infusion may cause abnormality of coagulation and bleeding diathesis and, rarely, transient renal insufficiency.

Monitoring should include regular assessment of vital capacity, respiratory and skeletal muscle weakness, serum sodium, potassium, magnesium, and creatinine. Prevention is best achieved with counseling about avoiding precipitating drugs, maintaining a high carbohydrate diet, and promptly treating infection (8).

Outcome

Clinical improvement with hemin therapy occurs within 1–2 days. However, if treatment is delayed, neurologic damage may be slow to recover and may occasionally leave residual weakness. Motor weakness usually resolves; occasionally, footdrop and wasting of intrinsic muscles of the hand are seen. The overall outcome has greatly improved over recent years, with better diagnosis, availability of hemin treatment, and prevention. Since the introduction of hemin therapy in 1971, case fatality rates have fallen from 10% to 52% before 1970 to up to 10% currently (2).

INTENSIVE CARE-ACQUIRED NEUROMUSCULAR DISORDERS (CRITICAL ILLNESS NEUROMUSCULAR ABNORMALITIES)

Critical illness neuromuscular abnormality (CINMA) is the term given to those NMDs that are acquired de novo during the treatment of critical illnesses other than primary neuromuscular conditions. This condition was first reported in adults with sepsis and multiorgan failure and was called *critical illness polyneuropathy* (CIP). Initially, CIP was considered an uncommon condition, but it is now considered to be one of the most common and severe complications in adult patients in the ICU. Intensive care-acquired NMDs are infrequent in children (43,56). A summary of the literature on CIP and myopathy in pediatric intensive care was published in 2007 (62).

At present, CINMA includes CIP, CIM (also known as *acute quadriplegic myopathy* or *acute myopathy of intensive care*), and prolonged neuromuscular blockades. Each of these categories may occur in pure form or in combination with others. The spectrum of illness varies from isolated nerve entrapment, which presents with focal pain or weakness, to severe myopathy or neuropathy with associated severe and prolonged weakness (43,56).

Incidence and Prevalence

The prevalence of CINMA is likely to be higher than generally recognized. Clinical assessment alone may not be sufficient to provide the true incidence. In a prospective, multicentered study in adults, clinical and electrophysiologic neuromuscular evaluation was performed in those who were ventilated for 7 days. Up to one-third of patients were diagnosed with clinically relevant acquired paresis (12,13). Prospective studies have found that CIP or CIM was present in 52%–57% of patients remaining in the ICU for >7 days (36) and in ~68%–100% of patients with sepsis or systemic inflammatory response syndrome (22). In children, the incidence of critical care illness-associated muscle weakness appears to be much lower (5).

Risk Factors

A number of factors increase the risk of CINMA, including sepsis, systemic inflammatory response, multiorgan failure, mechanical ventilation (7,12), corticosteroids, neuromuscular-blocking drugs (5,12), aminoglycosides (5), hyperosmolality, parenteral nutrition (22), and hyperglycemia (37).

Pathogenesis

The pathogenesis of CINMA is not fully understood. CIP is likely to be another end-organ manifestation of multiple-organ dysfunction. In this regard, various cytokines and inflammatory mediators may have a role in pathogenesis by damaging myelin, oligodendrocytes, and even axons. For example, nitric oxide maintains vascular tone and may contribute to paralysis of arteriolar vasoreactivity in septic shock. As blood vessels, supplying peripheral nerves lack autoregulation, impaired microcirculation may cause nerve energy failure. Both hypoxia and ischemia impair axonal transport of proteins. An alternative mechanism involves hyperglycemia and hyperosmolality, both of which increase endovascular resistance. Microvascular permeability may aggravate endoneural edema (43). It is of interest that in the adult studies of glycemic control in critical illness, tight glycemic control using insulin is associated with a reduction in CIP (59).

The mechanism that underlies CIM is not clear. Broadly, two types of acute quadriplegic myopathies are encountered. *Acute necrotizing myopathy* occurs in sepsis and multiorgan dysfunction. It is fulminant and is associated with increased serum creatine kinase, myoglobulinuria, and myopathic changes on electromyography. *Thick-filament myopathy* is associated with the use of corticosteroids, and concurrent use of neuromuscular blocking agents (NMBAs) augment damage. The toxicity of these drugs can be explained by upregulation of cytoplasmic receptors for corticosteroids in muscles as a result of immobilization and pharmacologic denervation. In some patients, thick-filament loss and myonecrosis may be present, which suggests a spectrum of muscle injury between the two types of acute quadriplegic myopathy.

Clinical Features

Prolonged Neuromuscular Transmission Blockade

Prolonged neuromuscular transmission blockade has been described in those who receive muscle relaxants for several days or weeks. These patients become ventilator-dependent and have persistent paralysis and areflexia long after the drug is discontinued. Renal failure or dysfunction is an important factor, as many commonly used NMBAs have significant clearance via the kidney. In a patient with renal failure, even only a few hours of NMBAs at high doses can result in prolonged (several days) neuromuscular blockade. Hypermagnesemia and metabolic acidosis are other risk factors in prolonging neuromuscular blockade.

Critical Illness Polyneuropathy

CIP is characterized by acute, generalized neuropathy occurring after overwhelming sepsis and multiorgan dysfunction. Approximately 70% of adults with sepsis demonstrate peripheral nerve dysfunction on electrophysiologic studies, but only 30% of these develop clinical symptoms. Clinical signs usually develop 2–3 weeks after the onset of sepsis. Rapid development of flaccid, quadriparesis or paraparesis with hyporeflexia/areflexia occurs. The symptoms of polyneuropathy are usually not identified early because these patients are usually sedated to facilitate mechanical ventilation. The problem is recognized when an obvious difficulty is encoun-

tered in weaning from mechanical ventilation. During recovery, some patients may complain of painful paresthesia and some may develop weakness after discharge. Loss of sensation in a glove-and-stocking distribution is seen. These patients fail to grimace or move their limbs in response a painful stimulus. Clinically, the cranial nerves appear to be spared, but they may show abnormal electrophysiology. Bladder and bowel function is usually preserved. Limb edema, a common occurrence in critically ill patients, may obscure distal atrophy.

Critical Illness Myopathy

Terms used to describe CIM include *acute quadriplegic myopathy, floppy-person syndrome, necrotizing myopathy of intensive care, thick-filament myopathy*, and *steroid-induced quadriparesis*. CIM is a more common cause of CINMA weakness than CIP (30). It was first described as acute myopathy in individuals with acute severe asthma treated with corticosteroids. Exposure to corticosteroids or NMBAs appears to be the major risk factor for developing CIM. Other risk factors include sepsis and multiorgan failure. Irrespective of age, the clinical features of CIM appear to be the same. Patients have flaccid tetraparesis or tetraplegia. Deep-tendon reflexes are either normal or diminished but usually are not completely lost. The cranial nerves are intact on examination, although facial weakness may be mild. Sensation is preserved. Painful stimulation elicits facial grimacing without limb withdrawal, unlike the finding in CIP. Weaning from mechanical ventilation is difficult.

Diagnosis

The diagnosis of CINMA is not easy, mainly because of limitations imposed by concurrent therapy and because the patient is usually deeply sedated and immobile. The laboratory findings are unhelpful, as these may merely reflect critical illness. Elevated creatine phosphokinase may suggest a possible toxic or inflammatory cause of myopathy. Guillain-Barré syndrome can be confused with CIP/CIM. However, it can be distinguished from these by careful observation of the clinical presentation, cranial nerve involvement, and any demyelination evident on nerve conduction studies.

Electrophysiologic Studies

Nerve conduction studies and electromyography can be performed at the bedside. CNS and non-neurologic causes can be excluded, and the cause of weakness can be localized to either muscle or nerve in most cases. In a cooperative patient, CIP can be distinguished from CIM with these procedures. Electrophysiologic testing may be difficult to perform in the acute stage of critical illness because access to nerve and muscle may be limited by dressings, intravascular catheters, splints, and peripheral edema. When the results of such tests are inconclusive, direct muscle stimulation may be necessary to differentiate between myopathy and neuropathy (57).

The salient features on electrophysiologic studies are:

- CIP—The features of CIP include decreased amplitude of CMAP in response to motor nerve stimulation, with preserved motor conduction velocity and some loss or absence of sensory nerve action potential on sensory nerve

TABLE 49.6

DIFFERENCES BETWEEN CRITICAL ILLNESS POLYNEUROPATHY AND CRITICAL ILLNESS MYOPATHY

	Critical illness polyneuropathy	Critical illness myopathy
Predisposing factor	Preceeding systemic inflammatory response syndrome, sepsis, or multiorgan failure	Often received nondepolarizing muscle blocking agent, high-dose corticosteroid or both
Clinical features	Sensory deficits present Weakness distal > proximal Tendon reflexes normal or ↓	No sensory deficit Weakness proximal > distal Tendon reflexes ↓or absent Weakness of muscles supplied by the cranial nerves may occur
Electrophysiology	Low amplitude/absent sensory action potentials Normal motor unit potentials. Reduced motor unit recruitment Normal muscle excitability. Features of axonopathy without demyelination.	Retained sensory nerve action potentials Small motor unit potentials Early motor unit recruitment Absent/reduced muscle excitability
Pathology	Axonal loss (sensory and motor nerve) Acute and chronic denervation of muscle	Loss of thick myosin filament. Type II fiber atrophy (type I less common) or severe muscle fiber necrosis

Adapted from Khan J, Burnham EL, Moss M. Acquired weakness in the ICU: Critical illness myopathy and polyneuropathy. *Minerva Anesthesiol* 2006;72:401–6.

stimulation, along with preserved sensory nerve conduction velocity. Phrenic nerve stimulation also yields reduced amplitude of diaphragm CMAP.

■ Electromyography findings may show fibrillation potentials or normal or large polyphasic motor unit potentials with a reduced recruitment pattern. Findings are suggestive of axonal loss only, most severe distally, without any features of demyelination (e.g., conduction blockade or temporal dispersion nerve slowing).

■ CIM—Nerve conduction is usually normal. However, CMAP may be reduced, with preserved sensory nerve action potential. The electromyography yields either no or a less-intense spontaneous fibrillation, but small motor unit potentials with an early recruitment pattern are seen.

■ Neuromuscular transmission defect—Pseudomyopathic findings with a decrement in response to repeated stimulation are seen.

Tissue Biopsy

Nerve biopsy and autopsy in patients with CIP show acute axonal degeneration that involves both sensory and motor nerve fibers and is more pronounced in distal rather than proximal segments. No features of inflammation are seen. In the chronic stage, the nerve shows severely reduced numbers of myelinated large-diameter fibers, thin myelin in almost all fibers, and cluster formation of myelinated small-diameter fibers, which indicates primary axonal degeneration with regeneration (42). Muscle biopsy from patients with CIP shows chronic denervation and myopathic changes. In CIM, atrophy of type II fibers is seen with occasional atrophy of type I fibers. Muscle fiber necrosis is also seen. Electron microscopy and immunohisto-

chemical studies demonstrate the loss of thick myosin filaments. The differences between CIP and CIM are summarized in **Table 49.6.**

Treatment and Prevention

No specific treatments have been recommended for CINMA. Early physiotherapy and good nutrition should help recovery. Studies have shown that glutamine, glutathione supplementation, and branched-chain amino acid supplementation is associated with improved survival and shorter ICU stay. Avoidance of prolonged immobilization and oversedation, strict glycemic control, and minimization of dosages and duration of corticosteroids and NMBAs can prevent, to some extent, the development of this devastating complication of critical illness that requires prolonged ICU stay.

Outcome

The development of CIP/CIM affects both the short- and long-term outcomes of critical illness, with increased duration of mechanical ventilation, prolonged ICU stay and hospitalization, and increased healthcare cost (12,21,34). Much of the data on outcome in CINMA are related to patients with CIP. Mortality is high in adults (50%–60%) and much lower in children (60). Chronic disability is a common finding in many patients after discharge from the ICU and hospital. Forty percent of pediatric cases had persistent neurologic sequelae (56). In adults, 68% recovered to the extent of being able to breathe spontaneously and walk without support. However, 28% were tetraplegic or paraplegic. Milder disabilities have been reported in patients with full functional recovery and include hypore-flexia or areflexia, sensory abnormalities, muscle atrophy, and footdrop (34,60). The time course of recovery varies greatly. Neuromuscular abnormalities may continue for 5 years after illness (12). Weakness and/or neuropsychologic changes may also persist for 5 years (16). Some patients may never become fully functional, which will have a major impact on their quality of life. Limited data are available regarding the outcome of CIM. If weakness occurs as a complication of severe asthma treated with steroids and NMBAs, recovery occurs within days to weeks. It is generally thought that patients with CIM recover faster and have better prognosis than do those patients with CIP (30).

DIAPHRAGMATIC PALSY

Diaphragmatic palsy can be bilateral or unilateral. Bilateral palsy is usually due to systemic illnesses, while unilateral palsy is due to injury to phrenic nerve (cervical motor neurons C3–C5) and is more common in infants and children than in adults.

Incidence and Causes

The most common causes of unilateral diaphragmatic palsy in children are birth trauma (due to difficult or breech delivery), congenital diaphragmatic eventration, and cardiothoracic surgery. The incidence of diaphragmatic palsy in children who underwent cardiac surgery in a large, prospective study was 4.9%; 5.4% following open surgery and 3.3% following closed heart surgery (1).

Pathophysiology

Unilateral palsy is often asymptomatic in older children but can cause severe respiratory compromise in newborn infants and young children because older children use the accessory muscles of respiration, while infants have a horizontal rib cage and weak intercostal muscles. A significant alteration in respiratory mechanics that occurs following diaphragmatic palsy is a paradoxic movement of the diaphragm on the affected side, with mediastinal shifting to the contralateral side during inspiration. This alteration causes decreased lung volumes, alveolar collapse, and atelectasis, which leads to dyspnea, failure to clear secretions, and pneumonia.

Clinical Features

Children with diaphragmatic palsy present with varied manifestations depending on their age and the underlying lung condition. Immediately after birth and during the first hours of life, tachypnea, increasing need for oxygen, hypercapnia, atelectasis, pneumonia, and a mediastinal shift are present. Over the next few days, the clinical condition may stabilize, only to recur days to weeks later; progression is often provoked by atelectasis or infection. In older children, uncomplicated diaphragmatic palsy may present as tachypnea, dyspnea on exertion, or

orthopnea. Patients with postsurgical phrenic nerve palsy experience pleural effusion, pneumonia, and difficulty in weaning from the ventilator or mechanical ventilation.

Diagnosis

Diaphragmatic palsy should be suspected in any child who has decreased breath sounds, fails to wean from a ventilator without a cardiac cause, and has a raised hemidiaphragm on chest x-ray. Chest x-ray shows an elevated affected hemidiaphragm, but this sign lacks sensitivity and specificity in the diagnosis of unilateral paralysis (15). Fluoroscopy on sniffing is a traditional method of diagnosing diaphragmatic movements. The normal diaphragm descends during a sniff. In the presence of unilateral diaphragmatic palsy, the affected diaphragm ascends. The sniff test is positive if a 2-cm or longer excursion is present and the whole leaf of the hemidiaphragm is involved. The sniff test is difficult to interpret if the hemidiaphragm is not completely paralyzed or when a child is on positive airway pressure. Electrical stimulation of the phrenic nerve that demonstrates delayed conduction time is more specific than fluoroscopy. Unilateral magnetic phrenic nerve stimulation is a reliable and sensitive alternative for diagnosing diaphragm paralysis (38).

Sonographic assessment of diaphragmatic motion can be used for diagnosis and to follow the progression of diaphragmatic function at the bedside. M-mode sonography has better results than the more commonly performed real-time, B-mode sonography. In a retrospective study of 278 children with diaphragmatic palsy and 742 hemidiaphragm elevations, M-mode ultrasound detected palsy correctly in all of the right-sided lesions and missed it in only 0.71% of the left-sided lesions (15).

CT scanning of the chest may be indicated in patients who have diaphragmatic palsy due to mediastinal pathology. MRI of the neck is advised in those who are suspected to have involvement of the spinal column or nerve roots that is causing diaphragmatic paralysis.

Management

The management of eventration of the diaphragm secondary to phrenic nerve injury in the newborn period invariably requires surgery. Plication of the diaphragm is also usually required in very young children with diaphragmatic palsy following cardiac surgery. Plication is required in diaphragmatic palsy due to arterial switch operation in as many as 100% of cases, due to Blalock-Taussig shunt in 58%, and due to correction of tetralogy of Fallot in 10% (1). In older children, phrenic nerve paralysis is thought to be potentially reversible; if the patient is asymptomatic, it may be managed conservatively, as spontaneous recovery of the affected hemidiaphragm has been reported in up to 90% of children.

Surgical plication is accepted as the effective treatment, but a controversy exists regarding its timing. Some authors advocate a proactive approach; others recommend plication surgery after 30 days of ineffective conservative therapy or if a child cannot be weaned from the ventilator even after 2 weeks (53). Some authors believe that the time between the diagnosis and surgical management of diaphragmatic palsy in children who have undergone cardiac surgery should not exceed 10 days, especially in infants (1).

Usual surgical procedures in diaphragmatic palsy are (a) open transthoracic plication of the noncontractive part of the paralyzed and elevated diaphragm, or (b) the thoracoscopic repair and fixation of the diaphragm. Some authors have used the laparoscopic approach, as it is minimally traumatic. The long-term outcome in these children is the same as with the conventional approach.

The aim of diaphragmatic plication is to decrease lung compression, stabilize the thoracic cage and mediastinum, and strengthen the respiratory action of intercostal and abdominal muscles, resulting in improved diaphragmatic recruitment that leads to better ventilation and lung volumes and improved respiratory functions (17). Diaphragmatic pacing through the placement of electrodes in the diaphragm to stimulate it to contract is being used in children with spinal cord injury or phrenic nerve injury. This procedure can be performed transthoracically, transabdominally, laparoscopically, or through thoracoscopy.

Outcome

Unless a potentially fatal comorbid illness threatens the prognosis of the patient with unilateral diaphragmatic paralysis, death from respiratory insufficiency does not occur if good ventilatory support is provided. Prognosis of unilateral diaphragmatic paralysis depends on etiology; it usually is excellent unless the patient has significant underlying pulmonary disease. The beneficial effect of diaphragmatic plication has been shown to be long-lasting and does not interfere with return of diaphragmatic function, which may occur within 18 months to 3 years (29).

CONCLUSIONS AND FUTURE DIRECTION

Improving our understanding of pathogenesis and pathophysiology of GBS, specifically with respect to bacterial and viral proteins, which share homologous epitopes to components of the peripheral nerves may help in developing more effective specific therapies. The role for immunomodulatory therapies must be defined further to optimize the long-term outcome.

The place for various immunosuppressants and immunomodulatory therapies in childhood MG is far from clear. In the future, the respective roles of various therapies in long-term management (especially of IVIG and newer immunosuppressants, mycophenolate mofetil and tacrolimus) should be clearly defined, and consensus should be reached on the role and timing of thymectomy in children with JMG.

With the advantage of well-understood pathogenesis of the porphyrias and an effective way to overcome the enzyme deficiencies, a cure for this disabling disease may be possible in the future using gene therapy.

We are in the early stages of understanding CINMA in children; therefore consensus should be developed regarding the terminology used and the diagnostic criteria. Interventions to prevent and treat CINMA should result from a better understanding of the epidemiology.

KEY POINTS

Guillain-Barré Syndrome

- GBS is the major cause of acute flaccid paralysis, with an incidence of 0.6–1.9 cases per 100,000 per year.
- GBS presents as a characteristically progressive, ascending, symmetric, areflexic weakness of more than one limb, with autonomic dysfunction occurring 1–3 weeks after nonspecific illness with viral symptoms.
- AIDP accounts for 85%–90% of cases of GBS; the remainder involve AMAN and AMSAN.
- Diagnosis is based on a characteristic clinical picture, nerve-conduction abnormalities, and CSF that shows albuminocytologic dissociation.
- Autonomic dysfunction is an important cause of death due to hemodynamic instability and arrhythmias.
- Autonomic instability and risk for succinylcholine-induced hyperkalemia/arrhythmia complicate the intubation of these patients.
- Treatment involves either plasma exchange (50 mL/kg) or IVIG 400 mg/kg/day for 5 days.
- IVIG may be preferable for young children whose line access for plasmapheresis is likely to be difficult.
- Plasmapheresis may be preferable for (a) patients with IgA deficiency who would be at risk for anaphylaxis with IVIG administration, (b) patients with congestive heart failure, or (c) those at risk of volume overload.

Myasthenia Gravis

- The prevalence of MG is 0.5–14.2 per 100,000.
- MG is characterized by weakness and fatigability, especially of ocular muscles.
- Diagnosis of MG is made with positive Tensilon test, AchR antibodies (in 85% of cases), decremental response to repetitive nerve stimulation, and abnormal single-fiber electromyogram.
- Myasthenic crisis, defined as respiratory failure (which occurs in 15%–20% patients), must be differentiated from cholinergic crisis.
- CEIs are first-line treatment for MG. Immunotherapy or steroids are generally second-tier treatment, and plasmapheresis or IVIG is third-tier treatment. Thymectomy is considered in indicated patients.

Acute Intermittent Porphyria

- The porphyrias comprise a group of disorders caused by an enzymatic defect in heme biosynthesis that leads to overproduction and accumulation of ALA and PBG.
- Clinical features include a triad of abdominal pain, changes in mental state, and peripheral neuropathy; respiratory paralysis and failure occur in up to 20% patients.
- Precipitating factors of AIP are drugs, starvation, hormonal factors, and infections.
- Treatment of an acute attack includes control of pain using opiate analgesics, hypertension using propranolol, seizures using diazepam, and gastrointestinal symptoms

using promethazine. Specific therapy is IV 10% glucose and hemin infusion at 3–4 mg/kg once daily for 4 days.

- Clinical improvement with hemin therapy is rapid, often noticeable within 1–2 days. Motor weakness usually resolves; occasionally, footdrop and wasting of the hand muscles are seen.

Critical Illness Neuromuscular Abnormalities

- In adults, CINMA is common and adds to ICU length of stay and cost of care.
- The spectrum of the disorder ranges from focal pain or weakness to severe myopathy or severe neuropathy, causing quadriparesis, prolonged weakness, and delayed weaning from ventilator. Sometimes, a combination of these factors may be present.
- The disorder is broadly categorized into CIP, CIM, and prolonged neuromuscular blockades.
- No specific treatments are recommended.
- Patients with CIM may recover faster and have better prognosis than will patients with CIP.

Diaphragmatic Paralysis

- Diaphragmatic palsy can be bilateral or unilateral. Unilateral palsy is more common in infants and children. Most common causes are birth trauma and cardiac surgery.
- Unilateral palsy is often asymptomatic in older children, but in newborn infants and young children, it can cause severe respiratory compromise.
- Fluoroscopy on sniffing is a traditional method of diagnosis. Sonographic assessment of diaphragmatic motion can be used for diagnosis and to follow the progression.
- Surgical plication is accepted as the effective treatment. Diaphragmatic palsy secondary to phrenic nerve injury in the newborn invariably requires surgery. Older children, if asymptomatic, may be managed conservatively.
- Prognosis of unilateral diaphragmatic paralysis depends on the etiology and age.

References

1. Akay TH, Ozkan S, Gultekin B, et al. Diaphragmatic paralysis after cardiac surgery in children: Incidence, prognosis and surgical management. *Pediatr Surg Int* 2006;22:341–46.
2. Anderson KE, Bloomer JR, Bonkovsky HL, et al. Recommendations for the diagnosis and treatment of the acute porphyrias. *Ann Intern Med* 2005;142:439–50.
3. Andrews PI. Autoimmune myasthenia gravis in childhood. *Semin Neurol* 2004;24:101–10.
4. Asbury AK, Cornblath DR. Assessment of current diagnostic criteria for Guillain-Barré syndrome. *Ann Neurol* 1990;27:S21–4.
5. Banwell BL, Mildner RJ, Hassal AC, et al. Muscle weakness in critically ill children. *Neurology* 2003;61:1779–82.
6. Batocchi AP, Evoli A, Palmisani MT, et al. Early onset myasthenia gravis: Clinical characteristics and response to therapy. *Eur J Pediatr* 1990;150:66–8.
7. Bednarik J, Vondracek P, Dusek L, et al. Risk factors for critical illness polyneuropathy. *J Neurol* 2005;252:343–51.
8. Chemmanur AT, Bonkovsky HL. Hepatic porphyrias: Diagnosis and management. *Clin Liver Dis* 2004;8:807–38.
9. Ciafaloni E, Massey JM. The management of myasthenia gravis in pregnancy. *Semin Neurol* 2004;24:95–100.
10. Cochen V, Arnulf I, Demeret S, et al. Vivid dreams, hallucinations, psychosis and REM sleep in Guillain-Barré syndrome. *Brain* 2005;128:2535–45.
11. Dalakas MC. Mechanism of action of IVIG and therapeutic consideration in treatment of acute and chronic demyelinating neuropathy. *Neurology* 2002;59(12Suppl 6):S13–1.
12. De Jonghe, Sharshar T, Lefaucheur JP, et al. Paresis acquired in the intensive care unit: A prospective multicenter study. *JAMA* 2002;288:2859–67.
13. de Letter MA, Schmitz PI, Visser LH, et al. Risk factors for the development of polyneuropathy and myopathy in critically ill patients. *Crit Care Med* 2001;29:2281–86.
14. Dombeck AT, Satonik RC. The porphyrias. *Emerg Med Clin N Am* 2005;23(3):885–99, x.
15. Epelman M, Navarro OM, Daneman A, et al. M-mode sonography of diaphragmatic motion: Description of technique and experience in 278 pediatric patients. *Pediatr Radiol* 2005;35:661–7.
16. Fletcher SN, Kennedy DD, Ghosh IR, et al. Persistent neuromuscular and neurophysiologic abnormalities in long term survivors of prolonged critical care illness. *Crit Care Med* 2003;31:1012–6.
17. Freeman RK, Wozniak TC, Fitzgerald EB. Functional and physiologic results of video-assisted thoracoscopic diaphragm plication in adult patients with unilateral diaphragm paralysis. *Ann Thorac Surg* 2006;8:1853–57.
18. Gajdos P, Chevret S, Clair B, et al. Clinical trial of plasma exchange and high-dose intravenous immunoglobulin in myasthenia gravis. *Ann Neurol* 1997;41:789–96.
19. Gajdos P, Chevret S, Toyka K. Plasma exchange for myasthenia gravis. *Cochrane Database Syst Rev* 2002;4:CD002275.
20. Gajdos P, Chevret S, Toyka K. Intravenous immunoglobulin for myasthenia gravis. *Cochrane Database Syst Rev* 2003;2:CD002277.
21. Garnecho-Montero J, Amaya-Villar R, Garcia-Garmendia JL, et al. Effect of critical illness neuropathy on the withdrawal from mechanical ventilation and the length of stay in septic patients. *Crit Care Med* 2005;33:349–54.
22. Garnecho-Montero J, Madrazo-Osuna J, Garcia-Garmendia JL, et al. Critical illness polyneuropathy: Risk factors and clinical consequences. A cohort study in septic patients. *Intensive Care Med* 2001;27:1288–96.
23. Gorson KC, Ropper AH, Muriello MA, et al. Prospective evaluation of MRI lumbosacral nerve root enhancement in acute Guillain-Barré syndrome. *Neurology* 1996;47:813–7.
24. Grob D, Arsura EL, Brunner NG, et al. The course of myasthenia gravis and therapies affecting outcome. *Ann NY Acad Sci* 1987;505:472–99.
25. Gronseth GS, Barohn RJ. Practice parameter: Thymectomy for autoimmune myasthenia gravis (an evidence-based review). Report of the Quality Standards Subcommittee of the American Academy of Neurology Neurology 2000;55:7–15.
26. Hughes RAC, Raphael JC, Swan AV, et al. Intravenous immunoglobulin for Guillain-Barré syndrome. *Cochrane Database Syst Rev* 2004;1:CD002063.
27. Hughes RAC, van der Meche FGA. Corticosteroids for Guillain-Barré Syndrome. *Cochrane Database Syst Rev* 2000;2:CD001446.
28. Hughes RAC, Wijdicks EFM, Benson E, et al. Supportive care for patients with Guillian Barré syndrome. *Arch Neurol* 2005;62:1194–8.
29. Huttl TP, Wichmann MW, Reichart B, et al. Laparoscopic diaphragmatic plication: Long-term results of a novel surgical technique for postoperative phrenic nerve palsy. *Surg Endosc* 2004;18:547–51.
30. Khan J, Burnham EL, Moss M. Acquired weakness in the ICU: Critical illness myopathy and polyneuropathy. *Minerva Anestesiol* 2006;72:401–6.
31. Korinthenberg R, Monting JS. Natural history and treatment effects in Guillain Barré syndrome: A multicentric study. *Arch Dis Child* 1996;74:281–7.
32. Korinthenberg R, Schessl J, Kirschner J, et al. Intravenously administered immunoglobulin in the treatment of childhood Guillian Barré syndrome: A randomized trial. *Pediatrics* 2005;116:8–14.
33. Kuwabara S. Guillain-Barré Syndrome: Epidemiology, pathophysiology, and management. *Drugs* 2004;64:597–610.
34. Latronico N, Shehu I, Seghlini E. Neuromuscular sequelae of critical illness. *Curr Opin Crit Care* 2005;11:381–90.
35. Lawn ND, Fletcher DD, Henderson RD, et al. Anticipating mechanical ventilation in Guillian Barré syndrome. *Arch Neurol* 2001;58:893–8.
36. Leijten FS, Harinck-de Weerd JE, Poortvliet DC, et al. The role of polyneuropathy in motor convalescence after prolonged mechanical ventilation. *JAMA* 1995;274:1221–5.
37. Louillet F, Colas F, Outin HD, et al. Neuromuscular abnormalities in critical illness. *Rev Neurol* 2005;161:1267–71.
38. Luo YM, Harris ML, Lyall RA, et al. Assessment of diaphragm paralysis with oesophageal electromyography and unilateral magnetic phrenic nerve stimulation. *Eur Respir J* 2000;15:596–9.
39. Mantegaazza R, Baggi F, Antozzi C, et al. Myasthenia gravis (MG): Epidemiological data and prognostic factors. *Ann NY Acad Sci* 2003;998:413–23.
40. Maramattom BV, Wijdicks EFM. Acute neuromuscular weakness in the intensive care unit. *Crit Care Med* 2006;34:2835–41.
41. McGrath TM, Percy AK. Guillain-Barré Syndrome. In: Scheld WM, Whitley RJ, Marra CM, eds. *Scheld's Infections of Central Nervous System.* Philadelphia: Lippincott Williams & Wilkins; 2004:287–304.
42. Ohto T, Iwasaki N, Ohkoshi N, et al. A pediatric case of critical illness

polyneuropathy: Clinical and pathological findings. *Brain Dev* 2005;27:535–8.

43. Petersen B, Schneider C, Strassburg HM, et al. Critical illness neuropathy in pediatric intensive care patients. *Pediatr Neurol* 1999;21:749–53.

44. Piastra M, Antonelli M, Caresta E. Noninvasive ventilation in childhood acute neuromuscular respiratory failure: A pilot study. *Respiration* 2006;73(6):791–8.

45. Rabinstein A, Wijdicks EFM. BIPAP in acute respiratory failure due to myasthenic crisis may prevent intubation. *Neurology* 2002;59:1647–9.

46. Raphael JC, Chevret S, Hughes RAC, et al. Plasma exchange for Guillain-Barré syndrome. *Cochrane Database Syst Rev* 2002;2:CD001798.

47. Rodriguez M, Gomez MR, Howard FM Jr. , et al. Myasthenia gravis in children: Long-term follow-up. *Ann Neurol* 1983;13:504–10.

48. Romi F, Gilhus NE, Aarli JA. Myasthenia gravis: Clinical, immunological, and therapeutic advances. *Acta Neurol Scand* 2005;111:134–41.

49. Sanders DB, El-Salem K, Massey JM, et al. Clinical aspects of MuSK antibody positive seronegative MG. *Neurology* 2003;60:1978–80.

50. Schneider-Gold C, Gajdos P, Toyka KV, et al. Corticosteroids for myasthenia gravis. *Cochrane Database Syst Rev* 2005;2:CD002828.

51. Seybold ME. Thymectomy in childhood myasthenia gravis. *Ann NY Acad Sci* 1998;841:731–41.

52. Sharshar T, Chevret S, Bourdain F, et al. Early predictors of mechanical ventilation in Guillian Barré syndrome. *Crit Care Med* 2003;31:278–83.

53. Simansky DA, Paley M, Refaely Y, et al. Diaphragm plication following phrenic nerve injury: A comparison of paediatric and adult patients. *Thorax* 2002;57:613–6.

54. Singhi SC, Jayshree M, Singhi P, et al. Intravenous immunoglobulin in very severe childhood Guillain-Barré syndrome. *Ann Trop Paediatr* 1999;19:167–74.

55. Sladky JT. Guillian-Barré syndrome in children. *J Child Neurol* 2004;19:191–200.

56. Tabarki B, Coffinieres A, van den Berg P, et al. Critical illness neuromuscular disease: Clinical, electrophysiological, and prognostic aspects. *Arch Dis Child* 2002;86:103–7.

57. Trojaborg W. Electrophysiologic techniques in critical illness associated weakness. *J Neurol Sci* 2006;15(242):83–5.

58. Vajsar J, Fehlings D, Stephens D. Long term outcome in children with Guillian Barré syndrome. *J Pediatr* 2003;142:305–9.

59. van den Bergh G, Wouters P, Weekers F, et al. Intensive insulin therapy in the critically ill patients. *N Engl J Med* 2001;345:1359–67.

60. van der Schaaf M, Beelen A, de Vos R. Functional outcome in patients with critical illness polyneuropathy. *Disabil Rehabil* 2004;26:1189–97.

61. Varelas PN, Chua HC, Natterman J, et al. Ventilatory care in myasthenia gravis crisis: Assessing the baseline adverse event rate. *Crit Care Med* 2002;30:2663–8.

62. Williams S, Horrocks IA, Ouvrier RA, et al. Critical illness polyneuropathy and myopathy in pediatric intensive care: A review. *Pediatr Crit Care Med* 2007;8(1):18–22.

63. Wollinsky K, Huiser P, Brinkmeier H, et al. CSF filtration is an effective treatment of Guillain-Barré syndrome: A randomized clinical trial. *Neurology* 2001;57:774–80.

64. Zhou SZ, Li WH, Sun DK. Myasthenia gravis in children: Clinical study of 77 patients. *Zhonghua Er Ke Za Zhi* 2004;42:256–9.

CHAPTER 50 ■ CHRONIC NEUROMUSCULAR DISEASE

JONATHAN GILLIS • MONIQUE M. RYAN

Children with chronic neuromuscular disease (NMD) may have recurrent admissions to the PICU and may have a disproportionate impact on use of healthcare resources. For the staff, these admissions often engender discussion about the appropriate use of intensive care support and the patient's quality of life. Management of these patients also highlights one of the major shortcomings of contemporary PICU practice: lack of continuity in care and long-term follow-up. In managing these patients, it is critical that the intensivist works with a neuromuscular neurologist who provides up-to-date information on diagnosis, disease trajectory, and prognosis, and who is able to develop a long-term care plan with the child and family. In most instances, this neurologist will remain the primary physician or an ongoing consultant to the general pediatrician after the child's discharge from the PICU.

OVERVIEW OF CHRONIC NEUROMUSCULAR DISEASES

Clinical Presentation and Differential Diagnosis

The presentation of chronic NMDs relates largely to their pathophysiology (**Table 50.1**). Diagnosis is based on clinical findings and ancillary investigations (e.g., serum creatine kinase, neurophysiology, and muscle and nerve biopsy). In this chapter, chronic NMDs will be discussed under the categories of disorders that primarily affect nerves, the neuromuscular junction, or muscles.

Nerve Disorders

Spinal Muscular Atrophy

Spinal muscular atrophy type 1 (SMA 1), the most common motor neuronopathy of childhood, is a devastating disease of childhood, with an incidence of 1 in 5,000 live births. SMA is caused by recessive mutations in the survival motor neuron gene on chromosome 5. The four clinical subtypes of SMA are defined on the basis of disease severity and progression. Infants with SMA 1 never sit unsupported, children with SMA type 2 sit but never stand, those with SMA type 3 are able to walk without assistance, and SMA type 4 is of adult onset (43). All forms of SMA have the same genetic basis. The variable rate of disease progression relates to variable expression of modifying genes.

Children with SMA type 1 present in the first months of life with hypotonia and decreased spontaneous movement. Progressive weakness causes loss of antigravity strength and increasing difficulty in breathing and feeding. Without ventilatory support, death from chronic respiratory insufficiency before the age of 2 is virtually universal (20,43). In some cases, noninvasive ventilatory support through nasal prongs or facemask has been successful in prolonging survival into the second decade of life (4), although others report less success (8,21). Invasive mechanical ventilation via tracheostomy does lead to long-term survival in SMA 1, and this form of support is used in Asia, Europe, and the US (5,12,21).

Congenital Neuropathies

The congenital hypomyelinating or demyelinating neuropathies generally present in the first few years of life with hypotonia, weakness, and absent deep-tendon reflexes, often in association with congenital or acquired joint contractures. Complications include respiratory insufficiency, gastroesophageal reflux, and vocal cord paresis (29). These rare disorders are most often related to dominant or recessive mutations in genes for myelin proteins, and they represent an extreme of the Charcot-Marie-Tooth disease spectrum. Classification into congenital hypomyelinating neuropathy, Déjérine-Sottas syndrome, or other forms of Charcot-Marie-Tooth disease is contingent on age at presentation and findings on nerve biopsy.

Neuromuscular Junction Disorders

Myasthenic Syndromes

The myasthenic syndromes are discussed in Chapter 49.

Muscle Disorders

Congenital Myopathies

The congenital myopathies are a heterogeneous group of rare disorders defined by distinctive histochemical or ultrastructural changes in muscle (28). The number of morphologically and genetically distinct congenital myopathies has grown rapidly in recent decades (**Table 50.2**). Clinical severity varies widely within each form of myopathy, and marked clinical overlap with other NMDs is observed. All may be associated with early-onset weakness, hypotonia and hyporeflexia, poor muscle bulk, dysmorphic features secondary to muscle weakness (e.g., pectus carinatum, scoliosis, foot deformities, high-arched palate, and elongated facies), and a distinguishing morphologic

TABLE 50.1

CHRONIC NEUROMUSCULAR DISORDERS OF CHILDHOOD

	Etiology	Age of onset	Course
ANTERIOR HORN CELL			
Spinal muscular atrophy	Genetic (AR)	Variable (infancy-adulthood)	Progressive
Poliomyelitis	Infectious	Variable	Static
Acid maltase deficiency	Genetic (AR)	Variable (infancy-adulthood)	Progressive
PERIPHERAL NERVE			
Congenital hypomyelinating neuropathy	Sporadic/genetic (AD/AR)	Neonatal	Static
Déjérine-Sottas disease	Sporadic/genetic (AD/AR)	Infancy	Static
Charcot-Marie-Tooth disease	Genetic (AD, AR, XL)	Childhood	Slowly progressive
Chronic inflammatory demyelinating polyneuropathy	Autoimmune	Variable (childhood)	Relapsing-remitting or progressive
NEUROMUSCULAR DISORDERS			
Congenital myasthenic syndromes	Genetic (AR, AD)	Neonatal or infancy	Static
Myasthenia gravis	Autoimmune	Variable (childhood)	Relapsing-remitting
MYOPATHIES			
Congenital myopathies	Genetic (AR, AD, XL)	Variable (infancy-adulthood)	Static or slowly progressive
Congenital muscular dystrophies	Genetic (AR)	Infancy-childhood	Static or slowly progressive
Myotonic dystrophy	Genetic (AD)	Variable (neonatal-adulthood)	Static or slowly progressive
Duchenne and Becker muscular dystrophies	Genetic (XL)	Childhood	Progressive
Other muscular dystrophies	Genetic (AD, AR)	Variable (infancy-adulthood)	Progressive

AR, Autosomal recessive; AD, autosomal dominant; XL, X-linked recessive

abnormality on muscle biopsy. Affected patients may present later in life with delayed motor milestones, frequent falls, or disease complications such as contractures, scoliosis, and respiratory insufficiency.

Muscle weakness in the congenital myopathies is generally static. Facial weakness is common. Distal as well as proximal weakness may be present. The respiratory muscles are usually involved, but cardiac involvement is rare (23,30). Respiratory muscle involvement in the congenital myopathies generally parallels the extent of limb weakness. Some disorders (e.g., myotubular myopathy and nemaline myopathy) may present at birth with severe hypotonia, little spontaneous movement, and respiratory insufficiency. In severely affected infants, death from respiratory insufficiency, aspiration, or pneumonia is common during the first weeks or months of life (30). However, some severely hypotonic infants survive with little residual disability (6). Increasing weakness of the axial musculature may cause spinal deformities, which can progress rapidly during periods of rapid skeletal growth, particularly adolescence. Paraspinal muscle rigidity and kyphoscoliosis frequently result in significant restriction of lung capacity and respiratory insufficiency (23).

Congenital Muscular Dystrophies

Muscle disorders include the congenital muscular dystrophies, some of which affect only muscle. Others are associated with structural abnormalities of the brain and eyes (**Table 50.3**). The muscular dystrophies are generally caused by genetic abnormalities of the muscle membrane. These conditions are associ-

ated with progressive weakness, raised serum creatine kinase, and dystrophic changes in muscle. Respiratory insufficiency is common. Some congenital muscular dystrophies are associated with a characteristic pattern of axial weakness, spinal rigidity, and early respiratory insufficiency with relative sparing of the limb muscles.

Myotonic Dystrophy

Myotonic dystrophy is caused by an abnormal expansion of a CTG trinucleotide repeat sequence in the myotonic protein kinase gene (DMPK) at 19q13. The size of the expanded repeat sequence corresponds with the severity of peripheral and respiratory muscle weakness. Normal individuals have 5–37 repeats; 50–350 repeats are seen in childhood- and adult-onset myotonic dystrophy, while infants with severe congenital myotonic dystrophy may have more than 2,000 repeats. The mother is the affected parent in cases of congenital myotonic dystrophy.

Infants with congenital myotonic dystrophy have congenital contractures, generalized hypotonia, and weakness. Facial weakness causes the characteristic tented upper lip and scaphoid temporal fossae. Swallowing difficulties are common; most children require gavage feeding. Respiratory insufficiency is common in children who present in the first few weeks of life and relates to lung hypoplasia caused by reduced intrauterine breathing movements, poor intercostal muscle action, and diaphragmatic hypoplasia (31). Bulbar weakness predisposes to aspiration. Preterm birth and asphyxia may exacerbate neonatal pulmonary hypertension and failure of central respiratory

TABLE 50.2

CONGENITAL MYOPATHIES

	Inheritance	Muscle biopsy findings	Natural history	Additional findings
Central core disease	AD	Type 1 fiber predominance Cores in type 1 muscle fibers	Weakness static or slowly progressive Most patients remain ambulant	Scoliosis Congenital hip dislocation Predisposition to malignant hyperthermia
Nemaline myopathy	Variable: AD, AR, sporadic	Type 1 fiber predominance Nemaline bodies on trichrome stain	Weakness static or slowly progressive Variable severity Respiratory insufficiency common Bulbar involvement common	Scoliosis Acquired joint contractures
Myotubular myopathy	X-linked	Central nuclei all muscle fibers	Severe congenital weakness Most patients are ventilator dependent Significant early mortality	Ptosis Ophthalmoplegia Macrocephaly Pyloric stenosis
Centronuclear myopathy	AD, AR	Central nuclei all muscle fibers	Variable weakness in childhood or later Most patients remain ambulant	Ophthalmoplegia in some Respiratory insufficiency may present late
Minicore myopathy	AR	Type 1 fiber predominance Multiple small cores in type 1 muscle fibers	Moderate weakness Most patients are ambulant Respiratory insufficiency in those with spinal rigidity	Ophthalmoplegia in some Spinal rigidity Hand involvement Cardiomyopathy in minority Predisposition to malignant hyperthermia
Congenital fiber-type disproportion	AD, AR, XL	Type 1 fiber predominance Type 1 fibers small	Variable weakness Respiratory insufficiency in some	Ophthalmoplegia in some Scoliosis common

AD, Autosomal dominant; AR, autosomal recessive; XL, X-linked recessive

control. Approximately 50% of patients with congenital myotonic dystrophy require ventilation at birth (31). Poor prognostic factors include continued requirement for ventilatory support at 30 days of age, prematurity, pulmonary hypertension, and a large number of CTG repeats (11). Children who require ventilation beyond the first month of life have 25% mortality in their first year (11). Most survivors become ambulant, with improved respiratory function with increasing age, but remain at risk for later respiratory deterioration, cardiac arrhythmia, complications of poor gastrointestinal motility, diabetes, and mental retardation (11,28).

Duchenne Muscular Dystrophy

Duchenne and Becker muscular dystrophies are related muscle disorders caused by mutations in the gene for dystrophin at Xp21. Duchenne muscular dystrophy (DMD) affects 1 in 3,000 boys and is the most common muscular dystrophy of childhood. DMD usually presents between 3 and 5 years of age with an abnormal ("waddling") gait and frequent falls. Progressive muscle weakness causes loss of independent ambulation between ages 8 and 13. Becker muscular dystrophy is less common (affecting ~1 in 30,000 boys), generally presents between 5 and 15 years of age, and is more slowly progressive. Long-term corticosteroid treatment slows the progression of DMD (7). Loss of ambulation is followed by the development of scoliosis and muscle contractures. Most young men with DMD die before the age of 20 because of respiratory in-

sufficiency (90%) or cardiomyopathy (10%) (14). Long-term survival is reported in men who are supported with mechanical ventilation via tracheostomy (37). Other findings in DMD include muscle pseudohypertrophy, which most commonly affects the calves, and static intellectual impairment in 30% of patients.

Other Muscular Dystrophies

The limb-girdle muscular dystrophies (LGMD) usually present in adulthood. These relatively uncommon neuromuscular conditions cause characteristic patterns of muscle weakness, preferentially affecting the pectoral and pelvic girdle muscles and generally sparing the face (Table 50.4). Respiratory muscle involvement is generally seen late in the disease course, but some LGMDs are associated with preferential involvement of the axial musculature and early respiratory insufficiency.

CLINICAL MANAGEMENT IN INTENSIVE CARE

Presentation to the Intensive Care Unit

Most presentations to the ICU by children with chronic NMDs will be for the management of respiratory compromise

TABLE 50.3

CONGENITAL MUSCULAR DYSTROPHIES

Site of defect	Protein defect	Disorder/inheritance	Natural history	Additional findings
Extracellular matrix protein	Laminin α2 (merosin)	Merosin-deficient CMD (CMD type 1A) (AR)	Severe muscle weakness Respiratory insufficiency common	Leukodystrophy Demyelinating neuropathy
	Collagen VI	Ullrich (AD, AR) and Bethlem (AR) CMDs	Mild-to-moderate muscle weakness Respiratory insufficiency by late childhood-adolescence	Proximal joint contractures Distal hyperlaxity Follicular keratosis
Sarcolemmal proteins	Integrin α7 (AR)		Congenital muscular dystrophy	
Glycosyltransferase enzymes	Fukutin (AR)	Fukuyama CMD (AR) Walker-Warburg disease (AR)	Severe muscle weakness Early respiratory insufficiency	Cerebellar dysgenesis Cobblestone lissencephaly Severe mental retardation
	POMGnT1	Muscle-eye-brain disease (AR)	Severe muscle weakness Early respiratory insufficiency	Cerebellar dysgenesis Cobblestone lissencephaly Severe mental retardation
	POMT1	Walker-Warburg disease (AR) LGMD with mental retardation (AR)	Severe muscle weakness Early respiratory insufficiency	Cerebellar dysgenesis Cobblestone lissencephaly Severe mental retardation
	Fukutin-related protein	CMD type 1C (AR) LGMD type 2I (AR)	Variable muscle weakness	Macroglossia Calf hypertrophy Cardiomyopathy
	LARGE	CMD type 1D (AR)	Moderately severe muscle weakness	Severe mental retardation Leukodystrophy
Endoplasmic reticulum protein	Selenoprotein 1 (*SEPN1*)	CMD with spinal rigidity (AR) Multiminicore disease (AR) Congenital fiber-type disproportion (AR)	Axial rigidity Axial weakness Respiratory insufficiency	Characteristic facies

CMD, congenital muscular dystrophy; AR, autosomal recessive; AD, autosomal dominant; LGMD, limb-girdle muscular dystrophy

because of intercurrent illness, surgery, or disease progression. The severity of pulmonary compromise in such patients depends on the pattern and severity of involvement of respiratory muscles, the development of secondary thoracic wall abnormalities, and resultant changes in lung compliance (3).

Inspiratory muscle weakness limits the ability to take deep breaths, which leads to peripheral airway collapse. Respiratory muscle weakness may also make coughing ineffective. The cough reflex involves an initial inhalation of gas followed by closure of the glottis, then generation of an expiratory force against a closed glottis and, finally, rapid expiratory flow once the glottis reopens (9). These steps require, in turn, inspiratory, bulbar, and expiratory muscles. Impairment of the cough reflex because of poor function of any of these muscles results in the inability to clear secretions and the development of atelectasis. Superimposed upper respiratory tract infections also increase the volume of secretions, leading to frequent and rapid development of pneumonia (25).

In children with DMD and congenital myopathies, weakness of the diaphragm develops at the same rate as weakness of the intercostal and abdominal muscles. Significant respiratory compromise may occur, although paradoxical breathing is absent. Diaphragmatic weakness may be accentuated by supine positioning, exacerbating respiratory compromise in sleep (16).

In children with SMA, the intercostal muscles are more affected than the diaphragm. As the descent of the diaphragm during inspiration generates negative intrathoracic pressure, the thoracic cage will collapse (because of weaker intercostal muscles) at a time when the abdomen is expanding. This abnormal pattern—paradoxical breathing—can lead to chest wall deformity and abnormal lung development.

Young children with neuromuscular diseases have abnormally high chest wall compliance because of hypotonia and loss of muscle bulk. Intercostal muscle weakness makes the rib cage less able to withstand the elastic recoil of the lungs, leading to low end-expiratory volume and atelectasis. With increasing age, cartilaginous ossification causes a reduction in chest wall compliance and increased chest wall rigidity. Thoracic kyphoscoliosis may develop because of weak paraspinal musculature. Scoliosis further reduces chest wall compliance and may lead to asymmetrical chest expansion. Together, these factors contribute to the development of ventilation-perfusion mismatch, increased work of breathing, and respiratory muscle fatigue.

Sleep apnea and episodes of hypoxemia are the usual initial manifestations of respiratory muscle compromise in children with NMDs, with later development of alveolar hypoventilation and respiratory failure. Two types of respiratory failure are seen. Type 1 respiratory failure is characterized by hypoxemia and a low to normal $PaCO_2$. It is corrected by supplemental inspired oxygen. Hypoxemia and carbon dioxide retention characterize type 2 respiratory failure. Patients in type 2 respiratory failure may adapt to chronic hypercapnia, relying on hypoxic drive to breathe. Administration of supplemental oxygen in

TABLE 50.4

THE LIMB-GIRDLE MUSCULAR DYSTROPHIES

Muscular dystrophy (inheritance)	Symbol	Gene location	Protein product	Clinical findings
Autosomal dominant	LGMD1A	5q22–q34	myotilin	Dysarthria, neuropathy, cardiomyopathy
	LGMD1B	1q11–q23	lamin A/C	Cardiomyopathy, conduction defects, proximal contractures
	LGMD1C	3p25	caveolin 3	Muscle cramps, calf hypertrophy
	LGMD1D	6q23	?	
	LGMD1E	7q	?	
Autosomal recessive	LGMD2A	15q15.1–q21.1	calpain 3	Scapular winging, calf hypertrophy, thigh abductors spared
	LGMD2B	2p13	dysferlin	Distal weakness, wasting posterior compartment calf
	LGMD2C	13q12	γ-sarcoglycan	Duchenne phenocopy, cardiomyopathy
	LGMD2D	17q12–q21.33	α-sarcoglycan (adhalin)	Duchenne phenocopy, cardiomyopathy
	LGMD2E	4q12	β-sarcoglycan	Duchenne phenocopy, cardiomyopathy
	LGMD2F	5q33–44	δ-sarcoglycan	Duchenne phenocopy, cardiomyopathy
	LGMD2G	17q11–q12	telethonin	Rare, marked clinical variability
	LGMD2H	9q31–34.1	E3 ubiquitin ligase (TRIM32)	Seen only in Manitoba Hutterites
	LGMD 2I	19q13.3	fukutin-related protein	Calf and tongue hypertrophy, variable course, cardiomyopathy
	LGMD2J	2q	titin	Rare, wasting posterior compartment calf
Emery-Dreifuss (X-linked)	EDMD	Xq28	emerin	Early proximal contractures, cardiac conduction defects
Emery-Dreifuss (AD)	EDMD-AD	1q11–q23	lamin A/C	Early proximal contractures, cardiac conduction defects
Facioscapulohumeral muscular dystrophy (AD)	FSHD1	4q35	?	Facial weakness, scapular winging, foot drop

LGMD, limb-girdle muscular dystrophy; EDMD, Emery-Dreifuss muscular dystrophy; AD, autosomal dominant

this instance may lead to respiratory depression. Children with type 2 respiratory failure often require ventilatory support to improve gas exchange (35,39).

Disease-specific Aspects of Respiratory Care

Spinal Muscular Atrophy

Patients with SMA types 1 and 2 are at risk of respiratory complications at an early stage, which may present as recurrent chest infections or failure to thrive (8,21).

Congenital Myopathies and Muscular Dystrophies

Respiratory problems are the primary cause of death in chronic NMDs. The degree of skeletal muscle weakness usually, but not always, reflects the severity of respiratory muscle involvement (30). Bulbar muscle involvement increases the risk of aspiration, and poor nutritional state may increase the susceptibility to respiratory infection (23). Most patients, even those who are asymptomatic, have restricted respiratory capacity and are at risk of insidious nocturnal hypoxemia (35). Sleep-related symptoms include sleep disturbance, nightmares, morning headache, daytime tiredness, and weight loss. Sudden respiratory failure

may be precipitated by intercurrent infection or anesthesia and can occur at any age (30,39).

All patients with congenital myopathy should have baseline evaluation of their respiratory function as part of routine clinical and preoperative care. Any child with a vital capacity <60% of the predicted value for age should be reviewed annually with lung function testing [forced vital capacity in the sitting and supine positions, forced expiratory volume in 1 second (FEV1), and maximal inspiratory and expiratory pressures], pulse oximetry, $Paco_2$ when awake and when asleep, and an assessment of bulbar function (39). Regular chest physiotherapy, postural drainage, and assisted coughing techniques may improve respiratory toilet in patients with bulbar weakness, reduced vital capacity, and recurrent aspiration. Respiratory infections should be treated early and aggressively (9,39).

Duchenne Muscular Dystrophy

The natural history of respiratory muscle involvement in DMD follows a characteristic pattern. First, an increase occurs in vital capacity (VC) that parallels somatic growth until the age of 10–12 years. After this age, for the next 2–4 years, patients lose the ability to walk unaided, and their respiratory function ceases to increase, gradually declining, with a fall in VC of

8.5% per year. Slower rates of deterioration, on the order of ~4.5% per year, are seen in children who achieve a maximum VC above 2.5 L (26). DMD is associated with characteristic patterns of respiratory dysfunction (26). Sleep-disordered breathing is associated with a VC that is <60% of that predicted for age. Sleep-disordered breathing and hypoventilation are associated with a VC that is <40% of that predicted for age. In adults, a VC of <1.5 L or cough peak flow of <160 L/min predicts risk of respiratory failure; a VC of <1 L is terminal unless respiratory support is offered (32).

Practical Issues During Intensive Care Admission

Children with chronic NMDs are particularly vulnerable to influenza, other viral respiratory infections, and aspiration. Pneumococcal and influenza vaccinations should be given routinely (25). Most children with chronic NMDs who are admitted to the PICU will recover and be discharged without needing prolonged invasive mechanical ventilation. At least 25%, however, will require noninvasive respiratory support (41). Sometimes, the episode that necessitates admission signifies the inevitable decline in the underlying illness. The major issue, therefore, is to decide when such ongoing respiratory support is required. On admission, the child's primary physician should be contacted and the following questions should be asked of both the family and the physician: What is the child's present level of respiratory and bulbar function? What is the present level, if any, of respiratory support? Have there been discussions about prognosis, and have previous decisions been made about the level of mechanical ventilation to be offered? Are other long-term providers, such as neurologists or pulmonologists, involved for respiratory management? Is a case worker providing the coordination of respiratory care and other multidisciplinary care involving physiotherapy, occupational therapy, social work, and home nursing staff?

ONGOING VENTILATORY SUPPORT

The indications for ongoing ventilatory support include CO_2 retention ($PaCO_2$ >50 mm Hg), chronic hypoxia (PaO_2 <90 mm Hg), VC <1 L, and recurrent pneumonia (39). The preferred method of home mechanical ventilation will depend on the clinical state of the patient and the rate of progression of the underlying disorder. The mode of support includes bilevel positive-airway pressure by nasal mask or mechanical ventilation via tracheostomy if noninvasive support is not feasible (39). Domiciliary oxygen is rarely indicated but may be necessary if oxygen saturation remains <90% once hypoventilation has been corrected. Home ventilation requires a large and ongoing support network for the patients and their families and may not be appropriate for all patients (42). Aggressive management is appropriate for the older child for whom assisted ventilation may result in marked improvement in quality of life (42).

During the ICU admission it is important to have a clear plan for weaning from mechanical ventilation that incorporates best practice in multidisciplinary care.

Long-Term, Noninvasive Ventilation for Chronic Neuromuscular Disease

Home noninvasive ventilation (NIV) is used increasingly in children with chronic NMDs because it decreases hospitalization rates (24,41,42) and improves respiratory function (33). NIV is not curative and does not prevent progression of the underlying NMD, but it may improve quality of life (42). The optimal time for introduction of NIV is controversial. In boys with DMD, daytime hypercapnia predicts death within 9 months unless ventilatory support is given (37). NIV should be considered in children with DMD and recurrent desaturation to <90%, increase in transcutaneous CO_2 by >15 mm Hg during rapid eye movement (REM) sleep, symptoms of sleep-disordered breathing, or more than 3 admissions per year for respiratory distress (39). The benefit of NIV before the development of respiratory insufficiency is not proven.

Delivery of Respiratory Support

Noninvasive ventilation can be delivered by a nasal mask, facemask, or mouthpiece connected to bilevel, pressure-targeted ventilators. Most bilevel pressure-targeted ventilators include a continuous positive-airway pressure (CPAP) mode in addition to spontaneous and timed bilevel support modes (36). In the CPAP mode, the ventilator delivers a flow of gas set at a constant positive pressure. CPAP is not helpful in the patient with frequent central apneas or hypoventilation. Bilevel positive-airway pressure ventilators also provide CPAP but allow independent control of expiratory and inspiratory muscles. NIV is contraindicated in patients with upper airway obstruction and uncontrollable airway secretions. Severe swallowing impairment secondary to bulbar involvement is a relative contraindication. Complications of NIV include pneumothorax, facial irritation, gastric distension and, in the long-term, midface hypoplasia (38).

Bulbar Dysfunction

NMDs that cause significant facial and bulbar weakness may result in feeding difficulties in infancy and, in older children, lead to recurrent aspiration, dysarthria, poor articulation, and poor control of secretions (28). In the PICU, poor control of oral secretions may delay extubation.

Feeding problems in the newborn period often necessitate gavage feeds. Insertion of a gastrostomy tube should be considered if problems persist after the first few months of life. Careful attention to nutrition is important, particularly during acute illnesses. Malnutrition can cause significant morbidity (30). Accelerated weight gain and improvement of respiratory function may follow gastrostomy.

Treatments for sialorrhea, such as anticholinergic agents and salivary gland botulinum toxin injections, may be effective but may cause increased viscosity of secretions and other side effects (10,30) (**Table 50.5**).

Orthopedic Complications

Scoliosis and kyphosis are common complications of chronic NMDs and can impact upon mobility and respiratory function.

TABLE 50.5

MANAGEMENT OF CHILDREN WITH CHRONIC NEUROMUSCULAR DISORDERS

Problem identified	Referral	Possible interventions

Skeletal muscle involvement
  Hypotonia
  Weakness
  Contractures
	Physiotherapy
	Occupational therapy
		Objective testing of muscle strength
		Regular exercise program
		Active and passive stretching
		Standing frame
		Orthotics/splinting—upper and lower limb
		Serial plaster casting
		Enhance mobility—walking frames or wheelchair
		Liaison with local services prior to discharge

Respiratory muscle involvement
  Reduced respiratory capacity
  Recurrent chest infections
  Aspiration
  Nocturnal hypoxia
  Respiratory failure
	Physiotherapy
	Lung-function tests
	Sleep study
	Respiratory physician
	Occupational therapy
		Breathing exercises
		Chest physiotherapy to clear secretions
		Seating assessment
		Influenza and pneumococcal vaccination
		Aggressive management of acute infections
		Nocturnal/daytime ventilation
		Liaise with local services

Bulbar involvement
  Feeding and swallowing difficulties
  Failure to thrive
	Speech pathologist
	Dietitian
	Gastroenterologist
		Speech therapy
		Modified barium swallow
		Caloric supplementation/thickened feed
		Gavage feeding or gastrostomy feeding

Bulbar involvement
  Dysarthria
  Excessive drooling
	Speech pathologist
	Surgeon
		Speech therapy
		Anticholinergic medications
		Pharyngoplasty
		Salivary duct surgery/botulinum toxin injections

Developmental or psychosocial delay	Occupational therapy Physiotherapy Speech pathology Psychologist Developmental physician	Developmental stimulation Home programs Reassessment if deterioration
Scoliosis	Physiotherapy Orthopedic surgeon	Spinal x-ray Monitoring of degree of curve Bracing Corrective surgery
Foot deformities	Physiotherapy Orthopedic surgeon	Splinting/serial casting Corrective surgery

Cardiac involvement
  Conduction defects
  Cardiomyopathy
  Cor pulmonale
	Cardiologist	Electrocardiogram, Holter monitor, cardiac echo
		Medication if indicated

Inability to perform activities of daily
  living
  Inability to achieve independence with
    bathing, toileting, dressing, feeding
  Difficulties with access
  Handwriting difficulties
	Occupational therapy
	Community nurse
		Aides for individual activities of daily living
		Wheelchair assessment
		Home nursing assistance
		Home and school modifications
		Typing and computer programs
		Car modifications
		Liaise with local services

Excessive weight gain
  Limits mobility and exacerbates
    weakness
	Dietitian
	Physiotherapy
		Calorie-controlled diet
		Exercise program

Inability to participate in sport/leisure activities	Physiotherapy Occupational therapy	Liaison with/visit schools Sporting organizations for people with disabilities Hydrotherapy
Constipation	Dietitian Physician Gastroenterologist	High-fiber diet Laxatives/enemas
Depression or behavioral problems	Psychologist	Individual or family therapy Medication

(Continued)

TABLE 50.5

(CONTINUED)

Problem identified	Referral	Possible interventions
Family financial and social difficulties	Social work Muscular Dystrophy Association Government assistance bodies	Disability allowance/pension Support groups Financial assistance with equipment and home modifications Transport and travel assistance
Planning future pregnancies	Geneticist Genetic counselor	Genetic counseling Planning prenatal diagnosis
Planning surgery	Consult with anesthesiologist Respiratory physician	Malignant hyperthermia precautions Lung function tests and pre-surgical physiotherapy
Planning future employment	Vocational counseling service Occupational therapy	Planning school studies Vocational planning Training, work placement and support
Coordination of care	Pediatrician, pediatric neurologist or rehabilitation specialist	Contact with general practitioner via telephone and letter Liaise with local services Arrange case conferences when necessary Determine timing of respiratory, orthopaedic, and palliative interventions

Thoracic bracing does not prevent or reverse spinal curvature but can improve stability during sitting. Spinal fusion halts progressive spinal deformity and preserves lung function. The introduction of segmental spinal instrumentation, with sublaminar wire fixation (incorporating Luque rods), has greatly eased the postoperative management in the PICU. The posterior surgical approach is considered best for preventing progression of spinal deformity. An anterior approach in patients reliant on anterior abdominal muscles and the diaphragm for respiration can lead to postoperative respiratory difficulty and long-term respiratory compromise. Postoperative complications are more common in children with VC of <30% predicted for age (22) and those with a spinal curve of >100 degrees (18).

Orthopedic surgery may also be needed for congenital and acquired contractures and pathologic fractures secondary to disuse osteopenia. Orthotics, splinting, and serial plaster casting may be necessary in children who are immobilized for long periods by illness or surgery, particularly for prevention of Achilles tendon and long-finger flexor contractures. Splinting must be undertaken in combination with passive stretching exercises to optimize benefit (27).

Cardiac Function

Symptomatic cardiac involvement is uncommon in the congenital myopathies and myasthenic syndromes, but cor pulmonale may be seen in those with advanced respiratory disease. Several of the congenital and limb-girdle muscular dystrophies (particularly CMD1C/LGMD 2I, LGMD 1A, and Emery-Dreifuss muscular dystrophy) are associated with cardiomyopathy and conduction defects. Patients with these conditions should undergo annual cardiac review.

Advanced DMD is commonly associated with cardiac conduction defects, resting tachycardia, and cardiomyopathy. Mitral valve prolapse and pulmonary hypertension may also occur. Subclinical or clinical cardiac involvement is present in ~90% of Duchenne or Becker muscular dystrophy patients but is the cause of death in only 20% of men with DMD and 50% of patients with Becker muscular dystrophy. Progression of cardiomyopathy in DMD or Becker muscular dystrophy may be slowed by treatment with β-blockers and angiotensin-converting enzyme inhibitors (14).

Myotonic muscular dystrophy is rarely associated with cardiomyopathy, but children with myotonic dystrophy commonly develop symptomatic or subclinical conduction disturbances that may cause left ventricular dysfunction. Patients with myotonic dystrophy require monitoring of cardiac conduction and may require a cardiac pacemaker (13).

Anesthesia

Patients with congenital myopathies and muscular dystrophies usually tolerate general anesthesia, but the potential exists for decompensation of respiratory function and rapid loss of muscle conditioning. Subclinical respiratory insufficiency may be unmasked by anesthesia and exacerbated by postoperative atelectasis and spinal instrumentation. For example, in a series of 143 patients with nemaline myopathy, 5 patients developed unexpected postoperative respiratory failure, 1 child had unexpected respiratory arrest 24 hrs after fundoplication, and another developed persistent lobar collapse (30). Preoperative assessment of respiratory state is important in helping to decide the timing of surgery. Patients should receive intensive preoperative physiotherapy, and they must be mobilized as soon as possible after surgery, as prolonged immobility may exacerbate muscle weakness.

Children with myotonic dystrophy may be extremely sensitive to anesthetics and analgesics, especially barbiturates and opiates, with a prolonged response to nondepolarizing muscle relaxants and a tendency to postoperative apnea and sedation (40).

Malignant hyperthermia is an autosomal-dominant, pharmacogenetic disorder characterized by an increase in skeletal muscle metabolism in response to certain inhalation anesthetics (particularly halothane) and depolarizing muscle relaxants (particularly succinylcholine). The triggering agent increases sarcoplasmic calcium concentrations, resulting in uncontrolled muscle contraction and hyperthermia, which may be fatal if untreated. Central core disease and minicore myopathy are associated with an increased risk of malignant hyperthermia. Malignant hyperthermia is less commonly associated with other congenital myopathies (1) and has been reported in DMD and other muscular dystrophies. Malignant hyperthermia precautions should be undertaken in all patients who are to undergo muscle biopsy for diagnostic purposes. Triggering anesthetics should be avoided.

QUALITY OF LIFE IN CHILDREN VENTILATED FOR CHRONIC NEUROMUSCULAR DISEASE

It is a common, if unstated, concern of intensive care staff that, once intubated for an acute episode of respiratory compromise, children with NMDs will not be able to be extubated and weaned from full ventilation. (9,17). This concern is not supported by the literature. In a 15-year review of children with chronic NMDs who were admitted to the PICU, most were discharged without the need for prolonged invasive ventilation; 9% of unplanned admissions ended in death (41). Nocturnal respiratory support was started in the PICU and continued after discharge in 23% of admissions. The authors concluded that "all children with underlying NMD should be provided with acute respiratory support in the anticipation that they are likely to recover. However, repeat admissions and chronic respiratory failure are likely and should be anticipated."

Most ventilator-dependent adults consider that their quality of life is reasonable (2,19). Relatively few studies have been undertaken in long-term, ventilated children, but the information available suggests that their quality of life is considered good (15,42).

CONCLUSIONS AND FUTURE DIRECTIONS

The complex ethical issues involved in the use of long-term ventilation in children with chronic NMDs have been reviewed recently (34). The clinical management of these children varies within and between countries. However, some fundamental guidelines should be followed:

- A specialist in neuromuscular diseases should be involved so that, as far as possible, up-to-date information on prognosis, function, and quality of life is available. This physician should be the one who usually cares for the child and family. and who has discussed ventilatory options and negotiated a proposed plan of care.
- The difficulty of being able to predict the exact clinical course should be acknowledged.

- Palliative care principles should always be followed, because most of these diseases cannot be cured. The treatment strategy should be to maintain as good a quality of life for as long as possible. It is important to stress to the child and family that their care will be actively continued even if they choose not to pursue artificial ventilation. The primary aim of treatment is maintenance of an acceptable quality of life.

Advances in the ICU management of children with chronic NMDs should be focused on improved management of respiratory impairment, better monitoring, and prevention of complications.

KEY POINTS

- NMDs are a common cause of significant chronic neurologic morbidity in childhood. Recent advances have improved clinical and genetic characterization of many of these conditions.
- NMDs are a common cause of admission to the PICU. Most acute complications of pediatric NMDs relate to respiratory insufficiency.
- It is important to consider the natural history in managing children with chronic NMDs. Although some disorders are progressive, inevitably causing increasing weakness and respiratory insufficiency, in many children, strength and ventilatory function stabilize and even improve with increasing age.
- Most children recover from their acute episode and are discharged. In some cases, however, respiratory decompensation heralds a deterioration in the child's condition and should trigger consideration of more aggressive respiratory support in the form of noninvasive ventilation or ventilation via tracheostomy.
- Supportive care of children with chronic NMDs includes physical therapy for stretching and maintenance of range of motion, optimization of upper-limb function with occupational therapy, orthopaedic management of contractures and scoliosis, and monitoring of swallow and nutrition.
- A case manager should be assigned to each patient early in his admission to coordinate the multidisciplinary team and provide consistent, clear, and comprehensive care.

References

1. Asai T, Fujise K, Uchida M. Anaesthesia for cardiac surgery in children with nemaline myopathy. *Anaesthesia* 1992;47:405–8.
2. Bach JR, Barnett V. Ethical considerations in the management of individuals with severe neuromuscular disorders. *Am J Phys Med Rehab* 1994;73: 134–40.
3. Bach JR, Niranjan V, Weaver B. Spinal muscular atrophy type 1: A noninvasive respiratory management approach. *Chest* 2000;117:1100–05.
4. Bach JR, Baird JS, Plosky D, et al. Spinal muscular atrophy type 1: Management and outcomes. *Pediatr Pulmonol* 2002;34:16–22.
5. Bach JR. There are other ways to manage spinal muscular atrophy type 1. *Chest* 2005;127:1463–4.
6. Banwell BL, Singh NC, Ramsay DA. Prolonged survival in neonatal nemaline myopathy. *Pediatr Neurol* 1994;10:335–7.
7. Biggar WD, Gingras M, Fehling DL, et al. Deflazacort treatment of Duchenne muscular dystrophy. *J Pediatr* 2001;138:45–50.
8. Birnkrant DJ, Pope JF, Martin JE, et al. Treatment of type I spinal muscular atrophy with noninvasive ventilation and gastrostomy feeding. *Pediatric Neurol* 1998;18:407–10.
9. Birnkrant DJ. The assessment and management of the respiratory complications of pediatric neuromuscular diseases. *Clin Pediatr* 2002;41:301–8.
10. Brei TJ. Management of drooling. *Semin Pediatr Neurol* 2003;10:265–70.

11. Campbell C, Sherlock R, Jacob P, et al. Congenital myotonic dystrophy: Assisted ventilation duration and outcome. *Pediatrics* 2004;113:811–6.
12. Chung BH, Wong VC, Ip P. Spinal muscular atrophy: Survival pattern and functional status. *Pediatrics* 2004;114:e548–53.
13. English KM, Gibbs JL. Cardiac monitoring and treatment for children and adolescents with neuromuscular disorders. *Dev Med Child Neurol* 2006; 48:231–5.
14. Finsterer J, Stollberger C. The heart in human dystrophinopathies. *Cardiology* 2003;99:1–19.
15. Frates RC, Jr., Splaingard ML, Smith EO, et al. Outcome of home mechanical ventilation in children. *J Pediatr* 1985;106:850–6.
16. Fromageot C, Lofaso F, Annane D, et al. Supine fall in lung volumes in the assessment of diaphragmatic weakness in neuromuscular disorders. *Arch Phys Med Rehab* 2001;82:123–8.
17. Gillis J, Rennick J. Affirming parental love in the pediatric intensive care unit. *Pediatr Crit Med* 2006;7:165–8.
18. Grossfeld S, Winter RB, Lonstein JE, et al. Complications of anterior spinal surgery in children. *J Pediatr Orthoped* 1997;17:89–95.
19. Hotes LS, Johnson JA, Sicilian L. Long-term care, rehabilitation, and legal and ethical considerations in the management of neuromuscular disease with respiratory dysfunction. *Clin Chest Med* 1994;15:783–95.
20. Iannaccone ST, Browne RH, Samaha FJ, et al. Prospective study of spinal muscular atrophy before age 6 years. *Pediatr Neurol* 1993;9:187–93.
21. Ioos C, Leclair-Richard D, Mrad S, et al. Respiratory capacity course in patients with infantile spinal muscular atrophy. *Chest* 2004;126: 831–7.
22. Jenkins JG, Bohn D, Edmonds JF, et al. Evaluation of pulmonary function in muscular dystrophy patients requiring spinal surgery. *Crit Care Med* 1982; 10:645–9.
23. Jungbluth H, Sewry C, Brown SC, et al. Minicore myopathy in children: A clinical and histopathological study of 19 cases. *Neuromuscul Disord* 2000; 10:264–73.
24. Katz S, Selvadurai H, Keilty K, et al. Outcome of non-invasive positive pressure ventilation in paediatric neuromuscular disease. *Arch Dis Child* 2004;89:121–4.
25. Keren R, Zaoutis TE, Bridges CB, et al. Neurological and neuromuscular disease as a risk factor for respiratory failure in children hospitalized with influenza infection. *JAMA* 2005;294:2188–94.
26. McDonald CM, Abresch RT, Carter GT, et al. Profiles of neuromuscular diseases: Duchenne muscular dystrophy. *Am J Phys Med Rehab* 1995; 74(5 Suppl):S70–92.
27. McDonald CM. Limb contractures in progressive neuromuscular disease and the role of stretching, orthotics and surgery. *Phys Med Rehab Clin North Am* 1998;9:187–211.
28. North KN, Ryan MM. The Congenital Myopathies. In: Noseworthy J, ed. *Neurological Therapeutics, Principles and Practice.* Rochester, NY: Martin Dunitz, 2006.
29. Ouvrier RA, Geevasinga N, Ryan MM. Autosomal recessive and X-linked forms of hereditary motor and sensory neuropathy in childhood. *Muscle Nerve* 2007, in press.
30. Ryan MM, Schnell C, Strickland CD, et al. Nemaline myopathy: A clinical study of 143 cases. *Ann Neurol* 2001;50:312–20.
31. Sarnat HB, O'Connor T, Byrne PA. Clinical effects of myotonic dystrophy on pregnancy and the neonate. *Arch Neurol* 1976;33:459–65.
32. Seddon PC, Khan Y. Respiratory problems in children with neurological impairment. *Arch Dis Child* 2003;88:75–8.
33. Simonds AK, Ward S, Heather S, et al. Outcome of paediatric domiciliary mask ventilation in neuromuscular and skeletal disease. *Europ Resp J* 2000;16:476–81.
34. Simonds AK. Ethical aspects of home long-term ventilation in children with neuromuscular disease. *Paediatr Resp Rev* 2005;6:209–14.
35. Smith PE, Edwards RH, Calverley PM. Mechanisms of sleep disordered breathing in chronic neuromuscular disease: Implications for management. *Q J Med* 1991;81:961–73.
36. Teague WG. Noninvasive ventilation in the pediatric intensive care unit for children with acute respiratory failure. *Pediatr Pulmonol* 2003;35: 418–26.
37. Vianello A, Bevilacqua M, Salvador V, et al. Long-term nasal intermittent positive pressure ventilation in advanced Duchenne's muscular dystrophy. *Chest* 1994;105:445–8.
38. Villa MP, Pagani J, Ambrosio R, et al. Mid-face hypoplasia after long-term nasal ventilation. *Am J Resp Crit Care Med* 2002;166:1142–3.
39. Wallgren-Pettersson C, Bushby K, Mellies U, et al. 117th ENMC workshop: Ventilatory support in congenital neuromuscular disorders—congenital myopathies, congenital muscular dystrophies, congenital myotonic dystrophy and SMA (II). 4–6 April 2003, Naarden, The Netherlands. *Neuromuscul Disord* 2004;14:56–69.
40. White RJ, Bass SP. Myotonic dystrophy and paediatric anaesthesia. *Paediatr Anaesth* 2003;13:94–102.
41. Yates K, Festa M, Gillis J, et al. Outcome of children with neuromuscular disease admitted to paediatric intensive care. *Arch Dis Child* 2004;89: 170–175.
42. Young HK, Lowe A, Fitzgerald DA, et al. Non-invasive ventilation in children with neuromuscular disease. *Neurology* 2007;68(3): 198–201.
43. Zerres K, Rudnik-Schoneborn S. Natural history in proximal spinal muscular atrophy. Clinical analysis of 445 patients and suggestions for a modification of existing classifications. *Arch Neurol* 1995;52:518–23.

CHAPTER 51 ■ DEVELOPMENTAL NEUROBIOLOGY, NEUROPHYSIOLOGY, AND THE PICU

LARRY W. JENKINS • PATRICK M. KOCHANEK

The emerging field of neurointensive care for infants and children is challenged with designing and implementing optimal therapies for complex insults, such as traumatic brain injury (TBI), asphyxial arrest, stroke, status epilepticus, and infections, for what is uniformly recognized as the most complex organ system—the central nervous system (CNS). The challenge is magnified in pediatrics by the need to accomplish this goal in an optimal manner, whether the patient is a newborn, infant, child, or adolescent. Salient differences in structural, biochemical, physiologic, and behavioral components of the brain from infancy to adolescence have been recognized, and an understanding of these factors may be important to the clinician when appropriately defining prognosis and/or guiding therapy. This chapter provides fundamental insights into this complexity and is organized around key concepts and developmental milestones that should provide useful constructs for understanding both developmental brain function and pathology in clinical practice. It provides basics in developmental neurobiology and neurophysiology that will help the reader navigate the chapters that follow. We recognize that, in several areas, a complete picture of developmental differences in neurobiology and neurophysiology across the PICU-relevant age spectrum is lacking—and extrapolation from data on newborns or adults is necessary. In some cases, only data from experimental animal models are available. Nevertheless, certain stages of development may be particularly resistant or vulnerable to PICU-relevant insults that may interfere with subsequent normal developmental progression. Key factors germane to pediatric intensive care that differentiate the newborn, infant, child, adolescent, and adult brain are discussed whenever possible. For more details, the reader is referred to several excellent reviews (1–4,7,8,12,19,21,22,30,32,34,36,38,39,42,46,52,53) to which much of this chapter is indebted.

CENTRAL NERVOUS SYSTEM DEVELOPMENT

Brain Development Timeline

CNS development occurs through the process of neurulation during embryogenesis. The neural plate is formed by ectodermal tissue at ~2 weeks of gestation. By the eighteenth day of gestation, the neural plate forms the neural groove, which in turn eventually fuses by the third gestational week, giving rise to the neural tube. Completed human neural tube formation occurs between 26 and 28 gestational days (46). Throughout the first month of human gestation, specific CNS regions, such as the forebrain, midbrain, and hindbrain, form due to neurogenesis and cellular migration. Concomitant with regional CNS development, neurogenesis and proliferation, migration, differentiation, synaptogenesis, apoptosis, and myelination occur and continue postnatally up to 10 years of age (Fig. 51.1). Major CNS developmental milestones in gestational weeks are as follows (32):

■ 3–4 weeks—Formation of the neural tube occurs.
■ 5–10 weeks—Hemispheres form.
■ 8–18 weeks—Neuronal proliferation is ongoing.
■ 12–24 weeks—Neuronal migration proceeds.
■ 25+ weeks—Neuronal arborization, synaptogenesis, programmed neuronal death, and neural connectivity occur.
■ 40+ weeks—Myelination is ongoing.

Aberrations in any of these brain developmental processes may produce congenital CNS defects, many of which can be life-threatening (46).

Development of Specific Brain Regions

Human brain size increases dramatically, beginning from early gestation and continuing for at least 2–3 postnatal years. CNS growth, based upon changes in gross brain size, peaks at around 4 months postnatally. However, specific brain regions have different growth time windows (Fig. 51.2) and periods of genetic and environmental vulnerabilities before and after birth (46). In general, the forebrain develops slower than the hindbrain, with the medial aspects of the hindbrain developing faster than the lateral. The neocortical and hippocampal structures grow mostly during the fetal period but do have some continuing neuronal and glial postnatal development. In contrast, the thalamus and hypothalamus develop during the early fetal and late embryonic periods, as does the mesencephalon. The pons and medulla of the hindbrain develop primarily during the embryonic period, which in humans encompasses weeks 3–7.5 of gestation (46).

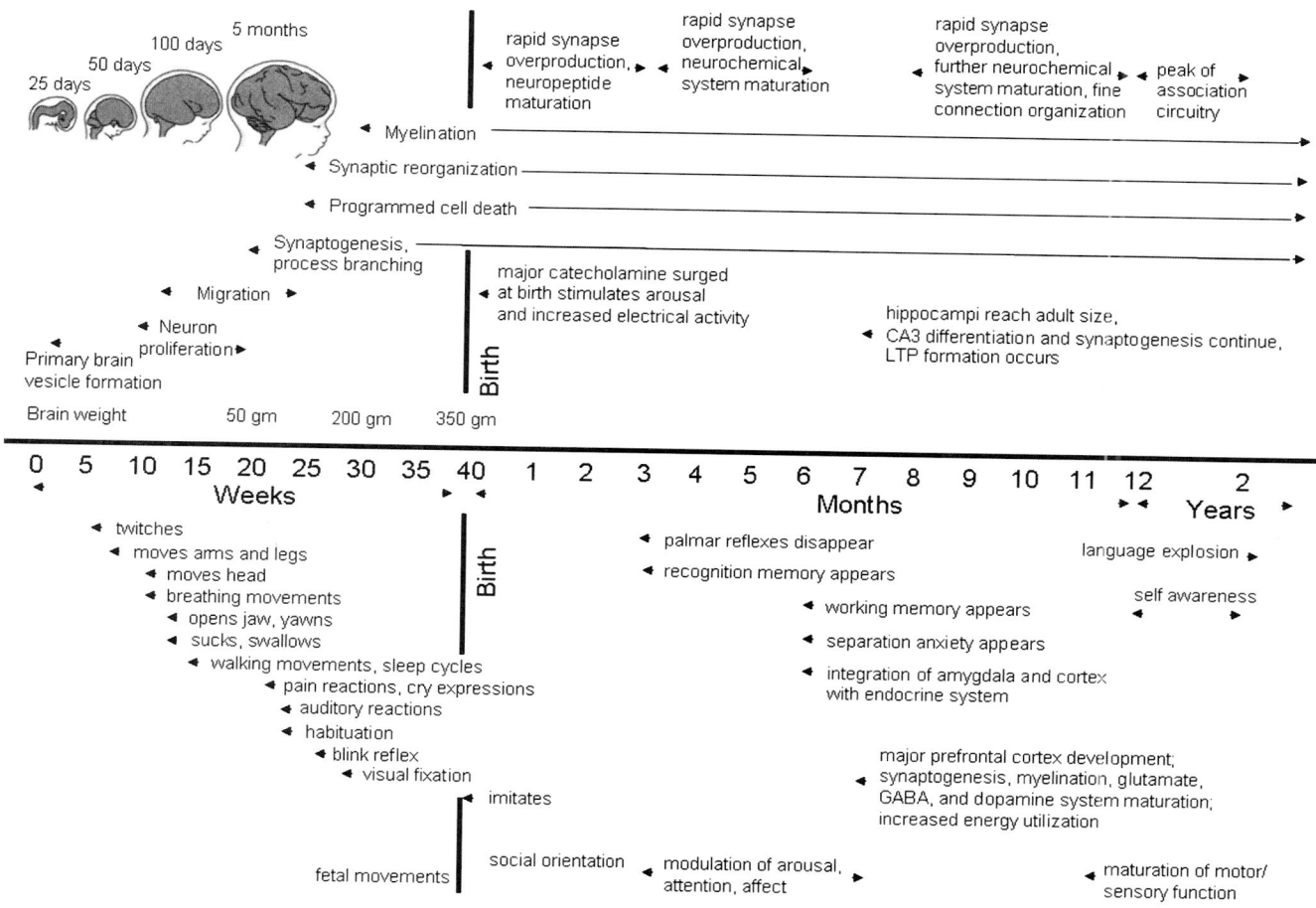

FIGURE 51.1. The key events of the human developmental timeline. The appearance of specific structural and functional developmental events is shown for the human fetus, infant, and young child up to 2 years of age. Modified from Lagercrantz H, Ringstedt T. Organization of the neuronal circuits in the central nervous system during development. *Acta Paediatr* 2001;90:707–15; additional data from Levitt P. Structural and functional maturation of the developing primate brain. *J Pediatr* 2003;143:S35–45; and from Herschkowitz N. Neurological bases of behavioral development in infancy. *Brain Dev* 2000;22: 411–16.

Neurogenesis and Proliferation

The neural tube is formed by the neuroectoderm, with neuroepithelial cells differentiating into various types of neurons and glia. The mature human brain contains an estimated 10^{10} neurons (37). Neural precursor cells from the epithelium form the developing CNS and undergo mitotic arrest at various times during development. Prior to becoming postmitotic cells, these cells determine their position within the embryonic axis and either reenter the cell cycle to increase the precursor pool or enter mitotic arrest (12). During development, neuronal populations within each brain region are highly regulated along a structured timetable. This regional variability appears conserved across species with regard to neuronal developmental patterns, but with species-specific timelines. For example, neurogenesis occurs within days in the rat compared to weeks in human. Environmental or genetic stress during neurogenesis is a particularly vulnerable time for regional brain development. However, the CNS is more resistant to such stressors following neurogenesis. Fetal alcohol syndrome is a classic example of environmental stress that can interfere with the developmental process of neurogenesis (46).

The prenatal stage of brain development is characterized by rapid cell division under the control of the cell cycle and, in turn, numerous cell signaling pathways, including at least nine different growth factor cascades (4). Cells also must duplicate their organelles and cellular molecules to maintain their size; thus, growth processes must also be coordinated with cellular replication. It has been estimated that ~200,000 new neurons are produced each minute at between 8 and 18 weeks of gestation. In contrast, it has been proposed that little neurogenesis occurs after birth, except in some select brain regions that continue into adulthood (32).

Programmed Cell Death

Neuronal cell type and number are regulated by apoptotic cell death during CNS development, which occurs in waves. Programmed cell death (PCD) begins in zones of proliferation and recurs as CNS remodeling proceeds based upon

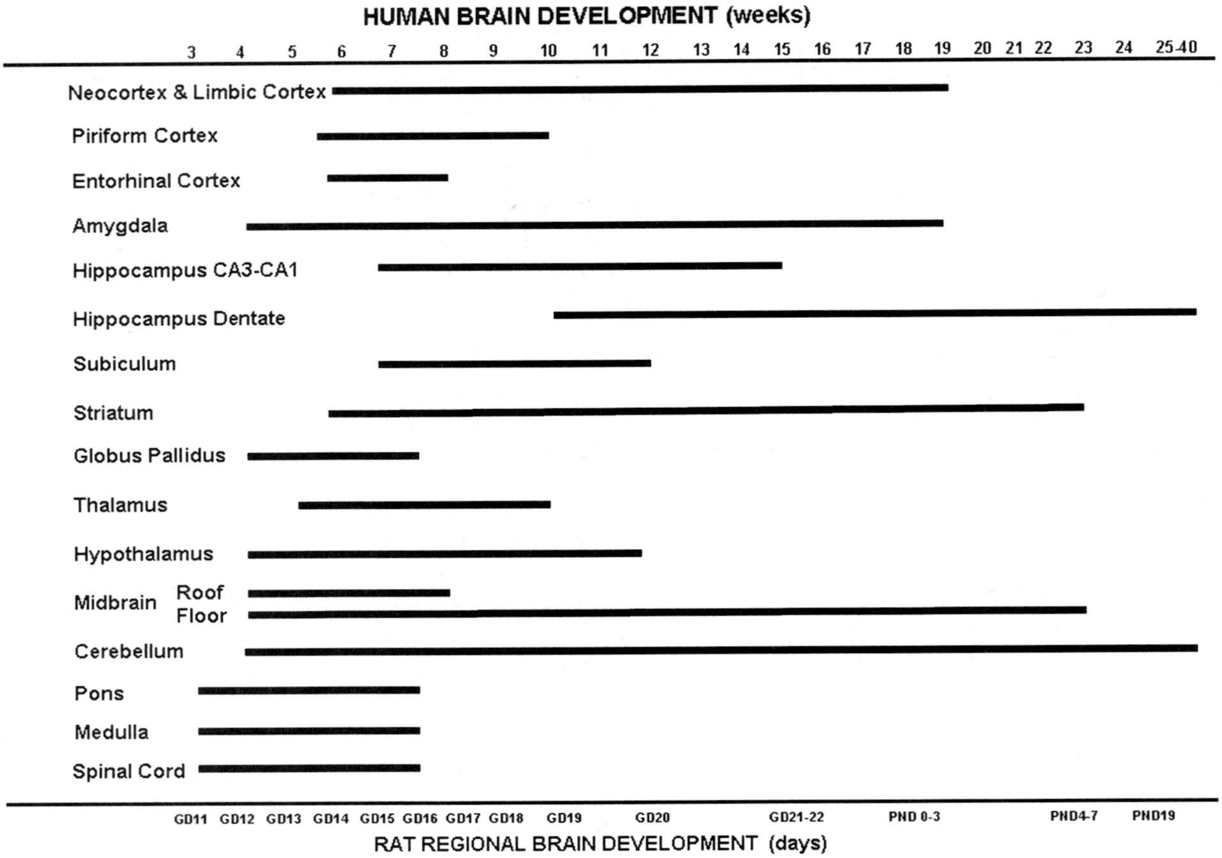

HUMAN BRAIN DEVELOPMENT (weeks)

FIGURE 51.2. Human regional brain development. The developmental timeline of selected human brain regions is shown in comparison to rat development timeline. The rat is the most commonly used species to study both normal and injury-related CNS development and thus has the most extensive normative database. GD, gestational day; PND, postnatal day. Modified from Rice D, Barone S, Jr. Critical periods of vulnerability for the developing nervous system: Evidence from humans and animal models. *Environ Health Perspective* 2000;108 Suppl 3:511–33, with permission.

the kind and number of connections made by each individual neuroblast and neuron (4). Furthermore, PCD persists postnatally due to continued CNS development. Two types of developmental PCD have been classified: (a) a proliferative apoptosis that affects morphogenetic processes involving neural precursor cells and postmitotic neuroblasts, and (b) a neurotrophic-related apoptosis that affects postmitotic neurons that fail to establish appropriate synaptic connections. Apoptotic regulation of neurons that undergo PCD prior to developing synaptic contacts (proliferative apoptosis) has been proposed to differ from target-dependent neuronal death pathways (neurotrophic-related apoptosis) (12) (**Fig. 51.3**). Proliferative neuronal apoptosis prevents premature and dysfunctional neurogenesis from occurring secondary to premature differentiation signals.

Interference in normal developmental neuronal death cascades by environmental or genetic stress can result in a number of different pathologies (4). In contrast to the trophin-mediated signals that promote growth and survival, extracellular signaling proteins exist that inhibit these processes. These survival and death signals, as will be seen in Chapter 52, appear to play a key role in the evolution of neuronal death after CNS injuries such as asphyxia, TBI, seizures, infections, and other PICU-relevant insults.

The Bcl-2 protein family, the adaptor protein Apaf1, and the cysteine-protease caspase family are the principal regulators of PCD (12). PCD pathways involve both intrinsic and extrinsic types of neuronal death. Intrinsic PCD signaling pathways involve a reduction in mitochondrial membrane potential, resulting in the release of cytochrome C by the activation of Apaf1 and caspase 9, with ultimate activation of caspase 3. Bcl-2 family proteins Bcl-2 and Bcl-XL are pro-survival molecules that inhibit the release of mitochondrial cytochrome C, whereas pro-death molecules, such as Bax and Bad, can directly affect mitochondrial membrane integrity.

In the extrinsic pathway, removal of neurotrophic factors leads to activation of the protein kinase c-Jun kinase (JNK). JNK can phosphorylate different substrates, including c-Jun, which in turn, activates transcription of Fas-L by binding to AP-1 sites in the gene promoter site (44). Fas modulates various effectors to activate caspases directly, to activate the stress-activated JNK pathway, or to inhibit the protein kinase B (PKB or Akt) survival pathway (44). Other receptor-coupled pro-death pathways also exist in developmental CNS PCD, but the mitochondrial apoptotic pathway is the most important (12) (**Fig. 51.3**). As many as 70% of developing neurons die via PCD during embryogenesis to eliminate excess cell numbers and to assist in neural tube closure. Due to the upregulation of

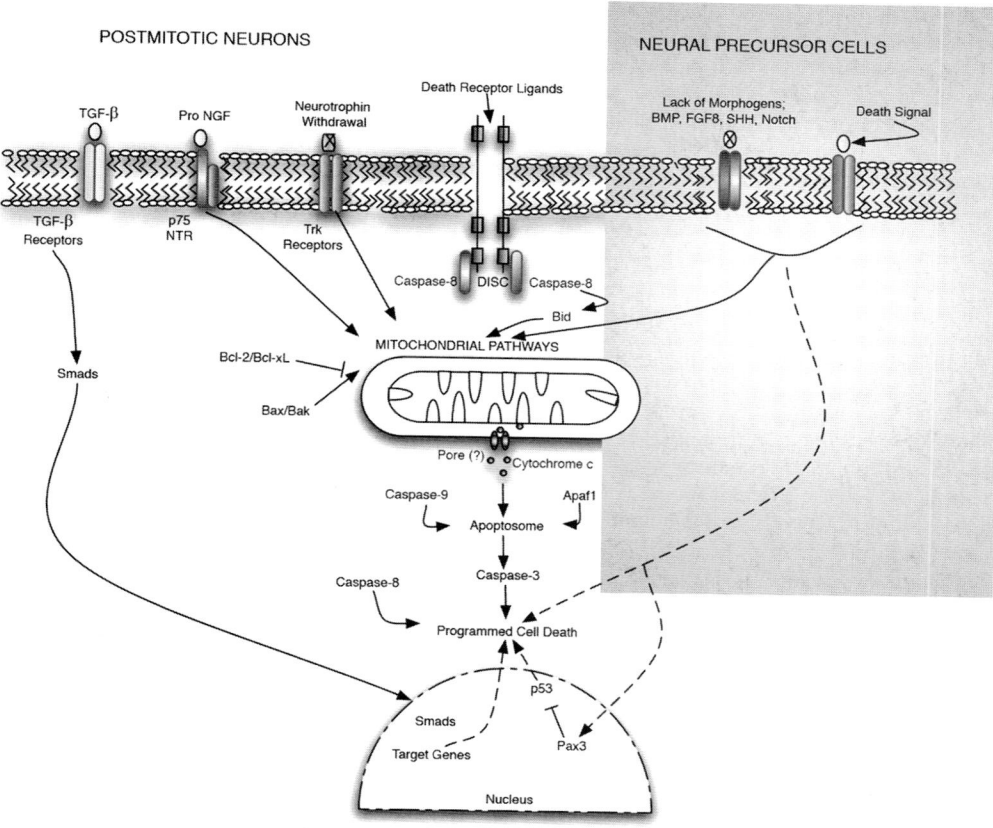

FIGURE 51.3. Both neural precursor cells and postmitotic neurons utilize mitochondrial pathways (cytochrome C and apoptosome) in PCD. BcL2 family proteins (BcL2, Bcl-X, Bax, and Bak) modulate and regulate the mitochondrial PCD pathway. Receptor-mediated PCD via caspase 8 has also been shown to participate in postmitotic neurons but not in neural precursor cells, which undergo PCD via the withdrawal of morphogens and regulation of the p53 pathway by the Pax3 transcription factor. Pax3 is a transcription factor that regulates neural development at the transcriptional level and can modulate the cell cycle via p53 to modulate PCD pathways. TGF-β and proNGF also stimulate PCD in postmitotic neurons. Smad proteins are regulators of transcription that are phosphorylated by activated TGF-β receptors and, in turn, activate gene expression patterns that modulate PCD and survival. Modified from De Zio D, Giunta L, Corvaro M, et al. Expanding roles of programmed cell death in mammalian neurodevelopment. *Semin Cell Dev Biol* 2005;16:281–94, with permission.

PCD machinery during development, the developing CNS may be more prone to injury-related PCD than is the adult brain. An especially sensitive age for injury-induced CNS PCD is in newborn infants in the PICU environment, discussed in greater detail in Chapter 52.

Migration, Differentiation, and Axonal Guidance

Neuronal migration occurs at between 12 and 24 gestational weeks in humans and is modulated by neurotransmitters such as glutamate. Importantly, glutamate *N*-methyl-D-aspartate (NMDA) receptor antagonists can inhibit neuronal migration and affect developmental neuronal apoptosis (32), which may have important effects upon developing CNS recovery and plasticity and, therefore, great relevance to the PICU.

The developmental processes responsible for the progression of neural lineages from stem cells to progenitors to postmitotic precursors and, ultimately, to mature neurons are con-

trolled by multiple pathways (17). Stem cell commitment to neuronal lineage and neuronal progenitor specification to a specific neural subtype are two distinct steps of neurogenesis. However, they are linked mechanistically by the same genes that regulate both processes (17). Both extracellular and intracellular signals modulate new gene expression that, in large part, determines neuronal and glial phenotypes. Differentiated neurons possess unique and characteristic sizes, shapes, polarities, and expressions of neurotransmitters, neurotrophins, and receptors, to name but a few differentiation attributes. Knowledge of this area of research is important, as both positive and negative experimental results have been reported concerning the potential of stem cells as therapy after brain injury, and this is sure to remain an active field of inquiry in the future.

Four primary types of signals guide axonal growth and target contact: chemoattractant, chemorepellent, contact attractive, and contact repellent. The first two classes of molecules are diffusible molecules that act over longer distances, while the latter two are within the extracellular matrix or membrane. Axonal pathfinding is most dependent upon repulsive cues and pioneer axons that reach targets early in development. Some of these guidance molecules also affect cell migration, as both developmental processes tend to share common mechanisms (32).

Synaptogenesis, Gliogenesis, and Myelination

Synaptogenesis is one of the most important developmental processes that occur during childhood and is an important potential mechanism of CNS injury and recovery in PICU-relevant injuries. Based upon nonhuman primate studies, a tentative timetable composed of five temporally distinct phases of synaptogenesis has been proposed for human development (32) (**Figs. 51.1** and **51.4**). At ~6–8 weeks of gestation, phase 1 of synaptogenesis is limited to the subplate. Beginning at ~12–17 weeks of gestation, synaptogenesis phase 2 remains somewhat limited to the cortical plate with most new synapses on neuronal dendritic shafts. Phase 3 is more rapid and dynamic; with up to 40,000 new synapses made per second, it begins at ~20–24 weeks of gestation and lasts up to 8 months postnatally. Similarly, phase 4 has a high rate of synaptogenesis, lasting until puberty. The third and fourth phases are more influenced by use-dependent experience. Lastly, phase 5 levels of synaptogenesis persist throughout adulthood to age 70, but with significant synapse loss during this period as well (32).

As a developing neuron reaches its destined position in the CNS, it extends dendrites and axons to distant targets via growth cones, which are guided by numerous extracellular molecules. Upon making target contact, presynaptic neurotransmitters or other secreted molecules diffuse and bind to the postsynaptic membrane and, along with other signals, induce postsynaptic receptor clustering and other elements of the synapse. Consequently, numerous proteins, molecules, and signal cascades play a role in synaptogenesis (37). Synaptic vesicle accumulation in the presynaptic terminal of a brain region is a helpful hallmark of the level of synapse maturation (33). A tremendous amount of synaptogenesis is ongoing in young chil-

dren that could have important implications for injury response and recovery in the PICU.

Glia are not passive participants in CNS development; rather, they exert significant influence over neuronal development. Glia include astrocytes, oligodendrocytes, radial glia, and microglia. Astrocytic development occurs well after neuronal migration and differentiation, and oligodendrocytic development occurs after that of axogenesis (46). Astrocytes have a multitude of functions in the CNS aside from the structural support of neurons. These functions include K^+ buffering, H^+ and Ca^{2+} ion homeostasis, ammonia detoxification, free radical scavenging, metal sequestration, growth factor production, immune response participation, and neuronal metabolic support functions (pH regulation, neurotransmitter uptake, supply of glycogen and tricarboxylic acid cycle intermediates, and provision of neurotransmitter precursors). Astrocytes also participate in synaptogenesis and neurogenesis in CNS development as well as in cognitive function (42). Protoplasmic astrocytes occur in gray matter, and fibrous astrocytes in white matter. An important feature of astrocytes is the use of the energy-dependent Na^+ gradient to uptake glutamate and K^+ and to regulate H^+ ions. As a result, excessive release of glutamate, energy failure, neuronal depolarization, or tissue acidosis in brain injury result in astrocytic swelling in both the perivascular and perineuronal astrocytic compartments, which can increase diffusion distances in the brain for metabolic gases (O_2 and CO_2), substrates, and waste products. It has been proposed that severe glial swelling may compress capillaries to reduce cerebral blood flow (CBF) and distort synaptic contacts, resulting in neuronal synaptic deafferentation. These changes can become important in a variety of CNS insults (see **Fig. 52.12**).

Microglia are CNS immune cells of myeloid origin that are similar to macrophages and represent 10% of the CNS cell populations in adults (52). They are normally in a resting state in normal brain, but with activation in response to infection or CNS injury, they morphologically (enlarge) and functionally change, resulting in the upregulation of cytokines and chemokines, as well as surface antigens. They have been implicated in the response to encephalitis, ischemia, TBI, and demyelinating diseases.

Oligodendrocytes produce myelin, modulate axonal function in the CNS, and are vulnerable to excitotoxic injury, decreased trophin levels, and oxidative stress conditions. Neurons and oligodendrocytes signal each other during myelination to modulate neurofilament spacing, phosphorylation, and axonal diameter. As myelination continues to occur until 10 years of age, injury to oligodendrocytes and altered myelination is an important consideration in the PICU in children who suffer brain injuries.

Myelination persists longer than most other CNS developmental processes, continuing through adolescence, making it, like synaptogenesis, another aspect of CNS development of special relevance to the PICU infant or child (46) (**Fig. 51.1**). In fact, myelination continues in humans until at least 30 years of age, and new evidence suggests that myelination may even be an important mechanism of activity-dependent plasticity (defined as both short- and long-term changes in synaptic strength stimulated by altered neural electrical activity via altered synaptic protein levels, protein posttranslational modifications, and nerve conduction velocity) (15). Several lines of evidence suggest that myelination is a process that is influenced by

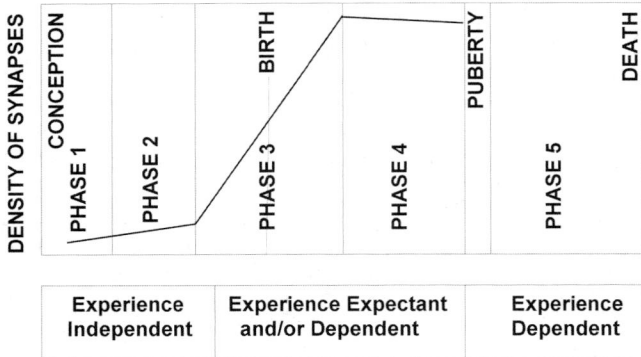

FIGURE 51.4. Synaptic changes (shown as relative densities based on a logarithmic scale) from data of the macaque monkey that has been extrapolated to humans. Phases of synaptogenesis that are predominately experience-dependent (require neural activity and are epigenetically regulated) or independent (genetically programmed) are indicated by the boxes along the X-axis. Modified from Lagercrantz H, Ringstedt T. Organization of the neuronal circuits in the central nervous system during development. *Acta Paediatr* 2001;90:707–15, with permission.

environmental factors. Neural activity also affects myelination. White matter development in children correlates with motor skill and increased cognitive function. MRI has shown a strong correlation between white matter development and cognitive function (intelligence quotient) in children and adolescents (15). While such data are correlative and do not prove an underlying relationship, it has been postulated that increased white matter conduction speed may have as strong an influence on synaptic amplitude, as do changes in pre- and postsynaptic elements and neurotransmitter function in plasticity paradigms, such as long-term potentiation (LTP), an electrophysiologic model of memory formation (15). Furthermore, neural activity may produce activity-dependent interactions between myelinating glia, neurons, and myelinated axons (15).

NEUROTRANSMITTER AND NEUROTROPHIN DEVELOPMENT

The synapse serves as the anatomical substrate for information flow between neurons and the point at which the release and response to neurotransmitters predominately occur within the nervous system (**Fig. 51.5**). The release of neurotransmitters from within presynaptic vesicles occurs by fusion with the presynaptic plasma membrane due to electrical depolarization and the influx of Ca^{2+} into the presynaptic bouton, which contains synaptic vesicles. Receptors in the postsynaptic membrane couple directly to ion channels or second messengers to mediate downstream effects. The removal of neurotransmitters that have been released occurs by glial uptake, enzymatic degradation, or transport proteins coupled to the Na^+ gradient established by synaptic and glial sodium and potassium adenosine triphosphate translocase enzymes (Na/K-ATPase). Neurotransmitter levels and receptor expression serve critical roles in synapse formation and in the circuitry

and networks necessary for behavioral function in the immature and mature CNS. Furthermore, synaptic activity mediated by neurotransmitters is a requirement for the survival of developing synaptic contacts in the immature brain (21). It is well documented that neurotransmitters both mediate synaptic transmission and have trophic functions (7,21,46). Neurotransmitters and neuromodulators that have been shown to play important roles in development include glutamate, γ-aminobutyric acid (GABA), acetylcholine, catecholamines, serotonin, and opioids. The human developmental neurotransmitter timeline displays considerable regional and temporal variation for various transmitter systems (46) (**Figs. 51.6 and 51.7**). These variations come into play when considering age- and regional-dependent injury, manipulations of the transmitter systems, and the possible effects of the transmitter systems on recovery. Insults to the brain at vulnerable developmental periods can produce long-term structural and functional CNS changes. Given the important neurotransmitter functions during CNS development, it is not surprising that a number of recent studies have implicated age-dependent adverse effects with the manipulation of neurotransmitter systems, especially the glutamatergic and GABAergic systems, using either commonly employed sedative and anesthetic agents or treatments with such agents after ischemia, status epilepticus, or TBI (7,26,27).

Preterm fetuses and newborn infants appear to be at particularly critical periods of developmental neurotransmitter vulnerability. Before birth, the majority of neuromodulators and neurotransmitters increase during synaptogenesis. At birth, increased brain activity and a surge of catecholaminergic activity are associated with arousal. A decrease in adenosine occurs, along with a desensitization of adenosine receptors during the first postnatal days (21). In addition, periods of developmental "switches" in neurotransmitter function occur at birth, and sensitivity to glutamate toxicity may be especially high and vulnerable at this time.

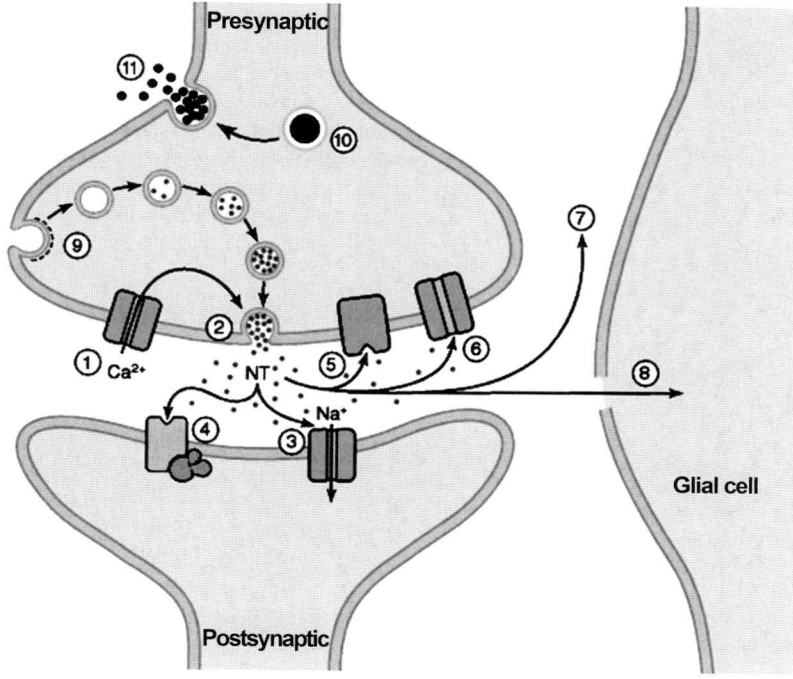

FIGURE 51.5. Schematic of a typical axodendritic synapse as seen at a dendritic spine. Calcium entry triggered by presynaptic terminal depolarization (1) induces neurotransmitter (NT)-containing synaptic vesicle exocytosis (2), which in turn, releases neurotransmitters into the synaptic cleft. NTs bind to their receptors at the postsynaptic density (concentration of postsynaptic proteins involved in synaptic function) of the postsynaptic membrane. These receptors modulate either ion channels (3) or on G-proteins that stimulate second-messenger production (4). Similar NT presynaptic receptors (5) are also activated, which can modulate subsequent NT presynaptic release. The uptake of many NTs occurs via a transport protein coupled to the sodium gradient at the presynaptic terminal (e.g., dopamine, norepinephrine, glutamate, and GABA) (6) or by degradation (acetylcholine) (7) or uptake by glia (glutamate) (8). Synaptic vesicle membranes are recycled by clathrin-mediated endocytosis (9). Large, dense core vesicles (10) that store protein and neuropeptides are released by repetitive stimulation at a more distant site from the postsynaptic density (11). From Holz RW, Fisher SK. *Basic Neurochemistry*, 6th ed. Philadelphia: Lippincott Williams & Wilkins, 1999, with permission (23).

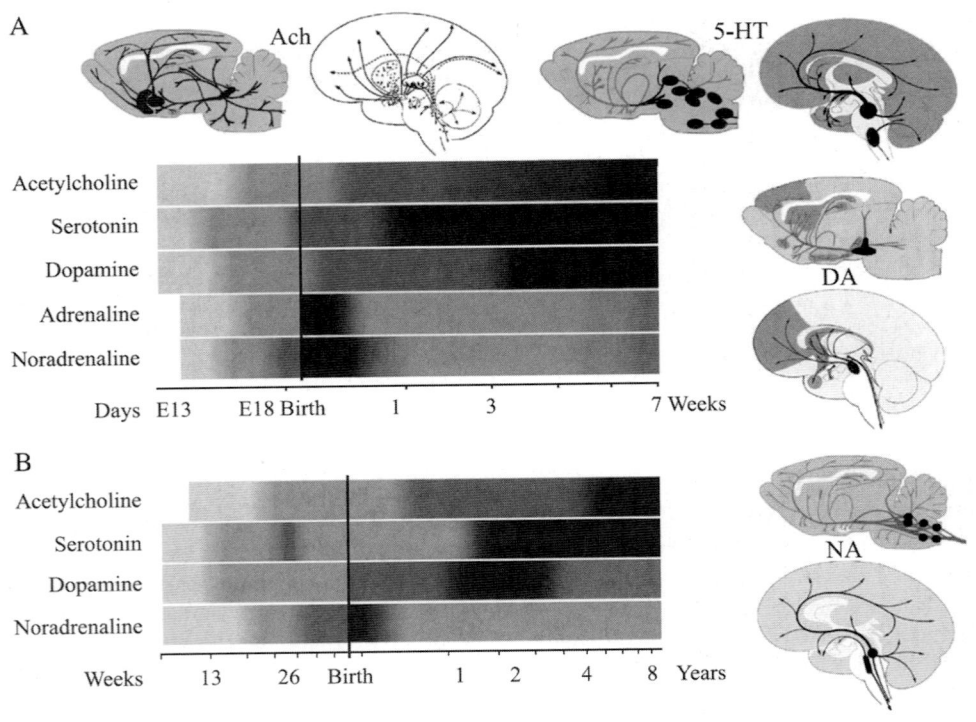

FIGURE 51.6. Comparison of rat (**A**) and human brain (**B**) timelines of the regional and temporal distribution of several major neurotransmitter levels during development. Ach, acetylcholine; 5-HT, serotonin; DA, dopamine; NA, noradrenaline. From Herlenius E, Lagercrantz H. Development of neurotransmitter systems during critical periods. *Exp Neurol* 2004;190 (Suppl 1):S8–21, with permission.

Glutamate and GABA

Amino acids are the most abundant neurotransmitters in the CNS and have important functions in brain development regarding neural networks, CNS structure, and plasticity. Glutamatergic and GABAergic neurotransmission play major roles in brain development. In fact, many of the CNS behavioral and functional milestones during development can be correlated with the maturation of these systems and their receptors (31).

Glutamate Receptor Development

Almost half of the synapses of the forebrain are glutamatergic, and excessive glutamate synapse creation occurs during the most active period of synaptogenesis in the first 2 years of postnatal human brain development. Each of the five types of major glutamate receptors contains various subtypes (21). Three general types of glutamate ionotropic receptors exist that couple to Na^+ and Ca^{2+}, namely, four alpha-amino-3-hydroxy-5-methyl-4-isoxazolepropionic acid (AMPA) receptor subtypes ($GluR_{1-4}$), five kainate receptor subtypes ($GluR_{5-7}$, KA_{1-2}), and seven NMDA receptor subtypes (NR_{1-3B}). Eight G-protein–coupled metabotropic glutamate receptors ($mGluR_{1-8}$) exist, which positively or negatively couple to phosphoinositide and cyclic nucleotide second messengers to varying degrees with pre- and postsynaptic and regional CNS distributions. AMPA receptors (which normally activate NMDA receptors) mature more slowly than NMDA receptors; thus, the NMDA receptor must depend on other systems (the immature $GABA_A$ receptor) to help depolarize immature neurons and activate the NMDA-coupled calcium channel. Immature NMDA receptors, which contain higher levels of the NR2B subunit, are relatively more excitable during early phases of development, to promote use-dependent plastic changes that are necessary for normal development and learning and memory (21). However, higher levels of NR2B make the brain more sensitive to excitotoxic insults, such as ischemia, TBI, and status epilepticus (7,21,27). In addition, the use of NMDA antagonists or anesthetic agents (e.g., ketamine), nitrous oxide, and isoflurane may also increase experimental developmental neuronal PCD in rodents (24,41), although some have challenged these laboratory findings (35). It is not yet clear if similar pathology occurs in humans and what the functional consequences might be, but it does appear that either too much or too little NMDA receptor activation can result in abnormal developmental processes and even neuronal death (21). A practical clinical example would be the use of nitrous oxide or ketamine (both NMDA receptor antagonist) in newborn infants. Although presently no definitive evidence indicates that NMDA receptor blockade triggers neural apoptosis in human infants, important research is necessary in this area, as it could have broad implications in the PICU.

GABA and the GABA Switch

In addition to its neurotransmitter role on neuronal excitability, GABA has trophic actions upon synaptic and neuritic outgrowth, as well as neuronal viability during development. An estimated 25%–40% of all CNS synapses contain GABA, and its deficiency is fatal to infants (21). GABAergic inhibition of excitatory synaptic CNS activity occurs by neuronal hyperpolarization via postsynaptic $GABA_A$ (outward chloride channel) and $GABA_B$ (G-protein–coupled inward potassium channel) receptors in the adult brain. The inhibitory actions of GABA are also mediated by a reduction of presynaptic excitatory neurotransmitter release via presynaptic $GABA_B$

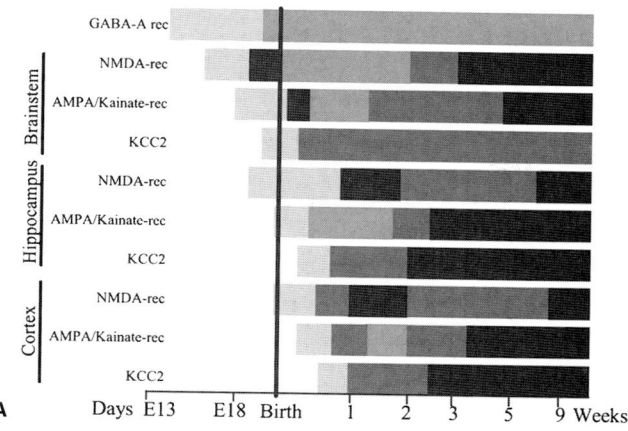

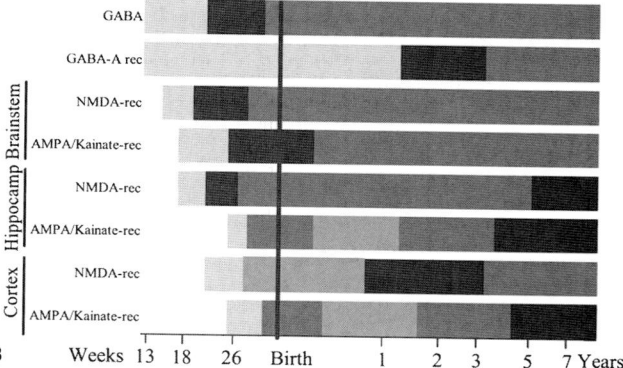

FIGURE 51.7. Comparison of rat (**A**) and human brain (**B**) timelines of the regional and temporal distribution of several major neurotransmitter receptor levels during development. rec, receptor. From Herlenius E, Lagercrantz H. Development of neurotransmitter systems during critical periods. *Exp Neurol* 2004;190 (Suppl 1):S8–21, with permission.

receptors (7). In contrast, GABA is an excitatory neurotransmitter during prenatal development prior to birth in humans. The GABA_A receptor binds barbiturates, benzodiazepines, and ethanol, which alter chloride (Cl⁻) flux thorough the channel (21). Thus, GABA is mainly excitatory during the fetal period but becomes inhibitory around birth in humans. The so-called "GABA switch" marks the point at which GABA becomes a inhibitory rather than excitatory neurotransmitter (20,21,32) (**Fig. 51.8**).

As discussed previously, glutamate synaptic transmission is initially based upon NMDA receptor function at developmental stages when the CNS lacks functional AMPA receptors and the GABA_A receptor stimulates NMDA receptor calcium influx, a role usually performed in the mature brain by the AMPA receptor. GABA_A receptor stimulation induces depolarization of immature neurons and increases NMDA-mediated intracellular Ca^{2+} during late human prenatal development. The switch from GABA excitation to inhibition that occurs at birth in humans is likely the result of a GABA-mediated induction of the expression and upregulation of the potassium-chloride cotransporter (KCC2), which serves to decrease the high Cl⁻ content of immature neurons (21,47). Several types of brain injury downregulate KCC2 and thus could affect the development of the GABA switch of the developing brain (21).

Adenosine

Adenosine is a neuronal, glial, and cerebrovascular transmitter that affects the excitability of neurons and the functional processes of oligodendrocyte progenitor proliferation and myelination during infancy and childhood (21). Four receptors—A_1, A_{2a}, A_{2b}, and A_3—have been identified with different regional and pre- and postsynaptic distributions. A_1 receptors are inhibitory and provide a line of defense against developmental excitotoxic cascades and, along with GABA, may be the most important inhibitory neurotransmitter-receptor system in the brain. A_{2a} receptors modulate dopaminergic D_2 receptor function and are highly concentrated in the basal ganglia (21). Due to the importance of adenosine receptor modulation of neuronal excitability and developmental processes, this system may be an important therapeutic target in brain injury (21).

Acetylcholine

Acetylcholine is one of the major excitatory transmitter systems of the CNS and is important in cognition and attention, motor function, and pain. Five muscarinic receptor subtypes have been identified, with $M_{1,2,5}$ coupled primarily to phosphoinositide turnover and $M_{2,4}$ coupled to cyclic AMP production. As with many receptors, some receptor subtypes couple to more than one second-messenger system. Cholinergic projections to the cortex from basal forebrain occur around 20 weeks in the human fetus. Abnormal cholinergic projections alter cortical development, plasticity, and function (21) and are critical to cognitive function in the infant and young child. In addition, cholinergic systems can also participate in toxic excitatory neurotransmitter cascades in epilepsy, TBI, and cerebral ischemia in children in the PICU.

Norepinephrine and Dopamine

Monoaminergic neurons form during telencephalic vesicle formation, and catecholamines are thought to play a significant role in early development. Norepinephrine is important in cognitive function, anxiety, arousal, and attention, and is necessary for normal brain development. Noradrenergic neurons appear at 5–6 weeks in humans, and adrenergic α_2 and β_1 receptors predominate in the CNS (21). In addition, as stated previously, a surge of catecholamine levels is associated with increased brain activity and arousal at birth (**Fig. 51.1**). Dopamine is also important in cognition, motor function, and addiction behavior. Five dopamine receptors have been identified (D_1–D_5), with the major CNS dopaminergic receptors being D_1 and D_2. Dopaminergic neurons begin to develop at 6–8 weeks in humans. D1 receptors, in particular, are critical for working memory function during the first year of life (21) (**Fig. 51.1**). The use of catecholamines for blood pressure support in the PICU in infants with immature or injury-altered blood-brain barrier (BBB) function warrants consideration due to the potent catecholinergic excitatory actions at birth, which in theory could be potentially excitotoxic at this critical developmental time. High dopamine concentrations have even been shown to exacerbate brain edema in adult animals after experimental TBI (6).

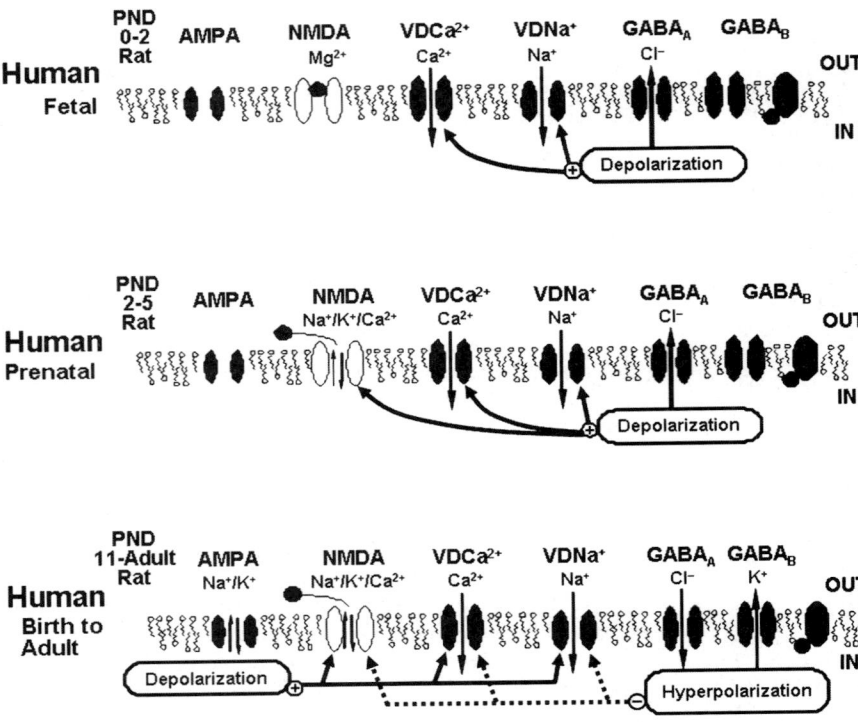

FIGURE 51.8. Comparison of the GABA switch in the human and the rat, which is well-documented in the rat and thought to occur in humans at birth. Prior to the switch of GABA$_A$ receptors from an outward gating depolarizing Cl$^-$ current to an inward hyperpolarizing Cl$^-$ current (**upper 2 panels**), the receptor is excitatory and helps to remove the magnesium (Mg^{2+}) block of the NMDA receptor channel, allowing calcium influx. Thus, GABA$_A$ receptors assume the excitatory role of nonfunctioning AMPA receptors during the developmental period prior to the switch. However, once AMPA receptors mature and the high Cl$^-$ content of developing neurons is reduced due to the upregulation of the potassium-chloride cotransporter (KCC2) (not shown), the GABA$_A$ receptor becomes inhibitory by gating an inward hyperpolarizing Cl$^-$ current (**lower panel**). Prior to the switch, GABA tone may contribute to excitotoxic glutamate cascades during brain injury (see Chapter 52). PND, postnatal day. Modified from Ben-Ari Y, Khazipov R, Leinekugel X, et al. GABA$_A$, NMDA and AMPA receptors: A developmentally regulated "menage a trois." *Trends Neurosci* 1997;20:523–29, with permission.

Serotonin

Serotonin (5-HT) neurons have extensive contacts and synchronize complex motor and sensory information, and at least fifteen 5-HT receptors are identified. The 5-HT$_1$ receptors, in general, inhibit cyclic AMP formation and open K$^+$ channels, while 5-HT$_2$ receptors stimulate phosphoinositide second messengers, release intracellular calcium, and are generally excitatory. Serotonin also modulates developmental proliferation, differentiation, migration, and synaptogenesis. Aberrations in serotonin levels during development and early childhood result in CNS connectivity malformations and may contribute to later psychiatric disorders (21).

Neurotrophins

Growth factors, both intrinsic and extrinsic to the CNS, play a major role in normal brain function, developmental processes, and in the injury and repair process. Nerve growth factor (NGF), brain-derived neurotrophic factor (BDNF), and neurotrophins 3–5 (NT3, NT4/5) are diffusible peptides that compose the neurotrophin family of trophic factors in mammalian brain. Receptors for the neurotrophin peptides are the tropomyosin kinase receptors (TrkA, TrkB, and TrkC) and the p75 neurotrophin receptor (p75 NTR), a member of the transforming growth factor (TGF) receptor family. NTs are critical for neuronal survival, and the loss of NT activity after CNS injury can contribute to neuronal death and loss of function. The role of neurotrophins in response to CNS injury is discussed in more detail in Chapter 52. NT precursors are called proneurotrophins and are cleaved by proteases to produce mature NTs. Proneurotrophins can also activate NT receptors and appear to be the preferred ligand for p75 NTR. ProNGF induces apoptosis via p75 NTR, and proNGF and NGF produce opposite responses—cell death and cell survival, respectively (9,11,12,33). NT receptors couple to a number of protein and lipid kinase intracellular pathways, such as the mitogen-activated proteins kinase (MAPK), the phosphoinositide 3-kinase (PI3K), and the PKB pathways. This coupling is extremely important to the regulation of neural survival or death after ischemia, TBI, or other CNS insults (see Chapter 52).

The regional distribution of NGF is highest in regions innervated by the cholinergic system of the basal forebrain, such as the neocortex and the hippocampus. Lower but significant levels are also seen in other brain regions (9). BDNF has a wider distribution than NGF, having been detected in the hippocampus, amygdala, thalamus, neocortex, cerebellum, and other brain regions (11). The adult hippocampus has the highest levels of both NGF and BDNF, which may be related to its important plasticity role in cognitive function (9). Obviously, any major change in neurotrophin systems during development by disease, injury, or treatment can have a dramatic impact on ongoing CNS development, especially at critical developmental periods.

SYNAPTIC AND BEHAVIORAL DEVELOPMENT

Due to ongoing developmental synaptogenesis, connectivity, wiring, and myelination, an associated increase and development of CNS electrical activity occurs. A measurable electrical encephalogram (EEG) develops and matures with gestational and postnatal age (31). However, birth is the point of significantly increased neural activity due to the arousal effects of neurotransmitters, neuromodulators, and neurotrophins. Preterm infants at ~32 weeks of gestation show quantitative changes in

EEG before and after birth, with up to a 30% increase in EEG amplitude and a 60% increase in continuity over the first post-natal weeks (40). Consistent changes are seen in quantitative EEG neurophysiologic measures over the first week after birth and, particularly, in measures of continuity over the first 4 days in normal preterm infants (54). Such behavioral and functional milestones also correlate with the development of glutamater-gic and GABAergic neurotransmission and synaptic maturity (55). As NMDA, AMPA, and GABA receptor (10) and neu-rotrophin (33) systems mature, LTP (an increase in synaptic strength of a population of neurons that may be an electro-physiologic and biochemical correlate of memory storage) and long-term depression (LTD, a decrease in synaptic strength of a population of neurons that may also be an electrophysiologic and biochemical correlate of memory storage) are established. Thus, LTP and LTD are likely associated with cognitive func-tion and definitively occur in cortical and hippocampal circuits within 2–3 weeks in the postnatal rat (50) and have been pro-posed to occur at 7–10 months in infants (22).

Primary behavioral and functional developments in the in-fant (**Fig. 51.1**) over the first 2 years:

- The cortical inhibition of brainstem reflexes due to matura-tion of GABA inhibition and myelination occurs postnatally at ~3 months. Excessive cortical inhibition of brainstem nu-clei, such as respiratory centers, may increase the risk for the sudden infant death syndrome (22).
- The development of recognition memory also takes place near the postnatal age of 3 months, which requires adequate hippocampal and cortical visual development (22).
- Working memory (recent past memory that enables one to solve a current cognitive task) develops in the infant over the latter half of the first year; it is dependent upon prefrontal cortical function and is modulated by glutamate, GABA, and dopamine (22). (d) Between 7–10 months, infant prefrontal cortices undergo dramatic maturation in synaptic density and neurotransmitter systems and have increased glucose utilization required for both growth and activity-dependent processes. Similarly, the hippocampus reaches adult size, and synaptogenesis, coupled with the maturation of neurotrans-mitter systems, makes LTP development possible. During this time of rapid growth and activity-dependent synaptoge-nesis and maturation, the infant brain is especially vulnera-ble to injury, resulting in either short- or long-term changes in behavioral function (22). For example, at 2 years of age, rapid language development and acquisition occur, which has been further linked to increased connections between prefrontal cortex and associational cortical regions with the limbic and motor systems. Significant synaptogenesis also occurs in many of these same brain regions (22).

These functions can be extremely vulnerable to injury and represent a critical period of developing brain vulnerability to injury-mediated, long-term dysfunction.

ANTIOXIDANT DEVELOPMENT

Free radicals are molecules that contain one or more unpaired electrons, such as superoxide, peroxynitrite, and hydroxyl rad-icals. Enzymes and low-molecular-weight antioxidants are the major brain antioxidant defense systems. Major enzyme sys-tems include peroxyredoxins, thioredoxins, superoxide dismu-

tase, catalase, and peroxidases that vary in concentration de-pending on species and brain regions. Glutathione, vitamin E, ascorbate, and coenzyme Q are water- or lipid-soluble low-molecular-weight antioxidants (5). Oxidative stress, produced by abnormal free radical generation in the brain, is at least par-tially quenched by these defense systems. The levels of these antioxidant enzymes and molecules in the brain vary with de-velopmental age (5,29). In general, lower levels occur during fetal development but increase at birth, as the transition from a low- to high-oxygen environment occurs (29). Based upon enzyme levels, catalase appears to be more of a contributor to antioxidant defenses in the immature brain, which may influ-ence the choice of antioxidant interventions in the developing brain after injury (5). Based upon the antioxidant enzyme pro-file during brain development, the immature CNS may be at greater risk than the adult brain for oxidative injury (5).

CEREBROVASCULAR AND METABOLISM DEVELOPMENT AND FUNCTION

Vascular Development

The CNS vascular system develops in three phases: vasculoge-nesis, angiogenesis, and barrier-genesis (13). Not surprisingly, the first functional organ developed in the human embryo is the cardiovascular system, with blood vessels generated by meso-dermal differentiated endothelial cells. These cells give rise to new blood vessels by a process called *vasculogenesis*, as com-pared to the generation of new blood vessels from existing vessels, called *angiogenesis* (45). The CNS developmental rate of angiogenesis is maximal around birth and early infancy and decreases thereafter (13). A major role for vascular endothe-lial growth factor and its endothelial receptors has been doc-umented for developmental CNS angiogenesis (13,45). Other trophic factors, especially some of the components of the TGF-β family, may also influence developmental CNS angiogenesis. These factors have been implicated in sprouting, vascular re-modeling, and perivascular cell recruitment (13). In addition, platelet-derived growth factor, as well as numerous adhesion molecules and factors/receptors that provide axonal cues, mod-ulate CNS vascularization (13,45). Immature blood vessels are stabilized by vascular mural cells, called *pericytes*, that are re-cruited to endothelial cells via some of these aforementioned factors (13,45). Tissue oxygen levels are very important in de-veloping CNS vasculature, as low levels stimulate angiogenesis and high oxygen levels inhibit this process (45).

Cerebral Blood Flow and Vascular Reactivity

Vascular reactivity of the cerebral circulation is an important neuroprotective mechanism whereby the CNS vessel diameter adjusts to physiologic changes (i.e., perfusion pressure, Pa_{O_2}, Pa_{CO_2}) to regulate CBF so that metabolic demands of the brain can be met. The ability of the cerebrovascular system to dilate or constrict has limits that are defined physiologically as the upper and lower limits of autoregulation. Impaired CBF au-toregulation and vascular reactivity are considered potential candidates in the etiology of secondary injury across the spectrum of age. For example, loss of pressure autoregulation could underlie, in part, the marked vulnerability of the acutely injured brain in a child to otherwise tolerable hypotension (see Chapter 52). Similarly, it is believed to contribute to periventricular hemorrhagic venous infarction in preterm infants. Most developmental studies of CBF and vascular reactivity have occurred in newborn infants and near-term and early postnatal laboratory animals.

Perfusion Pressure Autoregulation of Cerebral Blood Flow

Pressure autoregulation is the major cerebrovascular response to acute changes in perfusion pressure that result, at the extreme range, in either hypotension with hypoperfusion and tissue ischemia, or in hypertension and possible hyperemia and BBB disruption. Vascular tone in the cerebral circulation compensates for changes in cerebral perfusion pressure over a range of pressures to maintain CBF constant (between a cerebral perfusion pressure of ~40–160 mm Hg in adults) (**Fig. 51.9**). Cerebral perfusion pressure is equal to the difference between mean arterial pressure and intracranial pressure. Autoregulation occurs instantaneously and is believed to be mediated by changes in vascular smooth muscle tension by a direct myogenic mechanism; a review of this topic is available (36). Developmental studies of pressure autoregulation of CBF in newborns suggest a narrower perfusion pressure range, with a similar lower limit to that seen in adults—but an upper limit that is only ~90–100 mm Hg (19) (**Fig. 51.10**). Note that, for most of the studies in the normal state, intracranial pressure is generally assumed negligible, and cerebral perfusion pressure, which is thus approximated by mean arterial blood pressure, which is obviously not the case in the clinical setting of raised intracranial pressure. In both the term and preterm newborn lamb,

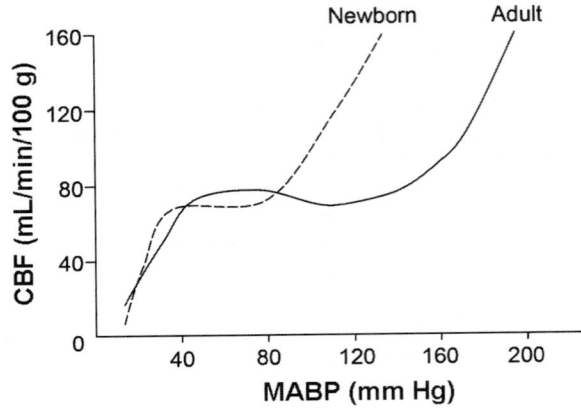

FIGURE 51.10. Comparison of the relative pressure: CBF autoregulatory curves from studies of subhuman primate newborns and adults. In the adult, CBF is maintained relatively constant when arterial blood pressure is between 50 and 160 mm Hg, while in newborns, CBF is maintained over a narrower range due to a reduced upper limit of CBF autoregulation. CBF autoregulation of newborns makes them more vulnerable to hypertensive episodes. MABP, mean arterial blood pressure. From Hardy P, Varma DR, Chemtob S. Control of cerebral and ocular blood flow autoregulation in neonates. *Pediatr Clin North Am* 1997;44:137–52, with permission.

the lower limit of pressure autoregulation is between 40 and 50 mm Hg. In contrast, the resting mean arterial blood pressure is substantially lower in the preterm than in the term newborn, demonstrating that the autoregulatory vascular reserve is much less in premature compared to term lambs (16). This finding suggests a greater risk for the preterm brain to a reduction in blood pressure. In addition, evidence suggests that, in critically ill infants, the autoregulatory responses may be absent or significantly impaired (25,28) and that early postnatal hypercapnia may further impair pressure autoregulation (49). Finally, pressure autoregulation of CBF is often disturbed after brain injury (8). The occurrence and consequences of impaired CBF autoregulation will be addressed in several of the following chapters across the spectrum of disorders in pediatric neurointensive care.

Cerebrovascular Response to Pao₂

The cerebrovascular response to changes in Pao_2 is mediated locally and results in vasodilation under reduced-oxygen conditions (hypoxic) and in vasoconstriction in high-oxygen conditions (hyperoxia) to maintain CBF constant over a range of po_2 values (**Fig. 51.9**). This curve is relatively flat, except at reduced Pao_2 levels (less than ~50 torr), at which a steep rise in CBF curve occurs to maintain cerebral oxygen delivery. At the end ranges of hypoxia and hyperoxia, the cerebrovascular response occurs in parallel with carotid body sensors that may also adjust systemic blood pressure and respiration to compensate for changes in blood oxygen levels. Consequently, the cerebrovascular response to oxygen and blood pressure interact and may not occur in isolation at the outermost values. These interactions, however, may be limited in some cases in the PICU, where ventilation and hemodynamics are often controlled in patients with severe brain injury. The dramatic increase in CBF (and cerebral blood volume) when Pao_2 is reduced to levels of ~50 torr or less provides the basis for meticulously avoiding even mild or moderate levels of hypoxemia in patients with

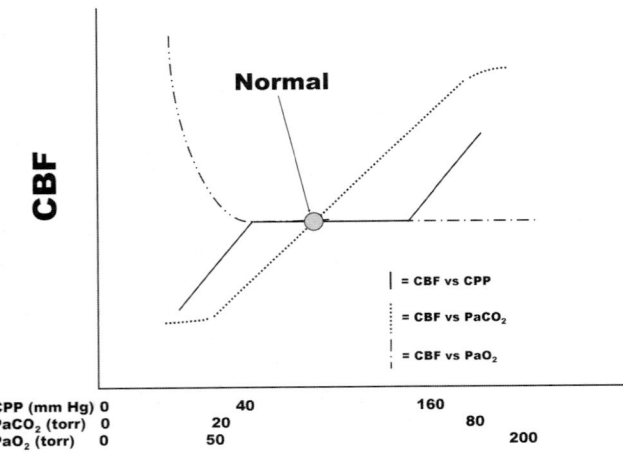

FIGURE 51.9. Relationships between CBF and cerebral perfusion pressure (CPP), $Paco_2$, and Pao_2 across therapeutic ranges generally encountered in the PICU. These values are provided based on normative data from adults. Pressure autoregulation maintains CBF constant between a CPP of between ~40 mm Hg and 160 mm Hg. CBF is linearly related to $Paco_2$, with an approximate 4% change in CBF per torr change in $Paco_2$ between ~20 torr and 80 torr. Below 20 torr, this curve dramatically flattens. Above ~80–100 torr, this relationship also more gradually flattens. The relationship between CBF and Pao_2 is relatively flat until a Pao_2 of ~50 mm Hg is reached, below which, a dramatic increase in CBF is observed.

reduced intracranial compliance, (discussed later in several of the chapters on specific disease entities in pediatric neurointensive care).

Cerebrovascular Response to PaCO$_2$

The cerebrovascular response to changes in PaCO$_2$ is mediated locally by changes in perivascular pH (51). However, in contrast to changes in perfusion pressure and PaO$_2$, a nearly linear relationship between PaCO$_2$ and CBF exists between the range of PaCO$_2$ values of 20 torr and 80 torr, with an approximate 4% per mm Hg change in PaCO$_2$ (8,36) (**Fig. 51.9**). At the ends of the spectrum (either hypocapnia or hypercapnia), the response is blunted, and these curves flatten. Consequently, vasodilation is seen with increasing arterial carbon dioxide concentration (hypercapnia) and vasoconstriction is seen with low arterial carbon dioxide concentration (hypocapnia). This vasoreactivity is the basis of hyperventilation-mediated reduction in CBF and the resultant reduction in cerebral blood volume that serves therapeutically to reduce intracranial hypertension. The CBF response to changes in PaCO$_2$ is generally related to the level of CBF at rest in a given brain region; thus, hyperventilation tends to equalize CBF throughout the brain (51). In addition, the CBF response to changes in PaCO$_2$ is transient, lasting less than 24 hrs for a given change (51) and is believed to be mediated by compensatory changes in brain interstitial bicarbonate concentration, which take time to manifest. When a hyperventilation-mediated reduction in PaCO$_2$ is used to reduce intracranial pressure, despite flattening of the CBF response to reduction in PaCO$_2$, relative ischemia has been suggested to occur, in part due to a reduction in CBF. Relative ischemia may also result from limited off-loading of oxygen from hemoglobin as the dissociation curve shifts to the left (36). Clinical utility and potential side effects of this therapy are discussed further in several of the chapters that follow, including Chapter 56. Carbon dioxide reactivity appears to be less vulnerable to injury than is pressure autoregulation (8). Altered CO$_2$ reactivity may suggest substantial damage to the brain region that is being assessed, and global loss of CO$_2$ reactivity is a concerning finding. Finally, CO$_2$ reactivity and pressure autoregulation are separate entities, as demonstrated by the fact that pressure autoregulation is maintained despite a new baseline CBF value when PaCO$_2$PaCO$_2$ is altered.

Cerebrovascular Regulation— Developmental Issues

Given that the most dramatic change facing the developing child is birth, going from a relatively hypoxic to an oxygen-rich environment, it is intuitive that the cerebrovascular system would normally be ready to respond to such challenges. However, even in normal term infants, it appears that several days are required for such vascular responses to further mature. Experimental studies in piglets have shown that CO$_2$ reactivity and pressure autoregulation are present but poorly developed at birth; however, both autoregulation and CO$_2$ reactivity mature rapidly over the first postnatal days. Resting CBF levels also increase over the first few postnatal days (18), and studies in preterm human infants have confirmed that CBF increases over the first 3 postnatal days (25,28). Similarly, CO$_2$ reactivity increases from birth to early postnatal age (25), as do EEG amplitude (54) and arterial blood pressure. However, during this postnatal period, CBF in infants is still lower than in adults. CBF further increases in children until 5–6 years of age,

when it may be as much as 50%–85% higher than in adults, then decreases to adult levels by 15–19 years of age (38) (**Fig. 51.11**). **Figure 51.11** shows the developmental changes in cerebral metabolism of glucose and CBF for both human and rat. Because of the higher fat content of rodent maternal milk, the growing rat fuels a large percentage of cerebral metabolism during the synthetic work related to early postnatal developmental growth spurts by utilizing ketone oxidation (38). In humans, CBF parallels glucose metabolism, and peak CBF and glucose metabolism occur between 3 to 9 years of age, corresponding to a very active growth period. However, it has been estimated that human infants also may utilize up to 20% of their energy needs from ketones during the postnatal period, when nourishment is based primarily on maternal milk.

Cerebral Blood Flow— Metabolism Coupling

In adults, a tight coupling of CBF to brain metabolism normally occurs and is termed "flow-metabolism coupling," as described previously. It has been shown that CBF-metabolism coupling appears intact in normal newborn infants (49). The peak in cerebral glucose utilization during development correlates with the density of glucose transport proteins (43). Postnatal changes in regional CBF and cerebral metabolism occur in parallel in the human infant, with the highest rates of local cerebral metabolic rate for glucose (LCMRg) and CBF occurring at between 3 and 9 years of age during the well-recognized period of rapid cognitive development (**Fig. 51.11**). Glucose is normally the lone cerebral substrate fueling active growth during this same period (38).

Cerebral Metabolism

Glucose serves as the major energy source for the developing brain. Glucose utilization through glycolytic and oxidative decarboxylation pathways parallels the energy demand of the developing brain. Consequently, LCMRg increases with developmental maturation and critical periods of growth and functional activity (53). Glucose entry into brain occurs via glucose transporter proteins (GLUTs). Of the five GLUTs (GLUT1–GLUT5), two (GLUT1 and GLUT3) are located in the brain, with GLUT1 found in the BBB and choroid plexus and GLUT3 found in neurons. GLUT5 is located in activated brain microglia. GLUT expression in the developing brain is proportional to energy demand, increases during maturation, and is highest during peak synaptogenesis (53). Peak GLUT protein expression correlates with glutamate receptor maturity and learning and memory development in the developing CNS.

Germane to the PICU is the fact that cerebral energy metabolism and blood flow peak between 3 and 8 years of age in humans (38). Glucose utilization in 5-week-old infants in most brain regions is 71%–93% of that in the adult brain. LCMRg increases over the next 3 months, especially in the basal ganglia and parietal, temporal, and occipital cortices. Frontal cortex LCMRg further increases by 8 months—at which time, cognitive function is rapidly developing (38). Adult levels of LCMRg are found by the time children are 2 years of age. LCMRg increases further until it reaches its highest levels, which are maintained until age 9 (**Fig. 51.11**). From this point

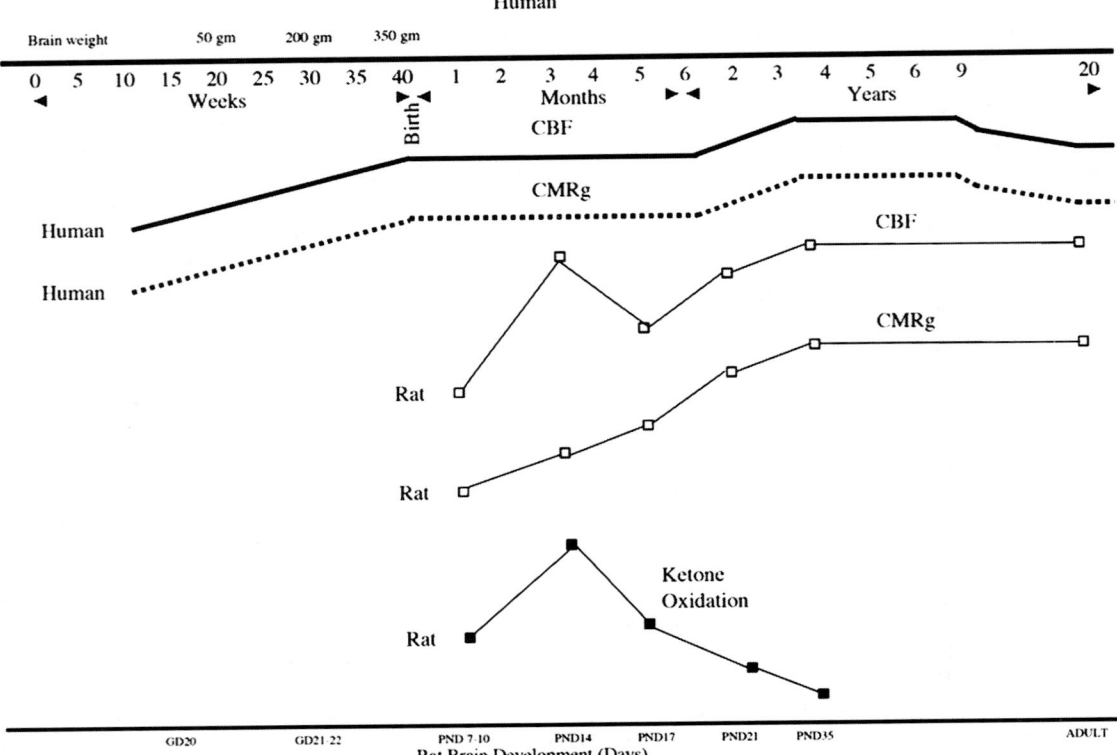

FIGURE 51.11. Developmental changes in cerebral metabolism of glucose (CMRg) and cerebral blood flow (CBF) for both human and rat. The rat fuels a large percentage of cerebral metabolism during the synthetic work related to early postnatal developmental growth spurts. In humans, peak CBF and CMRg occur between 3 to 9 years of age, corresponding to a very active growth period. GD, gestational day; PND, postnatal day. From Nehlig A. Cerebral energy metabolism, glucose transport and blood flow: Changes with maturation and adaptation to hypoglycaemia. *Diabetes Metab* 1997;23:18–29, with permission.

forward, LCMRg declines until about age 20 (38). Thus, the child's brain has considerable metabolic demand compared to adults.

In addition to the metabolism of glucose by the developing brain, the immature brain can utilize lactic acid, ketone bodies, and a large number of other metabolites, such as amino acids and free fatty acids (53). Monocarboxylate transporters for lactate and pyruvate develop over the midgestation period in the human brain, providing another significant energy source, using both extracellular lactate and pyruvate as substrates (14). Lactate and pyruvate have also been shown to modulate the LTP and LTD that may be involved in synaptic plasticity critical to cognitive development at later stages of brain maturation (55). Due to the high fat ingestion of infants secondary to milk intake, more ketones are available in infant blood than in adult blood and can represent up to 20% of the carbon skeletons used in energy production in infants (53). The BBB is quite permeable to ketones, and coupled with enhanced developmental brain enzymatic activity for ketone use compared to adults, ketones play a more important role in bioenergetics of the immature CNS (38). CNS substrate use of ketones may also be linked to amino acid and lipid biosynthetic pathway precursors, which are subsequently used in developmental membrane and myelin formation (38). However, as has been shown in rats (**Fig. 51.11**), once the child is no longer dependent on maternal milk, the use of ketones as a metabolic fuel decreases as well.

BLOOD-BRAIN BARRIER AND CHOROID PLEXUS DEVELOPMENT

Primary BBB functions serve to isolate brain blood compartments; provide selective transport of metabolites, ions, and molecules; and either metabolize or modify many blood- or brain-borne substances (3) (**Fig. 51.12**). The BBB is impermeable to hydrophilic molecules, ions, and proteins, while key metabolic substrates (e.g., glucose) enter via transport proteins (e.g., glucose transporter-1) and water passes through the BBB via aquaporin-4 channels (30). In addition, numerous metabolic barriers block the passage of molecules from blood to brain via the BBB, including P-glycoprotein (which involves energy-dependent movement of hydrophobic drugs out of the CNS) and enzymes (such as monoamine oxidase to metabolize catecholamines), which protect synaptic function (1,2).

The BBB is commonly thought to be "leaky" during fetal development and in the newborn infant. However, this issue remains a matter of debate (based upon experimental technical approaches), as evidence suggests that the fetal BBB is highly developed during the developmental period, including some mechanisms not found in the adult BBB (48). Tight junctions develop early during CNS maturation, and most proteins do not gain access to the extracellular compartment via the BBB during development. Cerebrospinal fluid (CSF) protein

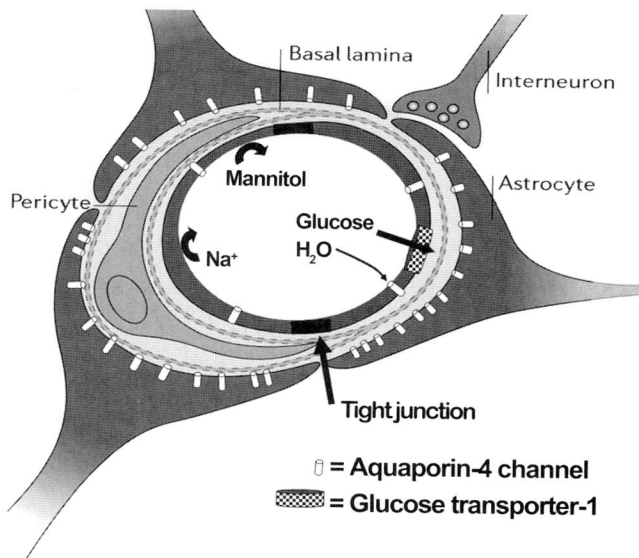

FIGURE 51.12. The structure of the mature BBB consists of endothelial cells connected by tight junctions, specialized supportive cells called pericytes, a basal lamina and perivascular astrocytic end feet. Modified from Abbott NJ, Ronnback L, Hansson E. Astrocyte-endothelial interactions at the blood-brain barrier. *Nat Rev Neurosci* 2006;7:41–53, with permission.

concentration is higher during early brain development and is thought to result from an immature choroid plexus; however, high CSF protein concentrations during development are not reflected in the extracellular space due to junctional complexes forming barriers at the CSF-brain interfaces that are not found in the adult brain (48). The BBB's permeability to ions and amino acids develops as transport systems mature in the brain; however, lipid-insoluble molecules are more permeable in the immature brain than in the adult brain (48). The majority view suggests that fetal BBB permeability to macromolecules is similar to adults, but small molecules enter the fetal brain more readily than in the adult CNS. Ion permeability decreases just before birth in large-animal experiments (13).

Small lipophilic molecules, such as CO_2, O_2, and ethanol, can readily pass through the BBB (1). However, the mature BBB is impermeable to many molecules and substances that are provided by cerebrovascular endothelial cell tight junctions, which form the complete zona occludens (30) (**Fig. 51.12**). Small polar molecules needed for brain function, such as glucose and amino acids, are transported across the barrier by carrier proteins (e.g., GLUT-1 for glucose and the L-system carrier L1 for large neutral amino acids, such as leucine) (1). Some small molecules and lipids are transported across the BBB by receptor-mediated endocytosis. The BBB is also able to remove hydrophobic molecules via p-glycoprotein—the energy-dependent, broad-spectrum efflux carrier, which plays a key role in BBB transport of a number of drugs. Finally, the cerebrovascular endothelial cells have an important metabolic function that is an integral component of the BBB. They contain monoamine oxidase and can defend brain synaptic function against circulating catecholamines (1). Abbott and Romero have characterized the BBB as having important "static and dynamic properties" (2). In addition, the barrier is surrounded by astrocyte foot processes, and these astrocytes can further modulate the entry and egress of substances across the BBB via their possession of various channels and transporters (such as the GLUTs previously discussed and the aquaporins, discussed later) and through intracellular metabolism (30). A complete discussion of astrocyte metabolic function is beyond the scope of this chapter.

A number of specific proteins mediate barrier functions at tight junctions (30). Germane to pediatric critical care medicine, cerebrovascular tight junctions effectively prevent the movement of hydrophilic substances, such as cations (Na+, K+) and osmolar agents (e.g., mannitol), along with proteins, among other molecules (30) (**Fig. 51.12**). Thus, the intact BBB is impermeable to salts and proteins, making osmolar gradients rather than oncotic gradients critical to water movement across the barrier (56) and serving as the theoretical basis for the use of hypertonic saline and mannitol in the treatment of intracranial hypertension (discussed in several later chapters). Water movement across the BBB is mediated via special water channels, termed *aquaporins*. In the BBB and astrocyte foot processes, water movement is facilitated specifically by aquaporin-4 channels (1). These are in relatively low concentration in the vascular endothelial cells and in higher concentration in the astrocytes, which use them for their rapid astrocytic influx of water during uptake of potassium, glutamate, and other substances (**Fig. 51.12**). The role of the BBB and astrocytes in CNS injury is discussed in detail in Chapter 52, as it relates to excitotoxicity and cellular swelling.

CEREBROSPINAL FLUID DYNAMICS

Two pathways of CSF circulation have been proposed—a minor and a major pathway (39) (**Fig. 51.13**). While the details of CSF dynamics during development remain unclear, it is classically thought that they differ in the developing brain compared to the adult. The major pathway of CSF absorption is via the arachnoid villi (arachnoid granulation) into the venous sinuses. The minor pathway includes drainage via ventricular ependyma, the interstitial and perivascular space, and perineural lymphatics (39). In adult humans, CSF production is around 500 mL/24 hrs, and the turnover may be three to four times a day. Interplay between the two drainage pathways maintains normal homeostasis and the neurochemical milieu in balance (39). The CSF circulation begins in development, with choroid plexus formation at around 40–60 days of gestation, depending on the ventricle. The arachnoid granulation appears just before birth, and CSF reabsorption occurs at later ages (**Fig. 51.13**). The minor CSF pathway is the major route for CSF dynamics in the developing immature human brain, with arachnoid granulation function occurring in the late infant stages. Radiologic evidence for the arachnoid granulation as a gross structure occurs around age 7 and continues to develop until age 20 (39).

CONCLUSIONS AND FUTURE DIRECTIONS

Fundamental aspects of normal brain biology and physiology have been reviewed in this chapter, with a focus on developmental issues. A number of important developmental

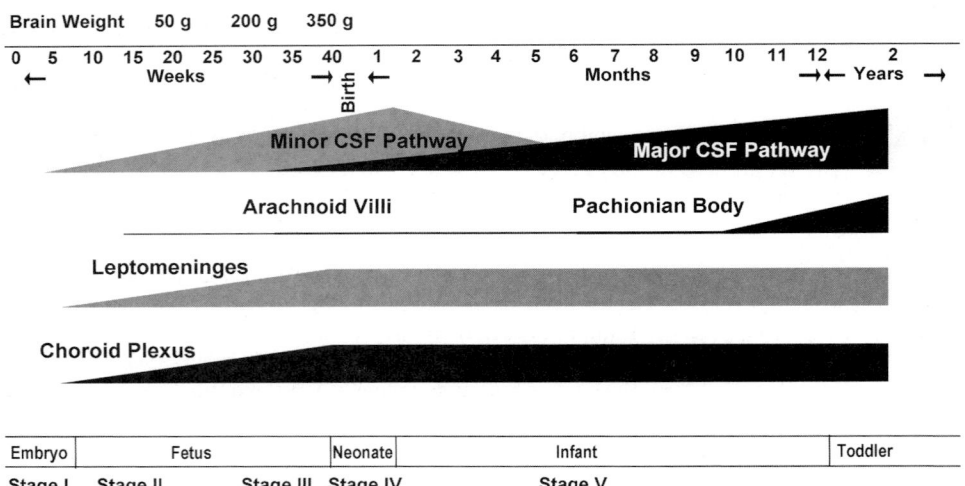

FIGURE 51.13. Cerebrospinal fluid (CSF) dynamics differ in the developing brain, compared to the adult. CSF absorption via the arachnoid villi (arachnoid granulation) into the venous sinuses is the major pathway. The minor pathway includes drainage via the ventricular ependyma, the interstitial and perivascular space, and the perineural lymphatics. In the developing immature human brain, the minor CSF pathway is the major route for CSF dynamics, with arachnoid granulation function not occurring until the late infant stages. From Oi S, Di Rocco C. Proposal of "evolution theory in cerebrospinal fluid dynamics" and minor pathway hydrocephalus in developing immature brain. *Childs Nerv Syst* 2006;22:662–9, with permission.

differences exist in the immature versus the adult brain relevant to pediatric neurointensive care. These differences span the gamut of biochemical, molecular, physiologic, and structural factors that influence current therapy on a daily basis and are likely to have an even greater impact on the future development of novel therapies that target brain injury in infants and children. This information also provides a foundation for the chapters that follow, which focus on the molecular biology of brain injury and the pathophysiology and treatment of key disorders in pediatric neurointensive care.

KEY POINTS

- Important biochemical, molecular, physiologic, and structural differences in CNS development influence treatment of brain injury in newborns, infants, children, adolescents, and adults.
- A unique aspect of PCD in the developing brain versus the adult brain is an imbalance between pro-death and pro-survival pathways induced by decreases in trophic and neurotransmitter neuronal input. Thus, the developing brain may be more sensitive to injuries that mimic regional developmental changes in trophin and neurotransmitter levels.
- Synaptogenesis is an active process that has a high rate of occurrence until puberty.
- Myelination persists longer than most other CNS developmental processes, continuing through adolescence.
- Around the time of birth, the neurotransmitter GABA switches from being excitatory to inhibitory in the CNS. The developing brain prior to this switch has enhanced sensitivity to excitotoxic injury.
- The lower limit of blood pressure autoregulation of CBF is similar in adults and infants, putting the developing brain at special risk for ischemia, as normal mean arterial pressure is age dependent.
- CBF and cerebral metabolic rate increase from birth and plateau between 3 and 9 years of age. This developmental progression mirrors synapse formation in the brain.
- Cerebrovascular tight junctions prevent movement of hydrophilic substances, osmotic agents, and proteins across the BBB.

ACKNOWLEDGMENTS

Supported by NIH grants NS42648 (LWJ) and NS38087 (PMK).

References

1. Abbott NJ. Astrocyte-endothelial interactions and blood-brain barrier permeability. *J Anat* 2002;200:629–38.
2. Abbott NJ, Romero IA. Transporting therapeutics across the blood-brain barrier. *Mol Med Today* 1996;2:106–13.
3. Abbott NJ, Ronnback L, Hansson E. Astrocyte-endothelial interactions at the blood-brain barrier. *Nat Rev Neurosci* 2006;7:41–53.
4. Altshuler K, Berg M, Frazier LM, et al. Critical periods in development: OCHP Paper Series on Children's Health and the Environment 2003; Paper 2.
5. Bayir H, Kochanek PM, Kagen VE. Oxidative stress in immature brain after traumatic brain injury. *Dev Neurosci* 2006;28:420–31.
6. Beaumont A, Hayasaki K, Marmarou A, et al. Contrasting effects of dopamine therapy in experimental brain injury. *J Neurotrauma* 2001;18:1359–72.
7. Ben-Ari Y, Khazipov R, Leinekugel X, et al. GABA$_A$, NMDA and AMPA receptors: A developmentally regulated "menage a trois." *Trends Neurosci* 1997;20:523–29.
8. Bouma GJ, Muizelaar, JP. Cerebral blood flow, cerebral blood volume, and cerebrovascular reactivity after severe head injury. *J Neurotrauma* 1992;9(Suppl 1):S333–48.
9. Connor B, Dragunow M. The role of neuronal growth factors in neurodegenerative disorders of the human brain. *Brain Res Brain Res Rev* 1998;27:1–39.
10. Constantine-Paton M, Cline HT. LTP and activity-dependent synaptogenesis: The more alike they are, the more different they become. *Curr Opin Neurobiol* 1998;8:139–48.
11. Das KP, Chao SL, White LD, et al. Differential patterns of nerve growth factor, brain-derived neurotrophic factor and neurotrophin-3 mRNA and protein levels in developing regions of rat brain. *Neuroscience* 2001;103:739–61.
12. De Zio D, Giunta L, Corvaro M, et al. Expanding roles of programmed cell death in mammalian neurodevelopment. *Semin Cell Dev Biol* 2005;16:281–94.
13. Engelhardt B. Development of the blood-brain barrier. *Cell Tissue Res* 2003;314:119–29.
14. Fayol L, Baud O, Monier A, et al. Immunocytochemical expression of monocarboxylate transporters in the human visual cortex at midgestation. *Brain Res Dev Brain Res* 2004;148:69–76.
15. Fields RD. Myelination: An overlooked mechanism of synaptic plasticity? *Neuroscientist* 2005;11:528–31.
16. Grant DA, Franzini C, Wild J, et al. Autoregulation of the cerebral circulation during sleep in newborn lambs. *J Physiol* 2005;564:923–30.
17. Guillemot F. Cellular and molecular control of neurogenesis in the mammalian telencephalon. *Curr Opin Cell Biol* 2005;17:639–47.
18. Haaland K, Karlsson B, Skovlund E, et al. Postnatal development of the cerebral blood flow velocity response to changes in CO_2 and mean arterial blood pressure in the piglet. *Acta Paediatr* 1995;84:1414–20.

19. Hardy P, Varma DR, Chemtob S. Control of cerebral and ocular blood flow autoregulation in neonates. *Pediatr Clin North Am* 1997;44:137–52.

20. Herlenius E, Lagercrantz H. Neurotransmitters and neuromodulators during early human development. *Early Hum Dev* 2001;65:21–37.

21. Herlenius E, Lagercrantz H. Development of neurotransmitter systems during critical periods. *Exp Neurol* 2004;190 (Suppl 1):S8–21.

22. Herschkowitz N. Neurological bases of behavioral development in infancy. *Brain Dev* 2000;22:411–16.

23. Holz RW, Fisher SK. *Basic Neurochemistry, 6th Edition.* Philadelphia: Lippincott Williams & Wilkins, 1999, Chapter 10.

24. Ikonomidou C, Bittigau P, Koch C, et al. Neurotransmitters and apoptosis in the developing brain. *Biochem Pharmacol* 2001;62:401–5.

25. Jayasinghe D, Gill AB, Levene MI. CBF reactivity in hypotensive and normotensive preterm infants. *Pediatr Res* 2003;54:848–53.

26. Johnston MV. Neurotransmitters and vulnerability of the developing brain. *Brain Dev* 1995;17:301–6.

27. Johnston MV, Nakajima W, Hagberg H. Mechanisms of hypoxic neurodegeneration in the developing brain. *Neuroscientist* 2002;8:212–20.

28. Kehrer M, Blumenstock G, Ehehalt S, et al. Development of cerebral blood flow volume in preterm neonates during the first 2 weeks of life. *Pediatr Res* 2005;58:927–30.

29. Khan JY, Black SM. Developmental changes in murine brain antioxidant enzymes. *Pediatr Res* 2003;54:77–82.

30. Kimelberg HK, Water homeostasis in the brain: Basic concepts. *Neuroscience* 2004;129:851–60.

31. Klebermass K, Kuhle S, Olischar M, et al. Intra- and extrauterine maturation of amplitude-integrated electroencephalographic activity in preterm infants younger than 30 weeks of gestation. *Biol Neonate* 2006;89:120–25.

32. Lagercrantz H, Ringstedt T. Organization of the neuronal circuits in the central nervous system during development. *Acta Paediatr* 2001;90:707–15.

33. Lessmann V, Gottmann K, Malcangio M. Neurotrophin secretion: Current facts and future prospects. *Prog Neurobiol* 2003;69:341–74.

34. Levitt P. Structural and functional maturation of the developing primate brain. *J Pediatr* 2003;143:S35–45.

35. Loepke AW, McCann JC, Kurth CD, et al. The physiologic effects of isoflurane anesthesia in neonatal mice. *Anesth Analg* 2006;102:75–80.

36. Michenfelder JD. *Anesthesia and the Brain.* New York: Churchill, Livingstone 1988, Chapter 1.

37. Munno DW, Syed NI. Synaptogenesis in the CNS: An odyssey from wiring together to firing together. *J Physiol* 2003;552:1–11.

38. Nehlig A. Cerebral energy metabolism, glucose transport and blood flow: Changes with maturation and adaptation to hypoglycaemia. *Diabetes Metab* 1997;23:18–29.

39. Oi S, Di Rocco C. Proposal of "evolution theory in cerebrospinal fluid dynamics" and minor pathway hydrocephalus in developing immature brain. *Childs Nerv Syst* 2006;22(7):662–9.

40. Olischar M, Klebermass K, Kuhle S, et al. Reference values for amplitude-integrated electroencephalographic activity in preterm infants younger than 30 weeks' gestational age. *Pediatrics* 2004;113:e61–6.

41. Olney JW, Young C, Wozniak DF, et al. Do pediatric drugs cause developing neurons to commit suicide? *Trends Pharmacol Sci* 2004;25:135–9.

42. Panickar KS, Norenberg MD. Astrocytes in cerebral ischemic injury: Morphological and general considerations. *Glia* 2005;50:287–298.

43. Pereira de Vasconcelos A, Ferrandon A, Nehlig A. Local cerebral blood flow during lithium-pilocarpine seizures in the developing and adult rat: Role of coupling between blood flow and metabolism in the genesis of neuronal damage. *J Cereb Blood Flow Metab* 2002;22:196–205.

44. Raoul C, Pettmann B, Henderson CE. Active killing of neurons during development and following stress: A role for p75(NTR) and Fas? *Curr Opin Neurobiol* 2000;10:111–17.

45. Ribatti D. Genetic and epigenetic mechanisms in the early development of the vascular system. *J Anat* 2006;208:139–52.

46. Rice D and Barone S, Jr. Critical periods of vulnerability for the developing nervous system: Evidence from humans and animal models. *Environ Health Perspective* 2000;108 Suppl 3:511–33.

47. Rivera C, Voipio J, Kaila K. Two developmental switches in GABAergic signalling: The K^+-Cl^- cotransporter KCC2 and carbonic anhydrase CAVII. *J Physiol* 2005;562:27–36.

48. Saunders NR, Habgood MD, Dziegielewska KM. Barrier mechanisms in the brain, II. Immature brain. *Clin Exp Pharmacol Physiol* 1999;26:85–91.

49. Taga G, Asakawa K, Hirasawa K, et al. Hemodynamic responses to visual stimulation in occipital and frontal cortex of newborn infants: A near-infrared optical topography study. *Early Hum Dev* 2003;75 (Suppl):S203–210.

50. Teyler TJ, Perkins AT, Harris KM. The development of long-term potentiation in hippocampus and neocortex. *Neuropsychologia* 1989;27:31–9.

51. Todd M, Shapiro HM, Obrist WD. Cerebral blood flow measurements and the critically ill patient. In: Grenvik A, Safar P, eds. *Brain Failure and Resuscitation.* New York: Churchill Livingstone, 1981, p. 135.

52. Town T, Nikolic V, Tan J. The microglial "activation" continuum: From innate to adaptive responses. *J Neuroinflammation* 2005;2:24.

53. Vannucci RC, Vannucci SJ. Glucose metabolism in the developing brain. *Semin Perinatol* 2000;24:107–15.

54. West CR, Harding JE, Williams CE, et al. Quantitative electroencephalographic patterns in normal preterm infants over the first week after birth. *Early Hum Dev* 2006;82:43–51.

55. Yang B, Sakurai T, Takata T, et al. Effects of lactate/pyruvate on synaptic plasticity in the hippocampal dentate gyrus. *Neurosci Res* 2003;46:333–7.

56. Zornow MH, Todd MM, Moore SS. The acute cerebral effects of changes in plasma osmolality and oncotic pressure. *Anesthesiology* 1987;67:936–41.

CHAPTER 52 ■ MOLECULAR BIOLOGY OF BRAIN INJURY

PATRICK M. KOCHANEK • HÜLYA BAYIR • LARRY W. JENKINS • ROBERT S.B. CLARK

Knowledge of the pathophysiology of central nervous system (CNS) injury, such as intracranial and cerebrovascular dynamics, has guided brain-oriented therapy since the inception of critical care medicine. Within each of the chapters in this section, the pathophysiology of each disease process is described, along with how it influences outcome and guides therapy. However, although therapy that is based solely on physiologic parameters, such as intracranial pressure (ICP) and cerebral blood flow (CBF), is important, it has limitations. For example, some patients with well-controlled cerebral hemodynamics still have poor outcome. The field of medicine is entering an exciting new era in which knowledge of the pathobiology of CNS injury is gaining importance for the intensivist and can augment pathophysiology-based therapy. Insight into secondary brain injury at the biochemical, cellular, and molecular levels has finally begun to yield dividends, with efficacy shown for several new therapies in ICU-relevant CNS injuries (10,44,60,90). This chapter builds on some of the material in several preceding chapters that address developmental issues of the CNS relevant to critical care (53–55). Where possible, this information on the bedside care of critically ill patients is linked with clinical data. It is hoped that this chapter and its counterpart (Chapter 51) aptly set the stage for the following chapters that discuss the individual CNS disorders encountered in the practice of pediatric critical care medicine.

INJURY RESPONSE IN THE IMMATURE BRAIN

Most research on developmental brain injury suggests that, in many ways, the immature brain is more resistant to injury and more capable of recovery than is the adult brain, as a result of enhanced plasticity (rewiring or repair). For example, despite similar impact parameters, the immature brain exhibits less neuronal death than the adult brain in experimental cerebral trauma. Similarly, tolerance of the immature brain to status epilepticus (SE) is greater than in the adult in experimental models (42). Classic studies of ablative brain lesions in laboratory models, such as hemispherectomy in cats, demonstrate that the earlier the brain lesion occurs in development, the better the outcome (99). Some suggest possible critical windows in development represent periods of the brain's enhanced vulnerability to specific developmental processes (34) (see Chapter 51). Some developmental aspects do predispose the immature brain to greater injury than the adult. For example, the small size of the infant skull may predispose to a more diffuse pattern of injury from a traumatic impact than does the adult skull (66). An injury that is more global than focal may yield a more profound disruption of function. Much of the controversy on this point results from the fact that outcomes from brain injury in infants and young children are often poorer than in adults (61). For example, outcome from out-of-hospital cardiac arrest is worse in children than in adults. However, the mechanism that underlies the cardiac arrest in children—asphyxia—is particularly injurious to the brain, compared to ventricular fibrillation (55). Similarly, reported outcomes in infants from severe traumatic brain injury (TBI) can be as bad as or worse than those in adults (61). This finding likely results from the contribution of inflicted childhood neurotrauma (child abuse) to severe TBI in infancy. Thus, although most data suggest that the developing brain exhibits both resistance and resilience to injury versus the adult, the mechanisms of injury are often severe in children. Our challenges for developing new therapies are no less than in adults.

PATHWAYS AND APPLICATIONS TO PEDIATRIC INTENSIVE CARE

Secondary Injury

The essence of neurointensive care is the prevention of secondary injury. Two distinct types of secondary injury are frequently lumped into a single concept. First, endogenous secondary injury cascades evolve in the minutes to days after the initial insult. Such processes as excitotoxicity, oxidative stress, and delayed neuronal death cascades, among others, kill neurons and injure other components of the CNS at varying rates. Emerging evidence supports the concept that these cascades can be abrogated in some cases, resulting in salvage of injured tissue and improved recovery of function. Efficacy in large, randomized, controlled clinical trials has been reported for mild hypothermia after both cardiac arrest from ventricular fibrillation in adults and perinatal asphyxia (10,44,90). Similarly, both thrombolytics and the antioxidant NXY-059 have shown efficacy in large, randomized, controlled clinical trials in stroke in adults (60). Although these therapies are being further evaluated and only beginning to be integrated into standard care, it is likely that additional therapies will follow. This chapter is focused on those events in injury evolution that may represent therapeutic targets.

In contrast to the endogenous secondary injury cascades, a parallel form of secondary injury involves the occurrence of secondary insults in critically ill patients in the field, emergency room, or ICU. These secondary insults produce adverse consequences on a CNS with enhanced vulnerability

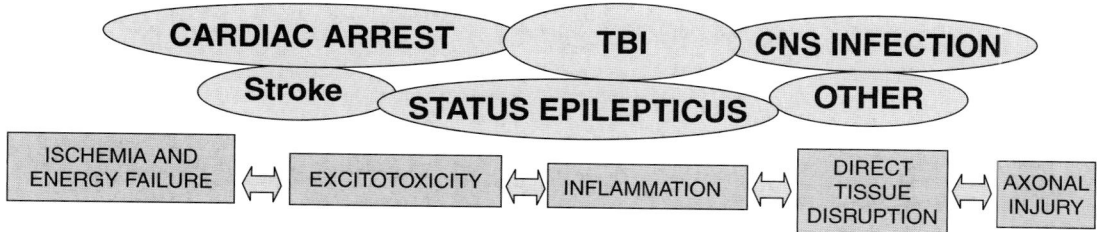

FIGURE 52.1. Overview of the major pathways of secondary injury after PICU-relevant insults to the CNS. Five categories of injury include ischemia and energy failure, excitotoxicity, inflammation, direct tissue disruption, and axonal injury.

after cardiac arrest, stroke, TBI, SE, or CNS infection. For example, hypoxemia, at a level tolerated by the normal brain, can have devastating effects after TBI. (Why the injured brain is highly vulnerable to secondary insults is discussed later.) Thus, in this chapter, the biochemical, cellular, and molecular aspects of endogenous damage evolution are discussed, followed by a discussion of the mechanisms that underlie enhanced vulnerability of the injured brain to secondary insults in the PICU.

Evolution of Secondary Injury

Presenting a complete synthesis of the mechanisms involved in the evolution of secondary damage after CNS injury is challenging, particularly when one considers that the concepts discussed in this chapter serve as the basis for all PICU-relevant CNS insults, i.e, cardiac arrest, TBI, stroke, SE, and CNS infection, among others. It is necessary to consider studies in models of CNS injury and, where possible, the relevant clinical conditions. We will focus on global cerebral ischemia/cardiac arrest, focal cerebral ischemia/stroke, and TBI. Where possible, insight into the relevance of these mechanisms in epilepsy and CNS infection will also be included.

Studies have begun to unravel those mechanisms producing secondary damage that are relevant to cardiac arrest, stroke, TBI, SE, CNS infection, and other insults. Five categories of mechanisms can be defined (**Fig. 52.1**): those associated with (a) ischemia and energy failure and (b) excitotoxicity, both initiating cell death cascades; (c) inflammation; (d) direct tissue disruption; and (e) axonal injury. Within each category, a constellation of mediators of secondary damage is involved (54). The quantitative contribution of each mediator to outcome and the interplay between these mediators remains unclear and varies with the insult. A sixth component of the response to brain injury will be discussed; namely, the role of endogenous neuroprotectants, repair, and regeneration. The ultimate result of the primary injury from TBI, which sets into motion these five cascade initiators, is summarized in **Figure 52.2**. The details of these initiators represent the crux of information to follow.

Study of the acute biochemical and molecular aspects of human brain injury has been limited, particularly in infants and children; however, several methods have been used, most commonly in TBI and occasionally in asphyxia. These include (a) the analysis of brain biochemistry and molecular biology using ventricular cerebrospinal fluid (CSF); (b) assessment of brain

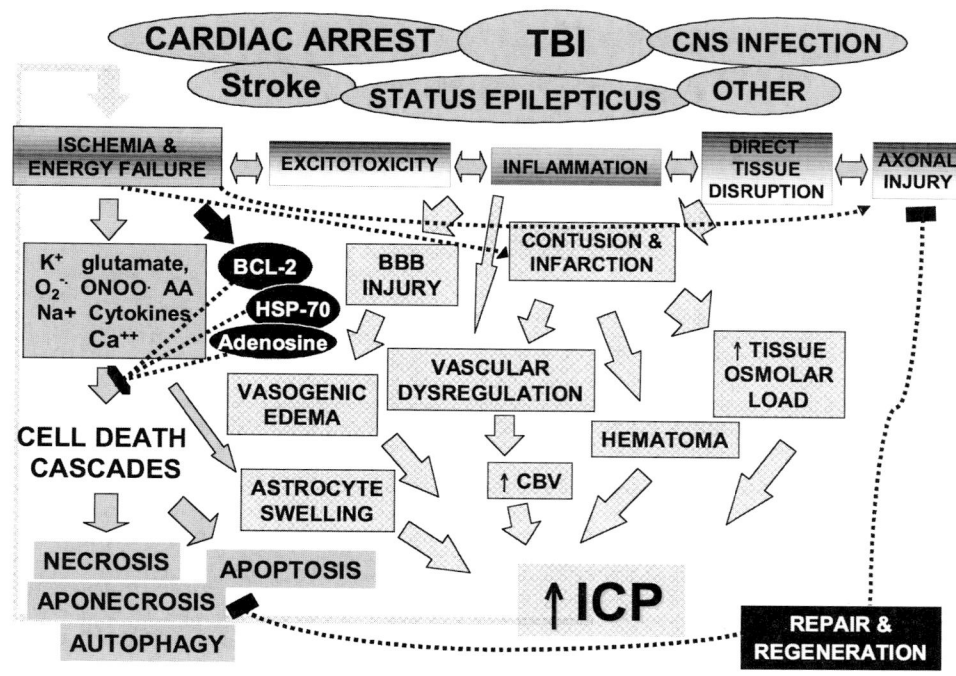

FIGURE 52.2. Secondary cascades triggered by the five initiators of secondary damage identified in **Figure 52.1** are shown for cell death cascades (gray), and for brain swelling-related process (**stippled gray**). In addition, a sixth category of endogenous neuroprotectants and repair and regeneration is initiated; the components of this cascade are shown in black. TBI, traumatic brain injury; O2-, superoxide anion; ONOO, peroxynitrite; AA, arachidonic acid; HSP-70, heat shock protein 70; CBV, cerebral blood volume; ICP, intracranial pressure.

interstitial fluid by cerebral microdialysis; (c) imaging-related tools, such as positron-emission tomography (PET) and MR spectroscopy; and (d) the assessment of molecular markers in brain tissue obtained from patients treated with surgical decompression. Assessment of postmortem brain tissue has provided molecular clues in some cases.

Ischemia

Global Cerebral Ischemia. The brain is exquisitely vulnerable to ischemia, which represents a unifying mechanism involved in the evolution of secondary damage across CNS insults. When CBF globally ceases, such as in cardiac arrest, a stereotypic time course of events occurs that is initiated by acute cellular energy failure. These changes are outlined in **Figure 52.3**. Phosphocreatine is depleted in 1 min, and the adenylate energy charge is depleted in ~5 min. After this time, no useful energy can be made available to ATP-requiring reactions (85). Membrane failure follows, with loss of ionic gradients, increases in intracellular calcium (Ca^{2+}) and sodium (Na^+), and a decrease in intracellular potassium (K^+). Free fatty acid release from the neuronal membrane also occurs, and electroencephalogram and evoked potentials fail. If energy failure is sustained beyond a critical period, an irreversible insult to neurons occurs and is believed to be manifest by acute necrotic death, with membrane failure, cellular Na and Ca accumulation, cellular swelling, and acute failure of organelles, such as mitochondria. However, during complete global brain ischemia, assessment of brain tissue with light microscopy reveals no obvious pathologic derangement,

and electron microscopy reveals only chromatin clumping (46). The resultant damage to neurons, glia, and white matter does not manifest until reperfusion, suggesting a critical role for reperfusion in the evolution of secondary damage, as well as the intriguing possibility that even prolonged periods of ischemia might be survived with good outcome if the deleterious consequences of reperfusion could be eliminated. At this writing, the duration of irreversibility for global cerebral ischemia in ventricular fibrillation cardiac arrest is believed to be between 5 and 10 min, although it can be modified by factors that include temperature, blood glucose concentration, and pH, among others. Although these principles generally hold true for cardiac arrest that results from asphyxia (the most common form in infants and children), some aspects are unique. A more comprehensive discussion of the specific pathophysiology of asphyxia is discussed in Chapter 58.

Focal Cerebral Ischemia. Unlike global brain ischemia, focal ischemic insults (strokes) produce brain regions with different degrees of blood-flow reduction related to the vascular anatomy surrounding the area of occlusion. The typical result is an ischemic core, in which flow reductions are profound, surrounded by penumbral brain regions that have less severe but still compromising CBF reductions. The consequences of penumbral CBF reductions on brain metabolism have been reviewed (43). The most sensitive biochemical or molecular event to CBF reduction in the ischemic penumbra is protein synthesis, which is inhibited by ~50% at a CBF of 55 mL/100 g/min and

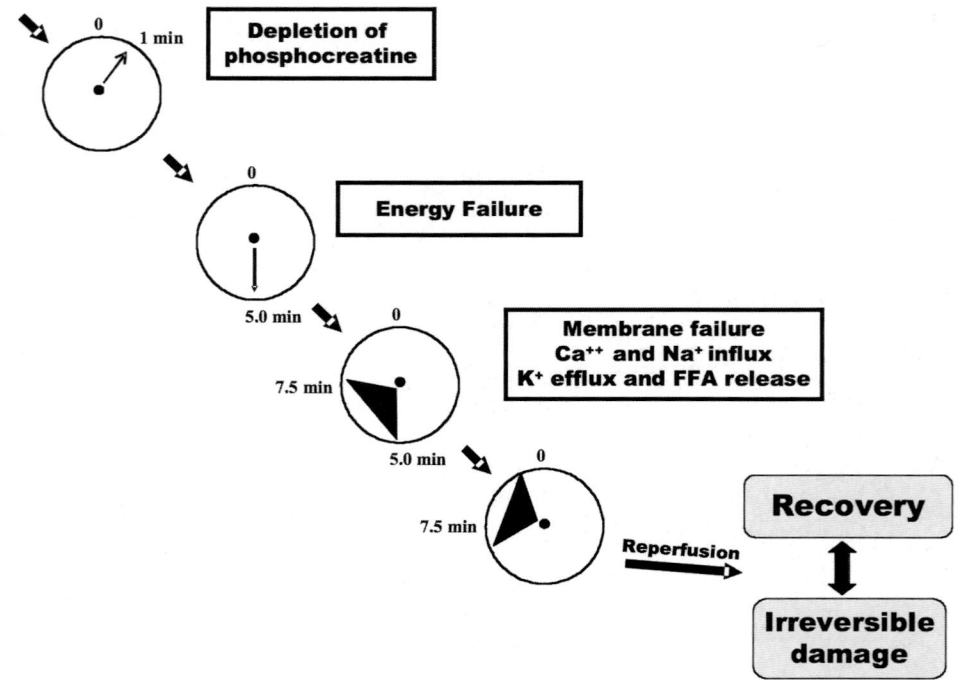

FIGURE 52.3. Temporal sequence of events that occurs in global cerebral ischemia, as seen with a "square-wave" ischemic brain insult, such as ventricular fibrillation cardiac arrest. Although ischemia rapidly sets the stage for damage, histology—even by electron microscopy—reveals little damage during the period of ischemia. With ischemic durations beyond 10 min at normothermia, considerable damage is manifest with reperfusion. FFA, free fatty acid.

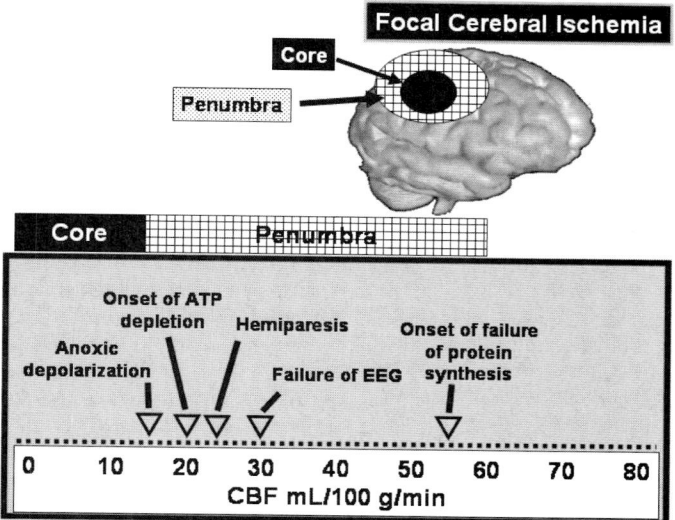

FIGURE 52.4. Cerebral blood flow (CBF, mL/100 g/min) thresholds of biochemical, electrophysiologic, and clinical failure of a number of key processes in the setting of focal cerebral ischemia (stroke). In focal ischemia, the core is the area with CBF below the threshold for anoxic depolarization and energy failure, while the penumbra has moderately reduced CBF, with levels above the threshold for energy failure. However, many processes are compromised in the penumbra (43). ATP, adenosine triphosphate; EEG, electroencephalogram.

generally fails below 35 mL/100 g/min (**Fig. 52.4**). Other homeostatic processes that fail at decreasing CBF thresholds in focal ischemia include glucose utilization below 25 mL/100 g/min and ATP depletion, beginning at a CBF less than ~20 mL/100 g/min. Peri-infarct depolarization waves occur at CBF levels of 50–70 mL/100 g/min and are postulated to contribute to damage in the penumbra by transiently increasing metabolic demands in this compromised zone. Electroencephalogram fails at a CBF of below ~30 mL/100 g/min, hemiparesis is seen at CBF thresholds of ~23 mL/100 g/min, and anoxic depolarization occurs at CBF values between 15 and 20 mL/100 g/min, resulting in ionic failure. These CBF thresholds for failure of molecular and cellular homeostasis represent estimates for the adult brain. Corresponding ischemic threshold values in the developing brain are less well established. Also, threshold values can be a moving target. For example, if neuronal metabolic demands are increased (i.e., hyperthermia, seizures), the CBF threshold value that would trigger neuronal death could be higher, consistent with enhanced vulnerability. Neuronal death in focal cerebral ischemia is suggested to involve necrosis in the regions of permanent energy failure and mixed or apoptotic phenotypes in penumbral regions. However, some biochemical footprints of apoptosis are seen even in core regions (92). Details of the specific cell death pathways are provided below.

Posttraumatic Ischemia. Early after severe TBI, the CBF, as assessed by stable xenon CT, is reduced in infants and young children (54), which mirrors studies in adults and suggests that early posttraumatic ischemia might represent a therapeutic target. Further supporting this possibility, early hypoperfusion or ischemia (CBF <20 mL/100 g/min) after severe TBI in infants and children was associated with poor outcome. Regional hypoperfusion is also commonly seen in contused brain regions. Mechanisms that underlie the early posttraumatic hypoperfusion may include a reduced vasodilatory response to nitric oxide (NO), cyclic guanosine monophosphate (cGMP), cyclic AMP (cAMP), and prostanoids, reduced NO production by endothelial NO synthase (NOS), and/or release of vasoconstrictors, such as superoxide anion or endothelin-1 (54). After TBI in children, increases in metabolic demands related to uptake

of the excitatory neurotransmitter glutamate, as reflected by increases in brain tissue lactate, have been reported (1) and are discussed below. Posttraumatic CBF will be further discussed in Chapter 56.

Ischemia in Other PICU-relevant Central Nervous System Insults. As discussed, ischemia is one unifying mechanism of secondary damage across PICU-relevant CNS insults. However, the role of ischemia in other disorders, such as meningitis and SE, is less well defined.

Meningitis. CBF was studied in 20 seriously ill children with meningitis, and reduced CBF was reported in seven (2). Global CBF was 26 ± 10 mL/100g/min in the reduced-flow group, and marked regional variability was seen. A role for ischemic damage in meningitis is suggested in focal cortical inflammatory lesions, where vasculitis and local infarction are seen, and in patients with venous sinus thrombosis (73). In contrast, increased flow velocity was reported in a study of 110 adults with meningitis (39). It is unclear if acute hyperemia contributes to herniation, which could importantly influence therapy. Vascular dysregulation in meningitis may be mediated by superoxide anion and the vasoconstrictor endothelin (73) and by disturbed regulation of NO production (40). The causes of hyperemia remain to be defined but inflammation-related mediators, such as inducible NOS (iNOS)-derived NO, could be involved.

Status epilepticus. In SE, clinical studies of CBF are limited; however, experimental work shows the anticipated early increases in CBF—as much as fourfold—in an attempt to meet increased metabolic demands (82). Although ischemic blood flows are generally not seen, in some models, the marked increase in CBF is not sustained (30), which might lead to relative ischemia and resultant neuronal injury, given that cerebral metabolic rate for oxygen and glucose are markedly increased during SE (85). Increases in CBF during SE likely result from metabolic coupling.

Cell Death Pathways

Selective Vulnerability. Neurons in certain regions are exceptionally vulnerable to injury in global brain ischemia, including the CA1 region of the hippocampus; cerebral cortex layers 3, 5, and 6; cerebellar Purkinje cells; and in infants, some brainstem nuclei (52, also reviewed in 22, 54). Approximately ≥5 mins of complete global brain ischemia can result in neuronal death in these regions when they are examined at or beyond 72 hrs after the insult. The mechanisms that underlie selective vulnerability of these neurons have been the topic of considerable research; however, a definitive answer remains elusive. These neurons do not have a unique vascular distribution; thus, intrinsic vulnerability is suggested. Nevertheless, insight has been gained from these studies into the question of how neurons die in cerebral ischemia.

A process known as *delayed neuronal death* causes these highly vulnerable neurons die after threshold insults. During ischemia, cellular membrane failure occurs, with Ca^+ and Na^+ accumulation and K^+ efflux. However, in threshold insults, these ionic disturbances can be reversed, and ionic gradients reestablished. In delayed neuronal death of selectively vulnerable neurons after global brain ischemia, electrophysiologic studies have revealed neuronal hyperexcitability in these regions after reperfusion, followed by a second wave of irreversible Ca^{2+} accumulation at ~48 hrs (52). The molecular cascades involved in delayed neuronal death in selectively vulnerable neurons are discussed below.

Although much has been written about selective vulnerability of the CA1 hippocampus after cardiac arrest, different neurons are selectively vulnerable after TBI. After experimental TBI, hippocampal neurons in the dentate hilus and the CA3 region of the hippocampus are most vulnerable (64) (**Fig. 52.5**). This pattern of neuronal vulnerability is shared with that seen in experimental models of epilepsy, as produced by systemic injection of the proconvulsant agent kainic acid. This finding suggests an important role for posttraumatic excitation in me-

diating neuronal death in CA3 and, consistent with that notion, neurons in the dentate gyrus and CA3 region of the hippocampus show regional excitation after TBI and mediate early posttraumatic seizures (35). In experimental SE, limbic structures, including not only hippocampus, but also the piriform cortex, temporal cortex, and amygdala, are vulnerable (101). Thus, which specific cells are most vulnerable after CNS insult depends on the type of insult; the intrinsic mechanisms involved in this vulnerability may differ. The optimal approach to treatment could thus differ in cardiac arrest, stroke, TBI, and other insults of the CNS. The pattern of neuronal death is also unique in meningitis. In experimental meningitis, the granular layer of the dentate gyrus of the hippocampus is highly vulnerable, particularly in regions closest to the CSF ventricular compartment (12). Selective vulnerability of the dentate was shown in acute bacterial meningitis in humans and may underlie learning deficits seen in this condition (74).

Necrosis, Apoptosis, and "Aponecrosis." Neuronal death can occur through multiple pathways including necrosis, programmed cell death (PCD) or apoptosis, and mixed phenotypes. Necrosis, which is characterized by denaturation and coagulation of cellular proteins, results from a progressive reduction in cellular ATP (22,54). Necrosis involves progressive derangements in energy and substrate metabolism that are followed by a series of morphologic alterations, including swelling of cells and organelles, subsurface cellular blebbing, amorphous deposits in mitochondria, condensation of nuclear chromatin and, finally, breaks in plasma and organellar membranes. It was assumed that all ischemic cell death occurred via this process, and that selective vulnerability represented a predilection for the development of necrosis in certain neurons. However, neuronal death after hypoxic-ischemic insults

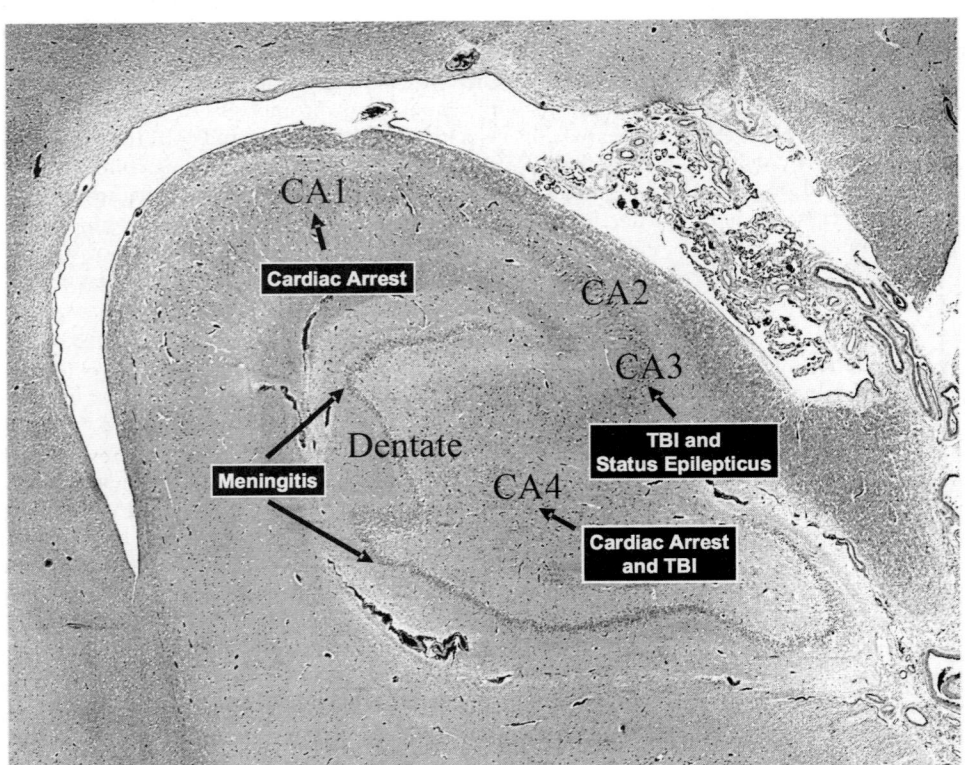

FIGURE 52.5. Horizontal section through the hippocampus of the human brain showing neuronal degeneration in the various hippocampal subfields; namely, CA1, CA2, CA3, CA4 (hilus), and dentate gyrus. The hippocampal subfields are some of the most selectively vulnerable brain regions to ischemic, traumatic, and infectious insults relevant to pediatric neurointensive care. The black boxes show the insults generally associated with damage in a given hippocampal subfield. The CA1 and CA4 regions are highly vulnerable to global ischemic insults, such as cardiac arrest. In contrast, the dentate gyrus is vulnerable in meningitis, while CA3 is vulnerable in TBI and SE. This Figure is not to suggest that all of these regions cannot be damaged by a given injury (for example, a prolonged cardiac arrest); rather, these injury patterns represent those seen with threshold insults. Hippocampal injury is important to disturbances in learning and memory, among other cognitive processes.

can also occur through PCD or apoptosis. More recently, it has been suggested that mixed phenotypes of neuronal death exist that have features of both necrosis and apoptosis. The development of PCD involves new protein synthesis and the activation of endonucleases, with a characteristic cleavage of DNA into nucleosomal fragments of double-stranded DNA, called "DNA laddering" on Southern blot analysis. PCD was classically described as being associated with cell death during embryogenesis (22,53). However, PCD is also involved in ischemia, TBI, meningitis, and epilepsy. Some reports indicate that selective vulnerable cell death in brain regions, such as the CA1 region of the hippocampus after transient global brain ischemia, occurs by an apoptotic mechanism. Delayed cell death of selectively vulnerable neurons was attenuated by inhibition of protein synthesis (93), and DNA extracted from the hippocampus of gerbils at 4 days after a threshold global ischemic insult showed a characteristic laddering pattern consistent with apoptosis (75). In contrast, it has also been reported that, after global cerebral ischemia in rats, delayed neuronal death occurred but exhibited necrotic features on electron microscopy (25).

PCD in the postischemic brain is not limited to scattered neuronal death in what have been traditionally deemed to be "selectively vulnerable regions," but it is also seen in penumbral regions around evolving cerebral infarcts (63). Apoptosis was evident in injured brain regions of infants who died from perinatal asphyxia between 3 and 7 days after birth, and was common in cortical layers I, II, and III, while necrosis was seen in deeper layers (28). Finally, cells with mixed phenotypes were seen in rat brain after experimental CNS injury that resulted from injection of excitatory amino acids (EAAs) (83). These mixed phenotypes include individual cells with features of both apoptosis and necrosis.

It is likely that the severity of the ischemic insult and other local factors determine whether an injured neuron recovers or dies from PCD or necrosis. After cardiac arrest, stroke, TBI, epilepsy, and CNS infections, a continuum from recovery to necrosis may exist in neurons; progress through this continuum depends on the severity and duration of the insult, the local milieu, and the given brain region. It is thus likely that an understanding of the mechanisms involved in both pathways will be necessary for development of novel therapies in CNS injury. The next section discusses the key initiators of neuronal death, followed by a brief discussion of the many cell-death effector pathways that have been defined to date.

Autophagy. An additional neuronal death process has been touted as potentially playing a role in the pathobiology of PICU-relevant CNS insults. Autophagy, a term from the Greek that means "self-eating," is a process that mediates normal turn-over of cellular constituents, such as organelles and membranes in autophagic vacuoles (20). It is associated with cell death during starvation. However, after ischemia and TBI, disruption of this process may lead to "autophagic stress" or "macroautophagy," with an accumulation of autophagic vacuoles resulting in cell death. The mechanisms by which accumulation of autophagic vacuoles leads to cell death remain unclear, but vacuole overload may enhance vulnerability to injury. This pathway may be operating in brain ischemia and trauma, and may be able to be inhibited by novel therapeutic agents.

Key Initiators

Energy failure. Energy failure sustained beyond a critical period produces neuronal membrane failure, Na^+ and Ca^{2+} accumulation, K^+ efflux, cellular swelling, and acute failure of organelles such as mitochondria and the endoplasmic reticulum (ER). Increases in intracellular Ca^{2+} mandate its sequestration, notably in mitochondria. Increases in intracellular Ca^{2+} result in mitochondrial dysfunction and ER stress. (See review of mitochondrial failure in CNS injury in 94). Three pathways are involved. First, Ca^{2+} activates several degradative enzymes (including calpain proteases and phospholipases) that modify mitochondrial proteins and lipids. Second, oxidative stress further modifies mitochondrial constituents. Finally, unchecked Ca^{2+} sequestration in mitochondria leads to mitochondrial permeability transition, which involves the formation of a large conductance pore in the inner mitochondrial membrane and produces uncoupling of oxidative phosphorylation, osmotic swelling, release of matrix metabolites, and ultimately, physical rupture. These processes can lead to neuronal necrosis, apoptosis, or mixed cellular phenotypes. Links between mitochondrial failure, excitotoxicity, and oxidative stress likely play a key role, as shown in **Figure 52.6**. Support for this hypothesis includes efficacy for cyclosporine-A in experimental cerebral ischemia and TBI. Cyclosporine-A blocks formation of the mitochondrial permeability transition pore and is neuroprotective in these models when its passage across the blood-brain barrier (BBB) is facilitated.

Parallel mechanisms underlying the role of disturbed Ca^{2+} homeostasis in the evolution of secondary damage after CNS injury involve the ER (81). The ER normally sequesters Ca^{2+}, and the resultant high concentration is important to its normal function in activating enzymes that control protein folding. Ischemia induces Ca^{2+} release from the ER when it is stimulated by inositol 1,4,5-triphosphate (IP3) or via activation of ryanodine receptors. IP3 is produced in the activation of metabotropic glutamate receptors in the excitotoxic process. Reduced ER Ca^{2+} concentration can trigger apoptosis, as discussed later.

An interesting biochemical finding that appears consistent across PICU-relevant CNS insults is the presence of sustained increases in brain tissue levels of lactate. Clinical studies that use MR spectroscopy have shown that brain tissue lactate levels are increased even at 1–2 weeks after cardiac arrest or TBI in infants and children, with poor outcome (1). The mechanisms involved may include chronic mitochondrial dysfunction/failure, sustained excitotoxicity, occult ischemia, or macrophage accumulation. This finding suggests chronic energy failure.

Excitotoxicity. Excitotoxicity is the process by which glutamate and other EAAs cause neuronal damage. Several cell injury mechanisms are linked to glutamate toxicity, which is also associated with neuronal damage in cardiac arrest, stroke, TBI, epilepsy, CNS infection, and hypoglycemia. Glutamate is the predominant excitatory neurotransmitter in the brain and acts through receptor types that are characterized according to specific EAA agonists. Glutamate levels increase in the brain early after ischemia or TBI as a result of release and/or failure of re-uptake (53,54). The three main ionotropic glutamate receptors are the N-methyl-D-aspartate (NMDA), kainate, and α-amino-3-hydroxy-5-methyl-4-isoxazoleproprionic acid (AMPA) receptors. NMDA receptors act primarily by allowing

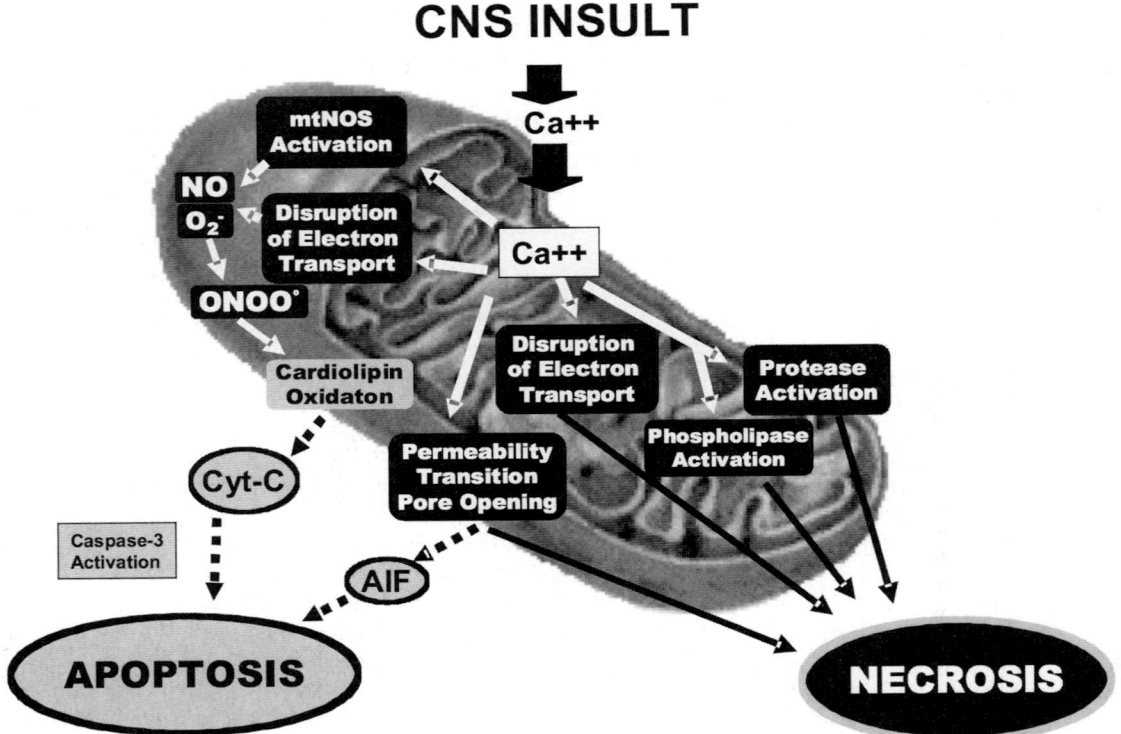

FIGURE 52.6. Mitochondrial cell death pathways resulting from calcium overload. Mitochondrial injury is one of the key pathways leading to either necrotic cell death (as a result of energy failure) or apoptotic cell death [as a result of release of apoptogenic factors (cytochrome-c and apoptosis inducing factor) from the mitochondrial membrane], along with death in cells with mixed necrotic and apoptotic phenotypes. mtNOS, mitochondrial nitric oxidase synthase; nNOS, neuronal nitric oxide synthase; NO, nitric oxide; $O2^{-}$·, superoxide anion; ONOO·, peroxynitrite; Cyt-c, cytochrome-c; AIF, apoptosis inducing factor.

Ca^{2+} influx, both directly and through voltage-gated channels, whereas the non-NMDA receptors mediate Na^{+} influx with secondary action on voltage-gated Ca^{2+} channels and reverse action of the Na^{+}/Ca^{2+} transporter. Glutamate also acts at metabotropic receptors, which trigger second messenger systems and increase intracellular Ca^{2+} levels by causing a release of intracellular stores. Increased intracellular Ca^{2+} triggers processes that can lead to cellular injury or death, including oxidative and nitrative stress, mitochondrial or ER failure, and activation of Ca^{2+}-dependent proteases (**Fig. 52.7**). These mechanisms are discussed later. EAAs other than glutamate may mediate excitotoxicity, and regional effects may depend on the local transmitter systems involved.

Two bodies of evidence link excitotoxicity to secondary brain injury: (a) demonstration of pathologic levels of glutamate after CNS insults at levels that are known to cause cell death in vitro, and (b) improvement in outcome with the use of EAA receptor antagonists in experimental models. Increased levels of EAAs in ventricular CSF from adult patients with TBI were first reported in 1994 (79). Glutamate levels were as high as 7 μM—sufficient to cause neuronal death in cell culture. Other investigators studied CSF and reported a dramatic excitotoxic response to TBI in infants and children (86). Victims of child abuse had particularly high and sustained increases in CSF glutamate. Most studies report maximal glutamate levels early after CA, stroke, or TBI, which may explain, in part, why human clinical trials that have targeted excitotoxicity have failed. Studies in experimental models have shown a distinct ad-

vantage to early versus delayed treatment with anti-excitotoxic therapies. The therapeutic window for this approach may be <1–2 hrs, making this mechanism most relevant to field and/or emergency room application.

Several therapies have antiexcitotoxic properties, including hypothermia, barbiturates, inhaled anesthetics, calcium-channel blockers, and anticonvulsants. Most clinical documentation of the antiexcitotoxic properties of these therapies has been in patients with severe TBI. In adults with severe TBI, researchers used intracerebral microdialysis and reported that induction of barbiturate coma was associated with a 59% reduction of glutamate and a 37% reduction of lactate concentration (36). Adults with severe TBI had lower CSF levels of glutamate when treated with 24 hrs of hypothermia (32°C) versus normothermia (67). It remains unclear if the antiexcitotoxic properties of these agents confer benefit. Other more novel drugs that have specific actions on glutamate physiology have been developed, including NMDA- and AMPA-receptor antagonists, glutamate release inhibitors, NMDA channel blockers, NMDA glycine-site antagonists (glycine is a co-agonist at the NMDA receptor), magnesium (which regulates NMDA receptor activation), and GABA agonists (which reduce glutamate release).

Although excitotoxicity is important after cardiac arrest, stroke, and TBI, differences exist that likely influence the effect of therapies. Excitotoxic damage seems to be largely mediated by NMDA-receptor stimulation after stroke and TBI. However, clinical trials have been performed to evaluate glutamate

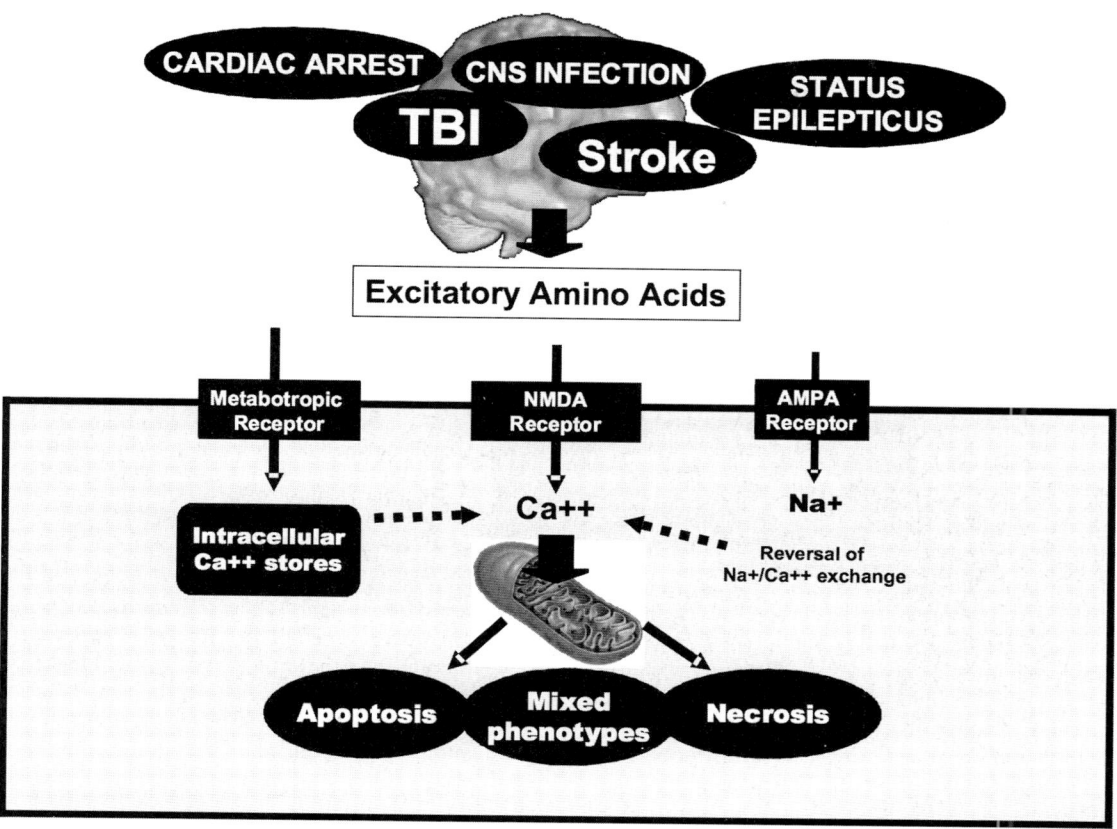

FIGURE 52.7. Receptors and key intracellular events resulting from excitotoxicity in neurons after PICU-relevant CNS insults. NMDA, N-methyl-D-aspartate; AMPA, α-amino-3-hydroxy-5-methyl-4-isoxazoleproprionic acid.

antagonists after stroke and TBI in adults, and none have proven successful. A limitation to studies of antiexcitotoxic therapies in human TBI is the variability of injuries. Bullock et al. (16), using microdialysis after TBI in adults, described four patterns of EAAs. Although many patients had prolonged increases in EAAs, others had only a brief period of increased concentrations. It is unlikely that antiexcitotoxic treatment would benefit patients without evidence of EAA increases, and future trials may need to be tailored to the patients' injuries.

Another relevant issue related to NMDA-receptor antagonists relates to developmental differences, as suggested in the preceding chapter. Apoptotic pathways appear to play a greater role in secondary neuronal death after injury in the developing versus the adult brain. A promising study in this regard demonstrated that the combination of xenon gas (an NMDA antagonist) with mild hypothermia was highly effective in preventing damage after a hypoxic-ischemic insult in developing rat pups (65). Some caution may be in order, as apoptotic neuronal degeneration was seen in neonatal rats after treatment with NMDA antagonists (45); however, controversy has arisen related to the possible role of unrecognized hypoglycemia in the injury in these studies. Additional studies are necessary.

Contrasting stroke and TBI, AMPA-receptor antagonists are an effective antiexcitotoxic strategy after experimental global ischemia. However, in a model of neonatal asphyxia in newborn piglets, the AMPA antagonist NBQX was detrimental rather than efficacious, suggesting developmental differences (11). Inhibition of plasticity by antiexcitotoxic therapies may

also limit their efficacy, especially during subacute periods. If antiexcitotoxic therapies are shown to be efficacious in clinical CNS injury, it is likely to be with early application.

Oxidative stress. Free radicals are generated during normal cerebral metabolism, with the normal reducing environment being maintained by a myriad of endogenous antioxidant systems. After cardiac arrest, stroke, and TBI, and in CNS infection, a number of biochemical pathways contribute to a marked increase in free radical production. Oxidative stress-mediated injury is of heightened importance in CNS because of the high level of polyunsaturation of lipids, high metabolic rate, and the association between excitotoxicity and free radical production (6). Excitotoxicity-mediated increases in intracellular Ca^{2+} are believed to contribute to mitochondrial sequestration of Ca^{2+}, disruption of electron transport, and the production of reactive oxygen species (ROS) either linked to, or independent of, opening of the mitochondrial permeability transition pore (19). Increases in cytosolic Ca^{2+} can activate neuronal NOS. Similarly, Ca^{2+} sequestration by mitochondria may also activate mitochondrial NOS, leading to NO production in neurons. Other sources of free radicals include cyclooxygenase-2, peroxidases (including myeloperoxidase and cytochrome-c), and both invading and resident inflammatory cells (**Fig. 52.8**). Free radicals cause lipid peroxidation, protein and DNA oxidation, protein dimerization, and activation of transcription factors with dysregulation of neuronal homeostasis. Free radicals can be grouped into ROS and reactive nitrogen species.

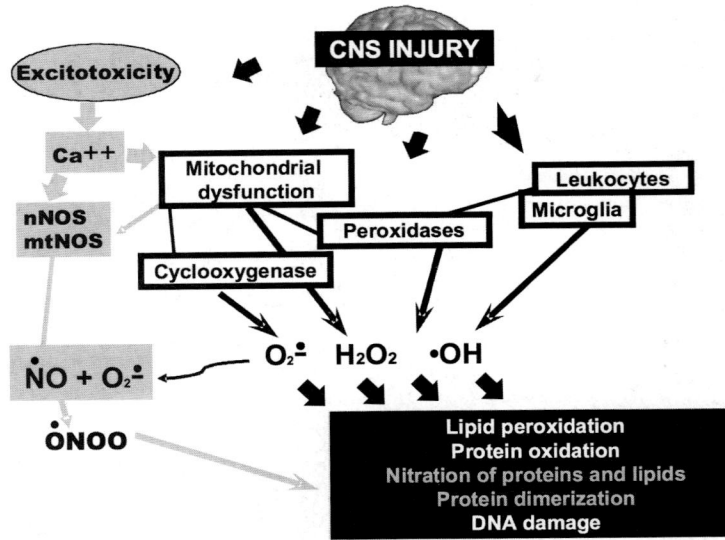

FIGURE 52.8. Pathways of oxidative and nitrative stress after CNS injury. Mitochondrial failure is a key participant with other pathways. Free radicals and other oxidants are generated, leading to lipid peroxidation, protein oxidation and dimerization, protein and lipid nitration, and DNA damage. mtNOS, mitochondrial nitric oxide synthase; n, neuronal; O_2^-, superoxide anion; ONOO·, peroxynitrite; ·OH, hydroxyl radical; H_2O_2, hydrogen peroxide.

ROS include superoxide anion, hydrogen peroxide, and hydroxyl radicals, the latter of which is highly reactive with almost every molecule in living cells. Among the reactive nitrogen species is NO, which is lipid soluble and readily crosses cell membranes. NO reacts with other free radicals and can inhibit lipid peroxidation and, in some settings, act as an endogenous antioxidant. However, the reaction of NO with superoxide anion leads to peroxynitrite formation, a highly reactive radical species that can produce lipid, protein, and DNA nitration. The final oxidation product of NO is nitrite, which is increased in the CSF of children with acute bacterial meningitis (96) and in adults after severe TBI and associated with injury severity and death.

Oxidative stress may serve as a key initiator of cell death cascades in cardiac arrest, stroke, TBI, epilepsy, and CNS infection. Oxidation of the abundant mitochondrial lipid cardiolipin leads to the release of cytochrome-c from the mitochondrial membrane and may serve as a seminal event that links oxidative stress and the intrinsic pathway of apoptosis (7). DNA damage from peroxynitrite in both the nucleus and mitochondria may also serve to activate the enzyme poly(ADP-ribose) polymerase (PARP), which can result in energy failure via the PARP-mediated cellular suicide pathway.

CNS insults are associated with evidence of free radical production and loss of antioxidant defenses. After experimental asphyxia, decreases are seen in a variety of antioxidants, including ascorbate, glutathione, thiols, and α-tocopherol in hippocampus at 10 min after reperfusion (50). In experimental cardiac arrest, hyperoxic resuscitation plays a critical role in the level of oxidative stress (97). Oxidation of the key enzyme pyruvate dehydrogenase was dramatic, with resuscitation on F_{IO_2} of 1.0 but minimal after room air resuscitation, and a beneficial effect on hippocampal neuronal death was seen with room air resuscitation. In stroke, a randomized, controlled clinical trial (60) in over 1600 adults reported benefit on 90-day functional outcome using the free radical spin trap NXY-059 versus vehicle. This is the only therapy other than thrombolytics shown to be efficacious in a large clinical trial of stroke therapy and supports an important role for oxidative stress in focal cerebral ischemia. Marked depletion of endogenous antioxidants, including ascorbate, glutathione, protein thiols, and

total antioxidant reserve, was seen in the CSF from infants and children with severe TBI (8). Studies in experimental cerebral ischemia indicate that mild hypothermia blocks cytochrome-c release (108). Finally, increases in the concentrations of markers of oxidative stress in CSF have also been reported in infants and children with both acute bacterial meningitis and seizures (51,96).

Trophic factor withdrawal. Another important trigger for neuronal death is trophic factor withdrawal, and this process likely has relevance in the evolution of secondary damage after CNS insults in pediatric neurointensive care. Neurotrophins, such as nerve growth factor, brain-derived neurotrophic factor, basic fibroblast growth factor, and others, are constitutively produced by neurons and glia, bind to receptors on target neurons, and are essential to survival and plasticity. Loss of trophic input to a target neuron via death of, or damage to, neuronal input from another brain region can trigger death of the target neurons. This process has been reported in experimental CNS injury models and is often manifest by apoptotic death of neurons in a brain region remote from the injury site at several days after injury. Neuronal death is mediated by loss of endogenous neuroprotectant signals, such as phosphoinositide 3-kinase (PI3K) and protein kinase B (PKB), which are otherwise constitutively produced. The details of these pathways are discussed in the section on cellular signaling pathways in this chapter.

Neuronal Death Effector Pathways. In mature tissues, PCD requires initiation by either intracellular or extracellular signals. These signals have been characterized in vitro and are becoming better characterized in vivo (53,54,56,105) (**Fig. 52.9**).

Intrinsic (mitochondrial) pathway of apoptosis. Intracellular signaling appears to be initiated in mitochondria, triggered by disturbances in cellular homeostasis, such as ATP depletion, oxidative stress, or calcium fluxes. Mitochondrial dysfunction leads to egress of cytochrome-c from the inner mitochondrial membrane into the cytosol. Cytochrome-c release can be blocked by antiapoptotic members of the bcl-2 family (bcl-2, bcl-xL, Mcl-1) and promoted by proapoptotic bcl-2 family members (bax, bad, bid) (105). Cytochrome-c in the presence

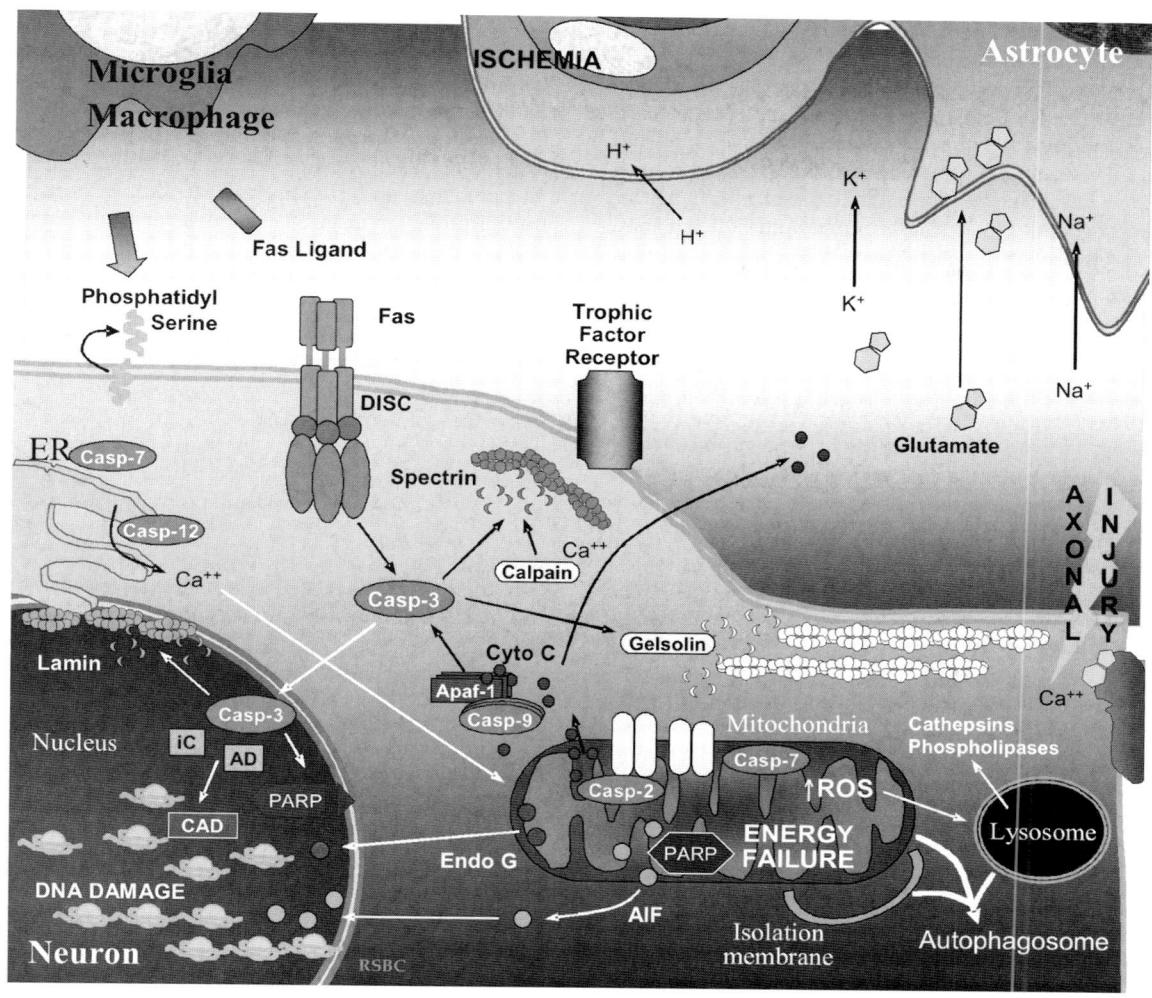

FIGURE 52.9. Neuronal death cascades resulting from necrosis, apoptosis [intrinsic, extrinsic, and apoptosis-inducing factor (AIF) pathways], and autophagy in CNS injury. Also see references 22, 53, and 105 for additional details. ER, endoplasmic reticulum; Casp, caspase; CAD, caspase activated deoxyribonuclease; Endo G, endonuclease G; ROS, reactive oxygen species; PARP, poly (ADP ribose) polymerase.

of dATP and a specific apoptotic-protease activating factor (Apaf-1) in cytosol activates the initiator cysteine protease caspase-9. Caspase-9 then activates the effector cysteine protease caspase-3, a key apoptosis effector that cleaves cytoskeletal proteins, DNA repair proteins, and activators of endonucleases (56). Evidence that supports a role for this pathway can be found across CNS insults, including global and focal ischemia, TBI, meningitis, and SE (17,33,41,71,105). Caspase inhibitors and mild hypothermia can attenuate neuronal death in experimental paradigms across these CNS insults (72,105,108).

Apoptosis-inducing factor (AIF) pathway. An additional intracellular cascade of PCD linked to mitochondrial injury is the AIF pathway (105). This caspase-independent pathway is activated by mitochondrial permeability transition and results in the release of AIF from the mitochondrial membrane. AIF release leads to large-scale DNA fragmentation (50–700 kilobase-pair in size). The AIF pathway is activated in experimental ischemia and TBI. A unique pathway for the induction of neuronal death via AIF release has been reported in experimental pneumococcal meningitis. This organism releases the toxin

pneumolysin, which creates membrane pores in lipid bilayers and triggers AIF release (13). To date, specific pharmacologic inhibitors of this pathway are lacking; however, this form of delayed neuronal death may represent an important therapeutic target.

Endoplasmic reticulum stress-triggered apoptosis. Another intracellular pathway that can trigger apoptosis independent of mitochondrial failure is through synthesis of unique proapoptotic factors associated with ER stress. The aforementioned reduction in ER Ca^{2+} concentration that results from IP3-mediated Ca^{2+} release from the ER leads to induction of proteins such as CHOP in neurons, which mediate apoptosis (95). Although additional details of this pathway remain to be clarified, selectively vulnerable CA1 hippocampal neurons are rich in IP3 receptors.

Extrinsic pathway apoptosis. Extracellular signaling of apoptosis occurs through the tumor necrosis factor (TNF) superfamily of cell surface death receptors, which include TNFR1 and Fas/Apo1/CD95 (reviewed in 105). Receptor-ligand binding of TNFR1–TNF-α or Fas-FasL promotes formation of a trimeric complex of TNF- or Fas-associated death domains, respectively. These death domains facilitate caspase recruitment. The proximity of multiple caspases (in this case, caspase-8) allows for activation of the effector cysteine protease, followed by activation of caspase-3, where the mitochondrial and cell-death receptor pathways converge. Clinical studies suggest that this mechanism may play a role in stroke and TBI. Fas and caspase-8 levels are increased in human cerebral contusions (106). Caspase-8 was seen predominantly in neurons.

Cellular signaling pathways. Neurotrophic factors, neurotransmitters, cytokines, and ROS activate multiple upstream signaling pathways linked to either pro-survival or pro-death activities (53). These receptors couple to signal transduction pathways, involving interactions and cross-talk between multiple serine/threonine and tyrosine protein kinase cascades. Many kinases involved in the cell-death process are serine/threonine protein kinases. Important participants in the cell-death cascades include the mitogen-activated protein kinases (MAPKs). MAPK cascades are complex and are mediated by successive protein kinases that sequentially activate each other by phosphorylation. They are linked to two key components of the cell-death cascade, jun kinase (JNK) and p38 MAPK (**Fig. 52.10**). JNK and p38 MAPK pathways activate caspase-3 (26). Activation of JNK leads to induction of pro-death genes, including FasL. The JNK increases p53 and Bax levels, which increase cell death. JNK and p38 function in different stress-signaling pathways, and both target similar nuclear transcription factors that can be activated by pro-death stimuli such as ROS (77). Studies in various injury models have documented changes in both JNK and p38 MAPK that may be related to cell death and functional impairment. MAPKs are also linked to survival signals through the extracellular signal-regulated kinase (ERK) pathway, highlighting the complex cross-talk between these cascades.

Several protein kinase cascades have a major survival role (**Fig. 52.10**). PI3-K, PKB, and protein kinase A (PKA) pathways are prototypic examples. PKB is also called akt; the complex nomenclature of these kinases has evolved across many disease processes. PI3K responds to neurotrophins and other pro-survival signals and activates PKB (76); PKB affects survival by a number of mechanisms, including the phosphorylation and inactivation of several pro-death mediators such as Bad. Bad, a member of the Bcl-2 family, is phosphorylated by PKB, resulting in Bad dissociation from Bcl-xL and binding to 14–3-3 proteins, thereby inhibiting cell death (24). cAMP-mediated activation of PKA can also lead to formation of the transcription factor cAMP response element binding protein (CREB), which is similarly associated with cell survival (48). Survival signals are exemplified by growth factors, cytokines, hormones, cell-cell interactions, and extracellular matrix adhesion molecules. Of course, inactivation of two pro-death members of the MAPK family, p38 and JNK/SAPK, has also been proposed as promoting survival by extracellular stimuli. Finally, activation of some PKC isoforms by PI3K can transduce pro-death signals, again highlighting the complexity of these kinase cascades. Thus, complex but important kinase pathways control neuronal death and plasticity. Recently, moderate hypothermia has been shown to preserve PKB activity in the brain after experimental cerebral ischemia (107), suggesting that this may mediate hypothermic neuroprotection. Further insight into these cascades may lead to the development of new therapies.

Poly(ADP-ribose) polymerase activation. Research has uncovered a unique cell death pathway related to activation of the enzyme PARP that plays a role in neuronal death in ischemia and TBI (29, reviewed in 55). PARP is found both in mitochondria and the nucleus and plays a homeostatic role in DNA repair in these two organelles. When activated by DNA damage, PARP catalytically adds poly(ADP ribose) units onto proteins in mitochondria and the nucleus, such as histones, to help direct DNA repair enzymes to sites of damage. However, a deleterious consequence of PARP activation in CNS injury is the consumption of large quantities of NAD, thus depleting mitochondrial energy stores. This paradoxic consequence of PARP activation has been labeled the "PARP cell suicide theory" and leads to mitochondrial failure and cell death, either from overwhelming energy failure or delayed neuronal death through release of cytochrome-c and/or AIF. This pathway may have clinical relevance, as PARP knock-out mice are highly protected from

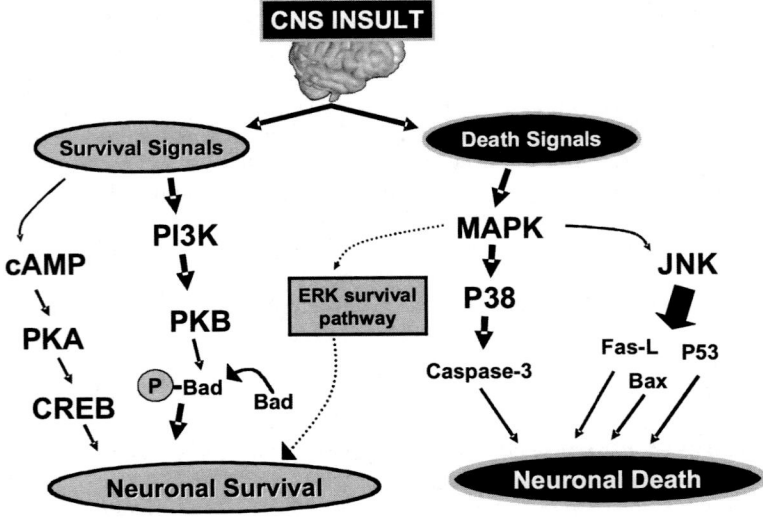

FIGURE 52.10. Cell survival and death signals in CNS injury. The protein kinase A and B pathways are associated with neuronal survival, while the MAPK pathway is associated generally with neuronal death. cAMP, cyclic adenosine monophosphate; PKA, protein kinase A; CREB, cAMP response element binding protein; PI3K, phosphoinositide 3 kinase; JNK, jun kinase; MAPK, mitogen-activated protein kinase pathway; FAS-L, fas ligand; ERK, extracellular signal-regulated kinase.

neuronal damage in experimental models of stroke and TBI (29, reviewed in 55).

Protease activation. In addition to the many consequences of Ca^{2+} homeostasis loss that have been discussed, increases in intracellular Ca^{2+} in neurons activates calpain proteases, which sets into motion a cascade of protease activation that has been referred to as the "calpain-cathepsin cascade" (103). Calpains (both mu and m isozymes) are located in dendritic regions and in axons and, when activated, cleave key cytoskeletal targets, such as spectrin, kinases, phosphatases, membrane receptors, and, importantly, lysosomes. Lysosomal rupture, believed to be mediated in part by calpains, leads to release of over 80 hydrolytic enzymes, of which cathepsins B, D, H, and L are believed to play a role in executing neuronal death. These pathways could have special importance in necrotic cascades. As discussed, failure or dysfunction of lysosomal degradation pathways may lead to an accumulation of autophagic vacuoles and result in cell death by autophagy.

Endogenous neuroprotectants. Studies have begun to define, in infants and children with CNS injury, the endogenous retaliatory response to these ischemic and excitotoxic insults. Due to space constraints, we focus here on selected examples of this cascade. The most extensive amount of clinical work on these pathways has been conducted in TBI (53,54) (**Fig. 52.2**).

Adenosine is an endogenous neuroprotectant produced in response to both ischemia and excitotoxicity. Adenosine antagonizes a number of events thought to mediate neuronal death (54). Breakdown of ATP leads to formation of adenosine, a purine nucleoside that decreases neuronal metabolism and increases CBF, among other mechanisms. Adenosine binding to A_1 receptors decreases excitation by increasing K^+ and Cl^- and decreasing Ca^{2+} conductances in the neuronal membrane. A_1 receptors are located on neurons in brain regions that are susceptible to injury (e.g., hippocampus) and are spatially associated with NMDA receptors. Thus, released adenosine minimizes excitotoxicity. Binding of adenosine to A_2 receptors (on cerebrovascular smooth muscle) causes vasodilation, although binding to A_{2a} receptors on neurons may be detrimental. In clinical studies, marked increases in CSF levels of adenosine have been shown in children with severe TBI, and brain interstitial levels of adenosine in adults with TBI were seen during episodes of jugular venous desaturation (secondary insults), thus supporting a role of adenosine as a "retaliatory" metabolite (54). Adenosine A_1 receptor knock-out mice develop lethal SE after experimental TBI, supporting an endogenous neuroprotectant effect (57).

Another endogenous neuroprotectant is HSP70, which is induced as part of the classic preconditioning response in brain and is increased in both CSF and brain tissue after severe TBI in children (53). HSP70 is believed to play an important role in optimizing protein folding as a molecular chaperone. It also inhibits proinflammatory signaling.

Bcl-2 is an important endogenous inhibitor of PCD in vitro (53). It is induced in experimental TBI and reduces cortical tissue loss. Bcl-2 is increased in injured brain after severe TBI in children (54). CSF levels of bcl-2 were increased approximately fourfold in TBI patients and associated with survival. Recent studies also suggest that nitrite may be a powerful cytoprotective molecule. Hypoxia-dependent bioactivation of nitrite reduces it to NO, S-nitrosothiols, N-nitrosamines, and iron-

nitrosylated heme proteins within 1–30 mins of reperfusion. These mediators appear to confer their protective effects on a number of systems (27). Thus, the brain mounts an important endogenous defense response to injury. Therapies designed to augment these pathways deserve further study.

Brain Injury Without Neuronal Death

It would be remiss to suggest that neuronal death is required for insults relevant to pediatric neurointensive care to produce important or even permanent impairment of neurologic function. Several processes that result from injury may lead to substantial functional impairments without cell death. These include synaptic damage, disturbances in cell signaling and glial-neuronal cross-talk, and alterations in neurotransmitter balance. Although these mechanisms are likely of principal importance to cognitive dysfunction in mild TBI, they are likely operating in damaged brain regions in severe TBI and may contribute to impaired recovery. For example, substantial synaptic loss in injured hippocampus and fiber degeneration remote from the impact has been reported in experimental models of TBI (38,87). These mechanisms may represent novel therapeutic targets in both the acute and chronic phases after injury. It is possible that these types of damage may be highly responsive to therapeutic interventions.

Brain Swelling

A unifying concept in brain injury is the occurrence of brain swelling. Cerebral swelling invariably develops, resulting from edema and/or increased cerebral blood volume (CBV), and can contribute to secondary ischemia from raised ICP, local compression, or the devastating consequences of herniation, as discussed in Chapter 56. Brain edema develops via three mechanisms: cellular swelling, BBB injury (vasogenic edema) (53–56), and/or osmolar swelling (**Fig. 52.11**).

Cellular Swelling

Astrocyte swelling. Cellular swelling, a term that has supplanted the traditional "cytotoxic edema," occurs predominantly in astrocyte foot processes and is less representative of a "toxic" rather than a homeostatic or mediator-driven process. For example, astrocyte-mediated reuptake of glutamate from the extracellular space is coupled to Na^+ and water accumulation. Similarly, acidosis, K^+, cytokines, and arachidonic acid mediate astrocyte swelling. The traditional concept of cytotoxic edema in neurons resulting from energy failure (the pump-leak model) is incomplete. Both perivascular and perineuronal astrocytes are involved (see Chapter 51). Cellular swelling is an important form of brain edema across insults but particularly so in ischemia and TBI. Cellular swelling may predominate after secondary insults. Using a model of diffuse TBI in rats, diffusion-weighted MRI was used to localize the increase in brain water (5). A decrease in the apparent diffuse coefficient after injury suggested predominantly cellular swelling, rather than vasogenic edema, in the development of intracranial hypertension.

Aquaporins. An additional molecular aspect of brain edema formation germane to astrocyte swelling that has recently been uncovered is the role of endogenous water channels called *aquaporins*. Aquaporins 1–9 represent a ubiquitous family of water channels that are integral membrane proteins that serve

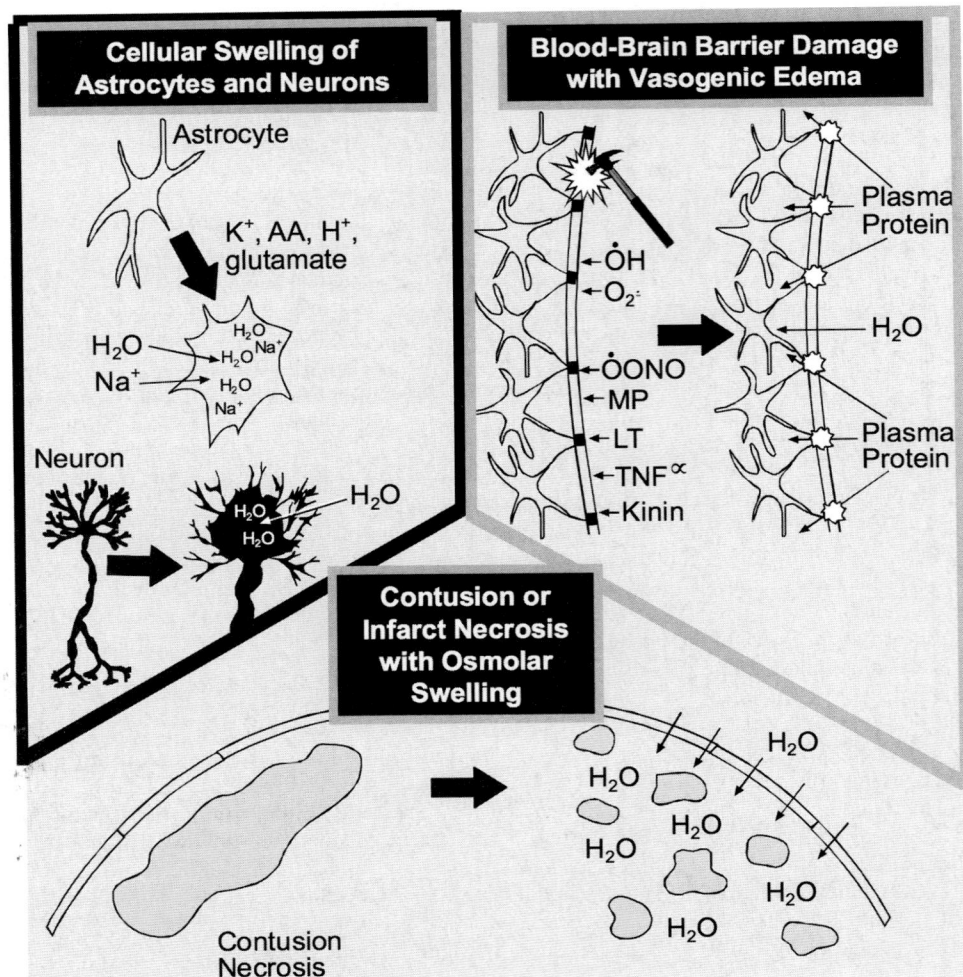

FIGURE 52.11. Three major mechanisms underlying the development of cerebral edema, including cellular swelling, BBB injury with vasogenic edema, and osmolar swelling that develops in both contusions and infarcts. AA, arachidonic acid; $O2^{-\cdot}$, superoxide anion; $ONOO\cdot$, peroxynitrite; $\cdot OH$, hydroxyl radical; MP, metalloproteinase; LT, leukotriene; TNF-α, tumor necrosis factor α.

as water transport pathways. For example, aquaporin-1 is involved in membrane transport of water across osmotic gradients, while aquaporins 4 and 9 are localized in astrocyte end-feet. Aquaporins also play an important role in production of CSF. Aquaporin-1 knock-out mice had markedly reduced ICP and improved survival after experimental brain injury (78). Astrocyte swelling may also play an important role in the pathogenesis of brain edema in CNS infections. Recent work in experimental meningitis has shown marked swelling of astrocyte foot processes that is mediated by aquaporin-4 (80). Aquaporin-4 knock-out mice exhibited substantially lower brain water content and ICP versus wild-type mice in experimental pneumococcal meningitis, supporting an important contribution of cellular swelling and water movement across the BBB even in meningitis. Thus, these water channels may represent a key new therapeutic target for control of raised ICP after TBI, ischemia, and CNS infections.

Vasogenic Edema

BBB permeability, with resultant vasogenic edema, can also contribute to secondary brain swelling; this is particularly true in CNS infections (70), stroke and, to some extent, in TBI. This mechanism is likely of less importance after cardiac arrest, although some studies of cardiac arrest in developing animals have suggested a role for BBB injury (89). Unfortunately, clini-

cal study of BBB permeability in pediatric neurointensive care has been limited.

In acute bacterial meningitis, the acute inflammatory cascade also contributes to BBB damage and includes cytokine-mediated induction of leukocyte-adhesion molecules, neutrophil accumulation, and related oxidative injury to vascular endothelium (70). In addition, an important role for matrix metalloproteinases (MMPs) has also been reported in experimental meningitis. MMPs are endoproteases that can degrade the extracellular matrix. CSF levels of MMPs were markedly upregulated and associated with poor outcome in children with acute bacterial meningitis (91). Similar increases in MMPs were not seen in viral meningitis (58). Hyaluronidase and pneumolysin also contribute to endothelial damage and BBB permeability.

Osmolar Swelling. A mechanism that appears to contribute greatly to the development of edema, particularly in TBI, is osmolar swelling in areas of contusion necrosis. Ironically, reconstitution of the injured BBB and/or development of an osmolar barrier around a necrotic focus may contribute to marked focal edema as the local osmolar load of the tissue increases, as macromolecules are degraded to constituents. This mechanism has been shown in adult TBI (49) and likely represents one of the underpinnings for the beneficial effects of osmolar

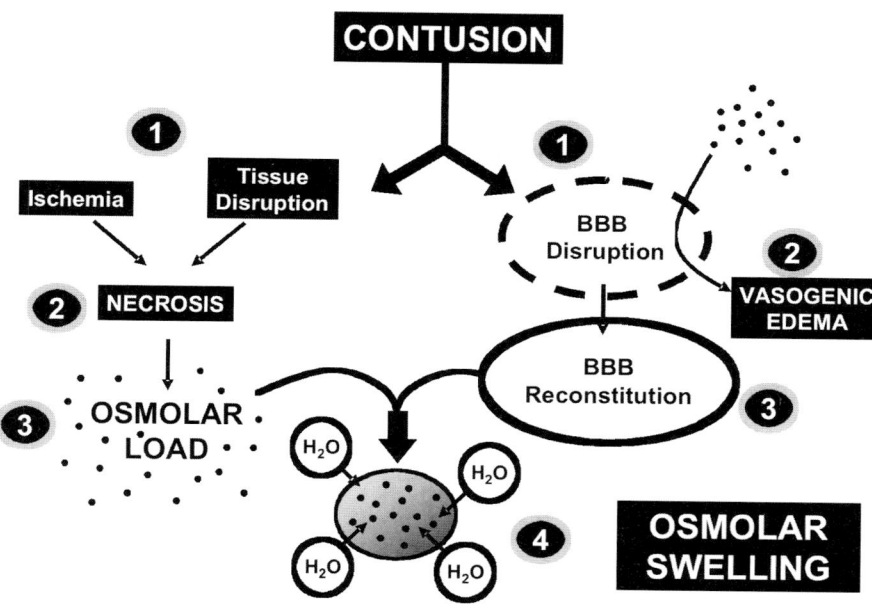

FIGURE 52.12. Temporal pathway involved in osmolar swelling in brain contusions or infarcts. Temporal profile shown by numbers 1–3. Necrotic brain regions generate a large osmolar load as they are degraded to constituent molecules. Early after the insult, BBB damage allows influx of additional proteins. With time, usually within 24–72 hrs, an osmolar barrier reforms, and water is then osmotically drawn from the surrounding brain regions into the contused or infarcted area resulting in expansion of the mass lesion, an event often appreciated on follow-up CT of the head in affected patients. BBB, blood-brain barrier.

therapy in the setting of cerebral contusion (**Fig. 52.12**). Osmolar swelling also likely underlies the development of compromising or potentially fatal mass lesions in the evolution of hemispheric stroke.

Mixed Edema Pictures. Vasogenic edema, cellular swelling from glutamate and hydrogen ion (H^+) uptake and opening of aquaporin channels, and tissue swelling from increased local osmolality all lead to brain edema in TBI. In asphyxial cardiac arrest, it is probably astrocyte swelling and vasogenic edema that predominate. In stroke, all three of these mechanisms likely operate, depending on the timing and location. For example, in stroke, early astrocyte swelling may occur in the infarct core, followed by vasogenic edema in injured but perfused penumbral regions, and then delayed osmolar swelling of the infarct as the macromolecules are degraded. In meningitis, vasogenic edema and cellular swelling likely contribute.

Cerebral Blood Volume. A role of increased CBV in brain swelling has long been suggested (54), particularly in pediatric brain injury. However, this notion was challenged in a comprehensive study in adult patients with severe TBI (68). Brain tissue water was increased in 76 adults with severe TBI; however, CBV was generally reduced. It is possible that increases in CBV contribute to secondary cerebral swelling in some patients; however, based on this study, the predominant mechanism of posttraumatic brain swelling is most likely edema rather than vascular engorgement. Similar studies should be conducted in children in pediatric neurointensive care, as hyperemia has been suggested to play a greater role in pediatric versus adult brain injury (54). A role for hyperemia in the pathogenesis of cerebral swelling in meningitis is controversial but is suggested in some studies. When an increase in CBV is seen after CNS injury, it may contribute to raised ICP and result from local increases in cerebral glycolysis—"hyperglycolysis" (9). In regions with increases in glutamate levels, such as in contusions, increased glycolysis is seen because astrocyte uptake of glutamate is coupled to glucose utilization. Hyperglycolysis

may also mediate a coupled increase in CBF and CBV and resultant local brain swelling. As glutamate uptake by astrocytes is coupled to Na^+ and water uptake, local cellular swelling is also seen (**Fig. 52.13**).

Additional clinical studies of brain swelling, edema, BBB permeability, and CBV are needed in infants and children with critical CNS insults. Also, as MRI and MR spectroscopy methods continue to develop and become applied to critically ill patients, our knowledge of the mechanisms involved in cerebral swelling should greatly advance. Although neuronal death is the key downstream event in insults relevant to pediatric neurointensive care, brain swelling (and the resultant raised ICP) is still the principal target for titration of therapy.

Inflammation and Regeneration

Except in the setting of CNS infections, inflammation traditionally was thought to be limited in the brain, as it was considered an immunologically privileged organ. However, that notion has changed greatly over the past 20 years. Currently, three major components are involved in the CNS inflammatory response to PICU-relevant insults: leukocytes, microglia, and regeneration. Contributions to secondary damage in the evolution of injury can be mediated by circulating leukocytes in the inflammatory response. However, an endogenous inflammatory response mediated by microglia—the macrophages of the CNS—along with neurons and astrocytes, has been recognized. Finally, the inflammatory response appears to have a delayed beneficial role, across insults, in the signaling of regenerative processes and neurogenesis. The contribution of each of these components to the evolution of damage and recovery appears to vary importantly with the specific insult.

Role of Inflammation in Secondary Injury. CNS infections are associated with robust acute inflammation, as discussed previously in the section on vasogenic edema. However, the inflammatory process also makes important contributions in stroke and TBI (4,53,54). Nuclear factor (NF)-κB activation, TNF-α, IL-1β, eicosanoids, neutrophils, and macrophages contribute

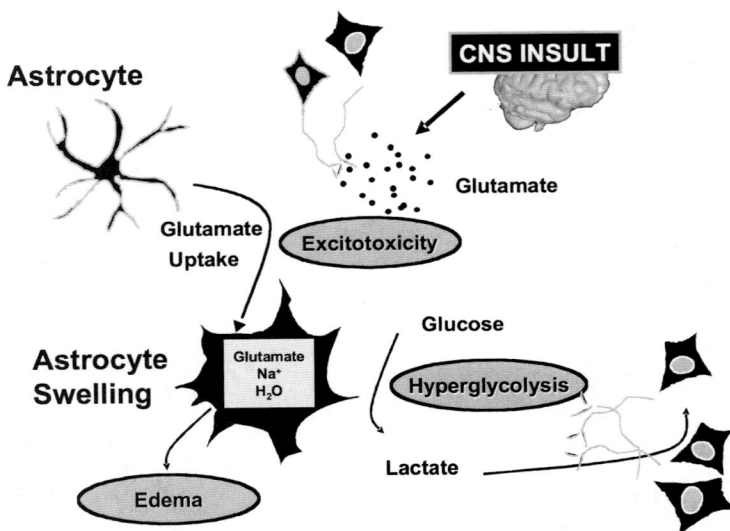

Astrocyte

Astrocyte Swelling

FIGURE 52.13. Cartoon depicting the phenomenon of "hyperglycolysis" and its potential relationship to brain swelling. In injured brain regions, astrocyte uptake of glutamate is coupled to Na^+ and water uptake and resultant astrocyte swelling. This process is exclusively dependent on glucose utilization by astrocytes, with local lactate generation. This lactate may either serve as a fuel for neurons or is washed out. If this local increase in glucose utilization is coupled to perfusion, it can result in an increase in CBV and thus exacerbate brain swelling by two mechanisms—astrocyte swelling and increased CBV.

to both secondary damage and repair. Clinical evidence for inflammatory cascade participation in PICU-relevant CNS injury has been shown best in TBI. Consistent with a role for IL-1β in the evolution of tissue damage in human TBI, Western analysis was performed on brain samples surgically resected from adults with refractory raised ICP secondary to severe contusion (21). IL-1–converting enzyme was activated, as evidenced by specific cleavage in patients with TBI. IL-1–converting enzyme activation, critical to the production of IL-1β, was not detected in patients who died of non-CNS etiologies, supporting the production of IL-1β, a pivotal proinflammatory mediator, in the injured brain in humans. A number of cytokines, including IL-6, IL-8, and IL-10, also increase in CSF after severe TBI in children (54). Contusion and local tissue necrosis, such as infarction in stroke, trigger upregulation of leukocyte-adhesion molecules and neutrophil influx, with additional secondary tissue damage. Neutrophil influx is accompanied by increases in brain iNOS levels, which can be detrimental early after injury, via NO production and its reaction with superoxide anion to produce peroxynitrite, as previously described. Evidence for this pathway in the human brain includes upregulation of iNOS in brain tissue in stroke (32) and increases in CSF levels of nitrites and nitrates after TBI. Macrophage infiltration then follows, with activation of resident microglia, both of which peak between 24 and 72 hrs (54). The circulating and endogenous acute and subacute inflammatory processes in the brain contribute to oxidative and nitrative stress and protease activation, with resultant BBB and neuronal injury.

The contribution of inflammation to cardiac arrest is more speculative. Traditional inflammatory pathways, such as leukocyte influx, do not appear to play an important role. However, endogenous inflammatory pathways may be important. NFκB is activated in selectively vulnerable CA1 neurons after experimental global cerebral ischemia (23), and administration of an NFκB decoy attenuates neuronal damage. However, hippocampal neurons from mice that lack the p50 subunit of NFκB show enhanced excitotoxic injury (104), suggesting a protective role. Similarly, although TNF-α is rapidly upregulated in mouse hippocampus after transient global cerebral ischemia, TNF-α gene-deficient mice do not have reduced damage (71).

Role of Inflammation in Repair and Regeneration. As indicated, possible beneficial aspects of inflammation have been observed in the CNS, particularly during the subacute or chronic injury phases. Two prototypic examples of the biphasic role of inflammation in CNS injury are seen when examining the role of TNF-α in experimental TBI (88). Mice deficient in TNF-α exhibit reduced brain edema and improved functional outcome (versus wild-type) early after TBI, supporting a detrimental role of this proinflammatory cytokine early after injury. However, the long-term consequences of TNF-α deficiency on functional and histologic outcome are detrimental, supporting a beneficial role for TNF-α in recovery and repair. For TNF-α, the transition from a beneficial to detrimental role occurs between 2 and 7 days after injury. Similarly, despite a detrimental role for iNOS early after cerebral ischemia (100), iNOS-deficient mice show impaired long-term outcome, versus controls, in experimental TBI (54). iNOS is important in neurogenesis and wound healing (18).

Regeneration and plasticity play important roles in mediating beneficial long-term effects on recovery, and these responses are linked to inflammation. Macrophage infiltration and differentiation of endogenous microglia into resident macrophages may link inflammation and regeneration, with elaboration of a number of trophic factors (e.g., nerve growth factor among others). A link has been reported between IL-6 and nerve growth factor production (59).

It remains unclear whether anti-inflammatory therapies will improve outcome in clinical CNS injury. If inhibition of the inflammatory response is considered, exacerbation of infection risk must also be anticipated, and any deleterious consequences on the link between inflammation and regeneration must be addressed. Finally, the potential role of an interaction between systemic aspects of inflammation and neuroinflammation could be important but remains to be explored.

Axonal Injury

Axonal injury plays an important role in TBI, and perinatal brain injury and white matter injury may also be important in stroke. Traumatic axonal injury (TAI) is the most established type of white matter damage in PICU-relevant CNS insults. The

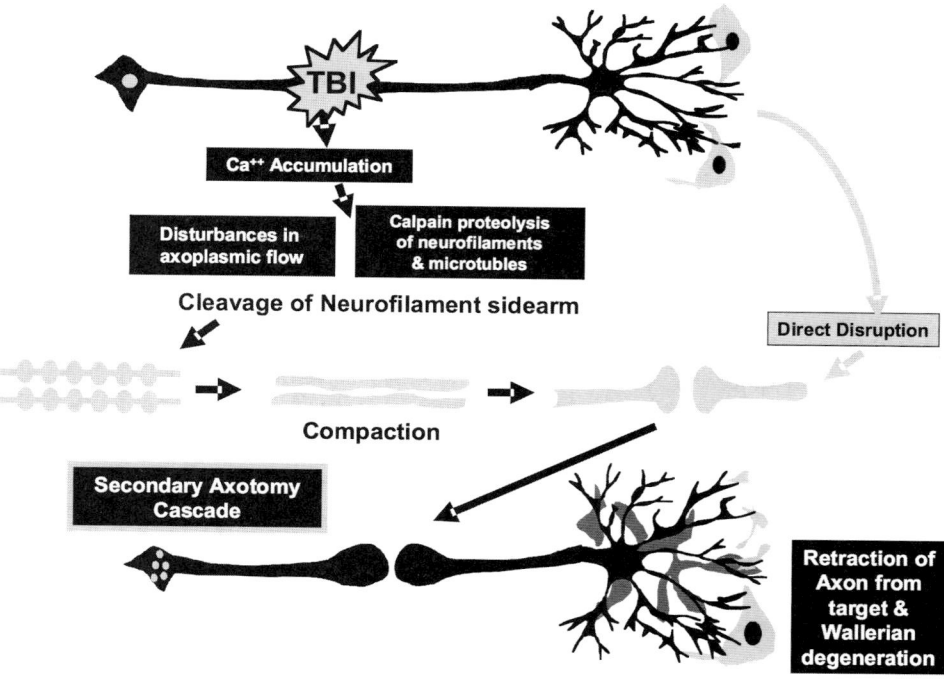

FIGURE 52.14. Cascades of axonal injury seen in either TBI or cerebral ischemia. Direct disruption of axons can occur in TBI, as shown on the right side of the figure. Believed to be more important, however, are two cascades of secondary axotomy related to either disturbances in axoplasmic flow or calcium-mediated proteolytic events, resulting in neurofilament compaction. These cascades may be responsive to some therapies, similar to those used to target neuronal death.

classic view that TAI occurs due to immediate physical shearing is represented primarily in severe injury, in which frank axonal tears occur. However, recent experimental studies suggest that TAI occurs by a delayed process termed "secondary axotomy" (**Fig. 52.14**) (84). Two hypothetical sequences have attempted to explain secondary axotomy, one attributing axolemmal permeability and calcium influx as the initiating event, the other suggesting a direct cytoskeletal abnormality that impairs axoplasmic flow (31,84). It has been posited that both forms of reactive axonal swelling take place but in different proportions, depending on the severity of injury. Superimposed on these theories is the finding that hypoxic-ischemic insults can also produce axonal swelling that resembles retraction balls. As a result, differing as well as unifying theories for axonal injuries in brain injury have been proposed (53). Common mechanistic features include focal ion flux, calcium dysregulation, and mitochondrial and cytoskeletal dysfunction. TAI contributes to the morbidity after TBI. Studies in experimental TBI models have shown that hypothermia and cyclosporin A can reduce TAI (14,15). Whether or not these therapies can minimize axonal damage in other CNS insults is uncertain. Another form of injury to white matter relates to the vulnerability of oligodendrocytes to excitotoxic injury from glutamate or other EAAs. However, the contribution of this pathway remains to be determined.

Mechanisms of Enhanced Vulnerability of Injured Brain

Hypotension and Hypoxemia

The injured brain is extremely vulnerable to secondary physiologic derangements that occur in the field, emergency department, or ICU, and hypotension and hypoxemia have

received the most investigation (18). For example, hemorrhagic shock exacerbates intracranial hypertension early after experimental TBI and worsens long-term functional outcome. The blood pressure threshold varies, depending on the injury severity and duration, but some reports suggest that hemorrhage with even minimal blood pressure reductions can be deleterious (69). Similarly, hypoxemia to $Pa\,O_2$ levels between 40 and 50 mm Hg for periods as short at 30 min can exacerbate neuronal death in experimental models of TBI. The period of enhanced vulnerability of the injured brain is not clearly defined; however, it is well described along the entire continuum of care in the critically ill. The mechanisms that underlie enhanced vulnerability are likely multifactorial and may differ over time. In the initial minutes to hours after cardiac arrest, TBI, and stroke, CBF is compromised, while metabolic demands are increased. Mechanical factors (e.g., thrombosis, vascular disruption, or vascular compromise from glial swelling), biochemical/molecular mechanisms (e.g., loss of endothelial NOS), or increases in levels of vasoconstrictors (e.g., endothelin-1) may mediate the inability of the vasculature to respond to additional challenges such as hypotension or hypoxemia. Similar mechanisms may also underlie the frequently observed loss of CBF blood pressure autoregulation that is seen in some insults (e.g., TBI). Increased metabolic demands early after these insults are substantial and result from both direct excitation of neurons, clinical or subclinical seizures, and increases in glucose utilization from glycolytic demands of astrocytes in EAA reuptake and mitochondrial dysfunction. During more delayed periods, such as in the ICU, the enhanced vulnerability of injured brain to secondary insults is typified by studies showing that a single jugular venous desaturation to <50% in adults with severe TBI doubled mortality rate (37). Enhanced vulnerability of the injured brain during the ICU phase may result from mechanisms other than those seen during acute injury, as cerebral metabolic demands several days after the insult are generally reduced. The most likely candidate for enhanced vulnerability during this phase is concomitant brain swelling, which generally peaks between 24 and 72 hrs. Hypotension or hypoxemia, even within the autoregulatory range, results in compensatory vasodilation with an increase in CBV, further increasing ICP and potentially leading to a vicious cycle. Compromised CBF can also impair protein syntheses as regeneration is beginning. Other mechanisms may also be important. Progressive loss of endogenous antioxidant defenses in CSF was shown over several days in children with severe TBI (8). This loss would place the injured brain at heightened risk for oxidative damage from an ischemia-reperfusion event. Finally, persistently increased levels of lactate, seen even weeks after brain injury in infants and children, may reflect chronic mitochondrial dysfunction or failure, which may represent an important underpinning for enhanced vulnerability of the brain to second insults in the PICU.

Hyperthermia

In experimental models of ischemia or TBI, hyperthermia has consistently been shown to exacerbate damage. Hyperthermia-mediated exacerbation of secondary brain injury is marked at the time of injury, but has been reported even days after experimental brain injury (3). The biochemical and molecular mechanisms involved have not been fully elucidated; however, exacerbation of the inflammatory response may be involved. Heightened metabolic demands in the injured brain with an inability to compensate with an appropriate increase in CBF could also be occurring. These experimental findings have served to support the need for fever prevention after cardiac arrest, stroke, and TBI, although this is less clear in CNS infections.

Hypoglycemia and Hyperglycemia

The vulnerability of the normal brain to hypoglycemia is well described in the classical experimental brain-injury literature (47). Using an insulin clamp in primates to produce hypoglycemia, a blood glucose level of 20 mg/dL sustained for 5 hrs produced severe neurologic injury and coma. Recent clinical data have suggested enhanced vulnerability to hypoglycemia in the injured brain; this would certainly be anticipated, as endogenous protective mechanisms, such as vasodilation, are often compromised after cardiac arrest, stroke, and TBI. Regional microdialysis measurements of interstitial brain glucose levels in adults with severe TBI have begun to shed some light on this issue. Brain glucose levels can reach critically low values after TBI (98). This finding may be particularly true in pericontusional brain regions in TBI, where astrocyte uptake of glutamate and mitochondrial dysfunction occur (9). Astrocyte-dependent homeostatic processes, such as uptake of excitatory neurotransmitters and pH regulation, are dependent on glycolytic rather than oxidative metabolism. Tight glucose control using insulin to achieve a serum glucose level between 90 and 120 mg/dL was associated with more frequent, critically low brain interstitial glucose levels than when serum glucose concentration was more loosely maintained at <150 mg/dL. Also concerning was the fact that tight glucose control was associated with increases in brain interstitial levels of glutamate and the lactate:pyruvate ratio, suggesting exacerbation of metabolic failure. Thus, it might be advisable to avoid tight glucose control in patients with brain injury, in favor of a more conservative approach.

Although care must be taken to avoid hypoglycemia after CNS insults, it is also well recognized that hyperglycemia can exacerbate CNS injury. This event has been most thoroughly investigated in experimental global cerebral ischemia, in which blood glucose concentrations >180 mg/dL achieved before the insult substantially exacerbate damage (62). The mechanisms involved in this exacerbation of ischemic brain injury by hyperglycemia include worsened brain swelling by lactate-mediated osmolar effects, along with greater local brain tissue acidosis following enhanced iron-catalyzed lipid peroxidation. It appears that before or after brain injury, marked hyperglycemia (>180 mg/dL) should be avoided or treated. Additional study of brain tissue glucose levels, as assessed by microdialysis, along with a study of regional glucose metabolism by PET are necessary to provide further guidance on optimal postinjury glucose management.

CONCLUSIONS AND FUTURE DIRECTIONS

Mechanisms involved in the evolution of secondary brain injury after CNS insults relevant to pediatric critical care medicine have been reviewed. Particular attention has been paid to studies at the bedside. Our understanding of the biochemical, cellular, and molecular responses has progressed following the application of molecular biology methods to human models. Future work should integrate these findings with bedside physiology and an improved assessment of outcome. Novel imaging and diagnostic methods, particularly MRI and MR spectroscopy, must be coupled with biochemical and molecular methods to clarify the mechanisms involved in secondary damage and the effects of novel therapies

KEY POINTS

- The two distinct types of secondary injury are (a) evolution of damage mediated by endogenous secondary injury cascades and (b) damage that results from secondary insults (e.g., hypotension) in the field, emergency department, or ICU.
- Ischemia is an important injury mechanism that plays varying roles across the spectrum of PICU-relevant CNS insults.
- Key cell-death pathways after CNS injury include necrosis, apoptosis, and autophagy. Some cells display mixed phenotypes with characteristics of two or more of these pathways.
- Key initiators of damage in the evolution of secondary injury include energy failure, excitotoxicity, oxidative stress, and trophic factor withdrawal.
- Apoptosis after CNS injury can result from activation of a number of mechanisms, including (a) an intrinsic (mitochondrial) pathway, (b) an apoptosis-inducing factor pathway, (c) an endoplasmic reticulum stress pathway, and (d) an extrinsic (extracellular signaling) pathway.
- An endogenous neuroprotectant response to CNS injury occurs and includes a variety of pathways: adenosine, heat shock proteins, and a variety of antiapoptotic proteins such as Bcl-2.

- Brain swelling after CNS injury results from cellular swelling, vasogenic edema, osmolar swelling, mixed edema patterns, and/or an increase in cerebral blood volume.
- Inflammation after CNS injury plays an important role in exacerbation of secondary damage and in initiating signals for repair and regeneration.
- Axonal injury involves a process that includes secondary axotomy after axonal stretch and/or ischemia.
- Key secondary extracerebral insults that adversely impact outcome across CNS injury etiologies include hypotension, hypoxemia, hyperthermia, and hypoglycemia/hyperglycemia.

ACKNOWLEDGMENTS

We thank the National Institutes of Health [NS38087 (PK), NS38620 (RC), NS 42648 (LJ), and NS30318 (PK, RC)], Centers for Disease Control (PK), and the American Heart Association (HB) for support. We thank Dr. R. Garman for assistance with **Figure 52.5**.

References

1. Ashwal S, Holshouser BA, Shu SK, et al. Predictive value of proton magnetic resonance spectroscopy in pediatric closed head injury. *Pediatr Neurol* 2000;23:114–25.
2. Ashwal S, Stringer W, Tomasi L, et al. Cerebral blood flow and carbon dioxide reactivity in children with bacterial meningitis. *J Pediatr* 1990;117:523–30.
3. Baena RC, Busto R, Dietrich WD, et al. Hyperthermia delayed by 24 hours aggravates neuronal damage in rat hippocampus following global ischemia. *Neurology* 1997;48:768–73.
4. Barone FC, Feuerstein GZ. Inflammatory mediators and stroke: New opportunities for novel therapeutics. *J Cereb Blood Flow Metab* 1999;19:819–34.
5. Barzo P, Marmarou A, Fatouros P, et al. Contribution of vasogenic and cellular edema to traumatic brain swelling measured by diffusion-weighted imaging. *J Neurosurg* 1997;87:900–7.
6. Bayir H. Reactive oxygen species. *Crit Care Med* 2005;33(12 Suppl):S498–S501.
7. Bayir H, Fadeel B, Palladino MJ, et al. Apoptotic interactions of cytochrome c: Redox flirting with anionic phospholipids within and outside of mitochondria. *Biochim Biophys Acta* 2006;1757:648–59.
8. Bayir H, Kagan VE, Tyurina YY, et al. Assessment of antioxidant reserve and oxidative stress in cerebrospinal fluid after severe traumatic brain injury in infants and children. *Pediatr Res* 2001;51:571–8.
9. Bergsneider M, Hovda DA, Shalmon E, et al. Cerebral hyperglycolysis following severe traumatic brain injury in humans: A positron emission tomography study. *J Neurosurg* 1997;86:241–51.
10. Bernard SA, Gray TW, Buist MD, et al. Treatment of comatose survivors of out-of-hospital cardiac arrest with induced hypothermia. *N Engl J Med* 2002;346:557–63.
11. Brambrink AM, Martin LJ, Hanley DF, et al. Effects of the AMPA receptor antagonist NBQX on outcome of newborn pigs after asphyxic cardiac arrest. *J Cereb Blood Flow Metab* 1999;19:927–38.
12. Braun JS, Novak R, Herzog KH, et al. Neuroprotection by a caspase inhibitor in acute bacterial meningitis. *Nature Med* 1999;5:298–302.
13. Braun JS, Sublett JE, Freyer D, et al. Pneumococcal pneumolysin and H$_2$O$_2$ mediate brain cell apoptosis during meningitis. *J Clin Invest* 2002;109:19–27.
14. Buki A, Koizumi H, Povlishock JT. Moderate posttraumatic hypothermia decreases early calpain-mediated proteolysis and concomitant cytoskeletal compromise in traumatic axonal injury. *Exp Neurol* 1999;159:319–28.
15. Buki A, Okonkwo DO, Povlishock JT. Postinjury cyclosporin A administration limits axonal damage and disconnection in traumatic brain injury. *J Neurotrauma* 1999;16:511–21.
16. Bullock R, Zauner A, Woodward JJ, et al. Factors affecting excitatory amino acid release following severe human head injury. *J Neurosurg* 1998;89:507–18.
17. Chan PH. Mitochondria and neuronal death/survival signaling pathways in cerebral ischemia. *Neurochem Res* 2004;29:1943–9.
18. Chesnut RM, Marshall LF, Klauber MR, et al. The role of secondary brain injury in determining outcome from severe head injury. *J Trauma* 1993;34:216–22.
19. Chinopoulos C, Adam-Vizi V. Calcium, mitochondria and oxidative stress in neuronal pathology. Novel aspects of an enduring theme. *FEBS J* 2006;273:433–50.
20. Chu CT. Autophagic stress in neuronal injury and disease. *J Neuropathol Exp Neurol* 2006;65:423–32.
21. Clark RSB, Kochanek PM, Chen M, et al. Increases in Bcl-2 and cleavage of caspase-1 and caspase-3 in human brain after head injury. *FASEB J* 1999;13:813–21.
22. Clark RSB, Lai Y, Hickey RW, et al. Hypoxic-ischemic Encephalopathy: Pathobiology and Therapy of the Postresuscitation Syndrome in Children. In: Fuhrman BP, Zimmerman J, eds. *Pediatric Critical Care*, 3rd ed. Philadelphia: Mosby Elsevier, 2006;904–28.
23. Clemens JA, Stephenson DT, Dixon EP, et al. Global cerebral ischemia activates nuclear factor-kappa B prior to evidence of DNA fragmentation. *Brain Res Mol Brain Res* 1997;48:187–96.
24. Coffer PJ, Jin J, Woodgett JR. Protein kinase B (c-Akt): A multifunctional mediator of phosphatidylinositol 3-kinase activation. *Biochem J* 1998;335:1–13.
25. Colbourne F, Sutherland GR, Auer RN. Electron microscopic evidence against apoptosis as the mechanism of neuronal death in global ischemia. *J Neurosci* 1999;10:4200–10.
26. Cross TG, Scheel-Toellner D, Henriquez NV, et al. Serine/threonine protein kinases and apoptosis. *Exp Cell Res* 2000;256:34–41.
27. Duranski MR, Greer JJ, Dejam A, et al. Cytoprotective effects of nitrite during in vivo ischemia-reperfusion of the heart and liver. *J Clin Invest* 2005;115:1232–40.
28. Edwards AD, Yue X, Cox P, et al. Apoptosis in the brains of infants suffering intrauterine cerebral injury. *Pediatr Res* 1997;42:684–9.
29. Eliasson MJ, Sampei K, Mandir AS, et al. Poly(ADP-ribose) polymerase gene disruption renders mice resistant to cerebral ischemia. *Nat Med* 1997;3:1089–95.
30. Engelhorn T, Doerfler A, Weise J et al. Cerebral perfusion alterations during the acute phase of experimental generalized status epilepticus: Prediction of survival by using perfusion-weighted MR imaging and histopathology. *AJNR Am J Neuroradiol* 2005;26:1563–70.
31. Fitzpatrick MO, Maxwell WL, Graham DI: The role of the axolemma in the initiation of traumatically induced axonal injury. *J Neurol Neurosurg Psychiatry* 1998;64:285–7.
32. Forster C, Clark HB, Ross ME, et al. Inducible nitric oxide synthase expression in human cerebral infarcts. *Acta Neuropathol* 1999;97:215–20.
33. Gianinazzi C, Grandgirard D, Imboden H, et al. Caspase-3 mediates hippocampal apoptosis in pneumococcal meningitis. *Acta Neuropathol* 2003;105:499–507.
34. Giza CC, Maria NS, Hovda DA. N-methyl-d-aspartate receptor subunit changes after traumatic injury to the developing brain. *J Neurotrauma* 2006;23:950–61.
35. Golarai G, Greenwood AC, Feeney DM, et al. Physiological and structural evidence for hippocampal involvement in persistent seizure susceptibility after traumatic brain injury. *J Neurosci* 2001;21:8523–37.
36. Goodman JC, Valadka AB, Gopinath SP, et al. Lactate and excitatory amino acids measured by microdialysis are decreased by pentobarbital coma in head-injured patients. *J Neurotrauma* 1996;13:549–56.
37. Gopinath SP, Robertson CS, Contant CF, et al. Jugular venous desaturation and outcome after head injury. *J Neurol Neurosurg Psychiatry* 1994;57:717–23.
38. Hall ED, Sullivan PG, Gibson TR, et al. Spatial and temporal characteristics of neurodegeneration after controlled cortical impact in mice: More than a focal brain injury. *J Neurotrauma* 2005;22:252–65.
39. Haring HP, Rotzer HK, Reindl H, et al. Time course of cerebral blood flow velocity in central nervous system infections. A transcranial Doppler sonography study. *Arch Neurol* 1993;50:98–101.
40. Hauck W, Samlalsingh-Parker J, Glibetic M, et al. Deregulation of cyclooxygenase and nitric oxide synthase gene expression in the inflammatory cascade triggered by experimental group B streptococcal meningitis in the newborn brain and cerebral microvessels. *Semin Perinatol* 1999;23:20–26.
41. Henshall DC, Clark RS, Adelson PD, et al. Alterations in bcl-2 and caspase gene family protein expression in human temporal lobe epilepsy. *Neurology* 2000;55:250–7.
42. Holmes GL, Ben-Ari Y. The neurobiology and consequences of epilepsy in the developing brain. *Pediatr Res* 2001;49:320–5.
43. Hossman KA. Pathophysiology and therapy of experimental stroke. *Cell Mol Neurobiol* 2006 26;1055–81.
44. Hypothermia after Cardiac Arrest Study Group. Mild therapeutic hypothermia to improve the neurologic outcome after cardiac arrest. *N Engl J Med* 2002;346:549–56.
45. Ikonomidou C, Bosch F, Miksa M, et al. Blockade of NMDA receptors and apoptotic neurodegeneration in the developing brain. *Science* 1999;283:70–4.
46. Jenkins LW, Povlishock JT, Lewelt W, et al. The role of postischemic recirculation in the development of ischemic neuronal injury following complete cerebral ischemia. *Acta Neuropathol* 1981;55:205–20.

47. Kahn KJ, Myers RE. Insulin-induced Hypoglycaemia in the Non-human Primate. I. Clinical consequences. In: Brierley JB, Meldrum BS, eds. *Brain Hypoxia*. London: Spastics International Medical, 1971:185–94.

48. Kaplan DR, Miller FD. Neurotrophin signal transduction in the nervous system. *Curr Opin Neurobiol* 2000;10:381–91.

49. Katayama Y, Kawamata T. Edema fluid accumulation within necrotic brain tissue as a cause of the mass effect of cerebral contusion in head trauma patients. *Acta Neurochir Suppl* 2003;86:323–7.

50. Katz L, Callaway C, Kagan V, et al. Electron spin resonance measure of brain antioxidant activity during ischemia/reperfusion. *Neuroreport* 1998;9:1587–93.

51. Kawakami Y, Monobe M, Kuwabara K, et al. A comparative study of nitric oxide, glutathione, and glutathione peroxidase activities in cerebrospinal fluid from children with convulsive diseases/children with aseptic meningitis. *Brain Dev* 2006;28:243–6.

52. Kirino T. Delayed neuronal death in the gerbil hippocampus following ischemia. *Brain Res* 1982;239:57–69.

53. Kochanek PM, Clark RSB, Jenkins LW. Traumatic Brain Injury: Pathobiology. In: Zafonte R, Zasler N, eds. *Brain Injury Medicine*, New York: Demos Medical Publishing, 2006.

54. Kochanek PM, Clark RSB, Ruppel RA, et al. Biochemical, cellular and molecular mechanisms in the evolution of secondary damage after severe traumatic brain injury in infants and children: Lessons learned from the bedside. *Pediatr Crit Care Med* 2000;1:4–19.

55. Kochanek PM, Clark RSB, Ruppel R, et al. Cerebral Resuscitation after Traumatic Brain Injury and Cardiac Arrest in Infants and Children in the New Millennium. In: Orlowski JP, ed. *Pediatric Clinics of North America*. Philadelphia: W.B. Saunders, Vol. 2001;48(3):661–81.

56. Kochanek PM, Forbes ML, Ruppel R, et al. Severe traumatic brain injury in infants and children. In: Fuhrman BP, Zimmerman J, eds. *Pediatric Critical Care, 3rd ed*. Philadelphia: Mosby Elsevier, 2006:1595–617.

57. Kochanek PM, Vagni VA, Janesko KL, et al. Adenosine A1 receptor knockout mice develop lethal status epilepticus after experimental traumatic brain injury. *J Cereb Blood Flow Metab* 2006;26:565–75.

58. Kolb SA, Lahrtz F, Paul R, et al. Matrix metalloproteinases and tissue inhibitors of metalloproteinases in viral meningitis: Upregulation of MMP-9 and TIMP-1 in cerebrospinal fluid. *J Neuroimmunol* 1998;84:143–50.

59. Kossmann T, Stahel PF, Lenzlinger PM, et al. Interleukin-8 released into the cerebrospinal fluid after brain injury is associated with blood-brain barrier dysfunction and nerve growth factor production. *J Cereb Blood Flow Metab* 1997;17:280–9.

60. Lees KR, Zivin JA, Ashwood T, et al. Stroke-Acute Ischemic NXY Treatment (SAINT I) Trial Investigators. *N Engl J Med* 2006;354:588–600.

61. Levin HS, Aldrich EF, Saydjari C, et al. Severe head injury in children: Experience of the Traumatic Coma Data Bank. *Neurosurgery* 1992;31:435–44.

62. Li PA, Siesjö BK. Role of hyperglycaemia-related acidosis in ischaemic brain damage. *Acta Physiol Scand* 1997;161:567–80.

63. Li Y, Chopp M, Jiang N, et al. Temporal profile of in situ DNA fragmentation after transient middle cerebral artery occlusion in the rat. *J Cereb Blood Flow Metab* 1995;15:389–97.

64. Lowenstein DH, Thomas MJ, Smith DH, et al. Selective vulnerability of dentate hilar neurons following traumatic brain injury: A potential mechanistic link between head trauma and disorders of the hippocampus. *J Neurosci* 1992;12:4846–53.

65. Ma D, Hossain M, Chow A, et al. Xenon and hypothermia combine to provide neuroprotection from neonatal asphyxia. *Ann Neurol* 2005;58:182–93.

66. Margulies SS, Thibault KL. Infant skull and suture properties: Measurements and implications for mechanisms of pediatric brain injury. *J Biomech Eng* 2000;122:364–71.

67. Marion DW, Penrod LE, Kelsey SF, et al. Treatment of traumatic brain injury with moderate hypothermia. *N Engl J Med* 1997;336:540–6.

68. Marmarou A, Barzo P, Fatouros P, et al. Traumatic brain swelling in head injured patients: Brain edema or vascular engorgement? *Acta Neurochir Suppl (Wien)* 1997;70:68–70.

69. Matsushita Y, Bramlett HM, Kuluz JW, et al. Delayed hemorrhagic hypotension exacerbates the hemodynamic and histopathologic consequences of traumatic brain injury in rats. *J Cereb Blood Flow Metab* 2001;21:847–56.

70. Meili DN, Christen S, Leib SL, et al. Current concepts in the pathogenesis of meningitis caused by streptococcus pneumoniae. *Curr Opin Infect Dis* 2002;15:253–7.

71. Murakami Y, Saito K, Hara A, et al. Increase in tumor necrosis factor-α following transient global cerebral ischemia do not contribute to neuron death in mouse hippocampus. *J Neurochem* 2005;93:1616–22.

72. Narkilahti S, Nissinen J, Pitkanen A. Administration of caspase 3 inhibitor during and after status epilepticus in rat: Effect on neuronal damage an epileptogenesis. *Neuropharmacology* 2003;44:1068–88.

73. Nau R, Bruck W. Neuronal injury in bacterial meningitis: Mechanisms and implications for therapy. *Trends Neurosci* 2002;25:38–45.

74. Nau R, Soto A, Bruck W. Apoptosis of neurons in the dentate gyrus in humans suffering from bacterial meningitis. *J Neuropathol Exp Neurol* 1999;58:265–74.

75. Nitatori T, Sato N, Waguri S, et al. Delayed neuronal death in the CA1 pyramidal cell layer of the gerbil hippocampus following transient ischemia is apoptosis. *J Neurosci* 1995;15:1001–11.

76. Nunez G, del Peso L. Linking extracellular survival signals and the apoptotic machinery. *Curr Opin Neurobiol* 1998;8:613–18.

77. Ono K, Han J. The p38 signal transduction pathway: Activation and function. *Cell Signal* 2000;12:1–13.

78. Oshio K, Watanabe H, Song Y, et al. Reduced cerebrospinal fluid production and intracranial pressure in mice lacking choroid plexus water channel Aquaporin-1. *FASEB J* 2005;19:76–8.

79. Palmer AM, Marion DW, Botscheller ML, et al. Increased transmitter amino acid concentration in human ventricular CSF after brain trauma. *Neuroreport* 1994;6:153–6.

80. Papadopoulos MC, Verkman AS. Aquaporin-4 gene disruption in mice reduces brain swelling and mortality in pneumococcal meningitis. *J Biol Chem* 2005;280:13906–12.

81. Paschen W, Doutheil J. Disturbance of endoplasmic reticulum functions: A key mechanism underlying cell damage? *Acta Neurochir Suppl* 1999;73:1–5.

82. Pereira de Vasconcelos A, Ferrandon A, Nehlig A. Local cerebral blood flow during lithium-pilocarpine seizures in the developing and adult rat: Role of coupling between blood flow and metabolism in the genesis of neuronal damage. *J Cereb Blood Flow Metab* 2002;22:196–205.

83. Portera-Cailliau C, Price DL, Martin LJ. Non-NMDA and NMDA receptor-mediated excitotoxic neuronal deaths in adult brain are morphologically distinct: Further evidence for an apoptosis-necrosis continuum. *J Comp Neurol* 1997;378:88–104.

84. Povlishock JT. Traumatically induced axonal injury: Pathogenesis and pathobiological implications. *Brain Pathol* 1992;2:1–12.

85. Rehncrona S, Siesjö BK. Metabolic and physiologic changes in acute brain failure. In: Grenvik A, Safar P, eds. *Brain Failure and Resuscitation*, New York: Churchill Livingstone, 1981:11–33.

86. Ruppel RA, Kochanek PM, Adelson PD, et al. Excitotoxicity amino acid concentrations in ventricular cerebrospinal fluid after severe traumatic brain injury in infants and children: The role of child abuse. *J Pediatrics* 2001;138:18–25.

87. Scheff SW, Price DA, Hicks RR, et al. Synaptogenesis in the hippocampal CA1 field following traumatic brain injury. *J Neurotrauma* 2005;22:719–32.

88. Scherbel U, Raghupathi R, Nakamura M, et al. Differential acute and chronic responses of tumor necrosis factor-deficient mice to experimental brain injury. *Proc Natl Acad Sci USA* 1999;96:8721–6.

89. Schleien CL, Koehler RC, Shaffner DH, et al. Blood-brain barrier disruption after cardiac resuscitation in immature swine. *Stroke* 1991;22:477–83.

90. Shankaran S, Laptook AR, Ehrenkranz RA, et al. Whole-body hypothermia for neonates with hypoxic-ischemic encephalopathy. *N Engl J Med* 2005;353:1575–84.

91. Shapiro S, Miller A, Lahat N, et al. Expression of matrix metalloproteinases, sICAM-1 and IL-8 in CSF from children with meningitis. *J Neurol Sci* 2003;206:43–8.

92. Sharp FR, Lu An, Tang Y, et al. Multiple molecular penumbras after focal cerebral ischemia. *J Cereb Blood Flow Metab* 2000;20:1011–32.

93. Shigeno T, Mima T, Takakura K, et al. Amelioration of delayed neuronal death in the hippocampus by nerve growth factor. *J Neurosci* 1991;11:2914–19.

94. Starkov AA, Chinopoulos C, Fiskum G. Mitochondrial calcium and oxidative stress as mediators of ischemic brain injury. *Cell Calcium* 2004;36:257–64.

95. Tajiri S, Oyadomari S, Yano S, et al. Ischemia-induced neuronal cell death is mediated by the endoplasmic reticulum stress pathway involving CHOP. *Cell Death Differ* 2004;11:403–15.

96. Tsukahara H, Haruta T, Todoroki Y, et al. Oxidant and antioxidant activities in childhood meningitis. *Life Sci* 2002;71:2797–2806.

97. Vereczki V, Martin E, Rosenthal RE, et al. Normoxic resuscitation after cardiac arrest protects against hippocampal oxidative stress, metabolic dysfunction, and neuronal death. *J Cereb Blood Flow Metab* 2006;26:821–35.

98. Vespa P, Boonyaputthikul R, McArthur DL, et al. Intensive insulin therapy reduces microdialysis glucose values without altering glucose utilization or improving the lactate/pyruvate ratio after traumatic brain injury. *Crit Care Med* 2006;34:850–6.

99. Villablanca JR, Burgess JW, Olmstead CE. Recovery of function after neonatal or adult hemispherectomy in cats. I. Time course, movement, posture and sensorimotor tests. *Beav Brain Res* 1986;19:205–26.

100. Wada K, Chatzipanteli K, Kraydieh S, et al. Inducible nitric oxide synthase expression after traumatic brain injury and neuroprotection with aminoguanidine treatment in rats. *Neurosurgery* 1998;43:1427–36.

101. Weise J, Englehorn T, Dörfler A, et al. Expression time course and spatial distribution of activated caspase-3 after experimental status epilepticus: Contribution of delayed neuronal cell death to seizure-induced neuronal injury. *Neurobiol Dis* 2005;18:582–90.

102. Yamasaki K, Edington HD, McClosky C, et al. Reversal of impaired wound repair in iNOS-deficient mice by topical adenoviral-mediated iNOS gene transfer. *J Clin Invest* 1998;101:967–71.

103. Yamashima T. Ca^{2+}-dependent proteases in ischemic neuronal death. A

conserved "calpain-cathepsin cascade" from nematodes to primates. *Cell Calcium* 2004;36:285–93.

104. Yu Z, Zhou D, Bruce-Keller AJ, et al. Lack of the p50 subunit of nuclear factor-kappaB increases the vulnerability of hippocampal neurons to excitotoxic injury. *J Neurosci* 1999;19:8856–65.

105. Zhang X, Chen Y, Jenkins LW, et al. Bench-to-bedside review: Apoptosis/programmed cell death triggered by traumatic brain injury. *Critical Care* 2005;9:66–75.

106. Zhang X, Graham SH, Kochanek PM, et al. Caspase-8 expression and proteolysis in human brain after severe head injury. *FASEB J* 2003;17:1367–9.

107. Zhao H, Shimohata T, Wang JQ, et al. Akt contributes to neuroprotection by hypothermia against cerebral ischemia in rats. *J Neurosci* 2005;25:9794–806.

108. Zhao H, Yenari MA, Cheng D, et al. Biphasic cytochrome c release after transient global ischemia and its inhibition by hypothermia. *J Cereb Blood Flow Metab* 2005;25:1119–29.

CHAPTER 53 ■ EVALUATION OF THE COMATOSE CHILD

NICHOLAS S. ABEND • SUDHA KILARU KESSLER • MARK A. HELFAER • DANIEL J. LICHT

Coma is a not a disease in itself, but rather it is the consequence of a range of insults to the central nervous system. The incidence of nontraumatic coma is 30/100,000 children per year (53), and the incidence of traumatic coma in children is 140/100,000 (28), with the most severe cases comprising 5.6/100,000 (33). The comatose child requires immediate evaluation and stabilization of vital functions, followed by a history and physical examination directed at identifying the underlying etiology of coma; this will direct specific management and allow for prognostication. The aims of this chapter are to (a) define coma and distinguish it from other states of altered consciousness, (b) review the underlying pathophysiology, (c) discuss a differential diagnosis of etiologies, (d) outline an approach to evaluation of a comatose child, (e) highlight potential complications of coma, and (f) review issues of prognosis.

DEFINITIONS

Consciousness is a state of wakefulness and awareness of self and surroundings. Coma is a state of altered consciousness with loss of both wakefulness (arousal, vigilance) and awareness of the self and environment, and it is characterized by sustained, pathologic, eyes-closed, unarousable unresponsiveness (35). Sleep-wake cycles are absent. Coma is a type of transitory state that can evolve toward recovery of consciousness, a minimally conscious state, a vegetative state, or brain death.

Between normal consciousness and coma is a spectrum of states of diminished consciousness, subdivided by convention into lethargy, obtundation, and stupor. *Lethargy* is a state of reduced wakefulness with attention deficits. *Obtundation* is characterized by blunted alertness and diminished interaction with the environment. *Stupor* is a state of unresponsiveness with little or no spontaneous movement, resembling deep sleep but differing from coma because vigorous stimulation induces temporary arousal. The descriptive terms listed here are not uniformly defined in the literature or by the physicians involved in a given patient's care; therefore, when describing a patient's state, especially in the acute setting in which tracking changes is important, a description of the patient's examination may convey more information than these one-word descriptors.

Other chronic states of altered neurologic function may resemble coma but must be clearly differentiated. A patient in a persistent vegetative state is awake but unaware and has sleep-wake cycles but no detectable cerebral cortical function. The eyes may be open, without visual fixation or pursuit. Generally this state is not diagnosed until 1 month after coma onset. A patient in a minimally conscious state has severely altered consciousness with minimal but definite behavioral evidence of self or environmental awareness, such as following simple commands or making simple nonreflexive gestures. *Akinetic mutism* is a condition of extreme slowing or absence of bodily movement with loss of speech. Wakefulness and awareness are preserved, but cognition is slowed. Causes include extensive bihemispheric disease and lesions that involve the inferior frontal lobes bilaterally, the paramedian mesencephalic reticular formation, or the posterior diencephalon. The *locked-in syndrome* is a state of preserved consciousness and cognition with complete paralysis of the voluntary motor system. Cortical function is intact, and electroencephalogram (EEG) patterns are normal. Locked-in syndrome may result from lesions of the corticospinal and corticobulbar pathways at or below the pons but may also arise with severe peripheral nervous system disease, such as Guillain-Barré syndrome, botulism, and critical illness polyneuropathy. Eye movements, most commonly vertical eye movements, may be preserved, allowing for some communication. *Delirium* is an acute confusional state characterized by changes in the level of consciousness, impaired attention, and a fluctuating course. It may occur with toxic-metabolic encephalopathy, focal lesions, or seizures. Coma must also be distinguished from brain death, which is the permanent absence of all brain activity, including brainstem function.

ANATOMY

The reticular activating system (RAS) constitutes the central core of the brainstem and extends from the caudal medulla to the thalamus and the basal forebrain. The RAS receives input stimulation from all sensory pathways and projects to vast areas of the cerebral cortex. The RAS activates the cortex and participates in feedback control that regulates incoming signals, which may account for the ability of certain signals to cause more arousal than other signals of equal electrical intensity.

The functional anatomy of the RAS can be partitioned broadly into medial and lateral zones. The medial RAS contains a mixture of large and small neurons. The most prominent cells in this region are the giant neurons, which have long ascending and descending axons. The ascending portions of the medial RAS emanate from the Raphe nuclei, which regulate sleep cycles and utilize serotonin as their major neurotransmitter. The descending pathways regulate automatic motor functions, including the automatic rhythms of breathing.

The lateral RAS projects to the reticular nucleus of the thalamus, which relays signals to the cortex, forming the ascending RAS, which maintains wakefulness. These projections are both *cholinergic* and *noradrenergic*. A second cholinergic pathway ascends through the hypothalamus to influence basal forebrain structures, including the *limbic* system, which influences conscious behavior. Lesions in this path are thought to be involved in the development of akinetic mutism. Noradrenergic pathways that originate in the *locus caeruleus* have an excitatory effect on most of the brain, mediating arousal and priming the brain's neurons to be activated by stimuli. Thus, wakefulness is maintained by the RAS, while awareness is dependent on the cortex and subcortical connections.

ETIOLOGIES OF COMA

The causes of coma are broad and are listed in **Table 53.1.** Many studies of pediatric coma make an initial division between traumatic and nontraumatic etiologies of coma. Nontraumatic subcategories include global derangements in homeostasis and discrete structural abnormalities. Multiple interrelated factors may be present in one patient. For example, status epilepticus (SE) may occur in the setting of encephalitis, infection that induces a catabolic state may produce decompensation in a child with an inborn error of metabolism, and hyponatremia or other electrolyte dysfunction may accompany brain injury and contribute to cerebral dysfunction.

In a population-based study, 278 of >600,000 children between the ages of 1 month and 16 years had 345 episodes of coma (53). Infection was the most common cause of nontraumatic coma, accounting for 38% of cases. Intoxication, epilepsy, and complications of congenital abnormalities each accounted for 8%–10% of cases. Nontraumatic accidents (such as smoke inhalation and drowning) and metabolic causes each accounted for 6% of cases.

EVALUATION OF THE COMATOSE CHILD

Coma is often a manifestation of life-threatening conditions. Therefore, initial evaluation of the child begins with assessment and stabilization of vital functions and identification of immediately reversible etiologies. Vital functions must be managed as the coma etiology is being investigated to prevent development of secondary brain injury. An algorithm for initial evaluation of coma is outlined in **Table 53.2** and discussed here. Guidelines based on an extensive literature review and expert consensus have been published online (www.nottingham.ac.uk/paediatric-guideline) by the Pediatric Accident and Emergency Research Group of the Royal College of Paediatrics and Child Health and the British Association for Emergency Medicine (1).

History

A detailed history may not always be available on initial evaluation of the comatose child, but historic information must be gathered as quickly as possible, as it may be crucial in identifying the cause of coma. The history must include a detailed description of events leading to coma, with particular attention to timing, exposures, and accompanying symptoms. Preceding somnolence suggests a metabolic or toxic cause. Sudden onset of coma without trauma suggests spontaneous

TABLE 53.1

ETIOLOGIES OF COMA

Trauma
Parenchymal injury
Intracranial hemorrhage
   Epidural hematoma
   Subdural hematoma
   Subarachnoid hemorrhage
   Intracerebral hematoma
Diffuse axonal injury

Nontraumatic causes
Toxic/metabolic
Hypoxic-ischemic encephalopathy
   Shock
   Cardiopulmonary arrest
   Near-drowning
   Carbon monoxide poisoning
Toxins
   Medications: narcotics, sedatives, antiepileptics,
      antidepressants, analgesics, aspirin
   Environmental toxins: organophosphates, heavy metals,
      cyanide, mushroom poisoning
   Illicit substances: alcohol, heroin, amphetamines, cocaine
Systemic metabolic disorders
   Substrate deficiencies
      Hypoglycemia
      Cofactors: thiamine, niacin, pyridoxine
   Electrolyte and acid-base imbalance: sodium, magnesium,
      calcium
   Diabetic ketoacidosis
   Thyroid/adrenal/other endocrine disorders
   Uremic coma
   Hepatic coma
   Reye syndrome
   Inborn errors of metabolism
      Urea cycle disorders
      Amino acidopathies
      Organic acidopathies
      Mitochondrial disorders
Infections/postinfectious/inflammatory
   Meningitis and encephalitis: Bacterial, viral, rickettsial,
      fungal
   Acute demyelinating diseases
      Acute disseminated encephalomyelitis
      Multiple sclerosis
Inflammatory/autoimmune
   Sarcoidosis
   Sjögren disease
   Lupus cerebritis
Mass lesions
   Neoplasms
   Abscess, granuloma
   Hydrocephalus
Paroxysmal neurologic disorders
   Seizures/SE
   Acute confusional migraine
Vascular
   Intracranial hemorrhage
   Arterial infarcts
   Venous sinus thromboses
   Vasculitis

TABLE 53.2

INITIAL EVALUATION OF COMA

Airway, breathing, and circulation assessment and stabilization
  Ensure adequate ventilation and oxygenation.
  Blood pressure management depends on considerations regarding underlying coma etiology.
    If hypertensive encephalopathy or intracranial hemorrhage, lower blood pressure. If
    perfusion-dependent state, such as some strokes or elevated intracranial pressure, reducing
    blood pressure may reduce cerebral perfusion.

Draw blood for glucose, electrolytes, ammonia, arterial blood gas, liver and renal function
  tests, complete blood count, lactate, pyruvate, and toxicology screen.

Neurologic assessment
  GCS score
  Assess for evidence of raised intracranial pressure and herniation.
  Assess for abnormalities that suggest focal neurologic disease.
  Assess for history or signs of seizures.

Administer glucose IV (in an adult, thiamine should be given first)

If concern for infection delays lumbar puncture, broad-spectrum infection coverage should be
  provided (including bacterial, viral, and possibly fungal).

Give specific antidotes if toxic exposures are known.
  For opiate overdose, administer naloxone.
  For benzodiazepine overdose, consider administering flumazenil.
  For anticholinergic overdose, consider administering physostigmine.

Identify and treat critical elevations in intracranial pressure.
  Neutral head position, elevated head by 20 degrees, sedation.
  Hyperosmolar therapy with mannitol 0.25–1 g/kg or hypertonic saline.
  Hyperventilation as temporary measure.
  Consider intracranial monitoring.
  Consider neurosurgical intervention.

Head CT (non-contrast)

Treat seizures with IV anticonvulsants. Consider prophylactic anticonvulsants.

Investigate source of fever and use antipyretics and/or cooling devices to reduce cerebral
  metabolic demands.

Detailed history and examination

Consider lumbar puncture, EEG or extended video EEG monitoring, MRI, metabolic testing
  (amino acids, organic acids, acylcarnitine profile), autoimmune testing (ANA panel,
  antithyroid antibodies), thyroid testing (TSH, T3, T4).

intracranial hemorrhage or seizure. Slowly progressive loss of consciousness suggests hydrocephalus, an expanding mass lesion, or indolent infection. Preceding headache with positional changes or Valsalva maneuver implies increased intracranial pressure (ICP) from hydrocephalus or a mass lesion. Headache with neck pain or stiffness suggests meningeal irritation from inflammation, infection, or hemorrhage. Fever suggests infection, but its absence does not exclude it, particularly in infants <3 months of age or in immunocompromised children. Recent fevers or illness suggest autoimmune processes, such as acute disseminated encephalomyelitis or possibly Reye syndrome, although this is uncommon. Questions about possible toxic ingestions should include a survey of medications and poisons kept in the places the child has recently been.

The child's past medical history may be valuable. A history of multiple episodes of coma, developmental delay, or other prior neurologic abnormalities suggests inborn errors of metabolism, but these are also risk factors for epilepsy, which may include nonconvulsive seizures or a postictal state. Toxic ingestions or inflicted childhood neurotrauma are also suggested by multiple episodes of coma. Recent weight changes or other constitutional abnormalities suggest endocrine dysfunction. Previously existing cardiac disease raises the possibility of dysrhythmia or cardiac failure, leading to hypoxic ischemic encephalopathy. Travel history may explain exposure to infections prevalent in certain areas, such as Lyme disease in the northeastern US. Exposure to kittens in a patient with axillary or inguinal lymphadenopathy may be a clue to infection with *Bartonella henselae*, which causes cat-scratch encephalopathy.

Eliciting a history of trauma, whether accidental or inflicted, is crucial. Understanding the mechanism of injury can direct further investigation. Intracranial lesions, such as epidural hematomas, may result in delayed loss of consciousness. Fractures at the base of the skull may compromise blood flow in the carotid artery or result in dissection of the artery as it enters the skull or travels through the petrous canal. Such arterial pathology can result in malignant middle cerebral artery syndromes.

Physical Examination

Numerically scored rating scales of consciousness levels allow objective description of a patient's degree of impairment and allow the patient's state to be tracked over time and conveyed quickly to other caregivers. The most widely used instrument is the Glasgow Coma Scale (GCS), which was initially developed to evaluate adults with head injury (48). Pediatric adaptations to the GCS, more developmentally appropriate for infants and children, include the Pediatric Coma Scale, the Children's Coma Scale, and the Glasgow Coma Scale-Modified for Children (**Table 53.3**) (18,37,39). The GCS and the pediatric adaptations categorize the patient based on measures of verbal response, eye opening, and movement. Combined with other modalities, the initial GCS score may have limited prognostic value. While the GCS allows efficient, standardized communication of a child's state, a more detailed description of the child's clinical findings is often more useful for relaying detailed information and detecting changes over time.

The general physical examination of the comatose child should focus on preventing secondary neurologic injury and identifying the etiology of coma. The general examination should start with vital signs determination. Hypotension due to sepsis, cardiac dysfunction (which may be secondary to severe neurologic injury in neurogenic stunned myocardium), toxic ingestion, or adrenal insufficiency, may lead to poor cerebral perfusion, resulting in diffuse or watershed hypoxic-ischemic injury. Hypertension may cause, or result from, coma-related conditions. Hypertension can be a physiologic response to in-

creased ICP that functions to maintain cerebral perfusion pressure (which is the difference between mean arterial pressure and ICP). In such a case, acutely lowering blood pressure may worsen the neurologic injury by reducing cerebral perfusion. Hypertension with bradycardia and a change in breathing pattern (Cushing triad) is an ominous sign of impending brain herniation. Management may require temporary emergent measures, such as hyperventilation (to reduce carbon dioxide and induce vasoconstriction) and hyperosmolar therapy, followed by more definitive neurosurgical therapy, to lower ICP. Hypertension in the setting of coma may also be the product of nonspecific sympathetic response or of stimulant intoxication. Primary or secondary hypertension may cause hypertensive encephalopathy that can manifest as coma. Primary hypertensive encephalopathy is suggested by a history of hypertension or renal disease, or by preceding headache, visual complaints, or seizures. Differentiating reactive/compensatory hypertension from a primary hypertensive encephalopathy may be difficult but is crucial in determining how to manage blood pressure.

Abnormalities in respiratory rate and breathing pattern may indicate pathology that originates in the lungs, acid-base derangement, or nervous system dysfunction. Cheyne-Stokes respiration describes a rhythmic pattern of accelerating hyperpnea followed by a fall in the amplitude of breathing and culminating in a decelerating rate of breathing and apnea. It is a nonspecific pattern seen with extensive bihemispheric cerebral dysfunction, diencephalic (thalamic and hypothalamic) dysfunction, or cardiac failure. Pontine or midbrain tegmental lesions may result in central neurogenic hyperventilation. Apneustic breathing, in its most common form, is characterized by a pause at the end

TABLE 53.3

GLASGOW COMA SCALE AND MODIFICATION FOR CHILDREN

Sign	Glasgow coma scale	Modification for children	Score
Eye opening	Spontaneous	Spontaneous	4
	To command	To sound	3
	To pain	To pain	2
	None	None	1
Verbal response	Oriented	Age-appropriate verbalization, orients to sound, fixes and follows, social smile	5
	Confused	Cries, but consolable	4
	Disoriented	Irritable, uncooperative, aware of environment	3
	Inappropriate words	Irritable, persistent cries, inconsistently consolable	
	Incomprehensible sounds	Inconsolable crying, unaware of environment or parents, restless, agitated	2
	None	None	1
Motor response	Obeys commands	Obeys commands, spontaneous movement	6
	Localizes pain	Localizes pain	5
	Withdraws	Withdraws	4
	Abnormal flexion to pain	Abnormal flexion to pain	3
	Abnormal extension	Abnormal extension	2
	None	None	1
Best total score			15

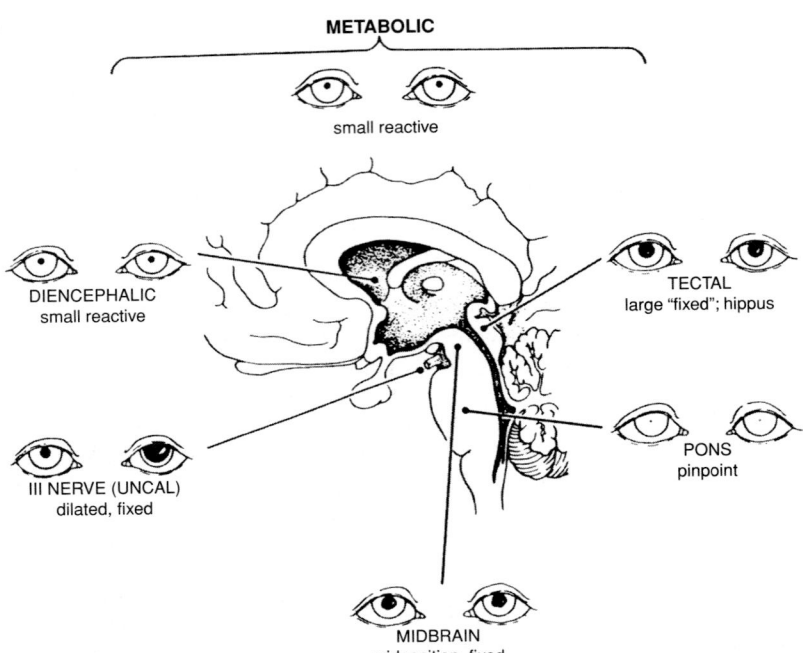

METABOLIC

small reactive

DIENCEPHALIC
small reactive

TECTAL
large "fixed"; hippus

III NERVE (UNCAL)
dilated, fixed

PONS
pinpoint

MIDBRAIN
midposition, fixed

FIGURE 53.1. Pupils in comatose patients. From Plum F, Posner JB. *The Diagnosis of Stupor & Coma*, 3rd ed. Philadelphia: F.A. Davis, 1982, with permission.

of inspiration and reflects damage to respiratory centers at the mid- or lower-pontine levels, at or below the level of the trigeminal motor nucleus. Apneusis occurs with basilar artery occlusion (leading to pontine infarction), hypoglycemia, anoxia, or meningitis. Ataxic breathing is completely irregular in rate and tidal volume and occurs with damage to the reticular formation of the dorsomedial medulla (35).

A complete general examination is important. Involuntary hip flexion with passive flexion of the neck (Brudzinski sign) and resistance to knee extension with hips flexed (Kernig sign) indicate meningeal inflammation/irritation. Skin examination provides information about trauma (bruises, lacerations), systemic disease (jaundice in liver failure, uremic frost, hyperpigmentation in adrenal insufficiency), and infection (superficial lacerations in cat-scratch fever, erythema migrans in Lyme disease, petechiae and purpura in meningococcemia). Organomegaly raises suspicion of metabolic, hematologic, and hepatic diseases.

The neurologic examination is directed toward localizing brain dysfunction, identifying coma etiology, and determining early indicators of prognosis. Evaluation of responsiveness must include vigorous auditory and sensory stimulation. Nailbed pressure, pinching, and sternal rubbing may be required. Responsiveness must be evaluated in terms of lack of verbal, motor, and cranial nerve responses. In a comatose child, much of the examination that requires patient cooperation (such as mental status and sensory testing) cannot be performed. Thus, the exam is aimed at assessing response to stimuli and function of the brainstem and motor systems.

A comatose child may be flaccid or may display an abnormal flexor or extensor posture. As originally described, *decorticate posturing* (flexion of the arms and extension of the legs) indicated supratentorial dysfunction and *decerebrate posturing* (extension and internal rotation of the arms and legs) indicated brainstem dysfunction. However, subsequent investigation proved this clinical anatomical correlation to be more complex. Plum and Posner (35) describe the following

guidelines for interpreting abnormal postures: flexor arm responses reflect more rostral and less severe supratentorial damage; extensor responses in the arm and leg correlate best with more severe but still supratentorial dysfunction; arm extension with leg flexion suggest pontine damage; and diffuse flaccidity correlates with brainstem damage below the pontomedullary level.

Examination of the cranial nerves in comatose patients allows investigation of both the brainstem and the cortical control of cranial nerve pathways. Funduscopic examination yields information about the retina and optic nerves. Papilledema may be seen with increased ICP. However, this may take hours or days to develop; thus, the absence of papilledema does not confirm that ICP is normal. Retinal hemorrhages may be seen in inflicted childhood neurotrauma. Flame-shaped hemorrhages and cotton-wool spots can be seen in hypertensive encephalopathy.

Pupils (**Fig. 53.1** and **Table 53.4**) are examined first by observing the size of both pupils in dim light and then by assessing reactivity to a bright light shined in each eye. Asymmetric pupils are caused either by disruption of the oculomotor nerve (cranial nerve III) or impairment of sympathetic fibers (Horner syndrome). Because the oculomotor nerve innervates the pupil constrictors, oculomotor nerve impairment results in an abnormally dilated pupil. Oculomotor nerve palsy also results in ptosis and ophthalmoparesis and may be a sign of uncal herniation. Horner syndrome describes disruption of the sympathetic innervation to the face, characterized by mild ptosis over an abnormally small pupil (miosis). In traumatic coma, Horner syndrome may be an important clue to dissection of the carotid artery, along which the sympathetic fibers travel, or an injury to the lower brachial plexus (C8–T1). Anisocoria (asymmetric pupils) is an important physical finding, and differentiating whether a pupil is abnormally large or abnormally small is crucial to identifying underlying pathology. In brief, in pupils that are more asymmetric in bright light, the pathology lies with the larger pupil and is likely the result of

TABLE 53.4

PUPIL ABNORMALITIES IN COMA

Etiology/localization	Pupil appearance
Metabolic	Small, reactive
Hypothalamic	Small, reactive
Tectal	Large, nonreactive, hippus
Pontine	Pinpoint
Midbrain	Mid-position, fixed
Oculomotor nerve, uncal herniation	Ipsilateral pupil dilated, fixed
Severe hypoxic-ischemic encephalopathy	Bilateral dilated, fixed
Opiate intoxication	Pinpoint
Anticholinergic poisoning	Dilated and fixed, unreactive to 1% pilocarpine

oculomotor palsy (cranial nerve III). Investigations to rule out uncal herniation or an aneurysm of the posterior communicating artery should follow. In pupils that are more asymmetric in darkness, the pathology lies with the smaller pupil. Investigation of the carotid artery, the low cervical-high thoracic spinal cord, or brachial plexus roots should follow to find causes of the Horner syndrome.

Abnormalities of eye position and motility may be signs of cortical, midbrain, or pontine dysfunction. Conjugate lateral eye deviation is caused by destructive lesions of the ipsilateral cortex or pons, or by focal seizures in the contralateral hemisphere. Rarely, thalamic lesions may cause "wrong-way eyes," in which the eyes deviate away from the side of the destructive lesion (26). Tonic down-gaze suggests dorsal midbrain compression. The complete dorsal midbrain syndrome of Parinaud includes pupillary light-near dissociation, lid-retraction, and convergence-retraction nystagmus.

Dysconjugate gaze suggests extraocular muscle weakness or, more commonly, abnormalities of the third, fourth, or sixth cranial nerves or nuclei. Unilateral or bilateral abducens nerve (cranial nerve VI) palsies are commonly seen in increased ICP, presumably because the nerve is stretched. This sign is therefore considered a "false localizing sign," as it suggests a focal brainstem lesion but, in fact, represents a more diffuse ICP change. An eye with oculomotor nerve (cranial nerve III) palsy is ptotic, depressed, and abducted, and has a dilated pupil. As discussed later, oculomotor nerve palsy in a comatose patient suggests uncal herniation with midbrain compression and requires urgent intervention. Trochlear nerve (cranial nerve IV) palsy causes hypertropia in the affected eye.

Roving eye movements are seen in comatose patients with intact brainstem function. Their disappearance may signal the onset of brainstem dysfunction. Periodic alternating gaze (ping-pong gaze) describes conjugate horizontal eye movements back and forth, with a pause at each end. It may be seen with extensive bilateral hemispheric, basal ganglia, or thalamic-midbrain damage with an intact pons and is thought to result from disconnection of cortical influences on oculovestibular reflex generators. It has also been reported in reversible coma from monoamine oxidase and tricyclic antidepressant toxicity.

Oculocephalic and oculovestibular reflexes are useful for assessing the integrity of the midbrain and pons in a comatose patient without spontaneous eye movements. To test oculo-

cephalic reflexes, the examiner holds the patient's eyelids open and quickly moves the head to one side. In a comatose patient with an intact brainstem, the eyes will move in the direction opposite the head motion. For example, if the head is moved to the right, the eyes will move conjugately to the left. After several seconds, the eyes may return to a neutral position. The head should be tested in both horizontal and vertical directions. Oculocephalic reflexes should not be tested if the patient has sustained cervical spine trauma or if the spine has not been cleared.

The oculovestibular reflex, commonly referred to as cold calorics, tests the function above the pontomedullary junction. The child must have an open external auditory canal with an intact tympanic membrane (including the absence of pressure equalization tubes), and visual inspection of the canal is an important first step. With the head elevated at 30 degrees, up to 120 mg of ice water is introduced in the ear canal with a small catheter. A conscious patient would experience nystagmus with slow deviation of the eyes toward the irrigated ear and a fast corrective movement away from the ear (the mnemonic COWS, *cold opposite, warm same,* applies to the fast phase). In a comatose patient, the fast correction mediated by the cortex is not seen. Instead, the eyes will deviate slowly toward the irrigated ear and remain fixed there. If the brainstem vestibular nuclei (located at the pontomedullary junction) are impaired, no movement will be seen. In brain death, in which brainstem function is nonexistent, no eye movement is seen with both ears tested. Five minutes should be allowed before the second ear is tested to allow return of temperature equilibrium between the two ears. Vertical eye movements may be tested by simultaneously irrigating both auditory canals with cold water, producing downward deviation in the comatose patient. Warm water irrigation produces upward gaze.

The remaining brainstem reflexes provide information about the integrity of lower regions of the brainstem. The corneal reflex is tested by tactile stimulation of the cornea, which should elicit bilateral eyelid closure. The afferent (sensory) signal is carried by the trigeminal nerve (cranial nerve V), and the efferent (motor) pathway is carried by the facial nerve (cranial nerve VII). Completion of the reflex loop requires intact trigeminal and facial nerve nuclei in the mid and lower pons. The cough reflex, which may be seen with stimulation of the carina when a patient is intubated or undergoes suctioning, is mediated by medullary cough centers; sensory and motor signals are carried by the glossopharyngeal (cranial nerve IX) and vagus (cranial nerve X) nerves. When the soft palate is stimulated, the gag reflex is elicited, manifested as elevation of the soft palate. As in the cough reflex, afferent and efferent signals are carried by the glossopharyngeal and vagus nerves, with processing in the medulla. Narcotics may suppress cough reflex, an important consideration for accurate assessment of brainstem function (30).

Laboratory, Imaging, and Electrophysiologic Investigation

Investigation should continue with laboratory, neuroimaging, and electrophysiologic testing. This area has been reviewed and is summarized in **Table 53.5** (23). Guidelines based on an extensive literature review and expert consensus have been

TABLE 53.5

INVESTIGATION OF NONTRAUMATIC COMA IN PEDIATRICS

Investigations	Indication/clinical clues	Possible abnormality	Further investigation if abnormal	Possible diagnoses	Action
Dextrostix	All	Low	Blood glucose	Hypoglycemia secondary to:	IV dextrose
Blood glucose			Liver function tests	Fasting	Fluids/insulin
			Blood ammonia	Severe illness	
			Blood lactate	Reye syndrome	
			Blood and urine amino acids	Organic aciduria	
			Urine organic acids	Fatty-acid oxidation defect	
				Hemorrhagic shock and encephalopathy	
				Diabetic ketoacidosis	
Blood sodium	Previous polydipsia/polyuria	High	Urinary sodium	Hypo/hypernatremia ± dehydration	Appropriate fluids
	All	Low			
Blood urea	All	High	Blood creatinine	Dehydration	Rehydrate
		High	Blood film	Hemolytic-uremic syndrome	Dialysis, plasmapheresis
Aspartate transaminase	All	High	Blood ammonia	Reye Syndrome	Sodium benzoate
				Hypoxia-ischemia	
Blood Ammonia	All (unless cause known)	High	Blood orotic acid	Urea cycle defect	
			Urine organic acids	Organic acidemia	
Full blood count and film	All	Low Hb	Hb electrophoresis	Anemia	Transfusion
		High WBC		Infection	3rd-generation cephalosporin
		Low platelets		DIC infection	
	Residence in endemic area	Sickle cells		Sickle cell disease	Dialysis, plasmapheresis
		Burr cells		Hemolytic-uremic syndrome	Quinine
		Parasites on thick/thin films		Malaria	Chelation
	Pica	Basophilic stippling	Wrist x-ray—lead line	Lead encephalopathy	Appropriate antibiotics
Blood culture	All				
Stool culture	All	Shigella, enteroviruses			
Mycoplasma IgG, IgM	All (unless cause known)		Chest x-ray	Mycoplasma encephalitis	Erythromycin, ?prednisolone
Viral titers	Analyze if unexplained		Repeat at discharge		
Urine for toxin screen	Analyze if unexplained		Blood film—basophilic stippling, wrist x-ray—lead line	Poisoning	Antidote
Blood lead	Analyze if unexplained				Chelation
CT scan without contrast	All (after resuscitation, afebrile patients should ideally be transferred for CT scan to a unit with neurosurgical facilities)	Blood:			
		Subdural	Skull x-ray/skeletal survey/clotting screen	Nonaccidental injury	Neurosurgical referral
					Child protection
		Extradural			Neurosurgical referral
		Intracerebral			
		Space-occupying lesion		Tumor	Neurosurgical referral
		Hydrocephalus:			
		Obstructive		?Space-occupying lesion	
		Communicating	CSF examination	?Meningitis, especially tuberculous	Antituberculous cover
		Abscess	Culture aspirate		Neurosurgical referral
			Contrast CT/MRI		Neurosurgical referral
		Swelling		Cerebral abscess, herpes simplex, stroke, ADEM	Anaerobic cover
		Focal low density			Mannitol 0.25 g/kg
		Abnormal basal ganglia	Plasma/CSF lactate, blood gas	Leigh syndrome, hypoxic-ischemic, striatal necrosis	

Investigation	Indication/detail	Finding	Additional test	Diagnosis	Treatment
Lumbar puncture	In febrile patient if no clinical or radiologic evidence of raised ICP (delay and treat if doubt)				
Pressure measurement		High			Mannitol, ventilate
Microscopy		High WBC	CT	Meningitis/e encephalitis	3rd-generation cephalosporin, acyclovir
Gram, bacterial culture		High RBC	CT (traumatic tap should clear by third bottle)	Hemorrhage/encephalitis/nonaccidental injury	Neurosurgical referral, acyclovir, child protection
Glucose		Low		Tuberculous meningitis	Immediate and prolonged antitubercular therapy
Protein		High		Tuberculous meningitis	Immediate and prolonged antitubercular therapy
PCR for viruses, TB					
Prolonged search for acid-fast bacilli, culture for TB on Lowenstein-Jensen	Prodrome >7 days, optic atrophy, focal signs, abnormal movements, CSF polymorphs <50%, hydrocephalus and/or basal enhancement on contrast CT			Tuberculous meningitis	Immediate and prolonged antitubercular therapy
Antibodies; e.g., herpes simplex, mycoplasma				Encephalitis	Acyclovir, erythromycin
Lactate	Abnormal breathing/eye movements, basal ganglia lucencies		Muscle biopsy	Leigh syndrome	
EEG	All, especially if ventilated or evidence of subtle seizures (nystagmus, tonic deviation of eyes, clonic jerking limbs)	Epileptiform discharges		Status epilepticus	IV benzodiazepines, phenytoin, thiopentone
		Asymmetrical foci of spikes or periodic lateralizing epileptiform discharges on slow background		Herpes simplex encephalitis (many patients do not have characteristic EEG)	High-dose IV acyclovir for 2 weeks
MRI	Unexplained encephalopathy	Frontotemporal abnormality; Thalamic abnormality	CSF for herpes simplex, PCR; CSF for EBV (arboviruses in endemic area)	Herpes simplex encephalitis	High-dose IV acyclovir for 2 weeks

hb, hemoglobin; WBC, white blood cell; CSF, cerebrospinal fluid; RBC, red blood cell; TB, tuberculosis; EEG, electroencephalogram; PCR, polymerase chain reaction; EBV, Epstein-Barr virus. From Kirkham FJ. Non-traumatic coma in children. *Arch Dis Child* 2001;85:303–12, with permission.

published online by the Pediatric Accident and Emergency Research Group of the Royal College of Paediatrics and Child Health and the British Association for Emergency Medicine (1). These guidelines can be printed, and provide detailed and easy-to-access flowcharts of the evaluation and management of a child with decreased consciousness. The guideline initially points out the importance of airway, breathing, and circulation, and the importance of continuous cardiopulmonary monitoring and frequent GCS assessment. Hypoxia, hypotension, hypoglycemia or hyperglycemia, hyperthermia or hypothermia, and anemia worsen the prognosis of coma and must be treated aggressively and quickly. Hypotonic fluids should not be administered, as doing so can worsen cerebral edema.

Core investigations should then occur. A Dextrostix reading should be taking on all children at the initial evaluation. Even if results are normal, laboratory glucose testing should be requested for confirmation, as hypoglycemia alone may cause coma, and hypoglycemia in association with other etiologies may worsen outcome. Hypoglycemia (capillary glucose <2.6 mmol/L) must be treated urgently with an IV dextrose infusion. Hyperglycemia may occur in diabetic ketoacidosis (capillary glucose >11 mmol/L, pH <7.3, and urine ketones). A blood gas should be performed on every patient. Electrolytes should be measured on all patients, as abnormalities may cause coma or may occur secondary to intracranial abnormalities. Liver function tests should be performed, as hepatic encephalopathy may cause coma, and liver injury can occur in the setting of systemic hypoxic ischemic injury. A complete blood count with differential is indicated in all patients to detect infection, anemia, disseminated intravascular coagulopathy, lead encephalopathy, or sickle cell disease. Blood, urine, and stool cultures should be obtained in most patients to investigate infectious etiologies. Toxin screens should be performed in all children and include acetaminophen, salicylate, and ethanol. Specific tests for medications found in the home should be conducted as necessary. Ammonia, lactate, and pyruvate tests may be performed in all patients to screen for metabolic disorders. If history is suggestive of metabolic disease, measurement of organic acids, amino acids, and acylcarnitine profile may be indicated.

After resuscitation, a head CT should be performed in all children to detect intracranial hemorrhage, space-occupying lesions (such as tumor or abscess), edema, focal hypodensities (such as acute disseminated encephalitis, herpes simplex encephalitis, infarct), or hydrocephalus. If a patient is febrile, infection is suspected, or no other etiology can be determined, then a lumbar puncture should be performed. If clinical or radiologic evidence is present for intracranial hypertension, lumbar puncture should be deferred and treatment should be initiated for possible infections (bacterial and viral). A normal CT does not rule out elevated ICP. Cerebrospinal fluid should be tested for cell count (both the first and last tubes should be tested to help differentiate true findings in the case of a traumatic tap), glucose, protein, Gram stain, bacterial culture, viral polymerase chain reaction, and additional cultures when suspected clinically (fungal or tubercular). An EEG may detect useful background changes (such as triphasic waves suggestive of metabolic encephalopathy or sharp waves associated with herpes simplex encephalitis) and may identify subclinical seizures. As described later, a prolonged EEG may be required to detect subclinical seizures. If the cause of coma remains unknown, additional studies may be directed at uncommon causes of coma in children, such as Hashimoto encephalitis (thyroid function tests and thyroid autoantibodies),

cerebral vasculitis (erythrocyte sedimentation rate, ESR; antinuclear antibody, ANA, panel; and possibly angiography), or paraneoplastic disorders. Once the patient has been stabilized and the etiology of coma remains unclear, a brain MRI may be performed for diagnostic and prognostic purposes.

COMPLICATIONS

The clinical course of a child in coma largely depends on the underlying illness and timing of treatment. Because the child's neurologic function will evolve over time, frequent serial examinations may be essential for diagnosis, identification of complications, and prognostication. Neurologic complications of coma include autonomic dysfunction, increased ICP, cerebral herniation, seizures, and metabolic derangements that may prolong the comatose state.

Increased Intracranial Pressure

Causes of increased ICP in coma include intracranial hemorrhage, space-occupying lesions, and cerebral edema. Cerebral edema may be vasogenic, cellular, or osmolar. Cellular swelling is predominantly astrocyte swelling as a consequence of homeostatic processes to control excitotoxicity or acidosis with sodium and water accumulation. Osmolar swelling can also occur in necrotic foci such as infarcts or contusions. Herniation syndromes often herald impending catastrophic deterioration and death unless ICP is lowered by medical or surgical means. Initial management of critically raised ICP includes IV hyperosmolar therapy (mannitol or sodium) and hyperventilation to achieve a Pco_2 of 35 mm Hg. Further reduction in Pco_2 may be necessary to achieve rapid but temporary reductions in cerebral blood flow and ICP, but excessive or prolonged hyperventilation may compromise cerebral perfusion, resulting in further hypoxic-ischemic injury. These initial measures may provide only temporary reductions in ICP. Barbiturate coma or hypothermia may reduce cellular energy requirements and may thus help protect the brain during periods of hypoxia and ischemia. Similarly, providing adequate sedation and paralysis may further reduce energy demand and prevent spikes in ICP. Maintaining a neutral neck position and elevating the head of the bed to 20–30 degrees may improve venous drainage. Surgical decompression may be required for more definitive therapy. Often a large craniectomy is performed with wide margins to allow space for brain expansion. If the margins are too small, fungating herniation may occur through the skull defect. The Cushing triad (hypertension, bradycardia, and a change in respirations) may occur with any type of increased intracranial hypertension, and more specific signs of herniation depend on the location of the herniation syndrome. These are summarized in **Table 53.6**. While neuroimaging will demonstrate the exact nature of the herniation, waiting for and transport to neuroimaging may be detrimental, and medical interventions should be implemented emergently prior to neuroimaging.

Seizures

Subclinical seizures in critically ill patients may be an underrecognized phenomenon; therefore, the index of suspicion in a

TABLE 53.6

HERNIATION SYNDROMES

Herniation syndrome	Location	Signs
Central herniation	Increased pressure in both cerebral hemispheres, causing downward displacement of the diencephalon through the tentorium, causing brainstem compression.	**Diencephalic stage:** withdraws to noxious stimuli, increased rigidity, or decorticate posturing; small, reactive pupils with preserved oculocephalic and oculovestibular reflexes; yawns, sighs, or Cheyne-Stokes breathing. **Midbrain-upper pons stage:** decerebrate posturing or no movement; mid-position pupils that may become irregular and unreactive; abnormal or absent oculocephalic and oculovestibular reflexes; hyperventilation. **Lower pons-medullary stage:** no spontaneous motor activity, but lower extremities may withdraw to plantar stimulation; mid-position fixed pupils; absent oculocephalic and oculovestibular reflexes; ataxic respirations. **Medullary stage:** generalized flaccidity; absent pupillary reflexes and ocular movements; slow irregular respirations, death.
Uncal herniation	Uncus of the temporal lobe is displaced medially over the free edge of the tentorium.	Ipsilateral third-nerve palsy (ptosis, pupil fixed and dilated, eye deviated down and out). Ipsilateral hemiparesis from compression of the contralateral cerebral peduncle (Kernohan notch). Other signs of brainstem dysfunction from ischemia secondary to compression of posterior cerebral artery.
Subfalcine (Cingulate) herniation	Increased pressure in one cerebral hemisphere leads to herniation of cingulated gyrus underneath falx cerebri.	Compression of anterior cerebral artery leads to paraparesis.
Tonsillar herniation	Increased pressure in the posterior fossa leads to brainstem compression.	Loss of consciousness from compression of reticular activating system. Focal lower cranial nerve dysfunction. Respiratory and cardiovascular function can be significantly affected early with relative preservation of upper brainstem function, such as pupillary light reflexes and vertical eye movements.

comatose child should be high. A recent study of nonresponsive children in an ICU demonstrated that 33% of children manifested electrographic patterns consistent with nonconvulsive status epilepticus (NCSE) (20). A second study demonstrated that 25% of children who presented to an emergency room with altered mental status were in NCSE (2). In another study, of 189 children (aged 1 day to 18 years; mean, 5 years) who were monitored with continuous EEG in the ICU, only 12.7% had convulsive seizures and 29.6% had nonconvulsive seizures. Of the patients with nonconvulsive seizures, 53% were detected within 1 hr, 87% were detected within 24 hrs, and 7% required longer than 48 hrs of continuous monitoring for detection (22). In a study of 570 consecutive patients with unexplained depressed levels of consciousness, 75 of whom were <18 years of age, continuous EEG monitoring detected subclinical seizures or seizures in 19% of patients (9). Importantly, age <18 years was associated with a higher incidence of electrographic seizures. Of the patients with seizures, 12% required monitoring for longer than 24 hrs to capture an event, emphasizing the importance of more prolonged monitoring. Other studies in adults have also demonstrated a similarly high incidence of subclinical seizures and NCSE.

Studies in adults have demonstrated that nonconvulsive seizure duration and time to detection predict outcome in patients with NCSE. When NCSE was diagnosed within 30 mins of onset, mortality was 36%, whereas when diagnosis was delayed for over 24 hrs, mortality increased to 75%. When NCSE lasted <10 hrs, 60% of patients returned home. However, when NCSE lasted >20 hrs none of the patients returned home, and 85% died (55). Studies have demonstrated that continuous electrographic discharges, even without clinical seizures, can be harmful, as evidenced by elevated neuron-specific enolase in children, known to be a marker of neuronal injury (31).

Other

Electrolyte abnormalities are common in comatose patients, occurring in more than half of patients in coma from severe head injury (34). The most commonly recognized metabolic derangement is hyponatremia that results from the syndrome of inappropriate antidiuretic hormone secretion or cerebral salt wasting. Other extracranial complications of coma include hypotension, hypoxemia, coagulopathies, and infections. In head trauma series, early complications, especially hypoxia and hypotension, predict poor outcome.

Further specific therapy of a comatose child depends entirely on the etiology of coma (see other chapters for specific etiologies).

PROGNOSIS

General Considerations

Coma is a nonspecific behavioral state that can be the consequence of multiple processes; therefore, the outcome of coma largely depends on the underlying etiology. It has been reported that, in 283 episodes of pediatric coma (defined as GCS <12 for at least 6 hrs), mortality at about 1 year ranged from 3% to 84%, depending on etiology (53). Causes that tended to produce structural brain changes, such as accidents [traumatic brain injury (TBI), smoke inhalation, strangulation, burns, drowning] and infections, had higher mortality rates (60%–85%) than did causes that were more reversible, such as metabolic changes (diabetic ketoacidosis, inborn errors of metabolism), epilepsy, and intoxication (3%–26%).

Two specific causes for coma, *hypoxic-ischemic* and *TBI*, are considered further in this section. Providing accurate prognostic information is extremely important and is one of the most frequent reasons for neurologic consultation in the PICU. In some cases, the child has already passed the most acute stages of illness, such that his current level of functioning and neurologic examination can be used to prognosticate. More commonly, the child has just experienced a traumatic or hypoxic-ischemic event resulting in coma, and the intensive care physicians and family need prognostic information to help determine the level of care that should be provided. Several types of data may be used in predicting outcome, including historic features of the event, physical signs, neurophysiologic studies (e.g., EEG and evoked potential testing), and neuroimaging.

An overly negative prediction may lead to withdrawal of treatment in a child with a potentially salvageable quality of life. Alternatively, providing an overly positive prediction in a child who has a high probability of never regaining consciousness may lead to survival past the acute stage, with return of spontaneous breathing and resultant prolonged persistent vegetative state, a condition that the child or family may not have wanted. From a systems perspective, given the significant costs involved in the care and rehabilitation of these patients, accurate outcome prediction aids in resource allocation, as more acute care and rehabilitative services could be provided for those patients most likely to benefit.

When applying data from studies of prognosis to individual patients, several complicating factors must be considered:

- Many studies provide little information regarding the exact definitions of terms such as "good" or "poor" outcome or "mild," "moderate," or "severe" neurologic disability. Boundaries between categories may be quite indistinct. Further, different families and patients have different concepts of good and poor outcome relating to their personal set of values. For some, a good outcome requires the child to be fully interactive and self-sufficient, while for others, a good outcome is a child who lives in any state. Some consider the

terms "poor/unfavorable" and "good/favorable," which are used as the outcome measures in most studies of coma prognosis, to be not descriptive of neurodevelopmental state but to convey judgment regarding quality of life (43). Being even severely disabled does not inherently equate with having a poor-quality life. Thus, while research may group patients into these categories, the terms must be redefined based on each family's perceptions. Further complicating the matter is that a family's perceptions may change over time as they live with the disabled child. Factors that children and their parents may have thought would portend a poor quality of life may, in fact, be adapted to and incorporated into a life that is meaningful and appreciated.

- Data suggests that improvement may continue for several years after injury; therefore, determining when to measure outcome is complicated. In children with severe TBI, the percent of children who were independent in all areas of function increased from 37% at discharge from the hospital to 65% at a median follow-up of 24 months (49). Further, a child's and family's ability cope with, and adapt to, a disability may improve with time. Thus, a family's judgment of outcome must be determined sufficiently after the initial event to allow time for these adaptive changes to occur. While data regarding prognosis are useful and needed, the goal may be to distinguish between a persistent vegetative state and some degree of consciousness (even with severe disability), as opposed to distinguishing between different levels of disability. Data on prognosis cannot be used in isolation to make judgments regarding quality of life, as so many factors (e.g., psychologic traits related to resilience, social support) beyond neurologic disability are intertwined.

- Some families may base decisions on averages, while others may base decisions on the hope for having an outlier outcome. The literature contains a few reports of patients who regained the ability to communicate after 4 months in coma, demonstrating that absolute statements regarding prognosis cannot be made to families. If the prognosis is unclear, or the family hopes for an outlier outcome, the physician must support the patient. Prognostic tests must foremost avoid falsely negative predictions and, therefore, must have a high specificity (percentage of patients who will not have a poor outcome and have a normal predictive test) and high positive predictive value (PPV, percentage of patients who will have a poor outcome and have an abnormal predictive test). The second goal is for tests to have high sensitivity (percentage of patients who will have a poor outcome and have an abnormal predictive test) to avoid providing costly care and extending family suffering when the patient will never recover. Further, it is important to consider the confidence interval surrounding these values.

- None of these studies is fully blinded. Testing results are used by treating clinicians to make clinical decisions, including how aggressively to treat the patient and when to withdraw care. For example, a given test result is thought to portend a poor outcome. If the results from this test are used clinically, and the family decides to withdraw care, the patient is then classified as a "poor" outcome. Thus, a study of this test could demonstrate an incorrect association between the test result and poor outcome. No studies of prognosis in children have described provision of maximal treatment for a predetermined duration with clinicians blind to test results.

- Many studies of prognosis have combined patients with coma due to multiple etiologies. As described later, studies have demonstrated that outcome in pediatric coma depends largely on etiology. Thus, defining a prognosis for coma in general is not possible or useful for a given patient, and data must be evaluated based on a particular etiology.

■ Prognosis may change as medical, neurologic, and neurosurgical care evolves. As new devices and management strategies (e.g., hypothermia induction, neuroprotective medications, improved ICP monitoring, and treatment) revolutionize care, outcome predictors must be periodically reassess. Recent studies in adults have started to compare such prognostic tests as somatosensory-evoked potential (SEP) in patients with or without hypothermia treatment.

Inciting Event

Several studies have demonstrated that cardiac arrests and longer periods of cardiopulmonary resuscitation (CPR) were associated with worse outcomes than were respiratory arrests. Mortality associated with cardiac arrest has been reported to be worse than that with respiratory arrest. One study demonstrated that, of 21 patients with respiratory arrest alone, 9 (43%) survived to hospital discharge (42). At 1-year follow-up, 5 were normal, 1 had a mild deficit, 1 had a moderate deficit, 2 had severe deficits, and 1 died. Of 80 patients with cardiac arrest, 6 (8%) survived to hospital discharge; at 1-year follow-up, 3 had moderate deficits, 2 were in a persistent vegetative state, and 1 died. Outcome assessment did not change between hospital discharge and 1-year follow-up. A study of 599 children with out-of-hospital cardiopulmonary arrest demonstrated survival in 8.6%, and one-third of the survivors had good neurologic recovery (56). Studies of in-hospital cardiopulmonary arrest demonstrated higher survival. In a study of 880 children with in-hospital pulseless cardiac arrest, 27% survived to hospital discharge; of the survivors, 65% had good neurologic outcome (pediatric cerebral performance category 1, 2, or 3) when evaluated at hospital discharge (29). Similarly, a study on the effect of hospital characteristics on outcomes of pediatric CPR demonstrated a 51% survival at 24 hrs after CPR (12). Survival was higher in hospitals with pediatric residents and in hospitals with a PICU. The odds ratio for survival was highest if the patient was younger than 1 year or in a monitored intensive care bed. Neurologic outcome was not reported. A study of inpatient cardiac arrest demonstrated that, of 602 children without any ventricular tachycardia or fibrillation, 27% survived to hospital discharge and 24% survived with good neurologic outcome (41). Of 272 patients with ventricular tachycardia or fibrillation on presentation, survival (35%) and neurologic outcome (33%) were better than in those who subsequently developed ventricular tachycardia or fibrillation (11% survived, 8% had good neurologic outcome).

The duration of CPR and the need for multiple doses of resuscitation medications also affect prognosis. CPR lasting >15 mins or the need for more than one bolus of epinephrine was shown to be associated with 100% mortality in one study (16). Another study demonstrated that no survivors with good neurologic outcome received more than three boluses of epinephrine or more than 31 mins of resuscitation (56). In a study of children who remained in coma 24 hrs after hypoxic-ischemic encephalopathy (HIE) with unclear outcome, CPR >10 mins had a 91% PPV for poor outcome (25).

Studies in pediatric near-drowning have demonstrated that children with spontaneous ventilation immediately after CPR

(21), who required <10 mins of CPR or arriving in the ER with a pulse (14) survived with little to no impairment. Conversely, children with no spontaneous ventilations, asystole, or requiring more than 25 mins of CPR (36) either died or had severe neurologic impairment.

An expert review of pediatric resuscitation by the International Liaison Committee on Resuscitation concluded that, while short duration of CPR is associated with better outcome, studies have reported good outcome despite in-hospital arrest that required 30–60 mins of CPR and excellent outcome after longer than 30 mins of cardiac arrest with ice-water submersion. The study states that "15 or 30 mins of CPR does not define the limits of cardiac or cerebral viability" (40).

In children with hypoxia-ischemia, a GCS score of <4–5 has been associated with a high risk of death or severe neurologic impairment (11,44). Complicating these prognostic indicators are studies that demonstrate that cold-water submersion for >15 mins (32) and an initial GCS score as low as 4 (11) may be associated with good recovery. In children with HIE-induced coma, a GCS score of <5 at 24 hrs has been associated with a PPV of 100% for poor outcome (25). In children with nonpenetrating TBI, a GCS score of <8 at 6 hrs after injury has been associated with high mortality (50), although some studies have shown that half of survivors who had a GCS score of <5 were independent at follow-up (49).

Monitoring of blood pressure during the acute phases of treatment for HIE or TBI has predictive value. Having a maximum systolic blood pressure of <90 mm Hg was associated with 100% mortality (50). Other studies have confirmed that even low normal blood pressure is associated with unfavorable outcome.

Studies in adults have demonstrated that seizures occur frequently following cardiac arrest (25%–44% of patients) but that seizures are not predictive of outcome. One group did not report on clinical seizures but demonstrated that epileptiform changes on EEG increased the relative risk of poor outcome (25).

Physical Examination

Many patients with severe brain injury receive paralytic or sedative medications that can affect the physical examination. The effect of these agents must be carefully considered before interpreting the potential significance of a comatose child's physical examination. A large meta-analysis of studies that assessed outcome in adult survivors of coma due to cardiac arrest demonstrated that absent corneal reflexes, absent pupillary reflexes, absent withdrawal to pain, and no motor response at 24 hrs after insult, combined with no motor response at 72 hrs after insult, strongly predicted death or poor neurologic outcome (51). Unfortunately, no signs were identified that allowed accurate prognostication within 24 hrs of cardiac arrest. The American Academy of Neurology published a practice parameter in adults that states certain clinical findings accurately predict poor outcome, including absence of pupillary responses and absent corneal reflexes within days 1–3 after CPR, as well as absent or extensor motor responses after 3 days (51). No similarly extensive studies have been conducted in children.

It has been demonstrated in children with HIE that the absence of spontaneous ventilation and absence of pupillary reflexes at 24 hrs after insult had a 100% PPV of poor outcome

(25). Admission signs were not predictive. A retrospective chart review study of children with near-drowning events demonstrated that children with purposeful movements and normal brainstem function at 24 hrs after resuscitation had a good outcome, while all children without purposeful movement and with abnormal brainstem signs had severe neurologic impairments or died (5). In another study of children with HIE, the sensitivity/specificity of motor response and pupillary response for unfavorable outcome were 93%/50% and 47%/100%, respectively (6). In children with TBI, the sensitivity/specificity of motor response and pupillary response for unfavorable outcome were 80%/85% and 75%/95%, respectively. In children with coma due to multiple etiologies, the absence of motor response to pain on day 3 after injury had PPV for unfavorable outcome of 100% (4). Together, these studies suggest that if not confounded by medications, the neurologic examination is quite predictive when performed >24 hrs after the inciting event. Falsely pessimistic predictions can be limited by using SEP in conjunction with the physical examination.

Evoked Potentials

When a sensory stimulus is delivered to nerves, neural structures along the particular sensory pathway produce electrical signals that can be detected by electrodes placed along the neural pathway and displayed as waves. Electrodes are placed peripherally (i.e., Erb point), along the spinal cord (i.e., third cervical level), and cortically (i.e., over the somatosensory cortex). Absent or delayed waves between the stimulus and recording electrode suggest anatomic disruption in the conduction pathways. Evoked potentials are not affected by sedative administration or environmental electrical noise and therefore may be useful in an ICU setting. However, intracranial lesions may alter the evoked potential signal.

In children with coma due to multiple etiologies, abnormal SEPs predicted unfavorable outcome with sensitivity of 75% and specificity of 92% (6). On initial testing, abnormal SEPs have a PPV for unfavorable outcome of 98% when absent bilaterally and a PPV for favorable outcome of 91% when present (4). All patients with favorable outcomes despite absent SEPs had structural lesions, such as subdural effusions or brainstem hemorrhage. In children with only HIE, in whom prognosis was unclear at 24 hrs after resuscitation, the finding of bilaterally absent N20 waves on the SEP had a 100% PPV for unfavorable outcome, with 63% sensitivity (25). Another study in children with HIE demonstrated that, of the 8 patients with absent responses, 6 died and 2 had neurologic deficits. Of 6 patients who had normal responses, 5 were normal and 1 died (24).

Brainstem auditory-evoked potentials (BAEP) use an auditory stimulus to evaluate brainstem but not cortical function. Thus, while they may be predictive of survival versus death, they lack utility in predicting neurocognitive outcome, which is based largely on cortical function. The neural structures that generate waves include the cochlear nerve (wave I), vestibular nucleus (wave II), superior olivary complex in the pons (wave III), and the lateral lemniscus and inferior colliculus in the midbrain (waves IV and V). Nine out of 10 brain-dead children in one study lacked all components of the BAEP, and 1 child had only wave I (45). Furthermore, 13 of 13 comatose children had at least waves I and V. Normal BAEP responses were reported in 5 infants in a persistent vegetative state after nontraumatic coma, all of whom had absent SEPs (15). Several reports have demonstrated that initially absent BAEP responses can return later. If wave I is abnormal, no conclusions can be drawn about further waves. Peripheral abnormalities altering wave I include preexisting deafness, middle ear fluid, cerumen, or cochlear damage (because of a temporal bone fracture or infarction).

Visual-evoked potentials (VEP) use a flickering light to activate the visual system. A study of 37 children in coma (including traumatic causes) found that all children with normal outcome had normal VEP, whereas all children who died had abnormal VEP (47). Contrary to this report, another study demonstrated that 15 children who eventually died following nontraumatic coma initially had normal VEPs (27). Preserved VEPs have been reported despite brain death.

Together, these studies suggest that bilaterally absent cortical SEP responses are predictive of death or severe disability but structural lesions must be excluded in children with TBI. The role of BAEP and VEP is less clear. The role of SEP in children with TBI is less clear, as these children are more likely to have structural lesions that may confound measurements.

Electroencephalogram

The EEG is a good indicator of thalamocortical function, but the utility of a single EEG is limited by the lack of specificity of findings. For example, a burst suppression pattern, which refers to an EEG background exhibiting alternating periods of low- and high-amplitude activity, may be seen in hypoxic-ischemic encephalopathy, metabolic encephalopathy, or with sedating medications. Thus, serial EEG recordings combined with clinical information may be required for prognostic purposes.

In adults with HIE, the presence of generalized burst suppression, profound background attenuation, or loss of reactivity to external stimuli are all predictive of poor prognosis, while the presence of normal posterior dominant rhythm and reactivity suggests a good prognosis. However, the only EEG finding reported to have 100% specificity for no recovery of consciousness is generalized suppression on an EEG performed at least 1 day after cardiac arrest (54). Several small studies of EEG in comatose children have been conducted. One study demonstrated that more than half of children with normal or slow activity on EEG had good outcomes (46). However, all patients in whom the worst EEG showed low amplitude or electrocerebral silence had a poor outcome. Another study demonstrated that the PPV for poor outcome was 100% with discontinuous activity and 96% with no reactivity or high-voltage slow waves (25). A third group studied 33 children who were comatose due to multiple etiologies (hypoxia in 36%) (38). Of 19 children with a nonreactive EEG pattern, 10 (53%) died, 3 (16%) had unfavorable outcome, and 6 (32%) had favorable outcome (although none were normal on follow-up). Of 14 children with a reactive EEG pattern, 3 (21%) were normal at follow-up, an additional 7 (50%) had a favorable outcome, and 4 (29%) died. Lack of reactivity had a 52.6% PPV for mortality. Several studies have demonstrated that response to stimulation and normal sleep patterns are associated with good prognosis.

Together, these studies demonstrate that mild slowing and rapid improvement of the EEG are associated with good outcome, while burst suppression, electrocerebral silence, and lack of reactivity are associated with poor outcome. Repeating the

TABLE 53.7

GENERAL GUIDELINES FOR NEUROIMAGING IN THE INITIAL EVALUATION OF SELECT CAUSES OF COMA

	Head CT	Diffusion-weighted Image	T2	T1	Echo gradient	Gadolinium contrast
Acute ischemia (Minutes to hours)	± (usually normal)	Bright signal indicates restriction of water diffusion (cytotoxic edema)	Hyperintense signal after several hours	Variable	May demonstrate petechial hemorrhage	− early + late (increasing after 3 days)
Subacute ischemia (3 days to 1 week)	Hypodense (dark)	Restriction of water will fade at 7–10 days	Hyperintense	Variable, hyperintense in neonate	Petechial or hemorrhagic transformation	+ enhancement
Acute hemorrhage (Hour to days)	Hyperdense (bright)	N/A	Very hypointense	Hypointense	Strongly positive	
Subacute hemorrhage (First several days)	Heterogeneous to hypodense	N/A	Very hypointense	Very hyperintense	Strongly positive	
Infection	Hypodense/ isodense	Restriction of water diffusion if abscess	Very hyperintense	Very hypointense	± petechial hemorrhage	+ enhancement

Intensity is relative to normal brain parenchyma (hypointense, dark relative to normal tissue; hyperintense, bright relative to normal tissue; isointense, same intensity of normal tissue).

EEG to determine whether improvement occurs is important, as is ensuring EEG changes are not pharmacologically induced or compromised by scalp edema or subdural collections. Prolonged EEG monitoring may be helpful to determine whether sleep-wake rhythms exist.

Neuroimaging

MRI, especially diffusion-weighted imaging (DWI), may be more sensitive to early HIE changes than is cranial CT (Table 53.7). However, MRI may be difficult to obtain in unstable ICU patients, as it frequently involves transport to the MRI facility, and access to the patient is limited during the study.

Injury to the basal ganglia or watershed regions has been demonstrated to have a sensitivity of 96% (patients with bad outcome have abnormal MRI), specificity of 50% (patients with good outcome have normal MRI), PPV of 82% (patients with abnormal MR have bad outcome), and negative predictive value (NPV) of 4% (patients with normal MR have bad outcome) for identifying poor outcome (8). Abnormal MRI on days 1–4 had 100% PPV and normal MRI on days 4–7 had 100% NPV. An example MRI of these findings in 2 patients with poor outcome is provided in **Figure 53.2.** In children rescued from near-drowning, abnormal signals in the cortex, basal ganglia, or brainstem were associated with persistent vegetative state or death with a specificity of 100% (13). On MR spectroscopy, elevated lactate (a marker of deficient aerobic energy metabolism) and reduced N-acetylaspartate (NAA, synthesized in neurons with reduced levels, suggesting neuron injury) were associated with poor outcome. Outcome was better predicted at 3–4 days than at 1–2 days.

In children with nonpenetrating TBI and a GCS score of <8, all patients with a normal admission CT survived. Nonsurvivors were more likely to have evidence of cerebral edema,

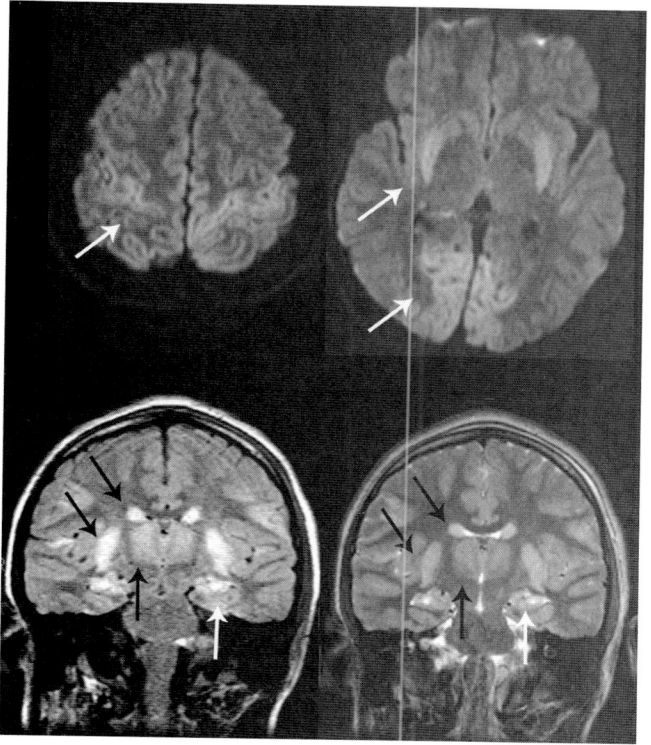

FIGURE 53.2. The MRIs of two teenage patients after severe hypoxic-ischemic encephalopathy. Diffusion-weighted images (DWI) show restriction in the central sulcus (*upper left, white arrow*), putamen and visual cortex (*upper right, white arrow*). Fluid-attenuated inversion recovery (*FLAIR, bottom left*) and T2 (*bottom right*) images demonstrate signal hyperintensity in the thalamus, putamen, and caudate (*black arrows*), as well as the hippocampus (*white arrows*).

TABLE 53.8

TESTS WITH HIGH PREDICTIVE VALUE FOR POOR NEUROLOGIC OUTCOME

Factor/sign/test	Result at ≥24 Hrs	PPV for unfavorable outcome	References
CPR	>10–15 mins	90%–100%	(5,24,44)
GCS	3–5	90%–100%	(10,24,44)
Pupillary Response	Absent	90%–100%	(5,24)
Respirations	Absent	100%	(24)
Motor Response	Absent	90%–100%	(3–5)
SEP N20	Absent bilaterally	90%–100%	(5,6,9,16)
EEG	Discontinuous/Silent/ Nonreactive	50%–100%	(24,38,46)
MRI	Watershed or Basal ganglia injury	80%–100%	(7,12)
MRI	Brainstem	100%	(12,52)

CPR, cardiopulmonary resuscitation; GCS, Glasgow Come Scale; SEP somatosensory-evoked potential; EEG, electroencephalogram

subarachnoid hemorrhage, or subdural hemorrhage. Among survivors, none of the findings correlated with the degree of disability (50). Lesions in the pons or caudal medulla were associated with 100% mortality (52). In children with TBI, even normal-appearing brain often had abnormal metabolite ratios, indicating diffuse axonal injury. Further, within the normally appearing brain, the NAA:Cr ratio was decreased more in children with poor outcome than in those with good outcome (19).

Newer MRI techniques have been useful in predicting outcome after TBI. Susceptibility-weighted MRI detects hemorrhagic diffuse axonal injury particularly well, and in children with TBI, the lesion volume using this technique accounted for 32% of the variance in cognitive performance (3). MR spectroscopy determines metabolic ratios in specific brain regions.

Combined Modalities

Several studies have suggested that multimodal findings may be more predictive than any single indicator. In a study of 102 children with TBI, it was demonstrated that, in children with HIE, combining abnormal SEPs with either abnormal motor or pupillary signs produced 100% specificity in predicting unfavorable outcome (6). Other investigators did not combine modalities in analysis but demonstrated that all children with good outcome despite bilaterally absent SEPs had structural lesions identifiable by neuroimaging that compromised accurate SEP measurements (4). Finally, a group that combined VEP, BAEP, and EEG findings to create an electrophysiology score demonstrated that a poor electrophysiologic score had a 100% PPV for poor outcome, while a good score had a 46% NPV for normal outcome (27).

CONCLUSIONS AND FUTURE DIRECTIONS

Coma refers to an abnormality in consciousness in which both wakefulness and awareness are disturbed. Coma has many etiologies, including lesions and abnormalities that affect the reticular activating system in the brainstem or the cortex diffusely. Coma is a medical emergency, in that some causes are reversible and secondary neurologic injury must be prevented. The history, examination, laboratory, imaging, and electrophysiologic evaluation may disclose the etiology of coma, allowing specific treatment. The prognosis in coma is more dependent on the specific etiology than on any other factor; thus, prognostic information cannot be provided for the family until the etiology is determined. Children may have multiple conditions that contribute to coma, and this must be considered. In children with HIE or TBI, abnormal exam signs (pupil reactivity and motor response), SEP (N20 wave absence bilaterally), EEG (electrocerebral silence not due to metabolic or medication etiology), and MRI (cortex and basal ganglia changes) each are highly predictive of poor outcome when performed at least 24 hrs after the inciting event. Combining these modalities improves the overall predictive value. SEPs are not commonly performed in children's hospitals, but data suggest that SEPs will become an increasingly important tool in guiding prognosis. Given that some prognostic tests have 100% PPV for unfavorable outcome when performed at 24 hrs, when decisions can be postponed, neurologic consultation and testing can provide quite definitive information. The tests that have high predictive value for poor neurologic outcome are summarized in **Table 53.8**. Findings were less predictive in the initial hours, suggesting that, during the initial period, honest statements to families must include statements regarding infrequent outliers who survived with better outcome than might have been predicted. Based on the current data, early decisions cannot be entirely evidence-based, and the course of care must depend on informed discussions with the family.

KEY POINTS

- Coma describes a state of altered wakefulness and awareness that is caused by multiple conditions that affect the brainstem or cortex diffusely.

- Coma is a medical emergency that requires rapid and accurate evaluation.
- Treatment is determined by coma etiology.
- Complications, such as elevated ICP and seizures, must be recognized and managed to prevent secondary neurologic injury.
- Providing accurate prognostic information requires evaluation for potential confounding factors and is enhanced when multiple prognostic features are combined and serially evaluated.

References

1. The Management of a Child (aged 0–18 years) with a Decreased Conscious Level. The Paediatric Accident and Emergency Research Group 2006; http://www.nottingham.ac.uk/paediatric-guideline/. Accessed on February 11, 2007.
2. Alehan FK, Morton LD, Pellock JM. Utility of electroencephalography in the pediatric emergency department. *J Child Neurol* 2001;16:484–7.
3. Babikian T, Freier MC, Tong KA, et al. Susceptibility weighted imaging: Neuropsychologic outcome and pediatric head injury. *Pediatr Neurol* 2005;33:184–94.
4. Beca J, Cox PN, Taylor MJ, et al. Somatosensory-evoked potentials for prediction of outcome in acute severe brain injury. *J Pediatr* 1995;126:44–9.
5. Bratton SL, Jardine DS, Morray JP. Serial neurologic examinations after near drowning and outcome. *Arch Pediatr Adolesc Med* 1994;148:167–70.
6. Carter BG, Butt W. A prospective study of outcome predictors after severe brain injury in children. *Intensive Care Med* 2005;31:840–5.
7. Carter BG, Taylor A, Butt W. Severe brain injury in children: Long-term outcome and its prediction using somatosensory evoked potentials (SEPs). *Intensive Care Med* 1999;25:722–8.
8. Christophe C, Fonteyne C, Ziereisen F, et al. Value of MR imaging of the brain in children with hypoxic coma. *AJNR Am J Neuroradiol* 2002;23:716–23.
9. Claassen J, Mayer SA, Kowalski RG, et al. Detection of electrographic seizures with continuous EEG monitoring in critically ill patients. *Neurology* 2004;62:1743–8.
10. De Meirleir LJ, Taylor MJ. Prognostic utility of SEPs in comatose children. *Pediatr Neurol* 1987;3:78–82.
11. Dean JM, Kaufman ND. Prognostic indicators in pediatric near-drowning: The Glasgow Coma Scale. *Crit Care Med* 1981;9:536–9.
12. Donoghue AJ, Nadkarni VM, Elliott M, et al. Effects of hospital characteristics on outcomes from pediatric cardiopulmonary resuscitation: A report from the national registry of cardiopulmonary resuscitation. *Pediatrics* 2006;119:995–1001.
13. Dubowitz DJ, Bluml S, Arcinue E, et al. MR of hypoxic encephalopathy in children after near drowning: Correlation with quantitative proton MR spectroscopy and clinical outcome. *AJNR Am J Neuroradiol* 1998;19:1617–27.
14. Fiser DH. Near-drowning. *Pediatr Rev* 1993;14:148–51.
15. Frank LM, Furgiuele TL, Etheridge JE, Jr. Prediction of chronic vegetative state in children using evoked potentials. *Neurology* 1985;35:931–4.
16. Gillis J, Dickson D, Rieder M, et al. Results of inpatient pediatric resuscitation. *Crit Care Med* 1986;14:469–71.
17. Goodwin SR, Friedman WA, Bellefleur M. Is it time to use evoked potentials to predict outcome in comatose children and adults? *Crit Care Med* 1991;19:518–24.
18. Hahn YS, Chyung C, Barthel MJ, et al. Head injuries in children under 36 months of age. Demography and outcome. *Childs Nervous System* 1988;4:34–40.
19. Holshouser BA, Tong KA, Ashwal S. Proton MR spectroscopic imaging depicts diffuse axonal injury in children with traumatic brain injury. *AJNR Am J Neuroradiol* 2005;26:1276–85.
20. Hosain SA, Solomon GE, Kobylarz EJ. Electroencephalographic patterns in unresponsive pediatric patients. *Pediatr Neurol* 2005;32:162–5.
21. Jacobsen WK, Mason LJ, Briggs BA, et al. Correlation of spontaneous respiration and neurologic damage in near-drowning. *Crit Care Med* 1983;11:487–9.
22. Jette N, Wittman J, Claassen J, et al. Time to first seizure in pediatric patients with nonconvulsive seizures on continuous EEG monitoring. *Annual Meeting of the American Epilepsy Society, New Orleans, Louisiana,* 2004;I.230.
23. Kirkham FJ. Non-traumatic coma in children. *Arch Dis Child* 2001;85:303–12.
24. Lutschg J, Pfenninger J, Ludin HP, et al. Brain-stem auditory evoked potentials and early somatosensory evoked potentials in neurointensively treated comatose children. *Am J Dis Child* 1983;137:421–6.
25. Mandel R, Martinot A, Delepoulle F, et al. Prediction of outcome after hypoxic-ischemic encephalopathy: A prospective clinical and electrophysiologic study. *J Pediatr* 2002;141:45–50.
26. Messe SR, Cucchiara BL. Wrong-way eyes with thalamic hemorrhage. *Neurology* 2003;60:1524.
27. Mewasingh LD, Christophe C, Fonteyne C, et al. Predictive value of electrophysiology in children with hypoxic coma. *Pediatr Neurol* 2003;28:178–83.
28. Michaud LJ, Rivara FP, Grady MS, et al. Predictors of survival and severity of disability after severe brain injury in children. *Neurosurgery* 1992;31:254–64.
29. Nadkarni VM, Larkin GL, Peberdy MA, et al. First documented rhythm and clinical outcome from in-hospital cardiac arrest among children and adults. *JAMA* 2006;295:50–7.
30. O'Connell F. Central pathways for cough in man—unanswered questions. *Pulm Pharmacol Ther* 2002;15:295–301.
31. O'Regan ME, Brown JK. Serum neuron specific enolase: A marker for neuronal dysfunction in children with continuous EEG epileptiform activity. *Eur J Paediatr Neurol* 1998;2:193–7.
32. Orlowski JP. Drowning, near-drowning, and ice-water submersions. *Pediatr Clin North Am* 1987;34:75–92.
33. Parslow RC, Morris KP, Tasker RC, et al. Epidemiology of traumatic brain injury in children receiving intensive care in the UK. *Arch Dis Child* 2005;90:1182–7.
34. Piek J, Chesnut RM, Marshall LF, et al. Extracranial complications of severe head injury. *J Neurosurg* 1992;77:901–7.
35. Plum F, Posner JB. *The Diagnosis of Stupor and Coma,* 3rd ed. Philadelphia: F.A. Davis Co., 1980.
36. Quan L, Wentz KR, Gore EJ, et al. Outcome and predictors of outcome in pediatric submersion victims receiving prehospital care in King County, Washington. *Pediatrics* 1990;86:586–93.
37. Raimondi AJ, Hirschauer J. Head injury in the infant and toddler. Coma scoring and outcome scale. *Child's Brain* 1984;11:12–35.
38. Ramachandrannair R, Sharma R, Weiss SK, et al. Reactive EEG patterns in pediatric coma. *Pediatr Neurol* 2005;33:345–9.
39. Reilly PL, Simpson DA, Sprod R, et al. Assessing the conscious level in infants and young children: A paediatric version of the Glasgow Coma Scale. *Childs Nervous System* 1988;4:30–3.
40. Resuscitation International Liaison Committee. Part 6: Paediatric basic and advanced life support. *Resuscitation* 2005;67:271–91.
41. Samson RA, Nadkarni VM, Meaney PA, et al. Outcomes of in-hospital ventricular fibrillation in children. *N Engl J Med* 2006;354:2328–39.
42. Schindler MB, Bohn D, Cox PN, et al. Outcome of out-of-hospital cardiac or respiratory arrest in children. *N Engl J Med* 1996;335:1473–9.
43. Shewmon DA. Coma prognosis in children. Part II: Clinical application. *J Clin Neurophysiol* 2000;17:467–72.
44. Spack L, Gedeit R, Splaingard M, et al. Failure of aggressive therapy to alter outcome in pediatric near-drowning. *Pediatr Emerg Care* 1997;13:98–102.
45. Steinhart CM, Weiss IP. Use of brainstem auditory evoked potentials in pediatric brain death. *Crit Care Med* 1985;13:560–2.
46. Tasker RC, Boyd S, Harden A, et al. Monitoring in non-traumatic coma. Part II: Electroencephalography. *Arch Dis Child* 1988;63:895–9.
47. Taylor MJ, Farrell EJ. Comparison of the prognostic utility of VEPs and SEPs in comatose children. *Pediatr Neurol* 1989;5:145–50.
48. Teasdale G, Jennett B. Assessment of coma and impaired consciousness. A practical scale. *Lancet* 1974;2:81–4.
49. Thakker JC, Splaingard M, Zhu J, et al. Survival and functional outcome of children requiring endotracheal intubation during therapy for severe traumatic brain injury. *Crit Care Med* 1997;25:1396–401.
50. White JR, Farukhi Z, Bull C, et al. Predictors of outcome in severely head-injured children. *Crit Care Med* 2001;29:534–40.
51. Wijdicks EF, Hijdra A, Young GB, et al. Practice parameter: Prediction of outcome in comatose survivors after cardiopulmonary resuscitation (an evidence-based review): Report of the Quality Standards Subcommittee of the American Academy of Neurology. *Neurology* 2006;67:203–10.
52. Woischneck D, Klein S, Reissberg S, et al. Prognosis of brain stem lesion in children with head injury. *Childs Nerv Syst* 2003;19:174–8.
53. Wong CP, Forsyth RJ, Kelly TP, et al. Incidence, aetiology, and outcome of non-traumatic coma: A population based study. *Arch Dis Child* 2001;84:193–9.
54. Young GB. The EEG in coma. *J Clin Neurophysiol* 2000;17:473–85.
55. Young GB, Jordan KG, Doig GS. An assessment of nonconvulsive seizures in the intensive care unit using continuous EEG monitoring: An investigation of variables associated with mortality. *Neurology* 1996;47:83–9.
56. Young KD, Gausche-Hill M, McClung CD, et al. A prospective, population-based study of the epidemiology and outcome of out-of-hospital pediatric cardiopulmonary arrest. *Pediatrics* 2004;114:157–64.

CHAPTER 54 ■ NEUROLOGIC MONITORING

BRAHM GOLDSTEIN • MATEO ABOY • ALAN GRAHAM

Increasing evidence demonstrates tangible benefits from neurologic monitoring in a variety of PICU patients. Continuous electroencephalogram (EEG) coupled with digital video monitoring for status epilepticus (SE) is routinely applied with good results in diagnosing nonconvulsive seizures and as part of a surgical approach for intractable seizures (47). Although sparse, evidence-based data show that intracranial pressure (ICP) monitoring in patients with severe traumatic brain injury (TBI) improves outcome (1,2). Intraoperative and postoperative neurophysiologic monitoring of children who undergo repair of congenital cardiac disease with near infrared spectroscopy (NIRS) technology has also demonstrated improvement in outcome (6). Thus, it is important for PICU personnel to understand the underlying engineering and physiologic principles of neuromonitoring. This chapter focuses on technologies currently in use for neuromonitoring of the critically ill and injured PICU patient.

SCIENTIFIC FOUNDATIONS

General Engineering Aspects of ICU Monitoring

Medical instrumentation systems are often composed of sensors, signal conditioning hardware and software, output displays, and auxiliary signals. Sensors are used to convert a physical measurand (i.e., a quantity, property, or condition of interest) into an electrical signal output. The sensors used for medical instrumentation purposes are designed to be minimally invasive and to respond to the source of energy present in the measure, while excluding all other sources as much as possible. Generally, the electrical signal produced by these sensors cannot be connected directly to the output display device. Signal conditioning and processing, such as amplification and analog filtering, are typically required (45). Additionally, the sensor outputs are analog signals and must be converted to digital form before they can be processed using more advanced digital signal processing techniques. Analog-to-digital (A/D) conversion involves signal conditioning, antialiasing filtering, uniform sampling, and quantization. (**Table 54.1** provides definitions for the engineering terms used in this chapter.) For an in-depth discussion of medical instrumentation, such as sensors, biopotential electrodes and amplifiers, blood pressure, flow, and volume measurement equipment, chemical biosensors, and imaging systems, the reader is referred to a general textbook on biomedical engineering (45).

Most signals are filtered with analog integrated circuits before A/D conversion. These frequency-selective filters are usually linear bandpass or highpass filters used to remove drift,

prevent aliasing, and reduce noise; they can distort the waveform morphology due to nonlinear phase in the passband or removal of signal frequencies.

During A/D conversion, analog signals are sampled at a rate determined by the manufacturer (i.e., the sampling rate or sampling frequency). To accurately represent the signal on patient monitor displays, the sampling rate must be high enough so that a linear interpolation between the sample points results in a visually smooth and representative signal. To achieve this, the sampling rate should be at least 10 times higher than the highest frequency component of the prefiltered signal. For most physiologic signals that vary with the cardiac and respiratory cycles, a sampling rate of 100 Hertz (Hz) is sufficient. Due to the impulsive nature of the QRS complex, electrocardiogram (ECG) signals have a higher bandwidth than most other physiologic signals encountered in the ICU and require a higher sampling rate of at least 250 Hz to accurately represent different segments of the ECG waveform. Electroencephalograms (EEGs) also require a higher sampling rate, although this signal is infrequently displayed directly on ICU patient monitors.

In addition to the sampling rate requirements, quantization requirements must be met to avoid quantization error. Each sample of the digital signal is represented by B bits and can only take one of 2^B levels. The quantization error is the error that results from using the quantized signal rather than the true signal amplitude.

Once the physiologic signals have been converted to digital form, more advanced digital signal processing algorithms are used to process these physiologic digital signals and extract clinically significant parameters. For instance, heart rate is estimated from the ECG signal using automatic QRS detection algorithms, and diastolic and systolic pressures are obtained from pressure signals. It is important for the clinician to understand that digital signal processing algorithms generally use a moving window of the physiologic signal to generate estimates. These moving-window segments (signal frames) range from 3–10 secs in duration. Consequently, the clinical parameters obtained represent an average over past values of the signal and cannot respond instantaneously to alarm conditions. Thus, patient monitors typically generate alarms *after* the alarm condition has persisted for several seconds. The obverse is also true. For example, after a successful resuscitation from cardiopulmonary arrest, the arterial oxygen saturation value will typically lag a few seconds after the patient's cyanosis has resolved.

Clinically Important Physiologic Systems and Signals

A limited number of physiologic systems may be monitored within the central nervous system (CNS). The EEG has been widely available for decades to record and quantitatively

TABLE 54.1

ENGINEERING TERMS AND DEFINITIONS

Aliasing – The apparent conversion of high-frequency signals to low-frequency signals due to an insufficient sample rate.

Analog-to-digital (A/D) conversion – The electrical conversion of an analog signal (often a voltage) to a digital representation that enables manipulation and processing by computers.

Bandpass filter – A filter that eliminates low- and high-frequency components of a signal, but retains an intermediate range.

Bandwidth – The range of frequencies spanned by a signal. When applied to bandpass filters, it describes the range of frequencies that are allowed to pass through the filter.

Capacitance – A measure of the ability of a circuit element to store electrical charge. Elements with a large capacitance dampen or resist rapid fluctuations in voltage.

Demodulation – The process of extracting an information-bearing signal from another signal; analogous to extracting a file of interest from a compressed or encrypted file.

Hertz (Hz) – A measure of frequency; equivalent to cycles per second (cps).

High-frequency noise – Many types of artifact in physiologic signals contain significant power at high frequencies. This noise is often emitted by medical equipment near the patient.

Highpass filter – A filter that eliminates low-frequency components of a signal but retains high-frequency components.

Inductance – A measure of the ability of a circuit element to store energy in a magnetic field. Elements with a large inductance dampen or resist rapid fluctuations in current.

Linear interpolation – The process of estimating a value of a signal or function between two intermediate values using a line between the two points.

Low-frequency noise – Some types of artifact in physiologic signals contain significant power at low frequencies. This noise is often caused by patient movement.

Lowpass filter – A filter that eliminates high-frequency components of a signal but retains low-frequency components.

Modulation – The process of embedding an information-bearing signal in another signal; analogous to creating an encrypted or compressed file that contains a file of interest.

Moving window – A technique for estimating an average quality of a signal continuously by averaging over period of the preceding 3–5 secs. For example, the systolic blood pressure is usually calculated by averaging the systolic peaks over a moving window of 3–5 secs.

Nonlinear – Any system or device the behavior of which is governed by a set of nonlinear equations.

Signal power – The power contained in a signal is generally defined as the square of the signal; often averaged over a moving window to create a smoothly varying continuous estimate.

measure the brain's electrical activity. Technology for monitoring ICP has also been available, and now is almost always accomplished with more accurate fiberoptic technology. The most recent advances, however, have occurred in our ability to monitor cerebral blood flow (CBF), both on a global and regional basis, using direct and indirect methods, such as ultrasound, tissue oxygenation, jugular venous oxygenation, and local blood flow and oxygenation indices. Additionally, monitoring of cellular and extracellular processes is beginning to progress from the research laboratory to the bedside, with the ability to measure regional brain tissue oxygen, carbon dioxide levels, pH, and extracellular fluid concentrations of glucose, lactate, and pyruvate. Finally, the term *multimodality neuromonitoring* refers to different combinations of these methods used simultaneously to provide a more complete physiologic picture of CNS activity from the cellular to the tissue to the organ level.

APPLICATION TO PEDIATRIC INTENSIVE CARE

Electroencephalogram

The EEG records the electrical activity of the brain observed via scalp electrical potentials. The EEG's sources are neurons located predominantly in the outermost layers of the cerebral cortex. Thus, the EEG is a spatial phenomenon that follows the spatial topography of the cortex.

Continuous Electroencephalogram

While a 1-hr EEG is often used in most clinical circumstances, the use of continuous 24-hr EEG or video-EEG monitoring is becoming increasingly commonplace in most ICUs for various clinical indications, such as monitoring SE and therapeutically induced coma in cases of refractory SE and TBIs. As well, 24-hr EEG has proven useful in the surveillance of patients at risk for subclinical seizures, persistent nonconvulsive SE, metabolic encephalopathies, and neurologic conditions that limit a patient's ability to respond (e.g., brainstem injuries, severe peripheral neuropathic syndromes) (35). The depth of impaired consciousness or coma can be immediately assessed, as can the degree to which ongoing electrographic seizures contribute to that state.

The most common pediatric EEG is a 20-lead EEG with continuous recording and simultaneous digital video recording, with clinical annotations made by bedside observers, usually the PICU nurse or parent. A variety of channel configurations (i.e., bipolar or reference montages) can be used, depending on the area of interest. A *channel* is simply a representation of the potential difference between two recording electrodes. Additional electrodes may include eye leads to discern ocular movements, electromyography, ECG, and a measurement of respiratory frequency. Current digital EEG technology has been used for the past 10 years, as increased computer power and storage capability phased out older, less flexible, and less information-rich analog, pen-and-paper systems.

Current digital acquisition systems record continuous EEG data to computer hard drives (1–1.5 GB/24 hrs/patient). Systems can acquire 32, 64, 128, or more channels, with higher numbers used for large arrays of electrodes, usually in patients who are undergoing intracranial recording for epilepsy surgery

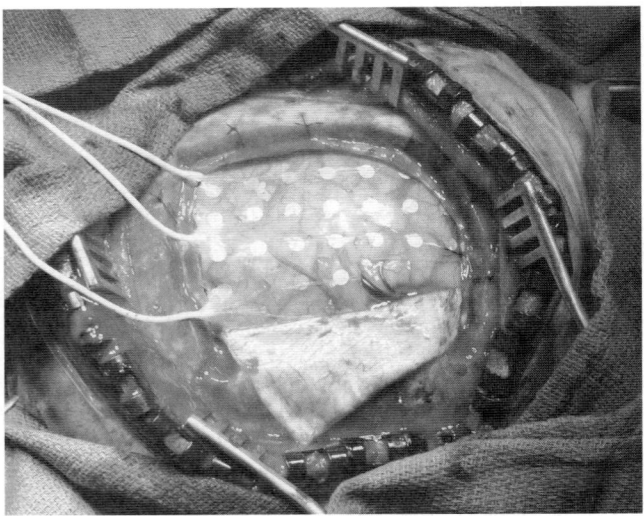

FIGURE 54.1. High-density subdural electrode grid placed intraoperatively over the frontotemporal region in a patient with intractable focal seizures. (Photo courtesy N. Selden, PhD, MD, Oregon Health & Science University, Portland, OR).

(**Figs. 54.1** and **54.2**) (47). Most patients require 32 or fewer channels. Sampling rates vary from 60 Hz to 257 Hz, and data can be instantly remontaged to allow better localization and interpretation of focal or generalized abnormalities.

A variety of software packages is available to interpret EEG data, often in real time. Specialized software can identify numerous epileptiform abnormalities and detect electrographic seizure activity. The parameters of these detection algorithms can be adjusted to increase yield and decrease false detections. Special software packages are available for the detection of neonatal seizures, while other packages can identify sleep stages. The systems can trigger alarms when a seizure or abnormality of interest is detected.

Most digital EEG monitoring systems can also acquire simultaneous digital video and audio signals. Temporal resolution is excellent, far surpassing analog video modalities. Data can be recorded from cart-mounted cameras and microphones in the patient's room, or remotely via wall- or ceiling-mounted devices. Digital video files can be large and, although file size can be decreased by reducing image resolution, video captures can occupy >12 GB/24 hr/patient using MPEG-2 format. Therefore, storage and transmission of data across hospital networks can be expensive and difficult. Many programs can automatically prune files into time samples based on preselected

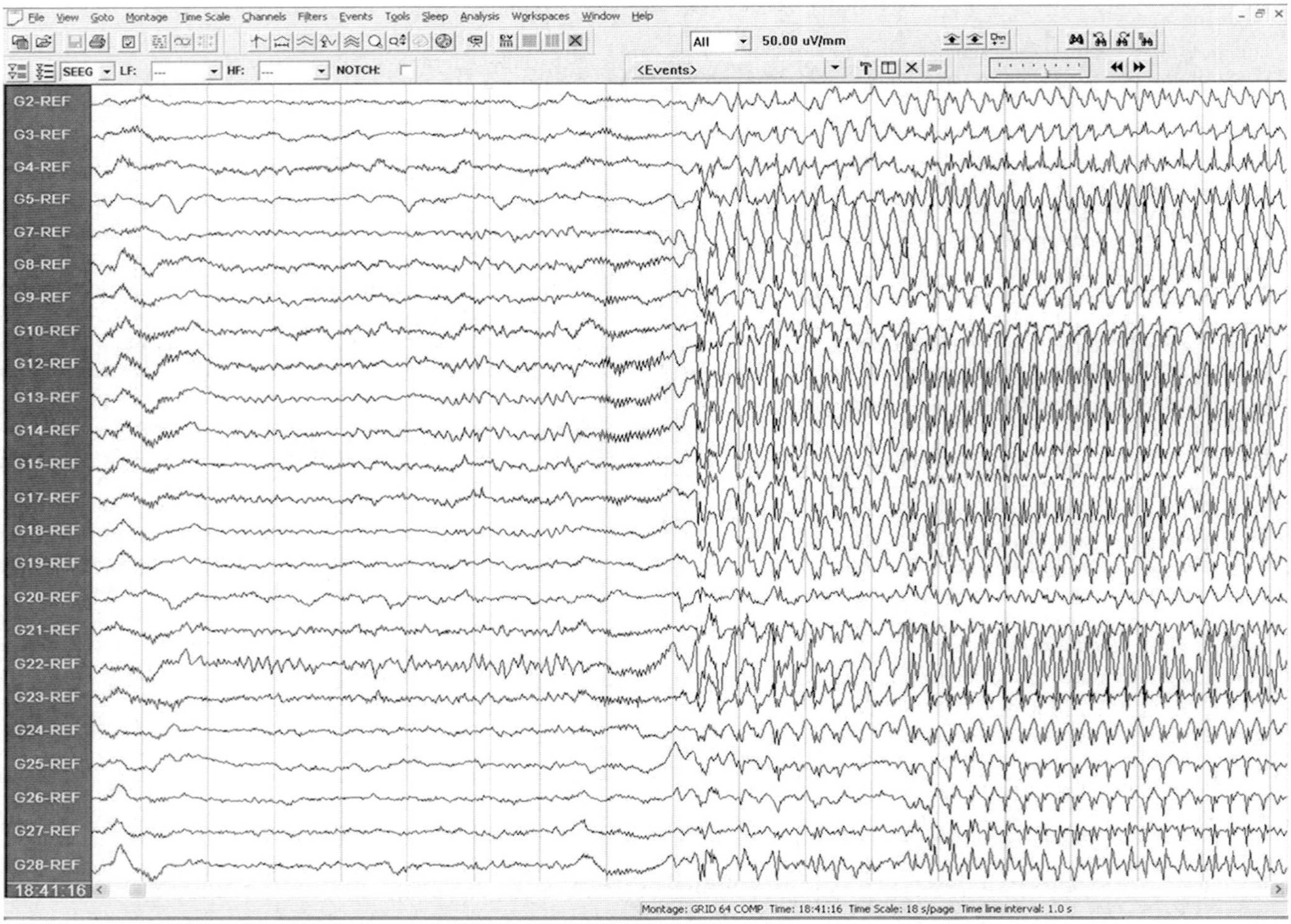

FIGURE 54.2. Intracranial EEG showing focal onset of a seizure with regional spread after 10 secs. (Photo courtesy N. Selden, PhD, MD, Oregon Health & Science University, Portland, OR).

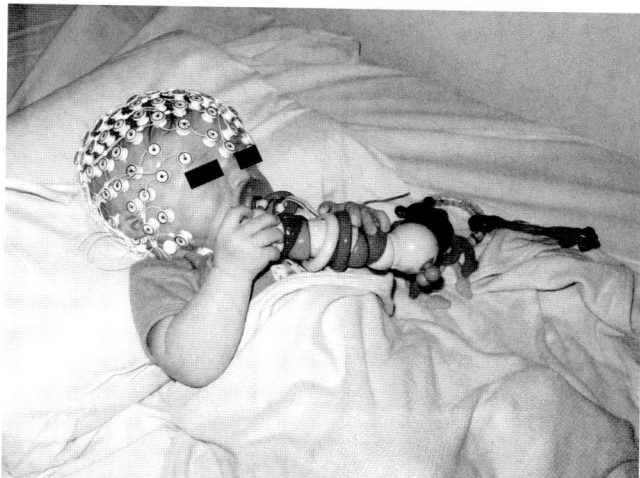

FIGURE 54.3. A 128-channel Geodesic Sensor Net for high-density EEG applied to a newborn. (Photo courtesy J. Quiring, PhD, Electrical Geodesics, Inc., Salem, OR).

criteria, saving only portions of every hour or time period, as well as computer-detected abnormalities. Compression algorithms may also be of use in creating smaller files for storage, transmission, or review via cable linkage to main workstations in the neuroepileptologist's laboratory.

The amount of useful clinical information gained through prolonged recordings, often involving simultaneous video monitoring, has proven far superior to brief routine EEGs. Prognostic information can be gained in patients with hypoxic-ischemic encephalopathies. Using continuous recording or serial studies, EEG monitoring can be used to confirm the diagnosis of brain death.

Newer technology includes various quantitative and graphic techniques, such as compressed spectral arrays and voltage maps, that can transform the EEG signal using a range of frequency and amplitude modulations and can be easily derived from EEG data to aid in the interpretation and source localization of abnormalities of interest (30). Recent advances in material sciences and engineering have led to new dense-array EEGs that can be specifically designed for children and infants (**Fig. 54.3**). The spatial information obtained from EEG data that is collected with standard electrode arrays is confounded by spatial aliasing error (38). However, a dense-array EEG allows sensors to be placed at more than 100 sample locations, making possible accurate measurement of the EEG as a time-varying, spatially distributed, electrical potential. Advantages of dense-array EEGs are that the time for electrode placement and removal is minimal, as the sensor net is only soaked in a solute bath, and the smell and potential skin irritation from collodion glue are eliminated.

Limitations of continuous EEG monitoring primarily involve the level of expertise required for data interpretation. In many cases, PICU staff can be taught to identify seizures and patterns of interest, but full review and analysis usually requires a neurophysiologist or neurologist. Although the amount of time required for interpretation has been reduced by technologic advances in digital acquisition, spike- and seizure-detection algorithms, and networked systems, it remains significant. Automatic detection software remains error prone and, if full analysis is to be delayed, many of the benefits of an-

ticipatory care may be lost. Additionally, the application and maintenance of electrodes usually require trained technologists. Lastly, prolonged electrode placement, usually with collodion, can cause scalp breakdown.

Bispectral Index

The bispectral index (BIS) monitor (Aspect Medical Systems, Natick, MA) (**Fig. 54.4**) integrates time domain, frequency domain, and higher-order spectral analysis of limited EEG signals to create a univariate descriptor of the level of sedation, which is represented as a dimensionless number ranging from 0 to 100. The BIS monitor was developed with data from adults, with the goal of decreasing the occurrence of awareness in the operating room (32). Using phase and power information, the bispectrum evaluates the coherence of sinusoidal frequencies. In the awake individual, multiple independent CNS signal generators produce a chaotic EEG. As deeper sedation occurs, phase coupling of different frequencies is thought to indicate a common source unifying some EEG signals. As phase angles for sinusoidal frequencies become coupled, the higher biocoherence is demonstrated by a large spike on the bispectrum display. The sequential signal processing from raw EEG to bispectrum is demonstrated in **Figure 54.5**.

To date, it is unclear whether BIS use improves patient outcomes and satisfaction, decreases cost and drug dosage, diminishes the incidence of withdrawal, or minimizes side effects of sedatives. Efforts to achieve optimal levels of sedation are challenging due to wide interpatient variability in the amount of sedative and analgesic medication required to achieve tolerance of mechanical ventilation and due to the difficulty in clinically assessing sedation in infants, young children, and those with developmental disabilities. Of note, BIS was developed using adult EEG data and was not designed to incorporate the developmental changes of the pediatric EEG, and it has been shown that BIS values vary significantly with age (11).

Limitations of BIS monitoring include a paradoxic increase in BIS score with some medications, including ketamine, chloral hydrate, hydroxyzine, and meperidine. Neuromuscular blockade in awake volunteers and ICU patients can result in a misleadingly low BIS score (45). Finally, it is important to understand that BIS scores do not reflect comfort (i.e., a patient-judged level of comfort) but rather a degree of sedation that is generally the result of medications that decrease

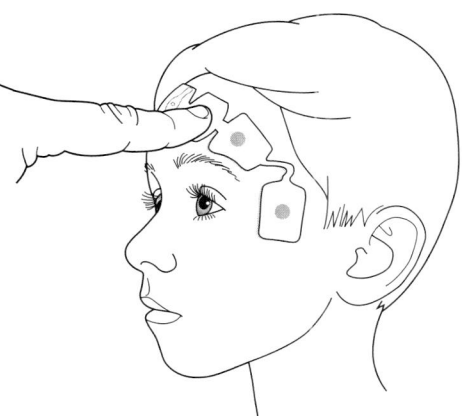

FIGURE 54.4. Illustration of BIS monitor leads placed over the forehead of a patient.

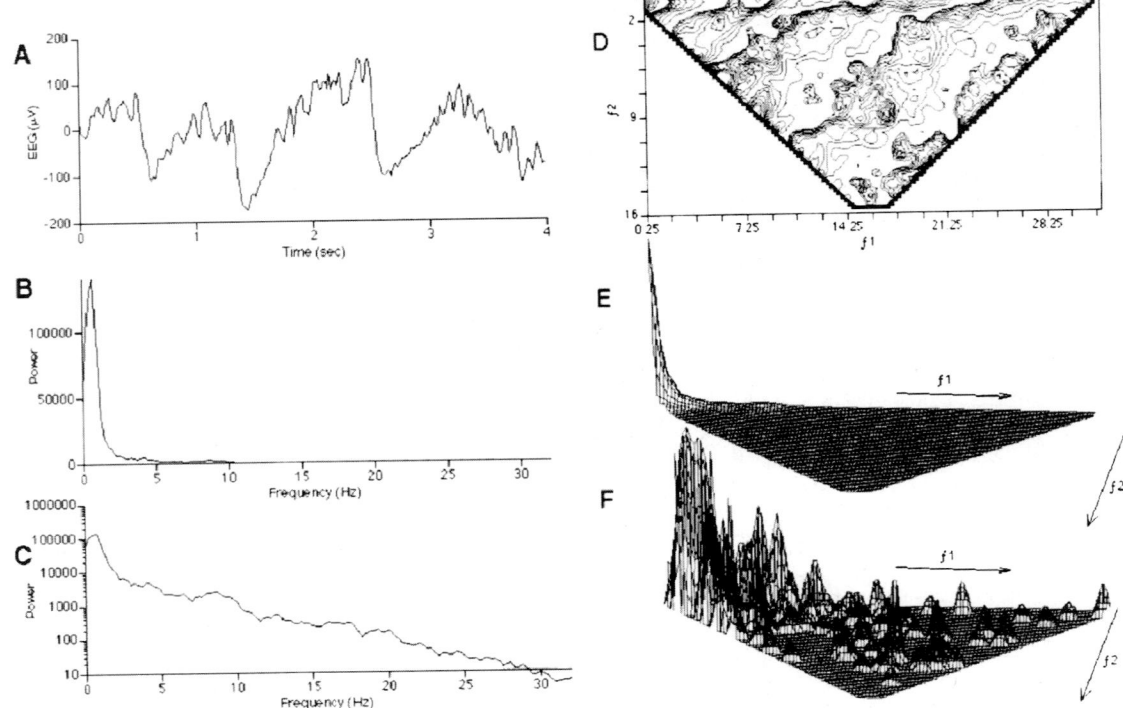

FIGURE 54.5. Examples of the processes of bispectral analysis. **A:** An epoch of raw EEG. **B:** The power spectrum after Fourier analysis of the epoch in part A. In this epoch, the large contribution from frequencies around 1 Hz overwhelms the contributions from higher frequencies. **C:** The same data that are in part B are plotted with a logarithmic power scale, allowing the contribution from faster waves to be identified despite the presence of large slow waves. **D:** After the complex spectrum for this epoch of data is computed, the bispectrum can be calculated. **E:** The same bispectral data plotted in three-dimensional perspective. **F:** Bicoherence plot with phase coherence features visible in a wide distribution of frequency. Adapted from Rampil IJ. A primer for EEG signal processing in anesthesia. *Anesthesiology* 1998;89:980–1002.

responsiveness. Thus, a fully awake patient may have a high BIS score and be alert and comfortable, while a sedated patient who has a low BIS score may experience pain.

Evoked Potentials: Visual, Auditory, Somatosensory, and Motor

Vision, hearing, sensory, and motor functions may all be discretely monitored to assess peripheral and CNS damage in patients with suspected injury. The integrity of the complete neural pathways may be assessed, with abnormalities assigned to specific levels or sites of injury. While these tests do not lend themselves to continuous monitoring in the PICU, one-time evaluations may prove useful for diagnostic or prognostic purposes (23).

Assessment of clinical conditions, including level of sedation, vegetative states, brain death, peripheral nerve damage, and stroke, may provide useful information. The main limitation is the limited clinical utility in an essentially one-time assessment of neural pathways versus continuous monitoring.

Intracranial Pressure

Raised ICP is the most common cause of death in neurosurgical patients, and is extremely common in patients who suffer from

severe head injury. Elevated ICP following TBI often results in secondary injury due to decreased cerebral perfusion pressure (CPP). Therapeutic interventions aimed directly at controlling abnormally elevated ICP have resulted in improved survival and neurologic outcomes. In other brain injuries, such as hypoxic and ischemic injuries, monitoring ICP has not been shown to improve outcome. The major aim of monitoring and managing elevated ICP is the prevention of cerebral ischemia. While expert opinions vary as to the value of invasive ICP monitoring, a recent evidence-based report on severe TBI in children provides strong support for the value of monitoring ICP, both in terms of outcome and in determining a treatment threshold (1,2).

The most common methods of ICP monitoring use either an intraventricular catheter or an intraparenchymal catheter. Of the two, the intraventricular catheter is more frequently used, is a more direct method, is believed to provide more accurate measurements, and results in the most satisfactory waveforms for off-line analysis. Additionally, the intraventricular catheter allows for removal of small amounts of cerebrospinal fluid to reduce ICP (5) and for the infusion of saline to determine the pressure-volume relationship of the brain, which can then be used to estimate cerebral compliance. From a safety point of view, intraventricular catheters present a risk of infection and are generally removed as soon as is practical (3).

Relatively recently, fiberoptic transducer-tipped catheters (FTCs) have been introduced into clinical practice and meet the standard of care in most PICUs. These devices monitor the variations in the amount of light reflected from a pressure-sensitive diaphragm located at the catheter tip. Several studies have been conducted to compare FTCs and conventional ICP monitors (3). Some of the key advantages of FTCs include versatility (FTCs can be placed into intraventricular, subarachnoid, or intraparenchymal regions), robustness to artifacts caused by patient movement or from fluid column sources, and the ability to drain cerebrospinal fluid and monitor simultaneously. Some of the drawbacks include the need for dedicated equipment for waveform display, as opposed to conventional ICP systems that use existing bedside monitoring devices. FTCs can exhibit a cumulative drift up to ±6 mm Hg over 5 days (10) and must be replaced if monitoring is in excess of several days, as FTCs cannot be recalibrated once inserted. FTCs are also considerably more expensive than conventional units.

Current methods of ICP monitoring rely on the analysis of discrete 3–5-sec, time-averaged parametric data that are numerically displayed next to the averaged parametric waveforms on the bedside monitors. In terms of engineering and signal processing, this type of monitoring, which is based on moving averages, is not as valuable as continuous ICP waveform monitoring at high sampling rates.

Cerebral Perfusion Pressure

The CPP is defined as the difference between the mean arterial pressure and the ICP. Because CPP drives the CBF and keeps oxygen and other essential nutrients flowing to the brain, it is believed that a certain CPP level must be maintained to avoid the risk of cerebral ischemia (4). CPP is a continuous calculation derived from the time-averaged difference between two physiologic signals: mean arterial pressure (MAP) and ICP (CPP = MAP – ICP). A recent evidence-based review of severe pediatric TBI found that CPP should be kept at a minimum of 40 mm Hg (4), while a similar review of adult TBI supports a minimum level of 70 mm Hg (9). Whether this minimum should be adjusted according to a child's age remains undetermined. Recent evidence suggests that age-dependent CPP values may be appropriate in TBI (see Chapter 52).

Jugular Venous Bulb Oxygen Saturation

Jugular venous bulb oxygen saturation ($SjvO_2$) refers to the oxygen saturation of the venous blood in the jugular bulb located at the base of the skull. Placement of a fiberoptic $SjvO_2$ catheter allows for continuous monitoring. The saturation normally ranges between 60% and 80%. The physiologic concept is that the difference between $SjvO_2$ and oxygen saturation of arterial blood (SaO_2) is an indirect measure of global CBF, as the $SO_2[a-v]$ is inversely proportional to the cerebral metabolic rate of oxygen. When CPP and CBF decrease, the brain has to extract the same amount of oxygen from a smaller amount of blood, causing the $SjvO_2$ to decrease. In general, $SjvO_2$ values of <50% are indicative of cerebral ischemia.

Abnormalities that increase oxygen consumption (e.g., fever or seizures) or that decrease oxygen delivery (e.g., increased ICP, hypotension, hypoxemia, hypocapnia, or anemia) may decrease $SjvO_2$ (48) (**Fig. 54.6**). Secondary insults that could contribute to the patient's neurologic injury may be identified

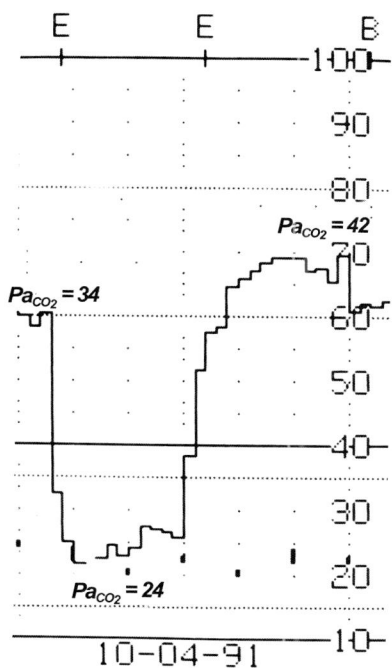

FIGURE 54.6. Jugular venous bulb oxygen saturation ($SjvO_2$) tracing that shows normal values of 60% in a patient with severe TBI who is stable on mechanical ventilation with a $PaCO_2$ = 34 mm Hg. However, during a period of inadvertent hyperventilation for routine pulmonary toilet, the patient is hyperventilated to a $PaCO_2$ = 24 mm Hg with significant cerebral hypoxemia, as shown by a $SjvO_2$ near 20%. The $SjvO_2$ value returns to normal when the $PaCO_2$ becomes 42 mm Hg after completion of pulmonary toilet.

early with $SjvO_2$ monitoring. Errors may be due to changes in head position or improper catheter placement, such as curling in the bulb or the catheter tip being adjacent to the vessel wall. Substantial differences between right and left jugular venous saturation can also be observed. Accuracy of $SjvO_2$ measurements of $SjvO_2$ is dependent upon precise in vivo calibration. Finally, while jugular venous bulb monitoring can be used to assess the adequacy of CPP and CBF, it is not capable of reliably assessing regional ischemia.

Transcranial Doppler

Transcranial Doppler (TCD) allows for portable, invasive, and repeatable measures of regional CBF. Although not strictly a continuous signal in terms of 24-hr availability, a multidirectional ultrasound probe has been constructed for simultaneous TCD of the middle cerebral artery, ophthalmic artery, and/or posterior cerebral artery (**Fig. 54.7**). The middle cerebral artery is the most commonly studied in children (7,39). TCD of the middle cerebral artery has been used in the postoperative management of pediatric cardiac surgery (6) and in severe brain injuries, cerebral arteriovenous malformation rupture, SE, and acute hydrocephalus.

Technical limitations of TCD include difficulty in locating adequate ultrasound windows through the bony skull, being able to view only medium- to large-sized vessels, variation in measurements between studies, poor correlation with other indices of CBF, and only actually measuring CBF velocity, while having to infer information about flow.

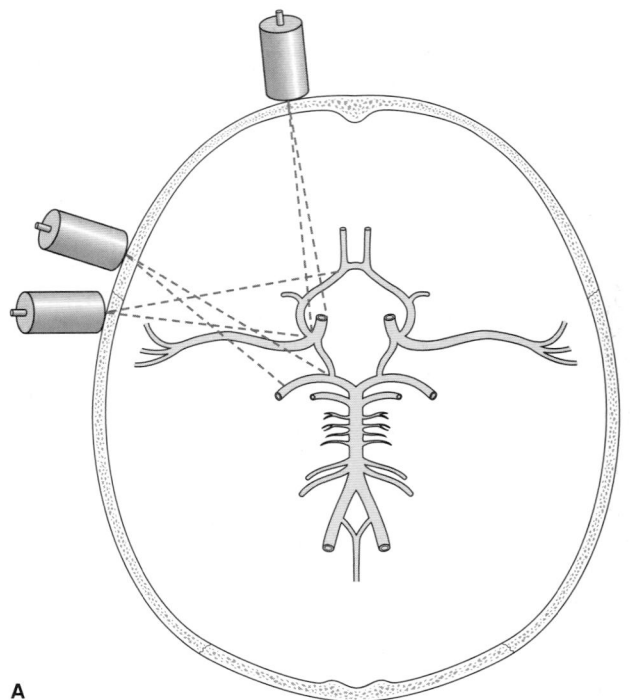

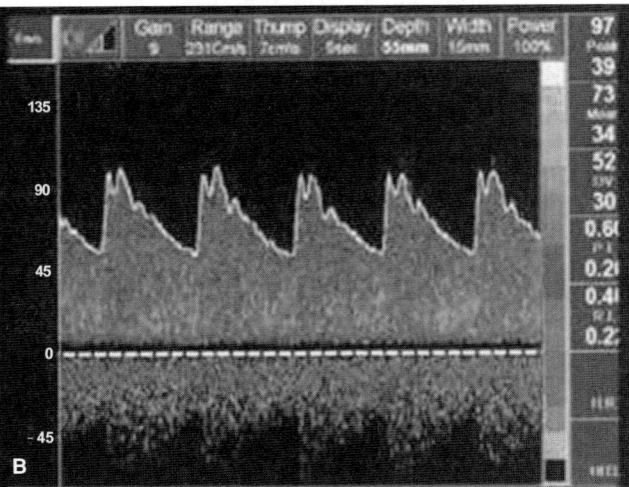

FIGURE 54.7. (A) Position of TCD probes of posterior cerebral artery (PCA), ophthalmic artery (OA), and middle cerebral artery (MCA), and (B) a sample tracing of normal MCA waveform.

Regional Brain Tissue Oxygenation Monitoring by Near-infrared Spectroscopy

NIRS technology uses a modification of the Beer-Lambert Law, which describes the relationship between absorption of light and the concentration of intravascular chromophores, such as deoxyhemoglobin (Hb), oxyhemoglobin (HbO_2), and the intracellular chromophore cytochrome aa_3. Key factors in the Beer-Lambert calculation are the absorption coefficient, tissue concentration of chromophore, distance between optodes, differential path length factor (described below), and scattering losses (37). NIRS technology differs from pulse oximetry in that it does not require a pulse; therefore, cerebral NIRS monitoring can be used during cardiopulmonary bypass.

The distance that the light travels, known as the optical path length, must be determined to obtain quantitative concentration changes from the light absorption data. The path length varies due to tissue scattering, which is reflected by the differential path length factor (DPF). The DPF is a correction factor that is multiplied by the interoptode distance to obtain the true path length.

NIRS can be accomplished by three mechanisms. A continuous-wave spectrometer is most commonly used in clinically available devices. Investigational devices exist that measure "time-of-flight," which has the added benefit of accurately measuring the path length of the light. Phase-resolved spectroscopy emits light that is modulated at a known frequency and assesses the phase shift of the transmitted light to derive the path length.

Commercially available NIRS monitors use two detector optodes at fixed distances (Fig. 54.8). The shorter interop-

tode distance is designed to represent extracranial (scalp and bone) tissue infrared absorption. In an effort to better represent intracranial brain tissue infrared absorption, the extracranial component is subtracted from the absorption data received by the longer interoptode distance (41). From the light absorption data generated via absorption of 730-nm (Hb) and 805-nm wavelengths (Hb + HbO_2), NIRS calculates regional cerebral oxygen saturation (rSO_2). A measurement of scaled absolute hemoglobin concentrations, reported as the tissue oxygenation index (TOI) is also available (40).

The range of baseline cerebral oxygen saturation values is very wide. In healthy children, cerebral oxygen saturations are reported to be 68% ± 10%, while in children with cyanotic heart disease, baseline values range from 38% to 57% (21). Current clinical usage of NIRS includes detection of superior vena cava occlusion during cardiopulmonary bypass (19) and assessing the effect of carotid ligation during initiation of venoarterial extracorporeal life support (14). Perhaps the most common application is in intraoperative neurophysiologic monitoring (combined with TCD and EEG) in children who undergo repair of congenital cardiac disease (6). Therapeutic changes as a result of NIRS have resulted in decreased rates of neurologic complications (6).

Some limitations of NIRS technology are its inability to account for patients' varying ratios of brain and extracranial tissues and the fact that DPF values vary with age and pathologic state (13,41). Icteric patients have depressed cerebral rSO_2 values, presumably due to absorption of light by bilirubin (24). Ongoing blood loss is associated with a decrease in rSO_2, despite a stable SjO_2, which may indicate that a changing Hb level confounds cerebral oximetry measurement (49). Furthermore, the reproducibility of cerebral oxygenation measurements in infants is poor (12). However, the major limitation is that no

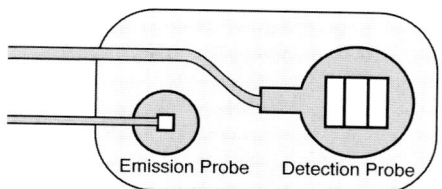

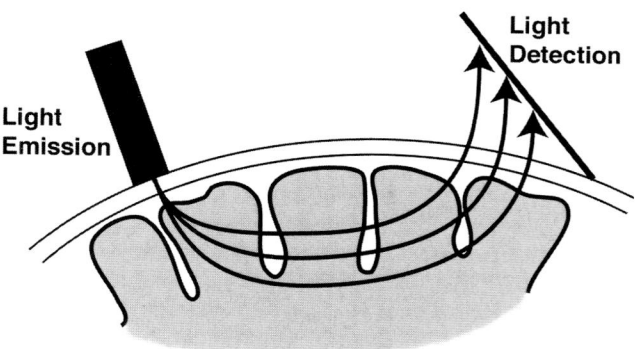

Light Emission

Light Detection

FIGURE 54.8. Near infrared spectroscopy uses light between 700 nm and 1000 nm wavelengths, similar to other forms of oximetry. The tissue oxygenation index can detect differences between the left and right frontal hemispheres of the brain at a tissue depth of 2–3 cm (illustration courtesy L. Ibsen, MD, MediaLab@Doernbecher).

"gold standard" exists with which to compare NIRS-derived rSo_2. Poor to moderate correlation is seen in comparing rSo_2 to global cerebral oxygenation measures, such as $Sjvo_2$ (27,35), central venous saturation (43,46), invasively monitored cortical brain tissue Po_2 (8), and postoperative elevation of the neuronal markers neuron-specific enolase and S-100 (29). A pediatric pilot study reported good agreement between NIRS and $Sjvo_2$ in a normal pediatric brain (36).

Laser-Doppler Flowmetry

Laser-Doppler flowmetry (LDF) measures the frequency shift of a laser light reflected off of red blood cells to calculate local CBF velocity in the cerebral cortex (39). LDF measures blood flow velocity in the microvessels of a small volume of brain tissue rather than in a large artery, such as with TCD. Flow is determined by multiplying the velocity by the volume of tissue. A small optical fiber that emits a laser light is placed in brain parenchyma through the same site as the ICP monitor. Limitations of this technique include: measurement reliability, movement artifact, inaccurate flow rates if the optical fiber is placed near a large blood vessel, and a decreased LDF signal if the hematocrit falls (20,22,25).

Regional Brain Tissue Oxygen ($Ptio_2$), Carbon Dioxide ($Ptico_2$), and pH

A tissue monitoring catheter (0.5 mm diameter) may be placed alongside the ICP catheter in the frontal cortex to a 2–3-cm depth to measure regional brain partial pressure tissue (Pti) changes in O_2, CO_2, and pH (16). The technology uses fluo-

rescent dyes that respond to O_2, CO_2, and pH, or it can be used with a Clark electrode for Po_2 measurements. A temperature probe may be added to obtain continuous brain tissue temperature measurements. Some limitations of this technology are measurements that reflect regional rather than global changes and a lack of correlation with other metabolic measures, such as $Sjvo_2$. Adult studies in TBI have suggested that differences between $Ptio_2$, $Ptico_2$, and pH are associated with outcome; however, pediatric experience is minimal (49).

Microdialysis

A microdialysis catheter may be inserted into brain tissue and connected to a microdialysis pump, which delivers perfusion fluid that equilibrates with extracellular brain tissue fluid through the dialysis membrane of the catheter. Fluid samples are collected approximately hourly and analyzed at the point of care with a special microdialysis analyzer. Changes in levels of glucose, lactate, pyruvate, and various amino acids in the interstitial fluid may be measured. Extracellular concentrations of lactate and glutamate have been reported to be increased during episodes of jugular venous desaturation (33). Recent adult studies have suggested that changes in these levels may precede the onset of symptomatic vasospasm in subarachnoid hemorrhage, may signal ischemia before detection by changes in either ICP or CPP, and may be predictive of outcome in TBI; studies also showed that increasing the Fio_2 results in decreased levels of lactate and glucose, suggesting a potential role for hyperoxygenation as an early therapy (17,18,34). A pediatric catheter is now available, but clinical experience is limited. A pediatric study in severe TBI reported that the extracellular glutamine:glutamate ratio may have some prognostic value and be linked to clinical outcome (32).

Multimodality Neuromonitoring

Preliminary evidence suggests that multiple neuromonitoring methods used in concert may improve overall patient outcome and reduce hospital length of stay (26). Additionally, multimodality neuromonitoring may help augment the clinical examination in patients with coma or other condition that confound physical findings (25). Although many PICUs are increasingly utilizing multimodality neuromonitoring, it remains to be seen which types and in what combinations these technologies may improve clinical outcomes.

CONCLUSIONS AND FUTURE DIRECTIONS

In conclusion, the past decade has seen significant technologic advances in the depth and breadth of neurologic monitoring of the PICU patient. However, caution must be exercised before widespread adoption of any new monitoring technology, as excessive or indiscriminate use may prove less effective and potentially detrimental if misinterpreted or acted on inappropriately (28). Whether these advances in neuromonitoring technology will affect clinical outcome remains to be studied and demonstrated, and careful evaluations, including risk to the patient, cost, avoidance of incorrect interpretations, and a clear association with improved outcome, must precede widespread adoption and use in the PICU (15,28). Understanding the pathophysiologic correlates of these neuromonitoring modalities, including the complex interrelationships between CBF, cerebral metabolism, cerebral autoregulation, and tissue and cellular states, will prove vital to fully utilizing the technologies to their best advantage.

KEY POINTS

- To understand the current and potential future application of neuromonitoring in the pediatric ICU, it is necessary to understand basic engineering and physiologic principles that underlie different monitoring technologies.

- Increasing evidence suggests that neuromonitoring with various modalities can improve diagnosis, treatment, and outcome in critically ill and injured children.

- Because digital signal processing algorithms generally use a moving window of the physiologic signal to generate estimates, the clinical parameters displayed on the bedside monitor represent an average over past values of the signal and cannot respond instantaneously to alarm conditions. Thus, in a deteriorating patient, monitors typically generate alarms after the alarm condition has persisted for several seconds and following resuscitation, will typically lag a few seconds after the patient's condition improves.

- Patient outcome in at least three disease states have been demonstrated to improve with the use of advanced neuromonitoring. These include continuous EEG coupled with digital video monitoring for SE in diagnosing nonconvulsive seizures and as part of a surgical approach for intractable seizures, intracranial pressure monitoring in patients with severe TBI, and intraoperative and postoperative neurophysiologic monitoring of children who undergo repair of congenital cardiac disease with NIRS technology.

- Preliminary evidence suggests that multimodality neuromonitoring may improve overall patient outcome, reduce hospital length of stay, and aid in the clinical examination of patients with coma.

References

1. Adelson PD, Bratton SL, Carney NA, et al. Guidelines for the acute medical management of severe traumatic brain injury in infants, children, and adolescents. Chapter 5. Indications for intracranial pressure monitoring in pediatric patients with severe traumatic brain injury. *Pediatr Crit Care Med* 2003;4:S19–24.
2. Adelson PD, Bratton SL, Carney NA, et al. Guidelines for the acute medical management of severe traumatic brain injury in infants, children, and adolescents. Chapter 6. Threshold for treatment of intracranial hypertension. *Pediatr Crit Care Med* 2003;4:S25–7.
3. Adelson PD, Bratton SL, Carney NA, et al. Guidelines for the acute medical management of severe traumatic brain injury in infants, children, and adolescents. Chapter 7. Intracranial pressure monitoring technology. *Pediatr Crit Care Med* 2003;4:S28–30.
4. Adelson PD, Bratton SL, Carney NA, et al. Guidelines for the acute medical management of severe traumatic brain injury in infants, children, and adolescents. Chapter 8. Cerebral perfusion pressure. *Pediatr Crit Care Med* 2003;4:S31–3.
5. Adelson PD, Bratton SL, Carney NA, et al. Guidelines for the acute medical management of severe traumatic brain injury in infants, children, and adolescents. Chapter 10. The role of cerebrospinal fluid drainage in the treatment of severe pediatric traumatic brain injury. *Pediatr Crit Care Med* 2003;4:S38–9.
6. Austin EH, 3rd, Edmonds HL, Jr., Auden SM, et al. Benefit of neurophysiologic monitoring for pediatric cardiac surgery. *J Thorac Cardiovasc Surg* 1997;114:707–15, 17; discussion 15–6.
7. Bissonnette B, Leon JE. Transcranial Doppler in pediatrics. *J Neurosurg Anesthesiol* 1991;3:77.
8. Brawanski A FR, Rothoerl RD, Woertgen C. Comparison of near-infrared spectroscopy and tissue p(O$_2$) time series in patients after severe head injury and aneurysmal subarachnoid hemorrhage. *J Cereb Blood Flow Metab* 2002;22:605–11.
9. Bullock R, Chesnut RM, Clifton G, et al. Guidelines for the management of severe head injury. Brain Trauma Foundation. *Eur J Emerg Med* 1996;3:109–27.
10. Crutchfield JS, Narayan RK, Robertson CS, et al. Evaluation of a fiberoptic intracranial pressure monitor. *J Neurosurg* 1990;72:482–7.
11. Davidson AJ, Huang GH, Rebmann CS, et al. Performance of entropy and bispectral index as measures of anaesthesia effect in children of different ages. *Br J Anaesth* 2005;95:674–9.
12. Dullenkopf A, Kolarova A, Schulz G, et al. Reproducibility of cerebral oxygenation measurement in neonates and infants in the clinical setting using the NIRO 300 oximeter. *Pediatr Crit Care Med* 2005;6:344–7.
13. Duncan A, Meek JH, Clemence M, et al. Measurement of cranial optical path length as a function of age using phase-resolved near infrared spectroscopy. *Pediatr Res* 1996;39:889–94.
14. Ejike JC, Schenkman KA, Seidel K, et al. Cerebral oxygenation in neonatal and pediatric patients during veno-arterial extracorporeal life support. *Pediatr Crit Care Med* 2006; Publish ahead of print.
15. Goldstein B. New technologies in the intensive care unit: A cautionary tale. *Pediatr Crit Care Med* 2005;6:378–9.
16. Haitsma IK, Maas AI. Advanced monitoring in the intensive care unit: Brain tissue oxygen tension. *Curr Opin Crit Care* 2002;8:115–20.
17. Hutchinson PJ, O'Connell MT, al-Rawi PG, et al. Clinical cerebral microdialysis—determining the true extracellular concentration. *Acta Neurochir Suppl* 2002;81:359–62.
18. Hutchinson PJ, O'Connell MT, Al-Rawi PG, et al. Clinical cerebral microdialysis: A methodological study. *J Neurosurg* 2000;93:37–43.
19. Ing RJ, Lawson DS, Jaggers J, et al. Detection of unintentional partial superior vena cava occlusion during a bidirectional cavopulmonary anastomosis. *J Cardiothorac Vasc Anesth* 2004;18:472–4.
20. Kirkpatrick PJ, Smielewski P, Czosnyka M, et al. Continuous monitoring of cortical perfusion by laser Doppler flowmetry in ventilated patients with head injury. *J Neurol Neurosurg Psychiatry* 1994;57:1382–8.
21. Kurth CD, Steven JL, Montenegro LM, et al. Cerebral oxygen saturation before congenital heart surgery. *Ann Thorac Surg* 2001;72:187–92.
22. Lam JM, Hsiang JN, Poon WS. Monitoring of autoregulation using laser Doppler flowmetry in patients with head injury. *J Neurosurg* 1997;86:438–45.
23. Limperopoulos C, Majnemer A, Rosenblatt B, et al. Multimodality evoked potential findings in infants with congenital heart defects. *J Child Neurol* 1999;14:702–7.
24. Madsen PL SC, Rasmussen A, Secher NH. Interference of cerebral near-infrared oximetry in patients with icterus. *Anesth Analg* 2000;90:489–93.
25. Miller JI, Chou MW, Capocelli A, et al. Continuous intracranial multimodality monitoring comparing local cerebral blood flow, cerebral perfusion pressure, and microvascular resistance. *Acta Neurochir Suppl* 1998;71:82–4.
26. Murkin JM. Perioperative multimodality neuromonitoring: An overview. *Semin Cardiothorac Vasc Anesth* 2004;8:167–71.
27. Nagdyman N, Fleck T, Schubert S, et al. Comparison between cerebral tissue oxygenation index measured by near-infrared spectroscopy and venous jugular bulb saturation in children. *Intensive Care Med* 2005;31:846–50.
28. Pinsky MR, Vincent J-L. Let us use the pulmonary artery catheter correctly and only when we need it. *Crit Care Med* 2005;33:1119–22.
29. Plachky J HS, Volkmann M, Martin E, et al. Regional cerebral oxygen saturation is a sensitive marker of cerebral hypoperfusion during orthotopic liver transplantation. *Anesth Analg* 2004;99:344–9.
30. Procaccio F, Polo A, Lanteri P, et al. Electrophysiologic monitoring in neurointensive care. *Curr Opin Crit Care* 2001;7:74–80.
31. Rampil IJ. A primer for EEG signal processing in anesthesia. *Anesthesiology* 1998;89:980–1002.
32. Richards DA, Tolias CM, Sgouros S, et al. Extracellular glutamine to glutamate ratio may predict outcome in the injured brain: A clinical microdialysis study in children. *Pharmacol Res* 2003;48:101–9.
33. Robertson CS, Gopinath SP, Goodman JC, et al. SjvO$_2$ monitoring in head-injured patients. *J Neurotrauma* 1995;12:891–6.
34. Sarrafzadeh AS, Sakowitz OW, Callsen TA, et al. Detection of secondary insults by brain tissue pO$_2$ and bedside microdialysis in severe head injury. *Acta Neurochir Suppl* 2002;81:319–21.
35. Scheuer ML. Continuous EEG monitoring in the intensive care unit. *Epilepsia* 2002;43 Suppl 3:114–27.
36. Shimizu N GF, Bissonnette B, Coles J, et al. Brain tissue oxygenation index measured by near infrared spatially resolved spectroscopy agreed with jugular bulb oxygen saturation in normal pediatric brain: A pilot study. *Childs Nerv Syst* 2005;21:181–4.
37. Soul JS, Du Plessis AJ. New technologies in pediatric neurology. Near-infrared spectroscopy. *Semin Pediatr Neurol* 1999;6:101–10.

38. Srinivasan R, Nunez PL, Silberstein RB. Spatial filtering and neocortical dynamics: Estimates of EEG coherence. *IEEE Trans Biomed Eng* 1998;45: 814–26.
39. Sudikoff S, Banasiak K. Techniques for measuring cerebral blood flow in children. *Curr Opin Pediatr* 1998;10:291–8.
40. Taillefer MC, Denault AY. Cerebral near-infrared spectroscopy in adult heart surgery: Systematic review of its clinical efficacy. *Can J Anaesth* 2005; 52:79–87.
41. Thavasothy M, Broadhead M, Elwell C, et al. A comparison of cerebral oxygenation as measured by the NIRO 300 and the IN-VOS 5100 near-infrared spectrophotometers. *Anaesthesia* 2002;57: 999–1006.
42. Tobias J. Cerebral oxygenation monitoring: Near-infrared spectroscopy. *Expert Rev Med Devices* 2006;3:235–43.
43. Tortoriello TA, Stayer SA, Mott AR, et al. A noninvasive estimation of mixed venous oxygen saturation using near-infrared spectroscopy by cerebral oximetry in pediatric cardiac surgery patients. *Paediatr Anaesth* 2005;15: 495–503.
44. Vivien B, Di Maria S, Ouattara A, et al. Overestimation of bispectral index in sedated intensive care unit patients revealed by administration of muscle relaxant. *Anesthesiology* 2003;99:9–17.
45. Webster J. *Medical Instrumentation: Application and Design*. New York: John Wiley & Sons, 1998.
46. Weiss M, Dullenkopf A, Kolarova A, et al. Near-infrared spectroscopic cerebral oxygenation reading in neonates and infants is associated with central venous oxygen saturation. *Paediatr Anaesth* 2005;15:102–9.
47. Wyllie E. Surgical treatment of epilepsy in children. *Pediatr Neurol* 1998; 19:179–88.
48. Yoshitani K, Kawaguchi M, Iwata M, et al. Comparison of changes in jugular venous bulb oxygen saturation and cerebral oxygen saturation during variations of haemoglobin concentration under propofol and sevoflurane anaesthesia. *Br J Anaesth* 2005;94:341–6.
49. Zauner A, Doppenberg EM, Woodward JJ, et al. Continuous monitoring of cerebral substrate delivery and clearance: Initial experience in 24 patients with severe acute brain injuries. *Neurosurgery* 1997;41:1082–91; discussion 91–3.

CHAPTER 55 ■ NEUROLOGIC IMAGING

DAVID JOSHUA MICHELSON • STEPHEN ASHWAL

Few aspects of patient care have been changed as substantially by recent advances in medical technology as has imaging for the noninvasive evaluation of central nervous system (CNS) injury (2). CT and MRI are the two most commonly used techniques, providing images with increasingly specific diagnostic and prognostic information for a wide variety of indications. This chapter discusses these techniques in detail, highlighting their value in selected clinical applications common in pediatric critical care.

TECHNIQUES

Computed Tomography

CT images, generated by the collection and analysis of x-ray beams as they are sent through tissues from multiple angles, are more than adequate for the identification of surgically remediable forms of acute neuropathology, such as fractures, tumors, large hemorrhages, and obstructive hydrocephalus. One major factor in favor of CT in comparison with MRI is that it can be quickly and easily obtained. Helical (spiral) scanners have so substantially shortened the acquisition times required for high-quality images that sedation for CT is unnecessary in the vast majority of infants and children who can refrain from moving briefly or who can be lightly restrained (37). One of the drawbacks of CT is radiation exposure, particularly of concern for young patients and those who require repeated studies, given the known dose-related risk of radiation-associated disease (20) and possible risk of developmental impairment (21). Considering this, alternative studies, such as ultrasound, MRI, or CT of lower-resolution (and thus lower radiation dose) may be preferable. Also, while the radiodense, iodinated contrast agents used in CT scanning are well tolerated by most children, acute allergic reactions can occur, particularly in older children and in children with a history of asthma.

Conventional Anatomic Imaging

Axial images of the head are routinely obtained with a slice thickness of 5 mm, although thinner slices can be obtained if greater detail is required, and images can be reformatted into other planes or into three dimensions. The brightness of each voxel [a pixel representing a three-dimensional (3-D) volume] on a CT image reflects tissue density. Fatty tissue, water, and air appear dark; soft tissues appear as intermediate shades of gray; and mineralized bone, concentrated blood, iodinated contrast, and metallic objects appear bright. CT is limited by streaking artifacts in areas around metal prostheses, fragments (such as dental fillings or gunshot pellets), and dense bone (such as the temporal petrous bones in the posterior fossa). Areas of abnormal signal on CT can be characterized as hypodense,

isodense, or hyperdense, relative to the normal neural tissue. The differential for hypodense parenchymal lesions includes edema, infarction, neoplasia, demyelination, inflammation, and cyst formation. Hyperdensity is found in areas of contrast enhancement, hemorrhage, calcification, and hypercellularity. Abnormal calcification can be seen with congenital or chronic infections, tumors and hamartomas, abnormal blood vessels, areas of ischemia, metabolic disorders, and endocrine disorders (11). Calcification of subependymal nodules in a patient with tuberous sclerosis complex is shown in **Figure 55.1**. Isodense lesions may be recognizable by their replacement of, or effect on, normal structures, unless they show abnormal contrast enhancement.

CT Angiography

CT angiography allows the vascular anatomy of the brain to be imaged fairly well by high-resolution CT scanning that is closely timed with an intravenous bolus of an iodinated contrast agent. A test bolus is initially given so as to determine the time delay required to capture images within either the arterial or venous phase, depending on the study desired. Thinly cut source images can be reformatted into 2- and 3-D images that are nearly as detailed as MR angiograms. As with anatomic imaging, the choice of CT depends on the constraints of radiation exposure, contrast sensitivity, and timing. CT angiography is faster that MR angiography and can usually be done without sedation in older children.

Magnetic Resonance Imaging

MR images are generated by analysis of signals produced by hydrogen nuclei of molecules in varying tissues as the spins of the nuclei are aligned in a strong external magnetic field and then perturbed by radiofrequency pulses. MRI is the modality of choice when resolution of fine anatomic detail is desired. Moreover, this technology also offers several specialized sequences that highlight metabolic changes within the brain and are applicable to a wide variety of diagnostic situations. MRI is also the imaging test of choice for spinal cord injury when neurologic deficits are present, as CT images of the spine, while superior for visualizing fractures and dislocations, do not allow for adequate assessment of the cord. MRI also allows for far more precise imaging of posterior fossa structures, as it is not subject to the artifact produced by the dense temporal petrous bones on CT.

The principal drawback of MR imaging is the long acquisition time, which frequently necessitates procedural sedation for most children <8 years old and for some who are older. An audiovisual system within the scanner greatly reduces the need for sedation in children >3 years of age (15). When intravenous

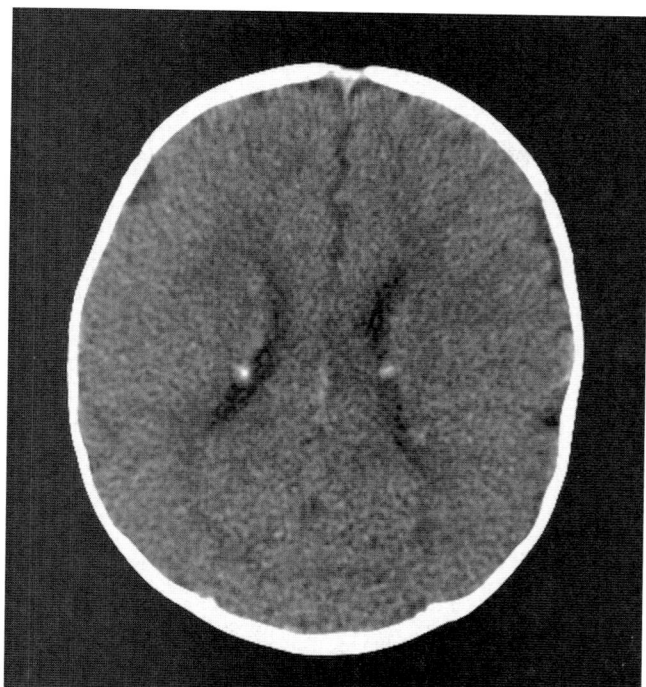

FIGURE 55.1. Four-month-old boy presenting with infantile spasms. Axial CT shows multiple bright nodules along the surface of the lateral ventricles due to subependymal hamartomas associated with tuberous sclerosis complex.

propofol is used for sedation, concentrations of supplemental O₂ above 60% can cause artifactual cerebrospinal fluid (CSF) hyperintensity within the sulci and cisterns that can be mistaken for subarachnoid hemorrhage.

Another drawback of MRI is the incompatibility of ferromagnetic materials with the strong electromagnetic field within the imaging suite. Plastic and aluminum MR-compatible monitors are available, and ventilator-dependent patients can be ventilated manually, but patients with metallic bullet fragments or implants, including cardiac pacemakers and neurostimulators, may not be able to undergo MRI safely. Information regarding the compatibility of an extensive list of implanted medical devices can be researched on the web site maintained

by Frank Shellock, Ph.D., at http://www.MRIsafety.com. Even when metallic objects pose no safety risk, they may create artifacts and distortions in the surrounding tissues.

Conventional Anatomic Imaging

As with CT, MR images are gray-scale maps, with the shade of each voxel reflecting the composition of the tissue it represents. The shade of a voxel on an MR image is referred to as its *intensity*, rather than its *density*, because it is determined by factors beyond proton density, including proton mobility (T1 relaxation) and local magnetic effects (T2 relaxation). Various sequences, such as spin echo (SE), gradient-recalled echo (GRE), and fluid-attenuated inversion recovery (FLAIR), use programmed pulses of radiofrequencies and gradient magnetic fields to produce images that highlight T1 or T2 signal effects. On T1-weighted images, fat, methemoglobin, and gadolinium-containing contrast agents appear bright (or hyperintense), while CSF, muscle, deoxyhemoglobin, and hemosiderin, appear dark. On T2-weighted images, CSF, edema, extracellular methemoglobin, and areas of hypercellularity, infarction, and demyelination appear bright, while muscle, cortical bone, deoxyhemoglobin, and hemosiderin appear dark.

Routine brain imaging in most institutions begins with a sagittal T1-weighted sequence that serves as a localizer for subsequent sequences and allows evaluation of the corpus callosum, pituitary gland, cerebellar vermis, and other midline structures. Axial T1- and T2-weighted images are also routinely acquired, although coronal images may be particularly helpful for investigation of the cerebellum, temporal lobes, and skull base. FLAIR sequences have improved sensitivity in older children for areas of abnormal intracranial T2 brightness in close proximity to CSF-filled spaces, such as the ventricles and sulci, which are bright in conventional T2 studies but dark on FLAIR images. High-resolution volumetric 3-D T1-weighted scans are particularly useful for patients who undergo evaluation of developmental abnormalities and for surgical planning.

Diffusion-weighted Imaging

The diffusion of water molecules can be measured along any 2-D plane to which a strong magnetic field gradient has been applied. Diffusion reflects random (Brownian) motion, capillary flow, and transcellular active transport. In standard diffusion-weighted imaging (DWI), bright areas reflect decreased or restricted movement of water along the studied plane. The

TABLE 55.1

THE EVOLVING APPEARANCE OF HEMORRHAGE ON CT AND MR IMAGING

Timing	Hyperacute (<1 day)	Acute (1–3 days)	Early subacute (3–7 days)	Late subacute (7–14 days)	Chronic (>14 days)
Blood product	OxyHb (intracellular)	DeoxyHb (intracellular)	MetHb (intracellular)	MetHb (extracellular)	Hemosiderin (extracellular)
CT image	Hyperdense	Hyperdense	Isodense	Isodense	Hypodense
MR image					
T1-weighted	Dark or gray	Dark or gray	Bright	Bright	Dark or gray
T2-weighted	Bright	Dark	Dark	Bright	Dark

Data from Bradley WG Jr. MR appearance of hemorrhage in the brain. *Radiology* 1993;189:15–2.

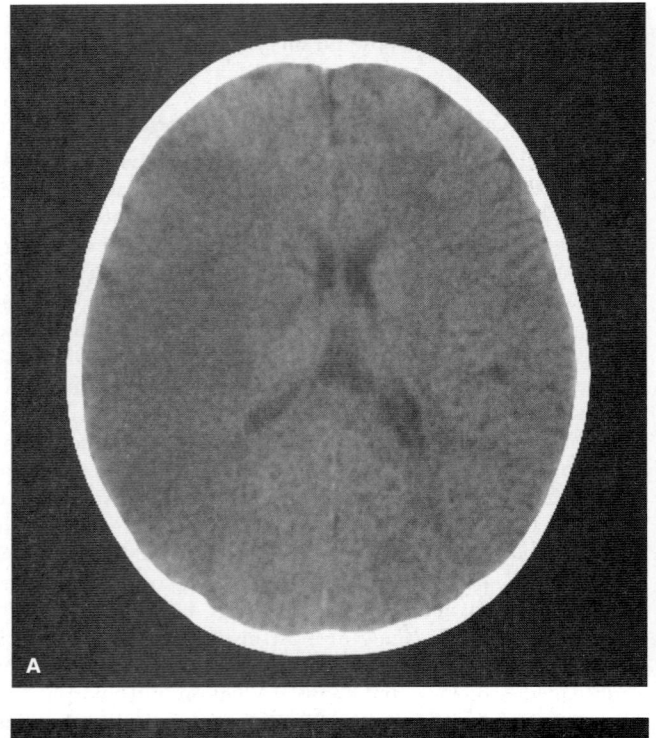

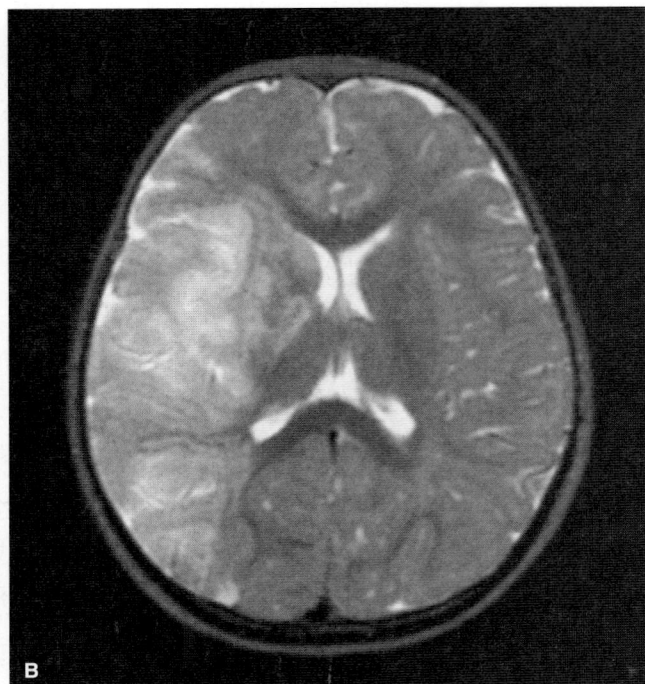

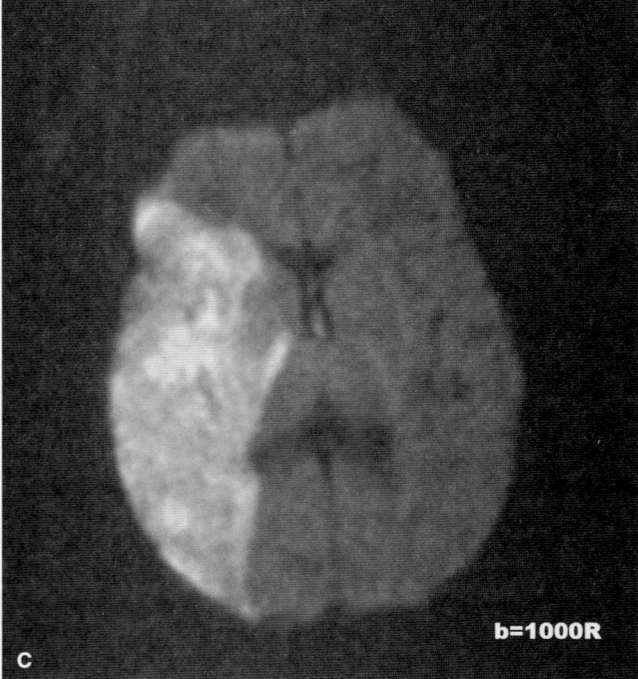

FIGURE 55.2. Two-year-old girl who awoke with left hemiparesis and right-gaze preference. (**A**) A wedge-shaped area of hypodensity is seen on axial CT. MRI shows (**B**) T2 hyperintensity and (**C**) corresponding diffusion restriction, indicative of an ischemic stroke in the distribution of the right middle cerebral artery.

apparent diffusion coefficient map summarizes the diffusion in all three orthogonal planes, such that areas of restriction appear dark. DWI is particularly useful in the early evaluation of ischemia, as diffusion restriction becomes apparent within minutes after cytotoxic injury is sustained (30). DWI is also used in the evaluation of brain tumors, helping to distinguish cystic tumors from epidermoid tumors and recurrent tumors from areas of peritumoral edema. Diffusion restriction is also seen within cerebral abscesses and empyemas (29); this

methodology is helpful when a suspected abscess cannot otherwise be distinguished radiologically from a tumor with central necrosis (28).

MR Angiography/Venography

Reconstructions of the arterial supply and venous drainage of the brain can be obtained from maximum intensity projections (MIP) from 2- or 3-D time-of-flight images that correlate with blood flow, rather than luminal diameter, and can exaggerate

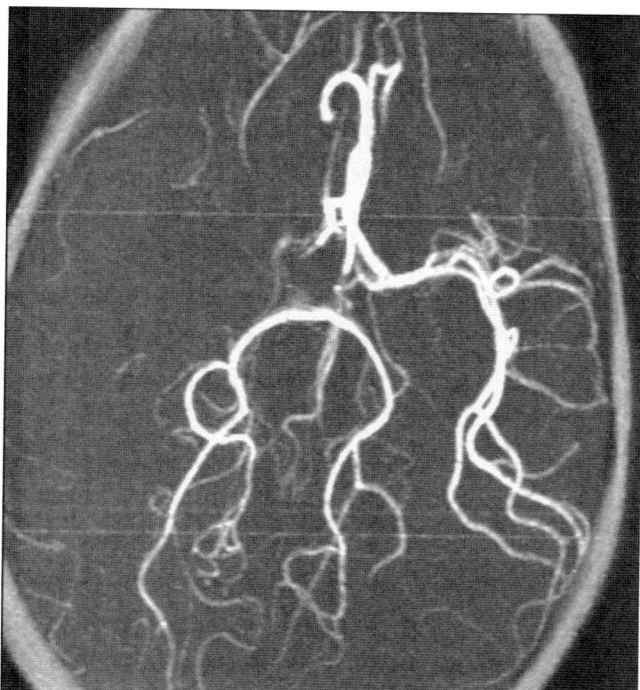

FIGURE 55.3. Maximum intensity projection from the MR angiogram of the patient with a right hemispheric stroke described in Figure 55.2, showing absent flow through the right middle cerebral artery.

the true degree of vascular stenosis. As the process of generating MIP images is also prone to producing artifacts, any suspected abnormality should be confirmed in the source images. Bolus infusion of contrast has been shown to improve the resolution of MR angiography in adults (48).

MR Spectroscopy

Spectroscopic imaging most often analyzes the signals generated by protons from a number of clinically important neuronal and glial metabolites, including N-acetyl aspartate (NAA), choline and phosphatidylcholine (Cho), creatine and phosphocreatine (Cre), myoinositol (mI), and lactate. Images can be generated using short, medium, or long echo relaxation times. The short echo images demonstrate a wider variety of metabolites and are useful for assessing inborn errors of metabolism (19). Longer echo times provide more accurate quantification of the principal brain metabolites, useful in the assessment of encephalopathy from trauma or ischemia (23) or in the evaluation of suspected tumor or tumor recurrence (6).

MR Perfusion

A number of MR methods have been developed for measuring cerebral perfusion. Fast imaging during paramagnetic contrast injection provides a purely qualitative picture of blood volume, relative regional blood flow, and perfusion delay. Alternatively, the protons within the blood entering the brain through the carotid arteries can be used as an endogenous contrast via spin labeling. It is anticipated that continuous arterial spin labeling will provide noninvasive and quantitative perfusion images. Applications for perfusion imaging include assessing the risk of ischemia in tissues with decreased perfusion, identifying the

decreased perfusion in primary and secondary vasculopathies, and grading the vascularity of tumors (24).

Susceptibility-weighted Imaging

Deoxygenated blood and such blood breakdown products as hemosiderin are weakly paramagnetic, and the artifacts that they produce on particular MR sequences can be exploited in the evaluation of patients for vascular abnormalities and small hemorrhages. Gradient echo T2-weighted images have been used for this purpose for some time and are widely available, but they are not nearly as sensitive as susceptibility-weighted imaging (SWI) that makes these same paramagnetic artifacts far more apparent (40).

SELECTED CLINICAL APPLICATIONS

Trauma

The initial workup of children with known or suspected head trauma will usually begin with a CT of the head and neck, looking for evidence of acute hemorrhage, fracture, or displacement of vertebrae out of their normal alignment. Young children who suffer traumatic brain injury are at particular risk of upper cervical spine injury (32) because of the relative weight of the cranium, weakness of the paraspinous muscles, elasticity and redundancy of the interspinous ligaments, and horizontal orientation of the incompletely ossified facet joints. Children <8 years of age have such mobility of their cervical spine as to have a normal atlantodental space as wide as 5 mm and anterior movement of C2 on C3 and of C3 on C4 of up to 4 mm. Alignment of the spinolaminar line is disrupted in true subluxation.

Spinal MRI should be considered in children, even when no evidence of misalignment or fracture of the vertebrae is seen on plain imaging in a neutral position, as soft tissue and cord edema, ischemia, and hemorrhage may only be visible on spinal MRI. The tendency of children to develop soft tissue and spinal cord injury without radiologic abnormality (SCIWORA) refers only to plain-film and CT imaging (36). As children reach adolescence, they are increasingly likely to sustain bony injuries with spinal trauma, but less severe injuries can still occur without plain-film evidence of fractures (9). Adolescents are also more likely than young children to present with lower cervical injuries and traumatic disc herniation.

MRI of the brain provides greater sensitivity than CT for brainstem injury (18), edema and petechial hemorrhages from axonal shearing (44), small extra-axial fluid collections, and older blood products (3) and is, therefore, the study of choice once a patient has been stabilized.

Imaging may find traumatic hemorrhage that is parenchymal, due to contusion or axonal shearing, or extraparenchymal, with the development of an epidural or subdural hematoma. On CT, hemorrhages appear hyperdense in the first week, isodense to brain between 1 and 3 weeks, and increasingly hypodense thereafter. Contrast administration causes enhancement of the outline of the hematoma, which becomes increasingly intense as the hemorrhage organizes (7,17). On MRI, hyperacute blood is dark on T1-weighted images and bright on T2-weighted images, in contrast to acute blood,

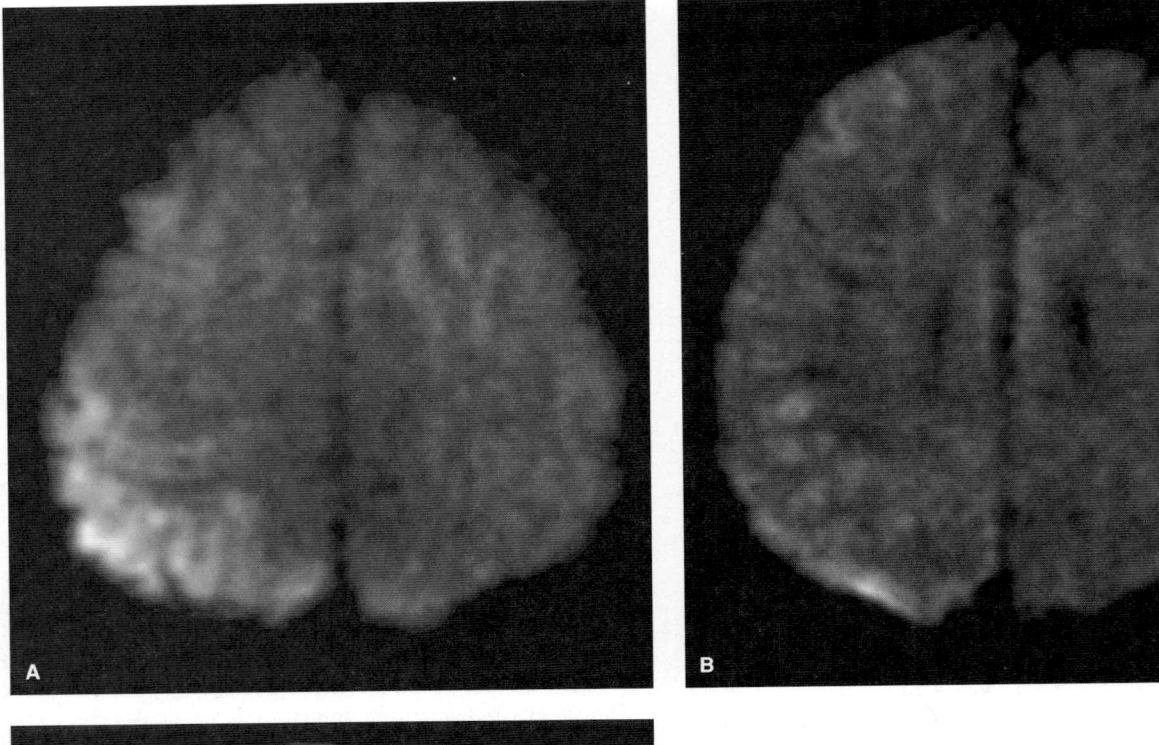

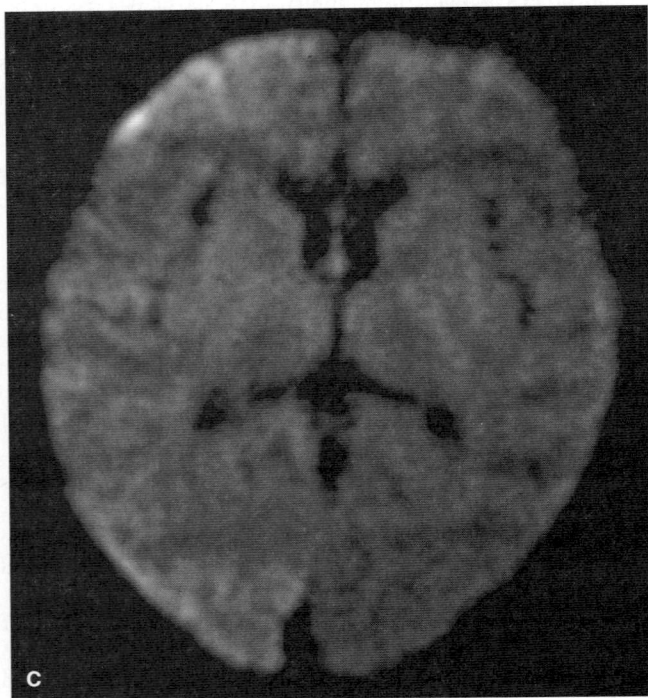

FIGURE 55.4. A–C. Thirteen-month-old boy presenting with pneumococcal meningitis and mild left-sided weakness. Diffusion-weighted image shows restriction within the interarterial or watershed regions of the right frontal and parietal cortex.

which is bright on T1-weighted images and dark on T2-weighted images. **Table 55.1** summarizes the evolution of the appearance of hemorrhage on CT and MRI. With layering of blood cells within a hematoma, the upper layer of fluid appears bright on T1- and T2-weighted images, while the bottom layer appears isodense to brain on T1-weighted images and dark on T2-weighted images (14). Finding signs of both old and new traumatic brain injury adds to the suspicion for nonaccidental trauma in infants, in whom nonaccidental trauma is 10–15 times more common than accidental trauma (39).

Subarachnoid hemorrhage due to trauma is most commonly seen layering along the falx cerebri in the posterior interhemispheric fissure or the tentorium cerebelli and is best detected in the acute stage by CT. Subacute hemorrhage can be detected by FLAIR sequences on MRI, although high signal intensity

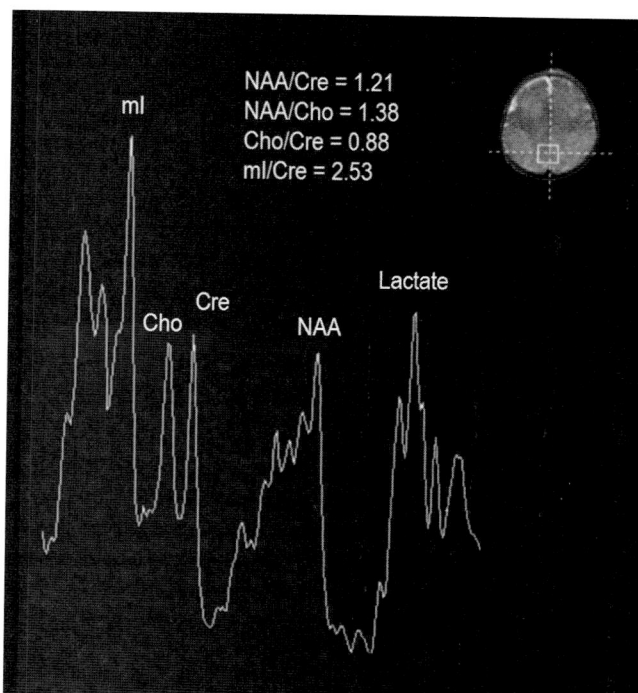

FIGURE 55.5. Two-year-old boy who underwent prolonged resuscitation after a near-drowning. The short echo proton MR spectroscopy of a voxel of cortex shows a very high myoinositol (*mI*) peak, an elevated choline (*Cho*) peak, a normal creatine (*Cre*) peak, a very low *N*-acetyl aspartate (*NAA*) peak, and a very large lactate peak. The metabolites are best described relative to Cre (*as shown*). The MR spectroscopy findings seen in this patient are highly predictive of a poor neurologic outcome.

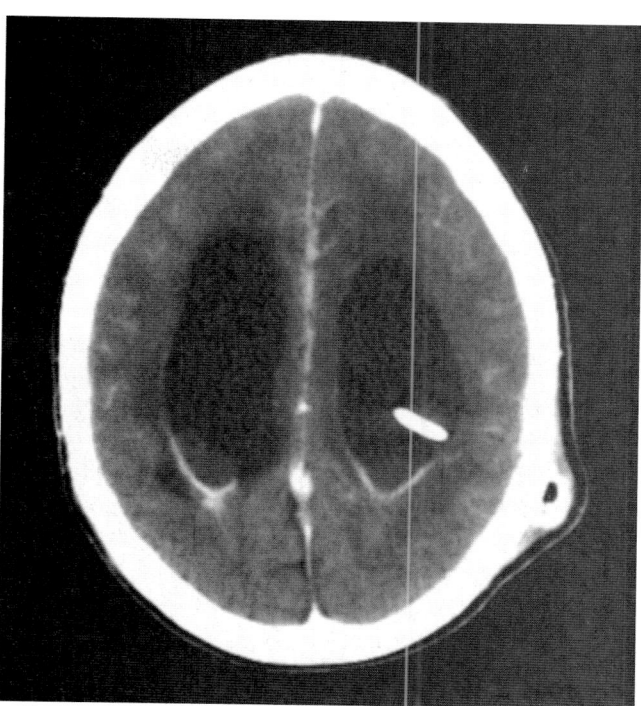

FIGURE 55.7. 13-year-old boy with lumbar myelomeningocele and congenital hydrocephalus presenting with fever and obtundation. Brain MRI with contrast shows expanded lateral ventricles due to shunt failure and contrast enhancement of the lining of the posterior horns of the ventricles due to ventriculitis and pseudomonas meningitis. A portion of the ventriculoperitoneal shunt is visible in the left lateral ventricle.

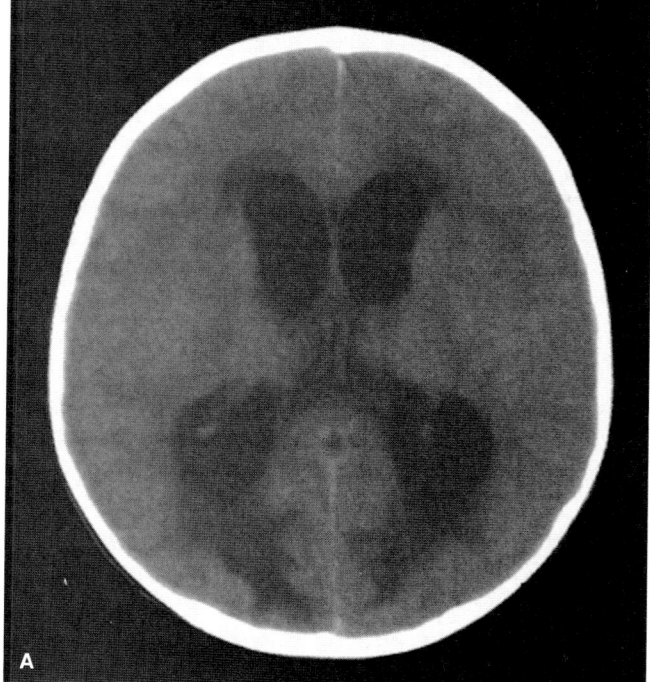

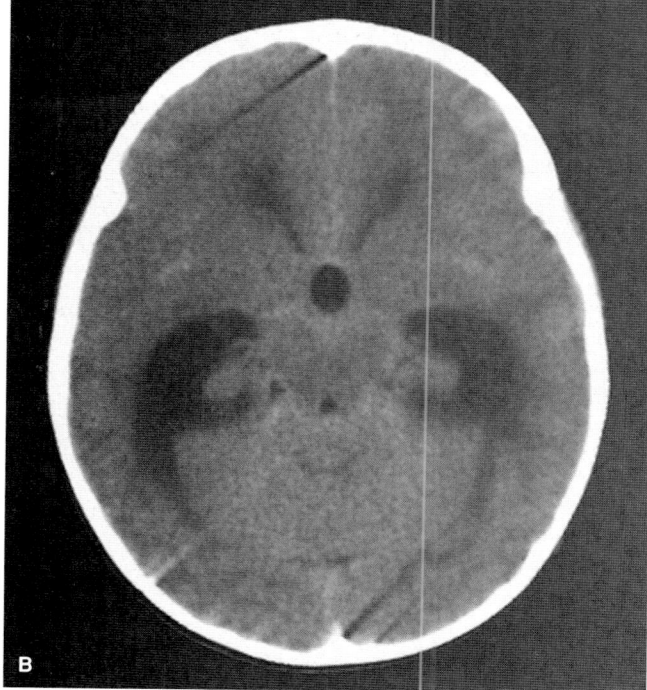

FIGURE 55.6. Eighteen-month-old boy with tuberculous meningitis who presented with obstructive hydrocephalus. Axial CT images show (**A**) marked enlargement of the lateral ventricles, periventricular hypodensity from transependymal edema, and effacement of the cerebral sulci and (**B**) hyperdense, purulent cerebrospinal fluid within the basal cisterns surrounding the midbrain.

on FLAIR can also be caused by rapid CSF flow, normally seen around the ventricular foramina, the aqueduct of Sylvius, and the prepontine cistern (35).

Children may have normal-appearing CT and MRI in the first 12 hrs after even severe traumatic brain injury, with severe cerebral edema becoming evident thereafter. Diffusion-weighted MRI can show areas of restricted diffusion due to cytotoxic edema within hours of injury. Proton spectroscopy is useful in determining the prognosis of children who are in a coma after head trauma, with poor outcome associated with decreased NAA levels and increased lactate and glutamate/glutamine levels in the first 2–4 days (42). The amount and depth of hemorrhage seen on SWI has also been shown to correlate with the duration of coma and long-term outcome in patients with severe diffuse axonal injury (1,45).

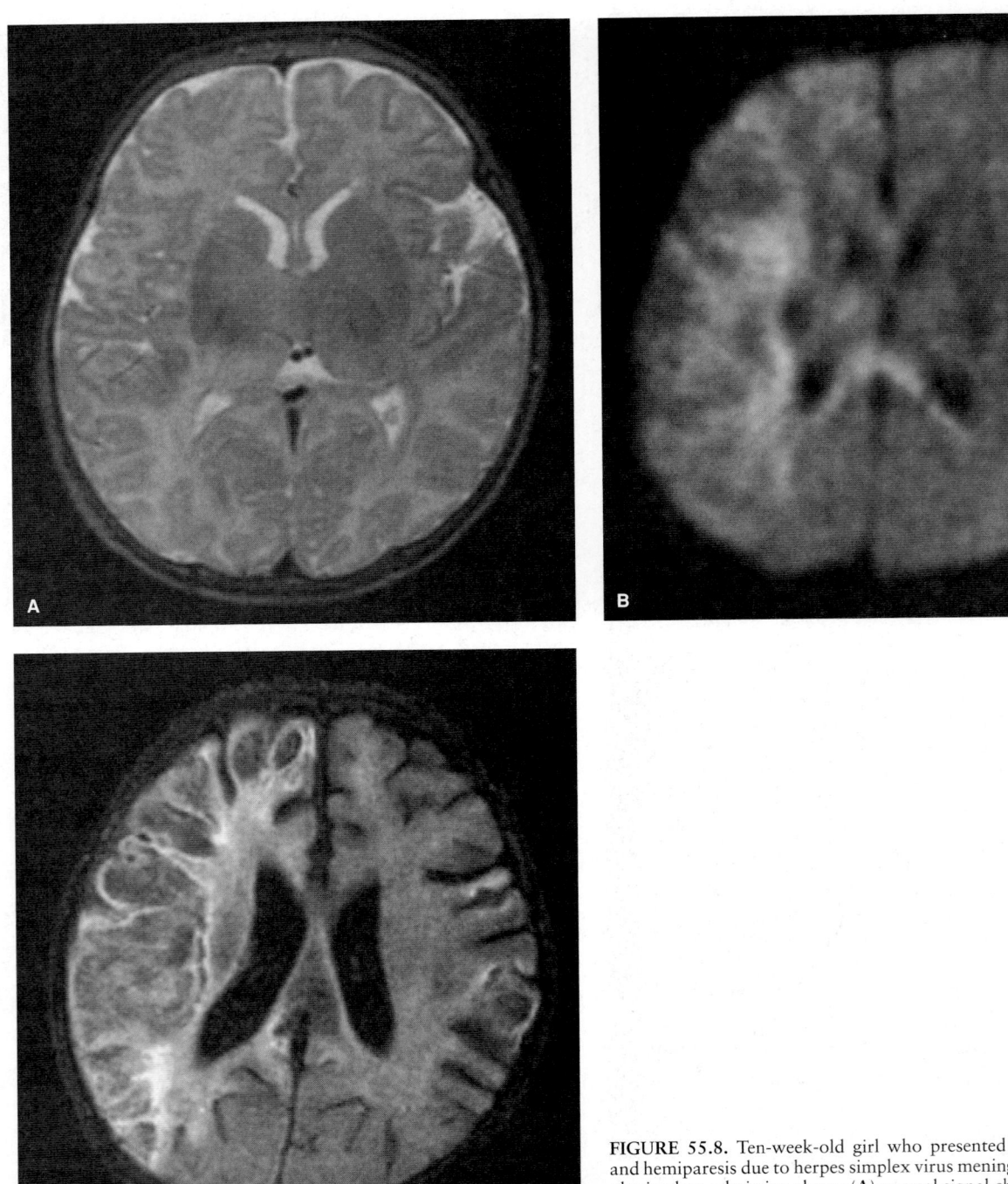

FIGURE 55.8. Ten-week-old girl who presented with focal seizures and hemiparesis due to herpes simplex virus meningoencephalitis. MRI obtained on admission shows (**A**) normal signal characteristics on T2-weighted images but (**B**) widespread right hemispheric diffusion restriction. MRI obtained 3 weeks later shows (**C**) corresponding extensive right hemispheric encephalomalacia on axial FLAIR image.

Hypoxic-Ischemic Injury

Stroke is increasingly recognized as a significant cause of morbidity and death in childhood (25). The imaging characteristics of infarctions depend more on the vascular distribution, degree, and duration of substrate deprivation than on the particular etiology and risk factors involved.

Infarction occurs in ~40% of children with cerebral sinovenous thrombosis, with accompanying hemorrhage in more than half of the patients (8). Presenting symptoms depend on the age of the child and the severity of the injury, but range from signs of focal injury, such as neurologic deficits and seizures, to diffuse signs of increased intracranial pressure, such as altered level of consciousness, headache, and vomiting. Superior sagittal sinus thrombosis can result in parasagittal infarction;

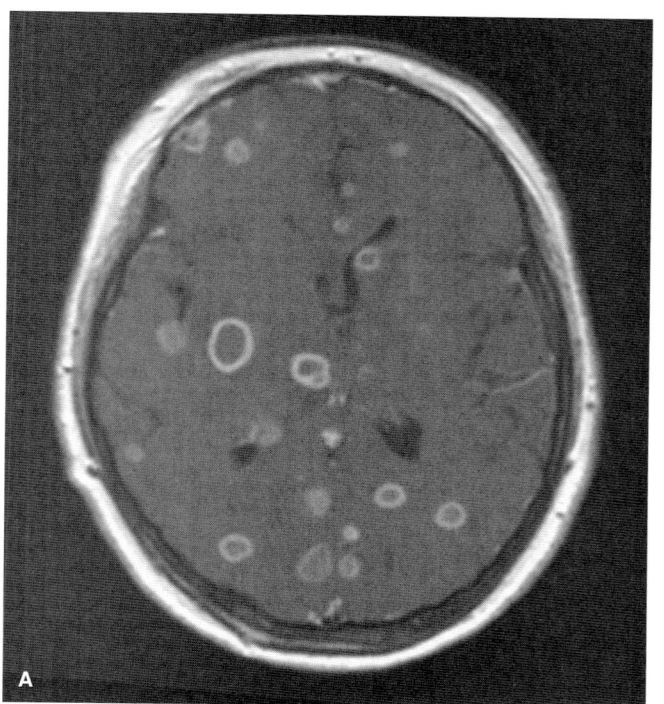

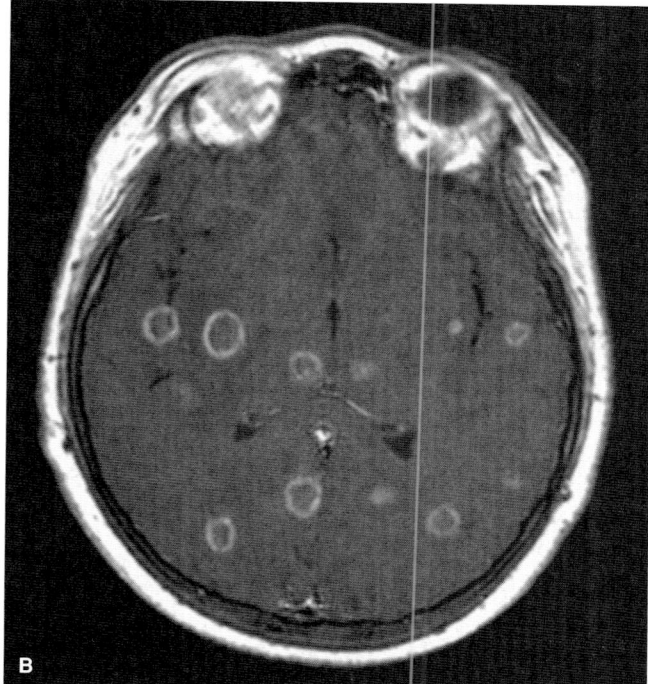

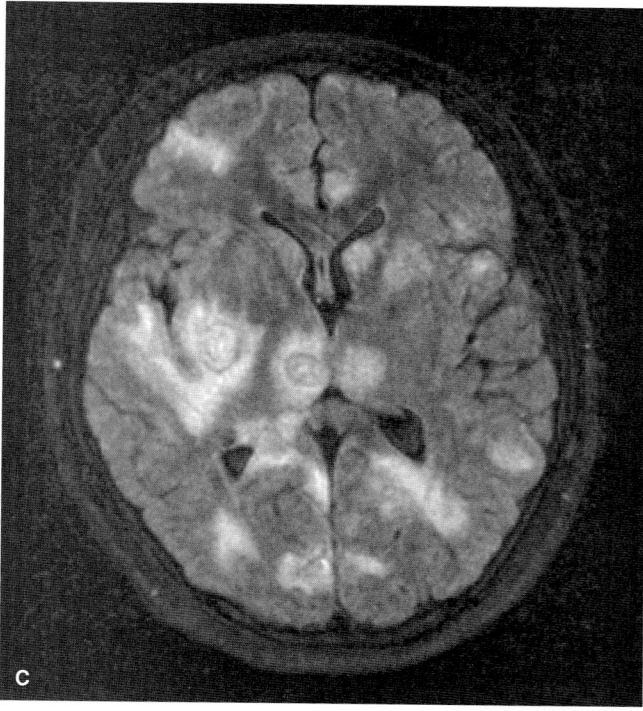

FIGURE 55.9. Twelve-year-old boy who presented with headaches and lethargy due to subacute amoebic meningoencephalitis from *Balamuthia mandrillaris*. **A,B:** Axial T1-weighted MR images with gadolinium contrast demonstrate multiple ring-enhancing lesions that show **(C)** surrounding T2 hyperintensity from vasogenic edema on axial FLAIR image.

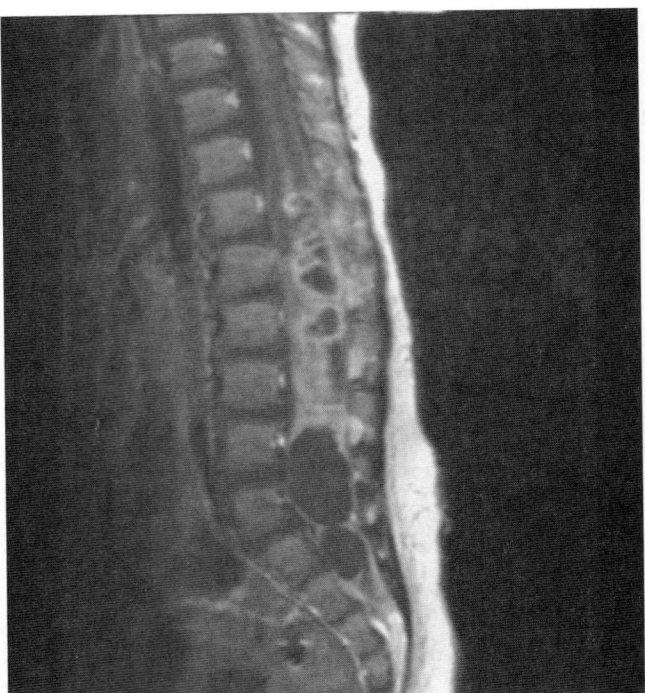

FIGURE 55.10. 14-month-old boy presenting with fever, irritability, and sudden refusal to walk. MRI of the thoracolumbar spine shows multiple loculated ring-enhancing abscesses within the spinal epidural space. Imaging also revealed a dural sinus tract associated with a small conus medullaris lipoma and tethering of the spinal cord.

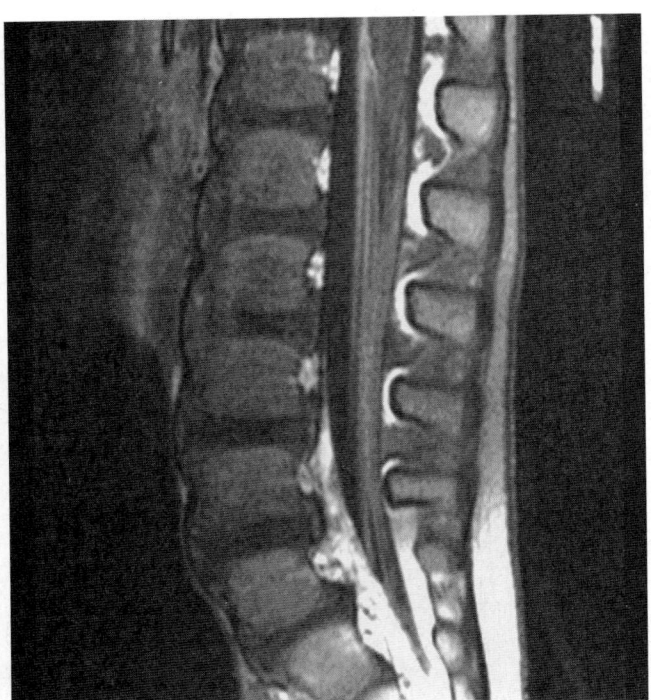

FIGURE 55.11. Eighteen-month-old boy who presented with refusal to walk and absent deep tendon reflexes 1 week after the resolution of a bout of infectious gastroenteritis. Sagittal T1-weighted MRI of the lumbar spine shows intense contrast enhancement of the dorsal and ventral nerve roots, consistent with his electrophysiologic diagnosis of Guillain-Barré syndrome.

transverse sinus and vein of Labbé thrombosis can result in temporal lobe infarction; and thrombosis of the deep cerebral veins, the straight sinus, or vein of Galen can result in thalamic infarction. Greater degrees of venous outflow reduction progressively cause vasogenic edema, infarction, and hemorrhage, all of which appear differently on neuroimaging. A CT scan may show areas of subcortical white matter hypodensity due to cerebral edema and areas of hyperdensity due to hemorrhage. Intravenous contrast is often necessary for detection of the venous thrombosis, with the flow of contrast around the thrombus described as the empty delta sign. MRI will show corresponding changes on routine T1- and T2-weighted images and is likely to visualize the thrombosis within the venous system, even without the use of contrast. MR venography can be useful when the diagnosis is suspected but uncertain. Diffusion-weighted imaging may show reduced, normal, increased, or mixed water movement, depending on the relative contributions of vasogenic and cytotoxic edema (50).

Focal arterial infarction appears on CT as a wedge-shaped area of hypodensity that involves the cortex and white matter supplied by the occluded artery (**Fig. 55.2A**). Posterior circulation infarctions may be particularly difficult to appreciate in infants whose temporal and occipital white matter normally appears hypodense. Gyriform contrast enhancement along the cortical injury is apparent between 5 days and 5 weeks following injury. MRI is even more sensitive than CT for the detection of ischemia-related cerebral edema (**Fig. 55.2B**), although both modalities may appear normal within the first 24 hrs after the appearance of clinical symptoms. Diffusion-weighted imaging, on the other hand, can show restricted wa-

ter movement from cytotoxic edema (**Fig. 55.2C**) in as little as 1 hr after injury (16). Angiography, using either CT or MR, can be used to assess the possibility of medium-to-large vessel abnormalities, such as occlusion, thrombosis, dysplasia, or dissection (**Fig. 55.3**). Neither method can exclude the type of small-vessel vasculopathy associated with systemic lupus erythematosus.

Diffuse hypoxic-ischemic injury can result from cardiopulmonary arrest or from severe hypotension or hypoxemia. A decrease in cerebral perfusion will initially cause shunting of blood flow to the posterior circulation, protecting the brainstem. The cortical areas supplied by branches of the carotid artery, especially the intervascular boundary zones, are vulnerable to ischemic injury, often resulting in a pattern referred to as a "watershed" distribution (**Fig. 55.4A–C**). More profound decreases in cerebral blood flow do not allow for preferential shunting and leave regions with the highest basal metabolic rate (including the thalami, basal ganglia, and sensorimotor cortex) most vulnerable to injury.

CT can be used for initial imaging of unstable patients, although scans within the first 24 hrs may be read as normal despite the presence of severe global ischemia. Even the earliest appreciable changes, such as basal ganglia hypodensity and effacement of the perimesencephalic cisterns, may be very subtle (13). Later CT scans will show clearer evidence of cerebral edema, with decreased differentiation between cortex and white matter, effacement of sulci and cisterns, and hypodensity of deep and cortical gray matter. Particularly ominous for prognosis is the "reversal sign," with white matter

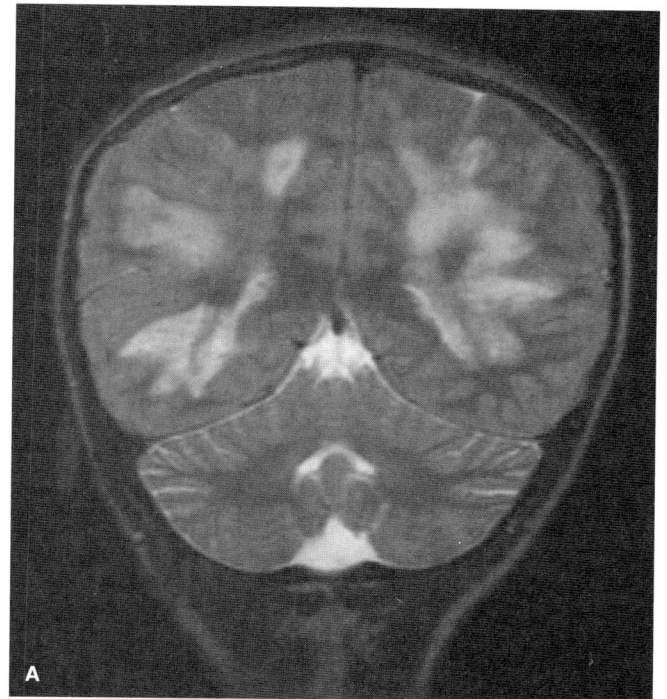

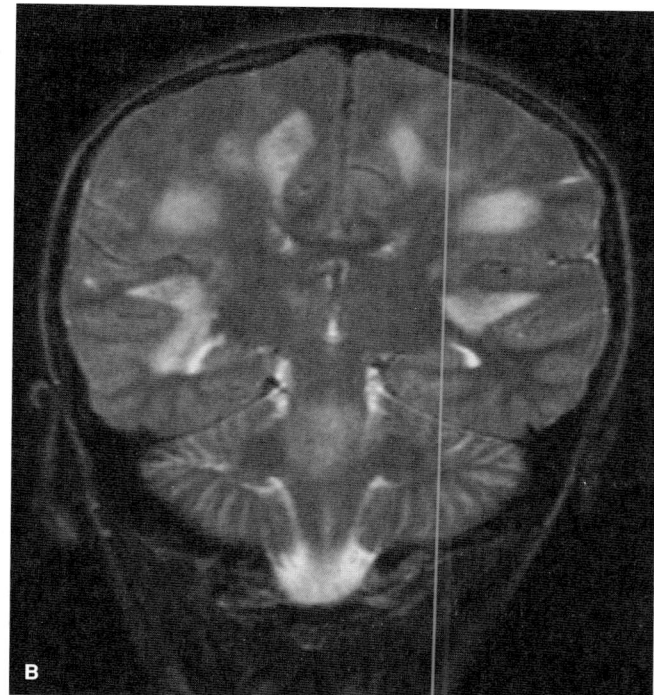

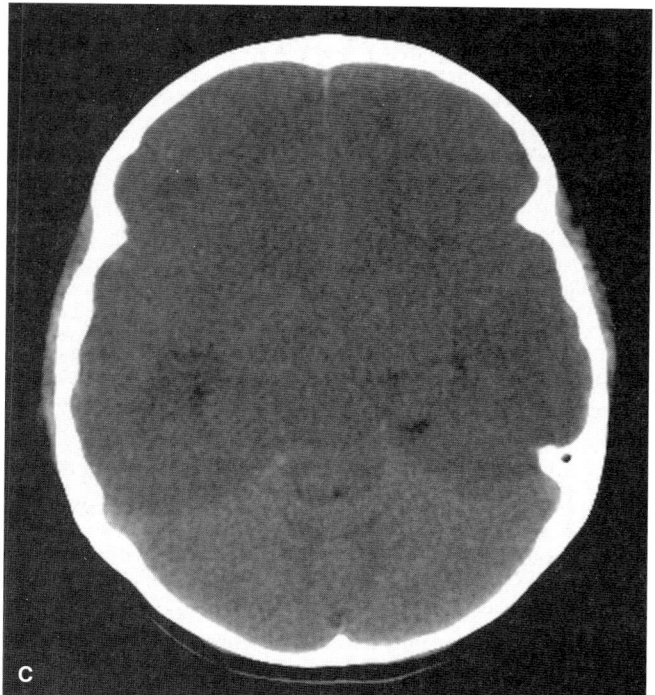

FIGURE 55.12. Seven-year-old girl who presented with hallucinations and obtundation due to acute disseminated encephalomyelitis. **A,B:** T2-weighted coronal MR images show diffuse T2 hyperintensity within the subcortical white matter, right thalamus, and pons. The patient deteriorated clinically despite aggressive immunomodulatory therapy. **C:** CT shows diffuse hypodensity of the supratentorial tissues with obliteration of the perimesencephalic cisterns. Autopsy showed diffuse cerebral edema and transtentorial herniation.

appearing denser than cortex, which may be due to impaired venous drainage (5).

Early changes of global ischemia can be as subtle on conventional MRI as they are on CT, although early diffusion restriction can be seen in areas of infarction, and proton MR spectroscopy can show a rise in glutamate and glutamine, with or without the presence of lactate. However, very early DWI can significantly underestimate the complete extent of ischemic injury (10). Prognosis is best assessed by the presence of lactate or of significantly reduced NAA:Cre ratios on MR spectroscopy obtained from 3 to 5 days after injury (Fig. 55.5).

Infection and Inflammation

Visualization of CNS infections is important for prompt diagnosis and treatment, as well as for monitoring the response to

TABLE 55.2

METABOLIC DISORDERS THAT PRODUCE GRAY MATTER IMAGING ABNORMALITIES

Cortical gray matter
  Neuronal ceroid lipofuscinoses
  Mucolipidosis I
Deep gray matter
  Striatal T2 hyperintensity
    Mitochondrial disorders (Leigh and MELAS syndromes)
    Juvenile Huntington disease
    Organic acidopathies
    Hypoxia-ischemia or hypoglycemia
  Globus pallidus T2 hypointensity
    Pantothenate kinase-associated neurodegeneration
      (PKAN)
    Oculodigital dental dysplasia
  Globus pallidus T2 hyperintensity
    Methylmalonic academia
    Toxins (carbon monoxide, manganese, cyanide)
    Kernicterus
    Succinate semialdehyde dehydrogenase deficiency
    Guanidoacetate methyltransferase deficiency
    Isovaleric academia

Adapted from Barkovich AJ. *Pediatric Neuroimaging.* Philadelphia: Lippincott Williams & Wilkins, 2005.

TABLE 55.3

METABOLIC DISORDERS THAT PRODUCE WHITE MATTER IMAGING ABNORMALITIES

Subcortical white matter
  Megalencephalic leukoencephalopathy with
    subcortical cysts
  Alexander disease
  Galactosemia
  Salla disease
  4-Hydroxybutyric aciduria
Deep white matter
  Krabbe disease
  GM1 or GM2 gangliosidosis
  X-linked adrenoleukodystrophy
  Metachromatic leukodystrophy
  Phenylketonuria
  Male syrup urine disease
  Lowe disease
  Sjögren-Larsson syndrome
  Hyperhomocysteinemia
  Radiation/chemotherapy
  Childhood ataxia with diffuse central nervous system
    hypomyelination
  Merosin-deficient congenital muscular dystrophy
  Dentatorubropallidoluysian atrophy
Lack of myelination
  Pelizaeus-Merzbacher disease
  Trichothiodystrophy
  18q- syndrome
  Salla disease
Nonspecific pattern of involvement
  Nonketotic hyperglycinemia
  Urea cycle disorders
  3-hydroxy-3-methylglutaryl-coenzyme A lyase deficiency
  Collagen vascular diseases
  Demyelinating diseases
  Viral infections

Adapted from Barkovich AJ. *Pediatric Neuroimaging.* Philadelphia: Lippincott Williams & Wilkins, 2005.

treatment and development of complications. When CNS infection is clinically suspected and a lumbar puncture is being contemplated, it is common practice to first obtain a CT of the head to determine whether a mass lesion is present that might predispose to cerebral herniation. Studies in adults have suggested that such routine imaging might not be necessary in patients with normal neurologic examinations (22) and that the presence of a mass lesion on CT is poorly predictive of the risk of imminent cerebral herniation, whether or not lumbar puncture is performed (38).

Meningitis

CT may show meningeal contrast enhancement when meningitis is present, especially in its later stages, and is important for investigating possible sources of infection such as mastoiditis, sinusitis, and skull-based fractures. Complications of meningitis, such as ischemic stroke from vasculitis, obstructive and communicating hydrocephalus, and hemorrhage from venous thrombosis, are also evaluated well by contrast-enhanced CT. Scans from a patient with obstructive hydrocephalus from tuberculous meningitis are shown in **Figure 55.6A,B**. MRI is more likely to show meningeal contrast enhancement in uncomplicated meningitis but has also been shown to predict the diagnosis of tuberculous meningitis when the meninges appear bright on precontrast T1-weighted magnetization transfer images (26). MRI with DWI is superior to CT in demonstrating some infectious and vasculitic complications of meningitis, including encephalitis, cerebritis, abscess, empyema, ventriculitis, and ischemia (**Fig. 55.7**).

Meningoencephalitis

CSF analysis is the principal method employed for diagnosing viral meningoencephalitis, but in children infected with the most common etiologic agent, herpes simplex virus (HSV) I, false negative polymerase chain reaction (PCR) testing is com-

mon when done within the first 72 hours of illness (46). MRI with DWI is highly sensitive for the detection of the cytotoxic edema and necrosis associated with this infection (43), and the presence and extent of such lesions are predictive of the long-term neurologic prognosis (41). **Figure 55.8A–C** shows an infant with evolving necrosis from HSV encephalitis. Imaging findings in encephalitis due to other viral agents, including enteroviruses and arboviruses, are often nonspecific and may be limited to subtle T2 hyperintensity within the cortical and subcortical gray matter. Ring-enhancing lesions should raise the possibility of unusual causes of meningoencephalitis, including fungi (cryptococcus, aspergillus, candida), parasites (toxoplasmosis, cysticercosis, amoebae), and mycobacterium tuberculosis. The differential is expanded in patients who are immunocompromised. A case of subacute amoebic meningoencephalitis is illustrated in **Figure 55.9A–C**.

Spinal Infections

Spinal CT with contrast enhancement has a higher detection rate for paraspinal infection than that of plain x-ray, which

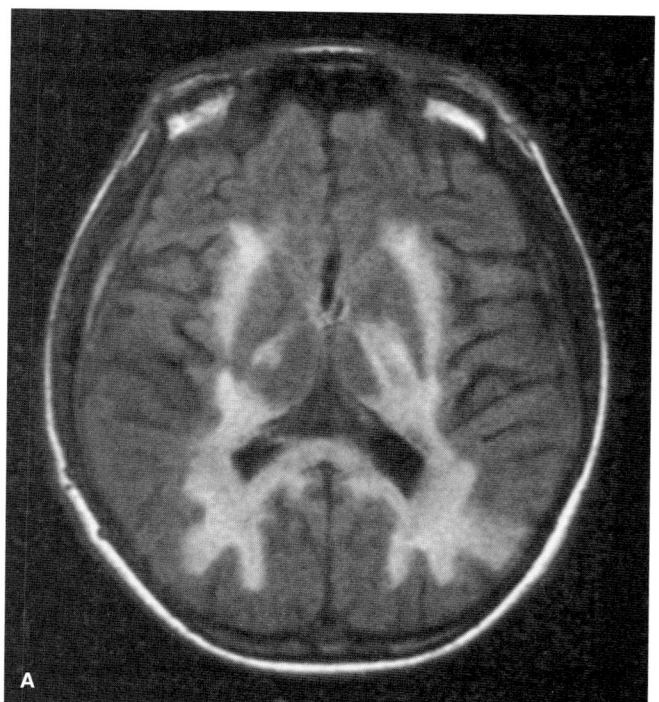
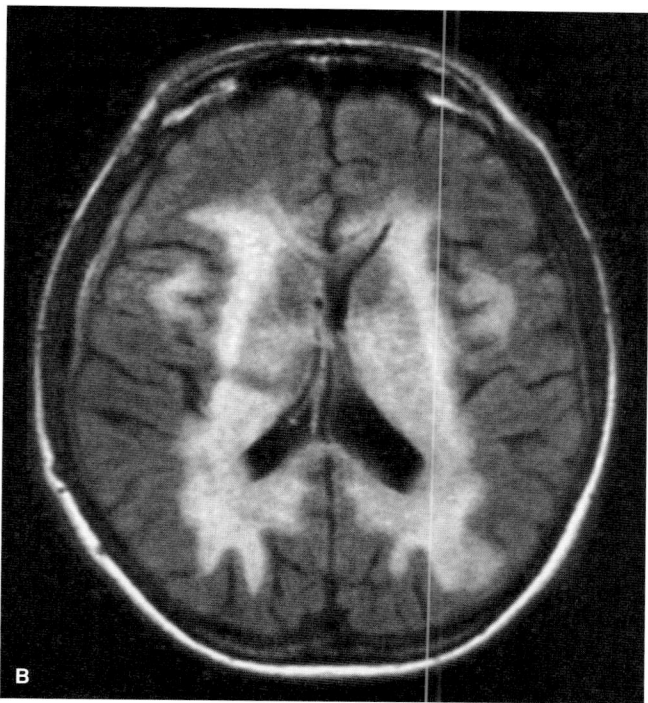

FIGURE 55.13. A,B. Seventeen-year-old boy with fulminant presentation of X-linked adrenoleukodystrophy, with MRI showing posteriorly predominant and confluent areas of hyperintensity within the periventricular and subcortical white matter on FLAIR imaging.

may only detect bony erosion and vertebral destruction, but it is insufficiently sensitive to exclude the presence of an early discitis or epidural abscess and does not directly assess the integrity of the spinal cord. Given the urgency with which surgical intervention might be needed to avoid permanent spinal cord injury, MRI should be performed early in the evaluation of all patients with suspected spinal infections if no contraindication exists (**Fig. 55.10**). In patients with spinal epidural abscesses that show no cord compression but have signs of severe neurologic impairment, neuroimaging can reveal cord ischemia due to vascular compression or thrombosis (47).

Postinfectious Encephalomyelitis

Inflammatory neuropathies with an autoimmune basis are thought to be triggered in most cases by infections, vaccinations, and traumatic injuries. Any portion of the central or peripheral nervous systems can be involved individually, as in such isolated syndromes as optic neuritis, acute cerebellar ataxia, transverse myelitis, and Guillain-Barré syndrome. **Figure 55.11** shows the cauda equina enhancement sometimes found in patients with Guillain-Barré syndrome. Alternatively, multiple areas of the nervous system can be involved at once with various manifestations of acute disseminated encephalomyelitis (ADEM). MRI is well suited for the detection of ADEM lesions within the brain and spinal cord, although patients may have severe optic neuritis without radiologic evidence of optic nerve involvement. The differential considered in some cases of ADEM includes atypical infection (e.g., cryptococcal meningitis), tumor (e.g., lymphoma), ischemic stroke, and recurrent demyelination from multiple sclerosis. MR spectroscopy and DWI may be particularly helpful in difficult cases in which biopsy would otherwise be considered necessary (31). Some clinical and radiologic features have been found to be

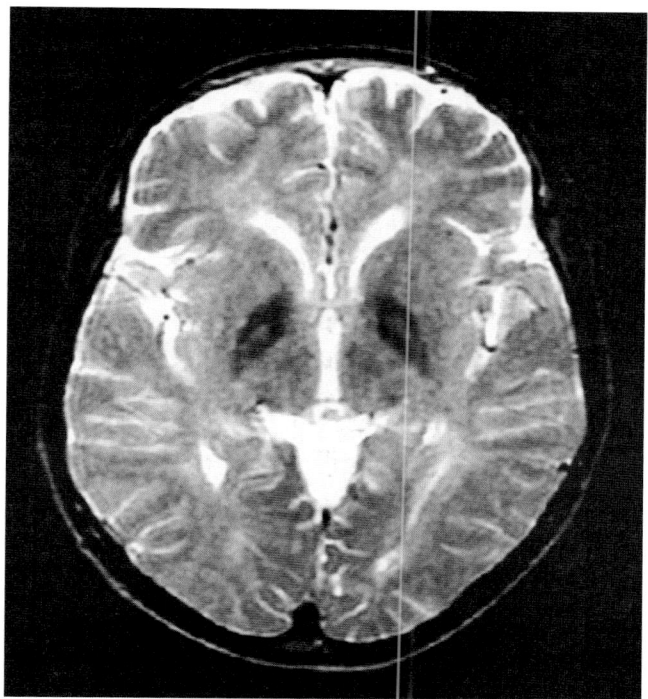

FIGURE 55.14. Fifteen-year-old boy presenting with tremor, dystonia, and dysarthria, diagnosed with pantothenate kinase associated neurodegeneration (PKAN) associated with mutation of the gene for pantothenate kinase 2. MR imaging was obtained using a 1.5 Tesla scanner. Axial T2-weighted image shows characteristic hypointensity within the globus pallidi bilaterally with a central high signal intensity focus, often described as the eye-of-the-tiger sign. Image courtesy of Dr. R. Nuri Sener of the Department of Radiology, Ege University Hospital, Bornova, Izmir, Turkey.

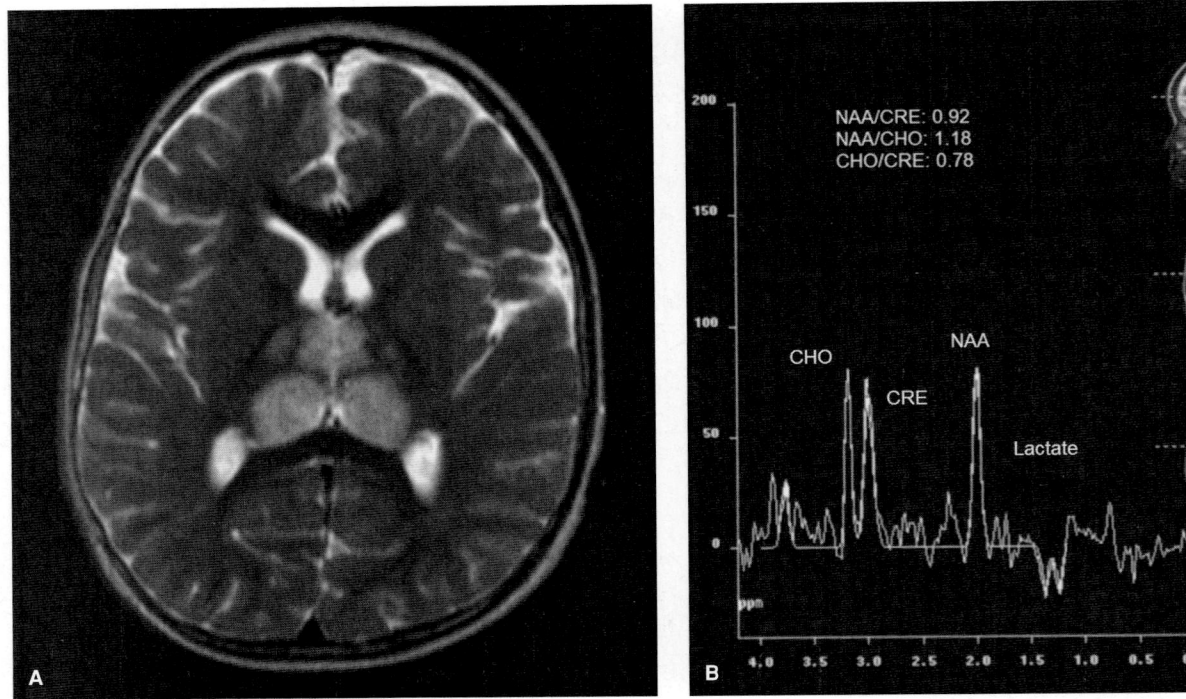

FIGURE 55.15. Eighteen-month-old boy who presented with coma after influenza vaccination. **(A)** MRI of the brain shows symmetrical bright T2-weighted signal within the thalami, and **(B)** long-echo proton MR spectroscopy of a voxel centered in the left thalamus shows a markedly low NAA:Cre ratio, indicating neuronal loss or dysfunction, and a high concentration of lactate, indicative of ischemia, consistent with a diagnosis of acute necrotizing encephalopathy.

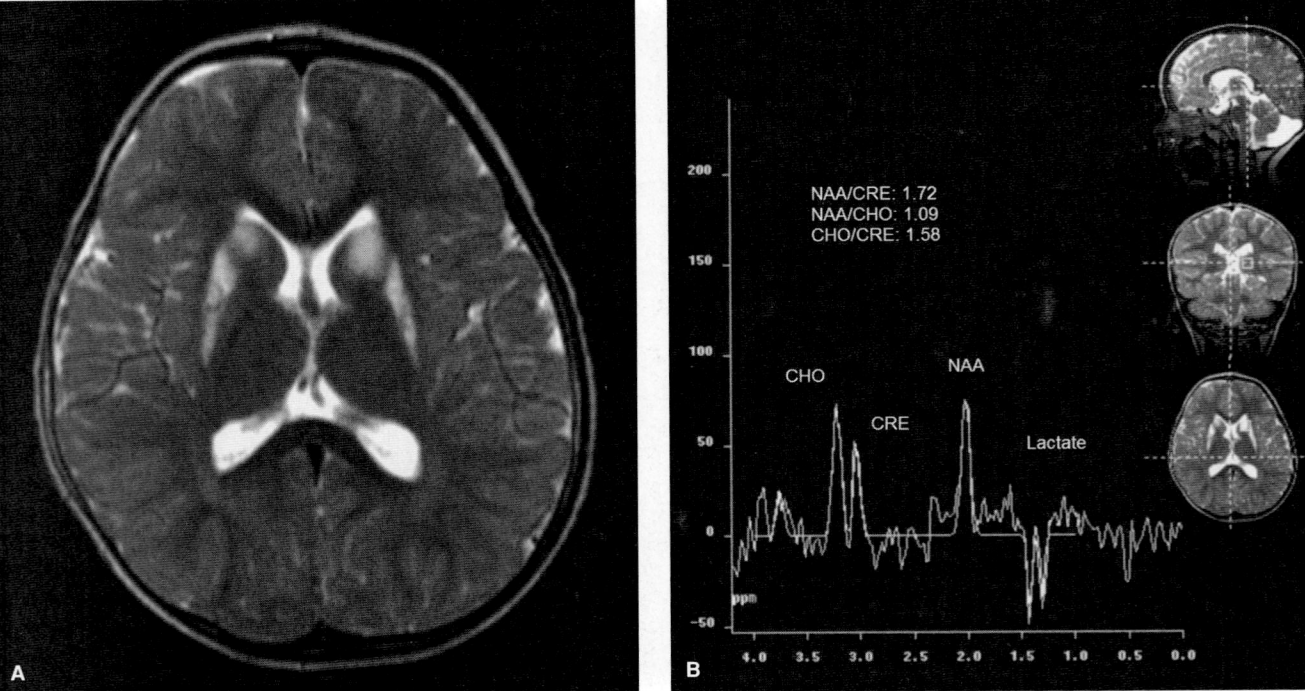

FIGURE 55.16. Sixteen-month-old boy who presented with slowly progressive ophthalmoplegia that acutely worsened during an otherwise mild febrile gastroenteritis. **(A)** MRI of the brain 9 months later shows persistent T2 hyperintensity within both caudate nuclei, and **(B)** long-echo proton MR spectroscopy of a voxel centered in the left caudate nucleus shows a low NAA:Cre ratio and a high concentration of lactate, consistent with a diagnosis of Leigh syndrome.

TABLE 55.4

TABLE 55.4

METABOLIC DISORDERS THAT PRODUCE GRAY AND WHITE MATTER IMAGING ABNORMALITIES

Cortical gray matter only
   Cortical dysgenesis
      Congenital CMV infection
      Congenital muscular dystrophy
      Peroxisomal disorders
   No cortical dysgenesis
      Mucopolysaccharidoses
      Lipid storage disorders

Deep gray matter
   Early thalamic involvement
      Krabbe disease
      GM1 or GM2 gangliosidosis
      Wilson disease
      Profound neonatal hypotensive encephalopathy
   Early globus pallidus involvement
      Canavan disease
      Kearn-Sayre syndrome
      Methylmalonic academia
      Toxins (carbon monoxide and cyanide)
      Maple syrup urine disease
      L-2-hydroxyglutaric aciduria
      Dentatorubropallidoluysian atrophy
      Urea cycle disorders
      Cree leukoencephalopathy
   Early striatal involvement
      Mitochondrial disorders (Leigh and MELAS syndrome)
      Wilson disease
      Organic acidurias
      Molybdenum cofactor deficiency
      β-Ketothiolase deficiency
      Biotinidase deficiencies
      Hypoxia-ischemia or hypoglycemia
      Cockayne syndrome
      Toxins

Adapted from Barkovich AJ. *Pediatric Neuroimaging.* Philadelphia: Lippincott Williams & Wilkins, 2005.

helpful in distinguishing between ADEM and early multiple sclerosis (49). A fulminant case of ADEM is presented in **Figure 55.12A–C.**

Toxic Metabolic Injury

A wide variety of metabolic disorders, from inborn errors of metabolism and acquired endogenous or exogenous toxins can have similar, nonspecific patterns of injury on neuroimaging. From an imaging perspective, these patterns can be characterized by whether they affect gray matter, white matter, or both (**Tables 55.2** through **55.4, Fig. 55.13**). Although CT is sometimes useful for the detection of the calcifications that can occur in these disorders, MRI is superior for identifying the pattern of injury and can, in some instances, provide a specific diagnosis, as with T2-weighted imaging in pantothenate kinase-associated neurodegeneration (**Fig. 55.14**) and with MR spectroscopy in leukodystrophies like Canavan disease (27).

While nonspecific, detection of otherwise unexplained deep gray-matter lactate contributes to the diagnosis of mitochondrial disorders (**Figs. 55.15** and **55.16**).

CONCLUSIONS AND FUTURE DIRECTIONS

The role of neuroimaging in clinical practice has grown in parallel with the tremendous technical innovations that have occurred in the last quarter century, with CT and MR having become indispensable to the diagnosis and management of most patients with neurologic disorders. Modifications of currently available MR techniques, such as chemical shift imaging and diffusion tensor imaging, are already showing great promise for clinical application.

CSI is generated by continuous MR spectroscopic sampling of an entire brain region and can be performed in two dimensions (e.g., an axial slice through the basal ganglia and thalami for a patient with hypoxic-ischemic injury) or three, providing far more information about the degree and distribution of injury than single-voxel studies. Ongoing research will allow correlation of these detailed metabolic maps to short- and long-term outcomes.

DTI expands on the principles used for DWI to generate imaging reflective of free water diffusion along the white matter tracts of the brain (4). DTI is being applied to study the normal development of white matter tracts in healthy children (34), abnormal development in neurologically impaired children (12), and acute disruption by traumatic, metabolic, or toxic injury (33).

The diagnostic and prognostic utility of imaging studies will continue to expand as further innovations allow us to use them to look ever more closely at the pathophysiology of neurologic disease.

KEY POINTS

- CT can be obtained with less time and need for sedation than MRI.
- MRI provides greater anatomic and metabolic detail than CT, without exposing patients to ionizing radiation and iodinated contrast.
- CT visualizes large traumatic hemorrhages that may need surgical intervention, and is ideal for identifying cervical spine fractures.
- MRI with SWI is superior for identifying and quantifying traumatic diffuse axonal injury and microhemorrhage.
- MRI of the cervical spine can show traumatic soft tissue and cord injury not visible on CT.
- CT may be normal up to 24 hrs after focal or global ischemic brain injury.
- MRI with DWI detects cytotoxic edema within hours of ischemic injury and can differentiate abscesses from necrotic tumors.
- MRI with proton spectroscopy can identify metabolic properties of tissues and improves the accuracy of prognosis in children with traumatic and ischemic brain injury.
- MRI can identify patterns of abnormalities associated with inborn errors of metabolism.

References

1. Babikian T, Freier MC, Tong KA, et al. Susceptibility weighted imaging: Neuropsychologic outcome and pediatric head injury. *Pediatr Neurol* 2005;33:184–94.
2. Barkovich AJ. *Pediatric Neuroimaging*. Philadelphia: Lippincott Williams & Wilkins, 2005.
3. Barkovich AJ, Atlas SW. MRI of intracranial hemorrhage. *Radiol Clin North Am* 1988;26:801–20.
4. Basser P, Matiello J, Le Bihan D. MR diffusion tensor spectroscopy and imaging. *Biophys J* 1994;66:259–67.
5. Bird CR, Drayer BP, Gilles FH. Pathophysiology of reverse edema in global cerebral ischemia. *AJNR Am J Neuroradiol* 1989;10:95–8.
6. Chernov M, Hayashi M, Izawa M, et al. Differentiation of the radiation-induced necrosis and tumor recurrence after gamma knife radiosurgery for brain metastases: Importance of multi-voxel proton MRS. *Minim Invasive Neurosurg* 2005;48:228–34.
7. Chuang SH, Fitz CR. CT of head trauma. In: Gonzales CF, Grossman CB, Masdeu JC, eds. *CT of the Head and Spine*. New York: Wiley, 1985;523–36.
8. deVeber G, Andrew M, Adams C, et al. Cerebral sinovenous thrombosis in children. *N Engl J Med* 2001;345:417–23.
9. Dickman CA, Rekate HL, Sonntag VKH, et al. Pediatric spinal trauma: Vertebral column and spinal cord injuries in children. *Pediat Neursci* 1989;15:237–56.
10. Dubowitz DJ, Bluml S, Arcinue E, et al. MR of hypoxic encephalopathy in children after near drowning: Correlation with quantitative proton MR spectroscopy and clinical outcome. *AJNR Am J Neuroradiol* 1998;19:1617–27.
11. Erdem E, Agildere M, Eryilmaz M, et al. Intracranial calcification in children on computed tomography. *Turk J Pediatr* 1994;36:111–22.
12. Fillipi C, Lin D, Tsiouris A, et al. Diffusion-tensor MR imaging in children with developmental delay: Preliminary findings. *Radiology* 2003;229:44–50.
13. Fitch SJ, Gerald B, Magill HL, et al. Central nervous system hypoxia in children due to near drowning. *Radiology* 1985;156:647–50.
14. Fobbin J, Grossman R, Atlas S. MR characterization of subdural hematomas and hygromas at 1.5T. *AJNR Am J Neuroadiol* 1989;10:687–93.
15. Forbes K, Pipe J, Karis J, et al. Brain imaging in the unsedated pediatric patient: Comparison of periodically rotated overlapping parallel lines with enhanced reconstruction and single-shot fast spin-echo sequences. *AJNR Am J Neuroradiol* 2003;24:794–8.
16. Gadian DG, Calamante F, Kirkham FJ, et al. Diffusion and perfusion magnetic resonance imaging in childhood stroke. *J Child Neurol* 2000;15:279–83.
17. Gean A. *Imaging of Head Trauma*. New York: Raven, 1994.
18. Gentry LR, Godersky JC, Thompson BH. Traumatic brain stem injury: MR imaging. *Radiology* 1989;171:177–87.
19. Grodd W, Krageloh-Mann I, Klose U, et al. Metabolic and destructive brain disorders in children: Findings with localized proton MR spectroscopy. *Radiology* 1991;181:173–81.
20. Hall E. Lessons we have learned from our children: Cancer risks from diagnostic radiology. *Pediatr Radiol* 2002;32:700–6.
21. Hall P, Adami HO, Trichopoulos D, et al. Effect of low doses of ionizing radiation in infancy on cognitive function in adulthood: Swedish population-based cohort study. *BMJ* 2004;328:19.
22. Hasbun R, Abrahams J, Jekel J, et al. Computed tomography of the head before lumbar puncture in adults with suspected meningitis. *N Engl J Med* 2001;345:1727–33.
23. Holshouser BA, Ashwal S, Shu S, et al. Proton MR spectroscopy in children with acute brain injury: Comparison of short and long echo time acquisitions. *J Magn Reson Imaging* 2000;11:9–19.
24. Huisman TA, Sorensen AG. Perfusion-weighted magnetic resonance imaging of the brain: Techniques and application in children. *Eur Radiol* 2004;14:59–72.
25. Jordan LC. Stroke in childhood. *Neurologist* 2006;12:94–102.
26. Kamra P, Azad R, Prasad KN, et al. Infectious meningitis: Prospective evaluation with magnetization transfer MRI. *Br J Radiol* 2004;77:387–94.
27. Kingsley PB, Shah TC, Woldenberg R. Identification of diffuse and focal brain lesions by clinical magnetic resonance spectroscopy. *NMR Biomed* 2006;19:435–62.
28. Leuthardt EC, Wippold FJ 2nd, Oswood MC, et al. Diffusion-weighted MR imaging in the preoperative assessment of brain abscesses. *Surg Neurol* 2002;58:395–402.
29. Lim CC, Lee W, Chng SM, et al. Diffusion-weighted MR imaging in intracranial infections. *Ann Acad Med Singapore* 2003;32:446–9.
30. Lovblad KO, Wetzel SG, Somon T, et al. Diffusion-weighted MRI in cortical ischaemia. *Neuroradiology* 2004;46:175–82.
31. Mader I, Wolff M, Nagele T, et al. MRI and proton MR spectroscopy in acute disseminated encephalomyelitis. *Childs Nerv Syst* 2005;21:566–72.
32. McGory BJ, Klassen RA, Chao EYS, et al. Acute fractures and dislocations of the cervical spine in children and adolescents. *J Bone Joint Surg [Am]* 1993;75:988–95.
33. McKinstry R, Miller J, Snyder A, et al. A prospective, longitudinal diffusion tensor imaging study of brain injury in newborns. *Neurology* 2002;59:824–33.
34. Mukherjee P, Miller J, Shimony J, et al. Normal brain maturation during childhood: Developmental trends characterized with diffusion-tensor MR imaging. *Radiology* 2001;221:349–58.
35. Noguchi K, Ogawa T, Seto H, et al. Subacute and chronic subarachnoid hemorrhage: Diagnosis with fluid-attenuated inversion recovery MR imaging. *Radiology* 1997;203:257–62.
36. Osenbach RK, Menezes AH. Spinal cord injury without radiographic abnormality in children. *Pediatr Neurosci* 1989;15:168–74.
37. Pappas JN, Donnelly LE, Frush DP. Reduced frequency of sedation of young children with multisection helical CT. *Radiology* 2000;215:897–9.
38. Pfister HW, Feiden W, Einhaupl KM. Spectrum of complications during bacterial meningitis in adults: Results of a prospective clinical study. *Arch Neurol* 1993;50:575–81.
39. Rivera FP, Kamitsuka MD, Quan L. Injuries to children younger than one year of age. *Pediatrics* 1988;81:93–7.
40. Sehgal V, Delproposto Z, Haacke EM, et al. Clinical applications of neuroimaging with susceptibility-weighted imaging. *J Magn Reson Imaging* 2005;22:439–50.
41. Sener RN. Herpes simplex encephalitis: Diffusion MR imaging findings. *Comput Med Imaging Graph* 2001;25:391–7.
42. Stinson G, Bagley LJ, Cecil KM, et al. Magnetization transfer imaging and proton MR spectroscopy in the evaluation of axonal injury: Correlation with clinical outcome after traumatic brain injury. *AJNR Am J Neuroradiol* 2001;22:143–51.
43. Teixeira J, Zimmerman RA, Haselgrove JC, et al. Diffusion imaging in pediatric central nervous system infections. *Neuroradiology* 2001;43:1031–9.
44. Tong K, Ashwal S, Holshouser B, et al. Hemorrhagic shearing lesions in children and adolescents with posttraumatic diffuse axonal injury: Improved detection and initial results. *Radiology* 2003;227:332–9.
45. Tong KA, Ashwal S, Holshouser BA, et al. Diffuse axonal injury in children: Clinical correlation with hemorrhagic lesions. *Ann Neurol* 2004;56:36–50.
46. Tyler KL. Update on herpes simplex encephalitis. *Rev Neurol Dis* 2004;1:169–78.
47. van de Warrenburg BP, Wesseling P, Leyten QH, et al. Myelopathy due to spinal epidural abscess without cord compression: A diagnostic pitfall. *Clin Neuropathol* 2004;23:102–6.
48. Willig DS, Turski PA, Frayne R, et al. Contrast-enhanced 3D MR DSA of the carotid artery bifurcation: Preliminary study of comparison with unenhanced 2D and 3D time-of-flight MR angiography. *Radiology* 1998;208:447–51.
49. Wingerchuk DM. The clinical course of acute disseminated encephalomyelitis. *Neurol Res* 2006;28:341–7.
50. Yoshikawa T, Abe O, Tsuchiya K, et al. Diffusion-weighted magnetic resonance imaging of dural sinus thrombosis. *Neuroradiology* 2002;44:481–88.

CHAPTER 56 ■ HEAD AND SPINAL CORD TRAUMA

ROBERT C. TASKER

The practicalities of critical care in children with traumatic brain injury (TBI) or spinal cord injury (SCI) are discussed in this chapter. The developmental neuroscience of acute neurotoxicity, vascular control, and cerebral hemodynamics and physiology is discussed in other chapters within this section of the book. The principal aim of this chapter is to review the recent clinical literature (in the main, between 2000 and 2006) toward informing the practice of neurocritical care. The focus of this chapter is TBI, but additional notes about inflicted TBI (iTBI), including what was previously called "shaken baby syndrome," and SCI are included when any areas of practice in these injuries differ from those of TBI.

Central to our understanding and treatment of TBI is the fact that mechanical forces at the time of accident—direct or contact force, acceleration and deceleration forces, and rotational or torsional forces—are responsible for primary injury. As a consequence of these forces, a variety of primary and secondary brain injuries occur (**Table 56.1**). The pathophysiology of these forms of injury is dealt with in Chapters 51 and 52. The first part of this chapter reviews core clinical science and information, to explain the rationale behind the author's clinical approach to head and spinal cord trauma.

EPIDEMIOLOGY

Traumatic Brain Injury

TBI is a major public health problem. In the US, it is estimated that TBI is sustained by 1.4 million people annually and that 90,000 experience the onset of long-term disability as a consequence. In the multistate TBI surveillance of the Centers for Disease Control and Prevention, the 2002 data estimated that 79 per 100,000 population were hospitalized with TBI-related diagnoses (40). In children, the data are equally alarming. TBI is the leading cause of death and disability in children, and in the US, 200,000 head injuries occur in children each year (68). Ten percent of children who are hospitalized with TBI have severe brain injury—as defined by a Glasgow Coma Scale (GCS) score <9 at presentation—and are usually admitted to a PICU.

In the UK, the prevalence rate for children (0–14 years of age) admitted to intensive care with TBI (the majority of whom are intubated and ventilated) is 5.4 per 100,000 population annually (129). Children admitted to the PICU with TBI come from more deprived households, and the commonest mechanism of injury is pedestrian accident. A significant summer peak in admissions is seen in children <10 years of age. Time of injury peaks in the late afternoon and early evening—a pattern that remains constant across the days of the week. Injuries that involve motor vehicles have the highest mortality rates (23% of vehicle occupants, 12% of pedestrians) compared with cyclists (8%) and falls (3%). In 65% of admissions, TBI is an isolated injury.

Inflicted Traumatic Brain Injury

iTBI includes one or more of the following features: shaking injury, cerebral lesions as a result of direct impact, compression, and penetrating injuries (24,37). Shaking injury is the most frequent form of iTBI in infants (birth to 12 months) (53). Population-based studies in Scotland indicate that the annual incidence is 24.6 per 100,000 children younger than 1 year [95% confidence interval (CI), 14.9–38.5] (24). In the US, in North Carolina, the incidence is 17 per 100,000 per person-year during the first 2 years of life (95% CI, 13.3–20.7) (95).

Spinal Cord Injury

SCI in children is uncommon and accounts for only 0.3%–10% of SCI in all ages (81). Bony fractures and dislocations of the pediatric spine are even less common. In Portugal and Sweden, in children up to 14 years old, the incidence of fatal injuries is 0.46 per 100,000 children per year. Across 19 countries throughout Europe, the estimated incidence of nonfatal injuries varies from 0.09 to 2.12 per 100,000 children per year (21).

HEAD INJURY PATTERNS

In general, head injuries conform to one of three types: *blunt* head injury, *sharp* head injury, or *compression* injury.

Blunt Head Injury

A blunt injury occurs when the head comes into forcible contact with a flat, smooth surface. This injury can be caused by a fall when the head hits the ground or a blow to the head by a blunt object. In both instances, the curvature of the skull at the point of impact tends to flatten. The area of impact is therefore spread over an area proportional to the deformation of the skull. If the deformity produces a fracture, its direction and extent will be related to the thickness of the scalp, the elasticity of the bone, and local weaknesses in the skull. In addition, the head and its contents will be subjected to either significant deceleration

TABLE 56.1

PRIMARY AND SECONDARY BRAIN INJURY

Primary brain injury	Secondary brain injury
Diffuse and focal axonal injury	Diffuse and focal hypoxic-ischemic injury
Diffuse and focal vascular injury	Diffuse and focal brain swelling
Focal brain contusion	Intracranial hypertension
Focal brain laceration	Hydrocephalus
	Infection and fever
	Seizures
	Metabolic disturbance, e.g., hyponatremia

in the case of a fall or significant acceleration in the case of a blow.

When the deformity of the skull exceeds the limit of tolerance, fracture lines begin. In children the unfused cranial sutures may be involved and produce the "bursting fracture" of childhood. When the distorting force is spent, the elasticity of the skull causes it to move back toward its original shape. The acceleration and deceleration produced by the changes in speed and direction of motion of the head are important factors in the production of brain damage. An immediate and steep rise in pressure occurs at the point of impact, while a fall in pressure that can equal a negative pressure of one atmosphere occurs at the opposite pole. The increased positive pressure may have little effect on the brain, but the negative pressure, if it exceeds one atmosphere, may produce small areas of cavitation and focal hemorrhages in the superficial cortex. The injury combinations that are likely to follow blunt head injury to the vault are summarized in **Table 56.2**.

Sharp Head Injury

The area of impact and extent of skull distortion is small in sharp head injury. Laceration of the scalp, local depression or fragmentation of the skull, tearing of the dura, and bruising and laceration of the underlying brain may be seen. An example of this injury is a blow by a thrown hard ball. When the area of impact is small, the effect upon the underlying bone is almost explosive; fragments may be sprayed out into the brain beneath. Intracerebral hemorrhage in these injuries usually arises from torn superficial vessels of the cortex.

Compression Head Injury

A compression or crush injury is unusual. Severe injuries may occur without initial loss of consciousness. Fractures tend to involve the foramina at the base of the skull, producing cranial nerve palsies (**Table 56.3**). Occasionally, the internal carotid artery is torn as it passes through the base of the skull, and fatal hemorrhage may occur. Less severe cases may be associated with vessel dissection and cerebrovascular stroke (see Chapter 58). Side-to-side compression causes fractures through the middle fossa across the sella turcica to the opposite side. In these cases, the pituitary is at risk from direct trauma.

Development and Head Injury Patterns

The stage of development of the skull, brain, and intracranial vasculature directly accounts for the types of injuries seen in different pediatric age groups. The infant's disproportionately large head and weaker neck muscles place them at more risk of rotational and acceleration-deceleration injuries (152). The relatively softer cranial vault, anatomy of the dura, and rich vascular supply of the subarachnoid space all place young children at risk for intracranial injury and bleeding—even when a skull fracture is not present. Last, the high water content and viscosity of the young brain means that it may be more at risk for axonal injury. With skull and brain maturation, adult patterns of intracranial injury are seen.

TYPES OF INTRACRANIAL INJURY

Blunt head injury is the most common reason for admission to the PICU. The three main mechanisms by which such injury can cause intracranial damage are (a) focal hemorrhagic and nonhemorrhagic lesion that mainly involve the cortical gray matter, (b) diffuse traumatic axonal injury (TAI), and (c) secondary injury caused by edema and space-occupying hemorrhages (**Table 56.1**).

Hemorrhage and Other Focal Brain Tissue Effects

Focal injury is thought to occur when the brain impacts against the rigid inner table of the skull, with resulting areas of direct cortical contusion. Focal brain injury may also produce mass effects from hemorrhage, contusion, or hematoma that can induce herniation and brainstem compression.

Epidural hematomas (EDH) complicate 2%–3% of all head injury admissions in children and are more frequent with advancing age; the peak is in the second decade. In infants, EDH of venous or bony origin is found in the posterior fossa adjacent to the venous sinuses. These venous EDHs often have a delayed presentation because the infant has significant intracranial reserve from unfused sutures and open fontanelles. In older children, EDH arises from arterial bleeding. Patients may have a short, lucid interval after injury, but they will deteriorate rapidly with an increasing intracranial mass.

Subdural hemorrhage (SDH) is a common problem in children, especially in those who suffer iTBI. The clinical presentation depends on the size and location of the hemorrhage and the presence of associated brain injuries. It is the associated brain injuries that account for immediate unconsciousness at the time of accident and any focal neurologic deficits (e.g., hemiparesis, pupillary abnormalities, and seizures). SDH associated with iTBI carries a high mortality.

Traumatic intraparenchymal hematomas, or contusions, are not common in children, but their frequency increases with age. These lesions most commonly involve white matter of the frontal and temporal lobes, the body and splenium of the corpus callosum, and the corona radiata. In the cortex, contusions frequently involve the inferior, lateral, and anterior aspects of the frontal and temporal lobes (69). These patterns and distribution of primary lesions are similar to those expected from

TABLE 56.2

FEATURES ASSOCIATED WITH VAULT FRACTURES IN BLUNT HEAD INJURY

Site of impact	Features associated with fracture lines
Mid-frontal	**Clinical** 　CSF rhinorrhea 　Meningitis, pneumocephalus 　Anosmia **Brain** 　General concussion 　Direct bruising of underlying cortex 　Laceration of subfrontal cortex **Hemorrhage** 　SAH, SDH
Lateral frontal or temporofrontal	**Clinical** 　CSF rhinorrhea and meningitis in anterior fractures 　Blindness in medial fractures 　EDH in posterior fractures **Brain** 　General concussion 　Motor aphasia from a blow to the left side **Hemorrhage** 　SAH, SDH, EDH
Lateral or temporoparietal	**Clinical** 　Movement of the brain is restricted by dural folds, but their sharp edges may cut into the brainstem. 　If fracture lines involve the base of the skull, cranial nerves V, VI, VII, and VIII may be involved, as well as the sella turcica. 　Involvement of middle meningeal vessels with EDH 　Middle-ear involvement with CSF otorrhea and meningitis **Brain** 　Concussion is not that severe in general 　Local contusions beneath impact may cause aphasia or contralateral weakness if the Rolandic fissure is involved. **Hemorrhage** 　SAH is uncommon. 　SDH follows small lacerations related to point of impact.
Posterolateral or occipitoparietal	**Clinical** 　CSF otorrhea, meningitis, and hearing loss when the petrous temporal bone is involved. **Brain** 　Concussion is severe. 　Distant injury with laceration of the frontal and temporal poles **Hemorrhage** 　EDH may occur in fractures in the middle fossa or posterior fossa. 　High risk of tearing of vessels: SAH and SDH formation
Midline posterior or occipital	**Clinical** 　Often associated fracture of cervical spine. 　Lower cranial nerve palsies **Brain** 　Concussion is severe. 　Distant subfrontal or temporal contusions and laceration **Hemorrhage** 　Subfrontal or temporal SAH and SDH

CSF, cerebrospinal fluid; SAH, subarachnoid hemorrhage; SDH, subdural hemorrhage; EDH, extradural hemorrhage

mechanical modeling (86,87) and are found as well in children with severe TBI (114). It is likely that occult, diffuse white-matter changes may also be present—even in regions of the brain that appear normal on conventional imaging. In a study of 19 head-injured patients, acute MRI and proton MR spectroscopy (^{1}H-MRS) studies 11 days after injury identified areas of white matter, ipsilateral to a contusion, which showed significant ^{1}H-MRS abnormalities (63). These findings are consistent with generalized cellular injury.

In adults, focal MRI-detected, white-matter abnormalities are also frequently associated with focal defects in cortical perfusion (159). Involvement of the frontal lobes (as part of a

TABLE 56.3

COMPRESSION FRACTURES

Type	Clinical problems
Side-to-side Fracture passes through the middle fossa across the sella turcica to the opposite side.	Injuries include: Anterior group of cranial nerves may be involved, in particular, 6th nerve. Internal carotid artery may be torn.
Front-to-back Wide fissures through the frontal sinus extending back through the cribriform and ethmoid regions	Disruption of: Frontal sinus Cribriform plate Roof of the orbit

focal frontal-lobe compartment syndrome) is also suggested by reports of frontal hypoperfusion using single photon emission tomography (134). This problem may also occur in children. A study of 14 children who sustained severe TBI and 14 matched controls with mild head injury at least 3 months after injury found diffuse prefrontal tissue loss even in the absence of focal brain lesions in this area (32). Another study found that gray matter loss in the frontal areas was primarily attributable to focal injury, whereas white matter loss in the frontal lobes was related to a combination of both diffuse and focal injury (162).

Diffuse Injury Involving Axons

Diffuse injury that involves axons results from shearing forces that act at interfaces of the brain with differing structural integrity, such as the gray-white matter boundaries. The neuronal axons that cross multiple brain regions are particularly vulnerable. TAI may vary from small foci of axonal injury to a more severe form of diffuse TAI, in which injury is widespread throughout the brain, including the brainstem. In fatal injuries, the extent and distribution of TAI throughout the brain appears to be similar in children and adults (3,73). Lesser degrees of TAI may be seen in those patients with less severe injury. In adults who survive 1–47 years after moderately severe TBI, diffuse TAI—but not of the severe type—was found in 6 of 20 patients (5). In an older study of 5 patients with concussive head injury, multifocal axonal injury in structures thought to be involved in consciousness and memory was demonstrated (35). In particular, involvement included the fornices, which are the major pathways projecting to the hippocampus.

TAI was thought to be a common finding in young patients with iTBI. Cranial CT imaging of TAI is variable in children. The extent and distribution of TAI depends on injury severity and category. In one report, 14 out of 117 children had cranial CT evidence of TAI, as evidenced by small intraparenchymal and/or intraventricular hemorrhage; intradural or extradural cerebral mass lesion, including EDH or SDH; or an open skull fracture (120). MRI is more sensitive to the white matter changes usually seen with TAI, but its value is limited, as such imaging provides no clear benefit to patient management.

TAI is difficult to discern at autopsy, particularly in the young. In a study that described 53 children who died of iTBI

(64), the principal finding was that diffuse TAI occurred infrequently in young children (i.e., 3 of 53 cases, 95% CI, 1%–16%). In all, 45 of 53 cases were found to have signs of impact to the head at autopsy in the form of either subscalp bruising or skull fracture. In the remaining 8 cases (all infants), neither bruising nor fracture was found at autopsy. These 8 infants were assumed victims of iTBI, and in one case, the care provider had confessed to having caused injury. In another report by the same group (using similar diagnostic criteria), of 37 infants <9 months of age, the authors found that the predominant histologic abnormality was diffuse hypoxic brain damage (65). Also, epidural cervical hemorrhage and focal axonal damage to the brainstem and spinal roots were seen in 11 cases, but not in controls. The authors' conclusion from these data was that the craniocervical junction is vulnerable in infant iTBI, the neuropathology being that of stretch injury from cervical hyperextension and flexion. This finding has also been reported in a Canadian series (140). The authors also concluded that the presence of diffuse hypoxic brain damage, rather than diffuse TAI, could be explained either by resistance to traumatic damage of unmyelinated axons in the immature brain or by the fact that shaking-type injuries are not of sufficient force to produce diffuse TAI (65). They suggested that craniocervical injury could lead to apnea and global hypoxia. This problem may be pertinent in infants without evidence of cerebral contusion or cranial impact injuries. Eleven of 37 infants in the second report had either trivial or no subscalp bruising and no skull fracture or contemporaneous extracranial injury. Three of these 11 infants had craniocervical axonal injury of varying severity (65–67). The remaining 8 had no evidence of such injury, implying either that the authors were unable to detect it or that their terminal hypoxic-cell encephalopathy was not caused by trauma. Taken together with the previously mentioned imaging and clinical reports, these findings are in keeping with a hypoxia- or ischemia-related problem. The authors discussed the potential significance of this pathophysiology in cases of iTBI without impact (66,67) and this issue has been debated in the literature (34,117,135). It is possible that iTBI contains an important component of both hypoxia-ischemia and axonal injury and that these factors likely vary with the spectrum of injury in this complex disorder (28).

Diffuse Swelling of the Cerebrum

Diffuse swelling occurs in two forms—swelling of one cerebral hemisphere and swelling of both cerebral hemispheres. During the early phase of posttraumatic coma in children, cerebral swelling develops and generally peaks between 24 and 72 hrs after injury. Diffuse swelling of one hemisphere may develop very rapidly, as was observed in 17 of 151 (11%) fatal nonmissile head injuries (3). The swelling was associated with acute SDH, even when this had been evacuated. Contusions in the ipsilateral hemisphere may also be related to such swelling. The incidence of diffuse brain swelling on initial head CT can be as high as 53% (61). However, the literature is inconclusive regarding the prognostic significance of this finding. A 1994 study found a mortality of 35% in adults and only 20% mortality in children (106).

In some instances, specific focal injury may occur in combination with diffuse injury. High-speed impact and acceleration-deceleration forces at the time of injury make the medial

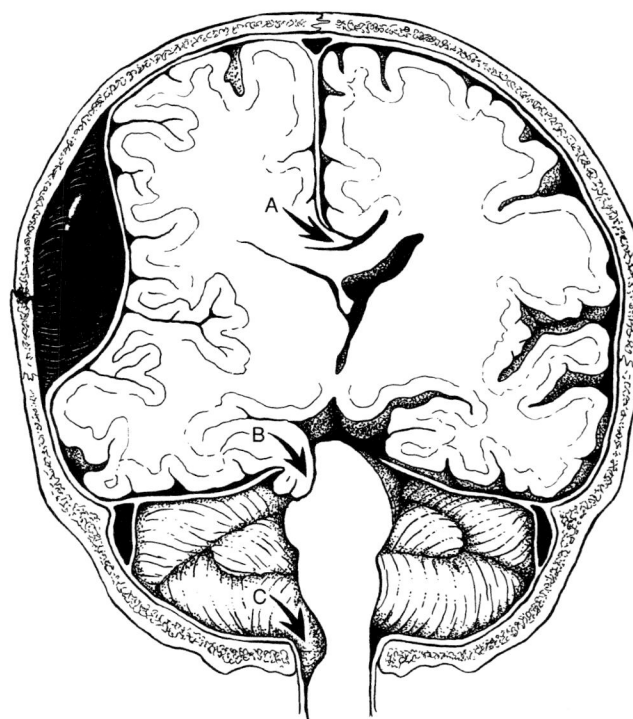

FIGURE 56.1. Herniation syndromes: (**A**) subfalcine and cingulate, (**B**) uncal, (**C**) foramen magnum (see Table 51.4). Subfalcine herniation occurs when one cerebral hemisphere is displaced under the falx cerebri across the midline (**A**). Uncal herniation refers to displacement of supratentorial structures inferiorly under the tentorium cerebelli, causing distortion and compression of the blood supply to infratentorial structures (**B**). Downward herniation of the cerebellum causes compression of the brainstem (**C**).

temporal lobe particularly vulnerable to mechanical deformation and contusion because of its position in the middle cranial fossa (4). Selective injury of the hippocampus may result from systemic vascular and metabolic perturbation—hypoxia, ischemia, seizures, and hypoglycemia—after injury (76,122,149). In TBI, the lesion found in the hippocampus most commonly consists of focal areas of selective neuronal loss in the CA1 subfield, similar to hypoxic insults. In the postacute period, hippocampal cell death may result from deafferentation or de-efferentation caused by transneuronal degeneration.

Focal and global brain swelling can act as a mass leading to shifts in brain tissue across neighboring intracranial compartments (**Fig. 56.1**). These tissue herniation syndromes can exist despite normal global intracranial pressure (ICP) (**Table 56.4**).

Posttraumatic Ischemia and Metabolism

In adults seen early after injury, cerebral blood flow (CBF) is reduced and secondary insults such as hypotension and hypoxemia have devastating effect. Brain swelling and any accompanying intracranial hypertension can contribute to this early secondary ischemia. Problems in CBF and metabolism are not exclusive to adults and are observed in infants and children. Infants with severe TBI commonly have cerebral hypoperfusion, and a global CBF of <20 mL/100 g/min was associated

with poor outcome (6). Following early posttraumatic hypoperfusion, CBF may increase to levels greater than metabolic demands, producing a state of relative hyperemia (102). Alternatively, a phase of increased cerebral metabolism of glucose may accompany posttraumatic hypoperfusion. In adults, monitoring parameters that reflect the coupling between CBF and metabolism (e.g., using brain microdialysis and oxygen probes) are being used increasingly, and the presence of key phenomena is influencing practice. As these phenomena may have some bearing on the optimum fluid and glucose management used in children, they are discussed here.

The brain tissue extracellular lactate-to-pyruvate ratio (LPR), obtained using cerebral microdialysis, has been considered a useful and sensitive marker of cerebral ischemia after TBI and subarachnoid hemorrhage (105,107). In metabolites, the use of a ratio, rather than absolute concentrations, means that an alteration in dialysate recovery rate does not result in spurious changes in LPR. A ratio of <20 suggests uncomplicated cerebral metabolism (130), and a rise in the ratio is a sensitive indicator of a fall in brain tissue partial pressure of oxygen ($P_{bt}O_2$) (99,100). In TBI, an increased ratio results from a 10- to 100-fold reduction in pyruvate concentration in association with a two- to fivefold increase in lactate concentration (158). However two reports of TBI suggest that the LPR (and levels of the components that make up the ratio) might be telling us more about other forms of cerebral metabolic perturbation in addition to ischemic crisis. One group found that in the first few hours after injury—at a time when $P_{bt}O_2$ was normal (i.e., nonischemic)—the LPR was increased because of low pyruvate concentration and not raised lactate (84). Later, when the $P_{bt}O_2$ was at its lowest level, signifying "hypoxia-ischemia," increased LPR was due to a combination of increased lactate and decreased pyruvate. Another group found that, even though raised lactate or LPR was present in 25% of cerebral microdialysis samples, cerebral ischemia—defined as raised lactate and LPR and low glucose—was much less frequent (~3%) (157). Furthermore, on combining these studies with positron emission tomography for assessing metabolism of oxygen, the incidence of high oxygen-extraction fraction (i.e., ischemia) was rare, at ~1%.

It has been suggested that the findings of these two clinical reports represent two metabolic states (82). Type 1, classical cerebral ischemia, is characterized by reduced microdialysis pyruvate and increased lactate, leading to increased LPR (in association with depressed $P_{bt}O_2$). This state is a result of overt lack of oxygen and glucose at the mitochondria (155). Type 2, cerebral metabolic perturbation, occurs when $P_{bt}O_2$ is normal (i.e., nonischemic), and a reduction in pyruvate is the sole change in dialysis metabolites. The rise in LPR in this state is "perhaps reflecting a limited glucose supply or an impairment of the glycolytic pathway." However, the mechanism of these early changes in pyruvate and later alterations in lactate are still not completely understood. One important difference between the two studies just discussed is the location of the monitoring probes. In the first study, the microdialysis probes were placed perilesional or pericontusional (84). In the second study, the microdialysis catheter was cited in the nondominant, normal-appearing, frontal lobe tissue (157). This difference is likely to be significant. A third group reported that microdialysis monitoring of normal-appearing tissue was not representative of perilesional tissue (57). Raised LPR persisted for at least 72 hrs in perilesional tissue. In the first 36 hrs, this rise was associated

TABLE 56.4

TYPES OF BRAIN TISSUE HERNIATION SYNDROMES

Syndrome	Mechanism	Clinical features
Foramen magnum	*Herniating tissue:* Downward mesial displacement of cerebellar hemispheres *Compression:* Unilateral or bilateral medulla by ventral parafollicular or tonsillae through foramen magnum	Episodic tonic extension with opisthotonic posturing, leading to quadriparesis Changes in blood pressure, heart rate, and arrhythmias Ataxic breathing Small pupils and disturbance of conjugate gaze
Central tentorial	*Herniating tissue:* Downward displacement of one or both cerebral hemispheres *Compression:* Diencephalon and midbrain through tentorial notch	ICP is usually raised Bilateral decorticate or decerebrate posturing An "upward" form of this syndrome may occur if supratentorial ventricles are decompressed in the presence of cerebellar mass
Uncal (lateral transtentorial)	*Herniating tissue:* Medial temporal lobe (uncus and parahippocampal gyrus) forced into the incisura *Compression:* Midbrain and posterior cerebral artery	ICP is usually raised Contralateral hemiparesis Ipsilateral pupillary dilatation and ptosis Unilateral or bilateral occipital lobe infarction Obstructive hydrocephalus from compression of aqueduct or perimesencephalic cistern Regions of necrosis and hemorrhage in tegmentum, subthalamus, midbrain, and upper pons
Cingulate	*Herniating tissue:* Cingulate gyrus herniates under the anterior falx *Compression:* Anterior cerebral artery	Infarction of regional tissue seen on imaging Contralateral lower extremity paresis

ICP, intracranial pressure

with raised lactate and raised pyruvate concentrations. After that time, raised LPR was a reflection of raised lactate with normal pyruvate concentrations. All microdialysis parameters were in the normal range in normal-appearing tissue.

Taken together, these observations suggest that perilesional tissue has features of type 1 (raised LPR, raised lactate, normal or low pyruvate) cerebral metabolic crisis. However, the absence of depressed $P_{bt}O_2$ suggests that the increased lactate occurs as a consequence of increased glycolytic activity, which may be due to perilesional spreading depression and depolarization (60,94). Such hyperglycolysis is marked by increased metabolism relative to utilization (164) and, post trauma, it represents an uncoupling between predominantly glycolytic and oxidative metabolism (29). Another instance when such a change in metabolism may be seen in TBI is in upregulation of an endogenous, cerebral, metabolic, protective response—the pentose-phosphate shunt—with or without depression in tricarboxylic acid cycle flux (27).

The importance and incidence of these metabolic and glycolytic problems in children is, as yet, unknown, as microdialysis and oxygen-probe monitoring are rarely undertaken in children. However, interest has been renewed in the type of IV fluid that should be used in TBI (e.g., lactate-containing or not, glucose-containing or not) and the potential role and risk of so-called "tight-glycemic control" in ICP management (154), which makes this discussion pertinent.

Hypothalamic-Pituitary Injury

The pituitary gland and its anatomic attachment to hypothalamic structures are vulnerable to injury following TBI, even though they are protected by the bony sella turcica. In blunt head injury, a lateral or temporoparietal fracture line may radiate down to the base of the skull and pass through the central area of the sella turcica to the opposite middle fossa (Table 56.2). In this instance, the pituitary stalk is at risk of trauma. In other forms of injury, the reason for pituitary vulnerability may be vascular or ischemic, as tissue swelling and edema cause compression of the hypophysial blood vessels within the restrictive space of the sella turcica. The hypophyseal-pituitary portal circulation is a rich network of blood vessels, predominantly supplied by the superior hypophysial arteries, which arise from the internal carotids. The long hypophysial blood vessels and the dense network of capillaries are vulnerable to rupture and hemorrhage, leading to subsequent ischemia and infarction of the anterior lobe of the pituitary gland.

Few studies directly link TBI with disruption and damage to the hypothalamic-pituitary structures. However, they provide convincing histopathologic evidence that lesions do occur in this part of the brain in severe TBI. Autopsy in 106 fatal TBI cases revealed hypothalamic lesions in almost 43% of adults (48). Lesions were typically suggestive of infarction and ischemia and consistent with either shearing of small per-forating blood vessels or with venous engorgement secondary to intracranial hypertension. In 28% of cases, pituitary lesions were also present and often associated with fracture of the middle cerebral fossa. Others have also reported traumatic infarction of the anterior pituitary gland, often in association with hemorrhage (49,80).

The key question is whether this form of injury is seen in nonfatal cases of TBI. The answer is yes, both acutely and on follow-up. A study of 50 adults admitted for intensive care following TBI found a high frequency of early posttraumatic endocrine abnormalities, in particular low basal cortisol levels with subnormal cortisol responses to a glucagon test, hypogonadism, and hyperprolactinemia (16,17). Another study confirmed the extent of these acute abnormalities, showing that 53% of patients demonstrate deficiency in at least one hormonal axis (146). Growth hormone deficiency has also been demonstrated in the acute setting, although growth-hormone resistance would be expected in critical illness. Low plasma insulin-like growth factor-I level is also found in association with decreased growth-hormone secretion. On follow-up, hypothalamic-pituitary dysfunction is being recognized increasingly. The literature on adults has flourished since 2000, and more recent reviews describe this subject area in detail (18,133). It appears that in moderate or severe TBI, the frequency of hypopituitarism is high, and subnormal responses, in at least one hypothalamic-pituitary axis, occur in 23%–69% of cases (2). Dynamic tests of anterior pituitary function reveal a high prevalence of previously undetected deficiencies in the growth hormone, adrenal, and thyroid axes. Serial neuroendocrine studies suggest that the natural history of post-TBI hypopituitarism involves an acute phase of transient abnormality, followed by a period of late presentation of endocrinopathy, even up to several years.

The literature concerning children and adolescents with TBI-related hypothalamic-pituitary dysfunction is much less detailed. To date, no comprehensive retrospective or prospective studies have been reported on this subject. A systematic review of the literature at this writing found only a few case reports, or small case series that highlighted a link between TBI and the occurrence of hypothalamic-pituitary hormone abnormality (1,2). The literature suggests that post-TBI–induced hypothalamic-pituitary dysfunction may be observed in children after a variety of mechanisms. Road traffic accidents, falls, and sport-related trauma appear to be the most common causes of TBI reported to have pituitary dysfunction, and it is often associated with loss of consciousness, SDH, or skull fracture. Post-TBI–induced hypopituitarism has also been reported after iTBI. A seminal paper on hypopituitarism reported on 3 children who had suffered acute trauma in infancy with loss of consciousness and SDH and were later diagnosed with multiple pituitary hormone deficiencies (116).

TRAUMATIC SPINAL CORD INJURY

Traumatic SCI is the result of primary and secondary injury mechanisms. The occurrence of some neurologic injury in association with vertebral column injury occurs in <50%, while complete SCI is seen in <25% cases (79). SCI is also a rare complication of intentional trauma, and its occurrence can be easily overlooked (70). At presentation, the damage from acute SCI is not fixed but, rather, evolves over hours or days. Post-SCI ischemia, related to failing autoregulation, blood pressure, cardiac output, and oxygenation, may contribute to worsening injury.

The clinician should be aware of the features and variety of spinal cord syndromes that may occur in the setting of trauma (Table 56.5). The pattern of SCI in children differs from that in adults in a number of ways because the child's spine is still developing. Children have wedge-shaped vertebral bodies, incomplete centers of ossification, and more lax ligaments (22). In children up to the age of 9 years, spinal injuries are more frequently seen in the atlas, axis, and upper cervical vertebrae

TABLE 56.5

SPINAL CORD SYNDROMES IN TRAUMA

Syndrome	Mechanism	Findings
Complete cord transection	Trauma Secondary vascular	Loss of all motor function Loss of sensory function Above C3—apnea and death
Brown-Sequard (cord hemisection)	Penetrating trauma	Ipsilateral loss of proprioception Ipsilateral loss of motor function Contralateral loss of pain and temperature sensation Suspended ipsilateral loss of all sensory modalities
Central cord	Neck hyperextension	Motor impairment greater in upper limbs than in lower limbs Suspended sensory loss in cervicothoracic dermatomes
Anterior cord	Hyperflexion Anterior spinal artery occlusion	Variable motor impairment Pain and temperature loss with sparing of proprioception
Conus medullaris	Direct trauma	Extension to lumbosacral roots may produce both upper and lower motor neuron signs Spastic paraparesis Sphincter dysfunction Lower sacral "saddle" sensory loss

(77). Ligamentous injuries that lead to atlanto-occipital dislocation are also more common than are bone injuries. After this age, an adult pattern of injury is seen, i.e., less involvement of the cervical spine (~55%).

Spinal Cord Injury Without Radiographic Abnormality

The anatomic characteristics of the younger child (i.e., lack of muscular development of the neck and the relatively large head size) also lead to the frequent occurrence of an entity known as spinal cord injury without radiographic abnormality (SCIWORA). That is, the elasticity of the immature spine may allow for significant distraction and flexion to injure the cord without resulting in either ligamentous or bone disruption and, hence, no apparent abnormalities on radiographic investigation (126,127). SCIWORA may occur in older children even though bone maturity is reached by age 9 years because ligamentous laxity continues into adolescence.

The possibility of SCIWORA should be considered in all pediatric TBI cases. The clinical features range from tingling dysesthesias or numbness to frank weakness or paralysis. MRI demonstrates five classes of post-SCIWORA cord findings: complete transection, major hemorrhage, minor hemorrhage, edema only, and normal (128). The neural findings are highly predictive of outcome. All patients with normal cord signals should make complete recovery. Patients with transection and major hemorrhage have very poor outcome, and intermediate outcomes are seen in the remaining grades of severity. A recent meta-analysis of 392 published cases found that complete recovery occurred in 39% of cases (108). Thoracic SCIWORA has also been identified as an important clinical entity in a subset of children who are usually victims of accidents that involve high-speed, direct impact, distraction from lap belts, and crush injury by slow-moving vehicles (128).

Traumatic Atlanto-occipital Dislocation

Atlanto-occipital dislocation is defined as disruption of the supporting ligaments such that displacement occurs in either the transverse or vertical direction. This lesion is rare in children and adolescents. Historically, most reported cases have been fatal, with the patient often not surviving initial cardiac arrest and apnea; however, the advent of modern prehospital care has led to an increase in survival following injury (88). Combined high-SCI and brainstem injuries must be suspected in this group (115).

INITIAL CLINICAL ASSESSMENT

History

It is important to know the mechanism of injury in cases of TBI because this information will help in anticipating potential patterns of injury and problems (Tables 56.2 and 56.3). The required details of an accident include the type of accident, the degree of force acting on the head, the position of the victim when found at the scene, and the victim's immediate state of consciousness. In cases of severe TBI resulting from child abuse, occult presentations may be recognized late. Brain edema may have already evolved to life-threatening levels, and other superimposed secondary insults (e.g., seizures and apnea) may complicate full understanding of the primary injury.

Primary Survey

The primary survey is a rapid, abbreviated, initial physical examination aimed at identifying and treating quickly any life-threatening injuries. The identification and correction of airway obstruction, inadequate ventilation, and shock take priority over detailed neurologic assessment. The full execution of this assessment and any intervention is described in detail in Chapter 23 and follows standard, internationally accepted guidelines. The following sections will focus on how the primary survey relates specifically to TBI. Where appropriate, reference will be made to the 2003 *Guidelines for the Acute Medical Management of Severe TBI in Infants, Children, and Adolescents* that were endorsed by the American Association for the Surgery of Trauma, the Child Neurology Society, the International Society for Pediatric Neurosurgery, the International Trauma Anesthesia and Critical Care Society, the Society of Critical Care Medicine, and the World Federation of Pediatric Intensive and Critical Care Societies (39). In this context, a *Standard* is an accepted principle of patient management that reflects a high degree of clinical certainty. A *Guideline* is a particular strategy or range of management that reflects a moderate degree of clinical certainty. Last, an *Option* is a strategy for which clinical certainty remains unclear. These terms will be used in the following sections to provide some idea about the weight of evidence in support of the accompanying recommendations.

Airway

The initial evaluation begins by demonstrating the presence of a patent, maintainable airway; the patient must be conscious, alert, and breathing spontaneously. At the scene of an accident, the issues concerning recommendations for endotracheal intubation are complex and likely to include the expertise of attending paramedics and the distance for transport. The aim is to prevent hypoxia or hypercarbia, which may lead to secondary brain injury (7). In adults the *Guideline* is that "hypoxemia must be avoided, if possible, or corrected immediately... by administering oxygen." An *Option* in adults is that the "airway should be secured in patients who have a severe head injury (GCS <9), inability to maintain an adequate airway, or hypoxemia not corrected by supplemental oxygen. Endotracheal intubation, if available, is the most effective procedure to maintain the airway." In children, the *Guideline* is that no evidence exists to support the use of endotracheal intubation over bag-valve-mask ventilation for the prehospital management of the airway. In fact, based on the available evidence, there is significant risk of major airway mishaps (7). Therefore, an *Option* in children, if prehospital endotracheal intubation is used, is to have specialized training for operators and to ensure that all intubated children have end-tidal carbon dioxide (E_tCO_2) detectors to document correct tracheal tube placement. One *Option* for when endotracheal intubation should be

TABLE 56.6

**INDICATIONS FOR INTUBATION IN THE
HEAD-INJURED CHILD**

Upper airway obstruction or loss of airway protective reflexes
    Loss of pharyngeal muscle activity and tone
    Inability to clear secretions
    Foreign body
    Direct trauma
    Seizures

Abnormal breathing due to
    Chest wall dysfunction
    Respiratory muscle dysfunction
    Pulmonary disease: aspiration, contusion, neurogenic
    Cervical spine injury

Apnea

Arterial partial pressure of carbon dioxide ($Paco_2$)
    Hypercarbia: $Paco_2$ >45 mm Hg
    Hypocapnia: spontaneous hyperventilation, causing $Paco_2$
    <25 mm Hg

Pupils
    Anisocoria >1 mm

Glasgow Coma Scale (GCS) score
    GCS <9
    Fall in GCS score of >3, irrespective of initial GCS

---

obtained in children is "a Glasgow coma score ≤8" so as "to avoid hypoxemia, hypercarbia, and aspiration" (8). Another *Option* for timing of intubation is the presence of hypoventilation (defined as ineffective respiratory rate for age, shallow or irregular respirations, frequent periods of apnea, or measured hypercarbia).

The range of indications for endotracheal intubation is listed in Table 56.6. Beyond the prehospital setting, any children who are unable to open their eyes or verbalize must be considered candidates for intubation because of concerns about absent or impaired airway protective reflexes. Similarly, an unconscious patient must be assumed to have an obstructed airway that requires immediate evaluation. Intracranial hypertension with impending herniation may be inferred from the presence of dilated, unresponsive pupils or a triad of symptoms that includes systemic hypertension, bradycardia, and an abnormal breathing pattern.

The recommended route of airway control is orotracheal intubation; nasotracheal intubation should be avoided because of the possibility of base of skull fractures. Precautions to protect the cervical spine and minimize the rise in ICP associated with intubation should be undertaken. The patient's neck should be maintained in a neutral position, with axial traction applied by a person whose only role is to maintain the position of the neck. All trauma patients with supraclavicular injury should be assumed to have cranial and cervical spine injuries until proven otherwise.

Ventilation

Several studies suggest that hypoxemia during prehospital care of children with severe TBI is common and that the proportion of patients with significant oxygen-hemoglobin desaturation

below 75% may be as high as 16% (7). In patients with SCI, the pattern of respiratory dysfunction depends on the level of injury (**Fig. 56.2**). Complete injury above C3 causes respiratory arrest and death unless immediate ventilatory assistance is given. Injury at the C3–C5 level leads to respiratory failure, but the onset might be delayed. The *Guideline* for severe TBI is that supplemental oxygen (100%) should be provided in the resuscitation phase of care for all patients with moderate-to-severe TBI to prevent, and immediately correct, hypoxia that could cause secondary brain injury.

The *Option* for monitoring is that "oxygenation and ventilation should be assessed continuously by pulse oximetry oxygen-hemoglobin saturation (Spo_2) and E_Tco_2 monitoring, respectively, or by serial blood gas measurements" (8). When hypoxia—defined as apnea, cyanosis, arterial Pao_2 of <60–65 mm Hg, or Spo_2 <90%—is identified, it should be corrected rapidly with oxygen.

Hypoventilation due to lung or neurologic causes is common in TBI. Hypercarbia is a potent cerebral vasodilator and should be avoided. Patients with physical findings suggestive of brainstem compression from brain tissue herniation should be hyperventilated with 100% oxygen as soon as possible to acutely lower ICP. The practice of aggressive hyperventilation therapy is considered an *Option* only when used "for brief periods in cases of cerebral herniation or acute neurologic deterioration" (12).

Circulation

After the airway and ventilation are confirmed as being adequate, the next step is assessment and optimization of the circulation. The injured brain is at risk from hypotension and inadequate perfusion, problems that have a number of potential causes. Blood loss may be present. Generally, blood loss sufficient to cause hypotension is not due to bleeding in the cranium, except in small infants in whom subgaleal hematomas can be life-threatening. Cardiogenic shock and arrhythmia may be present due to cardiac contusion. Alternatively, neurogenic shock may be present in cases of SCI above T4. This hemodynamic syndrome reflects sympathetic denervation of the heart (T1–T4) and vasculature, with resulting decreased inotropism, chronotropism, and arterial and venous dilation. It may be difficult to differentiate this syndrome from hypovolemia, but lack of compensatory tachycardia can be a useful diagnostic sign.

The initial assessment of circulatory function in patients with TBI includes the rapid determination of heart rate, blood pressure, quality of central and peripheral pulses, and capillary refill time. In children, hypotension is defined as systolic blood pressure below the 5th percentile for age or by clinical signs of shock. The 5th percentile for age of systolic blood pressure can be estimated from the formula: 70 mm Hg + (2 × age in years).

The *Guideline* for resuscitation of blood pressure in severe TBI is that "hypotension should be identified and corrected as rapidly as possible with fluid resuscitation" (8). However, the choice of resuscitation fluid is controversial. The current recommendation is 20 mL/kg isotonic crystalloid (0.9% sodium chloride solution) administered as soon as vascular access is obtained. Hypotonic fluid should not be used in the initial resuscitation phase, and subsequent doses of fluid should be guided by serial assessment of blood pressure, perfusion, and hematocrit.

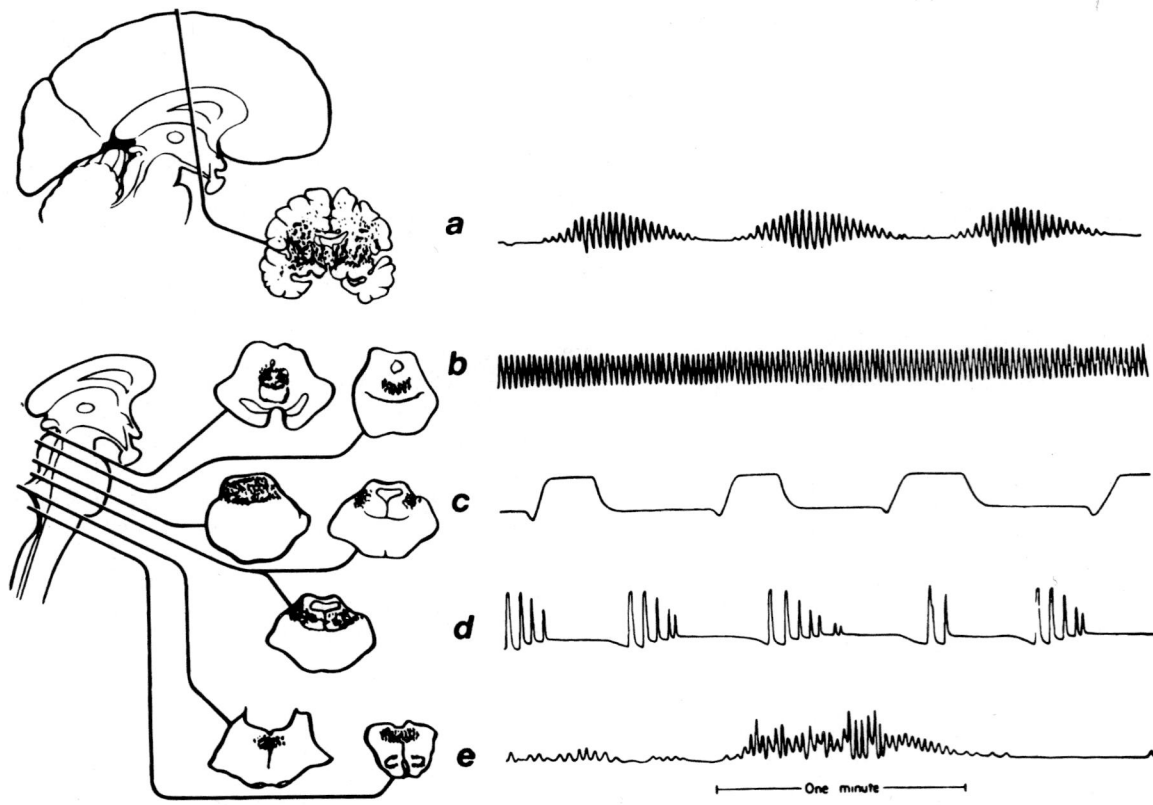

FIGURE 56.2. Abnormal breathing patterns due to lesions at different levels of the brain. Injury to different portions of the brain leads to distinctive abnormal breathing patterns that may help to localize the area of injury. A prolonged abnormal respiratory pattern may interfere with oxygenation and ventilation. From Mettler FA. *Neuroanatomy.* St. Louis: CV Mosby, 1948;816, with permission.

NEUROLOGY

The next step after adequate initial survey and stabilization is assessment of the neurologic examination. This process should be succinct and aimed primarily at diagnosing and treating life-threatening intracranial hypertension with imminent brain-tissue herniation (Table 56.4). A rapid assessment includes evaluation of the patient's pupillary size and its response to light, level of consciousness, and response in their extremities to a painful stimulus.

The pupillary response to light should be assessed first. This reflex consists of an afferent pathway through the optic nerve and an efferent pathway that involves both sympathetic and parasympathetic fibers. Transtentorial herniation causes compression of the parasympathetic fibers along the cranial nerve III and results in ipsilateral pupillary dilation with no response to direct or consensual stimulation. Bilateral dilated pupils that are unresponsive reflect, in the absence of medication or poisoning, bilaterally compressed cranial nerves III or severe cerebral hypoxia-ischemia. The presence of unilateral or bilateral dilated, unresponsive pupil is an indication for emergency hyperventilation, brain imaging, and surgical evacuation of a hematoma, if present.

The level of consciousness is assessed after the examination of the pupils, and it should be graded using the GCS. This descriptive scoring system evaluates performance in three areas: eye opening, which relates to the level of arousal; verbaliza-tion, which relates to content and mentation; and motor ability (**Table 56.7**). The GCS score has not been validated in children, and it is almost impossible to use in those <2 years of age. The "Infant Face Scale" may be of use in this regard, but it remains to be seen whether a score of 9–12 on this scale is equivalent to (and has the same implications as) a score of 9–12 on the GCS (54).

The motor component of the GCS score is the most important item to establish. The extremities are observed for the presence and symmetry of spontaneous movement. Reduced movement may be due to local or spinal cord injury. Mildly painful stimuli can be applied to the extremities by applying pressure on the nail bed. Central painful stimuli, such as sternal rub or supraorbital pressure, may elicit purposeful movement, decorticate posturing, or no response.

Secondary Survey

The aim of the secondary survey is to identify all traumatic injuries and to begin to prioritize treatment. A thorough physical examination is required; the areas of this survey that are especially important in TBI are discussed here.

Head

Examination of the head entails careful inspection for surface depressions, swellings, lacerations, or ecchymoses that

TABLE 56.7

GLASGOW COMA SCALE SCORE FOR CHILDREN AND INFANTS

Activity	Child response	Infant response	Score
Eye opening (E)	Spontaneous	Spontaneous	4
	To verbal stimuli	To verbal stimuli	3
	To pain	To pain	2
	None	None	1
Verbal (V)	Oriented	Coos and babbles	5
	Confused	Irritable cries	4
	Inappropriate words	Cries to pain	3
	Nonspecific sounds	Moans to pain	2
	None	None	1
Motor (M)	Follows commands	Normal spontaneous movement	6
	Localizes pain	Withdraws to touch	5
	Withdraws in response to pain	Withdraws to pain	4
	Flexion in response to pain	Abnormal flexion	3
	Extension in response to pain	Abnormal extension	2
	None	None	1

Total Score: Minimum 1E + 1V + 1M = 3; Maximum 4E + 5V + 6M = 15

would indicate underlying injury. Evidence of skull-base fracture includes Battle sign (i.e., retro-auricular ecchymosis), raccoon eyes (i.e., periorbital ecchymosis), cerebrospinal fluid (CSF) otorrhea, CSF rhinorrhea, and hemotympanum. Evidence of facial fracture includes instability of facial bones and zygoma (i.e., LeFort fracture) and facial step-off abnormality (i.e., orbital rim fracture). If any lacerations are present, they should be explored with a gloved finger so that underlying open or depressed skull fracture or foreign material can be identified.

In infants, the fontanelles and sutures should be palpated. The tone of the fontanelle (i.e., bulging, soft, or sunken) is an indication of ICP level. If possible, the head circumference should be measured and recorded. The mouth should be examined, and notation should be made as to whether the frenulum is torn or not. Last, evidence of extracranial vascular injury should be sought. Abnormal carotid neck pulses, bruits, and Horner syndrome indicate traumatic carotid dissection. Eye globe bruit indicates traumatic carotid cavernous fistula.

Neck

Injury to the cervical spine must be assumed to have occurred in any head-injured patient until such time as neck soft tissue or bony injury has been ruled out. The neck should be immobilized in an appropriately sized collar, and manipulation should be kept to a minimum. If the collar is removed for any reason, the neck should be held in midline position and gentle axial traction should be applied by a single operator. Obvious deformity, swelling, or ecchymosis of the neck should be visible on inspection. Palpation of the neck may show a malalignment, step-off, or splaying of the spinous processes, suggesting a ligamentous and unstable injury.

Thorax

The chest wall should be observed for the pattern and adequacy of ventilation. Specific patterns of breathing are seen with head injury and may have important localizing value (Fig. 56.2). Post-hyperventilation apnea indicates forebrain damage. Cheyne-Stokes respiration or alternating phases of hyperpnea are caused by dysfunction deep within the cerebral hemispheres or diencephalon. Hyperventilation or persistent, rapid breathing is caused by damage in the rostral brainstem or tegmentum. Apneustic breathing, or prolonged sustained end-inspiratory pauses, is caused by damage at the midpontine or caudal pontine level. Ataxic respiration, or completely random and irregular breathing, indicates damage to the medulla.

Spinal injury above the level of C4 results in paralysis of all muscles involved in breathing. These patients have poor-to-absent spontaneous respiratory effort. Injuries to the lower cervical spinal cord spare the diaphragm but abolish some of the accessory muscle strength, resulting in decreased vital capacity and retention of secretions. In adults, a direct relationship exists between the level of cord injury and the degree of respiratory dysfunction. With high lesions (i.e., C1 or C2) vital capacity is only 5%–10% of normal and cough is absent. With lesions at C3 through C6, vital capacity is 20% of normal and cough is weak and ineffective. With high thoracic cord injuries (i.e., T2 to T4), vital capacity is 30%–50% of normal and cough is weak. With lower cord injuries, respiratory function improves, and with injuries at T11, respiratory function, vital capacity, and cough should be near normal.

Neurology

Assessment of ocular signs and responses, the motor system, and functional integrity of the spine and spinal cord should be conducted and at least the following noted.

Ocular Responses. The position of the eyes at rest should be noted, and any deviation, conjugate or disconjugate, recorded. Spontaneous eye movements, including roving eye movements, ocular bobbing, or nystagmus, should be sought. Other noteworthy ocular phenomena are increased blinking, intermittent lid retraction, convergent or divergent spasms, and monocular nystagmus, most of which imply brainstem dysfunction. The corneal reflex should be tested, as its presence does relate to depth of coma.

Ocular motility should then be assessed with the "doll's eye maneuver" *but only if the cervical spine is known to be stable.* This maneuver, or oculocephalic reflex, is discussed in Chapter 53. The child's eyelids are held open while the head is briskly rotated first to one side and then the other. A positive response, indicating an intact pathway in the brainstem, is obtained by full conjugate eye deviation to the opposite side (i.e., if the head is rotated to the right, the eyes deviate to the left). Vertical eye movements are tested by briskly flexing and extending the neck. A positive response is observed when the eyes deviate upward with neck flexion and downward with neck extension. Further assessment of brainstem function by the "caloric" or oculovestibular response may cause discomfort and should only be performed in the deeply unconscious child. It is important to ensure that the tympanic membranes are intact before starting to instill up to 60 mL of iced saline.

Pupillary responses and the corneal reflex show a close correlation with severity of coma. The pupillary size at rest and reaction to light (both direct and consensual) will have been noted in the primary survey. Injury to the midbrain tectum may result in pupils that are at midposition and fixed to light but retain hippus, the ciliospinal reflex, and response to accommodation. Pinpoint pupils are associated with pontine lesions. Unilateral pupil dilation unreactive to direct stimulation but consensually reactive is caused by absent light perception in that eye or a deafferentated pupil. Alternately shining the light into each eye reveals the paradoxical dilation on the affected side with direct stimulation; this is the Marcus Gunn pupil and represents dilation of the affected side after consensually stimulated constriction. When light is shone into the deafferentated eye, both eyes perceive darkness and both eyes dilate accordingly. Ipsilateral pupillary constriction associated with ptosis and anhidrosis (i.e., Horner syndrome) may be an early sign of transtentorial herniation, damage to the hypothalamus with interruption of sympathetic pathways, or disruption of the cervical sympathetics.

Examination of the fundi is best left until other ocular signs and responses have been documented. Adequate fundal examination is important, but sometimes it can only be achieved through the use of short-acting mydriatics. The clinician should consider this decision judiciously and, when employed, the patient must be labeled as having received these drugs and the fact must be clearly documented. Other intracranial hemorrhages should be strongly suspected if retinal hemorrhages are seen, and the possibility of iTBI must be considered. Venous pulsations in the retinal vessels are a helpful sign, as their presence precludes any significant increase in ICP. Papilledema is the single most reliable sign of intracranial hypertension. With acute elevations in ICP, papilledema is rarely seen in the first 24–48 hrs, which may be a useful feature when assessing suspected iTBI.

Motor System. Asymmetry of the face should be noted, and the gag reflex elicited. Assessment of power is best achieved by observing movement in response to supraorbital or sternal pressure. Responses to stimulation of the limbs may be reflex and serve to confuse the picture. Focal weakness usually implies a structural lesion. Tone should be assessed in all 4 limbs. Pat-

terns of decerebration should be closely observed for, and not mistaken as, seizures. Whether they are unilateral or bilateral and whether they are spontaneous or occur only after stimulation must be assessed. In infants, "bicycling" movements of the upper and lower limbs may precede these episodes. In extensor hypertonus, the lower limbs are extended with internal rotation and, often, plantar flexion and scissoring. Positioning in the upper limbs may be one of two distinct types. In decorticate rigidity, the arms are flexed across the chest, while in decerebrate rigidity, the elbows are extended. Such rigidity may result from structural lesions and is often associated with a rise in ICP. It is generally considered that decorticate posturing is associated with cortical or hemisphere dysfunction, whereas the brainstem is more often damaged in children in whom the upper limbs show decerebrate patterns.

The patient should be observed for seizures. Generalized tonic-clonic seizures or myoclonic jerks will be easily identified, but the more subtle phenomena seen in infants, such as cyanosis and chewing movements, are less readily recognized as ictal.

Finally, the deep tendon reflexes should be elicited. Areflexia in combination with flaccidity that is not due to muscle relaxants is grave. Asymmetric reflexes may be helpful in lateralizing the injury. Bilateral hyperactive reflexes may be associated with TBI or SCI but should be symmetric and not associated with pathologic reflexes. Rapid, sustained dorsiflexion of each ankle to test for clonus should be performed. Stroking the sole of the foot with a firm object should cause a reflex of the great toe; a positive Babinski reflex occurs when the patient dorsiflexes his toe. Many infants retain this response and, in them, the test has little diagnostic value.

Functional Integrity of the Spine and Spinal Cord. The entire spine should be examined carefully. The patient should be log-rolled to perform this examination. Ecchymoses indicate trauma in the region and should be noted. The spinal column should be palpated, and widening of spaces between adjacent spinous processes, malalignment of the spine, or step-off of the spinous processes may indicate underlying distraction or dislocation.

The functional integrity of the spinal cord is evaluated by a thorough motor and sensory examination. The American Spine Injury Association (ASIA) recommends use of the following scale of findings for the assessment of motor strength in SCI: 0, no contraction or movement; 1, minimal movement; 2, active movement but not against gravity; 3, active movement against gravity; 4, active movement against resistance; 5, active movement against full resistance. The ASIA clinical scoring system records motor strength in 10 muscle groups and sensory function in 28 dermatomes. The motor level is defined as the lowest segment in which muscle strength is assessed as able to move and hold in an antigravity position (i.e., ≥3). The systematic examination required for formal assessment in SCI is best recorded using the ASIA charts (20). However, by way of summary, **Figure 56.3** and **Table 56.8** provide general criteria for determining sensory and motor level. Superficial reflexes, such as abdominal, cremasteric, and anal reflexes, are also helpful in localizing the level of injury. Absent or diminished superficial reflexes suggest corticospinal lesions above the segmental innervation of this reflex. The sensory level is described according to the lowest dermatome in which sensation to light touch and pinprick is normal.

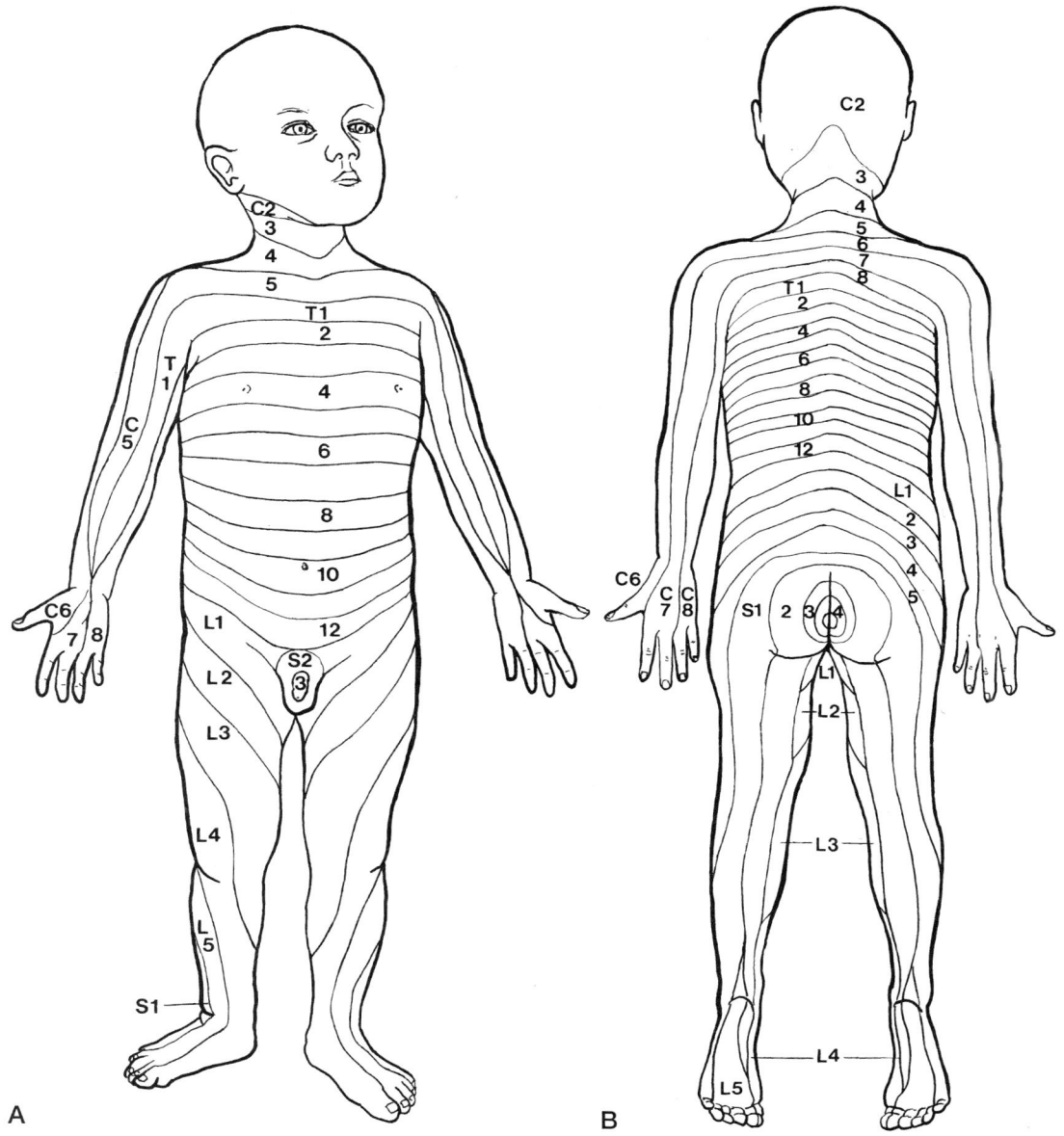

FIGURE 56.3. Segmental dermatomes are reproducible and helpful in identifying the level of spinal cord injury.

Complete injury is signified by loss of motor function, segmental reflexes, and sensation below a given level. The *zone of partial preservation* is an area adjacent to the neurologic level in which abnormal sensory and motor findings are noted. An area of abnormal findings that is not contiguous with the postulated level qualifies as *incomplete injury*. As this lesion has the potential for improvement, a reassessment is vital. The function that is classically retained is that of the sacral nerves, which means that perianal sensation and reflexes must be tested and documented. The sacral roots are assessed using perineal sensation to light touch and pinprick, bulbocavernosus reflex (S3, S4), anal wink (S5) and rectal tone, and evidence of urine retention or incontinence. Flaccid areflexic paralysis and anesthesia to all modalities characterize *spinal shock*. This problem is found in half of SCI patients and resolves within 24 hrs in >90%. SCI above the seventh thoracic vertebra may mask the tenderness normally associated with an intra-abdominal injury. Therefore, a high index of suspicion is needed in these patients to diagnose intra-abdominal bleeding.

INITIAL INVESTIGATIONS

The purpose of emergency laboratory and neuroradiologic investigations (along with the primary and secondary survey) in the child with TBI or SCI is to be able to respond to four key questions:

- Do any systemic metabolic or acid-base derangements require correction?
- Does this patient have intracranial pathology that requires emergency surgery?

TABLE 56.8

NERVE ROOTS UNDERLYING MUSCLE FUNCTION AND REFLEXES

Nerve root	Muscles and function	Reflexes
C4	Diaphragm Inspiration	
C5	Deltoid Shoulder flexion Shoulder abduction	Biceps (C5, C6)
C6	Biceps Elbow flexion	
C7	Extensor carpi radialis Wrist extension	Triceps (C7, C8)
C8	Flexor digitorum superficialis Finger flexion	
T1	Interossei Finger abduction Finger adduction	
T2–T7	Intercostals Expiration Forced expiration	
T8–T12	Abdominals Expiration Trunk flexion	Superficial abdominals
L2	Iliopsoas Hip flexion	Cremasteric (L1, L2)
L3	Quadriceps Knee extension	Knee (L3, L4)
L4	Tibialis anterior Foot dorsiflexion	
L5	Extensor hallucis longus Great toe extension	Hamstring (L5, S1)
S1	Gastrocnemius Foot plantar flexion	Ankle (S1, S2)
S2–S5	Anal sphincter Fecal continence	Bulbocavernosus (S3, S4) Anal wink (S5)

- Does this patient have an unstable spine that needs fixation?
- Does this patient require full investigation for suspected iTBI or shaken-baby syndrome?

Laboratory

A variety of blood and serum tests is required in children with TBI, SCI, or suspected iTBI. An overview of these investigations is discussed in Chapter 53. The forensic investigation of suspected iTBI should follow locally agreed professional standards of practice. Guidance can be found in reports from the American Academy of Pediatrics (19,92), the Royal College of Paediatrics and Child Health (137), and in standard textbooks (38,85). A summary of the essential baseline medical assessment of an infant with SDH and suspected iTBI is provided in **Table 56.9** (98).

Neuroradiology

A full account of neuroradiologic investigation is discussed in Chapter 55. This section will focus on some of the issues related to the process of patient care and management.

Head CT

An unenhanced head CT scan is the test of choice for patients who have moderate-to-high risk of injury after head trauma, as it reveals both hemorrhage and bony injury. The indications for head CT include GCS ≤ 14, progressive headache, decline in level of consciousness, seizure, unreliable history, vomiting, amnesia, signs of skull fracture or facial injury, penetrating skull injury, suspected iTBI, or focal or abnormal neurology. The initial head CT should include visualization of the craniocervical junction so that atlanto-occipital dislocation, rotatory subluxation of C1 on C2, and other craniocervical disruptions

ESSENTIAL BASELINE MEDICAL ASSESSMENT OF AN INFANT WITH SUBDURAL HEMORRHAGE AND SUSPECTED INFLICTED TRAUMATIC BRAIN INJURY

Assessment	Notes
Clinical history	Full case history Full documentation of all possible explanations for injury Identification of any previous concerns about unexplained injury Identification of relevant criminal record of care providers
Examination	Thorough general examination Documentation and clinical photographs of coexisting injury Head circumference, weight, and length plotted on centiles
Eyes	Ophthalmologist to examine both eyes through dilated pupils
Radiology	Initial cranial CT scan Repeat neuroimaging at 7 and 14 days Neuroradiologic report of all imaging Full skeletal survey; repeat at 10–14 days
Serology	Full blood count repeated over first 24–48 hrs Coagulation screen Urea and electrolytes, liver function tests, blood cultures
Follow-up investigations indicated by tests above	Exclude glutaric aciduria in cases with frontotemporal atrophy Lumbar puncture where meningitis is possible Save serum for viral serology

can be evaluated. Patients with negative CT scans and mild neurologic disturbances, such as posttraumatic seizures, vomiting, headache, irritability or GCS score of 12–15, can be observed. Children with normal examination or minimal neurologic deficit and small EDH, SDH, or intraparenchymal hemorrhage may also be closely observed. In the child with a lower GCS score, the absence of abnormalities on initial CT does not rule out ICP elevation (83). A skull x-ray is only helpful if head CT scan is not available.

Brain imaging provides some insight into the evolving mechanism of injury in the acute stage of iTBI. For example, patients with acute SDH (interhemispheric or convexity) can be categorized as those with diffuse cerebral hypoattenuation or those with focal cerebral hypoattenuation. Investigators found that such patterns of infarction fell into three groups: first, total hemisphere necrosis following acute hemisphere swelling subjacent to an ipsilateral convexity SDH (71); second, infarction related to acute brain swelling with CT findings of either infarction in the posterior cerebral artery distribution or in the distribution of the callosomarginal branch of the anterior cerebral artery; and third, infarction related to hypoperfusion—arterial border-zone distribution between anterior and middle, and middle and posterior cerebral arteries. Diffusion-weighted

imaging and apparent diffusion coefficient maps—forms of MRI sensitive to ischemia and cytotoxic edema—can be used to reveal nonhemorrhagic infarction much earlier than CT, in fact within hours. Diffusion-weighted imaging and apparent diffusion coefficient abnormalities were found in 16 of 18 (89%) patients with iTBI (144). These changes were more likely to involve posterior aspects of the cerebral hemispheres and, on review, severity of abnormality correlated significantly with poor outcome.

Spinal Imaging and Assessment of Stability

Imaging of the spine should be obtained in all patients with neck or back pain or tenderness, sensory or motor deficits, or an impaired level of consciousness, or in those with painful, distracting injuries outside of the spinal region. The goal of imaging is to rapidly identify injury of the spine that places neural tissue at risk. The majority of patients with traumatic SCI are found to have associated spine injury. The standard cervical radiographs include anteroposterior, lateral, and odontoid views. Technically adequate films allow visualization of the entire cervical spine to the C7 through T1 intervertebral space. Lateral views should be screened for changes in vertebral alignment, bony structure, intervertebral space, and soft tissue. Flexion-extension views are useful for detecting occult instability that results from ligamentous injury. This procedure is safe only in patients who are neurologically intact and in whom there is no subluxation greater than 3.5 mm on lateral films. Spinal CT scan is indicated when the spine has not been visualized adequately on standard films or if it appears abnormal. Spinal CT is very sensitive in detecting bony injury. Spinal MRI is highly sensitive to changes in the spinal cord, hemorrhage, and ligamentous injury, and is indicated in the presence of cord-related neurologic findings.

Spinal stability is defined as the capacity of the spine to withstand physiologic loading without neurologic injury, deformity, or pain. In practice, this state is predicted by clinical examination and imaging. In the thoracolumbar spine, instability is defined as injury to more than two CT-based "columns": the *anterior column,* which consists of the anterior longitudinal ligament and the anterior half of vertebral body or disc; the *middle column,* which consists of the posterior half of the body or disc and the posterior longitudinal ligament; and, the *posterior column,* which consists of the posterior arch and ligaments.

Clearance of the cervical spine as being stable is controversial. Some standards have been established for clearing the cervical spine in adults (78). Adults who are awake, alert, not intoxicated, and have no other distraction injuries, neck pain, or tenderness do not require any supplemental radiographic assessment to clear the cervical spine as being stable. These *Guidelines* can be used in children >9 years. In children with significant TBI or significant neck pain, a reasonable practice is to maintain cervical spine immobilization until an MRI can be performed to exclude ligamentous injury. However, no formal guidelines exist on this practice, and each unit should discuss its management strategy with neurosurgery, neuroradiology, and emergency medicine colleagues. In the conscious child, immobilization can be discontinued when the pain has resolved and flexion and extension radiographs reveal no apparent injury (51).

NEUROCRITICAL CARE MONITORING OF INTRACRANIAL PRESSURE

The forms of standard and advanced monitoring techniques for neurocritical care are described and discussed in Chapter 54. This section will focus on the use of ICP monitoring in TBI. Guidelines have been published regarding when ICP monitoring is indicated and what technology should be used (9,10). Unfortunately, the conclusion is that data are insufficient to support standards and guidelines on these topics. The *Options* are as follows. Children with severe TBI (GCS <9) and a mass lesion should have the mass removed and an ICP monitor inserted at the time of surgery. Nonsurgical children with GCS <9 or CT evidence of intracranial hypertension (e.g., swelling, shift, or cisternal compression) should also have ICP monitoring. Children with moderate head injury (GCS 9–12) merit careful observation. In these children, an open fontanelle may be used as a proxy for invasive monitoring. Deterioration warrants repeat head CT to rule out interval development or enlargement of a mass lesion and consideration for placement of an ICP monitor.

Traditionally, ICP monitoring is performed via a ventriculostomy. Newer technologies rely on fiberoptic monitoring, with the catheter sensor-tip placed in the brain parenchyma. The advantage of the ventriculostomy is that it enables CSF drainage as a treatment. However, it can be difficult to place and maintain function in the child with small, compressed, or distorted ventricles.

Intracranial Pressure and Cerebral Perfusion Pressure Target Levels

Normal ICP is usually <10 mm Hg in adults (93), varies between 3 and 7 mm Hg in younger children, and is <6 mm Hg in infants (119,160). In adults, the threshold for initiating treatment of intracranial hypertension is taken as 20–25 mm Hg. No standards exist for infants and children. However, it is likely that the ICP threshold for poorer outcome is similar across all ages (see Chapter 51). Four of five major studies, including more than 230 cases of severe pediatric TBI, reported that poor outcome was associated with ICP >20 mm Hg (52,58,132,141,142). The guidelines for severe pediatric TBI therefore state that, as an *Option*, "treatment should begin at an ICP ≥20 mm Hg" (9). Whether a lower threshold should be used in infants and newborns is unknown. This question is important in cases of iTBI, as raised ICP has been described in a number of case series of iTBI (23,36,44,62,96).

Cerebral perfusion pressure (CPP) is calculated as the difference between the mean systemic arterial pressure and the mean ICP. Two assumptions are made when using this calculation to guide treatment. The first assumption is that the mean systemic arterial pressure is a good reflection of brain surface arteriolar pressure, and this may not be the case. The second assumption is that both pressures contributing to the calculation are calibrated to the same level. In the case of ICP monitoring via ventriculostomy, the point for zero calibration can be adjusted, although few reports discuss the exact details of calibration and zeroing. This adjustment is not possible with the fiber-tip in-

traparenchymal devices, for which the pressure is recorded at the tip of the sensor. If, in the case of ventricular monitoring, the zero point for ICP is taken as the level of the external auditory meatus and the zero point for blood pressure is taken as the level of the right atrium, then the calculated CPP will overestimate "true" CPP by a factor proportional to the distance between the two zeroing points multiplied by the sine of the angle of elevation of the bed. In children, this overestimate will be on the order of 5 mm Hg. However, if an intraparenchymal fiber-tip device is used and the bed is elevated beyond 30 degrees, the error could be doubled. We should therefore be cautious about how the following data are interpreted, and perhaps be more conservative in the CPP limits we accept.

What target CPP should be maintained in children? A survey of PICUs in the UK showed that most units used age-dependent criteria (139). Reductions in CPP below specific threshold values are associated with poor outcome. In severe pediatric TBI, studies defined the CPP associated with poor outcome as between 40 and 65 mm Hg. In a study of 118 children (mean age 7 years), the overall mortality rate was 28%, and the CPP threshold associated with survival was >40 mm Hg (52). No further improvement in outcome was seen with mean CPP in deciles from 40 to 70 mm Hg. In contrast, in an epidemiologic study of 136 infants and children with severe TBI, it was reported that supranormal maximum systolic blood pressure (≥135 mm Hg) was associated with a 19-fold higher chance of survival (161). A retrospective study of children <16 years of age revealed no statistically significant difference in Glasgow Outcome Scale score when CPP was maintained between 40–49, 50–59, 60–69, or >70 mm Hg (90). A retrospective review using constructed receiver-operator curves suggests that children with CPP <40 mm Hg die (42). Those with CPP >45 mm Hg live. In iTBI, investigators found that, in 17 infants, poorer neurodevelopmental outcome was associated with lowest CPP and mean arterial pressure (23). However, on inspection of the data in the report, a relationship is not apparent between the quality of survival and level of CPP. In fact, blood pressure appears to be the major problem. The pediatric guideline for severe TBI is that "CPP >40 mm Hg should be maintained" (11). A modification of this recommendation is to titrate the CPP threshold according to age: thresholds of 40–50 mm Hg in infants and toddlers, 50–60 mm Hg in children, and >60 mm Hg in adolescents (103).

NEUROCRITICAL CARE TREATMENTS

Intracranial Pressure-directed Therapies

The guidelines for the management of children with severe TBI are summarized in **Table 56.10**. In general, intensivists follow a series of *Options* because of the paucity of the evidence-based data.

After endotracheal intubation and insertion of an ICP monitor, the first step used to reduce ICP is to ensure adequate sedation, analgesia, and neuromuscular blockade by using standard dosing of agents chosen by the treating physician. Propofol should not be used in children with severe TBI. Both the Center for Drug Evaluation and Research of the US Food and Drug Administration and the UK Committee on Safety of Medicine

TABLE 56.10

A SUMMARY OF GUIDELINES FOR ACUTE MEDICAL MANAGEMENT OF TRAUMATIC BRAIN INJURY

Guideline	A. Standard Accepted principles with certainty B. Guide Moderate clinical certainty	Notes Infants
Pediatric trauma center	A. Insufficient data B. Metropolitan area—transport to pediatric trauma center	
Prehospital airway management	A. Insufficient data B. Avoid hypoxia and correct immediately and use supplemental O_2. Endotracheal intubation is not better than bag-valve-mask ventilation.	
Prehospital resuscitation of blood pressure and oxygenation	A. Insufficient data B. Rapidly correct hypotension with fluid	Use infant-specific values
Indications for ICP monitoring	A. Insufficient data B. Insufficient data	Normal CT scan and open fontanelles and/or sutures do not rule out raised ICP.
Treatment threshold for raised ICP	A. Insufficient data B. Insufficient data	Herniation can occur at 25 mm Hg.
ICP monitoring	A. Insufficient data B. Insufficient data	
CPP	A. Insufficient data B. A CPP >40 mm Hg in children	Age-related differences are likely in optimal CPP goals.
Sedation and neuromuscular blockade	A. Insufficient data B. Insufficient data	
Cerebrospinal fluid drainage	A. Insufficient data B. Insufficient data	
Hyperosmolar therapy	A. Insufficient data B. Insufficient data	
Hyperventilation	A. Insufficient data B. Insufficient data	
Barbiturate coma	A. Insufficient data B. Insufficient data	May have deleterious effects on neurodevelopment.
Temperature control	A. Insufficient data B. Insufficient data	
Surgical treatment of ICP	A. Insufficient data B. Insufficient data	
Corticosteroids	A. Insufficient data B. Insufficient data	Recent adult study indicates worse outcome with steroids.

ICP, intracranial pressure; CPP, cerebral perfusion pressure. Data from Carney NA, Chesnut R, Kochanek PM. Guidelines for the acute medical management of severe traumatic brain injury in infants, children, and adolescents: Prehospital airway management. *Pediatr Crit Care Med* 2003;4:S9–11.

have stated that "Propofol is not indicated for pediatric intensive care unit sedation, as safety has not been established" (41,46). The other "first-tier" therapies include elevation of the head of the bed to 30 degrees and positioning of the head in the midline, ensuring no obstruction to cerebral venous return. If ICP remains elevated and a ventriculostomy tube is in place, CSF can be drained.

If ICP is still elevated after these initial measures, mannitol or hyperosmolar therapy using hypertonic saline can be instituted. Intermittent, IV infusions of mannitol, usually in the range of 0.25–0.5 g/kg, can be administered. Serum osmolality

should be assessed before redosing, and the mannitol infusion withheld if the serum osmolality is above 320 mOsm/L, as dehydration induced by mannitol can precipitate renal failure. Some centers use furosemide as an adjunct to mannitol to potentiate its effects as a diuretic. Hypertonic saline produces a 4-mm Hg decrease in ICP for 2 hrs post infusion and has been associated with fewer required interventions to maintain an ICP of <15 mm Hg (101,131). A continuous infusion of 3% saline (between 0.1 and 1.0 mL/kg/hr administered on a sliding scale) is effective. The minimum dose required to maintain ICP <20 mm Hg should be used. The use of hypertonic saline rather than mannitol makes sense during the initial phase of TBI management, when low volume status increases the risk of hypoperfusion. The greater volume status associated with hypertonic saline may also explain why few adverse reactions occur with sodium levels as high as 160 mmol/L. Infusions can be continued if serum osmolality is below 360 mOsm/L.

If the patient still continues to have raised ICP despite using all first-tier therapies, a number of "second-tier" therapies can be considered. If the basal cisterns are open on concurrent cranial CT scan and no significant mass or midline shift is present, a lumbar CSF drain can be considered by the neurosurgical staff (110). If the patient has no medical contraindications to using barbiturates, pentobarbital can be used to induce burst suppression and control elevated ICP by reducing cerebral metabolic activity. A commonly used protocol for pentobarbital is to use a loading dose of 10 mg/kg over 30 mins, followed by 5 mg/kg every hour for three doses, and then a maintenance infusion of 1 mg/kg/hr (56). The dose is titrated to the effect required (i.e., ICP control) while hypotension and unnecessary central nervous system depression are avoided. Alternatively, with evidence of brain swelling on CT scan, decompressive craniectomy can be considered (44,151). In one study children were randomized to receiving either early (within 6 hrs of enrollment), decompressive craniectomy or standard medical management if the ICP was sustained >20 mm Hg for >5 mins (151). ICP in the decompressive group was significantly decreased, and the patients required substantially less medical intervention to control ICP after decompression. The control group of 14 patients had 2 patients with favorable outcomes (normal or mildly disabled at 6-month follow-up), while the decompression group had 7 out of 13 with favorable outcomes using the same outcome criteria.

Other therapies that can be used as adjuncts to care include induced hypothermia (or at least maintenance of normothermia), controlled hyperventilation ($Paco_2$ 30–35 mm Hg) in those with cerebral hyperemia, and controlled arterial hypertension. In regard to induced hypothermia, the weight of evidence in TBI in adults points to no effect in improving outcome after TBI (45). (It bears noting that the results of a pediatric hypothermia study in TBI are pending, but preliminary presentation of the data also indicates that there is no effect.) In contrast to these findings in TBI, 2 studies in adults indicate that mild therapeutic hypothermia improves neurologic outcome after cardiac arrest (31,89). Also, evidence suggests that selective head cooling with mild systemic hypothermia could improve survival without severe neurodevelopmental disability in infants with moderate neonatal hypoxic-ischemic encephalopathy (72). Taken together with the previous discussion on pathophysiology of iTBI (i.e., a significant hypoxic component), such infants may be the next appropriate group for a randomized, controlled trial of hypothermia.

Individual units should discuss their local strategy for ICP control. Such protocols often evolve over the years, and it is imperative that therapies are audited to identify whether any unusual practices or variances in care are occurring (118). One way to document and measure therapies used to control ICP has been reported. The Pediatric Intensity Level of Therapy (PILOT) scale assigns scores to a variety of first- and second-tier treatments used in ICP control (**Table 56.11**) (143). The intensity of treatment in subgroups of patients and in different PICUs can be compared using this scale. It is the author's experience that, in those patients in whom intracranial hypertension

is a problem, the peak intensity of treatment occurs between days 3 and 4. Therefore, ICP treatments can be de-intensified in a stepwise process to ensure stability in adequate levels of ICP and CPP for at least 6–12 hrs between each reduction in therapy. Most patients are able to leave the PICU by day 7 post-injury.

Spinal Cord Injury-directed Therapies

In adults, high-dose methylprednisolone became the standard of care in the management of nonpenetrating acute SCI. This practice was based on the results of the National Acute Spinal Cord Injury Studies (NASCIS) II and III, a Cochrane review of all randomized clinical trials and other published reports that verified significant improvement in motor function and sensation in patients with complete or incomplete SCI who were treated with high doses of methylprednisolone within 8 hrs of injury. Since 1998, however, a number of authors have revisited these studies and questioned the validity of the results. Concerns have been raised about the study design, randomization, clinical end-points, and statistical analysis (121). In addition, the risks of steroid therapy were not, in retrospect, considered inconsequential; an increased incidence of infection and avascular necrosis was noted.

Therefore, a number of professional organizations have revised their recommendations concerning steroid therapy in SCI. The Canadian Association of Emergency Physicians no longer recommends high-dose methylprednisolone as the standard of care. The Congress of Neurological Surgeons states that steroid therapy "should only be undertaken with the knowledge that evidence suggesting harmful effects is more consistent than any suggestion of clinical benefit." The American College of Surgeons has modified their Advanced Trauma Life Support guidelines to state that methylprednisolone is "*a* recommended treatment" rather than "*the* recommended treatment." In a recent survey of spine surgeons, ~90% used steroids in SCI and followed the NASCIS II trial protocol, but only 24% believed that they were of any clinical benefit (55).

No studies have been conducted of methylprednisolone in children with acute SCI, and no official recommendations have been proposed for treatment. The decision to use steroids in acute SCI should therefore be made locally. If steroids are recommended, they should be initiated within 8 hrs of injury with the following protocol. Methylprednisolone 30 mg/kg bolus over 15 mins and an infusion of methylprednisolone at 5.4 mg/kg/hr for 23 hrs beginning 45 mins after the bolus, if the patient started therapy within 3 hrs of injury. If the patient starts treatment between 3 and 8 hrs after injury, the infusion can be continued for a total of 48 hrs.

Last, adults with SCI are at risk for deep vein thrombosis and venous thromboembolism. Current guidelines recommend that patients with SCI receive prophylaxis with low-molecular-weight heparin. Gastroparesis and paralytic ileus are also common, and treatment with prokinetics may be useful.

Seizures and Anticonvulsants

Seizures are the most common complication after a head injury. The standard definition for an early posttraumatic seizure is that it occurs within 1 week of trauma (91). The general

TABLE 56.11

PEDIATRIC INTENSITY LEVEL OF THERAPY (PILOT) SCALE

Variable	Score	Maximum score
Individual daily scored components are denoted "a", "b" or "c" in the scoring section		
General (at any time in previous 24 hrs)		
Treatment of fever (>38.5°C) or spontaneous temperature (<34.5°C)	1a	1a + 1b + 2c = 4
Sedation (opiates, benzodiazepines: any dose)	1b	
Neuromuscular blockade	2c	
Ventilation (most frequently observed $Paco_2$ in 24 hrs)		
Intubated/normal ventilation ($Paco_2$ 35.1–40 mm Hg)	1a	4
Mild hyperventilation ($Paco_2$ 32–35 mm Hg)	2a	
Aggressive hyperventilation ($Paco_2$ <32 mm Hg)	4a	
Osmolar therapy (total dose in 24 hrs)		
Mannitol ≤1 g/kg	1a	3a + 3b = 6
Mannitol 1.1–2 g/kg	2a	
Mannitol >2 g/kg	3a	
Hypertonic saline (any dose or rate, regardless of [Na])	3b	
Cerebrospinal fluid drainage (times in 24 hrs)		
0–11 times	1a	3
12–23 times	2a	
≥24 times or continuous	3a	
Barbiturates (total dose in 24 hrs; for score, 5 mg thiopental is equivalent to 1 mg pentobarbital)		4
Pentobarbital ≤36 mg/kg	3a	
Pentobarbital >36 mg/kg	4a	
Surgery (at any time in 24 hrs)		
Evacuation of hematoma	4a	4a + 5b = 9
Decompressive craniectomy	5b	
Other treatments (at any time in 24 hrs)		
Induced mild hypothermia (≥35°C–37°C)	2a	4 + 2 + 2 = 8
Induced moderate hypothermia (<35°C)	4a	
Lumbar drain	2b	
Induced hypertension (≥95th percentile for age)	2c	
Total possible score		4 + 4 + 6 + 3 + 4 + 9 + 8 = 38

Data from Shore PM, Hand LL, Roy L, et al. Reliability and validity of the pediatric intensity level of therapy (PILOT) scale: A measure of the use of intracranial pressure-directed therapies. *Crit Care Med* 2006;34:1981–7.

incidence of early seizures varies between 12% and 15% (43). The risk of long-term seizures in these patients is ~15%. The more severe the injury, the higher the incidence of seizures becomes. Severe TBI (GCS <9) has a 27% risk of seizures, while those patients who present with a GCS from 9–12 have a 12% risk, and those with a GCS of 13–15 have only a 2% risk (59). Seizures are more common in children who suffer an SDH or a depressed skull fracture.

In iTBI, evidence suggests that seizures are symptomatic of ischemia- or hypoperfusion-induced pathology, and therefore signify likely poor outcome. It was reported that 32 of 44 cases (73%) of iTBI had early posttraumatic seizures, and the mortality rate was 6% (25). The seizures were classified as being either responsive to medication without episodes of status epilepticus or unresponsive to medication (i.e., failure to respond to at least two anticonvulsant agents) with or without episodes of status epilepticus. In general, seizures that occur within 24 hrs of admission reached a peak severity and frequency by day 2 and resolved by 1 week. One-third of the patients had seizures

that were refractory to treatment. At follow-up, neurodevelopmental outcome correlated significantly with the presence and severity of the seizures. The authors' conclusion was that severity of primary brain injury was reflected in the severity of early seizures.

The acute treatment of seizures is discussed in Chapter 57. In patients who are refractory to treatment, which appears to be quite common in iTBI, continuous infusion of midazolam features most in the current pediatric intensive care literature (104,125). The alternative is high-dose phenobarbitone or anesthesia with short-acting barbiturates (47,147,148). The main problems with barbiturates are the zero-order kinetics once treatment is prolonged and the inability to assess clinical neurology.

Prophylactic anticonvulsants are recommended in adults with severe TBI, but their role in the management of children is controversial, as no prospective controlled trials have been conducted in children (138). In children, medications for seizure prophylaxis include phenytoin, phenobarbital, and carbamazepine. In some centers, the following approach is used: First, no treatment is undertaken for an isolated post-traumatic seizure, but a sustained or recurrent seizure is treated with phenytoin. After 6 months, phenytoin is weaned off and is restarted with evidence of clinical or electroencephalographic seizures. In these cases, the weaning of phenytoin is repeated after 1 year.

Posttraumatic Meningitis and Fever

Posttraumatic meningitis is a risk of mid-frontal, lateral-frontal, or temporofrontal fractures and posterolateral fractures (Table 56.2). It is best treated after an infective organism is cultured so that the antibiotic can be tailored appropriately. Initial empiric therapy after culture should cover *Streptococcus* and *Staphylococcus*. Ceftriaxone with or without vancomycin, depending on the local incidence of resistant Gram-positive organisms, is a reasonable choice until the specific organism is cultured.

Fever may be the earliest sign of meningitis but, in severe TBI, this is not always the cause. Early hyperthermia (i.e., temperature >38.5°C) within the first 24 hrs of admission occurs in ~30% of children admitted to PICU post-TBI; this phenomenon appears to be a function of severity of injury (120) and is to be expected in children with moderate degrees of subarachnoid hemorrhage. Generally, a rise in temperature of >39°C demands investigation, and the presence of a compound fracture, either internal or external, should serve to focus attention immediately upon the possibility of meningitis. Extracranial causes of fever are also possible (e.g., chest infection, fat embolism, wound infection) and must be sought. Neurogenic hyperthermia may be due to primary brain lesions associated with TAI and dysautonomia with storming episodes. Another possibility is dehydration. In a review of 93 severely injured children, it was found that episodes of fever occurred in 52% and, of these cases, almost half were due to infection (145). Irrespective of the cause, a rise in temperature must be controlled, as it may worsen neurologic outcome.

Fluids and Nutrition

Discussion about IV fluids has been a topic of many debates, and the reader should refer to Chapter 86 for more details about the issues in children with critical illness. It is clear that the use of low-sodium–containing crystalloids is associated with mortality and morbidity in children. However, prolonged use of IV 0.9% sodium chloride will inevitably cause hyperchloremia and acidosis. IV saline-induced hyperchloremic acidosis causes reduced urine flow, confusion, and increased morbidity in adults who undergo major surgery. Alexis Hartmann (1894–1964), a pediatrician, introduced Ringer's solution in an effort to avoid the development of life-threatening hyperchloremic acidosis following saline administration.

Glucose-containing IV solutions are not recommended in adults who have suffered TBI. In fact, the emphasis is on limiting glucose in the insulin-resistant critically ill, and on controlling blood glucose within a tight range by using supplemental insulin. This so-called tight glycemic control with intensive insulin therapy appears to be associated with better ICP control in TBI (154). However, brain microdialysis findings have questioned this approach. Intensive insulin therapy in 14 adults with TBI resulted in a net reduction in microdialysis glucose without altering glucose utilization or improving the LPR, when compared with controls (158). These authors had previously reported that low extracellular glucose was associated with poor outcome in TBI (156). Too few studies are available to consider the potential problems or merits of, respectively, glucose or no glucose in children with TBI. Traditionally, glucose-containing fluids have been used, particularly in the very young. Until more is known about the relationship between blood glucose, brain glucose, and outcome, it is advisable to continue with one's current fluid strategy. An option that circumvents these issues is to initiate enteral nutritional support by 72 hrs post-injury and aim for full nutritional replacement by day 7 (13).

Hypothalamic-Pituitary Dysfunction

In adults with moderate to severe TBI, the endocrine changes within the first few hours and days immediately after injury (14,50) share similarities with the changes in hypothalamic-pituitary-endocrine dysfunction observed in other critically ill patients (163). In particular, low basal cortisol levels with subnormal cortisol responses to stress test have been observed (16,17,146). Posterior pituitary dysfunction that leads to abnormalities in water homeostasis and results in either cranial (central) diabetes insipidus or syndrome of inappropriate antidiuretic hormone (SIADH) secretion is also commonly observed in the acute period after TBI (15,16). In the majority of cases, perturbations in water balance are usually transitory and resolve within a few days or weeks of the event. SIADH is manifest as hyponatremia (serum sodium ≤130 mmol/L), which will exacerbate cerebral swelling, worsen ICP, and cause seizures. Cerebral salt wasting may also cause hyponatremia. SIADH is treated with volume restriction, and cerebral salt wasting is treated with volume and sodium repletion. The differentiation between these entities can be difficult to discern, but the single, clear, differentiating factor is the patient's volume state. Patients with high volume status have SIADH, while those with low intravascular volume have cerebral salt wasting. In that patients with SIADH tend to make smaller amounts of highly osmolar urine, careful documentation of urine volume and urinary sodium concentration may assist in the diagnosis (30). Mineralocorticoids also have a role in facilitating sodium retention.

In view of the neuroendocrine studies in adults with TBI and what is known about pediatric TBI (see previous discussion), it seems likely that hypopituitarism is a neglected phenomenon in acute pediatric critical care. We therefore consider that, in the acute phase of illness, adrenal insufficiency should not be missed, because it can be life-threatening, and hypopituitarism must be identified early in the post-TBI period. An approach that is used in adults and is our practice in pediatric TBI cases with GCS scores 3–13 or cranial CT evidence of significant brain injury is summarized in Table 56.12 (1). A basal, early morning, cortisol concentration of <200 nmol/L suggests adrenocorticotropic hormone deficiency, and treatment with replacement doses of hydrocortisone is indicated until full endocrinologic assessment in the post-PICU phase. In patients with acute-phase basal cortisol concentrations between 200 and 400 nmol/L, we consider replacement therapy if the child has features that could be due to adrenal insufficiency

TABLE 56.12

SUGGESTED ALGORITHM FOR DIAGNOSIS OF ADRENAL INSUFFICIENCY IN PEDIATRIC TRAUMATIC BRAIN INJURY

Step 1	Consider testing in the following cases: Glasgow Coma Scale score 3 to 13 Cranial imaging that indicates significant brain injury Children who require inotropes or hyperosmolar therapy for intracranial pressure control
Step 2	Check morning cortisol Daily for the first 7 days post-injury
Step 3	Treat patients with the following levels of replacement hydrocortisone: Morning cortisol <200 nmol/L Morning cortisol ≥200 nmol/L but <400 nmol/L, and features of hypoadrenalism (i.e., hyponatremia, hypotension, or hypoglycemia)
Step 4	Refer patient to pediatric endocrinologist
Step 5	Endocrinologic assessment of anterior and posterior pituitary function in the postacute phase (usually 3–6 months)

Adapted from Acerini CL, Tasker RC. Traumatic brain injury-induced hypothalamic-pituitary dysfunction: A paediatric perspective. *Pituitary* 2007;10(4):373–80.

(e.g., hypotension, hyponatremia, or hypoglycemia). This indication may be difficult to assess in the patient who is receiving hyperosmolar therapy and inotropes for blood pressure support. Again, therapy is indicated until full endocrinologic assessment in the post-PICU phase. The reader should be aware that, at present, little prospective clinical evidence exists for this approach; therefore, replacement hydrocortisone should be viewed as an option. Also, recent reviews of steroid therapy in TBI indicate potential detrimental effects (Table 56.10) (39).

Assessment of growth hormone, gonadal, and thyroid axes is not necessary in the acute phase because, in adults, no evidence suggests that acute phase replacement of these hormones in the deficient patient improves outcome. These endocrine axes should be assessed in the post-PICU period, 3–6 months after injury.

OUTCOMES AND PROGNOSIS OF BRAIN INJURY

Lethal and Fatal Injuries

Instances do occur when a child can be deemed to have sustained a lethal head injury and intensive care, as described in this chapter, is not appropriate. The types of brain damage in such children who are >2 years of age are remarkably similar to those seen in adults (75). Postresuscitant children with GCS score of 3 and bilateral, fixed, and dilated pupils (not due to medication) are in this category. The methods and protocols by which regional and local emergency systems deal with such

patients should be decided locally. In our practice, we offer admission to the PICU to any child who has entered the emergency system; intensivists are best placed and best trained to deal with the issues surrounding brain death (see Chapter 61).

In any child with at least one pupil reactive to light, irrespective of the GCS score, all and full TBI-related interventions are offered. In our experience, it is impossible and inappropriate to use clinical features at the time of accident to predict survival. Such a child may well have sustained a fatal injury. If this should become evident over the course of intensive care, it should be assessed using appropriate technologies (see Chapters 54 and 61) and discussed in an environment in which parents and the family can be supported.

Long-term Outcome

After intensive care, children with severe TBI often face challenges when living at home, at school, and in the community. The prognosis for recovery after severe TBI may be due to a number of ictal and postacute factors. It is not an exact science, but it is important that intensivists be aware of their outcomes, not least because it is the only way to inform our understanding of what works and what the therapeutic targets should be. At present, we work on the assumption that uncontrolled intracranial hypertension and inadequate cerebral perfusion costs brain tissue, function, and potential. Below is some of the evidence.

Typically, children with TBI >4 years will have better outcomes than adults injured to a similar degree. Large series have repeatedly demonstrated a mortality rate of >45% in adults, compared with 25% in children. In children, ICP and admission neurology are the best predictors of outcomes (61). The survival of infants who suffer iTBI is similar to that of children with TBI. A review of a 16-case series that reported outcomes of iTBI found that the mortality rate in individual reports in the literature ranged from 13% to 36%, with the combined mortality being 20.6% (112 out of 544 cases) (26).

Regarding late outcome of TBI, a prospective study of 330 children with moderate or severe injury found that a considerable proportion had significant morbidity (113). Measurable declines in, and impairment of, health-related quality-of-life scores at 3 months (42% of children) and 12 months (40% of children) after injury were reported. In children <2 years of age, another study found that, of 112 children, most (67%) had mild disability or better 2 years later, with 45% functioning at an age-appropriate level (97). In contrast to the reports in TBI, morbidity in survivors of iTBI ranges from 59% to 100% (26). In fact, in a total of 317 survivors of iTBI, 74% had abnormal neurology.

The substrate for long-term deficits after TBI is undoubtedly the pathophysiologic problems that occur during the acute illness and how they impact on the white-matter architecture of the brain. A cross-sectional MRI study of 123 adults who survived TBI found a decrease in brain volume that continued for at least 3 years after injury at a rate greater than that seen with normal aging (33). Similar whole-brain atrophy, with decrease in brain parenchyma, also occurs after mild or moderate TBI in adults and is evident at an average of 11 months after trauma, particularly if the patient had loss of consciousness (112).

Some data in children with TBI do exist, and a few authors have reported similar findings in small series of children

TABLE 56.13

PICU SUMMARY POINTS ON HEAD AND SPINAL CORD TRAUMA

Resuscitation phase
  Quickly identify and treat life-threatening injuries
  Identify and correct airway obstruction, inadequate ventilation, and shock
  Assume that the cervical spine is unstable
  Identify intracranial hypertension with impending herniation, and use aggressive
    hyperventilation for a brief period if found

Secondary assessment phase
  Review all injuries and plan management with survey of head, neck, and thorax
  Assess ocular signs and responses
  Assess the motor system
  Assess the functional integrity of the spine and spinal cord

Investigation phase
  Head CT is the investigation of choice for bony and brain tissue injury
  Head CT should include visualization of the craniocervical junction
  Cervical radiographs include anteroposterior, lateral, and odontoid views; technically
    adequate films allow visualization of the entire cervical spine to C7–T1 intervertebral space
  Exclude metabolic or acid-base derangements that require correction
  Do not forget about iTBI; a retinal examination is mandatory

PICU intensification phase
After endotracheal intubation and insertion of ICP monitor target:
  ICP ≤20 mm Hg and CPP >40 mm Hg
  Temperature 35–37°C
  Normoxia, normocarbia, normotension, normoglycemia
  Head in the midline and 30-degree elevation position
First-tier TBI therapies include:
  Adequate sedation, analgesia and neuromuscular blockade
  Osmotherapy (mannitol or hypertonic saline)
Second-tier TBI therapeutic options to be considered are:
  Lumbar CSF drainage
  Barbiturates
  Decompressive craniectomy
  Controlled hyperventilation
  Controlled arterial hypertension
SCI management includes consideration of:
  Methylprednisolone
  Low-molecular-weight heparin
  Gastrointestinal prokinetics
Other neurocritical care issues include:
  Seizures and anticonvulsants
  Posttraumatic meningitis and fever
  IV fluids and nutrition
  Repeat imaging to rule out interval development or enlargement of mass
  Cortisol for those with adrenal insufficiency

Deintensification phase
  Wean ICP- and CPP-directed therapies in reverse order of escalation (see above)
  Involve rehabilitation services at an early stage in cases of SCI and severe TBI

Postacute phase
  Follow-up investigation of anterior and posterior pituitary function in those treated with
    hydrocortisone replacement

TBI, traumatic brain injury; CSF, cerebrospinal fluid; SCI, spinal cord injury; ICP, intracranial pressure; CPP, cerebral perfusion pressure

(74,109,124,150,153,162). In infants with iTBI, 4 case series have suggested an interference with head and brain growth following iTBI (36,111,123,136). The 2 largest series showed that 15 of 34 survivors of iTBI developed cerebral atrophy (136), and 15 of 16 iTBI children acquired microcephaly after injury (111). In 8 of the 15 children with microcephaly, the cause was cerebral atrophy. The period of ongoing volume loss late after TBI or iTBI may represent a variety of problems in children. Cerebral atrophy may be attributable to tissue loss at the time of injury. Alternatively, disruption of widely distributed neuronal circuits by TAI may result in gradual diminution of neuronal arborization. Last, it is also possible that, in addition to cerebral atrophy after TBI, loss of growth potential may occur in affected tissue.

CONCLUSIONS AND FUTURE DIRECTIONS

The care of the child who suffers severe TBI or SCI is a continuum that starts with at-the-scene resuscitation by bystanders and the emergency services, followed by hospital transfer, neurosurgery, PICU care, and lastly, rehabilitation in the community. This chapter has focused on one element within this continuum and the role of PICU therapies. Possible topics for future studies include the roles of hypoxia-ischemia and axonal injury in iTBI, the type of IV fluids that should be used in TBI (lactate-containing or glucose-containing, or not), the role and risk of "tight-glycemic control" in ICP management, TBI-related hypothalamic-pituitary dysfunction in children and adolescents, the use of hypothermia in infants with moderate iTBI and hypoxic-ischemic encephalopathy, and the use of steroids in children with acute SCI.

KEY POINTS

- The PICU aspect of head and spinal cord trauma care is summarized in Table 56.13.
- Hypotension and hypoxemia are strongly associated with poor outcome; the focus should be on these targets in resuscitation.
- Hypoventilation due to lung or neurologic causes is common in TBI and SCI.
- The mechanism and pattern of head and brain injury will help to anticipate meningitis, carotid dissection, and hypopituitarism.
- SCI is often overlooked and may be missed in the unconscious patient who presents with TBI or iTBI.
- Practitioners should develop a system of practice in which PICU treatments and outcomes are reviewed and contemporary TBI (http://www.braintrauma.org/) and SCI (http://www.asia-spinalinjury.org/) protocols are checked for new developments.
- Optimal brain and spinal cord trauma care requires multidisciplinary expertise.

References

1. Acerini CL, Tasker RC, Bellone S, et al. Hypopituitarism in childhood and adolescence following traumatic brain injury: The case for prospective endocrine investigation. *Eur J Endocrinol* 2006;155:663–9.
2. Acerini CL, Tasker RC. Traumatic brain injury-induced hypothalamic-pituitary dysfunction: A paediatric perspective. *Pituitary* 2007 (in press).
3. Adams JH, Graham DI, Scott G, et al. Brain damage in fatal non missile head injury. *J Clin Pathol* 1980;33:1132–45.
4. Adams JH, Graham DI, Gennarelli TA. Contemporary neuropathological considerations regarding brain damage in head injury. In: Becker DP, Povlishock JT, eds. *Central Nervous System Trauma Status Report.* Washington, DC: National Institutes of Health, 1985:65–87.
5. Adams JH, Graham DI, Jennett B. The structural basis of moderate disability after traumatic brain damage. *J Neurol Neurosurg Psychiatry* 2001;71:521–4.
6. Adelson PD, Clyde B, Kochanek PM, et al. Cerebrovascular response in infants and young children following severe traumatic brain injury: A preliminary report. *Pediatr Neurosurg* 1997;26:200–7.
7. Adelson PD, Bratton SL, Carney NA, et al. Guidelines for the acute medical management of severe traumatic brain injury in infants, children, and adolescents: Prehospital airway management. *Pediatr Crit Care Med* 2003;4:S9–11.
8. Adelson PD, Bratton SL, Carney NA, et al. Guidelines for the acute medical management of severe traumatic brain injury in infants, children, and adolescents: Resuscitation of blood pressure and oxygenation and prehospital brain-specific therapies for the severe pediatric traumatic brain injury patient. *Pediatr Crit Care Med* 2003;4:S12–18.
9. Adelson PD, Bratton SL, Carney NA, et al. Guidelines for the acute medical management of severe traumatic brain injury in infants, children, and adolescents: Indications for intracranial pressure monitoring in pediatric patients with severe traumatic brain injury. *Pediatr Crit Care Med* 2003;4:S19–24.
10. Adelson PD, Bratton SL, Carney NA, et al. Guidelines for the acute medical management of severe traumatic brain injury in infants, children, and adolescents: Intracranial pressure monitoring technology. *Pediatr Crit Care Med* 2003;4:S28–30.
11. Adelson PD, Bratton SL, Carney NA, et al. Guidelines for the acute medical management of severe traumatic brain injury in infants, children, and adolescents: Cerebral perfusion pressure. *Pediatr Crit Care Med* 2003;4:S31–3.
12. Adelson PD, Bratton SL, Carney NA, et al. Guidelines for the acute medical management of severe traumatic brain injury in infants, children, and adolescents: Use of hyperventilation in the acute management of severe pediatric traumatic brain injury. *Pediatr Crit Care Med* 2003;4:S45–8.
13. Adelson PD, Bratton SL, Carney NA, et al. Guidelines for the acute medical management of severe traumatic brain injury in infants, children, and adolescents: Nutritional support. *Pediatr Crit Care Med* 2003;4:S68–71.
14. Agha A, Rogers B, Mylotte D, et al. Neuroendocrine dysfunction in the acute phase of traumatic brain injury. *Clin Endocrinol* 2004;60:584–91.
15. Agha A, Thornton E, O'Kelly P, et al. Posterior pituitary dysfunction after traumatic brain injury. *J Clin Endocrinol Metab* 2004;89:5987–92.
16. Agha A, Sherlock M, Phillips J, et al. The natural history of post-traumatic neurohypophysial dysfunction. *Eur J Endocrinol* 2005;152:371–7.
17. Agha A, Sherlock M, Phillips J, et al. The natural history of post-traumatic hypopituitarism: Implications for assessment and treatment. *Am J Med* 2005;118:1416.
18. Agha A, Thompson CJ. Anterior pituitary dysfunction following traumatic brain injury (TBI). *Clin Endocrinol* 2006;64:481–8.
19. American Academy of Pediatrics Committee on Child Abuse and Neglect. Shaken baby syndrome: Inflicted cerebral trauma. *Pediatrics* 1993;92:872–5.
20. American Spinal Injury Association. Available at: http://www.asia-spinalinjury.org/.
21. Augutis M, Abel R, Levi R. Pediatric spinal cord injury in a subset of European countries. *Spinal Cord* 2006;44:106–12.
22. Bailey DK. The normal cervical spine in infants and children. *Radiology* 1952;59:712–9.
23. Barlow KM, Minns RA. The relation between intracranial pressure and outcome in non-accidental head injury. *Dev Med Child Neurol* 1999;41:220–5.
24. Barlow KM, Minns RA. Annual incidence of shaken impact syndrome in young children. *Lancet* 2000;356:1571–2.
25. Barlow KM, Spowart JJ, Minns RA. Early posttraumatic seizures in non-accidental head injury: Relation to outcome. *Dev Med Child Neurol* 2000;42:591–4.
26. Barlow K, Thompson E, Johnson D, et al. The neurological outcome of non-accidental head injury. *Pediatr Rehabil* 2004;7:195–203.
27. Bartnik BL, Sutton RL, Fukushima M, et al. Upregulation of pentose phosphate pathway and preservation of tricarboxylic acid cycle flux after experimental brain injury. *J Neurotrauma* 2005;22:1052–65.
28. Berger RP, Adelson PD, Richichi R, et al. Serum biomarkers after traumatic and hypoxemic brain injuries: Insight into the biochemical response of the pediatric brain to inflicted brain injury. *Dev Neurosci* 2006;28:327–35.
29. Bergsneider M, Hovda DA, Shalmon E, et al. Cerebral hyperglycolysis following severe traumatic brain injury in humans: A positron emission tomography study. *J Neurosurg* 1997;86:241–51.
30. Berkenbosch JW, Lentz CW, Jimenez DF, et al. Cerebral salt wasting syndrome following brain injury in three pediatric patients: Suggestions for rapid diagnosis and therapy. *Pediatr Neurosurg* 2002;36:75–9.
31. Bernard SA, Gray TW, Buist MD, et al. Treatment of comatose survivors of out-of-hospital cardiac arrest with induced hypothermia. *N Engl J Med* 2002;346:557–63.
32. Berryhill P, Lilly MA, Levin HS, et al. Frontal lobe changes after severe diffuse closed head injury in children: A volumetric study of magnetic resonance imaging. *Neurosurgery* 1995;37:392–9.
33. Blatter DD, Bigler ED, Gale SD, et al. MR-based brain and cerebrospinal fluid measurement after traumatic brain injury: Correlation with neuropsychological outcome. *AJNR Am J Neuroradiol* 1997;18:1–10.
34. Block RW. Fillers. *Pediatrics* 2004;113:432–3.
35. Blumbergs PC, Scott G, Manavis J, et al. Staining of amyloid precursor protein to study axonal damage in mild head injury. *Lancet* 1994;344:1055–6.
36. Bonnier C, Nassogne MC, Evrard P. Outcome and prognosis of whiplash shaken infant syndrome: Late consequences after a symptom-free period. *Dev Med Child Neurol* 1995;37:943–56.
37. Bonnier C, Nassogne MC, Saint-Martin C, et al. Neuroimaging of intraparenchymal lesions predicts outcome in shaken baby syndrome. *Pediatrics* 2003;112:808–14.
38. Byard RW. *Sudden Death in Infancy, Childhood, and Adolescence,* 2nd ed. Cambridge: Cambridge University Press, 2004.

39. Carney NA, Chesnut R, Kochanek PM. Guidelines for the acute medical management of severe traumatic brain injury in infants, children, and adolescents: Prehospital airway management. *Pediatr Crit Care Med* 2003; 4:S9–11.

40. Centers for Disease Control and Prevention (CDC). Incidence rates of hospitalization related to traumatic brain injury—12 states, 2002. *MMWR Morb Mortal Wkly Rep* 2006;55:201–4.

41. Center for Drug evaluation and Research. Available at http://www.fda.gov/cder/pediatric/labelchange.htm. Accessed April 12, 2007.

42. Chambers IR, Treadwell L, Mendelow AD. Determination of threshold levels of cerebral perfusion pressure and intracranial pressure in severe head injury by using receiver-operating characteristic curves: An observational study in 291 patients. *J Neurosurg* 2001;94:412–6.

43. Chiaretti A, De Benedictis R, Polidori G, et al. Early post-traumatic seizures in children with head injury. *Childs Nerv Syst* 2000;16:862–6.

44. Cho DY, Wang YC. Decompressive craniectomy for acute shaken/impact baby syndrome. *Pediatric Neurosurg* 1996;24:292–8.

45. Clifton GL, Miller ER, Choi SC, et al. Lack of effect of induction of hypothermia after acute brain injury. *N Engl J Med* 2001;344:556–63.

46. Committee on Safety of Medicine Propofol-Diprivan infusion: Sedation in children aged 16 years or younger contraindicated. *CSM* 2001; 27:10.

47. Crawford TO, Mitchell WG, Fishman LS, et al. Very-high-dose phenobarbital for refractory status epilepticus in children. *Neurology* 1988;38: 1035–40.

48. Crompton MR. Hypothalamic lesions following closed head injury. *Brain* 1971;94:165–72.

49. Daniel PM, Prichard MM, Treip CS. Traumatic infarction of the anterior lobe of the pituitary gland. *Lancet* 1959;2:927–31.

50. Della Corte F, Mancini A, Valle D, et al. Provocative hypothalamopituitary axis tests in severe head injury: Correlations with severity and prognosis. *Crit Care Med* 1998;26:1419–26.

51. Dias MS. Traumatic brain and spinal cord injury. *Pediatr Clin N Am* 2004;51:271–303.

52. Downard C, Hulka F, Mullins RJ, et al. Relationship of cerebral perfusion pressure and survival in pediatric brain-injured patients. *J Trauma* 2000;49:654–58.

53. Duhaime AC, Christian CW, Rorke LB, et al. Nonaccidental head injury in infants—the "shaken-baby syndrome." *N Engl J Med* 1998;338:1822–9.

54. Durham SR, Clancy RR, Leuthardt E, et al. CHOP Infant Coma Scale ("Infant Face Scale"): A novel coma scale for children less than two years of age. *J Neurotrauma* 2000;17:729–37.

55. Eck JC, Nachtigall D, Humphreys SC. Questionnaire survey of spine surgeons on the use of methylprednisolone for acute spinal cord injury. *Spine* 2006;31:250–3.

56. Eisenberg HM, Frankowski RF, Contant CF, et al. High-dose barbiturate control of elevated intracranial pressure in patients with severe head injury. *J Neurosurg* 1988;69:15–23.

57. Engstrom M, Polito A, Reinstrup P, et al. Intracerebral microdialysis in severe brain trauma: The importance of catheter location. *J Neurosurg* 2005;102:460–9.

58. Esparza J, M-Portillo J, Sarabia M, et al. Outcome in children with severe head injuries. *Childs Nerv Syst* 1985;1:109–14.

59. Ewing-Cobbs L, Kramer L, Prasad M, et al. Neuroimaging, physical, and developmental findings after inflicted and noninflicted traumatic brain injury in young children. *Pediatrics* 1998;102:300–7.

60. Fabricius M, Fuhr S, Bhatia R, et al. Cortical spreading depression and peri-infarct depolarization in acutely injured human cerebral cortex. *Brain* 2006;129:778–90.

61. Feickert HJ, Drommer S, Heyer R. Severe head injury in children: Impact of risk factors on outcome. *J Trauma* 1999;47:33–38.

62. Frank Y, Zimmerman R, Leeds NMD. Neurological manifestations in abused children who have been shaken. *Dev Med Child Neurol* 1985;27: 312–6.

63. Garnett MR, Blamire AM, Rajagopalan B, et al. Evidence for cellular damage in normal-appearing white matter correlates with injury severity in patients following traumatic brain injury: A magnetic resonance spectroscopy study. *Brain* 2000;123:1403–9.

64. Geddes JF, Hackshaw AK, Vowles GH, et al. Neuropathology of inflicted head injury in children. I. Patterns of brain damage. *Brain* 2001;124: 1290–8.

65. Geddes JF, Vowles GH, Hackshaw AK, et al. Neuropathology of inflicted head injury in children. II. Microscopic brain injury in infants. *Brain* 2001;124:1299–1306.

66. Geddes JF, Tasker RC, Hackshaw AK, et al. Dural haemorrhage in nontraumatic infant deaths: Does it explain the bleeding in "shaken baby syndrome"? *Neuropath Applied Neurobiol* 2003;29:14–22.

67. Geddes JF, Tasker RC, Adams GGW, et al. Violence is not necessary to produce subdural and retinal haemorrhage: A reply to Punt et al. *Pediatr Rehabil* 2004;7:261–5.

68. Gedeit R. Head injury. *Pediatr Rev* 2001;22:118–24.

69. Gentry LR, Godersky JC, Thompson B. MR imaging of head trauma: Review of the distribution and radiopathologic features of traumatic lesions. *AJR Am J Roentgenol* 1988;150:663–72.

70. Ghatan S, Ellenbogen RG. Pediatric spine and spinal cord injury after inflicted trauma. *Neurosurg Clin N am* 2002;13:227–33.

71. Gilles EE, Nelson MD. Cerebral complications of nonaccidental head injury in childhood. *Pediatr Neurol* 1998;19:119–28.

72. Gluckman PD, Wyatt JS, Azzopardi D, et al. Selective head cooling with mild systemic hypothermia after neonatal encephalopathy: Multicentre randomised trial. *Lancet* 2005;365:663–70.

73. Gorrie C, Oakes S, Duflou J, et al. Axonal injury in children after motor vehicle crashes: Extent, distribution, and size of axonal swellings using beta-APP immunohistochemistry. *J Neurotrauma* 2002;19:1171–82.

74. Grados MA, Slomine BS, Gerring JP, et al. Depth of lesion model in children and adolescents with moderate to severe traumatic brain injury: Use of SPGR MRI to predict severity and outcome. *J Neurol Neurosurg Psychiatry* 2001;70:350–58.

75. Graham DI, Ford I, Adams JH, et al. Fatal head injury in children. *J Clin Pathol* 1989;42:18–22.

76. Graham DI. Hypoxia and vascular factors. In: Adams JH, Duchen LW, eds. *Greenfield's Neuropathology*, 5th ed. London: Edward Arnold, 1992: 153–268.

77. Hachen HJ. Spinal cord injury in children and adolescents: Diagnostic pitfalls and therapeutic considerations in the acute stage. *Paraplegia* 1977;15:55–64.

78. Hadley MN. Radiographic assessment of the cervical spine in asymptomatic trauma patients. *Neurosurgery* 2002;50:S30–5.

79. Hamilton MG, Myles ST. Pediatric spinal injury: Review of 174 hospital admissions. *J Neurosurg* 1992;77:700–4.

80. Harper CG, Doyle D, Adams JH, et al. Analysis of abnormalities in pituitary gland in non-missile head injury: Study of 100 consecutive cases. *J Clin Pathol* 1986;39:769–73.

81. Heffez DS, Ducker TB. Fractures and dislocations of the pediatric spine. In: Pang D, ed. *Disorders of the Pediatric Spine*. New York: Raven Press, 1995:517–29.

82. Hillered L, Persson L, Nilsson P, et al. Continuous monitoring of cerebral metabolism in traumatic brain injury: A focus on cerebral microdialysis. *Curr Opin Crit Care* 2006;12:112–8.

83. Hirsch W, Beck R, Behrmann C, et al. Reliability of cranial CT versus intracerebral pressure measurement for the evaluation of generalized cerebral oedema in children. *Pediatr Radiol* 2000;30:439–43.

84. Hlatky R, Valadka AB, Goodman JC, et al. Patterns of energy substrates during ischemia measured in the brain by microdialysis. *J Neurotrauma* 2004;21:894–906.

85. Hobbs CJ, Hanks HGI, Wynne JM. *Child Abuse and Neglect: A Clinician's Handbook*, 2nd ed. New York: Churchill Livingstone Inc., 2000.

86. Holbourn AHS. Mechanics of head injuries. *Lancet* 1943;2:438–441.

87. Holbourn AHS. The mechanics of brain injuries. *Br Med Bull* 1945;3: 147–9.

88. Hosalkar HS, Cain EL, Horn D, et al. Traumatic atlanto-occipital dislocation in children. *J Bone Joint Surg Am* 2005;87:2480–8.

89. Hypothermia after Cardiac Arrest Study Group: Mild therapeutic hypothermia to improve the neurologic outcome after cardiac arrest. *N Engl J Med* 2002;346:549–56.

90. Jackson S, Piper IR, Wagstaff A, et al. A study of the effects of using different cerebral perfusion pressure (CPP) thresholds to quantify CPP "secondary insults" in children. *Acta Neurochir Suppl* 2000;76:453–6.

91. Jennett B, Teasdale G. Trauma as a cause of epilepsy in childhood. *Dev Med Child Neurol* 1973;15:56–72.

92. Kairys SW, Alexander RC, Block RW, et al. American Academy of Pediatrics. Committee on Child Abuse and Neglect and Committee on Community Health Services. Investigation and review of unexpected infant and child deaths. *Pediatrics* 1999;104:1158–60.

93. Kanter MJ, Narayan RK. Intracranial pressure monitoring. *Neurosurg Clin N Am* 1991;2:257–65.

94. Kawamata T, Katayama Y, Hovda DA, et al. Lactate accumulation following concussive brain injury: The role of ionic fluxes induced by excitatory amino acids. *Brain Res* 1995;674:196–204.

95. Keenan HT, Runyan DK, Marshall SW, et al. A population-based study of inflicted traumatic brain injury in young children. *JAMA* 2003;290:621–6.

96. Keenan HT, Nocera MA, Bratton SL. Frequency of intracranial pressure monitoring in infants and young toddlers with traumatic brain injury. *Pediatr Crit Care Med* 2005;6:537–41.

97. Keenan HT, Runyan DK, Nocera M. Longitudinal follow-up of families and young children with traumatic brain injury. *Pediatrics.* 2006;117:1291–7.

98. Kemp AM. Investigating subdural haemorrhage in infants. *Arch Dis Child* 2002;86:98–102.

99. Kett-White R, Hutchinson PJ, Czosnyka M, et al. Effects of variation in cerebral haemodynamics during aneurysm surgery on brain tissue oxygen and metabolism. *Acta Neurochir Suppl* 2002;81:327–9.

100. Kett-White R, Hutchinson PJ, Al Rawi PG, et al. Extracellular lactate/pyruvate and glutamate changes in patients during preoperative episodes of cerebral ischaemia. *Acta Neurochir Suppl* 2002;81:363–5.

101. Khanna S, Davis D, Peterson B, et al. Use of hypertonic saline in the treatment of severe refractory posttraumatic intracranial hypertension in pediatric traumatic brain injury. *Crit Care Med* 2000;28:1144–51.

102. Kochanek PM, Clark RS, Ruppel RA, et al. Biochemical, cellular, and

molecular mechanisms in the evolution of secondary damage after severe traumatic brain injury in infants and children: Lessons learned from the bedside. *Pediatr Crit Care Med* 2000;1:4–19.

103. Kochanek PM, Forbes ML, Ruppel R, et al. Severe traumatic brain injury in infants and children. In: Fuhrman BP, Zimmerman J, eds. *Pediatric Critical Care*, 3rd ed. 2006;1595–617.

104. Koul R, Chacko A, Javed H, et al. Eight-year study of childhood status epilepticus: Midazolam infusion in management and outcome. *J Child Neurol* 2002;17:908–10.

105. Landolt H, Langemann H, Mendelowitsch A, et al. Neurochemical monitoring and on-line pH measurements using brain microdialysis in patients in intensive care. *Acta Neurochir* 1994;60:475–8.

106. Lang DA, Teasdale GM, Macpherson P, et al. Diffuse brain swelling after head injury: More often malignant in adults than children? *J Neurosurg* 1994;80:675–80.

107. Langemann H, Alessandri B, Mendelowitsch A, et al. Extracellular levels of glucose and lactate measured by quantitative microdialysis in the human brain. *Neurol Res* 2001;23:531–6.

108. Launay F, Leet AI, Sponseller PD. Pediatric spinal cord without radiographic abnormality: A meta-analysis. *Clin Orthop Relat Res* 2005;433:166–70.

109. Levin HS, Benavidez DA, Verger-Maestre K, et al. Reduction of corpus callosum growth after severe traumatic brain injury in children. *Neurology* 2000;54:647–53.

110. Levy DI, Rekate HL, Cherny WB, et al. Controlled lumbar drainage in pediatric head injury. *J Neurosurg* 1995;83:453–60.

111. Lo TY, McPhillips M, Minns RA, et al. Cerebral atrophy following shaken impact syndrome and other non-accidental head injury (NAHI). *Pediatr Rehabil* 2003;6:47–55.

112. MacKenzie JD, Siddiqi F, Babb JS, et al. Brain atrophy in mild or moderate traumatic brain injury: A longitudinal quantitative analysis. *AJNR Am J Neuroradiol* 2002;23:1509–15.

113. McCarthy ML, MacKenzie EJ, Durbin DR, et al. Health-related quality of life during the first year after traumatic brain injury. *Arch Pediatr Adolesc Med.* 2006;160:252–20.

114. Mendelsohn D, Levin HS, Bruce D, et al. Late MRI after head injury in children: Relationship to clinical features and outcome. *Childs Nerv Syst* 1992;8:445–52.

115. Meyer PG, Meyer F, Orliaguet G, et al. Combined high cervical spine and brain stem injuries: A complex and devastating injury in children. *J Pediatr Surg* 2005;40:1637–42.

116. Miller WL, Kaplan SL, Grumbach MM. Child abuse as a cause of post-traumatic hypopituitarism. *N Engl J Med* 1980;302:724–8.

117. Miller M, Leestma J, Barnes P, et al. A sojourn in the abyss: Hypothesis, theory, and established truth in infant head injury. *Pediatrics* 2004;114:326.

118. Morris KP, Forsyth RJ, Parslow RC, et al. Intracranial pressure complicating severe traumatic brain injury in children: Monitoring and management. *Intensive Care Med* 2006;32:1606–12.

119. Munro D. Cerebrospinal fluid pressure in the newborn. *JAMA* 1928;90:1688–9.

120. Natale JE, Joseph JG, Helfaer MA, et al. Early hyperthermia after traumatic brain injury in children: Risk factors, influence on length of stay, and effect on short-term neurologic status. *Crit Care Med* 2000;28:2608–15.

121. Nesathurai S. Steroids and spinal cord injury: Revisiting the NASCIS 2 and NASCIS 3 trials. *J Trauma* 1998;45:1088–93.

122. Ng T, Graham DI, Adams JH, et al. Changes in the hippocampus and the cerebellum resulting from hypoxic insults: Frequency and distribution. *Acta Neuropathol* 1989;78:438–43.

123. Oliver JE. Microcephaly following baby battering and shaking. *Br Med J* 1975;2:262–4.

124. Onuma T, Shimosegawa Y, Kameyama M, et al. Clinicopathological investigation of gyral high density on computerized tomography following severe head injury in children. *J Neurosurg* 1995;82:995–1001.

125. Ozdemir D, Gulez P, Uran N, et al. Efficacy of continuous midazolam infusion and mortality in childhood refractory generalized convulsive status epilepticus. *Seizure* 2005;14:129–32.

126. Pang D, Wilberger JE. Spinal cord injury without radiographic abnormalities in children. *J Neurosurg* 1982;57:114–29.

127. Pang D, Pollack IF. Spinal cord injury without radiographic abnormality in children—the SCIWORA syndrome. *J Trauma* 1989;29:654–64.

128. Pang D. Spinal cord injury without radiographic abnormality in children, 2 decades later. *Neurosurgery* 2004;55:1342–3.

129. Parslow RC, Morris KP, Tasker RC, et al. Epidemiology of traumatic brain injury in children receiving intensive care in the UK. *Arch Dis Child* 2005;90:1182–7.

130. Persson L, Valtysson J, Enblad P, et al. Neurochemical monitoring using intracerebral microdialysis in patients with subarachnoid hemorrhage. *J Neurosurg* 1996;84:606–16.

131. Peterson B, Khanna S, Fisher B, et al. Prolonged hypernatremia controls elevated intracranial pressure in head-injured pediatric patients. *Crit Care Med* 2000;28:1136–43.

132. Pfenninger J, Kaiser G, Lutschg J, et al. Treatment and outcome of the severely head injured child. *Intensive Care Med* 1983;9:13–6.

133. Popovic V, Aimaretti G, Casanueva FF, et al. Hypopituitarism following traumatic brain injury. *Growth Horm IGF Res* 2005;15:177–84.

134. Prayer L, Wimberger D, Oder W, et al. Cranial MR imaging and cerebral 99mTc HM-PAO-SPECT in patients with subacute or chronic severe closed head injury and normal CT examinations. *Acta Radiol* 1993;34:593–9.

135. Punt J, Bonshek RE, Jaspan T, et al. The "unified hypothesis" of Geddes et al. is not supported by the data. *Pediatric Rehabilitation* 2004;7:173–84.

136. Rao P, Carty H, Pierce A. The acute reversal sign: Comparison of medical and non-accidental injury patients. *Clin Radiol* 1999;54:495–501.

137. Royal College of Paediatrics and Child Health working group on sudden unexpected death in infancy. RCPCH, 2004.

138. Schierhout G, Roberts I. Prophylactic antiepileptic agents after head injury: A systematic review. *J Neurol Neurosurg Psychiatry* 1998;64:108–12.

139. Segal S, Gallagher AC, Shefler AG, et al. Survey of the use of intracranial pressure monitoring in children in the United Kingdom. *Intensive Care Med* 2001;27:236–9.

140. Shannon P, Smith CR, Deck J, et al. Axonal injury and the neuropathology of shaken baby syndrome. *Acta Neuropathol* 1998;95:625–31.

141. Shapiro K, Marmarou A. Clinical applications of the pressure-volume index in treatment of pediatric head injuries. *J Neurosurg* 1982;56:819–25.

142. Sharples PM, Stuart AG, Matthews DSF, et al. Cerebral blood flow and metabolism in children with severe head injury. Part 1: Relation to age, Glasgow coma score, outcome, intracranial pressure, and time after injury. *J Neurol Neurosurg Psychiatry* 1995;58:145–52.

143. Shore PM, Hand LL, Roy L, et al. Reliability and validity of the pediatric intensity level of therapy (PILOT) scale: A measure of the use of intracranial pressure-directed therapies. *Crit Care Med* 2006;34:1981–7.

144. Suh DY, Davis PC, Hopkins KL, et al. Nonaccidental pediatric head injury: Diffusion-weighted imaging findings. *Neurosurgery* 2001;49:309–18.

145. Suz P, Vavilala MS, Souter M, et al. Clinical features of fever associated with poor outcome in severe pediatric traumatic brain injury. *J Neurosurg Anesthesiol* 2006;18:5–10.

146. Tanriverdi F, Senyurek H, Unluhizarci K, et al. High risk of hypopituitarism after traumatic brain injury: A prospective investigation of anterior pituitary function in the acute phase and 12 months after trauma. *J Clin Endocrinol Metab* 2006;91:2105–11.

147. Tasker RC, Boyd SG, Harden A, et al. EEG monitoring of prolonged thiopentone administration for intractable seizures and status epilepticus in infants and young children. *Neuropediatrics* 1989;20:147–53.

148. Tasker RC, Boyd SG, Harden A, et al. The clinical significance of seizures in critically ill young infants. *Neuropediatrics* 1991;22:129–38.

149. Tasker RC. Hippocampal selective regional vulnerability and development. *Dev Med Child Neurol* 2001;86:S6–7.

150. Tasker RC, Salmond CH, Gunn Westland A, et al. Head circumference and brain and hippocampal volume after severe traumatic brain injury in childhood. *Pediatr Res* 2005;58:302–8.

151. Taylor A, Butt W, Rosenfeld J, et al. A randomized trial of very early decompressive craniectomy in children with traumatic brain injury and sustained intracranial hypertension. *Childs Nerv Syst* 2001;17:154–62.

152. Thibault KL, Margulies SS. Age-dependent material properties of the porcine cerebrum: Effect on pediatric inertial head injury criteria. *J Biomech* 1998;31:1119–26.

153. Tomita H, Ito U, Saito J, et al. Cerebral atrophy after severe head injury. *Adv Neurol* 1990;52:553.

154. Van den Berghe G, Schoonheydt K, Beck P, et al. Insulin therapy protects the central and peripheral nervous system of intensive care patients. *Neurology* 2005;64:1348–53.

155. Verweij BH, Muizelaar JP, Vinas FC, et al. Impaired cerebral mitochondrial function after traumatic brain injury in humans. *J Neurosurg* 2000;93:815–20.

156. Vespa P, McArthur D, Glenn T, et al. Persistently low extracellular glucose correlates with poor outcome at 6 months after traumatic brain injury despite lack of increased lactate: A microdialysis study. *J Cereb Blood Flow Metab* 2003;23:865–77.

157. Vespa P, Bergsneider M, Hattori N, et al. Metabolic crisis without brain ischemia is common after traumatic brain injury: A combined microdialysis and positron emission tomography study. *J Cereb Blood Flow Metab* 2005;25:763–74.

158. Vespa P, Boonyaputthikul R, McArthur DL, et al. Intensive insulin therapy reduces microdialysis glucose values without altering glucose utilization or improving the lactate/pyruvate ration after traumatic brain injury. *Crit Care Med* 2006;34:850–6.

159. Vinjamuri S, O'Driscoll K. Significance of white matter abnormalities in patients with closed head injury. *Nucl Med Commun* 2000;21:645–9.

160. Welch K. The intracranial pressure in infants. *J Neurosurg* 1980;52:693–9.

161. White JR, Farukhi Z, Bull C, et al. Predictors of outcome in severely head-injured children. *Crit Care Med* 2001;29:534–40.

162. Wilde EA, Hunter JV, Newsome MR, et al. Frontal and temporal morphometric findings on MRI in children after moderate to severe traumatic brain injury. *J Neurotrauma* 2005;22:333–44.

163. Woolf PD. Hormonal responses to trauma. *Crit Care Med* 1992;20:216–26.

164. Yoshino A, Hovda DA, Kawamata T, et al. Dynamic changes in local cerebral glucose utilization following cerebral concussion in rats: Evidence of a hyper- and subsequent hypometabolic state. *Brain Res* 1991;561:106–19.

CHAPTER 57 ■ STATUS EPILEPTICUS

KIMBERLY D. STATLER • COLIN B. VAN ORMAN

Status epilepticus (SE) is a medical emergency of varied etiologies that requires prompt recognition and intervention. Children with prolonged seizures are at risk for brain injury and respiratory or hemodynamic compromise due to both prolonged convulsions and high anticonvulsant dosing. They may even suffer multiorgan dysfunction. Consequently, the pediatric intensivist must be familiar with the clinical presentation, causal pathophysiology, necessary clinical evaluation, potential complications, and goal-directed therapy of SE in infants and children.

DEFINITION

SE is classically defined as seizure activity, either continuous or episodic, without complete recovery of consciousness, that lasts for at least 30 mins. The evolution of SE can be conceptualized in stages (13,53): (a) *premonitory* or *prodromal SE*, characterized by an increasing frequency of serial seizures with recovery of consciousness between episodes; (b) *incipient SE*, defined as continuous or intermittent seizures that last up to 5 mins without full recovery of consciousness; (c) *impending* or *early SE*, marked by seizure activity that persists 5–30 mins; and (d) *established SE*, defined as seizures that last longer than 30 mins. When SE lasts longer than 30–60 mins, *subtle SE* usually develops. Subtle SE is characterized by progressive electromechanical dissociation, in which clinical signs diminish yet electroencephalographic (EEG) seizure activity persists. Finally, nonconvulsive SE (NCSE) refers to ongoing EEG seizure activity without associated clinical signs.

An operational treatment definition advocates defining SE as seizure activity that lasts longer than 5 mins, corresponding to initiation of therapy during impending or early SE. This operational definition is prudent, given that prompt intervention is crucial. In children, unprovoked, afebrile seizures typically last less than 4 mins, and seizures that last longer than 5 min are unlikely to remit spontaneously (51). Additionally, prolonged SE is associated with development of pharmacologic resistance and worse outcome (23). Indeed, children with SE that lasts longer than 30 mins are less likely to respond to anticonvulsants (23). Consequently, treatment recommendations in this chapter will be based on a definition of SE as either continuous or intermittent seizure activity that lasts at least 5 min without full recovery of consciousness.

CLASSIFICATION

SE is commonly classified by seizure type. For the purpose of the pediatric intensivist, SE can be considered as convulsive or nonconvulsive (**Table 57.1**). Additionally, the pediatric inten-

sivist should be familiar with the characteristics of *refractory SE* (RSE) and *neonatal SE*.

Generalized Convulsive Status Epilepticus

Generalized convulsive SE (GCSE) constitutes 73%–98% of pediatric SE (54) and is characterized by tonic, clonic, or tonic-clonic seizure activity that involves all extremities. In primary GCSE, seizure onset cannot be localized to one brain region by either clinical or EEG findings. In secondary GCSE, which is more common, seizures begin focally but spread to involve the entire brain. Early in the course, focal signs may persist on EEG; however, during prolonged GCSE, distinguishing secondary from primary GCSE often becomes difficult.

Focal motor SE, also called *simple complex SE*, *somato-motor SE*, or *epilepsy partialis continua*, is characterized by involvement of a single limb or side of the face. Focal motor SE is less common than GCSE and is frequently associated with focal brain pathology (**Table 57.2**).

Myoclonic SE is characterized by irregular, asynchronous, small-amplitude, repetitive myoclonic jerking of the face or limbs. Myoclonic SE is more common in comatose patients and is associated with several specific conditions, particularly anoxia or cardiac arrest (**Table 57.3**).

Nonconvulsive Status Epilepticus

NCSE is characterized by continuous nonmotor seizures and requires EEG confirmation for diagnosis. NCSE may occur in ambulatory or comatose patients. The most common type of NCSE in ambulatory children is *absence SE*, which is characterized by altered consciousness and a generalized 3-Hz symmetric spike-and-wave pattern on EEG. In contrast, *complex partial SE* in ambulatory patients is marked by altered consciousness and focal activity on EEG, usually involving the temporal lobe. In comatose patients, NCSE may be difficult to diagnose and should be considered in any patient with prolonged obtundation after seizure cessation or with coma of unclear etiology (17,21).

The diagnosis of NCSE in critically ill patients requires a high degree of suspicion and is probably under-recognized. Among critically ill patients who underwent continuous EEG monitoring for unexplained alterations in consciousness, 10% demonstrated NCSE (17). In this cohort, risk factors for NCSE included age <18 years, coma, convulsive seizures prior to EEG monitoring, and a history of epilepsy (17). Although the incidence of NCSE among critically ill children has not been well characterized, retrospective series document nonconvulsive seizures in 16% of PICU patients who were

TABLE 57.1

CLASSIFICATION OF STATUS EPILEPTICUS

Convulsive	Nonconvulsive
Generalized convulsive	Absence
Focal motor	Complex partial
Myoclonic	NCSE with coma
NCSE, nonconvulsive status epilepticus	

admitted with unexplained alterations in consciousness (46) and NCSE in 33% of children treated for SE (57). Nonconvulsive seizures and NCSE are more common among younger children, particularly those 1 month to 1 year of age, and are frequently associated with structural lesions (e.g., infarction, subdural hematoma, or intracerebral hemorrhage), anoxic injury, and acute infections (e.g., meningitis or encephalitis) (46,57). Although NCSE and nonconvulsive seizures occur in children with preexisting cerebral insults and epilepsy, over 40% of children with nonconvulsive seizures are previously healthy (46).

Refractory Status Epilepticus

SE of any classification that fails to remit despite treatment with adequate doses of two anticonvulsants is termed refractory SE (13). RSE develops in 30%–40% of adult patients and is associated with greater mortality than is more responsive SE (34,45). In children, 10%–25% of SE becomes refractory (14,23). Mortality for pediatric RSE is 20%–30%, and over 50% of survivors have neurologic sequelae (43,44). Almost half (46%) of neonates with SE develop RSE, and only 10% have good neurodevelopmental outcomes at 1 year of age (11).

TABLE 57.2

COMMON ETIOLOGIES OF FOCAL MOTOR STATUS EPILEPTICUS

Brain tumor
  Astrocytoma
  Oligodendroglioma
  Glioblastoma
Infection
  Brain abscess
  Viral encephalitis
  Cysticercosis
  Tuberculosis
Vascular
  Cortical vein thrombosis
  Arteriovenous malformation
  Cerebrovascular accident
Trauma
  Post traumatic cyst
  Chronic subdural hematoma
  Focal gliosis

TABLE 57.3

COMMON ETIOLOGIES OF MYOCLONIC STATUS EPILEPTICUS

Anoxic injury
  Cardiac arrest
  Cardiopulmonary bypass
  Carbon monoxide poisoning
  CO_2 narcosis
Infection
  Viral encephalitis
  Acute demyelinating encephalomyelitis
  Subacute sclerosing panencephalitis
  Opportunistic infection
Injury
  Heat stroke
  Lightning strike
  Intracranial hemorrhage
Metabolic
  Hepatic failure
  Renal failure
  Hypoglycemia
  Hyponatremia
  Nonketotic hyperglycemia
  Thiamine deficiency
Toxins
  Tricyclic antidepressants
  Anticonvulsants
  β-Lactam antibiotics
  Opiates
  Lithium
  Heavy-metal poisoning
Genetic/epilepsy syndromes
  Juvenile myoclonic epilepsy
  Lennox-Gastaut syndrome
  Absence epilepsy
  Degenerative myoclonus epilepsy
  Angelman syndrome

Neonatal Status Epilepticus

SE presents differently in neonates than in older infants and children. Neonates are unlikely to demonstrate GCSE or continuous seizure activity; however, frequent, serial seizures without recovery of consciousness can occur. Neonatal seizures are frequently poorly organized and polymorphic and may involve rapid extensor or flexor posturing, tremor of extended extremities, apnea, eye deviation, or automatisms (43,53). Because of such atypical manifestations, most types of bizarre or unusual transient events in the neonatal period may be seizures, particularly if they are stereotypic, insensitive to stimuli, unaltered by restraint or limb displacement, and recur periodically. Neonatal SE is difficult to diagnose, and both clinical and EEG criteria are often required (43). Conditions commonly associated with neonatal SE are presented in **Table 57.4.**

EPIDEMIOLOGY

Using the classic definition of continuous or intermittent seizure activity that lasts at least 30 mins without recovery of consciousness, reported incidences for SE in children aged 1 month

COMMON ETIOLOGIES OF NEONATAL STATUS EPILEPTICUS

Perinatal or acute insults
  Hypoxia-ischemia
  Intracranial hemorrhage
  Cerebral vascular accident
Infection
  Meningitis
  Encephalitis
  Abscess
Metabolic
  Hypoglycemia
  Hypocalcemia
  Hyponatremia
  Hypomagnesemia
  Bilirubin encephalopathy
Inborn errors of metabolism
  Phenylketonuria
  Nonketotic hyperglycemia
  Pyridoxine deficiency
  Histidinemia
  Hyperammonemia
  Homocitrullinemia
  Maple syrup urine disease
  Leucine-sensitive hypoglycemia
Toxins
  β-Lactam antibiotics
  Anesthetics
  Drug withdrawal
  Heavy-metal poisoning
Cerebral malformations
  Neuronal migration defect
  Neurocutaneous syndrome
Degenerative diseases
  Leigh encephalopathy
  Leukodystrophies
  Alpers disease
  Sandhoff disease
  Tay-Sachs disease
Benign familial syndromes
  Benign familial neonatal seizures
  Benign neonatal sleep myoclonus

to 16 years are 17–38 per 100,000 individuals per year (14,19,23). More than 40% of pediatric SE occurs in children <2 years of age (52). Reported age-specific incidences for SE are 51 per 100,000 for children <1 year of age, 29 per 100,000 for those 1–4 years old, 9 per 100,000 for those 5–9 years old, and 2 per 100,000 for those 10–15 year old (14). Racial influences may be important in SE, with a greater incidence in nonwhites than whites (19). Although mortality due to SE has decreased with improved supportive care, pediatric SE remains a medical emergency with overall mortality rates of 3%–7.2% (14,30,44).

Twenty-five percent to 40% of pediatric SE occurs in children with known epilepsy (4). In other words, 9.5%–27% of children with epilepsy will experience at least one episode of SE (7,54). Risk factors for SE in epileptic children include epilepsy induced by a known neurologic insult (symptomatic epilepsy) and previous episodes of SE (7). Other associated factors include use of multiple anticonvulsant medications, psy-

chomotor retardation, generalized background abnormalities on EEG, and tapering of anticonvulsant medications. That being said, 60% of SE episodes among epileptic children occur despite therapeutic anticonvulsant drug levels and without any identifiable inciting event, such as fever or concurrent illness (35).

Conversely, over half of SE occurs in patients without a prior diagnosis of epilepsy. In fact, 12% of children with new-onset unprovoked seizures present with SE (51,54). SE as the presentation of new-onset seizures is more common in younger children (52). Importantly, 17% of children with new-onset SE have associated, treatable inciting events, such as electrolyte abnormalities or central nervous system (CNS) infections (14).

Recurrent SE occurs in ~13%–55% of pediatric patients, usually within 2 years of the first SE episode (6,14,44,54). The median interval between the first episode and recurrence is 25 days (range, 0–463 days) (14). Risk factors for recurrent SE are age <6 years, focal seizures, and an acute or remote CNS injury (44,54). In fact, children with a preexisting neurologic abnormality are 3–24 times more likely than previously healthy children to experience recurrence (14,44).

No population-based data are available to estimate the incidence of neonatal SE. Seizure type and brain maturation are influenced by gestational age, and studies suggest that neonatal SE is more common in full-term than preterm infants (43). In neonates with asphyxial injury, the duration of seizures has been "independently associated with brain injury" (43), emphasizing the need for prompt recognition and treatment in neonates.

COMMON ETIOLOGIES

Although initial supportive and anticonvulsant therapies are similar regardless of cause, diagnostic tests and adjunctive treatments are guided by suspected etiology. The etiologies of SE are commonly classified as cryptogenic, remote symptomatic, febrile, acute symptomatic, or progressive encephalopathic (**Table 57.5**) (52). Etiologies for pediatric SE vary by report: 30%–50% febrile, 24%–28% remote symptomatic, 8%–28% acute symptomatic, 15% cryptogenic, and 1%–5% progressive encephalopathies (5,52). The etiology of pediatric SE is age dependent (52), and variations likely reflect different age distributions or sampling biases of the studies.

Febrile or acute symptomatic etiologies are most common in younger children and account for over 80% of SE among children <2 years of age (52). Two-thirds of episodes during the second year of life are due to febrile SE (52). In some cohorts, febrile SE continues to be a common etiology among children >3 years of age (5). However, cryptogenic and remote symptomatic etiologies account for more than 60% of SE in children >4 years of age (52). Tapering or withdrawal of anticonvulsant medications is a common inciting event among older children (30).

Central nervous system infection, metabolic abnormalities, traumatic brain injury, and anoxic brain injury are the most common specific etiologies of acute symptomatic pediatric SE (52). Other common inciting events are listed in **Table 57.6**. Meningitis is more frequent in infants. Anoxia is more common in children <5 years old. Among children who present with new-onset SE and fever, 12% have acute bacterial meningitis,

TABLE 57.5

ETIOLOGIC CLASSIFICATION OF STATUS EPILEPTICUS

Etiology	Definition
Cryptogenic (idiopathic)	Status epilepticus in the absence of an acute precipitating CNS insult or metabolic dysfunction in a patient without a preexisting neurologic abnormality
Remote symptomatic	Status epilepticus in a patient with a known history of a neurologic insult associated with an increased risk of seizures (e.g., traumatic brain injury, stroke, static encephalopathy)
Febrile	Status epilepticus provoked solely by fever in a patient without a history of afebrile seizures
Acute symptomatic	Status epilepticus during an acute illness involving a known neurologic insult (e.g., meningitis, traumatic brain injury, hypoxia) or metabolic dysfunction (e.g., hypoglycemia, hypocalcemia, hyponatremia)
Progressive encephalopathy	Status epilepticus in a patient with a progressive neurologic disease (e.g., neurodegeneration, malignancies, neurocutaneous syndromes)

Adapted from Shinnar S, Pellock JM, Moshe SL, et al. In whom does status epilepticus occur: Age-related differences in children. *Epilepsia* 1997;38:907–14.

and 8% have viral CNS infections (14). Hypoxic-ischemic injury is the most prevalent cause of neonatal SE in developed countries, but electrolyte abnormalities continue to be more common in developing regions (43).

MECHANISM OF DISEASE

The mechanisms of SE and the relationship between seizure activity, neuronal injury, and functional outcome are multifactorial and complex. Isolating the specific effects of seizures from those of underlying etiology and associated systemic influences remains difficult. Much of the current understanding of pathogenesis has been gleaned from experimental models. In many instances, experimental findings have been confirmed in patients with epilepsy.

Laboratory Models and Experimental Data

Experimental models of SE commonly use chemical convulsants or electrical stimulation to induce self-sustaining seizures. These models provide insight into the mechanisms of seizure initiation, propagation, and termination, as well as patterns of cerebral development that affect seizure development and SE.

Behavioral and Electroencephalographic Manifestations

The progression of both clinical and experimental convulsive status epilepticus (CSE) may be divided into five stages (60). The first stage is characterized by discrete seizures, which are typically focal with secondary generalization and manifest as generalized tonic-clonic convulsions. With time, the discrete seizures merge to produce an EEG pattern of asymmetric sharp and spike waves with waxing and waning amplitude accompanied by either generalized convulsions or serial tonic or clonic seizures involving one or more extremities. The third stage is characterized by continuous EEG seizure discharges and either clonic jerks or subtle clonic convulsive activity. In the fourth stage, flat periods of EEG activity interrupt continuous seizure discharges, and behavioral clonic convulsions may be overt, subtle, or absent. During the fifth stage, the EEG shows monomorphic, repetitive, sharp waves, called *periodic lateralized epileptiform discharges* (PLEDS), on a flat background, and accompanying motor manifestations are absent. In the immature (vs. the adult) brain, the EEG progression through all five stages is less consistent and behavioral manifestations less discrete (40). Treatment with anticonvulsants can interrupt both EEG and behavioral progression of SE.

Seizure Initiation and Progression

Seizure initiation and propagation involve a failure of γ-aminobutyric-acid (GABA)-mediated inhibition and/or an increase in glutamate-mediated excitation. A seizure begins with an intrinsically firing neuron, which, facilitated by inadequate inhibition, recruits adjacent neurons (71). Aberrant neuronal excitation commonly originates near regions of cerebral injury or scarring but may arise from uninjured neurons (12). As adjacent neurons begin firing, excitatory mediators, including glutamate, are released. Glutamate activates N-methyl-D-aspartate (NMDA) receptors and is thought to facilitate local neuronal synchronization, as well as seizure spread. In experimental models, NMDA antagonists block seizure progression (20).

The mechanisms that enable the self-sustained seizures necessary for SE remain poorly understood. Localized "feed-forward" excitatory circuits are identified in experimental models of self-sustaining hippocampal seizures (53). Aberrant excitatory circuits created by injury-induced axonal sprouting are associated with neuronal hyperexcitability and acquired epilepsy (12). The pathogenic contribution of such excitatory circuits to SE remains controversial, but they are unlikely to be a sufficient cause.

Other putative mechanisms that promote self-sustaining seizures include a reduction of inhibitory interneuron activity (12) and receptor trafficking changes that favor excitability (13). In seizure models, synaptic GABA$_A$ receptors are downregulated, whereas NMDA receptors are upregulated, promoting neuronal excitability (13). These seizure-induced alterations of GABA and glutamate activity may facilitate seizure continuation and spread, as well as hinder seizure termination.

A predominance of inhibition is required for seizure termination and may be achieved by augmenting inhibition or blocking excitation. Mechanisms implicated in seizure termination include a predominance of GABA activity, membrane

TABLE 57.6

POTENTIAL ETIOLOGIES OF ACUTE SYMPTOMATIC STATUS EPILEPTICUS

	Newborn	1–2 Months old	Infancy and childhood
Acute insult	Hypoxia-ischemia CNS infection Intracranial hemorrhage	CNS infection Subdural hematoma Anoxia VP shunt dysfunction	CNS infection Intracranial hemorrhage Anoxia VP shunt dysfunction

Genetic and metabolic	Hypoglycemia
	Hypernatremia
	Hyponatremia
	Hypocalcemia
	Hypomagnesemia
	Hyperbilirubinemia
	Organic acidemia
	Urea cycle defects
	    Nonketotic hyperglycemia
	    Congenital lactic acidosis
	Pyridoxine dependency
		Hypoglycemia
		Hypernatremia
		Hyponatremia
		Hypocalcemia
		Organic acidemia
		Urea cycle defects
		Phenylketonuria
		Riley-Day syndrome
			Hypoglycemia
			Hypernatremia
			Hyponatremia
			Hypocalcemia
			Lysosomal defects
			Urea cycle defects
			Uremia
			Hepatic failure

Malformation	Neuronal migration defect Chromosomal anomaly	Sturge-Weber syndrome Neurofibromatosis Tuberous sclerosis	

Other	Toxins
	Drugs
	Narcotic withdrawal
		Cocaine toxicity
		Drugs
		Narcotic withdrawal
			Febrile convulsion
			Drugs
			    Tricyclic antidepressants
			    Anticonvulsants
			    Calcineurin inhibitors
			    β-Lactam antibiotics
			    Opiates
			Narcotic withdrawal

CNS, central nervous system; VP, ventriculoperitoneal

stabilization by acidic extracellular pH, magnesium blockade of NMDA channels, activation of the Na/K-ATPase system, and activation of potassium (K^+) conductance to allow membrane repolarization (22). Adenosine, an endogenous neuroprotectant, is thought to regulate basal neural inhibition (9) and may also prove important for seizure termination. Treatment with adenosine antagonists, such as caffeine or aminophylline, is proconvulsive. Conversely, adenosine-releasing stem cells attenuate seizure activity in epilepsy models (27).

Refractory Status Epilepticus

The mechanisms that underlie the pharmacologic resistance that characterizes RSE remain unclear and are likely multifactorial. Putative mechanisms include alterations in anticonvulsant drug targets and failure to achieve efficacious drug levels in the brain (13,42). Changes in receptor composition or trafficking may be induced by prolonged seizure activity or chronic anticonvulsant therapy. For example, seizure-induced downregulation of GABA$_A$ receptors may reduce the efficacy of benzodiazepines in RSE (13). Similarly, extrusion of anticonvulsants across the blood-brain barrier (BBB) may limit anticonvulsant activity. Overexpression of the transporter's multidrug resistance gene-1 P-glycoprotein (MDR1) and multidrug resistance-associated protein 1 (MRP1) has been implicated in refractory epilepsy (42). Rats with pharmacologic-resistant seizures show marked overexpression of MDR1 and lower brain levels of

phenobarbital (42). In these models, co-administration of a P-glycoprotein inhibitor increases brain anticonvulsant levels and reduces pharmacologic resistance (42). Similarly, MDR1 and MRP1 are overexpressed in brain tissue from patients with refractory epilepsy (55); however, the relative contributions of MDR1 and MRP1 to RSE remain unknown.

Maturational Sequences in the Immature Brain

The immature brain is more susceptible to seizures than is the mature brain, likely due to maturational differences of excitatory and inhibitory systems (10). A predominance of excitatory activity guides early development. Consequently, the immature brain is more excitable, seizures generalize more rapidly, and the postictal refractory period is shorter. In rats, a mature balance of excitatory and inhibitory activity is achieved during the first 3 postnatal weeks (10). The corresponding timeline in humans is not clear; however, positron emission tomography studies suggest that functional GABA$_A$ activity reaches adult-like patterns during the teenage years (15).

Paradoxically, the immature brain is relatively resistant to seizure-induced cell death and synaptic reorganization (28). In contrast to the neuronal loss seen in adults, seizure-induced neurogenesis may occur in the immature brain (28). Despite a relative resistance to histologic injury, seizures during development can cause permanent, adverse effects, including cognitive impairment and lower seizure thresholds (10,28).

Cerebral Injury Induced by Status Epilepticus

Seizures that last 30–60 mins are sufficient to cause neuronal injury (24). Importantly, both CSE and NCSE may be injurious, and both must be controlled as efficiently as possible. Neuronal injury induced by SE is predominantly due to prolonged seizure activity, not to systemic complications, such as hypoxia, hypoglycemia, or hyperthermia. Autopsy study of 3 adult patients dying of focal motor SE without any systemic complications revealed neuronal loss in the piriform and entorhinal cortex, hippocampus, amygdala, and cerebellum (25). Similar injury patterns are reported in experimental models of SE induced by glutamate receptor agonists and in humans who accidentally ingested mussels that were contaminated with domoic acid, a potent glutamate receptor agonist (24,25).

These findings corroborate the hypothesis that seizure-induced cerebral injury is mediated by excitotoxicity. Excessive glutamate activates NMDA receptors, causing excessive calcium influx with resultant activation of intracellular proteases, nitric oxide production, free radical generation, oxidative injury, and ultimately cell death (24). Additionally, in cells that do not die, elevated intracellular calcium concentrations may alter calcium-dependent second-messenger effects, affecting neurogenesis, axonal sprouting, protein expression, gene regulation, and/or receptor-gated ion channel recycling (20). These alterations may promote the development of epilepsy and cognitive deficits after SE.

Clinically, patterns of cerebral involvement after pediatric SE are not well defined and likely vary by etiology. Febrile SE, which is the best studied, has been linked to hippocampal abnormalities. In a prospective comparison of acute MRI findings in 35 children with febrile or afebrile SE, febrile SE was associated with acute, vasogenic, hippocampal edema, which resolved 3–5 days after SE (48,50). Additionally, 24% of children with febrile SE had other abnormal findings, such as hippocampal asymmetry, an arachnoid cyst, and subtle loss of gray-white differentiation in the left middle temporal gyrus. In contrast, children with afebrile SE had no hippocampal enlargement, but roughly 60% had non-hippocampal abnormalities (e.g., delayed myelination, cerebral infarction, cortical dysplasia, and cerebral vasculitis) (48). Follow-up MRI in 23 children with febrile SE, performed at a mean interval of 5.5 months, showed reduced hippocampal volumes and increased hippocampal asymmetry, compared to the initial scan (49). Further, the expected age-dependent changes in hippocampal apparent diffusion coefficient measurements were not seen in children with febrile SE, which supports the hypothesis that they have underlying hippocampal abnormalities (50).

Increased Vulnerability with Concurrent Neurologic Insults

In the presence of an accompanying acute neurologic insult, the seizure duration necessary to cause neuronal injury may be shorter than 30–60 mins. Seizures increase glucose metabolism and intracranial pressure (ICP), placing vulnerable cerebral tissue at greater risk for injury. In adult patients with stroke, seizures are associated with worsening of cerebral edema and midline shift (64), as well as a threefold increase in mortality,

compared to patients who lack seizures (67). Similarly, seizures are an independent risk factor for poor outcome after severe traumatic brain injury (31,64). Posttraumatic seizures increase interstitial glutamate and glycerol concentrations, suggesting exacerbation of excitotoxicity, ischemia, and secondary neuronal injury (65,66). Among children <2 years of age, posttraumatic seizures portend a twofold increase in the risk of poor functional outcome (31). Importantly, subclinical seizures are common in patients with acute neurologic insults, yet diagnosis frequently requires a high degree of suspicion and continuous EEG monitoring (64).

CLINICAL PRESENTATION AND DIFFERENTIAL DIAGNOSIS

Common Presentations

Typical clinical presentations CSE and NCSE are described here. Representative EEG tracings for different classes of SE are shown in **Figure 57.1.**

Convulsive Status Epilepticus

Generalized Convulsive Status Epilepticus. GCSE may be tonic-clonic, clonic, or tonic in nature. Forty percent to 80% of GCSE in children presents as continuous seizures, most commonly with generalized tonic-clonic activity (4). In children with epilepsy, GCSE often starts as increasing frequency of serial seizures, with recovery of consciousness between episodes (premonitory SE), and prompt treatment during this stage may prevent progression (53). Serial seizures typically last 1–3 mins but tend to shorten as time elapses. Between seizures, patients are obtunded, showing autonomic signs, such as salivation, bradypnea, cyanosis, and arterial hypotension. In some cases, cardiovascular collapse may occur. Neurologic examination may reveal abnormal cranial nerve function and unilateral or bilateral Babinski responses (53). Cerebrospinal fluid pleocytosis as a consequence of GCSE has been documented in all ages.

Clonic Status Epilepticus. Clonic SE may persist hours or even days, waxing and waning in intensity, and a persistent postictal hemiplegia is usually observed. The behavioral manifestations of clonic SE are variable. Seizures tend to be continuous and may be generalized, unilateral, or restricted to one limb or segment. Fluctuations between different patterns of involvement may occur during a single episode of clonic SE. Additionally, the rhythm of jerks is variable and may also fluctuate. Clonic seizures in young children are predominantly unilateral; however, they may shift from side to side (4). Approximately 75% of patients with unilateral clonic seizures are 3 years of age or younger (4,53). Consciousness may be preserved during clonic SE, and autonomic involvement is generally less pronounced than with tonic-clonic seizures.

Tonic Status Epilepticus. Tonic SE is less common than tonic-clonic or clonic SE and occurs almost exclusively in children and adolescents with known epilepsy (4). Importantly, tonic SE has been precipitated by intravenous or oral benzodiazepine treatment of absence SE in children with Lennox-Gastaut syndrome (4,53). Tonic SE can persist for several days, much longer than other CSE types (4,53). Serial tonic seizures are

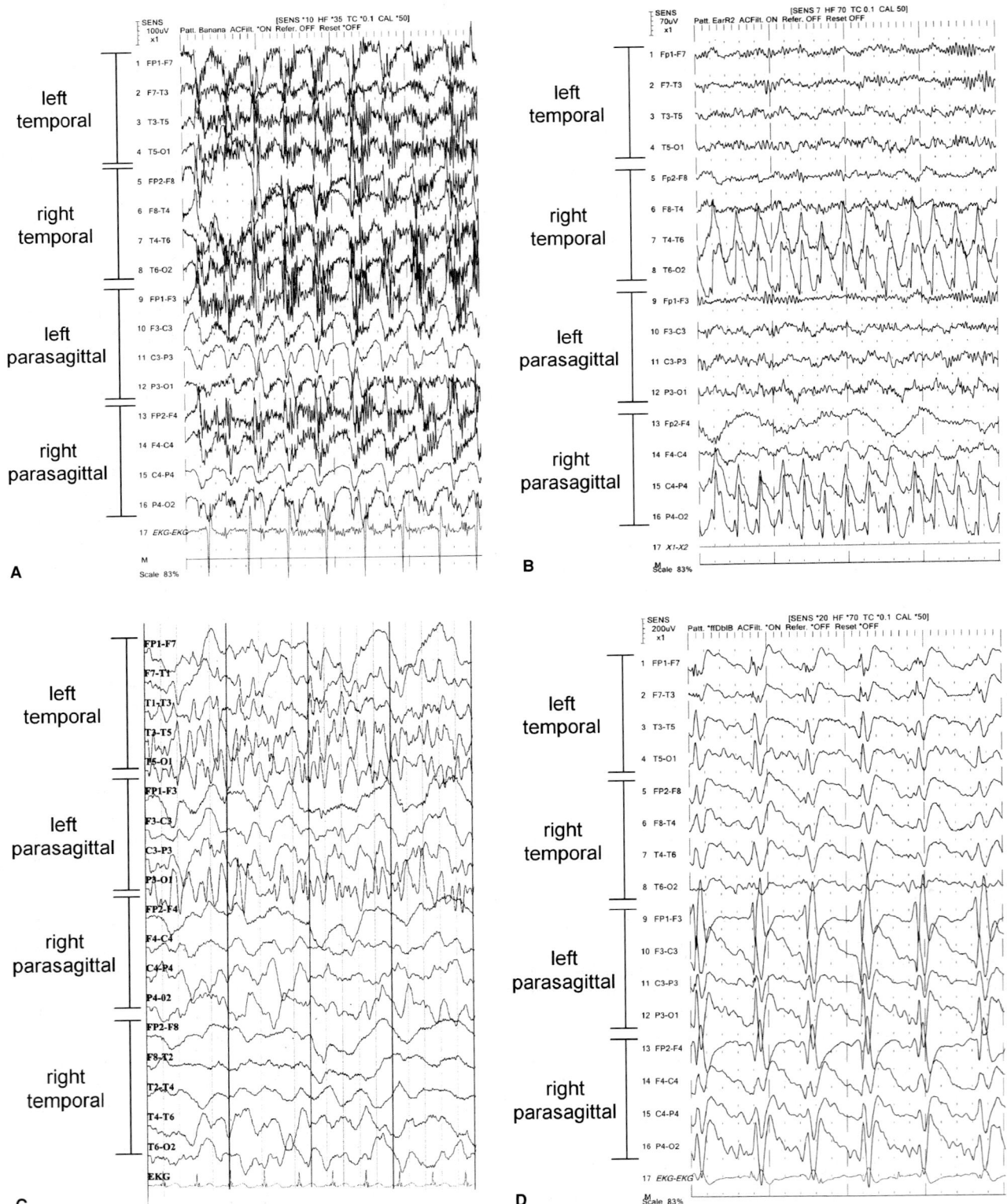

FIGURE 57.1. Representative EEG tracings that show status epilepticus. **A:** Generalized convulsive status epilepticus. Note the generalized spike and wave pattern, which is partially obscured by muscle artifact (heavy black tracings of fast activity), most prominent in the frontal and temporal leads. **B:** Focal motor status epilepticus in a patient with Sturge-Weber syndrome and a vascular lesion near the seizure focus. Note the repetitive spike-and-slow wave activity localized to the right posterior temporal and parietal leads. **C:** Complex partial status epilepticus arising from the left posterior temporal region. Note the rhythmic sharp wave activity in the left temporal leads with spread to the left occipital region. **D:** Nonconvulsive status epilepticus in a patient with Lennox-Gastaut syndrome. Note the bilateral symmetric spike-and-slow wave activity, which has maximal amplitude in the frontal leads.

typical, and autonomic manifestations, particularly increased bronchial secretions, may be pronounced. Over time, behavioral manifestations become limited to slight eye deviation, respiratory irregularities, and marked tracheobronchial obstruction due to hypersecretion. Consciousness is moderately to severely impaired, and a postictal confusional state may persist for days. The initial behavioral manifestations of tonic SE may be attenuated or even subclinical (4,53). In these cases, polygraphic monitoring is necessary to demonstrate the tachycardia, altered respiratory rhythm, occasional hypertonus of the trunk or neck muscles, and EEG activity indicative of tonic SE.

Focal Motor Status Epilepticus. Focal motor SE may affect children with acute inciting insults (Table 57.2) or those with known epileptic disorders. Focal motor SE due to an acute illness, such as encephalitis, typically develops into secondary GCSE. Conversely, in children with epilepsy, focal motor SE tends to have a more restricted distribution and may be manifest only as jerking of the corner of the mouth or cheek, salivation, swallowing difficulties, and absent speech. Even with narrowly localized seizures, autonomic disturbances and some impairment of consciousness may be present. Children who clinically appear to be in focal motor SE may be treated despite a lack of seizure activity on EEG (4,53).

Myoclonic Status Epilepticus. Myoclonic SE is characterized by the incessant repetition of massive myoclonic jerks. Acute hypoxic-ischemic encephalopathy is the most common cause of myoclonic SE among critically ill children. When associated with anoxic brain injury, myoclonic SE indicates severe diffuse brain damage and can be difficult to control. Myoclonic SE also occurs with metabolic insults, such as hypoglycemia, hepatic or renal failure, or heavy-metal intoxication (Table 57.3). Physical trauma or inflammatory disease rarely causes myoclonic SE. Importantly, myoclonic SE may be induced by high doses of β-lactam antibiotics, especially in patients with renal failure (4,53). Intrathecal administration of radiologic contrast agents is also associated with myoclonic SE, typically with a favorable prognosis (4,53). Finally, myoclonic SE also affects children with epilepsy (4,53) and has been described with Angelman syndrome (62).

Nonconvulsive Status Epilepticus

The diagnostic criteria for NCSE are in evolution, with no standard, uniformly accepted definitions or terminology. The classic definition of NCSE is tripartite: (a) prolonged (greater than 30 mins) alteration of consciousness or complex partial seizures without full recovery of consciousness, (b) epileptiform changes on the EEG that are different from the preictal state, and (c) prompt observable improvement in both the EEG and clinical state after administration of an IV antiepileptic medication.

Whether generalized or focal, NCSE can present with a variety of clinical features, including agitation and aggression, lethargy, confusion, delirium, fugue-like state, decreased speech, mutism, echolalia, blank staring with or without blinking, chewing and picking, tremulousness, subtle facial or limb myoclonus, rigidity or waxy flexibility, or vegetative features. NCSE is seen in children with epilepsy (Landau-Kleffner syndrome) and ring chromosome 20 (4,43). Additionally, critically ill patients with unexplained coma or prolonged obtundation after CSE may have NCSE (21).

Absence NCSE. Generalized NCSE is widely known as absence SE, although it has also been called *petit mal status* and *spike-wave stupor*. Absence SE typically occurs during the first decade of life, and 75% of cases occur before the age of 20 (4). Absence SE is characterized by a variable impairment of consciousness, ranging from mild slowing of higher cognitive functions to barely perceptible responsiveness. Complex automatisms may occur and motor manifestations (e.g., myoclonic eyelid and facial twitching, bilateral or unilateral limb myoclonus, and/or atonic phenomena that produce falls, head nods, knee buckling, or other alterations of posture) are seen in about half of the cases. Patients are totally or partially amnestic of these episodes. Of note, patients typically do not show the cycling in the clinical state that characterizes complex partial SE (4).

Complex Partial Status Epilepticus. Complex partial SE is also known as psychomotor status, focal NCSE, temporolimbic SE, or localized NCSE. It occurs less commonly in children but can be seen in the course of focal epilepsies (4). Complex partial SE can present as frequently recurring partial seizures without full recovery of consciousness between seizures or continuous long-standing episodes of mental confusion and behavioral disturbance with or without automatisms. Complex partial SE is often marked by cyclic alterations between unresponsive staring and partial responsiveness with quasi-purposeful reactive automatisms (4).

Nonconvulsive Status Epilepticus in Comatose Patients. NCSE should be considered in children with prolonged "postictal state" or unexplained alterations in consciousness. Nonconvulsive seizures are documented in 16% of PICU patients with unexplained alterations in consciousness (46), and NCSE occurs in 33% of children who were admitted to a neurologic monitoring unit, PICU, or NICU for SE (57). Importantly, in 85% of cases, NCSE was preceded by short, serial seizures that failed to meet classical criteria for CSE (57). Clinically, all children with NCSE exhibited acute confusion, stupor, or coma (57). Likewise, NCSE was documented in 10% of critically ill adults with altered mental status (17). Among adults with an apparently prolonged "postictal state" following convulsive seizures, 48% had persistent EEG seizures and 14% manifest NCSE after motor manifestations cease (21). Continuous (vs. short-duration) EEG monitoring is often necessary to verify the diagnosis of NCSE (15). Localized EEG findings are common and typically correlate with neuroimaging abnormalities (46,57) Additionally, consultation with a neurologist is imperative, as EEG interpretation can be difficult and determining EEG activity that requires treatment remains controversial.

Refractory Status Epilepticus

RSE may occur with any classification or etiology of SE and is associated with greater morbidity and mortality than more responsive SE (22). In a small case series of previously healthy children with RSE, all developed intractable epilepsy and functional disabilities (47). Although RSE typically has motor manifestations, it may begin as NCSE. Even in patients who present with GCSE, RSE frequently becomes subtle or nonconvulsive (NCRSE). Patients with acute structural lesions are at higher risk for NCRSE, and a high degree of suspicion with continuous EEG monitoring is required for timely and accurate diagnosis

(22). Additionally, continuous EEG monitoring is important to guide therapy in any patient with RSE.

Systemic Manifestations

Much of our knowledge of the systemic manifestations of SE comes from classic studies of GCSE in primates conducted during the early 1970s (38). GCSE can be divided into early and late phases. During early SE, compensatory mechanisms to attenuate seizure-associated injury are prominent. The transition from early to late SE occurs after ~30 to 45 mins of continuous seizure activity. Late SE is marked by failure of compensatory mechanisms and seizure-associated injury. Additionally, once the transition from early to late SE has occurred, SE is more difficult to terminate.

Autonomic and Metabolic Changes

The autonomic and metabolic changes seen during GCSE differ between early and late SE. During early SE, increased catecholamine levels result in tachycardia, hypertension, increased central venous pressures, and hyperglycemia. Cerebral blood flow (CBF) increases in response to increased cerebral metabolic demands. Lactic acidosis commonly results from continued, rigorous muscle activity. Mild hypoxemia and modest hypercarbia may occur, but patients usually maintain sufficient oxygenation and ventilation if the airway remains patent. Other autonomic signs, including diaphoresis, hypersecretion, and mydriasis, are frequent.

During late SE, compensatory reserves are exhausted, and marked hyperthermia, hypotension, and hypoglycemia may occur. Cerebrovascular autoregulation is lost and CBF becomes pressure-dependent, making prompt correction of hypotension crucial. Cerebral edema may accompany late SE and is more common in pediatric than in adult patients. Sustained motor convulsions may result in rhabdomyolysis and hyperkalemia. Hypoxia and hypercarbia are frequently more exaggerated during late SE. Respiratory compromise, associated with apnea or poor handling of secretions, is common. Pupillary and corneal reflexes may be absent in the ictal or postictal phases of both early and late SE.

Other Concerns

Rarely, disseminated intravascular coagulation and multiorgan failure may be induced by SE itself or by the inciting cause. Myoglobinuria or dehydration and shock may lead to renal failure. Hepatic insufficiency or failure may result from the underlying cause of SE, as a side effect of anticonvulsant therapy, or from hyperpyrexia. Finally, emesis is common, and patients with SE are at high risk for aspiration.

Differential Diagnosis

CSE is usually easy to diagnose and not readily confused with other disorders in a nonparalyzed patient. However, pseudostatus epilepticus can be confused with CSE on occasion, with disastrous results. Clinical signs suggestive of nonepileptic psychogenic seizures include motor movements that fluctuate in intensity, frequency, and/or distribution, with lack of facial muscle involvement and including pelvic thrusting. Vocalization, bizarre behavior, explosive emotional expression, and resis-

tance to examination are common. Although urinary incontinence, tongue biting, and cyanosis can occur, they are less common than in CSE. In pseudostatus epilepticus, the EEG is often obscured by muscle and movement artifact, and no postictal EEG changes occur. A well-developed α rhythm can be discerned during brief moments of movement cessation or on termination of pseudoseizures. In contrast, patients with CSE have both ictal and postictal EEG changes. Furthermore, the muscle artifact associated with pseudoseizures lacks the repetitive characteristics seen in true CSE.

In contrast, the seizure behavior associated with NCSE is nonspecific and may produce diagnostic confusion. Two common conditions that may simulate the seizure behaviors of NCSE are postictal drowsiness and anticonvulsant-induced sedation. Continuous EEG recordings may be necessary to accurately distinguish these disorders. Toxic-metabolic (including drug intoxication and drug withdrawal) and infectious (including para- and postinfectious) encephalopathies of numerous etiologies present with altered mental status and may be clinically indistinguishable from NCSE. Additionally, altered mental status that mimics NCSE can be caused by acute structural lesions, including traumatic brain injury, tumors, and stroke. Neuroimaging studies are helpful in differentiating these etiologies. Finally, psychiatric disorders should be considered in patients with behavioral changes not associated with appropriate ictal and interictal EEG changes.

CLINICAL MANAGEMENT

SE is a medical emergency that requires prompt intervention, as seizure duration is inversely associated with treatment responsiveness and favorable outcome. Management of the critically ill child with SE is directed toward rapid cessation of seizures, supportive care of associated systemic derangements or complications, treatment of causal or underlying conditions, and prevention of seizure recurrence.

Initial Stabilization

As with any critically ill child, the first priority of initial stabilization is to ensure airway patency and control. The patient should be positioned so that ongoing seizure activity will not cause physical harm. Nothing should be placed into the patient's mouth due to the risk of aspiration. Supplemental oxygen should be provided and respiration assisted as needed. Precautions should be taken to prevent aspiration.

In patients with hypoxia, hypoventilation, or a Glasgow Coma Scale score <8, rapid-sequence endotracheal intubation should be considered for airway protection and respiratory support. Data regarding the preferred induction agents for intubation are lacking. A short-acting barbiturate such as thiopental is commonly used, although dose-associated hypotension should be anticipated and avoided. Benzodiazepines or narcotics are also acceptable choices. If neuromuscular blockade is necessary to facilitate intubation, a short-acting, nondepolarizing agent such as rocuronium is preferable. In the absence of a known normal serum potassium level, succinylcholine should be avoided due to the risk of hyperkalemia associated with ongoing seizure activity. Repeated or continued neuromuscular blockade should also be avoided, as it may mask ongoing seizure activity.

Reliable IV access should be established as soon as possible. If placement of IV catheters is difficult or prolonged, an intraosseous catheter may be considered. Hypotension or dehydration should be treated with isotonic fluid resuscitation. Hypertension is common with ongoing seizure activity, and treatment should not be considered unless it persists after seizure activity has stopped.

Hypoglycemia should be considered as an inciting event, and the serum glucose level should be checked promptly. In the absence of rapid testing, empiric dextrose should be administered intravenously. Thiamine (50–100 mg IV) may be considered prior to dextrose administration in older children at risk of nutritional deficiencies. Electrolyte abnormalities, such as hyponatremia or hypocalcemia, should also be considered. Serum electrolytes should be checked and replaced appropriately. High-dose antibiotics should be administered empirically to all patients at risk of bacterial infection, as well as to those who present with new-onset SE and fever. Empiric acyclovir should also be considered for patients who present with new-onset SE and fever and who are at risk for herpetic infections.

Supportive Care for Associated Derangements

Prolonged seizure activity is associated with the development of metabolic acidosis, hyperthermia, and rhabdomyolysis. Metabolic acidosis usually corrects spontaneously after seizure cessation and appropriate hydration. Due to the potential for exacerbating cerebral injury, hyperthermia (>38.5°C) should be treated with surface and/or systemic cooling to promptly achieve normothermia. Precautions should be taken to prevent shivering associated with active cooling. If neuromuscular blockade is required, continuous EEG monitoring is indicated to assess for ongoing seizure activity.

Other supportive care is determined by the cause of SE and side effects of necessary anticonvulsant therapies. Empiric therapies targeted to the cause of SE should be initiated concurrently with attaining seizure control. Among children admitted to the PICU with SE, roughly 60% require intubation (31). The average duration of mechanical ventilatory support is 2 days (31). The typical PICU length of stay is 3 days; however, in patients with acute infectious etiologies, such as meningitis and encephalitis, length of stay is longer (31). For patients who require pharmacologically induced coma for RSE, continued respiratory, hemodynamic, and nutritional support are required. Vasoactive or inotropic agents are frequently needed to manage medication-induced hypotension or myocardial depression. Parenteral nutrition may be necessary due to development of ileus.

Diagnostic Tests

Swift cessation of seizures is crucial, and anticonvulsant therapy should not be delayed to facilitate diagnostic testing. All patients with SE should receive serum glucose and electrolyte testing. Further diagnostic tests are guided by probable or suspected etiology. Serum anticonvulsant medication levels should be measured in children on chronic therapy. Blood and urine

specimens should be obtained for culture, especially in febrile children. Serum and urine toxicology screening tests should be sent for patients with possible ingestions. After the seizures have stopped, a head CT scan is appropriate in patients with new-onset seizures or those at risk for anatomic abnormalities, mass intracranial lesions (e.g., brain tumor, brain abscess, intracranial hemorrhage), or cerebral edema. Once a mass intracranial lesion or cerebral edema has been excluded, lumbar puncture is indicated in patients at risk for meningitis or those with a new-onset seizure disorder. Due to the risk of downward herniation, lumbar puncture should be avoided in patients with evidence of increased ICP. Serum ammonia, lactate, and serum amino and urine organic acid levels should be checked in infants and children at risk for inborn errors of metabolism. More specific metabolic testing may be appropriate for certain patients and should be considered in consultation with a pediatric neurologist or geneticist.

Medications for Seizure Termination

Rapid cessation of SE is associated with improved response rates and clinical outcomes. Consequently, administration of anticonvulsants for SE should proceed along a defined timeline, with the goal of controlling SE within 30 mins of presentation (**Fig. 57.2**). The progression of treatment includes administration of a first-line agent, administration of a second-line agent, and initiation of pharmacologic coma for treatment of RSE.

Randomized clinical trials evaluating anticonvulsant efficacy in the pediatric population are lacking. Consequently, anticonvulsant choice is guided largely by clinician experience and expert opinion. Recently, the results of a comprehensive survey that investigated the anticonvulsant practices of ~40 pediatric neurologists who specialize in epilepsy have been published (68). The first- and second-line anticonvulsant recommendations in this chapter represent the preferred treatments identified by this survey. Suggestions of the National Institute for Clinical Excellence (1) and the Scottish Intercollegiate Guidelines Network (2) are also incorporated. Treatment of NCSE or RSE is based on clinical cohort or case studies, extrapolation from adult practice, and clinical experience.

First- and Second-Line Medications

First- and second-line medications for SE are determined by SE classification (**Tables 57.7** and **57.8**). Recommended medication doses are detailed in **Table 57.9**.

Benzodiazepines. Benzodiazepines bind the GABA$_A$ receptor complex and facilitate GABA action by increasing the frequency of channel opening, thereby increasing chloride permeability and leading to hyperpolarization. Commonly used benzodiazepines for SE include lorazepam, diazepam, and midazolam. In a retrospective, population-based study, 58% of children with convulsive seizures that lasted longer than 5 mins responded to benzodiazepines (39). However, benzodiazepines lose potency during prolonged SE (13,22,23), possibly related to seizure-induced GABA$_A$ receptor downregulation (13). Additionally, benzodiazepines may precipitate myoclonus in a small percentage of neonates or tonic seizures in patients with Lennox-Gastaut syndrome.

The IV administration of lorazepam is the first-line treatment for all types of convulsive SE except neonatal SE, for

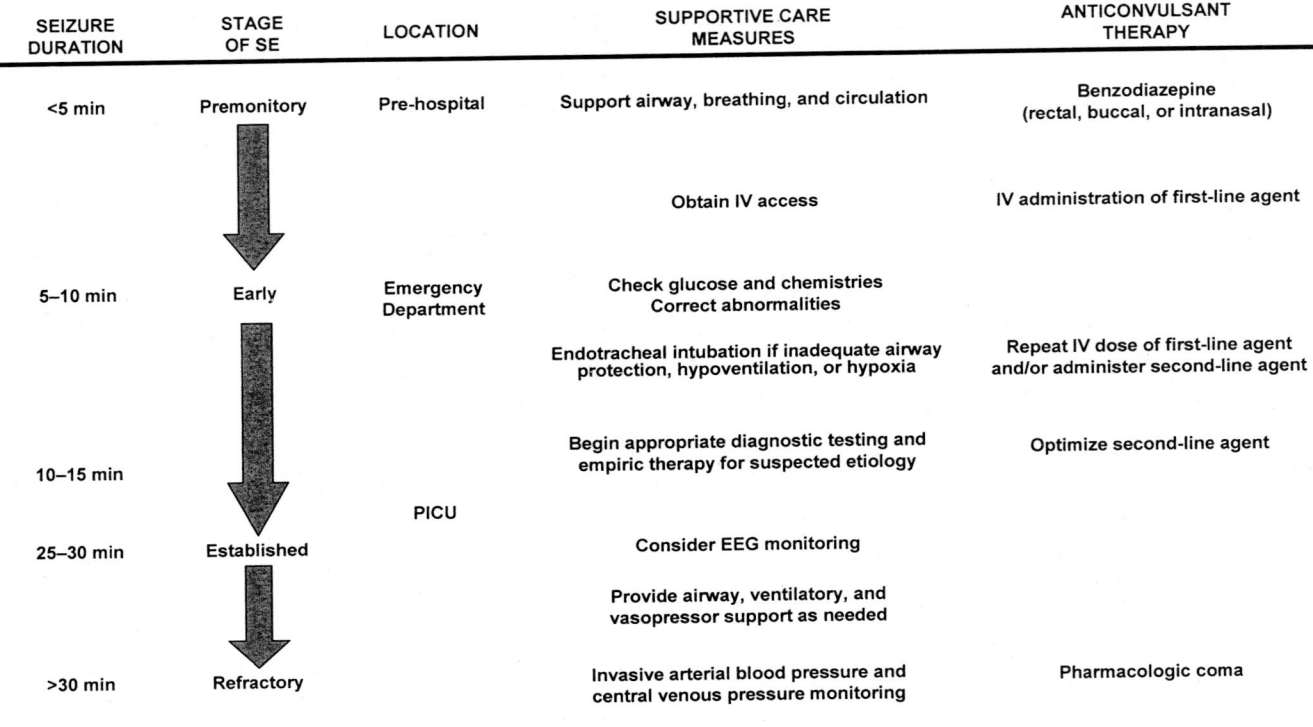

SEIZURE DURATION	STAGE OF SE	LOCATION	SUPPORTIVE CARE MEASURES	ANTICONVULSANT THERAPY
<5 min	Premonitory	Pre-hospital	Support airway, breathing, and circulation	Benzodiazepine (rectal, buccal, or intranasal)
			Obtain IV access	IV administration of first-line agent
5–10 min	Early	Emergency Department	Check glucose and chemistries Correct abnormalities	
			Endotracheal intubation if inadequate airway protection, hypoventilation, or hypoxia	Repeat IV dose of first-line agent and/or administer second-line agent
10–15 min			Begin appropriate diagnostic testing and empiric therapy for suspected etiology	Optimize second-line agent
25–30 min	Established	PICU	Consider EEG monitoring	
			Provide airway, ventilatory, and vasopressor support as needed	
>30 min	Refractory		Invasive arterial blood pressure and central venous pressure monitoring	Pharmacologic coma
			Continuous EEG monitoring	

FIGURE 57.2. Suggested algorithm for the goal-directed treatment of pediatric status epilepticus. Adapted from Chen JW, Wasterlain CG. Status epilepticus: Pathophysiology and management in adults. *Lancet Neurol* 2006;5:246–56 and Dhar R, Mirsattari SM. Current approach to the diagnosis and treatment of refractory status epilepticus. *Adv Neurol* 2006;97:245–54.

which it is a second-line agent. The peak effect of IV lorazepam occurs 15 mins after dosing, and the duration is 3–6 hrs. If a single dose is not effective, a second dose is recommended before or concurrent with administration of a second-line agent. Both diazepam and midazolam may be administered intravenously as well, but they have less favorable pharmacokinetic profiles than lorazepam (13). Given intravenously, both diazepam and midazolam have shorter durations than lorazepam (roughly 15–30 and 30–80 mins, respectively). Additionally, midazolam is metabolized by cytochrome P4503A4 enzymes and may have variable metabolism and more drug interactions.

Administration of diazepam per rectum (0.2–0.5 mg/kg) is acceptable for patients who receive prehospital care or for those without established IV access. The bioavailability of rectal diazepam is 90%, and peak effect occurs 1.5 hrs after adminis-

tration. Alternatively, midazolam may be given via intramuscular (0.1–0.15 mg/kg; max 0.5 mg/kg), buccal (0.3 mg/kg), or intranasal (0.2–0.5 mg/kg; max 0.5 mg/kg) administration in patients without IV access (37,58,70). The bioavailability of intramuscular midazolam is ~90%, and it is rapidly absorbed, with an average onset of 2–3 mins and peak plasma levels 30 mins after dosing. Buccal administration of midazolam is easy and safe, and it may be more efficacious than rectal diazepam (2,37). For buccal dosing, an appropriate dose of the IV preparation of midazolam is placed between the gum and cheek. In a randomized trial that compared seizure cessation after equipotent doses of buccal midazolam and rectal diazepam, buccal midazolam was effective in twice as many patients and had better seizure control, shorter onset of action, less need for IV lorazepam dosing, and less seizure recurrence (37). Similarly,

TABLE 57.7

PREFERRED MEDICATIONS FOR CONVULSIVE STATUS EPILEPTICUS

	GCSE	Focal motor	Myoclonic	Neonatal
First-line	Lorazepam	Lorazepam	Lorazepam	Phenobarbital
Second-line	Fosphenytoin	Fosphenytoin	Fosphenytoin Valproate	Fosphenytoin Lorazepam

GCSE, generalized convulsive status epilepticus. Data from Wheless JW, Clarke DF, Carpenter D. Treatment of pediatric epilepsy: Expert opinion, 2005. *J Child Neurol* 2005;20 Suppl 1:S1–56.

TABLE 57.8

PREFERRED MEDICATIONS FOR NONCONVULSIVE STATUS EPILEPTICUS

	Absence	Complex partial	NCSE with coma
First-line	Lorazepam	Lorazepam	Lorazepam
Second-line	Valproate	Fosphenytoin	Fosphenytoin Pharmacologic coma

NCSE, nonconvulsive status epilepticus. Data from Wheless JW, Clarke DF, Carpenter D. Treatment of pediatric epilepsy: Expert opinion, 2005. *J Child Neurol* 2005;20 Suppl 1:S1–56.

intranasal administration of midazolam has been shown to be safe in children and may be more efficacious than rectal diazepam (70).

Phenobarbital. Phenobarbital is the first-line agent for neonatal SE and a second-line agent for GCSE or complex partial SE. Phenobarbital is a barbiturate and acts by enhancing GABA$_A$ activity. The binding site for barbiturates differs from that of benzodiazepines, and reduced efficacy during prolonged SE has not been described. Interestingly, cerebral uptake of phenobarbital is increased by seizure activity, likely due to increased CBF and BBB permeability (53). Intravenous administration of phenobarbital results in an onset of action after roughly 5 mins and peak levels after 15 mins. Dose adjustment may be indicated in patients with severe renal or hepatic failure. Phenobarbital can cause dose-dependent respiratory and hemodynamic depression, and these potential side effects should be anticipated and avoided.

Fosphenytoin. Fosphenytoin is the second-line agent for GCSE, complex partial SE, and neonatal SE. Fosphenytoin is a pro-drug that is dephosphorylated to phenytoin. Phenytoin acts as an activity-dependent antagonist of voltage-dependent sodium (Na$^+$) channels. Fosphenytoin has similar efficacy and fewer administration side effects, such as local injection site irritation and arrhythmias, as compared to phenytoin. Still, EKG monitoring is indicated during administration of loading doses. Fosphenytoin is dosed as phenytoin equivalents (PE units), and peak levels of phenytoin are achieved roughly 20 mins after IV dosing. Phenytoin is highly protein bound and, in patients on chronic phenytoin therapy, fosphenytoin may displace phenytoin from albumin binding sites and rapidly raise free phenytoin levels. Similarly, valproate may displace phenytoin from albumin binding sites. Therapeutic total levels of roughly 20 mg/dL are typically targeted, although in patients with hypoalbuminemia or concurrent valproate therapy, total levels may underestimate free plasma concentrations. In these patients, free phenytoin levels should be followed.

Valproate. Valproate is the second-line agent for absence SE and may be useful as an adjunctive therapy for GCSE, complex partial SE, or myoclonic SE. The precise mechanism of action of valproate remains unclear, but it increases endogenous GABA levels, enhances GABA response, and may stabilize neuronal membranes. Larger loading doses may be required to achieve therapeutic levels in patients on liver enzyme-inducing drugs, such as phenobarbital, phenytoin, or carbamazepine. Therapeutic valproate levels are 50–150 mcg/mL; both efficacy and toxicity may be increased at higher doses. Valproate is generally well tolerated but may rarely cause hypotension during acute administration. Hepatotoxicity and hyperammonemia are associated with valproate use, and transaminase levels and liver function should be monitored during treatment. Additionally, valproate has been associated with thrombocytopenia and coagulation disorders, possibly due to decreased hepatic production of clotting factors, as well as pancreatitis.

Nonconvulsive Status Epilepticus

Treatment of NCSE in children is not well studied. Similar to CSE, medication choice is based on seizure type (**Table 57.7**).

TABLE 57.9

MEDICATION DOSING FOR STATUS EPILEPTICUS

Medication	Dose	Delivery rate	Comments
Lorazepam	0.05–0.15 mg/kg/dose IV (max 4 mg)	2 mg/min	Repeat in 5 min
Phenobarbital	15–20 mg/kg IV	60 mg/min	Repeat in 5-mg/kg dose PRN to ~40 mg/kg
Fosphenytoin	15–20 mg PE/kg IV	100 mg PE/min	
Valproate	15–20 mg/kg	20 mg/min	Repeat in 10-mg/kg doses PRN to ~40 mg/kg

PE, phenytoin equivalents

Treatment of NCSE in comatose children is identical to that used for RSE, with rapid progression to pharmacologic coma. Continuous EEG monitoring should be used to guide therapy; however, consensus regarding the optimal EEG end-point is lacking. The most controversial EEG discharges are PLEDs. Therapy for PLEDS in NCSE remains controversial, and consultation with a pediatric neurologist is recommended. Additionally, PLEDs are commonly seen with structural lesions or herpes encephalitis, and adjunctive therapies should target potential inciting insults.

Refractory Status Epilepticus

Due to the ongoing risk for seizure-induced cerebral injury and systemic complications, RSE, whether convulsive or nonconvulsive, should be treated urgently (**Table 57.10**). Regardless of the medication chosen for induction of pharmacologic coma in patients with RSE, invasive blood pressure and central venous pressure are generally indicated to guide titration of ventilatory, fluid, and vasopressor support and to minimize systemic side effects of prolonged SE and high anticonvulsant dosing. Typically, pharmacologic coma is continued for 24 hrs after seizure control before tapering. If seizures recur on a reduced dose of medication, coma can be reinstated for an additional 24 hrs. The recurrence of seizures on discontinuation of pharmacologic coma is usually a poor prognostic sign.

Pharmacologic coma is typically achieved using benzodiazepine or barbiturate infusions, guided by continuous EEG monitoring. The end-point of pharmacologic coma may be either cessation of EEG seizure activity or burst suppression. Unfortunately, a consistent association between EEG end-point and outcome is lacking. Consequently, while rapid seizure termination is desired, the most efficacious EEG end-point remains controversial. Historically, benzodiazepines are targeted to seizure cessation, while barbiturates are titrated to burst suppression (16). Therapeutic goals should be identified for individual patients in consultation with a pediatric neurologist.

Treatment of pediatric RSE is not well studied and is based largely on clinical experience and extrapolation from adult practice. Randomized, controlled trials of treatment efficacy in adults are also lacking; however, the three most common therapies—midazolam, pentobarbital, and propofol—have been compared by meta-analysis (16). Midazolam infusion, the most common therapy, is associated with the longest duration of therapy, the highest incidence of breakthrough seizures, and the greatest number of changes in therapy due to lack of efficacy, but with the least hemodynamic compromise. Conversely, pentobarbital is associated with the shortest duration of therapy, the lowest incidence of breakthrough seizures, the least changes in therapy, and the most hypotension. Outcomes were associated with etiology of RSE, not treatment choice, and were similar among therapies.

Midazolam. Midazolam infusions have been used to treat neonatal and pediatric RSE. In neonates, midazolam infusions were efficacious for RSE resistant to phenobarbital and phenytoin, and hypotension was a rare side effect (11). In cohorts of pediatric patients, mean midazolam infusion rates of 8.7–15 mcg/kg/min were required (29,41). In comparison, the mean effective midazolam infusion rate in adults was 8 mcg/kg/min (61). Mild, transient hypotension occurred in treated children but responded to fluid administration and did not require initiation or escalation of vasopressor support (29,41).

Due to GABA$_A$ resistance, some authors advocate that midazolam infusions may not be efficacious for RSE, particularly if therapeutic doses of other benzodiazepines have already been given or if the duration of SE is quite prolonged (13). However, aggressive, goal-directed midazolam therapy may be efficacious, even for prolonged RSE. In 17 PICU patients with RSE that lasted a median of 2.1 hrs (range 0.5–63 hrs), midazolam was aggressively titrated using a goal-directed algorithm: an initial loading dose of 0.5 mg/kg and an infusion rate of 2 mcg/kg/min, followed by an additional bolus dose of 0.5 mg/kg and escalation of the infusion to 4 mcg/kg/min if seizures persisted longer than 5 mins (41). Persistent or recurrent seizures were then treated with repeated bolus doses of 0.1 mg/kg, with increases of 4 mcg/kg/min in the infusion rate every 5 mins until seizures were controlled. Although most patients had been treated with benzodiazepines prior to initiation

TABLE 57.10

MEDICATION DOSING FOR REFRACTORY STATUS EPILEPTICUS

Medication	Dose	
	Loading	Infusion
Midazolam	0.2–0.5 mg/kg IV	0.05–4 mcg/kg/min[a]
Pentobarbital	10–15 mg/kg IV initially then 2–5 mg/kg q 5 min to stop seizure	1–3 mg/kg/hr
Thiopental	5 mg/kg IV initially then 1–2 mg/kg q 5 min to stop seizure	3–5 mg/kg/hr
Propofol	2–5 mg/kg IV	25–65 mcg/kg/min
Valproate	40 mg/kg IV	3 mg/kg/min
Ketamine	1.5 mg/kg IV	0.01–0.05 mg/kg/hr
Topiramate	25 mg/kg NGT	Increase by 5–10 mg/kg/d NGT

[a]Higher infusion rates may be used, as delineated in the text. NGT, nasogastric tube

of the midazolam algorithm, only 2 patients (12%) failed midazolam therapy. The mean time to control of SE was 0.3 hr (range 0.1–1.5 hrs). The median peak infusion rate was 4 mcg/kg/min (median 8.7 mcg/kg/min; range 2–32 mcg/kg/min). The median duration of midazolam infusion was 16 hrs (range 2–113 hrs). Adverse effects were minimal. Transient mild hypotension, which responded to modest fluid resuscitation, occurred in 12%, breakthrough seizures occurred in 47%, and relapse of SE after discontinuation of midazolam therapy occurred in 6%.

Pentobarbital and Thiopental. Barbiturate coma is a common therapy for RSE. Fluid resuscitation and low-dose vasopressor or inotropic support are frequently required due to the cardiovascular effects of high barbiturate doses. Although dosing is usually titrated to burst suppression, targeting the cessation of EEG seizure activity may provide similar efficacy with fewer side effects. Barbiturates suppress cerebral metabolism and may be beneficial for patients with increased ICP. In addition to cardiovascular toxicity, the adverse effects of high-dose barbiturates include hypothermia, ileus, and increased susceptibility to infections, especially ventilator-associated pneumonia (63).

Pentobarbital and thiopental are the most commonly used barbiturates. Dosing for either agent is titrated to effect, and higher infusion rates than those listed in **Table 57.10** are frequently necessary. Both agents tend to accumulate in fatty tissue, and recovery times may be prolonged. Drug clearance is usually more predictable with pentobarbital. The hepatic metabolism of thiopental exhibits saturation, resulting in increasing accumulation during high-dose infusions (53). Additionally, thiopental is metabolized to pentobarbital, which accounts for 10%–15% of active barbiturate levels during thiopental therapy (53). Due to the long elimination half-life, gradual tapering of pentobarbital or thiopental is usually not necessary.

Other Medications. Propofol, valproate, ketamine, topiramate, and volatile anesthetics have been used as adjunctive therapies for RSE. Propofol administration is common in adults and has shown promise in children, controlling 64% of SE in 1 pediatric case series (63). However, the use of prolonged propofol infusions is associated with propofol infusion syndrome, which is characterized by metabolic acidosis, lipidemia, arrhythmias, and cardiovascular collapse (32). Risk factors for propofol infusion syndrome include lean body mass, high dose, and greater than 24 hrs of administration (32). In response, propofol use for sustained sedation in children <16 years of age has been contraindicated in the US, Canada, and the European Union. Consequently, the use of propofol for RSE in children remains controversial, and the risks and benefits must be carefully weighed for each patient. If used, the infusion duration should be as short as possible, and the dose should not exceed 67 mcg/kg/min (18). During propofol therapy, patients should be closely monitored for the development of metabolic acidosis or lipidemia, and therapy should be stopped at the first indication of toxicity.

Valproate has been added as adjunctive therapy in adults and children with RSE. Case series show efficacy, but larger therapeutic trials are lacking (72). When administered as a continuous infusion, the mean efficacious dose is roughly 3 mg/kg/min (72). Of note, valproate may be particularly helpful in patients with myoclonic SE, absence SE, or Lennox-Gastaut syndrome.

Ketamine is an NMDA antagonist that is neuroprotective in experimental SE models and has been used in clinical RSE (13). As it acts as a glutamate antagonist, efficacy is preserved during prolonged RSE. Importantly, ketamine may increase intracranial pressure and should not be administered in the absence of neuroimaging that excludes mass intracranial lesions.

Topiramate is a newer anticonvulsant medication that potentiates GABA activity, reduces glutamate release, and provides activity-dependent blockade of voltage-gated sodium channels. Topiramate is typically used for chronic seizure control but has been administered to adult and pediatric patients with RSE via nasogastric tube (8,59). In adult patients, the initial topiramate dose was 25–100 mg twice daily, with rapid escalation to total doses of 300–1600 mg/day (59). In children, topiramate dosing was initiated at 2–5 mg/kg/day and increased by 5–10 mg/kg/day, to a maximum dose of 25 mg/kg/day (8). High-dose topiramate is also efficacious for infantile spasms. Finally, volatile anesthetics, such as isoflurane, may be used to treat RSE but have not been subject to clinical trials (53).

Surgical Treatment Options

RSE that fails to respond to high-dose suppressive therapy is associated with high morbidity and mortality in children. Most children are not surgical candidates; however, lobar resection or hemispherectomy can be considered in patients with discrete, localized seizure foci. In selected cases, surgical resection is effective and has a low morbidity and mortality in experienced hands. The largest case series reports on 10 children who underwent resection to treat RSE: 6 had functional hemispherectomies, and 4 had lobar or multilobar resections (3). All had acute control of the SE, and 7 remained seizure-free at follow-up. Epilepsy syndromes commonly amenable to resection include hemimegalencephaly, Rasmussen encephalitis, prenatal cerebral artery infarction, tuberous sclerosis, malformations of cortical development, and Sturge-Weber syndrome. Other surgical options may include multiple subpial transections, corpus callosotomy, and implantation of a vagal nerve stimulator (69). Surgical treatment of RSE requires focused evaluation, often including functional neuroimaging and surgical implantation of subdural grids to localize seizure foci; surgery must be considered in consultation with experienced pediatric neurosurgeons and neurologists.

OUTCOMES

Prognosis after SE is largely dependent on etiology and age. In general, children with acute symptomatic or progressive encephalopathic etiologies have greater risk for mortality and morbidity (6,36,44). Conversely, children with febrile or cryptogenic etiologies tend to fare better. The risk of adverse outcome is particularly high among infants with perinatal difficulties or neurologic abnormalities prior to the development of SE (6).

Mortality is 3%–7% overall (14,30) but varies greatly according to the etiology of the SE. Reported mortality with cryptogenic or febrile SE is 0%–2% (44). Conversely, among children with acute symptomatic etiologies, mortality increases to 12.5%–16% (36,44). Anoxia and acute bacterial meningitis carry particularly high risks of mortality (44). Similarly, the risk of mortality is higher for younger children, ranging 3%–22.5% for those <2 years of age (44).

Risk of Developing Epilepsy

Children in whom new-onset seizures present as SE may have a greater risk of developing epilepsy. In a prospective cohort study, the cumulative risk of epilepsy 5 years after new-onset seizures was 27% among children who presented with SE versus 3% among those who presented without SE (54). Additionally, afebrile, noncryptogenic etiologies of SE are associated with subsequent development of epilepsy (6,7). In fact, among children with acute or remote symptomatic SE, over half will develop epilepsy (44). Finally, intractable epilepsy is associated with young age at first SE episode and remote symptomatic etiology of SE (7).

Functional Disabilities

Cognitive or motor disabilities are reported after SE in 10%–35% of children (6,33,36). Risk factors for poor outcomes after SE include age <12 months, neuroimaging abnormalities, and acute symptomatic, remote symptomatic, or progressive encephalopathy etiology (6). While SE is associated with neurologic sequelae in many studies, other reports suggest a low incidence of morbidity after SE (39). Isolating the specific contributions of SE from those of seizure etiology is difficult, and similar functional outcomes are reported among epileptic children with or without SE (54). Additional longitudinal prospective studies are necessary to further clarify the specific effects of SE on cognitive and motor outcomes in children.

CONCLUSIONS AND FUTURE DIRECTIONS

Recent research in SE has begun to delineate differences between acute seizure management and prevention of epilepsy in the immature brain. Additionally, technologic advances hold promise for earlier and more reliable diagnosis of the underlying structural abnormalities in SE, which may have importance for recurrence or SE-related morbidities.

Status Epilepticus and Epileptogenesis

Newer anticonvulsant medications target the development of epilepsy (epileptogenesis), as well as acute seizure control. The process of epileptogenesis can be divided into three stages: the initial insult, a latency period, and development of chronic, unprovoked seizures. Interestingly, the processes that sustain SE may differ from those that promote epileptogenesis. Accordingly, experimental investigations suggest that therapies may have different efficacies for the control of acute SE and the prevention of subsequent epilepsy.

In a model of SE in immature (15- and 28-day-old) rats, administration of diazepam was more effective at stopping SE

than at preventing subsequent epilepsy (56). Conversely, administration of topiramate was more effective at preventing epilepsy than at stopping SE. Interestingly, rat age and SE duration affected the efficacy of both agents. Topiramate decreased cumulative seizure time more effectively in 28-day-old rats, yet had better efficacy for epilepsy prevention in 15-day-old rats. Diazepam decreased cumulative seizure time for both ages but was more efficacious in preventing epilepsy in 28-day-old rats. Not surprisingly, as seizure duration increased beyond 20 mins, the antiepileptogenic efficacy of both agents decreased. Further delineation of the effects of age, seizure duration, and medication administration on mechanisms of epileptogenesis may be used to tailor future therapeutic interventions in pediatric SE.

Application of Newer Neuroimaging Techniques

Recent advances in neuroimaging may provide better localization of epileptic foci and hold promise for earlier detection of SE-related structural abnormalities and associated morbidities. Peri-ictal imaging with MRI often reveals localized edema, gyri effacement, and diffusion restriction abnormalities. Unlike the diffusion restriction abnormalities commonly seen with cerebral ischemia, in SE they are often reversible and may indicate areas of hypermetabolism. More powerful MRI capabilities, such as 3-Tesla scanners, are able to detect more subtle structural lesions (26). In many cases, these lesions may be amenable to surgical resection, providing a viable treatment strategy for refractory or recurrent SE patients. Additionally, serial imaging can provide information about the regional rates of brain growth in patients with SE. Patterns of growth may provide clues to the risks or mechanisms for such comorbidities as attention deficit disorder or cognitive deficits (26).

Diffusion tensor imaging and diffusion spectral imaging are newer MRI techniques that can delineate white matter tracts based on the orientation of water diffusion in brain tissue. The diffusion of water is usually anisotropic (occurring in all possible directions) in brain tissue, but becomes more organized along mature white matter tracts (26). Changes in anisotropy, indicating alterations in white matter structure, are reported using diffusion tensor imaging in patients with temporal lobe epilepsy or tuberous sclerosis and cognitive disabilities (26). Diffusion tensor imaging is good for detecting changes in large white matter tracts but may miss localized, subtle alterations. Diffusion spectral imaging samples all water diffusion patterns in a region and generates a probabilistic map of white matter tract direction (26). Application of diffusion spectral imaging allows detection of more subtle differences and may be helpful for delineating patterns of development and cortical organization (26). Application of these newer techniques may advance the understanding of both normal brain development and structural abnormalities associated with SE.

KEY POINTS

- SE is a medical emergency that carries a mortality of 3%–7% in children.
- Survivors have a risk of morbidity, especially if SE is prolonged.

- Prompt, goal-directed therapy, including respiratory and hemodynamic support, rapid cessation of seizure activity, and treatment of underlying etiology, is indicated.
- The goal of therapy should be seizure cessation within 30 mins of presentation.
- Lorazepam is the preferred first-line anticonvulsant for most pediatric SE.
- Phenobarbital is the first-line agent for neonatal SE. Second-line agents include fosphenytoin, phenobarbital, and valproate.
- SE that fails to remit after treatment with two agents is considered refractory and carries a greater risk of morbidity and mortality.
- For RSE, pharmacologic coma should be induced promptly.
- Pentobarbital is the most commonly used agent to induce pharmacologic coma in children, although midazolam may be effective in some cases.
- The main determinant of outcome after SE is the underlying etiology, and acute inciting events must be sought and managed concurrent with attaining seizure control.

ACKNOWLEDGMENTS

Drs. Statler and Van Orman thank Dr. Susan Bratton for critical review of the manuscript. Dr. Statler is a Child Health Research Career Development Award recipient and a Primary Children's Medical Center Foundation Scholar. She is supported by the National Institutes of Health (K12-HD 01410-01), the Child Health Research Center at the University of Utah, and the Primary Children's Medical Center Foundation.

References

1. National Institute for Clinical Excellence. Clinical guideline 20, the epilepsies: The diagnosis and management of the epilepsies in adults and children in primary and secondary care. 2004; Accessed April 4, 2006; www.nice.org.uk.
2. Scottish Intercollegiate Guidelines Network. Guideline 81, diagnosis and management of epilepsies in children and young people: A national clinical guideline. 2005; Accessed April 4, 2006; www.sign.ac.uk.
3. Alexopoulos A, Lachhwani DK, Gupta A, et al. Resective surgery to treat refractory status epilepticus in children with focal epileptogenesis. Neurology 2005;64:567–70.
4. Arzimangoglou A, Guerrini R, Aicardi J. Aicardi's epilepsy in children. Philadelphia: Lippencott, Williams, & Wilkins, 2004.
5. Asadi-Pooya AA, Poordast A. Etiologies and outcomes of status epilepticus in children. Epilepsy Behav 2005;7:502–5.
6. Barnard C, Wirrell E. Does status epilepticus in children cause developmental deterioration and exacerbation of epilepsy? J Child Neurol 1999;14:787–94.
7. Berg AT, Levy SR, Novotny EJ, et al. Predictors of intractable epilepsy in childhood: A case-control study. Epilepsia 1996;37:24–30.
8. Blumkin L, Lerman-Sagie T, Houri T, et al. Pediatric refractory partial status epilepticus responsive to topiramate. J Child Neurol 2005;20:239–41.
9. Boison D. Adenosine and epilepsy: From therapeutic rationale to new therapeutic strategies. Neuroscientist 2005;11:25–36.
10. Brooks-Kayal AR. Rearranging receptors. Epilepsia 2005;46 Suppl 7:29–38.
11. Castro Conde JR, Hernandez Borges AA, Domenech Martinez E, et al. Midazolam in neonatal seizures with no response to phenobarbital. Neurology 2005;64:876–9.
12. Chang BS, Lowenstein DH. Epilepsy. N Engl J Med 2003;349:1257–66.
13. Chen JW, Wasterlain CG. Status epilepticus: Pathophysiology and management in adults. Lancet Neurol 2006;5:246–56.
14. Chin RF, Neville BG, Peckham C, et al. Incidence, cause, and short-term outcome of convulsive status epilepticus in childhood: Prospective population-based study. Lancet 2006;368:222–9.
15. Chugani DC, Muzik O, Juhasz C, et al. Postnatal maturation of human GABA$_A$ receptors measured with positron emission tomography. Ann Neurol 2001;49:618–26.
16. Claassen J, Hirsch LJ, Emerson RG, et al. Treatment of refractory status epilepticus with pentobarbital, propofol, or midazolam: A systematic review. Epilepsia 2002;43:146–53.
17. Claassen J, Mayer SA, Kowalski RG, et al. Detection of electrographic seizures with continuous EEG monitoring in critically ill patients. Neurology 2004;62:1743–8.
18. Cornfield DN, Tegtmeyer K, Nelson MD, et al. Continuous propofol infusion in 142 critically ill children. Pediatrics 2002;110:1177–81.
19. Delorenzo RJ. Epidemiology and clinical presentation of status epilepticus. Adv Neurol 2006;97:199–215.
20. Delorenzo RJ, Sun DA. Basic mechanisms in status epilepticus: Role of calcium in neuronal injury and the induction of epileptogenesis. Adv Neurol 2006;97:187–97.
21. Delorenzo RJ, Waterhouse EJ, Towne AR, et al. Persistent nonconvulsive status epilepticus after the control of convulsive status epilepticus. Epilepsia 1998;39:833–40.
22. Dhar R, Mirsattari SM. Current approach to the diagnosis and treatment of refractory status epilepticus. Adv Neurol 2006;97:245–54.
23. Eriksson K, Metsaranta P, Huhtala H, et al. Treatment delay and the risk of prolonged status epilepticus. Neurology 2005;65:1316–8.
24. Fujikawa DG. Prolonged seizures and cellular injury: Understanding the connection. Epilepsy Behav 2005;7 Suppl 3:S3–11.
25. Fujikawa DG, Itabashi HH, Wu A, et al. Status epilepticus-induced neuronal loss in humans without systemic complications or epilepsy. Epilepsia 2000;41:981–91.
26. Grant PE. Imaging the developing epileptic brain. Epilepsia 2005;46 Suppl 7:7–14.
27. Guttinger M, Fedele D, Koch P, et al. Suppression of kindled seizures by paracrine adenosine release from stem cell-derived brain implants. Epilepsia 2005;46:1162–9.
28. Holmes GL. Effects of seizures on brain development: Lessons from the laboratory. Pediatr Neurol 2005;33:1–11.
29. Igartua J, Silver P, Maytal J, et al. Midazolam coma for refractory status epilepticus in children. Crit Care Med 1999;27:1982–5.
30. Karasalihoglu S, Oner N, Celtik C, et al. Risk factors of status epilepticus in children. Pediatr Int 2003;45:429–34.
31. Keenan HT, Bunyan DK, Marshall SW, et al. A population-based comparison of clinical and outcome characteristics of young children with serious inflicted and noninflicted traumatic brain injury. Pediatrics 2004;114:633–9.
32. Kumar MA, Urrutia VC, Thomas CE, et al. The syndrome of irreversible acidosis after prolonged propofol infusion. Neurocrit Care 2005;3:257–9.
33. Lacroix J, Deal C, Gauthier M, et al. Admissions to a pediatric intensive care unit for status epilepticus: A 10-year experience. Crit Care Med 1994;22:827–32.
34. Mayer SA, Claassen J, Lokin J, et al. Refractory status epilepticus: Frequency, risk factors, and impact on outcome. Arch Neurol 2002;59:205–10.
35. Maytal J, Novak G, Ascher C, et al. Status epilepticus in children with epilepsy: The role of antiepileptic drug levels in prevention. Pediatrics 1996;98:1119–21.
36. Maytal J, Shinnar S, Moshe SL, et al. Low morbidity and mortality of status epilepticus in children. Pediatrics 1989;83:323–31.
37. Mcintyre J, Robertson S, Norris E, et al. Safety and efficacy of buccal midazolam versus rectal diazepam for emergency treatment of seizures in children: A randomised controlled trial. Lancet 2005;366:205–10.
38. Meldrum BS, Brierley JB. Prolonged epileptic seizures in primates. Ischemic cell change and its relation to ictal physiological events. Arch Neurol 1973;28:10–7.
39. Metsaranta P, Koivikko M, Peltola J, et al. Outcome after prolonged convulsive seizures in 186 children: Low morbidity, no mortality. Dev Med Child Neurol 2004;46:4–8.
40. Mikati MA, Werner S, Shalak L, et al. Stages of status epilepticus in the developing brain. Epilepsy Res 2003;55:9–19.
41. Morrison G, Gibbons E, Whitehouse WP. High-dose midazolam therapy for refractory status epilepticus in children. Intensive Care Med 2006;32:2070–6.
42. Oby E, Janigro D. The blood-brain barrier and epilepsy. Epilepsia 2006;47:1761–74.
43. Prasad AN, Seshia SS. Status epilepticus in pediatric practice: Neonate to adolescent. Adv Neurol 2006;97:229–43.
44. Raspall-Chaure M, Chin RF, Neville BG, et al. Outcome of paediatric convulsive status epilepticus: A systematic review. Lancet Neurol 2006;5:769–79.
45. Rossetti AO, Logroscino G, Bromfield EB. Refractory status epilepticus: Effect of treatment aggressiveness on prognosis. Arch Neurol 2005;62:1698–702.
46. Saengpattrachai M, Sharma R, Hunjan A, et al. Nonconvulsive seizures in the pediatric intensive care unit: Etiology, EEG, and brain imaging findings. Epilepsia 2006;47:1510–8.
47. Sahin M, Menache CC, Holmes GL, et al. Prolonged treatment for acute symptomatic refractory status epilepticus: Outcome in children. Neurology 2003;61:398–401.
48. Scott RC, Gadian DG, King MD, et al. Magnetic resonance imaging findings within 5 days of status epilepticus in childhood. Brain 2002;125:1951–9.
49. Scott RC, King MD, Gadian DG, et al. Hippocampal abnormalities after prolonged febrile convulsion: A longitudinal MRI study. Brain 2003;126:2551–7.

50. Scott RC, King MD, Gadian DG, et al. Prolonged febrile seizures are associated with hippocampal vasogenic edema and developmental changes. *Epilepsia* 2006;47:1493–8.

51. Shinnar S, Berg AT, Moshe SL, et al. How long do new-onset seizures in children last? *Ann Neurol* 2001;49:659–64.

52. Shinnar S, Pellock JM, Moshe SL, et al. In whom does status epilepticus occur: Age-related differences in children. *Epilepsia* 1997;38:907–14.

53. Shorvon S. *Status epilepticus: Its clinical features and treatment in children and adults.* Cambridge: Cambridge University Press, 1994.

54. Sillanpaa M, Shinnar S. Status epilepticus in a population-based cohort with childhood-onset epilepsy in Finland. *Ann Neurol* 2002;52:303–10.

55. Sisodiya SM, Lin WR, Harding BN, et al. Drug resistance in epilepsy: Expression of drug resistance proteins in common causes of refractory epilepsy. *Brain* 2002;125:22–31.

56. Suchomelova L, Baldwin RA, Kubova H, et al. Treatment of experimental status epilepticus in immature rats: Dissociation between anticonvulsant and antiepileptogenic effects. *Pediatr Res* 2006;59:237–43.

57. Tay SK, Hirsch LJ, Leary L, et al. Nonconvulsive status epilepticus in children: Clinical and EEG characteristics. *Epilepsia* 2006;47:1504–9.

58. Towne AR, Delorenzo RJ. Use of intramuscular midazolam for status epilepticus. *J Emerg Med* 1999;17:323–8.

59. Towne AR, Garnett LK, Waterhouse EJ, et al. The use of topiramate in refractory status epilepticus. *Neurology* 2003;60:332–4.

60. Treiman DM, Walton NY, Kendrick C. A progressive sequence of electroencephalographic changes during generalized convulsive status epilepticus. *Epilepsy Res* 1990;5:49–60.

61. Ulvi H, Yoldas T, Mungen B, et al. Continuous infusion of midazolam in the treatment of refractory generalized convulsive status epilepticus. *Neurol Sci* 2002;23:177–82.

62. Valente KD, Koiffmann CP, Fridman C, et al. Epilepsy in patients with Angelman syndrome caused by deletion of the chromosome 15q11–13. *Arch Neurol* 2006;63:122–8.

63. Van Gestel JP, Blusse Van Oud-Alblas HJ, Malingre M, et al. Propofol and thiopental for refractory status epilepticus in children. *Neurology* 2005;65:591–2.

64. Vespa P. Continuous EEG monitoring for the detection of seizures in traumatic brain injury, infarction, and intracerebral hemorrhage: "To detect and protect." *J Clin Neurophysiol* 2005;22:99–106.

65. Vespa P, Martin NA, Nenov V, et al. Delayed increase in extracellular glycerol with post-traumatic electrographic epileptic activity: Support for the theory that seizures induce secondary injury. *Acta Neurochir Suppl* 2002;81:355–7.

66. Vespa P, Prins M, Ronne-Engstrom E, et al. Increase in extracellular glutamate caused by reduced cerebral perfusion pressure and seizures after human traumatic brain injury: A microdialysis study. *J Neurosurg* 1998;89: 971–82.

67. Waterhouse EJ, Vaughan JK, Barnes TY, et al. Synergistic effect of status epilepticus and ischemic brain injury on mortality. *Epilepsy Res* 1998;29: 175–83.

68. Wheless JW, Clarke DF, Carpenter D. Treatment of pediatric epilepsy: Expert opinion, 2005. *J Child Neurol* 2005;20 Suppl 1:S1–56.

69. Winston KR, Levisohn P, Miller BR, et al. Vagal nerve stimulation for status epilepticus. *Pediatr Neurosurg* 2001;34:190–2.

70. Wolfe TR, Macfarlane TC. Intranasal midazolam therapy for pediatric status epilepticus. *Am J Emerg Med* 2006;24:343–6.

71. Young GB. Status epilepticus and brain damage: Pathology and pathophysiology. *Adv Neurol* 2006;97:217–20.

72. Yu Kt, Mills S, Thompson N, et al. Safety and efficacy of intravenous valproate in pediatric status epilepticus and acute repetitive seizures. *Epilepsia* 2003;44:724–6.

CHAPTER 58 ■ CEREBROVASCULAR DISEASE AND STROKE

JOHN PAPPACHAN • FENELLA KIRKHAM

Stroke and cerebrovascular disorders are an important cause of morbidity and mortality in children. Recent epidemiologic data suggest that ~3200 cases of stroke occur per year in the population aged between 30 days and 18 years in the US alone. Although outcome for stroke in children is significantly better than in adults, 20% die and 50%–80% are left with significant disability. This chapter concentrates on the presentation, pathophysiology, investigation, and treatment of children who present to the PICU with acute stroke syndromes. The most recent epidemiologic data are reviewed, and the pathogenesis of hemorrhagic and ischemic stroke syndromes, their risk factors, and conditions that predispose to stroke are described. Approximately half of the children who present with stroke have a previously recognized condition, most commonly congenital heart disease and sickle cell disease, and so the clinical context may provide clues about the likely pathophysiology. Trauma and infection (e.g., bacterial and tuberculous meningitis and varicella) are common triggers in the symptomatic as well as the cryptogenic groups. The pivotal role played by pediatric intensivists in facilitating and accelerating emergency medical and surgical intervention, preventing secondary damage, and minimizing morbidity and mortality, as well as risk of recurrence, is emphasized. The socioeconomic burden of this disease is highlighted, the clinical presentation described, and the diagnosis-specific and independent management strategies are explored.

Efficient transport and intensive care is essential, and patients may require emergency treatment for seizures and intracranial hypertension. Neurosurgical involvement may be required, particularly where level of consciousness is deteriorating, for drainage of intracerebral hemorrhage, hemicraniectomy for malignant middle cerebral infarction, or shunting for posterior fossa infarction. Urgent exchange blood transfusion for patients with ischemic stroke in the context of sickle cell disease (SCD) is reasonable, but no other specific treatment exists to limit the extent of infarction; thrombolysis cannot currently be recommended for children. Recurrent stroke affects ~10% of children with arterial ischemic stroke (AIS), and 6% of those with sinovenous thrombosis have a further cerebral or systemic thrombosis, so that early diagnosis and prophylaxis are important. Ideally, emergency neuroimaging should include MRI, MR angiography (MRA), MR venography (MRV), and fat-saturated, T1-weighted imaging of the neck for the diagnosis of vascular pathologies such as sinovenous thrombosis and extracranial arterial dissection, in which anticoagulation may be a better initial choice than aspirin. In addition, stroke mimics, such as demyelination, reversible posterior leukoencephalopathy (RPLS), border-zone ischemia, and hemispheric or focal edema in a nonvascular distribution, may be distinguished, and alternative management strategies commenced. Although the only randomized, controlled trial (RCT) data pertain to primary prevention of stroke in sickle cell anemia, consensus statements on the management of stroke in childhood have been published by the Seventh American College of Chest Physicians (ACCP) Conference on Antithrombotic and Thrombolytic Therapy (33) and by the Paediatric Stroke Working Group of the UK Royal College of Physicians (RCP) (39).

PRESENTATION, EPIDEMIOLOGY, DEFINITIONS, OUTCOMES, AND COSTS

Overview of Childhood Presentation with Stroke and Cerebrovascular Disease

Acute focal signs of stroke in childhood can be symptomatic of a variety of pathologies (Table 58.1). The World Health Organization definition of stroke is "rapidly developing clinical signs of focal (or global) disturbance of cerebral function, with symptoms lasting 24 hrs or longer, or leading to death, with no apparent cause other than of vascular origin." Patients whose signs resolve within 24 hrs have transient ischemic attacks (TIAs) by definition, but many have recent cerebral infarction or hemorrhage on imaging (20). Coma is a well-recognized presentation in children with subarachnoid hemorrhage (SAH) or intracerebral hemorrhage (ICH) (26), large middle cerebral artery (MCA) territory infarction, vertebrobasilar circulation stroke, sinovenous thrombosis, bilateral border-zone ischemia, and RPLS. Seizures or headache may herald stroke and cerebrovascular disease (CVD), particularly sinovenous thrombosis, in children (20,46). Silent infarction may be demonstrated in up to 25% of children with sickle cell anemia on MRI (28) and may affect other "at-risk" populations, such as those with congenital heart disease.

Epidemiology

Stroke and cerebrovascular disorders are relatively rare in children but cause disproportionate morbidity and mortality (16), particularly in those with critical illness (27). Already among the top 10 causes of childhood death, the prevalence is probably increasing as a consequence of increased recognition and improved sensitivity of diagnostic neuroimaging (MR/CT angiography), in addition to the therapeutic advances that now allow children with predisposing conditions such as SCD,

TABLE 58.1

DIFFERENTIAL DIAGNOSIS IN CHILDREN WHO PRESENT WITH ACUTE FOCAL NEUROLOGIC DEFICIT

- Primary hemorrhagic stroke +/– mass effect
- Acute Ischemic arterial stroke +/– hemorrhage +/– **mass effect**
- Acute venous stroke +/– hemorrhage +/– venous infarction +/– mass effect
- Postictal (As Todd paresis is of short duration, if persistent, neuroimaging is essential; children with prolonged seizures may develop permanent hemiparesis.)
- Hemiplegic migraine (but diagnosis of exclusion, as migrainous symptoms are commonly seen in cerebrovascular disease, e.g., dissection)
- Acute disseminated encephalomyelitis
- Brain tumor
- Nonaccidental injury (subdural hematoma, strangulation with compression of internal carotid artery)
- Encephalitis, e.g., secondary to herpes simplex (usually have seizures)
- Rasmussen encephalitis
- Posterior leukoencephalopathy (hypertension/hypotension or immunosuppression)
- Unilateral hemispheric/focal cerebral edema—e.g., secondary to metabolic
- Alternating hemiplegia

All stroke syndromes are potential neurosurgical emergencies and should always be discussed with a pediatric neurologist on presentation. Further management and any transfer must involve liaison with the nearest available PICU.

congenital heart disease, and malignancy to survive. Neonatal stroke affects 25–30 per 100,000 live births, while epidemiologic data have suggested incidence rates of between 2 and 13 per 100,000 children/year (16,53), with one-half to two-thirds being ischemic and the remainder being hemorrhagic or having alternative diagnoses (e.g., sinovenous thrombosis without parenchymal involvement). The more conservative estimates predict 3200 cases of stroke per year in a population aged between 30 days and 18 years of age in the US alone. Ischemic stroke peaks in the first year of life, while SAH is more common in teenagers. Boys are at higher risk, as are those of black ethnicity. Although childhood stroke is much more common in SCD (35), this condition does not entirely account for the ethnic disparity (16). The combined mortality rate is ~20% (640 annualized deaths in the US), and an additional 50%–80% of events will result in permanent cognitive or motor disability (5,11,18). Importantly, prognosis in pediatric stroke is significantly better than in the adult population. However, children who do not die acutely will probably survive beyond middle age, making the treatment of any resulting comorbidity extremely expensive. Thus, the health burden of this disease entity is very large (11).

Definitions, Outcomes, and Costs

Healthcare utilization is not adequately reflected by incidence figures. In 1996, the lifetime cost of a first stroke in an adult was estimated to be $90,981 (52). The diagnostic workup in children will be greater because of their more heterogeneous risk factors. Acute treatment costs may be smaller because of the paucity of proven acute interventions, but the long-term healthcare costs of rehabilitation and continued care and treatment of recurrent stroke might well be much greater.

The socioeconomic costs of a disease are most appropriately described by disease outcome. Ischemic stroke occurs commonly in an arterial distribution (20), but superficial infarcts in the parietal, occipital, or frontal lobes or the thalami may be venous (46) (**Figs. 58.1 and 58.2**). Mortality is 6%–20%, half of which is stroke related, and half is due to the underlying disease (21,27). Long-term disability may have decreased from approximately 85% to 50%–60% (11,18), probably due to the inclusion of children with a milder spectrum of disease due to increasing diagnostic sensitivity and perhaps related to the use of antithrombotic agents. Seizure disorders complicate 15%–20% of ischemic strokes. Predictors of poor outcome include the presence of multiple etiologic risk factors (31), seizures at onset, arterial stroke type rather than sinovenous thrombosis (11), and for sinovenous thrombosis, the presence of venous infarcts (11,46). The estimated rates of recurrent stroke for AIS are <5% for neonates and 6%–14% in older infants and children (21,50), with a further 20% experiencing recurrent TIAs (21). Recurrence rates are lower for sinovenous thrombosis in older infants and children—approximately 3%—although subsequent systemic thrombosis also occurs in a further 3% (12,27,46).

Hemorrhagic stroke includes ICH (4,26,32) (**Fig. 58.1A**), most commonly due to arteriovenous malformation (13), and SAH (4,26,32), often secondary to aneurysm, but sinovenous thrombosis may cause either (46). Mortality is 8%–40% if ICH and SAH are included (26), i.e., approximately twice that of ischemic stroke. While hemorrhage is predictive of death, the incidence of neurologic disability (33%–50%), seizures (5%–10%), and recurrence (10%–20%) is lower (4,32), although the risk of death at the time of recurrence is also high.

In summary, the available epidemiologic data indicate that stroke in children is increasing either the incidence or recognition of and leads to a significant burden in terms of mortality, neurologic disability, cognitive problems, and seizures. As children who survive stroke are expected to live a full lifespan, the burden of illness for an individual will last for several decades. While primary prevention is difficult, many children are initially admitted to the PICU, and the clinicians there have a very important role in preventing secondary damage and minimizing both morbidity and mortality by facilitating and accelerating emergency medical and surgical intervention and reducing the risk of early recurrence. Stroke in any population is devastating but is particularly so in a child: the potential for aggressive acute intervention in the inherently plastic and potentially recoverable pediatric brain must be explored. The pediatric intensivist is very commonly part of the team managing the acute insult and thus has an opportunity to change the evolution of this disease process and its ultimate cost to the individual and society. The discussion in this chapter concentrates on the presentation, pathophysiology, investigation, and treatment of children who present to the PICU with acute stroke syndromes.

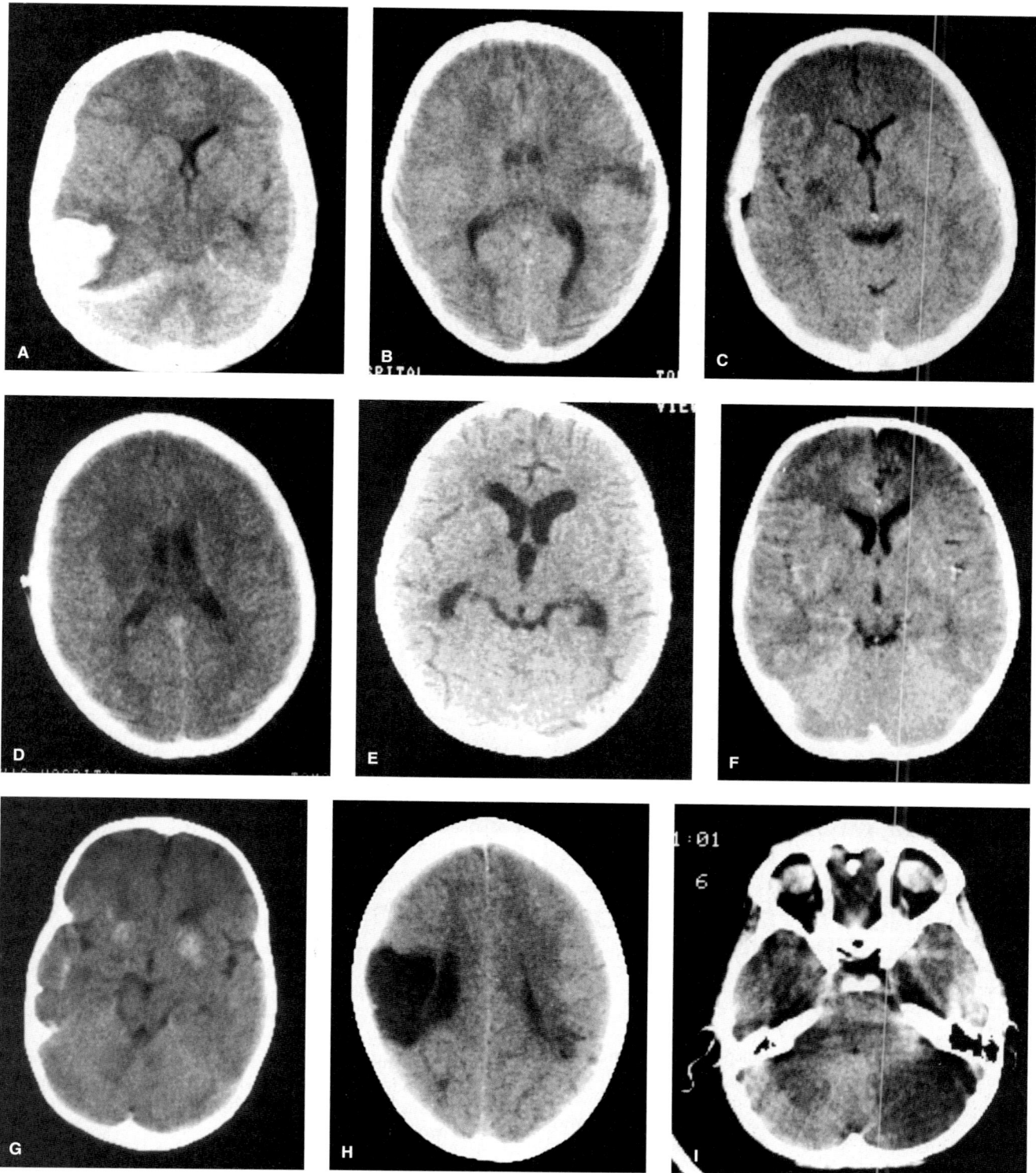

FIGURE 58.1. CT scans from children with hemorrhagic and ischemic (arterial and venous) stroke and its mimics. (**A**) Spontaneous intracerebral hemorrhage with midline shift. (**B**) Cortical ischemic stroke after minor head injury. (**C**) Small infarct associated with middle cerebral artery stenosis. (**D**) Larger infarct after recurrence of stroke in C. (**E**) Hydrocephalus and basal ganglia infarct in tuberculous meningitis. (**F**) Frontal infarction associated with moyamoya. (**G**) Calcification associated with moyamoya. (**H**) Old congenital infarct. (**I**) Cerebellar infarction in an unconscious boy. (*Continued*).

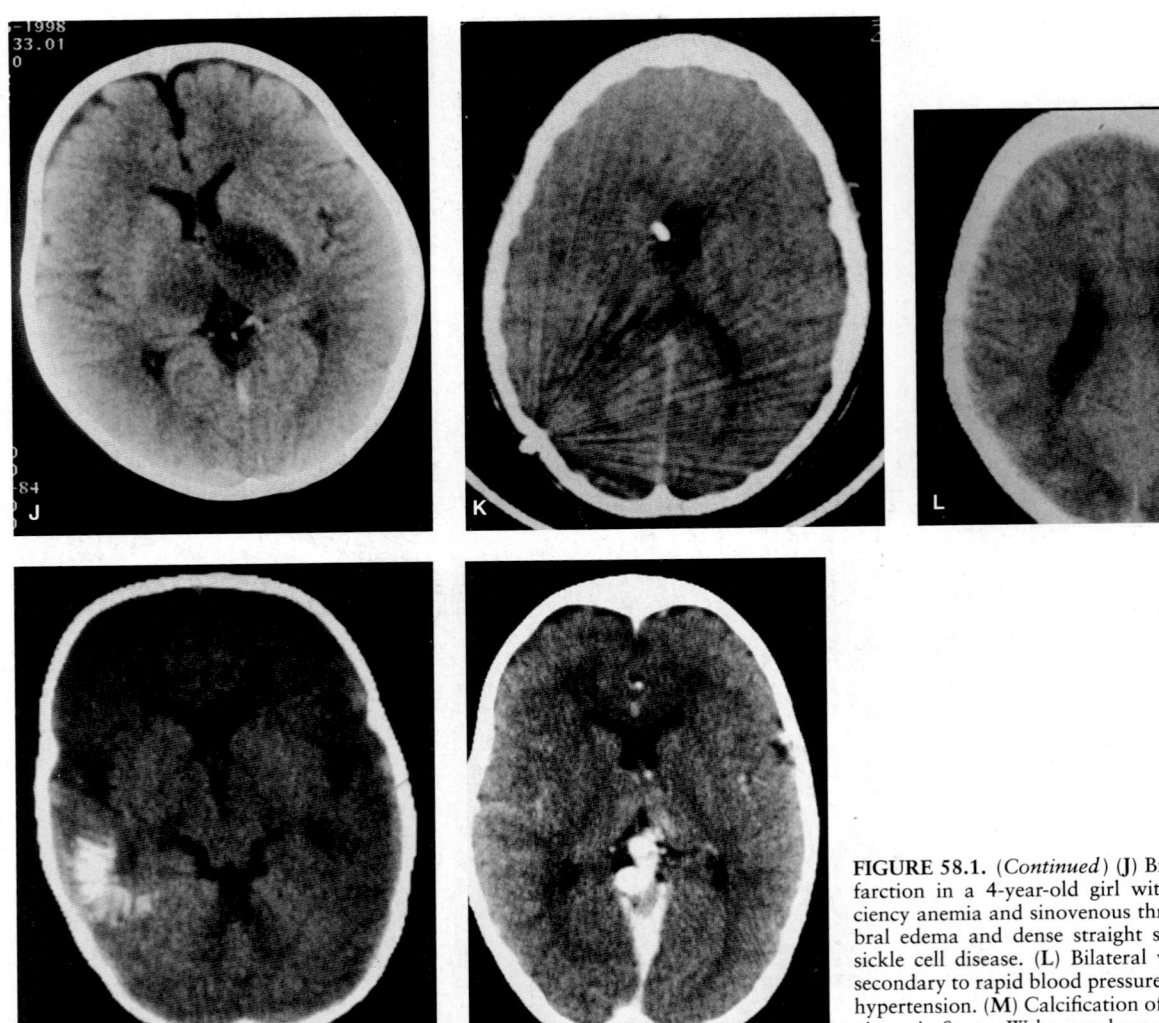

FIGURE 58.1. (*Continued*) (**J**) Bilateral thalamic infarction in a 4-year-old girl with severe iron deficiency anemia and sinovenous thrombosis. (**K**) Cerebral edema and dense straight sinus thrombosis in sickle cell disease. (**L**) Bilateral watershed ischemia secondary to rapid blood pressure reduction in severe hypertension. (**M**) Calcification of the frontal pial angioma in Sturge-Weber syndrome. (**N**) Vein of Galen malformation (contrast CT).

MECHANISM OF DISEASE: CORE PATHOPHYSIOLOGY

Risk Factors

Numerous inherited conditions predispose to CVD and stroke, but our understanding of the precise mechanisms has been limited until recently. Approximately half of the children with a first-ever AIS have a known predisposing cause; however, for the remainder, the stroke is, at least initially, unexplained (20). The most common predisposing conditions in childhood are heart disease (20,34) and anemias, including SCD (20,35) (Fig. 58.2J–L, Q–S). Other acquired conditions such as leukemia and brain tumor (**Fig. 58.2H, I**); chromosomal disorders, including Down syndrome; and genetic disorders such as neurofibromatosis are also usually obvious at the time of presentation (20). Those previously well may have a history of trauma or recent infection, e.g., with varicella (20,45) (**Figs. 58.2A** and **58.3A**), and investigation may often reveal a vasculopathy (20) and/or hereditary coagulopathy (34). They may also have single-gene disorders with a highly significant

predisposition to stroke (37), such as homocystinuria (7), Fabry disease (43), and Menkes disease (37), but these may not be obvious. However, most people with these conditions do not have stroke, and whether those who do experience stroke have additional genetic or environmental factors remains controversial. Hemorrhagic stroke and sinovenous thrombosis may also occur in the context of acquired illnesses or conditions with Mendelian inheritance (4,27,46), but data on family history are limited. As for adult stroke, genes that control intermediate risk factors such as hypertension (20) and hyperhomocysteinemia (40) may be important.

Phenotype of Childhood Stroke

Previously Recognized Diagnoses

Congenital Heart Disease. Cardiac embolism may occur, particularly at the time of interventions such as catheterization or surgery or secondary to infective endocarditis, but echocardiography often fails to reveal a source of clot (20); other pathophysiologies, including sinovenous thrombosis (28,38,46) (**Figs. 58.1J,K** and **58.2M–Q**) and primary cerebral

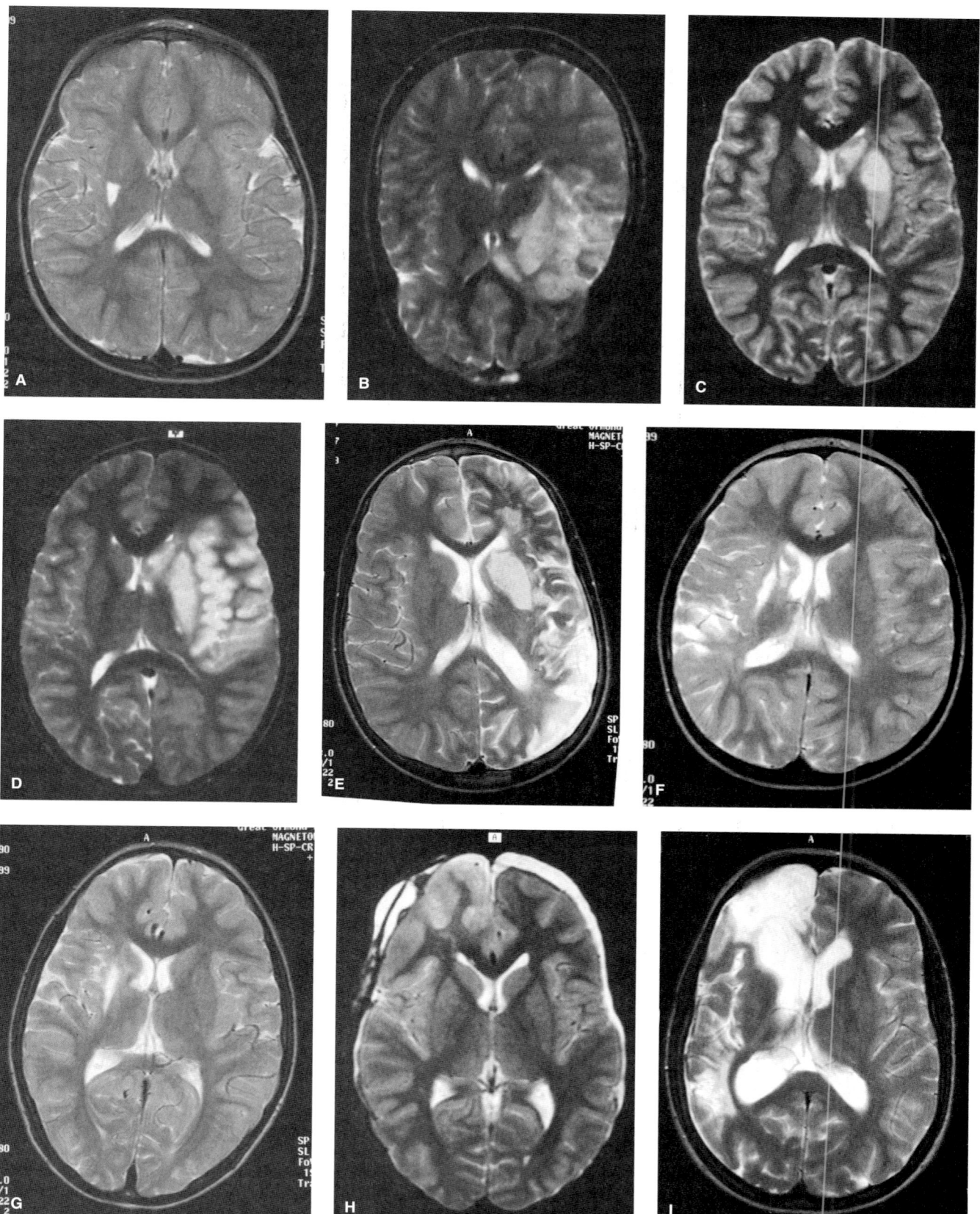

FIGURE 58.2. MRI scans from children with first and recurrent ischemic (arterial and venous) stroke and its mimics. (**A**) Basal ganglia infarct associated with transient cerebral arteriopathy after varicella. (**B**) Temporal infarction associated with dissection. (**C**) Small infarct associated with middle cerebral artery stenosis. (**D**) Larger infarct after recurrence of stroke in C. (**E**) Recurrent infarction after dissection. (**F**) "Silent" posterior watershed recurrent infarction after embolic occlusion. (**G**) Deep white matter infarct in *Haemophilus influenzae* meningitis. (**H**) Right frontal cortical edema after craniopharyngioma surgery. (**I**) "Silent" recurrent infarction in the posterior watershed territory in the same patient as in D. (*Continued*)

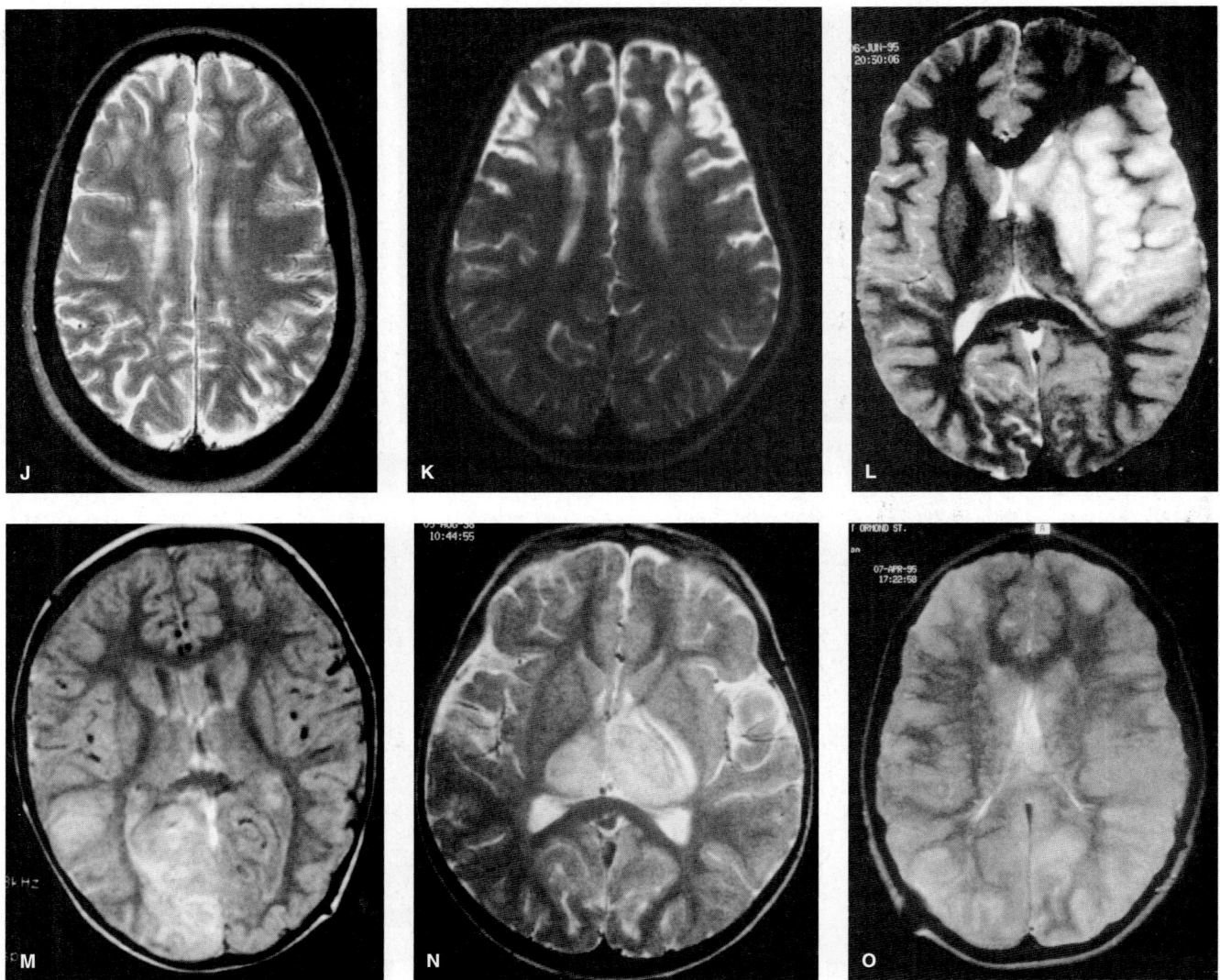

FIGURE 58.2. (*Continued*) (**J**) "Silent" infarction in the deep white matter in sickle cell anemia. (**K**) Bilateral frontal infarction in sickle cell anemia and moyamoya. (**L**) Large middle cerebral artery territory infarct in sickle cell anemia. (**M**) High signal in the right occipital lobe associated with straight sinus occlusion; subacute thrombus is seen as high signal on proton density images. (**N**) Bilateral thalamic infarction in sinovenous thrombosis (same patient as Fig. 58.1J). (**O**) Thrombus in the straight and left transverse sinuses on coronal T1-weighted MRI.

arterial disease (20) (**Figs. 58.3** and **58.4**), should be excluded. In contrast to studies in young adults, previously undiagnosed cardiac disease, such as patent foramen ovale, is relatively uncommon (20), but otherwise asymptomatic abnormalities of the aortic valve are associated with primary CVDs such as cervicocephalic dissection and moyamoya (**Figs. 58.3** and **58.4**) (20). Abnormalities of vascular embryogenesis at the time of neural crest development and associated inherited connective tissue diseases (e.g., Marfan syndrome) may thus be associated with CVD as well as cardiovascular disease.

Sickle Cell Disease. The best-studied population is that with sickle cell anemia, among whom most children with overt ischemic stroke (**Fig. 58.2L**) have intracranial, large-vessel disease (**Fig. 58.3D–F**) with intimal hyperplasia pathologically.

Twenty-five percent of patients have had a stroke by the age of 45 (35); ischemic stroke predominates in childhood, while the majority of adults have spontaneous ICH or SAH secondary to aneurysm (35), although hemorrhage secondary to hypertension and steroid use has been well documented in children, sinovenous thrombosis (**Figs. 58.1K** and **58.2Q**) (46), posterior leukoencephalopathy, and watershed ischemia (**Fig. 58.2R,S**) (23) have probably been previously under-recognized. This very complex, recessively inherited disease illustrates the need for a very careful description of the phenotype when attempting to look for epistatic genes for stroke and other neurologic complications. The predisposition to large- and small-vessel disease, "silent" (covert) and clinical (overt) infarction, seizures, and cognitive deterioration may be in part related to genetic makeup but is probably also linked to

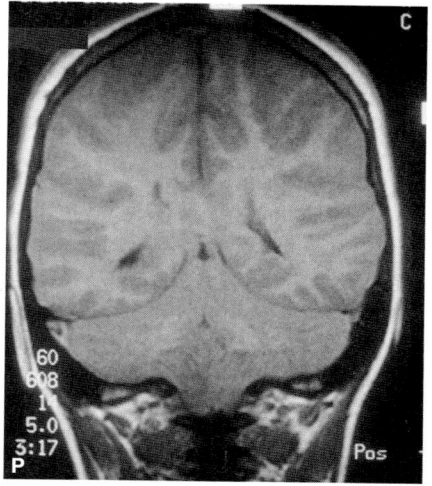
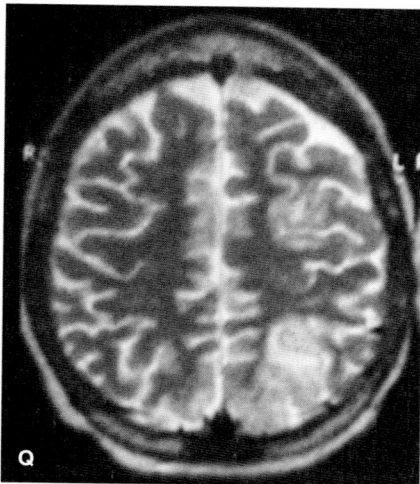
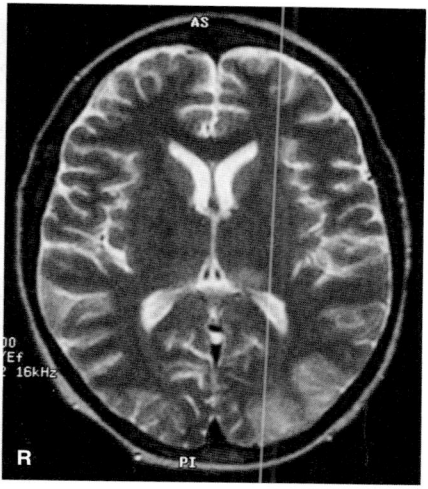
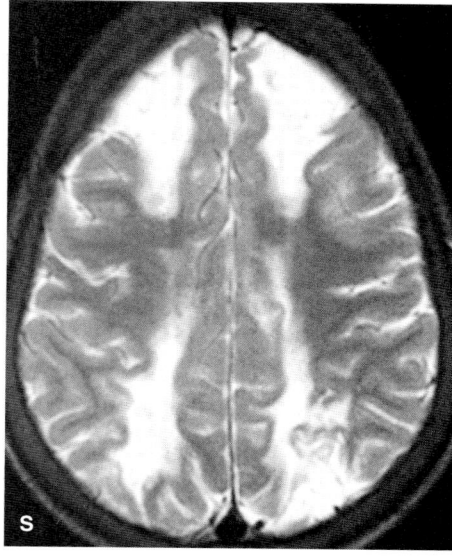

FIGURE 58.2. (*Continued*) (**P**) Widespread cortical and basal ganglia hypersignal on T2-weighted axial MRI (same patient with sickle cell disease as shown in Fig. 58.1K). (**Q**) T1-weighted coronal images showing marked swelling of the cerebral hemispheres and posterior fossa leading to tonsillar descent and brain death in same patient with sickle cell disease as shown in **Figs. 58.1K** and **58.2P**. High signal is seen in the right transverse sinus (delta sign) due to sinovenous thrombus. (**R**) Occipital edema in distribution compatible with reversible posterior leukoencephalopathy in sickle cell anemia and acute chest crisis. (**S**) Bilateral watershed infarction in sickle cell anemia and facial infection

environmental exposures, e.g., infection, poor nutrition, or hypoxemia (29).

Intermediate Risk Factors for Childhood Stroke

Infection, Inflammation, and Immune Deficiency. At least one-third of cases of childhood stroke occur in the context of infection (42). Bacterial and tuberculous meningitis are well-recognized associations (**Figs. 58.1E, 58.2G,** and **58.3B**) (20). Frank immunodeficiency, either inherited or acquired, also appears to be an occasional association (20). Recently, chickenpox within the previous year has been documented to be more common in otherwise cryptogenic stroke than in controls (45) (**Figs. 58.2A** and **58.3A**). In SCD, high leukocyte count is a risk factor for stroke, and cerebrovascular episodes are often precipitated by infections. This group of patients is also relatively immunodeficient, in part secondary to splenic autoinfarction or surgical removal of the spleen. High white cell count and immunodeficiency predict recurrent infarction, suggesting a role for chronic infection (21). Genetic modulators of the immune response may also be important in the development of CVD and stroke, and the host inflammatory response may also play

a role in, for example, determining levels of intermediary cytokines, which may have harmful effects on the endothelium.

Anemia. Stroke syndromes are well described in the hemolytic anemias, including intermediate forms of thalassemia, hereditary spherocytosis, and paroxysmal nocturnal hemoglobinuria, as well as SCD. Iron deficiency appears to be a risk factor for stroke in children with heart disease (38), sinovenous thrombosis (46), and probably for AIS in general (20).

Hyperhomocysteinemia. Classic homocystinuria (deficiency of cystathionine β-synthase) has long been recognized as an important cause of arterial vascular disease and infarction. Considerable evidence suggests that it is high levels of homocysteine that predispose to vessel abnormalities (40). Reduction in transcriptional activity of the 5,10-methylene tetrahydrofolate reductase gene results in decreased conversion of homocysteine to methionine by the gene product and, therefore, results in hyperhomocysteinemia. Homozygosity for the thermolabile variant of this gene appears to be a risk factor for neonatal and childhood AIS (34,40), sinovenous thrombosis (46), and

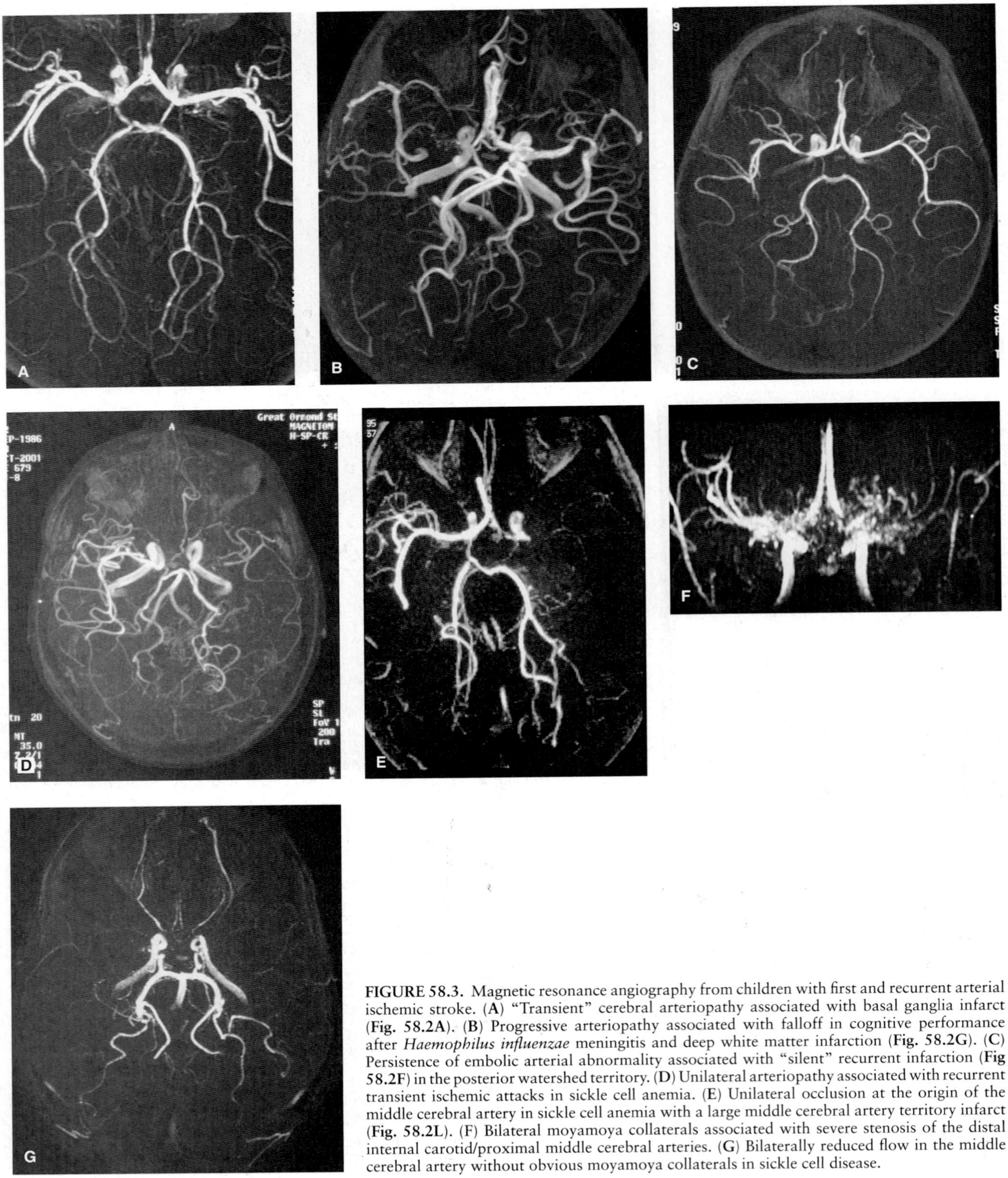

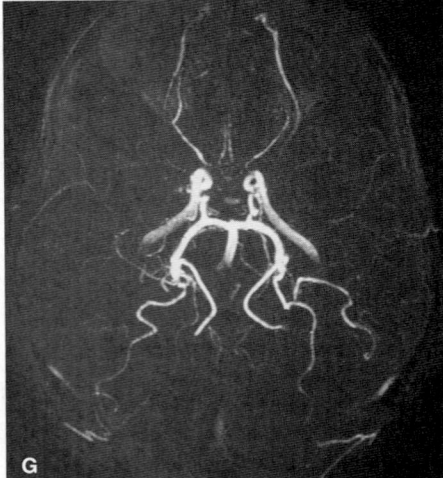

FIGURE 58.3. Magnetic resonance angiography from children with first and recurrent arterial ischemic stroke. (**A**) "Transient" cerebral arteriopathy associated with basal ganglia infarct (**Fig. 58.2A**). (**B**) Progressive arteriopathy associated with falloff in cognitive performance after *Haemophilus influenzae* meningitis and deep white matter infarction (**Fig. 58.2G**). (**C**) Persistence of embolic arterial abnormality associated with "silent" recurrent infarction (**Fig 58.2F**) in the posterior watershed territory. (**D**) Unilateral arteriopathy associated with recurrent transient ischemic attacks in sickle cell anemia. (**E**) Unilateral occlusion at the origin of the middle cerebral artery in sickle cell anemia with a large middle cerebral artery territory infarct (**Fig. 58.2L**). (**F**) Bilateral moyamoya collaterals associated with severe stenosis of the distal internal carotid/proximal middle cerebral arteries. (**G**) Bilaterally reduced flow in the middle cerebral artery without obvious moyamoya collaterals in sickle cell disease.

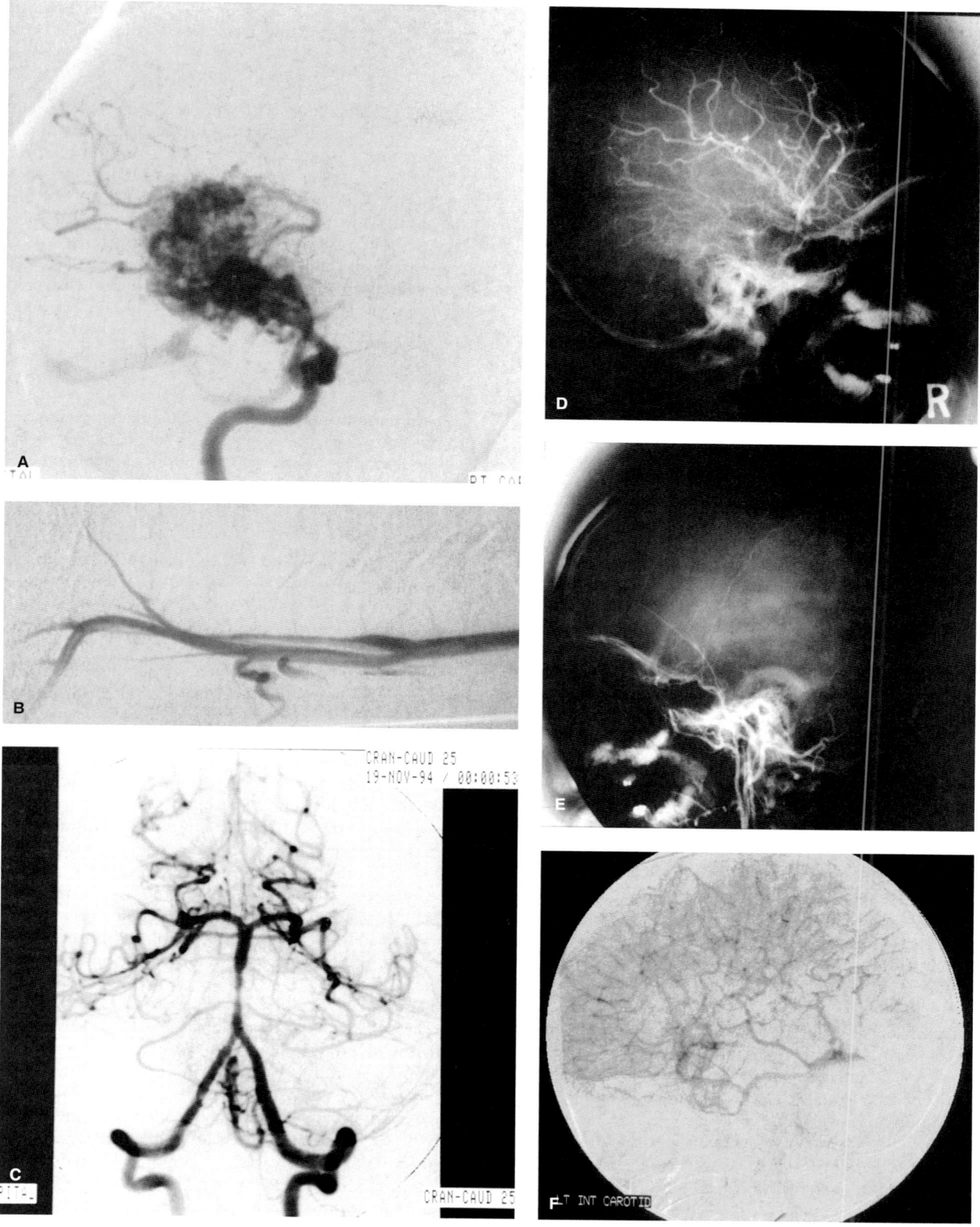

FIGURE 58.4. Conventional cerebral angiography from children with first and recurrent arterial and venous ischemic and hemorrhagic stroke. (**A**) Arteriovenous malformation in an 11-year-old boy presenting with a spontaneous intracerebral hemorrhage. (**B**) Typical "rat's tail" tapering occlusion in the internal carotid artery in dissection. (**C**) Irregularity of the midsegment of the basilar artery and the origins of both anterior inferior cerebellar arteries. (**D**) Right-sided moyamoya collaterals. (**E**) Paucity of vessels on the left side in the patient in D with right-sided moyamoya. (**F**) Venous phase demonstrating absence of flow in the occluded superior sagittal and straight sinus with multiple collateral vessels draining the hemisphere toward the cavernous sinus (**Fig. 58.2M**).

recurrence in childhood AIS (40). Apart from genetic predisposition, homocysteine levels are also influenced by the dietary intake of folate, vitamin B_{12}, and vitamin B_6. Supplementation may reduce homocysteine levels, although few available data support efficacy in stroke prevention, and a varied, healthy diet should provide adequate intake.

Hypertension. Hypertension is one of the most important risk factors for stroke in young adults and in the elderly but has largely been ignored in the pediatric literature. In one series, 54% of children with cryptogenic stroke and 46% of children with symptomatic stroke had systolic blood pressure >90th percentile and a significant association with cerebral arterial abnormalities (20), but at this writing, we have no evidence for an association with recurrence risk (21). The A3 and A4 alleles of the GT-repeat polymorphism of the angiotensinogen gene appear to be associated with a fourfold risk of clinical stroke in SCD, perhaps because of an effect on blood pressure.

Lipid Abnormalities. In a series of childhood stroke, 9% of those in whom random cholesterol was measured had high levels, while 31% had high triglyceride levels and 22% had high lipoprotein (a), a risk factor for atherosclerosis in adults (20). In another series, apolipoprotein abnormalities were seen more commonly in association with childhood stroke (1). High lipoprotein (a) was a risk factor for recurrent stroke in German children with AIS (50).

Disorders of Coagulation. Recognized disorders of coagulation occur acutely in a substantial proportion of children with childhood stroke (10,20,34), but up to half resolve within 3 months of the ictus, and the prevalence of inherited coagulopathies is ~10% in previously well patients. Factor V Leiden (which is common in Caucasian populations and is the most common cause of activated protein C resistance) and the prothrombin 20210 mutation are important risk factor for venous thrombosis in adults and may be associated with neonatal and childhood sinovenous thrombosis (46) and perhaps with AIS (34). A significant proportion of children with stroke have multiple prothrombotic disorders (20), and evidence exists for interaction between the factor V Leiden mutation and hyperhomocysteinemia. Although relatively rarely associated with childhood stroke, these prothrombotic disorders appear to be associated with recurrence (21,50), particularly in those with no previously diagnosed condition (21).

Vascular Adhesion. Adhesion of red and white cells and of platelets appears to be an important mechanism of endothelial damage in SCD and may play a role in stroke of other etiologies, such as moyamoya. Evidence has been reported that different molecular mechanisms are involved in the adhesion of red and white cells and platelets to the vascular endothelium in SCD. These mechanisms include adhesive ligands (e.g., von Willebrand factor) and molecules on the red blood cells and endothelial cell surfaces (e.g., vascular cell adhesion molecule).

Nitric Oxide. Nitric oxide is one of the most potent naturally occurring vasodilators and is a regulator of normal vascular tone, cell adhesion, and thrombosis, probably playing an important role in determining whether the endothelium is damaged (e.g., in SCD). A delicate balance exists between hypoxia-driven vasoconstriction and nitric oxide–driven vasodilatation in hypoxic conditions, and factors that affect nitric oxide biosynthesis may play a key role in the pathogenesis of vascular occlusion and stroke.

Arterial Disease

Up to 80% of children with AIS have abnormal conventional or magnetic angiographic studies (20) (**Figs. 58.3 and 58.4**). A nonabrupt onset of stroke is characteristic of those with arteriopathy (7). Typical abnormalities include internal carotid artery (ICA) or vertebral dissection, stenosis or occlusion of the distal ICA or MCA, moyamoya syndrome (bilateral severe stenosis or occlusion of the internal carotid arteries with collateral formation), and occasionally, rarer patterns such as small-vessel vasculitis (20). A diagnosis of vascular disease predicted recurrent stroke in a German cohort (50), and moyamoya is associated with recurrent stroke and TIAs in patients with and without SCD (14,21). Stenoses commonly improve or stabilize [transient cerebral arteriopathy (8)] but may progress (9); the field currently has aroused considerable interest, as it may have important implications for acute management strategies to prevent recurrence. Spontaneous hemorrhage is most commonly secondary to an arteriovenous malformation (4,13,26), but aneurysms occur, often in association with underlying conditions.

Extracranial/Intracranial Dissection. Among children, cervicocephalic dissections are reported in between 6.5% and 20% of any ischemic arterial stroke and in up to 50% of children with posterior circulation ischemic stroke (15,18), statistics that point to an estimated annual caseload of 56–173 children with stroke due to cervicocephalic dissections, or 1–3 cases per week in the US alone (15). Risk factors include minor trauma, infection migraine, hyperhomocysteinemia, and rare disorders such as fibromuscular dysplasia, Marfan or Ehlers-Danlos syndrome, and α_1-antitrypsin deficiency (15). Dissections are caused by blood penetrating and splitting the wall of an artery that supplies the brain. The most frequently affected artery is the ICA, followed by the vertebral artery. In children, anterior circulation dissections are frequently intracranial (60%) (15), affecting the intracranial ICA, MCA, and anterior cerebral artery, although circle of Willis involvement may be difficult to distinguish from transient cerebral arteriopathy (8). Approximately 80% of posterior circulation dissections are extracranial, and more than half are located within the vertebral artery at the level C1–C2. Multiple dissections are common and are seen in 8%–28% of children.

The origin of the dissection is likely to be a small intimal tear or primary intramural hemorrhage of the vasa vasorum. Arterial dissection results in an intramural hematoma and its variable extension along the course of that artery. The MRA is not usually diagnostic, but a lesion in the neck vessels may be suggested by reduced flow in the intracranial vessels (**Fig. 58.3H**). In many cases, the intramural hematoma may be demonstrated using fat-saturated T1-weighted MRI of the neck (**Fig. 58.5**), although conventional arteriography may sometimes be required to demonstrate the tapering partial occlusion of the artery ("rat's tail") (**Fig. 58.4B**). Head or neck trauma is a well-recognized cause of dissection, and it is worth noting that intraoral injuries (e.g., from a pencil carried in the mouth) can contuse the carotid artery in the peritonsillar area. Although an underlying arteriopathy has long been suspected, no single factor has been identified, and a variety of genetic and environmental factors are probably involved.

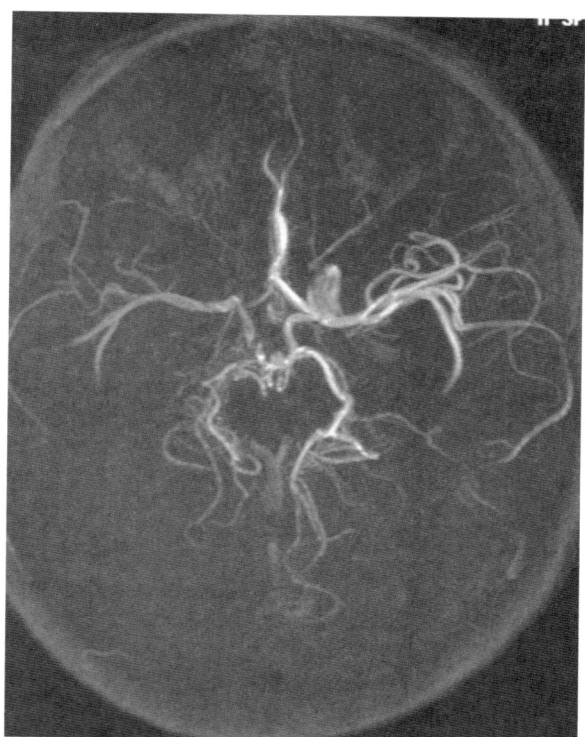

FIGURE 58.5. Axial fat-saturated, T1-weighted MRI of the neck in a patient presenting with an acute hemiparesis shows blood in the wall characteristic of dissection.

Local effects. The dissection may compress surrounding nerve structures, disrupting their nutrient blood supply. Subadventitial extension may lead to aneurysmal distension, which may either cause local compression or lead to thromboembolic phenomena. Extracranial aneurysms do not usually rupture, unlike intracranial dissections, which can lead to SAH. Subintimal dissection results in stenosis or occlusion of the arterial lumen, a potent thrombogenic stimulus.

Distant effects. Hemodynamic consequences of dissection may reduce oxygen delivery to substrate-dependent neuronal tissue. However, arterial-to-arterial thromboembolism is probably the most important pathogenetic mechanism in dissection-related stroke. The evidence that this is the case includes (a) the delay that often exists between the time of dissection and subsequent neurologic deficit; (b) angiographic evidence of distal embolization in 50% of children who present with cervicocephalic dissection; (c) patterns of stroke in ICA dissection that suggest the etiologic relevance of local hemodynamic effects in only 8% of cases (**Fig. 58.3G**); and (d) transcranial Doppler evidence that microemboli in the MCA downstream from the dissection correlate with stroke recurrence and are reduced with antithrombotic therapy, although no RCTs have yet looked at reduction of microemboli or clinical stroke rate.

Other Intracranial Arteriopathies

Moyamoya. Moyamoya (**Figs. 58.3F** and **58.4D,E**) derives from the Japanese word meaning "something hazy, like a puff of smoke drifting in the air" and describes the appearance of the collaterals (25) seen in association with bilateral severe stenosis or occlusion of the terminal ICAs in childhood. Collaterals arise from the anterior and posterior ethmoidal arteries and external carotid system or the middle meningeal/superficial temporal arteries via transdural vessels. Moyamoya may be idiopathic (moyamoya *disease*) or occur in the context of a wide range of other disorders (moyamoya *syndrome*) and is best considered an angiographically defined phenomenon rather than a pathologic entity (25).

Associations include SCD, where moyamoya syndrome predicts a higher recurrence risk (14), and Down syndrome, where a widespread vasculopathy may affect small and large vessels commonly associated with moyamoya collaterals. Moyamoya has been reported in Williams syndrome, a disorder known to involve mutations in the elastin gene, suggesting that abnormal vessel distensibility may lead to hypoperfusion and promote the development of collateral vessels. Other recognized associations include neurofibromatosis, cranial irradiation, and arteriopathies, including fibromuscular dysplasia. A genetic predisposition is probably associated with the otherwise idiopathic cases reported in Japan, with evidence for linkage to HLA AW24, AW46, BW54, and B51-DR4. Recently, familial cases of moyamoya syndrome have shown linkage to 17q25, adjacent to the NF1 gene on 17q11.2. Basic fibroblast growth factor, which is involved in proliferation of vascular endothelium and promotion of angiogenesis, is increased in the cerebrospinal fluid of Japanese patients with moyamoya syndrome.

"Transient" cerebral arteriopathy in previously well children. "Transient" cerebral arteriopathy may involve an inflammatory response to infections such as varicella, *Borrelia*, or tonsillitis (8). Cerebral imaging (**Figs. 58.2A** and **58.3A**) typically shows small subcortical infarcts located in the basal ganglia and internal capsule and on conventional arteriography, multifocal lesions of the arterial wall are seen, with narrowing in the distal ICA, and the proximal anterior, middle, or posterior cerebral arteries (8). Although the vasculopathy may stabilize or even disappear in many cases (8), progression is associated with recurrent stroke (9).

Intracranial Arteriopathy in Sickle Cell Disease. Narrowing of the distal ICA and proximal MCA and anterior cerebral artery is also characteristic of SCD (**Figs. 58.3D,E,G**), although in these patients, gradual progression to occlusion commonly occurs with or without moyamoya collaterals (14). Pathologic examination of these arteries shows endothelial proliferation, fibroblastic reaction, hyalinization, and fragmentation of the internal elastic lamina. The majority of clinical and silent infarcts occur in the MCA territory or in the border zones between the middle, anterior, and posterior cerebral territories.

Vascular Malformations

Arteriovenous malformations. The prevalence of arteriovenous malformations is 10–500 per 100,000 children (13). Arteriovenous malformations are defined by the presence of high-flow arteriovenous shunts through a nidus of abnormal thin-walled, coiled, and tortuous connections between feeding arteries and draining veins, without an intervening capillary network (**Fig. 58.4A**). The current view is that they represent abnormalities of developmental vascular remodeling. Compared to adults, arteriovenous malformations in children more commonly present with hemorrhage and occur in eloquent or deep areas of the brain (particularly basal ganglia and thalamus).

Capillary telangiectasias. Capillary telangiectasias are collections of dilated ectatic capillaries with normal intervening neural tissue, without smooth muscle or elastic fibers; they are not commonly associated with ICH or SAH.

Cavernous angioma. Cavernous angiomas (cavernomas) are vascular malformations that comprise thin-walled sinusoidal spaces lined with endothelial tissue and contain intravascular or intervascular calcifications, without any intervening parenchymal tissue. Multiple lesions are seen in 13% of sporadic cases and 50% of familial cases. It is thought that venous hypertension due to obstructed outflow results in the formation of the cavernoma. Cavernomas may present with symptoms related to frank ICH or with epilepsy, possibly secondary to intermittent leakage of blood around the cavernoma.

Venous angioma. Venous angiomas are thin-walled venous channels with normal intervening neural tissue that are associated with a very low risk of bleeding.

Sturge-Weber syndrome. Sturge-Weber syndrome (**Fig. 58.1M**) is a sporadic condition characterized by a venous angioma of the leptomeninges, a choroidal angioma, and a facial capillary hemangioma involving the periorbital area, forehead, or scalp (32) that probably result from a failure of regression of a vascular plexus around the cephalic portion of the neural tube at between 6 and 9 weeks of gestation. Epilepsy, hemiplegia, and learning disability, often progressive (32), are probably the result of an ischemic mechanism. The patient may be relatively well between episodes of status epilepticus or acute hemiparesis. Aspirin may reduce the frequency of stroke-like episodes (32). If intractable epilepsy cannot be controlled by medical means, hemispherectomy may be beneficial.

Vein of Galen Malformation. Vein of Galen malformation (17) (**Fig. 58.1N**) is an embryonic choroidal arteriovenous malformation. It can be diagnosed antenatally, has a male preponderance but no known genetic predisposition, and usually presents in the neonatal period as heart failure or, in older children with hydrocephalus, seizures, proptosis, or prominent scalp veins. Endovascular treatment is often offered at specialized centers and appears to provide good quality of life, particularly for older children not presenting in heart failure with mural, rather than choroidal, malformations (17).

Aneurysms. Arterial aneurysms are acquired lesions that are rare in children, who account for <5% of all cases. They are multiple in 2%–5% of children. Three-quarters of patients with arterial aneurysms present with ICH. Approximately 10%–15% of arterial aneurysms are posttraumatic; a similar proportion are mycotic and are associated with infection (e.g., *Staphylococcus*, *Streptococcus*, Gram-negative organisms, and HIV). Mycotic aneurysms may also arise secondary to embolization of infective thrombi into the intracranial circulation in patients with subacute bacterial endocarditis. Other associations with arterial aneurysms in children are polycystic kidney disease, SCD, tuberous sclerosis, Marfan syndrome, Ehlers-Danlos syndrome type IV, pseudoxanthoma elasticum, and hypertension,

but no underlying systemic disorder is found in a substantial proportion.

Cerebral Sinovenous Thrombosis

Anatomy. The venous drainage of the brain occurs through the "superficial" or "deep" cerebral sinovenous systems, which consist of a network of sinuses and veins. Flow is highly responsive to changes in mean arterial pressure, reductions in which can result in stasis or reversal of blood flow within the dural sinuses, and a relative reduction of thrombomodulin in cerebral venous endothelium exaggerates the prothrombotic tendency. The "superficial" venous system includes the cortical veins, which drain into the superior sagittal sinus and then mainly into the right lateral sinus. The "deep venous system" includes the inferior sagittal sinus and the paired internal cerebral veins, which join to form the vein of Galen and the straight sinus, draining predominantly into the smaller caliber left lateral sinus and jugular vein.

Pathophysiology of Sinovenous Thrombosis. In neonates, pathogenesis of sinovenous thrombosis (**Figs. 58.1J,K** and **58.4F**) may be related to mechanical distortion of the cranial bones during birth. In older children trauma, sepsis, and underlying illnesses such as malignancy or systemic inflammation play a larger role (12,28,46). Septic foci include the inner ear, mastoid, or air sinuses and lead to thrombophlebitic sinovenous thrombosis. Dehydration, anemia, and inherited prothrombotic disorders (congenital or acquired) are also recognized risk factors (10,28,46). Finally, positional alterations in flow dynamics can have a significant role in the pathogenesis of sinovenous thrombosis in neonates and older children with vascular malformations.

Venous Infarction. Cerebral infarction results when perfusion to the affected area of the brain is reduced to critical levels. In sinovenous thrombosis, "outflow" obstruction causes venous hypertension in the affected region of the brain, leading to focal cerebral edema (**Fig. 58.2M–Q**). When tissue hydrostatic pressure exceeds arterial inflow pressure, infarction, which may be hemorrhagic, ensues. Risk factors for venous infarction include rapid onset of sinovenous thrombosis, complete luminal occlusion, and thrombosis located at the entry points of cerebral veins into the sagittal sinus (**Fig. 58.6**).

Intracranial Hypertension. Sinovenous thrombosis leads to disruption of cerebrospinal fluid absorption within the superior sagittal sinus, resulting in diffuse cerebral swelling, communicating hydrocephalus, or pseudotumor cerebri (benign intracranial hypertension) (46).

Other Stroke Syndromes and Stroke Mimics in the Differential Diagnosis

Posterior Circulation Arterial Stroke. Arterial disease in association with posterior circulation infarction in the cerebellum (**Fig. 58.1I**), brainstem, and parieto-occipital lobes is much more common in boys than in girls (19). A positive diagnosis of dissection may require conventional angiography in the acute phase, as MRI and MRA commonly miss the diagnosis in the posterior circulation (**Fig. 58.7**). Etiologic factors include minor trauma, subluxation of the cervical spine at the extremes of flexion and extension, chiropractic manipulation, frequent neck movements (e.g., secondary to athetoid cerebral palsy),

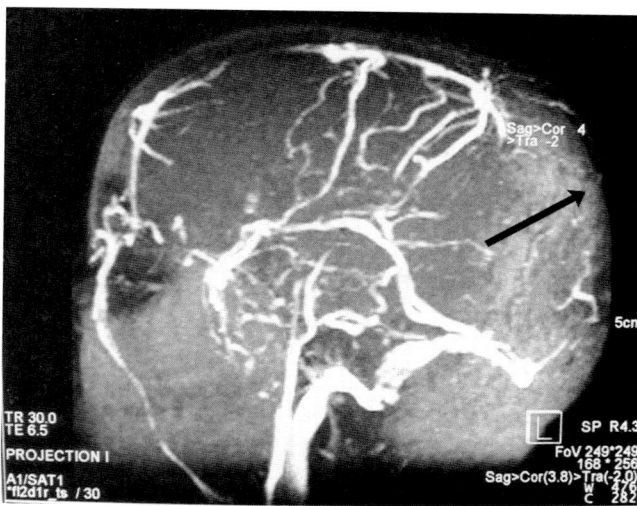

FIGURE 58.6. MR venogram in a teenager with systemic lupus erythematosus and a warm autoimmune hemolytic anemia showing chronic sagittal sinus thrombosis, with a flow void posteriorly.

hypertension, cardiac anomalies (19), and perhaps Fabry disease (43) (**Fig. 58.7**). Some patients with conventional risk factors for stroke (hypertension, hypercholesterolemia, hyperhomocysteinemia) have vascular imaging compatible with early atheroma (19) (**Figs. 58.4C and 58.7**).

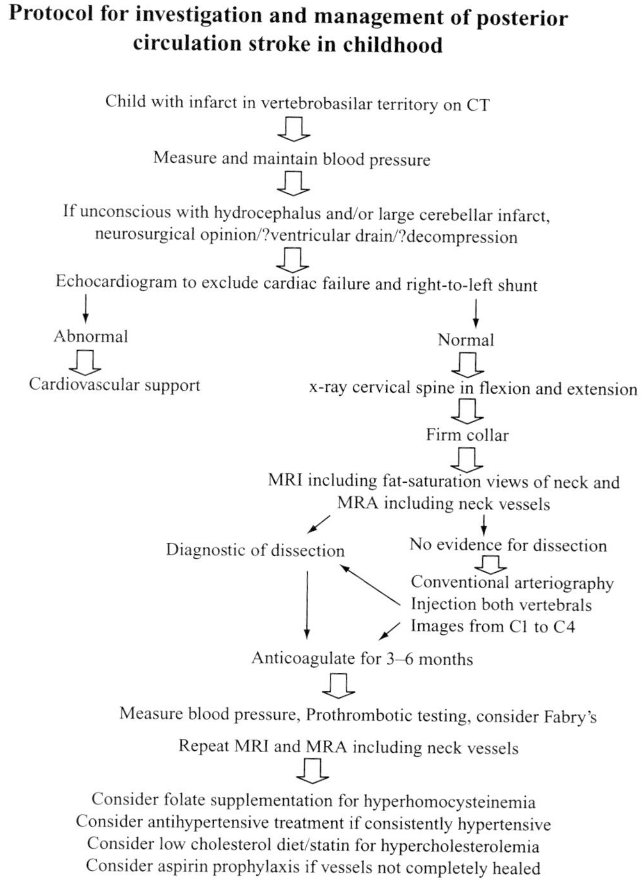

Protocol for investigation and management of posterior circulation stroke in childhood

Child with infarct in vertebrobasilar territory on CT

⇩

Measure and maintain blood pressure

⇩

If unconscious with hydrocephalus and/or large cerebellar infarct, neurosurgical opinion/?ventricular drain/?decompression

⇩

Echocardiogram to exclude cardiac failure and right-to-left shunt

Abnormal   Normal

⇩   ⇩

Cardiovascular support   x-ray cervical spine in flexion and extension

⇩

Firm collar

⇩

MRI including fat-saturation views of neck and MRA including neck vessels

Diagnostic of dissection   No evidence for dissection

⇩

Conventional arteriography
Injection both vertebrals
Images from C1 to C4

⇩

Anticoagulate for 3–6 months

⇩

Measure blood pressure, Prothrombotic testing, consider Fabry's

Repeat MRI and MRA including neck vessels

⇩

Consider folate supplementation for hyperhomocysteinemia
Consider antihypertensive treatment if consistently hypertensive
Consider low cholesterol diet/statin for hypercholesterolemia
Consider aspirin prophylaxis if vessels not completely healed

FIGURE 58.7. Algorithm for the management of posterior circulation stroke.

Reversible Posterior Leukoencephalopathy and Border-zone Ischemia. RPLS (**Fig. 58.2R**) is a cliniconeuroradiologic syndrome characterized by seizures, disorders of consciousness, altered mental status, visual abnormalities, and headaches, all of which are associated with predominantly posterior white matter abnormalities on CT and MRI examinations (36) but without arterial or venous disease. RPLS is a relatively common stroke mimic (47) and has been recognized in an increasing number of medical settings, including hypertensive encephalopathy, eclampsia, after acute chest crisis in SCD (23) and immunosuppression. Acute hypotension in the context of poor cardiac function and/or anemia may also cause occipital infarction without vascular disease (19). As treatments are different, it is essential to distinguish RPLS from posterior circulation embolic stroke secondary to vertebrobasilar dissection (19); the latter typically presents "out of the blue," is much more common in boys, and is typically associated with infarction in the cerebellum and/or brainstem as well as the occipitoparietal cortex, but MR and conventional arteriography may be required to make a positive diagnosis (19). It is also important to exclude sinovenous thrombosis, particularly of the sagittal and straight sinuses (**Figs. 58.1J,K and 58.2M–Q**), which may be associated with venous infarction in the parietal and occipital lobes as well as the thalami (**Figs. 58.1J,K and 58.2M–Q**).

The rapid resolution of clinical and neuroradiologic abnormalities in the majority of cases of RPLS suggests vasogenic cerebral edema, which is thought to result from impaired cerebrovascular autoregulation and endothelial injury. Most patients make a full clinical and radiologic recovery after conservative measures, including slow reduction of blood pressure and maintenance of normal oxygenation. Some patients with otherwise typical RPLS have additional imaging abnormalities anteriorly and/or in the gray matter, often in a distribution suggestive of border-zone ischemia (**Fig. 58.1I**), and the changes are not necessarily reversible in all cases (23). Patients with parieto-occipital infarction may have visual problems and epilepsy in the long term (36).

Acute Disseminated Encephalomyelitis. MRI may reveal demyelination in children who present with acute focal neurologic signs (20). Evidence suggests that IV methylprednisolone reduces the duration of the illness and perhaps improves long-term outcome.

Metabolic Stroke. Diabetes and inborn errors of metabolism can cause acute focal neurologic symptoms and signs (metabolic stroke) due to either vascular injury or direct tissue injury, which may be permanent or transitory (37).

Vascular injury. Homocysteine is a highly chemically reactive thiol amino acid that can cause direct endothelial injury. Inborn errors that affect three enzymes—5,10-methylenetetrahydrofolate reductase, methionine synthase, and cystathionine β-synthase—(or the synthesis of their vitamin cofactors) are known to cause homocystinuria and may present with arterial or venous stroke in infancy or childhood.

Fabry disease is a lysosomal storage disorder that causes accumulation of the glycosphingolipid globotriaosylceramide in blood vessel endothelial cells and, to some extent, in the vascular smooth muscle. It is an X-linked disorder caused by deficiency of the lysosomal hydrolase α-galactosidase A and is an important cause of cryptogenic stroke in the young, particularly those with vertebrobasilar territory infarction (43). Proteinuria may be a useful screen, but if the clinician has a strong index of suspicion, exclusion should be by enzyme diagnosis, as replacement is available.

Menkes disease is an X-linked disorder of copper transport caused by deficiency of a copper-transporting adenosine triphosphatase, which in turn, causes copper deficiency (37). Subdural hematomas, tortuosity, and obliteration of intracranial vasculature can result.

Nonvascular injury. In addition to diabetes, some organic acidemias, urea cycle disorders, and other inborn errors of metabolism can cause metabolic stroke (37). Female carriers with ornithine carbamoyl transferase deficiency may present with focal signs. Mitochondrial disorders can cause stroke-like episodes (such as mitochondrial encephalopathy with lactic acidosis and stroke-like episodes). The exact mechanisms by which these occur are unknown. In the organic acidemias and urea cycle disorders, it is likely that accumulation of a toxic metabolite causes infarction of a selectively vulnerable area of the brain. By contrast, mitochondrial disorders are liable to cause infarction because of deficient energy supply and by the generation of oxygen free radicals. As arginine supplementation may be beneficial (30), it is important to exclude mitochondrial disorders.

CLINICAL PRESENTATION AND DIFFERENTIAL DIAGNOSIS

Stroke and CVD can cause considerable anxiety to the pediatric intensivist at least in part because of the large number of individual conditions, each of which is relatively rare. The differential diagnosis includes a wide range of alternative pathologies (6,47), and protocols for investigation and treatment are not well defined. The important clinical clues for diagnosis are often (a) for symptomatic stroke, a preexisting diagnosis, and (b) for cryptogenic stroke, the trigger(s) (Figs. 58.7, 58.8, 58.9, and 58.10). As a result of controlled trials of thrombolysis, increased awareness of the need for rapid assessment and appropriate management of acute stroke in adults and the concept of "brain attack" have received widespread publicity. Thrombolysis must begin within 3 hrs; however, few children are triaged this quickly. Indeed, in many children the correct diagnosis is not made for days or weeks (6). Nevertheless, there is little doubt that stroke units save adult lives and improve outcome in survivors, in part because a team's experience may lead to rapid diagnosis and appropriate management of common and rare stroke syndromes. Currently, services for children are not organized in this way, and it has not yet proved possible to conduct large randomized trials of treatment in groups of children with similar pathologies. A number of "stroke mimics" exist that may be benign and require no treatment (47) (Fig. 58.10). On the other hand, patients may have potentially serious CVD, either venous or arterial, without infarction at presentation; timely intervention may prevent stroke. Comprehensive radiologic investigation is therefore essential, and increasing evidence suggests that emergency MRI provides information that may, in certain circumstances, guide management in the individual patient.

Children with stroke syndromes can present to the pediatric intensivist in a variety of ways. Unlike adult stroke, the vast majority of pediatric stroke victims will either present to, or be rapidly referred to, a tertiary center. PICU involvement will thus commence at the stage of resuscitation and retrieval and will continue to facilitate elective or emergency intervention (Fig. 58.11). The common clinical presentations are presented in Table 58.1. The importance of recognizing these as a medical/surgical emergency cannot be overstated.

Children may present with an immediate airway problem in coma, needing anesthesia and intubation for airway protection, with status epilepticus resistant to first-line therapy and requiring airway protection for second-line therapy (e.g., barbiturate coma) or with a reduced level of consciousness either requiring observation in the PICU or mandating airway protection for further investigation. Periprocedural admission to the PICU may also be required for planned intervention in children who have known intracranial pathology that predisposes to stroke (e.g., embolisation of arteriovenous malformation or aneurysm, extracranial-intracranial bypass for moyamoya). Children may also present with signs of intracranial hypertension or imminent central or uncal herniation (Fig. 58.12).

PICU MANAGEMENT AND INVESTIGATION

Diagnosis-independent Management

Basic Measures

Emergency management of children who present with coma, altered level of consciousness, or status epilepticus must follow standard resuscitation algorithms targeted at the maintenance of airway, breathing, and circulation. No studies have specifically examined the effect of the loss of cardiorespiratory integrity on stroke outcome in children. However, based on principles that would be applied to the care of any acutely ill child, as well as those from the evidence base in adults, the aim should be maintenance of oxygen saturation, cardiac output, systemic and cerebral perfusion pressure (CPP), normothermia, and careful avoidance of hypoglycemia and hyperglycemia. This section provides an overview of emergent neuroprotection in this context, but the controversies are discussed in more detail later in the chapter.

An intravenous/intraosseous catheter should be inserted for administration of isotonic fluids (crystalloid, colloid, or packed red blood cells). At the same time, blood should be taken for biochemical and hematologic analysis by the referring hospital [including a full coagulation profile and platelet count in case surgery or intracranial pressure (ICP) monitoring is required immediately after arrival at the tertiary center]. The presence of shock, as assessed by capillary refill time, tachycardia, base deficit, and plasma lactate, should be treated aggressively to normalize perfusion and systemic hemodynamics. The primary goal should be optimization of intravascular volume, stroke volume, and perfusion pressure with the appropriate use of aggressive volume loading. Any total body water deficit should be estimated using standard algorithms and corrected over 24–48 hrs. IV maintenance fluids should be titrated to age and initial plasma sodium (discussed later). A child who requires intubation and mechanical ventilation should have

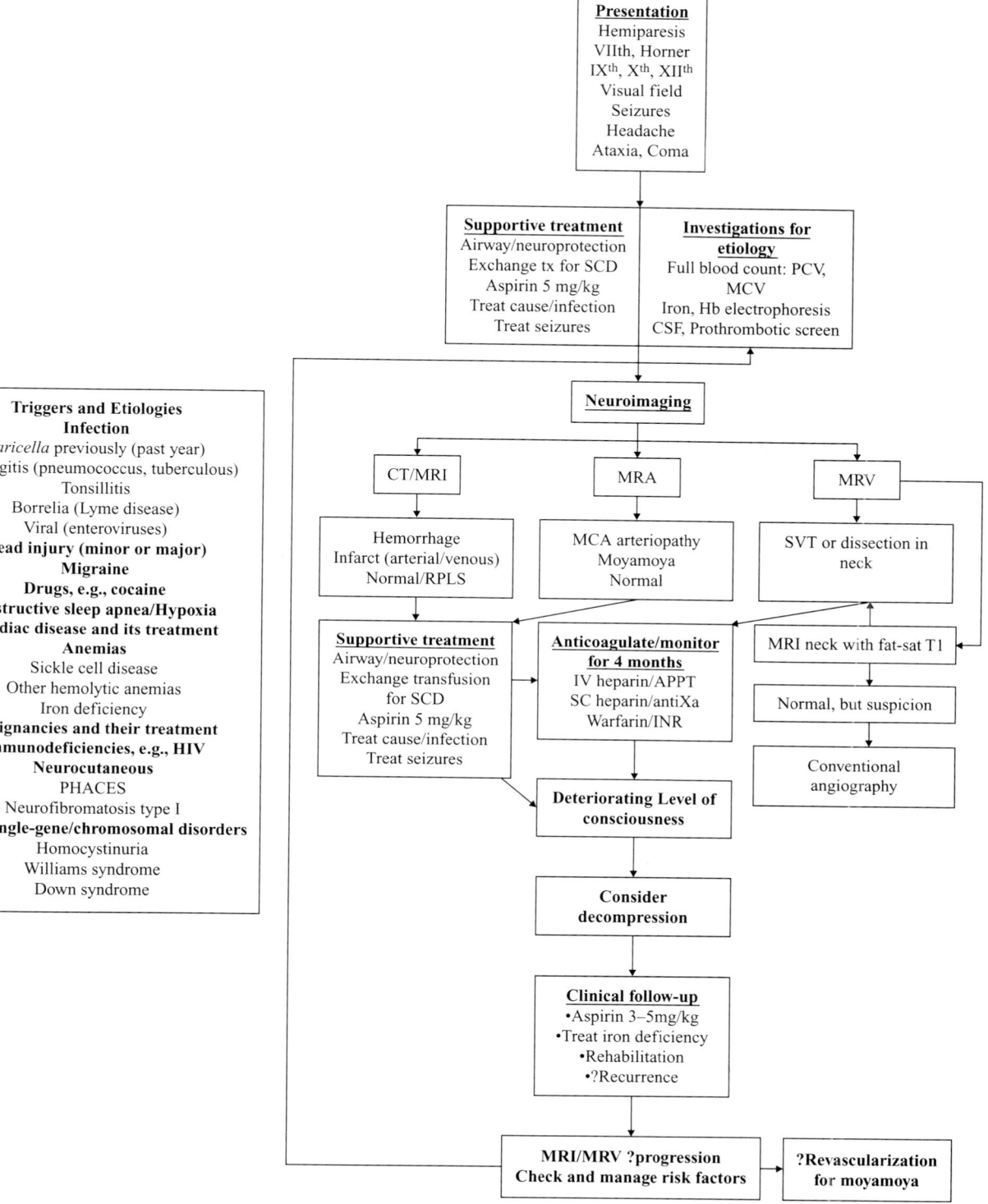

FIGURE 58.8. Algorithm for the diagnosis and management of arterial stroke.

invasive catheters inserted for the measurement of arterial and right atrial pressures.

In any unconscious child with a stroke syndrome, it is reasonable to assume a degree of intracranial hypertension (assumed ICP of 20 mm Hg) and target a minimum mean arterial pressure of ICP + 50 mm Hg to achieve a satisfactory CPP

(**Fig. 58.12**). Preload augmentation is probably best titrated to systolic pulse pressure variation, the target being a variance of <5 mm Hg. Subsequent perfusion pressure augmentation should be achieved, if required, with the use of centrally administered noradrenaline. It is important that this treatment protocol is started locally at the request of the tertiary center before

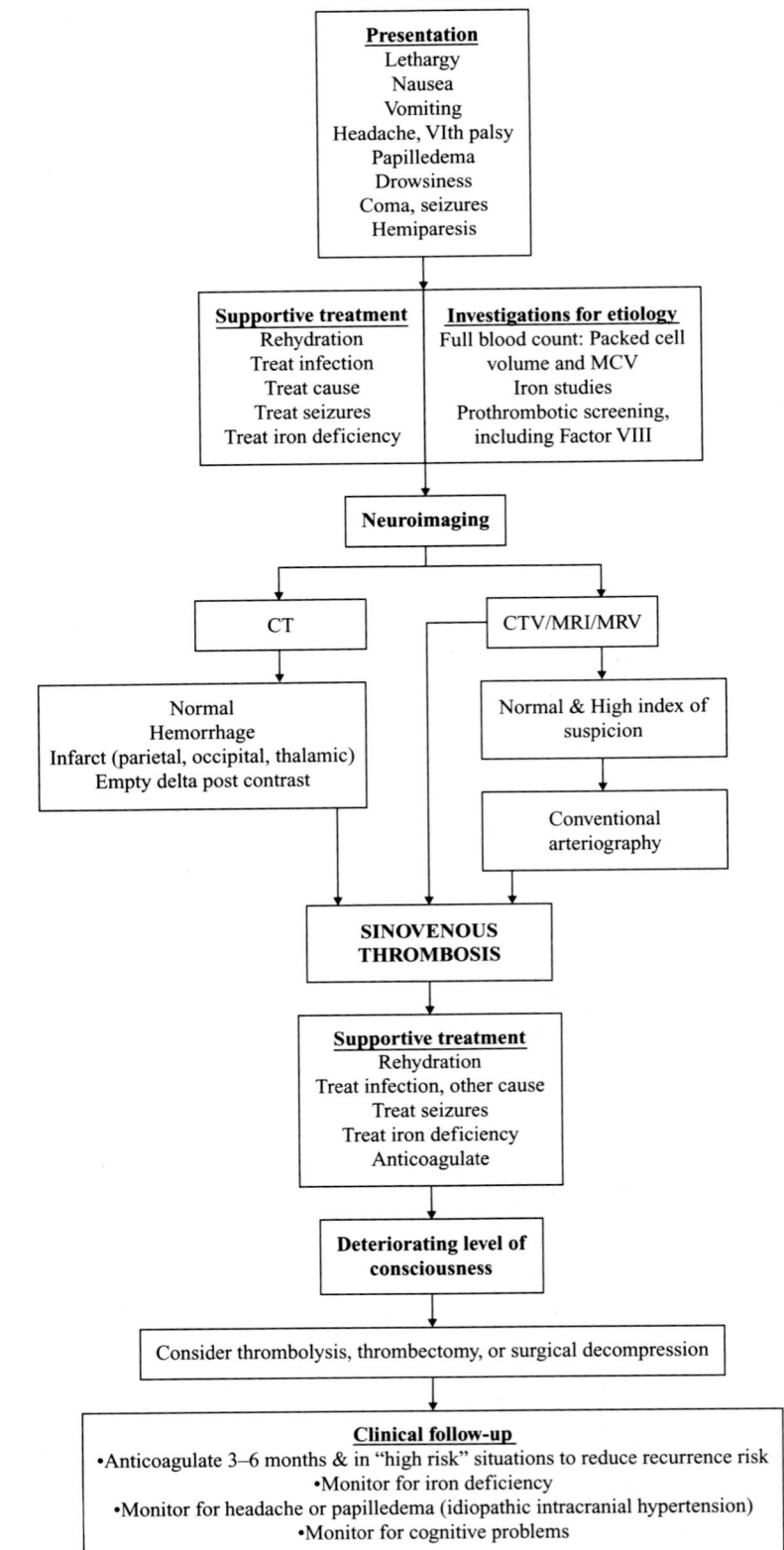

FIGURE 58.9. Algorithm for the management of sinovenous thrombosis.

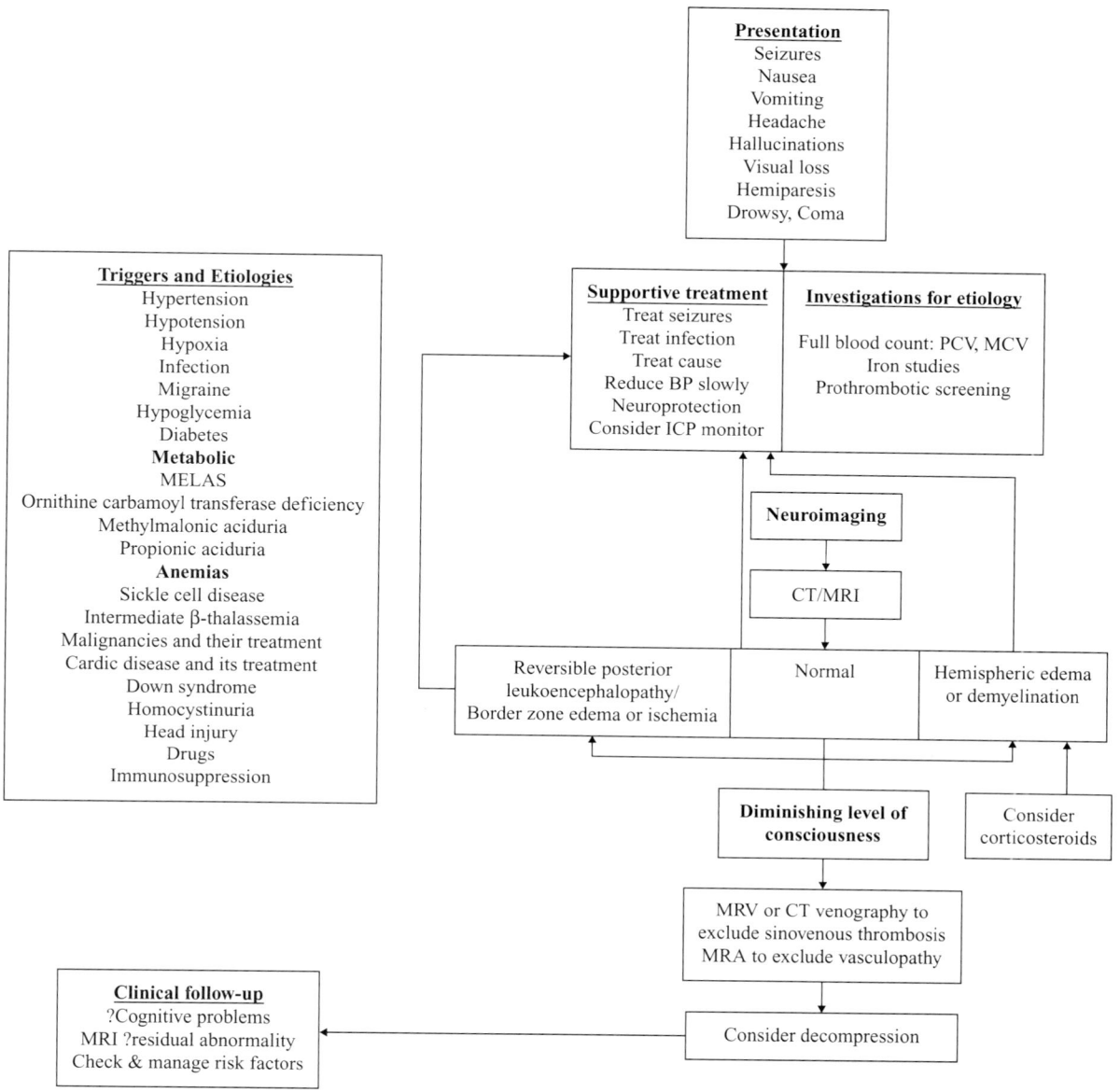

FIGURE 58.10. Algorithm for the management of stroke mimics.

transfer. Far too often, this does not occur, augmenting the potential for secondary neuronal loss.

Hypertension should be assumed to be physiologic (reflecting disrupted cerebral autoregulation in response to intracranial hypertension) and not treated, at least initially. In consultation with the treating neurosurgeon, hypertension following ICH associated with an arterial/arteriovenous malformation may require treatment, as the risk of rebleeding must be balanced against the need to maintain CPP. If a clear diagnosis of RPLS or watershed ischemia associated with hypertension has been made, blood pressure should be reduced slowly, over at least 48 hrs. Levels of hypertension that mandate intervention have not been established, and individual treatment decisions should be made after discussion with local pediatric neurologists and neurosurgeons.

Children who are not already intubated and whose level of consciousness deteriorates should be mechanically ventilated, and emergent neurosurgical consultation should be obtained in case they require drainage of a hematoma, ventriculostomy for hydrocephalus, or craniectomy for intractable intracranial hypertension. Seizures in the acute phase should be managed according to standard algorithms. Infarct volume and outcome appear to be related to body temperature during the first few days of the stroke; at present, the evidence is inconclusive in children and a direct causative effect remains unproven, but maintaining body temperature just below 37°C is unlikely to do harm (41). Similarly, hyperglycemia at presentation is associated with both increased mortality and worse functional outcome.

No RCT evidence exists at present to direct neuroprotective therapy in pediatric nontraumatic coma. However, reasonable nonrandomized data do exist to suggest that these children are prone to secondary damage after the initial insult and to the detrimental effects of subsequent intracranial hypertension,

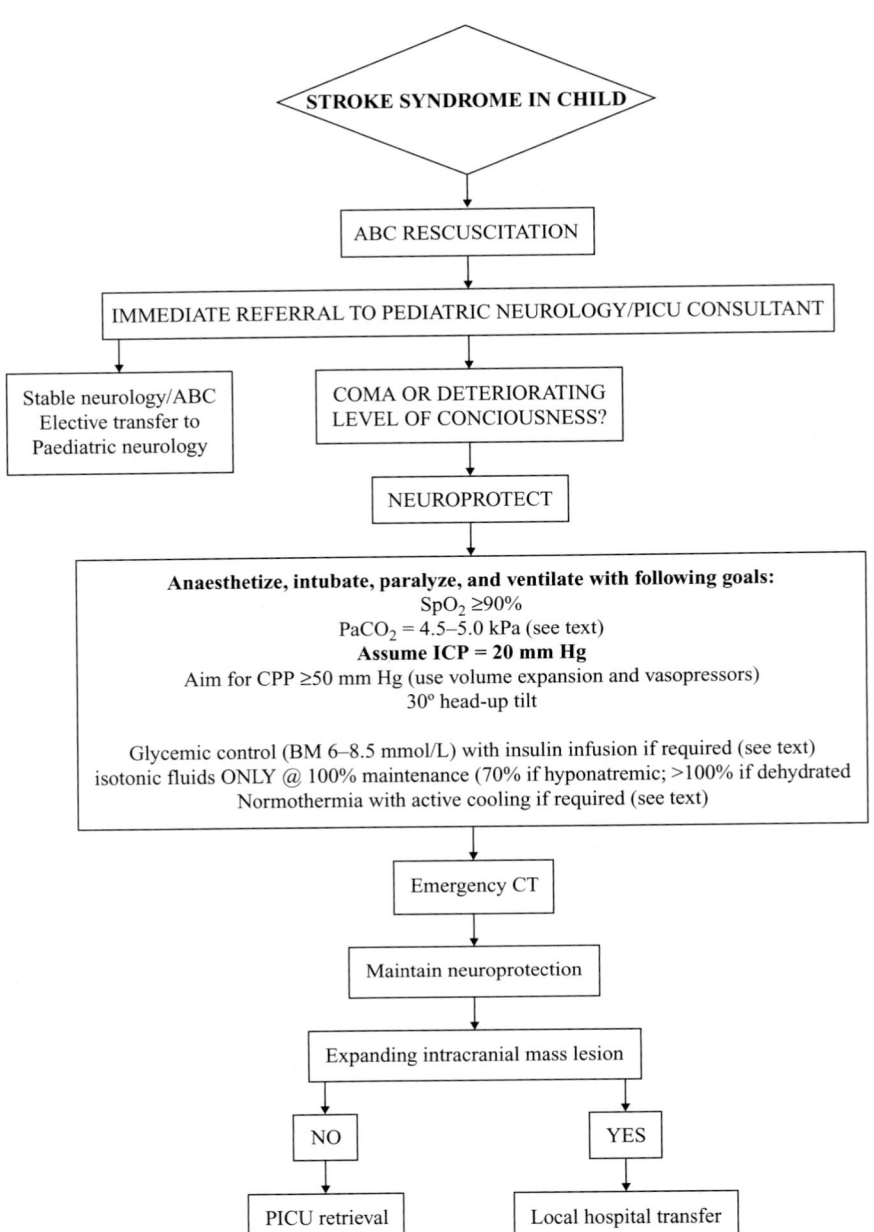

FIGURE 58.11. Emergency management of childhood stroke.

perhaps as a consequence of hydrocephalus or generalized or focal edema. It is therefore our practice to treat these children very much as we treat patients with closed-head injuries, employing general neuroprotective strategies as soon as possible (as summarized in **Fig. 58.11**), monitoring ICP invasively if indicated, and treating intractable intracranial hypertension using an algorithm such as is described in **Figure 58.12**. Obvious parallels exist between the management of traumatic and nontraumatic coma in children and that in adults, but inconsistencies exist for neuroprotective strategies, fluid management protocols, glycemic control, temperature control, transfusion in SCD, and the management of intracranial hypertension; strategies for the individual child must be carefully considered. The evidence base in each of these categories and our recommendations are detailed below.

Neuroprotection—Controversies and Recommendations

Intravenous Maintenance Fluids. Neonates, infants, and smaller children are at risk of hypoglycemia if isotonic glucose-free maintenance fluids are used prior to the successful initiation of enteral nutrition. We therefore recommend that this group of children receive isotonic normal saline with extra glucose added to achieve a final concentration of either 5% or 10%. For older children, glucose-free isotonic maintenance fluids using normal saline will normally suffice until enteral feeding is established. Traditionally, fluid restriction to 70% of calculated total requirements is recommended. This approach was promoted by the use of hypotonic maintenance fluids in patients at risk of developing a syndrome of inappropriate antidiuretic hormone secretion. The use of isotonic maintenance

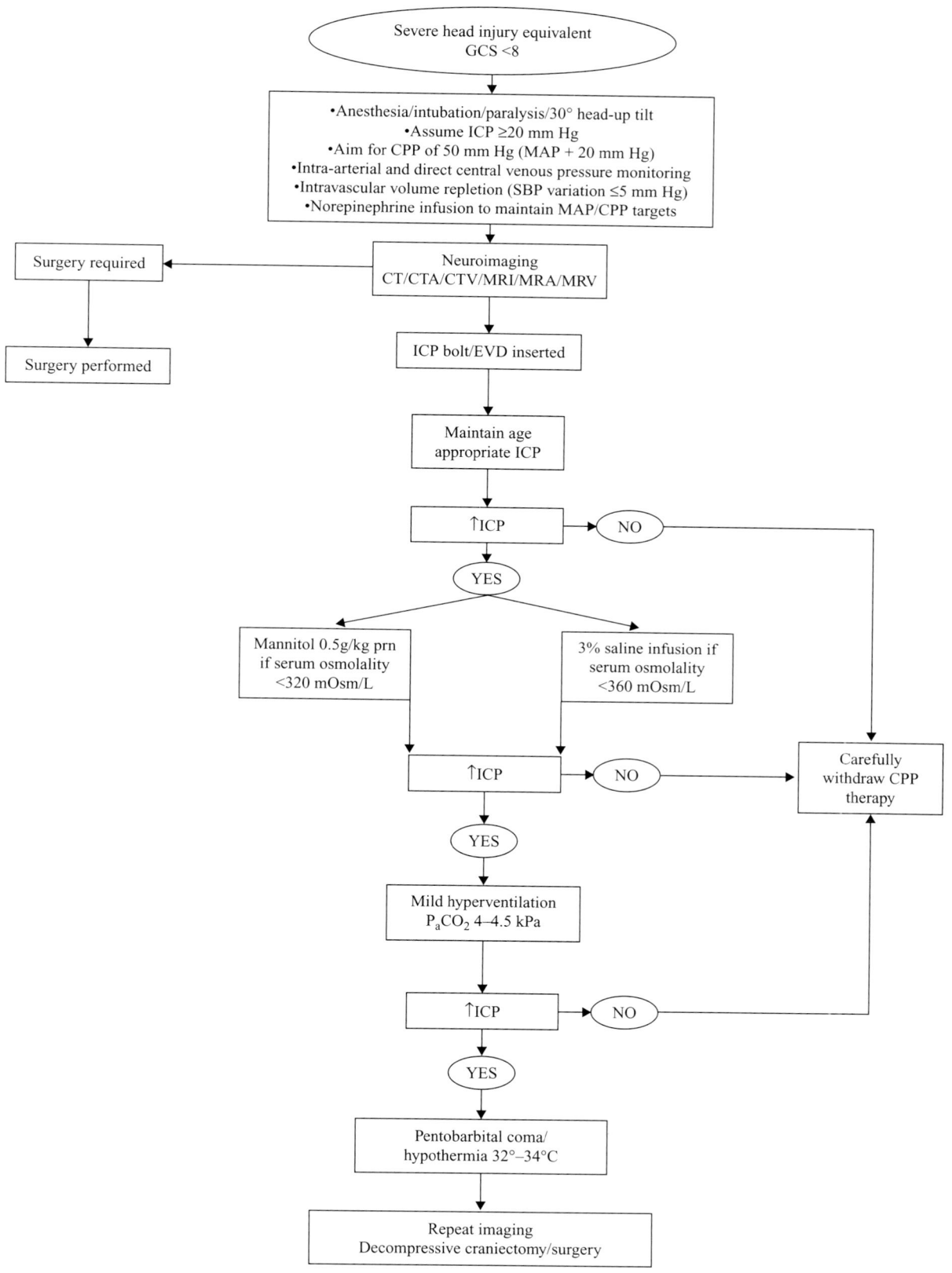

FIGURE 58.12. Neuroprotection in childhood stroke.

fluids greatly reduces the risk of hyponatremia in this setting. We would therefore recommend the use of 100% maintenance, except in children whose plasma sodium is below the normal range, in whom fluid restriction (70% of calculated requirements) should be used initially to hasten an elevation of plasma sodium. Enteral nutrition must be the gold standard, and perhaps more rigorous efforts should be made to establish post-pyloric feeding, either with radiologically (neonate, infant, and small child) or endoscopically (older child) placed nasogastric/orogastric jejunal feeding tubes. In the particular context of sinovenous thrombosis, when prothrombotic states and dehydration are common etiologic factors, it may even be necessary to rehydrate in addition to prescribing maintenance fluids.

Glycemic Control. The pivotal single-centered, RCT of tight-versus-loose glycemic control in adult cardiac intensive care patients has somewhat controversially changed adult intensive care practice. This, together with reasonable evidence from the pediatric and adult literature that initial posttraumatic brain injury hyperglycemia is associated with increased mortality and worse 6-month functional outcome, has led to a creeping practice of tighter glycemic control in the pediatric traumatic and nontraumatic population treated in the PICU. We feel it imprudent to recommend generalizing the levels of glycemic control suggested in the adult paper to the pediatric population with traumatic brain injury (TBI) and nontraumatic coma for three reasons.

1. The report is from a single center, regards only adults, and relates entirely to cardiac surgical patients.
2. No RCTs have been performed on PICU patients, although funding for such a trial coordinated by the UK Paediatric Intensive Care Society Study Group has recently been awarded. This trial will randomize children with requirements for ventilation and inotropes to tight or loose glycemic control and will enroll head injuries. Final recommendations must await the conduct and publication of such trials.
3. A study highlighted the potential dangers of tight (5–6.7 mmol/L) versus loose (6.7–8.3 mmol/L) glycemic control using a combination of microdialysis, positron electron tomography, and jugular venous bulb measurements of cerebral glucose concentrations, markers of cellular distress, and oxygen extraction ratios, respectively. Tight glycemic control was associated with a 70% decrease in microdialysis cerebral glucose concentrations, as well as significantly greater markers of cellular oxidative stress and oxygen extraction ratio.

Thus, although we would recommend attention to normoglycemia, tight glycemic control to the degree used in the adult study cannot be recommended at this stage. A compromise might be to aim for blood glucose levels between 6 and 8.5 mmol/L and certainly to treat levels above 10 mmol/L with a sliding scale of insulin. The pediatric population, especially neonates and infants, is at far greater risk of hypoglycemia than is the adult population, and an adequate glucose load of at least 4 mg/kg/hr of dextrose must accompany insulin infusions. A pertinent supplementary question is how long glycemic control should be continued. The strongest data relate to outcome and hyperglycemia at the time of initial presentation after pediatric stroke. In the context of critical illness, however, our inclina-

tion would be to recommend continuation of this strategy until the child is extubated.

Management of Intractable Intracranial Hypertension

Early referral to a PICU with access to neurosurgery is mandatory for children with stroke who have depressed or deteriorating consciousness level or other signs of raised ICP. It is our policy that the referring hospital transports the child after stabilization to minimize time delays.

ICP monitoring should be considered to guide CPP-directed therapy in these children. Neuroprotection is described in **Figure 58.12** and follows published guidelines (Chapter 56). Medical management steps include maximizing sedation (including thiopentone to achieve burst suppression as analyzed by a bedside cerebral function monitor), paralysis, elevating the head of the bed (30 degrees), a loading dose (18 mg/kg) and subsequent maintenance dose of phenytoin, a hypertonic 3% saline infusion to achieve a plasma osmolality ≥ 320 mOsm/L, hyperventilation to a $PaCO_2$ of 30–37.5 mm Hg (4.0–5.0 kPa) and active cooling to between 32° and 34°C (**Figs. 58.11 and 58.12**). Chronic hyperventilation cannot be recommended, but acute hyperventilation in the context of imminent herniation does rapidly decrease ICP. If intracranial hypertension persists (despite maximal medical management and cerebrospinal fluid drainage via an external ventricular drain) or if clinical evidence exists of impending central or uncal transtentorial herniation, the following options are available; however, the superiority of one over the other is not supported by RCT data.

Decompressive Craniectomy. Intractable intracranial hypertension of any stroke-related cause should also be a potential indication for surgical decompression. Again, no RCT data exist; however, case series suggest that this option may be of benefit, especially in the context of malignant MCA syndrome (22). Certainly, the inability to maintain CPP and persistently elevated levels of ICP (>20 mm Hg) are associated with poor outcome, and it would seem logical to at least consider a surgical option. A problem with decompressive craniectomy in the UK has been the inability to store resected bone, for regulatory reasons. This situation had previously mandated subsequent cranial reconstruction in survivors, using titanium plates, which not only has a significant cost implication but also introduces the risk of subsequent infection. The recently introduced practice of implanting bone flaps into the anterior abdominal wall, below the Scarpa fascia, for subsequent autologous reconstruction approximately 6 months after surgery, has obviated this problem. Patients with secondary hydrocephalus, as in the context of sinovenous thrombosis, may need ventriculostomy and/or surgical decompression.

Hypothermia. Hyperpyrexia undoubtedly increases the cerebral metabolic demand for oxygen and is thus likely to exacerbate penumbral injury adjacent to infarct zones, where microcirculatory disturbances are known to interfere with substrate demand coupling. Cerebral cooling could redress this balance and affect outcome. However, no studies in adults or children have been reported that confirm this theory, and the potential systemic side effects of hypothermia remain a concern. However, data do suggest that moderate hypothermia (32–34°C) after severe TBI in children is safe relative to standard normothermic management (3). Although decreased mortality was seen in the hypothermic groups (initiated rapidly within 6 hrs of injury or in a more delayed fashion <24 hrs of injury), an increased potential for dysrhythmias was also seen, although they were manageable with fluid administration or rewarming. Additionally, mean ICP decreased during the first 72 hrs after injury. Although functional outcome at 3 or 6 months did not differ between treatment groups, functional outcome tended to improve from the 3- to 6-month cognitive assessment in the hypothermia group. Thus, although hypothermia cannot be recommended for inclusion in standard neuroprotection protocols, it possibly has a place in the management of intractable intracranial hypertension. The study quoted here suggests that the systemic safety profile of hypothermia is acceptable, at least in the short term (24–48 hrs). Adult studies of out-of-hospital cardiac arrests that involve ventricular fibrillation have established the utility of this paradigm (3).

However, unless ICP is measured in unconscious children with stroke, these ICP/CPP-related emergencies will not be recognized, and a therapeutic opportunity will be missed.

Emergency Neuroimaging

Apart from the lack of RCTs, the major barrier to evidence-based practice for childhood stroke is the wide range of pathologies, for each of which the current optimal strategy may be different. Hemorrhagic stroke, which may require urgent neurosurgical intervention, must be excluded by emergency CT (**Fig. 58.1A**) or MRI (**Table 58.2**). If available, MRI is very useful in the acute situation, either in excluding alternative pathologies or confirming arterial disease (**Table 58.2**). A guide to differential diagnoses in children who present with acute focal neurologic deficit is provided in **Table 58.1**; many are obvious on MRI (**Fig. 58.2**, **Table 58.2**). In addition, it is important that the vascular pathology is defined so that conditions that require urgent management, such as arterial dissection, are not missed. Despite the need for general anesthesia in most cases, MRI has advantages over CT, as in addition to the essential

exclusion of hemorrhage, ischemia may be documented within minutes (using diffusion-weighted imaging) or hours (using T2-weighted imaging) rather than days. In adults, ischemic but uninfarcted tissue with "misery perfusion" on perfusion MRI is a target for emergency reperfusion with thrombolysis, usually within a 3-hr window, although for basilar artery thrombosis, evidence suggests benefit at least up to 12 hrs. The addition of MRA of the circle of Willis and of the neck vessels (**Fig. 58.3**), fat-saturated T1-weighted MRI of the neck (**Fig. 58.5**), and MRV (**Fig. 58.6**) allow definition of the vascular pathology, which often guides management (**Table 58.2**).

Sinovenous thrombosis may be accompanied by hemorrhagic or bland infarction—typically occipital, parietal, frontal, or thalamic (46) (**Figs. 58.1J,K** and **58.2M–Q**); although often missed on CT (**Fig. 58.1K**), the occluded sinus may be seen on MRI (**Fig. 58.2M**) or CT/MR venography (**Fig. 58.6**). Importantly, most of the conditions that mimic ischemic stroke (5,47), such as acute disseminated encephalomyelitis, metabolic disease, and posterior leukoencephalopathy (**Fig. 58.2R**), may be recognized on MRI, which may mean that a child is not exposed to the unnecessary risks of antithrombotic therapy but receives the appropriate evidence-based management strategy for the condition. Metabolic stroke is relatively rare, and clinical clues are often present (e.g., persistent vomiting; on neuroimaging, the infarcts are usually not in a typical vascular distribution). The demyelination associated with acute disseminated encephalomyelitis is usually obvious on MRI.

Approximately 80% of children with an infarct in an arterial territory have large-vessel disease, e.g., stenosis, occlusion, or dissection, demonstrable on MRA or MRI (20). Thrombosis in the large venous sinuses (sagittal, lateral, straight) may be diagnosed on MR (**Fig. 58.6**) or CT venography, which is essential in patients with thalamic or cortical infarcts (particularly parietal and occipital) (**Figs. 58.1J,K** and **58.2M–Q**) (46). Although a 1% risk of stroke exists, patients with a normal MRA and MRV and no evidence of dissection on fat-saturated MRI of the neck should undergo conventional angiography, which is usually required for the diagnosis of small-vessel vasculitis, cortical venous thrombosis, and sometimes, for the diagnosis of dissection (**Fig. 58.4B**), particularly in the posterior circulation (19).

Neurophysiology

Emergency electroencephalogram may be helpful in diagnosing hemiplegic migraine and electrical seizure activity in the unconscious patient. Epilepsy with postictal hemiparesis may be diagnosed on electroencephalogram. This study in hemiplegic migraine usually shows unilateral slow background activity, in addition to the evidence of edema on diffusion- or T2-weighted MRI (44).

Specific Measures

Hemorrhagic Stroke

Patients with hemorrhagic stroke require immediate transfer to a PICU with on-site neurosurgery in the event that craniectomy is required, but pediatric neurology and hematology consultations should also be obtained in view of the wide differential diagnosis (4,26) and high early mortality of up to 25%.

TABLE 58.2

EMERGENCY IMAGING FOR CHILDHOOD STROKE

Magnetic resonance imaging (MRI) (including diffusion and perfusion), arteriography (MRA), venography (MRV)
Exclude hemorrhage
Define extent and territory of infarct
MRA to define vascular anatomy of circle of Willis and neck vessels
T1-weighted spin echo of the neck with fat-saturation sequence to exclude dissection
MRV to exclude sinovenous thrombosis
Diffusion imaging to differentiate acute from chronic infarction
Perfusion imaging to demonstrate areas of tissue larger than demonstrated on diffusion imaging of abnormal cerebral blood flow, blood volume, and mean transit time

CT scan to exclude hemorrhage if MRI not available acutely
Conventional angiography if:
Hemorrhage without coagulopathy and cause is not obvious on MRA or MRV
Ischemic stroke, MRA normal, and fat-saturated T1-weighted MRI of the neck does not demonstrate dissection

Structural arterial disorders, specifically arteriovenous malformations, aneurysms and cavernomas, sinovenous thrombosis, developmental venous anomalies, and coagulopathies such as hemophilia, are the most common pathologies. In the acute phase, the main priorities are to prevent cerebral herniation if the blood collection is space-occupying, reverse any coagulopathy, exclude sinovenous thrombosis, and treat any associated vasospasm (e.g., SAH) with volume expansion and calcium-channel blockers such as nimodipine.

Underlying coagulopathy is particularly common in children <1 year of age. Hemorrhagic disease of the newborn should be treated with vitamin K, and disseminated intravascular coagulation should be treated with fresh frozen plasma or Beriplex™ (a prothrombin complex containing a concentrate of factors II, VII, IX, and X). Fresh platelet transfusion is required if the hemorrhage has occurred in the context of thrombocytopenia, and recombinant factor VIII is the treatment for hemophilia. The use of recombinant activated factor VII (rFVIIa) should be considered in hemorrhagic stroke with large clot volumes. An adult randomized controlled trial reported that three doses of recombinant activated factor VII given within 4 hrs after the onset of ICH limited the growth of the hematoma, reduces mortality, and improves functional outcomes at 90 days despite a small increase in the frequency of thromboembolic adverse events (49).

Emergency vascular imaging should include an MRV as well as an MRA, as 10% of hemorrhages in young adults are secondary to sinovenous thrombosis. The urgency for appropriate imaging is particularly acute, because the conditions that underlie hemorrhagic stroke caused by sinovenous thrombosis have a high mortality rate and may be treatable (46). The use of anticoagulants in the management of sinovenous thrombosis with hemorrhage in childhood has been controversial (28), but in two adult trials, outcome overall was better in the treated group and new hemorrhage was not documented (48). Heparin should certainly be considered in the presence of deterioration in clinical status, e.g., intractable seizures, coma, or CT/MR venography evidence of propagation of thrombus.

If an underlying arteriovenous malformation is present, the recurrence risk is 2%–3% per year for life if untreated, and a carefully considered decision regarding management (neurosurgery, neuroradiology with coils, or stereotactic radiotherapy) must be made once the patient has recovered from the acute phase (4,13,26). Although less common, aneurysms are associated with a significant rebleeding risk, particularly soon after presentation. A vascular team with considerable experience should evaluate these children so that an individual management strategy, targeted at preventing recurrence, can be implemented.

Ischemic Stroke

Approximately half of the children who present with AIS and a similar proportion of those with sinovenous thrombosis have a known predisposing condition (**Figs. 58.8 and 58.9**), particularly SCD, cardiac disease, bacterial meningitis, and malignancy. Some of these children are candidates for emergency management of the stroke, such as exchange transfusion for patients with SCD (24) or anticoagulation for venous sinus thrombosis (28,48). Ideally, neuroimaging to identify the pathology of the infarct and of the vascular disease should be performed either before or as therapy commences. As mentioned previously, the Seventh ACCP Conference on An-

tithrombotic and Thrombolytic Therapy developed guidelines for antithrombotic therapy in children, including those who had suffered an ischemic stroke (33). At about the same time, the Paediatric Stroke Working Group of the RCP produced guidelines that are freely available on the Internet (39). These 2004 guidelines were based on the available evidence at the time and largely agree on most issues, with a few differences, the main one being that the ACCP guidelines suggest anticoagulation in situations such as initial presentation with AIS, and the RCP guidelines favor aspirin. This variation largely reflects the lack of evidence, but it may also reflect differences in approach between pediatric neurologists (who often insist on comprehensive emergency neuroimaging to distinguish between arterial dissection and transient cerebral arteriopathy, as the current consensus is that treatment should be anticoagulation for the former and aspirin for the latter), and hematologists (who have more experience with anticoagulation in situations in which the diagnosis is uncertain).

Stroke Due to Sickle Cell Disease. Children with SCD are at high risk for stroke. In an RCT, children with high transcranial Doppler velocities (>200 cm/sec) had a 40% stroke risk over the subsequent 3 years. Primary prevention of stroke was possible if these children were screened appropriately and transfused indefinitely (2). However, therapy for acute stroke and secondary prevention has evolved through hematologic clinical experience rather than being subject to rigorous evaluation by RCT (24,33,39). Hemoglobin and sickle hemoglobin percentages should be measured at presentation with any neurologic complication, and packed red blood cells (20 mL/kg) should be cross-matched as quickly as possible. The accepted goal is to begin transfusion within 2–4 hrs of presentation, particularly if the deficit is persisting or progressing, although no randomized controlled data exist (33,39). If available, exchange (using a manual regime or an automated cell separator for erythrocytapheresis) transfusion is recommended rather than simple transfusion. In a retrospective analysis of this population, a fivefold increase in risk of recurrent stroke was observed in children who received initial and then chronic simple transfusion as opposed to exchange transfusion (24) at the time of initial stroke, suggesting that exchange transfusion should be used for emergency management. Over the first 48 hrs, the goal is to reduce the hemoglobin S percentage to <20% and raise the hemoglobin to 10–11 g/dL, with a hematocrit of >30%. Blood should be leukocyte-depleted and ABO, Rhesus D and K, Fy, Jk, and MNS red cell phenotype compatible with the recipient to minimize the risk of alloimmunization.

Historically, patients with stroke in the context of SCD have often been managed in local hospitals without access to neuroimaging or with access to CT only, although it has become clear that, as well as MCA territory and watershed infarction secondary to arterial stenosis, the pathology includes hemorrhage, sinovenous thrombosis, RPLS, acute necrotizing encephalitis, and arterial dissection, and that emergency MRI, MRA, and MRV may guide management (**Table 58.2, Figs. 58.2, 58.3, 58.5 and 58.6**). Controversy continues regarding the acute and long-term management of these alternative neurologic diagnoses, and the local hematologist and pediatric neurologist should be involved in decisions. Nevertheless, in the absence of clear contraindications, patients with SCD should be managed according to standard protocols for the pathology with which they present.

Thrombolysis with Tissue Plasminogen Activator. In adults with ischemic stroke, the main focus of recent studies has been in looking at the possibility of minimizing the effect of the initial stroke by promoting recanalization of the occluded artery using thrombolysis. One controlled study of IV tissue plasminogen activator (tPA) that was conducted in adults who could be randomized within 3 hrs showed significant benefit in terms of outcome at 3 months. However, thrombolysis in adults carries a 10% risk of hemorrhage, with considerable associated mortality. The results beyond a 3-hr window have been very disappointing, and only ~5% of patients fulfill the criteria for treatment. No randomized evidence supports the use of tPA in the acute treatment of stroke in children. Although children with a stroke often present to a physician within 3 hrs, the rarity of childhood stroke, the low sensitivity of CT for acute infarction, and the wide differential in this age group (6,47) result in a very low diagnostic rate in the time window described in adult thrombolytic trials. Due to the lower mortality in this age group, the lack of RCT data make recommendations for the acute use of thrombolysis difficult to justify in risk–benefit terms.

After detailed counseling and consultation with the family, very occasionally, thrombolysis with IV tPA within 3 hrs or intra-arterial tPA within 6 hrs may be considered for MCA infarction, or intra-arterial tPA within 12 hrs may be considered for basilar artery occlusion. Circumstances in which this may be justifiable include children known to be at risk (e.g., because of congenital heart disease) who stroke in the hospital. Acute thrombolysis has also been used in children with propagation of venous sinus thrombosis in whom clinical symptoms persist or deteriorate.

Prevention of Propagation of Thrombus and Early Recurrence. Except for those with SCD, the acute management of stroke in children remains controversial, and many physicians give no specific treatment. As outlined previously, unless emergency MRI is available, distinguishing sinovenous thrombosis from arterial stroke may be difficult, although clinical clues may help. Children with AIS referred to teaching centers have a recurrence risk for stroke of at least 10% and an even higher risk of additional TIAs (21,50). For sinovenous thrombosis, there may be spontaneous recanalization of thrombosed venous sinuses with general measures such as rehydration, antibiotics, and correction of hypoxemia but non-recanalization or propagation is a recognized problem that may influence prognosis (28,46).

Anticoagulation. The use of anticoagulation remains controversial. In unselected stroke, probably mainly arterial, one trial in adults suggested benefit, while others demonstrated that, although benefit in terms of functional outcome may be appreciated, it is counterbalanced by the increased mortality secondary to hemorrhage. As children are probably less at risk of hemorrhage, a case may be made for anticoagulation in AIS, but the only cohort series, in which physicians chose either low-molecular-weight heparin (LMWH) or aspirin for their patients, showed no advantage over aspirin (51). For sinovenous thrombosis in adults, a small, controlled trial of IV unfractionated heparin showed reduction in mortality, and a larger controlled trial of subcutaneous LMWH showed a trend for benefit in terms of death and dependency (48). In children with sinovenous thrombosis, anticoagulation acutely and for 3–6

months thereafter in high-risk situations (e.g., relapse of the underlying disorder) is associated with a reduced risk of recurrent systemic or cerebral thrombosis (28). For AIS, the ACCP guidelines recommend anticoagulation with unfractionated or LMWH for 5–7 days or until cardioembolic stroke and dissection are excluded (33), and they offer a practical regimen. This is a reasonable approach, particularly if comprehensive emergency neuroimaging and echocardiography are not available. Providing no hemorrhage is seen on imaging, anticoagulation for 3–6 months should certainly be considered in children with confirmed extracranial arterial dissection associated with AIS or cerebral sinus venous thrombosis, as recommended in both the ACCP and the RCP guidelines (33,39). The use of anticoagulation in patients with cardiac disease is more controversial (33,39) and may be influenced by the cardiac pathology and by neurologic and imaging findings, as embolism is often difficult to prove (20). Individual patient management should involve senior clinicians in cardiology and neurology. A case may also be made for anticoagulating patients with known prothrombotic abnormalities, as recurrence risk is higher in this group (21,50), although no evidence suggests that the risk is reduced with anticoagulation compared with aspirin, at least in part because the available pediatric studies involve cohorts in which the physicians were allowed to choose treatment (21,51), and no randomized data in children are available.

Antiplatelet Agents. In two very large controlled trials in adults, aspirin appeared to be associated with a modest improvement in outcome, probably because of a reduction in early recurrence and perhaps, in addition, via its antipyretic effect. The risk of hemorrhage appears to be lower than with anticoagulants. No strong evidence has reported a benefit from using aspirin in childhood stroke, but data from a German cohort suggest that a dose of 5 mg/kg/day is safe (51), and in the Great Ormond Street study, a trend for reduction of recurrence was seen, compared with no prophylaxis (21). The RCP guidelines suggest aspirin (5 mg/kg/day) be administered immediately following AIS, except in the presence of evidence of hemorrhage (39), followed by 1–5 mg/kg/day long term, whereas the ACCP guidelines recommend aspirin (2–5 mg/kg/day) once anticoagulation has been discontinued. The RCP guidelines suggest continuing aspirin at a dose of 1–5 mg/kg/day in children with cerebral arteriopathy other than dissection or moyamoya (39); however, if well tolerated, long-term, low-dose aspirin is probably a reasonable approach for all non-SCD children with AIS, in that although the risk of recurrence is greatest in the first year after stroke, risk is ongoing, even for those with cryptogenic stroke. In an attempt to produce a consistent approach, members of the International Paediatric Stroke Study have agreed to consistently use a dose of 3–5 mg/kg of aspirin as short- and long-term prophylaxis if they do not choose anticoagulation.

CONCLUSIONS AND FUTURE DIRECTIONS

Further multicentered, multinational studies of epidemiology and risk factors for primary and secondary stroke must be urgently performed. The results of these studies must be used to encourage and adequately power randomized interventional studies to establish appropriate evidence-based guidelines for the treatment of this particular, potentially salvageable pediatric emergency.

KEY POINTS

■ Up to 3200 children per year in the US alone will suffer a stroke.

■ Stroke and CVD are among the top 10 causes of childhood death.

■ Mortality is 6%–20%, and at least 50% of children have residual disability.

■ Morbidity and mortality are higher for children who present with stroke in the context of critical illness.

■ Ischemic strokes in children are most common in the neonatal period, while SAH is most common in teenagers, with boys at greater risk than girls for SAH.

■ Hemorrhagic and ischemic stroke peak in the first year of life.

■ Stroke is more common in children of black ethnicity, even after correcting for the influence of SCD.

■ Childhood stroke represents a significant socioeconomic health burden, as most survivors live for several decades.

■ Advances in imaging and increasing survival of children with predisposing disease probably account for the increasing prevalence of stroke.

■ 10% of patients with AIS suffer recurrent stroke, and recurrent TIAs and silent infarction are also common.

■ Following sinovenous thrombosis, children may suffer recurrent cerebral and systemic thrombosis.

■ Emergency neuroimaging, ideally MRI, to define diagnosis and direct diagnosis-specific intervention is good practice.

■ If anticoagulation can be undertaken, conditions for which it is indicated (sinovenous thrombosis and dissection) should be actively looked for

■ Stroke mimics, such as RPLS and acute disseminated encephalomyelitis, can usually be distinguished on MRI.

■ Patients with arterial stroke other than dissection should receive aspirin 5 mg/kg.

■ Aggressive therapeutic intervention, whether medical, surgical, or radiologic, may reduce morbidity and mortality.

■ Intracranial hypertension is a common feature of stroke, and CPP-targeted therapy should be considered.

■ Neurosurgical intervention may be required for drainage of intracerebral hematoma, craniectomy for malignant MCA, or cerebellar infarction or shunt for hydrocephalus.

■ Optimal treatment requires a multidisciplinary approach.

■ Childhood stroke carries a better prognosis than seen in adults.

ACKNOWLEDGMENTS

This work has benefited from R&D funding received from the NHS executive. FJK was supported by the Wellcome Trust (0353521 B/92/2) and Action Research and is currently supported by the Stroke Association (PROG4).

References

1. Abram H KE, Warty VS, Painter MJ. Natural history, prognosis and lipid abnormalities of idiopathic ischemic childhood stroke. *J Child Neurol* 1996;11:276–82.

2. Adams RJ MV, Hsu L, Files B, et al. Prevention of a first stroke by transfusions in children with sickle cell anemia and abnormal results on transcranial Doppler ultrasonography. *N Engl J Med* 1998;339:5–11.

3. Adelson PD, Ragheb J, Kanev P, et al. Phase II clinical trial of moderate hypothermia after severe traumatic brain injury in children. *Neurosurgery* 2005;56(4):740–54; discussion, 740–54.

4. Al Jarallah A, Riela AR, Roach ES. Nontraumatic brain hemorrhage in children: Etiology and presentation. *J Child Neurol* 2000;15:284–9.

5. Blom I, De Schryver EL, Kappelle LJ, et al. Prognosis of haemorrhagic stroke in childhood: A long-term follow-up study. *Dev Med Child Neurol* 2003;45:233–9.

6. Braun KP, Kappelle J, Kirkham FJ, DeVeber GA. Diagnostic pitfalls in paediatric ischaemic stroke. *Dev Med Child Neurol* 2006;48:985–90.

7. Braun KP, Rafay MF, Uiterwaal CS, et al. Mode of onset predicts etiological diagnosis of arterial ischemic stroke in children. *Stroke* 2007;38:298–302.

8. Chabrier S, Rodesch G, Lasjaunias P, et al. Transient cerebral arteriopathy: A disorder recognized by serial angiograms in children with stroke. *J Child Neurol* 1998;13:27–32.

9. Danchaivijitr N, Cox TC, Saunders DE, et al. Evolution of cerebral arteriopathies in childhood arterial ischemic stroke. *Ann Neurol* 2006;59:620–6.

10. DeVeber, G, Monagle, P, Chan, A, et al. Prothrombotic disorders in infants and children with cerebral thromboembolism. *Arch Neurol* 1998;55:1539–43.

11. DeVeber G, MacGregor D, Curtis R, et al. Neurologic outcome in survivors of childhood arterial ischemic stroke and sinovenous thrombosis. *J Child Neurol* 2000;15:316–24.

12. DeVeber G, Andrew M, Adams C, et al. Cerebral sinovenous thrombosis in children. *N Engl J Med* 2001;345:417–23.

13. Di Rocco C TG, Rollo M. Cerebral arteriovenous malformations in children. *Acta Neurochir* 2000;142:145–56.

14. Dobson SR, Holden KR, Nietert PJ, et al. Moyamoya syndrome in childhood sickle cell disease: A predictive factor for recurrent cerebrovascular events. *Blood* 2002;99:3144–50.

15. Fullerton H, Johnston SC, Smith WS. Arterial dissection and stroke in children. *Neurology* 2001;57:1155–60.

16. Fullerton HJ, Wu YW, Zhao S, et al. Risk of stroke in children: Ethnic and gender disparities. *Neurology* 2003;61:189–94.

17. Fullerton HJ, Aminoff AR, Ferriero DM, et al. Neurodevelopmental outcome after endovascular treatment of vein of Galen malformations. *Neurology* 2003;61:1386–90.

18. Ganesan V, Hogan A, Shack N, et al. Outcome after ischaemic stroke in childhood. *Dev Med Child Neurol* 2000;42:455–61.

19. Ganesan V, Chong WK, Cox T, et al. Posterior circulation stroke in childhood. *Neurology* 2002;59:1552–6.

20. Ganesan V, Prengler M, McShane MA, et al. Investigation of risk factors in children with arterial ischemic stroke. *Ann Neurol* 2003;53:167–73.

21. Ganesan V, Prengler M, Wade A, et al. Clinical and radiological recurrence after childhood arterial ischemic stroke. *Circulation* 2006;114:2170–7.

22. Gupta R, Connolly ES, Mayer S, Elkind MS. Hemicraniectomy for massive middle cerebral artery territory infarction: A systematic review. *Stroke* 2004;35:539–43.

23. Henderson JN, Noetzel MJ, McKinstry RC, et al. Reversible posterior leukoencephalopathy syndrome and silent cerebral infarcts are associated with severe acute chest syndrome in children with sickle cell disease. *Blood* 2003;101:415–9.

24. Hulbert ML, Scothorn DJ, Panepinto JA, et al. Exchange blood transfusion compared with simple transfusion for first overt stroke is associated with a lower risk of subsequent stroke: A retrospective cohort study of 137 children with sickle cell anemia. *J Pediatr* 2006;149:710–2.

25. Ikezaki K. Rational approach to treatment of moyamoya disease in childhood. *J Child Neurol* 2000;15:350–6.

26. Jordan LC, Hillis AE. Hemorrhagic stroke in children. *Pediatr Neurol* 2007;36:73–80.

27. Jordan LC, van Beek JG, Gottesman RF, et al. Ischemic stroke in children with critical illness: A poor prognostic sign. *Pediatr Neurol* 2007;36:244–6.

28. Kenet G, Kirkham F. For the European Thromboses Study Group. Risk factors for recurrent venous thromboembolism in the European collaborative paediatric database on cerebral venous thrombosis: A multicentre cohort study. *Lancet Neurol* 2007;6:595–603.

29. Kirkham FJ, Hewes DKM, Hargrave D, et al. Nocturnal hypoxaemia predicts CNS events in sickle cell disease. *Lancet* 2001;357:1656–9.

30. Koga Y, Akita Y, Junko N, et al. Endothelial dysfunction in MELAS improved by l-arginine supplementation. *Neurology* 2006;66:1766–9.

31. Lanthier S, Carmant L, David M, et al Stroke in children: The coexistence of multiple risk factors predicts poor outcome. *Neurology* 2000;54:371–8.

32. Maria BL, Neufeld JA, Rosainz LC, et al. Central nervous system structure and function in Sturge-Weber syndrome: Evidence of neurologic and radiologic progression. *J Child Neurol* 1998;13:606–18.

33. Monagle P, Chan A, Massicotte P, et al. Antithrombotic therapy in children: The Seventh ACCP Conference on Antithrombotic and Thrombolytic Therapy. *Chest* 2004;126 (3 Suppl):645S–87S.

34. Nowak-Göttl U, Sträter R, Heinecke A, et al. Lipoprotein (a) and genetic polymorphisms of clotting factor V, prothrombin and methylenetetrahydrofolate reductase are risk factors of ischaemic stroke in childhood. *Blood* 1999;94:3678–82.

35. Ohene-Frempong K, Weiner SJ, Sleeper LA, et al. Cerebrovascular accidents in sickle cell disease: Rates and risk factors. *Blood* 1998;91:288–94.

36. Pavlakis SG, Frank Y, Chusid R. Hypertensive encephalopathy, reversible occipitoparietal encephalopathy, or reversible posterior leukoencephalopathy: Three names for an old syndrome. *J Child Neurol* 1999;14:277–81.

37. Pavlakis SG, Bialer MG. Stroke in children: Genetic and metabolic issues. *J Child Neurol* 2000;15:308–15.

38. Phornphutkul C RA, Nadas A, Berenberg W. Cerebrovascular accidents in infants and children with cyanotic congenital heart disease. *Am J Cardiol* 1973;32:329–34.

39. Royal College of Physicians Paediatric Stroke Working Group. Stroke in childhood: Clinical guidelines for diagnosis, management and rehabilitation http://www.rcplondon.ac.uk/pubs/books/childstroke/childstroke_guidelines. pdf. Accessed August 2007.

40. Prengler M, Sturt N, Krywawych S, et al. Homozygous thermolabile variant of the methylenetetrahydrofolate reductase gene: A potential risk factor for hyperhomocysteinaemia, CVD, and stroke in childhood. *Dev Med Child Neurol* 2001;43:220–5.

41. Reith J, Jorgensen HS, Pedersen PM, et al. Body temperature in acute stroke: Relation to stroke severity, infarct size, mortality, and outcome. *Lancet* 1996;347:422–5.

42. Riikonen, RS, Santavuori, P. Hereditary and acquired risk factors for childhood stroke. *Neuropaediatics* 1994;25:227–33.

43. Rolfs A, Bottcher T, Zschiesche M, et al. Prevalence of Fabry disease in patients with cryptogenic stroke: A prospective study. *Lancet* 2005;366: 1794–6.

44. Sand T. EEG in migraine: a review of the literature. *Funct Neurol* 1991;6(1): 7–22.

45. Sébire G, Meyer L, Chabrier S. Varicella as a risk factor for cerebral infarction in childhood: A case-control study. *Ann Neurol* 1999;45:679–80.

46. Sébire G, Tabarki B, Saunders DE, et al. Venous sinus thrombosis in children. *Brain* 2005;128:477–89.

47. Shellhass RA, Smith SE, O'Tool E, et al. Mimics of childhood stroke: Characteristics of a prospective cohort. *Pediatrics* 2006;118:704–9.

48. Stam J, De Bruijn SF, DeVeber G. Anticoagulation for cerebral sinus thrombosis. *Cochrane Database Syst Rev* 2002;(4):CD002005.

49. Steiner T, Diringer MN, Schneider D, et al. Dynamics of intraventricular hemorrhage in patients with spontaneous intracerebral hemorrhage: Risk factors, clinical impact, and effect of hemostatic therapy with recombinant activated factor VII. *Neurosurgery* 2006;59(4):767–73;discussion, 773–4.

50. Sträter R, Becker S, von Eckardstein A, et al. Prospective assessment of risk factors for recurrent stroke during childhood—a 5-year follow-up study. *Lancet* 2002;360:1540–5.

51. Sträter R, Kurnik K, Heller C, et al. Aspirin versus low-dose low-molecular-weight heparin: Antithrombotic therapy in pediatric ischemic stroke patients: A prospective follow-up study. *Stroke* 2001;32:2554–8.

52. Taylor TN DP, Torner JC, Holmes J, et al. Lifetime cost of stroke in the United States. *Stroke* 1996;27:1459–66.

53. Zahuranec DB, Brown DL, Lisabeth LD, et al. Is it time for a large, collaborative study of pediatric stroke? *Stroke* 2005;36:1825–9.

CHAPTER 59 ■ HYPOXIC-ISCHEMIC ENCEPHALOPATHY

ERICKA L. FINK • MIOARA D. MANOLE • ROBERT S.B. CLARK

Simply put, hypoxic-ischemic encephalopathy (HIE) can be defined as damage to cells in the brain due to hypoxia. The clinical entity is much more complex, as HIE represents a broad spectrum of brain injury that results from hypoxemia and/or ischemia, with or without reperfusion, and can result from diverse etiologies. In newborns, infants, and children, HIE is very heterogeneous in terms of developmental stage at the time of insult, regional vulnerability, and etiology, making clinical management/treatment and outcome prediction quite difficult, let alone devising uniform and accepted guidelines and standards for management. These daunting hurdles deserve special scientific attention, as HIE is a major cause of morbidity and mortality in pediatric patients. It presents a heavy burden both for the patient and caregivers in terms of disability and quality of life in survivors, and for society in the form of the high costs associated with lifelong health care assistance. To date, no efficacious treatment for HIE exists; however, progress has been made in preventing HIE, demonstrated by (a) use of postresuscitative mild hypothermia in adults after ventricular tachycardia/fibrillation (VT/VF)-induced cardiac arrest and in newborns after birth asphyxia, and (b) early application of thrombolytics in adults after embolic stroke. The challenges for this millennium are to maximize HIE prevention and to discover and implement effective treatments for resuscitated pediatric victims who suffer insults that would otherwise result in HIE.

CORE PATHOPHYSIOLOGY AND PATHOBIOLOGY

Prolonged hypoxemia and ischemia leads to brain injury by triggering multiple pathologic cascades that can lead to cell death and loss of neurologic function. Interwoven with pathologic cascades are endogenous neuroprotective responses initiated to minimize damage. These cellular responses have similarities to other types of acute brain injury, such as traumatic brain injury (TBI), central nervous system (CNS) infections, stroke, and status epilepticus; these are covered in detail in Chapter 52. However, a few fundamental aspects of particular relevance to HIE warrant comment here.

Global and Focal Hypoxic-Ischemic Encephalopathy

HIE can result from multiple causes that can be roughly divided based on whether the result is global or focal disease.

Global HIE can result from respiratory arrest, cardiac arrest, strangulation, poisoning, or, rarely, other conditions such as sagittal sinus thrombosis or profound shock states. For global HIE in infants and children, asphyxial cardiac arrest is the most common diagnosis, which is in contrast to adult victims of cardiac arrest, in whom cardiac arrhythmias are the most common cause. Focal HIE can result from embolic or thrombotic stroke or intracerebral hemorrhage. Global and focal insults that result in HIE have some commonalities and some important differences.

As outlined in Chapter 52, the principal commonality is the interruption of oxygen and blood flow to brain cells. Whether this interruption is global due to cardiac arrest or focal due to vascular interruption of local cerebral blood flow (CBF), parenchymal cells—neurons, astrocytes, oligodendrocytes, and microglia—will not tolerate prolonged durations of ischemia. The degree of brain damage is directly and strongly correlated with the duration of no-flow; consequently, the clinical outcome is strongly and inversely correlated with the duration of no-flow. Thus, the common clinical goal is to restore CBF as rapidly as possible, whether by return of spontaneous circulation (ROSC), in the case of cardiac arrest, or by revascularization, in the case of stroke.

Final common pathways after critical global or focal ischemia include excitotoxicity from membrane failure, with increased release and decreased reuptake of excitatory amino acids such as glutamate and glycine; oxidative stress; mitochondrial dysfunction; energy failure; and initiation of cell death cascades (84) (**Fig. 59.1**). Neuronal and glial cell death can result from necrotic, apoptotic, and autophagic pathways (see Chapter 52). Each mechanism of cell death has a characteristic morphologic appearance and temporal pattern that can be observed at the microscopic and ultrastructural levels (56). *Necrosis* is a process characterized by immediate mitochondrial and energy failure, leading to cellular swelling, loss of membrane integrity, and a prominent inflammatory response in surrounding tissues. *Apoptosis* is an energy-requiring process that generally requires new protein synthesis. Enzymatic degradation of cytoskeletal proteins results in cell somal and nuclear shrinkage, and DNA is characteristically fragmented via endonucleases. In contrast to necrosis, apoptosis produces minimal inflammation. Autophagic stress can also result in cell death. Autophagy is an adaptive response to starvation, and results in autodigestion of cellular proteins and organelles to feed the cell. Triggering of autophagy after acute insults could potentially be beneficial or detrimental, likely depending upon the degree or duration of injury. The role of autophagy after cerebral ischemia is newly under investigation.

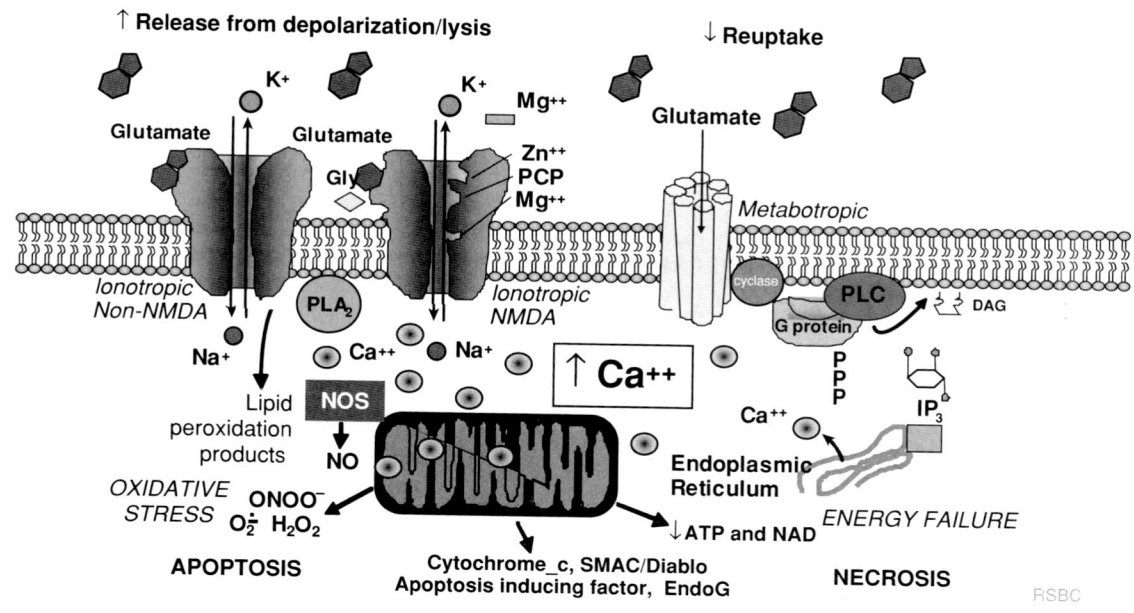

FIGURE 59.1. Cellular mechanisms resulting in cell death and hypoxic-ischemic encephalopathy. Prominent contributory mechanisms include excitotoxicity, disturbances in calcium homeostasis, oxidative stress, energy failure, and release of substances triggering cell-death pathways.

The obvious pathophysiologic difference between critical global and focal ischemia is the absence of systemic hypoxemia and ischemia before, during, and after focal insults. Multiorgan system failure, particularly cardiovascular failure, can profoundly contribute to the pathologic evolution in the postresuscitative phase, making cardiovascular and systemic stabilization a priority after cardiac arrest. Induction of both pathologic and protective hypoxia-inducible cell signaling pathways can occur prior to the insult in patients with cardiac arrest. These pathways can be triggered in all regions of the brain rather than in those downstream of vascular occlusion, as occurs during stroke. Thus, cell signaling pathways, both bad and good, may represent global therapeutic targets after hypoxia-ischemia from cardiac arrest.

Cardiac Arrest

Several clinical studies that examined cardiac arrest in children are outlined in **Table 59.1.** In contrast to adults, in whom most cardiac arrests are due to cardiac arrhythmia and intrinsic heart disease, most cardiac arrests in children, including in-hospital and out-of-hospital arrests, are due to asphyxia. A large meta-analysis showed that ROSC from all causes of cardiac arrest was achieved in 13% of pediatric patients. Where the cardiac arrest occurs—in-hospital or out-of-hospital—has a large impact on ROSC, which is achieved in 24% of children with in-hospital and 9% of children with out-of-hospital cardiac arrest (157). Mortality after cardiac arrest in children is very high, estimated to be greater than 90% and, despite the potential for plasticity in the developing brain, children who survive have dismally poor neurologic outcomes, similar to adults. This finding may be related in part to the prearrest hypoxemia and brain hypoperfusion prior to no-flow ischemia

seen during asphyxial cardiac arrest (**Fig. 59.2**). Morbidity is equally dismal. Of the survivors, over half will develop some degree of HIE.

Asphyxial cardiac arrest, accounting for ~80%–90% of pediatric cardiac arrests, begins with respiratory failure followed by hypoxemia, hypercarbia and acidosis, hypotension, pulseless electrical activity, then, ultimately, asystole. The most common clinical entities associated with asphyxial cardiac arrest include sudden infant death syndrome (SIDS), pneumonia, aspiration, and submersion injury (**Table 59.2**). Cardiac arrhythmias account for ~10% of pediatric cardiac arrest. Re-entrant arrhythmias, Wolfe-Parkinson-White syndrome, long-QT syndrome, congenital heart disease with postoperative arrhythmia, electrical injury, physical exertion, and trauma are the most frequent causes of arrhythmia in this cohort. Both adults and children who present with VT/VF as an initial rhythm have a higher incidence of good outcome compared with asphyxial arrest. For children who suffer out-of-hospital cardiac arrest, survival to hospital discharge for those who present with VT/VF is significantly higher than for those who present with asystole (30% vs. 5%, respectively) (156). This difference appears to be the case for in-hospital cardiac arrest as well, although it is less pronounced, as children with VT/VF-associated cardiac arrest had the highest survival to hospital discharge (35%), followed by pulseless electrical activity/asystole (27%), and finally late-onset VT/VF (11%). Late VT/VF was postulated to be a reperfusion arrhythmia (103). The incidence of asphyxial versus VT/VF cardiac arrest reverses with increasing age. A retrospective cohort study of 272 children with nontraumatic, out-of-hospital cardiac arrest showed that 7.6% of children between the ages of 1 and 7 years and 27.0% of those between the ages of 3 and 18 years presented with VT/VF (136). One type of congenital heart disease deserves specific mention as a salient cause of cardiac arrest in children. Hypertrophic

TABLE 59.1

REVIEW OF PEDIATRIC CARDIAC ARREST LITERATURE

Authors (year)	OH/IH	n	Age[a]	Male (%)	ROSC (%)	VT/VF (%)	Survival to d/c (%)	Good outcome (%)[b]	Predictors of good outcome	Predictors of poor outcome
RETROSPECTIVE STUDIES										
de Mos et al. (2006)	IH	91	4 yr		82	4	25	43	ECMO within 24 hrs	Renal failure; epinephrine gtt; calcium bolus during CPR
Engdahl et al. (2003)	OH	98	1 yr	52		8	5	60		
Gerein et al. (2006)	OH	503	5.6 yr	58	5	4	2			
Hickey et al. (1995)	OH	41	43 mo	68	56	22	27	73	ROSC in field; awake in ED	
Horisberger et al. (2002)	IH	89	6 mo		87 (IH) 57 (OH)		58	79		OH arrest; longer ROSC; trauma etiology
	OH									
Kuisma et al. (1995)	OH	79	2.9 yr	53	10	4		80	Witnessed arrest; near-drowning; bystander CPR; rapid ROSC	
Parra et al. (2000)	IH	32	3.5 mo		63		42	73	Mechanical support	
Pitetti et al. (2002)	OH	189	41 mo	64		4	2.6	0	Sinus rhythm in ED; fewer epinephrine doses	
Ronco et al. (1995)	OH	63	14 mo	65	39		9.5	17		1st ED rhythm non-VT/VF; ROSC >20 mins; >2 doses epinephrine
Schindler et al. (1996)	OH	80	1 yr	50	63		7.5	0	Rapid ROSC	
Slonim et al. (1997)	IH	205			24		13.7			Trauma etiology; longer ROSC; higher PRISM III
Suominen et al. (1997)	OH	50	1.2 yr		26	8	16	12	CPR <15 min	
PROSPECTIVE STUDIES										
Lopez-Herce et al. (2005)	OH	95	63 mo	64	47	9	28	82		ROSC >20 mins
Nadkarni et al. (2006)	IH	880	5.6 yr	54	63	14	27	65		No ROSC in field
Sirbaugh et al. (1999)	OH	300	9 mo	60	11	3	2	17	Witnessed arrest; PEA or VF as 1st rhythm	>3 doses epinephrine; ROSC >30 min; 1st rhythm asystole
Young et al. (2004)	OH	599		58	29	9	8.6	31		

[a]Mean or median age, depending upon the study

[b]Good outcome among survivors, defined as good outcome, mild disability, or unchanged from baseline at hospital discharge

OH, out-of-hospital; IH, in-hospital; ROSC, return of spontaneous circulation; VT/VF, ventricular tachycardia/fibrillation; d/c, discharge; ECMO, extracorporeal membrane oxygenation; CPR, cardiopulmonary resuscitation; ED, emergency department; PEA, pulseless electrical activity

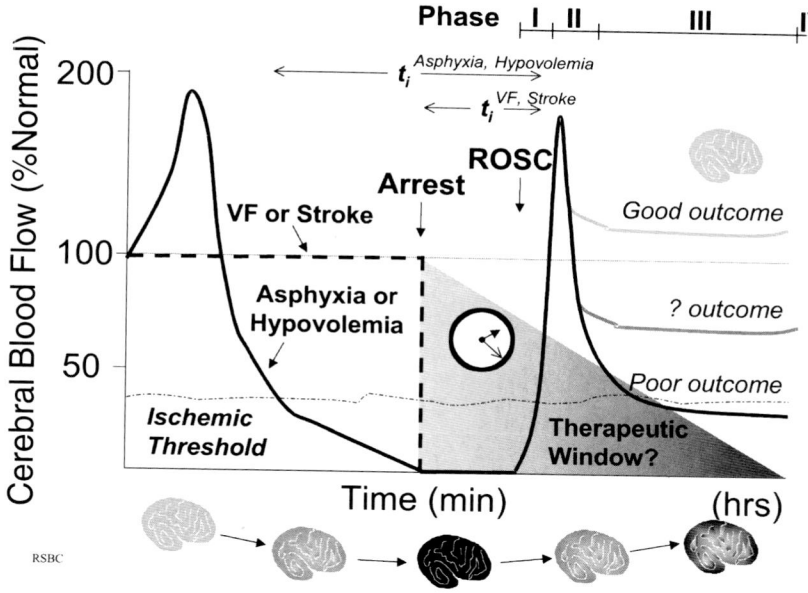

FIGURE 59.2. Typical patterns of CBF after cardiac arrest. Differences exist between CBF after asphyxial arrest (more predominant in children) and cardiogenic arrest (more prominent in adults). Four typical phases of CBF have been described, including no-flow (phase I), hyperemia (phase II), hypoperfusion (phase III), and recovery (phase IV).

cardiomyopathy accounts for approximately one-half of sudden cardiac deaths in children, and most occurred in previously well children (19).

Cerebral Blood Flow after Cardiac Arrest in Experimental Models

Age-related changes in CBF during normal development and key facets of CBF regulation are presented in Chapter 51 and serve as important background information for the sections that follow. The temporal pattern of CBF after cardiac arrest has been ascertained predominately from experimental models using adult animals and VT/VF cardiac arrest or global cerebral ischemia paradigms such as aortic or carotid occlusion. Studies that describe CBF after aphyxial cardiac arrest are few, particularly in models of "pediatric"-relevant ages. Asphyxial

TABLE 59.2

COMMON ETIOLOGIES OF OUT-OF-HOSPITAL CARDIAC ARREST IN INFANTS AND CHILDREN

Etiology	Frequency (%)	Survival to hospital discharge (%)
SIDS	23	0
Trauma	20	5
Respiratory	16	21
Submersion	12	17
Cardiac	8	8
Central nervous system	6	3
Burn	1	0
Poisoning	1	17
Other	10	10
Unknown	3	6

Adapted from Young KD, Seidel JS. Pediatric cardiopulmonary resuscitation: a collective review, *Ann Emerg Med* 1999;33:195–205.

cardiac arrest produces a physiologically different milieu compared with VT/VF arrest due to the fact that hypoxemia, acidosis, hypercarbia, and hypotension precede the cardiac arrest (Fig. 59.2). It has been reported that an asphyxial arrest of 7 mins produces severe impairment of neurologic function, comparable to a VT/VF arrest with a duration of 10 mins (34). Furthermore, compared head-to-head, asphyxial cardiac arrest in dogs resulted in more prevalent and prominent microinfarcts and petechial hemorrhage compared with VT/VF cardiac arrest of similar duration (149).

CBF during and after cardiac arrest is phasic in nature. During cardiac arrest, global ischemia occurs, with no-flow or low-flow if cardiopulmonary resuscitation is being provided. Immediately following reperfusion, a heterogenous return of CBF can occur despite normal or increased cerebral perfusion pressure, typically correlating with the duration of ischemia. Studies in adult animal models of cardiac arrest demonstrate that CBF in the postarrest period can be divided into four phases (Fig. 59.2): multifocal no reflow (Phase I), global hyperemia (Phase II), delayed hypoperfusion (Phase III), and restitution of normal blood flow (Phase IV) (8,46,68).

Initially described in 1968 in a global cerebral ischemia model, the existence of a multifocal, no-reflow phase is somewhat controversial (8). It has also been demonstrated that the hetereogenous brain reperfusion, or the "no-reflow" phenomenon, can also occur after VF cardiac arrest (46,83). This phase is characterized by localized areas of the brain that fail to reperfuse after ROSC. These areas are more extensive with increasing duration of cardiac arrest and are observed at a macroscopic and microscopic level. At a microscopic level, areas of "no reflow" are interspersed with areas of restored blood flow and microinfarcts. Brain regions that are selectively vulnerable include the thalamus, amygdala, hippocampus, and striatum. It is hypothesized that vasospasm, perivascular edema, and increased blood viscosity play a role in the development of this "no reflow" phenomenon.

The second phase of CBF after cardiac arrest is characterized by increased global CBF immediately after ROSC and is often referred to as the "hyperemia" phase. This phase is present for ~15–30 mins after ROSC. Global CBF during this phase is typically two to three times higher than baseline CBF. Investigators demonstrated that, during the hyperemia phase, local CBF was extremely heterogeneous, with some areas of no-flow present (68). Some believe that this hyperemic phase is essential for neuronal functional recovery (100). This opinion is based on studies that show that hypertensive reperfusion improves neurologic outcome, whereas postarrest hypotension worsens neurologic outcome (100,123,139). In addition to hypertensive reperfusion, hemodilution and thrombolysis in this phase have been shown to improve outcome in animal models (47,81).

The third phase of CBF after cardiac arrest begins ~15–30 mins after ROSC, can persist for several hours, and is often referred to as the "delayed-hypoperfusion" phase. During this phase, regional heterogeneity of the CBF is seen, with areas of high, normal, and low flow (8,46). The severity, or duration and degree, of delayed hypoperfusion is associated with more severe impairment of functional recovery, especially if not matched by a lower metabolic rate (34). Therefore, interventions that increase CBF and minimize delayed hypoperfusion during phase III after ischemia may improve neurologic recovery. A spectrum of temporal and regional reperfusion patterns occurs, depending on the duration of cardiac arrest. After milder insults, the hypoperfusion phases are characterized by shorter duration and less impairment of CBF. After a 9-min VF cardiac arrest in piglets, CBF was 10%–20% lower than baseline (108). In a global cerebral ischemia model in rats, ischemia of 3-min duration produced a 23% reduction of CBF, whereas 20 mins of ischemia produced a 50% reduction compared to baseline (133). Immature animals subjected to carotid artery ligation and hypoxia (Rice-Vannucci model) did not show hypoperfusion over the first 24 hrs after ROSC (99). Delayed hypoperfusion seems to occur consistently with durations of ischemia >15 mins (105,138).

Cerebral Blood Flow after Cardiac Arrest in Humans

Most available data on CBF patterns after cardiac arrest in humans are recorded >6 hrs after ROSC, as these patients need intensive stabilization during the initial first few hours. Furthermore, serial measurements of CBF have been rarely reported in these patients. The objective of most studies done to date has been to establish a relationship between CBF and ultimate outcome of the patient after cardiac arrest. Even less information exists regarding CBF values after cardiac arrest in infants and children. In neonatal asphyxia, CBF velocities have been estimated by Doppler ultrasonography and have suggested that the development of high CBF velocities after 24 hrs is predictive of poor prognosis (63). A study of CBF in 9 children in a persistent vegetative state several days after cardiac arrest (phase IV) of different etiologies (near-drowning, SIDS, postsurgery) showed CBF values that ranged from 12 to 56 mL/100 g brain tissue/min. In this series, CBF measurements in 2 children who were clinically brain dead at the time of the study were 0.2 and 2 mL/100 g brain tissue/min. CBF values of <10 mL/100 g brain tissue/min are thought to be reflective of brain death, and CBF of >10–15 mL/100 g brain tissue/min is associated with potential for patient survival (9).

Data from adults who were resuscitated from cardiac arrest show that at 24 hrs after ROSC patients can have low,

normal, or high CBF. In adult patients resuscitated from cardiac arrest, persistently high CBF values reflective of completely disrupted autoregulation (100–200 mL/100 g brain tissue/min) may indicate the onset of irreversible brain damage (37). Another study in adult patients showed that CBF <20 mL/100 g brain tissue/min is associated with death within days (29). In a study of hemispheric CBF in adult patients who were resuscitated from cardiac arrest, investigators found that patients with favorable outcomes had CBF values of 39 mL/100 g brain tissue/min, whereas patients with poor outcome had CBF values of 25 mL/100 g brain tissue/min (107). In the same study, it was shown that low hemispheric CBF (<30 mL/100 g brain tissue/min) and low reactivity to acetazolamide, an indicator of intact reactivity to changes in $PaCO_2$, are associated with poor outcome in adult patients with HIE. The ischemic threshold is considered to be 18–20 mL/100 g brain tissue/min for all ages in humans, although the true ischemic threshold may vary by age and may be relative to cerebral metabolism.

Cerebral Metabolism after Cardiac Arrest

Whether cerebral metabolism is coupled to CBF after cardiac arrest is controversial (32). Since the "luxury perfusion syndrome" was described in 1966, referring to a relative hyperemia in relationship to the brain's metabolic needs (79), several studies were conducted to determine if CBF and metabolism are truly coupled. One group compared cerebral metabolic rate for oxygen ($CMRO_2$) with CBF in a model of global cerebral ischemia without cardiac arrest (94). $CMRO_2$ increased immediately after ischemia during the hyperperfusion phase and decreased to values lower than control during the delayed hypoperfusion phase. The same authors manipulated $CMRO_2$ by altering brain temperature, and found that CBF increased parallel to $CMRO_2$ during hyperthermia (95). They concluded that CBF and metabolism are coupled and that delayed postischemic hypoperfusion is not an important determinant of neuronal injury, as CBF appears to be primarily determined by the cerebral metabolic demands. In contrast, another group found that $CMRO_2$ increased by 200% and remained at 160% of baseline values for several hours after ischemia, whereas CBF decreased by 40% compared to baseline (73). These results suggest that CBF is not coupled with $CMRO_2$ in the period of delayed hypoperfusion. Nonoxidative or anaereobic cerebral metabolism adds an additional level of complexity. Cerebral metabolic rates for glucose (CMR_{Glu}) have been shown to decrease during the hypoperfusion phase and are generally felt to be coupled with CBF after potassium-induced cardiac arrest in rats (24,104). $CMRO_2$ and CMR_{Glu} levels can be discordant after acute brain injury (20).

Data are limited regarding cerebral metabolic needs after cardiac arrest in humans. CBF and $CMRO_2$ were generally coupled in 11 patients resuscitated from cardiac arrest when measurements were taken >24 hrs after arrest (29). In 14 patients who were resuscitated from cardiac arrest, $CMRO_2$ and CBF were proportionally reduced to <50% of normal (17). In another study, nonsurviving patients gradually developed the "luxury-perfusion syndrome," likely secondary to significant necrosis of brain tissue (31). In this study, the authors found coupling of CBF and $CMRO_2$ in survivors. CMR_{Glu} level is also generally felt to be reduced in a magnitude similar to $CMRO_2$, after cardiac arrest in adult patients (121).

Systemic Variables That Affect Cerebral Blood Flow after Cardiac Arrest

As discussed in detail in Chapter 51, CBF is influenced by systemic physiologic variables, in particular, $Paco_2$, Pao_2, blood pressure, and temperature (**Fig. 59.3**). CBF is sensitive to changes in $Paco_2$, referred to as CO_2 reactivity. Low $Paco_2$ produces vasoconstriction and decreased CBF, and higher $Paco_2$ produces vasodilatation and increased CBF. Typically, for every 1 mm Hg change in $Paco_2$, CBF changes by 2%–6%. Cerebrovascular reactivity to CO_2 is often preserved in comatose patients who are resuscitated from cardiac arrest. Therefore, extreme hyperventilation and hypocarbia could exacerbate hypoperfusion and therefore should be avoided in the early postresuscitation period. However, defining the optimal $Paco_2$ early after resuscitation is complex and must also consider issues such as profound acidosis and response to catecholamines, among others. The level of Pao_2 has little effect on CBF until it is less than ~55 mm Hg, in which case CBF dramatically increases. A major controversy exists regarding the target Pao_2 for resuscitation and during the postresuscitation period, as an Fio_2 of 1.0 does not appear to hold clinical advantages over room air resuscitation (39) and may actually be deleterious related to increasing oxidative stress (150). A study from 2006 suggests that oximetry-guided resuscitation may be optimal (13). At present, it appears most logical to target normocarbia and normoxia in patients during and after cardiac arrest.

In general, CBF is maintained constant with the brain's ability for autoregulation over a range of cerebral perfusion pressure, ~50–150 mm Hg in adults. Normal autoregulatory curves are age-dependent, both in terms of lower and upper threshold limits and baseline CBF (see Chapter 51). For cerebral perfusion pressure above or below threshold values, CBF is directly correlative to cerebral perfusion pressure. Adults resuscitated from cardiac arrest may have compromised autoregulation, with either absent autoregulation or increased lower limits of autoregulation (range 80–120 mm Hg) (106,140). In experimental cardiac arrest studies, outcome was shown to be improved with induced arterial hypertension after ROSC (139). In humans, an association exists between blood pressure after ROSC and outcome. Patients with higher mean arterial pressure in the first 2 hrs after cardiac arrest are more likely to have better outcomes (100). The relationship between blood pressure autoregulation and outcome is not clear in infants and children after cardiac arrest.

Hypothermia, now a class IIb recommendation from the American Heart Association (AHA) for postresuscitation treatment of cardiac arrest, typically decreases CBF, but this occurs via a coupled reduction in cerebral metabolism (recent guidelines for resuscitation and use of hypothermia are shown in **Tables 59.3** and **59.4**). Hypothermia also has suppressive effects on excitatory neurotransmission and oxygen radicals. In animal studies, hypothermia and induced hypertension were associated with improved survival (54,124). Two randomized, multicentered, clinical trials in adult patients after primarily VT/VF cardiac arrest certainly support the use of hypothermia after cardiac arrest (3,22) and suggest that therapies that include metabolic suppression may have clinical utility.

Prolonged central hypoxia depresses ventilation, stimulating chemoreceptors and a vagal response, which produces bradycardia, followed by pulseless electrical activity or asystole (70). Oxygen stores are depleted after ~20 secs and loss of consciousness occurs. Glucose and ATP stores are depleted within 5 mins, whereupon the patient's brain crosses the threshold for cerebral ischemia (130). Following ROSC and reperfusion, typically a transient cerebral hyperemia occurs that lasts minutes and may be followed by global hypoperfusion. The duration and degree of postresuscitative hypoperfusion is proportional to the duration of the cardiac arrest, is related to ultimate severity of injury, and can last hours to several days (43); this period, during which the brain is at risk of secondary injury, may represent a therapeutic target.

Pathobiology after Reperfusion

With reperfusion after ROSC, a complex cascade of events is initiated that includes membrane depolarization; supraphysiologic accumulation of excitatory amino acids, primarily glutamate; calcium influx; acidosis; oxidative stress; mitochondrial dysfunction; and activation of lipases, proteases, and nucleases (**Fig. 59.1**). A detailed discussion of the mechanisms of secondary injury in the postischemic brain is presented in Chapter 52. Reperfusion and restoration of oxygen delivery to injured brain leads to profound increases in oxygen and nitrogen radicals, free radical damage to cells, and initiation of redox-sensitive cell signaling pathways (**Fig. 59.4**). Clinically, cellular hypoxia is manifest as depressed mental status, which is related to the depth and duration of hypoxia. The metabolic and electrical failure that is produced can result in coma, despite restoration of CBF, oxygen, and substrate delivery during reperfusion.

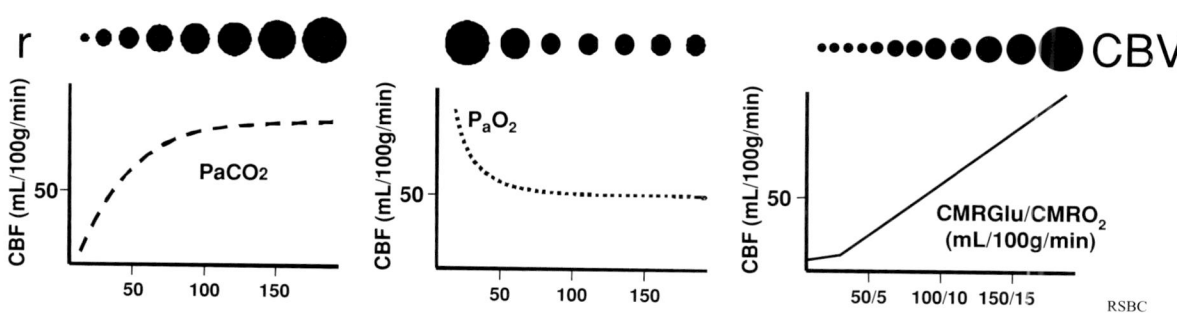

FIGURE 59.3. Physiologic factors affecting normal CBF. Under a constant cerebral perfusion pressure, CBF changes occur via changes in the diameter of the cerebral blood vessels (r = radius), resulting in changes in cerebrovascular resistance and cerebral blood volume (CBV).

TABLE 59.3

IMPORTANT CHANGES IN RECOMMENDATIONS FOR PEDIATRIC RESUSCITATION FROM THE INTERNATIONAL LIAISON COMMITTEE ON RESUSCITATION CONSENSUS ON SCIENCE, WITH TREATMENT RECOMMENDATIONS FOR PEDIATRIC AND NEONATAL PATIENTS: PEDIATRIC BASIC AND ADVANCED LIFE SUPPORT

Recommendation change	Classification*
Recommended chest compression-ventilation ratio:	IIa
For lone rescuers with victims of all ages: 30:2	
For health care providers performing two-rescuer CPR for infants and children: 15:2 (exception: 3:1 for neonates)	
Use of one shock followed by immediate CPR is recommended for each defibrillation attempt, instead of three stacked shocks	IIa
Biphasic shocks with an automated external defibrillator are acceptable for children >1 year of age. Attenuated shocks using child cables or activation of a key or switch are recommended in children <8 years old.	IIa
Routine use of high-dose IV epinephrine is no longer recommended.	III
Intravascular (IV and intraosseous) route of drug administration is preferred to the endotracheal route.	IIa
Cuffed endotracheal tubes can be used in infants and children provided correct tube size and cuff inflation pressure are used.	IIa
Exhaled CO_2 detection is recommended for confirmation of endotracheal tube placement.	I
Consider induced hypothermia for 12–24 hrs in patients who remain comatose following resuscitation.	IIb

*Class I: General agreement that a procedure or treatment is useful and effective
Class II: Conflicting evidence or divergence of opinion exists
Class IIa: Weight of evidence or opinion favors utility or efficacy of procedure or treatment
Class IIb: Weight of evidence or opinion is less well established
Class III: Evidence or general agreement that the procedure or treatment is either not useful or not effective or, in some cases, may be harmful
Increased emphasis on performing high-quality CPR: *"Push hard, push fast, minimize interruptions of chest compression; allow full chest recoil, and don't provide excessive ventilation."*
Adapted from The International Liaison Committee on Resuscitation (ILCOR) Consensus on Science with Treatment Recommendations for Pediatric and Neonatal Patients: Pediatric basic and advanced life support. *Pediatrics* 2006;117:e955–77.

Although all parenchymal cells in the brain are susceptible to hypoxia-ischemia, most attention has been directed toward neurons. Various neuronal populations are known to be selectively vulnerable to hypoxia-ischemia, including neurons within the CA1 region of the hippocampus, cerebral cortical layers 3 and 5, amygdaloid nucleus, basal ganglia, and cerebellar Purkinje cells, which have a predilection to undergo delayed neuronal death—even up to 5 days after injury (12). As discussed in Chapter 52, this hierarchy of neuronal vulnerability is of great importance in cardiac arrest because the ischemic insult in this setting is global. Unique aspects in cellular energy metabolism and connectivity are thought to play a role in this trait, as these regions in general do not have especially vulnerable microcirculatory patterns. That is not to say that watershed regions are not also selectively vulnerable to hypoxia-ischemia; although interestingly, watershed infarcts that appear

TABLE 59.4

EVIDENCE IN SUPPORT OF THE USE OF THERAPEUTIC HYPOTHERMIA (32–34°C FOR 12–24 hrs) IMMEDIATELY AFTER RESUSCITATION FROM CARDIAC ARREST

Evidence (references)	Level*
Two prospective, randomized studies of adults with VF arrest (18,95)	1,2
Two prospective, randomized studies of newborns with birth asphyxia (50,128)	2
Numerous animal studies of both asphyxial and VF arrest (146)	6
Acceptable safety profiles in adults (18,95) and neonates (50,128) treated with hypothermia for up to 72 hrs	7

*Level 1: Randomized clinical trials or meta-analysis of multiple clinical trials with substantial treatment effects
Level 2: Randomized clinical trials with smaller or less significant treatment effects
Level 3: Prospective, controlled, nonrandomized cohort studies
Level 4: Historic, nonrandomized cohort or case-controlled studies
Level 5: Case series: patients compiled in serial fashion, control group lacking
Level 6: Animal or mechanical model studies
Level 7: Extrapolations from existing data collected for other purposes, theoretical analyses
Level 8: Rational conjecture (common sense); common practices accepted before evidence-based guidelines
Adapted from The International Liaison Committee on Resuscitation (ILCOR) Consensus on Science with Treatment Recommendations for Pediatric and Neonatal Patients: Pediatric basic and advanced life support. *Pediatrics* 2006;117:e955–77.

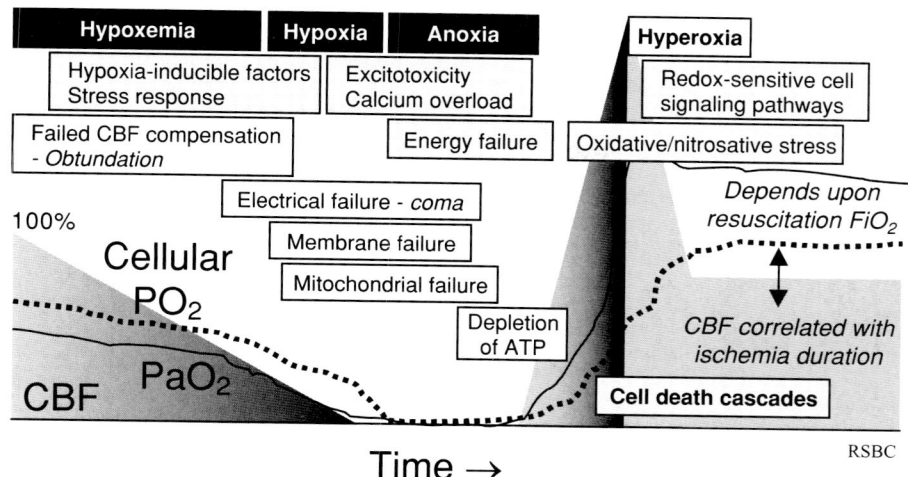

FIGURE 59.4. Pathobiology of asphyxial cardiac arrest. Hypoxemia triggers a stress response and induction of hypoxia-inducible factors and manifests clinically as obtundation. Prolonged hypoxemia can result in tissue hypoxia and eventually anoxia, with cell membrane and mitochondrial failure, energy failure, electrical failure, and coma. Reperfusion triggers oxidative stress and redox-sensitive signaling pathways and, if sufficiently prolonged, initiation of cell death cascades in selectively vulnerable brain regions.

pathologically as laminar necrosis are more common after VT/VF versus asphyxial cardiac arrest (149). After asphyxial cardiac arrest, microinfarcts and petechial hemorrhage are more common. Selectively vulnerable regions prone to the development of HIE after cardiac arrest are similar in rats (**Fig. 59.5**) and humans (**Fig. 59.6**).

CLINICAL ASPECTS OF HYPOXIC ISCHEMIC ENCEPHALOPATHY

Acute Management of Cardiac Arrest

The clinical goals for pediatric cardiac arrest are effective cardiopulmonary resuscitation (CPR), rapid ROSC, and preven-

tion of secondary injury. Time to initiation and quality of CPR can strongly impact survival and neurologic outcome. Community education in bystander CPR may influence outcome after out-of-hospital arrests (155). Many hospitals have brought this concept to in-hospital cardiac arrest and organized dedicated rapid-response teams (67,145). The AHA provides pediatric advanced life support guidelines (5), with supporting scientific review. Important new recommendations to these guidelines are shown in **Table 59.3**. While cardiopulmonary resuscitation techniques and algorithms have been standardized and supported by agencies such as the AHA, American Academy of Pediatrics, International Liaison Committee on Resuscitation, and others, few randomized, controlled trials have been reported to support these recommendations in children. An exception is the evaluation of high-dose versus standard-dose epinephrine, where no benefit, and perhaps even detriment, of

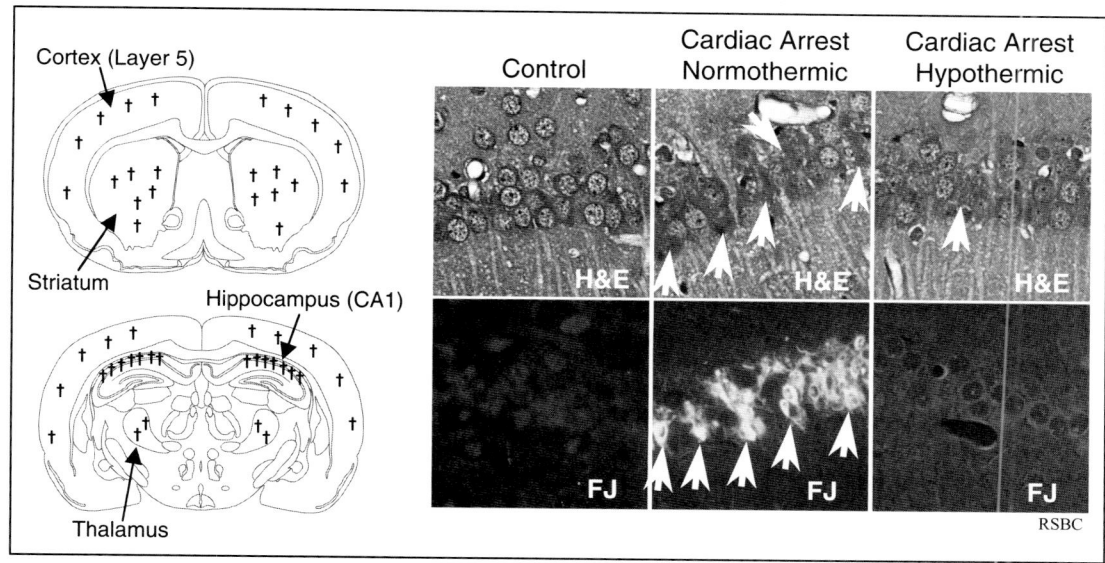

FIGURE 59.5. Selectively vulnerable brain regions after 8–9 mins of cardiac arrest in rats (†). Neurons in the CA1 region of the hippocampus are particularly vulnerable. Dying neurons are identified as condensed cells using hematoxylin and eosin (H&E) staining and using Fluoro-Jade B (FJ), which stains degenerating neurons (*arrows*). Photomicrographs depict coronal brain sections from postnatal day 17 rats after 8 mins of asphyxial cardiac arrest under normothermic (37°C for 1 hr) or hypothermic (32°C for 1 hr) conditions.

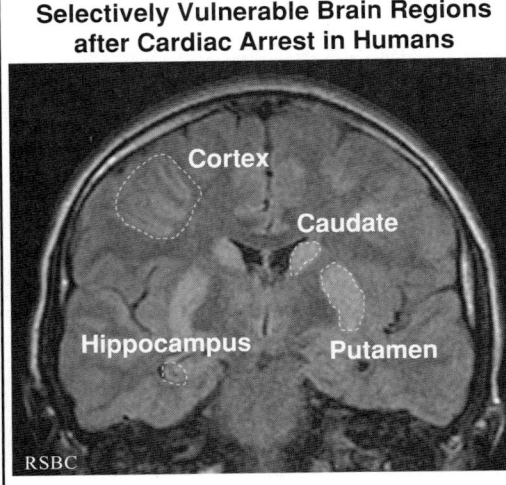

Selectively Vulnerable Brain Regions after Cardiac Arrest in Humans	Structure	Function	Clinical Consequence
	Basal ganglia Putamen Caudate	Motor control, cognition Learning, memory, behavior	Dystonia Impairments in motivation, executive function, attention, memory, chorea & dystonia
	Globus pallidus	Motor control	Akinetic-rigid syndrome, behavior
	Cortex (esp. Layers 3 and 5)	Cognition, learning, attention, consciousness, language/speech, higher-order processing, vision	Coma, persistent vegetative state, seizures, myoclonus, language, and executive impairment
	Watershed areas ACA-MCA MCA-PCA		Brachial diplegia Cortical blindness
	Cerebellum (esp. Purkinje cells)	Balance, gait, cognition	Dysmetria, fine movement disorder
	Hippocampus (esp. CA1 region)	Learning, memory, visual-spatial organization	Seizure, amnesia, memory deficit

FIGURE 59.6. Selectively vulnerable brain regions after cardiac arrest in humans. A T2-flair MRI image from a patient 1 week after asphyxial cardiac arrest due to anaphylaxis, with bilateral enhancement and edema seen in the caudate and putamen, hippocampus, and cerebral cortex. Table describing selectively vulnerable structures, their function, and clinical consequence. ACA, anterior cerebral artery; MCA, middle cerebral artery; PCA, posterior cerebral artery

high-dose versus standard-dose epinephrine has been demonstrated in separate randomized clinical trials in Brazil (112) and the US (111).

A treatment guideline algorithm based on the literature and protocols and practice at the Children's Hospital of Pittsburgh is provided in **Figure 59.7.** Resuscitation begins with airway, breathing, and circulation. Establishment of an open airway for ventilation and oxygenation is especially imperative to the pediatric population, as most arrests in infants and children have an asphyxial etiology, most commonly respiratory failure or shock. Head tilt, chin lift, and jaw thrust are generally sufficient for opening the airway, but jaw thrust is the only recommended maneuver for patients for whom there is concern for cervical spine injury (if trauma is suspected). Positive-pressure ventilation delivered by bag-valve-mask is as effective as intubation in many cases. If an artificial airway is necessary, rapid-sequence intubation technique should be used unless there is suspicion of increased intracranial pressure (ICP), in which case ventilation must be maintained to avoid CO_2 reactivity-associated increases in ICP. Conversely, hyperventilation should also be avoided unless signs and symptoms of brain herniation are present. Special attention should be paid to the prevention of aspiration by employing the Sellick maneuver. Early attention to airway and breathing diverges from adult CPR guidelines, whereby restarting the heart and chest compressions are now the first intervention, given that the nature of adult out-of-hospital cardiac arrest is frequently related to heart disease. Circulation should be addressed immediately during or following noninvasive or invasive attainment of the airway and breathing, with the performance of effectual chest compressions and rapid obtainment of vascular access. In the case of a shockable rhythm, automated external defibrillators are approved for use in children >1 year of age, especially if the unit contains a pediatric adaptor to deliver a smaller dose of energy. Data are insufficient to support their use in children

<1 year of age. Circulatory shock should be treated aggressively following published pediatric shock guidelines (Chapter 26) (33).

Outpatients should be transported to the nearest emergency department for stabilization. Health care providers should perform frequent and serial evaluations to assess cardiorespiratory stability, and attempts should be made to identify the underlying cause of cardiac arrest if not already apparent. After initial stabilization, it is useful to perform a quick neurologic assessment of the patient. At minimum, this should include an examination of pupillary responses and assignment of Glasgow Coma Scale (GCS) score. The GCS was first validated in patients with TBI, with the intention of providing some uniformity in the assignment of severity of injury, and it may provide useful information in the comatose patient after cardiac arrest. Some problems are associated with using the GCS in cardiac arrest patients. The use of sedatives and intubation (also a problem in patients with trauma) after cardiac arrest can hinder GCS interpretation, given that the score is based on a patient's verbal, motor, and eye-opening abilities. In addition, an infant or younger child may not have the ability to understand and follow commands. The motor score was found to be a more sensitive predictor for brain injury severity after trauma than was the full GCS (57), and deserves further study in children after cardiac arrest. Other groups have adapted the GCS for use in infants and children. One example is the Children's Hospital of Philadelphia infant coma scale ("Infant Face Scale"), validated for children <2 years of age (42).

Patients remain at significant risk of secondary brain injury after ROSC from hypotension, hypoxemia, seizures, hypoglycemia, and hyperthermia; therefore, efforts should be made to prevent these conditions or to treat them promptly should they occur. Measurement of blood gas tensions, pH, serum electrolytes, and glucose should be performed if resources are available. It is our opinion that all surviving pediatric patients be

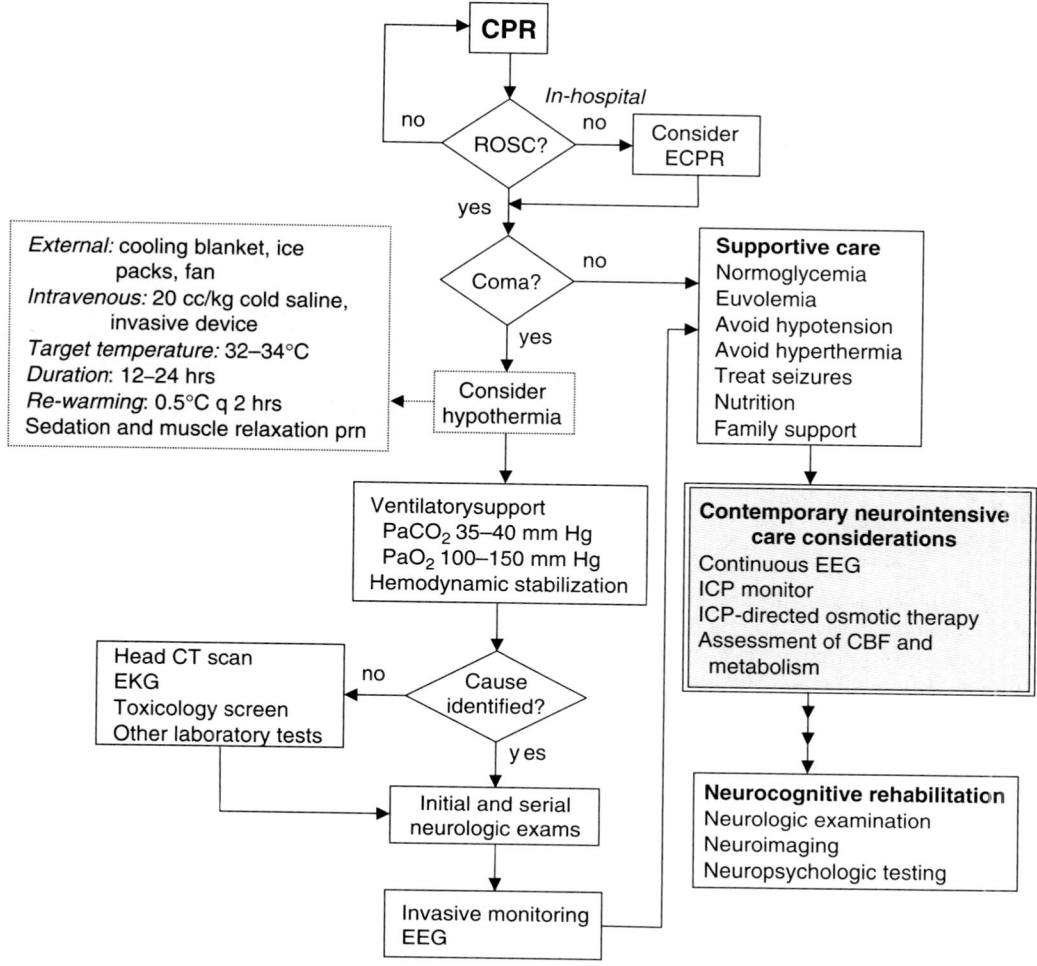

FIGURE 59.7. Algorithm for the management and treatment of post-circulatory arrest syndrome in infants and children. Guidelines based on medical literature and protocols and practice at the Children's Hospital of Pittsburgh. CPR, cardiopulmonary resuscitation; ROSC, return of spontaneous circulation; ECPR, extracorporeal cardiopulmonary resuscitation; EEG, electroencephalogram; ICP, intracranial pressure; CBF, cerebral blood flow; EKG, electrocardiogram

transferred to a tertiary-care center that specializes in the care of infants and children for further evaluation and treatment.

PICU Management

The PICU management of patients after cardiac arrest consists largely of supportive care and prevention of secondary insults. While not proven to be effective, invasive cardiopulmonary monitoring can be useful in the prevention and identification of physiologic instability and in reducing the incidence of or minimizing the effects of secondary insults. Certainly, placement of an arterial catheter for continuous blood pressure measurement and a central venous catheter for central venous pressure measurement and vasoactive drug delivery can be justified in patients who remain in coma after cardiac arrest.

The degree of cerebral edema is variable after cardiac arrest and reperfusion, although it is more common after asphyxial versus VT/VF arrest. It has been noted that patients with respiratory arrest followed by cardiac arrest more frequently had evidence of cerebral edema on CT scan 3 days after presentation

and poorer outcome at 1 week, versus arrhythmia-induced cardiac arrest patients (96). In general, ICP is increased after global ischemia and can be severe enough to cause intracranial hypertension and herniation syndrome if the period of ischemia is prolonged (124). However, monitoring of ICP, once a standard measurement after cardiac arrest, is no longer considered standard practice, largely because (a) case series performed in the 1980s showed that aggressively treating elevated ICP in children after submersion injury increased the number of surviving patients with severe disability and vegetative state (23,27), and (b) increased ICP is often a consequence, rather than the cause, of cerebral ischemia. However, revisiting the use of ICP monitoring, particularly in combination with concurrent monitoring of CBF, cerebral metabolism, and/or evolving neurologic injury, may be warranted.

A head CT scan is frequently the first radiologic test performed in comatose patients after cardiac arrest. CT can be rapidly obtained but may often be normal—including clear differentiation of white matter and gray matter with high fat and water content, respectively—acutely after cardiac arrest. However, findings of cerebral edema, such as loss of cortical gray/white matter density and interface, reversal sign, and/or cerebral swelling, indicate more severe injury and less favorable neurologic outcome (55). An initial CT may be helpful in situations in which the etiology of arrest is unclear or concomitant trauma may exist. Following cardiac arrest, serial head CT scans are indicated only if new or evolving pathology, such as hemorrhage, evolving mass lesion, or herniation, is suspected.

Contemporary Neurointensive Care Monitoring

Cerebral Blood Flow and Estimation of Cerebral Perfusion

Currently, CBF can be measured directly but intermittently using techniques such as stable Xenon CT, positron-emission tomography, or perfusion MRI (119). While these measurements appear to have utility in management of TBI, little has been reported related to the use of these modalities in patients after cardiac arrest, and available reports have focused on the temporal patterns of CBF and relationship to outcome rather than on the use of CBF measurements to guide clinical management. Surrogate measures reflecting CBF in humans, particularly those allowing continuous measurement, have been evaluated. Transcranial Doppler ultrasonography is a noninvasive, bedside method for estimating CBF and may be used to extrapolate effects of cerebral edema and ICP on CBF velocity (87,125). Transcranial Doppler measures middle cerebral artery blood flow velocity as a surrogate for CBF but does not provide a direct measurement. Another disadvantage of this method is that it provides no information about regional heterogeneity of CBF after cardiac arrest.

Cerebral Metabolic and Brain Activity Monitoring

Brain oxygenation can be measured using near infrared spectroscopy (NIRS), and can be used to noninvasively and continuously estimate cerebral oxygen extraction. Current disadvantages of NIRS include limited depth of penetration, which limits interrogation to millimeters beneath the brain surface; global rather than regional information; and lack of definitions of target and critical values. However, theoretically, NIRS measurement of continuous oxygen saturation on the brain surface can provide relative real-time alterations in brain oxygenation, which can be useful in terms of titration of therapies. NIRS performed in the first 48 hrs after neonatal asphyxia has been shown to be useful in predicting outcome at 3 months (148). Brain oxygenation can also be determined invasively using a fiberoptic catheter placed into brain parenchyma to measure brain tissue oxygen partial pressure ($Pbto_2$). While the utility of $Pbto_2$ is currently being studied in patients with TBI, its use in patients after cardiac arrest remains investigational.

Global cerebral metabolism can also be measured directly if a jugular bulb catheter is placed and CBF is measured simultaneously. Cross-brain extraction of oxygen—the arteriovenous difference of oxygen content ($AVDo_2$)—and glucose—arteriovenous difference of glucose ($AVD_{glucose}$)—can be used to calculate $CMRo_2$ and CMR_{Glu}, respectively. Examining jugular venous bulb oxygen saturation ($Sjvo_2$) as a reflection of cerebral metabolism also has potential utility, particularly if direct CBF measurements are not available and given that arterial oxygen saturations are typically at or near 100%. $Sjvo_2$ level is frequently employed to monitor patients with TBI, with normal values reported to be 55%–71% and values <50% considered the critical threshold for brain ischemia. Central venous saturation from the superior vena cava may not be a suitable substitute for $Sjvo_2$; the $Sjvo_2$ level was reported to be 10% lower than mixed venous saturation within 6 hrs after cardiac arrest and was later higher than the mixed venous saturation in nonsurvivors (31). Like $Pbto_2$ monitoring, $Sjvo_2$ monitoring in patients after cardiac arrest remains investigational.

An electroencephalogram (EEG) represents a real-time summation of an electrical signal, from a pool of spatially related neurons, that is displayed in 8 or 16 (or more) channels. EEG is a noninvasive bedside method increasingly being used after HIE to diagnose and monitor response to treatment of nonclinical seizures. The actual incidence of seizures in infants and children after cardiac arrest is unknown but is as high as 30% in adults after cardiac arrest. A newer indication is continuous monitoring during periods of muscle relaxation, especially during the induction of hypothermia, which is increasingly being used for post-resuscitation therapy in cardiac arrest patients (151). EEG, alone or in combination with other methods, has been used to predict outcome after pediatric cardiac arrest (91). Presence of a discontinuous EEG and epileptiform spikes or discharges correlated with poor outcome. Somatosensory-evoked potentials (SEPs) use electrical stimulation of peripheral nerves and record the response of somatosensory pathways. Absence of SEPs may be more sensitive and specific in predicting unfavorable outcome after cardiac arrest (91).

Cerebral microdialysis uses intermittent or continuous sampling of extracellular fluid to measure changes in brain chemistry and is based on the diffusion of small, water-soluble substances through a semipermeable membrane. It is invasive and involves insertion into the brain of a catheter equipped with a dialysis membrane. Molecules that are diffusible below 20,000 daltons and perhaps larger molecules up to 100,000 daltons may be measured, depending on the cutoff size of the semipermeable membrane (62). Concentrations of glucose, lactate, neurotransmitters, drugs, and markers of tissue damage and inflammation can be measured. Currently, cerebral microdialysis is also used as a research tool, and its place as a point-of-care monitor after cardiac arrest remains unclear (59).

Magnetic Resonance Imaging/Spectroscopy

MR imaging provides detailed information about ischemic brain injury, is noninvasive, and does not use ionizing radiation (15,30,142). Diffusion-weighted imaging uses differences in water diffusivity to acutely diagnose ischemia that may not be discernible on T2-weighted images and to describe regions of brain at risk for HIE. The disadvantages of MRI are a relatively longer scanning time compared with CT, the increased need for sedation or muscle relaxant to prevent motion artifact (vs. CT), and the restriction of metal objects (e.g., EEG leads). A scoring system, validated in infants, that combines MRI with neurologic examination has been used to predict outcome in HIE late after initial injury (53). MRI coupled with arterial spin labeling can be used to trace arterial and venous blood supply to the brain and quantify CBF and cerebral blood volume.

Brain MR spectroscopy (MRS) has been used experimentally to demonstrate the relationship of metabolites such as lactate, pyruvate, glutamate, N-acetylaspartate, and phosphocreatine to outcome in patients with HIE. Elevated lactate and decreased N-acetylaspartate are associated with worse neurologic outcome in neonates with asphyxial injury (10,76). Increased lactate may persist up to 1 week after asphyxial injury (11). Currently, both MRI and MRS are used primarily for outcome prediction and not minute-to-minute PICU management.

Biomarkers

No single clinical, laboratory, or imaging test exists to detect occult or evolving brain injury or to predict neurologic outcome with certainty after cardiac arrest in children (or adults). Serum and urine biomarkers are surrogates of brain injury that present a promising approach to these problems (**Fig. 59.8**). Ideal serum or urine biomarkers would be uniquely found in the brain, proportional to the degree of damage, and readily detectable in a point-of-care fashion. Most work has focused on neuron serum enolase (NSE, a glycolytic protein from neurons and neuroectodermal cells), S-100b (a calcium-regulated protein released by injured astrocytes to modulate differentiation of neurons and glia), and/or myelin basic protein (69). Serial cerebrospinal fluid sampling is an impracticable and possibly unsafe procedure for most patients with cardiac arrest, given the conceivable presence of cerebral edema and increased ICP. Serum NSE is felt to be a sensitive and specific indicator of neuronal injury when measured up to 72 hrs after cardiac arrest (48,127). Treatment with mild, induced hypothermia suppressed NSE concentration compared with normothermia, which was then associated with improved outcome after cardiac arrest in adult patients (144). Decreased NSE levels were postulated to be due to the neuroprotective effects of hypother-

mia and may be useful as a marker for future clinical trials. S100b may have neuroprotective characteristics at low concentrations but is associated with astroglial cell death at higher concentrations in animal models (85). Higher serum levels of S100b at 24 hrs after cardiac arrest are associated with death or poorer neurologic outcome (137). Higher glucose concentrations in the first 24 hrs after cardiac arrest were found to be an independent marker of poor outcome in one adult cardiac arrest study (101). Levels of NSE, S100B, and myelin basic protein in serum were studied after HIE in infants and children. HIE was defined as use of either rescue breaths or chest compressions. NSE was increased and showed a delayed peak over a period of days after the insult in many patients, suggesting the occurrence of delayed neuronal death. In contrast, S100B was increased only early after the insult, consistent with the fact that delayed astrocyte death has not been reported. Myelin basic protein was not increased, suggesting a limited role for axonal injury after asphyxia or asphyxial cardiac arrest (18).

Perhaps combining a panel of clinical findings with biomarkers will provide a more powerful early prediction of long-term neurologic outcome. A combination of GCS score, NSE, and S100b should predict vegetative state or death in adults after cardiac arrest with 100% specificity (113). Another study found increased predictability for poor neurologic outcome when serum NSE levels were combined with SEPs (93). Novel potential serum biomarkers are also under investigation for their ability to predict outcome after cardiac arrest. For example, procalcitonin, the precursor for the hormone calcitonin, predicts survival but not neurologic outcome in adults after cardiac arrest (49). Inflammatory markers such as IL-8 are also increased after adult cardiac arrest but are not predictive of outcome (102). Many other biomarkers and biomediators have been found to be increased after TBI; this finding may be relevant to HIE as well (72).

Therapies That Target the Prevention and Treatment of Hypoxic-Ischemic Encephalopathy

Therapeutic Hypothermia

Mild, induced hypothermia has come to the forefront as a promising strategy for improving survival and neurologic outcome after cardiac arrest in adult patients, but the benefits in pediatric patients remain to be determined. In a pediatric model of asphyxial arrest in rats, brief (1-hr) application of mild hypothermia resulted in improved neuronal survival versus normothermia assessed at 5 weeks after injury (45) (**Fig. 59.5**). Mechanisms of action for hypothermia include reduced levels of brain metabolic needs, excitotoxicity, oxidative stress, and inflammation. The AHA now endorses this therapy for comatose adult patients with VF/VT-induced cardiac arrest after two multicentered, randomized, controlled studies demonstrated its efficacy (3,22). Whole-body hypothermia or selective head cooling is now also endorsed in the neonatal population for reduction of morbidity and mortality after birth asphyxia (52,128). Whole-body cooling may be the more effective modality, given that deeper brain structures are cooled as well as superficial brain structures, and selective head cooling may not be as effective outside the neonatal period. Extrapolating

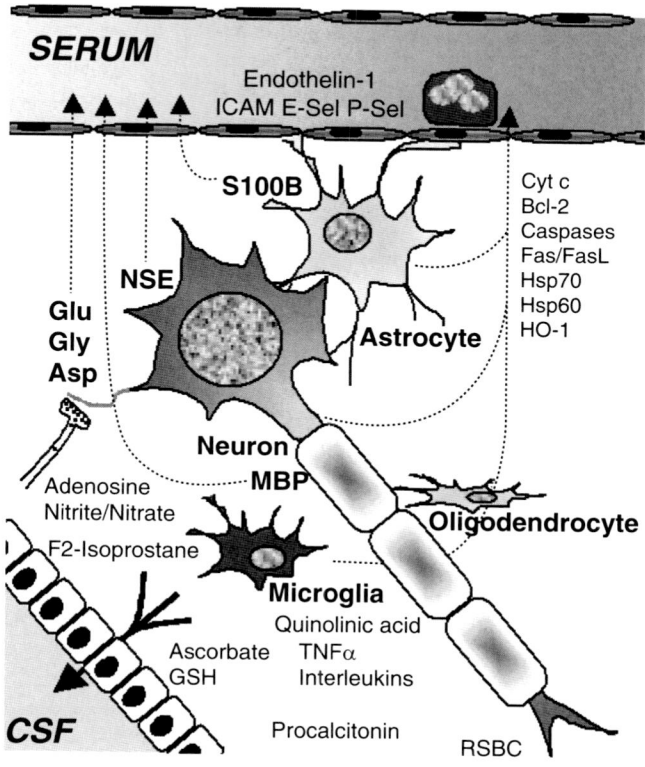

FIGURE 59.8. Potential biomarkers and biomediators for identifying and following brain injury, validating mechanisms of injury, and serving as targets for therapeutic drug monitoring.

from these and an abundance of experimental studies that showed the efficacy of induced hypothermia with a good safety profile, the AHA recommends considering induced hypothermia (32–34°C for 12–24 hrs) for comatose pediatric patients after cardiac arrest as a type IIb recommendation (**Table 59.4**) (4). During induction of hypothermia, particular attention should be paid to electrolyte abnormalities, volume status, shivering, coagulopathy, dysrhythmias, and effects on drug metabolism (60). Previous concerns about the potential adverse effects of hypothermia on successful defibrillation/cardioversion appear unfounded, as a recent laboratory study has shown that hypothermia increased the likelihood of successful cardioversion, compared with normothermic arrest (26). Based on experimental studies, hypothermia is most effective when initiated as early as possible. The multicentered clinical studies cited show that hypothermia is effective even when applied up to 6 hrs after cardiac arrest. These studies used a range of duration of hypothermia (12–72 hrs), time to rewarming (12–24 hrs), and temperature (32–34°C). Pilot studies that used iced saline to more rapidly achieve target temperature in adults after cardiac arrest suggested that it is effective, feasible, and without obvious adverse effects (21). Further study is necessary to define optimal timing, duration, degree of cooling, and rewarming intervals, and to demonstrate that patients stand to benefit from hypothermia.

Cutting-edge Strategies

Certain centers with the capability to provide extracorporeal membrane oxygenation are now applying it as a rescue therapy for in-hospital pediatric cardiac arrest or imminent cardiac arrest (called extracorporeal cardiopulmonary resuscitation, or ECPR) and for patients with impending heart failure post-cardiac surgery (97). ECPR reestablishes cardiac output, allows for heart-lung rest, and can be combined with hypothermia, as bypass enables rapid cooling and temperature control and alleviates concern for the arrhythmogenicity or myocardial depression of hypothermia. ECPR can be implemented during active CPR, although it requires significant resources and highly skilled personnel (97). One in-patient case series showed that good neurologic outcome was possible even with prolonged resuscitation and that the survival rate was higher in patients with isolated cardiac disease (97). It is likely that ECPR can be effective in select patients (92).

Other "cutting-edge" strategies to improve outcomes after prolonged cardiac arrest are currently under investigation. These include high-volume, continuous, venovenous hemofiltration, which improved neurologic outcome in a small, nonrandomized trial in adults after cardiac arrest (80). Thrombolytics, one of the only proven treatments for stroke, has a narrow therapeutic time window but may be useful during CPR in patients with cardiac arrest from myocardial infarction or pulmonary embolus (6). Coenzyme Q used with mild, induced hypothermia reduces mortality, versus hypothermia alone, after cardiac arrest in a pilot study (14). An examination of secondary outcomes of a large clinical trial showed that bicarbonate given during resuscitation in adults in cardiac arrest increased the likelihood of obtaining ROSC and improved long-term outcome, but treatment was not randomized (14). Failed clinical trials include magnesium with and without diazepam, calcium channel blockers, barbiturates, and corticosteroids (1,2,64,90).

Cognitive Rehabilitation

Experimentally, environmental enrichment and exercise have been shown to improve cognitive outcome in animal models of brain ischemia. Literature is scant on the effect of rehabilitation on pediatric neurocognitive outcome. Environmental enrichment increases the amount of dendritic branching and synapses (65) and may enhance neurogenesis (71). Because synaptogenesis occurs throughout childhood (peaking around 4 years of age) (118), rehabilitation could make a significant impact, particularly in younger children with mild-to-moderate disability. Treatment in the form of therapies that help with muscle tone and control, oral muscle development, and vision (in the case of cortical vision impairment) are simple but can make a significant impact on the patient's quality of life.

Outcome

Deaths after ROSC are most often due to brain death, multiorgan system failure, or withdrawal of support when the decision is based primarily on projected neurologic outcome. Patients who survive develop HIE and can have single or multiple neurologic disabilities of varying severity that evolve after the insult. Common manifestations of HIE include cerebral palsy, mental retardation, dysphagia, cortical vision impairment or blindness, hearing impairment or deafness, microcephaly, temperature instability, chronic lung disease, and seizures. Infants after hypoxic-ischemic injury may not demonstrate the clinical neurologic impairments of HIE until later in life, when developmental milestones are not met; therefore, this population deserves long developmental screening. Outcome after cardiac arrest is poor regardless of age. Of the children who attain ROSC, prediction of survival and neurologic outcomes after cardiac arrest is difficult at best. However, patient care or end-of-life decisions necessitate the delivery of timely and reliable information for clinicians and families; unfortunately, these data do not exist.

The Glasgow Outcome Scale was created in 1975 to assign outcome in patients after brain injury in a simplified fashion (143). Essentially, on this scale, 1 = dead, 2 = vegetative, 3 = severe disability, 4 = moderate disability, and 5 = normal. The Glasgow Outcome Scale provides a gross estimate of the degree of disability in patients after brain injury, but it is not designed to discern specific neurologic diagnoses, although it is often used to assess therapeutic efficacy in clinical trials (120). The King's Outcome Scale for Childhood Head Injury (KOSCHI) has been validated as a more sensitive method of classifying outcome in pediatric patients with TBI (38). This scale focuses on mild disabilities, which are difficult to detect in children during development. Because brain injury after cardiac arrest takes time to evolve, repair, and stabilize, the best time or times to assess outcome remain unclear.

Data are available from large studies on survival rates and the ability of clinical, radiologic, and/or other testing to predict poor neurologic outcome (**Table 59.1**). Outpatient survival rate to hospital discharge for children after cardiac arrest is poor at ~9%, with two-thirds of the survivors having neurologic impairment (157). Over half of patients are <1 year of age, with half of these being newly born and having the best survival rate (36%). Males comprise ~60% of pediatric cardiac arrest patients and survival rates are equal between genders. The use of three or more doses of epinephrine or a resuscitation duration >30 mins is associated with poor neurologic outcome in survivors (157). Patients with witnessed cardiac arrest have better outcomes than those with unwitnessed cardiac arrest, but prehospital CPR may not make a difference in overall survival rate. Based on data from the National Registry of CPR, survival rate to hospital discharge was higher for inpatient pediatric cardiac arrest patients (27%) versus out-of-hospital arrest patients (8%), with 65% of those survivors having good neurologic outcome. In that study, the mean time to initiation of CPR was <1 min and was provided by trained health care personnel (103).

In a study of patients who had cardiac arrests within a PICU, a hospital discharge rate of 13.7% was reported. For CPR durations of <15 mins, 15–30 mins, and >30 mins, the survival rates were 19%, 12%, and 6%, respectively. Only 2 of 35 patients who had a cardiac arrest prior to their PICU cardiac arrest survived to discharge. Severity of illness, as measured by the Pediatric Risk of Mortality III score, was found to be a significant predictor of survival (134). Another study of cardiac arrest in PICU patients had a similar hospital discharge rate to that previously reported for inpatient pediatric cardiac arrest and found that preexisting renal failure and requirement for epinephrine predicted poor outcome (40). One pediatric cardiac ICU reported successful CPR in 63% (24/38) of patients, with 20 having ROSC and 4 placed on mechanical cardiopulmonary support. All 4 of the mechanically supported patients and 10 ROSC patients survived to hospital discharge, and 11 remained alive at 6 months, 3 with neurologic impairment (110). A case series using ECPR showed that it has utility for in-hospital cardiac arrest and that implementation can take place during CPR, with surprisingly positive outcomes. Although patients had prolonged resuscitation times, good neurologic outcome was still possible, and survival was better in patients with isolated cardiac disease (97). A recent study in adults showed that clinical exam findings (absent corneal reflexes, pupillary response, withdrawal response to pain, and motor response) at 24 hrs after cardiac arrest can strongly predict death or poor neurologic outcome (28). A large systematic review supports this viewpoint, finding that pupillary light response, corneal reflexes, motor responses to pain, myoclonus, status epilepticus, serum NSE, and SEP studies assist in predicting outcome in adults after cardiac arrest (154). Additional data are necessary to address this issue in infants and children.

EMERGING THERAPIES

The first steps in improving outcome from cardiac arrest involve prevention of HIE and include optimizing CPR and developing tailored practice parameters for the PICU management of blood pressure, temperature, PaO_2 and $PaCO_2$, serum glucose, serum osmolality, and nutrition. Development of contemporary neurointensive care monitoring, with the identification of treatment goals and thresholds, is similarly imperative. Tailoring treatments based on the etiology of the insult, age and gender of the patient and, ultimately, genotype, is also vital and on the horizon. Optimization of hypothermia and when and when not to use ECPR also warrant further clinical evaluation, as do the development of several emerging therapies, some of which are discussed below and shown temporally in **Figure 59.9.**

Reestablishment and Maintenance of Cerebral Blood Flow

It is well recognized that hypotension after ROSC can worsen cerebral ischemia. Studies assessing strategies to improve perfusion abnormalities after resuscitation from cardiac arrest have focused on the postischemic hypoperfusion phase. The mechanism of postischemic hypoperfusion is not well understood, but it is postulated to be the result of vasospasm, tissue edema, and cell aggregation. Hemodilution (hematocrit to 25%) and hypertension in the immediate postresuscitation period can improve postischemic CBF and survival in animal models (81,124).

Pharmacologic agents for CBF promotion shown to be beneficial in animal studies include endothelin A antagonists, remifentanil, nitrous oxide, and nitric oxide donors. Studies in humans that assess improvement in neurologic function after treatment with these agents are lacking. The endothelin A receptor antagonist BQ485, administered shortly after ROSC, improves CBF, functional activity, and neurologic outcome after cardiac arrest in rats (75). Nitrous oxide and remifentanil are cerebral vasodilators and increase regional CBF when used as anesthetics in healthy volunteers (77,86). Nitrous oxide increases CBF preferentially in the gray matter, whereas remifentanil has a more pronounced effect in the basal ganglia and subcortical structures. Anesthesia with remifentanil and/or nitrous oxide could increase CBF and perhaps be beneficial after cardiac arrest. Administration of the nitric oxide donor DE-TANONOate has also been shown to reduce neurologic injury following hypoxia-ischemia in the newborn rat (153).

Antiexcitotoxic Strategies

Many antiexcitotoxic therapies have been tried in patients after cerebral ischemia. This is a logical treatment, given the pivotal influence of excitatory amino acid-induced neurotoxicity in the evolution of HIE (**Fig. 59.1**). Hypothermia, shown to be protective after adult VT/VF cardiac arrest and neonatal asphyxia, is thought to exert its effects, at least in part, by reducing excitotoxicity and cerebral metabolism. In contrast, pharmacologic, antiexcitotoxic strategies have not shown benefit in preventing or reducing HIE. Pentobarbital given after VF in a cat model decreased the frequency of seizures, but no overall difference in mortality or neurologic outcome was observed (147). Thiopental given after global ischemia in monkeys also showed no difference in neurologic outcome or mortality, and many animals that received thiopental had cardiac arrhythmias (51). However, barbiturates combined with halothane anesthesia improved neurologic outcome and reduced infarct size in a dog model of focal ischemia (135). A randomized clinical trial of thiopental has been performed, The Brain Resuscitation Clinical Trial I Study Group. This study of 262 adult comatose survivors of cardiac arrest that used otherwise identical postresuscitation protocols showed no difference in mortality in patients who received thiopental compared with controls, although patients receiving thiopental had double the incidence of hypotension (1). Novel antiexcitotoxic agents, including those targeting N-methyl-D-aspartate (NMDA) and α-amino-3-hydroxy-5-methyl-4-isoxazoleproprionic acid (AMPA) receptors, shown to be beneficial in animal models, have also

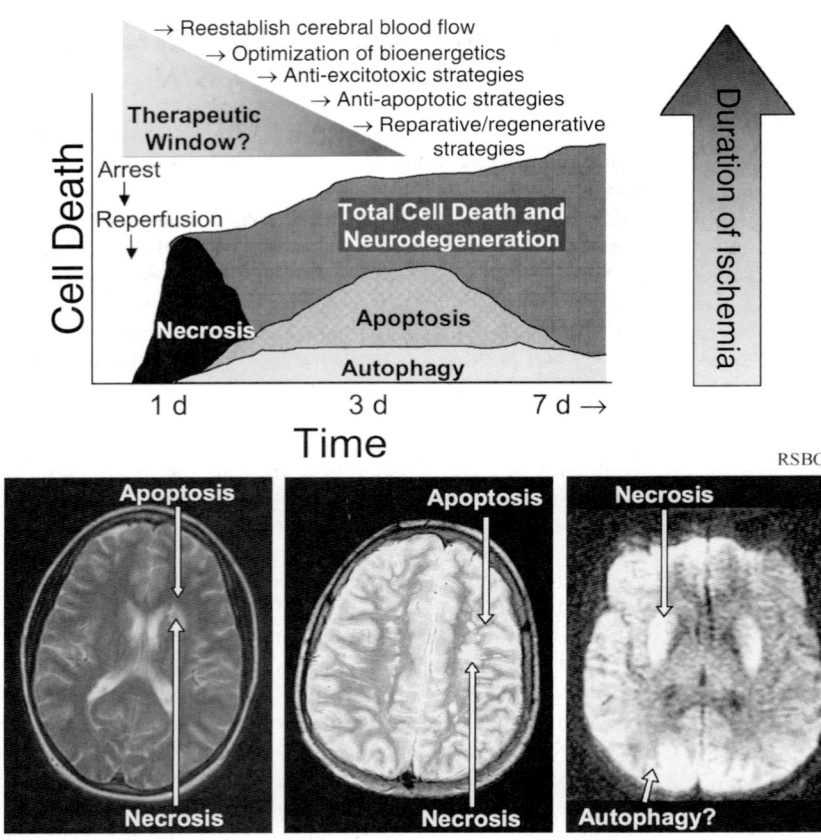

FIGURE 59.9. Futuristic treatment strategies targeting cell-death pathways (apoptosis, necrosis, and/or autophagy) that produce hypoxic-ischemic encephalopathy. The therapeutic windows for these novel strategies are likely temporally and regionally dependent.

failed in clinical trials. Many have not only shown lack of benefit, but also undesirable side effects (98).

Optimization of Bioenergetics and Preventing Energy Failure

Energy stores and fuel preferences evolve during development and differ between neurons, astrocytes, and other cell types. One study demonstrated that glycogen stores were decreased in the cerebral cortex of postnatal day 7 rats compared with adult rats and that, unlike adult rats, rat pups demonstrated a greater reliance on ketone bodies for energy, correlating with their high-fat milk diet (89). Not surprisingly then, enzymes involved with ketone metabolism are at maximal levels at preweaning and decrease by 50% afterward, and glycolytic enzymes reach adult levels after weaning, when the diet switches from high fat to primarily carbohydrates (36). A key enzyme in nonoxidative acetyl CoA metabolism, pyruvate dehydrogenase, matures during the weaning period, and its role in nonoxidative acetyl CoA can be inhibited by ketone and medium-chain fatty acid elements (78,122). The ability to metabolize fatty acids matures in parallel with glycolysis (116).

Cerebral metabolism is altered during brain ischemia. Within seconds of cessation of CBF, loss of consciousness and electrocerebral silence occur; ATP is depleted within 5 mins, and lactate is produced as cells switch to anaerobic respiration to preserve energy stores (131). Repletion of energy substrates and oxidative metabolism after ROSC may restore function to vulnerable but irreversibly injured cells. After reperfusion, selectively vulnerable neurons may have a second wave of ATP depletion at 24 hrs in the striatum and 48 hrs in the hippocampus that coincides with cell death mainly by apoptosis (114), possibly representing a window of opportunity in which optimizing energy balance and restoring energy supply may be effective in reducing brain damage.

The administration of ketones has shown promise in preventing energy failure and lactic acidosis after global ischemia in juvenile mice (141). Fats are converted to the ketone bodies β-hydroxybutyrate, acetoacetate, and acetone, which cross the blood-brain barrier via monocarboxylic transporters. In a rat model of forebrain ischemia, treatment with ketone bodies decreased neuronal damage if the duration of ischemia was 10 mins—but not 15 mins (132). Ketogenic diets (composed of 80%–90% fat) have also been tested in different models of brain injury (50,158).

Antiapoptotic Strategies

Developing neurons may be at higher risk of apoptotic cell death after brain injury, as demonstrated by their increased sensitivity to irradiation (129). Relative to adult rats, neonatal rats show increased apoptosis-inducing factor, caspase-3, and cytochrome c release from mitochondria after hypoxia-ischemia (159). In other words, the developing brain appears more primed for apoptosis after injury than does with the mature brain. Thus, antiapoptotic strategies may be more effective in infants and children than in adults. In a model of neonatal hypoxia-ischemia, systemic injection of a pan-caspase inhibitor decreased infarction size in the striatum, hippocampus, and cortex, versus vehicle treatment (35). Combining hypothermia (29°C) and intraventricular administration of a caspase inhibitor can also reduce histopathologic damage, versus control groups (7). Interestingly, the degree of apoptosis after cerebral ischemia may be gender dependent. Female rats treated with a caspase inhibitor after neonatal hypoxia-ischemia had smaller stroke volumes, whereas treatment was not effective in their male counterparts (117). This finding is consistent with both cell-culture (41) and clinical studies (126), suggesting that gender may play a prominent role in apoptosis and, therefore, response to antiapoptotic treatments after brain injury in the developing brain.

Regeneration and Repair

As outlined in Chapter 51, the third trimester of human gestation through toddler age is a time of explosive brain growth and development through neurogenesis, dendrite and synapse formation, axon lengthening, and myelination (74). The developing brain is more vulnerable to excitotoxicity and is biased toward programmed cell death, as the brain is avidly pruning synapses and creating memories. The adolescent brain continues to undergo modulation of cognitive function and anatomy (61,88). Studies in children have demonstrated superior adaptive plasticity (66), as seen in their ability to recover from epilepsy brain resection (25), ability learn multiple languages, and increased potential for gains in function with targeted rehabilitation compared with adults. Experimental models have been developed to mimic appropriate developmental age and clinically relevant scenarios (44,152). The juvenile mouse brain has been postulated to have more potential for neurogenesis than the neonatal brain after hypoxia-ischemia, implying that the neonatal mouse is already at maximal capacity for regeneration at baseline (115). Consequently, the young brain may be at greater risk of injury yet also have a greater potential for regeneration and repair (58).

Neurogenesis has been shown to occur postnatally in the dentate gyrus of the hippocampus and subventricular zones, peaking in the neonatal period (82,109). Stem cell proliferation and migration has been documented after hypoxia-ischemia in neonatal rats and mice in vivo (16), but neuronal phenotypes have limited survival compared to supporting cells. Neural stem cells reproduce throughout life, but their ability to replicate, migrate, and survive in areas of injury declines with age. In addition, the gradual changing of the cellular environment that occurs with aging does not favor regeneration. Cellular transplants and growth factor replacement remain potential adjuvant therapies after hypoxic-ischemic injury and require investigation. Agents such as erythropoietin are currently in clinical trials in TBI in adults. Finally, the disadvantages of these therapies are just beginning to become illuminated. For instance, abnormal axonal migration may cause seizures and promote the growth of tumors (82). Given that global cerebral ischemia causes extensive and diverse cellular injury in the brain, these therapies may not be tenable, although they may prove to be useful in more limited, focal brain injury. Further research is necessary.

CONCLUSIONS AND FUTURE DIRECTIONS

HIE in infants and children results in devastating consequences for the child and family. Certain etiologies are potentially preventable, such as near-drowning and SIDS (Back-to-Sleep program), and prevention strategies should be emphasized. Early recognition and urgent initiation of resuscitative efforts may prevent the development of HIE if ROSC is achieved before the irreversible ischemic threshold is reached. Future postresuscitation therapies and PICU management for pediatric patients at risk for developing HIE should target outcomes with both increased survival and improved quality of life in mind.

KEY POINTS

- HIE can be a consequence of multiple and diverse etiologies; the most common encountered in pediatric critical care include cardiac arrest, severe shock, and stroke. Cardiac arrest is primarily due to asphyxia in the pediatric-aged group, compared with cardiac arrhythmia in the adults.
- Characteristic CBF patterns that occur after cardiac arrest and reperfusion include the no reflow, hyperemic, delayed hypoperfusion, and recovery phases. The depth and duration of delayed hypoperfusion correlates with the duration of ischemia.
- Brain regions that are selectively vulnerable to HIE include the CA1 region of the hippocampus, cortical layers 3 and 5, basal ganglia, and cerebellar Purkinje cells.
- Following cardiac arrest, poor outcomes, defined as death or severe neurologic disability, are disappointingly high.
- Therapeutic hypothermia prevents HIE after VT/VF cardiac arrest in adults and birth asphyxia in neonates, but its efficacy after asphyxial cardiac arrest in infants and children remains to be proven.

ACKNOWLEDGMENTS

We appreciate generous support from the National Institutes of Health (K12 HD047349 ELF; T32 HD040686 MDM; NS38620, HD04568, and NS30318 RSBC) and the Laerdal Foundation.

References

1. Randomized clinical study of thiopental loading in comatose survivors of cardiac arrest. Brain Resuscitation Clinical Trial I Study Group. *N Engl J Med* 1986;314:397–403.
2. A randomized clinical study of a calcium-entry blocker (lidoflazine) in the treatment of comatose survivors of cardiac arrest. Brain Resuscitation Clinical Trial II Study Group. *N Engl J Med* 1991;324:1225–31.
3. Mild therapeutic hypothermia to improve the neurologic outcome after cardiac arrest. *N Engl J Med* 2002;346:549–56.
4. The International Liaison Committee on Resuscitation (ILCOR) Consensus on Science with Treatment Recommendations for Pediatric and Neonatal Patients: Pediatric basic and advanced life support. *Pediatrics* 2006;117:e955–77.
5. 2005 American Heart Association (AHA) guidelines for cardiopulmonary resuscitation (CPR) and emergency cardiovascular care (ECC) of pediatric and neonatal patients: Pediatric advanced life support. *Pediatrics* 2006;117:e1005–28.

6. Abu-Laban RB, Christenson JM, Innes GD, et al. Tissue plasminogen activator in cardiac arrest with pulseless electrical activity. *N Engl J Med* 2002;346:1522–8.

7. Adachi M, Sohma O, Tsuneishi S, et al. Combination effect of systemic hypothermia and caspase inhibitor administration against hypoxic-ischemic brain damage in neonatal rats. *Pediatr Res* 2001;50:590–5.

8. Ames A, 3rd, Wright RL, Kowada M, et al. Cerebral ischemia. II. The no-reflow phenomenon. *Am J Pathol* 1968;52:437–53.

9. Ashwal S, Schneider S, Thompson J. Xenon computed tomography measuring cerebral blood flow in the determination of brain death in children. *Ann Neurol* 1989;25:539–546.

10. Ashwal S, Holshouser BA, Tomasi LG, et al. 1H-magnetic resonance spectroscopy-determined cerebral lactate and poor neurological outcomes in children with central nervous system disease. *Ann Neurol* 1997;41:470–81.

11. Auld KL, Ashwal S, Holshouser BA, et al. Proton magnetic resonance spectroscopy in children with acute central nervous system injury. *Pediatr Neurol* 1995;12:323–34.

12. Back T, Hemmen T, Schuler OG. Lesion evolution in cerebral ischemia. *J Neurol* 2004;251:388–97.

13. Balan IS, Fiskum G, Hazelton J, et al. Oximetry-guided reoxygenation improves neurological outcome after experimental cardiac arrest. *Stroke* 2006;37:3008–13.

14. Bar-Joseph G, Abramson NS, Kelsey SF, et al. Improved resuscitation outcome in emergency medical systems with increased usage of sodium bicarbonate during cardiopulmonary resuscitation. *Acta Anaesthesiol Scand* 2005;49:6–15.

15. Barber PA, Darby DG, Desmond PM, et al. Identification of major ischemic change. Diffusion-weighted imaging versus computed tomography. *Stroke* 1999;30:2059–65.

16. Bartley J, Soltau T, Wimborne H, et al. BrdU-positive cells in the neonatal mouse hippocampus following hypoxic-ischemic brain injury. *BMC Neurosci* 2005;6:15.

17. Beckstead JE, Tweed WA, Lee J, et al. Cerebral blood flow and metabolism in man following cardiac arrest. *Stroke* 1978; 9:569–73.

18. Berger RP, Adelson PD, Richichi R, et al. Serum biomarkers after traumatic and hypoxemic brain injuries: Insight into the biochemical response of the pediatric brain to inflicted brain injury. *Dev Neurosci* 2006;28:327–35.

19. Berger S, Utech L, Hazinski MF. Sudden death in children and adolescents. *Pediatr Clin North Am* 2004;51:1653–77.

20. Bergsneider M, Hovda DA, Shalmon E, et al. Cerebral hyperglycolysis following severe traumatic brain injury in humans: A positron emission tomography study. *J Neurosurg* 1997;86:241–51.

21. Bernard S, Buist M, Monteiro O, et al. Induced hypothermia using large volume, ice-cold intravenous fluid in comatose survivors of out-of-hospital cardiac arrest: A preliminary report. *Resuscitation* 2003;56:9–13.

22. Bernard SA, Gray TW, Buist MD, et al. Treatment of comatose survivors of out-of-hospital cardiac arrest with induced hypothermia. *N Engl J Med* 2002;346:557–63.

23. Biggart MJ, Bohn DJ. Effect of hypothermia and cardiac arrest on outcome of near-drowning accidents in children. *J Pediatr* 1990;117:179–83.

24. Blomqvist P, Wieloch T. Ischemic brain damage in rats following cardiac arrest using a long-term recovery model. *J Cereb Blood Flow Metab* 1985;5:420–31.

25. Boatman D, Freeman J, Vining E, et al. Language recovery after left hemispherectomy in children with late-onset seizures. *Ann Neurol* 1999;46:579–86.

26. Boddicker KA, Zhang Y, Zimmerman MB, et al. Hypothermia improves defibrillation success and resuscitation outcomes from ventricular fibrillation. *Circulation* 2005;111:3195–201.

27. Bohn DJ, Biggar WD, Smith CR, et al. Influence of hypothermia, barbiturate therapy, and intracranial pressure monitoring on morbidity and mortality after near-drowning. *Crit Care Med* 1986;14:529–34.

28. Booth CM, Boone RH, Tomlinson G, et al. Is this patient dead, vegetative, or severely neurologically impaired? Assessing outcome for comatose survivors of cardiac arrest. *JAMA* 2004;291:870–9.

29. Brodersen P. Cerebral blood flow and metabolism in coma following cardiac arrest. *Rev Electroencephalogr Neurophysiol Clin* 1974;4:329–33.

30. Bruce DA. Imaging after head trauma: Why, when and which. *Childs Nerv Syst* 2000;16:755–9.

31. Buunk G, van der Hoeven JG, Meinders AE. Prognostic significance of the difference between mixed venous and jugular bulb oxygen saturation in comatose patients resuscitated from a cardiac arrest. *Resuscitation* 1999;41:257–62.

32. Buunk G, van der Hoeven JG, Meinders AE. Cerebral blood flow after cardiac arrest. *Neth J Med* 2000;57:106–12.

33. Carcillo JA, Fields AI. Clinical practice parameters for hemodynamic support of pediatric and neonatal patients in septic shock. *Crit Care Med* 2002;30:1365–78.

34. Cerchiari EL, Hoel TM, Safar P, et al. Protective effects of combined superoxide dismutase and deferoxamine on recovery of cerebral blood flow and function after cardiac arrest in dogs. *Stroke* 1987;18:869–78.

35. Cheng Y, Deshmukh M, D'Costa A, et al. Caspase inhibitor affords neuroprotection with delayed administration in a rat model of neonatal hypoxic-ischemic brain injury. *J Clin Invest* 1998;101:1992–9.

36. Clark JB, Bates TE, Cullingford T, et al. Development of enzymes of energy metabolism in the neonatal mammalian brain. *Dev Neurosci* 1993;15:174–80.

37. Cohan SL, Mun SK, Petite J, et al. Cerebral blood flow in humans following resuscitation from cardiac arrest. *Stroke* 1989;20:761–5.

38. Crouchman M, Rossiter L, Colaco T, et al. A practical outcome scale for paediatric head injury. *Arch Dis Child* 2001;84:120–4.

39. Davis PG, Tan A, O'Donnell CP, et al. Resuscitation of newborn infants with 100% oxygen or air: A systematic review and meta-analysis. *Lancet* 2004;364:1329–33.

40. de Mos N, van Litsenburg RR, McCrindle B, et al. Pediatric in-intensive-care-unit cardiac arrest: Incidence, survival, and predictive factors. *Crit Care Med* 2006;34:1209–15.

41. Du L, Bayir H, Lai Y, et al. Innate gender-based proclivity in response to cytotoxicity and programmed cell death pathway. *J Biol Chem* 2004;279:38563–70.

42. Durham SR, Clancy RR, Leuthardt E, et al. CHOP Infant Coma Scale ("Infant Face Scale"): A novel coma scale for children less than two years of age. *J Neurotrauma* 2000;17:729–37.

43. Edgren E, Enblad P, Grenvik A, et al. Cerebral blood flow and metabolism after cardiopulmonary resuscitation. A pathophysiologic and prognostic positron emission tomography pilot study. *Resuscitation* 2003;57:161–70.

44. Fink EL, Alexander H, Marco CD, et al. An experimental model of pediatric asphyxial cardiopulmonary arrest in rats. *Pediatr Crit Care Med* 2004;5:139–144.

45. Fink EL, Marco CD, Donovan HA, et al. Brief induced hypothermia improves outcome after asphyxial cardiopulmonary arrest in juvenile rats. *Dev Neurosci* 2005;27:191–9.

46. Fischer M, Hossmann KA. No-reflow after cardiac arrest. *Intensive Care Med* 1995;21:132–41.

47. Fischer M, Bottiger BW, Popov-Cenic S, et al. Thrombolysis using plasminogen activator and heparin reduces cerebral no-reflow after resuscitation from cardiac arrest: An experimental study in the cat. *Intensive Care Med* 1996;22:1214–23.

48. Fogel W, Krieger D, Veith M, et al. Serum neuron-specific enolase as early predictor of outcome after cardiac arrest. *Crit Care Med* 1997;25:1133–8.

49. Fries M, Kunz D, Gressner AM, et al. Procalcitonin serum levels after out-of-hospital cardiac arrest. *Resuscitation* 2003;59:105–9.

50. Gasior M, Rogawski MA, Hartman AL. Neuroprotective and disease-modifying effects of the ketogenic diet. *Behav Pharmacol* 2006;17:431–9.

51. Gisvold SE, Safar P, Hendrickx HH, et al. Thiopental treatment after global brain ischemia in pigtailed monkeys. *Anesthesiology* 1984;60:88–96.

52. Gluckman PD, Wyatt JS, Azzopardi D, et al. Selective head cooling with mild systemic hypothermia after neonatal encephalopathy: Multicentre randomised trial. *Lancet* 2005;365:663–70.

53. Haataja L, Mercuri E, Guzzetta A, et al. Neurologic examination in infants with hypoxic-ischemic encephalopathy at age 9 to 14 months: Use of optimality scores and correlation with magnetic resonance imaging findings. *J Pediatr* 2001;138:332–7.

54. Hachimi-Idrissi S, Corne L, Huyghens L. The effect of mild hypothermia and induced hypertension on long term survival rate and neurological outcome after asphyxial cardiac arrest in rats. *Resuscitation* 2001;49:73–82.

55. Han BK, Towbin RB, De Courten-Myers G, et al. Reversal sign on CT: Effect of anoxic/ischemic cerebral injury in children. *AJR Am J Roentgenol* 1990;154:361–8.

56. Harukuni I, Bhardwaj A. Mechanisms of brain injury after global cerebral ischemia. *Neurol Clin* 2006;24:1–21.

57. Healey C, Osler TM, Rogers FB, et al. Improving the Glasgow Coma Scale score: Motor score alone is a better predictor. *J Trauma* 2003;54:671–8; discussion 678–80.

58. Hickey RW, Painter MJ. Brain injury from cardiac arrest in children. *Neurol Clin* 2006;24:147–58.

59. Hillered L, Persson L. Neurochemical monitoring of the acutely injured human brain. *Scand J Clin Lab Invest Suppl* 1999;229:9–18.

60. Hovland A, Nielsen EW, Kluver J, et al. EEG should be performed during induced hypothermia. *Resuscitation* 2006;68:143–6.

61. Huang H, Zhang J, Wakana S, et al. White and gray matter development in human fetal, newborn and pediatric brains. *Neuroimage* 2006;33:27–38.

62. Hutchinson PJ, O'Connell MT, Nortje J, et al. Cerebral microdialysis methodology–evaluation of 20 kDa and 100 kDa catheters. *Physiol Meas* 2005;26:423–8.

63. Ilves P, Lintrop M, Metsvaht T, et al. Cerebral blood-flow velocities in predicting outcome of asphyxiated newborn infants. *Acta Paediatr* 2004; 93:523–8.

64. Jastremski M, Sutton-Tyrrell K, Vaagenes P, et al. Glucocorticoid treatment does not improve neurological recovery following cardiac arrest. Brain Resuscitation Clinical Trial I Study Group. *JAMA* 1989;262:3427–30.

65. Johansson BB. Functional outcome in rats transferred to an enriched environment 15 days after focal brain ischemia. *Stroke* 1996;27:324–326.

66. Johnston MV. Clinical disorders of brain plasticity. *Brain Dev* 2004;26:73–80.

67. Jones D, Bellomo R, Bates S, et al. Long term effect of a medical emergency team on cardiac arrests in a teaching hospital. *Crit Care* 2005;9:R808–15.

68. Kagstrom E, Smith ML, Siesjo BK. Local cerebral blood flow in the recovery period following complete cerebral ischemia in the rat. *J Cereb Blood Flow Metab* 1983;3:170–82.

69. Kandiah P, Ortega S, Torbey MT. Biomarkers and neuroimaging of brain injury after cardiac arrest. *Semin Neurol* 2006;26:413–21.

70. Kaplan JL, Gao E, De Garavilla L, et al. Adenosine A1 antagonism attenuates atropine-resistant hypoxic bradycardia in rats. *Acad Emerg Med* 2003;10:923–30.

71. Kempermann G, Kuhn HG, Gage FH. More hippocampal neurons in adult mice living in an enriched environment. *Nature* 1997;386:493–5.

72. Kochanek PM, Clark RS, Ruppel RA, et al. Biochemical, cellular, and molecular mechanisms in the evolution of secondary damage after severe traumatic brain injury in infants and children: Lessons learned from the bedside. *Pediatr Crit Care Med* 2000;1:4–19.

73. Kofke WA, Nemoto EM, Hossmann KA, et al. Brain blood flow and metabolism after global ischemia and post-insult thiopental therapy in monkeys. *Stroke* 1979;10:554–60.

74. Krageloh-Mann I. Imaging of early brain injury and cortical plasticity. *Exp Neurol* 2004;190 Suppl 1:S84–90.

75. Krep H, Brinker G, Schwindt W, et al. Endothelin type A-antagonist improves long-term neurological recovery after cardiac arrest in rats. *Crit Care Med* 2000;28:2873–80.

76. L'Abee C, de Vries LS, van der Grond J, et al. Early diffusion-weighted MRI and 1H-magnetic resonance spectroscopy in asphyxiated full-term neonates. *Biol Neonate* 2005;88:306–12.

77. Lagace A, Karsli C, Luginbuehl I, et al. The effect of remifentanil on cerebral blood flow velocity in children anesthetized with propofol. *Paediatric Anaesthesia* 2004;14:861–5.

78. Lai JC. Oxidative metabolism in neuronal and non-neuronal mitochondria. *Can J Physiol Pharmacol* 1992;70 Suppl:S130–7.

79. Lassen NA. The luxury-perfusion syndrome and its possible relation to acute metabolic acidosis localised within the brain. *Lancet* 1966;2:1113–5.

80. Laurent I, Adrie C, Vinsonneau C, et al. High-volume hemofiltration after out-of-hospital cardiac arrest: A randomized study. *J Am Coll Cardiol* 2005;46:432–7.

81. Leonov Y, Sterz F, Safar P, et al. Hypertension with hemodilution prevents multifocal cerebral hypoperfusion after cardiac arrest in dogs. *Stroke* 1992;23:45–53.

82. Lichtenwalner RJ, Parent JM. Adult neurogenesis and the ischemic forebrain. *J Cereb Blood Flow Metab* 2006;26:1–20.

83. Lin SR. Cerebral circulation after cardiac arrest. Angiographic and carbon black perfusion studies. *Radiology* 1975;117:627–32.

84. Liou AK, Clark RS, Henshall DC, et al. To die or not to die for neurons in ischemia, traumatic brain injury, and epilepsy: A review on the stress-activated signaling pathways and apoptotic pathways. *Prog Neurobiol* 2003;69:103–42.

85. Liu L, Li Y, Van Eldik LJ, et al. S100B-induced microglial and neuronal IL-1 expression is mediated by cell type-specific transcription factors. *J Neurochem* 2005;92:546–53.

86. Lorenz IH, Kolbitsch C, Hormann C, et al. The influence of nitrous oxide and remifentanil on cerebral hemodynamics in conscious human volunteers. *Neuroimage* 2002;17:1056–64.

87. Lowe LH, Bulas DI. Transcranial Doppler imaging in children: Sickle cell screening and beyond. *Pediatr Radiol* 2005;35:54–65.

88. Luna B, Thulborn KR, Munoz DP, et al. Maturation of widely distributed brain function subserves cognitive development. *Neuroimage* 2001;13:786–93.

89. Lust WD, Pundik S, Zechel J, et al. Changing metabolic and energy profiles in fetal, neonatal, and adult rat brain. *Metab Brain Dis* 2003;18:195–206.

90. Machado C. Randomized clinical trial of magnesium, diazepam, or both after out-of-hospital cardiac arrest. *Neurology* 2003;60:1868;author reply 1868–9.

91. Mandel R, Martinot A, Delepoulle F, et al. Prediction of outcome after hypoxic-ischemic encephalopathy: A prospective clinical and electrophysiologic study. *J Pediatr* 2002;141:45–50.

92. Massetti M, Tasle M, Le Page O, et al. Back from irreversibility: Extracorporeal life support for prolonged cardiac arrest. *Ann Thorac Surg* 2005;79:178–83.

93. Meynaar IA, Oudemans-van Straaten HM, van der Wetering J, et al. Serum neuron-specific enolase predicts outcome in post-anoxic coma: A prospective cohort study. *Intensive Care Med* 2003;29:189–95.

94. Michenfelder JD, Milde JH. Postischemic canine cerebral blood flow appears to be determined by cerebral metabolic needs. *J Cereb Blood Flow Metab* 1990;10:71–6.

95. Michenfelder JD, Milde JH. The relationship among canine brain temperature, metabolism, and function during hypothermia. *Anesthesiology* 1991;75:130–6.

96. Morimoto Y, Kemmotsu O, Kitami K, et al. Acute brain swelling after out-of-hospital cardiac arrest: Pathogenesis and outcome. *Crit Care Med* 1993;21:104–10.

97. Morris MC, Wernovsky G, Nadkarni VM. Survival outcomes after extracorporeal cardiopulmonary resuscitation instituted during active chest compressions following refractory in-hospital pediatric cardiac arrest. *Pediatr Crit Care Med* 1994;5:440–6.

98. Muir KW, Lees KR. Excitatory amino acid antagonists for acute stroke. *Cochrane Database Syst Rev*:CD001244, 2003.

99. Mujsce DJ, Christensen MA, Vannucci RC. Cerebral blood flow and edema in perinatal hypoxic-ischemic brain damage. *Pediatr Res* 1990;27:450–3.

100. Mullner M, Sterz F, Domanovits H, et al. Systemic and cerebral oxygen extraction after human cardiac arrest. *Eur J Emerg Med* 1996;3:19–24.

101. Mullner M, Sterz F, Domanovits H, et al. The association between blood lactate concentration on admission, duration of cardiac arrest, and functional neurological recovery in patients resuscitated from ventricular fibrillation. *Intensive Care Med* 1997;23:1138–43.

102. Mussack T, Biberthaler P, Kanz KG, et al. Serum S-100B and interleukin-8 as predictive markers for comparative neurologic outcome analysis of patients after cardiac arrest and severe traumatic brain injury. *Crit Care Med* 2002;30:2669–74.

103. Nadkarni VM, Larkin GL, Peberdy MA, et al. First documented rhythm and clinical outcome from in-hospital cardiac arrest among children and adults. *JAMA* 2006;295:50–7.

104. Nakashima K, Todd MM, Warner DS. The relation between cerebral metabolic rate and ischemic depolarization. A comparison of the effects of hypothermia, pentobarbital, and isoflurane. *Anesthesiology* 1995;82:1199–208.

105. Nemoto EM, Bleyaert AL, Stezoski SW, et al. Global brain ischemia: A reproducible monkey model. *Stroke* 1977;8:558–64.

106. Nishizawa H, Kudoh I. Cerebral autoregulation is impaired in patients resuscitated after cardiac arrest. *Acta Anaesthesiol Scand* 1996;40:1149–53.

107. Nogami K, Fujii M, Kato S, et al. Analysis of magnetic resonance imaging (MRI) morphometry and cerebral blood flow in patients with hypoxic-ischemic encephalopathy. *J Clin Neurosci* 2004;11:376–80.

108. Nozari A, Rubertsson S, Gedeborg R, et al. Maximisation of cerebral blood flow during experimental cardiopulmonary resuscitation does not ameliorate post-resuscitation hypoperfusion. *Resuscitation* 1999;40:27–35.

109. Ong J, Plane JM, Parent JM, et al. Hypoxic-ischemic injury stimulates subventricular zone proliferation and neurogenesis in the neonatal rat. *Pediatr Res* 2005;58:600–6.

110. Parra DA, Totapally BR, Zahn E, et al. Outcome of cardiopulmonary resuscitation in a pediatric cardiac intensive care unit. *Crit Care Med* 2000;28:3296–300.

111. Patterson MD, Boenning DA, Klein BL, et al. The use of high-dose epinephrine for patients with out-of-hospital cardiopulmonary arrest refractory to prehospital interventions. *Pediatr Emerg Care* 2005;21:227–37.

112. Perondi MB, Reis AG, Paiva EF, et al. A comparison of high-dose and standard-dose epinephrine in children with cardiac arrest. *N Engl J Med* 2004;350:1722–30.

113. Pfeifer R, Borner A, Krack A, et al. Outcome after cardiac arrest: Predictive values and limitations of the neuroproteins neuron-specific enolase and protein S-100 and the Glasgow Coma Scale. *Resuscitation* 2005;65:49–55.

114. Pulsinelli WA, Duffy TE. Regional energy balance in rat brain after transient forebrain ischemia. *J Neurochem* 1983;40:1500–3.

115. Qiu L, Zhu C, Wang X, et al. Less neurogenesis and inflammation in the immature than in the juvenile brain after cerebral hypoxia-ischemia. *J Cereb Blood Flow Metab*, Aug 2006 [epub ahead of print].

116. Reichmann H, Maltese WA, DeVivo DC. Enzymes of fatty acid beta-oxidation in developing brain. *J Neurochem* 1988;51:339–44.

117. Renolleau S, Fau S, Goyenvalle C, et al. Specific caspase inhibitor Q-VD-OPh prevents neonatal stroke in P7 rat: A role for gender. *J Neurochem* 2007;100:1062–71.

118. Rice D, Barone S, Jr. Critical periods of vulnerability for the developing nervous system: Evidence from humans and animal models. *Environ Health Perspect* 2000;108 Suppl 3:511–33.

119. Robertson CL, Hlatky R, Advanced Bedside Neuromonitoring. In: Fink MP, Abraham E, Vincent JL, et al. *Textbook of Critical Care*. Philadelphia: Elsevier Saunders, 2005:287–94.

120. Robertson CM, Joffe AR, Moore AJ, et al. Neurodevelopmental outcome of young pediatric intensive care survivors of serious brain injury. *Pediatr Crit Care Med* 2002;3:345–50.

121. Rudolf J, Ghaemi M, Ghaemi M, et al. Cerebral glucose metabolism in acute and persistent vegetative state. *J Neurosurg Anesthesiol* 1999;11:17–24.

122. Rust RS. Energy metabolism of developing brain, *Curr Opin Neurol* 1994;7:160–5.

123. Safar P, Stezoski W, Nemoto EM. Amelioration of brain damage after 12 minutes' cardiac arrest in dogs. *Arch Neurol* 1976;33:91–5.

124. Safar P, Xiao F, Radovsky A, et al. Improved cerebral resuscitation from cardiac arrest in dogs with mild hypothermia plus blood flow promotion. *Stroke* 1996;27:105–113.

125. Saliba EM, Laugier J. Doppler assessment of the cerebral circulation in pediatric intensive care. *Crit Care Clin* 1992;8:79–92.

126. Satchell MA, Lai Y, Kochanek PM, et al. Cytochrome c, a biomarker of apoptosis, is increased in cerebrospinal fluid from infants with inflicted brain injury from child abuse. *J Cereb Blood Flow Metab* 2005;25:919–27.

127. Schoerkhuber W, Kittler H, Sterz F, et al. Time course of serum neuron-specific enolase. A predictor of neurological outcome in patients resuscitated from cardiac arrest. *Stroke* 1999;30:1598–603.

128. Shankaran S, Laptook AR, Ehrenkranz RA, et al. Whole-body hypothermia for neonates with hypoxic-ischemic encephalopathy. *N Engl J Med* 2005;353:1574–84.
129. Shirai K, Mizui T, Suzuki Y, et al. Differential effects of x-irradiation on immature and mature hippocampal neurons in vitro. *Neurosci Lett* 2006;399:57–60.
130. Siesjo BK. Cell damage in the brain: A speculative synthesis. *J Cereb Blood Flow Metab* 1981;1:155–85.
131. Siesjo BK, Wieloch T. Cerebral metabolism in ischaemia: Neurochemical basis for therapy. BJA: *Brit J Anaesthesia* 1985;57:47–62.
132. Sims NR, Heward SL. Delayed treatment with 1,3-butanediol reduces loss of CA1 neurons in the hippocampus of rats following brief forebrain ischemia. *Brain Res* 1994;662:216–22.
133. Singh NC, Kochanek PM, Schiding JK, et al. Uncoupled cerebral blood flow and metabolism after severe global ischemia in rats. *J Cereb Blood Flow Metab* 1992;12:802–8.
134. Slonim AD, Patel KM, Ruttimann UE, et al. Cardiopulmonary resuscitation in pediatric intensive care units. *Crit Care Med* 1997;25:1951–5.
135. Smith AL, Hoff JT, Nielsen SL, et al. Barbiturate protection in acute focal cerebral ischemia. *Stroke* 1974;5:1–7.
136. Smith BT, Rea TD, Eisenberg MS. Ventricular fibrillation in pediatric cardiac arrest. *Acad Emerg Med* 2006;13:525–9.
137. Snyder-Ramos SA, Gruhlke T, Bauer H, et al. Cerebral and extracerebral release of protein S100B in cardiac surgical patients. *Anaesthesia* 2004;59:344–9.
138. Snyder JV, Nemoto EM, Carroll RG, et al. Global ischemia in dogs: Intracranial pressures, brain blood flow and metabolism. *Stroke* 1975; 6:21–7.
139. Sterz F, Leonov Y, Safar P, et al. Hypertension with or without hemodilution after cardiac arrest in dogs. *Stroke* 1990;21:1178–84.
140. Sundgreen C, Larsen FS, Herzog TM, et al. Autoregulation of cerebral blood flow in patients resuscitated from cardiac arrest. *Stroke* 2001;32: 128–32.
141. Suzuki M, Suzuki M, Sato K, et al. Effect of beta-hydroxybutyrate, a cerebral function improving agent, on cerebral hypoxia, anoxia and ischemia in mice and rats. *Jpn J Pharmacol* 2001;87:143–50.
142. Taylor SB, Quencer RM, Holzman BH, et al. Central nervous system anoxic-ischemic insult in children due to near-drowning. *Radiology* 1985;156:641–6.
143. Teasdale G, Jennett B. Assessment of coma and impaired consciousness. A practical scale. *Lancet* 1974;2:81–4.
144. Tiainen M, Roine RO, Pettila V, et al. Serum neuron-specific enolase and S-100B protein in cardiac arrest patients treated with hypothermia. *Stroke* 2003;34:2881–6.
145. Tibballs J, Kinney S, Duke T, et al. Reduction of paediatric in-patient cardiac arrest and death with a medical emergency team: Preliminary results. *Arch Dis Child* 2005;90:1148–52.
146. Tisherman SA, Sterz F. Therapeutic Hypothermia. In: Clark RSB, Carcillo JA, eds. *Molecular and Cellular Biology of Critical Care Medicine, Vol. 4.* New York: Springer, 2005.
147. Todd MM, Chadwick HS, Shapiro HM, et al. The neurologic effects of thiopental therapy following experimental cardiac arrest in cats. *Anesthesiology* 1982;57:76–86.
148. Toet MC, Lemmers PM, van Schelven LJ, et al. Cerebral oxygenation and electrical activity after birth asphyxia: Their relation to outcome. *Pediatrics* 2006;117:333–9.
149. Vaagenes P, Safar P, Moossy J, et al. Asphyxiation versus ventricular fibrillation cardiac arrest in dogs. Differences in cerebral resuscitation effects–a preliminary study. *Resuscitation* 1997;35:41–52.
150. Vereczki V, Martin E, Rosenthal RE, et al. Normoxic resuscitation after cardiac arrest protects against hippocampal oxidative stress, metabolic dysfunction, and neuronal death. *J Cereb Blood Flow Metab* 2006;26:821–35.
151. Vespa PM, Nuwer MR, Nenov V, et al. Increased incidence and impact of nonconvulsive and convulsive seizures after traumatic brain injury as detected by continuous electroencephalographic monitoring. *J Neurosurg* 1999;91:750–60.
152. Vexler ZS, Sharp FR, Feuerstein GZ, et al. Translational stroke research in the developing brain. *Pediatr Neurol* 2006;34:459–63.
153. Wainwright MS, Grundhoefer D, Sharma S, et al. A nitric oxide donor reduces brain injury and enhances recovery of cerebral blood flow after hypoxia-ischemia in the newborn rat. *Neurosci Lett* 2007 26;415(2): 124–9.
154. Wijdicks EF, Hijdra A, Young GB, et al. Practice parameter: Prediction of outcome in comatose survivors after cardiopulmonary resuscitation (an evidence-based review). Report of the Quality Standards Subcommittee of the American Academy of Neurology, *Neurology* 2006;67:203–10.
155. Wik L, Steen PA, Bircher NG. Quality of bystander cardiopulmonary resuscitation influences outcome after prehospital cardiac arrest, *Resuscitation* 1994;28:195–203.
156. Young KD, Seidel JS. Pediatric cardiopulmonary resuscitation: A collective review, *Ann Emerg Med* 1999;33:195–205.
157. Young KD, Gausche-Hill M, McClung CD, et al. A prospective, population-based study of the epidemiology and outcome of out-of-hospital pediatric cardiopulmonary arrest, *Pediatrics* 2004;114:157–64.
158. Yue Z, Horton A, Bravin M, et al. A novel protein complex linking the delta 2 glutamate receptor and autophagy: Implications for neurodegeneration in lurcher mice, *Neuron* 2002;35:921–33.
159. Zhu C, Wang X, Xu F, et al. The influence of age on apoptotic and other mechanisms of cell death after cerebral hypoxia-ischemia, *Cell Death Differ* 2005;12:162–76.

CHAPTER 60 ■ METABOLIC ENCEPHALOPATHIES IN CHILDREN

PHILLIPPE JOUVET • ANNE LORTIE • BRUNO MARANDA • ROBERT C. TASKER

Metabolic encephalopathies include a variety of disorders divided into three groups according to their pathophysiology (**Table 60.1**). In this chapter, we consider the pathophysiology, clinical presentation, neurologic aspects, and management of the metabolic encephalopathies commonly treated in PICUs, excluding metabolic status epilepticus (Chapter 57). For general details on each disease, refer to the respective chapters in this book.

MECHANISM OF DISEASE: CORE PATHOPHYSIOLOGY

The mechanisms responsible for neurologic impairment in metabolic encephalopathy are classified into three groups: (a) endogenous intoxication due to an accumulation of neurotoxic metabolite(s), (b) energy failure secondary to the lack of metabolites essential for brain function, and (c) acute water, electrolyte, and/or endocrine disturbances.

Encephalopathies with Endogenous Intoxication

Liver failure and several inborn errors of metabolism (IEM) in the catabolic pathway of amino acids may induce a metabolic encephalopathy by endogenous intoxication. In these diseases, intermediate products of amino acid catabolism are not detoxified by the liver (and/or the kidney), accumulate, and contribute to neurologic symptoms (**Fig. 60.1**). Cerebral edema, which is frequently associated with these disorders, is due mainly to cytotoxic mechanisms. As the encephalopathy is related to the accumulation of toxic metabolites, specific therapeutic strategies are required to decrease this accumulation and restore brain function.

Hyperammonemia and Liver Diseases

The neurotoxicity of ammonia has been studied extensively and represents a model of endogenous intoxication. Blood ammonia concentration of >300–500 μmol/L is associated with severe central nervous system (CNS) dysfunction, including cerebral edema and coma (34). Ammonia is mainly released by the intestine and muscles. When the hepatic urea cycle is not functional, ammonia is not transformed into urea, and ammonia free base (NH_3) is able to enter the brain across the blood-brain barrier (BBB). This barrier has a much lower permeability to the ammonium ion (NH_4^+), which implies that the diffusion of ammonia across the BBB depends partly on arterial blood pH (9,45,51). Once in the brain, ammonia is buffered by the formation of glutamine via the astrocytic enzyme glutamine synthetase. As this enzyme functions at near maximal capacity under normal physiologic conditions (12), the brain capacity to synthesize glutamine is easily exceeded and hyperammonemia rapidly ensues. The pathophysiology of disabling symptoms associated with hyperammonemia is not fully understood, but various mechanisms have been observed in patients and experimental models (2,6,12,17). High levels of ammonia in the brain may lead to cell swelling and cerebral edema through glutamine accumulation, which induces astrocyte swelling and disturbed function (4); increased cerebral blood flow (CBF) (32); and alteration in mitochondrial function, with the consequent changes in cerebral energy metabolism and reduced ATP concentration (31,41). A number of human disorders are associated with hyperammonemia. IEM with hyperammonemia include primary urea cycle enzyme defects and secondary inhibition of urea cycle by organic acidurias (propionic, methylmalonic aciduria) or fatty acid oxidation disorder (FAOD) (34).

Urea Cycle Disorders. The urea cycle is the final common pathway for the excretion of waste nitrogen in mammals. For more details on these diseases, see Chapter 98.

Reye Syndrome. Reye syndrome is characterized by the combination of liver disease and metabolic encephalopathy. In 1980, the US Centers for Disease Control defined Reye syndrome as an acute noninflammatory encephalopathy with microvesicular fatty metamorphosis of the liver confirmed by biopsy or autopsy and/or a threefold increase of transaminases and/or ammonia without cerebrospinal fluid pleocytosis and without reasonable explanation for the neurologic presentation of the hepatic abnormality (37). The last part of the definition requires clinical expertise; therefore, whether the diagnosis should be used when thorough screening for all infectious, metabolic, and toxic disorders have not been undertaken is the subject of debate (10). In this setting, some clinicians use the term "Reye-like" illness.

The clinical features and electron microscopy findings on liver biopsy in patients with Reye syndrome are compatible with hepatotoxicity caused by acute, reversible mitochondrial failure. Mitochondria provide most of the energy for liver cell function via oxidative phosphorylation fed by the tricarboxylic acid cycle and products of β-oxidation (19). The etiology of Reye syndrome is probably heterogeneous, but it is likely to involve a mechanism in which mitochondrial failure results in impaired glucose homeostasis, ammonia metabolism, and hepatocyte function.

CAUSES OF METABOLIC ENCEPHALOPATHIES CLASSIFIED ACCORDING TO PATHOPHYSIOLOGY

Endogenous intoxication
Hyperammonemia and liver disease
   Urea cycle disorders
   Reye syndrome
   Hepatic encephalopathy
Organic acids disorders: MSUD, PA, MMA, IVA, 3HiB-uria,
   GA type I
Ketoacidosis
Wilson disease

Energy failure
Hypoglycemia: hyperinsulinism, GSD
Mitochondrial defects: pyruvate dehydrogenase deficiency,
   pyruvate carboxylase deficiency, respiratory chain deficiency
Fatty acid oxidation disorders
Thiamine deficiency
Biotin-responsive basal ganglia disease

Water, electrolyte, and endocrine disturbances
Disorders of osmolality: Diabetic ketoacidosis and nonketotic
   hyperosmolar coma, hyponatremia, hypernatremia
Hypocalcemia
Hypercalcemia
Hypomagnesemia
Hypophosphatemia
Thyroid disorders
Intestinal diseases that induce encephalopathy
Burn encephalopathy

MSUD, maple syrup urine disease; PA, propionic aciduria; MMA, methylmalonic aciduria; IVA, isovaleric aciduria; 3HiB-uria, 3 hydroxyisobutyric aciduria; GA type I, glutaric aciduria type I; GSD, glycogen storage disorders

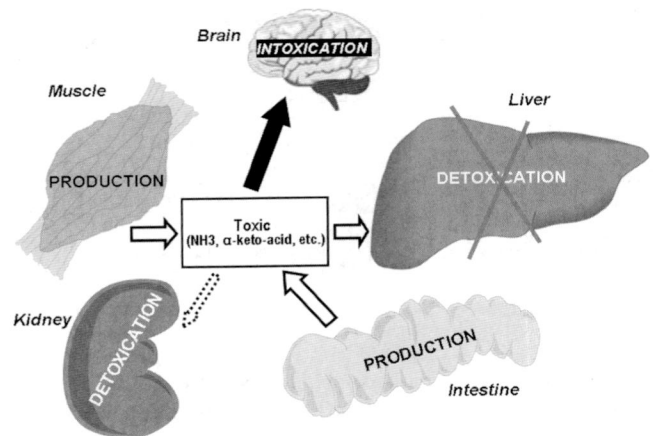

FIGURE 60.1. Endogenous intoxication model: impairment of nitrogen metabolism due to liver failure or inborn error of catabolic pathway of amino acids. The nitrogen produced by the intestine and muscle amino acid catabolism is not properly metabolized, resulting in toxic accumulation and brain damage. From D Rabier (Biochemical Laboratory, Necker Hospital, France), with permission.

reduction in cell respiration, probably due to the inhibition of respiratory chain complex I (23,44).

In patients with propionic and methylmalonic acidurias, symmetrical necrosis of the globi pallidi is observed during acute decompensation (13). Many toxic products accumulate in these two conditions, and their respective pathophysiologic brain toxicity is not known. Hyperammonemia is frequently observed.

Wilson Disease

Oxidative damage may be caused by an accumulation of copper in the basal ganglia (36). Wilson disease is associated with an initial neurologic presentation between the ages of 10 and 20 years in one-third of cases.

Encephalopathies with Energy Failure

Any mechanism that causes reduction in brain energy supply may lead to encephalopathy. This process occurs in hypoxemia-ischemia, when energy substrates are decreased for other reasons. Cerebral energy is supplied by mitochondria, and the principal metabolic substrate in the brain is glucose (**Fig. 60.2**). As the encephalopathy is secondary to energy deprivation, specific therapeutic strategies that decrease cerebral energy demands and increase energy production, when possible, are required to restore brain function.

Hypoglycemia

Under normal conditions, the brain derives its energy from glucose metabolism. Glucose must be transported across the BBB via the *GLUT-1* glucose transporter. Mutations in this gene are associated with hypoglycorrhachia without hypoglycemia. Glycogen storage disease, hyperinsulinism, and FAOD may present with severe hypoglycemia. Under conditions of prolonged fasting, the brain can switch to lactate oxidation and increase ketone uptake to partially restore energy balance. At a critical glucose concentration, however, the brain receives

Hepatic Encephalopathy. Hepatic encephalopathy is characterized by astrocytic swelling and cytotoxic brain edema (27,48). The mechanisms involved in hepatic encephalopathy include the combined toxic effect of accumulated ammonia, mercaptans, fatty acids, and phenol; changes in the γ-aminobutyric acid (GABA) benzodiazepine system; changes in the BBB; and disturbances in neurotransmission (6,35).

Amino and Organic Acids Disorders

Among the amino and organic acid disorders, those that most frequently cause patients to be admitted to the PICU for acute metabolic encephalopathy are maple syrup urine disease (MSUD), propionic acidurias, and methylmalonic acidurias. Hyperammonemia and/or the accumulation of intermediate metabolites (due to downstream enzyme defects) are involved in the pathophysiology of acute encephalopathy and are reversible with specific treatment.

In MSUD, acute encephalopathy is associated with a high risk for cerebral edema (42). The mechanism of brain edema is not completely understood. Plasma leucine concentration and duration of exposure to high leucine levels appear to correlate with encephalopathy (22). At the cellular level, α-keto isocaproic acid (a derivative product of leucine accumulated in MSUD) specifically induces apoptosis in rat glial and neuronal cells (23). Apoptosis has been reported to be associated with a

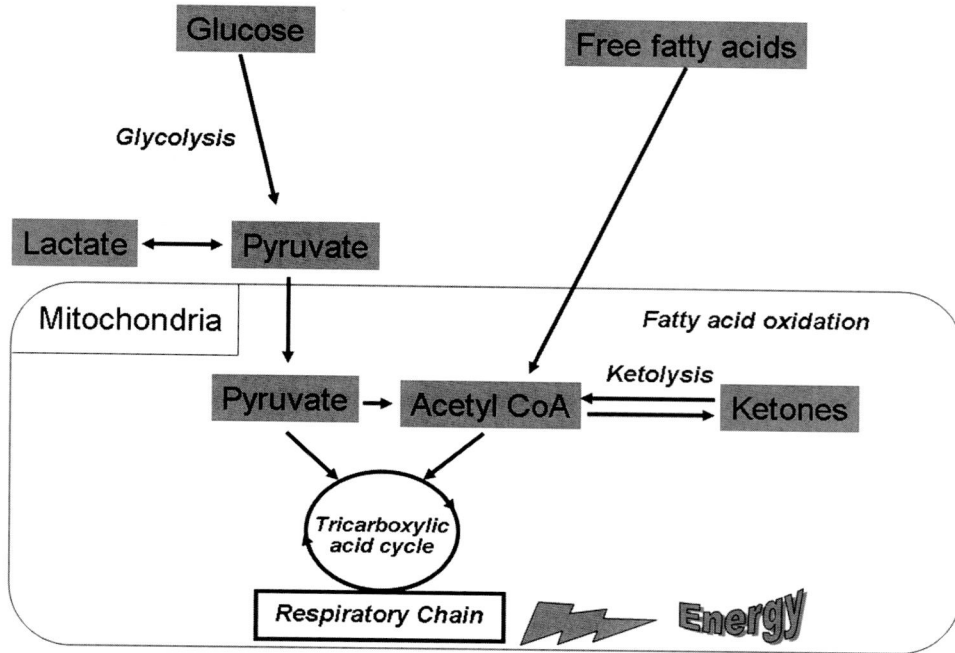

FIGURE 60.2. Energy failure model of metabolic encephalopathy. Hypoglycemia and any enzyme defect in mitochondrial energy production may result in metabolic encephalopathy. The pathophysiology of metabolic encephalopathy by fatty acid oxidation defect is multifactorial.

inadequate glucose to support its needs, which may result in metabolic encephalopathy (20). The exact mechanism to explain how hypoglycemia kills neurons is not yet elucidated, but it does not seem to be related only to energy failure (46).

Primary Mitochondrial Energy Metabolism Defects

Primary defects in mitochondrial energy metabolism include pyruvate dehydrogenase complex deficiency, tricarboxylic acid cycle deficiencies, and respiratory chain defects. All of these conditions may present with acute encephalopathy, which results from lack of energy production, despite normal brain oxygenation. These diseases are currently untreatable.

FAODs comprise another group of diseases with impaired mitochondrial energy metabolism. The encephalopathy observed in these diseases is not fully understood and may result from multifactorial insults, including limited fuel for the brain due to hypoglycemia concomitant with abnormally low ketones, hyperammonemia, and decrease in CBF due to circulatory failure (43).

Thiamine Deficiency

Thiamine (vitamin B_1) has an important role in several metabolic processes, including the decarboxylation of pyruvate and α-ketoglutarate (two steps of the tricarboxylic acid cycle), with magnesium as a cofactor, and in the conversion of five-carbon to six-carbon sugars by means of the enzyme transketolase. Thiamine deficiency, therefore, decreases the amount of energy available to the brain and increases the concentrations of several metabolites. Patients who receive total parenteral nutrition, chronic dialysis, or a high-carbohydrate diet during debilitating illness are at risk of thiamine deficiency, and Wernicke encephalopathy may be observed. In these settings, the features are highly variable and may manifest by sudden collapse and death or seizures, or by the classic, but extremely rare, triad of ataxia, confusion, and ocular abnormalities (49).

Encephalopathies with Acute Water, Electrolyte, and/or Endocrine Disturbances

Disorders of Osmolality

The osmolality of a solution is determined by the number of particles in the solution. Sodium, glucose, and urea are the primary osmoles of the extracellular space. Potassium is the primary osmole of the intracellular space. Because cell membranes are permeable to water, an osmotic equilibrium is maintained. That is, the volume of intracellular fluid is determined by the osmolality of the extracellular space. Hypernatremia and hyperglycemia are the major causes of serum hyperosmolality, and hyponatremia is the major cause of hypo-osmolality. Any modification of brain water volume may result in acute encephalopathy.

Diabetic Ketoacidosis and Nonketotic Hyperosmolar Coma. Cerebral edema in diabetic ketoacidosis (DKA) typically occurs within the first 12 hrs after the onset of treatment, but can be present before treatment initiation. The mechanism of cerebral edema is not well understood, with evidence for both osmotic and vasogenic edema. Cerebral water distribution and cerebral perfusion during treatment of uncomplicated DKA showed an expansion of the extracellular space relative to the intracellular space and increased cerebral perfusion (18). These findings are most consistent with a vasogenic mechanism (increase in cerebral capillary endothelial permeability) of edema formation rather than osmotic cell swelling, which is associated with expansion of the intracellular space. Hypotheses for vasodilation and consecutive vasogenic edema include ketone stimulation of the production of vasoactive peptides and/or reperfusion during rehydration therapy of ischemic cerebral tissues. On the other hand, Cameron et al. observed increased levels of brain taurine and myoinositol in DKA (7). Both of these endogenous osmolytes may be generated by brain cells in order to maintain adequate cell volume during the acute onset, and they may induce an osmotic edema during vigorous rehydration therapy. Regardless of the final mechanism, all authors agree that initial rehydration should be sufficient to restore hemodynamic stability and that subsequent volume repletion should occur over a 48-hr period.

Hyperosmolar hyperglycemic nonketotic coma is increasing in frequency in children as a result of the emerging problem with obesity in childhood and shares similar pathogenesis with DKA without ketone body contribution (8).

Hyponatremia. Osmotic disequilibrium between a low osmolality plasma compartment and higher osmotic pressure within glial cells will result in astrocytic water accumulation and brain edema. Rapid decrease in sodium concentration is much more likely to cause severe edema. Hyponatremia may result from water retention, sodium loss, or both. Water retention is often caused by inappropriate antidiuretic hormone secretion and sodium loss from renal disease, vomiting, and diarrhea. Both mechanisms of hyponatremia are worsened by infusion of hypotonic solutions. Conversely, a too-rapid correction of hyponatremia can induce central pontine myelinolysis. This syndrome is characterized by confusion, cranial nerve dysfunction and, when the lesion is larger, "locked-in" syndrome and quadriparesis (28).

Hypernatremia. Hypernatremia is associated with cellular dehydration, which affects brain function. Because the brain can compensate for slow or chronic changes in osmolality, acute changes, such as salt poisoning, should be treated quickly, while chronic changes should be treated slowly. Hypernatremia is usually caused by dehydration, in which water loss exceeds sodium loss or by overhydration with hypertonic saline solution.

Acute Uremic Encephalopathy—Dialysis Encephalopathy. The mechanism of acute uremic encephalopathy is multifactorial and does not strictly correlate with concentrations of blood urea nitrogen alone. Disturbed equilibrium of ions between the intracellular and extracellular spaces is an important mechanism. Hypertensive encephalopathy may be associated. The treatment is dialysis.

Dialysis encephalopathy—the rapid shift of fluids and electrolytes between intracellular and extracellular spaces due to dialysis—may be associated with acute transitory neurologic disturbances which usually occur toward the end of dialysis or up to 24 hrs later.

Calcium, Magnesium, and Phosphate Disorders

Calcium is the major divalent cation in the extracellular fluid. It is an important regulator of cellular function and is essential for numerous cellular processes, especially neurotransmission. Severe hypocalcemia and hypercalcemia may both induce encephalopathy. Magnesium is the second most abundant intracellular cation in the body and is required for the maintenance of normal activities. It is a cofactor of numerous enzymes that play vital roles in energy metabolism. Hypomagnesemia (usually in association with other electrolyte abnormalities, such

as hypocalcemia) and hypermagnesemia may both induce encephalopathy. Hypophosphatemia may also cause neurologic dysfunction.

Others

Thyroid disorders—both hyperthyroidism (thyrotoxicosis) and hypothyroidism—affect the CNS and may lead to coma.

In terms of intestinal diseases that can induce encephalopathy, intestinal intussusception and abdominal surgery in children may be associated with depressed levels of consciousness. This type of presentation may be explained either by a possible endogenous opioid poisoning by massive secretion of endorphins during paroxysms of pain or by gastrointestinal release of neurotoxic vasoactive peptides and neuroactive gut hormones.

In burn encephalopathy, a few days after severe burn injury, awareness and responsiveness may decline without any neurologic findings in the physical exam. The mechanism is not known. It may be related to outpouring of stress hormones and cytokines after the massive inflammatory response to the high doses of narcotics and/or to sleep deprivation.

CLINICAL PRESENTATION AND DIFFERENTIAL DIAGNOSIS

In some circumstances, the patient's diagnosis is clear at the time of admission to the PICU and clinical management can focus on specific treatment. This is the case in two-thirds of patients with IEMs who are admitted to the PICU (24). In the other cases, the challenge is to quickly diagnose treatable disorders so as to ensure prompt treatment and recovery. The diagnosis is suspected on the combination of clinical course and laboratory investigations. Metabolic encephalopathies must be considered in parallel with other common conditions, such as sepsis, hypoxic-ischemic encephalopathy, encephalitis, exogenous intoxication, and brain tumors.

Clinical Presentation of Metabolic Encephalopathies

Metabolic encephalopathy may present within hours or days with progressive confusion, diverse motor and sensory abnormalities, and, rarely, hallucinations. Patients must be assessed as soon as possible, and certainly before they deteriorate into coma. The selective central anatomic dysfunction of each metabolic disease is not well understood. Impaired consciousness is caused by a disorder diffusely affecting both cerebral hemispheres and the brainstem. Sometimes, lesions can be more specifically located, especially in the brainstem and basal ganglia. At a more advanced state, neurovegetative problems with respiratory abnormalities, hiccups, apnea, bradycardia, and hypothermia can occur.

A careful history easily guides the diagnosis in some circumstances—for example, the polyuria and polydipsia that preceed the encephalopathy in DKA, or an infusion of hypotonic solutions in the perioperative period in hyponatremic encephalopathy. In other circumstances, especially in the case of an IEM, the history is not obvious and requires specific details of the events that preceded any behavioral change. Drug exposure, personal history, and family history must be carefully reviewed.

Decompensation may occur at any age from the neonatal period to adulthood. Each attack can follow a rapid course that ends in either spontaneous improvement or unexplained death, despite supportive measures in the PICU. The following events may trigger acute decompensation.

Prolonged fasting. Children with endogenous intoxication and FAODs may deteriorate with fasting because, during this state, protein catabolism is increased and free fatty acid is the preferred fuel.

Anesthesia and surgery. Both anesthesia and surgery induce protein catabolism and increase energy demand.

Infections. Infections increase protein catabolism and increase energy demand (29). The most typical cause of acute onset in infants is gastrointestinal infection, which combines the infectious effect on metabolism and a fasting state.

Prolonged exercise. Patients with endogenous intoxication and FAODs may decompensate with prolonged exercise, as it creates protein catabolism and increases free fatty acid use (43).

Drugs. Valproic acid may worsen patients with urea cycle disorders (21) and respiratory chain disorders because of drug-induced enzyme inhibition. Steroids and adrenocorticotropic hormone (ACTH) increase protein catabolism.

High protein intake. Protein intake is restricted in patients with endogenous intoxication disorders. Noncompliance to the diet, typically seen surrounding holidays and parties, may lead to acute decompensation.

An IEM should be suspected when the following history is found: (a) recurrent coma, (b) unexplained death in the family or any neonatal death, even if it was attributed to another cause (e.g., sepsis, anoxia, etc.), (c) consanguinity. Although most genetic disorders are hereditary and transmitted as recessive disorders, the majority of cases appear sporadically in developed countries because of small family sizes.

The clinical features of metabolic encephalopathy are usually nonspecific, except in the following presentations. In the comatose state, characteristic changes in muscular tone and involuntary movements appear in some diseases. In MSUD, generalized hypertonic episodes with opisthotonos are frequent, and boxing or pedalling movements and slow limb elevations, spontaneous or upon stimulation, are observed. In organic aciduria, axial hypotonia and limb hypertonia with large amplitude tremors and myoclonic jerks (which are often mistaken for convulsions) are observed. Intracranial hypertension, secondary to cerebral edema and seizures, are frequent presenting symptoms in metabolic encephalopathies. Focal signs are sometimes seen, even within the context of a diffuse metabolic encephalopathy, such as hyponatremia or hypoglycemia. These focal signs can mimic a stroke in certain mitochondrial encephalopathies. Other patients with organic acidemias and urea cycle defects present with focal neuro-

logic signs and cerebral edema. These patients can be mistakenly diagnosed as having cerebrovascular accident or cerebral tumor.

Hepatomegaly may be observed, especially in organic academia, FAOD, Wilson disease, hyperinsulinism, and glycogen storage diseases. An *abnormal urine or body odor* is present in some diseases, in which volatile metabolites accumulate. In urine, an abnormal odor can be detected on a drying paper or by opening a container of urine that has been closed at room temperature for a few minutes. The three most important examples are the fruity smell of ketoacids in DKA, the maple syrup odor of MSUD, and the sweaty feet odor of isovaleric acidemia. *Myoglobinuria* is an indicator of FAOD.

Laboratory Investigations

General supportive measures and laboratory investigations should be undertaken as soon as metabolic encephalopathy is suspected. The initial approach for investigations is outlined in **Table 60.2**. It is important to perform these investigations as early as possible, and all laboratory tests should be obtained simultaneously, as most disorders may produce only intermittent abnormalities. The determination of plasma ammonia concentration is crucial when metabolic encephalopathy is suspected because hyperammonemia is life-threatening and necessitates urgent management. Venous blood should be collected in an ammonia-free, heparinized blood tube, placed on ice at the bedside, and transferred quickly to the laboratory, where the plasma should be separated immediately. By conducting immediate laboratory investigations, the encephalopathies caused by acute water and electrolyte disturbances are rapidly evaluated. For further discussion on the causes of these disturbances, see Chapters 92, 93, 94, and 98. IEM are more difficult to diagnose, and the following biologic signs should prompt consideration of such disorders (**Table 60.3**).

Metabolic acidosis with an increased anion gap is observed in intermediate acid accumulation, such as organic acid disorders (propionic and methylmalonic acid). Moderate *hyperammonemia* (80–150 μmol/L) is frequently observed in IEM due to a secondary blockage of the urea cycle. Severe hyperammonemia (>300 μmol/L) is observed in primary urea cycle defects, organic acid disorders, and FAOD. Hyperammonemia must be interpreted cautiously, as a falsely high level may be due to technical problems at the time of sampling and transfer to the laboratory. Two ammonia levels, obtained using the proper technique, are required to ensure the diagnosis. Hyperammonemia, with abnormalities in liver function tests, is seen in acute liver failure and Reye syndrome. Conditions that produce a Reye-like illness are detailed in **Table 60.4**.

Hyperlactatemia—elevated lactic acid levels—in the absence of sepsis or tissue hypoxia is a significant finding. Moderate elevation (3–6 mmol/L or 270–550 mg/L) is often observed in organic acid disorders. A level above 6 mmol/L (550 mg/L) is seen mainly in primary mitochondrial energy metabolism defects. In such circumstances, the simultaneous measurement of lactate-to-pyruvate ratio and 3-hydroxyburate:acetoacetate ratio (on a plasma sample that is immediately deproteinized at the bedside) is a useful tool to assess the cytoplasmic and mitochondrial redox states, respectively (40). *Hypoglycemia without ketonuria* is observed in FAOD and hyperinsulinism.

TABLE 60.2

LABORATORY INVESTIGATIONS IN METABOLIC ENCEPHALOPATHY

	Routine tests	Storage of samples and metabolic tests[a]
Urine	Smell (special odor) Look (special color) Acetone (Acetest) Ketoacids (DNPH)[b] pH Electrolytes (Na+, K+) Urea, creatinine	Fresh sample in the refrigerator, frozen sample at –20°C, for metabolic testing (AAC, OAC, orotic acid)
Blood	Electrolytes (Na+, K+, Cl−, HCO3−) Glucose, Ca2+, Mg2+, Phosphate Urea, creatinine Osmolality Blood gases Transaminases, bilirubin, GGT Ammonia Lactic acid Creatine kinase Blood cell count Prothrombin time	Plasma heparinized at –20°C (5 mL); Whole blood (10 mL) collected on EDTA at –20°C (for molecular biology studies); Plasma or blood on filter paper for acylcarnitine dosage; Redox status if lactate >10 mmol/L (AAC, OAC, acylcarnitnines)
Miscellaneous	CSF if no intracranial hypertension with concentration of lactate and pyruvate	CSF (1 mL) frozen for AAC *Other metabolic tests:* Skin biopsy for fibroblast culture; If death: liver and muscle biopsy

[a]Tests should be discussed with specialists in metabolic diseases.
[b]This test screens for the presence of α-keto acids, as occur in MSUD. It can be replaced by an amino acid chromatography, if available, in an emergency situation.
DNPH, dinitrophenylhydrazine test; AAC, amino-acid chromatography; OAC, organic acid chromatography; CSF, cerebrospinal fluid

Neurophysiology and Neuroimaging in Metabolic Encephalopathies

Neurophysiology

Regardless of etiology, an electroencephalogram (EEG) during an acute encephalopathic process usually shows varying degrees of slow activity. The severity of slowing is usually well correlated with the severity of the encephalopathy. This slowing is nonspecific and merely reflects cortical and subcortical dysfunction. Triphasic waves were initially considered specific to hepatic coma but are now recognized in different metabolic conditions. When clinical seizures occur, the EEG can provide information as to the severity of the epileptic condition. A burst-suppression pattern that is not due to medication is associated with poor prognosis. Seizures are easily recognized in metabolic encephalopathies, and, rarely, an EEG can also reveal subclinical epileptiform activity (26).

Neuroimaging

A cerebral CT scan is essential when evaluating a comatose patient (see Chapter 53). If any clinical signs of intracranial hypertension are present, a CT scan should be obtained after the patient has been stabilized (i.e., treatment of fluid and electrolyte imbalance, adequate oxygenation and perfusion, temperature control, etc.). The CT scan will help to evaluate the severity of cerebral edema. For example, the absence of cerebrospinal fluid spaces above the tentorium and obliteration of the basal cisterns are associated with high intracranial pressure (ICP) (47). Also, some specific lesions may be observed in white matter or basal ganglia in organic acid disorders and mitochondrial disorders, respectively (30) (see Chapter 55).

MRI of the brain is much more informative than CT scan, and specific abnormalities can suggest diagnosis of certain pathologies, such as mitochondrial encephalopathies (16). Occasionally, MRI study can even provide information with direct implication for treatment, such as in biotin-responsive basal ganglia disease. This rare disease appears as a subacute encephalopathy and seems to be related to a defect in a transporter of biotin across the BBB. MRI of the brain shows bilateral, symmetrically increased T2-signal intensity within the central part of the caudate nuclei and within parts, or all, of the putamen. No specific laboratory findings are associated with this disease. The symptoms may be reversed by providing biotin (38). MR spectroscopy can also provide clues to the underlying neurologic processes by evaluating brain tissue lactate concentration, thus avoiding the risk of lumbar puncture, especially in cases with cerebral edema (11,16).

Differential Diagnosis

The nonspecific clinical presentation, the many possible etiologies, and the presence of intermittent abnormalities may explain why metabolic encephalopathy is sometimes not

TABLE 60.3

ALGORITHM FOR THE DIAGNOSIS OF IEM REVEALED BY ENCEPHALOPATHY

Clinical presentation	Predominant metabolic disturbance	Associated metabolic/ neurologic disturbance	Most frequent diagnoses (disorder/enzyme deficiency)	Differential diagnosis
Metabolic coma without focal neurologic signs	Metabolic acidosis	With ketosis	Organic aciduria (MMA, PA, IVA, GA I, MSUD) PC MCD Ketolysis, Gluconeogenesis	Diabetes Exogenous intoxication Encephalitis
		Without ketosis	PDH Ketogenesis FAO FDP	
	Hyperammonemia	Normal glucose	Urea cycle defects	Reye syndrome Encephalitis Exogenous intoxication
		Hypoglycemia	FAO HMG CoA lyase	
	Hypoglycemia	With acidosis	Gluconeogenesis, MSUD, HMG CoA lyase FAO	
		Without acidosis	FAO Hyperinsulinism	
	Hyperlactatemia	Normal glucose	PC MCD Krebs cycle PDH Respiratory chain	
		Hypoglycemia	Gluconeogenesis FAO GSD	
Neurologic coma with focal signs, seizures, severe intracranial hypertension, strokes or stroke-like episodes	Biologic signs are variable, can be absent or moderate.	Cerebral edema	MSUD OTC	Cerebral tumor Migraine Encephalitis
		Hemiplegia or hemianopsia	MSUD OTC MMA PA	
		Extrapyramidal signs	MMA GA I Wilson Homocystinuria	
		Caudate nucleus and putamen necrosis	BBGD Urea cycle defect MMA PA IVA	
		Stroke-like	Respiratory chain CDG Thiamine responsive megaloblastic anemia	Moya moya syndrome, Vascular hemiplegia Cerebral sinus thrombosis Cerebral tumor

Treatable disorders appear in bold type.
MMA, methylmalonic academia; PA, propionic academia; IVA, isovaleric aciduria; GA I, glutaric aciduria type I; MSUD, maple syrup urine disease; PC, pyruvate carboxylase; MCD, multiple carboxylase deficiency; PDH, pyruvate dehydrogenase; FAO, fatty acid oxidation; FDP, fructose-1, 6-diphosphatase; HMG CoA lyase, 3-hydroxy-3-methylglutaryl coenzyme A lyase; GSD, glycogen storage disorders; OTC, ornithine transcarbamylase; BBGD, biotin-responsive basal ganglia disease; CDG, carbohydrate-deficient glycoprotein syndrome

TABLE 60.4

CONDITIONS THAT PRODUCE A REYE
SYNDROME-LIKE ILLNESS

Viral infection
Influenza A and B virus
Varicella zoster
Parainfluenza
Adenovirus
Coxsackie virus
Cytomegalovirus
Herpes simplex
Epstein-Barr virus

Inborns errors of metabolism
Urea cycle defect
Organic acidemias
Fatty acid oxidation defects
Others: Triple H syndrome (hyperammonemia,
  hyperornithinemia, homocitrullinuria), Biotinidase defect,
  HMG CoA lyase defect, FDP defect, fructosemia

Toxins and medications
Drugs: Salicylates, valproic acid, antiemetics, paracetamol,
  outdated tetracycline, zidovudine
Toxins: Aflatoxin, hypoglycin, ackee, pteridine, calcium
  hopantenate, isopropyl alcohol, methobromide, lead,
  margosa oil, diallyl acetate

diagnosed. In clinical practice, it is not rare to find a history
of previous unexplained coma in a patient hospitalized for a
recurrent attack (5).

Infection and Sepsis

An infection may be responsible for acute encephalitis, or it
may be the event that precipitates the acute metabolic deterioration.

Exogenous Intoxication: Poisons, Substance Abuse, Drug Overdoses

Most accidental poisonings occur in small children who ingest
common household products. The ingestion is usually discovered quickly. The differential diagnosis may be difficult in cases
of unrevealed intentional poisoning, such as in Munchausen
syndrome by proxy.

The diagnosis of metabolic encephalopathy should be suspected when vaguely defined and/or undocumented diagnoses,
such as encephalitis, basilar migraine, intoxication, poisoning,
or stroke are suggested, especially in the presence of moderate
ketoacidosis, hyperlactatemia, or hyperammonemia.

CLINICAL MANAGEMENT

The assessment and management of the infant or child with
an altered level of consciousness is a pediatric emergency. A
review of the appropriate clinical approach, including resuscitation and institution of initial therapy of the comatose child,
is discussed in Chapter 53. The basis of the neurologic support
includes attention to intracranial hypertension with fluid and
electrolyte balance, adequate oxygenation and perfusion, temperature control, seizure control, and prevention of infection.
The treatment of many of the diseases involved in metabolic encephalopathies is covered in other chapters of this book. How-

ever, in the context of a child referred with a presumed or identified metabolic encephalopathy, specific neurologic support is
necessary.

Management of Intracranial Hypertension in Metabolic Encephalopathies

Only in the presence of severe hyperammonemia (>300
μmol/L) does the management of intracranial hypertension differ from the usual recommendations. As explained in the pathophysiology section, the BBB has a much lower permeability to
NH_4^+ than to NH_3. For this reason, despite the lack of reported
clinical study, the authors suggest avoiding any aggressive hyperventilation and setting mechanical ventilation and sedation
to obtain a pH of 7.30–7.35 until a sustained decrease of hyperammonemia is achieved. It should be noted that hypocapnia
did not decrease CBF during hyperammonemia in one animal
study (3).

Intracranial pressure monitoring is not routinely performed
in metabolic encephalopathy because of the potential rapid improvement with the correct treatment. However, in some circumstances, ICP monitoring may be helpful to maintain an
adequate cerebral perfusion pressure. Using near-infrared
spectroscopy to noninvasively monitor cerebral oxygenation
and cerebral blood volume may detect changes in cerebral
hemodynamics in children with intracranial hypertension and
may be helpful in the management of metabolic encephalopathy (50).

Seizure Control

In the case of hyperammonemia or suspicion of mitochondrial
disorder, seizures should be appropriately treated; however,
valproic acid is contraindicated.

Temperature Control

A clinical trial on the neuroprotective effect hypothermia was
recently conducted in traumatic brain injury and did not show
clear benefit of hypothermia on outcome (1). No such clinical
trial in metabolic encephalopathy has been reported. However,
fever should be prevented or treated in the setting of raised
ICP; in cases of endogenous intoxication, the reduction of
metabolic rate induced by hypothermia may decrease toxic
production (52).

Specific Treatment

Many of the specific metabolic therapies oriented toward the
underlying process and etiology of encephalopathy are covered
elsewhere in the book. This discussion will be restricted to some
key therapeutic considerations.

Diabetic Ketoacidosis

When patients with DKA are clinically symptomatic of cerebral
edema, the rate of fluid administration should be reduced, and
mannitol (0.25–1 g/kg IV over 20 min) or hypertonic saline
(NaCl 3%, 5–10 mL/kg over 30 min) may be given (14).

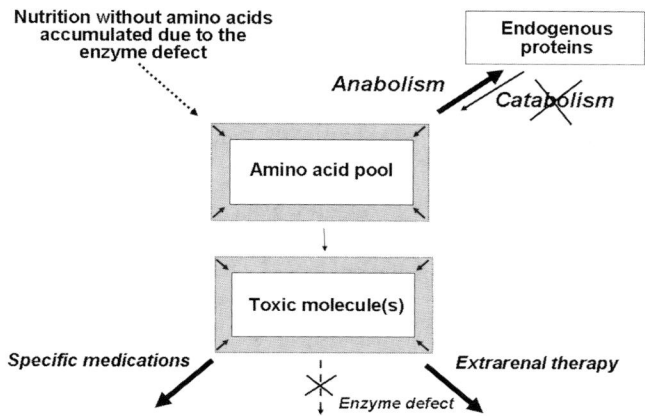

FIGURE 60.3. Schematic of the emergency treatment of IEMs with endogenous intoxication. After an increase in exogenous protein intake or protein catabolism, the toxic metabolites accumulate. According to the enzyme defect, treatment includes nutritional support without the amino acids that accumulate due to the enzyme defect (for example, in urea cycle disorders, all amino acids are excluded initially), promotion of protein anabolism by adequate caloric intake, specific medications (Table 60.5), and extrarenal therapy in the most severe cases.

Initial Treatment of Suspected Inborn Error of Metabolism

If an IEM is suspected, therapy must focus on treatable diseases. First, glucose (not protein or lipid) is infused to limit protein catabolism (which will treat endogenous intoxication). The rate of glucose infusion should be high, so that enough energy is generated via glycolysis. This therapy will also ap-

ply to FAODs and ketoacidosis. A central line is necessary to provide concentrated solutions of glucose, and the goal is to infuse 1000 kcal/m^2/d, which may require the addition of insulin infusion to avoid hyperglycemia.

As soon as an endogenous intoxication is diagnosed, nutritional support should be discussed with the specialist, and it can include the following (**Fig. 60.3**):

- Promotion of protein anabolism through administration of glucose and lipid, without proteins, preferably by enteral continuous feeding, with a caloric intake of at least 1,500 kcal/m^2/d. When the diagnosis is confirmed, special amino acid mixtures are used to supply nontoxic amino acids. For example, in MSUD, the enzyme defect involves the branched-chain amino acids (leucine, valine, and isoleucine). The mixtures used are initially free of these three amino acids.
- Avoidance of any factor that promotes protein catabolism, including steroid therapy.
- Specific medications in some IEM, such as ammonia removal drugs (see **Table 60.5**).
- Metabolite excretion: Small organic acids (methylmalonic, propionic, isovaleric, etc.) are excreted in urine, and hydration helps to decrease their concentration in blood and restore acid-base balance.
- Extrarenal therapy (see Chapter 37). When a high and/or prolonged toxic accumulation occurs, toxic removal by dialysis is necessary to prevent further brain damage. The criteria for dialysis and the optimal modality to use are not yet well established for each disease and are currently based on individual institutional experience. The decision is made using a multidisciplinary approach that involves intensivists,

---

TABLE 60.5

SPECIFIC TREATMENTS OF IEM

Drug	Effect	Indication(s)	Dose	Administration route
Sodium benzoate	Ammonia removal	NH$_3$ >200 mcmol/L	500 mg/kg/d	IV
Phenylbutyrate	Ammonia removal	NH$_3$ >200 mcmol/L	600 mg/kg/d	IV or PO
Arginine	Ammonia removal	NH$_3$ >200 mcmol/L	300 mg/kg/d	IVC
Carglumic acid	Ammonia removal	NAGS defect, MMA, PA, FAOD, and NH$_3$ >200 mcmol/L	50 mg/kg/6 hr	PO
Carnitine	Primary or secondary deficiency compensation	Organic aciduria Hyperlactacidemia FAOD	100 mg/kg/d	IVC or PO
Glycine	Increased urine	IVA	500 mg/kg/4 hr	IVC or PO
Vitamin B12	Enzyme cofactor	MMA	1–2 mg/d	IM
Metronidazole	Decreased toxin production by intestine bacteria	AMM, AP	20 mg/kg/d	PO
Biotin	PC cofactor	Hyperlactatemia, PA	10–20 mg/d	IV or PO
Riboflavin	Cofactor of acyl CoA dehydrogenase	FAOD	20–40 mg/d	IV or PO
Dichloroacetate or Dichloropropionate	PDHk inhibitor	Hyperlactatemia >10 mmol/L	25 mg/kg/12 hr	IV or PO

In suspected cases of IEM, the above specific treatments may be indicated in metabolic encephalopathy, after specialist consultation. Some therapies are specific for toxic accumulation (i.e., hyperammonemia) and some are specific for a particular disease.
IVC, continuous intravenous infusion; NAGS, N-acetylglutamate synthase; MMA, methylmalonic acidemia; PA, propionic acidemia; FAOD, fatty acid oxidation disorder; IVA, isovaleric acidemia; PC, pyruvate carboxylase; PDHk, pyruvate dehydrogenase kinase

specialists in metabolic diseases, and nephrologists. The challenge is to quickly remove the toxins without worsening the cerebral edema by hemodynamic and/or osmotic shifts. The greater the cerebral edema, the higher the risk of cerebral herniation during therapy, especially in cases of hyperammonemia. If neurologic deterioration is observed during extrarenal therapy, the toxic clearance should be reduced.

The efficacy of treatment is based on neurologic improvement, gastrointestinal tolerance that reflects that calories are being assimilated, and a decrease in blood levels of measurable toxic metabolites (e.g., amino acid chromatography in MSUD, ammonemia, pH in organic aciduria, etc.). In some instances, additional tests may be helpful. For example, if urinary ketones are initially positive, then their later absence reflects improvement. Also, in MSUD and organic acid disorders, decrease in urea/creatinine urinary ratio reflects protein catabolism in the absence of renal failure and protein intake (22).

OUTCOMES

Morbidity and mortality of patients with metabolic encephalopathies who are admitted to the PICU are difficult to assess due to the many associated etiologies, each with incidence rates that vary according to the population concerned and the admission policy of the PICU. In children, the incidence of cerebral edema in DKA is ~1% of acute episodes in the UK, with a mortality rate of 23%–24% and a morbidity rate of 15%–35% in survivors (15,33). Metabolic encephalopathy due to IEM represented 2% of admissions to a PICU that had a national reference center for metabolic diseases. The mortality rate of these patients was 28.6% (25). Given that the incidence of metabolic encephalopathy due to IEM is probably lower in PICUs that do not have access to a national reference center, it is difficult for practitioners in those PICUs to develop an expertise in treatment. Therefore, the development of a network among such referral centers may help to improve the outcomes of patients with these rare diseases.

CONCLUSIONS AND FUTURE DIRECTIONS

In the infant or child with an acute encephalopathy, a variety of metabolic causes may account for acute brain dysfunction. Given the highly selected population referred to intensive care, the intensivist should be aware of the more common differential diagnoses, necessary investigations, and therapeutic priorities. The future in the diagnosis and treatment of metabolic encephalopathies includes the following:

- Developing techniques that will speed the diagnosis of IEM, such as tandem mass spectrometry, which is a specific and sensitive method that may improve diagnosis of IEM in an emergency (39).
- Developing neuroprotective treatments that limit brain damage until specific treatment is obtained. Hypothermia is one such treatment, but its side effects may modify cerebral hemodynamics.
- Developing additional substitutive enzyme therapies for IEMs. Only a few IEMs can be treated with enzyme substitution. For example, carglumic acid (Carbaglu®, Orphan

Europe, France), an analog of *N*-acetylglutamate, treats hyperammonemia due to a defect in *N*-acetylglutamate synthase. The development of substitutive enzyme therapy for other IEMs should decrease the incidences of acute decompensation that require intensive care.

KEY POINTS

- Metabolic encephalopathies are caused by a large number of etiologies. A systematic investigation is necessary, including neuroimaging and laboratory tests (Table 60.2).
- The practitioner should be careful not to confuse a symptom or a syndrome (such as Reye syndrome) with an etiology.
- Diseases that are amenable to treatment should be considered first.
- Intracranial hypertension is frequently present in metabolic encephalopathy, and requires strict hemodynamic control.
- Specific treatments of endogenous intoxication must be started as soon as possible and conducted simultaneously with diagnostic investigations.

References

1. Adelson PD, Ragheb J, Kanev P, et al. Phase II clinical trial of moderate hypothermia after severe traumatic brain injury in children. *Neurosurgery* 2005;56:740–54.
2. Bachmann C, Braissant O, Villard AM, et al. Ammonia toxicity to the brain and creatine. *Mol Genet Metab* 2004;81 Suppl 1:S52–7.
3. Barzilay Z, Britten AG, Koehler RC, et al. Interaction of CO2 and ammonia on cerebral blood flow and O2 consumption in dogs. *Am J Physiol* 1985;248:H500–7.
4. Binesh N, Huda A, Thomas MA, et al. Hepatic encephalopathy: A neurochemical, neuroanatomical, and neuropsychological study. *J Appl Clin Med Phys* 2006;7:86–96.
5. Bodman M, Smith D, Nyhan WL, et al. Medium-chain acyl coenzyme A dehydrogenase deficiency: Occurrence in an infant and his father. *Arch Neurol* 2001;58:811–4.
6. Butterworth RF. Pathophysiology of hepatic encephalopathy: A new look at ammonia. *Metab Brain Dis* 2002;17:221–7.
7. Cameron FJ, Kean MJ, Wellard RM, et al. Insights into the acute cerebral metabolic changes associated with childhood diabetes. *Diabet Med* 2005;22:648–53.
8. Carchman RM, Dechert-Zeger M, Calikoglu AS, et al. A new challenge in pediatric obesity: Pediatric hyperglycemic hyperosmolar syndrome. *Pediatr Crit Care Med* 2005;6:20–4.
9. Carter CC, Lifton JF, Welch MJ. Organ uptake and blood pH and concentration effects of ammonia in dogs determined with ammonia labeled with 10 minute half-lived nitrogen 13. *Neurology* 1973;23:204–13.
10. Casteels-Van Daele M. Reye syndrome or side-effects of anti-emetics? *Eur J Pediatr* 1991;150:456–9.
11. Cecil KM. MR spectroscopy of metabolic disorders. *Neuroimaging Clin N Am* 2006;16:87–116, viii.
12. Cooper AJ, Plum F. Biochemistry and physiology of brain ammonia. *Physiol Rev* 1987;67:440–519.
13. de Sousa C, Piesowicz AT, Brett EM, et al. Focal changes in the globi pallidi associated with neurological dysfunction in methylmalonic acidaemia. *Neuropediatrics* 1989;20:199–201.
14. Dunger DB, Sperling MA, Acerini CL, et al. ESPE/LWPES consensus statement on diabetic ketoacidosis in children and adolescents. *Arch Dis Child* 2004;89:188–94.
15. Edge JA, Hawkins MM, Winter DL, et al. The risk and outcome of cerebral oedema developing during diabetic ketoacidosis. *Arch Dis Child* 2001;85:16–22.
16. Faerber EN, Poussaint TY. Magnetic resonance of metabolic and degenerative diseases in children. *Top Magn Reson Imaging* 2002;13:3–21.
17. Felipo V, Butterworth RF. Neurobiology of ammonia. *Prog Neurobiol* 2002;67:259–79.
18. Glaser NS, Wootton-Gorges SL, Marcin JP, et al. Mechanism of cerebral edema in children with diabetic ketoacidosis. *J Pediatr* 2004;145:164–71.
19. Glasgow JF, Middleton B. Reye syndrome—insights on causation and prognosis. *Arch Dis Child* 2001;85:351–3.

20. Herbel G, Boyle PJ. Hypoglycemia. Pathophysiology and treatment. *Endocrinol Metab Clin North Am* 2000;29:725–43.

21. Honeycutt D, Callahan K, Rutledge L, et al. Heterozygote ornithine transcarbamylase deficiency presenting as symptomatic hyperammonemia during initiation of valproate therapy. *Neurology* 1992;42:666–8.

22. Jouvet P, Jugie M, Rabier D, et al. Combined nutritional support and continuous extracorporeal removal therapy in the severe acute phase of maple syrup urine disease. *Intensive Care Med* 2001;27:1798–806.

23. Jouvet P, Rustin P, Taylor DL, et al. Branched chain amino acids induce apoptosis in neural cells without mitochondrial membrane depolarization or cytochrome c release: Implications for neurological impairment associated with maple syrup urine disease. *Mol Biol Cell* 2000;11:1919–32.

24. Jouvet P, Saudubray J-M, de Pascau L, et al. Décompensation aiguë des maladies héréditaires du métabolisme. In Lacroix J, Gauthier M, Beaufils F. eds. *Urgences et soins intensifs pédiatriques*. Montréal: Presse de l'Université de Montréal, 2006, pp in press.

25. Jouvet P, Touati G, Lesage F, et al. Impact of inborn errors of metabolism on admission and mortality in a pediatric intensive care unit. *Eur J Pediatr* Aug 2006, Epub ahead of print.

26. Kaplan PW. The EEG in metabolic encephalopathy and coma. *J Clin Neurophysiol* 2004;21:307–18.

27. Kato M, Hughes RD, Keays RT, et al. Electron microscopic study of brain capillaries in cerebral edema from fulminant hepatic failure. *Hepatology* 1992;15:1060–6.

28. Kleinschmidt-Demasters BK, Rojiani AM, Filley CM. Central and extrapontine myelinolysis: Then and now. *J Neuropathol Exp Neurol* 2006;65:1–11.

29. Klose DA, Kolker S, Heinrich B, et al. Incidence and short-term outcome of children with symptomatic presentation of organic acid and fatty acid oxidation disorders in Germany. *Pediatrics* 2002;110:1204–11.

30. Kolker S, Mayatepek E, Hoffmann GF. White matter disease in cerebral organic acid disorders: Clinical implications and suggested pathomechanisms. *Neuropediatrics* 2002;33:225–31.

31. Kosenko E, Kaminsky Y, Grau E, et al. Brain ATP depletion induced by acute ammonia intoxication in rats is mediated by activation of the NMDA receptor and Na+,K(+)-ATPase. *J Neurochem* 1994;63:2172–8.

32. Larsen FS, Gottstein J, Blei AT. Cerebral hyperemia and nitric oxide synthase in rats with ammonia-induced brain edema. *J Hepatol* 2001;34:548–54.

33. Lawrence SE, Cummings EA, Gaboury I, et al. Population-based study of incidence and risk factors for cerebral edema in pediatric diabetic ketoacidosis. *J Pediatr* 2005;146:688–92.

34. Leonard JV, Morris AA. Urea cycle disorders. *Semin Neonatol* 2002;7:27–35.

35. Mas A. Hepatic encephalopathy: From pathophysiology to treatment. *Digestion* 2006;73 Suppl 1:86–93.

36. Merker K, Hapke D, Reckzeh K, et al. Copper related toxic effects on cellular protein metabolism in human astrocytes. *Biofactors* 2005;24:255–61.

37. National Institutes of Health. Diagnosis and treatment of Reye's syndrome. *JAMA* 1981;246:2441–4.

38. Ozand PT, Gascon GG, Al Essa M, et al. Biotin-responsive basal ganglia disease: A novel entity. *Brain* 1998;121 (Pt 7):1267–79.

39. Piraud M, Vianey-Saban C, Bourdin C, et al. A new reversed-phase liquid chromatographic/tandem mass spectrometric method for analysis of underivatised amino acids: Evaluation for the diagnosis and the management of inherited disorders of amino acid metabolism. *Rapid Commun Mass Spectrom* 2005;19:3287–97.

40. Poggi-Travert F, Martin D, Billette de Villemeur T, et al. Metabolic intermediates in lactic acidosis: Compounds, samples and interpretation. *J Inherit Metab Dis* 1996;19:478–88.

41. Ratnakumari L, Qureshi IA, Butterworth RF. Effects of congenital hyperammonemia on the cerebral and hepatic levels of the intermediates of energy metabolism in spf mice. *Biochem Biophys Res Commun* 1992;184:746–51.

42. Riviello JJ, Jr., Rezvani I, DiGeorge AM, et al. Cerebral edema causing death in children with maple syrup urine disease. *J Pediatr* 1991;119:42–5.

43. Saudubray JM, Martin D, de Lonlay P, et al. Recognition and management of fatty acid oxidation defects: A series of 107 patients. *J Inherit Metab Dis* 1999;22:488–502.

44. Sgaravatti AM, Rosa RB, Schuck PF, et al. Inhibition of brain energy metabolism by the alpha-keto acids accumulating in maple syrup urine disease. *Biochim Biophys Acta* 2003;1639:232–8.

45. Stabenau JR, Warren KS, Rall DP. The role of pH gradient in the distribution of ammonia between blood and cerebrospinal fluid, brain and muscle. *J Clin Invest* 1959;38:373–83.

46. Tasker R, Poss B, Dean M. Reye syndrome and metabolic encephalopathies. In Rogers M, ed. *The Textbook of Pediatric Intensive Care*, 3rd ed. Baltimore: Williams & Wilkins, 1996:779–807.

47. Tasker RC, Matthew DJ, Kendall B. Computed tomography in the assessment of raised intracranial pressure in non-traumatic coma. *Neuropediatrics* 1990;21:91–4.

48. Traber PG, Dal Canto M, Ganger DR, et al. Electron microscopic evaluation of brain edema in rabbits with galactosamine-induced fulminant hepatic failure: Ultrastructure and integrity of the blood-brain barrier. *Hepatology* 1987;7:1272–7.

49. Vasconcelos MM, Silva KP, Vidal G, et al. Early diagnosis of pediatric Wernicke's encephalopathy. *Pediatr Neurol* 1999;20:289–94.

50. Wagner BP, Pfenninger J. Dynamic cerebral autoregulatory response to blood pressure rise measured by near-infrared spectroscopy and intracranial pressure. *Crit Care Med* 2002;30:2014–21.

51. Warren KS, Nathan DG. The passage of ammonia across the blood-brain-barrier and its relation to blood pH. *J Clin Invest* 1958;37:1724–8.

52. Whitelaw A, Bridges S, Leaf A, et al. Emergency treatment of neonatal hyperammonaemic coma with mild systemic hypothermia. *Lancet* 2001;358:36–8.

CHAPTER 61 ■ BRAIN DEATH

DANIEL L. LEVIN

To place the concept of brain death in proper perspective, one needs to review the history of the definition of death, the criteria used to determine death, and the tests used to determine that the criteria have been fulfilled. This review entails an exploration of the societal, cultural, and legal context in which the definition, criteria, and tests were created and the uncertainty and fears that prevailed concerning a misdiagnosis of death (23). Understanding the difficulty in defining and diagnosing death in combination with the development of whole-organ transplantation helps in explaining the need to create a concept of brain death as a criterion of death in a patient with a beating heart and an intact circulation. Although currently brain death is generally accepted as a criterion of death, we will examine the controversies that are associated with brain death, including whether brain death should be defined as whole brain, higher brain (neocortical), or brainstem death; whether brain death is equivalent to death; and whether the concept should be abandoned and a return to absence of circulation is appropriate.

DEATH

Definition of Death

Recent History

Confusion and anxiety over the diagnosis of death have been attributed to the availability of recently developed technology and its introduction into the modern ICU. Patients who previously would have died with the loss of respiration, heartbeat, and consciousness can now be supported so that ventilation and heartbeat are maintained, even in patients with a persistent, dense coma and the loss of neurologic functions that are clinically associated with death or brain death. Mollaret and Goulon in 1959 coined the term "coma depasse," or a state beyond coma (35), to describe these patients.

The importance of precisely defining death became more apparent in 1967, when at Groote Schuur Hospital in Cape Town, Dr. Christiaan Barnard successfully transplanted the heart of Denise Ann Darvall, a victim of an automobile crash, into Louis Washkansky, a man with terminal heart failure. The procedure was much different from the living related-donor kidney transplant of 1954 or the cadaveric kidney transplants of the 1960s. Denise Ann Darvall was a brain-dead, beating-heart, organ donor, and the transplant provoked a good deal of anxiety about medicine, doctors, and death. *Newsweek* headlined the story "When Are You Really Dead?" on December 18, 1967.

The anxiety over when death occurs has been an issue for a long time and is related to previous technologic advances and other social, professional, and ethical factors. Because of these multiple factors, death has never been completely definable in objective, technical terms. It has always been, at least in part, a subjective and value-based construct (39). The following historic material is derived, in large part, from Pernick (39).

Ancient History

In the past, everyone agreed that death occurred when a person's heartbeat and breathing stopped. However, it was not clear whether the absence of a heartbeat and/or respiration defined death or whether it was an indicator (i.e., criteria) of death. This debate was due in large part to the controversy over the difference between the death of the organism as a whole and the death of the individual parts of the organism. The difficulty was in understanding the distinction between the end of the physical nature of an organism and the end of the personal existence of that organism.

Historically, various observers, including surgeons, soldiers, butchers, and executioners, knew that an organism's body parts did not always die simultaneously and that certain specific organs were crucial to the life of the entire organism. Greek physicians believed that death could begin in the lungs, brain, or heart, but that the heartbeat distinguished between the living and the dead. Hippocrates attributed reason, sensation, and motion to the brain, but held that the heart was the sole indicator of life and death.

For the ancient Hebrews, *ruach,* or breath, was primary, often defined as constituting life itself; this was a dominant view in Christian life as well. Talmudic scholars, however, challenged this view, and some considered the heartbeat a valid indicator of life and death. Maimonides, a 12th-century rabbi and physician, asserted the vital importance of the head. For example, a decapitated body was dead, even if it still moved, because its motions lacked central direction, indicating the guidance of the soul.

Plato believed that both the vitality of the body and the identity of the individual depended on the presence of the immortal soul, distinct in nature from the body. Therefore, the person was the soul, and the body was a tool or vessel used by the soul, and the death of the body was not the same as the death of the soul. Aristotle believed that the person was the integration of the soul and body and that, therefore, the death of the body was the death of the soul. He distinguished two parts of the soul that were responsible for bodily vitality: the vegetative soul of nourishment and growth and the animated soul of motion and sensation.

Physicians not only disagreed on the definition and indicators of death, but also on their application, as well as on diagnostic errors. Pliny, an early observer of physicians, wrote, "That they cannot define even death itself." Galen described diagnoses that were confused with death, including hysteria, asphyxia, coma, and catalepsy. St. Augustine described a monk named Restitutus who could suspend his own heartbeat.

Maimonides thought that it was possible to survive protracted drowning, and Elijah restored breath to a corpse. The absence of a heartbeat and breath as a definition of death became questionable.

In that Hippocratic medical ethics prohibited the medical treatment of terminal patients, the doctor's duty was to forecast impending death and then withdraw without diagnosing or certifying death. Throughout most of Western history, the actual diagnosis of death was performed by individuals other than physicians, and it was important to protect against the misdiagnosis of death. The Talmud prescribed the Jewish tradition of visiting the corpse for 3 days and then checking for the presence of vital signs. During the Great Plague in the 14th century, however, this tradition conflicted with the need for early burial, which prompted a fear of premature internment or being buried alive—a fear almost as great as the fear as the plague itself.

Period of Enlightenment (1740–1850)

During the period of Enlightenment, scientific, social, and ethical factors combined to blur the boundary between life and death, making it frighteningly indistinct. In the 1600s, the Papal physician Paulus Zacchias wrote that no sign prior to the start of putrefaction could reliably distinguish the dead from the living. In 1740, Jacques Benigne Winslow published a dissertation entitled, "The Uncertainty of the Signs of Death and The Danger of Precipitate Internments and Dissections." The surgeon Antoine Louis stated that the onset of rigor mortis was a sufficient diagnostic sign of death.

By the middle of the 19th century, when Edgar Alan Poe wrote *The Fall of the House of Usher* and *The Premature Burial*, the public was panicked by the thought of premature internment. Poe wrote of,

> The unendurable oppression of the lungs—the stifling fumes of the damp earth—the clinging to the death garments—the rigid embrace of the narrow house—the blackness of the absolute Night, the silence like a sea that overwhelms—the unseen but palpable presence of the Conqueror Worm ... a degree of appalling and intolerable horror from which the most daring imagination must recoil.

Poe's descriptions were not merely literary license. Even in the 18th century, medical technology played an important part in fueling intense public concern about premature internment. Artificial respiration was pioneered in France in 1740 and, by 1767, humane societies taught artificial respiration for the resuscitation of drowning and suffocation victims. In the 18th century, resuscitation included the means to revive circulation, sensation, and motion, and drowning victims were given vigorous shakes and thumps to restore the motion of blood. Smelling salts were introduced in 1721 by Leyden, and electric shock was used by Giovanni Bianchi to resuscitate a dog in 1755. Electrical resuscitation of a human occurred in 1774. In a more bizarre experiment in 1803, Giovanni Aldini used electrification on the corpse of an executed convict to demonstrate twitching and wheezing. In 1808, Mary Shelley used Aldini as the source for her literary creation, Doctor Frankenstein. By 1846, the introduction of inhalation anesthesia, which induced a reversible, painless, motionless, coma-like state, added to the confusion of the understanding of life versus death. Public anxiety rose as the distinction between life and death became even more difficult to discern.

Other early technologic advances, long preceding the modern era of intensive care, caused social, scientific, and ethical confusion between the distinction of life and death. In 1701, Anton von Leeuwenhoek reported that many single-cell organisms could survive months of desiccation, and later, Baker and Spallanzani revived worms after several decades of suspended animation. Claude Bernard described "latent life" in plant seeds, while others showed the ability of reptiles and fish to survive long periods of complete freezing. John Hunter and Marshall Hall began to study the phenomenon of hibernation.

To add to the excitement and confusion, in Paris in the 1780s, Anton Mesmer induced in individuals a trance-like state during which the soul seemed to escape the body, leaving the body apparently lifeless or moving about in a zombie-like state. Mesmer actually claimed to restore the dead to life. Could loss of consciousness be added to the loss of breath and heartbeat as unessential to continued life? If so, what was death? Was a new definition of death necessary, or were new tests to establish the criteria of death needed?

Criteria of Death

Certainly if, up to this time, a definition of death could not be clearly established, universally accepted criteria to fulfill a definition were lacking. A variety of criteria, including lack of heart beat, breath, circulation, or consciousness, and cessation of vital functions, were accepted, and a variety of tests was utilized to fulfill these criteria.

Tests of Death

With the view that "when the vital functions cease, life is extinct," the medical community of the 18th century was compelled to develop better, more sensitive tests to detect vital functions. Investigations led to an evolution from tests for lack of respiration and circulation as criteria that fulfilled the definition of death to tests that explore brain death or lack of consciousness and central integrative function as criteria that fulfilled the definition of death. Tests for respiration included holding a mirror, candle, or feather to the nose, submerging the body in water and watching for bubbles, putting a bowl of liquid on the chest, auscultating with the recently invented stethoscope, or holding a hygrometer to the nose to test for the presence of humidity. Tests for circulation included palpating the pulse or listening to the pulse with a stethoscope, opening an artery, or looking for livid spots, pallid skin, depressed loins, and sunken eyeballs. A combination of a slack jaw, unblinking eye, and relaxed sphincters indicated a loss of muscular irritability. Coldness meant loss of "vital heat."

The application of chemicals that normally produced skin blisters but failed to do so on dead patients, showed the loss of the body's inflammatory response. Failure to respond to artificial ventilation gained acceptance as a test fulfilling the criterion of death. When proposed by Charles Kite in 1788 as a test to indicate death, the failure of the body to twitch in response to electrical stimulation may have been the distant ancestor of the flat electroencephalogram (EEG). Smelling salts and the blowing of a trumpet in the ears of patients who were assumed dead were tests that were also employed.

Toward Brain Death as a Criterion

The use of rigor mortis and putrefaction as tests of death were questioned by those individuals who believed that suspended animation might actually suspend life in a recoverable form. But in the 18th century, the Scottish physician William Cullen focused attention on the neurophysiologic work of Heller and concluded that "nervous sensibility" and "muscular irritability" were the principles of life and perhaps the essences of life itself. In 1774, he wrote, "The living state depends on a certain condition in the nerves and muscle fibres by which they are sensible and irritable. It is this condition, therefore, which may be properly called the vital principle in animals." This concept that life was sensorimotor potential and not cardiopulmonary action was the distant relation of brain death. The first case of "brain death" in an organism maintained on a "respirator" with a functioning circulation may have been described by William Harvey, who preserved the circulation and respiration of a decapitated rooster in 1627.

During the Age of Enlightenment, the separateness of the mind and body gained importance. For René Descartes, the human body and the human self were totally distinct. Descartes believed that the body died at the instant of its separation from the soul, located in the pineal gland, but that the soul survived beyond the body. Robert Whytt thought the soul to be dispersed throughout the nervous system. Georges Buffon further decentralized individual life by postulating that all living creatures were composed of living "molecules." Marie-Francois-Xavier Bichat distinguished "organic life"—the heart, lung, and other functions that maintain metabolism—from "animal life"—sensation and volition of the brain. He stated, "The patient may live internally for several days after he has ceased to exist beyond himself." But A.P.W. Philip singled out the body's powers of sensation and volition, which were located in the brain, as defining the life of the whole individual. Thus began the movement toward brain death as the criterion of death.

Technical difficulties, however, hampered the medical establishment from defining brain death at this point. The apparent privacy of other people's mental states left 19th-century physicians no practical way to invoke a definition of death based on the absence of mental activity. Even if they could agree on the loss of neurologic functions to define death, and even if the demonstration of the loss of this function could meet a criterion sufficient to meet such a definition, physicians still had no test to establish that the criterion was fulfilled.

Societal Considerations

Misdiagnosis of Death. The public was panicked at the thought of false diagnosis of death, not only because of its fear of premature burial, but because of its fear of premature withdrawal of life-giving resuscitation, therapy, or palliation. By contrast, the misdiagnosis of a dead person as alive would delay burying the dead and would spread disease. Saving a single individual from premature burial at the cost of exposing thousands to contagion from delayed internment was another concern. However, premature abandonment of a patient was considered equivalent to murder, and it was believed that the killing of one patient was far worse than continuing to treat a thousand corpses.

The fear of premature burial had a strong influence on the fear of misdiagnosis or falsely diagnosed death. Waiting periods for burial extended from religious tradition to law. In Munich, as well as other cities, bodies were placed in open caskets with a bell rope placed in their hands to signal if they awoke. The architecture of the building that kept these bodies permitted a centrally stationed guard to observe most of the guests, and individual examinations were performed twice each hour around the clock, with artificial resuscitation devices always at hand. Escapable, alarmed, and provisioned coffins that included signal bells and flags, speaking tubes, and even automated ejection devices were designed. A coffin invented by Russian Count Michael de Karnice-Karnicki and patented in Berlin in 1897 was triggered by a glass ball placed directly on the buried person's chest. Any movement of the ball activated a spring trigger, which in turn opened an air duct, turned on an electric lamp, rang a bell for half an hour, and raised a flag 4 feet above the ground. In order to prevent premature burial, blood letting, embalming, autopsy, cremation, and decapitation prior to burial became common practice. Religious, cultural, and national differences all came to play in the debate concerning premature burial.

The Experts. A component of professional self-interest became prominent in the late 19th century. Although it was not originally the physician's duty to diagnose and pronounce death, tests for death became increasingly more complicated for laymen to understand and verify. In addition to those tests already discussed, the stethoscope was improved, electrical tests became more sophisticated, and body temperature was measured. High-intensity lights were used to examine the skin between the fingers for signs of circulation, microphones amplified chest sounds, radiographic fluoroscopy searched for the motion of vital organs, and the ophthalmoscope was used to examine the circulation of the retina. Time-lapse photography could record the reaction of pupillary reflex irritability to atropine and belladonna. Ammonia was injected subcutaneously to see if preserved metabolic function turned the eyeballs bright green. A shiny, metal needle stuck into living muscle would rust. Skin was burned, a nipple pincher was used to test pain, and a long needle with a flag on it was jabbed into the heart to detect its motion. A gentleman ironically named Spilsbury favored opening a blood vessel to see if circulation remained.

To add to the technological difficulties, experts made new discoveries that blurred the boundaries of life and death even more. In 1880, Sidney Ringer showed that a heart removed from a frog could be kept alive in a salt solution. People wondered if all of the separate parts of an organism could be kept alive in vitro. Charles Scott Sherrington, the conceptual founder of modern neurophysiology, distinguished the life of an organism from the lives of its parts, in that the organism had the ability to integrate and coordinate these parts—a capability vertebrates exercise through their nerves.

Was all of the anxiety based on rational fears? Were false-positive diagnoses being made? Were people buried alive? It is an inherently untestable—nonfalsifiable—hypothesis. No study can be designed to prove that any testing method can prevent the possibility of making a false positive diagnosis of death.

The Modern Era: Transplantation. By the 1920s, Alexis Carrel showed the medical profession how to perform kidney transplants in animals, and blood transfusions were being performed in humans. The EEG was invented in 1929, and the Russians discovered that animals, including humans, could survive deep cold for more than 1 hr without vital signs. Cardiopulmonary resuscitation was introduced, Edward Drinker built the first mechanical respirator, and electrical defibrillation was invented. The first renal transplant between 2 living people occurred in 1954, and that returns us to Denise Ann Darvall.

Between 1967 and today, people have continued to be afraid of being wrongly declared dead as well as being wrongly declared alive. A patient can be in a coma, without a functioning heart, lungs, kidneys, or gastrointestinal tract, with a donor liver, a reversed coagulation system, a blocked immune system, and a paralyzed musculoskeletal system, and still be "alive." No wonder the public and the health profession are alarmed and confused. What does it mean to be dead? What are the criteria of death? What tests fulfill the criteria? Does the meaning of death change over time (39)?

BRAIN DEATH AS A CRITERION OF DEATH

Current Status

According to Bernat (12), the analysis of death should proceed in three phases: (a) the definition of death, which makes explicit the traditional implicit concept of death; (b) the measurable criterion of death that is both necessary and sufficient for death that can be employed in a death statute; and (c) the development and validation of tests for death to show conclusively that the criterion has been fulfilled. He argues that the definition is primarily philosophic, the criterion is both philosophic and medical, and the tests are primarily medical.

Definition of Death

Bernat proffers five assumptions concerning the definition of death (12):

- Death is a nontechnical word that is used broadly in common language, and any definition should capture this common understanding as a univocal term; for example, the death of a dog should have the same meaning as the death of a human being.
- Death is primarily a biologic phenomenon.
- Death is irreversible; for example, patients who undergo successful cardiopulmonary resuscitation have not returned from the dead, but from dying.
- Death is understood as an event and not as a process; death is not dying. When one is dead disintegration occurs.
- The event of death should be determinable by physicians (using tests to fulfill criteria) to have occurred at some specific time, at least in retrospect. Physicians should be able to distinguish a living organism from a dead one.

Brain Death as a Criterion of Death

In defense of the whole-brain concept as a criterion of death, Bernat and his colleagues define death as the permanent cessation of critical functions of the organism as a whole, not the whole organism. They refer to that set of vital functions of integration, control, and behavior that are greater than the sum of the parts of the organism and that operate in response to demands from the organism's internal and external milieu to support its life and maintain its health. Critical functions of the organism as a whole involve three distinct biologic categories: (a) vital functions of spontaneous breathing and autonomic control of the circulation, (b) integrating functions that assure homeostasis, and (c) consciousness, which is required for the organism to respond to requirements for nutrition, protection, and other needs. The critical functions of all three categories must be permanently lost for the organism to be dead. If this definition was met by certain criteria and tests were devised to fulfill the criteria, the circumstance could then exist in which death was nonoverlapping with life; they would be dichotomous and jointly exhausting. One is either alive or dead but not both (12).

According to Veatch (59), in his defense of the higher brain (neocortical) criterion of brain death, defining death, "Is not a trivial exercise in coining the meaning of a term. Rather it is an attempt to reach an understanding of the philosophic nature of man and that which is essentially significant to man which is lost at the time of death."

In an article entitled, "The Impending Collapse of The Whole Brain Definition of Death," Veatch argues that no one really believes that literally all functions of the entire brain must be lost for an individual to be dead and that a better definition of death involves a higher (neocortical) brain orientation (60). The persistence of some blood flow to the brain, some electrical activity on EEG, and some endocrine functions of the brain in individuals who have been tested and meet the whole-brain criterion of death creates doubt about the validity of the whole-brain criterion, which is why Bernat included the words *critical functions* in his definition. Veatch also states that the term "brain death" (his quotes) is ambiguous because it fails to distinguish between the biologic claim that the brain is dead and the social/legal/moral claim that the individual as a whole is dead because the brain is dead. Veatch believes that,

> It should be clear by now that the definition of death debate is actually a debate over the moral status of human beings. It is a debate over when humans should be treated as full members of the human community. When humans are living, full, moral, and legal rights accrue. Saying people are alive is simply short hand for saying they are bearers of such rights. That is why the definition of death debate is so important.

In contrast to the higher (neocortical) and whole-brain criteria, Pallis in the UK indicates that what is important is identifying what allows the brain to function as a unit, and that is the brainstem (37). In fact, the bedside clinical tests, which are considered by many sufficient to diagnose brain death, center on brainstem function. Although this view has wide acceptance in the UK, it is not generally accepted elsewhere.

In considering the validity of the whole-brain criteria of death, investigators wonder why the criteria and tests arbitrarily stop at the base of the skull (49,50,60). Why is the important role of the spinal cord in integrative functions of the central nervous system excluded? To add to this complicated debate about brain death, whether it be whole, higher, or stem, with or without the spinal cord, as a valid criterion of death, some agree with Shewmon, Taylor, and Truog that brain death is not equivalent to death (50,55,57). Shewmon argues that it is not and that, in fact, "... the notion of 'brain death' as bodily death is logically and physiologically incoherent, and that its replacement by something scientifically more credible would promote not only the sanctity of life, but ironically even transplantation as well" (50). He promotes a "circulatory-respiratory" criterion. Taylor argues that brain death is a social construct devised primarily for the utilitarian purpose of permitting organ transplantation (55). He supports a return to absence of circulation as the acceptable biologic definition of death. Truog also supports the position, calling the concept of brain death incoherent in theory and confused in practice and that the only purpose served by the concept is the facilitation of procurement of transplantable organs (57). Hanley agrees, stating that, while the consensus criteria for whole-brain death as the criterion for the definition of death are helpful, "They remain (perhaps of social necessity) without a prospective validation and are therefore prescriptive definitions rather than empirically validated criteria" (26). Cranford restates the question that many scholars pose, "...as to why brain death should be considered equivalent to cardiorespiratory death as the death of a human being" (18).

According to Schrader, and in contrast to Bernat and Veatch, what is lost at the time of death that is significant to man is personhood (52). However, the person is not simply a person but a biologic organism as well. If not, death of the neocortex in the biologically functioning organism (i.e., the persistent vegetative state) would be defined as death. Those who argue against the neocortical definition of death point out that if this were an accepted criterion for the definition of death, it would lead to dead individuals who are breathing either spontaneously (persistent vegetative state) or with mechanical assistance and could be buried as such. Would they be buried still attached to the mechanical ventilator? Several authors indicate that this would pose aesthetic problems and that breathing should be stopped probably with medications prior to burial. Alternatively, a person is not simply a biologic organism, but also a person. If not, the integrated function of the brain would be irrelevant, and the person in a persistent vegetative state would be a living, normal person (52). A human is a composite of two intimately related but conceptually distinguishable components. Human beings are biologic entities (*Homo sapiens*) and persons. As such, we are subject to more than one death: a death as a biologic entity and a death as a person, which is a different sort of death (52). This is in contrast to Bernat's position of a singular death.

Biologic death is the cessation of the processes of biologic synthesis and replication. Partial biologic death is the complete, irreversible cessation of function in a specific portion of the biologic organism. Complete biologic death is the complete, irreversible cessation of all biologic functions, including the synthetic (reproductive and transformative) operations of all organs and cells. The biologic death of the organism is the irreversible loss of integration of the biologic units, irrespective of the independent functioning and/or viability of some or all of those units. The death of a person occurs when the body ceases to be a person, to encase a person, or to be uniquely associated with a person (52).

Reasons for Having Criteria of Death

If we can understand as important and accept a definition of death, why have criteria for death? Criteria must be agreed upon so that tests can be used to fulfill the criteria and pronounce a patient dead. The pronouncement of death enables society to engage in death behavior. The public can regard the person as a corpse, the grieving process can begin, and religious rites, funerals, and burials can proceed. Legally, the pronounce-

ment of death allows for the reading of wills, distribution of inheritance and property, payment of insurance, remarriage, succession, and—if the criteria of brain death are fulfilled—organ donation (52).

Beyond awaiting the onset of putrefaction, or rigor mortis, the absence of heartbeat and/or respiration would be enough of a criterion (or criteria) to define biologic death, if it were not for technology and the medical need for viable, whole organs for transplantation. Even with the advances in technology over many decades, there would be little concern for establishing criteria to define death and devise tests to ensure that the criteria have been fulfilled if we could state that the human being has suffered either biologic death (partial or complete) or suffered the death of the person, then disconnect the human being from all support, await the cessation of heartbeat and/or respiration, and pronounce him dead (24). It could be that way, if not for organ transplantation. In fact, in one study in the US (62), diagnoses of brain death (23%) were less frequent than the discontinuation of support (32%) and do-not-resuscitate status (26%) and were similar to failed cardiopulmonary resuscitation (19%). This is similar to studies in European countries, but brain death is diagnosed less frequently in South American countries. Protocols have been developed for non-beating heart, whole-organ procurement and have gained increasing support recently. In most cases, successful organ transplantation for the recipient still depends on the hemodynamic stability of the beating-heart donor (46). What is needed is a criterion of death that allows a physician to perform tests to fulfill the criterion while the patient (i.e., donor) is still hemodynamically stable. We return to the earlier attempts to define death as the loss of both the organism's biologic life and the loss of personhood—and the integrative functions of that biologic life—which together make up a human being.

In 1968, the Harvard criteria were established (**Table 61.1**), and they were followed by several other sets of criteria, each with their own variations (1). All of these criteria were based on the concept of whole-brain death (which included the brainstem) and not neocortical death, with all or part of the brainstem left intact. Thus, patients in a persistent vegetative state were excluded.

The criteria of United Kingdom Royal Colleges and Faculties of medicine do not recommend any confirmatory tests (16) and, in an analysis of 25 moribund patients, it was concluded that brain death can be established solely on clinical grounds (34). In their review of brain death in the PICU, Rowland

---

TABLE 61.1

HARVARD CRITERIA FOR BRAIN DEATH (1968)

1. Unresponsiveness, temperature $>32.2°C$
2. Absence of depressant drugs
3. No spontaneous movements
4. Apnea off respirator for 3 mins at room air
5. Absence of brainstem reflexes, including
   Decerebrate or decorticate posturing
   Pupils-fixed and dilated
   No swallowing or vocalization
   No corneal or pharyngeal reflexes
   No stretch or deep tendon reflexes
6. Isoelectric electroencephalogram
7. All of the above should be repeated after 24 hrs

et al. supported the concept of brain death, using clinical criteria alone (45). In that all of the currently used ancillary studies have limitations and are not pathognomonic for brain death and, since brain death can be determined reasonably by clinical examination, we should not rely exclusively on unreliable tests to support diagnoses.

The apnea test is a clinical test that is commonly used. Although in the 1980s, several attempts were made to standardize the tests and prevent cardiorespiratory deterioration by giving 100% oxygen to the patient during the test, a great deal of variability seems to exist in the way the test is performed, and some authors have questioned the accuracy of the test and the consistency of its application (58).

No large prospective studies validate the clinical diagnosis of brain death. Therefore, clinical protocols are, even if logical, somewhat arbitrary. A major problem with using protocols to make the clinical diagnosis of brain death has been inconsistency in their use, even within institutions and ICUs. It is probably most important to have the clinicians agree upon a protocol and meticulously adhere to it.

The Harvard criteria applied mostly, although not exclusively, to adults, and the debate about whether they applied to children or infants (especially preterm infants) was put aside by the National Collaborative Study and the President's Commission (41,43), which excluded from the criteria children <5 yrs of age. Since 1968, much discussion has focused on four questions:

- Do the adult criteria apply to infants and children?
- Are ancillary tests necessary or even capable of establishing the criteria of brain death beyond the history, physical examination, and exclusion of confounding variables?
- Are there appropriate time intervals between triggering event(s), the physical examination of death, the ancillary tests, and the pronouncement of death?
- Is the whole-brain death definition of death the only acceptable one, or are there exceptions to this criterion?

Do the Adult Criteria of Brain Death Apply to Infants and Children?

Although some have suggested that the adult criteria do not apply to children (44), that children of different ages have different tests, or that the combination of differently aged children and different tests requires different waiting periods, most authors now generally agree that, except in very immature, preterm newborns, the same criteria of brain death apply to full-term newborns, infants >7 days of age, children, and adults (7,8,9). Those rare examples in which certain infants seem to recover after fulfilling the criteria and test for brain death are open to question. Only in premature infants and the newly born are the criteria not generally accepted.

The Special Task Force excluded infants of <1 week from its guidelines for brain death in infants and children (44). Volpe addressed the issue of making a diagnosis of brain death in the newborn (63). First, if the injury occurred in utero, the duration of the insult and severity may be difficult to establish. Second, the issue of hypotension as a regulator of brain function is difficult to assess, considering what normal systemic arterial blood pressure may be. Third, EEG and cranial ultrasound may not be 100% reliable in the newborn. Fourth, because

of immaturity, the clinical examination cannot be relied upon. At the time of examination, some of the brainstem reflexes may be in evolution or may not even have yet developed. The clinical courses of preterm and term infants <1 month of age in whom brain death was diagnosed were reviewed (9). Five preterm infants ranging in gestation from 29 to 36 weeks met the clinical criteria of brain death. However, 3 patients who had electrocerebral inactivity on EEG demonstrated cerebral blood flow (CBF) on radionuclide scanning. The other 2 patients had electrocerebral activity but absent CBF, and therefore, no correlation existed between EEG and isotope estimation of CBF. It was concluded that the diagnosis of brain death could be established in the preterm and term infant after a neurologic assessment, an EEG showing electrocerebral inactivity, and isotope estimation of CBF, followed by 24 hrs of observation. The accuracy of the clinical examination in small infants is questioned in a frequently quoted reference (38), which discusses a premature infant who sustained an intraventricular hemorrhage on day 2 of life and showed the absence of brainstem reflexes, apnea, and flaccidity, but was never clinically brain dead. However, except for the urgency of organ transplantation from anencephalic donors and a few isolated cases in other full-term newborns, the need to test and fulfill the criteria of death as brain death in small and young infants is relatively rare.

Ancillary Tests to Fulfill the Criteria of Brain Death

Although many authors believe that the clinical diagnosis of brain death based on history, physical examination, and an apnea test is sufficient, in some cases (e.g., barbiturate levels greater than the therapeutic range), one may wish to have ancillary tests available to expedite the ability to diagnose brain death.

Currently, various tests are used to document brain death and, as discussed previously, some tests (EEG, brainstem auditory evoked responses) may even have their roots in tests developed during the last century (Table 61.2). With the possible exception of a four-vessel cerebral angiography test showing no CBF, no test is absolutely confirmatory of brain death and can only be consistent with the diagnosis and, therefore, used to supplement the clinical impression, not to make the diagnosis. Frequently, examples of disparities can be found between the clinical examination and test results and between differing kinds of tests. In addition, specialists may disagree on the interpretation of the same test.

If one chooses to utilize ancillary tests to confirm the diagnosis of brain death, those tests available include all of the examinations indicated in **Table 61.2**, although EEG and radionuclide brain scanning are currently the two most frequently used tests.

Electroencephalography

The American Electroencephalographic Society's suggested guidelines for EEG are: the EEG must be performed over a 30-min period by a qualified technician, using a minimum of eight scalp- and ear-reference electrodes with interelectrode distances of 10 cm; the machine sensitivity must be >2 $\mu v/mm$, with electrode resistance between 100 and 10,000 ohms; the

TABLE 61.2

ANCILLARY TESTS TO CONFIRM BRAIN DEATH

Test	Clinical disparity
Electroencephalogram	Yes
Cerebral angiogram	Yes
Radionuclide angiogram	Yes
^{123}I-IMP and Tc-^{99}mHMPAO	Yes
Xenon CT	Yes
Brainstem evoked responses (somatic, visual, auditory)	Yes
P-31 MRI, PET	Yes
Doppler sonography	Yes
Intracranial pressure monitoring	Yes
Endocrinologic function of the brain	Yes

For detailed list of references to these tests, see Farrell MM, Levin DL. Brain death in the pediatric patient: Historical, sociological, medical, religious, cultural, legal, and ethical considerations. Crit Care Med 1993;21:1951.
^{123}I-IMP, N-isopropyl-(^{123}I) p-iodoamphetamine; Tc-^{99}mHMPAO, technetium-^{99}m hexamethyl-propyleneamine oxime; PET, positron emission tomography

auditory and photic stimuli and reactivity to pain must be tested during the recording; and the electrocerebral inactivity cannot be determined using telephone EEGs (4). Technically, the EEG may be difficult to perform on infants and small children, thus weighing against it as a confirmatory test of brain death. In the PICU, the EEG may show multiple artifacts, which are bizarre and difficult to identify and locate. Maintenance of an interelectrode distance of 10 cm may be difficult, resulting in failure to detect very low-voltage activity. An isoelectric EEG, when performed on a premature infant or asphyxiated newborn, must be interpreted with extreme caution. Ashwal and Schneider, in their experience of five neonates, found diffuse 2–4μv activity on EEG, despite absent radionuclide isotope bolus studies (6). These infants were clinically brain dead (comatose, apneic, absence of cephalic reflexes). In a review of 18 brain-dead neonates, 9 had electrocerebral inactivity on EEG (9). Electrocerebral inactivity resolved in one, who had an increased circulating phenobarbital level. Of the remaining 9 infants who had EEG activity, 5 developed electrocerebral inactivity, 3 continued to have activity, and 1 had cardiac arrest. They concluded that electrocerebral inactivity on an EEG in the absence of barbiturates, hypothermia, or cerebral malformations was confirmatory of brain death if the clinical findings remained unchanged throughout 24 hrs. In a review of 56 patients with a clinical diagnosis of brain death, on whom a total of 80 EEGs were performed, residual electrocerebral activity was observed in 11 (19.6%) patients for as long as 168 hrs after the onset of the clinical diagnosis. All clinically brain-dead patients died (25).

Drug intoxication from barbiturates, diazepam, meprobamate, methaqualone, trichloroethylene, and succinylcholine may specifically cause electrocerebral inactivity. In addition, there is a 3% discordance between those who interpret the records. Therefore, the validity of the EEG is in question, since the presence of EEG activity does not rule out the possibility of brain death any more than electrocerebral inactivity is unequivocal evidence of it. When a patient is clinically brain dead, the outcome is death, irrespective of the presence or absence of EEG activity.

Cerebral Arteriogram

Although the absence of CBF on four-vessel cerebral arteriography is irrefutable evidence of brain death, the converse is not true, and a patient can be brain dead and have demonstrable flow. Nonfilling cerebral vessels on two aortocranial injections of contrast media 25 mins apart is required by the Swedish Criteria for brain death (29). Even with all of the technical and logistical difficulties encountered in performing cerebral angiography, when the patient is in a barbiturate coma, only the arteriogram can be used to diagnose brainstem death without the necessity of waiting several days for barbiturate levels to fall below the upper limit of therapeutic levels. Angiography will detect CBF, even though it may be suppressed by as much as 40% during barbiturate coma. In all other circumstances, however, examination remains the "gold standard" for the diagnosis of brain death.

Radionuclide Brain Scanning

Radionuclide brain scanning consists of IV injection of ^{99}mTc pertechnetate, which passes through the cervical circulation into the intracranial vault. A tourniquet is placed around the patient's forehead to exclude detection of scalp circulation, and images are obtained with a portable γ-scintillation camera. Demonstration of the absence of intracranial circulation is confirmatory evidence of brain death.

The presence of sagittal sinus activity in the absence of intracranial arterial circulation does not exclude the diagnosis of brain death. This technique has the advantage of simplicity; however, its efficacy has not been proven in the premature infant and young child <2 months of age. Another disadvantage of this technique is that CBF in the premature infant may be only 12 mL/100 g/min, while the test assesses only flow to the cerebral hemispheres. In addition, the brainstem cannot be evaluated, and a negative radioisotopic bolus study implies only that cerebral perfusion is <24% of the normal predicted blood flow (29). Therefore, neither the EEG nor the radionuclide scan can replace examination of the cranial reflexes.

In a review of 18 preterm and term infants, 17 of whom underwent radionuclide scanning, two conclusions were drawn (9). First, in newborns, the combination of a negative radionuclide study and simultaneous electrocerebral inactivity is tantamount to brain death at the time of study. Second, imperfect correlation was noted between EEG and isotope studies in preterm infants. In a study of 18 pediatric patients who ranged in age from 6 months to 13 years, investigators reported absent flow in 8 patients, faint visualization of the sagittal sinus in 2 patients, and normal flow in 8 patients (28). All 8 patients with absent flow were clinically brain dead with electrocerebral inactivity on EEG. Of those patients who showed normal flow, 1 had full neurologic recovery, 1 persisted in a vegetative state, and the remaining 6 died. In another study of 9 brain dead children between 13 months and 13 yrs, 100% correlation was demonstrated between radionuclide cerebral imaging and four-vessel cerebral angiography (47).

Therefore, absent flow on radionuclide cerebral imaging in a clinically brain-dead patient who also shows electrocerebral inactivity on EEG is confirmatory of brain death. Radionuclide cerebral imaging is helpful only if it demonstrates the absence of flow.

Brainstem Auditory-Evoked Responses

Brainstem auditory-evoked responses have been used to test the integrity of the anatomic pathway of hearing. This test can be performed with portable equipment at the bedside, where electrodes are placed over the mastoids and the vertex, with sound delivered to each ear via headphones or tubal inserts. In normal individuals, waves I through V are visible. However, brain-dead patients demonstrate the absence of all waves, although the presence of wave I may not be incompatible with this diagnosis. Wave I indicates that the peripheral auditory mechanism is intact. A study of 23 comatose children, 10 of whom had clinical examinations consistent with brain death, demonstrated the absence of waves I through VII in 9 patients (54). Wave I was present in the remaining patient. All 10 patients died, and 13 patients who were comatose showed at least 2 identifiable waveforms. In their case report of 2 infants who suffered severe neurologic impairment with the absence of brainstem auditory-evoked responses but who subsequently recovered, Dear and Godfrey believed the absence of brainstem auditory-evoked responses was not a confirmatory test of brain death (20). We conclude that, at present, the use of brainstem auditory-evoked responses cannot confirm a diagnosis of brain death. Brainstem auditory-evoked responses may be abolished for several reasons in individuals who are not dead; for example, injury to the cochlear nerve from head trauma and various causes of sensorineural hearing loss, including meningitis.

The other methods of investigation, which include visualization of cerebral arterial pulsations by real time and cranial Doppler ultrasonography, xenon CT and CBF determination, assessment of cerebral metabolic function on MRI, positron emission tomography, and heart rate variability analysis (13), may be supportive of brain death but are not currently used in lieu of EEG, radionuclide scanning, or arteriogram.

Time Intervals of Observation and Testing

The Task Force recommended observation periods according to age (44). For infants ranging in age from 7 days to 2 months, it recommended two examinations and EEGs separated by at least 48 hrs. However, if one examination demonstrates the absence of flow on a radionuclide study, the second examination and EEG may be omitted. For infants >1 yr of age, an observation period of at least 12 hrs in the presence of an irreversible cause is necessary, although a longer period of 24 hrs may be required in certain instances (hypoxic-ischemic encephalopathy). As in infants ranging in age between 7 days and 2 months, however, if the EEG is isoelectric or the radionu-

clide study demonstrates no flow, the observation period may be shortened. The major consideration with all of these recommendations is that the physical examination must remain consistent with brain death throughout the observation. Ashwal and Schneider noted that term infants who were clinically brain dead for 2 days and preterm infants who were brain dead for 3 days did not survive despite EEG or CBF status (9).

In summary, three separate observation periods are recommended, depending on the child's age and the result of a laboratory test (**Table 61.3**). However, we question the existence of a distinct, definable difference between the brain of a 2-month-old and that of a 3-month-old, which justifies the recommendation to lengthen the evaluation period by 24 hrs. In addition, we believe brain death is a clinical diagnosis and, therefore, would not alter the length of the observation period based on the result of a laboratory test. Further, except for the preterm and newly born infant, age-related criteria may complicate the evaluation unnecessarily. The diagnosis of brain death usually takes place in the PICU, where it takes many hours to complete a thorough history and physical examination, achieve normothermia and normotension, and exclude toxic and metabolic disorders. As a practical matter, then, a 12-hr observation period seems a reasonable time to observe the patient. Some authors note an absence of valid data for all of the recommendations concerning time intervals, age, and tests therefore, the clinical examination is still the most important determination of brain death (24).

In that questions concerning infant versus adult criteria—which tests and at what intervals—remain so perplexing, a prospective study to answer them should be designed. However, Shewmon pointed out that designing a study to absolutely ensure the diagnosis of brain death with no possibility of a false diagnosis is difficult at best (48). He describes a hypothetical confirmatory study in which all of the patients who fulfilled the criterion of brain death as diagnostic of death did experience brain death (irreversibility). For this analysis, he used Bayesian methodology, which proves that, for N in the range of a large clinical study, estimations of prior probabilities are, for all practical purposes, irrelevant to the calculation of the posterior probabilities. The risk of a false-positive diagnosis for the next patient who meets the criterion is ~$1/(N+2)$. The chance of at least one false-positive diagnosis among the next $(N+1)$ patient who meets the criterion is ~50%. Thus, achievement of the requisite moral certainty of a declaration of death (irreversibility) necessitates an impossibly large N for the study. He stated, however, that, "This does not mean that one cannot diagnose death, but rather that the validity of the diagnostic criteria must be self-evident on a priori grounds, and that

TABLE 61.3

TIME INTERVALS NECESSARY FOR DIAGNOSING BRAIN DEATH

Age	Conditions/tests	Time interval
<7 days	N/A	N/A
>7 days–2 months	Physical exam, two electroencephalograms	48 hrs
>7 days–2 months	Physical exam, radionucleotide test with no flow	24 hrs
2 months–1 year	Physical exam: two electroencephalograms	24 hrs
>1 year	Physical exam: irreversible cause	12 hrs
>1 year	Physical exam; hypoxic-ischemic encephalopathy	24 hrs

confirmatory studies are necessarily inadequate or superfluous." In addition, Bernat (11) reminded us that, "One must be flexible and understand that even with the finest tools technology has to offer, the diagnosis of 'whole-brain' death is probably an approximation."

Why not try to do the study anyway? To return to Shewmon's Bayesian analysis, "to have a 99.999% certainty that P_{true} is at least 99.999%, we need a study with over 1 million patients who meet the criteria and who all have proven brain death (irreversibility)" (48).

In addition to the previously mentioned issue of residual brain blood flow, electrical activity, and endocrinologic function in patients diagnosed as brain dead by current testing, another interesting controversy lies in the acceptance of brain death as a criterion of death and acceptance of the Harvard criteria as valid tests to conclusively prove that brain death is equivalent to the death of a person. The controversy involves the idea of persistent or chronic brain death (51,53).

Even though it is frequently stated that patients who are clinically brain dead do not live for more than a few weeks, even with maximum support, prolonged survival of 175 patients for at least 1 week has been documented (51). Approximately 80 patients survived at least 2 weeks, ~44 survived at least 4 weeks, ~20 at least 2 months, and 7 at least 6 months. Fifty-six cases had sufficient individual information for a meta-analysis and calculation of actuarial survival curves; they were divided into 2 subgroups: those supported indefinitely with spontaneous cardiac arrest (36 cases and 1 still surviving) and those from whom treatment was withdrawn (19 cases). Survivals occurred up to 14.5 years. A rapid drop off in survival curves with a subsequent slow decline was seen, with the transition occurring at 5 to 6 months. The study concludes that cardiovascular instability in patients diagnosed as brain dead is not inevitable. "The tendency to asystole with brain death can be transient and is attributable more to systemic factors than to absence of brain function per se. If brain death is to be equated with death, it must be on some basis more plausible than loss of somatic integrative unit (51)."

Spike and Greenlaw documented a patient who, after a prolonged hypoxic episode secondary to status asthmaticus, was readmitted to the PICU 6 months after undergoing a valid evaluation and being diagnosed as brain dead (53).

Although Bernat (12) is probably correct that currently whole-brain death is generally accepted as a criterion of death and that the Harvard criteria and some ancillary testing fulfill the criterion of whole-brain death, it is certainly important to note that reasonable debate exists as to the validity of the argument for brain death including whole-brain death as a sufficient criterion of death.

CULTURAL, RELIGIOUS, AND LEGAL CONSIDERATIONS IN BRAIN DEATH

Cultural Consideration

In many societies, the concept of brain death is recognized and accepted as a sufficient criterion of death for medical and legal purposes. In many others, the concept is recognized but not accepted. Certainly it is not accepted as equivalent to the

death of a person in all societies. Even when accepted medically and legally, it is not the most common mode of declaring death in PICUs. In a study of 6000 patients, 300 died (62). The mode of death was discontinuation of support in 95 (32%), do-not-resuscitate status in 78 (26%), brain death in 70 (23%), and failed cardiopulmonary resuscitation in 57 (19%). The modes of death are remarkably similar in studies in European and North American countries (32), but not in South America (3,31). It is not known from these studies how many patients may have met brain death criteria but died in another way due to family or physician wishes and lack of acceptance of the concept of brain death.

Cultural differences certainly influence the acceptance of brain death as a criterion of death. These differences may be deep-seated and based in religion or societal norms, but they also may be as simple as the practical consideration of availability of resources. In some countries (e.g., Japan), brain death is officially recognized, but the public harbors a deep-seated resistance to it. This resistance is grounded in a different view of life and death in that the function of the child's brain is not of the utmost importance; rather, existence of the child in itself is meaningful and should be respected whether or not her brain is dead.

Religious Beliefs

Most religions have taken a stance on brain death. In Jewish orthodoxy, human life is sacred; therefore, premature termination of life is unacceptable. However, the determination of death by absent heartbeat is not always a prerequisite to death, since respiration can also be considered central to the maintenance of life. In a review of brain death and organ transplantation, brain death was described as analogous to physiologic rather than physical decapitation (61). Brain death can be declared in the absence of spontaneous respiration and brain function. Death of the brain at a cellular level for each and every brain cell is not necessary for confirmation of brain death. Once death has been confirmed by either the classic or brain-death criteria, no biblical obligation exists to maintain treatment or artificial support of the corpse. In 1987, the chief rabbinate of Israel accepted performance of heart transplantation based upon the declaration of brain death of the donor (42).

In Catholic teaching, according to which death occurs when the soul departs the body, the problem is determining the moment of death. Pope Pius XII addressed a group of anesthesiologists in 1957 on this issue, saying, "It remains for the doctor, and especially the anesthesiologist, to give a clear and precise definition of 'death' and 'the moment of death' of a patient who passes away in a state of unconsciousness" (40). Nothing in the Bible or in official church teaching prohibits using death of the entire brain as a reliable sign of the person's death (36). Concerning the terminally unconscious patient, Pope Pius XII stated, "It is incumbent on the physician to take all reasonable, ordinary means of restoring the spontaneous vital functions and consciousness, and to employ such extraordinary means as are available to him to this end. It is not obligatory, however, to continue to use extraordinary means indefinitely in hopeless cases" (40).

Among Protestants, no consistent stand on brain death has been taken, although the concept of brain death has been acknowledged and accepted by leading Protestant theologians.

Even though the concept of brain death has been recognized by Jewish, Roman Catholic, and Protestant theologians, some religious groups, primarily fundamentalist, do not equate brain death with death of the person.

With the large number of practitioners of the Muslim religion, it is difficult to make generalizations concerning their view of brain death; however, one interesting study sheds some light on the issue (2). Of 50 senior Muslim scholars surveyed in several countries, 32 responded. Twenty-nine of 32 (90.6%) allowed organ donation during lifetime, but only when absolutely necessary and no harm is caused to the donor; 28/32 (87.5%) allowed organ donation after death when it was absolutely necessary; and 29/32 (90.6%) initially rejected the brain death concept and did not allow for discontinuation of life support in brain-dead patients. Seven of 9 scholars who were approached directly to explain the concept of brain death changed their view and accepted the concept.

Buddhist and Shinto scholars seem to generally accept the concepts of both brain death and organ transplantation, although many stop short of formally endorsing them in writing (27).

Legal Definitions

When is a person legally dead? Sir Peter Medawar concluded that a man is legally dead "when he has undergone irreversible changes of a type that make it impossible for him to seek to litigate" (10). Black's *Law Dictionary* defines death as "the bodily condition of showing no response to external stimuli, no spontaneous movements, no breathing, no reflexes, and a flat reading (usually for a full day) on a machine that measures a brain's electrical activity, also termed legal death" (14).

In 1970, Kansas state legislature proposed the first statutory replacement for the common-law definition of death (which required total cessation of all vital functions), citing two definitions of death: either the absence of spontaneous respiratory and cardiac function or the absence of spontaneous brain function. In 1972, Capron proposed a model statute of death, which stated, "A person is dead when there is an irreversible cessation of spontaneous respiratory and circulatory functions or in the event that artificial means of support preclude a determination that these functions have ceased if there has been an irreversible cessation of brain functions" (15). A second model statute was proposed in 1975 by the American Bar Association and, in 1981, the Uniform Determination of Death Act was enacted and endorsed by both the American Bar Association and the American Medical Association (43). It states that "An individual who has sustained either (1) irreversible cessation of circulatory and respiratory functions, or (2) irreversible cessation of all functions of the entire brain, including the brain stem, is dead. A determination must be made in accordance with accepted medical standards."

Although brain death is not just a matter of facilitating organ transplantation, difficulties may arise without such legislation. In addition, the time of death is important in cases of inheritance and distribution of an estate, the circumstances of which may differ depending on whether a patient was declared dead on the basis of "classical criteria" or "brain-death criteria," as is the case, for example when a husband and wife are fatally injured in the same accident and survivorship and consequent inheritance may be determined by the physician's choice.

According to Veith, often people misconstrue brain death as a mechanism for acquiring organs for donation. No special definition of death exists for organ transplant donors (61). In an effort to alleviate the problem of demand for organs far exceeding the supply, in 1968, the US Congress enacted the Uniform Anatomical Gift Act, which recognized the legal status of donor cards, living wills, and the authority of the next of kin to make a donation on behalf of a loved one (46). The major limitation to widespread transplantation in the US is physician reluctance to discuss the topic with parents and next of kin. Many states now have a policy of "Required Request," which mandates that healthcare providers inquire regarding organ donation, regardless of the criteria used to define death. However, <5% of deaths meet brain-death criteria, and of those patients, <25% are possible organ donors.

ORGAN TRANSPLANTATION

An important reason to have brain-death criteria is to be able to end life support in an entirely hopeless group of patients; certainly, another important purpose for having a concept of brain death as a criterion of death is the practical issue of declaring a beating-heart, hemodynamically stable patient dead in order to procure whole organs for transplantation. Bernat argues that the whole-brain death criterion of death best suits, or maps onto, our common understanding of what death is and allows for beating-heart donor, whole-organ donation to proceed (12). Certainly, the higher brain (neocortical) criterion leads to the problem of spontaneously breathing patients (anencephalic infants and persistent vegetative state patients) being declared dead and becoming organ donors.

The University of Pittsburgh Medical Center protocol for donation after cardiac death in adult patients allows for whole-organ donation from terminally ill patients who's surrogate consents to (a) have support withdrawn, (b) wait 5 mins for cessation of heartbeat, and (c) be declared dead before having rapid organ procurement in an attempt to circumvent the tenants of the "dead donor" rule (no patient should be harmed in order to procure organs for another). Although this protocol has recently gained substantial acceptance and endorsement from institutions and medical societies, considerable debate continues on ethical grounds due to the uneasy feeling that patients may not be truly dead and could possibly be revived if resuscitated (12).

Exception to the Whole-brain Death Criterion

In that it is difficult to understand if whole-brain death is a sufficient criterion for death, and it is difficult to prove every brain cell is dead, can a distinction be made between death as the death of the whole organism and death of the organism as a whole (33)? Examination of the possible exceptions to the whole-brain death criterion may help to elucidate whether or not all organ donors must be dead or just irreversibly damaged. Some difficult situations and possible exceptions to examine are: the anencephalic baby, the preterm elective abortion, and the full-term infant diagnosed as having in utero brain death, as well as the brain-dead pregnant woman with a potentially viable fetus.

Anencephalic Fetus/Newly Born as Organ Donor

Proponents of the use of the anencephalic fetus/infant as a whole-organ donor have suggested that such an infant either does not meet the criteria of brain formation that requires a criterion of brain death or that one can be accepted as a donor prior to meeting the criterion (5). Successful organ procurement is difficult to achieve in anencephalic infants and, even with considerable effort, the success rate of defining brain death and procuring organ donation from anencephalic infants is very low (33). Proponents argue that an exception could be made in the whole-brain criterion of death for anencephalics because they have never had a brain; ergo, they do not require a criterion for death. They maintain that not requiring criteria in these cases also positively benefits society, the recipient, the recipient's family, and the donor's family. Last, they argue that these cases are so clear that no slippery-slope argument would apply.

Those who do not support the use of anencephalic infants as organ donors argue that the benefits would be small, in that a small, actual success rate in organ donation is achieved. Additional arguments include a possible undue pressure on the families to donate; an unnecessary use and, therefore, waste of resources best used elsewhere; the potential abuse of women to become pregnant to produce infants and their organs for transplantation; the mistrust of physicians and medicine by the public; and an altered definition of death being extended to others, especially those patients in a persistent vegetative state (33). On this slippery slope, persistent vegetative state could come to be viewed as adult-onset anencephaly. These arguments are based mostly on utilitarian concepts, however, and still may beg the issue. The concept that the Harvard criteria of whole-brain death were developed because of the need for organs has been rejected by some (33,61). In addition, from a deontologic point of view, anencephalic infants are persons; they are not dead persons. Viewed as such, the argument against using anencephalic infants would invoke the Kantian principle of not using persons solely as a means to an end.

Healthcare providers resist the temptation to change the rules to meet our perceived immediate needs, even though the pressures for change are great in our pluralistic society of multiple value systems (19). Such a debate is legitimate, but the final answer is not yet available.

Fetal Brain Death

Any discussion of the use of fetal organs and/or tissues segues into the extremely difficult area of diagnosing brain death/irreversibility in the fetus (22) and abortion. The arguments concerning early fetal demise (abortion) and induced late fetal demise (infanticide) are heavily emotional and extremely complex. Legitimate efforts based on sound ethical principles to make fetal tissues available for positive medical and scientific efforts must continue.

Brain Death in the Pregnant Woman

Unusual cases have occurred in which the biologic life of a brain-dead pregnant woman has been extended for days, weeks, or months in order to successfully deliver a viable fetus as an independent infant. The medical and ethical issues involved with such attempts are both difficult and interesting (52). However, with the fetus/infant viewed as a patient and not as a donor, these issues seem to be different from anencephalic and fetal donors being used as a means to an end and the dead donor rule. We shall leave this matter as another fascinating permutation of modern intensive care, which all the more necessitates understanding the ethical basis on which our decisions are made concerning care of patients.

Ethical Considerations

The patient must be declared dead prior to removal of organs, and it is never possible to allow someone to die in order that someone else may benefit. Ethically, in terms of distribution of scarce resources, it is also wrong to maintain a brain-dead patient on a ventilator with no chance to benefit the patient. This approach is an abuse of bed space, economic resources, and the time of highly qualified personnel. As Veith stated, "It confuses the person with his corpse" (61). In addition, keeping a brain-dead corpse on a ventilator constitutes a failure to accord respect for the dead and could be considered abuse of a corpse. Although it is unlikely that legal liability would result, one could also argue in terms of "wrongful life." In contrast, some argue that a dead patient should remain on mechanical ventilation for the sake of the family, especially when events have progressed rapidly, to give the family time to accept the outcome. However, allowing the family a decent amount of time to adjust to the death poses many new problems, including the following:

- What is a decent amount of time? An individual's adjustment to death of a loved one is highly variable.
- The family has no adjustment time in cases of sudden death.
- Brain death is usually not declared in the emergency room, but in the PICU, and the process may take several hours. Usually this time period is adequate to talk to the family and await the arrival of other family members. Prolonged requests for delay may seem at first to have reasonable bases, but alternatively may signal denial and bargaining.
- Last, prolonging mechanical support can interfere with the delivery of healthcare to other patients and demoralizes the staff.

CONCLUSIONS AND FUTURE CONSIDERATIONS

Although generally accepted, the debate concerning brain death as a criterion of death is fueled by medical, social, cultural, and religious factors. It is unlikely, in our diverse, multicultural society and world, that the debate will soon, if ever, be resolved, since it will be difficult to have one uniform, universally accepted definition of death met by brain-death criteria sufficient to meet all medical and legal requirements for pronouncing patients dead and procuring organs for donation.

The possibility of having patients or their families elect, in advance, which criterion they would choose for themselves to be diagnosed as dead already exists to some extent in law in New Jersey, to accommodate strictly orthodox Jewish patients. Emanuel describes "bounded zones" of death wherein the lower bound is cardiorespiratory activity and the higher bound is persistent vegetative state, suggesting that patients or their families could choose their own criterion for death within these bounded zones (21). Veatch's writings led to the idea that, if one chooses brain-death criteria, one could also choose which criterion she preferred—whole-brain, higher brain, or brainstem (60).

Truog considers the argument that, given the problems with both the whole-brain death criterion fulfilling the definition of death and the ethical considerations of the non-beating heart whole-organ donations procurement, perhaps the dead donor rule should be abandoned altogether, permitting organs to be harvested from patients who meet criteria, such as complete loss of all brain function or absence of all neocortical function (i.e., including anencephalic infants and patients in persistent vegetative state) even though they are not dead (57). Organ procurement could occur with consent of family or, in the case of persistent vegetative state, by previously stated wishes of the patient. A change in the law might be required to permit a form of legal killing for the greater good.

In the future, these very difficult medical, legal, and ethical considerations might be circumvented with the ongoing development and success of technologies that include transgenic organs from genetically engineered pigs, artificial organs, and stem cell research.

KEY POINTS

- The problem of defining death, developing sufficient criteria to fulfill that definition, and have decisive convincing tests to prove that the criteria are met is a long-standing one.
- The development of successful whole-organ transplantation has led to the development of whole-brain death as a criterion of death and the establishment of tests to fulfill that criterion.
- Controversies clearly exist as to the validity of brain death as a criterion of death, as well as controversies concerning different criteria of brain death. One day, patients and their families may be able to choose which criteria they wish to have used to diagnose their death.
- "What dies is the organism as a whole. It is this death, the death of the individual human being that is important for physicians and for the community, not the 'death' of organs or cells, which are mere parts (30)." We believe we must concern ourselves with the death of the organism as a whole, not the death of the whole organism (17).
- The physician must approach establishing the diagnosis in a cautious, compassionate, meticulous manner, and, if doubt regarding the diagnosis exists, a longer observation period or ancillary tests may be warranted.
- It may not be possible for the physician to completely divorce himself from the societal context in which this determination is being made.
- Delay and use of tests to avoid making the diagnosis of brain death is not in the best interest of the patient, the family, the ICU, or society (56).

ACKNOWLEDGMENTS

I would like to thank Mary M. Farrell, MD, and the many members of The Southern Methodist University-Children's Medical Center Dallas, University of Texas Southwestern Medical School Biomedical Ethic Study group, especially Tom Mayo, who contributed to the development of this material.

References

1. A definition of irreversible coma. Report of the As Hoc Committee of the Harvard Medical School to examine the definition of brain death. *JAMA* 1968;205:337.
2. Al Mousaw M, Hamed T, Al-Matouk H. Views of Muslim scholars on organ donation and brain death. *Transplant Proc* 1997;29:3217.
3. Althabe M, Cardigni, G, Vassallo JC, et al. Dying in the intensive care unit: Collaborative multicenter study about forgoing life-sustaining treatment in Argentine pediatric intensive care units. *Pediatr Crit Care Med* 2003;12:164–9.
4. American Electroencephalographic Society. Guidelines in EEG and evoked potentials. *J Clin Neurophysiol* 1986;3:131–68.
5. Ashwal S, Peabody JL, Schneider S, et al. Anencephaly: Clinical determination of brain death and neuropathologic studies. *Pediatr Neurol* 1990;6:233–9.
6. Ashwal S, Schneider S. Failure of electroencephalography to diagnose brain death in comatose children. *Ann Neurol* 1979;6:512–7.
7. Ashwal S, Schneider S. Brain death in children: Part I. *Pediatric Neurol* 1987;3:5–11.
8. Ashwal S, Schneider S. Brain death in children Part II. *Pediatric Neurol* 1987;3:69–77.
9. Ashwal S, Schneider S. Brain death in the newborn. *Pediatrics* 1989;84:429–37.
10. Beecher H. After the "definition of irreversible coma," *N Engl J Med* 1969;281:1070–1.
11. Bernat JL. How much of the brain must die in brain death? *J Clin Eth* 1992;3:21–6.
12. Bernat James L. A defense of the whole-brain concept of death. *Hastings Cent Rep* 1998;28:14–23.
13. Biswas AK, Scott WA, Sommerauer JF, et al. Heart rate variability after acute traumatic brain injury in children. *Crit Care Med* 2000;28:3907–12.
14. *Black's Law Dictionary*, 8th ed., Gardner B, ed., Stamford: Thomson West, 2006.
15. Capron A. Legal definition of death. *Ann NY Acad Sci* 1978;315:349–59.
16. Conference of Royal Colleges and Faculties of the United Kingdom. Diagnosis of brain death. *Lancet* 1976;2:1069.
17. Cowley LT, Young E, Raffin TA. Care of the dying: An ethical and historical perspective. *Crit Care Med* 1992;20:1473–82.
18. Cranford R. Even the dead are not terminally ill anymore. *Neurology* 1998;51:1530–1.
19. Cutter MAG. Moral pluralism and the use of anencephalic tissue organs. *J Med Philos* 1989;14:89–95.
20. Dear PRF, Godfrey DJ. Neonatal auditory brainstem response cannot reliably diagnose brainstem death. *Arch Dis Child* 1985;60:396.
21. Emanuel LL. Reexamining death: The asymptotic model and a bounded zone definition. *Hastings Cent Rep* 1995;25:27–30.
22. Engelhardt HT. Brain life, brain death, fetal parts. *J Med Philos* 1989;14:1–3.
23. Farrell MM, Levin DL. Brain death in the pediatric patient: Historical, sociological, medical, religious, cultural, legal, and ethical considerations. *Crit Care Med* 1993;21:1951.
24. Freeman JM, Ferry PC. New brain death guidelines in children: Further confusion. *Pediatrics* 1988;81:301–3.
25. Grigg MM, Kelly MA, Celesia GC, et al. Electroencephalographic activity after brain death. *Arch Neurol* 1987;44:948–54.
26. Hanley DF. Brain death: An update on the North American viewpoint. *Anesthesia and Intensive Care* 1995;3:24–5.
27. Hardacre H. Response of Buddhism and Shinto to the issue of brain death and organ transplantation. *Camb Q Healthc Ethics* 1994;3:585–601.
28. Holzman B, Curless R, Sfakianakis G. Radionuclide cerebral perfusion scintigraphy in determination of brain death in children. *Neurology* 1983;33:1027–31.
29. Ingvar D, Widen L. Brain death: Summary of a symposium. *Lakartidningen* 1972;69:3804–14.
30. Kass LP. Death as an event: Commentary on Robert Morison. *Science* 1971;173:698–702.
31. Delio JK, Jefferson PP, Pedro CRG, et al. Evolution of the medical practices and modes of death on pediatric intensive care units in southern Brazil. *Pediatr Crit Care Med* 2005;258–63.
32. Martinot A, Grandbasien Leteurtre S, et al. No resuscitation orders and withdrawal of therapy in French pediatric intensive care units. *Acta Paediatr* 1998;87:769–73.
33. May WF. Brain death: Anencephalics and aborted fetuses. *Transplant Proc* 1990;22:985–8.
34. Mohundas A, Chou S. Brain death: A clinical and pathological study. *J Neurosurg* 1971;35:211–8.
35. Mollaret P, Goulon M. Le coma depasses (memoire preliminaire). *Rev Neurol (Paris)* 1959;101:3–15.
36. Moraczawski A, Showalter J. *Determination of death: Theological, Medical, Ethical, and Legal Issues*. St. Louis: The Catholic Health Association of the United States, 1982:39.
37. Pallis Christopher. ABC of brain stem death: The arguments about the EEG. *Br Med J*, 1983;286:284–8.

38. Pasternak SF, Volpe JJ. Full recovery from prolonged brain stem failure following intraventricular hemorrhage. *J Pediatrics* 1979;95:1046–9.

39. Pernick MS. Back from the grave: Recurring controversies over defining and diagnosing death in history. In: Zaner RM, ed. *Death: Beyond Whole-Brain Criteria.* Norwell, MA: Kluwer Academic Publishers, 1988:17–74.

40. Pope Pius XIII. The prolongation of life. An address of Pope Pius XII to an international congress of anesthesiologists. *The Pope Speaks* 1958;4:393–8 (Acta Apostolicae Sedia 1957;49:17).

41. President's Commission for the Study of Ethical Problems in Medicine and Biomedical and Behavioral research: Defining death. Washington, DC: Government Printing Office, 1981.

42. Rappaport HZ, Rappaport I. Principles and concepts of brain death and organ donation: The Jewish perspective. *Childs Nerv Syst* 1998;14:381–3.

43. Report of the medical consultants on the diagnosis of death to the President's commission for the study of ethical problems in medicine and biomedical behavioral research: Guidelines for the determination of death. *Neurology* 1982;32:395–9.

44. Report of Special Task Force: Guidelines for the determination in the newborn. *Pediatrics* 1987;80:293–7.

45. Rowland TW, Donnelly JH, Jackson AH, et al. Brain death in the pediatric intensive care unit. *Am J Dis Child* 1983;137:547–50.

46. Sadler A, Sadler B, Stason E. Uniform anatomical gift act: A model for reform. *JAMA* 1968;206:2501–6.

47. Schwartz J, Baxter J, Brill D. Diagnosis of brain death in children by radionuclide cerebral imaging. *Pediatrics* 1984;73:14–8.

48. Shewmon DA. The probability of inevitability: The inherent impossibility of validating criteria for brain death or "irreversibility" through clinical studies. *Stat Med* 1987;6:535–53.

49. Shewmon DA. Commentary on guidelines for the determination of brain death in children. *American Neurological Association* 1988;24:789–91.

50. Shewmon DA. "Brainstem death," "brain death" and death: A critical reevaluation of the purported equivalence. *Issues in Law & Medicine,* 1998;14: 125–45.

51. Shewmon DA. Chronic "brain death": Meta-analysis and conceptual consequences. *Am Acad Neurol* 1998;51:1538–45.

52. Shrader D. On dying more than one death. *Hastings Cent Rep* 1986;16:12–7.

53. Spike J, Greenlaw J. Ethics consultation: Persistent brain death and religion: Must a person believe in death to die? *J Law Med Ethics* 1995;23: 291–4.

54. Steinhart, CM Weiss IP. Use of brainstem auditory evoked potentials in: Pediatric brain death. *Crit Care Med* 1985;13:560–62.

55. Taylor RM. Reexamining the definition and criteria of death. *Semin Neurol* 1997;17:265–70.

56. Truog RD, Fackler JC. Another point of view: Rethinking brain death. *Crit Care Med* 1992;20:1705–13.

57. Truog RD. Is it time to abandon brain death? *Hastings Cent Rep* 1997;1: 29–37.

58. Vardis R, Pollack MM. Increased apnea threshold in a pediatric patient with suspected brain death. *Crit Care Med* 1998;26:1917–19.

59. Veatch R. "Brain death: Welcome definition or dangerous judgment?" *Hastings Cent Rep* 1972;2:10–3.

60. Veatch RM. The impending collapse of the whole-brain definition of death. *Hastings Cent Rep* 1993;4:18–24.

61. Veith F. Brain death and organ transplantation. *Ann NY Acad Sci* 1978; 315:417–41.

62. Vernon DD, Dean M, Timmons OD, et al. Modes of death in the pediatric intensive care unit: Withdrawal and limitation of supportive care. *Crit Care Med* 1993;21:1798–1802.

63. Volpe JJ. Commentary: Brain death determination in the newborn. *Pediatrics* 1987;80:293–7.

CHAPTER 62 ■ CARDIAC ANATOMY

STEVEN M. SCHWARTZ • ZDENEK SLAVIK • SIEW YEN HO

Congenital heart disease is often simple to describe and understand, as in the case of an atrial or ventricular septal defect. However, when more comprehensive defects are present, it can be quite complex and even forbidding to those not well versed in the subtleties of cardiac anatomy. Significant controversies have persisted regarding the best overall approach to nomenclature of complex congenital heart disease, and many cardiologists frequently use various shorthand designations or colloquialisms to describe these lesions, leading many noncardiologists to consider it an exercise in semantics or hair-splitting that is best left to the pediatric cardiologist. In reality though, the intensive care physician must be familiar with the way in which such defects are described, as anatomy often dictates physiology, and physiology is the cornerstone of the clinical care of these patients. The common approaches to systematically and comprehensively categorizing the anatomy of congenital heart disease are reviewed in this chapter, with the intended goal of familiarizing the pediatric critical care physician with the basic schemes used in assigning specific terms to specific defects. This chapter is not intended to resolve controversies where they exist, nor is it proffered as a comprehensive review of any one particular approach; rather, it provides a practical framework for describing complex defects in an organized manner that helps the intensive care physician to understand "how the blood goes 'round" and sets the basis for better communication with cardiology and cardiac surgery colleagues.

SEGMENTAL APPROACH TO CONGENITAL HEART DISEASE

Even though many common lesions can be described directly, the underlying basis for complete description of any congenital heart lesion is a segmental approach to cardiac anatomy that requires analysis of each cardiac segment, its morphology, and its relationship to adjoining cardiac segments. This methodical approach can be used to consider each part of the heart in turn: atria, ventricles, and great arteries. The connections between the segments (atrioventricular and ventricular-arterial) are described, as are the atrial and ventricular septa, cardiac venous connections, and the position of the heart within the thorax. With the segmental approach, all congenital heart defects can be described in complete detail, and the physiology can be determined from the anatomy.

Two primary systems are currently in use for describing complex cardiac defects. Although the merit of one system or the other has been the subject of numerous scholarly papers and debates (1,12), in truth, they have more similarities than differences, and many cardiologists and cardiac surgeons use terms derived from both systems at different times. Robert Anderson is the primary advocate of the concept of *sequential segmental analysis*, which emphasizes morphology, connections, and relations of segmental components as the basis for nomenclature. Richard and Stella Van Praagh, building substantially on work by Maurice Lev, have advocated a system also based firmly in morphologic analysis of various segments, but with some significant differences in terms of specific nomenclature, analysis, and definition of connections or junctions between segments, and use of this system relies on cardiac embryology to understand the basic patterns of postnatal congenital heart disease. The advantage of the former system is that it allows description of any given situation with no need to speculate about unobserved embryologic events. The latter approach has inherent value in that almost all lesions can be recognized to be the result of incomplete or inaccurate steps in the transition of the heart from the embryonic heart tube to the mature four-chamber heart.

Both of these systems are based on the principles that (a) specific cardiac chambers have unique, distinguishing characteristics that allow them to be clearly identified even when their right/left relationships to each other or connections to adjoining structures are altered or absent, and (b) that the precise nature of these relationships and connections should be carefully and fully described.

Atrial Situs

The terms "right" and "left" atria refer to specific, distinguishing morphologic characteristics of each atrium, not to the side of the heart on which they are located or their accompanying venous or ventricular connections. Features that identify the *right* atrium include (a) a blunt atrial appendage with a wide connection to the smooth-walled part of the atrium, (b) the limbus of the fossa ovalis, and (c) remnants of the valves of the sinus venosus such as the Eustachian valve of the coronary sinus. The *left* atrium is characterized by (a) a hooked appendage with a more narrow connection to the smooth-walled portion of the chamber, (b) the flap valve of the fossa ovalis, and (c) no remnants of venous valves. Venous connections are not used to designate the morphologic right and left atria, as these connections can be variable in congenital heart disease (i.e., total anomalous pulmonary venous return, unroofed coronary sinus, bilateral superior vena cava).

Once the morphology of the atria has been identified, the atrial arrangement, or *situs*, can be defined. *Atrial situs* refers to the arrangement of the morphologic right and left atria within the heart. *Situs solitus* is the normal arrangement, wherein the right atrium is to the right and the left atrium is to the left. *Situs inversus* is the opposite arrangement; the right atrium is to the left and the left atrium is to the right. A major difference between the Anderson and Van Praagh approaches to nomenclature regards the recognition of the possibility of atrial isomerism. *Atrial isomerism* is defined as the presence of two morphologically left or two morphologically right atria rather than one of each. Van Praagh contends that having two right or left atria is an impossibility, and that atrial situs in all hearts can be described as solitus, inversus, or ambiguus, with ambiguus referring to the situation in which separate right and left atria cannot be differentiated (16). Using this approach, anatomic variants that would be considered cases of atrial isomerism are more generally defined in terms of heterotaxy syndromes, and extracardiac abnormalities of laterality often coexist with the congenital heart disease. *Polysplenia syndrome* is thus often used to mean the same thing as left atrial isomerism, and *asplenia syndrome* is often used to describe the same atrial arrangement as right atrial isomerism. Anderson argues that this approach is at times inaccurate, as not all patients with congenital heart disease congruent with polysplenia are actually polysplenic, and not all with cardiac anatomy consistent with asplenia are asplenic. Rather, the Andersonian system suggests that atrial situs can be identified in all cases as usual or solitus, mirror-image or inversus, right isomerism or left isomerism (8).

As suggested previously, the assignment of atrial situs can be assisted by observation of other asymmetrically distributed structures, and the identification of atrial isomerism can lead to investigations for malposition of noncardiac structures. The bronchi can be particularly helpful in identifying atrial situs because the right and left bronchi have characteristic features readily seen on chest x-ray and bronchial situs almost always reflects atrial situs (4). Specifically, the right main stem bronchus is shorter, more vertically oriented, and located directly behind the mediastinal segment of the right pulmonary artery. The left main stem bronchus is longer, more horizontally oriented, and below the left pulmonary artery. When the atria are inverted, the left-sided bronchus will usually have the orientation of a typical right bronchus, and the left lung may contain three lobes. The right-sided bronchus will then have a typical left main stem bronchus anatomy. Isomeric arrangement of the atria usually is reflected by a bilaterally symmetrical bronchial arrangement of either a right or left type. In heterotaxy syndromes (atrial isomerism), abdominal structures in addition to the spleen can be abnormally distributed. Right atrial isomerism or asplenia can be thought of as bilateral right-sidedness and can be associated with a midline liver and intestinal malrotation. Left atrial isomerism, or polysplenia syndrome, can be thought of as bilateral left-sidedness and is also associated with an intestinal malrotation.

The finding of atrial isomerism is also typically accompanied by certain predictably associated intracardiac defects. Right atrial isomerism, or asplenia syndrome, usually includes anomalies of pulmonary venous return and atrioventricular canal-type defects, along with double-outlet right ventricle (DORV) or transposition (7,9,15), whereas left atrial isomerism tends to be more commonly associated with abnormalities of systemic venous connections, particularly interrupted inferior vena cava and DORV or normally related great arteries. Polysplenia can also be associated with atrioventricular canal

defects and some abnormalities of pulmonary venous drainage but usually not to the degree that these are associated with asplenia. These associations are important for the cardiologist, in that they prompt complete assessment for these types of lesions; they are also important for the intensivist in terms of providing a mental framework for understanding and describing these complex anatomic variants.

The Atrial Septum

The atrial septum in its usual state contains a foramen ovale on the right side, and the flap valve of the foramen on the left. The foramen, when patent, allows right-to-left shunting of blood when the right atrial pressure exceeds the left, but it is closed by the flap valve when left atrial pressure is higher. The foramen ovale is the remnant of the ostium secundum; therefore, atrial septal defects (ASDs) in this area are referred to as *secundum ASDs*. The foramen primum is the embryologic opening between the early atrial septum (septum primum) and the area where the endocardial cushions ultimately form. The foramen primum is closed by endocardial cushion tissue, thus making primum ASDs a common component of atrioventricular canal (endocardial cushion) defects. The least common type of ASD is the sinus venosus ASD, which is found in the superior part of the atrial septum, where the sinus venosus is incorporated into the embryonic atrium. This type of defect is often associated with partial anomalous venous connection of the right upper pulmonary vein.

Ventricular Morphology and Topology

As with the atria, the right and left ventricles are identified by certain constant morphologic patterns, not by their location within the heart or the body. The morphologic right ventricle is heavily trabeculated, contains the moderator band of the septum, and has septal attachments of the associated atrioventricular valve. The left ventricle is smooth-walled, more bullet-shaped, and has no septal attachments of the atrioventricular valve. When two distinct atrioventricular valves exist, the tricuspid valve is *always* associated with the morphologic right ventricle and the mitral valve is *always* associated with the left ventricle.

The topology of the ventricles refers to the spatial anatomy of the ventricle with regard to the inflow and outflow. Determination of the "handedness" of a ventricle is made by considering the relationship of the inflow and outflow tracts of the ventricle when looking at the septal surface (**Fig. 62.1**). One can imagine placing the palm of the hand on the septal surface of the ventricle with the thumb extended toward the inflow and the fingers pointed toward the outflow. If this can be accomplished with the right hand, the ventricle is said to be "right-handed;" if it can be accomplished with the left hand, the ventricle is left-handed. In general, the right ventricle of a normal heart is said to have right-handed topology, and the left ventricle, left-handed topology. However, this terminology does not describe or identify the morphology of the ventricle, nor does it describe the location within the heart, although certain anatomic and morphologic arrangements are generally associated with specific handedness for the morphologic right and left ventricles (see following section).

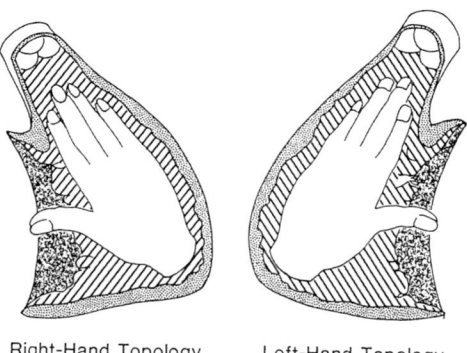

FIGURE 62.1. Ventricular topology is determined by imagining the palmer surface of the hand on the septal surface of the morphologically right ventricle, with the thumb pointing toward the inlet and the fingers pointing toward the outlet. Right-hand topology is present if this alignment can be accomplished with the right hand. Left-hand topology is present if this alignment requires use of the left hand. From Anderson RH. Nomenclature and Classification: Sequential Segmental Analysis. In: Moller JH, Hoffman JIE, eds. *Pediatric Cardiovascular Medicine.* Philadelphia: Churchill Livingstone, 2000:263–74, with permission.

Atrioventricular Connections, Junctions, and Alignments

The exact nature of the atrioventricular relationship can take many forms. Usually, two separate atrioventricular valves are present, one leading into each ventricle. Furthermore, the right atrium usually opens into the morphologic right ventricle and the left atrium into the left ventricle. Of course, in complex congenital heart disease, this is not always the case and, as such, precise description of the arrangement of this part of the heart is essential. For the purpose of clarity, it is helpful to consider both the type of atrioventricular connection and the mode of connection. The type of atrioventricular connection or alignment refers to the anatomic concordance or discordance of the atrium and ventricle. A normal heart has concordant atrial and ventricular connections, or alignments, in that the morphologic right atrium opens to the morphologic right ventricle and the left atrium opens to the morphologic left ventricle. A discordant connection or alignment is one in which the morphologic right atrium opens to the morphologic left ventricle and vice versa. When atrial isomerism is present, or when both atria open into one ventricle, the relationship can be described as *ambiguous* and reference can be made to the topology of the ventricles (**Fig. 62.2**) or to the looping pattern. Also, a single common atrioventricular valve that guards the opening between right and left atria above and right and left ventricles below can still be referred to in terms of concordant and discordant connections or alignments.

The mode by which the atria open into the ventricles, i.e., the precise morphology of the atrioventricular valve or valves, must also be described accurately. When the heart has two atria, two atrioventricular valves, and two ventricles, the tricuspid valve is always associated with the morphologic right ventricle, and the mitral valve is always associated with the morphologic left ventricle. When one of the valves is atretic and/or the ventricle is hypoplastic, there are still considered to be two atrioventricular valves in terms of assignment of

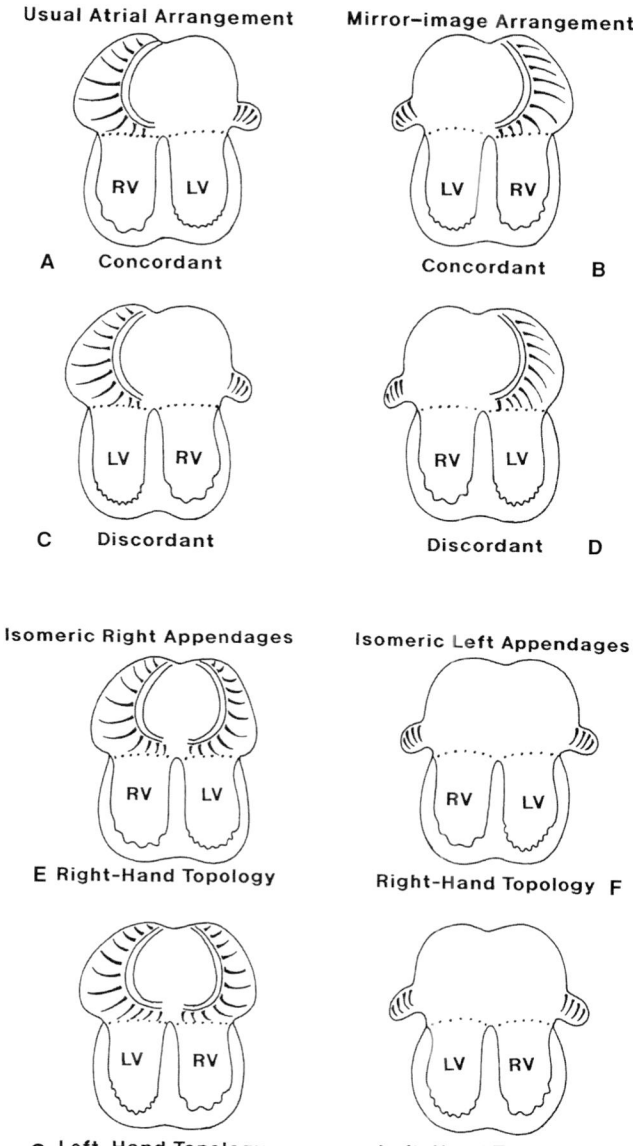

FIGURE 62.2. (A–D) The atrioventricular connection can be described as concordant or discordant when there are two morphologically different atria. (E–H) When atrial isomerism is present, the connection can be referred to by identifying the atrial morphology followed by the ventricular topology. RV, right ventricle; LV, left ventricle. Modified from Anderson RH. Nomenclature and Classification: Sequential Segmental Analysis. In: Moller JH, Hoffman JIE, eds. *Pediatric Cardiovascular Medicine.* Philadelphia: Churchill Livingstone, 2000;263–74, with permission.

anatomic diagnosis (e.g., tricuspid atresia or hypoplastic left heart). Nomenclature is more complex when there is a single, common atrioventricular valve, as in an atrioventricular canal-type defect, in which the two valves are not fully formed and distinct, or in the case of a double-inlet connection (both atrioventricular valves open into the same ventricle). In these types of anatomic situations, the atrioventricular valves are often referred to as right and left. The basis of this argument is that, as neither is a properly formed valve, use of the names "tricuspid" and/or "mitral" is technically inaccurate and referring to the valves on the basis of their respective position within the heart is most correct (1). Others have suggested that, even under these circumstances, the valves can and should be identified as mitral and/or tricuspid (12).

The nature of the atrioventricular connection can be further complicated when an inlet ventricular septal defect (VSD) is present. These types of VSDs often involve override or straddle of the atrioventricular valve. *Override* occurs when the annulus of the atrioventricular valve overrides the ventricular septum and thus allows the atrium associated with the overriding valve to empty into both ventricles. A *straddling atrioventricular valve* is one in which the chordal attachments of the valve cross the plane of the septum to attach to the contralateral ventricle. The left atrioventricular valve, for example, may have chordal attachments to the right side of the ventricular septum. Override and straddle are not mutually exclusive, and straddle is the far more complex problem to repair, which leads to consideration of single-ventricle-type palliation when significant straddle is present.

Ventricular Arrangements

Using the sequential segmental approach of Anderson, once the morphologic right and left atria and ventricles have been identified, and once the nature of the atrioventricular connection has been ascertained, the relationships between the atria and ventricles can be described by referring to concordance, discordance, and topology, as needed (3). *Topology* is determined by imagining the palm of the hand on the septal surface of the morphologic right ventricle. If the right hand allows the thumb to point through the inlet while the fingers point at the outlet, the heart has right-hand topology. If this alignment of the thumb and fingers requires the left hand to be used, left-hand topology is present. Single ventricles are described with reference to morphology of the ventricle. The nomenclature system proposed by Van Praagh is based on an embryologic approach to segmental anatomy (17). Understanding this system requires basic familiarity with the transition of the heart from the straight heart tube of the early embryo to the mature, four-chambered heart of the fetus and newborn (**Fig. 62.3**). The heart tube contains the progenitor areas for all four cardiac chambers. The most caudal areas of the heart tube, the sinus venosus and atrium, are destined to become the right and left atria. The embryologic atrium leads directly into the embryonic ventricle, the future left ventricle. Moving more rostrally, the ventricle opens into the bulbus cordis, the future right ventricle, which then gives rise to the outlet of the heart, the conus arteriosus, and arterial trunk. Transition from the straight heart tube requires the tube to loop, usually with the apex of the loop being rightward, referred to as a *dextro* or *d-loop*. The apex occurs at the junction of the ventricle and bulbus cordis. When d-looping occurs, the embryologic ventricle ends up leftward of the bulbus cordis, thus placing the left ventricle to the left of the right ventricle. When looping occurs abnormally, with the apex of the loop to the left, the morphologic left ventricle ends up rightward of the morphologic right ventricle. This arrangement is referred to as a *levo* or *l-looped* heart.

Obviously, it is impossible to replay the exact sequence of embryologic development when it is necessary to make a precise anatomic diagnosis in a fetus or newborn. The power of this particular nomenclature system, however, lies in its ability to predict comprehensive patterns of abnormalities, as much

congenital heart disease represents incomplete or improperly finished incidents in embryologic heart development. From a practical standpoint then, a heart in which the morphologic right ventricle is on the right side and the morphologic left ventricle is on the left side is d-looped, and a heart in which the morphologic right ventricle is on the left and the morphologic left ventricle is on the right is l-looped. This nomenclature system further requires that the lower cardiac chamber, in order to be called a ventricle, has an inlet from an atrium. This inlet can be atretic, but it must be present. A lower chamber with an outlet but not an inlet is referred to as an *outlet chamber*; lack of both an inlet and an outlet is the hallmark of a trabecular pouch. A lower chamber with an inlet but no outlet is still considered a ventricle. The position of outlet chambers and/or trabecular pouches combined with the morphology of the ventricle can be used to determine the looping pattern in single-ventricle anatomy. However, hypoplastic left-heart syndrome, for example, has two anatomic ventricles (both lower chambers with inlets, even if one is severely stenotic or atretic), so that it can be named using a system for biventricular hearts, even though the physiology is that of a single ventricle.

The Ventricular Septum

The ventricular septum is normally composed of an *inlet portion* formed by endocardial cushion tissue, a *trabecular* or *muscular portion* that represents the muscular area between the ventricle and bulbus cordis after looping is completed (sometimes described as having sinus and trabecular portions), and the *outflow* or *conal portion* of the septum. Malalignment defects, such as those that occur in tetralogy of Fallot or interrupted aortic arch, are generally located in this area because they represent failure of proper alignment of the portions of the ventricular septum. The junction between all of these parts is the *membranous septum*, the most common site of VSDs. Inlet defects occur posteriorly in the plane of the atrioventricular valves, muscular VSDs occur anywhere in the trabecular septum, and outlet VSDs are found in the conotruncal region. It is important to understand that the description of VSD location in many types of complex defects is more related to the position of the great arteries than to the VSD itself. In other words, two hearts with VSDs in the outlet septum may be called by different terms (e.g., subaortic versus subpulmonary) based on the arrangement of the great arteries.

The Great Arteries

The great arteries have relationships with the ventricles and with each other. The ventricular relationships are defined and determined by outflow tract anatomy and alignments. The relationship of one great artery to the other is considered in terms of anterior-posterior and left-right positioning. Normally, related great arteries occur when a heart has concordant ventriculo-arterial connections, with the aorta posterior and slightly rightward of the pulmonary artery (**Fig. 62.4A**). In ventriculo-arterial concordance, the aorta arises from the morphologic left ventricle, and the pulmonary artery arises from the morphologic right ventricle. Ventriculo-arterial discordance occurs when the aorta arises from the morphologic right ventricle and the pulmonary artery arises from the morphologic left ventricle.

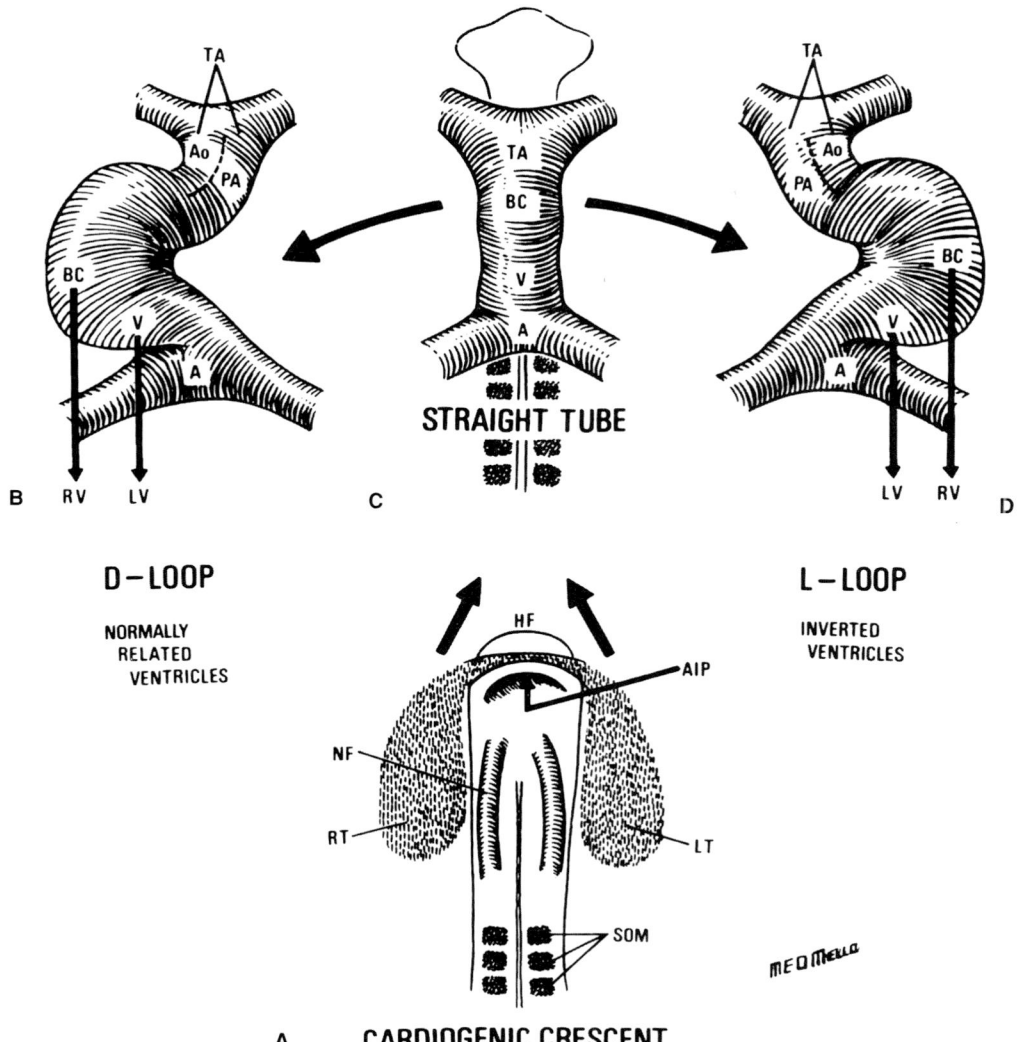

FIGURE 62.3. The embryologic cardiac crescent (**A**) contains the early precursors of the straight heart tube (**B**). The tube usually loops with the apex to the right, forming a d-loop (**C**) and bringing the future right ventricle to the right of the future left ventricle. When the apex of the loop is to the left, or l-looped (**D**), the morphologic right ventricle ends up leftward of the morphologic left ventricle, so-called *ventricular inversion*. HF, head fold; AIP, anterior intestinal portal; NF, neural fold; RT, right side of cardiac crescent; LT, left side of cardiac crescent; SOM, somites; A, atrium; V, ventricle (future left ventricle); BC, bulbus cordis (future right ventricle); TA, truncus arteriosus, LV, left ventricle; RV, right ventricle; Ao, aorta; PA, pulmonary artery. From Van Praagh R, Weinberg PM, Matsuoka R, et al. Malpositions of the heart. In: Adams FH, Emmanouilides GC, eds. *Moss' Heart Disease in Infants, Children and Adolescents, 3rd ed.* Baltimore: Williams & Wilkins, 1983;422–58, with permission.

Concordance and discordance can thus be considered to be synonymous with normally related and transposed great arteries, respectively (11,14), although some have suggested that the anterior-posterior relationship of the great arteries is the most definitive feature of transposition, at least from an historic perspective (1,10). Therefore, given the possibilities for confusion, some have argued that the terms "concordant" and "discordant" should be used to describe all situations in which two ventricles connect individually to two great arteries (1). When a heart has double-outlet ventriculo-arterial connection, one of the ventricles gives rise to both great arteries. In this case, or in the case of only a single great artery arising from a discordant ventricle, the artery with improper orientation can be said to

be malposed (11,14). The term *malposition* can also be used to describe anterior-posterior malposition in the presence of ventriculo-arterial concordance. The anatomic arrangement of the great arteries should be distinguished from their physiologic orientation in that deoxygenated blood can course from right atrium to morphologic left ventricle to transposed pulmonary artery, resulting in a physiologically normal situation.

Using the nomenclature system proposed by Anderson, each great artery is assigned to the ventricle to which it is more than 50% committed (1). This approach offers the benefit of simplicity that comes with the intuitiveness of the nomenclature. DORV, for example, occurs when the both great arteries are more than 50% committed to the right ventricle.

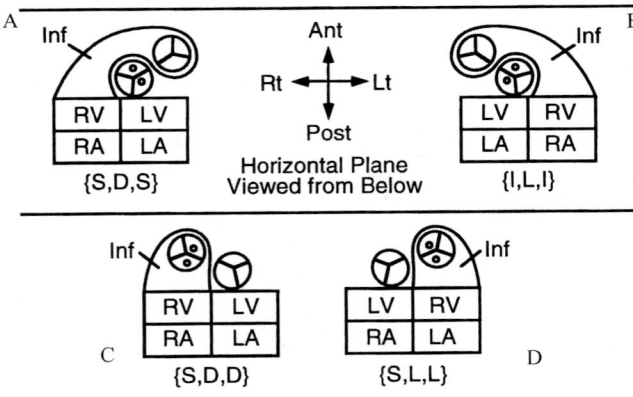

FIGURE 62.4. Schematic diagrams of normally related and transposed great arteries, using the segmental nomenclature scheme proposed by Van Praagh. (**A**) Normal heart: atrial situs solitus, d-loop, situs solitus normally related great arteries {S,D,S}. The heart has atrioventricular concordance and ventriculo-arterial concordance and a subpulmonary infundibulum (Inf) or conus. The aorta (designated by the coronary orifices on the diagram) is posterior (Post) and rightward (Rt). (**B**) Mirror image normal: atrial situs inversus, l-loop, situs inversus normally related great arteries {I,L,I}. The heart has atrioventricular and ventriculo-arterial concordance and a subpulmonary infundibulum or conus. The aorta is posterior and leftward (Lt) of the pulmonary artery. The difference from normal is that the right atrium (RA) and ventricle (RV) are on the left, the left atrium (LA) and ventricle (LV) are on the right, and the aorta is leftward of the pulmonary artery. (**C**) Usual form of transposition of the great arteries (d-TGA): atrial situs solitus, d-loop, d-transposition of the great arteries {S,D,D}. The heart has atrioventricular concordance, ventriculo-arterial discordance, and subpulmonary conus. The aorta is anterior (Ant) and rightward of the pulmonary artery. (**D**) Congenitally corrected transposition of the great arteries (l-TGA): atrial situs solitus, l-loop, l-transposition of the great arteries {S,L,L}. The heart has atrioventricular and ventriculo-arterial discordance and subpulmonary infundibulum. The aorta is anterior and leftward of the pulmonary artery. Modified from Foran RB, Belcourt C, Nanton MA, et al. Isolated infundibuloarterial inversion {S,D,I}: A newly recognized form of congenital heart disease. *Am Heart J* 1988;116:1337–50.

The relationship of the great arteries to each other must then be described, such as DORV with the aorta rightward of the pulmonary artery. Accuracy of this schema for assigning ventriculo-arterial relationships is highly dependent on obtaining standard echocardiographic views, as some rotation from the standard plane can make a normally placed aorta appear to override a perimembranous VSD by more than 50%, thus leading to an incorrect anatomic diagnosis.

Using the more embryologically based approach of Van Praagh, the great arteries are described as normally related, transposed, or malposed. With normally related vessels, the aorta is posterior to the pulmonary artery, and the relationship between them can be noted as *situs solitus* (s) when the aorta (aortic valve) is rightward of the pulmonary artery (pulmonary valve), or *situs inversus* (i) when the aorta is leftward of the pulmonary artery (**Fig. 62.4**). In transposition, the aorta is generally anterior to the pulmonary artery, and the relationship can be described as *dextro* (d) when the aorta is rightward or *levo* (l) when the aorta is leftward. When the connection between one of the ventricles and a great artery is identifiable but the semilunar valve is atretic, the relationship between that ventricle and the great artery in question can still be described. When the artery itself is atretic, with no connection to the heart, as

can occur in some forms of pulmonary atresia, the term *transposition* technically cannot be used, as only one artery arises improperly.

When the heart has a double-outlet connection, the great artery (usually the aorta) that is committed to the improper ventricle is said to be malposed. The definition of a double-outlet ventricle using this system is not based on the percent override of the artery; rather, it is based on the precise anatomy of the infundibulum or conus of the outflow tracts. The conus is a remnant of the conus arteriosus of the embryonic heart that persists into the more mature heart. During normal cardiogenesis, the great arteries each have subarterial conus separating the great arteries from the bulbus cordis. Because the bulbus cordis is the future right ventricle, the outlets are thus initially both aligned with the right ventricle. In the course of normal cardiac development, the subaortic conus is reabsorbed, and the aorta is brought down into continuity with the tricuspid and mitral valves. When viewed in the echocardiographic long axis, the continuity between the mitral and aortic valves can clearly be seen, even when there is a large perimembranous VSD. The absence of subaortic conus in this anatomy defines the aorta as being committed to the left ventricle. When the subpulmonary conus is reabsorbed and the subaortic conus persists, it is the pulmonary artery that is pulled into continuity with the mitral valve, and the resultant anatomy is a transposition of the great arteries. Incomplete reabsorption of either conus results in both great arteries remaining committed to the right ventricle (bulbus cordis), and the anatomic diagnosis is DORV.

Because either conus can be partially reabsorbed, the relationship of the great arteries to each other and to the VSD that inevitably occurs in double-outlet connections must still be described. The "d" and "l" terminology used to describe transposition can be used here, with d-malposition/transposition of the aorta describing an aorta that is rightward of the pulmonary artery and l-malposition/transposition defining a leftward aorta (with respect to the pulmonary artery). Physiologically, when the subaortic conus is incompletely reabsorbed, the aorta is generally positioned closer to the left ventricle than to the pulmonary artery and the VSD is described as subaortic, as the aorta tends to override the VSD (when it is an outlet VSD) and the pulmonary artery is completely committed to the right ventricle. The resultant physiology is that of a large VSD. This anatomy is described as DORV with d-malposition of the aorta (the left ventricular outflow tract and aorta is normally rightward of the right ventricular outflow tract and pulmonary artery at the level of the semilunar valves). When the subpulmonary conus is incompletely reabsorbed, the pulmonary artery tends to override an outlet VSD and preferentially receive oxygenated blood from the left ventricle. In this arrangement, the aorta is generally completely committed to the right ventricle and preferentially receives deoxygenated blood. The physiology is thus that of transposition of the great arteries, and the VSD is described as subpulmonary, even though it may be in the same location within the ventricular septum as the subaortic VSD just described; this would be DORV with l-malposition of the aorta. When the VSD is located in the inlet or trabecular septum in the presence of DORV, the VSD is said to be remote, and the surgical course is usually that of single-ventricle palliation due to an inability to baffle the two ventricles to separate outlets. In the rare circumstance that both parts of the embryologic conus are reabsorbed, the anatomy is double-outlet left ventricle. Subaortic conus can also persist in the face of ventriculo-arterial concordance in the rare anatomy known as *anatomically corrected malposition of the great arteries*. In this case, great arteries arise from the morphologically appropriate ventricles, but the aorta is anterior to the pulmonary artery due to the persistent subaortic conus (13).

SYSTEMIC AND PULMONARY VENOUS CONNECTIONS

The systemic and pulmonary venous connections are often abnormal in complex lesions. The nomenclature is fairly intuitive, but it is important to specify these anomalies when they exist, as many have clinical implications for central line placement, surgical intervention, or physiologic shunts. Abnormalities of systemic venous connections can include bilateral superior vena cava, left superior vena cava, or interrupted inferior vena cava. Furthermore, the site of major venous connections to the heart can be altered from normal such that a right-to-left shunt occurs. Pulmonary venous connections may be either partially or totally anomalous, returning to sites other than the left atrium. Usually, the important aspects of description include noting which pulmonary veins are anomalous and categorizing the connection as supracardiac, cardiac, or infracardiac. Again, it is best to completely specify the exact nature of the connections when describing hearts with these anomalies.

CARDIAC POSITION

Chest x-ray is very helpful in making the diagnosis of an abnormally positioned heart, but a complete assessment usually requires echocardiography to identify the location of the cardiac apex. *Levocardia* is the normal positioning of the heart and describes a situation in which the heart is on the left side of the thorax; *dextrocardia* occurs when the heart is located predominantly in the right chest, and mesocardia is an intermediate situation with a more midline position. The position of the heart within the thorax does not automatically reveal the location of the apex of the heart. For example, one may find dextrocardia in which the apex of the heart still points toward the left side of the body and levocardia in which the apex is to the right. In general, when describing cardiac position, it is probably best to specify the position of the apex.

CLINICAL EXAMPLES

Using the segmental approach to the description of cardiac anatomy, it can be seen that a normal heart has atrioventricular concordance, two atrioventricular connections, and ventriculo-arterial concordance. Alternatively, this anatomy can be referred to as *atrial situs solitus*, d-loop ventricles, and arterial situs solitus {S,D,S}. The most common form of transposition of the great arteries (d-TGA) has atrioventricular concordance and ventriculo-atrial discordance (**Fig. 62.4C**) and can be referred to as atrial situs solitus, d-loop ventricles, and d-transposition of the great arteries {S,D,D}. Getting slightly more complex, congenitally corrected transposition (**Fig. 62.4D**), also called *isolated ventricular inversion*, is that condition in which the morphologic right atrium opens into the right-sided morphologic left ventricle, which gives rise to

the transposed pulmonary artery. The morphologic left atrium opens into the left-sided morphologic right ventricle, which gives rise to the transposed aorta. The great arteries are considered anatomically transposed because they arise from the "wrong" morphologic ventricles, but they are, in fact, physiologically correct. The pulmonary artery still carries deoxygenated blood to the lungs, and the aorta brings oxygenated blood to the body. This anatomy can be described as atrioventricular discordance and ventriculo-arterial discordance or as atrial situs solitus, l-looped ventricles, and l-transposition of the great arteries {S,L,L}. The most common double-inlet connection occurs when both the right and left atria open into a right-sided morphologic left ventricle, which gives rise to the pulmonary artery. The aorta arises off of an anterior and leftward chamber that lacks an atrioventricular inlet. The connection between the left ventricle and the chamber that gives rise to the aorta is through a VSD that is, at least according to Van Praagh, most properly referred to as the *bulboventricular foramen*, as the lack of atrioventricular inlet precludes referring to this outlet chamber as a ventricle. This heart can be referred to as having situs solitus atrial arrangement, a double-inlet atrioventricular connection with single left ventricle with right-handed topology and ventriculo-arterial discordance. It can also be designated as situs solitus atria, l-loop, and l-transposition of the great arteries {S,L,L} with double-inlet left ventricle. A Taussig-Bing heart, which has a DORV, bilateral subarterial conus, and subpulmonary VSD (aorta completely committed to the right ventricle, pulmonary artery may override the septum) would be described as atrioventricular concordance, ventriculo-arterial discordance with double-outlet ventriculo-arterial connection—or as atrial situs solitus, d-loop, l-malposition of the aorta {S,D,L} with DORV and subpulmonary VSD. Thus, any type of cardiac anatomy can be described using either school of segmental anatomy or even a combination of the two, as both offer particular advantages in certain situations. Even the heterotaxy syndromes that involve right or left atrial isomerism are initially described as above with appropriate modifications based on the ventricular and great artery relationships.

CONGENITAL CARDIAC DEFECTS

The incidence of congenital heart defects is 6–8 per 1000 live births (1 in 130–145 live births). Approximately 25% of congenital heart lesions can be considered complex, and one-third will require intervention during infancy (2), thus requiring intensive care. These figures do not include the clinically silent bicuspid, nonstenotic aortic valve, or mitral valve prolapse, and they exclude the incidence of a patent ductus arteriosus (PDA) in those born prematurely. Congenital heart defects are the most common congenital malformations, resulting in 10% of all infant deaths (6) and 50% of deaths due to a congenital malformations (1). Twenty-five percent of neonates with congenital heart defects (6) have other associated congenital abnormalities. Despite this and due to advances in the evaluation and treatment of these fragile children by a multidisciplinary team of physicians that includes pediatric intensivists, cardiologists, surgeons, anesthesiologists, and other healthcare providers (nurses, respiratory therapists, nutritionists, etc.), up to 85% of neonates born with congenital heart disease are now expected to survive to adulthood (5).

Congenital Heart Defects with Left-to-Right Shunts

Ventricular Septal Defect

VSD is the most common congenital heart defect (30%). Depending on their position in various parts of interventricular septum, VSDs can be divided into *inlet*, *perimembranous*, *muscular*, and *outlet* (which may be subaortic, subpulmonic, or doubly committed) defects (**Fig. 62.5**). Their position has implications for spontaneous closure rate (highest in muscular defects) and function of surrounding valves (aortic and pulmonary valve incompetence in doubly committed defects, aortic and tricuspid valve incompetence associated with perimembranous defects). Multiple defects can be present mainly in the muscular part of interventricular septum. Most VSDs are small (<3 mm in diameter). The size of the defect is only one factor that influences the volume of left-to-right shunt, with relative right and left ventricular pressure and compliance and the ratio

of pulmonary and systemic vascular resistance also playing important roles. The high kinetic energy of the blood that reaches pulmonary circulation due a large left-to-right shunt through VSD represents a risk for early onset of pulmonary vascular disease, and timely (before 2 years of age) VSD closure is advocated. VSDs have a high rate of spontaneous closure, especially in isolated small defects (up to 90% by 6 years of age). They are frequently associated with other congenital heart defects (e.g., aortic coarctation), or the defect is part of a more complex congenital cardiac malformation (e.g., tetralogy of Fallot). Significant risk of infective endocarditis is associated with VSDs.

Atrial Septal Defects

Various parts of interatrial septum can be affected by defects and, according to their position, ASDs are divided into *secundum* (within oval fossa and around foramen ovale), *primum* (part of atrioventricular septal defect), and *sinus venosus* (superior or inferior adjacent to the orifice of the superior or inferior caval vein) (**Fig. 62.6**). The spectrum of secundum

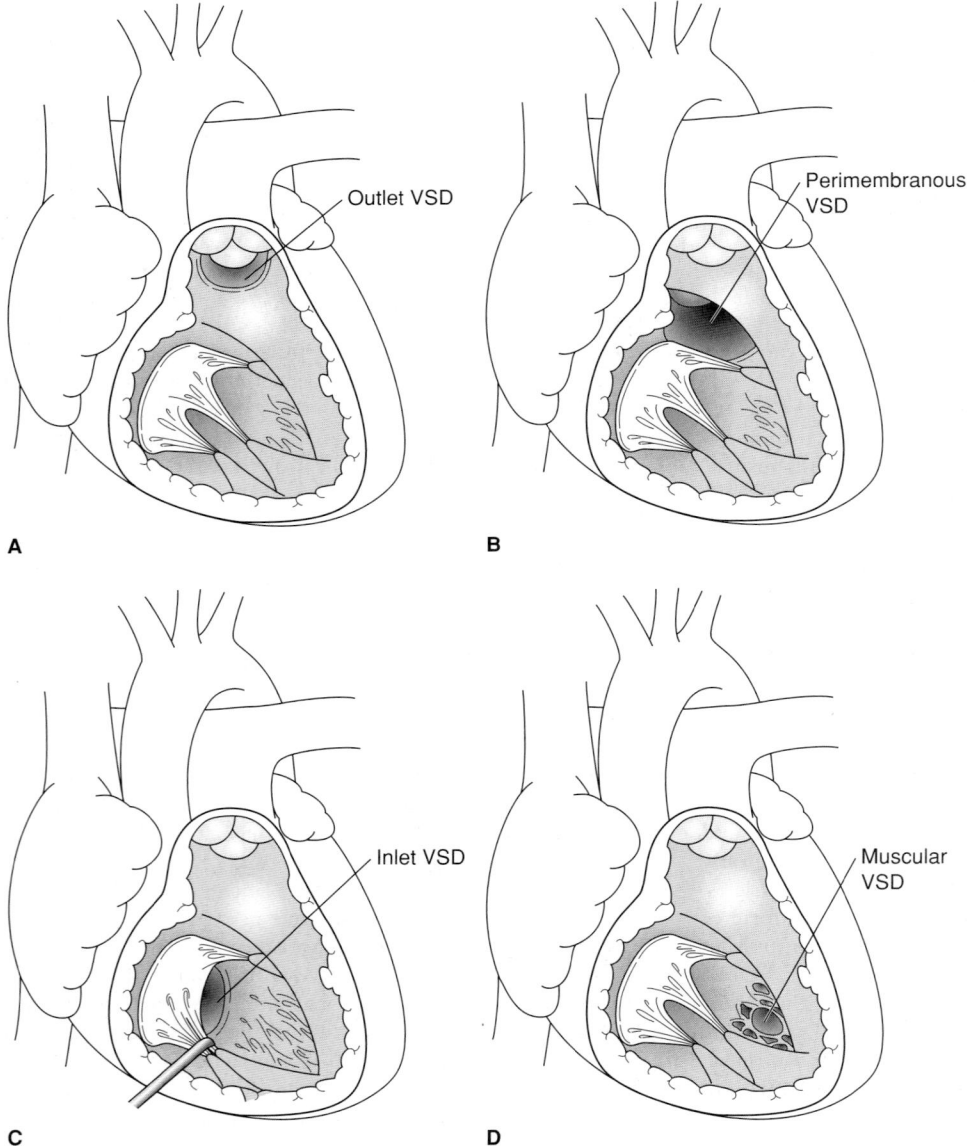

A

B

C

D

FIGURE 62.5. Various types of ventricular septal defects viewed from within the right ventricle. (**A**) outlet, (**B**) perimembranous, (**C**) inlet, (**D**) muscular or trabecular.

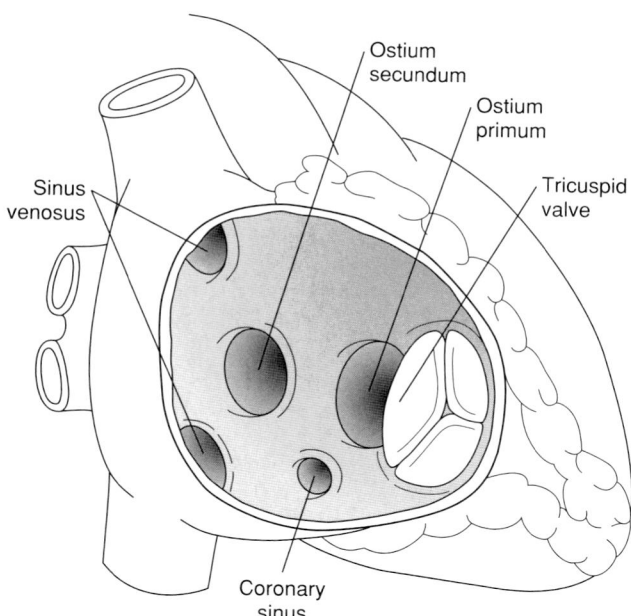

FIGURE 62.6. Various types of atrial septal defects (sinus venosus, ostium secundum, ostium primum) viewed through the right atrium. An unroofed coronary sinus may also act as an atrial septal defect.

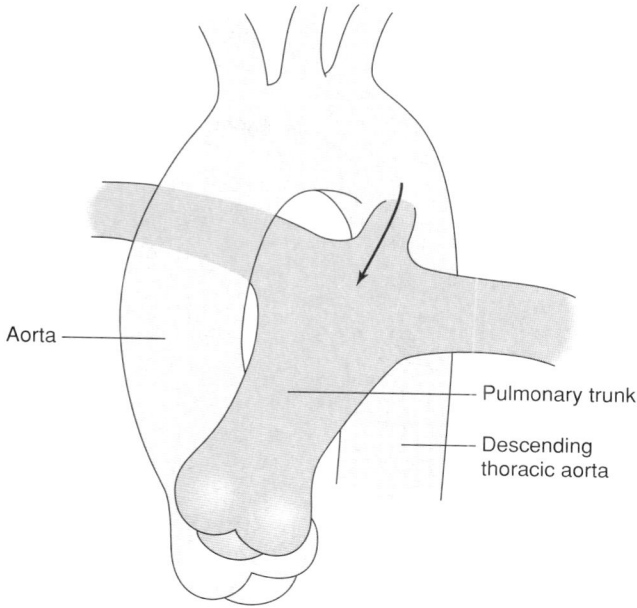

FIGURE 62.7. Patent ductus arteriosus (**arrow with left-to-right shunt**).

ASDs is dependent on the extent of missing septal wall. Small defects (<3–4 mm) are often considered part of the patent foramen ovale and may undergo spontaneous closure in some patients. Secundum ASDs are associated with other congenital heart defects (e.g., pulmonary valve stenosis). A sinus venosus superior defect is commonly associated with partial anomalous pulmonary venous drainage that involves the right upper pulmonary vein joining the superior vena cava. The volume of left-to-right shunt depends on the size of the defect and the relative compliance of right and left ventricles. The low kinetic energy of blood that reaches the pulmonary arteries makes the increase of pulmonary vascular resistance associated with isolated ASD in childhood very rare. Large ASDs left untreated until adulthood are associated with risk of atrial dysrhythmias and pulmonary vascular disease. Paradoxical embolism may occur regardless of ASD size, but it is rare in children. Antibiotic prophylaxis for infective endocarditis (subacute bacterial endocarditis prophylaxis) is not required in isolated secundum ASDs or 6 months after successful repair of an ASD.

Patent Ductus Arteriosus

The ductus arteriosus is part of the normal fetal circulation that joins the main pulmonary artery with the descending aorta. It allows for most of the blood that reaches the main pulmonary artery to bypass the lungs prenatally. The blood flow direction through the ductus arteriosus reverses postnatally, and the ductus arteriosus spontaneously closes in most neonates. Patency beyond 1 month of age (3 months in premature infants) is considered abnormal (**Fig. 62.7**). High rates of patency are common in preterm neonates. A PDA is mostly left-sided but right-sided or bilateral PDAs can be present. The PDA is the only source of pulmonary blood supply in some complex congenital heart defects (e.g., pulmonary valve atresia with intact ventricular septum), but it can be absent in others (e.g., most neonates with persistent truncus arteriosus) postnatally. Risk of

pulmonary vascular disease is high in a large PDA left untreated into childhood. Subacute bacterial endocarditis prophylaxis is required prior to surgical correction.

Atrioventricular Septal Defects

The complete form of an atrioventricular septal defect (AVSD) is characterized by the absence of the interatrial septum primum and inlet part of the interventricular septum, with concomitant malformation of the common atrioventricular valve and a variable degree of valvar incompetence (**Fig. 62.8**). This defect is often associated with trisomy 21 and can lead to the early development of pulmonary vascular obstructive disease. A *partial form* affects either the interatrial or interventricular septum, with variable abnormality of the atrioventricular (AV) valve apparatus.

Truncus Arteriosus

Truncus arteriosus (TA) is a single arterial trunk that is guarded by a single truncal valve that arises from the heart to bifurcate

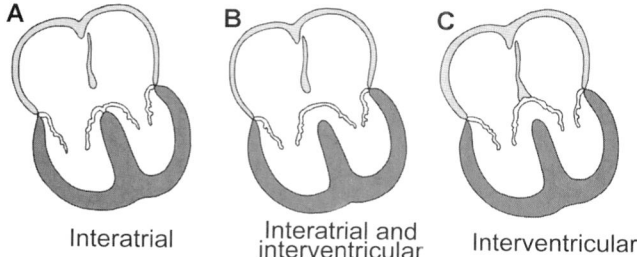

FIGURE 62.8. Atrioventricular septal defect (AVSD) due to deficiency between atrial and ventricular septal structures. (**A**) Shunting at atrial level (ostium primum ASD). (**B**) Shunting at both atrial and ventricular levels (complete AVSD). (**C**) Shunting at ventricular level only ("inlet VSD").

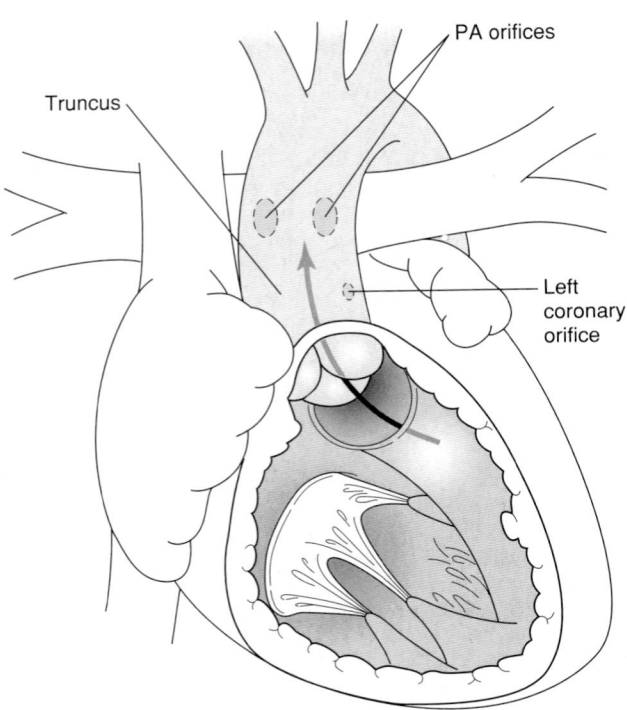

FIGURE 62.9. Truncus arteriosus Type II. The relationship of the truncal artery (truncus) to the truncal valve, left coronary ostium, and ventricular septal defect (**arrow**) is shown.

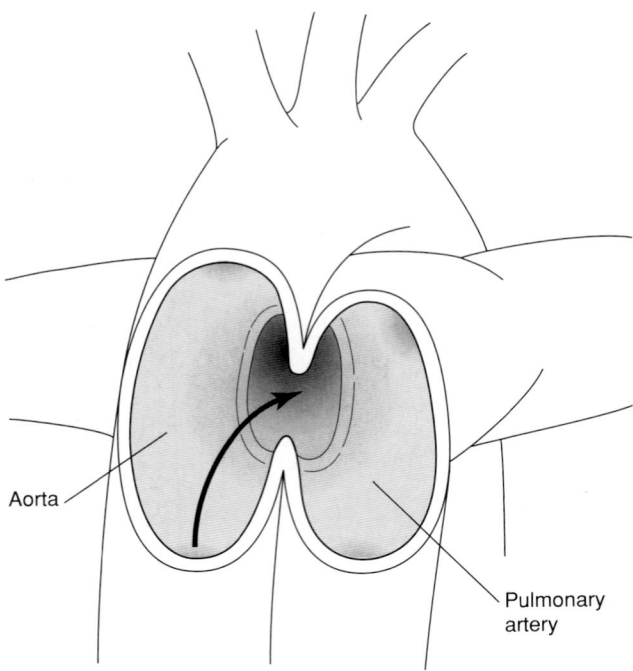

FIGURE 62.10. Aorta-pulmonary window.

into the ascending aorta and pulmonary arteries (type I) or to give rise to the branch pulmonary arteries at various locations (types II–IV) (**Fig. 62.9**). The truncal valve has a variable number of cusps and overrides the ventricular septal defect, thereby receiving blood from both the left and right ventricle. Stenosis and/or incompetence of the truncal valve occurs. The origin of the pulmonary arteries from the persistent truncus varies resulting in the different subtypes of the lesion. In TA type I the main pulmonary artery arises from the truncus and divides into the left and right pulmonary arteries. In TA type II, both left and right pulmonary arteries arise separately from the posterior aspect of the truncus, and in TA type III, the branch pulmonary arteries arise separately from the lateral walls. The large volume of pulmonary blood flow leads to early onset of congestive heart failure during the first days and weeks of life. The high kinetic energy of blood that reaches the pulmonary arterioles causes early pulmonary vascular obstructive disease in untreated patients. Cyanosis, which is typically mild, may be more significant in the presence of reduced pulmonary blood flow due to high pulmonary vascular resistance or pulmonary arterial stenoses. TA has a strong association with chromosome 22q11 microdeletion (DiGeorge syndrome).

Aortopulmonary Window

Direct, side-by-side communication is present between the ascending aorta and the main pulmonary artery in the form of an oval opening (**Fig. 62.10**). Separate aortic and pulmonary valves are found, distinguishing this lesion from TA. Free transmission of aortic blood pressure into pulmonary arteries represents a high risk of early onset of pulmonary vascular disease.

Partial or Total Anomalous Pulmonary Venous Connection

Abnormality in the pulmonary venous connections occurs when one (partial anomalous pulmonary venous connection, PAPVC) to all four (total APVC, TAPVC) pulmonary veins connect anomalously with the systemic venous system (inferior or superior vena cavae), right atrium, or coronary sinus (**Fig. 62.11**). The partial variety, involving the right upper pulmonary vein connected with the superior vena cava, is often associated with a superior sinus venosus ASD. Depending on the insertion of the anomalous connection, TAPVC can be *supracardiac* (with pulmonary venous drainage into the innominate vein or superior vena cava), *intracardiac* (with pulmonary venous drainage into coronary sinus or right atrium), or *infracardiac* (with pulmonary venous drainage into hepatic or portal veins). Obstruction of the anomalous pulmonary venous connection (mainly in the supracardiac and infracardiac forms) results in profound cyanosis with severe pulmonary hypertension postnatally. Unobstructed TAPVC presents with signs and symptoms of mild cyanosis with congestive heart failure from the increased pulmonary blood flow. Systemic blood flow depends on interatrial communication (atrial septal defect) and shunt from the right into the left atrium. Muscularization of the pulmonary venous wall and progressive narrowing of pulmonary veins have been described.

Cyanotic Congenital Heart Defects

Tetralogy of Fallot

Tetralogy of Fallot is the most common cyanotic congenital heart defect, named for a combination of *VSD* with *overriding aorta*, *right ventricular outflow tract obstruction*, and

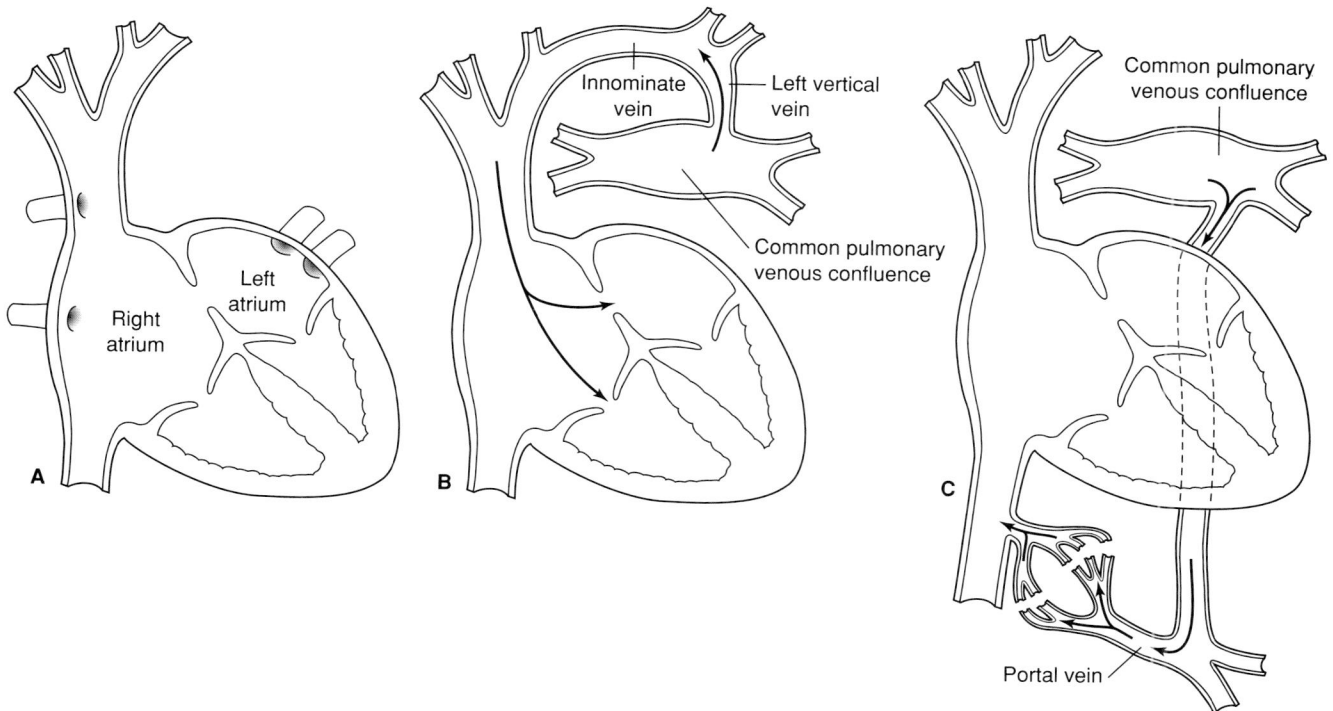

FIGURE 62.11. Variants of anomalous pulmonary venous connections. (**A**) Partial anomalous venous connection of the right pulmonary veins to the right atrium. (**B**) Supracardiac total anomalous pulmonary venous connection, with vertical vein to the innominate vein; (**C**) Infracardiac total anomalous pulmonary venous connection with vertical vein traversing the esophageal hiatus in the diaphragm and connecting to the inferior vena cava via the portal vein.

right ventricular hypertrophy (**Fig. 62.12**). Interventricular septal malalignment that involves superior and anterior shift of the outlet septum contributes to subvalvar pulmonary stenosis. Some degree of pulmonary annular and arterial hypoplasia is commonly present. Its severe form may involve pulmonary

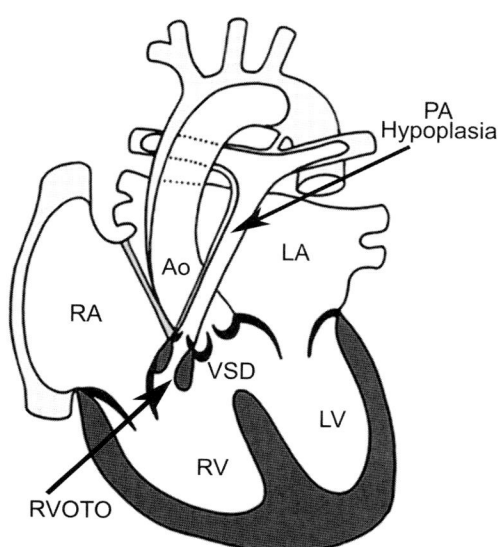

FIGURE 62.12. Tetralogy of Fallot. Ao, aorta; LA, left atrium; RA, right atrium; LV, left ventricle; RV, right ventricle; VSD, ventricular septal defect; RVOTO, right ventricular outflow tract obstruction; PA, pulmonary artery.

atresia and variable degrees of central pulmonary arterial hypoplasia, sometimes with additional aortopulmonary collateral arteries supplying different segments of the pulmonary circulation. AVSD, anomalous origin of the left anterior interventricular coronary artery from the right coronary artery, and/or right-sided aortic arch are the most common cardiac anomalies associated with tetralogy of Fallot. Chromosome 22q11 microdeletion (DiGeorge Syndrome), is common, especially if a right-sided aortic arch is found.

Pulmonary Atresia with Intact Ventricular Septum

Pulmonary atresia with intact ventricular septum results in a spectrum of hypoplasia of the right ventricle and tricuspid valve (**Fig. 62.13**). The pulmonary arteries are usually of normal size due to blood flow from an obligate PDA, which arises from the aorta in a reverse angle. Coronary arterial fistulae connecting with the right ventricular cavity are present in up to one-third of all cases. These can be associated with coronary arterial stenoses, which in combination can lead to coronary steal phenomenon and myocardial ischemia postnatally. The degree of right ventricular hypoplasia and presence of coronary anomalies determine suitability for a palliative or corrective surgical repair.

Transposition of Great Arteries

Ventriculo-arterial discordance leads to an aorta arising from the right ventricle and the pulmonary artery arising from the left ventricle, which results in systemic and pulmonary blood flow configured in parallel circuits rather than in series (**Fig. 62.14**). Postnatal survival depends on mixing of blood between

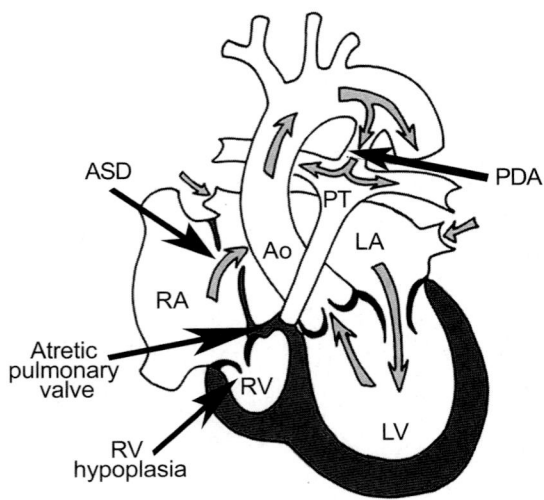

FIGURE 62.13. Pulmonary atresia with intact ventricular septum. ASD, atrial septum defect; Ao, aorta; PT, pulmonary trunk; PDA, patent ductus arteriosus; LA, left atrium; LV, left ventricle; RA, right atrium; RV, right ventricle.

the systemic and pulmonary circulations, usually at the atrial and ductal levels. VSD and/or pulmonary stenosis are the most frequent associated cardiac defects. Coronary artery anomalies are common, with an intramural course of a coronary artery being rare but most difficult for the surgeon to manage intra-operatively.

Obstructive Congenital Heart Defects

Pulmonary Valve Stenosis

A variable degree of commissural fusion between the valvar cusps is the most common cause of pulmonary stenosis (**Fig. 62.15**). Tethering of the superior cusp edges and dysplasia of cusps themselves are less common varieties of stenosis. Mild, isolated stenosis rarely progresses. Concomitant presence of right ventricular muscular hypertrophy depends on the hemo-

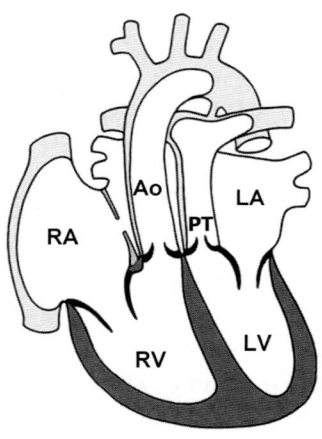

FIGURE 62.14. Transposition of the great arteries {S,D,D},with the pulmonary trunk arising from the left ventricle and the aorta arising from the right ventricle. RA, right atrium; Ao, aorta; PT, pulmonary trunk; LA, left atrium; RV, right ventricle; LV, left ventricle.

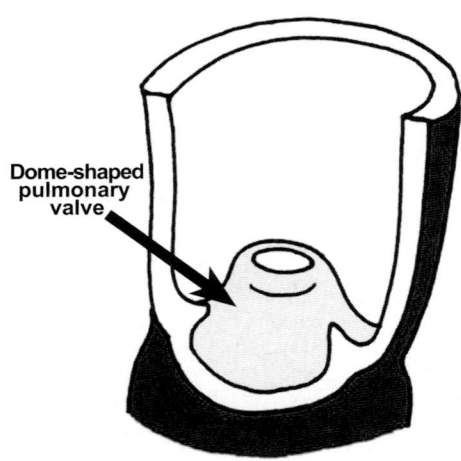

FIGURE 62.15. Pulmonary valve stenosis with dome-shaped valve.

dynamic significance of the stenosis. Severe forms of right ventricular hypertrophy may contribute to subvalvar stenosis. Supravalvar pulmonary stenosis that affects the main pulmonary artery or its branches may occur in isolation or in combination with valvar and subvalvar stenoses. This combination is seen as part of tetralogy of Fallot (see earlier description). ASDs and VSDs are the most common associated cardiac defects.

Aortic Valve Stenosis

Stenotic valves can be described as unicuspid, bicuspid, or tricuspid, depending on the number of functional commissures between valvar cusps (**Fig. 62.16**). Unicuspid valves are usually most severely stenosed. Bicuspid valves, on the other hand, may present without stenosis in childhood. Gross dysplasia of valvar cusps has been described in up to 10% of congenital aortic valve stenoses. Concomitant aortic valve regurgitation is more common in previously treated valves (i.e., after balloon and/or surgical valvuloplasty). Aortic coarctation is the most common associated defect. Any malformed aortic valve is likely to undergo calcification in adulthood.

Coarctation of the Aorta and Interruption of the Aortic Arch

In coarctation of the aorta, narrowing in the distal part of aortic arch around the aortic isthmus may be accompanied by variable degree and extent of aortic arch hypoplasia (**Fig. 62.17**). Aortic coarctation is closely associated with arterial ductal insertion into the aortic wall, and a discrete shelf inside the aortic lumen may become obvious only on ductal closure in some patients postnatally. Arterial ductal patency plays an important role in most cases with severe neonatal aortic coarctation, as it allows for blood flow to reach the lower part of the body. Collateral arteries that bridge the narrow aortic segment develop gradually during childhood in untreated patients. VSD, bicuspid aortic valve, and aortic and mitral valve stenoses are the most common associated anomalies. Systemic hypertension due to abnormal arterial wall structure and function and intracranial arterial aneurysms represent a long-term risk of severe complications, even in successfully treated patients.

In aortic arch interruption, a segment of the aortic arch is missing or replaced by a solid cord (**Fig. 62.18**). Depending

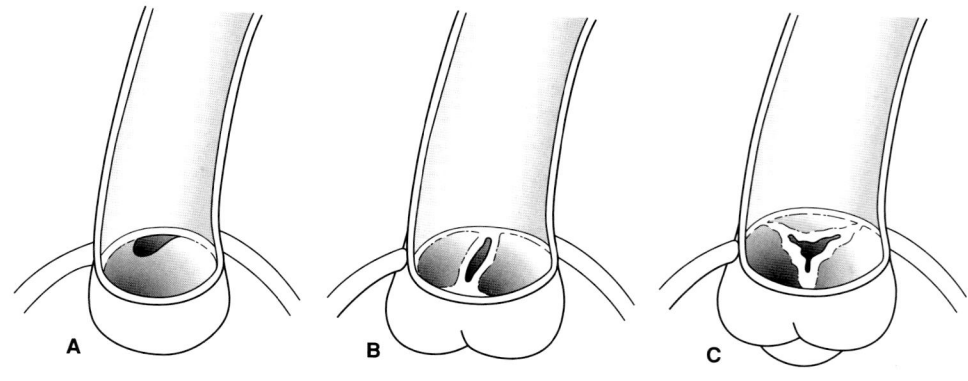

FIGURE 62.16. Different types of aortic valve stenosis with (A) unicuspid valve, (B) bicuspid valve, and (C) dysplastic valve.

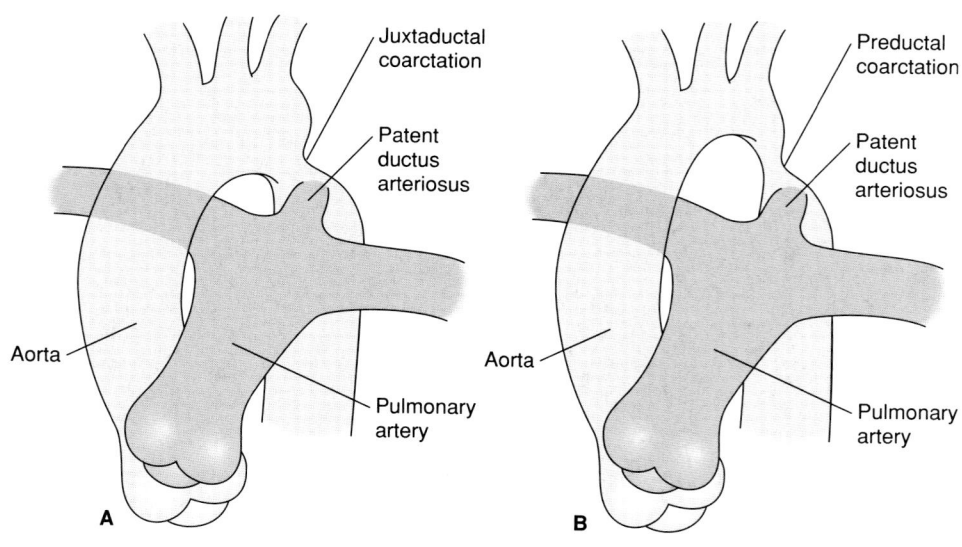

FIGURE 62.17. (A) Juxtaductal coarctation of the aorta. (B) Preductal coarctation associated with aortic arch hypoplasia.

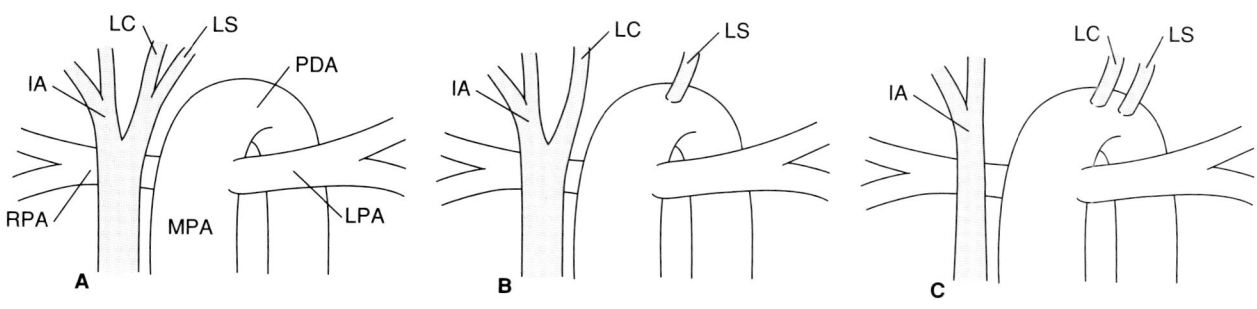

FIGURE 62.18. Interrupted aortic arch. (A) Type A interruption of the arch distal to the left subclavian artery. (B) Type B interruption of the arch distal to the left carotid artery and proximal to the left subclavian artery. (C) Type C interruption of the arch between the innominate artery and the left carotid artery. IA, innominate artery; LPA, left pulmonary artery; MPA, main pulmonary artery; PDA posterior descending artery; RPA, right pulmonary artery.

on the location of the missing aortic arch segment, the defect is categorized as type A, interruption distal to the left subclavian artery; type B (most common), interruption between the common carotid and left subclavian arteries; and type C, interruption between the two common carotid arteries. A PDA with right-to-left shunt is the only source of blood supply for body parts distal to the interruption. A VSD is the most common associated heart defect. Chromosome 22q11 microdeletion is strongly linked with type B interruption of the aortic arch.

Complex Congenital Heart Defects

Ebstein Anomaly of the Tricuspid Valve

Tricuspid valve malformation due to apical displacement of the septal and mural leaflet annular attachment is the leading underlying pathology of Ebstein anomaly. Annular attachment of the anterosuperior leaflet is usually normal. All leaflets of the valve may be larger or smaller than normal, contributing to the failure of all three leaflets to coapt successfully in ventricular systole. A variable degree of tricuspid valve incompetence is the most frequently encountered hemodynamic abnormality. Marked apical displacement of the tricuspid valve limits the size of the right ventricular cavity and may contribute to right ventricular outflow obstruction. An ASD is the most frequently associated anomaly. A wide spectrum of tricuspid valve malformations influences clinical presentation, from an asymptomatic child or adolescent presenting with supraventricular tachycardia or mild cyanosis (due to a right-to-left interatrial shunt) to a critically ill cyanotic neonate with severe obstruction to the right ventricular outflow and marked tricuspid regurgitation. Supraventricular tachycardia due to a manifest accessory connection (Wolff-Parkinson-White syndrome) can occur in utero, in infancy, in childhood, or in adolescence in patients with Ebstein anomaly.

Univentricular Hearts

A wide variety of congenital heart defects involves hypoplasia of one ventricle (right or left) and abnormality of the AV valves (tricuspid, mitral, or AVSD). The abnormality may be stenosis or atresia of the AV connection or both AV valves emptying into a dominant ventricle (i.e., double-inlet ventricle) (**Fig. 62.19**). A hypoplastic ventricle may communicate with the dominant ventricle through a VSD. Anomalies of systemic and pulmonary venous connections are common, as are anomalies of the ventriculo-arterial connections. The heterotaxy syndromes (asplenia/polysplenia) are strongly associated with these complex defects.

Hypoplastic left-heart syndrome is a common form of univentricular heart with variable but mostly severe degrees of hypoplasia that affects the mitral valve, left ventricle, aortic valve, and aortic arch, including coarctation. The left ventricle is unable to support the systemic circulation postnatally. Systemic arterial blood flow and survival depend on a PDA with a right-to-left shunt. As pulmonary vascular resistance drops after birth, systemic perfusion (Qs) decreases due to excessive pulmonary (Qp) blood flow (an increased Qp:Qs ratio). The right ventricle must sustain both pulmonary and systemic circulations. If the ASD is markedly restrictive, obstruction to pulmonary venous drainage occurs, which typically results in a very poor outcome. Anatomic anomalies of the central nervous system are common and should be investigated preoperatively, even in the absence of systemic hypoperfusion.

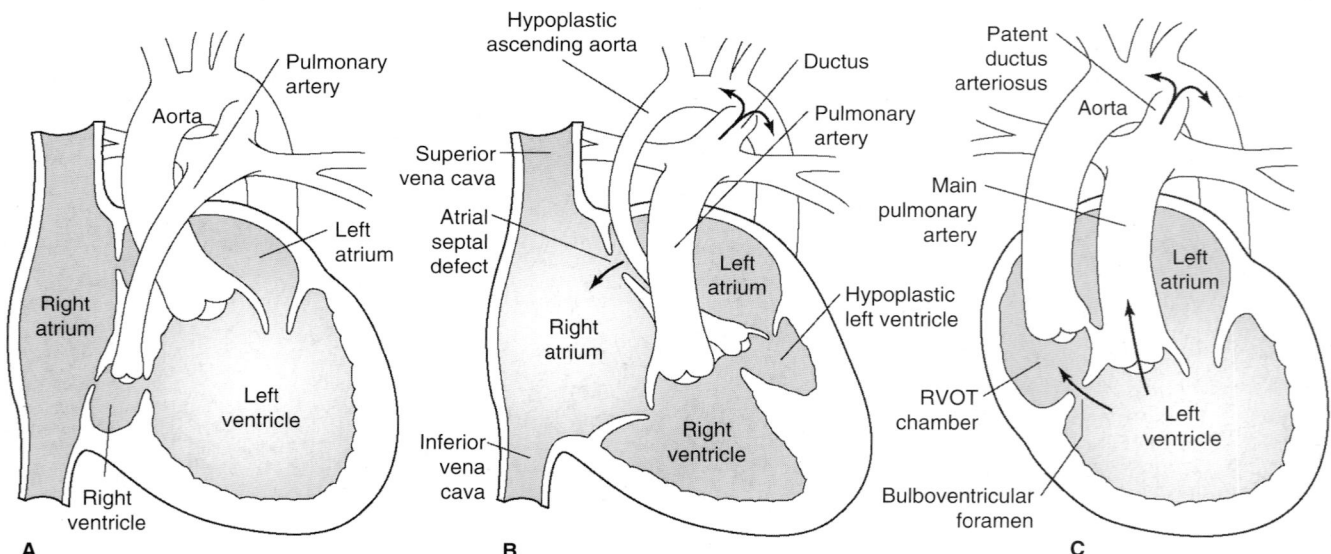

FIGURE 62.19. Common variants of "univentricular" hearts. (**A**) Tricuspid atresia with a small VSD and severely hypoplastic right ventricle. (**B**) Mitral atresia with a small VSD and severely hypoplastic left ventricle. Systemic blood flow is propelled by the right ventricle via the pulmonary artery and ductus arteriosus. Pulmonary venous return enters the left atrium and crosses the atrial septal defect into the right atrium. Systemic venous flow returns normally from the inferior vena cava and superior vena cava to the right atrium. (**C**) Double-inlet left ventricle with a small bulboventricular foramen and small outlet chamber. The aorta arises from a hypoplastic RV outflow (RVOT) chamber, producing subaortic stenosis. The main pulmonary artery connects with the left ventricle.

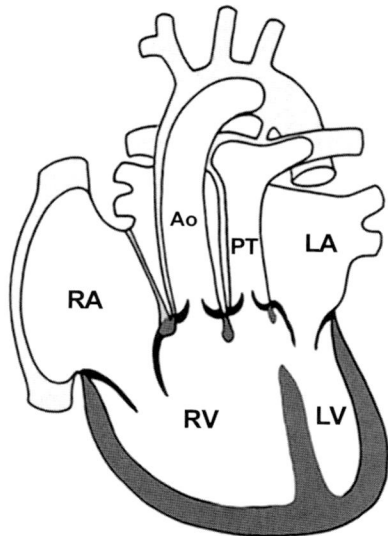

FIGURE 62.20. Double-outlet right ventricle with transposition physiology (aorta rightward and side-by-side with the pulmonary trunk). RA, right atrium; Ao, aorta; PT, pulmonary trunk; LA, left atrium; RV, right ventricle; LV, left ventricle.

Double-Outlet Right Ventricle

In DORV, both aorta and pulmonary artery arise from the morphologic right ventricle. A semilunar valve is committed to a ventricle when ≥50% of the valve arises from the ventricle. Thus, in DORV, the left ventricle ejects through a VSD into the semilunar valves (**Fig. 62.20**). The relative position of the VSD and the semilunar valves determines the distinctly divergent postnatal hemodynamics. A subaortic position of the VSD is more common and associated with pulmonary stenosis, which results in a tetralogy of Fallot-like situation. When the VSD is in a subpulmonary position, a transposition-like physiology results, with the left ventricle ejecting blood through the VSD back into the pulmonary artery.

CONCLUSIONS AND FUTURE DIRECTIONS

The future of understanding complex congenital heart disease lies in connecting the well-known phenotypes to the underlying genotypes and developmental anomalies that lead to the formation of the defect. Diagnosis of the cardiac defects into earlier stages of fetal life may lead to opportunities to intervene and correct—or at least modify—the cardiac defect. Advances in bioinformatics allow for caregivers in the PICU to visualize and review ultrasonographic images, MRIs, and angiograms, at the bedside to facilitate understanding and communication among the team members caring for the critically ill infant, child, or adolescent.

KEY POINTS

- The incidence of congenital heart defects is 6–8 per 1000 live births (1 in 130–145 live births).

- Approximately 25% of congenital heart lesions can be considered complex, and one-third will require intervention during infancy.
- Congenital heart defects are the most common congenital malformations, resulting in 10% of all infant deaths and 50% of deaths due to a congenital malformation.
- Twenty-five percent of neonates with congenital heart defects have other associated congenital abnormalities.
- The use of the segmental approach to the description of complex congenital heart disease systems allows a clear form of communication of all essential elements of the cardiac anatomy.
- The intensive care physician should be comfortable using this terminology to discuss congenital cardiac lesions with the cardiologists and cardiac surgeons on the team toward ensuring that all anatomic issues are clarified in the preoperative and postoperative ICU management of these complex patients.
- Congenital cardiac defects are broadly classified into four categories: left-to-right shunts, cyanotic defects, obstructive defects, and other complex congenital heart defects.

References

1. Anderson RH. Nomenclature and classification: Sequential segmental analysis. In: Moller JH, Hoffman JIE, eds. *Pediatric Cardiovascular Medicine.* Philadelphia: Churchill Livingstone 2000;263–74.
2. Anderson RH, Baker EJ, Macartney FJ, et al. eds. *Paediatric Cardiology,* 2nd ed. London: Churchill Livingstone, 2005.
3. Anderson RH, Becker AE, Tynan M, et al. The univentricular atrioventricular connection: Getting to the root of a thorny problem. *Am J Cardiol* 1984; 54:822–8.
4. Partridge JB, Scott O, Deverall PB, et al. Visualization and measurement of the main bronchi by tomography as an objective indicator of thoracic situs in congenital heart disease. *Circulation* 1975;51:188–96.
5. Perloff JK, Warnes CA. Challenges posed by adults with repaired congenital heart disease. *Circulation* 2001;103:2637–43.
6. Peterson S, Peto V, Rayner M. Congenital heart disease statistics 2003. British Heart Foundation Statistics Database 2003. www.heartstats.org. Accessed May 2007.
7. Sinzobahamvya N, Arenz C, Brecher AM, et al. Atrial isomerism: A surgical experience. *Cardiovasc Surg* 1999;7:436–42.
8. Uemura H, Ho SY, Devine WA, et al. Analysis of visceral heterotaxy according to splenic status, appendage morphology, or both. *Am J Cardiol* 1995; 76:846–9.
9. Uemura H, Ho SY, Devine WA, et al. Atrial appendages and venoatrial connections in hearts from patients with visceral heterotaxy. *Ann Thorac Surg* 1995;60:561–9.
10. Van Mierop LHS. Transposition of the great arteries. I. Clarification of further confusion? (editorial) *Am J Cardiol* 1971;28:735–8.
11. Van Praagh R. Transposition of the great arteries. II. Transposition clarified. *Am J Cardiol* 1971;28:739–41.
12. Van Praagh R. Nomenclature and classification: Morphologic and segmental approach to diagnosis. In: Moller JH, Hoffman JIE, eds. *Pediatric Cardiovascular Medicine.* Philadelphia: Churchill Livingstone, 2000;275–88.
13. Van Praagh R, Durnin RE, Jockin H, et al. Anatomically corrected malposition of the great arteries {S,D,L}. *Circulation* 1975;51:20–31.
14. Van Praagh R, Perez-Trevino C, Lopez-Cuellar M, et al. Transposition of the great arteries with posterior aorta, anterior pulmonary artery, subpulmonary conus, and fibrous continuity between aortic and atrioventricular valves. *Am J Cardiol* 1971;28:621–31.
15. Van Praagh S, Santini F, Sanders SP. Cardiac malpositions with special emphasis on visceral heterotaxy (asplenia and polysplenia syndromes). In: Fyler DC, ed. *Nadas' Pediatric Cardiology.* Philadelphia: Hanley & Belfus, 1991; 589–608.
16. Van Praagh R, Van Praagh S. Atrial isomerism in the heterotaxy syndromes with asplenia, or polysplenia, or normally formed spleen: An erroneous concept. *Am J Cardiol* 1990;60:1504–6.
17. Van Praagh R, Weinberg PM, Matsuoka R, et al. Malpositions of the heart. In: Adams FH, Emmanouilides GC, eds. *Moss' Heart Disease in Infants, Children and Adolescents,* 3rd ed. Baltimore: Williams & Wilkins, 1983;422–58.

CHAPTER 63 ■ CARDIOVASCULAR PHYSIOLOGY

PETER OISHI • DAVID F. TEITEL • JULIEN I. HOFFMAN • JEFFREY R. FINEMAN

The chief function of the cardiovascular system is to deliver essential products to the tissues in order to maintain normal metabolic function and to remove metabolic waste products from them. Derangements in normal cardiovascular function are integral to the pathophysiology of a wide array of critical disease processes in children. In addition, many therapies employed in the intensive care setting directly or indirectly impact the cardiovascular system in ways that may either improve or impede its function. Complicating matters further, components within the cardiovascular system may be differentially or, in fact, diametrically affected by specific therapies, requiring practitioners to reconcile these varying responses.

This chapter contains a review of the basic vascular anatomy and the fundamental hemodynamic principles that govern flow through the circulation, an examination of the general mechanisms that regulate vascular tone, and a review of some specific regional circulations in detail. In addition, the special circumstance of the fetal circulation and the perinatal transition are reviewed. An understanding of these concepts should assist the intensivist in caring for patients with cardiovascular compromise and in arbitrating the various needs of the regional circulations.

THE CARDIOVASCULAR CIRCUIT AND VASCULAR ANATOMY

The cardiovascular system is composed of a pump and a large network of tubes that carry blood with all of its metabolic substances to and away from the tissues. The pump is the heart, which is actually two pumps in series: the right ventricle, which pumps blood through the pulmonary circulation, and the left ventricle, which pumps blood through the systemic circulation. Some authors divide the circulation into the *central circulation*, which includes the pulmonary circulation and the large systemic arteries and veins, and the *peripheral circulation*, which includes the various regional vascular beds.

Vascular anatomy is suited to match its function within the circulation. Vessels are composed of concentric layers, which include, from inside to out, the intima, media, and adventitia, although some vessel types can lack some layers. The innermost layer of the intima is the vascular endothelium, which is responsible for critical vascular metabolic processes. In addition, it functions as a barrier to the movement into the interstitial space of fluid, gases, and solutes with varying degrees of permeability that depend upon the location within the circulation. In large arteries, the internal elastic lamina separates the intima from the media, which is composed mostly of smooth muscle cells. In addition, this interface contains varying amounts of nerves and perforating vessels that nourish the arteries themselves, termed *vasa vasorum*. The external elastic lamina separates the media from the adventitia, which contains nerves, vasa vasorum, and connective tissue. Smaller arteries have less elastic tissue, and the arterioles have even less. Smooth muscle cell contraction decreases the compliance of the vessel, making it stiffer, and decreases the luminal diameter. A number of factors cause vascular smooth muscle cells to contract or relax; the contractile state of the smooth muscle cells forms the basis of vascular tone. Capillaries are thin-walled vessels, essentially lacking all but the endothelial cell layer, which makes them suitable for transporting and receiving substances to and from the tissues that they supply. Veins have the same basic layers as arteries, but are less well organized and have thinner walls and larger luminal diameters as compared to arteries at similar locations in the circulation. In addition, many veins contain unidirectional valves, which prevent blood from moving backward away from the heart.

HEMODYNAMIC PRINCIPLES

The cardiovascular system does not conform precisely to simple physical models of fluid hemodynamics. However, a basic understanding of hemodynamic principles is essential in the care of critically ill patients with cardiovascular derangements.

Flow, Velocity, and Cross-Sectional Area

The velocity of blood through a segment of the circulation has units of distance and time (e.g., centimeters/second). The flow of blood through the circulation has units of volume and time (e.g., liters/minute). At a constant flow, the velocity of blood through a vessel relates to the cross-sectional area of the vessel, expressed by the equation:

$$v = Q/A$$

where v is velocity, Q is flow, and A is the cross-sectional area.

From this relationship, it can be seen that velocity is proportional to flow and inversely proportional to the cross-sectional area. Thus, peak velocity occurs in the aorta and reaches its nadir in the capillary beds, which have tremendous cross-sectional areas. Velocity increases again as blood moves from the capillaries toward the central veins.

Pressure, Flow, and Resistance

The primary determinants of flow (Q) through a vascular segment are the inflow pressure (P_i), the outflow pressure (P_o), and the vascular resistance (R). For Newtonian fluids moving with laminar flow through cylindrical tubes, the relationship of flow to various physical factors can be expressed by Poiseuille's law, which is:

$$Q = (P_i - P_o)\,\pi r^4/8\eta l$$

where r is radius, η is viscosity, and l is length.

Thus, flow through a vessel will increase as the pressure difference across the vessel increases. Furthermore, as the diameter of the vessel increases, so too will flow at any given pressure difference ($P_i - P_o$). Conversely, increases in viscosity and vessel length result in a decrease in flow.

Alterations in blood vessel diameter, resulting from changes in the contractile state of vascular smooth muscle, are central to the regulation of blood flow, particularly in the regional vascular beds. The relationship of pressure and flow to resistance can be understood by examining the hydraulic equivalent of Ohm's law:

$$R = (P_i - P_o)/Q$$

which states that the resistance to flow through a vessel is equivalent to the change in pressure across the vessel divided by the flow through the vessel. Again, for Newtonian fluids moving through cylindrical tubes, this relationship can be expressed by a rearrangement of Poiseuille's law to give the hydraulic resistance equation:

$$R = (P_i - P_o)/Q = 8\eta l/\pi r^4$$

Therefore, when Poiseuille's law is applied, the resistance to flow is determined solely by the dimensions of the vessel and the viscosity of the fluid. Moreover, as resistance changes with the fourth power of the radius, vascular contraction or relaxation has a profound impact on flow through a vessel.

Studies indicate that pressure within the vasculature decreases progressively from the aorta to the vena cava and that the largest drop occurs at the level of the arterioles (4). Thus, it follows from the relationships above that resistance is greatest at the level of the arterioles if blood flow is constant through the circulation. However, how do we reconcile this fact with the impact of vessel diameter on resistance, in that the internal diameter of a capillary is far less than an arteriole? These findings can be reconciled by understanding that capillary beds are vessels in parallel, while the arterial system feeding a particular capillary bed is in series. When calculating the resistance of a system composed of a set of resistors in series (e.g., aorta, large arteries, small arteries, arterioles), the total resistance is equal to the sum of the individual resistances. Conversely, when calculating the resistance of a system composed of a set of resistors in parallel, such as a capillary network, the total resistance is equal to the sum of the reciprocals of the individual resistances (1/R). Thus, for a capillary network, the total resistance is less than the resistance in any individual capillary.

In addition, organs may have a number of resistance vessels in parallel proximal to the capillary bed. These vessels may be patent or may be recruited with increased flow. Increased pulmonary blood flow that occurs with exercise, for example,

is in part accommodated by the recruitment of arteries that were previously closed. Thus, an additional factor, k, which represents these vessels or potential vessels can be added to the resistance equation:

$$R = 8\eta l/\pi r^4 k$$

From this equation, it can be seen that an increase in k will reduce resistance. In addition, the loss of these vessels—i.e., a reduction in k—that may occur with disease (such as the obliteration of distal pulmonary arteries in advanced pulmonary arterial hypertension) or the occlusion of vessels by intravascular emboli will result in increased resistance.

Finally, changes in pressure that occur in response to changes in flow and resistance can be expressed when Ohm's law is rearranged as:

$$P_i = QR + P_o$$

Thus, vascular pressure may increase when vascular resistance or blood flow increases. These factors are not independent, and pressure may remain constant with increased blood flow because the increased flow has caused vascular resistance to decrease, for example, by dilating or recruiting previously closed vessels; that is, if the product *QR* does not increase, neither will pressure.

Compliance

A change in intravascular pressure results in a proportional change in intravascular volume. The incremental change in volume (ΔV) per unit change in pressure (ΔP) defines the compliance (C) of a vessel, as indicated by the equation:

$$C = \Delta V/\Delta P$$

The walls of veins are thinner, less well organized, and contain less elastic tissue than those of arteries and thus are ~20 times more compliant. As a result, the majority of the circulating blood volume at any one time resides in the venous system, and therapeutic volume expansion has a disproportionate affect on venous, as opposed to arterial, volume.

Imprecision of Mathematical Models

The application of these mathematical relationships in the vasculature has important caveats. Blood is not Newtonian, although at normal hematocrits, this is probably of little consequence. Additionally, the walls of small arteries are neither smooth nor straight; rather they branch, curve, and taper. Furthermore, blood flow is pulsatile, so that additional energy (and therefore a higher pressure) is necessary to overcome inertia and to accelerate the blood at each ejection. Because of short distances between arterial branch points, laminar flow is unlikely in peripheral vascular beds, and viscous pressure losses would be greater than in a physical model. Arteries are also distensible, and continuously changing transvascular pressures alter their radii; therefore, pressure-flow relationships are not linear. Lastly, vascular beds are comprised of many blood vessels in parallel. These vessels are not all open all the time, and their radii vary. Despite these differences, the general principles of changes in physical factors such as viscosity and radius apply (19).

INTERACTION OF THE CARDIAC PUMP AND THE VASCULATURE

Cardiac output is determined by heart rate, contractility, preload, and afterload. The precise mechanisms relevant to the control of heart rate and contractility, which are properties directly related to the heart, are reviewed in Chapter 65. Preload and afterload are related to both the heart and properties of the vasculature. These interactions can be understood by examining the vascular function curve, the cardiac function curve, otherwise known as the Starling curve, and their interactions.

Vascular Function Curve

The vascular function curve describes how changes in cardiac output affect central venous pressure (CVP), or venous return (**Fig. 63.1**). To understand this relationship, a conceptual model can be used to partition the circulation into components, including a pump, an arterial compartment with a given compliance (C_a), a resistor (which represents the resistance through the arterioles, capillaries, and venules), and a venous compartment with a given compliance (C_v) (**Fig. 63.2**). The pump displaces blood from the venous compartment into the arterial compartment at some rate (Q) which in this model, is equivalent to the cardiac output. The compliance of the arterial compartment accommodates a portion of this volume before blood is propelled across the microvascular resistor into the venous compartment, which can accommodate a much larger volume than the arterial compartment due to its greater compliance. Increases in Q, will decrease the volume of blood that resides in the venous compartment and, hence, will decrease the pressure

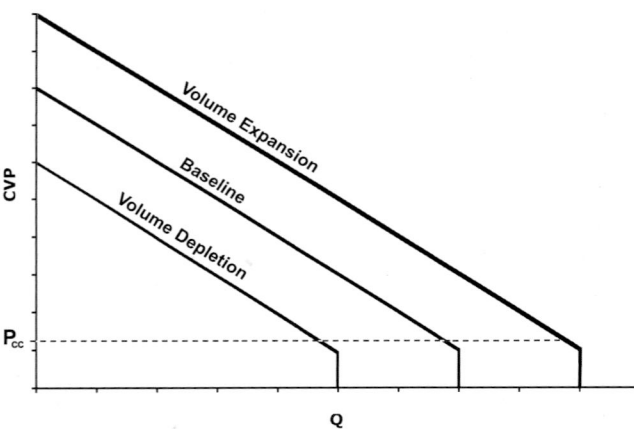

FIGURE 63.1. Vascular function curves shown at different intravascular volumes. The vascular function curve describes the effect of cardiac output (Q) on central venous pressure (CVP), or venous return. Increases in Q decrease CVP, while decreases in Q increase CVP. Maximal Q occurs at the critical closing pressure of the venous circulation, whereby reductions in the volume of blood in the venous compartment are not possible, representing the lowest possible CVP and highest possible Q for any given blood volume (P_{cc}, critical closing pressure). At zero Q, the system reaches equilibrium, where pressures within the arterial and venous compartments are determined solely by compliance for any given blood volume. Volume expansion and depletion result in respective parallel increases and decreases in the vascular function curve.

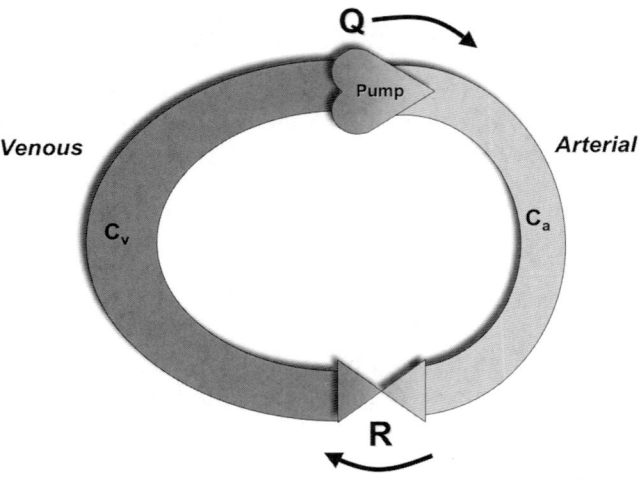

FIGURE 63.2. A conceptual model of the circulation. The circulation is partitioned into components, including a pump, an arterial compartment with compliance (C_a), a resistor (R), which represents the microvascular resistance of the arterioles, capillaries, and venules, and a venous compartment with compliance (C_v). The pump displaces blood from the venous compartment into the arterial compartment at rate (Q), which has units of volume and time (e.g., liters/minute). Increases in Q, will decrease the volume of blood residing in the venous compartment and thus will decrease central venous pressure (CVP). Conversely, decreases in Q will increase the volume of the venous compartment, which will increase CVP. CVP is determined by Q, R, and the ratio of C_a:C_v. As the compliance of the venous compartment is ~20 times that of the arterial compartment, the venous compartment contains a larger volume than the arterial compartment under normal conditions.

in the venous compartment, which is equivalent to the CVP. Conversely, decreases in Q will increase the volume of blood that resides in the venous compartment, which will increase CVP.

Important concepts can be seen at the extremes of the curve (**Fig. 63.1**). At some point, a maximal Q is achieved, whereby further reductions in the volume of blood in the venous compartment are not possible. Drawing blood from the venous compartment beyond this point would create a negative pressure within the venous compartment, which would tend to collapse the vessel walls. This point is termed the *critical closing pressure* (P_{cc}) and represents the lowest possible CVP and highest possible Q for any given blood volume. On the opposite extreme, when Q becomes zero, the system reaches a steady state, where pressures within the arterial and venous compartments are determined solely by compliance. In this situation, CVP would be at its maximum for any given blood volume. It is also important to note that the curve is affected by the blood volume, with parallel increases from baseline with expansion of the circulating volume (such that occur with blood transfusions) and decreases with volume depletion (such that occur with hemorrhage) (**Fig. 63.1**).

Cardiac Function Curve

The cardiac function curve is the reverse of the vascular function curve. That is, it examines how changes in CVP affect Q (**Fig. 63.3**). This relationship is based on Starling's law that describes increases in Q that result from increased stretch of the myocardium, which augments contractility (see Chapter 65).

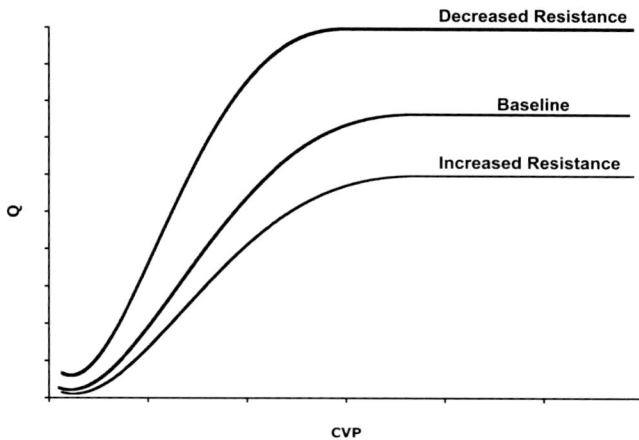

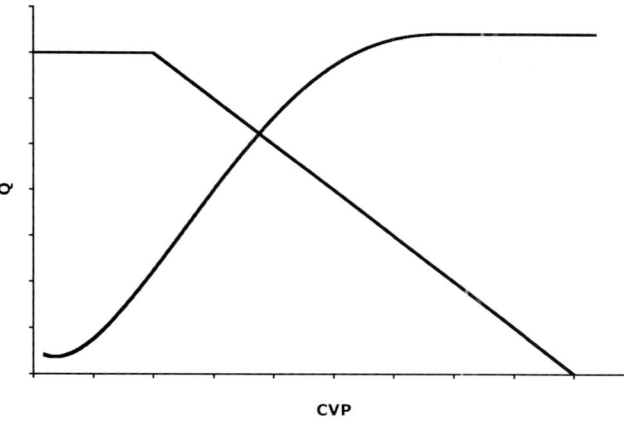

FIGURE 63.3. Cardiac function curves shown under conditions of varying degrees of systemic vascular resistance (afterload). The cardiac function curve describes how changes in central venous pressure (CVP) or venous return affect cardiac output (Q). On the steep portion of the curve, increases in CVP augment ventricular contractility. Increases in systemic vascular resistance (increased afterload) shift the curve downward, while decreases in systemic vascular resistance (decreased afterload) shift the curve upward.

FIGURE 63.4. The cardiovascular system operates at one theoretical point of intersection between the vascular and cardiac function curves. Deviations from this point are transient when the curves are accurate.

On the steep portion of the curve, increases in CVP, through increased venous return, distend the right ventricle (i.e., increase preload), which augments right ventricular contractility and flow through the pulmonary circuit. This then increases pulmonary venous return, which increases left ventricular preload and output. Although the cardiac function curve is directly related to CVP, it may also be affected by the other determinants of cardiac output, including afterload, contractility, and heart rate. For example, increases in systemic vascular resistance that increase afterload can result in a downward shift in the curve, while systemic vasodilation that decreases afterload will result in an upward shift in the curve (Fig. 63.3).

Interaction of Vascular and Cardiac Function Curves

At any given time, the cardiovascular system operates at one theoretical point of intersection between the vascular and cardiac function curves (Fig. 63.4). Deviations from this point are transient when the curves are accurate. For example, according to the simplified model presented here, if the pump suddenly ejected an increased volume of blood, volume and pressure would increase in the arterial compartment and decrease in the venous compartment, which would transiently shift the vascular function curve to the left. According to the cardiac function curve, subsequent ejection would decrease, as CVP was reduced. Over a short period of time, this decrease in Q would result in an increase in CVP in accordance with the vascular function curve, returning the system to the initial point of intersection.

The superimposition of these curves in various physiologic states is useful, as it illustrates important interactions between cardiac output, preload, peripheral resistance (or afterload), and blood volume. For example, from **Figure 63.5**, it can be seen that alterations in vascular resistance affect both the vascular and cardiac function curves, whereas changes in blood

volume only affect the vascular function curve (**Fig. 63.6**). Furthermore, it can be seen that whereas alterations in blood volume result in parallel changes in the vascular function curve (**Figs. 63.1** and **63.6**), alterations in resistance alter the slope of the curve but not the CVP at zero Q, because this point depends only on blood volume and compliance (**Fig. 63.5**). As the cardiovascular system operates at the point of intersection between the two curves, alterations in blood volume will shift the operative state of the system, even though it does not alter intrinsic cardiac function (**Fig. 63.6**). Critical illnesses with their attendant physiologic derangements will variably impact the cardiovascular system and may differentially affect the vascular and cardiac function curves. Likewise, therapies may also have differential effects. Thus, while the theoretical model described by the vascular and cardiac function curves is overly simplified, it is useful as a foundation with which to rationalize a therapeutic approach to various cardiovascular derangements.

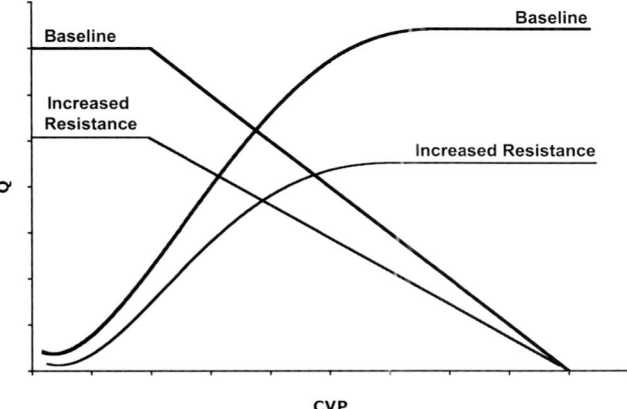

FIGURE 63.5. Effects of increased systemic vascular resistance on the vascular and cardiac function curves. Increased systemic vascular resistance (afterload) shifts both curves downward, moving the operating state of the system that occurs at the point of intersection between the two curves downward. Increased systemic vascular resistance does not alter the vascular function curve at zero Q, as the CVP at this point is determined solely by the compliance of the venous compartment, at any given volume.

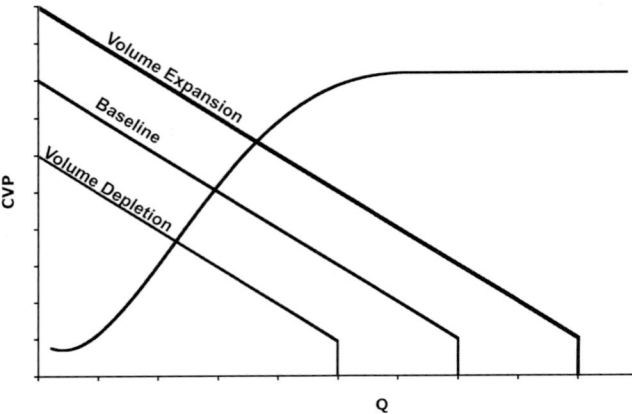

FIGURE 63.6. Effects of intravascular volume on the vascular and cardiac function curves. Intravascular volume expansion increases and intravascular volume depletion decreases the vascular function curve. The cardiac function curve is not altered by changes in intravascular volume. Because the cardiovascular system operates at the point of intersection between the two curves, the functional state of the system is affected by the volume status.

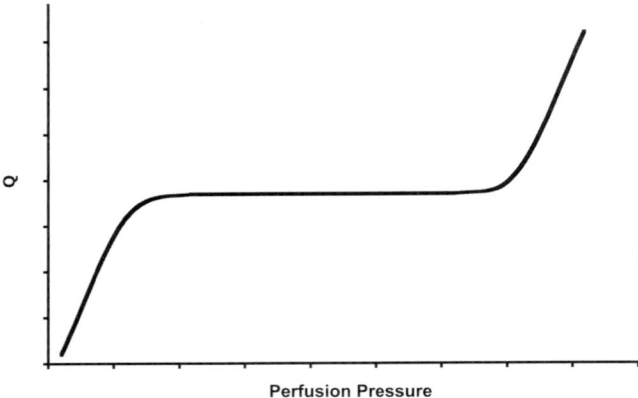

FIGURE 63.7. Autoregulation. Blood flow (Q) through most organs is maintained constant over a wide range of perfusion pressures. In general, decreases in perfusion pressure result in vasodilation, while increases in perfusion pressure result in vasoconstriction, thereby maintaining constant flow through alterations in vascular resistance. At the points of downward and upward inflection, maximal dilation or constriction have occurred, and constant blood flow can no longer be maintained in the face of decreased or increased perfusion pressures respectively.

REGULATION OF VASCULAR RESISTANCE

The contractile state of the vasculature is central to cardiovascular physiology because vascular resistance directly affects afterload, one of the four main determinants of cardiac output, and because alterations in resistance within and between vascular beds dictates flow within organs as well as the distribution of blood flow throughout the body. The main site of resistance within the circulation occurs at the level of the arterioles. However, larger arteries and veins of varying sizes also affect resistance and may become a primary site of resistance under various conditions. While a number of anatomic factors contribute to the resistance imposed by a vessel, smooth muscle cell tone is the predominant regulating mechanism.

Several mechanisms control the contractile state of vascular smooth muscle and, thus, vascular resistance, including: neural control, hormonal control, endothelial derived factors, myogenic processes, and local metabolic products. Autoregulation is a more general phenomenon that may involve several of these specific mechanisms.

Autoregulation

Blood flow to tissues remains relatively constant over a wide range of arterial blood pressures due to autoregulation (**Fig. 63.7**). The mechanisms of this phenomenon are largely unknown. Several hypothetical mechanisms exist, including local metabolic control, myogenic activity of vascular smooth muscle, and tissue pressure. These mechanisms may act alone or in combination. The metabolic hypothesis suggests that blood flow is closely linked to tissue metabolism. According to this theory, blood flow must be sufficient to support the metabolic demands of an organ. With increasing demands or with insufficient delivery of metabolic substrates, vasoactive substances are formed and/or released that result in vasodilation, which

increases blood flow. As flow rises, the metabolites are washed out, restoring their concentration to normal. In organs with high oxygen consumption, autoregulation of blood flow is largely dependent on tissue oxygenation. However, a number of substances may contribute to this process, including carbon dioxide, hydrogen ions, lactic acid, histamine, potassium ions, prostaglandin, endothelin (ET)-1, nitric oxide (NO), and adenosine. A second proposed mechanism of autoregulation is myogenic control (12). According to this theory, increased intravascular pressure stimulates vasoconstriction of vascular smooth muscle. A venous-arterial reflex has been described in which an increase in venous pressure causes arteriolar constriction, probably by a neurally mediated mechanism (12). Tissue pressure is another possible mechanism for autoregulation. By this proposed mechanism, increased tissue pressure in areas of encapsulated organs or in the brain leads to decreased blood flow to those areas. Autoregulation seems to play a more significant role in control of resting blood flow in vital organs such as the brain and heart and becomes significant in other areas during times of increased metabolic demand. In addition, various mechanisms may be specific for a given organ, such as macula densa signaling in the kidney.

Neural Control

Neural control of the circulation allows rapid regulation and provides simultaneous control of various regions within the circulation. Neural regulation consists of feedback (afferent limb) information provided by baroreceptors and cardiac stretch receptors and neurologic control (efferent limb) through the autonomic nervous system, which is composed of the sympathetic and parasympathetic systems. Nearly all blood vessels in the body are innervated by the autonomic nervous system; the effect of this control varies from one vascular bed to another.

The afferent limb of the neural control mechanisms consists of baroreceptors in arterial walls and stretch receptors within heart muscle. Baroreceptors are found in each carotid sinus and in the aortic arch. Two types of baroreceptors have been identified. Type 1 receptors control dynamic changes in blood pressure; type 2 receptors are responsible for control of resting blood pressure (7). These receptors respond to stretch of the arterial wall and send nerve impulses to cardioinhibitory and vasomotor centers of the medulla. Stimulation of carotid sinus receptors results in slowing of heart rate, vasodilation, and a decrease in arterial blood pressure. Smooth muscle in the walls of these baroreceptor regions is innervated by vasoconstrictor efferent fibers, suggesting that sympathetic activity may modify baroreceptor responses.

Stretch receptors are also found in the walls of the atria and ventricles. Atrial stretch receptors are located in the walls of both atria at the venoatrial junctions. Two kinds of atrial receptors have been described. Type A receptors fire during atrial contraction and respond to changes in atrial pressure, and type B receptors fire during ventricular systole and respond to changes in atrial volume. Type A receptors stimulate and type B receptors inhibit sympathetic activity. These stretch receptors provide feedback to the hypothalamus and inhibit secretion of antidiuretic hormone (vasopressin). Atrial stretch causes secretion of atrial natriuretic factor (ANF), which is discussed in more detail later. Atrial receptors also alter sympathetic stimulation of the renal circulation (7). By these mechanisms, atrial stretch receptors play an important role in regulation of intravascular volume. They are also responsible for stimulation of increased heart rate by the Bainbridge reflex.

Two types of stretch receptors are found in ventricular myocardium. The first type fire in a pulsatile manner in time with cardiac rhythm and are small in number. The second respond to mechanical stimulation and to various drugs and chemicals through nonmyelinated afferent nerves known as C *fibers*. Stimulation of C fibers, which are primarily located in the left ventricle, causes hypotension and bradycardia from parasympathetic stimulation and sympathetic inhibition. Evidence suggests that carotid baroreceptors are more important for control of sympathetic regulation of muscle blood flow, whereas cardiac receptors are more important in control of sympathetic regulation of kidney blood flow.

The efferent limb of neural control of the circulation, the autonomic nervous system, is divided into the sympathetic and parasympathetic systems. Two different types of sympathetic nerve fibers exist: vasoconstrictor and vasodilator. Sympathetic stimulation of the arterioles by vasoconstrictor fibers increases vascular resistance; these vessels are called *resistance vessels*. The nerve endings of these sympathetic vasoconstrictor fibers contain the vasoconstrictor norepinephrine, which is released upon nerve stimulation. Other substances present at the neurovascular junction, including monoamines, polypeptides, purines, and amino acids, can influence the release and the effects of norepinephrine (7). Impulses carried through vasoconstrictor fibers contribute the normal vascular tone or baseline constriction that is present at rest in most vascular beds. These vasoconstrictor fibers are more prevalent in skeletal muscles, where intrinsic tone is fairly high under resting conditions; they are much less prevalent in the cerebral and coronary beds. Sympathetic vasoconstriction of larger arteries and of veins changes their volume and thus changes the circulating volume; these vessels are known as *capacitance vessels*.

Sympathetic stimulation may also increase blood flow through activation of vasodilator fibers, which are primarily found in the vascular beds of skeletal muscle. The transmitter in vasodilator fibers is thought to be acetylcholine, although in primates it may be epinephrine. These vasodilator fibers may cause a small anticipatory increase of blood flow to the skeletal muscle; however, once muscle exercise begins, local vasodilation probably plays a more important role.

The parasympathetic system primarily controls heart function and rate and has a very limited role in control of the peripheral circulation. The transmitter stored in nerve endings of the parasympathetic system is acetylcholine. Parasympathetic vasodilator fibers are found in the cerebral circulation and in the bladder, rectum, and external genitalia.

Hormonal Control

Hormonal control of the peripheral circulation can best be described as vascular constriction or vasodilation in response to circulating hormones. The vasculature in the peripheral circulation is responsive to various circulating substances, including catecholamines, angiotensin II, vasopressin, eicosanoids, NO, neurokinins, and peptide hormones.

Catecholamines are the hormones of the adrenergic system. Adrenergic receptors to catecholamines are present in the smooth muscle throughout the peripheral vascular system and can be categorized as α- and β-receptors. Stimulation of α-receptors causes vascular smooth muscle to contract, causing vasoconstriction; stimulation of β-receptors causes vascular smooth muscle to relax, causing vasodilation. These receptors are responsive to both endogenous catecholamines and sympathomimetic drugs. Norepinephrine, an α-adrenergic agonist, is secreted by the adrenal medulla and is carried by the bloodstream to receptors in the peripheral vasculature. Preganglionic sympathetic fibers innervate the adrenal medulla and stimulate norepinephrine secretion. Therefore, this hormonal regulation is centrally controlled. Epinephrine is also secreted by the adrenal medulla, but it is a much weaker vascular stimulant and tends to exert a β-agonistic effect at physiologic concentrations.

Angiotensin II, a powerful vasoconstrictor, is produced by activation of the rennin-angiotensin-aldosterone system. The juxtaglomerular apparatus in the kidney secretes renin in response to decreased renal arterial pressure or a decrease in extracellular fluid volume. Renin, in turn, cleaves angiotensinogen to angiotensin I, which is then converted to angiotensin II by an angiotensin-converting enzyme (ACE) found in lung and vascular endothelium. Angiotensin II has direct vasoconstrictor properties, acts centrally to stimulate the vasoconstrictor centers of the brain, and stimulates the secretion of antidiuretic hormone (vasopressin). In addition, renin can be formed locally in many organs, which partially explains why angiotensin-receptor blockade has an additive clinical effect with ACE inhibitors. Antidiuretic hormone is synthesized in the hypothalamus and secreted by the posterior pituitary. It is a very potent vasoconstrictor but plays a minimal role in regulation of the circulation under resting conditions.

Prostaglandins and other eicosanoids play a small role in regulation of flow in the systemic circulation. ANF is another hormone that participates in regulation of the systemic circulation. This peptide hormone is released from atrial myocytes of both atria, and in smaller amounts from the ventricular myocytes. Ventricular production of ANF decreases with maturation; large amounts of ANF are produced in fetal ventricular myocardium, whereas in adults, the ventricles produce small amounts. ANF is released in response to stretch of either atrium; increased circulating levels of ANF are detected when left atrial pressure is elevated, even when the right atrial pressure is normal. In the kidney, ANF decreases tubular reabsorption of sodium. In the circulatory system, ANF has vasodilator and cardioinhibitory effects. Circulating levels of ANF are increased in certain pathophysiologic conditions, such as congenital heart disease associated with elevated atrial pressures, congestive heart failure, valve disease, hypertension, coronary artery occlusion, and atrial arrhythmias. In addition, B-type natriuretic peptide, which is produced by the ventricular myocytes in response to stretch, has natriuretic, diuretic, and vasoactive properties. Measurements of B-type natriuretic peptide are used in the diagnosis, risk stratification, and management of adult cardiac disease and are emerging in the clinical management of pediatric patients as well.

Endothelial-derived Factors

The vascular endothelial cells are capable of producing a variety of vasoactive substances, which participate in the regulation of normal vascular tone. These substances, such as NO and ET-1, are capable of producing vascular relaxation and/or constriction, modulating the propensity of the blood to clot, and inducing and/or inhibiting smooth muscle migration and replication (6,14) (**Fig. 63.8**). Increased understanding of the role of the vascular endothelium in regulating blood flow in health and disease has resulted in several treatment strategies that target the endothelium. These include inhaled NO for pulmonary hypertension, L-arginine supplementation for coronary artery disease and the pulmonary vasculopathy of sickle cell disease, phosphodiesterase inhibitors [i.e., sildenafil, which prevents the breakdown of guanosine $3'5'$-monophosphate (cGMP)] for pulmonary hypertensive disorders, endothelin-receptor antag-

onists for pulmonary hypertensive disorders and subarachnoid hemorrhage, and NO inhibitors for refractory hypotension secondary to sepsis and persistent patency of the ductus arteriosus. Indeed, many older therapies, such as nitrovasodilators, affect endothelial function, a fact which, until recently, was not fully appreciated.

NO is a labile humoral factor produced by NO synthase from L-arginine in the vascular endothelial cell. NO diffuses into the smooth muscle cell and produces vascular relaxation by increasing concentrations of cGMP, via the activation of soluble guanylate cyclase (**Fig. 63.8**). NO is released in response to a variety of factors, including shear stress (flow) and the binding of certain endothelium-dependent vasodilators (such as acetylcholine, ATP, and bradykinin) to receptors on the endothelial cell. Basal NO release is an important mediator of resting pulmonary and systemic vascular tone in the fetus, newborn, and adult, as well as a mediator of the fall in pulmonary vascular resistance that normally occurs at the time of birth (17).

ET-1 is a 21-amino acid polypeptide also produced by vascular endothelial cells (27). The vasoactive properties of ET-1 are complex, and studies have shown varying hemodynamic effects on different vascular beds. However, its most striking property is its sustained hypertensive action. In fact, ET-1 is the most potent vasoconstricting agent discovered, with a potency 10 times that of angiotensin II. The hemodynamic effects of ET-1 are mediated by at least two distinctive receptor populations, ET_A and ET_B. The ET_A receptors are located on vascular smooth muscle cells and mediate vasoconstriction, whereas the ET_B receptors may be located on endothelial and smooth muscle cells and mediate both vasodilation and vasoconstriction (**Fig. 63.8**). Individual endothelins occur in low levels in the plasma, generally below their vasoactive thresholds, suggesting that they are primarily effective at the local site of release. Even at these levels, they may potentiate the effects of other vasoconstrictors such as norepinephrine and serotonin. The role of endogenous ET-1 in the regulation of normal vascular tone is presently unclear.

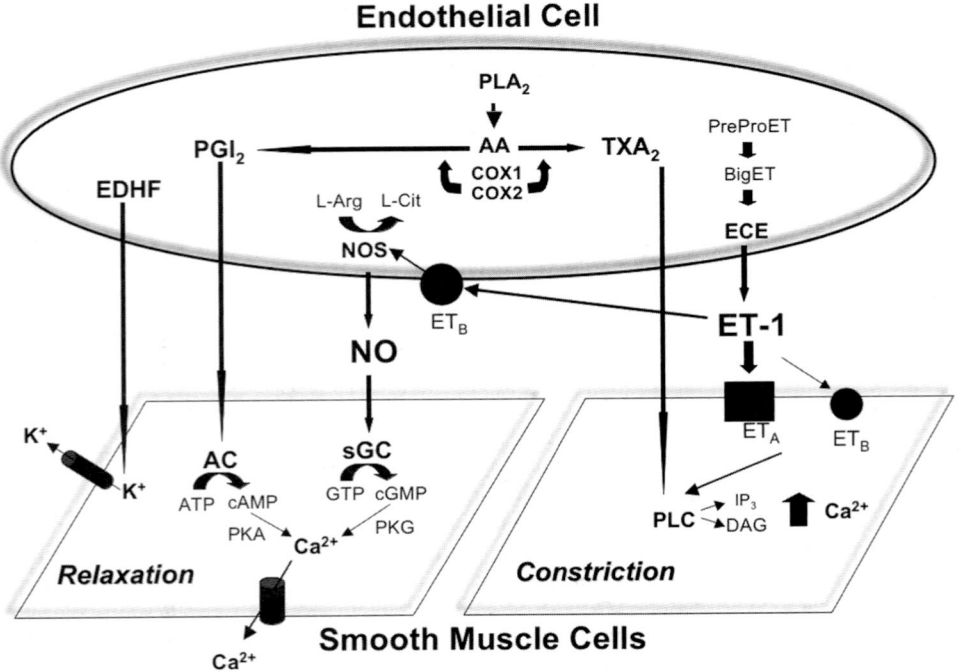

FIGURE 63.8. A schematic of some endothelial-derived factors, which may cause smooth muscle cell relaxation (**left**) and/or constriction (**right**). EDHF, endothelial derived hyperpolarizing factor; PGI_2, prostaglandin I_2; L-Arg, L-arginine; L-Cit, L-citrulline; PLA_2, phospholipase A_2; AA, arachidonic acid; COX1, cyclooxygenase-1; COX2, cyclooxygenase-2; TXA_2, thromboxane A_2; PrePro ET, PrePro endothelin; BigET, Big endothelin; NOS, nitric oxide synthase; ECE, endothelin-converting enzyme; ET_B, endothelin B receptor; NO, nitric oxide; ET-1, endothelin-1; K^+, potassium channels; AC, adenylate cyclase; sGC, soluble guanylate cyclase; ATP, adenosine-5′-triphosphate; cAMP, cyclic adenosine monophosphate; GTP, guanosine-5′-triphosphate; cGMP, cyclic guanosine-$3'$-$5'$ monophosphate; PKA, phosphokinase A; PKG, phosphokinase G; ET_A, endothelin A receptor; PLC, phospholipase C; IP_3, inositol triphosphate; DAG, diacylglycerol.

Nevertheless, alterations in ET-1 have been implicated in the pathophysiology of a number of disease states (25).

Endothelial-derived hyperpolarizing factor (EDHF), a diffusible substance that causes vascular relaxation by hyperpolarizing the smooth muscle cell, is another important endothelial factor. EDHF has not yet been identified, but current evidence suggests that the action of EDHF is dependent on potassium (K^+) channels (8) (**Fig. 63.8**). Activation of K^+ channels in the vascular smooth muscle results in hyperpolarization of the cell membrane, closure of voltage-dependent calcium (Ca^{2+}) channels, and ultimately, vasodilation. K^+ channels are also present in endothelial cells. Activation within the endothelium results in changes in Ca^{2+} flux and may be important in the release of NO, prostacyclin (PGI_2), and EDHF. K^+ channel subtypes include ATP-sensitive K^+ channels, Ca^{2+}-dependent K^+ channels, voltage-dependent K^+ channels, and inward-rectifier K^+ channels (8).

The breakdown of phospholipids within vascular endothelial cells results in the production of the important byproducts of arachidonic acid, including PGI_2 and thromboxane (TXA_2). PGI_2 activates adenylate cyclase, resulting in increased cyclic AMP production and subsequent vasodilation, whereas TXA_2 results in vasoconstriction via phospholipase C signaling (**Fig. 63.8**). Other prostaglandins and leukotrienes also have potent vasoactive properties.

In general, regional circulations regulate their flow so that they obtain required amounts of oxygen and nutrients, and all of the mechanisms described previously may be invoked. However, an overriding principle exists wherein shear rate must be kept constant within narrow limits to avoid endothelial damage. Any increase in local organ flow is sensed by endothelial integrins that trigger a cascade of responses that culminate in release of NO (22).

Myogenic Processes

In 1902, Bayliss described an intrinsic increase in vascular tone in response to elevated intravascular pressure. This myogenic response results in alterations in vascular tone following changes in transmural pressure or stretch (11). This response is especially important at the arteriolar level and is thought to participate in regional autoregulation. Increases in intravascular pressure and/or stretch result in an increase in arteriolar smooth muscle tone, while decreasing pressures have the reverse effect. The precise mechanisms that mediate this response are unclear, but a role for dynamic changes in intracellular Ca^{2+} and myosin light-chain phosphorylation has been documented (5). More recent work has focused on the role of tyrosine phosphorylation pathways in this response (16).

Local Metabolic Products

Tissues have the ability to regulate their own blood flow in response to changes in metabolic demands. The local chemical environment of arterioles can cause vasodilation or, to a lesser extent, vasoconstriction. For example, a decrease in Po_2, an increase in Pco_2, and an increase in hydrogen (H^+) or K^+ concentration each cause arteriolar vasodilation. Many tissues will release adenosine, a potent vasodilator, in response to increased

metabolism or decreased oxygen tension. Other mediators include lactic acid, histamine, prostaglandin, ET-1, and NO.

REGULATION OF REGIONAL CIRCULATIONS

Vascular resistance within each regional circulation dictates the distribution of blood flow to the individual organs. An understanding of the factors that regulate resistance within the specific regional vascular beds is essential in allowing the intensivist to combat cardiovascular derangements, while arbitrating the various, if not disparate, needs of the specific organs.

In addition, when caring for neonates, an understanding of the fetal circulation is critical, as a number of problems may occur when the normal transition from the fetal to postnatal circulation is compromised. While not a regional circulation, the fetal circulation is marked by important differences in regional blood flow from the postnatal situation.

Fetal Circulation

The presence of central shunts allows the fetal circulation to be remarkably efficient at distributing oxygen and substrate. The fetal ventricles primarily perform their postnatal functions as follows: the fetal right ventricle supplies the majority of its blood via the ductus arteriosus and descending aorta to the placenta for oxygen uptake, and the left ventricle supplies the majority of its blood via the ascending aorta to the heart and brain for oxygen delivery (**Fig. 63.9**). So that the central venous

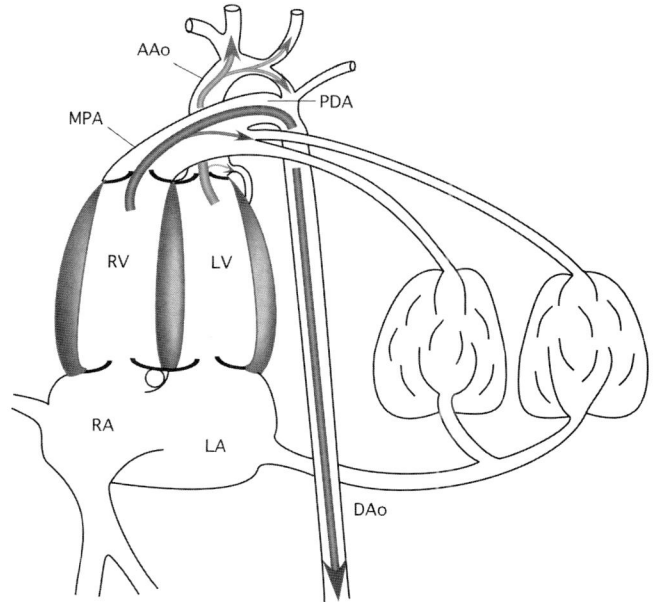

FIGURE 63.9. Preferential pattern of ventricular output. The left ventricle (LV) receives blood from the left atrium (LA) and directs the majority via the ascending aorta (AAo) to the highly metabolic heart and upper body. The right ventricle (RV) receives right atrial blood (RA) and ejects it via the main pulmonary artery (MPA) primarily down the ductus arteriosus (DAo) to the placenta for oxygen uptake. PDA, patent ductus arteriosus.

circulation can facilitate these tasks, the least saturated venous blood must be directed to the right ventricle and the most saturated blood must be directed to the left. To appreciate how this process is achieved, it is best to divide the central venous circulation into five components: the venous return from the upper body, the myocardium, the lungs, the lower body, and the placenta.

The least saturated blood returns from the upper body via the superior vena cava and from the myocardium via the coronary sinus. This blood is directed appropriately across the tricuspid valve to the right ventricle. The leftward and superior course of the Eustachian valve directs over 95% of the blood flowing caudally from the superior vena cava away from the foramen ovale and toward the tricuspid valve. In addition, the location of the coronary sinus caudad to the foramen causes venous blood from the myocardium to flow across the tricuspid valve to the right ventricle (**Fig. 63.9**). Blood returning from the lungs is not well saturated, but by the nature of the normal drainage of the pulmonary veins to the left atrium, preferential flow to the right ventricle is not possible. However, as the pulmonary blood flow represents no more than 8% of combined ventricular output, it does not have an appreciable effect on oxygen delivery.

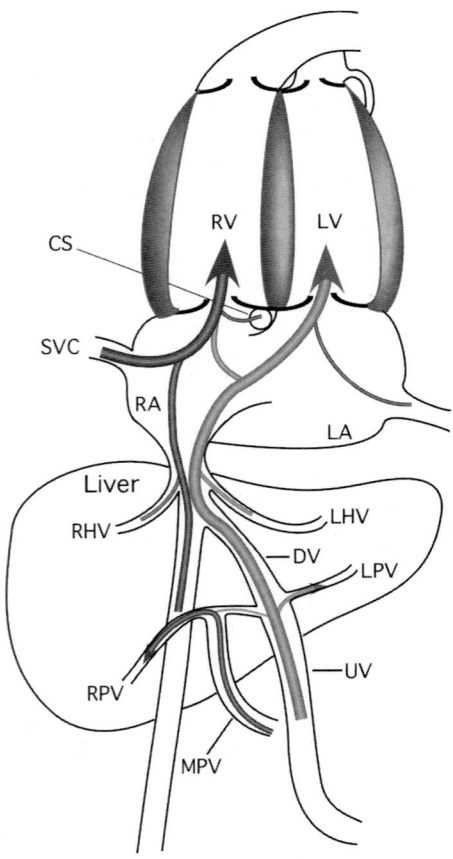

FIGURE 63.10. Preferential pattern of venous return to the right (RV) and left (LV) ventricles. Preferentially, higher-saturated blood from the umbilical vein (UV) passes via the ductus venosus (DV) and left hepatic vein (LHV) to the left atrium (LA) and left ventricle. Less-saturated blood from the lower body via the inferior vena cava (IVC), the right hepatic vein (RHV) (via the right portal vein), the coronary sinus (CS), and the superior vena cava (SVC) passes to the right atrium (RA) and then the right ventricle. MPV, main portal vein.

Inferior vena caval return comes from the remaining two sources, the lower body and the placenta. The majority of lower body flow, except that from the liver, ascends the distal inferior vena cava. This stream of relatively desaturated blood enters the lateral margin of the right atrium and is directed primarily across the tricuspid valve. Placental (umbilical venous) and liver venous return is more complicated (**Fig. 63.10**). Under normal conditions in the fetal sheep, ~55% of the highly saturated umbilical venous return ascends via the ductus venosus to the inferior vena cava-right atrium junction, where it preferentially crosses the foramen ovale. Slightly less than half of the remaining umbilical venous return enters the left lobe of the liver, from whence it reaches the left hepatic vein. The left hepatic vein joins the ductus venosus near the inferior vena cava, so that this highly saturated blood is also directed to the foramen ovale. The limbus of the foramen ovale helps to direct this blood into the left atrium. The remainder of the umbilical venous blood, along with over 95% of the poorly saturated portal venous blood, is directed to the right lobe of the liver. From the right lobe, this much-less saturated blood enters the right hepatic vein and tends to stream with the blood of the distal inferior vena cava to the tricuspid valve. In that the hepatic artery, which carries blood that is moderately well saturated, contributes <10% of hepatic blood flow in the fetus, it does not significantly contribute to oxygen supply. Hepatic arterial blood is distributed to both lobes of the liver, with the right lobe receiving somewhat more.

Thus, preferential streaming patterns among the various sources of venous return allow most of the poorly saturated blood from the upper body, myocardium, and lower body to reach the right ventricle and the more highly saturated umbilical venous return to reach the left ventricle. Although the separation of fetal ventricular output is not as efficient as the postnatal separation, it is quite remarkable in its ability to allow the right and left ventricles to perform their normal postnatal functions of delivery of blood for oxygen uptake and oxygen supply, respectively.

Transition from the Fetal to the Postnatal Circulation

The changes in the central circulation at birth are primarily caused by external events rather than by primary changes in the circulation itself. Most important of these external events are the rapid and large decrease in pulmonary vascular resistance and the disruption of the umbilical-placental circulation. The various mechanisms responsible for the decrease in pulmonary vascular resistance are discussed later. This decrease has profound effects on the central shunts in the systemic circulation. Abruptly, at birth, the ductus arteriosus, until it closes in the first hours or days of life, changes from a right-to-left conduit of blood to the descending aorta, to a left-to-right conduit of blood to the lungs. This shunt may be prolonged in the premature infant, causing a steal of blood from the regional vascular beds of greatest resistance.

As previously mentioned, the ductus venosus carries umbilical venous return primarily to the left heart. Although the amount of umbilical venous blood that enters the ductus venosus is variable and is greatly affected by stresses such as hypoxemia, changes in flow do not appear to be caused by active vasoconstriction of the ductus venosus; rather they occur passively in accordance with changes in umbilical blood flow. At birth, the umbilical-placental circulation is abolished, causing a marked reduction in ductus venosus flow and in flow to the left lobe of the liver. However, portal venous flow through the ductus venosus increases from <5% to >50% by 1 hr of age so that, despite an increase in portal venous flow at birth, hepatic flow actually decreases substantially. This shunt of portal venous blood through the ductus venosus is transient, generally lasting for 1 day to 2 weeks. The functional closure of the ductus venosus is probably a passive phenomenon, although it has been demonstrated that the isolated ductus venosus can respond to adrenergic stimulation and prostanoids. In the intact newborn lamb, it can dilate in response to prostaglandin E_1. Thus, its closure may be partly induced by the same hormonal changes that are implicated in the closure of the ductus arteriosus.

Although vasoactive processes are involved in the closure of the ductus arteriosus and may be involved in closure of the ductus venosus, closure of the foramen ovale at birth is entirely passive, secondary to alterations in the relative return of blood to the right and left atria. Prior to birth, direct left atrial return via the pulmonary veins is only ~8% of combined venous return. Thus, the pressure gradient from right to left maintains a large flow of blood across the foramen ovale, and its flap appears as a windsock bulging into the left atrium. With the onset of oxygen ventilation, the proportion of combined venous return that directly enters the left atrium via the pulmonary veins increases dramatically, to more than 50% (24), because of the marked increase in pulmonary blood flow, which includes a transient left-to-right shunt through the ductus arteriosus. Left atrial pressure thus exceeds right, and the redundant flap of tissue of the foramen ovale that previously bowed into the left atrium is now pressed against the septum. Small left-to-right shunts may be visualized in the newborn by color Doppler ultrasonography, but these shunts are not hemodynamically significant. Although patency of the foramen ovale may be present for several years, shunts of any significance occur only when the primum septum is deficient, thus forming a secundum atrial septal defect, or when an ostium primum defect is present.

Interaction of the Systemic and Pulmonary Circulations

The simplified model of the circulation outlined in **Figure 63.2,** describes resistance as a single resistor that lies between the large arteries and veins of the systemic circulation. In fact, total systemic vascular resistance represents the sum of the resistances of each regional vascular bed. The pulmonary vascular resistance, which is normally 10%–20% of the systemic vascular resistance, is distinct, as a separate pump (i.e., the right ventricle) propels blood through the pulmonary circuit. Therefore, under normal conditions, only the total systemic resistance need be considered as a factor that affects cardiac output. However, if the right ventricle fails, pulmonary vascular resistance is added in series to systemic vascular resistance. This effect is dramatically accentuated in the setting of right ventricular failure with elevated pulmonary vascular resistance. Thus, in various critical illnesses, consid-

eration of the systemic and pulmonary vascular resistance is required.

Pulmonary Circulation

The exact mechanisms involved in intrinsic relaxation and constriction of the pulmonary vascular smooth muscle are not completely understood, but recent advances have focused on the role of the pulmonary vascular endothelium in these processes. Changes in pulmonary vascular resistance can occur at various levels within the circulation, and vasoactive substances and their properties may change during passage through the pulmonary vascular bed as a result of metabolism by the lung.

Morphologic Development

The stage of morphologic development of the pulmonary circulation affects vascular responses to various stimuli in the perinatal period. In the fetus and newborn, small pulmonary arteries have a thicker medial smooth muscle layer in relation to diameter than do similar arteries in adults. This increased muscularity is partly responsible for the increased vascular reactivity and pulmonary vascular resistance in the neonate immediately after birth.

Studies in human lungs identify the small pulmonary arteries by their relationship to the airways. Arteries follow the airways toward the alveoli. When these vessels are traced distally, a point is reached at which the medial smooth muscle coat no longer completely encircles the vessels; rather, it gives way to a region of incomplete muscularization. In these partially muscularized arteries, the smooth muscle is arranged in a spiral or helix. The nonmuscularized portions of these vessels contain precursor smooth muscle cells. Under certain conditions, such as hypoxia, these precursor cells may rapidly differentiate into mature smooth muscle cells. Moving distally, the muscle disappears altogether in arteries that are still larger than capillaries. In these arteries, an incomplete pericyte layer is found within the endothelial basement membrane.

In the near-term fetus, only approximately half the precapillary arteries (those associated with respiratory bronchioli) are muscularized or partially muscularized, and the arteries that are associated with alveoli are free of smooth muscle. In the first 4–6 weeks following birth, progressive involution of the circumferential medial smooth muscle occurs, with overall reduction in medial muscular thickness of the walls of the small pulmonary arteries. In adults, circumferential muscularization extends peripherally along the intra-acinar arteries so that most are completely muscularized, although with only a very thin layer of smooth muscle; this pattern is reached at about puberty. A number of neonatal pulmonary vascular disorders (e.g., congenital heart disease with increased pulmonary blood flow) are associated with a failure of the normal involution of medial smooth muscle and/or a precocious progression to the adult morphologic state, with a developmentally inappropriate extension of muscularized arteries toward the periphery.

During fetal growth, the number of small arteries increases greatly. In humans, the main preacinar pulmonary arterial branches that accompany the larger airways are developed by 16 weeks of gestation; however, the intraacinar circulation follows alveolar development late in gestation and after birth, and arteries multiply as alveoli develop, a process generally complete by ~10 years of age (18).

Pulmonary Blood Flow in the Fetus

In the fetus, gas exchange occurs in the placenta and pulmonary blood flow is low, supplying nutritional requirements for lung growth and allowing the lung to serve a metabolic or paraendocrine function. Pulmonary blood flow in near-term fetal lambs represents ~8%–10% of combined ventricular output, as right ventricular blood is diverted away from the lungs through the widely patent ductus arteriosus to the descending thoracic aorta and the placenta for oxygenation (**Fig. 63.9**). Fetal pulmonary arterial mean blood pressure increases progressively with gestation and, at term, is ~50 mm Hg, exceeding mean aortic blood pressure by 1–2 mm Hg. Total pulmonary vascular resistance is extremely high relative to that in the infant or adult.

Regulation of Pulmonary Vascular Resistance in the Fetus

Pulmonary vascular resistance in the fetal lung is high and decreases slightly throughout the final third of gestation. Many factors, including mechanical effects, state of oxygenation, and the production of vasoactive substances, regulate the tone of the fetal pulmonary circulation. The most prominent factor associated with high fetal pulmonary vascular resistance is the low blood O_2 tension (pulmonary arterial blood P_{O_2}, 17–20 torr). The exact mechanism and site of hypoxic pulmonary vasoconstriction in the fetal pulmonary circulation remain unclear. In addition to the low-oxygen environment, many substances, such as α-agonists, TXA_2, and leukotrienes, constrict the pulmonary circulation of the fetus. However, their role, if any, in the maintenance of the high fetal pulmonary vascular resistance does not appear prominent. In addition to the production of vasoconstrictors, the fetal pulmonary circulation produces vasodilating substances that modulate the degree of vasoconstriction under normal conditions and may play a more active role during periods of fetal stress. NO appears to be especially important. In fetal lambs, inhibition of NO synthesis produces marked increases in resting fetal pulmonary vascular resistance and inhibits the oxygen-induced decrease in pulmonary vascular resistance. In addition, studies of intrapulmonary arteries and isolated lung preparations of the sheep reveal maturational increases in NO-mediated relaxation during the late fetal and early postnatal period.

Regulation of Pulmonary Vascular Resistance during the Perinatal Transition

At birth, with initiation of pulmonary ventilation, pulmonary vascular resistance decreases rapidly and is associated with an eight- to 10-fold increase in pulmonary blood flow. By the first day of life, mean pulmonary arterial blood pressure is generally half systemic. After the initial abrupt decrease in pulmonary vascular resistance and pressure, a slow, progressive decrease follows, with adult levels reached after 2–6 weeks (**Fig. 63.11**).

The mechanisms that regulate the fall in pulmonary vascular resistance and increase in pulmonary blood flow after birth are in large part related to the increase in alveolar oxygen tension and the physical expansion of the lung. The role of oxygen is supported by increased pulmonary flow with hyperbaric oxygenation without ventilation. The role of physical expansion is supported by pulmonary vasodilation that occurs by inflating the lungs with a low oxygen-containing gas mix-

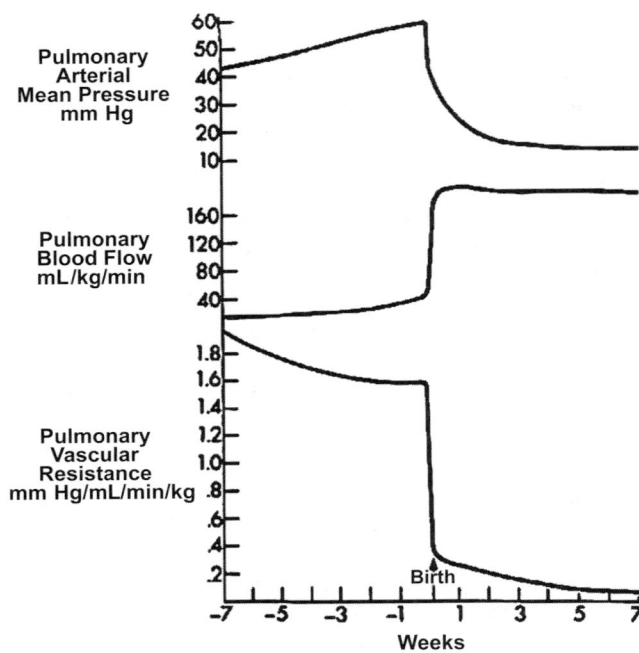

FIGURE 63.11. The changes in pulmonary arterial pressure, blood flow, and vascular resistance that occur around birth. Data from Morin FC III, Egan E. Pulmonary hemodynamics in fetal lambs during development at normal and increased oxygen tension. *J Appl Physiol* 1992;73:213–8; and Soifer SJ, FC Morin III, DC Kaslow, et al. The developmental effects of prostaglandin D2 on the pulmonary and systemic circulations in the newborn lamb. *J Dev Physiol* 1983;5:237–50.

ture that does not change arterial blood gas composition. The exact mechanisms of oxygen-induced pulmonary vasodilation during the transitional circulation remain unclear. The increase in alveolar or arterial O_2 tension may decrease pulmonary vascular resistance, either directly via K^+ channel activation or indirectly by stimulating the production of vasodilator substances such as PGI_2, bradykinin, adenosine, ATP, and NO. Lung inflation alone may lower pulmonary vascular resistance by either physical or chemical mechanisms. One mechanism operates through changes in alveolar surface tension. Another, more important, mechanism is the production and release of prostaglandins (predominantly PGI_2), which occurs either with mechanical stimulation of the lung or with rhythmic lung expansion (13).

NO has been implicated as an important mediator of the decrease in pulmonary vascular resistance at birth that is associated with increased oxygenation. For example, inhibition of NO synthesis attenuates the increase in pulmonary blood flow due to oxygenation of fetal lambs induced by either maternal hyperbaric oxygen exposure or in utero ventilation with oxygen. In utero ventilation without changing fetal blood gases increases endothelial NO synthase gene expression in lung parenchyma of fetal lambs; this is further increased by ventilation with 100% oxygen. In vitro data reveal a maturational increase in NO production from late gestation to the early postnatal period that is modulated, in part, by oxygen. Moreover, both acute and chronic inhibition of NO synthesis prior to delivery significantly attenuate the normal increase in pulmonary blood flow at birth. These data suggest an important role for NO activity during the transitional circulation. However, the immediate decrease in pulmonary vascular resistance minutes after birth is not attenuated by NO inhibition. Therefore, the decrease in pulmonary vascular resistance is due to the initiation of ventilation and oxygenation. First, pulmonary vasodilation is caused by physical expansion of the lung and the production of prostaglandins (PGD_2 and PGI_2), which are probably independent of fetal oxygenation and result in a modest increase in pulmonary blood flow and decrease in pulmonary vascular resistance. Second, further maximal pulmonary vasodilation is associated with fetal oxygenation that is independent of prostaglandin production; it is most likely caused by the synthesis of NO, although the exact stimuli for NO production have not yet been defined. Both components are necessary for the successful transition to extrauterine life.

Regulation of Postnatal Pulmonary Vascular Resistance

The successful transition from the fetal to the postnatal pulmonary circulation is marked by the maintenance of the pulmonary vasculature in a dilated, low-resistance state. Evidence suggests that basal NO release and the subsequent increase in smooth muscle cell cGMP concentrations, in part, mediate the low resting pulmonary vascular resistance of the newborn (20). Other vasoactive substances, including histamine, 5-hydroxytryptamine, bradykinin, and metabolites of arachidonic acid by the cyclooxygenase and lipoxygenase pathways, have also been implicated in mediating postnatal pulmonary vascular tone. However, their roles are not well elucidated. Two of the most important factors affecting pulmonary vascular resistance in the postnatal period are oxygen concentration and pH. Decreasing oxygen tension and decreases in pH elicit pulmonary vasoconstriction. Alveolar hypoxia constricts pulmonary arterioles, diverting blood flow away from hypoxic lung segments, toward well-oxygenated segments, thus enhancing ventilation-perfusion matching. This response to hypoxia, unique to the pulmonary vasculature, is greater in the younger animal than in the adult. Indeed, in most vascular beds (e.g., cerebral vasculature), hypoxia is a potent vasodilator.

The exact mechanism of hypoxic pulmonary vasoconstriction remains incompletely understood but likely involves changes in the local concentration of reactive oxygen species that, in turn, regulate voltage-gated K^+ channels and Ca^{2+} channels (15). Acidosis potentiates hypoxic pulmonary vasoconstriction, while alkalosis reduces it (21). The exact mechanism of pH-mediated pulmonary vascular reactivity also remains incompletely understood but appears to be independent of $Paco_2$. Data suggest that K^+ channels also play an important role in mediating these responses (3). Manipulating alveolar oxygen tension and systemic arterial pH are fundamental approaches to changing pulmonary vascular tone in the critical care setting. Alveolar hyperoxia and alkalosis are often used to decrease pulmonary vascular tone because they generally relieve pulmonary vasoconstriction with little effect on the systemic circulation as a whole. However, severe alkalosis is generally avoided due to the detrimental effects of severe hypocarbia or alkalosis on cerebral and myocardial blood flow (14).

Despite extensive innervation of the lung, neural input is not a major determinant of basal pulmonary vascular tone. However, given that pulmonary neurohumoral receptors are sensitive to α-adrenergic, β-adrenergic, and dopaminergic agonists, vasoactive agents that stimulate these receptors will affect the vascular tone of both the pulmonary and systemic circulations. As alterations in vascular tone in response to a given agent are dependent upon the relative tone of the vascular bed at a given time, the response to these agents is difficult to predict in an individual critically ill patient.

Postnatal Pulmonary Blood Flow

Several other factors, unique to the lung, influence pulmonary blood flow in addition to pulmonary vascular tone. In a standing position, due to gravity, mean pulmonary vascular pressures increase from the apex to the base of the lung, but alveolar pressure is relatively constant throughout the lung. Therefore, the relationship between intravascular pressures and alveolar pressures is not uniform; rather, it is a function of the height within the lung. This relationship is further complicated by the variable effects of lung inflation on pulmonary vascular pressures, which depend on the spatial relationship between the alveoli and the vessels. Pulmonary vessels are termed extra-alveolar, corner, or intra-alveolar. Extra-alveolar and corner vessels increase their size with lung expansion due to radial traction placed on their walls by the lung parenchyma. However, intra-alveolar vessels are directly associated with alveoli and thus are subject to compression with alveolar expansion.

To characterize this relationship, West divided the lung into three theoretical zones that move down the lung from the apex to the base and are based on the relationship between pulmonary artery pressure (PAP), or inflow pressure, alveolar pressure (P_{av}), and pulmonary venous pressure (P_{ven}), or outflow pressure. In theory, no blood flows to zone I because P_{av} exceeds PAP, or $P_{av} > PAP > P_{ven}$. In this zone, intra-alveolar vessels would be collapsed. Clinically, zone I conditions probably do not exist in a healthy lung, as pulmonary blood flow does occur at the apex. The fact that extra-alveolar and corner vessels are patent in this zone may help to maintain blood flow. In zone II, PAP exceeds P_{av} and blood flow occurs independent of outflow pressures, or $PAP > P_{av} > P_{ven}$. In this zone, blood flow increases down the lung, as PAP, but not P_{av}, is influenced by gravity. In zone III, blood flow is dictated by the normal relationship of PAP to P_{ven}, or inflow pressure minus outflow pressure. In this zone, blood flow does not change dramatically down the lung as it does in zone II because gravity affects PAP and P_{ven} equally, or $PAP > P_{ven} > P_{av}$. Subsequently, an additional zone, zone IV, has been described in which pulmonary blood flow decreases at the extreme base of the lung. This decrease occurs due to the impact of the weight of the lung on the extra-alveolar and corner vessels, which causes compression that increases resistance to flow and the decrease in ventilation that occurs at the base, resulting in areas of relative hypoxia with resultant hypoxic pulmonary vasoconstriction.

Under normal conditions, pulmonary blood flow is largely determined by zone III conditions. However, with disease, less favorable conditions can predominate. Particularly pertinent to pediatric critical care are the effects of positive-pressure ventilation with high levels of peak end-expiratory pressure. Increased alveolar pressure, may expand zone II and allow zone I conditions to be realized, resulting in mismatching of ventilation and perfusion and intrapulmonary shunting with hypoxia and hypercapnia. Likewise, pneumonia and pulmonary edema, along with other conditions, can increase zone IV conditions within the lung. Finally, hypotension from multiple etiologies, such as hemorrhage, can expand zone I and zone II conditions.

Coronary Circulation

Blood flow, and thus oxygen delivery, to the entire body is dependent on the cardiac pump. Increased needs of the body must be matched by increased delivery of metabolic substances, which often requires an increase in cardiac output and, thus, myocardial oxygen consumption. Myocardial oxygen demand is almost exclusively met by increased myocardial blood flow; in this way, coronary blood flow is, in fact, regulated not only by the needs of the heart but by the overall needs of the body at any given time.

Coronary Anatomy

Blood flow to the myocardium is supplied by the right and left coronary arteries, which arise from the sinuses of Valsalva, just behind the right and left coronary cusps of the aortic valve. The right coronary artery supplies the right atrium and ventricle, while the left coronary artery, which divides into the left anterior descending artery and the circumflex artery, supplies the left atrium and ventricle, although some redundancy does exist. Venous return to the right atrium occurs principally through the coronary sinus, with a lesser portion returning through the anterior coronary veins. In addition, arteriosinusoidal, arterioluminal, and thebesian vessels connect the coronary arterial system to the cardiac chambers, forming an extensive plexus of subendocardial vessels.

Regulation of Coronary Blood Flow

Coronary blood flow is regulated by physical forces that are related to the anatomic position of the coronary vessels within and around the dynamic myocardium, metabolic factors that couple coronary blood flow to oxygen demand, and neural factors. In that under normal conditions, the perfusion, or inflow, pressure of the coronary circulation does not change dramatically, alterations in coronary blood flow are largely determined by alterations in vascular resistance, brought about by changes in luminal size.

Physical Factors That Regulate Coronary Blood Flow. Coronary perfusion pressure is directly related to aortic pressure. Blood flow within the coronary vasculature is dynamic as the vessels are exposed to the varying pressures generated within the cardiac cycle. At the end of diastole, when the ventricle is relaxed, pressures in the intramural coronary arteries are similar to each other and to aortic pressure. At the beginning of systole, subendocardial tissue pressure rises to equal intracavitary pressure but then falls off linearly across the wall to ~10 mm Hg in the outer subepicardium. These pressures are transmitted to the coronary vessels. Thus, intravascular pressures in the inner subendocardial arteries exceed aortic pressure but are lower than aortic pressure in the outer subepicardial arteries. In fact, during early left ventricular systole, flow is transiently reversed by extravascular compression of the subendocardial arteries that supply the left ventricle. In early diastole, blood flows first into the subepicardial vessels that have not been compressed and then flows to the narrowed subendocardial vessels. Under normal conditions, subepicardial and subendocardial vessels are equally perfused during diastole. However, if diastole is excessively shortened, such as with severe tachycardia and/or if perfusion pressure is decreased, subendocardial ischemia can occur. On the other hand,

flow within the coronary vessels that perfuse the right ventricular myocardium is normally maintained during systole and diastole because of the lower afterload induced by the pulmonary circulation that results in lower right ventricular intracavitary pressures (2). Perfusion of the hypertrophied right ventricle of severe pulmonic stenosis or tetralogy of Fallot would be expected to resemble that of the left ventricle.

Myocardial Oxygen Demand-Supply Relationship. The left ventricle extracts an almost maximal amount of oxygen from the blood that passes through the myocardium, such that increases in myocardial oxygen demand must be met by increases in coronary blood flow. With maximal exertion, left ventricular oxygen consumption may increase fourfold, as does left coronary blood flow. Increased coronary perfusion pressures alone cannot increase flow to this extent, and thus the increased flow must be achieved by a decrease in coronary vascular resistance.

In fact, coronary blood flow is tightly coupled to the oxygen supply-to-oxygen demand ratio. Coronary blood flow increases when oxygen supply decreases and/or when oxygen demand increases. In this way, coronary blood flow is, in fact, linked to the overall oxygen needs of the body, as increases in cardiac output typically increase myocardial oxygen consumption. Likewise, when the body's metabolic needs decrease (e.g., during rest), myocardial oxygen consumption decreases, as does coronary blood flow. The mechanisms responsible for this coupling remain elusive. However, a number of substances known to influence vascular tone may participate, including adenosine, O_2, NO, H^+ ions, K^+, CO_2, and prostaglandins.

Coronary Reserve. Under normal conditions, coronary blood flow is autoregulated such that if perfusion pressure is raised or lowered, there is a range over which almost no change in flow occurs; a rise in pressure evokes vasoconstriction, and a fall in pressure evokes vasodilatation (10). At perfusion pressures above some upper limit, flow increases, probably because the pressure overcomes the constriction. More importantly, at low perfusion pressures, flow decreases, indicating that the coronary vasculature is beginning to reach maximal vasodilatation and can no longer decrease resistance to compensate for the decreased perfusion pressure. A further decrease in perfusion pressure will cause ischemia.

Under normal conditions, when flow through the coronary circulation is autoregulated, maximal flow for any given inflow or perfusion pressure is limited by active vasoconstriction. The difference between this autoregulated flow and the maximal potential flow that would occur in the absence of any vasoconstriction (i.e., complete coronary dilation) is termed *coronary flow reserve* (9). Coronary flow reserve indicates the amount of extra flow that the myocardium can receive at a given pressure to meet increased demands for oxygen; insufficient reserve occurs when increases in myocardial oxygen demand cannot be matched with increased supply, which will result in ischemia. Coronary flow reserve is normally lower in the subendocardium than in the subepicardium such that decreases in coronary flow reserve are always more profound in the subendocardium than in the subepicardium.

Coronary reserve can be affected in a number of ways. For example, if autoregulation is normal but the maximal flow is decreased, then coronary flow reserve will be reduced. Such a change can occur with (a) marked tachycardia; (b) a decrease in the number of coronary vessels due to small-vessel disease, as in some collagen vascular diseases, especially systemic lupus erythematosus; (c) increased resistance to flow in one or more large coronary vessels because of embolism, thrombosis, atheroma, or spasm; (d) impaired myocardial relaxation due to ischemia; (e) myocardial edema; (f) a marked increase in left ventricular diastolic pressure; (g) marked increase in left ventricular systolic pressure if coronary perfusion pressure is not also increased, as in aortic stenosis or incompetence; and (h) an increase in blood viscosity, most commonly seen with hematocrits over 65%.

Coronary flow reserve can also be reduced if maximal flows are normal but autoregulated flows increase, which can occur with exercise, tachycardia, anemia, carbon monoxide poisoning, leftward shift of the hemoglobin oxygen dissociation curve (as in infants with a high proportion of fetal hemoglobin), hypoxemia, thyrotoxicosis, acute ventricular dilatation (because of increased wall stress), inotropic stimulation by catecholamines, and acquired ventricular hypertrophy.

In addition, autoregulated flow and maximal flows may be reduced at the same time, such as with severe tachycardia or cyanotic heart disease with hypoxemia, ventricular hypertrophy, and polycythemia. Under these circumstances, coronary flow reserve can be drastically reduced. Furthermore, pericardial tamponade, a rise in right or left ventricular diastolic pressures, and α-adrenergic stimulation all raise the pressure at which autoregulation fails to compensate for decreased perfusing pressure.

Importantly, coronary reserve is also significantly reduced with ventricular hypertrophy. Myocardial wall stress is regulated within a fairly narrow range, with or without myocardial hypertrophy. Consequently, myocardial blood flow per unit mass is fairly constant. A close relationship exists between peak wall stress in systole and the ratio of left ventricular mass to volume (23,26). If hypertrophy does not occur, coronary flow reserve is normal, but it is reduced if the left ventricular mass is increased. Should the heart dilate acutely, the mass-to-volume ratio decreases, wall stress and myocardial oxygen consumption increase, and coronary flow reserve falls. Decreasing ventricular dilatation by afterload and preload reduction reverses these unfavorable events and is another reason for the resulting improvement in ventricular function.

Right Ventricular Myocardial Blood Flow. Right ventricular myocardial blood flow follows the general principles of coronary blood flow, but differences exist that are related to the low right ventricular systolic pressure and to the fact that alterations in aortic pressure change coronary perfusing pressure without altering right ventricular pressure work. For example, if the normal right ventricle is acutely distended by pulmonary embolism, right ventricular failure will eventually occur; the increased wall stress increases oxygen consumption, but the raised systolic pressure reduces the coronary flow, so that when supply cannot match demand, right ventricular myocardial ischemia results. Raising aortic perfusing pressure mechanically or with α-adrenergic agonists increases right ventricular myocardial blood flow, relieves ischemia, and restores right ventricular function to normal. Improved coronary flow is not the only mechanism of this improvement; the increased left ventricular afterload moves the ventricular septum toward the right ventricle and improves left ventricular performance (1). If right ventricular pressure is chronically elevated so that right ventricular hypertrophy occurs (as in pulmonic stenosis, many forms

of cyanotic congenital heart disease, and some chronic lung diseases), right ventricular myocardial blood flow behaves in the same way as left ventricular blood flow, with one exception. If aortic pressure is lowered, left ventricular pressure also decreases, as does left ventricular work and oxygen consumption. However, in the right ventricle, the workload may not be reduced (if no ventricular septal defect is present), so that an imbalance between myocardial oxygen supply and demand may occur. The worst imbalance occurs when aortic systolic pressure is maintained but coronary perfusing pressure decreases, and this can occur in a child with tetralogy of Fallot who has an aortopulmonary anastomosis (e.g., Blalock-Taussig shunt) that is too large. The high aortic and left ventricular systolic pressures mandate an equally high right ventricular systolic pressure, but the low diastolic aortic pressure reduces coronary perfusion pressure in diastole and can cause both left and right ventricular ischemia and failure.

Neural Factors. Coronary blood flow increases with sympathetic stimulation, but the mechanisms for this increase are not entirely straightforward. As sympathetic activation tends to increase myocardial oxygen consumption, in large part due to increases in contractility and heart rate, coronary blood flow increases in order to increase oxygen supply, as described previously. However, experiments that isolate the effects of sympathetic stimulation on the coronary arteries from alterations in myocardial work indicate that, in fact, vasoconstriction is the predominant effect of sympathetic activation of the coronary arteries. Even though α-receptors and β-receptors are located on coronary vessels, these studies indicate that coronary blood flow is most strongly influenced by local metabolic processes that match oxygen supply and demand.

CONCLUSIONS AND FUTURE DIRECTIONS

An understanding of the various components and mechanisms that comprise the cardiovascular system is critical, but is only useful when placed in the total context of any given clinical scenario. Various pathophysiologic conditions, as well as therapies, result in alterations within the various components of the cardiovascular system that are synthesized into one clinical condition, albeit ephemeral. These conditions move the cardiovascular system away from its homeostatic baseline and evoke compensatory responses. For example, sepsis may cause vascular dilation, with a reduction in arterial blood pressure. This condition is detected by baroreceptors and chemoreceptors and through various central and local feedback loops that increase sympathetic discharge, heart rate, contractility, and vascular tone. Blood flow to the skin, muscle, and splanchnic circulations is reduced, and blood reserves from the splanchnic circulation and muscle are mobilized. Autoregulatory mechanisms are enacted to preserve blood flow through other vital organs such as the brain and heart. Furthermore, renal mechanisms are set in motion to conserve salt and water in an effort to expand intravascular volume. These responses may transiently normalize the arterial pressure and may compensate for the initial insult. Of course, these mechanisms come at a physiologic cost and, with time, if the inciting stimulus remains, deleterious consequences may prevail. For example, with a prolonged reduction in flow, splanchnic ischemia may develop with subsequent translocation of enteric organisms into the bloodstream, myocardial oxygen demand may rise above supply with subsequent heart failure, and the renal compensatory mechanisms may result in renal failure. Thus, the clinician must have an appreciation for the primary derangement, the compensatory responses, and the impact of therapy on all of these systems.

Furthermore, some clinical scenarios have the potential of placing portions of the cardiovascular system in conflict. For example, infants with tetralogy of Fallot who suffer severe right ventricular outflow tract obstruction with hypoxemia may be treated with α-agonists (e.g., phenylephrine) to increase systemic vascular resistance and pulmonary blood flow. This therapy increases left ventricular afterload and thus decreases cardiac output. Whether oxygen delivery increases depends on whether the oxygen saturation increases sufficiently to overcome the decrease in cardiac output. This situation requires a thorough understanding of the overarching physiology, the goals of therapy, and the effects of therapy on the various regional vascular beds.

A progressive expansion in our understanding of the cardiovascular system has led to an increasing ability to support patients with various ailments. This support comes in many forms, including mechanical support and pharmacologic agents that alter cardiac performance and vascular function. The massive literature on cardiovascular physiology belies the fact that many fundamental processes, such as the central role of the vascular endothelium in vascular biology, were only recently uncovered. Thus, it is probable that ongoing and future investigations will result in novel therapies that will allow more specific targeting of the various components within the cardiovascular system, maximizing therapeutic intentions while minimizing the unintended consequences.

KEY POINTS

- The cardiovascular system delivers essential metabolic substances to the tissues and removes waste products from the tissues.
- Cardiovascular compromise is integral to a number of disease processes that result in critical illness, and many of the therapies used in delivering critical care are aimed at restoring cardiovascular function.
- Components within the cardiovascular system may be differentially, if not diametrically, affected by illness and therapy, requiring clinicians to reconcile these responses.
- The resistance to flow through the vasculature is central to cardiovascular function, as it is a major factor in determining cardiac output and the distribution of blood flow throughout the circulation.
- Interactions between vascular endothelial cells, which produce numerous essential vasoactive factors, and vascular smooth muscle cells regulate dynamic changes in vascular resistance.
- Neural, hormonal, myogenic, and local metabolic mechanisms are also integral to the regulation of vascular tone.
- The vascular and cardiac function curves and their interactions can be used as a theoretical model with which to understand cardiovascular performance under various physiologic and pathologic conditions. At any one time, the

cardiovascular system operates at the point of intersection between the vascular and cardiac function curves.
- Blood flow to most organs is autoregulated, such that blood flow remains constant over a wide range of perfusion pressures.
- In the fetus, the right ventricle supplies most of its blood via the ductus arteriosus and descending aorta to the placenta for oxygen uptake, and the left ventricle supplies most its blood to the brain and heart for oxygen delivery. Critical shunts within the fetal circulation enable this process.
- The most important events in the transition from the fetal to the postnatal circulation are the rapid and large decrease in pulmonary vascular resistance and the disruption of the umbilical-placental circulation.
- Under normal conditions, systemic vascular resistance is the principle factor that affects afterload and cardiac output, but under conditions of right ventricular failure, the state of the pulmonary vasculature is critical.
- The pulmonary vasculature is actively maintained in a dilated, low-resistance state. Alterations in this process are central to the pathophysiology of a number of pulmonary vascular disorders and can severely impact overall cardiovascular performance.
- Hypoxic pulmonary vasoconstriction is an essential and unique feature of the pulmonary vasculature, as it allows for the matching of ventilation and perfusion.
- Alterations in coronary blood flow support cardiac work in a manner that allows myocardial performance (oxygen delivery) to match the overall needs (oxygen demand) of the entire body.
- The left ventricle extracts an almost maximal amount of oxygen from blood passing through the myocardium such that increases in myocardial oxygen demand must be met by increases in coronary blood flow.
- Constriction and relaxation of the coronary arteries comprise the primary mechanism by which coronary blood flow is altered to match myocardial oxygen supply to meet demand.
- Various pathophysiologic conditions result in diverse alterations within the component circulations of the cardiovascular system but are synthesized into one clinical condition, albeit ephemeral.
- Management of critically ill patients requires a thorough understanding of the overarching physiology, the goals of therapy, and the effects of therapy on the various regional vascular beds.
- Future therapies should allow for more specific targeting of the various components within the cardiovascular system.

References

1. Belenkie I, Horne SG, Dani R, et al. Effects of aortic constriction during experimental acute right ventricular pressure loading. Further insights into diastolic and systolic ventricular interaction. *Circulation* 1995;92:546–54.
2. Berne RM, Levy MN. *Coronary Circulation, Cardiovascular Physiology.* Toronto: Mosby, 1986.
3. Cornfield DN, Resnik ER, Herron JM, et al. Pulmonary vascular K^+ channel expression and vasoreactivity in a model of congenital heart disease. *Am J Physiol Lung Cell Mol Physiol* 2002;283:L1210–9.
4. Davis MJ, Ferrer PN, Gore RW. Vascular anatomy and hydrostatic pressure profile in the hamster cheek pouch. *Am J Physiol* 1986;250:H291–303.
5. Davis MJ, Hill MA. Signaling mechanisms underlying the vascular myogenic response. *Physiol Rev* 1999;79:387–423.

6. Dinh-Xuan AT. Endothelial modulation of pulmonary vascular tone. *Eur Respir J* 1992;5:757–62.
7. Ebert TJ, Stowe DF. Neural and endothelial control of the peripheral circulation—implications for anesthesia: Part I. Neural control of the peripheral vasculature. *J Cardiothorac Vasc Anesth* 1996;10:147–58.
8. Faraci FM, Heistad DD. Regulation of the cerebral circulation: Role of endothelium and potassium channels. *Physiol Rev* 1998;78:53–97.
9. Hoffman JI. Problems of coronary flow reserve. *Ann Biomed Eng* 2000;28:884–96.
10. Hoffman JIE. Transmural myocardial perfusion. *Prog Cardiovasc Dis* 1987;29:429–64.
11. Johnson PC. The myogenic response. In: Bohr DF, Somlyo AP, Sparks HV, eds. *Handbook of Physiology. The Cardiovascular System.* Bethesda: American Physiologic Society, 1980.
12. Johnson PC. Autoregulation of blood flow. *Circ Res* 1986;59:483–95.
13. Leffler CW, Hessler JR, Green RS. The onset of breathing at birth stimulates pulmonary vascular prostacyclin synthesis. *Pediatr Res* 1984;18:938–42.
14. Moncada S, Higgs A. The L-arginine-nitric oxide pathway. *N Engl J Med* 1993;329:2002–12.
15. Moudgil R, Michelakis ED, Archer SL. Hypoxic pulmonary vasoconstriction. *J Appl Physiol* 2005;98:390–403.
16. Murphy TV, Spurrell BE, Hill MA. Cellular signalling in arteriolar myogenic constriction: Involvement of tyrosine phosphorylation pathways. *Clin Exp Pharmacol Physiol* 2002;29:612–9.
17. Palmer RM, Ashton DS, Moncada S. Vascular endothelial cells synthesize nitric oxide from L-arginine. *Nature* 1988;333:664–6.
18. Reid LM. The pulmonary circulation: Remodeling in growth and disease. The 1978 J. Burns Amberson Lecture. *Am Rev Respir Dis* 1979;119:531–46.
19. Roos A. Poiseuille's law and its limitations in vascular systems. *Med Thorac* 1962;19:224–38.
20. Rudolph AM, Yuan S. Response of the pulmonary vasculature to hypoxia and H^+ ion concentration changes. *J Clin Invest* 1966;45:399–411.
21. Schreiber MD, Heymann MA, Soifer SJ. Increased arterial pH, not decreased $PaCO_2$, attenuates hypoxia-induced pulmonary vasoconstriction in newborn lambs. *Pediatr Res* 1986;20:113–7.
22. Shyy JY, Chien S. Role of integrins in endothelial mechanosensing of shear stress. *Circ Res* 2002;91:769–75.
23. Strauer BE. Significance of coronary circulation in hypertensive heart disease for development and prevention of heart failure. *Am J Cardiol* 1990;65:34G–41G.
24. Teitel DF, Iwamoto HS, Rudolph AM. Effects of birth-related events on central blood flow patterns. *Pediatr Res* 1987;22:557–66.
25. Vane JR, Anggard EE, Botting RM. Regulatory functions of the vascular endothelium. *N Engl J Med* 1990;323:27–36.
26. Vogt M, Motz W, Strauer BE. Coronary haemodynamics in hypertensive heart disease. *European Heart Journal* 1992;13 Suppl D:44–9.
27. Yanagisawa M, Kurihara H, Kimura S, et al. A novel potent vasoconstrictor peptide produced by vascular endothelial cells. *Nature* 1988;332:411–5.

CHAPTER 64 ■ CARDIORESPIRATORY INTERACTIONS IN CHILDREN WITH HEART DISEASE

LARA SHEKERDEMIAN

The term *cardiorespiratory interactions* describes the physiologic inter-relationship between spontaneous or mechanical breathing and the cardiovascular system. These interactions can be exaggerated or abnormal in certain disease states. The complex interactions that are present in congenital heart disease, in particular in infants and children early after cardiac surgery, have formed the basis of extensive research, such that ventilation is now routinely used as a hemodynamic tool in some patient groups. This chapter includes an historic overview of the evolution of our understanding of cardiopulmonary physiology and a discussion of the interactions between ventilation and the cardiovascular system, with particular reference to infants and children with congenital and acquired heart disease who are in the PICU.

SCIENTIFIC FOUNDATIONS

An Historic Perspective

From the Breath of Life to Capillaries: The Ancient Greeks to the Renaissance

The most fundamental cardiopulmonary interaction is that of gas exchange, and its importance has been recognized for millennia. The ancient Greeks called the air that we breathe the "breath of life." Galen, who was probably the most respected Greek physician after Hippocrates, concluded that the lungs served to provide the blood with heat, from the inhaled air, which was then carried to the heart. He also described the functions of venous and arterial blood. The venous blood was responsible for nutrition, and arterial blood, which contained "pneuma" (or spirituous air), delivered vitality from the heart to the vital organs. The concept of the heart being a muscular pump was not yet realized; instead, the heart was thought to suck blood from the veins during an active diastolic phase and deliver it to the arteries through microscopic pores in the interventricular septum. Galenic physiology was based upon blood being "expended" at its destination and not returning to the heart; thus, the heart constantly produced blood.

Sixteenth-century physiologists challenged Galen's theories. Servetus, who was a Spanish doctor, accurately described the transit of blood from the pulmonary artery, through the lungs, to the pulmonary veins, during which time it changed color as it became mixed with inspired air. He wrote that expiration

cleansed the blood and that blood from the pulmonary veins was drawn to the left side of the heart by diastole. Servetus, therefore, provided the first accurate description of cardiopulmonary physiology and introduced the idea that the circulation of blood between the heart and lungs, and the contribution of ventilation to this, represented a continuum. In the early 1600s, William Harvey concluded that "energy" from the right and left ventricles drove blood in a pulsatile manner to the lungs and the body. He recognized that, in the lungs, some form of microscopic "communication" must occur between the arteries and veins, so that inspired air could be drawn into the blood that returns to the left heart. Similar communications in the other organs would enable the body's other tissues to expel their unwanted waste. However, Harvey was unable to define these channels himself (11). In the 1660s, Malpighi completed the loop when he identified the movement of blood through capillaries in the lung and other organs.

Thus, the mystery of the physiologic mechanisms that underlie gas exchange was unraveled several centuries ago. A discussion of how the study of heart-lung interactions has progressed well beyond the level of gas exchange follows.

Respiration and the Arterial Pulse: The 18th and 19th Centuries

With a clear understanding of the circulation and the mechanism of gas exchange in hand, scientists were set to explore the relationships between flow and pressure in blood vessels during respiration. In 1733, Reverend Stephen Hales, a veterinarian, observed the pulsatility of arterial blood through brass pipes that he inserted directly into the arteries of a live horse. He proposed that such a thing as blood pressure must exist, and he was subsequently the first person to measure it (20). Hales observed that the blood pressure fell during inspiration and increased during expiration in healthy animals.

In 1871, Kussmaul showed in 4 patients with tuberculous pericarditis that the radial pulse was absent during inspiration but returned during expiration (3,17). He suggested that this phenomenon should be named "pulsus paradoxus" in what was probably the earliest documentation of a pathologic cardiopulmonary interaction. Although the phrase *pulsus paradoxus* has been used ever since in this context, this phenomenon, which is also associated with cardiac tamponade, is not paradoxic but is, in fact, an exaggeration of normal physiology (47).

Measurement of Intravascular Pressures

Stephen Hales was the first to directly measure the pressure within a vessel. However, the large pipes that he used were clearly not suitable for use in humans or even small animals. Nearly two centuries later, during the mid-20th century, the advent of intravascular catheterization opened a "Pandora's box" for cardiovascular physiologists. Cardiac catheters enabled physiologists to continuously and relatively safely measure intravascular pressures, calculate flows and vascular resistances, and scientifically explore cardiopulmonary interactions in health and disease.

Invasive Study of Cardiorespiratory Interactions: The Contribution of Cournand

In some of the most important in vivo physiologic investigations of all time, André Cournand, Dickinson Richards, and their coworkers conducted an exhaustive series of several hundred studies of normal cardiorespiratory physiology and pathophysiology in healthy adults and in adults with cardiac failure. To describe in detail the full spectrum of Cournand and Richards' studies is beyond the scope of this chapter. However, some of their most significant findings with relation to children in the PICU are outlined in the following sections.

Differing Effects of Spontaneous Respiration on the Right and Left Ventricle in Man. One of Cournand's first physiologic investigations in humans was his study of the effect of spontaneous respiration on the right ventricular (RV) and left ventricular (LV) output in healthy adults. Spontaneous inspiration led to an increase in RV stroke volume and a reduction in LV stroke volume. The reverse occurred during spontaneous expiration (19). This finding reinforced that "pulsus paradoxus" is an exaggeration of a normal cardiopulmonary interaction.

Pulmonary Vasculature: Hypoxic Pulmonary Vasoconstriction and the Intrapulmonary Shunt. Hypoxic pulmonary vasoconstriction and the intrapulmonary shunt, a fundamental cardiopulmonary interaction that is also known as the Euler-Liljestrand mechanism, was one of the first to be elucidated using cardiac catheterization in the laboratory setting. In a detailed study of healthy anesthetized cats, von Euler and Liljestrand demonstrated that regional ventilation with an inspired oxygen fraction of 0.1 or with an inspired carbon dioxide fraction of 0.19 resulted in an increase in pulmonary artery pressure, with localized pulmonary vasoconstriction and shunt of deoxygenated blood away from that lung region (46). In 1947, Cournand et al. confirmed that hypoxic pulmonary vasoconstriction occurred in adult humans (30).

Positive-Pressure Ventilation and Cardiac Output. Based upon some anecdotal observations that positive-pressure ventilation (PPV) resulted in a fall in cardiac output, Cournand's group went on to uncover the relationship between airway (or pleural) pressure and cardiac output. They performed a series of investigations in invasively instrumented, healthy adults who were receiving noninvasive intermittent PPV via a mask. Cournand showed that during PPV with a higher airway pressure, which did not fall to atmospheric at any time during the respiratory cycle, the cardiac output fell by approximately 15%. However, in the same volunteers, the cardiac output was preserved when a lower mean airway pressure was used (6) (**Fig. 64.1**).

Positive Pressure Ventilation and Right Ventricular Filling. In their series of investigations in volunteers receiving "mask" PPV, Cournand's group uncovered the mechanism responsible for the change in cardiac output during PPV in healthy individuals. They showed that a rise in mean airway (or pleural) pressure produced a proportionate fall in RV filling pressure and that this was the key mechanism underlying the concomitant fall in cardiac output (6):

$$\text{Right ventricular filling pressure} = \text{RVEDP} - P_{pl}$$

where RVEDP is RV end-diastolic pressure and P_{pl} is pleural pressure.

Cournand recommended that, to minimize circulatory disturbance, intermittent PPV should provide "... a gradual increase in pressure during inspiration, a rapid drop in pressure

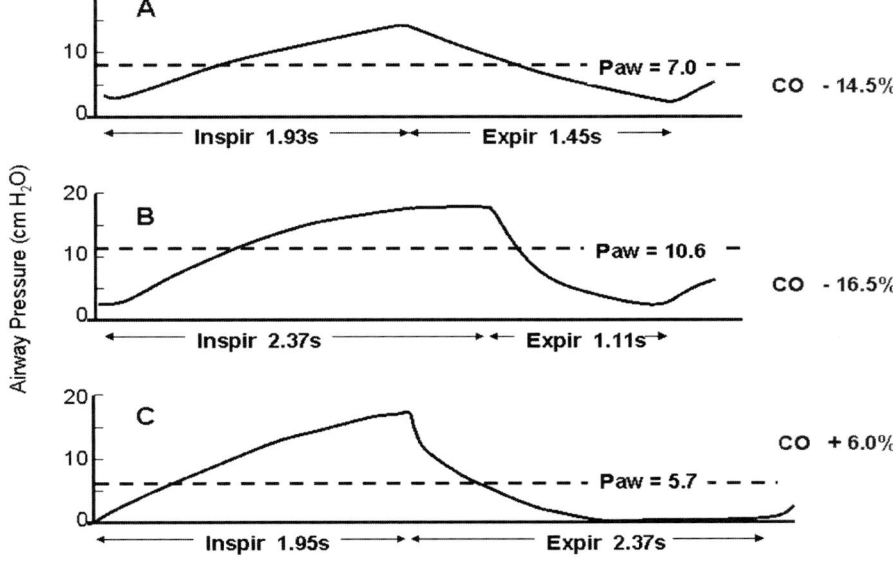

FIGURE 64.1. Cardiac output during three different patterns of "mask" PPV. **A,B:** The inspiratory-to-expiratory time ratio is inverse, and airway pressure never reaches atmospheric during expiration; both patterns are associated with a fall in cardiac output (CO). **C:** Inspiration is shorter than expiration, and the mean airway pressure (P_{aw}) is lower. Thus, cardiac output is preserved. Adapted from Cournand A, Motley HL, Werkö L, et al. Physiological studies of the effects of intermittent positive pressure breathing on cardiac output in man. *Am J Physiol* 1947;152:162–74.

after cycling occurs, and a mean pressure as near atmospheric as possible, and an expiratory time equal to or exceeding the inspiratory time" (6). These recommendations have largely stood the test of time and are now considered to be basic principles of PPV in adult and pediatric intensive care.

Determinants of Stroke Volume: The Right Heart

Under most conditions, RV stroke volume is primarily determined by RV filling (preload). Intrathoracic pressure is a key determinant of these conditions in health and in disease, and the mechanisms at work are explained here.

Intrathoracic Pressure and Right Ventricular Preload

Systemic venous return to the right heart is a passive phenomenon that relies on pressure gradients between the peripheral venous circulation, the extrathoracic great veins, and the right heart. At a simplistic level, the circulation can be considered a "three-compartment model," consisting of the thorax, the abdomen, and the peripheries (**Fig. 64.2**). The peripheries are subject to a relatively constant pressure, which approximates atmospheric pressure. The extrathoracic great veins (in the abdomen) are subject to respiratory variations, largely due to diaphragmatic movement; and the intrathoracic veins and the right atrium are subject to pleural pressure (35).

Spontaneous Inspiration and the Right Heart. During spontaneous inspiration, the pleural pressure becomes negative and the mean right atrial pressure falls. Also during inspiration, the diaphragm descends, thus increasing the pressure to which the extrathoracic great veins are subject. Therefore, venous return from the abdominal compartment and from the peripheral circulation increases during inspiration, as the gradients increase in favor of blood flow to the thorax (**Fig. 64.2**).

The interactions between venous return (which usually equals cardiac output), right atrial pressure, and pleural pressure are, in fact, very complex. Although the three factors are intimately related, they are also independent. For example, the increase in venous return as pleural pressure falls must not be limitless; otherwise, even in a healthy person, during deep breathing, the right heart would ultimately become volume-overloaded. The work of Arthur Guyton has served to advance our understanding of these interactions. In a landmark study in dogs, Guyton demonstrated a critical mean right atrial pressure below which no further increase in systemic venous return could occur (see Chapter 63). In health, this threshold is reached at a mean right atrial pressure of between 0 and −5 mm Hg. At lower atrial pressures, the intrathoracic great veins tend to collapse, thus mechanically limiting central venous return and preventing right heart volume overload (10). However, if, at a given pleural pressure, a bolus of fluid is given, the right atrial pressure and venous return (and therefore cardiac output) can be increased. Within normal physiologic boundaries, it is therefore the atrial pressure rather than pleural pressure that determines the *limits* of venous return (**Fig. 64.3**).

Positive Pressure Inspiration and the Right Heart. During PPV, the reverse occurs. As the intrathoracic pressure becomes

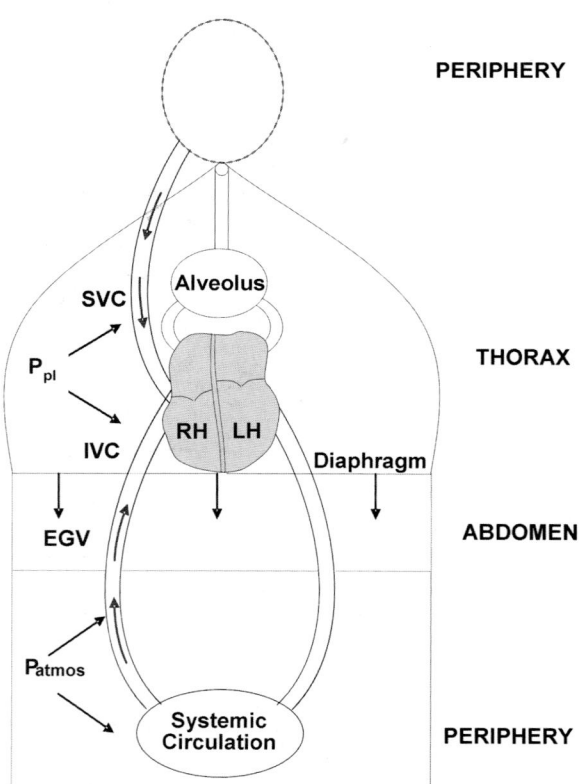

FIGURE 64.2. The "three-compartment" model of circulation. SVC, superior vena cava; IVC, inferior vena cava; EGV, extrathoracic great veins P$_{pl}$, pleural pressure; P$_{atmos}$, atmospheric pressure; RH, right heart; LH, left heart.

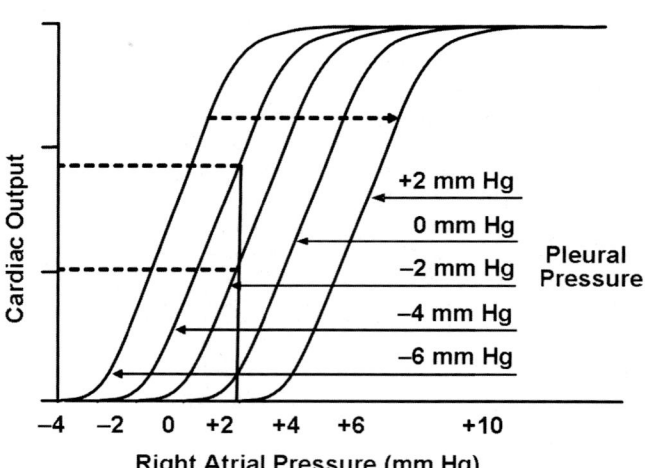

FIGURE 64.3. The relationship between right atrial pressure and cardiac output at varying pleural pressures in a healthy heart. This graph is based on the principles of the work of Guyton and illustrates interactions between pleural pressure, right atrial (filling) pressure, and cardiac output (or venous return) in healthy individuals. The solid vertical line shows how, at a given atrial pressure, cardiac output increases as pleural pressure becomes more negative. Conversely, for every 2-mm Hg increase in pleural pressure, the atrial pressure must also increase by 2 to maintain the cardiac output. The curves also show that, within limits, for a given pleural pressure, cardiac output can be augmented by increasing the atrial pressure (for example with volume administration).

increasingly positive, the right atrial pressure increases and the venous pressure gradient is reduced between the peripheries, the extrathoracic great veins, and right atrium. This reaction results in a fall in RV preload, and can theoretically compromise the RV stroke volume, which may fall. However, in the intact circulation, the use of sensible ventilatory strategies (applying the principles of Cournand), in tandem with intrinsic compensatory baroreceptor responses, largely mitigates against any overt clinical manifestations of these adverse effects. At higher intrathoracic pressures, at which cardiac output may become compromised even in the healthy heart, colloid administration can help to restore RV preload and cardiac output (**Fig. 64.3**).

Intrathoracic Pressure and Right Ventricular Afterload

If venous return were the only determinant of cardiac output during positive pressure ventilation, one would expect that, in the presence of normal myocardial function, volume expansion would preserve the cardiac output under conditions of increasing mean airway pressure; however, this is not always the case. In a landmark study in healthy dogs that received a peak end-expiratory pressure (PEEP) of 20 cm H_2O, Henning observed that RV stroke volume could not be normalized with colloid administration despite complete restoration of the RV preload. The mechanism underlying this observation is that higher intrathoracic pressures and lung volumes directly influence pulmonary vascular resistance and RV afterload and, hence, RV function (12).

Pulmonary interdependence describes the relationship between lung volumes (or alveolar distension) and the status of the pulmonary vessels (**Fig. 64.4**). As the lung volume is increased from residual volume to functional residual capacity, so the extra-alveolar pulmonary parenchymal vessels increase in diameter and "straighten"; thus, pulmonary vascular resistance falls. If a positive intrathoracic pressure is applied, and lung volumes increase above functional residual capacity, the alveolar capillaries become stretched and their luminal diameter falls; thus, pulmonary vascular resistance increases. In practice, this phenomenon is observed at high PEEP levels (usually well above 10 cm H_2O).

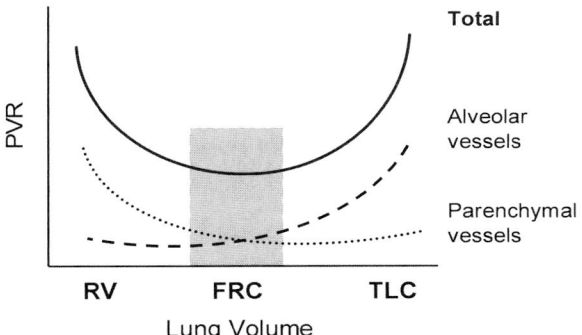

FIGURE 64.4. Lung volumes and pulmonary vascular resistance. Although lung volume has opposite effects on alveolar and parenchymal vessels, both types of vessels have the lowest pulmonary vascular resistance (PVR) at functional residual capacity (FRC). Hence, total PVR is lowest at FRC. RV, residual volume; TLC, total lung capacity.

A fall in lung volume below functional residual capacity is associated with an elevation of pulmonary vascular resistance and. at low lung volumes, this may be further compounded by hypoxic pulmonary vasoconstriction (**Fig. 64.4**). This combination can result in hemodynamic compromise in a number of pediatric patient groups. Pulmonary hypertension is associated with significant morbidity in infants early after surgical repair of large septal defects, totally anomalous pulmonary venous connection, or after the arterial switch operation (22,43).

Intrathoracic Pressure and the Left Ventricle

Left ventricular stroke volume is determined by its contractility and the impedance to LV ejection or afterload. In a healthy individual, spontaneous and mechanical ventilation primarily influence the right heart. However, ventilation also exerts subtle but important effects on LV afterload that can be of greater significance in certain pathologic states.

Spontaneous Ventilation and Left Ventricular Afterload

Left ventricular afterload is determined by its transmural pressure. Transmural pressure of an intrathoracic structure is the gradient "across" its wall and relates the measured pressure within the structure to the pressure surrounding it (the pleural pressure). Thus, for the left ventricle:

$$P_{LVTM} = P_{Ao} - P_{PL}$$

where P_{LVTM} is the LV transmural pressure, P_{Ao} is the aortic pressure, and P_{PL} is the pleural pressure.

As demonstrated by this equation, increased afterload can result from an increase in aortic (or arterial) blood pressure *or* from a fall in pleural pressure. During spontaneous inspiration, the intravascular aortic pressure may fall slightly, but the pleural pressure falls relatively more and becomes negative. Thus, the LV transmural pressure and afterload increase during spontaneous inspiration. In healthy individuals who are spontaneously breathing, respiration predominantly affects the right heart, and subtle changes in afterload of the left ventricle do not adversely affect ventricular function.

The impact of changes in pleural pressure on the left ventricle become much more significant if an exaggerated negative pleural pressure is applied. If healthy individuals perform a Mueller maneuver or an inspiratory threshold-loading maneuver, in which the pleural pressure falls to well below −20 cm H_2O, afterload increases significantly and LV ejection fraction falls (14). This interaction can occur in otherwise healthy individuals with normal hearts—the "negative pressure pulmonary edema," which can occur during a severe asthma attack (44) or with acute airway obstruction (29). It is likely that this mechanism contributes to the LV dysfunction in a number of important chronic disease states, including obstructive sleep apnea.

Positive Pressure Ventilation and Left Ventricular Afterload

PPV reduces the transmural LV pressure and, therefore, lowers the LV afterload (see previous equation), which may result in increased LV stroke volume and a lower end-diastolic volume. Although in health this cardiopulmonary interaction is of little clinical importance, it has important implications for the management of patients with acute and chronic heart failure.

CARDIORESPIRATORY INTERACTIONS IN CHILDREN WITH HEART DISEASE

Ventilation is a valuable although underutilized hemodynamic tool in pediatric cardiac intensive care. When used carefully and tailored according to a clinical situation, ventilation is often far more effective in manipulating the circulatory physiology than are cardiovascular pharmacologic agents. A number of common settings in which ventilation can be used in this way are discussed here and are summarized in **Table 64.1**.

Cardiorespiratory Interactions in Children with Heart Failure

Cardiopulmonary interactions play a major role in the symptomatology, hemodynamic manifestations, and the management of heart failure in the PICU.

Cardiorespiratory Interactions during Resting Ventilation

Heart failure with *systolic* ventricular dysfunction is commonly encountered in the PICU. The term "heart failure" covers a broad clinical spectrum that includes:

- Transient ventricular dysfunction after repair of congenital heart disease
- Severe, acute decompensated heart failure secondary to myocarditis, sepsis, arrhythmia, or ischemia
- Severe chronic (or acute-on-chronic) heart failure, secondary to dilated cardiomyopathy or congenital heart disease with systemic ventricular failure

Children with systolic heart failure are particularly susceptible to the interactions between spontaneous breathing and the heart for three main reasons:

- LV afterload is elevated at baseline due to activation of neurohumoral mechanisms, including the renin-angiotensin system and the intrinsic catecholamines.
- The work of breathing (WOB) is increased at baseline, compared to healthy individuals, and the negative inspiratory swings in pleural pressure are exaggerated due to reduced lung compliance and increased lung water secondary to elevated left atrial pressures.
- The right atrial pressure is increased, and cardiac output is reduced. The capacity of these patients to increase their cardiac output is greatly limited (**Fig. 64.5**).

During spontaneous inspiration, the afterload on the left ventricle and preload on the right ventricle will further increase. Whereas these cardiorespiratory interactions are well tolerated (or are even desirable) under normal circumstances, they are exaggerated and can further exacerbate ventricular dysfunction in children with systolic heart failure. These

---

TABLE 64.1

CARDIORESPIRATORY INTERACTIONS IN CHILDREN WITH HEART DISEASE DURING SPONTANEOUS AND POSITIVE-PRESSURE VENTILATION

	Key issues	Spontaneous respiration		Positive-pressure ventilation/CPAP	
Heart failure (acute, or chronic)	Elevated LV afterload Systolic LV dysfunction	Increased work of breathing Exaggerated negative intrapleural pressure swings	Increased LV afterload	Reduced work of breathing Obliterated negative swings in pleural pressure	Reduced venous return Reduced LV afterload Improved LV function
Postoperative—tetralogy of Fallot	Good systolic function Diastolic RV dysfunction Preload-dependent	Increased RV preload Improved diastolic pulmonary artery flow	Improved cardiac output	Reduced RV preload Reduced diastolic pulmonary artery flow	Reduced cardiac output
Postoperative—Fontan/BCPS	Good systolic function Preload dependent Cardiac output depends on pulmonary blood flow.	Increased preload Negative intrathoracic pressure improves pulmonary blood flow.	Improved cardiac output	Reduced preload Reduced pulmonary blood flow	Reduced cardiac output
Duct-dependent systemic flow	Excessive pulmonary flow, leading to reduced systemic flow	Tachypnea and oversaturation are common. Limited control of pulmonary flow	Possible excessive pulmonary flow and reduced systemic cardiac output	Better control of pulmonary flow, pH, and pulmonary resistance	Improved systemic cardiac output

CPAP, continuous positive airway pressure; BCPS, bidirectional cavopulmonary shunt; LV, left ventricle; RV, right ventricle

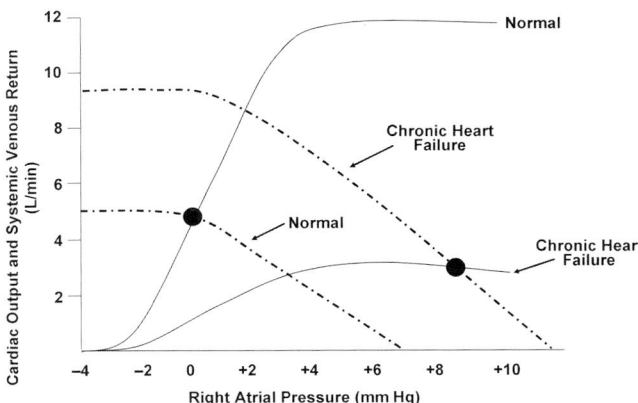

FIGURE 64.5. Relationship between venous return, cardiac output, and right atrial pressure in normal individuals and in patients with chronic systolic heart failure. This graph shows the cardiac output (**solid lines**) and systemic venous return (**broken lines**) in normal, healthy individuals and in those with chronic decompensated cardiac failure. The intersection of the venous return curve and the cardiac output curve, in health, produce a steady-state cardiac output of ~5 L/min, optimally operating at an atrial pressure that approximates atmospheric. In patients with untreated cardiac failure, cardiac output is reduced. The compensatory mechanisms for a reduced cardiac output result in partial restoration of cardiac output at the expense of a significantly elevated atrial pressure.

interactions become even more pronounced with exertion, stress or agitation—circumstances in which either or both of the WOB and vascular tone are increased.

Positive Pressure Ventilation in Heart Failure

PPV produces beneficial cardiopulmonary interactions in children with acute or chronic heart failure, through a number of mechanisms.

Positive-pressure respiratory support facilitates the unloading of respiratory muscles, resulting in reduced respiratory effort and WOB. By increasing the mean airway pressure and reducing the WOB, PPV prevents the exaggerated negative inspiratory swings in spontaneously breathing patients with severe heart failure.

A positive intrathoracic pressure lowers the pressure gradient between the thorax and the periphery and reduces the systemic venous return, resulting in reduced RV preload and RV end-systolic and end-diastolic volumes. Although this intervention may reduce stroke volume and cardiac output in the intact circulation, the reduced right heart volume load in the failing heart results in improved cardiac performance and in better ventriculoventricular interactions.

Through its effects on intrathoracic pressure and WOB, PPV reduces the LV transmural pressure (31), thereby reducing the LV afterload, which improves LV stroke volume and ejection fraction.

Patients with heart failure have elevated levels of endogenous catecholamines, increased myocardial oxygen consumption, and elevated cardiac sympathetic tone. These contribute to the elevated afterload and the increased stroke work of the impaired left ventricle. A positive intrathoracic pressure reduces the levels of norepinephrine in patients with chronic heart failure (5) and reduces cardiac sympathetic tone (15) and myocardial oxygen consumption (16).

The Treatment of Heart Failure with Positive-Pressure Ventilation

In an historic study in 1973, Beach observed that *some* postcardiotomy adult patients who met objective criteria for discontinuation of PPV responded to extubation with an unexpected and sudden fall in cardiac output without any disturbance in gas exchange (2). He noted that this deterioration was more likely in patients with impaired cardiac function.

Positive-Pressure Ventilation in Children with Postcardiotomy Systolic Ventricular Dysfunction. Open cardiac surgery inevitably results in significant, albeit largely transient, myocardial injury due to a number of intraoperative factors, including cardiopulmonary bypass, cross-clamp, temperature change, and cardiotomy. This injury is often associated with a degree of early postoperative systolic ventricular dysfunction. Most infants and children are intubated and ventilated with PPV when they are in the PICU early after open heart surgery. Therefore, part of their "hemodynamic" support routinely includes PPV, which produces desirable effects on RV preload, LV afterload, and WOB at this critical time. Indeed, some neonates and younger infants will benefit from the continuing hemodynamic benefit of a period of continuous positive-airway pressure (CPAP) immediately after endotracheal extubation.

Positive-Pressure Ventilation in the Nonsurgical Patient with Systolic Ventricular Dysfunction. PPV is clearly beneficial for children with ventricular dysfunction, but in the nonsurgical setting, these are patients in whom the process of intubation may itself cause significant hemodynamic compromise. However, PPV does not necessarily require endotracheal intubation; it can safely and effectively be delivered to children of all ages via a face mask or a nasopharyngeal tube.

Presently, no short- or long-term clinical trials have been conducted to study PPV in children with chronic heart failure, but its role in adults has been extensively researched. Noninvasive PPV [CPAP or bilevel positive airway pressure (BiPAP)], is now a mainstay of therapy in hospitalized adults with acute pulmonary edema secondary to decompensated heart failure. In these patients, noninvasive ventilation via CPAP or BiPAP results in symptomatic improvement, a reduced need for endotracheal intubation, and reduced early mortality (25,26). In adults with chronic congestive heart failure, CPAP improves cardiac volumes (28) and LV ejection fraction (24). Long-term CPAP also improves functional status, and quality of life in patients with end-stage heart failure (41,42). The use of noninvasive PPV in children with heart failure warrants prospective investigation.

Cardiorespiratory Interactions in Children with Congenital Heart Disease

In the field of pediatric intensive care, some unique cardiorespiratory interactions exist in infants and children with congenital heart disease, and these are of particular significance during the perioperative period. The management and manipulation of these interactions can profoundly influence the clinical course of these patients, either to their benefit or detriment. Discussed next are 4 specific patient groups for whom manipulation of

TABLE 64.2

NEWBORNS AND YOUNG INFANTS WITH FUNCTIONALLY UNIVENTRICULAR
CIRCULATION: DIAGNOSTIC GROUPS

Diagnostic group	Preoperative physiology	Postoperative physiology
Hypoplastic left heart syndrome (and variants)	Duct-dependent systemic circulation	Norwood-type physiology
Interrupted aortic arch and ventricular septal defect	Duct-dependent systemic circulation	Biventricular circulation[a]
Truncus arteriosus	Single outlet heart	Biventricular circulation[a]
Critically obstructed pulmonary circulation	Duct-dependent pulmonary circulation[a]	Neonatal systemic-pulmonary artery shunt

[a]Circulatory physiology, in which cardiopulmonary interactions do not fall within the scope of this chapter.

ventilation has a well-described role in hemodynamic therapy while they are in the PICU.

Cardiorespiratory Interactions in Functionally Univentricular Circulation

Neonates and young infants with functionally univentricular circulation represent a large group with a spectrum of complex diagnoses, including common arterial trunk, hypoplastic left heart syndrome, and postoperative Norwood patients (**Table 64.2**). The unifying feature of the preoperative and/or postoperative circulatory physiology of infants with functionally univentricular circulation is that the perfusion of the pulmonary and systemic (including coronary) circulations is from the output of a single (or functionally single) ventricle. Thus, the relative delivery of the ventricular output to the systemic and pulmonary vascular beds depends on the relative resistances of the two circulations. Most cardiac intensivists would agree that these infants present the greatest management challenge of all those with congenital heart disease. The key to limiting morbidity and maximizing intact survival of infants with functionally univentricular circulation lies in optimizing their systemic oxygen delivery from birth until the postoperative period after cardiac surgery.

Infants with a critically obstructed systemic circulation, such as hypoplastic left heart syndrome and its variants, have a duct-dependent systemic circulation at birth. Ductal patency requires pharmacologic treatment with prostaglandin. However, once the duct is wide open, the subsequent distribution of the cardiac output depends solely upon the resistance of the pulmonary and systemic circulations. If the systemic vasculature is constricted, blood preferentially flows to the lungs, compromising systemic and myocardial perfusion; this is clinically manifested as oversaturation, acidosis, end-organ dysfunction, and myocardial ischemia. Infants with truncus arteriosus or hypoplastic left heart syndrome are known to be the subgroup with congenital heart disease that is at greatest risk of neonatal necrotizing enterocolitis, which directly results from gut ischemia (27).

The Role of Ventilation in Optimizing Systemic Oxygen Delivery. The pulmonary vasculature of neonates is highly sensitive to the vasodilating effects of inspired oxygen and alkalosis and to the constricting effects of carbon dioxide and acidosis. Routine resuscitation and early neonatal care of the infant with known or suspected duct-dependent systemic

perfusion should include the avoidance, or cautious administration of, supplemental oxygen and the avoidance of alkalosis. In addition, pain and agitation should be avoided in all of these patients, so that sudden increases in systemic vascular resistance do not exacerbate systemic hypoperfusion (48).

Preoperative mechanical ventilation is commonly required in infants with functionally univentricular circulation, most frequently to optimize systemic perfusion. Ventilation can be used to control respiratory rate (and avoid respiratory alkalosis), control the oxygen saturation, optimize arterial carbon dioxide levels, enable the administration of sedating agents, and stabilize pulmonary vascular resistance.

In the early postoperative period following Norwood-type operations or placement of neonatal systemic-to-pulmonary artery shunts, ventilation should similarly be tailored to optimize systemic oxygen delivery using the same basic principles. Optimal systemic oxygen delivery occurs when the pulmonary-to-systemic flow ratio (Qp/Qs) is ~1:1, corresponding to a systemic oxygen saturation of ~80%. The use of supplemental nitrogen or carbon dioxide delivered with the ventilator gases to augment systemic oxygen delivery in the Norwood circulation has been investigated in the laboratory and clinical settings. Limited data suggest that, while supplemental nitrogen (to reduce the inspired oxygen fraction to ~0.17) does lower the systemic arterial oxygen saturations, it also reduces the mixed venous saturation and cerebral oxygen delivery (45). In contrast, the addition of 3% carbon dioxide to the ventilator circuit improves mixed venous saturation without changing systemic arterial saturation in both the preoperative (45) and postoperative (4) settings, suggesting that supplemental carbon dioxide, but not nitrogen, improves systemic oxygen delivery in the functionally univentricular circulation.

Previously, the beneficial cardiovascular effects of PPV in infants and children with heart disease were discussed. The following sections include a discussion of the important cardiorespiratory interactions that are present in children after right heart surgery and how even seemingly conservative PPV may have important detrimental cardiovascular effects in these patients.

Cardiorespiratory Interactions after the Fontan Operation

A low cardiac output state can complicate the early postoperative course of children after Fontan operations, but this is only rarely due to systolic dysfunction of the systemic ventricle. In these patients, the low output is most commonly secondary to abnormalities of diastolic function. This problem may seem out of place in a chapter about ventilation, but ventilation plays a critical role in the hemodynamic management of children in the PICU early after Fontan operations.

In the first report in the literature of the atriopulmonary connection in 3 adults with tricuspid atresia, Fontan observed a clinical improvement after extubation and wrote that PPV should be "stopped early because positive pressure prevents central venous return" (8). Several years later, Laks wrote that extubation resulted in a fall in right atrial pressure, which was "in general accompanied by some improvement in clinical condition" (18).

In Fontan patients, extubation results in a fall in central venous and, therefore, pulmonary artery pressures. A recent study showed that this reduction in pulmonary artery pressure was accompanied by an immediate and sustained improvement in systemic cardiac output (23), which supports the observations of Fontan and Laks (and most cardiac intensivists) that Fontan patients show a clinical and hemodynamic improvement once spontaneously breathing.

Pulmonary Blood Flow and Ventilation in the Fontan Circulation. Pulmonary blood flow is the key determinant of cardiac output in Fontan patients. In brief, the key elements of the Fontan circulation are that the systemic veins are in continuity with the pulmonary arteries, either through direct (cavopulmonary) anastomoses or via an atriopulmonary connection. The pulmonary venous return is to a pulmonary venous (left, or common) atrium. In the absence of a subpulmonary pumping chamber, pulmonary blood flow is a passive phenomenon that is driven by a sufficient pressure difference across the lungs— or between the systemic veins and the pulmonary venous atrium.

It is now easy to see how even seemingly minor changes in intrathoracic pressure may have significant influence on pulmonary blood flow. With these observations in mind, Penny and Redington sought to examine the influences of changes in intrathoracic pressure on pulmonary blood flow in spontaneously breathing patients after Fontan operations, and observed that pulmonary blood flow increased by nearly two-thirds during inspiratory cardiac cycles, as the pleural pressure became negative (33,34) (**Fig. 64.6**). Flow was reversed,

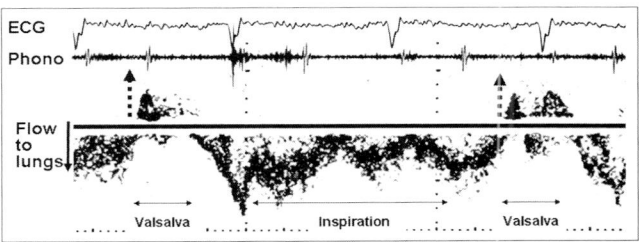

FIGURE 64.7. Pulsed-wave Doppler profile of pulmonary arterial flow during two brief Valsalva maneuvers in a Fontan patient. Blood flows toward the lungs during spontaneous inspiration (**solid arrow**). Flow is reversed (**dotted arrow**) during two brief Valsalva maneuvers. Thus, blood flows away from the lungs and cardiac output is lost during a sudden, substantial increase in intrathoracic pressure.

implying a brief complete cessation of cardiac output when these patients performed a Valsalva maneuver (**Fig. 64.7**). The question then arose as to whether (in children with good systolic function) negative-pressure ventilation (NPV) might augment cardiac output by mimicking spontaneous respiration, as an adjunctive tool in sicker Fontan patients in whom early extubation may not be possible. We performed a series of studies in which ventilated children early after Fontan operations received a brief period of NPV using a cuirass device. These children initially received PPV with a mean airway pressure of 6–9 cm H_2O; they then received cuirass NPV with a mean airway pressure of −6 to −9 cm H_2O. A brief period of NPV increased their pulmonary blood flow by 42% (36,39) (**Fig. 64.8**).

Therapeutic NPV has only been rarely used in Fontan patients. Most importantly, these studies have further reinforced our understanding of the important cardiopulmonary interactions in this group. The key message of these physiologic studies is that some basic principles should be followed in managing

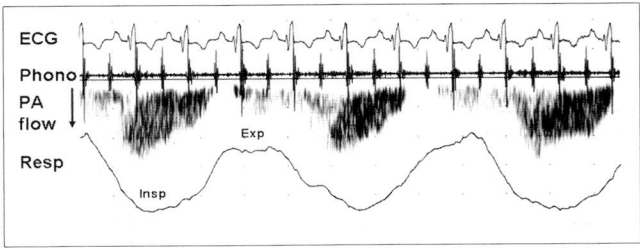

FIGURE 64.6. Pulsed-wave Doppler profile of pulmonary arterial flow in a spontaneously breathing Fontan patient. Pulmonary blood flow (**arrow**) bears no relationship to ventricular systole. Flow increases during spontaneous inspiration and is minimal during expiration. ECG, electrocardiogram; Phono, Phonocardiogram; PA, pulmonary artery; Resp, Respirometer trace; Insp, spontaneous inspiration; Exp, spontaneous expiration.

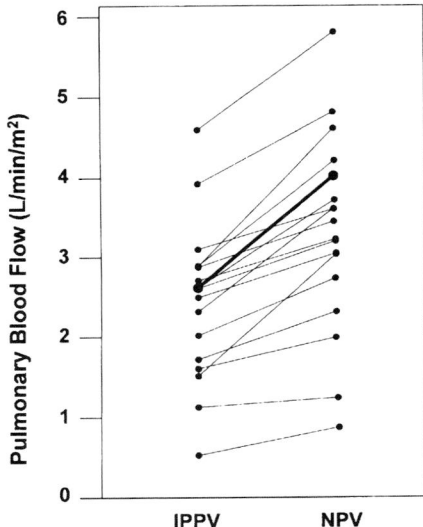

FIGURE 64.8. Pulmonary blood flow during PPV and after 15 mins of cuirass NPV in Fontan patients. Mean pulmonary blood flow increased from 2.4 L/min/m² to 3.5 L/min/m² after 15 mins of NPV ($p < 0.001$). IPPV, intermittent positive pressure ventilation; NPV, negative pressure ventilation.

ventilation of children immediately after Fontan operations. These are:

1. Establish spontaneous breathing early while intubated.
2. Maintain low PEEP (3–5 cm H_2O).
3. Minimize mean airway pressures.
4. Extubate early.

Thus, the majority of Fontan patients should be extubated within a few hours of returning from the operating room. In the modern era, the failure to successfully wean a Fontan patient from mechanical ventilation early should prompt a search for reasons why.

Cardiopulmonary Interactions after the Bidirectional Cavopulmonary Shunt

Pulmonary blood flow is the key determinant of systemic oxygen delivery in infants and children after a bidirectional cavopulmonary shunt (BCPS, or Glenn operation). Similar to Fontan patients, pulmonary blood flow in these patients is a passive phenomenon that depends on adequate venous return to a low-resistance pulmonary circulation. A unique feature of infants and children with a BCPS (but not of Fontan patients), is that pulmonary blood flow is entirely derived from upper body venous return. The systemic arterial oxygen saturations after a BCPS are highly predictive of pulmonary blood flow and systemic cardiac output. These patients are highly preload dependent, and simple colloid or blood transfusion can produce untold improvements in arterial saturation. In patients who have undergone a BCPS, significant elevations of central venous (pulmonary artery) pressure, related to venous obstruction, pulmonary hypertension, or the use of excessively high airway pressures, result in venous congestion of the upper body, usually associated with systemic desaturation and signs of reduced systemic oxygen delivery. Similar to Fontan patients, extubation of infants and children after a BCPS is associated with hemodynamic improvement, with an increase in systemic cardiac output increases and a fall in pulmonary artery pressure (23).

Ventilation and Systemic Oxygen Delivery after a BCPS. Routine postoperative ventilatory practice after a BCPS should be tailored to optimizing systemic oxygen delivery and cerebral blood flow. On returning from the operating room, these patients should routinely be cared for with elevation of the upper body to assist systemic venous drainage, thereby encouraging pulmonary blood flow. In these patients, an increase in mean airway pressure reduces the pulmonary blood flow and, hence, systemic cardiac output. It is therefore standard practice to manage these infants similarly to the Fontan patient, using conservative airway pressures and aiming for early extubation.

Recent studies suggest that a mild respiratory acidosis, induced by addition of carbon dioxide to the ventilator gases, may improve systemic oxygenation and reduce oxygen consumption in ventilated children after the BCPS. Given that cerebral blood flow (and upper body venous return) is the key determinant of pulmonary blood flow in these patients, a degree of hypercapnic cerebral vasodilation is likely to be the mechanism that underlies this phenomenon. Although, in general, acidosis increases pulmonary vascular resistance and hence decreases pulmonary blood flow, it is likely that the effects of mild hypercapnia on the cerebral vasculature outweigh those on the pulmonary vasculature after a BCPS. Thus, in venti-

lated patients with significant arterial hypoxemia early after a BCPS, a mild respiratory acidosis may result in improved oxygenation and systemic oxygen delivery (13,21). However, the strategy used to achieve this outcome is extremely important: alveolar derecruitment is highly undesirable, as it is likely to complicate subsequent ventilatory weaning. Similar to infants with hypoplastic left heart syndrome, therefore, a mild respiratory acidosis should be achieved through the addition of carbon dioxide to the inspired ventilator gases rather than by deliberate hypoventilation.

Cardiorespiratory Interactions in Patients with Diastolic Right Ventricular Dysfunction early after Tetralogy of Fallot Repair

In most institutions, mortality early after complete correction of tetralogy of Fallot repair is less than 3%. Most infants have a relatively uncomplicated postoperative course in the PICU and can be extubated within 24 hrs of surgery.

However, well known is the small subgroup of infants who develop a low cardiac output early after surgery, with elevated venous pressures and refractoriness to standard pharmacologic agents. In these patients, systolic ventricular function is usually well preserved, with the favorable echocardiographic appearance of the heart somewhat belying the poor appearance of the patients. In 1995, Cullen characterized the underlying problem by using Doppler echocardiography in a cohort of patients who received mechanical ventilation in the ICU early after tetralogy repair. He showed that a significant proportion of these patients had restrictive RV physiology early after tetralogy repair and that this was associated with the development of a low cardiac output state (7). The hallmark of restrictive physiology is diastolic anterograde flow into the pulmonary artery, coincident with atrial systole. Although abnormal, this antegrade diastolic pulmonary arterial flow represents an important source of cardiac output and limits the duration of pulmonary regurgitation within the cardiac cycle. It would follow that a reduction in, or loss of, this flow could precipitate further clinical decline in some patients, or conversely, that augmentation of the flow could confer a hemodynamic benefit. The cardiac output of children with restrictive RV physiology after tetralogy of Fallot repair is highly sensitive to changes in intrathoracic pressure.

Cardiac Output and Ventilation in Patients with Restrictive Right Ventricular Physiology. Several years before Cullen's study in children, Appleton demonstrated important pathological cardiorespiratory interactions in spontaneously breathing adults with restrictive cardiomyopathy who were undergoing cardiac catheterization. Half of these patients had characteristic diastolic antegrade pulmonary artery flow during atrial systole. The hemodynamic basis for this flow was that the RV diastolic pressure exceeded pulmonary artery diastolic pressure during atrial systole, which led to premature opening of the pulmonary valve. Of great relevance, this forward flow was only present during inspiratory cardiac cycles (1).

In children with restrictive physiology who were receiving PPV early after tetralogy repair, Cullen demonstrated that antegrade forward pulmonary artery flow was markedly reduced during the inspiratory phase but was relatively preserved during expiration, suggesting that an increasingly positive intrathoracic pressure caused a significant reduction in pulmonary blood flow and, hence, cardiac output. Combined with Appleton's observations, this finding suggests that spontaneous inspiration would augment diastolic pulmonary artery flow of infants with restrictive physiology. This hypothesis was confirmed in spontaneously breathing patients in the convalescent phase after tetralogy repair (9) and in our own investigation of the cardiovascular effects of NPV in this population.

In general, therefore, the principles of ventilatory management of children early after tetralogy repair should be similar to those in Fontan patients, with the use of conservative airway pressures and early establishment of spontaneous respiration. In most units, the majority of children can and should be extubated during the first 24 hrs after surgery (40). In the current era, not all children with diastolic RV dysfunction develop a low cardiac output state, but a low output state is still most commonly associated with restrictive physiology. The first step in managing a child with a low cardiac output after tetralogy repair is to perform a detailed echocardiogram. If this test confirms restrictive physiology, the appropriate ventilatory strategies—use of conservative mean airway pressures and early establishment of spontaneous respiration—should be applied, while minimizing the doses of inotropic agents.

As in the Fontan circulation, as understanding of cardiopulmonary interactions after right heart surgery improved, the question naturally arose as to whether they could be further exploited in children while in the PICU early after surgery. We hypothesized that NPV, by mimicking spontaneous respiration, would augment pulmonary blood flow in children early after tetralogy repair. In a series of studies that compare the cardiac output during conventional intermittent PPV and during cuirass NPV, we showed that NPV increased the cardiac output by a total of 67% (37) (**Fig. 64.9**). Echocardiographic study of these patients further supported the hypothesis, with augmentation of antegrade diastolic pulmonary arterial flow as the intrathoracic pressure became negative during negative-pressure inspiration (39). These studies showed that, as in Fontan patients, ventilatory management of children early after tetralogy repair should be considered integral to their routine hemodynamic therapy. Thus, although on occasions therapeutic NPV has been used with success (38), the key message of these investigations is that ventilation should be always be tailored to the physiology of children after tetralogy repair.

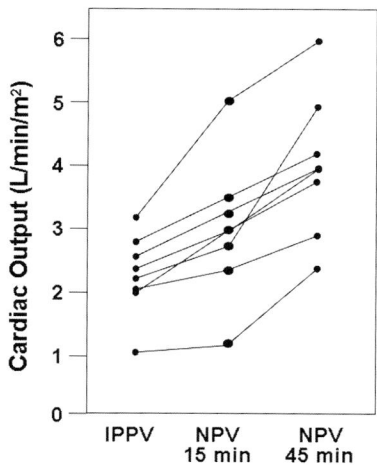

FIGURE 64.9. Cardiac output during PPV, and during NPV in children after tetralogy of Fallot repair. Cardiac output increased by 21% after 15 mins of NPV and by a further 38% between 15 and 45 mins. The total increase was 67% ($p < 0.0001$).

Cardiorespiratory Interactions Late after Tetralogy of Fallot Repair. Interestingly, restrictive RV physiology is not only an immediate postoperative phenomenon, but affects a proportion of children and adults late after surgery. It is also likely that early restrictive physiology predicts its presence later in life, with identical associated cardiopulmonary interactions (32). In a series of convalescent studies in patients late after tetralogy of Fallot repair, the presence of restrictive physiology predicts superior ventricular performance and exercise tolerance years later (9). It is therefore somewhat reassuring that infants with restrictive RV physiology, some of whom may spend longer in the PICU early after surgery, may indeed benefit from this phenomenon in the medium- and long-term.

CONCLUSIONS AND FUTURE DIRECTIONS

Cardiorespiratory interactions have been the subject of medical explorations for many centuries, and our current knowledge would not exist without the work of investigators prior to the 20th century. However, the invasive, exhaustive studies of physiologists in Europe and North America during the last century have enabled us to approach ventilation in a newer light: not only as a technique of achieving optimal gas exchange, but also as a hemodynamic tool.

Children in the PICU who have heart disease represent a complicated spectrum when their circulatory physiology and associated cardiorespiratory interactions are considered. For example, in one bed may be a child who requires noninvasive PPV as part of her treatment for cardiomyopathy; in the next bed may be a child who requires spontaneous ventilation early after a Fontan operation; and in the next bed may be a newborn infant with hypoplastic left heart syndrome who is receiving additional carbon dioxide to optimize systemic oxygen delivery. In all 3 patients, ventilation is being used to optimize their hemodynamic performance but via 3 very different approaches. An understanding of cardiorespiratory interactions is integral to good cardiac intensive care.

As in all areas of pediatric critical care, patient numbers are often a limiting factor in designing controlled trials that will definitively address whether a therapy improves outcome. However, this factor cannot always be used as a reason *not* to study a therapy in a scientific, systematic manner; an example would be evaluation of a possible role for long-term noninvasive positive-pressure respiratory support in children with end-stage heart failure. Over the past decade, the awareness of intensivists of the role of ventilation in optimizing the hemodynamics of infants and children with congenital heart disease has improved. Over the next decade, this concept must be even better addressed in routine practice so that, for some patients, adjustment of the ventilator is considered before the vial of a cardiovascular drug is opened.

KEY POINTS

■ Ventilation is an important determinant of systemic cardiac output.
■ In healthy individuals, spontaneous and mechanical ventilation primarily affect the right heart.

- Cournand's basic principles of mechanical ventilation should be routinely considered as a default in all patients who receive PPV.
- Ventilation has important effects on LV afterload in patients with systolic ventricular dysfunction, such that a negative intrathoracic pressure increases afterload and compromises stroke volume.
- PPV is beneficial for children with systolic heart failure, and it can be delivered by the noninvasive route.
- Some unique cardiorespiratory interactions are present in infants and children with congenital heart disease, in particular in infants with a functionally univentricular circulation or those after "right heart" surgery.
- Ventilation can be more useful than vasoactive drugs in optimizing systemic oxygen delivery in infants and children with congenital heart disease.
- Children with diastolic dysfunction after "right heart" surgery often benefit from early extubation.

References

1. Appleton CP, Hatle LK, Popp RL. Demonstration of restrictive ventricular physiology by Doppler echocardiography. *J Am Coll Cardiol* 1988; 11(4):757–68.
2. Beach T, Millen E, Grenvick A. Hemodynamic response to discontinuance of mechanical ventilation. *Crit Care Med* 1973;1(2):85–90.
3. Bilchick KC, Wise RA. Paradoxical physical findings described by Kussmaul: Pulsus paradoxus and Kussmaul's sign. *Lancet* 2002;359(9321):1940–2.
4. Bradley SM, Simsic JM, Atz AM. Hemodynamic effects of inspired carbon dioxide after the Norwood procedure. *Ann Thorac Surg* 2001;72(6):2088–93.
5. Bradley TD, Logan AG, Kimoff RJ, et al. Continuous positive airway pressure for central sleep apnea and heart failure. *N Engl J Med* 2005;353(19):2025–3.
6. Cournand A, Motley HL, Werkö L. Physiological studies of the effects of intermittent positive pressure breathing on cardiac output in man. *Am J Physiol* 1948;152:162.
7. Cullen S, Shore D, Redington A. Characterization of right ventricular diastolic performance after complete repair of tetralogy of Fallot. Restrictive physiology predicts slow postoperative recovery. *Circulation* 1995;91(6):1782–9.
8. Fontan F, Baudet E. Surgical repair of tricuspid atresia. *Thorax* 1971;26(3):240–8.
9. Gatzoulis MA, Clark AL, Cullen S, et al. Right ventricular diastolic function 15 to 35 years after repair of tetralogy of Fallot. Restrictive physiology predicts superior exercise performance. *Circulation* 1995;91(6):1775–81.
10. Guyton AC, Adkins LH. Quantitative aspects of the collapse factor in relation to venous return. *Am J Physiol* 1954;177(3):523–7.
11. Harvey W. *Anatomical Studies on the Motion of the Heart and Blood in Animals, 5th ed.* Leake C, translator. Springfield (IL): Charles C. Thomas, 1978.
12. Henning RJ. Effects of positive end-expiratory pressure on the right ventricle. *J Appl Physiol* 1986;61(3):819–26.
13. Hoskote A, Li J, Hickey C, et al. The effects of carbon dioxide on oxygenation and systemic, cerebral, and pulmonary vascular hemodynamics after the bidirectional superior cavopulmonary anastomosis. *J Am Coll Cardiol* 2004;44(7):1501–9.
14. Karam M, Wise RA, Natarajan TK, et al. Mechanism of decreased left ventricular stroke volume during inspiration in man. *Circulation* 1984; 69(5):866–73.
15. Kaye DM, Mansfield D, Aggarwal A, et al. Acute effects of continuous positive airway pressure on cardiac sympathetic tone in congestive heart failure. *Circulation* 2001;103(19):2336–8.
16. Kaye DM, Mansfield D, Naughton MT. Continuous positive airway pressure decreases myocardial oxygen consumption in heart failure. *Clin Sci (Lond)* 2004;106(6):599–603.
17. Kussmaul A. Über schwielige Mediastino-Perikarditis und den paradoxen Puls. *Berliner klinische Wochenschrift* 1873;10:433–64.
18. Laks H, Williams WG, Hellenbrand WE, et al. Results of right atrial to right ventricular and right atrial to pulmonary artery conduits for complex congenital heart disease. *Ann Surg* 1980;192(3):382–9.
19. Lauson HD, Bloomfield RA, Cournand A. The influence of the respiration on the circulation in man, with special reference to pressures in the right

auricle, right ventricle, femoral artery, and peripheral veins. *Am J Med* 1946;1:315.
20. Lewis O. Stephen Hales and the measurement of blood pressure. *J Hum Hypertens* 1994;8(12):865–71.
21. Li J, Hoskote A, Hickey C, et al. Effect of carbon dioxide on systemic oxygenation, oxygen consumption, and blood lactate levels after bidirectional superior cavopulmonary anastomosis. *Crit Care Med* 2005;33(5):984–9.
22. Lindberg L, Olsson AK, Jogi P, et al. How common is severe pulmonary hypertension after pediatric cardiac surgery? *J Thorac Cardiovasc Surg* 2002;123(6):1155–63.
23. Lofland GK. The enhancement of hemodynamic performance in Fontan circulation using pain free spontaneous ventilation. *Eur J Cardiothorac Surg* 2000;20(1):114–8.
24. Mansfield DR, Gollogly NC, Kaye DM, et al. Controlled trial of continuous positive airway pressure in obstructive sleep apnea and heart failure. *Am J Respir Crit Care Med* 2004;169(3):361–6.
25. Masip J, Betbese AJ, Paez J, et al. Non-invasive pressure support ventilation versus conventional oxygen therapy in acute cardiogenic pulmonary oedema: A randomised trial. *Lancet* 2000;356(9248):2126–32.
26. Masip J, Roque M, Sanchez B, et al. Noninvasive ventilation in acute cardiogenic pulmonary edema: Systematic review and meta-analysis. *JAMA* 2005;294(24):3124–30.
27. McElhinney DB, Hedrick HL, Bush DM, et al. Necrotizing enterocolitis in neonates with congenital heart disease: Risk factors and outcomes. *Pediatrics* 2000;106(5):1080–7.
28. Mehta S. Liu PP, Fitzgerald FS, et al. Effects of continuous positive airway pressure on cardiac volumes in patients with ischemic and dilated cardiomyopathy. *Am J Respir Crit Care Med* 2000;161(1):128–34.
29. Miro AM, Shivaram U, Finch PJP. Noncardiogenic pulmonary oedema following laser treatment of a tracheal neoplasm. *Chest* 1989;96:1430–1.
30. Motley HL, Cournand A, Werkö L, et al. The influence of short periods of induced acute anoxia upon pulmonary artery pressure in man. *Am J Physiol* 1947;130:315.
31. Naughton MT, Rahman MA, Hara K, et al. Effect of continuous positive airway pressure on intrathoracic and left ventricular transmural pressures in patients with congestive heart failure. *Circulation* 1995;91(6):1725–31.
32. Norgard G, Gatzoulis MA, Josen M, et al. Does restrictive right ventricular physiology in the early postoperative period predict subsequent right ventricular restriction after repair of tetralogy of Fallot? *Heart* 1998;79(5):481–4.
33. Penny DJ, Redington AN. Doppler echocardiographic evaluation of pulmonary blood flow after the Fontan operation: The role of the lungs. *Br Heart J* 1991;66(5):372–4.
34. Redington AN, Penny D, Shinebourne EA. Pulmonary blood flow after total cavopulmonary shunt. *Br Heart J* 1991;65(4):213–7.
35. Shekerdemian L, Bohn D. Current topic: Cardiovascular effects of mechanical ventilation. *Arch Dis Child* 1999;80:475–80.
36. Shekerdemian LS, Bush A, Shore DF, et al. Cardiopulmonary interactions after Fontan operations: Augmentation of cardiac output using negative pressure ventilation. *Circulation* 1997;96(11):3934–42.
37. Shekerdemian LS, Bush A, Shore DF, et al. Cardiorespiratory responses to negative pressure ventilation after tetralogy of Fallot repair: A hemodynamic tool for patients with a low-output state. *J Am Coll Cardiol* 1999;33(2):549–55.
38. Shekerdemian LS, Schulze-Neick I, Redington AN, et al. Negative pressure ventilation as haemodynamic rescue following surgery for congenital heart disease. *Intensive Care Med* 2000;26(1):93–6.
39. Shekerdemian LS, Shore DF, Lincoln C, et al. Negative-pressure ventilation improves cardiac output after right heart surgery. *Circulation* 1996;94(9 Suppl):II49–55.
40. Shekerdemian LS, Penny DJ, Novick W. Early extubation after surgical repair of tetralogy of Fallot. *Cardiol Young* 2000;10(6):636–7.
41. Sin DD, Logan AG, Fitzgerald FS, et al. Effects of continuous positive airway pressure on cardiovascular outcomes in heart failure patients with and without Cheyne-Stokes respiration. *Circulation* 2000;102(1):61–6.
42. Sin DD, Mayers I, Man GC, et al. Can continuous positive airway pressure therapy improve the general health status of patients with obstructive sleep apnea?: A clinical effectiveness study. *Chest* 2002;122(5):1679–85.
43. Soongswang J, Adatia I, Newman C, et al. Mortality in potential arterial switch candidates with transposition of the great arteries. *J Am Coll Cardiol* 1998;32(3):753–7.
44. Stalcup SA, Mellins RB. Mechanical forces producing pulmonary edema in acute asthma. *N Engl J Med* 1977;297:592–6.
45. Tabbutt S, Ramamoorthy C, Montenegro LM, et al. Impact of inspired gas mixtures on preoperative infants with hypoplastic left heart syndrome during controlled ventilation. *Circulation* 2001;104(12 Suppl 1):I159–64.
46. von Euler US, Liljestrand G. Observations on the pulmonary arterial blood pressure in the cat. *Acta Physiol Scand* 1946;12:301.
47. Wise RA, Robotham JL, Summer WR. Effects of spontaneous ventilation on the circulation. *Lung* 1981;159:175–86.
48. Wright GE, Crowley DC, Charpie JR, Ohye RG, Bove EL, Kulik TJ. High systemic vascular resistance and sudden cardiovascular collapse in recovering Norwood patients. *Ann Thorac Surg* 2004;77(1):48–52.

CHAPTER 65 ■ HEMODYNAMIC MONITORING

GILLIAN C. HALLEY • SHANE TIBBY

Understanding the principles and practice of hemodynamic monitoring is essential to the management of critically ill children. This area of medicine not only requires a detailed knowledge of patient physiology and pathophysiology, but demands an understanding of the physical principles that underpin the technology and awareness of the limitations and potential errors of the information gathered.

As the population of intensive care patients has grown in complexity and variability, clinicians have become increasingly dependent upon the information gathered by bedside monitoring systems, aware of our inability to quantify cardiac output using clinical examination alone (60), and aware that controversy exists regarding the reliability of information gathered from invasive monitoring and whether it has any potential to improve outcome (50). Likewise, certain monitoring tools have become almost obligatory in the ICU, but other promising technologic developments are not yet in widespread use. In truth, clinicians are firmly entrenched in a symbiotic relationship with the machines that they use and should ensure that training in critical care medicine emphasizes the importance of understanding the benefits, risks, and potential limitations of this technology.

THE IDEAL MONITORING SYSTEM

An ideal monitoring system would be noninvasive, safe, associated with no discomfort, and responsive to change in real time. The data collected would be reliable, accurate, repeatable, and continuously displayed, and the system would have the ability to store and retrieve information (53). As this ideal system does not yet exist, the potential benefits involved in monitoring patients must be balanced against the risks. As a general rule, the least invasive monitoring that is appropriate should always be used. The use of invasive monitoring should be reserved for those patients in whom it is essential for diagnosis, patient safety, or assessment of interventions or therapies.

Rapidly developing technology brings with it a risk of information overload, resulting in multiple conflicting data that confuse rather than assist the complex process of diagnosis and management. The risk of frequent false alarms associated with multiple alarm sources in the ICU has been highlighted (10), but as yet, no integrated, multiparameter, intelligent monitoring system is available for clinical use. Future advances in monitoring may include the integration of multiple signals into intelligent alarm systems, or computer-assisted interpretation of trends. Until these systems are realized, the clinicians/healthcare providers must perform the function of that gating system.

PHYSICAL EXAMINATION

In the PICU, examination and reassessment are used to continuously monitor patients (Table 65.1). Interpreting data in isolation from clinical signs and symptoms will increase the risk of error and may lead to management strategies that are inappropriate for the patient. Children in the PICU are necessarily surrounded by many monitors and alarm systems, and in this setting, it is often easy to take for granted the role of the experienced bedside diagnostician. Abnormal capillary refill time, temperature gradient, pulse volume, and signs of dehydration have been recognized as important features of "shock" that have been incorporated into advanced pediatric life-support guidelines (1). It is less clear how useful these measurements are in the postresuscitation or postoperative period, when many other hemodynamic factors and therapies will affect interpretation.

The human mind provides a sophisticated monitoring system that contains complex neural networks that have been trained to compute and integrate a wide variety of signals—aural, tactile, and visual—to create recognizable patterns and detect potential errors. This sifting and ordering of information is part of a complex process that leads to a carefully calculated conclusion. It includes sophisticated feedback mechanisms that allow for the data to be continually re-evaluated in the light of new information, or following response to an intervention. No artificial intelligence system has yet been designed that can carry out this level of complex analysis and decision making.

Clinical Pattern Recognition

No one value or measurement should determine a clinical diagnosis. For example, a consensus has been reached on the various clinical parameters that define shock (5). These include the presence of tachycardia, hypothermia, or hyperthermia; decreased mental status; signs of impaired perfusion (flash capillary refill) and bounding pulses (warm shock) or delayed capillary refill time >2 secs; cold peripheries and decreased pulse volume (cold shock); and urine output <1 mL/kg/hr.

Consider a postoperative cardiac surgical patient who has a cardiac output inadequate to meet the demands of the body, resulting in reduced end-organ perfusion. The diagnosis of low cardiac output syndrome may be considered to be a subjective one but is, in fact, a recognizable clinical pattern that is constructed after processing information from patient monitoring. In this example, clinical observation reveals pallor and a gray hue to the lips, suggestive of poor perfusion of the skin and mucous membranes. The patient is agitated and "difficult

CLINICAL MONITORING TOOLS FOR CARDIAC OUTPUT

Level of consciousness, activity, or agitation
State of hydration
Peripheral edema
Respiratory pattern
Peripheral perfusion/capillary refill time
Toe-to-core temperature gap
Heart rate and rhythm
Pulse characteristics
Urine output
Hepatomegaly
Jugular venous pressure
Pulmonary and cardiac auscultation

to sedate" secondary to cerebral underperfusion. Examination reveals cool extremities, with thready distal pulses, and delayed capillary refill time. The urinary catheter holds only a few drops of concentrated urine. A glance at the bedside monitor reveals a wide toe-to-core temperature gap, a sinus tachycardia, and a blood pressure trending down with a waveform that has a narrow, spiky character and a large volume swing with ventilation. The central venous pressure (CVP) is 2 mm Hg, and it has been difficult to get reliable trace on the saturation monitor. The arterial blood gas demonstrates an arterial oxygen saturation of 98%, a mixed venous saturation of 33%, and lactic acidosis. These signs, put together, are enough to confirm the diagnosis of low cardiac output syndrome.

Capillary refill, if measured correctly, can be a useful marker of hypovolemia during acute assessment and early resuscitation from shock or dehydration (5,38). The significance of capillary refill in the ICU is less clear (61). Toe-to-core temperature gap and capillary refill have not been shown to be related to adverse outcome following cardiac surgery in children. Common sense dictates that these clinical tests *in isolation* would not be indicative of low cardiac output or intravascular volume status; nor would they be predictive of clinical outcome due to the many confounding variables, such as fever, ambient temperature and lighting, surface cooling, vasoactive medication, choice of limb, inconsistency in technique, and interobserver variability, that affect their assessment. Assessment of peripheral perfusion, capillary refill and, possibly, trends in the toe-to-core temperature gap over time should alert the clinician to the need for a more detailed hemodynamic assessment of the patient. An exaggerated capillary refill time of >6 secs (rather than the usual standard of 2 secs) was shown to be more predictive of systemic vascular resistance in pediatric critical care patients (61).

Standard research methodology dictates that when an individual monitoring tool is tested, each variable must be evaluated independently, although in reality, best clinical practice is most likely to include a *combination* of clinical skills and noninvasive technologies that will allow the most efficient and least invasive real-time hemodynamic evaluation of the critically ill patient. It is not easy to study "best practice" in this way, but the role of clinical pathways, clinical audit, and multicentered, goal-directed protocol development may offer a practical substitute in the search for methods of reducing morbidity and mortality.

THE ELECTROCARDIOGRAM

Principles

The clinical electrocardiogram (ECG) was developed in Holland by Willem Einthoven in 1912, and the early electrodes were tubs of electrolyte solution (usually saline) in which the patients immersed their limbs. The modern day ECG uses skin electrodes to monitor the electrical activity of the heart. The signal is then boosted using an amplifier, filtered to remove noise, and displayed on an oscilloscope. A 12-lead ECG is required to fully assess an abnormal rhythm, but much information can be gained from a 3-lead ECG (right arm, left arm, and indifferent leads). A rhythm strip from lead II is useful for displaying dysrhythmias. The CM5 configuration is able to detect 89% of ST segment changes due to left ventricular (LV) ischemia. In the CM5 configuration, the right arm electrode is placed on the manubrium (chest lead from *m*anubrium), and the left arm electrode is on V5 position (5th interspace in left anterior axillary line). The indifferent lead is on the left shoulder or any other convenient position.

Practice

ECG interpretation can assist in the evaluation of heart rate and rhythm, ischemia, and conduction defects. It does not assist in the evaluation of cardiac output but may highlight areas where intervention could improve cardiac output (e.g., restoring atrioventricular synchrony). Due to the relatively small stroke volume and the nature of the neonatal myocardium, changes in the heart rate of an infant will have a greater impact on cardiac output compared to an older child or adult. The ECG can be used as a trend monitor following cardiac surgery when changes in heart rate can assist in management decisions regarding intravascular volume requirements or choice of inotrope. Continuous bedside ECG monitoring can alert to the presence of myocardial ischemia (ST segment changes) or hyperkalemia (peaked T waves). The ECG is important in assessing whether a postoperative tachycardia is a sinus rhythm in origin. In this setting, p-wave identification may be aided by recording the ECG at a higher speed (50 mm/sec) or by utilizing surgically placed, temporary atrial pacing wires that can be attached to the ECG leads.

Errors

Waveform artifact may arise if electrical interference occurs from the main power line or other equipment in the PICU. Electrocautery (diathermy) is the main source of electrical interference, and appears as 60-cycle interference. Use of an appropriate band-pass filter easily eliminates 60-cycle interference.

Muscle activity from shivering, seizures, or fasciculations may introduce waveform artifact. As display of the heart rate depends on detection of the R-wave and measurement of the RR interval, waveform artifact may lead to inaccurate heart rate display. The digital heart rate display must always be confirmed by inspection of the ECG waveform. Movement artifact can be minimized by placing the ECG electrodes over bony prominences.

Complications

Burns at the site of ECG electrodes have been reported when the surgical diathermy plate has been absent or improperly positioned, resulting in conductance of the diathermy current to the ECG electrodes.

NONINVASIVE BLOOD PRESSURE MONITORING

Systemic blood pressure (BP) is a fundamental cardiovascular parameter that varies with age, although the pressure obtained at any given time will also vary with the patient's underlying physiologic or pathophysiologic condition. The absolute value depends upon the methodology of measurement; therefore, it is useful to understand the strengths and weaknesses of the various techniques used to measure BP. Several methods of indirect arterial BP measurement have been developed, including the palpation method (Riva-Rocci), the auscultatory method (Korotkoff sounds), the oscillometric method, the rheographic method, the phase-shift method, and ultrasonic arterial wall motion detector. In 1896, Riva Rocci introduced a method for indirect measurement of BP, based on measuring the external pressure required to compress the brachial artery so that arterial pulsations could no longer be transmitted through the artery. In 1905, Korotkoff described the sounds created during this technique, and these five phases of change in sound continue to form the basis of indirect BP measurement.

Principles

Indirect BP is recorded by using a cuff placed around the arm or leg. The cuff is inflated above arterial pressure until pulsations are abolished. The cuff is then slowly deflated until pulsation returns.

The device used is called a *sphygmomanometer* and consists of a manometer, an inflatable bladder in a cuff, and an inflation-deflation device. The manometer is a mercury column set at zero before cuff inflation, or an aneroid device with an indicator needle that rotates around a circular, calibrated scale. The latter is susceptible to fatigue over time, which leads to falsely low readings and necessitates regular calibration. The cuff consists of an inflatable bladder within a restrictive cloth sheath and is connected to an inflation bulb that contains a control-release valve. In children, it is important that the center of the bladder (usually marked with an arrow) is placed directly over the artery. Turbulent blood flow, shock-wave formation, and instability of the arterial wall produce a series of audible frequencies (the Korotkoff sounds) as the external occluding pressure on a major artery is reduced (**Fig. 65.1**). Korotkoff sounds can be heard using a stethoscope or amplified using a Doppler device, which is particularly useful in infants and small children. The cuff is inflated above systolic blood pressure (SBP) (the pulse is abolished) and then deflated slowly (~2–3 mm Hg/sec). When the cuff pressure is less than systolic, the arterial wall is partly open, and turbulent blood flow becomes audible. When cuff pressure is below diastolic blood pressure (DBP), the sounds muffle or disappear completely, as flow is no longer obstructed.

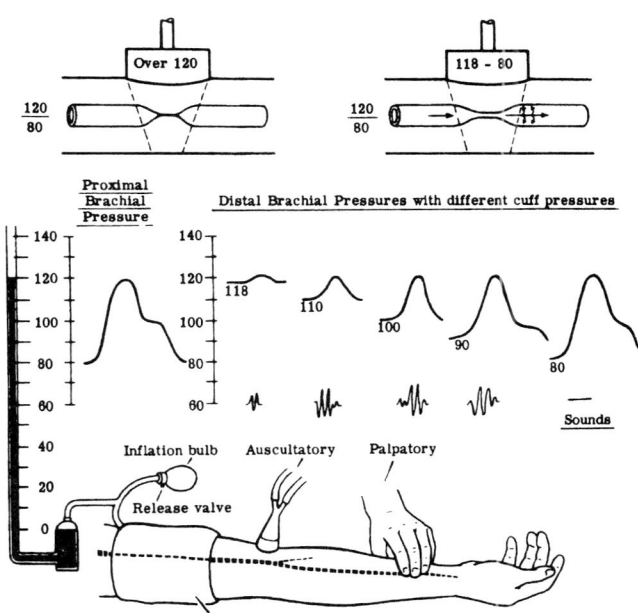

FIGURE 65.1. Method of obtaining blood pressure with a blood pressure cuff and Korotkoff sounds. From Abel FL, McCutcheon EP. Cardiovascular Function Principles and Applications. Boston: Little Brown, 1979;231, with permission.

- Phase I   Systolic value, first sound
- Phases II and III   Sound character changes
- Phase IV   Sound becomes muffled
- Phase V   Sound becomes absent

DBP is recorded at phase IV or V. In some pathophysiologic states (e.g., aortic regurgitation), phase V may never occur. Measurement of BP in infants and children presents particular problems due to lack of cooperation, a relative increase in the importance of cuff selection, and difficulty distinguishing the Korotkoff sounds, which can often be heard throughout the entire period of deflation. It is recommended that phase IV represent DBP in children <13 years old (46). Ultrasonic (Doppler) blood flow detectors are useful in children and will detect SBP at the first audible "swishing" sound made by return of blood flow to the extremity.

Automated BP devices such as Dinamap (*device for indirect noninvasive mean arterial pressure*) have reduced the incidence of error associated with the manual technique of measurement. These devices employ the oscillometric method and can measure heart rate as well as SBP, DBP, and mean BP (MBP). The principle is that blood flow through a vessel produces oscillations of the arterial wall, and these are transmitted to an inflatable cuff. As the cuff pressure decreases, a characteristic change in the magnitude of oscillations occurs, which generates SBP, DBP, and MBP. SBP is recorded when a rapid increase occurs in oscillation amplitude and, at this point, arterial pressure just exceeds cuff pressure. The mean pressure reading is taken at the maximum amplitude of oscillations during cuff deflation. The DBP coincides with a sudden decrease in oscillations. If large changes in BP occur over a short period of time, the readings may be inaccurate due to the nature of the automated cuff inflation, as the cuff is set to inflate at 35 mm Hg above the previous SBP.

Practice

In summary, noninvasive blood pressure monitoring is a noninvasive, safe, and minimally painful technique, which is simple to use and understand and readily available. The equipment is relatively cheap, reusable, and easy to maintain. It is technically difficult if access to the patient is limited or if the patient is small or uncooperative. It is reliable for trend analysis, although the absolute values obtained may differ from the gold standard of invasive arterial BP measurements. This inability to reflect true BP is more important in infants and young children, in whom a difference of 10 mm Hg of pressure is more significant than the same error in older children or adults. Noninvasive blood pressure monitoring is not an appropriate tool for children who are critically ill, hemodynamically unstable, or on vasoactive drugs, when even relatively minor inaccuracies in pressure can have significant clinical consequences and can impact on therapeutic decision making.

Errors

Measurement error during manual noninvasive blood pressure monitoring can be introduced due to poor sound transmission from long stethoscope tubing, poor hearing sensitivity of the operator, improper cuff size, and a too-rapid deflation rate. Calibration errors can occur due to manometer fatigue. One of the most important factors affecting the accuracy of measurement is the cuff size relative to the patient. A narrow cuff produces a higher pressure, and a wide cuff produces an artificially low pressure. The American Heart Association recommends that the width of the inflatable bladder be 40% of the mid-circumference of the limb and that the length should be twice the width. In children, the occluding bladder should be long enough to encircle the limb completely, as overlapping of the ends of the bladder in children does not appear to introduce an error in measurement (46). The accuracy of measurement is improved with slow cuff *deflation*, as this aids the detection of arterial pulsations. Rapid cuff *inflation* will help to avoid venous congestion. In shivering patients, muscle contraction around the artery lowers tissue compliance, which can raise the SBP artifactually ("pseudohypertension"). External pressure on the cuff or tubing can cause inaccurate reading. The accuracy is reduced in the presence of low cardiac output, significant hypotension, hypoperfusion, or vasoconstriction, dysrhythmias, or excessive body edema. In clinical states of reduced peripheral blood flow, the risk of poor recording or error in the pressure measurement will increase at a time when the importance of obtaining an accurate reading is also increased. The cuff pressure will tend to over-read in the presence of hypotension and under-read in the presence of is hypertension.

Complications

Complications are minimal but can include occlusion to venous outflow, which results in congestion and pain, or occlusion to arterial inflow, which can aggravate any potential ischemia in the peripheries. Peripheral nerve damage (e.g., ulnar nerve palsy) and petechial hemorrhage in the area under the cuff are more common when inflations are frequent (every 1–2 mins)

and can be reduced by rotating the cuff position or increasing the interval between cuff inflations ($\geq$ every 5 min). The risk of ulnar nerve palsy can be reduced if the cuff is sitting clear of the elbow.

Several devices have been developed that measure noninvasive blood pressure *continuously* (25,45). However, they have not entered routine clinical practice because of their tendency to underestimate true arterial BP and because of the potential for circulatory impairment.

ARTERIAL BLOOD PRESSURE MONITORING

In 1616, William Harvey announced that Galen was wrong in his assertion that the heart constantly produces blood; instead, he proposed that the body contains a finite amount of blood that circulates in one direction only. In 1733, the Reverend Stephen Hales, a British veterinarian, invasively recorded BP in a horse by inserting a brass pipe into an artery and using a connected glass tube to demonstrate the rise in pressure as a column of blood. It was not until 1847 that human BP was recorded using Carl Ludwig's kymograph, which consisted of a U-shaped manometer tube connected to an arterial brass pipe cannula.

Principles

Invasive measuring of BP will vary with the site of measurement because the pulse pressure undergoes natural amplification as it passes through the arterial tree, resulting in higher systolic readings at the pedal arteries compared to the aortic root. Pedal pressure is significantly higher than radial pressure in children. The equipment required for invasive BP monitoring includes an arterial cannula with a heparinized saline column and flushing device, a transducer, an amplifier, and an oscilloscope. A continuous column of fluid from the blood vessel lumen to the transducer diaphragm transmits variations in intraluminal pressure, causing changes in resistance and current that are converted into an electrical signal, which is amplified to display a waveform and digital pressure on the bedside monitor. Disposable transducers have diaphragms that contain silicon crystals that undergo a change in electrical resistance in proportion to the pressure applied to the diaphragm. To obtain an accurate measure of BP, the catheter manometer system must precisely reproduce the arterial waveform. The arterial pressure waveform is a complex sine wave that is a summation of a series of simple sine waves of different frequencies. The first harmonic, or *fundamental frequency*, is equal to the heart rate. The *natural frequency* of the system is the speed at which the system oscillates once set in motion (also called the *resonant frequency*) and should be at least 10 times the fundamental frequency. The heart rate in critically ill children is often high, which can cause problems with systolic overshoot, as the harmonic components of the pressure wave approach the resonant frequency of the system.

The natural (resonant) frequency of the arterial BP is directly related to the catheter diameter, inversely related to the square root of the system compliance, inversely related to the square root of the length of the tubing, and inversely related to the square root of the density of the fluid in the system.

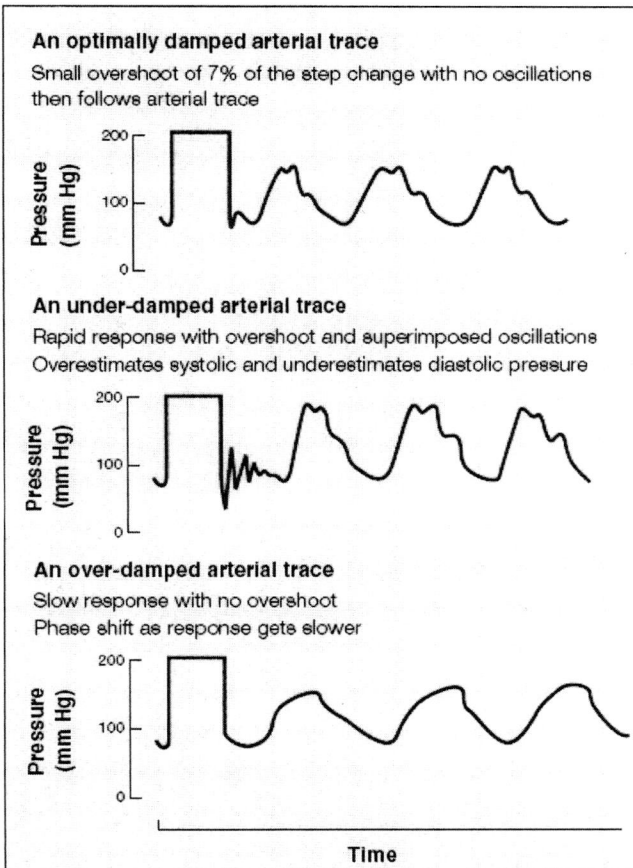

An optimally damped arterial trace
Small overshoot of 7% of the step change with no oscillations then follows arterial trace

An under-damped arterial trace
Rapid response with overshoot and superimposed oscillations
Overestimates systolic and underestimates diastolic pressure

An over-damped arterial trace
Slow response with no overshoot
Phase shift as response gets slower

FIGURE 65.2. Quantification of the degree of damping via the fast-flush test. Reproduced from: Anaesthesia UK web site http://www.frca.co.uk/article.aspx?articleid=100382, with permission. Accessed 08/02/07.

The optimal dynamic response is achieved with a system that contains a liquid with low viscosity and minimal air bubble trapping in tubing that is short and wide with stiff walls. It is possible to assess the dynamic response by delivering a fast-flush test, conducted during diastole (32). This test causes an abrupt pressure change, inducing a sinusoidal pressure wave that progressively decreases in amplitude and a frequency equal to the natural frequency of the system. Examination of this change allows determination of the natural frequency as well as the *coefficient of damping*, which describes how quickly the system will stop oscillating as a result of frictional forces. An optimal dynamic response results in one undershoot below baseline, followed by a much smaller overshoot above baseline, before returning to the underlying waveform (**Fig. 65.2**).

In an *underdamped* system, persistent resonant waves are seen after the fast-flush test, and a tall, narrow waveform occurs with an artificially high SBP and a notch in the arterial tracing immediately following the SBP. This pattern could be due to small air bubbles in the system or long tubing. Motion of the catheter within a vessel will also result in oscillations of the pressure tracing. With *overdamping*, a low return to baseline after the fast-flush test and a more rounded waveform are seen, with a slow upstroke, a poorly defined dicrotic notch, and a narrow pulse pressure. This pattern could be due to compliant catheters or tubing, or large air bubbles or a blood clot in

the system. The result is an artificially low SBP. In summary, overdamping lowers the SBP, raises DBP to a lesser extent, and reduces the pulse pressure. In both underdamping and overdamping, the MBP is relatively unaffected. The MBP can be determined from a pulse pressure tracing by calculating the area of the waveform and dividing it by the length of the base. The formula,

$$MBP = DBP + [(SBP - DBP)/3]$$

is useful only for adult patients with low heart rates ($\sim$60 bpm) in which one-third of the cardiac cycle is spent in systole.

Practice

Cannulation

Cannulation can be performed by the transfixation method or the direct threading technique (**Fig. 65.3**). When cannulating an artery, sufficient collateral blood should flow to the distal tissues perfused by the vessel to allow these tissues to remain viable should the catheter become thrombosed. The risk of distal limb ischemia is increased in end arteries, such as the brachial arteries, that have a very poor collateral circulation.

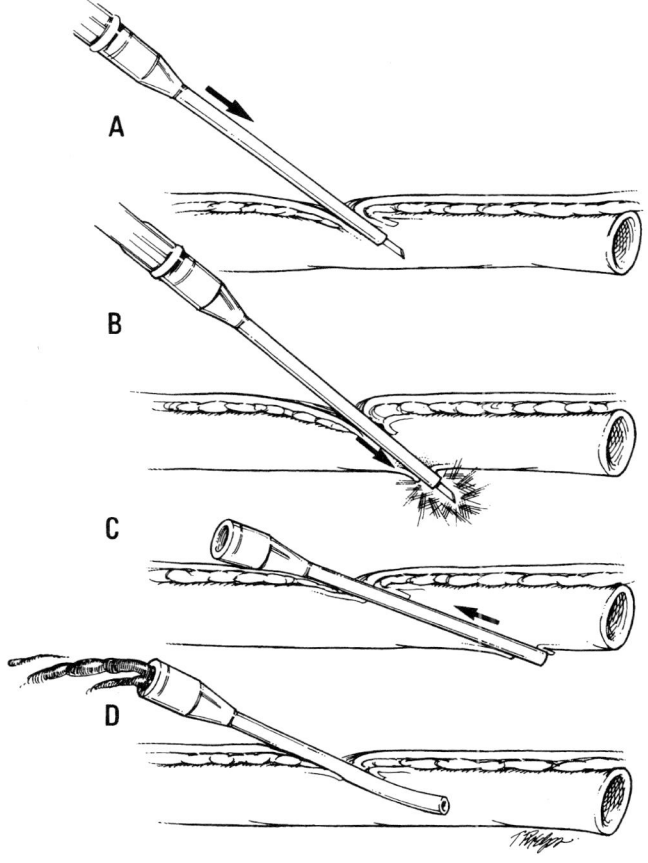

FIGURE 65.3. Radial artery cannulation. The catheter-over-needle unit is inserted into the artery (**A**). When arterial blood flow is seen in the needle hub, the catheter may be advanced over the needle into the artery. Another technique is to further advance the catheter and needle until blood flow ceases, thereby transfixing the artery (**B**), and to then remove the needle (**C**) and withdraw the catheter until blood flow is seen. The catheter is then advanced into the artery (**D**).

The radial artery is the most frequent site for cannulation, as this site is easy to access and has a low associated complication rate. The site of radial artery cannulation may be dictated by the underlying condition or operative plan. For example, the right radial should be used when the left subclavian artery is to be used for subclavian flap repair of aortic coarctation, and the left radial should be used when a right-sided subclavian artery-to-pulmonary artery shunt is planned. Early cannulation of the umbilical artery may enable preservation of femoral vessels in the newborn who will need subsequent catheter or surgical procedures. However, the risk of infection and necrotizing enterocolitis must be considered in this population, and early removal of umbilical catheters is prudent.

In infants with patent ductus arteriosus, it is worth remembering that the right radial arterial blood represents blood oxygen saturation to the brain, as the right subclavian, right common, and left common carotid arteries originate from the aorta proximal to the duct. The left subclavian and descending aorta represent the postductal oxygen saturation, which is lower in the presence of a right-to-left shunt through the patent ductus arteriosus.

Collateral blood flow to the hand can be assessed by the Allen test prior to inserting the catheter, although the predictive value and benefit in children is questionable. Other sites of cannulation include ulnar, femoral, axillary, dorsalis pedis, and posterior tibial arteries. The axillary artery is often cannulated in children. It has a good collateral supply, reducing the risk of ischemia with occlusion, but a theoretical risk of cerebral embolism due to flushing close to the aortic arch exists, as well as a potential risk of brachial plexus injury. Femoral catheters carry a risk of vascular problems or ischemia of the leg, as well as concern regarding fecal contamination and infection. Catheterization of the femoral vein and artery in the same leg may increase the risk of limb ischemia, especially in low-flow states or when potent vasoconstrictors are used. Access to the femoral arteries may be limited in patients who have had multiple cardiac catheterizations via the femoral vessels.

Vasospasm and thrombosis are the principal causes of arterial catheter failure. The addition of heparin (1 U/mL) and papaverine (a smooth muscle relaxant; 30 mg/250 mL) to the catheter infusion solution (0.9% or 0.45% NaCl) decreases the incidence of catheter failure (27). If arterial cannulation leads to thrombosis and early signs of circulatory compromise to an extremity, current guidelines recommend immediate catheter removal and systemic heparinization with unfractionated heparin (42). Approximately 70% of catheter-related arterial thromboses will resolve with these measures. However, thrombolytic therapy with tissue plasminogen activator may be added, if perfusion does not improve in 24 hrs. If all medical management fails, balloon thrombectomy via an arteriotomy can be employed to prevent limb loss.

Measurement

Direct BP measurement using arterial cannulation has the advantage of providing continuous monitoring, as well as providing access for blood sampling. A major advantage of invasive over noninvasive monitoring is the display of the *waveform* in addition to the BP value, allowing for recognition of the components of the signal (e.g., the dicrotic notch), assessment of the character of the waveform and the volume under the curve, and evaluation of the level of damping or resonance in the system. The waveform shape will alter, depending upon the site

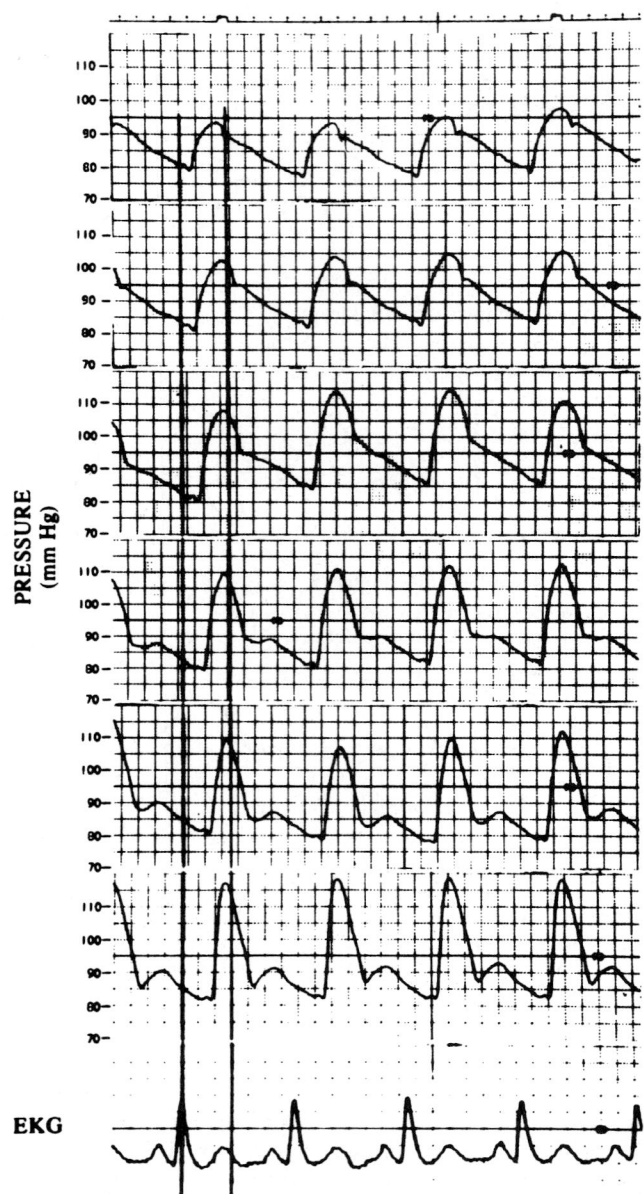

FIGURE 65.4. Examples of central versus peripheral arterial waveforms. From Abel FL, McCutcheon EP. *Cardiovascular Function Principles and Applications.* Boston: Little Brown, 1979;231, with permission.

of measurement (**Fig. 65.4**). It can also aid in monitoring other parameters in the cardiovascular system; for example, it can confirm the true heart rate in the presence of dysrhythmias or when double-counting or artifact from the ECG is encountered.

The area under the systolic portion of the waveform is proportional to the stroke volume; thus, a low pulse pressure may indicate diminished stroke volume. The diastolic downstroke is steeper and has a lower dicrotic notch in the presence of low systemic vascular resistance or hypovolemia. An increase in pulse pressure may indicate changes in systemic vascular resistance, as in septic shock. A low DBP can reflect excessive distal runoff, for example, in the presence of a large patent ductus arteriosus or collateral vessels. A sudden rise in DBP is usually seen on ligation of the patent ductus arteriosus.

A systolic upstroke with a steep gradient (dp/dt) implies good ventricular contractility. A less vertical upstroke can be due to suboptimal contractility, LV outflow obstruction, or peripheral vasoconstriction. In the presence of aortic stenosis, a slow rising upstroke, an anacrotic notch with a delayed peak, and reduced pulse pressure are seen. With aortic regurgitation, a steep upstroke, a bifid peak with low DBP, and an increased pulse pressure are characteristic.

Pulsus paradoxus is an exaggeration of the normal fall in SBP that occurs during the inspiratory phase of spontaneous breathing. During inspiration with spontaneous breathing, venous return to the right atrium and therefore right ventricular (RV) stroke volume increase, but venous return to the left atrium and LV stroke volume decrease. During positive-pressure breathing, pulsus paradoxus is reflected as an exaggerated SBP drop during the expiratory phase (see Chapter 64). Pulsus paradoxus is a classic sign of cardiac tamponade but can also be seen in constrictive pericarditis, early restrictive cardiomyopathy, or severe hyperinflation of the lungs, especially when combined with hypovolemia.

In addition to waveform interpretation, invasive BP monitoring also allows specific management strategies to be directed by changes in systolic, diastolic, or pulse pressure, rather than mean pressure alone. For example, in patients who have surgical repair to the aortic arch, it is important to avoid systolic hypertension in the early postoperative period, as this may put stress on the newly placed suture line. In newborns with shunt-dependent circulation, it may be crucial to know the DBP, as a high shunt runoff may increase the risk of gut underperfusion and necrotizing enterocolitis. DBP measurement is also important in a patient who has had surgery for LV outflow tract obstruction and has a hypertrophic myocardium with a critical coronary perfusion pressure.

Errors

A common source of error is an inaccurate transducer level. Zero reference, or atmospheric pressure, must be set with the transducer at the same level as the chamber being measured—in this case, the heart. Recordings should be made with the child in the supine position and the transducer at the level of the mid-chest or mid-axillary line. If the transducer is set lower than the reference level, the pressure readings are falsely high, and if it is set higher than reference, the pressure is falsely low. Raising or lowering the system can introduce errors of 7.5 mm Hg for each 10 cm change in position. Regular zeroing is required to counteract baseline drift. The effects of overdamping and underdamping have been described previously. Careful flushing of the catheter and pressure tubing to remove blood and air bubbles and choosing the shortest, stiffest, and largest catheter will minimize these errors.

Complications

The risks of invasive arterial monitoring include bleeding, infection, vascular compromise, nerve damage, and accidental injection of hyperosmolar solutions (**Table 65.2**). Important additional risk factors for distal limb ischemia in children are critical illness, low cardiac output states, use of vasopressors, and large catheter size relative to the dimensions of the artery.

TABLE 65.2

COMPLICATIONS OF INVASIVE BLOOD PRESSURE MONITORING

Bleeding
Thrombosis
Hematoma
Infection
Vascular compromise
Nerve damage
Accidental injection of air or thrombus
Digital necrosis
Arteriovenous fistulae
Carpal tunnel syndrome

In adults, it has been shown that the incidence of arterial occlusion (**Table 65.3**) increases linearly as the ratio of catheter outer diameter to vessel inner diameter increases, and this is even more important in children, in whom vessels are smaller; however, the catheter size cannot be reduced proportionally. The risk is increased in neonates compared to older children. Any intravascular catheter can result in infection. Risk factors for catheter-related infection of arterial lines include the use of an arterial system that permits backflow of blood into the pressure tubing and the duration of catheterization (8). Positive blood cultures without septicemia have been reported in 4% of children and 23% of adults with arterial catheters, and routinely changing the system does not seem to reduce the risk. Care should be taken during flushing of arterial lines, particularly with axillary arterial catheters due to the risk of cerebral embolization of air or debris.

CENTRAL VENOUS PRESSURE MONITORING

Central venous cannulation allows secure IV access in critically ill children who may require large-volume fluid infusions or parenteral nutrition, and it is essential for the infusion of vasoactive drugs such as epinephrine and norepinephrine. A central venous catheter is not only essential for monitoring CVP, which allows an indirect measurement of cardiac preload, but it also provides access for blood sampling for measurement of mixed venous saturation. The monitoring of trends in mixed venous saturation enables trending of cardiac output in the absence of other continuous cardiac output devices (Swan-Ganz catheter).

TABLE 65.3

FACTORS THAT INCREASE THE RISK OF ARTERIAL CATHETER THROMBOSIS

Larger catheter-to-vessel ratio
Prolonged cannulation
Multiple cannulation attempts
Presence of peripheral vascular disease
Venous and arterial femoral catheterization in single extremity
Younger age
Thrombogenic conditions

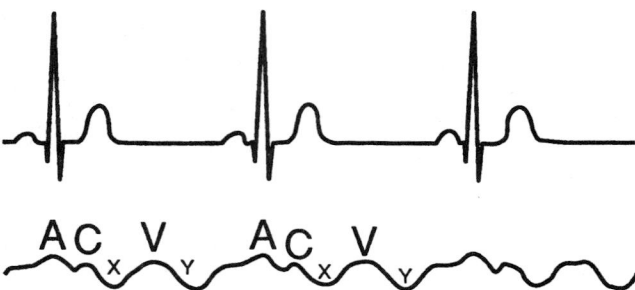

FIGURE 65.5. Central venous pressure trace with corresponding ECG. See text for explanation. From O'Rourke RA. The measurement of systemic blood pressure: Normal and abnormal pulsations of the arteries and veins. In: Hurst JW, ed. *The Heart.* New York: McGraw-Hill, 1990;159, with permission.

Principles

The normal CVP trace has three positive waves (*a, c,* and *v*) and two negative waves (*x* and *y*). The *a* wave is caused by atrial contraction (after the P wave on the ECG), the *c* wave is caused by ventricular contraction against a closed tricuspid valve, and the *v* wave is caused by atrial filling. The *x* descent is due to the tricuspid valve being pulled away from the right atrium by the contracting ventricle, while the *y* descent occurs as the tricuspid valve opens and blood enters the ventricle (**Fig. 65.5**). The pattern of this waveform can change in pathologic conditions, as with the cannon *a* waves seen in complete heart block. In common with all hemodynamic monitoring, the trend and response to therapeutic intervention is more important than a single value. In the presence of normal tricuspid valve function, the CVP is equal to the RV end-diastolic pressure, which is proportional to RV end-diastolic volume, which is the preload to the RV. The exact relationship between volume and pressure is compliance of the ventricle. It is important to avoid considering CVP purely as a reflection of "volume loading" of the ventricle, as ventricular compliance, afterload, and contractility will all affect the CVP. A change in CVP following a fluid challenge will depend on the state of venous filling and the compliance of venous capacitance vessels, as well as RV function and compliance. The CVP is measured using a catheter in a central vein with a reference point of the right atrium. Accurate zeroing is even more important than with the arterial system. The CVP will also vary with changes in intrapleural pressure that occur during spontaneous or positive-pressure breathing. The site of the catheter will affect the absolute values obtained. Although trend monitoring from a noncentral site (e.g., femoral venous catheter with a tip in the abdominal vena cava) is often used (9), elevated intrapleural pressures from high levels of positive-pressure ventilation (PPV) can lead to significant differences between intrathoracic and intra-abdominal CVP measurements.

Practice

Cannulation

The Seldinger technique is used for catheter placement, and common sites include the internal jugular, subclavian, and femoral veins (**Fig. 65.6**). ECG monitoring is essential during central line placement because of the risk of inducing dysrhyth-

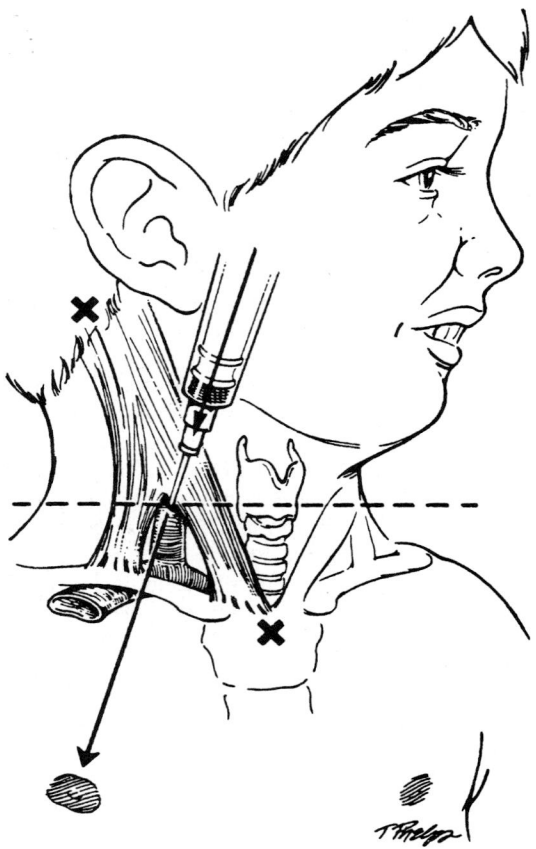

FIGURE 65.6. Internal jugular cannulation using the Seldinger technique. The head is turned to the opposite side, with needle puncture at the apex of the triangle formed by the heads of the sternocleidomastoid muscle (midway between the sternal notch and the mastoid process). The needle is aimed at the ipsilateral nipple. From Schleien CL. Cardiopulmonary Resuscitation. In: Nichols DG, Yaster M, Lappe DG, et al., eds. *Golden Hour—The Handbook of Advanced Pediatric Life Support.* St Louis: Mosby—Year Book, 1991;124, with permission.

mias when wires or catheters enter the heart. Careful positioning of the patient is important to the success of cannulation and to minimize the complications inherent in placement of a central venous catheter (**Table 65.4**). In infants who are <3 months of age and weigh <4 kg, the success rate for internal jugular cannulation is significantly decreased. Ultrasonic guidance can be useful, although this is technically more difficult in the small patient. The femoral vein is commonly used in pediatric patients but carries with it an infection risk that increases

TABLE 65.4

COMPLICATIONS OF CENTRAL LINE INSERTION

Arterial (carotid, subclavian, femoral) puncture
Local hematoma
Air embolism
Catheter malposition (to neck tissue, mediastinal, pericardial, or pleural cavities)
Pneumothorax
Hemothorax
Brachial plexus injury
Dysrhythmias

TABLE 65.5

COMPLICATIONS OF INDWELLING CENTRAL VENOUS CATHETERS

Infection
Local hematoma
Extravasation
Vascular thrombosis
Embolus (clot or air)
Intracardiac thrombus
Superior vena cava syndrome
Chylothorax
Local nerve damage

with duration in situ (8). Subclavian catheters carry a greater risk of pneumothorax, thoracic duct injury, and arterial cannulation. The risk of inadvertent arterial cannulation is increased in cyanosed patients with low cardiac output. This risk can be minimized by confirming three indicators of proper central venous placement in every patient: venous O_2 saturation, venous pressure waveform, and central vein location on x-ray.

Central venous catheters significantly increase the risk of infection in critically ill patients. They are also associated with long-term complications (**Table 65.5**) such as thrombosis (**Table 65.6**) in children who have had prolonged or repeated admissions to intensive care, repeated cardiac catheterizations, or repeated surgical procedures. However, these monitoring lines are so crucial to the clinical management of this patient group that they inevitably carry an overriding positive effect on survival by allowing the level of monitoring, sampling, and drug therapy that modern-day intensive care demands. With increasing awareness of the short- and long-term risks of intravascular catheters (Table 65.5), various strategies have been suggested to limit the associated morbidity. These include the use of heparin infusions or heparin-bonded catheters to reduce thrombosis risk, strategies to limit bacterial contamination with meticulous sterile techniques, antibiotic-impregnated catheters, and smaller-diameter catheters (8). In the cardiac surgical patient with single-ventricular physiology who will inevitably have multiple interventional and surgical procedures, the loss of central venous access due to thrombosis is particularly problematic. Thrombosis and occlusion of central veins (Table 65.6) may necessitate a higher-risk transhepatic approach for future cardiac catheterization and may even result in a patient becoming unsuitable for a further surgical procedure (i.e., bidirectional Glenn anastomosis). Alternative approaches use intracardiac catheters placed during the

TABLE 65.6

FACTORS THAT INCREASE THE RISK OF VASCULAR THROMBOSIS

Prolonged cannulation
Injection of hyperosmolar solutions
Underlying thrombogenic condition
Large catheter size
Multiple puncture attempts
Low-flow states

cardiac repair (21), umbilical venous lines in neonates, percutaneously inserted catheters (silicon catheters inserted centrally from the antecubital fossa), or surgically inserted Broviac (tunneled) catheters. Advances in echocardiography have reduced the numbers of patients who require a preoperative invasive cardiac catheterization study, thus decreasing the number of cannulations of the large venous vessels.

LEFT ATRIAL PRESSURE MONITORING

The CVP estimates the LV end-diastolic pressure when cardiac and pulmonary functions are normal; however, this does not commonly occur in the PICU. Therefore, a surgically placed left atrial catheter can be a very useful monitoring tool in the postoperative period (51), particularly when right atrial pressure is unlikely to reflect left atrial pressure, as in marked RV failure, pulmonary hypertension, and/or left failure.

Errors

As previously noted, trends are more important than isolated measurements. Inaccurate calibration can introduce errors as stated. Errors in left atrial pressure measurement can occur when the left atrial line is malpositioned, particularly when it traverses the mitral valve or enters into the jet of mitral regurgitation, which may be seen as an abnormal regurgitant v waveform.

Complications

The most devastating complication of left atrial lines is the introduction of air embolism or thromboembolism, which may lead to stroke, myocardial infarction, or necrotizing enterocolitis. These risks are minimized by avoiding blood draws and flushes through the left atrial line. These lines should be removed as soon as possible after cardiac surgery (generally within 2 days).

CARDIAC OUTPUT MEASUREMENT

Cardiac output is the volume of blood ejected by the systemic ventricle each minute, typically measured in L/min. It is customary in pediatrics to index this measurement to body surface area (L/min/m^2), which results in a common reference range throughout infancy and childhood: 3.5–5.5 L/min/m^2. Cardiac output is a core hemodynamic variable (**Table 65.7**) that is a major determinant of systemic oxygen delivery; yet, despite the availability of several methods, this variable is seldom measured in pediatric practice due to technical difficulty, potential for complications, perceived inaccuracy in infants, and the presence of anatomic shunts in many children with congenital heart disease. A common doubt expressed by clinicians is, "does cardiac output measurement improve patient outcome?" This is a reasonable question, given the lack of demonstrated benefit in pediatric and adult clinical trials (13,50).

Perhaps a more reasonable question would be whether cardiac output measurement allows for a more rational approach

TABLE 65.7

COMMON HEMODYNAMIC VARIABLES

Parameter	Formula	Normal range	Units
Cardiac index	CI = CO/body surface area	3.5–5.5	$L/min/m^2$
Stroke index	SI = CI/heart rate	30–60	mL/m^2
Systemic vascular resistance index	SVRI = 79.9 × (MAP – CVP)/CI	800–1600	$dyne\text{-}sec/cm^5/m^2$
Pulmonary vascular resistance index	PVRI = 79.9 × (MPAP – LAP)/CI	80–240	$dyne\text{-}sec/cm^5/m^2$
Left ventricular stroke work index	LVSWI = SI × MAP × 0.0136	50–62 (adult)	$g\text{-}m/m^2$
Right ventricular stroke work index	RVSWI = SI × MAP × 0.0136	5.1–6.9 (adult)	$g\text{-}m/m^2$
Arterial oxygen content	$CaO_2 = (1.34 \times Hb \times SaO_2) + (PaO_2 \times 0.003)$		mL/L
Oxygen delivery	$DO_2 = CI \times CaO_2$	570–670	$mL/min/m^2$
Fick principle	$CI = VO_2/(CaO_2 – CvO_2)$	160–180 (infant VO_2)	$mL/min/m^2$
		100–130 (child VO_2)	$mL/min/m^2$
Mixed venous oxygen saturation		65%–75%	
Oxygen extraction ratio[a]	$OER = (SaO_2 – SvO_2)/SaO_2$	0.24–0.28	

CI, cardiac index; CO, cardiac output; SI, stroke index; SVRI, systemic vascular resistance index; MAP, mean systemic arterial pressure (mm Hg); CVP, central venous pressure (mm Hg); PVRI, pulmonary vascular resistance index; MPAP, mean pulmonary arterial pressure; LAP, left atrial pressure; LVSWI, left ventricular stroke work index; RVSWI, right ventricular stroke work index; CaO_2, arterial oxygen content; Hb, hemoglobin concentration (g/L); SaO_2, arterial oxygen saturation; PaO_2, partial pressure of dissolved oxygen; DO_2, oxygen delivery; VO_2, oxygen consumption; CvO_2, mixed venous oxygen content; OER, oxygen extraction ratio; SvO_2, mixed venous oxygen saturation.
[a]The equation given for OER is only valid if the contribution from dissolved oxygen is minimal. If this is not the case, oxygen content (CaO_2, CvO_2) must be substituted for saturation (SaO_2, SvO_2).

to therapy in a subset of critically ill patients. These patients include those with shock, multiple organ failure, unexplained hypotension, severe cardiac disease, or those in whom significant cardiopulmonary interactions exist (58,63). The relevance of measuring cardiac output (and its derived parameters) is highlighted by the fact that hemodynamic profiles can change quickly in critical illness, myocardial failure is a common cause of death, and cardiac output cannot be estimated clinically (7,60). Once the decision is made to measure cardiac output, a suggested checklist for its interpretation includes:

A. Is flow adequate for *this* patient at *this* time?
B. If not, why?
C. Do regional perfusion deficits exist?
D. Which therapeutic regime is optimal?
E. How has the patient responded to the chosen therapy?

Principles

A. Is Flow Adequate for This Patient at This Time?

This statement incorporates several key principles: understanding the accuracy of the chosen measurement tool, the need to interpret cardiac output in tandem with other markers of adequacy of flow, recognition of the dynamic nature of the value of the variable and need for repeated measurement, and knowledge that cardiac output is both patient and disease specific.

Accuracy. *Accuracy* encompasses both bias and precision. Bias refers to how far the measured cardiac output is, *on average*, away from the true cardiac output (i.e., does the technique systematically underestimate or overestimate true cardiac output). *Precision* refers to the *repeatability* of the technique (the standard deviation, or scatter of results around the bias), and is

often expressed in percentage terms as the coefficient of variation (CV):

$$CV = 100 \times standard\,deviation/mean$$

The two measures of accuracy are sometimes expressed jointly as the mean squared error (MSE):

$$MSE = bias^2 + precision^2 \text{ (mathematically equivalent to } bias^2 + variance)$$

Accuracy is represented graphically in **Figure 65.7A**. Two hypothetical methods of cardiac output measurement are shown; both have a similar overall accuracy (MSE). However, method "X" systematically over-reads true cardiac output but is relatively repeatable (high precision, or low variance, CV = 8%), meaning that a change in cardiac output between two measurements is likely to represent a true change, albeit in relative terms. Conversely, technique "Y" has minimal bias but poor precision (CV = 30%). Consider a situation in which the true cardiac output decreases between two time points. Technique "X" is likely to track this change (**Fig. 65.7B**), whereas technique "Y" may not, or may even interpret the change as being in the opposite direction (**Fig. 65.7C**). To some extent, poor precision can be attenuated by averaging several consecutive measurements (provided the true cardiac output remains the same during this period).

Adequacy of Flow. *Adequacy of flow* relates to whether measured cardiac output is sufficient to meet the metabolic needs of the body and underscores the need to interpret this variable in terms of its contribution to the balance between oxygen delivery and oxygen consumption (**Fig. 65.8**) (63). Two common markers of adequacy of flow are blood lactate and mixed (or central) venous oxygen saturation (see the later section, "Markers of Adequacy of Flow"). Normally, the tissues will extract more oxygen when cardiac output is inadequate, resulting in a

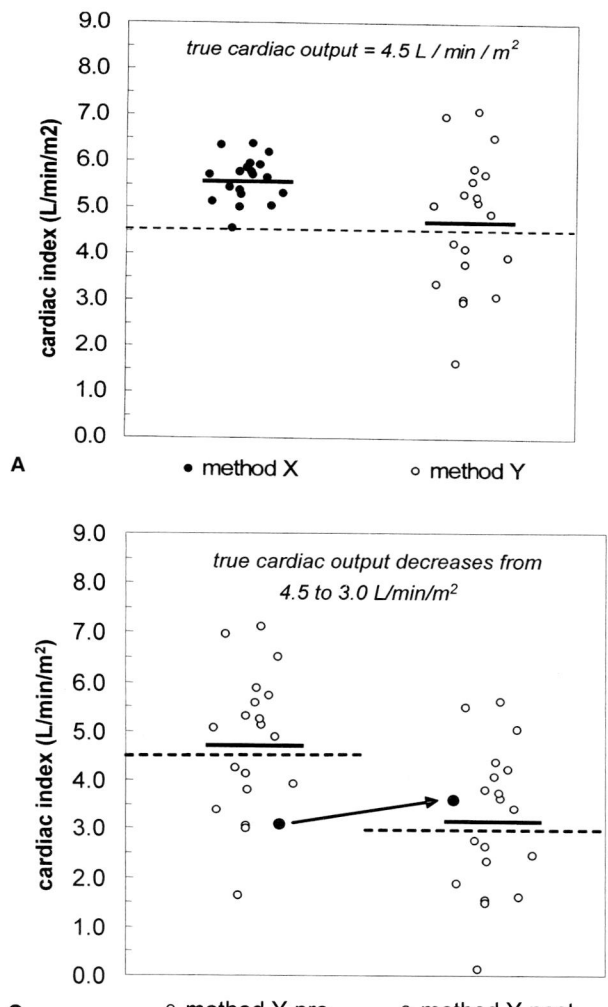

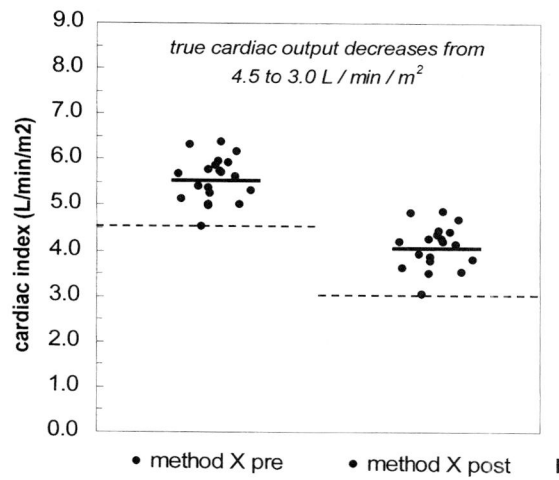

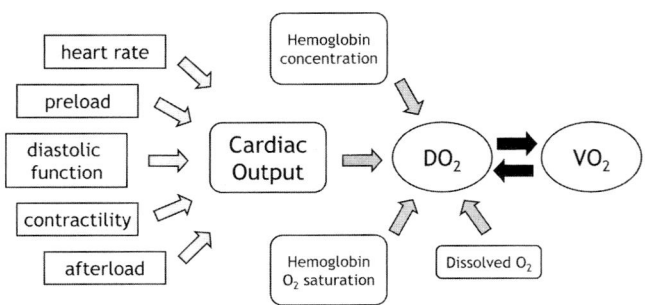

FIGURE 65.7. **(A)** Two methods of cardiac output are shown: method X (**black circles**) has a moderate bias but high precision; method Y (**white circles**) has minimal bias but low precision. The consequences are shown in **B** and **C**, where method X will track a change in cardiac output, but method Y may not. In fact, if a single reading is taken, it is conceivable that method Y may even track the change in cardiac output in the wrong direction (**red circles with arrow**).

FIGURE 65.8. Relationship between hemodynamic variables: cardiac output, oxygen delivery (Do_2), and oxygen consumption (Vo_2).

drop in mixed or central venous oxygen saturation; this can be regarded as an early compensatory mechanism. When extraction exceeds a critical limit, anaerobic respiration will occur, with a resultant rise in blood lactate, which is a sign of decompensation, as this form of energy generation is inefficient and unsustainable. Several important caveats must be remembered: (a) inadequate flow is but one cause of an elevated blood lactate level in critical illness, and (b) mixed venous oxygen saturation does not necessarily fall in inadequate flow states in patients with septic shock and/or anaphylaxis.

B. Why Is Flow Inadequate?

Cardiac output is the composite of five factors: preload, diastolic function, contractility, heart rate, and afterload (**Fig. 65.8**). The fact that all of these factors are interrelated complicates evaluation and stabilization of the patient. For example, hypovolemia results in decreased preload. As a compensatory mechanism, tachycardia and an increase in afterload occur, the latter having a negative impact on contractility. Thus, four of the five determinants of cardiac output are affected due to just one cause. The challenge is twofold: finding a technique to measure each of the five components of cardiac output and identifying the underlying etiology of inadequate flow.

C. Do Regional Perfusion Deficits Exist?

Cardiac output, blood lactate, and mixed venous oxygen saturations are global parameters that convey very little about regional perfusion or metabolic abnormalities. A clinical example may involve titrating the dose of an inoconstrictor (e.g., adrenaline) to maintain a desired BP and cardiac output at the expense of splanchnic hypoperfusion. Several techniques are available for measuring tissue bed perfusion (see the later section, "Regional Perfusion Measurement"); however, few are practical at the bedside due to issues of portability, accuracy, and clinical interpretation.

Initial hemodynamics   Therapy   Result

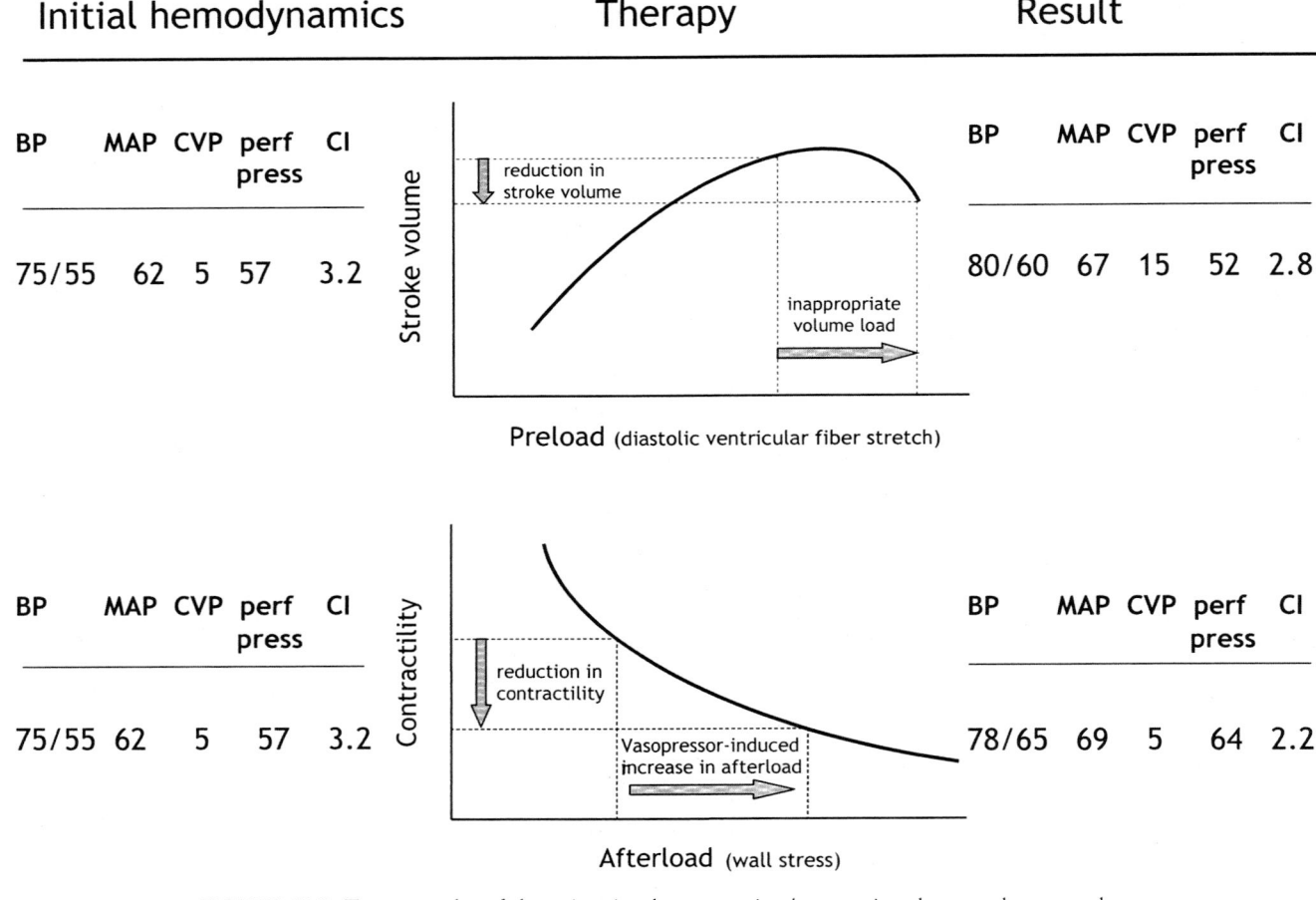

BP	MAP	CVP	perf press	CI
75/55	62	5	57	3.2

BP	MAP	CVP	perf press	CI
80/60	67	15	52	2.8

BP	MAP	CVP	perf press	CI
75/55	62	5	57	3.2

BP	MAP	CVP	perf press	CI
78/65	69	5	64	2.2

FIGURE 65.9. Two examples of therapies aimed at correcting hypotension that may have an adverse effect on cardiac output. In the top figure, an inappropriate volume load is given, resulting in an increase in blood pressure at the expense of a decrease in both cardiac output and perfusion pressure. In the bottom figure, the same initial hemodynamic profile is treated with vasoconstrictors, again increasing the mean blood pressure with a detrimental effect on cardiac output. BP, blood pressure; MAP, mean arterial blood pressure; CVP, central venous pressure; perf press, perfusion pressure (all mm Hg); CI, cardiac index $(L/min/m^2)$.

D. Which Therapeutic Regime Is Optimal? and E. How Has the Patient Responded to the Chosen Therapy?

An accurate measure of cardiac output and its associated determinants (preload, diastolic function, contractility, heart rate, afterload), together with a sound understanding of cardiovascular physiology may allow for an informed choice of therapy. In clinical practice, however, the BP is the most common hemodynamic variable used to titrate therapy. Although an adequate systemic perfusion pressure (mean arterial pressure − mean central venous pressure) is a prerequisite to maintaining organ function, it must be appreciated that perfusion pressure and cardiac output are interrelated variables. Systemic perfusion pressure = cardiac output × systemic vascular resistance. Thus, therapies instituted to correct hypotension are likely to have an effect on cardiac output, which may be detrimental despite correcting the BP. Two common examples are overzealous volume loading (**Fig. 65.9**, top) and excessive use of vasoconstrictors (**Fig. 65.9**, bottom).

In the first example (**Fig. 65.9**, top), inappropriate volume loading in a patient who is already operating at the top of

his Starling curve produces a small increase in arterial BP, a larger increase in CVP (the net effect being a slight decrease in perfusion pressure), but a larger detrimental decrease in cardiac output due to excessive diastolic ventricular fiber stretch. In the second example (**Fig. 65.9**, bottom), inappropriate use of a vasoconstrictor has corrected the hypotension but again adversely affected cardiac output because of the inverse relationship between contractility and afterload. Thus, it is vital that any change in therapy is evaluated serially and comprehensively, as many therapies aimed at maintaining BP may adversely affect cardiac function.

SPECIFIC TECHNIQUES

The Fick Method

The Fick method was first described by Adolph Fick in 1870, who applied the concept of mass balance to the measurement of blood flow. As such, it remains one of the most technically challenging, yet useful techniques for measuring cardiac output,

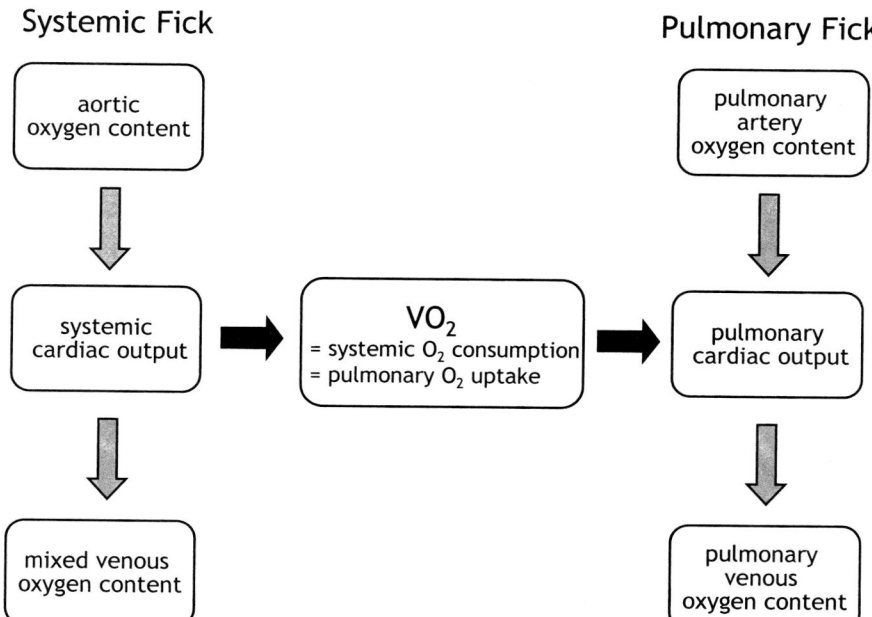

Systemic Fick

aortic oxygen content

↓

systemic cardiac output

↓

mixed venous oxygen content

Pulmonary Fick

pulmonary artery oxygen content

↓

pulmonary cardiac output

↓

pulmonary venous oxygen content

VO₂ = systemic O₂ consumption = pulmonary O₂ uptake

FIGURE 65.10. The Fick principle can be applied to both the systemic and pulmonary circulation.

not least because of its applicability to patients with anatomic shunts (20).

Principles

The Fick principle involves adding (or removing) an indicator and measuring the change in indicator concentration upstream and downstream of the point of indicator addition (or removal); flow can then be calculated via the formula:

Flow (volume/time) = indicator added (mass/time)/
change in indicator concentration (mass/volume)

For calculation of cardiac output, the most common measured indicator is oxygen consumption, although carbon dioxide production can also be utilized. For oxygen consumption, the Fick formula is:

$$\text{Cardiac output} = \frac{VO_2}{C_{aorta} - C_{mixed\ venous}}$$

where $V_{O_2} = \propto \frac{V_{O_2}}{O_2 sat_{aorta} - O_2 sat_{mixed\ venous}}$ oxygen consumption; C = oxygen content; O₂ sat = oxygen saturation.

A valuable aspect of the Fick principle is that it allows cardiac output to be calculated separately for the systemic (Q_s) and pulmonary (Q_p) circulations (**Fig. 65.10**). In the absence of an anatomic shunt, the cardiac output from both sides of the heart is essentially the same; thus Q_p:$Q_s = 1$ (ignoring the small amount of right-to-left shunt from thebesian and bronchial venous veins). However, in the presence of a shunt, the Fick equation can be rearranged to calculate the ratio of pulmonary-to-systemic blood flow (Q_p:Q_s).

$$Qp = \frac{VO_2}{C_{pulm\ vein} - C_{pulm\ artery}} \qquad Qs = \frac{VO_2}{C_{aorta} - C_{mixed\ venous}}$$

$$Qp:Qs = \frac{C_{aorta} - C_{mixed\ venous}}{C_{pulm\ vein} - C_{pulm\ artery}} \approx \frac{O_2 sat_{aorta} - O_2 sat_{mixed\ venous}}{O_2 sat_{pulm\ vein} - O_2 sat_{pulm\ artery}}$$

Care must be taken to sample at the correct anatomic site relative to the shunt. For example (**Fig. 65.11**), with a large

atrial septal defect exhibiting a pure left-to-right shunt, systemic venous blood must be measured upstream to the atrium. [One alternative is a weighted average of the superior and inferior vena caval saturations in proportion to the estimated venous return from the upper and lower body (70).]

Practice

The Fick technique requires a method for measuring oxygen consumption or carbon dioxide production, as well as access to the arterial and mixed venous circulations. Traditional methods for measuring oxygen consumption, such as the Douglas bag or spirometry, preclude measurement in the intensive care environment. However, these techniques have been advanced

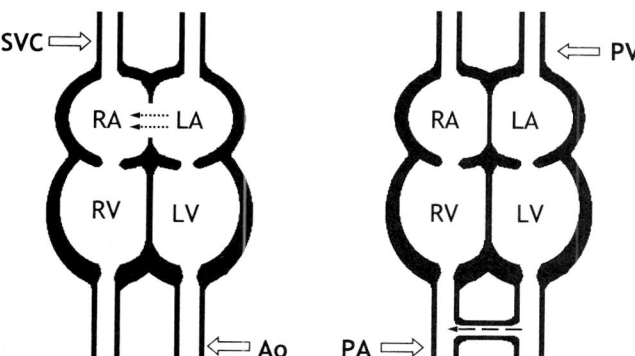

FIGURE 65.11. Calculation of pulmonary to systemic blood flow (Q_p:Q_s) in the setting of an anatomic shunt. The example on the left shows a large atrial septal defect with left-to-right shunt. In this setting, mixed venous blood should be sampled upstream of the shunt, for example, in the superior vena cava. On the right is a patent ductus arteriosus with pure left-to-right flow. Here, pulmonary artery blood should be sampled downstream of the shunt, to allow calculation of Q_p:Q_s. SVC, superior vena cava; RA, right atrium; LA, left atrium; RV, right ventricle; LV, left ventricle; Ao, aorta; PA, pulmonary artery; PV, pulmonary veins.

with portable metabolic monitors and/or mass spectrometry. Metabolic monitors utilize a gas-dilution principle to measure flow, a fast-response paramagnetic differential O_2 sensor to measure change in oxygen concentration, and an infrared CO_2 sensor. If flow and differential concentrations are known, content can be calculated via the Haldane transformation (3). Oxygen content in the arterial and mixed venous blood is measured using co-oximetry (saturation) and a routine blood gas analyzer (PaO_2), via the formula:

$$O_2 \text{ content (mL } O_2 \text{ per liter of blood)} = [1.34 \times \text{Hb (g/L)} \times \% \text{ saturation}/100] + [PaO_2(\text{mm Hg}) \times 0.003]$$

where Hb = hemoglobin.

If CO_2 is used, the formula is more complex, taking into account PCO_2, plasma solubility coefficient of CO_2, the apparent dissociation constant of the CO_2-HCO_3 system (pK), arterial O_2 saturation, hemoglobin concentration, and pH (56).

Errors

As the Fick technique is vulnerable to many sources of error at each measurement step, attention to detail is vital.

Errors in Measurement of Oxygen Consumption

Loss of Expired Gas. All expired gas must pass through the metabolic monitor to allow for an accurate estimation of expiratory tidal volumes. In the clinical setting, the most common reason for this necessity is leak around the endotracheal tube. Although a leak of up to 5% may produce an error that is within acceptable limits, quantification is difficult given the inaccuracies in tidal volume measurement inherent in many ventilators (particularly for infants) (6). Similarly, absence of an audible air leak is an unreliable clinical sign; thus, it is recommended that a cuffed endotracheal tube be used. A second source of air leak is via a pneumothorax; however, this contributes to measurement error only with a large and ongoing air leak, such as seen with a bronchopulmonary fistula.

High Fractions of Inspired Oxygen. Most metabolic monitors employ the Haldane transformation to estimate oxygen consumption. When the FIO_2 is very high, such as with severe lung disease, difference between the fractions of inspired and expired oxygen may be very small, creating an error in the denominator of the Haldane algorithm. Ideally the FIO_2 should be <0.60; at levels >0.85, the error is likely to be significant (65).

Violation of the Law of Mass Balance. The law of mass balance requires that oxygen consumption in the body be in equilibrium with oxygen uptake by the lungs. Although the lungs also consume oxygen, this largely comes from the systemic circulation via the bronchial arteries and is thus accounted for within the Fick equation. However, in the setting of severe pneumonia (37) or the early stages of chronic lung disease (52) (and perhaps also with acute lung injury from other causes), the lungs may consume significant oxygen directly from the inspired gas, producing a discrepancy between measured oxygen uptake and systemic oxygen consumption (the former being greater) and, hence, an overestimation of cardiac output.

Other Sources of Error

Gas volumes must be converted to standard conditions, and the partial pressure of water vapor within the system must be carefully controlled. However, both are routinely performed in modern metabolic monitors.

Errors in Arterial and Mixed Venous Oxygen Content Calculation

Venous oxygen saturation will be inaccurate if calculated via a nomogram in the blood gas analyzer; it must be measured directly using co-oximetry. Ignoring the contribution from dissolved oxygen may result in considerable error when the PaO_2 is elevated (70). Finally, mixed venous blood is seldom sampled from pediatric patients for technical reasons; central venous blood is often used as a surrogate, which poses a potential problem, as the oxygen saturation in the pulmonary artery, right atrium, and both vena cavae can be very different. A cardinal assumption is that the error from the chosen sampling site will remain relatively constant, allowing for accurate trending of the estimated cardiac output; again, this is not guaranteed in the critically ill patient.

Indirect Fick Method

The technique just outlined requires measurement of either O_2 or CO_2 content directly from the blood and is thus known as the *direct Fick method*. As discussed, one of the limitations is the requirement for invasive vascular access. An alternative (for CO_2) may be to estimate the Fick parameters indirectly from the inspired and expired gases using a CO_2 partial rebreathe technique, whereby the patient rebreathes a proportion of the exhaled CO_2 for a short period of time while mechanically ventilated—known as the *indirect Fick method*.

In common with many less invasive techniques, the indirect Fick method requires a series of assumptions, which may limit its validity in the ICU environment. Here, Q_p is not measured but rather pulmonary capillary blood flow (in essence, effective, or nonshunt, blood flow) is derived. By measuring change in the parameters before and at the end of the CO_2 rebreathing period, pulmonary capillary blood flow is calculated from the formula:

$$Q_{pcbf} = \frac{\Delta VCO_2}{\Delta C_{\text{mixed venous}} - \Delta C_{\text{pulmonary end capillary}}}$$

In this equation, (a) ΔVCO_2 is measured, (b) it is assumed that a brief partial re-breathe period does not change mixed venous CO_2, hence $\Delta C_{\text{mixed venous}}$ is zero, and (c) $\Delta C_{\text{pulmonary end capillary}}$ is estimated from alveolar CO_2 content, which is in turn, estimated from end-tidal PCO_2 via a correction factor. Intrapulmonary shunt flow is calculated from Nunn's iso-shunt diagrams and added to pulmonary capillary blood flow, giving Q_p, or total pulmonary blood flow.

Indicator Dilution Methods

All indicator dilution methods are based upon the original description by Stewart in 1897, with later refinements by Hamilton between 1928 and 1932. Perhaps the best known of these methods is thermodilution, which utilizes temperature (via an injection of saline at room temperature) as the indicator. With the introduction of the pulmonary artery (Swan-Ganz) catheter in 1970 (**Fig. 65.12**), pulmonary artery thermodilution became the first commercially available method of cardiac output

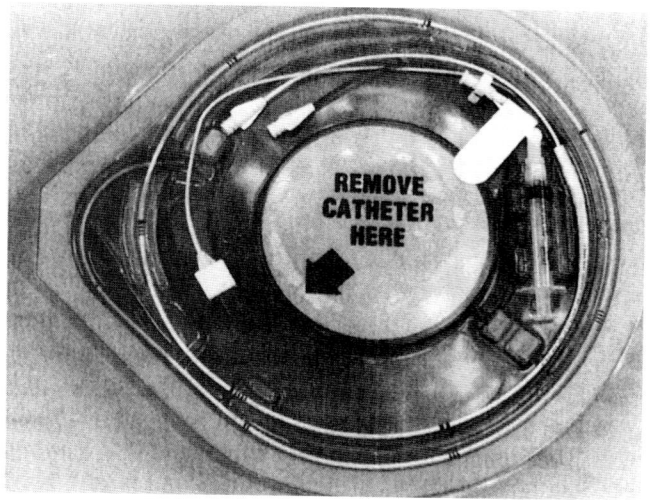

FIGURE 65.12. Quadruple-lumen pulmonary artery catheter (Swan-Ganz catheter).

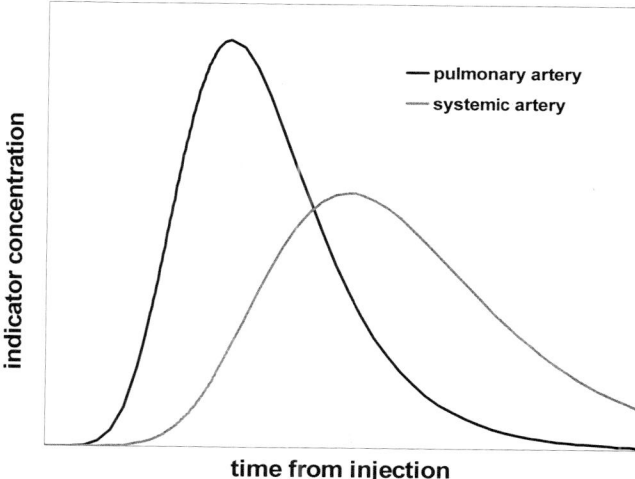

FIGURE 65.13. Dilution curves. The shape will vary according to the site of measurement. Measurement of injectate concentration nearer to the site of the central venous injection, such as seen within the pulmonary artery, will produce peaked curves with a relatively steep down slope. Conversely, measurements in a systemic artery will have first traversed the pulmonary circulation, left heart, and aorta and are thus less peaked with a prolonged down slope (partly due to superimposition of secondary and tertiary curves from recirculation).

measurement and has until recently been the generally used technique. Over the last decade, the popularity of this method has waned for a variety of reasons, including the growing perception that cardiac output measurement may not alter patient outcome and the introduction of cheaper and less technically challenging alternatives. Despite this, pulmonary artery thermodilution remains the most common benchmark against which new modalities are compared.

Principles

All dilution techniques follow a similar principle (71). An indicator is injected into a central vein, and cardiac output is calculated by measuring the change in blood indicator concentration over time at a point downstream of the injection. The method for sensing the indicator varies according to the injectate and may utilize a thermistor (temperature), densitometry or oximetry (dye), or an ion-selective electrode (lithium charge). The relationship is expressed mathematically as:

$$\text{cardiac output} = \frac{\text{amount of indicator injected}}{\int_0^\infty \text{conc}_\text{indicator}(t)\,dt}$$

The denominator represents the integral of the indicator concentration with respect to time—in other words, the area under the curve for indicator concentration versus time measured between the time of injection and infinity. The shape of the curve will differ according to where it is measured relative to the site of injection. For example, the transit time is brief when the indicator is measured within the pulmonary artery, resulting in peaked curves with a relatively short tail. However, if the indicator is measured in a systemic artery, it must first pass through the pulmonary circulation and left heart, resulting in a longer transit time and producing a curve that is less peaked with a prolonged tail (**Fig. 65.13**).

Calculation of the area under the curve is a fundamental challenge shared by all indicator methods, largely due to the problem of recirculation. Recirculation refers to the phenomenon in which the indicator within the initial portion of the concentration-time curve traverses the body and arrives back at the measurement site before the terminal portion of concentration-time curve has passed the measurement site, with

the net effect being a secondary (and sometimes tertiary) curve superimposed on the primary curve. Recirculation is more common when the site of measurement is further from the injection and in states of low cardiac output. Thus, calculation of cardiac output requires a mathematical means of separating the primary curve from the secondary/tertiary curves. The most accepted approach is the Stewart-Hamilton method, which assumes mono-exponential decay for the primary curve. Many other methods are used, including deconvolution and the fitting of log normal or γ distributions to the descending portion of the curve.

A useful property of indicator dilution curves is that they also allow for calculation of vascular volumes via the mean transit and exponential down-slope times. Several vascular volumes have been suggested as measures of preload (see the later section, "Components of Cardiac Output"). In addition, other calculations that relate to tissue volumes and liver function are possible, depending on the indicator used.

The main differences between the various dilution techniques are threefold: the choice of indicator (temperature, dye, ionic charge), the site of indicator measurement (pulmonary artery, large systemic artery, peripheral artery), and the algorithm used to calculate cardiac output (**Table 65.8**).

Errors

Indicator dilution is accurate, provided a series of conditions are met (44), including rapid and even indicator injection, complete mixing of the indicator and blood, no loss of indicator between injection and measurement, absence of dysrhythmias, no anatomic shunt, minimal valve regurgitation, and steady-state flow.

Of all the dilution methods listed in **Table 65.8**, pulmonary artery thermodilution remains the most technically challenging and perhaps error-prone, primarily due to difficulty in accessing the pulmonary artery percutaneously (as opposed to other dilution methods, which require central venous and arterial

TABLE 65.8

DILUTION METHODS FOR DETERMINING CARDIAC OUTPUT

Method	Advantages	Disadvantages	Additional variables measured
Thermodilution: (pulmonary artery sampling)	Proven track record; semicontinuous mode available	Variations in cardiac output with respiratory cycle; difficult access in small patients; inaccurate at low flow; low but significant morbidity: infection, bleeding, catheter knotting	Pulmonary pressure; wedge pressure; mixed venous oxygen saturation
Thermodilution: Transpulmonary (systemic artery sampling)	Easy access in small patients; repeatable; continuous if device is combined with arterial pulse contour method (combination commercially available)	Requires dedicated arterial line, safe length of insertion time unknown, frequent recalibration required if used in conjunction with pulse contour method	Intrathoracic blood volume (preload); cardiac function index (contractility); extravascular lung water; stroke volume variability (if used with pulse contour method)
Dye dilution	Accurate	Sequential measurements limited by dye clearance; commercial availability of dye and devices	
Lithium chloride dilution	Utilizes preexisting central venous and arterial lines; continuous if device is combined with arterial pulse contour method (combination commercially available)	Sequential measurements limited by lithium clearance; theoretical risk of toxicity; requires blood sample with each measurement; unlicensed in <40 kg; frequent recalibration required if used in conjunction with pulse contour method	Stroke volume variability (if used with pulse contour method)

access only). The left subclavian route is the preferred access point to encourage proper placement, although any of the major upper limb veins is appropriate. Complications of percutaneous pulmonary artery catheter placement include pneumothorax, hemothorax, sepsis, catheter malposition, catheter knotting, ventricular dysrhythmias, balloon rupture, embolization, pulmonary artery occlusion, and pulmonary infarction. Obviously, the first four complications can be seen with placement of any central venous line (29).

One source of error with pulmonary artery thermodilution that is not shared by other indicator methods is sensitivity to cyclical alterations in cardiac output produced by mechanical ventilation. PPV causes a transient drop in venous return during inspiration and, hence, preload to the RV, with a resultant fall in right heart stroke volume. Because the transit time between injection and temperature sensing in the pulmonary artery is very short, the measured cardiac output may vary depending on when the measurement is taken in relation to the ventilatory cycle. To account for this situation, three to four measurements should be taken at systematic intervals throughout the ventilatory cycle and then averaged, which will produce an estimate within +10% of the true cardiac output in adults (provided all other sources of inaccuracy are dealt with) (30). It has been estimated that a minimal change of 12%–15% between serial averaged thermodilution measurements must occur to represent a true change in cardiac output (55).

Transpulmonary thermodilution is a related technique that carries various sources of potential error (67). Here, temperature change is sensed in a large systemic artery, which means that considerable heat dissipation is possible, as the indicator traverses the pulmonary vasculature, left heart, and aorta before reaching the temperature sensor, a situation ameliorated by using a cooled indicator (typically 5% dextrose or normal saline at <10° centigrade). Surprisingly, doing so results in only a modest and relatively constant heat loss, which can be factored into the algorithm (2,59).

Dye and lithium dilution both share the limitation that the indicator remains in the circulation for some time (dye more so than lithium), which means that repeated injections cannot be given over a narrow time interval, thereby producing two limitations: rapid changes in cardiac output may not be sensed, and the variability of the technique cannot be assessed by averaging consecutive measurements.

Impedance Methods

Impedance is the opposition to the flow of an alternating current and was first applied to the measurement of cardiac output in 1966. Impedance-based techniques for cardiac output measurement are not used widely in the clinical setting because (a) invasive (intracardiac) impedance is too invasive, and (b) noninvasive modifications (thoracic impedance) currently lack sufficient accuracy in critically ill patients. Nonetheless, as many fundamental physiologic principles have been elucidated using intracardiac impedance, a basic understanding of this technique is recommended for ICU clinicians.

Principles

With impedance methods, the chest is regarded as a conductor whose impedance is altered by the changes in blood volume and velocity that occur with each heartbeat, from which stroke volume is calculated. Impedance is defined for pulsatile flow (equated with alternating current) using Ohm's Law in a similar manner as resistance for nonpulsatile flow (direct current):

$$\text{Resistance (R)} = \frac{\text{potential difference (V)}}{\text{direct current (I)}}$$

Measurement is via a series of voltage-sensing and current-transmitting electrodes. The site of electrode placement defines the type of impedance measurement, from the noninvasive (thoracic bioimpedance, where electrodes are placed on the chest) to the invasive (intracardiac, requiring electrode placement within the LV).

Practice

Intracardiac Impedance. Stroke volume is measured with multipolar catheters placed directly into the LV; these partition the ventricle into a series of cylindrical segments. The invasiveness of this technique means that its use in the ICU is limited to situations in which catheters are placed during cardiac surgery and as such, represents a research rather than a clinical tool. Combination with a pressure sensor allows simultaneous measurement of ventricular pressure-volume loops, the area enclosed by one cardiac cycle being defined as stroke work. In the experimental setting, it is possible to alter preload by placing a snare around the inferior vena cava. These alterations in preload generate a family of pressure-volume loops. The resultant pressure-volume relationships allow calculation of two measures of systolic function: end-systolic elastance or using preload-recruitable stroke work (**Fig. 65.14**).

Thoracic Impedance. The electrodes are placed around the chest wall. The standard formula for stroke volume measurement is:

$$\text{stroke volume} = \frac{L^3 \times VET \times dZ/dt_{max}}{4.25 \times Z_0}$$

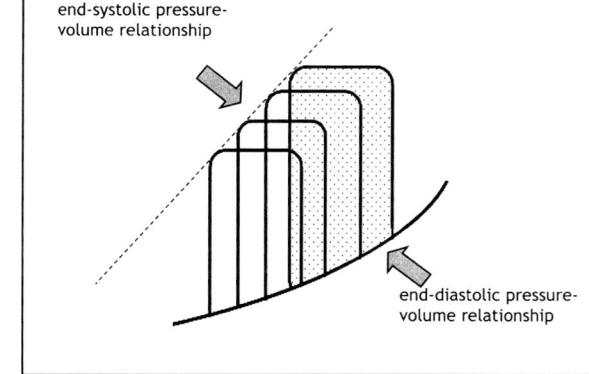

FIGURE 65.14. Pressure-volume loops measured via a conductance catheter. The area inside the pressure-volume loop is equal to stroke work (**hatched area**). If preload is progressively reduced, such as via caval snaring, then sequential pressure volume loops will diminish in size and migrate horizontally to the left. The slope of a line joining the upper left corner of each loop (this point being end-systolic pressure) represents end-systolic elastance (**dashed line**), a measure of contractility. A related measure, preload-recruitable stroke work, can also be derived from the pressure-volume loops. This represents the slope of a regression line from plotting end-diastolic volume against stroke work.

Where:

L = thoracic segment length
VET = ventricular ejection time
dZ/dt_{max} = maximum rate of impedance change
Z_0 = transthoracic baseline impedance.

However, it is now known that the volume change sensed by thoracic bioimpedance is almost exclusively extracardiac, as the myocardium tends to shield the electrodes from the impedance changes occurring within the ventricle. Thus, the change in impedance signal and, hence, stroke volume estimation comes predominantly from blood volume alterations within the systemic and pulmonary vessels inside the chest.

Errors

If used correctly, intracardiac impedance is very accurate. However, many authors have questioned the accuracy of thoracic bioimpedance in the ICU environment, particularly in states of low cardiac output, hypotension, and chest wall edema (22).

Doppler Ultrasound

Christian Doppler proposed his principle in 1842, which was subsequently applied to the measurement of blood flow by Franklin in 1961. Although the Doppler principle can be applied using sound, light, or any electromagnetic radiation, sound is the most common medium employed for measurement of blood flow. Doppler ultrasound can be used as a stand-alone technique but is more commonly employed as an integral adjunct to bedside echocardiography.

Principles

An ultrasound beam of known frequency is directed toward a moving column of blood, whereby a proportion of the beam is reflected back to the transmitter by the erythrocytes at a different frequency. The frequency shift will be proportional to the velocity of the reflecting blood cells, via the formula:

$$\text{Blood velocity} = \frac{\Delta \text{frequency} \times c}{2 \times f_t \times \cos\theta}$$

where:

Δfrequency = the frequency shift between transmitted and reflected signal
c = the sound velocity in blood
f_t = the transmitting frequency
θ = the angle of insonation (i.e., the angle between the path of the ultrasound beam and the linear direction of blood flow).

The resultant velocity-time signal can be represented spectrally, producing a characteristic triangular shape, which will differ slightly depending upon where blood flow is measured (**Fig. 65.15**). If flow is measured in the aorta, the velocity-time integral (area enclosed by the triangle) is known as *stroke distance*, which represents the distance that a column of blood will travel along the aorta in one cardiac cycle. Conversion of *stroke distance* to *stroke volume* (and hence cardiac output, by multiplying by the heart rate) requires multiplication by the area of the aortic valve, which is measured using either two-dimensional or M-mode echocardiography (62).

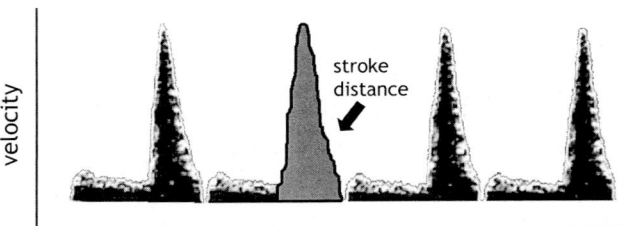

FIGURE 65.15. Typical descending aortic Doppler trace. The velocity time integral is known as stroke distance, which represents the distance that a column of blood will travel along the aorta in one cardiac cycle.

Practice

Stand-alone Doppler Ultrasound. If performed as a stand-alone technique, Doppler ultrasound requires only a modest amount of user expertise and training. The technique can be applied to any pulsatile vessel; however, measurement of cardiac output is typically performed in the aorta, either via the transthoracic or transesophageal routes. The transthoracic approach is noninvasive but intermittent. Typically, the probe is placed in the sternal notch and directed toward the aortic root. Optimal signal acquisition is often confirmed by the quality of both a visual and an auditory component. Signal acquisition may be compromised if the heart is malpositioned or the lung fields are hyperinflated. Conversely, the transesophageal approach is semi-invasive but potentially continuous. Here, a 5.5-mm flexible probe is inserted to the mid-esophagus, to a point where the esophagus lies adjacent and parallel to the descending aorta, with verification of signal optimization as for the transthoracic approach. Both techniques provide a range of Doppler-derived variables that may provide information on contractility, preload, and afterload (11).

Doppler Ultrasound with Echocardiography. Echocardiography can provide a vast amount of functional and morpho-logic information in addition to cardiac output measurement, including indices of diastolic dysfunction, regional wall abnormalities, valve regurgitation, pericardial effusion, chamber dilatation, and cardiac chamber interdependence (57). Newer associated modalities, such as three-dimensional echocardiography and Doppler tissue imaging, are emerging and may provide additional insights into cardiac function. The main disadvantage of echocardiography is the requirement for significant user expertise.

Errors

Doppler waves can be continuous or pulsed; both have advantages and limitations. Stand-alone Doppler techniques generally employ continuous-wave Doppler, which reacts to all blood flow within the path of the beam (i.e., not only flow across the aortic valve), resulting in range ambiguity. Range ambiguity is the inability of the imaging system to precisely localize the source (location) of the reflected signal in the heart, which is less likely when coupled with two-dimensional imaging techniques.

Pulsed-wave Doppler ultrasonography has an advantage over continuous wave Doppler in that it allows determination of the velocity of flow at a specific location (called a *gate*). However, it carries the disadvantage of "aliasing," in which the system cannot reliably calculate the speed and direction of high-velocity blood flow, especially with high-frequency probes (i.e., 12 MHz). High-frequency probes have higher imaging resolution, which is important in pediatric echocardiography but results in an inability to resolve high-velocity blood flow. Using a lower-frequency probe (3 MHz) allows measurement of higher-velocity blood flow but with lower imaging quality. Significant error may occur when the angle of insonation is >15 degrees, unless angle correction (for cos θ; see Equation, blood flow velocity formula) is employed. Ideally, perfect, parallel alignment of the ultrasound beam and blood flow should be sought. Lastly, probe position, particularly for transesophageal Doppler (**Fig. 65.16**), remains a concern. Small probe rotations

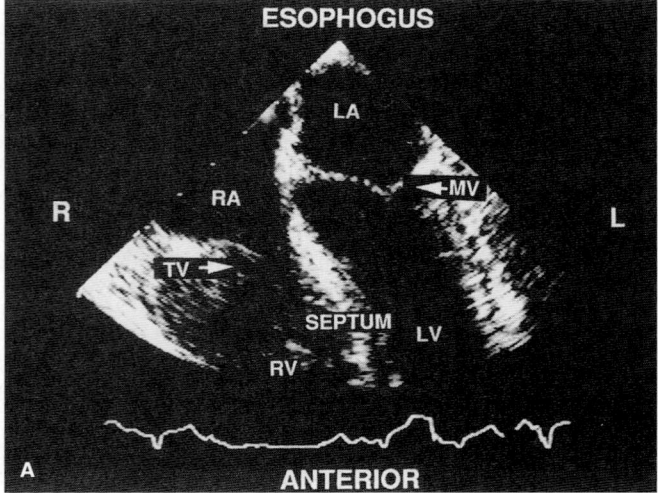

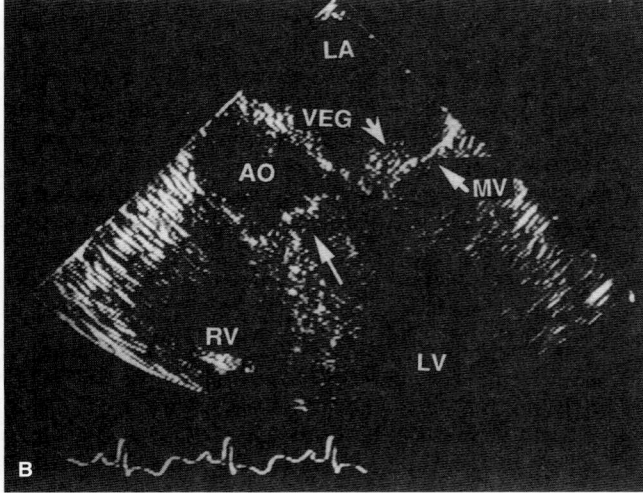

FIGURE 65.16. Two-dimensional transesophageal echocardiograms. (**A**) Four-chamber view showing left atrium (LA), right atrium (RA), right ventricle (RV), left ventricle (LV), with the septum and atrioventricular (AV) valves in the normal position. (**B**) Four-chamber view showing the aortic outflow (AO), LA, RV, and LV. In the center of the mitral valve (MV) is a highly echogenic vegetation (VEG). A subaortic membrane is also present (**arrow**).

or vertical movement can produce considerable changes in the measurement of the velocity of blood through the aortic valve and, hence, cardiac output calculations. In addition, risk exists for endotracheal tube displacement, particularly with neonates, which must be avoided.

Arterial Pulse Contour Methods

An association between stroke volume and arterial pulse contour was suggested by Erlanger over a century ago. Since that time, a variety of theories concerning the relationship between flow and pressure in the arterial tree have been postulated. Advances in microprocessor technology have allowed these to be transformed into bedside monitoring tools that measure beat-to-beat changes in stroke volume.

Principles

Arterial pulse contour methodology cannot be appreciated without an understanding of several basic physiologic concepts concerning arterial flow and pressure (43). Both flow and pressure are primarily pulsatile events in the proximal arterial system and do not achieve nonpulsatile or mean values until the level of the arterioles, which coincides with the point of greatest pressure drop. Resistance to flow occurs throughout the arterial tree; in the vessels that receive pulsatile flow, it is called *impedance*, while in those that receive nonpulsatile flow, it is designated as *resistance* (also known as systemic vascular resistance).

Arteries contain elastic tissue, and in the aorta, this results in dilatation during systole. In essence, a proportion of the stroke volume is stored in the aorta rather than being transmitted directly to the peripheral vasculature (Windkessel effect). This property is defined as *compliance*, or the unit change in volume per unit change in pressure. Compliance is followed by a period of elastic recoil during diastole, which partially explains the diastolic continuation of blood flow within small arteries. Aortic compliance is nonlinear (as is impedance), meaning that the pressure change for a given volume ejected by the heart will vary according to vascular volume status, diastolic arterial pressure (and hence systemic vascular resistance), and stroke volume. Compliance is also affected by a variety of factors, including age, disease, catecholamines, etc. All of these factors, as well as the pressure wave reflected from the periphery back to the aorta, influence the shape of the arterial waveform.

Practice

A variety of methods exist for continuous pulse-contour analysis, all of which utilize a combination of calculations for aortic impedance, aortic compliance, total or systemic vascular resistance, pressure wave reflection, and transfer function between large and small arteries, although not all components are included in every method (15). Perhaps the best known of these is the modified Windkessel approach (68), which describes the arterial pressure response to stroke volume as being a function of characteristic impedance of the proximal aorta, aortic compliance, and total systemic vascular resistance, the latter two variables being considered in parallel. Accuracy may be improved by (a) ultrasonic measurement of aortic cross-sectional area, which allows for a recalibration of the aortic compliance relationship for the individual patient (Modelflow™), or (b) a more sophisticated analysis of the pressure waveform that

takes into account the shape as well as the area of the pressure wave (PiCCO™).

An alternative method (LiDCO™plus) involves arterial pulse power analysis, but because it does not rely on waveform morphology, it is not, strictly speaking, a pulse contour method. All methods require an indwelling arterial catheter to measure changes in stroke volume, and all require an alternative method for cardiac output measurement (i.e., transpulmonary thermodilution) for (re)calibration.

Errors

Aortic valve incompetence will compromise the validity of these methods by providing an alternative route for diastolic runoff. Any degree of dampening of the arterial trace will also affect the estimation of stroke volume. Lastly, several of the pulse contour methods are based upon the premise of a relatively reproducible arc tangent relationship between change in aortic pressure and aortic cross-sectional area (and hence volume), and this carries three possible sources of error. First, this relationship has been derived from cadaveric studies in adults only, and whether the same association holds for children is unknown. Second, although the shape of the aortic cross-sectional area versus pressure curve is relatively constant, differing intercepts exist between individuals. Errors in estimating cross-sectional area, and hence compliance could result; therefore, cross-sectional area should be directly measured ultrasonically (17). Third, accuracy with the use of vasoconstrictors is largely unknown. To date, only preliminary evaluations of beat-to-beat analysis have appeared in the pediatric literature.

MARKERS OF ADEQUACY OF FLOW

Because of the technical difficulties of measuring cardiac output in clinical practice, several measures of adequacy of organ flow and oxygen delivery are employed.

Mixed Venous Oxygen Saturation

Mixed venous blood is defined when all sources of systemic venous return (superior vena cava, inferior vena cava, and coronary sinus) have merged, which occurs in the normal heart in the RV and pulmonary artery (4). Referring back to the Fick equation, it can be seen that mixed venous saturation will decrease when oxygen delivery falls or oxygen consumption increases. The normal mixed venous oxygen saturation is $\sim73\%$ (range, 65%–75%), but it is obviously less in cyanosed patients. The "typical" range for the arteriovenous oxygen saturation difference is 20%–33%, although this is highly variable and related to multiple factors (present in the Fick equation).

The oxygen extraction ratio can also be calculated as the following:

$$\text{oxygen extraction ratio} = (Sao_2 - Svo_2)/Sao_2$$

Normal values are between 0.24 and 0.28. Because of the difficulty in accessing mixed venous blood, central venous saturation has been suggested as an alternative in both pediatric and adult practice (69). Central venous blood should ideally be sampled from the superior vena cava just before it enters the right atrium because samples taken from a right atrial catheter may selectively draw blood from the coronary sinus, which is relatively desaturated (typical values 30%–37%). The superior vena cava is preferred over the inferior vena cava because of variability of oxygen saturation in the latter, depending upon the exact site of sampling, which is due to tissue beds with widely varying saturations draining into the inferior vena cava, ranging from muscle (60%–71%), to gut/liver (66%), to renal (92%) (4). Thus, if the inferior vena cava is used for central venous sampling, the catheter tip should lie above the hepatic veins.

One factor that may confound interpretation of pediatric central venous values is the proportionate difference in superior vena caval flow between adults and children. In adults, the superior vena cava carries ~35% of the total body venous return. In children, this is age dependent, typically being 50% in newborns, rising to a peak of 55% by 2.5 years, and decreasing to adult values by age 6.5 years (49). Furthermore, these merely represent average values in healthy children, with major differences occurring between individuals and disease states.

Data that quantify the relationship between central and mixed venous saturation in critically ill children are sparse. Immediately after cardiac surgery, central venous values are, on average, lower than mixed venous values by between 7% and 17%; however, this difference largely disappears by 24 hrs. Conversely, among adults with shock of varying etiology, central venous saturation is 7% higher (47), although differences within individual patients can be as high as 20% (18).

Importantly, differences between central and mixed venous saturations are less important than the fact that they both vary to the same degree in the majority (90%) of clinical scenarios (47). The value of central venous oxygen saturation monitoring has been demonstrated in one randomized, controlled trial, in which a reduction in mortality (30.5% versus 46.5%) was seen in adults with shock when this variable was incorporated into an algorithm for early goal-directed therapy (48).

Blood Lactate

Although historically, the standard explanation for the occurrence of an elevated blood lactate in critical illness was tissue hypoxia from inadequate oxygen delivery, it is now appreciated that this is an oversimplification, in that hyperlactatemia can have multiple etiologies (28). A common cause, *tissue dysoxia*, whereby the cells cannot utilize delivered oxygen, may be seen in states of mitochondrial dysfunction associated with sepsis, poisoning, and various inborn errors of metabolism. A second cause is accelerated aerobic glycolysis, in which lactate is generated predominantly from skeletal muscle (35). Here, the proposed mechanism is hyperstimulation of sarcolemmal Na/K-ATPase from excess catecholamines (both endogenous and exogenous). The energy supply for this enzyme is linked to the glycolytic and glycogenolytic pathways; thus, overstimulation produces pyruvate at a rate that outstrips the oxidative capacity of the mitochondria, resulting in lactate accumulation. A third reason may be due to administration of exogenous lactate at a rate faster than the body can metabolize it. Examples include administration of lactate-containing replacement fluids during high-volume hemofiltration and the use of "old blood" as a pump prime during neonatal cardiopulmonary bypass.

Fourth, acute hyperventilation can elevate blood lactate levels, perhaps secondary to increased splanchnic release of lactate during hyperventilation (31). A final concept that deserves a brief mention is the *lactate shuttle*. It is increasingly recognized that lactate may function as a currency for maintaining the redox potential both within and between cells (23). Regardless of the possible causes, the presence of a persistently elevated lactate level should always prompt a vigorous search for possible causes, as a significantly elevated lactate implies a poorer prognosis (26).

Regional Perfusion

Abnormalities of regional perfusion may not be appreciated by monitoring either central venous oxygen saturation or blood lactate, as both are global markers. Therefore, robust measures of regional perfusion are necessary.

Tissue P_{CO_2} Monitoring Using Tonometry

Tonometry is a technique designed to measure tissue hypoperfusion (33). It involves placement of a CO_2-permeable balloon adjacent to a mucosal surface. Tissue hypoperfusion should lead to inadequate clearance of products of cell respiration, resulting in a rise in intracellular CO_2, which will diffuse freely across the mucosal cell membrane and equilibrate with that inside the tonometer balloon. If this value is corrected for the P_{CO_2} in arterial blood, it is said to quantify the degree of tissue hypoperfusion.

The first application in critical illness was via gastric tonometry, which was used as a surrogate for splanchnic perfusion. The great enthusiasm that heralded this technique in the 1990s has not been sustained, partly due to inconsistent results concerning prognosis and the lack of benefit from therapies directed at correcting abnormal tonometric values. In retrospect, it may have been partly due to methodologic problems in many of the original studies, such as choice of tonometer medium (air being more accurate than saline), inaccuracy in saline-based P_{CO_2} measurement with blood gas analyzers, use of buffers in the tonometric medium, choice of tonometric variable (uncorrected versus arterial-corrected P_{CO_2}, derived pH, etc.), use of gastric acid blockers, and the influence of feeding.

Sublingual tonometry has been suggested as a more accessible alternative, particularly during the early phases of resuscitation (39).

Near Infrared Spectroscopy (Optical Monitoring Methods)

A variety of optical methods for measuring tissue perfusion are available, including laser Doppler flowmetry, near infrared spectroscopy (NIRS), orthogonal polarization spectral imaging, and the peripheral perfusion index. Among these techniques, NIRS has gained the most popularity. Some PICUs have recently added NIRS as a standard monitoring device for patients with potential hemodynamic instability or deficits in regional (primarily cerebral) perfusion. The NIRS technique is based on the principle that deoxygenated hemoglobin absorbs light in the range of 760 nm or lower, whereas both deoxygenated and oxygenated hemoglobin absorb light at ~800 nm. Thus, the passage of light at two different wavelengths can detect the changes in the concentrations of oxyhemoglobin and deoxyhemoglobin, which in turn, permits the calculation of the percent O_2 saturation in the tissue. Light in the near-infrared spectrum also has the desirable property of undergoing the least amount of absorption and scattering as it passes through tissue, allowing NIRS light to penetrate skin and skull, for instance, to measure O_2 saturation in brain parenchyma.

Practice. The commercially available NIRS device (INVOS® System, Somanetics, Troy, Michigan) utilizes a sensor placed over the forehead to emit and detect the near-infrared light. The algorithm is weighted to sample venous blood predominantly. Hence, the numerical display reflects the venous O_2 saturation of the region of the brain being sampled (Sro_2 index). Generally, sensors are placed on each side of the forehead to reflect right and left cerebral cortical venous O_2 saturation. Sro_2 correlates well with jugular bulb O_2 saturation and moderately well with mixed venous O_2 saturation. (64). The adequacy of regional cerebral perfusion should be investigated if the Sro_2 decreases 12–20 points from baseline, if Sro_2 is >30 points lower than the arterial O_2 saturation, or if the absolute Sro_2 index is <50 in a patient without an intracardiac shunt.

Errors and Complications. Because NIRS is noninvasive and easy to use, few technical errors or complications occur. The greater challenge involves interpretation of Sro_2 values. Since a significant decrease in Sro_2 from a baseline signifies the possibility of inadequate O_2 delivery to that region, the clinician must take careful note of which Sro_2 values should be taken to represent the baseline. In addition, important clinical conditions (such as mitochondrial dysfunction, distribution of flow to non-nutritive vessels, or brain death) may be associated with normal Sro_2.

COMPONENTS OF CARDIAC OUTPUT

Five elements contribute to cardiac output: heart rate, preload, diastolic function, contractility, and afterload. Of these, only heart rate is measured routinely, which is complicated by the fact that these elements are interdependent, meaning that an apparent abnormality in one (or more) of these variables may actually be caused by an aberration in another (or several others).

Heart Rate

The importance of heart rate, particularly sinus tachycardia, in critical illness is often overlooked. If measured via an ECG, heart rate is an objective clinical sign (in comparison to many others, such as work of breathing, capillary refill, level of consciousness). The presence of significant tachycardia in the absence of other causes (such as extreme fever or arrhythmia) suggests inadequate flow. Tachycardia will exacerbate diastolic dysfunction by reducing available ventricular filling time. Conversely, the existence of an inappropriately "normal" heart rate in the setting of severely deranged hemodynamics (narrow pulse pressure, thready central pulses, grossly prolonged capillary refill, drowsiness) suggests imminent cardiovascular collapse.

Preload

Preload relates to the net force that influences ventricular fiber stretch at the end of diastole. It is both difficult to measure at the bedside and influenced by many factors (**Table 65.9**). Rather than measuring preload, we are often more interested in addressing a related clinical question. The question really is: "Will the patient respond to a fluid bolus by increasing stroke volume?" Failure to do so can occur for three reasons: administration of inadequate volume, severely impaired contractility, and the patient is already functioning at the plateau of the Starling curve (**Fig. 65.9**).

Broadly speaking, measures of "preload" can be static or dynamic, with the latter more important in predicting fluid responsiveness (14). Two common static, pressure-based, measures of preload are CVP (or right atrial pressure) and pulmonary artery occlusion pressure (or left atrial pressure). Both are poor markers of volume status (36) because many factors compromise the ability of a pressure measurement to act as a surrogate for volume status, including venous capacitance, cardiac chamber compliance, cardiac valve competence, pulmonary artery pressure, and the ability of the lung to function as a Starling resistor with PPV. Nonetheless, CVP may be a reasonable trending measurement with a low value suggesting underfilling (54).

Two volume-based measures are derived from transpulmonary thermodilution: global end-diastolic volume and intrathoracic blood volume. Accurate measurement requires simultaneous thermodilution and dye dilution. In practice, these are derived following thermodilution via a regression equation. Although both have been evaluated favorably in adult practice, little data exist in children.

Echocardiographic measures of preload include measurement of LV end-diastolic volume. Measurement of RV end-diastolic volume is more difficult due to the complex anatomy of the RV. Corrected flow time is a Doppler-derived measurement that has been used successfully in adults to guide intraoperative volume replacement; however, it is also affected by afterload and contractility (11). Pediatric studies suggest that this variable has a better negative than positive predictive value (identifying patients who will not respond to volume, rather than those who will).

Dynamic measures of preload all relate to the cyclical fluctuations in stroke volume induced by changes in preload during PPV. Thus, any of the continuous measures of cardiac

---

TABLE 65.9

FACTORS THAT INFLUENCE PRELOAD

Blood volume
Venous capacitance
Intrathoracic pressure
Filling time
Atrioventricular synchrony
Diastolic function
Ventricular compliance
Pericardial restraint
Atrioventricular valve competency
Pulmonary artery pressure

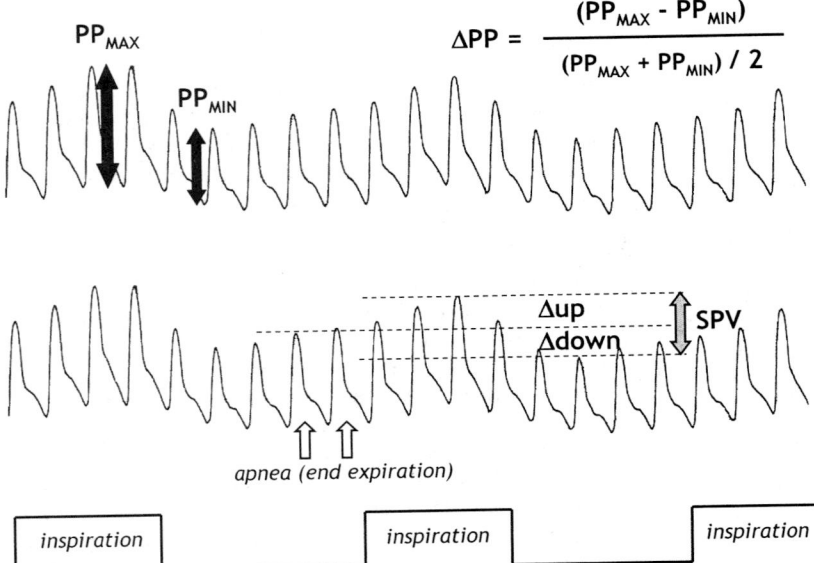

$$\Delta PP = \frac{(PP_{MAX} - PP_{MIN})}{(PP_{MAX} + PP_{MIN}) / 2}$$

FIGURE 65.17. Measures of arterial blood pressure variability during mechanical ventilation. Large variability of the arterial pressure suggests that measures to increase preload (e.g., fluid volume administration) will increase stroke volume. The **top panel** demonstrates the calculations for pulse pressure variability (ΔPP). The **bottom panel** shows calculations for systolic pressure variation. At commencement of inspiration with PPV, an initial rise in systolic blood pressure (Δup) occurs, possibly due to the emptying of pulmonary capacitance vessels and secondary to the effect of decreasing afterload. However, the positive-pressure breath also decreases systemic venous return and, thus, right-heart preload, which is transferred to the left heart by the end of the inspiratory breath and continues into early expiration. The net effect is a drop in systolic blood pressure ($\Delta down$), which will return to baseline by end of expiration. Systolic pressure variation (SPV) is merely the sum of Δup and $\Delta down$. PP_{MAX}, maximal pulse pressure, PP_{MIN}, minimal pulse pressure.

output (and hence stroke volume) may be used. It has been suggested that variations in the arterial BP trace can also be used in a similar way, although considerable debate ensues as to which of the three types of arterial variability is best. Pulse-pressure variation, SBP variation, and delta down (the downward portion of SBP variation from baseline) have all been studied (41). Regardless of the measure used, the interpretation is similar: greater variation suggests a higher probability of increasing stroke volume in response to fluid administration (Fig. 65.17).

One of the major difficulties in comparing these variability measures is the lack of standardization of the stimulus inducing the variation (PPV). Changes in preload are affected primarily by swings in pleural pressure, which in turn are affected by tidal volume and transmural pressure gradient across the lung (which are influenced by factors such as pulmonary edema, lung consolidation, etc.). Thus, potential exists for inducing both false-positive readings due to excessive ventilation as well as false-negative readings when low tidal volumes are used. For this reason, tidal volumes of at least 8 mL/kg (16) should be used.

Diastolic Function

The fact that heart failure may occur in the presence of preserved systolic function has been appreciated since the mid-1980s. Diastolic function is crucial to maintaining an adequate cardiac output; yet, measurement of this entity remains challenging. Diastole is defined as the period from the end of aortic ejection (aortic valve closure) until the onset of ventricular tension that occurs with the following beat. It is an energy-consuming process, which is influenced by both active and passive mechanisms (66). Active processes primarily influence relaxation, which largely center on regulation of cytosolic calcium (Ca^{2+}) levels. Passive processes affect ventricular stiffness and involve mainly external factors, including viscoelastic

properties of the extracellular matrix and changes in both diastolic load and afterload.

Intracardiac pressure and volume measurements allow quantification of the active and passive components of diastolic function. Active relaxation can be estimated by (a) the time constant of isovolumic pressure decline (the time for ventricular pressure to fall by approximately two-thirds), (b) the isovolumic relaxation time, or (c) the maximum rate of pressure decay (–dP/dt). Passive stiffness can be estimated by the diastolic slope of the pressure-volume curve (24).

Unfortunately, the ability to measure diastolic function at the bedside is limited in pediatric practice. The most common technique is Doppler echocardiography. A variety of Doppler-derived parameters can be used to estimate (a) and (b) above and to examine patterns of mitral valve and pulmonary venous flow during LV filling (including mitral E- and A-wave velocities). A related parameter is the myocardial performance index (Tei index), which is said to measure aspects of both systolic and diastolic function (19). Unfortunately, most of these measures are affected by many factors, including age, heart rate, afterload, volume status, and ventricular filling. Attention has focused toward Doppler tissue imaging indices (40); however, the utility of Doppler tissue imaging as a monitoring tool is in its infancy in pediatrics.

Contractility

Gold standard measures of contractility, such as end-systolic elastance and preload recruitable stroke work are measured using intracardiac impedance and are thus seldom used at the bedside (Fig. 65.14). Stroke work represents the area enclosed by the ventricular pressure-volume loop; however, this may be estimated by the product of stroke volume and arterial pressure measurements (Table 65.7). Although not a true measure of contractility, it allows some insight into cardiac reserve, namely, how stroke volume changes in the face of changing afterload.

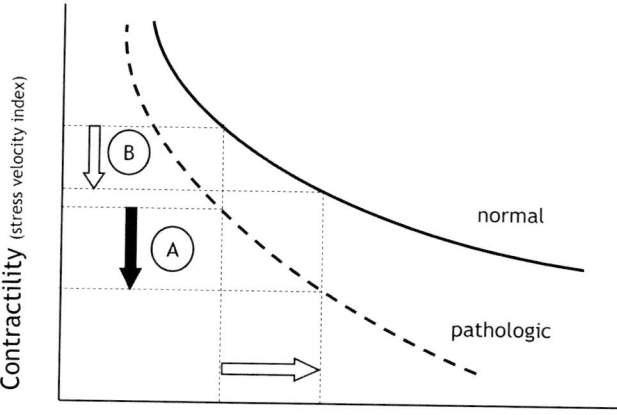

FIGURE 65.18. The contractility-afterload relationship can be estimated echocardiographically by plotting the stress velocity index (velocity of circumferential muscle fiber shortening corrected for heart rate) against wall stress. This relationship can change in acute illness in two ways: (a) the x-intercept can shift to the left, meaning that a reduction in absolute contractility occurs for a given afterload; and (b) the negative gradient can become steeper, meaning that a greater reduction in contractility is seen for a comparable increase in afterload. This is shown for the pathologic contractility afterload curve (**dashed**), where a given increase in afterload produces a larger reduction in contractility (**A**) than that seen under normal conditions (**B**).

Transpulmonary thermodilution allows for derivation of the cardiac function index, defined as stroke volume divided by global end-diastolic volume. Said to be a load-independent measure of contractility, little is known about its application in pediatric practice.

The echocardiographic stress velocity index (**Fig. 65.18**) elaborates on the contractility-afterload relationship by plotting stress velocity (contractility) against end-systolic wall stress (afterload). The slope of this relationship with changes in afterload helps to identify cardiac pathologies (12). Unfortunately, widespread adoption of this technique has been limited by the need for specialized software and significant user expertise.

The shortening fraction (SF), or percent change, in ventricular diameter is a convenient measure of global systolic function, such that:

$$SF = 100 \times (\text{end-diastolic dimension}$$
$$- \text{end-systolic dimension})/(\text{end-diastolic dimension})$$

Normal SF values are 29%–41%. SF is not a reliable measure of systolic function when ventricular geometry or regional wall motion is abnormal. Furthermore, SF is load dependent. Therefore, even though intrinsic ventricular contractility is identical in two different patients, the patient with decreased preload will evidence lower SF. The ejection fraction (EF) provides similar information as the SF but uses the percent change in end-diastolic *volume*, such that:

$$EF = 100 \times (\text{end-diastolic volume}$$
$$- \text{end-systolic volume})/(\text{end-diastolic volume})$$

The normal EF in children is 60% ± 7%.

Doppler tissue imaging is a relatively new modality that may provide information on contractility as well as diastolic function (40).

Afterload

Afterload is the net force opposing LV fiber shortening during ventricular ejection and is quantified as LV wall stress (34). Wall stress is best measured at end systole and requires measurement of transmural ventricular pressure, LV end-systolic dimension, and wall thickness. The latter two variables are measured using echocardiography. The LV transmural pressure (LV_{tm}) equals the difference between intraventricular and extraventricular pressures. LV intracavitary pressure (LV_{ic}) may be estimated from the MAP; however, accurate quantification of extraventricular pressure is difficult and may involve balloon measurement of esophageal or pleural pressure (P_{pl}). Understanding wall stress allows for an appreciation of how factors that increase intrathoracic pressure, such as PPV, result in a reduction in afterload. The following example illustrates this point. A child develops respiratory distress shortly after extubation on the second day following a cardiac surgical repair. The oxygen requirement increases while peripheral perfusion worsens, at which point the following pressures are noted:

$$MAP = (LV_{ic}) = 60 \text{ mm Hg}$$
$$P_{pl} = -20 \text{ mm Hg}$$
$$\text{hence, } LV_{tm} = LV_{ic} - P_{pl} = 60 - (-20) = 80 \text{ mm Hg.}$$

The child is promptly reintubated and placed on PPV. At the instant of reintubation, only P_{pl} increases, such that:

$$MAP = LV_{ic} = 60 \text{ mm Hg}$$
$$P_{pl} = 10 \text{ mm Hg}$$
$$\text{hence, } LV_{tm} = LV_{ic} - P_{pl} = 60 - (10) = 50 \text{ mm Hg.}$$

The sole act of reintubation has decreased LV_{tm} and, therefore, wall stress and afterload. The child's peripheral perfusion now improves steadily.

Systemic vascular resistance is a derived measure of small-vessel resistance to nonpulsatile flow. As such, it should be regarded as a *contributor to* rather than being *synonymous with* afterload. Systemic vascular resistance utilizes Ohm's law to measure the ratio of mean pressure drop across the systemic vascular bed to the flow via the formula:

$$SVRI = \frac{79.9 \times (MAP - CVP)}{\text{cardiac index}}$$

where SVRI = systemic vascular resistance index; and units of measurement are dyn-sec/cm^5/m^2).

CONCLUSIONS AND FUTURE DIRECTIONS

Intravascular pressure measurement remains the cornerstone of hemodynamic monitoring. However, technologic advances in the last decade have made available a variety of techniques for bedside measurement of cardiovascular function. Unsurprisingly, all have limitations; the choice of technique often represents a trade-off between invasiveness, accuracy, repeatability, response mode (continuous versus intermittent), risk, and user expertise.

It is likely that future developments will expand upon three current trends: (a) the provision of methods that are less invasive, continuous and require a modest amount of user expertise; (b) exploration of new measures of the components of cardiac output (heart rate, preload, diastolic function, contractility, and afterload); and (c) interpretation of these parameters in a clinical context, rather than as isolated numbers (for example, fluid responsiveness rather than preload).

KEY POINTS

- Clinical examination and an appreciation of cardiovascular physiological principles are vital prerequisites to hemodynamic monitoring. Pressure and flow measurements should be an adjunct to clinical examination and decision making based on the aggregate integrated information obtained over time.
- Pattern recognition plays an important role in interpretation of hemodynamic signals.
- An appreciation of the advantages and limitations of current monitoring technology is crucial.
- Measures of flow should always be interpreted with other markers of adequacy of flow.
- A small, but growing number of techniques for quantification of preload, diastolic function, contractility and afterload are now available and increasingly being deployed in the PICU.

References

1. American Heart Association. Pediatric Advanced Life Support 1997–1999. Emergency cardiovascular care programs. American Heart Association, 1997.
2. Arfors KE, Malmberg P, Pavek K. Conservation of thermal indicator in lung circulation. *Cardiovasc Res* 1971;5:530–4.
3. Behrends M, Kernbach M, Brauer A, et al. In vitro validation of a metabolic monitor for gas exchange measurements in ventilated neonates. *Intensive Care Med* 2001;27:228–35.
4. Bloos F, Reinhart K. Venous oximetry. *Intensive Care Med* 2005;31:911–13.
5. Carcillo JA, Fields AI. Clinical practice parameters for hemodynamic support of pediatric and neonatal patients in septic shock. *Crit Care Med* 2002;30:1365–78.
6. Castle RA, Dunne CJ, Mok Q, et al. Accuracy of displayed values of tidal volume in the pediatric intensive care unit. *Crit Care Med* 2002;30:2566–74.
7. Ceneviva G, Paschall JA, Maffei F, et al. Hemodynamic support in fluid-refractory pediatric septic shock. *Pediatrics* 1998;102:e19.
8. Centers for Disease Control and Prevention. Guidelines for the Prevention of Intravascular Catheter-Related Infections. *MMWR* 2002;51(RR-10):1–29.
9. Chait HI, Kuhn MA, Baum VC. Inferior vena caval pressure reliably predicts right atrial pressure in pediatric cardiac surgical patients. *Crit Care Med* 1994;22(2):219–24.
10. Chambrin, MC. Alarms in the intensive care unit: How can the number of false alarms be reduced? *Critical Care Medicine* 2001;5:184–8.
11. Cholley BP, Singer M. Esophageal Doppler: Noninvasive cardiac output monitor. *Echocardiography* 2003;20:763–9.
12. Colan SD, Borow KM, Neumann A. Left ventricular end-systolic wall stress-velocity of fiber shortening relation: A load-independent index of myocardial contractility. *J Am Coll Cardiol* 1984;4:715–24.
13. Connors AF Jr. , Speroff T, Dawson NV, et al. The effectiveness of right heart catheterization in the initial care of critically ill patients. SUPPORT Investigators. *JAMA* 1996;276:889–97.
14. Coudray A, Romand JA, Treggiari M, et al. Fluid responsiveness in spontaneously breathing patients: A review of indexes used in intensive care. *Crit Care Med.* 2005;33:2757–62.
15. Dart AM, Kingwell BA. Pulse pressure: A review of mechanisms and clinical relevance. *J Am Coll Cardiol* 2001;37:975–84.
16. De Backer D, Heenen S, Piagnerelli M, et al. Pulse pressure variations to predict fluid responsiveness: Influence of tidal volume. *Intensive Care Med* 2005;31:517–23.
17. De Vaal JB, de Wilde RB, van den Berg PC, et al. Less invasive determination of cardiac output from the arterial pressure by aortic diameter-calibrated pulse contour. *Br J Anaesth.* 2005;95:326–31.
18. Edwards JD, Mayall RM. Importance of the sampling site for measurement of mixed venous oxygen saturation in shock. *Crit Care Med* 1998;26:1356–60.
19. Eidem BW, O'Leary PW, Tei C, et al. Usefulness of the myocardial performance index for assessing right ventricular function in congenital heart disease. *Am J Cardiol* 2000;86:654–8.
20. Fishman AP. Respiratory gases in the regulation of the pulmonary circulation. *Physiol Rev* 1961;41:214–79.
21. Flori HR, Johnson LD, Hanley FL, et al. Transthoracic intracardiac catheters in pediatric patients recovering from congenital heart defect surgery: Associated complications and outcomes. *Crit Care Med* 2000;28(8):2997–3001.
22. Fuller HD. The validity of cardiac output measurement by thoracic impedance: A meta-analysis. *Clin Invest Med* 1992;15:103–12.
23. Gladden LB. Lactate metabolism: A new paradigm for the third millennium. *J Physiol* 2004;558:5–30.
24. Hamlin SK, Villars PS, Kanusky JT, et al. Role of diastole in left ventricular function, II: Diagnosis and treatment. *Am J Crit Care* 2004;13:453–66.
25. Hansen S, Staber M. Oscillometric blood pressure measurement used for calibration of the arterial tonometry method contributes significantly to error. *Eur J Anaesthiol* 2006;23(9):781–7.
26. Hatherill M, McIntyre AG, Wattie M, et al. Early hyperlactataemia in critically ill children. *Intensive Care Med* 2000;26:314–8.
27. Heulitt MJ, Farrington EA, O'Shea TM, et al. Double-blind, randomized, controlled trial of papaverine-containing infusions to prevent failure of arterial catheters in pediatric patients. *Crit Care Med* 1993;21(6):825–9.
28. James JH, Luchette FA, McCarter FD, et al. Lactate is an unreliable indicator of tissue hypoxia in injury or sepsis. *Lancet* 1999;354:505–8.
29. Janik JE, Conlon SJ, Janik JS. Percutaneous central access in patients younger than 5 years: Size does matter. *J Pediatr Surg* 2004;39:1252–356.
30. Jansen JRC, Schreuder JJ, Settels JJ, et al. An adequate strategy for the thermodilution technique in patients during mechanical ventilation. *Intensive Care Med* 1990;16:422–5.
31. Karlsson T, Stjernstrom EL, Stjernstrom H, et al. Lactate metabolism and hypocarbic hyperventilation. An experimental study in piglets. *Acta Anaesthesiol Scand* 1995;39(1):109–17.
32. Kleinman B. The fast-flush test—is the clinical comparison equivalent to its in vitro stimulation? *J Clin Monit Comput* 1998;14:485.
33. Kolkman JJ, Otte JA, Groeneveld AB. Gastrointestinal luminal PCO2 tonometry: An update on physiology, methodology, and clinical applications. *Br J Anaesth* 2000;84:74–86.
34. Lang RM, Borow KM, Neumann A, et al. Systemic vascular resistance: An unreliable index of left ventricular afterload. *Circulation* 1986;74:1114–23.
35. Levy B, Gibot S, Franck P, et al. Relation between muscle Na^+,K^+-ATPase activity and raised lactate concentrations in septic shock: A prospective study. *Lancet* 2005;365:871–5.
36. Lichtwarck-Aschoff M, Beale R, Pfeiffer UJ. Central venous pressure, pulmonary artery occlusion pressure, intrathoracic blood volume, and right ventricular end-diastolic volume as indicators of cardiac preload. *J Crit Care* 1996;11:180–8.
37. Light RB. Intrapulmonary oxygen consumption in experimental pneumococcal pneumonia. *J Appl Physiol.* 1988;64:2490–5.
38. Lima A, Bakker J. Noninvasive monitoring of peripheral perfusion. *Intensive Care Med* 2005;31:316–26.
39. Maciel AT, Creteur J, Vincent JL. Tissue capnometry: Does the answer lie under the tongue? *Intensive Care Med* 2004;30(12):2157–65.
40. Maclaren G, Kluger R, Prior D, Royse A, Royse C. Tissue Doppler, strain, and strain rate echocardiography: Principles and potential perioperative applications. *J Cardiothorac Vasc Anesth* 2006;20:583–93.
41. Magder S. Clinical usefulness of respiratory variations in arterial pressure. *Am J Respir Crit Care Med* 2004;169:151–5.
42. Monagle P, Chan A, Massicotte P, et al. Antithrombotic therapy in children: The Seventh ACCP Conference on Antithrombotic and Thrombolytic Therapy. *Chest* 2004;126(3 Suppl):645S–87S.
43. Nichols WW, O'Rourke MF, eds. *McDonald's Blood Flow in Arteries, 5th ed.* London: Arnold, 2005.
44. Nishikawa T, Dohi S. Errors in the measurement of cardiac output by thermodilution. *Can J Anaesth* 1993;40:142–53.
45. Parati G. Non-invasive beat-to-beat blood pressure monitoring: New developments. *Blood Press Monit* 2003;8(1):31–6.
46. Perloff, D, Grim C, Flack J, et al. Human blood pressure determination by sphygmomanometry. *Circulation* 1993;88:2460–70.
47. Reinhart K, Kuhn HJ, Hartog C, et al. Continuous central venous and pulmonary artery oxygen saturation monitoring in the critically ill. *Intensive Care Med* 2004;30:1572–8.
48. Rivers E, Nguyen B, Havstad S, et al. Early goal-directed therapy in the treatment of severe sepsis and septic shock. *N Engl J Med* 2001;345:1368–77.
49. Salim MA, DiSessa TG, Arheart KL, et al. Contribution of superior vena caval flow to total cardiac output in children. A Doppler echocardiographic study. *Circulation* 1995;92:1860–5.
50. Sandham JD, Hull RD, Brant RF, et al. A randomized, controlled trial of the use of pulmonary-artery catheters in high-risk surgical patients. *N Engl J Med* 2003;348(1):5–14.
51. Santini F, Gatti G, Borghetti V, et al. Routine left atrial catheterization for the post-operative management of cardiac surgical patients: Is the risk justified?. *Eur J Cardiothorac Surg* 1999;16(2):218–21.
52. Schulze A, Abubakar K, Gill G, et al. Pulmonary oxygen consumption: A hypothesis to explain the increase in oxygen consumption of low birth weight infants with lung disease. *Intensive Care Med* 2001;27:1636–42.
53. Shephard JN, Brecker SJ, Evans TW. Bedside assessment of myocardial performance in the critically ill. *Intensive Care Med* 1994;20:513–21.

54. Skinner JR, Milligan DW, Hunter S, et al. Central venous pressure in the ventilated neonate. *Arch Dis Child* 1992;67:374–7.

55. Stetz CW, Miller RG, Kelly GE, et al. Reliability of the thermodilution method in the determination of cardiac output in clinical practice. *Am Rev Respir Dis* 1982;126:1001–4.

56. Sun XG, Hansen JE, Stringer WW, et al. Carbon dioxide pressure-concentration relationship in arterial and mixed venous blood during exercise. *J Appl Physiol* 2001;90:1798–810.

57. Thomas JD, Popovic ZB. Assessment of left ventricular function by cardiac ultrasound. *J Am Coll Cardiol* 2006;48(10):2012–25.

58. Thompson AE. Pulmonary artery catheterization in children. *New Horiz* 1997;5:244–50.

59. Tibby SM, Hatherill M, Marsh MJ, et al. Clinical validation of cardiac output measurements using femoral artery thermodilution with direct Fick in ventilated children and infants. *Intensive Care Med* 1997;23:987–91.

60. Tibby SM, Hatherill M, Marsh MJ, et al. Clinicians' abilities to estimate cardiac index in ventilated children and infants. *Arch Dis Child* 1997;77:516–8.

61. Tibby SM, Hatherill M, Murdoch IA. Capillary refill and core-peripheral temperature gap as indicators of haemodynamic status in paediatric intensive care patients. *Arch Dis Child* 1999;80:163–6.

62. Tibby SM, Hatherill M, Murdoch IA. Use of transesophageal Doppler ultrasonography in ventilated pediatric patients: Derivation of cardiac output. *Crit Care Med* 2000;28:2045–50.

63. Tibby SM, Murdoch IA. Monitoring cardiac function in intensive care. *Arch Dis Child* 2003;88:46–52.

64. Tortoriello TA, Stayer SA, Mott AR, et al. A noninvasive estimation of mixed venous oxygen saturation using near-infrared spectroscopy by cerebral oximetry in pediatric cardiac surgery patients. *Paediatr Anaesth* 2005;15(6):495–503.

65. Ultman JS, Bursztein S. Analysis of error in the determination of respiratory gas exchange at varying FIO_2. *J Appl Physiol* 1981;350:210–6.

66. Villars PS, Hamlin SK, Shaw AD, et al. Role of diastole in left ventricular function, I: Biochemical and biomechanical events. *Am J Crit Care* 2004;13:394–403.

67. von Spiegel T, Hoeft A. Transpulmonary indicator methods in intensive medicine. *Anaesthesist* 1998;47:220–8.

68. Wesseling KH, Jansen JR, Settels JJ, et al. Computation of aortic flow from pressure in humans using a nonlinear, three-element model. *J Appl Physiol* 1993;74:2566–73.

69. Whyte RK. Mixed venous oxygen saturation in the newborn. Can we and should we measure it? *Scand J Clin Lab Invest* 1990;50(Suppl 203):203–11.

70. Wilkinson JL. Haemodynamic calculations in the catheter laboratory. *Heart* 2001;85(1):113–20.

71. Zierler K. Indicator dilution methods for measuring blood flow, volume, and other properties of biological systems: A brief history and memoir. *Ann Biomed Eng* 2000;28:836–48.

CHAPTER 66A ■ HEART FAILURE IN INFANTS AND CHILDREN: ETIOLOGY, PATHOPHYSIOLOGY, AND DIAGNOSIS OF HEART FAILURE

JEFFREY J. KIM • JOSEPH W. ROSSANO • DAVID P. NELSON • JACK F. PRICE • WILLIAM J. DREYER

Heart failure is a multifaceted syndrome that affects many patients in the PICU. This chapter is divided in to three sections that provide a detailed overview of: Etiology, Pathophysiology, and Diagnosis of Heart Failure (Section A), Cardiomyopathy (Section B), and Myocarditis (Section C). The treatment of heart failure is detailed in Chapter 67.

Heart failure in infants and children can be a difficult disease process to assess and treat. Many of the classic physical exam findings that students are taught in medical school, such as crackles, jugular venous pulsations, and pedal edema, frequently are not found on examination of a child with heart failure. Common adult risk factors and comorbidities such as smoking and diabetes are often not considered when taking the history of a child with ventricular dysfunction. No standard functional classification exists for children with left ventricular (LV) dysfunction and congestive heart failure (CHF). Despite the advances in understanding of heart failure management in adults, few large, randomized, placebo-controlled studies have been performed that assess the safety and efficacy of medical therapies for heart failure in children. Much accepted practice comes by way of adopting proven treatments used in adult. Even the terms used to describe heart failure in children seem inadequate for the disease processes that they represent.

A paradigm shift has occurred in the way heart failure is considered and defined. Previously, heart failure was described as a condition in which the heart was unable to maintain an adequate cardiac output to meet the metabolic demands of the body. Increased understanding of the important molecular and neurohormonal changes that occur in heart failure have engendered a new way to think about heart failure. Arnold Katz has defined heart failure as "a clinical syndrome in which heart disease reduces cardiac output, increases venous pressures, and is accompanied by molecular abnormalities that cause progressive deterioration of the failing heart and premature myocardial cell death" (35). If heart failure is a clinical syndrome, then it is not ventricular dysfunction, nor is it valvar insufficiency or pulmonary overcirculation. *Heart failure is a constellation of structural and functional abnormalities, elevated filling pressures, neurohormonal activation, and signs or symptoms.* When heart failure is mentioned in this section, the discussion is referring to this clinical syndrome of heart failure just described.

Reference to acute decompensated heart failure (DHF) includes acute cardiovascular failure and shock, as well as the situation of exacerbated preexisting heart failure symptoms. In adults, decompensated heart failure remains an enormous clinical burden to the population. According to statistics, >500,000 new cases of heart failure are diagnosed annually, with a lifetime risk of ~1 in 5 (43). Most of these patients will likely struggle with bouts of acute and, possibly, chronic decompensation (10). The incidence of decompensated heart failure in children is significantly lower than it is in adults. However, it is an important disease process and is becoming increasingly more common as survival of children with congenital heart disease and primary myocardial disease continues to increase. When decompensated heart failure persists, cardiac transplant is often required. The leading diagnosis that results in transplantation in pediatric patients is primary myocardial disorders, although palliated congenital heart disease is quickly becoming more frequent, emphasizing the evolving demographics of this patient population.

ETIOLOGY OF HEART FAILURE IN CHILDREN

Pediatric heart failure can manifest itself in both acquired and congenital forms with etiologies as disparate as structural, metabolic, and environmental in origin. The following are features of some of the more common causes of heart failure in childhood.

Heart Failure Due to Structural Heart Disease

Excessive Pulmonary Blood Flow

Symptomatic pulmonary overcirculation is a markedly different form of heart failure than the classic descriptions of CHF described in adults. Ventricular systolic function is usually preserved in lesions that are associated with a large net left-to-right shunt, and low cardiac output is not a typical finding in this situation. However, if heart failure is thought of as a clinical syndrome characterized by elevated filling pressures, compensatory activation of the neurohormonal system, and progressive symptomatology, however, pulmonary overcirculation certainly deserves to be recognized within the spectrum of heart failure.

As in heart failure due to LV dysfunction, circulatory adaptive mechanisms are employed in symptomatic pulmonary overcirculation to preserve cardiac output and end organ perfusion. The sympathetic nervous system is activated and plasma levels of *norepinephrine* increase, stimulating the renin-angiotensin-aldosterone system, causing peripheral vasoconstriction and increasing the heart rate. Plasma norepinephrine concentrations are elevated in infants and children with heart failure due to left-to-right shunting lesions, and these concentrations normalize after surgical repair of the structural defects. Likewise, plasma levels of *arginine vasopressin (antidiuretic hormone)*, a neurohormone that causes peripheral vasoconstriction and free water retention, are also increased in children with heart failure due to shunting lesions, as well as in situations of ventricular dysfunction (55). *Natriuretic peptides* are secreted by the atria and ventricles in response to myocardial stretch due to pressure or volume loads on the heart. Plasma levels of atrial natriuretic peptide and B-type natriuretic peptide (BNP) are elevated in children with congenital heart disease and correlate with $Q_p:Q_s$ in patients with left-to-right intracardiac shunts (42).

In acyanotic heart lesions such as ventricular septal defect and complete atrioventricular canal defect, signs and symptoms of heart failure usually develop during the first few weeks of life, after the pulmonary vascular resistance has fallen. Signs such as tachypnea, retractions, grunting, and diaphoresis with feeding usually herald this change in physiology. Other acyanotic lesions also associated with large left-to-right shunting include the patent ductus arteriosus, aortopulmonary window, and systemic arteriovenous malformations. These typical "run off" lesions may manifest with signs of heart failure in the first few days (in premature infants) or weeks of life, with bounding pulses in addition to signs of respiratory compromise. If left uncorrected, over time, these defects can lead to pulmonary vascular disease.

Cyanotic cardiac defects can also be associated with pulmonary overcirculation and heart failure, and include truncus arteriosus, total anomalous pulmonary venous connection, double-outlet right ventricle (RV) without pulmonary valvar stenosis, and single ventricle lesions (both palliated and unpalliated) without obstructed pulmonary blood flow. In these lesions, an admixture of highly oxygen-saturated and less-saturated blood occurs at the atrial, ventricular, or great arterial level, and the mixed blood is then sent to the pulmonary and systemic circulations, preferring the path of least resistance. Chest x-ray may reveal increased pulmonary vascular markings despite low systemic arterial oxygen saturations. Classic signs of heart failure are also seen in infants with unrepaired or nonpalliated forms of cyanotic pulmonary overcirculation and include cardiomegaly, hepatomegaly, tachypnea, and poor weight gain.

Pressure Overload

Some forms of congenital heart disease can manifest with signs of heart failure in the early newborn period (first 3 days of life). Infants with critical aortic stenosis may present shortly after birth with shock or cyanosis. Critical coarctation of the aorta or interrupted aortic arch may also present in the first few days of life as the ductus arteriosus closes. These left-sided obstructive lesions often coexist, and the clinical spectrum can vary between an isolated bicuspid aortic valve with minimal obstruction to hypoplastic left heart syndrome. The RV will

support the systemic circulation in the setting of a widely patent ductus arteriosus. When the ductus closes, however, the RV cannot adequately perfuse the systemic circulation, resulting in a profound metabolic acidosis and, if untreated, multiorgan system failure and death.

Ventricular dysfunction caused by systemic hypertension can also lead to heart failure. Although rare in children, system hypertension is thought to be the etiology of dilated cardiomyopathy (DCM) with depressed myocardial function in pediatric patients with neuroblastoma and Wilms tumor. In neuroblastoma, high levels of circulating catecholamines cause peripheral vasoconstriction and raise systemic vascular resistance. Additionally, norepinephrine is directly toxic to the myocardium, and a protracted period of high concentrations is thought to result in myocyte dropout and apoptosis. Patients with Wilms tumor may have high circulating levels of rennin, which also increases systemic vascular resistance. Treatment of these tumors can lead to reverse remodeling of the myocardium and improved ventricular function. Other causes of systemic hypertension (e.g., renal artery stenosis, nephritis) in children may also lead to ventricular dysfunction and heart failure, but these diseases usually initially manifest with ventricular hypertrophy.

Valvular Insufficiency

Pulmonary valvular insufficiency that causes RV dysfunction or progressive heart failure is usually a result of previous surgery or catheter-based interventions on the pulmonary valve. Congenital forms of pulmonary insufficiency are also recognized, such as absent pulmonary valve syndrome. Most patients who undergo surgical correction of tetralogy of Fallot are left with some degree of pulmonary insufficiency. In the previous surgical era, a great majority of patients who received a transannular incision of the RV outflow tract developed moderate-to-severe pulmonary insufficiency. Similarly, balloon valvuloplasty of a stenotic pulmonary valve can result in significant regurgitation. Most patients tolerate this volume load on the RV and do not develop symptoms until several years after onset of ventricular dilation. However, once symptoms develop, RV failure usually progresses to an end-stage in which treatment strategies are unlikely to promote reverse remodeling.

Acute and chronic aortic insufficiency can cause LV dysfunction and heart failure. Dilation of the aortic root is a frequent cause of chronic aortic insufficiency and can be seen in patients with Marfan syndrome and other congenital conditions. Aortic root dilation has also been identified as a late finding following surgery for transposition of the great arteries and tetralogy of Fallot (9,59). Patients with a bicuspid aortic valve are also at risk for eventual aortic root dilation and concomitant aortic insufficiency (51).

Acute aortic insufficiency can also result from dissection of the aorta or rupture of a sinus of Valsalva aneurysm, secondary to trauma or endocarditis. These patients are typically quite ill and may present in shock. In acute aortic insufficiency, aortic and LV pressures reach an equilibrium. LV dilation does not occur and, as the end-diastolic pressure acutely rises, pressure is transmitted back to the left atrium, leading to pulmonary edema (3) (**Fig. 66A.1**). Immediate surgical intervention is necessary for survival. In moderate-to-severe chronic aortic insufficiency, the increased volume and pressure load on the LV can lead to ventricular hypertrophy and dilation. Over time, chamber dilation progresses and myocardial dysfunction ensues with

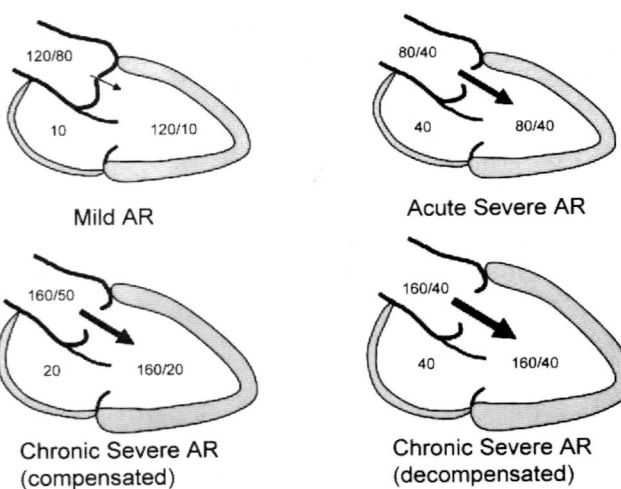

Mild AR

Acute Severe AR

Chronic Severe AR (compensated)

Chronic Severe AR (decompensated)

FIGURE 66A.1. Different stages of aortic regurgitation (AR). (**A**) In mild AR, LV size, function, and hemodynamics are normal. (**B**) In acute severe AR, there is equilibration of aortic and LV pressures (80/40 mmHg in this example). Left atrial pressure is elevated, leading to pulmonary edema. (**C**) In chronic severe, compensated AR, the LV may begin to dilate, but LV ejection fraction is often maintained in the normal range by increased preload. Systolic arterial hypertension and a wide pulse pressure are present. However, LV filling pressures are normal or only slightly elevated, such that dyspnea is absent. (**D**) In decompensated chronic severe AR, the LV is dilated and hypertrophied, and LV function is often depressed as a result of afterload excess. Forward output is decreased, leading to fatigue and other low-output symptoms. Fibrosis and hypertrophy decrease LV compliance, leading to increased filling pressures and dyspnea. From Bekeredjian R, Grayburn PA. Valvular heart disease: Aortic regurgitation. *Circulation* 2005;112:125–34, with permission.

a decrease in LV ejection fraction. In decompensated chronic aortic insufficiency, patients develop symptoms of heart failure as elevated left heart pressures are transmitted to the pulmonary veins, causing congestion and exertional dyspnea.

Tricuspid regurgitation is an uncommon cause of heart failure in children. Clinically significant tricuspid regurgitation is most often seen in patients with Ebstein anomaly, a congenital defect of the heart in which the annular attachments of the tricuspid valve are displaced toward the apex of the RV. The ventricle becomes divided into an "atrialized" inlet portion and functional apical and infundibular portions. The tricuspid valve leaflets fail to coapt, causing severe tricuspid regurgitation and right atrial enlargement. Prograde pulmonary blood flow may be significantly compromised, and RV function may eventually deteriorate. Patients diagnosed in the newborn or infant period have the most severe form of the disease and develop signs of heart failure early on. The mortality rate is high among patients who require surgical intervention at this age. Older individuals with less severe disease may develop symptoms of right heart failure, including hepatomegaly, jugular venous distention, peripheral edema, and dyspnea with exertion. Atrial arrhythmias are also common in this cohort. Other causes of significant tricuspid regurgitation include endocarditis and tricuspid valvar dysplasia.

Mitral regurgitation is a common finding in pediatric heart failure, usually as a consequence of ventricular dysfunction and LV enlargement, rather than as an isolated cause of heart failure. In the setting of DCM and heart failure, progressive cham-

ber dilation causes the mitral valve annulus to stretch. The mitral valve leaflets fail to coapt, and regurgitation of blood into the left atrium results. Symptoms of pulmonary venous congestion develop as LV filling pressures increase. Isolated mitral valve disease can occur due to ischemia/infarction of a papillary muscle, trauma, or inflammatory disease processes, or it may be congenital in origin. When mitral regurgitation is not a result of DCM, the LV progressively dilates as a result of the volume load, and contractility is usually maintained or increased, as afterload is decreased. Eventually, as the regurgitant volume increases, LV function deteriorates and symptoms of heart failure ensue. Symptomatic mitral regurgitation carries a poor prognosis in children, especially when associated with significant LV dysfunction.

Congenital and acquired *mitral stenosis* rarely affects pediatric patients. Parachute mitral valve, double-orifice mitral valve, and mitral arcade are all morphologic subtypes of the congenitally stenotic mitral valve. Symptoms generally develop from left atrial hypertension and pulmonary congestion. With advanced disease, systemic cardiac output may be limited.

Right Heart Failure

Right heart failure in children is usually a result of a chronic volume and/or pressure overload on the RV, which often occurs in patients who have undergone surgery on the RV outflow tract (e.g., tetralogy of Fallot, truncus arteriosus, pulmonary atresia with ventricular septal defect, etc.) and are left with significant residual regurgitation or stenosis. RV dysplasia, an inherited cardiomyopathy characterized by RV dysfunction and dysrhythmias, is an uncommon form of right heart failure in children.

Low Cardiac Output Syndrome Following Cardiac Surgery

The most common heart failure clinical scenario in the cardiac intensive care setting is the postoperative surgical patient with low cardiac output syndrome. Over the past few decades, significant advances in surgical techniques and pediatric cardiac intensive care have contributed to marked improvement in morbidity and mortality following pediatric heart surgery. Despite these improvements, patients remain at risk for low cardiac output and impaired systemic oxygen delivery, especially in the early postoperative period. This transient drop in cardiac output after cardiac surgery has been referred to as low cardiac output syndrome. In the early postoperative period, this syndrome is due primarily to transient myocardial dysfunction, compounded by acute changes in myocardial loading conditions, including postoperative increases in systemic and/or pulmonary vascular resistance. Residual cardiac abnormalities, even if minor, may further aggravate an underlying low output state. Surgical repair of cardiac malformations exposes the myocardium to periods of ischemia, resulting in transient myocardial stunning or damage. Cardiopulmonary bypass, which activates the complement and inflammatory cascades (25), also contributes to myocardial injury, alterations in pulmonary and systemic vascular reactivity, and pulmonary dysfunction (1,6). In addition, some repairs require ventriculotomy, which further exacerbates myocardial dysfunction.

Although advances in myocardial protection, cardioplegia, and perfusion techniques have dramatically reduced perioperative cardiovascular injury, even relatively simple cardiac procedures are still associated with measurable myocardial dysfunction.

Several studies have documented the predictable and reproducible fall in cardiac output after congenital heart surgery in neonates, infants, and young children (14,66). In an early study of neonates who underwent arterial-switch operation, the median decrease in cardiac index, which occurred typically 6–12 hrs after cardiopulmonary bypass, was 32%. Nearly 25% of these infants had a cardiac index nadir of <2 L/min/m^2 after surgery (66). This fall in output occurs without significant changes in atrial filling pressure or inotropic support, suggesting the presence of contractile dysfunction or increased ventricular afterload, as systemic vascular resistance rises during this same period. Wall-stress analysis in patients 1–2 weeks after surgery demonstrated that myocardial function was normalized or augmented, indicating that postoperative myocardial depression in these patients was a transient phenomenon (12). Data from the multicentered PRIMACORP study (*PR*ophylactic *I*ntravenous use of *M*ilrinone *A*fter *C*ardiac *O*perations in *P*ediatrics) indicate that the incidence of postoperative low cardiac output syndrome remains significant, ranging from 10% in treated patients to 27% in control patients (31). An extensive discussion about the management of the postoperative patient is found in Chapter 70.

PATHOPHYSIOLOGY OF HEART FAILURE

Molecular and Cellular Mechanisms of Myocardial Dysfunction

Heart failure alters the structure and function of the myocardium at both the molecular and cellular levels. In particular, calcium (Ca^{2+}) dysregulation can lead to maladaptive changes in the contractile apparatus as heart failure progresses. Also, disruption of sarcomeric proteins can threaten the structural integrity of the myocardium.

In the normal heart, cellular depolarization leads to voltage-gated Ca^{2+} influx into the myocyte cytoplasm, which in turn, triggers the release of Ca^{2+} stores from the sarcoplasmic reticulum (SR) via a receptor-mediated Ca^{2+} channel known as the ryanodine receptor (RyR) channel (15). The free Ca^{2+} then interacts with critical sarcomeric components that activate the excitation-contraction process. Myocyte relaxation results from closure of the RyR channel and the rapid removal of cytosolic calcium by reuptake into the SR via an SR Ca^{2+}/ATPase pump (SERCA). Efflux of Ca^{2+} is also mediated to some degree by a sarcolemmal Na$^+$/Ca^{2+} exchanger (NCX) and a sarcolemmal calcium ATPase pump. These processes are meticulously balanced so that no net gain or loss of cellular calcium occurs with each contraction-relaxation cycle.

This complex interplay of ion pumps and exchangers, along with various modulators, often becomes dysregulated in the presence of heart failure. The ultimate outcome of this dysregulation is a significant reduction in SR Ca^{2+} levels, which decreases both the amplitude and duration of Ca^{2+} release and results in a subsequent reduction in contractile force production.

One likely mechanism for SR Ca^{2+}-store depletion in heart failure is decreased SERCA activity, which results in reduced SR loading with Ca^{2+} (29,52). Decreased SERCA expression has been clearly demonstrated in patients with heart failure, and increased SERCA expression in animal models has been shown to improve ventricular function (48,58). Other mechanisms that have been implicated in heart failure-associated calcium depletion include an increase in NCX activity and altered RyR function. Increased NCX activity leads to enhanced efflux of Ca^{2+} from the cytosol and a resultant decreased availability of intracellular Ca^{2+} for uptake into the SR. NCX overexpression has been demonstrated in animal models of ventricular remodeling and heart failure (23). RyR hyperphosphorylation, which has also been demonstrated in models of heart failure, results in a modification of its channel-gating properties, which induces diastolic leak of Ca^{2+}, leading to blunted Ca^{2+}-induced Ca^{2+} release during systole and possibly causing triggered afterdepolarizations and subsequent ventricular dysrhythmias (28). The confluence of these molecular maladaptations, among others, culminates to form the cellular basis for cardiac dysfunction.

Sarcomeric proteins and the structural integrity of the myocardium have also been shown to be violated in the presence of heart failure. In the last several years, multiple investigators have demonstrated the role of cytoskeletal proteins in cardiomyopathies and cardiac dysfunction (63). Mutations in virtually any of the sarcomeric proteins can potentially result in the above-mentioned abnormalities, and acquired defects in these proteins (as in the troponin complex) have been implicated as well. The Z-line, in particular, has drawn substantial interest in recent years. The Z-line is a subsarcolemmal, multifunctional protein complex that acts to crosslink adjacent sarcomeres (38). It also appears to play a significant role as a signaling molecule. Z-line structural or signaling function impairment has been shown to lead to ventricular dilation and heart failure (7). Dystrophin is another protein that has been strongly implicated in models of heart failure. In the stable myocyte, dystrophin and its associated complex connects the sarcomere to the sarcolemma/extracellular matrix and plays a key role in the transduction of physical force. Dystrophin has been identified as the gene responsible for the muscular dystrophies and X-linked cardiomyopathy (30). Importantly, abnormalities in dystrophin have also been noted in the ventricular myocardium of patients with end-stage cardiomyopathy regardless of etiology (65). Mechanical unloading of the heart with a ventricular-assist device has subsequently been shown to lead to reverse remodeling of dystrophin, suggesting that dystrophin may be a common molecular mechanism in myocardial dysfunction and may even be a reliable marker for the progression of heart failure (64).

Ventricular Hypertrophy in Response to Chronic Heart Failure

Ventricular hypertrophy, an important part of myocardial remodeling, occurs in response to stimuli such as hemodynamic overload, mechanical stress, or disruption of myocyte structure and function. As expected, these changes are commonly seen in the presence of chronic heart failure. Although myocardial remodeling may initially be beneficial to cardiac function, ultimately, it can result in the progression of heart failure and has been linked to the pathogenesis of cardiac dysrhythmias and sudden death.

A major stimulus for myocardial remodeling and ventricular hypertrophy is mechanical stress secondary to hemodynamic overload. Exposure of cardiac myocytes to mechanical stress results in the activation of numerous molecular signaling cascades, as well as the reactivation of fetal gene programs, which leads to cellular growth, protein synthesis, and hypertrophic changes. This process is known as "mechano-transduction." Multiple signaling pathways have been implicated in the process of mechano-transduction, and they include humoral factors, G-protein–coupled receptors, changes in calcium signaling, and the activation of numerous kinases. The most prominent of the signaling pathways will be reviewed briefly here.

Neurohumoral factors have been shown to play an essential role in the induction of cardiac hypertrophy. The renin-angiotensin system is well documented to be activated in heart failure (34). Angiotensin II is produced as a result of this cascade and has been shown to be produced in direct response to mechanical stress on the cardiomyocyte (57). Activation of angiotensin II type-1 receptors results in the induction of fetal gene programs through the action of multiple signaling protein kinases that target genes such as c-fos, c-jun, and Elk1 in the nucleus, resulting in cell growth, hypertrophy, and apoptosis (47,60). Endothelin-1 is another vasoconstrictor peptide that is produced in increased amounts in the presence of hemodynamic overload and mechanical stretch, and it has been shown to be a potent inducer of cardiac hypertrophy, as evidenced by increased protein synthesis and cell size (33).

Several lines of evidence suggest that numerous growth factors also play a role in the development of cardiac hypertrophy in the presence of heart failure. The most prominent of these is transforming growth factor-β, but other growth factors, such as fibroblast growth factor, insulin-like growth factor, and epidermal growth factor, have been implicated as well. Their action is likely mediated via protein kinases that modulate cardiac hypertrophy by phosphorylation of nuclear transcription factors such as c-jun and fos (24).

Calcineurin, an intracellular Ca^{2+}-calmodulin-activated phosphatase, has been implicated in mechanisms of heart failure associated cardiac hypertrophy. Hemodynamic overload and neurohormonal activation lead to an acute increase in sarcoplasmic free Ca^{2+}, which results in the activation of calcineurin. In coordination with other signaling transduction pathways, this leads to a hypertrophic response in the cardiomyocyte. Transgenic mice overexpressing activated calcineurin develop hypertrophic cardiomyopathy (HCM), while administration of a calcineurin inhibitor such as cyclosporine prevents a hypertrophic response at the cellular level (49).

Neurohormonal Activation and Hemodynamic Defense Mechanisms in Heart Failure

Heart failure results in a baroreceptor-mediated increase in sympathetic tone, which leads to elevated levels of circulating catecholamines, such as epinephrine and norepinephrine. This high catechol state mediates several pathophysiologic responses, including tachycardia, increased myocardial contractility, and arterial and venous vasoconstriction. In the acute setting, exaggeration of circulating catechols results in the expected tachycardia and increased myocardial contractility via sympathetic stimulation. However, over time, chronic cardiac stimulation leads to a relative catechol depletion phenomenon and downregulation of adrenergic receptors. Also, high levels of circulating catechols (e.g., norepinephrine) have been shown to be directly toxic to myocardial cells via the induction of apoptosis, likely due to calcium overload. As an adjunct to this finding, norepinephrine levels have been shown to be useful biologic markers of heart failure and have even been linked to prognosis. These data point to the fact that chronic cardiac stimulation, which is known to accompany heart failure, does indeed ultimately result in maladaptive changes.

The renin-angiotensin-aldosterone system (RAS) acts in concert with the sympathetic nervous system and is also known to be activated in heart failure, as mentioned previously. In patients with progressive heart failure, marked increases in circulating levels of renin, angiotensin II, and aldosterone are found. Angiotensin II is a potent peripheral vasoconstrictor and works both by increasing sympathetic tone and by directly stimulating angiotensin II type-1 receptors in the vasculature. Aldosterone has potent sodium-retention properties and is secreted by the adrenal gland in response to angiotensin II, adrenocorticotropic hormone, and potassium. Activation of RAS therefore leads to increased ventricular afterload and significant salt and water retention, which is clearly counterproductive in the setting of heart failure. Both increased circulating catecholamines and the upregulation of RAS are now known to play a significant role in the progression of ventricular dysfunction and heart failure in adults. In addition to the maladaptive effects that these neurohormonal systems cause to cardiovascular hemodynamics in general, norepinephrine, angiotensin II, and aldosterone have all been found to have direct toxicity on myocytes (62). Clinical studies have corroborated these findings by demonstrating an association between elevated levels of these neurohormonal markers and poor prognosis (11,17).

Natriuretic peptides are hormones that have been shown to act as a counter-regulatory system to the aforementioned pathophysiologic processes by providing beneficial effects such as vasodilation and natriuresis. The observation that infusion of atrial tissue extracts resulted in natriuresis in rats was made in 1982. Since then, three distinct, major natriuretic peptides have been isolated and synthesized: atrial natriuretic peptide, BNP, and C-type natriuretic peptide. Although genotypically different, all three have functionally been found to have potent natriuretic, diuretic, and vasorelaxant properties via their action on guanylyl cyclase-linked membrane receptors (8,40). Myocardial stretch and chamber pressure appear to be the principal mechanisms by which the natriuretic peptides are activated.

BNP is synthesized predominantly in the cardiac ventricles and is released in response to certain pathophysiologic states such as heart failure. BNP has physiologic counter-regulatory effects that ultimately lead to systemic vasodilation and natriuresis. It suppresses RAS, reducing the overall extracellular fluid volume. It also causes a sum reduction in sympathetic tone, which leads to vasorelaxation and a blunted tachycardia response. BNP infusions in humans have been shown to promote natriuresis and inhibit RAS in a manner independent of blood pressure changes (32).

Heart Failure as an Inflammatory Process

It is now understood that heart failure is often associated with a generalized perturbation of the inflammatory cascade, thus influencing the process of myocardial function and cardiac remodeling. Inflammation in heart failure is a result of the coordinated activation of specific transcription factors in response to external stimuli (infection, oxidative stress, circulating neurohormones, etc.). The best understood of these transcription factors is nuclear factor (NF)-κB, which has been shown to play a role in both acute myocardial injury and chronic heart failure. Although most studies regarding NFκB in the cardiac inflammatory process have been in relation to myocardial infarction, multiple studies have suggested its involvement in the development of heart failure of diverse etiologies (19,27,68). It has therefore been postulated that NFκB plays a central role in the activation of the innate cardiac immune system.

Once activated, the inflammatory cascade leads to the production of numerous proinflammatory and anti-inflammatory mediators. Tumor necrosis factor (TNF) is produced endogenously by cardiac myocytes in response to stress or injury. TNF binds to cardiac TNF receptors and has been linked to detrimental effects such as myocyte hypertrophy, apoptosis, extracellular matrix alterations, and disturbance of calcium homeostasis, which leads to ventricular dilation and dysfunction. Ex vivo, elevated levels of TNF have been shown to depress myocardial function, and circulating concentrations of TNF similar to those measured in patients with heart failure were sufficient to produce negative inotropic effects detectable at the level of the cardiac myocyte. Subsequent studies in transgenic mice with targeted overexpression of TNF in myocardium revealed decreased LV ejection fractions as well (18).

IL-1 is another inflammatory mediator that, similar to TNF, is produced endogenously by cardiac myocytes in response to stressful stimuli. IL-1 is thought to be intimately involved in the progression of myocyte hypertrophy and in the altered calcium homeostasis seen in heart failure. IL-6 is produced in response to stimulation by cytokines such as IL-1 and TNF and has been implicated in maladaptive responses such as myocyte hypertrophy. However, unlike IL-1 and TNF, IL-6 has been postulated to have some protective effects on myocytes in regard to apoptosis. Imbalance in downstream regulation of IL-6–related pathways may determine its overall effect on the failing heart (54). From a clinical standpoint, both IL-1 and IL-6 have been shown to produce negative inotropic effects in various experimental models (37,41). Human studies have shown that plasma concentrations of IL-6 and IL-6–related cytokines are increased in patients with heart failure in direct correlation to decreasing functional status (67).

Another mediator thought to play an important role in the inflammatory cascade with respect to heart failure is nitric oxide (NO). NO mediates multiple signaling pathways in the heart, which have been shown to have both beneficial and toxic effects, depending on the setting. Beneficial effects of NO include improved relaxation, increased preload reserve, and de-

creased afterload, while detrimental effects include myocardial depression and β-adrenergic desensitization. DCM and CHF have been shown to be associated with enhanced nitric oxide synthase (NOS) activity and increased systemic NO production (13,26). Endomyocardial biopsies taken from patients with varying degrees of heart failure have revealed enhanced NOS activity (2). In vitro evaluation has also shown that upregulation of NOS in single cardiac myocytes induces contractile dysfunction (69). Although it has been speculated that NO may act directly as a negative inotrope, its exact role in the progression of heart failure and its precise mechanism of action have not been clearly elucidated.

In addition to the acute functional effects that inflammatory mediators may have on the heart, it is becoming increasingly clear that they also play an important role in the process of ventricular remodeling. As alluded to previously, many of the cytokines have been implicated in the development of myocyte hypertrophy, apoptosis, and even in alterations of fetal gene expression (69). Accumulating evidence demonstrates that certain inflammatory mediators also play a role in the progressive degradation of extracellular matrix, which leads to ventricular dilatation and its subsequent replacement with fibrous tissue (61).

Undoubtedly, a complex interplay occurs between molecular mechanisms, hypertrophic changes, neurohormonal activation, and inflammatory mediators in heart failure. Although adaptive at its core, the ultimate outcome of these complex responses is usually a maladaptive one. With a better understanding of the underlying mechanisms, we may be able to identify new preventative and therapeutic modalities, which, in the future, may become invaluable in the treatment of children with heart failure.

ACUTE DECOMPENSATED HEART FAILURE IN CHILDREN

Clinical Manifestations of Decompensated Heart Failure in Children

The clinical manifestations of DHF in children are somewhat dependent on the age at presentation. Therefore, the history and physical examination should be targeted for the appropriate clinical scenario. In neonates, common causes of DHF include perinatal asphyxia, toxemia, incessant tachyarrhythmias, neonatal myocarditis, severe anemia, or hyperviscosity syndrome. Certain types of CHD, such as hypoplastic left heart syndrome with a severely restrictive atrial septum, may manifest soon after birth as well, but not usually as isolated heart failure. The history should include questions regarding prenatal course, birth history, potential perinatal insults, and family history. The physical exam, as expected, should evaluate for signs of left- or right-sided heart failure. In neonates, findings may include rapid, shallow breathing, dyspnea, wheezing, resting tachycardia, hepatomegaly, jugular venous distension, or hydrops. Cardiac evaluation should assess for gallops; a single, second heart sound; murmurs; and abnormal pulses.

Beyond the immediate perinatal period, DHF in infants can be broadly categorized into causes more likely to occur in the first few weeks of life and causes more likely to occur in the first few months of life. During the first weeks of life, CHDs dependent on ductal blood flow may present. Defects dependent on ductal flow for systemic perfusion (i.e., hypoplastic left heart syndrome, critical aortic stenosis, interrupted aortic arch, etc.) often present with increasing tachycardia, tachypnea, diminished pulses, and worsening perfusion. On the other hand, defects dependent on ductal flow for pulmonary circulation (i.e., critical pulmonary stenosis, pulmonary atresia, etc.) often present with progressive cyanosis. Again, assessment for cardiac murmurs; single, second heart sounds; clicks; and pulses is critical. In this age group, evaluation of differential oxygen saturations (preductal and postductal) may also be of particular importance.

Lesions that present as DHF in infants beyond the first few weeks of life include those with increasing left-to-right shunting as pulmonary vascular resistance decreases. These shunting lesions include large ventricular septal defects, complete atrioventricular canal defects, aortopulmonary windows, truncus arteriosus, unobstructed total anomalous pulmonary venous return, and persistent patent ductus arteriosus, as covered previously. Of note, premature neonates with persistent patency of the ductus arteriosus may present earlier, particularly in infants who weigh <1500 g. Other important causes of DHF in infancy include primary myocardial diseases, myocarditis, and anomalous left coronary artery from the pulmonary artery (ALCAPA). In the pure sense, ALCAPA is a left-to-right shunting lesion that presents with heart failure secondary to LV ischemia, as flow in the left coronary system reverses with decreasing pulmonary vascular resistance (coronary steal). These infants may present with unique symptoms of intense irritability and angina, particularly during feeding.

Historic evaluation in all infants with suspected heart failure should include an accurate assessment of feeding (tachypnea with feeds, gagging, diaphoresis, time to complete feeding, etc.). It should also include an assessment of nutritional status and weight gain, as this may be the first manifestation of a failing heart (5). Along similar lines, physical examination in older infants should assess for cachexia and malnutrition, as well as the standard assessment for tachypnea, diaphoresis, and increased work of breathing. Precordial activity may be increased, and again, murmurs, gallops, or clicks may give important clues to etiology.

Older children are more likely to develop symptomatic heart failure from acquired or operated cardiac conditions, rather than newly recognized or unoperated CHD. Exceptions to this generalization include unrepaired large atrial septal defects, Ebstein anomaly of the tricuspid valve, or ventricular inversion. Patients with palliated CHD may develop DHF as a consequence of chronic pressure or volume overload. This population usually consists of patients with single-ventricle physiology, progressive valvular disease, or RV-dependent systemic circulations. As always, myocarditis or primary myocardial disorders can present at any age. Other potential etiologies of acquired heart failure in older children include rheumatic heart disease, hypothyroidism, or Kawasaki disease. The history in this age group should include questions regarding exercise capacity, easy fatigability, orthopnea, paroxysmal nocturnal dyspnea, and weight gain or weight loss. Physical examination should evaluate for resting tachycardia, tachypnea, hepatomegaly, jugular venous distension, ascites, edema, and diminished perfusion. Cardiac examination should focus on the presence of gallops, new murmurs, an RV impulse, and

perfusion deficits. In all age groups, a directed history and physical examination can provide valuable clues into the presence and possible etiologies of impending DHF.

Cardiorenal Syndrome

Renal insufficiency commonly occurs in patients with DHF. The pathophysiologic process in which combined cardiac and renal dysfunction amplifies progression of end-organ damage has been termed the cardiorenal syndrome. The physiologic interactions of the heart and kidney are complex and poorly understood; however, in simple terms, it is clear that dysfunction of one organ system frequently affects the other. The renal insufficiency that accompanies DHF is usually attributed to poor cardiac output and diminished renal perfusion. However, iatrogenic contributions from medication administration and other treatment strategies should not be overlooked. In addition, progressive renal insufficiency, with its resultant fluid retention and increased systemic vascular resistance, can aggravate heart failure symptoms and directly lead to worsening ventricular function. Therefore, a vicious circle of repetitive injury and insult is initiated. From a clinical standpoint, it has become clear that the coexistence of cardiac and renal dysfunction has a particularly poor prognosis. In adults, in the outpatient setting, even slight decreases in renal function have been correlated with a substantial increase in mortality associated with cardiac disease (20). Among patients hospitalized for DHF, worsening renal function and increasing serum creatinine levels have been associated with longer lengths of hospital stay, higher in-hospital costs, and increased risk of in-hospital mortality (16).

Dysrhythmias in Acute Decompensated Heart Failure

Dysrhythmias are common in association with heart failure. They can be the primary cause of ventricular dysfunction (tachycardia-induced cardiomyopathy), and patients with poor cardiac function are clearly prone to developing rhythm disturbances. Incessant atrial tachycardia, junctional tachycardia, accessory pathway-mediated tachycardia, and ventricular tachycardia have all been linked to the development of cardiomyopathy. Although the minimal heart rate necessary to develop cardiomyopathy is not known, studies suggest that patients who develop ventricular dysfunction typically have persistent heart rates in excess of 140 bpm (22). A thorough discussion of the diagnosis and management of arrhythmias is found in Chapter 68.

Children with DCM are also more likely to develop secondary arrhythmias, which can be either atrial or ventricular in origin and may put these children at risk for sudden death. The maladaptive remodeling and sarcomeric changes that occur in heart failure can predispose the myocardium to after-depolarizations, which may initiate ventricular arrhythmias. In adults, multiform premature ventricular contractions, ventricular couplets, and ventricular tachycardia were present in 80%–90% of patients with DCM and heart failure. The ventricular arrhythmias were noted to become more frequent and complex as ventricular function deteriorated (21).

Regardless of the scenario, DHF is becoming an ever-growing problem in the pediatric population. A clinician's index of suspicion must therefore remain high. Increasing familiarity with its manifestations should lead to significant improvements in the diagnosis and management of this disease in the near future.

Laboratory Evaluation of Decompensated Heart Failure

A comprehensive assessment of the child with DHF must include a thorough laboratory evaluation, including ancillary tests such as chest x-ray, electrocardiography (ECG), and echocardiography. Classic findings on blood work include metabolic and respiratory acidemia due to poor tissue perfusion and pulmonary congestion, hyponatremia and hypochloremia due to free water retention, and elevated creatinine levels due to poor renal perfusion and compromised renal function. A determination of hemoglobin should also be performed because severe anemia can precipitate high-output cardiac failure in itself, and any degree of anemia can accentuate heart failure of any cause. More elegant laboratory tests that assess neurohormonal markers in heart failure have evolved, and many have been found to have prognostic value. For example, elevated norepinephrine, aldosterone, angiotensin II, and vasopressin levels have all been linked to some degree to worse outcomes (17).

BNP measurement is one laboratory test that has taken a particularly prominent role in the assessment of heart failure. An assay for the evaluation of BNP levels was approved in 2000 by the US Food and Drug Administration, and it has subsequently been shown to be effective in diagnosing heart failure in numerous clinical scenarios (45). Measurement of serum BNP levels is clinically useful in differentiating pulmonary causes of dyspnea from cardiac causes of dyspnea (50). In children, BNP levels positively correlate with a clinical heart failure score and negatively correlate with ejection fraction (46). More importantly, elevated BNP levels in the setting of heart failure are related to increased morbidity and mortality (39).

Clinical Diagnostic Studies of Heart Failure

Chest Radiography

Chest x-ray invariably provides additional information in the assessment of DHF. An enlarged cardiac silhouette due to cardiomegaly is frequently found. A cardiothoracic ratio of >0.55 in infants and >0.5 in children is the standard for cardiomegaly. In one study, an enlarged cardiac silhouette on chest x-ray had 85% sensitivity and 95% specificity for the diagnosis of heart failure in the presence of CHD (53). In addition to cardiac size, the chest x-ray also allows for assessment of pulmonary congestion. In children with DHF, evidence of increased pulmonary vascular markings is usually seen. The left lower lobe of the lung may also be collapsed due to compression of the left lower lobe bronchus.

Electrocardiography

ECG can also be useful in the assessment of DHF. An ECG can provide information regarding atrial enlargement, ventricular hypertrophy, strain, and changes in ST-segment or T-wave morphology. However, these changes are usually nonspecific,

and their use in the diagnosis of heart failure is therefore limited. An exception to this may be in the cases of myocarditis, ALCAPA, or tachyarrhythmia-induced cardiomyopathy, in which pathognomonic ECG findings can sometimes be found. In patients with myocarditis, a pattern of myocardial infarction with wide Q waves and ST-segment changes may be seen. Ventricular tachycardia, supraventricular tachycardia, atrial fibrillation, or atrioventricular block occurs in some children.

The ECG is abnormal in 98% of children with restrictive cardiomyopathy (RCM). The most common abnormalities are right and/or left atrial enlargement; however, ST-segment depression and ST-T wave abnormalities are frequently present. RV and/or LV hypertrophy and conduction abnormalities can also be seen.

Echocardiography

The most precise way to quickly evaluate cardiac function and obtain a semiquantitative assessment of heart failure remains two-dimensional echocardiography. Not only is an echocardiogram indispensable in providing details regarding cardiac anatomy in CHD, but estimations of gradients, shunting, and cardiac output can also be made. LV systolic function can be quantified with either shortening fraction or ejection fraction. Although values vary with age, in general, normal values for shortening fraction range from 28% to 44%, while normal values for ejection fraction range from 56% to 78%. It is important to note that both of these classic measures of function are load-dependent. Newer modalities such as myocardial performance index and Doppler tissue imaging are load-independent measures and allow for more global assessments of ventricular function (including diastolic function) and regional wall motion abnormalities, respectively. Assessment of RV function has always been more challenging due to geometric restrictions, and myocardial performance index and Doppler tissue imaging have proved promising in this regard.

The characteristic findings in patients with a DCM include ventricular enlargement and globally decreased function. Color Doppler echocardiography can determine the presence and degree of semilunar valve or A-V valve regurgitation, while pulsed Doppler can assist in ruling out outflow tract obstruction (HCM) and assess the degree of diastolic dysfunction by atrioventricular valve inflow patterns. Serial echocardiography is useful in tracking changes in ventricular function over the course of time, which can also help to guide medical therapy.

Children with DCM have a dilated, dysfunctional LV on two-dimensional (**Fig 66A.2A**) and M-mode echocardiography. Segmental wall motion abnormalities are relatively common, but global hypokinesis is predominant. A pericardial effusion is frequently present. Doppler and color Doppler commonly demonstrate mitral regurgitation. Dilation of other chambers also may be seen. Cardiac output calculations may also be obtained and are frequently reduced. Coronary artery or structural abnormalities that could produce these features should be excluded. Improved techniques, particularly tissue Doppler imaging and myocardial velocity measurements, are being studied to better characterize tissue changes and monitor them over time.

The hallmark echocardiographic findings of HCM are asymmetric hypertrophy of the interventricular septum, with or without systolic anterior motion of the mitral valve (Fig. 66A.2B). Other segments of the LV, including the free wall and the apex, may be hypertrophied as well. The LV systolic

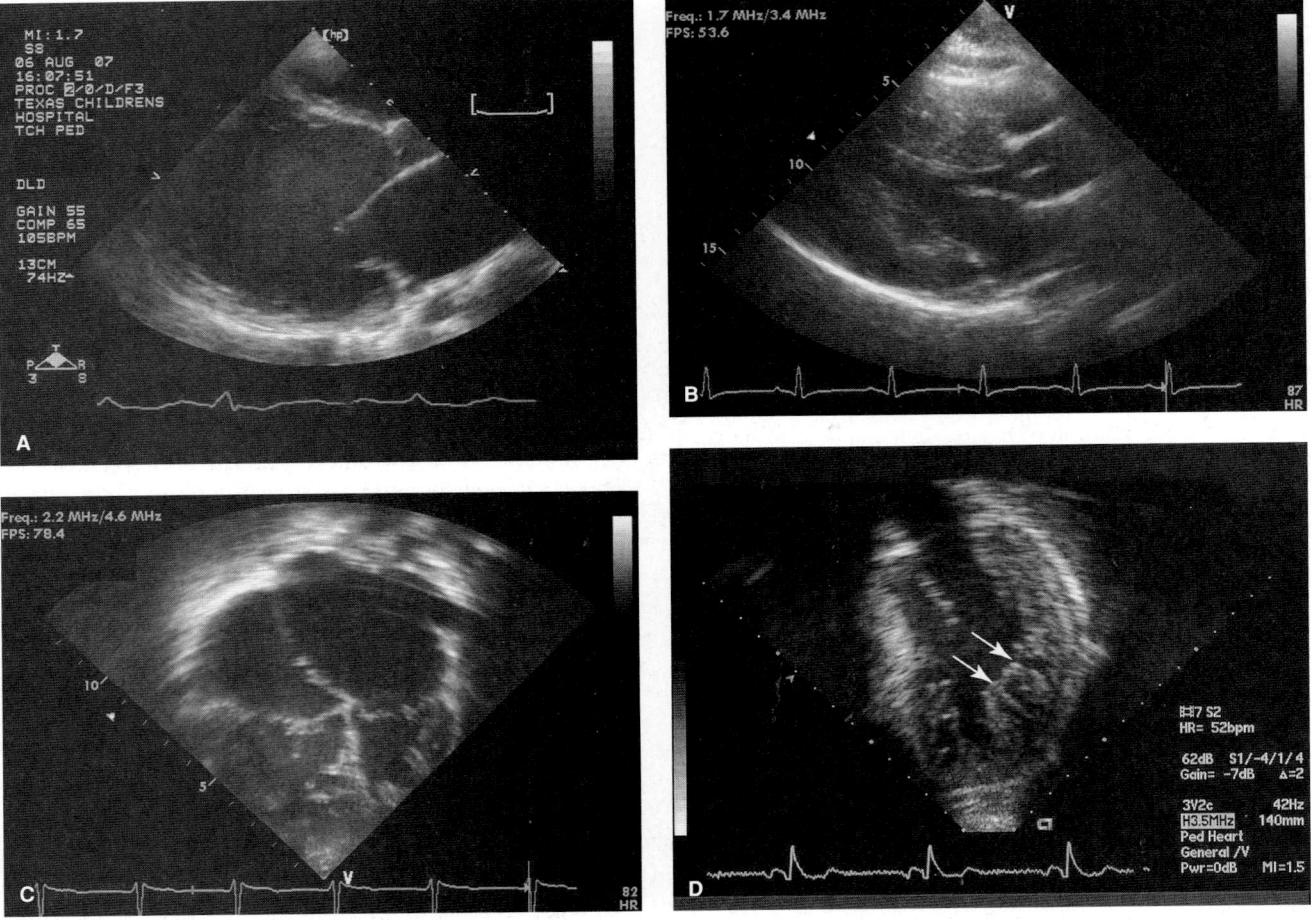

FIGURE 66A.2. Representative single-frame echocardiograms demonstrating the salient features of the four types of cardiomyopathy seen in pediatric patients. (**A**) Dilated cardiomyopathy, parasternal long axis view. Note the dilated left ventricular (LV) chamber and relatively thin LV posterior wall and septum. (**B**) Hypertrophic cardiomyopathy, parasternal long axis view. Note the thickened LV posterior wall and septum and the small LV chamber size. (**C**) Restrictive cardiomyopathy, apical four chamber view. Note the markedly dilated right and left atria. (**D**) LV noncompaction, apical four chamber view. Note the thickened LV myocardium and deep trabeculations indicated by the arrows.

function is typically hyperdynamic but may be normal. Evidence of outflow-tract obstruction can be determined by Doppler interrogation of the LV outflow tract. Assessment of diastolic function, which may be abnormal, can be performed utilizing Doppler tissue imaging and mitral inflow patterns.

The echocardiogram is diagnostic in children with RCM. On two-dimensional imaging, classic cases demonstrate markedly dilated atria, often dwarfing the size of the ventricles (Fig. 66A.2C). Typically, normal or nearly normal LV systolic function and absence of significant hypertrophy or dilatation are present. However, some degree of systolic dysfunction may be apparent at presentation or progress over time, with reported shortening fractions as low as the low 20s and ejection fractions as low as the upper 30s. In addition, as many as 40% of patients have, or develop, mild and sometimes progressive LV hypertrophy. Variable patterns of hypertrophy have been reported. The "mixed restrictive/hypertrophic phenotype" can result in a confusing clinical picture in terms of diagnosis, RCM versus HCM, and optimal therapeutic approaches. During two-dimensional imaging, thrombi should

be specifically sought. Thrombotic and embolic events have been described in ~21% of pediatric patients reported to have idiopathic RCM. Pericardial thickening on two-dimensional evaluation would suggest constrictive pericarditis rather than RCM. Doppler patterns of diastolic dysfunction have been well characterized in adults and pediatric data have also been reported.

Echocardiography is diagnostic in children with LV noncompaction (Fig. 66A.2D). Specific echocardiographic criteria have been established: (a) absence of coexisting cardiac abnormalities; (b) the existence of two layers, with a thin epicardial band and a much thicker noncompacted endocardial layer (a ratio of noncompacted to compacted layers of >2 being diagnostic); (c) predominant localization of the noncompaction to the mid-lateral, apical, and mid-inferior ventricular segments; and (d) evidence of color Doppler flow into the trabeculations (4). Pediatric patients will often fulfill most of these criteria, but the ratio may be <2. Also, it is well established that pediatric patients may have coexisting congenital heart disease.

Magnetic Resonance Imaging

In addition to providing an anatomic evaluation of the heart in failure, MRI can also provide accurate tissue characterization by measuring T1 and T2 relaxation times and spin densities (44). Relaxation time analysis provides a sensitive measure for acute myocarditis. Utilizing T1 spin-echo cine MR angiography and gadolinium-enhanced spin echo imaging, investigators demonstrated that focal myocardial enhancement combined with regional wall motion abnormalities strongly supported the diagnosis of myocarditis (56).

Cardiac Catheterization

Cardiac catheterization is an invasive procedure with inherent risks and potential complications, which sometimes limits its application for diagnostic purposes. Catheterization can help in the hemodynamic assessment of patients by directly measuring LV end diastolic, pulmonary capillary wedge, pulmonary artery, and central venous pressures. Also, a cardiac catheterization with coronary artery angiography may be necessary to exclude coronary artery anomalies (both congenital and acquired).

Cardiac catheterization is an important part of the evaluation in patients with RCM and should be performed at the time of diagnosis. Typically, filling of the ventricles reveals an early diastolic dip with a subsequent plateau pattern, also called the *square root sign*. In "classic" RCM, the LV end-diastolic pressure, left atrial pressure, and pulmonary capillary wedge pressure are markedly elevated and at least 4–5 mm Hg (preferably 10 mm Hg) greater than the right atrial pressure and RV end-diastolic pressure. In cases in which the pressures are essentially equal, volume loading may reveal the differences in pressure between the right and left sides. Pulmonary hypertension is frequently present at the time of initial catheterization, in addition to elevated LF and/or RV end-diastolic pressures (3,66).

CONCLUSIONS AND FUTURE DIRECTIONS

One of the greatest challenges in pediatric heart failure is the study of it. Data are minimal regarding the diagnosis, treatment, and monitoring of heart failure in children. Currently, the pediatric cardiologist is resigned to reading the adult literature and carefully applying recommended guidelines to pediatric patients. Large, multicentered, controlled trials are required to determine the safety and efficacy of cardiac medications and devices as well as the role of diagnostic tools in children with heart failure; without data from such trials, it is extremely difficult to make proper assessments in this population. The future of pediatric heart failure will depend on rigorous investigation, collaboration, and participation in multi-institutional studies.

Several promising tools are available for the diagnosis and monitoring of pediatric heart failure. Novel applications such as three-dimensional echocardiography and cardiac MRI appear to hold promise and will likely be utilized to expanding degrees in the assessment of cardiac function. The role of plasma BNP concentrations for risk stratification and assessment of treatment is still in its infancy. Near-infrared spectroscopy is now commonly used during cardiopulmonary bypass for car-diac surgery in children and may have a role in assessing cardiac output noninvasively in children with DHF. Likewise, arterial pulse-wave analysis, which is a validated method by which to determine real-time cardiac output in children, should be studied for a possible role in monitoring and treating patients with heart failure (36).

KEY POINTS

- Heart failure is a clinical syndrome characterized by elevated venous filling pressures, structural or functional abnormalities of the myocardium, and activation of the neurohormonal axis.
- Heart failure alters the structure and function of the myocardium at both the molecular and cellular levels.
- Although myocardial remodeling may initially be beneficial to cardiac function, ultimately, it can result in the progression of heart failure and has been linked to the pathogenesis of cardiac dysrhythmias and sudden death.
- Heart failure is often associated with a generalized perturbation of the inflammatory cascade, which influences the process of myocardial function and cardiac remodeling.
- Elegant laboratory tests that assess neurohormonal markers in heart failure have evolved, and many have been found to be prognostic.
- The most precise way to quickly evaluate cardiac function and obtain a quantitative assessment of heart failure remains two-dimensional echocardiography.

References

1. Asimakopoulos G, Smith PL, Ratnatunga CP, et al. Lung injury and acute respiratory distress syndrome after cardiopulmonary bypass. *Ann Thorac Surg* 1999;68:1107–15.
2. Balligand JL, Ungureanu-Longrois D, Simmons WW, et al. Cytokine-inducible nitric oxide synthase (iNOS) expression in cardiac myocytes. Characterization and regulation of iNOS expression and detection of iNOS activity in single cardiac myocytes in vitro. *J Biol Chem* 1994;269:27580–8.
3. Bekeredjian R, Grayburn PA. Valvular heart disease: Aortic regurgitation. *Circulation* 2005;112:125–34.
4. Bers DM, Perez-Reyes E. Ca channels in cardiac myocytes: Structure and function in Ca influx and intracellular Ca release. *Cardiovasc Res* 1999;42:339–60.
5. Buchorn R, Hammersen A, Bartmus D, et al. The pathogenesis of heart failure in infants with congenital heart disease. *Cardiol Young* 2001;11:498–504.
6. Chai PJ, Williamson JA, Lodge AJ, et al. Effects of ischemia on pulmonary dysfunction after cardiopulmonary bypass. *Ann Thorac Surg* 1999;67:731–5.
7. Chen J, Chien KR. Complexity in simplicity: Monogenic disorders and complex cardiomyopathies. *J Clin Invest* 1999;103:1483–5.
8. Cheung BM, Kumana CR. Natriuretic peptides—relevance in cardiovascular disease *JAMA* 1998;280:1983–4.
9. Chong WY, Wong WH, Chiu CS, et al. Aortic root dilation and aortic elastic properties in children after repair of tetralogy of Fallot. *Am J Cardiol* 2006;97:905–9.
10. Chung P, Hermann L. Acute decompensated heart failure: Formulating an evidence-based approach to diagnosis and treatment (Part I). *Mt Sinai J Med* 2006;64:506–15.
11. Cohn JN, Levine TB, Olivari MT, et al. Plasma norepinephrine as a guide to prognosis in patients with chronic congestive heart failure. *N Engl J Med* 1984;311:819–23.
12. Colan SD, Trowitzsch E, Wernovsky G, et al. Myocardial performance after arterial switch operation for transposition of the great arteries with intact ventricular septum. *Circulation* 1988;78:132–41.
13. de Belder AJ, Radomski MW, Why HJ, et al. Myocardial calcium-independent nitric oxide synthase activity is present in dilated

cardiomyopathy, myocarditis, and postpartum cardiomyopathy but not in ischaemic or valvar heart disease. *Br Heart J* 1995;74:426–30.

14. du Plessis AJ, Jonas RA, Wypij D, et al. Perioperative effects of alpha-stat versus pH-stat strategies for deep hypothermic cardiopulmonary bypass in infants. *J Thorac Cardiovasc Surg* 1997;114:991–1000.

15. Fill M, Copello JA. Ryanodine receptor calcium release channels. *Physiol Rev* 2002;82:893–922.

16. Forman DE, Butler J, Wang Y, et al. Incidence, predictors at admission, and impact of worsening renal function among patients hospitalized with heart failure. *J Am Coll Cardiol* 2004;43:61–7.

17. Francis GS, Cohn JN, Johnson G, et al. Plasma norepinephrine, plasma renin activity, and congestive heart failure. Relations to survival and the effects of therapy in V-HeFT II. The V-HeFT VA Cooperative Studies Group. *Circulation* 1993;87:VI40–8.

18. Franco F, Thomas GD, Giroir B, et al. Magnetic resonance imaging and invasive evaluation of development of heart failure in transgenic mice with myocardial expression of tumor necrosis factor-alpha. *Circulation* 1999;99:448–54.

19. Frantz S, Fraccarollo D, Wagner H, et al. Sustained activation of nuclear factor kappa B and activator protein 1 in chronic heart failure. *Cardiovasc Res* 2003;57:749–56.

20. Fried LF, Shlipak MG, Crump C, et al. Renal insufficiency as a predictor of cardiovascular outcomes and mortality in elderly individuals. *J Am Coll Cardiol* 2003;41:1364–72.

21. Galvin JM, Ruskin JN. Ventricular tachycardia in patients with dilated cardiomyopathy. In Zipes DP, Jalife J (eds.). *Cardiac Electrophysiology: From Cell to Bedside, 4th ed.* Philadelphia, WB Saunders 2004;575–87.

22. Gelb BD, Garson A Jr. Noninvasive discrimination of right atrial ectopic tachycardia from sinus tachycardia in "dilated cardiomyopathy." *Am Heart J* 1990;120:886–91.

23. Gias U, Ahmmed G, Hong Dong P, et al. Changes in Ca^{2+} cycling proteins underlie cardiac action potential prolongation in a pressure-overloaded guinea pig model with cardiac hypertrophy and failure. *Circ Res* 2000;86:558–70.

24. Gu X, Bishop SP. Increased protein kinase C and isozyme redistribution in pressure-overload cardiac hypertrophy in the rat. *Circ Res* 1994;75:926–31.

25. Hall RI, Smith MS, Rocker G. The systemic inflammatory response to cardiopulmonary bypass: Pathophysiological, therapeutic, and pharmacological considerations. *Anesth Analg* 1997;85:766–82.

26. Hare JM, Givertz MM, Creager MA, et al. Increased sensitivity to nitric oxide synthase inhibition in patients with heart failure: Potentiation of beta-adrenergic inotropic responsiveness. *Circulation* 1998;97:161–6.

27. Haywood GA, Tsao PS, der Leyen HE, et al. Expression of inducible nitric oxide synthase in human heart failure. *Circulation* 1996;93:1087–94.

28. Hersel I, Jung S, Mohacsi P, Hullin R. Expression of the L-type calcium channel in human heart failure. *Basic Res Cardiol* 2002;97:I4–10.

29. Hobai IA, O'Rourke B. Decreased sarcoplasmic reticulum calcium content is responsible for defective excitation-contraction coupling in canine heart failure. *Circulation* 2001;103:1577–84.

30. Hoffman EP, Brown RH, Jr., Kunkel LM. Dystrophin: The protein product of the Duchenne muscular dystrophy locus. *Cell* 1987;51:919–28.

31. Hoffman TM, Wernovsky G, Atz AM, et al. Efficacy and safety of milrinone in preventing low cardiac output syndrome in infants and children after corrective surgery for congenital heart disease. *Circulation* 2003;107:996–1002.

32. Hunt PJ, Espiner EA, Nicholls MG, et al. Differing biological effects of equimolar atrial and brain natriuretic peptide infusions in normal man. *J Clin Endocrinol Metab* 1996;81:3871–6.

33. Ito H, Hirata Y, Hiroe M, et al. Endothelin-1 induces hypertrophy with enhanced expression of muscle-specific genes in cultured neonatal rat cardiomyocytes. *Circ Res* 1991;69:209–15.

34. Jiang JP, Downing SE. Catecholamine cardiomyopathy: Review and analysis of pathogenetic mechanisms. *Yale J Biol Med* 1990;63:581–91.

35. Katz AM. Overview Definition, Historical Aspects. In: Katz AM, ed. *Heart Failure: Pathophysiology, Molecular Biology and Clinical Management.* Philadelphia: Lippincott Williams and Wilkins, 2000;3.

36. Kim JJ, Dreyer WJ, Chang AC, et al. Arterial pulse wave analysis: An accurate means of determining cardiac index in children. *Ped Cardiol* 2005;26:505.

37. Kinugawa K, Takahashi T, Kohmoto O, et al. Nitric oxide-mediated effects of interleukin-6 on $[Ca^{2+}]_i$ and cell contraction in cultured chick ventricular myocytes. *Circ Res* 1994;75:285–95.

38. Knoll R, Hoshijima M, Hoffman HM, et al. The cardiac mechanical stretch sensor machinery involves a Z disc complex that is defective in a subset of human dilated cardiomyopathy. *Cell* 2002;111:943–55.

39. Koglin J, Pehlivanli S, Schwaiblmair M, et al. Role of brain natriuretic peptide in risk stratification of patients with congestive heart failure. *J Am Coll Cardiol* 2001;38:1934–41.

40. Koller KJ, Goeddel DV. Molecular biology of the natriuretic peptides and their receptors *Circulation* 1992;86:1081–8.

41. Kumar A, Brar R, Wang P, et al. Role of nitric oxide and cGMP in human septic serum-induced depression of cardiac myocyte contractility. *Am J Physiol* 1999;276:R265–76.

42. Kunii Y, Kamada M, Ohtsuki S, et al. Plasma brain natriuretic peptide and the evaluation of volume overload in infants and children with congenital heart disease. *Acta Med Okayama* 2003;57:191–7.

43. Lloyd-Jones DM, Larson MG, Leip EP, et al. Lifetime risk for developing congestive heart failure: The Framingham Heart Study. *Circulation* 2002;106:3068–72.

44. Magnani JW, Dec GW. Myocarditis: Current trends in diagnosis and treatment. *Circulation* 2006;113(6):876–90.

45. Maisel AS, Krishnaswamy P, Nowak RM, et al. Rapid measurement of B-type natriuretic peptide in the emergency diagnosis of heart failure. *N Engl J Med* 2002;347:161–7.

46. Mir TS, Marohn S, Laer S, et al. Plasma concentrations of N-terminal pro-brain natriuretic peptide in control children from the neonatal to adolescent period and in children with congestive heart failure. *Pediatrics* 2002;110:e76.

47. Miyada S, Haneda T, Osaki J, et al. Renin-angiotensin system in stretch-induced hypertrophy of cultured neonatal rat heart cells. *Eur J Pharmacol* 1996;307:81–8.

48. Miyamoto MI, del Monte F, Schmidt U, et al. Adenoviral gene transfer of SERCA2a improves left ventricular function in aortic banded rats in transition to heart failure. *Proc Natl Acad Sci USA* 2000;97:793–8.

49. Molkentin JD, Lu JR, Antos CL, et al. A calcineurin-dependant transcriptional pathway for cardiac hypertrophy. *Cell* 1998;93:215–28.

50. Morrison LK, Harrison A, Krishnaswamy P, et al. Utility of a rapid B-natriuretic peptide assay in differentiating congestive heart failure from lung disease in patients presenting with dyspnea. *J Am Coll Cardiol* 2002;39:202–9.

51. Nistri S, Sorbo MD, Marin M, et al. Aortic root dilatation in young men with normally functioning bicuspid aortic valves. *Heart* 1999;82:19–22.

52. Piacentino VR, Weber CR, Chen X, et al. Cellular basis of abnormal calcium transients of failing human ventricular myocytes. *Circ Res* 2003;92:651–8.

53. Pickert CB, Moss MM, Fisher DH. Differentiation of systemic infection and congenital obstructive left heart disease in the very young infant. *Pediatr Emerg Care* 1998;14:263–7.

54. Podewski EK, Hilfiker-Kleiner D, Hilfiker A, et al. Alterations in Janus kinase (JAK)-signal transducers and activators of transcription (STAT) signaling in patients with end-stage dilated cardiomyopathy. *Circulation* 2003;107:798–802.

55. Price JF, Towbin JA, Denfield SW, et al. Arginine vasopressin levels are elevated and correlate with functional status in infants and children with congestive heart failure. *Circulation* 2004;109:2550–3.

56. Roditi GH, Hartnell GG, Cohen MC. MRI changes in myocarditis—evaluation with spin echo, cine MR angiography and contrast enhanced spin echo imaging. *Clin Radiol* 2000;55(10):752–8.

57. Sadoshima J, Xu Y, Slayter HS, et al. Autocrine release of angiotensin II mediates stretch-induced hypertrophy of cardiac myocytes in-vitro. *Cell* 1993;75:977–84.

58. Schmidt U, del Monte F, Miyamoto MI, et al. Restoration of diastolic function in senescent rat hearts through adenoviral gene transfer of sarcoplasmic reticulum Ca^{2+}-ATPase. *Circulation* 2000;1:790–6.

59. Schwartz ML, Gauvreau K, del Nido P, et al. Long-term predictors of aortic root dilation and aortic regurgitation after arterial switch operation. *Circulation* 2004;110(Suppl 1):II128–32.

60. Shah BH, Catt KJ. A central role of EGF receptor transactivation in angiotensin II-induced cardiac hypertrophy. *Trends Pharmacol Sci* 2003;24:239–44.

61. Sivasubramanian N, Coker ML, Kurrelmeyer K, et al. Left ventricular remodeling in transgenic mice with cardiac restricted overexpression of tumor necrosis factor. *Circulation* 2001;104:826–31.

62. Tan LB, Jalil JE, Pick R, et al. Cardiac myocyte necrosis induced by angiotensin II. *Circ Res* 1991;69:1185–95.

63. Towbin JA, Bowles NE. The failing heart. *Nature* 2002;227–33.

64. Toyo-Oka T, Kawada T, Nakata J, et al. Translocation and cleavage of myocardial dystrophin as a common pathway to advanced heart failure: A scheme for the progression of cardiac dysfunction. *Proc Natl Acad Sci* 2004;101:7381–5.

65. Vatta M, Stetson SJ, Perez-Verdia A, et al. Molecular remodeling of dystrophin in patients with end-stage cardiomyopathies and reversal in patients on assistance-device therapy. *Lancet* 2002;359:936–41.

66. Wernovsky G, Wypij D, Jonas RA, et al. Postoperative course and hemodynamic profile after the arterial switch operation in neonates and infants. A comparison of low-flow cardiopulmonary bypass and circulatory arrest. *Circulation* 1995;92:2226–35.

67. Wollert KC, Drexler H. The role of interleukin-6 in the failing heart. *Heart Fail Rev* 2001;6:95–103.

68. Wong SC, Fukuchi M, Melnyk P, et al. Induction of cyclooxygenase-2 and activation of nuclear factor-kappa B in myocardium of patients with congestive heart failure. *Circulation* 1998;98:100–3.

69. Yokoyama T, Nakano M, Bednarczyk JL, et al. Tumor necrosis factor-alpha provokes a hypertrophic growth response in adult cardiac myocytes. *Circulation* 1997;95:1247–52.

CHAPTER 66B ■ HEART FAILURE IN INFANTS AND CHILDREN: CARDIOMYOPATHY

JOHN LYNN JEFFERIES • SUSAN W. DENFIELD • WILLIAM J. DREYER

Cardiomyopathies are heart muscle disorders associated with significant morbidity and mortality, both in children and adults. These disorders have been classified by the World Health Organization and the International Society and Federation of Cardiology task force into five forms according to phenotype (35). The first form is dilated cardiomyopathy (DCM), in which the left ventricle (LV) or both ventricles are enlarged and hypocontractile to variable degrees. In general, systolic dysfunction is the main clinical feature, with resultant signs and symptoms of congestive heart failure (CHF). The second form is hypertrophic cardiomyopathy (HCM), also previously known as *idiopathic hypertrophic subaortic stenosis*, characterized by LV hypertrophy that may be asymmetric. Systolic function is usually preserved or hypercontractile, and symptoms may result from LV outflow tract obstruction, diastolic dysfunction, or arrhythmias resulting in sudden death. The third form is restrictive cardiomyopathy (RCM), which is recognized by markedly dilated atria with generally normal ventricular dimensions and systolic function (3). Diastolic filling is impaired, and symptoms result from pulmonary and right-sided systemic venous congestion. The fourth form is arrhythmogenic right ventricular dysplasia (ARVD) and is characterized by left-bundle-branch block, ventricular tachycardia, a dilated right ventricle (RV), and a dyskinetic RV outflow tract with replacement of myocardium by adipose tissue, beginning in the epicardium and extending to the endocardium. The above-mentioned organizations also recognize a fifth category of "other" cardiomyopathies. Left-ventricular noncompaction (LVNC) has gained considerable clinical attention as a "new" cardiomyopathy in this classification. In this form of cardiomyopathy, the LV wall is thickened with large spongiform trabeculations, and the LV is typically hypocontractile.

The most common form of cardiomyopathy is DCM, accounting for 51%–58% of pediatric cases. HCM is second most common, being identified in 25%–42% of patients, with the remaining forms of cardiomyopathy accounting for the remainder of pediatric cases (23,32). The importance of these disorders lies in the fact that they are responsible for a high proportion of cases of CHF and sudden death, as well as the need for cardiac transplantation.

DILATED CARDIOMYOPATHY

DCM represents a heterogeneous group of myocardial disorders that result in ventricular dilation and impaired systolic contractile function in the absence of coronary artery disease, valvular abnormalities, and pericardial disease. Mitral regurgitation is common, as are ventricular arrhythmias, particularly ventricular tachycardia, torsade de pointes, and ventricular fibrillation. Impaired contractile function generally culminates with chamber enlargement. The regulation of normal contractile function necessary to maintain an appropriate cardiac output is a complex process. It requires normal electrical conduction, normal intercellular and intracellular calcium signaling, appropriate energy production, sufficient force generation from the sarcomeric proteins, and adequate force transmission from the sarcomere through to the extracellular matrix via cytoskeletal proteins. A defect in any of the critical proteins that regulate or are actively involved in this pathway can theoretically lead to DCM.

Primary DCMs are disorders intrinsic to the myocardium that occur without a secondary cause and are presumably genetically transmitted diseases of one of the structural or regulatory proteins mentioned previously. DCM was initially believed to be inherited in only a small percentage of cases. However, it was demonstrated that ~20% of probands had family members with echocardiographic evidence of DCM when family screening was performed (30). Additionally, inherited, familial DCM has been shown to occur in >30% of cases (2,16). Autosomal-dominant inheritance is the predominant pattern of transmission, with X-linked, autosomal recessive, and mitochondrial inheritance less common. Multiple genes have been identified as associated with the DCM phenotype, and they appear to encode two major subgroups of proteins: cytoskeletal and sarcomeric (40). The cytoskeletal proteins identified to date include dystrophin, desmin, lamin A/C, δ-sarcoglycan, metavinculin, muscle LIM protein, and α-actinin. In the case of sarcomere-encoding genes, overlap occurs with HCM, i.e., defects in the same gene may encode for an abnormal protein, resulting in either the DCM or HCM phenotype. A new gene, cipher/ZASP, a Z-line protein, has also been identified with DCM (42). In addition, defects in two other genes encoding for proteins with unknown functions (phospholamban and G4.5/Tafazzin) are associated with the DCM phenotype. Primary DCMs are commonly found in association with neuromuscular disorders, as cardiac myocytes and skeletal muscle myocytes share many of the same contractile proteins.

Secondary DCMs occur due to extrinsic myocyte injury from a myriad of sources. These can include hypoxic events, infections, environmental or toxin exposures, autoimmune reactions, arrhythmias, nutritional deficiencies, or abnormal autonomic responses. Metabolic disorders that affect substrate utilization or energy production within the myocardium, even though they may have a known genetic cause, should also be included in this group of secondary, rather than primary, cardiomyopathies. Myocarditis is perhaps the most common

SECONDARY CAUSES OF DILATED CARDIOMYOPATHIES

Infections Viral Bacterial Fungal Protozoan (Chagas/toxoplasmosis) Rickettsial (Rocky Mountain spotted fever) Spirochetal (Lyme disease)	*Ischemia* Hypoxia Birth asphyxia Drowning Kawasaki disease Coronary artery malformation Premature coronary artery disease

Arrhythmias
Supraventricular tachycardia
  Atrial flutter
  Ectopic atrial tachycardia
Ventricular tachycardia
Bradycardia
	Toxins
	Anthracyclines
	Radiation
	Other chemotherapeutic agents
	Sulfonamide sensitivity
	Penicillin sensitivity
	Iron (hemochromatosis)
	Copper

Endocrine Hyperthyroidism/hypothyroidism Excess catecholamines (pheochromocytoma or neuroblastoma) Congenital adrenal hyperplasia	*Systemic disorders* Systemic lupus erythematosus Juvenile rheumatoid arthritis Polyarteritis Nodosa Kawasaki disease

Metabolic diseases
Disorders of glycogen metabolism
Disorders of lipid metabolism
Defects of B-oxidation enzymes
  Carnitine deficiency syndromes
  Fatty acid transport defects
	Osteogenesis imperfecta
	Peripartum cardiomyopathy
	Hemolytic uremic syndrome
	Leukemia
	Amyloidosis
	Sarcoidosis

Nutritional deficiencies Protein: kwashiorkor Thiamine: beriberi Vitamin E Selenium Phosphate	Reye syndrome

Adapted from Denfield SW, Gajarski RJ, Towbin JA. Cardiomyopathies. In: Garson A, Bricker JT, Fisher DJ, et al., eds. *The Science and Practice of Pediatric Cardiology, 2nd ed.* Baltimore: Williams & Wilkins, 1998.

cause of secondary ventricular dysfunction in both children and adults and is discussed later. Also, with pediatric cancer survival markedly improved, another common secondary cause of DCM is the treatment of cancer with anthracycline-derived chemotherapeutic agents and/or radiation. The secondary causes of DCM are listed in **Table 66B.1**.

Pathology

The gross pathologic appearance of DCM, regardless of etiology, is a globular heart with severe left or even biventricular dilation. Ventricular dilation and hypocontractile function lead to accumulation of blood within the ventricles (volume overload) and subsequently elevate end-diastolic pressures, leading to atrial enlargement. Due to stasis of blood, intramural thrombi are common. On gross inspection, the myocardium may appear pale. Endocardial sclerosis is common. The overall weight of the heart is increased due to compensatory hypertrophy, although the free walls of the ventricles may actually appear thin. Microscopic examination typically reveals myocyte hypertrophy, myocyte degeneration, and varying amounts of interstitial fibrosis.

Natural History and Long-term Prognosis

The natural history of DCM depends upon the underlying cause. Four potential outcomes are possible after the initial recognition of ventricular dysfunction: (a) complete resolution of the patient's ventricular dysfunction; (b) improved degree of dysfunction without complete resolution of disease (however, patients are managed medically and maintain a cardiac output sufficient for normal daily living); (c) progressive deterioration and ventricular dysfunction, leading to the need for cardiac transplantation; or (d) death. Traditional teaching suggests that approximately one-third of patients who present with DCM will recover completely, one-third will improve but be left with some degree of residual dysfunction, and one-third will die or require transplantation. In 2003, the Pediatric Cardiomyopathy Registry estimated the median age of diagnosis of patients with DCM in the US to be 1.8 years. Of these children, 12.7% required heart transplantation, and 13.6% died within 2 years of initial diagnosis (23). Primary DCMs are more likely than not to progress, although with a varying time course, despite aggressive medical management. DCMs from secondary causes may or may not be progressive, depending upon the specific etiology. Patients who progress to intractable heart failure may benefit from palliative surgical interventions such as mitral valvuloplasty or cardiac transplantation. Additionally, patients may be supported with such techniques as extracorporeal membrane oxygenation, intra-aortic counterpulsation, and LV assist devices. Such techniques have allowed patients who would otherwise have died to be bridged to cardiac transplantation and, in some cases, to eventual recovery.

HYPERTROPHIC CARDIOMYOPATHY

HCM is characterized by LV hypertrophy, a nondilated LV cavity, systolic hypercontractility, diastolic dysfunction, and, in ~20% of cases, obstruction to LV outflow (hypertrophic obstructive cardiomyopathy) secondary to mitral-septal contact during systole (see Chapter 66A, Fig. 66A.2B). In the past, this disease was known as *idiopathic hypertrophic subaortic stenosis*, but this nomenclature has been abandoned, as most patients do not have an outflow gradient or stenosis. HCM is associated with myofiber disarray and increased cardiac fibrosis. Other forms of cardiac disease have small amounts of myofiber disarray and fibrosis, but the higher amount seen in HCM is distinctive. In the absence of such findings, the diagnosis of HCM should be suspect. HCM differs from DCM in that the physiologic abnormality is one of diastolic dysfunction rather than systolic dysfunction. HCM is typically diagnosed by unexplained LV hypertrophy on echocardiogram. Unexplained LV hypertrophy is estimated to occur in 1 in 500 persons in the general population, with up to 60% of these being secondary to HCM (27). HCM is recognized as the most common genetic cardiovascular disease and is the most common cause of sudden cardiac death (SCD) in young healthy subjects in the US, particularly true with athletic activity, which accounts for approximately one-third of the deaths (26) (**Fig. 66B.1**). As such, careful assessment of an individual's risk for SCD is a critical component to patient management (**Fig. 66B.2**). Clinical predictors in adults have been reported that are associated with a higher risk of SCD and include SCD in a first-degree relative, unexplained syncope, significant amounts of ventricular

ectopy (usually documented by Holter monitoring), massive LV hypertrophy, and the presence of a "malignant" genotype (28). The presence of any of these predictors should raise the consideration of placing an implantable cardioverter defibrillator in appropriate individuals. In adult populations, the absence of all of these risk factors carries a prognosis of <1% of SCD annually (10).

Molecular Genetics of Hypertrophic Cardiomyopathy

Classically, HCM has been described as a disease with an autosomal dominant inheritance pattern. β-myosin heavy chain, located on chromosome 14, was the first gene identified as linked to HCM (12). More than 400 mutations in 11 genes have been identified. In all cases, these genes encode sarcomeric proteins and include cardiac actin, cardiac troponin I, cardiac troponin T, cardiac troponin C, α-tropomyosin, titin, myosin-binding protein C, the essential and regulatory myosin light chains, and muscle LIM protein. These mutations do not appear to have racial predilections. Some families with HCM mutations have a high incidence of SCD or heart failure. These mutations are often classified as "malignant." In addition, nonsarcomere, protein-encoding genes, including AMP kinase (1) and the α-iduronidase gene (which causes Fabry disease) (37), have also been identified.

Genetic testing may be performed in HCM patients. Identification of a sarcomeric mutation provides a diagnosis of HCM and may be useful in screening other members of the family who could be at risk of developing HCM. Specific gene mutations (genotype) associated with HCM are present at birth, but it may be years before the appearance of clinical evidence of disease (phenotype). Genotype-phenotype correlations were initially performed on β-myosin heavy-chain, α-tropomyosin, myosin-binding protein C, and cardiac troponin T, and differences in age of onset, severity of hypertrophy, and survival were reported (43,44). However, the studies were performed on a small number of genotyped individuals and may not be representative of the entire population of HCM patients. It

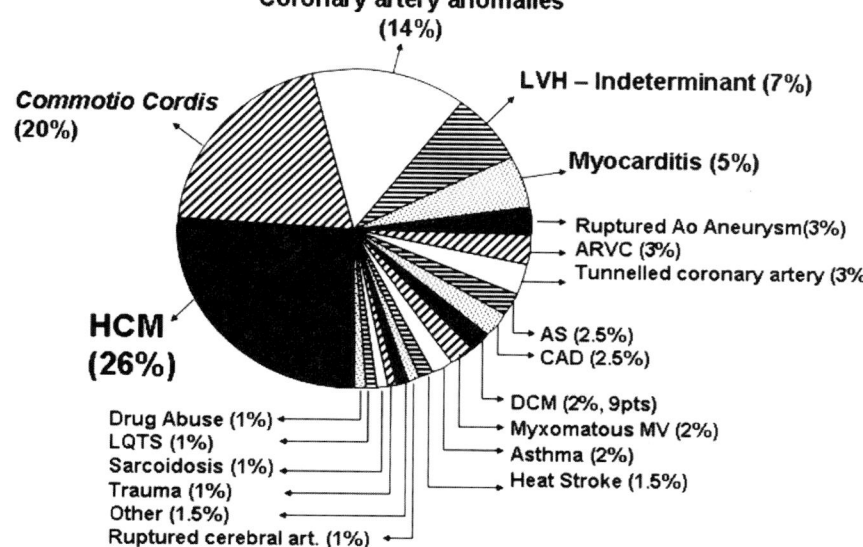

FIGURE 66B.1. Causes of sudden death in young competitive athletes, as reported to the Minneapolis Heart Institute Foundation national registry. Ao indicates aorta; art., artery; AS, aortic stenosis; CAD, coronary artery disease; DCM, dilated cardiomyopathy; LQTS, long-QT syndrome; LVH, LV hypertrophy; MV, mitral valve; and pts, patients. From Maron BJ, Pelliccia A. The heart of trained athletes: Cardiac remodeling and the risks of sports, including sudden death. *Circulation* 2006;114:1633–44, with permission.

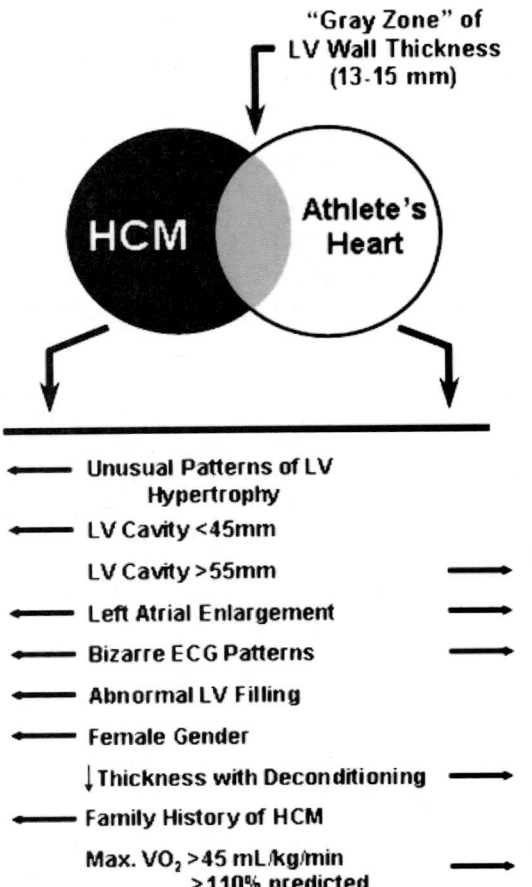

FIGURE 66B.2. Clinical criteria used to distinguish nonobstructive HCM from athlete's heart when maximal LV wall thickness is within shaded gray area of overlap, consistent with both diagnoses. From Maron BJ, Pelliccia A. The heart of trained athletes: Cardiac remodeling and the risks of sports, including sudden death. *Circulation* 2006;114:1633–44, with permission.

has been reported that many of these initial contributions were patient-specific and not gene- or mutation-specific, with clinical findings (phenotype) widely varying among individuals (41). Therefore, risk stratification on the basis of genotype may be ill advised. Certain phenotypes have very distinctive morphologies, e.g., apical HCM, in which hypertrophy is confined to the LV apex. Apical HCM is the result of mutations in the cardiac protein actin and can have complications such as atrial and ventricular arrhythmias. It must be remembered that genetic testing has limited utility in the evaluation of HCM. Currently, mutations in sarcomeric genes account for only ~60% of cases of inherited LV hypertrophy (18). Therefore, unless a specific mutation is known in a first-degree relative, genetic testing is not recommended for the routine evaluation of patients with HCM.

RESTRICTIVE CARDIOMYOPATHY

RCM is characterized by restrictive filling and reduced diastolic volume of either or both ventricles, with normal or near normal systolic function and wall thicknesses. Increased interstitial fibrosis may be present. It may be idiopathic or associated with

another disease. In children, RCM accounts for 2.5%–5% of the diagnosed cardiomyopathies (9,23). The average age at the time of diagnosis has been reported as 6 years, with a median of 5 years and a range from 0.1 to 19 years. No male or female predominance is associated with RCM. Sporadic and familial cases of RCM have been reported. In published cases, ~30% of patients have had a positive family history.

Etiology

RCM has multiple causes and may result from myocardial diseases, including noninfiltrative or infiltrative processes, storage diseases, endomyocardial diseases, myocarditis, and following cardiac transplantation (**Table 66B.2**). The pathology and histology vary with the underlying disease process. Endomyocardial fibrosis is the most common cause of pediatric RCM in the tropics. However, outside the tropics, idiopathic RCM is the most commonly reported cause of RCM in children. Endomyocardial fibrosis is most commonly biventricular, followed by purely LV involvement and, less commonly, purely RV. The histology of endomyocardial fibrosis is characterized by fibrosis of the endocardium of variable thickness. Histologic changes occur in predominantly three areas: the LV apex, the mitral valve apparatus, and the RV apex, which may extend to the supporting structures of the tricuspid valve. In severe cases, the process may extend to the outflow tracts. Loffler endocarditis, or the hypereosinophilic syndrome, is similar to endomyocardial

TABLE 66B.2

CAUSES OF RESTRICTIVE CARDIOMYOPATHIES IN CHILDREN AND ADULTS

Myocardial
Idiopathic
Familial
Scleroderma
Myocarditis
Cardiac transplantation
Pseudoxanthoma elasticum
Diabetic cardiomyopathy
Amyloidosis
Sarcoidosis
Gaucher disease
Hurler disease
Fatty infiltration
Hemochromatosis
Fabry disease
Glycogen storage diseases
Endomyocardial fibrosis
Hypereosinophilia syndrome (Löffler endocarditis)
Endocardial fibroelastosis
Carcinoid
Metastatic cancers
Radiation
Drugs
   Anthracyclines
   Serotonin
   Methysergide
   Ergotamine
   Mercurials
   Busulfan

fibrosis in many respects; debate is ongoing as to whether they are variants of the same disease. Although they have pathologic and clinical similarities, they also have important contrasts. Hypereosinophilic syndrome is typically seen in temperate climates and is more common in adult males. Usually, in this syndrome, a number of organs in addition to the heart are involved and may include the lungs, bone marrow, and brain. The cause of the eosinophilia is usually unknown but may be leukemic or secondary to parasitic, allergic, granulomatous, hypersensitivity, or neoplastic disorders. A number of metabolic disorders with specific enzyme deficiencies can also result in RCM, including lysosomal disorders such as Hurler syndrome, Gaucher disease, Fabry disease, and glycogen storage diseases that can be lysosomal disorders or result from cytoplasmic enzyme deficiencies.

RCM may result from hemochromatosis. Although a common cause of RCM in adults, amyloidosis is an extremely rare cause of RCM in children, as is sarcoidosis. Mediastinal radiation, anthracyclines, serotonin, methysergamide, ergotamine, mercurial agents, and busulfan have all been reported to cause RCM. To date, mutations in five genes have been identified that may result in a RCM phenotype (6,8,11,14,20,31,38). Desmin, Troponin I, and RSK2 mutations have been reported in children with RCM, while lamin A/C (Emery-Dreifuss muscular dystrophy) and transthyretin mutations have been reported to cause an RCM phenotype in adults. Outside the tropics, however, the idiopathic form of RCM is probably the most common form in children. Although the family history is positive in only ~30% of this population, a genetic basis or predisposition for the development of the disease is likely.

Pathophysiology

Diastolic function is primarily affected by ventricular compliance/stiffness and relaxation. In the normal heart, the phase of rapid or early filling occurs as the LV pressure drops below that in the left atrium, just after the mitral valve opens. In the classic description of RCM, ventricular filling is completed in early diastole, with little or no filling in late diastole. In this model, restrictive physiology results from increased myocardial stiffness with decreased compliance, causing a marked ventricular pressure rise with small changes in volume. The earliest phase of clinical diastole is isovolumic relaxation, which is an active energy-requiring process for the uptake of calcium ions into the sarcoplasmic reticulum. It is possible that restrictive hemodynamics may also be caused by dysfunction and delay of active relaxation of the ventricle rather than purely increased intrinsic stiffness of the ventricular wall (13). As diastolic diseases become better understood, it is likely that RCM will be found to result from either abnormal stiffness or abnormal relaxation or both, depending on the underlying cause of the disease and disease progression.

Natural History and Long-term Prognosis

The prognosis in children with RCM is poor. Half of the children die within 2 years of diagnosis. In RCM, heart failure-related deaths are the most common. SCD has also been reported to be a common cause of death in children with RCM (36). Patients who appear to be at greater risk for sudden

death include those who present with signs and symptoms of ischemia, such as syncope and chest pain (36). Prognostic factors for death from heart failure include cardiomegaly and pulmonary venous congestion on chest x-ray, age <5 years, thromboembolism, and elevated pulmonary vascular resistance index. The children with heart failure are at risk from ischemic complications as well (36).

ARRHYTHMOGENIC RIGHT-VENTRICULAR DYSPLASIA

ARVD, also referred to as *arrhythmogenic RV cardiomyopathy* (ARVC), is a form of cardiomyopathy that is characterized by fatty-fibrous replacement of the RV (24). ARVD has a prevalence of 1 in 5000 persons and is a well-recognized disease in Asia, Europe, and the US (33). This gradual process of replacement of normal myocardium with fatty and fibrous tissue predisposes patients to RV dysfunction and life-threatening ventricular arrhythmias. The disease has a predilection to affect only certain areas of the RV—the so-called "triangle of dysplasia," which consists of the RV outflow tract, the apex, and the subtricuspid area of the RV (25). In the early period of the disease, the RV is typically the only ventricle affected but, during the latter stages of the disease, fatty-fibrous tissue can progress in the LV in up to 50% of patients. Patients typically present in their 20s to early 40s with palpitations, nonsustained ventricular tachycardia, or sustained ventricular tachycardia of a left-bundle-branch morphology. SCD may be the initial presentation of the disease (7), and it appears to show a male predisposition.

Diagnosis is based on established criteria that take into account structural, electrocardiographic, histopathologic, and genetic factors (29). The electrocardiogram typically shows T-wave inversion in the precordial leads and a delayed S-wave upstroke. Echocardiography often shows dilation of the RV with segmental wall and/or global RV wall motion abnormalities. The RV outflow tract may be dilated, and an "echo-bright" moderator band and/or evidence of focal RV wall aneurysms may be seen. Cardiac MRI is now commonly used to further assess patients who are suspected of having ARVD. Cardiac MRI can be used to visualize fatty-fibrous replacement of the myocardium.

Emerging evidence suggests that the majority of ARVD cases have a genetic basis. ARVD appears to be a disease caused by desmosomal dysfunction. Desmosomes are a group of proteins that include junctional plakoglobin, plakophilin, desmoplakin, desmoglein, and desmocollin. These proteins function to bind the myocardial cells together (15). This contact allows for electrical conduction between myocytes as well as coordinated mechanical contraction. Six gene mutations have been linked to ARVD to date. Both dominant and recessive forms of ARVD have been linked to mutations in DSP, which encodes desmoplakin. These genes appear to have reduced penetrance and variable expressivity. Genes have been identified for Naxos disease and Carvajal syndrome, which are autosomal-recessive diseases in which patients have ARVD as well as woolly hair and palmoplantar keratodermas. Studies are ongoing to further delineate the genetic mechanisms of ARVD.

Intensive research has been employed to evaluate the latency of the disease (symptoms usually do not become evident until the third or fourth decade of life) and why ARVD has a striking incidence among in athletes (Fig. 66B.1). Many hundreds of thousands of myocardial contractions and changes in mechanical stress are required to disrupt myocardial cells. The RV is a thin ventricle compared to the LV and is more vulnerable to disruption. The thinnest part of the RV wall is in the region of the "triangle of dysplasia." In addition, patients who engage in sports activities have an increased frequency of myocardial contraction and increases in the mechanical stress placed on the myocardium, which results in myocardial disruption occurring at an earlier age. It has been shown that patients with ARVD who perform more intensive exercise routines have symptoms at a younger age and increased incidence of SCD as compared to less active patients with ARVD. As ARVD places patients at risk for dysrhythmias and SCD, the diagnosis precludes participation in competitive sports, and this may also apply to asymptomatic gene carriers (17). Management of patients with ARVD may consist of antiarrhythmic agents, but the therapy with survival benefit appears to be insertion of an implantable cardioverter defibrillator. In addition, therapies for heart failure may be instituted as the disease progresses and have included cardiac transplantation in some cases.

LEFT-VENTRICULAR NONCOMPACTION

LVNC is characterized by deep trabeculations in the LV endocardium (5,39). These trabeculations are seen particularly in the apex and free wall and are thought to represent an arrest in the normal process of myocardial compaction that occurs between weeks 5 and 8 of fetal life. Typically, apical hypertrophy with variable systolic dysfunction is also seen. This disorder, also identified as fetal myocardium, noncompaction of the LV myocardium, and spongiform myocardium, was considered to be a rare disorder in children but has been shown to occur more frequently than previously thought (34). The disorder has an unpredictable course, with some patients developing progressive heart failure, necessitating transplantation, and others developing an "undulating phenotype." The phenotypes display echocardiographic features that alternate between a DCM-like disorder and an HCM-like disorder, while others have primarily diastolic dysfunction (22). LVNC may be associated with systemic disorders such as Barth syndrome or mitochondrial or metabolic disorders (19,34). LVNC has also been associated with a variety of other diseases and syndromes, including Patau syndrome, Fabry disease, Melnick-Needles syndrome, and nail-patella syndrome.

The inheritance pattern in LVNC is variable. Most cases are transmitted as autosomal-dominant traits, but X-linked and mitochondrial transmission is also relatively common. Two autosomal-dominant genes have been reported thus far (α-dystrobrevin, ZASP) (19,42). An X-linked gene, G4.5 (4,19) in the Xq28 region, has been identified; this is the same gene that is linked with Barth syndrome.

The diagnosis of LVNC is typically made by noninvasive methods, although LV angiography can also be used. Echocardiography is the most frequently noted modality (see Chapter 66A, Fig. 66A.2D). Specific echocardiographic criteria for LVNC were discussed previously. It is well established that pediatric patients may have coexisting congenital heart disease

along with LVNC. Other modalities such as cardiovascular MRI are becoming more widely used in the diagnosis of LVNC. The use of specific imaging techniques such as delayed enhancement sequencing may provide further insight into the pathology of LVNC by identifying fibrosis and scarring that can be associated with this disease (21).

CONCLUSIONS AND FUTURE DIRECTIONS

Each of the cardiomyopathies described here has the potential to be a devastating disease for pediatric patients and their families. Each disease requires long-term follow-up care, and each has significant associated morbidity, including the possible need for cardiac transplantation and may even progress to death. Much additional information is still necessary to successfully diagnose and treat these disorders. Most cardiomyopathies are still classified as "idiopathic," although ongoing genetic research should shed additional light as to their true etiology. Multicentered clinical trials are necessary to guide medical therapy and to develop screening protocols for high-risk groups. In the future, genetic screening may be able to identify high-risk patients. In addition, gene-based treatments and/or myocyte progenitor cell transplantation may become therapeutic realities.

KEY POINTS

- Cardiomyopathies are the most common cause of heart failure and ventricular dysfunction in children and may be idiopathic, familial, or acquired.
- DCM represents a heterogeneous group of myocardial disorders that result in ventricular dilation, impaired systolic contractile function, mitral regurgitation, and ventricular arrhythmias in the absence of coronary artery disease, valvular abnormalities, and pericardial disease.
- HCM is characterized by LV hypertrophy, a nondilated LV cavity, systolic hypercontractility, diastolic dysfunction, and, in ~20% of cases, obstruction to LV outflow (hypertrophic obstructive cardiomyopathy) secondary to mitral-septal contact during systole.
- HCM is recognized as the most common genetic cardiovascular disease and is the most common cause of SCD in young healthy subjects, particularly athletes.
- RCM is characterized by restrictive filling and reduced diastolic volume of either or both ventricles, with normal or near-normal systolic function and wall thicknesses. The prognosis in children with RCM is poor. Half of the children die within 2 years of diagnosis. In RCM, heart failure-related deaths are the most common.
- ARVD, also referred to as *arrhythmogenic RV cardiomyopathy*, is a form of cardiomyopathy that is characterized by fatty-fibrous replacement of the RV. This gradual process of replacement of normal myocardium with fatty and fibrous tissue predisposes patients to RV dysfunction and life-threatening ventricular arrhythmias.
- LVNC is characterized by deep trabeculations in the LV endocardium. These trabeculations are seen particularly in the apex and free wall. Typically, apical hypertrophy with variable systolic dysfunction is also seen.

References

1. Arad M, Benson DW, Perez-Atayde AR, et al. Constitutively active AMP kinase mutations cause glycogen storage disease mimicking hypertrophic cardiomyopathy. *J Clin Invest* 2002;109:357–62.
2. Baig MK, Goldman JH, Caforio ALP, et al. Familial dilated cardiomyopathy: Cardiac abnormalities are common in asymptomatic relatives and may represent early disease. *J Am Coll Cardiol* 1998;31:195–201.
3. Bengur AR, Beekman RH, Rocchini AP, et al. Acute hemodynamic effects of captopril in children with a congestive or restrictive cardiomyopathy. *Circulation* 1991;83:523–7.
4. Bleyl SB, Mumford BR, Thompson V, et al. Neonatal, lethal noncompaction of the left ventricular myocardium is allelic with Barth syndrome. *Am J Hum Genet* 1997;61:868–72.
5. Chin TK, Perloff JK, Williams RG, et al. Isolated noncompaction of left ventricular myocardium. *A study of eight cases. Circulation* 1990;82:507–13.
6. Dalakas MC, Park K-Y, Semino-Mora C, et al. Desmin myopathy, a skeletal myopathy with cardiomyopathy caused by mutations in the desmin gene. *N Engl J Med* 2000;342:770–80.
7. Dalal D, Nasir K, Bomma C, et al. Arrhythmogenic right ventricular dysplasia: A United States experience. *Circulation* 2005;112:3823–32.
8. Delaunoy J, Abidi F, Zeniou M, et al. Mutations in the x-linked RSK 2 gene (RPS6KA3) in patients with Coffin-Lowry Syndrome. *Hum Mutat* 2001;17:103–16.
9. Denfield SW, Rosenthal G, Gajarski RJ, et al. Restrictive cardiomyopathies in childhood: Etiologies and natural history. *Tex Heart Inst J* 1997;24:38–44.
10. Elliott PM, Poloniecki J, Dickie S, et al. Sudden death in hypertrophic cardiomyopathy: Identification of high risk patients. *J Am Coll Cardiol* 2000;36:2212–18.
11. Facher JJ, Regier EJ, Jacobs GH, et al. Cardiomyopathy in Coffin-Lowry Syndrome. *Am J Med Genet* 2004;128A:176–8.
12. Fatkin D, Graham RM. Molecular mechanisms of inherited cardiomyopathies. *Physiol Rev* 2002;82:945–80.
13. Gewillig M, Mertens L, Moerman P, et al. Idiopathic restrictive cardiomyopathy in childhood. A diastolic disorder characterized by delayed relaxation. *Eur Heart J* 1996;17:1413–20.
14. Goldfarb LG, Park K-Y, CerveneKova L, et al. Missense mutations in desmin associated with familial cardiac and skeletal myopathy. *Nature Genet* 1998;19:402–3.
15. Green KJ, Gaudry CA. Are desmosomes more than tethers for intermediate filaments? *Nat Rev Mol Cell Biol* 2000;1:208–16.
16. Grunig E, Tasman JA, Kucherer H, et al. Frequency and phenotypes of familial dilated cardiomyopathy. *J Am Coll Cardiol* 1998;31:186–94.
17. Heidbuchel H, Corrado D, Biffi A, et al. Recommendations for participation in leisure-time physical activity and competitive sports of patients with arrhythmias and potentially arrhythmogenic conditions. Part II: Ventricular arrhythmias, channelopathies and implantable defibrillators. *Eur J Cardiovasc Prev Rehabil* 2006;13:676–86.
18. Ho CY, Seidman CE. A contemporary approach to hypertrophic cardiomyopathy. *Circulation* 2006;113:e858–62.
19. Ichida F, Tsubata S, Bowles KR, et al. Novel gene mutations in patients with left ventricular noncompaction or Barth syndrome. *Circulation* 2001;103:1256–63.
20. Jacobson R, Ittmann M, Buxbaum JN, et al. Transthyretin Ile 122 and cardiac amyloidosis in African-Americans: 2 case reports. *Tex Heart Inst J* 1997;24:45–52.
21. Jassal DS, Nomura CH, Neilan TG, et al. Delayed enhancement cardiac MR imaging in noncompaction of left ventricular myocardium. *J Cardiovasc Magn Reson* 2006;8:489–91.
22. Jenni R, Oechslin E, Schneider J, et al. Echocardiographic and pathoanatomical characteristics of isolated left ventricular non-compaction: A step towards classification as a distinct cardiomyopathy. *Heart* 2001;86:666–71.
23. Lipshultz SE, Sleeper LA, Towbin JA, et al. The incidence of pediatric cardiomyopathies in two regions of the United States. *N Engl J Med* 2003;348:1647–55.
24. Marcus FI. Update of arrhythmogenic right ventricular dysplasia. *Card Electrophysiol Rev* 2002;6:54–6.
25. Marcus FI, Fontaine GH, Guiraudon G, et al. Right ventricular dysplasia: A report of 24 adult cases. *Circulation* 1982;65:384–98.
26. Maron BJ. Hypertrophic cardiomyopathy: A systematic review. *JAMA* 2002;287:1308–20.
27. Maron BJ, Gardin JM, Flack JM, et al. Prevalence of hypertrophic cardiomyopathy in a general population of young adults. Echocardiographic analysis of 4111 subjects in the CARDIA Study. Coronary Artery Risk Development in (Young) Adults. *Circulation* 1995;92:785–9.
28. Maron BJ, Shen WK, Link MS, et al. Efficacy of implantable cardioverter-defibrillators for the prevention of sudden death in patients with hypertrophic cardiomyopathy. *N Engl J Med* 2000;342:365–73.
29. McKenna WJ, Thiene G, Nava A, et al. Diagnosis of arrhythmogenic right ventricular dysplasia/cardiomyopathy. Task Force of the Working Group Myocardial and Pericardial Disease of the European Society of Cardiology and of the Scientific Council on Cardiomyopathies of the International Society and Federation of Cardiology. *Br Heart J* 1994;71:215–8.
30. Michels VV, Moll PP, Miller FA, et al. The frequency of familial dilated cardiomyopathy in a series of patients with idiopathic dilated cardiomyopathy. *N Engl J Med* 1992;326:77–82.
31. Morgensen J, Kubo T, Duque M, et al. Idiopathic restrictive cardiomyopathy is part of the clinical expression of cardiac troponin I mutations. *J Clin Invest* 2003;111:209–16.
32. Nugent AW, Daubeney PE, Chondros P, et al. The epidemiology of childhood cardiomyopathy in Australia. *N Engl J Med* 2003;348:1639–46.
33. Peters S, Trummel M, Meyners W. Prevalence of right ventricular dysplasia-cardiomyopathy in a non-referral hospital. *Int J Cardiol* 2004;97:499–501.
34. Pignatelli RH, McMahon CJ, Dreyer WJ, et al. Clinical characterization of left ventricular noncompaction in children: A relatively common form of cardiomyopathy. *Circulation* 2003;108:2672–8.
35. Richardson P, McKenna W, Bristow M, et al. Report of the 1995 World Health Organization/International Society and Federation of Cardiology Task Force on the Definition and Classification of Cardiomyopathies. *Circulation* 1996;93:841–2.
36. Rivenes SM, Kearney DL, Smith EO, et al. Sudden death and cardiovascular collapse in children with restrictive cardiomyopathy. *Circulation* 2000;102:876–82.
37. Sachdev B, Takenaka T, Teraguchi H, et al. Prevalence of Anderson-Fabry disease in male patients with late onset hypertrophic cardiomyopathy. *Circulation* 2002;105:1407–11.
38. Sanna T, Dello Russo A, Toniolo D, et al. Cardiac features of Emery-Dreifuss muscular dystrophy caused by lamin A/C gene mutations. *Eur Heart J* 2003;24:2227–36.
39. Stollberger C, Finsterer J, Blazek G. Left ventricular hypertrabeculation/noncompaction and association with additional cardiac abnormalities and neuromuscular disorders. *Am J Cardiol* 2002;90:899–902.
40. Towbin, Bowles NE. The failing heart. *Nature* 2002;415:227–33.
41. Van Driest SL, Ackerman MJ, Ommen SR, et al. Prevalence and severity of "benign" mutations in the beta-myosin heavy chain, cardiac troponin T, and alpha-tropomyosin genes in hypertrophic cardiomyopathy. *Circulation* 2002;106:3085–90.
42. Vatta M, Mohapatra B, Jimenez S, et al. Mutations in cipher/ZASP in patients with dilated cardiomyopathy and left ventricular noncompaction. *J Am Coll Cardiol* 2003;42:2014–27.
43. Watkins H, McKenna WJ, Thierfelder L, et al. Mutations in the genes for cardiac troponin T and alpha-tropomyosin in hypertrophic cardiomyopathy. *N Engl J Med* 1995;332:1058–64.
44. Watkins H, Rosenzweig A, Hwang DS, et al. Characteristics and prognostic implications of myosin missense mutations in familial hypertrophic cardiomyopathy. *N Engl J Med* 1992;326:1108–14.

CHAPTER 66C ■ HEART FAILURE IN INFANTS AND CHILDREN: MYOCARDITIS

JOHN PHILIP BREINHOLT III • DAVID P. NELSON • JEFFREY A. TOWBIN

Clinically and histopathologically, myocarditis is most easily thought of in terms of myocardial inflammation. The first standardized diagnostic criteria for myocarditis were published in 1987, widely known as the Dallas criteria (2). Active myocarditis is characterized by an inflammatory cellular infiltrate of the myocardium with necrosis and/or degeneration of adjacent myocytes. Borderline myocarditis exhibits an inflammatory cellular infiltrate without evidence of myocyte injury. These findings are not typical of the ischemic damage that is associated with coronary artery disease. This definition does not take into account the underlying etiology (83). In addition, many cases of virus-induced cardiac dysfunction have little or no inflammation on histopathologic evaluation, calling into question whether the definition based on the Dallas criteria is broadly applicable.

ETIOLOGY

Most cases of myocarditis in the US and Western Europe result from viral infections (7). The epidemiology of myocarditis has undergone a shift over the past several decades. Throughout the 1970s and 1980s, enteroviruses (coxsackieviruses A and B, echovirus, poliovirus), particularly coxsackie B viruses, were the most commonly identified viruses; however, by the 1990s the most common causative viruses were adenovirus serotypes 2 and 5 (12,50), with coxsackievirus B (CVB) becoming less prevalent (**Table 66C.1**). Data demonstrate that parvovirus B19 (PVB19) has become the most commonly identified virus in subjects with suspected myocarditis since 2000 (6,15,32,48,62,63,78,79). This increase in PVB19 corresponds to a decrease in the incidence of adenovirus and enterovirus myocarditis. Although currently much less common, a wide variety of other viral causes of myocarditis (9) in children have been described, including cytomegalovirus (CMV), Epstein-Barr virus (EBV), hepatitis C, herpes simplex virus, human immunodeficiency virus (HIV), influenza, mumps, respiratory syncytial virus, rubella, and varicella. Other nonviral, infectious etiologies include bacteria, fungi, parasites, protozoa, rickettsia, and yeasts. Additional noninfectious causes include pharmaceutical agents (83,24), hypersensitivity reactions, autoimmune and collagen-vascular diseases, mixed connective tissue diseases, rheumatic fever, toxic reactions to infectious agents (57) (e.g., mumps or diphtheria), and other disorders such as Kawasaki disease and sarcoidosis (59,84). In many cases, the etiology is not identified.

EPIDEMIOLOGY

Myocarditis is an underdiagnosed disorder (7,83), with the incidence of the usual lymphocytic form ranging from 8.6% to 12% in young adults with sudden cardiac death (22,26) to as high as 16% to 21% in an autopsy series of children with sudden cardiac death (56). The multicentered Myocarditis Treatment Trial, based strictly on the Dallas criteria, reported a 9% incidence in adult patients (51). Moreover, myocarditis has been implicated as the cause of dilated cardiomyopathy (DCM) in 9% of patients in a large series from Johns Hopkins (30) and in up to 20% of DCM cases from other series (9).

Usually a sporadic disease, viral myocarditis can also occur as an epidemic. Epidemics usually are seen in newborns, most commonly in association with CVB. Another manifestation is in intrauterine myocarditis, which occurs either sporadically or during epidemics. Postnatal spread of coxsackievirus is via fecal/oral or air-borne transmission (33). The World Health Organization reports that this ubiquitous family of viruses results in cardiovascular sequelae in <1% of infections, although the rate increases to 4% when CVB is considered (36). Other important viral causes, such as adenovirus and influenza A, have an air-borne transmission (33). Although myocarditis can occur throughout the year, some etiologic agents are likely seasonal (e.g., coxsackievirus), while others are perennial (e.g., adenovirus, PVB19).

MECHANISM OF DISEASE: PATHOPHYSIOLOGY OF MYOCARDITIS

Immune Response to Viral Illness

The pathogenesis of myocarditis involves direct invasion by the cardiotropic virus that leads to activation of an immune response and local inflammation. This activation induces production of B cells, which results in myocytolysis and further interstitial inflammation and production of anti-heart antibodies (47).

The immunopathogenesis of CVB and encephalomyocarditis has been well described in mouse models. CMV, HIV, and adenovirus models also have been described. Viremia is present within 24–72 hrs of CVB infection and reaches maximum growth in the tissues at 72–96 hrs. Viral titers decline shortly

TABLE 66C.1

CAUSES OF MYOCARDITIS

Viruses	Nonviral infectious pathogens	Noninfectious etiologies
Adenovirus	**Bacteria**	**Pharmaceuticals**
Arbovirus	*Borrelia burgdorferi*	Acetazolamide
Cytomegalovirus	*Brucella melitensis*	Amphotericin B
Enterovirus	*Chlamydia pneumoniae*	Anthracyclines
▪ Coxsackie A and B	*Chlamydia psittaci*	Cephalosporins
▪ Echovirus	Clostridium	Cocaine
▪ Poliovirus	Klebsiella	Cyclophosphamide
	Legionella pneumophila	Digoxin
Epstein-Barr virus	Leptospira	Diuretics
Hepatitis A and B	Meningococcus	Dobutamine
Herpes simplex virus	Mycobacteria	Indomethacin
Human immunodeficiency	*Mycoplasma pneumoniae*	Isoniazid
virus	Salmonella	Methyldopa
Influenza A	Streptococcus species	Neomercazole
Measles	*Treponema pallidum*	Penicillin
Mumps	Tuberculosis	Phenylbutazone
Parvovirus B19	Typhoid	Phenytoin
Rabies		Sulfonamides
Respiratory syncytial	**Rickettsial**	Tetracycline
virus	*Rickettsia rickettsii*	Tricyclic Antidepressants
Rhinovirus	*Rickettsia tsutsugamushi*	
Rubella		**Hypersensitivity/Autoimmune**
Rubeola	**Fungi and yeasts**	Celiac disease
Varicella	Actinomyces	Diabetes mellitus
Vaccinia virus	Candida	Hashimoto thyroiditis
	Coccidiodes	Mixed connective tissue
Toxins and other	Histoplasma	disease
Scorpion venom		Myasthenia gravis
Diphtheria	**Protozoa**	Pernicious anemia
Smallpox vaccine	*Entamoeba histolytica*	Rheumatoid arthritis
Cornstarch	*Trypanosoma cruzi*	Rheumatic fever
Kawasaki disease	*Toxoplasma gondii*	Scleroderma
Sarcoidosis		Systemic lupus erythematosus
Scleroderma	**Parasites**	Takayasu arteritis
	Echinococcus granulosus	Thrombocytopenic purpura
	Heterophyiasis	Ulcerative colitis
	Plasmodium falciparum	Wegener granulomatosis
	Schistosomes	Whipple disease
	Taeniasis solium (Cysticercosis)	
	Toxocara canis	
	Trichinella spiralis	

thereafter, and essentially no organisms can be found by 7–10 days after inoculation. Antibody concentrations increase during this decline in viral titer, suggesting that antibody is integral to viral clearance. Macrophages appear 5–10 days after infection in the CVB model of myocarditis.

The natural killer (NK) cell is important in the pathogenesis of myocarditis. Animals depleted of their NK cells prior to infection with coxsackievirus develop a more severe myocarditis (34). NK cells are activated by interferon, which is an indirect modulator of myocardial injury. Murine skin fibroblasts serve as target cells for CVB-sensitized cytotoxic T cells. The NK cells specifically limit the nonenveloped virus infection by killing the virally infected cells. Male mice are less efficient in activating NK cells. It is presumed that a more efficient viral clearance results in a reduced amount of virally induced neoantigen production and decreased recogni-

tion by cytotoxic T lymphocytes. T cells generate injury by accumulation of activated macrophages; production of antibody and antibody-dependent, cell-mediated cytotoxicity; direct lysis by antibody and complement; and direct action of cytotoxic T cells. Myocardial injury is the result of direct viral myofiber destruction and T-lymphocyte cytolysis. Animals with absent or suppressed T-cell function have less myocardial injury.

In humans, antibody-mediated cytolysis was found among 30% of patients with suspected myocarditis, as well as in 18 of 19 patients with proven viral infections due to CVB, influenza A, or mumps virus (49). A muscle-specific, antimyolemmal antibody was found in these patients and correlated with the degree of in vitro-induced cytolysis of rat cardiocytes. Complementary DNA (to CVB2 RNA) cloning techniques were used to develop a CVB-specific complementary DNA hybridization probe that detected virus nucleic acid sequences in patients who were diagnosed as having active or healed myocarditis or DCM (10,11). As controls, they used patients with unrelated disorders and found that these patients had no virus-specific sequences (10), suggesting that in patients with congestive cardiomyopathy or healing myocarditis, viral particles persist even though viral culture is almost always negative. The findings imply a continual viral replication in cells, which may conceal the antigenicity by an immunologic process that prevents correct posttranslational processing of capsid proteins. Adult patients with myocarditis were found to have been exposed to a greater number of CVB1 to CVB6, as demonstrated by the number of positive and negative responses to neutralizing antibodies of those viruses (38). The investigators believed that immunization against several types of CVB was essential in the development of myocarditis. Although they postulated this cross-immunization theory, a few cases of myocarditis in their patients involved exposure to only one type of CVB, casting doubt on the validity of their theory.

Defective cell-mediated immunity occurs in patients with myocarditis and DCM as compared to healthy controls. The pathogenesis of adenoviral myocarditis differs from CVB (39). Specifically, the inflammatory infiltrate is substantially less in adenoviral infection (7,50,65). The number of CD2, CD3, and CD45ROT lymphocytes was significantly decreased in adenovirus-infected patients compared with those patients who had myocarditis not due to adenovirus (65). The adenoviruses have a number of strategies for modulating the immune response, which could impact the number of activated lymphocytes in the adenovirus-infected myocardium. Several adenovirus-encoded proteins can interact with host immune components, including proteins encoded by the E3 region, which can protect cells from tumor necrosis factor (TNF)-mediated lysis as well as downregulation of major histocompatibility complex class I antigen expression. The E1A proteins are capable of promoting the induction of apoptosis, inhibiting IL-6 expression, and interfering with IL-6 signal transduction pathways. These functions of E1A may be pertinent to the development of the myocardial pathology seen in DCM. First, IL-6 promotes lymphocyte activation, which is reduced in adenovirus-infected patients. Second, it has been shown that apoptotic cells occur in the myocardium of patients with DCM. Taken together, these events are likely to result in DCM.

Role of Autoimmunity in Myocarditis

Circulating autoantibodies that target contractile, mitochondrial, and structural proteins have been described in murine and human myocarditis. These autoantibodies have been detected in 25%–73% of patients with biopsy-confirmed myocarditis (64). Persistent viral infection of the myocardium is linked to induction of autoantibodies against the adenine nucleotide translocator (ANT) and myosin (64,68). ANT shuttles energy from the mitochondria to the cells, whereas myosin is a contractile protein.

Anti-ANT antibodies correlate with cardiac dysfunction (68). An increase in the ANT1 isoform was detected in patients together with a concomitant decrease in ANT2. Furthermore, in patients with enterovirus infection, this was more pronounced than in patients in whom no enterovirus was detected.

In animal models of CVB3 infection, nucleotide transport is inhibited. ANT1 transgenic mutant mice have a cardiomyopathic phenotype, supporting the concept that it is important in cardiac function.

Autoantibodies may have cytopathic effects on calcium homeostasis, energy metabolism, and signal transduction. They may also play a role in the activation of the complement cascade, leading to lysis of antibody-coated cells (42). Furthermore, novel autoantigens, including dihydrolipoamide dehydrogenase and sarcomere-specific creatine kinase, have been identified in patients with myocarditis (3,16,64). It is not clear, however, if these autoantigens are important pathogenetically. Nevertheless, in studies describing the use of immunoadsorption to remove circulating autoantibodies, cardiac function improved and myocardial inflammation decreased (27–29,72). Thus far, autoantibodies associated with persistent adenovirus infection of the myocardium have not been described.

Role of Cytokines in Myocarditis

Interest in the role of cytokines in the pathogenesis of myocarditis and DCM has grown considerably. Animal studies suggest a relationship between subclinical viral infection and the later development of DCM. This process is presumed to occur by an autoimmune-like mechanism triggered by the initial viral insult. Studies in murine models suggest that cytokine-mediated modulation of the immune response to viral infection may induce a chronic autoimmune myocarditis (43,53,60,69). Cytokines contribute to the regulation of antibody production and the maintenance of "self-tolerance." Susceptible murine strains, when infected with CVB3, develop myocyte necrosis and an acute inflammatory response. After the initial viral infection, resolution of inflammation eventually occurs. However, in other strains, a second autoimmune phase of myocarditis appears, with diffuse mononuclear cell infiltrates present in the heart. These mononuclear cells are a significant source of the cytokines IL-1 and TNF-α, and they release large amounts of TNF-α and IL-1b by human monocytes when exposed to CVB3. These cytokines participate in leukocyte activation, which may be beneficial in promoting a specific lymphocyte response to viral infection. However, they also may promote cardiac fibroblast activity. Therefore, it has been suggested that local secretion of cytokines in the myocardium perpetuates the inflammatory process, which subsequently leads to the fibrosis associated with DCM and ultimately the deterioration of cardiac function.

IL-1 and TNF-α are potential inhibitors of cardiac myocyte β-adrenergic responsiveness, and further studies have shown IL-1 and TNF-α to be the macrophage factors that mediate this effect (53). TNF-α levels are elevated in patients with chronic heart disease, myocarditis, or DCM (53,75). TNF-α can potentiate the immune response and induce apoptosis in cells, integral processes in the pathogenesis of myocarditis. Conversely, anti–TNF-α blocks or reduces the severity of myocarditis. Other inflammatory mediators, including IL-1 and granulocyte colony-stimulating factor, are also elevated in patients with myocarditis (53). Inflammatory cytokines may cause a direct negative inotropic response (14).

IL-2 limits myocardial damage when administered in the acute viremic stage, by enhancing NK cell activity (43,69). In contrast, IL-2 exacerbates the course and severity of the disease when given in the subacute, nonviremic stage, by increasing the number of infiltrating T cells. IL-12 protects mice from encephalomyocarditis virus-induced myocarditis (60). Further, IL-12 augments cytotoxic activity and induces Th1-specific immune responses.

Cytokines may act through inducible nitric oxide synthase (iNOS) (60). Nitric oxide can inhibit viral replication by targeting specific viral proteases, and the formation of peroxynitrate has potent antiviral effects. NOS-deficient mice have exhibited greater viral titers, higher viral mRNA loads, and more extensive myocyte necrosis (61). In a cardiac myosin-induced myocarditis model, NOS expression is induced in both macrophages and cardiomyocytes. However, NOS did not appear to be essential for the development of pathology, because myocarditis developed in mice that lacked interferon regulatory transcription factor (IRF)-1, a transcription factor that controls iNOS expression. Despite the failure to synthesize NOS in the myocardium, the prevalence and severity of disease in IRF-1–deficient animals were similar to results observed in control animals. In addition, no difference was detected in animals that lacked the IRF-2 gene, a negative regulator of IRF-1–induced transcription. However, in other studies of myosin-induced autoimmune myocarditis, NOS expression in cardiomyocytes and macrophages was associated with more intense inflammation, whereas NOS inhibitors were shown to reduce myocarditis severity (55).

In the rat model, nitric oxide expression is critical to the pathology of autoimmune myocarditis (60). Rats treated with aminoguanidine, an inhibitor of iNOS, had only focal mononuclear infiltration and a reduction of cardiomyocytes positive for iNOS. By comparison, untreated animals had considerable inflammatory infiltration and myocyte damage. In addition, serum levels of creatine kinase were significantly reduced in the treated animals, indicating reduced muscle damage. In a separate study, IL-2 levels appeared early, whereas IL-3, TNF-α, and iNOS were present later, during the period of peak inflammation. IL-10 was detected only after inflammation began to subside, and it persisted during recovery. These data support the notion that changes in the TH$_1$ and TH$_2$ responses are important for controlling outcome, as previously suggested for CVB3-induced myocarditis.

It is difficult to extrapolate the information obtained in animal models of myocarditis to human disease. Studies to clarify the role of cytokines and nitric oxide in the pathogenesis of myocarditis in humans are warranted, as is consideration of the potential efficacy of drugs to inhibit cytokine or iNOS expression. Further investigation is necessary to elucidate if viral persistence, combined with ongoing IL-6, IL-8, and TNF-α expression, in the absence of IL-10, leads to the progression from myocarditis to DCM.

Role of Cell Adhesion Molecules in Myocarditis

Cell adhesion molecules (CAMs) may also play a role in the pathogenesis of myocarditis. Intercellular adhesion molecule (ICAM)-1 is known to play a major role in cell-cell adhesion, particularly leukocyte adherence and transendothelial migration. ICAM-1 is a member of the immunoglobulin supergene family of CAMs and is a single-chain glycoprotein of 80–115 kDa with an extracellular domain that consists of five immunoglobulin-like repeats. ICAM-1 is predominantly expressed on endothelial cells but is also expressed on fibroblasts, epithelial cells, mucosal cells, lymphocytes, monocytes, and cardiac myocytes after inflammatory injury. Expression of ICAM-1 on endothelial cells is upregulated by cytokines such as IL-1 and TNF-α. Lymphocyte function-associated antigen (LFA)-1 is a well-established binding ligand of ICAM-1, and is part of the β_2 integrin family, consisting of a 180-kDa α subunit (CD11a) and a 95-kDa β subunit (CD18). LFA-1 is expressed on virtually all leukocytes, including monocytes. The adhesive interaction between LFA-1 and ICAM-1 mediates adhesion-dependent helper T-cell, cytotoxic T-cell, and NK-cell functions. Antibody to LFA-1 blocks the inflammatory response in animal models of myocarditis.

Cardiomyocyte Apoptosis

Apoptosis, or programmed cell death, has an important role in embryogenesis, tissue homeostasis, and regulation of immunologic responses, among normal physiologic processes, and is associated with the growth and regression of tumors. Cells that undergo apoptosis exhibit characteristic morphologic and biochemical features, including chromatin aggregation, nuclear and cytoplasmic aggregation, and formation of apoptotic bodies, resulting from the partition of the cytoplasm and nucleus into membrane-bound vesicles. These apoptotic bodies are rapidly phagocytosed by adjacent macrophages or epithelial cells without resulting in an inflammatory response. Apoptotic cells are detectable by terminal transferase labeling (terminal deoxynucleotide transferase-mediated biotin-deoxyuridine triphosphate nick end labeling, TUNEL) in myocardial tissue samples from patients with DCM.

A number of viruses have been implicated in the induction of apoptosis, including adenovirus, EBV, and HIV. Apoptotic cells are detected in adenovirus-associated myocarditis and DCM. In the areas of detected cells, up to 1% of cells may stain positive, including myocytes, infiltrating inflammatory cells, and endothelial cells. In tissue sections from control patients, either unstained or sporadically stained cells (one or two per section) may be detected. These data suggest a relationship between infection of the myocardium by adenovirus and the onset of apoptosis, which could result in pathologic processes associated with myocarditis and DCM (81). Furthermore, a number of inflammatory cells may be seen undergoing the apoptotic process. Although this could reflect a natural defense mechanism of the host against the virus, it also raises the possibility of virus-induced apoptosis as a mechanism of immune system avoidance. In tumors, infiltrating immune cells are destroyed by the induction of apoptosis through the expression of Fas ligand on the tumor cell that binds Fas on the lymphocyte.

Two of the adenovirus genes, E1A and E1B, regulate apoptosis via a p53-dependent pathway (19). The expression of E1A in cells results in the induction of apoptosis, but the coexpression of E1B (or the bcl-2 proto-oncogene) suppresses this effect and results in cell transformation. E1B encodes 19-kDa and 55-kDa proteins, either of which can suppress apoptosis. The 55-kDa protein of E1B binds to, and inhibits, p53, but the mechanism of suppression by the 19-kDa protein is unknown.

As previously noted, most models of experimental myocarditis have used CVB3 variants. It has been known for a number of years, however, that different variants induce different pathologic mechanisms and that different strains of mice are affected differently. Infection of BALB/c, MRL[+/+], or DBA/2 mice with a cardiotropic variant of CVB3 resulted in similar levels of inflammation, but only in DBA/2 mice was antiheart immunoglobulin G generated (34). Few CD8[+] T cells infiltrated the myocardium of MRL[+/+] and DBA/2 mice, but they are the major component of the T-cell response in BALB/c mice. The detection of apoptotic cells via TUNEL staining revealed no apoptotic cells in DBA/2 myocardium, inflammatory cells undergoing apoptosis in MRI[+/+] mice, or myocyte or inflammatory cell apoptosis in BALB/c mice (39). Ventricular contractility decreased in BALB/c mice with myocarditis, indicative of cardiomyopathy, whereas no change in DBA/2 mice was seen.

Long-term Sequelae of Myocarditis

In those cases in which resolution of cardiac dysfunction does not occur, chronic DCM results (31,54). It has been unclear what the underlying etiology of these long-term sequelae could be, but viral persistence and autoimmunity have been widely speculated. Enteroviral protease 2A directly cleaves the cytoskeletal protein dystrophin, resulting in dysfunction of this protein. Because mutations in dystrophin are known to cause an inherited form of DCM (as well as the DCM associated with the neuromuscular diseases Duchenne and Becker muscular dystrophies), it is likely that they are largely responsible for the chronic DCM seen in enteroviral myocarditis (13,76,77). Other viruses (e.g., adenoviruses), also have enzymes that cleave membrane structural proteins or result in activation or inactivation of transcription factors, cytokines, or adhesion molecules to cause chronic DCM (17). Therefore, it appears that a complex interaction between the viral genome and the heart occurs, resulting in the long-term outcome of affected patients.

As in mice, myocarditis in humans may have a genetic basis (58). Support for this theory includes the frequent finding of myocardial lymphocytic infiltrate in patients with familial and sporadic DCM, as well as the few reports of families in which two or more individuals have been diagnosed with myocarditis on endomyocardial biopsy. The identification of a common receptor for the four most common viral causes of myocarditis (CVB3 and CVB4 and adenoviruses 2 and 5) and the human coxsackievirus and adenovirus receptor (5,8,74) suggests that, if mutated, the result could be responsible for host differences leading to myocarditis.

The prognosis of acute myocarditis in newborns is especially poor (25). Mortality rates as high as 75% have been reported in infants (4); older infants and children have a better prognosis, with mortality rates between 10% and 25% (25). Most deaths occur in the first week of the illness. It is likely that other viral causes of myocarditis, such as adenovirus, have similarly poor outcomes as infants. Twenty-five percent of the patients continued to have an abnormal electrocardiogram or chest x-ray film even though they were clinically asymptomatic. Abnormalities in the resting electrocardiogram may not be seen but may be elicited with exercise (20). Adult patients who recover may be asymptomatic at rest or with light exertion but may

demonstrate a reduced working capacity with exercise stress testing.

Pathologic Findings of Myocarditis

Gross and Microscopic Findings

Pathologic findings are nonspecific, with similar gross and microscopic changes noted irrespective of the causative agent (33,83). The heart weight increases, and all four chambers are affected. The muscle is flaccid and pale, with petechial hemorrhages often seen on the epicardial surfaces, especially in cases of CVB infection. A hemorrhagic pericardial effusion also may develop relating to the often concomitant finding of pericarditis. The ventricular wall is frequently thin, although hypertrophy may be encountered. The valves and endocardium are not typically involved.

In cases of chronic myocarditis, the valves may appear glossy white, suggesting that endocardial fibroelastosis (EFE) may have resulted from an in utero viral myocarditis. When comparing myocarditis with EFE, children with myocarditis typically have symptoms for <2 weeks, whereas those with EFE have symptoms for >4 months. Mumps and CVB have been identified in the myocardium of infants with EFE (57). Mural thrombi occur in the left ventricle, and small emboli are often found in the coronary and cerebral vessels. Coronary emboli, although rare, may produce areas of ischemia or injury, with resultant production of the cardiac dysrhythmias that sometimes occur during the acute disease.

Bacterial myocarditis produces microabscesses and patchy focal suppurative changes. A combined perimyocarditis is also encountered frequently. Parasitic myocarditis caused by trichinella has a focal infiltrate with lymphocytes and eosinophils, but larvae are usually not identified.

An interstitial collection of mononuclear cells, including lymphocytes, plasma cells, and eosinophils, is typical of early myocarditis. Polymorphonuclear cells and viral particles are rarely encountered. Extensive necrosis of the myocardium, with loss of cross-striation in the muscle fibers and edema, is seen in severe infections, particularly with coxsackievirus. Perivascular accumulation of lymphocytes and plasma cells has been described with CVB myocarditis but is usually a minor finding. This accumulation is a much more prominent finding in myocardial infections from rickettsiae, varicella, trypanosomes, and other parasites, and in reaction to sulfonamides.

Diphtheria myocarditis is frequently complicated by dysrhythmias and complete atrioventricular block. Diphtheria exotoxin attaches to conductive tissue and interferes with protein synthesis by inhibiting a translocating enzyme in the delivery of amino acids. Triglyceride accumulates, producing fatty changes of the myofibers.

A severe myocarditis caused by *Trypanosoma cruzi* results in Chagas disease. Rare in North America, Chagas is endemic in South America, affecting up to 50% of the population. Microscopic examination reveals the organism as well as neutrophils, lymphocytes, macrophages, and eosinophils.

Sudden cardiac death in infancy may result from myocardial inflammation. A resorptive, degenerative process in the His bundle and left margin of the atrioventricular node was described in cases of infants who died in Northern Ireland (40). Ventricular tachycardia due to lymphocytic or granulomatous myocarditis may infrequently result in sudden cardiac death (23).

Giant cell myocarditis is a rare disease that results in progressive acute heart failure, is frequently fatal, and is recognized by multinucleated giant cells present on biopsy (18). It is associated with rheumatoid arthritis, rheumatic heart disease, sarcoidosis, syphilis, tuberculosis, ulcerative colitis, and fungal or parasitic infections (18,59,67,73). Giant cells also occur in idiopathic (Fiedler) myocarditis. Two types of giant cells have been characterized: cells that originate from the myocardium and cells that are derived from interstitial histiocytes.

CLINICAL MANIFESTATIONS OF MYOCARDITIS

In general, myocarditis should be considered in all children and adults with new-onset congestive heart failure (CHF) in whom no other etiology is found. Any cause of acute circulatory failure may mimic myocarditis. The differential diagnoses of CHF based on age range are listed in **Table 66C.2**. In many cases, an antecedent, nonspecific, flu-like illness or episode of gastroenteritis may precede the symptoms of CHF.

Distinct clinical presentations for myocarditis include acute, subacute, and fulminant forms of the disease (54). Patients with *acute* and *subacute myocarditis* present hemodynamically stable with no fever and requiring only low-dose inotropic support. *Subacute* presentation entails an indistinct onset of symptoms of heart failure that may have developed over weeks to months. Patients with *fulminant myocarditis* present with severe hemodynamic compromise with at least two of the following clinical features: fever, distinct onset of symptoms of heart failure (fatigue, dyspnea on exertion or at rest, acute-onset edema), and a history consistent with a viral illness within 2 weeks of presentation. These patients are typically in extremis on presentation and often require high-dose inotrope

TABLE 66C.2

DIFFERENTIAL DIAGNOSIS OF MYOCARDITIS BY AGE

Newborn and infant
Sepsis
Hypoxia
Hypoglycemia
Hypocalcemia
Structural heart disease
Left atrial myxoma
Idiopathic dilated cardiomyopathy
Barth syndrome
Endocardial fibroelastosis
Pompe disease
Anomalous left coronary artery from the pulmonary artery
Cerebral arteriovenous malformation

Child
Idiopathic dilated cardiomyopathy
X-linked dilated cardiomyopathy
Autosomal-dominant dilated cardiomyopathy
Anomalous left coronary artery from the pulmonary artery
Endocardial fibroelastosis
Chronic tachyarrhythmia
Pericarditis

and/or mechanical support. One other subtype of the fulminant form of clinical phenotype is the patient who presents acutely—like the fulminant myocarditis patient, with symptoms of severe DHF—but additionally manifests an infarct pattern on electrocardiogram that mimics that seen in anomalous left coronary artery from the pulmonary artery, including deep Q waves in leads I and aVL, and V4 through V6. Endomyocardial biopsy typically reveals significant necrosis with severe cellular edema and cell breakdown and typically identifies a coxsackievirus as the viral etiology, or no virus identification is made. Although not described in the literature, at one center, this presentation has been termed *fulminant necrotic myocarditis*. The potential value of delineating these clinical phenotypes is that long-term survival is typically better in patients with the fulminant forms of myocarditis; therefore, they are particularly excellent candidates for mechanical circulatory support as a bridge to recovery. Better outcomes were reported in patients with fulminant myocarditis, with 93% alive without heart transplant at 1 year and 93% alive without transplant at 11 years postinfection, whereas patients with acute myocarditis had a survival without transplant of 85% at 1 year and 45% at 11 years (54).

Age-specific Differences in Presentation

Differences in presentation are seen depending on the age of the child (i.e., newborn/infant versus child or adolescent), making the diagnosis challenging. Adults and adolescents present with similar findings.

Newborns or infants typically present with fever, irritability or listlessness, periodic episodes of pallor, tachypnea or respiratory distress, and diaphoresis. Poor appetite or vomiting is frequently seen. Sudden death may occur in this subgroup of children. On physical examination, pallor and mild cyanosis are commonly noted. The skin is usually cool and mottled, consistent with poor perfusion due to decreased cardiac output. Respirations are usually rapid and labored; grunting may be prominent, but rales are uncommon. The cardiovascular exam is consistent with CHF and includes resting tachycardia, a gallop rhythm, muffled heart sounds, and frequently an systolic regurgitant murmur due to mitral regurgitation. In some of these young children, particularly newborns, a tricuspid regurgitation murmur may also be identified. The pulses are usually thready, and hepatomegaly is usually obvious. Dysrhythmias (supraventricular or ventricular tachycardia) or atrioventricular block may also occur. It is important to remember that the younger the child, the more likely that intrauterine myocarditis has occurred and that the findings may be more associated with chronic disease than otherwise expected in acute disease.

Older children, adolescents, and adults commonly report a recent history of viral disease, generally 10–14 days prior to presentation. Initial symptoms include lethargy, low-grade fever, and pallor; the child usually has decreased appetite and often complains of abdominal pain. Diaphoresis, palpitations, rashes, exercise intolerance, and general malaise are common signs and symptoms. Later in the course of illness, respiratory symptoms become predominant. Physical exam findings are consistent with CHF. Unlike newborns, jugular venous distention and pulmonary rales may be found, and resting tachycardia is often prominent. Dysrhythmias, including atrial fibrillation, supraventricular tachycardia or ventricular tachycardia, and atrioventricular block, may occur. Syncope or sudden death may occur due to cardiac collapse.

DIAGNOSTIC TESTS

The diagnosis of myocarditis is often difficult to establish but should be suspected in any infant or child who presents with unexplained CHF or ventricular tachycardia. Appropriate diagnostic assessment includes chest x-ray, electrocardiogram, echocardiogram, and various laboratory studies.

Chest X-ray

As shown in **Figure 66C.1**, the chest x-ray on presentation usually demonstrates cardiomegaly with prominent pulmonary vascular markings that are suggestive of pulmonary edema, consistent with CHF. Comparisons over time may demonstrate significant improvement or normalization of the chest x-ray within a few months of presentation, suggesting a transient disease state (most typically, myocarditis).

Electrocardiogram

Sinus tachycardia with low-voltage QRS complexes (<5 mm total amplitude in all limb leads) with or without low-voltage

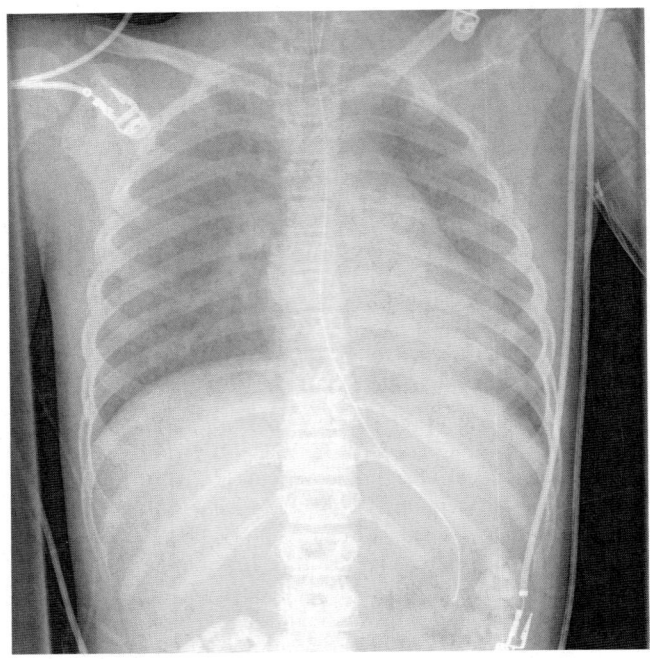

FIGURE 66C.1. Chest radiograph in a child with acute myocarditis. Presence of cardiomegaly and increased pulmonary vascular markings consistent with pulmonary edema.

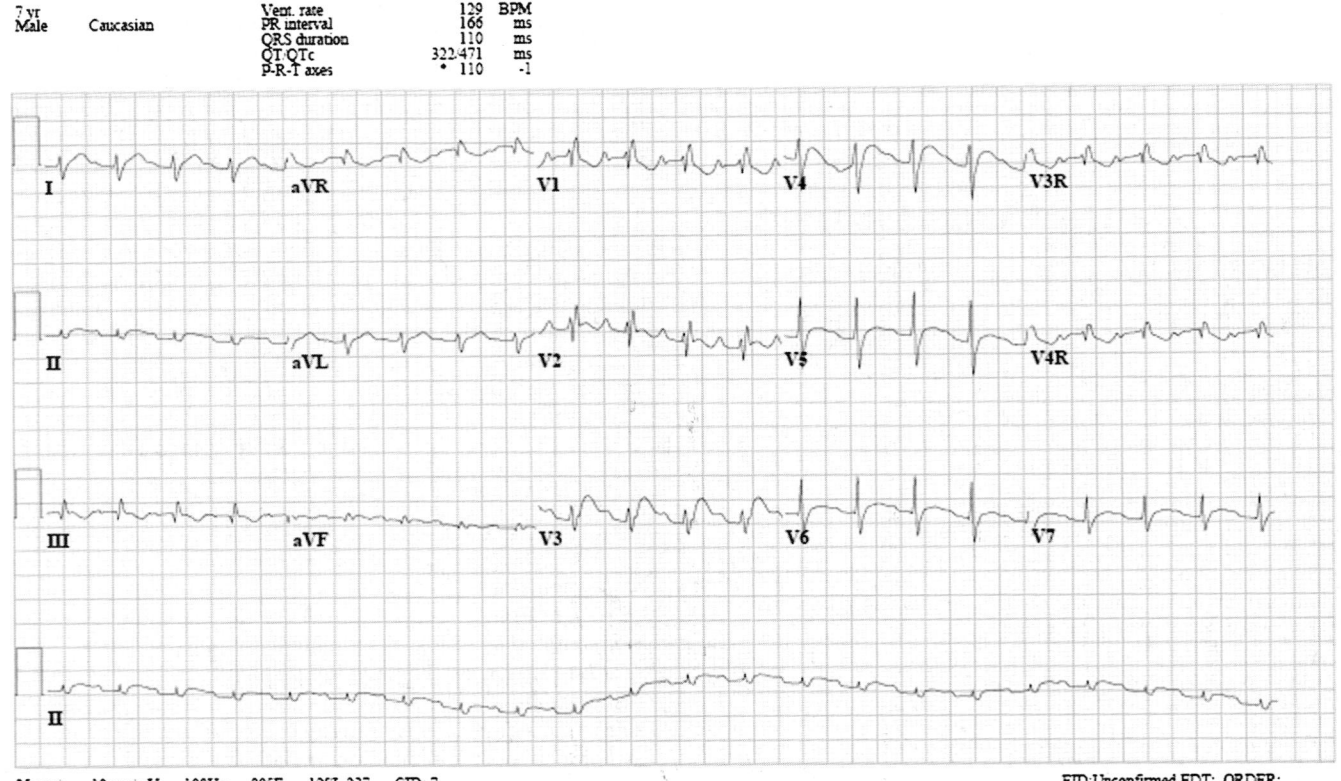

7 yr Male	Caucasian	Vent. rate	129	BPM
		PR interval	166	ms
		QRS duration	110	ms
		QT/QTc	322/471	ms
		P-R-T axes	• 110	-1

FIGURE 66C.2. Electrocardiogram in a case of myocarditis. Low-voltage QRS complexes with inverted T waves. Widened QRS complexes and ST-segment changes in the precordial leads consistent with ischemia noted throughout.

or inverted T waves are classically described. As shown in the example in **Figure 66C.2**, widened QRS complexes and ST-segment changes may be present. A pattern of myocardial infarction with wide Q waves (>35 msec) and ST-segment changes may also be seen in the fulminant necrotic presentation. Ventricular tachycardia, supraventricular tachycardia, atrial fibrillation, or atrioventricular block occurs in some children.

Echocardiogram

As shown in **Figure 66C.3**, a dilated and dysfunctional left ventricle consistent with DCM is seen on two-dimensional and M-mode echocardiography (i.e., left ventricle end-diastolic and end-systolic dimensions are increased; shortening and ejection fractions are decreased). Segmental wall motion abnormalities are relatively common, but global hypokinesis is predominant. Pericardial effusion frequently occurs. Doppler and color-Doppler commonly demonstrate mitral regurgitation (Fig. 66C.3). Dilation of other chambers may also be seen. Cardiac output calculations may be obtained and are typically reduced. Coronary artery or structural abnormalities that could result in these features should be excluded.

Viral Studies

Historically, a positive viral culture from the myocardium has been considered the diagnostic standard for myocarditis. Viral culture of peripheral specimens, such as blood, stool, or urine, is commonly performed but is unreliable at identifying the causative infection. A fourfold increase in antibody titer correlates with infection. However, these studies are nonspecific because prior infection with the causative virus is commonplace.

Cardiac Biomarkers and Immunologic Studies

In adults who present with suspected myocarditis, serum cardiac biomarkers (e.g., creatine kinase, troponin I and T) are routinely measured. Creatine kinase and erythrocyte sedimentation rate (35) have proven unhelpful, and troponin I and T have a low sensitivity, although both demonstrated a high specificity and reasonable positive predictive values of 82% (70) and 93% (46), respectively. The use of quantitative MHC antigen expression has been proposed, with conflicting results (37,82). These diagnostic studies are infrequently utilized in the pediatric population, although some data are emerging for their application in children (71).

Endomyocardial Biopsy

In acute myocarditis, a right ventricular endomyocardial biopsy can be performed, and samples (**Fig. 66C.4**) are evaluated histologically for inflammation. The inflammatory infiltrate is usually patchy and scattered within the ventricular myocardium. A mononuclear cell infiltrate is diagnostic of myocarditis, although this does not identify the etiology (**Fig. 66C.5**). The Dallas Criteria define myocarditis as "a process characterized by an inflammatory infiltrate of the myocardium with necrosis and/or degeneration of adjacent myocytes not typical of ischemic damage" due to coronary artery or other disease (2). At the time of initial biopsy, a specimen may be classified either as active myocarditis, borderline myocarditis, or no myocarditis, depending on whether (a) an inflammatory infiltrate occurs in association with myocyte degeneration or necrosis (active), or (b) too sparse of an infiltrate or no myocyte degeneration occurs (borderline) (2,51). Repeat endomyocardial biopsy may be appropriate in cases in which strong suspicion of myocarditis exists clinically. On repeat endomyocardial

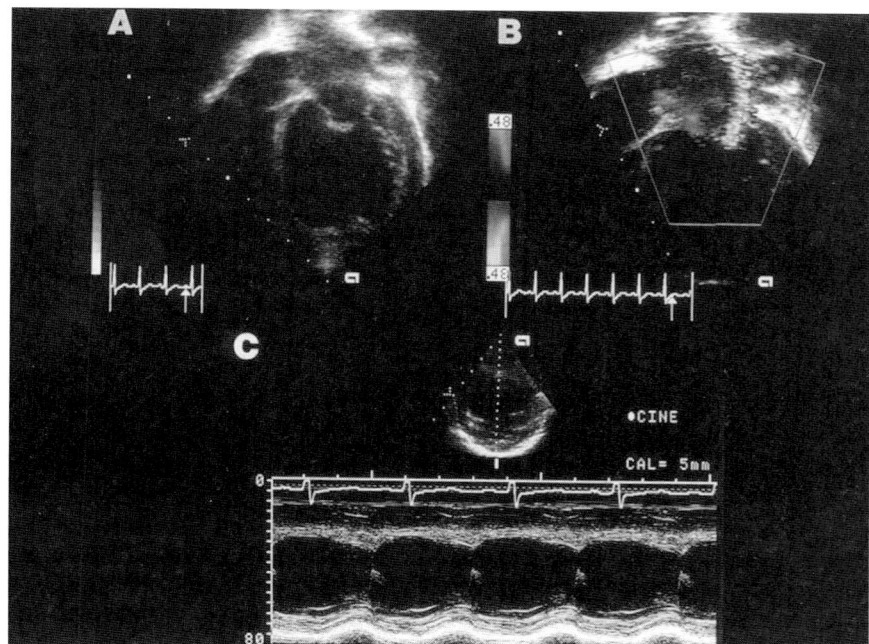

FIGURE 66C.3. Echocardiographic features of myocarditis. (**A**) Two-dimensional apical 4-chamber view demonstrating left ventricular dilation. (**B**) Color Doppler interrogation provides evidence of mitral regurgitation. (**C**) M-mode demonstrating systolic dysfunction with flattened interventricular septal motion, fair left ventricle (LV) posterior wall excursion, LV dilation with increased LV end-diastolic dimension, and reduced systolic function.

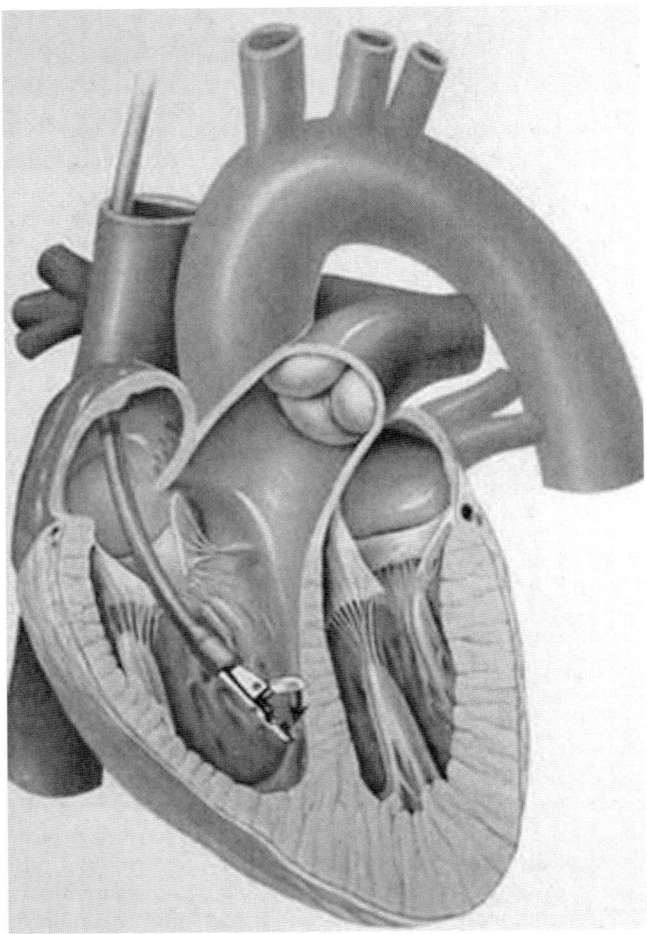

FIGURE 66C.4. Endomyocardial biopsy technique. The bioptome is advanced via the superior vena cava into the right atrium, across the tricuspid valve into the right ventricle, and finally situated against the interventricular septum, where the biopsy is performed. The bioptome also can be advanced via the inferior vena cava with similar results. From Towbin JA. Molecular genetic aspects of cardiomyopathy. *Biochem Med Metab Biol* 1993;49:285–320, with permission.

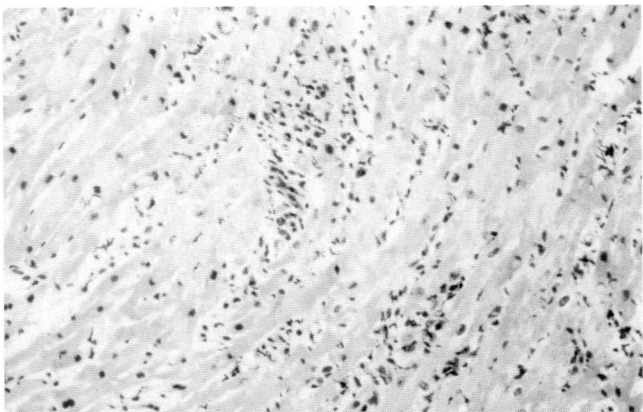

FIGURE 66C.5. Endomyocardial biopsy histology demonstrates lymphocytic infiltrates, myocardial edema, and necrosis.

biopsy, histology may be classified as ongoing myocarditis, resolving myocarditis, or resolved myocarditis. Because risk is associated with biopsy, particularly in young children or those with severe ventricular dilation, many centers have abandoned this procedure. With the availability of molecular diagnostic testing, the authors feel that biopsy is a useful test that allows confirmation of the diagnosis of myocarditis and is helpful, as it is often difficult to secure a diagnosis on patients with DCM.

Molecular Diagnostics

First reported in 1986, in situ hybridization was performed on myocardial tissue by using probes for coxsackievirus (10,11). Because this technique is difficult to use in a hospital setting, it lost favor and never gained widespread use. The polymerase chain reaction (PCR) amplification process, which identifies specific portions of a viral genome, is quite sensitive and specific (7,12,50). Approximately 20%–50% of cases were initially reported to identify enterovirus-positive results on PCR, although no other viral genome was analyzed in these early cases (1,41,80). PCR also has been used to screen for other viral genomes within cardiac tissue specimens. During the 1990s, adenovirus was demonstrated to be as prevalent as enterovirus in heart tissue specimens of patients with myocarditis or DCM (7,9,12,50). Additional viral genomes identified using PCR include CMV, EBV, herpes simplex virus, influenza A virus, PVB19, and respiratory syncytial virus (7,9,21,45). Mumps virus is responsible for EFE, a previously important cause of heart failure in children that has disappeared over the past 20 years (57). In Japan, hepatitis C virus has been shown to be a common etiologic agent (52). Over the past 3–4 years, PVB19 has become the predominant viral genome identified in the heart (9,32,48,62,63,78,79), with some evidence that PVB19 infects endothelial cells of small intracardiac arterioles and venules, which may be associated with endothelial dysfunction (78), injury to the myocardial microcirculation, and penetration of inflammatory cells in the myocardium (6). Use of more specific and sensitive diagnostic modalities, including real-time PCR or sequencing, will aid the detection, identification, and quantification of the causal virus toward predicting disease progression and developing future virus-specific treatment strategies (44,66).

CONCLUSIONS AND FUTURE DIRECTIONS

Areas that warrant future investigation are (a) the genetic basis of variable host susceptibility to myocarditis, (b) the causes of progression to DCM, (c) the evolving epidemiologic pattern of infecting viruses, and (d) the etiology-specific therapies, including responsive treatments and preventive vaccinations.

KEY POINTS

- Myocarditis is characterized by an inflammatory cellular infiltrate of the myocardium with necrosis and/or degeneration of adjacent myocytes.
- Data demonstrate that parvovirus B19 (PVB19) has become the most commonly identified virus in subjects with

suspected myocarditis since 2000. This increase in PVB19 corresponds to a decrease in the incidence of adenovirus and enterovirus myocarditis.

■ The prognosis of acute myocarditis in newborns is especially poor. Mortality rates as high as 75% have been reported in infants; older infants and children have a better prognosis, with mortality rates between 10% and 25%

■ Distinct clinical presentations for myocarditis include acute, subacute, and fulminant forms of the disease. Patients with *acute* and *subacute myocarditis* present hemodynamically stable with no fever and requiring only low-dose inotropic support.

■ Patients with *fulminant myocarditis* present with severe hemodynamic compromise with at least two of the following clinical features: fever, distinct symptoms of heart failure, and a history consistent with a viral illness within 2 weeks of presentation. These patients are typically in extremis on presentation and often require high-dose inotrope and/or mechanical support.

■ One other subtype of the fulminant form of clinical phenotype (*fulminant necrotic myocarditis*) is the patient who presents acutely—like the fulminant myocarditis patient, with symptoms of severe DHF—but additionally manifests an infarct pattern on electrocardiogram that mimics that seen in anomalous left coronary artery from the pulmonary artery, including deep Q waves in leads I and aVL, and V4 through V6. Endomyocardial biopsy typically reveals a coxsackievirus as the viral etiology, or no virus identification is made.

■ The potential value of delineating these clinical phenotypes is that long-term survival is typically better in patients with the fulminant forms of myocarditis; therefore, they are particularly excellent candidates for mechanical circulatory support as a bridge to recovery.

■ In those cases in which resolution of cardiac dysfunction does not occur, chronic DCM results.

References

1. Archard LC, Khan MA, Soteriou BA, et al. Characterization of Coxsackie B virus RNA in myocardium from patients with dilated cardiomyopathy by nucleotide sequencing of reverse transcription-nested polymerase chain reaction products. *Hum Pathol* 1998;29(6):578–84.
2. Aretz HT, Billingham ME, Edwards WD, et al. Myocarditis. A histopathologic definition and classification. *Am J Cardiovasc Pathol* 1987;1(1):3–14.
3. Baba A, Yoshikawa T, Ogawa S. Autoantibodies produced against sarcolemmal Na-K-ATPase: Possible upstream targets of arrhythmias and sudden death in patients with dilated cardiomyopathy. *J Am Coll Cardiol* 2002;40(6):1153–9.
4. Bengtsson E, Lamberger B. Five-year follow-up study of cases suggestive of acute myocarditis. *Am Heart J* 1966;72(6):751–63.
5. Bergelson JM, Cunningham JA, Droguett G, et al. Isolation of a common receptor for Coxsackie B viruses and adenoviruses 2 and 5. *Science* 1997;275(5304):1320–3.
6. Bock CT, Klingel K, Aberle S, et al. Human parvovirus B19: A new emerging pathogen of inflammatory cardiomyopathy. *J Vet Med B Infect Dis Vet Public Health* 2005;52(7-8):340–3.
7. Bowles NE, Bowles KR, Towbin JA. Viral genomic detection and outcome in myocarditis. *Heart Failure Clinics* 2005;1:407–17.
8. Bowles NE, Javier Fuentes-Garcia F, Makar KA, et al. Analysis of the coxsackievirus B-adenovirus receptor gene in patients with myocarditis or dilated cardiomyopathy. *Mol Genet Metab* 2002;77(3):257–9.
9. Bowles NE, Ni J, Kearney DL, et al. Detection of viruses in myocardial tissues by polymerase chain reaction. Evidence of adenovirus as a common cause of myocarditis in children and adults. *J Am Coll Cardiol* 2003;42(3):466–72.
10. Bowles NE, Richardson PJ, Olsen EG, et al. Detection of Coxsackie-B-virus-specific RNA sequences in myocardial biopsy samples from patients with myocarditis and dilated cardiomyopathy. *Lancet* 1986;1(8490):1120–3.
11. Bowles NE, Rose ML, Taylor P, et al. End-stage dilated cardiomyopathy. Persistence of enterovirus RNA in myocardium at cardiac transplantation and lack of immune response. *Circulation* 1989;80(5):1128–36.
12. Bowles NE, Towbin JA. Molecular aspects of myocarditis. *Curr Opin Cardiol* 1998;13(3):179–84.
13. Bowles NE, Towbin JA. Molecular aspects of myocarditis. *Curr Infect Dis Rep* 2000;2(4):308–314.
14. Bowles NE, Vallejo J. Viral causes of cardiac inflammation. *Curr Opin Cardiol* 2003;18(3):182–8.
15. Bultmann BD, Klingel K, Sotlar K, et al. Fatal parvovirus B19-associated myocarditis clinically mimicking ischemic heart disease: An endothelial cell-mediated disease. *Hum Pathol* 2003;34(1):92–5.
16. Caforio AL, Mahon NJ, Tona F, et al. Circulating cardiac autoantibodies in dilated cardiomyopathy and myocarditis: Pathogenetic and clinical significance. *Eur J Heart Fail* 2002;4(4):411–7.
17. Calabrese F, Thiene G. Myocarditis and inflammatory cardiomyopathy: Microbiological and molecular biological aspects. *Cardiovasc Res* 2003;60(1):11–25.
18. Cooper LT. Idiopathic Giant Cell Myocarditis. In: Cooper LT, ed. *Myocarditis: From Bench to Bedside*. New Jersey: Humana Press, 2003;405–20.
19. Davison AJ, Benko M, Harrach B. Genetic content and evolution of adenoviruses. *J Gen Virol* 2003;84(Pt 11):2895–908.
20. Dec GW. Introduction to Clinical Myocarditis. In: Cooper LT, ed. *Myocarditis: From Bench to Bedside*. New Jersey: Humana Press, 2003, 257–81.
21. Donoso Mantke O, Meyer R, Prösch S, et al. High prevalence of cardiotropic viruses in myocardial tissue from explanted hearts of heart transplant recipients and heart donors: A 3-year retrospective study from a German patients' pool. *J Heart Lung Transplant* 2005;24(10):1632–6.
22. Doolan A, Langlois N, Semsarian C. Causes of sudden cardiac death in young Australians. *Med J Aust* 2004;180(3):110–2.
23. Drory Y, Turetz Y, Hiss Y, et al. Sudden unexpected death in persons less than 40 years of age. *Am J Cardiol* 1991;68(13):1388–92.
24. Eckart RE, Love SS, Atwood JE, et al. Incidence and follow-up of inflammatory cardiac complications after smallpox vaccination. *J Am Coll Cardiol* 2004;44(1):201–5.
25. English RF, Janosky JE, Ettedgui JA, et al. Outcomes for children with acute myocarditis. *Cardiol Young* 2004;14(5):488–93.
26. Fabre A, Sheppard MN. Sudden adult death syndrome and other non-ischaemic causes of sudden cardiac death. *Heart* 2006;92(3):316–20.
27. Felix SB. Immunoadsorption in dilated cardiomyopathy. *Ernst Schering Res Found Workshop* 2006(55):353–61.
28. Felix SB, Staudt A, Dörffel WV, et al. Hemodynamic effects of immunoadsorption and subsequent immunoglobulin substitution in dilated cardiomyopathy: Three-month results from a randomized study. *J Am Coll Cardiol* 2000;35(6):1590–8.
29. Felix SB, Staudt A, Landsberger M, et al. Removal of cardiodepressant antibodies in dilated cardiomyopathy by immunoadsorption. *J Am Coll Cardiol* 2002;39(4):646–52.
30. Felker GM, Hu W, Hare JM, et al. The spectrum of dilated cardiomyopathy. The Johns Hopkins experience with 1278 patients. *Medicine (Baltimore)* 1999;78(4):270–83.
31. Felker GM, Jaeger CJ, Klodas E, et al. Myocarditis and long-term survival in peripartum cardiomyopathy. *Am Heart J* 2000;140(5):785–91.
32. Francalanci P, Chance JL, Vatta M, et al. Cardiotropic viruses in the myocardium of children with end-stage heart disease. *J Heart Lung Transplant* 2004;23:1046–52.
33. Friedman RA, Schowengerdt KO, Towbin JA. Myocarditis. In: Garson A, Bricker JT, Fisher DJ, et al., eds. *The Science and Practice of Pediatric Cardiology*. Baltimore: Williams & Wilkins, 1998;1777–94.
34. Godeny EK, Gauntt CJ. Murine natural killer cells limit coxsackievirus B3 replication. *J Immunol* 1987;139(3):913–8.
35. Greaves K, Oxford JS, Price CP, et al. The prevalence of myocarditis and skeletal muscle injury during acute viral infection in adults: Measurement of cardiac troponins I and T in 152 patients with acute influenza infection. *Arch Intern Med* 2003;163(2):165–8.
36. Grist NR, Reid D. General Pathogenicity and Epidemiology. In: Bendinelli M, Friedman H, eds. *Coxsackieviruses: A General Update*. New York: Plenum, 1988;241–52.
37. Herskowitz A, Ahmed-Ansari A, Neumann DA, et al. Induction of major histocompatibility complex antigens within the myocardium of patients with active myocarditis: A nonhistologic marker of myocarditis. *J Am Coll Cardiol* 1990;15(3):624–32.
38. Hori H, Matoba T, Shingu M, et al. The role of cell-mediated immunity in coxsackie B viral myocarditis. *Jpn Circ J* 1981;45(12):1409–14.
39. Huber SA. Coxsackievirus-induced myocarditis is dependent on distinct immunopathogenic responses in different strains of mice. *Lab Invest* 1997;76(5):691–701.
40. James TN. Sudden death in babies: New observations in the heart. *Am J Cardiol* 1968;22(4):479–506.
41. Jin O, Sole MJ, Butany JW, et al. Detection of enterovirus RNA in myocardial biopsies from patients with myocarditis and cardiomyopathy using gene amplification by polymerase chain reaction. *Circulation* 1990;82(1):8–16.
42. Kaya Z, Afanasyeva M, Wang Y, et al. Contribution of the innate immune system to autoimmune myocarditis: A role for complement. *Nat Immunol* 2001;2(8):739–45.

43. Kishimoto C, Kuroki Y, Hiraoka Y, et al. Cytokine and murine coxsackievirus B3 myocarditis. Interleukin-2 suppressed myocarditis in the acute stage but enhanced the condition in the subsequent stage. *Circulation* 1994;89(6):2836–42.

44. Klein RM, Jiang H, Niederacher D, et al. Frequency and quantity of the parvovirus B19 genome in endomyocardial biopsies from patients with suspected myocarditis or idiopathic left ventricular dysfunction. *Z Kardiol* 2004;93(4):300–9.

45. Klingel K, Sauter M, Bock CT, et al. Molecular pathology of inflammatory cardiomyopathy. *Med Microbiol Immunol (Berl)* 2004;193(2–3):101–7.

46. Lauer B, Niederau C, Kühl U, et al. Cardiac troponin T in patients with clinically suspected myocarditis. *J Am Coll Cardiol* 1997;30(5):1354–9.

47. Liu PP, Mason JW. Advances in the understanding of myocarditis. *Circulation* 2001;104(9):1076–82.

48. Maisch B, Ristic AD, Portig I, et al. Human viral cardiomyopathy. *Front Biosci* 2003;8:s39–67.

49. Maisch B, Trostel-Soeder R, Stechemesser E, et al. Diagnostic relevance of humoral and cell-mediated immune reactions in patients with acute viral myocarditis. *Clin Exp Immunol* 1982;48(3):533–45.

50. Martin AB, Webber S, Fricker FJ, et al. Acute myocarditis. Rapid diagnosis by PCR in children. *Circulation* 1994;90(1):330–9.

51. Mason JW, O'Connell JB, Herskowitz A, et al. A clinical trial of immunosuppressive therapy for myocarditis. The Myocarditis Treatment Trial Investigators. *N Engl J Med* 1995;333(5):269–75.

52. Matsumori A. Role of hepatitis C virus in cardiomyopathies. *Ernst Schering Res Found Workshop* 2006;(55):99–120.

53. Matsumori A, Yamada T, Suzuki H, et al. Increased circulating cytokines in patients with myocarditis and cardiomyopathy. *Br Heart J* 1994;72(6):561–6.

54. McCarthy RE 3rd, Boehmer JP, Hruban RH, et al. Long-term outcome of fulminant myocarditis as compared with acute (nonfulminant) myocarditis. *N Engl J Med* 2000;342(10):690–5.

55. Mikami S, Kawashima S, Kanazawa K, et al. Low-dose N omega-nitro-L-arginine methyl ester treatment improves survival rate and decreases myocardial injury in a murine model of viral myocarditis induced by coxsackievirus B3. *Circ Res* 1997;81(4):504–11.

56. Neuspiel DR, Kuller LH. Sudden and unexpected natural death in childhood and adolescence. *JAMA* 1985;254(10):1321–5.

57. Ni J, Bowles NE, Kim YH, et al. Viral infection of the myocardium in endocardial fibroelastosis. Molecular evidence for the role of mumps virus as an etiologic agent. *Circulation* 1997;95(1):133–9.

58. O'Connell JB, Fowles RE, Robinson JA, et al. Clinical and pathologic findings of myocarditis in two families with dilated cardiomyopathy. *Am Heart J* 1984;107(1):127–35.

59. Okura Y, Dec GW, Hare JM, et al. A clinical and histopathologic comparison of cardiac sarcoidosis and idiopathic giant cell myocarditis. *J Am Coll Cardiol* 2003;41(2):322–9.

60. Okura Y, Yamamoto T, Goto S, et al. Characterization of cytokine and iNOS mRNA expression in situ during the course of experimental autoimmune myocarditis in rats. *J Mol Cell Cardiol* 1997;29(2):491–502.

61. Padalko E, Ohnishi T, Matsushita K, et al. Peroxynitrite inhibition of Coxsackievirus infection by prevention of viral RNA entry. *Proc Natl Acad Sci U S A* 2004;101(32):11731–6.

62. Pankuweit S, Lamparter S, Schoppet M, et al. Parvovirus B19 genome in endomyocardial biopsy specimen. *Circulation* 2004;109(14):e179.

63. Pankuweit S, Moll R, Baandrup U, et al. Prevalence of the parvovirus B19 genome in endomyocardial biopsy specimens. *Hum Pathol* 2003;34(5):497–503.

64. Pankuweit S, Portig I, Lottspeich F, et al. Autoantibodies in sera of patients with myocarditis: Characterization of the corresponding proteins by isoelectric focusing and N-terminal sequence analysis. *J Mol Cell Cardiol* 1997;29(1):77–84.

65. Pauschinger M, Bowles NE, Fuentes-Garcia FJ, et al. Detection of adenoviral genome in the myocardium of adult patients with idiopathic left ventricular dysfunction. *Circulation* 1999;99(10):1348–54.

66. Pauschinger M, Kallwellis-Opara A. Frontiers in viral diagnostics. *Ernst Schering Res Found Workshop* 2006;(55):39–54.

67. Rosenstein ED, Zucker MJ, Kramer N. Giant cell myocarditis: Most fatal of autoimmune diseases. *Semin Arthritis Rheum* 2000;30(1):1–16.

68. Schultheiss HP, Schulze K, Dorner A. Significance of the adenine nucleotide translocator in the pathogenesis of viral heart disease. *Mol Cell Biochem* 1996;163-4:319–27.

69. Shioi T, Matsumori A, Nishio R, et al. Protective role of interleukin-12 in viral myocarditis. *J Mol Cell Cardiol* 1997;29(9):2327–34.

70. Smith SC, Ladenson JH, Mason JW, et al. Elevations of cardiac troponin I associated with myocarditis. Experimental and clinical correlates. *Circulation* 1997;95(1):163–8.

71. Soongswang J, Durongpisitkul K, Nana A, et al. Cardiac troponin T: A marker in the diagnosis of acute myocarditis in children. *Pediatr Cardiol* 2005;26(1):45–9.

72. Staudt A, Schäper F, Stangl V, et al. Immunohistological changes in dilated cardiomyopathy induced by immunoadsorption therapy and subsequent immunoglobulin substitution. *Circulation* 2001;103(22):2681–6.

73. Stoica SC, Goddard M, Tsui S, et al. Ventricular assist surprise: Giant cell myocarditis or sarcoidosis? *J Thorac Cardiovasc Surg* 2003;126(6):2072–4.

74. Tomko RP, Xu R, Philipson L. HCAR and MCAR: The human and mouse cellular receptors for subgroup C adenoviruses and group B coxsackieviruses. *Proc Natl Acad Sci U S A* 1997;94(7):3352–6.

75. Torre-Amione G, Kapadia S, Lee J, et al. Tumor necrosis factor-alpha and tumor necrosis factor receptors in the failing human heart. *Circulation* 1996;93(4):704–11.

76. Towbin JA, Bowles NE. The failing heart. *Nature* 2002;415(6868):227–33.

77. Towbin JA, Bowles NE. Dilated cardiomyopathy: A tale of cytoskeletal proteins and beyond. *J Cardiovasc Electrophysiol* 2006;17(8):919–26.

78. Tschope C, Bock CT, Kasner M, et al. High prevalence of cardiac parvovirus B19 infection in patients with isolated left ventricular diastolic dysfunction. *Circulation* 2005;111(7):879–86.

79. Wang X, Zhang G, Liu F, et al. Prevalence of human parvovirus B19 DNA in cardiac tissues of patients with congenital heart diseases indicated by nested PCR and in situ hybridization. *J Clin Virol* 2004;31(1):20–4.

80. Weiss LM, Liu XF, Chang KL, et al. Detection of enteroviral RNA in idiopathic dilated cardiomyopathy and other human cardiac tissues. *J Clin Invest* 1992;90(1):156–9.

81. White E. Regulation of apoptosis by the transforming genes of the DNA tumor virus adenovirus. *Proc Soc Exp Biol Med* 1993;204(1):30–9.

82. Wojnicz R, Nowalany-Kozielska E, Wodniecki J, et al. Immunohistological diagnosis of myocarditis. Potential role of sarcolemmal induction of the MHC and ICAM-1 in the detection of autoimmune mediated myocyte injury. *Eur Heart J* 1998;19(10):1564–72.

83. Wynne J, Braunwald E. The Cardiomyopathies and Myocarditides. In: E Braunwald, ed. *Heart Disease: A Textbook of Cardiovascular Medicine.* Philadelphia: WB Saunders Company, 2001;1751–806.

84. Yamamoto LG. Kawasaki disease. *Pediatr Emerg Care* 2003;19(6):422–4.

CHAPTER 67A ■ TREATMENT OF HEART FAILURE IN INFANTS AND CHILDREN: MEDICAL MANAGEMENT

JOSEPH W. ROSSANO • JACK F. PRICE • DAVID P. NELSON

Heart failure is a clinical syndrome characterized by a reduced ability of the heart to fill and/or eject blood to meet the body's metabolic demands. As noted in Chapter 66, this failure can occur secondary to a variety of conditions. The therapeutic options that exist in managing these complex patients will be discussed in this chapter, which is comprised of three sections: Medical Management (Section A), Mechanical Support (Section B), and Cardiac Transplantation.

PHARMACOLOGIC AGENTS USED FOR TREATMENT OF HEART FAILURE

Heart failure is generally a chronic, progressive disorder (51), though certain types of cardiomyopathy, such as left ventricular (LV) noncompaction, can have an undulating phenotype, with periods of improvement and/or deterioration in function (66). Another exception is acute myocarditis, especially the fulminate form, in which patients often have a complete recovery of function. Guidelines for the management of chronic heart failure in adults and children have been published by the International Society of Heart and Lung Transplant, the American College of Cardiology, and the American Heart Association (41,75). The primary aim of therapy is to reduce symptoms, preserve long-term ventricular performance, and prolong survival, primarily through antagonism of the neurohormonal compensatory mechanisms. As some of these medications may be detrimental during acute decompensation, the critical care physician should be knowledgeable of the medications and therapeutic goals of treatment of chronic heart failure. Furthermore, understanding the mechanisms of chronic heart failure may foster improved understanding of the treatment of decompensated heart failure.

Diuretics

Treating symptoms of "congestion" is critical to the management of heart failure in both acute and chronic settings (41). Diuretics are recommended for patients with symptoms of heart failure and evidence of volume overload. Although these are the most commonly used agents in the long-term management of heart failure patients, studies that demonstrate long-term benefits of diuretic treatment are lacking. Indeed, data from animal models of cardiomyopathy indicate that furosemide ac-

tivates the renin-angiotensin-aldosterone system (RAAS) and accelerates the decline of myocardial function (55). Furthermore, a retrospective study of adult heart failure patients identified increasing loop-diuretic dose as an independent predictor of mortality (29). Loop and thiazide diuretics remain the most commonly used diuretics. In adults, aldosterone antagonists, such as spironolactone, have been shown to improve mortality when added to standard heart failure management (68), though an increase in hyperkalemia may occur (67,91). These agents have not been well studied in children, but pediatric use is growing, likely secondary to the increased use in adults.

ANGIOTENSIN-CONVERTING ENZYME INHIBITORS/ ANGIOTENSIN-RECEPTOR BLOCKERS

Angiotensin-converting enzyme (ACE) inhibitors were the first agents to demonstrate improved survival in adults with symptomatic heart failure. These medications decrease the formation of angiotensin II, block the activation of the RAAS, and decrease adrenergic activity (15). Prospective, randomized, controlled trials of various agents within this class have demonstrated improvement in symptoms, with reduced progression of heart failure, decreased hospitalization, and improved survival. Mortality benefits are primarily due to decreased deaths from pump failure. Angiotensin-receptor blockers (ARBs), primarily used in adults who are not tolerant of ACE inhibitors, have also demonstrated an improvement in mortality that is comparable, and possibly superior, to ACE inhibitors (83). The combination of ACE inhibitors and ARBs may provide additional benefits of improved LV geometry, ejection fraction, and exercise capacity (101).

No large, randomized, controlled trials of ACE inhibitors in the treatment of pediatric heart failure have been conducted. The acute effects of captopril in patients with cardiomyopathy were demonstrated in the catheterization laboratory; with a single dose of 0.5 mg/kg, cardiac index and stroke volume increased by 22% and systemic vascular resistance (SVR) decreased without a significant decrease in mean aortic pressure (9). In a prospective study of 12 children with dilated cardiomyopathy (DCM), captopril (mean dose, 1.8 mg/kg/day) was instituted and, over a 3-month period, was associated with an improvement in LV end-diastolic volume and end-systolic volume indexes (89). Additionally, at 1 month, a decrease in aldosterone and plasma atrial natriuretic peptide was seen; however, these effects were not seen at 3 months. These echocardiographic results were similar to the prospective study that found that patients with volume-overloaded lesions (aortic regurgitation and mitral regurgitation) who were treated with ACE inhibitors had improved LV end-diastolic dimensions, mass, and shortening fraction over a mean time of 3.4 years (60). Although survival was not an end-point of these studies, an improvement in survival was demonstrated at 1 year in patients with DCM with treatment with an ACE inhibitor (48). This retrospective study failed to demonstrate a statistically significant increase in survival beyond 1 year of therapy. ACE inhibitors have been demonstrated to improve the $Q_p:Q_s$ ratio in some patients with large left-to-right shunting lesions (95); however, their efficacy in long-term management has not been demonstrated. Additionally, studies of ACE inhibition in Fontan patients failed to demonstrate an improvement in resting cardiac index, diastolic function, SVR, or exercise capacity (46).

β Blockers

As with ACE inhibitors, an accumulation of evidence from multiple randomized, controlled trials of β blockers in adult patients demonstrates benefits in symptoms, heart function, frequency of hospitalization, and survival (38,64,69). Although they possess negative inotropic properties, the presumed benefit of these agents is inhibition of the effects of the sympathetic nervous system. Data on β-blocker use in pediatric heart failure are limited, but supportive nonetheless. A review of the experience of metoprolol in 15 children with DCM at three centers in the US found that metoprolol was associated with a significant increase in fractional shortening and ejection fraction (82). Carvedilol use was reviewed in 46 patients with DCM (80%) or palliated congenital heart disease (20%) and was found to be associated with improvement in New York Heart Association functional class and fractional shortening at 3 months (16). A small, randomized, placebo-controlled study in 22 children with severe LV dysfunction found that patients given carvedilol had an improvement in ejection fraction and New York Heart Association class over a 3-month period (7). Additionally, 64% of the patients in the carvedilol group improved enough to be taken off of the cardiac transplantation list. A larger multicentered, prospective study of carvedilol has been completed, but the results have not been published at this writing.

Digoxin

Digoxin, one of the oldest medications used for the treatment of heart failure symptoms, improves contractility by inhibiting cardiac Na-K channels in the cardiac myocytes, leading to increased contractility (35). While digoxin is effective in alleviating symptoms of heart failure, it has not been shown to improve mortality, and higher doses are associated with an increase in mortality (72). Data on children have been extrapolated from adult studies, and the current recommendation of the International Society for Heart and Lung Transplantation is to use digoxin for symptomatic patients (75).

ELECTROPHYSIOLOGIC MANAGEMENT OF HEART FAILURE

Dysrhythmias are an important consequence and often unrecognized etiology of heart failure in children. Tachycardia-induced cardiomyopathy is uncommon, but reversible. Thus, an accurate diagnosis is essential. At Texas Children's Hospital, 21 patients presented over 10 years with tachycardia-induced LV dysfunction (6). Importantly, over 90% of these patients had resolution of LV dysfunction with medical therapy and/or radiofrequency ablation.

Antiarrhythmic Agents

Evidence is limited regarding the choice of antiarrhythmic agents in children with arrhythmias and heart failure. Metoprolol may be used, as it has efficacy for heart failure and as an antiarrhythmic for arrhythmias where β blockers would be indicated (e.g., re-entrant tachycardia, ectopic focus tachycardia, rate control for atrial fibrillation). The antiarrhythmic efficacy of carvedilol is not as well established but has been shown to decrease atrial and ventricular dysrhythmias in adults after myocardial infarction (56). Amiodarone is an effective antiarrhythmic medication for a variety of arrhythmias. It has been studied in adults with heart failure and has been found to decrease ventricular dysrhythmias but has not consistently improved survival, and some studies suggest a decrease in survival in patients treated with amiodarone (8,26,88). Patients with ventricular dysrhythmias and depressed LV function are at increased risk for sudden death, and consideration for implantable cardioverter-defibrillator (ICD) should be considered (see later discussion). An extensive discussion of the diagnosis and treatment of dysrhythmias can be found in Chapter 68.

Cardiac Resynchronization Therapy

Disturbances in the normal electrical conduction of the heart are common in chronic heart failure and often lead to dyssynchronous contraction. Although often due to left-bundle-branch block in adults, it is an uncommon pattern of conduction delay in children. Restoration of ventricular synchrony with synchronized biventricular pacing is referred to as *cardiac resynchronization therapy* (CRT). In appropriately selected adults, CRT results in reverse remodeling and improved symptoms of heart failure (3). When combined with an ICD, CRT may improve mortality (14). Data on CRT use in children are limited, but initial short-term results demonstrate improved ventricular function with CRT (28). CRT may prove useful for pediatric and adult patients with congenital heart disease and an intraventricular conduction delay, as often seen in patients with tetralogy of Fallot or functionally univentricular hearts.

Implantable Cardioverter-Defibrillator

Ventricular dysrhythmias and sudden cardiac death (SCD) occur with increased frequency in adults with heart failure.

Evidence is limited concerning the frequency of sudden death in children with heart failure, but available evidence suggests that sudden death and ventricular dysrhythmias occur much less frequently than in adult patients (24). The use of ICDs as primary prevention of SCD in adults with ventricular dysfunction has been demonstrated for both ischemic and nonischemic cardiomyopathy (36). From these studies, the Heart Failure Society of America recommends that prophylactic ICD placement should be considered for patients with an ejection fraction ≤30% with mild-to-moderate heart failure symptoms (30). There are no current guidelines regarding pediatric patients. At Texas Children's Hospital, ICD placement is strongly considered for children with cardiomyopathy and a history of ventricular arrhythmias. Due to the apparent reduced frequency of SCD in children with cardiomyopathy and to the increased frequency of inappropriate ICD shocks in children (18), ICD placement is not our current practice in children with isolated ventricular dysfunction.

MEDICAL MANAGEMENT OF ACUTE DECOMPENSATED HEART FAILURE

Etiology and Pathophysiology

No universally accepted definition for acute decompensated heart failure exists; however, it generally encompasses patients who are hospitalized for treatment of heart failure (4). An estimated 1 million hospitalizations occur annually for acute decompensated heart failure in adults (92), and it is the most common reason for hospital admission in patients >65 years of age. The burden of disease in the pediatric population is not known. Most admissions in children, as in adults, are for acute exacerbations of chronic heart failure. In contrast to adult patients, ischemic cardiomyopathy is rare in children, and idiopathic DCM is more common. Other important causes of acute decompensated heart failure in children include acute myocarditis, DCM secondary to other etiologies (e.g., anthracycline toxicity, anomalous coronary artery, inborn errors of metabolism), "high-output" cardiac failure from arteriovenous malformation, thyrotoxicosis or anemia, and tachycardia-mediated cardiomyopathy.

Irrespective of etiology, heart failure is thought to occur after an index event produces an initial decline in heart function (**Fig. 67A.1**), leading to compensatory mechanisms, including an activation of the sympathetic nervous system, salt and water preservation with activation of the RAAS system, and production of inflammatory cytokines (e.g., tissue necrosis factor, IL-1). These compensatory mechanisms often delay the onset of symptoms for months or even years. The compensatory mechanisms are generally counterproductive over time, however, contributing to progressive myocardial damage, LV remodeling, and eventual cardiac decompensation. The intensivist must be cognizant that the symptoms of heart failure seem to progress independently of the patient's hemodynamic status (52) and that, therefore, heart failure therapy should not be titrated simply based on echocardiographic and/or catheterization results.

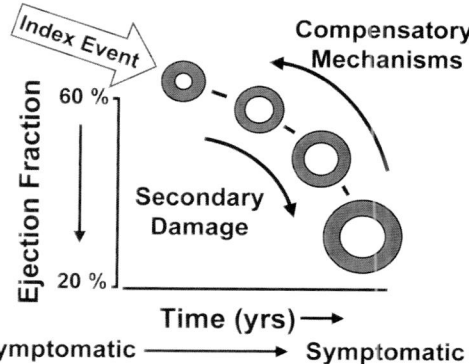

FIGURE 67A.1. Pathogenesis of heart failure. Heart failure begins after an index event produces an initial decline in pumping capacity of the heart. Following this initial decline, a variety of compensatory mechanisms are activated, including the adrenergic nervous system, the renin angiotensin system, and the cytokine system. In the short-term, these systems are able to restore cardiovascular function to a normal homeostatic so the patient remains asymptomatic. However, with time, the sustained activation of these systems can lead to secondary myocardial injury with pathologic left ventricular remodeling and subsequent cardiac decompensation. The progressive left ventricular remodeling and cardiac decompensation, will ultimately lead to a transition from asymptomatic to symptomatic heart failure. From Mann DL, Bristow MR. Mechanisms and models in heart failure. *Circulation* 2005;111:2837–49, with permission.

Algorithm for Rapid Assessment of Heart Failure

A useful tool to help guide management of the patient with acute decompensated heart failure is the rapid-assessment algorithm (37). Patients are characterized by the presence or absence of pulmonary or systemic congestion (i.e., elevated filling pressure) and the adequacy of perfusion. As shown in **Table 67A.1**, patients are classified according to signs of elevated filling pressures (wet or dry) and adequacy of perfusion (warm or cold). The goal is to maintain or transition a patient to the "warm and dry" category. Patients who present as "warm and wet" or "cold and wet" generally respond well to medical management. However, the "cold and dry" state is a dire condition that may require aggressive treatment such as mechanical support. It should be noted that this conceptual framework was designed for adults with heart failure. Although the benefit of this characterization for children with heart failure has not been validated, it is a useful conceptual framework with which to approach patient management.

Elevated Filling Pressures with Adequate Perfusion: "Warm and Wet"

Patients with congestion but adequate perfusion likely comprise the largest group of patients with acute decompensated heart failure, and the group that responds best to medial therapy. Diuresis, a critical component of the initial management of the patient with elevated filling pressures, may be the only therapy necessary to improve symptoms in the patient with adequate perfusion. In studies from adult patients, diuretics were found to increase stroke volume, decrease pulmonary capillary wedge pressure, and decrease SVR (100). Diuretics combined with vasodilators have also been shown to decrease mitral

TABLE 67A.1

PROFILE OF RESTING HEMODYNAMICS

	No congestion	Congestion
Adequate perfusion	"Warm and dry" A Optimal profile: focus on prevention of disease progression and decompensation	"Wet and warm" B Diuresis with continuation of standard therapy
Critical hypoperfusion	"Cold and dry" L Limited further options for therapy	"Wet and cold" C Diuresis and redesign of regimen with other standard therapies

Patients frequently progress from profile A to profile B or profile C. Profile "L" refers to patient's presenting with low output and no congestion. The letter L was chosen rather than the letter D to avoid the implication that this profile necessarily follows profile C or is a less desirable profile than C. From Grady KL, Dracup K, Kennedy G, et al. Team management of patients with heart failure: A statement for healthcare professionals from The Cardiovascular Nursing Council of the American Heart Association. *Circulation* 2000;102: 2443–56, with permission.

regurgitation and increase forward ejection fraction (90). Overdiuresis is a concern, as volume depletion and renal insufficiency may result. This process in which combined cardiac and renal dysfunction amplifies progression of end-organ damage has been termed the *cardiorenal syndrome* (see Chapter 66).

Assessment of systemic perfusion is essential in determining whether to continue chronic therapy for heart failure during acute exacerbations. If perfusion is adequate, β blockers and ACE inhibitors can generally be continued during hospitalization, but the negative inotropic effects of β blockers may necessitate discontinuation or dose reduction if perfusion is marginal. Some patients may not tolerate acute withdrawal from β blockade. In adults, continuance of chronic β-blocker therapy during hospitalization is associated with a decreased risk of death or rehospitalization (17). Initiation of β blocker is usually contraindicated while the patient is in a decompensated state of heart failure. Delaying initiation of a β blocker until the patient has been transitioned back to the "warm and dry" state is generally advised.

Elevated Filling Pressures with Poor Perfusion: "Cold and Wet"

Patients with congestion and poor perfusion represent a significant group of patients with acute decompensated heart failure admitted to the ICU. In one series of adult patients, 20% of patients admitted for heart failure were in this group, and they had a higher risk of death or need for urgent heart transplant compared with patients with adequate perfusion (61). The initial approach to these patients will depend upon the degree of circulatory compromise. The cornerstone of therapy for these patients is afterload reduction, as this is the more effective way to increase cardiac output in the failing heart than "whipping" it with inotropic agents. Vasodilators and diuretics alone may be adequate therapy for many patients. Avoiding inotropic agents when possible appears to be beneficial. A

review of over 15,000 adults hospitalized for heart failure observed higher in-hospital mortality in patients who were treated with dobutamine or milrinone than in patients treated with nitroglycerin or nesiritide (2). This finding is consistent with prior studies that have demonstrated that adult patients have increased mortality when treated with chronic milrinone (63) and more adverse events when treated with short-term milrinone (21). It is unclear whether these data from adult patients can be translated to pediatric patients with heart failure. At Texas Children's Hospital, milrinone is still first-line therapy for patients with decompensated heart failure in the "cold and wet" state, and we attempt to avoid using β-adrenergic agonists, especially at higher doses.

No pediatric data support the use of one vasodilator over another for acute decompensated heart failure. Nitroprusside is an effective vasodilator and has been used in the treatment of heart failure in adults for over three decades. The drug has a rapid half-life and can be quickly up-titrated to effect. Blood pressure must be monitored, as hypotension can develop. Cyanide toxicity is an important potential side effect, especially with chronic use or renal impairment. Pediatric experience is limited with other vasodilators, such as nitroglycerin, for heart failure treatment.

The human recombinant B-type natriuretic peptide nesiritide has been shown to have positive lusitropic properties, promote vasodilation, improve natriuresis, and inhibit renin and aldosterone. It has been demonstrated to rapidly improve symptoms in adults with acute decompensated heart failure. Long-term data are limited, and some concerns have been reported regarding renal toxicity and the effect on long-term survival (78,79). Experience with the use of nesiritide in children is limited. A study from our institution reported its use in 26 children who ranged in age from 3 weeks to 12 years. Urine output increased, mean central venous pressure decreased, and no episodes of hypotension were noted up to the maximum dose of 0.03 mcg/kg/min (42).

Inotropic agents may be required to improve perfusion in this group of patients. The decision to use inotropic agents should be based primarily on clinical assessment and not on echocardiographic results. Many patients with significant ventricular dysfunction will remain compensated, do not need, and are potentially harmed by, inotropes. Traditional inotropic agents used for decompensated heart failure include dobutamine, dopamine, and milrinone. Dobutamine, a β-adrenergic agonist, stimulates β_1 and β_2 receptors. Via the stimulation of β_1 receptors in the heart, dobutamine increases intracellular cyclic AMP (cAMP), which leads to increased calcium release from the sarcoplasmic reticulum and, thus, increased contractility. β_2 receptor activation results in peripheral vasodilation and decreased SVR, which may cause a reflex tachycardia, although this is rare. An increase in heart rate and contractility may result in an undesired increase in myocardial oxygen consumption. The use of dobutamine has been associated with improved symptoms, decreased filling pressures, increased ejection fraction, and improved exercise tolerance with short-term and intermittent infusions. However, tachycardia and dysrhythmias are common side effects. As stated previously, dobutamine use was associated with increased mortality in adult heart failure patients, compared to nesiritide or nitroglycerin; this was also the finding of the recently completed CASINO trial (1), which compared dobutamine with levosimendan or placebo. In this study, dobutamine use was associated with an increased 6-month mortality compared to levosimendan or placebo. For these reasons, routine use of dobutamine for heart failure has fallen out of favor. Other inotropes that have not been studied as extensively as dobutamine are also suspected of having similar detrimental effects for treatment of decompensated heart failure. As stated previously, afterload reduction is the cornerstone of treatment rather than inotropic support. *No trial of long-term therapy with a positive inotropic agent has demonstrated improved outcomes in patients with heart failure, and most trials have found increased mortality with positive inotropic agents.*

Dopamine is an endogenous catecholamine. At low doses (2–5 mcg/kg/min), dopamine receptors in the renal, cerebral, coronary, mesenteric, and pulmonary vasculature are stimulated. Higher doses of dopamine stimulate β-adrenergic receptors, increasing contractility and heart rate. At higher doses (≥10 mcg/kg/min), significant α-adrenergic stimulation occurs, resulting in vasoconstriction and increased SVR and pulmonary vascular resistance (PVR). No evidence supports the use of "renal" dose dopamine. The side-effect profile is similar to dobutamine, including the propensity for tachycardia, dysrhythmias, and increased myocardial oxygen consumption. Clinical trials of dopamine use for treatment of acute decompensated heart failure have not been conducted in adults or children. A trial of ibopamine, an oral dopaminergic drug, was prematurely stopped due to increased mortality in the ibopamine-treated patients. Dopamine continues to be the most common inotropic agent used in pediatric patients; thus, studies to evaluate its role in heart failure would be valuable.

Another commonly used agent for acute decompensated heart failure is milrinone, a phosphodiesterase (PDE) inhibitor with inotropic, lusitropic, and vasodilatory properties. Milrinone inhibits the breakdown of cAMP by the PDE III isozyme. By blocking break-down of intracellular cAMP, calcium transport into the cell is enhanced and myocyte contractility improved. In addition, reuptake of calcium is a cAMP-dependent process, so that these agents may enhance diastolic relaxation of the myocardium by increasing the rate of calcium reuptake

after systole. PDE inhibitors increase cardiac muscle contractility, vascular smooth muscle relaxation, and cardiac output without increasing myocardial oxygen consumption or ventricular afterload.

Although milrinone improves symptoms and decreases filling pressures in adult patients, it is not clear that it increases long-term survival in patients with heart failure. In a study that evaluated the short-term use of milrinone versus placebo in almost 1000 patients, no differences in mortality, hospital length of stay, or hospital readmission were found (21), but an increased incidence of hypotension and dysrhythmias in milrinone-treated patients was reported. A retrospective analysis of ischemic cardiomyopathy patients in this study correlated with increased short-term milrinone in-hospital mortality and with an increased rate of death or rehospitalization at 60 days (32). Interestingly, patients with nonischemic cardiomyopathy had a decreased rate of death or rehospitalization at 60 days. Other studies have also failed to demonstrate the long-term benefit of milrinone. A prospective study of oral milrinone for chronic heart failure found that milrinone-treated patients had increased hospitalization, overall mortality, and cardiovascular mortality (63). No trials of milrinone for pediatric patients with acute decompensated heart failure have been conducted. Milrinone has been evaluated in children postoperative from cardiac surgery and was found in a randomized, multicentered trial to decrease low cardiac output syndrome (LCOS) after surgery (39). Further investigation is necessary to assess the overall efficacy of milrinone in children with heart failure.

Levosimendan is a promising new agent in a new class of medications known as *calcium sensitizers*. As noted in the Chapter 66, calcium regulation in the failing myocardium is abnormal, with prolonged intracellular calcium transients and a decreased ability to restore low calcium levels in diastole. Expression of calcium channels in the sarcoplasmic reticulum is reduced, and myocardial contraction and relaxation depend primarily on calcium fluxes between the cytosol and extracellular fluid (43). Traditional inotropic agents that increase intracellular calcium are associated with increased oxygen consumption, impaired myocardial relaxation, and dysrhythmias (31). Levosimendan is novel in that it increases both inotropy and vasodilation without increasing calcium levels or myocardial oxygen demand (93). The enhancement of contractility occurs by binding to troponin C and increasing myofilament sensitivity to calcium. Levosimendan causes vasodilatation via opening of potassium-dependent ADT channels. The unique property of improving cardiac function without increasing intracellular calcium or myocardial oxygen consumption may prove to be a major breakthrough in the treatment of acute and chronic heart failure. Levosimendan has been used safely and effectively in adults, with recent studies demonstrating improved mortality. Isolated case reports have been published of its use in children with severe heart failure postoperatively and in the setting of a DCM (12,13). The drug is not currently available in the US.

Normal Filling Pressures with Poor Perfusion: "Cold and Dry"

Patients with inadequate perfusion and normal filling pressures represent a tenuous patient population. Vasodilators may not be beneficial and can worsen perfusion in patients with marginal blood pressure. Inotropic agents, such as those described previously, are often needed. In the setting of significantly compromised perfusion or cardiogenic shock, additional or alternative agents such as calcium chloride, epinephrine, or vasopressin may also be necessary. If perfusion can be improved by inotropic therapy, titration of vasodilation therapy may become feasible, but inotropic agents may not be sufficient to return the patient to an asymptomatic state. Furthermore, while these agents may be acutely life-saving, they may decrease long-term ventricular function and increase mortality. In the setting of increasing inotropic requirements to maintain adequate perfusion and lack of response to vasodilation therapy, it is our practice at Texas Children's Hospital to consider mechanical support.

Calcium chloride has been used to increase myocardial contractility in the post-arrest setting. In the adult heart, calcium released from the sarcoplasmic reticulum accounts for the majority of the calcium that binds to troponin C. In the neonate, as the sarcoplasmic reticulum is relatively sparse and undifferentiated, the neonatal myocardium is more dependent upon extracellular calcium stores for contractile function (80). Contractility is proportional to the level of ionized calcium in the blood. In contrast to catecholamines, calcium chloride does not induce tachycardia. In adult patients, calcium chloride infusions have been discouraged based on studies that implicate calcium with increased myocardial necrosis and worsening diastolic dysfunction (44,45). No studies have evaluated the use of chronic calcium chloride in pediatric patients for decompensated heart failure, but it has been used extensively in perioperative patients with congenital heart disease. The use of calcium chloride can acutely improve myocardial contractility and cardiac output without excessive tachycardia, especially in younger patients. Long-term safety and efficacy of calcium infusion in children have not been determined.

Epinephrine has dose-dependent actions on α- and β-adrenergic receptors. At low doses, β-adrenergic receptor response predominates, resulting in vasodilation, increased heart rate, and increased contractility. At higher doses, α-receptor stimulation mediates vasoconstriction and increased SVR. Although the increased SVR and contractility may acutely improve perfusion, it may occur at the expense of increased myocardial oxygen consumption and myocardial work. High-dose catecholamines for inotropic support can promote tachycardia and proarrhythmic effects, increase myocardial oxygen consumption, and depress the myocardial adrenergic response by downregulating β-adrenergic receptors. Furthermore, prolonged use of high-dose catecholamines may further amplify cardiomyocyte and sarcomeris injury, thus aggravating diastolic and systolic ventricular dysfunction (87). Long periods of epinephrine infusion are poorly tolerated by the failing myocardium.

The use of arginine vasopressin during and after cardiac arrest has been shown to improve return of spontaneous circulation and survival in some series (98). Vasopressin levels are elevated in pediatric patients with heart failure (71) but lower in patients after cardiopulmonary bypass (CPB). Vasopressin acts directly upon vascular smooth muscle to increase SVR, but does not have the associated tachycardia found with catecholamines. Vasopressin may also have direct effects on the myocardium by increasing cytosolic calcium via V_1 receptors.

The use of vasopressin in children to improve low cardiac output in postoperative catecholamine-resistant shock has been demonstrated. A study of vasopressin use in vasodilatory shock showed an improvement in stroke volume, an unexpected finding if arginine vasopressin acts only to increase afterload (76). This study suggests that vasopressin may have direct inotropic effects on the myocardium. Even if vasopressin has direct myocardial effects, the increased afterload with vasopressin is unlikely to be well tolerated for long periods in the failing myocardium.

In the setting of increased inotropic requirements for the failing myocardium, the situation is dire. Medical therapy is unlikely to return the patient to an asymptomatic state, and continuation of therapy will likely increase the stress on an already stressed myocardium. At this point, mechanical support should be considered to "rest the myocardium." In children, mechanical support in this setting has generally been used as a bridge to cardiac transplantation. In the setting of a potentially reversible process, such as myocarditis, mechanical support has been used as a bridge to recovery. Reducing the chronic mechanical stress in a failing heart may reverse some of the pathologic molecular changes characteristic of heart failure. For example, mechanical support has been associated with reversal of cytoskeletal abnormalities such as dystrophin proteolytic cleavage (94). In adult patients with severe heart failure who are not heart transplant candidates, mechanical support has been used as so-called *destination therapy*, or placing a patient on mechanical support without the intention of bridging the patient to cardiac transplantation or recovery of function. Mechanical support for this end is associated with increased survival and increased quality of life compared to medical therapy in adult patients with advanced heart failure (74). Options for mechanical support will be discussed later in this chapter but include short-term support with partial cardiopulmonary support from extracorporeal membrane oxygenation, medium-term support with centrifugal pump devices (e.g., Biomedicus), and long-term support with LV assist devices (e.g., Thoratec, Berlin Heart, DeBakey ventricular assist device). As heroic efforts such as mechanical support may not be available, appropriate, or desirable in many patients, palliative care and withdrawal of support may be appropriate.

Assessment of Therapeutic Efficacy

After therapy for heart failure is instituted, it is imperative that the effect of the therapy be continually evaluated. In adult patients, relief of symptoms correlates well with decreased filling pressures. As stated previously, it is unclear whether the use of the pulmonary artery for monitoring can improve outcome over clinical assessment. Although we advocate using superior vena cava (SVC) oxygen saturations for goal-directed therapy in patients with decompensated heart failure, this has also not been shown to improve outcomes. The clinical assessment should include determinants of overall cardiac output, pulmonary congestion, and systemic perfusion. Laboratory parameters such as B-type natriuretic peptide levels and high-resolution C-reactive protein have been demonstrated to correlate with heart failure severity. It is not clear that following these levels improves outcome when managing acute decompensated heart failure.

MEDICAL MANAGEMENT OF LOW CARDIAC OUTPUT AFTER CARDIAC SURGERY

Morbidity and mortality associated with LCOS following cardiac surgery are high. During earlier days of infant cardiac surgery, surgical mortality approached 20%. Although LCOS is associated with lower mortality in the current era, it results in increased hospital stay, increased resource utilization, and possible long-term cognitive dysfunction. Prompt recognition, diagnosis, and management of LCOS are fundamental to optimal cardiac intensive care and essential for optimal patient outcome. An extensive discussion of the management of the postoperative patient is found in Chapter 70.

Treatment of Low Cardiac Output after Surgery

Management of postoperative LCOS includes optimization of preload and afterload, prompt diagnosis of residual cardiac lesions, prevention of hypoxia, anemia, and acidosis, and administration of pharmacologic agents to improve myocardial contractile function (50). In addition, in low cardiac output associated with right heart failure, some children may benefit from creation or enlargement of an atrial-level shunt to allow right-to-left shunting.

Minimizing Oxygen Requirements

Reduced cardiac output and increased systemic oxygen consumption can adversely alter the systemic oxygen balance after CPB. One study of children aged 2 months to 15 years demonstrated a significant increase in oxygen consumption following CPB (49). Peak oxygen consumption correlated significantly with an increase in central temperature. Thus, fever in the setting of LCOS should be treated aggressively with antipyretic medication or surface cooling. A cooling blanket may be useful, but shivering should be avoided, as it may be associated with an increase in oxygen consumption. Total oxygen consumption can be decreased by the induction of heavy sedation, paralysis, or mild hypothermia that reduces the metabolic rate. Case reports of moderate hypothermia induction for patients with refractory LCOS suggest this may be a potential therapy for LCOS (22,23).

Ensuring Adequate Preload

Inadequate preload is common in postoperative cardiac surgical patients. Potential causes of postoperative hypovolemia include bleeding, excessive ultrafiltration, and vasodilation from rewarming or afterload reduction. Cardiac tamponade, which impairs preload by altering diastolic compliance, should also always be considered in patients showing signs of LCOS. Increased mediastinal pressure, with fluid or extrapleural air, can also lead to myocardial compression with LCOS and should be treated promptly. Myocardial swelling, which may limit myocardial filling and prevent adequate output, may necessitate sternal reopening.

Although true ventricular preload is the end-diastolic ventricular volume, preload assessment can be estimated from right and left atrial pressure. Continual reassessment of the optimal preload is essential, as ventricular compliance and subsequent preload needs often change postoperatively. **Figure 67A.2A** illustrates how preload determination is predominantly a "trial and error" process. When atrial pressure is low, fluid administration augments end-diastolic volume and increases stroke volume. With successive fluid administration, however, increases in stroke volume become limited due to the nonlinear nature of the ventricular diastolic compliance. Preload augmentation is also limited by elevations in LV end-diastolic pressure, which results in clinically significant edema formation and potential impairment of myocardial perfusion. Interpretation of hemodynamic pressure monitoring data should always be made with an understanding of the patient's underlying physiology. A poorly compliant ventricle, such as with right ventricular (RV) dysfunction after tetralogy of Fallot repair, would be expected to have higher end-diastolic and, thus, right atrial pressures than a normal heart, and may rely on higher filling pressures to generate adequate output. Patients with diastolic dysfunction may require more extensive postoperative volume administration to maintain preload and cardiac output. These patients will also benefit from lusitropic therapy intended to improve diastolic ventricular filling. **Figure 67A.2B**, illustrates how a change in ventricular diastolic compliance affects atrial pressure. Enhanced lusitropy should result in a greater stroke volume for a comparable atrial pressure.

Prompt Recognition of Dysrhythmias

Early recognition of postoperative dysrhythmias is imperative; therefore, a baseline postoperative surface electrocardiogram should always be obtained for comparison with preoperative and subsequent postoperative tracings. Continuous electrocardiographic monitoring during the postoperative period is also essential. Sinus bradycardia, bundle-branch block, and atrioventricular block can occur after many cardiac surgical procedures; thus, temporary atrial and ventricular pacing wires are typically placed to facilitate pacing, if necessary. Dysrhythmias occur frequently in postoperative cardiac surgical patients and may require overdrive pacing, cardioversion, or pharmacologic intervention (40). A review of the incidence of dysrhythmias in postoperative cardiac surgical patients showed the most common rhythm disturbances to be nonsustained ventricular and supraventricular tachycardia, with incidences of 22% and 12%, respectively. Sustained ventricular, junctional and supraventricular dysrhythmias were also common, with incidences of 6%, 5%, and 4%, respectively (40). Loss in atrioventricular synchrony can compromise preload, increase pulmonary congestion, and significantly diminish cardiac output; thus, maintenance of atrioventricular synchrony is essential (via pacing, if necessary).

Junctional ectopic tachycardia (JET) is a common tachyarrhythmia that usually occurs in the first 48 hrs following surgery, especially after procedures involving closure of a ventricular septal defect and in younger patients. It is generally poorly tolerated, especially in patients with unstable hemodynamics. Early recognition of JET and other dysrhythmias may be aided by careful surveillance of atrial pressure waveforms; loss of the distinct *a* and *v* waves, indicating loss of

i. Preload Recruitment

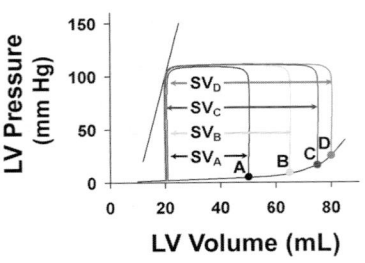
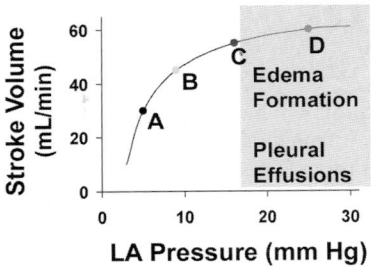

ii. Improve Diastolic Function (Positive Lusitropy)

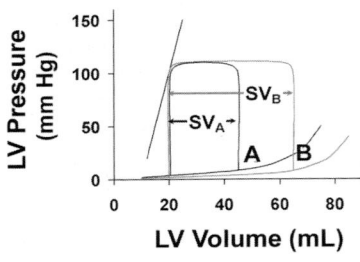
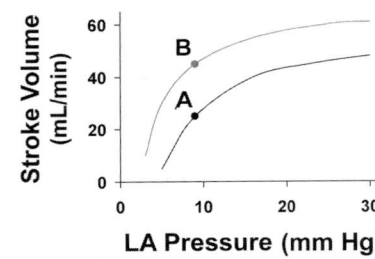

iii. Increase Contractility (Positive Inotropy)

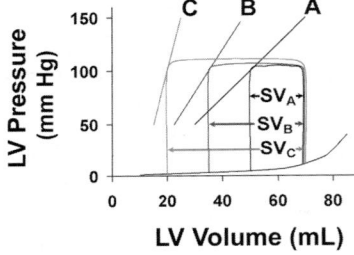
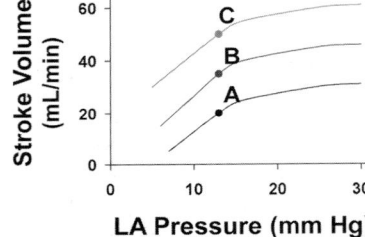

iv. Afterload Reduction

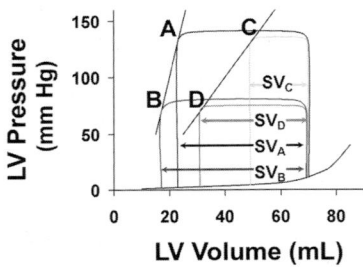
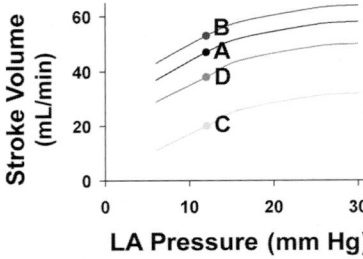

FIGURE 67A.2. Paired changes in pressure-volume and Starling relationships with isolated manipulations in preload (**i**), lusitropy (**ii**), contractility (**iii**), and afterload (**iv**). End-diastolic point A and stroke volume A (SV_A) for each pair of graphs represent the initial baseline hemodynamic condition. **Panel i** Demonstrates the effect of preload recruitment on the pressure-volume and Starling relationships. Fluid volume administration augments end-diastolic volume (EDV) from point A to point B, with the increase in stroke volume represented as the difference between SV_A and SV_B. As diastolic compliance is nonlinear, increases in stroke volume are progressively less with further fluid administration (SV_C and SV_D). End-diastolic volumes A, B, C, and D define the diastolic compliance relationship. Preload augmentation is limited by elevations in left ventricular end-diastolic pressure (EDP), which can lead to impaired myocardial perfusion and elevations in atrial pressure, with resultant transcapillary leak and edema formation. **Panel ii** demonstrates the beneficial effects of positive lusitropy on the pressure-volume and Starling relationships. Enhanced ventricular compliance corresponds to an increased EDV for the same EDP, thereby augmenting stroke volume without increasing atrial pressure. Enhanced lusitropy results in a greater stroke volume for a comparable atrial pressure. **Panel iii** demonstrates the beneficial effects of positive inotropy on the pressure-volume and Starling relationships. Increases in contractility are shown as enhancement of the end-systolic pressure-volume relationship (ESPVR), demonstrated by increases in the slopes of line A through line C in the left-hand graph. At constant preload, increased contractility enhances ejection during isovolumic contraction, decreasing the end-systolic volume and increasing stroke volume (from SV_A to SV_B to SV_C). Enhanced contractility results in a greater stroke volume for a comparable preload. **Panel iv** demonstrates the beneficial effects of afterload reduction on the pressure-volume and Starling relationships. From baseline conditions A or C, afterload reduction allows the heart to eject to a lower systolic pressure and volume (points B and D), enhancing ejection and augmenting stroke volume (SV_A to SV_B and SV_C to SV_D). At normal contractility (slope AB), the ventricle responds to altered afterload with only small changes in stroke volume (SV_A to SV_B). On the other hand, neonatal and failing hearts are particularly sensitive to alterations in afterload. Benefits of afterload reduction are therefore more pronounced in neonatal hearts and in the setting of poor contractility. With reduced contractility (as shown by the reduced slope of ESPVR CD), the increase in stroke volume is greater for a comparable change in afterload. Afterload reduction results in a greater stroke volume for a comparable preload.

atrioventricular synchrony, is often the first indication of dysrhythmia and/or atrioventricular dyssynchrony. Hypomagnesemia is a frequent occurrence after pediatric heart surgery and may contribute to the onset of JET. A recent study reported a reduction in the incidence of JET with administration of IV magnesium in the early postoperative period (25). Once diagnosed, treatment of JET is directed toward the reestablishment of atrioventricular synchrony. If the hemodynamics allow it, an effort should be made to discontinue adrenergic agents, which contribute to the onset of JET and increase the JET rate. Pac-

ing, either atrial (if atrioventricular conduction is preserved) or atrioventricular sequential, is the initial therapy of choice. If the junctional rate is too fast to allow pacing, the goal of pharmacologic therapy is to provide rate control to allow institution of atrial or dual-chamber pacing. While IV amiodarone is generally considered the drug of choice, induction of hypothermia and procainamide administration have also been shown to be effective. Finally, since common wisdom suggests that the risk of JET is greater in the presence of low output ("low cardiac output begets JET"), the diagnosis of JET should prompt the cardiac intensivist to search for other causes of LCOS, including other residual cardiac lesions.

Prompt Diagnosis of Residual Cardiac Lesions

Residual cardiac lesions in the postoperative patient can lead to LCOS and result in increased morbidity and mortality. Pressure and oximetry data from indwelling intracardiac catheters and transesophageal or surface echocardiography should be used to exclude residual structural lesions in patients with LCOS following CPB. Catheterization should be considered if LCOS persists and the etiology remains elusive. Careful evaluation for residual cardiac abnormalities is indicated especially when patients do not follow their expected postoperative course after heart surgery. Prompt diagnosis of residual structural lesions can help to direct medical management optimally or may prompt surgical or catheter-based intervention.

Treatment of Depressed Myocardial Contractility

As low cardiac output after pediatric heart surgery is often associated with some level of contractile dysfunction, inotropic support in the early postoperative period is usually necessary. **Figure 67A.2C** demonstrates the beneficial effects of positive inotropy on the pressure-volume and Starling relationships. At constant preload, increased contractility should enhance ejection during isovolumic contraction to increase stroke volume. Because inotropic agents have unwanted side effects, it is important to assess efficacy of these agents following initiation or dosage adjustment. The potential utility of Starling curves to assess efficacy of most hemodynamic interventions is illustrated in **Figure 67A.2D**. The Starling relationship specifies the therapeutic goal of all inotropic agents: enhanced contractility should result in a greater stroke volume for a comparable preload. As measurement of stroke volume is not routine in postoperative patients, an alternative to the true Starling relationship is illustrated in **Figure 67A.3**. In that stroke volume is not easily monitored, indirect measures of cardiac output (such as SVC saturation) or measures of end-organ perfusion (such as urine output) may be plotted against atrial pressure to attain a "modified" Starling relationship. Points A–C of **Figure 67A.3** indicate how preload recruitment is used to increase SVC saturation or urine output. However, in that preload recruitment is limited, inotropic agents are used to improve SVC saturation or urine output by shifting the Starling relationship leftward (point D). Using the modified Starling relationship, the therapeutic goal of enhanced contractility is improvement in systemic blood flow for a comparable preload (reflected as improved SVC saturation and enhanced organ perfusion).

Inotropic agents and vasodilators are routinely used in pediatric cardiac surgical patients to help reestablish adequate myocardial function during and after surgery. Support is often initiated with low-dose infusions of dopamine or dobutamine (3–5 mcg/kg/min). The infusion rate is usually titrated to optimize systemic blood flow and pressure. High doses of dopamine are rarely used because of increasing vasoconstric-

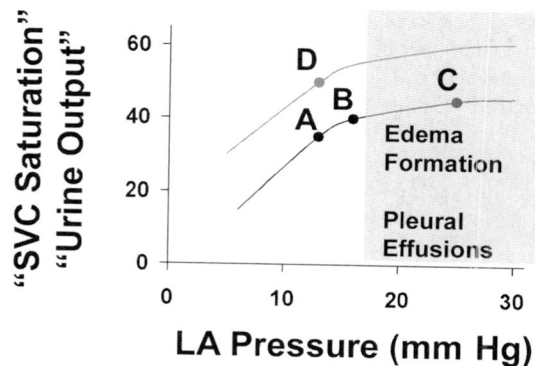

FIGURE 67A.3. Modified Starling relationship. As stroke volume is not easily monitored, indirect measures of cardiac output, such as superior vena cava (SVC) saturation, or measures of end-organ perfusion, such as urine output, may be plotted against atrial pressure to attain a "modified" Starling relationship. Fluid administration augments preload and leads to improvement in SVC saturation and end-organ perfusion (point A to point B). However, preload augmentation is limited; progressive fluid administration will ultimately lead to excessive atrial pressures, with resultant edema formation (point C). Alternate ways to improve SVC saturation or urine output include afterload reduction or improvements in lusitropy or inotropy, all of which shift the Starling relationship leftward (point D). The therapeutic goal of enhanced lusitropy, increased contractility, or afterload reduction is improvement in systemic blood flow for a comparable preload (reflected as improved SVC saturation and enhanced organ perfusion).

tor and chronotropic effects. Although some centers use higher doses of dobutamine, our practice is to add another agent if more support is necessary. Because of its greater myocardial α_1- and β_1-adrenergic effects, epinephrine is a more potent inotrope than is dopamine or dobutamine and is preferred for treatment of severe ventricular dysfunction. High-dose epinephrine (>0.1 mcg/kg/min) frequently results in tachycardia and systemic vasoconstriction. Epinephrine is often used in combination with IV vasodilators such as milrinone, sodium nitroprusside, and phenoxybenzamine to treat ventricular dysfunction and decrease systemic afterload (or at least attenuate the α_1-effects of epinephrine). Norepinephrine is pharmacologically similar to epinephrine but has more α_1-adrenergic effects. Because norepinephrine's potent vasoconstrictor effects result in marked increases in ventricular afterload, its use is usually avoided in children after congenital heart surgery.

The use of PDE inhibitors, which do not demonstrate many of the shortcomings common to catecholamine therapy, has increased considerably over the past few years. PDE inhibitors improve cardiac index by enhancing both systolic and diastolic function and by reducing SVR and PVR. In the pediatric population, milrinone is used more frequently than inamrinone because of its shorter half-life and lower incidence of thrombocytopenia (39,47).

The ability to achieve a rapid hemodynamic response upon initiation of milrinone is extremely important after separation from CPB, when uncompensated LCOS can quickly result in the deterioration of hemodynamic status and subsequent secondary organ dysfunction. For patients at high risk for LCOS, some centers prefer to load with milrinone during bypass to avoid potential hypotension associated with loading. As stated previously, the multicentered PRIMACORP study demonstrated that use of milrinone in children early after congenital heart surgery reduces the incidence of LCOS (39). As renal dysfunction results in delayed clearance of both milrinone and inamrinone, patients with renal insufficiency are at risk for toxicity due to excessive drug levels. Continuous infusion rates should thus be adjusted based on creatinine clearance to avoid excessive and prolonged vasodilation, especially in neonates.

Calcium supplementation and calcium sensitizing agents also warrant discussion. Cardiac contraction and relaxation are mediated by cyclic fluctuations in cytoplasmic calcium concentration. Hypocalcemia occurs frequently in the postoperative period and may be pronounced in patients with 22q11 deletion syndrome and in neonates with transient hypoparathyroidism. Transfusion of citrate-treated blood, which chelates calcium, and administration of loop diuretics may exacerbate the hypocalcemia. Ionized calcium, the physiologically active form of calcium, should be monitored frequently in the postoperative period, and normal or supernormal levels should be maintained with supplementation. Many centers routinely use calcium infusions in neonates after CPB to augment and stabilize extracellular ionized calcium, especially in patients with 22q11 deletion syndrome. Calcium-sensitizing agents, as described previously, have many potential advantages over traditional inotropic agents. The use of these agents, such as levosimendan, for LCOS has not been studied.

Although the mechanism remains unclear, investigators have advocated thyroid hormone therapy as a potential treatment for LCOS (10,19,70). During CPB, circulating levels of the thyroid hormones triiodothyronine (T₃) and thyroxine (T₄) are reduced; these deficiencies can persist for several days and may play a role in postoperative myocardial depression (70). One small study demonstrated hemodynamic improvement in infants with refractory LCOS when treated with T₃ (19). Another randomized study reported that children who were given postoperative T₃ supplementation had significantly higher cardiac output after surgery than those given placebo (10).

Arginine vasopressin has been advocated as a therapeutic option for pediatric patients with refractory hypotension after surgery to improve systemic arterial blood pressure when conventional therapies fail. CPB leads to decreased arginine vasopressin levels. Arginine vasopressin has been shown to be effective for refractory hypotension in patients on mechanical circulatory support (5,59), and it reverses phenoxybenzamine-related hypotension (62).

Both preoperative and postoperative patients can develop prolonged low cardiac output that requires escalating inotropic support and is refractory to other therapy. Recent data suggest that relative adrenal insufficiency contributes to morbidity in critically ill adult patients, and low-dose corticosteroid administration has been suggested as an option for patients with refractory LCOS. In a retrospective study of neonates who received escalating, high-dose epinephrine, inotrope requirements were observed to decrease significantly within 24 hrs of corticosteroid treatment (86). The results of this study are shown in **Figure 67A.4**. Some patients demonstrated low random cortisol levels with a normal adrenocorticotrophic hormone stimulation test, suggesting adrenal dysfunction. These data suggest that stress-dose hydrocortisone (50 mg/m²/day) may help to reduce inotropic requirements in pediatric patients with LCOS that is refractory to conventional therapy. The physiologic basis for the reduction in inotropic support after both arginine vasopressin and corticosteroid therapy remains obscure, but they may share a similar mechanism, as

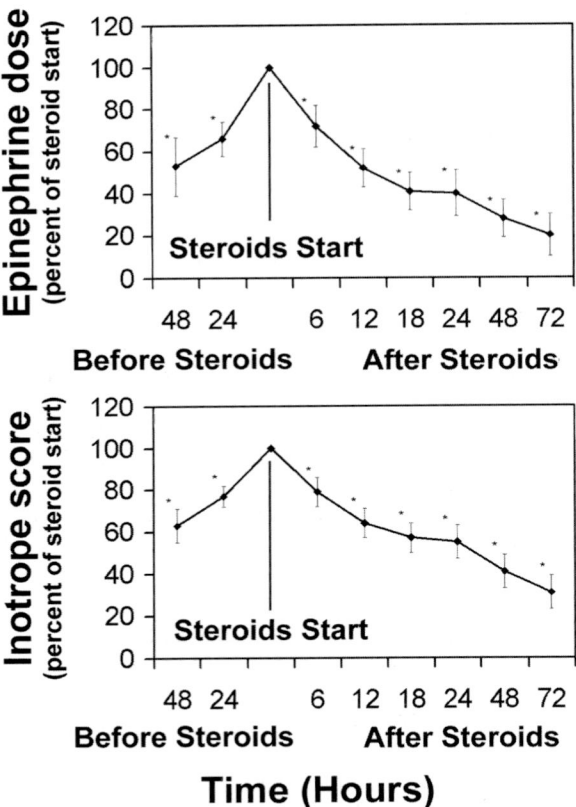

FIGURE 67A.4. Steroid use in critically ill infants after cardiac surgery. Epinephrine doses and inotropic scores in critically ill infants after heart surgery demonstrating significant decrease after administration of steroids. Values are plotted as a percentage of the baseline values at the time steroid administration was initiated. From Shore S, Nelson DP, Pearl JM, et al. Usefulness of corticosteroid therapy in decreasing epinephrine requirements in critically ill infants with congenital heart disease. *Am J Cardiol* 2000;88:591–94, with permission.

arginine vasopressin serves as a potent stimulus for adrenocorticotropin.

Afterload Reduction for Systemic Ventricular Failure

Elevated afterload is particularly detrimental to the neonatal heart, especially when compounded by postoperative myocardial dysfunction. Afterload reduction is thus often beneficial in postoperative patients who show signs of LCOS. Furthermore, if high-dose catecholamines cannot be avoided, afterload reduction/vasodilator therapy should be considered to counter catecholamine vasoconstrictor effects. The beneficial effects of afterload reduction on pressure-volume and Starling relationships are demonstrated in **Figure 67A.2D**; these graphs also demonstrates an important principle: benefits of afterload reduction are particularly pronounced in neonatal hearts and in the setting of poor contractility. With neonatal hearts or impaired contractility, afterload reduction is particularly useful to augment stroke volume and overall cardiac output. As with inotropic agents, it is important to assess efficacy of these agents following initiation or dosage adjustment, as vasodilator agents also have unwanted side effects. As shown in **Figure 67A.2,** the therapeutic goal of afterload reduction should be a greater stroke volume for a comparable preload. As noted previously, however, as measurement of stroke volume is not routine in postoperative patients, the modified Starling relationship can be used to assess efficacy of most hemodynamic interventions, including afterload reduction. As shown in **Figure 67A.3** the therapeutic goal of afterload reduction is improvement in systemic blood flow for a comparable preload (reflected as improved SVC saturation and enhanced organ perfusion).

Some centers advocate use of the potent vasodilator phenoxybenzamine, an α-adrenergic blocking agent, in selected pediatric patients after cardiac surgery. As phenoxybenzamine is a potent vasodilator with a very long half-life (>24 hrs), its use may be complicated by severe hypotension. For this reasons, many centers prefer to use sodium nitroprusside for afterload reduction and vasodilator therapy in patients with congenital heart disease. Although nitroprusside may be a slightly less effective vasodilator than phenoxybenzamine, its therapeutic effects are easier to titrate due to its very short half-life and rapid onset of action. Sodium nitroprusside has also been advocated in patients with excessive pulmonary blood flow after Norwood palliation. In such patients, the dual effects of nitroprusside include afterload reduction for improvement of myocardial performance and reduction of SVR to improve the balance of pulmonary and systemic blood flow. PDE inhibitors are also commonly used for afterload reduction in pediatric patients with congenital heart disease. These agents are particularly useful in the postoperative pediatric cardiac surgical patient because enhanced inotropic and lusitropic effects are combined with systemic and pulmonary vasodilation. In patients who require high doses of adrenergic agents, it is especially important to use one or more vasodilator agents simultaneously.

Management of Right-ventricular Failure

Right heart failure is a common complication of congenital heart surgery and, thus, one of the common causes of LCOS. Factors that contribute to postoperative RV dysfunction include difficulties with right heart myocardial protection and right ventriculotomy, which is required for the surgical correction of many congenital heart lesions. Patients who undergo right heart procedures, including tetralogy of Fallot and Fontan procedures, often demonstrate restrictive physiology (diastolic RV dysfunction), characterized by antegrade diastolic pulmonary arterial flow coinciding with atrial systole.

Children with acute RV restrictive physiology have a decreased cardiac index because the stiff RV has impaired diastolic filling. These patients typically have a slower postoperative recovery and a prolonged stay in the ICU, with longer periods of inotropic and ventilatory support. Alterations in LV filling may also occur due to the hypertensive RV. Alterations in ventricular compliance make patients with RV failure particularly sensitive to alterations in venous return caused by intrathoracic pressure changes. As discussed later, these patients benefit from ventilation strategies that minimize intrathoracic pressure (84). Patients with RV failure may benefit from manipulation of PVR to minimize RV afterload. PDE inhibitors are particularly beneficial in these patients due to the combined lusitropic and pulmonary vasodilatory effects.

The ability to maintain a right-to-left shunt at the atrial level is beneficial in patients with RV dysfunction. In patients who undergo the modified Fontan procedure, fenestration between the Fontan pathway and atrium is associated with reduced pleural effusion and significantly shorter hospital stays. In patients who undergo tetralogy of Fallot repair, a right-to-left atrial shunt can be similarly facilitated by maintaining the patency of the foramen ovale or by creating a small fenestration in the atrial septum.

Ventilation Strategies in Patients with Ventricular Dysfunction

Effects of Positive-pressure Ventilation in Left-ventricular Failure

As noted above, the ventilation strategy depends upon whether RV or LV dysfunction predominates. Positive intrathoracic pressure is often beneficial in patients with systemic ventricular dysfunction due to diminished LV afterload. In addition to optimal lung recruitment, higher levels of positive end-expiratory pressure may thus be hemodynamically beneficial in these patients. Tidal volumes should be maintained in the range of 8–10 mL/kg to avoid overdistension, which could increase PVR and RV afterload. Furthermore, evidence suggests that shorter inspiratory times may augment LV filling in patients with systemic ventricular dysfunction (58). Because alterations in thoracic pressure may have opposing hemodynamic effects, hemodynamic effects of all ventilatory maneuvers should be carefully evaluated with respect to systemic oxygen delivery.

Effects of Positive-pressure Ventilation in Right-ventricular Failure

As noted above, alterations in ventricular compliance make patients with RV failure particularly sensitive to changes in venous return caused by adjustments in intrathoracic pressure. Spontaneous inspiration enhances diastolic flow and, thus, overall cardiac output in these patients; therefore, early extubation can be beneficial. Due to the detrimental effects of positive-pressure ventilation on RV dynamics, alternative modes of ventilation such as negative-pressure or high-frequency jet ventilation have been studied. As high-frequency jet ventilation reduces mean airway pressure and PVR while maintaining a similar $PaCO_2$, it may be ideally suited to patients with RV dysfunction and/or pulmonary hypertension. In postoperative Fontan patients, high-frequency jet ventilation decreased mean airway pressure, reduced PVR, and increased cardiac index (57). Similarly, negative-pressure ventilation has been shown to augment cardiac output in patients with restrictive physiology after tetralogy of Fallot repair (85). Similar results were observed in patients with Fontan physiology (84). Although technical challenges associated with negative-pressure ventilation in postoperative cardiac surgery patients have prevented its widespread use, ventilation strategies used for patients with RV failure should aim to minimize mean airway pressure while maintaining lung volume at functional residual capacity, where lung function, PVR, and RV afterload are optimal. To ensure minimal RV afterload in patients with RV dysfunction, the ventilation strategy should be tailored to avoid increases in PVR.

MEDICAL MANAGEMENT OF MYOCARDITIS

Care of a patient who presents with a clinical picture and history suggestive of myocarditis varies, depending on the severity of myocardial involvement. Many patients present with relatively mild disease, with minimal respiratory compromise and only mild congestive heart failure. These patients require close monitoring to assess whether the disease will progress to dysrhythmias or worsening heart failure, with the need for intensive hemodynamic or antiarrhythmic support. Experimental animal studies suggest that bed rest may prevent an increase in intramyocardial viral replication in the acute stage (34); thus, it appears prudent to place patients under this restriction at the time of diagnosis. General supportive care is provided, such as preventing hypoxemia, maintaining cardiac output at levels that supply adequate tissue perfusion and prevent metabolic disturbances, using diuretics for removal of excess extracellular fluid volume, and using anticoagulation (aspirin, warfarin, and/or heparin) to reduce the likelihood of a thrombotic/embolic phenomenon.

As it is more effective to reduce the work on the heart than to "whip a failing heart," afterload reduction is the cornerstone of therapy for patients with myocarditis and clinically significant contractile dysfunction. Sodium nitroprusside is often used alone or in conjunction with other inotropic agents, especially if the patient requires an agent with vasoconstrictor properties. More recently, PDE inhibitors such as IV milrinone have been used to provide both inotropy and afterload reduction. In some circumstances, nesiritide may be beneficial (42). When chronic oral therapy is possible and hypotension is not present, an afterload-reducing drug such as captopril (0.3–3.0 mg/kg/day, divided every 8 hrs) or enalapril (0.2–0.4 mg/kg/day, divided every 12 hrs), may be used in addition to digoxin and diuretics (73). The addition of β blockers such as carvedilol or metoprolol also appears to enhance the normalization of cardiac function (11,81,99).

Because catecholamines generally aggravate myocardial injury, use should be carefully assessed and doses should be minimized. Low-dose dopamine or dobutamine (<5 mcg/kg/min) may provide some assistance in the presence of decreased ventricular function, but greater doses or addition of more potent catecholamines, such as epinephrine or norepinephrine, should prompt consideration for mechanical support. Although low-dose epinephrine may be temporarily necessary to maintain blood pressure and/or systemic perfusion, it is our practice to initiate mechanical circulatory support if prolonged or high-dose epinephrine (>0.03 mcg/kg/min) is necessary, as higher doses of catecholamines are likely to aggravate myocardial injury and are unlikely to improve outcome. These patients are at high risk for progressive shock or cardiac arrest. In that all inotropic agents have some detrimental effects, we strongly advocate goal-oriented therapy with mixed-venous or SVC saturation monitoring to guide inotrope and vasodilator therapy and especially to ensure that their use is beneficial.

Although the reduced use of high-dose catecholamines has reduced the frequency of dysrhythmias in these patients, they should be vigorously treated when they do occur. Antiarrhythmic therapy for supraventricular tachyarrhythmias may include β blockers procainamide or digoxin, although we tend to avoid digoxin in patients with suspected myocarditis. Ventricular dysrhythmias may respond to lidocaine. IV amiodarone may be preferable for refractory dysrhythmias or if ventricular function is severely depressed. Despite aggressive treatment of these dysrhythmias, rapid deterioration to ventricular fibrillation, especially in the very young, may occur and should be treated immediately by direct-current cardioversion. Complete atrioventricular block requires an immediate temporary transvenous pacemaker, with possible need for a permanent pacing system. Chronic dysrhythmias may persist long after the acute disease has subsided. Thus, children who recover from myocarditis should be followed long term.

Mechanical support is provided for patients unresponsive to medical therapy. Transplantation becomes necessary in patients who do not acutely recover despite medical and mechanical support of the failed myocardium.

Immune Modulation

Immunosuppression

The use of immunosuppressive agents in suspected or proven viral myocarditis is controversial (20,33,65,96). Some animal studies have suggested an exacerbation of virus-induced cytotoxicity in the presence of immunosuppressive drugs, possibly due to interference with interferon production. The Myocarditis Treatment Trial analyzed the use of immunosuppressive and steroid therapy in adult patients (54). No improvement was noted among patients treated with (a) azathioprine and prednisone versus (b) cyclosporine and prednisone, along with conventional medical therapy. Although immunosuppressive therapy has not been shown to be beneficial in most patients with histologically confirmed myocarditis, we advocate combined treatment with IV immunoglobulin and pulse-dose steroids for patients with the fulminant necrotic myocarditis phenotype of myocarditis. Due to anecdotal reports of benefit, patients with suspected fulminant necrotic myocarditis are treated with IV methylprednisolone (10 mg/kg body weight every 8 hrs for 3 total doses).

Antibody Therapy

A frequently used but unproven therapeutic option for children with myocarditis is IV δ-globulin, based on the observational, nonrandomized study that investigated its use in 21 of 46 children with myocarditis (27). Patients who received this drug had better LV function at follow-up. In addition, survival tended to be higher at 1 year, although the data did not reach statistical significance because of the small number of patients in the study. The experience at our institution is anecdotally similar. Patients are typically treated with 1–2 doses of 1 g/kg of IV immunoglobulin. A prospective, randomized trial is pending.

MEDICAL MANAGEMENT OF CARDIOMYOPATHIES

Treatment Strategies for Dilated Cardiomyopathy

Acute management of a child newly diagnosed with DCM should include an effort to rule out myocarditis or surgically correctable causes (i.e., anomalous left coronary artery arising from the pulmonary artery, aortic arch obstruction). The risk of complications such as thromboembolic events or dysrhythmia should be minimized, and supportive care of heart failure symptoms should be provided. If an intramural thrombus is detected by echocardiography, systemic anticoagulation is indicated. Dysrhythmias are a potential cause of sudden death in DCM patients. Thus, newly diagnosed patients should have inpatient telemetry and Holter monitoring performed. Electrolyte imbalances should be identified and corrected if present. If supraventricular or ventricular dysrhythmias are identified, they should be treated to improve an already diminished cardiac output. The choice of an antiarrhythmic agent should be balanced against its potential to further depress ventricular function. The short-term management of patients with heart failure arising from DCM should consist of the same supportive care as that used in the management of heart failure stemming from other conditions (see previous discussion). Typically, this includes IV diuretics for symptomatic relief from volume overload and venous congestion, as well as the administration of IV inotropes or PDE inhibitors to augment cardiac output. More recently, nesiritide, a recombinant form of B-type natriuretic peptide, has been useful in improving urine output and cardiac function. When the patient's acute decompensation has been controlled, however, the emphasis in treatment should shift to an oral regimen of ACE inhibitors, diuretics, and β blockers. The overall goal in management of patients with DCM is symptomatic treatment and optimization of long-term outcome.

Treatment Strategies for Hypertrophic Cardiomyopathy

Therapy of hypertrophic cardiomyopathy (HCM) is directed at reduction of symptoms, prevention of untoward complications, and prevention of SCD. All patients, when identified, should have risk assessment made regarding SCD (see Chapter 66). Risk stratification is challenging in children, yet it is important to try to identify patients at high risk of SCD who might benefit from placement of an ICD. In adults, patients who have survived a SCD episode or patients who have experienced one or more episodes of ventricular tachycardia are felt to be high risk and are thought to need an ICD. However, these patients comprise a small percentage of the total population of patients with HCM. Also in adults, the use of electrophysiologic testing is thought to have a low prognostic value in the evaluation of patients with HCM and is not considered useful in risk stratification (53). Currently, centers that treat children extrapolate from the adult data, as the risk factors in children are yet to be described. Medical therapy is the first-line approach to patients with HCM. Traditionally, β blockers or nondihydropyridine calcium-channel blockers, such as verapamil, have been used. Both groups of drugs reduce the heart rate, which improves ventricular filling by prolonging diastole. Disopyramide, a type I antiarrhythmic drug, has also been used to reduce symptoms and outflow tract obstruction. At our institution, β blockers are used first-line, with the addition of verapamil in patients with persistent symptoms and/or persistent severe LV outflow obstruction. Diuretics may alleviate symptoms in some patients but must be used with caution, as a reduction in preload could

result in increased outflow gradients. Likewise, the use of ACE inhibitors could result in altered loading conditions that could lead to worsening of the outflow gradient. A subset of patients will progress to end-stage HCM, characterized by decreased LV systolic function, thinning of the walls secondary to fibrosis, and LV dilation. These patients should be managed for heart failure with standard accepted medical and/or surgical therapy. Management of dysrhythmias may also be necessary with medical and/or invasive strategies. Not all arrhythmias are ventricular in nature, as up to 20% of adult patients with HCM will develop atrial fibrillation that may require antiarrhythmic therapy as well as anticoagulation. Nonmedical therapy consists of pacemaker therapy, surgical myomectomy, and alcohol septal ablation, although these options have been used primarily in adults. These therapies are directed at relieving outflow tract obstruction, and have varying degrees of success. Regardless of whether alcohol septal ablation or myomectomy is used, it must be remembered that these procedures do not reduce the risk of SCD secondary to ventricular dysrhythmias. Infective endocarditis is a relatively rare complication that occurs mainly in patients who have outflow tract obstruction, typically in the region of the thickened anterior leaflet of the mitral valve. Thus, prophylaxis for subacute bacterial endocarditis is required.

Therapeutic Strategies for Restrictive Cardiomyopathy

No consistent approach to therapy has been established for restrictive cardiomyopathy (RCM) in pediatric patients. A variety of medications have been administered in combinations, including digoxin, afterload-reducing agents, calcium-channel blockers, and β blockers. Due to the small number of patients in each study and the lack of uniformity of treatment within studies, the benefits or risks of these therapies cannot be determined. The risks and benefits of ACE inhibitors in pediatric RCM remain to be determined. It has been reported that captopril lowered aortic pressure by 24% without an increase in cardiac output when it was administered during cardiac catheterization to 4 pediatric patients with RCM (9). The investigators suggested that captopril should not be used in patients with RCM. However, in the studies that support the use of ACE inhibitors, acute decompensation was not reported, nor was therapeutic benefit established. Modulation of neurohumoral activation by ACE inhibitors may affect fibroblast activity, interstitial fibrosis, intracellular calcium handling, and myocardial stiffness. In adults with diastolic heart failure, the use of ACE inhibitors has been suggested, but data are limited. In adults with diastolic dysfunction, tachycardia is poorly tolerated; therefore, β blockers or calcium-channel blockers have been suggested as part of the treatment regimen. β-blocker therapy has been shown to blunt rapid heart rates in patients in whom significant ST segment depression occurred with increased heart rates (77). However, some children do not tolerate β-blocker therapy. At present, medical therapy remains supportive and should be initiated during an inpatient hospitalization. Diuretics are useful in patients with signs and symptoms of systemic or pulmonary venous congestion. Overdiuresis should be avoided because these patients are sensitive to alterations in preload. Due to a 21% incidence of thromboembolic events, antiplatelet therapy or anticoagulants should be administered. As current medical therapy appears to be ineffective, the development of pulmonary hypertension common, and mortality high, cardiac transplantation is the therapy of choice. When comparing survival of RCM patients with and without cardiac transplantation, it is evident that transplantation results in longer survival (97). Most patients should be evaluated and listed for transplantation at the time of presentation. While listed for transplantation, patients should have Holter monitoring performed every 6 months, or as symptoms dictate, to evaluate for signs of ischemia, ventricular dysrhythmias, or developing conduction disturbances. Implantable defibrillators should be considered for patients with evidence of ischemia and ventricular dysrhythmias. Strenuous physical activity should be avoided.

Therapeutic Strategies for Arrhythmogenic Right Ventricular Dysplasia

Management of patients with arrhythmogenic right ventricular dysplasia consists of antiarrhythmic agents, but the only therapy with survival benefit appears to be implantation of an ICD. In addition, therapies for heart failure may be instituted as the disease progresses toward a pattern similar to DCM. Cardiac transplantation is required in some cases.

Therapeutic Strategies for Left Ventricular Noncompaction

The treatment of LV noncompaction is dependent on associated comorbidities. Patients with the hypertrophic phenotype with or without depressed systolic function or the dilated phenotype should be treated as outlined previously. Aggressive anticoagulant therapy should be considered in cases of thrombus or systemic embolic events. In patients with associated mitochondrial myopathy, a combination of riboflavin, thiamine, coenzyme Q10, and carnitine may be considered. Serial Holter monitoring of patients with LV noncompaction should be considered, as these patients have an increased risk for dysrhythmias. Ventricular dysrhythmias have been associated with this condition and may prompt the placement of an ICD. Patients who are refractory to adequate medical therapy may require consideration for cardiac transplantation.

CONCLUSIONS AND FUTURE DIRECTIONS

Heart failure is commonly encountered in the care of critically ill children. Advances made in the treatment of heart failure over the last several decades have improved the outcome of patients, even those with severe ventricular dysfunction. Inhibition of the RAAS system and β blockade has become the cornerstone of management of chronic heart failure. Still, the field operates with a paucity of data on the treatment of acute decompensated heart failure in pediatric patients. Ventricular dysfunction and postoperative LCOS can often be managed with medical therapy, although mechanical support is increasingly utilized for severe cases.

KEY POINTS

- Heart failure is a clinical syndrome characterized by a reduced ability of the heart to fill and/or eject blood to meet the body's metabolic demand.
- ACE inhibitors and β blockers are the mainstays of chronic management due to their inhibition of the RAAS and the sympathetic nervous system. Diuretics are used for control of symptoms.
- Acute decompensated heart failure is commonly an exacerbation of chronic heart failure.
- An assessment of perfusion (warm or cold) and congestion (wet or dry) is useful in formulating management plans for patients with acute decompensated heart failure.
- The primary aim of acute decompensated heart failure therapy is to return the patient to a state of adequate perfusion (warm) and normal or near-normal filling pressures (dry).
- Catecholamine types of inotropic agents should be used with caution in the treatment of decompensated heart failure.
- In patients who fail to respond to medical therapies, mechanical support should be considered.
- LCOS in the early postoperative period is due primarily to transient myocardial dysfunction, compounded by acute changes in myocardial loading conditions, including postoperative increases in SVR and/or PVR.
- PDE inhibitors increase cardiac muscle contractility and vascular muscle relaxation without increasing myocardial oxygen consumption or ventricular afterload.
- Arginine vasopressin has been advocated as a therapeutic option for pediatric patients with refractory hypotension after surgery.
- Recent data suggest that relative adrenal insufficiency contributes to morbidity in critically ill adult patients, and low-dose corticosteroid administration has been suggested as an option for patients with refractory LCOS.

References

1. Aairis MN, Apostolatos C, Anastassiadis F, et al. Comparison of the effect of levosimendan, or dobutamine or placebo in chronic low output decompensated heart failure. Calcium Sensitizer or Inotrope or None in low output heart failure (CASINO) study (abstract). In: Program and abstracts of the European Society of Cardiology, Heart Failure Update 2004.
2. Abraham WT, Adams KF, Fonarow GC, et al. In-hospital mortality in patients with acute decompensated heart failure requiring intravenous vasoactive medications: An analysis from the Acute Decompensated Heart Failure National Registry (ADHERE). *J Am Coll Cardiol* 2005;46:57–64.
3. Abraham WT, Fisher WG, Smith AL, et al. Cardiac resynchronization in chronic heart failure. *N Engl J Med* 2002;346:1845–53.
4. Adams KF, Jr., Fonarow GC, Emerman CL, et al. Characteristics and outcomes of patients hospitalized for heart failure in the United States: Rationale, design, and preliminary observations from the first 100,000 cases in the Acute Decompensated Heart Failure National Registry (ADHERE). *Am Heart J* 2005;149:209–16.
5. Argenziano M, Choudhri AF, Oz MC, et al. A prospective, randomized trial of arginine vasopressin in the treatment of vasodilatory shock after left ventricular assist device placement. *Circulation* 1997;96:II-286–90.
6. Arora G, Cannon BC, Kim JJ, et al. Tachycardia-induced left ventricular dysfunction in infants and children (abstract). *Pediatr Cardiol* 2005;26:501.
7. Azeka E, Franchini Ramires JA, Valler C, et al. Delisting of infants and children from the heart transplantation waiting list after carvedilol treatment. *J Am Coll Cardiol* 2002;40:2034–8.
8. Bardy GH, Lee KL, Mark DB, et al. Amiodarone or an implantable cardioverter-defibrillator for congestive heart failure. *N Engl J Med* 2005;352:225–37.

9. Bengur AR, Beekman RH, Rocchini AP, et al. Acute hemodynamic effects of captopril in children with a congestive or restrictive cardiomyopathy. *Circulation* 1991;83:523–7.

10. Bettendorf M, Schmidt KG, Grulich-Henn J, et al. Tri-iodothyronine treatment in children after cardiac surgery: A double-blind, randomised, placebo-controlled study. *Lancet* 2000;356:529–34.

11. Blume ED, Canter CE, Spicer R, et al. Prospective single-arm protocol of carvedilol in children with ventricular dysfunction. *Pediatr Cardiol* 2006;27(3):336–42.

12. Braun JP, Schneider M, Dohmen P, et al. Successful treatment of dilative cardiomyopathy in a 12-year-old girl using the calcium sensitizer levosimendan after weaning from mechanical biventricular assist support. *J Cardiothorac Vasc Anesth* 2004;18:772–4.

13. Braun JP, Schneider M, Kastrup M, et al. Treatment of acute heart failure in an infant after cardiac surgery using levosimendan. *Eur J Cardiothorac Surg* 2004;26:228–30.

14. Bristow MR, Saxon LA, Boehmer J, et al. Cardiac-resynchronization therapy with or without an implantable defibrillator in advanced chronic heart failure. *N Engl J Med* 2004;350:2140–50.

15. Brunner-La Rocca HP, Vaddadi G, Esler MD. Recent insight into therapy of congestive heart failure: Focus on ACE inhibition and angiotensin-II antagonism. *J Am Coll Cardiol* 1999;33:1163–73.

16. Bruns LA, Chrisant MK, Lamour JM, et al. Carvedilol as therapy in pediatric heart failure: An initial multicenter experience. *J Pediatr* 2001;138:505–11.

17. Butler J, Young JB, Abraham WT, et al. Beta-blocker use and outcomes among hospitalized heart failure patients. *J Am Coll Cardiol* 2006;47:2462–9.

18. Cannon B, Friedman RA, Fenrich AL Jr., et al. Atrial leads and SVT discriminators do not decrease the incidence of inappropriate shocks in pediatric patients with implantable cardioverter-defibrillators (abstract). *Circulation* 2005;112:II–548.

19. Carrel T, Eckstein F, Englberger L, et al. Thyronin treatment in adult and pediatric heart surgery: Clinical experience and review of the literature. *Eur J Heart Fail* 2002;4:577–82.

20. Chan KY, Iwahara M, Benson LN, et al. Immunosuppressive therapy in the management of acute myocarditis in children: A clinical trial. *J Am Coll Cardiol* 1991;17(2):458–60.

21. Cuffe MS, Califf RM, Adams KF, Jr., et al. Short-term intravenous milrinone for acute exacerbation of chronic heart failure: A randomized controlled trial. *JAMA* 2002;287:1541–7.

22. Dalrymple-Hay MJ, Deakin CD, Knight H, et al. Induced hypothermia as salvage treatment for refractory cardiac failure following paediatric cardiac surgery. *Eur J Cardiothorac Surg* 1999;15:515–8.

23. Deakin CD, Knight H, Edwards JC, et al. Induced hypothermia in the post-operative management of refractory cardiac failure following paediatric cardiac surgery. *Anaesthesia* 1998;53:848–53.

24. Dimas VV, Denfield SW, Cannon BC, et al. Arrhythmias and sudden cardiac death in children with dilated cardiomyopathy (abstract). *Circulation* 2004;110:III–761.

25. Dorman BH, Sade RM, Burnette JS, et al. Magnesium supplementation in the prevention of arrhythmias in pediatric patients undergoing surgery for congenital heart defects. *Am Heart J* 2000;139:522–8.

26. Doval HC, Nul DR, Grancelli HO, et al. Randomised trial of low-dose amiodarone in severe congestive heart failure. Grupo de Estudio de la Sobrevida en la Insuficiencia Cardiaca en Argentina (GESICA). *Lancet* 1994;344:493–8.

27. Drucker NA, Colan SD, Lewis AB, et al. Gamma-globulin treatment of acute myocarditis in the pediatric population. *Circulation* 1994;89(1):252–7.

28. Dubin AM, Janousek J, Rhee E, et al. Resynchronization therapy in pediatric and congenital heart disease patients: An international multicenter study. *J Am Coll Cardiol* 2005;46:2277–83.

29. Eshaghian S, Horwich TB, Fonarow GC. Relation of loop diuretic dose to mortality in advanced heart failure. *Am J Cardiol* 2006;97:1759–64.

30. Executive summary: HFSA 2006 Comprehensive Heart Failure Practice Guideline. *J Card Fail* 2006;12:10–38.

31. Felker GM, Benza RL, Chandler AB, et al. Heart failure etiology and response to milrinone in decompensated heart failure: Results from the OPTIME-CHF study. *J Am Coll Cardiol* 2003;41:997–1003.

32. Felker GM, O'Connor CM. Inotropic therapy for heart failure: An evidence-based approach. *Am Heart J* 2001;142:393–401.

33. Frustaci A, Chimenti C, Calabrese F, et al. Immunosuppressive therapy for active lymphocytic myocarditis: Virological and immunologic profile of responders versus nonresponders. *Circulation* 2003;107(6):857–63.

34. Gauntt C, Huber S. Coxsackievirus experimental heart diseases. *Front Biosci* 2003;8:e23–35.

35. Gheorghiade M, Adams KF Jr. , Colucci WS. Digoxin in the management of cardiovascular disorders. *Circulation* 2004;109:2959–64.

36. Goldberger Z, Lampert R. Implantable cardioverter-defibrillators: Expanding indications and technologies. *JAMA* 2006;295:809–18.

37. Grady KL, Dracup K, Kennedy G, et al. Team management of patients with heart failure: A statement for healthcare professionals from The Cardiovascular Nursing Council of the American Heart Association. *Circulation* 2000;102:2443–56.

38. Hjalmarson A, Goldstein S, Fagerberg B, et al. Effects of controlled-release metoprolol on total mortality, hospitalizations, and well-being in patients with heart failure: The Metoprolol CR/XL Randomized Intervention Trial in congestive heart failure (MERIT-HF). MERIT-HF Study Group. *JAMA* 2000;283:1295–302.

39. Hoffman TM, Wernovsky G, Atz AM, et al. Efficacy and safety of milrinone in preventing low cardiac output syndrome in infants and children after corrective surgery for congenital heart disease. *Circulation* 2003;107:996–1002.

40. Hoffman TM, Wernovsky G, Wieand TS, et al. The incidence of arrhythmias in a pediatric cardiac intensive care unit. *Pediatr Cardiol* 2002;23:598–604.

41. Hunt SA, Abraham WT, Chin MH, et al. ACC/AHA 2005 Guideline Update for the Diagnosis and Management of Chronic Heart Failure in the Adult: A report of the American College of Cardiology/American Heart Association Task Force on Practice Guidelines. *Circulation* 2005;112:e154–235.

42. Jefferies JL, Denfield SW, Price JF, et al. A prospective evaluation of nesiritide in the treatment of pediatric heart failure. *Pediatr Cardiol* 2006;27(4):402–7.

43. Katz AM. Biochemical "defect" in the hypertrophied and failing heart: Deleterious or compensatory? *Circulation* 1973;47:1076–9.

44. Katz AM. Potential deleterious effects of inotropic agents in the therapy of chronic heart failure. *Circulation* 1986;73:III184–90.

45. Katz AM, Lorell BH. Regulation of cardiac contraction and relaxation. *Circulation* 2000;102:IV69–74.

46. Kouatli AA, Garcia JA, Zellers TM, et al. Enalapril does not enhance exercise capacity in patients after Fontan procedure. *Circulation* 1997;96:1507–12.

47. Latifi S, Lidsky K, Blumer JL. Pharmacology of inotropic agents in infants and children. 2000;12:57–79.

48. Lewis AB, Chabot M. The effect of treatment with angiotensin-converting enzyme inhibitors on survival of pediatric patients with dilated cardiomyopathy. *Pediatr Cardiol* 1993;14:9–12.

49. Li J, Schulze-Neick I, Lincoln C, et al. Oxygen consumption after cardiopulmonary bypass surgery in children: Determinants and implications. *J Thorac Cardiovasc Surg* 2000;119:525–33.

50. Lowes BD, Simon MA, Tsvetkova TO, et al. Inotropes in the beta-blocker era. *Clin Cardiol* 2000;23:III11–6.

51. Mann DL. Mechanisms and models in heart failure: A combinatorial approach. *Circulation* 1999;100:999–1008.

52. Mann DL. Heart failure as a progressive disorder. In: Mann DL, ed. *Heart Failure: A Companion to Braunwald's Heart disease 1st ed.*, vol. 1. Philadelphia: WB Saunders, 2004:123–8.

53. Maron BJ, McKenna WJ, Danielson GK, et al. American College of Cardiology/European Society of Cardiology clinical expert consensus document on hypertrophic cardiomyopathy. *J Am Coll Cardiol* 2003;42:1687–713.

54. Mason JW, O'Connell JB, Herskowitz A, et al. A clinical trial of immunosuppressive therapy for myocarditis. The Myocarditis Treatment Trial Investigators. *N Engl J Med* 1995;333(5):269–75.

55. McCurley JM, Hanlon SU, Wei SK, et al. Furosemide and the progression of left ventricular dysfunction in experimental heart failure. *J Am Coll Cardiol* 2004;44:1301–7.

56. McMurray J, Kober L, Robertson M, et al. Antiarrhythmic effect of carvedilol after acute myocardial infarction: Results of the Carvedilol Post-Infarct Survival Control in Left Ventricular Dysfunction (CAPRICORN) trial. *J Am Coll Cardiol* 2005;45:525–30.

57. Meliones JN, Bove EL, Dekeon MK, et al. High-frequency jet ventilation improves cardiac function after the Fontan procedure. *Circulation* 1991;84:III364–8.

58. Meliones J, Kocis K, Bengur AR, et al. Diastolic function in neonates after the arterial switch operation: Effects of positive pressure ventilation and inspiratory time. *Intensive Care Med* 2000;26:950–5.

59. Morales DL, Gregg D, Helman DN, et al. Arginine vasopressin in the treatment of 50 patients with postcardiotomy vasodilatory shock. *Ann Thorac Surg* 2000;69:102–6.

60. Mori Y, Nakazawa M, Tomimatsu H, et al. Long-term effect of angiotensin-converting enzyme inhibitor in volume overloaded heart during growth: A controlled pilot study. *J Am Coll Cardiol* 2000;36:270–5.

61. Nohria A, Tsang SW, Fang JC, et al. Clinical assessment identifies hemodynamic profiles that predict outcomes in patients admitted with heart failure. *J Am Coll Cardiol* 2003;41:1797–804.

62. O'Blenes SB, Roy N, Konstantinov I, et al. Vasopressin reversal of phenoxybenzamine-induced hypotension after the Norwood procedure. *J Thorac Cardiovasc Surg* 2002;123:1012–3.

63. Packer M, Carver JR, Rodeheffer RJ, et al. Effect of oral milrinone on mortality in severe chronic heart failure. The PROMISE Study Research Group. *N Engl J Med* 1991;325:1468–75.

64. Packer M, Coats AJ, Fowler MB, et al. Effect of carvedilol on survival in severe chronic heart failure. *N Engl J Med* 2001;344:1651–8.

65. Parrillo JE. Inflammatory cardiomyopathy (myocarditis): Which patients should be treated with anti-inflammatory therapy? *Circulation* 2001;104(1):4–6.

66. Pignatelli RH, McMahon CJ, Dreyer WJ, et al. Clinical characterization of left ventricular noncompaction in children: A relatively common form of cardiomyopathy. *Circulation* 2003;108:2672–8.

67. Pitt B, Williams G, Remme W, et al. The EPHESUS trial: Eplerenone in patients with heart failure due to systolic dysfunction complicating acute myocardial infarction. Eplerenone Post-AMI Heart Failure Efficacy and Survival Study. *Cardiovasc Drugs Ther* 2001;15:79–87.

68. Pitt B, Zannad F, Remme WJ, et al. The effect of spironolactone on morbidity and mortality in patients with severe heart failure. Randomized Aldactone Evaluation Study Investigators. *N Engl J Med* 1999;341:709–17.

69. Poole-Wilson PA, Swedberg K, Cleland JG, et al. Comparison of carvedilol and metoprolol on clinical outcomes in patients with chronic heart failure in the Carvedilol Or Metoprolol European Trial (COMET): Randomised controlled trial. *Lancet* 2003;362:7–13.

70. Portman MA, Fearneyhough C, Ning XH, et al. Triiodothyronine repletion in infants during cardiopulmonary bypass for congenital heart disease. *J Thorac Cardiovasc Surg* 2000;120:604–8.

71. Price JF, Towbin JA, Denfield SW, et al. Arginine vasopressin levels are elevated and correlate with functional status in infants and children with congestive heart failure. *Circulation* 2004;109:2550–3.

72. Rathore SS, Curtis JP, Wang Y, et al. Association of serum digoxin concentration and outcomes in patients with heart failure. *JAMA* 2003;289:871–8.

73. Rezkalla S, Kloner RA, Khatib G, et al. Beneficial effects of captopril in acute coxsackievirus B3 murine myocarditis. *Circulation* 1990;81(3):1039–46.

74. Rose EA, Gelijns AC, Moskowitz AJ, et al. Long-term mechanical left ventricular assistance for end-stage heart failure. *N Engl J Med* 2001;345:1435–43.

75. Rosenthal D, Chrisant MR, Edens E, et al. International Society for Heart and Lung Transplantation: Practice guidelines for management of heart failure in children. *J Heart Lung Transplant* 2004;23:1313–33.

76. Rosenzweig EB, Starc TJ, Chen JM, et al. Intravenous arginine-vasopressin in children with vasodilatory shock after cardiac surgery. *Circulation* 1999;100:II182–6.

77. Sachdev B, Takenaka T, Teraguchi H, et al. Prevalence of Anderson-Fabry disease in male patients with late onset hypertrophic cardiomyopathy. *Circulation* 2002;105:1407–11.

78. Sackner-Bernstein JD, Kowalski M, Fox M, et al. Short-term risk of death after treatment with nesiritide for decompensated heart failure: A pooled analysis of randomized controlled trials. *JAMA* 2005;293:1900–5.

79. Sackner-Bernstein JD, Skopicki HA, Aaronson KD. Risk of worsening renal function with nesiritide in patients with acutely decompensated heart failure. *Circulation* 2005;111:1487–91.

80. Schwartz SM, Duffy JY, Pearl JM. Cellular and molecular aspects of myocardial dysfunction. *Crit Care Med* 2001;29:S214–9.

81. Shaddy RE. Beta-adrenergic receptor blockers as therapy in pediatric chronic heart failure. *Minerva Pediatr* 2001;53(4):297–304.

82. Shaddy RE, Tani LY, Gidding SS, et al. Beta-blocker treatment of dilated cardiomyopathy with congestive heart failure in children: A multi-institutional experience. *J Heart Lung Transplant* 1999;18:269–74.

83. Sharma D, Buyse M, Pitt B, et al. Meta-analysis of observed mortality data from all-controlled, double-blind, multiple-dose studies of losartan in heart failure. Losartan Heart Failure Mortality Meta-analysis Study Group. *Am J Cardiol* 2000;85:187–92.

84. Shekerdemian LS, Bush A, Shore DF, et al. Cardiopulmonary interactions after Fontan operations: Augmentation of cardiac output using negative pressure ventilation. *Circulation* 1997;96:3934–42.

85. Shekerdemian LS, Schulze-Neick I, Redington AN, et al. Negative pressure ventilation as haemodynamic rescue following surgery for congenital heart disease. *Intensive Care Med* 2000;26:93–6.

86. Shore S, Nelson DP, Pearl JM, et al. Usefulness of corticosteroid therapy in decreasing epinephrine requirements in critically ill infants with congenital heart disease. *Am J Cardiol* 2001;88:591–4.

87. Singh K, Communal C, Sawyer DB, et al. Adrenergic regulation of myocardial apoptosis. *Cardiovasc Res* 2000;45:713–9.

88. Singh SN, Fletcher RD, Fisher SG, et al. Amiodarone in patients with congestive heart failure and asymptomatic ventricular arrhythmia. Survival Trial of Antiarrhythmic Therapy in Congestive Heart Failure. *N Engl J Med* 1995;333:77–82.

89. Stern H, Weil J, Genz T, et al. Captopril in children with dilated cardiomyopathy: Acute and long-term effects in a prospective study of hemodynamic and hormonal effects. *Pediatr Cardiol* 1990;11:22–8.

90. Stevenson LW, Brunken RC, Belil D, et al. Afterload reduction with vasodilators and diuretics decreases mitral regurgitation during upright exercise in advanced heart failure. *J Am Coll Cardiol* 1990;15:174–80.

91. Svensson M, Gustafsson F, Galatius S, et al. How prevalent is hyperkalemia and renal dysfunction during treatment with spironolactone in patients with congestive heart failure? *J Card Fail* 2004;10:297–303.

92. Thom T, Haase N, Rosamond W, et al. Heart disease and stroke statistics—2006 update: A report from the American Heart Association Statistics Committee and Stroke Statistics Subcommittee. *Circulation* 2006;113:e85–151.

93. Ukkonen H, Saraste M, Akkila J, et al. Myocardial efficiency during levosimendan infusion in congestive heart failure. *Clin Pharmacol Ther* 2000;68:522–31.

94. Vatta M, Stetson SJ, Perez-Verdia A, et al. Molecular remodelling of dystrophin in patients with end-stage cardiomyopathies and reversal in patients on assistance-device therapy. *Lancet* 2002;359:936–41.

95. Webster MW, Neutze JM, Calder AL. Acute hemodynamic effects of converting enzyme inhibition in children with intracardiac shunts. *Pediatr Cardiol* 1992;13:129–35.

96. Weller AH, Hall M, Huber SA. Polyclonal immunoglobulin therapy protects against cardiac damage in experimental coxsackievirus-induced myocarditis. *Eur Heart J* 1992;13(1):115–9.

97. Weller RJ, Weintraub R, Addonizo LJ, et al. Outcome of idiopathic restrictive cardiomyopathy in children. *Am J Cardiol* 2002;90:501–6.

98. Wenzel V, Krismer AC, Arntz HR, et al. A comparison of vasopressin and epinephrine for out-of-hospital cardiopulmonary resuscitation. *N Engl J Med* 2004;350:105–13.

99. Williams RV, Tani LY, Shaddy RE. Intermediate effects of treatment with metoprolol or carvedilol in children with left ventricular systolic dysfunction. *J Heart Lung Transplant* 2002;21(8):906–9.

100. Wilson JR, Reichek N, Dunkman WB, et al. Effect of diuresis on the performance of the failing left ventricle in man. *Am J Med* 1981;70:234–9.

101. Wong M, Staszewsky L, Latini R, et al. Valsartan benefits left ventricular structure and function in heart failure: Val-HeFT echocardiographic study. *J Am Coll Cardiol* 2002;40:970–5.

CHAPTER 67B ■ TREATMENT OF HEART FAILURE IN INFANTS AND CHILDREN: MECHANICAL SUPPORT

ANA LIA GRACIANO • JON N. MELIONES • KEITH C. KOCIS

Mechanical support of the failing circulation using extracorporeal life support (ECLS)—also referred to as ECMO (referring to the essential piece of the circuit, the extracorporeal membrane oxygenator) or ventricular assist devices (VADs)—is a new and expanding field of pediatric cardiac intensive care. The first use of ECLS in the operating room was accomplished by the pioneering work of John Gibbon in 1953, using a device of his own design to perform the first intracardiac repair with extracorporeal perfusion. Cardiopulmonary bypass (CPB) techniques have evolved tremendously since then and allow repairs of complex congenital heart defects that were previously lethal. Early visionary work by Barttlet and Hill led to the use of ECLS techniques outside of the operating room in the early 1970s, with Soeter et al. reporting the first prolonged use of ECMO to support a 4-year-old girl with severe hypoxemia after repair of tetralogy of Fallot (25). Since then, use of ECMO has grown tremendously, becoming a standard technique for refractory respiratory failure in the newborn, with overall survival exceeding 80%. Over the last decade, the use of ECLS for cardiac support has grown dramatically, in part due to the complex surgical repairs now being performed in neonates and infants with congenital heart disease. As of 2006, more than 30,000 pediatric patients have been managed on ECLS. Approximately 6000 patients were supported for primary cardiac causes, with an overall survival rate of ~40%, not significantly different from the earliest reports in the late 1980s. Despite the large increase in use of ECLS for cardiac support, overall outcomes remain modest. An alternate view is that the vast majority of these patients never would have survived without ECLS.

EXTRACORPOREAL LIFE SUPPORT

Extracorporeal life support is the term used to describe prolonged extracorporeal partial CPB, achieved by extrathoracic (via the carotid/vena cava or femoral vessels) or transthoracic (via the open sternum) cannulation. ECLS is the preferred and most common technique used for short-term cardiac support (3–14 days) of the neonate, infant, child, and adolescent with refractory heart failure.

Extracorporeal Life Support Circuit

Cardiac ECLS is provided with a now-standard system, most often consisting of a distensible venous drainage reservoir, a servoregulated roller pump, a membrane oxygenator in which gas exchange occurs, and a countercurrent heat exchanger to maintain blood temperature. The full technical details of this circuit are discussed in Chapter 36. Membrane oxygenators, which have greater longevity than do hollow-fiber oxygenators, are being used by most centers; however, hollow-fiber oxygenators are quickly and easily primed, making them very useful for rapid-deployment situations. Roller pumps are used by most of the ECLS centers, although centrifugal pumps are increasingly used. Centrifugal pumps have the advantage of maintaining venous inflow independent of gravity, which helps to maintain adequate venous return at higher flows. Crystalloid preprimed circuits are used at many large ECLS centers for rapid-deployment situations, while "dry circuits" can be rapidly primed on site while the patient is being cannulated. Patients are typically anticoagulated with heparin to prevent thrombosis within the circuit and to prevent the development of thromboemboli.

Indications

ECLS for refractory cardiac failure should be used in patients in whom cardiac function is *reversible and expected* to recover within a short period of time (5–14 days). Patient size, the reversibility of the underlying cause of heart failure, institutional resources, and expertise (medical, surgical, nursing) are among the complex issues that are taken into account when mechanical support is considered for the critically ill cardiac patient. Most institutions develop criteria that are specific for their institution. As of today, no randomized, controlled trial of ECMO has been performed for postoperative congenital cardiac patients with pump failure; thus, no universal selection criteria exist. Instead, the decisions as to when to consider ECLS and which patients should be selected are made at the bedside based on the clinician/team experience. These decisions represent the best of the "art" of medicine. The broadly defined indications and contraindications described in the following paragraphs represent a general consensus of ECMO centers and the individual experience of the authors in managing patients on ECLS.

Pediatric cardiac patients considered for ECLS fall essentially into two groups: surgical (postoperative) and medical (i.e., myocarditis). All candidates have clear evidence of low cardiac output syndrome with or without shock (hypotension, elevated filling pressures, low mixed venous oxygen saturations, decreased urine output, elevated lactic acid) that is refractory to maximal "standard medical" support (defined previously, in Chapter 67, Section A), including mechanical ventilation, vasoactive agents, analgesia, etc. As discussed previously, high-dose catecholamine infusions and/or cardiac arrest are neither desirable nor required prior to consideration of mechanical support. If it is anticipated that end-organ dysfunction will occur due to cardiac failure, the use of ECLS is indicated to support the vital organs while allowing the heart to recover (2,4,28).

In surgical patients, it is extremely important to exclude residual anatomic causes of postoperative myocardial dysfunction *before* considering ECLS. Significant residual hemodynamic lesions should be readdressed in the operating room, rather than placing these patients onto ECLS for "rest." Once these lesions are readdressed, ECLS may be necessary to recover the heart after the repeated and often prolonged CPB runs. Transport to the cardiac catheterization laboratory while on ECLS may be necessary in patients who fail to wean from ECLS in order to definitively rule out residual hemodynamically significant cardiac lesions. In fact, interventional cardiologists may be able to successfully manage some of these issues in the catheterization laboratory with balloon dilation, stents, coils, or closure devices. Multiple types of residual defects have been found during cardiac catheterization, including ventriculoseptal defects that require device closure, aortopulmonary collaterals that require coiling, and aortic valve and/or arch obstructions that require balloon valvuloplasty or angioplasty. If these defects cannot be managed in the catheterization lab, it is necessary to return the patient to the operating room.

Extracorporeal Life Support and Single-ventricle Physiology

Controversy still surrounds the use of ECLS in patients with single-ventricle physiology, such as hypoplastic left heart syndrome, as this was previously a contraindication for ECLS. Outcomes for patients with hypoplastic left heart syndrome on ECLS have improved during recent years at large centers with new techniques and strategies. One center reported experience with a group of 12 neonates who underwent stage I Norwood palliation and received ECLS during the perioperative period (19). Indications for support included dysrhythmia, low cardiac output, cardiac arrest, unbalanced circulation, and hypoxemia, with a mean duration of support of 68 hrs (range, 24–192 hrs). Eight patients were weaned off of support, and 6 (50%) were discharged home in good condition. As the authors conclude, "although the use of ECLS in patients with single-ventricle physiology still carries a significant risk, prompt initiation of support can improve the outcome in a group of patients with impaired cardiopulmonary function after stage I palliation" (26). A group that modified the standard ECMO system by eliminating the membrane oxygenator referred to it as "NOMO" (*no membrane oxygenator*) and thereby provided only roller-pump ventricular assist. In these cases, the infant's own lungs provided oxygenation by leaving the aortopulmonary shunt open, and full mechanical ventilation is continued. Since total flow [$(Q_t) =$ systemic $(Q_s) +$ pulmonary (Q_p) blood flow)] is supported by the ECLS, balancing pulmonary versus systemic flow is usually not complex (7,14). In the past, ligation of the aortopulmonary shunt [Blalock-Taussig

(BT) shunt] during ECLS was advocated, but this procedure has been abandoned due to increase mortality associated with ligation and subsequent complications (thrombosis of the BT shunt, pulmonary ischemia, etc). In addition, an alternative shunt is now being performed at many centers whereby the BT shunt is replaced by a right ventricular (RV)-to-pulmonary artery shunt (Sano shunt) (23). Patients with the Sano shunt may require increased ECLS flows to maintain adequate Q_p and systemic oxygen saturations. The use of ECLS for patients with single-ventricle physiology in the *preoperative* state remains dismal.

Extracorporeal Cardiopulmonary Resuscitation

Extracorporeal cardiopulmonary resuscitation relates to ECLS after cardiac arrest. Cardiac arrest constitutes almost 25% of all of the indications for ECLS in the pediatric cardiac population. Extracorporeal cardiopulmonary resuscitation has been used in >400 patients, with an overall survival to hospital discharge of 36%. Slightly improved survival is found in patients who have a witnessed cardiac arrest prior to ECLS. Recently, large centers have developed systems that allow rapid initiation of ECLS after cardiac arrest that does not quickly respond to conventional pediatric advanced life support therapy. These rapid-deployment systems provide fast, reliable support in patients with acute, sometimes "unexpected," deterioration leading to cardiac arrest. Preprimed circuits or modified, rapidly primed circuits are used with deployment and cannulation times of <1 hr.

Myocarditis Shock

Patients with *fulminant acute myocarditis* can have a rapidly progressive deterioration and fatal outcome if not managed aggressively with ECLS. ECLS has been shown to be beneficial in these patients by allowing time for recovery of cardiac function, with a hospital survival as high as 80%. Case reports detail the benefits of balloon atrial septostomy in these patients to decompress the left ventricle (LV) (similar to LV vents in postoperative patients). For long-term support, VADs (see later discussion) are theoretically preferred; however, patient size and institutional expertise may limit their use (6,9,18,24).

Extracorporeal Life Support as Bridge to Transplant

ECLS can be used as a bridge to heart transplantation. Acceptable posttransplant survival is seen in patients supported with ECLS for up to 2 weeks. Mortality then peaks if suitable organs are unavailable, thus necessitating a highly successful (and rapid) organ procurement program. Patients with dilated cardiomyopathy and post-heart transplant rejection fall predominantly into this group. Pre-ECMO cardiac arrest and renal insufficiency with the concomitant requirement for dialysis decrease the likelihood of survival before and after transplantation. Conceptually, VADs are the mechanical support system of choice for long-term support, but patient size and center expertise currently limit their use. Arkansas Children's Hospital reported their experience using ECLS as a bridge to transplant in 47 pediatric patients, with a mean duration of support of 242 hrs (22–1078 hrs). Improved survival was seen in patients with cardiomyopathy rather than those with typical congenital cardiac defects (59% vs. 20%, respectively) (12).

Contraindications

Contraindications for cardiac ECLS are similar to ECLS for respiratory failure and include prematurity (gestational age ≤34 weeks), weight <2 kg, irreversible cardiac failure without the option for transplantation, severe neurologic dysfunction, severe coagulopathy, multiorgan system failure, sepsis, and lethal congenital anomalies. As mentioned previously, cardiac arrest is *not* an absolute contraindication, assuming that the initial insult is reversible and rapid resuscitation is provided.

Patient Management Issues for the Pediatric Cardiac Patient on Extracorporeal Life Support

Optimum management of the cardiac ECLS patient requires an understanding of the general mechanics of an ECLS circuit, the effects of modifications made to the circuit for the individual patient (i.e., transthoracic cannulation), the patient's underlying cardiac anatomy and physiology, operative changes made to the patient's anatomy, presumed etiology of pump failure, and specific goals for recovering the patient's cardiac function to a level that allows removal of ECLS. These issues are generally quite unique for each patient placed on ECLS.

Venoarterial versus Venovenous Extracorporeal Life Support

Venoarterial ECLS provides biventricular and lung support for children with low cardiac output states and represents the preferred approach in most patients with ventricular dysfunction. Biventricular support is provided by draining blood from the right atrium into the ECLS circuit and returning it to the aorta, thus bypassing both ventricles and the lungs. Complete cardiac support *cannot* be provided while the patient is on venoarterial ECLS, as complete venous drainage of the heart by the venous cannula cannot be accomplished. Thus, some blood always remains (albeit small at high flows) that continues to circulate through the heart in a fashion dependent on the underlying anatomy of the patient. The importance of this non-bypassed blood, often ignored in respiratory failure, will be discussed in the following text.

Venovenous ECLS does not provide *direct* cardiac support; however, it can provide several indirect benefits to cardiac performance by perfusing the lungs and the coronary circulation with well-oxygenated, pH-balanced blood, without subjecting the patient to the risks of arterial cannulation. Patients *with reversible pulmonary artery hypertension* and secondary RV failure who do not respond to conventional therapies can sometimes be supported on venovenous ECLS, allowing pulsatile flow from the LV to the systemic circulation. Perfusion of the lungs with highly oxygenated, pH-balanced blood helps to decrease pulmonary vascular resistance, with subsequent im-

provement in RV output and, thus, LV output, which can lead to an overall hemodynamic improvement. This is not the case in instances of *irreversible* pulmonary vascular disease (i.e., Eisenmenger syndrome) with irreversible RV failure, in which case little improvement in hemodynamics is accomplished. Venovenous ECLS has several potential advantages over venoarterial ECLS, such as (a) not increasing LV afterload with the high-pressure aortic cannula in the aorta; (b) decreasing RV afterload with improvement in RV oxygen consumption (RV MVO_2); (c) improving the efficiency of LV filling, ejection, and function by decreasing RV overdistension and moving the interventricular septum into a more favorable position (interventricular dependence); and (d) improving regional oxygen delivery to the coronary circulation. Unfortunately, conversion to venoarterial ECLS is sometimes required when either RV or LV pump failure is significant, and this should be anticipated at the onset.

Cannulation

Venoarterial ECLS is typically accomplished with two cannulas, one arterial and one venous. The three primary routes for arterial/venous access are: transcervical (carotid artery/internal jugular vein), transthoracic (aorta, right atrium), and femoral (common femoral artery/vein). In small children, the transcervical approach is preferred, while femoral venoarterial cannulations can be used in older children in whom the risk of arterial ischemia is less. *Transthoracic cannulation* is the choice in patients who cannot be weaned from CPB in the operating room or in the immediate postoperative period. If the patient is placed on ECLS because of inability to wean from CPB, the cannulae placed in surgery are maintained. Although allowing for much greater venous return due to the size of the cannulae, the major disadvantages of this route include increased mediastinal bleeding, infection, and potential for cannulae dislodgment. Malpositions can occur with either arterial or venous cannulae. Misplacement of the arterial cannula can result in LV outflow tract obstruction, aortic insufficiency, dissection of the underside of the transverse aorta, or compromised cerebral or coronary blood flow. When not placed under direct vision, echocardiography should be utilized early on to ensure proper position. Venous cannula malpositions can result in cannula side holes backing out of the vein, resulting in a "venous airlock"; perforation of the right atrium with cardiac tamponade; tricuspid regurgitation; and difficulty in placement due to anatomic variations of the right atrium (juxtaposition of the atrial appendage). Small amounts of venous air can usually be "walked" into the venous reservoir, but massive airlock requires the patient to come off of ECLS support to remove the air from the circuit. Chest x-rays are routinely obtained after cannulation and daily on all patients. While this is helpful in determining the general location of the cannulae, echocardiography is preferred to assess exact cannulae position.

Coronary Perfusion and Extracorporeal Life Support

During the cardiac cycle of a normal four-chambered heart, the left coronary blood flow is highest during diastole, when

LV pressure is lowest. During systole, wall tension increases and coronary blood flow decreases or, in fact, reverses. Blood flow to the right coronary artery is highest during systole, although it continues throughout the entire cardiac cycle. Coronary blood flow is quite variable in patients with congenital heart disease, depending on which ventricle is providing systemic output and whether the other ventricle is pressure loaded (i.e., the RV with pulmonary hypertension). While on ECLS, coronary blood flow is nearly exclusively from the *non-bypassed blood* ejected from the systemic ventricle, except in unusual circumstances such as cardiac stun and aortic insufficiency. For this reason, lung rest strategies regularly employed in neonatal respiratory failure ECLS have the adverse effect of "hypoxemic and acidotic coronary perfusion." Currently, most centers maintain modest amounts of ventilatory support and oxygenation to the lungs while the patient is on ECLS to allow for improved myocardial oxygen delivery by improving the quality of the non-bypassed blood. As previously mentioned, venovenous ECLS offers several advantages over venoarterial ECLS for coronary blood flow.

Cardiac Stun

Cardiac stun refers to a transient state of profound myocardial dysfunction whereby the systemic ventricle is unable to generate sufficient pressure to open up the semilunar valve and eject blood into the aorta against the pressure generated by the ECLS aortic cannula. Cardiac stun is manifested by lack of pulsation in the aorta and resembles electromechanical dissociation. The heart is overdistended due to the lack of ejection, and coronary perfusion is extremely poor. It usually occurs within the first 6 hrs after initiation of flow and can last up to 2–3 days. The incidence of stun is ~5% in neonates. Several groups have described severe and prolonged LV dysfunction with the initiation of ECLS and have suggested ischemia-reperfusion injury and hypocalcemia as etiologies (8,16). Patients who develop cardiac stun are sicker, with more hypoxemia, hypercapnia, and acidosis, and have suffered more episodes of cardiac arrest prior to ECLS.

Left Atrial Decompression

In patients with poor LV function, left atrial decompression is required to prevent cardiac overdistension, mitral regurgitation, pulmonary edema or hemorrhage, and to improve coronary perfusion. Adequate decompression of the heart helps to decrease wall stress and myocardial oxygen consumption. Left-sided decompression procedures are important interventions necessary to improve the chances of recovery of cardiac function. The "venting" is performed via direct left atrial cannulation, with drainage through a connector to the venous cannula or through interventional cardiac catheterization procedures (balloon or blade atrial septostomy). Several reports have identified left atrial decompression as an important factor in the recovery of patients with myocarditis. Other indications for left atrial decompression consist of echocardiographic evidence of ventricular overdistension, with either massive pulmonary edema or pulmonary hemorrhage or the presence of cardiac stun.

Cardiac Preload/Afterload

Assessing the hemodynamic state of a patient on ECLS is more complex due to the necessity to consider the individual contributions from the ECLS circuit and the patient's native cardiac output in individually or jointly providing the systemic and pulmonary blood flow. For example, in a normal four-chambered heart, the amount of flow from the ECLS is easily determined from the circuit monitors, modified by any "shunt" in the circuit, such as an in-line dialysis catheter or continuous arterial blood gas analyzer. The non-bypassed blood, which is difficult to quantify, determines the pulmonary blood flow and then the native cardiac output from the patient, assuming that there is no stun. The total systemic output is the combination of these two flows. The arterial blood pressure is the product of the combined systemic output and the systemic vascular resistance, which is not directly measurable. As arterial blood pressure is monitored in these patients, it is important to understand how it can be modified. Increasing arterial blood can be accomplished by increasing ECLS flow, increasing native cardiac output, or increasing systemic vascular resistance. In patients with a single-ventricle physiology and a BT shunt, the combination of ECLS flow plus native cardiac output *minus* pulmonary blood flow through the shunt results in the total systemic output. Alteration of total systemic output and blood pressure must now take into consideration this factor: pulmonary blood flow.

Assessing adequacy of systemic output in ECLS patients usually requires a combination of indices, beginning with those just noted. In addition, mixed venous saturation is typically measured in the venous return of the circuit, with a goal of >75% in acyanotic patients. It must be remembered that if an LV vent is in place and ventilation is occurring with oxygen, there is a "left-to-right shunt," which will artificially increase the mixed venous saturation. In cyanotic patients, an arterial-venous oxygen saturation difference ($Sa-vo_2$) of 20%–25% is typically targeted. Lactate measurements can be helpful, although delay in clearance can occur after prolonged periods of extremely low cardiac output or cardiac arrest. Blood gases are obtained frequently to assess pH, Po_2, and Pco_2, which is necessary to adjust the ECLS circuit. Remember that a fresh membrane oxygenator is extremely efficient at removing CO_2 from the blood; therefore, it is often necessary to add back CO_2 to the blood returning to the patient. Once again, the systemic arterial CO_2 concentration will be the combination of CO_2 from the patient and the ECLS circuit, which can be modified by either altering the ventilator settings or the flow of gases to the membrane oxygenator.

Hypovolemia is common on ECLS for a variety of reasons. Large amounts of evaporative losses in the circuit and to the "exposed" patient occur, and capillary leak is common. Frequent blood draws for monitoring and bleeding require replacement of packed red blood cells. Coagulopathy is common, requiring replacement therapy. In addition, the systemic inflammatory response is highly activated, resulting in excess vasodilation. Systemic runoff with low diastolic (and, thus, mean) pressure can occur through either a BT shunt or systemic-to-pulmonary collaterals. Hypotension can occur as the result of mechanical problems with the circuit, such as inadequate venous drainage, cardiac tamponade, or tension pneumo- or hemothorax.

High plasma renin levels have been described in patients on ECMO and lead to systemic hypertension and increased systemic vascular resistance. Nonpulsatile flow has been described as a trigger for the rennin-angiotensin-aldosterone axis, leading to hypertension. High ECMO flows can also lead to systemic hypertension. Systemic hypertension should be aggressively treated, as decreasing afterload will decrease myocardial wall stress and improve native cardiac output. Vasoactive agents usually used to manage hypertension include nitroprusside, nitroglycerin, phenoxybenzamine, nicardipine, and milrinone. Recent reports have described the beneficial effect of fenoldopam, a new selective dopamine-1 receptor agonist that causes both systemic and renal arteriolar vasodilation. Arterial pressure should be maintained at appropriate ranges for age. Other factors that can lead to hypertension include hypervolemia, excessive inotropes, pain, agitation, hypothermia, and seizures.

Inotropic Support

Although inotropic agents are weaned rapidly after initiation of support, low-dose inotropes should be maintained to improve cardiac contractility and augment native cardiac output. These inotropes usually used include dopamine (3 mcg/kg/min), epinephrine (0.05 mcg/kg/min), milrinone (0.75 mcg/kg/min), and dobutamine (5 mcg/kg/min). The potential negative effects of high-dose catecholamines on cardiac recovery have been discussed previously. The presence of bradyarrhythmias or tachyarrhythmias has been correlated with poor outcome, and they should be aggressively treated, even though adequate output may be provided by the ECLS circuit alone. Tachyarrhythmias increase Mvo_2 and impair coronary perfusion, which delays or prevents recovery of cardiac function.

Coagulation Monitoring

Due to extracorporeal circulation, anticoagulation is nearly always required, though a few centers have reported short-term success without anticoagulation with the use of heparin-bonded circuits. When not utilizing anticoagulation, a fully primed ECLS circuit must be on immediate standby. Heparin is almost exclusively used, although use of hirudin and argatroban (thrombin inhibitors) has been reported in those patients who develop heparin-induced thrombocytopenia. Aminocaproic acid (Amicar) and heparin-bonded circuits are used to reduce bleeding in postoperative patients (13). Use of aprotinin, a serine protease inhibitor, is controversial due to reports of excessive thrombosis. Typically, the degree of anticoagulation is followed closely with the activated clotting time (ACT) test, a gross aggregate measure of total clotting ability. Although ACT is typically maintained at between 180 and 200 secs when on full flow, it may be decreased to 160 secs when active bleeding is occurring. A point-of-care, activated partial thromboplastin time test is now available and may replace ACT monitoring. Platelets, which are sequestered by the membrane oxygenator, should be transfused to maintain platelet counts above 100,000/mm³. Nonsurgical bleeding after cardiac surgery is usually related to heparin over-

dose, thrombocytopenia, and/or fibrinolysis. Clotting factors and fibrinogen levels must be maintained while the patient is on ECLS.

Ventilator Management

Ventilator management during ECLS remains complex, and differs from strategies for respiratory failure. The overall goal is to ventilate the lungs while minimizing the negative effects of positive-pressure ventilation, such as barotrauma, volutrauma, and oxygen toxicity. Adequate ventilation is necessary to avoid atelectasis, decrease pulmonary vascular resistance, and optimize the quality of the blood perfusing the coronary circulation (see previous discussion); this *cannot* be obtained with lung rest strategies. It is our preference to use a volume-target mode of ventilation with decelerating flow and modest degrees of support (e.g., pressure regulated volume control). Peak inspiratory pressures should be <30 cm H_2O, and positive end-expiratory pressures should be between 3 and 5 cm H_2O. Respiratory rates between 15 and 25 per minute are set, depending on the age of the patient. Chest x-rays are obtained to assess the adequacy of lung inflation, taking care to avoid over distension as well as collapse.

Fluid, Nutrition, and Renal Parameters

Most patients are managed with total parenteral nutrition, although trophic feeding can be started and advanced in select patients. Fluid balance is difficult to measure due to the large, insensible losses described previously. Diuretics (furosemide) are commonly used as the patient weans from mechanical support. In anuric or oliguric patients, early placement of a hemofilter into the ECLS circuit to provide continuous ultrafiltration, hemofiltration, or hemodialysis is recommended.

Analgesia, Sedation, and Neurologic Function

Adequate analgesia and sedation are essential for patients on ECLS. Morphine, fentanyl, and/or midazolam are usually used. Lorazepam can be used in intermittent doses, but infusions should not be used, as toxicity to propylene glycol has been reported. Neuromuscular blockade should be avoided, for it will limit clinical neurologic evaluation and induce both respiratory and generalized muscle weakness. Daily head ultrasounds should be obtained in neonates and young infants to assess for bleeding in the central nervous system. If no evidence for intracranial bleeding is seen on the initial head ultrasounds, many centers defer further studies, unless a change in clinical status occurs.

Infection

Patients on ECLS are at high risk of developing nosocomial infections, in particular via the multiple incisions in the skin (i.e., cannulation site, open chest, central venous lines, chest tubes, etc.). Daily surveillance cultures and broad-spectrum antibiotics are used in managing these patients. This area of patient care is decidedly very difficult to assess and manage and requires significant empiricism and clinical skill. Sepsis is a poor prognostic factor.

Thromboembolism

Many sources of emboli can occur during ECLS, such as air, fibrin, platelet aggregates, and blood microemboli. Air emboli may originate from areas of low or negative pressure within the ECLS system. Both roller and centrifugal pumps generate negative pressure when venous inflow is obstructed; other sources of air embolism are cracks in the tubing and loose stopcocks. Massive air embolism can be fatal. Thrombi during ECLS form in areas of cavitation, turbulence, stagnant flow, and connector seams. Thrombosis within the ECLS system is more common during periods of low flow, when heparin infusions are decreased, or during platelet transfusions.

Weaning Strategies from Extracorporeal Life Support

No minimal or maximal time exists for cardiac recovery while on ECLS. The ideal duration of cardiac support on ECLS is between 3 and 7 days, although ECLS data suggest that cardiac recovery may take as long as 2 weeks. ECLS has been used for long periods of time, though in general, survival is extremely rare after 14 days. If prolonged support is needed, patients should be converted to a VAD. The lack of return of any ventricular function within 72 hrs after surgery has been correlated with poor outcome (15).

As patients recover cardiac function and native cardiac output improves, ECLS flows can begin to be decreased. During this period, inotropic support may need to be increased but not to high levels, as discussed previously. Afterload reduction and improved contractility can be provided by a variety of agents, but most commonly milrinone. The amount of time that the patient is clamped off of the ECLS circuit (with cannulae being flashed so as to prevent thrombosis) is variable. Typically, the decision of the team to decannulate is made after an hour of relative hemodynamic stability. Echocardiographic assessment, either through the transthoracic or transesophageal route, is mandatory during these final weaning stages. Only at this point can the heart function be adequately assessed, with loading conditions that are now similar to what they will be off of ECLS.

Outcomes

From 1985 to January 2006, 6537 cardiac patients of all ages were supported by ECLS. Almost all were supported with venoarterial ECLS, with a survival rate of 38% for neonates, 43% for infants and children, and 31% for adults. Factors shown to be associated with decreased survival include single-ventricle physiology, inability to wean from CPB, and multiple organ system failure. Postoperative patients unable to be weaned after 200 hrs (~8.5 days) of extracorporeal support will rarely survive. Survival in patients with acute myocarditis is ~80% (15). Hospital survival for cardiac ECLS in patients with congenital heart disease is lower than for patients with

normal cardiac anatomy. One center's data showed an overall 39% survival to discharge, with risk factors for poor outcome identified as age <1 month, longer duration of mechanical ventilation before initiation of ECMO, renal failure, or hepatic failure. In another study, 81 children were placed on ECMO for cardiac causes; hospital survival was 49% with 7 late deaths. Factors that improved the odds of survival included initiation of ECMO in the operating room (64% vs. 29%) and absence of pulmonary hypertension. Important adverse factors for hospital survival were serious mechanical complications with the circuit, renal support, and residual cardiac lesions (5).

VENTRICULAR ASSIST DEVICES

VADs have been used in adults for several years with very good success; however, the use of these devices in children remains limited but expanding. Support for pediatric patients with body surface area of <0.7 m^2 is not possible with the devices designed for adults. Patients who have right, left, or biventricular dysfunction with adequate ability to oxygenate through their own lungs are ideally managed with a VAD. Long-term support (>30 days) is much more attainable and successful with a VAD than with ECLS. Technical challenges in designing a neonatal/pediatric-specific VAD involve the need to provide a wide range of stroke volumes in patients of widely varying sizes. In this section, we will review the types of devices available in Europe and the US and the current experience with these devices.

Classification

VADs are typically described in reference to their flow profile and can be divided into rotary/axial and pulsatile devices. These devices can be used as a bridge to recovery of heart function, as a bridge to heart transplant, or as permanent support of the failed heart. Cannulation differs depending on whether the device is being placed to support right (RVAD), left (LVAD), or biventricular (BiVAD) function. For an RVAD, the right atrium (venous drainage) and pulmonary artery (arterial return) are cannulated, while the left atrium (venous drainage) and aorta (arterial return) are cannulated for a LVAD. A BiVAD requires cannulation of the right atrium (venous drainage) and aorta (arterial return). Some devices are fully implantable, while others are paracorporeal, meaning the assist device chamber resides outside of the body and blood is transferred into and out of the device. These devices are powered pneumatically, electrically (including portable battery packs), or magnetically.

Rotary/Axial Ventricular Assist Devices

Centrifugal pumps are the most common type of VADs used in children. In reality, this VAD is essentially an ECLS circuit without an oxygenator in line. As a VAD, the centrifugal pump can be used to support right, left, or biventricular failure, and it is typically used for short-term support (<30 days). The centrifugal VAD system (e.g., BioPump, Medtronic Corporation, MN USA) is a nonpulsatile, extracorporeal, centrifugal pump that generates flow via a spinning rotor, which is magnetically coupled to a motor. Venous drainage depends on suction generated by the rotor and is *not* gravity dependent, as with the ECMO roller pump. Centrifugal pump output depends on the rotational speed of the pump, preload, and afterload. In other words, mean arterial pressure is maintained by varying intravascular volume and pump revolutions per minute (rpm). These pumps can generate large negative pressures whenever venous drainage is impaired, which can lead to cavitation and hemolysis. This problem is usually corrected by setting the flow at a lower speed or by adding volume. A flow probe is necessary to convert the rotational speed of these pumps into liters per minute output. The absence of an oxygenator and venous reservoir decrease heparin requirements and trauma to blood cells. Priming volumes for these circuits are smaller than those of roller pumps. If respiratory failure occurs, an oxygenator can be placed in line to provide pulmonary support (ECLS). Infants and children who weigh <6 kg can be supported with the centrifugal BioPump. Outcomes of 34 children (age, 2–258 days; weight, 1.9–6 kg) with congenital heart disease who required ventricular support after CPB were reported (27), with 63% (22/35) successfully decannulated and 31% surviving to hospital discharge.

The MicroMed DeBakey VAD (MicroMed Technology, Inc., Houston, Texas, USA) is the smallest VAD available (1×3 inches) and is the only implantable VAD available for children in the US. It creates flow through an axial rotor that spins at 7500–12,500 rpms, creating flows of up to 10 L/min. The apex of the LV is used as the inflow, and the ascending aorta as the outflow. The advantages of this device are the small size, relative ease of implant and explant, decreased infection risk, continuous flow that unloads the ventricle throughout the cardiac cycle, thereby minimizing stasis and risk of thrombus formation. The rapid impeller speed can lead to hemolysis. The MicroMed DeBakey child VAD has been granted "humanitarian device exemption" by the US Food and Drug Administration (FDA) and is currently approved for children ages 5–16 years with body surface area of between 0.7 and 1.5m^2. The device is restricted to patients who are in New York Heart Association class IV end-stage heart failure that is refractory to medical therapy and listed for heart transplant. Clinical trials in children are just beginning with this device.

Patient Management on a Centrifugal Ventricular Assist Devices

Indications for placement on a VAD are the same as for ECLS—typically, failure to wean from CPB but without the need for an oxygenator. The patient should be carefully evaluated to assess what type of support would be most suitable (LVAD, RVAD, BiVAD). Cannulation in patients who fail to wean from CPB is typically done through the mediastinum. Flows are maintained at 150 mL/kg/min. Anticoagulation is maintained with heparin infusions, with goal ACTs between 140 and 160 secs. Heparin-bonded circuits are being used at many centers. Plasma free hemoglobin should be <60 mg/dL and should be measured daily and, if values are higher (indicating high degree of hemolysis), pump replacement should be considered. Patients with single-ventricle physiology can also be managed with VADs. Troubleshooting technical difficulties is extremely important and must be done quickly. High arterial outlet pressure could be due to excessive flow for the cannula inserted, change in cannula position, clot in the cannula, high systemic vascular resistance, or LV ejection higher than the support provided by

the system, which will require weaning the flows. Low inlet pressure can be caused by hypovolemia or sometimes the atrial wall collapsing around the cannula.

Weaning from the centrifugal VAD is identical to the process followed with ECLS. When weaning flows, heparin infusions should be increased to maintain ACTs between 180 and 200 secs.

Pulsatile Ventricular Assist Devices

Pulsatile devices that can be used in larger children include HeartMate Left Ventricular Assist System, Thoratec Ventricular Assist Device System, Thoratec Implantable Ventricular Assist Device System (all three from Thoratec Corporation, Pleasanton, California, USA), the AB5000 Circulatory Support System, BVS 5000 (both from ABIOMED, Inc., Danvers, Massachusetts, USA), Novacor LVAS N 100 (WorldHeart, Oakland, California, USA), and the Excor pediatric blood pump (Berlin Heart AG Berlin, Germany).

The Thoratec systems are pneumatically powered, pulsatile assist devices that provide a stroke volume of 65 mL with a maximum output of 7 L/min. Both cannulas (arterial and venous) are exteriorized. Pediatric experience remains limited, but survival rates of almost 70% are reported (21). Pediatric outcomes with univentricular or biventricular assist have been reported in 29 children (mean age, 10 years; mean weight, 31 kg; mean body surface area, 1.07m^2), with better outcomes seen in patients with a diagnosis of cardiomyopathy or myocarditis (survival to hospital discharge of 72%). Unfortunately, only 1 of 7 patients with congenital heart disease survived. Significant neurologic complications were seen, predominantly in the congenital heart disease group (20,22).

The Excor pediatric blood pump is a paracorporeal system available in Europe, with compassionate use available in the US. The Excor pump comes in 5 sizes (10, 25, 30, 50, and 60 mL) and is the only pneumatically driven pulsatile device designed exclusively for neonates, infants, and children. The different sized pumps make this device suitable for patients ranging from neonates (2.5 kg) to adolescents. A multilayered, flexible membrane separates the blood and air chamber. The system is heparin coated, which reduces early complications related to thrombus formation. Most patients are managed with warfarin sodium. Survival with the Berlin Heart has been reported to be 52% in patients aged 6–16 years, with a mean support time of 17 days.

Other Forms of Mechanical Cardiac Support

Intra-aortic Balloon Pump

The intra-aortic balloon pump (IABP) has a balloon (0.75–10 mL) mounted on a 4 or 5 French (fr) catheter that inflates during diastole in the aorta to provide coronary blood flow augmentation and then deflates before cardiac ejection. This device has limitations in children due to the size of the aorta, greater elasticity and compliance of the aorta (which limits effective coronary augmentation), and difficulty in cardiac synchronization at rapid heart rates found in critically ill infants and children (17). Successful centers time balloon inflation to the rapid cardiac cycle by using echocardiography.

IABPs have been used in 14 children after cardiac surgery in which mechanical support was necessary for the treatment of refractory cardiac failure. The median age was 3 years (7 days to 13 years), with a median weight of 13.3 kg (3.5–51 kg). Ten of fourteen patients (71%) were successfully weaned from the IABP; 8 of those became long-term survivors (57%). The major IABP-related complication was mesenteric ischemia, which had a fatal outcome (1). Limb ischemia can be common and severe. IABPs are still of limited utility in small children.

Total Artificial Hearts

A few implantable, total artificial hearts (AbioCor™ and Jarvik 7) have been developed and are beginning to be used in adults.

CONCLUSIONS AND FUTURE DIRECTIONS

The future efforts toward improving treatment of heart failure in children will likely focus on the long-term treatment of patients with single and/or systemic right ventricles. It is probable that, as these patients live longer, significant heart failure will develop that will likely require heart transplantation. The increased use of mechanical support and the expansion of mechanical support to include destination therapy for pediatric or congenial heart disease patients may be possible. Paracorporeal and completely implantable pulsatile devices for children are the future of long-term cardiac support. The Pediatric Support Program of the National Heart, Lung, and Blood Institute is helping to address many of the current limitations in VADs for infants and children (3,10,11).

KEY POINTS

■ Patients with medically refractory heart failure can be supported using ECLS or VADs.

■ The advantages of ECLS support include the ability to use peripheral cannulation, support of both ventricles, use in small neonates, and extensive clinical experience with the technology.

■ The disadvantages of ECLS are the high number of complications and the relatively short duration of support.

■ The advantage of VADs is that prolonged cardiac assist can be successfully obtained.

■ The main disadvantage of VADs is that neonates and infants can only be supported by one device that has only compassionate-use indications by the FDA.

References

1. Akomea-Agyin C, Kejriwal NK, Franks R, et al. Intraaortic balloon pumping in children. *Ann Thorac Surg* 1999;67(5):1415–20.

2. Allan CK, Thiagarajan RR, Armsby LR, et al. Emergent use of extracorporeal membrane oxygenation during pediatric cardiac catheterization. *Pediatr Crit Care Med* 2006;7(3):212–9.

3. Baldwin JT, Borovetz HS, Duncan BW, et al. The National Heart, Lung, and Blood Institute Pediatric Circulatory Support Program. *Circulation* 2006;113(1):147–55.

4. Booth KL, Roths SJ, Perry SB, et al. Cardiac catheterization of patients supported by extracorporeal membrane oxygenation. *J Am Coll Cardiol* 2002;40(9):1681–6.

5. Chaturvedi RR, Macrae D, Brown KL, et al. Cardiac ECMO for biventricular hearts after paediatric open heart surgery. *Heart* 2004;90:545–51.

6. Chen YS, Yu HY, Huang SC, et al. Experience and result of extracorporeal membrane oxygenation in treating fulminant myocarditis with shock: What mechanical support should be considered first? *J Heart Lung Transplant* 2005;24(1):81–7.

7. Darling EM, Kaemmer D, Lawson DS, et al. Use of ECMO without the oxygenator to provide ventricular support after Norwood Stage I procedures. *Ann Thorac Surg* 2001;71(2):735–6.

8. Dickson ME, Hirthler MA, Simoni J, et al. Stunned myocardium during extracorporeal membrane oxygenation. *Am J Surg* 1990;160(6):644–6.

9. Duncan BW, Bohn DJ, Atz AM, et al. Mechanical circulatory support for the treatment of children with acute fulminant myocarditis. *J Thorac Cardiovasc Surg* 2001;122(3):440–8.

10. Duncan BW, Dudzinski DT, Noecker AM, et al. The PediPump: Development status of a new pediatric ventricular assist device. *Asaio J* 2005; 51(5):536–9.

11. Duncan BW, Lorenz M, Kopcak MW, et al. The PediPump: A new ventricular assist device for children. *Artif Organs* 2005;29(7):527–30.

12. Fiser WP, Yetman AT, Gunselman RJ, et al. Pediatric arteriovenous extracorporeal membrane oxygenation (ECMO) as a bridge to cardiac transplantation. *J Heart Lung Transplant* 2003;22(7):770–7.

13. Fortenberry JD, Meier AH, Pettignano R, et al. Extracorporeal life support for posttraumatic acute respiratory distress syndrome at a children's medical center. *J Pediatr Surg* 2003;38(8):1221–6.

14. Jaggers JJ, Forbess JM, Shah AS, et al. Extracorporeal membrane oxygenation for infant postcardiotomy support: Significance of shunt management. *Ann Thorac Surg* 2000;69(5):1476–83.

15. Kulik TJ, Moler FW, Palmisano JM, et al. Outcome-associated factors in pediatric patients treated with extracorporeal membrane oxygenator after cardiac surgery. *Circulation* 1996;94(9 Suppl):II63–8.

16. Martin GR, Short BL, Abbott C, et al. Cardiac stun in infants undergoing extracorporeal membrane oxygenation. *J Thorac Cardiovasc Surg* 1991;101(4):607–11.

17. Pantalos GM, Minich LL, Tani LY, et al. Estimation of timing errors for the intraaortic balloon pump use in pediatric patients. *Asaio J* 1999;45(3):166–71.

18. Pennington DG, Smedira NG, Samuels LE, et al. Mechanical circulatory support for acute heart failure. *Ann Thorac Surg* 2001;71(3 Suppl):S56–9; discussion S82-5.

19. Pizarro C, Davis DA, Healy RM, et al. Is there a role for extracorporeal life support after stage I Norwood? *Eur J Cardiothorac Surg* 2001;19:294–301.

20. Reinhartz O, Copeland JG, Farrar DJ. Thoratec ventricular assist devices in children with less than 1.3 m² of body surface area. *Asaio J* 2003;49(6):727–30.

21. Reinhartz O, Hill JD, Al-Khaldi A, et al. Thoratec ventricular assist devices in pediatric patients: Update on clinical results. *Asaio J* 2005;51(5):501–3.

22. Reinhartz O, Keith FM, El-Banayosy A, et al. Multicenter experience with the Thoratec ventricular assist device in children and adolescents. *J Heart Lung Transplant* 2001;20(4):439–48.

23. Sano S, Ishino K, Kado H, et al. Outcome of right ventricle-to-pulmonary artery shunt in first-stage palliation of hypoplastic left heart syndrome: A multi-institutional study. *Ann Thorac Surg.* 2004;78:1951–7.

24. Shekerdemian L. Nonpharmacologic treatment of acute heart failure. *Curr Opin Pediatr* 2001;13(3):240–6.

25. Soeter JR, Mamiya RT, Sprague AY, et al. Prolonged extracorporeal oxygenation for cardiorespiratory failure after tetralogy correction. *J Thorac Cardiovasc Surg* 1973;66:214–8.

26. Takatani S, Matsuda H, Hanatani A, et al. Mechanical circulatory support devices (MCSD) in Japan: Current status and future directions. *J Artif Organs* 2005;8(1):13–27.

27. Thuys CA, Mullaly RJ, Horton SB, et al. Centrifugal ventricular assist in children under 6 kg. *Eur J Cardiothorac Surg* 1998;13(2):130–4.

28. Wang SS, Ko WJ, Chen YS, et al. Mechanical bridge with extracorporeal membrane oxygenation and ventricular assist device to heart transplantation. *Artif Organs* 2001;25(8):599–602.

CHAPTER 67C ■ TREATMENT OF HEART FAILURE IN INFANTS AND CHILDREN: CARDIAC TRANSPLANTATION

STEVEN A. WEBBER

Transplantation offers the only hope for survival and improved quality of life for selected children with end-stage heart disease that is due to either acquired or congenital cardiac defects. The first pediatric transplant was performed by Kantrowitz and associates in December 1967, only a few days after Dr. Christian Barnard's pioneering operation in an adult. Interest in transplantation of the heart declined throughout the 1970s due to the high mortality that resulted primarily from lack of effective immunosuppressive medications. A resurgence of clinical activity developed in the early 1980s with the introduction of cyclosporine, the first oral immunosuppressive agent with relative specificity for inhibition of T lymphocytes, the primary mediators of allograft rejection. This therapy resulted in dramatic improvements in survival of all transplanted organs. With improvements in candidate and donor selection, preoperative management, surgical technique, and early postoperative care, ~95% of heart transplant recipients should leave the hospital alive and in good health after transplantation (18). Furthermore, pretransplantation mortality has fallen. This section provides an overview of the current state of the art of pediatric heart transplantation, focusing on issues of key interest to those who work in the PICU.

INDICATIONS FOR TRANSPLANTATION

Transplantation of the heart is generally considered to be indicated when expected survival is <2 years and/or when the patient has an unacceptable quality of life. Cardiomyopathy (predominantly dilated forms) and complex congenital heart defects remain the primary indications and together account for ~90% of transplantations undertaken in children (1). Worldwide transplant activity has remained constant over the last decade. Diagnoses that lead to transplantation are age-dependent, with congenital heart disease accounting for two-thirds of transplants in the infant age group and cardiomyopathy accounting for a similar proportion among adolescents (1).

The indications for heart transplantation in children were summarized in a 1999 report from the Pediatric Committee of the American Society of Transplantation and in a more recent report from 2007 (2,6). Perhaps the most controversial indication for heart transplantation is hypoplastic left heart syndrome and related pathologies in the newborn. Survival rates in excess of 80% at 1 year may be achieved at experienced centers, with either Norwood reconstruction or primary transplantation for this condition. Median waiting times for newborn heart transplant candidates are ~2 months in the US (and longer in other countries), resulting in very high costs of care prior to transplantation, significant pretransplant morbidities, and wait-list mortality as high as 25%. In light of these observations, most centers have moved away from transplantation and toward staged reconstruction for neonates with hypoplastic left heart syndrome. This strategy increases availability of organs for other infants with cardiac disease unsuitable for surgical palliation.

Relative and/or absolute contraindications include chronic infection with either hepatitis B or C, or HIV; prior nonadherence with medical therapy; recent or current treatment of malignancy with inadequate follow-up to ensure likely cure; active acute viral, fungal or bacterial infections; elevated and fixed pulmonary vascular resistance index (PVR) above 10 IU; inadequate intraparenchymal pulmonary vascular bed; diffuse pulmonary vein stenosis; and major extracardiac disease felt to be nonreversible with heart transplantation (e.g., severe systemic myopathy). Inevitably, some centers consider specific contraindications absolute, whereas others may feel they are relative. Decision-making is based on consensus discussion among all team members, including intensive care staff.

EVALUATION OF THE TRANSPLANT CANDIDATE

A vast number of children who undergo heart transplantation evaluation are hospitalized in the PICU. For many, the transplant will occur during the first hospital admission. Thus, the intensivist will be deeply involved in the transplant evaluation, which should include an assessment of expected survival without transplantation, the patient's current quality of life, the potential for alternate surgical or medical therapies, and the inherent risks of the transplant surgery itself. A typical evaluation protocol is shown in **Table 67C.1**.

Anatomic and Hemodynamic Considerations

The most complex anatomy may be transplanted, provided the lung vasculature is adequately developed and PVR is acceptable. Anatomic points of most interest to the surgeon include abnormalities of cardiac and visceral situs (especially anomalies of the systemic and pulmonary venous return) and the size and

EVALUATION OF CANDIDATES FOR HEART TRANSPLANTATION

History and physical examination

Required consultations
  Pediatric cardiologist, congenital cardiovascular surgeon, cardiac anesthesiologist, infectious disease specialist, psychiatrist or psychologist, transplant coordinator, social worker

Additional consultations (as required)
  Neonatology, genetics, neurology, dental, oncology, immunology, nephrology, nutritional services, physical/occupational therapy, developmental pediatrics, hospital finance

Cardiac diagnostic studies
  Chest radiograph, electrocardiogram, echocardiogram, cardiac catheterization
  In selected patients: exercise test, ventilation-perfusion scan, chest CT or MRI, pulmonary function tests

Blood type (ABO), anti-HLA antibody screen, complete blood count and white cell differential, platelet count, coagulation screen, blood urea nitrogen, serum creatinine, glucose, electrolytes, calcium, magnesium, liver function tests, lipid profile, brain natriuretic peptide.

Serologic screening for antibodies to the following pathogens: cytomegalovirus; Epstein-Barr; herpes simplex virus; varicella-zoster virus; HIV; hepatitis A, B, C, D, and measles; antibodies to *Toxoplasma gondii*

PPD/Mantoux tuberculosis test placement

Update immunizations including hepatitis B, pneumococcal and influenza (in season)

---

anatomy of the main and branch pulmonary arteries (including the presence of stenoses, distortions, and nonconfluence). Intracardiac anatomy is less important, as the bulk of the cardiac mass will be explanted. Abnormalities in the relation of the great arteries usually pose few problems. Extreme care on entry to the sternum must be taken when a right ventricular-pulmonary artery conduit or enlarged right atria (after Fontan procedure) is present. Cardiac catheterization is usually indicated pretransplant to assess PVR. Excessive fixed resistance will result in acute donor right ventricular failure. This situation would necessitate the need for a right ventricular assist device in the immediate postoperative period.

In general, children with indexed PVR (PVRI) ≤6 IU are considered low risk for acute donor right heart failure. If resistance is between 6 and 10 IU, the risks are higher, but transplantation is still generally not considered to be contraindicated. A PVRI in excess of 10 IU is usually considered a contraindication to isolated heart transplantation, unless a major fall is achieved (to well below 10 IU) with pulmonary vasodilator therapy (100% oxygen and/or nitric oxide). In borderline cases, restudy of hemodynamics after several days of inotropic and vasodilator therapy may be necessary. It should be noted, however, that a rapid fall in pulmonary resistance can lead to acute elevation in left atrial pressure in patients with very poor left ventricular function, even precipitating pulmonary edema.

Laboratory Investigations

The laboratory tests that should be conducted in a transplant candidate are summarized in **Table 67C.1**. Blood typing is necessary to ensure ABO compatibility with the transplanted organ, although infants and young children with absent or low anti-A and anti-B isohemagglutinin titers may be safely transplanted across traditional ABO barriers. This strategy was introduced by West et al. in Toronto (22) and is based on the principle that isohemagglutinins against blood group antigens do not normally develop until the latter part of infancy. Transplantation across blood group barriers prior to the development of naturally occurring anti-A and anti-B isohemagglutinins appears to result in outcomes comparable to ABO-compatible transplants (22). Furthermore, most of the transplanted infants did not form antibodies against donor blood group antigens during long-term follow-up, possibly due to the development of B-cell tolerance. This strategy has profound implications for PICU care, as use of blood products pre- and post-transplant must be carefully planned to avoid transfusion of blood products that contain inappropriate anti-A and anti-B antibodies.

Evaluation for the presence of preformed anti-HLA antibodies ("sensitized") is performed using panel-reactive antibody and solid-phase assays. Infectious disease evaluation includes serologic testing for cytomegalovirus (CMV), Epstein-Barr virus (EBV), varicella, herpes simplex virus, *Toxoplasma gondii*, HIV, measles, and hepatitis viruses A, B, C, and D. Serologic status for these agents may guide prophylaxis as well as the diagnostic evaluation of posttransplantation fever. The infectious disease evaluation should also include review of immunization history. Those candidates in whom transplantation is not likely to be imminent should undergo an update of appropriate immunizations at the time of the pretransplant evaluation.

Consultations

Each candidate is evaluated by a multidisciplinary team that includes the transplant cardiologist and surgeon, social worker, transplant coordinator, and infectious disease expert. A screening psychiatric/psychologic examination of the patient and the family is also very important. The primary purpose of this evaluation is to identify patients and families at high risk for poor psychosocial outcome while waiting for transplantation and after transplantation. Evaluation of past history of nonadherence to medical therapy is critical. Additional consultations may be required from specialist services such as hematology-oncology (when the patient has past history of malignancy), child development, genetics, neurology, and feeding/nutritional specialists. Patients with Fontan circulation require evaluation of the liver for evidence of cirrhosis, and may require formal hepatology consultation.

EVALUATION OF THE CARDIAC DONOR

Although the intensivist is not usually involved in the donor evaluation process (**Table 67C.2**), it is important for the PICU

TABLE 67C.2

EVALUATION OF THE CARDIAC DONOR

History
  Donor age, height, weight, and gender
  Cause of brain death
  History of cardiac arrest and length of resuscitation
  Evidence of chest trauma
  History of IV drug usage
  Past history of cardiovascular disease
  Distance from transplant center
  History of malignancy

Cardiovascular status
  Heart rate, blood pressure, central venous pressure
  Fluid balance
  Blood gas
  Types and doses of IV inotropes
  Inotropic support increasing or decreasing

Cardiovascular testing
  Electrocardiogram
  Chest radiograph
  Echocardiogram
  Cardiac enzymes

Other testing
  Infectious disease screen: CMV, EBV, *Toxoplasma gondii*,
    HIV-1, HIV-2, HTLV-1, HTLV-2, RPR, hepatitis B and C
  All culture results since admission to ICU

team to know about key aspects of the potential donor. Evaluation of the donor heart begins with a careful review of the history, including donor age and gender, body size, cause of death, presence of any chest trauma, need for cardiopulmonary resuscitation, length of resuscitation, and evaluation of the hemodynamic status of the donor (including blood pressure, heart rate, and central venous pressure, if available). The amount of inotropic support and trends in usage over time are also noted. A history of cardiopulmonary resuscitation is not, in itself, a contraindication to cardiac donation. It must be recognized that brain death results in dramatic physiologic disturbances in the donor, including temperature instability with hypothermia, circulatory volume changes (most commonly depletion), and neuroendocrine dysfunction, in addition to depletion of circulating thyroxine, cortisol, insulin, glucagon, and antidiuretic hormone.

To rule out structural abnormalities and to evaluate cardiac function, a complete echocardiogram should be performed. Most centers avoid the use of donor hearts whose systolic function is more than mildly impaired after treatment with inotropic agents or thyroid hormone (e.g., shortening fraction <26%, ejection fraction <50%). Some degree of atrioventricular valvar regurgitation is common after brain death and mild degrees do not constitute a contraindication to organ donation. Pericardial effusion may be indicative of myocardial contusion. A 12-lead electrocardiogram should be performed. Mild, nonspecific ST and T wave changes are commonly present and usually reflect central nervous system effects, electrolyte disturbances, or hypothermia; these do not contraindicate organ donation. Interpretation of cardiac enzymes may be difficult in the setting of generalized trauma. However, the elevation in cardiac troponin I levels in donor serum appears to be a useful predictor for acute graft failure after infant heart transplanta-

tion. Use of older donors (e.g., >35 years of age) for pediatric recipients is associated with high risk of posttransplant coronary disease and poor long-term survival (10).

Size matching is a critical issue in the selection of potential donors. Most centers avoid undersizing the donor below 75%–80% of recipient weight. Below this, cardiac output of the donor may be insufficient to meet the needs of the recipient. Use of oversized donors is common. Most candidates will have marked cardiomegaly, leaving ample room within the chest for an oversized donor heart. Use of donor-to-recipient weight ratios of 2.5:1 is common in pediatric practice, and ratios of 3:1 to 4:1 have been successfully used, especially in newborn and infant candidates. Marked oversizing often results in delayed sternal closure. In infant recipients, oversizing has been associated with a more prolonged ventilator course and increased risk of primary graft failure (7). Oversized donor hearts may also give rise to a postoperative syndrome characterized by a high-output state associated with systemic hypertension, raised intracranial pressure, and even mental status changes.

It has been suggested that oversizing of donors may improve outcome when the recipient has significant preoperative pulmonary hypertension. Certainly, undersizing should be avoided in the presence of recipient pulmonary hypertension. In adults, it has been shown that use of female donors is associated with higher perioperative mortality when recipient PVR is elevated.

All donors should be screened for CMV, EBV, HIV-1, HIV-2, human lymphotropic viruses 1 and 2 (HTLV-1, HTLV-2), and hepatitis viruses A, B, and C. Donors are also screened for syphilis and for antibodies to *T. gondii*. The presence of antibodies to CMV, EBV, or *T. gondii* does not constitute contraindication to transplantation but helps to guide posttransplantation therapy and surveillance. Evidence of donor retroviral infection (HIV or HTLV) is considered an absolute contraindication to heart transplantation. The presence of donor hepatitis B surface antigen is also usually considered an absolute contraindication to heart donation. The usage of hepatitis C-positive donors remains controversial.

SURGICAL TECHNIQUES OF GRAFT IMPLANTATION

A detailed review of surgical techniques is outside the scope of this text. They have been reviewed by Pigula and Webber (11). The *biatrial anastomosis* for cardiac transplantation has been applied to thousands of patients of all ages with excellent results. Despite the great success of this technique, the result is a nonanatomically correct one, with large atrial cavities. The resulting abnormal atrial geometry is thought to contribute to tricuspid valve dysfunction and sinus node dysfunction. For these reasons, many centers now perform *bicaval anastomosis* in children of all ages who undergo orthotopic heart transplantation. Some specific forms of congenital heart disease lend themselves particularly well to the bicaval technique, for example, in patients who have had previous Mustard or Senning operations or Glenn anastomoses. The bicaval technique may be associated with superior caval vein stenosis, especially in infants.

Transplantation for congenital heart disease is often performed after multiple palliative procedures and may present formidable surgical challenges. The anatomic substrate can be broadly classified as abnormalities of the systemic venous return, abnormalities of the pulmonary venous return, and abnormalities of the great vessels, including hypoplastic left heart syndrome. Surgical modifications of the two basic techniques are required for transplantation of these anatomic variants. Abnormalities of systemic venous return are among the most challenging anatomic variants to transplant. Fashioning unobstructed connections in a patient undergoing heart transplantation with left-sided cavae (e.g., in dextrocardia with situs inversus or in heterotaxy syndromes), requires special consideration and planning. Of key importance is procurement of generous sections of donor caval veins, including the innominate vein.

Increasing numbers of children come to heart transplantation after multiple palliative operations have been performed. Often, these operations have involved the pulmonary arteries in the form of systemic-to-pulmonary shunts, cavopulmonary anastomoses, or other procedures. In all cases, as much donor pulmonary artery as possible should be harvested. Most commonly, as is the case in bidirectional Glenn or Fontan operations, the cavopulmonary anastomosis is taken down, the pulmonary arteries are patched, and bicaval anastomoses are performed. Patch material may take the form of bovine pericardium, homograft, or donor or recipient discard. Repair is best accomplished after recipient cardiectomy and before organ implantation. In the case of discontinuous pulmonary arteries, the donor organ should be procured with the pulmonary bifurcation and pulmonary arteries intact. Direct left and right pulmonary artery anastomoses are then performed. Alternatively, excess donor aorta can be used to connect the right and left pulmonary arteries prior to implantation. Transplantation to a single lung is feasible when there is unilateral absence or severe hypoplasia of a pulmonary artery (8) and should only be performed when the dominant pulmonary artery is well developed and has low PVR.

Few centers currently perform primary transplantation for hypoplastic left heart syndrome. Because of the extensive arch hypoplasia, the donor surgeon must include the entire transverse and proximal descending aorta en bloc with the organ. While most centers perform transplantation of hypoplastic left heart syndrome under circulatory arrest, several techniques have been developed to minimize circulatory arrest time. Regional low-flow perfusion can eliminate the need for circulatory arrest. This technique employs a Gore-Tex tube graft (3.5 mm) anastomosed to the innominate artery, fashioned prior to bypass. Vascular isolation of the brachiocephalic vessels and the descending aorta allows continued perfusion of the brain during cardiectomy as well as graft implantation. This technique provides physiologic cerebral circulatory support and significant somatic circulatory support, such that circulatory arrest can be avoided completely (11).

POSTOPERATIVE MANAGEMENT AND EARLY COMPLICATIONS

Many of the fundamental principles of early postoperative management after heart transplantation are similar to those for pediatric patients who undergo other procedures with cardiopulmonary bypass (see Chapter 70, Section C). Aspects of care that are specific to the transplant recipient are discussed here.

Cardiovascular Considerations

Inotropic Agents

Abnormalities in cardiac function are inevitable due to the obligatory hypoxic-ischemic insult that the donor heart endures. Recovery of systolic function is usually rapid. However, abnormalities in diastolic function may persist for many weeks. Most heart transplant recipients will benefit from low-dose inotropic support in the immediate postoperative period, although often this is only required for 2–3 days. The choice of inotrope will reflect both physician preference and hemodynamic factors such as heart rate, PVR, and blood pressure. Low-dose dobutamine and isoproterenol are common choices. The latter is sometimes recommended because of its combined properties of chronotropy, inotropy, and pulmonary vasodilatation. The addition of a combined vasodilator/inotropic agent such as milrinone is logical in the presence of low cardiac output and evidence of high systemic vascular resistance.

Systemic Hypertension

In contrast to the nontransplant cardiac surgical patient, systemic hypertension is common. Many factors contribute to this, including vigorous function of an oversized donor organ and use of high-dose corticosteroids. It is not unusual to observe quite severe systolic hypertension within 24 hrs of a successful transplant procedure. Treatment with a variety of IV vasodilators, including β blockers, is necessary.

Pulmonary Vascular Resistance

The importance of PVR as a risk factor for acute donor right ventricular failure was discussed previously. Nitric oxide is begun in the operating room and is used to wean from cardiopulmonary bypass. Acidosis must be avoided, and high levels of inspired oxygen are provided. Generous sedation is provided in the early postoperative period. If necessary, prostaglandin E_1 can also be used. The right heart may require significant inotropic support, and sometimes epinephrine may be required in addition to milrinone and dobutamine. If right ventricular dysfunction persists with poor cardiac output despite this level of support, then mechanical assistance should be provided.

Cardiac Rate and Rhythm

Postoperative tachyarrhythmias and bradyarrhythmias have been observed in children following heart transplantation. The most common rhythm abnormality (other than sinus tachycardia) is sinus bradycardia, with or without an atrial or junctional escape rhythm. The denervated sinus node responds appropriately to exogenous chronotropic agents, and isoproterenol is useful in this respect. A simpler approach is atrial pacing, and all transplant recipients should have temporary pacing wires placed in the operating room. Ventricular ectopy and nonsustained ventricular tachycardia may occur in the first week or two after transplantation but rarely requires treatment.

The fresh cardiac allograft has limited ability to increase stroke volume; therefore, establishing an adequate heart rate is important for maintaining cardiac output. It is our practice to target a heart rate of 140–150 bpm in an infant, while a teenager should have a heart rate of 100 bpm. Atrial pacing is most commonly used to control the heart rate.

Primary Graft Failure

Both failure to wean from cardiopulmonary bypass and early postoperative graft failure are associated with high mortality. The term *primary graft failure* is often reserved for the finding of acute left ventricular or biventricular failure not due to elevated PVR. Poor donor selection, prolonged ischemic time, poor preservation technique, and hyperacute rejection should all be considered. The latter is extremely rare with routine recipient pretransplant screening for anti-HLA antibodies. When primary graft failure occurs, recovery is frequently possible if the circulation can be supported, which is usually achieved with extracorporeal membrane oxygenation (5). Retransplantation for early graft failure is generally associated with very poor outcomes (3), and many consider this a contraindication to retransplantation.

Respiratory Support

The principles of respiratory support do not differ from those of other pediatric open heart procedures. Early extubation should be the goal. The patient who has required prolonged preoperative mechanical ventilation will usually need more prolonged ventilatory support postoperatively, as retraining of respiratory muscles will be required. Infants with long-standing cardiomegaly will often have significant tracheobronchomalacia, and persistent or recurrent pulmonary atelectasis is not unusual.

Renal Function

The combination of chronic heart failure, cardiopulmonary bypass, and use of cyclosporine or tacrolimus all contribute to postoperative renal dysfunction, which is exacerbated with a low postoperative cardiac output state. Oliguria is common. Fortunately, acute renal failure is rare in children, and dialysis is seldom required. Persistent oliguria is managed with loop diuretics and low-dose dopamine (e.g., 3–5 mcg/kg/min). Low output is managed with inotropic agents, as discussed previously. Administration of a continuous furosemide infusion (up to 6 mg/kg/day) may be helpful. These maneuvers are usually successful in stimulating an adequate urine output (>1 mL/kg/hr). In some cases, particularly in neonates and infants, IV prostaglandin E_1 may also provide a diuretic effect. When urine output remains low, it may be necessary to decrease or hold calcineurin inhibitors (tacrolimus or cyclosporine), which can be facilitated by the use of IV induction agents as part of the early immunosuppressive regimen (see later discussion).

Gastrointestinal Considerations

Gastrointestinal complications are quite common early after pediatric heart transplantation (12). All patients should receive intravenous and, subsequently, oral H_2 antagonists to decrease the risk of stress ulcers in the early postoperative period. These are usually continued until corticosteroids have been weaned to low doses or discontinued. The nasogastric tube is removed as soon as the patient is extubated and able to take oral feeds and medications. Attention is paid to providing optimal calo-ries without use of excessive volumes, as most patients will tend to retain fluid in the early postoperative period. Pancreatitis is not uncommon following transplantation and should be sought in the presence of abdominal pain or unexplained feeding intolerance. Immunosuppressive regimens that avoid the use of azathioprine and corticosteroids may reduce this complication. Symptoms of gastrointestinal perforation may be subtle in small children on immunosuppressive medications, especially if corticosteroids are being used. Many children with chronic heart failure have gastroesophageal reflux disease; this should be aggressively managed but with knowledge that many drug interactions occur between immunosuppressant medications and drugs used for gastroesophageal reflux disease, including antacids, antihistamines, and prokinetic agents.

Infectious Precautions

Infections are a leading cause of death and morbidity in the first year following heart transplantation. Most severe infections occur during the initial hospitalization. During the first week after transplantation, invasive lines and drains are removed as soon as possible. A short course of antibiotics (e.g., 72 hrs) is given as prophylaxis against mediastinal and wound infection. Usually, a first-generation cephalosporin will suffice. Broader staphylococcal coverage (i.e., vancomycin) is given if the patient has had a prolonged ICU stay and has long-standing vascular catheters in place. Such lines are usually replaced in the operating room. Patients colonized with methicillin-resistant *Staphylococcus aureus* are also covered with vancomycin. Oral nystatin is started in the ICU, along with ganciclovir, if recipient or donor is seropositive for CMV. Patients at high risk for yeast infections (e.g., patients on pretransplant extracorporeal membrane oxygenation) are frequently given prophylaxis with fluconazole. However, it should be noted that all "azole" antifungals have a profound effect on calcineurin-inhibitor metabolism (via the cytochrome P450 system). A marked reduction in tacrolimus or cyclosporine dosing (50%–90% reduction) is required during concomitant use of an azole antifungal agent. Initiation of prophylaxis against *Pneumocystis carinii* can follow closer to the time of hospital discharge.

Immunosuppression and Early Acute Rejection

High-dose IV methylprednisolone (e.g., 15–20 mg/kg) is given in the operating room. A tapering course of corticosteroids is usually given over the next 1–2 weeks, with the majority of centers discharging patients on maintenance corticosteroid therapy (1). However, steroid-free immunosuppressive regimens are increasingly being used in pediatric practice. Cyclosporine or tacrolimus is commenced generally within 24–48 hrs of surgery once good urine output has been established. Both agents can be given intravenously or enterally. If anti-T-cell induction therapy is used (most commonly, polyclonal rabbit antithymocyte globulin; less often with an IL-2 receptor antagonist), then there is less urgency to introduce a calcineurin inhibitor in the immediate (first 1–2 days) posttransplant period. Cyclosporine or tacrolimus can then be commenced by the oral route rather than intravenously. Delay in commencement of these agents for several days (under coverage of induction

POTENTIAL COMBINATIONS OF MAINTENANCE IMMUNOSUPPRESSIVE DRUGS USED IN PEDIATRIC HEART TRANSPLANTATION

Number of agents	Potential combinations	Comments
Monotherapy	Tacrolimus or cyclosporine	Monotherapy rarely used with cyclosporine.
Dual therapy	Tacrolimus or cyclosporine *with* azathioprine *OR* mycophenolate mofetil *OR* sirolimus/everolimus or corticosteroids	Little experience with the mTOR (target of rapamycin) inhibitors sirolimus and everolimus in children. Steroid avoidance increasingly common in pediatric heart transplantation.
Triple therapy	Tacrolimus or cyclosporine *with* corticosteroids *with* azathioprine *OR* mycophenolate mofetil *OR* sirolimus/everolimus	In triple therapy regimens, mycophenolate mofetil is being used with increasing frequency in lieu of azathioprine.

therapy) may be particularly useful when urine output is low or renal function is deteriorating.

Numerous strategies are available for maintaining immunosuppression (13). All centers currently use a calcineurin inhibitor as the primary immunosuppressive agent, with approximate equal use of tacrolimus and cyclosporine at this writing. Most centers also use a second, adjunctive agent. More centers are using steroid avoidance regimens or early steroid weaning in children. The principles of maintenance therapy are summarized in **Table 67C.3**. In general, agents of similar classes are not given together, as they tend to enhance toxicities. Combination therapies use two or three agents of different classes with different mechanisms of action.

Careful daily assessment looking for signs of rejection is required, although severe rejection before 7–10 days is rare (except in the sensitized patient). Rejection is generally delayed with use of induction therapy. Infants and young children experience less acute rejection than do adolescents. Pallor, increasing tachycardia, abdominal pain, gallop rhythm, and oliguria all are suggestive of severe rejection. Ideally, rejection is identified by echocardiography and/or surveillance biopsy before such signs develop. The electrocardiogram may show reduced precordial voltages. The tempo of rejection can be quite abrupt in the early posttransplant period, and any deterioration in the patient's condition after initial recovery from surgery must be taken very seriously. If evidence of new graft dysfunction is unequivocal, empiric treatment of bolus intravenous corticosteroids is given. Endocardial muscle biopsy generally shows lymphocytic infiltrates (predominantly T cells) with varying degrees of edema and myocyte damage. Endomyocardial biopsies are graded according to an internationally agreed classification system developed by the International Society for Heart and Lung Transplantation (ISHLT) (16).

MEDIUM-TERM AND LATE COMPLICATIONS

A detailed discussion of all complications of heart transplantation beyond the immediate postoperative period is outside the scope of this text, and readers are referred to other reviews (15,18). This section focuses on those complications that the intensive care team will be required to manage from time to time.

Immunosuppressive therapy aims to prevent or minimize the immune response of the host to donor antigens, while avoiding complications of therapeutic immunosuppression. Immunologic complications of transplantation fall into two main groups—allograft rejection/graft dysfunction (both acute and chronic), reflecting inadequate or ineffective immunosuppression, and manifestations of non-specific immunosuppression, including infections and malignancy. Finally, nonimmune side effects of immunosuppressive therapy (i.e., tissue and organ toxicities) are an important cause of morbidity, and occasionally mortality, after heart transplantation in children.

Acute Rejection

Patients remain at risk for acute rejection indefinitely. No evidence exists that suggests that heart transplant recipients become truly tolerant to their allograft. The importance of acute rejection episodes becomes evident when causes of death after heart transplant are examined. Data from the ISHLT show that acute rejection is the most common cause of death between 30 days and 3 years after heart transplantation, accounting for almost 30% of all deaths (1). The peak hazard, or instantaneous risk, for first rejection is between 1 and 2 months after transplantation. By 1 year after transplantation, only 40% of pediatric heart recipients are free of acute rejection. Late acute rejection episodes (occurring beyond the first year after transplantation) appear to carry a particularly poor long-term prognosis (20), especially if associated with graft dysfunction. When any degree of systolic dysfunction is associated with acute rejection, rapid deterioration is common, even when the patient appears well. Thus, it is prudent to admit all patients with acute graft failure to the ICU for initiation of therapy. If systolic failure is more than mild, IV milrinone should be initiated, and the patient should be monitored for dysrhythmias. Unless graft failure is known to be due to coronary artery disease, treatment for acute rejection/graft dysfunction should be initiated with IV methylprednisolone (10–15 mg/kg, maximum 1 g) daily for 3–5 days. It is optimal to obtain an endomyocardial biopsy, as acute graft dysfunction may be associated with "acellular rejection" due to humoral rejection secondary to circulating anti-HLA antibodies. Additional therapies may then be required, including plasmapheresis. It should be emphasized that treatment of severe acute rejection should not be delayed while awaiting endomyocardial biopsy or biopsy results.

Acute rejection with hemodynamic compromise can be rapidly fatal. Unless specific contraindications exist, such patients should receive full hemodynamic support, including use of mechanical support, as the condition is generally reversible in nature.

Chronic Rejection or Posttransplantation Coronary Arterial Disease

The terms *chronic rejection* and *posttransplant coronary arterial disease* are generally used synonymously. Coronary disease subsequent to transplantation is an accelerated vasculopathy that is the leading cause of death among late survivors of pediatric heart transplantation (1). It accounts for ~40% of deaths in the 3–5 years after transplantation. The pathology differs somewhat from that of ischemic heart disease in the normal adult population. Typical allograft coronary arterial disease consists of myointimal proliferation that is generally concentric and involves the entire length of the vessel, including intramyocardial branches. Eventually, luminal occlusion occurs, often with associated inflammation. Both immune and non-immune mechanisms likely contribute to the development of graft vasculopathy, although immune mechanisms are probably of central importance in young children. Intriguing data have recently been published that show that persistence of viral genome of various viruses (especially adenovirus) detected in the myocardium of heart biopsy samples by polymerase chain reaction predict the development of coronary disease and late graft loss in children (14). Use of older donors, late acute rejection episodes, and older recipient age are all risk factors for the development of posttransplant coronary arterial disease (10). CMV infection may also contribute to the development of graft vascular disease (17).

Symptoms of ischemia are often absent, though some children experience episodes of abdominal pain and/or chest pain despite operative denervation of the heart. Syncope and sudden death are also common presentations of graft coronary disease in children. In the current era, the diagnosis is most often made during surveillance-selective coronary angiography. Intravascular ultrasound has much greater sensitivity for this diagnosis, though experience in children is much more limited than in adults.

Unfortunately, no curative treatment exists for established coronary arterial disease. Diastolic dysfunction tends to develop early and may be observed even with little evidence of epicardial coronary artery narrowing (9), which may be a reflection of diffuse small-vessel disease in many patients. Once overt systolic failure ensues, survival is poor, and consideration should be given to retransplantation. Outcomes for late retransplantation (beyond 6 months from primary transplant) are similar to those for primary transplantation (3). These patients sometimes require admission to the ICU for heart failure management. As with patients with ischemic myopathy, inotropic agents should be used with great caution. Patients with ischemia-induced syncope should receive automatic implantable cardioverter-defibrillators if they are to be discharged from the hospital. However, it may be more prudent to keep such patients in hospital until retransplantation can be performed. β blockers may be given for their anti-ischemic benefits if heart failure is not advanced and β agonists are not required.

Infections

An increased prevalence of all forms of infection is seen in patients after heart transplantation, compared to the general population of children. Most infections are caused by pathogens that also cause infection in the nonimmunocompromised host. Common examples include respiratory viruses, *Streptococcus pneumoniae*, and varicella virus. All infections that occur in nonimmunocompromised patients can cause greater disease severity in the recipient of a transplanted heart. Of particular note in this respect are infections due to CMV and EBV, which only rarely cause severe disease in the immunocompetent host. Rarely, opportunistic infections are seen due to *Pneumocystis jiroveci* (formerly *P. carinii*). Although most infections are well tolerated, infection is second only to graft failure as a major cause of death in the first 30 days after transplantation and second only to acute rejection as the main cause of death during the remainder of the first posttransplant year (1). On rare occasion, transplant recipients with severe infection require admission to the ICU. The principles of treatment are broadly the same as for severe infection/septic shock in the nonimmunocompromised host. Severe infection is often associated with immune paralysis; in general, if the child is sick enough to warrant admission to the ICU, maintenance immunosuppression should be temporarily withheld. However, corticosteroids should not be discontinued if they are being used chronically, and stress dosing may be indicated.

Broad-spectrum antibiotic coverage is required in any septic transplant recipient until an organism has been identified. *Streptococcus pneumoniae* infections occur with increased frequency, and antibiotics must be administered to cover this agent. When there is clinical and radiographic evidence of pneumonia and deteriorating clinical status, the clinician should maintain a low threshold for performing bronchoalveolar lavage to obtain deep cultures for viruses, fungi, and bacteria. *P. jiroveci* should be ruled out when hypoxia occurs and characteristic chest x-ray film changes are seen. Respiratory viral pathogens (e.g., respiratory syncytial virus, influenza, parainfluenza, adenovirus) should be sought when evidence of severe respiratory infection is seen in a heart transplant recipient. While viral respiratory disorders tend to be well tolerated in older children and further out from transplantation, acquisition of one of these respiratory viruses in the first few weeks after transplant can occasionally cause devastating disease, especially in infants.

Primary CMV infection is less problematic in heart transplant patients than in lung transplant recipients. In the former, pneumonitis is rare, whereas it is a common site of disease in lung and heart-lung recipients who develop primary infection posttransplantation. In heart recipients, gastroenteritis, hepatitis, and bone marrow suppression are relatively common findings. Diagnosis is facilitated by evaluation of peripheral blood by PCR or antigenemia (pp65) testing. Diagnosis of CMV *disease* remains a tissue diagnosis. When the diagnosis is made early, treatment with IV ganciclovir and/or oral valganciclovir is usually very effective.

EBV infection in the immunocompromised host can be asymptomatic or cause a nonspecific viral syndrome, mononucleosis, fulminant "viral sepsis," or posttransplant lymphoproliferative disorder (PTLD). The strongest risk factor for the development of PTLD is the development of primary EBV infection posttransplantation, although children who are seropositive for EBV at the time of transplant are not completely protected. A recent analysis of the Pediatric Heart Transplant Study (PHTS) database provides the most comprehensive analysis of PTLD in the pediatric heart population. This study identified 56 cases among 1184 primary transplants (4.7%) at 19 North American centers (19). Almost 90% were driven by EBV, and all but one was of B-cell origin. Most patients were treated with reduced immunosuppression, which resulted in complete remission in 75% of cases. However, relapse occurred in 19%, and the probability of survival after diagnosis was only 75%, 68%, and 67% at 1, 3, and 5 years, respectively. Therapeutic strategies include reduction or temporary cessation of immunosuppression, antiviral agents (without proven benefit), monoclonal antibodies against B-cell antigens (e.g., rituximab, a human/mouse chimeric monoclonal antibody directed against the CD20 antigen), chemotherapy, and, rarely, cellular (adoptive) immunotherapy. With the latter, patients are given infusions of autologous cytotoxic T lymphocytes (cultured ex vivo) directed against EBV-specific antigens. This experimental approach is under investigation in children at a small number of centers. Children with fulminant EBV sepsis and some with severe PTLD require admission to the ICU. The major role of the intensivist is general supportive care, recognition and treatment of comorbid infections, and monitoring of graft function that may be compromised at presentation or following therapeutic reduction in immunosuppression. Coordination of care among multiple specialists is an important aspect of the management of these sick patients in the ICU.

Nonimmune Complications

In addition to the consequences of over- or under-immunosuppression, transplant recipients experience a wide array of nonimmune toxicities of immunosuppressive therapies. These include systemic hypertension, hyperlipidemia, glucose intolerance, decreased bone mineral density, and bone marrow suppression (15). One complication worthy of particular attention is that of progressive renal dysfunction due to calcineurin inhibitor renal toxicity, which is becoming increasingly problematic as larger numbers of children survive long-term after heart transplantation. Some have already developed end-stage renal failure, requiring renal transplantation (4). It is important to carefully monitor renal function in all transplant recipients admitted to the ICU and to make appropriate dose adjustments to relevant medications based on estimates of creatinine clearance. It should be noted that estimates and direct measures of creatinine clearance overestimate glomerular filtration rate in this population and that the severity of renal disease is generally greater than perceived (4). Use of nephrotoxic drugs should be minimized when possible.

SURVIVAL

Parents and patients are interested in the chances of survival once a decision has been made to proceed with listing for transplantation. Despite this, emphasis is rarely given to pretransplant mortality and the optimal timing of transplantation. Premature transplantation results in exposure of the recipient to the hazards of transplantation and long-term immunosuppression. Excessive delay may result in death without transplantation or the development of comorbidities that may increase operative risk. These comorbidities include progressive end-organ dysfunction (especially renal), malnutrition associated with advanced heart failure, and progressive rise in PVR. These observations emphasize the importance of studying outcomes after listing the patient for transplantation—and not just after transplantation.

Data from the US Scientific Registry of Transplant Recipients reveal that children in all age groups have substantially shorter waiting times for heart transplants than do adults, but they have a greater risk of death while waiting. The highest death rate is among infants <1 year of age. The use of ABO-incompatible heart transplants may decrease wait-list mortality in infant heart transplant candidates (21). Several analyses of the PHTS database have focused on understanding risk factors for survival after listing for transplantation and for defining the optimal timing of transplantation. It has recently been shown that children awaiting transplant at the lowest urgency status (UNOS status 2 in the US) have a very low risk of sudden death while waiting if the underlying etiology is dilated cardiomyopathy. This statistic contrasts with the high risk of sudden death in adults with ischemic etiology who are on the transplant waiting list. These data suggest that routine use of automatic implantable cardioverter-defibrillators in all children awaiting transplant is not indicated, though certain subpopulations may benefit.

Data from the registries of the ISHLT, the US Scientific Registry of Transplant Recipients, and the PHTS all demonstrate important trends in posttransplant survival over the last decade. Importantly, significant improvements in outcome have occurred in recent years, with improved survival being most evident in the infant age group and at smaller volume centers. Most of the improvement appears to be due to reduction in early mortality. One-year survival is now ~90% at many centers, with only a relatively small drop over the following 3–4 years. The PHTS and the ISHLT databases continue to show a slightly higher perioperative and early mortality for infant recipients, but interestingly, these youngest recipients have the greatest conditional graft half-life based on analysis of 1-year survivors (1). It is likely that this reflects a lower incidence of posttransplant coronary artery disease in these very young recipients and a degree of immune privilege. The results of transplantation for congenital heart disease still lag slightly behind those of transplantation for cardiomyopathy; this difference is due to slightly higher perioperative mortality. Importantly, evidence of reduced survival has been noted among African American pediatric recipients compared to other racial groups.

Data from the US United Network for Organ Sharing from 1987 to 2004 shows that the median graft survival for African American recipients was only approximately half that for other recipients (5.3 versus 11.0 years).

CONCLUSIONS AND FUTURE DIRECTIONS

Despite advances in medical and surgical care from the pre-transplant through posttransplant periods, heart transplantation remains palliative, and all recipients are at risk for the adverse effects of nonspecific immunosuppression. Current immunosuppressive agents have narrow therapeutic windows and exhibit a wide array of organ toxicities, particularly in young patients. New immunosuppressive regimens have lowered the rates of acute rejection but appear to have had relatively little impact on the incidence of chronic rejection, the principal cause of late graft loss. The ultimate goal is to induce a state of donor-specific tolerance, wherein the recipient will accept the allograft indefinitely without the need for long-term immunosuppression. This quest is currently being realized in animal models of solid-organ transplantation and offers great hope for children undergoing heart transplantation in the future.

KEY POINTS

- The development of ABO-incompatible heart transplantation in infants may decrease wait-list mortality for this population and appears safe.
- A wide array of immunosuppressive regimens is used in children, but no large, randomized, controlled trials have been performed.
- Primary graft failure, infection, and acute rejection are the principal causes of death in the first year after transplantation.
- Graft coronary artery disease is the principal cause of late graft loss.
- Retransplantation is associated with poor results if performed early after primary transplantation but is associated with better results when performed for late indications.
- The "Holy Grail" of transplantation is the development of donor-specific graft tolerance.

References

1. Boucek MM, Edwards LB, Keck BM, et al. Registry of the International Society for Heart and Lung Transplantation: Eighth official pediatric report–2005. *J Heart Lung Transplant* 2005;24:968–82.
2. Canter C, Shaddy R, Bernstein D, et al. Indications for transplantation in pediatric heart disease. *Circulation* 2007;115(5):658–76.
3. Chin C, Naftel D, Pahl E, et al. Cardiac retransplantation in pediatrics: A multi-institutional study. *J Heart Lung Transplant* 2006;25:1420–4.
4. English RF, Pophal SA, Bacanu S, et al. Long-term comparison of tacrolimus and cyclosporine induced nephrotoxicity in pediatric heart transplant recipients. *Am J Transplant* 2002;2:769–73.
5. Fenton KN, Webber SA, Danford DA, et al. Long-term survival after pediatric cardiac transplantation and postoperative ECMO support. *Ann Thorac Surg* 2003;76:843–6.
6. Fricker FJ, Addonizio L, Bernstein D, et al. Heart transplantation in children: Indications. *Pediatric Transplantation* 1999;3:333–42.
7. Huang J, Trinkaus K, Huddleston CB, et al. Risk factors for primary graft failure after pediatric cardiac transplantation: Importance of recipient and donor characteristics. *J Heart Lung Transplant* 2004;23:716–22.
8. Lamour JM, Hsu DT, Quaegebeur JM, et al. Heart transplantation to a physiologic single lung in patients with congenital heart disease. *J Heart Lung Transplant* 2004;23:948–53.
9. Law Y, Boyle G, Miller S, et al. Restrictive hemodynamics are present at the time of diagnosis of allograft coronary artery disease in children. *Pediatr Transplant* 2006;10:948–52.
10. Pahl E, Naftel DC, Kuhn MA, et al. The impact and outcome of transplant coronary artery disease in a pediatric population: A 9-year multi-institutional study. *J Heart Lung Transplant* 2005;24:645–51.
11. Pigula FA, Webber SA. Donor Evaluation, Surgical Technique and Perioperative Management. Chapter 33. In: Fine R, Webber SA, Harmon W, et al., eds. *Pediatric Solid Organ Transplantation.* Oxford: Blackwell Publishing, 2007.
12. Rakhit A, Nurko S, Gauvreau K, et al. Gastrointestinal complications after pediatric cardiac transplantation. *J Heart Lung Transplant* 2002;21:751–9.
13. Russo L, Webber SA. Pediatric heart transplantation: Immunosuppression and its complications. *Curr Opin Cardiol* 2004;19:104–9.
14. Shirali GS, Ni J, Chinnock RE, et al. Association of viral genome with graft loss in children after cardiac transplantation. *N Engl J Med* 2001;344:1498–503.
15. Smith JM, Nemeth TL, McDonald RA. Current immunosuppressive agents: Efficacy, side effects, and utilization. *Pediatr Clin North Am* 2003;50:1283–300.
16. Stewart S, Winters GL, Fishbein MC, et al. Revision of the 1990 working formulation for the standardization of nomenclature in the diagnosis of heart rejection. *J Heart Lung Transplant* 2005;24:1710–20.
17. Webber SA. Cytomegalovirus infection and cardiac allograft vasculopathy in children. *Circulation* 2007;115(13):1701–2.
18. Webber SA, McCurry K, Zeevi A. Seminar: Heart and lung transplantation in children. *Lancet* 2006;368:53–69.
19. Webber SA, Naftel D, Fricker FJ, et al. Lymphoproliferative disorders after pediatric heart transplantation: A multi-institutional study. *Lancet* 2006;367:233–9.
20. Webber SA, Naftel DC, Parker J, et al. Late rejection episodes greater than 1 year after pediatric heart transplantation: Risk factors and outcomes. *J Heart Lung Transplant* 2003;22:869–75.
21. West LJ, Karamlou T, Dipchand AI, et al. Impact on outcomes after listing and transplantation, of a strategy to accept ABO blood group-incompatible donor hearts for neonates and infants. *J Thorac Cardiovasc Surg* 2006;131:455–61.
22. West LJ, Pollock-Barziv SM, Dipchand AI, et al. ABO-incompatible heart transplant in infants. *N Engl J Med* 2001;344:793–800.

CHAPTER 68 ■ CARDIAC CONDUCTION, DYSRHYTHMIAS, AND PACING

BRADLEY S. MARINO • JONATHAN R. KALTMAN • RONN E. TANEL

An understanding of the normal and abnormal cardiac conduction, dysrhythmia mechanisms, specific dysrhythmia diagnoses and management, the principles of temporary pacing, and antiarrhythmic drug classification and utilization is essential to caring for neonates, children, and adolescents with and without structural heart disease in the PICU.

THE CARDIAC CONDUCTION SYSTEM

The cardiac conduction system is composed of specialized myocardial cells that can create and propagate electrical depolarizations. The sinus node is the normal site of impulse formation in the heart. Propagation of the impulse then travels through the atrial myocardium to the atrioventricular (AV) node. Refractoriness of AV node cells is both voltage and time dependent. These characteristics result in slowing of conduction between the atrium and ventricle and potential filtering of rapid or closely coupled beats. From the AV node arises the bundle of His, which penetrates the interventricular septum and divides into right and left bundle branches (fascicles), and the left bundle further divides into an anterior and posterior fascicle. The fascicles propagate the depolarizing wave to the penetrating Purkinje fibers, which carry the electrical depolarization to the ventricular myocardium.

DYSRHYTHMIA MECHANISMS AND CLINICAL CATEGORIZATION

Tachyarrhythmias

Abnormally fast rhythms involve three electrophysiologic mechanisms: (a) *reentry*, (b) *increased automaticity*, and (c) *triggered automaticity*.

Reentry describes the phenomenon of an electrical wave front "reentering" cardiac tissue through which it has already traveled. Three essential elements are required for the existence of a reentrant circuit: two parallel pathways, unidirectional block in one pathway that indicates the different refractory properties of the two pathways, and slow conduction in the other pathway (Fig. 68.1). An electrical impulse will enter the circuit and begin to pass down the two pathways. If that impulse arrives in one limb of the pathway at such a time that the pathway with the longer refractory period has not recovered from the previous impulse, block will occur in that pathway. If the second pathway has recovered (shorter refractory period), the impulse will propagate down that second pathway. Propagation down that pathway may be slow enough to allow for the recovery of the first pathway, thus allowing the electrical impulse to travel in a retrograde fashion up the first pathway, thereby returning it to the original entry site into the circuit and establish a reentry circuit (a.k.a., *circus movement*). Reentrant arrhythmias typically have a regular rate with an abrupt onset and termination. In addition, this type of dysrhythmia can be provoked by an electrical stimulus, such as a premature atrial or ventricular contraction or by pacing maneuvers, and can be terminated by a variety of means, including pacing and direct-current cardioversion.

Automaticity refers to the ability of a cell or group of cells to spontaneously depolarize. When cells outside of the sinus node or AV node develop increased automaticity, they have the potential to suppress the sinus node if their rate of depolarization is greater than that of the sinus node. If these cells fire pathologically in a repetitive fashion, they result in a tachycardia. Automatic tachycardias typically have an irregular rate and a warm-up and cool-down phase, and they are sensitive to the adrenergic state. Unlike reentrant tachyarrhythmias, pacing and direct-current cardioversion do not convert these arrhythmias.

Triggered automaticity results from small oscillations of a cell's membrane potential during or after repolarization. If these oscillations are of sufficient amplitude to reach threshold, depolarization will occur. No direct evidence implicates triggered activity as a mechanism of clinically observed dysrhythmias. However, in vitro models of triggered activity clearly emulate certain clinical entities, such as torsades de pointes and arrhythmias seen with digoxin toxicity. Tachycardias derived from triggered activity share characteristics of both reentrant and automatic arrhythmias. For example, they may be induced or terminated with pacing maneuvers, have warm-up and cool-down phases, and are catecholamine sensitive.

Each mechanism of dysrhythmia may occur at any site in the heart. Reentrant circuits may involve only atrial tissue, giving rise to atrial flutter or atrial fibrillation. Postoperative reentrant pathways around surgical scars have been termed *intra-atrial reentrant tachycardia* (IART) or *incisional tachycardia*. Reentry may also involve pathways within or leading to the AV node, resulting in AV nodal reentrant tachycardia (AVNRT). Reentry that results in ventricular tachycardia (VT) usually involves circuits around areas of infarction, surgical scars, or anatomic obstacles. The most common reentrant tachycardias in the pediatric population are those that involve an *accessory pathway*, which is an anomalous electrical connection between atrial and ventricular myocardium across the AV groove. These AV reciprocating tachycardias (AVRT) use the accessory pathway

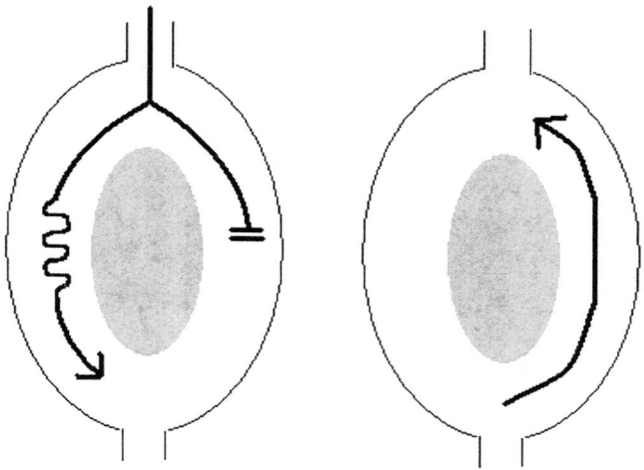

FIGURE 68.1. Schematic diagram representing a reentrant circuit. Requirements for reentry include two pathways, unidirectional block in one pathway (=) and slow conduction in the other pathway (~).

(usually the pathway with the longer refractory period) and the AV node (usually the pathway with slower conduction) as the two limbs of the reentrant circuit. Wolff-Parkinson-White (WPW) syndrome involves an accessory pathway that can support both antegrade and retrograde conduction. Concealed bypass tracts can only support retrograde conduction.

Automatic tachycardias may originate in any of the cardiac segments. Multifocal atrial tachycardia (MAT), or chaotic atrial rhythm, is derived from multiple atrial foci firing during the same time interval. Increased automaticity near the AV node gives rise to junctional ectopic tachycardia (JET). Finally, some rare types of VT may arise from isolated foci within the Purkinje fibers of the ventricle.

Diagnostic Approach to Tachyarrhythmias

A 12-lead electrocardiogram (ECG) with a long multilead rhythm strip, telemetry recording, or Holter monitor is necessary to determine the dysrhythmia mechanism (**Fig. 68.2**). Narrow-complex tachycardias imply conduction through the normal AV node and His-Purkinje system and are therefore supraventricular in origin. A wide-complex tachycardia should be assumed to be ventricular in origin but may also be due to a supraventricular tachycardia (SVT) with bundle-branch block, rate-dependent aberrancy, or antidromic reciprocating tachycardia (e.g., WPW). In reentrant tachycardias that involve an accessory pathway, a narrow-complex tachycardia results from antegrade (atria to ventricles) conduction down the AV node and retrograde (ventricles to atria) conduction up the accessory pathway, called *orthodromic reciprocating tachycardia.* When antegrade conduction occurs down the accessory pathway with

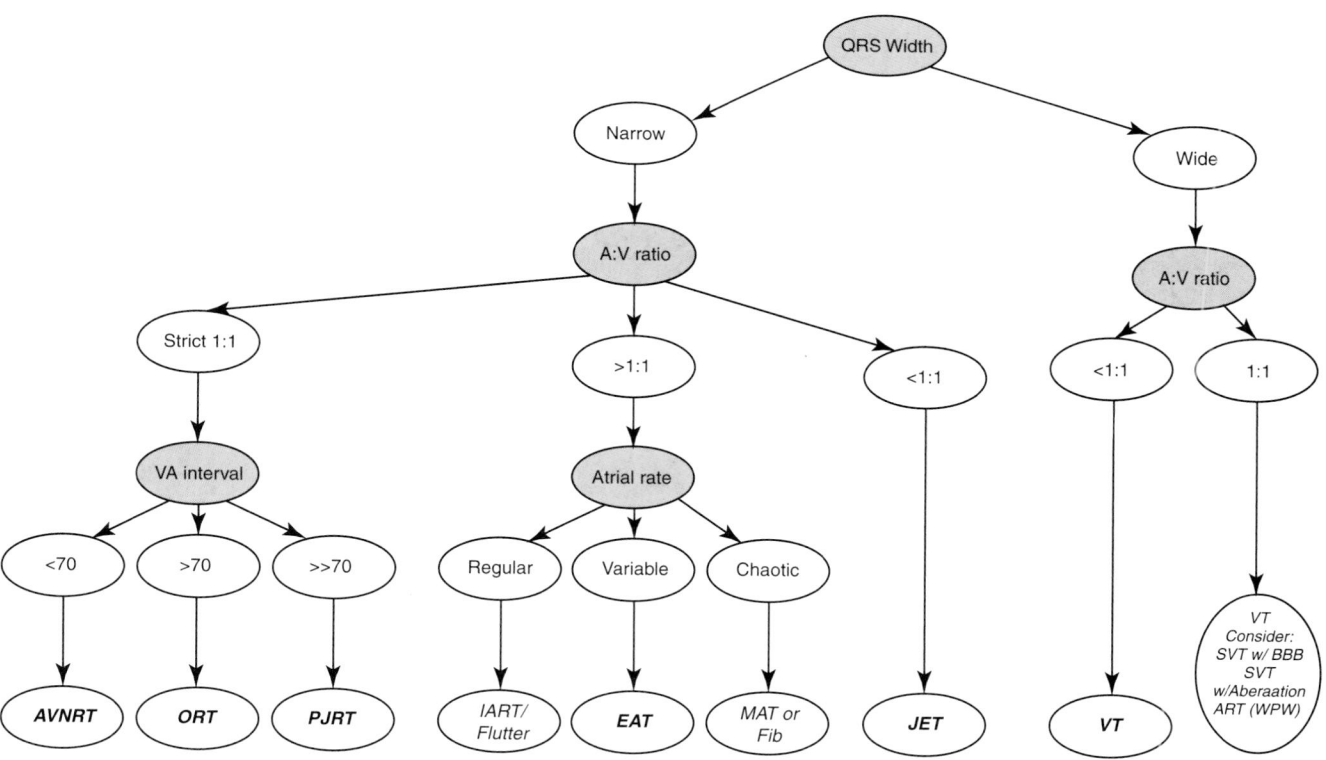

FIGURE 68.2. Diagnostic approach for determining tachycardia mechanism. ART, antidromic reciprocating tachycardia; AV, atrioventricular; AVNRT, atrioventricular nodal reentrant tachycardia; BBB, bundle branch block; EAT, ectopic atrial tachycardia; IART, intra-atrial reentrant tachycardia; JET, junctional ectopic tachycardia; MAT, multi-focal atrial tachycardia; ORT, orthodromic reciprocating tachycardia; PJRT, permanent junctional reciprocating tachycardia; SVT, supraventricular tachycardia; VA, ventriculo-atrial; VT, ventricular tachycardia; WPW, Wolff-Parkinson-White. From Walsh EP. Clinical Approach to Diagnosis and Acute Management of Tachycardias in Children. In: Walsh EP, Saul JP, Triedman JK, eds. *Cardiac Arrhythmias in Children and Young Adults with Congenital Heart Disease*, Philadelphia: Lippincott Williams & Wilkins, 2001, with permission.

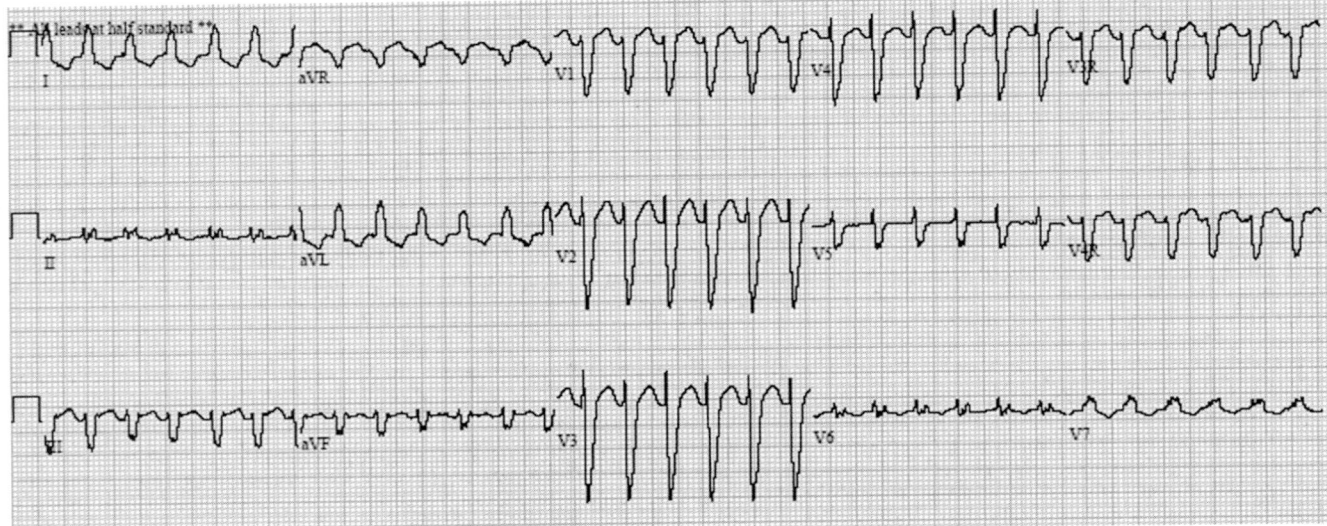

FIGURE 68.3. ECG showing supraventricular tachycardia conducted with aberrancy in a newborn.

retrograde conduction up the AV node, a wide-complex tachycardia, called *antidromic reciprocating tachycardia*, results.

The relationship of atrial to ventricular complexes is important to the determination of the tachycardia mechanism. If the ratio of P waves to QRS complexes is 1, then AVNRT or AVRT is likely. To differentiate AVNRT from AVRT, the retrograde VA conduction time (i.e., the time interval from the beginning of the QRS complex to the beginning of the retrograde P wave, RP interval) should be determined. If the VA time is <70 msecs, AVNRT is likely. If the VA time is >70 msecs, AVRT is the probable etiology. Sinus tachycardia may be differentiated from AVNRT or AVRT by a P-wave frontal plane axis of 0 to +90 degrees in a normal situs solitus heart. An A:V ratio >1 is diagnostic of a primary atrial tachycardia, although 1:1 AV conduction can also occur with a primary atrial tachycardia. If the atrial rate is regular, atrial flutter (or IART) is likely. An irregular atrial rate that has a single P-wave morphology different from the sinus P-wave morphology and the axis of which is outside of the 0 to +90-degree range suggests ectopic atrial tachycardia. Finally, an irregular atrial rate with three or more P-wave morphologies suggests MAT. JET may have 1:1 VA conduction or VA dissociation with occasional sinus capture and a ventricular rate greater than the atrial rate.

Wide-complex tachycardias should be assumed to be ventricular, until proven otherwise. A wide-complex tachycardia with AV dissociation (i.e., no relationship between P waves and QRS complexes) and a ventricular rate greater than the atrial rate is diagnostic of VT. A wide-complex tachycardia with an A:V ratio of 1 can be VT with retrograde conduction or SVT with aberrancy (**Fig. 68.3**), SVT with bundle-branch block, or antidromic SVT.

Bradyarrhythmias

Bradyarrhythmias result from abnormalities in impulse propagation or parasympathetic inhibition of the AV conduction system, resulting in sinus node dysfunction (SND), intraatrial block, AV node block, block within the bundle of His, or in-

traventricular fascicular block. When block occurs in the AV conduction system, depolarization may occur in an aberrant manner, a slower, subsidiary pacemaker may emerge, or myocardium distal to the obstruction to conduction may fail to depolarize.

Diagnostic Approach to Bradyarrhythmias

Review of the ECG recording can help to determine whether a bradyarrhythmia is due to SND or conduction block. Important features include the relationship of P waves to QRS complexes and the PR interval. If the ratio of P waves to QRS complexes is 1:1, the PR interval is normal, and the rhythm is atrially derived, then SND is present with sinus bradycardia or ectopic atrial bradycardia. If the PR interval is prolonged, then first-degree AV block is present. If the PR interval is prolonging beat to beat, culminating with a dropped QRS complex, then Mobitz type I (Wenckebach) second-degree AV block is present. Intermittent dropped QRS complexes without PR interval prolongation on prior beats indicates Mobitz type II second-degree AV block. Complete heart block, or third-degree AV block, is present when AV dissociation occurs and the ratio of atrial to ventricular complexes is greater than 1:1.

SPECIFIC DIAGNOSIS

Supraventricular Arrhythmias

The most common dysrhythmia in the pediatric population is SVT, with a reported incidence of 1 in 250–1000 (26). SVT may result from either reentry or enhanced automaticity; reentry is more common.

Atrioventricular Reciprocating Supraventricular Tachycardias

The most common type of reentrant SVT in children is AVRT, which requires participation of both the atrium and ventricle

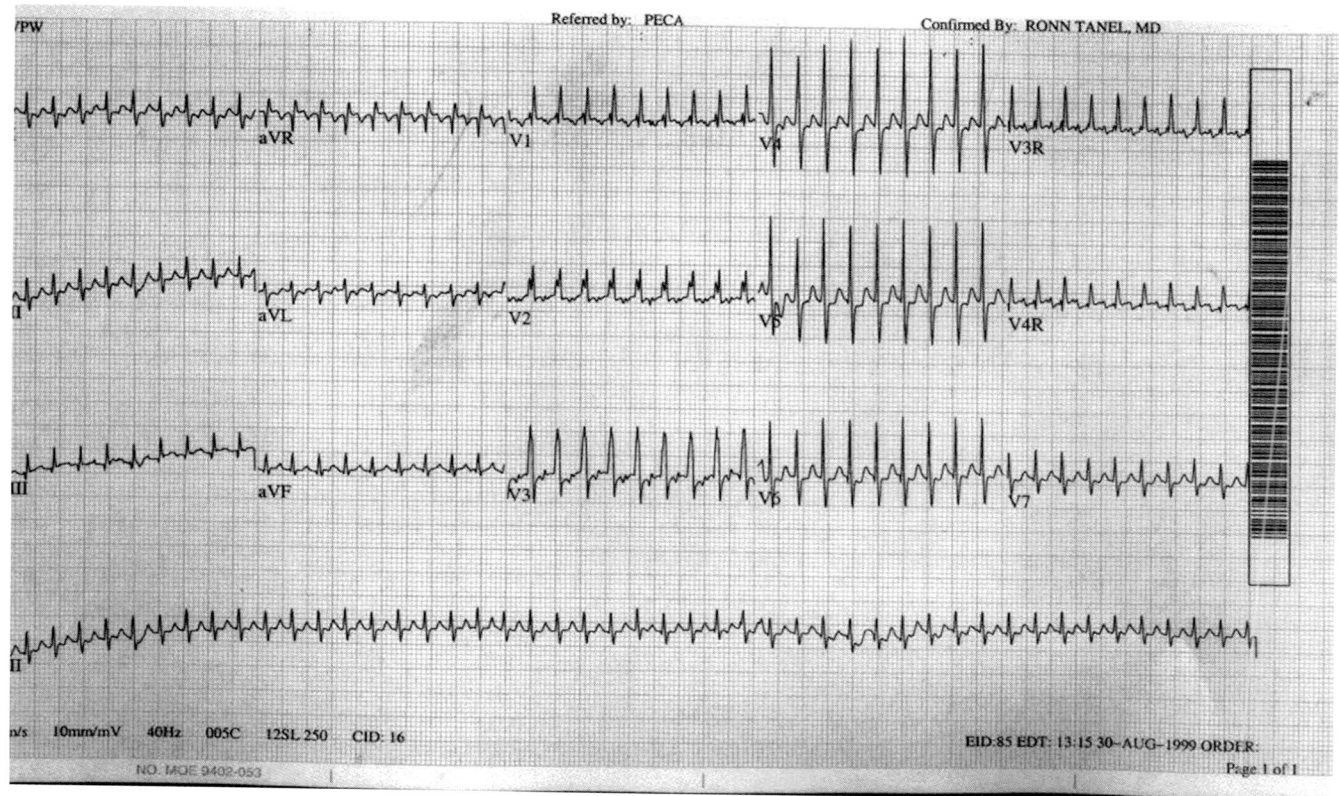

FIGURE 68.4. ECG showing AV reciprocating tachycardia.

in the reentrant circuit. AVRT utilizes accessory pathways and includes WPW syndrome, orthodromic tachycardia from concealed bypass tracts, and AVNRT (**Fig. 68.4**). SVT may present in the fetus or at any age during infancy and childhood. Accessory pathway-mediated tachycardias are more common in infants and young children, while AVNRT is more common in adolescents. Prolonged fetal tachycardia is one cause of nonimmune fetal hydrops. These infants frequently have symptoms of irritability and poor feeding. If SVT goes undetected, the patient may develop congestive heart failure, manifested as tachypnea, diaphoresis, pallor, and lethargy. Older children may complain of symptoms such as palpitations, chest pain, abdominal pain, or dizziness. Syncope may occur if the tachycardia rate is sufficiently fast to impair diastolic filling, resulting in hypotension and cerebral hypoperfusion.

Wolff-Parkinson-White Syndrome. WPW syndrome is characterized by a short PR interval and delta wave, which represents ventricular pre-excitation prior to normal activation of the AV node and His-Purkinje system (**Fig. 68.5**). WPW syndrome involves an accessory pathway that usually has both antegrade and retrograde conduction. SVT may be either orthodromic reciprocating tachycardia (down the AV node and up the accessory pathway) or antidromic reciprocating tachycardia (down the accessory pathway and up the AV node). Orthodromic reciprocating tachycardia is more common. Patients with WPW are at an increased risk of atrial fibrillation. If the accessory pathway supports rapid antegrade conduction of an atrial arrhythmia, hemodynamic instability and sudden death may re-

sult. In patients with WPW, the risk of sudden death is 1% every 10 years (3).

The incidence of WPW in childhood is ~1 in 1000 (28). Of patients who present during infancy, one-third continue to experience episodes of SVT after 1 year of age (6). Conversely, older patients have a greater chance for SVT recurrence. Some patients with WPW are asymptomatic, and the diagnosis is made incidentally. The risk of significant dysrhythmias, including sudden death, is unclear. The most precise method for risk stratification is invasive electrophysiologic testing, although clearly defined stratification guidelines for the pediatric population have not been created. Congenital heart disease occurs in association with WPW in ~20% of patients. Ebstein anomaly and L-transposition of the great arteries are the most common associated congenital anomalies.

Concealed Bypass Tract. Concealed bypass tracts only support retrograde conduction and orthodromic reciprocating tachycardia. Due to their inability to propagate extremely rapid atrial rates directly into the ventricle, concealed bypass tracts are less likely to cause hemodynamic instability or sudden death. Orthodromic reciprocating tachycardia in patients with WPW and concealed bypass tracts are indistinguishable. Differentiation is possible by evaluating the ECG in sinus rhythm, when the patient with a concealed bypass tract will have a normal PR interval without a delta wave and the patient with WPW will have a short PR interval and delta wave. This difference has important implications with regard to treatment. Patients with a concealed bypass tract present with SVT at

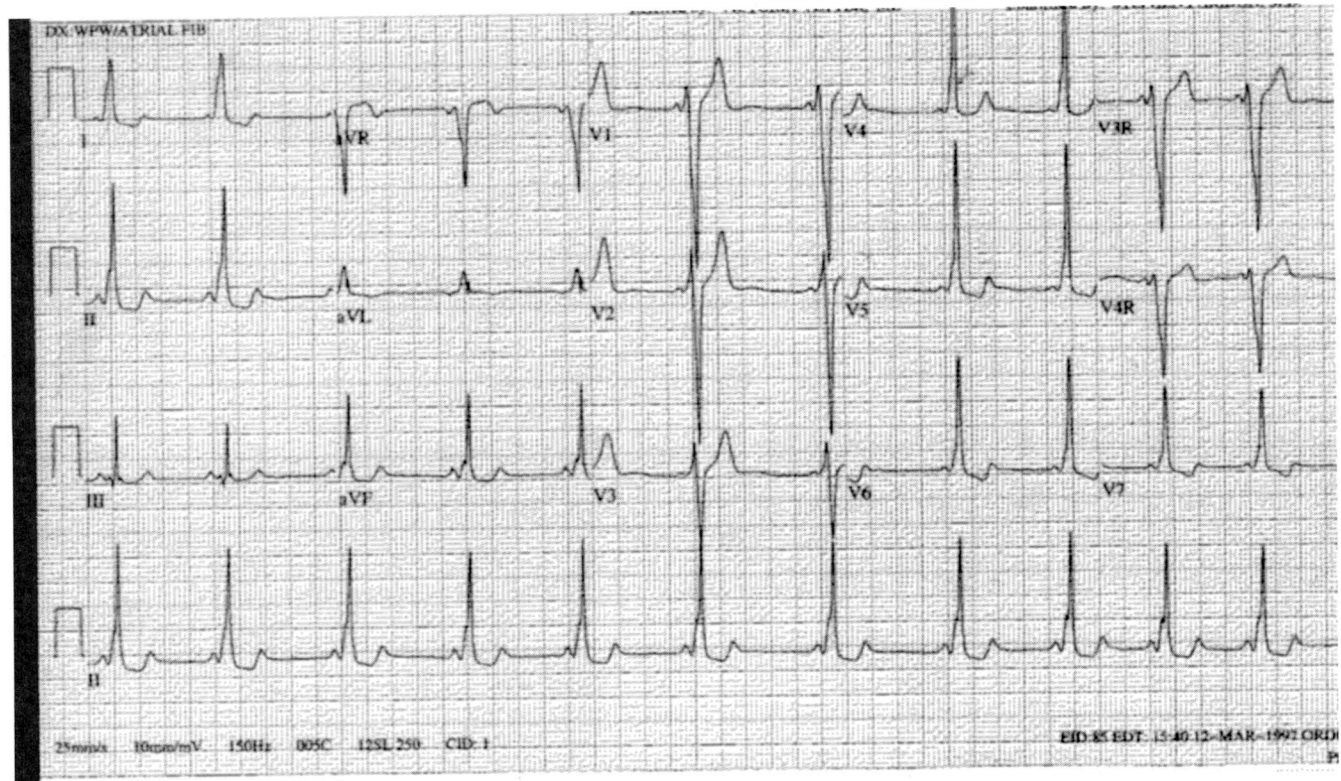

FIGURE 68.5. ECG from a child with Wolff-Parkinson-White syndrome. Note the short PR interval and delta wave.

any age from infancy through adolescence. An unusual type of SVT that involves a slowly conducting concealed bypass tract is the permanent form of junctional reciprocating tachycardia, which has a very long RP interval during the tachycardia, and the arrhythmia is frequently refractory to medical management.

Atrioventricular Nodal Reentrant Tachycardia. The two pathways used as substrate for the reentrant circuit in AVNRT are electrical approaches to the AV node located in the atrium. The "slow" pathway has slower conduction, a shorter refractory period, and is anatomically located in the mid-septal to posteroseptal region of the AV groove. The "fast" pathway has faster conduction, a longer refractory period, and is located in the anterior aspect of the atrial septum. Typical AVNRT involves conduction antegrade down the slow pathway and retrograde up the fast pathway. Atypical AVNRT involves the opposite sequence. The incidence of AVNRT increases with age and represents the most common type of reentrant SVT in adults. In the pediatric population, it is most commonly seen during adolescence. A possible explanation for this is that the AV node undergoes electrophysiologic alterations with age. In one study, dual AV node physiology was found in 15% of children <13 years of age and in 44% of children >13 years of age (5).

Treatment for Atrioventricular Reciprocating Tachycardia. The goal of acute therapy is to terminate the reentrant circuit and restore sinus rhythm. A patient who presents in shock should be treated with the ABCs of resuscitation (airway, breathing, and circulation). If vascular access cannot readily be obtained and/or the patient is in extremis, then direct-current cardioversion is indicated. Synchronized cardioversion should be performed with an energy dose of 0.5–1 joule/kg. The output can be doubled to a maximum of 6 joule/kg until the treatment is effective.

In the acute but stable patient with AVRT, first-line therapy is adenosine. Adenosine rapidly interrupts the reentrant circuit at the AV node. Due to its short half-life, adenosine should be administered through a large-bore intravascular catheter placed as close to the heart as possible. Digoxin is effective and especially useful in the patient with decreased myocardial function, but it may take several hours to achieve blood levels to provide pharmacologic cardioversion. Other IV pharmacologic therapies used in the acute setting include β blockers (e.g., esmolol), procainamide, and amiodarone. These medications should be used with caution, as they all have negative inotropic effects. Other therapeutic modalities include transesophageal pacing and vagal maneuvers. Vagal maneuvers for adolescents and older children include the Valsalva maneuver and the headstand. In infants, a bag of ice to the center of the face frequently terminates the SVT by eliciting the diving reflex. While IV calcium-channel blockers are an important therapy for SVT in adults, they are contraindicated in young children, especially in those children <1 year of age or who are receiving β blockers. Hemodynamic collapse and sudden death have been reported in infants treated with verapamil (9).

Chronic therapy attempts to prevent recurrences of SVT and depends upon the type of SVT. Digoxin and β blockers are first-line oral therapy for chronic prevention. Young children must be monitored for hypoglycemia and hypotension when β blockers are started.

Digoxin and calcium-channel blocker are contraindicated in patients with WPW because they may enhance antegrade conduction down the accessory pathway and allow for a more rapid ventricular response during atrial flutter or fibrillation. For SVT refractory to first-line therapy of adenosine or cardioversion, the Pediatric Advanced Life Support algorithm recommends amiodarone. Other agents such as flecainide, procainamide, sotalol, amiodarone, and verapamil can also be employed.

An increasingly popular therapeutic modality for recurrent SVT is catheter ablation, using either radiofrequency energy or cryoenergy. Radiofrequency ablation involves application of thermal energy via an electrode catheter to the arrhythmia substrate (i.e., accessory pathway or AV nodal slow pathway). Radiofrequency energy causes tissue heating and necrosis. Radiofrequency catheter ablation has been used successfully to cure various types of dysrhythmias in pediatric patients. The success rate for AVRT has been reported between 86% and 97%, depending upon the location of the accessory pathway, and >95% for AVNRT (15). Complication rates are low, with the most common serious complications being AV block, catheter perforation of the myocardium, and thromboembolism (15). Common indications for radiofrequency ablation of SVT include life-threatening dysrhythmias, medically resistant tachycardias, adverse drug reactions, tachycardia-induced cardiomyopathy, impending cardiac surgery, and patient choice. Recently, cryoablation has been introduced as an alternative means of destroying or altering the arrhythmia substrate. The theoretic advantage of cryoablation is that its effects can potentially be reversed, allowing for its safer use near the AV node.

Atrial Flutter/Intra-atrial Reentrant Tachycardia

Atrial flutter is observed in two distinct groups in the pediatric population: in newborns and in patients with congenital heart disease, especially following atrial surgery for congenital heart defects.

Atrial Flutter. Atrial flutter of infancy is rare. It may present in utero or during the newborn period. As congenital heart defects may coexist with the dysrhythmia, echocardiography is recommended to exclude most commonly atrial septal defect, aneurysm of atrial septum, or Ebstein anomaly. The reentrant circuit of atrial flutter of infancy is generally confined to the right atrium. Similar to typical adult atrial flutter, it may utilize the isthmus between the tricuspid valve and the inferior vena cava as the area of slow conduction. Characteristic saw-toothed flutter waves are usually present in leads II, III, and aVF. Atrial rates may reach over 400 bpm. AV block with 2:1 conduction results in a ventricular response rate of ≥200 bpm (**Fig. 68.6**). Conversion to sinus rhythm is often spontaneous, while persistent dysrhythmia is usually responsive to therapy.

Atrial flutter in the newborn is converted to sinus rhythm with medications, transesophageal pacing, or cardioversion. Medications include IV digoxin, procainamide, amiodarone, and sotalol. Procainamide should be used in conjunction with digoxin, as procainamide may slow the flutter rate, resulting in more rapid AV conduction. Digoxin is used to increase the degree of AV block in this setting. Once atrial flutter in the newborn period is converted to sinus rhythm, recurrence is uncommon.

Intra-atrial Reentrant Tachycardia. Atrial flutter in patients who have undergone surgery for congenital heart disease is referred to as IART or incisional atrial tachycardia to highlight its differences from typical atrial flutter (**Fig. 68.7**). The surgical procedures that predispose patients to IART generally involve surgery in the atria, including atrial septal defect repair, atrial baffling procedures (Senning or Mustard operation) for D-transposition of the great arteries, and the Fontan

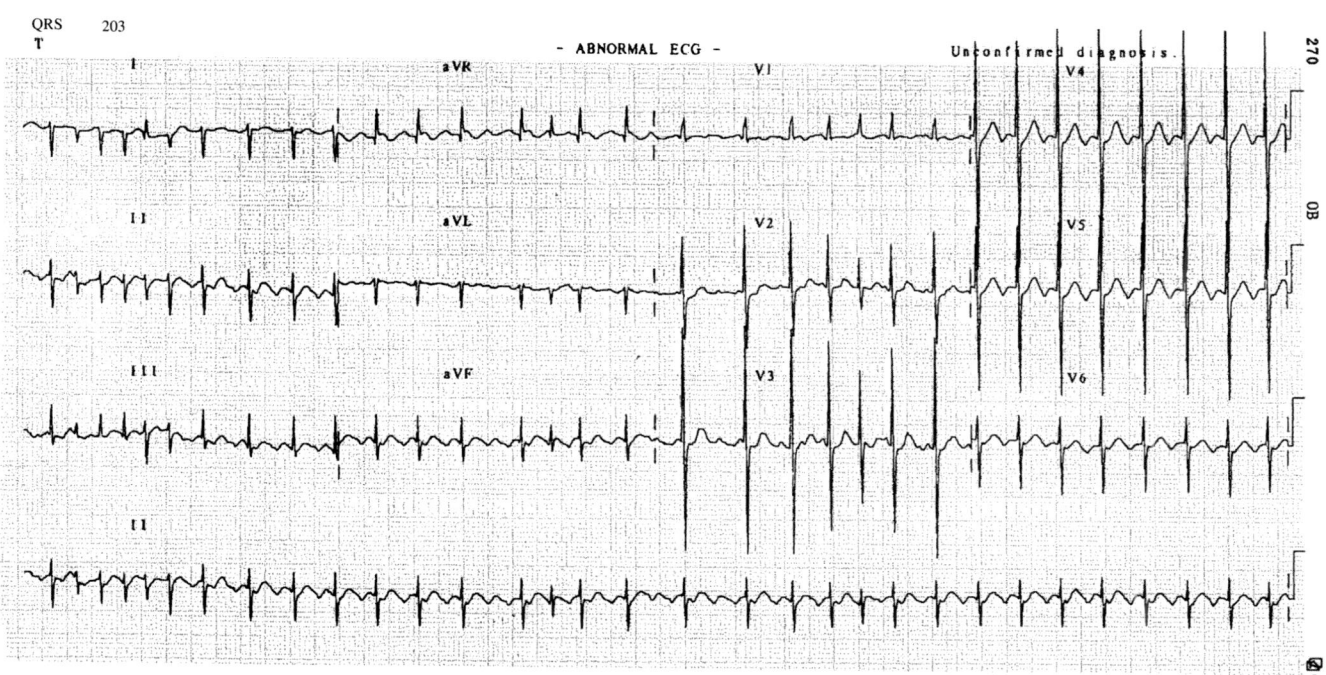

FIGURE 68.6. ECG showing atrial flutter with 2:1 conduction in a newborn. Note the typical flutter waves and "saw-tooth pattern" in leads II, III, and aVF.

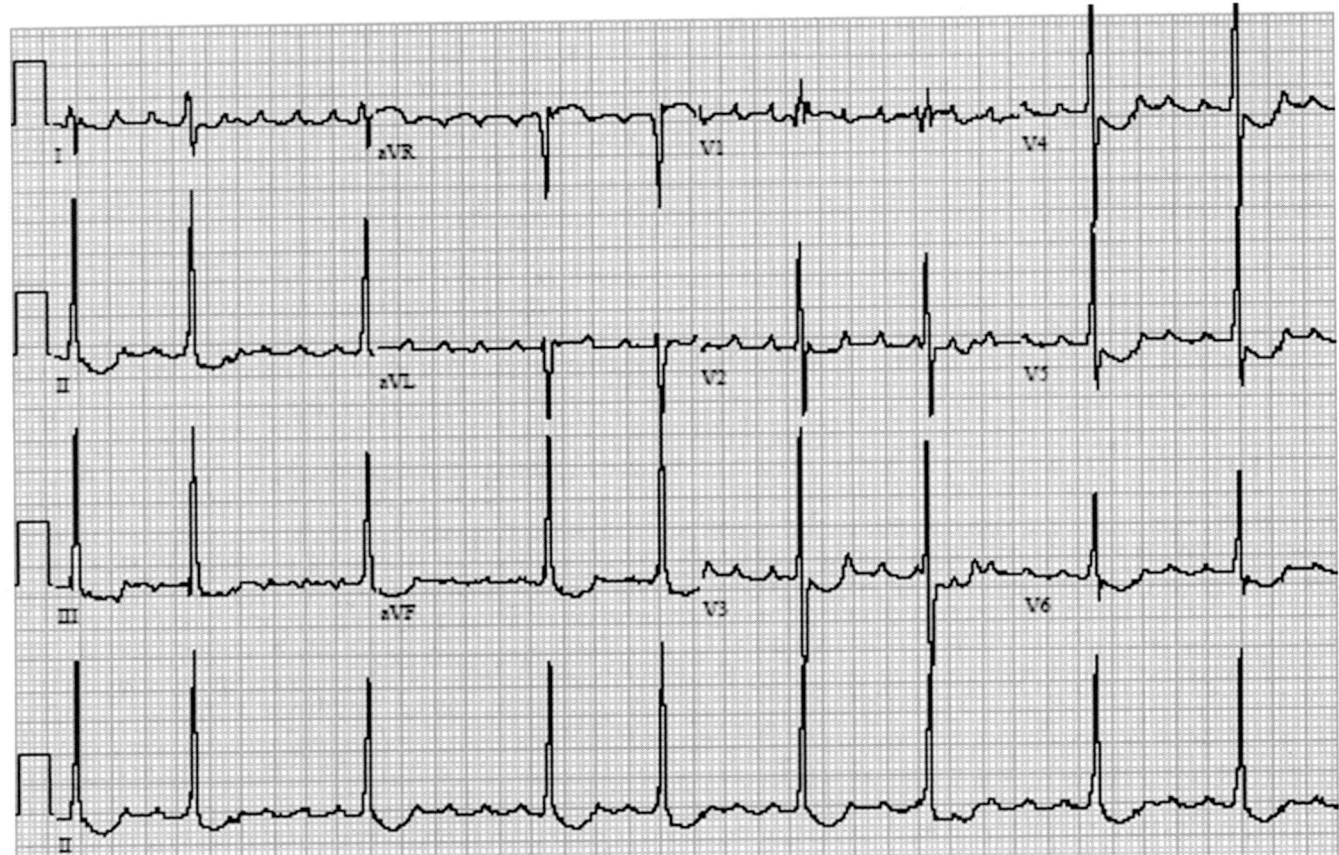

FIGURE 68.7. ECG showing intra-atrial reentrant tachycardia with variable conduction in a child with hypoplastic left heart syndrome status post-Fontan operation.

operation for the univentricular heart. The reentrant circuit may occur anywhere within the atria and frequently incorporates an anatomic barrier or surgical scar. During electrophysiology testing, more than one reentrant circuit may be defined. The typical saw-tooth flutter waves may not be apparent; therefore, the clinician must have a high index of suspicion for the diagnosis. The incidence of IART following congenital heart surgery increases with age. Predisposing factors include surgical scars within the atrium, elevated atrial pressure, abnormal atrial anatomy associated with the primary lesion, and SND (25). Atrial rates in IART vary considerably from 150 to 450 bpm, with variable conduction to the ventricle. Symptomatology is related to the ventricular response rate and myocardial function. A fast ventricular response may result in palpitations, syncope, or sudden death. A slower ventricular response rate may result in gradual fatigue or exercise intolerance, especially in the Fontan patient, as AV synchrony may be crucial for adequate cardiac output. If the ventricular response rate is slow enough, patients may be asymptomatic. Long-standing IART may result in sluggish blood flow in the atria or Fontan pathway and increase the risk for thrombus.

Prior to any attempts at converting IART to sinus rhythm, the presence of an atrial thrombus must be ruled out, which usually requires transesophageal echocardiography, especially in older children and adolescents, as transthoracic windows may be inadequate to visualize an intra-atrial thrombus. Acute therapy includes antiarrhythmic medications, transesophageal

pacing, and cardioversion. Medications that have been successful in this setting include procainamide, propafenone, amiodarone, and sotalol. An agent to slow AV nodal conduction, such as digoxin, should be used in conjunction with class IA antiarrhythmics, such as procainamide.

Chronic therapy for IART is often difficult, necessitating multiple medications and modalities. Digoxin may be used for rate control but generally has little direct effect on the arrhythmia substrate. Second-line medications include procainamide, flecainide, propafenone, amiodarone, and sotalol. Other modalities include overdrive atrial pacing techniques and radiofrequency ablation. Antibradycardia pacing may be useful in those patients with tachy-brady syndrome. Antitachycardia pacing devices have shown modest benefit (22). Radiofrequency ablation has been used to interrupt the reentrant circuit. Due to the presence of multiple reentrant circuits, complex atrial anatomy, and thick atrial muscle, success rates have been in the range of 70%–80%, with recurrence rates as high as 50% (25). New technologies, such as improved mapping systems and irrigated catheter tips, may help to improve success rates and decrease recurrence.

Automatic Supraventricular Tachycardia

Atrial automatic tachycardias tend to present in children <6 years of age but also occur in older children and adolescents. The heart rate is inappropriately high for the patient's level of activity and appears to be sensitive to the adrenergic state.

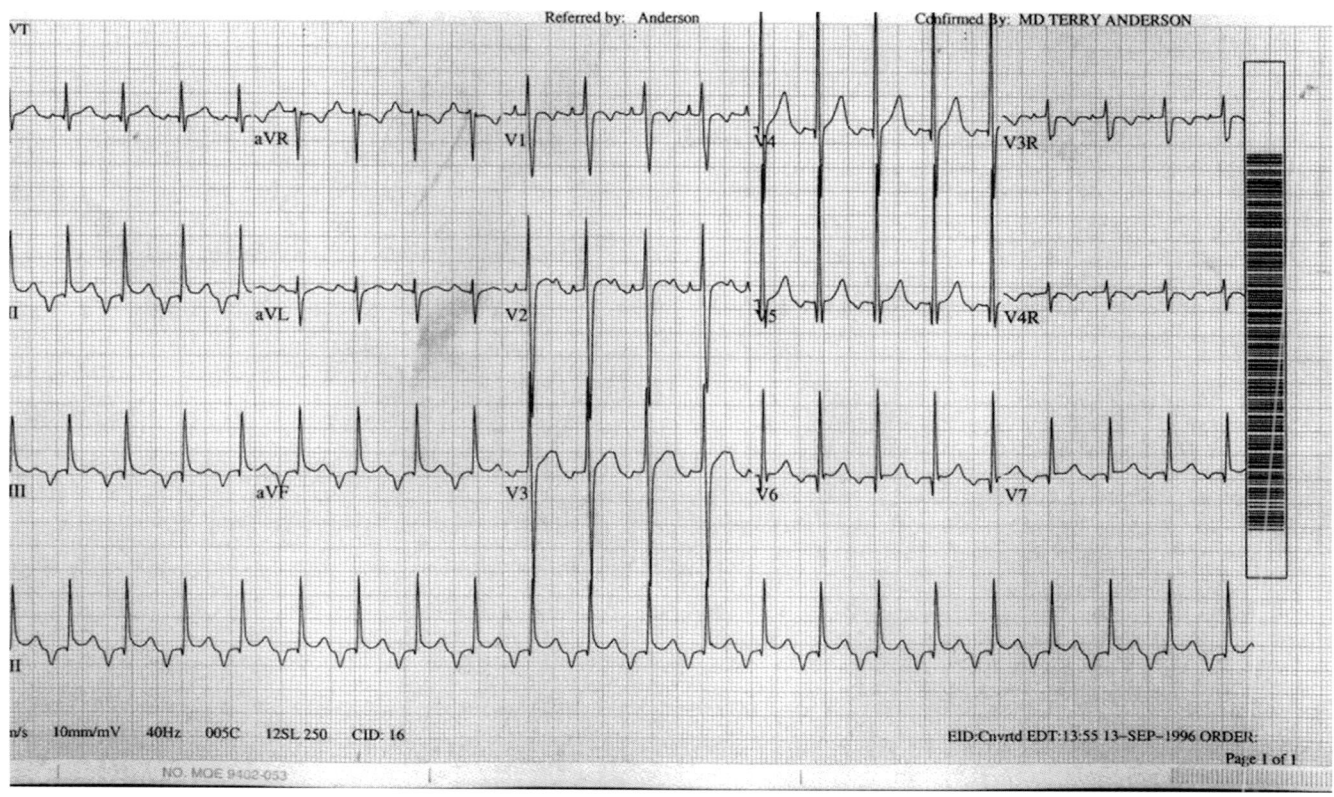

FIGURE 68.8. ECG showing ectopic atrial tachycardia. Note that the P wave is negative in leads II and aVF.

During sleep or under the influence of sedation, the rate will be slower or the tachycardia may even be suppressed by normal sinus node activity. These tachycardias tend to be chronic and incessant. At slower rates, they are often not perceived by the patient. Persistence of the tachycardia may eventually lead to a tachycardia-mediated cardiomyopathy. Presentation for many patients includes signs and symptoms of congestive heart failure.

Ectopic Atrial Tachycardia. *Ectopic atrial tachycardia* (EAT), or *automatic atrial tachycardia*, represents between 10% and 20% of the SVT seen in the pediatric population. EAT arises from a single focus of increased automaticity located within the atria. The firing rate of the ectopic focus is faster than that of the sinus node and overrides the normal sinus node activity. Heart rates can range from 130 to 210 bpm in children and adolescents, but can reach 300 bpm in infants (**Fig. 68.8**). The location of the ectopic focus is most commonly the atrial appendage or the orifices of the pulmonary veins in either atrium, with the right more common than the left. AV block may occur during the tachycardia but will not interrupt the atrial tachycardia. EAT is associated with conditions that result in atrial dilation, such as AV valve regurgitation and postoperative atrial surgery. In addition, the arrhythmia has been associated with

chronic cardiomyopathy and myocarditis. While some cases of EAT spontaneously resolve, most patients require chronic therapy.

Multifocal Atrial Tachycardia. MAT, or chaotic atrial rhythm, is rare and arises from multiple foci of increased automaticity located within the atria. The tachycardia is defined by the presence of three or more P-wave morphologies. MAT may be confused with atrial fibrillation because of the irregular rhythm and the variable P-wave morphologies (**Fig. 68.9**). The most common presentation is during the newborn period, with up to 50% of patients having an associated cardiac defect or other medical condition. Frequently, this type of tachycardia will spontaneously resolve during the first year of life.

Treatment of Ectopic Atrial Tachycardia/Multifocal Atrial Tachycardia. Treatment of an automatic SVT involves decreasing the ventricular response rate by slowing AV conduction and decreasing the automaticity of the abnormal focus or foci. Digoxin and calcium-channel blockers can slow conduction through the AV node, but they also have negative inotropic properties. Calcium-channel blockers should not be used in children <1 year of age. β blockers, which oppose adrenergic stimulation of the focus, may help suppress the tachycardia.

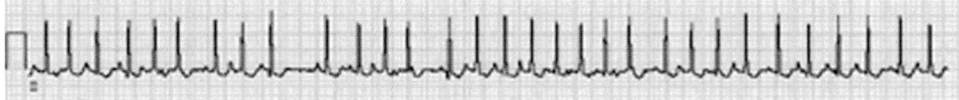

FIGURE 68.9. ECG from an infant with multifocal atrial tachycardia. Note the multiple P-wave morphologies.

Class IA agents, such as procainamide, and class IC agents, such as flecainide and propafenone, act by decreasing automaticity and prolonging refractoriness. Class III agents, such as amiodarone and sotalol, can slow conduction throughout the myocardium, including the abnormal focus. Radiofrequency ablation of the ectopic focus has become an effective means of curing EAT and is the treatment of choice for medically refractory dysrhythmia. Technical difficulties may arise, as the dysrhythmia is catecholamine-sensitive and may be suppressed by sedation. Of note, adenosine, overdrive pacing, and cardioversion will not be successful in converting automatic tachycardias to sinus rhythm.

Junctional Ectopic Tachycardia

JET occurs as a result of enhanced automaticity in the region of the AV node. JET is characterized by a narrow-complex tachycardia with AV dissociation and a ventricular rate faster than the atrial rate (**Fig. 68.10**). In the pediatric population, JET may be familial and congenital. Patients present during infancy, with some cases detected in utero. Congestive heart failure is frequently the presenting sign and is associated with higher heart rates (29). Medical therapy may be weaned after several months to years in some patients. In one follow-up study, patients who were weaned from their medications were either entirely in sinus rhythm or had intermittent episodes of a slow junctional ectopic rhythm (29). Sudden death has been reported in this population (29).

JET also occurs in the immediate postoperative period following surgery for congenital heart disease. Postoperative JET is usually transient, usually lasting up to 72 hrs. Despite its self-limited nature, postoperative JET can cause significant hemodynamic instability. The combination of depressed postoperative myocardial function, tachycardia rates as high as 250 bpm, and loss of AV synchrony may significantly impair cardiac output. With aggressive treatment, the ventricular rate can be slowed and the patient can be supported until the dysrhythmia resolves. Postoperative JET is most commonly seen following repairs that include a ventricular septal defect closure (30).

Treatment of Junctional Ectopic Tachycardia

For the congenital form of JET, digoxin may slow the tachycardia rate and support cardiac function. Often, a second-line agent is required, with amiodarone being the most successful. Antiarrhythmic therapy may result in enough SND that a pacemaker may be necessary. Ablation therapy is reserved for the most resistant cases of JET because of the high risk for the development of AV block. Postoperative JET can be treated pharmacologically with amiodarone. Digoxin and procainamide may be used rarely as second-line therapies. Other nonpharmacologic measures include controlling fever, hypothermia with core temperatures reduced to 35°C, and sedation. AV sequential pacing to restore AV synchrony and paired ventricular pacing to decrease the effective heart rate have been used to augment cardiac output.

Ventricular Tachycardia

Ventricular arrhythmias in the pediatric population are observed in a variety of patients and circumstances. Any wide-complex rhythm should first be considered ventricular in origin. It is inappropriate to use the rate of the tachycardia to determine whether the rhythm is supraventricular or ventricular in origin. Finally, in that many pediatric cardiac surgical

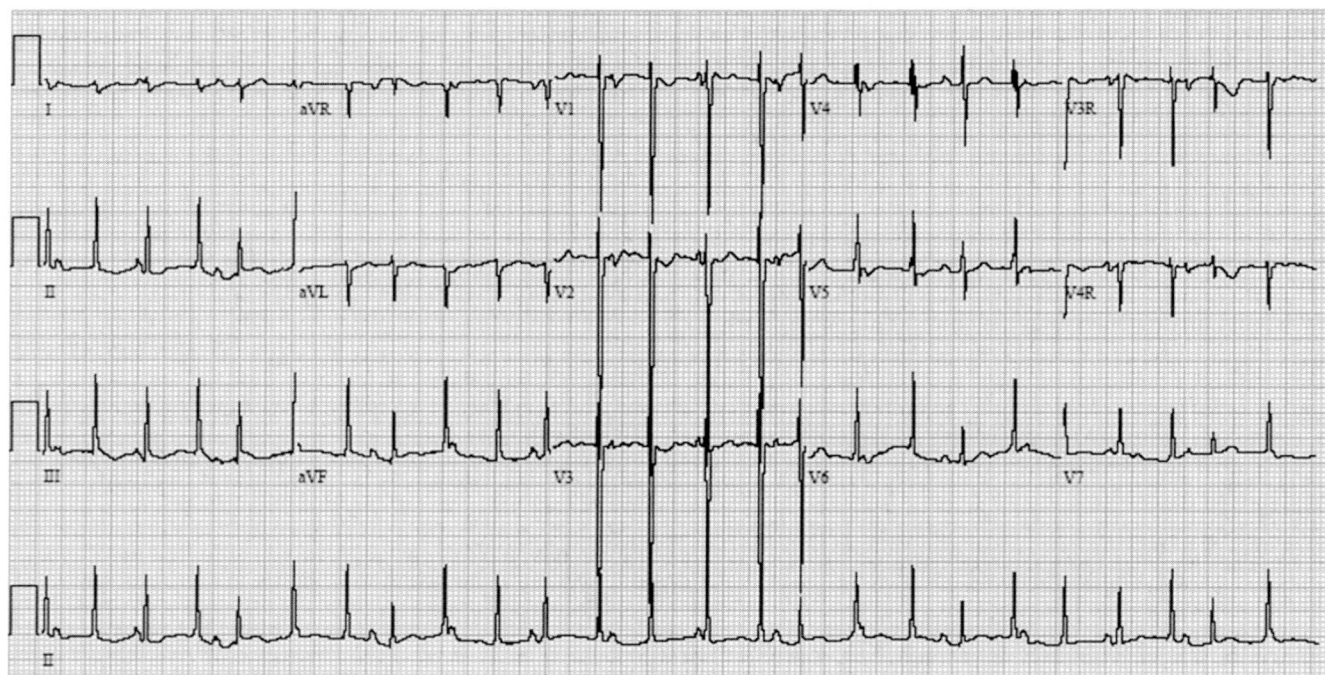

FIGURE 68.10. ECG showing congenital junctional ectopic tachycardia in a newborn. Note the narrow QRS complex with AV dissociation and a ventricular rate that is faster than the atrial rate.

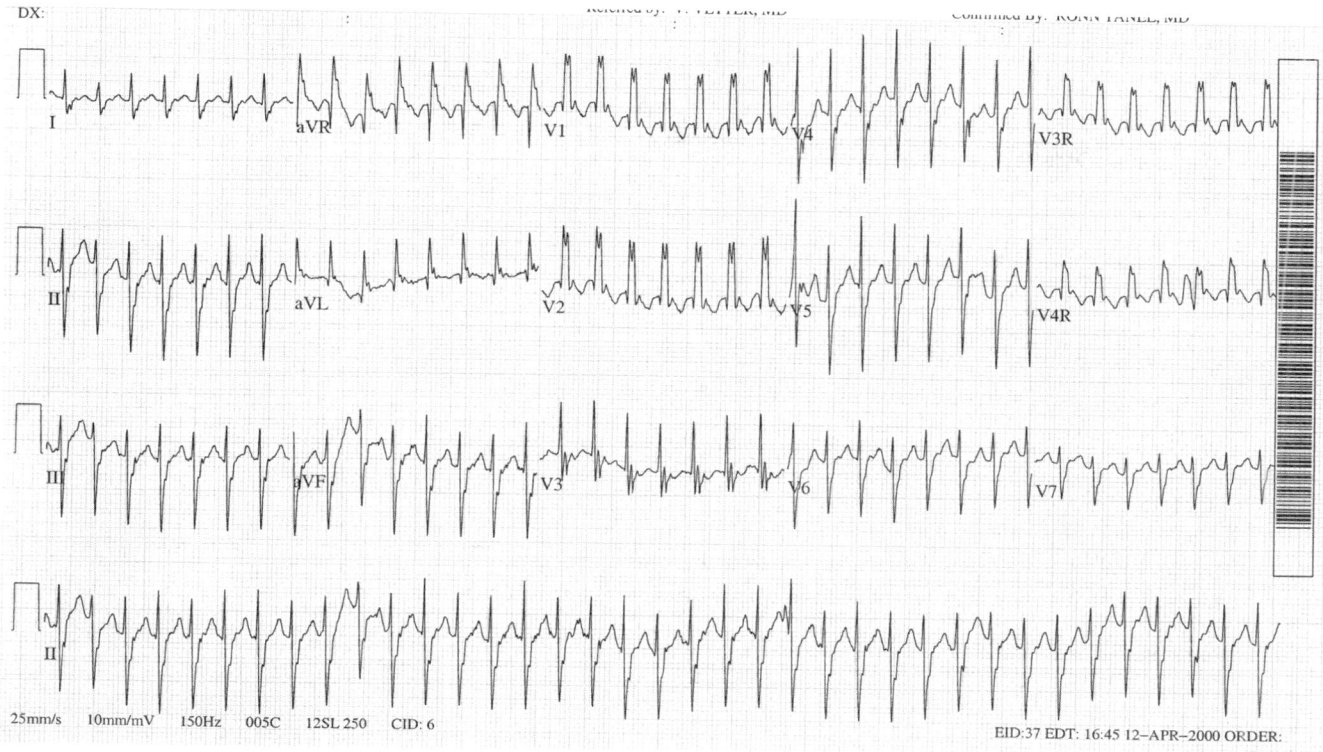

FIGURE 68.11. ECG from an infant with ventricular tachycardia.

procedures result in a prolonged QRS duration, usually with a right-bundle-branch block pattern, it is more difficult to determine the mechanism of a wide-complex tachycardia after congenital heart disease surgery.

During assessment of a wide-complex tachycardia, two important principles should be considered. The QRS complex should have a prolonged duration in VT, but this may be subtle in very young children, as normal measurements of the QRS duration vary with age (**Fig. 68.11**). In addition, VT typically has dissociation of the P waves and QRS complexes, with the QRS complexes occurring at a faster rate. However, children may have retrograde AV node conduction during VT, resulting in P waves (inverted) with a 1:1 relationship. If it is not possible to determine the P wave-to-QRS relationship by the surface ECG, recording the atrial activity with a transesophageal electrode catheter or temporary pacing lead placed at the time of cardiac surgery may be helpful. Other criteria used to evaluate wide-complex tachycardias in adults are often not helpful in children. Finally, symptoms and methods of terminating arrhythmias cannot definitively differentiate between supraventricular and VT since they are not specific. For example, rare types of VT can be sensitive to treatment with adenosine. The possible mechanisms of a wide-complex tachycardia are listed in **Table 68.1**.

The patient with a ventricular arrhythmia may be asymptomatic or may present with a cardiomyopathy or cardiac arrest. The patient may have prior history of heart disease, but VT may occur in a structurally normal heart. Ischemic heart disease, which is the basis for many of the ventricular arrhythmias noted in the adult population, is rare in pediatric patients. VT in pediatric patients may be associated with a prior surgical repair, myocarditis, cardiomyopathy of any cause, or primary

electrical disease. Some wide-complex rhythms may occur as a result of marked metabolic or pharmacologic effects on the normal conduction system. Although it is appropriate to manage a wide-complex rhythm as a ventricular arrhythmia, other noncardiac etiologies (i.e., hypoxia) should not be overlooked.

The mechanisms by which ventricular arrhythmias occur are the same as those that result in supraventricular arrhythmias: reentry, automaticity, and triggered automaticity. The patient should always be first evaluated clinically for signs of adequate perfusion and hemodynamic stability. If the situation allows, an ECG should be performed. ECG findings that should be noted during the evaluation of a wide-complex tachycardia are rate, variability of the R-R interval, QRS duration, QRS complex frontal plane axis, and QRS morphology (monomorphic versus polymorphic). The identification of characteristic features of certain types of VT may allow for more specific and directed therapy.

TABLE 68.1

MECHANISMS OF A WIDE QRS COMPLEX TACHYCARDIA

Orthodromic atrioventricular reciprocating tachycardia with aberration or bundle-branch block
Antidromic atrioventricular reciprocating tachycardia
Atrial tachycardia with bystander accessory pathway, allowing antegrade conduction (WPW)
Atrioventricular reciprocating tachycardia involving a Mahaim fiber
Ventricular tachycardia

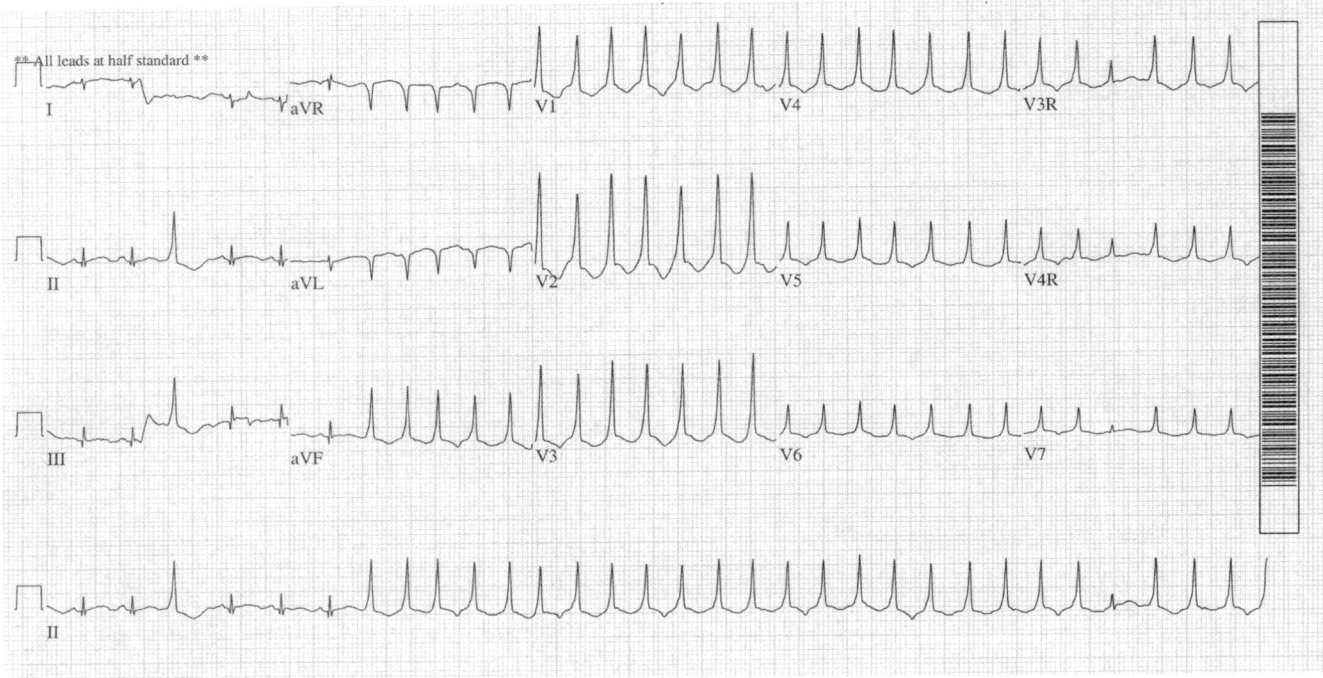

FIGURE 68.12. ECG from a newborn with accelerated ventricular rhythm.

Single, premature, ventricular complexes are not uncommon in children and are usually benign in the patient with a structurally normal heart (7,17), including patients who have ventricular ectopy in a pattern of bigeminy or trigeminy. Although these patterns may result in a relatively high frequency of ectopic beats, they need not be treated differently in the patient without underlying heart disease. On the other hand, the tenuous patient with complex congenital heart disease or a significant cardiomyopathy may be compromised by single, premature, ventricular complexes if ventricular filling is impaired. In this situation, an overall decrease in the number of perfusing beats may occur, which may be critical for a marginal patient. More importantly, this condition may be a harbinger of more serious dysrhythmias. The frequency, timing, and complexity of ventricular ectopy may help to predict the risk of future cardiac events in patients with underlying electrical or myocardial disease. Ventricular couplets may occur on rare occasion, but nonsustained and sustained runs of VT are unusual and generally pathologic.

Ventricular arrhythmias in the child or adolescent with a structurally and functionally normal heart are usually tolerated well. When a wide-complex tachycardia is irregular, occurs with a gradual onset and termination, and does not respond to cardioversion, an automatic mechanism should be suspected. The most common type of automatic ventricular arrhythmia in the structurally normal heart is that which arises from the right ventricular outflow tract, which may occur as single, premature, ventricular complexes, couplets, or runs of VT. The typical ECG pattern is that of a left-bundle-branch block morphology and inferior frontal plane axis. With a uniform QRS morphology and slower rate, the arrhythmia is frequently asymptomatic and is considered benign with respect to the risk of sudden cardiac events. The arrhythmia appears to arise from the ventricular conal septum, but a specific etiology has not been identified. If other cardiac disease can be excluded with certainty, the prognosis is excellent (19). Patients with a more incessant form of the arrhythmia that results in an elevated mean daily heart rate may be at risk for the development of a tachycardia-mediated cardiomyopathy. However, if the rate of the ventricular arrhythmia is <10% faster than the sinus rhythm rate, the rhythm is described as an accelerated ventricular rhythm (27) (**Fig. 68.12**). This rhythm is recognized in the newborn with a benign prognosis and usually results in spontaneous resolution of the arrhythmia substrate within the first year of life. Although automatic ventricular arrhythmias in the apparently structurally normal heart are generally benign, follow-up is indicated, as isolated instances of significant cardiac events have been reported (11) that probably represent a failure to identify underlying myocardial disease or other risk factors for sudden death (23).

Patients with an automatic VT may be treated with either medical therapy to suppress the focus or curative catheter-ablation therapy. The goal of medical therapy is to suppress the active focus or control the rate of the tachycardia. β blockers and verapamil may be very effective and have the benefit of being associated with a lower side-effect profile. Successful catheter-ablation therapy is performed with the arrhythmia focus usually located within the ventricular septum, which sometimes must be approached from the left ventricular side. However, indications for catheter ablation are not universal, especially in younger children, because many idiopathic ventricular arrhythmias in the structurally normal heart resolve spontaneously. Patients with a structurally normal heart can also develop a reentrant VT. Belhassen described an idiopathic left VT with a right-bundle-branch block pattern and superior frontal plane QRS axis (2) (**Fig. 68.13**). The arrhythmia is thought to be maintained by a reentry circuit involving one of the two fascicles of the left bundle (20,24). It is characteristically

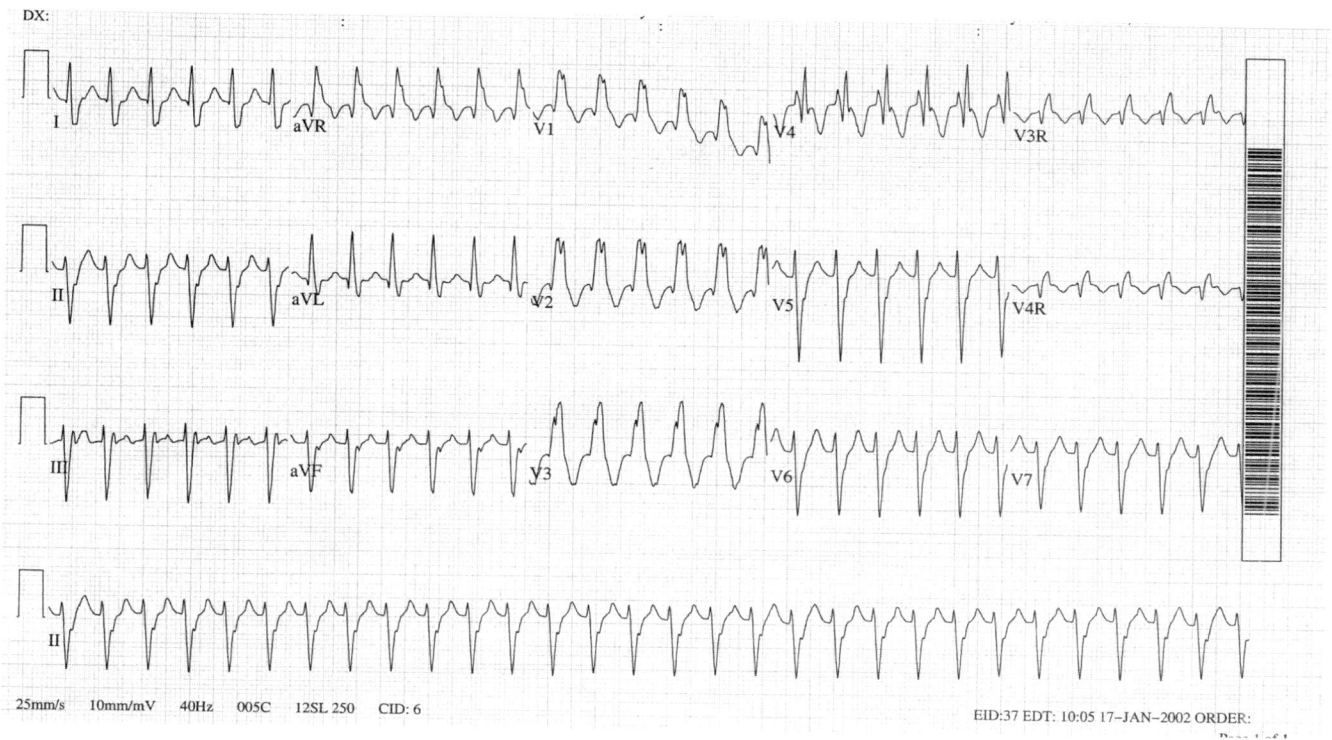

FIGURE 68.13. Idiopathic left ventricular tachycardia with a right-bundle-branch block and superior QRS frontal plane axis.

triggered by atrial or ventricular pacing and is particularly sensitive to treatment with verapamil or adenosine. This form of VT has been observed in children of all ages and is generally associated with an excellent long-term prognosis. If it does not resolve spontaneously or is refractory to medical therapy, the arrhythmia is amenable to catheter-ablation therapy.

In patients who have had prior surgical repair of congenital heart disease, a reentrant mechanism of VT is most commonly identified. The circuit typically occurs in those who have had a ventriculotomy as part of their surgical repair, but any anatomic scar or electrically abnormal area of myocardium may serve as a substrate. Surgical incisions and scar serve as a barrier around which the reentry circuit can travel. To effectively relieve the right ventricular outflow tract obstruction present in tetralogy of Fallot, the surgeon must almost always make a right ventricular outflow tract incision, augment the outflow tract region, and patch-repair the ventricular septal defect. An automatic mechanism can also occur at any ventricular site with enhanced excitability. Thus, the surgical procedures performed in these patients, in combination with long-term hemodynamic consequences, create a complex substrate for the development of arrhythmias.

The incidence of late sudden death after repair of tetralogy of Fallot has been reported to be ~6% (16). Extensive efforts have been made to identify patients with repaired tetralogy of Fallot who are at greatest risk for the development of VT and sudden death in follow-up. A number of demographic, hemodynamic, and electrophysiologic variables have been proposed as risk factors (**Table 68.2**), but the risk stratification of individual patients is still suboptimal. Programmed ventricular stimulation during an invasive electrophysiologic study has been used to help with risk stratification, although the prevalence of

inducible, sustained, monomorphic VT is high (13). This invasive tool appears to be of some diagnostic and prognostic value, but false-negative studies also occur at an unacceptably high rate (1). Although much of the assessment for sudden death in postoperative tetralogy of Fallot patients is focused on the cardiac rhythm, it is important to remember that electrophysiologic abnormalities are closely coupled to hemodynamic derangements. Therefore, anatomic and hemodynamic interventions may be as important as antiarrhythmic medications and devices in caring for these patients. Intracardiac electrophysiologic mapping of monomorphic VT in patients with repaired tetralogy of Fallot usually demonstrates a macro-reentrant circuit around the outflow tract patch or conal septum, which may be treated with catheter-ablation therapy (4).

TABLE 68.2

PROPOSED RISK FACTORS FOR VENTRICULAR TACHYCARDIA AND SUDDEN DEATH AFTER REPAIR OF TETRALOGY OF FALLOT

Late repair/older age at repair
Older age at follow-up/earlier surgical era
Prior systemic-to-pulmonary artery shunt
Transannular right ventricular outflow tract patch
Right ventricular pressure and/or volume overload
Residual ventricular septal defect
Ventricular arrhythmias
Atrial arrhythmias
Complete heart block
QRS duration >180 msecs

Patients with other cardiac lesions may also be at risk for ventricular arrhythmias. Patients enrolled in the Second Natural History study included those with aortic stenosis, pulmonary stenosis, and ventricular septal defect who had a higher frequency of premature ventricular complexes and higher-grade ventricular ectopy than the general population (31). Patients with aortic stenosis seem to be the highest risk group, with an increased mortality risk in patients with greater outflow tract gradients. Thus, all patients with repaired and unrepaired congenital heart disease should be considered at increased risk for ventricular arrhythmias and associated symptoms, including sudden death.

Arrhythmogenic right ventricular cardiomyopathy is another less common cause of VT in apparently healthy young people that is thought to be an under-recognized cause of sudden death. The pathologic findings may be subtle, and the patient frequently has a normal echocardiogram. The associated VT typically has the morphology of a left-bundle-branch block, as the arrhythmia generally arises form the right ventricular outflow tract. The baseline ECG is frequently normal. However, T-wave inversion in the right precordial leads, frequently a normal finding in pediatric patients, is sometimes observed. The QRS complex may be prolonged and characteristic low-voltage potentials (ε waves) may occur following the QRS complex. The cardiomyopathy involves aneurysmal dilatation and dyskinesis of the right ventricular outflow tract. Histologically, localized replacement or infiltration of with fibrous and adipose tissue is seen. Cardiac MRI has become the primary method of identifying the anatomic abnormalities. The diagnosis may be familial or sporadic, with molecular genetic studies showing that it is a disease of the cardiac desmosomes, resulting from defective cell adhesion proteins.

Patients with hypertrophic cardiomyopathy comprise another group with myocardial disease that is prone to ventricular arrhythmias. Left ventricular outflow tract obstruction may result in ventricular arrhythmias due to coronary artery insufficiency and myocardial ischemia. The histologic findings include disorganization of the cardiac muscle cells, which carries an arrhythmia potential itself. In fact, this microscopic finding seems to put patients at risk regardless of the degree of outflow-tract obstruction. Nonsustained VT is relatively common in adolescents with hypertrophic cardiomyopathy, but remains a poor marker of sudden death in pediatric patients. Other clinical risk factors include increased QRS duration, increased QT dispersion, myocardial bridging of the left coronary artery, ventricular wall thickness, exercise-induced hypotension, syncope, and family history of cardiac arrest.

Although cardiac tumors are rare, they are a source of ventricular arrhythmias with an automatic mechanism. Rhabdomyomas are the most common cardiac tumor in pediatric patients and are usually found in those with tuberous sclerosis. The tumors are usually multiple and are found in the ventricle and interventricular septum. Although many rhabdomyomas regress over time, young patients have been reported to die suddenly or develop congestive heart failure. Treatment of arrhythmias may include medications, catheter ablation, or surgical resection. Fibromas are usually single, large tumors of the ventricle that can be treated successfully with surgical resection. Hamartomas have been described as being associated with incessant VT in infants and have been treated with surgical resection and cryoablation in those refractory to medical therapy (32). However, if medical therapy results in successful arrhythmia suppression, the arrhythmia may spontaneously resolve over time.

Long-QT syndrome is due to one of several cardiac ion channelopathies and is associated with syncope, cardiac arrest, and sudden death. These symptoms are due to the polymorphic VT, torsades de pointes, that occurs as a result of a prolonged refractory period and increased "R-on-T" vulnerability. The electrical abnormality can occur as an inherited congenital problem or due to an acquired metabolic disturbance or medication exposure. As the presenting symptom can be that of a convulsion, all patients with a presumed seizure disorder should have a screening ECG. Other ECG findings include bradycardia, AV block, abnormal T-wave morphology, prominent U waves, and T-wave alternans. Other associations with the diagnosis are neurosensory hearing loss, Timothy syndrome, and Andersen syndrome. Although several genetic mutations have been recognized to cause long-QT syndrome, therapy continues to focus on the treatment and prevention of torsades de pointes. Effective therapies include pacing for bradycardia, isoproterenol infusion to avoid pause-dependent episodes of ventricular arrhythmia, lidocaine, magnesium, and β blockers. Long-term therapy is usually addressed with β blockers, mexiletine, pacemaker implantation, and consideration of implantable defibrillators. It is equally important to avoid cardiac stimulants and medications that are known to prolong the QT interval, such as some antiarrhythmic drugs, psychotropic medications, erythromycin, and many antifungal agents. It is important to screen family members, as the presenting symptom of long-QT syndrome may be a life-threatening arrhythmia.

Brugada syndrome is a familial, primary, electrical abnormality with ECG findings that consist of a right ventricular conduction delay and ST segment elevation in the anterior precordial leads (**Fig. 68.14**). Clinically, patients are young and present with syncope, ventricular arrhythmias, and sudden death. Several identified mutations affect the SCN5A gene, which encodes for the cardiac sodium channel. Some families do not have mutations in this gene, indicating that other genetic defects will be found, and that this is a genetically heterogeneous disease. Diagnostic testing includes a provocative drug challenge with a class I antiarrhythmic medication, which may reveal or enhance the characteristic ECG changes. The only effective treatment for Brugada syndrome is an implantable defibrillator. Catecholaminergic polymorphic VT has been associated with abnormalities in the cardiac ryanodine receptor, which is responsible for the release of calcium from the sarcoplasmic reticulum (12). It is thought that the increased calcium release is responsible for the development of arrhythmias. Patients develop polymorphic VT or bidirectional VT during exercise and other increased adrenergic states. β blockers and implantable defibrillators are the mainstay of therapy.

Polymorphic VT should be differentiated from monomorphic VT and is generally more poorly tolerated. Torsades de pointes (**Fig. 68.15**) is recognized by its characteristic pattern of positive and negative oscillations of the QRS complex around the isoelectric baseline, or "twisting of the points." It is a pause-dependent arrhythmia that is typically initiated by a premature ventricular complex that occurs during the vulnerable period of ventricular repolarization ("R-on-T phenomenon"). The arrhythmia is highly suggestive of the diagnosis of congenital or acquired long-QT syndrome. Causes for acquired long-QT syndrome should be considered, especially

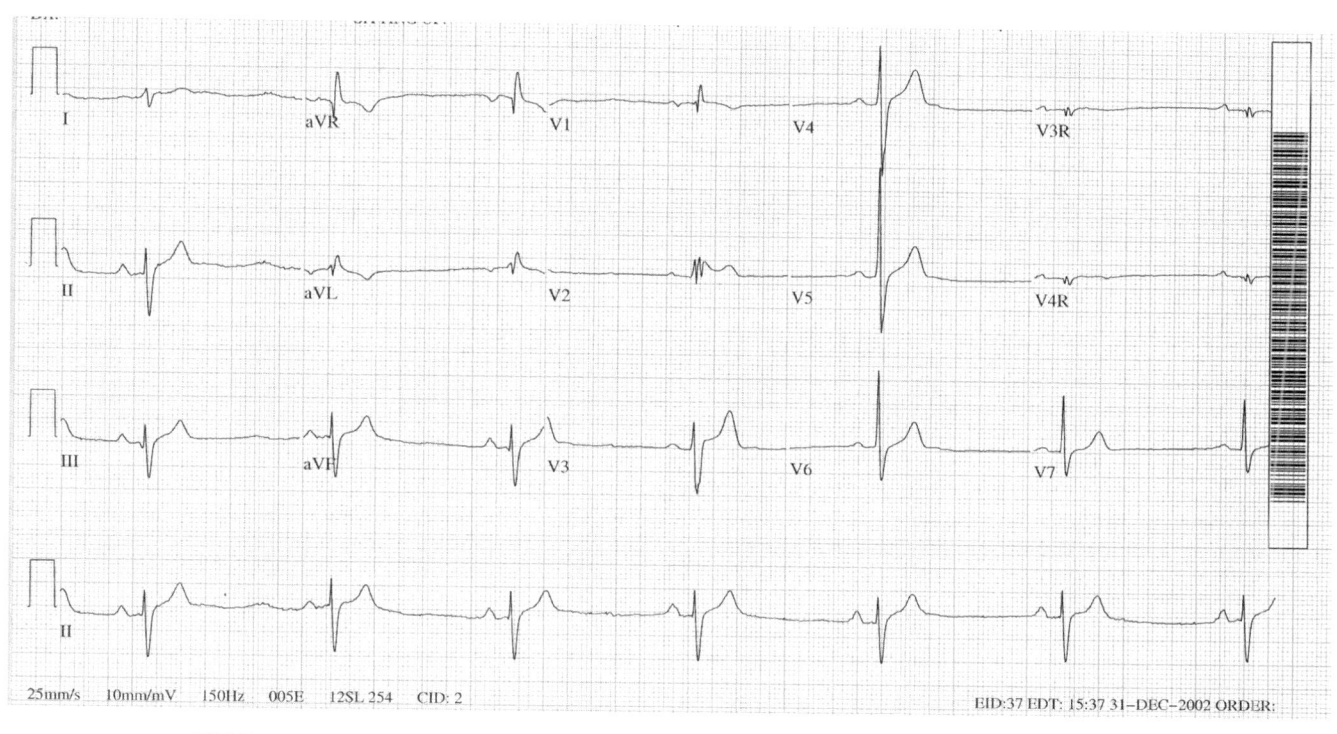

FIGURE 68.14. An ECG pattern observed in patients with Brugada syndrome. Note the right ventricular conduction delay and anterior precordial lead ST segment elevation.

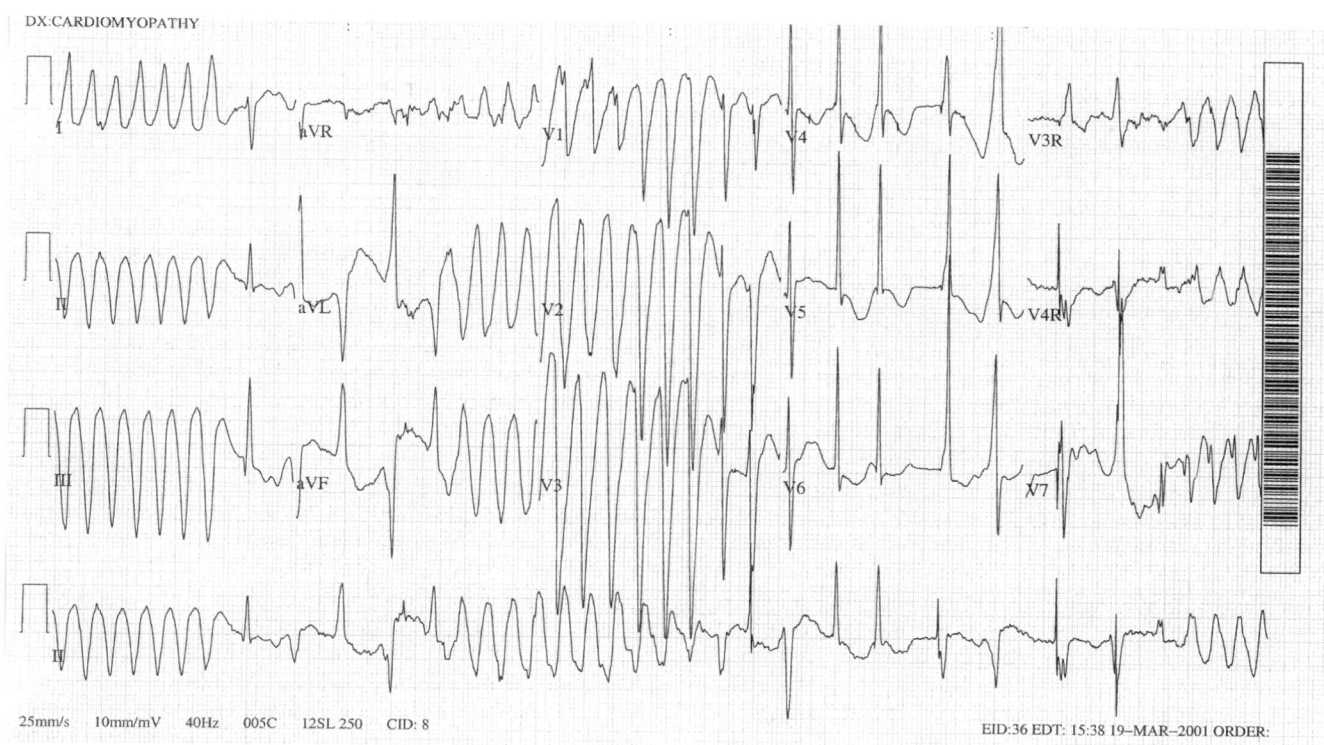

FIGURE 68.15. ECG showing torsades de pointes in a patient with long-QT syndrome.

QT-interval-prolonging drugs. Torsades de pointes should initially be treated with the withdrawal of any aggravating medications and correction of any metabolic abnormalities. Medical therapy should include magnesium supplementation, β blockers, and lidocaine. Although seemingly counterintuitive, isoproterenol may be beneficial by directly shortening myocardial repolarization times (21) and increasing the heart rate in order to avoid pause-dependent arrhythmias. Patients who experience sustained polymorphic VT with significant hemodynamic compromise despite maximal medical therapy may be candidates for circulatory support with extracorporeal membrane oxygenation. The arrhythmia must be reasonably controlled before the patient can be considered for an implantable defibrillator, as repeated therapies from a device could escalate arrhythmia activity. Bidirectional tachycardia, another type of polymorphic VT, is characterized by a beat-to-beat alternation of the QRS axis. Bidirectional VT is usually associated with digitalis toxicity or catecholamine-sensitive VT.

Ventricular arrhythmias may arise in several other specific and nonspecific situations. Any condition that can be associated with myocardial inflammation, ischemia, or infarction may result in an increased likelihood of ventricular arrhythmias. For example, myocarditis or a dilated cardiomyopathy of any cause can be associated with ventricular irritability. Coronary artery hypoperfusion, such as in Kawasaki disease or with an anomalous coronary artery, may manifest as a ventricular arrhythmia. Patients with pulmonary hypertension may be prone to the development of ventricular arrhythmias due to low cardiac output, coronary artery insufficiency, or a hypertensive right ventricle. Other patients frequently encountered in the ICU who may have an increased risk of ventricular arrhythmias include those with neuromuscular diseases and generalized myopathies, sepsis, and severe and long-standing hypertension.

Patients with neuromuscular diseases such as Duchenne muscular dystrophy seem to have more ectopy, as their skeletal muscle strength and myocardial contractility decrease. Patients with Becker muscular dystrophy do not appear to exhibit a similar correlation. Ventricular arrhythmias may occur in patients with myotonic dystrophy, another inherited disease, but this presentation does not usually occur until early adulthood. Rett syndrome is another neurologic disorder that is associated with sudden death. The diagnosis is usually made in school-aged and adolescent girls, who often have abnormalities of repolarization, including a prolonged QT interval, that seem to correlate with the severity of neurologic disease.

Wide-complex rhythms and ventricular arrhythmias are caused by an assortment of systemic causes (**Table 68.3**). Metabolic abnormalities can result in a wide-complex tachycardia. Hypoxia and metabolic acidosis can result in sinus tachycardia with delayed conduction through the His-Purkinje system. In addition, electrolyte abnormalities may have direct cellular effects on the myocardium that result in lengthening of the cardiac intervals. For example, hyperkalemia results in prolongation of the PR interval, QRS widening, and lengthening of the QT interval, with a terminal ECG that resembles a sinusoidal waveform (**Fig. 68.16**). Thus, for any critical care patient, the content of IV fluids, parenteral nutrition, and serum electrolytes should be carefully examined if ECG changes suggest an electrolyte abnormality. Physiologic causes of hyperkalemia include metabolic acidosis, such as in diabetic ketoacidosis or cellular death (as with bowel ischemia). The ECG changes seen with hyperkalemia respond promptly to imme-

TABLE 68.3

SYSTEMIC CAUSES OF VENTRICULAR ARRHYTHMIA

Metabolic	Hyperkalemia
	Hypokalemia
	Hypomagnesemia
	Hypocalcemia
	Hypoxia
	Acidosis
Ischemia	Kawasaki disease
Infectious	Systemic viral infections causing myocarditis
	Systemic bacterial infections causing endocarditis
Toxic	Cocaine/catecholamine infusions/stimulants
	Antiarrhythmic medications
	Digitalis toxicity
	Psychotropic medications
Traumatic	Commotio cordis
	Mechanical irritation/ central catheters

diate treatment with calcium, sodium bicarbonate, or glucose/insulin. Finally, drug overdoses (i.e., tricyclic antidepressants) may result in a wide-complex rhythm, some of which cause QRS-complex prolongation in association with tachycardia.

Medical management of acute ventricular arrhythmias is usually the first therapeutic option. A defibrillator should always be readily available in the event that the rhythm spontaneously deteriorates or responds adversely to the administration of a medication. Synchronized direct-current cardioversion may be used to treat a perfusing ventricular arrhythmia or a wide-complex arrhythmia with an organized electrical pattern. If the rhythm is pulseless or disorganized to the point that distinct QRS complexes cannot be recognized by the defibrillator, asynchronous defibrillation must be delivered immediately. Chronic therapy is warranted for most patients with spontaneous and sustained VT, unless a reversible and treatable cause is identified. The long-term medical treatment of VT generally involves careful follow-up and the suppression of any recurrences. The ultimate goal is to prevent potentially life-threatening events. Invasive electrophysiologic testing to exclude inducibility may be warranted in some patients and is probably the most accurate predictor of recurrence. However, sometimes the end-point of therapy is not easily determined, as aggressive treatment with some antiarrhythmic agents may result in more morbidity and mortality than the arrhythmia itself. Device therapy has become more commonly applied in children and is often necessary when symptoms are particularly concerning, significant risk factors exist, or the efficacy of medical therapy is in doubt.

In summary, ventricular arrhythmias are not uncommon in the PICU population and are more likely to be symptomatic if the tachycardia rate is very fast or if myocardial dysfunction is present. If the patient is relatively stable, medical attempts may be made to restore sinus rhythm after an ECG has been performed. Antiarrhythmic medications that affect the sodium and potassium channels of the ventricular myocardium, such as lidocaine, procainamide, sotalol, and amiodarone, may be most appropriate. Automatic and reentrant VT in both patients with and without congenital heart disease are amenable to treatment with catheter-ablation techniques. Finally, if patients

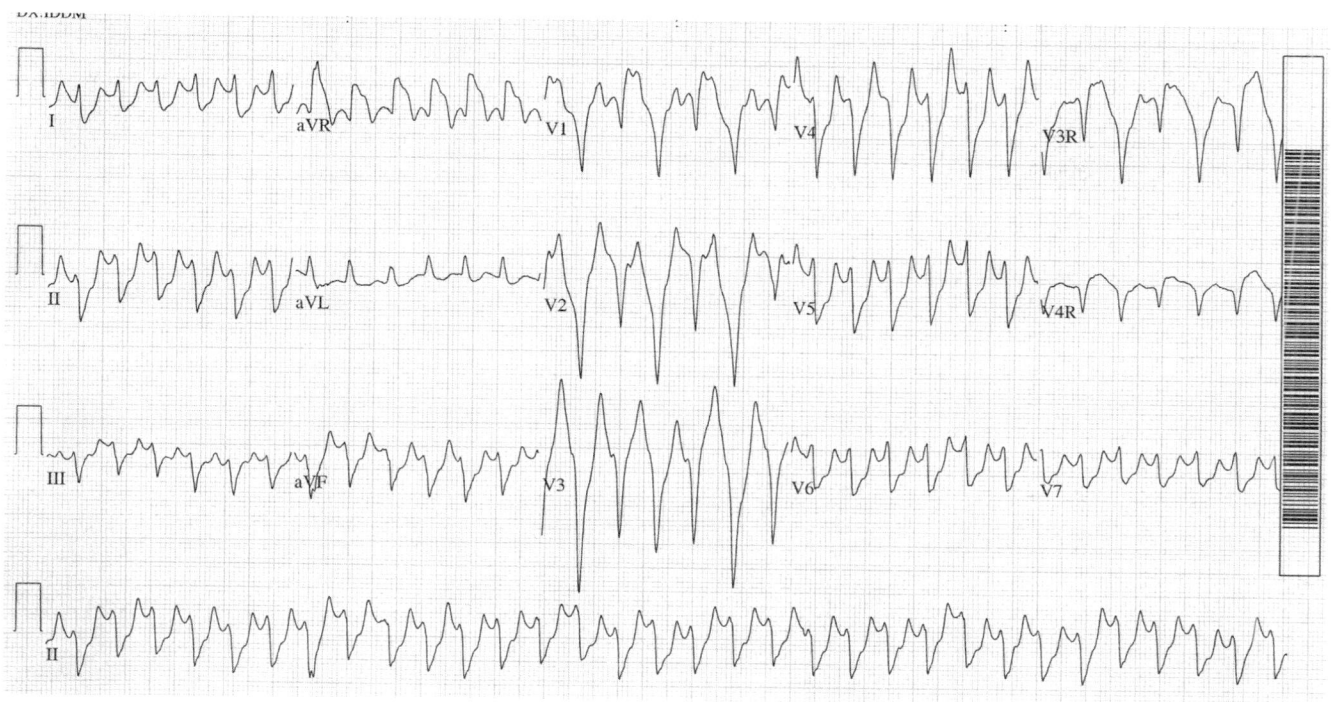

FIGURE 68.16. ECG findings observed with hyperkalemia.

are thought to be at significant risk for the development of life-threatening symptoms from VT, placement of an implantable defibrillator should be considered.

Bradyarrhythmias

Bradycardia due to SND may result in sinus bradycardia, junctional bradycardia, ectopic atrial bradycardia, and sinus pauses. Bradycardia may also be due to abnormalities of AV conduction, including first-, second-, or third-degree (complete) heart block. Second-degree heart block is further divided into Mobitz type I (Wenckebach), Mobitz type II, and fixed-ratio AV block. Sinus bradycardia may result from increased vagal tone, hypoxia, ischemia, central nervous system (CNS) disorders with increased intracranial pressure, hypothyroidism, hypothermia, drug intoxication (digoxin, β blockers, calcium-channel blockers), and prior atrial surgery. It is defined by heart rates <100 bpm in the neonate and <60 bpm in the older child. Sinus bradycardia may result in sinus pauses or escape rhythms, such as ectopic atrial bradycardia, junctional escape rhythm, or slow ventricular rhythm.

Sinus Node Dysfunction

The clinical manifestations of SND consist of pronounced sinus bradycardia, exercise-induced chronotropic incompetence, and sinus pauses (>2.5–3 secs while awake, dependent on age). When episodes of bradycardia are associated with SVT or atrial flutter or fibrillation, the situation is frequently referred to as "tachy-brady" syndrome. SND has intrinsic causes, including cardiomyopathy, myocarditis, trauma, ischemia, and infarction. A common cause of symptomatic SND in pediatric patients is prior surgery for congenital heart disease, especially the

atrial-switch operation, Fontan procedure, and repair of atrial septal defect. Extrinsic SND usually results from autonomic influences, such as neurally mediated syncope and carotid sinus hypersensitivity or cardioactive drugs. The assessment of sinus node function may involve an exercise stress test, ambulatory Holter monitor, pharmacologic challenge, or invasive electrophysiology test. Although medications have been used, the only reliable means by which to treat symptomatic SND is placement of an atrial pacemaker.

Abnormalities of Atrioventricular Conduction

Abnormalities of the AV conduction system can be described by the location of the block within the specialized conduction tissue (His bundle, AV node) or the pattern observed on the surface ECG. Clinically, it is useful to discuss these disorders based on the latter. First-degree heart block results from slowing of conduction at the level of the AV node and occasionally in the atrium or the His Purkinje system. It may be due to increased vagal tone, digoxin or β-blocker administration, viral myocarditis, Lyme disease, hypothermia, electrolyte abnormalities, congenital heart disease, rheumatic fever, or cardiomyopathy. First-degree AV block is characterized by PR-interval prolongation (**Fig. 68.17**). The rhythm is regular, originates in the sinus node, and has a normal QRS-complex morphology. First-degree AV block as an isolated event does not require investigation or treatment, but it may be the manifestation of an underlying disease state or conduction disturbance. Exclusion of higher-grade AV block may be indicated, depending on the clinical situation.

Second-degree heart block is the failure of an atrial impulse to traverse the AV node and infranodal conduction system and elicit a ventricular response. Mobitz type I, second-degree heart block, or Wenckebach, is defined by a progressive prolongation

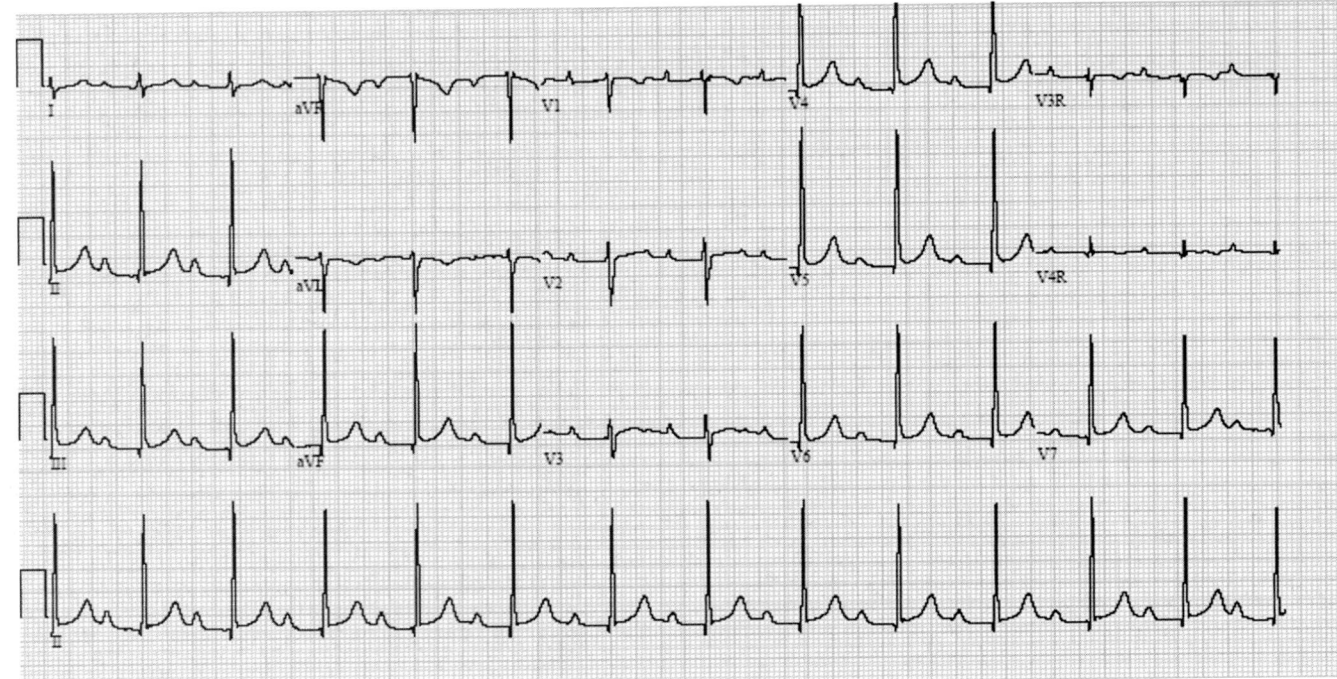

FIGURE 68.17. ECG showing first-degree AV block.

of the PR interval followed by a P wave that is not associated with a QRS complex (**Fig. 68.18**). The cycle may be repetitive and result in a pattern of periodicity. Mobitz type II, second-degree heart block is defined by intermittent loss of AV conduction without prior lengthening of the PR interval. This condition is always abnormal and may progress to complete heart block. High-grade second-degree heart block (frequent non-conducted P waves) can be associated with hemodynamic compromise and is treated with pacemaker implantation. Fixed-ratio AV block is a dysrhythmia in which sequential P waves have no subsequent QRS complex, and the repetitive nature results in a pattern of 2:1, 3:1, 4:1, etc., AV block. A normal PR interval with conducted beats is present. A slightly prolonged QRS complex may be seen. Fixed-ratio block results from either AV node or His-Purkinje disease, and intracardiac recordings are required to distinguish the site of injury. Patients may progress to complete heart block.

Third-degree heart block is the complete inability of an atrial impulse to be propagated to the ventricles. The ECG demonstrates AV dissociation (**Fig. 68.19**). The atrial rate is faster than the ventricular rate, and the atrial rhythm and rate

are normal for age. If an escape rhythm arises from the AV node (junctional rhythm), the QRS complex is narrow; however, if an escape rhythm arises from the distal His bundle or Purkinje fibers, the QRS complex is wide (idioventricular rhythm).

Complete heart block may be congenital or acquired. The incidence of congenital complete heart block has been estimated to be ~1 in 20,000 live births. Congenital complete heart block can be associated with L-transposition of the great arteries (congenitally corrected transposition of the great arteries), heterotaxy syndrome (left atrial isomerism), AV canal defect, or maternal systemic lupus erythematosus. Complete heart block due to maternal collagen vascular abnormality results from SS-A/Ro or SS-B/La antibodies crossing the placenta. Antibodies may cross the placenta as early as the sixteenth week of pregnancy. In over 60% of cases of congenital complete heart block, detectable autoantibodies can be found in the mother. The fetus and newborn with congenital complete heart block may develop hydrops fetalis. The spectrum of clinical symptoms depends on the ability of the ventricular rate to meet the patient's metabolic needs. The condition may first manifest during fetal life as persistent bradycardia or hydrops

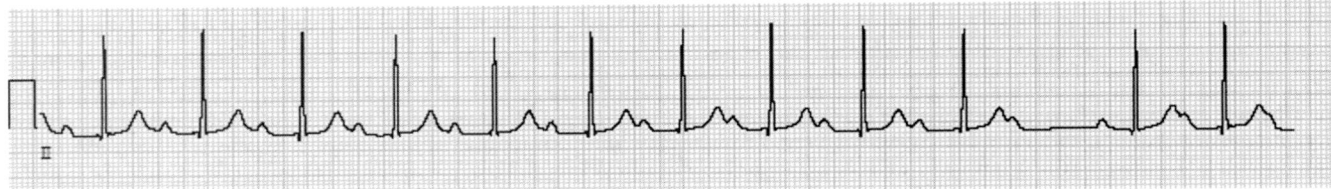

FIGURE 68.18. ECG showing second degree AV block, Mobitz type I, in a child. Note the progressive prolongation of the PR interval before the blocked P wave.

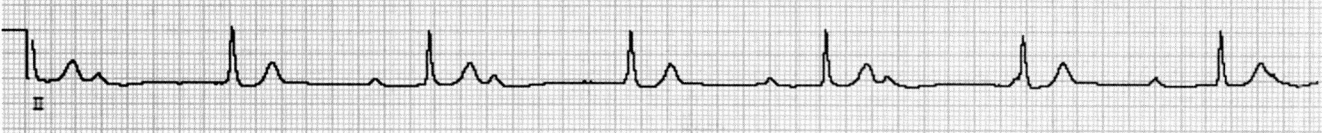

FIGURE 68.19. ECG showing complete heart block in an adolescent. Note the dissociation of the P waves and QRS complexes.

fetalis in severe cases. Postnatally, complete heart block may present with symptoms of reduced cardiac output and impaired exercise tolerance. A subset of patients may be at high risk for sudden death due to pause-dependent ventricular arrhythmias. The most common cause of transient and permanent acquired complete heart block is surgery near the AV node. Other causes of acquired complete heart block include cardiomyopathy and Lyme disease.

Treatment of Abnormalities of Atrioventricular Conduction

No intervention is necessary for sinus bradycardia if the cardiac output is maintained. Treatment for hemodynamically significant bradycardia is shown in **Table 68.4**. No treatment is necessary for first-degree or Mobitz type I second-degree heart block. Mobitz type II second-degree heart block, fixed-ratio AV block, and third-degree heart block are always pathologic and abnormal. It is most important to determine the appropriate time for referral for implantation of a permanent pacemaker. Some investigators have attempted to identify risk factors, instead of waiting for symptoms that may be dangerous and life-threatening.

If the child with complete heart block is hemodynamically unstable, transcutaneous or transvenous pacing can be performed acutely, and permanent transvenous or epicardial pacemaker placement can be performed later. Infants with congenital heart disease and complete heart block all require pacing, as the incidence of death in this group is as high as 29%. Patients with surgically acquired complete heart block are paced if the condition persists beyond the tenth postoperative day.

Third-degree heart block is managed with either ventricular-demand pacing or AV sequential pacing. In the fetus with maternal autoimmune disease, maternal treatment with corticos-

teroids and immunoglobulins has been attempted with varying degrees of success. Fetal hydrops should be treated with delivery of the baby if it is of a viable gestational age. Asymptomatic neonates and infants are usually paced if ventricular rates are below 55 bpm. Pacemaker implantation is recommended in an infant with congenital heart disease who has evidence of ventricular dysfunction, or if ventricular rates are <70 bpm. Severe bradycardia may be emergently treated with isoproterenol and temporary pacing. Older patients may be followed until they are symptomatic, develop very slow ventricular rates, have a wide-complex escape rhythm, or develop ventricular ectopy. Some patients with congenital complete heart block have ventricular dilatation and a clinical cardiomyopathy.

Principles of Temporary Pacing

Placement of temporary atrial and ventricular pacing wires is standard practice with most cardiothoracic surgical procedures that involve cardiopulmonary bypass. Temporary pacing wires are used for pacing patients with SND or AV block, recording atrial electrograms for diagnostic purposes, and overdrive pacing for termination of reentrant arrhythmias. Temporary pacemakers can be configured for either single- or dual-chamber pacing. Standard nomenclature is used to describe pacemaker function and programming. The first three letters of the program refer to the chamber paced, the chamber sensed, and the response to the sensed event, in that order (**Table 68.5**). The fourth and fifth letters refer to advanced programming options that are related to permanent implantable pacemakers with rate-responsive and antitachycardia features. Four types of pacemakers are available: asynchronous, single-chamber synchronous, double-chamber AV sequential, and programmable.

- Asynchronous or fixed-rate (AOO, VOO, DOO)—discharge is at a preset rate that is independent of the inherent heart rate.
- Single-chamber synchronous or demand (AAI, VVI)—discharge is at a preset rate only when the spontaneous heart rate drops below the preset rate.
- Dual-chamber AV sequential pacing (VDD, DVI, DDD)—usually uses two electrodes, one in the atrial appendage and one in the right ventricular apex. The atrium is stimulated to contract first; after an adjustable PR interval, the ventricle is stimulated.
- Programmable pacemakers—pacing rate, pulse duration, voltage output, and R-wave sensitivity are the most common programmable functions.

For instance, a VOO pacemaker paces the ventricle at the set rate with no regard to sensing, while a VVI pacemaker paces the ventricle, senses the ventricle, and inhibits pacing when an

---

TABLE 68.4

TREATMENT FOR HEMODYNAMICALLY SIGNIFICANT BRADYCARDIA

Trendelenburg position (supine with the head lower than the level of the pelvis and feet)
Volume expansion
Pharmacologic interventions
  Anticholinergic agents
    Atropine 0.02–0.04 mg/kg (maximum 1–2 mg)
  β-adrenergic agonists and activators of adenylate cyclase
    Isoproterenol infusion 0.01–2.0 mcg/kg/min
    Epinephrine IV bolus 0.01–0.5 mg/kg, infusion 0.1–
      0.5 mcg/kg/min
  Glucagon
Digoxin-specific antibody Fab fragments for digoxin toxicity
Temporary transcutaneous or transvenous pacing

TABLE 68.5

PACEMAKER CODES FROM THE NORTH AMERICAN SOCIETY OF PACING AND ELECTROPHYSIOLOGY AND BRITISH PACING AND ELECTROPHYSIOLOGY GROUP

Position 1	Position 2	Position 3
Chamber Paced	Chamber Sensed	Response to Sensed Event
O = none	O = none O	O = none
A = atrium	A = atrium	I = inhibited
V = ventricle	V = ventricle	T = triggered
D = dual (A + V)	D = dual (A + V)	D = dual (T + I)

The first two positions of this code are Chamber Paced and Chamber Sensed. The third position is described as follows:
D—(dual): In DDD pacemakers, atrial pacing is in the inhibited mode (the pacing device will emit an atrial pulse if the atrium does not contract). In DDD and VDD pacemakers, once an atrial event has occurred (whether paced or native), the device will ensure that an atrial event follows.
I—(inhibited): The device will pulse to the appropriate chamber, unless it detects intrinsic electrical activity. In the DDI program, AV synchrony is provided only when the atrial chamber is paced. On the other hand, if intrinsic atrial activity is present, no AV synchrony is provided by the pacemaker.
T—(triggered): Triggered mode is only used when the device is being tested. The pacing device will emit a pulse only in response to a sensed event.
Adapted from Miller RD. *Miller's Anesthesia, 6th ed*. Philadelphia: Elsevier, Inc., 2005.

intrinsic sensed ventricular event occurs, thus preventing an R-on-T phenomenon. A DDD pacemaker may pace the atrium, the ventricle, or both chambers, senses both chambers, and inhibits both the atrial and ventricular pacing chambers if an intrinsic sensed event occurs.

Mechanical contraction of the ventricles is most efficient when depolarization occurs down the normal conduction pathway of the His-Purkinje system with AV synchrony. The augmented preload as a result of atrial contraction at the end of ventricular diastole enhances cardiac output. For example, in patients with sinus bradycardia and intact AV conduction, atrial pacing is far more efficient than ventricular pacing alone due to important ventricular contractility mechanics and ventricular-ventricular interactions. Similarly, in patients with AV block, dual chamber pacing is superior to ventricular pacing alone due to the contribution of AV synchrony to the cardiac output.

Because temporary pacing wires deteriorate over a relatively short period of time, capture thresholds (the minimum amount of amperage required to depolarize the respective chamber of the heart) and sensitivity should be checked on a daily basis and the pacemaker output should be set to 2–3 times threshold value. If a child does not have a hemodynamically effective underlying rhythm and the pacing wires are deteriorating, new temporary pacing wires or implantation of a permanent pacemaker should be considered. Indications for permanent pacemaker implantation include SND, AV block, symptomatic hypervagal states, and long-QT syndrome with profound bradycardia and/or severe ventricular arrhythmias. Guidelines for pacemaker implantation are published by the American College of Cardiology, American Heart Association, and Heart Rhythm Society and are periodically updated, reflecting the current consensus opinion.

Antiarrhythmic Drugs

For children admitted to the PICU for arrhythmia and the initiation of antiarrhythmic drugs, five half-lives of the medication are required to achieve steady-state pharmacologic levels unless a loading dose is administered. During this time, families may be educated about the signs and symptoms of arrhythmia and how to appropriately dose the medication(s).

The antiarrhythmic drugs are distinguished by their effects on the two types of action potentials found in the cardiac tissues and on the autonomic nervous system. The fast-response action potential is rich with sodium channels and is found in atrial and ventricular myocytes, as well as in Purkinje fibers. The slow-response action potential is primarily mediated by the slow calcium channels and is present predominantly in the pacemaker regions of the heart (sinus node and the AV node).

The initial phase 0 of the fast-response action potential represents the rapid depolarization and results from the influx of sodium ions. The slope of the phase 0 depolarization influences the conduction velocity of cardiac tissue. Repolarization is the return of the action potential to the resting membrane potential and corresponds to phases 1 through 3, the width of the action potential. Repolarization results from inactivation of the inward sodium current and activation of the specialized potassium and calcium channels that direct current out of the cell. The period of repolarization determines the refractory period of the cardiac tissue (**Fig. 68.20**).

The Vaughn Williams classification of antiarrhythmic drugs, described in 1970, is based on pharmacologic effects on the types and phases of the cardiac-cell action potential. The drugs are categorized into four major groups, although many current medications have multiple (class) actions (**Table 68.6**).

Class I

The class I antiarrhythmic agents include a diverse group of medications that block the rapid sodium channel and delay the upstroke of the action potential, which results in lengthening of the QRS complex and QT interval. Because of the varying degrees of sodium-channel blockade and varying effects on the action-potential duration, the medications are further subclassified into subgroups IA, IB, and IC.

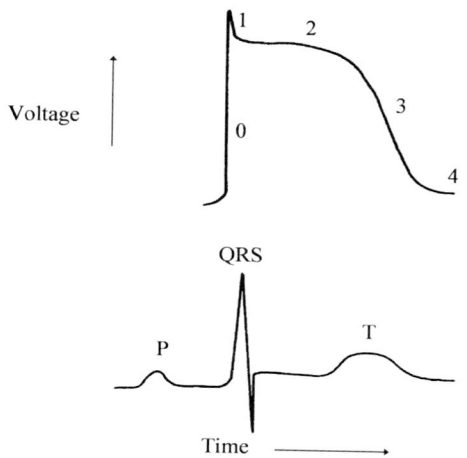

FIGURE 68.20. Fast-response cardiac-action potential and simultaneous correlation with surface ECG events. From Tanel RE, Levin MD. Pharmacologic Treatment of Heart Disease. In: Bell LM, Vetter VI, eds. *The Requisites in Pediatrics: Pediatric Cardiology.* Philadelphia: Elsevier Mosby, 2006:259, with permission.

Class IA. Class IA agents include procainamide, disopyramide, and quinidine. Medications in this group delay repolarization, resulting in slower conduction times and longer refractory periods. The class IA drugs are unique in their significant effects on the autonomic nervous system. Anticholinergic effects result in increased sinus node activity and more rapid AV node conduction. ECG changes that occur with this class of medications include widening of the QRS complex and prolongation of the QT interval. These medications are useful in treating atrial, ventricular, and AVRT. The class IA agents all carry a risk of proarrhythmia, with the aggravation of existing arrhythmias or the development of new atrial and ventricular arrhythmias, including torsades de pointes. As a result, some hesitate to use these drugs to treat arrhythmias in patients with structural heart disease or congestive heart failure.

Class IB. Medications in the class IB group include lidocaine, mexiletine, and phenytoin. These medications act by shortening the duration of the action potential. They are primarily used for treatment of ventricular arrhythmias. Lidocaine has

historically been used for the treatment of complex ventricular ectopy, VT, and ventricular fibrillation. It may also be useful for the emergent treatment of arrhythmias that occur in association with prolonged QT syndrome (torsades de pointes). Lidocaine has no significant effect on the autonomic nervous system and proarrhythmia is a rare adverse effect. Mexiletine is an oral medication that is used for chronic outpatient therapy in patients who are responsive to lidocaine.

Class IC. Class IC agents include flecainide, propafenone, and encainide. As with the class IA and class IB agents, these medications inhibit sodium channels in fast-response cells and have a profound depressant effect on conduction velocity, with little effect on the autonomic nervous system. As a whole, the group is used clinically to depress abnormal automaticity and prevent the induction of atrial muscle, ventricular muscle, and accessory pathway reentry circuits. The class IC agents have a relatively high potential for proarrhythmia. Proarrhythmia may lead to cardiac arrest and death, predominantly among patients with underlying heart disease (10,18).

Class II

Class II is designated for the β blockers, which include propranolol, esmolol, atenolol, nadolol, and carvedilol. These medications work by several mechanisms, primarily through competitive inhibition of the cardiac β-adrenergic receptor. By blocking endogenous catecholamines and decreasing sympathetic tone through an effect on the autonomic nervous system, the β blockers slow spontaneous discharge from the sinus node and abnormal automaticity from other cardiac tissues. In addition, AV nodal conduction is slowed. Direct cellular and membrane effects of the β blockers, seen with high chronic doses, include prolongation of the action-potential duration and an increase of the threshold for ventricular fibrillation. The medications are used to treat all arrhythmias of abnormal automaticity, especially those that are catecholamine driven. In addition, they may be used to treat reentry tachycardias by preventing the premature beats that act as initiating events or by affecting AV nodal conduction when that structure is part of the arrhythmia circuit. β blockers are an important part of the management of long-QT syndrome.

Many β blockers are currently available. Atenolol has more cardiac β-receptor selectivity, less CNS penetration, and a longer half-life. Nadolol requires less frequent dosing and has

TABLE 68.6

VAUGHN WILLIAMS'S CLASSIFICATION OF ANTIARRHYTHMIC DRUGS

Class	Effect	Drugs
I	Sodium-channel blockade	
Subclass IA		Procainamide, disopyramide, quinidine
Subclass IB		Lidocaine, mexiletine, phenytoin
Subclass IC		Flecainide, propafenone, encainide
II	β-adrenergic receptor blockade	Propranolol, esmolol, atenolol, nadolol, carvedilol
III	Potassium-channel blockade	Amiodarone, sotalol, bretylium
IV	Slow, inward, calcium-channel blockade	Verapamil, diltiazem, nifedipine
Other		Digoxin, adenosine

less penetration to the brain than other β blockers, making the incidence of CNS side effects low. Carvedilol and metoprolol have been approved in the US for the management of congestive heart failure in the adult population, but experience in pediatrics is limited. Patients with chronic congestive heart failure have increased sympathetic nervous system activity that is thought to be related to their clinical deterioration, and β-blocker therapy is thought to interfere with this debilitating neurohormonal pathway.

Class III

The class III agents include amiodarone, sotalol, and bretylium. By definition, class III antiarrhythmic agents prolong the action-potential duration through their actions primarily on potassium channels, with less of an effect on the phase 0 upstroke. These medications work primarily by prolonging the refractory period of myocardial tissue. Amiodarone and sotalol have additional effects on action-potential propagation and variable effects on the autonomic nervous system. Amiodarone is a potent antiarrhythmic agent that is usually reserved for the treatment of potentially life-threatening arrhythmias or arrhythmias that are refractory to other therapies. Amiodarone has been incorporated in advanced cardiac life support treatment algorithms after defibrillation and epinephrine for unstable VT or ventricular fibrillation (8,14). It is also the principal antiarrhythmic agent for junctional ectopic tachycardia. Sotalol is used in situations similar to those for amiodarone, but it has the advantage of a faster onset of action and a shorter duration of activity.

Amiodarone and sotalol are being used more commonly in pediatric practice, while bretylium has been removed from ACLS algorithms because of a high incidence of adverse events, the availability of safer agents, and its limited supply. Amiodarone has a number of serious noncardiac side effects that limit its long-term utility (e.g., nausea and emesis; photosensitivity; optic neuropathy and/or lens cataracts; hypothyroidism; pneumonitis; liver toxicity; neuropathy and neurocoordination issues, such as tremor and involuntary movements; poor coordination and gait abnormalities; and peripheral neuropathy). Many of these adverse effects are dose related, and may occur with greater frequency when there has been a higher total cumulative dose or longer duration of therapy. Cardiovascular side effects of amiodarone include diminished myocardial function, bradycardia, and in rare cases, proarrhythmia. Side effects of sotalol include proarrhythmia, including torsades de pointes, in 2%–4% of adult patients. Bretylium results in a biphasic norepinephrine response that can be associated with an initial worsening of arrhythmias.

Class IV

Class IV antiarrhythmic drugs are the calcium-channel blockers, specifically verapamil, diltiazem, and nifedipine. Of these, verapamil is used most frequently in pediatric practice for the treatment of arrhythmias. Verapamil and the other calcium-channel blockers block the slow, inward calcium current in slow-response cells of the sinus node and AV node. This cellular activity decreases sinus node automaticity, slows AV node conduction, and prolongs refractoriness, resulting in sinus bradycardia and prolongation of the PR interval. Verapamil is most valuable for the treatment of reentrant SVT that involves the AV node. It terminates the tachycardia by interrupting the reentrant circuit in the AV node. Verapamil should be avoided in

children <1 year of age based on reports of young infants who have responded to IV verapamil with cardiovascular collapse (9). Patients with WPW syndrome should not receive chronic verapamil therapy, as accessory pathway conduction may be enhanced while AV nodal conduction may be slowed, particularly during atrial tachycardias.

Diltiazem is frequently used for control of the ventricular rate during an atrial tachycardia by blocking conduction at the AV node. The calcium-channel blockers are widely used for long-term therapy of pulmonary hypertension, and nifedipine is preferred in those patients, as it has little effect on the sinus node, AV node, and cardiac contractility. Due to its potential for peripheral vasodilation, nifedipine is used for the acute management of hypertension.

Nonclassified Antiarrhythmic Medications

Digoxin. Digoxin is a cardiac glycoside that is useful for the treatment of both arrhythmias and congestive heart failure. Specifically, it is used to treat AVRT by blocking the AV node and interrupting the circuit. It is also used to achieve control of ventricular rate during an atrial tachycardia by blocking the response of the AV node to the atrial arrhythmia. Due to its ability to decrease automaticity, digoxin may be used for atrial tachycardia, atrial fibrillation, premature atrial complexes, and blocked premature atrial complexes. The mechanism of action is mediated by an increase in vagus nerve tone and decrease in sympathetic efferent activity. Cellular effects are due to binding of digoxin to sodium-potassium adenosine triphosphatase, which inhibits the sodium pump and ultimately increases intracellular calcium. Digoxin should not be used in patients with WPW syndrome due to its ability to block the AV node, shorten the accessory-pathway effective refractory period, and potentially enhance antegrade conduction across the accessory connection during an atrial tachycardia. Toxic concentrations can result in increased automaticity and triggered arrhythmias.

Digoxin toxicity can result in almost any type of arrhythmia, but the development of arrhythmias is generally a late indicator of toxicity. The ECG signs of digoxin toxicity are different in children as compared to adults. Infants more frequently present with sinus bradycardia and AV block. Older children also have bradyarrhythmias, but can also have atrial and junctional tachyarrhythmias. Pediatric patients, unlike adult patients, rarely develop ventricular tachyarrhythmias. For toxicity, the medication should be discontinued. Serum electrolyte abnormalities should be corrected, while atrial and ventricular arrhythmias can be treated with phenytoin or lidocaine. Atropine or a temporary pacemaker can be used to treat bradycardia or AV block. Digoxin-immune, antigen-binding Fab fragments are specific antibodies that may be used to bind digoxin and may be especially helpful in cases of potentially life-threatening toxicity.

Adenosine. Adenosine is an endogenous purine nucleoside that is useful for terminating SVT caused by a reentry mechanism. As adenosine blocks AV node conduction, it can be used to help differentiate between an AVRT and an automatic, ectopic, or reentrant atrial arrhythmia. It will terminate the reentrant circuit by abruptly blocking the AV node, but the atrial tachycardia will persist with block at the AV node, resulting in a ventricular response to the atrial arrhythmia of less than 1:1. The effects of adenosine are brief, as the drug is rapidly metabolized with a half-life of <10 secs. Caffeine and the methylxanthines cause competitive and reversible antagonism via the specific adenosine receptor, requiring higher doses of adenosine for clinical effect. Patients with orthotopic heart transplant have a denervation-induced supersensitivity to adenosine.

states, and long-QT syndrome with profound bradycardia and/or severe ventricular arrhythmias.

CONCLUSIONS AND FUTURE DIRECTIONS

Dysrhythmias due to a variety of mechanisms are frequently encountered in the critically ill pediatric patient. Both tachyarrhythmias and bradyarrhythmias may be due to intrinsic electrophysiologic abnormalities or may be the result of more systemic disease or iatrogenic treatments and procedures. It is important to have a systematic approach to the diagnosis and treatment of dysrhythmias, which includes knowledge of the possible mechanisms and available treatments. Only then will the acquisition of noninvasive and invasive ECG recordings be helpful in the management of these patients.

Current treatment options for dysrhythmias include electrical cardioversion, pharmacologic therapies, interventional procedures, and device implantation. These treatment strategies are the most likely areas of the field of dysrhythmia management to undergo significant change in the future. Medications have a role in the acute setting and are chronically used in patients who are not candidates for interventional therapies. The greatest opportunity for future research and development exists in the area of catheter-ablation therapy. New energy sources, catheter design, and modifications in the production of catheter-delivered lesions are all areas for potential improvement. Finally, implantable devices are almost constantly undergoing modification in an attempt to achieve functions that are as physiologic as possible. With these improvements, short- and long-term outcomes can be improved upon.

KEY POINTS

- The possible mechanisms of tachyarrhythmias are reentry, increased automaticity, and triggered activity.
- The most common dysrhythmia in children is SVT, specifically AVRT.
- The presenting symptoms of SVT are age dependent. Infants present with irritability, poor feeding, and possibly, signs of heart failure, while children present with complaints of palpitations, chest pain, nausea, and dizziness.
- Therapy for SVT is medical, with adenosine and/or synchronized cardioversion as first-line therapies. Digoxin or β blockers may also be used, as well as catheter ablation, in appropriate cases.
- Patients with WPW syndrome should never be chronically treated with digoxin or a calcium-channel blocker because these medicines enhance conduction through the accessory pathway.
- A wide-complex tachycardia should be considered VT until proven otherwise.
- Most symptomatic bradyarrhythmias are due to causes extrinsic to the specialized cardiac-conduction system, including conditions such as sepsis, drug overdose, intracranial lesions, and hypoxia.
- The general indications for pacemaker implantation in children include SND, AV block, symptomatic hypervagal

References

1. Alexander ME, Walsh EP, Saul JP, et al. Value of programmed ventricular stimulation in patients with congenital heart disease. *J Cardiovasc Electrophysiol* 1999;10:1033–44.
2. Belhassen B, Shapira I, Pelleg A, et al. Idiopathic recurrent sustained ventricular tachycardia responsive to verapamil: An ECG-electrophysiologic entity. *Am Heart J* 1984;108:1034–7.
3. Case CL. Diagnosis and treatment of pediatric arrhythmias. *Pediatr Clin North Am* 1999;46:347–54.
4. Chinushi M, Aizawa Y, Kitazawa H, et al. Successful radiofrequency catheter ablation for macro-reentrant ventricular tachycardias in a patient with tetralogy of Fallot after corrective surgery. *Pacing Clin Electrophysiol* 1995;18:1713–6.
5. Cohen MI, Wieand TS, Rhodes LA, et al. Electrophysiologic properties of the atrioventricular node in pediatric patients, *J Am Coll Cardiol* 1997;29:403–7.
6. Deal BJ, Keane JF, Gillette PC, et al. Wolff-Parkinson-White syndrome and supraventricular tachycardia during infancy: Management and follow-up. *J Am Coll Cardiol* 1985;5:130–5.
7. Dickinson DF, Scott O. Ambulatory electrocardiographic monitoring in 100 healthy teenage boys. *Br Heart J* 1984;51:179–83.
8. Dorian P, Cass D, Schwartz B, et al. Amiodarone as compared with lidocaine for shock-resistant ventricular fibrillation. *N Engl J Med* 2002;346:884–90.
9. Epstein ML, Kiel EA, Victorica BE. Cardiac decompensation following verapamil therapy in infants with supraventricular tachycardia. *Pediatrics* 1985;75:737–40.
10. Fish FA, Gillette PC, Benson DW, Jr. Proarrhythmia, cardiac arrest and death in young patients receiving encainide and flecainide. The Pediatric Electrophysiology Group. *J Am Coll Cardiol* 1991;18:356–65.
11. Garson A, Jr., Smith RT, Jr., Moak JP, et al. Incessant ventricular tachycardia in infants: Myocardial hamartomas and surgical cure. *J Am Coll Cardiol* 1987;10:619–26.
12. George CH, Higgs GV, Lai FA. Ryanodine receptor mutations associated with stress-induced ventricular tachycardia mediate increased calcium release in stimulated cardiomyocytes. *Circ Res* 2003;93:531–40.
13. Khairy P, Landzberg MJ, Gatzoulis MA, et al. Value of programmed ventricular stimulation after tetralogy of Fallot repair: a multicenter study. *Circulation* 2004;109:1994–2000.
14. Kudenchuk PJ, Cobb LA, Copass MK, et al. Amiodarone for resuscitation after out-of-hospital cardiac arrest due to ventricular fibrillation. *N Engl J Med* 1999;341:871–8.
15. Kugler JD, Danford DA, Houston KA, et al. Pediatric radiofrequency catheter ablation registry success, fluoroscopy time, and complication rate for supraventricular tachycardia: comparison of early and recent eras. *J Cardiovasc Electrophysiol* 2002;13:336–41.
16. Murphy JG, Gersh BJ, Mair DD, et al. Long-term outcome in patients undergoing surgical repair of tetralogy of Fallot. *N Engl J Med* 1993;329:593–9.
17. Nagashima M, Matsushima M, Ogawa A, et al. Cardiac arrhythmias in healthy children revealed by 24-hour ambulatory ECG monitoring. *Pediatr Cardiol* 1987;8:103–8.
18. Perry JC, Garson A, Jr. Flecainide acetate for treatment of tachyarrhythmias in children: Review of world literature on efficacy, safety, and dosing. *Am Heart J* 1992;124:1614–21.
19. Pfammatter JP, Paul T. Idiopathic ventricular tachycardia in infancy and childhood: A multicenter study on clinical profile and outcome. *J Am Coll Cardiol* 1999;33:2067–72.
20. Rodriguez LM, Smeets JL, Timmermans C, et al. Radiofrequency catheter ablation of idiopathic ventricular tachycardia originating in the anterior fascicle of the left bundle branch. *J Cardiovasc Electrophysiol* 1996;7:1211–6.
21. Sanguinetti MC, Jurkiewicz NK, Scott A, et al. Isoproterenol antagonizes prolongation of refractory period by the class III antiarrhythmic agent E-4031 in guinea pig myocytes. Mechanism of action. *Circ Res* 1991;68:77–84.
22. Stephenson EA, Casavant D, Tuzi J, et al. Efficacy of atrial anti-tachycardia pacing using the Medtronic AT500 pacemaker in patients with congenital heart disease. *Am J Cardiol* 2003;92:871–6.
23. Tada H, Ohe T, Yutani C, et al. Sudden death in a patient with apparent idiopathic ventricular tachycardia. *Jpn Circ J* 1996;60:133–6.
24. Thakur RK, Klein GJ, Sivaram CA, et al. Anatomic substrate for idiopathic left ventricular tachycardia. *Circulation* 1996;93:497–501.
25. Triedman JK, Saul JP, Weindling SN, et al. Radiofrequency ablation of intra-atrial reentrant tachycardia after surgical palliation of congenital heart disease, *Circulation* 1995;91:707–14.
26. Van Hare GF. Supraventricular tachycardia. In: Gillette PC, Garson A, eds. *Clinical Pediatric Arrhythmias*. Philadelphia: WB Saunders Company, 1999.
27. Van Hare GF, Stanger P. Ventricular tachycardia and accelerated ventricular rhythm presenting in the first month of life. *Am J Cardiol* 1991;67:42–5.

28. Vetter V. Arrhythmias. In: Moller JH, Hoffman JIE, eds. *Pediatric Cardio-vascular Medicine.* Philadelphia: Churchill Livingstone, 2000.

29. Villian E, Vetter VL, Garcia JM, et al. Evolving concepts in the management of congenital junctional ectopic tachycardia. *Circulation* 1990;81:1544–9.

30. Walsh EP, Saul JP, Sholler GF, et al. Evaluation of a staged treatment protocol for rapid automatic junctional tachycardia after operation for congenital heart disease, *J Am Coll Cardiol* 1997;29:1046–53.

31. Wolfe RR, Driscoll DJ, Gersony WM, et al. Arrhythmias in patients with valvar aortic stenosis, valvar pulmonary stenosis, and ventricular septal defect. Results of 24-hour ECG monitoring. *Circulation* 1993;87:I89–101.

32. Zeigler VL, Gillette PC, Crawford FA Jr. , et al. New approaches to treatment of incessant ventricular tachycardia in the very young. *J Am Coll Cardiol* 1990;16:681–5.

CHAPTER 69 ■ PREOPERATIVE CARE OF THE PEDIATRIC CARDIAC SURGICAL PATIENT

DAVID L. WESSEL • ALAIN FRAISSE

Among the causes of infant mortality in the US, congenital anomalies account for the largest diagnostic category (22). Structural heart disease leads the list of congenital malformations. Over 4 million children are born each year in the US, and nearly 40,000 of these have some form of congenital heart disease (CHD). Approximately half of these children appear for therapeutic intervention within the first year of life, the vast majority of whom require critical care expertise. Patients with congenital or acquired heart disease comprise a major diagnostic category for admissions to large PICUs across the country, comprising 30%–40% or more of ICU admissions in many centers.

In the past three decades, the development of surgical and catheter techniques for the diagnosis and treatment of critical heart disease in children has been paralleled by major advances in the field of intensive care. Increasingly, children with CHD are now managed in units specifically dedicated to pediatric intensive care or, in particular, pediatric *cardiac* intensive care (PCIC), rather than in surgical units that care primarily for adults following surgical management of acquired heart disease (4). Optimal care of these neonates, infants, and children requires an understanding of the subtleties of complex congenital cardiac anomalies, respiratory mechanics and physiology, the transitional circulation of the neonate, pharmacologic and mechanical support of the circulation, airway management, mechanical ventilation, treatment of multiorgan system failure, and the effects of cardiopulmonary bypass (CPB) on the heart, lungs, brain and abdominal organs.

Optimal preoperative care involves (a) initial stabilization, airway management, and establishment of vascular access; (b) a complete and thorough noninvasive delineation of the anatomic defect(s); (c) resuscitation with evaluation and treatment of secondary organ dysfunction, particularly the brain, kidneys, and liver; (d) cardiac catheterization if necessary—typically for physiologic assessment, interventional procedures such as balloon atrial septostomy or valvotomy, or anatomic definition not visible by echocardiography (e.g., coronary artery distribution in pulmonary atresia with intact ventricular septum or delineation of aorticopulmonary collaterals in tetralogy of Fallot with pulmonary atresia); and (e) surgical management when cardiac, pulmonary, renal, and central nervous systems are optimized. Crucial in this process is the continued communication among medical, surgical, and nursing disciplines.

Reliable tools or methods for preoperative risk stratification in pediatric cardiac surgery are essential to fully inform patients and their family, to compare institutions fairly, and to improve postoperative care in PCIC. Risk assessment is difficult and often requires collaboration between experienced clinicians and statisticians. Several scoring systems and biologic markers have been developed for predicting outcome and guiding perioperative therapy in pediatric cardiac ICUs (CICUs). Because of the complexity of congenital heart surgery, they have their inherent limitations. However, they share the common goal of the continued improvement in the quality of surgery and perioperative care of patients with CHD.

PATIENT DEMOGRAPHICS

Expanding the scope of reparative operations to the newborn and premature newborn has altered the demographic makeup of cardiac patients scheduled for surgery and admitted to the ICU. Admissions per year to a 24-bed CICU that is typical of other large American CICUs are shown in **Figure 69.1**. Half of the admissions were among patients <1 year of age, and in 2004, 23% of admissions were newborns. However, because of the complexity of illness among newborns, added diagnostic time preoperatively, and longer postoperative lengths of stay, the newborn population comprises nearly 50% of patient days. Nearly every other bed space is occupied by a newborn patient with heart disease. Thus, our clinical focus during the past two decades of cardiac intensive care has been on primary corrective surgery early in life (3).

MULTIDISCIPLINARY CARE

In addition to the important role of the surgeon in postoperative management, care is provided by those with expertise in critical care, including anesthetic principles, cardiac anatomy, and cardiac physiology. Moreover, clinicians must be versed both in the care of the neonate and premature neonate with CHD, and in the care of the adult with CHD, as these adult patients are often referred by their cardiologists back to a PCIC-based program. As few individuals can be expected to have such broad training (from newborn medicine through internal medicine), the challenge has been to develop truly multidisciplinary teams with leadership that can draw upon the expertise of many.

NEWBORN CONSIDERATIONS

Care of the critically ill neonate requires an appreciation of the special structural and functional features of immature organs, the interactions of the "transitional" neonatal circulation, and the secondary effects of the congenital heart lesion on other

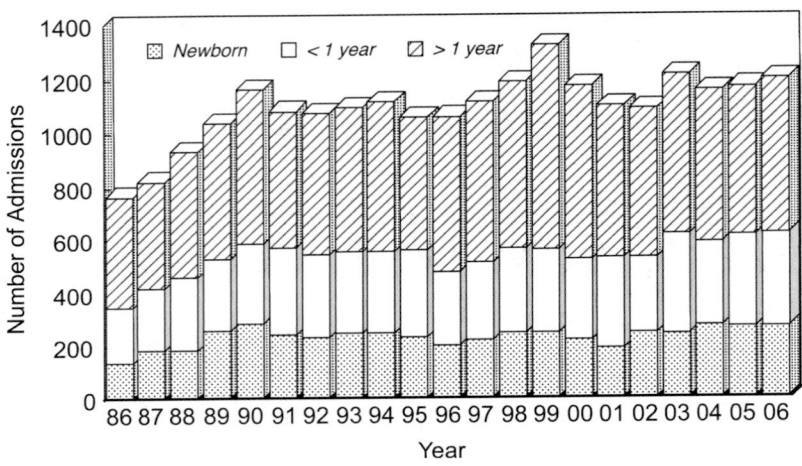

FIGURE 69.1. Number of annual admissions to the cardiac ICU at Children's Hospital Boston totals nearly 1200. It is typical of most pediatric cardiac ICUs that almost 25% of admissions are newborns; half are <1 year of age. Newborns account for 40%–50% of patient days.

organ systems (9,14,15,37,45). The neonate appears to respond more quickly and profoundly to physiologically stressful circumstances, which may be expressed in terms of rapid changes in pH, lactic acid, glucose, and temperature. Neonates have diminished fat and carbohydrate reserves. The higher metabolic rate and oxygen consumption of the neonate account for the rapid appearance of hypoxia when these patients become apneic. Immaturity of the liver and kidney may be associated with reduced protein synthesis and glomerular filtration, such that drug metabolism is altered and hepatic synthetic function is reduced. These issues may be compounded by the normally increased total body water of the neonate compared to the older patient, along with the propensity of the capillary system of the neonate to leak fluid from the intravascular space. This condition is especially prominent in the lung of the neonate, where the pulmonary vascular bed is nearly fully recruited at rest, and the lymphatic recruitment required to handle increased mean capillary pressures associated with increases in pulmonary blood flow may be unavailable (9,37). The neonatal myocardium is less compliant, less tolerant of increases in afterload, and less responsive to increases in preload than that of the older child. Younger age also predisposes the myocardium to the adverse effects of CPB and hypothermic ischemia implicit in surgical-support techniques utilized for reparative operations. These factors do not preclude intervention in the neonate but simply dictate that extraordinary vigilance be applied to the care of these children and that intensive care management plans emerge to account for the immature physiology.

The observed benefits of neonatal reparative operations in patients with two ventricles are numerous (**Table 69.1**). They will continue to dictate that care of the newborn with complex CHD after CPB is a central feature of cardiac intensive

care. Elimination of cyanosis and congestive heart failure early in life will optimize conditions for normal growth and development. Palliative procedures such as pulmonary artery bands and systemic-to-pulmonary artery shunts may not fully address cyanosis or congestive heart failure and may introduce their own set of physiologic and anatomic complications. Some examples of improved outcomes with a single reparative operation rather than staged palliation in a newborn are well known, supported by published literature, and evoke little controversy. Approaches that have been abandoned include banding the pulmonary arteries in truncus arteriosus (23), staging repair of type B interrupted aortic arch (34), and staging repair rather than single-session repair of transposition of the great arteries with interrupted aortic arch (40). In other conditions (such as the severely cyanotic newborn with tetralogy of Fallot), the risk and benefit of neonatal repair versus a palliative shunt are still debated (18).

Whereas the neonate may be more labile than the older child, many examples also exist of the enhanced neonatal resilience to metabolic or ischemic injury. In fact, the neonate may be particularly capable of coping with some forms of stress. Tolerance of hypoxia in the neonate is characteristic of many species (10), and the plasticity of the neurologic system in the neonate is well known. In neonates with transposition of the great arteries, severe hypoxemia that is sometimes associated with hemodynamic instability prior to balloon atrial septostomy may result in brain injury that is clinically unsuspected (36). Neonates with obstructive left heart lesions often present with profound metabolic acidosis but can be effectively resuscitated without persistent organ system impairment or sequelae as the rule rather than the exception. The pliability and mobility of vascular structures in the neonate improve the technical aspects of surgery. Reparative operations in neonates take best advantage of normal postnatal changes, allowing more normal growth and development in crucial areas such as myocardial muscle, pulmonary parenchyma, and coronary and pulmonary angiogenesis. Neonatal repair may obviate irreversible secondary organ damage arising from unrepaired or palliative approaches. Postoperative pulmonary hypertensive events are less common in the newborn and more common in the infant who has been exposed to weeks or months of high pulmonary pressure and flow (6,23), which seems especially true for such lesions as truncus arteriosus, complete atrioventricular canal defects, and transposition of the great arteries with

TABLE 69.1

ADVANTAGES OF NEONATAL REPAIR

Early elimination of cyanosis
Early elimination of congestive heart failure
Optimal circulation for growth and development
Reduced anatomic distortion from palliative procedures
Reduced hospital admissions while awaiting repair
Reduced parental anxiety while awaiting repair

ventricular septal defects. Finally, cognitive and psychomotor abnormalities associated with months of hypoxemia or abnormal hemodynamics may be diminished or eliminated by early repair. However, if early reparative surgery results in more exposures to CPB (e.g., repeated conduit changes), which may be associated with cognitive impairment or subtle adverse effects on motor function, then the risk-benefit assessment of early repair must be modified accordingly.

At most centers, the approach to neonates with CHD has been toward complete surgical correction rather than palliation in order to avoid the pathophysiologic consequences and limits on neonatal growth (3). This concept has been extended to include the premature newborns who now as a group are admitted to the CICU prior to surgical correction. One in ten newborns is premature. Despite improvements in ventilation, widespread use of surfactant, and prenatal administration of glucocorticoids, infants who are <30 weeks of gestation carry a significant risk of developing bronchopulmonary dysplasia. The coexistence of CHD and bronchopulmonary dysplasia may worsen the clinical course as a result of elevated pulmonary vascular resistance (PVR). Hence, palliative medical or surgical interventions were often preferred management options in premature infants with CHD. However, current experience with increased mortality after palliative surgery (35) supports the notion that early biventricular repair can be achieved with low mortality (44).

PREOPERATIVE MANAGEMENT AND CARE

Successful critical care management of patients with CHD is based on complete, accurate preoperative assessment and adequate preoperative patient preparation. The clinical and laboratory information routinely available preoperatively should be frequently reassessed and integrated with information from continuous monitoring during surgery and the immediate recovery phase. The perioperative team must be cognizant of the physical and laboratory findings that are of particular importance for CHD. Involvement by the intensivist in the preoperative preparation and early postoperative management provides a perspective on the pathophysiology that improves perioperative care.

Physical Examination and Laboratory Data

A complete history and physical examination are required, and when such information is obtained, attention should be directed to the extent of cardiopulmonary impairment, airway abnormalities, and associated extracardiac congenital anomalies (20,21). Upper and lower airway problems in patients with Down syndrome, calcium and immunologic deficiencies in patients with aortic arch abnormalities, and renal abnormalities in patients with esophageal atresia and CHD are a few of the associated congenital abnormalities with which the intraoperative team should be familiar. Intercurrent pulmonary infection is a common and significant finding in chronically overcirculated lungs. The presence, degree, and duration of hypoxemia are important details that, in the absence of iron deficiency, are reflected in a raised hematocrit. The nadir of physiologic anemia during infancy may contribute to left-to-right shunting by

| TABLE 69.2 |

TEN INTENSIVE CARE STRATEGIES TO DIAGNOSE AND SUPPORT LOW CARDIAC OUTPUT STATES

1. Know the cardiac anatomy in detail and its physiologic consequences.
2. Understand the specialized considerations of the newborn and implications of reparative rather than palliative surgery.
3. Diversify personnel to include expertise in neonatal and adult congenital heart disease.
4. Monitor, measure, and image the heart to rule out residual disease as a cause of postoperative hemodynamic instability or low cardiac output.
5. Maintain aortic perfusion and improve the contractile state.
6. Optimize preload (including atrial shunting).
7. Reduce afterload.
8. Control heart rate, rhythm, and synchrony.
9. Optimize heart-lung interactions.
10. Provide mechanical support when needed.

decreasing the relative PVR (32). Ten key features required to identify and treat low cardiac output states in the perioperative period are described in **Table 69.2**.

Chest radiography shows heart size, pulmonary vascular congestion, airway compression, and areas of consolidation or atelectasis. The electrocardiogram may reveal rhythm disturbances and demonstrate ventricular strain patterns (ST- and T-wave changes) characteristic of pathologic pressure or volume burdens on the ventricles. Electrolyte abnormalities caused by congestive heart failure and forced diuresis must also be evaluated preoperatively. Severe hypochloremic metabolic alkalosis may occur in some patients. It may be important to discontinue digoxin preoperatively and to avoid hyperventilation and administration of calcium to these patients during induction of anesthesia and preparation for the operating room. The alkalotic, hypokalemic, hypercalcemic, hypotensive, dilated, digoxin-bound myocardium fibrillates with ease.

Echocardiographic and Doppler Assessment

Advances in echocardiographic imaging have had an enormous impact on the diagnosis of CHD. Accurate anatomic diagnosis is now routine in children, without the need for cardiac catheterization. Echocardiography is the preferred imaging modality for assessment of intracardiac anatomic features in young children. However, the intensivist should be aware of the current limitations of echocardiographic and Doppler techniques so that alternative diagnoses can be considered when intraoperative or postoperative findings are inconsistent with the working echocardiographic diagnosis.

Skilled echocardiographers accurately interpret the alignment of cardiac chambers and great vessels but cannot always visualize an atrial septal defect or ventricular septal defect, although color flow-mapping techniques have vastly improved diagnostic capabilities. An atrial septal defect can be indirectly inferred from right ventricular volume overload and interventricular septal shift. Distal pulmonary artery architecture and conduits between a ventricle and a great artery are poorly imaged by echocardiography, and pressure gradients in these areas are not always measurable with Doppler techniques. Evaluation of atrioventricular valve regurgitation may be subjective and nonquantitative. Accuracy of echocardiographic diagnosis is limited by an inadequate window for imaging in the obese patient, the older child, and some postoperative patients. Techniques for three-dimensional echocardiography are available that may improve diagnostic capabilities, such as defining the mechanism of valve regurgitation.

Doppler measurements add greatly to noninvasive diagnostic capabilities. Measurements of pressure gradients across semilunar valves and other obstructions are frequently accurate but may not always correlate with peak systolic ejection gradients measured at catheterization. As good as echocardiographic diagnosis of anatomic defects and Doppler measurements of pressure gradients and valve function have become, the standard for assessment of physiology when other clinical information is ambiguous or contradictory remains cardiac catheterization.

Evaluation of left and right ventricular function in children with CHD is an essential component of the preoperative assessment. Quantitative assessment for left ventricular ejection fraction and shortening fraction is usually made by geometric modeling of the left ventricle, using the Simpson rule. However, this mathematical assumption can lead to markedly inaccurate estimations of ventricular volumes and dynamics. Moreover, the complex geometry of the right ventricle makes this a challenging task and necessitates the use of alternative methods. Developments in echocardiographic techniques, which use two-dimensional echocardiography, Doppler echocardiography, tissue Doppler imaging, and strain rate imaging, have enhanced our ability to accurately assess ventricular function. Doppler techniques offer unique advantages for left and right ventricular function, in that they are independent of geometry and relatively independent of loading conditions (13,49).

Cardiac Catheterization

When echocardiographic analysis with Doppler measurements and color flow mapping is complete and unambiguous, preoperative assessment may no longer require cardiac catheterization. Catheterization is not typically performed before infant or neonatal operations for ventricular septal defects, complete atrioventricular canal defects, tetralogy of Fallot, interrupted aortic arch, hypoplastic left heart syndrome, or coarctation of the aorta. However, in older patients with complex anatomy (e.g., a single ventricle), physiologic data from catheterization may be essential. This technique allows description of the direction, magnitude, and approximate location of intracardiac shunts. Intracardiac and intravascular pressures are measured to determine the presence of obstructions and whether shunt orifices are restrictive or nonrestrictive. Pressure gradients across sites of obstruction must be considered in light of simultaneous blood flow; a small pressure gradient measured at a time of low cardiac output is misleading.

Normally, oxygen saturation does not significantly change from vena cava to pulmonary artery. In the child with CHD, the superior vena cava gives the best indication of true Svo_2; an increase ("step-up") in saturation of $\geq5\%$ downstream from the superior vena cava suggests the presence of a left-to-right shunt (12), which would occur at the level of the right atrium with an atrial septal defect, in the right ventricle with a ventricular septal defect, and in the pulmonary artery with a patent ductus arteriosus. The magnitude of the left-to-right shunt can be calculated from the Fick equation (see Chapter 65). The oxygen consumption of the patient is usually measured by direct calorimetry, as are the saturation values, but subsequent flow and resistance calculations can be in error. The frequently used term Q_p/Q_s (pulmonary-to-systemic blood flow ratio) can be derived simply from the measured oxygen saturation values.

The patient whose aortic blood is fully saturated can be safely assumed to have no significant right-to-left shunting. However, when a right-to-left shunt is present, aortic blood is hypoxemic. Blood samples should also be obtained from the pulmonary veins, left atrium, and left ventricle for oxygen saturation determination and ascertainment of the source of desaturated blood. Pulmonary venous desaturation implies a pulmonary source of venous admixture (e.g., pneumonia, atelectasis, or other pulmonary disease). Intrapulmonary shunting may substantially alter the perioperative plan and the postoperative ventilatory requirements of the patient.

In the presence of a left-to-right shunt and elevated PVR, pressure and saturation measurements are often repeated, with the patient breathing 100% oxygen and/or inhaled nitric oxide to assess both the reactivity of the pulmonary vascular bed and any contribution of ventilation-perfusion abnormalities to hypoxemia. If breathing 100% oxygen increases pulmonary blood flow and dramatically increases Q_p/Q_s (with a fall in PVR), potentially reversible processes such as hypoxic pulmonary vasoconstriction are probably contributing to the elevated PVR. The patient with a high, unresponsive PVR and a small left-to-right shunt despite a large shunt orifice may have extensive pulmonary vascular damage from irreversible obstructive pulmonary vascular disease. If so, surgical repair is usually contraindicated (41).

During cardiac catheterization, anatomic abnormalities are identified angiographically. Special, angled views provide specific information about the location and extent of congenital defects (2,8). Ventricular function is assessed angiographically and physiologically (e.g., by pressure measurements). The calculated size of a cardiac chamber may have an important bearing on its ability to support the circulation of a child with hypoplastic ventricles.

Magnetic Resonance Imaging and Angiography

Following the development of electrocardiogram-gated MRI, MRI and MR angiography have emerged as important diagnostic modalities in the evaluation of the cardiovascular system. Image acquisition is triggered to the patient's electrocardiogram to counter motion artifacts and to acquire cine sequences that allow imaging of cardiac structures and visualization of blood flow throughout the cardiac cycle. In addition to providing excellent anatomic and three-dimensional images, particularly of the pulmonary veins and thoracic aorta, it is also possible with MR angiography to qualitatively assess valve and ventricular function and to quantify flow, ventricular volume, mass, and ejection fraction (5,17). While ferromagnetic implants near the region of interest might produce artifact, sternal wires and vascular clips produce relatively minor disturbances and therefore MRI can be performed in patients who have undergone previous cardiac surgery. Contraindications include patients with pacemakers, recently implanted endovascular or intracardiac implants, and aneurysm clips on vessels that will be exposed directly to the magnetic field. When MRI is contraindicated or when breath holds cannot be achieved easily in young, nonsedated children, CT scanning with three-dimensional imaging is an interesting alternative in the morphologic assessment of congenital cardiac anomalies. The radiation exposure can be reduced by decreasing the kilovoltage (30).

Assessment of Patient Status and Predominant Pathophysiology

Frequently, congenital heart defects are complex and can be difficult to categorize or conceptualize. Rather than trying to determine the management for each individual anatomic defect, a physiologic approach can be taken. The following questions should be asked:

1. How does the systemic venous return reach the systemic arterial circulation to maintain cardiac output? What intracardiac mixing, shunting, or outflow obstruction exists?
2. Is the circulation in series or parallel? Are the defects amenable to a two-ventricle or single-ventricle repair?
3. Is pulmonary blood flow increased or decreased?
4. Is there a volume load or pressure load on the ventricles?

Appropriate organization of preoperative patient data, preparation of the patient, and decisions about monitoring, anesthetic agents, postoperative care, sedation, and ventilations are best accomplished by focusing on a few major pathophysiologic problems, beginning with whether the patient is cyanotic, in congestive heart failure, or both. Most pathophysiologic mechanisms in the patient's disease that are pertinent to the perioperative plan and to optimal preparation of the patient will focus on one of the following major problems: severe hypoxemia, excessive pulmonary blood flow, congestive heart failure, obstruction of blood flow from the left heart, or poor ventricular function. Although some patients with CHD present with only one problem, many have multiple, interrelated problems.

Severe Hypoxemia

Many of the cyanotic forms of CHD present in the ICU with severe hypoxemia (PaO_2 <50 mm Hg) during the first few days of life, but without respiratory distress. Infusion of prostaglandin E_1 (PGE_1) in patients with decreased pulmonary blood flow maintains or reestablishes pulmonary flow through the ductus arteriosus, which may also improve mixing of venous and arterial blood at the atrial level in patients with transposition of the great arteries (11). Consequently, neonates rarely require surgery while they are severely hypoxemic. During preoperative preparation with PGE_1, neurologic examination and blood chemistry analysis of renal, hepatic, and hematologic function are necessary to assess the effects of severe hypoxemia during or after birth on end-organ dysfunction.

Cyanotic patients who present for surgery after infancy require adequate preoperative and postoperative hydration to prevent the thrombotic problems caused by their high hematocrits. The perioperative team should prepare for significant coagulopathy in the cyanotic patient. Premedication must be given cautiously to avoid causing hypoventilation in these patients.

PGE_1 dilates the ductus arteriosus of the neonate with life-threatening ductus-dependent cardiac lesions and improves the patient's condition before surgery. PGE_1 can reopen a functionally closed ductus arteriosus for several days after birth, or it can maintain patency of the ductus arteriosus for an extended period (11,50). The common side effects of PGE_1 infusion—apnea, hypotension, fever, excitation of the central nervous system—are easily managed in the neonate when normal therapeutic doses of the drug (0.02–0.05 mcg/kg/min) are used (31). However, as PGE_1 is a potent vasodilator, intravascular volume frequently requires augmentation. Patients with intermittent apnea resulting from administration of PGE_1 may require mechanical ventilation preoperatively.

PGE_1 usually improves the arterial oxygenation of hypoxemic neonates who have poor pulmonary perfusion due to obstructed pulmonary flow (critical pulmonic stenosis or pulmonary atresia). By providing pulmonary blood flow from the aorta via the ductus arteriosus, an infusion of PGE_1 improves oxygenation and stabilizes the condition of neonates with these lesions. The improved oxygenation reverses the lactic acidosis that may have developed during episodes of severe hypoxia. PGE_1 administration for 24 hrs usually markedly improves the condition of a severely hypoxemic neonate with restricted pulmonary blood flow (7).

Neonates with transposition of the great arteries must have adequate mixing of oxygenated and deoxygenated blood at the atrial level to achieve appropriate oxygen delivery. To accomplish this, balloon atrial septostomy has been applied for over 40 years to create or enlarge an interatrial septal defect (43), using echocardiographic guidance in most patients. Hence, balloon atrial septostomy is often performed at the patient's bedside rather than in the catheterization laboratory. It may also be of considerable value in creating an atrial septal defect in any neonate with left atrial obstruction such as hypoplastic left heart syndrome with intact atrial septum. For such patients, fenestration of the atrial septum with an intra-atrial stent is sometimes necessary to maintain patency (19).

Excessive Pulmonary Blood Flow

Excessive pulmonary blood flow is frequently the primary problem of patients with CHD. The intensivist must carefully evaluate the hemodynamic and respiratory impact of a left-to-right shunt and the extent to which it contributes to the perioperative course in the ICU. Children with left-to-right shunts may have chronic low-grade pulmonary infection and congestion that cannot be eliminated despite optimal preoperative preparation. If so, surgery should not be postponed further. Respiratory syncytial virus infections are particularly prevalent in this population, but improvements in intensive care have markedly improved outcome with this and other viral pneumonias (38).

Aside from the respiratory impairment caused by increased pulmonary blood flow, the left heart must dilate to accept pulmonary venous return that is several times normal. If the body requires more systemic blood flow, the heart responds inefficiently. Most of the increment in cardiac output is recirculated to the lungs. Eventually, symptoms of congestive heart failure appear.

Children with failing hearts increase endogenous cate-cholamine production and redistribute cardiac output to fa-vored organs by their increased heart rate and decreased ex-tremity perfusion (47). In the most severe cases, the evaluation reveals a child whose body weight is below the third percentile for age and who is tachypneic, tachycardic, and dusky in room air. The child may have intercostal and substernal retractions and skin that is cool to the touch. Capillary refill may be pro-longed. Expiratory wheezes are usually audible. Medical man-agement with digoxin, vasodilators, and diuretics may improve the patient's condition, but the diuretics may induce a profound hypochloremic alkalosis and potassium depletion, which may persist after surgery.

These clinical signs and symptoms suggest that profound pathophysiologic alterations have occurred. This informa-tion, combined with the anatomic description from the two-dimensional echocardiogram and the physiologic data from cardiac catheterization, permits accurate assessment of the severity of the illness and formulation of an anesthetic plan, a surgical or catheter intervention, and a predictable postoper-ative course.

Obstruction of Left Heart Outflow

Patients who require surgery to relieve obstruction to outflow from the left heart are among the most critically ill children for whom the intensivist must care. These lesions include interrup-tion of the aortic arch, coarctation of the aorta, aortic stenosis, and mitral stenosis or atresia as part of the hypoplastic left heart syndrome (see later discussion). These neonates present with in-adequate systemic perfusion and profound metabolic acidosis. The initial pH may be below 7.0 despite a low $PaCO_2$. Systemic blood flow is largely or completely dependent on blood flow into the aorta from the ductus arteriosus.

Ductal closure in the neonate with these problems causes dramatic worsening of the patient's condition. The patient be-comes critically ill or even moribund and requires PGE_1 in-fusion (see above) for survival. PGE_1 allows blood flow into the aorta from the pulmonary artery because it maintains the patency of the ductus arteriosus (7,26,39), thus creating a systemic circulation in the neonate that depends on right ventricular contractile function and ductal patency. Acidosis, metabolic derangements, and renal failure arise if systemic per-fusion is inadequate. PGE_1 infusion restores perfusion and aer-obic metabolism such that surgery can be deferred until the patient's condition improves. In addition to PGE_1 infusion, other supportive measures include ventilatory and inotropic support, as well as correction of metabolic acidosis, hypo-glycemia, hypocalcemia, and other electrolyte abnormalities. The stabilization period also allows assessment of the magni-tude of end-organ dysfunction caused by the preceding period of inadequate systemic perfusion. Adequacy of resuscitation, rather than severity of illness at presentation, appears to influ-ence postoperative outcome (25).

Ventricular Dysfunction

Ideally, the intensivist should participate in the presentation of all preoperative patients who have a planned admission to the ICU, thereby providing an opportunity to understand the extent of ventricular dysfunction preoperatively and provid-ing considerable insight into intraoperative and postoperative events. Although patients with large shunts may have com-plete mixing of systemic and venous blood and only mild-to-

moderate hypoxemia as a result of their excessive pulmonary blood flow, the price paid for near-normal arterial oxygen sat-uration is chronic ventricular dilation and dysfunction as well as pulmonary vascular obstructive disease. Consequently, nar-rowing the shunt or a staged approach to single-ventricle re-pair may be indicated before any other elective surgery can be undertaken. Older patients with CHD and poor ventricu-lar function due to chronic ventricular volume overload (aortic or mitral valve regurgitation or long-standing pulmonary-to-systemic arterial shunts) present a different problem, which may be amenable to afterload reduction to some extent. How-ever, in all of these circumstances, when the heart is dilated and volume overloaded, a propensity for ventricular fibrillation during sedation, anesthesia, and/or intubation of the airway is seen.

Assessment should include an estimation of the patient's functional limitation as an indicator of myocardial perfor-mance and reserve, quantification of the degree of hypoxia and the amount of pulmonary blood flow, and evaluation of PVR. For patients with increased Q_p/Q_s, systemic blood flow should be optimized prior to and during induction of anesthesia but without further augmenting pulmonary blood flow. However, during maintenance and emergence from anesthesia, retraction of the lung, positional changes, and abdominal distension may increase the hypoxemia and compromise the function of a di-lated, poorly contractile ventricle. If this sequence occurs dur-ing surgery, the management must be altered to improve pul-monary blood flow.

In addition, systolic function of the ventricle may be im-paired by intrinsic myopathic abnormalities related to drug toxicity (e.g., Adriamycin), inborn enzyme deficiencies, or ac-quired inflammatory or infectious disease. Patients with such dilated cardiomyopathies require optimization of ventricular performance, with emphasis on inotropic support and after-load reduction. At many centers, these patients are admitted to the ICU for inotropic support and optimization of hemo-dynamic state prior to a planned surgical intervention. The evidence supporting this practice is not well established in chil-dren.

Preoperative Management of Patients with a Single Ventricle

Single-ventricle Anatomy and Physiology

For a variety of anatomic lesions, the systemic and pulmonary circulations are in parallel, with a single ventricle effectively supplying both systemic and pulmonary blood flow. The rela-tive proportion of the ventricular output to either pulmonary or systemic vascular bed is determined by the relative resistance to flow in the two circuits. The pulmonary artery and aortic oxygen saturations are equal, with mixing of the systemic and pulmonary venous return within a "common" atrium. Assum-ing adequate mixing with normal cardiac output and normal pulmonary venous oxygen saturation, an SaO_2 of 80%–85% with an SvO_2 of 60%–65% indicates a Q_p/Q_s of ~1 and hence a balance between systemic and pulmonary flows. Although "balanced," the single ventricle is still required to receive and eject twice the normal amount of blood: one part to the pul-monary circulation and one part to the systemic circulation. A Q_p/Q_s of >1 implies an intolerable volume burden on the heart. While each of the defects associated with single-ventricle physiology involves specific management issues, they all share common management considerations in balancing flow and augmenting systemic perfusion.

Preoperative Management

Changes in PVR have a significant impact on systemic perfusion and circulatory stability, especially preoperatively, when the ductus arteriosus is widely patent. In preparation for surgery, it is important that systemic and pulmonary blood flow be as well balanced as possible to prevent excessive volume overload and ventricular dysfunction that reduces systemic and end-organ perfusion. For example, a newborn with hypoplastic left heart syndrome who has an arterial oxygen saturation of >90%, tachypnea, oliguria, cool extremities, hepatomegaly, and metabolic acidosis has severely limited systemic blood flow. Even though ventricular output is increased, the blood flow that is inefficiently partitioned back to the lungs is unavailable to the other vital organs. Immediate interventions are necessary to prevent imminent circulatory collapse and end-organ injury. In this "over circulated" state, PVR is falling as it should in the normal postnatal state, and the ductus arteriosus is maintained widely patent with prostaglandin infusion to permit unrestricted blood flow from the single right ventricle across the ductus to the systemic bed. Blood flow manipulation of mechanical ventilation and inotrope support may temporarily stabilize the patient (see later discussion), but surgery should not be delayed. Often, the newborn's spontaneous, unassisted ventilatory pattern provides a more stable cardiorespiratory condition than the injudicious use of positive-pressure ventilation and excessive use of vasoactive agents.

Similarly, in a patient with pulmonary atresia and an intact ventricular septum, for example, pulmonary blood flow depends on left ventricular contractile function and ductal patency. As PVR falls, pulmonary blood flow will be excessive and will eventually steal from the systemic circulation. Preoperative management should focus on an assessment of the balance between pulmonary (Q_p) and systemic flow (Q_s), which is best achieved by a thorough and continuous reevaluation of clinical examination for cardiac output state and perfusion, an evaluation of chest radiograph for cardiac size and pulmonary congestion, imaging with echocardiography to assess ventricular function and atrioventricular valve competence, and a review of laboratory data for alterations in gas exchange, acid-base status, and end-organ function. A central venous line positioned in the proximal superior vena cava may be useful to monitor volume status and sample for mixed venous oxygen saturation as a surrogate of cardiac output and oxygen delivery. Central venous lines are not necessary in all circumstances; they may have significant complications in small newborns and do not substitute for clinical examination.

Initial resuscitation involves maintaining patency of the ductus arteriosus with a PGE_1 infusion at a rate of 0.02–0.05 mcg/kg/min. Intubation and mechanical ventilation are not necessary in all patients. Patients are usually tachypneic, but provided the work of breathing is not excessive and systemic perfusion is maintained without a metabolic acidosis, spontaneous ventilation is often preferable to achieve an adequate systemic perfusion and balance of Q_p and Q_s. A mild metabolic acidosis and low bicarbonate level may be present, but this may

not specifically indicate poor perfusion and lactic acidosis. If the presentation involved circulatory collapse and end-organ dysfunction, then a period of days may be required to establish stability and return of vital organ function prior to surgery.

Patients require intubation and mechanical ventilation due to apnea secondary to PGE_1 or the presence of a low cardiac output state, or for manipulation of gas exchange to assist balancing pulmonary and systemic flows. An SaO_2 of >90% indicates pulmonary overcirculation, i.e., Q_p/Q_s >1.0. PVR can be increased with controlled mechanical hypoventilation to induce a respiratory acidosis, often necessitating sedation and neuromuscular blockade, and with a low FIO_2 to induce alveolar hypoxia. Ventilation in room air may suffice, but occasionally a hypoxic gas mixture is necessary and is achieved by adding nitrogen to the inspired gas mixture, thereby reducing the FIO_2 to 0.17–0.19. While these maneuvers are often successful in increasing PVR and reducing pulmonary blood flow, it is important to remember that these patients have limited oxygen reserve and may desaturate suddenly and precipitously. Controlled hypoventilation in effect reduces the functional residual capacity and, therefore, oxygen reserve, which is further reduced by the use of a hypoxic inspired gas mixture. An alternate strategy is to add carbon dioxide to the inspiratory limb of the breathing circuit, which will also increase PVR; however, because an hypoxic gas mixture is not used, systemic oxygen delivery is maintained (42,46). In practice, manipulating inspired gas concentrations is rarely needed in the current era. Patients who have continued pulmonary overcirculation with high SaO_2 and reduced systemic perfusion despite these maneuvers require early surgical intervention to control pulmonary blood flow. At the time of surgery, a snare may be placed around either branch pulmonary artery to effectively limit pulmonary blood flow.

Decreased pulmonary blood flow in preoperative patients with a parallel circulation is reflected by hypoxemia with an SaO_2 of <75%. Preoperatively this may be due to restricted flow across a small ductus arteriosus, increased PVR secondary to parenchymal lung disease, or increased pulmonary venous pressure secondary to obstructed pulmonary venous drainage or a restrictive atrial septal defect. Sedation, paralysis, and manipulation of mechanical ventilation to maintain an alkalosis may be effective if PVR is elevated. Nitric oxide may also be used in this situation as a specific pulmonary vasodilator. Systemic oxygen delivery is maintained by improving cardiac output with inotropes and maintaining the hematocrit at >40%. Among some newborns with hypoplastic left heart syndrome, pulmonary blood flow may be insufficient because the mitral valve hypoplasia in combination with the occasional finding of a restrictive or nearly intact atrial septum severely restricts pulmonary venous return to the heart. The newborn is intensely cyanotic and has a pulmonary venous congestion pattern on chest x-ray. Urgent interventional cardiac catheterization with balloon septostomy or dilation (or stent placement) of a restrictive atrial septal defect may be necessary (1,48). Immediate surgical intervention and palliation may be preferred at some centers.

Systemic perfusion is maintained with the use of volume and vasoactive agents. Inotropic support is often necessary because of ventricular dysfunction secondary to shock states associated with a closing ductus arteriosus at the time of presentation. Systemic afterload reduction with agents such as phosphodiesterase inhibitors (e.g., milrinone) may improve systemic perfusion and reduce atrioventricular valve regurgitation in volume-loaded hearts. However, milrinone may also decrease PVR and thus not fully address the imbalance of pulmonary and systemic flows. Oliguria and a rising serum creatinine level may reflect renal insufficiency from a low cardiac output. Necrotizing enterocolitis is a risk secondary to splanchnic hypoperfusion, and the authors prefer not to enterally feed newborns with a wide pulse width and low diastolic pressure (usually <30 mm Hg) prior to surgery, especially in the context of obstructive left heart lesions. It is important to evaluate end-organ perfusion and function, and optimize the patient's condition prior to surgery.

RISK STRATIFICATION IN PEDIATRIC CARDIAC SURGERY

Because the field congenital heart surgery encompasses ~200 diagnoses and 150 procedures, it is difficult to estimate risk for individual patients. Hence, a global score such as the Physical Status Classification Scheme of the American Society of Anesthesiology is not a valid measure for estimating perioperative risk in congenital heart surgery because age and underlying diagnoses are not taken into account (33). Several risk models have been established over the last 5 years to more specifically quantify perioperative risk after pediatric cardiac surgery (24,29). The Risk Adjustment in Congenital Heart Surgery (RACHS-1) classification, which has been shown to predict hospital mortality, classifies 79 open- and closed-heart operations into six risk categories (24). Evaluation of the RACHS-1 classification at a single institution allowed identification of independent risk factors for mortality: age, RACHS-1 risk category, and bypass time. However, this study also showed that the RACHS-1 lacks precision, with failure to classify some cases, whereas some other cases were open to variable interpretation (e.g., repair of double outlet right ventricle) and subsequent misclassification (27). Another international method, called the Aristotle Score, is based on the potential for mortality, the potential for morbidity, and the anticipated technical difficulty. Such a score adjusts the complexity to the specific patient characteristics, using the equation *complexity × survival = performance*. This complexity-adjustment method allowed precise scoring of the complexity for 145 congenital heart surgical procedures (29).

Besides methods and scoring that evaluate risk as well as quality of care, a valuable addition to the preoperative evaluation would be a blood marker capable of acutely predicting postoperative morbidity and mortality after congenital heart surgery. Preoperative N terminal pro-brain natriuretic peptide (BNP) plasma levels may provide a novel advance in estimating the risk of open heart surgery in children with CHD. Natriuretic peptides, in particular BNP, are cardiac hormones that are released by ventricular myocytes in response to ventricular dysfunction and wall stress. Increased preoperative plasma levels of N-terminal pro-BNP (NT-proBNP) are associated with prolonged postoperative inotropic drug therapy in children who undergo low-risk open-heart surgery. Thus, NT-proBNP levels appear to reflect the severity of heart failure, regardless of the type of CHD. However, the prognostic value of NT-proBNP levels is limited, especially in newborns, because of physiologically elevated levels in infants who are <3 months of age (16).

CONCLUSIONS AND FUTURE DIRECTIONS

The CICU has become the epicenter of activity in large cardiovascular programs. Nowhere are collaborative practices and multidisciplinary skills more valued or necessary. A curriculum in cardiac intensive care is now formally incorporated into cardiology training; pediatric intensive care training programs have a mandate to include curriculum and experience in management of postoperative cardiac patients (28). Specialists in this field must have in-depth training in cardiology and must be well versed in diagnosis and management of multiorgan system dysfunction; this is vital to the discipline of intensive care. Increased complexity of disease, advances in technology and applied research, shortened lengths of stay, and improved survival all describe the fast-paced, specialized environment that has accompanied the development of the new specialty of PCIC. While the dramatic reduction in mortality has been gratifying in cardiac intensive care (**Fig. 69.2**) and is attributable to many factors, achieving 100% survival with minimal morbidity remains our elusive goal. It will challenge the next generation of practitioners.

In the future, new imaging modalities will continue to give us better anatomic and physiologic information.

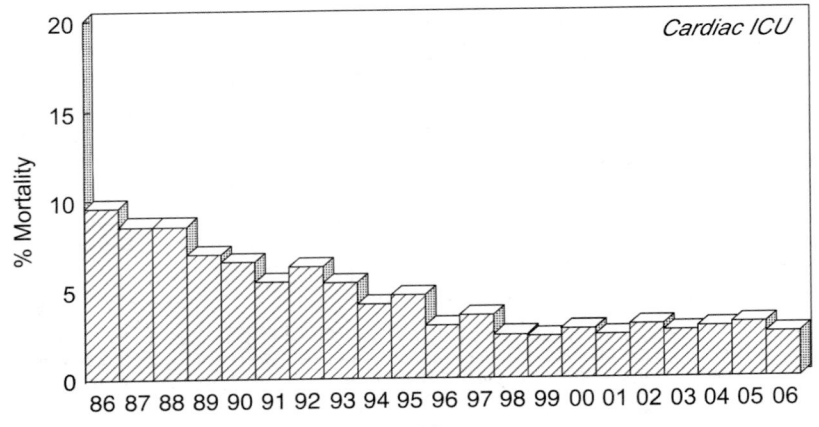

FIGURE 69.2. Mortality for all patients in the cardiac ICU at Children's Hospital Boston declined dramatically through the 1990s and was 2.5% in 2004, including surgical mortality <2%. Although this is common worldwide in many major pediatric cardiovascular centers, the goal of zero mortality remains elusive.

Three-dimensional imaging will one day be the precise, complete standard imaging in CHD. The ways in which the genetic make-up of patients influence outcome will be a focus of future research, along with a clearer understanding of polymorphisms as they relate to risks of CPB. Sophisticated pharmacogenetics will guide drug therapies in the ICU. Increasing clinical trial data will likely guide future patient assessment, and increasing pharmacokinetic data will inform dosage and duration of drug therapies. Discovery and innovation in the basic sciences will lead to new therapies, as it has with treatment of pulmonary hypertension and new inotropic support of the heart. Mechanical support devices that are more suitable for pediatrics will almost certainly be better developed in the future and provide options to support patients for longer or even indefinite periods of time, either as bridges to transplantation or even destination therapy. Undoubtedly, clinical teams will continue to become more highly specialized and propel PCIC to even higher standards, greater patient safety, and better outcomes.

KEY POINTS

Preoperative Care

- Pediatric cardiac intensive care has emerged as an important and necessary subspecialty.
- The complexity of heart disease and the expertise necessary to treat these patients require multidisciplinary training and collaborative, integrated care.
- Expertise is required for care of premature and full-term newborns, infants, and children, as well as rapidly growing numbers of adults with long-term survival and continuing need for care of their CHD.
- Reparative surgery in the newborn is the objective of advanced cardiovascular programs whenever feasible.
- Diagnosis is usually based on echocardiography and physical examination, with catheterization reserved usually for complex cases or interventional procedures.
- Adequate resuscitation of preoperative patients is essential to good outcomes.
- Balancing single-ventricle physiology and maintaining adequate cardiac output is important to achieving preoperative stabilization.
- Risk stratification and identification of biologic markers are maturing as useful tool sets to guide therapy and benchmarks for outcomes.
- Therapies for the future will target genetic factors and tailor treatments to the polymorphisms and individual inherited profiles of patients.
- Fetal diagnosis will increasingly continue to provide advanced knowledge, counseling, and therapeutic planning and eventually eliminate unanticipated postnatal circulatory collapse.

References

1. Atz AM, Feinstein JA, Jonas RA, et al. Preoperative management of pulmonary venous hypertension in hypoplastic left heart syndrome with restrictive atrial septal defect. *Am J Cardiol* 1999;83(8):1224–8.
2. Bargeron LMJR, Elliot LP, Soto B. Axial cineangiography of congenital heart disease. *Radiology* 1977;56:1075.
3. Castaneda AR, Mayer JE, Jr. , Jonas RA, et al. The neonate with critical congenital heart disease: Repair-a surgical challenge. *J Thorac Cardiovasc Surg* 1989;98(5 Pt 2):869–75.
4. Chang AC. How to start and sustain a successful pediatric cardiac intensive care program: A combined clinical and administrative strategy. *Pediatr Crit Care Med* 2002;3:107–11.
5. Chung T. Assessment of cardiovascular anatomy in patients with congenital heart disease by magnetic resonance imaging. *Pediatr Cardiol* 2000;21:18–26.
6. Clapp S, Perry BL, Farooki ZQ, et al. Down's syndrome, complete atrioventricular canal, and pulmonary vascular obstructive disease. *J Thorac Cardiovasc Surg* 1990;100:115–21.
7. Donahoo JS, Roland JM, Ken J. Prostaglandin E_1 as an adjunct to emergency cardiac operation in neonates. *J Thorac Cardiovasc Surg* 1981;81:227.
8. Fellows KE, Keane JF, Freed MD. Angled views in cineangiography of congenital heart disease. *Radiology* 1977;56:485.
9. Feltes TF, Hansen TN. Effects of an aorticopulmonary shunt on lung fluid balance in the young lamb. *Pediatr Res* 1989;26:94–7.
10. Fisher DJ, Heymann MA, Rudolph AM. Fetal myocardial oxygen and carbohydrate consumption during acutely induced hypoxemia. *Am J Physiol* 1982;242:H657–61.
11. Freed MD, Heymann MA, Lewis AB. Prostaglandin E_1 in infants with ductus arteriosus-dependent congenital heart disease. *Circulation* 1981;64:889–905.
12. Freed MD, Miettinen OS, Nadas AS. Oximetric detection of intracardiac left-to-right shunts. *Br Heart J* 1979;42:690–4.
13. Friedberg MK, Rosenthal DN. New developments in echocardiographic methods to assess right ventricular function in congenital heart disease. *Curr Opin Cardiol* 2005;20:84–8.
14. Friedman WF. The intrinsic physiologic properties of the developing heart. *Prog Cardiovasc Dis* 1972;15:87–111.
15. Friedman WF, George BL. Treatment of congestive heart failure by altering loading conditions of the heart. *J Pediatr* 1985;106:697–706.
16. Gessler P, Knirsch W, Schmitt B, et al. Prognostic value of plasma N-terminal pro-brain natriuretic peptide in children with congenital heart defects and open-heart surgery. *J Pediatr* 2006;148:372–6.
17. Geva T. Introduction: Magnetic resonance imaging. *Pediatr Cardiol* 2000;21(1):3–4.
18. Gladman G, McCrindle BW, Williams WG, et al. The modified Blalock-Taussig shunt: Clinical impact and morbidity in Fallot's tetralogy in the current era. *J Thorac Cardiovasc Surg* 1997;114:25–30.
19. Gossett JG, Rocchini AP, Lloyd TR, et al. Catheter-based decompression of the left atrium in patients with hypoplastic left heart syndrome and restrictive atrial septum is safe and effective. *Catheter Cardiovasc Interv* 2006;67:619–24.
20. Greenwood RD. Cardiovascular malformations associated with extracardiac anomalies and malformation syndromes. *Clin Ped* 1984;23:145–51.
21. Greenwood RD, Rosenthal A, Parisi L. Extracardiac abnormalities in infants with congenital heart disease. *Pediatrics* 1975;55:485–92.
22. Hamilton BE, Minino AM, Martin JA, et al. Annual summary of vital statistics: 2005. *Pediatrics* 2007;119:345–60.
23. Hanley FL, Heinemann MK, Jonas RA, et al. Repair of truncus arteriosus in the neonate. *J Thorac Cardiovasc Surg* 1993;105:1047–56.
24. Jenkins KJ, Gauvreau K, Newburger JW, et al. Consensus-based method for risk adjustment for surgery for congenital heart disease. *J Thorac Cardiovasc Surg* 2002;123:110–8.
25. Jonas RA, Hansen DD, Cook N, et al. Anatomic subtype and survival after reconstructive operation for hypoplastic left heart syndrome. *J Thorac Cardiovasc Surg* 1994;107:1121–7.
26. Jonas RA, Lang P, Mayer JE, et al. The importance of prostaglandin E_1 in resuscitation of the neonate with critical aortic stenosis. *J Thorac Cardiovasc Surg* 1985;89:314–5.
27. Kang N, Cole T, Tsang V, et al. Risk stratification in paediatric open-heart surgery. *Eur J Cardiothorac Surg* 2004;26:3–11.
28. Kulik T, Giglia TM, Kocis KC, et al. ACCF/AHA/AAP recommendations for training in pediatric cardiology. Task force 5: Requirements for pediatric cardiac critical care. *J Am Coll Cardiol* 2005;46:1396–9.
29. Lacour-Gayet F, Clarke D, Jacobs J, et al. The Aristotle score: A complexity-adjusted method to evaluate surgical results. *Eur J Cardiothorac Surg* 2004;25:911–24.
30. Lambert V, Sigal-Cinqualbre A, Belli E, et al. Preoperative and postoperative evaluation of airways compression in pediatric patients with 3-dimensional multislice computed tomographic scanning: Effect on surgical management. *J Thorac Cardiovasc Surg* 2005;129:1111–8.
31. Lewis AB, Freed MD, Heymann MA. Side effects of therapy with prostaglandin E1 in infants with critical congenital heart disease. *Circulation* 1981;64:893–8.
32. Lister G, Hellenbrand WE, Kleinman CS, et al. Physiologic effects of increasing hemoglobin concentration in left-to-right shunting in infants with ventricular septal defects. *N Engl J Med* 1982;306:502–6.
33. Mak PHK, Campbell RCH, Irwin MG. The ASA Physical Status Classification: Inter-observer consistency. American Society of Anesthesiologists. *Anaesth Intensive Care* 2002;30:633–40.
34. McCrindle BW, Tchervenkov CI, Konstantinov IE, et al. Risk factors associated with mortality and interventions in 472 neonates with interrupted

aortic arch: A Congenital Heart Surgeons Society study. *J Thorac Cardiovasc Surg* 2005;129:343–50.

35. McMahon CJ, Penny DJ, Nelson DP, et al. Preterm infants with congenital heart disease and bronchopulmonary dysplasia: Postoperative course and outcome after cardiac surgery. *Pediatrics* 2005;116:423–30.

36. McQuillen PS, Hamrick SEG, Perez MJ, et al. Balloon atrial septostomy is associated with preoperative stroke in neonates with transposition of the great arteries. *Circulation* 2006;113:280–5.

37. Mills AN, Haworth SG. Greater permeability of the neonatal lung. Postnatal changes in surface charge and biochemistry of porcine pulmonary capillary endothelium. *J Thorac Cardiovasc Surg* 1991;101:909–16.

38. Moler FW, Khan AS, Meliones JN, et al. Respiratory syncytial virus morbidity and mortality estimates in congenital heart disease patients: A recent experience. *Crit Care Med* 1992;20:1406–13.

39. Norwood WI, Lang P, Hansen DD. Physiologic repair of aortic atresia-hypoplastic left heart syndrome. *N Engl J Med* 1983;308:23–6.

40. Planche C, Serraf A, Comas JV, et al. Anatomic repair of transposition of great arteries with ventricular septal defect and aortic arch obstruction. One-stage versus two-stage procedure. *J Thorac Cardiovasc Surg* 1993;105(5):925–33.

41. Rabinovitch M. Pulmonary Hypertension. In: Adams FH, Emmanouilides GC, eds. *Moss' Heart Diseases in Infants, Children and Adolescents.* Baltimore: Williams & Wilkins, 1983;669.

42. Ramamoorthy C, Tabbutt S, Kurth CD, et al. Effects of inspired hypoxic and hypercapnic gas mixtures on cerebral oxygen saturation in neonates with univentricular heart defects. *Anesthesiology* 2002;96(2):283–8.

43. Rashkind WJ, Miller WW. Creation of an atrial septal defect without thoracotomy. A palliative approach to complete transposition of the great arteries. *JAMA* 1966;196:991–2.

44. Reddy VM, McElhinney DB, Sagrado T, et al. Results of 102 cases of complete repair of congenital heart defects in patients weighing 700 to 2500 grams. *J Thorac Cardiovasc Surg* 1999;117(2):324–31.

45. Romero TE, Friedman WF. Limited left ventricular response to volume overload in the neonatal period: A comparative study with the adult animal. *Pediatr Res* 1979;13:910–5.

46. Tabbutt S, Ramamoorthy C, Montenegro LM, et al. Impact of inspired gas mixtures on preoperative infants with hypoplastic left heart syndrome during controlled ventilation. *Circulation* 2001;104(12 Suppl 1):I159–64.

47. Talner NS. Heart Failure. In: Adams FH, Emmanouilides GC, eds. *Moss' Heart Diseases in Infants, Children and Adolescents.* Baltimore: Williams & Wilkins, 1983;708.

48. Vlahos AP, Lock JE, McElhinney DB, et al. Hypoplastic left heart syndrome with intact or highly restrictive atrial septum: Outcome after neonatal transcatheter atrial septostomy. *Circulation* 2004;109:2326–30.

49. Weidemann F, Eyskens B, Sutherland GR. New ultrasound methods to quantify regional myocardial function in children with heart disease. *Pediatric Cardiology* 2002;23:292–306.

50. Yokota M, Muraoka R, Aoshima M, et al. Modified Blalock-Taussig shunt following long-term administration of prostaglandin E1 for ductus-dependent neonates with cyanotic congenital heart disease. *J Thorac Cardiovasc Surg* 1985;90(3):399–403.

CHAPTER 70A ■ POSTOPERATIVE CARE OF THE PEDIATRIC CARDIAC SURGICAL PATIENT: GENERAL CONSIDERATIONS

DAVID L. WESSEL • ALAIN FRAISSE

Improvements in diagnostic accuracy, surgical techniques, and intensive care management have all contributed substantially to reduction in mortality among patients with congenital heart disease (CHD). However, postoperative mortality continues to be high in high-risk populations that undergo surgical procedures. Additionally, patients who undergo high-risk corrective operations or complex neonatal palliative procedures may experience considerable morbidity that further challenges the intensive care physician to improve care and outcome.

Especially for high-risk patients, the postoperative period is laden with rapid and dynamic change in physiologic condition. Anticipation of hemodynamic events and good care are the keys to success. Randomized, controlled trials to evaluate new therapies or to better assess existing practice are often lacking. Evidence-based medicine for CHD treatment is now emerging and will represent the standard for clinical decision-making in the future. Important initiatives include a pediatric heart network sponsored by the National Institutes of Health, which is charged to properly design and execute clinical trials for children with heart disease. This, combined with a surge in industry-sponsored trials of drug therapy in children and rigorous review of large European and North American CHD surgical databases, will increasingly inform decision-making in the future. In the meantime, the field relies heavily on experience and reason, combined with frank discussion of paradigms for best practice. This chapter on postoperative care of the patient with CHD is divided into three sections: General Considerations (Section A), Lesion-Specific Management (Section B), and Effects of Cardiopulmonary Bypass (Section C).

ASSESSMENT

When the clinical course of patients after cardiac surgery deviates from the usual expectation of uncomplicated recovery, the first priority is to verify the accuracy of the preoperative diagnosis and the adequacy of the surgical repair. For example, a young infant who is acidotic, hypotensive, and cyanotic after surgical repair of tetralogy of Fallot may tempt the clinician to ascribe these findings to the vagaries of ischemia-reperfusion injury related to cardiopulmonary bypass (CPB) or transient, postoperative stiffness of the right ventricle (RV). However, the real culprit may be an additional ventricular septal defect (VSD) that was undetected preoperatively and therefore not closed, a residual VSD around the surgical patch, or residual RV outflow obstruction. Any of these anatomic issues can produce serious adverse outcomes. Achieving the correct postoper-

ative assessment is therefore imperative, and treatment follows accordingly. Evaluation of the postoperative patient relies on examination, monitoring, interpretation of vital signs or other bedside data, and on imaging (**Table 70A.1**). When the accuracy of the diagnosis and adequacy of the repair are established, a low cardiac output state can be presumed and treatment optimized. Treating low cardiac output states and preventing cardiovascular collapse are often the central features of pediatric cardiac intensive care. They will be the focus of this section, without detailing the specific considerations for each lesion.

Each strategy to improve cardiac output will have benefits as well as risks. Optimizing preload involves more than just giving volume to a hypotensive patient. Fluid balance is associated with numerous considerations involving types of isotonic fluid, ultrafiltration in the operating room, optimal hematocrit, and the use of furosemide, thiazides, and possibly newer drugs such as fenoldopam or nesiritide. Fluid itself can be detrimental if excess extravascular water results in interstitial edema and end-organ dysfunction of vital organs such as the heart lungs and brain. Perhaps permitting a right-to-left shunt at the atrial level will optimize preload to the left ventricle (LV) in some conditions (see following text). Maintaining aortic perfusion after CPB and improving the contractile state of the heart with higher doses of catecholamines are reasonable goals that may have particularly deleterious consequences in the newborn myocardium after hypothermic CPB. The benefits of afterload reduction are well known but, in excess, afterload reduction may lead to hypotension and cardiovascular collapse or renal or cerebral insufficiency. Pacing the heart can stabilize the rhythm and hemodynamics but may also contribute to dyssynchronous, inefficient contraction of the heart or induce other dysrhythmias. Finally, mechanical support of the failing myocardium in the form of extracorporeal membrane oxygenation (ECMO) or ventricular assist devices, while lifesaving in many instances, has its own specific constraints and complications. It must be recognized that almost every treatment approach has its own set of adverse effects that may be damaging.

Assessment of a child following cardiac surgery begins with review of the operative findings, including details of the operative repair and CPB, particularly total CPB or myocardial ischemia (aortic cross-clamp) times, concerns about myocardial protection, recovery of myocardial contractility, typical postoperative systemic arterial and central venous pressures, findings from intraoperative transesophageal echocardiogram, and vasoactive medication requirements. This information will guide subsequent examination, which should focus on the

TABLE 70A.1

SIGNS OF HEART FAILURE OR LOW CARDIAC OUTPUT STATES

Signs
  Cool extremities/poor perfusion
  Oliguria and other end-organ failure
  Tachycardia
  Hypotension
  Acidosis
  Cardiomegaly
  Pleural effusions
Monitor and measure
  Heart rate, blood pressure, intracardiac pressure
  Extremity temperature, central temperature
  Urine output
  Mixed venous oxygen saturation
  Arterial blood gas pH and lactate
  Laboratory measures of end-organ function
  Echocardiography

quality of the repair or palliation plus a clinical assessment of cardiac output (**Table 69.2**). In addition to a complete cardiovascular examination, a routine set of laboratory tests should be obtained, including a chest x-ray, 12- or 15-lead electrocardiogram, blood gas analysis, serum electrolytes and glucose, an ionized calcium level, complete blood count, and coagulation profile.

Several biologic markers have been described that aid in delineating postoperative risk assessment. Serum lactate, a conventional indicator of tissue hypoxia, has predictive value for postoperative mortality. In 85 infants <6 weeks old and undergoing CPB, lactate concentration of <7 mmol/L on admission or <8 mmol/L at postoperative day 1 predicted survival with 82% sensitivity, 83% specificity, 97% positive-predictive value, and 43% negative-predictive value ($p <0.01$) (18). Others have observed that an intraoperative rise in lactate is predictive of survival (60). Several authors have suggested the use of serial plasma lactate measurements—although they are nonspecific indicators of inadequate oxygen delivery—to guide medical therapy in children following cardiac surgery (43).

A biologic marker protein, cardiac troponin T, is documented to reflect myocardial damage and clinical outcome after adult and pediatric cardiac surgery. In a retrospective cohort study on 1001 children having cardiac surgery, a level of troponin T >5.9 mcg/L on the first postoperative day was a strong independent predictor of death (56). However, the value of troponin T level might be limited, as it is correlated more with the degree of myocardial damage than with the complexity of surgery or patient condition. Hence, only prospective studies will provide a more specific interpretation of change with this biologic marker.

Monitoring

The level of appropriate bedside monitoring depends upon each patient's cardiac diagnosis, the type of repair or palliation, and anticipated requirements for hemodynamic and respiratory data. All patients should have continuous monitoring of their heart rate and rhythm by electrocardiogram, systemic ar-

terial blood pressure (invasive or noninvasive), oxygen saturation by pulse oximetry, and respiratory rate. Breath-to-breath end-tidal CO_2 monitoring is often routinely used in mechanically ventilated patients to monitor for possible disconnection, misplacement, or obstruction of the endotracheal tube. It is also a useful indicator for acute changes in pulmonary blood flow.

Monitoring central venous pressure following cardiac surgery is essential for many patients, except those who undergo the least complex procedures. For example, many do not routinely place a central venous catheter in patients who undergo thoracic procedures, such as coarctation of the aorta, vascular ring, and patent ductus arteriosus ligation, or in patients who undergo cardiotomy with a short period of mildly hypothermic CPB, such as repair of atrial septal defect. In many centers a percutaneous central venous catheter is placed electively after induction of anesthesia, especially if postoperative infusion of vasoactive drugs is anticipated. Intracardiac or transthoracic left atrial (LA) catheters are often used to monitor patients after complex reparative procedures. Pulmonary artery (PA) catheters are now seldom used but may be particularly useful if the postoperative management anticipates a problem such as: (a) a residual lesion producing an intracardiac left-to-right shunt (e.g., multiple VSDs); (b) residual RV outflow tract obstruction, as a catheter "pullback" can be performed to measure the RV-to-PA pressure gradient; and (c) pulmonary hypertension, thereby allowing rapid detection of pressure changes and assessment of the response to interventions.

LA catheters are especially helpful in the management of patients with ventricular dysfunction, coronary artery perfusion abnormalities, and mitral valve disease. The mean LA pressure is typically 1–2 mm Hg greater than mean right atrial (RA) pressure, which generally varies between 2 and 6 mm Hg in non-postoperative pediatric patients who undergo cardiac catheterization. In postoperative patients, mean LA and RA pressures are both often >6–8 mm Hg. However, they should generally be <15 mm Hg. The compliance of the RA is greater than that of the LA, except in the newborn; therefore, pressure elevations in the RA of older patients with two ventricles are typically less pronounced.

Possible causes of abnormally elevated LA pressure are listed in **Table 70A.2**. In addition to pressure data, intracardiac catheters in the RA (or a percutaneously placed central

TABLE 70A.2

COMMON CAUSES OF ELEVATED LEFT ATRIAL PRESSURE AFTER CARDIOPULMONARY BYPASS

1. Decreased ventricular systolic or diastolic function
    Myocardial ischemia
    Dilated cardiomyopathy
    Systemic ventricular hypertrophy
2. Left atrioventricular valve disease
3. Large left-to-right intracardiac shunt
4. Chamber hypoplasia
5. Intravascular or ventricular volume overload
6. Cardiac tamponade
7. Dysrhythmia
    Tachyarrhythmia, junctional rhythm
    Complete heart block

TABLE 70A.3

CAUSES OF ABNORMAL RIGHT ATRIAL, LEFT ATRIAL, OR PULMONARY ARTERY OXYGEN SATURATION

Location	Elevated O₂ saturation	Reduced O₂ saturation
RA	Atrial level left-to-right shunt Anomalous pulmonary venous return Left ventricular-to-right atrial shunt ↑ dissolved O_2 content ↓O_2 extraction Catheter tip position (e.g., near renal veins)	↑ V_{O_2} (e.g., low CO, fever) ↓ Sa_{O_2} saturation with a normal AV O_2 difference Anemia Catheter tip position (e.g., near CS)
LA	Does not occur	Atrial level right-to-left shunt ↓ Pv_{O_2} (e.g., parenchymal lung disease)
PA	Significant left-to-right shunt Small left-to-right shunt with incomplete mixing of blood Catheter tip position (e.g., PA "wedge")	↑ O_2 extraction (e.g., low CO, fever) ↓ Sa_{O_2} saturation with a normal AV O_2 difference Anemia

RA, right atrium; V_{O_2}, oxygenation consumption; CO, cardiac output; Sa_{O_2}, arterial oxygen saturation; AV, arteriovenous; CS, coronary sinus; LA, left atrium; Pv_{O_2}, pulmonary vein oxygen tension; PA, pulmonary artery

venous catheter), LA, and PA can be used to monitor the oxygen saturation of systemic venous or pulmonary venous blood.

The causes of abnormally high or low RA, LA, and PA oxygen saturations, which can be measured at the bedside in the ICU, are listed in **Table 70A.3**. Following reparative surgery, patients with no intracardiac shunts and an adequate cardiac output may have a mild reduction in RA oxygen saturation to ~60%. Lower RA oxygen saturation does not necessarily indicate low cardiac output. If a patient has arterial desaturation (common mixing lesions, lung diseases, etc.), the arteriovenous oxygen difference may be normal at 25%, and this could represent appropriate oxygen delivery and extraction. Elevated RA oxygen saturation is often due to left-to-right shunting at the atrial level (e.g., from the LA, from an anomalous pulmonary vein, or from an LV-to-RA shunt). Blood in the LA is normally fully saturated with oxygen (i.e., ~100%). The two chief causes of reduced LA oxygen saturation are an atrial level right-to-left shunt and pulmonary venous oxygen desaturation from abnormal gas exchange (i.e., lung disease).

In the absence of left-to-right shunts, the PA oxygen saturation is the best representation of the "true" mixed venous oxygen saturation (Sv_{O_2}), because all sources of systemic venous blood should be thoroughly combined as they are ejected from the RV. When elevated, this saturation is useful in the identification of residual left-to-right shunts following repair of VSDs. The absolute valve of the PA oxygen saturation is a predictor of significant postoperative residual shunt. In patients following repair of tetralogy of Fallot or VSD, a PA oxygen saturation >80% within 48 hrs of surgery with supplemental oxygen at a fractional inspired oxygen concentration (F_{IO_2}) <0.5 has been shown to be a sensitive indicator of a significant left-to-right shunt (Q_p:Q_s >1.5) 1 year after surgery (61). Determination of the PA oxygen saturation can also be useful in patients with systemic-to-PA collaterals because flow from these vessels into the pulmonary arteries can increase the oxygen saturation.

Low Cardiac Output Syndrome

Although some causes of low cardiac output after CPB are attributable to residual or undiagnosed structural lesions,

progressive low cardiac output states (LCOS) do occur. A number of factors have been implicated in the development of myocardial dysfunction following CPB, including the inflammatory response associated with CPB, the effects of myocardial ischemia from aortic cross-clamping, hypothermia, reperfusion injury, inadequate myocardial protection, and ventriculotomy (when performed). The expression and prevention of reperfusion injury after aortic cross-clamping on CPB is currently the subject of intense investigation. We have previously shown the typical decrease in cardiac index in newborns following an arterial switch operation (**Fig. 70A.1**) (85). In this group of 122 newborns, the median maximal decrease in cardiac index, which occurred typically 6–12 hrs after separation from CPB, was 32%. A quarter of all of these newborns reached a nadir of

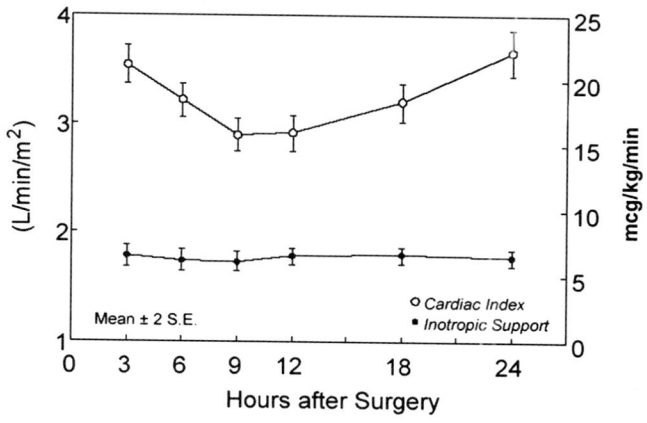

FIGURE 70A.1. Cardiac index (**left axis**) measured in infants following the arterial switch operation (ASO) for transposition of the great arteries (TGA) declined during the first 12 hrs and was not due to any reduction in inotropic support (**right axis**). A quarter of the patients reached a value <2.0 L/min/m². The median reduction in cardiac index on the first night is 33%. Adapted from Wernovsky G, Wypij D, Jonas RA, et al. Postoperative course and hemodynamic profile after the arterial switch operation in neonates and infants. A comparison of low-flow cardiopulmonary bypass and circulatory arrest. *Circulation* 1995;92:2226–35.

cardiac index that was <2 L/min/m² on the first postoperative night. LCOS does occur in the postoperative patient, but appropriate anticipation and intervention can do much to avert morbidity or the need for mechanical support. Signs of low cardiac output are listed in Table 70A.1. Mixed venous oxygen saturation, whole blood pH, and lactate, are laboratory measures commonly used to evaluate the adequacy of tissue perfusion and, hence, cardiac output.

Volume Adjustments

After CPB, the factors that influence cardiac output, such as preload, afterload, myocardial contractility, heart rate, and rhythm, must be assessed and manipulated. Volume therapy (increased preload) is commonly necessary, followed by appropriate use of inotropic and afterload-reducing agents. Atrial pressure and the ventricular response to changes in atrial pressure must be evaluated. Ventricular response is judged by observing systemic arterial pressure and waveform, heart rate, skin color and peripheral extremity temperature, peripheral pulse magnitude, urine flow, core body temperature, and acid-base balance. The relative merits of colloid or crystalloid solutions for fluid administration are hotly debated. While 5% albumin solution remains a popular choice because it remains within the vascular compartment longer than does crystalloid, its use may be limited by cost, availability, and risk of transfusion-related events and other morbidities. Alternatives that have recently gained popularity include crystalloid solutions such as 0.9% sodium chloride, balanced electrolyte solutions such as Ringer's lactate, and starch-polymer artificial colloids.

Preserving and Creating Right-to-Left Shunts

Selected children with low cardiac output may benefit from strategies that allow right-to-left shunting at the atrial level in the face of postoperative RV dysfunction. A typical example is early repair of tetralogy of Fallot, when the moderately hypertrophied, noncompliant RV has undergone a ventriculotomy and may be further compromised by an increased volume load from pulmonary regurgitation secondary to a transannular patch on the RV outflow tract. In these children, it is very useful to leave the foramen ovale patent to permit right-to-left shunting of blood, thus preserving cardiac output and oxygen delivery despite the attendant transient cyanosis. If the foramen is not patent or is surgically closed, RV dysfunction can lead to reduced LV filling, low cardiac output, and, ultimately, LV dysfunction. In infants and neonates with repaired truncus arteriosus, the same concerns apply and may even be exaggerated if RV afterload is elevated because of PA hypertension.

Right Ventriculotomy and Restrictive Physiology

RV "restrictive" physiology in infants and children who have undergone congenital cardiac surgery has been described by echocardiography as persistent antegrade diastolic blood flow into the pulmonary circulation following reconstruction of the RV outflow, and it occurs in the setting of decreased RV compliance as a result of diastolic dysfunction with an inability

to relax and fill during diastole. The RV is usually not dilated in this circumstance, and pulmonary regurgitation is limited because of the higher diastolic pressure in the RV (23,70).

The term "restrictive" RV physiology is also commonly used in the immediate postoperative period in patients who have a stiff, poorly compliant and sometimes hypertrophied RV. Poor RV compliance has several detrimental effects. It restricts RV filling during diastole; therefore, the underfilled RV ejects a smaller stroke volume, which, in turn, limits the preload to the LV. The poorly compliant RV also leads to an increase in RV end-diastolic pressure and RA pressure, which causes systemic venous hypertension. If RV end-diastolic pressure is sufficiently elevated, the septal position shifts to the left, which decreases LV compliance and function (ventricular interdependence). The causes of diastolic dysfunction include factors such as lung and myocardial edema following CPB, inadequate myocardial protection of the hypertrophied ventricle during surgery, coronary artery injury, residual outflow tract obstruction, and volume load on the ventricle from a residual VSD or pulmonary regurgitation and dysrhythmias. An LCOS with increased right-sided filling pressure (usually >10 mm Hg) is the common feature of neonatal restrictive RV physiology. As a result of the LCOS, patients often have cool extremities, are oliguric, and may have a metabolic acidosis. As a result of the elevated RA pressure, hepatic congestion, ascites, increased chest tube losses, and pleural effusions may be evident. These patients may be tachycardic and hypotensive, with a narrow pulse pressure. Preload must be maintained, despite elevation of the RA pressure. Significant inotrope support is often required (typically dopamine 5–10 mcg/kg/min and/or low-dose epinephrine <0.05 mcg/kg/min), and a phosphodiesterase inhibitor such as milrinone is beneficial because of its lusitropic properties. Sedation and even paralysis for a period of 24–48 hrs may assist by minimizing cardiorespiratory work.

Patients with restrictive physiology may be desaturated initially following surgery (typically, 75%–85%) because of right-to-left shunting at the atrial level. As RV compliance and function improve (usually within 2–3 postoperative days), the amount of shunt decreases, and both antegrade pulmonary blood flow and SaO₂ increase.

Mechanical ventilation may have a significant impact on RV afterload. Both underinflation and overinflation of the lungs raise pulmonary vascular resistance (PVR) and RV afterload, thereby increasing the amount of pulmonary regurgitation. In addition, an increase in PVR because of hypothermia, acidosis, and either hypoinflation or hyperinflation of the lung will also increase afterload on the RV and pulmonary regurgitation. Intermittent positive-pressure ventilation with the lowest possible mean airway pressure consistent with achieving adequate ventilation and maintenance of lung volume should be the goal.

The concept of preserving right-to-left shunting at the atrial level has been extended to older patients with single-ventricle physiology who are at high risk after Fontan operations (13). The Fontan circulation relies on passive flow of blood through the pulmonary circulation without benefit of a pulmonary ventricle. If an atrial septal communication or fenestration is left at the time of the Fontan procedure, the resulting right-to-left shunt helps to preserve cardiac output. These children have fewer postoperative complications (50). It is better to shunt blood right to left, accept some decrement in oxygen saturation, and maintain LV filling and cardiac output, than to have high oxygen saturation but low blood pressure and low cardiac output.

Pharmacologic Support

Catecholamines

Preload adjustments often do not suffice to provide adequate cardiac output. Use of pharmacologic agents to support cardiac output is common (12,87). Common vasoactive drugs used for cardiac patients in the ICU, along with their actions, are listed in **Tables 70A.4** and **70A.5**. Many prefer to use dopamine first in doses of 3–10 mcg/kg/min; >15 mcg/kg/min is rarely used because of the known vasoconstrictor and chronotropic properties of dopamine at very high doses. However, extreme biologic variability in pharmacokinetics and pharmacodynamics defies placing narrow limits on recommended dosages. Dopamine is of no benefit in the prevention or treatment of renal failure. Alternatives to dopamine include dobutamine and low-dose epinephrine (<0.05 mcg/kg/min) (42). The significant chronotropic effect and increased oxygen consumption induced by isoproterenol have also increasingly limited its use in

neonates and infants. Higher-dose epinephrine is occasionally useful for short-term therapy when high systemic pressures are sought, provided that the temporary increase in peripheral vascular resistance can be tolerated. High doses of epinephrine are occasionally necessary to increase pulmonary blood flow across significantly narrowed systemic-to-pulmonary artery shunts when oxygen saturations are low and falling.

Norepinephrine and arginine vasopressin have been advocated for states of refractory vasodilation associated with low circulating vasopressin levels, as may rarely occur after CPB in children (75). Vasopressin has been used to treat low systemic blood pressure in postoperative pediatric cardiac patients with pulmonary hypertension, where it may ameliorate hypoxic pulmonary vasoconstriction and attenuate pulmonary hypertension (77).

In the past, the side effects of inotropic support of the heart with catecholamines seemed a lesser concern in children than in adults with an ischemic, noncompliant heart. Tachycardia, an increased end-diastolic pressure and afterload, or increased myocardial oxygen consumption, despite their undesirable side effects, were tolerated by most children in need of inotropic support after CPB. However, with increasing perioperative

---

TABLE 70A.4

SUMMARY OF SELECTED VASOACTIVE AGENTS—NONCATECHOLAMINES

Agent	Doses (IV)	Peripheral vascular effect	Cardiac effect	Conduction system effect
		Noncatecholamines		
Digoxin (Total digitalizing dose)	premature, 20 mcg/kg neonate (0–1 mo), 30 mcg/kg infant (<2 yr), 40 mcg/kg child (2–5 yr), 30 mcg/kg child (>5 yr), 20 mcg/kg	Increases peripheral vascular resistance 1–2+; acts directly on vascular smooth muscle.	Inotropic effect 3–4+; acts directly on myocardium.	Slows sinus node slightly; decreases A-V conduction more.
Calcium chloride	10–20 mg/kg/dose (slowly)	Variable; age dependent. Vasoconstrictor	Inotropic effect 3+; depends on ionized Ca^{2+}.	Slows sinus node; decreases AV conduction.
Calcium gluconate	50–100 mg/kg/dose (slowly)			
Nitroprusside	0.5–5 mcg/kg/min	Donates nitric oxide group to relax smooth muscle and dilate pulmonary and systemic vessels.	Indirectly increases cardiac output by decreasing afterload.	Reflex tachycardia
Nitroglycerin	0.5–10 mcg/kg/min	Primarily venodilator. As a nitric oxide donor, may cause pulmonary vasodilation and enhance coronary vasoreactivity after aortic cross-clamping	Decreases preload; may decrease afterload. Reduces myocardial work related to change in wall stress.	Minimal
Milrinone	50–75 mcg/kg loading dose 0.25–1.0 mcg/kg/min maintenance	Systemic and pulmonary vasodilator	Diastolic relaxation (lusitropy); measurable inotropic effect	Minimal tachycardia
Vasopressin	.003–.002 U/kg/min	Potent vasoconstrictor	No direct effect	None known

TABLE 70A.5

SUMMARY OF SELECTED VASOACTIVE AGENTS—CATECHOLAMINES

Agent	Dose range	Catecholamines				Comment
		α	β_1	β_2	Dopa	
Phenylephrine	0.1–0.5 mcg/kg/min	4+	0	0	0	Increases systemic resistance; no inotropy; may cause renal ischemia; useful for treatment of tetralogy of Fallot spells.
Isoproterenol	0.05–0.5 mcg/kg/min	0	4+	4+	0	Strong inotropic and chronotropic agent; peripheral vasodilator; reduces preload; pulmonary vasodilator. Limited by tachycardia and oxygen consumption.
Norepinephrine	0.1–0.5 mcg/kg/min	4+	2+	0	0	Increases systemic resistance; moderately inotropic; may cause renal ischemia.
Epinephrine	0.03–0.1 mcg/kg/min	2+	2–3+	1–2+	0	Beta$_2$ effect with lower doses; best for blood
	0.2–0.5 mcg/kg/min	4+	4+	0	0	pressure in anaphylaxis and drug toxicity.
Dopamine	2–4 mcg/kg/min	0	0	0	2+	Splanchnic and renal vasodilator; may be
	4–8 mcg/kg/min	0	1–2+	2+	2+	used with isoproterenol; increasing doses
	>10 mcg/kg/min	2–4+	1–2+	0	0	produce increasing alpha effect.
Dobutamine	2–10 mcg/kg/min	1+	3–4+	2+	0	Less chronotropy and fewer dysrhythmias at lower doses; effects vary with dose, similar to dopamine; chronotropic advantage compared with dopamine may not be apparent in neonates.

experience in neonates and young infants, the adverse effects of vasoactive drugs have become more evident. The less compliant neonatal myocardium, like the ischemic adult heart, may raise its end-diastolic pressure during higher-dose infusions of catecholamines, further impairing ventricular compliance and further reducing ventricular filling. Actual myocardial necrosis caused by high doses of epinephrine infusions has been identified in neonatal animal models after CPB (14,15). Many of the complex corrective procedures performed in neonates and small infants are accompanied by transient postoperative dysrhythmias that are either induced or exacerbated by catecholamines. Nevertheless, the predictable and often significant decrease in cardiac output documented by many investigators after CPB in infants and older children continues to justify the practice of judiciously using catecholamines to support the heart and circulation while weaning patients from CPB and during the immediate postoperative period.

Phosphodiesterase III Inhibitors

Phosphodiesterase III inhibitors, such as milrinone, have emerged as important vasoactive agents for use in children after open-heart surgery (8,16,45). They are nonglycosidic, noncatecholamine, inotropic agents with additional vasodilatory and lusitropic properties. Used extensively in adults for treatment of heart failure, milrinone has been introduced to pediatric practice. These inhibitors exert their effects by inhibiting phosphodiesterase III, the enzyme that metabolizes cyclic AMP (cAMP). By increasing intracellular cAMP, calcium transport into the cell is favored, and the increased intracellular calcium stores enhance the contractile state of the myocyte. In addition, the reuptake of calcium is a cAMP-dependent process, and these agents may therefore enhance diastolic relaxation of the myocardium by increasing the rate of calcium reuptake

after systole (lusitropy). Milrinone also appears to work synergistically with low doses of β agonists and has fewer side effects than other catecholamine vasodilators, such as isoproterenol. In critically ill postoperative newborns, milrinone increased cardiac output, lowered filling pressures, and reduced PA pressures (16).

The PRIMACORP trial investigated the efficacy and safety of prophylactic milrinone use to prevent LCOS after cardiac surgery in high-risk pediatric patients (45). The study was a multicentered, randomized, double-blinded, placebo-controlled trial that used three parallel treatment groups (low-dose, 25-mcg/kg bolus over 60 mins followed by a 0.25-mcg/kg/min infusion for 35 hrs; high-dose, 75-mcg/kg bolus followed by 0.75 mcg/kg/min, or placebo). The composite endpoint of death or the development of LCOS was evaluated at 36 hrs and at the follow-up visit. Among 238 treated patients, the prophylactic use of high-dose milrinone significantly reduced the risk of death or the development of LCOS relative to placebo with a relative risk reduction of 55% ($p = 0.023$) in the treated patients. Patients who developed LCOS had a significantly longer cumulative duration of mechanical ventilation and hospital stay in comparison to those who did not develop LCOS. The authors concluded that the prophylactic use of high-dose milrinone following pediatric congenital heart surgery reduces the risk of LCOS. Dopamine or low-dose epinephrine and milrinone have emerged as the most commonly used vasoactive combinations of drugs to maintain cardiac output in postoperative patients.

Thyroid Hormone

LCOS typically overlaps with the time that free and total triiodothyronine (T$_3$) levels are significantly suppressed following the stress of surgical reconstruction, i.e., during the first

24–48 hrs postoperatively. This is a significant observation, as T_3 is the predominant form of biologically active thyroid hormone and is known to improve cardiac output by improving the inotropic state of animal and human hearts, while decreasing systemic vascular resistance. Limited studies of T_3 supplementation after cardiac surgery have been performed in children. In one study, two bolus doses of T_3 were given after the Fontan procedure to 10 children, and compared with a historic control group, the T_3 patients had a significantly shorter period of mechanical ventilation (54). In a study that randomized 40 children undergoing a wide variety of cardiac procedures to receive bolus dosing of T_3 or placebo, cardiac output was reported to be higher in the treatment group but was estimated by echocardiography (11). Another group randomized 28 children aged 0–18 years to a 5-day continuous infusion of T_3 (0.05–0.15 mcg/kg/hr) or placebo (19). Among neonates, the T_3 group had lower severity of illness scores and lower inotrope requirements. The T_3 group also had a trend toward higher SvO_2, fewer days of mechanical ventilation, and a shorter postoperative length of stay. No adverse effects of T_3 administration were recorded in any of these small series.

A randomized, double-blinded, placebo-controlled pilot study enrolled 42 neonates to evaluate the effect of T_3 replacement after either a Norwood procedure or two-ventricle repair of interrupted aortic arch and VSD. Patients were assigned to receive 0.05 mcg/kg/hr of T_3 or placebo for 72 hrs after CPB. The primary end-points were a composite clinical outcome score and cardiac index at 48 postoperative hrs. This analysis did not show improvement in cardiac output but did suggest better blood pressure and fluid balance in treated patients, even though urine output was not greater in the treatment group (51).

In summary, trials of T_3 supplementation are inconclusive, and its routine use cannot be recommended. Larger trials with more rigorous trial design are under way and may address whether certain subgroups at particular risk for LCOS may benefit from T_3 administration (25,67).

Other Afterload-reducing Agents

When systemic blood pressure is elevated and cardiac output appears low or normal, a primary vasodilator is indicated to normalize blood pressure and decrease systemic vascular resistance and therefore afterload on the LV. This situation is most often true for the newborn myocardium, which is especially sensitive to changes in afterload and tolerates elevated systemic resistances poorly. Nitroprusside is a potent vasodilator that possesses a short biologic half-life, rendering it readily titratable—a useful property in an unstable postoperative child. The use of nitroprusside may be associated with generation of the toxic metabolites cyanide and thiocyanate, which are produced in a dose-related manner. Nitroglycerin is a less potent vasodilator than nitroprusside, and its use is not associated with cyanide toxicity. Phosphodiesterase III inhibitors such as milrinone, although not pure vasodilators, have potent vasodilatory properties and, as discussed elsewhere, are widely used in the management of postoperative low cardiac output. Inhibitors of angiotensin-converting enzyme have proven to be important adjuvants to chronic anticongestive therapy in pediatric patients. IV forms are available and may be useful in treatment of systemic hypertension immediately after coarctation repair or when afterload reduction with these inhibitors would benefit patients unable to receive oral medications. Sudden hypotension with the IV forms may limit use their among infants and will persist even if the infusion is discontinued. Intensivists may prefer shorter-acting drugs such as nitroprusside or nitroglycerin.

The natriuretic hormone system is an important regulator of neurohumoral activation, vascular tone, diastolic function, and fluid balance. Preliminary data suggest that the endogenous biological activity of the natriuretic hormone system is decreased following pediatric CPB. In theory, infusions of brain natriuretic peptide could oppose the neurohumoral mechanism associated with vasoconstriction and fluid retention after pediatric CPB. In randomized adult studies following CPB, natriuretic hormone infusions suppress the renin-angiotensin-aldosterone axis and improve cardiac loading conditions, cardiac index, and urine output (20,58,68,91). We have increasing experience with nesiritide infusions in children. Nesiritide (synthetic B-type natriuretic peptide) was prescribed in an open-label fashion to 30 children after congenital heart surgery or with primary heart failure. Administration of nesiritide was well tolerated and associated with improvement in diuresis and fluid balance (53).

Fenoldopam is a new dopaminergic agent useful in the treatment of systemic hypertension and may have salutary effects on renal blood flow. It causes systemic vasodilatation, increased renal output, and increased tubular sodium secretion. It has no known chronotropic or inotropic effects on the heart but reduces afterload and may augment urine output in critical ill newborns after cardiac surgery. Few reports are available in children. The addition of fenoldopam to diuretic therapy was shown to improve urine output in postoperative oliguric children (22). However, the possible adverse effects of drugs with dopaminergic properties have been highlighted, and this agent requires further clinical investigation before its use can be endorsed in postoperative cardiac care.

Levosimendan is a calcium sensitizer that enhances the contractile state of the ventricle by increasing myocyte sensitivity to calcium, and it induces vasodilation. It increases cardiac output by increasing stroke volume and is independent of cAMP pathways that characterize the mechanism of action of both the catecholamines and the phosphodiesterase III inhibitors. Levosimendan binds to myocardial troponin C to improve the efficiency of the contractile apparatus. The improvement in myocardial performance and systolic function is accomplished without an increase in intracellular cAMP or intracellular calcium, thus avoiding well-known adverse effects of catecholamines on cardiac relaxation and diastolic function (80). Levosimendan also stimulates ATP-sensitive potassium (K^+) channels and induces vasodilation. Levosimendan has potential cardioprotective effects through mitochondrial actions linked to preconditioning in response to oxidative stress. In humans, it reduces circulating proinflammatory markers and soluble apoptosis mediators in patients with decompensated heart failure (1). The appeal of a drug that increases cardiac output, decreases cardiac filling pressures, reduces afterload on the ventricles, and has anti-inflammatory properties is enormous in pediatrics.

Levosimendan was administered in an open-label, named-patient (compassionate use) basis to 15 children, ages 7 days to 18 years who had severe heart failure and ventricular dysfunction and were refractory to dobutamine therapy (61). Remarkably, levosimendan allowed for discontinuation of catecholamine infusions in 10 of the 15 patients and permitted a reduction of catecholamine dose in three additional patients. No adverse effects were attributable to the drug. For patients in whom quantitative measures of LV function could be obtained echocardiographically, marked overall improvement in ejection fraction was observed. Perhaps the most heartening observation, consistent with the prolonged duration of action of the drug, was that improvement of ventricular function was sustained for some days even after completion of the 24-hr infusion. When viewed in conjunction with adult physiologic data in patients with severe heart failure, where levosimendan increased cardiac output and lowered pulmonary capillary wedge pressure more than dobutamine (32), this report provides a hopeful basis for designing trials in children. With its positive inotropic effects, levosimendan may be of value as adjunctive therapy to other inotropic drugs in patients who are refractory or tachyphylactic to other forms of inotropic support (32,80). Disappointingly, levosimendan provided no apparent improvement in LV ejection fraction among patients with end-stage heart failure. This is arguably the group in greatest need of new therapies (88). Levosimendan's hemodynamic effect in children is uncertain, but its pharmacokinetic profile seems similar to that seen in adults (82).

Other Strategies

Newer strategies to support low cardiac output associated with cardiac surgery in children include the use of atrio-biventricular pacing for patients with complete heart block or prolonged interventricular conduction delays and asynchronous contraction (47). Appreciation of the hemodynamic effects of positive- and negative-pressure ventilation may facilitate optimization of cardiac output by adjustments to ventilation. Avoidance of hyperthermia and even induced hypothermia may provide end-organ protection during periods of low cardiac output. Anti-inflammatory agents, including monoclonal antibodies, competitive receptor blockers, inhibitors of complement activation, and preoperative preparation with steroids, are being actively investigated in an effort to prevent, and protect major organs from, ischemic injury imposed by CPB and the reperfusion injury associated with the recovery period.

In children with LCOS who are resistant to catecholamine administration, a relative adrenal insufficiency has been proposed as a causative factor. Some retrospective studies have reported successful use of hydrocortisone to reduce inotropic requirement. Improved ventricular function, decreased inotropic support, reduction of serum lactate, and a shorter duration of mechanical ventilation after open-heart surgery in neonates has been shown (5,81).

Diastolic Dysfunction

Occasionally, an alteration of ventricular relaxation occurs which is an active energy-dependent process that reduces ventricular compliance. This event is particularly problematic in a patient with a hypertrophied ventricle who is undergoing surgical repair, e.g., tetralogy of Fallot or Fontan surgery, and, in some neonates, following CPB, when myocardial edema may significantly restrict diastolic function (i.e., "restrictive physiology") (23,70). The ventricular cavity size is small, and

the stroke volume is decreased. β-adrenergic antagonists and calcium-channel blockers add little to the treatment of this condition. In fact, hypotension or myocardial depression produced by these agents frequently outweigh any gain from slowing the heart rate. Calcium-channel blockers are relatively contraindicated in neonates and small infants because of their dependence on trans-sarcolemmal flux of calcium to both initiate and sustain contraction.

A gradual increase in intravascular volume to augment ventricular capacity, in addition to the use of low doses of inotropic agents, has proven to provide modest benefit in patients with diastolic dysfunction. Tachycardia must be avoided to optimize diastolic filling time and to decrease myocardial oxygen demands. If low cardiac output continues despite the above-outlined treatment, therapy with vasodilators can be carefully attempted to lower systolic wall tension by reducing afterload, thereby facilitating ventricular ejection. Because the capacity of the vascular bed increases after vasodilation, simultaneous volume replacement is often indicated. Milrinone or enoximone is useful under these circumstances, as these agents are noncatecholamines—so-called *inodilators*—with vasodilating and lusitropic (improved diastolic state) properties, in contrast to other inotropic agents. In the future, nesiritide may prove to have a particularly important role to play in lowering LV filling pressures in patients with heart failure.

Managing Acute Pulmonary Hypertension in the ICU

Children with many forms of CHD are prone to develop perioperative elevations in PVR, which may complicate the postoperative course, when transient myocardial dysfunction requires optimal control of RV afterload (86).

Although one often presumes that postoperative patients with pulmonary hypertension have active and reversible pulmonary vasoconstriction as the source of their pathophysiology, the critical care physician is obliged to explore anatomic causes of mechanical obstruction that impose a barrier to pulmonary blood flow. Elevated LA pressure, pulmonary venous obstruction, branch PA stenosis, or surgically induced loss of the vascular tree will all raise RV pressure and impose an unnecessary burden on the right heart. Similarly, a residual or undiagnosed left-to-right shunt will raise PA pressure postoperatively and must be addressed surgically. Extended use of pulmonary vasodilator strategies will only augment residual or undiagnosed shunts and increase the volume load on the heart.

Several factors peculiar to CPB may raise PVR; pulmonary vascular endothelial dysfunction, microemboli, pulmonary leukosequestration, excess thromboxane production, atelectasis, hypoxic pulmonary vasoconstriction, and adrenergic events have all been suggested to play a role in postoperative pulmonary hypertension. Postoperative pulmonary vascular reactivity has been related not only to the presence of preoperative pulmonary hypertension and left-to-right shunts, but also to the duration of total CPB. The incidence of postoperative pulmonary hypertension is lower in the current era of "early" corrective surgery, and its clinical management is now well understood (**Table 70A.6**).

TABLE 70A.6

CRITICAL CARE STRATEGIES FOR POSTOPERATIVE TREATMENT OF
PULMONARY HYPERTENSION

Encourage	Avoid
1. Anatomic investigation	1. Residual anatomic disease
2. Opportunities for right-to-left shunt as "pop off"	2. Intact atrial septum in right heart failure
3. Sedation/anesthesia	3. Agitation/pain
4. Moderate hyperventilation	4. Respiratory acidosis
5. Moderate alkalosis	5. Metabolic acidosis
6. Adequate inspired oxygen	6. Alveolar hypoxia
7. Normal lung volumes	7. Atelectasis or overdistension
8. Optimal hematocrit	8. Excessive hematocrit
9. Inotropic support	9. Low output and coronary perfusion
10. Vasodilators	10. Vasoconstrictors/increased afterload

Pulmonary Vasodilators

Many IV vasodilators have been used with variable success in patients with pulmonary hypertensive disorders who require critical care. Vasodilators historically reported as useful in pulmonary hypertension (e.g., tolazoline, phenoxybenzamine, nitroprusside, and isoproterenol) had little biologic basis for selectivity or enhanced activity in the pulmonary vascular bed (26). However, if myocardial function is depressed and the afterload-reducing effect on the LV is beneficial to myocardial function and cardiac output, these drugs may have some value. In addition to drug-specific side effects, they all have the limitation of potentially causing profound systemic hypotension, critically lowering right (and left) coronary perfusion pressure, and simultaneously increasing intrapulmonary shunt. Even with selective infusions of rapidly metabolized, intravenously administered, vasoactive drugs into the pulmonary circulation, systemic drug concentrations and systemic hemodynamic effects can be appreciable.

Prostacyclin appears to have somewhat more selectivity for the pulmonary circulation, but high doses can precipitate profound systemic hypotension in unstable postoperative patients with refractory pulmonary hypertension. While the drug's short half-life makes its titration easy, it is mainly used for chronic outpatient therapy in severe forms of primary pulmonary hypertension (10,74,92). Agents that improve ventricular function in addition to reducing afterload (e.g., phosphodiesterase III inhibitors) are more appealing when cardiac output is low.

As an alternative approach to nonspecific vasodilators, it seems logical to target vasoconstrictors known to be associated with pathologic states or critical events. In this regard, endothelin, a potent vasoconstrictor that is elevated in persistent pulmonary hypertension of the newborn, in children with CHD, and in patients after CPB, seems a likely candidate for investigation of specific receptor blockers. Promising amelioration of postoperative pulmonary hypertension associated with CPB has been shown in animal models of increased pulmonary blood flow (from intracardiac shunts) when pretreated with endothelin-A receptor blockers (66).

Nitric oxide (NO) is a selective pulmonary vasodilator that can be breathed as a gas and distributed across the alveoli to the pulmonary vascular smooth muscle (36,37). It is formed by the endothelium from L-arginine and molecular oxygen in a reaction catalyzed by NO synthase (NOS). It then diffuses to the adjacent vascular smooth muscle cells, where it induces vasodilation through a cyclic guanosine monophosphate-dependent pathway (46). As NO exists as a gas, it can be delivered by inhalation to the alveoli and then to the blood vessels that lie in close proximity to the ventilated lung. Because of its rapid inactivation by hemoglobin, inhaled NO (iNO) may achieve selective pulmonary vasodilation when pulmonary vasoconstriction exists. It has advantages over intravenously administered vasodilators that cause systemic hypotension and increase intrapulmonary shunting. iNO lowers PA pressure in a number of diseases without the unwanted effect of systemic hypotension, particularly dramatic in children with cardiovascular disorders and postoperative patients with pulmonary hypertensive crises (6,49,86,89).

Therapeutic uses of iNO in children with CHD abound in the ICU. For example, newborns with total anomalous pulmonary venous connection frequently have obstruction of the pulmonary venous pathway as it connects anomalously to the systemic venous circulation. When pulmonary venous return is obstructed preoperatively, pulmonary hypertension is severe and demands urgent surgical relief. Increased neonatal pulmonary vasoreactivity, endothelial injury induced by CPB, and intrauterine anatomic changes in the pulmonary vascular bed in this disease contribute to postoperative pulmonary hypertension. iNO dramatically reduces pulmonary hypertension without change in heart rate, systemic blood pressure, or vascular resistance.

Patients with total anomalous pulmonary venous connection, congenital mitral stenosis, and other pulmonary venous hypertensive disorders associated with low cardiac output appear to be among the most responsive to NO. These infants are born with significantly increased amounts of smooth muscle in their pulmonary arterioles and veins. Histologic evidence of muscularized pulmonary veins and pulmonary arteries suggests the presence of vascular tone and capacity for change in resistance at both the arterial and venous sites. The increased responsiveness to NO seen in younger patients with pulmonary venous hypertension may result from pulmonary vasorelaxation at a combination of precapillary and postcapillary vessels.

Successful use of iNO in a variety of other congenital heart defects following cardiac surgery has been reported by several groups. It may be especially helpful when administered during a pulmonary hypertensive crisis (49). Descriptions of use after Fontan procedures (41) and following VSD repair, along with a variety of other anatomic lesions have been described. Prophylactic use of iNO in patients at risk of developing postoperative pulmonary hypertensive crises is thought by some to reduce the duration of mechanical ventilation (57). Infants who are excessively cyanotic after a bidirectional Glenn anastomosis do not generally improve pulmonary blood flow and oxygen saturation in response to iNO. Increasing cardiac output and cerebral blood flow may have a much greater impact on arterial oxygenation by increasing flow through the Glenn shunt and into the pulmonary arteries. Elevated pulmonary vascular tone is seldom the limiting factor in the hypoxemic patient after the bidirectional Glenn operation (4).

iNO can also be used diagnostically in neonates with RV hypertension after cardiac surgery to discern those with reversible vasoconstriction. Failure of the postoperative newborn with pulmonary hypertension to respond to NO successfully discriminated anatomic obstruction to pulmonary blood flow from pulmonary vasoconstriction. Failure of the postoperative newborn to respond to NO should be regarded as strong evidence of anatomic and, possibly, surgically remediable obstruction (2).

If withdrawal of NO is necessary before resolution of the pathologic process, hemodynamic instability may be expected. We have previously suggested that the withdrawal response to iNO can be attenuated by pretreatment with the type V phosphodiesterase inhibitor sildenafil (Viagra) (7,62). In 29 ventilated infants who received ≥10 ppm NO and were randomized to receive 0.4 mg/kg of sildenafil or placebo 1 hr before discontinuing NO, rebound pulmonary hypertension occurred in 10/14 placebo patients and 0/15 sildenafil patients ($p < 0.001$). In addition, duration of ventilation was significantly reduced for sildenafil patients (62).

Sildenafil inhibits the inactivation of cGMP within the vascular smooth muscle cell and has the potential to augment the effects of endogenous or exogenously administered NO to relax vascular smooth muscle. Sildenafil can be administered in oral or IV forms and has been shown to have somewhat selective pulmonary-vasodilating capacity while lowering the LA pressure and providing a modest degree of afterload reduction in some postoperative children. Chronic oral administration of sildenafil to adults with primary pulmonary hypertension improves the exercise capacity, perhaps suggesting an important therapeutic application of the IV preparation in postoperative congenital heart surgery. Unfortunately, the IV form is no longer in development, but the need for an IV preparation of this class of agent is clear.

Undoubtedly, in that the causes of pulmonary hypertension in the intensive care setting are frequently multifactorial, the "best" therapy will be multiply targeted. Adding phosphodiesterase inhibitors to prostacyclin infusions, endothelin blockers, thromboxane inhibitors, and iNO may have individual and combined merit, with synergism-enhancing efficacy.

Cardiac Tamponade

Cardiac tamponade may occur following cardiac surgery due to compression of the heart within the thorax following blood or serous fluid collection or because of swelling of intrathoracic tissues in response to a perioperative systemic inflammatory response. The infant's small mediastinum makes compression of the heart and cardiac tamponade ever-present possibilities after chest closure, despite patent mediastinal drainage tubes and surgical resection of the anterior pericardium. The warning signs of tamponade are frequently subtle in small children, even minutes before cardiovascular collapse from tamponade. Any significant deterioration in hemodynamics after chest closure should be first attributed to tamponade if ventilation and cardiac rhythm are adequate. The signs of tamponade include tachycardia, hypotension, narrow pulse pressure, pulsus paradoxus, and high filling pressures on both the left and right sides of the heart.

Acute myocardial perforation with tamponade occasionally occurs during interventional cardiac catheterization procedures. Prompt support of the circulation with volume infusions and pressor support, along with immediate catheter drainage of the pericardial space, are essential in the event of this complication. Hemopericardium after ventricular puncture is usually self-limited, as the muscular ventricle seals the perforation after the responsible wire or catheter is removed. However, laceration of the more thin-walled atrium may require suture repair under direct vision in the operating room.

Other causes of cardiac tamponade are seen in patients with CHD, and treatment requires the intensivist to perform a pericardiocentesis or provide sedation and monitoring for the pericardiocentesis. Postoperative tamponade from bleeding immediately after operation, as previously discussed, is best handled by facilitation of chest tube drainage or reopening the sternotomy. These patients are usually still anesthetized and mechanically ventilated, so that new anesthetic considerations and choices are limited. However, some children develop pericardial effusions at other phases of their illness, owing to hydrostatic influences (e.g., patients with modified Fontan operations) or postpericardiotomy syndrome. Fluid in the pericardial space may accumulate under considerable pressure, and filling of the heart is impaired. If this problem is left unattended, the transmural pressure in the atria diminishes as the intra-atrial pressures rise, and diastolic collapse of the atria can be observed echocardiographically. The patients become symptomatic with narrow pulse pressure, pulsus paradoxus, tachycardia, respiratory distress, abdominal pain progressing to decreased urine output, hyperkalemia, metabolic acidosis, and hypotension with tremendous endogenous catecholamine response. Serial echocardiographic monitoring up to 5 weeks postoperatively is warranted, especially in selected high-risk patients, such as those who undergo Fontan-type procedures.

In summary, aggressive identification and treatment of low cardiac output conditions after cardiac surgery are central to the critical care of children with CHD. Successful application of these strategies and thoughtful use of pharmacologic intervention has undoubtedly contributed to the remarkable decline in mortality associated with congenital heart surgery in the past two decades. However, despite these interventions, additional (mechanical) support is sometimes necessary as a bridge to recovery.

MECHANICAL SUPPORT OF THE CIRCULATION

Despite the expanding options for pharmacologic support, the circulation cannot be adequately supported in some patients in either preoperative or postoperative situations. Mechanical assist devices have an important role in providing short-term circulatory support to enable myocardial recovery and the potential for longer-term support while the patient awaits cardiac transplantation. A variety of assist devices is available for adult-sized patients; however, ECMO is the predominant mode of support for children, although some centers have significant experience in the use of paracorporeal ventricular assist devices in children.

According to the Extracorporeal Life Support Registry, over 300 children per year receive ECMO for cardiac support, with the majority placed on ECMO following cardiotomy (27,30,90). While >50% of these patients are decannulated from ECMO, the overall survival to discharge has only been between 35% and 40% of reported cases over the past decade. However, this experience is gradually changing. At Children's Hospital Boston, ECMO has been utilized to support the circulation in nearly 300 patients. Neonates comprise 41% of all cardiac ECMO, with a survival rate to discharge of 50%. The pediatric group (infants through 16 yrs) comprises 55% of the total experience, with an improved survival rate to discharge of 59%.

Substantial institutional variability in patient selection for ECMO makes comparison of published experience difficult. Centers with an efficient and well-established ECMO service are more likely to utilize this form of support in patients with low cardiac output. Furthermore, surgical technique and bypass management are additional confounding factors that make comparisons of the use and indications for ECMO between institutions difficult to interpret. Nevertheless, this form of mechanical support can be life-saving, and it can be argued that ECMO should be available when needed for selected patients following congenital heart surgery. ECMO for pediatric resuscitation (rapid deployment during active cardiopulmonary resuscitation in a pulseless circulation) remains a controversial issue. Several centers have successfully implemented rapid-deployment teams for ECMO-assisted resuscitation (24). A rapid-response ECMO system was started at Children's Hospital Boston in 1996 (28); among nearly 300 cardiac ECMO patients, 50% were cannulated during active cardiopulmonary resuscitation (rapid-response system), and 55% of these patients were successfully discharged from the hospital. General indications for ECMO support of the circulation in patients with CHD are summarized in **Table 70A.7**. Mechanical support of the circulation for patients with congenital and acquired heart disease has become a major component of standard practice in pediatric cardiac intensive care. Further details on mechanical support of the circulation, including use of ECMO and ventricular assist devices, are provided in Chapter 36.

Cardiopulmonary Interaction

Altered respiratory mechanics and positive-pressure ventilation may have significant influence on hemodynamics following congenital heart surgery (73) (**Table 70A.8**). Therefore, the approach to mechanical ventilation should not only be directed at achieving a desired gas exchange, but also influenced by the potential cardiorespiratory interactions of mechanical ventilation and method of weaning. The mode of ventilation must be matched to the hemodynamic status of each patient in order to achieve adequate cardiac output and gas exchange. Fre-

TABLE 70A.7

TYPICAL INDICATIONS FOR EXTRACORPOREAL MEMBRANE OXYGENATION

I. Inadequate oxygen delivery
　A. Low cardiac output
　　1. Chronic (cardiomyopathy)
　　2. Acute (myocarditis)
　　3. Failure of weaning from CPB
　　4. Need for preoperative stabilization
　　5. Progressive postoperative failure
　　6. Refractory pulmonary hypertension
　　7. Refractory dysrhythmias
　　8. Cardiac arrest
　B. Profound cyanosis
　　1. Intracardiac shunting and cardiovascular collapse
　　2. Acute shunt thrombosis
　　3. Acute respiratory failure exaggerated by underlying heart disease
　　4. CHD complicated by other newborn indications for ECMO, such as meconium aspiration syndrome, PPHN, pneumonia, sepsis, respiratory distress syndrome

II. Support for intervention during cardiac catheterization

CPB, cardiopulmonary bypass; CHD, congenital heart disease; PPHN, persistent pulmonary hypertension of the neonate

quent modifications to the mode and pattern of ventilation may be necessary during recovery after surgery, with attention to changes in lung volume and airway pressure. Changes in lung volume have a major effect on PVR, which is lowest at the lung's functional residual capacity, while either hypoinflation or hyperinflation may result in a significant increase in PVR because of altered traction on alveolar septae and extra-alveolar vessels. The subject is fully discussed in Chapter 64.

Special Problems for the Cardiac Patient

Diaphragmatic paresis (reduced motion) or paralysis (with paradoxical movement) may precipitate and promote respiratory failure, particularly in the neonate or young infant who relies on diaphragmatic function for breathing more than do older infants and children (who can recruit accessory and intercostal muscles if diaphragmatic function proves inadequate). Injury to the phrenic nerve, usually the left, may occur during operations which require dissection of the branch pulmonary arteries well out to the hilum (e.g., tetralogy of Fallot, arterial switch operation), arch reconstruction from the midline (e.g., Norwood operation), manipulation of the superior vena cava (Glenn shunts), takedown of previous systemic-to-pulmonary shunts, or after percutaneous central venous access. Phrenic injury may occur more frequently at reoperation, when adhesions and scarring may obscure landmarks. Topical cooling with ice during deep hypothermia may also cause transient phrenic palsy. Increased work of breathing on low ventilator settings, increased PCO_2, and a chest x-ray that reveals an elevated hemidiaphragm, are suggestive of diaphragmatic dysfunction. However, the chest x-ray may be falsely negative if it is taken during peak positive-pressure ventilation. Ultrasonography or fluoroscopy is useful for identifying diaphragmatic motion or paradoxical excursion. Recovery of diaphragmatic

TABLE 70A.8

CARDIORESPIRATORY INTERACTIONS OF A POSITIVE-PRESSURE MECHANICAL BREATH

	Afterload	Preload
PULMONARY VENTRICLE	ELEVATED Effect: ↑ RVEDp ↑ RVp ↓ Antegrade PBF ↑ PR and/or TR	REDUCED Effect: ↓ RVEDV ↓ RAp
SYSTEMIC VENTRICLE	REDUCED Effect: ↓ LVEDp ↓ LAp ↓ Pulmonary edema ↑ Increase cardiac output	REDUCED Effect: ↓ LVEDV ↓ LAp

RVEDp, right ventricle end-diastolic pressure; RVEDV, right ventricle end-diastolic volume; RVp, right ventricle pressure; RAp, right atrial pressure; PBF, pulmonary blood flow; PR, pulmonary regurgitation; TR, tricuspid regurgitation; LVEDp, left ventricle end diastolic pressure; LVEDV, left ventricle end diastolic volume; LAp, left atrial pressure

contraction usually occurs; however, if a patient fails to tolerate repeated extubations despite cardiovascular and nutritional status being optimized, and if diaphragmatic dysfunction persists with volume loss in the affected lung, then the diaphragm may need to be surgically plicated. Infants with diaphragmatic paralysis often benefit from plication, whereas older children may better tolerate a paretic diaphragm (48). The avoidance of collapse of the lung may provide the critical advantage, as plication prevents the paralyzed diaphragm from being drawn into the thorax during spontaneous inspiration.

Increased airway resistance arises from several pathologic changes alone or in combination: secretions (either excessive in quantity or viscosity), swelling of the mucosa due to hyperemia or edema (most often resulting from trauma or infection), hyperactive bronchial smooth muscle, extrinsic compression by neighboring structures, or diminished forces pulling the conducting passages open. Patients who have secretions from the tracheal aspirate that have many visible organisms and polymorphonuclear cells on microscopy, together with fever, an elevated white cell count, and consolidation on the chest x-ray require treatment with appropriate antibiotics.

Postextubation stridor may be due to mucosal swelling of the large airway. A nebulized, inhaled α agonist (e.g., racemic epinephrine) promotes vasoconstriction and decreases hyperemia and, possibly, edema. If reintubation is necessary, a smaller endotracheal tube should be used if possible, along with diuresis and, often, a short-term administration of steroids prior to a subsequent attempt at extubation in 24–36 hrs. An evaluation for vocal cord dysfunction should be considered, especially in patients with surgery near the recurrent laryngeal nerve (e.g., Norwood operation, patent ductus arteriosus ligation).

Bronchospasm may be treated by inhaled or systemically administered bronchodilators, but they must be used with caution in light of their chronotropic and tachyarrhythmic potential. If all of these maneuvers fail to improve the patient, the minimum tidal volume and frequency that provide sufficient mechanical minute ventilation to satisfactorily supplement spontaneous ventilation and minimize overinflation of the lungs are determined and utilized during the recovery phase. As increased lung water is frequently one of the culprits in causing bronchospasm, diuresis is often an effective treatment.

Pulmonary edema, pneumonia, and *atelectasis* are the most common causes of lower airway and alveolar abnormalities, which interfere with gas exchange. If a bacterial pathogen is identified, therapy includes antibiotics and pulmonary toilet. If the cause is pulmonary edema, therapy is aimed toward lowering the LA pressure through diuresis and pharmacologic means to reduce afterload and improve the lusitropic state of the heart. For infants, fluid restriction is frequently incompatible with adequate nutrition, and, therefore, an aggressive diuretic regimen is preferable to restriction of caloric intake. Adjustment of end-expiratory pressure and mechanical ventilation serve as supportive therapies until the alveoli and pulmonary interstitium are cleared of the fluid that interferes with gas entry.

Pleural effusions and *ascites* may occur in patients after a Fontan operation or reparative procedures that require a right ventriculotomy (e.g., tetralogy of Fallot, truncus arteriosus) with transient RV dysfunction. Especially in young patients, pleural effusions and increased interstitial lung water may be a manifestation of right heart failure; this seems logically related to raised systemic venous pressure impeding lymphatic return to the venous circulation. The lymphatic circuit is often functioning at full capacity in these children. Fluid in the pleural space or peritoneum and intestinal distention compete with intrapulmonary gas for thoracic space. Evacuation of the pleural space or drainage of ascites and decompression of the intestinal lumen allow the intrapulmonary gas volume to increase.

A summary of factors that should be considered in the patient who fails to wean from mechanical ventilation is presented in **Table 70A.9**.

Weaning from Mechanical Ventilation

Early tracheal extubation of children following congenital heart surgery is not a new concept but has received renewed attention with the evolution of "fast-track" management for cardiac surgical patients. Early extubation generally refers to tracheal extubation within a few hours (i.e., 4–8 hrs) after surgery, although in practice it means the avoidance of routine, overnight mechanical ventilation. Factors to consider when

TABLE 70A.9

FACTORS THAT CONTRIBUTE TO THE INABILITY TO WEAN FROM MECHANICAL VENTILATION AFTER CONGENITAL HEART SURGERY

Residual cardiac defects
  Volume and/or pressure overload
  Myocardial dysfunction
  Low cardiac output state
Restrictive pulmonary defects
  Pulmonary edema
  Pleural effusion
  Atelectasis
  Chest wall edema
  Phrenic nerve injury
  Ascites/hepatomegaly
Airway
  Subglottic edema and/or stenosis
  Retained secretions
  Vocal cord injury
  Extrinsic bronchial compression
  Tracheobronchomalacia
Metabolic
  Inadequate nutrition
  Sepsis
  Stress response

planning early extubation are listed in **Table 70A.10.** A number of reports have been published that describe successful tracheal extubation in neonates and older children following congenital heart surgery, either in the operating room or soon after in the CICU, without significant compromise of patient care and with a low incidence for reintubation or hemodynamic instability. This fast-track strategy has been extended to routine,

early (within 24 hrs of surgery) discharge from the hospital. Although overzealous attempts to achieve this goal can have a negative impact on patients and families (e.g., discharge at 24 hrs to hotel with chest tube still in place), the practice has served to streamline care of these children and highlight the advances in perioperative care that now permit hospital discharge of infants and older children within 24 hrs of repair of congenital heart defects on CPB (83).

Failed extubation can be a significant problem in the postoperative period. The main reasons for failed extubation or inability to wean from mechanical ventilation are respiratory insufficiency, circulatory failure, or frequently, a combination of both in a nutritionally deprived newborn or infant. Upper airway obstruction with stridor accounts for ~25% of the total failures. The use of corticosteroids for upper airway obstruction is controversial, especially as a prophylaxis strategy. Cyanosis, increased work of breathing, or both may necessitate reintubation of the trachea. Although ventilation-perfusion abnormalities may exist in isolation, it is likely that some hemodynamic factor, such as significant residual heart disease, the insult of CPB, or raised atrial pressure associated with increased lung water, is a major contributor. Careful hemodynamic evaluation and echocardiographic assessment to rule out residual lesions are mandatory in these patients (44).

Finally, an additional airway malformation should be ruled out postoperatively after failure of early postoperative extubation (e.g., tracheobronchial malacia, long-segment tracheal stenosis, bilateral vocal cord paralysis, tracheal hemangioma). Diagnosis is made by bronchoscopy or MRI.

Central Nervous System

The dramatic reduction in surgical mortality in recent decades has been accompanied by a growing recognition of adverse

TABLE 70A.10

CONSIDERATIONS FOR PLANNED EARLY EXTUBATION AFTER CONGENITAL HEART SURGERY

Patient factors	Risk factors associated with anatomy and planned surgery
	Limited cardiorespiratory reserve of the neonate and infant
	Pathophysiology of specific congenital heart defects
	Timing of surgery and preoperative management
Anesthetic factors	Premedication
	Hemodynamic stability and reserve
	Drug distribution and maintenance of anesthesia on bypass
	Postoperative analgesia
Surgical factors	Extent and complexity of surgery
	Residual defects
	Risks for bleeding and protection of suture lines
Conduct of bypass	Degree of hypothermia
	Level of hemodilution
	Myocardial protection
	Extent of the inflammatory response and reperfusion injury
Postoperative management	Myocardial function
	Cardiorespiratory interactions
	Neurologic recovery
	Analgesia management

neurologic sequelae in some survivors (35,84). Abnormalities of the central nervous system (CNS) may be a function of coexisting brain abnormalities or acquired events unrelated to surgical management (e.g., paradoxical embolus, brain infection, effects of chronic cyanosis), but CNS insults appear to occur most frequently during or immediately after surgery. In particular, support techniques used during neonatal and infant cardiac surgery—CPB, profound hypothermia, and circulatory arrest—have been implicated as important causes of brain injury (63).

During hypothermic CPB, multiple perfusion variables might influence the risk of brain injury. These include (but are probably not limited to) the total duration of CPB, duration and rate of core cooling, pH management during core cooling, duration of circulatory arrest, type of oxygenator, presence of arterial filtration, and depth of hypothermia (9). Undoubtedly, interaction occurs between these elements, and CNS injury following CPB is most likely multifactorial. Early postoperative studies (in the ICU) revealed a higher incidence of neurologic perturbation in patients who undergo circulatory arrest, including a higher incidence of clinical and electroencephalographic seizures, a longer recovery time to the first reappearance of electroencephalographic activity, and greater release of the brain isoenzyme of creatine kinase. Neuron-specific enolase, a marker for cerebral cell damage was elevated during and 4 hrs after CPB in 35 neonates who underwent arterial switch operation. Half of these neonates had abnormal cranial ultrasound findings in the early postoperative period. Although most of these pathologic scans normalized within 2 weeks, intraventricular hemorrhage findings remained in 17% of the patients, and 4 neonates (11%) experienced seizures within the first week after operation (79).

Seizures

Seizures are the most frequently observed neurologic consequence of cardiac surgery, with an incidence of 4%–25% in older studies. Although the incidence of seizures in the ICU has dramatically declined in recent years, we treat seizures aggressively when they do occur, using benzodiazepines, phenobarbital, or phenytoin. Importantly, we have eliminated a number of practices that may have been associated with brain injury after CPB, including rapid cooling during CPB, use of prolonged hypothermic circulatory arrest, extreme α-stat strategy of intraoperative pH management, extreme hemodilution to hematocrits <20, applying heat lamps to infants on arrival at the ICU, hypocapnic hyperventilation, and prolonged muscle relaxation (masking seizure observations). Hyperthermia to any degree must be avoided in the early postoperative period.

Intraventricular Hemorrhage

Intraventricular hemorrhage, which may occur as a consequence of perinatal events or circulatory collapse in the first few days of life, is commonly associated with prematurity. Our approach has been to screen all premature infants or asphyxiated babies with a head ultrasound prior to CPB, which of course involves extensive anticoagulation, hemodynamic perturbation, and risk that bleeding will extend. Surgical intervention is delayed for several days if intraventricular bleeding is documented. By deferring operations in very premature newborns for 5–7 days after birth, a low incidence of intraven-

tricular hemorrhage in these high-risk patients can be achieved despite use of CPB (69).

Renal Function and Postoperative Fluid Management

Risk factors for postoperative renal failure include preoperative renal dysfunction, prolonged bypass time, low cardiac output, and cardiac arrest. In addition to relative ischemia and nonpulsatile flow on CPB, angiotensin II-mediated renal vasoconstriction and delayed healing of renal tubular epithelium has been proposed as one mechanism for renal failure. Postoperative sepsis and nephrotoxic drugs may cause further damage to the kidneys.

Because of the inflammatory response to bypass and significant increase in total body water, fluid management in the immediate postoperative period is critical. Capillary leak and interstitial fluid accumulation may continue for the first 24–48 hrs following surgery, necessitating ongoing volume replacement with colloid or blood products. A fall in cardiac output and increased antidiuretic hormone secretion contribute to delayed water clearance and potential prerenal dysfunction, which could progress to acute tubular necrosis and renal failure if an LCOS persists.

During CPB, optimizing the circuit prime, hematocrit, and oncotic pressure; attenuating the inflammatory response with steroids and protease inhibitors such as aprotinin (21); and using modified ultrafiltration techniques have all been recommended to limit interstitial fluid accumulation (29). During the first 24 hrs following surgery, maintenance fluids are usually restricted and volume replacement titrated to appropriate filling pressures and hemodynamic response.

Oliguria in the first 24 hrs after complex surgery and CPB is common in neonates and infants until cardiac output recovers and neurohumoral mechanisms abate. While diuretics are commonly prescribed in the immediate postoperative period, the neurohumoral influence on urine output is powerful. Diuresis will usually occur as time elapses after CPB (~24 hrs) and as cardiac output is enhanced through intravascular volume and pharmacologic adjustments.

Peritoneal dialysis, hemodialysis, and continuous venovenous hemofiltration provide alternate renal support in patients with severe oliguria and renal failure (64). Besides enabling water and solute clearance, maintenance fluids can be increased to ensure adequate nutrition. The indications for renal support vary, but include blood urea nitrogen >100 mg/dL, life-threatening electrolyte imbalance such as severe hyperkalemia, ongoing metabolic acidosis, fluid restrictions that limit nutrition, and increased mechanical ventilation requirements secondary to persistent pulmonary edema or ascites.

A peritoneal dialysis catheter may be placed into the peritoneal cavity at the completion of surgery or later in the ICU. The indications for peritoneal catheter placement in the ICU include the need for renal support and the need to reduce intra-abdominal pressure from ascites that may be compromising mechanical ventilation. Peritoneal drainage may be significant in the immediate postoperative period as third-space fluid losses continue. Replacement with albumin and/or fresh frozen plasma may be necessary to treat hypovolemia and hypoproteinemia.

Gastrointestinal Issues

Following cardiac surgery in neonates and children, adequate nutrition is exceedingly important. These critically ill children often have decreased caloric intake and increased energy demand after surgery; the neonate in particular has limited metabolic and fat reserves. Total parenteral nutrition can provide adequate nutrition in the early hypercatabolic phases of the early postoperative period.

Upper gastrointestinal bleeding and ulcer formation may occur following the stress of cardiac surgery in children and adults. Even though reports of the efficacy of histamine H_2 anti-receptors, sucralfate, or oral antacids in pediatric cardiac patients are limited, their use is common in many ICUs. Hepatic failure may occur after cardiac surgery (particularly after the Fontan operation) and is typically characterized by elevated liver enzymes and coagulopathy.

Necrotizing enterocolitis, although typically a disease of premature infants, is seen with considerable frequency in neonates with CHD. Risk factors include: (a) left-sided obstructive lesions (b) umbilical or femoral arterial catheterization/angiography, (c) hypoxemia, and (d) lesions with wide pulse pressures (e.g., systemic-to-pulmonary shunts, patent ductus arteriosus, especially in transposition of the great arteries, and severe aortic regurgitation, all of which may produce retrograde flow in the mesenteric vessels during diastole). Frequently, multiple risk factors exist in the same patient, making a specific etiology difficult to establish. Treatment includes continuous nasogastric suction, parenteral nutrition, and broad-spectrum antibiotics. Bowel exploration or resection may be necessary in severe cases.

Infection

Low-grade (<38.5°C) fever during the immediate postoperative period is common and may be present for up to 3–4 days, even without a demonstrable infectious etiology. However, several reports describe increased susceptibility to infection after CPB. CPB may activate complement and other mediators of inflammation but can also lead to derangements of the immune system and increase the likelihood of infection. Fever of <38.5°C in the immediate postoperative period is usually the result of a systemic inflammatory reaction to surgery rather than active infection, but its course should be closely observed.

Sepsis and nosocomial infection after cardiac surgery contribute substantially to overall morbidity. Despite the increased use of broad-coverage, third-generation cephalosporins, these agents do not seem to be more effective in decreasing postoperative infections. Meticulous catheter insertion and daily care routines, along with early removal of indwelling catheters in the postoperative patient may potentially reduce the incidence of sepsis.

Mediastinitis occurs in up to 2% of patients who undergo cardiac surgery; risk factors may include delayed sternal closure, early re-exploration for bleeding, or reoperation. Mediastinitis is characterized by persistent fever, purulent drainage from the sternotomy wound, instability of the sternum, and leukocytosis. *Staphylococcus* is the most common offending organism. Treatment usually involves debridement and irrigation with parenteral antibiotic therapy. Duration of therapy seldom exceeds 2 weeks.

POSTOPERATIVE MANAGEMENT OF PATIENTS WITH A SINGLE VENTRICLE AFTER NEONATAL PALLIATIVE SURGERY

The First Stage of Palliation

Management of patients following the first stage of single-ventricle reconstruction (stage I Norwood operation) is complex; intensive monitoring is essential, as the clinical status may change abruptly with rapid deterioration (**Table 70A.11**). Persistent or progressive metabolic acidosis is a bad prognostic sign and must be aggressively managed. Ideally, the pH should be 7.40, $PaCO_2$ should be 40 mm Hg, and PaO_2 should be 40 mm Hg in room air, with an SvO_2 of 60%, reflecting a well-balanced circulation. Higher saturations can be achieved if the systemic circulation is well dilated without compromising perfusion pressure. Frequent changes in mechanical ventilation settings and FIO_2 may be less important in the first few hours after surgery than previously thought, but thoughtful adjustment of the ventilator remains an important aspect of care. Manipulation of FIO_2 in the face of a restrictive 3.5-mm shunt may have less impact on pulmonary blood flow than would systemic vasodilation (59). Leaving the sternum open after surgery may help to facilitate lower filling pressures, a balanced circulation, and stable ventilation pattern.

Deep sedation for several hours, or even muscle paralysis and anesthesia, are sometimes continued following surgery to minimize the stress response until the patient has a stable circulation and gas exchange. This approach has its advocates and critics. Inotropic support with dopamine and, occasionally, low doses of epinephrine are often required, titrated to systemic pressure and perfusion. However, high doses of epinephrine are often detrimental, especially if patients with a modified Blalock-Taussig shunt have too much relative pulmonary blood flow. Afterload reduction with milrinone as a second-line agent is beneficial to reduce myocardial work and improve systemic perfusion. Monitoring superior vena cava oxygen saturations, as a measure of SvO_2 and cardiac output is useful in this assessment (72). Volume replacement to maintain preload is essential, aiming for a common atrial pressure that approximates 10 mmHg.

The type, diameter, length, and position of the shunt will also affect the balance of pulmonary and systemic flows. Generally, a 3.5-mm Blalock-Taussig shunt from the distal innominate artery will provide adequate pulmonary blood flow without excessive steal from the systemic circulation for most full-term neonates. Nevertheless, if the shunt results in a low diastolic pressure (<30 mm Hg), that, in turn, will decrease perfusion to other vascular beds (in particular coronary, cerebral, renal, and splanchnic perfusion). This may contribute to a prolonged and difficult postoperative course.

Overcirculation in the immediate postoperative period with an SaO_2 of >90% may reflect a low PVR, or increased flow across the shunt if the shunt size is too large or the shunt perfusion pressure is increased from residual aortic arch obstruction distal to the shunt insertion site. The increased volume load

TABLE 70A.11

MANAGEMENT CONSIDERATIONS FOR PATIENTS FOLLOWING A NORWOOD PROCEDURE

Scenario	Etiology	Management
Sao_2 ~80% Svo_2 ~60% Normotension	**BALANCED FLOW** $Q_p = Q_s$	No intervention

Sao_2 >90%
Hypotension
	Overcirculated
	$Q_p > Q_s$
	Low PVR
	Large BT Shunt
	Residual arch obstruction
		Raise PVR:
		    Controlled hypoventilation
		    Low Fio_2 (0.17–0.19)
		    Add CO_2 (3%–5%)
		Increase systemic perfusion:
		    Afterload reduction, vasodilation,
		        inotropic support
		    Surgical shunt revision

Sao_2 <75%
Hypertension
	UNDER CIRCULATED
	$Q_p < Q_s$
	High PVR
	Small, kinked, thrombosed BT shunt
		Lower PVR:
		    Controlled hyperventilation
		    Alkalosis
		    Sedation/paralysis
		Increase cardiac output:
		    Inotrope support
		Hematocrit >40%
		Surgical intervention

Sao_2 <75% Hypotension Low Svo_2	**LOW CARDIAC OUTPUT** Ventricular failure Myocardial ischemia Residual arch obstruction AV valve regurgitation	Minimize stress response Inotropic support Surgical revision Consider mechanical support Consider transplantation

Sao_2, arterial oxygen saturation; Svo_2, mixed venous oxygen saturation; Q_p, pulmonary blood flow; Q_s, systemic blood flow; PVR, pulmonary vascular resistance; Fio_2, inspired oxygen concentration; BT, Blalock-Taussig

on the systemic ventricle results in congestive cardiac failure and progressive systemic hypoperfusion with cool extremities, oliguria, and possibly metabolic acidosis. While manipulation of mechanical ventilation and inspired oxygen concentration along with systemic vasodilation may help limit pulmonary blood flow, surgical revision to reduce the shunt size may be necessary.

If significant systemic steal through a large shunt occurs, coronary perfusion may be reduced, leading to ischemia, low output, and dysrhythmias. Rhythm disturbances are uncommon in the immediate postoperative period following a Norwood operation, and a sudden loss of sinus rhythm, and in particular heart block or ventricular fibrillation, should increase the suspicion of myocardial ischemia.

In the immediate postoperative period, mild hypoxemia with an Sao_2 of 70%–75% and Pao_2 of 30–35 mm Hg is preferable to an overcirculated state with high systemic oxygen saturations and falling Svo_2. Pulmonary blood flow often increases on the first postoperative day as ventricular function improves and PVR falls during recovery from CPB. Pulmonary venous desaturation from parenchymal lung disease such as atelectasis, pleural effusions, and pneumothorax requires aggressive management.

Persistent desaturation and hypotension may reflect low cardiac output from poor ventricular function, thereby decreasing the perfusion pressure across the shunt. The Svo_2 is low (often <40%), and treatment is directed first at augmenting contractility with inotropic agents and subsequently at reducing afterload with a vasodilator. This is a serious clinical problem, with a high mortality rate after a Norwood operation. The related myocardial ischemia and acidosis further impair myocardial function and systemic perfusion, leading to circulatory collapse.

Atrioventricular valve regurgitation and residual aortic arch obstruction are important causes of persistent low cardiac output and the inability to wean from mechanical ventilation. Echocardiography is useful to assess valve and ventricular function, although it is less accurate for assessing the degree of residual arch obstruction. Cardiac catheterization is sometimes necessary and will enable fine tuning of hemodynamic support or balloon dilation of a hypoplastic segment of narrowed aorta. Occasionally, surgical revision of the aortic arch or atrioventricular valve is necessary, although this is seen more commonly in the interval before the bidirectional cavopulmonary shunt.

A modification to the Norwood procedure has been introduced that involves placement of a conduit from the RV to the PA confluence (also called a ventriculopulmonary shunt or Sano modification) (52,76). The primary advantage for this procedure in the immediate postoperative period is improved diastolic perfusion without runoff across an aortopulmonary shunt. Ventricular function is less likely to be compromised after surgery because the volume load to the ventricle is reduced from a lower Q_p:Q_s ratio, along with a reduced risk for myocardial ischemia because of improved coronary perfusion. Perfusion to cerebral, renal, and splanchnic circulations is also likely to be improved with the lack of diastolic runoff to the pulmonary circulation, and this may also enhance postoperative recovery. Because pulmonary blood flow occurs only during ventricular systole across the RV-to-PA conduit, a critical reduction in pulmonary blood flow and excessive hypoxemia may occur, especially during periods of low cardiac output or if dynamic obstruction to flow occurs at the ventricular insertion site. Efforts to overcome this limitation by creating a larger RV incision run the longer-term risk of ventricular dysfunction or aneurysm formation. The short-term survival advantage of the Sano modification of the Norwood operation at centers where mortality for the Norwood procedure was already below 15% will be difficult to demonstrate. Results from a Pediatric Heart Network randomized trial of Sano versus Blalock-Taussig shunt for patients with hypoplastic left heart syndrome are anxiously awaited.

Bidirectional Cavopulmonary Anastomosis

The bidirectional cavopulmonary anastomosis is the follow-up surgical procedure in infants after neonatal palliation of single-ventricle anatomy. In this procedure, also known as a bidirectional Glenn (BDG) shunt, the superior vena cava is transected and connected end-to-side to the right PA, but the pulmonary arteries are left in continuity. Therefore, flow from the superior vena cava is bidirectional into both left and right PAs. This is the only source of pulmonary blood flow, and inferior vena cava blood returns to the common atrium. Performed at between 3 and 6 months of age, the BDG has proven to be an important early staging procedure for patients with single-ventricle physiology because the volume and pressure load is relieved from the systemic ventricle, yet effective pulmonary blood flow is maintained. Q_p:Q_s is always <1, and the volume load to the single RV is relieved, compared to the volume load with a systemic-to-pulmonary artery shunt. However, the BDG is impractical in the newborn whose pulmonary cross-sectional area is inadequate to accommodate sufficient passive pulmonary blood flow for tolerable oxygenation.

The BDG is usually performed on CPB using mild hypothermia with a beating heart. The complications related to CPB and aortic cross-clamping are therefore minimal, and patients can be weaned and extubated in the early postoperative period (17). Systemic hypertension is common following a BDG. The etiology remains unclear, but possible factors include improved contractility and stroke volume after the volume load on the ventricle is removed and brainstem-mediated mechanisms secondary to the increased systemic and cerebral venous pressure. Treatment with vasodilators may be necessary during the immediate postoperative period and during the weaning process.

Following the BDG anastomosis, arterial oxygen saturation should be in the 80%–85% range. Persistent hypoxemia is often secondary to an LCOS and low Svo_2. Treatment is directed at improving contractility, reducing afterload, and ensuring that the patient has a normal rhythm and hematocrit. Increased PVR is an uncommon cause of hypoxemia, and iNO is rarely beneficial in these patients, which is not surprising because the PA pressure and resistance and vascular tone are simply not high enough following this surgery to see a demonstrable benefit from NO (3). Persistent, profound hypoxemia should

be investigated in the catheterization laboratory to evaluate hemodynamics, to look for residual anatomic defects that may be limiting pulmonary flow (e.g., PA stenosis or a restrictive atrial septal defect) or significant venovenous collaterals. Venovenous collaterals decompress the PA tree and divert blood flow away from the pulmonary capillary bed. The treatment consists of occluding venous collateral flow by inserting coils into the collateral vessels during cardiac catheterization.

Fontan Procedure

Since the original description in 1971 (33), the Fontan procedure and subsequent modifications have been successfully used to treat a wide range of simple and complex single-ventricle congenital heart defects. The repair is "physiologic" in that the systemic and pulmonary circulations are in series and cyanosis is corrected. However, given the current long-term outcome data, the repair should perhaps be viewed as palliative rather than curative (34,39). The morbidity and mortality associated with this surgery have declined substantially over the years, and many patients with stable single-ventricle physiology are able to lead normal lives (38). Factors that contribute to a successful cavopulmonary connection are shown in **Table 70A.12**. A systemic venous pressure of 10–15 mm Hg and a LA pressure of 5–10 mm Hg (i.e., a transpulmonary gradient of 5–10 mm Hg) are ideal.

Intravascular volume must be maintained and hypovolemia treated promptly. Venous capacitance is increased as patients rewarm and vasodilate following surgery, and a significant volume requirement of ~30–40 mL/kg on the first postoperative night is not unusual. Changes in mean intrathoracic pressure and PVR have a significant effect on pulmonary blood flow, which has been shown to be biphasic following the Fontan procedure, and earlier resumption of spontaneous ventilation is recommended to offset the detrimental effects of positive-pressure ventilation (65,71). Using Doppler analysis, it has been demonstrated that pulmonary blood flow predominantly occurs during inspiration in a spontaneously breathing patient, i.e., when the mean intrathoracic pressure is subatmospheric. Therefore, the method of mechanical ventilation following a Fontan procedure requires close observation. A delivered tidal volume of 10–12 mL/kg with the lowest possible mean airway pressure is appropriate. While it is preferable to wean from positive-pressure ventilation in the early postoperative period, hemodynamic responses must be closely monitored.

If appropriate selection criteria are followed, patients who undergo a modified Fontan procedure will have a low PVR without labile pulmonary hypertension. Therefore, vigorous hyperventilation and induction of respiratory and/or metabolic alkalosis is often of little benefit in this group of patients, and the related increase in mechanical ventilation requirements may be detrimental. A normal pH and a $Paco_2$ of 40 mm Hg should be the goal, and depending on the amount of right-to-left shunt across the fenestration, the arterial oxygen saturation is usually in the 80%–90% range.

However, PVR may increase following surgery, particularly secondary to acidosis, hypothermia, atelectasis, hypoventilation, vasoactive drug infusions, or stress response. Any acidosis must be treated promptly. If the cause is respiratory, ventilation must be adjusted. Metabolic acidosis reflects poor cardiac output and treatment directed at the potential causes, including reduced preload to the systemic ventricle, poor contractility, increased afterload, and loss of sinus rhythm.

MANAGEMENT CONSIDERATIONS FOLLOWING A MODIFIED FONTAN PROCEDURE

	Aim	Management
Baffle (right side) Pressure 10–15 mm Hg	Unobstructed venous return	→ or ↑ Preload Low intrathoracic pressure
Pulmonary circulation	PVR <2 Wood units/m^2 Mean PAp <15 mm Hg Unobstructed pulmonary vessels	Avoid increases in PVR, such as from acidosis, hypo- and hyperinflation of the lung, hypothermia, and excess sympathetic stimulation. Early resumption of spontaneous respiration.
Left atrium Pressure, 5–10 mm Hg	Sinus rhythm Competent AV valve Ventricle: Normal diastolic function Normal systolic function No outflow obstruction	Maintain sinus rhythm. → or ↑ rate to increase CO → or ↓ afterload → or ↑ contractility PDE inhibitors useful because of vasodilation and inotropic and lusitropic properties.

PAp, pulmonary artery pressure; PVR, pulmonary vascular resistance; CO, cardiac output; AV, atrioventricular; PDE, phosphodiesterase

The use of positive end-expiratory pressure continues to be debated. The beneficial effects of an increase in functional residual capacity, maintenance of lung volume, and redistribution of lung water must be balanced against the possible detrimental effect of an increase in mean intrathoracic pressure. A positive end-expiratory pressure of 3–5 cm H$_2$0, however, rarely has hemodynamic consequence or substantial effect on effective pulmonary blood flow.

Alternative methods of mechanical ventilation have also been employed for these patients. High-frequency ventilation has been used successfully, although the hemodynamic consequences of the raised mean intrathoracic pressure must be continually evaluated (55). Negative-pressure ventilation can be beneficial by augmenting pulmonary blood flow (78). The development of new negative-pressure ventilators has increased the interest in this mode of ventilation for this group of patients, but experience remains relatively small, and indications are not defined. Application of the negative-pressure ventilator cuirasse is cumbersome.

Nonspecific pulmonary vasodilators, such as sodium nitroprusside, glycerol trinitrate, PGE$_1$, and prostacyclin, have been used to dilate the pulmonary vasculature in an effort to improve pulmonary blood flow after a Fontan procedure; however, results vary. PVR may fall and pulmonary blood flow may increase. However, the increase in pulmonary blood flow may reflect a reduction of systemic afterload and improved ventricular function rather than pulmonary vasodilation. The response to iNO is also variable, and the improvement may relate to changes in ventilation-perfusion matching rather than to a direct fall in PVR.

Afterload stress is poorly tolerated after a modified Fontan procedure because of the increase in myocardial wall tension and end-diastolic pressure. The phosphodiesterase inhibitors, such as milrinone, are particularly beneficial due to their inotropic and lusitropic actions and vasodilating properties.

Specific Complications after the Fontan Procedure

Pleuropericardial Effusions. The incidence of recurrent pleural effusions and ascites has decreased since the introduction of the fenestrated baffle technique. (The baffle is the conduit that connects the inferior vena cava to the Glenn shunt, resulting in the "completion" Fontan. Fenestration creates a hole in the medial wall of the baffle to allow flow of some systemic venous blood directly into the atrium and ventricle rather than into the pulmonary circuit, which results in lower systemic venous pressures.) Despite the lower systemic venous pressures, for some patients, effusions remain a major problem, with associated respiratory compromise, hypovolemia, and possible hypoproteinemia. Reevaluation with cardiac catheterization may be indicated to investigate persistent elevation of systemic venous pressure.

Rhythm Disturbances. Atrial flutter and/or fibrillation, heart block, and less commonly, ventricular dysrhythmia, may have a significant impact on immediate recovery, as well as long-term outcome (31,40). Sudden loss of sinus rhythm initially causes an increase in left atrial and systemic ventricular end-diastolic pressure and a fall in cardiac output. The superior vena cava or PA pressure must be increased, usually with volume replacement, to maintain the transpulmonary gradient. Prompt treatment with antiarrhythmic drugs, pacing, or cardioversion is necessary.

Premature Closure of the Fenestration. Not all patients require a fenestration for a successful, uncomplicated Fontan operation. Those with ideal preoperative hemodynamics often maintain an adequate pulmonary blood flow and cardiac output without requiring a right-to-left shunt across the baffle. Similarly, not all Fontan patients who have received a fenestration will use it to shunt right-to-left in the immediate postoperative

TABLE 70A.13

ETIOLOGY AND TREATMENT STRATEGIES FOR PATIENTS WITH LOW CARDIAC OUTPUT IMMEDIATELY FOLLOWING THE FONTAN PROCEDURE

Low cardiac output	Etiology	Treatment
Increased TPG Baffle >20 mm Hg LAp <10 mm Hg ↑ TPG >>10 mm Hg **Clinical state:** High SaO$_2$/Low SvO$_2$ Hypotension/Tachycardia Core temperature high Poor peripheral perfusion SVC syndrome with pleural effusions and increased chest tube drainage Ascites/Hepatomegaly Metabolic acidosis	Inadequate pulmonary blood flow and preload to left atrium: Increased PVR Pulmonary artery stenosis Pulmonary vein stenosis Premature fenestration closure	Volume replacement Reduce PVR Correct acidosis Inotropic support Systemic vasodilation Catheter or surgical intervention
Normal TPG: Baffle >20 mm Hg LAp >15 mm Hg TPG normal 5–10 mm Hg **Clinical state:** Low SaO$_2$/Low SvO$_2$ Hypotension/Tachycardia Poor peripheral perfusion Metabolic acidosis	Ventricular failure: Systolic dysfunction Diastolic dysfunction AVV regurgitation and/or stenosis Loss of sinus rhythm ↑ Afterload stress	Maintain preload Inotrope support Systemic vasodilation Establish sinus rhythm or AV synchrony Correct acidosis Mechanical support Surgical intervention, including takedown to BDG and transplantation

LAp, left atrial pressure; TPG, transpulmonary gradient; PVR, pulmonary vascular resistance; SaO$_2$, systemic arterial oxygen saturation; SvO$_2$, SVC oxygen saturation; SVC, superior vena cava; AVV, atrioventricular valve; BDG, bidirectional Glenn anastomosis.

period. These patients are fully saturated following surgery and may have an elevated right-sided filling pressure but nevertheless maintain an adequate cardiac output. The problem is predicting which patients are at risk for low cardiac output after a Fontan procedure and who will benefit from placement of a fenestration; even patients with ideal preoperative hemodynamics may manifest a significant low-output state after surgery. Therefore, essentially all patients who undergo a Fontan procedure are fenestrated at some centers.

Premature closure of the fenestration may occur in the immediate postoperative period, leading to an LCOS with progressive metabolic acidosis and large chest-drain losses from high right-sided venous pressures (**Table 70A.13**). Patients may respond to volume replacement, inotrope support, and vasodilation; however, if hypotension and acidosis persist, cardiac catheterization and removal of thrombus or dilation of the fenestration should occur urgently.

Persistent Hypoxemia. Arterial O$_2$ saturation levels may vary substantially following a modified Fontan procedure. Common causes of persistent arterial O$_2$ desaturation of <75% include a poor cardiac output with a low SvO$_2$, a large right-to-left shunt across the fenestration, or additional "leak" in the baffle pathway, producing more shunting. An intrapulmonary shunt and venous admixture from decompressing collateral vessels draining either from the PA to the systemic venous circulation

or from a systemic vein to the pulmonary venous system are additional causes. Re-evaluation with echocardiography and cardiac catheterization may be necessary.

Low Cardiac Output State. Elevated LA pressure after a modified Fontan procedure may reflect poor ventricular function from decreased contractility or increased afterload stress, atrioventricular valve regurgitation, or loss of sinus rhythm (Table 70A.13). The right-sided filling pressure must be increased to maintain the transpulmonary (PA – atrial) pressure gradient, which may be accomplished with inotropic drugs and vasodilators to increase ventricular output. Rising RA and LA pressures with decreasing arterial blood pressure, along with rising blood urea nitrogen and elevated liver function tests, are markers of the failing Fontan circulation. If a severe low-output state with acidosis persists, take-down of the Fontan operation and conversion to a BDG shunt or other palliative procedure is life-saving.

CONCLUSIONS AND FUTURE DIRECTIONS

Postoperative care of the cardiac surgical patient requires extended training and a broad knowledge base of cardiovascular anatomy and physiology. Specialists in this field must have in-depth knowledge of pediatric cardiology as well as the principles of "general" pediatric intensive care. In view of the intensive interventions required in cardiac intensive care children, the expertise in procedural skills of cardiac anesthesiologists may also be extremely useful in the pediatric cardiac ICU team.

Increased complexity of disease, advances in technology and applied research, shortened lengths of stay, and improved survival all describe the fast-paced, specialized environment that has accompanied the development of the new specialty of pediatric cardiac intensive care. While the dramatic reduction in mortality in cardiac intensive care has been gratifying and is attributable to many factors, achieving 100% survival with minimal morbidity remains the elusive goal that will challenge the next generation of practitioners.

In the future, new imaging modalities will continue to provide better anatomic and physiologic information. Three-dimensional imaging will one day be the precise, complete standard imaging in CHD. The ways in which the genetic make-up of patients influence outcome will be a main focus of future research, along with a clearer understanding of polymorphisms as they relate to risks of CPB. Sophisticated pharmacogenetics will guide drug therapies for postoperative support in the ICU. In the future, more clinical trial data will likely guide patient assessment, and increased pharmacokinetic data will guide dosage and duration of drug therapies. Discovery and innovation in the basic sciences will lead to new therapies, such as they have with treatment of pulmonary hypertension and new inotropic support of the heart. It is likely that advances in tissue engineering will provide new and better bioprosthetic materials. Mechanical support devices that are more suitable for pediatrics will almost certainly be better developed in the future and provide options to support patients for longer or even indefinite periods of time, as either bridges to transplantation or even destination therapy. Refinements in CPB techniques and better understanding of the ischemia-reperfusion injury and inflammatory response to bypass will continue to reduce morbidity and improve postoperative end-organ function. Hybrid techniques will bring the catheterization laboratory and its interventional techniques to the operating room, and vice versa, so that boundaries between interventional cardiologists and surgeons will continue to blur. Fetal interventions for disease conditions such as restrictive atrial septum in hypoplastic left heart syndrome will likely alter the natural history of this disease and confront critical care practitioners with new management issues. Undoubtedly, clinical teams will continue to become even more highly specialized and propel pediatric cardiac intensive care to even higher standards, greater patient safety, and better outcomes.

KEY POINTS

- Know the anatomy and surgical procedure in detail.
- Search systematically for residual disease in the postoperative patient.
- Anticipate low cardiac output.
- Preserve right-to-left shunts for transient postoperative benefit in select patients.
- Optimize afterload reduction and avoid high doses of catecholamines.

- Appreciate heart-lung interactions and effects of positive-pressure breathing.
- Understand limitations and opportunities to manipulate single-ventricle physiology.
- Estimate the limit of cardiac reserve at the nadir of postoperative cardiac output.
- Embrace mechanical support of the circulation as a vital tool for bridge to recovery, bridge to transplantation as well as destination therapy.

ACKNOWLEDGMENT

The authors wish to thank Dr. Peter Laussen for his thoughts and contributions to this chapter, especially regarding early extubation and heart-lung interactions.

References

1. Adamopoulos S, Parissis J, et al. Effects of levosimendan versus dobutamine on inflammatory and apoptotic pathways in acutely decompensated chronic heart failure. *Am J Cardiol* 2006;98:102–6.
2. Adatia I, Atz AM, Jonas RA, et al. Diagnostic use of inhaled nitric oxide after neonatal cardiac operations. *J Thorac Cardiovasc Surg* 1996;112(5):1403–5.
3. Adatia I, Atz AM, Wessel DL. Inhaled nitric oxide does not improve systemic oxygenation after bidirectional superior cavopulmonary anastomosis. *J Thorac Cardiovasc Surg* 2005;129:217–9.
4. Ando M, Park IS, Wada N, et al. Steroid supplementation: A legitimate pharmacotherapy after neonatal open heart surgery. *Ann Thorac Surg* 2005;80:1672.
5. Atz AM, Wessel DL. Inhaled nitric oxide in the neonate with cardiac disease. *Semin Perinatol* 1997;21:441–55.
6. Atz AM, Wessel DL. Sildenafil ameliorates effects of inhaled nitric oxide withdrawal. *Anesthesiology* 1999;91(1):307–10.
7. Bailey JM, Miller BE, Lu W, et al. The pharmacokinetics of milrinone in pediatric patients after cardiac surgery. *Anesth* 1999;90:1012–8.
8. Bailey LL, Gundry SR, Razzouk AJ, et al. Bless the babies: One hundred fifteen late survivors of heart transplantation during the first year of life. *J Thorac Cardiovasc Surg* 1993;105:805–15.
9. Barst RJ, Rubin LJ, Long WA, et al. A comparison of continuous intravenous epoprostenol (prostacyclin) with conventional therapy for primary pulmonary hypertension. The Primary Pulmonary Hypertension Study Group. *N Engl J Med* 1996; 334:296–302.
10. Bettendorf M, Schmidt KG, Grulich-Henn J, et al. Tri-iodothyronine treatment in children after cardiac surgery: A double-blind, randomised, placebo-controlled study. *Lancet* 2000;356:529–34.
11. Bohn DJ, Poirer CS, Demonds JF. Efficacy of dopamine, dobutamine, and epinephrine during emergence from cardiopulmonary bypass in children. *Crit Care Med* 1980;8:367–73.
12. Bridges ND, Mayer JE, Jr. , Lock JE, et al. Effect of baffle fenestration on outcome of the modified Fontan operation. *Circulation* 1992;86:1762–9.
13. Caspi J, Coles JG, Benson LN, et al. Age-related response to epinephrine-induced myocardial stress. A functional and ulstrastructural study. *Circulation* 1991;84(suppl III):394–9.
14. Caspi J, Coles JG, Benson LN, et al. Effects of high plasma epinephrine and Ca^{2+} concentrations on neonatal myocardial function after ischemia. *J Thorac Cardiovasc Surg* 1993;105:59–67.
15. Chang AC, Atz AM, Wernovsky G, et al. Milrinone: Systemic and pulmonary hemodynamic effects in neonates after cardiac surgery. *Crit Care Med* 1995;23:1907–14.
16. Chang AC, Hanley FL, Wernovsky G, et al. Early bidirectional cavopulmonary shunt in young infants. Postoperative course and early results. *Circulation* 1993;88(5 Pt 2):II149–58.
17. Cheung PY, Chui N, Joffe AR, et al. Postoperative lactate concentrations predict the outcome of infants aged 6 weeks or less after intracardiac surgery: A cohort follow-up to 18 months. *J Thorac Cardiovasc Surg* 2005;130:837–43.
18. Chowdhury D, Parnell VA, Ojamaa K, et al. Usefulness of triiodothyronine (T3) treatment after surgery for complex congenital heart disease in infants and children. *Am J Cardiol* 1999;84:1107–9, A10.
19. Colucci WS, Elkayam U, Horton DP, et al. Intravenous nesiritide, a natriuretic peptide, in the treatment of decompensated congestive heart failure. Nesiritide Study Group. *N Engl J Med* 2000;343:246–53.
20. Costello JM, Backer CL, de Hoyos A, et al. Aprotinin reduces operative closure time and blood product use after pediatric bypass. *Ann Thorac Surg* 2003;75(4):1261–6.

21. Costello JM, Thiagarajan RR, Dionne R, et al. Initial experience with fenoldopam after cardiac surgery in neonates with an insufficient response to conventional diuretics. *Pediatr Crit Care Med* 2006;7:28–33.
22. Cullen S, Shore D, Redington A. Characterization of right ventricular diastolic performance after complete repair of tetralogy of Fallot. Restrictive physiology predicts slow postoperative recovery. *Circulation* 1995;91:1782–9.
23. de Mos N, van Litsenburg RRL, McCrindle B, et al. Pediatric in-intensive-care-unit cardiac arrest: Incidence, survival, and predictive factors. *Crit Care Med* 2006;34:1209–15.
24. Dimmick S, Badawi N, Randell T. Thyroid hormone supplementation for the prevention of morbidity and mortality in infants undergoing cardiac surgery. *Cochrane Database Syst Rev* CD004220, 2004.
25. Drummond WH, Gregory GA, Heymann MA, et al. The independent effects of hyperventilation, tolazoline, and dopamine on infants with persistent pulmonary hypertension. *J Pediatr* 1981;98:603–11.
26. Duncan BW, Hraska V, Jonas RA, et al. Mechanical circulatory support in children with cardiac disease. *J Thorac Cardiovasc Surg* 1999;117:529–42.
27. Duncan BW, Ibrahim AE, Hraska V, et al. Use of rapid-deployment extracorporeal membrane oxygenation for the resuscitation of pediatric patients with heart disease after cardiac arrest. *J Thorac Cardiovasc Surg* 1998;116:305–11.
28. Elliott M. Modified ultrafiltration and open heart surgery in children. *Paediatr Anaesth* 1999;9:1–5.
29. Extracorporeal Life Support Organization. ECLS Registry Report: International Summary. Ann Arbor, MI: Extracorporeal Life Support Organization, 2002.
30. Fishberger SB, Wernovsky G, Gentles TL, et al. Factors that influence the development of atrial flutter after the Fontan operation. *J Thorac Cardiovasc Surg* 1997;113:80–6.
31. Follath F, Cleland JGF, Just H, et al. Efficacy and safety of intravenous levosimendan compared with dobutamine in severe low-output heart failure (the LIDO study): A randomised double-blind trial. *Lancet* 2002;360:196–202.
32. Fontan F, Baudet E. Surgical repair of tricuspid atresia. *Thorax* 1971;26:240–8.
33. Fontan F, Kirklin JW, Fernandez G, et al. Outcome after a "perfect" Fontan operation. *Circulation* 1990;81:1520–36.
34. Freedom RM. Neurodevelopmental outcome after the Fontan procedure in children with the hypoplastic left heart syndrome and other forms of single ventricle pathology: Challenges unresolved. *J Pediatr* 2000;137:602–4.
35. Frostell CG, Fratacci MD, Wain JC, et al. Inhaled nitric oxide: A selective pulmonary vasodilator reversing hypoxic pulmonary vasoconstriction. *Circulation* 1991;83:2038–47.
36. Furchgott RF, Zawadzki JV. The obligatory role of endothelial cells in the relaxation of arterial smooth muscle by acetylcholine. *Nature* 1980;288:373–6.
37. Gentles TL, Gauvreau K, Mayer JE, Jr. , et al. Functional outcome after the Fontan operation: Factors influencing late morbidity. *J Thorac Cardiovasc Surg* 1997;114:392–403.
38. Gentles TL, Mayer JE, Jr., Gauvreau K, et al. Fontan operation in five hundred consecutive patients: Factors influencing early and late outcome. *J Thorac Cardiovasc Surg* 1997;114:376–91.
39. Gewillig M, Wyse RK, De Leval MR, et al. Early and late arrhythmias after the Fontan operation: Predisposing factors and clinical consequences. *Br Heart J* 1992;67:72–9.
40. Goldman AP, Delius RE, Deanfield JE, et al. Pharmacological control of pulmonary blood flow with inhaled nitric oxide after the fenestrated Fontan operation. *Circulation* 1996;94(9 Suppl):II44–8.
41. Habib DM, Padbury JF, Anas NG, et al. Dobutamine pharmacokinetics and pharmacodynamics in pediatric intensive care patients. *Crit Care Med* 1992;20:601–8.
42. Hannan RL, Ybarra MA, White JA, et al. Patterns of lactate values after congenital heart surgery and timing of cardiopulmonary support. *Ann Thorac Surg* 2005;80:1468.
43. Harkel ADJT, van der Vorst MMJ, Hazekamp MG, et al. High mortality rate after extubation failure after pediatric cardiac surgery. *Pediatr Cardiol* 2005;26:756–61.
44. Hoffman TM, Wernovsky G, Atz AM, et al. Efficacy and safety of milrinone in preventing low cardiac output syndrome in infants and children after corrective surgery for congenital heart disease. *Circulation* 2003;107(7):996–1002.
45. Ignarro LJ, Buga GM, Wood KS, et al. Endothelium-derived relaxing factor produced and released from artery and vein is nitric oxide. *Proc Natl Acad Sci U S A* 1987;84:9265–9.
46. Janousek J, Vojtovic P, Hucin B, et al. Resynchronization pacing is a useful adjunct to the management of acute heart failure after surgery for congenital heart defects. *Am J Cardiol* 2001;88:145–52.
47. Joho-Arreola AL, Bauersfeld U, Stauffer UG, et al. Incidence and treatment of diaphragmatic paralysis after cardiac surgery in children. *Eur J Cardiothorac Surg* 2005;27:53–7.
48. Journois D, Pouard P, Mauriat P, et al. Inhaled nitric oxide as a therapy for pulmonary hypertension after operations for congenital heart defects. *J Thorac Cardiovasc Surg* 1994;107:1129–35.
49. Lemler MS, Scott WA, Leonard SR, et al. Fenestration improves clinical outcome of the Fontan procedure: A prospective, randomized study. *Circulation* 2002;105:207–12.
50. Mackie AS, Booth KL, Newburger JW, et al. A randomized, double-blind, placebo-controlled pilot trial of triiodothyronine in neonatal heart surgery. *J Thorac Cardiovasc Surg* 2005;130:810–6.
51. Maher KO, Pizarro C, Gidding SS, et al. Hemodynamic profile after the Norwood procedure with right ventricle to pulmonary artery conduit. *Circulation* 2003;108(7):782–4.
52. Mahle WT, Cuadrado AR, Kirshbom PM, et al. Nesiritide in infants and children with congestive heart failure. *Pediatr Crit Care Med* 2005;6:543–6.
53. Mainwaring R, Lamberti J, Nelson J, et al. Effects of tri-iodothyronine supplementation following modified Fontan procedure. *Cardiol Young* 1997;7:194–200.
54. Meliones JN, Bove EL, Dekeon MK, et al. High-frequency jet ventilation improves cardiac function after the Fontan procedure. *Circulation* 1991;84:III364–8.
55. Mildh LH, Pettila V, Sairanen HI, et al. Cardiac troponin T levels for risk stratification in pediatric open heart surgery. *Ann Thorac Surg* 2006;82:1643–8.
56. Miller OI, Tang SF, Keech A, et al. Inhaled nitric oxide and prevention of pulmonary hypertension after congenital heart surgery: A randomised double-blind study. *Lancet* 2000;356:1464–9.
57. Mills RM, LeJemtel TH, Horton DP, et al. Sustained hemodynamic effects of an infusion of nesiritide (human b-type natriuretic peptide) in heart failure: A randomized, double-blind, placebo-controlled clinical trial. Natrecor Study Group. *J Am Coll Cardiol* 1999;34(1):155–62.
58. Mosca RS, Bove EL, Crowley DC, et al. Hemodynamic characteristics of neonates following first-stage palliation for hypoplastic left heart syndrome. *Circulation* 1995;92(suppl II):267–71.
59. Munoz R, Laussen PC, Palacio G, et al. Changes in whole blood lactate levels during cardiopulmonary bypass for surgery for congenital cardiac disease: An early indicator of morbidity and mortality. *J Thorac Cardiovasc Surg* 2000;119:155–62.
60. Namachivayam P, Crossland DS, Butt WW, et al. Early experience with Levosimendan in children with ventricular dysfunction. *Pediatric Critical Care Medicine* 2006;7:445–8.
61. Namachivayam P, Theilen U, Butt WW, et al. Sildenafil prevents rebound pulmonary hypertension after withdrawal of nitric oxide in children. *Am J Respir Crit Care Med* 2006;174:1042–7.
62. Newburger JW, Jonas RA, Wernovsky G, et al. Perioperative neurologic effects of hypothermic arrest during infant heart surgery. The Boston Circulatory Arrest Study. *N Engl J Med* 1993;329:1057–64.
63. Paret G, Cohen AJ, Bohn DJ, et al. Continuous arteriovenous hemofiltration after cardiac operations in infants and children. *J Thorac Cardiovasc Surg* 1992;104:1225–30.
64. Penny DJ, Redington AN. Doppler echocardiographic evaluation of pulmonary blood flow after the Fontan operation: The role of the lungs. *Br Heart J* 1991;66:372–4.
65. Petrossian E, Parry AJ, Reddy VM, et al. Endothelin receptor blockade prevents the rise in pulmonary vascular resistance after cardiopulmonary bypass in lambs with increased pulmonary blood flow. *J Thorac Cardiovasc Surg* 1999;117:314–23.
66. Portman MA, Fearneyhough C, Karl TR, et al. The Triiodothyronine for Infants and Children Undergoing Cardiopulmonary Bypass (TRICC) study: Design and rationale. *Am Heart J* 2004;148:393–8.
67. Publication Committee for the VMAC Investigators (Vasodilatation in the Management of Acute CHF). Intravenous nesiritide vs. nitroglycerin for treatment of decompensated congestive heart failure: A randomized controlled trial. *JAMA* 2002;287:1531–40.
68. Reddy VM, McElhinney DB, Sagrado T, et al. Results of 102 cases of complete repair of congenital heart defects in patients weighing 700 to 2500 grams. *J Thorac Cardiovasc Surg* 1999;117(2):324–31.
69. Redington AN, Penny D, Rigby ML. Antegrade diastolic pulmonary arterial flow as a marker of right ventricular restriction after complete repair of pulmonary atresia with intact ventricular septum and critical pulmonary valve stenosis. *Cardiol Young* 1992;2:382–6.
70. Redington AN, Penny D, Shinebourne EA. Pulmonary blood flow after total cavopulmonary shunt. *Br Heart J* 1991;65:213–7.
71. Riordan C, Randsbaek F, Storey J. Balancing pulmonary and systemic arterial flows in parallel circulations: The value of monitoring systemic venous oxygen saturations. *Cardiol Young* 1997;7:74–9.
72. Robotham JL, Lixfeld W, Holland L, et al. The effects of positive end-expiratory pressure on right and left ventricular performance. *Am Rev Respir Dis* 1980;121:677–83.
73. Rosenzweig EB, Kerstein D, Barst RJ. Long-term prostacyclin for pulmonary hypertension with associated congenital heart defects. *Circulation* 1999;99(14):1858–65.
74. Rosenzweig EB, Starc TJ, Chen JM, et al. Intravenous arginine-vasopressin in children with vasodilatory shock after cardiac surgery. *Circulation* 1999;100:II182–6.
75. Sano S, Ishino K, Kawada M, et al. Right ventricle-pulmonary artery shunt in first-stage palliation of hypoplastic left heart syndrome. *Sem Thorac Cardiovasc Surg Ped Card Surg Ann* 2004;7:22–31.

76. Scheurer MA, Bradley SM, Atz AM. Vasopressin to attenuate pulmonary hypertension and improve systemic blood pressure after correction of obstructed total anomalous pulmonary venous return. *J Thorac Cardiovasc Surg* 2005;129:464–6.

77. Shekerdemian LS, Bush A, Shore DF, et al. Cardiopulmonary interactions after Fontan operations: Augmentation of cardiac output using negative pressure ventilation. *Circulation* 1997;96:3934–42.

78. Sigler M, Vazquez-Jimenez JF, Grabitz RG, et al. Time course of cranial ultrasound abnormalities after arterial switch operation in neonates. *Ann Thorac Surg* 2001;71:877–80.

79. Slawsky MT, Colucci WS, Gottlieb SS, et al. Acute hemodynamic and clinical effects of levosimendan in patients with severe heart failure. Study Investigators. *Circulation* 2000;102:2222–7.

80. Suominen PK, Dickerson HA, Moffett BS, et al. Hemodynamic effects of rescue protocol hydrocortisone in neonates with low cardiac output syndrome after cardiac surgery. *Pediatr Crit Care Med* 2005;6:655–9.

81. Turanlahti M, Boldt T, Palkama T, et al. Pharmacokinetics of levosimendan in pediatric patients evaluated for cardiac surgery. *Pediatr Crit Care Med* 2004;5:457–62.

82. Vricella LA, Dearani JA, Gundry SR, et al. Ultra fast track in elective congenital cardiac surgery. *Ann Thorac Surg* 2000;69:865–71.

83. Wernovsky G, Stiles KM, Gauvreau K, et al. Cognitive development after the Fontan operation. *Circulation* 2000;102(8):883–9.

84. Wernovsky G, Wypij D, Jonas RA, et al. Postoperative course and hemodynamic profile after the arterial switch operation in neonates and infants. A comparison of low-flow cardiopulmonary bypass and circulatory arrest. *Circulation* 1995;92:2226–35.

85. Wessel DL. Current and future strategies in the treatment of childhood pulmonary hypertension. *Prog Ped Cardiol* 2001;12:289.

86. Wessel DL. Managing low cardiac output syndrome after congenital heart surgery. *Crit Care Med* 2001;29:S220–30.

87. Wessel DL. Testing new drugs for heart failure in children. *Ped Crit Care Med* 2006;7:493–4.

88. Wessel DL, Adatia I, Giglia TM, et al. Use of inhaled nitric oxide and acetylcholine in the evaluation of pulmonary hypertension and endothelial function after cardiopulmonary bypass. *Circulation* 1993;88(5 Pt 1):2128–38.

89. Wessel D, Almodovar M, Laussen P. Intensive Care Management of Cardiac Patients on Extracorporeal Membrane Oxygenation. In: Dunan B, ed. *Mechanical Support for Cardiac and Respiratory Failure,* 2000:75–111.

90. Yancy CW, Saltzberg MT, Berkowitz RL, et al. Safety and feasibility of using serial infusions of nesiritide for heart failure in an outpatient setting (from the FUSION I trial). *Am J Cardiol* 2004;94(5):595–601.

91. Zobel G, Dacar D, Rodl S, et al. Inhaled nitric oxide versus inhaled prostacyclin and intravenous versus inhaled prostacyclin in acute respiratory failure with pulmonary hypertension in piglets. *Pediatr Res* 1995;38:198–204.

CHAPTER 70B ■ POSTOPERATIVE CARE OF THE PEDIATRIC CARDIAC SURGICAL PATIENT: LESION-SPECIFIC MANAGEMENT

STEVEN M. SCHWARTZ • JOHNNY MILLAR

In addition to the general consequences of surgery and cardiopulmonary bypass, lesion-specific problems can occur following surgery for congenital heart disease. It is very important that the intensive care physician has precise knowledge of the preoperative anatomy and details of surgical procedures performed in each case to allow for anticipation, prompt and appropriate investigation, and treatment of complications. In this section, commonly performed surgical procedures are categorized, and associated problems that might be anticipated in the postoperative period are listed, followed by a discussion of investigation and management of specific complications, based on their pathophysiologic features.

COMPLICATIONS AFTER COMMON CARDIAC SURGICAL PROCEDURES

Repair of Left-to-Right Shunt Lesions

General Complications

Residual Lesions. These result in variable degrees of left-to-right shunting.

Pulmonary Hypertension. Most likely seen in three types of patients: (a) children in whom pulmonary vascular disease has had time to develop, (b) newborns, and (c) patients following relief of pulmonary venous obstruction.

Dysrhythmias. Any dysrhythmia may occur, regardless of the type of surgery performed; however, patients following surgery involving repair of a ventricular septal defect (VSD) are at increased risk of junctional ectopic tachycardia, and complete heart block may complicate repair of VSD or atrioventricular (AV) canal.

Specific Complications

- Atrial septal defect repair
  - Sinoatrial node dysfunction
  - Acute left ventricular (LV) failure in older children and adults
- VSD repair
  - Pulmonary hypertension
  - Dysrhythmias—junctional ectopic tachycardia, complete heart block
- AV canal repair

- Pulmonary hypertension
- Dysrhythmias—junctional ectopic tachycardia, complete heart block
- Left AV valve insufficiency or stenosis
- Ligation of patent ductus arteriosus
  - Recurrent laryngeal nerve damage
  - Damage to, or ligation of, surrounding vessels (left pulmonary artery, aorta)
- Truncus arteriosus repair
  - Pulmonary hypertension
  - Truncal valve stenosis or regurgitation
  - RV dysfunction
- Aortopulmonary window repair
  - Pulmonary hypertension
- Anomalous pulmonary venous drainage repair
  - Pulmonary hypertension
  - Dysrhythmias
  - Residual stenosis of pulmonary veins or anastomosis
  - High LV filling pressure due to small LA or LV

Repair of Right-sided Obstruction

General Complications

- Residual obstruction or regurgitation
- Right ventricular dysfunction. Both systolic and diastolic dysfunction may occur. The latter is more likely in a hypertrophied, noncompliant right ventricle (RV), particularly if repair has necessitated the use of a ventricular incision.

Specific Complications

- Tetralogy of Fallot repair (and variants)
  - RV dysfunction
  - Dysrhythmias—junctional ectopic tachycardia, complete heart block
  - Residual pulmonary stenosis
  - Pulmonary valve regurgitation
  - Residual VSD
- Absent pulmonary valve syndrome
  - Tracheobronchomalacia
- Pulmonary atresia, intact ventricular septum
  - RV dysfunction
  - Myocardial ischemia (if RV-dependent coronary circulation)
  - "Circular shunt" (if both Blalock-Taussig shunt and RV outflow tract patch)

Repair of Left-sided Obstruction

General Complications

- Residual obstruction
- Hypertension
- LV diastolic dysfunction

Specific Complications

- Aortic stenosis repair
  - Valvotomy
    - Residual stenosis
    - Aortic regurgitation
  - Ross procedure
    - Coronary ischemia
  - Konno procedure
    - Coronary ischemia
    - RV outflow tract obstruction
    - Dysrhythmias
- Subaortic stenosis repair
  - Residual stenosis
  - Mitral valve injury
  - Dysrhythmias
- Supravalvar aortic stenosis repair
  - Residual stenosis
  - Aortic regurgitation
  - Coronary ischemia
- Coarctation repair
  - Residual obstruction
  - Paraplegia
  - Post-coarctectomy syndrome
  - Unmasking of valvar atrial stenosis
  - Recurrent laryngeal nerve damage
- Interrupted aortic arch repair
  - Residual obstruction
  - Left main bronchus compression by aorta
  - Hypocalcemia if associated with DiGeorge syndrome
- Mitral stenosis repair
  - Pulmonary hypertension
  - Residual stenosis
  - Mitral regurgitation
  - LV dysfunction

Palliative Procedures

Systemic-to-Pulmonary Artery Shunt (Blalock-Taussig, Modified Blalock-Taussig, Central Shunts)

- Excessive pulmonary blood flow
- Systemic hypotension
- Serous leak, seroma/effusion
- Shunt thrombosis

Pulmonary Artery Banding

- Cyanosis
- Excessive pulmonary blood flow

Single-ventricle Staged Palliation

- Stage I "Norwood" (Blalock-Taussig shunt or RV-PA conduit)
  - Low cardiac output

- High $Q_p:Q_s$
- Low $Q_p:Q_s$
- Residual aortic arch obstruction
- AV valve dysfunction

Bidirectional Cavopulmonary Anastomosis (Glenn)

- Cyanosis
- Hypertension
- Superior vena cava syndrome

Fontan Procedure

- Large third-space fluid losses
- Cyanosis
- Low cardiac output
- Dysrhythmias

Miscellaneous

- Arterial switch operation
  - Ischemia
  - Neoaortic regurgitation
  - Transient LV dysfunction
- Intra-atrial Switch (Mustard or Senning)
  - Pulmonary or systemic venous obstruction
  - Dysrhythmias
- Repair of anomalous coronary artery from pulmonary artery
  - Myocardial failure
  - Mitral insufficiency
- Mitral valve surgery
  - Residual stenosis or insufficiency
  - Pulmonary hypertension

Approach to Investigation and Management

Residual Left-to-Right Shunt

Residual left-to-right shunts can occur after operations that involve repair of septal defects, when preoperative shunts are left unrepaired, or when unrecognized or untreated systemic-to-pulmonary artery shunts (aortopulmonary collaterals) exist. Because of the resultant increase in pulmonary blood flow, residual left-to-right shunts may lead to pulmonary edema, pulmonary hypertension, volume overload of the systemic ventricle, and, in certain circumstances, limitations of systemic cardiac output. Common signs or symptoms include a pulmonary outflow or VSD murmur, high systemic atrial pressure, hepatomegaly, and a large heart with increased pulmonary vascularity on chest x-ray.

Atrial level shunts are rarely a problem, unless they are associated with factors that cause left atrial hypertension, which increases left-to-right shunt flow and pulmonary artery pressure. Congestive heart failure and pulmonary overcirculation secondary to an atrial left-to-right shunt should therefore lead the clinician to carefully evaluate the patient for mitral stenosis or insufficiency, inadequate systemic ventricular size, poor systemic ventricular function, or systemic ventricular outflow tract obstruction with elevated end-diastolic pressure.

Ventricular and vascular shunts are more often problematic, as they are always associated with systemic ventricular volume overload and, often, with pulmonary hypertension. In general, shunts of Q_p:Q_s less than 1.5:1 to 2:1 without pulmonary hypertension are well tolerated, but larger shunts result in the clinical syndrome of congestive heart failure. Patients with large preoperative left-to-right shunts generally tolerate residual shunts better than those who were cyanotic before surgery. For example, a patient with a residual VSD following repair of tetralogy of Fallot has gone from a situation in which the LV was essentially volume "underloaded" preoperatively (due to the contribution of the RV to preoperative cardiac output) to one in which the LV is now volume overloaded.

Making the diagnosis of a residual shunt should lead to a discussion of the risk-benefit balance of attempting further repair, either surgically or in the catheterization lab for lesions with which this is an option. Some lesions are not repairable, and the patient must be managed in such a way as to minimize the adverse consequences of the shunt, which may include avoiding therapy that minimizes pulmonary resistance or that increases systemic resistance, either of which may aggravate the shunt. Examples of treatment that may be counterproductive include high levels of supplemental oxygen or hyperventilation that lower pulmonary resistance or high doses of α-adrenergic agonists that will increase systemic resistance. Prolonged inotropic support, mechanical ventilation, afterload reduction, and relatively large doses of diuretics are often necessary. As the heart recovers from the acute detrimental effects of surgery, the residual shunt may become better tolerated, allowing weaning of support.

Residual Systemic Ventricular Outflow Tract Obstruction

Residual systemic ventricular outflow tract obstruction should be looked for after all surgery to relieve outflow obstruction (such as repair of subaortic stenosis, aortic stenosis, or coarctation). Additionally, systemic ventricular outflow obstruction can occur after repair of AV canal defects or after other operations that remove large volume loads from the systemic ventricle when the underlying anatomy includes subvalvar hypertrophy; for example, when a patient with double-inlet LV is converted from a shunted circulation to a Glenn or Fontan. The volume unloading of the ventricle may cause the systemic outflow tract through the bulboventricular foramen to become narrowed. Signs and symptoms of systemic outflow obstruction include an ejection murmur and elevated systemic atrial pressure.

Relatively mild residual obstruction is usually well tolerated, but more severe lesions can significantly impair cardiac output. Interpretation of diagnostic studies, including Doppler ultrasound and cardiac catheterization, must focus on the anatomy in the presence of low cardiac output, as low flow across even a severe obstruction will not produce a large gradient. Unlike adults with systemic ventricular outflow obstruction, use of β-adrenergic agonists is not usually associated with myocardial ischemia, as long as cardiac output and myocardial oxygen delivery are actually improved. Particular caution is necessary, however, when the obstruction is dynamic (i.e., increased obstruction during systole). Increased contractility can actually worsen this type of lesion; therefore, inotropic drugs may be contraindicated. Unfortunately, the presence of systemic ventricular outflow obstruction limits the ability to use vasodilating agents for afterload reduction. The problem is that the afterload on the systemic ventricle is essentially fixed at the level of the obstruction, and distal vasodilation may

cause hypotension because of the inability to increase cardiac output.

Patients who have had effective relief of significant systemic ventricular outflow obstruction are often hypertensive due to continued hyperdynamic performance of the heart. It is particularly important to treat hypertension in the first postoperative 24 hrs to protect the surgical repair and to minimize the chances of bleeding from aortic suture lines. Effective treatments include vasodilators, β blockers, and angiotensin-converting enzyme (ACE) inhibitors.

Tricuspid or Mitral Valve Dysfunction

Residual AV valve dysfunction, either insufficiency or stenosis, can occur after any attempted valve repair or when closure of a septal defect unmasks valvar stenosis on one side of the heart. AV valve insufficiency is associated with high atrial pressures on the affected side of the heart. If atrial pressure is being directly monitored, very prominent v waves on the tracing will often be observed, and a regurgitant murmur will be heard. Because of the associated ventricular volume overload, signs or symptoms of ventricular failure may be present. AV valve stenosis is also associated with high atrial pressure but with prominent ("cannon") a waves. Peripheral (right-sided) or pulmonary (left-sided) edema is common with stenotic lesions, and pulmonary hypertension occurs with mitral stenosis. When severe, either stenosis or insufficiency can limit cardiac output.

As with other residual lesions, discussion regarding the possibility of further intervention is warranted. Medical management of AV valve insufficiency is focused on afterload reduction, with inotropic support when needed. Systemic vasodilators promote antegrade cardiac output in the face of mitral (or even aortic) insufficiency, whereas diuretics may be useful in either stenotic or regurgitant lesions. AV valve stenosis is, in general, not particularly amenable to medical management, although its consequences (e.g., pulmonary hypertension) may require aggressive medical treatment.

Right- or Left-ventricular Diastolic Dysfunction

Ventricular diastolic dysfunction should be an expected complication of any operation in which significant ventricular hypertrophy occurs, which most commonly happens after relief of obstructive lesions or in the presence of preexisting diastolic dysfunction. Operations that require a right ventriculotomy in an already hypertrophied RV represent a particularly high risk for postoperative diastolic dysfunction. A ventriculotomy can impair either systolic or diastolic function, and the anterior location of the RV makes myocardial preservation difficult because the RV is relatively exposed to ambient temperature in the operating room.

Diastolic dysfunction is marked by elevated atrial pressure and has many of the same features as seen in AV valve disease. The presence of a residual atrial shunt in this setting compounds the adverse effects of *left*-sided disease by promoting pulmonary overcirculation. Conversely, an atrial defect can help to maintain cardiac output when the *right* ventricle is noncompliant, although associated cyanosis will occur. The need to maintain high pressure to promote adequate ventricular filling results in hydrostatic pressure that favors extravasation of fluid and leads to pulmonary edema in the case of left-sided problems and third-space losses of fluid in the case of RV diastolic dysfunction.

In general, the first-line treatment for diastolic dysfunction is to use fluid to maintain adequate preload, although inotropic agents (such as milrinone) that reduce afterload can also improve diastolic function (14). Fluid administration can be limited by impairment of oxygenation and lung function with progressive pulmonary edema, or by complications of peripheral edema and third-spacing of fluid. Right-sided lesions in particular often respond very well to initial fluid boluses, but the hydrostatic forces in combination with diminished lymphatic drainage due to high venous pressure lead to ascites and to pleural effusions or large amounts of chest tube drainage (4). If a peritoneal drainage catheter is not present, progressively higher airway pressure may be necessary to compensate for increased abdominal pressure on the diaphragm and/or loss of effective lung volume. The high airway pressure is transmitted to the pulmonary vasculature because the pulmonary parenchyma is relatively healthy; this, in turn, increases pulmonary vascular resistance (PVR), thereby increasing afterload on the already poorly functioning RV. Raised intra-abdominal pressure and low cardiac output also result in decreased renal perfusion and, eventually, renal failure, further complicating fluid management. A downward spiral thus develops in which cardiac output cannot be readily restored and pulmonary gas exchange as well as fluid and electrolyte management cannot be adequately maintained. Effective treatment can include drainage of effusions or ascites followed by further fluid resuscitation. In severe cases, mechanical support with an RV assist device or ECMO may be necessary. In general, RV diastolic function often improves over several days as the ventricle heals from surgery and becomes more compliant, assuming that the initial operation effectively restored near-normal RV systolic pressure. LV diastolic dysfunction may similarly resolve but is more likely to be associated with prolonged heart failure and/or the need for transplantation.

Pulmonary Hypertension

The incidence of postoperative pulmonary hypertension has decreased as the fields of pediatric cardiology and cardiac surgery have moved toward earlier repairs of the left-to-right shunt lesions most often associated with chronic pulmonary vascular changes. Nevertheless, CPB can provoke pulmonary hypertension in those patients with significant underlying risk (13). Neonates, patients with pulmonary venous obstruction or mitral valve disease, and those with elevated preoperative pulmonary resistance are at particularly high risk, especially when associated with pain, agitation, suctioning, or hypoventilation. Signs and symptoms of pulmonary hypertension depend on the acuity of the change in resistance and on the underlying anatomy, particularly with regard to the existence of residual shunts. Chronic pulmonary hypertension that is not acutely worsened as a result of CPB can be well tolerated in the postoperative period, whereas acute pulmonary hypertensive crises can precipitate life-threatening symptoms. The presence of a patent foramen ovale, atrial septal defect, VSD, or systemic-to-pulmonary artery shunt causes the main clinical consequence of acute elevations in PVR to be cyanosis because of an increase in right-to-left shunting. Pulmonary hypertension without shunting can cause acute RV failure and low cardiac output without significant changes in saturation. A sudden fall in either blood pressure or saturation in a patient with known pulmonary vascular disease or with significant risk of postoperative pulmonary hypertension should prompt immediate consideration

of this diagnosis and institution of treatment when appropriate. The presence of a pulmonary artery pressure-monitoring catheter can help to establish the diagnosis of pulmonary hypertension. Most commonly, the systemic pressure falls while the pulmonary artery pressure remains unchanged. The increased ratio of pulmonary to systemic arterial pressure is diagnostic of an increase in PVR.

In addition to hypotension or cyanosis, a pulmonary hypertensive crisis in the absence of a right-to-left shunt is usually associated with an acute increase in right atrial pressure because the increase in RV afterload raises diastolic pressure. This pressure increase can also result in shift of the ventricular septum into the LV and a subsequent increase in left atrial pressure despite the decreased filling of the left side of the heart. Tachycardia is a common feature as the heart struggles to maintain systemic cardiac output with a diminished stroke volume. Other clinical manifestations can include a sudden decrease in lung compliance and/or onset of bronchospasm. As pulmonary hypertension is exacerbated by hypoxia and hypercarbia, these manifestations can be especially troublesome.

The most effective treatment strategy for those at significant risk of postoperative pulmonary hypertension is prevention. Maintenance of adequate analgesia and sedation, particularly during noxious stimuli such as suctioning, is important. Induction of respiratory alkalosis can be helpful in an acute pulmonary hypertensive crisis, but maintaining a pH above 7.5 for prolonged periods may have adverse consequences for cerebral perfusion. Therefore, a more practical approach is to avoid common problems that lead to hypoxia and respiratory acidosis, such as pneumothorax, right main stem bronchus intubation, or mucous plugging, and to maintain a pH between 7.4 and 7.5. It is generally appropriate to try to normalize the pH and reduce sedation on a daily basis while carefully observing the patient for symptoms associated with increased pulmonary artery pressure. Continued problems with pulmonary hypertension for more than 4–7 days suggest important residual lesions or more chronic pulmonary vascular disease.

When prophylactic therapy fails, more aggressive treatment with inhaled nitric oxide (iNO), sildenafil, bosentan, or even mechanical support may be helpful. Most studies have shown that low doses of NO (2–20 ppm) are as effective as higher doses (40–80 ppm) but are less likely to be associated with complications such as methemoglobinemia. Sildenafil and bosentan can be used to transition from iNO to chronic oral therapy for patients with chronic pulmonary vascular disease, as exogenous NO can lead to inhibition of endogenous production. Numerous other IV vasodilators, including calcium-channel blockers, nitrovasodilators, and prostaglandins, have been used but are often limited by the occurrence of systemic hypotension because of lack of pulmonary selectivity. Prostacyclin has shown promise as an agent that may reverse pulmonary vascular changes previously thought to be permanent.

Single-ventricle Lesions—Stage I Palliation

Single-ventricle lesions encompass distinctly different physiologies, depending on the stage of palliation. After stage I palliation procedures that involve a systemic-to-pulmonary artery shunt or pulmonary artery banding, the pulmonary-to-systemic blood flow ratio (Q_p:Q_s) is dependent on the systemic vascular resistance, size of the connection to the pulmonary artery, and to a lesser degree, the PVR. Arterial saturation is essentially an average of the pulmonary and systemic venous saturations weighted by the Q_p:Q_s, so that anything that decreases mixed venous saturation, pulmonary venous saturation, or Q_p:Q_s can result in increased cyanosis. Problems in the postoperative period that can lead to diminished oxygen delivery include low systemic cardiac output and/or excessive cyanosis. It is important to determine if the problem is primarily related to a low total cardiac output, disadvantageous partitioning of the cardiac output (low or high Q_p:Q_s), or to problems with pulmonary venous saturation. Poor systemic perfusion or an increased gradient between arterial and mixed venous oxygen saturation suggests a primary problem with total cardiac output or high Q_p:Q_s. Cyanosis with preserved hemodynamics suggests either low Q_p:Q_s or a primary pulmonary problem.

One of the most important principles to grasp in the management of the postoperative infant with this type of singe-ventricle stage I palliation is that increases in systemic vascular resistance can increase blood pressure, Q_p:Q_s, and arterial saturation at the expense of systemic perfusion. Therefore, a good blood pressure should not be taken, in and of itself, as a sign of adequate systemic perfusion. Many studies now suggest that higher blood pressure is, in fact, associated with lower systemic oxygen delivery, so that it has become common practice to use afterload reduction with phenoxybenzamine, milrinone, or nitroprusside to maximize perfusion (5,7). Blood pressure can be kept in an acceptable range by improving total cardiac output with β agonists such as low-dose epinephrine or even norepinephrine.

Another essential principle regarding management of these patients is that adequate oxygen delivery is best maintained by maximizing total cardiac output, and further adjustments can be made by manipulation of Q_p:Q_s. Again, this supports the use of afterload reduction, which can increase stroke volume and counteract pulmonary overcirculation. Therapeutic strategies aimed at maximizing PVR are of limited value in practice, particularly because the largest component of the pulmonary resistance occurs at the site of the band or shunt.

Single-ventricle Lesions—Stage II (Bidirectional Glenn) and Stage III (Fontan) Palliation

Second- and third-stage palliation for single-ventricle lesions are unique in that they result in pulmonary blood flow that is dependent on nonpulsatile venous flow. A unique aspect of the physiology of the bidirectional cavopulmonary anastomosis (Glenn) is that pulmonary blood flow is largely dependent on the resistance of two highly but differentially regulated vascular beds—the cerebral and pulmonary circulations. Both cerebral and pulmonary vasculatures have opposite responses to changes in carbon dioxide, acid-base status, and oxygen, which can make treatment of elevated pulmonary resistance or low arterial saturation particularly challenging. Hyperventilation and alkalosis, for example, may have limited utility in this setting. Although they are effective pulmonary vasodilators, hyperventilation and alkalosis cause cerebral vasoconstriction. As pulmonary blood flow is dependent on venous return via the superior vena cava (largely made up of cerebral blood flow), maneuvers that limit cerebral blood flow may decrease pulmonary flow and exacerbate hypoxemia. Hyperventilation following bidirectional cavopulmonary anastomosis does, in fact, impair cerebral blood flow and decrease arterial saturation (1). Other frequently used techniques for decreasing pulmonary resistance (such as deep-sedation/anesthesia) may also reduce

cerebral blood flow and therefore fail to increase pulmonary blood flow, even if they successfully reduce resistance. iNO, which acts selectively on the pulmonary vasculature, has been reported to be effective in reducing the transpulmonary pressure gradient for patients after a bidirectional cavopulmonary anastomosis (6) and may therefore work well in combination with mild hypoventilation for high pulmonary resistance and cyanosis. When the degree of cyanosis is not prohibitive, expectant management with good hemodynamic support and maintenance of hemoglobin will often suffice, because saturation tends to slowly improve in the first few days following surgery and again at the time of extubation as long as no intervening airway or pulmonary issues occur. Persistent cyanosis should prompt a search for lesions, such as decompressing venovenous collaterals, that divert superior vena cava blood away from the pulmonary circulation.

Systemic hypertension is a common phenomenon following the Glenn operation (3), perhaps a response to increased cerebral venous pressure or improved output from a ventricle that has had some of its volume load removed. Acute treatment with vasodilators is often necessary, and blood pressure tends to fall to normal levels over the first few postoperative days. A proportion of patients require more long-term treatment with ACE inhibitors.

Residual left-to-right shunts such as aortopulmonary collateral vessels can also be problematic following cavopulmonary anastomoses operations (12). They have been associated with persistent pleural effusions, high central venous pressures, and low cardiac output (11). Once significant aortopulmonary collaterals are identified, they should be occluded using the coil embolization technique.

It is important to recognize that changes in ventricular geometry occur, particularly with the bidirectional Glenn procedure, because of reduction in left-to-right shunt after ligation of the Blalock-Taussig or central shunt. When systemic outflow is dependent on flow through a VSD or bulboventricular foramen, acute decreases in ventricular dimension may precipitate effective subaortic stenosis. The appearance of an ejection murmur in a patient with susceptible anatomy following bidirectional cavopulmonary anastomosis should prompt a complete assessment for this phenomenon.

Fontan physiology is a hybrid of bidirectional Glenn and normal cardiovascular physiology. Like the bidirectional Glenn, pulmonary blood flow is dependent on systemic venous pressure, and all pulmonary flow is effective. If the Fontan baffle is fenestrated (2), a right-to-left shunt may still exist, causing some mild systemic arterial desaturation, but the systemic and pulmonary circulations are largely separated, as with a normal heart. Important issues for the intensive care physician arise when pulmonary artery pressure is elevated, which can occur because the pulmonary resistance is high, in the presence of mechanical pulmonary artery obstruction, or when myocardial dysfunction raises pulmonary venous atrial pressure. Numerous studies demonstrate that elevated pulmonary artery pressure (>10–15 mm Hg) is associated with poor outcome in Fontan patients, largely because it is very difficult to maintain central venous pressure in this range without large third-space losses of fluid. As these fluid losses progress, patients often develop pleural effusions, ascites, and peripheral edema. It then becomes necessary to increase ventilator pressures to maintain adequate functional residual capacity and tidal volume in the face of a full abdomen, heavy chest wall, and smaller effective pleural cavities. Increased airway pressure, particularly in the absence of parenchymal lung disease, effectively raises pulmonary resistance and thus necessitates even higher venous pressures to maintain cardiac output. Furthermore, as central venous and intra-abdominal pressures rise, renal perfusion pressure decreases, especially in the face of low cardiac output and borderline hypotension, as is often the case in this scenario. In general, Fontan fenestration can lower the risk of some of these complications by providing a source of systemic blood flow that is not dependent on passing through the pulmonary circulation (2). Fenestration can also decrease pulmonary artery pressure enough to reduce third-space losses of fluid (8).

When an individual with Fontan physiology is in a low cardiac output state, it is essential to determine and treat the underlying cause. It is common for postoperative Fontan patients to need large amounts of volume in the first day after surgery. Persistently low central venous and left atrial pressures strongly suggest the need for volume. Pulmonary artery obstruction should be considered as the cause of low output when left atrial pressure is low and central venous pressure is high. If central venous pressure is not monitored, large third-space fluid losses with a low or normal left atrial pressure should raise the suspicion of pulmonary artery obstruction. Even in the presence of a fenestrated Fontan, the capability of the fenestration to preserve cardiac output in the face of anatomic or physiologic obstruction to pulmonary blood flow is significantly limited compared to the situation after the bidirectional cavopulmonary anastomosis. Therefore, limited pulmonary flow can result in low cardiac output and, when a fenestration is present, significant cyanosis. Cyanosis can also result from intrapulmonary arteriovenous malformations (such as occur after the Glenn operation (9) or ventilation-perfusion mismatch related to low cardiac output.

If high pulmonary resistance is responsible for the elevation of central venous pressure, institution of the standard therapies of supplemental oxygen, hyperventilation, and alkalosis are indicated. However, as with the bidirectional Glenn patient, the use of high positive pressures to achieve these ends may be counterproductive. Negative-pressure ventilation can augment stroke volume and cardiac output (10) and high-frequency jet ventilation may lower $Paco_2$ at low mean airway pressures. Intravenous vasodilators such as prostacyclin or PGE should be used with caution because of the risk of systemic vasodilation with limited cardiac output. iNO has been reported to be effective in lowering the transpulmonary pressure gradient (6).

Low cardiac output with high left atrial and central venous pressures indicates myocardial dysfunction in the patient with Fontan physiology. Myocardial dysfunction can occur from ischemia-reperfusion injury if aortic cross-clamping and cardioplegia are used to create the Fontan baffle. It may also be related to poor preoperative myocardial function. The only effective long-term therapy for low cardiac output with ventricular dysfunction following a Fontan operation is to improve cardiac output and reduce left atrial pressure. The use of inotropic agents that do not increase ventricular afterload, such as phosphodiesterase inhibitors, dobutamine and low dose

epinephrine (≤ 0.05 mcg/kg/min) may be helpful. If systemic blood pressure will tolerate it, aggressive afterload reduction with vasodilating agents may also lower left atrial pressure significantly. If there is good reason to believe the insult to ventricular function is reversible, mechanical circulatory support can also be effective therapy. Because persistent aortopulmonary collateral vessels can be associated with hemodynamics similar to those of ventricular dysfunction, aggressive assessment and embolization of these vessels may be useful in this situation.

CONCLUSIONS AND FUTURE DIRECTIONS

The management of the postoperative pediatric cardiac surgical patient requires a comprehensive understanding of the basic principles of oxygen delivery, cardiovascular physiology, and the anatomy and physiology of congenital heart disease. Signs and symptoms of low cardiac output syndrome should be treated aggressively, and diagnostic and therapeutic strategies should address both universal and lesion-specific problems.

References

1. Bradley SM, Simsic JM, Mulvihill DM. Hyperventilation impairs oxygenation after bidirectional superior cavopulmonary connection. *Circulation* 1998;98:II372–6.
2. Bridges ND, Lock JE, Castaneda AR. Baffle fenestration with subsequent transcatheter closure. Modification of the Fontan operation for patients at increased risk. *Circulation* 1990;82:1681–9.
3. Chang AC, Hanley FL, Wernovsky G, et al. Early bidirectional cavopulmonary shunt in young infants. Postoperative course and early results. *Circulation* 1993;88:II149–58.
4. Cullen S, Shore D, Redington A. Characterization of right ventricular diastolic performance after complete repair of tetralogy of Fallot: Restrictive physiology predicts slow postoperative recovery. *Circulation* 1995;91:1782–9.
5. DeOliveira NC, Ashburn DA, Khalid F, et al. Prevention of early sudden circulatory collapse after the Norwood operation. *Circulation* 2004;110:II133–8.
6. Gamillscheg A, Zobel G, Urlesberger B, et al. Inhaled nitric oxide in patients with critical pulmonary perfusion after Fontan-type procedures and bidirectional Glenn anastomosis. *J Thorac Cardiovasc Surg* 1997;113:435–42.
7. Hoffman GM, Tweddell JS, Ghanayem NS, et al. Alteration of the critical arteriovenous oxygen saturation relationship by standard afterload reduction after the Norwood procedure. *J Thorac Cardiovasc Surg* 2004;127:738–45.
8. Lemler MS, Scott WA, Leonard SR, et al. Fenestration improves clinical outcome of the Fontan procedure. *Circulation* 2002;105:207–12.
9. McFaul RC, Tajik AJ, Mair DD, et al. Development of pulmonary arteriovenous shunt after superior vena cava-right pulmonary artery (Glenn) anastomosis. *Circulation* 1977;55:212–6.
10. Shekerdemian LS, Bush A, Shore DF, et al. Cardiopulmonary interactions after Fontan operations: Augmentation of cardiac output using negative pressure ventilation. *Circulation* 1997;96:3934–42.
11. Spicer RL, Uzark KC, Moore JW, et al. Aortopulmonary collateral vessels and prolonged pleural effusions after modified Fontan procedures. *Am Heart J* 1996;131:1164–8.
12. Triedman JK, Bridges ND, Mayer JEJ, et al. Prevalence and risk factors for aortopulmonary collateral vessels after Fontan and bidirectional Glenn procedures. *J Am Coll Cardiol* 1993;22:207–15.
13. Wessel DL, Adatia I, Giglia TM, et al. Use of inhaled nitric oxide and acetylcholine in the evaluation of pulmonary hypertension and endothelial function after cardiopulmonary bypass. *Circulation* 1993;88:2128–38.
14. Yano M, Kohno M, Ohkusa T, et al. Effect of milrinone on left ventricular relaxation and Ca^{2+} uptake function of cardiac sarcoplasmic reticulum. *Am J Physiol Heart Circ Physiol* 2000;279:H1898–905.

CHAPTER 70C ■ POSTOPERATIVE CARE OF THE PEDIATRIC CARDIAC SURGICAL PATIENT: EFFECTS OF CARDIOPULMONARY BYPASS

S. ADIL HUSAIN • MARK S. BLEIWEIS

The concept of hypothermia was first introduced to cardiac surgery in 1950, when Bigelow reported that canines cooled to 20°C could survive up to 15 mins of total circulatory arrest (3,4). Lewis and Taufic were the first to report the application of hypothermia with inflow occlusion in the repair of an atrial septal defect in 1952 (27). The attempt to save a pregnant woman from pulmonary embolus set the stage for the first approaches to employing extracorporeal circulation with surgical intervention. The sentinel work of Gibbon led to the first successful use of extracorporeal circulation in the open cardiac surgical repair of an atrial septal defect in a young woman in 1953 (15). Because the subsequent early experiences with the concept of cardiopulmonary bypass (CPB) were dismal, most surgical pioneers sought alternatives.

Arguably the most innovative advance in all of surgery followed, as Dr. Walton Lillehei and associates began using compatible adults as pump oxygenators to repair congenital heart defects. In this manner, controlled cross-circulation using human beings was employed as a mechanism of CPB. Although initial results were impressive (28 of the 47 patients survived operation), this technique had obvious limitations and risks (28,29). Bubble oxygenators were first produced in the early 1960s, and they revolutionized the concept of CPB. By the early 1970s, when coronary and valve surgery was becoming more commonplace, membrane oxygenators became favored due to their increased safety with longer exposure times.

Advances in both technique and hardware technology have made CPB applicable to all age groups. In addition, improvements in myocardial and cerebral protection and strategies to address systemic inflammatory response mechanisms have directly led to better outcomes for even the most complex congenital anomalies. Following is a review of the basic principles of CPB and its definitions and physiologic implications. With a better understanding of CPB and its systemic effects, the pediatric intensivist will be better prepared to care for postoperative patients with surgically treated congenital heart disease.

THE EXTRACORPOREAL CIRCUIT

Although the CPB circuit may differ between surgical centers, basic concepts are uniform. Blood drains from the patient via the right atrium or from both cavae into a cardiotomy reservoir. This drainage is dependent on gravity or can be assisted by a vacuum. Once in the reservoir, blood is pumped through a membrane oxygenator that incorporates a heat exchanger. Subsequently, this oxygenated blood is returned to the patient's systemic bloodstream, usually via a cannula in the aorta, arch vessel, axillary artery, or femoral artery. A filter is usually employed within this arterial line to prevent any embolization of air or other debris into the systemic circulation. In many instances, a hemofilter is used within the circuit for ultrafiltration of the patient's blood volume (**Fig. 70C.1**).

Cannulae

Discussions of cannulae employed in congenital cardiac surgery center around the sizes of tubing employed and the locations where they are placed. Differences are often matters of surgical preference. In general, drainage cannulae are placed within the right atrium and, even more commonly, in the superior and inferior vena cavae. As a result, the right atrium can be kept clear of most blood for the variety of anomalies that are repaired via entrance into this chamber. Arterial inflow into the body is achieved via a cannula placed directly into either the ascending aorta or any other large arterial branch such as the femoral artery. In the pediatric population, the ascending aorta is most commonly employed; however, variations may be necessary, depending upon the patient's anatomy and required repair (**Fig. 70C.2**). For example, the innominate artery may be cannulated for aortic arch cases in which low-flow continuous bypass is utilized during arch repair to avoid circulatory arrest. More than one arterial cannula may be necessary. For example, in an interrupted aortic arch, the innominate artery can be cannulated directly to perfuse the proximal aorta, and a second arterial cannula can be placed in the ductus or main pulmonary artery to perfuse distal to the interruption.

Prime

The prime constitutes the volume within the CPB circuit. Modern trends in CPB are to miniaturize its components to minimize the amount of prime. This goal is particularly important in neonates and small infants. Miniaturization creates an environment in which the infant's blood volume is exposed to foreign surfaces for the least amount of time and overall in smaller amounts, which is relevant in the context of blood exposure and inflammatory response. In a neonate, the priming volume may exceed the blood volume by as much as 200%–300% (18).

High prime volumes will lower the infant's hematocrit. The lowest acceptable hematocrit for a patient on bypass is

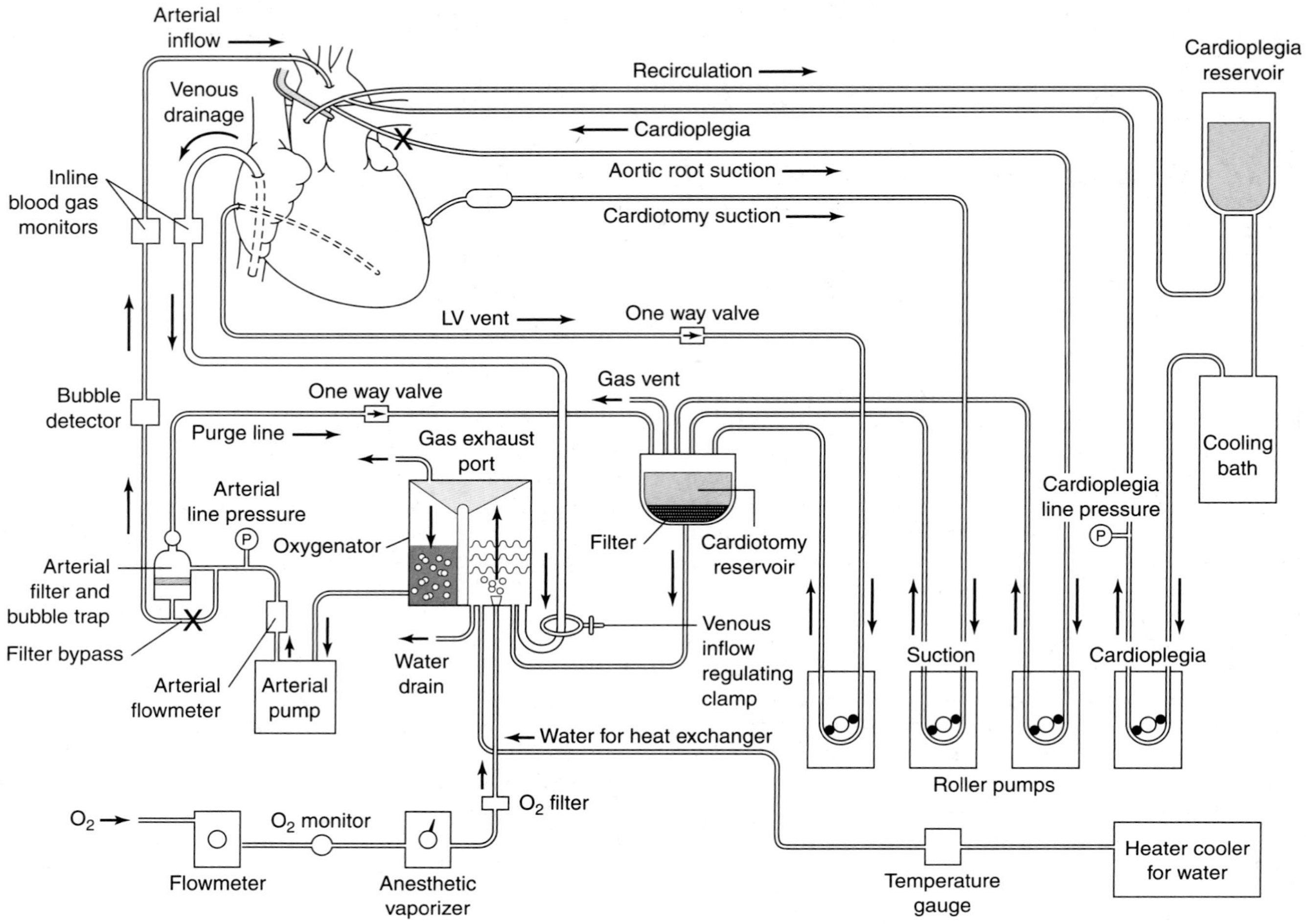

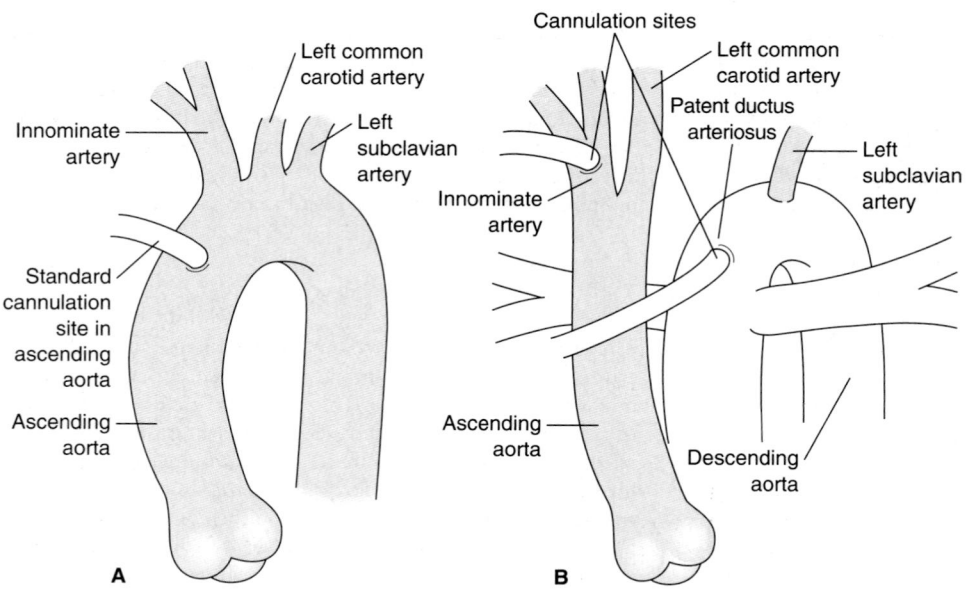

FIGURE 70C.1. Extracorporeal cardiopulmonary bypass circuit.

FIGURE 70C.2. Arterial cannulation sites during cardiopulmonary bypass. (**A**) Standard cannulation site in ascending aorta. (**B**) For type B interrupted aortic arch, cannulae placed directly into the innominate artery and the ductus arteriosus.

debatable and depends on the temperature, pH, and flow rate employed. A generally accepted clinical practice has been to maintain a higher hematocrit when using higher-temperature CPB, with the hematocrit target approximately the same as the minimum temperature during CPB. A minimal hematocrit of ~25% is usually acceptable for any CPB situation and thus often demands the use of donor blood within the prime (22). The use of donor blood has potential risks, such as complement activation, transfusion reaction, viral transmission, and electrolyte abnormalities. Hemodilution reduces clotting factors and colloid osmotic pressure and, in turn, promotes the release of stress hormones and inflammatory mediators (40). As a result of all of these physiologic sequelae, priming volumes should be kept to a minimum, and transfusions avoided. The optimum level of hemodilution is also directly correlated with degree of hypothermia and the overall impact on adequate oxygen delivery. Some groups advocate a more aggressive approach with target hematocrit of 35%, based on a potential association with improved neurologic outcomes (20).

Institutional differences exist in the use of packed red blood cells versus whole blood for priming solutions. Although whole blood improves colloid oncotic pressure, as well as levels of circulating clotting factors, it also contains a much higher glucose content. The resulting hyperglycemia has been delineated as a risk factor for neurologic injury. Colloid solutions, such as fresh frozen plasma and albumin, are commonly used. Priming solutions also contain electrolytes, glucose, calcium, lactate, and buffers (tris hydroxymethyl aminomethane or sodium bicarbonate, THAM). Buffer is added to help maintain appropriate pH. Agents such as mannitol and steroids may also be added to help with osmotic diuresis and as prophylaxis against systemic inflammatory responses.

Oxygenators

Oxygenators function as the gas-exchanging component of the CPB circuit. Their significance is found in their ability to maintain this exchange over a wide range of temperatures and flow rates. Bubble oxygenators were the first employed for CPB and functioned by allowing fresh microbubbles to mix with circulating blood, all within an oxygenation column. This direct interface created a traumatic environment for red blood cells, which led to increased hemolysis, platelet microaggregation, and an increased release of inflammatory mediators (46). Membrane oxygenators minimized this interface issue via the use of microporous hollow fibers. Micropores improve gas exchange within a smaller membrane surface area, thus decreasing the area upon which the circulating blood is exposed (41). Newer micropore hollow-fiber oxygenators also require very low prime volumes.

Pumps

A pumping mechanism is used during CPB to propel the blood through the circuit and back to the infant, and two forms are used—roller pumps and centrifugal pumps. Roller pumps are most widely used in the infant population and consist of two rollers oriented 180 degrees from one another. Blood is displaced in a forward manner, in a continuous nonpulsatile fashion. Forward displacement is the product of partial occlusion

of the pump tubing between the rollers and their associated casing apparatus. The second roller pump acts as a valve to minimize back flow.

The centrifugal pump system functions by entrapping blood against spinning curved blades that create a vortex. This mechanism is advantageous as another method to minimize priming volume and to minimize general red cell trauma. The vortex functions in removing any air that could be a source of embolization once the blood returns to the arterial circulation (21). These pumps are also capable of producing pulsatile flow, which may improve the overall flow through both infant and circuit.

Tubing

As with other components within the CPB circuit, a delicate balance must be achieved with the tubing employed. The tubes themselves are constructed with polyvinyl chloride and must be large enough to support appropriate flow rates but small enough to minimize pump prime and exposure surface area of the circulating blood. In neonates, 3/16-inch tubing is used for the arterial limbs of the circuit, and 1/4-inch tubing is used for the venous limbs. Progressively larger tubing is employed for heavier patients to appropriately support required flow rates. Heparin-bonded tubing has been utilized by some centers to improve the interface with circulating blood and to reduce the extent of anticoagulation required to safely maintain an infant on CPB. In addition, many have felt that its use impacts the degree of inflammatory response following CPB. Thus, heparin-bonded tubing has gained more intense favor, and investigation of its use within the pediatric population appears promising (13).

CARDIOPULMONARY BYPASS IN INFANTS VERSUS ADULTS

Significant differences exist in the management of infants and adults who are placed on CPB, including prime volume, temperature and hemodilution, and the anatomic and associated physiologic differences within congenital heart disease. In comparison with adults, infant anatomic abnormalities may involve interrupted aortic arch anatomy, presence of intracardiac shunts, and aortopulmonary collateral circulation. These differences require changes in both CPB strategy and in cannulation location and techniques.

As previously described, infants have lower circulating blood volumes, which, coupled with their increased oxygen consumption rates, requires careful attention to bypass flows. Infants require much higher flow rates, often 200 mL/kg/min (**Table 70C.1**). The structure and function of the underlying organ systems are not as mature in infants, and thus their response to CPB is also altered. For example, decreased liver function results in a diminished production of vitamin K-dependent clotting factors, making these patients subject to a bleeding diathesis. Also, as infants have a poor ability to thermoregulate under stress, close temperature monitoring is critical.

The immaturity of other organ systems may be beneficial to infants who require CPB. For example, the immature brain tolerates oxygen deprivation much better, thereby allowing for longer periods of hypothermia and circulatory arrest. The

TABLE 70C.1

PUMP FLOW RATES FOR CARDIOPULMONARY BYPASS

Patient weight (kg)	Pump flow rate (mL/kg/min)
<3	150–200
3–10	125–175
10–15	120–150
15–30	100–120
30–50	75–100
>50	50–75

immaturity of other organ systems can be detrimental to children who undergo CPB. The lungs of a neonate are extremely fragile and, at birth, only contain ~10% of functioning alveoli compared to an adult (22). Renal function may be impaired due to higher vascular resistance, with preferential blood flow away from the cortex. Subsequently, electrolyte balance may be compromised. The immune system is also immature, and complement generation is impaired, with dysfunctional mononuclear cells being evident (25). Numerous other derangements exist that are beyond the scope of this chapter. Needless to say, diminishing the overall morbidity and mortality associated with congenital cardiac surgery is accomplished by organizing a highly skilled multidisciplinary team to care for these patients in the perioperative as well as the hypercritical intraoperative period.

INITIATION OF CARDIOPULMONARY BYPASS

Definitions

For infants who require CPB for operative repair of congenital disease, the initial strategy consists of entering the mediastinum and preparing to initiate CPB. The pericardium is entered, and sutures are placed in the various sites where cannulae will be inserted to attach the infant to the CPB circuit. Heparin must be utilized during CPB, and a bolus dose of 300–400 units/kg is administered. Heparin and its effects upon anticoagulation are monitored intraoperatively by measuring the patient's activated clotting time (ACT). The goals set for ACT values are controversial and differ institutionally, as well as in cases in which heparin-bonded tubing is employed. An ACT of >350–400 secs is generally accepted (26). Heparin resistance may occur in patients with low levels of antithrombin III, and administration of fresh frozen plasma may be employed to counteract this clotting deficiency.

Prior to heparinization, extensive dissection is performed, including removal of the thymus gland for maximal operative exposure, as well as isolation of previously placed shunts, known aortopulmonary connections, or a patent ductus arteriosus. Following heparinization and cannulation, CPB is instituted and blood begins to drain from the patient's heart. Venous drainage is dependent upon the height difference between patient and circuit, the diameter of the venous cannula and line tubing, and whether vacuum assistance is used. Ar-

terial cannula pressure is continuously monitored and may be elevated in cases of a malpositioned or kinked arterial cannula.

Once CPB has been instituted without concerns at the cannula level or elsewhere in the circuit, the heat exchanger within the oxygenator can be cooled and the patient core body temperature can be lowered. Some degree of hypothermia is implemented in most congenital cardiac surgical procedures that require CPB. Tourniquets are generally placed around the superior and inferior vena cavae to allow for compression of the vessel walls around the cannulae. In this manner, all venous return now drains into the oxygenator and any airlock formation within the circuit is avoided. At this point, the anesthesia team withdraws ventilatory support, and the lungs collapse and become ischemic.

Cardiac Arrest—Myocardial Protection/Ischemia

Infants who require intracardiac repairs will have their heart arrested via two sequenced maneuvers. A small cardioplegia cannula placed in the ascending aorta distal to the aortic valve serves as an entry pathway for cardioplegia solution to be administered to the patient. Cardioplegia is an extremely cold (4–8°C) and highly potassium enriched solution, which allows for myocardial cells to be "protected" during periods of ischemia (33). Because of the high potassium concentration, the decompressed heart is arrested in diastole and, thus, has low myocardial oxygen and metabolic demands. An aortic cross-clamp is placed between the cardioplegia cannula and the aortic inflow cannula coming from the CPB circuit such that flow from the circuit to the body and cardioplegia flow to the coronary arteries can be separated. Induction cardioplegia is delivered at 30 mL/kg toward the competent aortic valve and into the coronary ostia. Some surgeons place ice or cold solution on the heart to ensure a hypothermic environment, thereby further diminishing metabolic demands and increasing myocardial protection, although risk of thermal injury to the phrenic nerves and other nearby structures exist.

Hypothermic Circulatory Arrest and Low-flow Cardiopulmonary Bypass

Flow rates on CPB are best determined by evaluating the size of the infant, degree of hypothermia, and technical requirements of the surgical procedure to be performed. Hypothermia reduces the metabolic rate and allows the surgeon and perfusionist to lower the perfusion flow rates accordingly. The concept of complete circulatory arrest—actually stopping pump flow—defines the extreme of low-flow rates during CPB. Certain surgical procedures, such as those that involve the aorta and its arch, are often performed with circulatory arrest, producing a completely bloodless field and permitting the surgeon to remove all cannulae from the operative field to maximize exposure and repair complex defects. A modification to this concept is that of low-flow perfusion where the inflow rates from the CPB circuit are dramatically reduced but not completely discontinued, all within the setting of aggressive hypothermia. This technique maintains some cerebral perfusion and theoretically provides better cerebral protection. Generally accepted correlations exist between flow rates and degree of hypothermia in regard to full-flow CPB, low-flow CPB, and finally, complete hypothermic circulatory arrest.

GENERAL PHYSIOLOGIC CONSIDERATIONS OF CARDIOPULMONARY BYPASS

To gain a comprehensive understanding of the physiologic, organ system-based effects of CPB and circulatory arrest, one must first understand the overall metabolic effects of hypothermia and the impact of flow dynamics. These topics are discussed here, followed by a discussion of the impact to each organ system, with a focus on intraoperative and postoperative management scenarios.

Hypothermia

As mentioned previously, hypothermia and its physiologic consequences are a key component of CPB and circulatory arrest. The rationale for hypothermia centers on its impact upon reduction in overall metabolic rate and molecular movement (35). The effect upon metabolic rate is described using the nomenclature of Q_{10}, which is defined by the difference in metabolic rate (oxygen consumption) at two temperatures, 10 degrees apart. It has been reported that infants have a higher Q_{10} than do adults and thus have a greater metabolic suppression and impact upon oxygen consumption (17). This would indicate that infants have the ability to withstand longer periods of altered blood flow and perfusion than adults at similar levels of hypothermia.

The technique of deep hypothermic circulatory arrest (DHCA) is beneficial for highly complex intracardiac or aortic arch repairs, especially in the neonatal population. Arrest times of 30 mins at temperatures of 18–20°C have been described with overall minimal clinically evident neurologic injury (13). The risk of neurologic injury rises with increasing arrest times, especially with arrest periods of >45–60 mins. Tympanic, esophageal, and/or rectal temperatures can be measured and followed during cooling. Surface cooling measures such as placement of ice bags around the patient's head and the use of cooling blankets are also widely employed.

Low-flow continuous bypass with deep hypothermia is another operative strategy that is based on the premise that some cerebral blood flow is better than no flow. Low-flow bypass in neonates and infants at ~30–50 mL/kg/min can be used in certain surgical scenarios to allow for improved surgical visualization while maintaining cerebral blood flow. Almost all complex congenital cardiac operations can be completed with avoidance of circulatory arrest, but this perfusion strategy requires careful planning and surgical technique for cannulation. The use of low-flow continuous CPB versus DHCA is an area of controversy, and bias of individual surgeons or centers still dictates the technique employed (36). More definitive evidence is necessary to scientifically confirm the superiority of one technique over the other.

In evaluating the published data regarding to neurologic sequelae, developmental issues and incidence of seizure activity have been well described. Early postoperative seizure activity has been found to be associated with the duration of DHCA. In addition, seizure activity itself has been associated with lower developmental test results at 1 year. In contrast, other studies have described minimal evidence of functional or anatomic injury after DHCA in both canine and human models (45). Greeley showed that the recovery of cerebral metabolism after CPB with DHCA is delayed compared to the recovery of cerebral metabolism after hypothermic CPB with continuous flow (18).

Despite its cerebral protective effects, hypothermia can significantly negatively impact other organ systems and strongly influence the postoperative course and management. Hypothermia has a profound impact upon tissue fluid sequestration, third spacing, and hemodilution (42). Changes in capillary permeability result from activation of the systemic inflammatory response. Respiratory compliance and function are significantly altered, and ventilatory support may be necessary until compliance improves. The fluid shifts associated with hypothermic CPB will focus attention on intravascular volume replacement early in the postoperative course, followed by diuresis later in the course.

Pulsatile versus Nonpulsatile Flow

The issue of pulsatile versus nonpulsatile flow was introduced previously in the section describing the different forms of pumps employed in CPB. The goal of pulsatile perfusion has been discussed extensively in literature of the Extracorporeal Life Support Organization. Studies have described a decrease in systemic vascular resistance and therefore diminished workload upon the post-CPB myocardium when using pulsatile flow (44). In addition, an increased production of nitric oxide has been associated with pulsatile flow, with resultant reduced right-heart strain and improved systemic oxygenation (37). The major benefit of pulsatile flow seems to be linked to a reduction in circulating vasoconstrictors following CPB. Improved regional perfusion to end organs seems to occur. However, the overall use of pulsatile pumps is limited, and the benefits described experimentally, although logical, are still largely unproven in the clinical setting.

Managing Acid-Base/Respiratory Physiology: α-stat and pH-stat

The oxygenator portion of the CPB circuit is responsible for gas exchange, i.e., oxygen introduction and carbon dioxide removal. The optimal management of acid-base balance during CPB (i.e., pH and carbon dioxide levels) remains a source of great debate and investigation. Two main strategies for managing pH are described: α-stat and pH-stat.

The α-stat strategy maintains a pH of 7.40 measured without correction for temperature (37°C), whereas pH-stat recognizes that temperature, more specifically, hypothermia has a significant impact upon pH. With hypothermia, blood pH becomes more alkalotic, and carbon dioxide is added to the circuit (and thus to the patient) to maintain a temperature-corrected pH of 7.40. However, this addition of carbon dioxide increases the intracellular pH and leads to a loss of electrochemical neutrality. More specifically, hydrogen and hydroxyl ions are impacted due to this change in intracellular pH. Cellular enzyme function is thus impacted when using pH-stat (43).

Studies that compare the α-stat and pH-stat strategies on oxygen consumption have revealed conflicting results. It has been suggested that alkaline pH during hypothermia (α-stat) prior to circulatory arrest is associated with less neurologic protection (23). Others, however, favor the α-stat strategy when myocardial preservation during ischemia is considered (2). Although the subject remains controversial, most agree that cerebral blood flow is increased when using the pH-stat method; however, overall cerebrovascular autoregulation is better maintained when α-stat is employed.

Myocardial Protection

As the goal of complete neonatal repair of complex congenital cardiac defects has been realized, the need for maximal intraoperative myocardial protection has become paramount. Complex and lengthy procedures are now performed with an ever-decreasing patient morbidity and mortality. In spite of these advances, primary myocardial failure still accounts for up to 50% of early deaths and remains prevalent within the pediatric population (8). Clearly, the surgical management of complex congenital heart disease is a product of both precise technical surgical repair and adequate myocardial protection.

Physiologic differences between the pediatric and adult myocardium exist, and they have implications for perioperative management. The pediatric heart is less compliant, resulting in a limited range of acceptable diastolic filling on the Starling curve. In addition, the neonate may be more sensitive to anesthetic agents, often requiring a judicious use of inotropic agents. The increased reliance of the newborn on normal glucose and calcium metabolism is well documented (6), yet, the role that hyperglycemia plays in the morbidity and mortality among pediatric cardiac patients is unknown. The normal neonatal myocardium is more tolerant of ischemic episodes; however, the impact of cyanosis, as well as pressure and/or volume loading, on myocardial mechanics is generally unknown.

The primary goal of cardioplegia is to achieve and maintain a complete electromechanical arrest in a nondistended, decompressed heart. Arrest of the heart in diastole due to the high potassium concentration in cardioplegia solution produces the most significant reduction in myocardial oxygen demand. Distribution of cardioplegia must be uniform and complete. Cardioplegia can be delivered in an antegrade (via the aorta or directly in the coronary arteries) or retrograde (via the coronary sinus) fashion. Antegrade cardioplegia delivered to the aortic root and directed toward the coronaries after placement of an aortic cross-clamp is by far the most common approach employed in the pediatric population. Retrograde cardioplegia delivered via the coronary sinus is also effective, even in small neonates. In neonates, infants, and children, it is best to place the retrograde catheter under direct vision when possible and to secure it in place with a purse string suture around the coronary sinus os. With this technique, the distribution to the right coronary artery territory is improved, particularly important when aortic insufficiency is present. Typically, an initial induction dose of

30 mL/kg is delivered at 4°C with a high potassium concentration (15–30 mEq/L) (31). Ventricular decompression is also critical during this phase, as the pressure within the ventricular free wall will impact coronary perfusion while the patient is on bypass.

Maintenance cardioplegia is achieved by repeat dosing at 15–20-min intervals throughout the period of desired arrest. The primary goal is to limit any myocardial ischemia during the arrest period. As has been emphasized, one of the principal protective mechanisms relates to cardiac hypothermia. The overall reduction in myocardial oxygen demand is achieved by a combination of electromechanical arrest, hypothermia, and mechanical decompression (7). Intermittent delivery ensures continuous arrest, allows for improved myocardial oxygen delivery, maintains metabolic substrates, and continues to assist in the overall hypothermic environment.

Intramyocardial air is a critical factor in myocardial dysfunction following cardiac surgery. It is reported that 4% of 350 patients were shown to have intramyocardial air detected immediately after CPB (16). This finding was confirmed via echocardiographic imaging despite the use of routine and aggressive de-airing maneuvers prior to removal of the aortic cross-clamp. In many of these cases, no obvious clinical sequelae were observed. The distribution of air was most often localized to the right coronary artery distribution due to the anterior position of the ostium within the proximal aorta. Therapy is focused upon increasing perfusion pressures via CPB to propel the air particles through the capillary bed. In addition, phenylephrine has been employed to aid in the removal of air from the coronary tree. Unfortunately, the impact of intramyocardial air may not be observed until the patient has left the operating room setting, and these scenarios can be quite concerning for surgeons and intensivists alike.

ORGAN SYSTEM EFFECTS OF CARDIOPULMONARY BYPASS

Altered Neurologic Function Due to Cardiopulmonary Bypass

The brain has the lowest tolerance of ischemia in comparison to other organs, and a very real incidence of neurologic injury has been observed with CPB. These observations have fueled intensive analysis of the impact of CPB and various operative techniques on neurologic function. In some series, the incidence of associated neurologic injury has been 10%–25% (11). An understanding of this issue is complicated by the difficulties in assessment of possible neurologic injury, as post-bypass neuropsychologic changes can be subtle and transient. In addition, neurologic deficits may involve a wide spectrum of issues, from subtle learning disabilities, behavioral disorders, seizures, and motor abnormalities to choreoathetosis.

The risk of abnormal neurologic development ranges from 2% to 10% for a variety of congenital heart defects and may be related to preoperative abnormalities in anatomy, oxygenation, or cerebral blood flow (12). Several factors are associated with cerebral protection and the avoidance of neurologic injury. Although these include rate of cooling, arterial blood pressure, cerebral blood flow, management of acid-base balance, and the presence of aortopulmonary collaterals, perhaps the most significant associated issue is that of microemboli and procedures that involve the systemic side of the heart. The use of membrane oxygenators, arterial filters, and appropriate anticoagulation within the CPB circuit has led to a decreased incidence of microembolic events. Treatment options include hypothermia and hyperbaric oxygen therapy, both of which have been found to reduce the size of microemboli, thus allowing them to pass through capillary beds (5).

Altered Renal Physiology Due to Cardiopulmonary Bypass

Renal dysfunction is a critical cause of morbidity and mortality following CPB. Post-CPB low cardiac output states are the most common cause for oliguria or anuria following congenital cardiac surgery. Preoperative renal dysfunction and congestive heart failure are also significant risk factors for postoperative renal insufficiency. Hypothermia has been shown to decrease renal perfusion. Elevated vasopressin release, resulting in fluid sequestration, is also a byproduct of CPB (39). Cortical blood flow is altered, and the renin-angiotensin system is activated to increase aldosterone production while patients are on CPB. Intraoperative use of "renal"-dose dopamine has not been shown to impact the incidence of renal insufficiency postoperatively. When renal failure occurs, a temporary peritoneal dialysis catheter may be useful, especially in neonates and small infants. Other forms of renal replacement therapy have also been utilized, such as continuous venovenous hemodialysis.

Altered Pulmonary Physiology Due to Cardiopulmonary Bypass

Preoperative pulmonary insufficiency is common in the neonatal population, and younger patients have been shown to be at risk for postoperative dysfunction (24). The basis of the pulmonary dysfunction after CPB is the result of many factors, including increased pulmonary vascular resistance from endothelial injury and lung deflation. Also, reduced compliance results in increased airway pressures needed to inflate the lungs, which may lead to volutrauma and barotrauma. Finally, activation of the inflammatory cascade during ischemia and reperfusion may result in increased airway resistance. During CPB, the lungs undergo a period of hypoxia and ischemia despite the membrane oxygenator's ability to replace lung function. However, the lung parenchyma does receive some blood supply from the bronchial arteries during bypass.

Patients with a large ventricular septal defect, truncus arteriosus, pulmonary vein stenosis, mitral stenosis, etc. often have pulmonary hypertension preoperatively, which presents a challenging intraoperative and postoperative management dilemma. These patients are more likely to have increased pulmonary vascular reactivity that leads to postoperative pulmonary hypertensive crises. Ventilatory management strategies to avoid periods of hypoxia and lung collapse are the mainstay of therapy, although secondary therapies such as inhaled nitric oxide, IV pulmonary vasodilators (milrinone, prostaglandins, etc.), and enteral sildenafil, among others, may be helpful.

Altered Endocrine Effects Due to Cardiopulmonary Bypass

CPB initiates a systemic inflammatory response and has significant impact on the endocrine system. It is associated with a tremendous increase in catecholamines, in particular, epinephrine and norepinephrine, as a result of many factors including ischemia, surgical stress, pain, and acid-base disturbances. Metabolism of catecholamines in the lungs is altered during CPB, resulting in increases in circulating levels, particularly of norepinephrine. Hypothermia results in both increasing production and decreasing metabolism of catecholamines. Circulating catecholamine levels do fall once CPB is discontinued and reperfusion occurs (30).

Hypothermia and CPB also impact insulin levels and peripheral responses to insulin. As a result, hyperglycemia occurs during the intraoperative period and persists during the postoperative recovery process. In addition, growth hormone and glucagon generally increase following CPB (25). Thyroid hormone levels [triiodothyronine (T_3) and thyroxine (T_4)] decrease immediately during CPB and for the first several days following surgery. Thyroid hormone levels often remain abnormal for 5–7 days. Alterations in thyroid regulation have been hypothesized to cause myocardial dysfunction, with attempts made to correct this imbalance by the administration of IV T_3 (34).

Systemic Inflammatory Response Due to Cardiopulmonary Bypass

The interaction of blood with nonendothelialized surfaces within the CPB circuit initiates the release of many substances, leading to a general systemic inflammatory response. Neutrophils and the complement system play integral roles in this response. The key dysfunction involves endothelial injury, leading to increased capillary permeability ("leak"). Capillary leak is greatest in neonates and infants. The resulting tissue edema can lead to poor wound healing and increased risks of infection.

Neutrophil release of superoxide free radicals, lysosomal enzymes, peroxides, etc. has been shown to induce endothelial cell injury (9). Levels of plasma cytokines such as IL-6 and IL-8 are known to increase with CPB. These cytokines act as chemoattractants for neutrophil-induced endothelial cell injury.

Attempts to manage the systemic inflammatory cascade include use of heparin-bonded circuits and administration of anti-inflammatory agents (Solu-Medrol) and antioxidants. The CPB circuit can be altered to limit the exposure of blood to nonendothelialized surfaces by miniaturizing the circuit and reducing priming volumes. Although the exact timing of administration is still not well established, preoperative steroids are known to reduce complement activation and decrease complement-mediated neutrophil adhesion and degranulation.

MANAGEMENT OF ANTICOAGULATION

Precise management of the clotting cascade intraoperatively and postoperatively is critical to the success of CPB and a

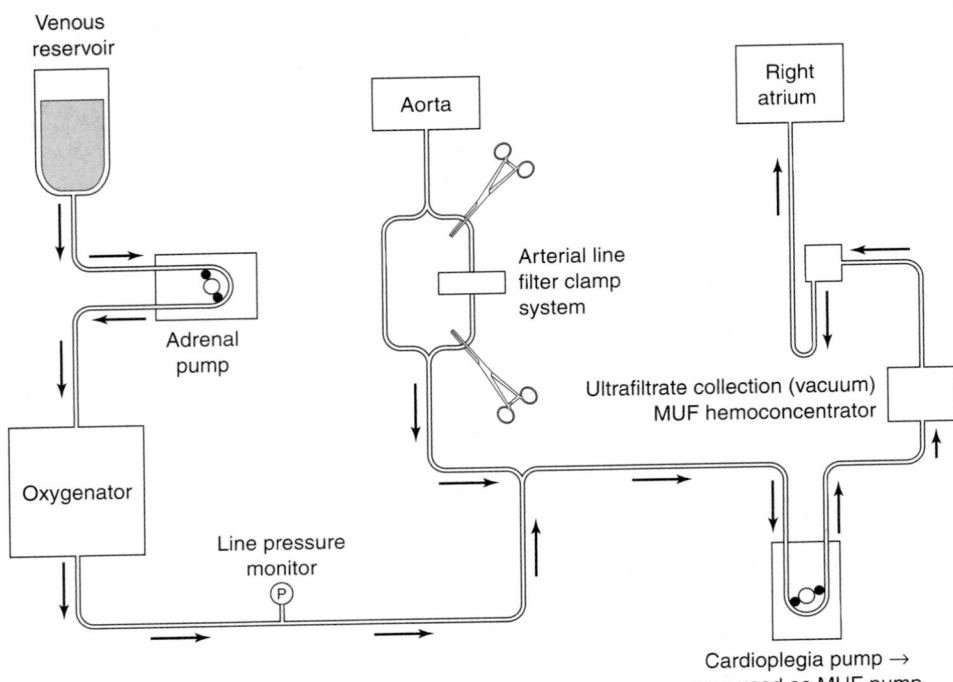

FIGURE 70C.3. Modified ultrafiltration for cardiopulmonary bypass. This technique removes excess free water, cytokines, and other small molecules, and it hemoconcentrates the patient's blood. MUF, modified ultrafiltration.

potentially significant problem in the PICU setting. ACT is the standard variable measured in the operating room to gauge levels of anticoagulation once systemic heparin has been administered. The pediatric population requires an ACT of at least 350–450 secs to maintain appropriate anticoagulation while on CPB. ACTs are measured by perfusion teams throughout the operative procedure to ensure that a safe interface is achieved between blood and circuit, thus avoiding circuit and/or oxygenator malfunction.

Coagulation factors are significantly altered by CPB. Initially, hemodilution from the priming volume of the circuit and initiation of CPB impact the quantity of factors. Secondly, ongoing activation of the extrinsic clotting system can result in a consumptive process. Both a quantitative and qualitative platelet dysfunction occurs as these cells are consumed in large numbers and activation occurs, with contact with the surface of the circuit and membrane oxygenator. Hypothermia following separation from bypass may also play a role in platelet dysfunction and the clotting impairment.

Protamine sulfate is a heparin antagonist that is administered (1–1.5 mg/100 units of circulating heparin) in the operating room to reverse the anticoagulation required for CPB. Protamine often results in a transient systemic vasodilatation, which can occasionally produce hypotension and hemodynamic instability. Although rare, more severe protamine reactions can result in severe pulmonary hypertension and may require urgent return to CPB until the process reverses.

Vigilant correction of coagulation parameters, platelet dysfunction and counts, and core temperature is critical in the aggressive treatment of postoperative bleeding. When coagulation or bleeding issues are of concern, appropriate communication between surgeon, perfusionist, anesthesiologist, and intensivist allows for a better transition from operating room to ICU.

MODIFIED ULTRAFILTRATION

As discussed previously, the systemic inflammatory response from CPB and cardiac surgery leads to a marked increase in total body water. This, in turn, can lead to marked tissue edema and increased risk of end-organ dysfunction. Modified ultrafiltration (Fig. 70C.3) is a technique to remove excess free water, cytokines, and other small molecules, with an additional benefit of hemoconcentrating the patient's blood. In this technique, blood is routed from the aortic cannula and passed through a hemofilter and a heat exchanger. Hemoconcentrated blood is then returned to the venous reservoir, thereby decreasing the need for transfusion of red blood cells. Modified ultrafiltration has been shown to improve cardiac function post-bypass and to reduce the incidence of postoperative pulmonary hypertensive crises (1).

CONCLUSIONS AND FUTURE DIRECTIONS

Many of the general principles and issues discussed regarding CPB also apply to the initial management strategies within the ICU setting. In most instances, the derangements described remain in an evolving process toward recovery as the patient is undergoing initial postoperative evaluation. CPB, low-flow continuous bypass, and DHCA have become technically and physiologically proficient tools in allowing surgical teams to repair complex congenital cardiac lesions. In spite of improving technology, the impact upon end-organ systems, coagulation cascades, and the systemic inflammatory response creates challenges for both intraoperative and postoperative management. A thorough understanding of these principles as well as continued research into their etiology and management is imperative to allow for the repair of these lesions with minimal sequelae.

KEY POINTS

■ Significant differences exist in the management of infants on CPB, including prime volume, temperature, hemodilution, and cannulation techniques.

■ Hypothermia reduces the metabolic rate and allows the surgeon and perfusionist to lower the perfusion flow rates.

■ Deep hypothermic circulatory arrest is utilized in surgery that involves the aorta and its arch, permitting the surgeon to remove all cannulae from the operative field to maximize exposure and repair complex defects.

■ Low-flow perfusion, where flow rates are dramatically reduced but not completely discontinued, maintains a level of cerebral blood flow that appears to be advantageous to neurologic function.

■ The primary goal of cardioplegia is to achieve and maintain a complete electromechanical arrest in a nondistended, decompressed heart.

■ Managing acid-base balance in a patient on CPB occurs along two separate lines of strategy. The α-stat strategy maintains a pH of 7.40, measured without correction for temperature, whereas pH-stat corrects the alkalotic pH that occurs with hypothermia with carbon dioxide gas.

■ The interaction of blood with non-endothelialized surfaces within the CPB circuit initiates the release of many substances, leading to a general systemic inflammatory response. Neutrophils and the complement system play integral roles in this response. The key dysfunction involves endothelial injury, leading to increased capillary permeability ("leak").

■ A quantitative and qualitative platelet dysfunction occurs after CPB, as these cells are consumed in large numbers and activation occurs with contact with the surface of the circuit and membrane oxygenator.

■ Modified ultrafiltration has essentially become a standard technique employed to help to reverse some of the adverse physiologic consequences induced by CPB.

References

1. Bando K, Vijay P, Turrentine MW, et al. Dilutional and modified ultrafiltration reduces pulmonary hypertension after operations for congenital heart disease: A prospective randomized study. *J Thorac and Cardiovasc Surg* 1998;115(3):517–25.
2. Becker H, Vinten-Johansen J, Buckberg GD, et al. Myocardial damage caused by keeping pH 7.40 during systemic deep hypothermia. *J Thorac Cardiovasc Surg* 1981;82:810–20.
3. Bigelow WG, Callaghan JC, Hopps JA. General hypothermia for experimental intracardiac surgery: The use of electrophrenic respirations, an artificial pacemaker for cardiac standstill, and radio-frequency rewarming in general hypothermia. *Ann Surg* 1950;132:531–9.
4. Bigelow WG, Lindsay WK, Greewood WF. Hypothermia: Its possible role in cardiac surgery: An investigation of factors governing survival in dogs at low body temperatures. *Ann Surg* 1950;132:849–66.
5. Blauth C, Smith P, Newman S, et al. Retinal microembolism and neuropsychiatric deficit following clinical CPB: Comparison of a membrane and a bubble oxygenator. *Eur J Cardiothorac Surg* 1989;3:135–8.
6. Boucek RJ Jr, Citak M, Graham TP, et al. Postnatal development of calcium release from cardiac sarcoplasmic reticulum. *Pediatr Res* 1984;18:119.
7. Buckberg GD. Myocardial temperature management during aortic clamping for cardiac surgery. *J Thorac Cardiovasc Surg* 1991;102:895–903.
8. Bull C, Cooper J, Stark J. Cardioplegia protection of the child's heart. *J Thorac Cardiovasc Surg* 1984;88:287–93.
9. Butler J, Rocer GM, Westaby S. Inflammatory response to cardiopulmonary bypass. *Ann Thoracic Surg* 1993;55:552–9.
10. Chai PJ, Williamson JA, Lodge AJ, et al. Effects of ischemia on pulmonary dysfunction after CPB. *Ann Thorac Surg* 1999;67:731–5.
11. Ferry PC. Neurologic sequelae of open-heart surgery in children. An "irritating question." *Am J Dis Child* 1990;144:369–73.
12. Fessatidis IT, Thomas VL, Shore DE, et al. Brain damage after profoundly hypothermic circulatory arrest: Correlations between neurophysiologic and neuropathologic findings: An experimental study in vertebrates. *J Thorac Cardiovasc Surg* 1993;106:32–41.
13. Finn A, Jaik S, Klein N, et al. Interleukin 8 release and neutrophil degranulation after pediatric cardiopulmonary bypass. *J Thorac Cardiovasc Surg* 1993;105:234–41.
14. Gaynor JW, Kern FH, Greeley WJ, et al. Management of Cardiopulmonary Bypass in Infants and Children. In: Baue AE, Geha AS, Laks H, et al., eds. *Glenn's Thoracic and Cardiovascular Surgery.* Stamford, CT: Appleton & Lange, 1996.
15. Gibbon JH Jr. Application of mechanical heart and lung apparatus to cardiac surgery. *Minn Med* 1954;37:171–85.
16. Greeley WJ, Kern FH, Ungerleider RM, et al. Intramyocardial air causes right ventricular dysfunction after repair of congenital heart defect. *Anesthesiology* 1990;73:1042–6.
17. Greeley WJ, Kern FH, Ungerleider RM, et al. The effect of hypothermic CPB and total circulatory arrest on cerebral metabolism in neonates, infants, and children. *J Thorac Cardiovasc Surg* 1991;101:783–94.
18. Greeley WJ, Ungerleider RM, Smith LR, et al. The effects of deep hypothermic cardiopulmonary bypass and total circulatory arrest on cerebral blood flow in infants and children. *J Thorac Cardiovasc Surg* 1989;97:737–45.
19. Grossi EA, Kallenbach K, Chau S, et al. Impact of heparin bonding on pediatric cardiopulmonary bypass: A prospective randomized study. *Ann Thorac Surg* 2000;70:191–6.
20. Gruber EM, Jonas RA, Newburger JW, et al. The effect of hematocrit on cerebral blood velocity in neonates and infants undergoing deep hypothermic CPB. *Anesthesiology* 1999;89:322–7.
21. Horton A, Wutt W. Pump-induced haemolysis: Is the constrained vortex pump better or worse than the roller pump?. *Perfusion* 1992;7:103–6.
22. Jaggers J, Ungerleider RM. Cardiopulmonary Bypass in Infants and Children. In: Mavroudis C, Backer CL, eds. *Pediatric Cardiac Surgery, 3rd ed.* Philadelphia: Mosby, 2003.
23. Jonas RA, Bellinger DC, Rappaport LA, et al. Relation of pH-strategy and developmental outcome after hypothermic circulatory arrest. *J Thorac Cardiovasc Surg* 1993;106:362–8.
24. Kanter RK, Bove EL, Tobin JR, et al. Prolonged mechanical ventilation of infants after open heart surgery. *Crit Care Med* 1986;14:211–4.
25. Kirklin JW, Barrat-Boyes BG. *Cardiac Surgery, 3rd ed.* Philadelphia: Churchill Livingstone, 2003.
26. Lazar HL, Buckberg GD, Manganaro AM, et al. Myocardial energy replenishment and reversal of ischemic damage by substrate enhancement of secondary blood cardioplegia with amino-acids during reperfusion. *Surgery* 1980;88(5):702–9.
27. Lewis FJ, Taufic M. Closure of atrial septal defects with the aid of hypothermia: Experimental accomplishments and the report of one successful case. *Surgery* 1953;33:52–9.
28. Lillehei CW, Cohen M, Warden HE, et al. Direct vision intracardiac surgery: By means of controlled cross circulation or continuous arterial reservoir perfusion for correction of ventricular septal defects, atrioventricularis communis, isolated infundibular pulmonic stenosis, and tetralogy of Fallot. In: Lam C, ed. *Proceedings of Henry Ford Hospital Symposium.* Philadelphia: WB Saunders, 1955.
29. Lillehei CW, Varco RL, Cohen M, et al. The first open-heart repairs of ventricular septal defects, atrioventricularis communis, and tetralogy of Fallot using extracorporeal circulation by cross circulation: A 30-year follow-up. *Ann Thorac Surg* 1986;41:4–21.
30. Lodge AJ, Undar A, Daggett CW, et al. Regional blood flow during pulsatile CPB and after circulatory arrest in an infant model. *Ann Thorac Surg* 1997;63:1243–50.
31. Mankad PS, Chester AH, Yacoub MH. Role of potassium concentration in cardioplegic solutions mediating endothelial damage. *Ann Thorac Surg* 1991;51:89–93.
32. Mault JR, Ohtake S, Klingensmith ME, et al. Cerebral metabolism and circulatory arrest: Effects of duration and strategies for protection. *Ann Thorac Surg* 1993;55:57–64.
33. Mayer J. Cardiopulmonary Bypass. In: Chang AC, Hanley FL, Wernovsky G, et al., eds. *Pediatric Cardiac Intensive Care.* Baltimore: Williams and Williams, 1998.
34. Mitchell JM, Pollock JCS, Jamieson MPG, et al. The effects of cardiopulmonary bypass on thyroid function in infants weighing less than five kilograms. *J Thorac and Cardiovasc Surg* 1992;103:800–5.

35. Moore FD Jr., Warner KG, Assousa S, et al. The effects of complement activation during cardiopulmonary bypass: Attenuation by hypothermia, heparin and hemodilution. *Ann Surg* 1988;208:95–103.

36. Newburger JW, Jonas RA, Wernovsky G, et al. A comparison of the perioperative neurologic effects of hypothermic circulatory arrest versus low-flow cardiopulmonary bypass in infant heart surgery. *N Engl J Med* 1993;329:1057–64.

37. Noris M, Morigi M, Donadelli R, et al. Nitric oxide synthesis by cultured endothelial cells is modulated by flow conditions. *Circ Res* 1995;76:536–43.

38. Paret G, Cohen AJ, Bohn DJ, et al. Continuous arteriovenous hemofiltration after cardiac operations in infants and children. *J Thorac Cardiovasc Surg* 1992;104:1225–30.

39. Philbin DM, Levine FH, Emerson CW, et al. Plasma vasopressin levels and urinary flow during CPB in patients with valvular heart disease: Effect of pulsatile flow. *J Thorac Cardiovas Surg* 1979;78:779–83.

40. Ratcliffe JM, Elliott MJ, Wyse RKH, et al. The metabolic losses in stored blood. *Implications for major transfusions in infants. Arch Dis Child* 1986;61:1208–14.

41. Sade RM, Barles DM, Dearing JP, et al. A prospective randomized study of membrane versus bubble oxygenators in children. *Ann Thorac Surg* 1980;29:502–11.

42. Schubert T, Vetter H, Owen P, et al. Adenosine cardioplegia: Adenosine versus potassium cardioplegia: Effects on cardiac arrest and postischemic recovery in the isolated rat heart. *J Thorac Cardiovasc Surg* 1989;98:1057–65.

43. Skaryak LA, Chai PJ, Kern FH, et al. Combining alpha-stat and pH-stat blood gas strategies during cooling prior to circulatory arrest provides optimal recovery of cerebral metabolism. *Circulation* 1993;88(Suppl I):335.

44. Taylor KM. Cardiopulmonary Bypass. In: Taylor KM, ed. *CPB: Principles and Management*. Baltimore: Williams and Williams, 1987.

45. Tharion J, Johnson DC, Celermajer JM, et al. Profound hypothermia with circulatory arrest: Nine years clinical experience. *J Thorac Cardiovasc Surg* 1982;84:66–72.

46. Van Oeveren W, Kazatchkine MD, Descamps-Latscha B, et al. Deleterious effects of CPB: A prospective study of bubble versus membrane oxygenation. *J Thorac Cardiovasc Surg* 1985;89:888–99.

CHAPTER 71 ■ NEUROHORMONAL CONTROL IN THE IMMUNE SYSTEM

KATHRYN A. FELMET

For most of the last century, scientists have considered the immune system an autonomous, self-regulating system even while popular thought acknowledged the idea that the mind influences recovery from disease. Neurally integrated pathways that generate fever, increase pain sensation, and alter behavior are evident to the layperson and make this connection intuitive. The power of the mind to alter the course of illness in response to placebo has been recognized for hundreds of years, but it was not until the 1930s that the power of the placebo effect factored into the study of medical intervention. We now know that mental expectations and classical conditioning are capable of producing naloxone-reversible analgesia, mimicking side effects of analgesics, producing hormone release, and even suppressing the immune system (4).

THE NEUROHORMONAL RESPONSE TO ACUTE STRESS

Outgoing signals from the brain to the immune system were first understood under the paradigm of the stress response. Acute stress causes activation of the sympathetic nervous system (SNS), which leads to epinephrine release; activation of the hypothalamic-pituitary-adrenal (HPA) axis, which leads to cortisol release; and activation of endogenous opioids. Together these systems prepare a body for action by putting growth and housekeeping functions on hold, making fuel substrates available, and supporting blood pressure and intravascular volume. The immunosuppressive effects of adrenal steroids were discovered decades ago; more recently, endogenous epinephrine and opioids have also been found to have immunosuppressive effects.

The proinflammatory and immune-supportive influence of pituitary peptide hormones on immune function was recognized in the 1970s. These proinflammatory peptides, such as vasopressin and prolactin, are also released as a part of the stress response. Dozens of molecules produced by the brain or released from nerve terminals have been discovered to have immunomodulatory properties.

Although the complex interplay of all of these signaling molecules remains poorly understood, the profusion of neuroendocrine immune (NEI) mediators suggests that the brain provides guidance and fine-tuning for the immune response (Fig. 71.1). To do so, the central nervous system (CNS) monitors immune function with high acuity, being sensitive to low levels of inflammatory cytokines and to very early mediators of inflammation. Immune-derived cytokines that circulate in the bloodstream and afferent sensory pathways that are carried via peripheral nerves influence CNS signal output and are capable of activating the central stress response.

Shared Chemical Language of Neuroendocrine and Immune Systems

The neuroendocrine and immune systems share a chemical language. Immune cells express receptors for neurotransmitters and hormones. Endocrine cells, peripheral nerves, and cells of the CNS express receptors for immune-derived cytokines. Immune cells also produce hormones and signaling molecules classically thought of as neurotransmitters. Brain cells produce a wide variety of cytokines (6). The significance of the production of these receptors and signaling molecules is not fully understood. Taken together, these facts add to the body of evidence that supports functional cross-talk between cells of the nervous, endocrine, and immune systems.

The Immune System as a Sensory Organ

This cross-talk between cells of the nervous, endocrine, and immune systems is not a static pattern of feedback loops but a complex, integrated system sensitive to environmental signals perceived by both the brain and the immune system. The immune system can be thought of as a sensory organ that perceives microscopic threats. Day-to-day activities result in wear and tear on epithelial barriers, leading to microbial and other nonself invasion. These peripheral stresses activate immune cells and initiate a cascade of humoral and neural signals that amplify the initial signal and moderate the immune response. Input from other sensory organs can also modulate immunoregulatory responses in the CNS, the simplest example of this being *classical conditioning*. When animals are preconditioned by pairing of an immunosuppressive stimulus (antilymphocyte serum) with a neutral stimulus (a flavored drink), the resulting immune suppression can be later reproduced with the flavored drink alone (5).

RECENT NEUROENDOCRINE IMMUNE MEDIATORS APPLIED TO CRITICAL ILLNESS

Our understanding of NEI interactions is still limited, but it is clear that perturbations to any single pathway in this intricate

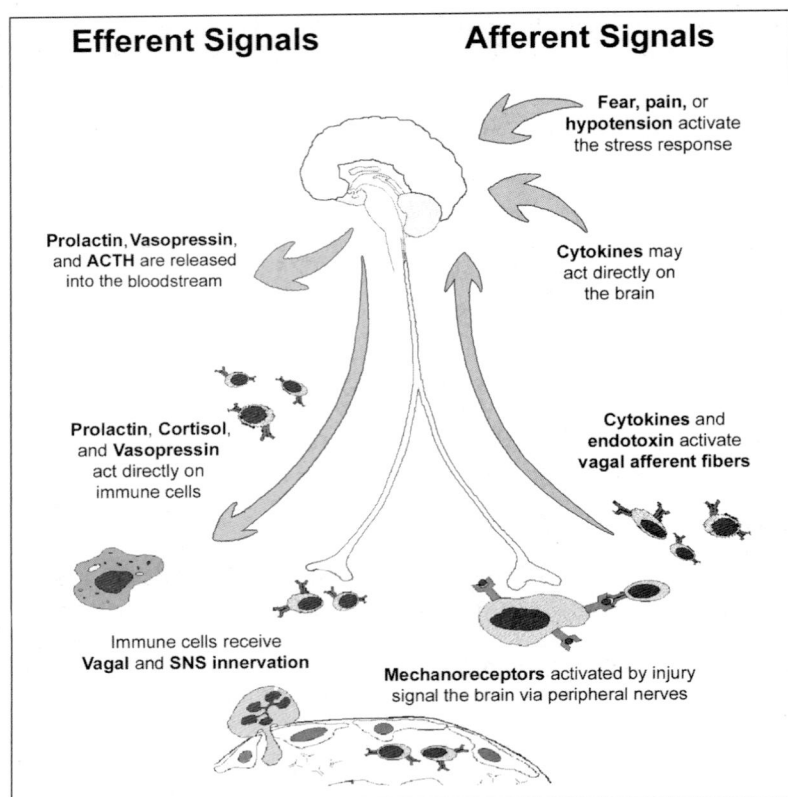

Efferent Signals

Afferent Signals

Fear, pain, or **hypotension** activate the stress response

Prolactin, Vasopressin, and **ACTH** are released into the bloodstream

Cytokines may act directly on the brain

Prolactin, Cortisol, and **Vasopressin** act directly on immune cells

Cytokines and **endotoxin** activate **vagal afferent fibers**

Immune cells receive **Vagal** and **SNS** innervation

Mechanoreceptors activated by injury signal the brain via peripheral nerves

FIGURE 71.1. Bidirectional NEI communication. Stimulation of the acute stress response generates immunosuppressive signals (activation of the hypothalamic-pituitary-adrenal axis, the sympathetic nervous system, and endogenous opioids) and immune-supportive signals (release of proinflammatory peptides such as vasopressin and prolactin). A threat to the homeostatic milieu, in the form of trauma or infection, activates the immune system. Activated immune cells produce cytokines (e.g., TNF-α, IL-1, IL-6), which signal the CNS by stimulating peripheral fibers of the vagus nerve or by circulating directly to the brain. Vagal nerve activity delivers anti-inflammatory signals in response to immune activation. ACTH, adrenocorticotropic hormone; SNS, sympathetic nervous system.

system may have distant reverberations. Because therapies used in critical care interfere with or mimic many of these pathways, it is incumbent upon the intensivist to pay attention to developments in the field of NEI interactions. In the past few years, corticosteroids, growth hormone, and vasopressin—all NEI mediators with immunomodulatory effects—have been proposed as therapeutic agents in the treatment of ICU patients.

Adrenal Replacement Therapy May Have Immunomodulatory Affects

A large, prospective, placebo-controlled, randomized clinical trial in adults with septic shock demonstrated that treatment with hydrocortisone and fludrocortisone reduced time on vasopressors and hospital mortality in patients with relative adrenal insufficiency (1). Adrenal replacement therapy has gained wide acceptance for its effects on response to circulating catecholamines. Corticosteroids are known to have immunosuppressive effects; however, it is unclear whether the small doses used for adrenal replacement will increase patients' susceptibility to nosocomial infection. Recovery from severe sepsis requires a balance between control of inflammation and activation of the specific or adaptive immune response. Studies of adrenal replacement therapy published to date have yet to consider the impact of these drugs on immune function.

Treatment with Growth Hormone Increases Mortality Due to Sepsis

The hypercatabolic state seen in critically ill patients has been attributed in part to growth hormone dysfunction. Trauma,

sepsis, and surgery are thought to induce a state of growth-hormone resistance (11,41). The hyperglycemic, catabolic state induced by growth-hormone depletion and resistance is compounded by the normal stress response, the effects of immune-derived cytokines, and inadequate calorie delivery in the ICU (11). Accordingly, exogenous growth hormone was proposed to preserve muscle and improve healing. In small studies, exogenous growth hormone given to postoperative patients and burn patients improved nitrogen balance and protein synthesis, increased muscle strength and lean body mass, and increased the rate of healing (11,23).

Unfortunately, use of exogenous growth hormone in critically ill patients is associated with increased mortality. In two large European studies of growth hormone use in critically ill adults, patients treated with growth hormone had a 1.9–2.4-fold relative risk of mortality, mostly because of multiorgan dysfunction syndrome, shock, or uncontrolled infection (50). The reasons behind this unexpected outcome may relate to growth hormone's effect in immune function. At physiologic levels, growth hormone is immunostimulatory, but it has immunosuppressive effects at supraphysiologic levels in vitro (25).

Vasopressin Infusion in Vasodilatory Shock

Vasopressin has been proposed as a replacement or adjunct to epinephrine in the resuscitation of cardiac arrest and catecholamine-unresponsive shock (49,57). Adults with septic shock have low levels of circulating vasopressin, and some evidence suggests that restoring high normal levels of vasopressin may be beneficial in vasodilatory shock (43,57). Children appear to have normal to high vasopressin levels (36).

Randomized clinical trials to evaluate the safety and efficacy of low-dose vasopressin infusions in septic shock are in process. As vasopressin has immunosuppressive effects when present in the CNS and immune-supportive effects when present in peripheral tissues (7), it is difficult to predict which effect would predominate during vasopressin infusion in the ICU.

PATHWAYS OF COMMUNICATION

Efferent Signals: How the Central Nervous System Communicates with the Immune System

This section summarizes the available data that describe the efferent pathways by which the brain communicates with the immune system, the afferent pathways by which the immune system informs the brain, and the impact of this communication on the function of immune cells. The vast majority of these data have been generated in vitro and in animal models that experimentally impair isolated NEI pathways. From these data, a sense of the overall impact of NEI pathways on the immune system and the critically ill patient as a whole may be synthesized.

Signals can travel between the brain and immune system on peripheral nerves or in the form of circulating chemical signals such as hormones or cytokines. Due to the relative ease of experimental modeling, more is known about the humoral control of immune responses than about the signals that travel along nerves. The paucity of data may give the false impression that innervation of the immune system plays a secondary role in control of immune responses. In fact, neural control has several advantages over humoral control. Direct neural control of immune function can be extremely rapid, discrete in location, and brief in duration (52). Humoral control occurs when molecules diffuse to and from the site of action; thus, these signals are slower in onset and termination.

The Cholinergic Anti-inflammatory Pathway

The importance of neural pathways in NEI communication is highlighted by the elegant work of Dr. Kevin Tracey, who demonstrated that the vagus nerve senses and regulates inflammation using simple and rapid feedback loops. Recognizing the role of the vagus nerve, the primary controller of involuntary life functions, in modulating immune function serves as a reminder of the importance of NEI communication. The brain not only manages immune function during infectious and inflammatory crises, but also maintains homeostasis in the face of routinely encountered antigens.

Vagal efferent fibers, distributed throughout the reticuloendothelial system, modulate the immune response to endotoxin through cholinergic signaling. Endotoxin (lipopolysaccharide) induces macrophages to release cytokines that promote local inflammation and potentiate activation of the specific immune response (30).

In vitro, through nicotinic receptors on immune cells, acetylcholine decreases tumor necrosis factor (TNF)-α release in response to endotoxin stimulation in a concentration-dependent manner (52). Acetylcholine also decreases expression of other endotoxin-inducible proinflammatory cytokines (IL-1β, IL-6, and IL-18) but does not alter release of the anti-inflammatory

cytokine IL-10 (52) (**Table 71.1**). Acetylcholine-dependent downregulation of inflammation is reproduced by stimulation of the vagus nerve. Transection of the vagus nerve results in increased TNF-α production by macrophages in response to endotoxin (52).

Vagal nerve activity seems to impact both local and systemic inflammation. Vagotomized animals release more TNF-α, IL-1, and IL-6 into the circulation during endotoxemia (52). Relative to sham-operated controls, these animals develop more severe local inflammation and are more sensitive to the lethal effects of endotoxin. Evidence suggests that vagally mediated inhibition of inflammatory responses to routinely encountered antigens is an important protection from autoimmune disease. Nicotine, which binds to nicotinic acetylcholine receptors, has been shown to inhibit inflammation in inflammatory bowel disease (IBD) and has been proposed as an adjunct in the treatment of sepsis (52).

Sympathetic Innervation of the Spleen: The Noradrenergic Pathway

The SNS also innervates the immune system. Bone marrow, thymus, spleen, lymph nodes, and gut-associated lymphoid tissue receive adrenergic, dopaminergic, and peptidergic input (6).

The splenic nerve contains 98% sympathetic fibers. The concentration of noradrenergic fibers in the spleen is concentrated in the white pulp around a central artery. These fibers play a role in controlling blood flow to these organs and thus may regulate lymphocyte traffic (18). Noradrenergic fibers also continue into lymphoid tissue without blood vessels. Norepinephrine release from peripheral nerves may impact immune cells nonsynaptically by diffusion from nerve fiber varicosities to the nearby cells of interest (18). During development, immune-derived neurotrophic factors may direct the growth of innervating fibers (59).

The main targets of noradrenergic innervation are T cells, macrophages, and mast cells. Lymph-node cortical and paracortical zones, where T cells reside, are supplied by noradrenergic fibers. B-cell germinal centers are not well innervated (18). T cells and other immune cells have β-adrenergic receptors as well as specific receptors for dopamine and a variety of neuropeptides (acetylcholine, substance P, neuropeptide Y, somatostatin, and prolactin) (6). Our knowledge about the functional significance of these neural inputs is limited in part because in vitro data cannot distinguish the effects of adrenergic innervation from the effects of circulating catecholamines (discussed in the following text).

In vitro, activation of β-adrenoceptors inhibits the endotoxin-induced release of the proinflammatory cytokines IL-1β, TNF-α, IL-12, and interferon (IFN)-γ and increases the release of the anti-inflammatory cytokines IL-10 and IL-6 in response to endotoxin (9,52). Stimulation of α-adrenoceptors may have the opposite effect (9,52). In general, catecholamines are believed to favor Th-2 cytokines and inhibit cellular immunity by suppressing type T helper cell (Th)-1 cytokine production (9,18). It is interesting to note that, in the NEI system, the sympathetic and parasympathetic nervous systems may act synergistically rather than in opposition.

Other Neurotransmitters

Researchers are still discovering new neurotransmitters, hormones, and cytokines, and continue to recognize new NEI roles for well-known molecules. The molecules described here are

TABLE 71.1

PROINFLAMMATORY AND ANTI-INFLAMMATORY CYTOKINES

	Produced by	Actions on immune cells	Relevance in critical illness
Proinflammatory cytokines			
TNF-α	APCs, NK cells, T-cells	Local inflammation, endothelial activation	An early mediator of inflammation and shock
IL-1β	APCs, epithelial cells	T-cell activation, macrophage activation	Causes fever and acute-phase protein production
IL-12	B cells, macrophages	Activates NK cells, induces CD4 T-cell differentiation into Th-1-like cells	Suppresses Th-2
IFNγ	Th-1 cells, NK cells	Potent macrophage activation, suppresses Th-2 responses	Low levels associated with increased risk of infection
GM-CSF	Macrophages, T cells	Stimulates growth and differentiation of granulocytes and monocytes	Increases HLA-DR expression, may be clinically useful as an immune stimulant
Anti-inflammatory cytokines			
IL-4	Th-2 cells, mast cells	B-cell activation, suppresses Th-1 cells, IGE switch	Suppresses Th-1 response
IL-10	Th-2 cells, APCs	Potent suppressor of macrophage functions	Suppresses Th-1response
Other important cytokines			
IL-2	T cells	T-cell proliferation, supports Th-1 cells	Most important proliferative factor for T-cells
IL-6	T cells, macrophages, endothelial calls	T- and B-cell growth and differentiation	Causes fever, and acute-phase protein production levels are related to severity of systemic inflammation
IL-8	Monocytes, endothelial cells	Chemotactic for neutrophils	Levels are related to severity of systemic inflammation
GCSF	Fibroblasts and monocytes	Stimulates neutrophil growth and differentiation	Exogenous GCSF safely increases neutrophil counts but does not alter mortality

APCs, antigen-presenting cells; NK, natural killer; GM-CSF, granulocyte-macrophage colony-stimulating factor; HLA-DR, human leukocyte antigen-DR; GCSF, granulocyte colony-stimulating factor

examples of this interface and add layers of complexity to the NEI system. These substances may function as neurotransmitters in neural pathways or as circulating messengers in humoral pathways.

Opioids. Exogenous opioids and endogenous endorphins have immunosuppressive effects. Opioids induce immune suppression at analgesic doses by binding to classical, naloxone-sensitive opioid receptors in the brain. In addition, immune cells have both classical and nonclassical opioid receptors, but it is unclear to what extent morphine interacts directly with these cells to cause immune suppression in vivo (31,47). Acutely, centrally acting morphine activates the sympathetic nervous system, and most of the observed immunosuppressive effects of morphine may occur via this pathway (10,27). Morphine also activates the HPA axis, which may lead to cortisol-mediated immune suppression, particularly during chronic administration.

In vitro, morphine has clear immunosuppressive effects. It decreases B-cell antibody production, reduces the T-cell proliferative response to mitogen, suppresses IL-2 gene expression, increases T-cell apoptosis, and decreases IL-6 levels. It is uncertain to what extent this mechanism is important in vivo (31,37). Acute and chronic exposure to morphine decreases splenic and peripheral natural-killer (NK)-cell activity in

animals (47). Treatment with morphine for as little as 36–72 hrs impairs macrophage response to monocyte colony-stimulating factor in mice and affects phagocytosis and superoxide production ex vivo (47).

Somatostatin. Somatostatin analogs (Octreotide) are used in the treatment of gastrointestinal hemorrhage. In addition to decreasing splanchnic blood flow, somatostatin inhibits the release of insulin and decreases secretion and absorption in the gastrointestinal tract (25). Somatostatin has direct immunosuppressive effects in vitro. Somatostatin receptors are expressed on peripheral T and B lymphocytes, on activated monocytes, and in hematopoietic precursors (35). In the bone marrow, somatostatin inhibits proliferation, particularly in response to granulocyte colony-stimulating factor (44). Somatostatin strongly inhibits IFNγ production by T cells, thereby decreasing macrophage activation and antigen presentation (6). Somatostatin also decreases prolactin release by the pituitary, and some of its immunosuppressive effects may occur via this mechanism. The effect of Octreotide infusions on immune function in critically ill patients has not been studied.

Other Neuropeptides. Substance P, a neuropeptide present in afferent nerves in the dorsal horn of the spinal column, was originally discovered to be a mediator of pain sensation. Substance P is powerfully proinflammatory via TNF-α and IL-12 and plays a role in chronic inflammation. In vitro and in vivo, substance P counteracts glucocorticoid-mediated apoptosis (16). Substance P is one of a growing group of neuropeptides that have been shown to have immunoregulatory function. Others include calcitonin gene-related peptide, neuropeptide Y, vasoactive intestinal peptide, pro-opiomelanocortin-related peptides, and β-endorphins (5). At the time of this writing, little is known about their function in the normal state or the stress response. Currently, no therapeutic agents are known to be directed at them. Further research may prove the importance of these molecules.

Humoral Efferent Pathways

The Hypothalamic-Pituitary-Adrenal Axis

Activation of the HPA axis begins with release of corticotrophin-releasing hormone (CRH) from the hypothalamus in response to cortical signals generated by fear, pain, or hypotension, or in response to immune-derived signal molecules, especially IL-1β, TNF-α, and IL-6 (60). CRH leads to adrenocorticotropic hormone (ACTH) release by the pituitary, which, in turn, causes cortisol release by the adrenal gland. Cortisol inhibits growth and generally increases catabolism while it enhances protein synthesis in the liver, where acute-phase reactants are generated. Cortisol potentiates the vasoconstrictive action of catecholamines and regulates the distribution of total body water (25). In the immune system, corticosteroids reduce circulating numbers of lymphocytes, monocytes, and eosinophils by stimulating apoptosis. Corticosteroids stabilize lysosomal membranes, decrease capillary permeability, impair demargination of white blood cells and phagocytosis, and decrease the release of IL-1, preventing fever. Steroids also support a Th-2 (humoral immunity) over a Th-1 (cellular immunity) phenotype (24).

Peptide Hormones: Prolactin and Vasopressin

Prolactin and vasopressin are the immunostimulatory hormones associated with the CNS response to stress. Release of these hormones occurs simultaneously with HPA-axis activation and SNS activation and thus represents an important counterbalance to the immunosuppressive effects of the stress response.

Prolactin, although best known for its role in promoting milk secretion, directly opposes many of the actions of corticosteroids. Prolactin release is stimulated by suckling, IL-1β, IL-2, IL-6, oxytocin, serotonin, and thyrotropin-releasing hormone. Prolactin levels are highest in newborns and lactating mothers but may be suppressed in response to hemorrhage, particularly in the peri-partum period (12,32). A prolactin-secretory response to psychological and physical stress has been reported (13,22). In the normal state, prolactin secretion is tonically inhibited by hypothalamic dopamine.

In the immune system, prolactin supports circulating lymphocyte numbers as a necessary cofactor for IL-2 and mitogen-stimulated proliferation (13) by opposing glucocorticoid-induced apoptosis (21). Prolactin increases IL-2 production by T cells and is a necessary cofactor for expression of the IL-2 receptor. Prolactin increases antibody production by B cells and increases cytokine-release capacity of macrophages and NK cells (13). The immunosuppressive drug cyclosporine exerts its effect through the prolactin receptor on lymphocytes (26).

Vasopressin is released in response to hypotension and increased serum osmolarity. Vasopressin has different immunomodulatory effects in the periphery than in the CNS. Circulating or local vasopressin enhances lymphocyte reactions and potentiates primary antibody responses. Peripheral vasopressin favors Th-1 responses (7). Vasopressin can also potentiate the release of prolactin (14). Acting centrally, vasopressin causes release of CRH, but it also has effects on the immune system independent of its effect in stimulating the HPA axis. When given intraventricularly to rats, vasopressin decreases the T-cell response to mitogen, probably via the sympathetic nervous system (48).

Afferent Signals: Alerting the Central Nervous System to a Microbial Threat

The immunoregulatory actions of pituitary hormones, vagal nerve activity, and SNS activation do not occur randomly but in response to information about the current state of immune function that is generated by classical sensory organs and the immune system and synthesized by the brain. The brain is alerted to a microbial threat via both humoral and neural pathways. Cytokines, particularly TNF-α and IL-1β, can act directly, reaching the brain via the bloodstream, or indirectly, by stimulating peripheral afferent nerves (52).

Immune Activation of Afferent Peripheral Nerves

Afferent nerves provide a surveillance system to allow the CNS to monitor immune function. The neural pathway of immune-to-brain communication centers on the vagus nerve; 70% of vagal fibers are sensory. TNF-α and IL-1 released from dendritic cells and macrophages have been shown to stimulate vagal afferents, even at concentrations too low to reach the brain via the bloodstream (52). Lymphocytes produce growth hormone, prolactin, and ACTH; mast cells and eosinophils produce vasoactive intestinal peptide and substance P. In that the concentrations of these signaling molecules are too low to reach the brain via the bloodstream, the target receptors are probably on peripheral nerves or other immune cells (6).

Afferent pathways also collect information about infection and injury independent of immune cells. Vagal afferents can be directly stimulated by endotoxin, a bacterial product that leads to TNF-α release. Receptors sensitive to mechanical, thermal, and osmolar changes may also activate vagal sensory fibers, suggesting that the brain can anticipate injury and the resulting inflammation (52). Circulating cytokines can also stimulate sensory nerves.

Inflammation-sensing pathways terminate in the dorsal vagal complex, which consists of the nucleus tractus solitarius (NTS) and the area postrema. The NTS, which receives the main portion of the vagal afferent signal, communicates with the paraventricular nucleus, the site of production of CRH (52). Inflammation sensed by the vagus nerve increases inflammation-suppressing signals traveling back down the vagus and activates humoral responses via the HPA axis.

Circulating Cytokines

Humoral pathways of immune-to-brain communications revolve around circulating cytokines. Receptors or receptor mRNA in the brain have been found for IL-1α, IL-1β, IL-2, IL-4, IL-6, TNF-α, IFN-γ, macrophage colony-stimulating factor, and stem cell factor (6). Endocrine glands also contain receptors for immune-derived cytokines. Receptors for IL-1α, IL-1β, IL-2, and IL-6 have been described in pituitary, thyroid, pancreas, ovary, and testis (6).

The existence of the blood-brain barrier (BBB) complicates our understanding of humoral pathways of immune-to-brain communication. Proinflammatory cytokines are large lipophobic molecules; therefore, their diffusion into the brain is physically limited (38). Despite this limitation, blockade of brain receptors for proinflammatory cytokines effectively prevents the adaptive behaviors associated with infection, collectively termed *the sickness response*. Transport proteins carry cytokines across the BBB into the brain. Saturable carriers for IL-1 and TNF-α that are active only at high concentrations have been shown to exist (52).

Cytokines may also bind to cell surface receptors on the endothelium of brain capillaries, causing a release of soluble mediators such as nitric oxide and prostaglandin (52). Soluble mediators may then diffuse into the brain parenchyma and modulate neuron activity. Intracerebral prostaglandins have been proposed as mediators of the febrile response and HPA axis activation.

Circumventricular organs, in which the BBB is weak, are also possible sites of immune-to-brain communication. Evidence for this kind of communication is strongest for the area postrema. At these sites, cytokine binding to receptors may generate the production of soluble mediators or directly increase the firing rates of neurons with connections within the brain. In particular, the vagal anti-inflammatory pathway can be activated by direct cytokine signaling of the area postrema (52).

Peripheral Responses: The Effects of Neuroimmunomodulation

The brain receives information about potential and ongoing immune responses and sends out signals that modulate these responses. Unfortunately for clinicians, more is understood about pathways of communication than about the nature and effect of the communication itself.

A great many publications address the impact of various NEI mediators on cytokine production by individual cells. Rather than a summary of these data, what follows is a review of the immunology central to our current understanding of NEI modulation and a description of the impact of NEI mediators in cases in which their effect on functional systems is understood. As our ability to understand the impact of NEI regulation is limited by our ability to assess the function of the immune system, discussion will be necessarily guided by the scientific methods currently available for evaluation of immune function. At this time, we have tools to assess the impact of NEI mediators on (a) nonspecific immune responses, including behavior and inflammation; (b) on the phenotypes of specific immune responses, particularly Th-1 and Th-2 responses; and (c) on growth and survival of immune cells.

The Sickness Response

The most obvious result of CNS integration of signals from the immune system is a combination of physiologic changes and behaviors associated with recovery, collectively known as the *sickness response*. In response to illness signaled mainly by TNF-α and IL-1, the CNS initiates physiologic changes, including fever, increased white blood cell count, production of acute-phase proteins in the liver, and increased slow-wave sleep, as well as behavioral changes, including decreased feeding and drinking and reductions in activity and social interaction (38). Alterations in pain sensation are also a part of the sickness response. In the acute phase, the stress response rapidly induces analgesia, presumably by a neural route. Later, inflammatory cytokines induce hyperalgesia, signaling the individual to care for a wound. These changes are not specific to individual pathogens and occur across a wide range of species (38).

Inflammation and Phagocytosis

The *nonspecific immune response*, comprised mainly of inflammation and phagocytosis, is even more evolutionarily conserved than the sickness response. Nonspecific immunity is initiated rapidly by microbial invasion or trauma and serves to limit tissue damage and infection to the wound or site of entry. Inflammation and phagocytic cells comprise the first line of defense and recognition. The inflammatory response leads to vasodilation, increased capillary permeability, and an influx of phagocytes, including blood monocytes, neutrophils, and tissue macrophages. Local coagulation limits hematogenous spread of infection. Phagocytic cells recruited by inflammation produce proinflammatory cytokines, primarily IL-1, IL-6, and TNF-α, amplifying the immune response locally (30).

Chemical mediators of the inflammatory response can have systemic effects. The vasodilation, increased capillary permeability, coagulation, and phagocyte diapedesis that prevent local spread of disease can be disastrous globally, causing hypovolemic shock, disseminated intravascular coagulation, and acute respiratory distress syndrome. Consequently, the prevailing paradigm in sepsis research has been that sepsis results from an unbridled hyperinflammatory response. In animal models of sepsis in which large inoculums of bacteria or large doses of lipopolysaccharide are administered, subjects die in the acute phase of their illness from proinflammatory cytokine storm. In these models, anti-inflammatory therapies improve survival.

Corticosteroids, vagal nerve stimulation, SNS activation, and circulating catecholamines are anti-inflammatory (30,34,42,52.) Inflammation is potentiated by prolactin and vasopressin (13,7). Opioids and corticosteroids suppress phagocytosis. Although excessive inflammation can be deadly, anti-inflammatory agents do not improve mortality in human sepsis, in which early death from cytokine storm is usually prevented by medical intervention and the relevant outcome is long-term survival. Recovery from sepsis depends on a balance between pro- and anti-inflammatory signals.

Inflammation recruits phagocytic cells, some of which are responsible for the initiation of the specific immune response. Antigen-presenting cells, such as macrophages and dendritic cells, engulf foreign matter and bacteria, break them down into large molecules, and present these molecules as antigens to T lymphocytes. Antigen presentation is the crucial step in initiating adaptive immunity: impaired antigen presentation is associated with mortality and secondary infection (58). Anti-inflammatory therapies, by virtue of the fact that they mimic pluripotent NEI pathways, tend to have effects beyond simple downregulation of proinflammatory cytokines. Anti-inflammatory therapies can cause immune cell apoptosis and modulate the specific immune response in ways that may not be favorable for overall survival.

Humoral versus Cellular Immunity

An antigen-specific immune response begins when a T lymphocyte recognizes its specific antigen on the surface of an antigen-presenting cell. The T cell begins to activate and proliferate. Each generation of proliferation takes 8–12 hrs; therefore, the generation of a specific immune response takes several days, during which time the organism is dependent on the nonspecific immune response for protection (38). T-cell proliferation is suppressed by catecholamines and supported by prolactin.

The population of T cells that results from this proliferation is not a homogeneous group, as different types of infection require different killing strategies. For instance, as viruses commandeer cellular machinery for their own replication, overcoming a viral infection requires killing of the infected cell. Most viral infections stimulate replication of cytotoxic T cells.

Helper T cells (Th cells) make cytokines that support other cells. The two lines of helper cells, Th-1 and Th-2, are mutually inhibitory and direct different types of immune responses. Th-1 cells are stimulated by pathogens, such as *Mycobacterium tuberculosis, Helicobacter pylori,* and *Pneumocystis carinii,* that accumulate inside the vesicles of macrophages and dendritic cells. A Th-1 or cell-mediated immune response promotes the microbicidal properties of the macrophage and supports the production of immunoglobulin (Ig) G, an opsonizing antibody that facilitates uptake of these pathogens. Cytokines associated with Th-1 responses, IFN-γ, IL-12, and TNF-α are proinflammatory (30). A Th-1 proinflammatory phenotype is associated with autoimmune disease (9).

Extracellular spaces are protected by the Th-2 or humoral immune response. In response to extracellular pathogens (e.g., *Staphylococcus* species), Th-2 cells initiate the humoral immune response by activating naïve antigen-specific B cells to produce IgM antibodies. Viruses and intracellular pathogens that travel through these spaces may be neutralized by the binding of specific antibodies. Antibody binding also facilitates uptake of pathogens by phagocytes. The cytokine profile associated with Th-2 humoral immune response is anti-inflammatory, with IL-4 and IL-10 predominating (30). The catecholamine and cortisol excess seen in the stress response favors Th-2 responses (9,24). The impact of vagal nerve activity and other hypothalamic hormones on the Th-1–Th-2 balance is not known.

Septic patients tend to have increased numbers of Th-2 cells relative to the normal Th-1–Th-2 balance and relative to nonseptic, critically ill controls. Whether this funding represents augmentation of humoral immunity or a suppression of cell-mediated immunity is not known. Additionally, this finding has not been correlated with outcomes from sepsis (20). A stress-induced shift to a Th-2 phenotype could be unfavorable in patients infected with a primarily intracellular pathogen.

Apoptosis and Lymphocyte Proliferation

A few days into an episode of sepsis, the catecholamine and cortisol excess of the acute phase suppresses the initial hyper-

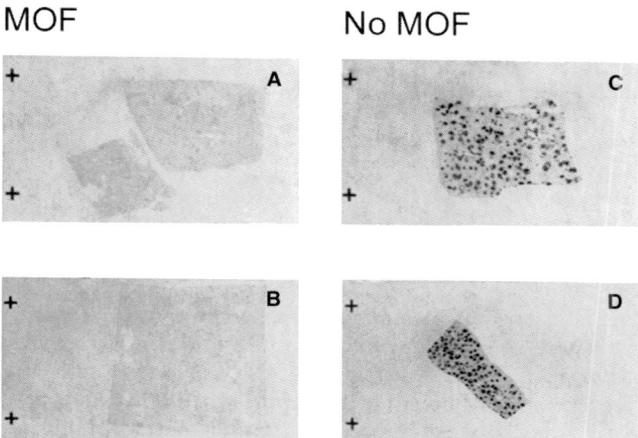

FIGURE 71.2. Depletion of lymphoid elements in patients who died with and without multiorgan failure (MOF). Immunohistochemical staining for B cells in autopsy samples of spleen from patients who died with and without MOF reveals lymphoid depletion that is visible to the naked eye. These are unmagnified images of slides of spleen stained for B cells (CD20). The number and size of lymphoid follicles (**dark spots**) are dramatically decreased in the patients with MOF. Patients A and B died with normal lymphocyte counts and without MOF; patients C and D died with prolonged lymphopenia (absolute lymphocyte count <1000 for more than 1 week) and MOF. Staining for DNA changes associated with apoptosis revealed increased apoptosis in patients with lymphoid depletion (not shown).

inflammatory state, replacing it with a state of relative immune suppression. Ideally, immune cells are protected by a balance of the proapoptotic forces of adrenal steroids and the antiapoptotic effects of serum prolactin. Once the acute phase of critical illness has passed, the normal pattern of pituitary hormone release and the normal adrenal response to ACTH are disrupted. As a result, cortisol levels often remain elevated (54,56). The balance between proapoptotic and antiapoptotic forces may be further upset in the ICU when patients are treated with prolactin-suppressing dopamine and steroids.

Apoptosis of B and T lymphocytes and dendritic cells has been demonstrated in autopsies of patients who died with sepsis and multiorgan failure (**Fig. 71.2**). A syndrome of immune paralysis, which consists of lymphoid depletion, deactivation of antigen-presenting cells, and production of anti-inflammatory cytokines, has been described in the same patients (58). The factors that converge to create the immune paralysis of critical illness are only partly understood, but apoptotic death of immune cells is a causative factor.

Immune-cell apoptosis was once thought to be clinically significant only as a marker of immune function; evidence now suggests that apoptosis has functional significance beyond the removal of effector cells (B and T lymphocytes) from the circulation. In vitro, uptake of apoptotic cells by surviving macrophages impairs antigen presentation and potentiates release of the anti-inflammatory cytokine IL-10, while suppressing release of the proinflammatory cytokine IL-12. Adoptive transfer of apoptotic lymphocytes increases mortality from sepsis in animal models, and blocking lymphocyte apoptosis improves survival (28). Clinical trials designed to test inhibitors of apoptosis in sepsis are planned.

IMMUNE COMPETENCE AND FAILURE IN THE P ICU

The Acute and Prolonged Phases of Critical Illness

We have alluded to a distinction between the NEI milieu in the first hours or days of critical illness and that seen after several days have elapsed (**Fig. 71.3**). The acute phase of critical illness is characterized by supranormal release of neuroendocrine mediators from the hypothalamus and pituitary. This secretory activity ensures that short-term goals of blood pressure support and mobilization of fuel substrates are met at the expense of neglecting homeostatic mechanisms, immune function, and cell growth and repair. When a patient's own fight-or-flight response is insufficient to maintain perfusion, shock ensues. During this phase, the anti-inflammatory effect of steroids and catecholamines may be beneficial in many patients. Although clinical trials of anti-inflammatory therapies in sepsis have generally been disappointing, a subset of patients may have a robust inflammatory response that puts them at increased risk of early death from septic shock. During the prolonged phase of critical illness, the effects of fight-or-flight mediators, whether endogenous or exogenous, may be harmful. The body's response to stress has mostly been studied as an acute event that occurs in normal, healthy people. The state of prolonged stress is not well understood, but it is likely that the hormonal milieu associated with survival in the acute phase of resuscitation, that of catecholamine and cortisol excess, may not be appropriate later on. Critically ill patients need a balance between immunosuppressive and immune-supportive signals, between a short-term improvement in blood pressure and long-term cell growth and repair.

Neuroendocrine Immune Failure

Decreased levels of anterior pituitary hormones and loss of the normal pattern of pulsatile release of these hormones characterize the prolonged phase of critical illness (53). ACTH, growth hormone, thyroid-stimulating hormone, prolactin, and luteinizing hormone are all similarly affected. Cortisol levels remain elevated in chronic critical illness despite a fall in ACTH release (56). The metabolic consequence of this neuroendocrine milieu is an impaired ability to use fatty acids as fuel substrates and a tendency to store fat and to waste protein from muscle and organs. The immune consequences are impaired lymphocyte and monocyte function and increased lymphocyte apoptosis. In patients who fail to recover but go on to develop multiorgan dysfunction, the state of catabolism and immune suppression persists even in the absence of exogenous dopamine, glucocorticoids, or other well-known suppressors of the somatotropic axis. Whether the hormonal milieu of prolonged critical illness represents neuroendocrine exhaustion or an adaptive response to chronic stress is unknown. It is also impossible to distinguish NEI failure from iatrogenic effects of the many ICU drugs derived from NEI mediators.

As dysfunction of normal homeostatic mechanisms may occur independently of ICU therapies, it may be tempting to label the neuroendocrine profile of chronically critically ill patients "normal." In fact, prolonged critical illness does not occur without medical intervention and, in the natural state, these patients would not survive. In the ICU, an appropriate hormone level cannot be judged with reference to norms established in healthy people. Instead, the appropriate hormonal milieu is that associated with the best outcomes, including recovery of organ function, effective wound healing, and freedom from nosocomial infection.

Immunomodulatory Effects of ICU Therapies

Many of the drugs used in the ICU, particularly during resuscitation, owe their potency to native pathways of chemical signaling. Some of these—catecholamines, glucocorticoids, and opioids—have clearly demonstrable immunosuppressive actions. An immunoregulatory role for other drugs (e.g., metoclopramide, Octreotide, and vasopressin) is hypothesized based on in vitro data but has not been extensively studied (**Fig. 71.4**).

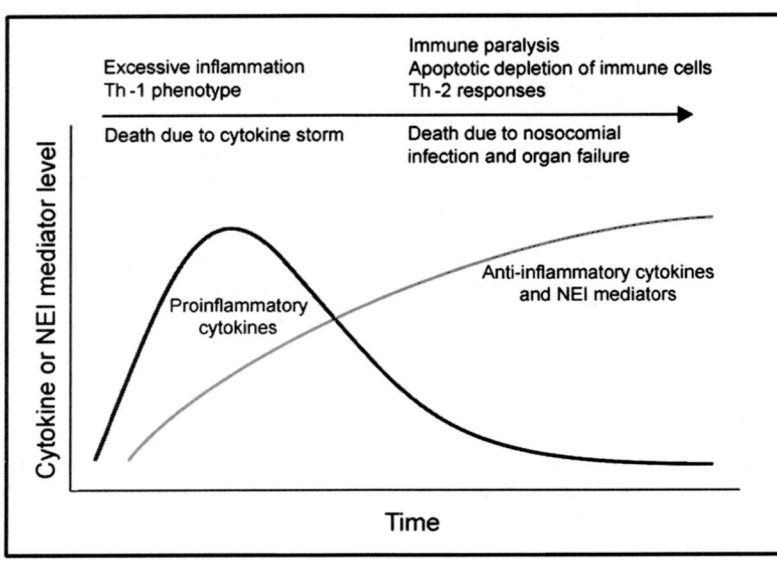

FIGURE 71.3. The acute and prolonged phases of critical illness and sepsis. Early death in sepsis can occur due to overwhelming inflammation with cytokine storm, which causes shock and tissue injury. Therapies directed at decreasing inflammation may be considered during this phase. Resuscitation medications used during this phase, including catecholamines and corticosteroids, are anti-inflammatory. During the prolonged phase of critical illness, patients developed immune paralysis with depletion of lymphoid elements due to apoptosis and decreased antigen-presenting capacity. During this stage, patients are at high risk for secondary infection. Therapies that enhance immune function by activating antigen-presenting cells or by blocking lymphocyte apoptosis may be considered in the future.

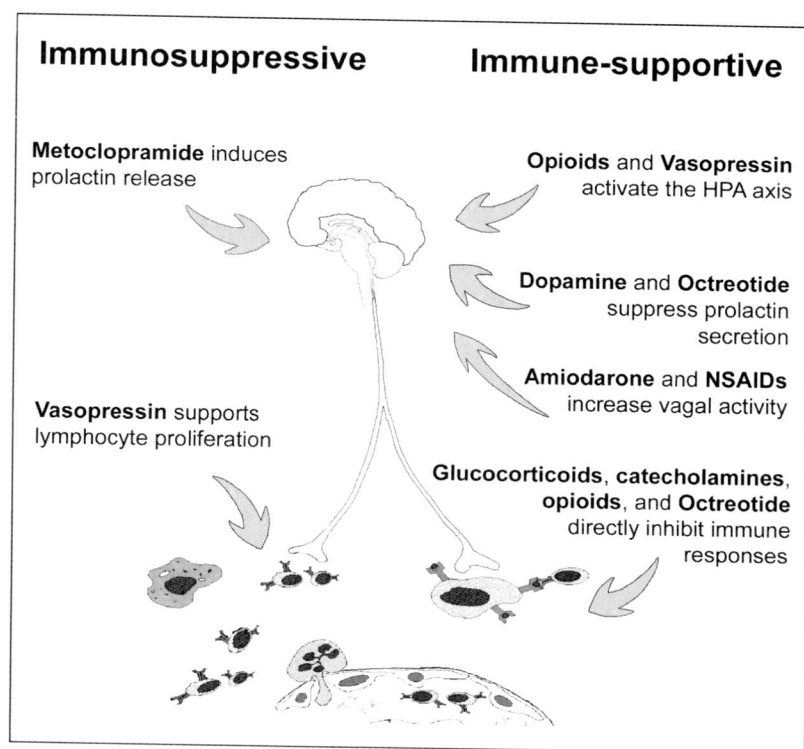

Immunosuppressive   Immune-supportive

Metoclopramide induces prolactin release

Opioids and **Vasopressin** activate the HPA axis

Dopamine and **Octreotide** suppress prolactin secretion

Amiodarone and **NSAIDs** increase vagal activity

Vasopressin supports lymphocyte proliferation

Glucocorticoids, catecholamines, opioids, and **Octreotide** directly inhibit immune responses

FIGURE 71.4. Drugs used in the ICU influence immune function. These commonly used ICU drugs can alter neuroendocrine secretory activity and can bind to immune cells directly. Circulating catecholamines and corticosteroids promote Th-2 type immune responses and are broadly anti-inflammatory and immunosuppressive. Opioids and vasopressin activate the HPA axis, leading to cortisol release. Dopamine and octreotide block the release of the immune-supportive hormone prolactin. Opioids and Octreotide also have direct effects on immune cells, decreasing lymphocyte proliferation and function of antigen-presenting cells. Amiodarone and nonsteroidal anti-inflammatory drugs (NSAIDs) may increase vagal activity, thus increasing anti-inflammatory signals. The only immune-supportive therapies commonly used in the ICU are vasopressin, which supports lymphocyte function, and metoclopramide, which induces prolactin release. HPA, hypothalamic-pituitary-adrenal.

Circulating Catecholamines

The effects of catecholamines on the immune system are complex and have mostly been observed in vitro. The extent to which these drugs mimic or suppress the effects of SNS activity on the immune system is not known. In general, catecholamines exert an immunosuppressive effect. Circulating catecholamines have been shown to modulate lymphocyte traffic and circulation in vivo. Within 30 mins of exogenous administration of catecholamines, lymphocytes and natural killer (NK) cells are mobilized, followed by an increase in circulating granulocytes and relative lymphopenia at 3–4 hrs (18). Prolonged infusion of β-agonists may have the opposite effect, reducing numbers and activity of NK cells (18). In vitro, catecholamines inhibit Th-1 and favor Th-2 responses and may inhibit the IL-2–mediated T-cell proliferative response (42).

Catecholamines in pharmacologic doses impact the release of other NEI mediators in vivo. Dopamine at doses as low as 1 mcg/kg/min has a powerful inhibitory effect on release of the proinflammatory mediator prolactin and has been shown to decrease lymphocyte proliferation (15,54). Dopamine-associated hypoprolactinemia has been associated with decreased T-cell response to mitogen ex vivo and with decreased circulating lymphocyte numbers and increased risk of secondary infection in the ICU (15,19). Dopamine inhibits pulsatile release of growth hormone and thus contributes to the catabolic state observed in critical illness (54).

Opioids

Opioid use is ubiquitous in critical care. As discussed previously, opioids have well-documented inhibitory effects on lymphocyte function and survival and on NK cell and macrophage growth and activity. Opioid abusers and their animal-model counterparts have increased susceptibility to infection (8).

Studies of the effects of opioids in critically ill patients are limited as in these patients, immune suppression and increased susceptibility to infection is multifactorial.

Glucocorticoids and Adrenal Support

In general, critically ill patients have elevated cortisol, and cortisol levels correspond to the severity of illness. In the acute phase of critical illness, adequate cortisol is necessary for the maintenance of vascular tone and for normal catecholamine responsiveness (55). Even without exogenous steroids, in the face of ongoing stress, cortisol levels in critically ill patients tend to remain elevated despite a decline in ACTH levels (56). Sustained cortisol production may be due to (a) direct autonomic innervation of steroidogenic cells, (b) paracrine action of the products of the adrenal medulla, or (c) the action of cytokines, which can directly stimulate cortisol production (17,51). Decreased cortisol clearance by the liver may contribute to elevated cortisol levels in prolonged critical illness (56).

In some critically ill patients, the HPA axis seems to have failed. These patients have a cortisol level that is inadequate to their degree of illness or inadequate relative to the ACTH levels measured in their blood. The incidence of relative adrenal insufficiency varies according to author and definition criteria. The incidence has been reported to range from 0% to 75%. Relative adrenal insufficiency is associated with poor outcomes in adults and children (2,3,31). Adrenal replacement therapy has been advocated in patients with catecholamine-resistant shock.

Both endogenous and exogenous steroids suppress fever, promote an anti-inflammatory cytokine profile, cause immune cell apoptosis, and promote a Th-2/humoral immunity phenotype. The impact of adrenal replacement therapy on immune function and susceptibility to nosocomial infection has not been studied; however, immune suppression almost certainly plays a role in the increased mortality seen in patients with sepsis treated with high-dose glucocorticoids.

The Vagus Nerve

We are only beginning to understand the function of the vagus nerve in modulating the immune system. Little data exist to describe the function of the cholinergic anti-inflammatory pathway in the ICU. Nonsteroidal anti-inflammatory drugs and the antiarrhythmic amiodarone are known to increase vagal activity (52). Vagal tone can be measured using spectral analysis of the oscillation frequencies in heart-rate variability. Beat-to-beat analysis indicates that, among septic patients, nonsurvivors have less variability—thus less vagal tone—than survivors (52).

Patients with vagal nerve stimulators and patients with transplanted organs have disruptions in their cholinergic anti-inflammatory pathways. Vagus nerve stimulators are occasionally used to control intractable seizures. These devices are generally recognized to be safe and have not been associated with increased risk of infection; however, the impact of this therapy on TNF-α synthesis and inflammation has not been investigated. Vagus nerve stimulation has been proposed as a mechanism to treat inflammation in IBD (52).

In abdominal-transplant patients, portions of the vagus nerve have been transected. In animal models, vagotomy increases vulnerability to endotoxin-induced septic shock (52). Intestinal transplant patients may be particularly sensitive to this phenomenon, as their graft may have increased permeability to translocated endotoxin and bacteria. Without the effect of the vagus nerve to inhibit TNF-α production in response to endotoxin, these patients may have intermittent elevations in inflammatory cytokines. Elevations in TNF-α, also known as *cachexin*, may impact the ability of these patients to gain weight. Rejection of an intestinal graft is often accompanied by bacterial translocation from the gut lumen. Sepsis in intestinal transplant patients may evolve more rapidly and may be associated with more profound shock than in other patients.

Assessment and Treatment of Immune Suppression Due to Critical Illness

Because good tests for immune function are not available, it is important to maintain vigilance for the immune suppression of critical illness. Strategies to limit exposure to nosocomial infection, such as isolation when appropriate, protocols to minimize catheter-related sepsis, and removal of ICU devices as soon as possible, may be beneficial in all patients. In addition, withdrawal of unnecessary immune suppressants, monitoring of subtle immune dysfunction, and compensation with suppressive antibiotics may minimize the risk for nosocomial infection.

Withdrawal of Unnecessary Immune Suppressants

After the initial period of stabilization, it is important to begin to think about restoring the capacity to grow, heal wounds, build muscle, and fight infection. The intensivist's first step should be to remember the immunosuppressive effects of the drugs that were necessary during resuscitation. Drugs that mimic the acute stress response, such as catecholamines and

steroids, should be tapered as soon as hemodynamics or underlying conditions allow. In situations in which catecholamines have no proven benefit, it may be appropriate to consider whether the negative effects on the immune system and on metabolism outweigh the potential benefits of the drug. Intensivists should carefully consider the use of "renal dose" dopamine, which inhibits release of prolactin, one of the very few antagonists to the overwhelmingly immunosuppressive effects of the stress response.

Morphine and other opioids should be used no more than necessary to control a patient's pain. As no analgesic is known to have an efficacy comparable to that of opioids, they remain the analgesic of choice in most situations. Antinociceptive action is closely linked with opioid-induced immune suppression, and affinity at the μ-receptor correlates with degree of effect on immune function (8). Opioids specific for the χ- or ∂-receptors may induce less immune suppression; therefore, methadone and fentanyl may be slightly less immunosuppressive than morphine (8). Studies of receptor affinity predict that buprenorphine, hydromorphone, oxycodone, oxymorphone, and tramadol are the least immunosuppressive (8). Opioids given locally, as in epidural analgesia, avoid the immunosuppressive complications of systemic administration (8). When the desired effect is anxiolytic, nonopioid alternatives should be considered.

Immune Monitoring and Future Therapies

Once active immune suppressants have been withdrawn to the extent possible, the degree of immune suppression that remains can be assessed. Vascular access, ventilation, surgical wounds, and exposure to antibiotic-resistant organisms place the ICU patient at extremely high risk for infection. The duration of immune suppression correlates strongly with the incidence of related infection so that, over time, even low-grade immune suppression may become clinically significant.

We are not yet able to monitor the state of the stress response activation or interpret the cytokine milieu in these patients, and no NEI mediators are currently available as therapies to support immune function. At this time, the intensivist can only compensate for the immune suppression that exists. The readily clinically available tests to monitor immune function are limited.

Lymphopenia and monocyte deactivation (impaired antigen presentation) have been associated with increased risk of poor outcomes, including nosocomial infection, prolonged hospital stay and mechanical ventilation, multiorgan dysfunction, and death (19,40,58). Lymphopenia can be assessed with a daily complete blood count. When the absolute lymphocyte count is persistently less than 1,000, indicators of T- and B-cell function may be measured. T-cell subsets will help identify patients with low CD4 counts who may benefit from early prophylaxis against fungus or *Pneumocystis carinii* pneumonia.

Patients with impaired B-cell function, as evidenced by low immunoglobulin levels, may benefit from IV immunoglobulin. Investigational therapies that target lymphopenia may be available in the near future. Recombinant human prolactin may have therapeutic potential to reverse lymphopenia observed in the ICU and to speed hematopoietic reconstitution after bone marrow transplant (45). Metoclopramide and vasopressin increase pituitary prolactin release (22). Clinical trials of metoclopramide to increase prolactin release in lymphopenic patients are under way.

Monocyte deactivation may be assessed by either flow-cytometric evaluation of human leukocyte antigen-DR expression or by ex vivo, endotoxin-stimulated TNF-α production. These tests are still investigational but are being used in clinical trials to assess a patient's immune phenotype for targeted intervention. Patients with persistent infection or documented monocyte deactivation may be candidates for immune stimulants, including granulocyte colony-stimulating factor (GCSF), granulocyte-monocyte colony-stimulating factor (GM-CSF), and IFNγ. Large clinical trials of GCSF in septic patients were disappointing (46). Granulocyte-macrocyte colony-stimulating factor stimulates cells of monocyte lineage and restores antigen-presenting capacity, the crucial initiating event of the specific immune response (58).

The cholinergic anti-inflammatory pathway may be amenable to pharmacologic intervention. CN1493, a drug currently in phase II trials for the treatment of IBD, may be a prototype for a new class of centrally acting anti-inflammatory agents (39,52). Whether activation of the cholinergic anti-inflammatory pathway could ameliorate symptoms of sepsis and critical illness has yet to be studied.

CONCLUSIONS AND FUTURE DIRECTIONS

The field of NEI interactions is still in its infancy. Sophisticated manipulation of NEI pathways to ameliorate the hyperinflammatory response of acute sepsis or the acquired immune suppression of critical illness remains out of our reach. NEI pathways have the potential to generate promising drugs for treatment of sepsis. At present, we must be attentive to the immune-modulating consequences of ICU therapies and of the neuroendocrine disarray of prolonged critical illness. We should be vigilant for new therapies aimed at restoring immune function. Perhaps most importantly, we must learn to assess investigational therapies with respect to their potential to impact NEI function. In the evaluation of new drugs, the effects of which derive from their similarity to neurotransmitters or hormone mediators, the possibility of unintended or unrecognized effects on immune function must be considered.

KEY POINTS

- The CNS monitors and regulates the immune system in clinically relevant ways.
- The immunosuppressive effects of the stress response, characterized by catecholamine and glucocorticoid excess, are balanced by the proinflammatory mediators prolactin and vasopressin.
- In the acute phase of septic shock, inflammation predominates, but during prolonged critical illness, many patients are immune-suppressed.
- Clinically significant immune suppression may result from failure of the NEI system or from the immunosuppressive side effects of NEI mediators used as ICU therapies.
- Catecholamines, glucocorticoids, somatostatin, and opioids have their immunosuppressive side effects and should be tapered as soon as clinical conditions allow.

- Future therapies may target the acquired immune suppression of critical illness.
- Studies of NEI mediators should include an assessment of their impact on immune function.

References

1. Annane D, Sebille V, Charpentier C, et al. Effect of treatment with low dose hydrocortisone and fludrocortisone on mortality in patients with septic shock. *JAMA* 2002;288(7):862–87.
2. Annane D, Sebille V, Troche G, et al. A 3 level prognostic classification in septic shock based on cortisol levels and cortisol response to corticotropin. *JAMA* 2000;283(8):1038–45.
3. Beishuizen A, Thijs LG. Relative adrenal failure in intensive care: An identifiable problem requiring treatment?. *Best Pract Res Clin Endocrinol Metab* 2001;15(4):513–31.
4. Benedetti, F, Mayberg, HS, Wager, TD, et al. Neurobiological mechanisms of the placebo effect. *J Neuroscience* 2005;25(45):103390–402.
5. Berczi I, Chalmers IM, Nagy E, et al. Immune effects of neuropeptides. *Baillieres Best Pract Res Clin Rheumatol* 1996;10(2):227–59.
6. Besedovsky HO, Del Rey A. Immune-neuroendocrine interactions: Facts and hypotheses. *Endocr Rev* 1996;17(1):64–102.
7. Bell J, Adler MW, Greenstein JI. The effect of arginine vasopressin on autologous mixed lymphocyte reactions. *Int Immunopharmacol* 1992;14:93–103.
8. Budd K. Pain management: Is opioid immunosuppression a clinical problem?. *Biomed Pharmacother* 2006;60(7): 310-7.
9. Calcagni E, Elenkov I. Stress system activity, innate and T helper cytokines and susceptibility to immune related diseases. *Ann NY Acad Sci* 2006;1069:62–76.
10. Carr DJ, France CP. Immune alterations in chronic morphine treated rhesus monkeys. *Adv Exp Med Biol* 1993;335:35–9.
11. Carroll P. Treatment with growth Hormone and insulin-like growth factor-1 in critical illness. *Best Pract Res Clin Endocrinol Metab* 2001;15(4):435–51.
12. Chaudry IH, Ayala A, Ertel W, et al. Hemorrhage and resuscitation: Immunological aspects. *Am J Physiol* 1990;259(4 Pt 2):R663–78.
13. Chicanza IC. Prolactin and immunomodulation: In vitro and in vivo observations. *Ann N Y Acad Sci* 1999;876:119–30.
14. Chikanza IC, Petrou P, Chrousos G. Perturbations of arginine vasopressin secretion during inflammatory stress, pathophysiologic implications. *Ann N Y Acad Sci* 2000;917:825–34.
15. Devins SS, Miller A, Herndon BL, et al. Effects of dopamine on T-lymphocyte proliferative responses and serum prolactin concentration in critically ill patients. *Crit Care Med* 1992;20(12):1644–49.
16. Dimri R, Sharabi Y, Shoham J. Specific inhibition of glucocorticoid-induced thymocyte apoptosis by substance p. *J Immunol* 2000;164(5):2479–86.
17. Ehrhart-Bornstein M, Hinson JP, Bornstein SR, et al. Intra-adrenal interactions in the regulation of adrenocortical steroidogenesis. *Endocr Rev* 1998;19:101–43.
18. Elenkov IJ, Wilder RL, Chrousos GP, et al. The sympathetic nerve–an integrative interface between two supersystems: The brain and the immune system. *Pharmacol Rev* 2000;52(4):595–638.
19. Felmet KA, Hall MW, Clark RS, et al. Prolonged lymphopenia, lymphoid depletion, and hypoprolactinemia in children with nosocomial sepsis and multiple organ failure. *J Immunol* 2005;174(6):3765–72.
20. Ferguson NR, Galey HF, Webster NR. T helper cell subset ratios in patients with severe sepsis. *Intensive Care Med* 1999;25:106–9.
21. Fletcher-Chiappini SE, Compton MM, La Voie HA, et al. Glucocorticoid-prolactin interactions in NB2 lymphoma cells: Anti-proliferative versus anticytolytic effects. *Pro Soc Exp Biol Med* 1993;202:345–52.
22. Freeman ME, Kanycska B, Lerany A, et al. Prolactin: Structure, function and regulation of secretion. *Physiol Rev* 2000;80(4):1523–631.
23. Gilpin DA, Barrow RE, Rutan RL, et al. Recombinant human growth hormone accelerates wound healing in children with large cutaneous burns. *Ann Surg* 1994;220:19–24.
24. Greenspan FS, Strewler GJ, eds. *Basic and Clinical Endocrinology*, 2nd ed. Stamford: Appleton and Lange, 1997.
25. Guyton AC, Hall JH. *Textbook of Medical Physiology*. Philadelphia: WB Saunders, 1996.
26. Russell DH, Kibler R, Matrisian L, et al. Prolactin receptors on human T and B lymphocytes: Antagonism of prolactin binding by cyclosporine. *J Immunol* 1985;134(5):3027–31.
27. Hall DM, Suo JL, Weber RJ. Opioid-mediated effects on the immune system: Sympathetic nervous system involvement. *J Neuroimmunol* 1998;83(1-2):29–35.
28. Hotchkiss RS, Nicholson DW. Apoptosis and caspases regulate death and inflammation in sepsis. *Nat Rev Immunol* 2006;6:813–22.
29. Houghtling RA, Mellon RD, Tan RJ, et al. Acute effects of morphine on blood lymphocyte proliferation and plasma IL-6 levels. *Ann N Y Acad Sci* 2000;917:771–7.

30. Janeaway CA, Travers P, Walport M, et al. *Immunobiology,* 5th ed. New York: Garland, 2001.

31. Joosten KF, de Kleijn ED, Westerterp M, et al. Endocrine and metabolic responses in children with meningococcal sepsis: Striking differences between survivors and non-survivors. *J Clin Endocrinol Metab* 2000;85(10): 3746–53.

32. Kohm AP, Sanders VM. Norepinephrine and (-2 adrenergic receptor stimulation regulate CD4+ T and B lymphocyte function in vitro and in vivo. *Pharmacol Rev* 2001;53(4): 487-525.

33. Kusnecov A, Sivyer M, King M, et al. Behaviorally conditioned suppression of the immune response by anti-lymphocyte serum. *J Immunol* 1983;130:2117–20.

34. Levite M. Nerve-driven immunity: The direct effects of neurotransmitters on T-cell function. *Ann N Y Acad Sci* 2000;917:307–21.

35. Lichtenauer-Kaligis EG, van Hagen PM, Lamberts SW, et al. Somatostatin receptor subtypes in human immune cells. *Eur J Endocrinol* 2000;143:S21–S25.

36. Lodha R, Vivekanandhan S, Sarthi M, et al. Serial circulating vasopressin levels in children with septic shock. *Pediatr Crit Care Med* 2006;7(3):220–4.

37. Madden JJ, Whaley WL, Ketelsen D. Opiate binding sites in the cellular immune system: Expression and regulation. *J Neuroimmunol* 1998;83(1-2):57–62.

38. Maier, SF, Watkins, LR. Cytokines for psychologists: Implications of bidirectoral communication for understanding behavior, mood, and cognition. *Psychol Rev* 1998;105:83–107.

39. Matthay MA, Ware LB. Can nicotine treat sepsis?. *Nat Med* 2004;10(11):1161–2.

40. Menges T, Engel J, Welters I, et al. Changes in blood lymphocyte populations after multiple trama: Association with posttraumatic complications. *Crit Care Med* 1999;27(4):733–40.

41. Noel GL, Suh HK, Stone JG, et al. Human prolactin and growth hormone release during surgery and other conditions of stress. *J Clin Endocrinol Metab* 1972;35:840–51.

42. Oberbeck R, Schmitz D, Wilsenack K, et al. Adrenergic modulation of survival and cellular immune functions during polymicrobial sepsis. *Neuroimmunomodulation* 2004;11(4):214–23.

43. Orozco H, Arch J, Medina-Franco H, et al. Molgramostim (GM-CSF) associated with antibiotic treatment in nontraumatic abdominal sepsis: A randomized, double-blind, placebo-controlled clinical trial. *Arch Surg.* 2006;141(2):150–3.

44. Oomen SP, Hofland LJ, van Hagen PM, et al. Somatostatin receptors in the haematopoietic system. *Eur J Endocrinol* 2000;143:S9–14.

45. Richards SM, Murphy WJ. Use of human prolactin as a therapeutic protein to potentiate immunohematopoietic function. *J Neuroimmunol* 2000;109: 56–62.

46. Root RK, Lodato RF, Patrick W, et al. Multicenter, double-blind, placebo-controlled study of the use of filgrastim in patients hospitalized with pneumonia and severe sepsis. *Crit Care Med* 2003;31(2):367–73.

47. Roy S, Loh HH. Effects of opioids on the immune system. *Neurochem Res* 1996;11:1375–86.

48. Shibasaki T, Hotta S, Wakabayashi I. Brain vasopressin is involved in the stress induced suppression of immune function in the rat. *Brain Res* 1998;808:84–92.

49. Stiell IG, Hebert PC, Wells GA, et al. Vasopressin versus epinephrine for in-hospital cardiac arrest: A randomized controlled trial. *Lancet* 2001;359: 105–9.

50. Takala J, Ruokonen E, Webster NR, et al. Increased mortality associated with growth hormone treatment in critically ill adults. *N Engl J Med* 1999;341:785–92.

51. Toth IE, Hinson JP. Neuropeptides in the adrenal gland: Distribution, localization of receptors, and effects of steroid hormone synthesis. *Endocr Res* 1995;21:39–51.

52. Tracey KJ. The inflammatory reflex. *Nature* 2002;420:853–9.

53. Van den Berghe G. The neuroendocrine response to stress is a dynamic process. *Best Pract Res Clin Endocrinol Metab* 2001;15(4):405–19.

54. Van den Berghe G, de Zegher F. Anterior pituitary function during critical illness and dopamine treatment. *Crit Care Med* 1996;24(9):1580–90.

55. Vermes I, Beishuizen A. The hypothalamic-pituitary-adrenal response to critical illness. *Best Pract Res Clin Endocrinol Metab* 2001;15(4):494–507.

56. Vermes I, Beishuizen A, Hampsink RM, et al. Dissociation of plasma adrenocorticotropin and cortisol levels in critically ill patients: Possible role of endothelin and atrial natriuretic hormone. *J Clin Endocrinol Metab* 1995;80:1238–42.

57. Vincent JL. Vasopressin in hypotensive and shock states. *Crit Care Clin* 2006;22(2):187–97.

58. Volk HD, Reinke P, Krausch D, et al. Monocyte deactivation-rationale for a new therapeutic strategy in sepsis. *Intensive Care Med* 1996;Suppl 4: S474–81.

59. Yang H, Wang L, Huang CS, et al. Plasticity of GAP-43 innervation of the spleen during immune response in the mouse: Evidence for axonal sprouting and redistribution of the nerve fibers. *Neuroimmunomodulation* 1998;5: 53–60.

60. Zaloga GP, Marik P. Hypothalamic-pituitary-adrenal insufficiency. *Crit Care Clin* 2001;17(1):25–41.

CHAPTER 72 ■ THE IMMUNE SYSTEM

MEREDITH L. ALLEN • NIGEL J. KLEIN • MARK J. PETERS

The immune system plays a role in every admission to the PICU, either as a component of the initial insult itself or as a consequence of the insult and the supportive care provided. The basic concepts of how host immune mechanisms operate during critical illness are well-appreciated. However, less is understood about how these mechanisms contribute to the clinical course seen in the ICU because of the complexity generated by; variability in the timing, location, and balance of different parts of the immune response. Interactions between the environment and host genetics are also a huge source of variability that is only now being investigated. A review of the ways in which developments in our understanding of childhood immunologic conditions have shed light on some of the immunologic mechanisms operating in critically ill children is provided in this chapter.

THE IMMUNE SYSTEM

The immune system consists of two arms. The *innate* arm of the immune system is present at birth. It is the more ancient of the two arms, and provides host defense against a vast array of microbes. The recognition systems employed are targeted against highly conserved structures common to large groups of microorganisms. This targeting is achieved through interactions between host-derived pattern recognition receptors and pathogen-associated molecular patterns on microbes.

The *adaptive* immune system develops after birth and provides highly specific recognition of both host and foreign antigens, allowing for effective handling of a multitude of microorganisms and for the generation of targeted immunologic memory. While the adaptive and innate systems are often considered as separate entities, the fact that the adaptive immune system has evolved in the presence of the innate system indicates that the two systems are linked, which is exemplified by the shared usage of a number of effector cells and soluble mediators. The key features of the innate versus adaptive immune system are outlined in **Table 72.1**.

IMMUNODEFICIENCY AND INTENSIVE CARE

A number of patients are admitted to the PICU as a result of infectious complications from congenital or acquired immune deficiencies [human immunodeficiency virus (Chapter 74), severe combined immunodeficiency disease, (Chapter 76), opportunistic infections (Chapter 84), Epstein-Barr virus-driven lymphoproliferative disease (Chapter 89), tumor lysis syndrome and neutropenic fever (Chapter 100), and idiopathic pneumonitis syndrome, post-bone marrow transplant respira-

tory failure, and veno-occlusive disease (Chapter 102)]. In addition to these severe defects, a number of conditions have been recognized, many originating from single gene deletions or polymorphisms, that are providing valuable insights into the complex processes of inflammation. Immunodeficiencies are listed in **Tables 72.2** and **72.3**.

BALANCE OF SUSCEPTIBILITY VERSUS SEVERITY: CLUES FROM THE IMMUNE SYSTEM

The importance of an intact immune system for protecting children from infection is not in doubt. However, even in patients with profound immunodeficiencies, the frequency, nature, and severity of infectious and inflammatory complications are variable. These factors are, at least in part, determined by the host's remaining functional immune system. Such dysregulated immunity can be seen in a number of scenarios, including in patients with severe combined immunodeficiency early in the process of immune restoration following stem cell transplantation, or in those with *Cryptosporidium* infections and CD40L deficiency. The relationship between infectious susceptibility and severity of the ensuing inflammatory response is complex and frequently determines the clinical course of critically ill patients. A number of defects in the immune system highlight the *balance* between risk of infection and severity of the host response. Four immune networks have been chosen to illustrate this point: complement system, mannose-binding lectin (MBL), endotoxin recognitions, and cytokines.

Complement System

Complement pathways play a critical role in the destruction of invading microorganisms. Working in concert with the adaptive immune system, activation of the three complement pathways (**Fig. 72.1**) leads to the construction of membrane attack complexes that cause direct lysis and death of the microorganisms (14). During activation, opsonic and chemotactic factors are also generated that facilitate the removal of live and dead organisms from the circulation and from tissues. The importance of these pathways is indicated by the facts that (a) many potentially harmful organisms have mechanisms for avoiding recognition by, or activation of, the complement system, (b) rare complement deficiencies exist in which patients are more vulnerable to infection, and (c) reduced levels of complement proteins in neonates and in the low-protein states of liver disease and nephrotic syndrome may contribute to the susceptibility to infection.

Inherited deficiencies of complement proteins are rare, but affected individuals suffer from an increased risk of bacterial

TABLE 72.1

CHARACTERISTICS OF THE INNATE VERSUS ADAPTIVE IMMUNE SYSTEM

Innate immune system	Adaptive immune system
Older phylogenetically—present in all multicellular organisms	Evolved later—present only in vertebrates
Present from birth	Learned response
Does not require previous exposure	Slower but more definitive
No memory	Memory specific to antigen
Cellular components—phagocytic system (monocytes, macrophages, dendritic cells) and natural killer cells	Cellular components—T and B lymphocytes
Soluble components—cytokines, complement, and acute-phase proteins	Soluble components—immunoglobulins

infections. Patients with terminal complement component deficiencies are particularly susceptible to *Neisserial* sp., including *N. meningitidis* (36); however, paradoxically, these episodes of infection are generally less severe than in normal populations. It appears that complement activation, while critical for host defense against meningococci, leads to more inflammation and clinical deterioration (33). Although the impact of complement deficiencies on the burden of clinical disease in the pediatric population is negligible, such immune defects serve to demonstrate the complex relationship that exists between susceptibility to, and severity from, an infectious insult.

Mannose-binding Lectin

MBL is a liver-derived plasma protein that recognizes repeating sugar arrays on the surface of many bacteria, fungi, viruses, and parasites. MBL binds to microbes, such as *Staphylococcus aureus* and *N. meningitides,* and activates complement in an antibody- and C1-complex–independent fashion. In contrast to most complement defects, MBL deficiency is common in the population. Three polymorphisms (codons 52, 54, and 57 in exon 1 of *MBL-2* gene) are associated with a deficiency of circulating functional MBL. Promoter polymorphisms also contribute to levels of the protein. Approximately one-third of the population is deficient in MBL, with 10% having a profound deficiency.

Children with reduced levels of MBL are at an increased risk for many minor infections of childhood and for more frequent and severe infections in the presence of coexisting immunodeficiencies, such as that caused by chemotherapy for the treatment of cancer. Intensive care is an environment in which many of the most basic defenses against infection are compromised: breaches in skin and airway, poor nutrition, gut hypoperfusion, and acquired "immunoparalysis." MBL deficiency appears to be influential in this environment. Children who are admitted to intensive care following infection, trauma, or surgery have a greatly increased risk of developing the systemic inflammatory response syndrome (SIRS) within the first 48 hrs of PICU admission if they have MBL deficiency [odds ratio (OR) 7.1; 95% confidence interval (CI) 2.9–19; $p = 0.0001$]. This is true for both infectious (OR, 11; 95% CI, 2–57; $p = 0.001$) and noninfectious illness (OR, 5; 95% CI, 1.5–19; $p = 0.018$) (14) (**Fig. 72.2**). Adults with MBL deficiency and SIRS also have a more severe clinical course and higher risk of death (21,24). At least one mechanism by which tight glycemic control may be beneficial in critically ill individuals is through the reduction of secondary infections; this may be related to MBL deficiency (27).

These data suggest that in many cases, residual infection may be contributing the development of systemic inflammation (17). In order for MBL deficiency to persist despite evolutionary pressure, there must be survival advantages in other situations afforded by these mutations. An advantage of MBL deficiency in some intra-cellular infections is possible but recently these genotypes have been shown to attenuate ischemia-reperfusion injury (64). Reduced production of C3a and C5a from this non-infectious stimulus reduces the secondary inflammation. Both mechanisms are active during sepsis so therapeutic targeting of this pathway would require very detailed understanding of the balance of effects in an individual patient at a particular time point.

TABLE 72.2

SEVERE COMBINED IMMUNODEFICIENCY SYNDROMES

Disorder	Mutated gene	Molecular defect
SCID-X1	Common g-chain	Absence of receptors for IL-2, IL-4, IL-7, IL-9, IL-15, IL-21
JAK3 deficiency	*JAK3*	Defect of signalling via IL-2, IL-4, IL-7, IL-9, IL-15, IL-21
IL-7 receptor deficiency	IL-7 receptor a	Absence of IL-7 receptor α
RAG-1, RAG-2 deficiency	*RAG-1* and *RAG-2*	Defective VDJ recombination
Artemis deficiency	Artemis	Defective VDJ recombination; radiation sensitivity
Ligase IV deficiency	Ligase IV	Defective VDJ recombination; radiation sensitivity
Cernunnos deficiency	Cernunnos	Defective VDJ recombination; radiation sensitivity
Adenosine deaminase deficiency	*ADA*	Block in purine salvage metabolism
Purine nucleoside phosphorylase deficiency	*PNP*	Block in purine salvage metabolism
T-cell receptor deficiencies	CD3ϵ/δ/γ	Defective T-cell signalling
ZAP70 deficiency	*ZAP70*	Defective T-cell signalling
ORAI-1	*ORAI-1*	Defective T-cell signalling
CD45 deficiency	*CD45*	Defective T- and B-cell signalling

TABLE 72.3

OTHER CONGENITAL IMMUNODEFICIENCY SYNDROMES

Disorder	Chromosome	Gene	Function/defect	Diagnostic tests
X-linked chronic granulomatous disease	Xp21	*gp91phox*	Component of phagocyte NADPH	Nitroblue tetrazolium test *gp91phox* by oxidase-phagocytic respiratory burst immunoblotting; mutation analysis
X-linked agammaglobulinemia	Xq22	Bruton's tyrosine kinase (*Btk*)	Intracellular signalling pathways essential for pre-B-cell maturation	*Btk* by immunoblotting or FACS analysis and mutation analysis
X-linked hyper-IgM syndrome (CD40 ligand deficiency)	Xq26 (**CD154**)	CD40 ligand	Isotype switching, T-cell function	CD154 expression on activated T cells by FACS analysis mutation analysis
Wiskott-Aldrich syndrome	Xp11	*WASP*	Cytoskeletal architecture formation, immune-cell motility and trafficking	*WASP* expression by immunoblotting; mutation analysis
X-linked lymphoproliferative syndrome	Xq25	*SAP*	Regulation of T-cell responses to EBV and other viral infections	Mutation analysis *SAP* expression—under development
Properdin deficiency	Xp21	properdin	Terminal complement component	Properdin levels
Leukocyte-adhesion deficiency type 1	21q22	CD11/CD18	Defective leucocyte adhesion and migration	CD11/CD18 expression by FACS analysis; mutation analysis
Chronic granulomatous disease (recessive)	7q11 1q25 16p24	*p47phox* *p67phox* *p22phox*	Defective respiratory burst and phagocytic intracellular killing	*p47phox, p67phox, p22phox,* expression by immunoblotting; mutation analysis
Chédiak-Higashi syndrome	1q42	*LYST*	Abnormalities in microtubule-mediated lysosomal protein trafficking	Giant inclusions in granulocytes; mutation analysis
MHC class II deficiency	16p13 19p12	*CIITA (MHC2TA)* *RFXANK*	Defective transcriptional regulation of MHC II molecule expression	HLA-DR expression; mutation analysis
RFX5			13q13	*RFXAP*
Autoimmune lymphoproliferative syndrome	10q24	*APT1* (Fas)	Defective apoptosis of lymphocytes	Fas expression; apoptosis assays; mutation analysis
Ataxia telangiectasia	11q22	*ATM*	Cell-cycle control and DNA damage responses	DNA radiation sensitivity; mutation analysis
Inherited mycobacterial susceptibility	6q23 5q31 19p13	Interferon g-receptor IL-12 p40 IL-12 receptor b1	Defective IFN-g production and signalling function	Interferon-g receptor expression; IL-12 expression; IL-12 receptor expression; mutation analysis

EBV, Epstein-Barr virus; WASP, Wiskott-Aldrich syndrome protein; MHC, major histocompatibility complex

Endotoxin Recognition

Perhaps the ultimate "danger-signal" on an invading pathogen is endotoxin or lipopolysaccharide (LPS). Nonspecific protection against LPS can be provided by antibodies directed against the core of endotoxin (EndoCAb). All adults have these antibodies, but observed levels vary within populations by more than 80-fold. Higher preoperative levels of IgM EndoCAb are associated with better outcomes following surgery, while higher IgG EndoCAb levels have been linked to survival in sepsis. In one study in children admitted to intensive care after head injury, following surgery, or for other noninfectious reasons, lower levels of IgG EndoCAb were seen in those who went on to develop the SIRS early in their PICU course than in those who did not suffer this complication (59).

Recognition of LPS is complex and involves multiple receptors and mediators. Functional mutations and polymorphisms of proteins involved in LPS recognition and signaling—including TLR4, CD14, MyD88, interleukin receptor-activated kinase (IRAK)-4, and nuclear factor (NF)-κB—have been identified. The pattern of disease susceptibility in relationship to these genetic variants is complex. A number of studies have

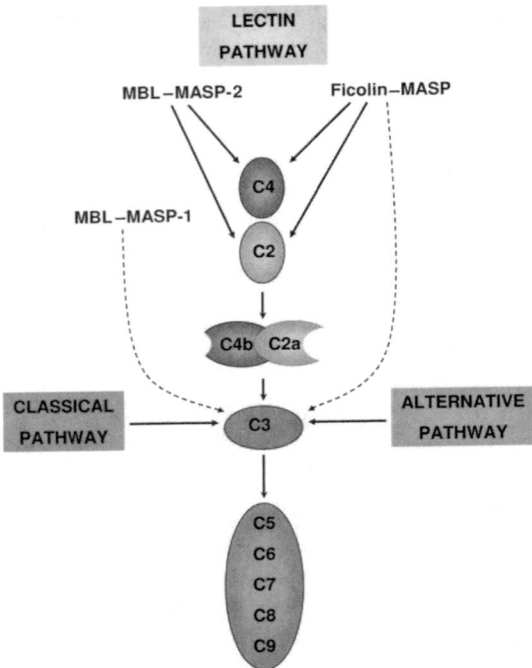

FIGURE 72.1. The complement and lectin pathways. The lectin pathway of complement is activated by MBL and ficolins. On binding to appropriate targets, MBL–MASP-2 complexes cleave C4 and C2 to form C3 convertase (C4bC2a). MBL–MASP-1 complexes may activate C3 directly. Ficolins also work in combination with the MASPs. The classic and alternative pathways also generate C3 convertase enzymes, which cleave C3. The lytic pathway (C5–C9) is common to all three routes of C3 cleavage. MBL, mannose-binding lectin; MASP, MBL-associated serine proteases; MASP-1, MBL-associated serine protease-1; MASP-2, MBL-associated serine protease-2. From Dommett RM, Klein N, Turner MW. Mannose-binding lectin in innate immunity: Past, present and future. *Tissue Antigens* 2006;68(3):193–209, with permission.

shown some relationship between reduced responsiveness to LPS and increased susceptibility to bacterial infection and sepsis. However, some benefit may be associated with having a reduced responsiveness to LPS, as such individuals appear to be protected from developing atherosclerosis.

Cytokines

Over the last decade, many studies have found associations between polymorphisms in genes that control levels of immune-system cytokines and susceptibility to, and severity of, critical illness. Results from these studies are complex, partially due to the phase of the condition under investigation. This is exemplified by IL-10, an anti-inflammatory cytokine, the levels of which are critical in the modulation of the proinflammatory/anti-inflammatory balance. Inter-individual differences in IL-10 levels are caused in part to a number of polymorphisms in the promoter region, found on chromosome 1, including those at positions −1082 (A/G), −819 (C/T), and −592 (C/A). The promoter polymorphism at position −1082 has been most associated with severity of infection (53,55). A small study showed that patients admitted to ICU with A alleles at this locus had an increased *susceptibility* to sepsis; however, once sepsis was established, the presence of the G allele was associated with higher IL-10 levels and increased

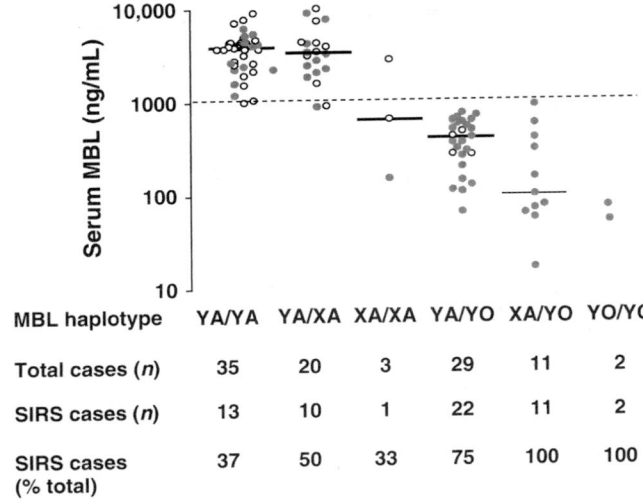

MBL haplotype	YA/YA	YA/XA	XA/XA	YA/YO	XA/YO	YO/YO
Total cases (*n*)	35	20	3	29	11	2
SIRS cases (*n*)	13	10	1	22	11	2
SIRS cases (% total)	37	50	33	75	100	100

FIGURE 72.2. Serum MBL levels, MBL short haplotype and development of SIRS. Log_{10}[MBL]serum is displayed against MBL haplotype (exon 1 and promoter polymorphisms) from those associated with the highest (YA/YA) to the lowest serum levels (YO/YO). A clear relationship exists between Log_{10} [MBL]serum and genotype (one-way analysis of variance, $p < 0.0001$ after correction for multiple comparisons). Filled circles represent cases that developed SIRS; open circles represent cases that did not develop SIRS. The odds ratios (95% CI) for the development of SIRS for each haplotype are shown, as is the risk of mortality derived from the maximum calculated PELOD score. MBL, mannose-binding lectin; SIRS, systemic inflammatory response syndrome; PELOD, Pediatric Logistic Organ Dysfunction. From Dommett RM, Klein N, Turner MW. Mannose-binding lectin in innate immunity: Past, present and future. *Tissue Antigens* 2006;68(3):193–209, with permission.

mortality (58). Similarly, children with the G allele were more likely to exhibit immunoparalysis and increased complications post-cardiac surgery (1).

Functional polymorphisms exist in a number of other genes, the products of which are thought to be important in sepsis, including cytokines such as tumor necrosis factor (TNF), IL-1, and IL-6, and proteins involved in hemostasis and thrombosis, such as plasminogen activator inhibitor 1 and angiotensin converting enzyme, which has multiple functions, including inflammatory modulation. How, when, and why such genetic variations influence the course and outcome of both infectious and noninfectious conditions are unclear. It is increasingly apparent that a balance exists between the effective recognition of potentially harmful microbes and the generation of an appropriate host response. Susceptibility to some infections may be balanced by a more benign course as a result of a less vigorous inflammatory response.

THE BALANCE BETWEEN PROINFLAMMATION AND ANTI-INFLAMMATION

Systemic Inflammatory Response Syndrome

SIRS can be induced by any major insult that does not result in immediate death. It is typically defined in terms of alterations in simple clinical or laboratory parameters that arise

TABLE 72.4

DEFINITIONS OF SYSTEMIC INFLAMMATORY RESPONSE SYNDROME, INFECTION, SEPSIS, SEVERE SEPSIS, AND SEPTIC SHOCK

SIRS

The presence of at least 2 of the following 4 criteria, *one of which must be abnormal temperature or leukocyte count:*

Core temperature of $\geq 38.5°C$ or $\leq 36°C$.

Tachycardia, defined as a mean heart rate $\geq SD$ above normal for age in the absence of external stimulus, chronic drugs, or painful stimuli;

OR otherwise unexplained persistent elevation over a 0.5–4-hr time period

OR for children <1 yr old: bradycardia, defined as a mean heart rate <10th percentile for age in the absence of external vagal stimulus, β-blocker drugs, or congenital heart disease, or otherwise unexplained persistent depression over a 0.5-hr time period

Mean respiratory rate ≥ 2 SD above normal for age or mechanical ventilation for an acute process not related to underlying neuromuscular disease or the receipt of general anesthesia

Leukocyte count elevated or depressed for age (not secondary to chemotherapy-induced leukopenia) or $\geq 10\%$ immature neutrophils

Infection

A suspected or proven (by positive culture, tissue stain, or polymerase chain reaction test) infection caused by any pathogen

OR a clinical syndrome associated with a high probability of infection. Evidence of infection includes positive findings on clinical exam, imaging, or laboratory tests (e.g., white blood cells in a normally sterile body fluid, perforated viscus, chest x-ray consistent with pneumonia, petechial or purpuric rash, or purpura fulminans)

Sepsis

SIRS in the presence of, or as a result of, suspected or proven infection

Severe sepsis

Sepsis plus one of the following: cardiovascular organ dysfunction

OR acute respiratory distress syndrome

OR two or more other organ dysfunctions. Organ dysfunctions are defined in **Table 72.5.**

Septic shock

Sepsis and cardiovascular organ dysfunction as defined in **Table 72.5.**

---

from this insult (23,34) (**Tables 72.4** and **72.5**). In brief, SIRS is defined by two or more of the following: (a) hyperthermia or hypothermia, (b) tachycardia or bradycardia, (c) tachypnea, and (d) a pathologic alteration in white cell count. When SIRS is the result of suspected or proven infection, it is termed *sepsis*; however, noninfectious causes, such as burns, trauma, surgery, and pancreatitis, can also cause this clinical picture.

SIRS remains a clinical diagnosis despite advances in the laboratory measurement of hundreds of inflammatory mediators, probably reflecting the complexity of the acute inflammatory response in which multiple mediators have overlapping actions and no single measurement quantifies the inflammatory response effectively. Simple biochemical assessments of end-organ function (platelet count, coagulation times, blood urea nitrogen and creatinine concentrations, hepatic enzymes, arterial blood gases, and lactate) form part of the assessment of organ failure that arises from SIRS—but not of SIRS itself (**Table 72.6**).

SIRS and its sequelae represent a continuum of clinical and pathophysiologic severity. Mild-to-moderate SIRS is most likely beneficial; for example, both a raised temperature and production of the cytokine TNF facilitate killing of microorganisms. However, a similar response may cause harm, either by being too severe or by spilling over into body compartments where they are not required. Examples include excessive body temperatures raising tissue oxygen demand beyond the available supply and causing rhabdomyolysis, while pathways that

involve TNF or IL-6 may contribute to unwelcome myocardial depression (23,34).

Excessive Proinflammation?

Overwhelming sepsis, such as that seen during the acute presentation of meningococcal septicemia, is a powerful reminder to the clinician of the effects of acute immune activation (**Fig. 72.3**). The view that sepsis-induced multiorgan failure results exclusively from an excessive, unchecked proinflammatory response typified by mediators such as TNF and IL-1 was widely held through the 1980s and early 1990s. This response overlaps with the predominantly proinflammatory T-helper-1 (Th-1) pattern of immunity associated with cytotoxic T-cell and macrophage activation and suppression of humoral responses. Therefore, initial efforts to find novel therapies for severe sepsis and septic shock focused on blocking elements of this "excessive" proinflammatory response. Important to this concept was the idea of compartmentalization of inflammation: inflammation at the site of infection is critical to infection control, but systemic overflow of inflammation leads to a systemic inflammatory response and secondary organ failure. However, expensive failures of numerous clinical trials of agents designed to block the acute proinflammatory response prompted a reassessment (**Fig.72.4**) (68). In 1996, Roger

TABLE 72.5

ORGAN DYSFUNCTION CRITERIA

Cardiovascular dysfunction
Despite administration of isotonic IV fluid bolus ≥40 mL/kg in 1 hr
Decrease in BP (hypotension) ≤5th percentile for age or systolic BP ≤2 SD below normal for age (**Table 72.6**)
OR Need for vasoactive drug to maintain BP in normal range (dopamine ≥5 mcg/kg/min, or dobutamine, epinephrine, or norepinephrine at any dose)
OR Two of the following:
Unexplained metabolic acidosis: base deficit >5.0 mEq/L
Increased arterial lactate >2 times upper limit of normal
Oliguria: urine output <0.5 mL/kg/hr
Prolonged capillary refill: >5 secs
Core to peripheral temperature gap >3°C

Respiratory
PaO_2/FIO_2 <300 in absence of cyanotic heart disease or preexisting lung disease
OR $PaCO_2$ >72 torr or 20 mm Hg over baseline $PaCO_2$
OR Proven need for >0.5 FIO_2 to maintain saturation >92%
OR Need for nonelective invasive or noninvasive mechanical ventilation

Neurologic
GCS ≤11 (57)
OR Acute change in mental status with a decrease in GCS ≥3 points from abnormal baseline

Hematologic
Platelet count <80,000/mm³ or a decline of 50% in platelet count from highest value recorded over the previous 3 days (for chronic hematology/oncology patients)
OR International normalized ratio >2

Renal
Serum creatinine level >2 times upper limit of normal for age or twofold increase in baseline creatinine

Hepatic
Total bilirubin >4 mg/dL (not applicable for newborn)
OR ALT 2 times upper limit of normal for age

BP, blood pressure; GCS, Glasgow Coma Scale; ALT, alanine aminotransferase

Bone suggested that the proinflammatory response does not occur in isolation and that a compensatory anti-inflammatory response syndrome (CARS) is always initiated at the same time (8). This "arm" of the immune response is typified by such mediators as IL-10, and shares many characteristics with the T-helper-2 (Th-2) response, involving the suppression of macrophage activation and promotion of antibody production.

This important insight raised the concept that wide variability might exist between patients in the nature of the immune response: a predominantly proinflammatory SIRS/Th-1 response in some, and predominantly anti-inflammatory CARS/Th-2 response in others. These responses may lead to multiorgan failure and death via different routes (**Fig. 72.5**), but the impact of agents that inhibit the proinflammatory processes will be opposite in the two groups. In short, any reduction in early

TABLE 72.6

AGE-SPECIFIC VITAL SIGNS AND LABORATORY VARIABLES

| Age group | Heart rate (beats/min) | | Respiratory rate (breaths/min) | Leukocyte count (x 10³/mm) | Systolic blood pressure (mm Hg) |
	Tachycardia	Bradycardia			
0 days–1 wk	>180	<100	>50	>34	<72
1 wk–1 mo	>180	<100	>40	>19.5 or <5	<75
1 mo–1 yr	>180	<90	>34	>17.5 or <5	<100
2–5yrs	>140	NA	>22	>15.5 or <5	<94
6–12yrs	>130	NA	>18	>13.5 or <4.5	<105
13–<18 yrs	>110	NA	>14	>11 or <4.5	<117

Lower values correspond to 5th percentile; upper values correspond to 95th percentile.
NA, not applicable

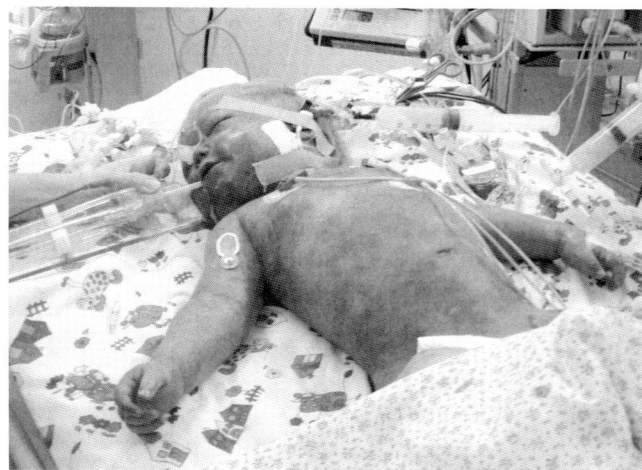

FIGURE 72.3. A child with fulminant meningococcal sepsis-induced multiorgan failure. This acute, severe process is an example of an excessive proinflammatory response that may be rapidly fatal.

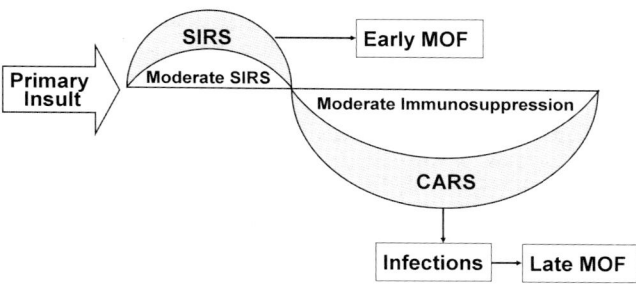

FIGURE 72.5. Immune response in critical illness. Following a primary insult, the patient mounts both a proinflammatory and anti-inflammatory response. An extreme inflammatory response in either direction will result in cellular and organ injury and death.

Balance of Proinflammatory and Anti-inflammatory Response

While clinical studies suggest that the proinflammatory and anti-inflammatory responses probably occur simultaneously following an insult, it is useful to think of the systemic immune response to an insult (septic or nonseptic) as a biphasic response (**Fig 72.5**). In most cases, the patient's compensatory anti-inflammatory response is proportional to the proinflammatory response and homeostasis is rapidly restored.

While a small number of children still die from profound cardiovascular collapse early in the course of sepsis, many of those admitted to intensive care have a brief self-limiting period of SIRS that can be adequately supported using modern intensive care therapy. In patients whose critical condition cannot be reversed with a short intensive care stay, the risk of nosocomial infection influences the morbidity and mortality

mortality obtained by anti-inflammatory therapies may be negated by increased late deaths in the CARS subgroup of patients. In support of this hypothesis, several studies of anti-inflammatory therapies undertaken in adult septic cohorts demonstrated a reduction in early deaths, which was offset by increased mortality in the subsequent days to weeks. One randomized study that attempted to target an anti-inflammatory agent (monoclonal antibody fragment to TNF) showed that a subgroup of patients with high levels of circulating IL-6 (a predominantly proinflammatory cytokine) may have benefited from TNF blockade, while the others did not (48).

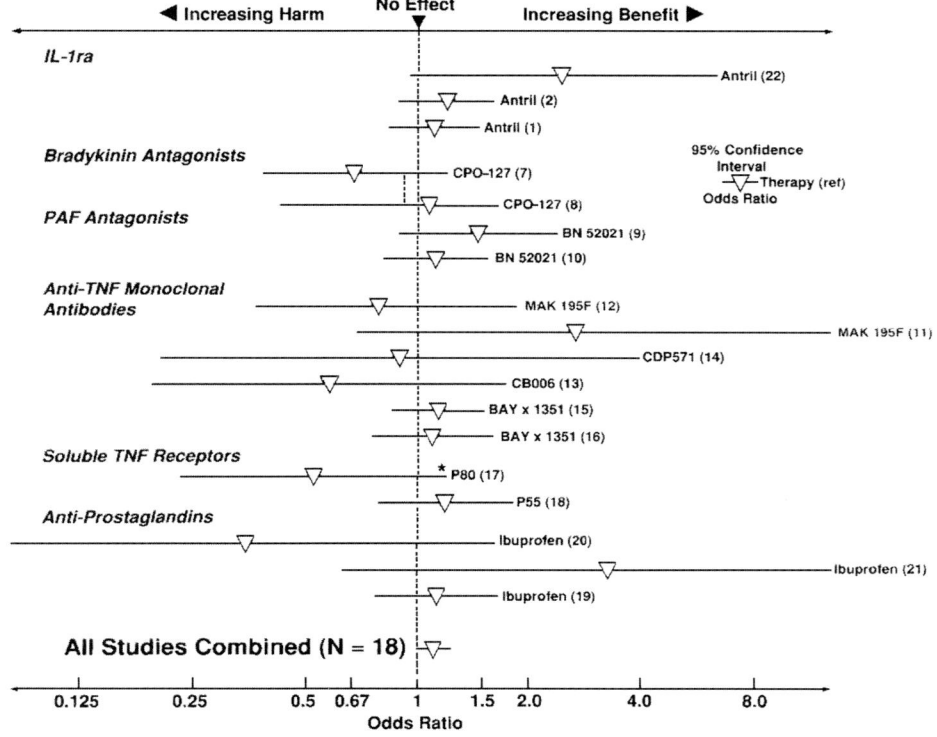

FIGURE 72.4. Odds ratios and 95% confidence intervals for survival in 18 clinical trials of nonglucocorticoid anti-inflammatory agents in adult patients with sepsis and septic shock. From Zeni F, Freeman B, Natanson C. Anti-inflammatory therapies to treat sepsis and septic shock: A reassessment. *Crit Care Med* 1997;25:1095–100, with permission.

associated with their stay. Mortality associated with nosocomial infection in PICUs has been documented to be as high as 10%. The incidence of nosocomial infection varies according to reports but averages around 14 per 1000 patient days. This figure is significantly higher in PICUs (23 per 1000 patient days). The latest available (2004) National Nosocomial Infection Surveillance report from the Centers for Disease Control in Atlanta demonstrates central line- and ventilator-related infection rates of 3–8 and 0.9–4.8, respectively, per 1000 device days in North American PICUs (interquartile range). The reason for the high incidence of nosocomial infection is unclear but does not appear to correlate with patients' initial admitting severity score. It may be that, in an attempt to restore the equilibrium following a proinflammatory SIRS response, some patients generate an excessive anti-inflammatory response.

Excessive Anti-inflammation: "Acquired Immunoparalysis"

An excessive compensatory anti-inflammatory response, or CARS, to the primary insult leaves patients in a state of *acquired immunoparalysis*, in which they are unable to produce an adequate immune response to a new threat, such as a nosocomial infection. In part, this inadequacy is attributable to apoptosis of dendritic cells and lymphocytes in response to the CARS/Th-2 mediators. Further infection during this phase of the patient's illness is likely to progress rapidly, contributing further to organ dysfunction, late multiorgan failure, and death. Failure of clinical trials directed against excessive proinflammation, along with recognition of the biphasic nature of the inflammatory response, has resulted in a general acknowledgment that any future trials should be appropriately targeted to the immune state of the individual patient. Several laboratory tests are being used to classify and monitor the immune status of critically ill patients (12,32). Most studies use two assays to define *acquired immunoparalysis*. One measures the capacity of host monocytes to produce TNF in response to stimulation with endotoxin, while the other measures surface expression of the major histocompatibility complex class II molecule on circulating monocytes (usually the human leukocyte antigen HLA-DR) by flow cytometry. As expression of this molecule is tightly controlled by a large number of pro- and anti-inflammatory mediators, surface expression levels reflect the balance between pro- and anti-inflammatory responses. Indeed, monocyte HLA-DR expression appears to correlate with in vitro cytokine production in response to bacterial antigens, lymphocyte proliferation in response to recall antigens, and the ability to present new antigens. While clinical studies have shown a contemporaneous relationship between reduced HLA-DR expression and circulating levels of the anti-inflammatory cytokines, to date they have failed to show a direct association between HLA-DR expression and circulating levels of the cytokines TNF-α, IL-10, or transforming growth factor-β.

Reduced monocyte surface expression of HLA-DR occurs in critically ill patients over the first few days of ICU admission following surgery, trauma, or sepsis. While levels between survivors and nonsurvivors do not appear to be significantly different at this stage, lower levels of HLA-DR expression have been found in patients who subsequently develop nosocomial infections. Repeated studies indicate that *persistent* downregulation

(>5–7 days) of surface HLA-DR expression on monocytes following an inflammatory insult appears to be associated with late mortality, while HLA-DR expression is restored promptly to premorbid levels in survivors following an inflammatory insult.

Ongoing physiologic insults, such as nosocomial infection, endocrine abnormalities, and repeated tissue trauma, propagate a state of immunoparalysis by attenuating recovery of HLA-DR expression, leaving the patient at risk of further infection, late morbidity, and mortality (**Fig. 72.6**).

RESOLUTION VERSUS PERSISTENCE OF THE INFLAMMATORY RESPONSE

The balance between those elements of the immune system determining the susceptibility to infective organisms and the severity of the resultant illness, as well as the pattern of pro- and anti-inflammatory responses in determining the clinical course have been discussed. It may be useful to consider the balance between processes that act to resolve acute inflammation and those that cause it to persist. An overlap obviously exists between this analysis and that discussed previously, with SIRS/Th-1 responses tending to prolong inflammation and CARS/Th-2 responses tending to resolve it, but further elements outside of this axis will be considered.

A key element in resolving the immune response is effective clearance of microorganisms. This requires the presence of activated polymorphonuclear cells (PMNs, or neutrophils) and other phagocytic cells in the appropriate tissue at the appropriate time, with intact cellular processes for killing and disposing of the bacteria. These cells are powerful agents for resolution of the inflammatory response because bacteria that have been recognized, ingested, and killed by PMNs no longer present an inflammatory stimulus. Inability of PMNs to get to the right place at the right time, or to achieve effective killing of bacteria, leads to persistence of the inflammatory response from unresolved infection. Autopsy studies from the Children's Hospital of Pittsburgh suggest that persistent or unrecognized infections are common in children with sepsis-induced multiorgan failure (2).

Defects in the Removal of Microorganisms

As stated previously, an important function of PMNs is to get to the right place at the right time and to achieve effective killing of bacteria. Conditions in which dysfunctions occur in these steps are associated with severe and often prolonged infections and provide clues as to the value of these processes in resolving infections and restoring homeostasis.

Neutropenia
Chemotherapy-induced neutropenia clearly demonstrates the importance of PMNs. More than 90% of cases of childhood acute leukemia suffer one or more episodes of febrile illness, and deaths related to infection account for two-thirds of treatment-related deaths in acute myeloid leukemia. Restoration of neutrophil counts is required to clear many infections but (in a paradox similar to the balance of susceptibility versus severity discussed previously) is often associated with a clinical

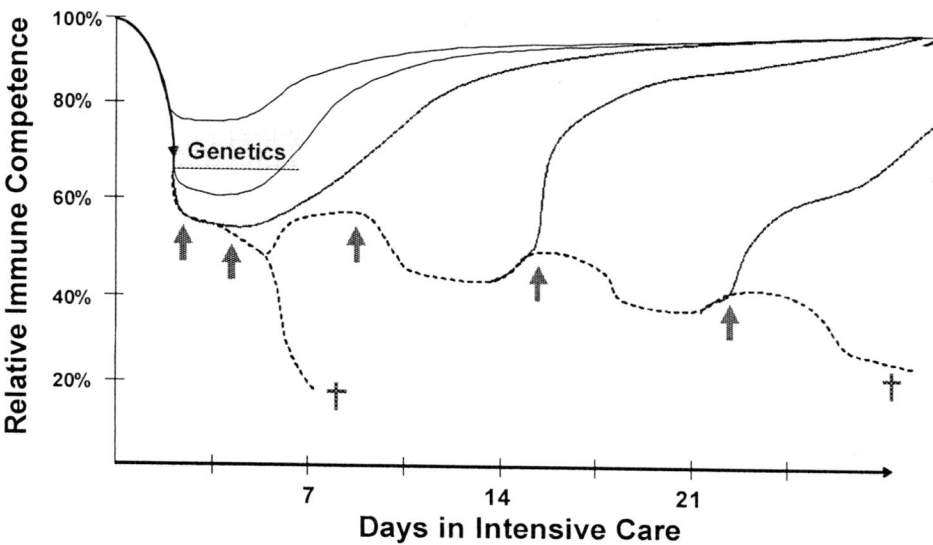

FIGURE 72.6. Possible immune response to primary inflammatory insult and the detrimental effect of secondary insults. Primary insult results in admission to a PICU, which leads to a relative fall in the patient's immune competence. Over the initial week, an attempt is made by the body to restore competency. Genetics (such as cytokine and receptor polymorphisms) may influence the effectiveness by which homeostasis is restored. Further insults (↑) to the patient (line sepsis, translocation of bacteria, additional operative procedures) delay recovery of the immune system, prolonging PICU stay and increasing likelihood of a fatal outcome (†).

deterioration as the systemic inflammatory response worsens. For example, worsening of acute lung injury following bone marrow transplantation engraftment is well recognized.

Leukocyte Adhesion

The mechanisms by which activated leukocytes are recruited into inflamed tissues have been studied in detail (**Fig. 72.7**). This multistep process is modulated by adhesion molecules present on whole cells, such as neutrophils, platelets, and endothelial cells. The importance of these molecules in the inflammatory cascade that may develop into the systemic inflammatory response is supported by animal and human data and by observations in patients who are deficient in elements of this sequence. Several rare conditions exist in which leukocytes do not migrate adequately from the circulation into tissues due to absence or dysfunction of these adhesion molecules.

Type 1 leukocyte adhesion deficiency results from a lack of expression of the surface protein CD18, which is necessary for the formation of the β_2 integrin heterodimers that are involved in firm adhesion. Failure of leukocytes to migrate into tissues results in delayed clearance of bacteria. Patients with

<1% expression of CD18 present early in life with recurrent bacteremias, progressing to life-threatening infections and requiring bone marrow transplantation for long-term survival. Patients with a moderate phenotype (2.5%–6% of the normal concentrations of protein) have peritonitis, delayed wound healing, and skin infections. However, while complete absence of CD18 is clearly detrimental in the local control of acute infection and inflammation, therapeutic blockade of CD18 is still being investigated as a treatment option in a number of chronic inflammatory conditions (20,25).

It has been recognized that leukocytes can form either complexes with themselves or with other cell types, including platelets and cell fragments, or "microparticles." These complexes then present a wider array of adhesion molecules than either cell alone. As such, these complexes have a greater capacity to bind to endothelial cells and migrate to tissues. In health, these complexes are constantly forming and dissociating and may act to provide a more activated subpopulation of cells for clearance of bacteria within the circulation or more ready recruitment into tissues. In sepsis, these circulating platelet-neutrophil complexes are reduced, probably due to selective binding to the endothelium and/or migration

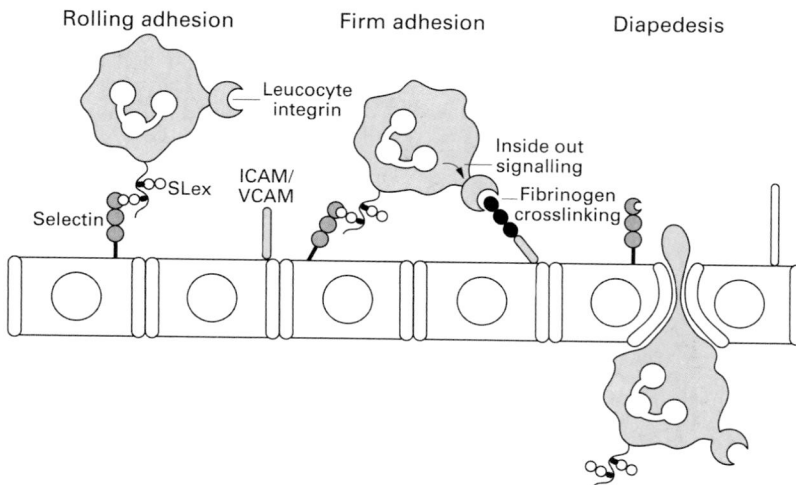

FIGURE 72.7. Mechanism of leukocyte-endothelial interaction. Rolling adhesion mediated by sialyl Lewis[x] and other glycosylated structures and selectins. Firm adhesion and diapedesis is mediated by integrins and molecules of the immunoglobulin superfamily (chemokines). ICAM, intercellular cell adhesion molecule; VCAM, vascular cell adhesion molecule.

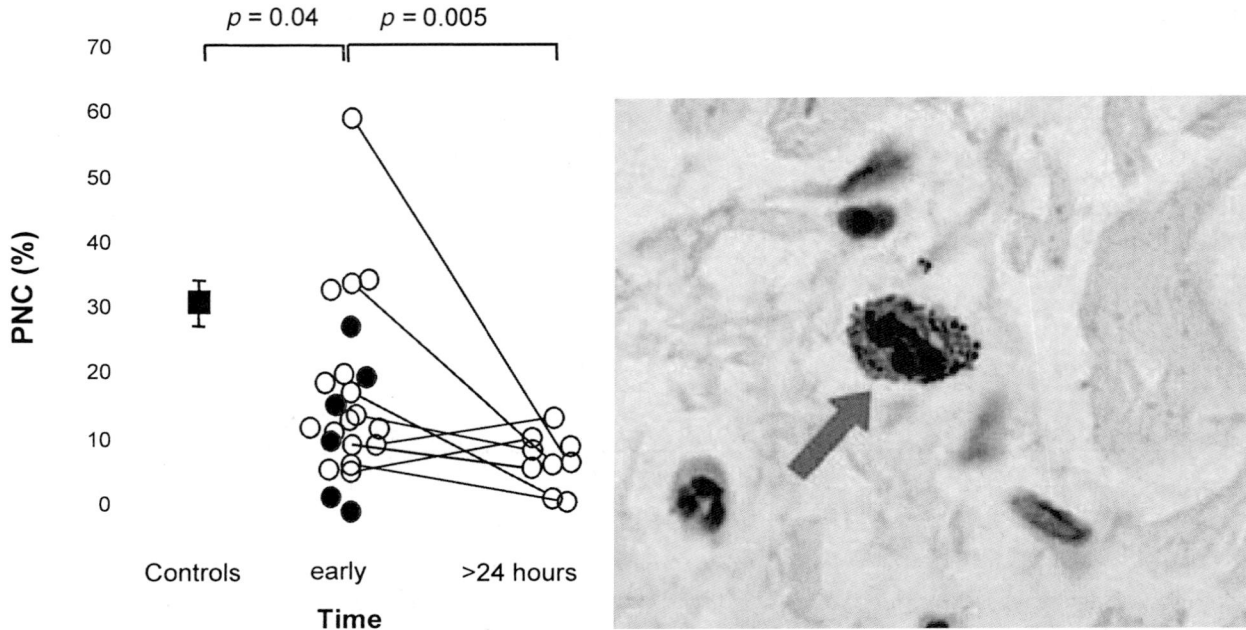

FIGURE 72.8. Platelet neutrophil complexes (PNC) in 23 cases of acute meningococcal sepsis. Control values for PNC (mean and 95% CIs are shown) were observed in PICU control patients ($n = 20$). Solid circles represent nonsurvivors; open circles represent survivors. The reduced level of PNC on presentation reduced further between 24 and 48 hrs. Skin biopsies demonstrated PNC in perivascular infiltrates (CD41 stained).

into the tissues (30) (**Fig. 72.8**). The potential for these primed platelet-neutrophil complexes to cause tissue injury and initiate thrombus formation is considerable and may explain why the combination of low platelets and neutrophils is a good predictor of poor outcome in meningococcal sepsis (49).

Bacterial Killing

Chronic granulomatous disease is a rare condition in which a patient's leukocytes lack the capacity to generate bacterial killing. These patients are deficient in the enzyme NADPH oxidase, which is required for production of the toxic conditions that effect bacterial killing. These patients suffer stubborn infections similar to those seen in patients with leukocyte adhesion deficiency or neutropenia. Interestingly, killing is now thought not to be dependent upon oxidative free radical production but on protease activity and local charge conditions in the vacuole, which cause compensatory ion shifts that disrupt bacterial membranes (54). Granuloma formation probably represents a failure to adequately remove microbial products. These lesions paradoxically may necessitate the use of steroids to reduce the ensuing inappropriate inflammatory response.

Effective Removal of Prokaryote and Eukaryote Material for Resolution of Infection and the Inflammatory Response

All of the steps just discussed are required for the effective killing of invading microorganisms and the inflammatory response that they generate. However, for the inflammatory response to resolve, an effective removal of cellular (both host

and microbial) debris must also occur without further release of proinflammatory elements, such as endotoxin. Importantly, "spent" PMNs undergo apoptosis (programmed cell death) after they have performed these useful functions—and therefore die "silently" without leaving inflammatory cellular debris. Typically, these apoptotic PMNs are, in turn, phagocytosed by tissue macrophages. The processes of apoptosis are significantly altered during systemic inflammation. Several lines of evidence suggest that PMN apoptosis is delayed in sepsis or SIRS. As with all of the systems discussed, this may be beneficial in appropriate circumstances, but harmful in others. Delayed PMN apoptosis may be of benefit by enabling further bacterial clearance, but it may also result in necrotic cell death, which provides a further inflammatory stimulus to the clearing macrophage. The balance between appropriate resolution and harmful persistence of the immune response is, therefore, complex and likely to be very dependent on local factors.

Similarly, apoptosis of lymphocyte subpopulations is differentially affected in both sepsis and SIRS. Insight into the importance of these processes may be gained by considering a condition in which apoptosis is severely abnormal.

Hemophagocytic Lymphohistiocytosis

Hemophagocytic lymphohistiocytosis (HLH) describes a mix of congenital and acquired conditions in which high fever, lymphadenopathy, hepatosplenomegaly, pancytopenia, liver dysfunction, and central nervous system dysfunction are often prominent (**Table 72.7**). Typically, these findings are within the context of an acute infection. Abnormally large and activated cells of myeloid origin (hemophagocytes) are typically found on examination of bone marrow. While these complex conditions are described elsewhere in this text, recent

CRITERIA FOR THE DIAGNOSIS OF HEMOPHAGOCYTIC LYMPHOHISTIOCYTOSIS

The diagnosis of HLH is established by fulfilling either or both of the following criteria:

1. A molecular diagnosis consistent with HLH (e.g., PRF mutations, SAP mutations, etc.)

AND/OR

2. Having ≥5 of the following:
   a. Fever
   b. Splenomegaly
   c. Cytopenia (affecting 2 cell lineages, hemoglobin <9 g/dL (or 10 g/dL for infants <4 wks of age), platelets <100,000/μL, neutrophils <1000 μL
   d. Hypertriglyceremia (>272 mg/dL) and/or hypofibrinogenemia (<150 mg/dL)
   e. Hemophagocytosis in the bone marrow, spleen, or lymph nodes without evidence of malignancy
   f. Low or absent NK cell cytotoxicity
   g. Hyperferritinemia (>500 ng/mL)
   h. Elevated soluble CD25 (IL-2Ra chain >2400 U/mL)

HLH, hemophagocytic lymphohistiocytosis

advances in the understanding of the pathogenesis and prevalence of these conditions offer insight into the resolution of the systemic inflammatory response syndrome and sepsis.

HLH represents a sustained, systemic inflammatory response following a variety of primary insults (viral, bacterial, or fungal) similar to the way in which SIRS represents a nonspecific final pathway after infection, trauma, burns, and pancreatitis (63). In fact, some reports indicate that HLH and SIRS overlap and coexist in individual cases. An autopsy study of adults who died while in the ICU found evidence of hemophagocytosis on bone marrow examination in 72% of cases; this rose to 83% of cases with sepsis (60). Similarly, children who died of H5N1 influenza virus pneumonia had evidence of hemophagocytosis on lung histology (28). An important distinction is that the outcome for children with active HLH who are in intensive care with multiorgan failure is dismal and much worse than the outcome of those with sepsis-induced multiorgan failure (43,47).

Several cellular mechanisms of congenital predispositions to HLH have been elucidated. Mutations in the genes for perforin are especially important, occurring in 20%–40% of HLH cases. Perforin is a protein found in granules of cytotoxic effector cells, including natural killer cells and activated lymphocytes. Perforin polymerizes in the membranes of target cells to allow entry of the variety of cytotoxic enzymes that cause target cell death via apoptosis. As described previously, apoptosis allows efficient packaging of toxic material (e.g., infected cells) for phagocytosis while causing the minimum amount of inflammatory stimulus. Lack of perforin prevents access of these enzymes, and the inflammatory stimulus of the infected target cell persists. Other defects in this process have been identified, including mutations to the *MUNC13-4* and *STX 11* genes, which act to prevent the normal release of these same enzymes from cytotoxic T-lymphocytes by preventing granule fusion to the plasma membrane. The multiorgan failure seen in HLH, therefore, at least in part, reflects the failure of the normal clearance

mechanisms to deal with the toxic debris of microorganisms and infected cells (69).

A possible overlap between HLH and SIRS is that they both reflect extreme examples of powerful proinflammation that have avoided the normal mechanisms for contracting the immune response. Similar failures of toxic substance clearance may occur in sepsis as a result of dysregulated apoptosis. In other words, both prolonged sepsis and HLH conditions can be viewed as relative failures of the host mechanisms to contract the immune response. With a severe or persistent insult (e.g., H5N1 infection), a close similarity may exist between HLH and SIRS, whereas in cases in which the primary insult can be removed rapidly, such as cardiopulmonary bypass or trauma, SIRS should normally diminish rapidly.

THERAPIES FOR THE SYSTEMIC INFLAMMATORY RESPONSE IN THIS FRAMEWORK

Several axes within the immune system have been described; patients with systemic inflammation will vary according to their individual position within this continuum. This variation may occur between individuals, in different episodes of infection, or even with time during the same episode of infection. Intensivists are well familiar with titrating therapies to the needs of an individual patient at a particular point in time in terms of respiratory and cardiovascular support. However, to date, therapies have not targeted and adjusted for SIRS in the same way. The framework described previously may represent ways of describing individual cases of sepsis/SIRS and targeting therapies to a patient's individual needs. We suggest that existing therapies may yet provide significant advances in the care for such children, if they can be targeted at those individuals with the greatest potential for benefit and the least likelihood of harm.

Therapies That Can Modulate the Balance Between Effective Microbial Killing and the Resultant Inflammatory Response

A proportion of patients who are admitted to the PICU will subsequently be found to have a major defect in their immune system. The vast majority of patients, however, who are either admitted with an infection or who develop an infectious complication while in the PICU, will not have been noted to be at an increased risk of either infection or an excessive inflammatory response prior to admission. The complex nature of how genetic polymorphisms are likely to act in the critical care setting makes therapies targeted at the inflammatory consequences of microbial destruction difficult and potentially dangerous. However, limited data indicate that, in *Staphylococcal* and *Streptococcal* toxic shock syndromes, the use of IV immunoglobulin and clindamycin could be beneficial. Both agents act to neutralize the effect of exotoxins—IV immunoglobulin by binding to the exotoxins and clindamycin by inhibiting the production of exotoxins. Data on how these agents may act in other conditions are limited.

A recombinant version of MBL is being developed for therapeutic use and may provide an opportunity for combining antimicrobial activity with inflammatory modulation. It will be interesting to see how this will operate in clinical practice (personal communication, R. Dormett, 2006). Bactericidal permeability increasing protein (BPI) is an antibacterial molecule with antiendotoxin properties. A recombinant form of this protein, rBPI$_{21}$, may provide a means of killing Gram-negative bacteria, while limiting the potentially harmful inflammatory effects of endotoxin. Clinical studies to date have been disappointing.

Possible Therapies for Acute Severe Proinflammation

High-dose Corticosteroids

The effects of exogenous steroids on the immune system are complex and vary according to type, dose, duration, and state of the immune system at the time of administration. Glucocorticoids bind to cytoplasmic glucocorticoid receptors and, via NFκB, act at a transcription level to modulate pro- and anti-inflammatory cytokine levels. Glucocorticoids inhibit production of the proinflammatory cytokines TNF-α, IL-1α, IL-1β, interferon (IFN)-γ, IL-6, IL-8, IL-12, and granulocyte-macrophage colony-stimulating factor (GM-CSF). In addition, glucocorticoids increase transcription of IL-1ra and IL-10, inhibit neutrophil activation, and suppress the synthesis of phospholipase A$_2$, cyclooxygenase, and inducible nitric oxide synthase. These broad-spectrum anti-inflammatory effects led to their investigation in sepsis.

Large doses of synthetic glucocorticoids (methylprednisolone or dexamethasone) have been investigated in unselected severe sepsis in adults (57). While some favorable cardiovascular changes were observed, an overall trend toward decreased survival, with high rates of nosocomial infection, was also observed. This effect may be secondary to a steroid-induced state of temporary hyperglycemia. Evidence suggests that uncontrolled hyperglycemia in critically ill patients is associated with a higher mortality rate, largely through sepsis-driven multiorgan dysfunction (62). The practice of high-dose steroids in sepsis has largely ceased. One meta-analysis observes that studies of steroids in adult sepsis after 1997 have shown a benefit when pooled, whereas pre-1989 studies tended to show harm (38). While these findings might reflect later studies using lower doses, it might also be explained by improved care of the side effects of steroid therapy, while retaining the benefits. Within the framework presented in this chapter, steroids might represent an effective intervention against excessive proinflammation that may worsen the risk of excessive anti-inflammation.

The option of high-dose steroids is being reconsidered in pediatric catecholamine-resistant septic shock, in which the risk of early cardiovascular collapse is greater than that of secondary infection. Observational studies suggest that relative adrenal insufficiency may be common and intensive cardiovascular support alone may be insufficient without replacing adequate doses of hydrocortisone (3). If this option is taken forward, any success is likely to be highly dependent on selecting only cases at very high risk of early (proinflammatory) death from cardiovascular failure. It would also require techniques to limit potentially harmful excessive immunosuppressive effects, including rapid reduction in dosage and great care to reduce the risks of nosocomial sepsis.

The impact of steroid therapy in a less-than-overwhelming episode of systemic inflammation may be reflected in their use perioperatively in elective cardiac surgery. While the intention was to suppress the post-bypass SIRS response (and indeed a reduction in plasma levels of proinflammatory cytokines has been observed), it remains unclear if suppression of SIRS is clinically beneficial in these patients. While very little evidence suggests that the use of steroids reduces the morbidity or mortality associated with cardiac surgery, some evidence does suggest that steroids may increase the duration of ventilation and worsen outcome (10,22,39), perhaps reflecting an excessive immunosuppressive result that leads to an anti-inflammatory state. Indeed, increased IL-10 production has been associated with perioperative steroid use.

Physiologic Doses of Corticosteroids

At physiologic levels, cortisol supports the vascular adrenergic receptor function and inhibits cytokine-induced nitric oxide synthase, thus potentiating vasoconstriction and myocardial contractility. The use of glucocorticoids has been reconsidered with evidence that adrenal failure or *relative adrenal insufficiency* is common in critically ill adults and children. Two reviews of randomized, controlled trials in septic patients have shown that physiologic doses of corticosteroids over 5–7 days improve systemic hemodynamics, shorten the duration of shock, and improve survival rates (4,38). A similar protocol has also shown to be beneficial in low cardiac output states. It is not clear if these steroid doses have significant anti-inflammatory effects.

Activated Protein C

Recombinant human activated protein C (rhAPC) possesses anticoagulant, profibrinolytic, and anti-inflammatory properties. It is still the only agent to have a positive outcome in a phase III sepsis trial. The PROWESS (Recombinant Human Activated Protein C Worldwide Evaluation in Severe Sepsis) randomized, controlled trial of 1690 critically adults with severe sepsis demonstrated that treatment with rhAPC was associated with a reduction in the relative risk of death of 19.4% (95% CI, 6.6–30.5) and an absolute reduction in the risk of death of 6.1% ($p = 0.005$) (7). It is interesting to speculate that rhAPC may have been more successful than other agents because of its lack of specificity or multiple sites of activity. As discussed previously, a very specific therapy with a "pure" anti-inflammatory action may harm a proportion of cases, while rhAPC has several targets and therefore may benefit a higher proportion of cases than it harms. At present, rhAPC is approved for use only in adult patients with severe sepsis who have a high risk of mortality, as determined by an Acute Physiology and Chronic Health Evaluation II (APACHE II) score of ≥ 25. However, a similar study in nearly 500 children with sepsis-induced cardiovascular and respiratory failure did not show any benefit of rhAPC above placebo for either mortality or time to resolve sepsis-induced organ failures (42). The low control group mortality and the very wide variability in the clinical features of patients in this study may have hidden the potential for benefit or harm in subgroups of patients.

Anticytokine Therapies—Monoclonal Antibodies

Agents that cause effective blockade of TNF are still being assessed in clinical trials (51). We suggest that, unless patients are selected prior to treatment on the basis of some laboratory or clinical parameters that have good positive predictive value for identifying an excessive proinflammatory response, any such agent is likely to fail in phase III studies.

Possible Therapies for Immunoparalysis

Aggressive Deintensification of Patients

Acquired immunoparalysis will only present a problem if the patient's immune system is challenged beyond the residual capacity to respond. Simple best practices of critical care may reduce this risk dramatically and should not be forgotten during the quest for more innovative solutions. Priority should be given to removal of invasive monitoring lines, endotracheal tubes, and urinary catheters at the earliest possible time in the PICU stay to reduce the risk of transient bacteremias in these vulnerable patients.

Stimulating Factors

In one of the landmark studies in sepsis, possible beneficial effects of administration of the proinflammatory cytokine IFN-γ to cases of severe sepsis established the principle that the anti-inflammatory state of acquired immunoparalysis exists and may cause harm following a systemic insult (13). At the time of this writing, no large-scale trials of the targeted use of IFN-γ in patients with acquired immunoparalysis have been reported.

GM-CSF and granulocyte colony-stimulating factor are naturally occurring cytokines that stimulate the number and antimicrobial functions of both neutrophils and monocytes. To date, they have a clear clinical use in the treatment of neutropenia, where their use has been shown to reduce the number of documented infections but not infection-related mortality (61). Interest has extended from their use in accelerating myeloid cell recovery to take advantage of their immune-enhancing properties. In animal models of sepsis, cotreatment with GM-CSF has been shown to enhance pathogen eradication and decrease morbidity and/or mortality (29). However, the outcome in clinical trials has been less clear. Administration of GM-CSF appears to have minimal side effects, to restore monocyte HLA-DR expression and function, and to assist in reducing sepsis episodes, but to date, it has not been shown to affect mortality (5,44,46,52). The effects are even less clear in randomized, controlled, neonatal trials (9). The value of GM-CSF may be greatest if subpopulations with evidence of acquired immunoparalysis are targeted.

A possible role of immunonutrients (arginine, glutamine, eicosapentaenoic acid, ω-3 fatty acids) as immunomodulating agents has gained attention. Glutamine is an abundant free amino acid in humans, critical for the integrity and function of metabolically active tissues. Under normal conditions, glutamine is a nonessential amino acid. However, in critical illness, glutamine levels in the body decrease, and its endogenous supply cannot match the increased demand. In vivo, circulating glutamine levels have been shown to be significantly reduced in both adults and children following surgery or trauma and to be associated with higher rates of infection (16).

Glutamine has immunomodulatory properties in vitro, with several actions on the immune system, including potentiation of the nonspecific cell-defense mechanisms of heat shock protein (Hsp) production in response to endotoxin and ischemia-reperfusion injury (66). Glutamine infusions enhance Hsp expression in multiple vital organs (heart, lung, and gut) in rat models of intestinal ischemia-reperfusion injury. In models of sepsis and injury, glutamine supplementation has been shown to increase survival, improve immune function, reduce bacteremia, increase gut barrier function, and decrease gastrointestinal mucosal atrophy. In vivo, parenteral supplementation with glutamine in adults has been associated with preservation of monocyte HLA-DR expression, decreases in infectious complications, and shortened hospital stay (6,26,45,56,65).

However, for each study in which glutamine administration to critically ill patients appears to show benefit, a similar study exists with no effect. While this may be attributable to the formulation and dose of glutamine chosen or the route of administration, it may also be that glutamine supplementation is beneficial only when appropriately targeted.

A mortality benefit has been suggested for enteral feeding with eicosapentaenoic acid, γ-linolenic acid, and antioxidants in adult septic shock cases (50). These observations are perhaps consistent with our framework, despite the lack of patient selection, because these lipids are reported to have both pro- and anti-inflammatory actions (37).

Removal of Inhibitory Plasma Mediators

Addition of IL-10 monoclonal antibodies has been shown to attenuate the inhibitory effect of serum drawn from critically ill patients on control monocyte phenotype and function (19). While IL-10 appears to play an important role in acquired immunoparalysis, it is not the only soluble factor that appears to be acting (19,41). Attempts to eliminate a wide range of different inhibitory factors (as well as possible proinflammatory mediators) have resulted in case reports of hemofiltration, apheresis, and plasmapheresis in critically ill patients. The ability of any of these therapies to change the level of circulating mediators depends on the method used. Conventional plasma exchange does not consistently affect plasma levels of IL-6, IL-6R, TNF-α, TNF-αR, or C-reactive protein. At present, this therapy remains experimental (67). By comparison, continuous hemofiltration has been shown to minimally reduce inflammatory mediators (complement activation, plasma thromboxane, and proinflammatory cytokines at high-volume filtration) (11,31,40). Retrospective, single-centered studies suggest that the use of continuous renal hemofiltration in critically ill children improves outcome. The mechanism by which this may be acting is uncertain, and while it may be through an immunomodulating effect, it may also be acting to remove free water, improve fluid balance, and correct acid-base status.

Possible Therapies for Failure of Resolution or Persistence of the Inflammatory Response

Treatments for Neutropenia

Granulocyte colony-stimulating factor and GM-CSF are now included in protocols to reduce the length of periods of neutropenia, hence, the risk of serious infections in cancer patients. It is less clear if they should be used in the acute phase of neutropenic sepsis to aid resolution, but this has become widespread practice. Infusion of granulocytes is also being more widely used, in particular to aid clearance of deep-seated and fungal infections. Case reports support this practice, but randomized trial data are not available (35).

Antiadhesion Molecules

Monoclonal antibodies that block either early rolling adhesion (anti-CD62E) or later firm adhesion (anti-CD18) of leukocytes remain under investigation in acute systemic inflammation and in related conditions (18). No role for these agents is yet apparent.

Therapies for Hemophagocytosis

Treatments for HLH are well established and consist of high-dose steroid, etoposide, and cyclosporin. No consensus exists as to the use of these drugs for hemophagocytosis that occurs as part of systemic inflammation in the ICU. It has been proposed that these drugs should be considered in persistent, acute inflammatory conditions, especially following severe viral infections, such as severe acute respiratory syndrome or H5N1 (28). These immunosuppressive drugs have the potential to cause significant harm, and currently, no data to support their use exists. Interferon-α and intravenous immunoglobulin (IVIG) have been reported as effective in the treatment of HLH (15).

Antiapoptotic Drugs

The exciting and potentially rewarding area of investigation into antiapoptotic drugs could also have been described previously under the section on therapies for immunoparalysis, as increased lymphocyte and dendritic cell apoptosis probably represents key consequences of the CARS/Th-2 response. While a number of agents for inhibiting apoptosis (caspase inhibitors, CD95 inhibitors, and protease inhibitors) are promising in animal models, none have passed into human trials. If an effective agent can be found, it is likely to face the same challenge as anti-TNF therapies—the need to identify cases most likely to benefit—in addition to the further challenge of balancing the impact of delaying apoptosis on different cells types (e.g., PMNs) versus lymphocytes.

CONCLUSIONS AND FUTURE DIRECTIONS

Critical illness (whether infective or noninfective in origin) evokes an immune response that influences the patient's intensive care course. Unlike other vital systems, no accepted physiologic variable or biochemical test exists with which to monitor the complexity and variability of this response. While the immune response has evolved to limit the harmful stimulus, an excessive or unchecked response can result in significant cellular and organ damage.

Biologic systems within the body are designed to both respond to a stressful event and to act to restore physiologic homeostasis. The immune system is no different. For every proinflammatory response, there appears to be a balancing anti-inflammatory response. Under ideal conditions, the inflammatory response is short lived, appropriately sized, and

effective during critical illness, and the patient recovers well with limited intensive care support. However, in many clinical scenarios, a balanced immune response is not seen, perhaps due to an inappropriate host immune response (too much or too little) or to the medical management instituted. Broad applications of immunomodulatory agents to patients with critical illness have failed spectacularly, probably because therapies have been administered to patients who vary in their timing, location, and relative balance of immune response.

Future therapeutic trials should target therapy appropriate to the individual inflammatory response of the critically ill patient. To do this, the treating clinician must be able to identify the patient's immunocompetence and inflammatory, as well as infectious, status. Only by understanding the immune response of an individual patient will the clinician be able to more judiciously use antimicrobials and immunomodulating therapies in the setting of critical illness.

KEY POINTS

■ The immune system is a phenomenally complex biologic system.

■ Critical illness (both septic and nonseptic) elicits an immune response that is designed to protect the body.

■ An unbalanced immune response may worsen the overall clinical state and exacerbate the level of organ dysfunction.

■ Many examples of congenital immunodeficiency provide the clinician with important insight into infection susceptibility, mechanisms of systemic inflammation, and multiorgan dysfunction.

■ To date, no interventional trial of immune modulation in critically ill children has been of proven benefit, perhaps due to a failure of appropriate targeting.

■ Future clinical trials must evaluate the patient's immunocompetence and inflammatory and infectious status.

■ Therapeutic trials of immunomodulative agents should be appropriately targeted to the immune state of the individual.

References

1. Allen ML, Hoschtitzky JA, Peters MJ, et al. Interleukin-10 and its role in clinical immunoparalysis following pediatric cardiac surgery. *Crit Care Med* 2006;34:2658–65.
2. Amoo-Lamptey A, Carcillo J. Comparative pathology of children with sepsis, isolated pneumonia, and organ failure without infection. *Pediatr Res* 2001;49:251.
3. Aneja R, Carcillo JA. What is the rationale for use of hydrocortisone therapy for infection related adrenal insufficiency and septic shock?. *Arch Dis Child* 2007;92(2):165–9.
4. Annane D, Bellissant E, Bollaert PE, et al. Corticosteroids for severe sepsis and septic shock: A systematic review and meta-analysis. *BMJ* 2004;329:480–9.
5. Azoulay E, Delclaux C. Is there a place for granulocyte colony-stimulating factor in non-neutropenic critically ill patients?. *Intensive Care Med* 2004;30:10–7.
6. Bastian L, Weimann A. Immunonutrition in patients after multiple trauma. *Br J Nutr* 2002;87 Suppl 1:S133–4.
7. Bernard GR, Vincent JL, Laterre PF, et al. Efficacy and safety of recombinant human activated protein C for severe sepsis. *N Engl J Med* 2001;344: 699–709.
8. Bone RC. Sir Isaac Newton, sepsis, SIRS, and CARS. *Crit Care Med* 1996;24:1125–8.
9. Carr R, Modi N, Dore C. G-CSF and GM-CSF for treating or preventing neonatal infections. *Cochrane Database Syst Rev* 2003;CD003066.
10. Chaney MA. Corticosteroids and cardiopulmonary bypass: A review of clinical investigations. *Chest* 2002;121:921–31.

11. Cole L, Bellomo R, Davenport P, et al. Cytokine removal during continuous renal replacement therapy: An ex vivo comparison of convection and diffusion. *Int J Artif Organs* 2004;27:388–97.

12. Cross AS, Opal SM. A new paradigm for the treatment of sepsis: Is it time to consider combination therapy?. *Ann Intern Med* 2003;138:502–5.

13. Docke WD, Randow F, Syrbe U, et al. Monocyte deactivation in septic patients: Restoration by IFN-gamma treatment. *Nat Med* 1997;3: 678–81.

14. Dommett RM, Klein N, Turner MW. Mannose-binding lectin in innate immunity: Past, present and future. *Tissue Antigens* 2006;68:193–209.

15. Estlin EJ, Palmer RD, Windebank KP, et al. Successful treatment of non-familial haemophagocytic lymphohistiocytosis with interferon and gamma-globulin. *Arch Dis Child* 1996;75(5):432–5.

16. Exner R, Tamandl D, Goetzinger P, et al. Perioperative GLY-GLN infusion diminishes the surgery-induced period of immunosuppression: Accelerated restoration of the lipopolysaccharide-stimulated tumor necrosis factor-alpha response. *Ann Surg* 2003;237:110–5.

17. Felmet KA, Hall MW, Clark RS, et al. Prolonged lymphopenia, lymphoid depletion, and hypoprolactinemia in children with nosocomial sepsis and multiple organ failure. *J Immunol* 2005;174:3765–72.

18. Friedman G, Jankowski S, Shahla M, et al. Administration of an antibody to E-selectin in patients with septic shock. *Crit Care Med* 1996;24: 229–33.

19. Fumeaux T, Pugin J. Role of interleukin-10 in the intracellular sequestration of human leukocyte antigen-DR in monocytes during septic shock. *Am J Respir Crit Care Med* 2002;166:1475–82.

20. Gardinali M, Borrelli E, Chiara O, et al. Inhibition of CD11-CD18 complex prevents acute lung injury and reduces mortality after peritonitis in rabbits. *Am J Respir Crit Care Med* 2000;161:1022–9.

21. Garred P, Strom J, Quist L, et al. Association of mannose-binding lectin polymorphisms with sepsis and fatal outcome, in patients with systemic inflammatory response syndrome. *J Infect Dis* 2003;188:1394–403.

22. Gessler P, Hohl V, Carrel T, et al. Administration of steroids in pediatric cardiac surgery: Impact on clinical outcome and systemic inflammatory response. *Pediatr Cardiol* 2005;26(5):595–600.

23. Goldstein B, Giroir B, Randolph A. International pediatric sepsis consensus conference: Definitions for sepsis and organ dysfunction in pediatrics. *Pediatr Crit Care Med* 2005;6:2–8.

24. Gordon AC, Waheed U, Hansen TK, et al. Mannose-binding lectin polymorphisms in severe sepsis: Relationship to levels, incidence, and outcome. *Shock* 2006;25:88–93.

25. Gottlieb A, Krueger JG, Bright R, et al. Effects of administration of a single dose of a humanized monoclonal antibody to CD11a on the immunobiology and clinical activity of psoriasis. *J Am Acad Dermatol* 2000;42:428–35.

26. Griffiths RD, Allen KD, Andrews FJ, et al. Infection, multiple organ failure, and survival in the intensive care unit: Influence of glutamine-supplemented parenteral nutrition on acquired infection. *Nutrition* 2002;18:546–52.

27. Hansen TK, Thiel S, Wouters PJ, et al. Intensive insulin therapy exerts antiinflammatory effects in critically ill patients and counteracts the adverse effect of low mannose-binding lectin levels. *J Clin Endocrinol Metab* 2003;88:1082–8.

28. Henter JI, Chow CB, Leung CW, et al. Cytotoxic therapy for severe avian influenza A (H5N1) infection. *Lancet* 2006;367:870–3.

29. Hubel K, Dale DC, Liles WC. Therapeutic use of cytokines to modulate phagocyte function for the treatment of infectious diseases: Current status of granulocyte colony-stimulating factor, granulocyte-macrophage colony-stimulating factor, macrophage colony-stimulating factor, and interferon-gamma. *J Infect Dis* 2002;185:1490–501.

30. Inwald DP, Faust SN, Lister P, et al. Platelet and soluble CD40L in meningococcal sepsis. *Intensive Care Med* 2006;32:1432–7.

31. Jiang HL, Xue WJ, Li DQ, et al. Influence of continuous veno-venous hemofiltration on the course of acute pancreatitis. *World J Gastroenterol* 2005;11:4815–21.

32. Kox WJ, Volk T, Kox SN, et al. Immunomodulatory therapies in sepsis. *Intensive Care Med* 2000;26 Suppl 1:S124–8.

33. Lehner PJ, Davies KA, Walport MJ, et al. Meningococcal septicaemia in a C6-deficient patient and effects of plasma transfusion on lipopolysaccharide release. *Lancet* 1992;340:1379–81.

34. Levy MM, Fink MP, Marshall JC, et al. 2001 SCCM/ESICM/ACCP/ATS/SIS International Sepsis Definitions Conference. *Crit Care Med* 2003;31:1250–6.

35. Liang DC. The role of colony-stimulating factors and granulocyte transfusion in treatment options for neutropenia in children with cancer. *Paediatr Drugs* 2003;5:673–84.

36. Mathew S, Overturf GD. Complement and properidin [*sic*] deficiencies in meningococcal disease. *Pediatr Infect Dis J* 2006;25:255–6.

37. Mayer K, Gokorsch S, Fegbeutel C, et al. Parenteral nutrition with fish oil modulates cytokine response in patients with sepsis. *Am J Respir Crit Care Med* 2003;167:1321–8.

38. Minneci PC, Deans KJ, Banks SM, et al. Meta-analysis: The effect of steroids on survival and shock during sepsis depends on the dose. *Ann Intern Med* 2004;141:47–56.

39. Morariu AM, Loef BG, Aarts LP, et al. Dexamethasone: Benefit and prejudice for patients undergoing on-pump coronary artery bypass grafting: A study on myocardial, pulmonary, renal, intestinal, and hepatic injury. *Chest* 2005;128:2677–87.

40. Morgera S, Slowinski T, Melzer C, et al. Renal replacement therapy with high-cutoff hemofilters: Impact of convection and diffusion on cytokine clearances and protein status. *Am J Kidney Dis* 2004;43:444–53.

41. Mueller A, Kreuzfelder E, Nyadu B, et al. Human leukocyte antigen-DR expression in peripheral blood mononuclear cells from healthy donors influenced by the sera of injured patients prone to severe sepsis. *Intensive Care Med* 2003;29:2285–90.

42. Nadel S, Goldstein B, Williams, MD, et al. Drotrecogin alfa (activated) in children with severe sepsis: a multicentre phase III randomised controlled trial. *Lancet* 2007;369:836–43.

43. Nahum E, Ben-Ari J, Stain J, et al. Hemophagocytic lymphohistiocytic syndrome: Unrecognized cause of multiple organ failure. *Pediatr Crit Care Med* 2000;1:51–4.

44. Nierhaus A, Montag B, Timmler N, et al. Reversal of immunoparalysis by recombinant human granulocyte-macrophage colony-stimulating factor in patients with severe sepsis. *Intensive Care Med* 2003;29:646–51.

45. Novak F, Heyland DK, Avenell A, et al. Glutamine supplementation in serious illness: A systematic review of the evidence. *Crit Care Med* 2002;30:2022–9.

46. Orozco H, Arch J, Medina-Franco H, et al. Molgramostim (GM-CSF) associated with antibiotic treatment in nontraumatic abdominal sepsis: A randomized, double-blind, placebo-controlled clinical trial. *Arch Surg* 2006;141:150–3.

47. Ouachee-Chardin M, Elie C, de Saint BG, et al. Hematopoietic stem cell transplantation in hemophagocytic lymphohistiocytosis: A single-center report of 48 patients. *Pediatrics* 2006;117:e743–50.

48. Panacek EA, Marshall JC, Albertson TE, et al. Efficacy and safety of the monoclonal anti-tumor necrosis factor antibody F(ab')2 fragment afelimomab in patients with severe sepsis and elevated interleukin-6 levels. *Crit Care Med* 2004;32:2173–82.

49. Peters MJ, Ross-Russell RI, White D, et al. Early severe neutropenia and thrombocytopenia identifies the highest risk cases of severe meningococcal disease. *Pediatr Crit Care Med* 2001;2:225–31.

50. Pontes-Arruda A, Aragao AM, Albuquerque JD. Effects of enteral feeding with eicosapentaenoic acid, gamma-linolenic acid, and antioxidants in mechanically ventilated patients with severe sepsis and septic shock. *Crit Care Med* 2006;34:2325–33.

51. Rice TW, Wheeler AP, Morris PE, et al. Safety and efficacy of affinity-purified, anti-tumor necrosis factor-alpha, ovine fab for injection (CytoFab) in severe sepsis. *Crit Care Med* 2006;34:2271–81.

52. Rosenbloom AJ, Linden PK, Dorrance A, et al. Effect of granulocyte-monocyte colony-stimulating factor therapy on leukocyte function and clearance of serious infection in nonneutropenic patients. *Chest* 2005;127: 2139–50.

53. Schaaf BM, Boehmke F, Esnaashari H, et al. Pneumococcal septic shock is associated with the interleukin-10-1082 gene promoter polymorphism. *Am J Respir Crit Care Med* 2003;168:476–80.

54. Segal AW. How neutrophils kill microbes. *Annu Rev Immunol* 2005;23:197–223.

55. Shu Q, Fang X, Chen Q, et al. IL-10 polymorphism is associated with increased incidence of severe sepsis. *Chin Med J (Engl)* 2003;116:1756–9.

56. Spittler A, Sautner T, Gornikiewicz A, et al. Postoperative glycyl-glutamine infusion reduces immunosuppression: Partial prevention of the surgery-induced decrease in HLA-DR expression on monocytes. *Clin Nutr* 2001;20:37–42.

57. Sprung CL, Caralis PV, Marcial EH, et al. The effects of high-dose corticosteroids in patients with septic shock. *A prospective, controlled study. N Engl J Med* 1984;311:1137–43.

58. Stanilova SA, Miteva LD, Karakolev ZT, et al. Interleukin-10-1082 promoter polymorphism in association with cytokine production and sepsis susceptibility. *Intensive Care Med* 2006;32:260–6.

59. Stephens RC, Fidler K, Wilson P, et al. Endotoxin immunity and the development of the systemic inflammatory response syndrome in critically ill children. *Intensive Care Med* 2006;32:286–94.

60. Strauss R, Neureiter D, Westenburger B, et al. Multifactorial risk analysis of bone marrow histiocytic hyperplasia with hemophagocytosis in critically ill medical patients-A postmortem clinicopathologic analysis. *Crit Care Med* 2004;32:1316–21.

61. Sung L, Nathan PC, Lange B, et al. Prophylactic granulocyte colony-stimulating factor and granulocyte-macrophage colony-stimulating factor decrease febrile neutropenia after chemotherapy in children with cancer: A meta-analysis of randomized controlled trials. *J Clin Oncol* 2004;22: 3350–6.

62. van den BG, Wouters P, Weekers F, et al. Intensive insulin therapy in the critically ill patients. *N Engl J Med* 2001;345:1359–67.

63. Verbsky JW, Grossman WJ. Hemophagocytic lymphohistiocytosis: Diagnosis, pathophysiology, treatment, and future perspectives. *Ann Med* 2006;38:20–31.

64. Walsh MC, Bourcier T, Takahashi K, et al. Mannose-binding lectin is a regulator of inflammation that accompanies myocardial ischemia and reperfusion injury. *J Immunol* 2005;175:541–6.

65. Wischmeyer PE, Lynch J, Liedel J, et al. Glutamine administration reduces Gram-negative bacteremia in severely burned patients: A prospective, randomized, double-blind trial versus isonitrogenous control. *Crit Care Med* 2001;29:2075–80.

66. Wischmeyer PE, Riehm J, Singleton KD, et al. Glutamine attenuates tumor necrosis factor-alpha release and enhances heat shock protein 72 in human peripheral blood mononuclear cells. *Nutrition* 2003;19:1–6.

67. Yekebas EF, Eisenberger CF, Ohnesorge H, et al. Attenuation of sepsis-related immunoparalysis by continuous veno-venous hemofiltration in experimental porcine pancreatitis. *Crit Care Med* 2001;29:1423–30.

68. Zeni F, Freeman B, Natanson C. Anti-inflammatory therapies to treat sepsis and septic shock: A reassessment. *Crit Care Med* 1997;25:1095–100.

69. zur SU, Schmidt S, Kasper B, et al. Linkage of familial hemophagocytic lymphohistiocytosis (FHL) type-4 to chromosome 6q24 and identification of mutations in syntaxin 11. *Hum Mol Genet* 2005;14:827–34.

CHAPTER 73 ■ THE POLYMORPHONUCLEAR LEUKOCYTE IN CRITICAL ILLNESS

M. MICHELE MARISCALCO

The phagocytic leukocytes play a central and critical role in the acute phase of the inflammatory response. They are rapidly mobilized to sites of infection or injury and release an array of cytotoxic molecules to nonspecifically eliminate microbes. Phagocytes are also critical to the normal repair of tissue injury. Individuals with deficits in phagocyte function or number have impairment in wound healing. Phagocytes include polymorphonuclear leukocytes (PMNLs), monocytes/macrophages, and dendritic cells. The PMNL system refers to neutrophils, basophils, and eosinophils. PMNLs are grouped together because of their common nuclear morphology and granule content; hence, the name *granulocytes*. In this chapter, discussion focuses on the neutrophil. While it maintains a central role in the innate immune system, the neutrophil is also critically involved in many of the pathologic processes that bring patients to the ICU: sepsis, ischemia-reperfusion injury, acute respiratory distress syndrome (ARDS), transfusion-related acute lung injury (ALI), and traumatic injury. A concise review of normal neutrophil physiology and function is provided first. Several outstanding reviews have been written (14,25,33). Those diseases in which neutrophil function "goes awry" as they relate to the critically ill infant and child, as well as therapies that affect neutrophil function are discussed in the remainder of the chapter.

As a way of clarification, leukocytes, other cells of hematopoietic origin, and other cells, such as endothelium and fibroblasts, are often characterized by proteins found on their surface. These proteins may have multiple names, often provided by the group that initially identifies them. However, these proteins may also be formally identified as human cell differentiation molecules (HCDM) and given a unique CD (cluster of differentiation) number, nomenclature that was first proposed in 1982. It is thought that the 350 HCDM now identified are only a small fraction of the possible cell-surface proteins. (The interested reader is referred to the most current list of HCDM at www.hla.org, accessed 1/3/2007).

NEUTROPHIL PHYSIOLOGY

Granulopoiesis, Marrow Release, and Margination

Fifty percent to 60% of the bone marrow, an organ 70% larger than the liver, is dedicated to producing neutrophils. Approximately 100 billion neutrophils leave the bone marrow each day in a healthy adult. The normal ratio of neutrophils to erythroid cells ranges from 2:1 to 3:1. As cells differentiate from hematopoietic stem cells, they undergo five divisions, from myeloblast to promyelocyte to myelocyte. After the myelocyte stage, they no longer undergo meiosis but remain in the large storage pool (Fig. 73.1). They mature in the storage pool for ~5 days under normal conditions. The nucleus contracts from the large, ovoid shape of the promyelocyte to the "band" and, finally, to the three- to five-lobed nucleus of the mature neutrophil. After release in the bloodstream, neutrophils circulate for up to 12 hrs.

The elimination of foreign microorganisms through phagocytosis, generation of reactive oxygen metabolites, and release of microbicidal substances is dependent on the mobilization of neutrophilic granules and secretory vesicles. The mature neutrophil contains four granule populations. These granules share common structural features, such as a phospholipid bilayer and an intragranular matrix that contains proteins destined for exocytosis or delivery to the phagosome. Proteins synthesized at the same stage of myeloid cell development localize to the same granule (17). The first granule, the primary or azurophil, forms during the myeloblast and promyelocyte stage and contains myeloperoxidase and neutrophil elastase (Fig. 73.1 and Table 73.1). Production of myeloperoxidase ceases at the promyelocyte-to-myelocyte stage. Secondary (specific) granules contain high concentrations of lactoferrin and low concentrations of gelatinase (matrix metalloproteinase 9, MMP-9) and form in myelocytes and metamyelocytes. Tertiary granules (gelatinase) form in band cells and segmented neutrophils and are low in lactoferrin and high in gelatinase. The secretory vesicles form in segmented neutrophils. Their membranes contain cytochrome b_{558} (one of the components of the NADPH-oxidase system), receptors for complement [CD35 (complement receptor 1, CR1), CD11b/CD18 (Mac-1, CR3)], receptor for complement component 1q (C1qR), and receptors for monovalent and polyvalent immunoglobulin (CD32, CD64, CD16) and for bacterial lipopolysaccharide (CD14). Exocytosis of granules occurs in reverse order, with secretory granules being the easiest to mobilize and the primary granule the least easy, requiring strong phagocytic stimuli.

The primary granule, formed in the myeloblast and promyelocyte (Table 73.1), contains a number of antimicrobial peptides: the four α-defensins (human neutrophil peptide 1 through 4), bactericidal/permeability increasing protein (BPI), and serprocidins (serine proteases with microbicidal activity: proteinase-3, cathepsin G, and elastase). The α-defensins have microbicidal activity against a broad range of fungi, bacteria, enveloped viruses, and protozoa. They exert their effect through the formation of transmembrane pores. Neutrophil defensins induce chemotaxis of monocytes and lymphocytes (54). BPI is highly cationic, kills Gram-negative bacteria

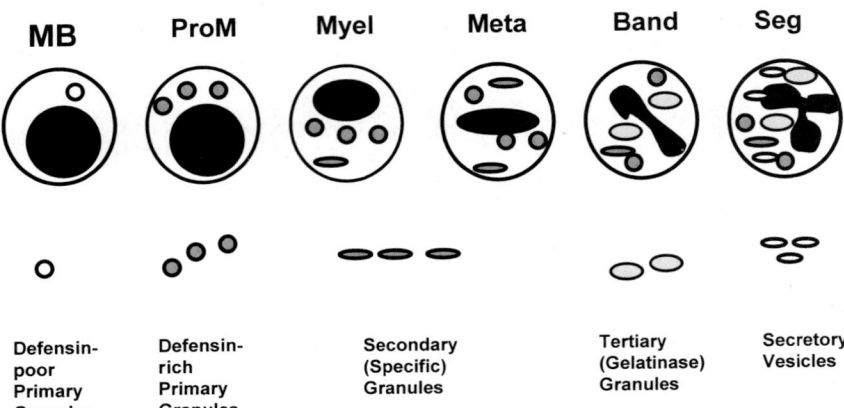

FIGURE 73.1. Neutrophil maturation. Note that granules develop during neutrophil maturation. No further cell division occurs beyond the myelocyte stage. MB, myeloblast; ProM, promyelocyte; Myel, myelocyte; Meta, Metamyelocyte; Seg, segmented (mature) neutrophil.

at nanomolar concentrations, and neutralizes lipopolysaccharide. A recent study examined the use of recombinant BPI (rBPI) as adjunctive treatment for children with severe meningococcemia (28). No effect on mortality was observed, but patients treated with rBPI had fewer multiple severe amputations and improved functional outcome (28). The serprocidins are cationic polypeptides with proteolytic activity against a variety of extracellular matrix proteins, such as elastin, fibronectin, laminin, type IV collagen, and vitronectin. Unrestrained

release of elastase is currently believed to play a crucial role in the pathogenesis of pulmonary emphysema. The serine proteases have a number of inhibitors: those found in the systemic circulation (α1-antitrypsin, also known as α1-proteinase inhibitor, and α2-macroglobulin) and those produced by the epithelial and immune cells (secretory leukoproteinase inhibitor and elafin) (19).

The specific and gelatinase granules are formed in the metamyelocyte stage and continue through maturation until the

TABLE 73.1

NEUTROPHIL GRANULE CONTENTS

Protein	Primary (Azurophil)	Secondary (Specific)	Tertiary (Gelatinase)	Secretory Vesicle
Membrane proteins				
Cytochrome b_{558}			+	+
CD11b/CD18 (CR3)		+	+	+
fMLF-R		+	+	+
Alkaline phosphatase				+
CD10				+
CD14				+
CD16 (FcγRIIIb)				+
CD35 (CR1)				+
C1qR				+
Enzymes				
Myeloperoxidase	+			
Proteinase-3	+			
Leukolysin		+	+	+
Collagenase		+		
Gelatinase		+	+	
Antimicrobial peptides				
Lysozyme	+	+	+	
Defensins	+			
BPI	+			
Cathepsins	+			
Lactoferrin		+		
Others				
Haptoglobin		+		
α_1-Antitrypsin	+			
β_2 Microglobulin		+	+	

CD, cluster of differentiation; CR3, complement receptor 3; fMLF-R, formylmethionine-leucine-phenylalanine receptor; BPI, bacterial permeability increasing factor formation of segmented neutrophils. Specific granules are larger and rich in antibiotic substances. More difficult to mobilize than gelatinase granules, they release their contents into the phagolysosome or the exterior of the cell. Gelatinase granules are smaller and more easily exocytosed. They are important primarily as a reservoir of matrix-degrading enzymes and membrane receptors required during neutrophil extravasation. Neutrophils contain three metalloproteinases (MMPs): neutrophil collagenase (MMP-8), gelatinase (MMP-9), and leukolysin (MMP-25) (17) (**Table 73.1**). The MMPs are able to degrade major structural components of the extracellular matrix and are important for the extravasation of neutrophils.

The secretory vesicles are endocytic and constitute a reservoir of membrane-associated receptors required at the earliest phases of neutrophil localization. The secretory vesicles are mobilized in response to a wide variety of inflammatory stimuli. The membranes are rich in CD11b/CD18 (Mac-1, CR3), CD35 (CR1), and receptors for the formylated bacterial peptide [formylmethionyl-leucyl-phenylalanine (fMLF), CD14 and CD16, (FcγRIIIb receptor)].

More than 40 different growth factors, cytokines, and chemokines regulate PMNL proliferation and differentiation and cell fate. The most clinically useful is granulocyte colony-stimulating factor (GCSF). GCSF specifically promotes neutrophil proliferation and maturation and enhances neutrophil microbicidal activity when administered in vivo. GCSF interacts with relatively late hematopoietic progenitors that have already committed to the neutrophil lineage and serves to support their growth and final maturation into functional neutrophils. Granulocyte-macrophage colony-stimulating factor (GM-CSF) acts on progenitors that are committed to produce either neutrophils or monocytes but can also act on granulocyte precursors directly. As with GCSF, it can enhance neutrophil reactivity when given in vivo.

Neutrophils continuously egress from the sinusoids of the bone marrow. Within the circulation, about half of the neutrophils are in the flowing stream; the other half are inaccessible to phlebotomy. This half is called the *marginating pool*. In response to stress, exercise, or IV epinephrine, the neutrophils in the marginating pool are released into the circulating pool. The marginating pool of neutrophils is in the postcapillary venules in major organs and in the capillaries of the lungs. As a result of longer transit times of neutrophils compared to erythrocytes, in normal lungs, the concentration of neutrophils within the pulmonary capillary blood is ~40–80 times higher than it is within the blood in large vessels. Neutrophils travel in "hops" through the lung microvasculature, moving quickly through larger capillary segments but stopping and deforming for entry into smaller segment; hence, the longer transit times.

Neutrophilia occurs after the administration of glucocorticoids. Approximately 60% of the neutrophilia is due to mobilization from the marginated pool, 10% is due to increased bone marrow release, and 30% is due to lengthened half-life in circulation. The administration of GCSF shortens the transit time of neutrophils through the marrow, particularly in the postmitotic pool. GCSF has no effect on demargination but delays clearance of neutrophils by inhibiting apoptosis.

In response to inflammatory stimuli or infection, neutrophil production and release significantly increase. Neutrophil release from the bone marrow initially exceeds production, causing a temporary decrease in the bone marrow neutrophil pool. Once the bone marrow neutrophil pool is reestablished,

release from the marrow increases and neutrophil count rises. In those individuals with limited neutrophil pool reserves, such as those with drug-induced neutropenia or those who have received chemotherapy, and in infants, neutrophil count may remain low while the neutrophil pool replenishes.

IL-6, one of the major regulators of the acute-phase response, induces demargination of intravascular neutrophils and shortens the neutrophil transit in the marrow. However, those neutrophils that are released preferentially sequester in the lung microvessels, are less deformable, and have increased F-actin (46). Neutrophil deformability is mediated by a rapid assembly of filamentous F-actin from soluble G-actin at the cell periphery. "Mature" neutrophils released from the bone marrow have altered function after infection, compared to cells produced during the "noninfected" state. They demonstrate decreased chemotaxis, decreased phagocytosis, and an impaired ability to upregulate CD10, a neutral endopeptidase that is present on only mature granulocytes. These cells generate greater stimulus-induced intracellular calcium flux (38).

Neutrophil Localization in Infection

The body has a highly coordinated and regulated response to microbes. The first defense is local immunity. The epithelial surface itself functions as a physical barrier. Antimicrobial peptides are released from the epithelium, and secretory IgA is released from submucosal plasma cells. Microbes may be eliminated or controlled at the source; however, if the microbial burden exceeds these processes, then neutrophil recruitment is required to control the infection. Epithelial-bacteria interactions result in the release of cytokines, specifically IL-1 and tumor necrosis factor (TNF)-α, and chemokines, such as IL-8, CXCL8, and GCSF (40). These activate the macrophages that reside in submucosa, which in turn amplify the proinflammatory signal with additional release of proinflammatory chemokines and cytokines.

The endothelium of the nearby postcapillary venule, under the immunologic pressure of proinflammatory cytokines, transforms from a nonadhesive surface to one that is proadhesive through the expression of specific ligands on the endothelial surface (**Table 73.2**). Selectins are responsible for the initial capture of the neutrophil from the free-flowing stream and their rolling on the endothelial surface. Selectins are present on both neutrophils (L-selectin, CD62-L) and on the endothelial surface (E- and P-selectin, CD62-E and CD62P, respectively) (45) (**Table 73.2**). Members of the immunoglobulin superfamily (IgSF), intercellular adhesion molecule-1 (ICAM-1) and vascular cell adhesion molecule (VCAM) are critical for neutrophil slowing, arrest, and migration on the cell surface. (**Fig. 73.2**) The receptors on the neutrophil surface for the IgSF are the β_2 integrins: Mac-1 (CD11b/CD18, CR3), LFA-1 (CD11a/CD18), and the β_1 integrin VLA-4 (CD49d/CD29) (**Table 73.2**). The leukocyte integrins are heterodimers comprised of α and β subunits. The β subunit may be shared by multiple members of a subfamily, while the α subunit confers specificity. The leukocyte integrins are generally functionally in an "inactive state." Through a process known as *inside-out signaling*, the integrins change their conformation and become "active," and ligand recognition can now occur. The endothelial surface secretes a number of chemokines and lipid-derived products, such as CXCL8 (IL-8) and platelet-activating factor (PAF), which

TABLE 73.2

ADHESION MOLECULES FOR NEUTROPHIL LOCALIZATION TO INFLAMMATORY SITES

Name	CD classification	Cell expression	Constitutive/Inducible	Ligand
Integrin family				
β_1 Integrins				
$\alpha_2\beta_1$ (VLA-2)	CD49b/CD29	Neutrophil	C/I?	Coll I, Coll IV, LN
$\alpha_4\beta_1$ (VLA-4)	CD49d/CD29	Neutrophil	C/I?	FN, VCAM, JAM2
$\alpha_5\beta_1$ (VLA-5)	CD49e/CD29	Neutrophil	C/I?	FN, Tsp
$\alpha_6\beta_1$ (VLA-5)	CD49f/CD29	Neutrophil	C/I?	LN
$\alpha_9\beta_1$		Neutrophil	C/I?	VCAM-1, osteopontin
β_2 Integrins				
$\alpha_L\beta_2$ (LFA-1)	CD11a/CD18	Neutrophil	C	ICAM-1, ICAM-2, ICAM-3, JAM-1
$\alpha_M\beta_2$ (Mac-1, CR3)	CD11b/CD18	Neutrophil	C/I	ICAM-1, C3b, C3bi, Fg, FN, Factor X
$\alpha_x\beta_2$ (p150,95)	CD11c/CD18	Neutrophil	C/I	C3bi, GPIb-IX-V
β_3 Integrins				
$\alpha_V\beta_3$ (Vitronectin Receptor)	CD51/CD61	Neutrophil	C	vWf, VN, FN, Fg, PECAM-1, Tsp, LN, Osp, Coll I, Coll IV
Immunoglobulin gene superfamily (IGSF)				
ICAM-1	CD54	T and B cell; Endo; Epi; hepatocytes, pneumocytes, fibroblasts	C/I	LFA-1, Mac-1
VCAM-1	CD102	Endo	I	$\alpha_4\beta_1$, $\alpha_9\beta_1$
JAM-1		Endo, Epi	C	LFA-1, JAM-1
Selectins and selectin ligands				
L-selectin	CD62-L	Neutrophil	C	Unknown endo ligand, PSGL-1,
P-selectin	CD62-P	Platelet, Endo	C/I	PSGL-1, E-selectin, GPIb-IX-V
E-selectin	CD62-E	Endo	I	PSGL-1
P-selectin-glycoprotein Ligand 1 (PSGL-1)	CD162	Neutrophil	C	P-selectin, E-selectin, L-selectin

Note that this table focuses primarily on adhesion molecules specifically for neutrophil localization to inflammatory sites.
Inducible adhesion molecules: While ICAM-1 is constitutively expressed on many cell types, its expression can also be induced by the cytokines TNF, IL-1, and IFN-γ after only a brief period (3–4 hrs). E-selectin and P-selectin can be induced on endothelial cells by TNF and IL-1 after 3–4 hrs of stimulation. VCAM-1 is present on endothelial cells only after cytokine stimulation. Its appearance is delayed compared to the other adhesion molecules. Both endothelial cells (Weibel-Palade bodies) and platelets (α granule) contain an intracellular pool of P-selectin, which can be mobilized to the surface after cell activation. Similarly, Mac-1 and p150,95 are constitutively present on neutrophils, but pools are also present in secretory vesicles that can be easily mobilized.
VLA, very late antigen; Coll I, collagen type I; Coll IV, collagen type IV; LN, laminin; FN, fibronectin; VCAM, vascular cell adhesion molecule; JAM, junctional adhesion molecule; Tsp, thrombospondin; LFA, leukocyte functional antigen; ICAM, intercellular adhesion molecule; Fg, fibrinogen; GPIb-IX-V, glycoprotein complex present on platelet surface; vWF, von Willebrand factor; Vn, vitronectin; PECAM-1, platelet-endothelial cell adhesion molecute-1; Osp, osteopontin; Endo, endothelial cell; Epi, epithelial cells

can activate the neutrophil through specific receptors (**Table 73.3**). This step is critical for mediating the transition from rolling to arrest. Once the leukocyte has arrested, it polarizes then "crawls" through the endothelial lining of the vessel, known as *diapedesis*. Neutrophils migrate toward chemotactic factors released by (a) the bacteria itself (bacterial peptide, fMLF), (b) anaphylatoxins (C5a, C3a) produced after complement activation, and (c) chemokines and arachidonic acid metabolites produced by macrophages and fibroblasts present in the subendothelial matrix (**Fig. 73.2**). Locomotion through the subendothelial matrix requires additional integrins present on the neutrophils, which recognize matrix proteins, including fibronectin, collagen, vitronectin, and vimentin. Locomotion results in the release of both gelatinase granule and secretory

vesicle contents. The presence of a continued source of cell membrane receptors incorporated into the plasma membrane after vesicle exocytosis allows the neutrophil to establish firm contact with the activated vascular endothelium and presents complement receptors and receptors for bacterial products to assist in microbe opsonophagocytosis. The release of metalloproteinases in the gelatinase granules facilitates the migration of the neutrophil through the extracellular matrix.

In many situations, neutrophil recruitment to the vascular endothelium does not occur in the sequential manner just described. Neutrophils or platelets already recruited to an inflammatory focus can recruit other neutrophils. In vascular beds, such as the liver, kidney, and lung, geometric constraints affect neutrophil localization. In the lung, neutrophil recruitment

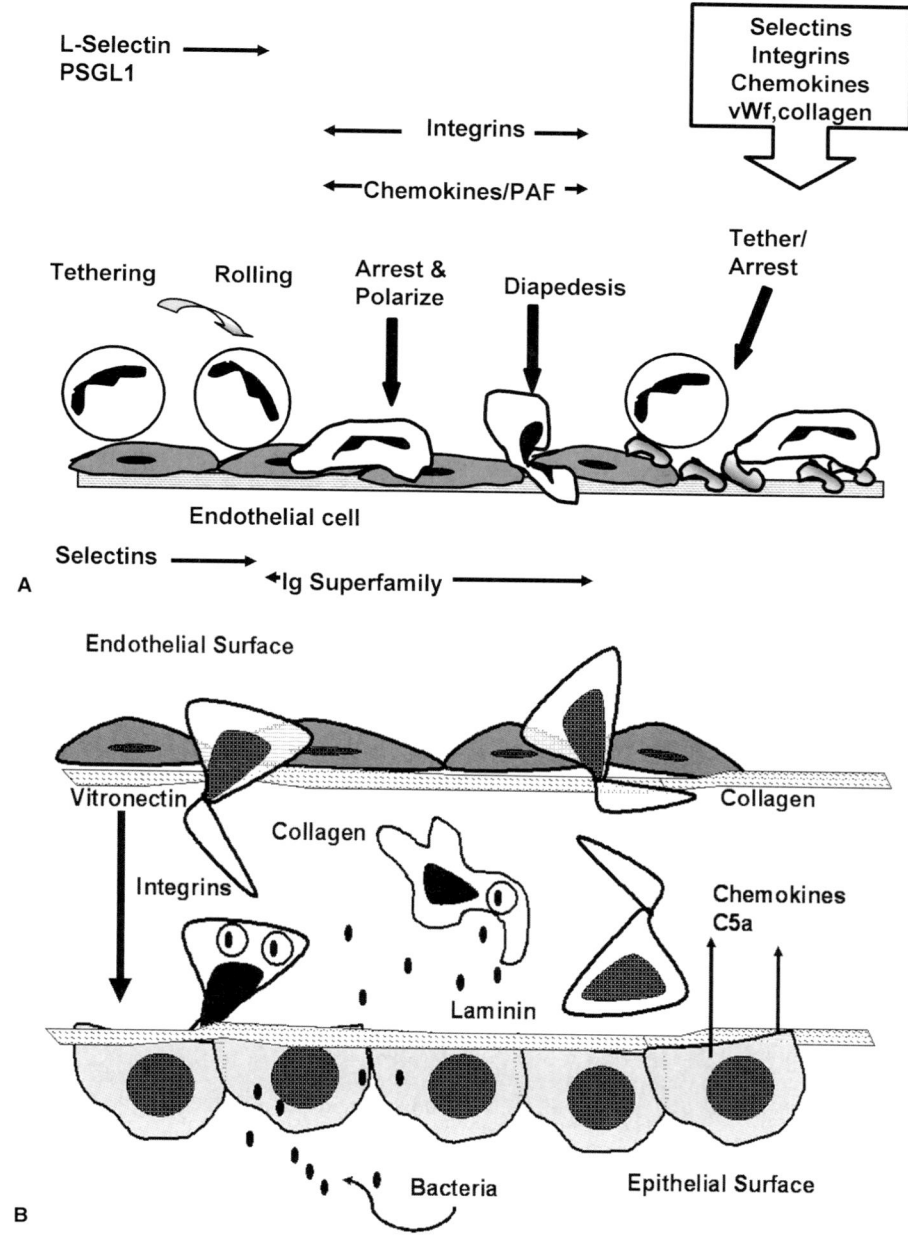

L-Selectin ——→
PSGL1

←—— Integrins ——→

←—Chemokines/PAF —→

Selectins
Integrins
Chemokines
vWf,collagen

Tethering   Rolling   Arrest &   Diapedesis   Tether/
                        Polarize   Arrest

Endothelial cell

Selectins ——→
A   ←Ig Superfamily ——————→

Endothelial Surface

Vitronectin   Collagen

Collagen

Integrins

Chemokines
C5a

Laminin

Bacteria   Epithelial Surface

B

FIGURE 73.2. Neutrophil localization. **A:** In an inflammatory focus, the endothelium, which is normally nonadhesive, becomes proadhesive as a result of activation by cytokines, such as IL-1β and TNF. Neutrophils are tethered from the free-flowing stream and roll on the endothelial lining of the blood vessel, an interaction mediated by all 3 members of the selectin family. The neutrophils slow, arrest, and change shape (polarize). Integrins and their ligands, the immunoglobulin gene superfamily, mediate the transition from rolling to arrest. This transition is also dependent on the production of activating agents by the endothelial surface, such as platelet-activating factor and IL-8. The neutrophils then crawl over the surface of the endothelium until they migrate through the endothelial monolayer. A neutrophil may be tethered by adherent platelets or another adherent leukocyte. Platelets themselves release chemokines, which activate neutrophils. Platelets may bind directly to von Willebrand factor (vWF) on the endothelial surface or on the basement membrane; alternatively, they may bind to collagen or fibronectin on the exposed basement membrane. **B:** Neutrophil localization in response to bacterial challenge. Bacteria present on the epithelial surface activate the epithelium to produce neutrophil chemokines NAP-2 (CXCL7) and ENA 78 (CXCL5); complement is activated, and the chemotactic factor C5a is produced. The epithelial surface also produces TNF-α and/or IL-1β, promoting the transition of the adjacent endothelial surface from an anti-adhesive to a proadhesive surface. Neutrophils emigrate out of the blood vessel across the endothelial cell lining and crawl through the basement membrane and along the connective tissue. This is mediated by members of the β_1-integrin family and CD11b/CD18 (Mac-1, $\alpha_M\beta_2$). These integrins interact with their specific epitopes in the basement membrane structural proteins (e.g., laminin and vitronectin) and collagen. Neutrophils can continue to emigrate across the epithelial surface. Upon encountering bacteria, neutrophils surround them with plasma membrane, forming a phagolysosome. In the phagolysosome, both oxygen-dependent and oxygen-independent mechanisms are operative, resulting in bacterial killing.

occurs in the capillary bed; in the liver, it occurs in the sinusoids. Using intravital microscopy, neutrophils appear to "hop" through the capillaries and sinusoids, rather than roll. They spend considerable periods of time in stationary contact with capillary endothelium, and this contact predisposes to adhesive interactions between the neutrophil and the endothelium. As neutrophils are exposed to inflammatory mediators, such as occurs in sepsis, they become more rigid. They are more easily trapped in lung capillaries and hepatic sinusoids (6). Though neither Mac-1 nor LFA-1 is required for neutrophils to localize to the bed, these adhesion molecules do mediate transmigration into the alveolus. However, the physical trapping of an activated neutrophil alone may be sufficient to result in injury, as described in following sections.

Opsonophagocytosis and Microbial Killing

The ingestion and disposal of microbes is a major aspect of neutrophil function. To facilitate recognition of microbes by neutrophils, these targets are covered with serum opsonins, which include proteolytic fragments derived from complement cascade and specific immunoglobulins. Receptors that recognize opsonized bacteria are present on the neutrophil surface (**Table 73.4**). These receptors include complement receptor 1 (CR1, CD35), CR3 (Mac-1 or CD11b/CD18), and receptors that recognize the Fc portion of immunoglobulin (FcRγ). Three Fcγ receptors recognize either monomeric IgG or complexed IgG. Neutrophils express FcRγII and FcRγIIIb, CD32 and CD16, respectively. These are low-affinity receptors and require

TABLE 73.3

CHEMOTACTIC FACTORS FOR NEUTROPHIL LOCALIZATION

Activating agent	Neutrophil ligand	Source
PAF	PAF receptor	Monocytes, endothelial cells
LTB$_4$	LTB$_4$ receptor	Monocytes, neutrophils
C5a	C5a receptor	Anaphylatoxin from complement activation
fMLF	fMLF receptor	Bacteria
C-X-C and CC chemokines		
IL-8 (CXCL8)	CXCR1, CXCR2	Endothelial cells, monocytes, neutrophils, T cells, epithelial cells
GRO-α, MGSA-α (CXCL1)	CXCR2>CXCR1	Epithelial cells
NAP-2 (CXCL7)	CXCR2	Epithelial cells
ENA-78 (CXCL5)	CXCR2	Epithelial cells
MIP-1α (CCL3)	CCR5, CCR1	T cells, monocytes
MIP-1β (CCL4)	CCR5	T cells, monocytes
RANTES (CCL5)	CCR1, CCR3, CCR5	T cells

Chemokines regulate cell trafficking of all types of leukocytes. Chemokines interact with a subset of seven-transmembrane spanning, G-protein-coupled receptors on the neutrophil surface. Chemokines for neutrophils are subdivided into major subfamilies based on the arrangement of the two amino-terminal cysteine residues CXC and CC. The CXC family has an amino acid between the two cysteine residues; the CC family does not.
PAF, platelet activating factor; LTB$_4$, leukotriene B$_4$; fMLF, formylmethionyl-leucyl-phenylalanine; CXCL, CXC chemokine ligand; CXCR, CXC chemokine receptor; GRO, growth regulating protein; MGSA, melanocyte growth stimulating activity; NAP, neutrophil activating peptides; ENA, epithelial derived neutrophil attractant; MIP, macrophage inflammatory peptide; CCL, CC chemokine ligand; CCR, CC chemokine receptor; RANTES, regulated on activation, normal T-cell expressed and secreted

IgG in a complex to signal the cell. As described in a previous section, CD16 is present in the gelatinase granules, and exocytosis of these granules results in upregulation of CD16. FcγRI (CD64) is a high-affinity Fcγ receptor. Neutrophils express little CD64; however, neutrophils treated with GCSF or interferon-γ, or neutrophils obtained from patients with bacterial infection, have dramatically increased amounts of CD64.

Ligation of FCγ and/or complement receptors initiates a cascade of biochemical events that results in the exocytosis of granules, the respiratory burst, and phagocytosis. As neutrophil receptors are activated, the plasma membrane "ruffles" and assumes a bipolar configuration, with the formation of a "head," or pseudopod, and "tail," or uropod. The pseudopod surrounds the microbe and fuses at the distal end to form a phagolysosome. The particle is internalized and generally completely surrounded by plasma membrane. Granules join this newly formed vacuole and discharge their contents within seconds. Release of myeloperoxidase from the primary granule is important for oxygen-dependent killing. Release of other granule contents, such as BPI, lactoferrin, and defensins, is critical for oxygen-independent killing.

The respiratory burst refers to the coordinated consumption of oxygen and production of metabolites that occur when neutrophils are confronted with appropriate stimuli, actions that are the basis of all oxygen-dependent killing by neutrophils and other phagocytes. The NADPH oxidase system is a transmembrane electron system in which NADPH, the primary electron donor on the cytoplasmic side of the membrane, reduces oxygen in the extracellular fluid or within the phagolysosome to form superoxide (O_2^-) (**Fig. 73.3**). In turn, two molecules

of O_2^- can spontaneously (or enzymatically through superoxide dismutase) form hydrogen peroxide (H_2O_2). While both H_2O_2 and O_2^- can directly kill bacteria, it is the hydroxyl radical (OH$^\bullet$) and hypohalous acids produced from O_2^- and H_2O_2, respectively, that are the most injurious to microbes and to healthy tissue/cells, if directly exposed. Myeloperoxidase released from primary granules forms hypochlorous acid (HOCl) from chloride ion and H_2O_2, which is directly toxic to microbes. Hypochlorous acid can react with amines to form N-chloroamines (RNHCl). RNHCl are lipophilic and can readily penetrate cellular membranes. HOCl and RNHCl can inactivate heme proteins, other proteins, and amino acids, and can oxidize DNA. OH$^\bullet$ formed in the presence of iron ions (Fe^{3+}) from O_2^- is a strong oxidant. HOCl, H_2O_2, and OH$^\bullet$ can participate in killing the microbe in the phagocytic vacuole. However, such reactive oxidants also activate latent neutrophilic metalloproteinases, such as collagenase and gelatinase, and inactivate plasma antiproteinases.

Modulation of the Immune Response

The mature neutrophil was thought of as an "end-stage" cell. However, a large body of work over the last 15 years demonstrates that the neutrophil retains its capacity for inducible gene expression and protein synthesis even after release from the marrow cavity. Mature neutrophils can synthesize a variety of cytokines, such as IL-1, IL-6, TNF-α, GM-CSF, macrophage colony-stimulating factor (M-CSF), and IL-8, all of which can influence the microenvironment. Production of these proteins occurs under conditions similar to those experienced by an

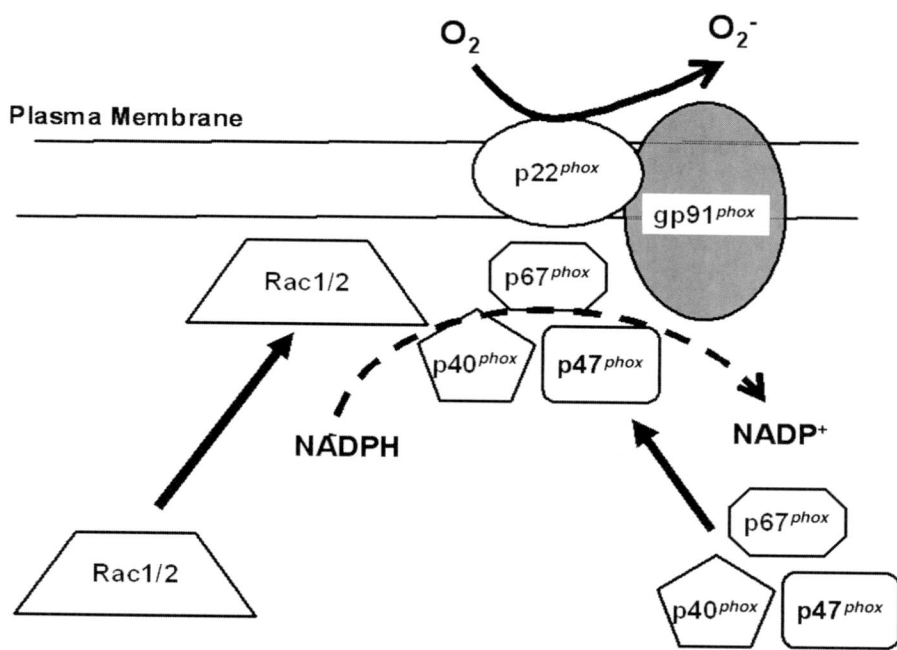

FIGURE 73.3. NADPH oxidase components and activation. On activation of the neutrophil, the 3 cytosolic components of the NADPH oxidase (p67^{phox}, p47^{phox}, and p40^{phox}) plus either Rac1 or Rac2 are translocated to the membrane of the phagocytic vacuole. The p47^{phox} binds to the membrane component of the NADPH oxidase, cytochrome b_{558} (gp91^{phox} plus p22^{phox}). The NADPH oxidase transfers an electron from NADPH to O_2 to form superoxide (O_2^-). The unstable superoxide is converted to hydrogen peroxide, either spontaneously or by superoxide dismutase.

emigrated neutrophil. While the amount of protein produced by an individual neutrophil is small compared to a monocyte/macrophage, for example, the amount produced by the large number of emigrated neutrophils is substantially greater. In addition, an emigrated neutrophil may continue to function for many days before it ultimately undergoes apoptosis.

Recent work has demonstrated that neutrophils have unique pathways that can afford control of gene product at the translational level in response to signals from the environment. Rapid protein synthesis without requirement for new transcription is one of several biologic advantages of "signal-dependent" translation of mRNA that is stored or silent in the basal state (29). For example, neutrophils contain constitutive mRNA for soluble IL-6 receptor-α (IL-6R-α) and retinoic acid receptor-α (RAR-α). After stimulation with PAF under the control of a specialized translational regulator, IL-6Rα and RAR-α protein is produced. IL-6Rα can result in *trans*-signaling events of the endothelial cell through the GP130-IL-6 complex on the endothelial surface. RAR-α is a nuclear hormone receptor and transcription factor that can regulate gene transcription of other products, such as IL-8 (29).

Preformed proteins released from granules can have profound influence on the microenvironment. Haptoglobin, an acute-phase protein, has been recently identified in the specific granules of neutrophils (49). Haptoglobin binds free hemoglobin, and haptoglobin-hemoglobin complexes are cleared by macrophages. Free hemoglobin serves as a source of iron, which may enhance bacterial growth and virulence or may participate in the generation of reactive oxygen species (ROS) (see preceding discussion regarding formation of OH$^•$). In addition to being antimicrobial, defensins released from the primary granule are also chemotactic for lymphocytes and monocytes, thus contributing the secondary wave of leukocytes required for resolution of infection. Neutrophils also produce vascular endothelial growth factor. While this growth factor is important in vascular proliferation, it also has a role in the develop-

ment of sepsis and in the progression of coronary artery lesions in acute Kawasaki disease (23,56).

Clearance of Neutrophils

The half-life of neutrophils is very short, less than 12 hrs in the circulation. Circulating neutrophils undergo apoptosis (programmed cell death) and are removed by the reticuloendothelial system of the spleen and bone marrow. In patients with sepsis, circulating neutrophils have profoundly delayed apoptosis (48).

Neutrophils that migrate to an inflammatory source have a prolonged half-life and increased function. However, these neutrophils do undergo apoptosis and are cleared from the tissue by inflammatory monocytes that have transformed to macrophages. Two apoptotic signal pathways have been characterized: the death receptor and the mitochondrial pathways. Both pathways ultimately result in the activation of caspase 3 and subsequent DNA fragmentation, chromatin condensation, and formation of the apoptotic body (27). Neutrophils can undergo apoptosis through either mechanism.

The induction of ligands on the apoptotic neutrophil results in recognition by the inflammatory tissue macrophages as an "eat me" signal. One signal, phosphatidylserine (PS), is formed during the early stages of apoptosis, as PS is relocated from the inner to the outer surface of the plasma membrane. PS is recognized by a specific PS receptor on the macrophage (22). Proteinases released by bacteria provide novel mechanisms for an "eat me" signal from the apoptotic neutrophil (22). The rapid influx of neutrophils must be followed swiftly by monocytes that mature into inflammatory macrophages. These macrophages can then either emigrate from the tissue into the lymphatics or proliferate and secrete reparative cytokines, such as transforming growth factor-β1 (TGFβ1), resolving the neutrophil accumulation and inflammatory process.

DEFECTS IN NEUTROPHIL NUMBER AND/OR FUNCTION

Neutrophils are important to the host defense at the epidermal/epithelial surface, which is continuously exposed to bacteria. Children with neutrophil defects will generally have recurrent bacterial infections of the skin, lung, oropharynx, and perirectal area. New defects in neutrophil function are continuously being identified. The following discussion focuses on several of the more prevalent defects. The reader is referred to scholarly treatises regarding this group of diagnoses (14,15,42).

Congenital and Developmental

Congenital Neutropenias

Congenital neutropenias encompass a diverse group; however, all are characterized by low neutrophil count (<200 neutrophils/μl). *Severe congenital neutropenia* (Kostmann syndrome) appears after birth, with 90% of all children symptomatic within 6 months. Several genetic defects are responsible for this phenotype. That which is associated with the GCSF receptor gene defect is also associated with increased susceptibility to infection. In these children, bone marrow arrest occurs at the promyelocyte or myelocyte stage. Omphalitis is often the presenting sign, but these children can also have upper and lower respiratory infections and skin and liver abscesses.

In children with *cyclic neutropenia/cyclic hematopoiesis*, a cyclic fluctuation occurs in all hemapoietic lines, though that of the neutrophil line is most marked. Neutrophil counts cycle at an average of 21 days, including periods of severe neutropenia that are 3–10 days in duration. In these children, oral ulcerations, gingivitis, pharyngitis, and tonsillitis are most common.

In both of these diseases, the use of GCSF has dramatically improved the outcome. GCSF has improved survival in children with Kostmann syndrome, and morbidity is improved in children with congenital neutropenia. However, in the latter, infections and hospitalizations naturally lessen with age. This is an important observation and reinforces the critical role that neutrophils play in younger children.

Defects of Oxidative Metabolism

The most widely recognized and most prevalent defect of neutrophil function is chronic granulomatous disease (CGD), a heterogeneous disease that is characterized by recurrent life-threatening infections with bacteria, fungi, and the formation of abnormal granulomata. The defect is in the NADPH oxidase, the enzyme system responsible for the oxidative burst. The NADPH oxidase is a six-protein complex that has two components—a membrane-bound complex embedded in the walls of the secondary granule (cytochrome b_{558}) and a distinct cytoplasmic component (**Fig. 73.3**). The cytochrome b_{558} is composed of a 91-kDa glycosylated β chain (gp91^{phox}) and a 22-kDa nonglycosylated α chain (p22^{phox}). The cytoplasmic components are p47^{phox}, p67^{phox}, p40^{phox}, and *rac*. The most common genotype of the CGD is the X-linked mutations of

gp91^{phox}, accounting for 70% of US cases. Males are affected, and females are carriers. With heavy lionization of the functional gene, an X-linked form of CGD has been reported in females. Defects in p47^{phox} occur in 25% of US cases, and defects in p22^{phox} and p67^{phox} occur in <5%. Clinically, CGD is quite variable and the age at presentation ranges from infancy to late adulthood. Typically, most affected individuals are diagnosed as toddlers and young children. The most frequent sites of infection are lung, lymph nodes, and liver. Of 360 patients in the CGD national registry in 2000, 80% had pneumonia and 68% had an abscess. Osteomyelitis, perianal abscess, and gingivitis are also common (53).

The functional defect is the inability of the NADPH complex to generate superoxide (O_2^-) and the downstream ROS, H_2O_2 and OH$^\bullet$, resulting in defective microbial killing and recurrent infections with catalase-positive bacteria. Organisms that produce their own H_2O_2 but do not degrade it (those that are catalase negative) supply the substrate for the formation of hypohalous acid by the myeloperoxidase released into the phagolysosome by the neutrophil. Note that other granule functions in the CGD neutrophils are intact. The metabolites of superoxide appear to be the mediators of bacterial killing in themselves. However, evidence suggests that the ROS are required for the activation of the primary granule serine proteases cathepsin G and elastase. Thus, ROS may be involved in other antimicrobicidal pathways in addition to producing a direct microbicidal effect. The overwhelming majority of infections result from *Aspergillus* (40%), *Staphylococcus aureus* (12%), *Burkholderia cepacia* (8%), *Nocardia* (7%), and *Serratia marcescens* (5%) (53). As many as 32% of those with CGD have gastrointestinal involvement, and 38% have urogenital involvement.

The cornerstone of treatment of CGD is trimethoprim/sulfamethoxazole prophylaxis. Since its institution, major infections have been reduced from 1 per year to 1 per 3.5 years; observations include fewer staphylococcal and skin infections and no increases in fungal infections. Itraconazole prophylaxis is routinely recommended in patients with CGD, regardless of age or previous fungal infections (42). A large, multicentered trial of interferon (IFN)-γ demonstrated 70% fewer infections, compared to placebo. It is unclear exactly how IFN-γ supports neutrophil function, as no difference in superoxide generation, bactericidal activity, or cytochrome b_{558} could be identified. A cohort of 80 patients in the original study, who had been on a regimen of IFN-γ for a mean of 9 years, demonstrated continued low incidence of serious infections (0.3 infections/patient year), with mortality rate of 1.5% per patient year (32).

Management of infections in these patients is critical to decrease morbidity and reduce mortality. Microbial diagnosis is critical. In severe infections, granulocyte infusions have been used; while they are potentially life saving, they may also complicate the ICU course (see later discussion on granulocyte transfusions). As the deletion for X-linked CGD is encoded next to the Kell blood antigen, deletion of the Kell locus may also occur, resulting in CGD with the McLeod phenotype. Hence, a potential transfusion hazard may exist in X-linked CGD patients. If Kell blood antigen-negative individuals are transfused with Kell-positive blood products (or granulocytes), antibodies to Kell antigen may develop. Therefore, all patients with CGD should be screened for Kell antigen. If they are found to be Kell negative, transfusion is best avoided, or Kell-negative erythrocytes or granulocytes should be used.

Glucose-6-phosphate dehydrogenase (G6PD) is the most common enzyme defect in humans, with ~400 million people affected worldwide. G6PD is involved in NADPH production through the hexose monophosphate pathway. As neutrophils have relatively few mitochondria, they rely on hexose monophosphate shunt activity for production of NADPH and energy formation. If NADPH is limited, impairment in respiratory burst may result. However, neutrophil dysfunction in patients with G6PD is less common than anticipated, as most individuals have >20% of G6PD activity in neutrophils, sufficient to maintain the respiratory burst in the normal range.

Defects of Leukocyte Adhesion and Trafficking

As outlined previously, it has been recognized for more than a century that leukocyte movement from the bloodstream toward inflammatory sites is critical for preventing and fighting infections. If neutrophils cannot localize to an inflammatory site, infections result. Children with recurrent, necrotic bacterial infections, impaired pus formation, and impaired wound healing were first described almost 30 years ago. Leukocyte adhesion deficiency-1 (LAD-1) with defects in the β_2 integrins was identified ~25 years ago; however, several new defects that lead to recurrent infections with defective neutrophil localization have been identified recently.

LAD-1 is an autosomal recessive disorder with mutations in the common chain of the β_2 integrin CD18 (33), which results in a deficiency in number or function of adhesion molecules Mac-1 (CD11b/CD18), LFA-1 (CD11a/CD18), and p150,95 (CD11c/CD18) on the cell surface. Neutrophils cannot adhere and transmigrate to the inflammatory focus. In addition, as Mac-1 is also the complement receptor 3, severely reduced complement-mediated phagocytosis occurs (**Tables 73.2** and **73.4**). Several clinical phenotypes are seen. Some patients have <1% of expression of these adhesion molecules. With this severe type, children usually present within the first months of life with omphalitis and delayed cord separation. They have severe infections, impaired pus formation, and impaired wound healing. They have neutrophilia at baseline, but with infections, the neutrophil count may rise >100,000/mcL. Recurrent infections of the skin, upper and lower airways, bowel, and perirectal area are common and are usually due to *S. aureus* or Gram-negative bacilli. Pathognomonic for neutrophil-adhesion defects, the skin lesions are necrotic, and almost no pus is seen surrounding them. An absence of neutrophil invasion is found on histopathology. In patients with a moderate phenotype, β_2-integrin expression may be up to 30% of normal adult controls. Infections are less ominous, but periodontal disease, leukocytosis, and delayed wound healing are still the rule. In an increasing number of LAD-1 variants, the quantity of β_2-integrin expression is normal, but functional defects occur. Treatment for these children is early and aggressive antibiotics. Bone marrow transplantation is the only definitive treatment for children with LAD-1.

In LAD-2 or congenital disorder of glycosylation IIc (CDGIIc), defects occur in glycosylation. Selectins must be appropriately glycosylated for full function (**Fig. 73.2A** and **Table 73.2**). In these children, neutrophils cannot be captured from the free-flowing stream; therefore, transition to an arrested cell—a critical step in leukocyte emigration—cannot occur. While these children do have severe recurrent infections, they also have associated neurodevelopmental defects due to glycosylation abnormalities.

TABLE 73.4

RECEPTORS FOR PHAGOCYTOSIS ON NEUTROPHILS

Receptor	CD classification	Ligand
FcγRI	CD64	Fc portion of IgG (high-affinity receptor)
FcγRIIA	CD32	Fc portion of IgG (low-affinity receptor)
FcγRIIIB	CD16	Fc portion of IgG (low-affinity receptor)
FcαRI		Fc of IgA
CR1	CD35	C3b>C4b>C3bi
CR3 (Mac-1)	CD11b/CD18	C3bi
C1qR		C1q

Complement fragments of C3: C3b, C3bi; complement fragment of C4: C4b; C1q is the q subunit of the complement complex 1.
CD, cluster of differentiation

Developmental Defects in Neutrophil Function

Bacterial infection is a major cause of death and long-term morbidity in preterm neonates. Infection rates among neonates who receive care in the NICU range from 25% to 50%. The large rate of infection is due to immaturity of bactericidal mechanisms. Clinical evidence demonstrates that the neonate's (and, in particular, the preterm infant's) immune incompetence closely patterns that observed in adult patients with profound neutropenia.

Newborn infants, whether born at term or very premature, have peripheral blood counts similar to older children and adults. However, they differ dramatically from adults in their response to sepsis. The profound, sustained neutrophilia with sepsis seen in adults is not found in neonates and premature infants. Instead, neonates and premature infants frequently become neutropenic during infection due to low neutrophil cell mass and an apparent inability to increase the proliferation of the early progenitor pool (7).

Neutrophils isolated from neonatal cord blood have diminished chemotaxis due, in part, to a decreased amount of Mac-1 that is mobilizable from the secretory vesicles and gelatinase granules. They also have diminished L-selectin (CD62-L) and P-selectin glycoprotein ligand-1 (PSGL-1), the ligand for P-selectin. Thus, at least in vitro, neonatal neutrophils have difficulty in being captured from the free-flowing stream, transitioning from a rolling to an arrested cell, and ultimately emigrating across the endothelial cell of the blood vessel (33). While term infants rapidly establish normal chemotactic function within 1–2 weeks, premature infants, whose chemotactic defect remains for weeks, do not.

In contrast, if bacteria are sufficiently opsonized, neonatal neutrophils demonstrate normal phagocytosis, although phagocytosis for *Candida* is decreased compared to adult neutrophils. As is true for term neonates, neutrophils from preterm infants are equally able to phagocytose fully opsonized bacteria. Critical is the fact that term or preterm plasma is unable to fully opsonize bacteria. Even adult neutrophils have defective phagocytosis if infant plasma is used for opsonization. However, while a therapeutic rationale exists for the use of IV gammaglobulin in neonates with established sepsis, no studies to date support the use of gammaglobulin to treat established infections or to prevent infections in the neonate.

Acquired Defects in Neutrophil Function: Malnutrition

Defects in phagocyte function are present in children with protein calorie malnutrition. While chemotaxis has been reported to be affected, bacterial ingestion and killing are consistently reduced. Decreases in several components of complement contribute to impaired neutrophil function. In addition, these children have defects in the mucous membranes of the respiratory, gastrointestinal, and urinary tract, making neutrophil function particularly critical for host defense (13).

NEUTROPHILS AND CRITICAL ILLNESS

Neutrophil Function in Critical Illness

It has been well recognized for several decades that neutrophils obtained from individuals with infection have diminished chemotactic function, compared to neutrophils from those same individuals after the infection has resolved. In human sepsis, neutrophil chemotaxis to the bacterial product fMLF and leukotriene B_4 (an arachidonic acid-derived chemotactic factor) is diminished. In patients with sepsis and multiple organ failure, chemotactic response to the chemokine IL-8 is also reduced. The loss of motility corresponds to reduction in the surface expression of the receptor for IL-8 and CXCR2, but not CXCR1 (11). Neutrophil Mac-1 (CD11b/CD18) was upregulated in the patients with sepsis and correlated with increased levels of IL-8, compared to normal volunteers (11). Increased Mac-1, CD64 ($Fc\gamma RI$), and "activation markers" were also found on neutrophils from patients with sepsis and were lower on patients who ultimately died (34). Neutrophil elastase was found in the serum of patients with severe sepsis and was correlated with disseminated intravascular coagulation (20). Neutrophil rigidity was increased overall in patients with sepsis. In those patients who recovered, rigidity returned toward normal, whereas in those individuals who did not improve, neutrophils remained rigid (16). In patients with sepsis and ALI, those who had diminished activation of the neutrophil transcription factors nuclear factor-κB and/or Akt had less time on the ventilator and improved survival compared to those who had increased activation of these transcription factors (55). Neutrophils from patients with sepsis have increased spontaneous oxidative burst activity. In traumatized patients, chemotaxis is delayed, spontaneous oxidative burst activity is increased, oxidative activity is diminished with further stimulation, and opsonophagocytosis is decreased.

Critical is the fact that circulating neutrophils from infected or traumatized patients are not the "same" as neutrophils from the same individual in the noninflamed or injured state. In many ways, these neutrophils appear to have already been stimulated. However, they may also be more prepared to fight infections. The high-affinity receptor for immunoglobulin, $Fc\gamma R1$ (CD64), is usually present in low amounts on neutrophils; however, in patients with sepsis, $Fc\gamma R1$ is upregulated dramatically. It is also possible that these differences in neutrophils in patients with sepsis or severe infections may be due to an increased pro-

portion of "aged" cells. Neutrophils have a limited lifespan in the circulation and, after 12 hrs, undergo spontaneous apoptosis. L-selectin (CD62L), which is critical to the initial "tether" of the neutrophil to the inflamed endothelium, decreases as they remain in circulation. L-selectin is markedly diminished in cells as these cells enter into apoptosis. In infection and trauma, circulating neutrophils have decreased markers of apoptosis and decreased L-selectin. Thus, the proportion of aged cells that would normally undergo apoptosis under noninflamed conditions decreases in those individuals with infections. GCSF and IL-6 increase transit time of neutrophils in the maturational pools and delay apoptosis, and they are both dramatically elevated in sepsis. GCSF administered to individuals with delayed wound healing demonstrated decreased neutrophil chemotaxis and decreased degranulation. However, respiratory burst and phagocytic activity were increased (21). Thus, the effects of critical illness on the neutrophil may not be due as much to the "illness" per se, but rather the release of factors which themselves result in a pool of neutrophils with increased inflammatory characteristics.

Neutrophils produced and circulating under such conditions contribute to organ injury. Strong evidence exists in animal models that trauma or ischemia results in "activated" neutrophils, and these neutrophils can sequester in remote organs, leading to injury. The evidence in humans is at least supportive of this hypothesis, if not as conclusive. Neutrophils from adults with pneumonia had increased ROS and content of elastase compared to neutrophils from adults with pulmonary edema (5). Furthermore, neutrophils obtained from the arterial circulation have decreased production of ROS compared to neutrophils from the central venous blood in patients with pneumonia, which is not the case in patients with pulmonary edema. It appears that neutrophils that are more "reactive" can be trapped in the human lung (2).

In adult neutropenic patients with respiratory failure and pneumonia, as many as one-third develop ARDS during their recovery from neutropenia (3). In a cohort of premature infants with respiratory distress who had early-onset neutropenia after birth, more were more likely to require greater inflation pressures on the ventilator and increased concentrations of inspired oxygen at 12 hrs, more required mechanical ventilation by 1 week, and more had pulmonary interstitial emphysema, intraventricular hemorrhage, and chronic lung disease, as compared to the cohort of premature infants with lung disease without neutropenia (18). Such examples are compelling evidence that, while neutrophils are critical to the host response, they are also involved in many of the diseases in the ICU.

Transfusion-related Acute Lung Injury

The neutrophil is the effector cell in transfusion-related ALI (TRALI). The animal models and human studies suggest that, for TRALI to develop, two "hits" must occur (44). The first results in activation of the endothelium, and a normal antiadhesive surface becomes proadhesive for neutrophils. Neutrophils become activated and sequestered in the lung. This first hit can occur from sepsis, trauma, and massive blood transfusion. The second hit is the infusion of specific antibodies directed against antigens on the neutrophil surface and/or biologic modifiers in the stored blood component, which activate the adherent or trapped neutrophils in the lung, causing neutrophil-endothelial injury, capillary leak, and ALI (44). Differentiating TRALI from transfusion-associated circulatory overload (hydrostatic pulmonary edema) may be difficult and may require more invasive studies, such as measurement of the left atrial pressure. Blood component and donor management strategies have been suggested to prevent TRALI, including the avoidance of blood products from individuals with known leukocyte antibodies, leukoreduction of blood components, shortening the storage time of cellular components to reduce accumulation of cytokines and other biologic response modifiers, and washing cellular components prior to transfusion.

Neutropenia and the ICU

Neutropenia clearly disposes patients to bacteremia, fungemia, and sepsis, but its effect on outcome in patients in the ICU is not completely clear. In adult critically ill patients with cancer, neutropenia does not affect the outcome, even in those individuals with sepsis (41). In a recent Cochrane Review, the use of colony-stimulating factors in patients with febrile neutropenia due to cancer chemotherapy reduced the amount of time spent in the hospital and time for neutrophil recovery, but no clear survival benefit was seen (12). Well-controlled trials of either GCSF or GM-CSF in neutropenic patients in the ICU have not been conducted. In small, noncontrolled cohorts of neutropenic patients in the ICU, use of colony-stimulator factors did not reduce the duration of neutropenia, the length of ICU stay, or survival.

In adult critically ill cancer patients, one-third experienced ARDS during neutrophil recovery (3). These patients were more likely to have leukemia/lymphoma, pneumonia, and prolonged neutropenia (>10 days duration) (3). In adult patients with neutropenia, respiratory status deterioration is associated with GCSF administration, in particular if individuals have pulmonary infiltrates during neutropenia. Even healthy adults can experience transient respiratory disturbances if they receive GCSF for granulocyte mobilization for blood progenitor cell transplantation. In such individuals, respiratory disturbances are minimized by use of continuous-infusion GCSF, rather than bolus injection. Under such conditions, equal numbers of granulocytes were obtained, but less neutrophil activation was observed (43).

The effect of neutropenia on children in the ICU is even less clear (47). In a large, multicentered study in a cohort of 359 ICU pediatric oncology patients, neutropenia was not associated with increased mortality, though fungal infections and higher Pediatric Risk of Mortality scores were associated with increased mortality. In another multicentered study of pediatric oncology patients, those with bacteremia and neutropenia had increased mortality (15%), compared to those who did not have neutropenia (4%, p <0.05) (51). As with adult patients, fungal infections in children with cancer are particularly problematic. Aggressive antineoplastic treatment, severe and long-lasting neutropenia, and/or lymphocytopenia are associated with fungal infections, but mortality is lower in children, compared to adults overall. In children, risk of death was almost fourfold higher if the patients were already receiving antifungals at the time of diagnosis (9). To date, no studies have been conducted in children to examine changes in lung function with the use of GCSF. Therefore, recommendations regarding the use of GCSF in neutropenic, critically ill patients must be individualized. In those neutropenic children with proven or suspected fungal infections in whom mortality is high, GCSF appears prudent. If neutropenic patients have sepsis (bacteremia and organ failure) along with neutropenia, again, GCSF would be indicated. However, those who have pneumonia or another pulmonary process and neutropenia may be at risk of developing worsening respiratory status with the use of GCSF. Therefore withholds GCSF or alternatively administering GCSF via continuous infusion should be considered.

In a meta-analysis that examined all studies in neonates who received either GCSF or GM-CSF in addition to antibiotics as treatment for serious infection, no survival benefit was seen at 14 days (8). A subgroup analysis (from 3 studies) of 97 infants who also had neutropenia showed a significant reduction in mortality by day 14. No benefit was observed from the use of prophylactic GM-CSF in decreasing sepsis; however, 1 study suggested that GM-CSF may provide protection against infection when given to preterm infants who are neutropenic or at high risk of becoming neutropenic (8).

Use of Colony-stimulating Factors in Non-neutropenic ICU Patients

Even though a number of studies have been conducted in both neonates (discussed previously) and adults, none contain conclusive evidence that either GCSF or GM-CSF improves outcome in the non-neutropenic patient. In a meta-analysis of 6 studies that enrolled ~2000 non-neutropenic adults with pneumonia, GCSF did not improve outcome (10). However, it is also clear that no excessive morbidity or mortality was associated with GCSF in this high-risk population. It is also important to highlight that GCSF and GM-CSF cannot be used interchangeably. GCSF differs from GM-CSF in its specificity of action on developing and mature neutrophils, its effects on neutrophil kinetics, and its toxicity profile. GM-CSF results in priming of monocytes/macrophages and release of inflammatory cytokines. GCSF also results in production of anti-inflammatory factors. In patients with sepsis, GCSF is markedly increased in the serum, while GM-CSF levels are equal to control or lower (35). GCSF or GM-CSF in the non-neutropenic ICU patient should only be used in the context of therapeutic trials.

Use of Granulocyte Transfusion in the ICU

In light of the previous descriptions of the use of GCSF to mobilize granulocytes for transfusion, it is hardly surprising that the use of granulocyte transfusions all but disappeared during the 1980s and 1990s. Little therapeutic benefit was observed, and reports surfaced regarding adverse pulmonary responses with granulocyte transfusions. At least some of the modest therapeutic effect appears to have been due to insufficient doses of granulocytes used and inability to harvest large quantities from donors. At least in adults, the use of GCSF and corticosteroid to stimulate increased cell counts for harvesting is well tolerated in general, though donors complain of bone ache, headache, and/or insomnia. Transfused granulocytes are able to localize to sites of infection in neutropenic subjects. Approximately 5% of transfusions had adverse pulmonary reactions in one study (39). All studies in adults have included a limited number of patients, and the trials were conducted prior to the availability of antifungal drugs that are more effective and less toxic than amphotericin B. A multicentered trial is now under way for adults.

In a meta-analysis of trials in neonates with confirmed or suspected sepsis and neutropenia (44 neonates), no benefit of granulocyte transfusion compared to placebo was observed (1). In one trial of granulocyte transfusion compared to IV immunoglobulin, a reduction in mortality was associated with granulocyte transfusion (1).

Critical Care Therapies and Neutrophil Function

Mechanical Ventilation

Since the early 1990s, studies have demonstrated that "mechanical stretch" of the lung results in lung injury. Ventilator-induced lung injury moved from the bench to the bedside with the ARDS network trial of low tidal volume versus high tidal volume. Mechanical stretch of the alveolar epithelium can lead to production of proinflammatory cytokines, in particular chemokines for neutrophils. In animal models of ventilator-induced lung injury, if neutrophils are depleted, ventilator-induced lung injury can be abrogated. However, in animal models, neutrophil activation occurs early in ventilator-induced lung injury, and injurious ventilation (high tidal volume) results in pulmonary neutrophil sequestration and decreased neutrophil deformability, but not to changes in adhesion molecule expression (30). In humans with ALI, the use of conventional ventilation strategy (compared to a protective ventilation strategy) for as little as 36 hrs resulted in increased production of plasma IL-6 and bronchoalveolar fluid, which activated donor neutrophils. In premature infants, the use of mechanical ventilation resulted in activation of circulating neutrophils and monocytes, as measured by increased CD11b/CD18 compared to infants treated with nasal CPAP (50).

Hypothermia

Mild hypothermia (32–34°C) is advocated in adult patients after cardiac arrest and possibly for traumatic brain injury. However, several lines of evidence suggest that hypothermia increases mortality in patients with sepsis and trauma and that hypothermia favors wound infections (31). Hypothermia decreases neutrophil motility, respiratory burst, and phagocytosis, thus potentially decreasing secondary inflammatory injury at the cost of increasing infection risk. In head-injured patients who were treated with hypothermia and pentobarbital, GCSF reversed the respiratory burst and phagocytosis abnormalities. It is unclear if GCSF would protect against nosocomial infections.

Cardiopulmonary Bypass

In cardiopulmonary bypass, interaction of the blood elements with the oxygenator membrane and the mechanical stress of the circuit on the cells result in an acute inflammatory process that is dependent on complement activation, production of platelet-activating factor and other arachidonic intermediates, and activation of the kallikrein system. Neutrophils are activated with increased oxidative burst, and myeloperoxidase, elastase, and lactoferrin are found in the plasma. This cellular activity is also true in extracorporeal membrane oxygenation (ECMO). Blood neutrophils from neonates who are being treated with ECMO are activated, and increased neutrophil elastase is found in the plasma, compared to those same neonates before ECMO is initiated. In addition, lung injury worsened once they were placed on ECMO. Leukocyte filtration systems for cardiopulmonary bypass or leukocyte depletion of blood used in ECMO circuits are useful to prevent injury induced by activated leukocytes.

Drug Effects

Barbiturates and Anesthetics. Barbiturates, midazolam, and propofol all have profound effects on neutrophils. All inhibit respiratory burst, and barbiturates inhibit chemotaxis, opsonophagocytosis, and intracellular killing. While anesthesia-relevant concentrations may have minimal effects, the considerably higher concentrations used in the ICU place patients potentially at risk for increased infections.

Pentoxifylline and Cyclic AMP Modulators. Pentoxifylline, a xanthine derivative, is a phosphodiesterase inhibitor used in adult patients for treatment of claudication. With the discovery that it also decreases *TNF* gene transcription in sepsis, pentoxifylline has attracted fresh attention as an anti-inflammatory agent. It has numerous functions, including preventing the development of necrotizing enterocolitis in neonates by preserving small-vessel function, preventing endothelial dysfunction in sepsis, enhancing prostacyclin release, and attenuating the release of thromboxane. Pentoxifylline increases erythrocyte and leukocyte deformability, presumably by increasing cyclic AMP levels. Methylxanthines suppress neutrophil chemotaxis, superoxide anion production, phagocytosis, and degranulation. In a meta-analysis of two single-centered, randomized, placebo-controlled trials of pentoxifylline in neonatal sepsis as an adjunct to antibiotics, all-cause mortality was reduced with the use of pentoxifylline, and no adverse events were found (24). Although the data are still limited, pentoxifylline should be considered in neonates with sepsis as an adjunct to antibiotic therapy.

The elevation of intracellular cyclic AMP results in decreased neutrophil adhesion, demonstrated with type IV phosphodiesterase inhibitors (rolipram) and the β_2 agonist isoproterenol, but not with type III phosphodiesterase inhibitors (milrinone). Neutrophils, monocytes, eosinophils, and mast cells have β_2-adrenergic receptors. Activation of neutrophil β_2-adrenergic receptors results in decreased IL-8-induced chemotaxis (52). Catecholamines, including epinephrine, norepinephrine, dobutamine, and dopamine, depress neutrophil phagocytic ability and production of ROS. Thus, many of the agents used commonly in the ICU can have direct suppressive effects on neutrophil function at the pharmacologic doses achieved.

Corticosteroids. The main anti-inflammatory effects of corticosteroids result from changes in the function of macrophages, monocytes, and granulocytes, including the decreased production of anti-inflammatory cytokines, inhibition of arachidonic acid metabolism, and decreased granulocyte adherence and migration. Lymphocyte number and function are also markedly affected by corticosteroids.

Modulating Neutrophil Function

Anti-integrin Therapy

With the critical role of neutrophils in pathophysiologic diseases, such as shock, ARDS, and ischemia-reperfusion injury, a number of therapies to block neutrophil adhesive function have been proposed and produced. Numerous animal studies have demonstrated that antiadhesive strategies are, in fact, successful. At least in theory, such strategies should also be beneficial in critically ill humans. Initial enthusiasm with this paradigm has given way to a number of negative human studies and a cautious reappraisal of the concept. Studies in traumatic shock, stroke, burns, myocardial infarction, and transplant have demonstrated no benefit of β_2-integrin, LFA-1, or ICAM-1 blockade in humans (57). Use of anti-α_4 or anti-$\alpha_4\beta_7$ therapy in inflammatory bowel disease, asthma, multiple sclerosis, and anti-$\alpha_L\beta_2$ in psoriasis has been more successful. These latter therapies do not target neutrophils per se, but other leukocytes—primarily lymphocytes (57).

Platelet Activating Factor Inhibition

PAF is a potent phospholipid synthesized by a large number of cells. Its functions are mediated through receptors that are located on a surface of a variety of cells, including the neutrophil. PAF is implicated in necrotizing enterocolitis in infants, asthma, systemic lupus erythematosus, rheumatoid arthritis, and Crohn disease. Neither the use of PAF acetylhydrolase (which increases the breakdown of PAF) nor the use of a PAF receptor antagonist has been demonstrated to decrease mortality in severely septic patients, although a substantial reduction in organ dysfunction has been achieved (37).

Neutrophil Elastase Inhibition

When neutrophils have reduced deformability, such as occurs in sepsis, severe trauma, and ALI, they potentially are trapped in capillaries. These neutrophils may then secrete neutrophil elastase, reactive oxygen products, and other soluble mediators of tissue injury. A selective inhibitor of neutrophil elastase, sivelestat, attenuates leukocyte adhesion in pulmonary capillaries and attenuates the decreased neutrophil deformability in animal models of sepsis. In humans with ALI, sivelestat infusion for 5 days also attenuated diminished neutrophil deformability. In a phase III multicentered, randomized, controlled trial of sivelestat in adult patients with ALI, no difference between sivelestat and placebo was seen in mortality or ventilator-free days at 28 days (58). An increase in mortality in the sivelestat group at 180 days was seen.

Activated Protein C

Despite multiple clinical trials of immunomodulatory therapies in severe sepsis through the years, only one has significantly affected outcome in adult patients. Surprisingly, that drug is the activated form of the naturally occurring anticoagulant protein C [drotrecogin alpha (activated), Vigris™]. Activated protein C (APC) decreased death by 20% in the PROWESS (Recombinant Human Activated Protein C Worldwide Evaluation in Severe Sepsis) trial, which included 1690 patients (4). If administered on day 1 of multiorgan failure, the drug had a greater effect on survival than if administered on day 2. In patients with sepsis and single-organ failure, APC did not improve outcome, and an increased risk of bleeding was associated with APC. A trial of APC in children with severe sepsis was halted early, as no benefit was detected with its use, although serious bleeding events were not greater with its use.

That the PROWESS trial demonstrated a benefit in adult patients with severe sepsis, but other anticoagulant therapy trials have had no effect, suggests that the role of APC may reside less in its role as an antithrombotic and more in its role as an anti-inflammatory. In human models of endotoxemia, at best an incomplete model of sepsis, APC had minimal effect on hemodynamics, inflammation, thrombin generation, and fibrinolysis. However, it inhibited leukocyte accumulation in the air spaces of subjects who received intrabronchial administration of endotoxin (36). Neutrophils express the endothelial protein C receptor (EPCR) on their plasma membrane. Treatment of neutrophils in vitro with APC inhibited neutrophil chemotaxis but had no effect on respiratory burst, bacterial phagocytosis, or apoptosis. Incubation of neutrophils and platelets in plasma from patients with sepsis resulted in increased adhesion to endothelial monolayers and self-aggregation, compared to incubation in plasma obtained from normal subjects. The addition of APC abrogated this increase in adhesion and aggregation, and the effect could be reversed by low-dose heparin (26).

CONCLUSIONS AND FUTURE DIRECTIONS

Many questions remain regarding the manipulation of neutrophil number and function in the PICU population. The neutrophil is at the foundation of the innate immune system. It is absolutely required for maintenance of the organism during the ongoing onslaught by environmental microbes and, in general, is sufficient to control invasion. However, neutrophil function can be compromised in the PICU in a number of circumstances, either by a limitation in number, as occurs with medication or genetic defect, or limitation in function. Some questions that should be addressed for the care of critically ill children are: (a) As neutrophils are activated in transfused blood, should all transfused blood be leukocyte-depleted for patients with ALI or those who are at risk of lung injury? (b) As pentoxifylline is a useful adjunct in neonates with sepsis, will it be useful in the older infant and child? Why has pentoxifylline not had increased use in the septic neonate? (c) Should GCSF be used in all critically ill neutropenic children or only in those without evidence of lung injury? Should GCSF be used in the subpopulation of patients who undergo therapies known to induce neutrophil dysfunction, i.e., barbiturate infusion and hypothermia? (d) Is the incidence of TRALI in children equal to that in adults? (e) APC has not been shown to improve outcome in infants and children with septic shock, though it has in adults. Is this due to inherent differences in adults and children in coagulation and/or inflammation? Can potential peptide mimetics be produced that provide the anti-inflammatory effects of APC without affecting hemostasis?

KEY POINTS

- Neutrophils are uniquely designed to deal with the host's interaction with microbes at mucosal and epithelial surfaces.
- Neutrophils released from the bone marrow during times of acute infection and injury function differently than neutrophils released during periods of normal hematopoiesis.
- Neutrophils released under such conditions are more rigid and more "sticky" and spontaneously produce increased amounts of ROS. It is thought that these cells may

contribute to organ dysfunction by being trapped in the capillary bed.

■ Neutrophils are critical to host immunocompetence, as is demonstrated by marked recurrent infections in individuals with congenital, developmental, or acquired defects in neutrophil function or number.

■ While the use of GCSF decreases hospitalization time of neutropenic patients, its use in the ICU population is far from clear. GCSF use and recovery from neutropenia may result in lung injury.

■ Transfusion-related ALI is more common than previously thought and should be considered in any patient with acute deterioration in lung injury. The effector cell is the neutrophil.

■ Granulocyte transfusion and the transfusion of activated neutrophils with blood cell transfusion may contribute to increased organ dysfunction, particularly pulmonary dysfunction. Leukocyte depletion of blood prior to use in ECMO circuits or use of leukocyte depletion filters in patients in cardiopulmonary bypass should be strongly considered.

■ Pentoxifylline appears to have a role in the care of neonates with sepsis.

■ The use of APC does not appear to be of benefit in children with severe sepsis, or in adults with single-organ failure and sepsis. It is of benefit in adults with severe sepsis.

References

1. Abraham E, Laterre PF, Garbino J, et al. Lenercept (p55 tumor necrosis factor receptor fusion protein) in severe sepsis and early septic shock: A randomized, double-blind, placebo-controlled, multicenter phase III trial with 1,342 patients. *Crit Care Med* 2001;29:503–10.
2. Azoulay E, Attalah H, Yang K, et al. Exacerbation with granulocyte colony-stimulating factor of prior acute lung injury during neutropenia recovery in rats. *Crit Care Med* 2003;31:157–65.
3. Azoulay E, Darmon M, Delclaux C, et al. Deterioration of previous acute lung injury during neutropenia recovery. *Crit Care Med* 2002;30:781–6.
4. Bernard GR, Vincent JL, Laterre PF, et al. Efficacy and safety of recombinant human activated protein C for severe sepsis. *N Engl J Med* 2001;344: 699–709.
5. Braun J, Pein M, Djonlagic H, et al. Production of reactive oxygen species by central venous and arterial neutrophils in severe pneumonia and cardiac lung edema. *Intensive Care Med* 1997;23:170–6.
6. Burns AR, Smith CW, Walker DC. Unique structural features that influence neutrophil emigration into the lung. *Physiol Rev* 2003;83:309–36.
7. Carr R. Neutrophil production and function in newborn infants. *Br J Haematol* 2000;110:18–28.
8. Carr R, Modi N, Dore C. G-CSF and GM-CSF for treating or preventing neonatal infections. *Cochrane Database Syst Rev* 2003;CD003066.
9. Castagnola E, Cesaro S, Giacchino M, et al. Fungal infections in children with cancer: A prospective, multicenter surveillance study. *Pediatr Infect Dis J* 2006;25:634–9.
10. Cheng AC, Stephens DP, Currie BJ. Granulocyte-colony stimulating factor (G-CSF) as an adjunct to antibiotics in the treatment of pneumonia in adults. *Cochrane Database Syst Rev* 2004;CD004400.
11. Chishti AD, Shenton BK, Kirby JA, et al. Neutrophil chemotaxis and receptor expression in clinical septic shock. *Intensive Care Med* 2004;30:605–11.
12. Clark OA, Lyman G, Castro AA, et al. Colony-stimulating factors for chemotherapy induced febrile neutropenia. *Cochrane Database Syst Rev* 2003;CD003039.
13. Cunningham-Rundles S, McNeeley D, Anaworanich J. Immune responses in malnutrition. In: Stiehm ER, Ochs HD, Winkelstein JA, eds. *Immunologic Disorders in Infants and Children.* Philadelphia: Elsevier, Saunders, 2004;761–84.
14. Dinauer MC. The Phagocyte System and Disorders of Granulopoiesis and Granulocyte Function. In: Nathan D, Orkin S, Ginsberg D, Look A, eds. *Nathan and Oski's Hematology of Infancy and Childhood.* Philadelphia: W.B. Saunders, 2003;923–1010.
15. Dinauer MC, Lekstrom-Himes JA, Dale DC. Inherited neutrophil disorders: Molecular basis and new therapies. *Hematology (Am Soc Hematol Educ Program)* 2000;303-18.
16. Drost EM, Kassabian G, Meiselman HJ, et al. Increased rigidity and priming of polymorphonuclear leukocytes in sepsis. *Am J Respir Crit Care Med* 1999;159:1696–702.
17. Faurschou M, Borregaard N. Neutrophil granules and secretory vesicles in inflammation. *Microbes Infect* 2003;5:1317–27.
18. Ferreira PJ, Bunch TJ, Albertine KH, et al. Circulating neutrophil concentration and respiratory distress in premature infants. *J Pediatr* 2000;136: 466–72.
19. Fitch PM, Roghanian A, Howie SE, et al. Human neutrophil elastase inhibitors in innate and adaptive immunity. *Biochem Soc Trans* 2006;34: 279–82.
20. Gando S, Kameue T, Matsuda N, et al. Serial changes in neutrophil-endothelial activation markers during the course of sepsis associated with disseminated intravascular coagulation. *Thromb Res* 2005;116:91–100.
21. Gerber A, Struy H, Weiss G, et al. Effect of granulocyte colony-stimulating factor treatment on ex vivo neutrophil functions in nonneutropenic surgical intensive care patients. *J Interferon Cytokine Res* 2000;20:1083–90.
22. Guzik K, Bzowska M, Smagur J, et al. A new insight into phagocytosis of apoptotic cells: Proteolytic enzymes divert the recognition and clearance of polymorphonuclear leukocytes by macrophages. *Cell Death Differ* 2007;14(1):171–82.
23. Hamamichi Y, Ichida F, Yu X, et al. Neutrophils and mononuclear cells express vascular endothelial growth factor in acute Kawasaki disease: Its possible role in progression of coronary artery lesions. *Pediatr Res* 2001;49: 74–80.
24. Haque K, Mohan P. Pentoxifylline for neonatal sepsis. *Cochrane Database Syst Rev* 2003;CD004205.
25. Johnston RJ, Babior BM. The Polymorphonuclear Leukocyte System. In: Stiehm ER, Ochs HD, Winkelstein JA, eds. *Immunologic Disorders in Infants and Children.* Philadelphia: Elsevier Saunders, 2004;109–28.
26. Kirschenbaum LA, Lopez WC, Ohrum P, et al. Effect of recombinant activated protein C and low-dose heparin on neutrophil-endothelial cell interactions in septic shock. *Crit Care Med* 2006;34:2207–12.
27. Kissoon N, Duckworth L, Blake K, et al. Exhaled nitric oxide measurements in childhood asthma: Techniques and interpretation. *Pediatr Pulmonol* 1999;28:282–96.
28. Levin M, Quint PA, Goldstein B, et al. Recombinant bactericidal/permeability-increasing protein (rBPI21) as adjunctive treatment for children with severe meningococcal sepsis: A randomised trial. rBPI21 Meningococcal Sepsis Study Group. *Lancet* 2000;356:961–7.
29. Lindemann SW, Weyrich AS, Zimmerman GA. Signaling to translational control pathways: Diversity in gene regulation in inflammatory and vascular cells. *Trends Cardiovasc Med* 2005;15:9–17.
30. Lionetti V, Recchia FA, Ranieri VM. Overview of ventilator-induced lung injury mechanisms. *Curr Opin Crit Care* 2005;11:82–6.
31. Mantz J, Paugam-Burtz C. Hypothermia, sepsis, and the granulocytes: Lessons to learn beyond the cytokines. *Crit Care Med* 2004;32:1974–5.
32. Marciano BE, Wesley R, De Carlo ES, et al. Long-term interferon-gamma therapy for patients with chronic granulomatous disease. *Clin Infect Dis* 2004;39:692–9.
33. Mariscalco MM. Integrins and Cell Adhesion Molecules. In: Polin RA, Fox WW, Abman SH, eds. *Fetal and Neonatal Physiology.* Philadelphia: Elsevier Saunders, 2004;1572–91.
34. Muller Kobold AC, Tulleken JE, Zijlstra JG, et al. Leukocyte activation in sepsis: Correlations with disease state and mortality. *Intensive Care Med* 2000;26:883–92.
35. Napolitano LM. Immune stimulation in sepsis: To be or not to be?. *Chest* 2005;127:1882–5.
36. Nick JA, Coldren CD, Geraci MW, et al. Recombinant human activated protein C reduces human endotoxin-induced pulmonary inflammation via inhibition of neutrophil chemotaxis. *Blood* 2004;104:3878–85.
37. Opal S, Laterre PF, Abraham E, et al. Recombinant human platelet-activating factor acetylhydrolase for treatment of severe sepsis: Results of a phase III, multicenter, randomized, double-blind, placebo-controlled, clinical trial. *Crit Care Med* 2004;32:332–41.
38. Orr Y, Taylor JM, Bannon PG, et al. Circulating CD10-/CD16 low neutrophils provide a quantitative index of active bone marrow neutrophil release. *Br J Haematol* 2005;131:508–19.
39. Price TH. Granulocyte transfusion therapy. *J Clin Apher* 2006;21:65–71.
40. Prince AS, Mizgerd JP, Wiener-Kronish J, et al. Cell signaling underlying the pathophysiology of pneumonia. *Am J Physiol Lung Cell Mol Physiol* 2006;291:L297–300.
41. Regazzoni CJ, Irrazabal C, Luna CM, et al. Cancer patients with septic shock: Mortality predictors and neutropenia. *Support Care Cancer* 2004;12: 833–9.
42. Rosenzweig SD, Uzel G, Holland SM. Phagocyte Disorders. In: Stiehm ER, Ochs HD, Winkelstein JA, eds. *Immunologic Disorders in Infants and Children.* Philadelphia: Elsevier Saunders, 2004;618–51.
43. Sato Y, Goto Y, Sato S, et al. Continuous subcutaneous injection reduces polymorphonuclear leukocyte activation by granulocyte colony-stimulating factor. *Am J Physiol Lung Cell Mol Physiol* 2004;286:L143–8.
44. Silliman CC. The two-event model of transfusion-related acute lung injury. *Crit Care Med* 2006;34:S124–31.
45. Springer TA. Traffic signals on endothelium for lymphocyte recirculation and leukocyte emigration. *Annu Rev Physiol* 1995;57:827–72.

46. Suwa T, Hogg JC, Klut ME, et al. Interleukin-6 changes deformability of neutrophils and induces their sequestration in the lung. *Am J Respir Crit Care Med* 2001;163:970–6.
47. Tamburro R. Pediatric cancer patients in clinical trials of sepsis: Factors that predispose to sepsis and stratify outcome. *Pediatr Crit Care Med* 2005;6:S87–S91.
48. Taneja R, Parodo J, Jia SH, et al. Delayed neutrophil apoptosis in sepsis is associated with maintenance of mitochondrial transmembrane potential and reduced caspase-9 activity. *Crit Care Med* 2004;32:1460–9.
49. Theilgaard-Monch K, Jacobsen LC, Nielsen MJ, et al. Haptoglobin is synthesized during granulocyte differentiation, stored in specific granules, and released by neutrophils in response to activation. *Blood* 2006;108:353–61.
50. Turunen R, Nupponen I, Siitonen S, et al. Onset of mechanical ventilation is associated with rapid activation of circulating phagocytes in preterm infants. *Pediatrics* 2006;117:448–54.
51. Viscoli C, Castagnola E, Giacchino M, et al. Bloodstream infections in children with cancer: A multicentre surveillance study of the Italian Association of Paediatric Haematology and Oncology. *Supportive Therapy Group-Infectious Diseases Section. Eur J Cancer* 1999;35:770–4.
52. Wenisch C, Parschalk B, Weiss A, et al. High-dose catecholamine treatment decreases polymorphonuclear leukocyte phagocytic capacity and reactive oxygen production. *Clin Diagn Lab Immunol* 1996;3:423–8.
53. Winkelstein JA, Marino MC, Johnston RB, Jr., et al. *Chronic granulomatous disease. Report on a national registry of 368 patients. Medicine (Baltimore)* 2000;79:155–69.
54. Yang D, Chertov O, Oppenheim JJ. Participation of mammalian defensins and cathelicidins in anti-microbial immunity: Receptors and activities of human defensins and cathelicidin (LL-37). *J Leukoc Biol* 2001;69:691–7.
55. Yang KY, Arcaroli JJ, Abraham E. Early alterations in neutrophil activation are associated with outcome in acute lung injury. *Am J Respir Crit Care Med* 2003;167:1567–74.
56. Yano K, Liaw PC, Mullington JM, et al. Vascular endothelial growth factor is an important determinant of sepsis morbidity and mortality. *J Exp Med* 2006;203:1447–58.
57. Yonekawa K, Harlan JM. Targeting leukocyte integrins in human diseases. *J Leukoc Biol* 2005;77:129–40.
58. Zeiher BG, Artigas A, Vincent JL, et al. Neutrophil elastase inhibition in acute lung injury: Results of the STRIVE study. *Crit Care Med* 2004;32:1695–702.

CHAPTER 74 ■ THE IMMUNE SYSTEM AND VIRAL ILLNESS IN THE CRITICALLY ILL

LESLEY DOUGHTY

The focus of this chapter will be the impact of common viral infections on immune function. Viral infections such as human immunodeficiency virus (HIV) deplete lymphocyte subsets, thereby creating vulnerability to opportunistic pathogens. The immune defects progressively worsen until death. As such, HIV represents the most extreme example of immunomodulation induced by viral infection. The effect of this viral infection on immune function is well understood; however, the effect of common viral infections, such as influenza A and B, respiratory syncytial virus (RSV), parainfluenza, adenovirus, enterovirus, and cytomegalovirus (CMV), on host immunity is less well appreciated and will be discussed in this chapter. Disruption of the mucosal/epithelial protective barriers important for tissue homeostasis and infection prevention can provide a portal of entry for bacteria. This aspect of viral infection has long been appreciated and thought to be the critical event in creating a permissive state for secondary bacterial infection. Research during the 1990s has identified that many alterations in immune function also occur during common viral infections and contribute to the evolution and severity of secondary bacterial infection.

In addition to increasing the risk of bacterial infection, viruses have been implicated in exacerbations of, and morbidity from, diseases such as asthma and a variety of autoimmune diseases. The data also suggest that viral infection may alter immune function, setting the stage for disease exacerbation, which can often lead to critical illness. Acute primary and reactivated latent viral infections, such as CMV in the immunosuppressed population, can be life-threatening; aggressive prophylaxis and/or treatment is used in transplant recipients. Reactivation of such viruses also occurs in critical illness, and the contribution of this viral activity on critical illness and immune function is not clear. This contribution to a number of disease states will be discussed to introduce the concept that viral infection can have more far-reaching effects on the host than simply acute infection-related symptoms. Given the frequency of infection and the duration of the immune response to common respiratory and gastrointestinal viruses in infancy and childhood, it is possible that these pathogens contribute significantly to vulnerability to, and morbidity from, critical illness in the pediatric population.

APPLICATION TO PEDIATRIC CRITICAL CARE

The frequency of viral infections in the pediatric population warrants consideration of the impact of viral infection on immunity in this population. For the most part, the viral illness can directly cause critical illness due to primary infection (bronchiolitis, croup, and influenza). However, the relationship between viral infection and serious bacterial infection is not often considered, except in post-influenza pneumonia and reactivation of latent viruses such as CMV in the immunosuppressed population (post-transplant and congenital immunodeficiency). A significant amount of data in the adult literature and, to a lesser degree, in the pediatric literature describe relative immunocompromise during critical illness of several etiologies. Some data demonstrate that CMV reactivation in critically ill adults worsens the outcome of critical illness. This finding has not been studied in critically ill children, who are not traditionally considered immunosuppressed. Given the adult data (discussed later), this association should be studied in children to evaluate the presence of, and potential contribution from, reactivated latent viruses in pediatric critical illness.

Children who suffer from asthma exacerbations are a constant presence in the PICU, due in part to the prevalence of serious asthma in children. Frequently, asthma exacerbations are preceded by viral symptoms. Antiviral immunity, including susceptibility to viral infections in the asthmatic, the mechanisms that lead to viral destabilization of asthma, and the synergy between allergen exposure and viral infection in this setting, has not been commonly considered and has essentially been unexplored in the critically ill asthmatic. All patients with status asthmaticus are essentially treated with the same strategies, including steroids, β agonists, and, in some cases, magnesium for bronchospastic symptoms. The potential use of immune strategies to reduce the exacerbating effect viral infection on bronchospastic symptoms in the most severe cases has not been explored.

Autoimmune disease leading to critical illness is not a common problem; however, when it does occur, it can be life-threatening and difficult to manage. For the most part, the role of viral infection in this setting has not been examined in children (except in new-onset type 1 diabetes mellitus). As in asthma, a thorough knowledge of the association between viral infections and exacerbation (and in some cases, etiology) of autoimmune disease may provide potential targets for interrupting the influence of viral infection in these settings.

The discussion here will present what is known epidemiologically and mechanistically about the impact of viral infection on immune function and its consequences. Given the frequency with which viral infection precedes critical illness, these data are pertinent to pediatric critical care.

SCIENTIFIC FOUNDATIONS

Immune Response to Viral Infection

Mucous membrane surfaces, respiratory epithelium, and skin are portals of entry for many viruses. As viral infections depend on host cellular machinery for survival and replication, entry into cells is a critical early step. Entry into cells is accomplished via a variety of mechanisms, some of which are common to many viruses, whereas others are virus specific. Examples of mechanisms that are shared by multiple viruses are fusion with cell membrane (enveloped viruses) and/or endocytosis after binding to cell-surface molecules. Many cell-surface molecules are exploited by viruses to gain entry into cells to facilitate viral replication. Expression of such molecules is cell-type specific and can determine tissue tropism for certain viruses. Examples of exploited host cell-surface molecules include CD4, CCR5, and CXCR4 for HIV; sialic acid residues for influenza; heparan sulfate and proteoglycans for herpesviruses and coxsackie adenovirus receptor; and B-cell receptors CD21 and C3d for Epstein-Barr virus (EBV).

Once viruses are in contact with cells, viral replication and the host response to viral infection begin. Viral replication can directly injure mucosal and epithelial protective barriers by causing cell lysis upon replication and release (**Table 74.1**). Via killing of virus-infected cells and expression of inflammatory mediators, the antiviral immune response can cause further mucosal injury. The immune response to microbial pathogens consists of several phases. The earliest and least specific is the innate immune response, followed by a pathogen-specific

adaptive immune response that leads to immunologic memory. These phases of immune response include activation of diverse cellular and humoral mediators, many of which are common to many types of infections. The immune response to viral infection involves mechanisms similar to immune responses to bacterial infections, as well as unique mechanisms. Recognition of viruses by the innate immune system begins by the host recognition of viral pathogen-associated molecular patterns (PAMPs) through their interaction with pattern recognition receptors (PRRs) such as the Toll-like receptors (TLRs), thereby initiating the immune response. Viral PAMPs include virion proteins, hemagglutinin, double-stranded RNA produced during replication of many viruses, F protein from RSV, single-stranded RNA, and viral DNA (1,9). TLRs 2, 3, 4, 7, 8, and 9 have been implicated in responses to viral PAMPs (1). In fact, the initial cellular reactions to viral PAMPs are very similar to those initiated by bacterial PAMPs (1) (**Figs. 74.1** and **74.2**). The innate response is critical for containment of viral particles and initiation of the adaptive, or antigen-specific, immune response that is necessary for viral eradication and immunologic memory. Binding to TLRs initiates intracellular signal transduction, which leads to production of inflammatory cytokines, including interferons (IFN)-α and -β (IFN-α/β), IFN-γ, tumor necrosis factor (TNF)-α, IL-12p70, IL-10, and many chemokines that facilitate trafficking of cells to sites of viral invasion (39). TLR-independent mechanisms for cytoplasmic viral detection also exist, including but not limited to, activation of the helicases retinoic-acid-inducible protein (RIG-1) by intracellular viral dsRNA produced during the replication of many viruses. This pathway is critical for induction of interferons, which are essential antiviral cytokines (1). These pleiotropic cytokines can affect viral replication by reduction of "viral receptor" molecule expression on the host cell surface and inhibition of transcription and translation of viral proteins through IFN-stimulated genes, such as Mx protein, 2′5′-oligoadenylsynthase, and double-stranded RNA kinase, and eukaryotic initiation factor-α (eIF-2α) thereby inhibiting viral replication (9).

IFNs activate natural killer (NK) cells and macrophages, induce maturation of dendritic cells, and upregulate proteins that are important in antigen presentation to T cells that are critical for antigen-specific immunity. Macrophages and dendritic cells can bind de novo synthesized intracellular viral peptides via the major histocompatibility complex (MHC) I and extracellular viral peptides via MHC II. Once activated by viruses, these cells mature as they migrate to draining lymph nodes, where they present viral antigens to CD4 T cells via MHC I and II. Antigen-activated CD4 and dendritic cells are critical for stimulation of CD8 cytotoxic T cells and B cells. Dendritic cells can present viral antigens to CD8 T cells via MHC I molecules, inducing an antigen specific proliferation of CD8 T cells. Cytotoxic CD8 T cells can eliminate virus (a) by further induction of another essential antiviral cytokine, IFN-γ, (b) by lysis of virus-infected cells via the release of perforin (a membrane pore-forming protein important for cytotoxicity), and (c) by induction of apoptosis through Fas ligand with Fas (CD95) on the virus-infected cells (9). A result of this immune cascade is eradication of the virus, production of antibodies specific for multiple viral peptides, and creation of memory T cells and B cells important in protection against subsequent infection with the same virus.

TABLE 74.1

MECHANISMS OF BACTERIAL ADHERENCE TO HOST CELLS DURING VIRAL INFECTION

Respiratory epithelial disruption	Loss of mucociliary function
	Basement membrane exposure
Bacterial features	Fimbriae
	Capsule
Expression of viral glycoproteins	Neuraminidase (influenza/ parainfluenza)
	Hemagglutinin (influenza/ parainfluenza)
	Glycoproteins F and G (RSV)
Upregulation of host cell receptors	CD14, CD15, and CD18
	PAFR
	Complement protein C3
	Fimbriae-associated receptors
	IgA translocating receptor
	Pentameric IgM
Proteins from injured ECM	Fibrinogen
Other	Coupling bacteria to epithelium by RSV
	Altered bacterial adhesins

RSV, respiratory syncytial virus; PAFR, platelet activating factor receptor;ECM, extracellular matrix. Adapted from Hament JM, Kimpen JL, Fleer A, et al. Respiratory viral infection predisposing for bacterial disease: A concise review. *FEMS Immunol Med Microbiol* 1999;26:189–95.

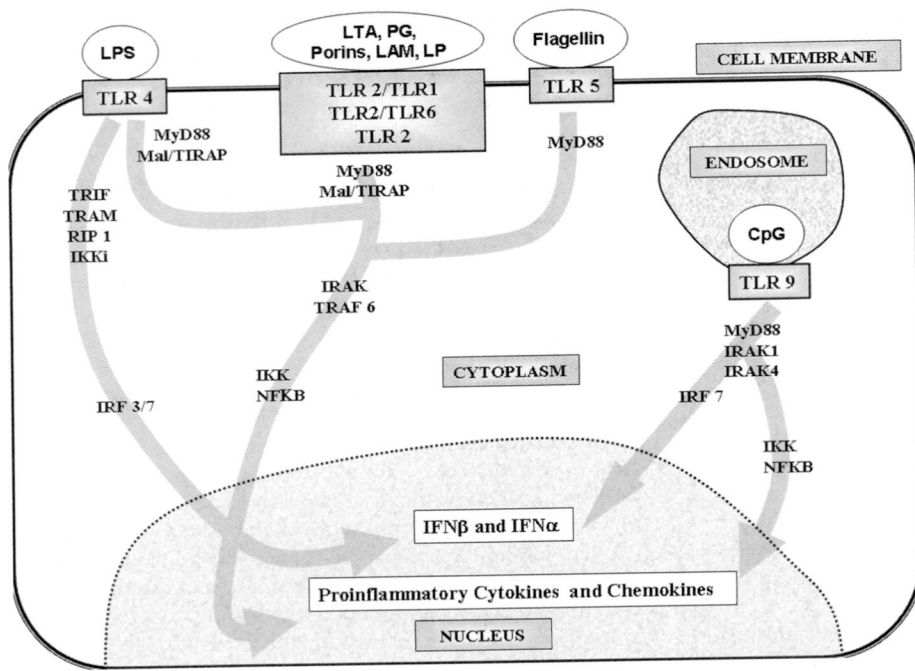

FIGURE 74.1. Early signaling initiated by bacterial pathogen-associated molecular patterns (PAMPs). Pattern recognition receptors (PRRs) recognize many components of bacteria, providing early signaling to initiate inflammatory responses to invading pathogens. The signaling pathways are shared by many Toll-like receptors (TLRs); however, the specificity of each differs, providing the ability to respond to a diverse range of pathogens. Considerable overlap between signaling pathways exists, leading to common endpoints, such as nuclear factor κB (NFκB) activation, which leads to induction of inflammatory cytokines and chemokines. Induction of IFN-α, IFN-β, and other interferon-inducible genes occurs by binding of TLR-2, -4, and -9 ligands. Adapted from Akira S, Uematsu S, Takenchi O. Pathogen recognition and innate immunity. *Cell* 2006;124:783–801

IMPACT OF VIRAL INFECTION ON ANTIBACTERIAL DEFENSE

Many reports present evidence that viral infection can compromise antibacterial function, thereby creating a permissive state for bacterial superinfection (**Table 74.2**). The antibacterial functions of many immune cell types are altered during and/or after viral infections. Examples of these effects are listed in **Table 74.2** (16,29,35,37). These effects have been elucidated using several viral infection models, including RSV, influenza, hepatitis B, CMV, EBV, HIV, and measles virus. Some induced immune defects are shared, and some are unique to specific viral infections. In addition, the duration of these defects is variable but usually transient, with the exception of those caused by HIV.

Many experimental examples of immune dysfunction induced by viral infection have been described both in vitro and

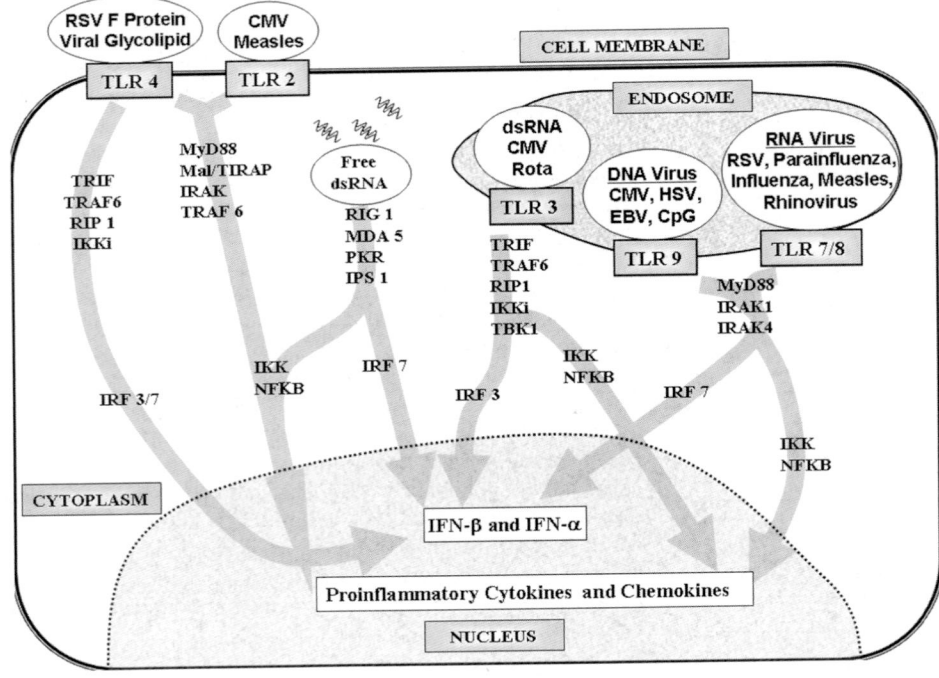

FIGURE 74.2. Early signaling initiated by viral PAMPs. Many viruses are recognized by TLR viral PAMPs, such as the fusion protein of respiratory syncytial virus (F protein), dsRNA, DNA, hemagglutinin protein, and envelope proteins. The PAMPs that are associated with many viruses that are capable of signaling through TLRs have not been identified. Intracellularly, many of the adaptor molecules and kinases activated by TLRs are shared and, as with bacteria, ultimately initiate similar inflammatory cascades via NFκB- and IFN-β-mediated signaling. Both of these pathways are important in containment of viral infections. As many aspects of the signaling pathways activated by both viral and bacterial PAMPs are shared, the impact of sequential signaling (e.g., viral followed by bacterial) has not been well characterized. Adapted from Akira S, Uematsu S, Takenchi O. Pathogen recognition and innate immunity. *Cell* 2006;124:783–801.

TABLE 74.2

IMMUNOMODULATORY EFFECTS OF VIRAL INFECTIONS

Cell type	Decreased	Increased
Macrophages	MHC expression	Inflammatory cytokines
	Activation and recruitment Phagocytosis Bacterial killing Antigen presentation	
Neutrophils	Bacterial killing	TLR-2 expression Apoptosis
Dendritic Cells	Altered IFN-α/β production Altered IFN-γ signaling MHC expression Antigen presentation	Apoptosis
NK Cells	Activation	
T Cells	CD4 proliferation CD8 cytotoxicity Th-2 cytokines Regulatory T-cell activation DTH response	Th-1 cytokines Apoptosis
Other	Bone marrow suppression Complement activation	

MHC, major histocompatibility complex; TLR, Toll-like receptor; DTH, delayed-type hypersensitivity

in vivo. Both RSV and influenza have been shown to significantly depress binding of bacteria, phagocytosis, and bactericidal activity in a monocyte cell culture system as well as in alveolar macrophages from virus-infected mice (33,42). Another such example describes a mouse model of pneumococcal pneumonia induced by nasal inoculation on day 14 after influenza infection (virus eradicated by day 14), resulting in significant enhancement of lethality, increased pulmonary pneumococcal counts, and significantly increased proinflammatory and anti-inflammatory cytokine levels (49). This study demonstrated two important points: (a) continued presence of live virus is not required for enhancement of lethality from secondary bacterial infection; and (b) this effect occurred 2 weeks post viral infection, demonstrating a prolonged effect on the host defenses. The duration of this effect is not known, as later time points were not tested.

Other less common viruses that are implicated in inducing a state of immunosuppression include measles, CMV, herpes viruses, and HIV. Many mechanisms of viral-induced immune suppression are thought to contribute to immune evasion and, in some, to have the ability to establish latency rather than be eradicated.

Measles continues to contribute significantly to childhood morbidity and mortality worldwide, and its complications have been implicated in more than 1 million deaths annually (32,43). Measles infection suppresses many aspects of the immune response, leading to profound vulnerability of the host to secondary infections. This immune modulation can persist many weeks (up to 6 months in some cases) after resolution of the acute measles infection and presence of the virus (32). The significance of this prolonged effect is evident by the frequency of complications that occur after measles infection. Most of the secondary infections result in pneumonia and diarrhea caused by other viral, bacterial, and parasitic infections as a result of immunosuppression. The mechanisms reported include depressed delayed-type hypersensitivity reactions, poor antigen presentation, poor lymphocyte proliferative response to mitogens, accelerated apoptosis of DCs and lymphocytes, bone marrow suppression, altered IFN-α/β production and signaling, and diminished DC IL-12p70 production, with a long-lasting shift toward a Th-2 response and sustained elevated levels of IL-4 (32). As with other viral infection, triggers for these effects include expression of measles viral proteins, including hemagglutinin, fusion proteins H and F, measles virus nucleoprotein, and the nonstructural proteins C and V. Measles can also initiate signaling through host cell receptors such as CD46 and CD150, both of which are important in regulating complement activation and T-cell and macrophage activation, and in sustaining the Th-2 cytokine profile. The consequence of these factors is prolonged immunosuppression from a transient viral infection, resulting in a high frequency of secondary infections.

Human CMV is an important pathogen and is endemic throughout the world. The infection often occurs in childhood, with 30%–40% incidence within the first year of life. In most immunocompetent people, CMV causes asymptomatic or very mild illness, and, in some, it causes a mononucleosis-like syndrome. In immunosuppressed individuals, it can cause severe or even fatal disease involving liver, lung, gastrointestinal tract, and central nervous system. In addition to its direct pathology, CMV is a virus capable of modulating the immune response, permitting its persistence in a latent state. It is likely that strategies important to CMV's ability to evade the immune system are also responsible for the generalized state of immune suppression seen during and transiently after acute infection (11). Multiple studies have described numerous alterations in host immune function, including loss of delayed-type hypersensitivity response to recall antigens, reduced lymphoproliferative responses and NK-cell activity, and suppressed bone marrow myelopoiesis compared to noninfected immunosuppressed individuals (11). CMV can infect dendritic cells and, in doing so, modulate the function of this critical aspect of host defense and contribute to viral persistence and subsequent immunosuppression. Expression of MHC molecules on the surface of CMV-infected DCs is diminished, reducing antigen presentation and T-cell proliferation and increasing DC-mediated apoptosis of activated T cells experimentally (40). Many of these findings have also been confirmed using monocyte-derived dendritic cells from immunocompetent adults infected with CMV (11). In recipients of orthotopic liver transplant, CMV disease (primary or reactivated) frequently preceded bacteremia and/or invasive fungal disease. This association was very strong, and CMV disease was statistically predictive for these two post-transplant complications. The use of anti-CMV treatments (ganciclovir or anti-CMV IgG) post-transplant reduced the incidence of invasive fungal disease. These data demonstrate the importance of the immunosuppressive effects of CMV disease even in a pharmacologically induced immunosuppressed state (12).

In addition to suppressing elements of the immune response, antecedent viral infection has also been shown experimentally to potentiate the response to secondary inflammatory challenges. Several reports cite synergy of viral infection, including adenovirus, influenza, CMV, and lymphocytic choriomeningitis virus, with an aseptic (lipopolysaccharide) or septic challenge (bacterial pneumonia or cecal ligation and puncture). This sequence of insults (viral infection followed by bacterial challenge) resulted in a potentiated inflammatory cytokine response, increased macrophage and neutrophil migration into infected tissues, and heightened lethality (7,10,11,26). Another mechanism for influenza-induced potentiation of the response to bacterial infection involves upregulation of TLR-2 on neutrophils, leading to increased respiratory burst activity in response to TLR-2 ligands, such as peptidoglycan from Gram-positive bacteria. This study also demonstrated increased phagocytosis of bacteria followed by enhanced neutrophil apoptosis, demonstrating significant alterations in neutrophil function after the onset of viral infection (23). These experiments highlight the importance of dysregulated inflammatory responses combined with poorly contained bacterial growth leading to heightened morbidity and mortality of bacterial superinfection following viral infection. It is very likely, although not yet proven, that this effect contributes to the severity of post-viral pneumonias, post-varicella toxic shock syndrome (TSS), and necrotizing fasciitis by facilitating a high bacterial burden with a potentiated inflammatory response. Given the epidemiologic data, it is also possible that these mechanisms contribute to severe presentations with high-grade bacteremia in such entities as meningococcemia, suggesting an association between viral infection and meningococcemia.

Viral and Bacterial Coinfection

The association between viral infection and bacterial infection has been repeatedly described for the following sequences: respiratory viruses such as influenza, RSV, and parainfluenza with a secondary bacterial pneumonia; varicella with TSS or necrotizing fasciitis; measles with bacterial pneumonia; and influenza with meningococcemia or toxic shock. Other viruses, including rotavirus and enterovirus, have also been associated with bacterial coinfection. Data that demonstrate important associations of antecedent/coincident viral infection complicated by serious bacterial disease include epidemiologic, human clinical studies, and experimental animal studies.

Several reports have described temporal epidemiologic associations between recent influenza infection and meningococcal disease outbreaks. Some reports cite the simultaneous seasonal peaks of both diseases, and others describe discrete outbreaks of meningococcal disease preceded by influenza outbreaks (18,24). Although these reports did not establish causality, the association was quite marked.

Antecedent and/or concurrent influenza infection has also been strongly associated with secondary bacterial pneumonia, which has historically carried with it severe morbidity and high mortality (38). A study of 154 children who were admitted with serious pneumonia demonstrated that the etiology in 23% of patients was bacterial and viral combined. The viruses present in this coinfected group included mostly influenza A or B, followed by RSV, parainfluenza 1–3, and adenovirus. This dually infected group had the longest hospital stay, the most pleural effusions, the most mechanically ventilated patients, and the only mortalities (28). Another study identified a small group of children with severe pneumonia and empyema who required chest tube placement, decortication, and in some, lobectomy. Many of these were pneumococcal in origin, and 77% of these had convalescent serum positive for the H1N1 influenza A strain several weeks after admission. The incidence of positive convalescent serum was higher in this group than in healthy control children from the same season, suggesting that antecedent influenza may have contributed to the severity and complications of the bacterial pneumonia (34). Many other studies support this association, demonstrating a 3%–45% incidence of coincident viral and bacterial pneumonia (48). In fact, some authors speculate that the seasonal fluctuation of invasive pneumococcal disease, which peaks in the winter months, may be related to winter virus exposure, including influenza and RSV (46). In addition, a possible role is emerging for antecedent viral infections, including influenza in severe community-acquired, methicillin-resistant *Staphylococcal aureus* pneumonia (13). Multiple studies also note that the incidence of severe group A β hemolytic streptococcal disease (GAβHS) also occurs coincident with influenza epidemics (36).

Studies that specifically examined infants with severe RSV (admitted to PICU) revealed a high incidence (38%–44%) of bacterial coinfection in mechanically ventilated infants whose tracheal aspirates were sent for culture. The incidence of coinfection may even be higher but not identifiable due to significant numbers of infants being pretreated with antibiotics. In these reports, the trend was toward a higher number of ventilator days in the coinfected groups. Although the incidence of respiratory viral and bacterial coinfection was common, very few cases of sepsis/septic shock, bacteremia, or meningitis were seen in infants with severe RSV (21,47). Other studies have not confirmed this finding. Unfortunately, the number of ventilated, nonpretreated infants whose aspirates were cultured for bacterial coinfection was low in some studies and may not be representative of the most worrisome RSV-infected infants (8,41). In addition, culture results were typically obtained only at admission and, as such, did not reflect the risk of secondary bacterial infection seen during the PICU course.

Numerous reports demonstrate serious bacterial superinfection as a complication of varicella. Case reports and epidemiologic studies cite many types of bacterial complications, including necrotizing fasciitis, TSS, epiglottitis, spinal epidural abscess, pyogenic arthritis, osteomyelitis, meningitis, orbital cellulitis, and subdural empyema. The primary bacterial culprits are GAβHS and *S. aureus*. In addition to varicella, influenza has also been associated with TSS (3,22,31).

Profound immunosuppression during measles infection has been long appreciated. During and for several weeks following measles infection, bacterial and/or other viral infections are common, contributing to the significant morbidity and mortality of measles in developing countries. In many cases, mortality is considered a result of the secondary infection and represents another situation in which viral immunomodulation has significant ramifications (43).

The previously mentioned data support the concept that common viral infections likely play an important causal role and may contribute to the severity of serious bacterial illness. The mechanisms have not been completely elucidated; however, many potential mechanisms have been demonstrated experimentally. Knowledge of the immune response to viral infections is important in understanding how aspects of viral infection and the host antiviral response diminish the quality of antibacterial defenses. In this regard, vigilance for the presence of coinfection in the critically ill with viral infections is essential.

Impact of Viral Infection on Bacterial Adherence

As discussed previously, serious bacterial superinfection or coinfection can occur during or following viral infections of many types, and several likely mechanisms for the process have been described. The first significant change induced by viral infection is often disruption of protective epithelial barriers as a result of diversion of cell machinery to intracellular viral formation and replication, often with direct lysis of infected cells (16). When protective epithelial barriers are disrupted, protective mucous and mucociliary dysfunction can occur, as can exaggerated bacterial adherence to exposed basement membrane elements, permitting penetration into deeper tissues (Table 74.1). This concept was demonstrated in experimental human inoculation with influenza followed by the development of detectable colonization with *S. pneumoniae* 6 days after inoculation (2). In addition, several studies have demonstrated a significant increase in nasopharyngeal colonization with commensal organisms during viral infection (parainfluenza, RSV, adenovirus) when compared to baseline colonization in the same children (2). Specifically, bacterial adherence is facilitated in areas where epithelium has been denuded, as has been seen in many experimental settings with cell culture and in vivo animal models. In addition, *S. aureus* in the lungs, specifically that adherent to areas of denuded tracheobronchial epithelium, was directly visualized postmortem during the 1957 influenza epidemic (14,16,38).

Mechanisms of bacterial adherence to infected or disrupted epithelium can be nonspecific, as exemplified by bacteria binding to fibrinogen and fibronectin-binding protein of the exposed extracellular matrix, seen with GAβHS in influenza A infection models (14). Some mechanisms for increased bacterial adherence during viral infection can be specific for bacterial features. For example, enhanced fimbriae-mediated and capsule-mediated binding of nontypeable *Haemophilus influenzae*, GAβHS, and *Neisseria meningitidis* to alveolar epithelial cells infected with RSV or influenza A has been demonstrated. These data indicate that viral infection can alter host cell membranes to favor binding to specific bacterial cell-wall elements (36).

Native host cell-surface protein/receptor expression [including platelet-activating factor receptor (PAFR), CD14, CD15, and CD18] can be upregulated during many viral infections. PAFR, CD14, CD15, complement protein C3, and the polymeric receptor responsible for translocating dimeric IgA or pentameric IgM have been associated with increased adherence of *N. meningitidis* and pneumococci to virus-infected epithelial cells. In some reports, these host proteins facilitate translocation of bacteria across nasopharyngeal mucosa (16).

In addition to altering expression of native host cell proteins/receptors, viral infection can result in the host cell expression of viral glycoproteins. The best characterized glycoproteins are hemagglutinin and neuraminidase (NA), which are expressed on the host cell surface during influenza and parainfluenza infections. Hemagglutinin binds to sialic acid residues

of host glycoproteins on the host cell surface, permitting internalization of virus and fusion of viral envelope with cell membrane, which leads to penetration into host cells. NA is critical for replication of influenza and parainfluenza because it cleaves sialic acid residues from host glycoproteins during viral budding from infected cells, thus facilitating release of newly synthesized virus (38). These sialic acid residues on host proteins provide protection against bacterial adherence, and once cleaved by NA, bacteria can adhere and invade. Formation of aggregates of mucin from respiratory epithelium with newly released viruses reduces infectious free viral particles. This formation is prevented by the sialidase activity of NA increasing the number of infectious viral particles to infect more epithelium and cleave more sialic acid residues (38). Different strains of influenza possess NA of varying potency, and the NA activity is thought to be a key determinant of the virulence of a given strain and, therefore, a determinant of the severity of an epidemic. Historically, NA activity of various influenza epidemics has paralleled the associated mortality, demonstrating the important role of NA in influenza pathology. Antihemagglutinin antibodies prevented bacterial superinfection in influenza experimental models. These data support an important role for these virus-induced glycoproteins in the susceptibility to bacterial superinfection in the setting of influenza and parainfluenza, which are highly dependent on hemagglutinin and NA for successful infection.

Other viral glycoproteins implicated in susceptibility to bacterial superinfection include glycoproteins F and G, which are inserted into the host cell membrane during RSV infection. Expression of glycoprotein G was shown experimentally to be involved in exaggerated binding of *N. meningitidis* to RSV-infected epithelial cells (14). In addition, RSV virions themselves bound pneumococci to form complexes that exhibited enhanced adherence to uninfected epithelial cell layers. In this way, RSV directly acted as a coupling agent between bacteria and host cells. In an in vivo model, sequential infection with RSV followed by pneumococcus (both intranasal) yielded significantly higher bacteremia compared to pneumococcal infection alone, suggesting that, through these just-described mechanisms, RSV virions may facilitate the penetration of bacteria from the mucosa to the bloodstream (14). Many factors, induced during viral infection that promote bacterial adherence and facilitate invasion are listed in **Table 74.1.**

VIRAL INFECTIONS AND ASTHMATIC EXACERBATIONS

Recent studies have demonstrated that respiratory viral infections can precipitate up to 60%–85% of acute asthma exacerbations in children. This association has become significantly stronger in more recent studies that employ polymerase chain reaction (PCR) virus detection (19) and with the identification of metapneumovirus. A causal relationship between viral infection and asthma exacerbation is most strongly suggested by an adult study that identified viral infection in 76% of patients with asthma exacerbations. Sputum from these individuals contained increased evidence of neutrophil activation and epithelial cell injury compared to those with noninfected asthma exacerbations. These markers of inflammation and cell injury correlated well with asthma exacerbation severity. The viruses identified in this study were mostly RSV and influenza, both of which can cause substantially lower respiratory infection. Rhinovirus and parainfluenza less commonly affect the lower airways and have been shown in clinical studies to have a significant impact on asthma exacerbations. Experimental rhinoviral infections in asthmatic human volunteers have been extensively studied to examine this relationship (19,50). Although rhinovirus infection is not thought to affect the lower airways, recent data suggest that this theory may not be correct in asthmatics. Increased severity of rhinoviral infection, more protracted lower-airway symptom duration, and a greater decline in lung function were reported in asthmatics compared to controls. These data demonstrate that, at least in the asthmatic, rhinovirus can extend beyond the upper respiratory tract. Furthermore, several studies have shown that rhinovirus can be detected in 30%–40% of infants hospitalized with "bronchiolitis," indicating that rhinovirus infection, as well as RSV, parainfluenza, and influenza, can be a significant contributor to hospitalization of infants and children with wheezing (15).

A number of findings have been described that suggest that the antiviral response is weakened in asthmatics, compared to nonasthmatic controls, even when studies have controlled for the use of inhaled corticosteroids and included mild asthmatics (no use of inhaled corticosteroids) (15,50). Asthmatics are more susceptible to rhinoviral infections, and viral repli-

cation in bronchial epithelial cells obtained from asthmatics is increased. Greater than 40% of a cohort of 50 asthmatic children had RNA evidence of rhinovirus that persisted up to 6 weeks after viral infection, which was much longer than the persistence of rhinovirus RNA in stable asthmatics. Asthma exacerbations were more severe in the children with persistence of viral RNA, suggesting that the severity of asthma exacerbations may be linked to prolonged and more severe rhinoviral infection (20). Induction of apoptosis of virus-infected host cells is a critical event in the innate antiviral response, because early apoptosis of virus-infected host cells prevents establishment and spread of virus and promotes phagocytosis of infected cells (50). Type 1 interferons are also critical to viral containment and to activation of other aspects of the innate and acquired immune response. Altered antiviral functions displayed in rhinovirus-infected bronchial epithelial cells from asthmatics include impaired type 1 interferon production and impaired early virus-induced apoptosis, which result in increased viral replication (50). Induction of proinflammatory cytokine responses was similar in both asthmatic and healthy bronchial epithelial cells, suggesting that all antiviral pathways were not deficient. Other studies demonstrated a reduced IFN-γ response to rhinovirus in peripheral blood mononuclear cells from asthmatics, suggesting another defect in a critical antiviral mediator (25). It has been suggested that in the presence of an

A. Normal Host

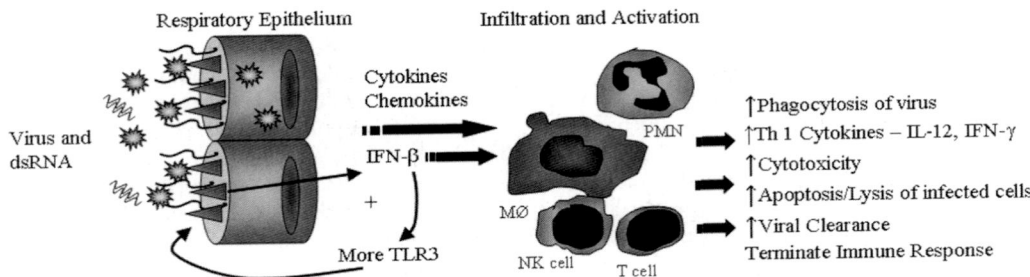

B. Asthmatic Host

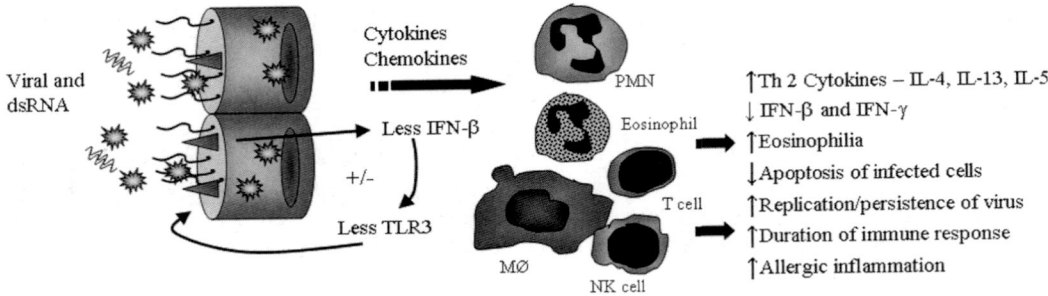

FIGURE 74.3. The antiviral immune response in asthma. Viruses infect respiratory epithelium and dsRNA (released during replication of most viruses) signals through TLR-3, which is constitutively expressed on epithelial cells. Both lead to production of a multitude of cytokines and chemokines, including IFN-β by epithelial cells. IFN-β upregulates TLR-3, leading to further induction of IFN-β. IFN-β also induces IFN-α both of which are pleiotropic cytokines that activate a multitude of inflammatory cells, kinases, and regulatory proteins critical for viral containment. **A:** Under normal circumstances, activation and infiltration of inflammatory cells lead to a proinflammatory response, including Th-1 cytokines, which are also important for viral clearance. Effective killing/apoptosis of infected cells occurs, promoting viral clearance and resolution of inflammation. **B:** Respiratory epithelial cells from asthmatics produce less IFN-β and TLR-3. Inflammatory cell stimulation is different with infiltration of eosinophils, a Th-2 response with less IFN-γ, longer survival of infected cells, and delayed viral clearance. Adapted from Message SD, Johnston SL. The immunology of virus infection in asthma. *Eur Respir J* 2001;18:1013–25.

impaired interferon response, a more vigorous inflammatory response (other mediators) may be necessary for virus eradication and, in this way, may contribute to asthma exacerbation (50). The asthmatic airway is characterized by the presence of eosinophils and T cells that express Th-2 cytokines, including IL-4, IL-5, and IL-13. It is hypothesized that this environment may contribute to ineffective antiviral responses that lead to more viral pathology, upregulation of mediators, and activation of cells (e.g., IgE and eosinophil) that are associated with asthma exacerbations (15) (**Fig. 74.3**).

Viral infection can synergize with allergen exposure, thereby precipitating more severe asthma exacerbations in atopic individuals. Exaggerated wheezing and eosinophil influx into the lower airway resulted from challenging atopic individuals with both experimental viral infection and allergen, compared to viral infection alone. It is hypothesized that chronic airway inflammation from atopy can predispose individuals to more adverse response to respiratory viral infection (15).

VIRAL INFECTIONS AND AUTOIMMUNE DISEASE EXACERBATIONS

Viral infection has been thought to be among the triggers for exacerbation of autoimmune disease, as well as a potential etiology, and has been extensively investigated. The viruses most closely associated with autoimmune phenomenon include CMV, herpes simplex virus (HSV), EBV, human herpes virus 6 and 7 (HHV-6 and HHV-7), hepatitis C, parvovirus B19, and measles (45). Viruses that are implicated in autoimmune diseases are listed in **Table 74.3**. The association has been identified either by direct identification of viral presence by PCR, detection of virus-specific proteins in serum or affected tissues (e.g., synovium, skin, neurons, and bowel mucosa), or positive IgM serology that indicates very recent infection at the time of exacerbation or presentation of autoimmune disease (45). Many of these viruses can remain in the host in a latent fashion and can become activated during stress or systemic inflammation by proinflammatory cytokines. It is unclear whether

reactivation of these viruses from their latent state is a product of the inflammatory response activated during an autoimmune exacerbation or if viral reactivation is provocative of autoimmune exacerbations. Most of the existing evidence is correlative rather than causal, in that evidence of these viruses can be found during exacerbations or onset of the diseases. Considerable data also support an association between coxsackie B4 (CB4) and type 1 diabetes mellitus. This association may be causal because more newly diagnosed type 1 diabetics have increased anti-coxsackie B4 antibodies and enteroviral RNA in peripheral blood mononuclear cells than do controls (5). In addition, "diabetogenic strains" of CB4 that have been identified from new-onset diabetics are capable of transferring pancreatic β-cell destruction to animal models (5). These data present a strong case for CB4 as one etiologic factor in the development of type 1 diabetes.

Several mechanisms for aggravation of autoimmune diseases by these just-discussed viruses have been proposed. A frequently hypothesized mechanism is referred to as *molecular mimicry*, in which the immune response to viral infection cross-reacts with self-antigens, resulting in activation of T and B cells, which causes formation of self-reactive auto-antibodies that are capable of mediating tissue injury. Alternatively, viruses such as CMV, during primary or reactivated disease, can activate antigen-presenting cells and/or virus-specific T cells, inducing cytokines and chemokines that can activate preexisting autoreactive T cells in susceptible individuals. This phenomenon is called *bystander activation*. *Epitope spreading* is another putative mechanism that involves exposure of damaged self-proteins during viral infection, resulting in anti-self-immune responses to proteins that, prior to damage, are not considered foreign (45).

IFN-α is a key antiviral cytokine produced during the immune response to most viruses. A considerable amount of data implicates IFN-α in the development of autoimmune diseases such as systemic lupus erythematosus (SLE), thyroid disease, and type 1 diabetes. Patients with SLE have high circulating IFN-α levels and evidence of activation of IFN-α-regulated genes. In addition, many reports describe patients receiving therapeutic IFN-α for diseases such as hepatitis C who develop autoimmune phenomena, such as SLE, type 1 diabetes, psoriasis, inflammatory arthritis, or Sjögren syndrome (4). IFN-α is known to potentiate immune responses through differentiation of monocytes to macrophages, augmented capacity for antigen presentation, and increased T-cell stimulation and survival. These effects may promote survival of autoreactive T cells and B cells, leading to autoantibody-mediated tissue damage. As viral infections also potently induce IFN-α, it is possible that the presence of IFN-α (administered exogenously or produced endogenously) is responsible for the association of viral infections with autoimmune exacerbations (4).

Generally, the therapy for autoimmune exacerbations includes pulse steroids and adjustment of other anti-inflammatory regimens. Viral infections, either primary or reactivated, are known to be significant pathogens in the context of immunosuppressed states (bone marrow and solid organ transplants). It may be prudent to evaluate the host fully by serum PCR for new or reactivated viral infection when an autoimmune exacerbation occurs. Results would guide and define a potential role for antiviral treatment during autoimmune exacerbations that require augmentation of immunosuppressive regimens.

TABLE 74.3

VIRAL INFECTIONS ASSOCIATED WITH AUTOIMMUNE DISEASES

Autoimmune disease	Virus
Type 1 diabetes mellitus	Coxsackie B4, enteroviruses, rotavirus
Multiple sclerosis	Measles, EBV, HHV-6
Rheumatoid arthritis	CMV, parvovirus B19
Sjögren syndrome	EBV, CMV, HHV-6, hepatitis C
Systemic lupus erythematosus	CMV, EBV, hepatitis C, parvovirus B19
Inflammatory bowel disease	CMV, EBV, measles

EBV, Epstein-Barr virus; HHV, human herpes virus; CMV, cytomegalovirus. Adapted from Soderberg-Naucler C. Does cytomegalovirus play a causative role in the development of various inflammatory diseases and cancer? *J Intern Med* 2006;259:219–46.

VIRAL REACTIVATION IN THE CRITICALLY ILL

As described previously, reactivation of latent viral infections, such as CMV, EBV, HSV, HHV-6, and HHV-7, can occur during stressed states, particularly in the presence of inflammatory cytokine production. Pathology caused by reactivation of these viruses is well described in transplant recipients (bone marrow and solid organ). Typically, categorization of an immunosuppressed state includes those receiving immunosuppressive therapies for autoimmune diseases, those who are post transplantation, those with immune-cell deficiencies (chemotherapy related and HIV), and those with primary immunodeficiency syndromes. Immune function in critical illness from a variety of mechanisms has been extensively studied, and a great deal of evidence identifies significant immune perturbations after the onset of critical illness that involves systemic stress, septic shock, trauma, surgery, brain injury/surgery, and post-transfusion, as well as other entities such as poor nutritional status and certain medications with unintended immunosuppressive side effects. These immune defects include impairment of both the innate and the adaptive immune responses and are listed in **Table 74.4** (6). Given these data, it may be reasonable to consider critically ill patients relatively immunosuppressed rather than immunocompetent, once the disease process has begun. The immunosuppression may not be as severe as that seen in transplant recipients, malignancy, and AIDS; however, the list in **Table 74.4** cites numerous immune defects for each category of illness once the illness/injury has begun. Additional evidence supporting this concept comes from emerging data that demonstrate reactivation of several latent viruses, which is a phenomenon common to those receiving pharmacologic immunosuppression and/or those awaiting bone marrow reconstitution.

Despite evidence of reactivation of latent viruses in "immunocompetent" critically ill adults, their contribution to critical illness has not been well defined. Numerous reports describe evidence of HSV reactivation in the critically ill, including burn patients, surgical patients, and nonsurgical patients, with prevalence ranging from 15%–23%. HSV-1 culture result correlation with morbidity is inconsistent; thus, HSV-1 reactivation may represent a marker of severe illness and relative immunosuppression from critical illness rather than a contributor to severity of illness. The data that suggest a contribution from CMV reactivation to severity of illness are more compelling. Reactivated CMV (diagnosed by CMV antigenemia, culture, and/or PCR from blood and/or bronchoalveolar lavage fluid) has been identified in 17%–35% of critically ill patients, many of whom had more severe morbidity and mortality, compared to CMV-negative critically ill patients. In some reports, CMV was associated with more comorbidity, sepsis at admission, steroid use, hepatic dysfunction, and nosocomial infection (17). Another latent virus known to reactivate during immunosuppression is HHV-6, with prevalence ranging from 48%–62% (44). In transplant/malignancy/AIDS, HHV-6 is known to cause fever, rash, pneumonitis, encephalitis, and bone marrow suppression. Frequently, it is found concomitantly with CMV and, in these cases, is associated with altered graft function, rejection, and graft-versus-host disease. As with CMV, HHV-6 has also been reported in immunocompetent critically ill patients (medical and surgical) with a prevalence of 65%. To date,

TABLE 74.4

IMMUNE DYSFUNCTION IN CRITICAL ILLNESS STATES, INCLUDING TRAUMA/POST-SURGICAL, BURN INJURY, SEPTIC SHOCK, BRAIN INJURY, MALNUTRITION, AND MULTIPLE TRANSFUSIONS

Affected immune cells	Immune defect
Macrophage/ dendritic cells	Increased anti-inflammatory cytokines Decreased proinflammatory cytokines Decreased HLA-DR Decreased antigen presentation Decreased phagocytosis Decreased NO and ROI Decreased PBMC response to LPS
Neutrophils	Decreased adhesion molecules Decreased NO, PAF, ROI Decreased chemotaxis Decreased phagocytosis Decreased degranulation Decreased lysosomal activity
NK cells and lymphocytes	Th-1 to Th-2 shift Poor response to mitogens Increased apoptosis Decreased cytotoxicity Decreased Ig production Anergy

HLA-DR, human leukocyte antigen-DR; NO, nitric oxide; ROI, reactive oxygen intermediates; PBMC, peripheral blood mononuclear cells; LPS, lipopolysaccharide; PAF, platelet activating factor; Ig, immunoglobulin. Adapted from Doughty L. Modulation of the Immune Response in Critical Illness/Injury. In Doughty L, Linden P, eds. *Immunology and Infectious Disease.* Norwell, MA: Kluwer Academic Publishers, 2003;115–54.

the literature only contains one study that shows no association between HHV-6 and worsened outcome. HHV-6 reactivation has also been implicated in drug-induced hypersensitivity syndrome, characterized by eosinophilia, mononucleosis-like symptoms, rash, atypical lymphocytosis, hepatic dysfunction, and lymphadenopathy. Reactivation of latent viruses in the herpes family can be present in critically ill patients who do not receive classic immunosuppressive medications, probably as a result of the immune defects acquired in the setting of critical illness and severe stress. The contribution of this phenomenon to morbidity is controversial in the adult literature. It has not been studied in critically ill children, and deserves more thorough investigation to determine whether latent viruses are reactivated in this setting and whether treatment might affect outcome, as it has in the transplant/malignancy/AIDS setting (44).

POTENTIAL THERAPEUTIC/DIAGNOSTIC STRATEGIES

Unfortunately, the paucity of successful antiviral therapies makes treatment of many viral infections impossible, with the exception of the herpes family viruses. Data has emerged over the last several years to support the use of some antivirals, with the hope of diminishing the contribution of viral infection to critical illness. The use of neuraminidase inhibitors (NI) is an important therapeutic strategy for the treatment of influenza. Multiple large studies have demonstrated reduction in length of illness by 1–4 days if an NI is begun within the first several hours of influenza symptoms. Prophylactic use has also been effective for high-risk populations and recently exposed individuals. It has also become clear from these studies that NI treatment has reduced the incidence of otitis media by 44%, lower respiratory tract complications that require antibiotics by 55%, and hospitalizations for any cause by 59% (30). These clinical data confirm mouse data that show that treatment with an NI improved survival in a model of secondary pneumococcal pneumonia created 7 days after influenza infection. Improvement was seen even when the NI was administered as late as 5 days after the onset of influenza. NI treatment did not reduce viral titers but did reduce bacterial adherence. These data suggest that inhibition of neuraminidase decreases neuraminidase-mediated changes in respiratory epithelium that are permissive for bacterial colonization and establishment of pneumonia (26). A diagram of a potential mechanism by which NI diminishes bacterial adherence/infection is depicted in **Figure 74.4**. These data support the use of NI agents both to reduce morbidity from influenza and to reduce secondary bacterial infection in high-risk children. Currently, chemoprophylaxis recommendations are for NI use in high-risk children and their close contacts. As these drugs are not approved by the US Food and Drug Administration for use in infants <1 year of age, further work must be accomplished to establish the safety and efficacy in that age group.

Given data that describe multifaceted immune compromise during viral infection, constant vigilance for the presence of coinfection at the time of presentation or superinfection later during the viral illness is prudent. Recent data demonstrate that lower respiratory bacterial coinfection is common in influenza, RSV, and parainfluenza infections (23%) in immunocompetent children at presentation (28). No data exist that describe the incidence of superinfection related to these viruses developing during a critical illness course or in high-risk infants and children. It could be surmised that the incidence of either coinfection or superinfection developing later in a viral course in high-risk children, critically ill presentations, or stalled clinical improvement situations might be even higher than in immunocompetent children. Perhaps it is prudent to consider that viral infection in such settings may not be the unifying and sole diagnosis and that further workup may be warranted at presentation and, if needed, later during the course of the viral infection. Certainly, further study is necessary to effectively answer this question and to appropriately guide care in the most vulnerable infants and children.

Data clearly support increased the incidence of adverse bronchospastic complications of respiratory viral infections in asthmatics and especially in those with atopic characteristics. Aggressive management of allergic airway inflammatory symptoms with multimodal therapy, including inhaled steroids (pulmonary and possibly nasal) combined with leukotriene inhibitors and possibly anti-IgE antibodies to minimize the atopic symptoms, may decrease the synergistic contribution of allergen exposure to viral infection-induced asthma exacerbations. Aggressive antiviral prophylaxis (vaccine and neuraminidase inhibitors) will likely complement these efforts to decrease the complications of viral infection in this population. Given the interesting data that show innate immune defects in asthmatics, strategies to augment innate and acquired immune function should also be explored toward altering the exaggerated immune vulnerability to complicated viral infection (26).

Data indicate that reactivation of human herpes virus of many types (CMV, EBV, HSV, HHV) can occur with fairly high

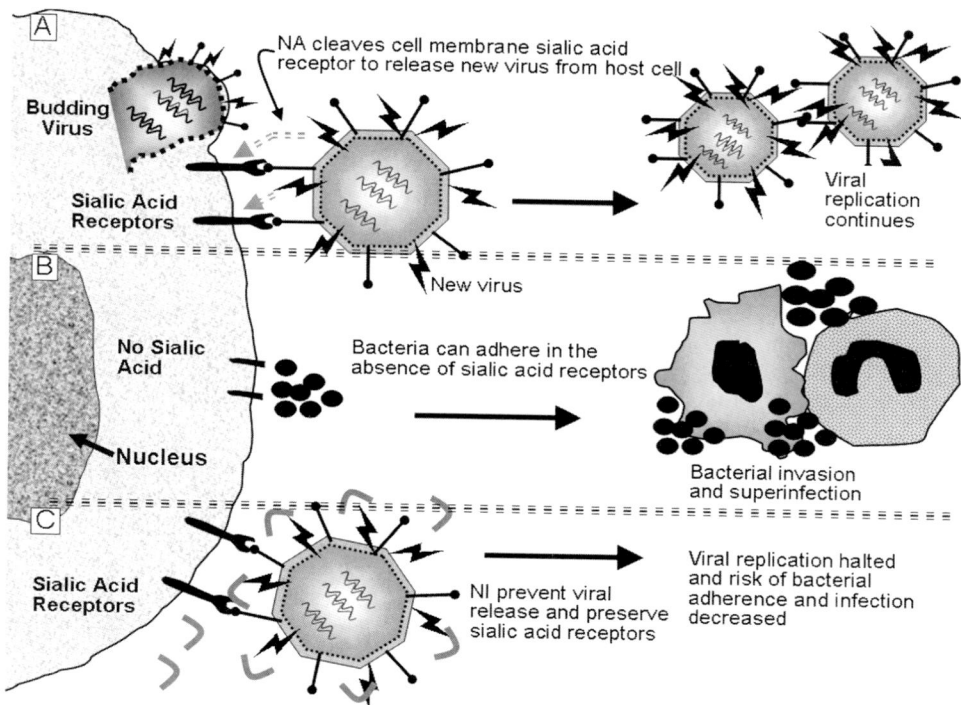

FIGURE 74.4. Mechanism of action of neuraminidase inhibitors. **A:** New virus is released from the cell surface by neuraminidase cleavage of hemagglutinin bound to sialic acid cell receptors. New virus continues to replicate, leading to destruction of infected tissue and clinical symptomatology. **B:** Bacteria such as pneumococcus can adhere to cell surfaces in the absence of sialic acid residues, leading to bacterial superinfection. **C:** Neuraminidase inhibitors block the release of new viruses, limiting viral replication and spread to other cells. Also, by limiting neuraminidase activity, protective sialic acid residues are preserved, decreasing bacterial adherence and invasion. ↙, neuraminidase; ●, hemagglutinin ⌒, neuraminidase inhibitor; ⬎, neuraminidase activity. Adapted from Moscona A. Neuraminidase inhibitors for influenza. *N Engl J Med* 2005;353:1363–73.

prevalence in critically ill patients who have been traditionally considered immunocompetent, as well as in the immunosuppressed populations. Life-threatening complications from reactivation of some of these viruses are well documented in the immunosuppressed; therefore, aggressive monitoring, prophylaxis, and/or treatment with ganciclovir, high-titer anti-CMV IgG, or acyclovir for HSV are commonly used at times of maximal immunosuppression. The contribution of reactivation of various herpes family viruses in the critically ill has not been unequivocally proven; however, given the current understanding of immune defects due to critical illness, this concept requires further investigation. It is possible that the immune defects secondary to critical illness permit viral reactivation and that viral reactivation may contribute to such things as multiple organ failure, acute respiratory distress syndrome, and hepatic and renal dysfunction. It is estimated that 60%–100% of young adults have evidence of prior CMV infection (CMV IgG), that 50%–60% of children are infected by 1 year of age, and that most children have been infected by 3 years of age (45). HSV-1 infection also usually occurs commonly in children, indicating that many critically ill children may be subject to herpes family virus reactivation. The prevalence of latent viral reactivation in critically ill children has not been studied at all. If frequent reactivation is found to occur in critically ill children as it does in adults, it may be reasonable to periodically screen for viral antigenemia/DNA and/or consider prophylaxis in the most vulnerable patients. Solid data will be required to justify this treatment due to the significant associated side effects (e.g., bone marrow suppression from medications such as ganciclovir).

CONCLUSIONS AND FUTURE DIRECTIONS

Viral infection is a constant nemesis in children. Data have emerged over the last 10 years to support the concept that viral infections may have a more pronounced and far-reaching effect on the host than previously understood. The data presented here are meant to introduce the consequences of some common viral infections on host immunity, including viral infections not previously thought to contribute to host defense alteration, such as rhinovirus and influenza. Bacterial superinfection of viral infection has traditionally been ascribed to disrupted protective barriers, such as respiratory epithelium, without an understanding of the transient alteration of immune function present during and after many common viral infections. Certainly, the data suggest that both issues exist and, with more mechanistic understanding of the impact of viral infection on both of these mechanisms, better strategies for prophylaxis against viral infection and prevention of superinfection should be forthcoming. In addition, better understanding of the contribution of viral infection to exacerbations of asthma and autoimmune diseases may provide insight into critical immune interactions and pathways to target in an effort to maintain the diseases described in a stable, uncomplicated state. In the case of viral reactivation in critical illness, prevention and/or treatment of these pathogens, when present, may eliminate unrecognized obstructions to new therapies and may improve the outcome of critical illness.

KEY POINTS

- Viral infections can alter host immune function and contribute to bacterial superinfection, asthma exacerbations, autoimmune disease exacerbations, and reactivation of latent viruses during critical illness.
- Viral infection can alter many aspects of the innate and acquired immune response, leading to vulnerability to bacterial superinfection.
- Viral and bacterial coinfection occurs frequently in children and may have a role in critical complications of the viral or bacterial disease.
- Viral infection can result in increased bacterial adherence to protective mucosal/epithelial barriers.
- Asthmatics, particularly with atopy, are more susceptible to viral infections and have heightened morbidity from exacerbations caused by viral infection.
- Autoimmune disease exacerbations have been linked to several viral infections—some acute and some from reactivated viruses.
- Reactivated herpes-family viruses (CMV, HSV, EBV, HHV-6, and HHV-7) have been found in critically ill immunocompetent individuals and may contribute to outcome in the critically ill.

ACKNOWLEDGMENTS

This work was supported by National Institutes of Health 5K08GM71568–03.

References

1. Akira S, Uematsu S, Takeuchi O. Pathogen recognition and innate immunity. *Cell* 2006;124:783–801.
2. Bakaletz LO. Viral potentiation of bacterial superinfection of the respiratory tract. *Trends Microbiol* 1995;3:110–4.
3. Chuang YY, Huang YC, Lin TY. Toxic shock syndrome in children: Epidemiology, pathogenesis, and management. *Paediatr Drugs* 2005;7:11–25.
4. Crow MK, Kirou KA. Interferon-alpha in systemic lupus erythematosus. *Curr Opin Rheumatol* 2004;16:541–7.
5. Devendra D, Eisenbarth GS. Interferon alpha-A potential link in the pathogenesis of viral-induced type 1 diabetes and autoimmunity. *Clin Immunol* 2004;111:225–33.
6. Doughty L. Modulation of the Immune Response in Critical Illness/Injury. In Doughty L, Linden ed. *Immunology and Infectious Disease.* Norwell, MA: Kluwer Academic Publishers, 2003;115–54.
7. Doughty LA, Carlton S, Galen B, et al. Activation of common antiviral pathways can potentiate inflammatory responses to septic shock. *Shock* 2006;26:187–94.
8. Duttweiler L, Nadal D, Frey B. Pulmonary and systemic bacterial co-infections in severe RSV bronchiolitis. *Arch Dis Child* 2004;89:1155–7.
9. Ertl H. Viral Immunology. In Paul WE, ed. *Fundamental Immunology.* Philadelphia: Lippincott Williams & Wilkins 2003;1201–28.
10. Fejer G, Szalay K, Gyory I, et al. Adenovirus infection dramatically augments lipopolysaccharide-induced TNF production and sensitizes to lethal shock. *J Immunol* 2005;175:1498–506.
11. Frascaroli G, Varani S, Mastroianni A, et al. Dendritic cell function in cytomegalovirus-infected patients with mononucleosis. *J Leukoc Biol* 2006;79:932–40.
12. George MJ, Snydman DR, Werner BG, et al. The independent role of cytomegalovirus as a risk factor for invasive fungal disease in orthotopic liver transplant recipients. *Boston Center for Liver Transplantation CMVIG-Study Group. Cytogam, MedImmune, Inc. Gaithersburg, MD. Am J Med* 1997;103:106–13.
13. Gonzalez BE, Hulten KG, Dishop MK, et al. Pulmonary manifestations in children with invasive community-acquired *Staphylococcus aureus* infection. *Clin Infect Dis* 2005;41:583–90.

14. Hament JM, Kimpen JL, Fleer A, et al. Respiratory viral infection predisposing for bacterial disease: a concise review. *FEMS Immunol Med Microbiol* 1999;26:189–95.

15. Heymann PW, Platts-Mills TA, Johnston SL. Role of viral infections, atopy and antiviral immunity in the etiology of wheezing exacerbations among children and young adults. *Pediatr Infect Dis J* 2005;24:S217–22, discussion S20-1.

16. Hussell T, Williams A. *Menage a trois* of bacterial and viral pulmonary pathogens delivers *coup de grace* to the lung. *Clin Exp Immunol* 2004; 137:8–11.

17. Jaber S, Chanques G, Borry J, et al. Cytomegalovirus infection in critically ill patients: Associated factors and consequences. *Chest* 2005;127:233–41.

18. Jensen ES, Lundbye-Christensen S, Samuelsson S, et al. A 20-year ecological study of the temporal association between influenza and meningococcal disease. *Eur J Epidemiol* 2004;19:181–7.

19. Johnston SL. Overview of virus-induced airway disease. *Proc Am Thorac Soc* 2005;2:150–6.

20. Kling S, Donninger H, Williams Z, et al. Persistence of rhinovirus RNA after asthma exacerbation in children. *Clin Exp Allergy* 2005;35:672–8.

21. Kneyber MC, Blusse van Oud-Alblas H, van Vliet M, et al. Concurrent bacterial infection and prolonged mechanical ventilation in infants with respiratory syncytial virus lower respiratory tract disease. *Intensive Care Med* 2005;31:680–5.

22. Laupland KB, Davies HD, Low DE, et al. Invasive group A streptococcal disease in children and association with varicella-zoster virus infection. Ontario Group A Streptococcal Study Group. *Pediatrics* 2000;105:E60.

23. Lee RM, White MR, Hartshorn KL. Influenza A viruses upregulate neutrophil toll-like receptor 2 expression and function. *Scand J Immunol* 2006;63:81–9.

24. Makras P, Alexiou-Daniel S, Antoniadis A, et al. Outbreak of meningococcal disease after an influenza B epidemic at a Hellenic Air Force recruit training center. *Clin Infect Dis* 2001;33:e48–50.

25. Martin JG, Siddiqui S, Hassan M. Immune responses to viral infections: Relevance for asthma. *Paediatr Respir Rev* 2006;7(Suppl 1):S125–7.

26. McCullers JA. Insights into the interaction between influenza virus and pneumococcus. *Clin Microbiol Rev* 2006;19:571–82.

27. Message SD, Johnston SL. The immunology of virus infection in asthma. *Eur Respir J* 2001;18:1013–25.

28. Michelow IC, Olsen K, Lozano J, et al. Epidemiology and clinical characteristics of community-acquired pneumonia in hospitalized children. *Pediatrics* 2004;113:701–7.

29. Mobbs KJ, Smyth RL, O'Hea U, et al. Cytokines in severe respiratory syncytial virus bronchiolitis. *Pediatr Pulmonol* 2002;33:449–52.

30. Moscona A. Neuraminidase inhibitors for influenza. *N Engl J Med* 2005;353:1363–73.

31. Moss RL, Musemeche CA, Kosloske AM. Necrotizing fasciitis in children: Prompt recognition and aggressive therapy improve survival. *J Pediatr Surg* 1996;31:1142–6.

32. Naniche D, Oldstone MB. Generalized immunosuppression: how viruses undermine the immune response. *Cell Mol Life Sci* 2000;57:1399–407.

33. Nickerson CL, Jakab GJ. Pulmonary antibacterial defenses during mild and severe influenza virus infection. *Infect Immun* 1990;58:2809–14. vfill

34. O'Brien KL, Walters MI, Sellman J, et al. Severe pneumococcal pneumonia in previously healthy children: the role of preceding influenza infection. *Clin Infect Dis* 2000;30:784–9.

35. Okamoto S, Kawabata S, Nakagawa I, et al. Influenza A virus-infected hosts boost an invasive type of Streptococcus pyogenes infection in mice. *J Virol* 2003;77:4104–12.

36. Okamoto S, Kawabata S, Terao Y, et al. The *Streptococcus pyogenes* capsule is required for adhesion of bacteria to virus-infected alveolar epithelial cells and lethal bacterial-viral superinfection. *Infect Immun* 2004;72: 6068–75.

37. Panuska JR, Merolla R, Rebert NA, et al. Respiratory syncytial virus induces interleukin-10 by human alveolar macrophages. *Suppression of early cytokine production and implications for incomplete immunity.* J Clin Invest 1995;96:2445–53.

38. Peltola VT, McCullers JA. Respiratory viruses predisposing to bacterial infections: Role of neuraminidase. *Pediatr Infect Dis J* 2004;23:S87–97.

39. Perry AK, Chen G, Zheng D, et al. The host type I interferon response to viral and bacterial infections. *Cell Res* 2005;15:407–22.

40. Raftery MJ, Schwab M, Eibert SM, et al. Targeting the function of mature dendritic cells by human cytomegalovirus: A multilayered viral defense strategy. *Immunity* 2001;15:997–1009.

41. Randolph AG, Reder L, Englund JA. Risk of bacterial infection in previously healthy respiratory syncytial virus-infected young children admitted to the intensive care unit. *Pediatr Infect Dis J* 2004;23:990–4.

42. Raza MW, Blackwell CC, Elton RA, et al. Bactericidal activity of a monocytic cell line (THP-1) against common respiratory tract bacterial pathogens is depressed after infection with respiratory syncytial virus. *J Med Microbiol* 2000;49:227–33.

43. Schneider-Schaulies S, ter Meulen V. Modulation of immune functions by measles virus. *Springer Semin Immunopathol* 2002;24:127–48.

44. Seishima M, Yamanaka S, Fujisawa T, et al. Reactivation of human herpesvirus (HHV) family members other than HHV-6 in drug-induced hypersensitivity syndrome. *Br J Dermatol* 2006;155:344–9.

45. Soderberg-Naucler C. Does cytomegalovirus play a causative role in the development of various inflammatory diseases and cancer?. *J Intern Med* 2006;259:219–46.

46. Talbot TR, Poehling KA, Hartert TV, et al. Seasonality of invasive pneumococcal disease: Temporal relation to documented influenza and respiratory syncytial viral circulation. *Am J Med* 2005;118:285–91.

47. Thorburn K, Harigopal S, Reddy V, et al. High incidence of pulmonary bacterial co-infection in children with severe respiratory syncytial virus (RSV) bronchiolitis. *Thorax* 2006;61(7):611–5.

48. Tsolia MN, Psarras S, Bossios A, et al. Etiology of community-acquired pneumonia in hospitalized school-age children: Evidence for high prevalence of viral infections. *Clin Infect Dis* 2004;39:681–6.

49. van der Sluijs KF, van Elden LJ, Nijhuis M, et al. IL-10 is an important mediator of the enhanced susceptibility to pneumococcal pneumonia after influenza infection. *J Immunol* 2004;172:7603–9.

50. Wark PA, Johnston SL, Bucchieri F, et al. Asthmatic bronchial epithelial cells have a deficient innate immune response to infection with rhinovirus. *J Exp Med* 2005;201:937–47.

CHAPTER 75 ■ IMMUNE MODULATION AND IMMUNOTHERAPY IN CRITICAL ILLNESS

MARK W. HALL

The immune response and its proper regulation by the host is critical for the mounting of a successful defense against invading pathogens and for facilitating healing and repair of injured tissues. Much of the morbidity seen in the ICU, however, is a direct consequence of abnormal regulation of this immune response. The classic example of this maladaptive scenario is the case of septic shock, whereby an overly robust proinflammatory response causes far more tissue damage than the original infection that initiated it. At the same time, it is important to appreciate that pathology also occurs when the pendulum swings in the other direction. It is intuitive that children with underactive immune systems as the result of chemotherapy or treatment with immunosuppressive medications are at high risk for the development of infectious complications. Perhaps less intuitive is the notion that an overactive endogenous compensatory anti-inflammatory immune response can follow a proinflammatory insult and can result in significant morbidity and mortality *without* the influence of exogenous immunosuppressants. The restoration and maintenance of a responsive immune system with a homeostatic balance between pro- and anti-inflammatory forces should be a goal of modern critical care medicine and has, thus far, proven difficult to achieve.

Historically, attempts at immunomodulation in the ICU have been largely focused on the abrogation of the proinflammatory response in such conditions as sepsis and acute respiratory distress syndrome (ARDS). It should be remembered that a great many patients suffer from iatrogenic immunosuppression as the result of treatment for malignancy, transplantation, or autoimmune disease. The history and role of immunomodulation and special considerations for the management of immunocompromised patients are reviewed in this chapter.

TARGETING PROINFLAMMATION

A detailed review of the immunology of inflammation can be found elsewhere in this text. To briefly review, the cytokines tumor necrosis factor (TNF)-α, IL-1β, and interferon (IFN)-γ are proinflammatory cytokines released by innate immune cells (TNF-α, IL-1β) and lymphocytes (IFN-γ) in response to an inflammatory stimulus. The signaling pathways associated with the production of proinflammatory cytokines in immune cells include the mitogen-activated protein kinase and nuclear factor (NF)-κB pathways. The cytokine that has been most reliably associated with adverse outcomes in the setting of proinflammatory disease is IL-6, likely because IL-6 is released in response to more potent proinflammatory cytokines and, therefore, serves as a *marker* for inflammation. IL-6, while an inducer of the acute phase response, has significant anti-inflammatory proper-

ties of its own. More potent anti-inflammatory cytokines, produced by both innate and adaptive immune cells, include IL-10 and transforming growth factor (TGF)-β. Innate immune cells include neutrophils, monocytes, macrophages, and dendritic cells, while adaptive immune cells include T and B lymphocytes.

Severe Sepsis and Septic Shock

The classic signs and symptoms of severe septic disease, including fever, altered vascular tone, and increased capillary permeability, are largely the result of the effects of proinflammatory cytokines rather than the offending pathogen itself. It is not difficult to understand, therefore, why a great deal of time and energy was spent during the 1980s and 1990s developing and testing regimens to target proinflammatory mediators in severe sepsis and septic shock.

Antiendotoxin Strategies

The first studies performed in this area focused on Gram-negative lipopolysaccharide (LPS). First using pooled antisera rich in anti-LPS activity (1,13), then using monoclonal anti-LPS antibodies (10,28), investigators tried in vain to consistently demonstrate a survival benefit in septic adults. One phase III trial was stopped after interim analysis demonstrated a trend toward *higher* mortality in treated patients (37). Recombinant bactericidal/permeability-increasing protein (BPI), an endogenous antimicrobial peptide capable of neutralizing endotoxin, was recently evaluated in a phase III trial in children with meningococcemia. While recombinant BPI conferred no improvement in survival, functional outcome was better in the treated group (34).

Anticytokine Strategies

Recombinant IL-1 receptor antagonist (IL-1ra), a naturally occurring IL-1β antagonist, underwent 2 large phase III trials, both of which failed to show improvement in adult sepsis survival (25,46). TNF-α has been similarly targeted with neutralizing monoclonal antibody therapy. Four major anti-TNF antibody studies have been performed in septic adults to date, including the North American Sepsis (NORASEPT) I and II trials and the International Sepsis (INTERSEPT) trial (3,4,15), which demonstrated no improvement in 28-day survival in the treatment arms. More recently, the Monoclonal Anti-TNF: A Randomized Clinical Sepsis (MONARCS) trial showed a slight but statistically significant reduction in 28-day mortality in the subgroup of patients with plasma IL-6 levels of >1000 pg/mL (47), suggesting that the most profoundly inflamed patients may benefit from TNF-α depletion. Antagonists of bradykinin (deltibant) and platelet activating factor (lexipafant) have also failed to show survival benefit in adults (23,56).

Activated Protein C

It should be noted that significant overlap exists between the inflammatory and hemostatic pathways. Activated protein C (APC) is an endogenous protein with antithrombotic, profibrinolytic, and anti-inflammatory properties. Recombinant human (rh) APC (rhAPC) has recently been studied in adults and children who had severe sepsis, with mixed results. In the subset of adults with the most severe illness (APACHE II scores ≥25 or ≥2 organ failure *and* an absence of risk factors for severe bleeding, including recent surgery), rhAPC was shown to significantly reduce mortality, compared to placebo (17). The pediatric phase III trial that followed, with resolution of organ failure as the primary outcome variable, was stopped at its planned interim analysis for lack of efficacy (27). No widely accepted indication currently exists for the use of rhAPC in pediatric septic disease.

Corticosteroids

The last decade has seen a paradigm shift in the role of corticosteroids in adult and PICUs. It was once thought that methylprednisolone or dexamethasone would, by virtue of their anti-inflammatory properties, have beneficial effects in the setting of the proinflammatory storm of sepsis. Two meta-analyses published in the mid-1990s concluded that the use of these drugs was associated with an *increased* risk of mortality from sepsis in adults (16,33). In retrospect, it appears that investigators chose the wrong drugs. Two more recent meta-analyses demonstrated a survival *benefit* associated with the use of a 5–7-day course of low-dose hydrocortisone (200–300 mg/day) in adults with severe sepsis or septic shock (6,41). The benefits of hydrocortisone are likely due to the fact that it has far less glucocorticoid (immunosuppressive) activity and far more mineralocorticoid (hemodynamic supporting) activity than either methylprednisolone or dexamethasone (**Table 75.1**).

Extracorporeal Therapies

Another approach to the restoration of immunologic homeostasis is the bulk removal of inflammatory mediators through hemofiltration, membrane adsorption, plasmapheresis, or plasma exchange (38). An advantage of most of these techniques is that no single mediator is targeted; rather, large concentrations of cytokines can be removed at once. Disadvantages include the need for dedicated large-bore IV access, exposure to blood products (plasma exchange), and the likely need for relatively long-term therapy. In fact, most prospective studies of extracorporeal therapies in sepsis have been small, involved

short-term treatment (1–2 days), and have been largely unsuccessful in demonstrating improved outcomes. Of these therapies, plasmapheresis and plasma exchange have shown the most promise in prospective trials, perhaps because plasma exchange involves the replacement of patient plasma with donor plasma, thereby both removing unwanted mediators and replacing potentially deficient ones (12,58,60).

Acute Respiratory Distress Syndrome

Glucocorticoids are the immunomodulators that have been studied most extensively in the setting of ARDS. Reduction of inflammation and inhibition of the fibroproliferative phase of ARDS seem to be reasonable therapeutic goals in the management of this syndrome. In 1998, improved pulmonary function, reduction in organ failure, and improved survival were demonstrated in adults with unresolving ARDS at 7 days who received a prolonged course of methylprednisolone (40). Recent studies have questioned these findings, including a prospective study of 180 adults that failed to show a survival benefit and, in fact, showed *increased* mortality rates in patients whose methylprednisolone was started more than 14 days after the onset of ARDS (55). While the use of glucocorticoids in patients without infection who have unresolving ARDS is still defensible (particularly in the second week of illness), the practice is currently being viewed with considerable equipoise. To date, no studies have been performed to address this question in the pediatric population.

Cardiopulmonary Bypass

Exposure of leukocytes and complement to the tubing and membranes associated with extracorporeal procedures, including cardiopulmonary bypass (CPB), is known to induce a potent proinflammatory response. While significant advances have been made in the development of less bioreactive coatings for these devices, many practitioners continue to rely on systemic anti-inflammatory agents to attenuate this response (53). The administration of glucocorticoids to the patient and/or bypass pump has been shown to reduce neutrophil activation and proinflammatory cytokine release. The serine protease inhibitor aprotinin is frequently used to mitigate postoperative bleeding after CPB. Aprotinin has also been shown to reduce proinflammatory cytokine production post-bypass, with a potentially synergistic effect with glucocorticoids. Attempts to effect bulk removal of proinflammatory cytokines through modified ultrafiltration during CPB have yielded variable results. It should be noted that the impact of these strategies, aimed at reducing the proinflammatory response to CPB, on patient outcomes is far from clear. Recent evidence suggests that a prolonged, severe anti-inflammatory innate immune response following pediatric CPB may, in fact, be harmful (5).

IMMUNOPARALYSIS

The recurrent failure of treatments that target proinflammation is coincident with burgeoning experimental and clinical evidence that an overactive anti-inflammatory response frequently predominates in the ICU, is often occult, and can be

TABLE 75.1

RELATIVE POTENCIES OF CORTICOSTEROIDS

Drug	Anti-inflammatory (immunosuppressive)	Mineralocorticoid
Dexamethasone	30	0
Methylprednisolone	5	1
Hydrocortisone	1	5

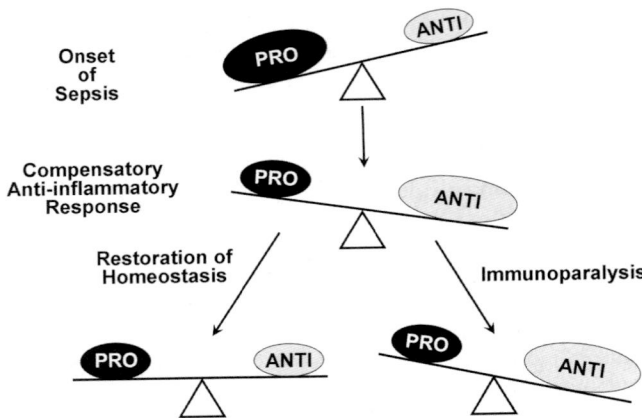

FIGURE 75.1. Schematic of the development of immunoparalysis following a proinflammatory insult.

highly pathologic. For more than 20 years, it has been known that a major inflammatory insult typically results in a compensatory anti-inflammatory response syndrome characterized by reduction in cell-surface marker expression on innate immune cells and increased production of anti-inflammatory cytokines, including IL-10 (35,49) (**Fig. 75.1**). During the 1990s, investigators began associating prolonged, severe depression of innate immune function with adverse outcomes following trauma, sepsis, and transplantation (9,20,50,59). This phenomenon, termed *immunoparalysis*, has been quantified in two major ways. First, surface expression of the class II major histocompatibility complex molecule HLA-DR, important in antigen presentation, has been shown to be reduced in circulating monocytes from patients with the compensatory anti-inflammatory response syndrome. Severe reduction in HLA-DR expression, such that <30% of circulating monocytes are strongly HLA-DR+ by flow cytometry, is characteristic of immunoparalysis. A more functional measure of innate immune capability is the ex vivo LPS-induced TNF-α production assay. In this test, an aliquot of whole blood is incubated with a standard concentration of LPS, and TNF-α production is measured in the supernatant. Patients with immunoparalysis will demonstrate a severe, prolonged reduction in their ability to make TNF-α ex vivo. Specific cutoffs for the definition of immunoparalysis by this method will vary, depending on the type and dose of LPS used, the volume of blood tested, and the duration of incubation.

Although the specific causes of immunoparalysis are not known, it is becoming clear that patients with this syndrome exhibit skewing toward a Th-2-like immune phenotype with high levels of circulating IL-10. In fact, anti–IL-10 neutralizing antibodies have been shown to partially reverse experimental immunoparalysis induced by incubation of healthy monocytes with plasma from septic adults (26). Immunoparalysis has also been reported in the context of post-transplantation immunosuppressive regimens, although it is unclear if this represents a direct drug effect or a downstream effect of lymphocyte inhibition (7,50).

Significance

The laboratory measures of immunoparalysis just described represent evidence that some patients' compensatory anti-

inflammatory response, while initially an adaptive attempt to restore immunologic homeostasis, can progress to a maladaptive state which can be thought of as a type of secondary immunodeficiency. It appears that the duration of immunoparalysis is crucial. If transient immunoparalysis is present for only 1 or 2 days, most authors agree that it is well tolerated. If severe, innate immune dysfunction persists for as little as 3–5 days, however, numerous prospective reports have shown an association with the development of secondary infection and death in adult and pediatric critical illness (29,42,59).

It is tempting to think that immunoparalysis is an epiphenomenon associated with severe illness rather than being directly contributory to outcome, but tantalizing evidence suggests that this is not so. It is possible to reverse immunoparalysis with beneficial effects on clinical outcomes through the use of immunostimulatory agents or through the tapering of exogenous immunosuppression. Dramatic improvement has been demonstrated in monocyte function and survival rates in adult transplant patients with sepsis and immunoparalysis when immunosuppression was tapered (with no coincident increase in graft rejection) (59). The drugs IFN-γ, granulocyte-macrophage colony-stimulating factor (GM-CSF), and, more recently, flt3-ligand (61) have been shown to reverse experimental immunoparalysis. Two small, uncontrolled case series have demonstrated reversal of immunoparalysis and suggested improved survival in adult septic patients following in vivo treatment with IFN-γ and GM-CSF, respectively (19,43). In 2005, improved monocyte function and enhanced clearance of infection were demonstrated in a prospective, randomized, controlled trial of GM-CSF in 40 non-neutropenic septic adults (52).

Across-the-board administration of immunostimulating agents to critically ill patients is unlikely to yield improvements in outcomes. For example, a recent Cochrane Database meta-analysis suggested that, while safe, drugs like GM-CSF have no proven benefit in the treatment or prevention of systemic infections in the NICU when given without the benefit of immune monitoring data (14). The disadvantage of the majority of interventional studies on this subject to date is that most were performed with no a priori knowledge of the patient's immune state. It is quite likely that the most benefit from IFN-γ or GM-CSF therapy, for example, would be seen in the subpopulation of patients with immunoparalysis. To give these agents to a child with a robust innate immune response could conceivably be harmful. Unfortunately, no overt marker of immunoparalysis can be detected on the basis of physical exam or blood counts. It is therefore critically important that standardized assays of innate immune function be employed to survey for immunoparalysis and to target those patients who may benefit from inclusion in prospective trials of immunostimulatory agents.

PATIENTS WITH OVERT IMMUNOSUPPRESSION

Impairment of immune function in the ICU is frequently the result of overt iatrogenic or endogenous inhibition of the immune response. Immunosuppressive medications continue to be the mainstay of treatment for children with cancer, transplantation, autoimmunity, and other chronic inflammatory diseases

TABLE 75.2

COMMONLY USED NON–ANTIBODY-BASED IMMUNOSUPPRESSIVE AGENTS

Class	Drug	Target	Nonimmune toxicities
Glucocorticoids	Methylprednisolone Dexamethasone Prednisone	Inhibition of proinflammatory and cell-proliferation gene transcription in lymphocytes and other immune cells	Hypertension, hyperglycemia, impaired wound healing, neuromuscular weakness, growth impairment
Calcineurin inhibitors	Tacrolimus (FK506) Cyclosporine A (CsA)	Inhibition of T-cell signaling pathways	Nephrotoxicity, CNS toxicity (including seizures), tremor, hypertension, hyperglycemia (FK506), hirsutism (CsA)
TOR protein kinase inhibitor	Sirolimus	Inhibition of T- and B-cell proliferation	Hyperlipidemia, hypertension, thrombocytopenia, rash
Antimetabolite	Azathioprine Mycophenolate mofetil	Purine synthesis inhibition	Bone marrow suppression, diarrhea, cholestasis

(Table 75.2). Accordingly, these patients are known to be at high risk for morbidity and mortality due to infection complications. Similarly, children with primary (congenital) and secondarily acquired (e.g., human immunodeficiency virus, HIV) immunodeficiencies pose a management challenge for the ICU practitioner. An overarching principle in the care of children with overt immunodeficiency is to remove the offending immunosuppressive agent whenever possible and/or to administer the appropriate immunologic supplementation to the deficient child. Obvious examples of this principle include the withholding of chemotherapy from a child with sepsis and the administration of IV immunoglobulin (IVIG) to a hypogammaglobulinemic child. It is sometimes the case, however, that the clinical situation precludes these options (chemotherapy has already been given, transplant rejection is a concern, or no specific immunologic supplementation is available). Three common scenarios in which overt immunosuppression is a concern are discussed in the next sections.

The Neutropenic Patient

Severe, prolonged neutropenia most commonly results from the administration of myelosuppressive chemotherapy in the context of cancer treatment but can also be seen with infection-induced marrow failure and as an unintended side effect of numerous drugs, including antibiotics. It has been understood for decades that an absolute neutrophil count (ANC) of <500 cells/mm³ is associated with increased incidence of sepsis and death in patients with malignancy. Prophylaxis against pneumocystic pneumonia and candidal infections with trimethoprim/sulfamethoxazole and fluconazole, respectively, should be considered in this population when patients are critically ill. Use of the drug granulocyte colony-stimulating factor (GCSF) has become the standard of care in the treatment of cancer patients with fever and neutropenia. Administration of GCSF results in increased myelopoiesis and neutrophil maturation. The National Comprehensive Cancer Network now advocates the use of a colony-stimulating factor in patients with a 20% risk of developing this condition (39). Another therapeutic option for the treatment of severely neutropenic children with life-threatening infection is the administration of donor leukocytes via granulocyte transfusion. This approach requires an element of planning, as a suitable donor is typically pretreated with GCSF for a period of time prior to leukapheresis. Further complicating this approach is the fact that donor leukocytes can induce a potent proinflammatory response following infusion. A 2005 Cochrane Database meta-analysis concluded that evidence to support or contraindicate the use of granulocyte transfusion therapy is inconclusive, but subgroup analysis suggested that patients who received >1 × 10¹⁰ cells per dose fared better than those receiving lower doses (54). In sum, while neutropenia may not be avoidable, safe and effective approaches can reduce its effect on morbidity and mortality.

The Lymphopenic Patient

Lymphopenia frequently accompanies critical illness and has been associated with increased risk of death in the settings of adult sepsis (32) and pediatric multiorgan dysfunction syndrome (MODS) (24). It is especially important to note that the definition of lymphopenia varies by age, with infants and toddlers requiring more robust lymphocyte numbers to remain immunocompetent (Table 75.3). However, some authors have chosen an absolute lymphocyte count (ALC) <1000 cells/mm³ as diagnostic of clinically relevant lymphopenia across all age groups (24). Causes of lymphopenia in the PICU include drug-related marrow failure (including chemotherapy), infection-induced bone marrow suppression, HIV infection, and lymphocyte loss via chylothorax drainage.

The HIV pandemic has taught numerous lessons about the importance of lymphocyte function in protecting against infection. Chief among them is the importance of appropriate antimicrobial prophylaxis in the setting of prolonged lymphopenia. CDC recommendations currently include the administration of trimethoprim/sulfamethoxazole, dapsone, or pentamidine for pneumocystic pneumonia prophylaxis in children with severe reductions in CD4+ T cell count (2).

Although the number of circulating lymphocytes may not necessarily be representative of cell numbers within lymphoid organs, such as the spleen and lymph nodes, numerous investigators have demonstrated apoptotic lymphocyte depletion in these organs at autopsy following critical illness (24,32).

TABLE 75.3

CENTERS FOR DISEASE CONTROL DEFINITIONS OF SEVERE REDUCTIONS IN CD4$^+$ COUNT IN CHILDREN

Age	CD4$^+$ count (cells/mm^3)
<1 year	<750
1–5 years	<500
6–12 years	<200

Adapted from *MMWR Recomm Rep* 1995;44(RR-4):1–11.

As such, the clinician must be suspicious of total-body lymphocyte depletion when peripheral lymphopenia is seen in the ICU. One potential consequence of lymphocyte depletion is a lack of antibody production by B cells. Assessment of quantitative immunoglobulin levels can identify patients with hypogammaglobulinemia who may benefit from replacement with IVIG. While the role of IVIG in the empiric management of critical illness in the *absence* of low IgG levels is somewhat controversial, as detailed below, the use of IVIG in the treatment of hypogammaglobulinemia in the ICU is not.

It is noteworthy that many therapies commonly used in the practice of critical care medicine may themselves promote or exacerbate lymphopenia. Glucocorticoids, for example, are potent inducers of lymphocyte apoptosis. Dopamine use has similarly been associated with the development of lymphopenia, presumably through its inhibitory effect on the neuroendocrine axes, most notably prolactin, which is known to be a necessary growth factor for lymphocytes (24). Currently, no lymphocyte-specific colony-stimulating factors are available that can be used to bolster lymphocyte numbers; however, elimination of lymphopenia-inducing agents when possible should be strongly considered, especially when suitable alternatives exist (e.g., another catecholamine or fenoldopam in place of dopamine).

The Transplant Patient

Patients who have undergone transplantation are placed in the double bind of taking medicines that place them at high risk for the development of infection, without which they are likely to reject their allograft. Multidrug regimens, including calcineurin inhibitors, corticosteroids, and other immunosuppressives (e.g., mycophenolate or azathioprine), are frequently employed to shut down the adaptive immune response against the transplanted organ, often with significant systemic toxicities. The suppressive effects of these regimens are not limited to the adaptive immune response, inhibiting the innate response as well, with reductions in monocyte function associated directly or indirectly with calcineurin inhibition. Lastly, most transplant regimens rely on plasma drug levels and end-organ toxicity to drive dose titration rather than on direct measures of immune function.

Several strategies can be employed to promote improved outcomes in the transplant patient with critical illness. First, antimicrobial prophylaxis is crucial for the prevention of secondary infection. Perhaps the most comprehensive set of recommendations in this regard comes from the Centers for Disease Control Guidelines for Preventing Opportunistic Infection in Hematopoietic Stem Cell Transplant Recipients (21) (Table 75.4). Although not necessarily generalizable to all transplant populations, these guidelines highlight the scope of the problem and identify a rational approach to prophylaxis. Second, the

TABLE 75.4

ROUTINE PREVENTIVE REGIMENS FOR PEDIATRIC HEMATOPOIETIC STEM CELL TRANSPLANT RECIPIENTS

Infection	Indication	First-line drug
Bacterial infections	Severe hypogammaglobulinemia (serum IgG level <400 mg/dL) at <100 days after transplant	IVIG 400 mg/kg/mo (or as needed to keep IgG level >400 mg/dL)
Candida species	Allogeneic recipients or high-risk autologous recipients from transplant to engraftment or until 7 days after ANC >1000 cells/mm^3	Fluconazole 3–6 mg/kg/day PO or IV (6 mo–13 yrs); or 400 mg PO or IV daily (>13 yrs). Max dose 600 mg/day
Cytomegalovirus	All patients from engraftment through day 100	Ganciclovir 5 mg/kg/dose IV every 12 hrs for 5–7 days, followed by 5 mg/kg/dose IV daily for 5 days/week
Pneumocystis jirovecii pneumonia	Allogeneic recipients or high-risk autologous recipients until 6 months post-transplant (longer if immunosuppression continued or GVHD)	Trimethoprim/sulfamethoxazole (TMP/SMX; 150 mg TMP/ 750 mg SMX) PO twice daily 3 times weekly. [Alternative regimens available; see *MMWR Recomm Rep* 2000;49(RR10):1–128.]
Herpes simplex virus	Seropositive patients from the beginning of conditioning therapy until engraftment	Acyclovir 250 mg/m^2/dose IV every 8 hrs or 125 mg/m^2/dose IV every 6 hrs
Varicella zoster virus	Post-exposure prophylaxis in actively immunosuppressed patients	Varicella-zoster immunoglobulin 125 units/10 kg body weight IM (max dose 625 units)
Methicillin-resistant *Staphylococcus aureus*	Known MRSA carriers	Mupirocin calcium ointment 2% to nares twice daily for 5 days or to wounds daily for 2 weeks

Recommendations include vaccination against influenza, respiratory syncytial virus, *Streptococcus pneumoniae*, and *Haemophilus influenzae* type b. IgG, immunoglobulin G; IVIG, IV immunoglobulin; ANC, absolute neutrophil count; GVHD, graft-versus-host disease; IM, intramuscularly; MRSA, methicillin-resistant *Staphylococcus aureus*. Adapted from *MMWR Recomm Rep* 2000;49(RR10):1–128.

use of antibody-based immunosuppressive regimens, including anti–IL-2 receptor antibodies, has been shown to be an effective antirejection strategy without the systemic toxicity profiles of drugs such as cyclosporine and tacrolimus (18). Lastly, the ICU practitioner can rapidly taper the exogenous immunosuppression to allow for a more robust immune response in the setting of suspected or proven infection. The impressive effect of this strategy was displayed by Volk et al., who, in the mid-1990s, demonstrated 90% patient survival (with 98% graft survival in that group) in immunoparalyzed adult transplant patients with sepsis when they underwent rapid tapering of immunosuppression. Immunoparalyzed patients who did not undergo rapid tapering experienced an 8% survival rate (59).

A major impediment to the optimal titration of immunosuppressive therapy in transplant patients is the reliance on drug levels as the primary indicator of immunosuppression. While plasma tacrolimus levels of <10 ng/mL and cyclosporine A levels of <200 ng/mL can be generally thought of as mildly to moderately immunosuppressive, functional assays of the immune response, such as ex vivo LPS-induced TNF-α production capacity, have the potential to serve as more relevant targets for titration of these potent drugs.

INTRAVENOUS IMMUNOGLOBULIN

Polyclonal IVIG has been administered to adults and children *without* preexisting hypogammaglobulinemia in the context of sepsis, with mixed results. A recent meta-analysis of IVIG use for the treatment of suspected or proven infection in critically ill neonates showed no effect on mortality with empiric use. It did show, however, that mortality risk was lowered when IVIG was used in the setting of proven infection (45). A 2004 meta-analysis of high-quality adult studies failed to show a reduced mortality risk when IVIG was empirically used in the treatment of sepsis (48). However, in a 2005, prospective, randomized, controlled trial in children <2 years of age with sepsis, 3 days of polyclonal IVIG treatment resulted in improved survival to discharge and in shorter durations of PICU stay (22). Interestingly, it appears that IVIG may be of particular benefit in the setting of severe, invasive group A strep infection (44).

A subset of IVIG trials has employed a product that is enriched in the IgM fraction of immunoglobulin. Evidence suggests that IgM-enriched IVIG may be beneficial in postoperative sepsis in adult patients, though a multicentered, randomized, controlled trial failed to show benefit in the setting of chemotherapy-induced neutropenic sepsis (30,51).

IMMUNONUTRITION

Another approach that has been taken to effect immunomodulation in the ICU is through immunonutrition. With this strategy, patients are provided with nutritional supplementation that, in the course of metabolism, has an effect on the immune response. The two substrates that have been the focus of the most investigation are the ω-3 polyunsaturated fatty acids (PUFA) and the amino acid arginine.

The ω-3 PUFAs, including docosahexaenoic, eicosapentaenoic, and α-linoleic acid, are thought to promote an antiinflammatory immune state through at least two mechanisms.

By incorporating into the cell's phospholipid membrane, ω-3 PUFAs compete with arachidonic acid precursors, resulting in lower arachidonic acid production. The ω-3 PUFAs are themselves less favorable substrates for eicosanoid formation. In addition, ω-3 PUFAs directly inhibit nuclear receptors, including PPARγ, which results in impairment of the propagation of the inflammatory response. Administration of ω-3 PUFAs has been shown in vitro and in vivo to be associated with Th-2 polarization, reduced innate and adaptive immune function, and reduced plasma concentrations of proinflammatory cytokines, although no mortality benefit has been definitively shown (36).

Arginine, by contrast, is thought to promote a more vigorous immune response through augmentation of intracellular killing and lymphocyte function. A 2001 meta-analysis of 22 studies in critically ill adults concluded that arginine supplementation resulted in *higher* mortality in treated patients, though its use was associated with a lower overall infection rate (31). More recent studies have explored the use of combined formulas, including both ω-3 PUFAs, arginine, and other supplements, in critically ill adults and children (11). While subtle differences in cytokine profiles have resulted, a significant impact on clinical outcomes has yet to be reliably demonstrated. Although it is important to note that these studies did not employ a priori measures of immune function to screen for such conditions as immunoparalysis, routine use of immunonutrition cannot currently be recommended.

THE IMPACT OF CRITICAL ILLNESS ON INFLAMMATION

In addition to overt immunosuppression with drugs (e.g., tacrolimus) and endogenous phenomena (e.g., immunoparalysis), the ICU practitioner must be aware of the profound immunologic effects of many of the drugs routinely used in the ICU. Catecholamines, for example, can enhance (α receptors) or inhibit (β receptors) the immune response. Bacteriocidal antibiotics can transiently exacerbate the inflammatory response due to release of bacterial components at the time of cell death. Conversely, β-lactams can lead to immunodeficiency through bone marrow suppression, while macrolides are known to impair proinflammatory cytokine production. Opioids are inducers of lymphocyte and macrophage apoptosis and can induce the anti-inflammatory cytokine TGF-β. Insulin is thought to have significant anti-inflammatory properties both through reduction of hyperglycemia-induced proinflammatory cytokine production and through direct inhibition of the NFκB pathway. Even furosemide is thought to be immunologically active, resulting in attenuation of the inflammatory response in mononuclear cells.

Concomitant organ failure and other conditions associated with critical illness further complicate the picture. Hepatic failure, with its associated impairment of cytokine clearance, is frequently associated with a proinflammatory state. Uremic plasma from patients with renal failure has been shown to induce apoptosis in innate and adaptive immune cells. As noted previously, extracorporeal therapies, including hemodialysis and continuous venovenous hemofiltration, can promote the inflammatory state through immune reactions to plastic tubing and membranes. Hyperglycemia, the control of which is now the target of prospective clinical trials in the PICU, has been clearly shown to be a potent activator of the NFκB pathway in innate immune cells. Conversely, the endogenous stress-induced cortisol response, although less immuno-suppressive than some exogenous glucocorticoids, inhibits proinflammatory cytokine production in leukocytes. These examples illustrate that the effects of these competing forces in a critically ill child can be confusing at best, but they also illustrate the need for assessment of the overall immune phenotype of the patient in determining the proper course of therapy (**Fig. 75.2**).

EXPERIMENTAL DIRECTIONS

The regulation of the immune response in critical illness is the subject of numerous intriguing research initiatives. For example, Tracey et al. have elegantly shown that innate immune cells bear nicotinic receptors, which, when stimulated, exert a suppressive effect. Activation of these receptors through vagal nerve stimulation or the use of nicotinic receptor agonists has the potential to offer new therapeutic options for immunomodulation (8). We are also gaining broader insight into the cast of characters involved in the immune response. The nuclear protein high mobility group box 1 (HMGB1) has recently been shown to be detectable in the serum following a proinflammatory insult and may mediate the late effects of inflammation. Anti-HMGB1 antibodies have been successful in improving mortality in animal models of established sepsis (62). Another molecule, ethyl pyruvate, has been shown to have similar benefit in experimental sepsis models, likely through abrogation of NFκB activity in inflammatory cells (57). As described previously, several small studies have suggested that an overactive anti-inflammatory response should also be the target of ongoing investigation. Large-scale, controlled trials of immunostimulatory agents for the treatment of immunoparalysis are as yet lacking.

CONCLUSIONS AND FUTURE DIRECTIONS

From the proinflammatory storm of sepsis to the anti-inflammatory dominance of immunoparalysis, it is clear that ICU patients span a spectrum of immune activity. It is naïve to assume that one type of immunotherapy will be suitable for all patients with a given condition. As such, the success or failure of any therapy directed at the restoration of immunologic homeostasis is likely to be dependent on the right patient receiving the right therapies at the right time. To that end, a program of immune monitoring is essential for directing treatments to patients who are most likely to benefit from them. Innate immune monitoring, through quantification of monocyte HLA-DR expression or ex vivo TNF-α production capacity, is relatively easy to accomplish but is in need of standardization across the critical care community. Along with this type of monitoring, the practitioner should continue to be vigilant in following absolute neutrophil and lymphocyte counts, instituting appropriate prophylactic therapy when indicated, and wisely titrating medications that have immunologic effects, both overt and subtle.

Perhaps the most important method of immunomodulation is that achieved through immunization. Prevention of disease, rather than its treatment, should continue to be the highest goal of the medical community. We should therefore continue to advocate for routine immunization against organisms such as *Haemophilus influenzae*, *Streptococcus pneumoniae*, and *Neisseria meningitis*. Similarly, high-risk children should receive prophylaxis against respiratory syncytial virus and influenza. The development of new vaccine programs, including immunization against *Pseudomonas* species in high-risk populations, holds promise to further extend this umbrella of protection.

Lastly, as is apparent from the previous discussion, the vast majority of data that describe the relationships between immune function and critical illness have come from adult

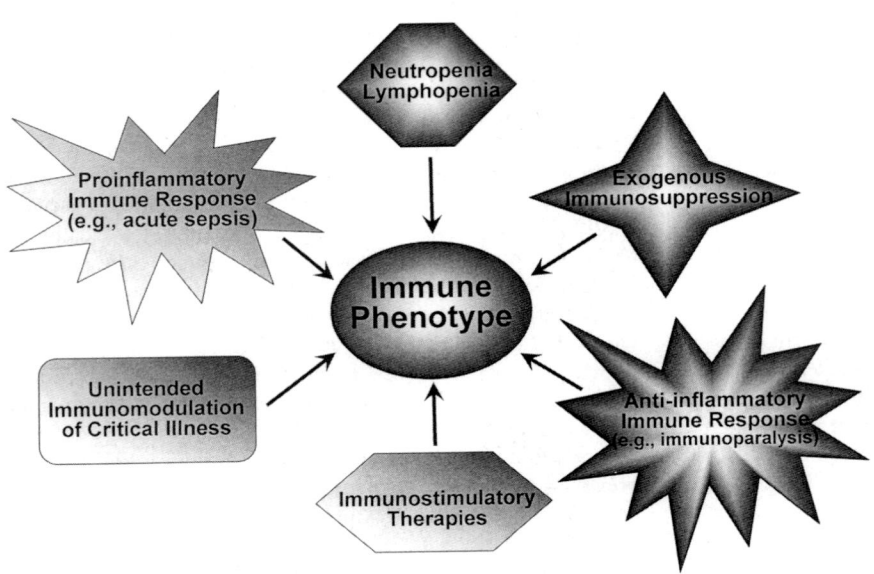

FIGURE 75.2. The patient's overall immune phenotype is determined by the net effects of pro- and anti-inflammatory forces acting to influence the inflammatory balance. Many of these forces are occult, necessitating immune monitoring.

studies. Significant developmental influences, most of which remain unknown, very likely immunologically differentiate infants from older children and adolescents. Multicentered descriptive and interventional studies are necessary to address this major gap in the literature and promote immunologic homeostasis in the PICU.

KEY POINTS

■ Abnormal regulation of the immune response— overactivity *or* underactivity of the immune system—is the cause of adverse outcomes in many forms of critical illness.

■ Therapies aimed at reducing levels of proinflammatory mediators in human sepsis by specifically targeting LPS, TNF-α, IL-1β, and others have been overwhelmingly unsuccessful in improving outcomes. The use of low-dose hydrocortisone in this setting, however, has been shown to impart clinical benefit.

■ The role of methylprednisolone in the treatment of ARDS continues to be controversial, with recent evidence suggesting that its use beyond the second week of ARDS may be harmful.

■ Innate immune function is dynamic following a proinflammatory insult, such as trauma or sepsis. A transient compensatory downregulation of innate immune function can be expected. More persistent reduction in innate immune function (beyond 3–5 days) is pathologic and is termed immunoparalysis.

■ Immunoparalysis can be quantified through measurement of HLA-DR expression on circulating monocytes, with increased risks of adverse outcomes if <30% of monocytes are HLA-DR$^+$. Another important measure of innate immune function is the capacity of whole blood to produce TNF-α when stimulated ex vivo. Persistent reduction in the ex vivo TNF-α response is similarly associated with adverse outcomes.

■ Immunoparalysis can be reversed through the use of immunostimulatory agents including IFN-γ or GM-CSF, or by withholding exogenous immunosuppression, likely with beneficial effects of outcome.

■ Critically ill patients with persistent neutropenia should be treated with GCSF, and consideration should be given to the use of prophylactic therapy for pneumocystic pneumonia and fungal infections.

■ Lymphopenia is associated with increased risk of death in sepsis and MODS. Use of appropriate prophylaxis against pneumocystic pneumonia and fungal infections, avoidance of lymphotoxic drugs, and treatment of hypogammaglobulinemia with IVIG are important aspects of care for the critically ill lymphopenic patient.

■ To date, immunonutrition with ω-3 polyunsaturated fatty acids or arginine has no role in the PICU.

■ Critical illnesses themselves, and most of the drugs used to treat critically ill children, have effects on the immune response. The development of routine immune monitoring protocols, including measurement of cell counts *and* immune function (e.g., HLA-DR expression or ex vivo TNF-α response), will be crucial to the identification of patients with overactive or underactive immune systems so that individualized treatment plans can be implemented.

References

1. Prophylactic intravenous administration of standard immune globulin as compared with core-lipopolysaccharide immune globulin in patients at high risk of postsurgical infection. The Intravenous Immunoglobulin Collaborative Study Group. *N Engl J Med* 1992;327:234–40.
2. 1995 revised guidelines for prophylaxis against *Pneumocystis carinii* pneumonia for children infected with, or perinatally exposed to, human immunodeficiency virus. National Pediatric and Family HIV Resource Center and National Center for Infectious Diseases, Centers for Disease Control and Prevention. *MMWR Recomm Rep* 1995;44:1–11.
3. Abraham E, Anzueto A, Gutierrez G, et al. Double-blind randomised controlled trial of monoclonal antibody to human tumour necrosis factor in treatment of septic shock. *NORASEPT II Study Group. Lancet* 1998;351:929–33.
4. Abraham E, Wunderink R, Silverman H, et al. Efficacy and safety of monoclonal antibody to human tumor necrosis factor alpha in patients with sepsis syndrome. *A randomized, controlled, double-blind, multicenter clinical trial. TNF-alpha MAb Sepsis Study Group. JAMA* 1995;273:934–41.
5. Allen ML, Hoschtitzky JA, Peters MJ, et al. Interleukin-10 and its role in clinical immunoparalysis following pediatric cardiac surgery. *Crit Care Med* 2006;34:2658–65.
6. Annane D, Bellissant E, Bollaert PE, et al. Corticosteroids for severe sepsis and septic shock: A systematic review and meta-analysis. *BMJ* 2004;329:480.
7. Baehr RV, Volk HD, Reinke P, et al. An immune monitoring program for controlling immunosuppressive therapy. *Transplant Proc* 1989;21:1189–91.
8. Bernik TR, Friedman SG, Ochani M, et al. Pharmacological stimulation of the cholinergic antiinflammatory pathway. *J Exp Med* 2002;195:781–8.
9. Bone RC. Immunologic dissonance: A continuing evolution in our understanding of the systemic inflammatory response syndrome (SIRS) and the multiple organ dysfunction syndrome (MODS). *Ann Intern Med* 1996;125:680–7.
10. Bone RC, Balk RA, Fein AM, et al. A second large controlled clinical study of E5, a monoclonal antibody to endotoxin: Results of a prospective, multicenter, randomized, controlled trial. *The E5 Sepsis Study Group. Crit Care Med* 1995;23:994–1006.
11. Briassoulis G, Filippou O, Kanariou M, et al. Temporal nutritional and inflammatory changes in children with severe head injury fed a regular or an immune-enhancing diet: A randomized, controlled trial. *Pediatr Crit Care Med* 2006;7:56–62.
12. Busund R, Koukline V, Utrobin U, et al. Plasmapheresis in severe sepsis and septic shock: A prospective, randomised, controlled trial. *Intensive Care Med* 2002;28:1434–9.
13. Calandra T, Glauser MP, Schellekens J, et al. Treatment of Gram-negative septic shock with human IgG antibody to Escherichia coli J5: A prospective, double-blind, randomized trial. *J Infect Dis* 1988;158:312–9.
14. Carr R, Modi N, Dore C. G-CSF and GM-CSF for treating or preventing neonatal infections. *Cochrane Database Syst Rev* 2003;CD003066.
15. Cohen J, Carlet J. INTERSEPT: An international, multicenter, placebo-controlled trial of monoclonal antibody to human tumor necrosis factor-alpha in patients with sepsis. International Sepsis Trial Study Group. *Crit Care Med* 1996;24:1431–40.
16. Cronin L, Cook DJ, Carlet J, et al. Corticosteroid treatment for sepsis: A critical appraisal and meta-analysis of the literature. *Crit Care Med* 1995;23:1430–9.
17. Dhainaut JF, Laterre PF, Janes JM, et al. Drotrecogin alfa (activated) in the treatment of severe sepsis patients with multiple-organ dysfunction: Data from the PROWESS trial. *Intensive Care Med* 2003;29:894–903.
18. Di Filippo S. Anti-IL-2 receptor antibody vs. *polyclonal anti-lymphocyte antibody as induction therapy in pediatric transplantation. Pediatr Transplant* 2005;9:373–80.
19. Docke WD, Randow F, Syrbe U, et al. Monocyte deactivation in septic patients: Restoration by IFN-gamma treatment. *Nat Med* 1997;3:678–81.
20. Doughty L, Carcillo JA, Kaplan S, et al. The compensatory anti-inflammatory cytokine interleukin 10 response in pediatric sepsis-induced multiple organ failure. *Chest* 1998;113:1625–31.
21. Dykewicz CA. Summary of the guidelines for preventing opportunistic infections among hematopoietic stem cell transplant recipients. *Clin Infect Dis* 2001;33:139–44.
22. El-Nawawy A, El-Kinany H, Hamdy El-Sayed M, et al. Intravenous polyclonal immunoglobulin administration to sepsis syndrome patients: A prospective study in a pediatric intensive care unit. *J Trop Pediatr* 2005;51:271–8.
23. Fein AM, Bernard GR, Criner GJ, et al. Treatment of severe systemic inflammatory response syndrome and sepsis with a novel bradykinin antagonist, deltibant (CP-0127). *Results of a randomized, double-blind, placebo-controlled trial. CP-0127 SIRS and Sepsis Study Group. JAMA* 1997;277:482–7.
24. Felmet KA, Hall MW, Clark RS, et al. Prolonged lymphopenia, lymphoid depletion, and hypoprolactinemia in children with nosocomial sepsis and multiple organ failure. *J Immunol* 2005;174:3765–72.
25. Fisher CJ, Jr., Dhainaut JF, Opal SM, et al. *Recombinant human interleukin 1 receptor antagonist in the treatment of patients with sepsis syndrome.*

Results from a randomized, double-blind, placebo-controlled trial. Phase III rhIL-1ra Sepsis Syndrome Study Group. JAMA 1994;271:1836–43.

26. Fumeaux T, Pugin J. Role of interleukin-10 in the intracellular sequestration of human leukocyte antigen-DR in monocytes during septic shock. *Am J Respir Crit Care Med* 2002;166:1475–82.

27. Goldstein B, Nadel S, Peters M, et al. ENHANCE: Results of a global open-label trial of drotrecogin alfa (activated) in children with severe sepsis. *Pediatr Crit Care Med* 2006;7:200–11.

28. Greenman RL, Schein RM, Martin MA, et al. A controlled clinical trial of E5 murine monoclonal IgM antibody to endotoxin in the treatment of Gram-negative sepsis. *The XOMA Sepsis Study Group. JAMA* 1991;266:1097–102.

29. Hall MW, Volk HD, Carcillo JA. Immune paralysis in pediatric multiple organ dysfunction syndrome. *Pediatr Res* 2000;47:57A.

30. Hentrich M, Fehnle K, Ostermann H, et al. IgMA-enriched immunoglobulin in neutropenic patients with sepsis syndrome and septic shock: A randomized, controlled, multiple-center trial. *Crit Care Med* 2006;34:1319–25.

31. Heyland DK, Novak F, Drover JW, et al. Should immunonutrition become routine in critically ill patients? A systematic review of the evidence. *JAMA* 2001;286:944–53.

32. Hotchkiss RS, Tinsley KW, Swanson PE, et al. Sepsis-induced apoptosis causes progressive profound depletion of B and CD4+ T lymphocytes in humans. *J Immunol* 2001;166:6952–63.

33. Lefering R, Neugebauer EA. Steroid controversy in sepsis and septic shock: A meta-analysis. *Crit Care Med* 1995;23:1294–303.

34. Levin M, Quint PA, Goldstein B, et al. Recombinant bactericidal/permeability-increasing protein (rBPI21) as adjunctive treatment for children with severe meningococcal sepsis: A randomised trial. *rBPI21 Meningococcal Sepsis Study Group. Lancet* 2000;356:961–7.

35. Livingston DH, Appel SH, Wellhausen SR, et al. Depressed interferon gamma production and monocyte HLA-DR expression after severe injury. *Arch Surg* 1988;123:1309–12.

36. Mayer K, Gokorsch S, Fegbeutel C, et al. Parenteral nutrition with fish oil modulates cytokine response in patients with sepsis. *Am J Respir Crit Care Med* 2003;167:1321–8.

37. McCloskey RV, Straube RC, Sanders C, et al. Treatment of septic shock with human monoclonal antibody HA-1A. *A randomized, double-blind, placebo-controlled trial. CHESS Trial Study Group. Ann Intern Med* 1994;121:1–5.

38. McMaster P, Shann F. The use of extracorporeal techniques to remove humoral factors in sepsis. *Pediatr Crit Care Med* 2003;4:2–7.

39. McNeil C. NCCN guidelines advocate wider use of colony-stimulating factor. *J Natl Cancer Inst* 2005;97:710–1.

40. Meduri GU, Headley AS, Golden E, et al. Effect of prolonged methylprednisolone therapy in unresolving acute respiratory distress syndrome: A randomized controlled trial. *JAMA* 1998;280:159–65.

41. Minneci PC, Deans KJ, Banks SM, et al. Meta-analysis: The effect of steroids on survival and shock during sepsis depends on the dose. *Ann Intern Med* 2004;141:47–56.

42. Monneret G, Lepape A, Voirin N, et al. Persisting low monocyte human leukocyte antigen-DR expression predicts mortality in septic shock. *Intensive Care Med* 2006;32:1175–83.

43. Nierhaus A, Montag B, Timmler N, et al. Reversal of immunoparalysis by recombinant human granulocyte-macrophage colony-stimulating factor in patients with severe sepsis. *Intensive Care Med* 2003;29:646–51.

44. Norrby-Teglund A, Ihendyane N, Darenberg J. Intravenous immunoglobulin adjunctive therapy in sepsis, with special emphasis on severe invasive group A streptococcal infections. *Scand J Infect Dis* 2003;35:683–9.

45. Ohlsson A, Lacy JB. Intravenous immunoglobulin for suspected or subsequently proven infection in neonates. *Cochrane Database Syst Rev* 2004;CD001239.

46. Opal SM, Fisher CJ, Jr., Dhainaut JF, et al. *Confirmatory interleukin-1 receptor antagonist trial in severe sepsis: A phase III, randomized, double-blind, placebo-controlled, multicenter trial. The Interleukin-1 Receptor Antagonist Sepsis -REF>Investigator Group. Crit Care Med* 1997;25:1115–24.

47. Panacek EA, Marshall JC, Albertson TE, et al. Efficacy and safety of the monoclonal anti-tumor necrosis factor antibody F(ab')2 fragment afelimomab in patients with severe sepsis and elevated interleukin-6 levels. *Crit Care Med* 2004;32:2173–82.

48. Pildal J, Gotzsche PC. Polyclonal immunoglobulin for treatment of bacterial sepsis: A systematic review. *Clin Infect Dis* 2004;39:38–46.

49. Polk HC, Jr., Wellhausen SR, Regan M. *A systematic study of host defense processes in badly injured patients. Ann Surg* 1986;204:282–97.

50. Reinke P, Volk HD. Diagnostic and predictive value of an immune monitoring program for complications after kidney transplantation. *Urol Int* 1992;49:69–75.

51. Rodriguez A, Rello J, Neira J, et al. Effects of high-dose of intravenous immunoglobulin and antibiotics on survival for severe sepsis undergoing surgery. *Shock* 2005;23:298–304.

52. Rosenbloom AJ, Linden PK, Dorrance A, et al. Effect of granulocyte-monocyte colony-stimulating factor therapy on leukocyte function and clearance of serious infection in nonneutropenic patients. *Chest* 2005;127:2139–50.

53. Rubens FD, Mesana T. The inflammatory response to cardiopulmonary bypass: A therapeutic overview. *Perfusion* 2004;19 Suppl 1:S5–12.

54. Stanworth SJ, Massey E, Hyde C, et al. Granulocyte transfusions for treating infections in patients with neutropenia or neutrophil dysfunction. *Cochrane Database Syst Rev* 2005;CD005339.

55. Steinberg KP, Hudson LD, Goodman RB, et al. Efficacy and safety of corticosteroids for persistent acute respiratory distress syndrome. *N Engl J Med* 2006;354:1671–84.

56. Suputtamongkol Y, Intaranongpai S, Smith MD, et al. A double-blind placebo-controlled study of an infusion of lexipafant (Platelet-activating factor receptor antagonist) in patients with severe sepsis. *Antimicrob Agents Chemother* 2000;44:693–6.

57. Ulloa L, Ochani M, Yang H, et al. Ethyl pyruvate prevents lethality in mice with established lethal sepsis and systemic inflammation. *Proc Natl Acad Sci U S A* 2002;99:12351–6.

58. van Deuren M, Santman FW, van Dalen R, et al. Plasma and whole blood exchange in meningococcal sepsis. *Clin Infect Dis* 1992;15:424–30.

59. Volk HD, Reinke P, Krausch D, et al. Monocyte deactivation-rationale for a new therapeutic strategy in sepsis. *Intensive Care Med* 1996;22 Suppl 4:S474–81.

60. Westendorp RG, Brand A, Haanen J, et al. Leukaplasmapheresis in meningococcal septic shock. *Am J Med* 1992;92:577–8.

61. Wysocka M, Montaner LJ, Karp CL. Flt3 ligand treatment reverses endotoxin tolerance-related immunoparalysis. *J Immunol* 2005;174:7398–402.

62. Yang H, Ochani M, Li J, et al. Reversing established sepsis with antagonists of endogenous high-mobility group box 1. *Proc Natl Acad Sci U S A* 2004;101:296–301.

CHAPTER 76 ■ IMMUNOLOGY OF CANCER AND PRIMARY IMMUNE DEFICIENCY SYNDROMES

BRANDT P. GROH • JENNIFER A. McARTHUR • SACHIN S. JOGAL • ROBERT F. TAMBURRO

PRIMARY OR CONGENITAL IMMUNE DEFICIENCY DISORDERS

The pediatric intensivist is frequently confronted with severe and life-threatening infections. Although the majority of these infections can be attributed to environmental risk factors and invasive monitoring, immune deficiency is a consideration in select cases. The incidence of well-defined congenital immune deficiency is estimated to be only 1 in 10,000 live births, but these children are over-represented at tertiary care centers, where expert immunologic care is available. The intensivist should recognize the child who presents with his second invasive bacterial infection, an opportunistic infection, or an infection slow to respond to conventional therapy as a child in need of an immunologic workup. With antibody defects being the most prevalent immune deficiencies (**Table 76.1**), laboratory evaluation should generally focus first on the possibility of humoral deficiency. Specific pathogens and characteristic host responses, however, may indicate the likelihood of a cellular, phagocytic, or innate immune defect. The clinical features common to the majority of congenital immune deficiencies are presented in **Table 76.2**. A summary of the diseases addressed in this chapter can be found in **Table 76.3**. Excellent reviews of primary immune deficiency are readily available and have been published previously (8,71).

DISORDERS PREDOMINANTLY AFFECTING IMMUNOGLOBULINS

Defects predominantly affecting antibody production and function comprise 65% of the congenital immune-deficient population. Included within this category are defects of questionable clinical significance such as isolated immunoglobulin (Ig) M deficiency, isolated IgA deficiency, and IgG subclass deficiencies. Only the disorders that involve quantitative total IgG deficiency and predictable immunologic consequences are discussed here. Antibody defects predispose patients to sinopulmonary infections with encapsulated organisms, such as *Streptococcus pneumoniae* and *Haemophilus influenzae*. The patient who presents with a severe pneumonia that has been poorly responsive to antibiotic therapy deserves quantitative assessment of immunoglobulin levels. Bacterial sepsis would be a less common presentation of an antibody defect, but poor responsiveness to therapy might again raise this concern.

X-linked Agammaglobulinemia

Since the original description of X-linked agammaglobulinemia (XLA) in 1952 by Colonel Ogden Bruton, significant advances have facilitated the accurate diagnosis and effective therapy of XLA. This defect occurs at an estimated incidence of 1 in 50,000 live births. Due to the persistence of maternal immunoglobulin, most XLA patients are not diagnosed until after the first 6 months of life. Surprisingly, adults with some residual IgG production have also been reported within this spectrum of disease. Although infection symptoms peak at around 7 months of age, 40% of boys are asymptomatic at 1 year, and the majority present between 3 and 5 years of age. A presentation with recurrent and refractory sinopulmonary infections is the rule, usually involving extracellular pyogenic bacteria, such as pneumococci, streptococci, meningococci, *H. influenzae*, and *Pseudomonas aeruginosa*. Infections with fungal pathogens and even *Pneumocystis jiroveci* (formerly *Pneumocystis carinii*) are occasionally reported (12). In addition, children with XLA have a unique susceptibility to enteroviral infections; poliomyelitis was a significant risk for these children in the era of oral polio vaccine.

Recognition of hypoplastic lymphoid tissue in the setting of invasive infection should heighten suspicion of a disorder such as XLA, in which mature B cells are absent from both lymphoid tissues and the circulation. Mature B cells, which comprise the bulk of tonsillar and lymphoid follicular tissue, are virtually absent from the circulation (<1% of circulating lymphocytes). Plasma cells and immunoglobulins are consequently also lacking, such that immunoglobulin levels are <10% of normal and antigen-specific responses cannot be demonstrated. An early clue to immunoglobulin deficiency is the finding of a low total protein level in the presence of a normal albumin level on routine blood analysis, as gammaglobulin comprises the largest fraction of the total protein measurement. The genetic defects of XLA are mutations in the Bruton's tyrosine kinase (BTK) gene at Xq22. A diagnosis can be supported by genotyping, but the absence of mature B cells in the peripheral blood, demonstrated by flow cytometry analysis of B-cell surface markers (CD19 and/or CD20) in the presence of normal T-cell numbers, is virtually diagnostic of XLA in a male. The finding of protein antigen unresponsiveness by specific titers to diphtheria and tetanus toxoid post-vaccination in conjunction with normal T-cell function (demonstrated by delayed-type hypersensitivity testing or lymphocyte proliferation assays), lends additional

TABLE 76.1

CLASSIFICATION AND FREQUENCY OF THE PRIMARY IMMUNE DEFICIENCY DISORDERS

Immune deficiency	Approximate % of total
Predominantly antibody defects	65
Predominantly cellular defects	5
Combined antibody and cellular defects	15
Complement defects	5
Phagocytic defects	10

From Stiehm ER, Ochs HD, Winkelstein JA. *Immunologic Disorders in Infants and Children, 5th ed*. Philadelphia: Elsevier Saunders, 2004, with permission.

TABLE 76.2

CLINICAL FEATURES COMMON IN IMMUNODEFICIENCY

Usually Present
Recurrent upper respiratory infections
Severe bacterial infections
Persistent infections with incomplete or no response to therapy

Often Present
Failure to thrive or growth retardation
Paucity of lymph nodes and tonsils
Infections with unusual organisms
Skin lesions (e.g., rash, telangiectasias, abscesses, warts)
Recalcitrant thrush
Clubbing
Diarrhea and malabsorption
Persistent sinusitis, mastoiditis
Recurrent bronchitis, pneumonia
Autoimmune disorders
Hematologic abnormalities (aplastic anemia, hemolytic anemia, neutropenia, thrombocytopenia)

Occasionally Present
Weight loss, fevers
Chronic conjunctivitis
Periodontitis
Lymphadenopathy
Hepatosplenomegaly
Severe viral disease
Adverse reaction to vaccines
Bronchiectasis
Urinary tract infections
Delayed umbilical cord separation (>30 days)
Chronic stomatitis
Granulomas
Lymphoid malignancies

From Stiehm ER, Ochs HD, Winkelstein JA. *Immunologic Disorders in Infants and Children, 5th ed*. Philadelphia: Elsevier Saunders, 2004, with permission.

diagnostic certainty such that genotyping is not necessary in the majority of cases.

Therapy has evolved from intramuscular gammaglobulin replacement to IV replacement to the relatively new option of subcutaneous replacement (30). In the intensive care setting, gammaglobulin replacement therapy can be helpful in the control and clearance of severe infections, and IV administration at physiologic replacement doses of 400–500 mg/kg is most appropriate. Concurrent IgA deficiency mandates the use of IgA-depleted IV immunoglobulin (IVIG) to minimize the risk of anaphylaxis. Children with a known diagnosis of IgG deficiency may benefit from supplementary gammaglobulin at the time of infection (49). Despite consistent IgG replacement therapy, a significant proportion of XLA patients progress to bronchiectasis, and chronic antibiotic therapy is recommended for this subset of patients (54). With currently available treatment, most patients lead productive and relatively infection-free lives.

Common Variable Immunodeficiency

Common variable immunodeficiency (CVID) describes an XLA-like condition with later onset, generally during the second or third decades of life, although earlier presentations may occur throughout the pediatric age range. Total IgG levels in CVID are less than 2 standard deviations below the mean for age, but generally not as low as those found in XLA. Also in contrast to XLA, IgM and IgA levels may be normal. The incidence of CVID is estimated to be between 1 in 25,000 and 1 in 66,000 individuals. Patients present in a fashion similar to XLA, with recurrent sinopulmonary disease related to encapsulated organisms. Sarcoidosis-like pulmonary granulomas and lymphoid hyperplasia may complicate the interpretation of pulmonary infections. Malabsorptive symptoms should prompt a work-up to exclude *Giardia lamblia* infection and autoimmune enteritis, similar to celiac enteropathy and/or inflammatory bowel disease (IBD). Autoimmune cytopenias are found in 10% of CVID patients, and multiple other autoimmune disease manifestations are reported. Nearly half of these patients manifest mild cellular immune deficiency characterized by chronic viral and yeast infections. Impaired cellular immunity probably underlies the 8- to 13-fold increase in total malignancies in this population and the 438-fold increase in lymphomas among females with CVID (19). Again, immunoglobulin levels are not typically as low as those in XLA, and mature B cells are detected by flow cytometry. Impaired vaccine responses, in particular to diphtheria and tetanus toxoid antigens, are most helpful in defining this disorder. Treatment involves antibody replacement, again with care to use IgA-depleted products in IgA-deficient patients. Patients with granulomatous disease have been treated with corticosteroids and, more recently, with etanercept after careful consideration of malignant and infectious etiologies (40). The +448A polymorphism of the tumor necrosis factor (TNF)-α gene has been associated with granuloma formation in CVID patients (47). The CVID population has significant genetic heterogeneity. The largest subgroup (10%) identified thus far relates to mutations in the transmembrane activator and calcium-modulating and cyclophilin ligand interactor (TACI) gene (15). A smaller subgroup has been found to have mutations in the inducible T-cell costimulator gene (ICOS). Occasionally, patients with mutations in genes

TABLE 76.3

SUMMARY OF PRIMARY IMMUNE DEFICIENCY DISORDERS

Category	Name	Type of deficiency	Gene	Primary organisms	Usual sites	Treatment	Associated findings
Humoral	1. X-linked agammaglobulinemia	Absent or low levels of all immunoglobulins	BTK	Encapsulated bacteria Enteroviruses	Sinopulmonary GI	IVIG, Antibiotics as needed ? gene therapy	Respiratory failure Bronchiectasis Sepsis, Diarrhea
	2. Common variable immunodeficiency	Low levels of IgG ± low IgA, IgM	ICOS, TACI	Encapsulated bacteria	Sinopulmonary GI	IVIG, Antibiotics as needed	T-cell dysfunction Autoimmunity
	3. Transient hypogammaglobulinemia	Low levels of immunoglobulins until age 4 years	Unknown	Encapsulated bacteria	Sinopulmonary	None	None
	4. Hyper IgM	Low levels of IgG and IgA Neutropenia	CD154, CD40 AICDA, UNG NEMO	Encapsulated bacteria, PCP Cryptosporidium	Sinopulmonary Lymph nodes GI, Liver	IVIG, Antibiotics as needed TMP-SMX	PCP, Autoimmunity Chronic liver disease, Cancer
Cellular	22q11.2 Deletion syndrome (DGS / velocardiofacial syndrome)	Thymic hypoplasia Absence of mature T-cells	T-box 1 (?)	Candida, Viruses PCP	MM Skin Lung	Antifungals as needed, TMP-SMX, ? thymic transplant	Congenital heart disease, Hypoparathyroidism Hypocalcemia
Combined Disorders	1. Severe combined immunodeficiency	Dysplastic thymus, low or absent levels of immunoglobulins Lymphopenia	IL2R gamma JAK3, RAG1/2 ZAP-70, PNP ADA, IL-7	Encapsulated bacteria Candida, Viruses PCP	Sinopulmonary MM Skin Liver, GI Blood	IVIG, TMP-SMX Antibiotics, Anti-virals, Antifungals HSCT ? gene therapy	Fatal without HSCT, enzyme replacement or gene therapy
	2. Wiskott-Aldrich syndrome	Low levels of IgA and IgM B- and T-cell dysfunction	WASP	Encapsulated bacteria, PCP Candida, Viruses	Sinopulmonary MM Skin	IVIG, Antibiotics as needed HSCT	Eczema, Bleeding Thrombocytopenia HSM, Malignancy Autoimmunity
	3. Ataxia telangiectasia	Low levels of IgA and IgG₂ Cutaneous anergy	ATM	Encapsulated bacteria	Sinopulmonary	IVIG, Antibiotics as needed	Muscle weakness Ataxia Malignancy Telangiectasias
	4. X-linked lymphoproliferative disorder	T- and B-cell dysfunction, low immunoglobulins	SH2D1A	EBV	Sinopulmonary Lymph nodes Liver	Rituximab or Etoposide Acutely IVIG HSCT	Lymphadenopathy Hepatic necrosis HLH, Malignancy
	5. Immune deficiency, polyendocrinopathy, X-linked (IPEX)	T- regulatory cell dysfunction	FoxP3	Staph, gram (-) bacteria, PCP Candida, CMV	Sinopulmonary MM, Skin GI	Steroids, Sirolimus Antibiotics as needed, ? HSCT	Growth failure IDDM, Eczema rash Autoimmunity
	6. Immuno-osseous dysplasias	Variable T- and B-cell defects	Unknown	Viral, primarily varicella	Skin Lung	IVIG, Antibiotics as needed ? HSCT	Autoimmunity

(continued)

TABLE 76.3

(*continued*)

Category	Name	Type of deficiency	Gene	Primary organisms	Usual sites	Treatment	Associated findings
Neutropenia	1. Severe congenital neutropenia	Neutrophil maturation defect	ELA2?	Pyogenic bacteria	Skin, MM Lymph node Blood	GCSF	Agranulocytosis MDS/AML
	2. Cyclic neutropenia	Neutrophil maturation defect	ELA2?	Pyogenic bacteria	Skin, MM Lymph node	GCSF	Periodic fevers Aphthous ulcers
	3. Primary autoimmune neutropenia	Antibody directed against neutrophil	Unknown	Pyogenic bacteria	Sinopulmonary Skin	Antibiotics TMP-SMX, GCSF	URI, May resolve by age 3
	4. Schwachman-Diamond syndrome	Neutropenia, T-, B-, and NK-cell abnormalities	SBDS	Pyogenic bacteria	Sinopulmonary	GCSF, Antibiotics as needed	Pancreatic insufficiency Leukemia Skeletal anomalies Pancytopenia, MDS
Neutrophil Dysfunction	1. LAD-1/LAD-2	Abnormal neutrophil migration	CD18/Sialyl-Lewis X	Staph species gram (-) bacteria, Fungi	Skin, Lymph node, MM Liver, Bone	Antimicrobials HSCT Oral fucose-LAD2	Gingivitis, Impaired wound healing, UC separation delayed
	2. Hyper-IgE syndrome	Impaired chemotaxis T-, B-cell dysfunction	Unknown	Staph species, Strep species	Skin, Lung (abscesses with pneumatoceles)	Staph prophylaxis, Antibiotics as needed, ? IVIG	Skeletal/connective tissue abnormalities Eczema, ↑eosinophil
	3. Chronic granulomatous disease	Oxidative burst and bactericidal activity impaired	gp91phox p-22phox p47-phox p67-phox	Staph species Catalase (+) bacteria Fungi	Sinopulmonary Lung, Bone Liver, GI Skin, MM	Antifungal prophylaxis, TMP-SMX, IFN-γ HSCT	Intestinal and bladder obstruction Osteomyelitis Liver abscesses
	4. Chediak-Higashi syndrome	Abnormal degranulation	LYST	Pyogenic bacteria	Sinopulmonary Skin	Ascorbic acid, Folate, Antibiotics as needed	Bleeding, albinism, HLH, Peripheral neuropathy
Complement	1. Hereditary angioedema	Low C2, C4 and C1-INH	C1-INH	None	GI, Upper respiratory tract	Steroids, C1-INH replacement, FFP	Abdominal crises Airway obstruction
	2. C1, C2, C3, C4	Low component levels	C1, C2, C3, C4	Encapsulated organisms	Skin Blood	Antibiotics as needed	Lupus-like syndrome
	3. C5-9	Absent membrane attack complex	C5-9	Meningococci	Blood Meninges	Vaccination, Early antibiotic therapy	Recurrent meningitis
	4. Properdin deficiency	Unstable C3 and C5 convertases	PFC	Meningococci	Blood Meninges	Vaccination, Early antibiotic therapy	Recurrent meningitis
	5. Mannan binding lectin deficiency	Impaired MASP-activation	MBL	Various bacteria	Sinopulmonary Meninges Blood	Antibiotics as needed	Autoimmunity ↑ SIRS/severity ? Kawasaki disease
Toll-like Receptors	EDA–ID IRAK-4 deficiency	Impaired TLR signaling	NEMO IRAK-4	Gram (+) bacteria	Sinopulmonary Blood	Antibiotics as needed	Recurrent sepsis

BTK, Bruton's tyrosine kinase; GI, gastrointestinal; IVIG, IV immunoglobulin; Ig, immunoglobulin; ICOS, inducible T-cell costimulator gene; TACI, transmembrane activator and calcium-modulating and cyclophilin ligand interactor; AICDA, activation-induced cytidine deaminase; UNG, uracil DNA glycosylase; NEMO, nuclear factor κB essential modulator; PCP, *Pneumocystis jiroveci* pneumonia; MM, mucous membrane; TMP-SMX, trimethoprim-sulfamethoxazole; PNP, polynucleotide phosphorylase; ADA, adenosine deaminase; HSCT, hematopoietic stem cell transplant; WASP, Wiscott-Aldrich syndrome protein; HSM, hepatosplenomegaly; EBV, Epstein-Barr virus; CMV, cytomegalovirus; HLH, hemophagocytic lymphohistiocytosis; IDDM, insulin-dependent diabetes mellitus; GCSF, granulocyte colony-stimulating factor; MDS/AML, myelodysplastic syndrome/acute myelocytic leukemia; SBDS, Shwachman Bodian Diamond syndrome; URI, upper respiratory infections; UC, umbilical cord; C1-INH, C1 esterase inhibitor; MBL, binding lectin; SIRS, systemic inflammatory response syndrome; TLR, Toll-like receptor; IRAK, IL-1-receptor-associated kinase associated with more classical immunodeficiencies, such as BTK and SH2D1A (mutated in X-linked lymphoproliferative disorder), have been described (8).

Transient Hypogammaglobulinemia of Infancy

A number of premature and, occasionally, term infants develop an exaggerated hypogammaglobulinemia at the natural nadir of maternal immunoglobulin between 6 and 9 months of age. Although immunoglobulin values in these infants overlap with those of immune-deficient infants, normal antigen responses can eventually be demonstrated, and most of these infants mature to have normal immunologic function. Normalization of IgG levels can be expected at between 2 and 4 years of age (71). Upper respiratory infections are common in these infants, and only rarely can IVIG use be justified to treat more invasive infections. The occurrence of invasive infections and the need for IVIG therapy should prompt reconsideration of a mild XLA phenotype, early onset CVID, or a combined immunodeficiency.

Hyper-IgM Syndrome

The occurrence of hypogammaglobulinemia with normal-to-high IgM levels was first recognized in males. It is now clear that both an X-linked defect in the CD40 ligand (CD154) and autosomal defects in CD40, activation-induced cytidine deaminase (AICDA), uracil DNA glycosylase (UNG), and nuclear factor (NF)-κB essential modulator (NEMO) lead to the hyper-IgM phenotype (24). The resultant immunologic dysfunction with these mutations is defective CD40 signaling by B-cells, affecting class switch recombination and somatic hypermutation. The X-linked form accounts for 65%–70% of all cases. These males generally present in infancy with upper and lower respiratory tract infections, and up to 40% will present with interstitial pneumonitis from *P. jiroveci* infection. Diarrhea is another common presenting symptom, often associated with *Cryptosporidium* infection. Cytopenias, lymphoid hyperplasia, IBD disease, and seronegative arthritis are not infrequent manifestations of autoimmune disease in hyper-IgM patients, reflecting T-cell dysfunction. For that reason, many authors classify the Hyper-IgM syndrome as a combined immune deficiency. Significant early mortality from chronic liver disease and malignancy has justified trials of stem cell transplantation for these patients.

DISORDERS PREDOMINANTLY AFFECTING CELLULAR FUNCTION

Defects localized within the T-cell compartment that affect either maturation of T cells or specific T-cell functions are discussed in this section. Dysgammaglobulinemia, as in the Hyper-IgM syndrome, is a frequent consequence of T-cell dysfunction, given the necessary role of T-cell signaling for immunoglobulin class switching and affinity maturation. Thus, some degree of antibody deficiency will accompany most cellular defects. The cardinal clinical features of T-cell dysfunction are yeast overgrowth, chronic viral infections, opportunistic infections, autoimmune disorders, and malignancies.

22q11.2 Deletion Syndrome

Infants with DiGeorge syndrome (DGS) and velocardiofacial syndrome have a characteristic 22q11.2 deletion and frequently manifest T-cell deficiency due to lack of normal thymic development. The frequency of these deletion syndromes is ~1 in 4000 persons. Genes within the characteristic deletion on chromosome 22 direct neural crest migration into the third and fourth pharyngeal arches, and the absence of these genes results in conotruncal cardiac defects, parathyroid hypoplasia, and thymic hypoplasia. The most common cardiac anomalies in DGS, in order of prevalence, are interrupted aortic arch type B (IAA type B), persistent truncus arteriosus, tetralogy of Fallot, right aortic arch, ventricular septal defect, and patent ductus arteriosus. Of all patients with IAA type B, 68% have DGS. Of all patients with persistent truncus arteriosus and tetralogy of Fallot, 33% and 2%, respectively, have DGS (76).

The characteristic deletion can be demonstrated by fluorescence in situ hybridization (FISH) probe in 90% of infants with the DiGeorge phenotype and a smaller percentage of infants with the velocardiofacial phenotype (71). Of the many genes contained in the deleted region, Tbx1 may be the most relevant to the human phenotype based on a murine model of DGS (41). Most DGS infants are recognized during the neonatal period because of the presence of congenital heart defects and/or hypocalcemia symptoms, such as tetany or seizures. However, poor correlation is seen between genotype and phenotype, particularly in regard to thymic hypoplasia. For example, even in the presence of the characteristic 22q11.2 deletion clinical syndrome of cardiac defects, hypocalcemia, and facial dysmorphology, complete thymic absence (complete DiGeorge) occurs in no more than 5% of affected infants. The remainder have variable degrees of thymic hypoplasia, altered T-cell kinetics, and occasional increased susceptibility to infection. In one series of 195 patients defined by the 22q11.2 deletion, only minimal difficulties with bacterial infections were noted, whereas a significant incidence of autoimmune disease, such as juvenile rheumatoid arthritis and immune thrombocytopenic purpura, was reported (36).

In the immediate postnatal period, absolute CD3 counts below 500 predict poor T-cell function and the potential need for immune reconstitution with either a thymic or hematopoietic stem cell transplant (HSCT) (71). Spontaneous improvement in T-cell numbers and function has been documented, and serial T-cell counts are necessary to distinguish complete DGS from delayed T-cell maturation. Infants with absolute CD3 counts below 1500 at birth should receive *P. jiroveci* prophylaxis. In addition, only cytomegalovirus (CMV)-negative and irradiated blood products should be transfused to avoid risk of infection and graft-versus-host disease (GVHD). Perioperative corticosteroid treatment may confound the immunologic workup in those infants who require immediate cardiac surgery; thus, repeat flow cytometry studies should be considered at ~1 month of age.

Defects in the Interferon γ-IL–12 Axis

Other predominantly cellular defects include defects in the interferon gamma (IFN-γ)–IL-12 axis, chronic mucocutaneous candidiasis, idiopathic CD4 lymphopenia, and natural killer (NK) cell dysfunction (8). The IFN-γ–IL-12 axis is an important component of the defense against intracellular organisms, such as *Mycobacteria*, *Salmonella*, and *Listeria*. Systemic infections with atypical *mycobacteria* and fatalities after bacille Calmette-Guérin immunizations have been described in patients with abnormalities of this axis. Defects that cause increased susceptibility to mycobacterial infections have been described in various portions of the IFN-γ receptor, the IL-12 receptor, and IL-12. This group of disorders has been referred to as *Mendelian susceptibility to mycobacterial disease*. The severity of infections and response to IFN-γ therapy depends upon the location and severity of the defect (39). Patients who have the most severe form of the disease, complete IFN-γ receptor 1 deficiency, may be candidates for HSCT. Unlike the other disorders within this group, these patients will have no response to IFN-γ therapy because they have a complete deficiency of the IFN-γ receptor (61).

IMMUNODEFICIENCY WITH COMBINED ANTIBODY AND CELLULAR DEFECTS

Combined immune deficiencies (CID), in general, are characterized by early-onset viral and yeast infections, usually resulting in growth failure. *P. jiroveci* pneumonia in an infant nearly always indicates CID. Maternal-fetal or transfusion-acquired GVHD is another prominent feature in infants with CID.

Severe Combined Immunodeficiency Disease

Severe combined immunodeficiency disease (SCID) is the prototype of combined immunodeficiencies. The incidence of SCID is estimated to be 1 in 100,000 to 1 in 150,000 individuals. These infants usually present in the first month of life with refractory oral candidiasis and persistent viral infections.

P. jiroveci is a frequent cause of morbidity and mortality in this group of infants. Absolute lymphopenia below 2000 cells/mm^3 is a common laboratory finding, even on cord blood specimens (32). Flow cytometry will generally indicate very low absolute CD3 or T-cell numbers. Maternal T-cell engraftment, however, may dramatically affect the fetal T-cell population; thus, clinical suspicion of SCID can justify lymphocyte proliferation assays regardless of lymphocyte counts. B cells and NK cells may be present or absent, depending on the specific defect. The classification of SCID subtypes is depicted in **Table 76.4**.

T(–)B(+) SCID is the largest subtype of SCID and is most commonly related to mutations in the IL2R gene on the X chromosome, which encodes the cytokine receptor gamma chain (γ_c) common to multiple cytokine receptors. Janus kinase 3 (JAK3) mediates γ_c signal transduction; therefore, JAK3 mutations result in a similar phenotype, although the pattern of inheritance is autosomal recessive (AR). T(–)B(–) SCID, in 50% of the cases, relates to mutations in the genes (*RAG1/2*) that regulate the somatic recombination of immunoglobulin and T-cell receptor genes during B- and T-cell development. Partial function of RAG1 or RAG2 is one cause of Omenn syndrome, which is characterized by erythroderma, eosinophilia, lymphoid hyperplasia, and hypogammaglobulinemia (78). Circulating lymphocytes in RAG1/2-deficient patients are primarily NK-cells. Metabolic defects in the purine salvage pathway do not spare NK-cells; thus, patients who present with adenosine deaminase (ADA) deficiency often have the most profound lymphopenia. Multiple skeletal abnormalities, including dysplasia of vertebral bodies and flaring of the costochondral junctions may be seen in up to 50% of these infants. Reticular dysgenesis is another T(–)B(–) form of SCID, which additionally involves a block in myeloid differentiation. Other cytokine and major histocompatibility complex (MHC) defects associated with a SCID phenotype are listed in **Table 76.4**.

The intensive care of an infant suspected or known to have SCID should include strict isolation and the use of only irradiated, CMV-negative, and leukocyte-depleted blood products. The intensivist should maintain a high index of suspicion for *P. jiroveci* infection, and both respiratory secretions and stool should be tested for a variety of pathogens. The infant with SCID may benefit from aggressive antiviral therapies in addition to antibiotics and IVIG. An immunologist or hematologist should be involved early in the care of these infants to facilitate arrangements for HSCT, which remains the most successful

TABLE 76.4

LYMPHOCYTE-PHENOTYPES CHARACTERISTICALLY ASSOCIATED WITH FORMS OF SEVERE COMBINED IMMUNODEFICIENCY DISEASE

Form of SCID	T-cells			B-cells	NK-cells
	CD3	CD4	CD8		
X-linked, JAK3, IL-2R, IL-7R	↓	↓	↓	Normal	↓
RAG1/2	↓	↓	↓	↓	Normal
ADA	↓	↓	↓	↓	↓
MHC II	Normal	↓	Normal	Normal	Normal
ZAP-70, MHC I	Normal	Normal	↓	Normal	Normal

From Bonilla FA, Geha RS. Primary immunodeficiency diseases. *J Allergy Clin Immunol* 2003;111:S571–81.

therapy for SCID. Survival rates of greater than 90% can be accomplished with HLA-matched sibling donor transplants, and even haploidentical transplants from a parent are reported to be successful in at least 75% of cases (13).

CID at the less severe end of the spectrum involves variable degrees of T- and B-cell dysfunction. Nezelof syndrome describes patients with predominant T-cell defect(s) and a lesser degree of B-cell dysfunction. MHC Class I and Class II deficiencies involve mild and more severe defects in both T- and B-cell function, respectively. Several immuno-osseous syndromes combine skeletal abnormalities with variable degrees of CID and include ADA deficiency as described previously, short-limbed dwarfism with and without ectodermal dysplasia, cartilage hair hypoplasia, CID with metaphyseal dysplasia, and Schimke immuno-osseous dysplasia.

Wiskott-Aldrich Syndrome

Wiskott-Aldrich syndrome (WAS) is an X-linked disorder that often presents with the classic triad of eczema, thrombocytopenia, and immunodeficiency. Boys present with bleeding within the first year of life, often in the nursery, with bloody diarrhea or prolonged oozing from a circumcision. Platelets in WAS patients are abnormally small and defective, as compared to the relatively large and functionally normal platelets seen in immune thrombocytopenic purpura. The intensivist caring for a WAS patient must be cognizant of both the bleeding and infection risks. Infections often involve encapsulated organisms related to the inability to produce antibodies in response to polysaccharide antigens. IgM levels are typically low, as reflected by low isohemagglutinin (blood group) antibodies. B-cell dysfunction is apparent early, while T-cell dysfunction is progressive over time. The mutated WAS protein (WASP) connects T-cell signaling to critical cytoskeletal regulatory mechanisms necessary for T-cell activation (70). Minor dysfunction of WASP may be associated with X-linked thrombocytopenia in some families, and a single case of a WASP mutation in a patient with X-linked neutropenia has been reported (7). Autoimmune phenomena are common manifestations of T-cell dysfunction in WAS. Although IVIG therapy and splenectomy may help to maintain platelet counts and minimize infections, an HLA-matched HSCT from a sibling or from a cord blood bank offers the best chance of long-term survival.

Ataxia Telangiectasia

Patients with ataxia telangiectasia present with delayed ambulation and speech, followed by deterioration of gross and fine motor skills. Cerebellar ataxia and oculocutaneous telangiectasias become evident at ~7 years of age. Frequent pulmonary infections may be related to subtle antibody defects or swallowing dysfunction and aspiration. Deficiencies in both humoral and cellular immunity have been reported. Median survival in the Ataxia Telangiectasia Clinical Center at Johns Hopkins Medical Institutions has recently been reported to be 25 years, with mortality frequently attributed to malignancy (18). Mutations in the ATM gene increase sensitivity to ionizing radiation and lead to lack of DNA double-strand break recognition and repair. The 10%–30% lifetime prevalence of malignancies is attributable to this defective DNA repair mechanism (see later discussion).

X-linked Lymphoproliferative Disease

The often life-threatening presentation of X-linked lymphoproliferative disease (XLP), or Duncan disease, represents an abnormal immune response to Epstein-Barr virus (EBV) infection. In most cases, it is related to mutations in the SH2D1A signal transduction protein. The frequency of XLP is undoubtedly underestimated because of the variability of clinical presentations. Classically, patients present with massive lymphadenopathy, hepatic necrosis, and bone marrow failure, much like posttransplant lymphoproliferative disease. This acute presentation of XLP is responsible for the reported 70% mortality by age 10. The remaining 30% may present late, with varying degrees of immune deficiency, ranging from mild hypogammaglobulinemia to CID. As many as one-third of long-term survivors will eventually develop a lymphoreticular malignancy; a 200-fold increased risk of lymphomas is seen in XLP. The diagnosis of XLP is facilitated by positive EBV serology and, more specifically, blood or tissue polymerase chain reaction assays. Bone marrow examination will often indicate hemophagocytosis. Rapid diagnosis is now available by flow cytometry, which documents the absence of intracellular SH2D1A staining in CD3$^+$CD8$^+$ cells (74). Etoposide and rituximab have proven useful in the therapy of acute lymphoproliferation in patients diagnosed prior to EBV exposure (45).

Immune Deficiency, Polyendocrinopathy, X-linked Syndrome

The defining clinical characteristics of immune deficiency, polyendocrinopathy, X-linked (IPEX) syndrome are enteropathy, eczematoid rash, and early endocrinopathy, most often, diabetes mellitus. Up to 50% of patients will present prior to diagnosis with a serious infection, usually *Staphylococcus*, *Candida*, or CMV. Autoimmune cytopenias and splenomegaly are also frequently noted at presentation. Therapy with sirolimus may be more effective than other forms of immunosuppression for the autoimmune manifestations of this disorder (6). Immunologic studies are surprisingly normal in most patients because the responsible *FoxP3* gene mutations on Xp11.23 impair the normal function of CD4$^+$CD25$^+$ regulatory T-cells without otherwise impairing T- or B-cell function. Survival beyond age 2 is unusual, although milder phenotypes have been reported. The value of HSCT for this disorder remains unclear.

NEUTROPHIL DISORDERS

Disorders of polymorphonuclear leukocytes (neutrophils) are also relatively uncommon. Patients with these disorders are at increased risk of serious infections that may result in the need for critical care services. It is important for the intensivist to be familiar with these disorders, as prompt identification and referral to a hematologist, oncologist, or clinical immunologist may facilitate early diagnosis and institution of appropriate adjunctive therapy. Early recognition and therapy may result in improved outcomes for these high-risk patients.

For neutrophils to effectively combat invading pathogens, they must be able to perform a number of complex functions. First and foremost, they must be able to proliferate and mature in the bone marrow. During their maturation, neutrophils form granules that contain bactericidal and hydrolytic proteins that are important for killing pathogens. Once mature, they must emigrate from the bone marrow into the systemic circulation. There, they must undergo several complex processes. The first is *rolling*, a process in which the neutrophil rolls loosely along the endothelial surface. Once it approximates its target, it binds tightly to the endothelial surface and becomes flattened through a process termed *adhesion*. Finally, the neutrophil must migrate across the endothelium via a process termed *diapedesis*. For rolling, adhesion, and diapedesis to occur, the neutrophil must communicate with the endothelial surface through the use of cell-surface proteins, including selectins, integrin, intercellular adhesion molecule (ICAM)-1, and platelet-endothelial cell adhesion molecule (PECAM)-1. Once through the endothelial membrane, the neutrophil is attracted to the invading pathogen by chemotactic factors including lipopolysaccharide, IL-1, TNF-α, and IFN-γ via a process called *chemotaxis*. Upon reaching the appropriate site, the neutrophil digests the offending pathogen through *opsonization* and *phagocytosis*. Opsonization is the process in which opsonins (such as IgG or C3b) are bound to the pathogen. These opsonins then bind to their receptors on the neutrophil (Fc receptors and complement receptors), allowing the neutrophil to phagocytose (digest) the pathogen [71]. These various complex interactions between neutrophils, endothelial cells, and other components of the immune system provide many opportunities for neutrophil function to be impaired. In general, neutrophil disorders can be divided into two broad categories: diseases associated with decreased numbers of neutrophils (neutropenia) and those with impaired neutrophil function.

Disorders Associated with Primary Neutropenia

Severe Congenital Neutropenia and Cyclic Neutropenia

In addition to the more common acquired forms of neutropenia, such as that secondary to cancer and its therapy, congenital causes of neutropenia must be considered. Severe congenital neutropenia, also known as Kostmann syndrome, and cyclic neutropenia are examples of inherited neutropenic disorders. Both of these conditions have been associated with mutations in the gene encoding neutrophil elastase, *ELA2*. Several heterozygous mutations of *ELA2* have been described in all patients with cyclic neutropenia and in most patients with severe congenital neutropenia, the exception being in families with AR severe congenital neutropenia [2]. However, the role that these *ELA2* mutations play in the pathophysiology of these disorders has not been well established [66]. Myeloid precursor cells from patients with these disorders demonstrate an abnormal response to hematopoietic growth factors. However, both conditions commonly respond to treatment with granulocyte colony-stimulating factor (GCSF), which decreases the degree of neutropenia, and therefore, the rate of serious infection [39]. Patients with severe congenital neutropenia have profound neutropenia [an absolute neutrophil count (ANC) of <500 neutrophils/m^3], and they experience recurrent bacterial infections beginning in the first year of life. Infections are commonly caused by *S. aureus* and *P. aeruginosa*. Pathophysiologically, this disease is characterized by a maturational failure of promyelocytes to myelocytes [39]. Clinically, these children have a risk of death from sepsis of 0.9% per year and a significant risk of malignant transformation to myelodysplastic syndrome or acute myelocytic leukemia (MDS/AML). The risk of development of MDS/AML increases with time, ranging from 2.9% per year during the first 6 years of therapy with GCSF up to 8.0% per year after 12 years of treatment [62].

Cyclic neutropenia is a rare autosomal dominant (AD) disorder. Patients with cyclic neutropenia experience recurrent episodes of severe neutropenia that lasts 3–6 days and occurs in cycles of every 14–36 days. Although these patients may be asymptomatic, during neutropenic cycles they may develop aphthous ulcers, gingivitis, stomatitis, and cellulitis, and they are at increased risk of mortality from serious infection [39]. In contrast to patients with severe congenital neutropenia, these patients do not appear to be at increased risk for the development of MDS/AML [66].

Autoimmune Neutropenia

Autoimmune neutropenia must also be considered in the differential diagnosis of neutropenia. These neutropenias may be either primary or secondary. Secondary autoimmune neutropenias are associated with inflammatory diseases, such as rheumatoid arthritis (i.e., Felty syndrome) and systemic lupus erythematosus (SLE). Often, these patients will have additional hematologic abnormalities, such as thrombocytopenia and/or hemolytic anemia. Successful treatment and control of the underlying disease is the most effective therapy for the neutropenia.

Primary autoimmune neutropenia most commonly begins in the newborn period and is frequently diagnosed within the first several months of life. These patients have significant neutropenia at presentation, with an ANC often <500–1000 neutrophils/m^3. However, severe infections such as pneumonia, sepsis, and meningitis, are relatively uncommon, occurring in ~10% of these children. Most patients present with relatively benign infections, such as otitis media, upper respiratory infections, and dermatitis, and the disease commonly resolves spontaneously by 2 to 3 years of age. Autoimmune neutropenia, as its name implies, is caused by antibodies directed against the neutrophil. These antibodies are frequently directed against the HNA-1a and HNA-1b antigens, although antibodies to the CD11/CD18 complex, CD35, and FcγRIIb have been described. Testing for these antibodies is often falsely negative; thus, repeat testing is indicated if the diagnosis is strongly suspected. In patients with a serious clinical course, a maturational arrest in the myelocyte/metamyelocyte stage may be detected upon examination of the bone marrow. This stage arrest is thought to occur because the antibodies directed toward the mature neutrophils also attack their precursors in the bone marrow. The treatment for patients with a benign form of autoimmune neutropenia may simply be antibiotics as needed to treat infections or antibiotic prophylaxis with such agents as trimethoprim-sulfamethoxazole. For patients with serious infections, GCSF has been found to be beneficial and is considered first-line therapy. Although corticosteroids and IVIG have been utilized, they do not appear to be as beneficial as GCSF [14,71].

Shwachman-Diamond Syndrome

Shwachman-Diamond syndrome is also associated with neutropenia. It is a rare autosomal disorder associated with neutropenia, exocrine pancreatic insufficiency, skeletal abnormalities, recurrent infections, and occasionally, pancytopenia; it is caused by a mutation in the gene encoding the Shwachman-Bodian-Diamond syndrome protein. The neutropenia associated with this disorder may be persistent or cyclic. Moreover, in addition to neutropenia, these patients may also have abnormalities of T-, B-, and NK-cell lymphocytes (71). GCSF therapy is useful in this condition to reduce the risk of serious infection. These children are at increased risk of myelodysplasia and leukemia independent of the use of GCSF (39).

Disorders of Neutrophil Function

Defects of Neutrophil Adhesion

In addition to disorders associated with an absolute decrease in the number of neutrophils, several conditions have been identified in which neutrophil function is compromised. For example, in leukocyte adhesion disorders, neutrophils are unable to bind appropriately to the endothelial surface, complete diapedesis, and migrate to the site of infection. First described in the 1980s, leukocyte adhesion deficiency type 1 (LAD-1) is an AR disorder caused by genetic mutations encoding CD18, the γ-subunit of the neutrophil adhesion molecule LFA-1. The neutrophils of patients with this disorder are unable to adhere appropriately to the endothelial surface and, therefore, are unable to migrate toward the site of infections. Patients often present with recurrent, severe infections and may have a history of delayed umbilical cord separation. The most frequent pathogens are enteric gram-negative bacteria, *S. aureus*, *Candida*, and *Aspergillus* species. These patients also exhibit impaired wound healing and have elevated neutrophil counts in the peripheral blood because their neutrophils are not able to marginate (39). Although rare, other types of leukocyte adhesion disorders have been described. Patients with LAD type 2 have impaired fucose metabolism, which can affect the expression of fucosylated receptors on the neutrophil that are important for leukocyte rolling along the vessel wall. Patients with this disorder are characterized by immunologic deficiencies, mental retardation, short stature, and distinctive facies, and may benefit from oral fucose therapy (71). A mutation involving RAC2, a neutrophil GTPase important for the function of the neutrophil actin cytoskeleton, has also been described, with the patient having a similar phenotype to patients with LAD-1 and being treated successfully with a matched, related HSCT (71).

Hyper-IgE Syndrome (Job Syndrome)

Hyper-IgE syndrome (HIES or Job syndrome) is an immunodeficiency first described by Buckley et al. in 1972. The classic form of the disease is characterized by recurrent staphylococcal infections, eczema, recurrent respiratory infections with persistent pneumatoceles, elevated IgE levels, eosinophilia, abnormal cytokine and chemokine expression, and T-cell dysfunction. Neutrophil chemotaxis may be impaired in some patients. Patients have been described as having coarse facial features, joint hyperextensibility, osteopenia, and prolonged retention of primary teeth, but the features may be quite variable. The causative genetic defect is unknown, as is the exact cause of the increased susceptibility to infection (71). Sporadic AD and AR forms have been described, with the sporadic and AD forms fitting the classical description. The AD form appears to have incomplete penetrance, and some cases appear to map to chromosome 4. The AR form differs significantly from the sporadic and AD cases. These patients lack the connective tissue findings of the AD form, have a high incidence of complications of the central nervous system (CNS), and have a higher frequency of complications from varicella-zoster and herpes simplex viral infections (59). The only treatment known to be of clear benefit is antibiotic prophylaxis against staphylococcal infections, although IVIG may be of benefit in individual patients (5).

Defects of Phagocytosis

Impaired phagocytic function has also been identified as a condition associated with increased risk of infection. Neutrophils have Fcγ receptors on their surface that bind IgG and signal the cell to phagocytose invading pathogens. A number of genetic polymorphisms have been described within the different classes of Fcγ receptors that influence this function. In vitro studies have demonstrated impaired phagocytosis in individuals with a particular genotype of the FcγRII receptor. This same genotype has been detected with increased frequency in patients with severe meningococcal disease when compared with healthy controls (21), a finding that may have potential implications for genetic screening and prophylactic immunization of family members of patients with severe meningococcal disease.

Defects of Intracellular Killing

Chronic granulomatous disease (CGD) is caused by a mutation in any of the four structural genes (gp91^{phox}, p22^{phox}, p47^{phox}, and p67^{phox}) of the NADPH oxidase apparatus. The majority of cases are inherited in an X-linked recessive manner (gp91^{phox}), whereas the others are AR. The disease is characterized by recurrent infections of the skin, lungs, and liver, as well as by excessive granuloma formation that can obstruct the gastrointestinal or genitourinary tract. Most infections are caused by *S. aureus*, *Burkholderia cepacia*, *Aspergillus* species, *Nocardia* species, and *Serratia marcescens*. *S. aureus* liver abscesses are highly suspicious for the diagnosis of CGD. Patients with CGD are most susceptible to catalase positive microorganisms.

The diagnosis of CGD can be made by laboratory tests that analyze superoxide formation, such as the nitroblue tetrazolium test, or by flow cytometry with dihydrorhodamine dye (39). The defect in NADPH oxidase causes an inability of the neutrophil to produce superoxide and its metabolites, thereby impairing the ability of the neutrophil to kill ingested microorganisms. Patients with CGD are commonly treated with the prophylactic antimicrobials trimethoprim-sulfamethoxazole and itraconazole to prevent bacterial and fungal infections, respectively. IFN-γ therapy has also been found to be effective for these patients, reducing infection rates by 70% when compared to placebo. HSCT has been curative in this patient population; however, transplant-related complications require careful consideration before this procedure is undertaken (63). Two additional disorders to consider in the differential of CGD include severe glucose-6-phosphate dehydrogenase deficiency and myeloperoxidase deficiency, both of which present with a milder phenotype.

Disorders of Neutrophil Granules

Immunodeficiencies may also result from defective formation of neutrophil granules. Chediak-Higashi syndrome, an AR disorder, is the best characterized of these disorders. The genetic mutation that causes Chediak-Higashi syndrome involves the *LYST* gene. This gene encodes a protein involved with the formation and function of vacuoles. The severity of the phenotype varies with the type of mutation (83). Neutrophils from these patients have impaired chemotaxis, and they are characterized by large perinuclear granules. In addition, elastase and cathepsin G may be absent from their neutrophil granules.

Patients with Chediak-Higashi disease have abnormalities in both the hematologic and neurologic systems. Clinical features include recurrent bacterial infections, peripheral nerve disorders, mental retardation, autonomic dysfunction, partial albinism, silver-colored hair, and platelet dysfunction. Patients often die in the first decade of life of a lymphoproliferative process, termed the *accelerated phase*, which is similar to hemophagocytic lymphohistiocytosis. If patients survive into the second or third decade of life, they often develop a debilitating peripheral neuropathy and eventually die of infection. Although HSCT appears to prevent the accelerated phase, it does not prevent the neurologic sequelae (39,83).

Neutrophil-specific granular deficiency is a rare autosomal disorder that is characterized by the absence of neutrophil granules. Patients with this disease may have recurrent severe infections, particularly with *S. aureus, S. epidermidis,* and enteric bacteria. The neutrophils of these patients are not able to migrate properly. Similar to patients with severe neutropenia, the severity of these infections may be underestimated by clinical exam because their neutrophils are unable to migrate properly to the site of infection and create visible suppuration and inflammation. Therefore, aggressive treatment with antibiotics and early consideration of surgical management are indicated (39,63).

COMPLEMENT DEFICIENCY

Normal Function

The complement system is a key component of innate immunity, acting to protect the host from microorganisms (31). Complement may be activated via three distinct pathways, all of which require activation of the complement protein C3 (20) (**Fig. 76.1**). The classical pathway is activated by antigen-antibody complexes derived from acquired immunity. The alternative pathway is triggered by the recognition of pathogen-associated molecular patterns (PAMPs) on the surface of bacteria by small amounts of C3 activated by spontaneous hydrolysis. Finally, complement may be activated by the lectin pathway, beginning with the detection of bacterial surface carbohydrates (i.e., mannose) by mannose-binding lectin (MBL) protein (also known as mannan-binding protein), resulting in the induction of MBL-activated serine proteases (MASP) and activation of the complement cascade. A clear understanding of the complement cascade and the biologic functions of the individual

components provides insight into the clinical manifestations of complement deficiencies.

Complement C1, a complex macromolecule, initiates activation of the classical pathway and plays a significant role in host defense against pathogens (31). C1 is composed of a recognition protein, C1q, in association with a tetramer composed of two proteases, C1r and C1s (31). The C1q recognition protein mediates the binding of C1 to a target cell or molecule. The binding of C1 results in the subsequent activation of C4, C2, and, ultimately, C3. Of note, all three pathways of complement activation converge at C3 and lead to the formation of C3a and C5a and the terminal membrane attack complex, C5b–C9 (31). Activated C3 is critical to opsonization. Activated C5 has numerous effects important in the pathogenesis of sepsis, with C5b initiating the formation of the terminal membrane attack complex (20,31). The terminal membrane attack complex functions to lyse the cell membrane of the target cell. The classical pathway may be initiated without antigen-antibody complexes by the direct binding of bacteria, viruses, and apoptotic cells to C1q and subsequent activation of the cascade.

The alternative complement pathway is critical to innate immunity and serves to activate complement in the absence of antibody. C3 is again the pivotal component. Under normal physiologic conditions, C3 in the plasma is activated via slow hydrolysis and interaction with alternative pathway proteins. Once C3 is activated, the pathway progresses identically to the classical pathway (**Fig. 76.1**). Of note, the alternative pathway C3 convertase is highly unstable and requires properdin for stability.

MBL is the initiating protein for the lectin pathway of complement activation. MBL recognizes specific carbohydrate sequences on the surface of microbes. Once bound to these surfaces, MBL activates two proteases, MASP-1 and MASP-2, which share structural homology with C1r and C1s. MASP-2 triggers the complement cascade by activating C4, whereas MASP-1 is believed to activate C3 directly.

Regulation

The complement system is critical to the host defense system, as it damages invading organisms and produces tissue inflammation. However, strict control of the complement system is essential to prevent complement-mediated destruction of host tissues. Many regulatory proteins exist that function in this role. For example, C1 esterase inhibitor (C1-INH) is a glycoprotein that recognizes and inactivates activated C1r and C1s. Because it is consumed during the process of inactivation, high levels of C1 inhibitor must be produced, requiring the activation of two gene sites (20). In fact, deficiency of C1-INH results in hereditary angioedema (described later). Several other regulatory proteins function at different points of the complement cascade to balance the destruction of invading microbes, while at the same time minimizing destruction of host tissues; it is believed that this occurs as a result of protected sites on microorganisms. When C3b binds to the membrane of microbes, it is positioned in such a way that regulatory protein factors H and I cannot reach it and, therefore, cannot inactivate it. On the other hand, when C3b binds host tissues, it is not protected from factors H and I; therefore, it can be quickly degraded (20).

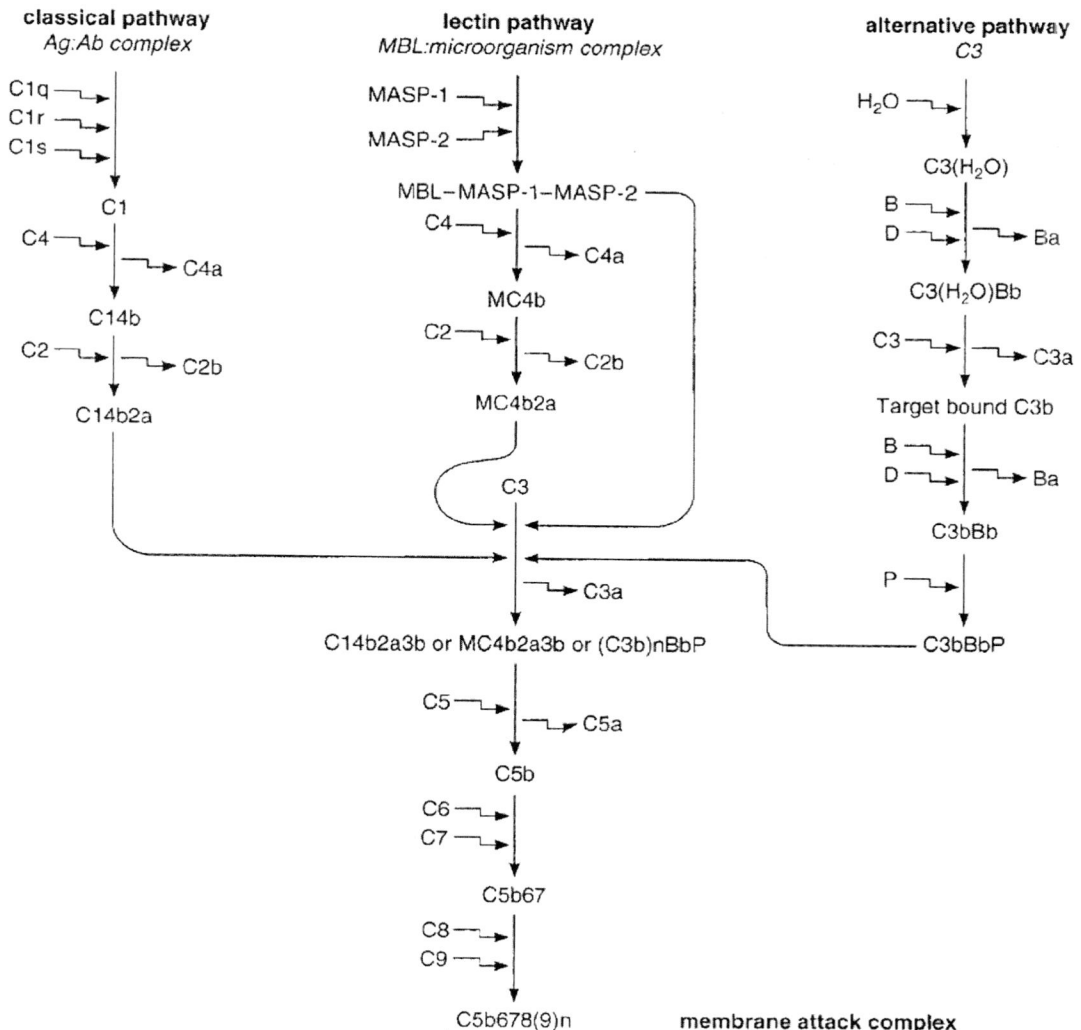

FIGURE 76.1. Activation of the complement cascade. The figure depicts the complement components involved in activation of the three pathways of the complement cascade. From Cunnion KM, Wagner E, Frank MM. Complement & Kinin. In: Parslow TG, Stites DP, Terr AI, Imboden JB, eds. *Medical Immunology.* New York: McGraw-Hill, 2001;175–88, with permission.

Deficiencies and Disease

The association of complement deficiencies with disease states is not well established because of difficulties in estimating the prevalence of complement deficiencies (68). However, an association with a defect in the complement system has clearly been demonstrated in some disorders. Rheumatologic disorders (especially SLE), an increased susceptibility to invasive infections (notably recurrent meningococcal disease), and hereditary angioedema represent the most common pediatric clinical settings in which complement deficiency is suspected (68).

Hereditary Angioedema

Hereditary angioedema is a rare AD disorder with an estimated frequency of 1 in 50,000 individuals (10,80). Children present with recurrent episodes of subcutaneous or submucosal angioedema that primarily affects the upper respiratory or gastrointestinal tracts (10,80). Clinical manifestations of this edema include limb swelling, painful abdominal crises, and life-threatening airway obstruction. The edema usually takes several hours to develop, although the literature contains one report of a child dying from asphyxiation within 20 mins of the onset of symptoms (9). The edema generally persists for 1–5 days. In one report, 40% of patients with hereditary angioedema died secondary to upper airway obstruction, often during the initial episode of upper airway edema (9). In fact, the edema tends to involve the intestines more frequently than the larynx.

Although episodes during childhood may be less frequent than in adulthood, hereditary angioedema usually presents in childhood, with 40% of patients having their first attack before age 5 (10). Hereditary angioedema is primarily the result of a deficiency in the C1-INH protein caused by a deletion, duplication, or mutation in the *C1-INH* gene (9,10,80). Two primary forms of hereditary angioedema (HAE) have been characterized: HAE type I, characterized by a reduced concentration of C1-INH, and HAE type II, characterized by a dysfunctional C1-INH. Type I accounts for 80%–85% of patients (9,10,80).

Without effective treatment, the disease has a high mortality, and diagnosis may be delayed in the absence of a family history (10,80). A high index of suspicion must be maintained by the intensive care practitioner, as distinguishing HAE from acquired angioedema facilitates treatment (10). Simple complement determinations are appropriate for the screening and diagnosis of the disorder. Analysis of C1-INH levels, both antigenic and functional, are most commonly used to establish the diagnosis. Analysis of C1q levels can help to differentiate between hereditary and acquired angioedema. Genetic testing may also be helpful in distinguishing hereditary and acquired angioedema in patients with no family history and in patients whose C1q level is equivocal (10).

The scenario in which the critical care provider is most likely to encounter hereditary angioedema is in the setting of acute laryngeal edema causing upper airway obstruction or with intestinal obstruction (80). In both instances, rapid resolution of symptoms is vital. Treatment options include antifibrinolytic agents, C1-INH-concentrate infusions, and fresh-frozen plasma, if C1-INH is not available (80). C1-INH concentrate is not currently available in the US, pending results of phase III clinical trials. Where it is available, C1-INH concentrate infusion appears to be the treatment of choice for acute upper airway obstruction or severe gastrointestinal symptoms secondary to hereditary angioedema (10). In a double-blinded, crossover study, nearly 70% of hereditary angioedema episodes responded within 30 min of a single infusion of C1-INH concentrate; 95% of these episodes resolved within 4 hrs (80). In children with suspected hereditary angioedema, *any* upper airway symptom merits treatment with C1-INH concentrate, if available (10). Moreover, in treating intestinal obstruction from hereditary angioedema, failure of clinical improvement following C1-INH infusion warrants consideration of alternative diagnoses for the abdominal symptomatology (10).

Infection

An increased susceptibility to invasive infection is a prominent feature of many patients with inherited complement deficiencies (26,68,71). Although complement protects against a variety of pathogens, patients with complement deficiency are most susceptible to bacterial infections (26,68,71). Moreover, the specific type of infection tends to be associated with the component of the complement cascade that is deficient. For example, children deficient in C3, important for opsonization, tend to be at increased risk for infections from encapsulated organisms, in which opsonization is the critical component of host defense. In fact, 80% of C3-deficient individuals have significant infections, as compared to 42% of C1-deficient, 33% of C4-deficient, and 50% of C2-deficient individuals (26,71). The lower incidence of infections in the three latter groups would appear to be related to their intact alternative pathway and the ability to activate C3 through this alternative mechanism.

The terminal components of the complement cascade, C5 through C9, form the membrane attack complex that is responsible for bacterial lysis and death (71). However, because C3 is not deficient, opsonization remains intact, and these patients are not excessively susceptible to encapsulated bacteria. Instead, these patients display increased susceptibility to

Neisseria infections, in which bactericidal activity is critical to host defense. *Neisseria meningitides* is also the most common pathogen among patients with X-linked properdin deficiency (68).

In addition to an increased incidence of meningococcal infections among patients with a terminal membrane attack complex complement deficiency, these children may also present with unusual patterns of infection. For example, types of meningococci commonly considered avirulent may cause fulminant sepsis or meningitis in these children (71). Infections from *Neisseria* serogroups W-135 and Y have been reported with increased frequency among patients deficient in the terminal components of the complement lectin cascade (68). Interestingly, a few studies suggest that meningococcal disease may have less morbidity and lower mortality in complement-deficient patients (26,71). Vaccination against meningococcal disease may be important for these patients (68). Not only do they appear to mount normal antibody responses to the administration of the tetravalent meningococcal vaccine but, because the median age for meningococcal disease in terminal complex deficiency and properdin deficiency is late adolescence, there is usually time for effective vaccination (26,68). Vaccination with the tetravalent meningococcal vaccine may be particularly important for properdin-deficient patients (68).

Rheumatologic Disorders

In addition to an increased susceptibility to infections, complement-deficient patients are at increased risk for rheumatologic disorders, most notably, SLE. The association between SLE and inherited C2 deficiency was recognized over 30 years ago. C2-deficient SLE is quite similar to genuine SLE, although antinuclear and dsDNA antibody levels are low or undetectable (37,52,68). Also, it is now known that SLE may be even more common among patients with a complete deficiency of C1 or C4 than among those with a C2 deficiency (37,52).

Mannan-binding Lectin Deficiency

In addition to deficits in the classical complement pathway, deficiencies in MBL may also contribute to disease states relevant to the pediatric critical care provider. MBL is a soluble pathogen-recognizing molecule that is capable of binding to microbes and activating complement via MASPs. Low levels of MBL have been reported in children deficient in opsonizing activity and with increased susceptibility to infection (72,75). Moreover, low levels appear to predispose to infection among cancer patients undergoing chemotherapy (75). In fact, among cancer patients who underwent gastrointestinal surgery, MBL levels were significantly lower in those who developed sepsis, systemic inflammatory response syndrome, or pneumonia (67,82). This association has not been found in all studies and is less apparent in patients who undergo intensive chemotherapy in which phagocytic function is strongly suppressed, such as treatment for AML and/or conditioning for allogeneic HSCT (75).

Among critically ill patients, MBL deficiency appears to increase susceptibility to sepsis and septic shock and may be associated with worse outcomes. In a post hoc analysis of Van den Berghe's landmark study of intensive insulin therapy in critically ill patients, conventionally treated nonsurvivors had significantly lower MBL levels on admission, at day 5, and at conclusion of the study, than did conventionally treated survivors (33). Moreover, among the subset of these patients with bacteremia, lower MBL levels were again detected among nonsurvivors. In another report, MBL genotype variant alleles were associated with a greater risk of sepsis, severe sepsis, septic shock, and mortality among 272 critically ill adults (29). In that study, serum MBL concentrations were inversely related to the severity of the sepsis. However, in a similar study, genotypes that resulted in low MBL levels were associated with an increased risk of bacterial infections, but not with an increased rate of sepsis, septic shock, or mortality in adults admitted to an ICU (73).

In a pediatric study, both MBL genotypes and MBL levels were evaluated in 100 consecutive admissions to a tertiary care PICU (25). Children with an MBL variant allele had an eightfold increased risk of developing systemic inflammatory response syndrome, as compared to those with a wild-type genotype, after adjusting for age, sex, and ethnicity. In this study, an association was also noted between the severity of the systemic response to infection and MBL variant alleles. MBL serum levels closely correlated with the MBL genotype; thus, low MBL levels (<1000 ng/mL) identified children at increased risk of systemic inflammatory response syndrome. In contrast, in a study of very low-birth-weight infants, MBL genotypes were not associated with an increased risk of sepsis (1).

In addition to sepsis, data suggests that low MBL levels and MBL variant genotypes may be related to a number of other disorders. For example, autoimmune disorders, such as SLE, rheumatoid arthritis, celiac disease, and IBDs have all been associated with low levels of MBL, although the data is far from conclusive (75). Data also suggests that low levels of MBL may be associated with the occurrence and the disease pattern of Kawasaki disease. In a Dutch study, children with Kawasaki disease were more likely to exhibit MBL variant genotypes, as compared to controls (4). In fact, among children <1 year of age, MBL variant genotypes were associated with a higher incidence of coronary artery involvement (4). In a study of Chinese patients with Kawasaki disease, MBL genotypes were found to modulate arterial stiffness, which is an important cardiovascular risk factor in children with Kawasaki disease (17). In that study, however, MBL genotype distributions did not differ between patients and controls or between patients with and without coronary artery aneurysms (17). MBL deficiency has also been associated with a number of other conditions, including rejection among heart transplant recipients, atherosclerosis, myocardial infarction, recurrent spontaneous abortions, and other obstetric and gynecologic complications (75).

Treatment for MBL deficiency is currently being investigated (75). The safety of infusing MBL, both purified from donor plasma and clinical-grade recombinant MBL, has been established in phase I trials. Clinical trials that test the potential benefits of MBL reconstitution in deficient individuals remain to be performed.

TOLL-LIKE RECEPTORS

Impaired Toll-like receptor (TLR) signaling has also been reported to be associated with immunodeficiency. TLRs are surface and intracellular pattern recognition receptors critical to the identification of invading microbes by recognizing the PAMPs of the microorganisms. The TLR-PAMP interaction triggers a complex signaling cascade that ultimately results in the activation of NFκB and activated protein-1. These two factors regulate the transcription of a multitude of genes encoding proinflammatory cytokines critical to the innate host defense (48).

Recently, three rare primary immune deficiencies associated with impaired TLR signaling have been described in humans (56). First, X-linked anhidrotic ectodermal dysplasia with immunodeficiency is caused by mutations in the *NEMO* gene. These patients may present with absent or conical teeth, dry skin due to absence or decreased number of eccrine sweat glands, and hypohidrosis with sparse scalp and eyebrow hair due to abnormal development of ectoderm-derived structures (56). In addition, these children experience an increased susceptibility to a wide variety of severe infections. Their overall prognosis is poor, with approximately half dying of overwhelming infection during childhood (23,55). The presence of conical incisors in a male with unusual infections suggests the need to assess for *NEMO* mutations (38). A second, AD form of anhidrotic ectodermal dysplasia with immunodeficiency has also been reported in association with a mutation of the gene encoding IκBα (56). IκBα is critical in the regulation of NFκB. This condition, phenotypically similar to the X-linked form, is characterized by abnormal development of ectoderm-derived structures and associated with multiple severe infections. The clinical features of the autosomal form, however, appear more severe and include severe T-cell dysfunction (23,55). HSCT has recently been used to successfully treat the immunodeficiency of AD anhidrotic ectodermal dysplasia; however, HSCT did not prevent the abnormalities of ectodermal dysplasia (23).

The third immunodeficiency associated with aberrant TLR signaling is caused by a mutation in the IL-1-receptor-associated kinase (IRAK)-4 gene (51,55). Patients with this AR mutation have recently been noted to have an increased susceptibility to infection. IRAK-4 acts upstream from the IκB-kinase complex in the Toll/IL-1 receptor (TIR) signaling pathway. These children have a very different clinical course than the anhidrotic ectodermal dysplasia patients. For example, they do not have developmental defects, and their increased susceptibility to infections appears limited to primarily pyogenic, encapsulated, gram-positive bacteria (e.g., *S. pneumoniae* and *S. aureus*). Their infections occur early in life, and the condition appears to improve as they age (51,55).

HEMOPHAGOCYTIC LYMPHOHISTIOCYTOSIS AND MACROPHAGE ACTIVATION SYNDROME

Hemophagocytic lymphohistiocytosis (HLH) and macrophage activation syndrome (MAS) comprise a spectrum of disorders related to defective NK-cells or cytotoxic T-cells. Both disorders have similar clinical features. MAS is typically seen in patients with autoimmune disease, and often resolves with aggressive treatment of the underlying autoimmune disorder. HLH requires much more aggressive therapy, often including HSCT.

HLH is often divided into *familial* HLH and *acquired* HLH. Clinically, the different types are often indistinguishable, with the exception that the familial forms present at <1 year of age in 70%–80% of the cases, whereas the acquired forms may present at any age. Familial forms of HLH may also be associated with an immunodeficiency, most notably Chediak-Higashi syndrome, Griscelli syndrome type 2, and XLP. HLH is a frequent but not absolute component of these disorders. Although acquired HLH is usually associated with infections, it may also occur with malignancy, inborn errors of metabolism, and after HSCT (35).

Several genetic mutations have been discovered in familial HLH. Between 20% and 50% of families have a defect in the perforin gene (*PRF*). This defect results in the production of a nonfunctional (defective) perforin protein. Perforin is secreted by cytotoxic T- and NK-cells. Perforin protein functions to perforate the cell membrane of target cells, thereby enabling the entry of granzymes into the target cell. This process ultimately results in apoptosis of the target cell (34). A mutation in the *MUNC 13-4* gene accounts for familial HLH in up to 20% of patients. Patients with this defect are unable to release granules from cytotoxic T-cells in a normal manner (77). A third genetic loci has been described in familial HLH patients that involves the syntaxin 11 (*STX11*) gene. Syntaxin 11 is a protein believed to be important in intracellular trafficking. Patients with mutations that involve this gene may have a slightly milder phenotype than the other forms of familial HLH. However, they may also be at more risk for myelodysplastic syndrome, acute myelocytic leukemia, and developmental delay (64).

Patients with the underlying immunodeficiencies that frequently develop HLH (Chediak-Higashi syndrome, Griscelli syndrome, and XLP) have also been found to have genetic mutations associated with impaired cytotoxic abilities. Patients with Chediak-Higashi syndrome have been found to have mutations in the *CHSI/LYST* gene. The LYST protein is involved in fusing granules to cell membranes. Patients with Griscelli syndrome who develop HLH have been noted to have mutations in the *RAB27A* gene. RAB27A plays a role in vesicle movement. Patients with these defects have been found to have poor cytotoxic function. XLP is associated with defects in the *SAP/SH2D1A* gene. The protein encoded for by this gene is important for the recruitment of signaling molecules involved in cytotoxic immunity (77).

Patients with HLH typically present with high and prolonged fevers associated with hepatosplenomegaly. Neurologic symptoms, a rash, and lymphadenopathy may also occur. An infectious source may or may not be found. The infections typically associated with HLH are viruses, especially EBV, but bacteria and protozoa have also been described as triggering agents (35). At first presentation, these patients may not appear to be critically ill. However, their condition may rapidly deteriorate into a life-threatening illness if HLH is not diagnosed and appropriate treatment is not initiated promptly. The Histiocyte Society has devised diagnostic guidelines to account for variability of presentation (**Table 76.5**).

Patients who do not receive timely therapy develop a severe systemic inflammatory response syndrome, which is characterized by end-organ damage. Although it is disconcerting for an intensivist to administer chemotherapy to critically ill children with this syndrome, these patients will not improve until appropriate treatment is initiated, and time is of the essence. Prompt initiation of therapy is crucial to successful treatment.

Treatment for HLH initially involves controlling the exuberant inflammatory response and treating any underlying infec-

---

TABLE 76.5

DIAGNOSTIC GUIDELINES FOR HLH

The diagnosis of HLH can be made by one of the following:
1. Molecular diagnosis consistent with HLH (*PRF* mutation, *MUNC13-4* mutation, etc.)
   OR
2. Having 5 of the following 8 criteria:
   a. Fever
   b. Splenomegaly
   c. Cytopenias affecting $\geq$ two cell lines
      Hemoglobin <9 g/dL, ($\leq$10g/dL for infants <4 weeks of age)
      Platelet count <100,000/mcL
      Neutrophils <1000/mcL
   d. Hypertriglyceridemia ($\geq$265 mg/dL) and/or hypofibrinogenemia ($\leq$150 mg/dL)
   e. Hemophagocytosis in bone marrow, spleen or lymph nodes without evidence of malignancy
   f. Low or absent NK-cell activity
   g. Hyperferritinemia ($\geq$500 mcg/L)
   h. Elevated soluble CD25 (IL-2Rα chain) $\geq$2400 U/mL

Adapted from Hentor JI, Horne A, Arico M, et al. HLH-2004: Diagnostic and therapeutic guidelines for hemophagocytic lymphohistiocytosis. *Pediatric Blood Cancer* 2007;48:124–31.

---

tion or malignancy. Corticosteroids are used to help decrease cytokine and chemokine production. Dexamethasone was chosen by the Histiocyte Society for their current protocol, HLH-2004, as it crosses the blood-brain barrier, and patients with HLH may have CNS involvement. Cyclosporine A is used for its ability to inhibit activation of T-lymphocytes. Etoposide is used for its toxicity to monocytes and histiocytes (35). These three medications are the mainstay of therapy in the HLH-2004 protocol. Intrathecal therapy is also utilized for patients with disease in the CNS. Once patients are in remission, those with known familial disease or genetic mutation, those with severe persistent disease, or those with reactivation of their disease go on to HSCT when an appropriate donor is identified. For patients who achieve remission and do not have a known genetic disease, therapy is discontinued to avoid the need for HSCT, if possible (34).

MAS has the same clinical presentation as HLH, but MAS is more responsive to immunosuppressive therapies. While most reports of MAS involve patients with systemic onset juvenile idiopathic arthritis (SOJIA), the literature does contain case reports of MAS in the context of several other connective tissue and autoinflammatory diseases (60). In addition, one of the authors of this chapter has personal experience with 3 children on hyperalimentation for short-gut syndrome who developed MAS. In this setting, MAS resolved once intralipid infusions were reduced to the minimum fatty acid requirements.

Management of MAS involves withdrawal of potentially hepatotoxic medications, including nonsteroidal anti-inflammatory medications, administration of high-dose pulse corticosteroids (methylprednisolone 30 mg/kg, maximum 1 g/day), and additional treatment with cyclosporine A for rapidly progressive and refractory cases (46). Criteria for early identification of MAS have been proposed. A decrease in platelet count combined with a coagulopathy similar to disseminated intravascular coagulopathy and hepatic dysfunction form a very sensitive and specific triad of the diagnosis of MAS. Clinical criteria, which are less specific, include CNS dysfunction, evidence of hemorrhage, and hepatomegaly. The demonstration of hemophagocytosis is not required for diagnosis, but hemophagocytosis in a bone marrow aspirate from a patient with SOJIA is virtually diagnostic of MAS (57). Perforin mutations are found in only a small minority of SOJIA patients who experience MAS. NK-cell function also tends to be normal in these patients. The excessive activation and proliferation of T-cells and macrophages that results in unrestricted release of inflammatory cytokines is clearly the result of an aberrant inflammatory response. Recent laboratory and therapeutic experiences indicate that IL-1 dysregulation may be at the heart of MAS occurring in the context of SOJIA (50).

IMMUNODEFICIENCY AND CANCER PREDISPOSITION

As described previously, several inherited immunodeficiency disorders have an increased risk of cancer, including WAS, ataxia telangiectasia, SCID, Kostmann syndrome, and XLP. In addition, patients with acquired immunodeficiencies, such as those with the acquired immunodeficiency syndrome and those receiving immunosuppressive therapy following organ transplantation also have an increased susceptibility to cancer. This association of immunodeficiency with a predisposition to cancer suggests that an intact immune system provides a surveillance mechanism to eliminate transformed cancer cells from the body. This theory of immune surveillance against malignant cells is supported by laboratory studies in which mice deficient in the IFN-γ receptor developed tumors more frequently and more rapidly upon exposure to carcinogens than did control mice (53).

On the other hand, the hypothesis for immune surveillance against cancer would appear to only partially explain the association between immunodeficiency and malignancy. For example, patients with severe immunodeficiencies are at increased risk for developing only specific types of cancers, mainly lymphoid malignancies (leukemias and lymphomas). The lack of increased risk for most other forms of cancer suggests that other factors must contribute to the development of malignancy. Moreover, in some immunodeficient conditions, cells have an increased susceptibility to genetic disruption and survive to be transformed into a malignant phenotype. For example, in patients with ataxia telangiectasia, disruption of the ATM gene increases the risk for DNA damage from radiation and, therefore, predisposes cells to become malignant independent of the immunodeficient state of this disease. In addition, immunodeficiency states are associated with an increased risk for infections that may contribute to the malignant transformation of cells. EBV infection, which has been linked to the evolution of lymphomas or lymphoproliferative disorders in post-transplant patients, represents one such example.

In sum, although the association between immunodeficiency states and a predisposition to cancer has been established, the mechanisms that contribute to this association are not completely understood and are likely multifactorial in origin.

IMMUNOLOGIC EFFECTS OF CANCER AND ITS TREATMENT

Predisposition to Immunodeficiency Associated with Cancer

In addition to immunodeficiency states that predispose to cancer, it is also widely accepted that most cancer patients are immunocompromised as a result of their underlying disease and/or their antineoplastic therapy. Many of these patients present with some degree of immunocompromise even prior to receiving cytotoxic therapy (53). For example, patients with acute leukemia are often pancytopenic at the time of diagnosis, and leukemia and lymphoma patients have long been known to have impaired neutrophil function. Additionally, both sarcoma and lymphoma patients have been found to present with reduced peripheral blood B- and T-cell populations (44,53). Further, functional impairments from intracranial and other solid tumors may predispose cancer patients to infection prior to therapy for a variety of reasons. Thus, oncology patients are likely to be immunocompromised prior to any cytotoxic cancer treatment. However, in addition to this underlying predisposition, antineoplastic therapy further compromises the immune function of these patients and places them at increased risk of severe infection. Several treatment-related factors, including neutropenia, loss of mucosal integrity, and T-cell dysfunction, contribute to an increased susceptibility of invasive infections in pediatric cancer patients.

Dating back to Bodey's landmark study of 1966, treatment-induced neutropenia has been established as one of the most significant risk factors for severe infection among cancer patients. In fact, the more severe the neutropenia, both in terms of absolute number and duration, the greater the risk of infection. In terms of absolute number, most bacteremias and bacterial pneumonias occur when the ANC is <100 cells/mm^3 (53). In terms of duration, treatment-induced neutropenia that persists for more than a week is associated with increased risk of infection (53). In fact, the prompt return of neutrophils following cytotoxic therapy portends a favorable outcome, even in the setting of a documented infection (53).

Although neutropenia clearly predisposes oncology patients to bacteremia and sepsis, its impact on outcome is less well established. Among pediatric cancer patients with severe sepsis who required both mechanical ventilation and inotropic support, no difference between survivors and nonsurvivors was reported in the percentage of patients with neutropenia (ANC <500 cells/mm^3) (68% and 72%, respectively, $p = 0.824$) (27). In contrast, another study noted a difference in mortality based on the presence or absence of neutropenia (ANC <1000 cells/mm^3) among children with cancer and a documented bloodstream infection (15% vs. 4%, respectively, $p = 0.03$) (79). A third study reported that the crude mortality rate for neutropenic patients was 36%, as compared to 31% for those without neutropenia among 2340 adult patients with cancer and a nosocomial bloodstream infection ($p = 0.053$) (81).

In addition to neutropenia, the impact of antineoplastic therapy on other effector cell lines of the immune system further impedes normal immune function. The impact of T-cell dysfunction is particularly detrimental and is the subject of much recent study. As with other hematopoietic cell subtypes,

T-cells are depleted following cytotoxic cancer therapy. The regeneration of T-cells, however, is often prolonged and incomplete. Therefore, cancer patients are susceptible to viral, fungal, and parasitic infections long after the end of their therapy and neutrophil recovery. In fact, $CD4^+$ T-cell subpopulations are more severely depleted in relation to their $CD8^+$ counterparts in patients who receive intensive chemotherapy regimens, rendering these patients even more susceptible to opportunistic infection (44,53). In addition to the viral, fungal, and parasitic infections, these patients may also have an increased susceptibility to some bacterial infections, including *Legionella*, *Listeria*, *Salmonella*, *Mycobacterium tuberculosis*, and atypical *Mycobacteria* (42). Moreover, T-cell dysfunction has been attributed to an increased risk of EBV-associated lymphoproliferative disorder and post-transfusion GVHD. Patients who have received protracted intensive chemotherapy and/or undergone allogeneic HSCT are at highest risk of complications related to T-cell deficiency states.

In addition to the impact on essential cell lines of the immune system, antineoplastic therapy also increases the risk of infection in pediatric cancer patients in a number of other ways. For example, the gastrointestinal tract has many rapidly dividing cells, placing it at risk for significant toxicity from antineoplastic therapy. This toxicity includes disruption of the mucosal barrier, fostering the systemic spread of pathogens. Severe oral mucositis exemplifies this toxicity and has been associated with a significantly increased risk of α-hemolytic streptococcal bacteremia in oncology patients and HSCT recipients (65). Moreover, the pain and discomfort of mucositis often interferes with normal nutrition, resulting in an increased risk of malnutrition and the need for parental alimentation. Both of these conditions have been associated with an increased risk of infection and/or impaired immune function. In addition, disruptions of the integumentary barrier, including the placement of indwelling catheters and the inherent risk of infection associated with these lines, further predispose these children to sepsis. Functional impairments induced by antineoplastic therapy (e.g., generalized weakness, swallowing difficulties, skin breakdown, etc.) may also increase susceptibility to infectious pathogens.

IMMUNE DYSFUNCTION ASSOCIATED WITH HEMATOPOIETIC STEM CELL TRANSPLANT

As described previously, immunosuppression is common with most antineoplastic therapy; however, it would appear to be most severe in the setting of allogeneic HSCT, due primarily to the fact that the process requires the near-complete replacement of the host lymphohematopoietic system. For replacement to successfully occur, intense immunosuppression of the host is required—a host who is likely immunocompromised as a result of underlying disease and previous therapy. Thus, HSCT patients will be profoundly immunocompromised until effective immune reconstitution occurs. Immune reconstitution, however, is a complex and prolonged process. In fact, although neutrophil engraftment may occur early in the post-transplant period, complete immune reconstitution requires months to years.

In terms of immune reconstitution, children differ from adults in two potentially important ways (3). First, the presence of a thymus greatly enhances both the kinetic and functional recovery of adaptive immunity in the pediatric transplant patient, which results in several beneficial effects, including improved recovery of naïve T-cells. Faster recovery of $CD4^+$ T-cell levels has been associated with a decreased risk of opportunistic infection following HSCT engraftment (3,69). Second, the incidence of GVHD appears to be lower in children than in adults. The presence of GVHD contributes significantly to immunosuppression by both impeding immune restoration and requiring further immunosuppressive therapy (3,28).

Immune reconstitution following HSCT is influenced by patient-, disease-, and transplant-related factors that include patient age, underlying disease and disease status, transplant type (autologous vs. allogeneic), preparative regimen, the presence of infection, HLA compatibility, GVHD, and the stem cell source, mobilization, and manipulation techniques (3). In addition, it is important to note that cellular reconstitution does not necessarily correlate with functional recovery, and innate immunity reconstitution precedes that of adaptive immunity (3).

Innate Immunity Recovery

Natural Killer Cells

The reconstitution of NK-cells has been extensively evaluated in the post-transplant period. NK-cell levels appear to return to normal within 1–2 months following HSCT, seemingly independent of transplant type, stem cell source, patient age, and GVHD (3). Also, it appears as though functional recovery occurs simultaneously with the return of NK cellularity, which is potentially very important to the recipient, given the antimicrobial and anti-tumor effects of these cells.

Neutrophils, Macrophages, and Monocytes

Granulocytes and monocytes also recover early in the post-transplant period, with neutrophil recovery preceding that of monocytes and tissue macrophages (3). However, recovery of these cells differs from that of NK-cells in two important ways. First, their recovery is influenced by transplant-related factors, such as stem cell source and GVHD. For example, an unmanipulated matched sibling stem cell graft will have more differentiated precursors, allowing quicker recovery of these subsets of cells than will a graft composed entirely of the more primitive $CD34^+$ stem cell. Second, in both animal and human studies, recovery in cellularity does not necessarily correspond with functional recovery (3). For example, reconstituted phagocytes have impaired bactericidal activity for at least 2 months following allogeneic HSCT, placing the child at increased risk of pyogenic infection and infection-related mortality (3).

Dendritic Cells

Dendritic cell recovery also occurs relatively early in the post-HSCT setting (3). In addition, much like neutrophil recovery, manipulations in the stem cell source appear to influence the speed of dendritic cell recovery (3). Although the relationship between cellular and functional recovery of these cells has not been well established, data do suggest that early dendritic cell recovery may serve to protect the transplant recipient against infection (22). Low levels of dendritic cells during the peri-engraftment period have also been associated with an increased risk of relapse, acute GVHD, and death (58).

Adaptive Immunity Recovery

Reconstitution of Humoral Immunity

In the early post-HSCT period, it is primarily the host plasma cells, which have survived the preparative regimen, that produce IgG (28). Progenitor cells contained in the allograft begin to give rise to naïve B-cells, resulting in production of IgM, 4–6 months after the transplant. Isotype switching, resulting in production of IgG and, subsequently, IgA, can only occur with CD^+4 T-helper cells, and thus occurs much later (3,28). In fact, IgG levels may remain abnormal for up to 1 year following transplant, and IgA levels for as long as 2 years (3,28). Even when normal levels of IgG are achieved, an oligoclonal pattern may be present, limiting their utility (28). The presence of severe acute GVHD or chronic extensive GVHD has been associated with reduced numbers of B-cells and diminished availability of $CD4^+$ T-helper cells, thereby further impeding reconstitution of humoral immunity (28). In general, B-cell recovery tends to occur before T-cell reconstitution (3).

T-cell Recovery

T-cell reconstitution is critical for immune competency and is believed to occur via two pathways. The first is a thymic-independent pathway termed *homeostatic peripheral expansion* (HPE), which merely involves the expansion of mature T-cells that survived the preparative regimen, were contained within the allograft, and/or were given via donor lymphocyte infusions (28). These T-cells are both quantitatively and qualitatively deficient. Also, HPE results in a T-cell pool limited to cells activated by the antigenic milieu of the host, with negligible numbers of cells having activity for antigens absent at the time of expansion (43). This limited repertoire significantly impedes the ability to generate effective clonal T-cell responses against microbes and tumor cells (3).

Recovery of thymic function, therefore, provides the optimal pathway for T-cell reconstitution. Unfortunately, thymic recovery does not generally occur for several months following allogeneic HSCT (3,28). Thymic recovery is limited by age-related decrements in thymic function, as well as by cytotoxic-, radiation-, and/or GVHD-induced thymic injury (28). As a result, recovery of normal T-cell number and function often does not occur within the first year following HSCT (3,28).

GVHD is particularly detrimental to immune reconstitution (28). First, the process is directly toxic to the thymic microenvironment. GVHD may also impair negative selection of T-cells that react to host antigens. This combination both results in decreased thymic function and recovery and fosters further GVHD. In addition, by causing widespread apoptosis, GVHD limits the effectiveness of HPE, thereby hindering thymic-independent immune restoration (11). Finally, the immunosuppressants necessary to treat GVHD further diminish both thymic function and HPE. Thus, both the pathophysiology of GHVD and the immunosuppression required to treat this condition prolong the course of immune reconstitution following HSCT.

CONCLUSIONS AND FUTURE DIRECTIONS

As described in this chapter, several specific genetic mutations have recently been identified as the cause of most of the well-defined immunodeficiency conditions. For several disorders, notably CVID, various mutations may lead to the same phenotype. The genetic basis of more subtle cytokine signaling defects and molecular pattern recognition deficits awaits clarification. Polymorphisms in cytokine signaling pathway may clarify minor variations in immune function that are presently unexplained. Therapeutic advances in the future are likely to include even more convenient and effective methods of IgG replacement. Enhancement of cellular immune function may be feasible with available cytokine therapies. For children with severe defects that justify HSCT, strategies for enhancing immune tolerance should allow for chimerism following stem cell "mini" transplants, thereby lessening the risks of postablation infection and GVHD. The ultimate therapeutic goal for single gene defects, however, is gene replacement therapy. The initial enthusiasm for the successful replacement of the γ_c gene in X-linked SCID and the ADA gene in ADA deficiency has been tempered by the development of leukemia in 3 of ~20 patients treated with this therapy worldwide (16). Improved control of vector integration sites should ultimately lessen, if not eliminate, this risk of malignancy.

KEY POINTS

- Although relatively rare, the pediatric critical care provider needs a sound working knowledge of primary immunodeficiencies, as prompt identification and diagnosis of these disorders allows for early institution of appropriate therapy and, potentially, improved outcomes among these high-risk patients.
- The intensivist should recognize a child presenting with his second invasive bacterial infection, an opportunistic infection, and/or an infection slow to respond to conventional therapy as a patient in need of an immunologic workup.
- Antibody defects are the most prevalent primary immune deficiency; thus, laboratory evaluation should generally first focus on the possibility of humoral deficiency.
- Antibody defects most commonly predispose patients to sinopulmonary infections with encapsulated organisms.
- An early clue to an immunoglobulin deficiency is the finding of a low total protein level in the presence of a normal albumin level on routine blood analysis.
- Gammaglobulin therapy may be helpful in the control and clearance of severe infections in patients with known immunodeficiency, and IV administration at physiologic replacement doses of 400–500 mg/kg is most appropriate.
- Although less common than antibody defects, predominantly cellular immune defects may also be encountered by the pediatric intensivist. Infants with DGS and velocardiofacial syndrome have a characteristic 22q11.2 deletion and frequently manifest T-cell deficiency. The 22q11.2 deletion syndrome is the most common cellular immune defect that is likely to present to the pediatric intensivist as a result of congenital heart disease and/or hypocalcemia.

■ The cardinal clinical features of T-cell dysfunction are yeast overgrowth, chronic viral infections, opportunistic infections, autoimmune disorders, and malignancies.

■ Dysgammaglobulinemia is a frequent consequence of T-cell dysfunction, given the necessary role of T-cell signaling for immunoglobulin class switching and affinity maturation.

■ Combined antibody and cellular immune deficiencies are generally characterized by the early onset of viral and yeast infections, usually resulting in growth failure.

■ The intensive care of an infant suspected or known to have SCID should include strict isolation and the use of only irradiated, CMV-negative, and leukocyte-depleted blood products.

■ The infant with SCID should be screened for *P. jiroveci* infection, and both respiratory secretions and stool should be tested for a variety of other pathogens.

■ The infant with SCID may benefit from aggressive antiviral therapies in addition to antibiotics and IVIG. An immunologist or hematologist should be involved early in the care of these infants to facilitate arrangements for HSCT, which at this date, remains the most successful therapy for SCID.

■ HSCT has also proven valuable for a number of other immune deficiencies, including WAS and CGD.

■ Primary neutrophil disorders may also be encountered by the intensivist and may be divided into two broad categories: diseases associated with decreased numbers of neutrophils (neutropenia) and those with impaired neutrophil function.

■ GCSF therapy may play a role in the treatment of neutropenic disorders. Prophylactic antibiotics, IVIG, and IFN-γ may be useful in the treatment of some functional neutrophil disorders.

■ Complement deficiencies are likely to present to the intensivist in the form of either hereditary angioedema, invasive infections (most notably meningococcal disease), or rheumatologic disorders, especially SLE.

■ C1-INH concentrate infusion therapy, where available, may be life-saving for children with acute upper airway obstruction or severe gastrointestinal symptoms secondary to hereditary angioedema.

■ In addition to deficits in the classical complement pathway, deficiencies in MBL may also contribute to disease states relevant to the pediatric critical care provider, including sepsis, Kawasaki disease, and autoimmune disorders.

■ Primary immunodeficiencies associated with impaired TLR signaling have been described.

■ In addition to primary immune deficiencies, it is important to recognize that cancer is commonly associated with immune deficiency. Not only are several primary immune deficiencies, including WAS, ataxia telangiectasia, SCID, Kostmann syndrome, and XLP, being associated with an increased risk of cancer, most cancer patients are immunocompromised as a result of their underlying disease and/or their anti-neoplastic therapy.

■ Several cancer treatment-related factors, including neutropenia, loss of mucosal integrity, and T-cell dysfunction, contribute to this immunocompromised state.

■ Immune suppression is most severe among those patients who receive an allogeneic HSCT. The replacement of the functional lymphohematopoietic system of the host with that of a donor requires intense immunosuppression, often in a patient whose underlying disease has rendered them immunocompromised.

■ HSCT patients remain profoundly immunocompromised until effective immune reconstitution occurs, which is a complex and prolonged process that requires months to years.

■ Immune reconstitution following HSCT is influenced by patient-, disease-, and transplant-related factors. Importantly, cellular reconstitution does not necessarily correlate with functional recovery.

■ The occurrence of GVHD in the HSCT patient will significantly impede the recovery of normal immune function.

ACKNOWLEDGMENT

The authors wish to express their gratitude to Dr. William Grossman for his expertise and insight in the writing of this chapter.

References

1. Ahrens P, Kattner E, Kohler B, et al. Mutations of genes involved in the innate immune system as predictors of sepsis in very low birth weight infants. *Pediatr Res* 2004;55:652–6.

2. Ancliff PJ, Gale RE, Liesner R, et al. Mutations in the ELA2 gene encoding neutrophil elastase are present in most patients with sporadic severe congenital neutropenia but only in some patients with the familial form of the disease. *Blood* 2001;98:2645–50.

3. Auletta JJ, Lazarus HM. Immune restoration following hematopoietic stem cell transplantation: An evolving target. *Bone Marrow Transplant* 2005;35:835–57.

4. Biezeveld MH, Kuipers IM, Geissler J, et al. Association of mannose-binding lectin genotype with cardiovascular abnormalities in Kawasaki disease. *Lancet* 2003;361:1268–70.

5. Bilora F, Petrobelli F, Boccioletti V, et al. Moderate-dose intravenous immunoglobulin treatment of Job's syndrome. *Case report. Minerva Med* 2000; 91:113–6.

6. Bindl L, Torgerson T, Perroni L, et al. Successful use of the new immune-suppressor sirolimus in IPEX (immune dysregulation, polyendocrinopathy, enteropathy, X-linked syndrome). *J Pediatr* 2005;147:256–9.

7. Bonilla FA, Geha RS. 12. Primary immunodeficiency diseases. *J Allergy Clin Immunol* 2003;111:S571–81.

8. Bonilla FA, Geha RS. 2. Update on primary immunodeficiency diseases. *J Allergy Clin Immunol* 2006;117:S435–41.

9. Bork K, Siedlecki K, Bosch S, et al. Asphyxiation by laryngeal edema in patients with hereditary angioedema. *Mayo Clin Proc* 2000;75:349–54.

10. Boyle RJ, Nikpour M, Tang ML. Hereditary angio-oedema in children: A management guideline. *Pediatr Allergy Immunol* 2005;16:288–94.

11. Brochu S, Rioux-Masse B, Roy J, et al. Massive activation-induced cell death of alloreactive T cells with apoptosis of bystander postthymic T cells prevents immune reconstitution in mice with graft-versus-host disease. *Blood* 1999;94:390–400.

12. Buckley RH. Immunodeficiency diseases. *JAMA* 1992;268:2797–806.

13. Buckley RH, Schiff SE, Schiff RI, et al. Hematopoietic stem-cell transplantation for the treatment of severe combined immunodeficiency. *N Engl J Med* 1999;340:508–16.

14. Capsoni F, Sarzi-Puttini P, Zanella A. Primary and secondary autoimmune neutropenia. *Arthritis Res Ther* 2005;7:208–14.

15. Castigli E, Wilson SA, Garibyan L, et al. TACI is mutant in common variable immunodeficiency and IgA deficiency. *Nat Genet* 2005;37:829–34.

16. Check E. Gene-therapy trials to restart following cancer risk review. *Nature* 2005;434:127.

17. Cheung YF, Ho MH, Ip WK, et al. Modulating effects of mannose-binding lectin genotype on arterial stiffness in children after Kawasaki disease. *Pediatr Res* 2004;56:591–6.

18. Crawford TO, Skolasky RL, Fernandez R, et al. Survival probability in ataxia telangiectasia. *Arch Dis Child* 2006;91:610–1.

19. Cunningham-Rundles C, Siegal FP, Cunningham-Rundles S, et al. Incidence of cancer in 98 patients with common varied immunodeficiency. *J Clin Immunol* 1987;7:294–9.

20. Cunnion KM, Wagner E, Frank MM. Complement & Kinin. In: Parslow TG, Stites DP, Terr AI, et al., eds. *Medical Immunology.* New York: McGraw-Hill, 2001;175–88.

21. Dahmer MK, Randolph A, Vitali S, et al. Genetic polymorphisms in sepsis. *Pediatr Crit Care Med* 2005;6:S61–73.

22. Damiani D, Stocchi R, Masolini P, et al. Dendritic cell recovery after autologous stem cell transplantation. *Bone Marrow Transplant* 2002;30:261–6.

23. Dupuis-Girod S, Cancrini C, Le DF, et al. Successful allogeneic hemopoietic stem cell transplantation in a child who had anhidrotic ectodermal dysplasia with immunodeficiency. *Pediatrics* 2006;118:e205–11.

24. Etzioni A, Ochs HD. The hyper IgM syndrome–an evolving story. *Pediatr Res* 2004;56:519–25.

25. Fidler KJ, Wilson P, Davies JC, et al. Increased incidence and severity of the systemic inflammatory response syndrome in patients deficient in mannose-binding lectin. *Intensive Care Med* 2004;30:1438–45.

26. Figueroa JE, Densen P. Infectious diseases associated with complement deficiencies. *Clin Microbiol Rev* 1991;4:359–95.

27. Fiser RT, West NK, Bush AJ, et al. Outcome of severe sepsis in pediatric oncology patients. *Pediatr Crit Care Med* 2005;6:531–6.

28. Fry TJ, Mackall CL. Immune reconstitution following hematopoietic progenitor cell transplantation: Challenges for the future. *Bone Marrow Transplant* 2005;35(Suppl 1):S53–S57.

29. Garred P, Strom J, Quist L, et al. Association of mannose-binding lectin polymorphisms with sepsis and fatal outcome, in patients with systemic inflammatory response syndrome. *J Infect Dis* 2003;188:1394–403.

30. Gaspar J, Gerritsen B, Jones A. Immunoglobulin replacement treatment by rapid subcutaneous infusion. *Arch Dis Child* 1998;79:48–51.

31. Goldfarb RD, Parrillo JE. Complement. *Crit Care Med* 2005;33:S482–4.

32. Hague RA, Rassam S, Morgan G, et al. Early diagnosis of severe combined immunodeficiency syndrome. *Arch Dis Child* 1994;70:260–3.

33. Hansen TK, Thiel S, Wouters PJ, et al. Intensive insulin therapy exerts antiinflammatory effects in critically ill patients and counteracts the adverse effect of low mannose-binding lectin levels. *J Clin Endocrinol Metab* 2003;88:1082–8.

34. Henter JI, Horne A, Arico M, et al. HLH-2004: Diagnostic and therapeutic guidelines for hemophagocytic lymphohistiocytosis. *Pediatr Blood Cancer* 2007;48:124–31.

35. Janka GE. Familial and acquired hemophagocytic lymphohistiocytosis. *Eur J Pediatr* 2007;166:95–109.

36. Jawad AF, Donald-Mcginn DM, Zackai E, et al. Immunologic features of chromosome 22q11.2 deletion syndrome (DiGeorge syndrome/velocardiofacial syndrome). *J Pediatr* 2001;139:715–23.

37. Jonsson G, Truedsson L, Sturfelt G, et al. Hereditary C2 deficiency in Sweden: Frequent occurrence of invasive infection, atherosclerosis, and rheumatic disease. *Medicine (Baltimore)* 2005;84:23–34.

38. Ku CL, Dupuis-Girod S, Dittrich AM, et al. NEMO mutations in 2 unrelated boys with severe infections and conical teeth. *Pediatrics* 2005;115:e615–9.

39. Lekstrom-Himes JA, Gallin JI. Immunodeficiency diseases caused by defects in phagocytes. *N Engl J Med* 2000;343:1703–14.

40. Lin JH, Liebhaber M, Roberts RL, et al. Etanercept treatment of cutaneous granulomas in common variable immunodeficiency. *J Allergy Clin Immunol* 2006;117:878–82.

41. Lindsay EA, Vitelli F, Su H, et al. Tbx1 haploinsufficiency in the DiGeorge syndrome region causes aortic arch defects in mice. *Nature* 2001;410:97–101.

42. Mackall CL. T-cell immunodeficiency following cytotoxic antineoplastic therapy: A review. *Stem Cells* 2000;18:10–8.

43. Mackall CL, Bare CV, Granger LA, et al. Thymic-independent T cell regeneration occurs via antigen-driven expansion of peripheral T cells resulting in a repertoire that is limited in diversity and prone to skewing. *J Immunol* 1996;156:4609–16.

44. Mackall CL, Fleisher TA, Brown MR, et al. Lymphocyte depletion during treatment with intensive chemotherapy for cancer. *Blood* 1994;84:2221–8.

45. Milone M. Use of B-cell directed therapy to treat primary Epstein-Barr virus (EBV) infection in patients with X-linked lymphoproliferative disease. *Immunology Reviews* 2005;203:994–6.

46. Mouy R, Stephan JL, Pillet P, et al. Efficacy of cyclosporine A in the treatment of macrophage activation syndrome in juvenile arthritis: Report of five cases. *J Pediatr* 1996;129:750–4.

47. Mullighan CG, Fanning GC, Chapel HM, et al. TNF and lymphotoxin-alpha polymorphisms associated with common variable immunodeficiency: Role in the pathogenesis of granulomatous disease. *J Immunol* 1997;159:6236–41.

48. Netea MG, Van der GC, Van der Meer JW, et al. Toll-like receptors and the host defense against microbial pathogens: Bringing specificity to the innate-immune system. *J Leukoc Biol* 2004;75:749–55.

49. Orange JS. Congenital immunodeficiencies and sepsis. *Pediatr Crit Care Med* 2005;6:S99–S107.

50. Pascual V, Allantaz F, Arce E, et al. Role of interleukin-1 (IL-1) in the pathogenesis of systemic onset juvenile idiopathic arthritis and clinical response to IL-1 blockade. *J Exp Med* 2005;201:1479–86.

51. Picard C, Puel A, Bonnet M, et al. Pyogenic bacterial infections in humans with IRAK-4 deficiency. *Science* 2003;299:2076–9.

52. Pickering MC, Botto M, Taylor PR, et al. Systemic lupus erythematosus, complement deficiency, and apoptosis. *Adv Immunol* 2000;76:227–324.

53. Pizzo PA, Poplack DG. *Principles and Practice of Pediatric Oncology*, 4th ed. Philadelphia: Lippincott Williams and Wilkins, 2002.

54. Plebani A, Soresina A, Rondelli R, et al. Clinical, immunological, and molecular analysis in a large cohort of patients with X-linked agammaglobulinemia: An Italian multicenter study. *Clin Immunol* 2002;104:221–30.

55. Puel A, Picard C, Ku CL, et al. Inherited disorders of NF-kappaB-mediated immunity in man. *Curr Opin Immunol* 2004;16:34–41.

56. Puel A, Yang K, Ku CL, et al. Heritable defects of the human TLR signalling pathways. *J Endotoxin Res* 2005;11:220–4.

57. Ravelli A, Magni-Manzoni S, Pistorio A, et al. Preliminary diagnostic guidelines for macrophage activation syndrome complicating systemic juvenile idiopathic arthritis. *J Pediatr* 2005;146:598–604.

58. Reddy V, Iturraspe JA, Tzolas AC, et al. Low dendritic cell count after allogeneic hematopoietic stem cell transplantation predicts relapse, death, and acute graft-versus-host disease. *Blood* 2004;103:4330–5.

59. Renner ED, Puck JM, Holland SM, et al. Autosomal recessive hyperimmunoglobulin E syndrome: A distinct disease entity. *J Pediatr* 2004;144:93–9.

60. Rigante D, Capoluongo E, Bertoni B, et al. First report of macrophage activation syndrome in hyperimmunoglobulinemia D with periodic fever syndrome. *Arthritis Rheum* 2007;56:658–61.

61. Roesler J, Horwitz ME, Picard C, et al. Hematopoietic stem cell transplantation for complete IFN-gamma receptor 1 deficiency: A multi-institutional survey. *J Pediatr* 2004;145:806–12.

62. Rosenberg PS, Alter BP, Bolyard AA, et al. The incidence of leukemia and mortality from sepsis in patients with severe congenital neutropenia receiving long-term G-CSF therapy. *Blood* 2006;107:4628–35.

63. Rosenzweig SD, Holland SM. Phagocyte immunodeficiencies and their infections. *J Allergy Clin Immunol* 2004;113:620–6.

64. Rudd E, Goransdotter EK, Zheng C, et al. Spectrum and clinical implications of syntaxin 11 gene mutations in familial haemophagocytic lymphohistiocytosis: Association with disease-free remissions and haematopoietic malignancies. *J Med Genet* 2006;43:e14.

65. Ruescher TJ, Sodeifi A, Scrivani SJ, et al. The impact of mucositis on alpha-hemolytic streptococcal infection in patients undergoing autologous bone marrow transplantation for hematologic malignances. *Cancer* 1998;82:2275–81.

66. Sera Y, Kawaguchi H, Nakamura K, et al. A comparison of the defective granulopoiesis in childhood cyclic neutropenia and in severe congenital neutropenia. *Haematologica* 2005;90:1032–41.

67. Siassi M, Hohenberger W, Riese J. Mannan-binding lectin (MBL) serum levels and post-operative infections. *Biochem Soc Trans* 2003;31:774–5.

68. Sjoholm AG, Jonsson G, Braconier JH, et al. Complement deficiency and disease: An update. *Mol Immunol* 2006;43:78–85.

69. Small TN, Avigan D, Dupont B, et al. Immune reconstitution following T-cell depleted bone marrow transplantation: Effect of age and posttransplant graft rejection prophylaxis. *Biol Blood Marrow Transplant* 1997;3:65–75.

70. Stewart DM, Tian L, Nelson DL. Linking cellular activation to cytoskeletal reorganization: Wiskott-Aldrich syndrome as a model. *Curr Opin Allergy Clin Immunol* 2001;1:525–33.

71. Stiehm ER, Ochs HD, Winkelstein JA. *Immunologic Disorders in Infants and Children*, 5th ed. Philadelphia: Elsevier Saunders, 2004.

72. Super M, Thiel S, Lu J, et al. Association of low levels of mannan-binding protein with a common defect of opsonisation. *Lancet* 1989;2:1236–9.

73. Sutherland AM, Walley KR, Russell JA. Polymorphisms in CD14, mannose-binding lectin, and Toll-like receptor-2 are associated with increased prevalence of infection in critically ill adults. *Crit Care Med* 2005;33:638–44.

74. Tabata Y, Villanueva J, Lee SM, et al. Rapid detection of intracellular SH2D1A protein in cytotoxic lymphocytes from patients with X-linked lymphoproliferative disease and their family members. *Blood* 2005;105:3066–71.

75. Thiel S, Frederiksen PD, Jensenius JC. Clinical manifestations of mannan-binding lectin deficiency. *Mol Immunol* 2006;43:86–96.

76. Van Mierop LH, Kutsche LM. Cardiovascular anomalies in DiGeorge syndrome and importance of neural crest as a possible pathogenetic factor. *Am J Cardiol* 1986;58:133–7.

77. Verbsky JW, Grossman WJ. Hemophagocytic lymphohistiocytosis: Diagnosis, pathophysiology, treatment, and future perspectives. *Ann Med* 2006;38:20–31.

78. Villa A, Santagata S, Bozzi F, et al. Partial V(D)J recombination activity leads to Omenn syndrome. *Cell* 1998;93:885–96.

79. Viscoli C, Castagnola E, Giacchino M, et al. Bloodstream infections in children with cancer: A multicentre surveillance study of the Italian Association of Paediatric Haematology and Oncology. *Supportive Therapy Group-Infectious Diseases Section. Eur J Cancer* 1999;35:770–4.

80. Waytes AT, Rosen FS, Frank MM. Treatment of hereditary angioedema with a vapor-heated C1 inhibitor concentrate. *N Engl J Med* 1996;334:1630–4.

81. Wisplinghoff H, Seifert H, Wenzel RP, et al. Current trends in the epidemiology of nosocomial bloodstream infections in patients with hematological malignancies and solid neoplasms in hospitals in the United States. *Clin Infect Dis* 2003;36:1103–10.

82. Ytting H, Christensen IJ, Jensenius JC, et al. Preoperative mannan-binding lectin pathway and prognosis in colorectal cancer. *Cancer Immunol Immunother* 2005;54:265–72.

83. Zarzour W, Kleta R, Frangoul H, et al. Two novel CHS1 (LYST) mutations: Clinical correlations in an infant with Chediak-Higashi syndrome. *Mol Genet Metab* 2005;85:125–32.

CHAPTER 77 ■ PRINCIPLES OF ANTIMICROBIAL THERAPY

PHILIP TOLTZIS • JEFFREY L. BLUMER

CATEGORIES OF INFECTION IN THE PICU

The pediatric intensivist encounters a wide variety of infections in the PICU. The first task in selecting an appropriate anti-infective agent is to determine the causative organism. Unfortunately, the precarious condition of the infected ICU patient frequently precludes delaying therapy until culture and susceptibility testing is completed. Consequently, in many instances empiric therapy must be initiated while awaiting culture results, then revised if and when the offending organism is isolated and tested. The best choice of empiric therapy is driven by knowledge of the pathogens that are most likely to be encountered in a given clinical situation and the susceptibility patterns of those pathogens.

The importance of selecting the correct anti-infective agent for initial empiric therapy in the critically ill patient is underscored by observations that document the consequences of choosing wrongly. Most of the relevant studies that address this issue have examined the outcomes of ICU patients treated initially with antibiotics to which the responsible organism proved resistant (5). Among adult ICU patients who experience ventilator-associated pneumonia, mortality rates are increased in subjects who initially receive ineffective therapy when compared with patients for whom the initial selection proved correct (5). Similarly, delayed therapy of healthcare-associated methicillin-resistant *Staphylococcus aureus* (MRSA) infection is an independent predictor of mortality and prolonged hospitalization (5).

Three categories of infected patients are typically found in the PICU: those whose infections were acquired in the community, those whose infections were nosocomially acquired, and those with a compromised immune system. The list of potential pathogens grows successively broader with each of these categories (**Table 77.1**).

The pathogens that are likely responsible for community-acquired infections can be inferred from the focus of the infection and the age of the child. Most patients who are admitted to the PICU with community-acquired infection experience blood-borne infection and sepsis, meningitis/meningoencephalitis, or pneumonia. In the youngest patients, aged newborn to 2 months, the same pathogens frequently cause infection in all of these foci simultaneously. Severe community-acquired infections in children aged ≥2 months are almost exclusively caused by bacteria and respiratory viruses. The predominant causes of bacteremia with sepsis and menin-

gitis are *Streptococcus pneumoniae* and *Neisseria meningitidis*. Less frequently, the child with community-acquired sepsis is infected with *S. aureus* or group A streptococcus; in these children symptoms may reflect the elaboration of exotoxins, which produce vasomotor instability and end-organ dysfunction. The variety of organisms that cause community-acquired pneumonia is broad and includes primarily the bacterium *S. pneumoniae* and community respiratory viruses, although *Bordetella pertussis* and the atypical bacteria (e.g., *Mycoplasma*, *Chlamydia*) may be encountered as well.

A greater array of potential pathogens is encountered in the child who has acquired nosocomial infection while in the PICU. The most frequent sites of nosocomial infection are those whose sterility has been compromised by hospital-related procedures, including infections of the bloodstream, potentiated by the placement of intravascular catheters; the lungs, by endotracheal intubation; the urinary tract, by placement of a bladder catheter; and the subcutaneous tissues, as a consequence of surgical wounds.

The broadest variety of potential pathogens is encountered in immunocompromised children, who include those with chemotherapy-induced neutropenia, children whose T-cell function is suppressed pharmacologically after stem cell or solid-organ transplantation, and those who are afflicted by one of the many congenital or acquired immune deficiencies. The list of potential infecting pathogens in these patients is usually extensive and depends, to some extent, on the nature of the immune defect and the apparent focus of infection.

FOUNDATIONS OF ANTIMICROBIAL THERAPEUTICS

Therapeutics is the discipline within pharmacology dealing with the use of drugs in the prevention or treatment of disease. Essential to the practice of anti-infective therapeutics is an understanding of the elements of effective therapy. From a pharmacologic perspective, three key determinants of effective therapy exist: pharmacokinetics, pharmacodynamics, and pharmaceutics (**Fig. 77.1**). In a given clinical situation, if a drug can be identified that has favorable characteristics in each of these three areas, it will virtually always provide effective therapy (20).

Pharmacokinetics is that aspect of pharmacology that relates drug administration to the concentration-time profile that the drug achieves in body fluids. It quantitatively describes the processes of drug absorption, distribution, metabolism, and

TABLE 77.1

MICROORGANISMS COMMONLY IMPLICATED IN INFECTIONS IN THE PICU

Type of infection	Microorganisms
Community-acquired	Bacteria: *Streptococcus pneumoniae, Neisseria meningitidis., Staphylococcus aureus, Streptococcus pyogenes, Bordetella pertussis*, group B streptococcus[a], *Listeria*[a], enteric Gram-negative bacilli[a,b], atypical respiratory tract bacteria Viruses: Herpes simplex[a], enterovirus[a], respiratory viruses
Nosocomial	Bacteria: Coagulase-negative staphylococcus, *S. aureus*, Enterobacteriaceae, *Pseudomonas, Acinetobacter, Nocardia, Clostridium difficile* Fungi: *Candida* Viruses: Respiratory and enteric viruses
Immunocompromised host	Bacteria: Coagulase-negative staphylococcus, *S. aureus*, viridans streptococcus, *Corynebacteria*, Enterobacteriaceae, *Pseudomonas, Acinetobacter* Fungi: *Candida, Aspergillus*, non-*Aspergillus* molds, *Cryptococcus*, endemic fungi, *Pneumocystis jiroveci* Viruses: Herpes virus family, adenovirus, respiratory viruses Parasites: Toxoplasma, enteric parasites

[a]Seen in infants <2 months of age.
[b]Primarily associated with urosepsis.

excretion. Pharmacokinetics plays a central role as a determinant of anti-infective efficacy. In most cases, the spectrum of activity of a given agent is known (pharmacodynamics), and the formulation to be used is known to be safe and appropriate for the patient to be treated (pharmaceutics) prior to drug administration. Therefore, almost any deviation from the expected clinical outcome must have a pharmacokinetic basis.

Most pharmacokinetic data that describe the biodisposition of anti-infectives in infants and children have been ascertained in relatively healthy subjects. These parameters can be altered significantly in the face of disease or may be affected by drug-drug interactions. Both of these confounders are common problems in the PICU (27,28). The doses and dosing intervals of many anti-infectives must be adjusted in the face of hepatic or renal functional impairment. In that the function of these organs is often changing during a stay in the PICU, frequent adjustments are required to ensure that therapy remains both effective and safe. Virtually all PICU patients are receiving multiple therapeutic agents. Each amplifies the potential for drug-drug interactions that may have an impact on anti-infective disposition.

Pharmacodynamics is that discipline within pharmacology that links drug exposure to the resulting concentration-effect relationships. In the context of antimicrobial agents, it deals with the mechanisms of anti-infective action and the drug's safety profiles. A number of procedures are available for testing the in vitro susceptibility of various microorganisms to anti-infective drugs (7). These procedures have been well established for bacteria, less so for fungi, and poorly developed for other infectious agents. These in vitro studies can serve as powerful surrogates for anti-infective action, as they provide potential targets for the anti-infective concentrations that must be achieved in vivo in order to ensure an optimal therapeutic response (14). Susceptibility to the antibacterial effects of

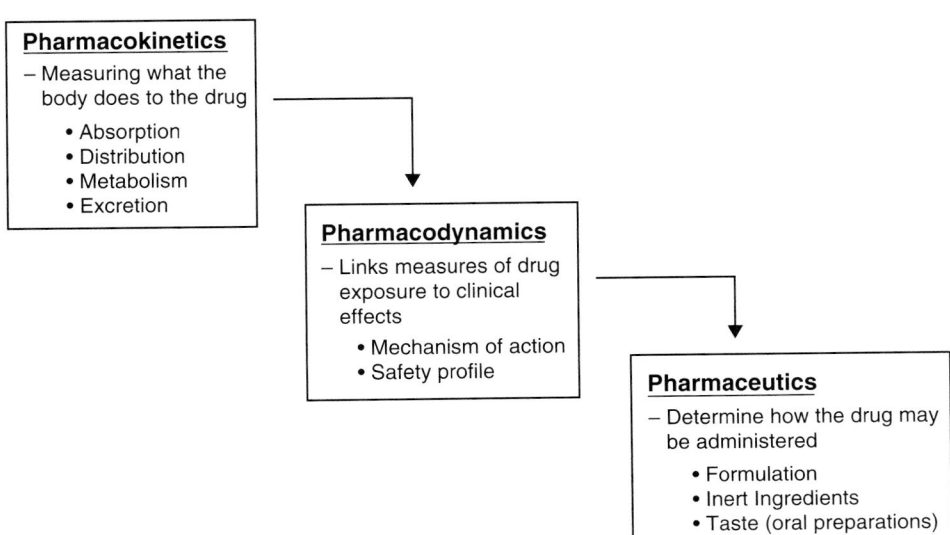

FIGURE 77.1. Determinants of effective anti-infective therapy.

TABLE 77.2

EXAMPLES OF CLINICALLY IMPORTANT UNUSUAL SIDE EFFECTS ASSOCIATED WITH ANTI-INFECTIVE AGENTS

Drug(s)	Adverse event
Aminoglycosides	Apnea; respiratory depression
Thiomethyltetrazole-containing cephalosporins	Hypoprothrombinemia
Carboxypenicillins and acylureidopenicillins	Inhibition of platelet aggregation
Metronidazole	Peripheral neuropathy
Amphotericin	Hyponatremia
Amphotericin	Anemia
Ceftriaxone	Biliary sludge/colic
Carboxy- and acylureidopenicillins	Exacerbation of CHF
Vancomycin	Hypotension 2° histamine release
Ganciclovir, acyclovir	Crystalluria
Sulfonamides, voriconazole	Stevens-Johnson syndrome
Chloramphenicol	Cardiogenic shock
Azoles	Liver failure
Acyclovir	Neutropenia

antibiotics is usually assessed by determining the minimal concentration of drug required to inhibit bacterial growth, termed the *minimum inhibitory concentration*, or MIC. MIC values provide some indication of the potency of the antibiotic against the infecting bacterial pathogen. As such, these values reflect the pharmacodynamic correlates of antibiotic effectiveness. Nevertheless, they must be interpreted with some caution. Hospital microbiology laboratories routinely provide an interpretation of the MIC value, indicating that the infecting organism is either "susceptible" or "resistant" to the anti-infective in question. These interpretations reflect only whether the antibiotic concentration, with routine, nontoxic dosing, exceeds the MIC in the blood compartment. If infection is identified in a compartment poorly penetrated by the antibiotic, the concentrations in the infected space may not exceed the MIC, and the interpretation rendered by in vitro susceptibility testing can be misleading.

The other dimension of pharmacodynamics deals with the safety profiles of the various anti-infective agents. Overall, toxicity has rarely limited the treatment of pediatric patients with these agents. Most of the anti-infective drugs employed in children were either synthesized or adopted for use, with the principle of selective toxicity as a guiding premise; that is, they were designed to injure invading organisms with little, if any, injury to the host cells. Consequently, very few side effects of significance have been reported. For those that do occur, it is essential to understand that they exist and to create an effective monitoring plan that is likely to identify problems at an early stage. Although anti-infective adverse events remain rare, in critically ill infants and children, some of the more unusual side effects of these drugs can assume enormous clinical importance (Table 77.2).

Pharmaceutics deals with the formulation of the drug actually administered to the patient. In the PICU, this most often refers to an agent that is administered by IV injection or infusion. Knowledge of any counter ions present, any excipients used as diluents or solubilizing agents, the concentration of the active moiety in the solution, its ability to be further diluted or concentrated, and the compatibility of the anti-infective with other parenteral agents that must be administered through the same IV line are significant considerations. For some drugs, enteral administration is essential, and emerging experience suggests that it can be accomplished effectively in most critically ill patients.

APPLICATION OF THE PHARMACOKINETIC-PHARMACODYNAMIC INTERFACE TO ANTIBIOTIC THERAPEUTICS

Contrary to usual practice, effective antibiotic treatment requires more than simply matching a drug with a microorganism (29). The key is the integration of the unique disposition characteristics of the drug selected in the individual patient (i.e., pharmacokinetics) with an understanding of the determinants of clinical activity of a drug already known to be effective in vitro (i.e., pharmacodynamics) (Table 77.3). Four crucial issues must be considered: (a) the expected variability in response when the same dose of drug (normalized to body weight) is administered to all patients, (b) the pharmacodynamic variables that are linked to microbiologic effect, (c) the amount of free fraction of drug that reaches the site of infection, and (d) the overarching effect of resistance (12,13).

Variability in Response to the Same Dose

When the pharmacokinetics of antibiotics is studied in healthy infants and children, given a fixed weight-adjusted dose, the results are always characterized by large interindividual variations in key pharmacokinetic parameter estimates, such as apparent volume of distribution, area under the plasma

TABLE 77.3

THE IDEAL ANTI-INFECTIVE AGENT FOR CRITICALLY ILL INFANTS AND CHILDREN

Selective and effective in its anti-infective activity
Capable of tissue penetration in concentrations that exceed by several fold the amount required to kill the infecting pathogen
High affinity for site of action
Resistant to inactivation of microbial enzymes, tissue fluids, or products of inflammation
Must not readily stimulate microbial resistance
Long elimination half-life
Devoid of drug-drug interactions
Absence of major organ system toxicity
Absence of developmental or behavioral toxicity
Formulated to administer in a manner commensurate with its mode of action (e.g., time >MIC; AUC/MIC, etc.)

MIC, minimum inhibitory concentration; AUC, area under the plasma concentration-versus-time curve

concentration-versus-time curve (AUC), and clearance. These interindividual variations, in turn, result in wide ranges in elimination half-life ($t_{1/2}$) and maximum and minimum plasma concentrations (C_{max} and C_{min}). The variability seen in these relatively healthy patients without end-organ dysfunction can often exceed tenfold. Thus, at a given dose of antibiotic, it is likely that a population of children exists for whom either the peak concentration is too low or the time that the effective concentration remains above the MIC for the suspected or documented pathogen is too short. In each case, in the absence of actually monitoring drug concentrations, a built-in failure rate appears to be associated with the use of "standard" dosing regimens. In clinical practice, failure occurs less frequently than one would predict solely on a pharmacokinetic basis because of the powerful impact of the innate immune mechanisms that augment the activity of the drugs employed.

In the PICU, these effects are amplified further. The changes in body water compartments that accompany serious illness and injury can markedly affect the volume of distribution for many antibiotics and may be influenced further by local inflammatory changes (e.g., bacterial meningitis) that can transiently alter the access of antibiotics to certain sanctuary sites within the body. Antibiotic clearance is dependent largely upon hepatic and renal function. The extent to which these are affected by the patient's underlying disease may profoundly affect the in vivo antibiotic exposure. Lastly, innate immunity is often impaired in the critically ill.

Pharmacodynamic Variables that are Linked to Microbiologic Effect

Inherent to the study of pharmacology is the dose-response relationship. It is generally anticipated that the pharmacologic effect will increase in proportion to the dose administered. Contrary to these expectations, antibiotic activity is subject to certain pharmacodynamic subtleties that modulate these predictions. The antibiotics in use currently sort themselves into two mechanistically distinct groups based upon their pharmacologic interactions with bacteria; they are either *time-dependent* or *concentration-dependent* killers. The activity of the first group is determined by the time that the antibiotic concentration at the site of the infection exceeds the MIC for the infecting bacteria (denoted T>MIC). For the second group, the functional activity is driven by the relationship between the concentration achieved at the site of the infection relative and the MIC (**Table 77.4**).

The first evidence of time-dependent killing was noted as early as the late 1940s and early 1950s, when Eagle et al. demonstrated that, in treating streptococcal pharyngitis, clinical efficacy was determined by the amount of time the concentration of penicillin exceeded the MIC for the group A streptococcus. Moreover, once the drug concentration exceeded the MIC by four- to sixfold, increasing the dose resulted in no greater clinical benefit. It is now clear that for all β-lactam

TABLE 77.4

MODE OF ANTIBACTERIAL ACTION: THE PHARMACOKINETIC-PHARMACODYNAMIC INTERFACE

Drug class	Mode of bacterial killing	Pharmacodynamic determinant
β-Lactams Linezolid Macrolides Clindamycin	Time-dependent	T>MIC
Aminoglycosides Fluoroquinolones Metronidazole	Concentration-dependent	C_{max}/MIC
Fluoroquinolones Glycopeptides Azithromycin	Concentration-/time-dependent	AUC/MIC

MIC, minimum inhibitory concentration; AUC, area under the plasma concentration-versus-time curve

TABLE 77.5

OPTIMAL TIME > MINIMUM INHIBITORY CONCENTRATION FOR VARIOUS β-LACTAM ANTIBIOTICS

	Stasis	Lysis
	% of Dosing interval	
Penicillins	30–40	60–70
Cephalosporins	30	50
Carbapenems	20	40

antibiotics, clinical efficacy correlates with T>MIC. Importantly, it has also been established that the concentration of free drug did not have to remain above the MIC for the entire dosing interval (7). In fact, to achieve the maximal antimicrobial effect, the various members of the β-lactam family needed to be above the MIC for different fractions of the dosing interval (Table 77.5).

The time dependence of β-lactam antibiotic killing is rooted in the origin of their antimicrobial effects through acylation of their molecular target, the penicillin-binding proteins (PBPs). Studies have demonstrated that the inhibition of peptidoglycan synthesis caused by this acylation process occurs only after most of the available sites have been covalently modified, a phenomenon that is achieved with concentrations of drug only slightly above the MIC. Hence, further increases in drug concentration do not result in greater killing. Moreover, a delay occurs between the times when maximal acylation is achieved and when bacterial stasis occurs, accounting for the requirement that drug be present in the infected space over an extended time to achieve its antibacterial effect.

For drugs such as the aminoglycosides, fluoroquinolones, azithromycin, and vancomycin, the concentration that reaches the site of infection appears to drive clinical efficacy. In some instances, killing correlates best with C_{max}/MIC (e.g., the aminoglycosides), whereas in others (e.g., the fluoroquinolones and azithromycin), effect is more strongly correlated to AUC/MIC. Common to all concentration-dependent antibiotics is that they are relatively slowly bactericidal but have a persistently suppressive effect on bacterial growth, even when the drug concentration falls below the MIC. The latter is termed a *postantibiotic effect*. Increasing the AUC/MIC ratio, a state functionally achieved by increasing the dose, can increase the apparent duration of the postantibiotic effect.

The Amount of Free Fraction of Drug

For both time-dependent and concentration-dependent antibiotics, it is the free form of the drug that is active. Protein binding to albumin is not a major determinant of drug action until it exceeds 90% of the total drug. Ceftriaxone, a commonly used third-generation cephalosporin, is a time-dependent killer that is >90% protein bound. The free drug concentration at the site of infection is low but adequate in most cases because of its potency. However, infections caused by organisms such as *S. aureus* and strains of *S. pneumoniae* that have decreased susceptibility to penicillin may not respond clinically, as predicted

by in vitro susceptibility testing, because of this pharmacokinetic characteristic. Similarly, the aminoglycoside antibiotics are potent agents against Gram-negative nonfermenting bacteria and are the quintessential concentration-dependent killers. Nevertheless, these drugs have proven to be inadequate as monotherapy for Gram-negative pneumonia because they bind avidly to cell debris and the free DNA that is released from dying neutrophils.

The Overarching Effect of Resistance

The fourth principle that emerges directly from existing experimental and clinical data relates to the dependence of each of the modes of antibiotic action on the MIC of the infecting pathogen. Antibiotic resistance poses a constant threat to effective therapy. Changes in antibiotic susceptibility patterns, particularly common in organisms associated with nosocomially acquired bacteria in the ICU, may crucially influence both the choice of antibiotic and the dose employed. As the MIC increases, the duration of time that the drug concentration at the site of infection remains above that MIC is shortened, and the ratios of the C_{max}/MIC and AUC/MIC are diminished. The end result is an adverse impact on clinical efficacy.

ANTIBACTERIAL AGENTS

The antibacterial drugs revolutionized medicine in the 20th century. Within several decades, agents were discovered that could safely and effectively eradicate virtually every bacterium with human pathogenic potential. The principles that underlie the use of the families of antibacterial drugs with the greatest utility in the PICU are described here (2).

The β-Lactams

The β-lactams are among the most useful drugs available to the clinician who cares for children. In general, these agents are bactericidal and have an excellent record for safety. As a result, they are often the first choice for empiric therapy of both hospital- and community-acquired infections. β-lactam antimicrobial agents include the penicillins, cephalosporins, carbapenems, and monobactams. All have a β-lactam ring, with variable rings and side chains. When bacteria develop resistance to β-lactam antibiotics, it is most often due to their ability to elaborate a β-lactamase enzyme that is able to cleave the β-lactam ring. β-lactamase-stable β-lactams appear to protect the β-lactam ring through the configuration of the side chain at the 6 position of the penicillins and the 7 position of the cephalosporins.

The ring structure defines the family of the agent. The penicillins, for example, contain a thiazolidine ring attached to the β-lactam ring; the cephalosporins contain a dihydrothiazine ring attached to the β-lactam ring. The nature of the side chains added to the ring structure is responsible for both the antibacterial spectrum of the compound and its pharmacokinetic properties.

The Penicillins

Spectrum of Activity

The introduction of penicillins into clinical practice began with the serendipitous observation by Fleming in 1928 that the mold, *Penicillium chrysogenum*, produced a substance (dubbed penicillin because of its origin) that inhibited the growth of *S. aureus* in culture. In 1939, Florey, Chain, and associates at Oxford began a concerted effort to extract, purify, and synthesize penicillin from broth cultures of the mold. The early crude materials were found to have a remarkable spectrum of antimicrobial activity and a low order of toxicity. None of the components was found to be superior to the benzylpenicillin that was designated penicillin G.

The precise mechanism responsible for the bactericidal effect of the penicillins is unknown. The notion that they simply inhibit the final steps in peptidoglycan cross-linking in the bacterial cell wall is clearly overly simplistic. Cell wall assembly in bacteria requires at least 30 steps. Some of the enzyme activities involved in this cell wall synthesis are found in a group of proteins called *penicillin-binding proteins*. Different classes of penicillins interact with different PBP groups. These interactions tend to be covalent and, in some bacterial species, are thought to unleash bacterial autolysins, which actually cause cell death.

The emergence of penicillin resistance among *S. aureus* due to elaboration of an enzyme that cleaved the β-lactam bond, a penicillinase, stimulated the development of the penicillinase-resistant penicillins (e.g., methicillin). The clinical efficacy of the natural penicillins in the treatment of Gram-positive infections resulted in the emergence of certain Gram-negative rods as important human pathogens, which led to the development of the aminopenicillins (e.g., ampicillin). These drugs retained all of the Gram-positive activity of the natural penicillins and, at the same time, were effective against enterococci and selected Gram-negative rods, but they remained susceptible to inactivation by bacterial β-lactamases. About the time that the aminopenicillins became widely used in the late 1960s, *Pseudomonas. aeruginosa* emerged as an important hospital-acquired pathogen. These observations stimulated the synthesis and introduction of the antipseudomonal penicillins (e.g., ticarcillin) into clinical practice. In essence, these drugs were aminopenicillins with anti-pseudomonal activity. They do have some additional enhanced Gram-negative activity but sacrifice some of the Gram-positive potency of the natural penicillins. The quest for broader-spectrum drugs led to further structural modifications in the penicillin nucleus. These produced the extended spectrum penicillins (e.g., piperacillin), which are drugs that retain the Gram-positive potency of the natural penicillins while providing adequate coverage for a broad spectrum of Gram-negative pathogens, including all of those covered by the amino- and anti-pseudomonal penicillins, as well as *Klebsiella* spp., *Acinetobacter*, *Morganella*, *Providencia*, and *Enterobacter* spp.

During the 1970s, it became apparent that, as each new penicillin was introduced, bacterial strains rapidly acquired β-lactamases with the ability to hydrolyze them; this was especially a problem among Gram-negative bacteria. A different strategy was adopted to address this problem. A group of β-lactam compounds, many of which were devoid of antibacterial activity, was synthesized as β-lactamase inhibitors (e.g., clavulanic acid). It was found that these could be combined with β-lactam antibiotics, resulting in a combination that was therapeutically active against β-lactamase-producing organisms.

Metabolism and Disposition

The penicillins vary markedly in biodisposition from drug to drug. Those used in the PICU are not well absorbed from the gastrointestinal tract; therefore, for most infections, they are administered parenterally. Protein binding varies markedly from a low of ~17% for ampicillin to >90% for nafcillin. Few of these drugs undergo any significant metabolism, although some, including ampicillin, nafcillin, ticarcillin, mezlocillin, and piperacillin, display significant hepatic elimination. However, most excretion is via the kidney, which employs processes of both filtration and tubular secretion. Because the elimination of the penicillins is mainly renal, significant developmental changes occur in elimination half-life during the first year of life. In addition, disease-associated alterations in renal function necessitate dosing modifications. Virtually all of the parenteral penicillins penetrate into the cerebrospinal fluid (CSF) in concentrations that are adequate to treat meningitis when a meningeal inflammation is present. In the absence of inflammation, very little penetration occurs.

The penicillins have short elimination half-lives. As with all β-lactam antibiotics, the drug concentrations must remain above the MIC for the infecting organism in order for the drug to be effective. Therefore, parenteral penicillins must be administered on a very frequent basis, usually every 4 hrs or by prolonged infusions (e.g., 2–3 hrs) for serious infections.

Adverse Effects

Adverse events occur very rarely but can be extremely varied in their presentation. The major toxic effects associated with the penicillins are allergic reactions. The mechanisms responsible for these allergic reactions relate to the ability of penicillins to act as haptens and combine with proteins. The most important antigenic component of the penicillins is the penicilloyl determinant, which is produced by opening the β-lactam ring, permitting amide linkage to proteins. Other breakdown products include the penicillanic acid derivatives that form in solution at high temperature or low pH. Finally, a number of minor determinants, including benzyl penicillin itself, can act as sensitizing agents or elicit major allergic reactions themselves. Anaphylactic reactions to penicillin occur in 0.2% of courses of treatment, with death resulting in 0.001%. It is often possible to substitute other β-lactam agents for a penicillin with minimal risk of cross-reactivity.

Other adverse events are rare and include alterations in platelet function by carbenicillin and ticarcillin; interstitial nephritis, noted especially with the penicillinase-resistant antistaphylococcal penicillins; hypokalemia and platelet functional impairment seen with the antipseudomonal and extended spectrum penicillins; and bone marrow suppression, particularly neutropenia, observed with prolonged use of virtually all of the penicillins.

Drug Interactions

Few drug-drug interactions of clinical significance are reported with the penicillins. The only one of note is that with probenecid, which competes with the penicillins for renal tubular secretion. This interaction is employed clinically to prolong the elimination half-life of penicillin or ampicillin when it is used to treat certain sexually transmitted diseases. The antipseudomonal penicillins and, to some extent, the extended-spectrum penicillins, have been shown to interact in solution with the aminoglycosides, causing degradation of the latter. This interaction is seen when the two are mixed in the same infusion solution for administration or in vivo in the face of renal failure.

The Cephalosporins

Spectrum of Activity

Immediately following World War II, the search intensified for active broad-spectrum antibiotics. In Italy, Professor Guiseppi Brotzu began a search for antibiotic-producing microorganisms, and the result of his efforts was the isolation of the fungus *Cephalosporanium acremonium* from the sewage extruded from an outlet into the sea near Kaglara, Sardinia. Crude filtrates of these fungal cultures were found to inhibit the growth of a variety of Gram-positive and Gram-negative bacteria. Cephalosporin C, one of the originally isolated compounds, underwent acid hydrolysis to 7-aminocephalosporanic acid, which has served as the starting material for the synthesis of four generations of cephalosporin antibiotics.

As with the penicillins, the precise mechanism of action of the cephalosporins is unknown. These agents bind to and inactivate specific PBPs, inhibiting the final synthetic steps of the bacterial cell wall. Various cephalosporins have differing affinities for the various PBPs, and the particular PBPs that are inactivated by the cephalosporin that determine the actual toxic effect on the bacterium.

The antibacterial activity of the various cephalosporins depends largely on their generation of origin. Unlike the natural penicillins, the first-generation cephalosporins are active against both Gram-positive and Gram-negative bacteria, as well as being acid stable and resistant to β-lactamase hydrolysis by the early β-lactamases. The activity of these agents against Gram-negative rods is somewhat variable. They are most commonly used for surgical prophylaxis and skin and orthopedic infections. Members of this generation include cephalothin and cephalexin.

The second-generation cephalosporins, such as cefuroxime and cefprozil, were synthesized to broaden coverage against respiratory pathogens and to provide some additional Gram-negative activity. For infections of the respiratory tract, they possess therapeutic activity against *S. pneumoniae, Streptococcus pyogenes, Haemophilus influenzae,* and *Moraxella catarrhalis.* For the latter two organisms, they provide adequate coverage whether or not the organism is a β-lactamase producer. In addition, they are active against *S. aureus* in the treatment of skin and skin-structure infections and reliable against *Escherichia coli* for urinary tract infections.

Around the same time that the second-generation cephalosporins were being developed, the cephamycin group of antibiotics was isolated from certain streptomyces species. These drugs are structurally similar to the cephalosporins but contain a methoxy group at the 7 position of the β-lactam ring. This group includes the drugs cefoxitin and cefotetan, which are generally less potent than the second-generation cephalosporins against respiratory pathogens but have clinically significant anaerobic activity.

The search for broader-spectrum antibiotics in the mid 1970s and early 1980s resulted in the synthesis of a group of parenteral third-generation cephalosporins, including ceftriaxone, cefotaxime, and ceftazidime. These have become among the most widely used drugs for the empiric treatment of infants and children with moderate-to-severe infections. They have greatly improved activity against Gram-negative organisms. Unfortunately, with the increased Gram-negative spectrum and potency, these agents have less Gram-positive potency than the first-generation cephalosporins. Nevertheless, they are clinically effective in treating most infections due to susceptible Gram-positive organisms. The exception is ceftazidime, which is the only member of the group with activity against *Pseudomonas* and has only marginal activity against Gram-positive pathogens.

Cefepime is the most widely available of the fourth-generation cephalosporins in the US. It has the Gram-positive potency of a first-generation cephalosporin and the Gram-negative spectrum of a third-generation cephalosporin, including *P. aeruginosa.* It is stable in the presence of many broad-spectrum β-lactamases active against the third-generation cephalosporins.

As the cephalosporins gain wider acceptance and use in pediatrics, it is important to remember that a number of organisms exist for which the cephalosporins currently available do not have reliable activity, most notably enterococci, MRSA, coagulase-negative staphylococci, and *Listeria monocytogenes.* However, newer agents under development will provide coverage for most of these pathogens.

Metabolism and Disposition

The cephalosporins vary markedly in biodisposition with patient age. They demonstrate varying degrees of protein binding, ranging from ~10% for cefazolin to >90% for ceftriaxone. The latter displays rather unique protein-binding characteristics. In addition to conferring a long elimination half-life, its binding shows saturation when the drug is administered in its usual therapeutic doses. Therefore, by administering ceftriaxone as a single daily dose, an initial bolus of free drug distributes rapidly to tissues due to the saturation of the protein-binding sites, followed by a continual release of active drug from bound reservoirs over 24 hrs. Of the four generations of cephalosporins, only the drugs in the third and fourth generations penetrate into the CSF reliably so that they can be used to treat bacterial meningitis.

Few of the cephalosporins undergo any significant metabolism. Several of those in the third generation have sufficient biliary excretion to make them useful in the treatment of hepatobiliary infections. Most excretion, however, is renal via glomerular filtration. Because the elimination of the cephalosporins is mainly renal, significant developmental changes occur in elimination half-life during the first year of life. Disease-associated alterations in renal function necessitate dosing modifications. In addition, because of its high degree of protein binding and related concerns about bilirubin displacement, ceftriaxone is not recommended for the treatment of infants in the first month of life.

Adverse Effects

The cephalosporins are the safest class of antibiotics and perhaps the safest class of drugs available in medicine today. Virtually no cephalosporin side effects occur in >7% of patients who receive the drugs, and they are even less frequent in infants and children. Gastrointestinal side effects are most common. Allergic reactions also occur but are not as frequent as those seen with the penicillins. The cross-reactivity of cephalosporins in patients with documented penicillin allergy is somewhat higher than in the general population. When cephalosporins were given to patients in whom penicillin allergy was documented by skin testing, only 1 of 99 developed a clinically significant reaction.

Other adverse reactions that have been associated with cephalosporins include positive Coombs reactions, bone marrow suppression, thrombocytosis, acute tubular necrosis, and mild transaminase elevations; these are all rare. Ceftriaxone has been associated with the formation of biliary sludge in the gallbladder, which, in some critically ill patients, may lead to signs and symptoms of cholecystitis. Finally, the cephalosporins that contain the thiomethyltetrazole ring (e.g., cefoperazone and cefotetan) have been implicated in bleeding due to hypoprothrombinemia.

Drug Interactions

Few drug-drug interactions of any significance have been reported with the cephalosporins.

Clinical Indications

The cephalosporins are the drugs of choice for the empiric treatment of infants and children with moderate-to-severe infections. In the newborn period, ampicillin plus cefotaxime has become a standard regimen for the treatment of infants with suspected sepsis and/or meningitis. Ceftriaxone has become the standard therapeutic intervention for such children admitted to the hospital beyond the first month of life. Ceftazidime and cefepime have become standard agents for empiric therapy in critically ill children, those with fever and neutropenia, and those with nosocomially acquired infections in the ICU.

The Monobactams: Aztreonam

Spectrum of Activity

Aztreonam is currently the only member of the monocyclic β-lactam antibiotic family that is referred to as *monobactams*. The drug interferes with bacterial cell wall synthesis in a manner similar to other β-lactam antibiotics, binding to PBP3. The spectrum of antibacterial activity of aztreonam is limited to aerobic Gram-negative bacteria. Thus, it resembles the aminoglycoside antibiotics in its activity.

Metabolism and Disposition

Aztreonam is administered parenterally by intramuscular (100% bioavailable) or IV administration. It is well distributed into most body fluids and tissues, including achieving effective antibacterial concentrations in the CSF of patients with bacterial meningitis. Approximately 30%–50% of the drug is bound to plasma protein. Aztreonam is eliminated from the body by both hepatic and renal mechanisms. Approximately 70% of an administered dose is excreted unchanged in the urine.

Clinical Indications

Aztreonam is not at this writing considered first-line therapy for any infections in pediatric patients. Nevertheless, it may have a role in situations in which an aminoglycoside antibiotic is indicated and the patient has impaired renal function or is concurrently receiving other potentially nephrotoxic agents.

Adverse Effects

Adverse effects associated with aztreonam use are similar to those described after the administration of other β-lactams. The drug is weakly immunogenic and does not precipitate allergic reactions in patients allergic to penicillin.

Carbapenems

Spectrum of Activity

The carbapenem antibiotics were discovered in the 1970s during a systematic screening program for β-lactamase inhibitors. The first carbapenems, the olivanic acids, were identified as part of the research program that yielded the discovery of clavulanic acid. Almost simultaneously, another research group discovered thienamycin from *Streptomyces cattleya*. A derivative of thienamycin, imipenem is available for clinical use in the US. Subsequently, two other agents were approved in the US, meropenem and ertapenem.

Imipenem, the prototype carbapenem, binds to all of the PBPs but possesses greatest affinity for PBP1 and PBP2. These drugs possess a broad spectrum of antibacterial activity against aerobic and anaerobic Gram-positive and Gram-negative pathogens. As such, they arguably are among the broadest antibacterial agents currently available. The carbapenems are highly resistant to degradation by both plasmid and chromosomally mediated β-lactamases, although bacteria expressing carbapenemases have emerged. *Pseudomonas* spp., in particular, may acquire resistance to the carbapenems through multiple mutations after sustained exposure to the drug, and *Stenotrophomonas* isolates usually are intrinsically resistant.

Metabolism and Disposition

None of the currently available carbapenems are absorbed after oral administration, and they are available only for parenteral administration. Like other β-lactam antibiotics, these drugs are well distributed in most body fluids and tissues, including the central nervous system (CNS) in patients with meningitis. Approximately 20% of imipenem and meropenem are bound to plasma proteins, while ertapenem is highly and saturably protein bound. Imipenem and meropenem are excreted by the kidney primarily by glomerular filtration. Unlike meropenem and ertapenem, imipenem is efficiently degraded by a proximal tubular brush border enzyme, dehydropeptidase I, resulting in urinary concentrations that are ineffective in treating serious urinary tract infections. Thus, for clinical use, imipenem is administered along with a competitive inhibitor of dehydropeptidase I, cilastatin. Meropenem and ertapenem are resistant to degradation by the dehydropeptidase enzyme.

Adverse Effects

The adverse effect profile of carbapenems is similar to other β-lactam antibiotics. Additionally, seizures have been reported in some patients with reduced renal function who are receiving high-dose therapy with imipenem. Patients with an underlying seizure disorder should receive carbapenems with caution. The overall incidence of these effects with meropenem is the same or somewhat lower than that seen with imipenem/cilastatin, and seizures have been rarely reported with ertapenem.

Drug Interactions

None identified.

Clinical Indications

The carbapenems are very broad-spectrum agents that provide rational and effective empiric antimicrobial coverage in most clinical situations. While they have been demonstrated to be safe and effective in pediatric patients with community-acquired respiratory tract infections, skin and soft tissue infections, uncomplicated urinary tract infections, and intra-abdominal infections, the real strength of these agents is in the treatment of serious infections in hospitalized patients. As such, they offer a therapeutic alternative for the treatment of Gram-negative bacterial sepsis in the immunocompromised patient, the treatment of nosocomial infections in critically ill children, and in the treatment of patients who have failed therapy with other broad-spectrum antibiotics or antibiotic combinations. The one exception is the lack of antipseudomonal coverage by ertapenem.

Resistance to β-lactams

Resistance to the β-lactams is a frequent and important problem in the critically ill child with serious infection and is mediated by one of two principal mechanisms: the production of β-lactamase enzymes capable of hydrolyzing the β-lactam ring and alteration of the target bacterial molecules, namely, the PBPs.

The β-lactamases constitute a broad array of enzymes expressed in both Gram-positive and Gram-negative bacteria. In the former, the enzyme is secreted into the cell-free environment, while in the latter, most enzyme is concentrated in the periplasmic space between the cell wall and the outer membrane. Hundreds of β-lactamases have been characterized, and no doubt many more exist. They have been variously categorized according to substrate preference, isoelectric focus, whether they are encoded on the bacterial chromosome or an episome, according to their ability to be inhibited by clavulanate, and according to their molecular structure. Two groups of β-lactamases are important for the pediatric intensivist. The Group 1 enzymes (also referred to as "AmpC" β-lactamases) hydrolyze virtually all β-lactam antibiotics except the carbapenems and are resistant to inhibition by clavulanate. These enzymes are chromosomally encoded on a sequence labeled *ampC* in *P. aeruginosa*, *Enterobacter cloacae*, *Serratia marcescens*, *Citrobacter freundii*, and *Morganella morganii*. Spontaneous mutations in the bacterial genome, producing so-called "de-repressed" mutant strains, can result in constitutive, large-quantity production of the AmpC β-lactamase. The Group 2 β-lactamases include a wide variety of enzymes that are primarily encoded on plasmids, which also commonly contain resistance determinants to other antibiotic classes. The Group 2 enzymes include the extended spectrum β-lactamases, which have become particularly problematic in both pediatric and adult ICUs and are especially prevalent in *Klebsiella* and *E. coli*. Both Group 1 and 2 β-lactamases are promoted by, and resistant to, the third-generation cephalosporins, and organisms expressing them are most reliably treated with a carbapenem.

Three organisms important in the PICU express β-lactam resistance based upon the alteration of PBPs: penicillin-resistant *S. pneumoniae*, MRSA, and most hospital-acquired coagulase-negative staphylococci. In both penicillin-resistant *S. pneumoniae* and MRSA, the molecular events that lead to the expression of PBPs with low affinity for the β-lactam drugs are rare. Consequently, most isolates are derived from finite groups of internationally disseminated clones. In penicillin-resistant pneumococcus, many strains are only mildly resistant to β-lactams, and cure can be achieved with high doses of β-lactam plus, in the case of meningitis, the addition of vancomycin. The β-lactam resistance in MRSA and coagulase-negative staphylococci is high grade and must be treated with an alternative class of drug.

The Aminoglycoside Antibiotics

Spectrum of Activity

The aminoglycosides available for clinical use in the US include amikacin, gentamicin, kanamycin, neomycin, netilmicin, streptomycin, and tobramycin. Streptomycin was the first aminoglycoside antibiotic discovered, isolated in 1944 from the soil actinomycetes *Streptomyces griseus*. The discovery of streptomycin launched three decades of investigative endeavors that yielded neomycin, kanamycin, gentamicin, and tobramycin. Gentamicin and netilmicin are both derived from species of the *Micromonospora*, which accounts for the difference in the spelling of their names (e.g., "micin") as compared with other available agents derived from *Streptomyces* (which are spelled as "mycin"). In 1972, a semisynthetic derivative of kanamycin—amikacin—was introduced that represented the first attempt to design an aminoglycoside that was resistant to inactivation by bacterial enzymes known to metabolize aminoglycosides.

The aminoglycoside antibiotics inhibit bacterial protein synthesis by irreversibly binding primarily to the 30S ribosomal subunit. Some agents, including gentamicin, kanamycin, and tobramycin, bind to multiple sites on both ribosomal subunits. The aminoglycosides are bactericidal against most aerobic Gram-negative bacilli. Cellular uptake of an aminoglycoside is an oxygen-dependent, active transport process; thus, anaerobic bacteria are universally resistant. While not clinically useful when used alone against Gram-positive bacteria, aminoglycosides exhibit synergistic activity with other antimicrobial agents against staphylococci, streptococci, and enterococci.

Bacterial resistance to newer aminoglycoside antibiotics is uncommon despite their extensive clinical use. Bacterial enzymes capable of inactivating aminoglycosides by acetylation, adenylation, or phosphorylation are the most common mechanisms of bacterial resistance to an aminoglycoside. The genes encoding these inactivating enzymes are transferred on plasmids. The most stable aminoglycoside against the effects of these inactivating enzymes is amikacin, followed by tobramycin and gentamicin.

Metabolism and Disposition

After oral administration, the aminoglycoside antibiotics are poorly absorbed into systemic circulation. Thus, for the treatment of systemic infections, these drugs must be administered either intramuscularly or intravenously. The aminoglycosides are not metabolized by the body and are excreted completely unchanged by the kidney via glomerular filtration. Hepatic disease does not interfere with the elimination of aminoglycosides whereas renal dysfunction will directly influence the aminoglycoside clearance. As the aminoglycosides do not cross the blood-brain barrier well, concentrations in the CSF are low and variable. Aminoglycosides should, therefore, not be used as single agents to treat meningitis.

Serum drug concentrations have often been suggested as objective parameters to direct aminoglycoside dosing when combined with improvement in physical exam and bacterial cultures. However, the identification of "therapeutic" concentration ranges for aminoglycoside antibiotics is based on limited numbers of patients, and the majority of studies involved adult subjects only. As a result, the true relationship between serum aminoglycoside concentration and clinical outcome is questionable.

Adverse Effects

The most commonly recognized adverse effects associated with aminoglycoside administration are ototoxicity and nephrotoxicity. The incidence of these adverse events in children is unknown. In adult patients, the incidence of ototoxicity has been estimated to range from 2% to as high as 25%, depending upon the patient population studied, method employed to determine eighth nerve function, and specific aminoglycoside administered. The incidence of ototoxicity with the use of newer agents (e.g., gentamicin, tobramycin, amikacin) approximates 2%. Animal and human studies have demonstrated aminoglycoside accumulation in the perilymph and endolymph of the inner ear. Hearing impairment results from the progressive destruction of vestibular or cochlear sensory hair cells, which are very aminoglycoside sensitive.

Aminoglycoside associated nephrotoxicity has been reported to occur in ~8%–26% of patients who receive these drugs. The mechanism responsible for this nephrotoxicity appears to result from proximal tubular necrosis causing subsequent compromise in glomerular function. Most cases of nephrotoxicity are reversible, reflecting the regenerative capacity of the primary cellular target.

Allergic reactions, including rash, fever, and eosinophilia, are uncommon and occur in ~1%–3% of patients who receive an aminoglycoside. Aminoglycoside-associated neuromuscular blockade causing weakness of skeletal muscles is a very uncommon adverse reaction but may precipitate respiratory depression. The exact mechanism responsible for this adverse effect is unknown, but may be due to competitive antagonism of acetylcholine activity at the neuromuscular junction. Patients at particular risk to experience aminoglycoside-induced neuromuscular blockade include those with myasthenia gravis, severe hypocalcemia, or infantile botulism, or those who have recently received neuromuscular-blocking agents. IV infusion of a calcium salt (e.g., $CaCl_2$) will successfully antagonize this adverse drug effect.

Drug Interactions

Clinically significant drug-drug interactions with aminoglycoside antibiotics are rare. The most commonly implicated compounds involve those that possess some inherent propensity to induce ototoxicity or nephrotoxicity.

Clinical Indications

The aminoglycoside agents are used predominately to treat serious infections by aerobic Gram-negative bacilli, including those caused by more resistant organisms, such as *Pseudomonas spp.* Because of their significant toxicities, aminoglycosides are used frequently as initial therapy and are discontinued after a clinical response is obtained or when a safer class of drugs is identified to treat the infection. However, continuing aminoglycoside use along with a β-lactam antibiotic is common practice in treating severe infections or highly resistant organisms. This practice is based on the premise that combination therapy for Gram-negative bacilli provides synergy and, theoretically, a better outcome. Clinical evidence for this is best for infections due to *P. aeruginosa.* Data with this organism in the immunocompromised host show a better survival and cure rate in patients who are treated with an aminoglycoside and an antipseudomonal β-lactam. Another argument for two-drug therapy is the possibility that induction of resistance is less likely to occur when an aminoglycoside is used with the β-lactam agent. Evidence that both supports and refutes this contention exists.

Aminoglycosides also are indicated in the treatment of serious enterococcal infections. While not susceptible to the aminoglycosides alone, many enterococci are killed synergistically when an aminoglycoside is added to penicillin or ampicillin. The levels of aminoglycoside necessary to produce synergy may not be as high as those required when the drugs are used alone to treat Gram-negative infections. The specific isolate should be tested in vitro for high-level aminoglycoside resistance as an indicator of the likelihood that synergy will occur. Synergy between an aminoglycoside and a β-lactam or glycopeptide drug can also be exploited in the treatment of serious infections due to other Gram-positive organisms, including viridans streptococci, group B streptococci, *S. aureus*, and coagulase-negative staphylococci. In these circumstances, the aminoglycoside may be employed early, until clinical stability is achieved, and then discontinued.

Glycopeptides and Other Antibiotics for Gram-positive Bacteria

Spectrum of Activity

Vancomycin, the prototype glycopeptide antibiotic, was discovered as part of a coordinated search for drugs effective against penicillin-resistant staphylococci. In the early 1950s, a missionary walking along a jungle path in Borneo collected a soil sample and forwarded it to a friend at Lilly Research Laboratories. This soil sample was found to contain *Streptomyces orientalis*, which, following picric acid precipitation, yielded vancomycin. Early preparations contained numerous impurities and were associated with a number of important adverse effects. Newer, purified forms have been available since 1986.

The glycopeptide antibiotics, like the β-lactam antibiotics, inhibit cell wall formation by inhibiting peptidoglycan synthesis. These drugs complex with the terminal amino acyl-D-alanyl-D-alanine portion of bacterial cell wall building blocks, thereby inhibiting peptidoglycan polymerase and the transpeptidation reactions. This interference with cell wall synthesis occurs during the second stage of peptidoglycan synthesis, which is a site different from the site of action for penicillins. These drugs are bactericidal against most Gram-positive bacteria, with the exception of the enterococci, against which it is bacteriostatic. The large molecular weight of vancomycin prevents it from passing across the membrane of Gram-negative bacteria to reach the cell wall; therefore, the drug has no utility in the treatment of Gram-negative bacterial infections.

Since the late 1980s, the prevalence of vancomycin-resistant enterococci has risen alarmingly. The molecular basis for vancomycin resistance in enterococci results from the complex, coordinated interactions of multiple genes usually encoded on a single transposon. The *vanA* gene, the most important of these, encodes a ligase that results in the formation of the peptidoglycan precursor UDP-MurNAc-L-Ala-D-Glu-L-Lys-D-Ala-D-Lac, whose C-terminus has profoundly reduced affinity for vancomycin.

Metabolism and Disposition

The glycopeptide antibiotics are not absorbed after oral administration. This pharmacokinetic characteristic of poor oral bioavailability is exploited with the drug's oral use in the treatment of *Clostridium difficile* antibiotic-associated colitis. As the drug is irritating when given intramuscularly, it must be given intravenously for systemic use. Approximately 55% of vancomycin is bound to plasma protein. Vancomycin distributes to most body fluids and tissues although, because of its large molecular size, penetration into some infected spaces, particularly devitalized wounds, may be marginal. Vancomycin penetration into the CNS is poor in patients with uninflamed meninges, although adequate concentrations for the treatment of bacterial meningitis are achieved in the presence of meningeal inflammation. The glycopeptide antibiotics are not metabolized and are excreted unchanged from the body by the kidney.

Adverse Effects

A large number of adverse effects have been associated with vancomycin administration, but most have been attributed to impurities in earlier pharmaceutical formulations. Newer, more pure formulations are safer. The "red-man syndrome," characterized by flushing, pruritus, tachycardia, and an erythematous rash, is associated with the rapid IV administration of vancomycin. The syndrome is due to vancomycin-induced histamine release. Pretreatment with antihistamine and slowing the vancomycin infusion rate reduce the frequency and severity of this reaction.

Ototoxicity and nephrotoxicity have long been attributed to vancomycin therapy, but the true incidences of these adverse effects are very low. Current estimates suggest that the incidence of vancomycin-associated ototoxicity and nephrotoxicity approximates 2% and 5%, respectively, and their occurrences are dependent upon the presence of other confounding variables such as concurrent administration of known ototoxic and nephrotoxic drugs, patient age, and severity of disease.

Therapeutic Drug Monitoring

For decades, the monitoring of serum peak and trough vancomycin concentrations has been advocated. As with the aminoglycoside antibiotics, the data that support routine monitoring of vancomycin concentrations are very limited, particularly in pediatric patients; therefore, routine monitoring can no longer be recommended (3,16,32). Rather, data support the monitoring of vancomycin serum concentrations only in those pediatric patients who are not responding to usual doses or who suffer from compromised renal function and in those undergoing dialysis procedures.

Drug Interactions

Drug interactions with vancomycin include the possible additive ototoxic and nephrotoxic effects with other drugs known to cause these toxicities.

Clinical Indications

Vancomycin therapy is indicated for the treatment of infections caused by MRSA and coagulase-negative staphylococci. The drug may also be used as an alternative to β-lactam therapy in the treatment of streptococcal and staphylococcal infections in children who are allergic to penicillin. The penetration of β-lactam antibiotics into most body spaces is superior to that of vancomycin, and the former are preferred if the infecting organism is susceptible to both classes of drugs. The use of vancomycin as part of an empiric antibiotic regimen in the treatment of the febrile immunocompromised or critically ill patient remains controversial. While it is clear that Gram-positive organisms account for an increasing number of infections in this patient population, no benefit has been demonstrated with the empiric use of vancomycin, as contrasted with adding it after an infection with a susceptible organism has been established.

Alternative Antibacterial Agents for Gram-Positive Infections

Several alternatives to vancomycin have been developed for the treatment of MRSA and other multiple-drug-resistant, Gram-positive pathogens. The semisynthetic lipoglycopeptide dalbavancin possesses more potent in vitro activity against many Gram-positive organisms compared with vancomycin and has a very prolonged terminal half-life that allows once-per-week IV dosing. Daptomycin, a parenteral lipopeptide, likewise has in vitro activity against virtually all clinical isolates of *S. aureus*, coagulase-negative staphylococci, and enterococci (including vancomycin-resistant enterococci) tested to date, but published experience describing its use in children is limited. Linezolid, the first licensed agent of the oxazolidinone family of bacterial protein-synthesis inhibitors, also possesses activity against most isolates of Gram-positive bacteria. Linezolid is available in both a parenteral and oral preparation, the latter allowing convenient, effective home therapy once clinical stability has been achieved in the appropriate patient.

Macrolide/Azalide Antibiotics

Spectrum of Activity

Erythromycin, the first macrolide, was isolated from a strain of *Streptomyces erythreus* found in soil collected in the Philippine Archipelago. First reported in 1952, this new class of drugs was referred to as "macrolides" due to their large macrocyclic ring structure. In the 1980s and 1990s, two new analogs were commercially released: the macrolide clarithromycin and the azalide azithromycin. Both of these agents have a broader spectrum of activity than erythromycin but cause fewer gastrointestinal side effects.

The macrolide antibiotics competitively bind to the 50S ribosomal subunit, antagonizing bacterial protein synthesis by interfering with translocation of tRNA and peptide bond formation. The binding site on the 50S ribosome subunit is the same target bound by other antibiotics, most notably the lincosamides (including clindamycin) and the streptogramins. This similarity in site of antibacterial action for these different drug classes may result in antibacterial antagonism if coadministered to the same patient and cross-resistance if the site is modified. The macrolides are active against many community-acquired respiratory pathogens, most notably pneumococcus, *Mycoplasma*, *Legionella*, and *Chlamydia*. They have less activity against *H. influenza*, although the newer macrolides are superior to erythromycin in this regard. They are the drugs of choice for eradication of *B. pertussis*.

Two types of resistance to macrolide antibiotics have been characterized. The first is related to methylation of the 23S ribosomal subunit encoded by a family of related genes, labeled *erm* (erythromycin resistance methylases). This mechanism confers absolute resistance to this class of drugs. A genetically transferable efflux pump mediates the second form of resistance. The *mef* (macrolide efflux) genes are included on transposons and encode a number of associated functions that work in a coordinated fashion to pump drug out of the bacteria. This resistance mechanism may be overcome by increasing the drug concentration.

Metabolism and Disposition

Erythromycin and azithromycin both are available in oral and IV preparations; clarithromycin is available only in tablet or suspension. Once in the bloodstream, these agents are widely distributed throughout the body. Serum protein binding is modest and variable. Moreover, in contrast to the β-lactam and aminoglycoside antibiotics, significant amounts of these drugs are found in the intracellular, as contrasted with the extracellular, fluid space. In fact, for azithromycin, >95% of all drug in the body is intracellular. These unusual disposition characteristics have important clinical consequences. The large volume of distribution results in relatively low serum and extracellular fluid concentrations. Thus, even though all of these agents are very potent in vitro against a wide range of bacterial pathogens, they are not always clinically effective against these same organisms (e.g., *H. influenzae*) because of the low free-drug concentrations achieved in the blood and extracellular fluid. In contrast, their high intracellular concentrations enhance their effectiveness against intracellular pathogens such as *Chlamydia* and *Legionella*.

Adverse Effects

The incidence of serious adverse effects with the use of these drugs is rare. The most common adverse effect associated with erythromycin use is gastrointestinal discomfort. Nausea, vomiting, severe abdominal cramping, and epigastric distress have all been reported in varying frequencies with the use of erythromycin, and the occurrence of these symptoms is the most common reason patients discontinue therapy. The basis for this toxicity rests in erythromycin's mimicry of the promotility gastrointestinal polypeptide motilin.

More serious adverse effects associated with erythromycin administration include hepatic toxicity, ototoxicity, and cardiac toxicity. The clinical course of erythromycin-associated hepatotoxicity is suggestive of a hypersensitivity reaction. Signs and symptoms usually manifest after 2–3 weeks of erythromycin therapy in patients who have never received the drug, whereas symptoms may occur within 1–2 days in patients who have taken erythromycin in the recent past. Erythromycin-associated ototoxicity and cardiac toxicity appear to occur most frequently after parenteral administration, often associated with high doses. Bilateral sensorineural hearing loss occurs most commonly in elderly patients. In reported cases, complete normalization of hearing deficits occurs promptly after the drug is discontinued. In contrast, erythromycin-associated cardiac toxicity represents a very serious and life-threatening adverse effect that has been described in both children and adults. Prolongation of the QT interval and ventricular tachyarrhythmias are most common manifestation. None of these more serious side effects have been noted with clarithromycin or azithromycin.

Drug Interactions

A number of important drug-drug interactions have been reported to occur in patients who receive erythromycin. Drugs that are reported to result in clinically important drug interactions with macrolides include carbamazepine, corticosteroids, cyclosporine, warfarin, and theophylline. Erythromycin appears to competitively interfere with the hepatic metabolism of drugs that are metabolized within the cytochrome CYP450 enzyme system. Coadministration of a chronic medication metabolized by this enzyme system usually results in the accumulation of the chronic medication, often leading to adverse drug effects.

Clinical Indications

Use of both oral and parenteral erythromycin has been largely replaced by use of azithromycin, which is most commonly used as part of a combination regimen for the treatment of community-acquired infections of the respiratory tract.

Quinolones

Spectrum of Activity

The fluoroquinolone agents that are currently marketed are not labeled for use in patients <18 years of age because of cartilage toxicity seen during preclinical testing. Nevertheless, their unique properties may offer important and perhaps life-saving therapy for selected pediatric patients. Discovered in a distillate from chloroquine synthesis in the search for new antimalarial compounds, nalidixic acid is the precursor to an increasing number of newer quinolone derivatives. The new fluoroquinolones are potent antibiotics that possess a broad spectrum of in vitro antibacterial activity. The second-generation quinolones ciprofloxacin and levofloxacin are effective against many Gram-negative pathogens, including *P. aeruginosa*, and indeed were the first oral antibiotics available for *Pseudomonas* infections. However, they have marginal activity against *S. pneumoniae*, limiting their use in pneumonia. Newer-generation quinolones have largely maintained their activity against Gram-negative bacteria but have improved their activity against pneumococcus. They also have activity against the atypical respiratory pathogens *Mycoplasma pneumoniae* and *Chlamydia pneumoniae*, rendering them excellent choices for both community- and hospital-acquired respiratory tract infection.

The quinolones inhibit bacterial DNA topoisomerase, often referred to as DNA-gyrase, which is necessary for bacterial DNA replication and some aspects of transcription and repair. Although mammalian cells contain a DNA gyrase similar to the one found in bacteria, fluoroquinolones do not interact with this enzyme at concentrations achieved after routine dosing. Bacterial resistance to quinolones is most commonly a result of mutations that alter quinolone binding to DNA-gyrase. Bacterial resistance is more often a chromosomal-mediated process than a plasmid-mediated process and, when it occurs, it usually confers cross-resistance to other fluoroquinolones. Cross-resistance by this mechanism does not usually occur between fluoroquinolones and other antibiotic drug classes (e.g., aminoglycosides or β-lactams). Resistance also is conferred by expression of multidrug efflux pumps that extrude the antibiotic from the bacterial cell.

Metabolism and Disposition

Because of restricted labeling, only limited data are available regarding the pharmacokinetics of fluoroquinolones in infants and children. The quinolones are available in both IV and oral formulations. Oral bioavailability approaches 100%, offering the clinician an enteral option for the treatment of serious Gram-negative bacterial infections in the patient who lacks IV access. These drugs are primarily metabolized by the liver and do not require substantial dose adjustments in patients with mild-to-moderate renal functional impairment. In contrast, dosage adjustments may be necessary for most quinolone drugs in patients with liver disease.

Adverse Effects

Adverse effects associated with the clinical use of quinolone antibiotics are usually mild and transient in nature. Nausea, abdominal distress, headache, and dizziness appear to be the most common adverse events in adults. Less common adverse effects have included skin rash, photosensitivity reactions, and CNS manifestations, including depression, hallucinations, and seizures. Some quinolones have been associated with prolongation of the QT interval. The most important quinolone-associated adverse effect pertinent to pediatric patients is the possibility of drug-induced arthropathy. Preliminary toxicity studies in rodent and juvenile canine models described destructive lesions of cartilage following the administration of quinolone antibiotics, particularly nalidixic acid and ciprofloxacin. Reports of joint complaints in teenage patients with cystic fibrosis who receive ciprofloxacin have appeared in the literature, but the incidence of true quinolone-associated arthropathy in young children is unknown.

Drug Interactions

Concomitant enteral administration of quinolones with divalent and trivalent cation-containing antacids, sucralfate, and iron substantially reduces the oral absorption of quinolone antibiotics. This decreased absorption is most likely due to chelation of the quinolone by these cations, forming a poorly soluble complex. Similarly, the presence of food in the stomach (either from meals or tube feedings) may delay the rate and overall extent of quinolone absorption. If these agents must be prescribed for the same patient, the time interval between administration of the two drugs should be as long as possible. In contrast, no interference with oral quinolone absorption is observed when these drugs are coadministered with oral histamine H_2-receptor antagonists.

An increased incidence in adverse effects involving the CNS has been described in patients who receive quinolones in combination with certain nonsteroidal anti-inflammatory drugs. In 1986, the Japanese Ministry of Health reported an increased frequency of convulsions in patients who received fenbufen and enoxacin. The true significance of this possible interaction with other nonsteroidal anti-inflammatories is unknown, but caution should be exercised with their combined use.

ANTIFUNGAL AGENTS

The use of antifungal agents presents challenges not encountered with antibacterial drugs. Most serious fungal infections occur in compromised patients with significantly diminished immune function. Survival depends on the global improvement in the patient's condition and immunity as well as the institution of the correct therapy. In many circumstances, the outcome is poor regardless of the antimicrobial choice. Moreover, in vitro susceptibility testing for antifungal drugs, only recently standardized, does not predict successful outcome with the same accuracy as antibacterial susceptibility testing. Additionally, large clinical trials to define the superiority of one agent over another in a defined setting frequently are lacking. Definition of the efficacy of therapy is further hampered by the uncertainty inherent in diagnosing invasive fungal infection, particularly those caused by filamentous fungi. Finally, many of the newer antifungal agents have been incompletely studied in children.

These issues notwithstanding, antifungal therapy has made substantial advances over the past 15 years with the introduction of new classes of drugs that are more effective and less toxic than older options. It should be emphasized that the field of antifungal therapy is very active, and future therapeutic recommendations will evolve accordingly.

Polyenes

The polyenes in current use include nystatin and colloidal and lipid-associated amphotericin B. Amphotericin B is a macrocyclic antimicrobial derived from *Streptomyces*. It is solubilized by the addition of sodium deoxycholate, with which it forms a colloidal dispersion. The drug was introduced in the late 1950s, after it was demonstrated in open-labeled, non-comparative studies to be effective in treating a broad variety of serious fungal infections. Over nearly 50 years of use, amphotericin B has remained a cornerstone of treatment for virtually all significant fungal infections, including those caused by *Candida*, *Aspergillus*, non-*Aspergillus* molds, *Cryptococcus*, and the endemic fungal pathogens such as *Histoplasma*, *Blastomyces*, *Coccidioides*, and *Sporothrix*. Only a small number of fungal pathogens are typically resistant to amphotericin. These include the yeast *Candida lusitaniae* and the molds *Aspergillus terreus* and *Pseudallescheria boydii*.

Amphotericin B acts by binding to ergosterol, the principal sterol component of the fungal cell membrane, which leads to the loss of intracellular constituents and ultimately to cell death (17,26). The drug further generates oxidative species that damage fungal mitochondria (31).

Amphotericin B is not absorbed from the gastrointestinal tract and must be given intravenously. The drug distributes widely in tissues. The organs with the highest concentrations of amphotericin are liver, kidney, and lung, with little drug detectable in bronchial secretions and brain. Nevertheless, amphotericin B has been used successfully for selected fungal infections of the CNS, particularly those due to *Cryptococcus* and *Coccidiomycosis*, although advanced cases frequently require intraventricular instillation of drug. The mechanisms of elimination of amphotericin B are unknown. Only a small amount of the injected dose is detectable in the urine, and less than half can be recovered in bile. Blood levels therefore are not influenced by renal or hepatic insufficiency.

Amphotericin B use is associated with significant toxicities in the host (17), although broad experience indicates that the drug is better tolerated in children than in adults. Two categories of amphotericin B toxicity have been described: infusion-related and dose-related. The infusion-related toxicities include fever, chills, rigors, nausea and vomiting, arthralgias, and myalgias. These toxicities are uncomfortable but usually not dangerous, although occasionally they may be associated with hypotension and dysrhythmias. Small studies have supported the administration of antipyretics and meperidine prior to amphotericin B infusion, and hydrocortisone with the amphotericin itself, to reduce infusion-related symptoms (17).

Dose-related toxicities correlate with cumulative end-organ exposure to drug and include nephrotoxicity, which is reflected both by a decline in glomerular filtration rate and a tubulopathy, resulting in potassium, magnesium, and bicarbonate wasting, and anemia. Observational studies suggest that the incidence of nephrotoxicity can be lessened by sodium loading prior to infusion. Some authorities suggest that renal toxicity can be reduced further by converting dosing to every other day once the infection has been stabilized, but this strategy remains unproven.

As a response to the toxicities inherent in amphotericin B deoxycholate, lipid-associated formulations of the drug have been introduced to enable higher dosing with fewer side effects. The addition of the lipid carrier has little effect on the in vitro antifungal activity of amphotericin (6). The three available lipid formulations are liposomal amphotericin B (LAmB), amphotericin B colloidal dispersion (ABCD), and amphotericin B lipid complex (ABLC). LAmB encases amphotericin in a true liposome, ABCD surrounds the drug in a lipid disc, and ABLC complexes the drug within a lipid sheet. Typically, the lipid formulations are infused at a dose several-fold higher than that employed with conventional amphotericin B deoxycholate (3–5 mg/kg/dose versus 0.5–1 mg/kg/dose of the conventional drug). The amphotericin remains complexed to the lipid in the bloodstream and is released in the site of infection. The lipid formulations do not have as wide a distribution as conventional amphotericin B and concentrate particularly in the liver and spleen, major repositories of the reticuloendothelial system.

By design, the lipid-complexed amphotericins consistently demonstrate decreased toxicity when compared with amphotericin B deoxycholate. The incidence of infusion-related reactions is reduced with LAmB but is less convincingly with the other lipid formulations. Dose-related toxicities, on the other hand, are substantially decreased for all of the lipid formulations. Typically, the incidence of elevation of serum creatinine twofold or more above baseline is reduced by nearly half.

Azoles

The azoles represent a major advance in antifungal therapy due to their broad activity and their relatively mild toxicity compared with the polyenes. A series of azole agents has been introduced in the last 25 years, with the first, miconazole and ketoconazole, replaced by the less toxic fluconazole and itraconazole. A new generation of broad-spectrum azoles is emerging into clinical use. Voriconazole is commercially available, while posaconazole is awaiting approval by the US Food and Drug Administration (FDA). All of the azoles share the same mechanism of actions, namely, the inhibition of the enzyme lanosterol 14α-demethylase. This enzyme is necessary for the synthesis of the key fungal cell membrane element ergosterol, the molecular target of the polyenes. Inhibition of this enzyme results in ergosterol depletion, along with the accumulation of methylated sterol precursors, which in turn, results in inhibition of fungal cell growth and death. The improved spectrum of the newer azoles appears to result from their increased inhibitory potency against the lanosterol 14α-demethylase in an ever-broader variety of fungal species.

Lanosterol 14α-demthylase is part of the fungal microsomal CYP450 complex, and all of the azoles have some, albeit lower, activity against the homologous eukaryotic enzymes. Consequently, drug-drug interactions with other agents metabolized by certain CYP450 isoforms are prominent and common to all of the azoles. They are especially prominent with voriconazole. Several of the interactions are clinically important in the patient who is likely to require antifungal therapy, including those receiving benzodiazepines, long-acting barbiturates, phenytoin, tacrolimus, sirolimus, cyclosporine, warfarin, rifampin, omeprazole, calcium-channel blockers, and hydrochlorothiazide (4). Scrupulous monitoring of the serum concentrations or the potential toxicities of the concomitant medication is essential. Other untoward side effects of the azoles are mild and are composed primarily of constitutional symptoms such as nausea, abdominal pain, and headache (4). Mild elevations of hepatic transaminases are common, but significant elevations occur infrequently and, unlike with ketoconazole, fulminant hepatitis with the newer azoles is rare (4). Voriconazole is associated with distinct side effects not noted with other azoles. The more common of these, visual disturbance, occurs in up to one-third of patients who are exposed to voriconazole and are experienced most frequently during the first week of therapy. They are neither permanent nor usually dose limiting. Voriconazole also is occasionally associated with rash and, rarely, with Stevens-Johnson syndrome or toxic epidermal necrolysis (19).

The new azole agents possess some differences in their pharmacological properties. All of the newer azole compounds are available as both IV and oral preparations, except for itraconazole and posaconazole, which have only oral formulations. Itraconazole, voriconazole, and posaconazole are cleared almost exclusively by the liver, and no dose adjustment is required for renal insufficiency. However, the sulfobutylether-β-cyclodextrin sodium (SBECD) vehicle for IV administration of voriconazole are cleared via glomerular filtration, and both should be avoided in patients with significant renal insufficiency. Fluconazole is cleared by the kidneys, and dose adjustment in renal failure is necessary. These agents also differ in their degree of protein binding. Itraconazole and posaconazole are highly protein bound; consequently, neither is dialyzed or enters the CNS efficiently. It is uncertain if this latter characteristic precludes their use in infections of the CNS, but caution should be exercised in this setting until clinical data regarding efficacy are available. In adults, voriconazole exhibits nonlinear pharmacokinetics thought to result from saturable clearance (19). Indeed, its metabolism is mostly dependent upon CYP2C19, a polymorphic enzyme. As many as 20% of non-Indian Asians may achieve voriconazole levels fourfold higher than other subjects because of these genetic polymorphisms.

Mechanisms of azole resistance have been defined, particularly in *Candida* spp. These include (a) overexpression of multidrug efflux pumps with subsequent extrusion of the drug from the intracellular environment of the fungus, and (b) alterations of the target enzyme lanosterol 14α-demthylase or other enzymes in the synthetic pathway for ergosterol. In many of these resistant isolates, two or more mechanisms of resistance are coexpressed. Resistance to a more narrow-spectrum azole does not necessarily imply coresistance to others. Fluconazole-resistant isolates of *Candida*, for example, usually remain susceptible to voriconazole and posaconazole.

Fluconazole remains the major alternative to amphotericin in the treatment of serious infections due to *Candida* spp. It has a wide distribution with excellent penetration into virtually all body compartments, including the CNS. The principal limitation of fluconazole is its relatively narrow spectrum, which is confined to *Candida* spp. With the broad use of this agent throughout the 1990s and 2000s, resistance to selected *Candida* spp. has become more frequent. *C. krusei* is intrinsically resistant to fluconazole, as are some isolates of *C. glabrata*, and worldwide, the incidence of infection from both of these species has increased since the introduction of fluconazole. Acquired fluconazole resistance in *C. albicans* and other non-albicans species, such as *C. tropicalis* and *C. parapsilosis*, remains uncommon but has been documented. Fluconazole has no clinically relevant activity against *Aspergillus* or other molds.

In contrast to fluconazole, itraconazole possesses in vitro activity against most *Aspergillus* spp. and the endemic fungi. However, the bioavailability of the original capsule formulation was low and variable. An oral solution of itraconazole was developed that solubilizes the drug by complexing it with cyclodextrin, thereby increasing the drug's bioavailability substantially, although the vehicle may cause an osmotic diarrhea.

Voriconazole is a synthetic derivative of fluconazole with a superior spectrum of activity as compared with the parent drug. Voriconazole has in vitro activity against virtually all *Candida* spp., including those resistant to fluconazole; against *Aspergillus* spp., including the polyene-resistant species *A. terreus*; and most of the endemic fungi. It also is active against some but not all of the non-*Aspergillus* molds. Notably, voriconazole is not active against Zygomycetes (19). Currently, the drug is used most prominently in the treatment of invasive aspergillosis, a clinical entity that historically has proven exceedingly difficult to cure.

Posaconazole is structurally similar to itraconazole. It possesses the broadest activity of all of the azoles, including virtu-ally all *Candida* spp., cryptococcus, nearly all *Aspergillus* spp., and non-*Aspergillus* molds, including many *Fusarium* spp. and *P. boydii*. It is also active against Zygomycetes, including *Rhizopus* and *Mucor*, making it the only azole to date effective against these organisms. It has strong activity against the important endemic fungi as well.

Echinocandins

The echinocandins are a novel class of antifungal agents. They share a superior safety profile and lack significant drug-drug interactions. Presently, three echinocandins have been licensed by the FDA: caspofungin, micofungin, and anidulafungin. All three agents have a very similar spectrum of activity.

The echinocandins are semisynthetic compounds derived from natural products of molds. They inhibit 1,3-β-D-glucan synthase, the enzyme responsible for the production of the polysaccharide 1,3-β-D-glucan, a component of the fungal cell wall. Organisms exposed to the echinocandins lose their rigidity and produce truncated, abnormal hyphae. They ultimately swell and lyse under osmotic pressure. The antifungal spectrum of the echinocandins is limited to *Candida* and *Aspergillus* spp. Nevertheless, these drugs have demonstrated in vitro activity against all isolates within these groups, including *C. krusei* and *C. glabrata*, which are intrinsically resistant to fluconazole, and *C. lusitaniae*, which is intrinsically resistant to the polyenes. The echinocandins also have excellent in vitro activity against non-albicans candidal species with acquired resistance to the azoles. To date, resistance to the echinocandins among clinical isolates of *Candida* and *Aspergillus* is very rare.

1,3-β-D-glucan of *Cryptococcus* has a conformation that does not bind the echinocandins, and these drugs have no activity against species included in this genus (11). The drugs also lack activity against a number of molds of clinical importance, particularly Zygomycetes, *Fusarium*, and *Pseudallescheria* and its asexual form *Scedosporium*. The echinocandins also are not active against *Trichosporin*. The drugs are effective in vitro against the mycelial forms of several of the dimorphic endemic pathogens but are only weakly active against the yeast forms.

The echinocandins are rational choices for patients with suspected or proven disease caused by *Candida* or *Aspergillus*, especially those who are failing more conventional therapy. They have also been tested as empiric antifungal therapy in febrile neutropenia. In this setting, the drugs are safe and at least as effective as amphotericin and fluconazole in preventing invasive fungal infections. The drugs' effectiveness in established fungal disease is less well proven. Open-label trials have documented success rates that exceed 80% in patients with newly diagnosed *Candida* infection or in those with disseminated candidiasis that is refractory to other therapies. When compared in a double-blinded, randomized trial to amphotericin, caspofungin performed equally in invasive candidal disease and was less toxic than the comparator drug (24). Most of the experience in the treatment of invasive aspergillosis has been collected in open-label studies directed toward patients who are unresponsive to or intolerant of other agents. Clinical response in this context, either when used alone or with voriconazole, approximates 50%.

Although minor differences in the pharmacology exist among the three approved echinocandins, none are absorbed orally and all are available only as IV preparations (11). They are highly protein bound and have poor penetration into the CNS (11). Caspofungin and micofungin are both metabolized in the liver and excreted in an inactive form in the bile and urine. Dosage adjustment is suggested for moderate-to-severe hepatic insufficiency. Only a very small proportion of active drug is excreted in the kidneys, and dosing need not be altered for renal failure. By contrast, anidulafungin is slowly degraded in human plasma, and the degradation products are then excreted in the bile. Preliminary studies indicate that this drug may be safely dosed in both renal and hepatic insufficiency without adjustment. The echinocandins are poor substrates for the cytochrome CYP450 enzymes, with relatively few drug-drug interactions (11).

1,3-β-D-glucan is not a component of eukaryotic cells, accounting for the excellent safety profile of the echinocandins. The most frequent attributable adverse effect is pain and phlebitis at the injection site. Significant adverse effects such as peripheral blood cytopenia or liver or kidney toxicity do not occur.

Combination Antifungal Therapy

The difficulty inherent in curing a patient of invasive fungal disease suggests that combinations of agents may be superior to single-agent therapy. Some theoretical concerns have given pause to this strategy. In particular, the use of azoles decreases the synthesis of ergosterol, the molecular target of the polyenes, suggesting that the combination may be antagonistic. Clinical experience suggests that such antagonism is uncommon and that combination of one class with another usually leads to synergistic or additive effects (31). However, these issues remain largely unresolved, and the ideal combinations of agents for a given pathogen have not been determined.

ANTIVIRAL AGENTS

Antiviral chemotherapy differs in key ways from antibacterial therapy. Viruses are obligate intracellular organisms, and antiviral drugs work intracellularly. Therefore, traditional pharmacokinetic studies that measure the pattern of drug in the intravascular compartment may not reflect the more relevant intracellular kinetics. Moreover, in contrast to antibacterial drugs, in vitro susceptibility tests are not standardized for antiviral agents and, in many instances, they correlate poorly with clinical efficacy. The response of the host to an antiviral agent is more strongly associated with the integrity of the host immune system than with the intrinsic properties of the drug.

Three acyclic nucleoside analogs with antiviral activity are in frequent use and likely to be encountered by the pediatric intensivist. These include acyclovir, ganciclovir, and cidofovir. A fourth drug, foscarnet, is a pyrophosphate analog commonly used when resistance is encountered to the nucleoside analogs.

Acyclovir

Mechanism and Spectrum

Acyclovir is an analog of deoxyguanosine with in vitro and clinical activity against herpes simplex virus type 1 (HSV-1), HSV

type 2 (HSV-2), and varicella-zoster virus (VZV). The drug was discovered in the mid-1970s and came into wide clinical use by the 1980s. A similar compound with nearly identical activity, penciclovir, was identified in the 1980s (1). Both acyclovir and penciclovir require triphosphorylation for antiviral activity. Addition of the first phosphate group is mediated by viral thymidine kinase (TK). Monophosphorylation occurs very inefficiently in the absence of this enzyme, accounting for the selectivity of acyclovir and penciclovir for virally infected cells (25). Subsequent addition of the second and third phosphate group is mediated by host cellular enzymes. The triphosphorylated drugs serve as substrates for viral DNA polymerase, acting primarily as chain terminators of nascent DNA. Neither drug is recognized by cellular DNA polymerases to any significant degree.

In vitro, acyclovir suppresses the growth of HSV-1 and HSV-2 at low concentrations. Approximately twice the amount of drug is required to suppress the growth of VZV. Cytomegalovirus (CMV) and Epstein-Barr virus (EBV), which do not encode TK, are inhibited in cell culture only by very high concentrations of drug. Acyclovir has no in vitro or in vivo activity against viruses outside of the herpes virus group.

Acyclovir generally is well tolerated. Its principal toxicity is renal impairment, which results from crystallization of drug in the renal tubules, a phenomenon that is potentiated by rapid infusion. Slow administration while maintaining adequate hydration is usually adequate to avoid nephrotoxicity (25). Occasionally, patients experience disorders of the CNS such as agitation, confusion, or hallucinations. These findings are most frequently noted in severely ill patients or in those with underlying CNS disease. Acyclovir generally is not associated with bone marrow suppression. However, two trials in infants suggest that acyclovir can produce neutropenia when administered to this young age group (21). In both circumstances, the neutropenia was self-limiting and responded to dose reduction or cessation.

Indications

In addition to its confirmed utility in severe, non–life-threatening herpetic infections, acyclovir has demonstrated utility in the treatment of two particularly dangerous herpes simplex infections that afflict the normal host: HSV encephalitis and neonatal herpes. It is also the treatment of choice for HSV infections in immunocompromised patients. The drug also has been effective in the treatment of VZV infection in the immune-suppressed patient, a condition marked by widespread disease that involves the lungs and abdominal viscera.

Additionally, acyclovir has proved to be very effective in suppressing reactivation of latent HSV when given prophylactically to selected hosts, including HSV-seropositive bone marrow transplant patients (18) who are at high risk of experiencing severe HSV mucositis from reactivated virus within the month after transplantation. Several investigators have demonstrated at least some effectiveness of acyclovir in suppressing newly acquired or reactivated CMV infection in solid-organ transplant patients, an unexpected finding given the drug's marginal activity against CMV in vitro. Even with HSV and VZV, the drug does not eradicate latent virus in ganglia cells, and recurrence rates return to baseline after suppressive therapy has been withdrawn.

Resistance

The majority of resistant isolates encountered in clinical practice have been isolated from immunocompromised subjects. Most have a mutated TK gene, resulting in virus with undetectable TK activity (labeled TK deficient, or TK^D, mutants) (1). In rare circumstances, resistance is mediated by alterations of the viral DNA polymerase. Response to acyclovir frequently is slow in immune-suppressed patients, even when they are infected with acyclovir-susceptible virus, but infection with TK^D HSV is associated with nearly absent response or with progression of the lesions despite 5–7 days of therapy. When the drug resistance of a virus is mediated by altered TK activity, the virus does not respond to increased doses of acyclovir or to penciclovir or ganciclovir, both of which likewise require phosphorylation by TK for their antiviral effect. The largest experience in treating TK^D HSV is with foscarnet. The rare cases of infection by acyclovir-resistant HSV that is mediated by altered DNA polymerase may be coincidentally resistant to foscarnet or cidofovir, but resistance patterns in these isolates are difficult to predict.

Ganciclovir

Mechanism and Spectrum

Ganciclovir is an acyclic nucleoside analog of deoxyguanosine with activity against several pathogenic human herpes viruses, specifically, HSV-1, HSV-2, VZV, CMV, and human herpes virus 6 (HHV-6). Like the other antiviral acyclic nucleosides, the drug requires intracellular phosphorylation to be active (23). After cell entry, ganciclovir monophosphate is synthesized by viral-specific enzymes. As with acyclovir, for HSV-1, HSV-2, and VZV, this step is catalyzed by viral TK (9). For CMV, the compound is monophosphorylated by a phosphotransferase encoded in the viral open reading frame UL97. Second and third phosphate groups are then added by host cellular kinases. Ganciclovir triphosphate selectively inhibits the activity of viral DNA polymerases.

Neutropenia is the most frequently encountered adverse effect of ganciclovir and the most common reason for premature cessation of therapy. The incidence of neutropenia is dependent upon the route of administration, the underlying disease, and whether other bone marrow suppressive drugs are given concomitantly. Bone marrow transplant patients appear particularly prone to suffering from neutropenia after exposure to the drug. Other bone marrow cell lines, particularly platelets, can also be suppressed by ganciclovir. Both neutropenia and thrombocytopenia are reversible if the dose is reduced or if the drug is discontinued. The neutropenia from ganciclovir can be mitigated by the administration of granulocyte-stimulating factor, which may allow prolongation of the antiviral therapy. Other adverse events are less prominent. Impaired renal function has been reported in a number of trials of ganciclovir, but recipients frequently have received other nephrotoxic agents. CNS complaints, including confusion and headache, have also been recorded, particularly among patients with renal insufficiency.

Indications

Ganciclovir is the established agent of choice in the treatment of CMV infections. Like all herpes viruses, CMV converts to a state of latency after the initial infection and may reactivate throughout the life of the host. In otherwise healthy patients, both primary and reactivated CMV infections usually cause asymptomatic or self-limiting illness. In immunocompromised individuals, asymptomatic infection may progress to serious and sometimes life-threatening disease. In the compromised host with established, systemic CMV infection, initial ganciclovir therapy usually is comprised of an intensive, IV induction phase for several weeks, followed by a maintenance phase after symptoms of the infection have abated. In some patients, particularly those with CMV pneumonitis, ganciclovir therapy is augmented with IV immune globulin with high titers of antibody against CMV.

Recent emphasis has been placed on using ganciclovir as prophylaxis against multiorgan infection in transplant recipients. Two preventative strategies have been employed (30). In the first, termed *universal prophylaxis*, IV or oral ganciclovir is administered to high-risk patients for the first 3–6 months after transplantation. The second, termed *preemptive therapy*, involves screening the patient at regular intervals for asymptomatic CMV infection, usually by testing blood for CMV protein or DNA, and then instituting ganciclovir therapy immediately after virus is detected. Both strategies are effective in preventing disseminated disease.

Ganciclovir is the first-line therapy for disseminated HHV-6 disease. HHV-6 is a ubiquitous human herpes virus that produces disseminated infection, including severe encephalitis, in immunocompromised persons, particularly recipients of bone marrow and solid-organ transplants. Although large therapeutic trials are lacking, anecdotal reports indicate that ganciclovir frequently produces a virologic and clinical response in transplant patients with HHV-6 encephalitis and other organ disease. Ganciclovir has clinical effectiveness against HSV-1, HSV-2, and VZV infection in humans. Because its therapeutic index is lower than that for acyclovir, acyclovir is preferred as the first-line agent in these infections.

Resistance

Resistance to ganciclovir has been reported in both HSV and CMV. Those with HSV infection unresponsive to acyclovir are frequently infected with a thymidine kinase-deleted mutant. As viral thymidine kinase is responsible for synthesis of ganciclovir monophosphate, such isolates are considered resistant to ganciclovir as well. CMV isolates resistant to ganciclovir primarily possess mutations in the UL97 sequence encoding the CMV phosphotransferase. Isolates whose resistance emanates from TK or UL97 mutations are generally susceptible to foscarnet and cidofovir, as neither of these agents requires an initial phosphorylation step from a virus-specific enzyme. CMV resistance to ganciclovir also has resulted from mutations in the UL54 region of the genome encoding the viral DNA polymerase.

Cidofovir

Mechanism and Spectrum

Like acyclovir and ganciclovir, cidofovir is an acyclic nucleoside analog. In contrast to most other nucleoside analogs, cidofovir possesses a phosphonate group on its broken ring and does not depend on viral kinase for monophosphorylation (10). Two additional phosphate groups are then added to the phosphonate moiety by host cellular enzymes to form the active triphosphorylated compound. The lack of requirement for viral phosphorylating enzymes to produce active compound renders the drug inhibitory to a wide variety of DNA viruses. The triphosphorylated molecule serves as a competitive inhibitor of viral polymerase and as a DNA chain terminator, similar to other acyclic antiviral drugs. The selectivity of cidofovir derives from its profound potency against viral polymerases. In vitro, the drug is ~1000-fold more inhibitory against viral DNA synthesis than it is against any of the cellular DNA polymerases.

Cidofovir possesses in vitro antiviral activity against all of the HHVs, namely, HSV-1 and HSV-2, CMV, VZV, EBV, HHV-6, HHV-7, and HHV-8, including most that are resistant to acyclovir, ganciclovir, and foscarnet. Additionally, it is active against adenovirus, the human papilloma and polyoma viruses, and the poxviruses, including monkeypox, smallpox, and vaccinia.

Pharmacology and Toxicity

Several active metabolites of cidofovir are formed intracellularly, and some have extremely long half-lives, which supports dosing weekly or every other week. Cidofovir accumulates in renal tubular cells aided by an organic ion transporter. Accumulation leads to nephrotoxicity, a risk that may be reduced by the administration of probenecid before and at 3 hrs and 8 hrs after cidofovir infusion and by generous IV hydration.

Indications

The use of cidofovir most likely to be encountered by the pediatric intensivist is for evolving or established adenovirus infection in immunocompromised patients, particularly those who have received bone marrow transplant. Adenovirus infection in these children frequently presents as fever and diarrhea ~1–2 months after transplantation and, left untreated, commonly disseminates to multiple organs, with death occurring in over half of patients. Several open-label trials with small numbers of subjects have demonstrated eradication of virus and cessation of symptoms in patients with adenovirus-infected bone marrow transplants who were treated with cidofovir (10). Cidofovir also has been used in infants and toddlers with pediatric laryngeal papillomatosis. Drug usually is injected directly into the lesions under direct laryngoscopy over several months, resulting in long-term and possibly permanent remission of the disease. In adults, cidofovir has been used widely and with success for CMV retinitis in patients with acquired immune deficiency syndrome. The drug should also be considered for any serious herpetic or CMV infections that are resistant to other antiherpetic drugs.

Resistance

Clinically apparent resistance to cidofovir is infrequent. Cidofovir-resistant viruses have mutations in their polymerase genes. Reports have suggested diminished response to cidofovir after prolonged therapies with other antiviral nucleoside analogs in some patients with CMV disease who have acquired immune deficiency syndrome or who have had bone marrow transplant.

Foscarnet

Mechanism and Spectrum

Foscarnet is the sodium salt of phosphonoformic acid, a pyrophosphate analog. It has activity against the DNA poly-

merase genes of several HHVs, including HSV-1 and HSV-2, VZV, CMV, and HHV-6, as well as hepatitis B virus. It also has activity against the HIV-1 reverse transcriptase. Normally, the addition of a nucleoside triphosphate to the growing DNA chain results in the cleavage of a pyrophosphate group, so that only one of the three nucleotide phosphate groups remain. Foscarnet binds to the element of the polymerase molecule that mediates this cleavage, inhibiting further synthesis of the nascent chain (8). The inhibitory effect on cellular polymerase requires drug concentrations >100-fold higher than those required to inhibit viral replication. In vitro and, presumably, in vivo viral inhibition is readily reversible, with viral cytopathic effect restored within several days after removal of drug from the culture medium. This latter property is ascribed to the readiness with which the drug crosses the cell membrane in both directions because, in contrast to the acyclic nucleotide analogs, the molecule is not trapped intracellularly by phosphorylation (22).

Pharmacology and Toxicity

Foscarnet has poor oral bioavailability and must be administered intravenously. The drug has a large volume of distribution and adequate CNS penetration. Parent drug is excreted by the kidneys through both glomerular filtration and tubular secretion. Dosing adjustment is required for patients with diminished renal function. Pharmacokinetic determinations are extremely variable due to the substantial deposition of drug into cartilage and bony matrix. Foscarnet subsequently slowly leaches out of bone, resulting in an extremely long terminal half-life.

The principal toxicity of foscarnet is renal impairment. Early studies identified nephrotoxicity in over 25% of adult patients with acquired immune deficiency syndrome and more than half of bone marrow transplant recipients exposed to the drug. Renal toxicity usually is reversible after cessation of therapy, especially in those with normal pre-existing renal function. The nephrotoxicity can be reduced by hydration prior to and during infusion. A second commonly reported side effect of foscarnet is derangement of calcium, phosphate, potassium, and magnesium. The most frequently reported side effects are depression of ionized calcium and hyperphosphatemia. Penile and vulvar ulcerations have been reported during foscarnet therapy, possibly due to exposure of these surfaces to high concentrations of active drug in the urine

Indications

Foscarnet has demonstrated clinical effectiveness against disease caused by HSV-1, HSV-2, VZV, CMV, HHV-6, and HIV-1. Its principal therapeutic role, however, has centered on its use as a second-line agent in herpes viral disease that is unresponsive to less toxic drugs, particularly acyclovir and ganciclovir. Unlike these acyclic nucleoside compounds, foscarnet does not depend upon phosphorylation by viral enzymes to achieve activity. Thus, herpes viruses that have emerged resistant to acyclovir and ganciclovir as a result of altered TK or CMV UL97 remain susceptible to foscarnet (15).

Resistance

Resistance to foscarnet can be promoted by serial passage in medium-containing drug and has been documented in clinical samples. The resistance is conferred by mutations in the viral polymerase gene, although several loci associated with foscarnet resistance have been identified. Cross-resistance to other antiviral agents is variable and unpredictable.

CONCLUSIONS AND FUTURE DIRECTIONS

Infection remains one of the major challenges in the PICU. It is the cause of admission for many patients and complicates the ICU course of others. Safe and effective treatment with anti-infective agents remains the cornerstone of the management of these problems. A thorough understanding of how existing antibacterials, antifungals, and antiviral agents work and the spectrum of their activities is one of the two major prerequisites to their rational and effective use. The other is an intimate awareness of the impact that physiologic derangements associated with serious illness and injury impose on the biodisposition of these agents. Armed with this knowledge, healthcare providers in the PICU can safely and effectively manage most infections with existing drugs.

Despite this optimism, a tipping point has been reached in the use of these agents. As we continue to rely on the current anti-infective armamentarium, pathogenic organisms are developing resistance with increasing frequency. At the same time, the development of newer agents has slowed to a mere trickle. Nevertheless, some news is promising. First, the agents under development appear to target the emerging "chinks in our armor." Drugs with potent activity against methicillin-resistant staphylococci, coagulase-negative staphylococci, Gram-negative organisms protected by extended-spectrum β-lactamases, and various *Pseudomonas* spp. are in development. In addition, newer antifungals agents with potent activity against *Aspergillus* spp. as well as some of the more difficult-to-treat candidal isolates are on the horizon. However, the greatest excitement remains in the arena of natural immunity. As our knowledge and understanding in this arena grows, targets for pharmacologic modulation are increasingly identifiable. In this context, a number of new natural products that have been isolated and studied in animal-model systems appear wholly protective in the face of significant pathogen burden and have no anti-infective activity in vitro. It is entirely conceivable that our rich heritage of anti-infective therapy will soon give way to an era of routine, effective immune modulation.

KEY POINTS

- PICU patients experience infections with a variety of community-acquired and nosocomially acquired pathogens.
- Anti-infective agents, including antibiotics, antifungals and antivirals, are the cornerstones of the management of infections in the PICU.
- Key to the effective use of these agents is a thorough understanding of their in vitro activity along with recognition of the translation of their molecular mechanisms of action into useful clinical dosing regimens.
- The physiologic derangements associated with critical illness or injury may dramatically alter the biodisposition of anti-infective agents requiring individualization of dosing strategies.

- Three families of anti-infectives are in common use in the PICU: antibacterials, antifungals, and antivirals. This chapter provides a brief overview of the activity, biodisposition, and safety profiles of the agents used most commonly in the PICU.
- Among the antibacterials there are essentially two modes of bacterial killing: time-dependent and concentration-dependent. Recognition of these modes of action is a major determinant of dosing.
- The antibacterial agents most commonly used in the PICU include the β-lactams, aminoglycosides, glycopeptides, macrolide/azalides, and fluoroquinolones.
- The antifungal agents discussed include the polyene, amphotericin B, the azoles, and the echinocandins.
- Discussion of the antivirals is limited to the acyclic nucleosides because of their activity against HSV, CMV, and to some extent, adenovirus, as well as foscarnet.

References

1. Bacon TH, Levin MJ, Leary JJ, et al. Herpes simplex virus resistance to acyclovir and penciclovir after two decades of antiviral therapy. *Clin Microbiol Rev* 2003;16:114–28.
2. Bryskier A, ed. *Antimicrobial Agents*. Washington, DC: ASM Press, 2005.
3. Cantu TG, Yamanaka NA, Lietman PS. Serum vancomycin concentrations: Reappraisal of their clinical value. *Clin Infect Dis* 1994;18:533–43.
4. Charlier C, Hart E, Lefort A, et al. Fluconazole for the management of invasive candidiasis: Where do we stand after 15 years? *J Antimicrob Chemother* 2006;57:384–410.
5. Cosgrove SE. The relationship between antimicrobial resistance and patient outcomes: Mortality, length of hospital stay, and health care costs. *Clin Infect Dis* 2006;42(Suppl 2):S82–9.
6. Coukell AJ, Brogden RN. Liposomal amphotericin B. Therapeutic use in the management of fungal infections and visceral leishmaniasis. *Drugs* 1998;55:585–612.
7. Craig WA, Ebert SC. Killing and regrowth of bacteria in vitro: A review. *Scand J Infect Dis Suppl* 1990;74:63–70.
8. Crumpacker CS. Mechanism of action of foscarnet against viral polymerases. *Am J Med* 1992;92:3S–7S.
9. Crumpacker CS. Ganciclovir. *N Engl J Med* 1996;335:721–9.
10. De Clercq E. Clinical potential of the acyclic nucleoside phosphonates cidofovir, adefovir, and tenofovir in treatment of DNA virus and retrovirus infections. *Clin Microbiol Rev* 2003;16:569–96.
11. Denning DW. Echinocandin antifungal drugs. *Lancet* 2003;362:1142–51.
12. DeRyke CA, Lee SY, Kuti JL, et al. Optimising dosing strategies of antibacterials utilising pharmacodynamic principles: Impact on the development of resistance. *Drugs* 2006;66:1–14.
13. Drusano GL. Antimicrobial pharmacodynamics: Critical interactions of 'bug and drug.' *Nat Rev Microbiol* 2004;2:289–300.
14. Ebert SC, Craig WA. Pharmacodynamic properties of antibiotics: Application to drug monitoring and dosage regimen design. *Infect Control Hosp Epidemiol* 1990;11:319–26.
15. Erice A, Gil-Roda C, Pérez JL, et al. Antiviral susceptibilities and analysis of UL97 and DNA polymerase sequences of clinical cytomegalovirus isolates from immunocompromised patients. *J Infect Dis* 1997;175:1087–92.
16. Freeman CD, Quintilliani R, Nightengale CH. Vancomycin therapeutic drug monitoring: Is it necessary? *Ann Pharmacother* 1993;27:594–8.
17. Gallis HA, Drew RH, Pickard WW. Amphotericin B: 30 years of clinical experience. *Rev Infect Dis* 1990;12:308–29.
18. Gluckman E, Lotsberg J, Devergie A, et al. Prophylaxis of herpes infections after bone-marrow transplantation by oral acyclovir. *Lancet* 1983;2:706–8.
19. Johnson LB, Kauffman CA. Voriconazole: A new triazole antifungal agent. *Clin Infect Dis* 2003;36:630–7.
20. Kearns GL, Abdel-Rahman SM, Alander SW, et al. Developmental pharmacology–drug disposition, action, and therapy in infants and children. *N Engl J Med* 2003;349:1157–67.
21. Kimberlin DW, Lin CY, Jacobs RF, et al. Safety and efficacy of high-dose intravenous acyclovir in the management of neonatal herpes simplex virus infections. *Pediatrics* 2001;108:230–8.
22. Lietman PS. Clinical pharmacology: Foscarnet. *Am J Med* 1992;92:8S–11S.
23. McGavin JK, Goa KL. Ganciclovir: An update of its use in the prevention of cytomegalovirus infection and disease in transplant recipients. *Drugs* 2001;61:1153–83.

24. Mora-Duarte J, Betts R, Rotstein C, et al. Comparison of caspofungin and amphotericin B for invasive candidiasis. *N Engl J Med* 2002;347:2020–9.

25. O'Brien JJ, Campoli-Richards DM. Acyclovir. An updated review of its antiviral activity, pharmacokinetic properties and therapeutic efficacy. *Drugs* 1989;37:233–309.

26. Ostrosky-Zeichner L, Marr KA, Rex JH, et al. Amphotericin B: Time for a new "gold standard." *Clin Infect Dis* 2003;37:415–25.

27. Pinder M, Bellomo R, Lipman J. Pharmacological principles of antibiotic prescription in the critically ill. *Anaesth Intensive Care* 2002;30:134–44.

28. Power BM, Forbes AM, van Heerden PV, et al. Pharmacokinetics of drugs used in critically ill adults. *Clin Pharmacokinet* 1998;34:25–56.

29. Roberts JA, Lipman J. Antibacterial Dosing in Intensive Care: Pharmacokinetics, Degree of Disease and Pharmacodynamics of Sepsis. *Clin Pharmacokinet* 2006;45:755–73.

30. Sia IG, Patel R. New strategies for prevention and therapy of cytomegalovirus infection and disease in solid-organ transplant recipients. *Clin Microbiol Rev* 2000;13:83–121, table of contents.

31. Steinbach WJ, Stevens DA, Denning DW, et al. Combination and sequential antifungal therapy for invasive aspergillosis: Review of published in vitro and in vivo interactions and 6281 clinical cases from 1966 to 2001. *Clin Infect Dis* 2003;37(Suppl 3):S188–224.

32. Thomas MP, Steele RW. Monitoring serum vancomycin concentrations in children: Is it necessary? *Pediatr Infect Dis J* 1998;17:351–3.

CHAPTER 78 ■ BACTERIAL SEPSIS AND MECHANISMS OF MICROBIAL PATHOGENESIS

NEAL J. THOMAS • ROBERT F. TAMBURRO • MARK W. HALL • SURENDER RAJASEKARAN • JOHN S. VENGLARCIK

Bacterial sepsis is a major cause of morbidity and mortality in children and a leading reason for medical admissions to the PICU. Worldwide, sepsis is the most common cause of deaths in infants (preferentially in males), as it can occur secondary to pneumonia, diarrhea, malaria, and other invasive bacterial diseases. Conversely, whereas death from bacterial sepsis was the routine even 40 years ago, great progress has been made in the treatment of this heterogeneous, infectious condition, and now the vast majority of children with bacterial sepsis survive in developed countries. This chapter will serve to identify the epidemiology, etiology, pathophysiology, clinical presentation, clinical management, outcomes, and future direction of bacterial sepsis in children.

DEFINITIONS

In 1989, Bone et al. initially described the "sepsis syndrome" in an attempt to identify patients who displayed evidence of a systemic response to infection but did not uniformly demonstrate classic signs of infection. The constellation of signs and symptoms included elevated temperature, tachycardia, tachypnea, abnormal peripheral white blood cell count, and evidence of organ dysfunction (9). A formal consensus conference was subsequently convened in 1991 to further this work by providing a framework to define the systemic inflammatory response to infection. The definitions that resulted, which included systemic inflammatory response syndrome (SIRS), sepsis, severe sepsis, and septic shock, were further refined in the 2001 International Sepsis Definitions Conference (41). Unfortunately, these definitions used parameters that were specific to adults, which limited their utility in children. A variety of definitions of pediatric sepsis and its associated organ dysfunction ensued in the literature; however, none provided comprehensive and age group-specific definitions that could be used in future clinical studies. Thus, an International Consensus Conference on Pediatric Sepsis and Organ Dysfunction was convened to develop pediatric-specific definitions for SIRS, sepsis, severe sepsis, and septic shock, which were published in 2005 (59) (Table 78.1).

SIRS was defined as the presence of at least two of four criteria, one of which is an abnormal temperature or leukocyte count. Upper and lower limits of these four SIRS criteria for the six specific age groups were also identified, by consensus, during the conference. Sepsis is defined as SIRS in the presence of, or as a result of, a suspected or proven infection. Severe sepsis and septic shock are defined as sepsis plus the presence of organ dysfunction. The consensus group also defined criteria for specific organ dysfunction (59). In addition to a proinflammatory response, the body mounts a compensatory anti-inflammatory reaction syndrome (CARS) that is important in the sepsis process. Although not as extensively described as SIRS, CARS, if sufficiently severe, may result in an increased susceptibility to infection and is believed to be an important predisposing factor to sepsis in a number of clinical settings commonly encountered in the PICU, including trauma and postoperative cardiopulmonary bypass.

Although sepsis, severe sepsis, and septic shock have been defined in the pediatric population, a precise characterization and staging of patients with sepsis is still lacking. In light of this, a new conceptual framework for analyzing sepsis was proposed as part of the 2001 International Sepsis Definitions Conference (41). Known by the acronym "PIRO," this classification scheme for sepsis stratifies patients on the basis of their *p*redisposing conditions, the nature and extent of the *i*nsult (in the case of sepsis, infection), the nature and magnitude of the host *r*esponse, and the degree of concomitant *o*rgan dysfunction (see also Chapter 21 and **Table 21.1**). This concept of PIRO is rudimentary, and testing and refinement are needed before it is ready for routine application in clinical practice.

EPIDEMIOLOGY

Bacterial sepsis, as defined and outlined by the previously mentioned clinical criteria, is a worldwide problem that is confounded by the multiple etiologies and multiple host defense issues. The most comprehensive study to examine the epidemiology of severe sepsis in the US reported that, in 1995, >42,000 cases of severe sepsis occurred in children who were <19 years of age, with an incidence of 0.56 cases per 1000 population annually (74). This incidence was greatest in children <1 year of age (5.16 per 1000) and decreased to a low of 0.20 per 1000 in children 10–14 years of age. However, it is important to recognize that the highest rate of sepsis in this youngest age group was due to the inclusion of low-birth-weight infants. Males (0.60/1000) have higher rates of sepsis compared to females (0.52/1000), and this gender discrepancy is most obvious in the youngest age groups. Despite this wide disparity in incidence across age groups, mortality was fairly consistent at ~10% for all age groups (74).

ETIOLOGY

The pathogens that cause severe sepsis vary by age; yet, across all age groups, gram-positive bacteria, mainly *Staphylococcus* and *Streptococcus* species, are the most prevalent, with specific etiologies as outlined in **Table 78.2** (74). Geographic location

TABLE 78.1

DEFINITIONS OF SYSTEMIC INFLAMMATORY RESPONSE SYNDROME, INFECTION, SEPSIS, SEVERE SEPSIS, AND SEPTIC SHOCK

SIRS
The presence of at least 2 of the following 4 criteria, one of which must be abnormal temperature or leukocyte count:
- Core temperature of >38.5°C or <36°C.
- Tachycardia, defined as a mean heart rate >2 SD above normal for age in the absence of external stimulus, chronic drugs, or painful stimuli;

  OR otherwise unexplained persistent elevation over a 0.5- to 4-hr period
  OR for children <1 yr old: bradycardia, defined as a mean heart rate <10th percentile for age in the absence of external vagal stimulus, β-blocker drugs or congenital heart disease; or otherwise unexplained persistent depression over a 0.5-hr period.

- Mean respiratory rate >2 SD above normal for age or mechanical ventilation for an acute process not related to underlying neuromuscular disease or the receipt of general anesthesia.
- Leukocyte count elevated or depressed for age (not secondary to chemotherapy-induced leukopenia) or >10% immature neutrophils.

Infection
A suspected or proven (by positive culture, tissue stain, or PCR test) infection caused by any pathogen OR a clinical syndrome associated with a high probability of infection. Evidence of infection includes positive findings on clinical exam, imaging, or laboratory tests (e.g., white blood cells in a normally sterile body fluid, perforated viscus, chest x-ray consistent with pneumonia, petechial or purpuric rash, or purpura fulminans).

Sepsis
SIRS in the presence of, or as a result of, suspected or proven infection.

Severe Sepsis
Sepsis plus one of the following: cardiovascular organ dysfunction OR ARDS OR 2 or more other organ dysfunctions.

Septic Shock
Sepsis and cardiovascular organ dysfunction.

From Goldstein B, Giroir B, Randolph A; International Consensus Conference on Pediatric Sepsis. International pediatric sepsis consensus conference: Definitions for sepsis and organ dysfunction in pediatrics. *Pediatr Crit Care Med* 2005;6:2–8, with permission.

TABLE 78.2

OCCURRENCE AND CASE FATALITY OF SELECT PATHOGENS AMONG CHILDREN WITH SEVERE SEPSIS BY AGE

	Age group					
	<1 Year		1–10 Years		11–19 Years	
Organism	Cases (%)	Case fatality (%)	Cases (%)	Case fatality (%)	Cases (%)	Case fatality (%)
Meningococcus	0.3	20.0	8.0	10.4	2.3	15.1
H. influenza	1.6	4.2	2.4	1.6	1.9	6.8
Pseudomonas	3.6	14.6	7.7	12.4	6.9	9.4
Staphylococcus (all types)	22.7	8.6	11.2	7.9	14.4	7.8
Staphylococcus aureus	2.3	5.7	2.9	0	3.5	3.8
Streptococcus (all types)	12.1	10.2	9.8	13.9	6.9	8.8
Pneumococcus	1.7	12.8	4.0	19.1	2.0	6.4
Group A *streptococcus*	0.3	0	0.7	5.0	0.2	0
Group B *streptococcus*	3.1	7.6	0.1	50.0	0.8	5.6
Fungus	10.0	10.8	13.3	16.8	10.4	11.6

From Watson RS, Carcillo JA, Linde-Zwirble WT, et al. The epidemiology of severe sepsis in children in the United States. *Am J Respir Crit Care Med* 2003;167:695–701, with permission.

and host immunologic status are also important influences in the etiology of sepsis. Moreover, interventions such as chemoprophylaxis and immunization exert an important impact on the bacteria linked to sepsis in the pediatric population.

Streptococcus agalactiae (group B streptococcus) was the predominant organism associated with neonatal sepsis in the first 3 days of life until the widespread adoption of intrapartum chemoprophylaxis in the early 1990s. The rate of other bacteria that cause early-onset sepsis, including *Escherichia coli*, *Listeria monocytogenes*, enterococcus, non-group D α-hemolytic streptococci, and nontypable *Haemophilus influenzae*, has remained constant (6). Presently, *Staphylococcus* is the most common infecting organism among neonates, causing 25.7% of all cases of neonatal sepsis (74) and reflecting the impact of nosocomial infections in this age group. Approximately 90% of these episodes were due to coagulase-negative staphylococcus, with *S. aureus* implicated in the other 10%. *Pseudomonas aeruginosa*, gram-negative enteric bacteria, and environmental bacilli are also significant causes of nosocomial-acquired sepsis. Low birth weight is a significant risk factor for severe sepsis, and respiratory and cardiovascular diseases are commonly observed underlying conditions in newborn sepsis.

As passive maternal immunity declines, the infant becomes exposed to bacteria in the community. In the recent past, septicemia due to *Haemophilus influenzae type-b* (Hib), *Streptococcus pneumoniae*, and *Neisseria meningitidis* was common. However, the prevalence of these organisms has significantly changed due to the advent of conjugated vaccines for Hib and *S. pneumoniae* in developed countries. Invasive disease in a healthy, immunized population due to Hib is virtually nonexistent, and the rates of invasive pneumococcal disease have declined dramatically (36). Under certain circumstances and in certain populations and locations, *S. aureus* and *Salmonella* spp. can cause invasive disease. After the first month of life, age-related differences become less distinct. In infants between 1 and 3 months of age, disease can be due to either the neonatal or community-associated pathogens, and both groups of organisms deserve consideration for treatment in the infant with signs of infection. Infants tend to have a primary bacteremia as compared to older children who have infections of the respiratory tract (73).

In otherwise healthy school-aged children, sepsis unassociated with a focus of infection becomes uncommon; meningococcemia is the most common example of this clinical scenario. However, meningococcemia will also be impacted by immunization strategies. College freshmen (many of whom will be 17 or 18 years old) who reside on campus in a dormitory are at increased risk for disseminated *N. meningitidis* infections (29), and most colleges and universities now require meningococcal immunization for this group of students. Although a polysaccharide meningococcal vaccine has been available for quite some time, a new conjugated vaccine is now routinely recommended for use in adolescents >11 years of age. Rickettsial infections can also manifest as sepsis. In endemic areas of the US, *Rickettsia rickettsiae* causes Rocky Mountain spotted fever and initially may present similarly to meningococcemia with fever, shock, and petechial rash. Human ehrlichioses (human monocytic ehrlichiosis due to *Ehrlichia chaffeensis*, human granulocytic anaplasmosis due to *Anaplasma phagocytophila*, and granulocytic ehrlichiosis due to *Ehrlichia ewingii*) can be mistaken for Rocky Mountain

TABLE 78.3

CLINICAL CONDITIONS THAT PREDISPOSE THE HOST TO SPECIFIC BACTERIA

Condition	Bacteria
Asplenia	*Streptococcus pneumoniae*
Polysplenia	*Salmonella*
Sickle cell disease	*Streptococcus pneumoniae*
	Salmonella
Nephrotic syndrome	*Streptococcus pneumoniae*
HIV/AIDS	*Streptococcus pneumonia*
	Haemophilus influenzae type b
	Staphylococcus aureus
	Pseudomonas aeruginosa
Complement deficiencies	*Neisseria meningitidis*
C5, C6, C7, C8, C9	*Neisseria gonorrhoeae*
Iron overload	*Yersinia enterocolitica*
	Listeria monocytogenes
	Vibrio vulnificus
Neutropenia	*Streptococcus viridans*

HIV, human immunodeficiency virus; AIDS, acquired immune deficiency syndrome

spotted fever (66). Human monocytic ehrlichiosis is more likely to have a rash, and skin manifestations are unusual in human granulocytic anaplasmosis. It is important to recognize that ehrlichiosis may be a life-threatening infection in patients who are coinfected with human immunodeficiency virus (HIV).

Disseminated streptococcal and staphylococcal infections can be seen in children ≥6 years of age but are usually related to a focus. In the case of *S. aureus*, the focus can be bone and joint, lung, heart, or brain. Disseminated group A streptococcal infections may be associated with pharyngitis or soft tissue infections. Patients with compromised integrity of the skin and mucous membranes due to instrumentation and indwelling catheters, and children and adolescents with primary and secondary immune deficiencies are all at risk for sepsis from a variety of common and uncommon bacteria. Certain conditions predispose to sepsis with certain bacteria (**Table 78.3**). Children with inherent or acquired predisposition to sepsis are discussed later in this chapter.

MECHANISM OF DISEASE: CORE PATHOPHYSIOLOGY

Gram-Positive and Gram-Negative Bacteria

The structural simplicity of bacteria makes it easier for them to adapt and change in response to threats; this is most obvious clinically by their ability to develop resistance to antibiotics. The patterns of infection constantly change in response to the complex interaction between bacteria and man. We develop new antibiotics, extend vaccination schedules and add new modalities of care, based on the knowledge that, potentially, any bacterial infection in a suitable host can develop into sepsis. This interaction led to the results of an epidemiologic survey of sepsis that indicated that gram-positive bacteria are now the predominant pathogens in sepsis in the US (44). Worldwide, the incidence of gram-positive sepsis is also increasing (5). Additionally, in transplant patients or those ICU patients who develop sepsis as a result of central venous line or soft tissue infections, gram-positive organisms account for the majority of infections. Complicating these infections are the increasing rates of multi-antibiotic resistance such as vancomycin-resistant *S. aureus* and enterococcus.

In recent decades, research into gram-negative bacteria and their role in the pathogenesis of sepsis has been substantial. Only now are we beginning to realize that significant differences exist in the infective process and pathophysiology of sepsis that are based on the causative organism. The conventional view of the molecular mechanisms of septic shock was derived from extensive basic medical investigations into the pathogenesis of lipopolysaccharide (LPS)-mediated endotoxic shock. The primary cause of shock after bloodstream infection with gram-negative bacteria is endotoxin. This complex macromolecule is common to the outer membrane of essentially all clinically significant aerobic gram-negative bacteria found in human infections. Endotoxin alone is sufficient to induce shock when given experimentally. Substantial evidence suggests that endotoxin triggers the complement, clotting, fibrinolytic, and kinin pathways, and rapidly induces the production of various cytokines from monocytes and macrophages, leading to the production of the potent vasodilator nitric oxide (NO), which appears to be responsible for hypotension. Bradykinin and complement enhance endothelial permeability, which, along with the disruption of normal coagulation homeostasis, can lead to microvascular thrombosis and disseminated intravascular coagulation (DIC). The traditional view has been that gram-negative bacteria are the most important cause of septic shock in patients. The convenience of using a single molecule such as LPS in experimental settings has considerably advanced our understanding of the pathogenesis of gram-negative sepsis but does not explain why gram-positive bacteria and other pathogens, including protozoan parasites, mycogens, and viruses, also induce a syndrome that is hemodynamically indistinguishable from endotoxemia (51). One could conclude that the nature of the infective organism does not matter as much as the body's response to the infection. In the past, this was the scientific premise around which much basic and clinical research was designed. However, we are beginning to appreciate the clear differences that exist in sepsis pathophysiology, depending on the invading organism.

Microbial Factors

It is frequently taught that one of the fundamental differences between gram-positive and gram-negative bacteria is the way in which they initiate disease. Gram-positive bacteria depend on the production of powerful exotoxins (e.g., tetanus, botulism, diphtheria); with gram-negative bacteria, it is principally the cell wall component LPS of the outer envelope that is implicated in pathogenesis of sepsis. Gram-positive bacteria also harbor endotoxin-like cell wall components, lipoteichoic acid (LTA) and peptidoglycan, but the bacterial components responsible for the induction of sepsis by gram-positive organisms are only recently beginning to be characterized. Gram-positive sepsis differs from gram-negative sepsis in that the organisms often arise from skin, soft-tissue structures, and catheter sites rather than from enteric or genitourinary sources. Additionally, gram-positive organisms require a highly orchestrated host response with intracellular killing by neutrophils and macrophages, as opposed to gram-negative pathogens, which may be readily killed in the extracellular space by antibody and complement.

Cell Wall Components

Most of the toxicity of endotoxin resides in the innermost core region, which consists of lipid A. The structure of lipid A is remarkably well conserved in most common gram-negative bacteria, irrespective of the species. Indeed, the clinical features of sepsis caused by *Escherichia coli* are no different than those caused by *Klebsiella* spp. (51). Complicating research into the mechanisms of gram-positive sepsis is the fact that gram-positive cell wall shows more structural variability than in a gram-negative organism. In gram-positive bacteria, the cell wall contains a thick (20–80 nm) layer of peptidoglycan (**Fig. 78.1**), which lies directly over the plasma membrane. Embedded in the peptidoglycan are molecules of LTA. LTA resembles LPS in certain respects and can therefore be considered the gram-positive counterpart of LPS. It contains a diacylglycerol lipid moiety instead of a phospholipid-like structure, as well as highly charged glycerophosphate repeating units. In vitro studies have demonstrated that these structural components of gram-positive cell walls are able to mimic some of the properties of endotoxin. LTA and peptidoglycan do not require their active secretion to induce proinflammatory

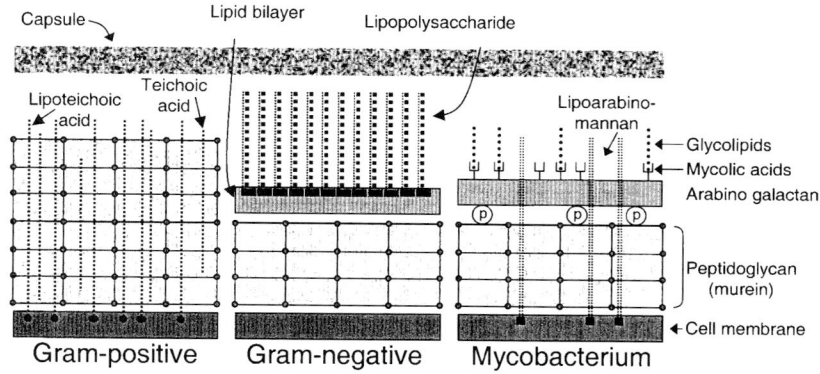

FIGURE 78.1. Cell wall structure of bacteria. All types of bacteria contain a cell membrane surrounded by a PGN-containing layer. LTA and LAM are inserted into the cell membrane of gram-positive bacteria. LPS forms the outer layer of the outer membrane of gram-negative bacteria. The mycobacteria also contain a carbohydrate shell, but not all bacteria contain a capsule. From Van Amersfoort ES, Van Berkel TJC, Kuiper J. Receptors, mediators, and mechanisms involved in bacterial sepsis and septic shock. *Clin Microbiol Rev* 2003;16:379–414, with permission. PGN, peptidoglycan; LTA, lipoteichoic acid; LAM, lipoarabinomannan; LPS, lipopolysaccharide.

cytokines from mononuclear cells. Rather, their release occurs as a result of treatment or immune lyses. Furthermore, data from work with *S. aureus* suggest that a complex synergistic relation exists between peptidoglycan and LTA in their ability to cause shock. The ability of gram-positive cell wall to induce multiorgan dysfunction has been demonstrated by the cell wall constituents inducing NO production, organ injury, and resistance to norepinephrine. Clinical data in humans is lacking, but it appears as if, during either immune-mediated or antibiotic-induced bacterial lysis, these endotoxins are released and exert their effect by inducing endothelial dysfunction and clinical deterioration (39). Moreover, mycobacterial cell wall components such as lipoarabinomannan can also induce myeloid cells to produce cytokines.

Soluble Factors

The production of soluble extracellular toxins is one of the hallmarks of disease caused by some gram-positive bacteria. The list is extensive, but examples include the toxins of clostridial species (gas gangrene, antibiotic-associated colitis), diphtheria (*Corynebacterium diphtheriae*), food poisoning (*Bacillus cereus, S. aureus*), and anthrax (*Bacillus anthracis*). The mode of action of many of these toxins is highly specific and well understood. In the etiology of gram-positive sepsis, different components of the bacteria seemed to be involved. The prime example is toxic shock syndrome toxin-1, a so-called superantigen (SAg). Concentrations of <0.1 pg/mL of a bacterial SAg are sufficient to stimulate the T lymphocytes in an uncontrolled manner, resulting in fever, shock, and death (58). The literature now describes 41 bacterial SAgs (58). SAgs are unusual because they do not require previous processing or highly specific presentation by antigen-presenting cells. Thus, they are able to bind to and activate more lymphocytes than conventionally processed antigens; hence, the term superantigen. SAgs are characterized by their ability to bind both major histocompatibility complex (MHC) class II molecules and T-cell receptors, which occurs promptly and in sequential fashion. The sole purpose of SAgs appears to be to bring these two critical molecules together to activate as many T cells as possible (58). The net result is the release of a large and sudden bolus of cytokines, which causes the acute condition. The range of microbic products thought to act as SAgs is somewhat wide: it includes the staphylococcal enterotoxins, streptococcal pyrogenic exotoxins, and the *Yersinia pseudotuberculosis* toxin. SAgs may also play a role in conditions such as Kawasaki disease. Many microbial products are T-cell mitogens, but some are remarkable because they activate only those lymphocytes that express particular variable β chains in the T-cell receptor, to which they bind with high affinity. Attempts have been made to modulate T-cell activation in experimental models of SAg-induced injury with glucocorticoids or antibodies directed against SAgs. Various methods of filtering blood to remove SAgs or the cytokines have been tried with some success. CTR (a novel hydrophobic organic compound with a hexadecyl alkyl chain) adsorbent beads were found to have adsorption rates of 50%–90% for enterotoxins, toxic shock syndrome toxin-1, and cytokines such as tumor necrosis factor (TNF)-α and IL-6. In vivo, the rat mortality rates at 8 hrs after endotoxin injection were 92%, 92%, and 14% for the endotoxemic, control column, and CTR treatment groups, respectively (67). This is currently a promising area of research.

Specific Bacteria/Syndromes

Streptococcus Pneumoniae

The capsular polysaccharide of *S. pneumoniae* is responsible for much of the virulence associated with this organism, with those strains that produce the largest quantity of capsular polysaccharide being considered the most virulent. Once inside the bloodstream of the host, encapsulation allows *S. pneumoniae* to escape neutrophil phagocytosis and avoid classic complement-mediated bactericidal activity. The teichoic acid and TLA of the cell wall induce the production of IL-1 and TNF-α, which then mediate a systemic response. The lack of type-specific antibody due to splenic dysfunction, such as in individuals with sickle cell disease, prevents opsonization and contributes to delayed clearance of *S. pneumoniae*.

Toxic Shock Syndrome (Staphylococcal and Streptococcal)

Cases of menstruation-associated staphylococcal infection in young women called attention to a syndrome of fever and profound shock, often followed by conjunctival hyperemia and desquamation, subsequently termed toxic shock syndrome. Toxic shock syndrome toxin-1, a 194-amino acid protein produced by certain strains of *S. aureus*; enterotoxins A, C, D, E, and H, also produced by *S. aureus*; as well as streptococcal pyrogenic exotoxin A, B, and C are the SAgs that mediate toxic shock syndrome by stimulating the production of IL-1 and TNF-α, resulting in capillary leak, loss of intravascular volume, poor peripheral vascular resistance, and hypotension.

Other Gram-Positive Bacteria (Enterococci, Viridans Streptococci, Clostridium)

Enterococci possess several virulence factors. Perhaps the most important in the ICU setting is antimicrobial resistance, which contributes greatly to the appearance of infection in the context of broad-spectrum antibiotic coverage. Other factors that lead to this virulence are an adhesion-promoting surface carbohydrate and a hemolysin-bacteriocin that lyse human erythrocytes. Some viridans group streptococci, *S. mutans, S. sanguis, S. mitis,* and *S. bovis,* produce extracellular dextran. The dextran both promotes adherence to the heart valves and makes the organism somewhat resistant to penicillin. *S. mutans* also produces extracellular glucan, which mediates adherence to dental enamel and accounts for its role in dental caries. Viridans group streptococci do not possess the vast array of virulence factors that other streptococci contain, which accounts for the relatively low potential for these organisms to cause an infection in a healthy person. Clostridium species produce a large number of exotoxins and other virulence factors. In fact, *Clostridium perfringens* produces 12 recognized toxins. In the context of myonecrosis, the α toxin of *C. perfringens* possesses phospholipase and sphingomyelinase activity that is critical for the development of gas gangrene.

Meningococcemia

For *N. meningitidis* to cause disease, the organism must first colonize the epithelial cells. An immunoglobulin A1 protease active against human immunoglobulin A1 plays an important role in enhancing colonization. The capsular polysaccharide impairs phagocytosis and promotes dissemination.

Meningococcal LPS is largely responsible for the induction of SIRS. Furthermore, meningococcal endotoxin is a potent inducer of the Shwartzman reaction and appears to account for the endothelial damage that results in a high rate of hemorrhagic skin lesions with meningococcemia. Complement-dependent bactericidal activity is of paramount importance in the prevention of disseminated disease. Therefore, individuals with complement deficiency, especially terminal complement components C5 through C8, and properdin deficiency are susceptible to chronic and recurrent invasive meningococcal disease. A family history of recurrent or chronic meningococcemia should raise the suspicion of these deficiencies. These individuals should receive meningococcal vaccine to induce high titers of antibodies, which will promote clearance by the reticuloendothelial system and reduce the risk of serious disease. Group B *N. meningitidis* is not as immunogenic as other strains due to expression of surface sialic acid, which has structural similarities to human intercellular adhesion molecules. As a consequence, group B *N. meningitidis* is not included in any of the current meningococcal vaccines and is particularly resistant to serum-mediated and phagocytic killing.

Haemophilus Influenzae Type b

As with *N. meningitidis*, Hib produces an immunoglobulin A1 protease that, along with the lipid A component (lipooligosaccharide) of Hib LPS, facilitates colonization. Translocation to the blood involves disruption of the endothelial barrier and loosening of the tight junctions, with bacterial migration to the subendothelial space. In the absence of specific antibody, the capsular polysaccharide of Hib provides resistance to the bactericidal activity of serum and interferes with phagocytosis, thus promoting dissemination. Hib is a more potent stimulator of intercellular adhesion molecule-1 and IL-8 than of IL-1 and TNF-α.

Pseudomonas Species

As pseudomonas requires minimal nutritional support and possesses intrinsic resistance to many antibiotics, it is well suited to proliferate in environments that put selective pressure on competing flora, especially those moist environments in the healthcare setting in which broad-spectrum antibiotics are administered. Species other than *Pseudomonas aeruginosa* are being implicated in outbreaks, including *P. putida*, *P. fluorescens*, and *P. stutzeri*.

Pseudomonas produces a variety of virulence factors: exotoxins A, S, and U; elastase; alkaline protease; cytotoxins; phospholipase C; phenazines; and cell-bound organelles, such as pili, flagella, and membrane-bound LPS. The pili and flagella promote attachment, colonization, and invasion. Intravascularly, LPS triggers the cytokine pathway that causes sepsis. The wide variety of toxins is more important to local damage than in the development of systemic disease.

Fusobacterium, Salmonella, Yersinia, Vibrio Vulnificus

The invasiveness of *Fusobacterium necrophorum* in the context of Lemierre syndrome, also called postanginal sepsis, can be explained by the production of the proteolytic enzymes endotoxin, leukocidin, and hemagglutinin. Disruption of the mucosal barrier of the oropharynx leads to hypoxia and tissue destruction, which creates the oxygen-free environment required to maintain the low oxidation-reduction potential necessary for bacterial proliferation. Furthermore, the family to which *Fusobacterium* belongs has been associated with thromboembolic phenomena that are a consequence of the lipid A moiety of their LPS. The pathogenesis of postanginal sepsis then can best be understood in terms of the Virchow triad, specifically that damage to the endothelium of the internal jugular vein, alteration of normal blood, and blood hypercoagulability lead to vascular thrombosis. The anatomy of the lateral pharyngeal space allows invasion of the internal jugular vein either by direct extension or by lymphatic or hematogenous spread from the peritonsillar vessels.

Salmonella initially access the submucosal space via adherence and invasion of specialized epithelial cells. The bacteria can survive and proliferate in the macrophages of Peyer patches and then spread to the bloodstream, resulting in production of a heat-labile, cholera-like enterotoxin that stimulates cAMP and causes the efflux of electrolytes and water into the gut lumen. Multiple genes code for virulence factors involved in this process. The Vi antigen of some serotypes interferes with C3 binding, whereas other strains have virulence factors that prevent the formation and fusion of the C5b-9 membrane attack complex. All *Yersinia* share some common virulence factors that are outer-membrane proteins that facilitate adherence and invasion of the organism to the gut mucosa, platelet aggregation, blockade of phagocytosis, and impairment of complement-mediated killing. Expression of the virulence genes is affected by environmental conditions such as temperature. Once the organism has invaded, *Yersinia* localizes in lymphoid tissue in the gut and regional lymph nodes and in extraintestinal sites such as the liver, spleen, and meninges. *Y. enterocolitica* is a sideorophoric organism; therefore, iron-overload conditions, such as liver disease, hemochromatosis, and thalassemias, have been associated with an increased risk of invasive yersiniosis.

Virulence of *Vibrio vulnificus* has been associated with the presence of a polysaccharide capsule. *V. vulnificus* also contains LPS, but it is not a strong trigger for release of cytokines associated with sepsis syndrome despite the fact that the capsular polysaccharide may provoke cytokine release. Bradykinin may play a role in dissemination, which may be inhibited by a bradykinin antagonist. The organism requires iron for growth, which may account for the clear increase in susceptibility of patients with hemochromatosis to serious infections with this organism.

Rocky Mountain Spotted Fever

Virulence in *R. rickettsii* can vary strikingly from strain to strain and is affected by the feeding status of the tick, inoculum, and host factors. Once the organism has been introduced into the bloodstream by the tick, it attaches to endothelial cells and invades the cytosol, where it reproduces and ultimately exits the cell. The damage to the endothelial cell is mediated by a variety of proteins. The end result of endothelial damage is accumulation of inflammatory cells, leading to a lymphohistiocytic vasculitis, which progresses to hemorrhage, edema, widespread organ dysfunction, and shock.

Ehrlichia

Clear understanding of the pathophysiology of *Ehrlichia* infections has not been described. The limited knowledge that we have comes from a handful of postmortem specimens. The organism infects specific lymphocytes and may lead to their death.

Infected lymphocytes can be seen in perivascular inflammatory infiltrates, but *Ehrlichia* does not cause the endothelial damage or the vasculitis associated with other Rickettsial species.

Other Bacteria

While most adult infections with *Listeria monocytogenes* occur after ingestion, infants are infected after transplacental spread from a bacteremic mother. The organism directly enters cells by means of specific cellular proteins. Listeriolysin O, a major virulence factor, allows the microbe to escape from the phagosome and avoid intracellular killing. Once intracellular, *L. monocytogenes* can utilize the actin-based cellular contractile mechanism for moving from cell to cell without exposing itself to the extracellular environment, thus evading the immune response. *L. monocytogenes* is also a siderophore, and increased susceptibility to infection can be seen in hemochromatosis and transfusion-induced iron overload.

Host Defense

The Innate and Adaptive Immune Systems

The interaction of host leukocytes with bacterial pathogens is essential for the mounting of an effective immune response to infection but is also responsible for many of the harmful clinical features associated with the sepsis syndrome. To understand the immunologic response in sepsis, one must first have an appreciation for the cell types involved in its generation and propagation. Immune cells can be divided into components of the innate or adaptive immune systems (see Chapter 72). Most innate immune cells (monocytes, macrophages, dendritic cells, natural killer cells, neutrophils) constitutively express receptors that are capable of sensing molecules that are frequently expressed by pathogenic organisms. These bacterial pathogen-associated molecular patterns (PAMPs) include ligands such as LPS, LTA, and peptidoglycan. The initiation of an innate immune response typically does not require the interaction of an innate immune cell with other leukocytes. Additionally, activation of an innate immune cell does not require previous exposure to a PAMP, or priming. Each exposure has the potential to result in a robust response, thus standing in contrast to the adaptive immune system, which responds to repeat exposures to the same antigen with increasing speed and vigor. PAMP recognition and subsequent activation of the inflammatory response occur via several groups of intracellular and extracellular receptors, the best characterized being the Toll-like receptors (TLRs) (2). This family, named for its homology to receptors important for fungal immunity in *Drosophila*, contains at least nine receptors that sense PAMPs expressed on a wide variety of pathogens (bacteria, viruses, fungi) (**Table 78.4**). These receptors can be found on the cell surface or within endosomes. Binding of a ligand to the TLR complex (the TLR itself plus costimulatory molecules found at or near the cell membrane) results in the initiation of a cascade of intracellular protein phosphorylation, ultimately resulting in the translocation of transcription factor nuclear factor (N)-κB to the nucleus, where transcription of proinflammatory gene elements is initiated. Cell surface receptors that are specific for mannose and the Fc portion of immunoglobulin are also frequently found on innate immune cells.

Another family of molecules has recently been described that is structurally similar to the TLRs; they contain leucine-rich repeat (LRR) regions thought to be important in PAMP binding, but are located in the intracellular compartment. Variously termed NLRs (NACHT-LRRs) (45) and CATERPILLARs (69), this family contains the NOD subfamily of intracellular receptors that are known to bind to diaminopimelic acid found in gram-negative bacteria (NOD1) and muramyl dipeptide seen in gram-positive species (NOD2). Ligation of these receptors is thought to promote assembly and activation of a cytoplasmic protein complex known as the *inflammasome*, which is important in the processing and release of proinflammatory cytokines and augmentation of signaling via the NFκB pathway, thus illustrating how innate immune cells can respond to pathogens that invade either the extracellular *or* intracellular space.

Activation of phagocytic innate immune cells results in enhancement of pathogen internalization and intracellular killing and in the release of cytokines and chemokines that modulate the inflammatory response. Another critical function of innate immune cells is to effect antigen presentation to elements of the adaptive immune system. After phagocytosis of a PAMP-expressing pathogen, cells such as macrophages and dendritic cells break down the foreign proteins and load the resulting peptides onto MHC molecules for subsequent display on the cell surface. They then migrate to lymphoid organs, where activation of the adaptive immune system takes place. Activated innate immune cells are also capable of producing proinflammatory cytokines, including TNF-α, IL-1β, IL-12, and IL-18. Interestingly, these cells can and do make anti-inflammatory cytokines as well. These molecules, including IL-10, transforming growth factor (TGF)-β, and IL-1 receptor antagonist, are frequently released by innate immune cells following a proinflammatory insult as a means to restore homeostasis. The role of IL-6 in this context is the subject of current investigation. IL-6 is made by immune cells and endothelium in response to proinflammatory stimuli and, in fact, is the cytokine whose levels are most correlated with adverse clinical outcome following an inflammatory insult. In vitro and in vivo evidence suggests that IL-6 may itself have anti-inflammatory properties, including induction of endogenous glucocorticoid production and promotion of an anti-inflammatory T-cell response. Imbalance between proinflammatory and anti-inflammatory forces has been clearly linked to adverse outcomes in the setting of human septic disease.

The adaptive immune system is composed of T and B lymphocytes. The initiation and propagation of an adaptive immune response is different from that of the innate immune system in several ways. First, each lymphocyte is programmed through gene rearrangement to respond to a distinct antigenic stimulus, in contrast to monocytes, for example, which are all capable of sensing LPS through their TLR4 receptor complexes. Second, the activation of lymphocytes typically requires assistance in the form of antigen presentation by innate immune cells. Third, the adaptive immune response is frequently characterized by the development of memory cells that are capable of generating a more rapid and robust antibody response upon repeat exposure to a given antigen. The relevance of the adaptive immune response to critical illness is highlighted by an association between apoptosis in lymphoid organs and sepsis mortality (34). Prolonged lymphopenia and apoptosis-associated depletion of lymphoid organs has also been demonstrated to be strongly associated with death from nosocomial sepsis in the

TABLE 78.4

TOLL-LIKE RECEPTORS AND THEIR LIGANDS

Receptor	Ligand	Origin of ligand
TLR1	Triacyl lipopeptides	Bacteria and mycobacteria
	Soluble factors	*Neisseria meningitidis*
TLR2	Lipoprotein/lipopeptides	Various pathogens
	Peptidoglycan	gram-positive bacteria
	Lipoteichoic acid	gram-positive bacteria
	Lipoarabinomannan	Mycobacteria
	Phenol-soluble modulin	*Staphylococcus epidermidis*
	Glycoinositolphospholipids	*Trypanosoma cruzi*
	Glycolipids	*Treponema maltophilum*
	Porins	*Neisseria meningitidis*
	Atypical lipopolysaccharide	*Leptospira interrogans*
	Atypical lipopolysaccharide	*Porphyromonas gingivalis*
	Zymosan	Fungi
	Heat-shock protein 70	Host
TLR3	Double-stranded RNA	Viruses
TLR4	Lipopolysaccharide	gram-negative bacteria
	Taxol	Plants
	Fusion protein	Respiratory syncytial virus
	Envelope protein	Mouse mammary-tumor virus
	Heat-shock protein 60	*Chlamydia pneumoniae*
	Heat-shock protein 70	Host
	Type III repeat extra domain A of fibronectin	Host
	Oligosaccharides of hyaluronic acid	Host
	Polysaccharide fragments of heparin sulphate	Host
	Fibrinogen	Host
TLR5	Flagellin	Bacteria
TLR6	Diacyl lipopeptides	*Mycoplasma*
	Lipoteichoic acid	gram-positive bacteria
	Zymosan	Fungi
TLR7	Imidazoquinoline	Synthetic compounds
	Loxoribine	Synthetic compounds
	Bropirimine	Synthetic compounds
	Single-stranded RNA	Viruses
TLR8	Imidazoquinoline	Synthetic compounds
	Single-stranded RNA	Viruses
TLR9	CpG-containing DNA	Bacteria and viruses
TLR10	ND	ND
TLR11	ND	Uropathogenic bacteria

From Akira S, Takeda K. Toll-like receptor signalling. *Nat Rev Immunol* 2004;4:499–511, with permission. ND, not determined

setting of pediatric multiorgan dysfunction syndrome (MODS) (22).

A detailed review of the immunobiology of T cells and antibody-producing B cells is beyond the scope of this chapter, but the role of T lymphocytes in the modulation of the immune response deserves mention. T cells can be generally thought of as belonging to one of two classes, CD4+ helper T cells (Th) and CD8+ cytotoxic T cells. Over the last decade, it has become clear that helper T cells can assume different phenotypes depending on the cytokine milieu in which their activation takes place. In the presence of proinflammatory mediators, naïve T cells typically develop into Th-1 cells, which promote the proinflammatory response through the production of cytokines such as interferon (IFN)-γ, IL-2, and granulocyte-macrophage colony-stimulating factor (GM-CSF). In the pres-

ence of anti-inflammatory mediators, T-cell differentiation is skewed toward the Th-2 phenotype. Th-2 cells elaborate cytokines, including IL-4, IL-10, and IL-13, which inhibit the innate immune response and promote the production of antibodies by B cells. Thus, similar to the innate immune system, the adaptive immune response must achieve a balance between proinflammation and anti-inflammation.

It is likely that many other groups of T cells contribute to the overall immune response, but the regulatory T cell (Treg) is a cell type that has been the subject of increasing interest. This subpopulation of CD4+ cells is present in both naturally occurring and inducible forms (13). Their cell surface markers are distinct from those expressed by Th-2 cells, but they share their ability to produce anti-inflammatory mediators. In fact, upon activation, Tregs produce copious amounts of IL-10 and TGF-β and are capable of downregulating both the innate and adaptive immune responses. Tregs may be resistant to sepsis-induced apoptosis and may potentiate a pathologic anti-inflammatory response in some patients.

Inflammatory Imbalance and the Sepsis Syndrome

In large part, it is the action of the immune system, not the bacteria themselves, that is responsible for morbidity and mortality from bacterial sepsis. When confined to a local region, the effects of proinflammatory cytokines, such as vasodilation and increased capillary permeability, are beneficial in that they allow for recruitment and activation of effector immune cells to eliminate infection. When the immune response is overly robust, these mediators spill over into the systemic circulation, resulting in the classic signs and symptoms of bacterial sepsis. Attenuation of this inflammatory response has been the target of numerous clinical trials in adult sepsis over the past two decades, almost all of which have demonstrated either no benefit or increased harm (see later discussion). The proinflammatory storm, although occurring predominantly early in the course of sepsis, frequently gives way to a potentially harmful compensatory anti-inflammatory immune response with impairment of innate immune function and increased levels of circulating IL-10. When profound and persistent, this state is referred to as *immunoparalysis* (Fig. 78.2) (see Chapter 75 for more detail).

Host Risk Factors

Genetic Predisposition

Many factors, both inherited and acquired, may influence an individual's susceptibility and response to an infectious process. An ever-growing body of literature suggests that the genetic composition of an individual influences the risk of developing sepsis and the outcome from that septic process (59). Perhaps this genetic predisposition was best demonstrated by analyzing death from infection in adopted children (64), where the death of a biologic parent before the age of 50 from an infectious etiology correlated with an over fourfold relative risk of premature death from an infectious etiology in the adoptee. No

such association was found between the risk of death due to infection in adopted children and their adoptive parents (64). Recently, a host of polymorphisms have been identified that code for inflammatory molecules and protein products essential for host defense (59), including polymorphisms for TNF-α, TNF-β, Fc-γ receptors, mannose-binding lectin, TLRs, IL-1, IL-1RA, IL-6, IL-10, plasminogen activator inhibitor (PAI)-1, and heat shock proteins (59). Current work is attempting to identify associations between these polymorphisms and sepsis severity.

The assessment of TNF-α polymorphisms and infectious processes is illustrative of this line of investigation. Studies have demonstrated a strong association between the TNF-α polymorphisms, TNF-α production, and the clinical presentation and/or outcome for a variety of infectious diseases, with the less common A allele at the TNF-α-308 found more frequently in those who died (47). The same allele was also associated with death in children with meningococcal disease (49). It should be noted that not all studies have demonstrated an association between these polymorphisms and clinical outcomes. In fact, of the 10 studies that evaluate the TNF-α-308 polymorphism for its association with mortality from sepsis, 4 found a positive association and 6 did not (59). These findings highlight many of the difficulties in assessing the role of polymorphisms in a complex, multifactorial process. Functional phenotypic assessment of candidate polymorphisms remains controversial because the same variant not infrequently has very different effects in different populations (42). Moreover, the traditional approach of case-control designs is limited by the potential for confounding or spurious associations that result from correlation with the true risk factor and by the potential for population stratification (42). Therefore, any conclusions regarding associations between disease state and polymorphic alleles must be tempered until confirmed in additional populations by independent investigators. Despite these limitations, large-scale studies may be critical in developing a clear understanding of the genetic determinants of sepsis, particularly if attention is paid to the criteria necessary for conducting high-quality gene association studies (59).

Race/Ethnicity/Gender/Age Differences

Other factors, such as race, ethnicity, gender, and age may influence the incidence and outcomes from sepsis. Several large epidemiologic adult studies have demonstrated that blacks are more likely to be hospitalized for severe sepsis than are whites. Unfortunately, much less data are available on children, although among newborns, data suggest worse outcomes among blacks for a number of conditions, including sepsis. Moreover, the effect of gender on sepsis has been investigated. In a large, pediatric epidemiologic study of sepsis, males had a significantly higher incidence of severe sepsis than did females. This difference was largest among infants, present among 1–9 year olds, but not appreciated among children 10–18 years of age (74). This difference in incidence and outcomes among the sexes may be secondary to differences in the immune response. Data suggest that both humoral and cell-mediated immune responses to antigen challenge are enhanced in females as compared to males. Numerous studies also support the view that hormones of the endocrine system, including different concentrations of sex steroids, contribute to the difference in immunologic response among the sexes. Moreover, age clearly

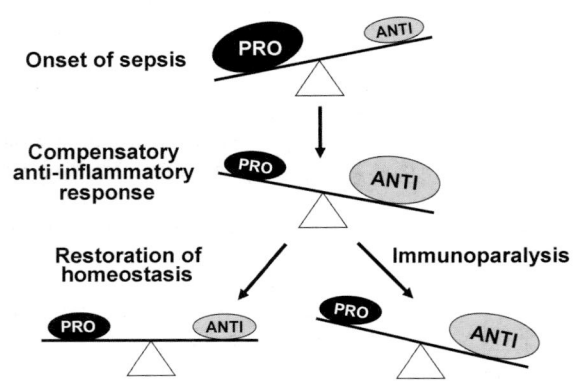

FIGURE 78.2. The balance between proinflammatory and anti-inflammatory mediators frequents shifts from a proinflammatory state to a compensatory anti-inflammatory response in the first days following the onset of sepsis. If persistent, this dominance of the anti-inflammatory response is pathologic and is termed immunoparalysis.

TABLE 78.5

ANNUAL INCIDENCE, CASE FATALITY, AND NATIONAL ESTIMATES OF SEVERE SEPSIS BY AGE

Age	Incidence (per 1,000) population)	National estimate of cases	Case fatality (%)	National estimate of deaths
<1 year	5.16	20,145	10.6	2135
0–28 days	3.60	14,049	10.3	1361
29–364 days	1.56	6096	13.5	774
1–4 years	0.49	7583	10.4	786
5–9 years	0.22	4168	9.9	413
10–14 years	0.20	3836	9.6	368
15–19 years	0.37	6633	9.7	644
All children	0.56	42,364	10.3	4383

From Watson RS, Carcillo JA, Linde-Zwirble WT, et al. The epidemiology of severe sepsis in children in the United States. *Am J Respir Crit Care Med* 2003;167:695–701, with permission.

influences the incidence and outcome of sepsis, even among pediatric subgroups (74) (**Table 78.5**).

Comorbidities

The presence of a comorbidity predisposes significantly to both the incidence and outcome of pediatric sepsis. Nearly half of all children with severe sepsis have an underlying comorbidity; the most common being neuromuscular, cardiovascular, and respiratory disorders (74). The most common neuromuscular conditions appear to be seizure disorders, cerebral palsy, and developmental abnormalities. Septic children with a comorbid condition also have higher hospital mortality rates than children who do not have such a coexisting condition. Children with neoplastic disease account for the greatest number of sepsis-related deaths among all children and have the highest case fatality rate among children <1 year of age. Among older children, cardiovascular conditions have the highest case fatality rate of all comorbid conditions. In addition, the risk of death from sepsis increases with increasing numbers of organ dysfunction.

Environmental Risk Factors

Any device that breaches the skin barrier and remains in place creates the potential for contamination of the device and subsequent bacteremia. Most endemic transmission follows the route of nose to hand to device from either the patient or the healthcare worker.

Central Venous Lines

The widespread but often necessary use of indwelling central venous catheters in the ICU lends itself to a large number of nosocomial bloodstream infections. Gram-positive bacteria, largely *Staphylococcus*, are usually present on the patient's skin before placement of the device. In contrast, healthcare workers introduce gram-negative organisms present on their hands during manipulation of IV devices. More than half of all catheter-related infections are due to *S. aureus* and coagulase-negative *Staphylococcus* (77). Gram-negative organisms (*E. coli*,

Klebsiella spp., *Pseudomonas* spp., *Enterobacter* spp., *Serratia* spp., and *Acinetobacter*) account for another 21%; enterococcus accounts for 9%, and *Candida* accounts for 6%. Factors associated with an increased risk for catheter-related infection include the very young, the chronically ill, and those with poor nutritional status, loss of skin integrity, and neutropenia.

Urosepsis

Virtually all closed-system urinary catheters are colonized by 7 days after placement, and open systems are colonized much sooner. Although pyelonephritis and secondary sepsis can occur, isolated episodes of cystitis are far more common. Organisms can contaminate the catheter at placement by ascending between the urethral wall and the outside of the catheter or through the internal lumen. Higher rates of infection are associated with diarrhea, low urine flow, and urinary stasis. The most common bacteria associated with infection are *E. coli*, other gram-negative bacilli, *Enterococcus*, and *Candida*.

Surgical Site Infections

Surgical-site infections are the third most commonly reported infection, accounting for ~15% of all infections. Risk factors for these infections include: contaminated procedure, surgery longer than 2 hrs, abdominal or thoracic procedure, and presence of ≥3 discharge diagnoses. *S. aureus* and coagulase-negative *Staphylococcus* account for 37% of pediatric surgical-site infections, but gram-negative organisms are becoming more prominent (72).

Osteomyelitis

Contiguous or nonhematogenous osteomyelitis is uncommon in children. The most common cause is an open fracture, but facial infections, implanted devices, and chronic open ulcers are also associated with contiguous osteomyelitis. *S. aureus* is the typical pathogen, but enteric gram-negative organisms and anaerobic bacteria reflect the environmental contamination on exposed bone. Bone biopsy with culture is the correct method of diagnosis.

Endocarditis

Right-sided endocarditis is being diagnosed more often with the increased use of indwelling venous catheters. Endocarditis that occurs within 2 months of surgery (early postoperative endocarditis) develops as a consequence of thrombi forming at sites of denuded endothelium and exposed sutures. These sites can become infected with bacteria introduced via the bypass pump, from a surgical wound infection, secondary to a catheter-associated infection, or from an exposed pacemaker wire. Data reporting early postoperative endocarditis reveal that *S. aureus* and coagulase-negative *Staphylococcus* account for approximately half of the infections, with one-fifth of the infections due to gram-negative bacilli. Fungi are becoming increasingly important.

Hemodialysis

Arteriovenous catheters used in hemodialysis are at risk for contamination and infection with each episode of dialysis. *S. aureus* causes most of the infections of dialysis grafts, which can lead to bacteremia, sepsis, and death. Measures taken to lessen the risk of infection, including topical and systemic antibiotics, have met with some success, although routine weekly

ENVIRONMENTAL CONDITIONS THAT PREDISPOSE THE HOST TO SPECIFIC BACTERIA

Organism	Environmental source
Listeria monocytogenes	Food, especially dairy and pork products
E. faecium	Commercial chicken and meat products
Clostridium perfringens	Soil
Salmonella	Poultry, pork, beef, egg, and dairy products
Yersinia	Pork, chitterlings (pork intestines) and dairy products
Vibrio vulnificus	Seawater and undercooked seafood (clams, oysters, and mussels)

dosing of an antibiotic presents concern for increasing the risk of an antibiotic-resistant infection.

Other Environmental Risk Factors

Some bacteria associated with sepsis are linked to exposure to specific environmental sources (**Table 78.6**). Identifying a source can be difficult but is important in preventing other cases.

Bacterial Pathogenesis

Translocation

The gastrointestinal tract is a complex system, the primary function of which is the digestion and absorption of nutrients. However, in addition to this function, the intestinal tract must also serve as a barrier to prevent the spread of intraluminal bacteria and endotoxin to other organs of the body (43). In critically ill patients, increased intestinal permeability has been demonstrated in a number of settings, leading to translocation of the bacteria of the intestinal lumen, as well as their toxins, into the bloodstream. The normal intestinal physiologic barrier is primarily maintained by the mechanical cell barrier that is created by tight intercellular junctions and the normal microbial flora (17). Alterations in the components of the intestinal barrier may result in bacterial and toxin translocation. In sepsis and other critical illnesses, the intestinal mucosa requires increased oxygen secondary to an elevated metabolic rate (17). However, these clinical conditions are also often characterized by splanchnic hypoperfusion and a reduction in oxygen delivery. This imbalance of oxygen requirements and availability results in anaerobic glycolysis and intracellular acidosis, which promote increased intestinal mucosa permeability. Moreover, the injury to the mucosa caused by ischemia may be exacerbated by reperfusion, with increased formation of reactive oxygen species, which may result in further intestinal injury and increased intestinal permeability (17). Given the fact that the distal small bowel and colon contain massive amounts of bacteria and endotoxin (10^{10} anaerobes, and 10^5–10^8 each of gram-positive, gram-negative aerobic, and facultative microorganisms per gram of tissue), it is plausible that increased gut permeability results in bacterial transloca-

tion into the bloodstream. This theory is supported by animal models, in which the passage of bacteria from the intestinal lumen to the systemic circulation has been conclusively demonstrated (17).

The human data for translocation are less definitive. First, clinical studies have demonstrated that bacteria isolated from patients with systemic infections are often of the same strain as bacteria predominantly present in the fecal flora. Another more direct method used to document bacterial translocation in humans in a variety of clinical conditions is the assessment of mesenteric lymph node cultures. Surgical reports have demonstrated (by culture of intestinal serosa and mesenteric lymph nodes) bacterial translocation in 10%–15% of patients who undergo surgery, with postoperative sepsis occurring two to three times more commonly in patients with translocation. Two other lines of evidence have been offered in support of the concept of bacterial translocation. First, data suggest that the risk of infectious complications caused by enteric bacteria is higher among patients with clinical conditions associated with splanchnic hypoperfusion and ischemia-reperfusion of the intestine. Second, the incidence of infectious complications and overall prognosis in critically ill patients may be reduced by the administration of antibiotics for selective gut decontamination and other therapeutic measures directed at intestinal dysfunction (17). Alternatively, a body of evidence questions the significance of bacterial translocation in humans. Increased intestinal permeability in a variety of clinical settings has not demonstrated a relationship with disease severity or sepsis, and simultaneous culturing of portal vein and systemic blood found very little correlation. Animal modeling has also supported the argument against bacterial translocation, in that systemic injection of the quantity and species of translocated bacteria into healthy or stressed animals results in little systemic inflammation, no organ failure, and complete recovery (3). However, whether this condition can be compared to the status of a critically ill child is unknown.

Thus, the role of bacterial translocation in sepsis requires further clarification. Clearly, data suggest that critical illness is associated with loss of intestinal integrity, which appears to be associated with the sepsis syndrome and poor outcomes. Nevertheless, dissimilar findings by other investigators have prompted a re-evaluation of the theory of intestinal bacterial translocation. Recent theories have been offered that may unify these seemingly disparate findings (18). It has been suggested that splanchnic hypoperfusion and other insults that cause intestinal mucosal injury and promote bacterial translocation may be able to induce an intestinal inflammatory response, even when the translocated bacteria are destroyed by the immunologic and nonimmunologic cells of the intestine. Shock, trauma, or sepsis-induced intestinal injury may promote cytokine generation from the intestines, and the mesenteric microcirculation may serve as a priming bed for circulating neutrophils (18). It has been suggested that the intestinal lymphatics are the major route by which intestinal-derived proinflammatory or toxic factors reach the systemic circulation (18). This theory is supported by several lines of evidence. First, animal data suggest that the mesenteric lymph nodes are the first and, often, only tissue to contain translocating bacteria. Second, higher levels of endotoxin are detected in the thoracic duct as compared to the portal vein; portal vein endotoxin levels do not exceed the postulated endotoxin-filtrating capacity of the liver, and elevated levels of endotoxin are identified in the thoracic duct before their subsequent detection in the portal circulation (17,18). Moreover, in a model of hemorrhagic shock, increases in lung permeability and alveolar apoptosis were prevented by dividing the major lymph duct exiting the gut (18). These findings, not extensively studied in humans, support the role of lymphatic transport in the development of systemic endotoxemia.

In summary, bacterial translocation, once believed to be the simple movement of bacteria and toxins across the lining of the intestines into the systemic circulation secondary to increased intestinal permeability, is now known to be a much more complex process. Although the exact mechanisms remain unclear, it appears that splanchnic hypoperfusion and intestinal injury can result in the gut becoming a cytokine-generating organ. These nonbacterial, inflammatory mediators then access distant organ systems via mesenteric lymphatics, rather than the portal circulation. Additionally, injury to intestinal mucosa results in the production of mediators that are capable of activating systemic neutrophils. This cascade of proinflammatory events results in SIRS. Clearly, further study is indicated to better understand the relationship between splanchnic hypoperfusion, increased intestinal permeability, intestinal injury, sepsis, and MODS.

Selective Decontamination

Selective decontamination, aimed at minimizing the risk of nosocomial infection, involves the use of oral nonabsorbable and systemic antibiotics to eliminate potentially pathogenic, aerobic bacteria from the oropharynx, stomach, and intestines, while at the same time causing minimal effect on indigenous anaerobic flora (17). In this way, potentially pathogenic bacteria that may be colonizing the gastrointestinal tract are eradicated, while the indigenous flora remain, which provides further protection against secondary colonization. Although its efficacy remains controversial, meta-analyses have demonstrated a decrease in nosocomial respiratory infections after selective decontamination. The impact on nosocomial bacteremia and mortality is less well established. Data suggest that the combination of oral and systemic antibiotics is more effective. Limited data from critically ill children suggest that selective decontamination may lead to fewer nosocomial infections. In specific, high-risk populations, selective decontamination may be of greater benefit.

Physiology and Pathophysiology of Sepsis

Host Factors

A detailed discussion of the physiologic host responses to bacteria is beyond the scope of this review. In this section, we will examine the downstream signaling processes that differentiate gram-negative from gram-positive sepsis. Evidence suggests that, in gram-negative infections, it is the monocyte-macrophage that first responds to endotoxin (51). Endotoxin first binds to LPS-binding protein, an acute-phase protein produced by the liver. The endotoxin-LPS-binding protein complex acts as the ligand for CD14 (a cell-surface receptor on mononuclear cells), and signal transduction results in monocyte/macrophage activation, leading to cytokine release. It has become clear that gram-positive processing is more complex. Several human proteins have the ability to bind endotoxin, which is "shuttled" between them and CD14. It appears

that the CD14 mechanism is not limited to endotoxin-LPS-binding protein but that it is a pattern-recognition molecule that can also respond to components of the gram-positive bacterial cell wall, such as peptidoglycan and LTA. Less is known about signal-transduction pathways after activation of CD14, but data suggest that staphylococcal peptidoglycan and LPS produce different patterns of protein kinase [extracellular receptor kinase (ERK), p38, and c-Jun kinase (JNK)] activation. Thus, recognition of a variety of microbial components by CD14 initiates a different pattern of intracellular transcription factors from gram-positive and gram-negative organisms.

Chemokine Activation

The activation of monocytes by gram-positive components leads to the production of the proinflammatory cytokines, particularly TNF-α and IL-1, and then to other mediator cascades, including the complement and coagulation pathways, inflammatory prostanoids, and production of reactive oxygen intermediates. Both gram-positive and gram-negative microbial components bind to pattern recognition receptors such as the TLRs. The ways in which gram-positive and gram-negative organisms initiate this process subtly differ. Whereas LPS in combination with LPS binding protein interacts with CD14 and the trimolecular complex binds with TLR4, LTA interacts with TLR-2 (14). The result of this binding is usually the activation of several intracellular pathways that lead to the activation of transcription proteins (e.g., NF$\kappa\beta$ and activator protein-1) that are implicated in the expression of widespread effector molecules such as cytokines. Proinflammatory molecules such as interleukins and TNF-α seek to eradicate invading microorganisms by stimulating inflammation, accomplished by orchestrating cellular and humoral responses that lead to increasing vascular permeability, increasing adherence to endothelium, and exerting chemotactic effects, all of which encourage migration of leukocytes to the primary site of infection. In addition, cytokines stimulate the proliferation of B- and T-cell lymphocytes. Most attention has focused on the ability of these bacteria to cause cytokine release, with IL-8 being the most abundant cytokine produced in response to the exotoxins, and endotoxin being most active in inducing IL-1, IL-6, and TNF-α. Although in vitro studies show clear differences in cytokine responses, they do not necessarily reflect what happens in the more complex situation of an intact host. Animal models of gram-positive infection present a more varied picture. IV injection of S. epidermidis produced a shock-like state and a cytokine response similar to that seen with gram-negative bacteremia, although considerably larger inocula were associated with the gram-positive organism.

Perhaps surprisingly, few data compare cytokine levels in septic patients with gram-positive or gram-negative infections. Some small studies found no apparent differences. In contrast, larger analyses note that patients with gram-negative sepsis tend to have higher TNF-α and IL-6 levels (51). Also, clinical trials of various antimediators have shown that responses differ on exposure to interventions between gram-positive and gram-negative organisms. More research is required to study the qualitative and quantitative differences between the two types of bacteria in the responses to antichemokine adjunct. In the future, knowledge of the causative agent may help optimize antimediator therapy.

Differential Responsiveness to Anti-Inflammatory Agents

Many clinical trials in patients with severe sepsis have been undertaken with anticytokine and other anti-inflammatory treatment strategies. These trials have been predicated on the hypothesis that SIRS is deleterious in sepsis and that blockade of the critical mediators of sepsis would improve clinical outcome. It was assumed that gram-positive-induced and gram-negative-induced SIRS were similar. Therefore, therapeutic strategies directed toward the host inflammatory response should equally benefit septic patients, regardless of the causative organism. This central hypothesis on which anti-inflammatory therapy for sepsis is based is an attractive concept of "a single bullet that hits all" because the identity of the causative organism is frequently not known at the onset of sepsis. Some clinical responses present compelling evidence of the differential responses of human subjects based on the etiology of the organisms. The most remarkable demonstration of the potential differential effects of anticytokine therapy in septic patients is the study of soluble type II (p75) TNF receptor:Fc fusion protein. In a phase II clinical trial of septic shock, a statistically significant worsening of outcome was observed in patients with gram-positive sepsis (23). Although these disturbing results have several potential explanations, the detrimental effects of treatment were not seen in patients with documented gram-negative infections. This variation in outcome was not observed with the type I (p55) soluble TNF receptor:immunoglobulin molecule; treatment appeared to benefit patients with both gram-positive and gram-negative sepsis (1). Because the anti-inflammatory agents in these trials were similar in structure and immunologic action, the explanation for this difference is not clear. It may be explained by the differential binding characteristics of the two TNF receptors (p55 and p75) for the TNF-α ligand in the systemic circulation (1,23). Favorable trends in survival have been observed in a variety of clinical trials of sepsis with anti-inflammatory agents. The potential differences in responsiveness to antimediator strategies between gram-positive and gram-negative sepsis are depicted in **Figure 78.3.** Anti-inflammatory agents for sepsis generally appeared to benefit patients with gram-negative organisms as the cause of sepsis, which is not surprising, as the laboratory research behind the development of clinical trials has often focused on using LPS or gram-negative organisms as the research tool. The therapies that have evolved as a result of these investigations will benefit gram-negative sepsis. This finding is less consistent with anti-TNF strategies than with other anti-inflammatory agents.

Two-hit Theory

Components from gram-positive organisms may potentiate a deleterious immune response initiated by gram-negative organisms or vice versa, which leads to the possibility of a "two-hit" phenomenon of one agent priming the host to have an amplified response to infection and, hence, a worse outcome. In animal models, SAgs and LPS very efficiently synergize in the induction of lethal shock, and synergism between peptidoglycan and LPS

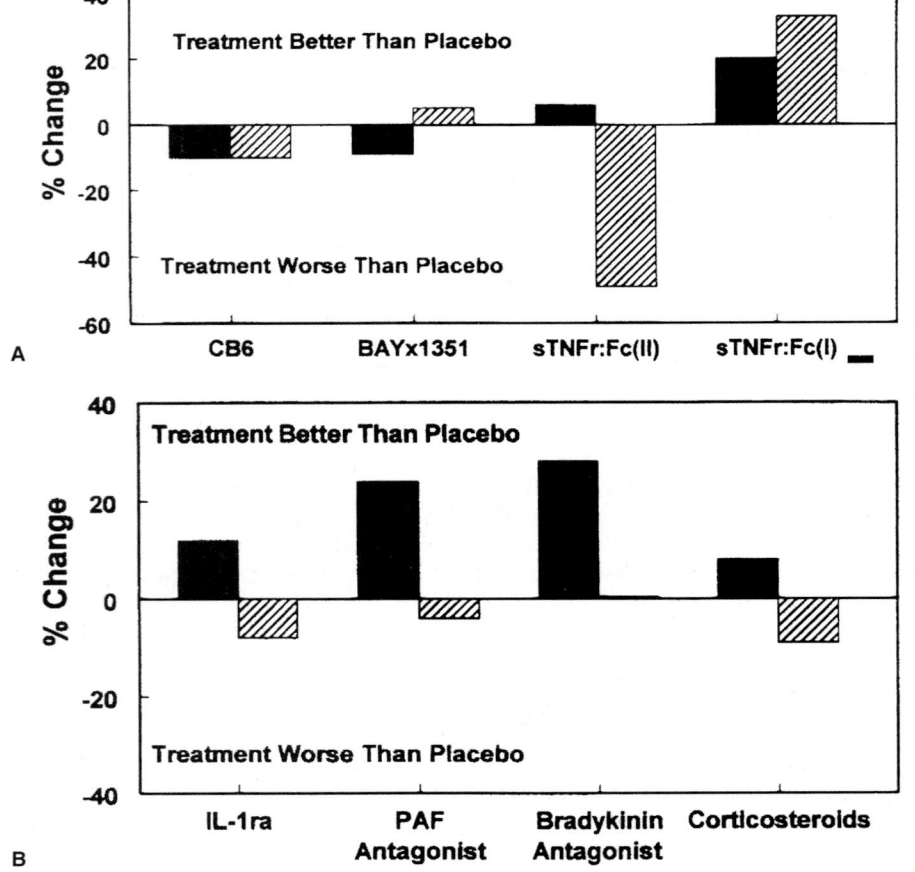

FIGURE 78.3. A: The difference in mortality between placebo and highest-dose treatment groups in sepsis trials with anti-TNF agents based on the type of infecting microorganism. CB6, anti-TNF murine monoclonal antibody; BAYx1351, anti-TNF murine monoclonal antibody sTNFr:Fc(II), soluble TNF receptor type II Fc fusion protein sTNFr:Fc(I), soluble TNF receptor type I Fc fusion protein: *solid bars*, gram-negative pathogens; *hatched bars*, gram-positive pathogens. **B:** The difference in mortality between placebo and highest-dose treatment groups in sepsis trials with anti-inflammatory agents based on the type of infecting microorganism. IL-1ra, IL-1 receptor antagonist; PAF, platelet-activating factor bradykinin antagonist, deltibant (CP 0127) corticosteroids, steroids. *Solid bars,* gram-negative pathogens; *hatched bars,* gram-positive pathogens. From Opal SM, Cohen J. Clinical gram-positive sepsis: Does it fundamentally differ from gram-negative bacterial sepsis? *Crit Care Med* 1999;27:1608–16, with permission.

leads to increased mortality and MODS. This synergism may partly explain (a) the high mortality associated with mixed bacterial infections, and (b) the deleterious effects of translocation of bacteria or their cell-wall components from the gut lumen in patients with sepsis. However, it has not been proven that this is a relevant model of human sepsis or gut translocation leading to a new infection.

Cellular Pathophysiology of Septic Shock

Shock is defined as a state of inadequate perfusion and oxygenation of the body and its organs. The cytochemical disruption of the endothelium is responsible for most of the cardiovascular manifestation of sepsis. The endothelium is a thin layer of flat cells that form the interface between circulating blood and tissue. Endothelial cells line the interior surface of the entire circulatory system and are responsible for a variety of physiologic responses that include the control of the vasodilatation, vasoconstriction, and coagulation pathways. The invading microorganisms and/or toxins activate signaling pathways that involve both humoral and cellular components. These cytokines and cells interact with the endothelium, which then becomes the tissue mediator and executor of the systemic response to the invading organism. The entire response is actually directed toward protection of the body from the invading microbe, but its overt nature leads to tissue damage both generally as a "bystander phenomenon" and specifically as receptor-targeted injury. The first cells to come in contact with bacterial components once they gain entry into the vasculature are white blood cells. The activation of cells such as neutrophils and macrophages is thought to be among the earliest steps in sepsis. The result of this activation leads to the increased production of enzymes such as phospholipase 2, and neutrophils from septic patients have increased phospholipase 2 activity. Phospholipase converts membrane phospholipids to arachidonic acid and platelet-activating factor. The arachidonic acid is subsequently metabolized by the lipoxygenase pathway, leading to the production of more inflammatory molecules that cause further tissue damage and increase microvascular permeability. Sepsis involves the production of cytokines by the activation of neutrophils, monocytes, and microvascular endothelium. The damaged endothelium then activates both the procoagulant and anticoagulant pathways. This entire process involves the release of a wide variety of humoral and inflammatory mediators. The interaction of these different mediators with various target receptors leads to a microvascular injury that characterizes the increased vascular permeability.

Cellular Response

The macrophages are among the first cells to come in contact with the pathogen. Macrophages play a critical role in the inflammatory response subsequent to a microbial challenge. The excessive, unregulated, prolonged stimulation of the macrophage in conjunction with other active cells, such as the leukocyte and the endothelium, leads to the release of proinflammatory mediators such as TNF-α and IL-1. The neutrophils are the central effector cells that are responsible for the destruction of bacteria. Hence, they are capable of producing a wide variety of cytotoxic molecules which include proteases, cytokines, and toxic oxygen radicals (**Fig. 78.4**). In normal conditions, very little interaction occurs between the endothelium and the neutrophils. When activated systemically or in the presence of endothelial damage, they become me-

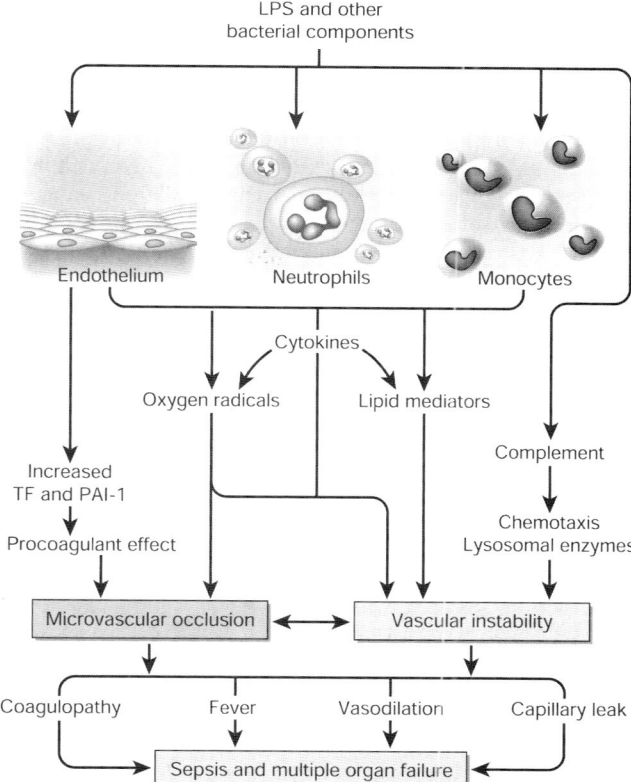

FIGURE 78.4. Pathogenic networks in shock. Lipopolysaccharide (LPS) and other microbial components simultaneously activate multiple parallel cascades that contribute to the pathophysiology of ARDS and shock. The combination of poor myocardial contractility, impaired peripheral vascular tone, and microvascular occlusion leads to tissue hypoperfusion and inadequate oxygenation and, thus, organ failure. From Cohen J. The immunopathogenesis of sepsis. *Nature* 2002;420:885–91, with permission.

diators of microvascular injury. Distinct phases occur during this process, which include rolling, firm adhesion, activation, aggregation, and migration through cell junction into tissue (70). In the latter phase of sepsis, neutrophil dysfunction has been noted, characterized by markedly depressed chemotaxis and altered neutrophil metabolic function and microbial killing activity, all of which render the neutrophils ineffective in defending against invading organisms. Occlusion of postcapillary venules causes relative tissue hypoxia, and proteases and oxygen radicals add to the endothelial damage, increasing vascular permeability.

Microvascular Changes

Endothelial dysfunction is a sentinel event in the pathogenesis of septic shock. The dysfunction is a result of injury that occurs due to production of oxygen free radicals, arachidonic acid metabolites, complement activation, platelet aggregation, and monocyte production of cytokines. In addition, the endothelium is capable of generating its own inflammatory mediators in a process known as "activation of the endothelium" (27), which involves a change from anticoagulant to procoagulant and the production of vasoactive substances such as NO along with adhesion molecules. These changes result in increased microvascular permeability, edema, and eventually, systemic hypotension from fluid losses. The production of NO, kinins, and vasoactive peptides leads to peripheral vasodilation, which causes decreased vascular resistance or "warm shock" (27).

Myocardial Dysfunction

Myocardial dysfunction, once considered a preterminal event, is common in sepsis (12,15). Human septic myocardium is characterized by reversible biventricular dilation, increased end-diastolic volume, decreased ejection fraction, and diminishing response to volume resuscitation and catecholamine resistance. Humoral factors, including TNF-α and IL-1β, in synergy with NO, are largely responsible for this phenomenon (15).

Metabolic Response

The clinical manifestation of sepsis and the ensuing organ failure are traditionally ascribed to the effect of inflammatory mediators that induce circulatory changes, with resulting tissue hypoxia and widespread cellular damage. However, this effect has not been completely proven to be the case, considering that histologic appearances of the failed organs are often normal, with minimal or no apoptosis or necrosis (33). Recognition of elevated mixed venous oxygen saturation (SvO$_2$) and a concurrent lactic acidosis in sepsis spawned the concept of altered oxygen supply dependency and a heavily promoted strategy of driving the circulation with fluids and high-dose inotropes to achieve "supranormal" levels of oxygen delivery and consumption. Outcomes were adverse when applied to critically ill patients with organ failure.

Septic shock includes signs of bioenergetic derangements, with increases in mixed venous oxygen saturation (SvO$_2$) and lactate. Because increasing severity of sepsis may be associated with a progressive fall in tissue oxygen consumption with a rise in tissue oxygen tension, the bioenergetic derangement is likely one of reduced cellular use of oxygen rather than tissue hypoxia. The SvO$_2$ reflects the balance between local oxygen supply and demand. The elevated values found in sepsis imply abnormally reduced cellular utilization of oxygen, thereby accounting for the elevation in SvO$_2$. It is now also appreciated that sepsis-induced lactic acidosis may arise from increased activity of muscle Na/K-ATPase pumps, rather than from anaerobic metabolism secondary to inadequate tissue perfusion (40). Skeletal muscle has been shown to be a leading source of lactate production through exaggerated aerobic glycolysis rather than through tissue hypoxia.

The mitochondria control the amount of oxygen consumed by the cells via the process of oxidative phosphorylation. Mitochondrial activity is controlled by numerous extrinsic factors, including levels of ATP, local partial pressure of oxygen, and reactive oxygen species. Numerous hormonal influences (e.g., thyroid hormones, leptin, catecholamines, and corticosteroids) also mediate their actions partly through influencing mitochondrial respiration. NO and its metabolite peroxynitrite are potent inhibitors of the electron transport chain, with variable duration of effects depending on the levels produced. Sepsis is the classic condition in which large amounts of NO are generated systemically. Indeed, numerous studies have confirmed an inhibitory effect of NO on mitochondria in both septic patients and in laboratory models that is probably responsible for the cellular inability to utilize oxygen. Apart from respiratory complex inhibition, physical damage to mitochondria occurs that varies across organs and depends on sepsis severity.

Immunoparalysis

Neutralization of proinflammatory cytokines, such as TNF-α and IL-1, decreases mortality in animal models of sepsis but not in humans. In contrast to animals, which succumb to shock during the first 72 hrs, many patients die much later, with signs of opportunistic infections accompanied by downregulation of their monocytic human leukocyte antigen (HLA)-DR expression and reduced ability to produce LPS-induced TNF-α (20). This phenomenon of monocyte deactivation in septic patients with fatal outcome shows similarities to experimental monocytic refractoriness induced by LPS desensitization. A study in pediatric patients confirmed this theory, in that children with MODS had significantly reduced HLA-DR expression (54) (**Fig. 78.5**). Decreased TNF-α activity is thought to lead to immunoparalysis, and blockade by drugs such as etanercept and infliximab, now being utilized in children with collagen vascular diseases and after transplantation, can create features of immunoparalysis and decreased TNF-α activity, which may account for an increased susceptibility to infections in these patients.

CLINICAL PRESENTATION AND DIFFERENTIAL DIAGNOSIS

Clinical Presentation

To effectively treat sepsis, it must be rapidly recognized by pediatric healthcare providers. A very high index of suspicion is

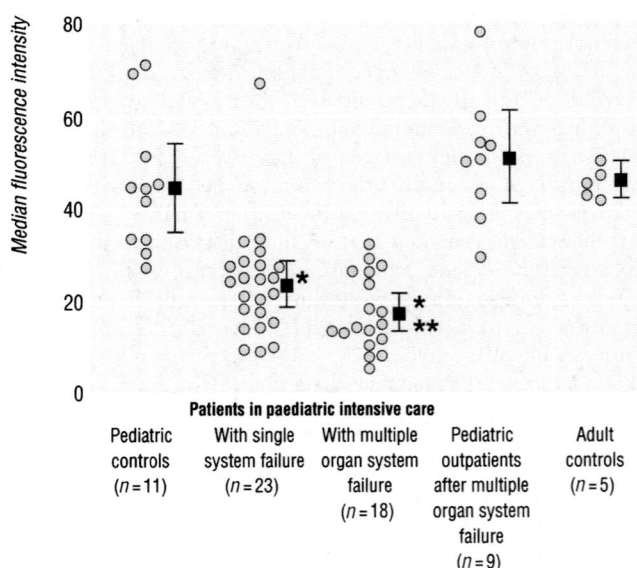

FIGURE 78.5. Median fluorescence intensity of monocyte HLA-DR expression in control pediatric outpatients, cases in PICU because of single- or multiple-organ system failure, pediatric patients receiving outpatient follow-up after multiple system failure, and healthy adults. Individual values and means with 95% confidence intervals (*bars*) are shown for each group (*p <0.05, analysis of variance v control groups). HLA-DR expression was also significantly lower in children with multiple-organ system failure than in those with single-system failure (**p <0.05). From Peters M, Petros A, Dixon G, et al. Acquired immunoparalysis in paediatric intensive care: Prospective observational study. *Br Med J* 1999;319:609–10, with permission.

required from the onset of symptoms, as the diagnosis of severe sepsis is a clinical one, made by signs of decreased tissue and organ perfusion on physical examination. The clinical presentation can vary widely, depending on many factors, including the timing of the infection, the organism responsible for the shock state, and the patient's previous state of health. The classic triad of clinical signs of sepsis that can be determined at any level of healthcare is change in temperature (either hyperthermia or hypothermia), tachypnea and tachycardia, and change in mental status. It is important to recognize the lack of hypotension in this triad. Children can have severe sepsis and septic shock without hypotension. The addition of basic laboratory parameters can help to confirm the diagnosis but are unnecessary at the initial stages of resuscitation.

Septic shock, most commonly a combination of distributive, hypovolemic, and cardiogenic shock, by definition, requires manifestations of decreased organ perfusion. Whereas a change in mental status is the most obvious symptom to note on a brief physical examination, other symptoms include decreased urine output, delayed capillary refill, or an increased base deficit, most likely representing an increased serum lactate. This decrease in organ perfusion leads to systemic symptoms that affect organs of the entire body. The cardiovascular response to severe infection will be reviewed in detail in the following section. The respiratory system usually is a source of buffering, with tachypnea leading to a respiratory alkalosis that is compensatory in nature in the face of metabolic acidosis. However, if the myocardial dysfunction and capillary leak that accompany bacterial sepsis are severe, pulmonary edema and acute respiratory distress syndrome (ARDS) may lead to an impairment of this compensatory mechanism. The central nervous system (CNS) may be affected by both changes in mental status (including both somnolence and agitation) and, if the decreased cerebral perfusion is severe, by seizures. Both the renal and hepatic systems are also injured by this decreased organ perfusion. Aside from oliguria or anuria, these organs are routinely monitored by laboratory parameters. Hematologic failure can occur either in the form of DIC or thrombocytopenia, which may cause purpura or petechiae. Peripheral perfusion can be determined by the examination of capillary refill, the presence of peripheral cyanosis or mottling, and weak or absent pulses. In the face of certain bacteria or toxins, dermatologic manifestations of infection are common, as discussed previously.

Hemodynamic Data

The hemodynamic alterations that can occur with bacterial sepsis are varied. As the ages of children cared for in the PICU range from newborns to young adults, children must be categorized to determine parameters that signify abnormal. Recent definitions published by the International Consensus Conference on Pediatric Sepsis (24) stratified children into the age groups listed in **Table 78.7**, based on defining categories of children that are clinically and physiologically meaningful (24). The use of these categories is essential in determining if a child meets certain definitions of sepsis. Variability in heart rate can be great, and most commonly is represented as tachycardia. However, bradycardia may signify severe infection, particularly in the neonatal period; bradycardia in older children usually signifies a near-terminal event. As stated, the presence of hypotension is not required for the diagnosis of sepsis or septic shock due to the fact the children, through multiple compensatory mechanisms, will maintain their blood pressure remarkably well until decompensation. Definitions of systemic hypotension, based on systolic blood pressure are also outlined in **Table 78.7** (24).

It is clear that sepsis in children is much different than in adults. While certain children, especially those in whom sepsis is recognized early in the course of infection, can present with the classic adult picture of "warm," vasodilated shock signified by an increase in cardiac output and a decrease in systemic vascular resistance, most children will present with "cold" shock, with an increase in systemic vascular resistance and a decrease in cardiac output, requiring inotropic support as opposed to a vasopressor. However, children often change during their course of sepsis, and therapies that may have been appropriate on one day of sepsis may not be beneficial, or may even be harmful, on another (12). Therefore, obtaining proper hemodynamic data, including those that presently can only be obtained with a pulmonary artery catheter (PAC), may be more important in pediatric sepsis due to its changing features. The importance of obtaining this information was eloquently demonstrated in children with fluid-refractory septic shock who had PACs placed. Numerous additions or changes in therapy occurred in this cohort based on the initial evaluation of cardiac index and systemic vascular resistance. Almost 20% of these children were receiving the wrong class of cardiovascular support altogether, and 36% needed the

TABLE 78.7

AGE-SPECIFIC VITAL SIGNS AND LABORATORY VARIABLES

Age group	Heart rate, beats/min		Respiratory rate, breaths/min	Leukocyte count, leukocytes × 10³/mm	Systolic blood pressure, mm Hg
	Tachycardia	Bradycardia			
0 days–1 wk	>180	<100	>50	>34	<65
1 wk–1 mo	>180	<100	>40	>19.5 or <5	<75
1 mo–1 yr	>180	<90	>34	>17.5 or <5	<100
2–5 yrs	>140	NA	>22	>15.5 or <6	<94
6–12 yrs	>130	NA	>18	>13.5 or <4.5	<105
13 to <18 yrs	>110	NA	>14	>11 or <4.5	<117

Lower values for heart rate, leukocyte count, and systolic blood pressure are for the 5th percentile, and upper values for heart rate, respiration rate, or leukocyte count for the 95th percentile. From Goldstein B, Giroir B, Randolph A; International Consensus Conference on Pediatric Sepsis. International pediatric sepsis consensus conference: Definitions for sepsis and organ dysfunction in pediatrics. *Pediatr Crit Care Med* 2005;6:2–8, with permission.

addition of a different class of cardiovascular therapy to reverse persistent septic shock (12).

Laboratory Abnormalities

Cytokine production causes a variety of abnormalities. A leukocytosis occurs due to demargination of polymorphonuclear cells (PMNs) and increased production and release of immature PMNs from the bone marrow. Neutropenia develops when the PMNs are consumed peripherally as they attach to endothelial cells and become ensnared in peripheral capillaries. Platelet count is likely to decrease early due to increased peripheral consumption and increase later as a result of reactive thrombocytosis. Proteins synthesized by the liver are variable. Acute-phase proteins, including C-reactive protein, amyloid, α_1-acid glycoprotein, haptoglobin, fibrinogen, ceruloplasmin, and α_1-antitrypsin, are produced in response to IL-1 and IL-6 stimulation. The levels of albumin, prealbumin, transferrin, and retinol-binding protein fall. As these factors are produced in proportion to the cytokine stimulation, they will mirror the intensity of the process. Due to uptake of iron and zinc by liver cells and inflammatory cells, serum levels fall, while copper levels increase in response to higher concentrations of ceruloplasmin. The low iron will manifest as a mild anemia that can be seen in individuals with considerable inflammation. Sepsis places considerable stress on the host. Accelerated use of energy sources leads to an increase in free fatty acids, hyperglycemia, and the catabolism of amino acids. Coagulation abnormalities are common. Fibrinogen, factor V, and factor VIII levels are decreased. Prothrombin time is prolonged in 50%–75% of patients with DIC, the partial thromboplastin time is prolonged in 50%–60% of cases, fibrin degradation products are present in most patients with DIC, and D-dimer is elevated in 90% of patients and is more specific than fibrin degradation products (8). The peripheral smear will demonstrate microangiopathic changes.

Differential Diagnosis

During the first 3 months of life, *E. coli* and *S. agalactiae* are the most common causes of sepsis, with the risk of *E. coli* declining each month. *L. monocytogenes* has a much lower incidence than the other two. Other agents to be considered include enterococcus, coliforms, and nontypable *H. influenzae*. Rarely, Hib and *S. pneumoniae* can also be seen in this age group. In the context of the PICU, *S. aureus* and *Pseudomonas* should be considered. Candidemia is common in premature infants but unusual in otherwise healthy infants. Viruses can also present in a fashion indistinguishable from a bacterial process in young infants, especially herpes simplex. Varicella, influenza, adenovirus, and respiratory syncytial virus can cause serious, life-threatening infections. In certain circumstances, a TORCH complex (toxoplasma, rubella, cytomegalovirus, and herpes simplex virus) agent should be considered. Rarely, SIRS can be seen with the intravascular infusion of lipids alone. In older, otherwise healthy children and adolescents, *S. pneumoniae* and *N. meningitidis* are the most commonly seen bacterial causes of sepsis, with Hib now quite rare. *Salmonella* species should be considered in the presence of significant diarrhea, and *S. aureus* or Group A streptococcus should be

considered in the presence of cellulitis, a skeletal infection, or indwelling catheter. *P. aeruginosa* should be suspected with erythema gangrenosum, and a variety of gram-negative bacilli can be isolated in the patient with impaired immunity. In patients with a history of a tick bite, Rocky Mountain spotted fever and *Ehrlichia* should be suspected. Certain foods are linked with pathogens (**Table 78.6**). Other unusual pathogens such as *Sphingomonas paucimobilis* are being seen more frequently. A child with acquired immune deficiency syndrome and disseminated *Mycobacterium avium* complex may develop sepsis syndrome. Abdominal catastrophes should raise the possibility of an anaerobic infection. Leptospirosis, brucellosis, and tularemia are rare and linked to specific exposures.

Fungal infections have become much more common as a cause for sepsis and are associated with a high mortality rate. In the immunocompromised patient, a variety of viral entities can present as a life-threatening infection, such as primary herpes simplex, disseminated varicella, and adenovirus. Rabies virus must be considered, especially if the patient had contact with a bat or raccoon. Bioterrorism has resurrected the threat of smallpox (see Chapter 30). Severe Kawasaki disease, Steven-Johnson syndrome, drug reactions, juvenile rheumatoid arthritis, pancreatitis, and systemic lupus erythematosus can all masquerade as sepsis. Other causes of SIRS include trauma, burns, and autoimmune disorders. Nothing can replace a thorough history and complete physical exam when looking for noninfectious causes of SIRS. Past problems and procedures, recent medications, travel, and potential exposures can all aid in the diagnosis. Children with neutropenia often manifest symptoms consistent with SIRS without being infected.

Diagnosis

The most important aspect of the evaluation of the patient with suspected sepsis is the procurement of adequate bacterial cultures from all possible, relevant sources—blood; cerebrospinal fluid (CSF, meningitis, and encephalitis); urine (urosepsis); stool (enteric fever); respiratory secretions and pleural fluid (pneumonia and empyema); skin lesions (cellulitis and abscesses); vaginal (toxic shock syndrome), synovial (arthritis and osteomyelitis), and peritoneal (ruptured viscus) fluid—preferably before the administration of antimicrobial agents. Care must be taken in the techniques used to obtain these cultures, as inappropriate collection and handling of specimens is a major cause of false-negative cultures. It is never appropriate to delay treatment of a critically ill child while waiting to obtain cultures. One blood culture set is rarely advisable or sufficient, two blood culture sets are usually adequate when bacteremia is due to a pathogen not likely to be a contaminant, three blood culture sets are usually adequate when a continuous bacteremia is suspected, and four blood culture sets are reasonable when the anticipated pathogen is likely to be a common contaminant such coagulase-negative staphylococci. However, the total volume is far more important than the number of cultures. More important is the appropriate dilution of blood to broth; the ideal is 1:5 dilution to decrease the effect of sodium polyanetholesulfonate, which inhibits phagocytosis and serum bactericidal activity but can also decrease the growth of some pathogens. The recommended amount of blood per culture for different age groups is as follows: 1–2 mL in neonates, 2–3 mL in infants, 3–5 mL in children, and 10–20 mL in adolescents. Viral cultures can yield significant information if obtained with the appropriate method and materials. Sites suitable for sampling include conjunctiva, nasopharynx, urethra, vagina, and vesicles or ulcers on skin and mucous membranes. Blood and CSF can be sent for viral culture, but results are usually disappointing and better detection methods are available. The one exception would be a blood culture for HIV in a newborn.

DNA amplification by polymerase chain reaction (PCR) is revolutionizing the diagnosis of infectious diseases. It is particularly useful in detecting herpes simplex infection of the CNS in newborns by examining CSF for viral DNA. Similarly, a PCR test is available for enterovirus in the CSF. This technology is helpful in diagnosing bacterial infections that take a long time to grow in culture, such as *Mycobacterium tuberculosis* and *Borrelia burgdorferi*, and in diagnosing rickettsial infections, in which treatment is needed acutely but antibodies may take weeks to develop in the serum. This is a field in which new assays will continue to be developed, and it holds the real possibility of changing microbiology labs forever.

CLINICAL MANAGEMENT/TREATMENT

Importance of Early Intervention

Early diagnosis and intervention in the treatment of bacterial sepsis is crucial to achieve optimal outcomes, particularly in high-risk patients who may not be able to mount an effective immune response. This population includes children with primary immunodeficiency, transplantation, malignancy, chemotherapy-induced leukopenia, and other secondary immunodeficiencies. While not necessarily immunosuppressed, children with other comorbidities, including chronic lung disease or congenital heart disease, may not be able to tolerate the cardiorespiratory derangements associated with sepsis. Accordingly, these special populations deserve close monitoring and consideration for early referral to a tertiary care center.

The first hours following the diagnosis of severe sepsis in any patient represent a unique opportunity for intervention to reverse shock and prevent organ dysfunction. Perhaps the best illustration of this principle is the report that demonstrated that fluid resuscitation with >40 mL/kg (average 60 mL/kg) in the first hour of treatment conferred a dramatic survival advantage to children with septic shock, compared to those who received less fluid in the same time frame (10). This notion of early and aggressive resuscitation was replicated in adults patients in whom goal-directed therapy on outcomes from severe sepsis and septic shock was examined (61). Another example of the timeliness of a therapy being related to its efficacy can be found in the use of antibiotics. While it should be made clear that administration of antibiotics should *in no way* take precedence over proper management of the airway, breathing, and circulation, recent evidence strongly suggests that the early use of appropriate empiric antimicrobial agents can significantly reduce morbidity and mortality from severe sepsis. While this may seem intuitive, debate continues regarding the use of empiric broad-spectrum antibiotics versus the concomitant desire to reduce patient exposure to broad-spectrum agents for fear of promoting antibiotic resistance. Numerous studies have

demonstrated reduced mortality when empiric antibiotic selection has ultimately been the correct therapeutic course in the settings of adult sepsis, pneumonia, intra-abdominal infection, and neonatal nosocomial bacteremia. It is now generally recommended that a de-escalating approach to the use of empiric antimicrobial agents be adopted, with broad-spectrum agents being transitioned to the narrowest possible spectrum drugs once culture and sensitivity data are known. Empiric antibiotic therapy must be tailored to provide coverage for community-acquired or nosocomial pathogens (for children who have been hospitalized for >48 hrs or who are at high risk for developing nosocomial infection), taking into account regional, hospital, and unit-specific resistance patterns.

Guidelines for Clinical Management

The American College of Critical Care Medicine (ACCM) published clinical practice parameters for hemodynamic support of pediatric and neonatal patients in septic shock in 2002 (11). This important document was based upon review of the medical evidence and consensus expert opinion and fulfills the essential role as the standardization of pediatric sepsis treatment. This section will serve as a review of these guidelines. The ACCM clinical practice parameters define shock by clinical parameters (hypothermia *or* hyperthermia, altered mental status, and abnormal peripheral vasodilation *or* vasoconstriction), hemodynamic variables (inadequate organ perfusion pressure), and oxygen-use measures (SvO_2). A detailed algorithm is provided that is notable for its rigorous time line (11). Within the first 5 mins of the diagnosis of shock, the child's airway and breathing should be maintained and IV access established. Continuous pulse oximetry, cardiorespiratory monitoring, urine output measurement, and frequent vital-sign assessment are necessary. Isotonic fluid boluses (normal saline or colloid) should be administered IV in 20 mL/kg aliquots up to and over 60 mL/kg in the next *15 mins*, while the patient is monitored for hypoglycemia and hypocalcemia if the shock state is not reversed. If shock persists despite the administration of 60 mL/kg of IV fluid, the authors recommend establishing arterial and central venous access and initiating therapy with a dopamine infusion. If the shock state is not reversed with a dopamine dose of 10 mcg/kg/min, it is recommended to transition to an epinephrine infusion in the setting of vasoconstrictive (cold) shock or norepinephrine for vasodilatory (warm) shock. The former is characterized by poor peripheral pulses, prolonged capillary refill, and diminished peripheral pulses compared to central pulses. Patients with warm shock demonstrate bounding peripheral pulses, erythematous skin, and instantaneous capillary refill. Children with septic shock, in contrast to adults, frequently present in cold shock with low cardiac output and high systemic vascular resistance, and children who present in warm shock often transition to cold shock over the first 48 hrs of illness (12). Thus, titration of inotropic or vasopressor support should be based upon frequent reassessment of the child's hemodynamic state.

Should either type of shock state be persistent despite adequate intravascular volume status and an appropriate inotrope or vasopressor regimen, the authors recommend consideration of the use of hydrocortisone for empiric treatment of adrenal insufficiency. This topic has been the source of controversy in the literature over the last decade. Use of highly potent glucocorticoids was associated with increased mortality in the setting of adult sepsis, but subsequent work suggested that a short course of low-dose hydrocortisone is associated with improved mortality and more rapid shock reversal in adult severe sepsis and septic shock (4,48), perhaps due to the fact that hydrocortisone has less glucocorticoid effect and more mineralocorticoid effect than drugs that were previously studied. Risk factors that favor the use of hydrocortisone include prior corticosteroid use, purpura fulminans, HIV infection, and chronic pituitary or adrenal abnormalities. A great deal of evidence suggests that a state of relative adrenal insufficiency can develop in the context of a severe inflammatory insult. It is postulated that this is due to inhibitory effects of high levels of proinflammatory cytokines at the hypothalamic, pituitary, adrenal, and target tissue levels. Specific definitions for the diagnosis and management of relative adrenal insufficiency continue to be ardently debated. Most authors agree that both a random cortisol level (which should be elevated in the shock state) and a cortisol level 1 hr post-ACTH stimulation should be obtained to optimally evaluate the adrenal axis. A random cortisol level <15–25 mcg/dL and/or a difference of ≤9 mcg/dL between pre- and post-ACTH stimulation are abnormal, but the association between these values and the efficacy of hydrocortisone replacement therapy remains unclear. In the ACCM guidelines, a random cortisol level of <18 mcg/dL with shock is consistent with adrenal insufficiency. The guidelines indicate that this point in the algorithm should be reached *within 60 mins* of the diagnosis of shock if it is not reversed with fluid and catecholamine therapy.

Should shock continue to be present in the second hour of resuscitation, the ACCM guidelines recommend therapies based upon the patient's clinical, hemodynamic, and oxygen-use phenotype. Patients with normal blood pressure who demonstrate cold shock and an Svo$_2$ of <70% should be treated with afterload reduction with careful attention to preservation of preload. Children who demonstrate low blood pressure, cold shock, and an Svo$_2$ of <70% should be treated with titration of epinephrine and ongoing optimization of volume status. Lastly, children who are hypotensive but are persistently vasodilated should undergo additional volume loading, with consideration given to the use of vasopressin as an adjunct vasoconstrictor. Should these maneuvers fail to reverse shock, the authors recommend placement of a PAC to direct ongoing therapy to maintain normal perfusion pressure and maintain the cardiac index between 3.3 and 6 L/min/m^2. For children with refractory shock a final recommendation is given to consider the use of extracorporeal membrane oxygenation (ECMO) as a rescue therapy for life-threatening septic shock. Numerous case series describe the successful use of this treatment for sepsis from organisms including meningococcus and Hantavirus, and survival rates with ECMO in the treatment of refractory pediatric septic shock have been reported to be as high as 50%.

Other Therapies for Acute Management of Sepsis

A number of treatments aimed at attenuating the inflammatory response during sepsis have been the subject of prospective research in humans as adjunctive therapy. Activated protein C (APC) is an endogenous molecule with antithrombotic, profibrinolytic, and anti-inflammatory properties. It was hypothesized that APC's ability to ameliorate microvascular thrombosis and blunt the inflammatory response would lead to improved survival and organ function in severe sepsis. The use of recombinant human (rh) APC has, in fact, been associated with a significant reduction in mortality in a specific subset of adults with severe sepsis in a large prospective, randomized, doubleblinded, placebo-controlled study (19). However, a pediatric phase III follow-up study aimed at promoting resolution of organ dysfunction was stopped at its planned interim analysis due to lack of efficacy (25). Currently no widely accepted pediatric indication exists for rhAPC in the treatment of pediatric bacterial sepsis.

Extracorporeal therapies such as hemofiltration, plasmapheresis, and plasma exchange represent another approach to the acute restoration of inflammatory homeostasis in sepsis. These treatments are predicated upon bulk removal of inflammatory mediators through diffusion, convection, or membrane adsorption (46). Plasma exchange offers the additional advantage of replacement of plasma proteins that may become depleted in sepsis, e.g., von Willebrand's factor cleaving protease inhibitor. Data from large, randomized, controlled trials are lacking. However, several small, controlled trials suggest a survival benefit associated with prolonged treatment with plasmapheresis or plasma exchange.

The IV administration of polyclonal IV immunoglobulin (IVIG) has also been studied in the context of sepsis in both children and adults. Supplementation of the adaptive immune response in this way has resulted in conflicting results. A recent meta-analysis of IVIG use for the treatment of neonatal infection showed no effect on mortality with empiric use but did show a reduction in mortality risk when used in the context of proven infection (50). These data were supported when a metaanalysis of IVIG use in adult sepsis failed to show a reduction in mortality risk (55). A prospective, randomized, controlled trial of 100 children who were <2 years of age and had sepsis showed that 3 days of polyclonal IVIG therapy resulted in improved survival to discharge and shorter length of ICU stay (21). A subset of IVIG trials has used a product that is enriched in the IgM fraction of immunoglobulin. Both retrospective and prospective evidence suggests that IgM-enriched IVIG may be beneficial in adult postoperative patients with severe sepsis.

Subacute Management

Management in the PICU

Septic shock requires immediate resuscitation, and children with septic shock should be treated in a PICU. A wellcoordinated and integrated approach directed at rapidly restoring systemic oxygen delivery and improving tissue perfusion has been shown to improve survival significantly in adults with septic shock (61), and the goal should be similar in children. Although the initial approach may differ based on priorities and available resources, critical elements should be integrated into any resuscitative effort. Therapy should be guided by tissue and organ perfusion parameters. Fluid infusion should be vigorous and titrated to clinical end-points of volume repletion. Systemic oxygen delivery should be supported by ensuring arterial oxygen saturation, maintaining adequate concentrations of hemoglobin, and using vasoactive agents directed to physiologic and clinical end-points, as described previously. In addition to support of the airway and breathing, continuous electrocardiographic monitoring and pulse oximetry should be performed for detection of rhythm disturbances and perfusion. Urine output should be monitored continuously.

Multiorgan Dysfunction

Once admitted to the PICU, the goals of therapy include assessing the adequacy of the fluid resuscitation, reviewing the choice of antibiotic coverage, and completing a thorough history and physical. It is also important to assess the degree of organ dysfunction and to aggressively support perfusion of each vital organ. Although the progression of sepsis to MODS is poorly understood, it is highly likely that poor perfusion, hypoxia, hyperglycemia, and acidosis all contribute to the process. Detailed attention to organ system support is essential because the cumulative burden of organ system failure increases the likelihood of mortality, with the risk of mortality increasing with each additional organ system failure. Lung dysfunction, which commonly accompanies sepsis, tends to occur early and persists, in contrast to shock, which also occurs early but tends to either resolve rapidly or progress rapidly to death (**Fig. 78.6**). Serious abnormalities of liver function, coagulation, and CNS function tend to occur hours to days after the onset of sepsis and to persist. In addition to the number of organ failures, the severity of each failure affects the prognosis. Fortunately, the majority of organ failures resolve within 1 month in survivors of sepsis (75).

Ventilation Strategies

Nearly 50% of all adult patients with severe sepsis will develop ARDS, and the prevalence in children is likely similar. The response to sepsis often requires a high minute ventilation in the face of this inflammatory process that decreases compliance of

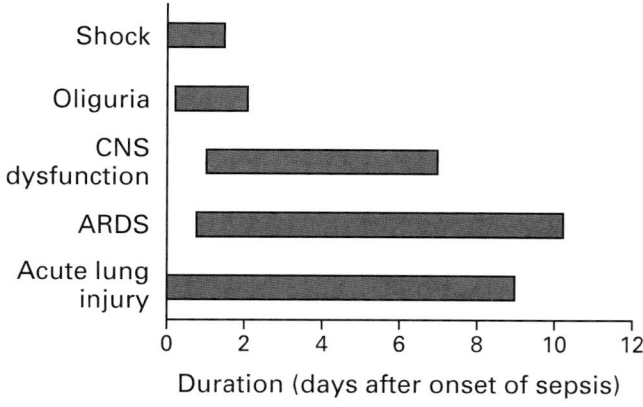

FIGURE 78.6. Onset and resolution of organ failure in patients with severe sepsis. The bars show the duration of organ failure, with the timing of the onset and resolution of organ failure shown at the left and right ends of the bars, respectively. Acute lung injury—or its more severe form, ARDS—develops early and is long-lived, with a mean duration of nine days. Shock and oliguria are similar in the timing of their onset, and the duration of both is brief, averaging <2 days. In contrast, CNS dysfunction has a delayed onset and an intermediate duration. From Wheeler AP, Bernard GR. Treating patients with severe sepsis. *N Engl J Med* 1999;340:207–14, with permission.

the respiratory system, increases airway resistance, and impairs muscle efficiency (75). Timely intubation and mechanical ventilation based on clinical parameters rather than laboratory indices are crucial, as intubation and mechanical ventilation reduce respiratory-muscle oxygen demand and decrease the risk of aspiration and cerebral anoxia from a catastrophic event. Based on data from adult patients, lung-protective ventilation should be used. Multiple trials have now shown the benefit of a high positive end-expiratory pressure and low-tidal-volume approach. The goal of mechanical ventilation is to maintain a reasonable level of oxygenation while keeping the fraction of oxygen in inspired gas (FiO$_2$) below 0.6, allowing from some hypercapnia with the buffered pH >7.25. Nonconventional modes of ventilation, such as airway-pressure-release ventilation and high-frequency ventilation, may be required to support oxygenation and minimize lung toxicity.

Renal Replacement Therapy

Acute renal failure frequently accompanies severe sepsis and portends a poor prognosis, with increased mortality in children with sepsis. In septic shock, with its attendant hemodynamic instability, continuous venovenous hemofiltration is better tolerated than traditional dialysis (see Chapter 37). Moreover, some evidence suggests that hemofiltration can clear some mediators of inflammation and, thus, may be beneficial even in the absence of acute renal failure. In high-cutoff hemofiltration, a high-flux hemofilter with an in vivo cutoff point of ~60 kDa is used, which allows for clearance of molecules up to that size. In addition, it has been shown that monocyte activation is suitably downregulated by this mode of renal replacement. Preventing fluid overload and the consequential cellular injury is also beneficial. A recent study of children with MODS demonstrated that survivors had less fluid overload than nonsurvivors, with the resultant recommendation of early initiation of hemofiltration (26).

Cardiac Monitoring

In bacterial sepsis, early diagnosis and intervention will result in improved outcomes. Compromised perfusion can often be diagnosed clinically by poor perfusion and signs of decreased organ function. However, the variable and dynamic clinical presentation of children with sepsis, with the likelihood of an underlying comorbidity, often complicates patient management. In septic shock, the use of cardiac monitoring may complement the clinical detection of compromised perfusion as well as assist in decision making regarding interventions. Certain variables are essential to making informed clinical decisions in the management of sepsis. In any system, flow varies directly with dP/R, where dP is the *perfusion pressure* and R is the *resistance*. Applying this concept to systemic perfusion:

Perfusion = (mean arterial pressure − central venous pressure)/ systemic vascular resistance

The goal of treating septic shock is to maintain the perfusion pressure above the critical point at which blood flow to varied organs is compromised. In this regard, maintenance of mean arterial pressure with norepinephrine has been shown to improve urine output and creatinine clearance in hyperdynamic sepsis. Cardiac monitoring allows for better assessment of the hemodynamic status of the patient. For example, monitoring of the central venous pressure allows for the assessment of the adequacy of fluid resuscitation. Fluid-refractory shock is defined as the persistence of signs of shock after the administration of sufficient fluids to achieve a central venous pressure of 8–12 mm Hg. In addition, the monitoring of SvO_2 may provide insight as to the adequacy of oxygen delivery. Decreased mixed venous saturations may reflect a cardiac output insufficient to meet the metabolic demands of the tissues. Alternatively, sepsis is also associated with abnormalities in oxygen extraction or utilization, resulting in elevated mixed-venous saturations. It is difficult to assess these functional parameters without knowledge of the cardiac output or pulmonary pressures, particularly in light of a dynamic process such as bacterial sepsis (12).

The PAC is used to diagnose disease states with cardiovascular relevance, and to monitor the progress of critically ill patients to guide the selection and adjustment of medical therapy. Despite the widespread use of these devices, data about their utility are conflicting. The majority of nonrandomized studies in critically ill patients have suggested that the PAC is associated with increased morbidity and mortality. Conversely, some investigators feel that an inherent bias is involved because only very sick patients will require a PAC. A recent study of over 3000 adults, including patients with sepsis, demonstrated no statistical difference in mortality or morbidity when controlling for severity of illness (62). The goal of resuscitation is to restore the normal balance between oxygen supply and demand. In fact, using a supranormal cardiac index as a goal has failed to show an overall difference in outcome in adults with shock. The ACCM task force recommends the use of PACs in dopamine-resistant patients (11), based on studies that demonstrated safety and some benefit, including one study which demonstrated that a large number of subjects were receiving incorrect cardiovascular therapy after fluid resuscitation (12). Given the concerns regarding PACs and the improvements in echocardiography, it is possible that echocardiography will assume an expanding role in the management of septic shock. However, no trial has demonstrated the usefulness of echocardiography in bacterial sepsis.

Transfusion

In addition to optimizing myocardial function, several other therapeutic interventions may influence outcomes from septic shock. For example, in that oxygen delivery is dependent on the concentration of hemoglobin, optimizing hemoglobin levels may improve outcomes from sepsis. However, the transfusion of packed red blood cells must be implemented judiciously and with caution, as evidence suggests that a liberal transfusion practice in adults is associated with a higher mortality (31,71). Similarly, a randomized, controlled trial in stable, critically ill children found that a restrictive transfusion threshold of hemoglobin 7 g/dL did not increase adverse outcomes compared to the more liberal threshold of hemoglobin 9 g/dL (37). The results of these and other trials may influence the opinions of the ACCM task force, which currently recommends transfusion if the hemoglobin is <10 mg/dL. Importantly, patients with cardiovascular disease, low cardiac output, severe arterial hypoxemia, low mixed-venous saturation, and/or persistent lactic acidosis may need higher hemoglobin despite lack of data to support this practice. Reassessment should be made based on emerging evidence.

Nutrition

Any critical illness, including sepsis, will increase the nutritional requirements of the body. These conditions promote a catabolic state and negative nitrogen balance, and this effect may be accentuated by exogenous steroids. Prolonged bed rest and inactivity also produce a negative nitrogen balance in healthy individuals. Thus, a hypermetabolic state such as sepsis, in concert with bed rest and inactivity, may result in malnutrition. Following the initial resuscitation of the critically ill patient, the nutritional status should be assessed and a plan of nutritional management developed. It is best to utilize the enteral route if possible. Enteral nutrition has been advocated as a means of reducing villous atrophy with increased intestinal permeability, with consequent reduction in the incidence of gut translocation and septic complications. However, this paradigm has not been substantiated with a meta-analysis that showed no benefit to enteric feeding in critically ill adults. In fact, patients with acute sepsis exhibit increased gastrointestinal permeability and decreased gastrointestinal functional absorptive capacity in comparison with healthy control subjects (35). Despite this, studies have shown that early enteral feeding of critically ill children on vasoactive drugs and mechanical ventilation is feasible and well tolerated. Patients with sepsis who require pressors and narcotics often have a degree of gastroparesis and thus may benefit from transpyloric feeding, which may be associated with a shorter time interval to full-strength feeds and a decreased incidence of nosocomial pneumonia. The European Society of Parenteral and Enteral Nutrition recommends that if critically ill patients are not expected to be feeding within 3 days, enteral nutrition should be commenced. Enteral feedings have many theoretical advantages, including gastric pH buffering, avoidance of the use of parenteral-nutrition catheters, preservation of gut mucosa, avoidance of the introduction of bacteria and toxins from the gastrointestinal tract into the circulation, a more physiologic pattern of enteric hormone secretion, the ability to administer a complete, nutritional mixture that includes fiber, and lower costs (75). While generally thought to be beneficial in critically ill patients, it is important to note that enteral immunonutrition with L-arginine, ω-3 fatty acids, zinc, and selenium has proven to be harmful in severe sepsis (7).

Glycemic Control

Hyperglycemia with insulin resistance is common in critically ill children. Hyperglycemia is associated with activation of the protein kinase C pathway, polyol pathway, and reactive oxygen species, which leads to alteration in protein expression and, eventually, to cell damage (65). The increased serum glucose is probably an adaptive mechanism that provides for the brain, red blood cell, and immune system hypermetabolism. However, maintaining a tight control on serum glucose has been shown to be beneficial in a number of adult studies. A tighter glycemic control is thought to lead to improvements in white blood cell function and phagocytosis and to suppress the hepatic acute-phase response. A study in children revealed that when the glycemic profile of PICU admissions was examined, nonsurvivors had a higher duration of hyperglycemia and a higher peak serum glucose (65). The etiology of the hyperglycemia is unclear, as hyperglycemia in pediatric septic shock has been shown to be due to hypoinsulinemia rather than insulin resistance. Children are generally more prone to hypoglycemia when treated with insulin; therefore, insulin therapy should be used cautiously. The impact of tight glucose control in critically ill children is presently undergoing study.

Identifying the Source of Infection and Source Control of Infection

In patients with sepsis, it is crucial to attempt to make a microbiologic diagnosis and institute appropriate therapy early. Although the focus of infection can sometimes be difficult to detect in patients who present with sepsis, a careful history and physical exam may help to narrow the suspected sources. For example, a history of travel or contact with wild animals can suggest infections with atypical and uncommon organisms such as the *Rickettsial* spp. These intermediate organisms cause a clinical syndrome that is similar to sepsis but requires a different diagnostic and treatment approach. Obvious sources of infection, such as surgical wounds and indwelling foreign bodies (central venous catheters, ventriculoperitoneal shunts, urinary catheters, etc.) should be carefully scrutinized. Blood cultures should be obtained for all patients with sepsis. If the patient has a central line, both peripheral and catheter cultures should be sent to the lab. The length of time to bacterial growth and the colony count often determine if the catheter is the infectious source. A colony count that is 5–10 times greater from the catheter compared to the peripheral blood is indicative of an infected device. A quantitative culture that yields at least 100 CFu/μL is diagnostic of a central venous catheter infection. If bacteremia persists with appropriate antibiotics, the catheter should be removed.

In cases of immunocompromised states, intra-abdominal infections, or oral/neck infections, anaerobic cultures should also be considered. If antibiotics have already been given, blood culture should be obtained immediately prior to the next scheduled dose to minimize blood drug level. A lumbar puncture should be considered in patients with signs of meningitis or neurologic symptoms. A lumbar puncture should ideally be performed prior to administration of antibiotics, but this may not be practical for all children. Hemodynamic instability or raised intracranial pressure will require deferral of the lumbar puncture until the patient is more stable. As obtaining sputum samples in children is difficult, the predominant strategy is to provide empiric antibiotic therapy. In children who have required endotracheal intubation, however, it is important to send a tracheal aspirate for culture. If a pleural fluid or empyema is present, a diagnostic thoracentesis may be performed for fluid culture. Exudate from sites of soft-tissue infection should be cultured. If the patient has an abscess, aspiration may be indicated for diagnostic purposes. Aside from the Gram stain, none of the studies will impact initial antimicrobial selection.

Source control of infection encompasses all of the adjunctive physical measures that can control a focus of infection and modify factors that promote microbial growth or impair host antimicrobial defenses. Every child who presents with sepsis should be evaluated for a source of infection. The evaluation can vary from a thorough physical exam to complex imaging, based on the clinical assessment. Source control predominantly includes the drainage of infected fluid collections, debridement of infected tissue, and removal of devices or foreign bodies. Examples of source control include the removal of a central venous line in a patient with persistent bacteremia in spite of appropriate antibiotics being infused. The prompt identification of necrotizing soft-tissue infections requires immediate surgical debridement.

Antimicrobial Control of Infection

Antibiotics should be started within the first hour of recognition of sepsis. If obtaining a specific culture is delayed, antibiotics should not be withheld. A third-generation cephalosporin will usually provide sufficient empiric coverage as first-line therapy. A β-lactam antibiotic with an aminoglycoside is also as efficacious. If an anaerobic infection is suspected, the addition of metronidazole or clindamycin is appropriate. For children with indwelling catheters, prosthetic materials, or potential infections with methicillin-resistant *S. aureus*, vancomycin should be added. Vancomycin is also indicated in the treatment of bacterial meningitis or sepsis in areas with high levels of penicillin-resistant pneumococcus and in neutropenic patients with fever in whom coagulase-negative staphylococci and *Streptococcus viridans* are predominant pathogens. If a CNS infection is suspected, appropriate dosing is indicated to allow CNS penetration. The choice of empirical antibiotic coverage therapy is variable and depends on several factors related to the patient's history, previous pathogens isolated, known colonization, the presence of an underlying disease or foreign body, and the susceptibility patterns of microorganisms in the hospital and community. If patients exhibit clinical deterioration or have persistent bacteremia 72 hrs after the start of antibiotic, reassessment is necessary.

Hyperbaric Oxygen

Hyperbaric oxygen is the administration of 100% oxygen at two to three times the atmospheric pressure at sea level in a chamber, which can result in arterial oxygen tension in excess of 2000 mm Hg and oxygen tension in tissue of almost 400 mm Hg.

Local hypoxia disrupts neutrophil-mediated killing of bacteria by free radicals. Hyperbaric oxygen restores this defense against infection and even increases the rate of killing of some common bacteria by phagocytes. In addition, hyperbaric oxygen alone is bactericidal for certain anaerobes, bacteriostatic for certain species of *Escherichia* and *Pseudomonas*, and suppresses clostridial production of α toxin (68). Hyperbaric oxygen has been used as an adjunct to wound care and infection control in myonecrosis, necrotizing fasciitis, and refractory osteomyelitis. Treatment protocols vary depending on the pathology; however, for treatment of wounds that do not respond to debridement or antibiotics, most protocols average 90 mins with 20–30 treatments.

Prevention of Sepsis

Nosocomial Infection

As with most diseases, successful treatment of sepsis may be more effectively accomplished with prevention than with the most effective of therapies. Given that nearly half of the children who develop sepsis have an underlying comorbidity and will likely require frequent hospitalization, successful prevention may be highly dependent on eliminating nosocomial infections. Nosocomial infections contribute significantly to hospital-associated morbidity, mortality, and costs (60,63). In the PICU, bloodstream infections account for 21%–28% of all nosocomial infections (60,63), and the rate of catheter-related bloodstream infections has been reported at 7.3 per 1000 catheter days. In light of this, much attention has been directed to decrease the incidence of nosocomial catheter-related bloodstream infections. In 2002, the Society of Critical Care Medicine, in collaboration with multiple other organizations, published guidelines intended to provide evidence-based recommendations for preventing catheter-related infections. These guidelines emphasized the following areas: (a) educating and training healthcare providers who insert and maintain catheters; (b) using maximal sterile barrier precautions during central venous catheter insertion; (c) using a 2% chlorhexidine preparation for skin antisepsis; (d) avoiding routine replacement of central venous catheters as a strategy to prevent infection; (e) using antiseptic/antibiotic-impregnated, short-term central venous catheters if the rate of infection is high despite adherence to other strategies; and (f) removing the catheter as soon as possible. Paramount to the success of this process is the identification of risk factors for the development of catheter-related bloodstream infections. Critically ill children may have an increased risk of catheter-related sepsis for a variety of reasons, including their immune status, the number and location of the catheters, and the content of their infusates. A number of studies have demonstrated an association between catheter-related bloodstream infections and the use of total parenteral nutrition (16) (see Chapter 81 for further discussion of nosocomial infection).

High-risk Patient Populations

Along with decreasing nosocomial infections, another important strategy is the early identification of high-risk patient populations who may be at increased risk for sepsis from both nosocomial and non-nosocomial sources.

Burns. Improved resuscitation and respiratory support of burn victims has resulted in reduced rates of early death from shock in this patient population but a concomitant increase in late mortality from infection. Infection rates in children hospitalized for burns appear to be higher than in critically ill nonburn patients and approximate rates of other immunocompromised groups. Data suggest increased rates of central catheter infections, ventilator-related pneumonia, and urinary catheter-related urinary tract infections in children with burns. Burn patients are predisposed to sepsis for a number of reasons: (a) a global decrease in cellular immune function is associated with burns; (b) neutropenia is common, neutrophil function is depressed, and T-cell transcription is altered; (c) these patients are at risk for increased gut permeability; and (d) bacteremia may occur with wound manipulations.

Trauma. Trauma is another significant risk factor for sepsis (52). Traumatically injured children are at risk for both injury-related and nosocomial infections. Injury-related infections are primarily wound, intra-abdominal, and CNS infections, while nosocomial infections include respiratory, bloodstream, and urinary tract infections (53). The nosocomial infections are most common among mechanically ventilated trauma victims, head-injured patients, and those who require prolonged immobilization or hospitalization (76). The propensity for nosocomial infection fits well with the currently accepted paradigm of the immune response to traumatic injury in which traumatic injury and the initial resuscitation are followed by SIRS, which may lead to early MODS. In most instances, the seriously injured patient will survive the initial SIRS response without

developing MODS. However, after a period of relative clinical stability, the patient may manifest CARS with suppressed immunity and diminished resistance to infection, leading to a high risk of sepsis and subsequent MODS.

Human Immunodeficiency Virus. HIV-infected children are also at increased risk of viral, bacterial, and fungal sepsis, and the case fatality rate for nonopportunistic infections may be greater for them than in non–HIV-infected children. Pathophysiologically, apoptosis of CD4 T lymphocytes and functional abnormalities of T lymphocyte T-helper 1 clonal maturation patterns, with defective IL-2 and IF-γ production, render patients susceptible to viral and intracellular organisms (32). In addition, associated defects of B-lymphocyte function, natural killer cell activity, neutrophil bactericidal activity, and defective antigen-specific immunoglobulin production, despite an increase in total globulin fraction, predispose children to bacterial sepsis (32). Prior to the advent of highly active antiretroviral therapy (HAART), reported primary bacterial infection rates and nosocomial infection rates were very high. The use of HAART in many parts of the world has resulted in an ever-growing cohort of clinically stable HIV-infected children, with low viral loads and normal CD4 T-lymphocyte counts. Access to HAART has markedly decreased the rate of progression to acquired immune deficiency syndrome, the prevalence of organ-specific complications of HIV, the risk of recurrent sepsis, and the high early childhood mortality from HIV infection (30). The impact of the initiation of HAART on morbidity during acute episodes of sepsis has not been established.

Asplenia. Children born without a spleen or who have impaired splenic function secondary to disease or splenectomy are at significantly increased risk of life-threatening bacterial sepsis. Thus, effective caregiver and patient education, appropriate immunizations, and prophylactic antibiotics must be implemented to prevent these infections. Vaccination guidelines for the prevention of pneumococcal, meningococcal, and Hib disease have been established for these children. Annual influenza immunization is also recommended for asplenic children and their household contacts to minimize the risk of secondary bacterial infections (57). In addition to appropriate immunization, antimicrobial prophylaxis is recommended for all children <5 years of age and for at least 2 years after splenectomy. Half of all cases of postsplenectomy sepsis occur within the first 2 years after splenectomy (57).

Patients with Cancer and Hematopoietic Stem Cell Transplant. Children with neoplasia account for nearly 13% of all cases of severe sepsis in children who are 1–9 years of age and ~17% of cases in children who are 10–19 years of age (74). However, oncology patients should not be considered a homogeneous group, as significant differences exist in their predisposition to sepsis. Leukemia/lymphoma patients have diseased bone marrow and tend to receive more intensive myeloablative therapy, resulting in disruption of normal immune function. As a result of these factors, neutropenic bacteremia appears to occur more frequently among leukemia patients. Patients with solid tumors may also receive myeloablative therapy; however, usually less so. Anatomic obstruction and functional impairment tend to predispose these children to sepsis. In addition to the type of cancer, the state of the disease and its treatment may influence the predisposition to sepsis. Not surprisingly, infection rates are significantly higher in patients who receive more intensive protocols. Moreover, hematologic parameters, particularly neutropenia (absolute neutrophil count <500), have long been used to identify oncology patients at risk for sepsis, with a well-established relationship between decreased leukocytes and an increased risk of infection. It has been shown that temperature >39.0°C in neutropenic cancer patients increases the likelihood that the patient is bacteremic (see Chapter 100). In addition to neutropenia, the absolute monocyte count appears to be useful in identifying high-risk patients. Furthermore, the presence of a comorbidity has been found to predispose children with cancer to sepsis and contribute to the severity of the illness.

Sickle Cell Disease. Children with sickle cell disease are at high risk of serious bacterial infection, in large part from functional asplenia. Recommended immunizations and the prophylactic use of antibiotics are successful in decreasing the risk of infection in these children. (See Chapter 104 for further discussion.)

Prophylaxis

Prophylaxis is the use of antimicrobial drugs in the absence of suspected or documented infection to decrease the incidence of infection in high-risk populations. Antimicrobial agents are commonly prescribed to prevent infections in children despite the fact that the efficacy of this practice is unsubstantiated for most conditions. The use of prophylactic antibiotics has been categorized into three major indications. First, antibiotic prophylaxis may be indicated for children because of exposure to specific pathogens such as *N. meningitides*. The risk of contracting invasive meningococcal disease among contacts of infected individuals is essential in determining the need for antimicrobial prophylaxis. Close contacts of all people with invasive meningococcal disease are at high risk and should receive prophylaxis, ideally within 24 hrs of diagnosis of the primary case. For most children, rifampin is the drug of choice. Rifampin chemoprophylaxis may also be indicated for close contacts of invasive Hib disease. The second major indication for antimicrobial prophylaxis is to prevent infections of vulnerable body sites, which is most effectively achieved if the period of risk is defined and brief, the expected pathogens have predictable antimicrobial susceptibilities, and the site is accessible to antimicrobial agents. The periprocedure use of antibiotics to prevent bacterial endocarditis in children with specific cardiac lesions is a well-established example of this form of prophylaxis. The importance of this practice is emphasized by the fact that endocarditis is associated with the highest case fatality rate of all forms of pediatric sepsis (74). Other examples of this form of prophylaxis include the use of antibiotics following specific types of animal bites and in children with documented vesicoureteral reflux, although this latter practice is currently being reevaluated. The final form of prophylactic antibiotic use is to prevent infections in high-risk patient populations. For example, the use of antibiotic prophylaxis is recommended for all asplenic children <5 years of age, regardless of immunization status (57). Children with sickle cell disease and children with HIV also should be treated with prophylactic antibiotics.

OUTCOMES

Estimates as to the precise number of childhood deaths that are attributable to sepsis are greatly limited by the inexact information that is available. However, estimates in the US in 1995 place sepsis as the fourth highest cause of death in infants and second (behind accidents) in children 1–14 years of age. In the largest study performed to examine the scope of pediatric sepsis and outcomes from this disease process, the case fatality rate is fairly consistent at ~10% for all age groups (74) (**Table 78.5**). A follow-up study that used data from 1999 reported an increase in the incidence of severe sepsis, but a decrease in mortality to 9.0% (73). This mortality rate, although high, is much lower compared to the overall rate of mortality in adults (17.9%) during a similar time period (44). Moreover, it is much lower than the 57% mortality reported in children with septic shock in 1985 (56). Clearly, great progress has been made in making survival the rule rather than the exception in pediatric sepsis. Worldwide, severe sepsis is an even more daunting issue. According to the World Health Organization Report of 2005, 10.6 million children die each year before reaching their fifth birthday, and almost three-fourths of deaths each year occur as a result of infectious diseases, such as severe infections, acute respiratory infections, and diarrheal diseases. One of the goals of the World Health Organization is to implement the movement of knowledge to developing countries worldwide toward decreasing these preventable deaths (**Fig. 78.7**).

Clearly, outcomes from pediatric sepsis are linked to the state of the child prior to the infectious insult. Children with preexisting medical conditions have a much higher chance of succumbing to sepsis compared to previously healthy hosts. The case-fatality rate is higher in every age group in children with comorbidities (74) (**Fig. 78.8**), and mortality increased from sepsis in children when it occurred after surgical procedures. Mortality from sepsis appears to be linked to the severity of MODS, given the collective increase in the risk of death associated with increasing severity of organ dysfunction when a scaled and weighted pediatric MODS score is used. Each unit increase in the pediatric logistic organ dysfunction (PELOD) score multiplied the hazard ratio by 1.1, leading to a sharp rise in mortality as the PELOD score increased (38) (**Fig. 78.9**). A similar trend was seen in a distinct cohort of children in whom mortality increased from 7% in those with single-organ failure to 53% in those with 4 or more organs failing (74). Mortality from sepsis also varies according to the infecting organism. Case fatality rates appear highest from *Meningococcus, Pseudomonas,* and *Streptococcus* and appear somewhat less with *H. influenza* and *Staphylococcus*; however, mortality can also be dependent on the age of the child and the treatment protocols used for outlining therapy (**Table 78.2**). Gender only influences mortality rates in infants, where infant boys have a higher mortality rate than infant girls.

The cost of severe sepsis is substantial, the estimated cost in the US being over $47,000 per hospital stay, for an average length of stay of 31 days (74)—a cost that exceeds those associated with any other diagnoses. In the US, it is estimated that children with severe sepsis cost in excess of $1.9 billion per year. Lengths of stay and hospital costs were higher in surgical patients, and no gender difference was noted in these outcomes. Despite similar lengths of stay, nonsurvivors had significantly higher hospital costs (74).

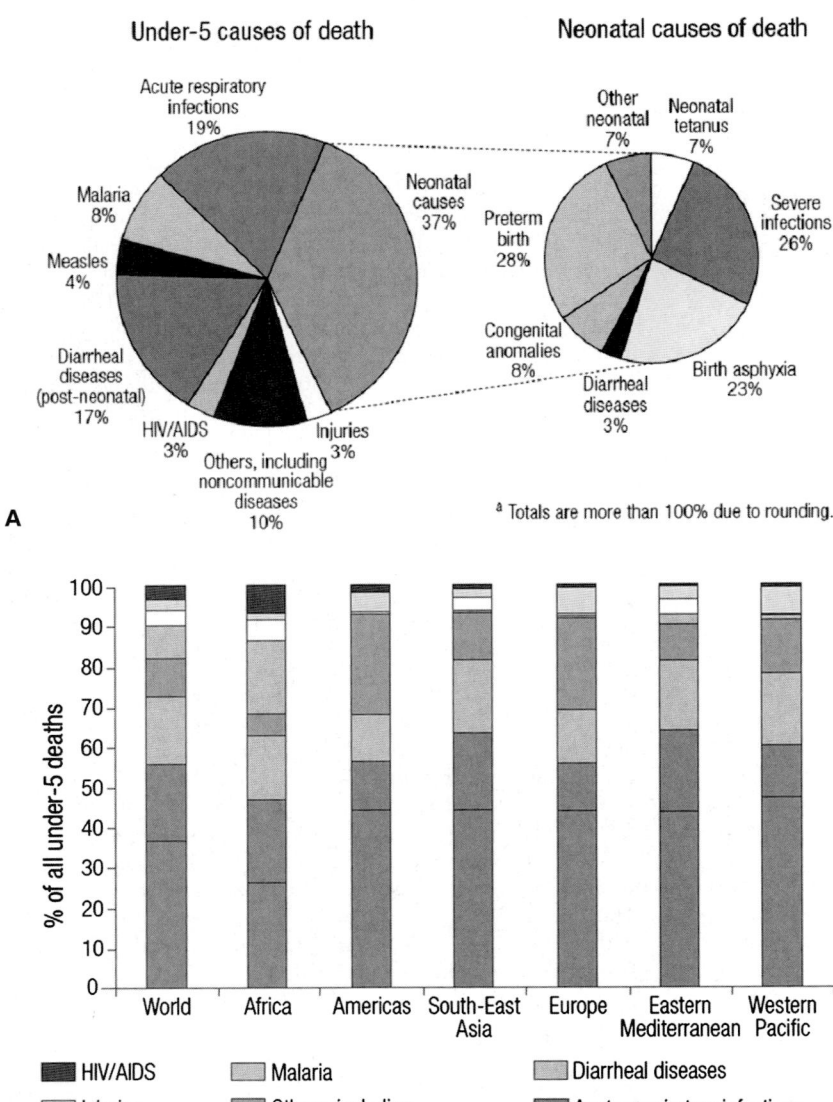

A

^a Totals are more than 100% due to rounding.

B

FIGURE 78.7. A: The causes of death in children <5 years of age worldwide. **B:** Major causes of death among children <5 years of age, by WHO region. (Note that totals sum to more than 100% due to rounding.) Despite the substantial reductions in the number of deaths observed in recent decades, around 10.6 million children still die every year before reaching their fifth birthday. Almost all of these deaths occur in low- and middle-income countries. From *The World Health Report* 2005, WHO, Geneva Switzerland, with permission.

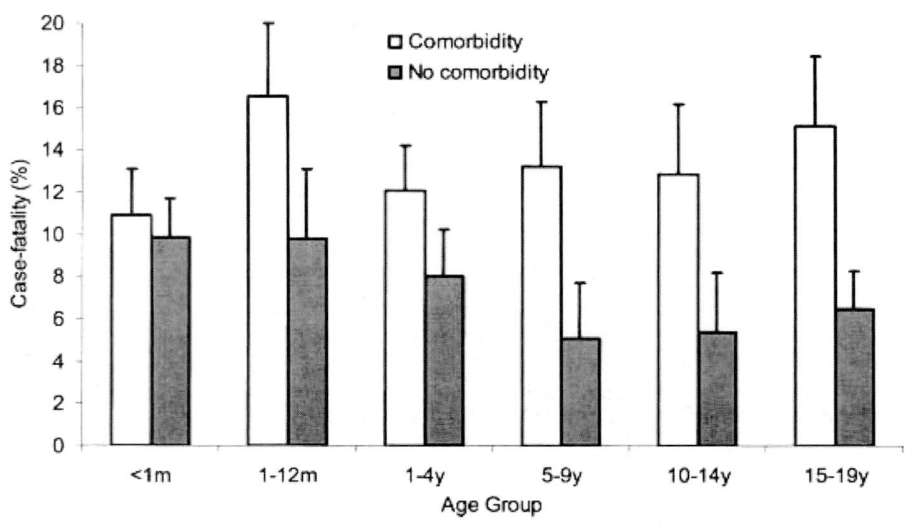

FIGURE 78.8. Case fatality of children with severe sepsis by age and comorbidity. Case fatality was highest in children 1–12 months old and was significantly higher among children with any underlying disease. Results for children who were <1 month old and 1–12 months old are from the five states (Massachusetts, Maryland, New Jersey, New York, and Virginia) in which neonates could be identified (*n* = 6349, or 66% of the entire seven-state cohort). Results for children >1 year of age are from the entire seven-state cohort (*n* = 9675); 95% confidence intervals are shown by *error bars*. From Watson RS, Carcillo JA, Linde-Zwirble WT, et al. The epidemiology of severe sepsis in children in the United States. *Am J Respir Crit Care Med* 2003;167:695–701, with permission.

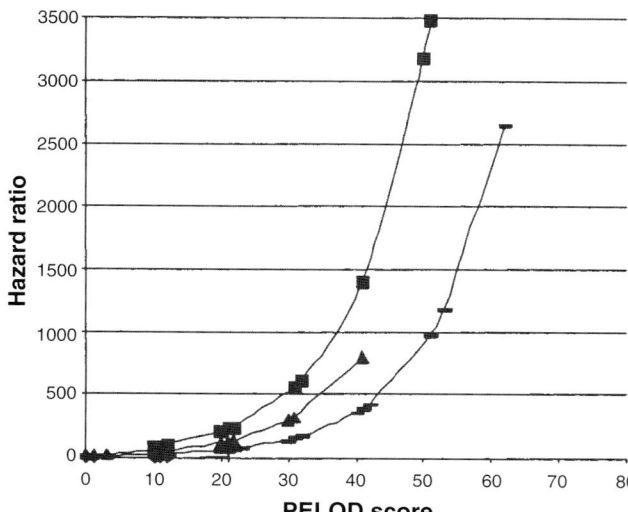

FIGURE 78.9. Observed cumulative hazard ratios (HR) of death of the PELOD score (which may range from 0 to 71) and the diagnostic category of septic state in the study population (593 children); HR of death is calculated by multiplying HR of the pediatric logistic organ dysfunction (PELOD) score (1.096 PELOD score) by HR of diagnostic category; i.e., no systemic inflammatory response syndrome (SIRS) (*diamond*); SIRS, sepsis (*dash*); severe sepsis (*triangle*); and septic shock (*square*). From Leclerc F, Leteurtre S, Duhamel A, et al. Cumulative influence of organ dysfunctions and septic state on mortality of critically ill children. *Am J Respir Crit Care Med* 2005;171:348–53, with permission.

CONCLUSIONS AND FUTURE DIRECTIONS

An exciting group of therapies is the subject of ongoing research in the area of bacterial sepsis and septic shock. Some continue to explore ways by which to interrupt the proinflammatory surge characteristic of early sepsis. An agent that shows particular promise in this regard is ethyl pyruvate, a molecule which has been shown to globally reduce proinflammatory cytokine production in both in vitro and in vivo models of endotoxemia (28). Another drug deserving of study in this setting is pentoxifylline, a nonspecific phosphodiesterase inhibitor that has been shown to inhibit proinflammatory cytokine production by innate immune cells and increase production of anti-inflammatory mediators such as IL-10. Data suggest that pentoxifylline, as an adjunctive therapy, reduces mortality from neonatal sepsis with no adverse effects, though its role in the PICU is unclear. Expressed later in the course of sepsis compared to TNF-α is the high-mobility gene box 1 (HMGB1) protein, also thought to be a mediator of proinflammation. This nuclear protein is now known to be released into the circulation in the late phase of sepsis and is associated with persistence of the inflammatory state. Administration of HMGB1-neutralizing antibodies has been shown to confer protection in animal models of established sepsis (78).

Enthusiasm for the promotion of an anti-inflammatory phenotype in response to sepsis has been dampened by the appreciation of immunoparalysis as a potentially harmful sequela of sepsis. The across-the-board use of proinflammatory agents such as granulocyte colony-stimulating factor and GM-CSF as immunostimulatory agents following sepsis has been shown to be safe but of questionable efficacy. Many investigators endorse the measurement of innate immune parameters to identify the subset of patients who are functionally immunosuppressed as a result of immunoparalysis (20). Tapering of exogenous immunosuppression or administration of GM-CSF or IF-γ has been used to reverse immunoparalysis with beneficial effects. The benefits of immunomodulation targeted specifically to the reversal of immunoparalysis (normalization of monocyte HLA-DR expression and TNF-α production capacity) have yet to be evaluated in large-scale clinical trials.

Perhaps the best way to manage sepsis is to prevent its occurrence in the first place. For this reason, the most effective sepsis-related public health measure continues to be routine vaccination. Experimental evidence suggests that a protective immune response to endotoxin can be induced from vaccines made from *E. coli* or *Pseudomonas* species. Such vaccines could be of particular benefit to children with chronic illnesses who are at high risk for the development of nosocomial sepsis. Prevention of translocation of bacteria through the intestine is another area of ongoing research interest. Early enteral nutrition is thought to promote intestinal barrier function and reduce septic complications from burns and other forms of critical illness, but it is clear that much more knowledge regarding this intervention remains to be learned. Recombinant human IL-11, an endogenous anti-inflammatory cytokine with particular efficacy in the promotion of gut mucosal integrity, has been shown to prevent secondary bacterial infection in small cohorts of adults with hematologic malignancy.

The vast majority of large-scale prospective, randomized, controlled trials of sepsis therapies have been performed in adults. The relative infrequency of severe sepsis and septic shock in children and the relatively low pediatric mortality compared to adults make the design and implementation of these studies difficult. As care becomes more standardized across PICUs, with the assistance of evidence-based recommendations such as the ACCM clinical practice parameters, collaborative interventional research should be more feasible. Despite this progress, it is likely that investigators will find it necessary to emphasize primary outcome measures other than mortality (length of stay, resource utilization) when conducting trials in the pediatric population.

KEY POINTS

Clinical

■ The constellation of symptoms of the sepsis syndrome includes elevated temperature, tachycardia, tachypnea, abnormal peripheral white blood cell count, and evidence of organ dysfunction.

■ Treatment in the first hour:
  ■ Follow ABCs of resuscitation.
  ■ Aggressive 20 mL/kg normal saline boluses until perfusion improves.
  ■ If no improvement after 60 mL/kg normal saline, arterial line and central venous line are inserted and dopamine administration is started.
  ■ If no improvement after dopamine and fluids, epinephrine is administered for cold shock, and norepinephrine for warm shock.

- If no improvement, hydrocortisone should be considered for suspected adrenal insufficiency.
- Cultures and antibiotics as soon as possible in the first hour:
  - Cultures should be obtained: blood (2–3 mL in infants, 3–5 mL in children, and 10–20 mL in adolescents), urine, tracheal secretions. Spinal fluid should be obtained if patient is hemodynamically stable and increased intracranial pressure is not suspected.
  - Broad-spectrum antibiotics are given based on regional, hospital, or unit resistance patterns (e.g., third-generation cephalosporin OR ampicillin/gentamicin).
  - Vancomycin is added or substituted for suspected methicillin-resistant *S. aureus*, penicillin-resistant *S. pneumoniae*, or in a neutropenic patient with fever.
- Intubation and mechanical ventilation of children with sepsis reduces respiratory-muscle oxygen demand and decreases the risk of aspiration and cerebral anoxia from a catastrophic event.
- Estimates of deaths due to severe sepsis in the US place sepsis as the fourth highest cause in infants and second in children 1–14 years of age. The case fatality rate is fairly consistent at ~9%–10% for all age groups.
- According to the World Health Organization Report, 10.6 million children die each year before reaching their fifth birthday and almost three-fourths of deaths each year occur as a result of infectious diseases, such as severe infections, acute respiratory infections, and diarrheal diseases.

Basic Science

- LTA can be considered the gram-positive counterpart of LPS.
- Superantigens are produced by gram-positive organisms and can bring together MHC class II molecules and T-cell receptors, resulting in the release of a large and sudden bolus of cytokines.
- The interaction of host leukocytes with bacterial pathogens is essential for the mounting of an effective immune response to infection but is also responsible for many of the harmful clinical features associated with the sepsis syndrome.
- Imbalance between proinflammatory and anti-inflammatory forces has been clearly linked to adverse outcomes in the setting of human septic disease.
- The action of the immune system is responsible for morbidity and mortality from bacterial sepsis, not the bacteria themselves.
- The cytochemical disruption of the endothelium is responsible for most of the cardiovascular manifestation of sepsis.

References

1. Abraham E, Glauser MP, Butler T, et al. p55 Tumor necrosis factor receptor fusion protein in the treatment of patients with severe sepsis and septic shock. A randomized controlled multicenter trial. Ro 45–2081 Study Group. *JAMA* 1997;277:1531–8.
2. Akira S, Takeda K. Toll-like receptor signalling. *Nat Rev Immunol* 2004;4:499–511.
3. Alverdy JC, Laughlin RS, Wu L. Influence of the critically ill state on host-pathogen interactions within the intestine: Gut-derived sepsis redefined. *Crit Care Med* 2003;31:598–607.
4. Annane D, Bellissant E, Bollaert PE, et al. Corticosteroids for severe sepsis and septic shock: A systematic review and meta-analysis. *Br Med J* 2004;329:480–8.
5. Babay HA, Twum-Danso K, Kambal AM, et al. Bloodstream infections in pediatric patients. *Saudi Med J* 2005;26:1555–61.
6. Baltimore RS, Huie SM, Meek JI, et al. Early-onset neonatal sepsis in the era of group B streptococcal prevention. *Pediatrics* 2001;108:1094–8.
7. Bertolini G, Iapichino G, Radrizzani D, et al. Early enteral immunonutrition in patients with severe sepsis: Results of an interim analysis of a randomized multicentre clinical trial. *Intensive Care Med* 2003;29:834–40.
8. Bick RL. Disseminated intravascular coagulation current concepts of etiology, pathophysiology, diagnosis, and treatment. *Hematol Oncol Clin North Am* 2003;17:149–76.
9. Bone RC, Fisher CJ, Jr., Clemmer TP, et al. Sepsis syndrome: A valid clinical entity. Methylprednisolone Severe Sepsis Study Group. *Crit Care Med* 1989;17:389–93.
10. Carcillo JA, Davis AL, Zaritsky A. Role of early fluid resuscitation in pediatric septic shock. *JAMA* 1991;266:1242–5.
11. Carcillo JA, Fields AI. Clinical practice parameters for hemodynamic support of pediatric and neonatal patients in septic shock. *Crit Care Med* 2002;30:1365–78.
12. Ceneviva G, Paschall JA, Maffei F, et al. Hemodynamic support in fluid-refractory pediatric septic shock. *Pediatrics* 1998;102:e19.
13. Chatila TA. Role of regulatory T cells in human diseases. *J Allergy Clin Immunol* 2005;116:949–59.
14. Cohen J. The immunopathogenesis of sepsis. *Nature* 2002;420:885–91.
15. Court O, Kumar A, Parrillo JE, et al. Clinical review: Myocardial depression in sepsis and septic shock. *Crit Care* 2002;6:500–8.
16. de Jonge RC, Polderman KH, Gemke RJ. Central venous catheter use in the pediatric patient: Mechanical and infectious complications. *Pediatr Crit Care Med* 2005;6:329–39.
17. De-Souza DA, Greene LJ. Intestinal permeability and systemic infections in critically ill patients: Effect of glutamine. *Crit Care Med* 2005;33:1125–35.
18. Deitch EA. Bacterial translocation or lymphatic drainage of toxic products from the gut: What is important in human beings? *Surgery* 2002;131:241–4.
19. Dhainaut JF, Laterre PF, Janes JM, et al. Drotrecogin alfa (activated) in the treatment of severe sepsis patients with multiple-organ dysfunction: Data from the PROWESS trial. *Intensive Care Med* 2003;29:894–903.
20. Docke WD, Randow F, Syrbe U, et al. Monocyte deactivation in septic patients: Restoration by IFN-gamma treatment. *Nat Med* 1997;3:678–81.
21. El-Nawawy A, El-Kinany H, Hamdy El-Sayed M, et al. Intravenous polyclonal immunoglobulin administration to sepsis syndrome patients: A prospective study in a pediatric intensive care unit. *J Trop Pediatr* 2005;51:271–8.
22. Felmet KA, Hall MW, Clark RS, et al. Prolonged lymphopenia, lymphoid depletion, and hypoprolactinemia in children with nosocomial sepsis and multiple organ failure. *J Immunol* 2005;174:3765–72.
23. Fisher CJ, Jr., Agosti JM, Opal SM, et al. Treatment of septic shock with the tumor necrosis factor receptor:Fc fusion protein. The Soluble TNF Receptor Sepsis Study Group. *N Engl J Med* 1996;334:1697–702.
24. Goldstein B, Giroir B, Randolph A. International pediatric sepsis consensus conference: Definitions for sepsis and organ dysfunction in pediatrics. *Pediatr Crit Care Med* 2005;6:2–8.
25. Goldstein B, Nadel S, Peters M, et al. ENHANCE: Results of a global open-label trial of drotrecogin alfa (activated) in children with severe sepsis. *Pediatr Crit Care Med* 2006;7:200–11.
26. Goldstein SL, Somers MJ, Baum MA, et al. Pediatric patients with multi-organ dysfunction syndrome receiving continuous renal replacement therapy. *Kidney Int* 2005;67:653–8.
27. Hack CE, Zeerleder S. The endothelium in sepsis: Source of and a target for inflammation. *Crit Care Med* 2001;29:S21–S27.
28. Han Y, Englert JA, Yang R, et al. Ethyl pyruvate inhibits nuclear factor-kappaB-dependent signaling by directly targeting p65. *J Pharmacol Exp Ther* 2005;312:1097–105.
29. Harrison LH, Dwyer DM, Maples CT, et al. Risk of meningococcal infection in college students. *JAMA* 1999;281:1906–10.
30. Hatherill M. Sepsis predisposition in children with human immunodeficiency virus. *Pediatr Crit Care Med* 2005;6:S92–S98.
31. Hebert PC, Wells G, Blajchman MA, et al. A multicenter, randomized, controlled clinical trial of transfusion requirements in critical care. Transfusion Requirements in Critical Care Investigators, Canadian Critical Care Trials Group. *N Engl J Med* 1999;340:409–17.
32. Hogan CM, Hammer SM. Host determinants in HIV infection and disease. Part 1: Cellular and humoral immune responses. *Ann Intern Med* 2001;134:761–76.
33. Hotchkiss RS, Swanson PE, Freeman BD, et al. Apoptotic cell death in patients with sepsis, shock, and multiple organ dysfunction. *Crit Care Med* 1999;27:1230–51.
34. Hotchkiss RS, Tinsley KW, Swanson PE, et al. Sepsis-induced apoptosis causes progressive profound depletion of B and CD4+ T lymphocytes in humans. *J Immunol* 2001;166:6952–63.
35. Johnston JD, Harvey CJ, Menzies IS, et al. Gastrointestinal permeability and absorptive capacity in sepsis. *Crit Care Med* 1996;24:1144–9.
36. Kaplan SL, Mason EO, Jr., Wald ER, et al. Decrease of invasive pneumococcal infections in children among 8 children's hospitals in the United States

after the introduction of the 7-valent pneumococcal conjugate vaccine. *Pediatrics* 2004;113:443–9.

37. Lacroix J, Hebert PC, Hutchison JS, et al. Transfusion strategies for patients in pediatric intensive care units. *New Engl J Med* 2007 19;356(16):1609–19.
38. Leclerc F, Leteurtre S, Duhamel A, et al. Cumulative influence of organ dysfunctions and septic state on mortality of critically ill children. *Am J Respir Crit Care Med* 2005;171:348–53.
39. Lepper PM, Held TK, Schneider EM, et al. Clinical implications of antibiotic-induced endotoxin release in septic shock. *Intensive Care Med* 2002;28:824–33.
40. Levy B, Gibot S, Franck P, et al. Relation between muscle Na+K+ ATPase activity and raised lactate concentrations in septic shock: A prospective study. *Lancet* 2005;365:871–5.
41. Levy MM, Fink MP, Marshall JC, et al. 2001 SCCM/ESICM/ACCP/ATS/SIS International Sepsis Definitions Conference. *Crit Care Med* 2003;31:1250–6.
42. Lin MT, Albertson TE. Genomic polymorphisms in sepsis. *Crit Care Med* 2004;32:569–79.
43. Magnotti LJ, Deitch EA. Burns, bacterial translocation, gut barrier function, and failure. *J Burn Care Rehabil* 2005;26:383–91.
44. Martin GS, Mannino DM, Eaton S, et al. The epidemiology of sepsis in the United States from 1979 through 2000. *N Engl J Med* 2003;348:1546–54.
45. Martinon F, Tschopp J. NLRs join TLRs as innate sensors of pathogens. *Trends Immunol* 2005;26:447–54.
46. McMaster P, Shann F. The use of extracorporeal techniques to remove humoral factors in sepsis. *Pediatr Crit Care Med* 2003;4:2–7.
47. Mira JP, Cariou A, Grall F, et al. Association of TNF2, a TNF-alpha promoter polymorphism, with septic shock susceptibility and mortality: A multicenter study. *JAMA* 1999;282:561–8.
48. Morel J, Venet C, Donati Y, et al. Adrenal axis function does not appear to be associated with hemodynamic improvement in septic shock patients systematically receiving glucocorticoid therapy. *Intensive Care Med* 2006;32:1184–90.
49. Nadel S, Newport MJ, Booy R, et al. Variation in the tumor necrosis factor-alpha gene promoter region may be associated with death from meningococcal disease. *J Infect Dis* 1996;174:878–80.
50. Ohlsson A, Lacy JB. Intravenous immunoglobulin for suspected or subsequently proven infection in neonates. *Cochrane Database Syst Rev* 2004;CD001239.
51. Opal SM, Cohen J. Clinical gram-positive sepsis: Does it fundamentally differ from gram-negative bacterial sepsis? *Crit Care Med* 1999;27:1608–16.
52. Osborn TM, Tracy JK, Dunne JR, et al. Epidemiology of sepsis in patients with traumatic injury. *Crit Care Med* 2004;32:2234–40.
53. Patel JC, Mollitt DL, Pieper P, et al. Nosocomial pneumonia in the pediatric trauma patient: A single center's experience. *Crit Care Med* 2000;28:3530–3.
54. Peters M, Petros A, Dixon G, et al. Acquired immunoparalysis in paediatric intensive care: Prospective observational study. *Br Med J* 1999;319:609–10.
55. Pildal J, Gotzsche PC. Polyclonal immunoglobulin for treatment of bacterial sepsis: A systematic review. *Clin Infect Dis* 2004;39:38–46.
56. Pollack MM, Fields AI, Ruttimann UE. Distributions of cardiopulmonary variables in pediatric survivors and nonsurvivors of septic shock. *Crit Care Med* 1985;13:454–9.
57. Price VE, Dutta S, Blanchette VS, et al. The prevention and treatment of bacterial infections in children with asplenia or hyposplenia: Practice considerations at the Hospital for Sick Children, Toronto. *Pediatr Blood Cancer* 2006;46:597–603.

58. Proft T, Fraser JD. Bacterial superantigens. *Clin Exp Immunol* 2003;133:299–306.
59. Randolph AG. International sepsis forum on sepsis in infants and children. *Pediatr Crit Care Med* 2005;6:S1–S164.
60. Richards MJ, Edwards JR, Culver DH, et al. Nosocomial infections in pediatric intensive care units in the United States. National Nosocomial Infections Surveillance System. *Pediatrics* 1999;103:e39.
61. Rivers E, Nguyen B, Havstad S, et al. Early goal-directed therapy in the treatment of severe sepsis and septic shock. *N Engl J Med* 2001;345:1368–77.
62. Sakr Y, Vincent JL, Reinhart K, et al. Use of the pulmonary artery catheter is not associated with worse outcome in the ICU. *Chest* 2005;128:2722–31.
63. Singh-Naz N, Sprague BM, Patel KM, et al. Risk assessment and standardized nosocomial infection rate in critically ill children. *Crit Care Med* 2000;28:2069–75.
64. Sorensen TI, Nielsen GG, Andersen PK, et al. Genetic and environmental influences on premature death in adult adoptees. *N Engl J Med* 1988;318:727–32.
65. Srinivasan V, Spinella PC, Drott HR, et al. Association of timing, duration, and intensity of hyperglycemia with intensive care unit mortality in critically ill children. *Pediatr Crit Care Med* 2004;5:329–36.
66. Stone JH, Dierberg K, Aram G, et al. Human monocytic ehrlichiosis. *JAMA* 2004;292:2263–70.
67. Taniguchi T, Hirai F, Takemoto Y, et al. A novel adsorbent of circulating bacterial toxins and cytokines: The effect of direct hemoperfusion with CTR column for the treatment of experimental endotoxemia. *Crit Care Med* 2006;34:800–6.
68. Tibbles PM, Edelsberg JS. Hyperbaric-oxygen therapy. *N Engl J Med* 1996;334:1642–8.
69. Ting JP, Davis BK. CATERPILLER: A novel gene family important in immunity, cell death, and diseases. *Annu Rev Immunol* 2005;23:387–414.
70. Tsiotou AG, Sakorafas GH, Anagnostopoulos G, et al. Septic shock: Current pathogenetic concepts from a clinical perspective. *Med Sci Monit* 2005;11:RA76–85.
71. Vincent JL, Baron JF, Reinhart K, et al. Anemia and blood transfusion in critically ill patients. *JAMA* 2002;288:1499–507.
72. Wallace WC, Cinat ME, Nastanski F, et al. New epidemiology for postoperative nosocomial infections. *Am Surg* 2000;66:874–8.
73. Watson RS, Carcillo JA. Scope and epidemiology of pediatric sepsis. *Pediatr Crit Care Med* 2005;6:S3–5.
74. Watson RS, Carcillo JA, Linde-Zwirble WT, et al. The epidemiology of severe sepsis in children in the United States. *Am J Respir Crit Care Med* 2003;167:695–701.
75. Wheeler AP, Bernard GR. Treating patients with severe sepsis. *N Engl J Med* 1999;340:207–14.
76. White JR, Dalton HJ. Pediatric trauma: Postinjury care in the pediatric intensive care unit. *Crit Care Med* 2002;30:S478–88.
77. Wisplinghoff H, Bischoff T, Tallent SM, et al. Nosocomial bloodstream infections in US hospitals: Analysis of 24,179 cases from a prospective nationwide surveillance study. *Clin Infect Dis* 2004;39:309–17.
78. Yang H, Ochani M, Li J, et al. Reversing established sepsis with antagonists of endogenous high-mobility group box 1. *Proc Natl Acad Sci U S A* 2004;101:296–301.

CHAPTER 79 ■ CRITICAL VIRAL INFECTIONS

RAKESH LODHA • SUNIT C. SINGHI • JAMES D. CAMPBELL

Various types of viral infections may pose a challenge to the pediatric intensivist. Dengue hemorrhagic fever (DHF) occurs in more than 100 countries and requires early recognition and aggressive management to reduce the adverse outcomes. Various other viral hemorrhagic fevers occur in specific geographic areas; however, the likelihood does exist that these agents could be used in bioterrorism. Human immunodeficiency virus (HIV) infection is on the rise in many developing countries and is likely to have significant implications for child health. Measles infection is still a major problem in many developing countries. Herpes viruses can also be responsible for serious illnesses that require intensive care. This chapter discusses these infections, with emphasis on the more severe infections.

DENGUE HEMORRHAGIC FEVER AND DENGUE SHOCK SYNDROME

Background

Dengue fever (DF) is an acute febrile illness caused by viruses that belong to the Flaviviridae family and is characterized by biphasic fever, myalgia, arthralgia, and rash. DHF is characterized by abnormalities in hemostasis and marked leakage of plasma from the capillaries; the latter may lead to dengue shock syndrome (DSS).

Epidemiology

The global incidence of dengue has grown dramatically in recent decades, with the infection now endemic in more than 100 countries in Africa, the Americas, the Eastern Mediterranean, Southeast Asia, and the Western Pacific. Southeast Asia and the Western Pacific are most seriously affected. Before 1970, only nine countries had experienced DHF epidemics, a number that increased more than fourfold by 2005. Nearly 2.5 billion people are at risk to contract dengue, and the World Health Organization (WHO) currently estimates that 50 million cases of dengue infection occur worldwide annually.

During epidemics of dengue, attack rates among those susceptible are often 40%–50%, but may reach 80%–90%. Of the estimated 500,000 cases of DHF around the world that require hospitalization each year, a very large proportion are children. Approximately 2.5% of hospitalized patients die, although case fatality ratios may be underestimated and may be up to twice as high. Without proper treatment, DHF case fatality rates can exceed 20%. With modern intensive supportive therapy, such rates can be reduced to less than 1%.

Virus

DF and DHF are caused by infection due to any of the four serotypes of dengue viruses, which are arboviruses that belong to the family Flaviviridae. These viruses are spherical particles ~50 nm in diameter. Dengue RNA has ~11,000 nucleotides. The envelope protein bears epitopes that are unique to the serotypes; the antibodies to these unique epitopes neutralize by interfering with the entry of the virus into the cells. Other epitopes are shared between dengue viruses (dengue subgroup antigens) and other flaviviruses (group antigens). Four well-defined types of dengue virus have been identified and are labeled Den 1, Den 2, Den 3, and Den 4; they have distinctive genetic makeup, allowing the use of genotyping to trace the movement of dengue viruses between different geographic regions.

Transmission

Dengue viruses are transmitted to humans through the bites of infective female *Aedes vexans* mosquitoes. After virus incubation of 8–10 days, an infected mosquito is capable, during probing and blood feeding, of transmitting the virus to susceptible individuals for the rest of its life. Infected female mosquitoes may also transmit the virus to their offspring by transovarial (via the eggs) transmission. Humans are the main amplifying host of the virus, although studies have shown that, in some parts of the world, monkeys may become infected and perhaps serve as a source of virus for uninfected mosquitoes. The virus circulates in the blood of infected humans for 2–7 days, at approximately the same time that they have fever.

Importance of the Disease to the Intensivist

The severe forms of DHF and DSS require management in a critical care setting. Affected children require very careful monitoring and aggressive fluid therapy to improve their outcomes. In view of significant capillary leak, fluid therapy is challenging and requires frequent modification. Respiratory distress, due to extensive pleural effusions, myocardial dysfunction, or extensive bleeding, is potentially life-threatening. Multiorgan failure may occur in a few children. Given the occurrence of these infections in a large part of the world and the increase in international travel, pediatric intensivists in both endemic and nonendemic parts of the world must be able to recognize and manage DHF and DSS.

Pathophysiology of the Infection and Its Consequences

Virus is inoculated into the human by the mosquito, spreads to regional lymph nodes and the reticuloendothelial organs, multiplies, and enters the bloodstream. The major pathophysiologic changes that determine the severity of disease in DHF and differentiate it from DF are plasma leakage (capillary permeability with resultant hypovolemia) and abnormal hemostasis. These problems lead, in turn, to rising hematocrit values, moderate-to-marked thrombocytopenia, and varying degrees of bleeding manifestations (45).

The dendritic cells (DCs) in the tissues internalize the virus, where it resides in cystic vacuoles, vesicles, and endoplasmic reticulum. After the phagocytosis and antigen processing, the DCs release a number of cytokines, including tumor necrosis factor (TNF)-α and interferon (IFN)-α, which lead to activation of other virus-infected and virus-uninfected DCs in a paracrine manner. IFN-γ is an important second signal for secretion of bioactive IL-12 from DCs in addition to its effect on expression of molecules that are involved in stimulating antigen-specific T-cell response. During a secondary dengue infection, memory T cells produce early IFN-γ and CD40L in the DC microenvironment, leading to greater DC activation and subsequent T-cell stimulation and cytokine release, especially IL-12. The viremia may be cleared, but the cascade of events initiated by the early, poorly controlled type 1 cytokine response contributes to the pathogenesis of DHF/DSS. Various studies have shown higher levels of TNF-α, soluble TNF-α receptor, and IFN-γ levels in patients with DHF/DSS as compared to those with DF.

The mechanism of antibody-dependent enhancement has been proposed (29). It has been observed that sequential infection with any two of the four serotypes of dengue virus results in DHF/DSS in an endemic area. Serotype cross-reactive antibodies generated from previous primary infection with a particular dengue viral serotype are not highly specific for the other serotypes involved in secondary infections. Hence, they bind to the virions but do not neutralize them. Such antibody-coated virions are taken up more rapidly than uncoated virus particles, leading to enhanced antigen presentation by the infected dendritic cells to the T cells, resulting in more rapid activation and proliferation of memory T cells. The cytokines produced by the activated T cells have several important effects that lead to the pathogenesis of the DHF/DSS.

Complement activation mediated by nonstructural viral protein NS1 leads to local and systemic generation of anaphylatoxins and SC5b-9, which may contribute to the pathogenesis of the vascular leakage that occurs in patients with DHF/DSS.

Cytokines are implicated in the pathogenesis of vascular compromise and hemorrhage in dengue virus infection. The release of cytokines in response to dengue viral infection includes both inflammatory and inhibitory cytokines, and the net outcome will depend on the balance between various cytokine actions. An overall increase occurs in the levels of T-cell activation markers, such as soluble IL-2 receptor, soluble CD4 and CD8, IL-2 and IFN-γ, as well as increases in monokines, such as TNFα, IFN-β, and granulocyte-macrophage colony-stimulating factor (GM-CSF), and these levels are consistently higher in those with DHF/DSS than in those with DF. Dengue patients with shock have significantly higher levels of IL-6 at admission, compared to normotensive patients. Elevated IL-6 is also associated with a higher incidence of ascites. Similarly, high levels of IL-8 can be recovered from serum and pleural fluid of patients with DSS.

Endothelial cells also undergo apoptosis, which causes disruption of the endothelial cell barrier, leading to the syndrome of generalized vascular leakage. The mast cells may play a role in the initiation of chemokine-dependent host responses to dengue virus infection. Assessment of microvascular leakage using strain-gauge plethysmography in children with DHF and DSS found that, although the coefficient of microvascular permeability (K_f) was higher in children with either DHF or DSS as opposed to that in healthy controls, no significant difference existed between the 2 groups (DHF, DSS), suggesting a similar pathogenetic mechanism (11).

Dengue viral infection is commonly associated with thrombocytopenia; one postulated mechanism is molecular mimicry. Antibodies against dengue virus proteins, especially NS1, cross-react with platelet surface proteins and thus, cause thrombocytopenia. These antibodies, in addition to causing platelet lysis via complement activation, also inhibit adenosine diphosphate-induced platelet aggregation. The titre of these immunoglobulin M (IgM) antibodies has been found to be much higher in patients with DHF/DSS than in those with DF. Dengue virus infection can also activate blood clotting and fibrinolytic pathways. Mild disseminated intravascular coagulation (DIC), liver injury, and thrombocytopenia together contribute to hemorrhagic tendency. Central nervous system (CNS) involvement also has been identified and has been attributed to direct neurotropic effect of dengue virus.

The risk factors for DHF/ DSS are:

- Virus strain—Epidemic potential, risk of DHF is greatest for Den 2 followed by Den 3, Den 4, and Den 1.
- Preexisting anti-dengue antibody is present.
- Age of host—Younger children are at increased risk.
- Secondary infection is present.
- Genetic predisposition (51) is present.
- Hyperendemicity—Two or more virus serotypes may be circulating simultaneously at high level.

Pathology

Usually, no gross or microscopic lesions account for death, except when massive gastrointestinal or intracranial bleeding is found. Presence of viruses in tissues mainly leads to hemodynamic alterations with generalized vascular congestion, increased permeability, and mast-cell recruitment in lungs. Variable hepatic involvement has been reported: diffuse hepatitis with mid-zonal necrosis and steatosis, focal areas of necrosis, and normal histology in some children. Dengue virus antigen can be detected using immunohistochemistry in hepatocytes from necrotic areas.

Clinical Manifestations

The clinical manifestations of dengue virus infection vary from asymptomatic to severe life-threatening illness in the form of DHF/DSS (44). Most dengue infections in young children are mild and indistinguishable from other common causes of febrile illnesses. Fever, headache, myalgia, arthralgia, skin rashes, and malaise characterize the illness (44). Some people develop such severe myalgia and arthralgias that dengue is sometimes called "breakbone fever." Skin eruptions are reported in >50% of laboratory-confirmed dengue cases, more commonly in children and adults with primary infections. A flushing of the face, neck, and chest may initially occur in the febrile period, a centrifugal maculopapular rash may arise on the third or fourth day, a confluent petechial rash with round pale areas of normal skin may occur later, or a combination of these manifestations may be seen.

Typically, after an incubation period of 4–6 days, patients may develop abrupt onset of high-grade fever (often 39°C–40°C and usually continuous), facial flushing, headache, and retro-orbital pain. Anorexia, vomiting, abdominal pain, and tenderness over the right costal margin are common. Varying degrees of tender hepatomegaly may be appreciated; the spleen is less commonly enlarged. All DHF/DSS patients have some hemorrhagic phenomena in the form of a positive tourniquet test, petechiae, bruising at venipuncture sites, bleeding from the gums, epistaxis, hematemesis, or melena. Occasionally, adolescent girls may have vaginal bleeding that mimics menstrual bleeding. Rarely, bleeding from the external auditory canals, muscle hematomas, hematuria, or intracranial hemorrhage may occur. Fever usually subsides after 2–7 days. At this stage, the child may show varying degrees of peripheral circulatory failure, characterized by excessive sweating, restlessness, and cold extremities.

The four warning signs for impending shock are intense, sustained abdominal pain; persistent vomiting; restlessness or lethargy; and a sudden change from fever to hypothermia, with sweating and prostration. Initially, the pulse pressure is narrow; later, the blood pressure may start falling, and untreated, may progress to unrecordable blood pressure and irreversible shock. If not appropriately treated, a child may die within 12–24 hrs after the first signs of DHF emerge. Prior to the child becoming afebrile, thrombocytopenia and a rise in hematocrit occur; these features are characteristic of the disease and may help to distinguish it from other endemic febrile diseases. Unusual manifestations of DHF/DSS include encephalitis and glomerulonephritis (44). Acute hepatic failure is uncommon, although many children have evidence of hepatic involvement.

In some patients, infection with dengue virus may mimic Reye syndrome. In general, when children have involvement of the CNS, it is manifested as encephalopathy. True encephalitis, though reported, is very rare. Patients may have lethargy, confusion, alteration of consciousness/coma, nuchal rigidity, convulsions, and paresis. The CNS involvement is frequently associated with prolonged shock and the resultant metabolic acidosis and severe DIC that lead to intracranial bleeding, electrolyte imbalances (e.g., hyponatremia, hypocalcemia), and metabolic disturbances (e.g., hypoglycemia). Myocardial dysfunction has also been reported (35). Most reported cases of renal disease associated with dengue virus infections are associated with late acute hepatic failure. The risk factors for renal failure are use of nephrotoxic drugs, intravascular hemolysis (e.g., G-6-PD deficiency), and an underlying hemoglobinopathy.

Case Definition and Grading of Dengue Hemorrhagic Fever

The presence of thrombocytopenia with concurrent hemoconcentration differentiates DHF from DF. On the basis of clinical features, DHF is classified into four grades of severity. Grades III and IV define DSS (6) (**Table 79.1**).

Some patients with dengue infection have varying degrees of mucosal and cutaneous bleeding with some degree of thrombocytopenia. These patients may not demonstrate other criteria for diagnosis of DHF/DSS (i.e., hemoconcentration or objective evidence of fluid leak, such as ascites and pleural effusion); they are classified as having *dengue fever with unusual bleeding* and may be seen in significant numbers in epidemics. As hypovolemia and hypotension do not occur in this group, fluid requirement is less than in those with DHF (34). It is, therefore, important to distinguish these children from classical DHF.

Diagnosis

Diseases that may mimic DHF/DSS include those that may cause influenza-like illnesses followed by severe manifestations. Examples include infections due to Gram-negative bacteria such as *Neisseria meningitidis* (meningococcemia), *Salmonella*

TABLE 79.1

GRADING OF DENGUE HEMORRHAGIC FEVER

Grade	Clinical features	Bleeding manifestations	Hemodynamic status
Grade I	Fever accompanied by nonspecific constitutional symptoms	A positive tourniquet test and or easy bruising	Tachycardia ± normal BP, pulse pressure
Grade II	Fever accompanied by nonspecific constitutional symptoms	Spontaneous bleeding, usually in the form of skin or other hemorrhages	Tachycardia ± normal BP, pulse pressure
Grade III (DSS)	Same as Grades I/II, may present with cold peripheries	Spontaneous bleeding may be present	Circulatory failure manifested by a rapid, weak pulse, narrowing of pulse pressure, or hypotension, with cold clammy skin and restlessness
Grade IV (DSS)	Same as Grades I/II; may present with cold peripheries. May have features suggestive of organ hypoperfusion	Spontaneous bleeding may be present	Profound shock with undetectable blood pressure or peripheral pulse

DSS, dengue shock syndrome; BP, blood pressure

typhi (typhoid, enteric fever), and *Yersinia pestis* (plague). Occasionally, malaria caused by *Plasmodium falciparum* may manifest with fever and bleeding but is distinguished by the presence of splenomegaly and significant pallor. Chikungunya, Rift Valley Fever, sandfly fever, hepatitis, and rickettsial diseases may be difficult to distinguish from DF.

The following features are useful for making a provisional diagnosis of DHF/DSS when a child lives in, or has recently traveled from, an endemic area (44). *Clinical criteria*: Acute onset high fever, hemorrhagic manifestations (at least a positive tourniquet test), hepatomegaly, and shock. *Laboratory criteria*: Thrombocytopenia (less than 100,000 cells/mm^3), hemoconcentration (hematocrit elevated at least 20% above the standard for age, sex, and population baseline or baseline hematocrit). Two clinical observations and one laboratory finding (or at least a rising hematocrit) are sufficient to establish a provisional diagnosis of DHF. A rise in hematocrit of 20% over the baseline can be documented if the hematocrit is monitored regularly from the early stages of illness. As patients are likely to present with symptoms suggestive of DHF, a drop in hemoglobin or hematocrit of more than 20% following volume replacement therapy can be taken as an indication of previous hemoconcentration. Hematocrit can, however, be affected by various factors, including baseline anemia, time of hematocrit estimation during illness, and blood loss. In monitoring hematocrit, the possible effects of preexisting anemia, severe hemorrhage, or early volume replacement therapy should be considered. In a patient with suspected DHF, the presence of shock suggests the diagnosis of DSS.

Laboratory Investigations

Either demonstration of dengue virus on culture or demonstration of antibodies against dengue virus is required for confirming dengue infection (**Table 79.2**). Viral isolation is recommended if the blood sample is taken within 5 days of the onset of fever, while serologic methods are used if blood samples are taken after defervescence or during convalescence (7). Meticulous attention must be paid to sample collection and transport of clinical samples for virus isolation. Samples may be inoculated either in suckling mice or in various tissue cultures of mammalian or mosquito origin.

TABLE 79.2

DIAGNOSTIC TESTS FOR DENGUE HEMORRHAGIC FEVER

Period	Tests
Within first 5 days of onset of fever	Viral isolation from blood (inoculated either in suckling mice or in various tissue cultures of mammalian or mosquito origin)
After defervescence/in convalescent phase	Serologic tests: IgM: MAC ELISA, strip test IgG: hemagglutination inhibition test, strip test

IgM, immunoglobulin M; MAC-ELISA, IgM antibody-capture enzyme-linked immunosorbent assay; IgG, immunoglobulin G

Commonly used serologic tests to detect antibodies include IgM antibody-capture enzyme-linked immunosorbent assay (MAC-ELISA) test and hemagglutination inhibition test. The MAC-ELISA test measures dengue-specific IgM antibodies and suggests recent infection with dengue virus. The hemagglutination inhibition test measures immunoglobulin G (IgG) antibodies. It is a simple, sensitive, and reproducible test but requires paired sera collected at an interval of 1–2 weeks. Positive test results indicate a recent infection due to a flavivirus, but cross-reactivity occurs across this group of viruses. A commercially available strip test requires a drop of serum and gives results within few minutes. Quantitation of the IgG and IgM antibodies may help in differentiating between primary and secondary dengue virus infections. IgG antibodies will be abundant in secondary infection but not in primary infection.

Use of the polymerase chain reaction (PCR) may shorten the time required for result (17). PCR can also detect viruses inactivated by improper storage or by complexing with neutralizing antibody. However, the PCR test is still experimental.

Other Investigations

During the course of illness, children with DHF/DSS show increasing hematocrit, decreased platelet counts, and increased white cell counts with relative lymphocytosis; however, they may have leukopenia. The peripheral smear may show transformed/atypical lymphocytes. In severe illness with prolonged shock, laboratory evidence may show DIC. Blood chemistry tests may show reduced levels of total protein and albumin. These disturbances are more marked in patients with shock. Levels of transaminases are raised frequently. A higher increase in levels of AST than ALT suggests the possibility of DHF rather than hepatitis due to another virus. In more severe cases, hyponatremia, acidosis, and an increase in blood urea and creatinine may be present.

Chest x-rays may show varying degrees of pleural effusion, commonly on the right side, occasionally bilateral. Pleural effusion index (the proportion of the width of the right hemithorax occupied by a pleural effusion seen on chest x-ray taken in the right lateral decubitus position) may be used as an objective measure of plasma leakage. Ultrasonography of the abdomen may show an enlarged gall bladder due to wall edema and ascites due to generalized vascular leaks. Abnormal electrocardiogram and myocardial dysfunction on echocardiogram have also been reported.

Treatment

Dengue Fever

The treatment of DF is symptomatic and consists of fever management, fluid replacement, and close monitoring for clues to progression to DHF/DSS. No specific antiviral drugs have been shown to be efficacious. Fever may be treated with paracetamol or acetaminophen. Salicylates and other nonsteroidal anti-inflammatory drugs should be avoided, as these may predispose a child to mucosal bleeds, and salicylates have been associated with Reye syndrome. In an epidemic setting, all patients with DF require regular monitoring by a primary care physician for early detection of DHF. The primary care physician/healthcare worker should monitor the patient for clinical features of DHF/DSS along with hematocrit and platelet counts, if possible. Any patient who develops cold extremities, restlessness, acute abdominal pain, decreased urine output, bleeding, or hemoconcentration should be admitted to a hospital. Children with a rising hematocrit and thrombocytopenia without clinical symptoms should also be admitted. Children should be encouraged to improve their oral fluid intake, when possible. Electrolyte/carbohydrate solutions, such as WHO oral rehydration salt solutions, are preferred over plain water or other fluids.

Dengue Hemorrhagic Fever/Dengue Shock Syndrome

The management discussed here is based on guidelines issued by the WHO (12). Early recognition of these conditions is crucial for decreasing case fatality rates. As no specific antiviral medications exist for dengue infections, supportive and aggressive fluid therapy is the cornerstone of management.

In the hospital, children without hypotension (DHF grades I and II) should be given Ringer's lactate infusion at the rate of 7 mL/kg over 1 hr. After 1 hr, if the hematocrit decreases and vital parameters improve, fluid infusion rate may be decreased to 5 mL/kg over the next hour and to 3 mL/kg/hr for 24–48 hrs. When the patient is stable, as indicated by normal blood pressure, satisfactory oral intake, and urine output, the child can be discharged (**Fig. 79.1**). If at 1 hr, the hematocrit is rising and vital parameters do not show improvement, fluid infusion rate is increased to 10 mL/kg over the next hour. In case of no improvement, the fluid infusion rate is further increased to 15 mL/kg over the third hour. If no improvement is observed in vital parameters and hematocrit at the end of 3 hrs, administration of plasma infusion (10 mL/kg) or colloids should be initiated (**Fig. 79.2**). Once the hematocrit and vital parameters are stable, the infusion rate is gradually reduced and discontinued over 24–48 hrs.

In children with hypotension (DSS grade III), Ringer's lactate solution at 10–20 mL/kg is infused over 1 hr or given as bolus if blood pressure is unrecordable (DSS grade IV). The bolus may be repeated twice if no improvement occurs. If no improvement occurs in vital parameters and hematocrit is rising even after repeated boluses of crystalloids, colloids (10 mL/kg) are rapidly infused. If the hematocrit is falling without improvement in vital parameters, blood is transfused, presuming that lack of improvement is due to occult blood loss (9) (**Fig. 79.2**). Once improvement starts, fluid infusion rate is gradually decreased. In addition to fluids, oxygen should be administered to all patients in shock.

A few studies have evaluated the efficacy of different types of fluids in DHF/DSS (i.e., crystalloids and various colloids) (43,57). Irrespective of the fluid choice, mortality was low and

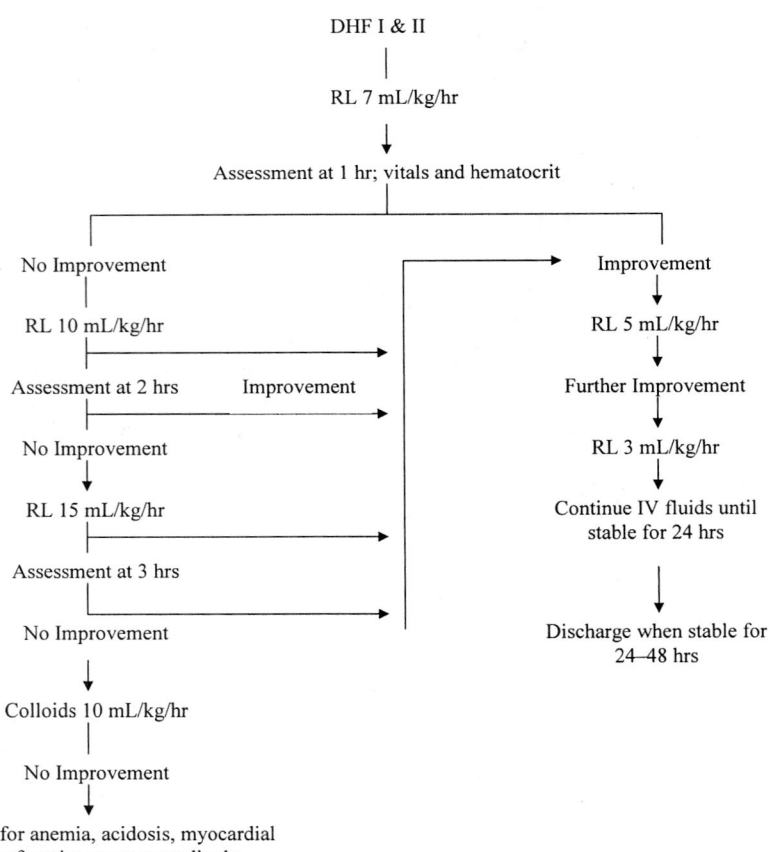

DHF, Dengue hemorrhagic fever; RL, Ringer's lactate

FIGURE 79.1. Intravenous fluid infusion in dengue hemorrhagic fever.

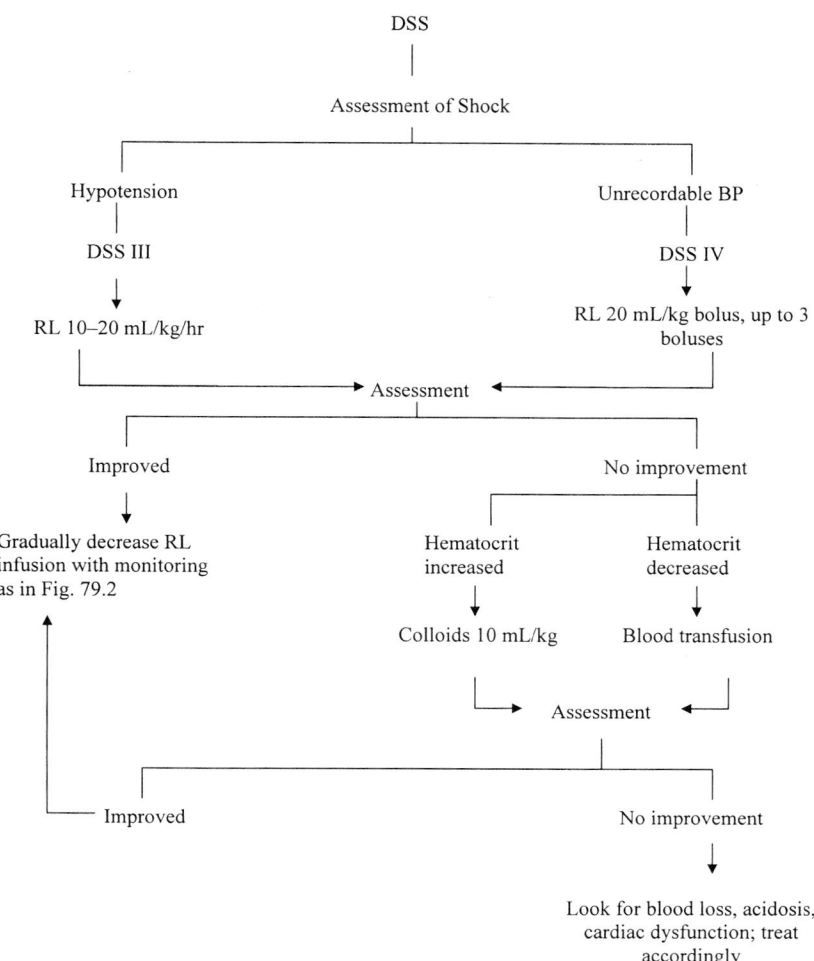

DSS, Dengue shock syndrome; BP, blood pressure, RL, Ringer's lactate;

FIGURE 79.2. Treatment of dengue shock syndrome.

similar with all fluids evaluated. Minor advantages were reported with hydroxyethyl starch, and it may be preferred in severe shock. Dextran was associated more often with severe allergic-type reactions.

The WHO guidelines are useful in that they offer an algorithmic approach to fluid resuscitation of DHF and DSS. However, the usefulness of these guidelines is limited beyond the immediate resuscitation because they do not address the treatment of complicated forms of the disease, including fluid overload and multiple organ function failure, which likely result in disability or death. In an evaluation of a new protocol in patients with DHF and DSS that was intended to prompt earlier recognition of the disease, aggressive management of shock, and early aggressive diuresis or dialysis in the event of extensive edema, the authors suggest that aggressive shock management and possibly the use of judicious fluid removal may decrease mortality rates in the severest forms of DSS (49). However, this study had major drawbacks—high mortality and use of retrospective controls. In most cases, it may be appropriate to give just enough fluid to maintain blood pressure and hematocrit.

For uncontrolled bleeding in DHF or DSS, the role of plasma or platelet infusion remains unclear. In a small study in which

children with severe thrombocytopenia were included, platelet infusion did not alter the outcome (33). Infusion of fresh frozen plasma and platelet concentrates may be beneficial in patients with DIC. Treatment with methylprednisolone did not show any benefit in a double-blinded, placebo-controlled trial in patients with DSS.

Monitoring

In view of the rapidly changing course in DHF and DSS, close monitoring of the patient is crucial in the first few hours of illness. Heart rate, respiratory rate, blood pressure, and pulse pressure should be measured frequently, continuously, or at least every 30 mins until the patient is stable and, thereafter, at least every 2–4 hrs. Central venous pressure monitoring is desirable, when possible, in all children who develop hypotension. Laboratory monitoring includes hematocrit measurement every 2 hrs for the first 6 hrs or until stable. Absolute platelet counts may be conducted once per day until they show a rising trend. Platelet counts are repeated and coagulation studies performed if uncontrolled bleeding is present. If insertion of a central line is not feasible, clinical and hematocrit monitoring every 30 mins may guide the rate of fluid infusion. It is emphasized that infusion rates decrease rapidly in the first 6 hrs following intervention in most uncomplicated cases of DSS and DHF (33).

Prognosis

If DHF or DSS is left untreated, the mortality may be as high as 40%–50%. The causes of death include prolonged shock, massive bleeding, fluid overload, and acute hepatic failure with encephalopathy. The mortality may be higher in settings that lack experienced medical teams. Early recognition of illness, careful monitoring, and appropriate fluid therapy have resulted in reduction in mortality to 1%–5%. Early recognition of shock is of paramount importance, as the outcome in DSS depends on the duration of shock. If shock is identified when pulse pressure begins narrowing and IV fluids are administered, the outcome is excellent. Recovery is fast, and the majority of patients recover in 24–48 hrs without sequelae. The outcome may not be as good once the patient develops cold extremities. The prognosis is grave in patients with prolonged shock and when blood pressure is not recordable at the time of presentation.

Recent Advances in Therapy

The compounds that have shown promising results in experimental settings include anti-TNF-α antibody, ribavirin, amantadine, peptide inhibitors of dengue virus infectivity, castanospermine and deoxynojirimycin, and sulfated polysaccharides obtained from the red seaweeds *Gymnogongrus griffithsia* and *Cryptonemia crenulata* (28).

Vaccines

The first vaccine to combat dengue viruses was developed at Mahidol University in Bangkok, Thailand, and licensed by Sanofi Pasteur. It produces 80%–90% seroconversion rates to all four serotypes after the administration of two doses in young children. Efforts are underway to develop newer vaccines.

Conclusions and Future Directions

DHF and DSS are the serious manifestations of dengue virus infections. The great need for better understanding of the pathogenesis of DHF/DSS may pave the way for new therapies. Prevention of dengue infections by efficient vector control is also needed. Development of an effective vaccine may reduce the disease burden. Given the worldwide prevalence of the disease, development of antiviral drugs active against dengue should be a priority.

VIRAL HEMORRHAGIC FEVERS

Viral hemorrhagic fevers (VHF) compose a group of clinical syndromes that are characterized by hemorrhagic manifestations. Disseminated intravascular coagulopathy appears to be the common pathogenetic feature of these illnesses.

The pathogenic viruses are from the Flaviviridae family (Kyasanur Forest disease, Omsk, dengue, and yellow fever viruses), Bunyaviridae family (Congo, Hantaan, and Rift Valley fever viruses), the Arenaviridae family (Junin, Machupo, Guanarito, and Lassa viruses), and the Filoviridae family (Ebola and Marburg viruses) (Table 79.3). The dengue viruses, Rift

TABLE 79.3

VARIOUS VIRAL HEMORRHAGIC FEVERS

Disease	Virus	Vector	Geographic areas
Crimean-Congo hemorrhagic fever	Congo virus	Ixodid Ticks (Hyalomma)	Bulgaria, western Crimea, Rostov-on-Don and Astrakhan regions, Pakistan, Afghanistan, Arabian Peninsula, South Africa, Oman, southern Russia
Kyasanur Forest disease	Kysanur forest disease virus	Ticks	Mysore State, India
Omsk hemorrhagic fever	Omsk virus	Ticks	South central Russia, northern Romania
Rift Valley fever	Rift valley fever virus	Mosquitoes	North, Central, East, and South Africa, Saudi Arabia, Yemen
Argentine hemorrhagic fever	Junin virus	Rodent	Argentina
Bolivian hemorrhagic fever	Machupo virus	Rodent	Amazonian Bolivia
Lassa fever	Lassa virus	Rodent (*Mastomys*)	Nigeria, Sierra Leone, Liberia
Marburg disease	Marburg virus	Unknown	Congo Republic, Germany, Yugoslavia Zimbabwe, Kenya, South Africa
Ebola hemorrhagic fever	Ebola virus	Unknown	Northern Zaire, southern Sudan, Uganda, Central and West Africa
Hemorrhagic fever with renal syndrome	Hanta virus	Rodents (Apodemus agrarius, Clethrionomys glareolus, Apodemus flavicollis)	Japan, Korea, Far Eastern Siberia, north and central China, European and Asian Russia, Scandinavia, Czechoslovakia, Romania, Bulgaria, Yugoslavia, Greece
Yellow fever	Yellow fever virus	Mosquitoes (Aedes and Haemogogus)	Tropical areas of Africa and the Americas

Valley fever virus, and yellow fever virus are transmitted by mosquitoes. Ticks are responsible for transmission of Omsk, Kysanur forest disease, and Congo viruses. Human infection may occur from infected animals or materials in case of Junin, Lassa, Marburg, Ebola, and Hanta viruses. Some viruses that cause hemorrhagic fever, such as Ebola, Marburg, Lassa, and Crimean-Congo hemorrhagic fever viruses, can spread from one person to another. This type of secondary transmission of the virus can occur directly, through close contact with infected people or their body fluids. It can also occur indirectly, through contact with objects contaminated with infected body fluids. For example, contaminated syringes and needles have

---

TABLE 79.4

CLINICAL FEATURES OF VIRAL HEMORRHAGIC FEVERS

Disease	Incubation period	Clinical features	Case fatality
Crimean-Congo hemorrhagic fever	3–12 days	Fever, severe headache, myalgia, abdominal pain, anorexia, nausea, and vomiting; erythematous facial or truncal flush and injected conjunctivae; hemorrhagic enanthem on the soft palate and a fine petechial rash on the chest and abdomen. Large areas of purpura and bleeding from gums, nose, intestine, lungs, or uterus may be seen. Hepatomegaly in absence of icterus. In severe illnesses, CNS symptoms and signs may be seen	2%–50%
Kyasanur Forest disease	3–8 days	Severe myalgia, prostration, and bronchiolar involvement. Often presents without hemorrhage but occasionally with severe gastrointestinal bleeding, bronchopneumonia, acute renal failure, and focal liver damage, meningoencephalitis	3%–10%
Omsk hemorrhagic fever	3–8 days	Moderate epistaxis, hematemesis, and a hemorrhagic enanthem but no profuse hemorrhage, bronchopneumonia	1%–10%
Rift Valley fever	3–6 days	Fever, headache, prostration, myalgia, anorexia, nausea, vomiting, conjunctivitis, and lymphadenopathy, purpura, epistaxis, hematemesis, and melena	~1%
Argentine, Venezuelan, and Bolivian hemorrhagic fever and Lassa fever	~7–14 days	Fever, headache, diffuse myalgia, anorexia, sore throat, dysphagia, cough, oropharyngeal ulcers, nausea, vomiting, diarrhea, pains in chest, abdomen, pleuritic chest pain; tourniquet test may be positive. Hypovolemic shock may be accompanied by pleural effusion and renal failure; respiratory distress (airway obstruction, pleural effusion, or congestive heart failure); neurologic symptoms, seizures	10%–40%
Marburg disease and Ebola hemorrhagic fever	4–7 days	Headache, malaise, drowsiness, lumbar myalgia, vomiting, nausea, and diarrhea. Maculopapular eruption, often hemorrhagic, dark red enanthem on the hard palate, conjunctivitis, and scrotal or labial edema. Gastrointestinal hemorrhage in severe illness. Hypotension and coma in severe cases. DIC and thrombocytopenia are seen in most patients.	Marburg disease: 25% Ebola hemorrhagic fever: 50%–90%
Hemorrhagic fever with renal syndrome (Hanta, Puumala)	9–35 days	Fever, petechiae, mild hemorrhagic phenomena, mild proteinuria. Thrombocytopenia, petechiae, proteinuria. Hypotension may follow defervescence. Hemoconcentration, ecchymoses, oliguria. Confusion, extreme restlessness. Fatal cases may manifest retroperitoneal edema and marked hemorrhagic necrosis of the renal medulla.	5%–10%
Yellow fever	3–6 days	Abrupt onset. Fever, headache, severe myalgias, diarrhea, vomiting, severe prostration, conjunctival suffusion, photophobia, cervical and axillary adenopathy, and more rarely, splenomegaly or hepatosplenomegaly. Papulovesicular lesions involving the soft palate and pulmonary manifestations are frequent during the first stage of the illness. The second stage of the illness is associated with neurologic involvement. Hemorrhagic manifestations are similar to those observed with other viral hemorrhagic fevers.	<10%

played an important role in spreading infection in outbreaks of Ebola hemorrhagic fever and Lassa fever. These illnesses may be seen in patients who have traveled to the endemic areas.

Clinical Features

The clinical features of different types of viral hemorrhagic fevers are summarized in **Table 79.4** (12,48).

Diagnosis

Healthcare providers must have a high index of suspicion for VHF in endemic areas. In nonendemic areas, histories of recent travel, recent laboratory exposure, or exposure to an earlier case should evoke suspicion of a viral hemorrhagic fever. In all VHF, the virus can be recovered during the early febrile stage. Bunyaviruses can be recovered from acute-phase serum by inoculation into tissue culture or living mosquitoes. Argentine, Bolivian, and Venezuelan hemorrhagic fever viruses can be isolated from acute-phase blood or throat washings by inoculation intracerebrally into guinea pigs, infant hamsters, or infant mice. Lassa virus may be isolated from acute-phase blood or throat washings by inoculation into tissue cultures. For Marburg disease and Ebola hemorrhagic fever, acute-phase throat washings, blood, and urine may be inoculated into tissue culture, guinea pigs, or monkeys. The viruses are readily identified by electron microscopy, with a filamentous structure that differentiates them from all other known agents.

Specific complement-fixing and immunofluorescent antibodies appear during convalescence. The viruses of hemorrhagic fever with renal syndrome (HFRS) can be recovered from acute-phase serum or urine by inoculation into tissue culture. A variety of antibody tests using viral subunits are becoming available.

Serologic diagnosis depends on demonstrating seroconversion—a fourfold or greater increase in immunoglobulin G antibody titer in acute and convalescent serum samples taken 3–4 weeks apart. Viral RNA may also be detected in blood or tissues, using reverse-transcriptase PCRs.

Handling blood and other biologic specimens is hazardous, and must be performed by specially trained personnel. For those hemorrhagic fever viruses that can be transmitted from person to person (Ebola, Marburg, Lassa, and Crimean-Congo hemorrhagic fever viruses), avoiding close physical contact with infected people and their body fluids is the most effective way of controlling the spread of disease. Infection-control techniques include barrier nursing, isolating infected individuals, and wearing protective clothing. Other infection-control recommendations include proper use, disinfection, and disposal of instruments and equipment (needles, thermometers, etc.) used in treating or caring for patients with VHF.

VHF isolation precautions include:

- Isolating the patient (universal, contact, droplet).
- Wearing protective clothing in the isolation area, in the cleaning and laundry areas, and in the laboratory; protective gear should include a scrub suit, gown, apron, two pairs of gloves, mask, head cover, eyewear, and rubber boots.

- Cleaning and disinfecting spills, waste, and reusable equipment safely.
- Cleaning and disinfecting soiled linens and laundry safely.
- Using safe disposal methods for nonreusable supplies and infectious waste.
- Providing information about the risk of VHF transmission to health facility staff.
- Reinforcing use of VHF isolation precautions with all health facility staff.

Differential Diagnosis

Mild cases of hemorrhagic fever are similar to many self-limited systemic bacterial or viral infections. In severe cases, the differential diagnoses include typhoid fever, typhus, leptospirosis, or a rickettsial spotted fever.

Treatment

Ribavirin administered IV is effective in reducing mortality in Lassa fever and HFRS (41). The principle involved in management of all of these diseases, especially HFRS, is the reversal of dehydration, hemoconcentration, renal failure, and protein, electrolyte, or blood losses. The management of hemorrhage should be individualized. Transfusions of fresh blood and platelets are frequently given. Good results have been reported in a few patients after the administration of clotting factor concentrates. The efficacy of other modalities, such as corticosteroids, ε-aminocaproic acid, pressor amines, or α-adrenergic blocking agents has not been established. Sedatives should be selected with regard to the possibility of kidney or liver damage. The successful management of HFRS may require renal dialysis. Although extensive study of vaccines for VHF is ongoing, and some vaccines are in advanced stages of development, no vaccines are currently available for most of these diseases (12).

Prognosis and Prognostic Factors

The case fatality rates are shown in **Table 69.4**. The presence of significant volume depletion, coupled with hemodynamic instability, is a poor prognostic sign in patients with VHF infection. In the largest case study of Ebola-Zaire infection, terminally ill patients typically presented with signs of severe volume loss, including obtundation, anuria, and shock (13). In these patients, tachypnea was the most significant criterion that differentiated between fatal and nonfatal outcomes. Tachypnea was associated with bleeding from mucosa and puncture sites, anuria, and hiccups; the tachypnea preceded death by only a few days. Impaired consciousness and splenomegaly have been reported as independent predictors of mortality in Crimean-Congo hemorrhagic fever.

Conclusions and Future Directions

VHF can be caused by a variety of viruses, which could be used for bioterrorism. Better understanding of the pathogenesis and evaluation of antiviral drugs and other therapeutic modalities is necessary to improve outcomes.

HIV INFECTION IN THE CRITICALLY ILL CHILD

HIV infection has become an important contributor to childhood morbidity and mortality, especially in many developing countries. The pandemic has undone many of the significant gains in child health. Increasing numbers of infants and children with HIV infection/AIDS are being admitted to PICUs, particularly in certain geographic areas, and a significant proportion of these patients may be first diagnosed during their PICU stay. Most patients are admitted because of respiratory infections and respiratory failure, septic shock, and CNS disorders (20,59). As the number of children receiving antiretroviral therapy increases, severe complications of therapy may also become indications for PICU admission (50). In addition to patient-specific issues, the unique stresses on medical and nursing staff members who care for HIV-infected children require attention and management. Specific infection control, nutritional, and medicolegal strategies will facilitate safe, effective delivery of care to HIV-infected infants and children in the PICU.

Epidemiology

The WHO estimated that, at the end of 2005, more than 40.3 million persons worldwide were living with HIV infection; 2.3 million of these were children under 15 years of age. In 2005 alone, 3.1 million people were estimated to have died due to AIDS, including 570,000 children. More than 90% of HIV-infected individuals live in developing nations. Sub-Saharan Africa accounts for nearly 90% of the world's total population of HIV-infected children. India and Thailand dominate the epidemic in Southeast Asia, with more recent expansion into Vietnam, China, and Cambodia. Worldwide, it is estimated that 660,000 children, including 270,000 children between 0 and 18 months of age, require antiretroviral treatment and that 4 million HIV-infected and HIV-exposed infants and children require cotrimoxazole prophylaxis from 6 weeks of age to prevent *Pneumocystis jiroveci* pneumonia. Without access to antiretroviral therapy, 20% of children who are infected by their mothers (i.e., vertically infected) will progress to AIDS or death during their first year of life, and more than half of HIV-infected children will die before their fifth birthday.

In the US, virtually all HIV infections in children who are under 13 years of age are the result of vertical transmission from an HIV-infected mother. A minority of children (2%) was infected through receipt of contaminated blood products and/or clotting factors. Vertical transmission is also the major mode of transmission in other parts of the world, but blood, blood products, and unsafe injections contribute to pediatric HIV infection, as well.

HIV-1 and HIV-2

HIV-1 and HIV-2 are members of the Retroviridae family and belong to the *Lentivirus* genus. The HIV-1 genome is single-stranded RNA that is 9.2 kb in size. Long terminal repeats at both ends contain the regulation and expression genes of HIV. The genome has three major sections: the gag region, which encodes the viral core proteins (p24, p17, p9, p6, all derived from the precursor p55); the pol region, which encodes the viral enzymes [reverse transcriptase (p51), protease (p10), and integrase (p32)]; and the env region, which encodes the viral envelope proteins (gp120 and gp41, both derived from the precursor gp160). The other products of the genome are regulatory proteins such as tat (pl4), rev (p19), nef (p27), vpr (p15), and vif (p23) (39).

The major external viral protein of HIV-1 is a heavily glycosylated gp120 protein that is associated with the transmembrane glycoprotein gp41. The gp120 contains the binding site for the CD4 molecule, the most common T lymphocyte surface receptor for HIV. Several chemokines serve as coreceptors for the envelope glycoproteins, permitting membrane fusion and entry into the cell. Most HIV strains have a specific tropism for one of the chemokines: the fusion-inducing molecule CXCR-4, which has been shown to act as a coreceptor for HIV attachment to lymphocytes, and CCR-5, a β-chemokine receptor that facilitates HIV entry into macrophages. Other mechanisms of attachment of HIV to cells are non-neutralizing antiviral antibodies and complement receptors. Following viral attachment, gp120 and the CD4 molecule undergo conformational changes, allowing gp41 to interact with the fusion receptor on the cell surface. Viral fusion with the cell membrane allows entry of viral RNA into the cell cytoplasm. Viral DNA copies are then transcribed from the virion RNA through viral reverse transcriptase enzyme activity, and duplication of the DNA copies produces double-stranded circular DNA. Because the HIV-1 reverse transcriptase is error-prone, many mutations arise, creating wide genetic variation in HIV-1 isolates, even within an individual patient. The circular DNA is transported into the cell nucleus, where it is integrated into chromosomal DNA; this is called the *provirus*. The provirus can remain dormant for extended periods.

HIV-1 transcription is followed by translation. A capsid polyprotein is cleaved to produce, among other products, the virus-specific protease (p10). This enzyme is critical for HIV-1 assembly. The RNA genome is then incorporated into the newly formed viral capsid. As the new virus is formed, it buds through the cell membrane and is released.

HIV diversity, leading to multiple viral groups [groups M (main), O (outlier), N (non-M, non-O)], probably originated from multiple zoonotic infections found in primates in different geographic regions. Group M then diversified to several subtypes (or clades A to H). In each region of the world, certain clades predominate. For example, clade B is found in South America, clade E in Thailand, and clade C in South Africa. Clades are mixed in some patients due to HIV recombination, and some crossing between groups (i.e., M and O) has been reported.

HIV-2 is a rare cause of infection in children. It is most prevalent in Western and Southern Africa. If HIV-2 is suspected, a specific test that detects antibody to HIV-2 peptides should be used.

Transmission

Transmission of HIV-1 occurs via sexual contact, parenteral exposure to blood, or vertical transmission from mother to child. The primary route of infection in the pediatric population is vertical transmission, accounting for virtually all new cases in developed countries. Most large studies in the US and Europe have documented mother-to-child transmission rates in untreated women to be between 12%–30%. In contrast, transmission rates in Africa and Asia are higher, up to 50%. Perinatal treatment of HIV-infected mothers with antiretroviral drugs has dramatically decreased these rates (27).

Vertical transmission of HIV can occur during the intrauterine or intrapartum periods or through breast-feeding. Up to 30% of infected newborns are infected in utero. The highest percentages of HIV-infected children acquire the virus intrapartum. Breast-feeding is an important route of transmission, especially in developing countries. A meta-analysis of prospective studies found that the additional risk of transmission through breast-feeding in women with HIV infection before pregnancy was 14%, compared with a 29% increase in breast-feeding women who acquired HIV postnatally (22). The risk factors for vertical transmission include preterm delivery (<34 weeks gestation), a low maternal antenatal CD4 count, use of illicit drugs during pregnancy, >4 hr duration of ruptured membranes, and birth weight <2500 g (27).

Transfusions of infected blood or blood products have accounted for a variable proportion of all pediatric AIDS cases. Heat treatment of factor VIII concentrate and HIV antibody screening of donors has virtually eliminated HIV transmission to children with hemophilia. Blood donor screening has dramatically reduced, but not eliminated, the risk of transfusion-associated HIV infection. In many developing countries, where screening of blood donors is not uniform, the risk of transmitting HIV infection via transfusion is still significant.

Although HIV can be isolated rarely from saliva, it is in very low titers (<1 infectious particle/mL) and has not been implicated as a transmission vehicle. In younger children, sexual transmission is infrequent, but a small number of cases that resulted from sexual abuse have been reported. In contrast, sexual contact is a major route of transmission in the adolescent population, accounting for most cases.

Pathogenesis

When the mucosa is the portal of entry for HIV, the first cells to be infected are the dendritic cells, which process the antigens introduced and transport them to the lymphoid tissue. In the lymph node, HIV selectively binds to cells expressing CD4 molecules on their surface, primarily helper T lymphocytes (CD4 cells), and cells of the monocyte-macrophage lineage. Other cells bearing CD4, such as microglia, astrocytes, oligodendroglia, and placental tissue containing villous Hofbauer cells, may also be infected by HIV. CD4 lymphocytes migrate to the lymph nodes that house infected cells, where they become activated and proliferate, making them highly susceptible to HIV infection. This antigen-driven migration and accumulation of CD4 cells within the lymphoid tissue may contribute to the generalized lymphadenopathy characteristic of the acute retroviral syndrome in adults and adolescents. HIV preferentially infects the very cells that respond to it (i.e., HIV-specific memory CD4 cells), which accounts for the progressive loss of response by these cells and the subsequent loss of control of HIV replication. Usually within 3–6 weeks from the time of infection, a burst of plasma viremia occurs. With establishment of a cellular and humoral immune response within the following 2–4 months, the viral load in the blood declines sub-

stantially, and patients enter a phase that is characterized by a lack of symptoms and a return of CD4 cells to only moderately decreased levels (39). Unlike in adults, early HIV-1 replication in children has no apparent clinical manifestations. The viral load increases by 1–4 months, and almost all HIV-infected infants have detectable HIV-1 in peripheral blood by 4 months of age.

In adults and teenagers, the long period of clinical latency (often up to 8–12 years) is not indicative of viral latency. In fact, a very high turnover of virus and CD4 lymphocytes (more than 1 billion cells per day) occurs, which gradually causes deterioration of the immune system, evidenced particularly by depletion of CD4 cells. These cells may be destroyed by multiple mechanisms: HIV-mediated single-cell killing, formation of multinucleated giant cells of infected and uninfected CD4 cells (syncytia formation), virus-specific immune responses, superantigen-mediated activation of T cells (rendering them more susceptible to infection with HIV), and programmed cell death (apoptosis). The viral burden in the lymphoid organs is greater than that in the peripheral blood during the asymptomatic period. Cell-mediated and humoral responses occur early in the infection. The CD8 T cells play an important role in containing the infection. HIV-specific cytotoxic T lymphocytes (CTLs) develop against both the structural (i.e., env, pol, gag) and regulatory (e.g., tat) viral proteins. The CTL cells control the infection by killing HIV-infected cells before new viruses are produced and by secreting potent antiviral factors that compete with the virus for its receptors (e.g., CCR5). Neutralizing antibodies appear later during the infection and seem to help in the continued suppression of viral replication during clinical latency (39).

Before highly active antiretroviral therapy (HAART) was available, three distinct patterns of disease were described in children. Approximately 10%–20% of HIV-infected newborns in developed countries presented with a rapid disease course, with onset of AIDS and symptoms during the first few months of life and, if untreated, death from AIDS-related complications by 4 years of age (40). In resource-poor countries, >85% of the HIV-infected newborns may have such a rapidly progressing disease.

It has been suggested that if intrauterine infection coincides with the period of rapid expansion of CD4 cells in the fetus, it could effectively infect the majority of the body's immunocompetent cells. Most children in this group have a positive HIV-1 culture and/or detectable virus in the plasma within the first 48 hrs of life. This early evidence of viral presence suggests that the newborn was infected in utero. In contrast to the viral load in adults, the viral load in infants remains high for at least the first 2 years of life.

The majority of perinatally infected newborns (60%–80%) present with a second pattern—a much slower progression of disease with a median survival time of 6 years. Many patients in this group have a negative viral culture or PCR in the first week of life and are therefore considered to be infected intrapartum. In a typical patient, the viral load rapidly increases by 2–3 months of age (median, 100,000 copies/mL) and then slowly declines over a period of 24 months. This observation can be explained partially by the immaturity of the immune system in newborns and infants. The third pattern of disease (i.e., long-term survivors) occurs in a small percentage (<5%) of perinatally infected children who have minimal or no progression of disease with relatively normal CD4 counts and very low viral loads for longer than 8 years.

HIV-infected children have changes in the immune system that are similar to those in HIV-infected adults. CD4 cell depletion may be less dramatic because infants normally have a relative lymphocytosis. Therefore, for example, a value of 750 CD4 cells/mm^3 in children <1 year of age is indicative of severe CD4 depletion and is comparable to <200 CD4 cells/mm^3 in adults. Lymphopenia is relatively rare in perinatally infected children and is usually only seen in older children or those with end-stage disease.

B-cell activation occurs in most children early in the infection, as evidenced by hypergammaglobulinemia associated with high levels of anti-HIV-1 antibody. This response may reflect both dysregulation of T-cell suppression of B-cell antibody synthesis and active CD4 enhancement of B-lymphocyte humoral responses. CD4 depletion and inadequate antibody responses lead to increased susceptibility to various infections, and the clinical manifestations vary with the severity of immunodeficiency.

Clinical Manifestations

The clinical manifestations of HIV infection vary widely among infants, children, and adolescents. In most infants, physical examination at birth is normal. Initial signs and symptoms may be subtle and nonspecific, such as lymphadenopathy, hepatosplenomegaly, failure to thrive, chronic or recurrent diarrhea, interstitial pneumonia, or oral thrush, and they may be distinguishable from other causes only by their persistence. Whereas systemic and pulmonary findings are common in the US and Europe, chronic diarrhea, wasting, and severe malnutrition predominate in Africa. Symptoms found more commonly in children than in adults include recurrent bacterial infections, chronic parotid swelling, lymphocytic interstitial pneumonitis (LIP), and early onset of progressive neurologic deterioration. The HIV classification system is used to categorize the stage of pediatric disease via two parameters: clinical status (**Table 79.5**) and degree of immunologic impairment (**Table 79.6**).

The Spectrum of Diseases in the PICU

The reasons for PICU admission among HIV-infected children may or may not be related to their HIV infection. The causes of PICU admission unrelated to the HIV infection are usually similar to those found in non–HIV-infected children of comparable age. Many children with clinically unsuspected HIV infection are treated in PICUs. In the early stages of the illness, when the immunosuppression is not severe, the children are likely to respond to standard management. In patients with significant immunosuppression, the prognosis is determined by its severity.

The most common HIV-related diseases that lead to PICU admission are respiratory infections and respiratory failure, septic shock, and disorders of the CNS (20,59). Acute respiratory failure secondary to *Pneumocystis jiroveci* or bacterial infections is the most important cause of PICU admission. Pneumocystic pneumonia is common in HIV-infected children with severe immunodeficiency, and if untreated, is universally fatal.

Respiratory Diseases Complicating HIV Infection

While acute respiratory failure secondary to pneumocystic pneumonia remains one of the most frequent causes of PICU admission among HIV-infected children, the initial diagnostic evaluation of HIV-infected children with respiratory distress should always consider the other causes of infectious pneumonitis: bacterial, fungal, mycobacterial, and viral infections.

Pneumocystis Jiroveci Pneumonia. *P. jiroveci* (previously *P. carinii*) pneumonia (PCP) is the opportunistic infection that led to the initial description of AIDS. PCP is one of the commonest AIDS-defining illnesses in children in the US and Europe. However, data regarding the incidence of PCP in children in other parts of the world are scarce. The majority of the cases occur at between 3 and 6 months of life (1). For further details, refer to Chapter 84.

Even if a child develops PCP while on prophylaxis, therapy may be started with trimethoprim/sulfamethoxazole, as the prophylaxis may have failed because of poor compliance or unusual pharmacokinetics. Drug resistance may also be the cause, in which case the use of one of the alternative drugs is recommended. Untreated, PCP is universally fatal. With the use of appropriate therapy, the mortality decreases to less than 10%. The risk factors for mortality are the severity of the episode and the severity of the immunosuppression.

Recurrent Bacterial Infections. Both cell-mediated and humoral immunity fail as HIV infection progresses. Despite hypergammaglobulinemia, HIV-infected children are at risk for severe and recurrent bacterial infections. Delay in clearing infections may also be caused by the usual pathogens. In various studies from developing countries, up to 90% of HIV-infected children had history of recurrent pneumonias. Initial episodes of pneumonia often occur before the development of significant immunosuppression. As the immunosuppression increases, the frequency increases. The common pathogens for community-acquired pneumonia in these children are *Streptococcus pneumoniae*, *Haemophilus influenzae*, and *Staphylococcus aureus*. However, in children with severe immunosuppression and in hospital-acquired infections, Gram-negative organisms, such as *Pseudomonas aeruginosa*, gain importance. The clinical features of pneumonia in HIV-infected children are similar to those in uninfected children. However, in severely immunocompromised children, the signs may be subtle. Often, the response to therapy is slow, and the relapse rates are high. Bacteremia may be more common, seen in up to 50%.

While attempts should be made to isolate the causative organism, such efforts should not delay empirical therapy. Sick children with pneumonia should be treated with parenteral antibiotics. Choices of appropriate antibiotics are often made based on local patterns of etiologies and susceptibilities. In many settings, an appropriate choice would be a combination of a broad-spectrum cephalosporin and an aminoglycoside. In areas where a large proportion of *S. aureus* isolates are resistant to antistaphylococcal antibiotics (MRSA or methicillin-resistant *S. aureus*), the empiric inclusion of vancomycin, clindamycin, linezolid, or other drugs to which community-acquired MRSA is usually susceptible should be considered. Children with nonsevere pneumonia can be managed as outpatients with a second- or a third-generation cephalosporin or a combination, such as amoxicillin-clavulanic acid. As

TABLE 79.5

CLINICAL CATEGORIES OF HUMAN IMMUNODEFICIENCY VIRUS INFECTION

Clinical category N
Children who have no signs or symptoms considered to be the result of HIV infection or who have only one of the conditions listed in Category A

Clinical category A
Children with 2 or more of the conditions listed below but none of the conditions listed in Categories B and C
Lymphadenopathy ($\geq$0.5 cm at more than 2 sites; bilateral = 1 site
Hepatomegaly
Splenomegaly
Dermatitis
Parotitis
Recurrent or persistent upper respiratory infection, sinusitis, or otitis media

Clinical category B
Children who have symptomatic conditions other than those listed for Category A or C that are attributed to HIV infection. Examples of conditions in clinical Category B include but are not limited to:
Anemia (<8 g/dL), neutropenia (<1000/mm^3), or thrombocytopenia (<100,000/mm^3) persisting for at least 30 days
Bacterial meningitis, pneumonia, or sepsis (single episode)
Candidiasis, oropharyngeal (thrush), persisting for more than 2 months in children >6 months of age
Cardiomyopathy
Cytomegalovirus infection, with onset before 1 month of age
Diarrhea, recurrent or chronic
Hepatitis
HSV stomatitis, recurrent (more than two episodes within 1 year)
HSV bronchitis, pneumonitis, or esophagitis, with onset before 1 month of age
Herpes zoster (shingles) involving at least two distinct episodes or more than 1 dermatome
Leiomyosarcoma
Lymphoid interstitial pneumonia
Nephropathy
Nocardiosis
Persistent fever (lasting >1 month)
Toxoplasmosis, onset before 1 month of age
Varicella, disseminated

Clinical category C
Serious bacterial infections, multiple or recurrent (i.e., any combination of at least two culture-confirmed infections within a 2-year period), of the following types: septicemia, pneumonia, meningitis, bone or joint infection, or abscess of an internal organ or body cavity (excluding otitis media, superficial skin or mucosal abscesses, and indwelling catheter-related infections)
Candidiasis, esophageal or pulmonary (bronchi, trachea, lungs)
Coccidioidomycosis, disseminated (at site other than, or in addition to, lungs or cervical or hilar lymph nodes)
Cryptococcosis, extrapulmonary
Cryptosporidiosis or isosporiasis with diarrhea persisting >1 month
Cytomegalovirus disease, with onset of symptoms at age >1 month (at a site other than liver, spleen, or lymph nodes)
Encephalopathy (at least one of the following progressive findings present for at least 2 months in the absence of a concurrent illness other than HIV infection that could explain the findings):
(a) failure to attain or loss of developmental milestones, or loss of intellectual ability, verified by standard developmental scale or neuropsychologic tests;
(b) impaired brain growth or acquired microcephaly demonstrated by head circumference measurements or brain atrophy demonstrated by CT or MRI (serial imaging is required for children <2 years of age);
(c) acquired symmetric motor deficit manifested by two or more of the following: paresis, pathologic reflexes, ataxia, or gait disturbance
HSV infection causing a mucocutaneous ulcer that persists for >1 month; or bronchitis, pneumonitis, or esophagitis for any duration affecting a child >1 month of age
Histoplasmosis, disseminated (at a site other than, or in addition to, lungs or cervical or hilar lymph nodes)
Kaposi sarcoma
Lymphoma, primary, in brain
Lymphoma, small, noncleaved cell (Burkitt syndrome), or immunoblastic or large cell lymphoma of B-cell or unknown immunologic phenotype
Mycobacterium TB, disseminated or extrapulmonary
Mycobacterium, other species or unidentified species, disseminated (at a site other than, or in addition to, lungs, skin, or cervical or hilar lymph nodes)
Mycobacterium avium complex or *M. kansasii*, disseminated (at site other than, or in addition to, lungs, skin, or cervical or hilar lymph nodes)
Pneumocystis jiroveci pneumonia
Progressive multifocal leukoencephalopathy
Salmonella (nontyphoid) septicemia, recurrent
Toxoplasmosis of the brain with onset at >1 month of age
Wasting syndrome in the absence of a concurrent illness other than HIV infection that could explain the following findings:
(a) persistent weight loss more than 10% of baseline, *OR*
(b) downward crossing of at least two of the following percentile lines on the weight-for-age chart (e.g., 95th, 75th, 50th, 25th, 5th) in a child at least 1 year of age, *OR*
(c) <5th percentile on weight-for-height chart on two consecutive measurements at least 30 days apart, *PLUS*
    (i) chronic diarrhea (i.e., at least two loose stools per day for >30 days), OR
    (ii) documented fever (for at least 30 days, intermittent or constant)

HIV, human immunodeficiency virus; HSV, herpes simplex virus; TB, tuberculosis. From Centers for Disease Control and Prevention. 1994 Revised classification system for human immunodeficiency virus infection in children less than 13 years of age. *MMWR* 1994;43:6–8.

IMMUNOLOGIC CATEGORIES BASED ON AGE-SPECIFIC CD-4 T LYMPHOCYTE COUNTS IN CHILDREN WITH HIV INFECTION

		Age of child					
		<12 mo		1–5 yrs		6–12 yrs	
	Immunologic categories	Cells/mm³	%	Cells/mm³	%	Cells/mm³	%
1	No evidence of Suppression	≥ 1500	≥ 25	≥ 1000	≥ 25	≥ 500	≥ 25
2	Moderate Suppression	750–1499	15–24	500–999	15–24	200–499	15–24
3	Severe Suppression	>750	<15	<500	<15	<200	<15

From Centers for Disease Control and Prevention. 1994 Revised classification system for human immunodeficiency virus infection in children less than 13 years of age. *MMWR* 1994;43:6–8.

P. jiroveci pneumonia cannot be excluded at the outset in most HIV-infected children with severe respiratory infections, cotrimoxazole should be added unless another diagnosis has been definitively made. The principles of supportive care of HIV-infected children admitted to PICU with severe pneumonia are similar to those in non–HIV-infected children.

Tuberculosis. With the spread of the HIV infection, a resurgence in tuberculosis (TB) has occurred. Coexistent TB and HIV infections accelerate the progression of both diseases. HIV-infected children are more likely to have extrapulmonary and disseminated TB; the course is also likely to be more rapid. An HIV-infected child with tubercular infection is more likely to develop the disease than a child without HIV infection. The overall risk of active TB in children who are infected with HIV is at least five- to tenfold higher than that in uninfected children (16) (see Chapter 84).

All HIV-infected children with active TB should receive long-duration antitubercular therapy; a 9–12-month therapy is preferred. The American Academy of Pediatrics recommends a total duration of 12 months of anti-TB therapy for children infected with HIV, while the American Thoracic Society/Centers for Disease Control recommend a total of 6 months of therapy, regardless of HIV status (5,6). A close follow-up is essential to diagnose nonresponse/drug resistance early.

Infection with Mycobacterium avium-intracellulare. Pulmonary disease with *Mycobacterium avium-intracellulare* is uncommon in children with HIV infection, despite immunosuppression. The common symptoms and signs include persistent fever, failure to thrive, night sweats, lymphadenopathy, organomegaly, and refractory anemia. The pulmonary lesions are usually limited to lymphadenopathy and localized parenchymal lesions. The diagnosis of disseminated disease primarily depends on isolation of the organism from blood. Current therapy for disseminated *M. avium-intracellulare* infection involves use of a combination of clarithromycin or azithromycin with ethambutol.

Viral Infections. Infections caused by respiratory syncytial virus (RSV), influenza, and parainfluenza viruses result in symptomatic disease more often in HIV-infected children, in comparison to noninfected children. Infections with other viruses, such as adenovirus and measles virus, are more likely

to lead to serious sequelae than are the previously mentioned viruses. As RSV infection most often occurs in children in the first 2 years of life, during which many may not be severely immunocompromised, the severity of illness may not be different from the non–HIV-infected children. In children with AIDS, disseminated cytomegalovirus is a known opportunistic infection, but pneumonia caused by this virus is rare. The principles of diagnosis and treatment of these infections in HIV-infected children are similar to those in non–HIV-infected children.

Fungal Infections. Pulmonary fungal infections usually present as a part of disseminated disease in immunocompromised children. Primary pulmonary fungal infections are uncommon. Pulmonary candidiasis should be suspected in any HIV-infected child with lower respiratory tract infection that does not respond to the common therapeutic modalities. A positive blood culture supports the diagnosis of invasive candidiasis. For other fungal infections, refer to Chapter 84.

Lymphoid Interstitial Pneumonitis. Lymphoid interstitial pneumonitis (LIP) has been recognized as a distinctive marker for pediatric HIV infection and is included as a Class B condition in the revised CDC criteria for AIDS in children. In the absence of antiretroviral therapy, nearly 20% of HIV-infected children develop LIP. The etiology and pathogenesis of LIP are not well understood. Suggested etiologies include an exaggerated immunologic response to inhaled or circulating antigens and/or primary infection of the lung with HIV, Epstein-Barr virus (EBV), or both. LIP is characterized by nodule formation and diffuse infiltration of the alveolar septae by lymphocytes, plasmacytoid lymphocytes, plasma cells, and immunoblasts. No involvement of the blood vessels or destruction of the lung tissue occurs.

LIP is usually diagnosed in children with perinatally acquired HIV infection when they are >1 year of age, unlike with PCP. Most children with LIP are asymptomatic. Tachypnea, cough, wheezing, and hypoxemia may be seen when children present with more severe manifestations; crepitations are uncommon. Clubbing is often present in advanced disease. These patients can progress to chronic respiratory failure. Long-standing LIP may be associated with chronic bronchiectasis. The presence of a reticulonodular pattern, with or without hilar lymphadenopathy, that persists on chest x-ray for 2 months or greater and that is unresponsive to antimicrobial therapy is considered presumptive evidence of LIP. Care should be taken to exclude other possible etiologies. A definitive diagnosis of LIP can only be made by histopathology. Children with LIP have a relatively good prognosis compared to other children who meet the CDC surveillance definition of AIDS. However, children with severe disease are likely to manifest with respiratory failure.

Early disease is managed conservatively. The effect of antiretrovirals on LIP is probably limited. Steroids are indicated if children with LIP have symptoms and signs of chronic pulmonary disease, clubbing, and/or hypoxemia. Treatment usually includes an initial 4–12-week course of prednisolone (2 mg/kg/day), followed by a tapering dose, using oxygen saturation and clinical status as a guide to improvement. This treatment is then followed by chronic low-dose prednisolone.

Gastrointestinal Diseases

The pathologic changes in the gastrointestinal tract of children with AIDS are variable and can be clinically significant. However, only a few conditions may be indications for admission to a PICU. A variety of microbes can cause gastrointestinal disease, including bacteria (*Salmonella, Campylobacter, M. avium-intracellulare* complex), protozoa (*Giardia, Cryptosporidium, Isospora,* microsporidia), viruses (cytomegalovirus, herpes simplex virus, rotavirus), and fungi (*Candida*). The protozoal infections are most severe and can be protracted in children with severe immunosuppression. Children with cryptosporidium infestation can have severe diarrhea that leads to hypovolemic shock, which may merit admission to the PICU. AIDS enteropathy, a syndrome of malabsorption with partial villous atrophy not associated with a specific pathogen, is probably the result of direct HIV infection of the gut.

HIV-infected children with marked failure to thrive who are admitted to the PICU primarily for other indications may require supplemental enteral feedings; in some, placement of a gastrostomy tube for nutritional supplementation may be necessary. Few children may need total parenteral nutrition.

Chronic liver inflammation is relatively common in HIV-infected children. In some, hepatitis caused by cytomegalovirus, hepatitis B or C viruses, or *Mycobacterium avium* complex (MAC) may lead to liver failure and portal hypertension. It is important to recognize that several of the antiretroviral drugs (e.g., didanosine) and protease inhibitors may also cause reversible elevation of transaminases. Pancreatitis is uncommon in HIV-infected children, perhaps the result of drug therapy (e.g., didanosine, lamivudine, nevirapine, or pentamidine). Rarely, opportunistic infections (e.g., *M. avium* complex or cytomegalovirus) may be responsible for acute pancreatitis. The principles of management of these conditions are similar to those in non–HIV-infected children.

Neurologic Diseases

The incidence of CNS involvement in perinatally infected children may be more than 50% in developing countries but lower in developed countries, with a median onset at about 1.5 years of age. The most common presentation is progressive encephalopathy with loss or plateau of developmental milestones, cognitive deterioration, impaired brain growth that results in acquired microcephaly, and symmetric motor dysfunction. CNS infections (meningitis due to bacterial pathogens, fungi, such as *Cryptococcus,* and a number of viruses) may be

responsible for clinical presentations that are indications for PICU admission. CNS toxoplasmosis is exceedingly rare in young infants but may occur in HIV-infected adolescents; the overwhelming majority of these cases have serum IgG antitoxoplasma antibodies as a marker of infection. The management of these conditions is similar to that in non–HIV-infected children; the response rates and outcomes may be poorer.

Cardiovascular Involvement

Cardiac abnormalities in HIV-infected children are common, persistent, and often progressive; however, most are subclinical. In a recently published study of HIV-infected children, left ventricular (LV) structure and function progressively deteriorated in the first 3 years of life, resulting in subsequent persistent mild LV dysfunction and increased LV mass. Chronic mild depression of LV function and elevated LV mass were associated with higher all-cause mortality (25). Children with encephalopathy or other AIDS-defining conditions have the highest rate of adverse cardiac outcomes. Resting sinus tachycardia has been reported in up to nearly two-thirds, and marked sinus arrhythmia in one-fifth, of HIV-infected children. Gallop rhythm with tachypnea and hepatosplenomegaly appear to be the best clinical indicators of congestive heart failure in HIV-infected children; anticongestive therapy is generally very effective, especially when initiated early. Electrocardiography and echocardiography are helpful in assessing cardiac function before the onset of clinical symptoms.

Renal Involvement

Nephropathy is an unusual presenting symptom of HIV infection, more commonly occurring in older symptomatic children. Nephrotic syndrome is the most common manifestation of pediatric renal disease, with edema, hypoalbuminemia, proteinuria, and azotemia with normal blood pressure. Polyuria, oliguria, and hematuria have also been observed in some patients. Hypertension is unusual in these children.

Diagnosis

All infants born to HIV-infected mothers test antibody-positive at birth because of passive transfer of maternal HIV antibody across the placenta. Most uninfected infants lose maternal antibody between 6 and 12 months of age. As a small proportion of uninfected infants continues to have maternal HIV antibody in the blood for up to 18 months of age, positive IgG antibody tests cannot be used to make a definitive diagnosis of HIV infection in infants who are younger. In a child >18 months, demonstration of IgG antibody to HIV by a repeatedly reactive enzyme immunoassay (EIA) and confirmatory test (e.g., Western blot or immunofluorescence assay) can establish the diagnosis of HIV infection.

Although serologic diagnostic tests were the most commonly used in the past, tests that allow for earlier definitive diagnosis in children have replaced antibody assays as the tests of choice for the diagnosis of HIV infection in infants. Specific viral diagnostic assays, such as HIV DNA or RNA PCR, HIV culture, or HIV p24 antigen immune dissociated p24 (ICD-p24), are essential for diagnosis of young infants born to HIV-infected mothers. By 6 months of age, the HIV culture and/or PCR identifies all infected infants, who are not having any continued exposure due to breast-feeding. HIV DNA PCR is the preferred virologic assay in developed countries. Plasma HIV RNA assays may be more sensitive than DNA PCR for early diagnosis, but data are limited. HIV culture has similar sensitivity to HIV DNA PCR; however, it is more technically complex and expensive, and results are often not available for 2–4 weeks, compared to 2–3 days with PCR. The p24 antigen assay is less sensitive than the other virologic tests.

Antiretroviral Therapy

Decisions about antiretroviral therapy for pediatric HIV-infected patients are based on the magnitude of viral replication (i.e., viral load), CD4 lymphocyte count or percentage, and clinical condition. The indications for initiation of HAART are detailed in **Table 79.7**. In the developed world, the decision to initiate HAART is based on clinical, immunologic, and virologic parameters. In contrast, in settings in which access to laboratory tests is limited, the decision to treat may be based only on clinical symptoms.

Availability of antiretroviral therapy has transformed HIV infection from a uniformly fatal condition to a chronic infection, with which children can lead a near-normal life. The currently available therapy does not eradicate the virus and cure the child; it rather suppresses the virus replication for extended periods of time. The three main groups of drugs are nucleoside reverse transcriptase inhibitors (NRTI), non-nucleoside reverse transcriptase inhibitors (NNRTI), and protease inhibitors (PI). HAART is a combination of two NRTIs with a PI or an NNRTI. The details of antiretroviral drugs are shown in **Table 79.8**.

Some complications of antiretroviral therapy, such as lactic acidosis, severe pancreatitis, and Stevens-Johnson syndrome, may require care in the PICU. The therapy for these conditions includes discontinuing the offending drug, when possible, and supportive care similar to the care provided for these problems in non–HIV-infected children.

Outcome

Published literature is limited regarding the outcomes after initiation of antiretroviral treatment in critically ill HIV-infected children. In a recently published report from South Africa, it was observed that the majority of HIV-infected children survived to discharge from the PICU, but only half survived to

hospital discharge (21). Limitation of intervention decisions, usually made in the PICU, directly influenced short-term survival and the opportunity to commence HAART. Although few critically ill HIV-infected children in developing countries survived to become established on HAART, the long-term outcome of children on HAART remains encouraging.

Prevention of Transmission in the PICU

The staff in the PICU should always adhere to universal precautions, regardless of the presence or absence of known or suspected HIV infection in their patients. Staff may have a greater likelihood of exposure to HIV-contaminated body fluids in the PICU, as compared to other healthcare settings, due to the increased number of invasive procedures performed in the PICU. In case of exposure, the staff should follow the standard guidelines for post-exposure prophylaxis (PEP) (54). The majority of HIV exposures will warrant a two-drug regimen, using two NRTIs [zidovudine and lamivudine or emtricitabine (FTC)] or one nucleotide reverse transcriptase inhibitor and one NRTI (tenofovir and lamivudine or emtricitabine). The US Public Health Service now recommends that expanded PEP regimens be PI based. The PI preferred for use in expanded PEP regimens is lopinavir/ritonavir (LPV/RTV). Other PIs acceptable for use in expanded PEP regimens include atazanavir, fosamprenavir, ritonavir-boosted indinavir, ritonavir-boosted saquinavir, and nelfinavir. Although side effects are common with NNRTIs, efavirenz may be considered for expanded PEP regimens, especially when resistance to PIs in the source person's virus is known or suspected. Caution is advised when efavirenz is used in women of childbearing age because of the risk of teratogenicity. PEP should be initiated as soon as possible, preferably within hours rather than days of exposure. If a question exists concerning which antiretroviral drugs to use or whether to use a basic or expanded regimen, the basic regimen should be started immediately rather than delay PEP administration. PEP should be administered for 4 weeks, if tolerated.

Conclusions and Future Directions

HIV infection in children is a serious problem in many developing countries. The severe manifestations of HIV infection, conditions resulting from severe immunosuppression, and drug toxicities may require intensive care. Development of a vaccine

---

TABLE 79.7

INDICATIONS FOR INITIATION OF HIGHLY ACTIVE ANTIRETROVIRAL THERAPY IN HIV-INFECTED CHILDREN

Clinical category		CD4 percentage		Plasma viral load	Recommendation
AIDS (clinical category C)[a]	OR	15% (immune category 3)[b]		Any value	Initiate HAART
Mild-to-moderate symptoms (clinical category A or B)[a]	OR	15%–25% (immune category 2)[b]	OR	>100,000 copies/mL	Consider initiating HAART
Asymptomatic (clinical category N)[a]	AND	>25% (immune category 1)[b]	AND	<100,000 copies/mL	Usually HAART is deferred, and the child is monitored.

[a]See table 79.5.
[b]See Table 79.6. HAART, highly active antiretroviral therapy. From Working Group on Antiretroviral Therapy and Medical Management of HIV-Infected Children. *Guidelines for the Use of Antiretroviral Agents in Pediatric HIV Infection.* National Institutes of Health (NIH). US. Nov. 3, 2005.

TABLE 79.8

ANTIRETROVIRAL DRUGS COMMONLY USED IN CHILDREN

Drug	Dose	Side effects
Nucleoside reverse transcriptase inhibitors		
Abacavir	3 mo–13 yrs: 8 mg/kg/dose q 12 hrs >13 yrs: 300 mg/dose q 12 hrs (max: 300 mg/dose)	Hypersensitivity
Didanosine	0–3 mo: 50 mg/m^2/dose q 12 hrs 3 mo–13 yrs: 90–150 mg/m^2 q 12 hrs (max: 200 mg/dose) >13 yrs: <60 kg: 125 mg tablets q 12 hrs >13 yrs: >60 kg: 200 mg tablet q 12 hrs (higher dose for powder preparations)	Peripheral neuropathy, pancreatitis, abdominal pain, diarrhea
Lamivudine (3TC)	1 mo–13 yr: 4 mg/kg q 12 hrs >13 yrs: <50 kg: 4 mg/kg/dose q 12 hrs >13 yrs: >50 kg: 150 mg/kg/dose q 12 hrs	Pancreatitis, neuropathy, neutropenia
Stavudine (d4T)	1 mo–13 yrs: 1 mg/kg q 12 hrs >13 yrs: 30–60 kg: 30 mg/dose q 12 hrs >13 yrs: >60 kg: 40 mg/dose q 12 hrs	Headache, gastrointestinal upset, neuropathy
Zalcitabine	<13 yrs: 0.01 mg/kg/dose q 8 hrs >13 yrs: 0.75 mg q 8hrs	Rash, peripheral neuropathy, pancreatitis
Zidovudine	Neonates: 2 mg/kg q 6 hrs 3 mo–13 yrs: 90–180 mg/m^2 q 6–8 hrs >13 yrs: 200 mg q 8 hrs or 300 mg q 12 hrs	Anemia, myopathy
Non-nucleoside Reverse Transcriptase Inhibitors		
Nevirapine (NVP)	2 mo–13 yrs: 120 mg/m^2 (max 200 mg) q 24 hrs for 14 d, followed by 120–200 mg/m^2 q 12 hrs *OR* <8 yrs: 7 mg/kg q 12 hrs >8 yrs: 4 mg/kg q 12 hrs >13 yrs: 200 mg q 24 hrs for 14 d; then increase to 200 mg q 12 hrs if no rash or other side effects	Skin rash, Steven Johnson syndrome
Efavirenz	>3 yrs: 10–<15 kg: 200 mg q 24 hrs 15–<20 kg: 250 mg q 24 hrs 20–<25 kg: 300 mg q 24 hrs 25–<32.5 kg: 350 mg q 24 hrs 32.5–<40 kg: 400 mg q 24 hrs >40 kg: 600 mg q 24 hrs	Skin rash, central nervous system symptoms, increased transaminase levels
Protease inhibitors		
Amprenavir	4–16 yrs & <50 kg: 22.5 mg/kg q 12 hrs (oral solution) *OR* 20 mg/kg q 12 hrs (capsules) >13 yrs & >50 kg: 1200 mg q 12 hrs (capsules)	
Indinavir	500 mg/m^2 q 8 hrs >13 yrs: 800 mg q 8 hrs	Hyperbilirubinemia, nephrolithiasis
Lopinavir/ ritonavir	6 mo–12 yrs: 7–<15 kg: 12 mg/kg lopinavir *OR* 3 mg/kg ritonavir q 12 hrs with food; 15–40 kg: 10 mg/kg lopinavir *OR* 2.5 mg/kg ritonavir q 12 hrs with food >12 yrs: 400 mg lopinavir *OR* 100 mg ritonavir q 12 hrs with food	Diarrhea, fatigue, headache, nausea, and increased cholesterol and triglycerides
Nelfinavir	<13 yrs: 50–55 mg/ kg q 12 hrs >13 yrs: 1250 mg q 12 hrs (max 2000 mg)	Diarrhea, abdominal pain
Ritonavir	<13 yrs: 350–400 mg/m^2 q 12 hrs (starting dose: 250 mg/m^2) >13 yrs: 600 mg q 12 hrs (starting with 300 mg)	Bad taste, vomiting, nausea, diarrhea, rarely, hepatitis
Saquinavir	50 mg/kg q 8 hrs >13 yrs: soft gel capsules, 1200 mg q 8 hrs	Diarrhea, headache, skin rash

Data from Working Group on Antiretroviral Therapy and Medical Management of HIV-Infected Children. *Guidelines for the Use of Antiretroviral Agents in Pediatric HIV Infection.* Bethesda, Maryland: National Institutes of Health, Nov. 3, 2005.

to prevent HIV infection is a high priority. More efficacious antiretroviral drugs that have fewer adverse effects are also necessary. Making available antiretroviral therapy at an affordable cost remains a considerable challenge. In the short term, finding effective ways to control vertical transmission from mother to child may help in substantial reduction in childhood HIV infection load.

MEASLES

Measles remains an important cause of death among young children, despite the availability of a safe and effective vaccine for nearly four decades. Unlike in many industrialized countries, measles remains a common illness in many developing countries, where >95% of measles deaths occur. More than 30 million people are affected each year by measles. In 2003, an estimated 530,000 measles deaths occurred globally, most of them in children (30). In countries where measles has been largely eliminated, cases imported from other countries are now the most important source of infection. Unimmunized children, even in prosperous countries, remain at risk of acquiring the infection. Measles infections can run a severe course, even in children living in prosperous countries (55). Severe measles is particularly likely in poorly nourished young children, especially those who do not receive sufficient vitamin A or whose immune systems have been weakened by HIV/AIDS or other diseases.

Description of Organism

Measles virus is a large, pleomorphic RNA virus (100–300 nm in diameter) belonging to the *Paramyxoviridae* family. The virus genome is a linear strand of RNA that contains ~15,900 nucleotides (molecular weight: 4.5×10^6 Daltons). The virus can easily be inactivated by heat, ultraviolet light, lipid solvents, and extremes of pH. All measles strains are antigenically homogeneous.

Transmission

The measles virus is spread from an infected individual to a new host by the respiratory route via aerosolized droplets of respiratory secretions. Close person-to-person contact can facilitate transfer of nasal secretions of a patient to the nose of the host. There is no known animal reservoir, and asymptomatic carriers are unknown.

Pathogenesis and Pathophysiology

The primary site of initial infection is the respiratory epithelium of the nasopharynx. The virus multiplies locally and then spreads to the regional lymphoid tissue. A primary viremia follows (day 2–3 after infection), leading to seeding of the reticuloendothelial system and extensive replication. Between the days 5 and 7 of infection, an extensive secondary viremia occurs and infection in the skin, conjunctivae, and the respiratory tract is established; the clinical syndrome of measles becomes evident at this time. The viral burden reaches its maximum height between the days 11 and 14 and, thereafter, rapidly declines. Immunologically compromised patients may have defective clearing of the virus and increased severity of organ involvement. Malnourished children often experience more severe measles infections than do well-nourished children. In Africa, the mortality rate for measles infection is 25%–50% in infants and young children with edematous malnutrition (8).

Widespread distribution of multinucleated giant cells is the characteristic pathologic feature of measles. Of the various organ systems involved, the most prominent are the lungs and the brain. In fatal cases, a striking proliferation of the respiratory epithelia, with formation of peribronchiolar fibroepithelial nodules and cystic transformation of tracheobronchial glands, has been demonstrated. The lung tissues may show marked interstitial pneumonitis with diffuse endothelial cell and pneumocyte degeneration. The brain sections show a paucicellular inflammatory infiltrate with diffuse neuronal damage. However, these findings are found in severe cases and cannot be considered representative of the pathology in all cases of measles.

Clinical Features

The incubation period of measles is about 8–12 days. The first sign of infection is usually high fever, which begins about 8–12 days after exposure and lasts 1–7 days. During this initial stage, the child may develop coryza (runny nose), cough, red and watery eyes, and an enanthem—small white Koplik spots usually found on the buccal mucosa near the molars. Children are usually very irritable. After several days of fever, a rash develops, usually beginning on the face (often in the hairline) and upper neck. The rash is initially erythematous and maculopapular; typical of measles rash is the coexistence of discrete and confluent red maculopapules. Microvesicles may be seen on the top of the erythematous base. Over a period of about 3 days, the rash proceeds downward, eventually reaching the hands and feet. The rash lasts for 5–6 days and then fades. The rash occurs, on average, at day 14 after exposure to the virus, with a range of 7–18 days. Pharyngitis, cervical lymphadenopathy, diarrhea, vomiting, laryngitis, and croup may also occur during the illness.

Atypical measles, a clearly defined clinical syndrome that occurred in previously vaccinated individuals (specifically those who received a killed measles vaccine that is no longer available) after exposure to natural measles, is no longer seen. This illness was characterized by high fever, petechial rash, and pneumonitis and was caused by immune complex deposition. It had a different progression of the rash (cephalad from the extremities).

Some children infected with measles develop complications and can present with a rapidly progressive illness.

Pneumonia

Primary viral involvement of the lungs is common with measles infections. It is characterized by hyperinflation and fluffy perihilar infiltrates. Unilateral, segmental involvement has also been observed. Infants with measles-associated lower respiratory tract infections may present with features suggestive of bronchiolitis. Extensive infection may lead to significant hypoxemia. Children with defects in cell-mediated immunity are particularly prone to develop severe pneumonia. Although measles virus itself can lead to severe pulmonary disease, secondary bacterial pneumonias are also responsible for some measles-related complications and deaths. Children with measles infections have an increased susceptibility to bacterial infections. This propensity may be due to multiple causes: disruption of the respiratory tract epithelium; nonspecific suppression of immune responses by measles infection, and vitamin A deficiency. The bacterial pneumonias are usually due to common respiratory pathogens: *H. influenzae*, *S. pneumoniae*, and *S. aureus*. In some studies, coinfection with viruses (parainfluenza and adenovirus) has been reported. Depending on the setting, ~5%–10% of children hospitalized with measles will require intensive care. One study reported that 15 of 237 children hospitalized with measles required intensive care (2); severe respiratory distress that required mechanical ventilation was the reason for the PICU admission in all cases in this series. Acute respiratory distress syndrome and air leaks are examples of complications among the children in this series (2).

Other respiratory complications include otitis media, mastoiditis, laryngitis, and laryngotracheobronchitis, including severe laryngotracheobronchitis. In developing countries, where latent TB infection is common, immune suppression during measles infection may lead to development of reactivation disease.

Neurologic Involvement

Neurologic involvement is not uncommon in children, with the reported incidence of encephalitis being about 0.5–1.0 per 1000 measles cases. Measles virus can result in 3 different forms of CNS infections (46): acute progressive infectious encephalitis, acute postinfectious encephalitis, and subacute sclerosing panencephalitis (SSPE). The acute progressive form of brain disease, also referred to as inclusion body encephalitis, reflects a direct attack by the virus under conditions of yielding cell-mediated immunity. The postinfectious acute disease is interpreted to reflect an autoimmune reaction. Symptoms of encephalitis usually develop in the second week of illness. Some children may have rapid deterioration, and marked increase in intracranial pressure and herniation may occur. Cerebellar ataxia, myelitis, and motor deficits have been reported. Survivors may have sequelae, such as seizures, deafness, and motor deficits. SSPE is a rare CNS disease with progressive degenerative loss of intelligence, behavioral difficulties, and seizures.

Other *unusual complications* of measles include myocarditis and pericarditis; clinical consequences of such involvement are rare. Some children infected with measles virus may have bleeding manifestations related to thrombocytopenia. Severe disease may lead to DIC.

Differential Diagnosis

The differential diagnosis of measles includes all illnesses in which erythematous maculopapular rash occurs, such as rubella, erythema infectiosum, roseola infantum, enteroviral infections, infectious mononucleosis, *Mycoplasma pneumoniae* infections, and drug reactions. The typical course and pattern of rash usually allow the diagnosis to be made clinically.

Diagnosis

In endemic areas, the diagnosis is usually clinical. For confirmation, demonstration of specific antimeasles IgM antibody in serum is the most commonly used modality. Other means of making the diagnosis include rise in IgG antibodies to measles (acute and convalescent sera) and isolation of the virus from urine, blood, throat, or nasopharyngeal secretions.

Treatment

The treatment for mild infections is supportive. Children who require hospitalization must be managed for the complications. Randomized clinical trials have demonstrated reduction in morbidity and mortality in severe measles with use of vitamin A (32). These findings led to the recommendation to treat all children who require hospitalization with a dose of 200,000 IU of vitamin A. The WHO and UNICEF recommend vitamin A for all children with measles in regions where vitamin A deficiency is a problem or the case fatality ratio for measles is 1% or more. The dose should be repeated after 24 hrs.

In a recently published systematic review, no significant reduction in the risk of mortality in the vitamin A group was seen when all of the studies were pooled, using the random-effects model [relative risk (RR), 0.70; 95% confidence interval (CI), 0.42–1.15] (31). However, using megadoses of vitamin A (200,000 IU) on 2 consecutive days was associated with a reduction in the risk of mortality in children <2 years of age (RR, 0.18; 95% CI, 0.03–0.61) and a reduction in the risk of pneumonia-specific mortality (RR, 0.33; 95% CI, 0.08–0.92). The literature includes a few reports of successful use of inhaled and IV ribavirin in severe infections (52), but no controlled trials have been conducted. The associated bacterial infections should be managed with appropriate antimicrobials. Supportive care and monitoring are important in severe infections, as multiple organ systems may be affected.

Prognosis

The complication rates are higher in malnourished children, immunocompromised children, and in those with vitamin A deficiency. Patients with measles who require intensive care have a high risk for death or long-term complications, even when treated in a modern PICU (2). One study reported 26% mortality in 15 children with measles who were admitted to the PICU (2). Acute respiratory distress syndrome, air leaks, and bacteremia were the most severe complications in these patients.

Conclusions and Future Directions

Measles, a vaccine-preventable infection, is an important cause of death among young children in developing countries. The conditions that may require intensive care include pneumonia, laryngotracheobronchitis, and CNS infections. Vitamin A may be helpful in reducing the morbidity and mortality due to measles. No proven antiviral drugs for measles are available. Improving the availability of vaccine and ensuring adequate immunization of susceptible children are the most important challenges in prevention of measles-associated mortality. Development and evaluation of antiviral agents that are effective against measles virus are required. In the short-term, identification of children who may benefit the most from early intensive care is essential and will aid in early institution of intensive care and in prioritizing the available resources.

NONPOLIO ENTEROVIRAL INFECTIONS

Enteroviruses are nonenveloped, single-stranded RNA viruses in the Picornaviridae family; the subgroups are polioviruses, coxsackieviruses, and echoviruses. Newer enteroviruses are classified by numbering. Although more than 60 different serotypes have been identified, 11 account for the majority of disease. Enteroviruses are ~30-nm particles that consist of a naked, protein capsid and dense central core of RNA. Enterovirus capsids are composed of four proteins: VP1, VP2, VP3, and VP4; the first three are surface proteins, and the last lies on the inner surface. These proteins are the determinants of host range and tissue tropism. The genetic material of the enteroviruses is a single-stranded, positive-sense RNA molecule. Cleavage of a long polyprotein that is translated from the genome leads to formation of four capsid proteins and seven nonstructural proteins.

In the US, enteroviruses have been found to be responsible for 33%–65% of acute febrile illnesses and 55%–65% of hospitalizations for suspected sepsis in infants during the summer and fall, and 25% year-round. In tropical and semitropical areas, enteroviruses frequently circulate year-round. Large outbreaks of enterovirus infections can occur. Outbreaks of hand-foot-and-mouth disease associated with severe CNS and/or cardiopulmonary disease due to enterovirus 71 have occurred in recent years in Australia, Japan, Malaysia, and Taiwan, and community outbreaks of enterovirus meningitis have been reported (14). Factors associated with increased incidence and/or severity of enterovirus infection include young age, male sex, poor hygiene, overcrowding, and low socioeconomic status; more than 25% of symptomatic enterovirus infections occur in infants. Breast-feeding reduces the risk of infection in infants.

Pathogenesis

After the initial contact of the virus with oral or respiratory mucosa, implantation occurs in the pharynx and the gastrointestinal tract. Within 24 hrs, the infection spreads to regional lymphoid tissue. Minor viremia occurs thereafter, usually on day 3, leading to infection of many secondary sites; this phase coincides with onset of clinical symptoms. Multiplication of the virus at secondary infection sites leads to major viremia, which often lasts until day 7 of infection. CNS infection may occur, along with infection of secondary sites or during the phase of major viremia. With the appearance of antibody in the blood, viremia ceases and the viral load in the secondary infection sites decreases. However, virus may continue to replicate in the gastrointestinal tract for many weeks.

Clinical Features

Enteroviral infections vary from mild to fatal illnesses. The spectrum of mild illnesses includes nonspecific febrile illness, common cold, pharyngitis, herpangina, stomatitis, and parotitis. Croup may be caused by coxsackie and echovirus infections; however, this illness is milder when compared to croup caused by influenza and parainfluenza viruses. The respiratory tract infection may result in bronchitis, bronchiolitis or pneumonia; these are caused by coxsackie and echovirus infections. Some of these infections may be severe, and the child may require intensive care. Pleurodynia, characterized by fever and spasmodic chest and upper abdominal muscular pain, is rarely diagnosed now. The major etiologic agents in epidemic pleurodynia were coxsackie B3 and B5. Gastrointestinal manifestations occur commonly in coxsackie and echoviral infections;

manifestations other than diarrhea and vomiting include peritonitis, mesenteric adenitis, appendicitis, hepatitis, and pancreatitis.

Various serotypes of coxsackie and echoviruses have been implicated in causation of pericarditis and myocarditis. These are often associated with involvement of other organ systems. Neurologic illness is a frequent manifestation of infection with enteroviruses; the most common illness is aseptic meningitis. Encephalitis, paralytic disease due to infection of anterior horn cell infection, Guillain-Barré syndrome, transverse myelitis, and cerebellar ataxia may occur. The genitourinary manifestations include nephritis, orchitis, and epididymitis. Arthritis and myositis may be caused by coxsackie virus infections. Skin rashes are common with enterovirus infections and may be maculopapular, morbilliform, petechial, or small vesicles. A common distribution is on the palms, soles, and oral mucosa, leading to the so-called hand-foot-mouth syndrome.

Laboratory Diagnosis

As highlighted in the previous section, enteroviral illnesses have a wide range of manifestations, and therefore, one must have a high index of suspicion to make the diagnosis. The clinical presentation may be mistaken for bacterial infections or other viruses that cause similar illnesses. The diagnosis of enterovirus infection can be confirmed by virus isolation and detection. The samples may be collected from the nasopharynx, throat, stool, rectal swab, blood, urine, and cerebrospinal fluid (CSF). Viral isolation in culture usually takes less than a week. The virus may be detected in the body fluids by nucleic acid techniques: cDNA and RNA probes and PCR. Serology is usually not used for diagnosis.

Treatment

The mainstay of care is supportive treatment. IV immunoglobulin has been used in neonates with severe disseminated infection and is used for children with persistent CNS infection due to immune deficiencies that cause hypogammaglobulinemia. The antiviral drug pleconoril was evaluated for treatment of severe enteroviral infections, particularly neurologic infections, myocarditis, and infections in immunodeficient patients (47); however, it is no longer being manufactured. In absence of any evidence indicating any benefit, corticosteroids should be avoided in severe illnesses. Children with enteroviral infections require universal and contact precautions when admitted to healthcare facilities.

Conclusions and Future Directions

Nonpolio enteroviruses are responsible for variety of illnesses. Some of the respiratory, myocardial, and CNS infections may be severe enough to require intensive care. The mainstay of care is supportive treatment. The challenges that impact control of nonpolio enteroviruses include development and evaluation of simpler and rapid diagnostic methods, antiviral drugs, and cost-effective supportive care.

SEVERE VARICELLA INFECTIONS

Varicella (chickenpox) is a common and usually self-limited exanthematous illness of childhood. However, primary varicella can result in severe manifestations, such as pneumonia, hepatitis, encephalitis, and DIC, particularly in certain groups: neonates, pregnant women, adolescents, adults, and the immunocompromised. Varicella-zoster virus (VZV) establishes life-long latency in the dorsal root ganglia after the primary infection. Reactivation of virus leads to zoster (shingles), which is usually characterized by a pruritic vesicular rash in a dermatomal pattern in immunocompetent patients. Zoster may manifest as a more severe illness in immunocompromised patients and can involve multiple dermatomes and viscera. Up to 3.5% of children may have a complicated course (26). Deaths are uncommon, with the reported figure less than 2 deaths per 100,000 in children between 1 and 14 years of age (23).

Description of Virus

VZV is a member of the Herpes viridae family and consists of viral DNA inside an icosahedral nucleocapsid surrounded by lipid envelope. Primary infection with VZV presents as varicella (chickenpox), while reactivation presents as localized cutaneous infection, called zoster (shingles). VZV produces cytopathic effects in cells that are indistinguishable from those produced by herpes simplex viruses.

Clinical Features

Transmission of varicella occurs by either airborne droplets or contact with secretions or infected vesicular fluid. The incubation period is typically 2 weeks, with a range of 10–21 days. Chickenpox is characterized by a rash, low-grade fever, and malaise. Patients may have prodromal constitutional symptoms 1–2 days before the onset of rash. The rash, which evolves from maculopapules to pruritic vesicles to crusts, often initially appears on the trunk or face and spreads over days to involve the entire body. Groups, or crops, of skin lesions, which number on average 250–500 in the unvaccinated child, progress from macules to vesicles to crusts. Simultaneously having lesions in various stages of evolution is a clinical hallmark of chickenpox. Most patients with varicella make an uneventful recovery after ~1 week. However, some patients may develop the complications described in the next sections.

Bacterial Superinfection

Secondary bacterial complications can occur in skin, soft tissues, and other sites and is often caused by group A *Streptococcus* (GAS) and *Staphylococcus aureus*. Varicella is a particularly important risk factor for severe invasive GAS infections in previously healthy children and, in recent years, an increasing proportion of these cases in the US have been associated with varicella. A GAS infection should be considered in any child with varicella who also has localized skin findings of erythema, warmth, swelling, or induration, and in any child with varicella who becomes febrile after having been afebrile, who has a temperature of >39°C beyond day 3 of illness, or who has any fever beyond day 4 of illness. When present, GAS infections are usually painful, and initially, the amount of pain is frequently out of proportion to the clinical findings (4).

Pneumonia

VZV pneumonia is the most serious complication of disseminated VZV infection, with mortality rates of 9%–50%. Reported prevalence of VZV pneumonia has varied from less than 5% to up to 50% of all varicella infections in adults (24). Most cases of VZV pneumonia have been reported in immunocompromised adults and in those with chronic lung disease.

Varicella pneumonia usually presents 1–6 days after the onset of the rash and is associated with tachypnea, chest tightness, cough, dyspnea, fever, and occasionally, with pleuritic chest pain and hemoptysis. Chest symptoms may start before the appearance of the skin rash. Physical findings are often minimal, and chest x-rays typically reveal nodular or interstitial pneumonitis. Findings of VZV pneumonia on chest x-ray consist of multiple 5–10-mm, ill-defined nodules that may be confluent and fleeting. Hilar lymphadenopathy and pleural effusion are unusual. The small, round nodules usually resolve within a week after the disappearance of the skin lesions but may persist for months. Usually resolving in 3–5 days in milder disease, the small nodules may persist for several weeks in widespread disease. The lesions calcify and can persist as numerous, well-defined, randomly scattered, 2–3-mm dense calcifications (36).

High-resolution CT of the chest in patients with varicella pneumonitis usually shows 1–10-mm, well-defined and ill-defined nodules that are diffuse throughout both lungs. Nodules with a surrounding halo of ground-glass opacity, patchy ground-glass opacity, and coalescence of nodules are also seen. These findings disappear concurrently with healing of skin lesions after antiviral chemotherapy (36).

Encephalitis

Encephalitis is another serious complication of varicella infection. See Chapters 80 and 84 for more details.

Disseminated Varicella and Zoster

Disseminated varicella and zoster with multivisceral involvement is classically described in immunocompromised patients, particularly those with deficient cell-mediated immunity, bone marrow and renal transplant recipients, and AIDS patients. Even with treatment, the disease carries a very high mortality. Less common complications include transverse myelitis, Guillain-Barré syndrome, purpura fulminans, myocarditis, arthritis, and fulminant hepatic failure. Please refer to Chapter 84 for diagnosis and management.

Conclusions and Future Directions

Varicella (chickenpox) is a common and, usually, self-limited exanthematous illness. However, primary varicella can result in severe manifestations, such as pneumonia, hepatitis, encephalitis, and DIC. The challenge is to achieve and improve vaccine availability at affordable cost and wider immunization coverage. Doing so may help to provide an overall reduction in severe varicella infection and mortality. Identification of the profile of children who may benefit the most from early intensive care may help in early institution of intensive supportive care. The role of corticosteroids in severe varicella pneumonia should be investigated.

SEVERE HERPES SIMPLEX VIRUS INFECTIONS

Herpes simplex virus (HSV) infection is one of the most common human viral infections and frequently involves the skin, mucous membranes, and the genitalia. CNS and pulmonary involvement, although less frequent, carry high morbidity and mortality. Immunocompetent patients with HSV infection usually have asymptomatic or mild disease, while immunocompromised patients have a higher risk of disseminated disease, with involvement of multiple organ systems. HSV infection in neonates tends to be severe, with high chances of CNS and visceral dissemination and subsequent morbidity and mortality. Neonatal HSV infection, caused by HSV-2 in ~70% of cases, is estimated to occur in ~1 in 4000 newborns in the US (19). Herpes simplex encephalitis (HSE) is the most commonly identified cause of sporadic viral encephalitis beyond 6 months of age. Estimated frequency varies from 4 per million per year in the US to 2.5 per million per year in Sweden (53).

Description of the Virus

HSV is an enveloped virus with double-stranded linear DNA genome, which is enclosed in a regular icosahedral protein capsid; the outer envelope is acquired from the nuclear membrane of host cells and contains various viral glycoproteins. Two distinct strains of HSV, which differ by 50% in their DNA structure, are recognized. HSV-1 which causes orolabial, ocular, and CNS infection, is more prevalent than HSV-2, which is the predominant cause of genital infections, neonatal infections, and aseptic meningitis.

Pathogenesis

Primary oropharyngeal HSV-1 infection results in axoplasmic transport of virus to the trigeminal sensory ganglion, where it establishes latency. Latent HSV-1 is detectable in the trigeminal ganglia of virtually all seropositive individuals. The majority of cases of HSE are due to reactivated virus from dorsal root ganglia, but virus can also reach the CNS via olfactory bulbs during viremia of primary infection. Evidence also suggests persistence of HSV genome in the CNS of asymptomatic individuals. Whether this latent virus could reactivate and cause encephalitis is not clear (53). Neonatal infection is most frequently acquired during the intrapartum period, and primary infection in the mother, rupture of membranes >6 hrs, and fetal invasive monitoring appear to increase the risk.

Clinical Features

HSV infections commonly involve oral and genital skin and mucosa. Visceral involvement in herpes is not common, but it carries high morbidity and mortality.

Infections of the Central Nervous System

HSE is a life-threatening manifestation of HSV infection of the CNS. Although HSE is rare, mortality rates reach 70% in the absence of therapy, and only a minority returns to normal function (53). This dreaded manifestation of HSV infection can occur within weeks after birth (neonatal HSV disease) or in childhood or adulthood (HSE). Most cases of neonatal HSV disease are caused by HSV-2, whereas virtually all cases of HSE are caused by HSV-1. HSV encephalitis is discussed in detail in Chapter 80.

Pneumonia

HSV pneumonia is classically seen in immunocompromised patients, but a few case reports describe its occurrence in immunocompetent individuals. HSV pneumonia, particularly in immunocompromised patients, carries a high mortality. The diagnosis of this and other infections caused by the herpes virus family are made difficult by the phenomenon of latency. In that these viruses can be found in healthy people previously infected and in that many of these viruses commonly infect humans, distinguishing the presence of latent virus in people with infections due to other causes and infection caused by the virus itself is difficult.

Disseminated Involvement

Extensive cutaneous and visceral dissemination of HSV is seen in certain children with immune deficiencies, such as severely malnourished children, transplant recipients, patients with malignancies or other conditions that require immunosuppression, patients on high-dose steroid therapy, AIDS patients, burns patients, or patients with other immunodeficiencies, particularly those affecting T lymphocytes. Disseminated disease in these patients may manifest as a sepsis-like syndrome with fever or hypothermia, leukopenia, hepatitis, DIC, and shock and often results in death. This form of herpes has a high mortality, even with appropriate therapy.

Neonatal Herpes

Neonatal herpes may manifest in one of three ways. The least severe form is disease limited to skin, eyes, and mucous membranes (SEM disease), which presents usually between days 5 and 19 of life. Disseminated HSV is rapidly progressive and has a high mortality rate. It also usually has onset before the third week of life. Neonatal HSV disease may also be localized to the CNS. Clinicians may fail to make an early diagnosis because children often have no associated cutaneous findings (37). Most surviving infants with CNS or disseminated disease have neurologic sequelae, and the mortality rate in the absence of therapy is very high (80%) for babies in the latter category. Early recognition and treatment may improve outcome (56). As the clinical features may be nonspecific, the diagnosis is often not considered and administration of therapy is delayed.

Diagnosis

Cutaneous HSV infections can be diagnosed rapidly by microscopic examination of stained scrapings from the vesicles for giant cells and intranuclear inclusions (Tzanck smear). This method, when compared to viral culture, has a specificity of ~90% and sensitivity of 80% in males and 50% in females (42). HSV PCR has been found to be as sensitive as viral culture for diagnosis of cutaneous HSV infection and has the advantage of allowing rapid diagnosis (18).

PCR of the CSF is the method of choice for diagnosis of HSE, but CSF PCR results can be negative in the first 72 hrs following illness onset. CSF virus culture is of little value in all patients. For details of the role of neuroimaging, see Chapter 80.

Neonatal herpes may occur in the absence of skin lesions; therefore, if the infection is suspected, swabs of the mouth, nasopharynx, conjunctiva, rectum, skin lesions, mucosal lesions, and urine should be promptly taken and submitted for virus culture. Evidence of disseminated or CNS infection should be sought using liver function tests, complete blood cell count, CSF analysis, and chest x-ray, if respiratory abnormalities are present. Microscopic examination, culture, and PCR assay of bronchoalveolar lavage fluid may help in the diagnosis of HSV pneumonia.

Management

Serious HSV infections require treatment with IV acyclovir. The recommended dose for HSE is 10 mg/kg every 8 h for 21 days. It is also recommended that all patients with HSE undergo a CSF PCR for HSV at the end of 14 days to document elimination of replicating virus. Neonatal and disseminated forms of HSV also require treatment with IV acyclovir. The dose recommended for neonatal HSV encephalitis and neonatal disseminated infection is 20 mg/kg every 8 hrs for 21 days, while SEM disease requires treatment for 14 days (38). Emergence of acyclovir-resistant strains has been particularly reported in immunocompromised patients on acyclovir therapy. The drug of choice for acyclovir-resistant HSV strains is IV foscarnet.

Prognosis

With therapy, most infants with SEM HSV infection improve. The mortality rate is significantly higher in the neonates with disseminated infection and encephalitis. The risk of death is increased in neonates who are in or near coma at presentation, have disseminated intravascular coagulopathy, or are premature. In babies with disseminated disease, HSV pneumonitis is also associated with greater mortality. For HSV infection limited to the skin, eyes, or mouth, the presence of ≥ 3 recurrences of vesicles has been reported to be associated with an increased risk of neurologic impairment, as compared with ≤ 2 recurrences (56).

Conclusions and Future Directions

HSV infections of the lungs and brain can be severe, having high morbidity and mortality. Immunocompromised children are at a higher risk for severe infections. Neonates are at a greater risk for severe disease. Acyclovir is the mainstay of therapy. However, HSV diagnosis often goes unsuspected. Given the difficulty in making the clinical diagnosis of HSV, the growing worldwide prevalence, and the availability of effective antiviral therapy, the need to develop rapid, accurate laboratory diagnosis of patients with HSV is clear, as is the need to evaluate the benefit of early administration of acyclovir in patients with suspected severe HSV infection without waiting for virologic confirmation. Development of a vaccine to prevent HSV infection should receive high priority for eventual control of HSV infection.

KEY POINTS

Dengue Hemorrhagic Fever and Dengue Shock Syndrome

■ Dengue infection is now endemic in more than 100 countries. It is caused by dengue virus (four serotypes) that belongs to Flaviviridae family.

■ The clinical manifestations of dengue virus infection vary from asymptomatic to severe, life-threatening DHF and DSS that require intensive care.

■ DHF and DSS are characterized by profound capillary leak and thrombocytopenia.

■ Suggested pathogenic mechanisms include increased replication of a serotype of dengue virus enhanced by the presence of non-neutralizing antibodies, complement activation, and increased cytokine levels.

■ Laboratory findings include hemoconcentration and thrombocytopenia.

■ The diagnosis is confirmed by viral culture (initial 5 days of illness) or demonstration of specific IgM antibodies (after first 5 days of illness).

■ Supportive care and aggressive fluid therapy are the cornerstones of management. Fluid therapy is guided by clinical response and monitoring of hematocrit.

■ No specific antiviral drugs for dengue infection are available.

■ Early detection and aggressive fluid therapy can reduce case fatality rates to <1%.

Viral Hemorrhagic Fevers

■ VHF, caused by various viruses belonging to the Flaviviridae family (Kyasanur Forest disease, Omsk, dengue, and yellow fever viruses), the Bunyaviridae family (Congo, Hantaan, and Rift Valley fever viruses), the Arenaviridae family (Junin, Machupo, Guanarito, and Lassa viruses), and the Filoviridae family (Ebola and Marburg viruses), are characterized by hemorrhagic manifestations.

■ Ebola, Marburg, Lassa, and Crimean-Congo hemorrhagic fever viruses can spread from person to person.

■ Viruses that cause hemorrhagic fevers can be used in bioterrorism.

■ The clinical manifestations of these syndromes are quite similar.

■ The severity is variable, and the case fatality rates may be up to 90%. The diagnosis can be confirmed by viral isolation or serologic tests.

■ The principle involved in management of all of these diseases, especially HFRS, is the reversal of dehydration, hemoconcentration, renal failure, and protein, electrolyte, or blood losses.

■ IV ribavirin administered is effective in reducing mortality in Lassa fever and HFRS.

HIV Infection

■ HIV infection has become an important contributor to childhood morbidity and mortality, especially in many developing countries.

- Children with HIV infection may need admission to PICUs because of respiratory infections and respiratory failure, septic shock, and CNS disorders.
- Severe complications of therapy may also become indications for admission into the PICU.
- The PICU staff should be aware of postexposure prophylaxis.

Measles

- Measles, a vaccine-preventable infection, is an important cause of death among young children.
- The conditions associated with measles that may require intensive care include pneumonia, laryngotracheobronchitis, and CNS infections.
- Vitamin A may be helpful in reducing the morbidity and mortality due to measles.
- No proven antiviral drugs for measles are available.

Nonpolio Enteroviruses

- Nonpolio enteroviruses are responsible for a variety of illnesses.
- Some of the respiratory, myocardial, and CNS infections may be severe enough to require intensive care.
- The mainstay of care is supportive treatment.

Severe Varicella Infections

- Varicella (chickenpox), a common and usually self-limited exanthematous illness, may result in severe manifestations, such as pneumonia, hepatitis, encephalitis, and DIC.
- The diagnosis can usually be made on the basis of clinical features and can be confirmed by virologic studies.
- Acyclovir is the drug of choice; valacyclovir, famciclovir, and foscarnet are newer alternatives.
- Recommendations have been made for routine varicella vaccination for all healthy children between 12 and 18 months and to all susceptible children before their 13th birthday, in addition to catch-up vaccination in older children and those who are at high risk of transmission and exposure.

Severe HSV Infections

- HSV infections of the lungs and brain can be severe, having high morbidity and mortality.
- Immunocompromised children and neonates are at a higher risk of severe infections.
- Acyclovir is the mainstay of therapy.

References

1. Abrams EJ. Opportunistic infections and other clinical manifestations of HIV disease in children. *Pediatr Clin N Am* 2000;47:79–108.
2. Abramson O, Dagan R, Tal A, Sofer S. Severe complications of measles requiring intensive care in infants and young children. *Arch Pediatr Adolesc Med* 1995;149:1237–40.
3. American Academy of Pediatrics. Committee on Infectious Diseases. Severe invasive group a streptococcal infections: A subject review. *Pediatrics* 1998;101:136–40.
4. American Academy of Pediatrics. Tuberculosis. In: Pickering LJ, editor. *Red Book Report of the Committee on Infectious Diseases*, 25th ed. Elk Grove Village, IL: American Academy of Pediatrics, 2000;593–613.
5. American Thoracic Society/Centers for Disease Control and Prevention/Infectious Diseases Society of America. Treatment of tuberculosis. *Am J Respir Crit Care Med* 2003;167:603–62.
6. Anonymous. Clinical diagnosis. In: *Dengue Haemorrhagic Fever, Diagnosis, Treatment, Prevention and Control*, 2nd ed. Geneva: World Health Organization, 1997;12–23.
7. Anonymous. Laboratory diagnosis. In: *Dengue Haemorrhagic Fever, Diagnosis, Treatment, Prevention and Control*, 2nd ed. Geneva: World Health Organization, 1997;34–47.
8. Anonymous. Severity of measles in malnutrition. *Nutr Rev* 1982;40:203–5.
9. Anonymous. Treatment. In: *Dengue Haemorrhagic Fever, Diagnosis, Treatment, Prevention and Control*, 2nd ed. Geneva: World Health Organization, 1997;24–33.
10. Becroft DM, Osborne DR. The lungs in fatal measles infection in childhood: Pathological, radiological, and immunological correlations. *Histopathology* 1980;4:401–12.
11. Bethell DB, Gamble J, Loc PP, et al. Noninvasive measurement of microvascular leakage in patients with dengue hemorrhagic fever. *Clin Infect Dis* 2001;32:243–53.
12. Bossi P, Tegnell A, Baka A, et al. Bichat guidelines for the clinical management of haemorrhagic fever viruses and bioterrorism-related haemorrhagic fever viruses. *Euro Surveill* 2004;9:E1–8.
13. Bwaka MA, Bonnet MJ, Calain P, et al. Ebola hemorrhagic fever in Kikwit, Democratic Republic of the Congo: Clinical observations in 103 patients. *J Infect Dis* 1999;179(Suppl 1):S1–7.
14. Cardosa MJ, Perera D, Brown BA, et al. Molecular epidemiology of human enterovirus 71 strains and recent outbreaks in the Asia-Pacific region: Comparative analysis of the VP1 and VP4 genes. *Emerg Infect Dis* 2003;9:461–8.
15. Centers for Disease Control and Prevention. 1994 Revised classification system for human immunodeficiency virus infection in children less than 13 years of age. *MMWR* 1994;43:6–8.
16. Chan SP, Birnbaum J, Rao M, et al. Clinical manifestations and outcome of tuberculosis in children with acquired immunodeficiency syndrome. *Pediatr Infect Dis J* 1996;15:443–7.
17. Chien LJ, Liao TL, Shu PY, et al. Development of real-time reverse transcriptase PCR assays to detect and serotype dengue viruses. *J Clin Microbiol* 2006;44:1295–304.
18. Cohen PR. Tests for detecting herpes simplex virus and varicella-zoster virus infections. *Dermatol Clin* 1994;12:51–68.
19. Committee on Fetus and Newborn, Committee on Infectious diseases, American Academy of Pediatrics. Perinatal herpes simplex virus infections. *Pediatrics* 1980;66:147–9.
20. Cooper S, Lyall H, Walters S, et al. Children with human immunodeficiency virus admitted to a paediatric intensive care unit in the United Kingdom over a 10-year period. *Intensive Care Med* 2004;30:113–8.
21. Cowburn CA, Hatherill M, Eley B, et al. Short-term mortality and implementation of antiretroviral treatment for critically ill HIV-infected children in a developing country. *Arch Dis Child* 2006 May 2;[Epub ahead of print].
22. Dunn DT, Newell ML, Ades AE, et al. Risk of human immunodeficiency virus type 1 transmission through breastfeeding. *Lancet* 1992;340:585–8.
23. Fairley CK, Miller E. Varicella-zoster virus epidemiology - a changing scene? *J Infect Dis* 1996;174:S314–19.
24. Feldman S. Varicella-zoster virus pneumonitis. *Chest* 1994;106:22–27.
25. Fisher SD, Easley KA, Orav EJ, et al. Mild dilated cardiomyopathy and increased left ventricular mass predict mortality: The prospective P2C2 HIV Multicenter Study. *Am Heart J* 2005;150:439–47.
26. Fornaro P. Epidemiology and cost analysis of varicella in Italy: Results of a sentinel study in the pediatric practice. Italian Sentinel Group on Pediatric Infectious Diseases. *Pediatr Infect Dis J* 1999;18:414–9.
27. Fowler MG, Simonds RJ, Roongpisuthipong A. Update on perinatal HIV transmission. *Pediatr Clin North Am* 2000;47:21–38.
28. Guglani L, Kabra SK. T-cell immunopathogenesis of dengue virus infection. *Dengue Bulletin* 2005;29:58–69.
29. Halstead SB. Pathogenesis of dengue: Challenges to molecular biology. *Science* 1988;239:476–81.
30. http://www.who.int/mediacentre/factsheets/fs286/en. Accessed November 2006.
31. Huiming Y, Chaomin W, Meng M. Vitamin A for treating measles in children. *The Cochrane Database Systematic Reviews* 2005;4:CD001479.
32. Hussey GD, Klein MA. Randomized, controlled trial of vitamin A in children with severe measles. *N Engl J Med* 1990;323:160–4.
33. Kabra SK, Jain Y, Madhulika, et al. Role of platelet transfusion in dengue hemorrhagic fever. *Indian Pediatr* 1998;35:452–4.
34. Kabra SK, Jain Y, Pandey RM, et al. Dengue hemorrhagic fever in children in the 1996 Delhi epidemic. *Trans Royal Society Trop Med Hygiene* 1999;93:294–8.
35. Kabra SK, Juneja R, Madhulika, et al. Myocardial dysfunction in children with dengue haemorrhagic fever. *Natl Med J India* 1998;11:59–61.

36. Kim EA, Lee KS, Primack SL, et al. Viral pneumonias in adults: Radiologic and pathologic findings. *Radiographics* 2002;22:S137–49.

37. Kimberlin DW. Neonatal herpes simplex infection. *Clin Microbiol Rev* 2004;17:1–13.

38. Kimberlin DW, Lin C-Y, Jacobs RF, et al. Natural history of neonatal herpes simplex virus infections in the acyclovir era. *Pediatrics* 2001;108:223–9.

39. Luzuriaga K, Sullivan JL. Viral and immunopathogenesis of vertical HIV-1 infection. In Pizzo PA, Wilfert CM. *Pediatric AIDS*, 3rd ed. Philadelphia: Lippincott Williams & Wilkins, 1998;89–104.

40. Luzuriaga K, Sullivan JL. Viral and immunopathogenesis of vertical HIV-1 infection. *Pediatr Clin North Am* 2000;47:65–78.

41. McCormick JB, King IJ, Webb PA, et al. Lassa fever. Effective therapy with ribavirin. *N Engl J Med* 1986;314:20–6.

42. Nahass GT, Goldstein BA, Zhu WY, et al. Comparison of Tzanck smear, viral culture, and DNA diagnostic methods in detection of herpes simplex and varicella-zoster infection. *JAMA* 1992;268:2541–4.

43. Nhan NT, Phuong CXT, Kneen R, et al. Acute management of dengue shock syndrome: A randomized double-blind comparison of 4 intravenous fluid regimens in the first hour. *Clin Infect Dis* 2001;32:204–13.

44. Nimmannitya S. Clinical manifestations of dengue/dengue hemorrhagic fever. In: *Monograph on Dengue/Dengue Hemorrhagic Fever.* New Delhi: World Health Organization, 1993;48–54.

45. Nimmannitya S. Dengue fever/dengue haemorrhagic fever: Case management. *Trop Med (Nagasaki)* 1994;36:249–56.

46. Norrby E, Kristensson K. Measles virus in the brain. *Brain Res Bull* 1997;44:213–20.

47. Nowak-Wegrzyn A, Phipatanakul W, Winkelstein JA, et al. Successful treatment of enterovirus infection with the use of pleconaril in 2 infants with severe combined immunodeficiency. *Clin Infect Dis* 2001;32:E13–4.

48. Piggot DC. Hemorrhagic fever viruses. *Crit Care Clin* 2005;21:765–83.

49. Ranjit S, Kissoon N, Jayakumar I. Aggressive management of dengue shock syndrome may decrease mortality rate: A suggested protocol. *Pediatr Crit Care Med* 2005;6:412–9.

50. Rey C, Prieto S, Medina A, et al. Fatal lactic acidosis during antiretroviral therapy. *Pediatr Crit Care Med* 2003;4:485–7.

51. Sakuntabhai A, Turbpaiboon C, Casademont I, et al. A variant in the CD209 promoter is associated with severity of dengue disease. *Nat Genet* 2005;37:507–13.

52. Stogner SW, King JW, Black-Payne C, et al. Ribavirin and intravenous immune globulin therapy for measles pneumonia in HIV infection. *South Med J.* 1993;86:1415–8.

53. Tyler KL. Herpes simplex virus infections of the central nervous system: Encephalitis and meningitis, including Mollaret's. *Herpes* 2004;11:57A–64A.

54. Update US Public Health Service Guidelines for the Management of Occupational Exposures to HIV and Recommendations for Postexposure Prophylaxis. *MMWR (RR 9)* 2005;54:1–19.

55. Van Den Hof S, Smit C, Van Steenbergen JE, et al. Hospitalizations during a measles epidemic in the Netherlands, 1999 to 2000. *Pediatr Infect Dis J* 2002;21:1146–50.

56. Whitley R, Arvin A, Prober C, et al. Predictors of morbidity and mortality in neonates with herpes simplex virus infections. The National Institute of Allergy and Infectious Diseases Collaborative Antiviral Study Group. *N Engl J Med* 1991;324:450–4.

57. Wills BA, Nguyen MD, Ha TL, et al. Comparison of three fluid solutions for resuscitation in dengue shock syndrome. *N Engl J Med* 2005;353:877–89.

58. Working Group on Antiretroviral Therapy and Medical Management of HIV-Infected Children. *Guidelines for the Use of Antiretroviral Agents in Pediatric HIV Infection.* Bethesda, Maryland: National Institutes of Health, Nov. 3, 2005.

59. Zar HJ, Apolles P, Argent A, et al. The etiology and outcome of pneumonia in human immunodeficiency virus-infected children admitted to intensive care in a developing country. *Pediatr Crit Care Med* 2001;2:108–12.

CHAPTER 80 ■ CENTRAL NERVOUS SYSTEM INFECTIONS

PRATIBHA D. SINGHI • SUNIT C. SINGHI • CHARLES R.J.C. NEWTON • JAKUB SIMON

Infections of the central nervous system (CNS) are among the most devastating infectious diseases, causing death and disability worldwide. They often present as serious medical emergencies, and institution of early, appropriate intensive care is of utmost importance in reducing mortality and morbidity. This chapter is structured to familiarize the intensivist with common CNS infections, help generate differential diagnoses, and develop an appropriate treatment plan. It does not attempt to cover all possible infections that may affect the CNS.

A discussion on meningitis—bacterial, aseptic, and tubercular—is followed by sections on encephalitis and myelitis, with special emphasis on herpes, Japanese encephalitis (JE), and acute disseminated encephalomyelitis (ADEM). A section on brain abscess and epidural abscess, with emphasis on aspects relevant to the intensivist, is also included. Cerebral malaria, being an important problem for intensivists in developing countries, is also discussed.

ANATOMY AND PHYSIOLOGY

As important aspects of CNS anatomy and physiology are discussed in Chapter 51, specific implications of anatomic and/or physiologic issues will be identified in this chapter as they pertain to the specific infections under discussion.

PATHOGENESIS

To cause CNS infections, pathogens must gain access either to the subarachnoid space to cause meningitis or to the brain and spinal cord parenchyma to cause encephalitis, myelitis, or a CNS abscess. Most infections spread to the CNS through the bloodstream; however, different pathogens go to different anatomic locations. The organisms that typically cause bacterial meningitis rarely cause brain abscess, and those found in brain abscesses rarely cause meningitis. At times, the CNS may be infected by direct spread of organisms from an infective focus adjacent to the brain (otitis media, sinusitis, dental abscess) or from a cerebrospinal fluid (CSF) shunt or skull fracture.

CLINICAL PRESENTATION

The main features of CNS infections are fever, headache, and altered sensorium. Focal neurologic signs may also be seen. However, these symptoms and signs are nonspecific and can be seen in noninfectious CNS syndromes as well. Hence, a comprehensive evaluation is necessary to narrow the differential diagnosis. Epidemiologic risk factors for CNS infections and physical examination may provide etiologic clues. Broadly, a child with CNS infections may present with any of the following syndromes.

Acute Meningitis Syndrome

Acute meningitis syndrome presents as acute onset over a few hours to a few days of fever, headache, vomiting, photophobia, neck stiffness, and altered sensorium. An acute upper respiratory tract infection may precede the onset of meningitis by a few days. Examples of CNS infections that present with an acute meningitis syndrome include bacterial and viral meningitis.

Subacute or Chronic Meningitis Syndrome

Onset is usually gradual, often without any evident predisposing condition. Fever is often present but tends to be lower than in acute meningitis. Progression is slower over a few weeks. Examples of CNS infections that present with a subacute or chronic meningitis syndrome include tuberculous and fungal meningitis.

Acute Encephalitis Syndrome

Acute encephalitis may be diffuse or focal. In diffuse encephalitis, alteration of sensorium is predominant and occurs earlier in the course of disease than in acute meningitis. Seizures are seen more frequently than with meningitis and often during the initial phase of disease. Focal encephalitis reflects tropism of some viruses for specific locations in the CNS, such as temporal lobe infection by herpes simplex virus (HSV).

Encephalopathy with Systemic Infection

Many systemic infections involve the CNS, and CNS symptoms may be the presenting feature in some cases. For example, shigellosis, typhoid fever, malaria, rickettsial diseases, and infective endocarditis may involve the CNS. It is therefore important to consider systemic infection as a possible underlying cause in children with encephalopathy.

Postinfectious Syndromes

ADEM, transverse myelitis, optic neuritis, and multiple sclerosis (MS) are disorders of demyelination of the CNS (collectively referred to as *idiopathic inflammatory diseases of the CNS*) that may present global or focal neurologic deficits days to weeks after recovery from an infectious illness, suggesting an autoimmune phenomenon triggered by infection or vaccine.

DIAGNOSIS

A general diagnostic approach to a patient with suspected CNS infection must include a thorough history and physical. Chronicity of signs and symptoms will help to categorize the illness according to one of the just-mentioned syndromes. Significant history, such as ill contacts, trauma, surgery, travel, insect bites, contact with animals, and sexual activity, may help to determine etiology. Premorbid or comorbid conditions, such as prior viral illness, immunodeficiency, presence of CSF shunt, associated diarrhea, respiratory illness, sinusitis, rash, arthritis, and other associated signs and symptoms, are important. Laboratory tests may include general assessment with complete blood count, chemistry panel, C-reactive protein (CRP), liver function tests, urine analysis, and other testing to assess systemic illness. Specific testing of blood, including blood culture, thick and thin blood smears, polymerase chain reaction (PCR), antigen testing, and serology, may be indicated. General assessment of the CNS, including CSF opening pressure, white and red blood cell counts, protein, and glucose, is most often indicated; the usual CSF characteristics of meningitis are listed in **Table 80.1.** Specialized studies on CSF, including Gram stain with aerobic and anaerobic bacterial culture, fungal stain, and fungal culture, acid-fast bacilli stain, and mycobacterial culture, should be considered. CSF inspection for parasites, viral culture, PCR, antigen testing, and serology may also be indicated. Neuroimaging, electroencephalogram (EEG), and other studies may add to the diagnosis. Drainage of abscesses and obtaining CNS tissue for histopathology are occasionally required.

MANAGEMENT

As with any other serious illness, management starts with the primary survey to ensure immediate attention to the basic airway, breathing, and circulation (ABCs) of life support before looking for an etiologic diagnosis. A secondary survey, with particular attention to the neurologic examination, meningeal signs, and assessment of the severity of coma, if present, is then undertaken. The physical examination in a child with meningitis is mainly geared toward excluding focal neurologic pathology, determining whether the child has clinically significant elevation of intracranial pressure (ICP), finding any source of infection elsewhere in the body (e.g., sinusitis, otitis, pneumonia), and identifying any other etiologic clues, such as rashes or skin lesions.

Children with a Glasgow Coma Scale score of <8, pharyngeal hypotonia, poor gag reflex, and loss of swallowing reflex require intubation and supplemental oxygen. Appropriate techniques should be used to minimize potential increases in ICP associated with endotracheal intubation (see Chapter 22). Clinical signs and laboratory data that warrant admission of a child with meningitis to the PICU are listed in **Table 80.2.** Antimicrobial therapy must be administered promptly and, due to limited penetration into the CSF, at high doses. Details of antimicrobial therapy are discussed in later sections in which specific etiologies of CNS infection are described.

Any evidence of shock, such as poor perfusion, hypovolemia, and/or hypotension, requires aggressive treatment with normal saline boluses and inotropes, if necessary, to maintain normal blood pressure. Shock in CNS infection may be septic, neurogenic, hypovolemic, or a combination of these.

With increasing severity of illness and raised ICP, the cerebral blood flow (CBF) decreases, especially in the subcortical white matter. The level of impairment of consciousness correlates well with decreased cerebral perfusion, and mortality and sequelae are inversely related to the cerebral perfusion pressure and CBF. ICP, therefore, must be maintained within a narrow range in children with meningitis. Although ICP monitoring is not routinely recommended, it may be considered in those children with CNS infection who have clinical signs of moderate-to-severe increase in ICP. The approach to control of ICP in patients with CNS infection follows the same algorithm as in other etiologies of intracranial hypertension.

Seizures are controlled with IV benzodiazepines, generally diazepam or lorazepam. Approximately half of the patients with seizures progress to refractory status epilepticus (SE). SE associated with intracranial infections is more difficult to treat and has a poor outcome (36). The overall approach to the treatment of SE is discussed in Chapter 57.

Alterations in fluid and electrolyte homeostasis are often seen with CNS infection and may be life-threatening if not corrected in a timely fashion. An accurate record of fluid intake

TABLE 80.1			

CEREBROSPINAL FLUID CHARACTERISTICS IN MENINGITIS

Characteristics	Viral	Bacterial	Tubercular
WBC/mm³	N (<5) or raised to 10–100	Raised 100 to >1000	Raised 100–1000
Predominant cell type	Lymphocytes	Neutrophils	Lymphocytes
Glucose CSF: serum	N (<0.6) or decreased to <0.4	Decreased to <0.4 or much lower	Decreased to <0.4 or lower
Protein mg/dL	N (<50) or up to 100	Raised 100 to >500	Raised 100–500

WBC, white blood cell; N, normal; CSF, cerebrospinal fluid

TABLE 80.2

CHECKLIST OF CLINICAL SIGNS AND METABOLIC DATA THAT WARRANT ADMISSION OF A CHILD WITH MENINGITIS TO THE PICU

Clinical signs	Metabolic data
Glasgow Coma scale <8	Significant metabolic acidosis
Airway instability	Hypoxemia
Poor/irregular respiratory effort	Hypercapnia
Respiratory distress	Hyponatremia
Hyperventilation	Anemia
Poor perfusion/ hypotension	Neutropenia
Oliguria/anuria	Other falciparum parasitemia >5%
Hypertension/bradycardia	
Abnormal posturing	
Impaired pupillary response	
Deranged liver/renal functions	
Abnormal doll's eye movements	
Abnormal motor response	
Focal neurodeficits	
Cranial nerve palsy	
Seizures	
Purpura/bleeding diathesis	

and output and monitoring of electrolytes is essential. Fever, diminished intake, and vomiting may lead to significant dehydration and hypovolemia. Capillary leak secondary to sepsis can further add to hypovolemia. Diabetes insipidus may rapidly lead to hypovolemia and hypernatremia due to urinary free-water loss. The syndrome of inappropriate secretion of antidiuretic hormone may lead to free-water retention, hypo-osmolality, and hyponatremia. These conditions must be recognized early to ensure appropriate management.

Fluid restriction to two—thirds of normal maintenance has historically been practiced with the hope that it reduces cerebral edema, presumably aggravated by the syndrome of inappropriate secretion of antidiuretic hormone. However, it has been contended that a raised antidiuretic hormone level is an appropriate response to fluid deficit as it returns to normal on fluid administration. A prospective randomized trial of fluid restriction versus maintenance fluids with a clinical outcome (37) showed that restriction of fluids does not improve the outcome in children with meningitis. The increased fluid volume and mild systemic hypertension in children with meningitis may represent a compensatory mechanism to overcome raised ICP and to maintain adequate CBF and perfusion. Restriction of fluids and, thereby, extracellular volume may adversely affect cerebral perfusion and may worsen the outcome. Empiric fluid restriction in children with CNS infection is therefore not justified. A meta-analysis of fluid therapy trials found evidence to support the use of IV maintenance fluids in preference to restricted fluids in the first 48 hrs in settings with high mortality rates and in which patients present late, but it found insufficient evidence to guide practice when children present early and mortality rates are lower (25). Fluid therapy should be aimed at maintaining normovolemia and normal blood pressure, thereby maintaining adequate cerebral perfusion.

Careful monitoring of hydration status, intravascular volume, electrolytes, and osmolality should guide fluid management.

Hyponatremia should be identified early and corrected slowly over 36–48 hrs with normal saline or, occasionally, with 3% saline, after calculating the sodium deficit. It is important to prevent and/or treat hyponatremic seizures. Children with meningitis are also prone to develop hypokalemia due to gastrointestinal losses, hemodilution, osmotherapy, diuretic therapy, and associated septicemia.

BACTERIAL MENINGITIS

Etiology

Worldwide, three major meningeal pathogens (*Haemophilus influenzae*, *Neisseria meningitidis*, and *Streptococcus pneumoniae*) account for the majority of cases, but the proportion caused by each organism is somewhat variable by region and age.

Haemophilus spp. are small, Gram-negative, pleomorphic coccobacilli that are either encapsulated or unencapsulated. Encapsulated strains are classified into six types, designated *a* through *f*. Nearly all invasive *H. influenzae* infections are caused by serotype b (Hib). Hib strains have been further classified according to their outer membrane polysaccharides (omps), which are useful for epidemiologic studies. Presently, almost all invasive disease worldwide is caused by nine clones of Hib, although nontypeable *H. influenzae* may rarely cause meningitis.

Neisseria species are non–spore-forming, nonmotile, kidney-shaped, Gram-negative cocci that often appear in pairs (diplococci). Meningococci are classified by serogroups, which have important epidemiologic and prevention-related implications. Although 13 serogroups are recognized, most meningococcal disease is caused by organisms in serogroups A, B, C, Y, and W135. The virulence of meningococci is determined by their capsular polysaccharide, pili, immunoglobulin (Ig) A protease, lipopolysaccharide (endotoxin), omps, and outer membrane vesicles. All isolates from invasive infections are encapsulated (serogroup positive), whereas 20%–90% of those isolated from carriers are unencapsulated (nontypeable).

Pneumococci are non–spore-forming, nonmotile, small, Gram-positive streptococci that are generally seen in pairs or chains. They are classified into serotypes on the basis of antigenic differences among capsular polysaccharides, which are essential for pneumococcal virulence. Approximately 90 pneumococcal serotypes have been characterized; however, only some of these cause invasive pneumococcal infections. Capsular types 1, 4, 6, 9, 14, 18, 19, and 23 cause ~85% of serious infections in children, a pattern different from that observed in adults. The serotypes that cause meningitis have a strong correlation with those that cause pneumonia and bacteremia.

Gram-negative bacilli can also be implicated in meningitis. Most cases of neonatal meningitis and sepsis due to Gram-negative bacilli are caused by *Escherichia coli* strains that bear the K1 capsular polysaccharide antigen, a marker of neurovirulence. In addition to the K1 capsule, many other potential virulence factors for meningitis have been documented. Gram-negative bacterial meningitis in children beyond the neonatal period is generally nosocomial or may be associated with other conditions, such as gut infections, head trauma, neurosurgical procedures, and immunodeficiency. Other *Enterobacteriaceae* can cause meningitis, including *Klebsiella, Salmonella, Enterobacter,* and *Pseudomonas* spp.

Group B streptococci are the most common cause of invasive neonatal disease in many countries. They are classified into six main serotypes; type III is responsible for most cases of neonatal meningitis. A decrease in the incidence of neonatal invasive group B streptococcal disease has been seen in developed countries, secondary to treatment of pregnant women with vaginal colonization at the time of delivery.

Listeria monocytogenes is a Gram-positive, non–spore-forming, catalase-positive, aerobic rod. An important cause of neonatal meningitis, its source is generally the genital tract infection of the mother. However, nosocomial infection may also occur, particularly in low-birth-weight babies in long-term intensive care.

Staphylococci are Gram-positive organisms that are generally seen in pairs or clusters. *Staphylococcus aureus* is a virulent organism that is coagulase positive and causes pneumonia, sepsis, endocarditis, osteomyelitis, and meningitis. It is generally seen in malnourished children with staphylococcal skin lesions, dermal sinuses, or CSF shunts. Secondary meningitis may also be seen in children with head trauma, neurosurgical procedures, or sinusitis.

Anaerobic meningitis may occur in certain conditions, such as rupture of brain abscess; chronic otitis, mastoiditis, or sinusitis; head trauma; neurosurgical procedures; congenital dural defects; gastrointestinal disease; suppurative pharyngitis; CSF shunts; and immunosuppression. *Bacteroides fragilis, Fusobacterium* spp., and *Clostridium* spp. are anaerobic pathogens that may cause meningitis.

Epidemiology

Hib remains the leading cause of bacterial meningitis in countries where Hib vaccine has not been introduced, with endemic annual incidence rates as high as 100 per 100,000 (40). Approximately 80% of cases develop in unvaccinated children <2 years of age, and nearly all cases occur in children <5 years. Meningitis caused by Hib in the first 2 months of life is rare, presumably because of placental transfer of protective maternal bactericidal antibodies. Natural immunity develops after 3 years of age, and concentrations of polyribosylribitol phosphate antibodies reach adult values by 7 years of age (29). The two main factors that determine risk for disease are nasopharyngeal carriage and the concentration of circulating anticapsular antibody. High-risk factors for invasive Hib infection include sickle cell anemia, asplenia, CSF fistulas, and chronic pulmonary infections. If children >6 years have Hib meningitis, such underlying conditions as otitis media, sinusitis, CSF leaks, and immunodeficiency states, including splenectomy, should be excluded.

Meningococcal meningitis occurs primarily in children and young adults. A wide geographic variation exists between the serotypes of meningococci that are endemic and those that cause epidemics. In developed countries, most cases are due to serogroups B and C. However, serogroup A is responsible for large-scale epidemics in many developing countries, including Africa, India, Nepal, and Saudi Arabia. Age-specific incidence of meningococcal infection is inversely proportional to the

presence of serum bactericidal antibodies against serogroups A, B, and C. More than 50% of infants possess bactericidal antibody at birth as a result of transplacental transfer; hence, meningococcal meningitis is rarely seen in the first 3 months of life. An intact complement system is also an important host defense against invasive meningococcal disease. Recurrent or chronic neisserial infections have been associated with rare isolated deficiencies of late complement components (C5, C6, C7, or C8, and perhaps C9) due to the role of complement in opsonophagocytosis. Deficiency or dysfunction of properdin, which is a stabilizing factor of C3 convertase in the alternate complement pathway, also predisposes to meningococcal infections. The time from nasopharyngeal acquisition to bloodstream invasion is short (usually 10 days). The incubation period may also be short, because "secondary" cases commonly occur within 1–4 days of the index case.

Pneumococcal meningitis occurs in all age groups, but maximum incidence rates are seen at the extremes of age. The common predisposing factors include pneumonia, otitis media, sinusitis, CSF fistulas or leaks, head injury, sickle cell disease, and thalassemia major.

Enterobacteriaceae, group B streptococci, and *Listeria,* cause meningitis predominantly in neonates. *Enterobacteriaceae* are normal gut flora, 25% of women are colonized with group B streptococci in the developed world, and *Listeria monocytogenes* may infect or colonize the female gastrointestinal tract, predominantly in the developing world. Aspiration of contaminated secretions, pneumonia, and hematogenous seeding of the meninges result in early-onset meningitis incidence of ~10 per 100,000 (22).

Vaccines against Hib, *S. pneumoniae,* and *N. meningitidis* have decreased the disease burden by 99%, 94%, and 90%, respectively, in countries where vaccines are available. Due to the lack of vaccine availability worldwide, the global disease burden has been reduced by a mere 2%.

Pathogenesis

The development of childhood bacterial meningitis typically progresses through phases that include nasopharyngeal colonization and vascular invasion, meningeal invasion and multiplication in the subarachnoid space, induction and progression of inflammation in the subarachnoid space with associated pathophysiologic alterations, and damage to the CNS.

Nasopharyngeal Colonization and Vascular Invasion

Most organisms that cause bacterial meningitis are transmitted by the respiratory route. They colonize the nasopharyngeal mucosa by adherence to the mucosal epithelium and evasion of mucosal host defense mechanisms. Adherence is mediated through adhesins of the bacterial surface that help surface binding to epithelial cell receptors and differs in various organisms. In *N. meningitidis,* adherence depends on the binding of fimbriae on the bacterial cell wall, whereas in *S. pneumoniae,* it depends mainly on the cell wall components. Host secretory IgA antibodies inhibit adherence and penetration of pathogens. The organisms secrete highly specific endopeptidases that cleave the heavy chains of secretory IgA and impair specific mucosal immunity, allowing the organisms to colonize.

Infection of the nasopharyngeal cells causes injury to the ciliated epithelial cells of the respiratory tract, resulting in loss of protective ciliary activity. Bacteria penetrate the mucosal barrier either through transepithelial or paraepithelial means. A number of bacterial factors help the process of invasion, including pili and lipo-oligosaccharides on the outer membranes of *N. meningitidis* and *H. influenzae* and the binding of *S. pneumoniae* to the polymeric immunoglobulin receptors on the mucosa. Pneumolysin and hyaluronidase of the pneumococci also facilitate mucosal invasion.

To survive in the bloodstream, the pathogens must overcome the host defense systems of circulating antibodies, complement-mediated bacterial killing, and neutrophil phagocytosis. The bacterial polysaccharide capsule operates against these mechanisms. In the absence of specific anticapsular antibodies, nonspecific activation of the alternative complement pathway is the main host defense against encapsulated bacteria. Persons with impaired alternative complement pathways and asplenia are at particular risk for overwhelming sepsis and meningitis by these encapsulated bacteria.

Meningeal Invasion

The blood-brain barrier (BBB) normally protects against meningeal invasion. Penetration of BBB depends on various neurotropic and virulence factors, including capsule characteristics, fimbriae, surface proteins of bacteria, and, perhaps, a critical magnitude of bacteremia.

After penetrating the meninges, the bacteria multiply freely in the CSF, which has diminished host defense mechanisms. The bacterial capsular polysaccharides have high antiphagocytic properties, and the CSF has a very low concentration of specific antibody. The bacteria thus multiply rapidly and spread over the entire surface of the brain and spinal cord along penetrating vessels.

Inflammation of the Subarachnoid Space

The multiplication and autolysis of bacteria in the CSF lead to the release of bacterial components, including fragments of cell wall and lipopolysaccharide that trigger a strong inflammatory response in the subarachnoid space by inducing the production and release of inflammatory cytokines and chemokines. These cytokines can be produced by many brain cells including astrocytes, glia, endothelial cells, ependymal cells, and macrophages. Early-response cytokines include IL-1β, IL-6 and tumor necrosis factor (TNF), which then trigger a cascade of inflammatory mediators, including other interleukins, chemokines, platelet-activating factor, matrix metalloproteinases, nitric oxide (NO), and free oxygen radicals. Increase in cytokines enhances permeability of the BBB and recruits leukocytes from the blood into CSF, leading to CSF pleocytosis. These mediators also affect CBF and cerebral metabolism and contribute to the development of cerebral edema and neurologic sequelae.

Pathophysiology

Disruption of the Blood-Brain Barrier and Changes in Cerebral Blood Flow

Loss of autoregulation leads to changes in CBF, which increases in the early phase and decreases in the later phase of meningitis. The increase in CBF in early meningitis is secondary to the va-

sodilatory effect of NO. Later, the CBF progressively declines, most likely as a result of vasospasm. Loss of autoregulation also makes cerebral perfusion dependent on the systemic blood pressure, and the cerebral perfusion pressure drops when blood pressure drops.

In addition to the global cerebral hypoperfusion, focal hypoperfusion can occur due to vasculitis of large and small arteries crossing the inflamed subarachnoid space, which can cause ischemic damage that leads to permanent neurologic sequelae. Occlusion or severe stenosis of the intracranial internal carotid artery or of the middle and anterior cerebral arteries or involvement of the large vessels at the base of the brain can lead to stroke and result in paresis.

Neuropathology

Bacterial meningitis includes inflammation of the subarachnoid space, inflammatory involvement of the cerebral blood vessels, and parenchymal brain damage. Histologic examination reveals loss of neurons, generally focal, particularly in patients who have a late mortality. Cerebral edema in bacterial meningitis may be vasogenic, cytotoxic, or interstitial. Vasogenic cerebral edema occurs as a result of increased BBB permeability, which leads to extravasation of large molecules and serum into the brain parenchyma. Cytotoxic edema occurs because of an increase in intracellular water that is secondary to alterations of the cell membrane permeability and loss of cellular homeostasis, with influx of potassium and calcium into the cell. Interstitial edema occurs due to an increase in CSF volume, which may occur due to increased CSF production secondary to increased blood flow in the choroid plexus. Associated decrease resorption of the CSF may also occur because of increased outflow resistance across the arachnoid villi of the sagittal sinus. Interstitial edema is probably the main cause of obstructive hydrocephalus in meningitis. Severe brain edema can cause herniation of brain tissue and compression of the brainstem due to increased ICP. The ICP may also increase because of excessive intracerebral hypertension, including the development of obstructive hydrocephalus, cerebritis, cerebral infarction and cerebral venous thrombosis, SE, and syndrome of inappropriate secretion of antidiuretic hormone. Death from meningitis may occur because of critically raised ICP, extensive cerebral infarction, disseminated intravascular coagulation (DIC), and/or circulatory failure resulting from septic shock and refractory SE.

Clinical Presentation

The clinical presentation of meningitis is variable and is determined by the age of the child, the infecting organism, host resistance, and length of time between onset of illness and first evaluation by a physician. The onset is usually sudden but may occasionally be insidious.

The presentation in neonates and infants is generally nonspecific with fever, poor feeding, vomiting, lethargy, irritability, high-pitched cry, and seizures. Fever may be absent in very small infants and in severely malnourished babies. On examination, the anterior fontanel is full and often bulging and separation of sutures may be seen. The typical presentation in older children is with acute onset of fever, headache, vomiting, anorexia, photophobia, and altered sensorium. A history of preceding upper respiratory or gastrointestinal infection is often present. Children who are <3 years of age may not be able to complain of headache and may only present with irritability.

On examination, signs of meningeal irritation (stiffness and pain on flexion of the neck), a positive Kernig sign, and positive Brudzinski sign are seen. Older children may adopt a tripod posture with arms held back and straight on sitting surface. Meningeal signs are usually attenuated or absent in malnourished children, neonates, young infants, and deeply comatose children.

Seizures may be the presenting feature in almost 1 in 6 children with meningitis and may recur. Meningitis is a common cause of convulsive SE with fever, and the classic symptoms and signs of meningitis may be absent in such children. Children with fever and seizures should prompt a high index of suspicion for bacterial meningitis in. Raised ICP is common in bacterial meningitis. It often manifests with progressive impairment of sensorium with deepening coma, headache, vomiting, and Cushing triad (hyperventilation, hypertension, bradycardia). Papilledema is uncommon at presentation; if it is present, a CT scan must be obtained to exclude a mass lesion or a complication.

Focal signs are seen in ~14% cases and may be due to subdural collection, cortical infarction, or cerebritis. The progression of symptoms generally depends upon the pathogen. Most cases of *H. influenzae* and pneumococcal meningitis have an acute or subacute progression. Pneumococcal meningitis may start as nonspecific sepsis and progress to meningitis. A fulminant picture with manifestations of sepsis, shock, and rapid progression to death is characteristic for meningococcemia, a syndrome more distinct from meningococcal meningitis.

Associated findings vary according to the organism; patients with meningococcemia may present with a maculopapular rash, which rapidly progresses into a petechial rash. Rashes can occasionally be seen in *H. influenzae* or pneumococcal meningitis. The presence of a petechial rash is highly suggestive of meningococcemia. A child with meningitis should also be examined for other sites of infections, such as pneumonia, otitis media, endocarditis, sinusitis, pyoderma, or joint infections.

Differential Diagnosis

The clinical differential diagnosis in a child with meningitis depends mainly on the age of the child and the clinical syndrome at presentation. Meningitis in neonates and very young infants may present as nonspecific septicemia, without any symptoms and signs of CNS involvement. Lumbar puncture (LP) should be done in all such cases to exclude meningitis. In older infants, febrile seizures are the most important differential diagnosis. In the absence of meningeal signs, meningitis may be missed in these babies. LP should be done in all infants <6 months of age and in all children who present with febrile seizures, who have irritability and/or lethargy, or who look toxic. In children with acute onset fever and neck rigidity, the differential diagnosis includes aseptic meningitis, pneumonia, and other infections that may cause meningism, such as retropharyngeal abscess, typhoid fever, cervical lymphadenitis, and, rarely, spinal epidural abscess. A good physical examination and appropriate studies help in excluding most of these conditions. In children with a subacute onset of fever and neck rigidity, causes of chronic meningitis, such as tubercular, fungal, and para-

sitic infection, must be excluded. A predominantly encephalopathic presentation must be differentiated from encephalitis, Reye syndrome, metabolic problems, hepatic encephalopathy, intoxications, and other causes of coma. Cerebral malaria is an important differential diagnosis in developing countries, particularly in endemic regions. Its evaluation and treatment are discussed later. In children with raised ICP and focal signs, cerebral abscess, focal encephalitis, such as herpes, intracranial bleeds, and other space-occupying lesions must be excluded. Urgent neuroimaging is warranted in such cases.

Diagnosis

Early recognition of bacterial meningitis is important for optimal outcome. However, published data suggests that the diagnosis is often missed on initial evaluation. The World Health Organization (WHO) Integrated Management of Childhood Illness referral criteria for meningitis include lethargy, unconsciousness, inability to feed, stiff neck, and seizures. These were found to have a sensitivity of 98% and a specificity of 72% to predict meningitis.

Laboratory

Definitive diagnosis of meningitis is made by analysis and culture of the CSF. If there is a clinical suspicion of meningitis, an LP should be done at the earliest opportunity. Considerable controversy has arisen regarding the safety of the LP in children with CNS infections because of the risk of cerebral herniation following LP. However, a temporal relationship does not necessarily imply causality, and very sick children with meningitis may have herniation even if an LP is not performed. Delay in LP can delay the diagnosis of meningitis and thereby often delay administration of appropriate therapy. LP both provides confirmatory diagnosis and helps in organism identification, which is invaluable for selection of the most appropriate antibiotics, deciding the duration of therapy, and avoiding empiric antimicrobial therapy that most children with CNS infections would otherwise receive. It is recommended that LP be undertaken in all cases of suspected meningitis unless one of the following contraindications is present: raised ICP (unequal pupils, blood pressure/heart rate changes, abnormal respiratory pattern, deep coma/deteriorating consciousness), focal neurologic symptoms or signs (obtain a CT to exclude space-occupying lesion), shock/cardiorespiratory instability, thrombocytopenia (platelet count <40,000/mm³/coagulation disorder), or local infection at LP site.

Antibiotics should, however, be administered in all cases of suspected meningitis even if the LP is delayed. Delay in the administration of antibiotics is associated with increased mortality and morbidity in adults and children. Early antibiotic administration may decrease the yield on culture and Gram stain but does not significantly alter the cellular and biochemical parameters of the CSF.

Obtaining a CT scan before performing the LP is not routinely recommended. A proper history and clinical examination are sufficient in most cases to decide the safety of performing an LP. A CT scan should be obtained only in select cases in which focal neurologic symptoms or signs, clinical evidence of critically raised ICP, or papilledema are observed, or when doubt exists regarding the diagnosis and a mass lesion or a complication such as a brain abscess is suspected. CT is normal in most cases of bacterial meningitis, including those with subsequent herniation. It must be remembered that a normal CT does not rule out raised ICP.

The characteristic CSF findings in bacterial meningitis are increased opening pressure, polymorphonuclear pleocytosis, decreased glucose, and increased protein concentration. A cloudy CSF under pressure can be considered diagnostic of bacterial meningitis. Normal CSF in children has zero to five mononuclear cells/mm^3 (lymphocyte and monocytes); polymorphonuclear cells are very rarely seen. Presence of a single polymorphonuclear cell in the clinical setting of meningitis should be considered significant. In neonates, the upper limit of normal extends to a white blood cell (WBC) count of 20–30 WBC/mm^3, although the mean count is generally 5–10 WBC/mm^3. The CSF glucose is <40 mg/dL in 50%–60% cases. A ratio of serum to blood glucose of <0.4 was 80% sensitive and 98% specific for diagnosis of bacterial meningitis in children >2 months of age; in term neonates, a ratio of <0.6 is considered abnormal. The CSF may occasionally be completely normal in early stages of bacterial meningitis; a repeat LP after a few hours may show abnormalities. Antibiotic therapy must therefore be started in all cases with a strong suspicion of bacterial meningitis.

The LP may occasionally be traumatic; a grossly traumatic CSF can be used for culture alone. With less traumatic LPs, prediction of meningitis can often be made. A predicted CSF white cell count is calculated using the formula:

$$CSF WBC (predicted) = CSF red blood cell (RBC)$$
$$\times (blood WBC / blood RBC)$$

The observed WBC count divided by the predicted WBC gives the observed-to-predicted ratio. The specificity and positive predictive value of an observed-to-predicted ratio of ≤0.01 and a WBC:RBC ratio of ≤0.01 were 100% reliable (95% confidence interval, 74–100 and 91–100, respectively) in predicting the absence of disease.

The Gram stain is a quick, inexpensive, accurate method for organism identification. The positivity of the Gram stain depends on the number of organisms in the CSF. The lower limit for detection is ~10^5 colony-forming units/mL of CSF, which corresponds to a positive smear in 70%–80% of cases of untreated bacterial meningitis. In case of a clear CSF, smears for Gram stain should be obtained from centrifuged sediment, whereas the fresh, uncentrifuged specimen can be used if the CSF is cloudy. The likelihood of having a positive Gram stain also depends on the specific bacterial pathogen: 90% of cases caused by *S. pneumoniae*, 86% by *H. influenzae*, 75% by *N. meningitides*, 50% by Gram-negative bacilli, and approximately one-third of cases caused by *L. monocytogenes* have positive Gram-stain results. False-positive Gram stain may rarely result from observer misinterpretation, or reagent or skin flora contamination.

Acridine orange stain is a fluorochrome that stains the nucleic acid of some bacteria so that they appear bright red orange when seen under a fluorescent microscope. It stains the intracellular bacteria better than the Gram stain and may be positive even when the Gram stain is negative.

CSF culture is positive in the majority of untreated cases of meningitis. Ideally, freshly obtained CSF should be directly plated, and enriched thioglycolate media should be used. The yield is poor in developing countries because of pretreatment with antibiotics, delayed plating, and inadequate storage and transport. Blood culture, pleural fluid, and aspiration of other

sterile sites (e.g., petechiae in suspected meningococcemia) can be helpful.

It has been suggested that in the absence of other tests, empiric diagnosis of bacterial meningitis can be made if the CSF shows cells >300/mm^3 with polymorphs >60% and sugar <50% of the blood level, or an absolute value of <30 mg/dL. This method has a sensitivity of 80% and specificity of 56%. The presence of a polymorphic response with hypoglycorrhachia in an acutely sick and toxic-looking child favors the diagnosis of bacterial meningitis. Most cases of viral meningitis have a lymphocytic response; in some cases, however, an initial polymorphic response may occur. The CSF sugar is generally normal; occasionally, it may be low but is rarely below 30 mg/dL. On the other hand, ~10% of cases with bacterial infection have an initial lymphocytic predominance. Other clinical parameters, such as a viral prodrome (with the child not looking very toxic), a rash, lymph node, or parotid gland enlargement, may favor the diagnosis of viral meningitis. Although tubercular meningitis may occasionally have an acute presentation, generally the symptoms are more prolonged; evidence of tuberculosis (TB) elsewhere in the body, such as lungs, abdomen, and fundus for choroid tubercles, should be investigated.

It is not always possible in children to differentiate between viral and bacterial meningitis based on clinical symptoms or even after blood or CSF analysis using routine investigations. Rules for clinical decision-making that are based on certain clinical and laboratory parameters have been devised for this purpose, and some of them have been found to be 100% sensitive and reasonably specific. However, such rules should only be applied after a complete validation process, on patients with the same characteristics as those used for their derivation and validation and, importantly, should not replace the clinician's skill (10). Rapid diagnostic tests that detect the pathogen by counter-current immunoelectrophoresis, enzyme-linked immunosorbent assay (ELISA), and latex agglutination are useful in providing early diagnosis in such cases, as well as in suspected cases of partially treated bacterial meningitis. The latex agglutination test is more sensitive than counter-current immunoelectrophoresis. The latex agglutination test for *S. pneumoniae* and *N. meningitidis* has a specificity of 96% and 100%, respectively, but has a lower sensitivity, varying from 69% to 100% for *S. pneumoniae* and from 37% to 70% for *N. meningitidis*. However, a negative bacterial antigen test result does not exclude infection caused by a specific meningeal pathogen.

PCR assays detect the nucleic acids of the common organisms that cause meningitis and are very specific. A PCR sensitivity and specificity of over 90% has been shown for patients with suspected meningococcal disease. The DNA load in PCR has also been correlated with the incidence of mortality in patients with meningococcal disease. PCR for pneumococcus is sensitive and specific in the CSF; however, in blood, it may be false positive because of nasopharyngeal carriage. Broad-range bacterial PCRs that can rapidly detect a number of viable and nonviable organisms have shown a sensitivity of 100%, a specificity of 98.2%, a positive predictive value of 98.2%, and a negative predictive value of 100%. These can therefore be used for screening; a subsequent PCR would be needed to identify the specific bacteria. These tests are expensive and not easily available in most developing countries. They are generally used to differentiate partially treated bacterial meningitis from viral meningitis when the Gram stain is negative. To prove tubercular, herpetic, or cryptococcal infection, special staining techniques/tests may be required.

Serum and CSF CRP levels can help in discriminating between bacterial and viral meningitis with high probability and in making a diagnosis of bacterial meningitis in children with fever without focus. However, diagnostic value of serum CRP was not perfectly discriminant in several studies. Raised serum CRP >50 mg/L is a nonspecific indicator of bacterial infection; it falls to normal after 1–2 days of antibiotic therapy. In the presence of CSF pleocytosis, elevated serum CRP levels of >20 mg/L in children <6 years of age and >50 mg/L in older children have a high sensitivity and specificity in distinguishing bacterial from viral meningitis. A CRP level of <40 mg/L may be found in bacterial meningitis; however, in the presence of a normal serum CRP level of <10 mg/L, the diagnosis of bacterial meningitis is highly unlikely. An elevated peripheral WBC count is suggestive of infection but may not be seen in all cases of meningitis and is, therefore, a poorly discriminating criterion for deciding on the need for LP in a sick child. CSF cytokines are highly sensitive and specific markers of bacterial infection. Increased CSF levels of lactate, Limulus amebocyte lysate, procalcitonin, and various cytokines have been reported in bacterial meningitis but have not been substantiated in multiple studies or standardized; determination of these levels is not routinely done for diagnosis of meningitis.

Complications

Several complications may occur with meningitis, either as an acute, early, often reversible phenomenon or as late events that generally result in permanent sequelae. Common complications are listed in **Table 80.3**.

Raised ICP is present at the time of admission in most patients hospitalized for bacterial meningitis and must be managed aggressively. In a 2004 study, almost half of the children with meningitis who required PICU care had raised ICP. Signs of raised ICP were seen either at admission or developed within 48 hrs of admission (35). The increase in ICP is associated with deepening coma and pupillary, respiratory, and blood pressure changes. Cerebral herniation was seen on autopsy in 30% of children dying of meningitis. Children with Glasgow Coma Scale score of <7 have high incidence of raised ICP.

Seizures, which often occur in the first 2–3 days and cease within 1–3 days, are due to cortical irritation secondary to the inflammatory process and fever and, at times, because of electrolyte disturbances. If an EEG performed at the end of

TABLE 80.3

COMPLICATIONS OF BACTERIAL MENINGITIS

Raised ICP
Seizures
Subdural empyema
Infarcts
Cerebritis
Hydrocephalous
Cranial nerve involvement
Brain abscess
Sensorineural deafness
DIC

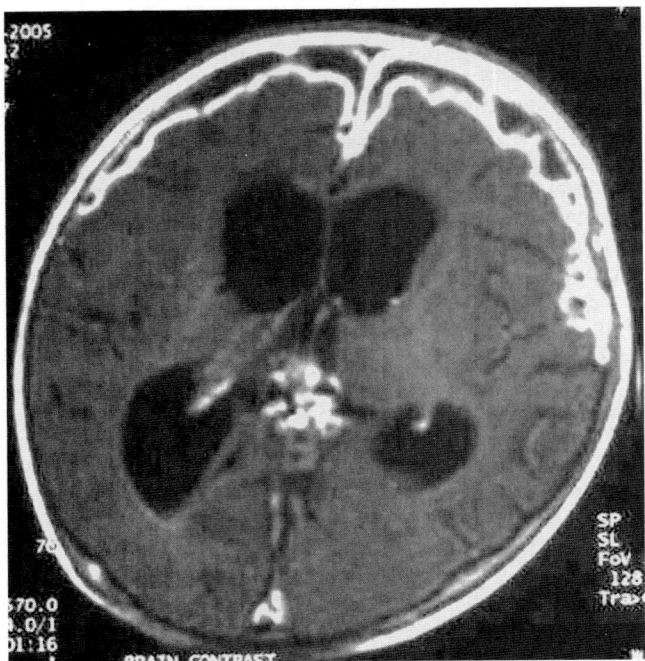

FIGURE 80.1. Contrast MRI showing subdural collections along frontal, parietal convexities and along interhemispheric fissure, with enhancement of dura and parenchymal surface suggestive of subdural empyema.

antibiotic therapy is normal, the anticonvulsant therapy can be gradually withdrawn. However, if seizure onset is later in the course of illness and is associated with underlying structural damage (e.g., an infarct), anticonvulsant therapy may be required for a longer period.

Subdural effusions are a common complication of meningitis, particularly in Hib meningitis, and may occur in almost half of cases. They are often benign, resolve spontaneously, and do not require any intervention. However, in a child with subdural effusion and persistent or recurrent fever, associated raised ICP, focal signs, or the presence of subdural empyema (**Fig. 80.1**), a subdural tap is indicated. Subdural effusion was found in 25% of patients; only 6 of 22 required drainage for raised ICP (35).

Cerebritis and infarction present with new focal features and occur because of involvement of the blood vessels in the inflammatory exudate or direct spread of infection from the subarachnoid space to the brain. Cerebritis and infarction may progress to form a cerebral abscess and are associated with a poor outcome.

Ventriculitis, which may occur, particularly in neonates and infants, presents with persistent fever and is diagnosed by CT and ventricular tap. Prolonged systemic antibiotic therapy is necessary in such cases. Drainage of CSF and/or intraventricular administration of antibiotics may also be required. Cranial nerve involvement may occur directly or secondary to raised ICP; the third, sixth, and eighth nerves are commonly involved. Sensorineural deafness occurs in 5%–30% cases, especially with pneumococcal meningitis, because of bacterial involvement of the cochlea through the internal auditory canal or via hematogenous spread. It may be transient or permanent and is associated with low CSF glucose and use of ototoxic antibiotics. Abnormalities in the brainstem-evoked responses occur within days and generally recover at the end of the first 2 weeks, although major deficits may persist. Hearing (brainstem-evoked responses or audiometry) must be formally assessed at the time of discharge.

DIC may occur with fulminant meningococcal and Gram-negative infections and requires aggressive therapy. Spread of infection leading to pneumonia, pericarditis, arthritis, and osteomyelitis rarely occurs.

Neuroimaging

The diagnosis of meningitis is made by clinical presentation and CSF analysis. In the early stages of meningitis, a CT scan is often normal. Later, CT may show meningeal enhancement and widening of basal cisterns. However, these findings do not affect therapeutic decisions. A CT scan at presentation is necessary to exclude other pathologies in a child with focal neurologic signs. Later in the illness, CT scan is performed to look for complications if a child does not show clinical improvement or has sudden unexplained deterioration, new-onset seizures or focal neurologic signs, signs of raised ICP, persistent fever, or enlarging head. Routine ultrasound of the head in infants with open fontanel has been found to detect most complications early.

Treatment

If bacterial meningitis is suspected, treatment should be instituted without delay. CSF, blood, and pertinent cultures should ideally be taken before starting antibiotics, but if specimens are difficult to obtain, therapy should be started and specimens obtained later. Most deaths because of bacterial meningitis occur during the first 48 hrs of hospitalization. Coma, raised ICP, seizures, and shock have been identified as significant predictors of death and morbidity. In a study from India, 40% of children with bacterial meningitis required admission to the PICU for one or more indications (35). All children with suspected bacterial meningitis must be kept under vigilant observation and monitoring so that complications (e.g., shock or raised ICP) can be recognized and managed early.

Initial empiric antibiotic therapy should be broad enough to cover all of the likely organisms according to the age of the child and the predisposing condition, and it should be based on sound knowledge of epidemiologic patterns of organisms and resistance patterns. Bactericidal antibiotics are preferred, as they cause more effective sterilization of CSF and improve survival in comparison to bacteriostatic drugs. Targeted antimicrobial therapy is based on organism identification by Gram stain and confirmation on culture. The Infectious Disease Society of America guidelines for empirical and specific antimicrobial therapy and the recommended dosages of the antimicrobials are shown in **Tables 80.4, 80.5,** and **80.6** (44).

In the US and other countries where pneumococci resistant to third-generation cephalosporins have emerged, vancomycin is added to the initial empiric regimen. The antimicrobials are given IV; if IV access cannot be secured, intramuscular administration is an acceptable alternative until IV access can be secured. In developing countries, a combination of ampicillin

---

TABLE 80.4

RECOMMENDATION FOR EMPIRICAL ANTIMICROBIAL THERAPY FOR PURULENT MENINGITIS BASED ON PATIENT AGE AND SPECIFIC PREDISPOSING CONDITION

Predisposing factor	Common bacterial pathogens	Antimicrobial therapy
Age \<1 month	*Streptococcus agalactiae, Escherichia coli, Listeria monocytogenes, Klebsiella* spp.	Ampicillin plus cefotaxime or ampicillin plus an aminoglycoside
1–23 months	*S. pneumoniae, N. meningitidis, S. agalactiae, H. influenzae, E. coli*	Vancomycin plus a third-generation cephalosporin[a,b]
2–50 years	*N. meningitidis, S. pneumoniae*	Vancomycin plus a third-generation cephalosporin[a,b]
\>50 years	*S. pneumoniae, N. meningitides, L. monocytogenes;* aerobic Gram-negative bacilli	Vancomycin plus ampicillin plus a third-generation cephalosporin[a,b]
Head trauma Basilar skull fracture	*S. pneumoniae, H. influenzae,* group A β–hemolytic streptococci	Vancomycin plus a third-generation cephalosporin[a]
Penetrating trauma	*S. aureus,* coagulase-negative staphylococci (especially *S. epidermidis*), aerobic Gram-negative bacilli (including *P. aeruginosa*)	Vancomycin plus cefepime, vancomycin plus ceftazidime, or vancomycin plus meropenem
Post-neurosurgery	Aerobic Gram-negative bacilli (including *P. aeruginosa*), *S. aureus,* coagulase-negative staphylococci (especially *S. epidermidis*)	Vancomycin plus cefepime, vancomycin plus ceftazidime, or vancomycin plus meropenem
CSF shunt	Coagulase-negative staphylococci (especially dermidis), *S. aureus,* aerobic Gram-negative bacilli (including *P. aeruginosa*), *Propionibacterium acnes*	Vancomycin plus cefepime[c], vancomycin plus ceftazidime[c], or vancomycin plus meropenem[c]

[a]Ceftriaxone or cefotaxime.
[b]Some experts would add rifampin if dexamethasone is also given.
[c]In infants and children, vancomycin alone is reasonable unless Gram stains reveal the presence of Gram-negative bacilli.
From Tunkel AR, Hartman BJ, Kaplan SL, et al. Practice guidelines for the management of bacterial meningitis. *Clin Infect Dis* 2004;39:1267–84, with permission.

TABLE 80.5

RECOMMENDATION FOR SPECIFIC ANTIMICROBIAL THERAPY IN BACTERIAL MENINGITIS BASED ON ISOLATED PATHOGEN AND SUSCEPTIBILITY TESTING

Microorganism; susceptibility	Standard therapy	Alternative therapies
Streptococcus pneumoniae Penicillin MIC	Penicillin G or ampicillin	Third-generation cephalosporin[a], chloramphenicol
<0.1 mcg/mL		
0.1–1.0 mcg/mL[b]	Third-generation cephalosporin[a]	Cefepime (B-II), meropenem (B-II)
≥2.0 mcg/mL	Vancomycin plus a third-generation cephalosporin[a,c]	Fluoroquinolone[d] (B-II)
Cefotaxime or ceftriaxone MIC ≥1.0 mcg/mL	Vancomycin plus a third-generation cephalosporin[a,c]	Fluoroquinolone[d] (B-II)
Neisseria meningitis; Penicillin MIC	Penicillin G or ampicillin	Third-generation cephalosporin[a], chloramphenicol
<0.1 mcg/mL		
0.1–1.0 mcg/mL	Third-generation cephalosporin[a]	Chloramphenicol, fluoroquinolone, meropenem
Listeria monocytogenes	Ampicillin or penicillin G[e]	Trimethoprim-sulfamethoxazole, meropenem (B-III)
Streptococcus agalactiae	Ampicillin or penicillin G[e]	Third-generation cephalosporin[a] (B-III)
Escherichia coli and other Enterobacteriaceae[g]	Third-generation cephalosporin (A-II)	Aztreonam, fluoroquinolone, meropenem, trimethoprim-sulfamethoxazole, ampicillin
Pseudomonas aeruginosa[g]	Cefepime[e] or ceftazidime[e] (A-II)	Aztreonam[e] ciprofloxacin[e] meropenem[e]
Haemophilus influenzae; β-Lactamase-negative	Ampicillin	Third-generation cephalosporin[a], cefepime, chloramphenicol, fluoroquinolone
β-Lactamase-positive	Third-generation Cephalosporin (A-I)	Cefepime (A-I), chloramphenicol, fluoroquinolone
Staphylococcus aureus; Methicillin-susceptible	Nafcillin or oxacillin	Vancomycin, meropenem (B-III)
Methicillin-resistant	Vancomycin[f]	Trimethoprim-sulfamethoxazole, linezolid (B-III)
Staphylococcus epidermidis	Vancomycin[f]	Linezolid (B-III)
Enterococcus spp.; Ampicillin-susceptible	Ampicillin plus gentamicin	—
Ampicillin-resistant	Vancomycin plus gentamicin	—
Ampicillin- and vancomycin-resistant	Linezolid (B-III)	—

All recommendations are A-III, unless otherwise indicated.
[a]Ceftriaxone or cefotaxime.
[b]Ceftriaxone, cefotaxime-susceptible isolates.
[c]Consider addition of rifampin if the MIC of ceftriaxone is >2 mcg/mL.
[d]Gatifloxacin or moxifloxacin.
[e]Addition of an aminoglycoside should be considered.
[f]Consider addition of rifampin.
[g]Choice of a specific antimicrobial agent must be guided by in vitro susceptibility test results. MIC, minimal inhibitory concentration.
From Tunkel AR, Hartman BJ, Kaplan SL, et al. Practice guidelines for the management of bacterial meningitis. *Clin Infect Dis* 2004;39:1267–84, with permission.

and chloramphenicol may be used if financial constraints prevent the use of cephalosporins (27). However, increasing resistance of *H. influenzae* to ampicillin and chloramphenicol, and of pneumococci to penicillin and chloramphenicol, is being reported from Africa and Asia. The mechanism of resistance varies in pathogens; resistance of *H. influenzae* to ampicillin is mediated by a β-lactamase in most cases; therefore, a combination of a β-lactam with a β-lactamase inhibitor may be effective. On the other hand, such a combination would not be effective in pneumococci and meningococci, in which most of the resistance is mediated by change in penicillin binding proteins.

Meropenems and newer fluoroquinolones, such as gatifloxacin, moxifloxacin, and trovafloxacin, have been found

to be as effective as cephalosporins for treatment of bacterial meningitis; however, they are not included as first choice in standard recommendations. Meropenem may be useful in patients with meningitis caused by resistant Gram-negative bacilli that produce extended-spectrum β-lactamases.

The duration of antibiotic therapy depends on the organism isolated. The standard recommendation has been 7 days for *N. meningitides* and *H. influenzae*, 10–14 days for *S. pneumoniae*, and a minimum of 3 weeks for Gram-negative, group B streptococcus, and *Listeria* meningitis. Shorter durations of ceftriaxone have been found effective in children >3 months of age with uncomplicated meningitis; however, these are not yet accepted as standard recommendations.

TABLE 80.6

RECOMMENDED DOSAGES OF ANTIMICROBIAL THERAPY IN PATIENTS WITH BACTERIAL MENINGITIS (A-III)

	Total daily dose (dosing interval in hours)			
	Neonates, age in days			
Antimicrobial agent	0–7[a]	8–28[a]	Infants and children	Adults
Amikacin[b]	15–20 mg/kg (12)	30 mg/kg (8)	20–30 mg/kg (8)	15 mg/kg (8)
Ampicillin	150 mg/kg (8)	200 mg/kg (6–8)	300 mg/kg (6)	12 g (4)
Aztreonam	—	—	—	6–8 g (6–8)
Cefepime	—	—	150 mg/kg (8)	6 g (8)
Cefotaxime	100–150 mg/kg (8–12)	150–200 mg/kg (6–8)	225–300 mg/kg (6–8)	8–12 g (4–6)
Ceftazidime	100–150 mg/kg (8–12)	150 mg/kg (8)	150 mg/kg (8)	6 g (8)
Ceftriaxone	—	—	80–100 mg/kg (12–24)	4 g (12–24)
Chloramphenicol	25 mg/kg (24)	50 mg/kg (12–24)	75–100 mg/kg (6)	4–6 g (6)[c]
Ciprofloxacin	—	—	—	800–1200 mg (8–12)
Gatifloxacin	—	—	—	400 mg (24)[c]
Gentamicin[b]	5 mg/kg (12)	7.5 mg/kg (8)	7.5 mg/kg (8)	5 mg/kg (8)
Meropenem	—	—	120 mg/kg (8)	6g (8)
Moxifloxacin	—	—	—	400 mg (24)[d]
Nafcillin	75 mg/kg (8–12)	100–150 mg/kg (6–8)	200 mg/kg (6)	9–12 g (4)
Oxacillin	75 mg/kg (8–12)	150–200mg/kg (6–8)	200 mg/kg (6)	9–12 g (4)
Penicillin G	0.15 mU/kg (8–12)	0.2 mU/kg (6–8)	0.3 mU/kg (4–6)	24 mU (4)
Rifampin	—	10–20 mg/kg (12)	10–20 mg/kg (12–24)[e]	600 mg (24)
Tobramycin[b]	5 mg/kg (12)	7.5 mg/kg (8)	7.5 mg/kg (8)	5 mg/kg (8)
TMP-SMZ[f]	—	—	10–20 mg/kg (6–12)	10–20 mg/kg (6–12)
Vancomycin[g]	20–30 mg/kg (8–12)	30–45 mg/kg (6–8)	60 mg/kg (6)	30–45 mg/kg (8–12)

[a]Smaller doses and longer intervals of administration may be advisable for very low-birth weight neonates (<2000 g).
[b]Peak and trough serum concentrations must be monitored.
[c]Higher dose recommended for patients with pneumococcal meningitis.
[d]No data on optimal dosage required in patients with bacterial meningitis.
[e]Maximum daily dose of 600 mg.
[f]Dosage based on trimethoprim component.
[g]Maintain serum, though concentrations of 15–20 mcg/mL. TMP-SMZ. trimethoprim-sulfamethoxazole.
From Tunkel AR, Hartman BJ, Kaplan SL, et al. Practice guidelines for the management of bacterial meningitis. *Clin Infect Dis* 2004;39:1267–84, with permission.

With appropriate antibiotic therapy, the CSF culture and Gram stain become negative within 24–48 hrs. The CSF glucose generally normalizes over 72 hrs. The increase in cells and proteins may persist for several days. Fever generally decreases within a week, although it may last for up to 10 days in uncomplicated *H. influenzae* meningitis. Fever that persists for >10 days is considered "persistent," and fever that recurs after 24 hrs of an afebrile period is considered "recurrent." Persistent fever may be due to thrombophlebitis, spread of infection (e.g., arthritis), occurrence of complications (e.g., subdural empyema, cerebritis, or ventriculitis), intercurrent viral infections, and, rarely, drug fever. Secondary fever is most often due to nosocomial infections or complications.

A repeat LP during treatment and at the end of therapy is not routinely necessary if the child has improved and is afebrile. Test-of-cure LP is recommended in neonates with Gram-negative meningitis.

Indications for repeat LP on appropriate antibiotic therapy are as follows: lack of clinical improvement after 3–4 days, appearance of new symptoms or signs, initial CSF grows resistant/unusual organisms and no clinical improvement occurs within 24–48 hrs of specific therapy, and Gram-negative meningitis in a neonate.

The inflammatory cascade in patients with bacterial meningitis can lead to tissue damage and worsen the neurologic sequelae. It is believed that antibiotic therapy exaggerates the inflammatory response by causing bacterial lysis and endotoxin release. Steroid therapy has been shown to reduce indices of inflammation, including cerebral edema, elevated ICP, and CSF outflow obstruction in experimental meningitis. A systematic review has shown that dexamethasone, if given prior to or with the first dose of antibiotic therapy, has beneficial effects in patients with meningitis due to *H influenzae* and pneumococci (46). The American Academy of Pediatrics recommends the use of dexamethasone in *H. influenzae* meningitis. A dose of 0.4 mg/kg, 12 hourly for 2 days, has been found to be as effective as 0.15 mg/kg/dose, 6 hourly for 4 days. However, in developing countries, most children receive antibiotics before a diagnosis of meningitis is made, and corticosteroid administration before or with the first dose of antibiotics is rarely possible. As dexamethasone may mask the presentation of underlying infections (e.g., brain abscess, tubercular meningitis, or meningitis due to resistant bacteria), delaying their diagnosis and treatment, routine administration of steroids cannot be recommended in developing countries. Benefit of steroids has not been established in neonatal meningitis.

Several nonsteroidal anti-inflammatory agents have shown beneficial effects in experimental meningitis. Indomethacin inhibits prostaglandin synthesis by inhibition of cyclooxygenase and has been shown to reduce indices of inflammation and cerebral hyperemia in early phases of meningitis. Pentoxifylline, a methylxanthine phosphodiesterase inhibitor, has several anti-inflammatory properties and has been shown to reduce TNF-α production and indices of CSF inflammation. Platelet activating factor inhibitors have shown to reduce cerebral edema in experimental pneumococcal meningitis. Recombinant bactericidal permeability-increasing protein and recombinant protein C may help to reduce severity of sepsis but have poor penetration in CSF and, as such, are unlikely to reduce meningeal inflammation.

The use of human IV immunoglobulin is particularly important for children who have immunoglobulin deficiencies and for neonates who have a limited immunologic response, such as those with group B streptococcus meningitis. Monoclonal antibodies directed at the molecules responsible for leukocyte-endothelial adhesion can be used to reduce CSF leukocytosis and other indices of CSF inflammation.

Prognosis

The mortality rates of meningitis continue to be as high as 15%–20%. Neurologic sequelae are common and include hydrocephalous, spasticity, visual and hearing loss, cognitive deficits, and developmental delay. High serum cortisol levels (420 ng/mL) and high systolic blood pressure were found to be significant predictors of neurologic and hearing sequelae (38). Coma, raised ICP, SE, shock, and respiratory depression are important predictors of morbidity and mortality in children with acute bacterial meningitis (35). Early recognition and prompt management of these factors, preferably in an intensive care setting, are important. Delay in diagnosis is an avoidable adverse prognostic factor.

Prevention

Isolation of children with meningitis caused by *H. influenzae* or *N. meningitidis* until they have received effective antimicrobial therapy for 24 hrs is recommended to prevent spread of infection. For *H. influenzae* meningitis, rifampin prophylaxis (20 mg/kg once daily for 4 days) is recommended for all household contacts if at least one unvaccinated contact is <4 years old; rifampin prophylaxis for the index case is not needed if ceftriaxone was used but is needed if ampicillin and/or chloramphenicol were used, as they do not eradicate *H. influenzae*.

In treating meningococcal disease, rifampin prophylaxis (10 mg/kg, 12 hourly for 2 days) is recommended for household and daycare contacts to prevent secondary cases and to reduce nasopharyngeal carriage. A single intramuscular dose of ceftriaxone (125 mg for children <12 yrs and 250 mg for older children and adults) has been found to be better than oral rifampin for eliminating meningococcal group A nasopharyngeal carriage. A single oral dose of 500 mg of ciprofloxacin or 500 mg of azithromycin may be used for adults.

Universal immunization against *H. influenzae* has virtually wiped out *H. influenzae* meningitis from developed countries; however, this protocol must still be implemented in many developing countries. Conjugate vaccines for pneumococci and meningococci used for mass immunization in some countries have been shown to reduce disease prevalence dramatically.

Until such time that a similar situation becomes feasible, they could be used in special high-risk situations in developing countries. Universal efforts at introducing mass immunization programs against the common pathogens that cause meningitis in resource-poor countries is the way to prevent this deadly disease.

ASEPTIC MENINGITIS

Aseptic meningitis is a clinical syndrome of meningeal inflammation in which common bacterial agents cannot be identified in the CSF. In general, aseptic meningitis is characterized by a benign clinical course and a lack of long-term sequelae; however, some cases may be associated significant morbidity.

Etiology

Although most cases of aseptic meningitis are caused by viral infections, some may be caused by nonviral pathogens, including fungi, some unusual bacteria and mycoplasma, autoimmune diseases, malignancies, and drug reactions. The majority of organisms that can cause meningitis can also penetrate into the brain parenchyma and cause encephalitis (**Table 80.7**). In the past, aseptic meningitis was commonly seen with mumps virus, lymphocytic choriomeningitis virus, and poliovirus. These are uncommon causes in developed countries today, but continue to be important causes in many developing countries. Enteroviruses are the most common etiologic agents for aseptic meningitis in both the developing and developed world, but will not be discussed in this chapter because of the relatively benign course in an immunocompetent individual. Other viruses, including arboviruses, herpesviruses, paramyxoviruses, and orthomyxoviruses, will be discussed in more detail in the following encephalitis section. Tuberculous meningitis, although grouped under aseptic meningitis by some, actually has an entirely different clinical presentation, pathogenesis, and outcome and will be discussed separately.

TUBERCULAR MENINGITIS

Tubercular meningitis (TBM) is the most serious complication of TB, especially in children. It is fatal without effective treatment and is associated with significant morbidity even with treatment. CNS TB may take a number of forms, including TBM, tuberculomas, tubercular abscesses, and, rarely, myeloradiculopathy. TBM is the most common.

Etiology

TBM is caused by *Mycobacterium tuberculosis*; meningitis due to *M. bovis* or atypical mycobacteria, such as *M. avium-intracellulare*, is extremely rare in children.

Epidemiology

A resurgence of TB is being seen both in developing countries and in developed countries due to the association with human

TABLE 80.7

COMMON INFECTIOUS CAUSES OF ASEPTIC MENINGOENCEPHALITIS

| Organism | Disease | | | Diagnosis | | |
| | Infectious | | Postinfectious | Culture | PCR | Serology |
	Parenchyma	Meninges				
Virus						
Adenoviruses	+	+		Y		Y
Arboviruses	++	+				Y
Enteroviruses	+++	++++	+	Y	Y	
Herpesviruses	+++	+	+	Y	Y	Y
Human immunodeficiency viruses	+	+		Y	Y	Y
Influenza A and B viruses	++	+		Y	Y	
Japanese encephalitis virus	++	+	+			Y
Lymphocytic choriomeningitis virus	+	+				Y
Measles	+	+	+	Y		Y
Mumps	++	+	+	Y		Y
Rubella	+	+	+	Y		Y
Rabies	+	+		Y		
Bacteria						
Bartonella henselae	+	+		Y	Y	Y
Bordetella pertussis	+	+		Y	Y	Y
Borrelia burgdorferi (Lyme disease)	++	+			Y	Y
Brucella spp.	+	+		Y		Y
Chlamydia spp.	+	+		Y	Y	Y
Ehrlichia spp.	+	+			Y	Y
Leptospira spp.	++	+		Y	Y	Y
Mycobacteria spp.	++	+		Y	Y	
Mycoplasma spp.	++	+	+	Y	Y	Y
Rickettsia spp.	++	+				Y
Treponema pallidum	++	+			Y	Y
Fungi						
Aspergillus fumigatus	+	+		Y	Y	Y
Blastomyces dermatitidis	+	+		Y		Y
Candida spp.	+	++		Y		
Cryptococcus neoformans	+	+		Y		Y
Coccidioides immitis	+	+		Y		Y
Histoplasma capsulatum	+	+		Y		Y
Others						
Toxoplasma gondii	+	+			Y	Y
Entamoeba histolytica	+	+			Y	Y
Acanthamoeba	+	+		Y		Y
Trichinella	+	+				Y
Naegleria	+	+		Y		

Y, yes; + denotes relative frequency of involvement

immunodeficiency virus (HIV) infection. In addition, multidrug resistance is increasingly common. With estimates of 2 billion (one-third of the world's population) infected, 10% are expected to progress to a diseased state (24). Children, with their relatively compromised cell-mediated immunity, suffer, with TBM annual incidence rates as high as 32/100,000.

Pathogenesis

Involvement of the CNS mostly occurs during a primary infection in children, whereas in adults, it may occur during reactivation. Tubercular meningitis usually results from the hematoge-nous spread of bacteria to the CNS from a primary focus elsewhere in the body, usually the lungs. A caseous lesion forms in the cerebral cortex or meninges, increases in size, ruptures, and discharges tubercle bacilli into the subarachnoid space, leading to the formation of a thick gelatinous exudate that infiltrates the corticomeningeal blood vessels and causing inflammation and obstruction of vessels and subsequent infarction of the cerebral cortex. The brainstem and various cranial nerves, particularly nerves III, VI, and VII, are surrounded by the exudates (**Fig, 80.2B**). The exudate accumulates mostly at the base of the brain and interferes with the normal flow of CSF, leading to hydrocephalus. Vasculitis (**Fig. 80.2D**), infarction, and hydrocephalus result in severe brain damage. Occasionally,

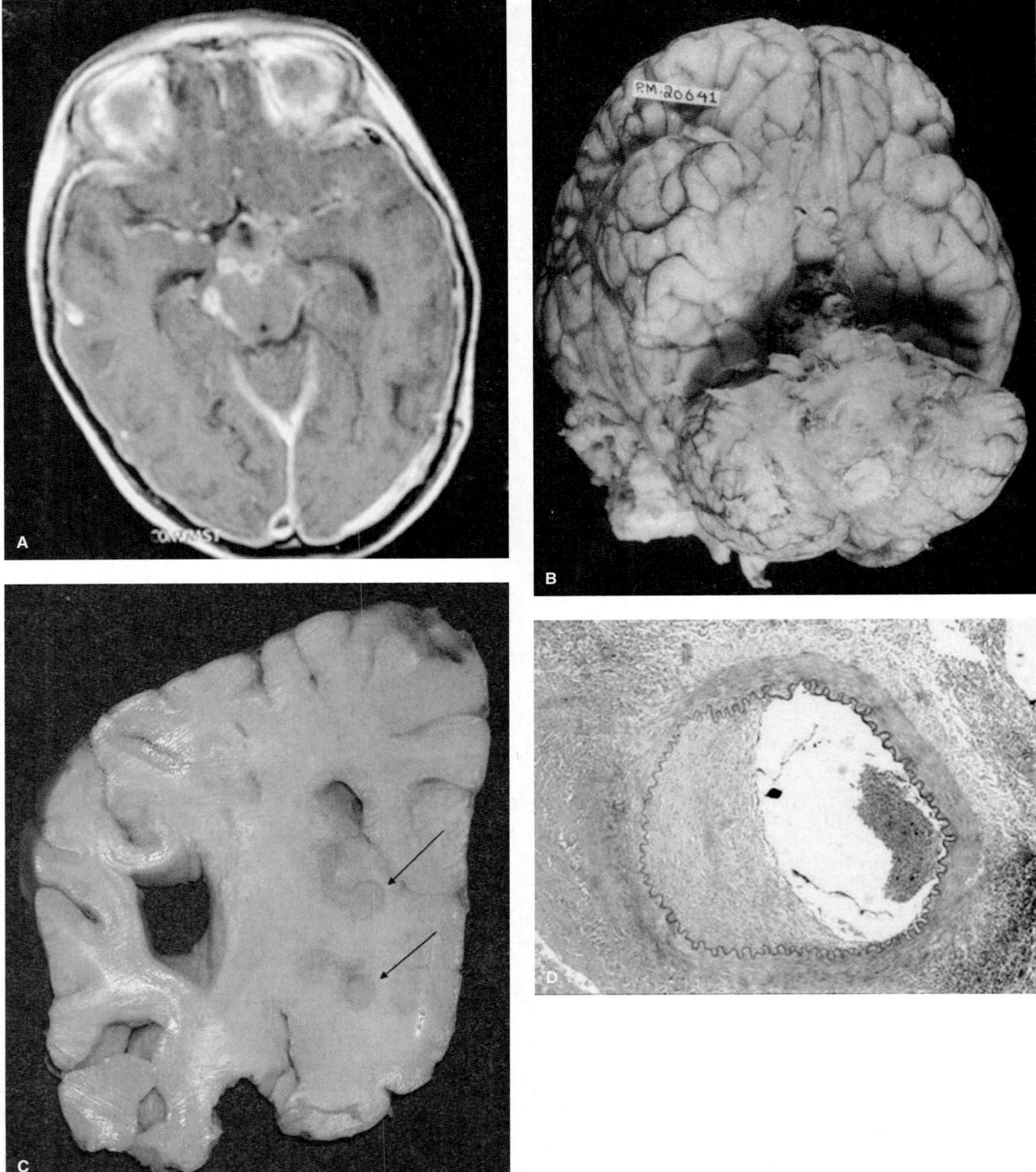

FIGURE 80.2. A: Contrast MRI showing paradoxic development of multiple tuberculomas in a child with tubercular meningitis shunted for hydrocephalous and on antitubercular therapy. **B:** On autopsy, the brain showed thick basal exudates encasing the cranial nerves. **C:** Slices of the brain showing two tuberculomas. **D:** Histopathology showing intense vasculitis with occlusion of the vessel lumen.

tubercular meningitis occurs many years after the primary infection when rupture of one or more of the subependymal tubercles discharges tubercle bacilli into the subarachnoid space.

Clinical Presentation

The clinical presentation of TBM is variable. The onset is generally insidious, with low-grade fever, poor feeding, irritability, headache, and vomiting, followed by neck rigidity and altered sensorium. Occasionally it may be rapid, particularly in infants and young children, who may experience symptoms for only a few days before the onset of acute hydrocephalus, seizures, and cerebral edema. More commonly, the signs and symptoms progress slowly over several weeks and can be divided into three stages (Table 80.8). Although the staging system brings objectivity in data comparisons, the progression is not necessarily in a smooth continuum in an individual patient. The main presenting clinical symptoms and signs in children include alteration in consciousness (79%), focal neurologic signs (66%), fever (66%), and seizures (53%). Contact with an infected adult can be found in approximately half of cases. No significant difference has been observed in the neurologic findings in HIV-infected and uninfected children (47).

Diagnosis

The diagnosis of tubercular meningitis may be difficult because of its nonspecific and variable presentation. In endemic areas, TBM must be considered in the diagnosis of any child with a meningoencephalitic presentation. Differentiation of TBM from partially treated bacterial meningitis is a common problem in developing countries. The CSF is generally clear or straw colored in TBM, with a cell count of 10–500 cells/mm³, predominantly lymphocytes, although in a few cases polymorphonuclear leukocytes may be present. A "cobweb" formation in the CSF on prolonged standing is highly suggestive of TBM.

TABLE 80.8

CLINICAL STAGING OF PATIENTS WITH TUBERCULOUS MENINGITIS

Stage I (early) (days to weeks)	Nonspecific symptoms and signs (fever, headache, irritability, malaise)
	Lethargy or alteration in behavior
	No neurologic deficits
	No clouding of consciousness
Stage II (intermediate) (weeks to months)	Meningeal irritation
	Minor neurologic deficits (cranial nerve deficits)
Stage III (late) (months to years)	Abnormal movements
	Convulsions
	Stupor or coma
	Severe neurologic deficits (hemiplegia, paraplegia, decerebration)

The CSF glucose is typically <40 mg/dL, the protein is elevated (generally up 150–200 mg/dL, but may increase to 1000–2000 mg/dL). Low CSF chloride is no longer considered diagnostic of TBM. Identification or isolation of mycobacterium on smear or culture is the gold standard for diagnosis of TBM. Successful isolation is possible in as many as 80% of cases if multiple samples are processed; however, in general, the yield is much lower. The yield may be increased by using the cobweb or sediment from a large volume of CSF. Radiometric culture (BACTEC) gives early results. CSF PCR, adenosine deaminase levels, ELISA, and other antigen or antibody detection tests have been reported to be useful with varying degrees of sensitivity and specificity. Positive results support, but negative results do not exclude, the diagnosis of TBM. The rare "serous" or sterile TBM with a CSF that resembles aseptic meningitis is considered an immunologic reaction to tuberculoprotein. The CSF is often normal in children with tuberculomas.

Neuroimaging

Neuroimaging is extremely valuable in the diagnosis of tubercular meningitis, particularly because isolation of acid-fast bacilli is not possible in many cases. The CT scan characteristically shows thick basilar enhancement, parenchymal enhancement, hydrocephalus, cerebral edema, early focal ischemia, or infarcts and, sometimes, silent tuberculomas. MRI scan shows similar findings and may detect additional posterior fossa lesions, which may not be detected by CT. Brain involvement has been shown in MRIs of patients with miliary TB without symptoms or signs of CNS involvement. CT or MRI of the brain may, however, be normal during early stages of disease. CT signs of TBM were found to be less prominent in HIV-infected versus noninfected children (47). Corroborative evidence of TB elsewhere in the body, especially pulmonary involvement on chest x-ray and choroid tubercles on funduscopy, gastric aspirates for acid-fast bacilli, and family screening for identification of contact, may aid in the diagnosis. The tuberculin skin test is positive in 30%–50% of cases, and a pulmonary focus on chest x-ray is detected in 50%–87% of patients. The diagnosis of TBM depends upon a high degree of clinical suspicion, supportive evidence, and specific investigations. Even if the diagnosis is not confirmed, antitubercular therapy should be considered in the presence of meningitis with thick basal exudates.

Treatment

Most children with TBM of insidious onset will not come to the attention of the intensivist; however, some children with an acute, rapidly progressive course and those with serious complications, such as deep coma, stroke, and marked increase in ICP, will need intensive care.

Specific antitubercular therapy should have good BBB penetration and should be directed against both intracellular and extracellular organisms (33). As in other forms of TB, multiple drugs should be used to avoid the emergence of resistance. Initial treatment regimens have varied, using either three or four drugs. All regimens include isoniazid and rifampicin. The third drug used is generally pyrazinamide, but sometimes it is ethambutol or streptomycin. In the four-drug regimen, isoniazid + rifampicin + pyrazinamide + either ethambutol or streptomycin are used. Although clinical trials have shown that the efficacy of streptomycin is approximately equal to that of ethambutol in the initial phase of treatment, the increasing frequency of resistance to streptomycin worldwide has made the drug less useful. Thus, streptomycin is not recommended as being interchangeable with ethambutol unless the organism is known to be susceptible to the drug or the patient is from a population in which streptomycin resistance is unlikely (3). On the other hand, as ethambutol has a poor penetration across the BBB, the WHO recommends that streptomycin be used instead of ethambutol in the initial therapy of cases of TBM (49).

The initial regimen is given either daily or twice or thrice weekly for 2 months, followed by a continuation phase generally with two drugs. Pyridoxine is recommended for infants, children, and adolescents who are being treated with isoniazid and who have nutritional deficiencies or symptomatic HIV infection (3). Although different regimens are recommended by various expert groups, in general, certain principles are commonly agreed upon for treatment of CNS TB: in the initial phase, four drugs are preferred and a longer duration of continuation phase is advocated. The efficacy of short-course treatment regimens using intermittent supervised therapy has been proven for pulmonary and non-CNS extrapulmonary TB in adults and in children. Although the WHO recommends a 4-month continuation phase for TBM in its Guidelines for National Programmes, current data are inadequate support short-course regimens for CNS TB.

The regimens recommended by the WHO (49), the American Thoracic Society (3), and the Indian Academy of Pediatrics for CNS TB are listed in **Table 80.9**. These regimens are used when the organisms are susceptible to standard antituberculous agents. However, resistant strains are being reported from both developed and developing countries, particularly in association with HIV and malnutrition. Resistance to isoniazid or streptomycin is most common; multidrug resistance is seen in 1.4% of cases. Inappropriate or inadequate treatment is the main cause of resistance. Noncompliance is a major issue and is compounded by inappropriate prescribing practices by physicians.

In children, drug resistance in CNS TB is rare and is difficult to establish because of the low rates of organism isolation. It may be suspected if neurologic worsening or absence of clinical or radiologic improvement is seen after adequate therapy for several weeks. In cases where an adult contact has been identified, results of culture susceptibility of specimens obtained from that contact may be used to "confirm" the diagnosis of resistance and to guide the choice of drugs. Most of the data available for resistant TB are from adults. Drug resistance has been reported in some children with TBM. Management of resistant cases is a challenge. Several second-line drugs are available; most of them are expensive. Two or more of these drugs must be introduced simultaneously. The duration of treatment of multidrug-resistant TB is at least 18–24 months. In spite of aggressive treatment, the outcome is not favorable.

Corticosteroids are used with antitubercular therapy, as they reduce the neurologic sequelae of all stages of TBM, especially when they are administered early in the course of disease.

TABLE 80.9

RECOMMENDED TREATMENT REGIMENS FOR CENTRAL NERVOUS SYSTEM TUBERCULOSIS

Therapy	WHO	American Thoracic Society	Indian Academy of Pediatrics
Initial Continuation Phase	HRZS Daily for 2 months HR for 4 months	HRZE daily for 2 mo **OR** daily for 2 weeks followed by twice weekly[a] for 6 weeks HR daily **OR** twice weekly for 10 months	HRZE or (HRZS) daily for 2 months HRE daily for 10 months

Doses for antitubercular drugs for children[b]		
	Daily dose mg/kg/24hrs	**Twice weekly dose mg/kg/dose**
Isoniazid (max)	10–15 (300 mg)	20–30 (900 mg)
Rifampin (max)	10–20 (600 mg)	10–20 (600 mg)
Pyrazinamide (max)	15–30 (2.0 g)	50–70 (2 g)
Ethambutol (max)	15–25 (1.0 g)	50 (2.5 g)
Streptomycin (max)	20–40 (1.0 g)	25–30 (1.5 g)

[a] All intermittent therapies to be monitored by directly observed therapy (DOT) for the duration of therapy.
H, isoniazid; R, rifampicin; Z, pyrazinamide; S, streptomycin; E, ethambutol
[b] WHO recommends somewhat lower doses; it does not recommend twice weekly doses.

Corticosteroids have been found to significantly improve the survival rate and intellectual outcome of children with TBM. Enhanced resolution of basal exudates and tuberculomas has been reported with the use of steroids, although no significant effect on the ICP or the incidence of basal ganglia infarctions was found. In very sick children, dexamethasone is administered IV for the first few days, followed by 1–2 mg/kg/day oral prednisolone, generally given for an initial 6 weeks and tapered off over 2–3 weeks.

Shunt surgery is often necessary in children with TBM who develop hydrocephalous (1). External ventricular drainage has been used by some as an alternative to shunt surgery. In cases that present with life-threatening ICP secondary to hydrocephalous, an emergency ventricular tap is life saving until shunt surgery is done. Shunt surgery in HIV-positive TBM patients has been associated with a poor outcome.

Children with TBM need periodic clinical and radiologic monitoring. Despite adequate antitubercular therapy, improvement in clinical status may take several days, depending upon the stage of disease. Some children in deep coma with severe neurodeficits may take several weeks to improve. Corticosteroid administration is often associated with some clinical improvement within several days. Alleviation of raised ICP after shunt may result in improvement in sensorium within 48–72 hrs. A postoperative CT is advised in all cases within 1 week after shunt surgery, or earlier in cases with clinical deterioration or no improvement. The CSF parameters may take months to normalize; CSF glucose returns to normal in 50% cases within 2 months and in the vast majority by 6 months. CSF cellular response and CSF protein levels may take 6 months to normalize.

Paradoxic response, including development of tuberculomas in children (**Fig 80.2 A,C**), is known even after up to 1 year on standard treatment for TBM (19). The cause and nature of these tuberculomas are poorly understood, but they do not represent failure of drug treatment. This possibility should be considered whenever a child with tuberculous meningitis deteriorates or develops focal neurologic findings while on treatment. The clinical signs and symptoms may sometimes be severe; corticosteroids are helpful in such cases. Rarely, drug resistance may develop during treatment and is suspected when a patient with TBM shows worsening or cord involvement. Additional antitubercular drugs and steroids are used.

Prognosis

The outcome of TBM correlates most closely with the clinical stage of illness at the time treatment is initiated. The majority of patients in stage 1 have a good outcome, whereas most patients in stage 3 who survive have permanent disabilities, including blindness, deafness, paraplegia, epilepsy, or mental retardation.

ENCEPHALITIS AND MYELITIS

The term *encephalitis* denotes inflammation of brain parenchyma. Encephalitis caused by direct infection of the CNS is called *primary encephalitis*. Clinically, symptoms and signs of cortical or brainstem involvement, such as seizures and altered sensorium, are seen. Pathologically, the brain parenchyma shows (a) inflammation and destruction of neurons, and (b) pathogen detected by direct visualization, tissue staining, immunostaining, or nucleic acid detection. Acute inflammatory demyelination that occurs in temporal association with a systemic viral infection or immunization but without direct viral invasion in the CNS is called *postinfectious encephalitis*. As the spinal cord may also be involved, it is referred to as ADEM. Clinically, symptoms and signs of white matter involvement in addition to gray matter involvement are often seen. Pathologically, demyelination and perivascular aggregation of immune cells in the CNS are noted but not evidence of virus or viral antigen, suggesting an autoimmune etiology. The term *encephalopathy* refers to signs of diffuse cerebral dysfunction and can involve dysfunction that does not have an inflammatory component.

Viral encephalitis may be sporadic or may occur in epidemics. Although epidemic encephalitis has declined in developed countries as a result of improvements in living conditions and mass immunization against many of the childhood exanthems, such as measles, mumps, and rubella, large epidemics of encephalitis, with devastating consequences, continue to occur in many developing countries. Most children with encephalitis are critically ill and require urgent management in the ICU.

Etiology

The most common cause of neonatal encephalitis is HSV, most often HSV type 2 (HSV-2). Other viruses, such as enterovirus or adenovirus, may also cause encephalitis in the neonate. Intrauterine infections, such as cytomegalovirus (CMV), rubella, and toxoplasma, may involve the brain but generally do not present as acute encephalitis.

In childhood, the most common causes of epidemic encephalitis are arthropod-borne viruses (arboviruses) and enteroviruses. Eastern equine encephalitis (EEE) and western equine encephalitis are caused by Alphaviridae. St. Louis encephalitis, West Nile virus encephalitis, and JE are caused by Flaviviridae. Colorado tick fever is caused by an orbivirus, a member of the family Reoviridae. Enteroviruses are viruses that infect primarily the enteric tract and include polio, echo, coxsackie, and other enteroviruses. Adenovirus, Epstein-Barr virus (EBV), measles, mumps, varicella, and the bacterium *Bartonella henselae* also cause sporadic cases. Subacute sclerosing panencephalitis is a chronic, persistent infection of the measles virus, also quite rare due to the widespread use of measles vaccine. Tick-borne bacterial diseases, such as borreliosis, rickettsial diseases, and ehrlichiosis, may also cause encephalitis. The common etiologies of acute encephalitis are listed in **Table 80.7** and vary by geographic region.

Epidemiology

In a large number of cases of encephalitis, the etiologic agent may not be identified due to lack of investigative facilities. Herpes simplex encephalitis is the most common cause of sporadic and severe encephalitis throughout childhood. Two-thirds of the population is infected with HSV type 1 (HSV-1), and 1 out of 4 individuals is infected with HSV-2. Approximately, 80% of infections are asymptomatic, and transmission occurs from asymptomatic shedding of virus or via contact with lesions. The majority of encephalitis beyond the neonatal period is caused by HSV-1, although HSV-6 can cause some cases. Most cases of HSV encephalitis are caused by reactivation of latent virus. This topic is discussed in detail later in this chapter.

Arbovirus encephalitis in North America generally occurs in the late summer and fall. St. Louis encephalitis virus and West Nile virus are common vector-transmitted causes of aseptic meningitis and encephalitis throughout America. Birds are the reservoirs, and multiple species of mosquitoes are the principal vectors. Exposure to these mosquitoes may be more likely to occur indoors, as poorly sealed residences appear to be a risk factor. The majority of infections with St. Louis encephalitis and West Nile virus are asymptomatic, but significant neurologic findings, including extrapyramidal signs, optic neuritis, cranial nerve abnormalities, polyradiculitis, myelitis, and seizures may occur. EEE and western equine encephalitis also utilize the bird as reservoir and mosquito as the vector, but horses and humans are dead-end hosts. EEE is the most severe of the four common arboviral encephalitides just discussed, with a fatality rate as high as 50%.

Enteroviruses are endemic in the developed and developing world, with higher transmission rates in summer and fall. Most enteroviral infection is asymptomatic, and meningitis is more common than encephalitis. The only enterovirus against which a vaccine is available is polio, which is slated to follow smallpox in eradication efforts. Target vaccination campaigns address outbreaks in countries where polio transmission occurs, including Nigeria and Pakistan. JE is the leading cause of epidemic encephalitis in many developing countries and will be discussed separately. Rabies, mumps, and measles encephalitis are now rarely seen in developed countries but continue to be seen in many developing countries.

Pathogenesis

Viruses gain access to the CNS by either the hematogenous or the neuronal route. The mechanism of spread to the CNS by either of these routes depends on various viral factors, site of entry, and viral replication in intermediate cells. The host factors that prevent this access include local immune response at the site of entry, systemic immune responses, and protection offered by the BBB (4). The mechanism of spread to the CNS and the host response influence the clinical manifestations of neurologic disease.

Hematogenous spread is the main pathway of viral spread in human beings. Enteroviruses and arboviruses represent viruses that spread to the CNS through viremia, although their site of entry differs. The virus first replicates at the local site of entry and causes primary viremia. It then infects secondary tissue and undergoes secondary replication, causing an extensive viremia that seeds the CNS. Viral entry into the epithelium is prevented by protective layers of keratin; breaks in this defensive layer can result in increased risk of infection by viral entry into the subepithelial layer or directly into the blood. The conjunctival, respiratory, oral, and nasopharyngeal epithelial layers are nonkeratinized and allow easy entry for viruses that spread through the respiratory route or by large droplets.

After crossing the epithelial barrier and entering a receptive cell, primary replication occurs. The virus can then reach a lymph node and replicate there, or it can bypass the lymph node and enter the bloodstream, causing primary viremia, which leads to seeding of other organs and often marks the onset of clinical illness. In the blood, the virus may circulate freely in the plasma or be attached to or inside cells. Most viruses undergo secondary replication in the liver and spleen, which are highly vascular structures. Secondary viremia follows, and high titers of virus are released in the bloodstream for prolonged periods, leading to the seeding of target organs. As the CNS is protected by the BBB, large numbers of viruses are required to gain access to the brain cells or CSF. The exact mechanisms of viral transport from blood to brain and of viral endothelial cell tropism are not well known. The viruses enter the endothelial cells of arteries, arterioles, and capillaries and cause damage that leads to vasculitis, hemorrhage, and thrombosis. The viruses then enter the CSF and may either involve the meninges alone or may enter the brain parenchyma and cause encephalitis.

Viruses can also spread to the CNS via neurons. Viremia and neuronal spread to the CNS can occur concurrently and are not mutually exclusive. Rabies and HSV represent viruses that reach the brain by peripheral neuronal spread, which occurs along peripheral or cranial nerves. Rabies virus classically infects by the myoneural route; however, very rarely, infection can occur from corneal transplantations and via aerosolized route. Following a bite by a rabid animal, rabies virus replicates locally in the soft tissue. It then enters the peripheral nerve and travels by anterograde and retrograde intra-axonal transport to infect neurons in the brainstem and hippocampus and throughout the brain. Cranial nerves, particularly the olfactory nerve, may also provide a pathway for viral access to the CNS. The olfactory neurons are not protected by the BBB and, therefore, provide easy neuronal access to the brain. HSV can infect the brain through the olfactory system and the trigeminal nerve. The inferomedial temporal lobe, which has direct connection with the olfactory bulb, is the initial site of early HSV encephalitis.

After gaining access to the CNS, the virus attaches itself to the host cells. The capsid or envelope proteins bind with receptors of host cells. The mechanism of cell entry varies among enveloped and nonenveloped viruses. Enveloped viruses enter the cell either by direct fusion or receptor-mediated endocytosis. Nonenveloped viruses may undergo structural changes or proteolysis; the capsid protein then fuses with the cell membrane and releases the viral genome into the cytoplasm. Once the viral genome enters the cell, viral replication occurs in the nucleus or the cytoplasm. Positive-stranded viral mRNA is produced, and gene products are subsequently translated. When viral protein synthesis begins, the host protein synthesis decreases, and host cell functions are affected. Within the brain, spread from one cell to another may involve multiple mechanisms.

A number of host and viral factors, including the route of infection, genetic composition of the virus, receptor differences, etc., may influence neurotropism.

Host factors, such as age, sex, immunity, and genetic differences, also influence the extent, location, and severity of viral CNS disease. Viral infections in very young children are often much more serious, with a higher morbidity and mortality than in older children. Enterovirus infections in children <2 weeks can produce a severe systemic infection, including meningitis or meningoencephalitis, with high morbidity and mortality. In contrast, older children rarely have severe disease or significant morbidity. Physical activity may increase the risk of acquisition or severity of viral infection. Exercise has been associated with increased risk of paralytic poliomyelitis and may result in an increased incidence of enteroviral myocarditis and aseptic meningitis.

The host resists viral infections via both cellular and systemic immune defense mechanisms. Certain enzymatic pathways are activated that destroy viral nucleic acid transcripts and stimulate secretion of interferons (4). Interferons inhibit viral penetration, replication, translation, and assembly. However, some viruses have developed resistance to interferons, and, occasionally, the inflammatory response itself may cause damage to brain tissue with destruction of the infected neurons. In postinfectious encephalitis, the immune response is misdirected against the brain itself and causes immune-mediated demyelination.

Clinical Manifestations

The clinical manifestations of encephalitis vary according to the site, severity of parenchymal involvement, and a number of host factors. Most viruses that cause encephalitis simultaneously involve the meninges, causing "meningoencephalitis," while some viruses (e.g., rabies) do not have significant meningeal involvement.

In neonates, encephalitis generally presents with nonspecific symptoms and signs of systemic sepsis, including fever, poor feeding, irritability, lethargy, seizures, or apnea. History of maternal fever in the peripartum may be present in some cases of enterovirus or adenovirus infections. History of maternal genital herpes is seen in only 20%–27% of infants with herpes infection. Hence, an absence of parental history of HSV infection does not exclude neonatal HSV infection. Skin lesions in the neonate are seen in some cases of neonatal herpes encephalitis. Focal neurologic signs may be present in some but not all neonates. As specific signs of encephalitis may not be present, strong consideration should be made to performing HSV PCR in neonates with suspected sepsis from whom CSF is obtained for bacterial culture.

The usual presentation of encephalitis in older children is with acute-onset fever, headache, seizures, behavioral changes, and rapid alteration in sensorium, progressing to coma. A prodromal illness with myalgias, fever, anorexia, and lethargy, reflecting the systemic viremia may be seen in some cases. Alteration in sensorium, the hallmark of encephalitis, generally occurs early and progresses rapidly, as compared to meningitis. Seizures are common and may be generalized or focal. The neurologic symptoms may vary from subtle to severe, and depending on the degree of meningeal involvement, symptoms and signs of meningitis, including photophobia, vomiting, and stiff neck, may be present. Other symptoms and signs depend on the neuroanatomic site of involvement. Cortical involvement may lead to disorientation and confusion, basal ganglia involvement to movement disorders, and brainstem involvement to cranial nerve dysfunction. Associated spinal cord involvement (myelitis) may cause flaccid paraplegia with abnormalities of the deep tendon reflexes.

A careful physical and neurologic examination is essential. A quick neurologic evaluation includes Glasgow Coma Scale and evaluation for any life-threatening signs of raised ICP. Subsequently, a detailed examination of sensory, motor, and cerebral function can be undertaken to elicit any focal neurologic signs.

Etiologic differentiation of encephalitides may not be possible on the basis of clinical features and usual laboratory tests. However, certain diagnostic clues can be obtained from the history and examination and from epidemiology. A history of recent travel, exposure to persons with infections, and insects or animal bites should be obtained. A history of focal seizures, personality changes, and aphasia suggests herpes encephalitis. Fever with severe pharyngitis and fatigue may indicate EBV encephalitis. Fever, parotitis, and dysphagia suggest mumps encephalitis. Fever, conjunctivitis, and the characteristic rash of measles indicate measles encephalitis. History of a dog bite or bat exposure with characteristic behavioral changes and predominant bulbar involvement suggests rabies. The furious type of rabies with agitation, characteristic hydrophobia, or hypersalivation is much more common than the "paralytic" or "dumb" type with flaccid ascending paralysis. Exposure to kittens suggests *Bartonella henselae* (cat-scratch) encephalitis. Encephalitis in summer with a suggestive rash is seen with Rocky Mountain spotted fever (petechial), enteroviruses, arboviruses (maculopapular), and Lyme disease (erythema migrans). Epidemics of JE generally occur after the rainy season during mosquito breeding periods; signs and symptoms of basal ganglia involvement are further diagnostic clues.

Differential Diagnosis

Encephalitis must be differentiated from other causes of encephalopathy and coma. Bacterial meningitis may present with encephalopathic components due to the pathophysiology discussed previously, increased ICP, and global CNS dysfunction. Cerebral malaria is an important, eminently treatable condition that must be differentiated urgently in many developing countries. This subject is discussed in detail in a separate section of the chapter. Other febrile encephalopathies, such as those caused by *Salmonella* and *Shigella*, would generally have suggestive symptoms and signs of the primary illness. Fever and the presence of focal signs help in distinguishing encephalitis from encephalopathies secondary to metabolic problems and toxins. Children with Reye syndrome present with afebrile encephalopathy following a prodrome of nausea and vomiting. They have mild hepatomegaly, hypoglycemia, some elevation of liver transaminases with mild hyperbilirubinemia (serum bilirubin <5 mg/dL), and elevated blood ammonia levels.

A biphasic illness, with antecedent viral illness, rash, or immunization followed by sudden onset meningoencephalitis with multifocal motor deficits indicates ADEM (see later section). Several differential diagnoses that should be considered in a child with an encephalitic presentation are listed in Table 80.10.

Diagnosis

Given the more significant outcome of encephalitis, compared to aseptic meningitis, aggressive determination of etiology is often sought. The CSF can be obtained by LP once the child is hemodynamically stable, the ICP is not significantly elevated, and focal lesions have been excluded. In general, CSF findings in encephalitis are nonspecific and CSF abnormalities seldom correlate with clinical or histologic severity of encephalitis.

TABLE 80.10

DIFFERENTIAL DIAGNOSIS OF ACUTE ENCEPHALITIS/MENINGOENCEPHALITIS ACUTE DISSEMINATED ENCEPHALOMYELITIS

Infectious
Bacterial meningitis
Tuberculous meningitis
Cerebral malaria
Cryptococcal meningoencephalitis
Brain abscess

Metabolic
Hepatic coma
Reye syndrome
Uremia
Hypoglycemia
Hyposmolar or hypersomolar states
Organic acidemias
Amino acidopathies
Urea cycle defects
Fat oxidation defects
Mitochondrial disorders
Acute intermittent porphyria

Toxic
Shigellosis
Salmonella
Drugs
Lead encephalopathy
Carbon monoxide poisoning
Pertussis

Vasculitic
Systemic lupus erythematosus
Polyarteritis nodosa

Other
Benign raised intracranial pressure
Trauma
Nonconvulsive status epilepticus
Neoplasms
Cerebrovascular accidents

CSF analysis is helpful only in a few cases. Generally, the CSF is clear and colorless; the opening pressure may be high in children with raised ICP. CSF cell count and protein are generally slightly elevated or may be normal, and the glucose concentration is often normal. CSF pleocytosis (>5 WBC/mm^3) is seen in $>95\%$ of cases of acute viral encephalitis and is typically lymphocytic. In the early phase of infection, a mixed pleocytosis that consists of both polymorphonuclear and mononuclear cells and later becomes lymphocytic may be seen. A polymorphonuclear predominance may persist throughout the illness in some types of infection, notably EEE. Atypical lymphocytes in the CSF may occasionally be seen in EBV and CMV encephalitis. Evaluation of the CSF early in the course of acute encephalitis may yield few or no cells. Such a finding does not exclude the diagnosis, and a repeat LP after 1–2 days is often helpful in subsequently demonstrating pleocytosis. CSF pleocytosis >500 WBC/mm^3 may be seen in $\sim 10\%$ cases. Vasculitis or tissue necrosis causes extravasation of red blood cells into CSF and elicits CSF leukocytosis with increased polymorphonuclear cells. Red blood cells in the CSF may be seen in late stages of HSV encephalitis. The possibility of a traumatic LP

must be excluded. Very rarely, subarachnoid hemorrhage from occult trauma or a vascular malformation may be considered. A very low CSF glucose is unusual in viral encephalitis, and other causes, including bacterial and tubercular meningitis, must be considered.

Confirmatory diagnosis is performed by culture, rapid diagnostic tests (including antigen detection and PCR), demonstration of rise in specific antibody titer, and direct visualization of the organism (41). The need for biopsy is less common now than in the past, but may be an option of last resort. An etiologic agent is identified in a variable number of cases, but rarely exceeds 60%.

Success of viral culture depends on cells inoculated and is highly dependent on the capabilities of the virology laboratory, the quality of the sample provided, and information provided by the clinician that allows laboratory personnel to perform specific testing. PCR has replaced viral culture for identification of HSV and enteroviruses from the CSF and is available for CMV, EBV, varicella zoster virus (VZV), human herpesvirus (HHV)-6, HIV, influenza, adenovirus, *Mycoplasma*, *Mycobacteria*, *Rickettsia*, and others. PCR assays are usually highly sensitive and specific. However, false positives may occur because of contamination of laboratory specimens, and false negatives may occur because the infectious encephalitis process may not be near enough to the meninges or CSF or because of the presence of inhibitory factors in the CSF. As the viral genomic material remains in the CSF from weeks to months, its detection helps in confirming the antecedent viral infection in cases of postinfectious encephalitis. Quantitative as well as qualitative DNA amplification techniques may be of value.

Isolation of pathogens from sites other than the CNS may provide a clue to diagnosis. Culture from sites of entry and primary viral replication, such as conjunctivae, nasopharynx, and rectum are useful in identifying enteroviruses and adenoviruses. CMV is readily cultured from urine.

Rapid diagnostic tests provide a diagnosis before diagnosis by culture. Direct fluorescence antibody staining can be performed on cells scraped from the base of lesions (HSV or VZV).

Serology may be helpful if high titers are identified acutely or at least a fourfold rise is noted when measured 3–4 weeks later. An antibody index (measure of specific antibody in CSF compared to the serum) may be useful to determine if infection is localized to the CNS. Serologic tests may lack specificity, and tests for antibodies vary in their quality. Attention should be paid to which antibody detection method has highest sensitivity and specificity (ELISA or other), as well as to the antibody (IgG, IgM, other, or both) being tested. Elevated levels of myelin basic protein in the CSF suggest demyelinating injury as in ADEM. Intrathecal oligoclonal bands are seen occasionally in postinfectious encephalitis, in contrast to MS, in which they are often present.

EEG may be complementary to neuroimaging in the diagnosis of encephalitis and may help in distinguishing generalized from focal encephalitis. In generalized encephalitis, the EEG typically shows diffuse slowing with high voltage slow waves; occasionally, spikes and spike wave activity may be seen. In focal encephalitis, focal EEG abnormalities, including focal slow waves or spikes, may be seen. The EEG is particularly helpful in HSV encephalitis, wherein characteristic periodic lateralized epileptiform discharges (PLEDS) may be seen. However, it must be remembered that PLEDS are not seen in all cases of HSV encephalitis and that the presence of PLEDS is not sine quo non with HSV encephalitis, as PLEDS are also seen in other conditions, including infarcts and other focal lesions.

Before the advent of rapid diagnostic tests, brain biopsy for histologic examination, viral culture, and fluorescent antibody staining was a diagnostic option. This process is now rarely used for the specific diagnosis of encephalitis.

Other tests that may provide diagnostic clues include the peripheral blood smear, which generally shows lymphocytosis. Marked leukocytosis may be seen in EEE. Leukopenia and thrombocytopenia are seen in rickettsial infection, measles, and viral hemorrhagic fever. Characteristic cytoplasmic inclusions in monocytes, known as *morulae*, are seen in ehrlichiosis. Finding of malarial parasites in the smear helps to confirm a diagnosis of cerebral malaria.

Chest x-ray may help in the diagnosis of TB, mycoplasma, or legionella. A full-thickness skin biopsy from the nape of the neck, where numerous hair follicles are located, has a high sensitivity (50%–90%) and a specificity of almost 100% for diagnosis of rabies.

Neuroimaging

Children with suspected encephalitis are often critically ill and have raised ICP; therefore, an LP cannot be performed at presentation in some cases. Neuroimaging is the most important urgent investigation required in such cases.

MRI is a sensitive method of diagnosing encephalitis that detects brain inflammation and edema in the cerebral cortex, the gray-white matter junction, the basal ganglia, or the cerebellum. Specific areas of involvement may suggest the etiology, as with involvement of the inferomedial temporal lobe and frontal lobes in HSV; bilateral thalamic and basal ganglia involvement in JE; hippocampal, cerebellar, and mesencephalic areas in rabies; and disseminated lesions in brainstem and basal ganglia in EEE.

MRI is the diagnostic modality of choice in differentiating acute infectious encephalitis from ADEM. In ADEM, the MRI shows multiple patchy areas of involvement of the white matter and, at times, the deep gray matter of the brain; the spinal cord may also be involved in some cases. Demyelination is best seen in T2-weighted and FLAIR images. Gadolinium contrast enhancement of lesions may be seen in some cases. Lyme disease and MS may also involve diverse areas of brain, brainstem, and spinal cord. Gadolinium also confirms that the multifocal areas of demyelination in ADEM are all of the same stage, in contrast to MS, in which the lesions are of different stages. However, acute presentation of MS that requires management in the PICU is rarely seen in children.

MRI may be insensitive in detecting encephalitis early, especially in neonates with higher brain water content. The CT scan may help to exclude a bleed or a space-occupying lesion in a suspected case, but is not significantly useful for the diagnosis of encephalitis.

Treatment

Acute encephalitis is a neurologic emergency. All children with altered sensorium and a clinical suspicion of encephalitis should be admitted to the PICU for management of life-threatening problems, observation and monitoring of the course of illness, and differentiating from other causes of coma.

CNS infections, particularly meningoencephalites, are the most common cause of refractory SE in the PICU (36) and must be managed energetically. Continuous EEG and cerebral function monitoring is warranted. Specific antimicrobial therapy should be initiated as soon as an etiologic agent is reasonably suspected or identified. Bacterial, fungal, and parasitic etiologies of encephalitis require specific antimicrobial therapy. Antiviral therapy is important for treatment of HSV encephalitis and must be administered promptly in all suspected cases (see later section on herpes encephalitis). Acyclovir is not effective for CMV encephalitis, for which ganciclovir or foscarnet must be used (41). Amantadine and rimantadine are effective against influenza A, whereas oseltamivir and zanamivir are effective against both influenza A and B. Highly active antiretroviral therapy is available for HIV infection. No specific antiviral therapy is available for enteroviral and arboviral encephalitis. Passive immunity in the form of IV immune globulin may be helpful in immunocompromised individuals who cannot mount an effective immune response. The role of high-dose steroid therapy has not been established in acute viral encephalitis. High-dose dexamethasone was not found to be useful in a study of JE.

Prognosis

The immediate and long-term outcome in encephalitis is determined by several factors, including etiology, host factors (e.g., age and immune status), severity of illness, level of consciousness at presentation, early intensive management, and institution of specific therapy. Most arboviral encephalitides except EEE and JE have a good prognosis in children. The prognosis of HSV encephalitis has improved significantly with use of early acyclovir therapy. Children with severe encephalitis and/or delayed therapy may be left with permanent neurodeficits.

HERPES ENCEPHALITIS

HSV is the most common cause of fatal sporadic encephalitis in childhood. Human disease can be caused by any of the eight herpes viruses: HSV-1, HSV-2, VZV, CMV, HHV-6 and HHV-7, EBV, and Kaposi sarcoma herpes virus (HHV-8). Also, one simian herpes virus, B virus (cryptotetia-crypta) rarely causes serious human disease that involves the CNS. All of these viruses have similar biologic characteristics, can remain latent for long periods of time, and can become reactivated. However, most herpes simplex encephalitis (HSE) beyond the neonatal period is caused by HSV-1 and, occasionally, HSV-6; most neonatal HSE is caused by HSV-2.

Epidemiology

HSE occurs worldwide, in developed and developing countries. It occurs sporadically at any time of the year and does not occur in epidemic form. Humans are the sole reservoirs of the virus. HSV remains latent in most cases and is transmitted during reactivation. The acquisition of HSV-1 is influenced by geographic location, socioeconomic factors, and age. Primary infection occurs early in children from developing countries and lower socioeconomic strata, whereas it is generally delayed until adolescence in more affluent populations from developed countries.

HSV-2 is generally acquired in adults by sexual contact and may either cause genital infection or be excreted asymptomatically during primary or recurrent infections. Neonates acquire the infection from infected mothers. HSE can occur at any age; both sexes are equally affected. Primary infection often occurs in childhood.

Pathogenesis

HSV is acquired by respiratory droplets or by direct contact with infectious secretions through close contacts with a person excreting HSV. The virus is transported from the abraded skin or mucous membrane by retrograde axonal flow to the dorsal root ganglia, where it replicates. It may cause primary infection with viremia at this time or become latent, as a result of host-virus interaction. The primary infection may disseminate to various organ sites in neonates and children with poor immunity. The latent virus can become spontaneously reactivated at any time. Stress, exercise, fever, immune suppression, and tissue damage are some of the known risk factors for reactivation.

Encephalitis can be caused by both primary and recurrent HSV infection. The route of primary CNS infection is thought to be the olfactory and trigeminal nerves, which explains the neurotropism of HSV to the temporal lobe. Whether reactivation of virus occurs within a previously infected brain tissue or in the olfactory or trigeminal nerves with subsequent passage to the brain is not yet fully understood. The role of host immunity is also poorly defined.

Fetal or neonatal disease is generally acquired from the infected mother, rarely in utero, and more commonly during birth through direct contact with infected secretions in the genitalia. Postnatal contact with HSV accounts for a small number of cases. The disease may present either in a disseminated form, isolated CNS involvement, or with involvement of skin, eyes, and mouth. In the disseminated form, the CNS is most likely infected via the hematogenous route, whereas isolated encephalitis probably occurs through intraneuronal spread.

Clinical Presentation

Neonates

Intrauterine infection may manifest in the neonate with skin vesicles or scarring and involvement of the eyes (e.g., chorioretinitis or optic atrophy) and brain (e.g., microcephaly or encephalomalacia). Clinical presentation of disseminated disease is similar to bacterial sepsis. Symptoms start approximately a week after birth and include poor feeding, lethargy, irritability, and seizures and may sometimes progress to shock with multiorgan failure. Herpetic lesions of the skin or mucosa are seen in 20%–30% cases and provide a clinical clue to diagnosis. In neonates with isolated encephalitis, the clinical symptomatology of encephalitis is similar to that of encephalitis with

disseminated disease; skin lesions are often seen after ~2 weeks of age.

Children

HSE in children generally presents acutely with fever, headache, vomiting, and focal seizures, followed within a few days by alteration in sensorium. Neck stiffness may occur in some cases. At times, preceding nonspecific influenza like symptoms of malaise, lethargy, or mild irritability may be present. Behavioral and personality changes and difficulty with speech may be noted in some children. Focal neurologic abnormalities develop in most cases, generally reflecting involvement of the temporal or frontal lobes. Raised ICP with papilledema, transtentorial herniation, and hemodynamic instability follows. Focal signs and personality changes may provide etiologic clues. HSE has no other specific clinical markers. Presence of herpetic skin lesions has no correlation with concurrent encephalitis. The course of HSE is generally rapid and may be fatal unless specific therapy is started early. Early diagnosis is therefore essential.

Differential Diagnosis

It may not be possible to differentiate HSE from other causes of encephalitis on the basis of clinical features alone. Comparison of positive versus negative findings in brain biopsies revealed that most of the "positive" cases presented with features of focal encephalitis. Presence of focal seizures and frontotemporal signs, including behavioral changes and speech difficulties, are clues but are not specific for HSE.

A number of conditions may mimic HSE, including other viral encephalitis, such as EEE, JE, western equine encephalitis, St. Louis encephalitis, EBV, and other viral infections. The differential diagnosis should also include bacterial and fungal infections (e.g., early brain abscess) and other infections, including tubercular, rickettsial, toxoplasma, and collagen vascular diseases.

Diagnosis

In the absence of skin lesions, making a clinical diagnosis of herpes is problematic (7), particularly in neonates. Swab cultures from conjunctiva, nasopharynx, and rectum may detect early infection. The MRI is not as helpful in neonates as in older children because of diffuse involvement and high brain-water content of the neonatal brain. PLEDS on EEG, if seen, add to the diagnosis but are not specific for herpes.

Laboratory Diagnosis

Identification of HSV in the CSF by PCR is a rapid, highly sensitive (95%) and specific (almost 100%) test that has become the gold standard for diagnosis of HSE. Antibodies to HSV in the CSF take a few days to develop; hence, immunologic tests to detect them are not helpful for early diagnosis of HSE. A fourfold rise in antibody titer over a few weeks may be helpful for a retrospective diagnosis. Antibodies in the CSF are not specific for HSE and, per se, are not helpful in diagnosis. Isolation of the virus from the CSF by culture is possible in less than half of cases with HSE. Identification of virus at sites other than

CSF by direct fluorescence antibody, PCR, or culture in the context of clinical symptomatology suggestive of encephalitis is adequate to make the diagnosis of HSE. CSF shows variable pleocytosis predominantly polymorphic in the first 24–48 hrs, followed by a lymphocytic response. RBCs may be seen secondary to the necrotizing nature of HSE; at times, the CSF may be xanthochromic. Mild elevation of protein with normal glucose levels is usually seen. As with all other encephalitides, in a small number of cases the CSF may be normal in the early phase of illness.

Characteristic EEG findings in HSE are aforementioned PLEDS, often seen arising from the involved temporal region. With progression of disease, they may spread to the other temporal lobe within a few days. PLEDS and/or focal temporal slowing were seen in 90% of PCR-positive patients at symptom onset, compared with only 30% of the PCR-negative group. Sensitivity of the EEG recordings decreases after 48 hrs (2). However, PLEDs may be seen in conditions other than HSE, such as other focal encephalitides, infarct, and hypoxic-ischemic injury.

Brain biopsy was once the most important diagnostic test for diagnosis of HSE when PCR and sophisticated neuroimaging facilities were not available. Currently, with a combination of MRI, CSF PCR, and EEG a diagnosis of HSE can be made with reasonable accuracy.

Neuroimaging

MRI is often the first diagnostic investigation, as LP may be contraindicated in children with raised ICP and focal signs. Involvement of inferofrontal and mediotemporal lobes with gyral swelling and cerebral edema is characteristic (**Fig. 80.3**). The MRI is much more sensitive than CT and detects changes earlier than CT in cases of HSE. If an MRI facility is not immediately available, a CT scan may be obtained. Low-density areas in a unilateral medial temporal lobe and insular cortex are seen. Small areas of hemorrhage may also be seen in these regions. The CT may appear normal in very early phases of the disease and abnormalities may be visible only after 4–5 days of illness.

Treatment

A child with suspected HSV should be managed on an urgent basis in the ICU with prompt administration of acyclovir. In children, 30 mg/kg/day divided every 8 hrs for 14–21 days is the treatment of choice, whereas for neonatal HSE, 60 mg/kg/day divided every 8 hrs for 21 days is recommended; negative PCR is often obtained prior to discontinuation of therapy. Oral acyclovir or valacyclovir prophylaxis for 3–6 months after neonatal infection has also been advocated by some experts to prevent relapses. Newer antiviral agents, such as famciclovir, ganciclovir, vidarabine, and foscarnet, have also been tried in HSE. No evidence suggests that any of these is better than acyclovir unless resistance is documented. Corticosteroid administration concurrent with acyclovir was a significant predictor of favorable outcome at 3 months after infection in a retrospective study of adults with HSE (18). However, the effectiveness of corticosteroids in HSE remains to be determined by prospective, randomized, controlled studies.

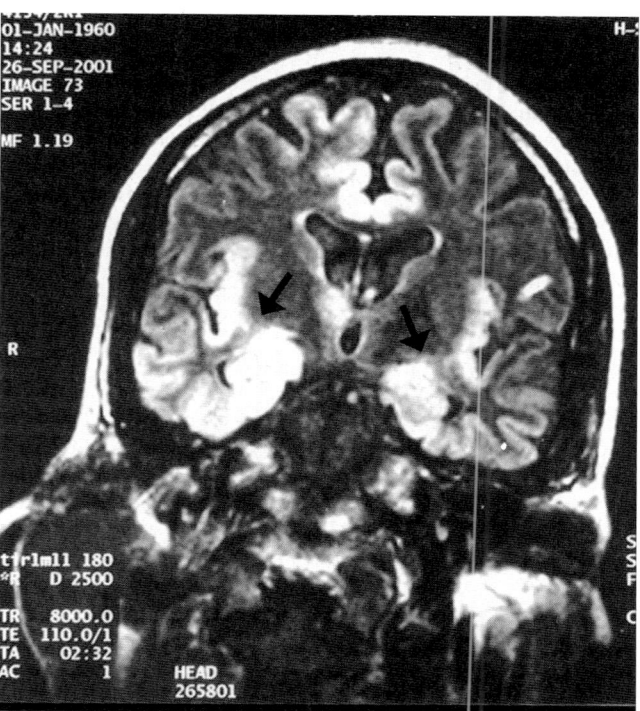

FIGURE 80.3. Coronal FLAIR-MRI showing hyperintense signal involving bilateral temporal lobes and cingulate gyri in a case of herpes encephalitis.

Prognosis

Early administration of acyclovir has considerably reduced the morbidity and mortality associated with HSE. Relapse of HSE has been documented in 12% of acyclovir-treated adult patients and is considered to be secondary to immunologically mediated pathogenicity (40). Outcome is poor in neonates with disseminated disease, with a 50% mortality rate and 50% of survivors with neurologic sequelae. Mortality is lower (~14%) in neonates with isolated encephalitis.

JAPANESE ENCEPHALITIS

JE is an important arthropod-borne encephalitis endemic in Asia, particularly India, Nepal, Philippines, Thailand, Cambodia, Vietnam, Myanmar, and some parts of China. Approximately 3 billion people live in endemic regions, and ~50,000 cases, with 10,000 deaths, reported annually. JE is the most common form of epidemic and sporadic encephalitis in the tropical region of Asia. The epidemics generally occur after the rainy season in rural areas with rice fields.

Etiology

The JE virus is an enveloped, single-stranded, RNA flavivirus that is antigenically related to St. Louis encephalitis virus, West Nile virus, and Murray Valley virus. It was first isolated in Japan in 1933 and contains several polypeptides encoded by a single, long, open-reading frame. Genomic sequencing of a number of isolates that originate from various geographic regions is known.

JE is a zoonotic disease maintained by a pig-mosquito-pig and bird-mosquito-bird cycle. Pigs and wild birds are the natural hosts of the virus. Pigs serve as amplifier hosts. Bats can also carry the virus for a long time. Humans are incidental dead-end hosts and acquire the disease by the bite of mosquitoes that have fed upon infected pigs and birds. The vector mosquitoes are generally *Culex* spp. and breed in rice fields and stagnant water.

Pathophysiology

Following a bite by an infected mosquito, the initial viral replication may occur in regional lymph nodes. The CNS involvement occurs via the hematogenous route. Viremia lasts for 4–5 days. The binding of JE virions to the cells in the CNS is possibly assisted by certain neurotransmitter receptors. Basal ganglia involvement is usually seen.

Clinical Presentation

JE affects mainly children and young adults. The incubation period is 5–15 days, and most infections are either asymptomatic or mildly symptomatic. JE infection that progresses to encephalitis often starts acutely with fever, headache, tiredness, nausea, vomiting, and diarrhea and progresses within a few days to confusion, irritability, and coma. The onset may be abrupt, with high fever, chills, and seizures, with rapid progression to altered sensorium and neurodeficits. Seizures occur in ~75% of children but are less common in adults. Meningism and headache are more common in adults than in children. Extrapyramidal signs, including mask-like facies, rigidity, tremor, and choreoathetosis, are seen in some cases. Dystonia is more common in children as compared to adults (17). Upper-motor neuron facial palsy occurs in ~10% of cases. In a small number of cases, the illness may start with flaccid paralysis of one or more limbs, generally the legs, with no loss of consciousness. Subsequently, altered sensorium may occur in approximately one-third of cases. Rise in ICP may occur and lead to cerebral herniation.

Differential Diagnosis

The differential diagnosis of JE is similar to that of other encephalitides. During an epidemic, JE should be suspected in any child with sudden onset fever and altered sensorium. The presence of extrapyramidal symptoms and signs in a child with encephalitis strongly suggests the diagnosis of JE. However, laboratory confirmation is essential.

Diagnosis

The diagnosis of JE is made based on clinical presentation, epidemiologic risk factors, and supporting laboratory data. If CSF can be obtained safely, lymphocytic pleocytosis with moderate elevation of protein and a normal glucose may be seen. The CSF may be acellular or show polymorphonuclear pre-

dominance in early stages. The virus can be isolated from the CSF by inoculating into 2–4-day-old mice or by infection of cell cultures. Viral antigens can be detected in the CSF by indirect immunofluorescence assay. Viral antibodies can be detected by rapid serologic assays, such as IgM-capture ELISA (MAC-ELISA) and IgG-ELISA. IgM is more specific early in infection and is positive in nearly all patients at ~7 days, IgG increases later in the course of illness. Monoclonal antibodies (mabs) have also been used for diagnosis, and real-time PCR for JE is available (16) but not yet routinely used. Virus detection in mosquitoes can also be analyzed by ELISA, and viral isolation can be done by insect bioassay. Diffuse slowing is commonly seen on EEG. Theta and delta coma, burst suppression, and, occasionally, epileptiform activity are suggestive.

Neuroimaging

CT scans show hypodense areas in the thalamus, basal ganglia, midbrain, and brainstem in approximately half of JE cases. MRI scans are more sensitive. Abnormal signals that are hypointense on T1-weighted and hyperintense on T2-weighted images that involve the thalami and basal ganglia bilaterally are characteristic (**Fig. 80.4**). The cerebral hemispheres and cerebellum may also show abnormal signals.

Treatment

Children with symptomatic JE are usually seriously ill and require urgent intensive and supportive care. No specific

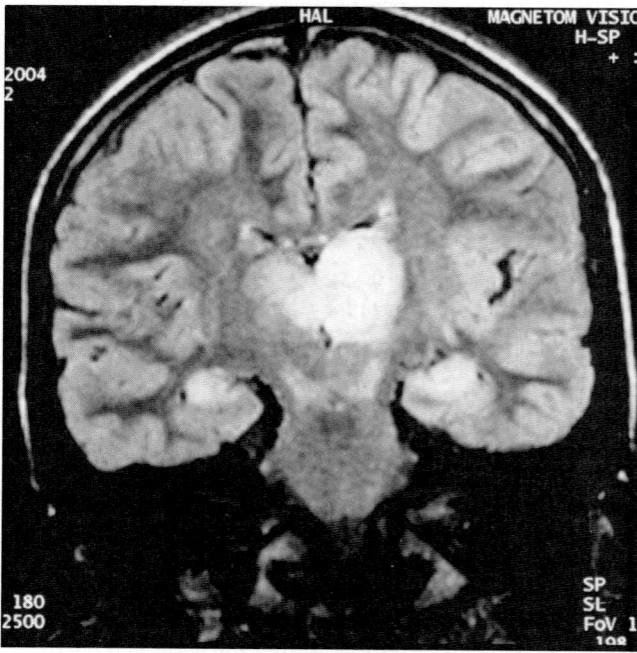

FIGURE 80.4. Coronal FLAIR-MRI showing bilateral hyperintense signal involving the hippocampus, thalamus, and midbrain in a case of Japanese encephalitis.

therapy exists for JE. Use of recombinant interferon is investigational.

Prognosis

Approximately 25%–30% cases are fatal and almost half of those who survive have residual neurologic sequelae. Focal neurologic deficits and altered sensorium at presentation have been correlated with neurologic sequelae.

Prevention and Control

Vaccination against JE is the most effective way of preventing epidemics. Currently a mouse-brain-derived, inactivated vaccine is being used and is recommended for people living in or traveling to endemic areas for >30 days. Three doses of the vaccine are generally advised; however, two doses have been found to be equally protective. A single dose may provide some protection and may be beneficial for countries with limited resources. A live, attenuated vaccine is also available and found to be effective. Use of vaccine has considerably reduced the number of JE cases in Japan, China, and Korea.

Mosquito control measures that employ larvicidal and adulticidal techniques have been used. Water management systems with alternate drying and wetting in rice fields and the use of neem-based products as fertilizers suppress the breeding of culicine vectors. Personal protective measures to reduce mosquito bites are important.

ACUTE DISSEMINATED ENCEPHALOMYELITIS

ADEM is an inflammatory demyelinating disorder of the CNS that usually follows infections or, less frequently, immunization. It is most frequently seen in children and young adults and is usually a monophasic illness; occasionally, it can be multiphasic, at which time it must be differentiated from MS (6). The common preceding infections are respiratory and gastrointestinal viral illnesses; however, ADEM has been reported following many viral and bacterial infections. Postimmunization encephalomyelitis occurs most commonly after measles, mumps, rubella, and rabies vaccination.

Pathogenesis

The essential feature of ADEM is an inflammatory patchy demyelination with preservation of axon cylinders, perivenular round cell inflammation, and prominence of microglial cells in the inflammatory exudate. The exact mechanism of the demyelination is incompletely understood because most patients with ADEM recover completely. It is mainly extrapolated from experimental allergic encephalomyelitis and is considered to occur secondary to immunodysregulation in susceptible individuals. T-helper cells become sensitized to autoantigens, such as myelin proteins, leading to a complex inflammatory cascade, with release of lymphokines and other mediators of inflammation, as well as disruption of the BBB. Typically, the subcortical

white matter is affected; sometimes additional gray matter lesions are seen.

Epidemiology

ADEM is increasingly being reported from both developed (20) and developing countries (32), possibly due to increased availability of MRI; however, an actual increase may also have occurred. ADEM is more common in the winter months. Typical cases of ADEM occur 5–20 days after an infectious illness or, sometimes, immunization. Risk factors are incompletely identified but may include genetic susceptibility, pathogen characteristics, immunization, and other factors. The overall annual incidence of ADEM is ~0.4/100,000 (20). The incidence of severe forms of ADEM (e.g., hemorrhagic encephalomyelitis) that may follow measles has diminished in developed countries because of widespread immunization.

Clinical Presentation

ADEM can occur at any age but is generally seen in young children. The mean age at presentation is ~7 years, with a slight male preponderance. Most cases have an acute meningoencephalitic presentation with fever, headache, and irritability, progressing rapidly to altered sensorium and, often, an abrupt multifocal neurodeficit (32). However, evolution of signs may occur over a few days in a small number of cases. Seizures are seen in ~25%–33% of cases and may be focal or generalized. A history of preceding infectious illness or immunization 1–3 weeks prior to the illness can be elicited in most but not all cases. Although any part of the CNS may be involved, the common sites include the white matter tracts, deep gray matter, spinal cord, and optic nerves. Hemiparesis or quadriparesis may be present. Ataxia is predominant in some cases and extrapyramidal symptoms, such as choreoathetosis or dystonia, may occur in others. In the affected limbs, the muscle tone is generally increased with increased stretch reflexes, upgoing plantar reflexes, and, at times, clonus. Predominant brainstem involvement may occasionally be seen. Simultaneous involvement of the spinal cord may present with a transverse myelitis-like presentation. When optic neuritis occurs, it is usually bilateral; however, involvement of the second eye may follow involvement of the first eye. Other cranial nerve palsies may also occur. Mental or psychiatric disturbances have also been reported. A fulminant presentation with rapid deterioration may occur in a few cases, particularly in children <3 years of age.

Differential Diagnosis

Because of the variability of presentation, a number of conditions may warrant consideration. It is important to exclude infectious meningoencephalitis by CSF examination in suspected cases. Characteristic neuroimaging and exclusion of other diagnoses are necessary to establish the diagnosis.

Diagnosis

A clinical definition of ADEM has recently been put forth by the Brighton collaboration of the Centers for Disease

Control and Prevention (http://www.brightoncollaboration.org/internet/en/index.html). One of three levels of diagnostic certainty may be established with the presence of encephalopathy or focal/multifocal CNS findings on MRI imaging that are consistent with ADEM. Relapse and alternate diagnoses detract from diagnostic certainty.

CSF may show pleocytosis or may be normal and is not helpful in making a diagnosis of ADEM. Red blood cells may be seen in cases of hemorrhagic encephalitis. Elevated CSF HSV or Lyme titers do not exclude the possibility of associated ADEM. Oligoclonal bands are positive in ~10% cases. CSF myelin basic protein concentration, reflecting demyelination, may be elevated. The EEG may show focal or generalized slowing and, at times, spikes or sharp waves or rhythmic δ activity. Elevation of WBC, platelet, CRP, and sedimentation rates may be seen occasionally.

Neuroimaging

The CT scan shows low-density abnormalities in approximately half of cases and is far less sensitive than MRI. The MRI scan is the diagnostic modality of choice. The lesions are best visualized on T2-weighted or proton density sequences. Multiple large confluent centrifugal white matter lesions seen generally at the junction of deep cortical gray and subcortical white matter are characteristic (**Fig. 80.5**). The lesions are generally patchy in distribution but may be fairly symmetric.

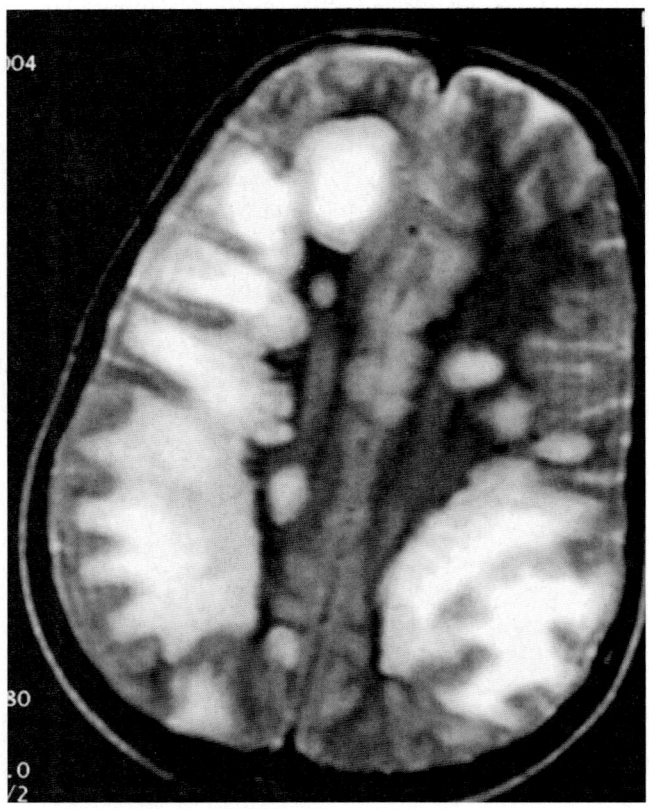

FIGURE 80.5. T2-weighted axial image showing large bilateral asymmetric areas of T2 white matter hyperintensities in ADEM.

Lesions may also be seen in deep gray matter, basal ganglia, and thalami in a third of cases. The brainstem, optic nerves, cerebellum, and spinal cord may also be involved. Periventricular and corpus callosum lesions are less common in childhood ADEM, as compared to MS. Gadolinium enhancement, which is typically uniform and usually not very dense, is variably seen. In fulminant cases, areas of hemorrhage may be seen. The lesions of ADEM are typical but not pathognomonic; variations in the character or distribution of lesions may occasionally be seen and necessitate differentiation from other conditions, such as HSV-2 encephalitis, Lyme disease, stroke, and MS. Ring enhancement of lesions or mass effect sometimes found in ADEM may suggest abscess, neurocysticercosis, or tumor. Certain features on MRI, such as large, ill-defined, subcortical white matter lesions, or involvement of deep gray matter sparing of corpus callosum, may help to differentiate the initial presentation of ADEM from MS (6). Rarely, the MRI may be normal on initial presentation and may show lesions characteristic of ADEM if repeated several weeks later, even though patients may be showing clinical improvement, suggesting that a normal initial scan does not necessarily exclude the diagnosis of ADEM and that the appearance of new lesions during recovery from ADEM may not necessarily represent worsening.

Other imaging methods, such as magnetization-transfer MRI, single-photon emission CT scanning, or nuclear MR spectroscopy, have been tried, but none is pathognomonic. Diagnosis of ADEM should be made on clinical grounds in conjunction with neuroimaging.

Treatment

The mainstay of treatment is IV methylprednisolone given in a dose 20–30 mg/kg/day for 3–5 days. Improvement may be observed in some cases within hours but usually occurs over several days. Generally, a taper of oral steroids for 3–6 weeks is used. Concern over treatment with steroids in light of HSE in the differential is occasionally raised. Currently, no evidence is convincing that the use of steroid in the context of HSV infection treated with acyclovir is harmful; clinical judgment regarding the most likely diagnosis must be used.

Plasmapheresis and IV immune globulin 2 g/kg/day for 2–3 days have also been used, especially in cases in which meningoencephalitis cannot be excluded and it is feared that corticosteroids might worsen the course of infection. To date, no evidence is convincing that treatment with a combination of IV corticosteroids and IV immune globulin is better than either modality alone.

Prognosis

Most children with a mild to moderate illness who receive appropriate therapy show good recovery. Acute mortality is rare. Fulminant cases, particularly in children <2 years, are at higher risk. Residual deficits are seen in approximately one-third of cases and include motor, visual, autonomic, and intellectual deficits, as well as epilepsy. Children with transverse myelitis may have residual bladder and bowel dysfunction and motor deficits. MRI lesions resolve slowly over a period of several months, and most disappear by 6 months (32). A small number of children may have recurrent ADEM during the taper of corticosteroid therapy. This condition usually responds to increasing the corticosteroid dose and prolonging the therapy. Others may have recurrent attacks of ADEM after complete clinical and radiologic recovery. These children often respond to a repeat course of methylprednisolone and oral steroids. Among those who have recurrence, most have a single attack of ADEM; some children may have two or three attacks in a year or two following the initial attack and then do not have further recurrences for several years. A very small number may have repeated recurrences, such that they cannot be weaned off of steroids. Nonsteroidal immunosuppressants have been tried in such cases. These patients do not manifest the immunologic changes of MS, but whether they represent an overlap between the two remains to be determined.

BRAIN AND SPINAL CORD ABSCESS

Abscess in the brain and spinal cord can occur as a primary event or, occasionally, as a complication of bacterial meningitis. Although uncommon in most developed countries, brain abscesses are not infrequently seen in developing countries. CNS abscesses are important to the intensivists, as they represent an eminently treatable form of serious, potentially fatal, localized CNS infection.

Etiology

The common pathogens include anaerobic bacteria, Gram-negative organisms, streptococci, and staphylococci. Many unusual aerobic and anaerobic organisms may also cause brain abscess. Except in neonates, where Gram-negative organisms (particularly *Citrobacter diversus, Enterobacter sakazakii,* and *Proteus mirabilis*) are the most common pathogens, the specific organism is determined mainly by the underlying cause of the brain abscess. In children with cyanotic heart disease, the most common organisms are the α-hemolytic streptococci. In cases with subacute bacterial endocarditis, streptococci and *S. aureus* are common. In posttraumatic cases, *S. aureus* is the most common pathogen. In children with otitis or sinusitis, anaerobic or aerobic streptococci, *Bacteroides fragilis, Proteus* spp., Pseudomonas, or *H. influenzae* spp. may be isolated. Polymicrobial involvement is seen in approximately a third of cases. In cases secondary to meningitis, the etiologic organisms are those that caused the meningitis.

Pathogenesis

Infection of the brain parenchyma may occur because of hematogenous spread or direct spread from an adjacent infected focus. Hematogenous spread may occur in any child with bacteremia but is common in children with predisposing factors. Cyanotic congenital heart disease, particularly tetralogy of Fallot, is the most common underlying condition. Polycythemia with increased blood viscosity possibly leads to microinfarcts, which make the cerebral parenchyma vulnerable to bacterial seeding. Chronic pulmonary infection, subacute bacterial endocarditis, and immunocompromised status are other predisposing factors. Direct spread of infection may occur from

chronic otitis, mastoiditis, a sinusitis, after penetrating trauma, and after neurosurgical procedures. Congenital defects such as dermal sinuses, epidermoid cysts, and encephaloceles, may become infected and rarely may lead to brain abscess or intramedullary abscess of the spinal cord (30). Brain abscess secondary to meningitis is rare if early appropriate therapy is initiated. However, in neonates and in children with Gram-negative meningitis, particularly with *Citrobacter, Enterobacter,* and *Proteus* infections, brain abscess is not uncommon.

Following hematogenous infection, the pathogens localize, generally at the gray-white matter junction in the brain, and cause cerebritis. Poor vascular supply in the white matter and at the gray-white interface allows organisms to affect these areas. The inflammation and edema progress over a few days to weeks, leading to central necrosis with formation of a surrounding capsule of inflammatory granulation tissue. This progression occurs in four stages. The first stage of "early cerebritis" consists of leukocytic infiltration and focal brain edema, not clearly demarcated from normal brain parenchyma. This stage lasts 1–3 days and is followed by "late cerebritis," in which central liquefaction necrosis is surrounded by an area of neovascularization and fibroblastic infiltration, forming an ill-defined beginning of a capsule. This phase lasts from day 4 to day 9 and is followed by a phase of early capsule formation. The necrotic center shrinks, and the fibroblastic capsule becomes well formed. The fourth phase is late capsule formation, in which a dense fibrous capsule is surrounded by reactive astrocytes and glial cells, marked edema, and neovascularization. This phase generally occurs after 2 weeks of infection. Progression from the onset of early focal cerebritis to late capsule formation may take from 4–6 weeks. In some cases, however, the progression may be rapid and rupture of the abscess may occur into the ventricular system.

Although most often seen in the cerebral hemisphere, brain abscesses may occur in the cerebellum as well as in the brainstem. In the cerebral hemispheres, the distribution of abscess in the frontal, parietal, and temporal lobes is almost equal. The site of abscess is often determined by the etiologic factors. Abscesses secondary to ear infection are located generally in the unilateral temporal lobe or cerebellum, and those following sinusitis are located in the frontal lobe. In children with cyanotic heart disease, abscesses are generally seen in the distribution of the middle carotid artery. Intramedullary abscess of the spinal cord is seen at the site of an anatomic spinal defect in the majority of patients. Hematogenous spread from a urogenital, gastrointestinal, or other source can also occur. The abscess may be solitary or multiple. Multiple abscesses are particularly seen in infections with Gram-negative organisms and *S. aureus* and in neonates.

Clinical Presentation

The presentation is generally subacute, with fever, headache, vomiting, altered sensorium, seizures, and focal neurodeficits. However, the classic triad of fever, headache, and vomiting seen in adults is seen in only half of childhood cases. Seizures may be focal or generalized and are seen in almost half of cases. A bulging fontanelle and increasing head size may be seen in infants, and neck rigidity may be seen in older children. Papilledema, sixth-nerve palsy, and occasionally, cerebral herniation syndromes may occur secondary to raised ICP. Focal deficits are determined by the site of the abscess but may not necessarily be seen, especially in neonates and young infants. Meningismus, pyramidal signs, and cranial nerve palsies are often associated with a brainstem abscess. Hydrocephalus may develop due to mass effect. Occasionally, the presentation may be acute or even abrupt if the abscess ruptures in the ventricles or if hemorrhage occurs in the abscess cavity.

Diagnosis

A high index of suspicion is essential, particularly in children with high risk factors. The differential diagnosis includes neoplasms, focal encephalitis, subdural hematoma, and other mass lesions. An LP is often contraindicated in a child with brain abscess because of the risk of cerebral herniation. Examination of the CSF is not required for making a diagnosis in cases with typical neuroimaging findings. Occasionally, in carefully considered cases, in which doubt in diagnosis remains even after neuroimaging, an LP may be performed. The CSF is generally under pressure and shows a mild-to-moderate pleocytosis, elevation of protein, and normal glucose. In some cases, it is possible that no cells are seen. Marked pleocytosis (in thousands/mm^3) may be seen if the abscess has ruptured into the ventricles, as may occur in some neonates. Gram stain and culture are generally negative, unless the abscess has ruptured.

Confirmation of the etiologic organism is achieved by aspiration of the abscess and analysis and culture of the aspirated contents. Other sources of organism identification, such as blood culture or aspiration from sinuses or mastoids, should also be considered. The EEG may show focal slowing or, occasionally, spikes over the region of the abscess. Periodic lateralizing discharges or diffuse slowing may also be seen. The EEG may be normal in some cases.

Neuroimaging

A CT scan or MRI with contrast is warranted in all suspected cases. Contrast-enhanced CT scan shows a characteristic ring-enhancing lesion with central hypodensity and surrounding edema in a mature abscess (**Fig. 80.6**). In early cases of cerebritis, the ring enhancement may be incomplete. Mass effect with midline shift may be seen. The MRI is more sensitive than CT in diagnosis of cerebritis. Rarely, a radionuclide ^{99m}TC-pertechnetate scan may be necessary to identify early focal cerebritis. In countries where TB is endemic, a pyogenic abscess must be differentiated from a tubercular abscess. Tubercular abscesses are generally seen at the base of the brain, especially in the cerebellum (**Fig. 80.7**). MR spectroscopy may sometimes be necessary to differentiate an abscess from a neoplasm.

Treatment

Antibiotic therapy with surgical drainage or excision of the abscess is required in most cases. In children, aspiration

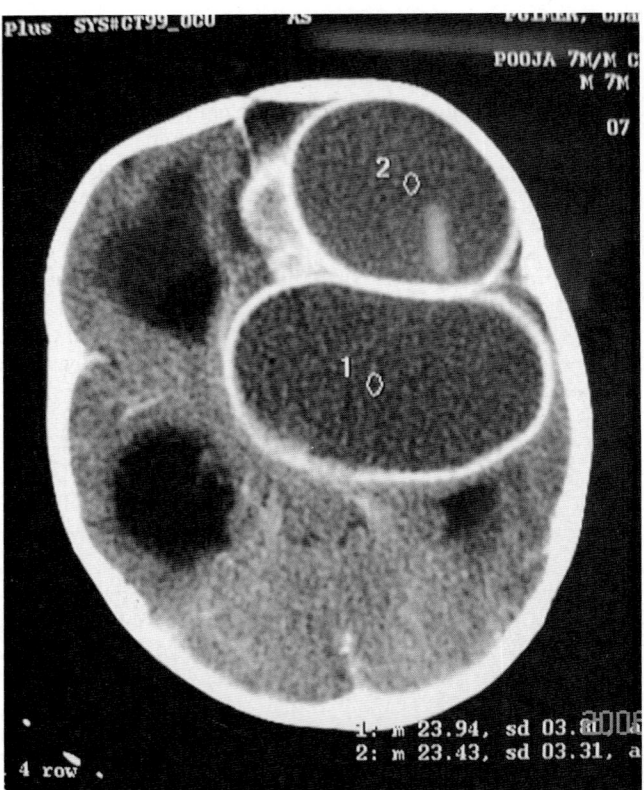

FIGURE 80.6. Contrast-enhanced CT showing multiple staphylococcal brain abscesses with ring enhancement and midline shift.

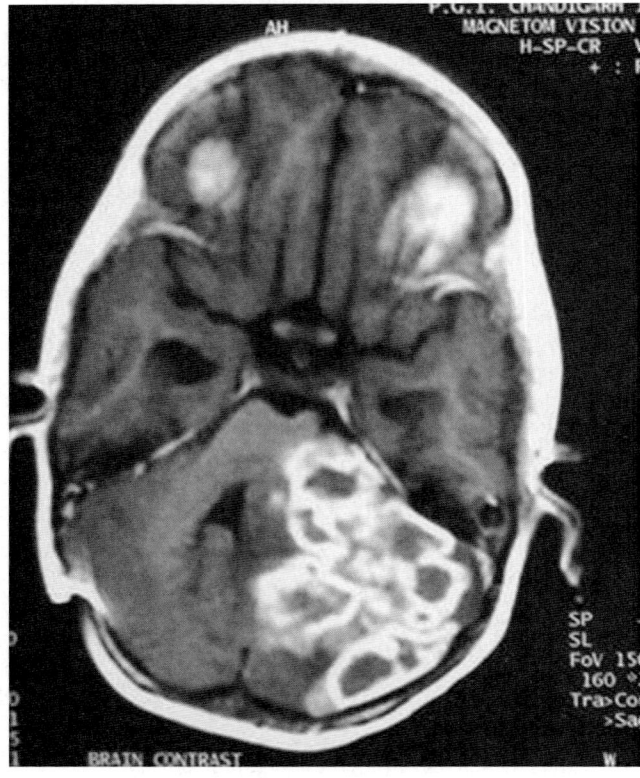

FIGURE 80.7. Contrast MRI showing multiple, conglomerate tubercular abscesses with thick, enhancing, irregular margins and surrounding edema in the cerebellum.

under CT guidance is used more frequently because of the low mortality and morbidity associated with the procedure. Multiple aspirations are often required. Excision is undertaken if no clinical improvement ensues despite multiple aspirations and antibiotics. Very small abscesses or those in critical areas of the brain may be managed with medical treatment alone. The choice of antibiotics depends upon the suspected causative organism. Empiric antibiotic therapy before organism identification typically consists of a broad-spectrum combination of agents to cover anaerobic, Gram-negative, and staphylococcal species. Cefotaxime or any other third- or fourth-generation cephalosporin with metronidazole is generally used. If *S. aureus* is suspected or identified, vancomycin should be added. It may be modified according to the underlying predisposing condition and the immune status of the child. Definitive antibiotic therapy is dictated by the organism identified. IV antibiotics in highest doses are required for at least 6 weeks in most cases. Corticosteroids given IV at presentation help to reduce cerebral edema and raised ICP. The fear that they may reduce penetration of antibiotics in the abscess cavity has not been substantiated. Follow-up scans are done periodically after surgical drainage/excision to determine the response.

Prognosis

Mortality is high in newborns and young infants and in children with multiple large abscesses and cyanotic heart disease; children with intramedullary abscess of the spinal cord have higher morbidity than children with subdural abscesses, epidural abscesses, or adults. Rupture of brain abscess into the ventricular system can be a life-threatening event unless managed immediately and aggressively. Outcome is poor in cases with low Glasgow Coma Scale score, Gram-negative organisms, and associated sepsis (43). Intramedullary abscess of the spinal cord can result in necrosis of the spinal cord, resulting in permanent neurologic deficit. Brain and spinal cord abscesses, if detected late, are associated with significant neuromorbidity. The residual deficits depend on the site of the abscess and may include hemiparesis, cranial nerve palsies, cognitive deficits, and epilepsy. Increasing availability of imaging procedures has helped in early identification and better management of brain and spinal cord abscesses and has led to significant decrease in mortality and morbidity. Early decompression is associated with improved outcome.

SUBDURAL EMPYEMA

Subdural empyema is a suppurative collection in the subdural space. It is an important focal intracranial infection that is often a complication of acute bacterial meningitis and may require early intensive management.

Etiology

In children in whom subdural empyema is a complication of meningitis, the organisms are those that cause meningitis. In others, the organisms are similar to those that cause brain abscess.

Pathogenesis

Spread of infection to the subdural space may occur either as a complication of meningitis or, occasionally, by direct spread from infected sinuses or otitis media, osteomyelitis of skull bones, or head trauma. The emissary veins that traverse the subdural space become infected, and as the subdural space is not limited by attachment, pus collection can be large. Most subdural collections are seen over the cerebral hemispheres, but some may involve the parafalcine region. The majority of subdural empyemas are unilateral; infants may have bilateral involvement. Large collections behave like space-occupying lesions and may cause dangerous elevations of ICP and extensive involvement of brain parenchyma.

Clinical Presentation

The onset is subacute, with fever, headache, vomiting, and, often, seizures. Neck rigidity and focal signs may be present. Infants present with poor feeding, irritability, fever, full fontanelle, and an enlarging head. Persistent or recurrent fever in a child who has bacterial meningitis with focal seizures or other focal neurologic signs suggests a subdural empyema.

Diagnosis

The diagnosis of a subdural empyema is made by neuroimaging. A contrast-enhanced, crescent-shaped, hypodense lesion, at times with loculations, is characteristic. The enhancement is generally linear, along the dura; at times enhancement of underlying brain parenchyma may also be seen (**Fig. 80.1**). MRI is more sensitive than CT for detecting small collections and for differentiating from cerebritis and thrombosis. The density difference of the collection can distinguish sterile from purulent collections. Purulent collections are hyperintense to the CSF in both T1- and T2-weighted images.

Analysis of the subdural fluid obtained by subdural tap or surgical drainage reveals a purulent fluid with marked leukocytosis. Organism identification can be performed by Gram stain and culture. An LP is often contraindicated. Peripheral blood leukocytosis is not specific.

Treatment

Removal of the purulent collection and IV administration of appropriate antibiotic therapy in high doses for 3–6 weeks in warranted. Antibiotics are chosen according to the suspected source of infection. Surgical removal of an adjacent source of infection, such as chronic otitis media or osteomyelitis, is also necessary. Repeat scans are required periodically to assess the possibility of reaccumulation and to monitor the course. Supportive therapy is provided on the same principles as for meningitis or brain abscess.

Prognosis

The morbidity and mortality associated with subdural empyema has declined significantly with the use of early appropriate medical and surgical intervention. Common residual deficits after large subdural empyemas include hemiparesis and focal seizures.

EPIDURAL ABSCESS

A cranial epidural abscess is a collection of suppurative material between the dura and the cranium. Spinal epidural abscesses also occur, although not commonly in children.

Etiology

The common causative organisms include staphylococci, streptococci, and some anaerobic organisms, such as *Bacteroides fragilis*. In spinal epidural abscesses, *S. aureus* is the most common organism. Other organisms, such as pneumococci, streptococci, and salmonellae, may be responsible in some cases. The spread of infection is usually hematogenous but may occasionally occur by local spread of an adjacent infection or secondary to spinal trauma. Over half of spinal epidural abscesses are located in the thoracic or lumbar regions, often on the posterior aspect of the cord.

Pathophysiology

In the case of cranial epidural abscess formation, the pathogens enter the extradural space either by direct spread from a contiguous site of infection or secondary to trauma or a neurosurgical procedure. In spinal epidural abscesses, the spread of infection is usually hematogenous. Progression of inflammation leads to spinal cord ischemia and even infarction. Inflammation of blood vessels causes vasculitis and venothrombophlebitis; increase in size of abscess causes spinal compression. A combination of these factors causes ensuing spinal dysfunction.

Clinical Presentation

Children with a cranial epidural abscess present with fever, headache, vomiting, neck rigidity, focal seizures, and focal neurodeficits, including hemiparesis. Children with spinal epidural abscess present with fever, back pain, and symptoms and signs of spinal cord compression. Localized tender swelling may be found at the site of the pain. Progression may lead to bladder and bowel involvement. A sensory level may be seen in late cases. The rate of progression is variable; generally, an interval of few days passes from the onset of symptoms to complete paraplegia. However, in some cases the child may be paralyzed within hours, resembling acute transverse myelitis. In infants, the initial presentation may be nonspecific and similar to sepsis, resulting in late detection after deficits have already occurred.

Diagnosis

An LP is contraindicated, as it is associated with risk of accidentally spreading infection to the CSF and spinal herniation in cases of complete spinal block. If done, CSF may show leukocytosis, elevated protein, and hypoglycorrhachia. As with sub-

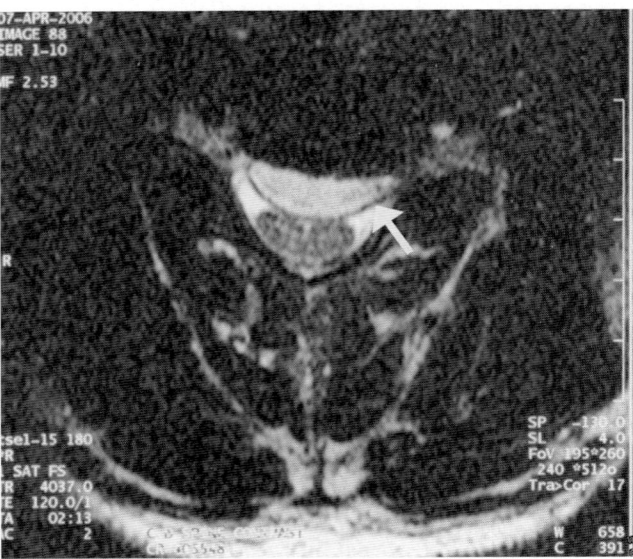

FIGURE 80.8. Contrast MRI at the cervical level showing a well-defined hyperintense extradural collection in the spinal canal, causing cord compression.

dural abscesses, the diagnosis of epidural abscess is made by neuroimaging. MRI is more sensitive than CT and shows an enhancing lenticular collection between the dura and the cranium or the cord (**Fig. 80.8**). If spinal epidural abscess is suspected, the entire spine should be scanned, as multiple abscesses may be present. Plain radiographs of the spine and contrast myelography have no role in diagnosis.

Treatment

Treatment involves surgical drainage, appropriate antibiotics, and supportive management. As *S. aureus* is a common pathogen, the initial antibiotic therapy consists of a combination of antibiotics to cover staphylococci and Gram-negative organisms. Once the abscess is drained and the organism identified, the appropriate antibiotic therapy is administered IV for 4–6 weeks. No scientific evidence supports the use of corticosteroids.

Prognosis

Early appropriate management has lead to a significant decrease in mortality and morbidity. The outcome is determined by the severity of neurodeficits, particularly paralysis, at the time of presentation. As with intramedullary and subdural abscesses, the urgency with which decompression is accomplished is critical. Paralysis for >36 hrs before intervention is associated with a poor prognosis. Complete recovery may be expected in children who do not have paralysis at presentation.

CERBROSPINAL FLUID SHUNT INFECTION

CSF shunts are placed by neurosurgeons to relieve pressure from CSF accumulation and brain parenchymal displacement when hydrocephalus is present. CSF shunts may direct CSF from the ventricles to the peritoneum (ventriculoperitoneal), atrium (ventriculoatrial), or to the outside world (externalized). Ventriculoperitoneal shunts are the most common.

Etiology

More than two-thirds of all shunt infections are caused by staphylococcal species. In a number of series, *Staphylococcus epidermidis* has been most frequently isolated (45), whereas in others, *S. aureus* and other coagulase-negative staphylococci have predominated. Gram-negative enteric organisms, usually *E. coli*, *Klebsiella*, *Proteus*, and *Pseudomonas* species are responsible for 6%–20% of infections. Streptococcal species are found in 8%–10% of infections. Multiple organisms are cultured in 10%–15% of infections. The traditional meningitic pathogens (*H. influenzae*, *Streptococcus pneumoniae*, *Neisseria meningitidis*) have been described in 5% of shunt infections. Other less common organisms, such as fungi and commensal microbes (e.g., diphtheroids) may rarely be responsible.

Epidemiology

The incidence of shunt infection has declined over the years to <4%. Several factors, including more refined shunt materials, improvement in operating room facilities and surgical techniques, pretreatment of shunt assembly in bacitracin solution, and a reduction in preshunting invasive studies (e.g., pneumoencephalography), are some of the factors responsible. Shunt infections generally occur in a bimodal distribution from the time of last shunt surgery. Almost, 70%–85% of the infections occur within 6 months of surgery. The second peak of infections occurs after 12 months.

Pathogenesis

Shunt devices act as foreign bodies and interfere with natural host defense mechanisms, such as chemotaxis and phagocytosis. Shunt catheters have been shown in vitro to decrease the motility of neutrophils, hindering their ability to phagocytose bacteria in effective numbers. In addition, staphylococci form an extracellular mucoid biofilm called "slime," which increases bacterial adherence to the shunt and decreases susceptibility to antibiotics. Shunt infection is more common in infants <6 months of age at the time of surgery, most likely because of a relatively deficient immune response to bacterial infection or a higher skin bacterial density. Shunts may become infected by several mechanisms: colonization at the time of surgery; breakdown of the surgical wound or of the skin that overlies the shunt, which allows direct access of microbes to the shunt; retrograde infection from the distal end through transluminal passage of bacteria; and hematogenous seeding and infection of CSF shunts, which occurs infrequently.

Clinical Presentation

Most children present with fever, headache, vomiting, lethargy, irritability, and change in mental status. Occasionally, seizures,

cranial nerve palsies, visual deficits, and neck rigidity may be seen. The classic symptoms of infection, such as fever and pain, may be absent in some cases. The infected intact surgical wound or cellulitis along the shunt may be associated with local pain and erythema. Infection of the proximal end may result in meningitis or ventriculitis in ~30% cases; however, intracranial empyemas and abscesses are rarely seen. Spread of infection to the distal end may cause peritonitis with abdominal pain and distension.

Diagnosis

A high degree of suspicion for infection helps in early diagnosis. The prerequisites for a diagnostic label of shunt infection are no meningitis/ventriculitis and a sterile CSF culture at the time of shunt placement, shunt in place for at least 24 hrs, and a positive CSF culture obtained from the shunt/LP. The gold standard for diagnosis of shunt infection is the isolation of organism from culture of the shunt or of the fluid in contact with it. The risk of infection after a single diagnostic shunt tap appears to be low, and obtained CSF can be evaluated for infection. A high WBC count in the CSF is highly correlated, but sometimes the CSF counts may be normal. CSF glucose may be low or normal; CSF protein levels are typically not raised. Certain patients, even in the absence of infection, may have an elevated CSF white count, generally eosinophilic, probably due to a hypersensitive reaction to the presence of shunt tubing. A positive CSF Gram stain and culture are diagnostic and extremely important in deciding the course of treatment. Culture of CSF obtained from the shunt more often identifies the causative organism, as compared with CSF from the LP or ventricular tap. Antibiotic administration before obtaining CSF decreases the yield. The peripheral WBC count and blood cultures are usually not helpful. Ultrasonography in neonates and young infants may show ventriculitis or a "CSFoma," which strongly suggest infection. A CT scan or MRI is useful if early postoperative scans are available for comparison. An increase in ventricular size because of associated shunt malfunction is often seen. Patients with infection of the distal end may show abdominal pseudocysts around the shunt.

Treatment

Various management regimens have been used, but a combination of antibiotics, shunt removal, and external drainage is perhaps most effective. Some authors recommend shunt removal only if the infection is severe or nonresponsive to antibiotics. Ventriculitis associated with shunt infection appears to clear more quickly with external drainage. The drainage tube should be changed every few days and placed preferably at different sites to avoid repeated discharge of organisms due to colonization of drainage tube lying in the infected ventricle. External drainage provides access to CSF, which can be examined daily to help monitor infection and allows administration of intraventricular antibiotics. The antibiotics used for staphylococcal coverage include cloxacillin or vancomycin, often in conjunction with aminoglycosides. Rifampicin can be added to augment the therapy. Third-generation cephalosporins and aminoglycosides can be used for Gram-negative bacteria. Because it is bacteriostatic, chloramphenicol is not recommended in the treatment of shunt infections. Intraventricular therapy with vancomycin and aminoglycosides (gentamicin, amikacin, and netilmicin) has also been used; whether this is more effective than IV therapy alone is not established. The duration of therapy is dependent on the organism isolated, the extent of infection as determined by cultures obtained after externalization and CSF chemistries, and cell count. Generally, 2–3 weeks of therapy are required; once the CSF is sterile for several consecutive days, a new shunt is inserted.

Prevention

Use of prophylactic antibiotics before and after surgery helps in reducing subsequent shunt infection if infection rates at an institution are higher than 5%. However, centers vary in their practice.

FUNGAL INFECTIONS OF THE CENTRAL NERVOUS SYSTEM

Most patients with a fungal infection of the CNS have some predisposing deficiency in immune response, very often caused by neutropenia, lymphoreticular malignancy, lymphoma, malnutrition, use of immunosuppressive drugs, potent broad-spectrum antibiotic therapy, or acquired immunodeficiency syndrome (AIDS) due to HIV. Direct inoculation may occur during neurosurgical procedures, such as ventriculoperitoneal shunt placement, or following head injury.

Etiology

The large number of fungi that can infect the CNS can be divided into those that can cause disease in a healthy host (*Cryptococcus, Histoplasma, Blastomyces, Coccidioides immitis, Sporothrix* spp., etc.) and those that cause opportunistic infection in immunocompromised host (*Candida* spp. *Aspergillus* spp., Zygomycetes, and *Trichosporon* spp). In recent times, opportunistic fungal infections in immunologically compromised hosts have increased worldwide. The fungal infections that may be suspected according to underlying predisposing factors are shown in **Table 80.11**.

Epidemiology

The true incidence of fungal CNS infection is unknown. *Candida* and *Aspergillus* spp. are ubiquitous and disseminate from endogenous sources. *Candida neoformans,* an encapsulated yeast, is an environmental fungus and is found in soil and bird droppings. The incidence of cryptococcal meningitis has risen with the increased prevalence of HIV infection, and is currently estimated at ~1 per 100,000. Of the varieties of *C. neoformans,* variety *grubii,* having type A serotype, and variety *neoformans,* having type D serotype, are worldwide in distribution, while variety *gatti* has BC serotypes and is found in tropical and subtropical regions (Australia, Southeast Asia, central Africa, and California), particularly on flowering eucalyptus trees. *Coccidioides, Histoplasma,* and *Blastomycosis* have been reported in

TABLE 80.11

FUNGAL INFECTIONS THAT MAY BE SUSPECTED IN PRESENCE OF VARIOUS PREDISPOSING FACTORS

Predisposing factor	Fungi most likely to cause infection
Prematurity	*Candida albicans*
Primary immunodeficiency (e.g., CGD, SCID)	*Candida, Cryptococcus, Aspergillus*
Corticosteroids	*Cryptococcus, Candida*
Cytotoxic agents	*Aspergillus, Candida*
Secondary immunodeficiency (e.g., AIDS)	*Cryptococcus, Histoplasma*
Iron chelator therapy	Zygomycetes
Intravenous drug abuse	*Candida,* Zygomycetes
Ketoacidosis, renal acidosis	Zygomycetes (*Mucor*)
Trauma, foreign body	*Candida*

CGD, chronic granulomatous disease; SCID, severe combined immunodeficiency; AIDS, acquired immunodeficiency syndrome

different parts of US. Zygomycetes and *Trichosporon* also have a ubiquitous distribution (**Table 80.12**).

Pathogenesis

With the exception of mucormycosis, the primary site of infection is usually in the lungs and rarely in skin, from which hematogenous spread occurs to the CNS (**Table 80.12**). Pulmonary infection occurs from inhalation of fungal particles (yeast or basidiospores of *cryptococci,* arthroconidia of *coccidioidosis,* and spores of *Histoplasma* and *Blastomycosis*). The pulmonary infection often remains subclinical or asymptomatic. Sometimes, it may cause pneumonia of varying severity, including diffuse interstitial pneumonia in immunocompromised patients. Dissemination from lung is rare in *Coccidioides* and *Histoplasma. Blastomycosis* causes a granulomatous lung lesion, which may disseminate in up to one-third of patients and involve the CNS.

Zygomyces (*Mucor* spp.) spread directly into the CNS from paranasal sinuses through tissue planes and blood vessels; *Aspergillus* may also spread through this route. *Candida* and *Aspergillus* spread to the CNS primarily through the hematogenous route. Direct inoculation of *Candida* may occur during head injury or neurosurgical procedure, such as ventriculostomy and ventriculoperitoneal shunt placement. Rarely, direct spread occurs from osteomyelitis of skull or vertebrae.

Pathology

Clinical manifestations may be due to meningitis, meningoencephalitis, or focal lesion infarction and abscess. Fungal meningitis predominantly involves the base of the brain. *Coccidioides immitis* causes widespread basal meningitis. *Candida* occasionally causes meningitis. *Cryptococcus neoformans,* when disseminated, may involve the CNS in up to 90% of cases, causing infection of the subarachnoid space. The basic lesion is a combination of suppurative and granulomatous inflammation. The chronic inflammatory response leads to thickening

TABLE 80.12

GEOGRAPHIC DISTRIBUTION, PREDISPOSING HOST CHARACTERISTICS, PRIMARY PATHOGENIC MECHANISM AND PREDOMINANT CLINICAL SYNDROME OF VARIOUS FUNGAL CENTRAL NERVOUS SYSTEM INFECTIONS

Fungus	Distribution	Primary pathogenesis	Predisposing host characteristics	Usual clinical syndrome
1. *Cryptococcus neoformans* variety *neoformans*, variety *gatti*, variety *grubii*	Worldwide Common in Australia, Southeast Asia, Central Africa, California.	Pulmonary infection from inhalation of small yeast (basidiospore) Dissemination involves CNS in 30%–50%; often meningitis	Impaired cell-mediated immunity	Meningitis Meningoencephalitis Cryptococcoma
2. Coccidioides (*C. immitis*)	South and Central America, Southern US Occasional	Pulmonary infection from inhalation of arthroconidia. Dissemination in 0.2%; Up to 30% have meningitis; Also involves thoracic and lumber spine	Impaired cell-mediated immunity	Meningitis
3. Histoplasma (*H. capsulatum*)	Parts of US Rare	Inhalation of spores, dissemination rare; of these, 10%–25% have CNS infection, more in patients with AIDS	Impaired cell-mediated immunity	Meningitis
4. Blastomycosis (*B. dermatitidis*)	Parts of US Rare	Inhalation of spores from soil leads to primary granulomatous lesion of lung, skin: Dissemination in up to one-third of patients.	No prominent risk factor or immune defect	Meningitis
5. Candida (*C. albicans, C. tropicalis,* & others)	Normal flora of body Common	Pulmonary or GI primary, Hematogenous dissemination, CNS involvement in 50% with dissemination; most often leads to meningitis in infants. Direct inoculation via trauma, VP shunt placement, indwelling catheter	Patients with impaired cell-mediated immunity, neutropenia, prematurity, broad-spectrum antibiotics, corticosteroid therapy, hyperalimentation, malignancy, indwelling catheters, diabetes, abdominal surgery, thermal injury	Meningitis commonly, Abscess
6. Aspergillus (*A. fumigatus, A. flavus, A. terreus*)	Ubiquitous Occasional	Hematogenous spread in immunocompromised host from pulmonary primary. Direct extension from paranasal sinus or following head trauma. Surgery	Immunocompromised host (graft-versus-host disease, neutropenia)	Infarct, Abscess
7. Zygomycosis (*Mucor*)	Ubiquitous Infection only in immunocompromised occasional	Direct extension to CNS from nasal or paranasal sinuses through tissue plains leading to rhinocerebral disease. Hematogenous, rarely. Angioinvasive, causes cerebrovascular occlusion and infarction.	Diabetes, diabetic ketoacidosis, Immunosuppressive therapy, IV drug users, malignancy, deferoxamine chelation therapy, renal acidosis.	Infarct, Abscess

CNS, central nervous system; AIDS, acquired immune deficiency syndrome; VP, ventriculoperitoneal

of meninges, hydrocephalus, arteritis, cranial nerve palsies, and infarction. *Cryptococcus neoformans* and *Candida* often cause meningoencephalitis. In cryptococcosis, clusters of organisms spread through the brain, with little or no surrounding inflammatory responses, predominantly involving basal ganglia and cortical grey matter. The typical cystic lesion contains gelatinous polysaccharide, which can be detected in CSF. *Aspergillus,*

Zygomycetes, Blastomyces, and candidiasis cause focal lesions. Disseminated candidiasis, especially *C. albicans*, and *C. tropicalis*, and disseminated aspergillosis (**Fig. 80.9 A,B**) produce microabscesses. Vasculitis predisposes to infarction and hemorrhage. *Aspergillus* (all species—*A. fumigatus, A. flavus, A. terreus*) is the most common cause of CNS focal infections in organ-transplant recipients.

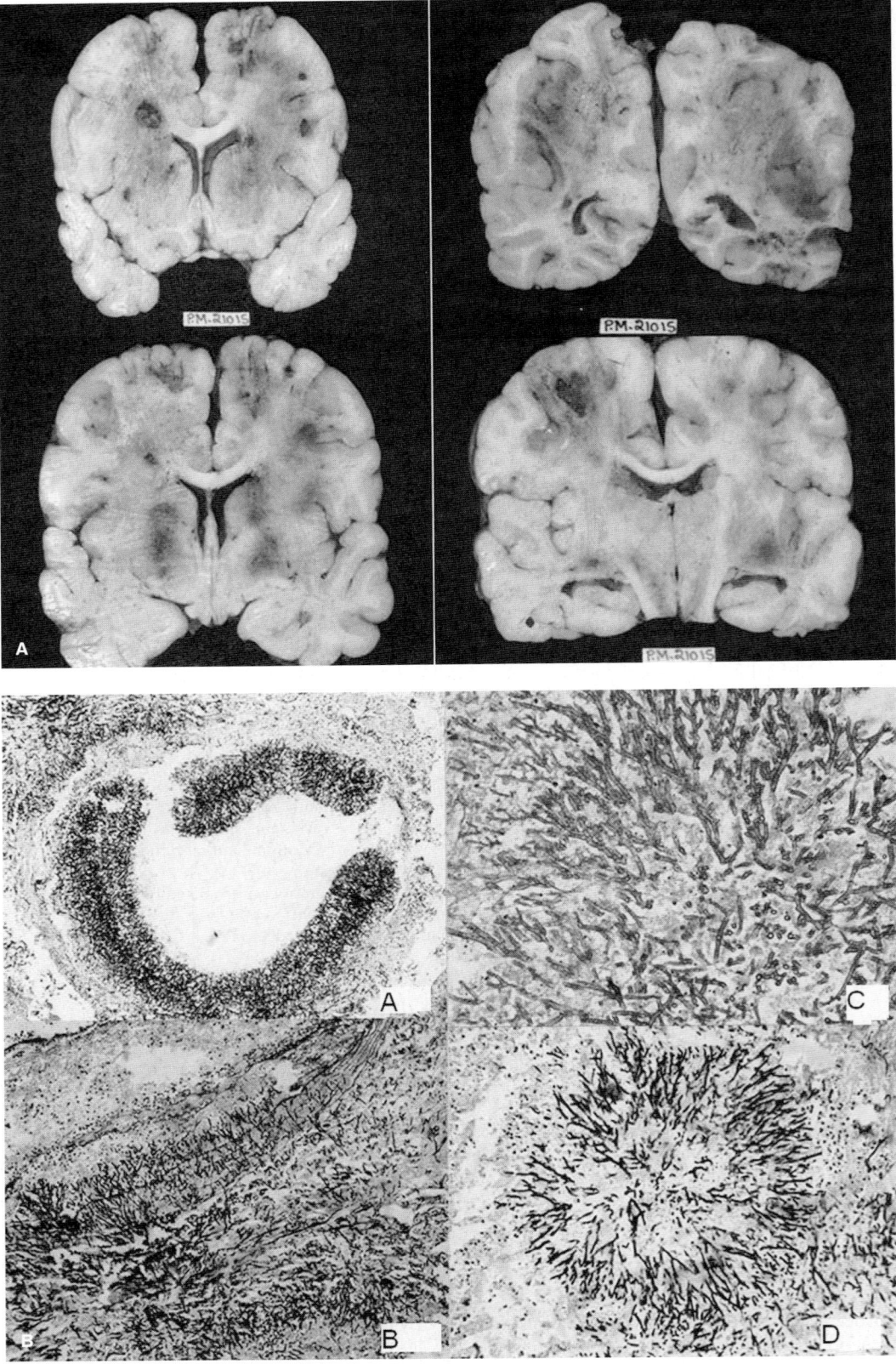

FIGURE 80.9. A: Cut sections of the brain showing multiple necrotic lesions caused by *Aspergillus* in a child with disseminated aspergillosis. **B:** Histopathology showing (*A*) ulcerated bronchial mucosa with many fungal hyphae (GMS stain), (*B*) invasion of vessel wall by fungal hyphae, and centrifugal spread with acute angle dichotomous branching of *Aspergillus hyphae*, as seen with PAS stain (*C*) and GMS stain (*D*).

Clinical Features

These infections have no pathognomonic signs and symptoms. However, some characteristic clinical features, such as new-onset seizures and insidious onset may help. The literature contains many reports of patients who presented with new-onset seizures and deteriorated or died before a fungal cause was diagnosed. Fungal infection should be included in the differential diagnosis of new-onset seizures, especially when associated with predisposing factors.

FUNGAL MENINGITIS

The common causes are *C. neoformans*, *C. immitis*, *Candida*, and *Aspergillus*. Clinical manifestations of fungal meningitis are less stereotyped than the manifestations of bacterial meningitis (5). Cryptococcal meningitis is often acute or subacute in HIV-infected children (14) and in those with T-cell suppression. Patients usually present with some combination of fever, headache, lethargy, nausea, vomiting, neck rigidity, impaired mental status, convulsion, and focal neurologic deficits (14). Raised ICP may develop acutely or during progression of the disease. Severe symptoms and signs may develop within days in patients with cryptococcal meningitis who are receiving high-dose corticosteroid therapy or in those with HIV infection. Fungal meningitis should always be a consideration in the differential diagnosis of a patient with a subacute or chronic meningitis syndrome (26).

Rhinocerebral syndrome is a major presentation of zygomycosis (*Rhizopus* and *Mucor* spp.), often in patients with poorly controlled diabetes. It presents with orbital pain, nasal discharge, and facial edema. Proptosis and visual loss may occur. Involvement of carotids may cause hemiparesis. Subsequently, trigeminal nerve and adjacent brain may be involved—classically found in mucormycosis, in which blackish necrotic areas are seen in the palate and nasal turbinates. Aspergillosis or mucormycosis may produce sudden onset of neurodeficit due to vasculitis. Rarely, subarachnoid hemorrhage occurs due to mycotic aneurysmal bleed.

Diagnosis

It is important to suspect fungal infections in a given clinical context. In the presence of a predisposing condition, such as HIV infection, children who present with fever with or without CNS signs should have an LP for CSF analysis and culture. CSF examination usually reveals high proteins, low glucose, and mononuclear leukocytosis ranging between 20–500 cells/mm³. Polymorphonuclear leukocytes are more likely to be seen in *Aspergillus*, Zygomycetes, or *Blastomyces*. Cell count may be normal or <20 cells/mm³ in patients with AIDS or those on high dose corticosteroid therapy.

Direct microscopic examination of CSF mixed with India ink on a slide is helpful in identification of encapsulated cryptococci in >50% cases. In patients with AIDS, the yield may be up to 80%.

CSF cultures are frequently negative. Sometimes fungi require days to weeks to grow in culture medium. *Candida* takes several days, and *Cryptococci* 3–10 days, while *Histoplasma*

and *Coccidioides* may take up to 6 weeks. Cisternal CSF may yield organism when lumbar CSF is negative. *C. neoformans* has the best yield on culture; it is positive in up to 90% patients, especially in those with AIDS. *Blastomyces* and *Histoplasma capsulatum* rarely yield positive culture. In coccidioidal meningitis, culture may be positive in ∼50%. Methenamine silver stain of a direct aspirate or biopsy is very helpful in identification of *Aspergillus* and Zygomycetes, which cause tissue invasion and infarction.

Latex agglutination test using CSF is positive (titer 1:8 or more) in up to 90% and is highly specific for cryptococcal meningitis. The test is diagnostic and may be positive early in the infection, even when culture is negative (26). False-negative results are uncommon and repeated negative tests over 1 month exclude the diagnosis (26).

Complement fixating antibody titer of ≥1:32 is found in CSF of 90% of coccidioidomycosis cases. CSF complement fixating antibody titers are diagnostic of meningitis; the test is negative, even in presence of high serum complement fixating antibody titers, when in absence of meningitis.

Diagnosis of *Aspergillus* infection can be made by assaying serum or CSF galactomannan, a polysaccharide marker on *Aspergillus* cell wall. A galactomannan index value of >0.5 in serum has a sensitivity and specificity exceeding 80%. Immunologic tests to detect specific antibodies in CSF are also available for *Histoplasma*, Zygomycetes, and *Sporothrix*, but these are not very specific. Serologic tests available for diagnosis of *Candida* and *Aspergillus* have not been evaluated specifically for CNS infection using CSF. PCR has shown promise in diagnosis of fungal meningitis, but requires further studies.

Neuroimaging

CT and MRI scans show the basal involvement, associated abscess, and areas of infarction. Cryptococcomas may be seen as small enhancing lesions.

Treatment

Amphotericin B remains the most used and successful drug for fungal infections of CNS (**Table 80.13**), although concentrations of the drug in the CSF is generally low or even immeasurable. For this reason, some clinicians use an intrathecal dose (0.25–0.5 mg/kg) as a last resort. It may cause vasculitis and arachnoiditis. Lipid formulation of Amphotericin B, such as Liposomal amphotericin B (AmBisome) 4 mg/kg/day or more, may be a better alternative to conventional amphotericin B, especially in the setting of renal dysfunction.

Flucytosine penetrates well into CSF and achieves concentrations that approach 75% of simultaneous serum concentrations. However, administering flucytosine alone for treatment of CNS fungal infections is associated with a high risk of treatment failure because of development of in vitro and in vivo resistance. When flucytosine is administered in combination with amphotericin B or fluconazole, relapse rate is lower when compared with amphotericin B alone.

Of the azoles, fluconazole is effective against *Cryptococcus* and *Candida*. It crosses the BBB easily and has a long half-life in the CNS. However, CSF sterilization is slower as compared to an amphotericin B-containing regimen. Itraconazole has potent

TABLE 80.13

ANTIFUNGAL THERAPY RECOMMENDED IN COMMON FUNGAL CENTRAL NERVOUS SYSTEM INFECTION

Fungus	Antifungal agent	Dose	Route	Duration
Cryptococcus neoformans	Amphotericin B[b]; + 5-FC, then Fluconazole	0.7–1 mg/kg/day q 24 hrs 100–150 mg/kg/day q 6 hrs 10 mg/kg/loading, then 5–6 mg/kg/day daily	IV PO PO PO	2 wks 2 wks 8–10 wks HIV patients: indefinite Non-HIV patients: 6 mos–1 yr
Candida albicans & other	Amphotericin B ± 5-FC then Fluconazole	0.7–1 mg/kg/day q 24 hrs 100–150 mg/kg/day q 6 hrs 10 mg/kg loading, then 5–6 mg/kg/day daily	IV PO PO/IV	2 wks 4–6 wks
Aspergillus fumigatus	Amphotericin B ± 5-FC or Voriconazole	1–1.5 mg/kg/day q 24 hrs 100–150 mg/kg/day q 6 hrs 6 mg/kg, 2 doses 12 hrs apart, then 4 mg/kg q 12 hr[a]	IV PO IV/PO	initial 6 mos to 1 yr
Coccidioides immitis	Amphotericin B, then fluconazole	0.7–1 mg/kg/day 10 mg/day loading then 5–6 mg/kg/day	IV PO	4 wks life-long

[a]By IV infusion, 5 mg/mL strength, maximum rate 3 mg/kg/hr. 5-FC levels should be monitored 2–4 hrs after oral dose after 3–4 days, with target peak 40–60 mcg/mL.

antifungal activity against a broad spectrum of fungi, including *Aspergillus*. Although it has very limited penetration into the CSF, it has been successful in the treatment of cryptococcal meningitis in patients with AIDS.

Voriconazole is a new broad-spectrum triazole with remarkable activity against *Aspergillus, Fusarium, Scedosporium,* and dematiaceous fungi. Penetration into the CSF and early favorable clinical experience make voriconazole the drug of choice in CNS aspergillosis and scedosporiosis.

Caspofungin, a new antifungal and first in a new class of echinocandins, works by blocking the synthesis of glucan, a major component of the fungal cell wall. Caspofungin is fungicidal against *Candida* spp. and active against *Aspergillus*. Activity against *Fusarium, Rhizopus,* and *Trichosporon* is limited. Case series and retrospective reports suggest that caspofungin is effective alone or in combination with polyenes, such as amphotericin, for refractory invasive *Candida* infection and in combination with voriconazole in refractory CNS infection due to *Aspergillus* spp.

In cryptococcal meningitis, amphotericin B plus flucytosine has proven successful. This combination sterilizes CSF within 2 weeks. Amphotericin B alone produces cures in >50% of patients, with a risk of considerable drug-related toxicity. Amphotericin B at a dose of 0.7 mg/kg/day is used with flucytosine 100 mg/kg/day for at least 2 weeks, followed by fluconazole (12 mg/kg/day) for 8–10 weeks. In patients with AIDS, a repeat LP should be performed 2 weeks after starting amphotericin to ensure that CSF pressure is normal and CSF is sterile before shifting to maintenance fluconazole, which is continued indefinitely as suppressive therapy to prevent relapses. Intraventricular amphotericin B has been used successfully in cases with a poor prognosis.

Cryptococcomas in the brain parenchyma are much less common than meningeal disease. In small and multiple lesions, antifungal chemotherapy alone is generally successful, although fluconazole may be needed for an extended period of up to 2 years. Large cryptococcomas (<3 cm) located in surgically accessible areas may be considered for surgical removal.

In CNS cryptococcal infection, corticosteroid administration should be discontinued; if it is not possible to do so, the dose must be reduced rapidly and as far as the underlying disease permits. Relapse rate is very high in patients with underlying AIDS, well above 50%, and in non-AIDS patients, it is ~15%–25%. Most relapses occur in the first 3–6 months after cessation of therapy; hence, the need for prolonged suppressive therapy in patients with AIDS. Data in adults suggest that patients with control of their HIV infection (CD4 count >100 cells/μL on a regimen of highly active antiretroviral therapy) and who have been asymptomatic after 2 years of treatment may be considered for cessation of antifungals (23). Unexpected deaths or loss of vision during the first 1–2 weeks of treatment may occur in some patients with AIDS and cryptococcal meningitis. These patients deteriorate suddenly and may manifest a dramatic increase in ICP (13). The pathogenesis of such an event is not fully understood. External CSF drainage should be considered in these patients.

In coccidioidal meningitis after initial treatment with amphotericin B (0.5–0.7 mg/kg/day) for 4 weeks, control of meningitis is achieved through the use of fluconazole or intrathecal amphotericin-B. Fluconazole (12 mg/kg/day) is tried first, and intrathecal amphotericin B is used only as an alternative regimen, beginning with 0.01 mg/day, increased as tolerated up to 0.5 mg per day. The need for continuing therapy may be guided by monitoring CSF cells and glucose; the target is 10 cells/mm^3 or less with normal CSF glucose concentrations for at least 1 year. A lowering of the CSF antibody titer is also considered a good prognostic sign.

In *Candida* meningitis, amphotericin B is the primary therapeutic agent, preferably in combination with flucytosine, as it has synergistic activity against *Candida*. It is followed by fluconazole.

Aspergillus infections of the CNS are very difficult to eradicate. High doses of amphotericin B have rarely been successful in arresting the infection. Voriconazole may be considered as a first choice for *Aspergillus* meningitis because it has both IV and oral formulations and early studies suggest that 25% of patients may respond. Aforementioned retrospective data in adults support addition of caspofungin to voriconazole for invasive aspergillosis. In patients with Zygomycetes (*Rhizopus, Mucor*) or *Aspergillus* infection with invasion of blood vessels and resultant infarction, in addition to high-dose amphotericin B (1.5 mg/kg/day) or liposomal amphotericin (5–7.5 mg/kg/day), direct surgical removal of infected tissue should be undertaken if lesions are accessible

The management of fungal brain abscesses is not well standardized. *Blastomyces* and *Histoplasma* abscesses have been successfully removed surgically, with concomitant amphotericin B treatment. Dematiaceous fungi that cause brain abscesses are surgically removed or debulked as primary therapy for cure, along with antifungal agents.

If *Candida* or cryptococcal meningitis develops in a patient with a shunt in place, eradication of infection is best achieved by removing the shunt and treating with antifungal agents.

Prognosis

The most important determinant of the outcome of fungal CNS infections is the causative fungus and the patient's underlying condition. The outcome of cryptococcal CNS infection is usually better than that of other forms of fungal meningitis. In cryptococcal meningitis, convulsions and focal neurologic deficits are independent predictors of in-hospital mortality in HIV-infected children (14). Poor prognostic factors associated with failure of amphotericin B therapy or relapse after therapy include an initial positive CSF India ink test result, high CSF opening pressure, low CSF leukocyte counts (<20 cells/mm^3), cryptococci isolated from extraneural sites, absent anticryptococcal antibody, initial CSF or serum cryptococcal antigen titer of 1:32 or more or post-treatment titers of 1:8 or more, corticosteroid therapy, lymphoreticular malignancy, and a CSF glucose concentration that remains abnormal during 4 weeks or more of therapy (13,26). Very high CSF antigen titers (≥1:1024), low serum albumin concentration, and low CD4 cell count (<5 cells/mL) and increased ICP in excess of 250 mm H$_2$O predict failure to rapidly sterilize CSF in patients with AIDS (26).

The mortality with *Candida* meningitis is 10%–20%. Children may be left with permanent neurologic or mental deficits. Poor prognostic factors for patients with *Candida* meningitis include diagnosis made more than 2 weeks after symptom onset, CSF glucose concentrations <35 mg/dL, and development of intracranial hypertension and focal neurologic deficits (26).

Among patients with coccidioidal meningitis, only 50% survive initial treatment, and most have extremely high risk of relapse and frequently require life-long suppressive therapy.

Prevention

A cryptococcal vaccine has been developed but is not yet licensed. Fluconazole therapy for ≥1 year can reduce the number of cryptococcal meningitis cases in HIV-infected patients. The use of azoles as prophylactic agents to prevent histoplasmosis and coccidioidomycosis in HIV-infected patients is under investigation.

PARASITIC INFECTIONS

Once considered limited to the tropics, parasitic infections are being widely reported across the world. Increasing travel and immigrating populations are responsible for this change. A large number of parasites can affect the CNS. Most of them cause chronic or subacute involvement; however, some may present acutely either with a meningoencephalitic presentation or as a mass lesion with marked cerebral edema and raised ICP. These cases would present to the intensivist. A discussion of all parasitic CNS infections is beyond the scope of this chapter. Some of the parasites that can involve the CNS and their clinical manifestations are listed in **Table 80.14**. Cerebral malaria and neurocysticercosis are discussed separately.

TABLE 80.14

COMMON PARASITIC CENTRAL NERVOUS SYSTEM INFECTIONS

Parasite	Clinical manifestations
Protozoa	Cerebral malaria
Plasmodium falciparum	Meningitis/meningoencephalitis
Amoeba	Meningitis/meningoencephalitis
Entamoeba histolytica	Meningoencephalitis
Acanthamoeba	
Naegleria	
Trypanosoma	
brucei (*rhodesiense* or *gambiense*)	
cruzi	
Toxoplasma gondii	
Helminths (*worms*)	
Cestodes (flatworms)	
Taenia solium (neurocysticercosis)	Seizures/meningoencephalitis
	Mass lesion with raised ICP
Echinococcus (hydatid cyst) (multilocularis/ granulosus)	Solitary/multiple
	Seizures
Nematodes (roundworms)	
Trichinella	Meningoencephalitis
Strongyloides	Meningoencephalitis
Ascaris	Seizures

Etiology

In any case of suspected parasitic infection, the most important etiologic clue is obtained by a detailed history, particularly related to travel to, or immigration from, endemic areas. Some parasitic infections, such as falciparum malaria, manifest clinically within a few days, whereas others, such as neurocysticercosis, may manifest several months or even years after infection. It is important to inquire about both recent travel and past travel to endemic areas. History of suggestive mode of acquisition, such as blood transfusion for malarial parasite, bathing in a pond for *Naegleria*, exposure to tsetse fly for African trypanosomiasis, or Reduviid bug for American trypanosomiasis, is also important. Underlying immune status of the child, such as HIV-positive status, corticosteroid therapy, and asplenia, may indicate possible specific opportunistic parasitic diseases, such as toxoplasmosis.

Epidemiology

Amoeba have a worldwide distribution. *Entamoeba histolytica*, transmitted by the fecal-oral route, is carried by ~0.5 billion individuals worldwide, causing symptoms in 500 million and death in 100,000 each year. Disseminated disease with CNS involvement occurs in a fraction of this subset. Free-living amoeba, including *Acanthamoeba* and *Naegleria*, are found in fresh or brackish water, and disease occurs in warm months, when exposure is increased. Trypanosoma are transmitted by vectors, including the tsetse fly in Africa and Reduviid bug in Central and South America. *T. brucei* is the etiologic agent of African trypanosomiasis (also known as African sleeping sickness), with *T. brucei rhodiense* causing East African trypanosomiasis and *T. brucei gambiense* causing West African trypanosomiasis. *T. cruzi* is the etiologic agent of American trypanosomiasis (Chagas disease). It is estimated that ~700,000 cases of American trypanosomiasis and 400,000 cases of African trypanosomiasis occur each year. Exact incidence rates of CNS trypanosomiasis are not known, but increase with length of illness. *Toxoplasma gondii* is acquired most commonly by ingestion of oocysts present in cat feces or through ingestion of tissue cysts of contaminated meat that is undercooked. Seroprevalence of toxoplasmosis varies from several percent in countries such as Thailand to 90% in France. The largest disease burden is in neonates born to mothers with primary toxoplasmosis during gestation and in immunocompromised individuals. Echinococcosis is caused by a larval form of the tapeworm *Taenia echinococcus*. Cystic echinococcosis is caused by *Echinococcus granulosus*, found worldwide in association with sheep herding. *Echinococcus multilocularis* involves the CNS less often, is associated with exposure to wild rodents and foxes, and is only found in the northern hemisphere. Nematodes, such as *Trichinella* and *Ascaris*, are found in soil in tropical areas with poor sanitation. *Strongyloides* is also endemic in tropical climes with poor sanitation, but infection occurs by penetration through exposed skin.

Pathogenesis

Infection by the parasite (e.g., *E. histolytica*, *Acanthamoeba*, *Toxoplasma*, *Echinococcus*, and *Ascaris*) typically occurs through the gastrointestinal tract, via a vector (e.g., malaria, trypanosomiasis), or by skin penetration (*Strongyloides*). The parasite typically undergoes a stage of multiplication, followed by hematogenous seeding of the CNS. *Naegleria* penetrates via the nasal mucosa and spreads via olfactory nerves to the CNS.

Clinical Presentation

The clinical presentation of parasitic CNS disease varies considerably based on the causative agent. Symptoms of acute meningitis or meningoencephalitis are most typical, with fever, headache, vomiting, photophobia, neck stiffness, and altered sensorium. New-onset seizures are another common clinical presentation, as in neurocysticercosis (NCC). Cystic echinococcal infection may present insidiously over years with a slowly enlarging cyst, causing headache and progressing toward neurologic deficit and herniation.

Diagnosis

The CSF may be diagnostic in certain cases, such as finding of free-floating amoebae in the case of *Naegleria* or Giemsa stain for trypanosomiasis. A positive serology in serum or CSF may suggest NCC; rise in specific IgM titer for toxoplasmosis is highly suggestive. PCR studies are also available for some parasites. Various investigations may be of use in diagnosis, such as blood film for malaria or presence of eosinophilia for helminths.

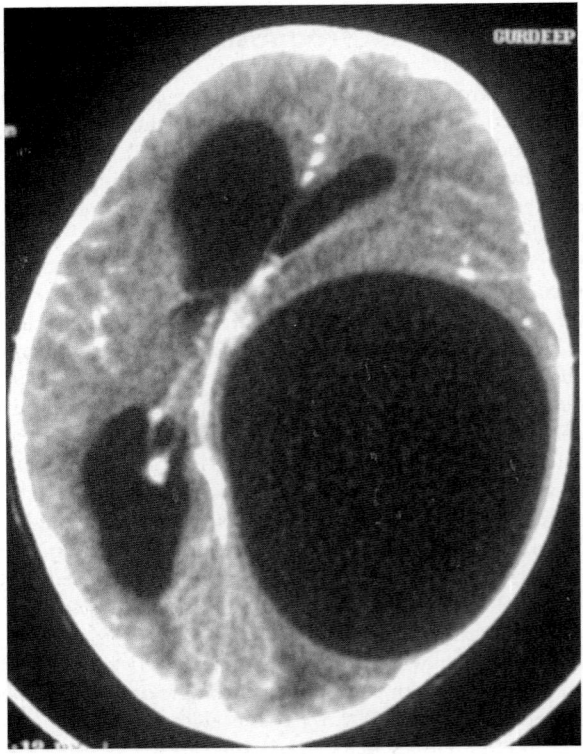

FIGURE 80.10. CECT showing a large, rounded cystic lesion with imperceptible walls with midline shift and mass effect, causing ventricular dilatation on the opposite side—hydatid cyst.

Neuroimaging

Neuroimaging may reveal characteristic findings, such as a scolex seen within the cyst in NCC. The presence of a round, thin-walled cyst filled with fluid isointense to CSF suggests hydatid due to *Echinococcus*, (**Fig. 80.10**), whereas small, ring-enhancing lesions (particularly in deep gray matter) in a child with HIV suggest toxoplasmosis.

Treatment

The supportive management in the ICU is principally similar to other CNS infections. Specific antiparasitic therapy would depend on the etiologic organism. Surgical removal of large cysts is indicated in some cases. Rupture of the cyst should be avoided, as it can induce anaphylactic shock.

NEUROCYSTICERCOSIS

NCC is the most common parasitic infection of the CNS and an important cause of epilepsy in the tropics. The clinical presentations are variable and depend on the stage and location of cysts. Most cases present with seizures, and approximately one-third of cases have symptoms and signs of raised ICP. Generally, the presentation is not serious enough to warrant admission to the PICU; however, some cases may present with significant cerebral edema, leading to either an encephalitic presentation or a mass effect.

Etiology

NCC is caused by infestation of the CNS with encysted larvae of *Taenia solium*. Humans acquire intestinal infection (taeniasis, tapeworm) from pigs by ingestion of undercooked pork infected with *T. solium* cysticerci. In the intestine, cysticerci develop into adult worms and release thousands of eggs that are extremely contagious. Open defecation and inadequate sewerage cause contamination of soil with infected stools. The intermediate host is the pig that becomes infected by grazing on soil contaminated with parasitic eggs. The eggs hatch into larvae, invade the intestinal mucosa, and reach the muscles or the brain, where they mature into cysticerci over a period of 3 weeks to 2 months. When humans consume undercooked pork that contains the cysts, the life cycle of the parasite is completed.

Cysticercosis in humans is acquired through the feco-oral route by ingestion of contaminated raw vegetables or food prepared by carriers of tapeworms; rarely, it is due to autoingestion of ova in patients who have intestinal tapeworms. After ingestion of *T. solium* eggs, larvae (oncospheres) form and penetrate the intestinal mucosa, with subsequent migration throughout the body and penetration of the CNS, skeletal muscle, subcutaneous tissue, and the eyes, where mature cysts form.

Epidemiology

Cysticercosis is endemic in Latin America, Mexico, India, sub-Saharan Africa, and China. NCC is not limited to develop-ing countries but is also seen in many developed countries, mainly because of increasing number of immigrants from endemic areas. It is estimated that >1000 new cases of NCC are diagnosed in the US each year. Approximately 20 million people are infected worldwide, and ~50,000 die from the disease every year.

Pathogenesis

Cysticerci may live within host tissues for years without causing any inflammation or disease, as they have various mechanisms for evading host response, including inhibition of complement activation and suppression of cellular immune response.

The cyst has four stages: The *vesicular (metacestode)* stage marked by is a fluid-filled cyst with a thin wall and an eccentric opaque scolex. This cyst degenerates to the *colloidal stage,* when gelatinous material appears in cyst fluid, followed by the *granular nodular stage* in which the cyst contracts and the walls are replaced by focal lymphoid nodules and necrosis. Finally, in the *nodular calcified stage*, the granulation tissue is replaced by collagenous structures and calcification. Symptomatology most often occurs when the cyst transitions from the living vesicular to the dying colloidal stage, releasing inflammatory mediators. Inflammation and (less commonly) subsequent calcification serve as a nidus for seizure activity.

Clinical Manifestations

The clinical presentation of NCC is variable and depends on the stage and location of the cysts; it is classified into parenchymal and extraparenchymal types.

Parenchymal Neurocysticercosis

The common clinical manifestations include:

- Seizures in 70%–90% cases, more frequent in children as compared to adults. In a large series of 500 children, seizures were reported in 95% cases (34). Most seizures are complex partial; approximately one-fourth are simple partial. Generalized seizures are less common. Seizures are generally brief; SE has been reported in 2%–32% cases.
- Raised ICP with headache and vomiting in almost one-third of cases. Papilledema has been reported in 2.3%–6.6% of children.
- Focal neurodeficits in 4% of children are determined by the location of the cysts.
- Encephalitis: children and adolescents with numerous cysts and marked diffuse cerebral edema may occasionally present with severe acute raised ICP and an encephalitic picture. They are difficult to treat and have a poor prognosis.

Extraparenchymal Neurocysticercosis

Extraparenchymal involvement is rare in children and includes (a) ventricular involvement, presenting as obstructive hydrocephalous or chronic meningitis; (b) subarachnoid involvement, presenting as basilar arachnoiditis or chronic meningitis; cysts may enlarge, become racemose, and cause mass effects; (c) spinal involvement, with cysts that may be located in the leptomeningeal space or within the cord; radicular pain, paresthesias and spinal cord compression may occur; intramedullary cysts may present as transverse myelitis with paraplegia and sphincteric disturbances; and (d) ophthalmic involvement, which may affect the subretinal space, vitreous humor, subconjunctiva, or anterior chamber, and may cause visual deficits, sudden blindness, and similar symptoms.

Other presentations of NCC include hydrocephalous, vasculitis, and stroke. Stroke is due to vasculitis secondary to cysticercus arachnoiditis at the base of the brain. The infarcts are generally small, and lacunar; occasionally, large infarcts due to occlusion of middle cerebral or internal carotid artery may occur. Numerous unusual presentations, including dorsal midbrain syndrome, papillitis, ptosis, and cerebral hemorrhage, may also be seen. Fever is unusual in NCC.

Diagnosis

The gold standard for diagnosis of NCC is pathologic confirmation through biopsy or autopsy. Practically, the diagnosis rests mainly on neuroimaging. Immunologic tests have not proven to be very sensitive or specific for diagnosis of NCC, particularly for single lesions. Low positivity from 17% to 25% has been reported in children with NCC (34). ELISA of CSF and serum shows high false-positive and false-negative reactions. Enzyme-linked immunoelectrotransfer blot assay using purified glycoprotein antigens from *T. solium* cysticerci was reported to be highly specific and nearly 100% sensitive for patients with either multiple active parenchymal cysts or extraparenchymal NCC. However, sensitivity is less for patients with either single cysts or calcifications. A crude soluble extract ELISA was found to be more sensitive and specific than dot blot assay. Peripheral eosinophilia is variably reported. CSF is normal in parenchymal NCC; in NCC meningitis, it may show mild pleocytosis with some elevation of protein and hypoglycorrhachia. The cellular response may be polymorphonuclear or lymphocytic. Diagnostic criteria for human cysticercosis and neurocysticercosis were revised to make them specific for the diagnosis of NCC. In clinical practice, it may not be feasible to apply these diagnostic criteria. In view of the pleomorphism of the disease, NCC should be kept in the differential diagnosis of a wide variety of neurologic disorders, particularly seizures, and appropriate neuroimaging studies should be undertaken to confirm the diagnosis.

Neuroimaging

The characteristic CT picture consists of small, low-density, ring or disc-enhancing lesions, with perilesional edema. The scolex appears as a bright, high-density, eccentric nodule in these cysts and is pathognomonic of NCC. Enhancing lesions represent degenerating (colloidal vesicular) cysticerci. In most cases, the lesions (termed *single, small, enhancing CT lesions*) are single and <20 mm in size (**Fig. 80.11A**). Some may have multiple lesions; NCC with numerous cysts produces the "starry-sky" appearance typical of NCC. Calcifications are few millimeters in size and may be single or multiple. Vesicular cysts appear as small, round, nonenhancing lesions with CSF-density cystic fluid; the wall is isodense to the brain parenchyma.

In subarachnoid NCC, the CT findings include hydrocephalous, tentorial enhancement, and occasionally, infarcts. Cystic hypodense lesions, representing racemose cysts, may rarely be seen in the sylvian fissure or cerebellopontine angle. Intraventricular NCC manifests as hydrocephalous; rarely, intraventricular cysts may be identified.

MRI is more sensitive than CT for visualization of extraparenchymal cysts and identification of scolex. On T1-weighted images, live cysts are seen as round lesions, either isointense or slightly hyperintense to the CSF, with a scolex that is hyperintense or isointense to white matter. On T2-weighted images, the cysts are isointense to CSF and the perilesional edema appears bright (**Fig. 80.11B**). The scolex may not be seen because of the high intensity cystic fluid. The scolex is better seen on proton density-weighted images. Gadolinium-enhanced MRI shows ring enhancement of lesion (**Fig. 80.11C**). Calcified lesions appear hypointense on all MR imaging sequences and may at times be missed.

Proton MR spectroscopy is under investigation for evaluation of inflammatory granulomas. Presence of lipid peak reportedly indicates a tuberculoma; low levels of metabolites with a poor signal-to-noise ratio could indicate NCC. MR spectroscopy may also help in differentiating NCC from a neoplasm.

Other Imaging

Radiographs of skeletal muscles to look for calcified cysts and stool examination for tapeworms are rarely positive. If a subcutaneous nodule is detected in a child with suspected NCC, it should be biopsied to corroborate the diagnosis.

Differential Diagnoses

Parenchymal Neurocysticercosis

In a child with a single, small, enhancing CT lesion, if the scolex is not visualized, the differential diagnoses include:

- Tuberculoma, particularly in developing countries. Raised ICP, progressive focal neurodeficit, size of CT lesion >20 mm, lobulated irregular shape, and marked edema, causing midline shift favor the diagnosis of tuberculoma but are not absolute criteria. Tests for exclusion of TB (e.g., Mantoux skin test and chest x-ray) should be done in all cases.
- Other parasitic granulomas, such as toxoplasmosis and, rarely, schistosomiasis, sparganosis, and paragonimiasis.
- Neoplasms, such as low-grade astrocytoma or cystic cerebral metastasis
- Microabscess
- Fungal lesion, particularly cryptococcosis, and rarely, histoplasmosis or sarcoidosis

Most of these are rare in children.

Extraparenchymal Neurocysticercosis

Hydrocephalous with racemose NCC in the subarachnoid space may simulate a low-density tumor. Meningitis due to NCC must be differentiated from other causes of meningitis, particularly tubercular and fungal meningitis.

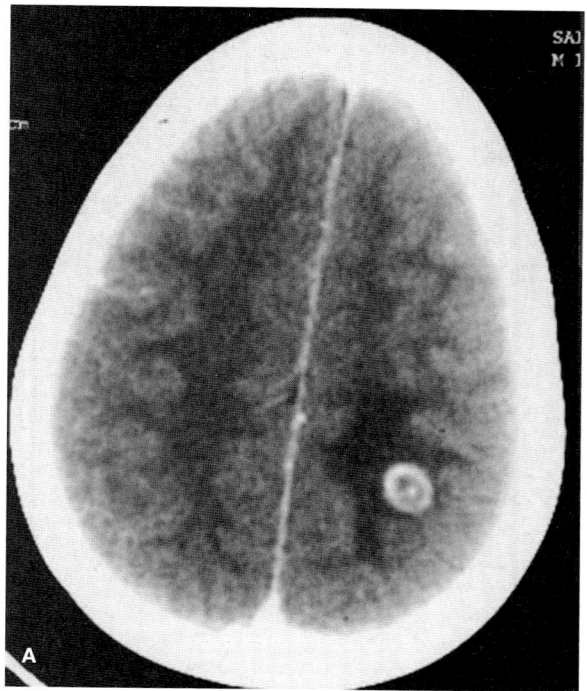

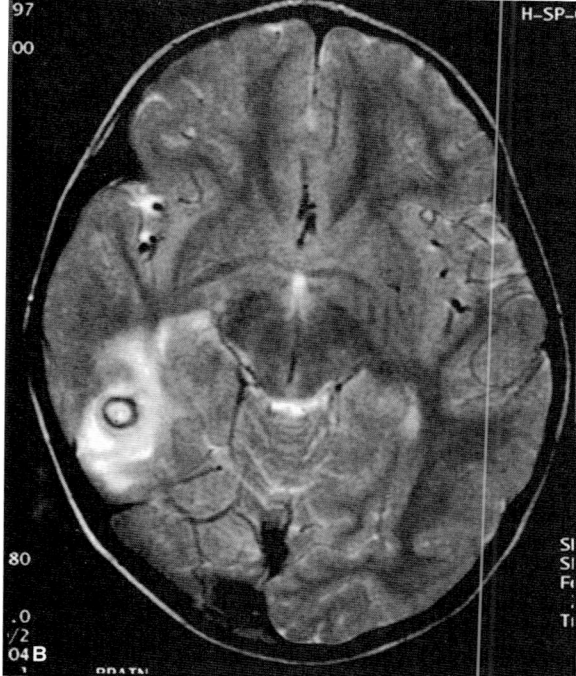

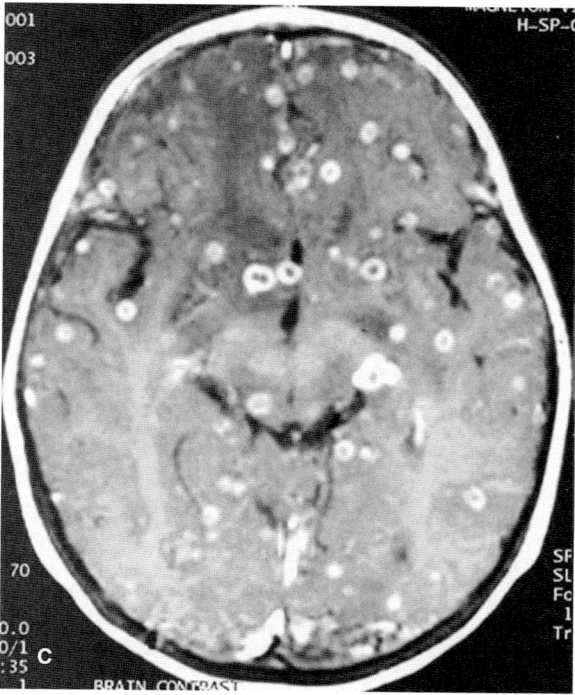

FIGURE 80.11. Neurocysticercosis (NCC). **A:** CECT showing a single, small, ring-enhancing lesion (SSECTL) with a well-defined eccentric scolex, and perilesional edema. **B:** T2-weighted MRI showing a single NCC lesion with a scolex and bright perilesional edema. **C:** Contrast MRI showing multiple, ring-enhancing NCC lesions in a small, multiple NCC.

Treatment

A child with an encephalitic presentation requires intensive care management similar to any other encephalitis. IV steroids are used to reduce the cerebral edema, and anticonvulsants to control the seizures. Cysticidal therapy is not used in the acute phase, as it may provoke a further inflammatory response and worsen the edema. It may be considered later in select cases once the edema subsides and the child is stable. Praziquantel and albendazole are the two drugs that have been found effec-

tive against *T. solium* cysticerci. Albendazole has been found to be more efficacious, less expensive, and better tolerated than praziquantel. It has better penetration into the subarachnoid space, its bioavailability increases with coadministration of steroids, and it is currently the drug of choice for treatment of NCC (8). It has been used in a dose of 15 mg/kg/day in two to three divided doses for 28 days. Shorter durations of 14 days to 8 days have also been used. In a placebo-controlled trial of 1 week versus 4 weeks of albendazole therapy in children with one to three enhancing lesions, both regimens were found to be equally effective (31). Praziquantel is used in a dose of 50 mg/kg/day for a period of 15 days. However, a single-day praziquantel therapy (25 mg/kg/dose every 2 hrs × three doses) has been reported to be effective and comparable to 7-day treatment with albendazole.

Cysticidal therapy should not be used in the following cases: (a) markedly raised ICP, particularly in disseminated NCC, as sudden elevations of ICP may occur secondary to the host inflammatory response; such cases should be treated with steroids alone; (b) ophthalmic NCC, as the host response may cause damage to the eye; and (c) calcified lesions, as the parasite is already dead. Consensus guidelines for the treatment of NCC (11) recommend that treatment should be individualized. Seizures due to NCC are usually well controlled with a single anticonvulsant. Carbamazepine or phenylhydantoin are commonly used. Recurrence of seizures after discontinuation of antiepileptic drugs is less (10.5%) in children than in adults (50%). Generally, antiepileptic drugs have been used for approximately a 2-year seizure-free interval. Shorter durations of antiepileptic drugs may be sufficient. A controlled study found no difference in seizure recurrence when antiepileptic drugs were given for a 1-year versus a 2-year seizure-free interval. Seizure recurrence correlated significantly with an abnormal CT (persistence or calcification of lesion) and an abnormal EEG at the time of withdrawal. Children with both CT and EEG abnormalities had a significantly higher risk of seizure recurrence. Thus, anticonvulsant therapy may be withdrawn after a 1-year seizure-free interval in those children in whom the lesion has disappeared and the EEG is normal prior to withdrawal. Children with persistent or calcified lesions may require longer therapy.

Corticosteroids are used for short periods of time to reduce cerebral edema, generally concomitantly with anticysticercal therapy, if given, to prevent or ameliorate the adverse reactions that may occur due to the host inflammatory response. Oral prednisolone 1–2 mg/kg or IV dexamethasone is used if cerebral edema is seen on neuroimaging. Corticosteroids are the mainstay of therapy in the encephalitic form of NCC.

Surgery for cyst removal has been used in ophthalmic NCC. Shunt placement is necessary in cases with hydrocephalous; use of steroids and albendazole reduces shunt failure. Endoscopic removal of cysts from the ventricles may obviate the need for shunt placement. Successful medical treatment of subarachnoid, spinal, and other forms of extraparenchymal NCC has led to a decrease in the role of surgery in NCC. Follow-up must be individualized. A repeat CT after 3–6 months is generally indicated to determine whether the lesions have resolved partially or completely, are persisting, or have calcified.

Prognosis

The outcome depends upon the type of NCC, cyst location, and the number of cysts. Patients with NCC who present with seizures and single parenchymal cysts generally have a good prognosis; seizures are well controlled in most cases, and lesions disappear within 6 months in over 60% cases. Risk of seizure recurrence is low. Patients with multiple lesions, particularly disseminated NCC and calcifications, have frequent seizure recurrences. NCC encephalitis has a guarded prognosis.

Prevention

Proper animal husbandry, hygiene, and sanitation can eradicate transmission of *T. solium* from pigs to humans. Mass treatment of the population with praziquantel did not show lasting benefits.

CEREBRAL MALARIA

Cerebral malaria (CM) is a clinical syndrome characterized by CNS dysfunction associated with *Plasmodium falciparum* infection. Although falciparum malaria is one of the major causes of death in children living in malaria endemic areas of sub-Saharan Africa, where they are exposed to infections from birth; it is increasingly being encountered in developed countries due to the increase in international travel and migration from endemic areas. There are differences in the pathophysiology of severe malaria in children growing up in malaria endemic areas compared to those unexposed to infections (nonimmune).

Etiology

Malaria is caused by protozoan parasites, of which only four species infect humans. *P. falciparum* is responsible for almost all of the life-threatening disease. The parasites are transmitted by anopheline mosquitoes. Sporozoites enter into the bloodstream when the mosquito feeds and undergo a stage of development in the liver before invading the erythrocytes. In the erythrocytes, the *P. falciparum* undergo a 48-hr cycle, which causes clinical symptoms. *P. falciparum* is unique, in that the late trophozoites and schizonts are sequestered in the microcirculation of vital organs. Sequestration may obstruct blood flow and impair metabolism of surrounding parenchymal cells, thereby causing the severe complications of falciparum malaria such, as cerebral involvement.

Epidemiology

Malaria is endemic in much of the developing world in tropical areas where mosquito eradication programs have not been successfully implemented. Over 3 billion people (more than half of the world's population) live in endemic areas, including Southeast Asia, Central and South America, and Africa. Globally, it is estimated that 300–500 million cases and 1.5–3 million deaths occur annually, making malaria one of the top 3 infectious disease killers worldwide, along with TB and HIV.

Pathogenesis

The pathophysiology of severe falciparum malaria in nonimmune individuals appears to be different from that in African children who are exposed to the parasites from birth. Hypoglycemia, lactic acidosis, and severe anemia occur in both groups, but concomitant bacterial infections, pulmonary edema, and renal failure are much more common in nonimmune individuals.

Plasmodial infections stimulate monocytes to produce cytokines, principally TNF, IL-1, and IL-6. TNF production significantly increases with schizont rupture, and TNF is probably the mediator of fever associated with schizogony. TNF stimulates the synthesis of NO, which in turn has been proposed as a central mediator in the pathogenesis of CM, as it interferes with neuronal transmission by inhibiting glutamate-induced excitatory synaptic activity (12). Furthermore, NO is a potent vasodilator, which may increase the cerebral blood volume.

ICP is elevated in almost all African children with CM. Severe intracranial hypertension is associated with neurologic sequelae, transtentorial herniation, and death. However, in nonimmune adults, transtentorial herniation is not a common postmortem feature, and opening LP pressures are normal in most patients.

Raised ICP is probably caused by an increase in cerebral blood volume, secondary to an increase in CBF and/or from the sequestration of cells within the cerebral microvasculature. Cerebral edema does not appear to play a major role in raising the ICP in most immune and nonimmune patients; however, cytotoxic edema is associated with severe intracranial hypertension. The BBB appears to be mildly impaired in most patients.

Although the pathogenesis of CM is not well understood (15), the mechanisms of neurologic dysfunction are likely to be multifactorial. The most favored hypotheses for the development of impaired consciousness are the mechanical obstruction of the microvasculature by the sequestered parasites and/or the effect of toxic substances. Obstruction of blood flow through microvessels could reduce the delivery of oxygen and other substrates, causing a reduction in metabolism and level of consciousness. Cerebral lactate production is increased, possibly as a result of anaerobic glycolysis in the brain secondary to hypoxia. However, global ischemia is not a feature, as CBF is not decreased and most patients survive without sequelae.

A number of genes have been associated with protection against severe falciparum malaria, of which sickle cell disease is the most widely recognized. More recently, polymorphisms associated with susceptibility have been described. Several polymorphisms in the TNF promoter region are associated with increased risk of CM and death. A common intercellular adhesion molecule (ICAM)-1 polymorphism (ICAM-1[Kilifi]) that alters protein binding to infected red blood cells (IRBC) was associated with CM in Kenyan children.

The pathologic hallmark of CM is engorgement of the cerebral capillaries and venules with IRBC. This feature is not pathognomic, as it is also present in patients with noncerebral malaria, but the degree of sequestration is much greater in CM. Cerebral edema is found postmortem but is rarely detected by CT during life. The sequestration of erythrocytes that contain mature stages of *P. falciparum* in the microvasculature of the brain is attributed to cytoadherence, the specific binding of the IRBC to the endothelial cells of the vessels. Other factors, such as erythrocyte rosette and aggregate formation and reduced erythrocytic deformability, may also play a role in the pathophysiology.

Clinical Presentation

CM should be suspected in any child who has visited or even transiently landed at an airport in an endemic area and develops CNS symptoms, such as headache and mental status changes.

Children with malaria usually have a history of fever, headache, irritability, restlessness, or drowsiness. Vomiting and, to a lesser extent, diarrhea are common and may contribute to dehydration or electrolyte depletion. Children may also complain of abdominal pain, and some are constipated. Fever is usually present, although its absence does not exclude the diagnosis. In most children, the temperature is $>39°C$, often continuous or irregular, and without any definite pattern. Mild icterus is common. Meningism may be present, such that CM cannot be differentiated clinically from bacterial meningitis. Seizures are common and often precipitate the lapse into unconsciousness. Brainstem signs, including dysconjugate eye movement and decerebrate posturing, also occur. Falciparum malaria is associated with a distinctive retinopathy, which includes retinal hemorrhages, retinal whitening, color changes in the vessels, and less frequently papilledema. These features are associated with sequestration in the brain and help to differentiate CM from other causes of encephalopathy (42). Seizures are an important presenting feature of CM, especially in African children, and are associated with a poor outcome. Focal motor and generalized tonic-clonic convulsions are most commonly seen, but subclinical seizures that are only evident on electroencephalography are also present.

The liver is often enlarged and may be slightly tender. Splenic enlargement, which may not be present on admission, usually occurs a few days into the illness. Spontaneous bleeding from the gastrointestinal tract occurs in nonimmune individuals. Hypoglycemia is a common complication of severe falciparum malaria, particularly CM. In African children, it is significantly associated with neurologic sequelae and death. In nonimmune adults, nonketotic hypoglycemia is caused by hyperinsulinemia, particularly during pregnancy and after the administration of quinine (48). In African children, hypoglycemia appears to be caused by impaired hepatic gluconeogenesis, resulting from either reduced hepatic blood flow or lactate inhibiting the uptake of amino acids by the liver.

Metabolic acidosis, a prominent feature of CM in both nonimmune adults and African children, is mainly caused by lactic acid, but other acids also contribute. Lactate concentrations are increased in CSF and blood, with higher concentrations measured in fatal cases, compared with survivors. Both in African children and nonimmune adults, admission CSF lactate concentrations are a good predictor of outcome in CM. Lactate may be produced by anaerobic glycolysis of the IRBC and/or the human host. In particular, impaired perfusion caused by hypovolemia and impaired microcirculatory flow contribute. Hypovolemia appears to be more common in some children. Hemolytic anemia that results from the destruction of IRBC is an inevitable consequence of a falciparum malaria infection. Severe anemia is one of the life-threatening complications of *P. falciparum* in African children, either in the presence or absence of CM or acidosis. Besides destruction of the red blood cells by the spleen, anemia may be caused by failure of the bone marrow to produce erythrocytes (manifesting as dyserythropoiesis) and immune-mediated intravascular hemolysis of both infected and noninfected red blood cells.

Diagnosis

The WHO (48) has adopted the following strict criteria for the diagnosis of CM: (a) a patient is unable to localize a painful stimulus (such as pressure on the sternum) at least 1 hr after last seizure; (b) asexual parasites are present in the peripheral blood; and (c) other causes of encephalopathy (e.g., meningitis, encephalitis, or hypoglycemia) are excluded. Although this definition is suitable for research purposes, any child with *P. falciparum* infection and disturbed consciousness should be evaluated and treated for CM.

CSF is usually acellular, and other diagnoses, such as encephalitis, should be entertained if a pleocytosis is found; however, CM cannot be excluded. CSF lactate concentrations are raised, but total protein and glucose concentrations are usually normal. Blood cultures may reveal an occult septicemia, particularly caused by Gram-negative organisms, and urine cultures should be done to detect concurrent urinary tract infections. The parasite count in severe falciparum malaria varies considerably, ranging from a barely detectable parasitemia to >20% erythrocytes parasitized. The lack of a detectable parasitemia does not exclude the diagnosis of CM, since the parasites may be sequestered within the deep vascular beds or chemoprophylaxis may have suppressed the parasitemia. Thus, blood smears must be examined every 6 hrs for 48 hrs to exclude this infection. Rapid diagnostic tests, such as the immunochromatographic test for *P. falciparum* histidine-rich protein 2 and lactate dehydrogenase, may be helpful, particularly in the absence of positive blood smear. Parasite mRNA or DNA PCR testing is more sensitive than microscopy, but it is expensive, more laborious, and does not estimate parasite load. Anemia, usually with evidence of hemolysis (raised unconjugated bilirubinemia, low haptoglobin concentration), is almost always present. Thrombocytopenia is common but rarely severe enough to cause bleeding. Fibrin degradation products are raised, but laboratory features of frank DIC are uncommon.

Hypoglycemia and a lactic acidosis (21) are the major metabolic complications. Hypoxemia is associated with pulmonary edema and infections. Renal impairment is common. Hyponatremia is mainly caused by salt depletion, but some cases may be caused by inappropriate antidiuretic hormone secretion. Hypoalbuminemia is also common and may result in low plasma calcium concentrations. Hypophosphatemia is a feature of severe malaria and may be exacerbated by glucose therapy.

Treatment

Any child with severe falciparum malaria should be admitted to the ICU. The management of a child with CM should consist of three components: management strategies for a child with impaired level of consciousness, supportive care, and antimalarial therapy.

Antimalarial therapy is complicated by the emergence of parasites that are resistant to various antimalarial drugs and the difficulty of obtaining specific antimalarial drugs in various countries. A combination of antimalarials with different actions should be used to prevent the emergence of resistant parasites. Any child with features of severe falciparum malaria should be treated with parenteral antimalarial therapy (**Table 80.15**). At present, the drugs of choice for treatment of severe falciparum malaria are the cinchona alkaloids (quinine and its diastereomer quinidine) and the artemisinin compounds. The artemisinin compounds are more parasiticidal but are currently not licensed in North America. Since quinine for IV administration is unavailable in the US, quinidine is used. Cinchona alkaloids are effective against the latter erythrocytic stages. Most authorities recommend a loading dose to rapidly achieve high therapeutic levels, but this should be avoided in children who have been given cinchona alkaloids or mefloquine within the last 24 hrs. Side effects are common, particularly cinchonism (tinnitus, hearing loss, nausea, restlessness, blurred vision). Serious cardiovascular side effects, such as hypotension and cardiac arrhythmias, may occur if the drugs are administered undiluted and too rapidly. The Q-T interval should be monitored during the infusion. Artemisinin compounds (artesunate, artemether, arteether) are fast-acting and act against all blood stages, reducing the time to parasite clearance and fever resolution in comparison to the cinchinoid alkaloids. Artesunate is the favored drug, as it can be administered IV or intramuscularly and is associated with less neurotoxicity in animal models. A randomized trial found less mortality and better tolerability of artesunate, as compared with IV quinine in adults with severe falciparum malaria (9).

A second antimalarial drug should be combined with the parenteral antimalarial to prevent the emergence of resistance to the former. They can be used in parasites that are relatively resistant to the cinchinoids, to shorten the course of therapy, or for the treatment of nonsevere falciparum malaria. Atovaquone-proguanil (Malarone^{TM}) is useful in this context. Antibiotics (e.g., clindamycin) are effective against the blood stages but should not be used as primary antimalarial drugs. Mefloquine can be used, although parasite resistance is increasing. The spread of chloroquine-resistant strains of *P. falciparum* has severely limited the use of chloroquine, and it should not be used in the treatment of severe falciparum malaria. Likewise, the spread of resistance to the sulfonamides (sulfadoxine, sulfalene, cotrimoxazole) have limited their usefulness. The biguanides (proguanil and chlorproguanil) are useful prophylactic drugs. Halofantrine is an effective drug, but its cardiovascular toxicity has limited its use.

Supportive treatment is important, as most children die within 24 hrs, before the antimalarials have time to work. Children with severe falciparum malaria should be monitored closely. Blood glucose and fluid balance should be measured every 6 hrs, parasitemia and hematocrit every 12 hrs. Electrolytes, tests of renal function, albumin, calcium, phosphate, and blood gases should be performed at least daily during the acute stages. Hyperpyrexia should be treated with standard modalities for lowering temperature, although paracetamol is associated with decrease parasite clearance. Fluid balance is critical in severe malaria, as many children are hypovolemic, but overaggressive fluid therapy can precipitate pulmonary edema and aggravate intracranial hypertension. Recent studies suggest that albumin may improve outcome. Renal function must be carefully monitored because acute renal failure is a common cause of death in nonimmune patients. Patients with pulmonary edema or acute respiratory distress syndrome require supplemental oxygen and positive pressure ventilation, with positive end-expiratory pressure to maintain adequate oxygenation and diuretics or hemofiltration to correct the fluid overload. Blood transfusions should be considered when the hematocrit falls toward 20%, or the child has evidence of cardiovascular compromise. The role of exchange transfusions in the management of CM is controversial. However, most authorities recommend exchange

TABLE 80.15

PARENTERAL ANTIMALARIAL TREATMENT OF CEREBRAL MALARIA

Drug	Route	Loading dose	Maintenance dose
Quinidine gluconate	IV	15 mg *base*/kg (24 mg/kg *salt*) in normal saline over 4 hrs **OR** 6.25 mg *base*/kg (10 mg *salt*/kg) over 2 hrs	7.5 mg *base*/kg (12 mg *salt*/kg) infused over 4 hrs, every 8–12 hrs with ECG monitoring **OR** 0.0125 mg *base*/kg/min (0.02 mg *salt*/kg/min) as a continuous infusion for 24 hrs
Quinine dihydrochloride	IV	20 mg *salt*/kg over 2–4 hrs	10 mg *salt*/kg over 2–4 hrs every 8–12 hrs until able to take orally
Quinine dihydrochloride	IM	20 mg *salt*/kg (dilute IV formulation to 60 mg/mL) given in two injection sites (anterior thigh)	10 mg *salt*/kg every 8–12 hrs until able to take orally
Artemether	IM	3.2 mg/kg	1.6 mg/kg/day for a minimum of 5 days
Artesunate	IV/IM	2.4 mg/kg	1.2 mg/kg after 24 hrs, then 1.2 mg/kg/day for 7 days

Parenteral therapy should be given for at least 72 hrs before changing to oral medication. Total therapy should be at least 7 days, and a parenteral antimalarial should be used in conjunction with another antimalarial of a different class. IV, intravenous; IM, intramuscular

transfusion in patients who have a parasitemia in excess of 10% (http://www.cdc.gov/Malaria/diagnosis_treatment/tx_clinicians. htm) or who are deteriorating in spite of conventional treatment. Vitamin K and cryoprecipitate should be administered if a patient has a bleeding diathesis. Seizures must be treated promptly with benzodiazepines, and a prophylactic anticonvulsant, such as phenytoin or phenobarbital, should be used if seizures recur. A CT or MRI scan should be completed to exclude brain swelling before an LP is performed. If brain swelling is detected, ICP monitoring should be considered. Steroids appear to be deleterious, increasing the incidence of bleeding without any beneficial effect on outcome. Secondary bacterial infections should always be suspected and broad-spectrum antimicrobial treatment should be started as soon as a complicating infection is suspected. Severe falciparum malaria is a multisystem disease, and advice from hematologists, infectious disease specialists, and nephrologists may be needed. A reference center, such as the Centers for Disease Control in Atlanta, should be contacted for current information (http://www.cdc.gov/Malaria/diagnosis_treatment/tx_clinicians. htm) about antimalarial therapy.

Prognosis

The mortality in nonimmune individuals ranges from 15% to 26%, with patients usually dying within the first 4 days of the illness from renal failure or pulmonary edema. In African children, the mortality is similar, but most children die within 24 hrs of admission with brainstem signs suggestive of herniation, metabolic acidosis, severe hypoglycemia, or anemia. Neurologic sequelae occur in ~5% of nonimmune individuals and include cranial nerve lesions, extrapyramidal tremor, polyneuropathy, epilepsy, or psychiatric manifestations. In African children, sequelae are more common and more severe. Hemiparesis, ataxia, and cortical blindness are the most common sequelae, but some children are left in a vegetative state. More recently, it has been demonstrated that epilepsy is associated with exposure to CM. Impairment of a wide range of cogni-

tive functions has been documented, particularly in memory, executive functions, and language.

Prevention

Currently, no vaccine is available for malaria. Prophylaxis for travelers involves taking an oral antimalarial such as mefloquine or atovaquone-proguanil. Mefloquine is started 1 week before departure, taken weekly, and continued for 4 weeks after return from endemic areas. Although licensed in North America for children who weigh >5 kg and are older than 6 months, the WHO advocates mefloquine use in children who weigh <5 kg or are 6 months of age if travel cannot be avoided. Atovaquone-proguanil is started 1–2 days before departure, taken daily, and continued for 1 week after return. Atovaquone-proguanil is licensed in North America for children who weigh >11 kg. Protection from mosquito bites by mosquito-eradication programs and use of bed nets, protective clothing, and insect repellant is advocated for both travelers and individuals who live in malaria-endemic regions.

CONCLUSIONS AND FUTURE DIRECTIONS

In summary, CNS infections have varied etiology, clinical presentation, treatment course, and prognosis. It is important that the intensivist is familiar with the clinical syndromes and the epidemiology, so that an appropriate differential diagnosis may be generated, diagnostic tests obtained, and empiric and specific treatment initiated. Future directions in the understanding, diagnosis, and management of CNS infection will undoubtedly include improved molecular diagnostic techniques, including PCR, for a larger number of etiologic agents, which will enhance the understanding of the epidemiology of CNS infections, as well as their etiology. Advances in molecular microbiology and immunology will also enhance the understanding of pathogenesis and allow for the development of improved therapeutic and preventive measures.

KEY POINTS

Meningitis

- Meningitis is inflammation of the meninges that presents acutely when bacterial or viral and subacutely when mycobacterial or fungal.
- Bacterial meningitis is a serious bacterial infection that is often missed clinically, and CSF should be obtained when suspected.
- CSF in bacterial meningitis has elevated polymorphonuclear neutrophils, low glucose, and high protein.
- Bacterial meningitis must be treated emergently with a broad-spectrum antibiotic.
- The top three causes of bacterial meningitis include *H. influenzae*, *N. meningitidis*, and *S. pneumoniae*; all three can be prevented with available vaccines.
- Aseptic meningitis has high PMNs initially and then high lymphocyte counts.
- Aseptic meningitis is mainly caused by viruses but is also caused by TB and other agents.

Encephalitis and Myelitis

- Encephalitis is inflammation of brain parenchyma, and myelitis is the inflammation of the spinal cord.
- Most agents that cause meningitis may spread to the brain and spinal cord.
- Arboviruses are the most common cause of epidemic encephalitis.
- Herpes simplex is the most common cause of sporadic encephalitis.
- HSE must be treated promptly with acyclovir.
- JE can be prevented with vaccination.
- ADEM is a postinfectious autoimmune reaction treated with high-dose steroids.

Abscess

- LP is often contraindicated when a brain abscess is suspected.
- Antimicrobial therapy with drainage is often necessary in treating CNS abscesses.

Shunt Infection

- Most shunt infections are due to *Staphylococcus* species— *S. epidermidis* and *S. aureus*.
- Antibiotics, shunt removal, and external drainage are often required for appropriate management of shunt infections.

Fungal Infection

- Fungal CNS infection often has an insidious onset.
- Most fungal CNS infection is due to hematogenous spread from the lung.
- Mucormycosis occurs via direct spread from sinuses.
- Amphotericin B remains an appropriate initial empiric antimicrobial for most suspected fungal infections of CNS.

Parasitic Infections

- Most parasitic infections of the CNS are subacute, but some (e.g., cerebral malaria) can be acute and severe.
- The most important etiologic clue to parasitic infection is living in or visiting an endemic area.

ACKNOWLEDGMENT

Some of the figures are courtesy Prof. N. Khandelwal and Prof. R.K. Vasishta from the Departments of Radiodiagnosis & Imaging and Histopathology, PGIMER, Chandigarh.

References

1. Agrawal D, Gupta A, Mehta VS. Role of shunt surgery in pediatric Tubercular Meningitis with hydrocephalus. *Indian Pediatr* 2005;42:245–50.
2. Al-Shekhlee A, Kocharian N, Suarez JJ. Re-evaluating the diagnostic methods in herpes simplex encephalitis. *Herpes* 2006;13:17–9.
3. American Thoracic Society, Centers for Disease Control and Prevention, Infectious Disease Society of America. Treatment of tuberculosis. *Am J Resp Crit Care Med* 2003;167:603–62.
4. Cassady KA, Whitley RJ. Pathogenesis and pathophysiology of viral central nervous system infections. In: Scheld WM, Whitley RJ, Durack DT, eds. *Infection of the Central Nervous System.* Philadephia: Lippincott-Raven, 2004;57–74.
5. Chen TL, Chen HP, Fung CP, et al. Clinical characteristics, treatment and prognostic factors of candidal meningitis in a teaching hospital in Taiwan. *Scand J Infect Dis* 2004;36:124–30.
6. Dale RC, Branson JA. Acute disseminated encephalomyelitis or multiple sclerosis: Can the initial presentation help in establishing a correct diagnosis? *Arch Dis Child* 2005;90:636–9.
7. De Tiege X, Rozenberg F, Burlort K, et al. Herpes simplex encephalitis: Diagnostic problems and late relapse. *Dev Med Child Neurol* 2006;48:60–3.
8. Del Brutto OH, Roos KL, Coffey S, et al. Meta Analysis: Cysticidal drugs for neurocysticercosis: Albendazole and praziquantel. *Ann Int Med* 2006;145:43–51.
9. Dondorp A, Nosten F, Stepniewska K, et al. Artesunate versus quinine for treatment of severe falciparum malaria: A randomised trial. *Lancet* 2005;366:717–25.
10. Dubos F, Lamotte, Bibi-Triki F, et al. Clinical decision rules to distinguish between bacterial and aseptic meningitis. *Arch Dis Child* 2006;91:647–50.
11. Garcia HH, Evans CAW, Nash TE, et al. Current consensus guidelines for treatment of neurocysticercosis. *Clin Microbiol Rev* 2002;15:747–56.
12. Gimenez F, Barraud dL, Fernandez C, et al. Tumor necrosis factor alpha in the pathogenesis of cerebral malaria. *Cell Mol Life Sci* 2003;60:1623–35.
13. Graybill JR, Sobel J, Saag M, et al. Diagnosis and management of increased intracranial pressure in patients with AIDS and cryptococcal meningitis. *Clin Infect Dis* 2000;30:47–54.
14. Gumbo T, Kadzirange G, Mielke J, et al. Cryptococcus neoformans meningoencephalitis in African children with acquired immunodeficiency syndrome. *Pediatr Infect Dis J* 2002;21:54–6.
15. Idro R, Jenkins NE, Newton CR. Pathogenesis, clinical features, and neurological outcome of cerebral malaria. *Lancet Neurol* 2005;4:827–40.
16. Kabilan L, Ramesh S, Srinivasan S, et al. Hospital and laboratory-based investigations of hospitalized children with central nervous system-related symptoms to assess Japanese encephalitis virus etiology in Cuddalore district, Tamil Nadu, India. *J Clin Microbiol* 2004;42:2813–5.
17. Kalita J, Misra UK, Pandey S, et al. A comparison of clinical and radiological findings in adults and children with Japanese encephalitis. *Arch Neurol* 2003;60:1760–4.
18. Kamei S, Sekizawa T, Shiota H, et al. Evaluation of combination therapy using acyclovir and corticosteroid in adult patients with herpes simplex virus encephalitis. *J Neurol Neurosurg Psychiatry* 2005;76:1544–9.
19. Kumar R, Prakash M, Jha S. Paradoxical response to chemotherapy in neurotuberculosis. *Pediatr Neurosurg.* 2006;42:214–22.
20. Leake JA, Albani S, Kao AS, et al. Acute disseminated encephalomyelitis in childhood: Epidemiology, clinical, and laboratory features. *Pediatr Infect Dis J* 2004;23:756–64.
21. Maitland K, Newton CR. Acidosis of severe falciparum malaria: Heading for a shock? *Trends Parasitol* 2005;21:11–6.
22. May M, Daley AJ, Donath S, et al. Australasian Study Group for Neonatal Infections Early onset neonatal meningitis in Australia and New Zealand, 1992–2002. *Arch Dis Child Fetal Neonatal Ed* 2005;24:533–7.

23. Mussini C, Pezzotti P, Miro JM, et al. International Working Group on Cryptococcosis. Discontinuation of maintenance therapy for cryptococcal meningitis in patients with AIDS treated with highly active antiretroviral therapy: An international observational study. *Clin Infect Dis* 2004;38: 565–71.

24. Njoku AK. Tuberculosis: Current trends in diagnosis and treatment. *Niger J Clin Pract* 2005;8:118–24.

25. Oates-Whitehead RM, Maconochie I, Baumer H, et al. Fluid therapy for acute bacterial meningitis. *Cochrane Database Sys Rev* 2005;3:CD004786.

26. Perfect JR. Fungal meningitis. In: Scheld WM, Whitley RJ, Marra CM, eds. *Infections of the Central Nervous System*, 3rd ed. Philadelphia: Lippincott Williams and Wilkins, 2004;691–712.

27. Prasad K, Singhal T, Jain N, Gupta PK. Third-generation cephalosporins versus conventional antibiotics for treating acute bacterial meningitis. *Cochrane Database Sys Rev* 2004;2:CD001832.

28. Ramers C, Billman G, Hartin M, et al. Impact of a diagnostic cerebrospinal fluid enterovirus, PCR test on patient management. *JAMA* 2000;283: 2680–5.

29. Saez-Leorens X, McCracken GH. Bacterial meningitis in children. *Lancet* 2003;361:2139–48.

30. Simon JK, Lazareff JA, Diament MJ, et al. Intramedullary abscess of the spinal cord in children: A case report and review of the literature. *Pediatr Infect Dis J* 2003;22:186–92.

31. Singhi P, Devi D, Khandelwal N. One week versus four weeks of albendazole therapy for neurocysticercosis in children: A randomized, placebo-controlled, double-blind trial. *Pediatr Infect Dis J* 2003;22:268–72.

32. Singhi P, Ray M, Singhi S, et al. Acute disseminated encephalomyelitis in North Indian Children. *J Child Neurol* 2006;21:851–7.

33. Singhi P, Singhi S. Central nervous system tuberculosis. *Curr Treat Options Infect Dis* 2001;3:481–92.

34. Singhi P, Singhi S. Neurocysticercosis in children. *J Child Neurol* 2004;19:482–92.

35. Singhi S, Khetarpal R, Baranwal AK, et al. Intensive care needs of children with acute bacterial meningitis: A developing country perspective. *Ann Trop Pediatr* 2004;24:133–40.

36. Singhi S, Murthy A, Singhi P, et al. Continuous midazolam versus diazepam infusion for refractory status epilepticus. *J Child Neurol.* 2002;17: 106–10.

37. Singhi S, Singhi P, Srinivas B, et al. Fluid restriction does not improve the outcome of acute meningitis. *Pediatr Infect Dis J* 1995;14: 495–503.

38. Singhi SC, Bansal A. Serum cortisol levels in children with acute bacterial and aseptic meningitis. *Pediatr Crit Care Med* 2006;7:74–8.

39. Skoldenberg B, Aurelius E, Hjalmarsson A, et al. Incidence and pathogenesis of clinical relapse after herpes simplex encephalitis in adults. *J Neurol* 2006;253:163–70.

40. Sow So, Diallo S, Campbell JD, Tapia MD, et al. Burden of invasive disease caused by Haemophilus influenzae type b in Bamako, Mali: Impetus for routine infant immunization with conjugate vaccine. *Pediatr Infect Dis J* 2005;24:533–7.

41. Steiner I, Budka H, Chaudhuri A, et al. Viral encephalitis: A review of diagnostic methods and guidelines for management. *Eur J Neurol* 2005;12: 331–43.

42. Taylor TE, Fu WJ, Carr RA, et al. Differentiating the pathologies of cerebral malaria by postmortem parasite counts. *Nat Med* 2004;10:143–5.

43. Tseng JH, Tseng MY. Brain abscess in 142 patients: Factors influencing outcome and mortality. *Surg Neurol* 2006;65:557–62.

44. Tunkel AR, Hartman BJ, Kaplan SL, et al. Practice guidelines for the management of bacterial meningitis. *Clin Infect Dis* 2004;39:1267–84.

45. Turgut M, Alabaz D, Erbey F, et al. Cerebrospinal fluid shunt infections in children. *Pediatr Neurosurg.* 2005;41:131–6.

46. Van de Beek D, de Gans J, McIntyre P, et al. Corticosteroids for acute bacterial meningitis. *Cochrane Database Sys Rev* 2003;3:CD004405.

47. Van der Weert EM, Hartgers NM, Schaff HS, et al. Comparison of diagnostic criteria of tuberculous meningitis in human immunodeficiency virus-infected and uninfected children. *Pediatr Infect Dis J* 2006;25:65–9.

48. WHO. Severe falciparum malaria. *Trans Royal Soc Tropic Med Hygiene* 2000;94 (Suppl 1):S1–1–S1–74.

49. WHO. *Treatment of Tuberculosis. Guidelines for National Programmes.* Geneva, World Health Organization. WHO/TB 2003;313.

CHAPTER 81 ■ NOSOCOMIAL INFECTIONS IN THE PEDIATRIC INTENSIVE CARE UNIT

JOHN P. STRAUMANIS

Since the beginning of medical practice, clinicians have been challenged by nosocomial infections—the transmission of infection from medical practitioner or hospital environment to patient. It was not until medical procedures became increasingly invasive, and the potential for curing infections with antibiotics became a reality, that the topic of nosocomial infections became an area of interest in the medical field. Well before that time, even before Louis Pasteur's germ theory, Ignaz Semmelweis made an important clinical observation and correlation in terms of preventing nosocomial infections in 1847. He realized that his close friend and colleague died of symptoms identical to puerperal fever after his finger was cut during an autopsy on a woman who died of puerperal fever. Semmelweis further noted that a midwife-run obstetric ward had a rate for puerperal fever of only 2%, a stark contrast to his ward, run by physicians, which had an infection rate of >12%. The physicians performed autopsies in the morning on women who had died of puerperal fever before examining their patients on the obstetric ward. Semmelweis instituted the practice of making the students wash their hands with a chlorinated lime solution prior to examining their patients. As a result, the infection rate dropped to <2% the following year. To this day, hand washing remains one of the most important safeguards in preventing nosocomial infection (42).

Nosocomial infections are important to consider, treat, and, most importantly, prevent in any hospital setting, but especially in the ICU. Hospital-acquired infections can lead to significant morbidity and mortality, and infection-control measures can greatly impact these outcomes. It is equally important to prevent the infection of hospital personnel in order to diminish the risk of spreading infection to other patients and to other personnel, thereby preventing missed days from work, which could impact the ability to staff the PICU. Additional financial costs are associated with nosocomial infections, including hospital costs, loss of productivity of healthcare personnel, and loss of income to families from missing time at work.

DEFINITIONS

An understanding of several definitions is important. A *nosocomial infection* is any infection that a patient acquires within the hospital setting that is not present at admission. Even if symptoms develop after discharge, such infections should be considered nosocomial. *Community-acquired infections* are those present at the time of admission, even if they do not necessarily cause symptoms at the time of admission. The differentiation between community-acquired and nosocomial infections may

take some investigation and is dependent on normal incubation times as well as ancillary testing such as sensitivities and genetic typing of the organism. *Surgical site infections* (SSIs) are associated with the surgical procedure itself, including the wound and the direct surgical field exposed during the procedure. Other infections at distant sites, even though the surgical procedure or anesthesia for the procedure put the patient at risk for such an infection, are considered nosocomial but not SSIs. *Colonization* is the growth or presence of potentially infectious organisms in a cavity, on a surface, in tissue, in body fluids, or even associated with a medical device, without causing a host reaction, a clinically adverse event, or disease.

The ways in which to report nosocomial infection rates vary widely. They may be noted as a percentage of patients, number of infections per 100 patients, or number of infections per 1000 device days. The National Nosocomial Infection Surveillance (NNIS) System of the Centers for Disease Control and Prevention (CDC) reports SSIs in terms of number of infections per 100 procedures. The SSIs are further classified as superficial, or incisional and deep, or involving the organ space involved in the operation. Where possible, this chapter will report rates using these standards.

OVERVIEW AND EPIDEMIOLOGY

The CDC reports 2 million nosocomial infections in the US annually, which lead to increased mortality and an associated $4.5 billion in excess healthcare costs (36). While it is not possible to eliminate all nosocomial infections, at least one-third could be prevented with implementation of organized infection-control programs. Given the incidence, morbidity, mortality, and cost of nosocomial infections, those that could be prevented but were not may be considered a source of medical error. Despite even the best infection-control program, the risk of nosocomial infection will always be present in the ICU due to the unique nature of the critically ill or injured patient.

The risk of nosocomial infection depends on a variety of factors. The location within the hospital plays an important role, with the highest rates typically occurring in the ICU. Even the type of ICU influences the nosocomial infection rate, with different rates seen in medical, surgical, trauma, burn, neurologic/neurosurgical, and cardiac ICUs. The PICU is unique in that it typically cares for all of these subsets of patients over the pediatric age range. Another unique factor in the PICU is that different aged patients will have different incidence patterns of the various types of hospital-acquired infections. For children <5 years of age, the top three nosocomial infections are bloodstream infections, pneumonia, and urinary tract

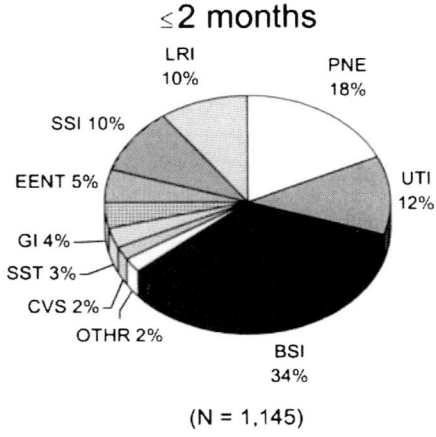

≤2 months

(N = 1,145)

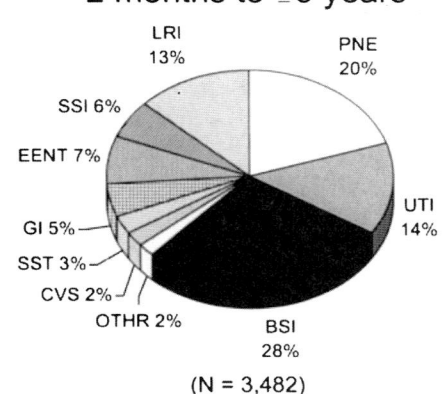

>2 months to ≤5 years

(N = 3,482)

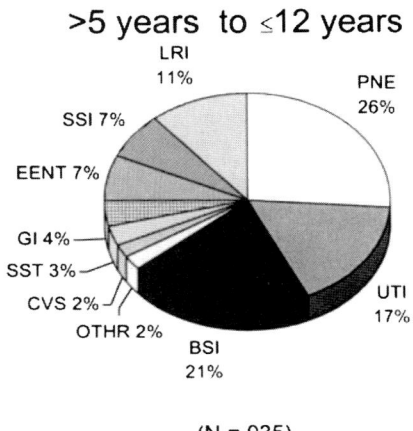

>5 years to ≤12 years

(N = 935)

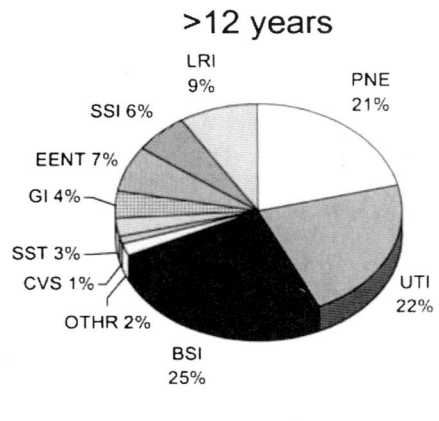

>12 years

(N = 728)

FIGURE 81.1. LRI, lower respiratory tract infection other than pneumonia; PNE, pneumonia; UTI, urinary tract infection; BSI, bloodstream infection; CVS, cardiovascular infection; SST, skin or soft tissue infection; GI, gastrointestinal infection; EENT, eye, ear, nose, throat infection; SSI, surgical site infection; OTHR, other infection. From Richards MJ, Edwards JR, Culver DH, et al. Nosocomial infections in pediatric intensive care units in the United States. National Nosocomial Infections Surveillance System. *Pediatrics* 1999;103(4):e39, with permission.

infections (UTIs). In children between 5 and 12 years of age, the top three acquired infections are pneumonia, bloodstream infections, and UTIs. In the adolescent population, bloodstream infections are followed by UTIs and then pneumonia in incidence (**Fig. 81.1**). The location of the hospital also plays a role, with an increased risk of nosocomial infection being noted in developing nations. One study reported that all types of nosocomial infections, when standardized to device days, were increased in the ICUs of developing nations. The device utilization rates were noted to be similar in the developed and developing nation ICUs, making the increased infection rate more likely to be secondary to factors within the ICUs, hospitals, or national healthcare systems (38,39) (**Table 81.1**).

General Risk Factors

In addition to the location within the hospital and the type of ICU, general risk factors exist that are independent of the type of nosocomial infection. Although these risk factors can influence the likelihood of contracting a nosocomial infection, only a few can be realistically altered to impact nosocomial infection rates.

The age of the patient can affect the risk of nosocomial infection. Typically, younger children, particularly neonates, have the highest risk in the pediatric population. The relative immaturity of the immune system in the neonate, coupled with

common ICU interventions that bypass the physical barriers to infection such as skin and mucosal surfaces, is responsible for the increased risk. The use of parenteral nutrition with high glucose concentrations and lipids is an additional risk factor for infection. The fact that premature infants are impacted the most by these factors explains why NICUs have higher nosocomial infection rates than PICUs. Patients who are immunosuppressed from chemotherapy, human immunodeficiency virus infection, or steroid use are similarly at an increased risk for developing a nosocomial infection.

Severity of illness as predicted by the Pediatric Risk of Mortality score has been correlated to the risk of nosocomial infections; in one study, a score above 13 predicted nosocomial infection in a Brazilian PICU with 78.9% sensitivity, 64.4% specificity, 21.8% positive-predictive value, and 96.1% negative-predictive value. Independent risk factors of developing a nosocomial infection were length of stay, prior antimicrobial therapy, and device utilization ratios, with the latter two factors being the best predictors of nosocomial infection risk (3).

Understaffing is an independent risk factor for acquiring nosocomial infections, most likely due to the fact that adherence to good hand hygiene has been shown to be inversely correlated to workload. Understaffing increases workload and therefore nosocomial infection risk (6).

Red blood cell transfusions have been found to be an independent risk factor for the development of nosocomial

TABLE 81.1

COMPARISON OF DEVICE USE AND RATES OF DEVICE-ASSOCIATED INFECTION IN THE ICUs OF THE US NATIONAL NOSOCOMIAL INFECTION SURVEILLANCE SYSTEM AND THE INTERNATIONAL NOSOCOMIAL INFECTION CONTROL CONSORTIUM

Variable	US NNIS ICUs 1992–2004	INICC ICUs 2002–2005
Rate of device use[a]		
Mechanical ventilators	0.43 (0.23–0.62)	0.38 (0.19–0.64)
CVCs	0.57 (0.36–0.74)	0.54 (0.22–0.97)
Urinary catheters	0.78 (0.65–0.90)	0.73 (0.48–0.94)
Rate per 1000 device[a]		
Ventilator-associated pneumonia	5.4 (1.2–7.2)	24.1 (10.0–52.7)
CVC-associated bloodstream infection	4.0 (1.7–7.6)	12.5 (7.8–18.5)
Catheter-associated UTI	3.9 (1.3–7.5)	8.9 (1.7–12.8)
Proportion of device-associated infections with resistance, %[b]		
MRSA	59	84
Ceftriaxone-resistant *Enterobacteriaceae*	19	55
Ciprofloxacin-resistant *Pseudomonas aeruginosa*	29	59
Vancomycin-resistant enterococci	29	5

[a]Overall (pooled) and 10th to 90th percentile range for US NNIS teaching hospitals; overall (pooled) and range of individual countries for the INICC hospitals; [b]Overall (pooled) data from NNIS, 1992–2004 (300 hospitals) and from INICC, 2002–2005. Data from National Nosocomial Infections Surveillance (NNIS) System Report, data summary from January 1992 through June 2004, issued October 2004. *Am J Infect Control* 2004;32:470–85. NNIS, National Nosocomial Infection Surveillance System; INICC, International Nosocomial Infection Control Consortium; CVC, central venous catheter; UTI, urinary tract infection; MRSA, methicillin-resistant *Staphylococcus aureus*. From Rosenthal VD, Maki DG, Salomao R, et al. Device-associated nosocomial infections in 55 intensive care units of 8 developing countries. *Ann Intern Med* 2006;145(8):582–91, with permission.

infections in critically ill adult ICU patients. In a single-centered prospective, observational study, the incidence of nosocomial infection was 14.3% in transfused patients and 5.8% in nontransfused patients. Each unit of packed red blood cells administered increased the risk of developing a nosocomial infection by 9.7%. Increasing severity of illness did not affect the risk of developing a nosocomial infection. However, within each quartile of probability of survival, the transfused group had a higher rate of nosocomial infection, which was significant in all but the most severely ill patients, with a probability of survival of <25%. Those patients with >25% probability of survival had higher mortality rates, longer ICU stays, and longer hospitalizations compared to nontransfused patients (43) (**Fig. 81.2**).

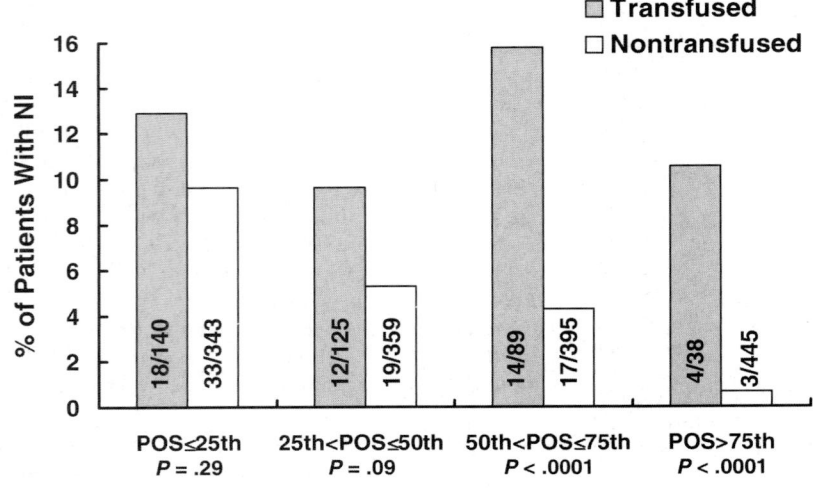

FIGURE 81.2. Nosocomial infection (NI) rates adjusted for probability of survival (POS). The overall rate of NI in transfused patients was significantly higher than in nontransfused patients (p <0.0001; Cochran-Mantel-Haenszel test). Numbers within the bars indicate the number of patients with NI/total in each group. The p values beneath each bar refer to the significance level of the within-group comparisons (Student's t-tests). From Taylor RW, O'Brien J, Trottier SJ, et al. Red blood cell transfusions and nosocomial infections in critically ill patients. *Crit Care Med* 2006;34(9):2302–8, with permission.

Isolation Precautions

Prevention of nosocomial illness can be in large part facilitated through the use of isolation precautions, which can be divided into two categories: standard and transmission-based precautions. *Standard precautions* should be used at all times and are designed to prevent the practitioner from coming in contact with potentially infectious bodily fluids. The most important standard precaution is hand hygiene. Soap and water hand washing is considered the gold standard. Use of waterless antiseptic agents is appropriate, except in the presence of visible dirt, proteinaceous bodily fluids such as blood, or when contamination with spores is likely. Soap and water is necessary under these circumstances. Hand hygiene must be practiced both before and after patient contact, even if gloves are worn. Barriers such as gloves, masks, eye protection, and nonsterile gowns should be worn when contact with bodily fluids or secretions is likely.

Transmission-based precautions are aimed at protection against transmission of infectious organisms from patients with documented or suspected infection, as well as from those colonized with specific organisms. These additional precautions are over and above the standard precautions and are based on route of transmission: contact, droplet, or air-borne transmission. Common organisms that require each type of isolation are listed in **Table 81.2.** *Contact precautions* are used for a wide variety of organisms that spread by direct contact with the patient or indirect contact via fomites such as toys, stethoscopes, and unwashed hands. Contact isolation should include single-patient rooms or cohorting, gowns, and gloves in addition to standard precautions. *Droplet precautions* are used for organisms that spread short distances (<3 feet away) from the patient via coughing or sneezing. Droplet isolation includes single-patient rooms or cohorting of patients with the same organism. Healthcare providers should wear masks with eye shields in addition to following standard precautions. Organisms such as adenovirus and influenza require both contact and droplet precautions. *Air-borne precautions* include additional safeguards to be taken for organisms such as tuberculosis, measles, and varicella that are transmitted by air currents. Patients should be in private rooms with negative air flow. For measles and varicella isolation, susceptible healthcare providers should avoid contact if possible. For other organisms that require air-borne precautions, a fitted respirator should be worn by all who enter in the patient's room. Isolation should be based on the clinical symptoms or conditions present at admission, and should always begin even before the organism is isolated (2) (**Table 81.3**).

For protection against air-borne infections, selecting the correct type of respirator and ensuring a proper fit are crucial.

TABLE 81.2

TRANSMISSION-BASED ISOLATION RECOMMENDATIONS FOR SPECIFIC INFECTIOUS ORGANISMS AND ILLNESSES

Contact precautions	Droplet precautions	Air-borne precautions
Clostridium difficile	Adenoviruses	*Mycobacterium tuberculosis*
Conjunctivitis, viral and hemorrhagic	Diphtheria	Rubeola (measles) virus
Diphtheria (cutaneous)	*Haemophilus influenzae* type b (invasive)	Varicella-zoster virus
Enteroviruses	Hemorrhagic Fever viruses	During aerosol-generating
Escherichia coli O157:H7 and other Shiga toxin-producing *E. coli*	Influenza	procedures such as intubation, nebulized therapy, and
Hepatitis A virus	Mumps	bronchoscopy
Herpes simplex virus (neonatal, mucocutaneous, or cutaneous)	*Mycoplasma pneumoniae*	Severe acute respiratory syndrome
Herpes zoster (localized with no evidence of dissemination)	*Neisseria meningitidis* (invasive)	Viral hemorrhagic fevers
Impetigo	Parvovirus B19 during the phase of illness before onset of rash in immunocompetent patients	Consider for influenza
Major (noncontained) abscess, cellulitis, or decubitus ulcer	Pertussis	
Multidrug-resistant organisms as determined by local infection control	Plague (pneumonic)	
Parainfluenza virus	Respiratory syncytial virus (beneficial during large outbreaks)	
Pediculosis (lice)	Rubella	
Respiratory Syncytial Virus	Severe acute respiratory syndrome	
Rotavirus	Streptococcal pharyngitis, pneumonia, or scarlet fever	
Scabies		
Shigella		
Staphylococcus aureus (cutaneous or draining wounds)		
Viral hemorrhagic fevers (Ebola, Lassa, or Marburg)		

Some organisms may include more than one type of isolation. This list is not all inclusive.
Data from American Academy of Pediatrics. Infection Control for Hospitalized Children. In: Pickering LK, Baker CJ, Long SS, et al, eds. *Red Book: 2006 Report of the Committee on Infectious Diseases.* 27th ed. Elk Grove Village: American Academy of Pediatrics, 2006;153–64.

TABLE 81.3

CLINICAL SYNDROMES OR CONDITIONS THAT WARRANT PRECAUTIONS IN ADDITION TO STANDARD PRECAUTIONS TO PREVENT TRANSMISSION OF EPIDEMIOLOGICALLY IMPORTANT PATHOGENS PENDING CONFIRMATION OF DIAGNOSIS[a]

Clinical syndrome or condition[b]	Potential pathogens[c]	Empiric precautions[d]
Diarrhea		
Acute diarrhea with a likely infectious cause	Enteric pathogens[e]	Contact
Diarrhea in patient with history of recent antimicrobial use	*Clostridium difficile*	Contact
Meningitis	*Neisseria meningitidis*	Droplet
Rash or exanthems, generalized, cause unknown		
Petechial or ecchymotic with fever	*N. meningitidis*	Droplet
Vesicular	Varicella virus	Air-borne and contact
Maculopapular with coryza and fever	Measles virus	Air-borne
Respiratory tract infections		
Pulmonary cavitary disease	*Mycobacterium tuberculosis*	Air-borne
Paroxysmal or severe persistent cough during periods of pertussis activity in the community	Bordetella pertussis	Droplet
Viral infections, particularly bronchiolitis and croup, in infants and young children	Respiratory syncytial virus or parainfluenza virus	Contact and droplet
Risk of multidrug-resistant microorganisms[f]		
History of infection or colonization with multidrug-resistant organisms	Resistant bacteria	Contact
Skin, wound, or urinary tract infection in a patient with a recent hospital or nursing home stay in a facility in which multidrug-resistant organisms are prevalent	Resistant bacteria	Contact
Skin or wound infection		
Abscess or draining wound that cannot be covered	*Staphylococcus aureus*, group A streptococcus	Contact

[a]Infection-control professionals are encouraged to modify or adapt this table according to local conditions. To ensure that appropriate empiric precautions are implemented, hospitals must have systems in place to evaluate patients routinely according to these criteria as part of their preadmission and admission care.

[b]Patients with the syndromes or conditions listed may have atypical signs or symptoms (e.g., pertussis in neonates, absence of paroxysmal or sever cough in adults). The clinician's index of suspicion should be guided by the prevalence of specific conditions in the community and clinical judgment.

[c]The organisms listed in this column are not intended to represent the complete or even most likely diagnoses but, rather, possible causative agents that require additional precautions beyond Standard Precautions until they can be excluded.

[d]Duration of isolation varies by agent (see Garner JS. Hospital Infection Control Practices Advisory Committee. Guidelines for isolation precautions in hospitals. *Infect Control Hosp Epidemiol* 1996;17:53–80.)

[e]These pathogens include shiga toxin-producing *Escherichia coli* including *E. Coli* O157:H7, *Shigella* organisms, *Salmonella* organisms. *Campylobacter* organisms, hepatitis A virus, enteric viruses including rotavirus, and *Cryptosporidium* organisms.

[f]Resistant bacteria judged by the infection-control program on the basis of current state, regional, or national recommendations to be of special clinical or epidemiologic significance.

From American Academy of Pediatrics. Infection Control for Hospitalized Children. In: Pickering LK, Baker CJ, Long SS, et al, eds. *Red Book: 2006 Report of the Committee on Infectious Diseases, 27th ed*. Elk Grove Village: American Academy of Pediatrics, 2006, with permission.

Respirators can be either air-supplying or air-purifying. The air-supplying respirators provide the greatest protection but are expensive and require high amounts of maintenance to ensure proper functioning. Air-purifying respirators filter air through a cartridge that must be selected based on the type of hazard (bacterial or chemical) to which the wearer will be exposed. These respirators are protective, but not to the same degree as the air-supplying devices. Disposable respirators are air-purifying or filtering devices. The N95 respirators are the most commonly used in healthcare settings. The letter designates the mask's reaction to oil. "N" means not oil-proof. If exposed to oil, the filtering efficiency of the mask may not be maintained. Oil-resistant masks and oil-proof masks are designated "R" and "P," respectively. The number indicates the filtering efficiency of the mask with an adequate seal; "95" identifies the mask as having the ability to filter at least 95% of particles, with a median diameter of 0.3 microns or greater. Most respirators have limitations when used by individuals with facial hair, and specialized devices may be necessary (26).

The personal protective equipment that should be worn is determined by the organism being isolated. To ensure the maximal effect of the protective equipment, it must be donned and removed in the proper order. After performing hand hygiene, the gown should be donned first, followed by the mask or respirator, ensuring proper fit. The face shield or goggles are placed on after the mask, and finally, the gloves are donned. When removing the protective items, the following sequence should be followed to prevent self-inoculation or exposure to infectious particles. The gloves are removed first by pulling them off away from the body, and the outer surface of the glove should be considered contaminated. With one gloved hand, the other glove is removed by pulling on the outer surface. The removed glove is kept in the gloved hand, and the ungloved fingers are placed under the cuff of the remaining glove, pulling it off inside out, with the first glove inside the second. The gloves are properly discarded. The face shield or goggles are removed next by touching only the sides or headband, as the outer, forward-facing surface is potentially contaminated; these are discarded or stored for appropriate cleaning. The gown is removed by pulling down and away from the body, touching only the inside of the gown because the front and sleeves are contaminated. The gown is rolled into a bundle, with the inner surface of the gown on the outside of the bundle, and discarded. Finally, the mask is removed without touching the front surface by pulling on the straps or ties from behind; the mask is discarded. Lastly, hand hygiene is performed (7).

Prevention of nosocomial infections occurs not only at the bedside or by practitioners directly involved with patient care. Institutional and structural levels of infection control should exist at all healthcare facilities. The CDC has additional evidence-based recommendations for healthcare facilities available at: www.cdc.gov/ncidod/dhqp/pdf/guidelines/Enviro_guide_03.pdf.

Compliance with Hand Hygiene

Despite 150 years having passed since Semmelweis nearly eradicated the transmission of nosocomial infections on his obstetric ward, present-day practitioners wash their hands less than half of the time. The best practice is to wash with soap and water before and after patient contact. Even with the alcohol-based hand sanitizers placed near patient care areas, the compliance rate remains low. Observational studies put the usage rate of any hand hygiene at 14%–48%. An improvement from 48% to 66% in hand hygiene compliance was noted with the initiation of an educational program at one institution (35). Over the course of the program, the nosocomial infection rates decreased from 16.9% to 9.9%. Differences in the compliance rate exist among various practitioners. Interestingly, those with less medical training have better compliance rates. Healthcare assistants were 64% compliant, followed by nurses and nursing students (49%), ancillary personnel (including dieticians, therapists, and phlebotomists) (46%), with physicians and medical students performing the worst, with only a 26% hand-hygiene compliance rate. Factors that can impact hand hygiene include workload, staffing shortages, and the availability of sinks. Alcohol-based sanitizing solutions provide a resolution to the latter factor, as their use does not require sinks or running water. Additional factors that may help to improve compliance are that the alcohol-based preparations tend to cause less irritation and drying of the hands and they save the practitioner time when compared to soap and water. Studies have proven that the alcohol-based solutions are effective against infection, including viruses, as long as hands are not visibly soiled. For visible soilage or when *Clostridium* spores are potentially present, soap and water must be used (6,19,37,47).

The presence of an active infection-control and surveillance program can lower nosocomial infection rates by as much as one-third when compared to hospitals without such programs. Surveillance programs enable hospitals to monitor trends and allow for interventions when indicated (15).

Surveillance Cultures

The increasing incidence of resistant organisms colonizing and infecting people in the community impacts the risk of developing a nosocomial infection in the hospital. As the incidence rises in the community, the risk increases of falsely identifying a community-acquired infection as nosocomial and of transmitting these community infections to other patients, thus causing a true nosocomial infection. In communities that have high levels of resistant organisms, it may be worth screening for these infections at admission. This approach has most notably been used with screening for methicillin-resistant *Staphylococcus aureus* (MRSA). The first step in screening is to identify those patients at high risk for MRSA to both prevent false positives on screening and to control cost. Patients considered to have an increased risk of MRSA colonization or infection include (a) patients with a prior MRSA infection or identified colonization; (b) patients who have been frequently hospitalized, particularly if they have been admitted in the prior 6 months; (c) interhospital transfers from high-incidence regions; (d) residents of chronic-care facilities; and (e) patients with chronic skin lesions. All patients with a high risk of carriage of MRSA should be screened at admission and/or admitted to isolation. The admission screening is most commonly performed by culturing the anterior nares, but other sites such as wounds or skin lesions, catheter sites, tracheostomies, and the umbilicus in neonates can be used. Following admission screening, surveillance screening is performed to identify new, hospital-acquired infections. The frequency of such screening varies from weekly to monthly, depending on the local prevalence of MRSA. Discussions with infection-control personnel can aid in determining the necessary frequency of screening, as well as which areas or patients in the hospital warrant such monitoring. Screening in the ICU is beneficial due to the high incidence of patients at risk for MRSA colonization, the high frequency of use of invasive devices that can increase the risk of nosocomial transmission, and the ability to prevent spread to a population that can ill afford an additional infection. The use of routine screening in other areas of the hospital should be determined based on the recommendations of the local infection-control officer. The routine screening of medical staff is not currently recommended. However, it may be considered in difficult-to-control outbreaks. Once a patient is identified as being colonized with MRSA, she should be isolated, informed of her colonization status, and considered for treatment to clear the colonization (9). This approach has been used for MRSA colonization and infections but could be used for a variety of organisms if the frequency in the community or hospital warrants such an approach and when adequately specific and sensitive screening tests are available.

Once screening or other surveillance measures have been used to identify patients with organisms that are likely to be spread by nosocomial transmission, cohorting of patients with the same organism and the staff caring for them may be beneficial. The theory is that, after contact with one infected patient, the next contact of the healthcare worker would be a patient with the same organism, thus diminishing the spread of infection to a naïve patient. Standard precautions still must be used to prevent infection or colonization of the healthcare worker and to minimize the risk of spreading infection. This approach has proven successful for MRSA and vancomycin-resistant enterococci in a variety of settings. The Dutch have used such a strategy for 20 years in patients known to have MRSA to decrease the prevalence of infections to <2% despite a high prevalence in the surrounding countries. Similar techniques have been used for MRSA in Finnish nursing homes and in statewide surveillance in Rhode Island, as well as for vancomycin-resistant enterococci, using a regional approach in the US (6).

CATHETER-RELATED BLOODSTREAM INFECTIONS

Intravascular catheters are essential in the critical care setting. They provide stable and secure access for caloric-dense nutrition, medications, fluids, and blood products, as well as a means by which to monitor laboratory values, assess treatments, measure vital pressures, and aid in diagnosis and direct therapies. Typically, tunneled central venous catheters have a lower risk of infection compared to percutaneously inserted lines. Tunneled lines, with or without cuffs, are generally used for long-term access of at least several weeks, usually require surgical placement, and are not the commonly used line in ICUs.

Published guidelines from the CDC have set criteria for diagnosing bloodstream infections that involve intravascular catheters. A *catheter-related bloodstream infection* is either a bacteremia or fungemia documented with at least one peripherally obtained blood culture that is obtained from a vein and not a catheter. Clinical evidence of an infection, including a host response, must be present that cannot be attributed to any source other than the catheter. The growth of an organism in the bloodstream must be documented by (a) positive semiquantitative or quantitative cultures of a catheter segment with an organism identical in species and antibiogram as isolated from a peripheral blood culture, (b) simultaneously drawn peripheral and line quantitative blood cultures with greater than a 5:1 ratio in catheter blood versus peripheral blood colony counts, or (c) a differential in timing of culture positivity of >2 hrs between the catheter and peripheral blood culture, where the catheter culture is positive first. A *catheter-associated bloodstream infection* has less rigorous criteria and requires the presence of a central line being in place during the 48 hrs prior to the drawing of the positive culture and compelling evidence that the infection is related to the line. This definition is helpful for surveillance but can overestimate the true incidence of bloodstream infections (33).

Approximately 15 million central venous catheter days occur in the US annually. Assuming a rate of 5.3 central venous catheter infections per 1000 catheter days for ICUs, ~80,000 nosocomial central venous line infections occur each year. Various adult and pediatric studies from individual units have placed the additional cost to the hospital admission of a nosocomial bloodstream infection to be in the range of $34,000–$56,000 (15,33).

Coagulase-negative staphylococci are the most common cause of pediatric nosocomial bloodstream infections, accounting for 20% to nearly 50% of isolates. gram-negative bacteria account for 25% of PICU nosocomial bloodstream infections. *S. aureus* and *Candida* spp. are responsible for ~10% each throughout the pediatric age range. Other organisms that cause nosocomial bloodstream infections are dependent upon the age

of the child and other clinical factors. β-hemolytic streptococci are more prevalent in the neonatal population, causing 8.5% of the hospital-acquired infections in this age group. Bimodal peak is reported for enterococcal infections seen in infants and patients 13–65 years of age, with 9.4% and 8.5% of isolates, respectively. At 7.3%, *Klebsiella* spp. are the third most common isolates behind coagulase-negative staphylococci and *S. aureus* in the pediatric oncology population (4,33,44).

The cause of central venous line infection can be from many sources, depending upon the conditions under which the line was placed (emergently versus in a controlled situation), experience of the operator, site selection, ongoing line care, and other extrinsic factors. The most common route of infection for percutaneous lines in the ICU is migration of skin organisms down the external surface of the catheter to the bloodstream; this can be greatly influenced by catheter care and the patient's own bacterial flora. Other sources of line-associated infection can be grouped into the following categories: (a) hematogenous spread from distant sites with increased risk due to biofilm and clot formation on the catheter surface, which is influenced by type of catheter material and the presence of antiseptic or antibiotic coatings; (b) infection via contaminated infusate, which is rare in the US but may be more prominent in developing nations; (c) colonization of the catheter hub, especially with long-term catheters; (d) transducer or IV tubing contamination; or (e) contamination of the catheter prior to insertion, which can occur in the manufacturing process due to use of expired catheters, or by contamination at the time of insertion through operator error or improper site preparation (29,33,40) (**Fig. 81.3**).

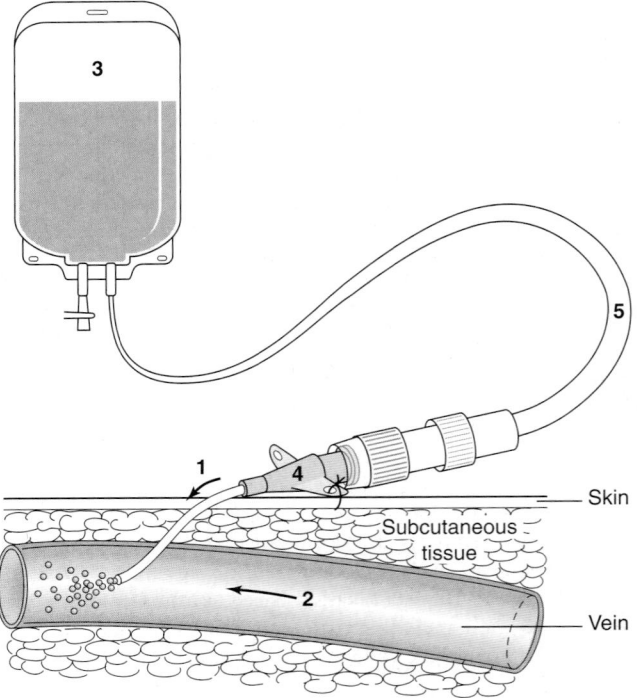

FIGURE 81.3. Mechanisms of nosocomial bloodstream infection. (1) Migration of skin bacteria down external surface of catheter; (2) Hematogenous spread from distal sites; (3) Contaminated infusate; (4) Colonization of catheter hub; (5) Contamination of transducer or IV tubing.

Diagnosis and Treatment of Catheter-Related Infections

Definitive diagnosis of a catheter-related infection can be difficult, which certainly complicates management decisions regarding catheter removal. Most symptoms such as fever, chills, and rigors have poor specificity; as a result, central venous catheters should not be removed for fever alone. Site inflammation with or without purulence and positive bloodstream cultures has better specificity but low sensitivity. As a result, surveillance cultures are not recommended, and cultures should only be obtained when a catheter-related bloodstream infection is suspected. Use of clinical judgment is important and, if the patient has fever with only mild-to-moderate symptoms, the catheter should not be routinely removed. Cultures positive for common nosocomial bloodstream infections, such as coagulase-negative staphylococci, *S. aureus*, and *Candida* spp. without an identified source of infection and in the presence of a central venous catheter should raise suspicion for the possibility of a catheter-related bloodstream infection (29).

Two blood cultures should be obtained when a catheter-related infection is suspected, and at least one, if not both, should be drawn percutaneously. When paired central and peripheral cultures are sent, it is recommended that they either be quantitative cultures or qualitative cultures with continuously monitored differential time to positivity to aid in the diagnosis of a catheter-related bloodstream infection. A differential time to positivity at least 2 hrs earlier for the central-line culture compared to the peripheral culture is indicative of a central venous line infection, with a sensitivity of 91% and a specificity of 94%. This method is simpler for most hospital laboratories and is at least as accurate as quantitative cultures. Once the decision has been made to remove the line, the catheter tip should be sent for quantitative or semiquantitative cultures; qualitative broth cultures are not recommended (**Fig. 81.4**). The skin should be prepped prior to catheter removal, then the catheter removed with sterile forceps, the distal portion cut and sent for culture. For pulmonary artery catheters, the most likely positive portion of the apparatus is the tip of the introducer rather than the tip of the catheter. Exchanging the catheter over a guidewire minimizes the risks associated with the placement of the line at a new site; however, it does not lower the risk of infection. For those patients with suspected line infections and mild-to-moderate symptoms, a change over a guidewire may be an alternative while awaiting blood and catheter tip cultures. Once a catheter-related bloodstream infection has been verified, if the line was exchanged over a guidewire, the line should be removed and replaced at a different site. Nontunneled catheters may be replaced once appropriate antibiotic therapy has been instituted. It may not be necessary to remove the catheter in patients without evidence of persistent bloodstream infection or if there is a culture-positive, coagulase-negative staphylococcal

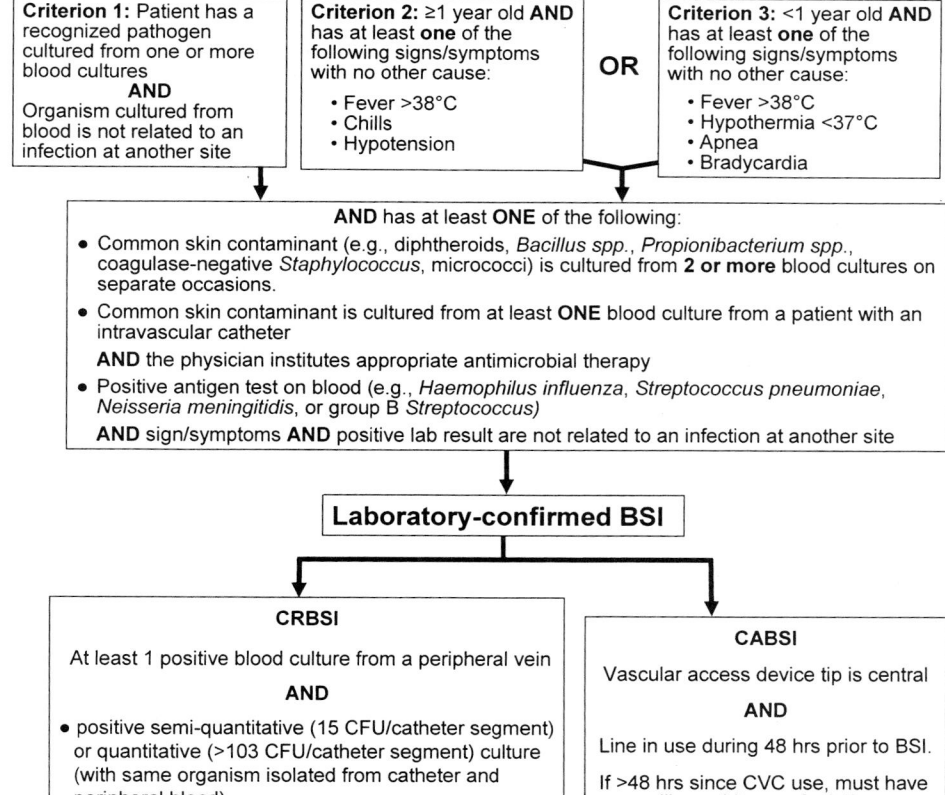

FIGURE 81.4. Bloodstream infection (BSI) diagnostic flow diagram. A catheter-related BSI (CRBSI) can also be confirmed with at least one positive blood culture from a peripheral vein and a differential time to positivity at least 2 hrs earlier for a central-line culture. CABSI, Catheter-associated BSI; CFU, colony-forming units; CVC, central venous catheter. From Stockwell JA. Nosocomial infections in the pediatric intensive care unit: affecting the impact on safety and outcome. *Pediatr Crit Care Med.* 2007;8(2 Suppl):S21–37, with permission.

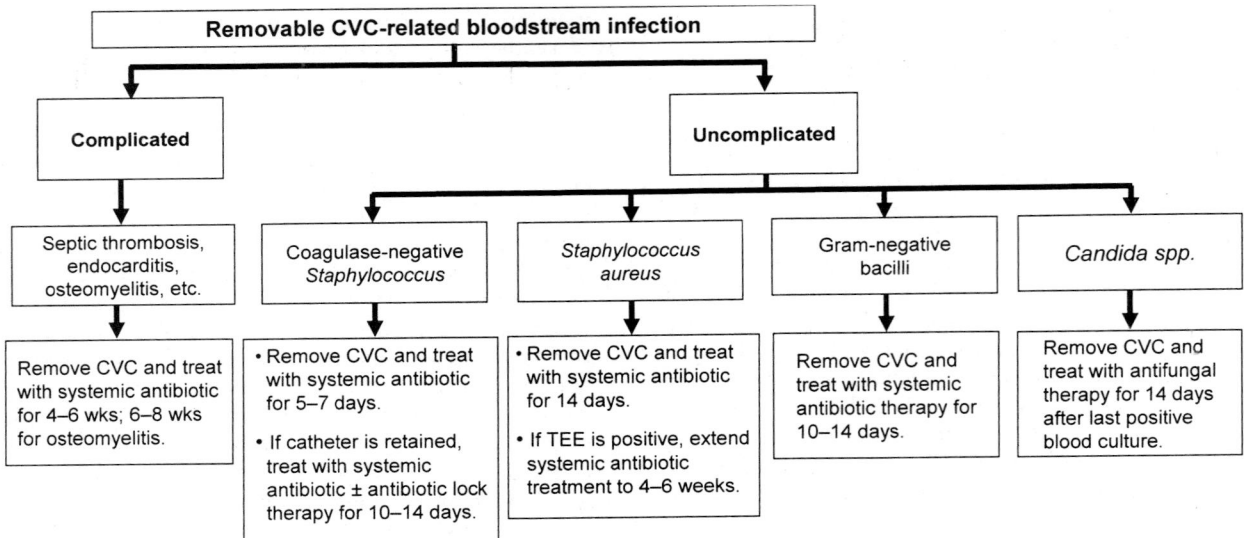

FIGURE 81.5. Approach to the management of patients with nontunneled central venous catheter (CVC)-related bloodstream infection. Duration of treatment will depend on whether the infection is complicated or uncomplicated. The catheter should be removed, and systemic antimicrobial therapy should be initiated, except in some cases of uncomplicated catheter-related infection due to coagulase-negative staphylococci. For infections due to *Staphylococcus aureus*, transesophageal echocardiography (TEE) may reveal the presence of endocarditis and help to determine the duration of treatment. From Mermel LA, Farr BM, Sherertz RJ, et al. Guidelines for the management of intravascular catheter-related infections. *Clin Infect Dis* 2001;32(9):1249–72, with permission.

infection in the absence of local or metastatic infectious complications. For both conditions, appropriate antibiotic therapy is indicated (**Fig. 81.5**). Persistent bacteremia or lack of clinical improvement after removal of the colonized catheter with the patient on antimicrobial therapy should prompt a thorough evaluation for infective endocarditis, septic thrombosis, and other distant sites of infectious seeding, especially if symptoms are present >3 days after catheter removal (13,29, 33,40).

Placing a new line in children may be difficult compared to placing it in adults, and some authors have reported successful treatment of central line infections without removal of the device. Such management should include close observation of the clinical condition, with prompt removal if clinical deterioration occurs. Initial therapy should be broad-spectrum and aimed at organisms likely to be causing the infection, based on typical isolates for the hospital as well as predominant sensitivity patterns. Typical empiric coverage should include gram-positive and gram-negative coverage. It is important to cover for MRSA, with its increasing presence in both the hospital and the community. Initial therapy is usually vancomycin along with a third-generation cephalosporin or aminoglycoside. For severe infections in patients who are immunosuppressed or for yeast species that are isolated or highly suspected, the addition of antifungal coverage is appropriate. Once an isolate's sensitivities are known, the antibiotic regimen should be appropriately adjusted to prevent the selection of resistant organisms. Success rates in treating infections with the offending line in place are successful in up to 90% of coagulase-negative infections, using a minimum of 10–14 days of treatment. As infections caused by fungi or gram-negative organisms are extremely resistant to treatment if the catheter is left in place, all central

lines should be removed under these circumstances and treatment should be a minimum of 14 days. Removal of the catheter in coagulase-negative staphylococci infections requires only a 5–7-day course of therapy. Regardless of the culture results, if the child does not respond or worsens within the first 3 days of antibiotic therapy, the line should be removed (13,29).

Prevention of Catheter-related Infections

Many strategies can be practiced to prevent catheter-related infections both at the time of line insertion and during care of the site after insertion. Thorough hand washing prior to insertion is basic clinical practice. Skin preparation should be performed with a 2% aqueous chlorhexidine gluconate solution. Chlorhexidine has been proven to lower catheter-related infections compared to both 10% povidone-iodine and 70% alcohol. Where a 2% solution of chlorhexidine is not available, povidone-iodine or 70% alcohol should be used. Chlorhexidine preparations should not be used on infants <2 months of age due to possible absorption through the immature skin. After adequate skin preparation, full barrier precautions, which include a large sterile or full-body drape, long-sleeved sterile gown, cap, mask, and sterile gloves, should be taken. Use of full barrier precautions reduces the risk of infection compared to standard precautions, which consist of a small drape and sterile gloves. Once the line is secured, a dressing should be applied. The use of transparent, semipermeable, polyurethane dressings further secures the device; allows for visual inspection of the catheter and insertion site; allows for bathing; and, through less frequent dressing changes, can save personnel time. These points favor use, even though studies have yet to find improvement in catheter infection rates compared to standard gauze and tape dressings.

Regardless of the type of dressing utilized, it should be replaced when damp, soiled, loosened, or visual inspection of the site is necessary. Early studies of a chlorhexidine-impregnated sponge dressing at the site of catheter insertion of arterial and central venous lines revealed a threefold decrease in bloodstream infections. The chlorhexidine-impregnated sponge is only effective in preventing extraluminal surface infections and not the intraluminal infections, which are more common in long-term indwelling catheters. Data are limited regarding the use of this product in patients who are <16 years of age. One minor risk is a local dermatitis, which is more common in neonates, making its use not yet warranted in this population. Antiseptic ointments, such as povidone-iodine, applied at the catheter insertion site may be used and are superior to no ointment being used. Antibiotic ointments should not be used at the insertion site due to a potential risk of developing resistance and an increased risk of colonization with *Candida* spp. A catheter hub containing 3% iodinated alcohol in an antiseptic chamber is available in Europe. Studies have shown a fourfold reduction in the incidence of catheter infections. Devices have been modified to prevent small amounts of iodinated alcohol from entering the bloodstream, which occurred in earlier models. The use of antibiotic lock prophylaxis and systemic antibiotic prophylaxis with vancomycin and other antibiotics is not recommended due to the risk of creating antibiotic resistance (8,13,15,28,33,40).

One of the most underrated means of reducing catheter-related infections is prompt removal of the catheter once it is no longer needed. Additionally, placing a line with only the number of lumens required for care decreases the risk of infection; conversely, a higher number of lumens increases infection risk. In children who require multiple-lumen catheters in the PICU, the lines are typically manipulated frequently, which increases infection risk (13).

Polyvinyl chloride and polyethylene catheters are less likely to impede bacterial adherence to the catheter and, as a result, are not usually available from manufacturers in the US. Teflon and polyurethane catheters are associated with fewer line-related infections. Additional antimicrobial resistance can be imparted by coating or impregnating central venous catheters with antiseptics or antibiotics. Various catheters are approved by the US Food and Drug Administration for use in children who weigh >3 kg. Chlorhexidine- and silver sulfadiazine-coated catheters have been shown to reduce infection risk compared to standard catheters. These studies have only examined catheters with the coating on the external catheter surface. The antimicrobial activity decreases over time and has a half-life against *Staphylococcus epidermidis* of 3 days. The beneficial infection-control aspects of the catheter should be realized over the first 14 days. Despite treated catheters being more expensive than nontreated catheters, a cost savings of $68–$391 per catheter was found in one study, provided that a high infection rate exists even though other more economical interventions are first implemented. An infection rate >3.3 per 1000 catheter days may favor the added cost in adults where the average NNIS bloodstream-infection rate ranges from 2.9–5.9 infections per 1000 catheter days. With an average NNIS pediatric bloodstream-infection rate of 7.6 per 1000 catheter days in the US, a benefit may also be appreciated in the pediatric population. Preliminary studies have found improved

anti-infective activity with catheters that have antiseptic coating on both the external and luminal surface. Resistance to chlorhexidine has been seen in vitro but not noted in clinical use. The literature contains rare reports of anaphylaxis to chlorhexidine/sulfadiazine catheters; nearly all of these have been in Japan and, as a result, these catheters are not commercially available there (28,33). Catheters impregnated internally and externally with the antibiotics minocycline and rifampin have shown lower infection rates when compared to externally coated chlorhexidine/sulfadiazine catheters in a randomized, multicentered trial. The half-life of antimicrobial activity against *S. epidermidis* is 25 days, and the catheters begin showing beneficial effects after 6 days of use. As with the antiseptic catheters, bacterial resistance is possible and has been seen in vitro; however, minocycline/rifampin-resistant organisms have yet to be reported in clinical use. As with antiseptic catheters, antibiotic-impregnated catheters should be reserved for patient populations in whom the catheter infection rate exceeds 3.3 per 1000 catheter days (33).

Literature from adult studies initially suggested the need for central-line replacement every few days due to the higher cumulative risk of catheter infection over time. More recent data from randomized, controlled studies have disproved these earlier findings. Replacement at a new site carries all of the risks associated with insertion and does not lower the cumulative risk of infection. Replacement of the catheter over a guidewire has a higher risk of infection compared to leaving the line in place or replacing at a new site. Benefits of changing a catheter over a guidewire include less discomfort to the patient, lower mechanical complication risk, and preserving access in patients who have limited access options (15,33). The pediatric literature is quite different from the adult literature on this topic. For peripheral venous catheters, no increase in phlebitis risk is associated with increased duration of catheter use, as long as the catheter was placed under aseptic conditions. With peripheral arterial catheters, which include femoral and axillary arterial lines, risk of infection increases with longer catheter placement and if the system permits backflow into the pressure tubing. However, the risk of infection is constant at 6.2% from day 2 to day 20 following insertion. Therefore, routine replacement of arterial lines is not recommended. The routine replacement of central venous catheters is not recommended due in part to the limited number of vascular sites in children. This finding is substantiated by one large study ($n = 397$ catheters) in which no relationship was found between the length of time of catheter use and the daily probability of infection. Routine replacement of tubing and infusion sets has been proven to decrease the risk of catheter infection. Tubing for peripheral and central lines should be changed no more frequently than every 72 hrs for routine fluids. Infusion sets used for blood, blood products, and lipid infusions should be changed within 24 hrs of starting the infusion. For arterial lines, the tubing and the transducer should be changed at 96-hr intervals. Stopcocks that are used inline with the tubing and catheter are commonly contaminated up to 50% of the time. The impact of stopcock microbial growth on catheter infections is unknown, and no recommendation exists for frequency of replacement. Common sense would dictate changing stopcocks with tubing changes and when soiled or potentially contaminated (13,33).

In adult studies, the subclavian site has significantly lower infection risk than does the internal jugular site. However, this risk must be balanced by the increased risk of complications as well as operator experience and expertise. Observational studies on dialysis lines have found internal jugular lines to have a lower infection rate. A higher colonization rate at the femoral site with an increased risk of catheter infection has been reported in the adult population but has not been found in studies of pediatric patients, in which femoral sites were associated with fewer mechanical complications and had an equivalent infection rate when compared to catheters at other sites. When selecting a catheter site for the pediatric patient, the infectious risks, the risks of insertion, and the skills of the operator should be weighed. In the pediatric population, the femoral site is a viable option as long as nonfemoral sites are considered and utilized in older pediatric patients because they likely have similar infection risks compared to adults (13,15,33). The type of line inserted must be determined by the patient's needs and the infectious risks associated with the line (Table 81.4).

Extracorporeal Membrane Oxygenation

The risk factors identified for nosocomial infections associated with extracorporeal membrane oxygenation (ECMO) are prolonged ECMO support, support for cardiac disease, undergoing a major surgical procedure immediately prior to or while on ECMO, and having an open chest while on ECMO. The reported nosocomial infection rates for children on ECMO is 11% for all patients who require support, with subgroup infection rates of 8% for neonates and 13.5% for patients on ECMO for cardiac diagnoses. The nosocomial infections associated with ECMO include wound infections of the neck and chest, bloodstream infections, UTIs, and respiratory infections. Potential reasons for the increased risk of infection while on ECMO include loss of the skin barrier to infection, especially for those patients who require an open chest; alteration of lymphocyte subsets; decrease in peripheral natural killer cells; and

TABLE 81.4

DESCRIPTION OF VASCULAR ACCESS DEVICES AND RISK OF INFECTION

Catheter type	Entry site	Length	Comments
Peripheral venous catheters (short)	Usually inserted in veins of forearm or hand	<3 in	Phlebitis with prolonged use; rarely associated with bloodstream infection
Peripheral arterial catheters	Usually inserted in radial artery; can be placed in femoral, axillary, brachial, posterior tibial arteries	<3 in	Low infection risk; rarely associated with bloodstream infection
Midline catheters	Inserted via the antecubital fossa into the proximal basilic or cephalic veins; does not enter central veins	3–8 in	Anaphylactoid reactions have been reported with catheters made of elastomeric hydrogel; lower rates of phlebitis than short peripheral catheters
Nontunneled CVCs	Percutaneously inserted into central veins (subclavian, internal jugular, or femoral)	8 cm or longer, depending on patient size	Account for most CRBSIs
Pulmonary artery catheters	Inserted through a Teflon introducer in a central vein (subclavian, internal jugular, or femoral)	30 cm or longer, depending on patient size	Usually heparin-bonded; similar rates of bloodstream infection as CVC; subclavian site preferred to reduce infection risk
PICCs	Inserted into basilic, cephalic, or brachial veins and enter the superior vena cava	20 cm or longer, depending on patient size	Lower rate of infection than nontunneled CVCs
Tunneled CVCs	Implanted into subclavian, internal jugular, or femoral veins	8 cm or longer, depending on patient size	Cuff inhibits migration of organisms into catheter tract, lower rate of infection than nontunneled CVC
Totally implantable	Tunneled beneath skin and have devices that are subcutaneous-port accessed with a needle; implanted in subclavian or internal jugular vein	8 cm or longer, depending on patient size	Lowest risk for CRBSI; improved patient self-image; no need for local catheter site care; surgery required for catheter removal
Umbilical catheters	Inserted into either umbilical vein or umbilical artery	6 cm or less, depending on patient size	Risk for CRBSI similar to catheters placed in umbilical vein versus artery

CVC, central venous catheter; CRBSI, catheter-related bloodstream infection; PICC, peripherally inserted central catheters
From O'Grady NP, Alexander M, Dellinger EP, et al. Guidelines for the prevention of intravascular catheter-related infections. The Hospital Infection Control Practices Advisory Committee, Center for Disease Control and Prevention, US. *Pediatrics* 2002;110(5):e51, with permission.

decreased total B-cell counts. Yeast infections are noted as well and are believed to be due to use of broad-spectrum antibiotics (34).

NOSOCOMIAL RESPIRATORY INFECTIONS

If infections of eye, ear, nose, and throat with pneumonia are included, respiratory tract infections are the most common site of nosocomial infections for nearly all ages of patients in the PICU (38). Much attention has been placed on ventilator-associated pneumonia (VAP) as a common and potentially preventable nosocomial infection. Other hospital-acquired respiratory infections include sinusitis, otitis media, and tracheitis. Respiratory syncytial virus (RSV) can be an important pathogen in nosocomial infections due to its annual outbreaks in the community and the number of children hospitalized as a result. However, practitioners must be cognizant of the possibility of other organisms with similar signs and symptoms entering the PICU and being a potential nosocomial infection, such as severe acute respiratory syndrome (SARS) and avian flu.

The sources of nosocomial respiratory infections in the PICU are multiple and may come from the hospital environment, therapeutic and diagnostic equipment, hospital staff, family members, and even other patients. Environmental sources include (a) fomites such as toys and cribs improperly cleaned between patient use, and (b) contamination of hospital water sources with organisms such as *Legionella*. Contamination of the patient's respiratory tract can occur from devices in direct contact with the patient, such as endotracheal tubes, nasoenteric tubes, suction catheters, and bronchoscopes, as well as those with indirect contact, such as mechanical ventilators, ventilator tubing, nebulizers, and oxygen delivery devices. The human vector most likely to transmit infection to the patient is the hospital staff. Poor hand hygiene, improper isolation practices, and fomites such as stethoscopes are the most common risk factors. Family members and other patients can also transmit an infection to the PICU patient. All of these factors must be considered and controlled to minimize nosocomial respiratory tract infections.

Ventilator-associated Pneumonia

Nosocomial pneumonia is the second most common site of hospital-acquired infection in the PICU after catheter-related bloodstream infections. Nosocomial pneumonia can occur in any patient but is more common in infants, young children, and patients over 65 years of age. Those at highest risk for acquiring pneumonia in the PICU are patients who require intubation and mechanical ventilation. The increased risk is due to the bypassing and alteration of the host defenses in part because the vocal cords are stented open, which increases the risk of aspirating gastrointestinal contents. The risk of nosocomial pneumonia is increased 6–20-fold in patients who require mechanical ventilation when compared to those patients not ventilated. The definition of VAP is the development of a new pneumonia at least 48 hrs after initiation of mechanical ventilation. Independent risk factors for the development of VAP in children are immunodeficiency, immunosuppression, and neuromuscular blockade. Additional risk factors include genetic syndromes

with neuromuscular weakness, burns, steroid administration, and use of total parenteral nutrition. As in adults, children are at higher risk for VAP with antibiotic use, longer ICU lengths of stay, use of indwelling catheters due to hematogenous spread, use of H_2-receptor-blocker therapy, reintubation, and transport out of the ICU while intubated. The presence of a nasoenteric tube increases risk because it provides a direct route from the upper gastrointestinal tract to the oropharynx. Other associated therapies that affect risk of nosocomial pneumonia include in-line nebulizers and manipulation of ventilator circuits. The VAP rate in children accounts for 10%–26% of nosocomial infections. The pediatric NNIS VAP rate (January 1992 through June 2004 data) is 2.9 episodes per 1000 ventilator days. The number of hospitalized patients who acquire nosocomial pneumonia ranges from 16% to 29%. The incidence of pediatric nosocomial pneumonia by hospital location is highest in the NICU, followed by the PICU, and then the pediatric ward. Nosocomial pneumonia has the highest mortality rate of all pediatric nosocomial infections, with rates ranging from 20% to 70%. Although length of time with an endotracheal tube in place increases the risk of nosocomial pneumonia, the greatest risk is during the first 2 weeks of intubation. Nearly all intubated children will have colonization of their endotracheal tube with hospital-acquired organisms by a mean of 5 days (45,47).

VAP rates for adult ICUs in developing countries range from 10.0 to 52.7 per 1000 ventilator days, with an overall rate calculated with data from 55 ICUs in eight countries of 24.1 VAP infections per 1000 ventilator days. This rate is dramatically higher than the reported US adult rates of 5.4 per 1000 ventilator over the same time period. The most common organisms isolated in the developing countries were *Enterobacteriaceae* spp. (26%), of which 58% were resistant to ceftriaxone; *Pseudomonas aeruginosa* (26%), with 60% resistant to fluoroquinolones; *S. aureus* (22%), with 84% methicillin resistant; and *Acinetobacter* spp. (20%) (39).

The bacterial organisms identified most often are gram-negative bacilli, with *P. aeruginosa* being the most common species identified in PICUs. Other important organisms in this group are *Escherichia coli*, *Klebsiella pneumoniae*, and *Enterobacter* spp., which are being reported with an increased frequency in PICUs in the US. The second most common bacterial etiology of pediatric nosocomial pneumonia is the gram-positive organisms. The frequently isolated bacteria are *S. aureus* and coagulase-negative staphylococci. The mortality rate is less than that seen with the gram-negative organisms. *S. epidermidis* nosocomial pneumonia is a common cause in the NICU population and is typically the result of hematogenous spread. Anaerobic nosocomial pneumonia is rare in the pediatric population but accounts for 23% of nosocomial pneumonias in adults, perhaps in part be due to the difficulty in isolating the organisms and the inability to obtain protected brush specimens in children. Viruses, predominantly RSV, are the most common cause of nosocomial respiratory infections. Fungal infections are exceedingly rare but may occur in children who are immunosuppressed, especially if they frequently receive broad-spectrum antibiotics (47).

Symptoms and Diagnosis of Ventilator-associated Pneumonia

The diagnosis of VAP in children can be made on clinical grounds without the use of bronchoscopy. The set clinical

TABLE 81.5

CLINICAL CRITERIA FOR DIAGNOSING VENTILATOR-ASSOCIATED PNEUMONIA BY AGE

	All patients	**1–12 years of age**	**<12 months of age**
Chest film	At least 2 serial CXR with new or progressive and persistent infiltrate or consolidate or cavitation that develops later than 48 hrs post initiation of mechanical ventilation		
Additional Criteria	At least one of the shaded criteria *AND* at least two of the non-shaded criteria	At least 3 of the criteria below	Worsening gas exchange *AND* at least 3 of the criteria below
Temperature	>38°C without other recognized cause	>38.4°C or <37°C without other recognized cause	Temperature instability without other recognized cause
WBC count	<4000/mm³ OR >12,000/mm³	<4000/mm³ OR >15,000/mm³	<4000/mm³ OR >15,000/mm³ and band forms >10%
Altered mental status	If >70 years of age without other recognized cause	N/A	N/A
Sputum/Secretions	New onset purulent sputum *OR* change in the character of sputum *OR* increased respiratory symptoms		
Respiratory Symptoms	New onset or worsening of cough, dyspnea, or tachypnea		Apnea, tachypnea, increased work of breathing, or grunting
Auscultation findings	Rales or bronchial breath sounds		Wheezing, rales, or ronchi
Cough	N/A as separate criteria	N/A as separate criteria	+
Worsening oxygenation or ventilation	Present	Present	Required criteria
Heart rate	N/A	N/A	<100 beats/min OR >170 beats/min

CXR, chest x-ray film, WBC, white blood cell count; N/A, not applicable
Modified from Wright ML, Romano MJ. Ventilator-associated pneumonia in children. *Semin Pediatr Infect Dis* 2006;17(2):58–64.

diagnostic criteria and the alternate criteria, which vary by age, are listed in **Table 81.5**. The presence of pneumatoceles on chest film in children who are <12 months of age also meets the radiographic criteria for pneumonia noted in the table. The diagnosis of VAP can be made on clinical and radiographic grounds, but determination of the causative organism is necessary to direct antibiotic therapy. However, determination remains difficult because endotracheal tube cultures are inaccurate due to colonization of the endotracheal tube and upper airway with gram-negative bacilli and staphylococci, which occurs within a few days of intubation. For adults and older children, bronchoalveolar lavage and protected-specimen brush collection has been used with success. However, the protected-specimen brush samples cannot be obtained in young children because of the size of bronchoscope required, and bronchoalveolar lavage performed directly has a high incidence of contamination. Recognized methods to determine the causative organism include positive blood cultures that cannot be attributed to another source, positive cultures from pleural fluid, a positive bronchoalveolar lavage specimen despite its limitations, >5% of cells from bronchoalveolar lavage containing intracellular bacteria, a positive culture of lung parenchyma, or histopathologic evidence of fungal hyphae (45). Once nosocomial pneumonia is suspected, empiric treatment should be started, covering the most likely organisms with consideration of the hospital's resistance patterns. When a specific causative is identified, antibiotic coverage should be adjusted. If the diagnostic workup is negative and a viral etiology is suspected, the discontinuation of antibiotics may be considered.

Prevention of Ventilator-associated Pneumonia

Ventilator-associated Pneumonia Bundle. In 2004, the Institute for Healthcare Improvement launched their campaign to save 100,000 lives, which included an evidence-based approach to lower mortality in six different areas, one of which was VAP. To achieve this goal, an evidence-based set of guidelines was developed to aid practitioners in decreasing mortality. The evidence was based on research conducted in adults, and at the time, it was unknown how this could or should be applied to critically ill children. The adult VAP bundle consists of the following interventions: (a) elevation of the patient's head of bed between 30 and 45 degrees; (b) daily sedation holidays, a break in the administration of sedatives, and a daily readiness for extubation assessment; (c) stress ulcer prophylaxis; and (d) deep vein thrombosis prophylaxis. The application of such a bundle can reduce the incidence of VAP by as much as 45%, even though the last two items do not directly address nosocomial pneumonia but are designed to treat complications commonly seen in sedate, sedentary, adult ICU patients. Data are minimal as to whether the use and effectiveness of these interventions

TABLE 81.6

COMMONLY UTILIZED PEDIATRIC VENTILATOR-ASSOCIATED PNEUMONIA BUNDLE ITEMS

Items to prevent iatrogenic spread of infection
  Adherence to good hand hygiene practices
  Use of universal precautions
  Use of appropriate isolation techniques based on infectious
    organism (proven or suspected)

Items to prevent aspiration of gastric contents
  Elevate the head of the bed between 30 and 45 degrees
  Monitor/drain gastric contents

Items to improve oral hygiene
  Oral rinsing/cleaning with chlorhexidine (0.12%)
  Use of toothbrush and oral swabs in daily oral care

Items to decrease endotracheal tube risk factors
  Use of in-line suction equipment where appropriate and
    available
  Suction of the hypopharynx prior to endotracheal
    suctioning and repositioning

Items to avoid contamination of respiratory equipment
  Dedicated oropharyngeal suction equipment
  Prevention of accumulation of respiratory circuit
    condensates
  Prevention of contamination of ventilation equipment

Items to decrease the duration of mechanical ventilation
  Daily readiness for extubation trials
  Neuromuscular blockade holidays

Adapted from Curley MA, Schwalenstocker E, Deshpande JK, et al. Tailoring the Institute for Health Care Improvement 100,000 Lives Campaign to pediatric settings: The example of ventilator-associated pneumonia. *Pediatr Clin North Am* 2006;53(6):1231–51.

affect the incidence of pediatric VAP. As a result, many centers have implemented only the low-risk interventions such as elevating the head of the bed, performing the readiness to extubate test, and using stress ulcer prophylaxis. Interventions such as sedation holidays are untested and, at least theoretically, are risky in younger patients, who may be at higher risk for unintended extubation (11).

Studies have not yet been performed on the effectiveness of implementing a pediatric VAP bundle, but in centers that apply a coordinated effort to decrease VAP, it appears that its frequency can be decreased. Items frequently utilized in pediatric centers are aimed at specific risk factors (**Table 81.6**). As with any infection-prevention regimen, adherence to infection-control practices to prevent the iatrogenic spread of infection is critical. Hand hygiene with either alcohol-based solutions or soap and water, along with use of universal precautions and appropriate isolation are the most effective and least utilized infection control practices. Elevation of the head of the bed prevents aspiration of gastric contents. This risk can be further minimized by gastric decompression with gastric tubes and the routine monitoring of gastric residuals. The importance of oral hygiene is becoming more evident. The American Dental Association recommends that routine oral care begin in infancy, well before the emergence of dentition. The guideline to use oral swabs and brush the teeth of critically ill patients stems from this recommendation and the fact that dental plaque consisting of predominantly gram-negative bacteria forms within 48 hrs of ICU admission. In adult studies, the use

of a 0.12% chlorhexidine oral rinse solution in patients in surgical intensive care was associated with a decreased incidence of VAP.

Adult studies provide increasing evidence that subglottic drainage of secretions significantly diminishes the risk of VAP. These specialized endotracheal tubes are both expensive and not yet available for the majority of the pediatric population because of size limitations. The findings of these studies have led to the practice of suctioning the hypopharynx to clear secretions in pediatric patients. This suctioning should be performed (a) prior to suctioning the endotracheal tube to prevent aspiration of hypopharyngeal secretions should the patient cough, and (b) prior to the manipulation of the endotracheal tube during retaping or repositioning. A few centers have also instituted the practice of clearing these secretions before moving the patient in bed. The use of in-line suctioning may not have direct effects on the rate of VAP, but use of the closed system has been shown to be cost effective and may have the added benefit of preventing the contamination of the suctioning equipment. The type of heater-humidification or heat and moisture exchangers in ventilator circuits has not been found to influence the incidence of VAP. However, if condensation should occur in the ventilator circuit, it could potentially become contaminated and theoretically cause an infection. Therefore, the condensate should be routinely removed from the circuit through the use of a trap. Staff should be conscientious and avoid contamination of respiratory equipment such as the end of the ventilator circuit, the resuscitation bag, and suction equipment to further diminish the risk of VAP (10,11,16).

Minimizing the length of time that the patient requires mechanical ventilation is important in preventing nosocomial pneumonia. Prompt treatment and reversal of the condition that necessitated mechanical ventilation must occur. A mechanism should be established by which to assess the patient's readiness to be extubated once the underlying condition is resolved. Adult VAP bundles have included sedation holidays to assess patients' respiratory strength and to ensure that patients are not excessively sedated. For most children in the PICU, sedation holidays are impractical, as they could potentially result in unintended extubations, particularly in children who are too young to cooperate or comprehend the necessity of the critical care interventions to which they are being subjected. Instead, the use of constant, high-dose sedation should be avoided and appropriate sedation scales should be used. If neuromuscular blockade is being used, it is reasonable to intermittently hold the paralyzing agents if clinically appropriate. Another potential, albeit unproven, element of a pediatric VAP bundle should be the daily assessment as to whether or not the patient can be extubated (**Fig. 81.6**). This should be done on a daily basis from the day of intubation to the day of successful extubation, unless a clinical contraindication is present. One of the main benefits of the readiness-for-extubation test is that it occurs regardless of whether the patient is thought by the clinicians to be ready for extubation. The method noted in the figure is one example of an extubation-readiness test; individual modifications may be required based on institutional practices (11).

While minimizing the duration of mechanical ventilation is important in preventing VAP, it is the presence of the endotracheal tube that imparts the risk of VAP and not the positive-pressure ventilation commonly associated with it. In a meta-analysis of 12 studies that examined pneumonia rates in adult patients who received noninvasive or invasive ventilation, a benefit was found to noninvasive ventilation in terms of

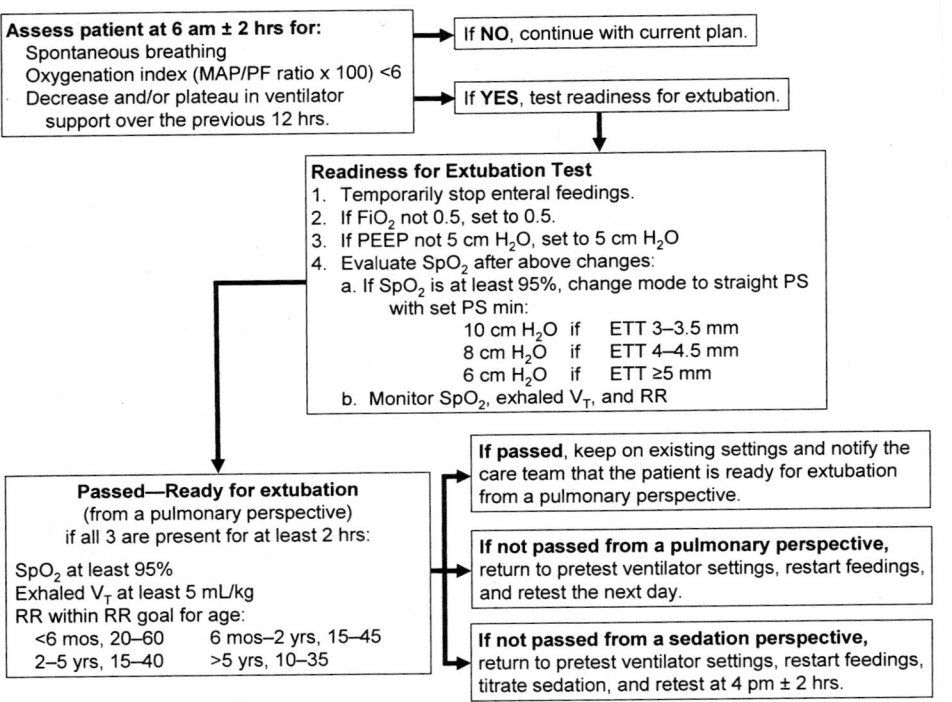

Assess patient at 6 am ± 2 hrs for:
Spontaneous breathing
Oxygenation index (MAP/PF ratio x 100) <6
Decrease and/or plateau in ventilator
support over the previous 12 hrs.

If **NO**, continue with current plan.

If **YES**, test readiness for extubation.

Readiness for Extubation Test
1. Temporarily stop enteral feedings.
2. If FiO₂ not 0.5, set to 0.5.
3. If PEEP not 5 cm H₂O, set to 5 cm H₂O
4. Evaluate SpO₂ after above changes:
   a. If SpO₂ is at least 95%, change mode to straight PS
     with set PS min:
       10 cm H₂O if   ETT 3–3.5 mm
       8 cm H₂O if   ETT 4–4.5 mm
       6 cm H₂O if   ETT ≥5 mm
   b. Monitor SpO₂, exhaled V$_T$, and RR

Passed—Ready for extubation
(from a pulmonary perspective)
if all 3 are present for at least 2 hrs:

SpO₂ at least 95%
Exhaled V$_T$ at least 5 mL/kg
RR within RR goal for age:
  <6 mos, 20–60   6 mos–2 yrs, 15–45
  2–5 yrs, 15–40   >5 yrs, 10–35

If **passed**, keep on existing settings and notify the care team that the patient is ready for extubation from a pulmonary perspective.

If **not passed from a pulmonary perspective**, return to pretest ventilator settings, restart feedings, and retest the next day.

If **not passed from a sedation perspective**, return to pretest ventilator settings, restart feedings, titrate sedation, and retest at 4 pm ± 2 hrs.

FIGURE 81.6. Daily test for patient readiness for extubation. In this model, prescreening for suitability for extubation is assessed over a 2-hr period. If prescreening criteria are met, feeds are held and the patient is brought to low ventilator settings for a trial on pressure support ventilation. If the patient does well based on preset criteria, extubation is considered. MAP, mean arterial pressure; PF ratio, PaO₂/FiO₂ ratio; PEEP, positive end-expiratory pressure; ETT, endotracheal tube; PS, pressure support; V$_T$, tidal volume; RR, respiratory rate. From Curley MAQ, Arnold JH, Thompson JE, et al. Clinical trial design: Effect of prone positioning on clinical outcomes in infants and children with acute respiratory distress syndrome. *J Crit Care* 2006;21:23–32; with permission.

lessening the risk for developing pneumonia [relative risk, 0.31; 95% confidence interval (CI), 0.16–0.57; $p = 0.0002$]. Studies have also found that patients managed with noninvasive ventilation have a shorter ICU length of stay and a decreased mortality rate. When appropriate, noninvasive ventilation should be considered as a potential method by which to decrease VAP risk (16,20).

Sinusitis

Sinusitis is a risk factor for the development of pneumonia. Patients in intensive care are uniquely at risk for developing a nosocomial sinus infection because of supine positioning, decreased sinus drainage due to positive-pressure ventilation, and nasal placement of therapeutic devices that obstruct sinus drainage. Using the criteria of having purulent secretions and radiological evidence of sinusitis, the incidence of nosocomial sinusitis has been estimated to be in the range of 5%–35%. In a study of adult ICU patients who did not have radiologic evidence of sinusitis prior to intubation and were randomized to nasotracheal or orotracheal intubation, 95% of the nasotracheally intubated group developed radiographic evidence of sinusitis compared to 22.5% in patients who were intubated orally. Prospective studies of ICU patients found the sinusitis rate to be 15.7 cases per 1000 patient days when a nasoenteric tube was in place compared to 1.6 cases per 1000 days for those patients without such a device. These rates were independent of whether or not the patient received mechanical ventilation. Although it may be impossible to avoid placing nasoenteric devices because they are necessary to provide vital nutrition to critically ill patients, nasotracheal tubes should be used for specific and well-defined reasons. Additional risk factors of sinusitis can be addressed through the use of VAP bundles, which include elevation of the head of the bed and attention to good oral hygiene (14).

Respiratory Syncytial Virus

RSV is one of the most common etiologies of pediatric nosocomial respiratory tract infections in the PICU and is the most common nosocomial infection overall on pediatric wards. Forty percent of these nosocomial RSV infections occur in the lower respiratory tract. RSV is different from other organisms that cause nosocomial infections in that although those children with underlying cardiopulmonary disease may have more severe infections, healthy children more commonly contract nosocomial RSV infections. The risk factors of contracting an RSV nosocomial infection are young age, especially neonates; underlying chronic illness such as cardiac or pulmonary disease; a long hospitalization; overcrowding or staff shortages; and most importantly, hospitalization during the RSV endemic season. An additional source of nosocomial RSV infection is healthcare workers. It is estimated that half of the staff on pediatric wards during an RSV season become infected. The symptoms that the staff experiences vary from mild to significant, and up to 20% may have an asymptomatic infection. Reinfection is common, even in the same season, because immunity to RSV is incomplete. Immunocompromised patients deserve special mention for two reasons. First, depending on the degree of immunosuppression, the illness can be quite severe. Reports from transplant units place mortality from RSV lower respiratory tract infections anywhere from 20% to 100%. Second, immunosuppressed neonates and children who receive corticosteroids can be considered in this group; they have prolonged shedding of active virus even if asymptomatic. Shedding of virus can continue up to 3 weeks in these patients (19,47).

Prevention of nosocomial RSV responds to simple infection-control measures. The most common modes of transmission of RSV from one person to another are via either large-droplet aerosols or adherence to fomites. As large droplets can only travel short distances (<1 meter), they require close person-to-person contact. Fomites pose the greatest risk of transmission in a hospital setting. RSV can survive and remain infectious on nonporous surfaces for 6–12 hrs. RSV could theoretically be spread by small-droplet aerosol, but studies have found this to not be the case. The virus can spread distances up to 7 meters, but it is thought that this mode of transmission is inefficient and therefore unlikely. Studies of transmission in multibed rooms have found a 3% transmission rate from infected to uninfected patients (19). Factors other than small-droplet transmission, such as staff or fomites, most likely account for many of these infections.

Influenza and Other Respiratory Viruses

Most respiratory viruses can be transmitted and contained using the methods described for RSV. SARS deserves special attention and is discussed in the next section. A very effective method of preventing the nosocomial transmission of influenza is through the annual immunization of healthcare workers.

Severe Acute Respiratory Syndrome

Evaluation of infection-control practices during the SARS outbreak in 2003 reveals a great deal about the effectiveness of these practices for SARS and other respiratory pathogens. Personal protective equipment appeared to be quite effective in preventing acquisition of SARS. It was found that consistent wearing of either a simple surgical mask or an N95 respirator was more effective than inconsistent use, with a 13% versus 56% infection rate respectively. A trend, albeit not statistically significant, of better protection was found with the N95 respirator compared to a surgical mask. However, in Vietnam, at least one hospital with documented SARS cases controlled the spread with only surgical masks during the first 3 weeks of the outbreak. Potential reasons for this equality of protection include the fact that the N95 respirators were not properly fitted and thus no better than surgical masks or that the healthcare workers may not have removed personal protective equipment in the proper order. Additional infection-control measures used to prevent large-droplet transmission of infectious agents during the SARS outbreak included "physical space interventions" such as separation of patients, methods to decrease infectious aerosols during at-risk therapies, and environmental decontamination and containment. It was noted that certain procedures seemed to increase the transmission of SARS in instances in which it is postulated that smaller droplets, which can travel further distances, are formed. These procedures included intubation, continuous positive-airway pressure, and nebulization therapy (17).

NOSOCOMIAL URINARY TRACT INFECTIONS

In incidence studies of nosocomial infections, including patients of all ages and in all hospital locations, UTIs are the most frequent, accounting for approximately one-third of infections. Nosocomial UTIs account for 13%–20% of all hospital-acquired infections in the PICU, making them the third most common nosocomial infection behind bloodstream and respiratory infections. The actual rate of catheter-associated UTIs in ICUs varies based on the type of unit and ranges from 3.0

to 6.7 per 1000 catheter days. The higher incidence rates have been described in burn units. The NNIS system notes the PICU nosocomial urinary tract rate to be 4.0 infections per 1000 catheter days. Secondary urosepsis is uncommon in the PICU population, with an incidence of 3%. A study of PICU patients with nosocomial UTIs found that 58% were female, the mean age in the infected group was 4.6 years, all patients had urinary catheters in place for at least 3 days, and 26.9% were catheterized for 8 days or longer. The infected group had a trend toward increased mortality. Multiple regression analysis in this study found having prior cardiac surgery as the only significant risk factor. Additional studies found through multivariate analysis that the nosocomial UTI risks are increased based on duration of catheterization, female sex, absence of systemic antibiotics, and disconnection of the catheter-collecting tube junction. Most infections are caused by a single organism, with 82% identified as gram-negative bacteria or yeast species. Twenty percent of nosocomial UTIs have antibiotic resistance. In the PICU, a UTI can be challenging to diagnose, as the patient will not have the typical symptoms (e.g., frequency and dysuria) due to the severity of the critical illness or due to a catheter being in place and masking these symptoms. Strategies to prevent or decrease nosocomial UTIs include minimizing exposure to urinary catheters by using them only when truly indicated, using a sterile insertion technique, maintaining uninterrupted use of a closed collection system, and removing the device as soon as possible—ideally in <3 days. One center lowered its nosocomial UTI rate from 1.4 to 0.12 infections per 100 admissions after initiating a policy that dictated catheter removal after 48–72 hrs of use. No pediatric studies have been reported, but silver alloy-coated catheters have been shown to be effective in decreasing infections (23,27,38).

NOSOCOMIAL GASTROINTESTINAL INFECTIONS

Nosocomial diarrhea is defined as loose stools that occur > 48 hrs after admission, a stool frequency of at least two per 12 hrs, and no identified noninfectious cause of the loose stools. In general, nosocomial diarrhea accounts for up to 35% of all pediatric hospital-acquired infections. The reported PICU rate is 4%–5%. Outside the PICU, viral etiologies as a group predominate and are usually organisms similar to those seen in the community, such as rotavirus, adenovirus, and Norwalk virus. The single most common organism isolated in the PICU and on the general ward is *Clostridium difficile*. *C. difficile* is almost exclusively isolated as a cause of diarrhea in children >1 year of age. It is believed that, although present in the gastrointestinal tract of newborns, *C. difficile* does not typically cause disease in neonates and young infants. The organisms responsible for nosocomial diarrhea are typically spread by the fecal-oral route, which may explain the fact that most children with at least viral etiologies of their diarrhea are incontinent (i.e., diapered). Infection control techniques are important in preventing and controlling nosocomial diarrhea. Good hand hygiene and contact precautions are paramount to this effort. The viruses that cause diarrheal illnesses can survive on fomites and other surfaces for several hours, and the spores of *C. difficile* can survive for more than a day on such inanimate surfaces. With attention to hydration and electrolyte status, mortality from nosocomial diarrhea is rare, but dehydration is always a concern, especially in young children (24,38).

Necrotizing Enterocolitis

The etiology of necrotizing enterocolitis is multifactorial; however, nosocomial, epidemic outbreaks do occur in NICUs. In a review of epidemics, investigators found that they last ~8–10 weeks, with an average of 10.5 cases per epidemic, and common organisms were identified in nearly half of the epidemics. The mortality rate of recent cases was <10%. Affected centers used infection-control measures that focused on preventing orofecal transmission to limit the epidemic, including strict use of hand washing, the use of gloves, isolation of the infected newborns, cohorting of cases, and the closing of some units. The proposed mechanism is either orofecal transmission to susceptible premature infants, increased virulence of the organism, or the synergistic action of two microorganisms. Identified organisms in outbreaks have been *E. coli, K. pneumoniae, Enterobacter cloacae, Clostridium butyricum, C. difficile, S. epidermidis,* coronavirus, rotavirus, and echovirus. Often, the causal organism is not identified. Controversy exists as to whether *Clostridia* spp. are causative organisms, as they may be part of the normal intestinal flora (5).

SURGICAL SITE INFECTIONS

The NNIS system tracks SSIs for a variety of surgical procedures. This data is sorted by site or, when enough data is available, by specific operation. The rates are further stratified by risk index category. The risk index is determined by the anesthetic risk based on preoperative assessment scores of the American Society of Anesthesiologists, whether or not the surgical field is contaminated, and duration of the operative procedure as benchmarked against a preset standard for each operation. The NNIS SSI rates include data from adult and pediatric patients. Causative organisms of pediatric SSIs are most commonly *S. aureus* (20% of all reported infections), although these are more commonly seen in patients who are ≤2 months of age. Coagulase-negative staphylococci and *P. aeruginosa* account for ~14% each of all pediatric SSIs. *P. aeruginosa* is isolated more commonly from SSIs in children >2 months of age (38).

Nosocomial Infections of the Central Nervous System

Nosocomial infections of the central nervous system usually involve a surgical site or the presence of a foreign body. The pooled mean rates for craniotomy reported by the NNIS are 0.91, 1.72, and 2.41 infections per 100 operations for zero, one, and either two or three risk index categories, respectively. The risk of a SSI from a ventricular shunt with zero risk categories is 4.42 per 100 operations, whereas it is 5.36 per 100 if one or more risk index categories are present. Other central nervous system operations have a combined SSI rate of 1.53 per 100 operations (31).

A review of children who underwent 281 intracranial surgeries found an incidence of 3.2 SSIs per 100 operations. No superficial infections where noted in this retrospective study. Of the 9 reported infections, two were deep incisional infections that involved the fascial and muscular layers, and seven

involved deeper structures such as the bone and dura. Several risk factors for infection were identified in this population and included repairs of syndromic craniosynostosis and an oblique facial cleft. With a more complicated preoperative diagnosis, the infectious risk was increased [odds ratio (OR), 13.0; 95% CI, 2.6–64.4]. Additional factors increasing risk of nosocomial infection included an increased duration of surgery (OR, 12.1; 95% CI, 2.4–59.9), closure of the overlying skin under tension (OR, 12.5; 95% CI, 3.0–52.6), and the presence of more than four surgeons during the operative procedure (OR, 6.3; 95% CI, 1.2–32.0). Demographics such as age and gender as well as associated medical conditions and previous surgical procedures, including tracheotomy and ventriculoperitoneal shunt were not associated with higher rates of infection (46).

A prospective analysis was performed of 1000 parenchymatously placed monitors at a single center over an 8-year period; it included but was not exclusive of pediatric patients. Two-thirds of the devices were placed in patients with traumatic head injury. Probe tip cultures were obtained in 547 cases, with 91.5% of the cultures negative for bacterial growth. Forty-six (8.5%) of the cultures were positive. *S. epidermidis* grew in nearly half of the positive cultures (47.8%). Other organisms isolated included *E. coli* (19.7%), *Corynebacterium* (10.9%), and *S. aureus* (6.6%). Incidence of positive culture probe tips was similar regardless of whether the device was placed in the ICU or operating room. No patients had evidence of infection at the insertion site (18).

Epidural catheters are often used in the ICU to manage pain. The reported infection rates in these catheters range from 0% to 0.7% in published studies. A study of 1458 pediatric patients with postoperative epidural catheters found no epidural abscesses over a 6-year period. Local superficial infections are not frequently reported, but the rate appears similar to those of intravascular lines. The proposed mechanism of infection is similar to IV lines as well. Possible sources of epidural catheter infection include skin contamination, introduction of bacteria by the needle or catheter, hematogenous spread, or contamination of the infusate. Risk of infection can be reduced in the same manner as with the placement of intravascular lines. Attention to aseptic technique during placement, adequate skin preparation and disinfection prior to placement, and maintenance of appropriate dressings are important safety measures to prevent infection of the catheter and the epidural space. The duration of catheter use also influences the risk of infection as is seen in intravascular catheters. The longer the catheter is in place, the higher the risk of infection. However, most infections occur within the first 5 days after insertion (12). In a prospective study of 210 children who received short-term epidural analgesia, no serious systemic infections, such as meningitis or epidural abscess, were noted. The incidences of dressing contamination, cellulitis, and bacterial colonization were more common in caudally placed catheters than in lumbar catheters. Little difference was reported in the incidence of gram-positive organism positive cultures between the two sites. Caudal catheters were much more likely to be contaminated with gram-negative organisms, 16% versus 3% (22).

Selected Surgical Site Infections

Adult rates of SSIs following cardiovascular surgery are between 1.5 and 2.3 infections per 100 operations. Retrospective studies assessed the rate in children to be 0.5–5 infections per 100 operations. The low rate of 0.5 may have been an underestimate due to study design. Two other prospective pediatric studies placed the rate at 2.3–3.4 infections per 100 operations. In these studies, the wound infection rate ranged from 1 to 1.5 per 100 operations, while the organ space infections (sternal osteomyelitis and mediastinitis) ranged from 0.8 to 2.4 infections per 100 surgeries. Over half of the infections in children were caused by *S. aureus*, followed in frequency by coagulase-negative staphylococci, enterococci, and *Enterobacter* spp. These organisms accounted for nearly 90% of the isolated bacteria in the two studies. Debridement when appropriate and IV antibiotics were the therapies administered to these patients. Risk factors for SSI have been identified and can be divided into preoperative, intraoperative, and postoperative categories. Preoperative risks include younger age at time of surgery, a higher American Society of Anesthesiologists score, a longer preoperative inpatient length of stay, a prior sternotomy, and an elevated leukocyte band count. Intraoperative factors that affect the incidence of SSIs are the duration of the surgery, cardiopulmonary bypass, and circulatory arrest. Postoperative factors associated with infection risk include failed primary closure of the chest, low cardiac output, infection at another site, and the duration of use of mechanical ventilation, central venous line, and urinary catheter. In a multivariable analysis, a longer duration of surgery (OR, 1.4; 95% CI 1.2–1.8) and <1 month of age at the time of surgery (OR, 14; 95% CI 3.3–58.4) were independently associated with pediatric cardiovascular SSI. Patients without a SSI had a median surgical time of 150 mins (range, 45–450 mins), while those children with a wound infection had a median duration of 233 mins (range, 80–600 mins). Children with sternal osteomyelitis or mediastinitis had a median surgery length of 270 mins (range, 135–450 mins; $p = 0.0005$, compared to those patients without infection). In another study, the incidence of SSI based on age was 7.6% for <1 month, 3.9% for 1–12 months, 3.5% for 1–4 years, and 1.6% for children >4 years of age. Children > 1 year of age were more likely than younger children to be bacteremic with positive blood cultures (73% versus 17%; $p = 0.001$) (1,30).

Mediastinitis

Mediastinitis, defined by purulent discharge in the mediastinal space necessitating surgical debridement, positive cultures from the mediastinal space, or sternal instability in the presence of positive blood cultures, is rare in the PICU population. The incidence ranges from 0.04% to 3.9%, with most studies placing the rate at ~1% in the post-cardiac surgery population, despite IV perioperative prophylaxis. Gram-positive organisms account for approximately two-thirds of infections, with *S. aureus* causing most and the remainder nearly all due to coagulase-negative *Staphylococcus*. A third of the cases are due to gram-negative bacteria, with *P. aeruginosa* responsible for half of the infections. Polymicrobial infections are infrequent, and fungal infections are rare. Mediastinitis occurs at a mean of 11 days following sternotomy, with gram-positive infections occurring later than gram-negative infections—13 versus 6.5 days, respectively. Concurrent bacteremia is found in 40%–50% of patients with mediastinitis. Gram-positive mediastinitis has positive blood cultures 67% of the time, and gram-negative mediastinitis has positive cultures in 18% of cases. In a multivariable analysis, delayed sternal closure was

found to be an independent risk factor for the development of gram-negative mediastinitis (25).

VECTOR-BORNE INFECTIONS

Nosocomial transmission of traditionally vector-borne infections, such as malaria and dengue fever, is possible in the hospital setting. Malaria has been reported to be transmitted via blood transfusions, organ transplantation, needle-stick injuries, improper use and cleaning of medical devices such as glucometers and catheters, misuse of multidose vials, and open wounds. Malaria is highly infectious, with nosocomial transmission possible with even a small amount of blood, as a single milliliter of blood may contain millions of red blood cell that harbors *Plasmodium* species (21). Dengue fever has been transmitted by needle-stick injuries and bone marrow transplantation. Nosocomial transmission of vector-borne infections should be considered if the patient has not traveled to endemic areas of the world (32).

CONCLUSIONS AND FUTURE DIRECTIONS

Nosocomial infections are an important and, in large part, preventable cause of morbidity and mortality in the PICU. Although not all nosocomial infections can be eliminated due in part to the unique nature of the PICU patient, the incidence can be dramatically reduced through the use of infection-control measures. Simple interventions such as consistent use of hand hygiene, isolation practices, adherence to sterile technique, elevating the head of the bed, and judicious use and prompt removal (when no longer required) of central lines, urinary catheters, and endotracheal tubes can dramatically affect nosocomial infection rates. Use of care bundles can increase effectiveness of these and other measures by standardizing the approach to nosocomial infection prevention. Although all nosocomial infections may not be preventable, the goal of the pediatric critical care practitioner should be zero. Consistent use and monitoring the effectiveness of infection-control measures will go a long way toward achieving the goal.

The medical community must take action on reducing and preventing nosocomial infections. Future efforts should be directed toward differentiating community-acquired infection from nosocomial infections, reducing the development of resistant organisms through judicious use of antibiotics to render nosocomial infections less problematic, designing ICUs to allow for proper isolation practices and to facilitate hand hygiene, and developing constraint design or forcing functions to ensure compliance with hand hygiene and infection control bundles. Pay for performance and loss of reimbursement from insurers may be the eventual impetus for change in healthcare systems toward eradicating hospital-acquired infections.

KEY POINTS

- Adherence to infection-control practices, including hand hygiene, is still one of the most beneficial but overlooked methods by which to prevent nosocomial infections.
- Isolation precautions are critical to the prevention of transmission of infections within the hospital and must be put

in place at the time of patient admission based on the likely pathogenic organisms or disease process.

■ Surveillance cultures at the time of patient admission can decrease nosocomial spread of resistant organisms and should be considered if the infection rate or carrier state in the community is high.

■ Prevention of catheter-related bloodstream infections begins at the time of placement, with adherence to sterile technique. Care of the catheter site and use of antiseptic- or antibiotic-impregnated catheters can further decrease the risk of infection.

■ Routine removal or rotation of central venous catheters does not reduce the risk of catheter-related bloodstream infections.

■ Prevention of VAP is facilitated by the use of a bundled protocol that includes elevation of the head of the bed and daily assessment of readiness for extubation.

References

1. Allpress AL, Rosenthal GL, Goodrich KM. Risk factors for surgical site infections after pediatric cardiovascular surgery. *Pediatr Infect Dis J* 2003;23(3):231–4.
2. American Academy of Pediatrics. Infection Control for Hospitalized Children. In: Pickering LK, Baker CJ, Long SS, et al, eds. *Red Book: 2006 Report of the Committee on Infectious Diseases.* 27th ed. Elk Grove Village: American Academy of Pediatrics, 2006;153–64.
3. Arantes A, Carvalho Eda S, Medeiros EA, et al. Pediatric risk of mortality and hospital infection. *Infect Control Hosp Epidemiol* 2004;25(9): 783–5.
4. Biedenbach DJ, Moet GJ, Jones RN. Occurrence and antimicrobial resistance pattern comparisons among bloodstream infection isolates from the SENTRY Antimicrobial Surveillance Program (1997–2002). *Diagn Microbiol Infect Dis* 2004;50(1):59–69.
5. Boccia D, Stolfi I, Lana S, et al. Nosocomial necrotising enterocolitis outbreaks: Epidemiology and control measures. *Eur J Pediatr* 2001;160(6):385–91.
6. Bonten MJ. Infection in the intensive care unit: Prevention strategies. *Curr Opin Infect Dis* 2002;15(4):401–5.
7. CDC. http://www.cdc.gov/ncidod/sars/pdf/ppeposter148.pdf. Vol. 2007.
8. Coffin SE, Zaoutis TE. Infection control, hospital epidemiology, and patient safety. *Infect Dis Clin North Am* 2005;19(3):647–65.
9. Coia JE, Duckworth GJ, Edwards DI, et al. Guidelines for the control and prevention of methicillin-resistant Staphylococcus aureus (MRSA) in healthcare facilities. *J Hosp Infect* 2006;63(Suppl 1):S1–44.
10. Collard HR, Saint S, Matthay MA. Prevention of ventilator-associated pneumonia: An evidence-based systematic review. *Ann Intern Med* 2003;138(6):494–501.
11. Curley MA, Schwalenstocker E, Deshpande JK, et al. Tailoring the Institute for Health Care Improvement 100,000 Lives Campaign to pediatric settings: The example of ventilator-associated pneumonia. *Pediatr Clin North Am* 2006;53(6):1231–51.
12. Dawson S. Epidural catheter infections. *J Hosp Infect* 2001;47(1):3–8.
13. de Jonge RC, Polderman KH, Gemke RJ. Central venous catheter use in the pediatric patient: Mechanical and infectious complications. *Pediatr Crit Care Med* 2005;6(3):329–39.
14. Eggimann P, Pittet D. Infection control in the ICU. *Chest* 2001;120(6):2059–93.
15. Farr BM. Preventing vascular catheter-related infections: Current controversies. *Clin Infect Dis* 2001;33(10):1733–8.
16. Flanders SA, Collard HR, Saint S. Nosocomial pneumonia: State of the science. *Am J Infect Control* 2006;34(2):84–93.
17. Gamage B, Moore D, Copes R, et al. Protecting health care workers from SARS and other respiratory pathogens: A review of the infection control literature. *Am J Infect Control* 2005;33(2):114–21.
18. Gelabert-Gonzalez M, Ginesta-Galan V, Sernamito-Garcia R, et al. The

19. Hall CB. Nosocomial respiratory syncytial virus infections: The "Cold War" has not ended. *Clin Infect Dis* 2000;31(2):590–6.
20. Hess DR. Noninvasive positive-pressure ventilation and ventilator-associated pneumonia. *Respir Care* 2005;50(7):924–9; discussion 929–31.
21. Jain SK, Persaud D, Perl TM, et al. Nosocomial malaria and saline flush. *Emerg Infect Dis* 2005;11(7):1097–9.
22. Kost-Byerly S, Tobin JR, Greenberg RS, et al. Bacterial colonization and infection rate of continuous epidural catheters in children. *Anesth Analg* 1998;86(4):712–6.
23. Langley JM. Defining urinary tract infection in the critically ill child. *Pediatr Crit Care Med* 2005;6(3 Suppl):S25–9.
24. Langley JM, LeBlanc JC, Hanakowski M, et al. The role of *Clostridium difficile* and viruses as causes of nosocomial diarrhea in children. *Infect Control Hosp Epidemiol* 2002;23(11):660–4.
25. Long CB, Shah SS, Lautenbach E, et al. Postoperative mediastinitis in children: Epidemiology, microbiology and risk factors for gram-negative pathogens. *Pediatr Infect Dis J* 2005;24(4):315–9.
26. Martyny J, Glazer CS, Newman LS. Respiratory protection. *N Engl J Med* 2002;347(11):824–30.
27. Matlow AG, Wray RD, Cox PN. Nosocomial urinary tract infections in children in a pediatric intensive care unit: A follow-up after 10 years. *Pediatr Crit Care Med* 2003;4(1):74–7.
28. Mermel LA. New technologies to prevent intravascular catheter-related bloodstream infections. *Emerg Infect Dis* 2001;7(2):197–9.
29. Mermel LA, Farr BM, Sherertz RJ, et al. Guidelines for the management of intravascular catheter-related infections. *Clin Infect Dis* 2001;32(9):1249–72.
30. Nateghian A, Taylor G, Robinson JL. Risk factors for surgical site infections following open-heart surgery in a Canadian pediatric population. *Am J Infect Control* 2004;32(7):397–401.
31. National Nosocomial Infections Surveillance (NNIS) System Report, data summary from January 1992 through June 2004, issued October 2004. *Am J Infect Control* 2004;32 (8):470–85.
32. Nemes Z, Kiss G, Madarassi EP, et al. Nosocomial transmission of dengue. *Emerg Infect Dis* 2004;10(10):1880–1.
33. O'Grady NP, Alexander M, Dellinger EP, et al. Guidelines for the prevention of intravascular catheter-related infections. The Hospital Infection Control Practices Advisory Committee, Center for Disease Control and Prevention, US. *Pediatrics* 2002;110(5):e51.
34. O'Neill JM, Schutze GE, Heulitt MJ, et al. Nosocomial infections during extracorporeal membrane oxygenation. *Intensive Care Med* 2001;27(8):1247–53.
35. Pittet D, Hugonnet S, Harbarth S. Effectiveness of a hospital-wide programme to improve compliance with hand hygiene. *Lancet* 2000;356:1307–12.
36. Public health focus: Surveillance, prevention, and control of nosocomial infections. *MMWR Morb Mortal Wkly Rep* 1992;41(42):783–7.
37. Randle J, Clarke M, Storr J. Hand hygiene compliance in healthcare workers. *J Hosp Infect* 2006;64(3):205–9.
38. Richards MJ, Edwards JR, Culver DH, et al. Nosocomial infections in pediatric intensive care units in the United States. National Nosocomial Infections Surveillance System. *Pediatrics* 1999;103(4):e39.
39. Rosenthal VD, Maki DG, Salomao R, et al. Device-associated nosocomial infections in 55 intensive care units of 8 developing countries. *Ann Intern Med* 2006;145(8):582–91.
40. Slaughter SE. Intravascular catheter-related infections. Strategies for combating this common foe. *Postgrad Med* 2004;116(5):59–66.
41. Stockwell JA. Nosocomial infections in the pediatric intensive care unit: Affecting the impact on safety and outcome. *Pediatr Crit Care Med* 2007;8(2 Suppl):S21–37.
42. Tan SY, Brown J. Ignac Philipp Semmelweis (1818–1865): Hand washing saves lives. *Singapore Med J* 2006;47(1):6–7.
43. Taylor RW, O'Brien J, Trottier SJ, et al. Red blood cell transfusions and nosocomial infections in critically ill patients. *Crit Care Med* 2006;34 (9):2302–8.
44. Wisplinghoff H, Bischoff T, Tallent SM, et al. Nosocomial bloodstream infections in US hospitals: Analysis of 24,179 cases from a prospective nationwide surveillance study. *Clin Infect Dis* 2004;39(3):309–17.
45. Wright ML, Romano MJ. Ventilator-associated pneumonia in children. *Semin Pediatr Infect Dis* 2006;17(2):58–64.
46. Yeung LC, Cunningham ML, Allpress AL, et al. Surgical site infections after pediatric intracranial surgery for craniofacial malformations: Frequency and risk factors. *Neurosurgery* 2005;56(4):733–9; discussion 733–9.
47. Zar HJ, Cotton MF. Nosocomial pneumonia in pediatric patients: Practical problems and rational solutions. *Paediatr Drugs* 2002;4(2):73–83.

Camino intracranial pressure device in clinical practice. Assessment in a 1000 cases. *Acta Neurochir (Wien)* 2006;148(4):435–41.

CHAPTER 82 ■ INTERNATIONAL AND EMERGING INFECTIONS

TROY E. DOMINGUEZ • CHITRA RAVISHANKAR • MIRIAM K. LAUFER

Infections are the leading cause of death among children worldwide. Some of the most common infections (e.g., pneumonia and gastrointestinal infections) occur in both developing and industrialized countries. Yet, some life-threatening infections are predominantly transmitted in developing countries due to poor sanitation, the absence of adequate public health infrastructure, and a high density of disease-carrying vectors. Several of the "international" infections discussed in this chapter, such as leptospirosis and hantavirus, have also been known to occur in North America.

When a child who has been abroad is evaluated for an illness, many infections cannot be distinguished on clinical grounds alone. Most of the illnesses described in this chapter have a protean presentation, including fever and abdominal and/or respiratory complaints. In addition to the standard ICU evaluation, a careful travel history along with a detailed account of potential water, food, and animal exposures can help to narrow the differential diagnosis and point toward the appropriate diagnostic assays and empiric therapy (**Table 82.1**). Most studies of illnesses among returned travelers have focused on the adult population. Diarrhea is one of the most common complaints following travel and frequently requires hospitalization among children (82). Among international travelers, gastroenteritis rarely requires intensive care management.

Emerging infections that originated outside the US will be discussed. West Nile virus reached the east coast of the US in the late 1990s and has subsequently spread throughout the country. Avian influenza, an infection with the potential for a global pandemic, is currently concentrated in Asia but is spreading via migratory birds throughout the world. Although potentially no longer a major problem, severe acute respiratory syndrome (SARS) will be discussed as an example of an emerging disease with potential for worldwide public health implications.

INTERNATIONAL INFECTIONS

Malaria

Mechanism of Disease

Epidemiology. Malaria is the most significant parasitic disease in humans. An estimated 300–500 million infections occur each year, and these result in 1–3 million deaths. Most severe infections and deaths occur in children <5 years of age in Africa. In developed countries, malaria is also the most common cause of febrile illness without localizing signs in returned travelers from developing countries (29).

Malaria is transmitted by a bite from the female anopheline mosquito. The areas of highest transmission are found in sub-Saharan Africa, although transmission also occurs in many regions of South Asia, Southeast Asia, the South Pacific, and Central and South America (**Fig. 82.1**). Local outbreaks of malaria in the US occur almost every year due to imported malarial cases infecting local anopheline mosquitoes (25).

Four species of *Plasmodium* cause malaria infections in humans: *P. falciparum*, *P. vivax*, *P. malariae*, and *P. ovale*. Worldwide, infection with *P. falciparum* is most common and is exclusively responsible for nearly all life-threatening malaria disease. The second most common species is *P. vivax*.

Repeated exposure to malaria infection, as experienced by individuals who live in malaria-endemic areas, causes a state of "semi-immunity." Patients are still at risk for infection, but their immune systems are able to control the level of parasitemia, and severe disease is extremely rare. In the areas of highest transmission, semi-immunity occurs around the age of 5 years. In areas of lower transmission, it is delayed or absent. Semi-immunity is lost within 6–12 months of leaving an endemic area (14), which is a particular concern for people born in malaria-endemic areas who are living in developed countries. They may return to their country of origin expecting to still be protected from severe disease and fail to take preventive measures, when in fact they are nearly as susceptible as any malaria-naïve traveler.

Hemoglobinopathies commonly found in African and Asian populations are thought to be the result of evolutionary pressure exerted by malaria over time (83). Red blood cell polymorphisms, including hemoglobins S, C, and E, glucose-6-phosphate dehydrogenase deficiency, pyruvate kinase deficiency, and α-thalassemia, are associated with decreased risk of severe malaria disease. The Duffy antigen located on the surface of the red blood cell is necessary for invasion by *P. vivax*. Most Africans lack this antigen, and, as result, *P. vivax* is extremely rare in Africa.

Etiology. All human *Plasmodia* species follow a similar life cycle. The *Anopheles* mosquito injects sporozoites into the human during the process of taking a blood meal. The sporozoites immediately travel to the liver. In the hepatic stage, which lasts 1–2 weeks, the parasites undergo asexual reproduction and become schizonts; no symptoms are associated with this exo-erythrocytic life-cycle stage. When the schizonts in the liver rupture, merozoites emerge into the bloodstream and begin the erythrocytic stage of infection that is associated with clinical disease. Merozoites infect erythrocytes and mature into trophozoites; these become schizonts. Rupture of infected red

TABLE 82.1

CAUSES OF SYSTEMIC FEBRILE ILLNESS AMONG RETURNED TRAVELERS

Diagnosis	Caribbean	Central America	South America	Sub-Saharan Africa	South or Central Asia	Southeast Asia
Malaria	+	++	++	+++	++	++
Dengue	++	++	++	–/+	++	++
Mononucleosis	+	+	+	+	+	+
Rickettsia	–	–	–	+*	+/–	+
Typhoid fever	+	+	+	–/+	++	+

Adapted from Freedman DO, Weld LH, Kozarsky PE, et al. Spectrum of disease and relation to place of exposure among ill returned travelers. *N Engl J Med* 2006;354:119–30.

cells that contain the schizont forms produces more merozoites capable of invading more red blood cells.

The cycle of multiplication, infection, and rupture results in the clinical manifestations of malaria. The burden of malarial parasites multiplies 12–15-fold with each erythrocytic cycle. With *P. falciparum*, these cycles of asexual reproduction last ~48 hrs. Some merozoites differentiate into male or female gametocytes that can be taken up during a blood meal by an *Anopheles* mosquito and undergo sexual reproduction in the mosquito midgut. The offspring of the sexual reproduction phase enter the mosquito salivary glands as sporozoites, ready to be transferred to a human host.

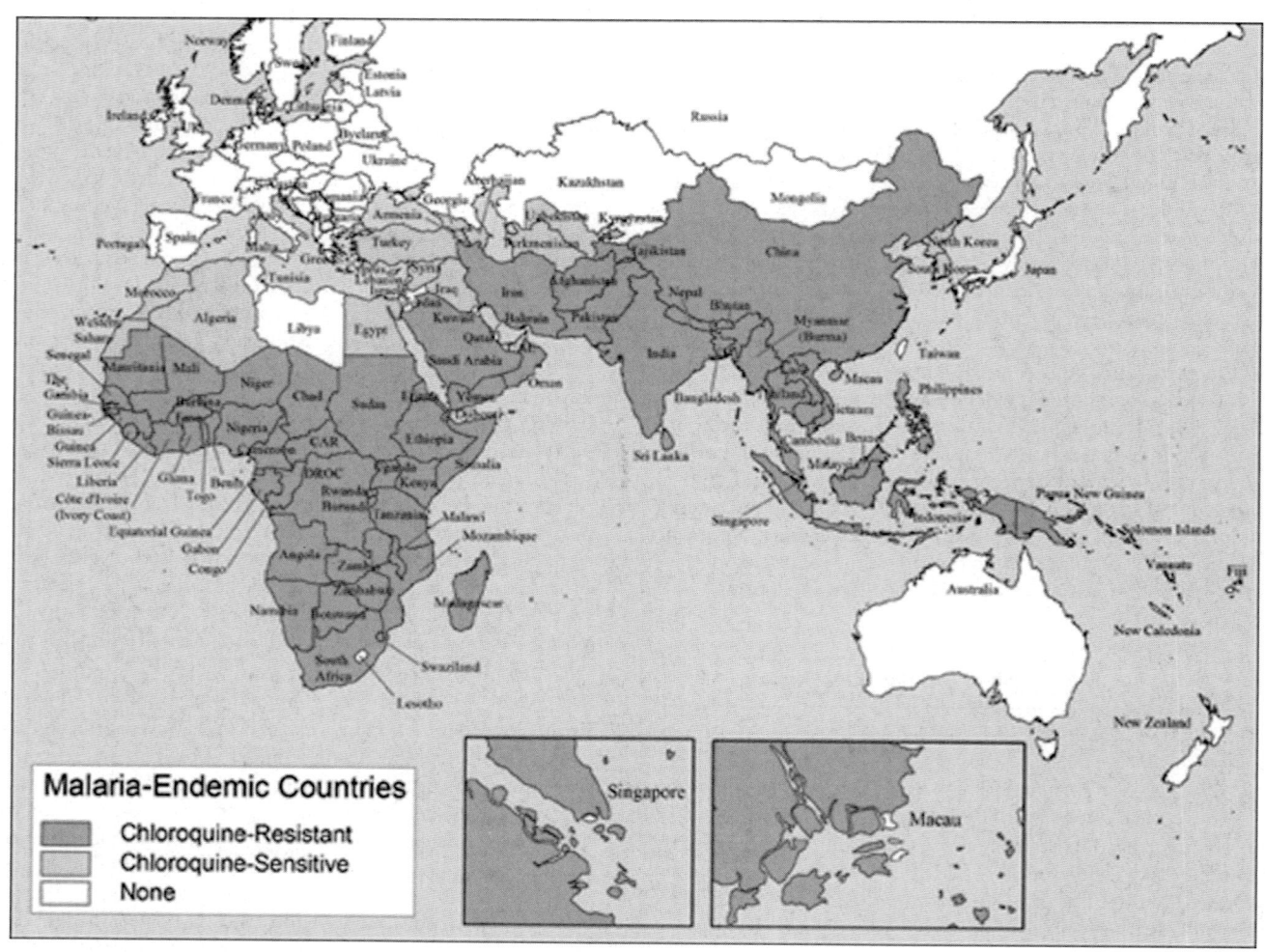

Malaria-Endemic Countries
- Chloroquine-Resistant
- Chloroquine-Sensitive
- None

A

FIGURE 82.1. Distribution of malaria (all species). From the US Centers for Disease Control and Prevention, http://wwwn.cdc.gov/travel/yellowBookCh4-Malaria.aspx. (*continued*)

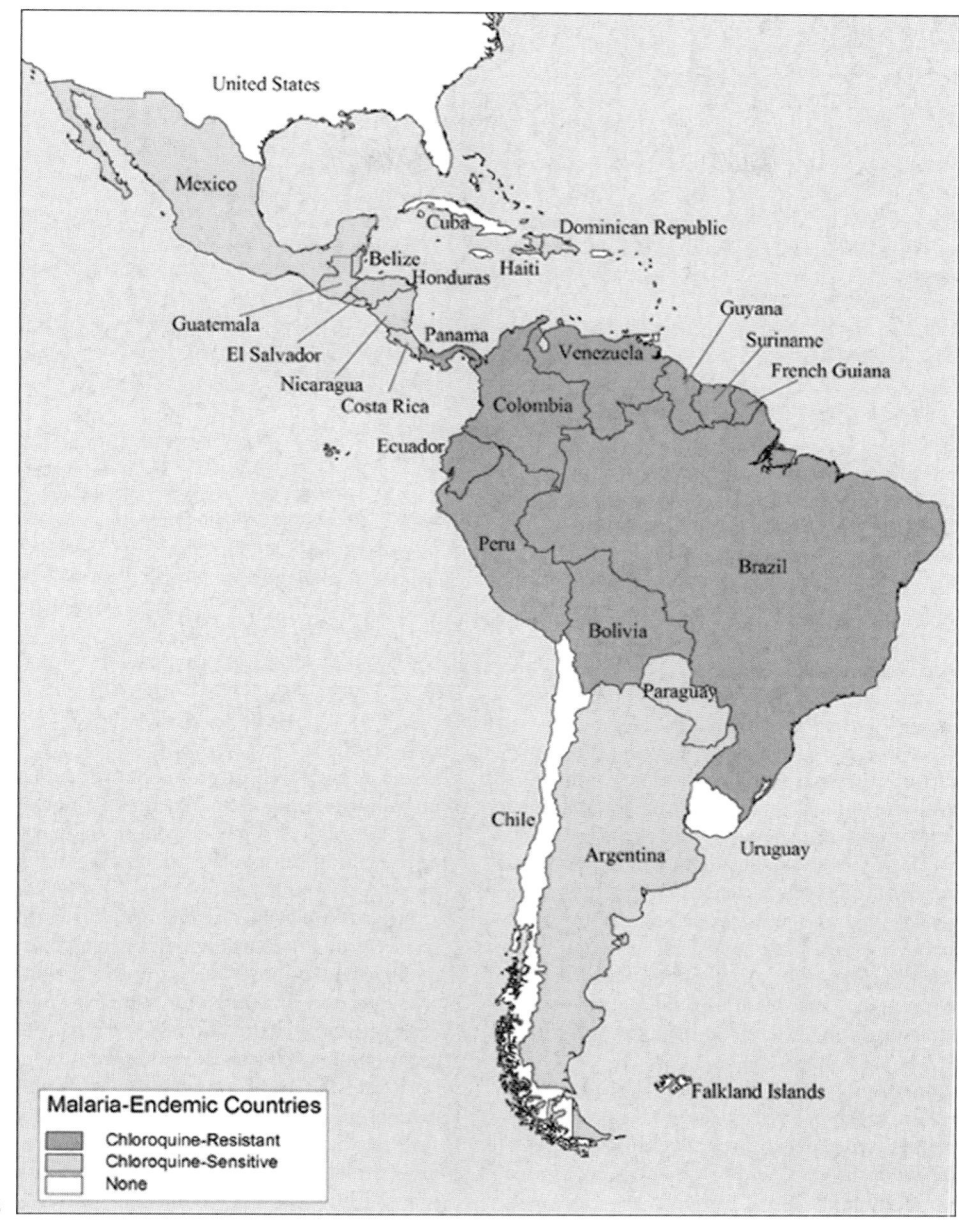

B

FIGURE 82.1. (*continued*)

Severe disease from *P. falciparum* infection is thought to be due to the ability of infected red cells to adhere to the vessel walls in the microvasculature, a process called *sequestration*, which is associated with end-organ damage. Sequestration in the brain microcirculation is associated with the most dreaded complication of infection—cerebral malaria. Sequestration occurs in other organs. In children in endemic areas, sequestration is prominent in the gastrointestinal tract and the skin (73).

Clinical Presentation and Differential Diagnosis

The initial presentation of uncomplicated malaria is a nonlocalizing febrile illness with fever, chills, headache, and diaphoresis. The fevers may be paroxysmal, reflecting the replicating cycle of the parasites, although the pattern of fever cycles is more common among the non-falciparum species. Other common symptoms include nausea, vomiting, diarrhea, malaise, myalgias, dizziness, diarrhea, and dry cough.

Patients without sufficient antimalarial immunity who present with uncomplicated infection can rapidly deteriorate and develop severe disease, or they may initially present with severe disease. The World Health Organization (WHO) has suggested that the following clinical features help to identify patients at high risk of death: prostration, impaired consciousness, acidotic breathing, multiple convulsions, circulatory collapse, pulmonary edema, abnormal bleeding, jaundice, and hemoglobinuria. Laboratory results that are associated with severe disease include severe anemia, hypoglycemia, acidosis, renal impairment, hyperlactatemia, and hyperparasitemia. The definitions for each of these criteria are listed in **Table 82.2.**

TABLE 82.2

DEFINITION OF POOR PROGNOSTIC SIGNS IN SEVERE MALARIA

Prostration	Inability to sit in a child who was previously able to sit. In infants, can be defined as unable to feed.
Impaired consciousness	Coma that lasts at least 30 mins after a seizure, with no other cause identified (e.g., meningitis, hypoglycemia). Impairment may be less severe.
Respiratory distress (acidotic breathing)	In the absence of abnormalities on auscultation or radiography, normal oxygen saturation
Multiple convulsions	>2 in 24 hrs
Circulatory collapse	Hypotension with cold, clammy skin
Pulmonary edema	Not due to volume overload
Abnormal bleeding	Spontaneous mucosal bleeding or laboratory evidence of disseminated intravascular coagulopathy
Jaundice	Detected clinically or >3 g/dL (50 mcmol/L)
Hemoglobinuria	Macroscopic
Severe anemia	Normocytic anemia with hemoglobin <5 g/dL or hematocrit <15%
Hypoglycemia	<40 g/dL or 2.2 mmol/L
Acidosis	Arterial or capillary pH <7.3 or bicarbonate <15 mmol/L
Renal impairment	Urine output <0.5 mL/kg/hr, failure to respond to rehydration, creatinine >3.0 mg/dL
Hyperlactatemia	>5 mmol/L
Hyperparasitemia	>4%–5% in nonimmune children and adults

The classic syndrome of severe disease among children is cerebral malaria, as discussed in detail in Chapter 80. Patients with any impairment of consciousness should be treated as if they have cerebral malaria. Severe malarial anemia is an important, life-threatening form of severe disease in young children from endemic areas. Hypoglycemia, acidosis, and pulmonary edema also complicate severe disease and are associated with a poor outcome. The severe manifestations that are more common in adults are jaundice and hepatic dysfunction, acute respiratory distress syndrome (ARDS), and renal dysfunction.

An important feature and marker of disease severity in children with severe malaria is the presence of a metabolic acidosis that reflects several metabolic derangements. The acidosis is commonly found in children with cerebral malaria but is also associated with anemia, hypoglycemia, or hypovolemia. An elevated plasma lactate is often seen with the acidosis. Studies in adults have demonstrated increased production of lactate and elevated lactate-to-pyruvate ratios, suggesting impaired tissue substrate delivery. Hypovolemia that leads to tissue hypoperfusion may be a common cause of metabolic acidosis in children, although experts disagree about this. In patients with severe anemia, the low oxygen-carrying capacity may lead to oxygen consumption and delivery mismatch, with anaerobic metabolism and metabolic acidosis.

Hypoglycemia occurs in 10%–30% of children with severe disease. Parasitized red blood cells consume glucose and increase the demand for glucose in the host. Impairment in the gluconeogenic pathway has been observed in adults with severe malaria and may be an important contributor to the pathogenesis of hypoglycemia and lactic acidosis (68). In addition, the hypoglycemia in adults frequently occurs after the initiation of therapy and is associated with hyperinsulinism. Treatment with quinine is thought to stimulate insulin secretion. In children, hypoglycemia is frequently seen on presentation and is usually associated with appropriately low insulin levels. Hypoglycemia may be present in the absence of high-parasite-density parasitemia on blood smear because the parasites that are present in the blood and not visualized on the smear consume large quantities of glucose.

Severe malarial anemia presents with profound pallor. It more frequently occurs in highly endemic areas due to repeated malarial infections. The etiology is multifactorial. Causes include increased destruction with lysis of cells by malarial parasites, decreased production of red blood cells mediated by the inflammatory cascade, and immune-mediated hemolysis of both infected and uninfected cells. Lung and renal disease are rarely found among children with severe malaria. The progression to acute lung injury or ARDS may be rapid, and happen even after treatment and parasite clearance. The etiology of renal failure in severe malaria is not well understood.

Other severe complications include hypotension with shock, splenic rupture in children with hypersplenism, and disseminated intravascular coagulation (DIC). Hypersplenism is seen in areas of endemicity and is known as *hyper-reactive malarial splenomegaly* or *tropical splenomegaly syndrome*. It is thought to be the result of an abnormal immune response to malaria that leads to stimulation of B lymphocytes. Rhabdomyolysis has rarely been reported. Blackwater fever (hemoglobinuria, hemolysis, renal failure) and algid malaria (cardiovascular collapse, shock, hypothermia) are rarely seen in children.

Laboratory findings in patients with severe malaria include thrombocytopenia, hyperbilirubinemia, anemia, and elevated hepatic transaminases. The white blood cell count can be normal or low with a left shift. Other nonspecific markers of inflammation such as C-reactive protein and erythrocyte sedimentation rate are usually elevated. Coagulation abnormalities may be present due to DIC. Hypokalemia is seen in ~40% of patients after admission and is thought to be caused by renal potassium loss (52).

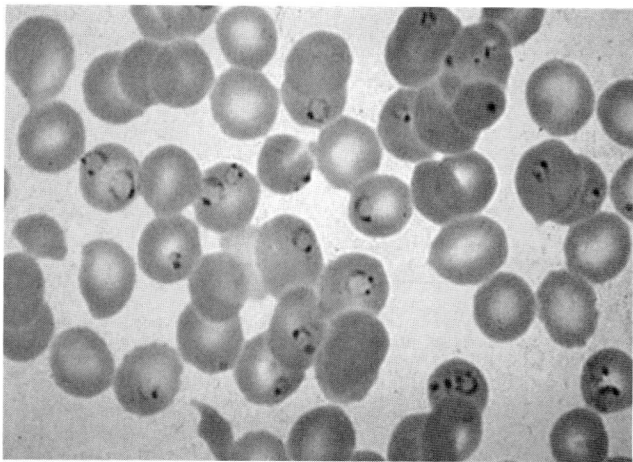

FIGURE 82.2. Malaria thin smear showing parasites within erythrocytes. Courtesy of Dr. Terrie Taylor.

In patients returning from an endemic area with a febrile illness, a high suspicion for malarial infection is needed. The initial presentation is often mistaken for influenza. For travelers returning from tropical countries, a variety of nonspecific febrile illnesses might be considered, including typhoid fever, dengue, leptospirosis, and rickettsial diseases. It may be difficult to rule out bacterial sepsis as the etiology of the illness until the blood culture results are available.

Diagnosis. The diagnosis of malaria is established by examining thick and thin blood smears stained with a 3% Giemsa stain. In thick smears, parasites are identified after lysis of the red blood cells. This method is more sensitive than a thin smear (limits of detection, 5–20 parasites/mcL vs. 50–200 parasites/mcL, respectively, for an experienced microscopist). In a thin smear, the parasites are visualized within the erythrocytes (**Fig. 82.2**). This method is useful for determination of species, as the morphology of the parasites and of the infected cells can be appreciated, and for quantification of very high parasitemias if the thick smear is too dense. A single negative set of malaria smears does not rule out the diagnosis of malaria, as parasites move between the bloodstream and sequestration within organs and tissues. Three sets of thick and thin smears 12–24 hrs apart have been recommended for establishing a diagnosis in patients with a high likelihood of malaria. Rapid testing with dipstick immunoassays can be used to diagnose malaria or to identify species, although none is approved for use in the US at this time.

To assess the full extent of the disease, all patients should be assessed for severe disease. Blood glucose, pH, or bicarbonate level, creatinine, and complete blood count must be measured to help classify severity. Blood cultures should also be obtained to evaluate the possibility of a concomitant bacteremia (6,10).

Clinical Management

Specific Antimalarial Therapy. For uncomplicated malaria, the decision for specific antimicrobial therapies depends upon the infecting species and the geographic source of the infection. The appropriate therapies for uncomplicated disease are listed in **Table 82.3**. Although medication can be administered orally,

it is recommended that patients remain in the hospital until parasite clearance can be documented, allowing providers to ensure compliance with the medication and monitor for any deterioration in the clinical status.

Patients with any signs of severe disease should initially be treated with parenteral therapy. Quinine is the mainstay of therapy in endemic areas, although it is not available in the US. Quinidine is the recommended drug in the US. As its use as an antiarrhythmic agent is becoming obsolete, PICUs should identify a source of quinidine so that they can be prepared for a patient with severe malaria. If no quinidine can be located in an emergency situation, providers can contact Eli Lilly Company (800-821-0538) to obtain the needed supply.

The antimalarial treatment regimen for quinidine has not been well studied, and many recommendations are based on recommended dosing of quinine. A loading dose of quinidine is given at the initiation of treatment if the patient did not receive mefloquine in the previous 12 hrs or over 40 mg/kg of quinidine in the previous 48 hrs. The treatment regimen is listed in **Table 82.3**. Once the level of parasitemia falls below 1% and the child is able to take oral intake, oral quinidine may be administered at the same dose to complete a total 3–7-day course. Clindamycin, tetracycline, or doxycycline is usually administered at the same time as the quinidine. These drugs can be administered orally if the patient can tolerate oral medication and should be continued for 7 days.

Cardiac monitoring is essential during IV quinidine administration due to the risk of prolonged QT, widening of the QRS, and hypotension. An electrocardiogram should be obtained at baseline prior to beginning the medication. The quinidine infusion should be decreased or stopped if an increase of >50% in the width of the QRS complex, prolongation of the QTc to >0.6 secs or >25%, or hypotension is seen.

Malaria smears should be repeated every 8 hrs when patients have signs or symptoms of severe disease. Quinine and quinidine are slow-acting medications, and it is common for parasites to increase in the blood for the first 24 hrs after initiation of therapy. Once the patient has had a good clinical response and has a parasite density <1%, malaria smears can be obtained once or twice daily.

Outside the US, artemisinin-derivatives are being used to treat severe disease. They are more rapid-acting than quinine and quinidine and have significantly less adverse effects. At this time, these drugs are not available in the US. IV artesunate may be available on a compassionate-use basis through the Centers for Disease Control and Prevention (CDC) for patients who cannot tolerate quinidine.

Supportive Care. In addition to the specific antimalarial therapy, adequate supportive care is essential to survival. Hypoglycemia is a common complication that leads to increased morbidity and mortality. If hypoglycemia is present, it should be corrected with dextrose infusions. Maintenance fluid administration should include dextrose concentrations sufficient to prevent the development of hypoglycemia in patients with normal glucose levels at presentation.

Fluid and electrolyte management is especially important in children with severe malaria. Metabolic acidosis can often be corrected with volume replacement. In patients with impaired consciousness or any other suspicion of cerebral malaria, volume resuscitation should proceed cautiously, as cerebral edema is common. Albumin has been shown to be more beneficial

TABLE 82.3

TREATMENT OF UNCOMPLICATED AND SEVERE MALARIA

Diagnosis	Therapy
Uncomplicated malaria with *P. falciparum* or unknown species: chloroquine sensitive (*only* Central America west of the Panama Canal, Haiti, Dominican Republic)	**Chloroquine phosphate** 10 mg base/kg initial dose, followed by 5 mg base/kg at 6, 24, and 48 hrs Total dose 25 mg base/kg Maximum adult dose: 1500 mg base
Uncomplicated malaria with *P. falciparum* or unknown species: chloroquine resistant (all regions except for those mentioned above)	**Quinine sulfate** 8.3 mg base/kg PO TID for 3–7 days Maximum adult dose: 542 mg base/dose *PLUS* one of the following for 7 days **Doxycycline** 2.2 mg/kg PO BID Maximum adult dose: 100 mg/dose **Tetracycline** 25 mg/kg/day divided QID Maximum adult dose 250 mg/dose **Clindamycin** 20 mg/kg/day divided TID **Atovaquone-proguanil** Adult tabs: 250 mg atovaquone/100 mg proguanil Pediatric tablets: 62.5 mg atovaquone/25 mg proguanil Doses given once per day for 3 days: 5–8 kg: 2 pediatric tabs 9–10 kg: 3 pediatric tabs 11–20 kg: 1 adult tab 21–30 kg: 2 adult tab 31–40 kg: 3 adult tabs >40 kg: 4 adult tabs **Mefloquine** 15 mg salt/kg PO initial dose, followed by 10 mg salt/kg PO 6–12 hrs after initial dose. Total dose: 25 mg salt/kg Maximum adult dose: 1250 mg salt
Complicated/severe malaria	**Quinidine gluconate** *Continuous infusion*: 6.25 mg base/kg IV over 1–2 hrs, followed by 0.0125 mg base/kg/min continuous infusion for at least 24 hrs *Every 8-hr dosing*: 15 mg base/kg over 4 hrs, followed by 7.5 mg base/kg every 8 hrs Switch to oral therapy when parasite density is <1%. Complete 3–7 days of quinidine therapy *PLUS* **doxycycline, tetracycline, or clindamycin** as above. If patient cannot tolerate oral medication, doxycycline or clindamycin may be administered intravenously.

than saline among comatose children with severe malaria (1). In the absence of intrinsic renal disease, renal output is a good measure of fluid status. Children who remain oliguric after a total of 40-mg/kg bolus infusion of saline should have a central catheter placed to monitor intravascular status (51). Potassium levels may fall during treatment due to an improvement in acid-base status and rise in pH.

The treatment of oliguric renal failure can be accomplished using hemodialysis/hemofiltration or peritoneal dialysis. In a study of adult patients with infection-associated acute renal failure, patients undergoing hemofiltration had a more rapid resolution of acidosis, shorter duration of renal replacement

therapy, and lower mortality rate than those treated with peritoneal dialysis (65). The use of dopamine or epinephrine infusions to improve renal blood flow has not been shown to be of benefit (23).

Transfusion. Packed red blood cell transfusions are indicated for patients with symptomatic anemia. The role of exchange transfusion is controversial. No adequate comparative trials have been performed to document a benefit. Anecdotal experience suggests that in cases of high parasite density (>10%) or severe end-organ damage that does not improve with antimalarial therapy, exchange transfusion may be of benefit.

The CDC recommends considering exchange transfusion if the parasite density is >10% or in the presence of cerebral malaria, non-volume overload pulmonary edema, or renal insufficiency. The exchanges continue until the parasitemia falls below 1%. The risk of the procedure, including bleeding, volume overload, transfusion reactions, blood-borne infection, and catheter-related infections, must be considered when making this decision.

Outcomes

The global mortality rate for patients with severe malaria is 15%–30% with most of the deaths occurring within 24 hrs of admission. In malaria-endemic areas, where resources are somewhat limited, impaired consciousness and respiratory distress are strongly associated with death. Among returned travelers who were treated in Europe for *P. falciparum*, the mortality rate was found to be 5%–10% (13). Where malaria is not endemic, increased morbidity and death is often associated with the failure to initially diagnose malaria.

P. falciparum infection has no chronic phase. Once the infection has resolved, it does not emerge again. Recurrence of parasitemia in a patient living in a nonendemic area is due to failed initial therapy. The only long-term sequelae of *P. falciparum* infection that has been well described is the neurologic impairment following cerebral malaria, as described in Chapter 80.

Future Directions—Malaria

The artemisinin-based therapies are derived from the Chinese medicinal plant, *Artemisia annua*. These drugs are more rapid-acting than most previously developed antimalarial agents. In addition, resistance to these drugs has not been detected. They are being used as part of combination therapy to treat malaria in malaria-endemic countries and are becoming more widely available with the support of international donors. These drugs (including artesunate, artemether, and dihydroartemisinin) are not yet approved by the US Food and Drug Administration (FDA). The combination of artemether-lumefantrine is sold in Europe as Riamet.

Vaccination against malaria has been very challenging. The only vaccination model that has ever been successful in preventing malaria has been the injection of irradiated sporozoites. This strategy cannot be replicated on a large scale, as it requires mosquito salivary gland dissection, parasite culture, and multiple doses, while only conferring short-lived immunity. Phase I and phase II trials of subunit vaccines are underway throughout the world.

Typhoid

Mechanism of Disease

Epidemiology. Typhoid fever is an enteric fever syndrome caused by *Salmonella enterica* serotype Typhi and occasionally by *S. enterica* serotype Paratyphi. These organisms are only carried by humans, and transmission usually occurs via contaminated food or water. Typhoid fever can be found in many tropical developing countries, as it is a result of poor water sanitation. Perhaps 10–20 million new cases are reported each year. The highest burden is in Asia, followed by Latin America and Africa (22). Over half of returned travelers who have typhoid fever report travel to the Indian subcontinent (4).

The disease afflicts people living in endemic areas as well as travelers to the area due to food and water-borne exposure. Children <5 years of age are more likely to develop severe forms of the illness and require hospitalization.

Etiology. *S. typhi* is a Gram-negative rod in the family *Enterobacteriaceae*. The organism is ingested, passes through the intestine into the mesenteric lymph nodes, and may travel to the liver and spleen. The organisms replicate in these tissues, usually for 7–14 days, until they enter the bloodstream. The symptoms of typhoid fever begin with the bacteremic phase. The bacteria travel through the blood to cause secondary infections in the liver, spleen, gall bladder, bone marrow, and Peyer patches of the terminal ileum. Although *S. typhi* produces exotoxin, typhoid fever has a remarkably low case fatality rate of <1%. Mortality is a result of unusual complications of the infection.

Clinical Presentation and Differential Diagnosis

The typical presentation of typhoid fever is fever, chills vomiting, anorexia, myalgia, and nonfocal abdominal pain. The fever rises slowly, and as it reaches its peak, it is sustained, unlike the paroxysms of fever typical of malaria. Diarrhea is found in 8%–35% of cases and is more common in children. Although this is a disease that begins with an enteric exposure, constipation may be a presenting complaint.

Physical examination often reveals hepatosplenomegaly and abdominal pain. Rose spots are the typical rash of typhoid fever. They are 2–4 mm wide blanching erythematous papules usually found on the trunk. They are frequently transient and may be difficult to see on individuals with dark skin. Relative bradycardia in the face of high fever is typically associated with typhoid fever, although this is not a reliable finding.

Central nervous system (CNS) manifestations are variable. An "apathetic affect" is common, and intermittent episodes of confusion can occur in the absence of direct infection of the CNS. Altered mental status is a manifestation of typhoid encephalopathy, one of the severe complications of typhoid fever. Seizures may occur in young children.

Laboratory findings are nonspecific. The white blood cell count is often slightly low, although young children may have leukocytosis. Mild increases in liver function tests are common. In severe disease, coagulopathy may be present, with thrombocytopenia and signs of DIC.

Complications of typhoid fever usually occur late in the course of the illness, 1–2 weeks after the onset of symptoms in 10%–15% of patients. Gastrointestinal bleeding is common, but severe bleeding that requires transfusion and possibly surgery is a rare but life-threatening form of the disease. Intestinal perforation usually occurs in the ileum, as this is the site of the greatest bacterial replication. Typhoid encephalopathy is usually accompanied by shock and carries a very high mortality rate.

The differential diagnosis depends on the precise travel and exposure history of the patient. Malaria is frequently the leading alternative diagnosis because typhoid and malaria coexist in many regions, and they are among the leading causes of fever without localizing signs in returned travelers. The pattern of fever may distinguish the two diseases: in typhoid, the fever rises gradually and is sustained, while malaria is associated with sudden-onset paroxysms of fever. However, treatment for both infections may be indicated as evaluation is under way. Other diseases to consider include bacterial sepsis of other etiologies, leptospirosis, rickettsial disease, dengue, hepatitis, Epstein-Barr virus, typhus, brucellosis, and tularemia.

Diagnosis. The diagnosis of typhoid fever is challenging. The sensitivity of blood culture has been reported to be as low as 40% and as high as 80%. The best sensitivity is achieved when large-volume specimens are collected and during the first week of illness. Bone marrow culture is more sensitive than standard blood culture. It remains positive beyond the first week of illness, even after the initiation of antimicrobial therapy.

In endemic areas, the Widal serologic test is used to diagnose typhoid fever. The test is neither reliable nor specific and is therefore not recommended for use in developed countries where other options are available (17,59). Currently, no approved rapid tests exist to diagnose typhoid fever.

Clinical Management

Fluoroquinolones and third-generation cephalosporins are the medications of choice for empiric therapy for typhoid fever. If cultures are positive and the susceptibility patterns are known, treatment may be tailored to the susceptibility pattern of the specific organism. However, the advantage of completing therapy with a fluoroquinolone is that a decreased incidence of chronic intestinal carriage is seen with this class of treatment. For fluoroquinolone-susceptible infections, 5-day duration is sufficient for therapy of uncomplicated disease.

The emergence of fluoroquinolone-resistant *S. typhi* has complicated the treatment of typhoid fever. The problem is most prominent in South Asia and Southeast Asia. Infections with organisms that demonstrate in vitro resistance to the quinolone nalidixic acid and have minimum inhibitory concentrations of fluoroquinolones, such as ciprofloxacin, within the susceptible range, have diminished clinical response to fluoroquinolone therapy. Therefore, organisms that are nalidixic acid-resistant should be managed as fluoroquinolone-resistant infections (37). Treatment of resistant infections requires 10–14 days of therapy with fluoroquinolones at the maximum dose or third-generation cephalosporins. Azithromycin for 5–7 days has shown to be effective against fluoroquinolone-resistant *S. typhi* and successfully eliminates intestinal carriage (19, 62). Recommended therapies for typhoid fever are listed in **Table 82.4.**

Hospitalization is required for young children, as they are at higher risk for complication, and for any patients who are suspected of having complicated disease. Persistent vomiting and severe diarrhea are also indications for hospitalization. It may be prudent to hospitalize most patients with typhoid fever for parenteral therapy until the antimicrobial susceptibility is known and an acceptable oral therapy can be selected.

Severe disease requires parenteral therapy for a minimum of 10 days. Controlled clinical trials have demonstrated a benefit of the addition of dexamethasone for treatment of severe typhoid with delirium, obtundation, or shock (3 mg/kg infusion over 1 hr, followed by 1 mg/kg every 6 hrs for 8 doses) (35). If dexamethasone is administered, providers should be aware that further intestinal complications may be masked. Severe intestinal bleeding or perforation requires hemodynamic stabilization and surgery. In cases of perforation, the intestine should be explored for additional sites of perforation.

Outcomes

Relapse occurs in 5%–10% of appropriately treated infections. The organism is generally identical to the initial infection, although the symptoms are more mild. The same treatment can be repeated. Relapse is more common with fluoroquinolone-resistant infections.

Excretion of *S. typhi* can persist beyond the clinical illness. Chronic carriage is defined as excretion for greater than 3 months. This is a rare occurrence among children. If it occurs, prolonged treatment with ciprofloxacin or the combination of amoxicillin and probenecid is recommended for eradication.

Future Directions—Typhoid

The fact that *S. paratyphi* is becoming an increasingly important cause of typhoid fever is of concern because the current typhoid fever vaccines have no activity against *S. paratyphi*.

Chagas Disease

Mechanism of Disease

Trypanosoma cruzi, the etiologic agent of Chagas disease, is one of the most common parasitic infections in humans. The WHO estimates that 100 million people are at risk for the infection and that 18 million people are infected throughout

---

TABLE 82.4

TREATMENT OF TYPHOID FEVER

	Drug	Dose	Duration
Empiric	Ceftriaxone	60 mg/kg/day	7–14
Fully susceptible	Ciprofloxacin or ofloxacin	15 mg/kg/day	5–7 days
	Amoxicillin (second line)	75–100 mg/kg/day	14 days
	Trimethoprim-sulfamethoxazole (second line)	8/40 mg/kg/day	14 days
Multidrug resistant	Ceftriaxone	60 mg/kg/day	10–14 days
	Azithromycin	8–10 mg/kg/day	7 days
	Ciprofloxacin or ofloxacin (nalidixic acid *susceptible* infection)	15 mg/kg/day	5–7 days
	Ciprofloxacin or ofloxacin (nalidixic acid *resistant* infection)	20 mg/kg/day	10–14 days

Mexico, Central America, and South America. The reduviid bug (kissing bug) is responsible for transmitting the disease to human via feces contamination after a bite or through feces contamination of conjunctiva or mucosa. Housing conditions are important for disease transmission, as the reduviid bugs usually live in the cracks within the walls of mud and straw houses found in rural and poor urban areas. Transfusion-associated *T. cruzi* is another important mode of disease transmission in countries (e.g., Brazil) with a high prevalence of disease. Screening of the blood supply has been established in many endemic areas. The FDA has recently approved an enzyme-linked immunosorbent assay (ELISA) to screen blood, organ, and tissue donations. Screening has been adopted by the American Red Cross and other organizations in the US (8).

Clinical Presentation and Differential Diagnosis

The initial symptoms of infection with *T. cruzi* are nonspecific and often unrecognized. Beginning 6–10 days after exposure and lasting up to 2 months, patients may develop general malaise. Other associated physical findings may include hepatosplenomegaly, lymphadenopathy, rash, and edema. The reduviid bug has a predilection for biting on exposed areas during sleep, so that the bite occurs in the periorbital or perioral areas and can produce a characteristic swelling of the eyelid and face called *Romaña sign*. Romaña sign may be present in half of the patients with clinically apparent acute disease.

Abnormalities in the heart can develop during the acute illness, and abnormalities on electrocardiogram and chest radiography are common although generally do not produce symptomatic disease. The changes are due to the inflammatory response to parasites that have a tropism for the cardiac muscle. Life-threatening illness is extremely rare during the acute phase of the infection, although meningitis and myocarditis have been reported.

After acute infection, most patients enter a prolonged asymptomatic period, known as the *indeterminate phase*, and remain in this phase for the rest of their lives. Approximately 15%–30% of patients with indeterminate infection will eventually develop end-organ damage, typically decades after the initial infection. In normal hosts, chronic infection can occur in the myocardium or the esophagus and colon.

Chagas cardiomyopathy is consistent with a diffuse process. Patients present with chest pain, dizziness, and peripheral edema. Chest x-rays show cardiomegaly in all chambers of the heart. The typical electrocardiographic finding is a right-bundle-branch block. Other conduction abnormalities may also be seen.

Megaviscera syndrome, due to neuronal loss in the gastrointestinal tract, leads to megaesophagus and megacolon. The presenting symptom of megaesophagus is dysphagia, although this occurs late in the disease. The finding on upper gastrointestinal contrast studies is diagnostic (**Fig. 82.3**). Megacolon is associated with constipation and the palpation of a fecaloma on examination. Barium enema can be used to confirm the diagnosis.

Reactivation of *T. cruzi* infection can occur in immunocompromised patients, including those with human immunodeficiency virus (HIV) infection or those receiving immunosuppressive therapy, and in children who are infected before 2 years of age (26). The CNS is the most common site of reactivation. Trypanosome invasion of the brain forms chagoma masses, causing patients to present with headache, fever, cog-

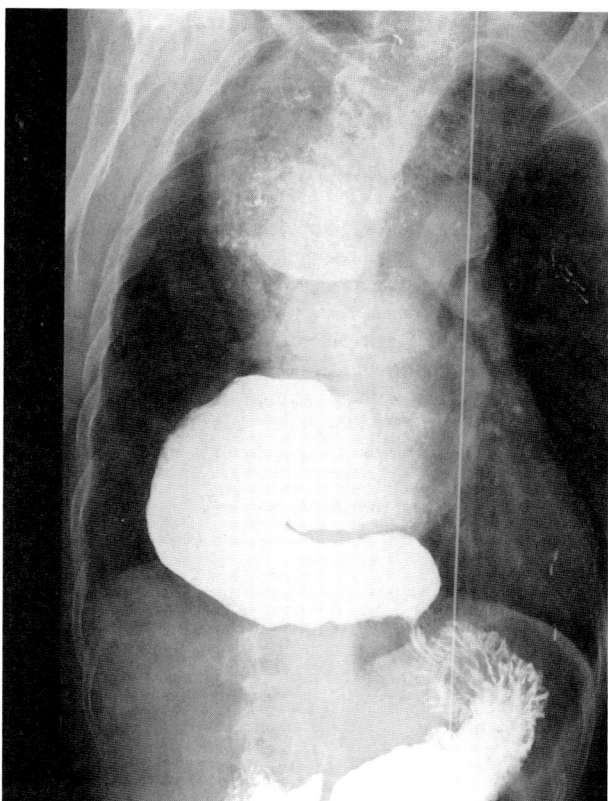

FIGURE 82.3. Megaesophagus due to chronic Chagas disease. Courtesy of Dr. Igor Laufer.

nitive changes, focal neurologic impairment, and seizures. The second site most commonly affected during reactivation is the heart. Cardiac reactivation manifests as acute myocarditis or cardiomyopathy. In patients who already have cardiac damage due to chronic infection, reactivation can lead to new, acute inflammation or worsening congestive heart failure. Reactivation of cardiac disease may occur with or without neurologic disease.

Diagnosis. During the acute phase, parasitemia can be detected in the bloodstream on stained smears or microscopic examination of anticoagulated blood or buffy coat. Organisms may also be visualized in infected organs, including lymph nodes, bone marrow, and pericardial fluid. Xenodiagnosis and blood culture in specific liquid medium may be more sensitive than direct visualization, but the facilities are rarely available and the tests require 2–8 weeks to achieve a diagnosis.

During the indeterminate, chronic phase, the diagnosis can be made by serology. A positive IgM does not differentiate acute from chronic infections, as intermittent rises in IgM are common in chronic infections. A serologic diagnosis can be made using an anti-*T. cruzi* IgG ELISA test, complement fixation, hemagglutination, or indirect immunofluorescence. Because of the poor specificity of these tests, experts generally recommend obtaining two serologic tests to confirm the diagnosis. Clinical diagnostic tests are available through the CDC. Polymerase chain reaction (PCR) is a very sensitive method by which to detect the low-level infection present during chronic infection, although it is not yet widely available.

Clinical Management

Treatment of Chagas disease is most beneficial during the acute phase of the infection. For those with end-organ damage due to chronic infection, treatment has not been demonstrated to improve outcomes. The two effective treatment regimens are nifurtimox (8–10 mg/kg/day, divided 3 times per day) for 90–120 days or benznidazole (5–10 mg/kg/day in 2 divided doses) for 30–90 days. Patients who weigh <40 kg require higher doses—up to 12 mg/kg/day of nifurtimox and 7.5 mg/kg/day of benznidazole. Common side effects include hypersensitivity, bone marrow suppression, and peripheral neuropathy and may require suspension of treatment with benznidazole. Weight loss, gastrointestinal distress, and psychiatric disturbance may result from treatment with nifurtimox (72). Availability of these drugs varies by country. Only nifurtimox, produced by Bayer in Germany, is available in the US through the Drug Service of the CDC. Treatment is considered to be successful when both parasitemia is cleared and serology is negative.

During the acute illness, patients may require intensive care for treatment of pancarditis that can result with *T. cruzi* infection. Patients are managed according to the requirement of their cardiomyopathy. Thromboembolism is common, and some suggest the use of anticoagulants for individuals in atrial fibrillation or other thrombogenic arrhythmias. Clinically significant pericardial effusions can occur. Chronic sequelae of Chagas disease, such as cardiomyopathy, megaesophagus, and megacolon, are rare among children. Symptomatic management is required.

For patients with *T. cruzi* reactivation, specific antitrypanosomal treatment is indicated, although survival is uniformly poor. The restoration of the immune system, such as the institution of highly active antiretroviral therapy in patients immunocompromised due to HIV, is important to control the infection.

Outcomes

Patients who are treated during the acute phase achieve a "cure," defined as the disappearance of IgG, in 30%–80% of cases. For those with severe cardiac disease, heart transplant may be an effective long-term solution of Chagas cardiomyopathy, despite the risk of reactivation of chronic infection due to transplant-associated immunosuppression. Sudden death occurs in 38% of patients with Chagas cardiomyopathy, often without a recognized change in cardiac status. Risk factors for death include New York Heart Association stage III or IV heart failure, cardiomegaly on chest x-ray and left ventricular dysfunction on echocardiogram (71). Immunocompromised individuals with reactivation CNS infection rarely survive beyond 3 months.

Human African Trypanosomiasis

Mechanism of Disease

The WHO estimates that 500,000 people are infected with *Trypanosoma brucei*, with an estimated 50,000 deaths per year from human African trypanosomiasis (HAT). Within Africa, two forms of HAT exist: West African sleeping sickness and East African sleeping sickness, which are caused by infection with *T. brucei gambiense* and *T. brucei rhodesiense*, respectively. Areas with high infection rates include The Congo and

Uganda. Outbreaks have been reported in areas of conflict because control activities are abandoned. East African HAT is endemic at a very low rate in Kenya, Mozambique, Zambia, Tanzania, and Malawi. HAT is extremely rare in travelers.

The transmission to humans occurs after a bite from the tsetse fly that results in wound contamination by infected saliva. The habitat and species of tsetse fly are also different for the two regions, with a habitat of forested rivers and shores in western and central Africa and the savannah being the habitat in eastern and southern Africa. Other mechanisms of disease transmission in both areas include blood transfusions, contaminated needles, or congenital transmission.

Trypanosoma are parasitic protozoa that are single-celled flagellates transmitted by biting insect vectors. The life cycle involves both the vector stage and the mammalian host stage when the infective trypomastigote is injected into the bloodstream and is able to reach the CNS.

Clinical Presentation and Differential Diagnosis

In general, the presentation of HAT can be divided into an early, or hemolymphatic, stage and a late, or encephalitic, stage. The difference between the two stages is the presence of CNS involvement. In West African HAT (caused by *T. b. gambiense*), a prolonged asymptomatic period may occur, followed by a febrile stage, in which trypanosomes can be found in the blood and lymphatic systems. During this time, patients develop a nonspecific illness characterized by intermittent fever, myalgia, malaise, and fatigue. Most patients have lymphadenopathy. Pruritus and transient facial edema are rare but may be clues to the diagnosis when present. The late-stage West African HAT occurs after several months of the early febrile illness, although progression to CNS disease is more rapid in children. Headaches and somnolence with night-time insomnia can occur. Developmental delay is more common than somnolence in children. Extrapyramidal signs, cerebellar ataxia, and hemiparesis may occur.

Eastern African HAT (caused by *T. b. rhodiense*) has a more acute presentation. A chancre at the site of inoculation can occur 5–15 days after the bite, with surrounding cellulitis or regional adenopathy. Disease can progress rapidly. Myocarditis is rare, but patients may die due to dysrhythmia or cardiac failure before the neurologic disease becomes clinically apparent.

Lumbar puncture demonstrates an increased number of monocytes and an elevated protein level. A white blood cell count >5 cells/mcL is considered positive for CNS disease. Occasionally foamy plasma cells, the pathognomonic Mott morula cells, are found in the cerebrospinal fluid (CSF). CSF total IgM levels may be beneficial in establishing a diagnosis, as they have been found to be elevated in patients with sleeping sickness.

Brain imaging may show basal ganglia involvement such as seen in Parkinson disease, ventriculomegaly, and asymmetric white matter abnormalities. Electroencephalography in encephalopathic patients may be abnormal, but findings are not pathognomonic. The differential diagnosis includes malaria, tuberculosis, HIV, leishmaniasis, toxoplasmosis, typhoid, and viral encephalitis.

Diagnosis. Definitive diagnosis is made by visualizing trypomastigotes in the blood or tissue. Aspiration of enlarged lymph nodes has a high yield. Thick and thin blood smears are prepared with Giemsa stains, similar to malaria smear preparation. If parasitemia is low, repeated specimens should be examined over different days to increase the sensitivity of diagnosis. In advanced cases, trypanosomes may be easier to visualize in the CSF than in the peripheral blood. To maximize the utility of the CSF direct examination, 6–8 mL of CSF should be double-centrifuged and the sediment examined

Clinical Management

Treatment regimens vary based on the infecting organism and stage of illness. *T. b. gambiense* can usually be distinguished from *T. brucei rhodesiense* based on the patient's travel or exposure history. Any patient with evidence of trypanosomiasis and a CSF white blood cell count >5 cells/mm^3 is considered to have late disease, regardless of clinical neurologic status. First-line treatment of the hemolymphatic stage is parenteral pentamidine for *T. brucei gambiense* and IV suramin for *T. brucei rhodesiense*. As use of suramin carries a risk of anaphylactic shock, a test dose must be given first. Eflornithine is only useful for late *T. brucei gambiense* disease; however, convulsions may occur in 6%–7% of treated patients, and bone marrow toxicity is common. For CNS disease, IV melarsoprol is effective for both varieties of HAT. The treatment is highly effective but extremely toxic, with death rates of 4%–6%. Encephalopathy, generalized seizures, coma, and neurogenic pulmonary edema can complicate therapy. Prednisone can be used to decrease these adverse effects without impairment of the treatment efficacy. Polyneuropathy may lead to permanent weakness unless thiamine is administered, and treatment is suspended until symptoms resolve.

Outcomes

HAT is fatal if untreated. Patients are usually followed up to 2 years after treatment, with periodic lumbar punctures performed to evaluate recurrence of CNS disease. Recurrences require different treatment regimens or higher doses. Long-term prognosis depends on the stage of disease when treatment is initiated and the recurrence of disease, as significant injury to the CNS can occur with disease progression. Significant CNS disease can lead to demyelination, cortical and subcortical atrophy, and multifocal deep white matter lesions. Additionally, hypoxic-ischemic injury may occur as a result of seizures.

Future Directions—Human African Trypanosomiasis

Much of the research on HAT has focused on identification of appropriate targets for drug development. With the genome of *T. brucei* nearly completed, more opportunities will be available to explore new pathways to exploit with antitrypanosomal drugs. Vector control, which had been achieved in the 1960s but lost in the recent past, will be a key factor in the control of this disease.

Leptospirosis

Mechanism of Disease

Leptospirosis is a bacterial disease caused by the spirochete, *Leptospira interrogans*. Infections can range from being asymptomatic, to causing an influenza-like illness, to causing hemorrhage, renal failure, and death. Leptospires are carried by a variety of wild and domestic animals, including rodents, dogs, and livestock. In most cases, these animals have chronic renal infection with *Leptospira* without any symptoms, and they shed the organisms in their urine. Once excreted, the leptospires survive for months in moist, warm conditions. Transmission frequently occurs due to contact with infected water or moist soil. The most common scenario is flooding of urban areas or fields, leading to the spread of infected excreta and exposure of the human population. Leptospirosis can occur in urban and rural areas of developing countries, as well as through exposures in poor, urban settings in developed countries, recreational and sporting exposures, and through adventurous travel.

The precise burden of the disease is difficult to assess due to frequent under-reporting from developing countries. The clinical presentation mimics other diseases, and cases of leptospirosis are often attributed to other causes. For example, in Southeast Asia, leptospirosis is responsible for 13% of nonmalarial fever (40), and it is frequently the etiology of illnesses suspected to be dengue (11,41).

Leptospires are coiled, thin, and flagellated in appearance microscopically and are obligate, slow-growing anaerobes. The bacterial cell wall has a double-membrane architecture and shares features of both Gram-positive and Gram-negative organisms. Cell wall lipopolysaccharide contains antigens to which natural immunity is targeted and is the basis for serovar grouping.

Once gaining entry into the bloodstream, *Leptospira* cause disease through direct infection and through the host immune response. The organisms are highly motile and are able to penetrate and infect a wide variety of organs, including the liver, kidney, lungs, brain, and eyes. A disseminated vasculitis occurs with endothelial damage and inflammatory infiltrates in these end organs.

Clinical Presentation and Differential Diagnosis

Most infections caused by *Leptospira* result in an asymptomatic or mild infection, which is unlikely to come to the attention of a critical care specialist. Severe disease, however, is life-threatening. The clinical course of leptospirosis has been described as being biphasic consisting of an acute (septicemic) phase that usually lasts 1 week, followed by an immune phase. The biphasic nature may not be detected clinically, as patients often come to medical attention after the first phase or may have overlapping syndromes. During the acute phase, the most common symptom is fever, often with chills, and other common symptoms include headache, conjunctival suffusion, myalgia, nausea, and vomiting. Myalgias can be severe. Mild changes in mental status may occur without meningitis. A pretibial papular rash may develop. Jaundice occurs in less than half the identified cases of leptospirosis during the acute phase.

The immune phase is associated with the resolution of these acute symptoms, with an increase in antibody production and excretion of the leptospires in the urine. Typical manifestations of the immune phase are aseptic meningitis and anterior uveitis. CSF analysis reveals a lymphocytic pleocytosis and a high opening pressure. Focal neurologic findings are rare.

The severe icteric form of the disease, Weil disease, may develop as a progression from the initial febrile episode or as a distinct separate phase from the first. It is characterized by jaundice, renal failure, and hemorrhage. Serum bilirubin levels are elevated out of proportion to transaminase levels. Renal failure usually occurs during the second week of the illness. Pulmonary symptoms occur irregularly and may take the form of dyspnea or cough or may be severe with hemorrhage and ARDS. Thrombocytopenia is common but is not usually associated with DIC.

Hemorrhagic complications can occur in severe disease that is either icteric or anicteric. Purpura, petechiae, epistaxis, and mild hemoptysis are the most frequent manifestations. The pathognomonic sign of leptospirosis, conjunctival suffusion, is due to conjunctival hemorrhage and scleral icterus. Pulmonary hemorrhage can also occur.

In anicteric disease, the white blood cell count may be low, normal, or elevated. Neutrophil predominance is typical. In contrast, lymphocytosis is a hallmark of Weil disease. Elevations in the serum level of muscle enzymes occurs in most cases.

Patchy infiltrates seen on chest x-ray are thought to represent areas of intra-alveolar and interstitial hemorrhage. The areas involved are usually at the lung bases and periphery, with bilateral involvement. Histologically, these findings represent endothelial damage and hemorrhage, not inflammatory exudate. Disease can progress to diffuse alveolar infiltrates and radiographic evidence of ARDS.

The differential diagnosis includes other viral infections that are prevalent in the area where the patient resides and/or has traveled and may include common infections in the US, such as influenza, Ebstein-Barr virus, hepatitis viruses, and community-acquired pneumonia. Other vector-borne infections should be considered based on the appropriate epidemiology and include malaria, dengue, Hantavirus, typhoid fever, rickettsial infections, and arborvirus disease. Toxic shock syndrome may also mimic leptospirosis.

Diagnosis. The most common diagnostic method is serology using the microscopic agglutination test. The patient's serum agglutinates with leptospira antigen suspensions of known serovars to determine titers. A fourfold increase in antibody titers or conversion from seronegative to a titer >1:100 is considered diagnostic. Rapid tests to detect IgM are under development.

Diagnosis of leptospirosis can be made through direct visualization of the organism or by serologic evaluation. Culture of the organism from the CSF or blood during the first week of illness or from the urine during the immune phase is not a dependable method for diagnosis, as it has poor sensitivity and requires 6–8 weeks for growth. Real-time PCR can detect *Leptospira* from clinical samples and may be a rapid, reliable strategy where the assay is available. The added advantage of the real-time PCR is that it offers a quantitative assessment of the bacterial load, which may be associated with prognosis (78).

Clinical Management

The benefit of antibiotic therapy on the outcome of leptospirosis has not been definitively demonstrated. However, some reports suggest that treatment decreases the duration of illness and, in children, it has been observed that antibiotics reduce the duration of thrombocytopenia and extent of renal failure (54). Treatment of severe disease is recommended. Antimicrobials with demonstrated in vivo efficacy against leptospirosis are penicillin, doxycycline, ceftriaxone, and cefotaxime.

Doxycycline has typically been reserved for mild or moderate disease. However, in areas endemic for both leptospirosis and rickettsiosis, cephalosporin or doxycycline therapy may be preferable to penicillin therapy because of their activity against coinfecting rickettsia (76). For children in developed countries, initial empiric therapy with an IV cephalosporin should be initiated while the investigation of the etiology is under way. As the Jarisch-Herxheimer reaction (release of endotoxin from large-scale death of bacteria that can follow administration of an antimicrobial in certain diseases) can occur with the initiation of β-lactam therapy, patients should be closely monitored during the first doses.

Aside from antibiotic therapy, management of severe leptospirosis is supportive. Acutely, patients should have prompt treatment of hypovolemia and/or shock and should be assessed for pulmonary involvement and the need for respiratory support. Electrolyte disturbances may also need to be corrected.

Patients with prerenal azotemia should respond well to fluid hydration and electrolyte correction. Most often, the oliguria seen with leptospirosis responds to fluid treatment. In patients with acute, intrinsic renal failure, prompt treatment with renal replacement therapy has been suggested to reduce mortality. Peritoneal dialysis has been demonstrated to be inferior to venovenous hemofiltration in treating patients with infection associated with renal failure (65). Improvement in mean arterial blood pressure, lowering of heart rate, and normalization of systemic vascular resistance was seen in a small series of patients who underwent hemofiltration for renal failure associated with severe leptospirosis (75).

In patients in whom mechanical ventilation is necessary, lung-protective strategies based upon low tidal volumes (4–6 mL/kg) and high positive end-expiratory pressure to maximize lung recruitment improve outcomes. Inotropic support may be necessary in many of these patients. To evaluate heart function in adult cases of ARDS and circulatory failure, pulmonary artery catheterization has been performed. A common finding is an elevated cardiac output with low systemic vascular resistance, as seen in early septic shock. Furthermore, red blood cell transfusion and correction of thrombocytopenia and coagulopathy with platelet and fresh frozen plasma transfusion may be necessary. Extracorporeal membrane oxygenation (ECMO) has been successful in some severe cases.

Outcomes

Case fatality rates for severe disease range from 5% to 40%. Death has usually been caused by acute renal failure due to acute tubular necrosis and pulmonary hemorrhage. However, mortality rates have been noted to decline in some areas where the use of hemodialysis has become more common.

Among survivors, normalization of glomerular filtration rate occurred by 6 months, although some had a mild persistent defect in urinary concentrating ability. Hepatic function usually returns to normal, although elevated bilirubin levels may persist for weeks. Chronic visual disturbances may persist after other organ system recovery, and anterior uveitis may present several weeks or longer after the acute stage (45).

Future Directions—Leptospirosis

Vaccines are under development for human leptospirosis. Animal immunization with killed vaccine is widely used, but immunity is short lived and the formulations have high rates of adverse side effects. The mechanism of protection from infection is not yet well enough understood to develop a subunit vaccine.

Hantavirus

Mechanism of Disease

Over 20 types of Hantaviruses, part of the Bunyavirus family, have been identified in many different rodent populations throughout the world. These infections are associated with two major groups of diseases: the "Old World" viruses in Europe and Asia, which cause hemorrhagic fever with renal syndrome (HFRS), and "New World" viruses found in the Americas, characterized by cardiopulmonary disease and called Hantavirus pulmonary syndrome (HPS). Each virus has a specific rodent reservoir. The host rodent develops asymptomatic infection and can excrete infectious virus in urine, feces, and saliva. Excretion can continue even after the resolution of viremia. Transmission is thought to occur through inhalation of hantavirus aerosols found in rodent feces, although infection may occur through exposure to urine and saliva. No arthropod vectors are necessary.

Human disease begins with inhalation of infected particles that reach the bronchioles or alveoli. Viremia develops with damage to the characteristic endothelial surfaces. On histologic examination, no direct cytopathic effect is seen. The cellular damage of the lung and kidney capillary endothelium, as well as the myocardial depression, is thought to be due to the cytokine response.

Hantavirus was first recognized in the US in the "Four Corners" region in the southwest in 1993, with a cluster of deaths associated with pulmonary edema presenting with hypotension (24). When the viral strain responsible for this outbreak was identified, it was called the *Sin Nombre Hantavirus*. It is carried by a deer mouse. The infection is rare, with under 500 cases reported in the US since 1993, and children account for <10% of cases nationwide (32). The states with the highest incidence rates are New Mexico, Montana, Utah, Nevada, Arizona, and Colorado, but cases have been reported from Canada to Mexico.

After identification of the Sin Nombre virus in the US, cases of HPS due to Hantaviruses were identified throughout South America. The most common species in South America HPS is the Andes virus. In Chile, ~500 cases have been reported (56). The seroprevalence of antibodies against the Latin American Hantaviruses shows extensive geographic diversity. For example, the seropositive rates in Venezuela, Brazil, and Paraguay are 1.7%, 14.3%, and 42.7%, respectively (66), suggesting that nonvirulent strains frequently circulate in the same region or that the development of disease requires both the virus and an additional factor that is likely environmental.

In Latin America, disease frequently occurs in family clusters and children are often infected. Transmission from person to person is rare but has been reported with the Andes virus in Argentina (55).

The most severe forms of HFRS are cases of the Hantaan virus on the Korean peninsula and the Dobrava virus in the Balkans. A milder disease is caused by the Seoul virus in Southeast Asia. The Puumala virus, found in Scandinavia, Western Europe, and Russia can cause a benign illness called *nephropathia epidemica* that causes an interstitial nephritis but has also been associated with HFRS.

Clinical Presentation and Differential Diagnosis

Hemorrhagic Fever with Renal Syndrome. HFRS is characterized by fever, renal failure, and hemorrhage. Symptoms usually begin 2–3 weeks after exposure, but incubation may be from 2 days to 6 weeks. The disease has been described to have five phases:

- *Febrile.* The onset of fever may be sudden and accompanied by headache, back and abdominal pain, vomiting, myalgias, weakness, and chills. Flushing and dermatographism may be prominent. This phase lasts an average of 5 days.
- *Hypotensive.* Shock develops. Hemorrhage, capillary leak, proteinuria, leukocytosis, thrombocytopenia, and hypotension may occur. On examination, petechiae and hemorrhage may be noted. Other common findings include hepatosplenomegaly, conjunctivitis, and change in vision.
- *Oliguric.* The oliguric phase usually begins with the return of blood pressure to normal or even hypertension and may last 3–7 days before improvement in urine output. This is the period with the highest risk of death because patients with fatal disease develop severe hemorrhagic manifestations. Milder cases are associated with nausea and vomiting.
- *Diuretic.* The diuretic phase follows and may last several weeks.
- *Convalescent.* Convalescence may be asymptomatic or associated with some renal abnormalities such as polyuria or hyposthenuria. Permanent renal damage may be a long-term sequela.

Laboratory results show worsening thrombocytopenia and leukocytosis in the febrile and hypotensive phases. Toward the end of this phase, proteinuria can develop, followed by renal insufficiency and electrolyte imbalance during the oliguric phase. Most clinically ill patients have enlarged kidneys on ultrasound, and some have ascites or pleural effusion.

The differential diagnosis is broad and depends on the exposure history of the patient. For patients who have traveled to Asia, rickettsial disease, Dengue virus, and leptospirosis are possible infectious causes. The mild noninfectious etiologies, including renal disease and renal vein thrombosis, might not be easy to differentiate from mild common viral illnesses.

Hantavirus Pulmonary Syndrome

The incubation period for HPS due to the Sin Nombre virus is usually 1–2 weeks but may be much shorter or longer after exposure to infected excreta (56). HPS consists of three phases: a prodromal phase that lasts 3–6 days, a cardiorespiratory phase that lasts 7–10 days, and a convalescent phase. In the prodromal phase, patients usually have nonspecific symptoms of fever, myalgia, and headache. Abdominal pain and diarrhea may also be present. Sore throat is common in children. Patients frequently seek medical care during this time, but the lack of severe disease does not warrant hospitalization. During the cardiopulmonary phase, hospitalization and intensive care are often required. This phase develops rapidly, with most patients having cough, shortness of breath, tachypnea, and tachycardia. Initially, auscultation of the lungs may reveal only mild abnormalities. As the disease progresses, hypotension and hypoxemia develop. Renal insufficiency and bleeding/petechiae have not been seen in children in the US but are commonly seen in children in South America with Andes virus infection (67).

The most consistent laboratory evaluation abnormality is thrombocytopenia. Other abnormalities include leukocytosis, hemoconcentration (more common in the South American form), myelocytosis, lack of granulation of neutrophil, and >10% lymphocyte with immunoblast appearance (27). DIC may develop. Renal impairment is common in South American HPS and may require dialysis (56).

The initial chest x-ray most commonly demonstrates interstitial edema, and many also have airspace disease. Pleural effusion is common and may help to differentiate HPS from other causes of ARDS (39).

The differential diagnosis includes community-acquired bacterial and viral pneumonias, septic shock with ARDS, initially acute gastroenteritis, leptospirosis, septicemic plague, Colorado tick fever, tularemia, relapsing fever, Rocky Mountain fever ("spotless"), Legionnaire disease, ehrlichiosis, Q fever, coccidioidomycosis, and histoplasmosis. Cardiac shock with high peripheral vascular resistance points toward a viral hemorrhagic fever rather than septic shock (64). Rash with HPS has not been reported in North American children, although petechial rash can be seen in South American infections. A history of peridomestic and/or recreational contact with rodent-infested structures is present in most cases. Severe HFRS may be confused with hemolytic uremic syndrome, but the former lacks a microangiopathic, hemolytic anemia.

Diagnosis

The diagnosis of any Hantavirus infection is based on the presence of antibody in a region of the nucleocapsid that is conserved among all species. IgM is almost always present at the time of clinical symptoms, and IgG levels rise early and peak during the first week of illness. A fourfold rise in IgG can distinguish previous exposure from acute infection. An ELISA is available to state health departments through the CDC. In patients from regions where baseline seroprevalence is high, a reverse transcriptase PCR may be required for acute diagnosis. Viral isolation is rarely successful.

Clinical Management

For all serious hantaviral disease, most treatment is supportive. Patients with severe HFRS or HPS require intensive care monitoring and resuscitation to reverse shock and treat circulatory failure, mechanical ventilation for respiratory failure, and the use of renal replacement therapies in some circumstances. The patients require management of increased capillary permeability, myocardial dysfunction, and elevated systemic vascular resistance. The use of ionotropic support with dobutamine has been recommended in the ICU (31). In both children and adults, ECMO has been used in severe cases, and experts recommend the following criteria: cardiac index <2.3 L/min/mm^2, Pao$_2$/Fio$_2$ <50 or unresponsive to conventional support. However, these clinicians often begin ECMO prior to achieving these criteria because decompensation can be so rapid (56).

Although ribavirin is active against Hantaviruses in vitro, a small blinded, controlled trial did not demonstrate any benefit of ribavirin in the treatment of HPS (57). Administration of ribavirin within 4 days of onset of illness reduced the incidence of renal failure in HFRS in China. Although end-organ damage is mediated by the host inflammatory response, the use of steroids to mitigate the extent of the damage has not been studied in severe disease.

Outcomes

In patients with HFRS, the outcome depends on the type of infecting virus. Dobrava and Hantaan viruses are associated with more severe disease and have reported mortality rates between 5% and 10%, whereas Seoul virus and Puumala virus have reported mortality rates of 1%–2% and <0.2%, respectively. In severe cases, 15%–20% of the children require renal replacement therapy. Renal insufficiency resolves in most cases.

The overall case fatality for HPS in the US is 35% in 453 cases as of September 2006. For children in this population, the overall mortality rate is 33%, and an elevated prothrombin time was associated with mortality (61,70). Reported mortality rates are higher with Andes virus infection (47%) and may be related to the occurrence of hemorrhage or renal insufficiency (67). Most deaths with HPS are the result of hypoxemia, ventricular dysfunction with hypotension, and arrhythmias (31).

Poliomyelitis

Epidemiology

Poliomyelitis was the first enteroviral disease to be recognized, and a clinical description of the disease was first given in the late 18th century by a London pediatrician. The peak incidence of the disease was during the 1950s, with over 20,000 cases per year occurring in the US and a large epidemic occurring in Denmark. With vaccination programs, the incidence of disease declined markedly. In the US, no cases of wild-type poliovirus have been reported since 1979, and vaccine-associated poliomyelitis has not been acquired since 1999. In 2006, endemic cases worldwide were confined to Africa (western, central, and horn), India, Pakistan, and Afghanistan, with two-thirds of the cases occurring in Nigeria and one-quarter in India (18).

The peak incidence of poliovirus infections occurs in the summer and fall in temperate climates, with infections occurring year-round in tropical climates. Most infections occur in children <5 years of age. However, in areas of recurrent epidemics, the age distribution shifts to older children and younger adults.

Four types of infection with poliovirus occur: inapparent infection, abortive infection, nonparalytic infection, and paralytic poliomyelitis. Most infections are inapparent and account for 90%–95% of infections. Abortive infections are seen in 4%–8% and result in a mild, nonspecific illness. Aseptic meningitis without evidence of paralysis is seen in 1%–2% of cases. Finally, paralytic poliomyelitis is seen in <1% of infections (69).

Risk factors for paralytic disease with poliovirus infection include older age, pregnancy, recent diphtheria/pertussis/tetanus vaccination, physical exercise at the time of infection, trauma at the time of infection, and tonsillectomy. In areas of endemicity, children <5 years of age account for the vast majority of cases of paralytic polio, as they have most of the infections. Tonsillectomy is a risk factor for the development of the bulbar form of poliomyelitis. Older children and adults, as well as immunodeficient individuals, are at higher risk for vaccine-associated paralytic poliomyelitis. An additional risk factor for vaccine-associated paralytic poliomyelitis is recent intramuscular injection after oral poliovirus vaccination (18,69).

Etiology

Polioviruses are in the enterovirus subgroup of the family *Picornaviridae*. Other enteroviruses include coxsackievirus and echovirus. The viruses are small, single-stranded, positive-sense, RNA viruses with three serotypes. Immunity to one serotype does not confer immunity to the others. The viral genome encodes for four capsid proteins and seven nonstructural proteins. Neutralizing antibodies are made to the capsid proteins. Humans are the only known hosts of poliovirus, although other animals are known to be hosts for other enteroviruses. After infection, viral components and virions are formed intracellularly (18,69).

Infection is spread primarily via the fecal-oral route, although transmission by oral-oral contact may occur as well. After the virus is transmitted to an uninfected individual, it enters the mucosa of the pharynx and upper alimentary tract and replicates (alimentary phase). The infection then spreads to lymph tissue (tonsils, lymph nodes, and Peyer patches), where the virus undergoes further multiplication, leading to a minor viremia and seeding of other organs over the next few days (lymphatic phase). By days 3–7, replication in secondary infection sites produces a major viremia with possible CNS infection (viremic phase). By 1 week, specific antibody formation clears the viremia although the virus continues to be shed from the lower intestinal tract for several weeks (18,69).

Replication of poliovirus in the CNS may damage the anterior and dorsal horn cells of the spinal cord and medulla (cranial nerve nuclei and reticular formation), producing the manifestations of paralytic polio. Other affected areas potentially include the midbrain, portions of the hypothalamus and thalamus, and the vermis and midline nuclei of the cerebellum. The white matter of the cerebral cortex and spinal cord are usually spared. The CNS lesions can be more widespread than the clinical manifestations of disease suggest and may be partially reversible (18,69).

Presentation and Differential Diagnosis

Nonparalytic cases of poliomyelitis have evidence of CNS injury without paralysis, including meningismus, muscle spasms, and CSF that suggests aseptic meningitis. In general, these patients should not require intensive care. Paralytic poliomyelitis is life-threatening in children in the event that respiratory insufficiency develops during the disease course. The incubation period is ~3–5 days for minor illness and 1–2 weeks for CNS involvement. However, the incubation time for paralysis may extend up to 1 month. In children, the disease often progresses in two phases: a minor phase with prodromal symptoms, followed by CNS disease. These symptoms are nonspecific and consist of sore throat, fever, nausea, vomiting, abdominal discomfort, rash, constipation, and flu-like symptoms (18,69).

The paralytic symptoms may not begin for several days after the prodrome. Signs such as toxicity, irritability, higher fever, anxiousness, and the presence of diminished superficial reflexes may herald the onset of paralysis. Weakness may progress over a period of 3–5 days to flaccid paralysis with loss of deep tendon reflexes. The time course can also be of rapid onset with progression over several hours. Transient fasciculations may be observed during disease progression. In general, the lower extremities are more commonly affected than the upper. Muscle spasm may be present prior to the onset of paralysis. As weakness progresses, the patient may have a weak cough, weak cry, and nasal flaring. With severe disease, quadriplegia and respiratory failure occur. In patients with brainstem disease, bulbar symptoms may be present. These signs include pharyngeal hypotonia, hoarseness, deviation of the soft palate, diminished swallowing, increased secretions, aphonia, and "rope" sign (hypotonia of hyoid muscles). Neuronal damage in the brainstem can cause autonomic dysfunction manifest by paralytic ileus, bladder paralysis, cardiac arrhythmias, and systemic hypertension (18,69).

Patients with paralytic poliomyelitis are classified into 3 clinical groups. Those children with pure spinal poliomyelitis do not have cranial nerve involvement but have muscular weakness and/or paralysis. Respiratory failure, when present, is due to weakness or paralysis of thoracic muscles and diaphragm. This form is most commonly seen and represents 79% of the cases. The second group includes individuals with pure bulbar poliomyelitis that have weakness or paralysis of cranial nerves IX, X, and/or XII primarily. These patients may show signs of agitation or delirium and may have evidence of cardiac dysrhythmias or hypertension, hypothermia, and disordered control of breathing. The respiratory failure in this group of patients is due to extrathoracic airway obstruction and lack of airway clearance of secretions that can lead to aspiration. Pure bulbar poliomyelitis is uncommon and represents 2% of the cases. Those patients with bulbospinal disease account for the remaining 19% of the cases and demonstrate a combination of features. Rarely do patients present with encephalitic poliomyelitis manifest by high fever, mental status changes, spasticity, seizures, and bulbar signs (18,69).

The diagnosis of poliomyelitis is confirmed by poliovirus recovery from the stool and/or oropharynx. The virus may also be isolated from the CSF in some circumstances. Further typing is then performed to rule out a vaccine strain. Serology for the three poliovirus serotypes is problematic in that high titers of neutralizing antibody may be present at the time of presentation. However, the presence of IgM antibodies suggests acute infection (18,69).

The differential diagnosis includes Guillain-Barré syndrome, other enterovirus infections, acute disseminating encephalomyelitis, rabies, botulism, West Nile virus, Ebstein-Barr virus, and other causes of aseptic meningitis or encephalitis (18,69). The presence of flaccid paralysis and lack of significant sensory changes is helpful in ruling out other diseases.

Treatment

Treatment of children with paralytic poliomyelitis is primarily supportive. The focus in the ICU is on the monitoring and management of associated respiratory failure. In patients with bulbar or bulbospinal poliomyelitis, maintenance of airway patency with suctioning and positioning is of importance to ensure adequate ventilation and prevent aspiration of secretions and pneumonia. Close assessment of adequacy of gas exchange by arterial blood gases and noninvasive monitors can help to prevent hypoxia and the consequences of hypoventilation. With airway obstruction or high risk of aspiration, tracheal intubation and mechanical ventilation are necessary. Patients with spinal poliomyelitis who have significant weakness or paralysis of the muscles of respiration may require mechanical ventilation as well. Respiratory failure occurs more frequently in those patients with bulbar poliomyelitis. Given the prolonged time to recovery or residual paralysis that occurs in some patients, tracheostomy may be necessary to provide a stable airway and long-term mechanical ventilation.

No known specific antiviral therapy effectively treats poliovirus infection. Pleconaril is an new oral antiviral agent that has been used to treat enterovirus infections. Use of pleconaril to treat poliomyelitis patients has been reported, but the efficacy is unknown (50). The drug is thought to diminish viral replication by inhibiting viral capsid uncoating.

Analgesia may be necessary in those patients with significant myalgia or headaches. Constipation can also be problematic and require the use of laxatives (18,69). Physical and occupational therapists and physiatrists should be involved to assist with proper positioning, splinting, and therapies to facilitate recovery and prevent contractures. In addition, neurologists, pulmonologists, and infectious disease experts may be of benefit in the evaluation and treatment of severe cases.

Outcomes

Patients with mild weakness may have a complete recovery, although those patients with flaccid paralysis will likely have persistent weakness. If recovery occurs, on average 60% recovery will occur by 3 months and 80% by 6 months. The time period for improvement does not usually extend beyond 18 months, so that any residual deficits that exist at that time are likely permanent. The mortality rate in paralytic poliomyelitis may be as low as 4% but is higher in adults and in those patients with bulbar disease. The mortality rates in bulbar disease may be as high 25%–75%. Post-poliomyelitis syndrome occurs in ~25%–40% of patients with a history of paralytic poliomyelitis after a 30–40-year time period from infection.

These patients have an exacerbation of existing or new weakness and muscle pain (18,69).

Future Directions—Poliomyelitis

With appropriate immunization programs, polio can be eradicated worldwide. Travelers to regions where infection remains endemic should be certain that they are fully immunized prior to arrival.

EMERGING INFECTIONS

West Nile Virus

Mechanism of Disease

The first recognized case of West Nile virus (WNV) infection occurred in 1937 in a febrile woman in the West Nile province of Uganda and was isolated from children in Egypt during acute febrile illnesses in the 1950s. WNV infections were subsequently associated with outbreaks in Israel, France, South Africa, and India, most commonly causing febrile illness and, rarely, encephalitis or meningitis. In the late 1990s, several outbreaks of encephalitis and meningitis were seen in Russia, Israel, and Romania. The first outbreak in the western hemisphere occurred in 1999 in New York City. Since that time, WNV has rapidly spread in the US, with over 4000 cases of WNV infection in 2002 and 45 states reporting WNV infections in 2003. Only Alaska and Hawaii have not reported human or animal cases of WNV (**Fig. 82.4**).

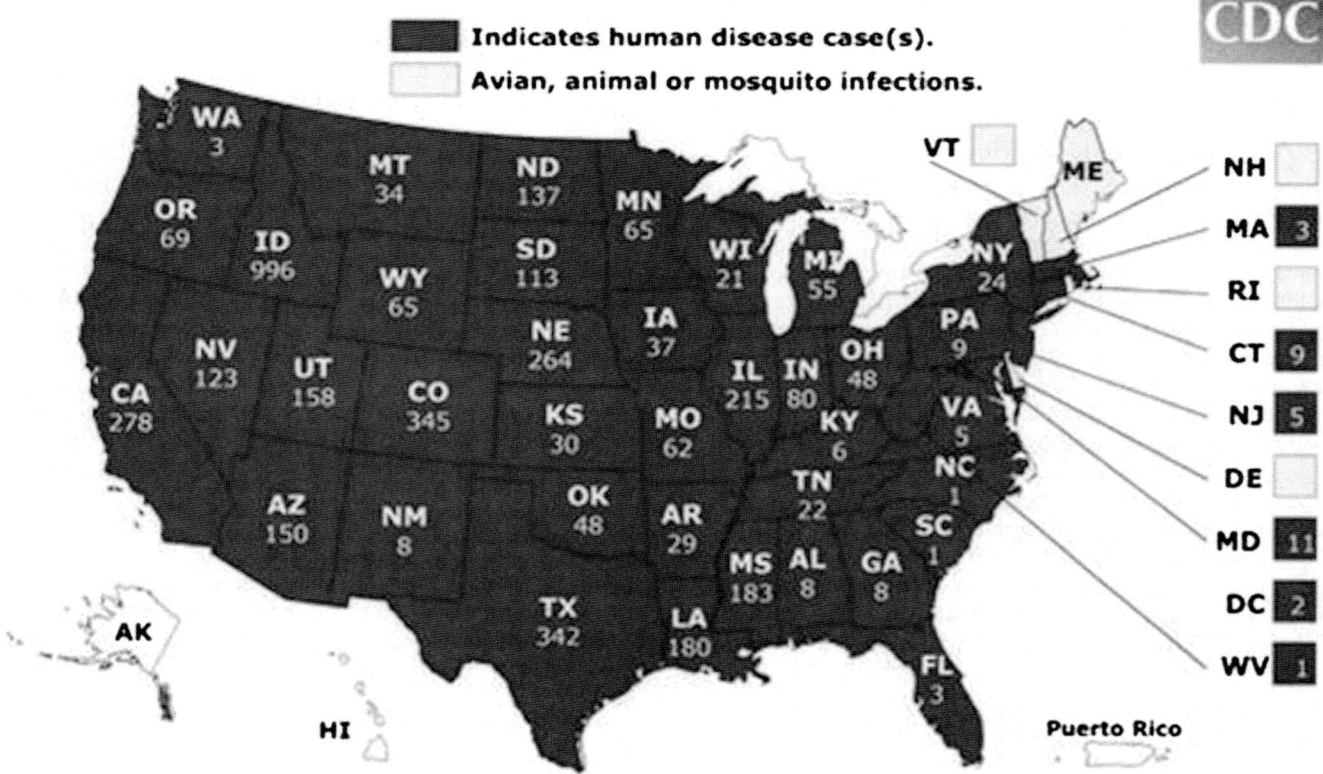

FIGURE 82.4. Distribution of West Nile Virus in the US in 2006. From the US Centers for Disease Control and Prevention, http://www.cdc.gov/ncidod/dvbid/westnile/Mapsactivity/surv&control06Maps.htm.

The basis for the increasing incidence and severity of WNV infections is unclear but is potentially related to increasing virulence, changes in host factors, or predisposing chronic disease. Based upon statistics from the New York epidemic, ~1 in 5 patients develop a febrile illness, and 1 in 150 patients develop severe neurologic disease. Most infections with WNV occur during late August to September, with the peak transmission time being between mid-July and December.

The strongest risk factor for the development of West Nile neuroinvasive disease (WNND) and death is advanced age (age >70 years) (30). WNND is also associated with disruption of the blood-brain barrier and immunosuppression and occurs less frequently in children than in adults. Although children may have less exposure to mosquitoes that transmit the disease, it is thought that children likely have more asymptomatic infections or milder disease.

With the increasing prevalence of the WNV, other modes of viral transmission have been identified, including blood transfusion, breast-feeding, organ transplantation, and transplacental infection. No adverse effects of viral transmission to infants have been documented (28,33). At this writing, screening for WNV is being performed on blood components in the US, using WNV nucleic acid amplification tests to reduce this risk.

WNV is a single-stranded RNA virus from the *Flavivirus* family. WNV is similar to other *Flaviviruses* in the Japanese encephalitis virus complex, including St. Louis encephalitis virus and Japanese encephalitis virus, among others. WNV is sustained through an enzootic cycle between birds and mosquitoes. Mosquitoes of the order *Culex* are important vectors for transmitting WNV infections. Perching birds (sparrows, blue jays, crows, and magpies) are thought to be important hosts for WNV, as they develop a high level of viremia. Viral amplification occurs through bird-mosquito-bird infection cycles, which increases the likelihood of transmission of infection to humans when they are bitten by infected mosquitoes. Humans are believed to be "dead-end" hosts because they develop an insufficient viremia to infect feeding mosquitoes. After human inoculation by feeding mosquitoes infected with WNV, the virus replicates in dendritic cells and ascends to regional lymph nodes, with dissemination to the bloodstream and other organs.

Clinical Presentation and Differential Diagnosis

The incubation period is usually 2–6 days (range, 2–14 days), with prolonged incubations of up to 3 weeks seen in some immunocompromised patients. WNV has been isolated in the blood of immunocompetent individuals 2 days before the onset of symptoms, with clearing of the viremia after ~4 days. In immunocompromised hosts the viremia can be prolonged and extend up to 1 month after onset. Symptomatic infection associated with WNV has been categorized as West Nile fever and WNND.

In West Nile fever, an abrupt onset of fever occurs, with symptoms that may include headache, myalgia, nausea, vomiting, abdominal pain, or diarrhea. Additionally, sore throat, cough, and maculopapular rash have been described. Most cases have resolution of symptoms within 1 week, but milder symptoms of malaise and fatigue may persist for several weeks.

WNND develops in fewer than 1% of those infected. In reported cases of pediatric patients in California with WNND, ~50% had meningitis and most commonly presented with headache, nuchal rigidity, and fever. Also, ~50% of the patients had a rash, and one-third had muscle weakness. In those cases with encephalitis, most patients had fever, headache, nuchal rigidity, and alteration in consciousness. Muscle weakness is a prominent part of the clinical manifestation of WNV encephalitis and was seen in ~80% of these patients. Of note, none of these patients had a rash. Patients with encephalitis may have bulbar findings and hyperreflexia as well. Several of the children with encephalitis were also noted to be immunocompromised. All patients with encephalitis were admitted to the PICU (28). Rare extraneurologic complications include myocarditis, pancreatitis, and hepatitis.

Laboratory evaluation may reveal a mild leukopenia or leukocytosis. Hyponatremia can occur in patients with WNND. In patients with WNND, CSF findings can include a mild pleocytosis with lymphocytes, mild-to-moderate protein level elevation, and normal glucose levels. CT and MRI imaging of the brain may initially be normal or show only mild leptomeningeal enhancement despite significant neurologic findings. Follow-up neuroimaging with MRI later in the disease course may show gray matter abnormalities. When performed, electromyography and nerve conduction studies may be consistent with a motor axonal polyneuropathy and demonstrate evidence of anterior horn cell injury.

In patients with WNND, other causes of aseptic meningitis should be considered, including infections with enterovirus and other viruses in the *Flavivirus* family. The presentation with acute muscle weakness may suggest a diagnosis of Guillain-Barré syndrome. Other treatable infections, including herpesvirus infection or bacterial meningoencephalitic, should be considered as well.

Diagnosis. The presence of WNV nucleic acid can be detected using reverse-transcriptase PCR and provides strong evidence of infection. However, WNV nucleic acid often cannot be detected after the viremia has resolved, 3–5 days after the symptoms appear. An IgM ELISA can be performed on the serum or CSF. IgM is detectable 3–5 days into illness. WNV IgM is cross-reactive with other *Flaviviruses*. Therefore, further testing may be required to improve the specificity of the diagnosis. IgM antibody has been known to be detectable in patients up to 1 year after WNV infection.

Clinical Management

Treatment is mainly supportive. Endotracheal intubation may be necessary for airway protection in severe cases of encephalitis. Although rare, seizures may occur, and must be treated aggressively. WNV replication and cytopathogenicity are inhibited by ribavirin and interferon-α in vitro; however, clear benefit has not been demonstrated in patients with WNND, and no controlled trials have been performed.

Outcomes

Overall case mortality in patients with WNV meningoencephalitis has been recently reported to range between 4% and 14%, with virtually all deaths occurring in patients with encephalitis. Children appear to be spared the most severe outcomes: the youngest fatality was in a 19-year-old (33,58).

In adults, half of patients have reported that they have not recovered physically, functionally, or cognitively at 12 months post-illness. Clinical details regarding the course of pediatric patients with WNV encephalitis are less well studied, given the infrequency of the disease in children. Prolonged neurologic recovery has been reported, with some children having neurologic symptoms for >6 months (28,33).

Future Directions—West Nile Virus

Studies are ongoing to investigate potential therapies for WNV infection (21). Of particular interest is the use of pooled high-titer anti-WNV antibody. A clinical trial of interferon-α is also underway.

Avian Influenza

Mechanism of Disease

Influenza pandemics have swept the world in the past, most notably the "Spanish flu" of 1918–1919 that killed 20–40 million people. Given the pandemic potential, concern about new influenza viruses giving rise to devastating worldwide infection have always been a concern. In 1997, an avian influenza virus strain H5/N1 spread from chickens to humans in Hong Kong. It was only controlled after culling every chicken on the island (15). In 2003, an outbreak of H5/N1 infection spread throughout southeast Asia. The infection has spread beyond its origin in southeast Asia, to central Asia, Africa and eastern Europe, likely via the migration of wild birds. Spread to domestic poultry in eastern Europe has occurred rarely.

The outbreak that began in 2003 was unique for several reasons. It is an extremely virulent strain of the virus, causing very high rates of death in both wild and domestic birds. Whereas previously identified avian influenza strains were not found to be spread efficiently by migrating birds, these wild birds are now clearly linked to the spread of infection. This strain of virus has been extremely difficult to control. It has persisted and even spread despite having killed of 150 million infected or exposed birds. Humans have primarily been infected by contact with poultry, although several cases are thought to have occurred through contact with dead wild birds. By the end of 2006, 258 human cases were reported, with 154 deaths. The countries where human cases of avian influenza have occurred as of March 2007 are: Azerbaijan, Cambodia, China, Djibouti, Egypt, Indonesia, Iraq, Laos, Nigeria, Thailand, Turkey, and Vietnam (85). The activities that have been associated with human cases of avian influenza include handling of diseased birds, playing with infected poultry (especially ducks), and consumption of uncooked poultry (86). Human-to-human transmission has been suspected in several cases (5,38,79); however, sustained human-to-human transmission has not been documented. In addition, nosocomial transmission to healthcare workers has not occurred (2).

Influenza A viruses belong to the family of *Orthomyxoviridae*. Antigenic subtypes are defined by two major surface glycoproteins: hemagglutinin and neuraminidase (NA). *Antigenic drift*, defined as changes within the same viral subtype, is responsible for the annual occurrence of influenza epidemic, whereas antigenic shift, with the circulation of a new subtype, has led to pandemics. The reservoir for influenza type A viruses is wild waterfowl. In these birds, influenza A viruses usually cause asymptomatic infection in the gastrointestinal tract, and the virus is transmitted through the fecal-oral route.

Several factors limit the spread of avian influenza to humans. Host-specific infection is mediated by binding to receptors on cells, a necessary step to allow for replication and propagation of infection. Avian viruses tend to bind to α-2,3-Gal-terminated saccharides found on avian intestinal epithelium, and human viruses bind to α-2,6-Gal-terminated saccharides on human respiratory epithelium. Some 2,3-Gal-terminated saccharides are found in the lower respiratory tract and may account for the small number of human cases (80). However, even if infection occurs in a human, it is poorly transmitted because upper respiratory shedding is the most conducive to transmission (74).

Clinical Presentation and Differential Diagnosis

The presenting signs and symptoms may vary, depending on the specific type of avian influenza viral infection. For the H5/N1 virus, the incubation period ranges from 2 to 8 days. The earliest symptoms are high fever and an influenza-like illness with lower respiratory involvement. Upper respiratory symptoms only occur occasionally. Gastrointestinal symptoms, including diarrhea (with or without blood), vomiting, and abdominal pain, are common and may precede the respiratory illness, although the degree of gastrointestinal involvement may vary by clade. Patients usually reach medical attention at the time of the respiratory illness. Almost all patients have signs and symptoms of pneumonia, including dyspnea, increased respiratory rate, and crackles on auscultation. In a comparison of cases of mild versus severe disease, hypoxia never occurred in mild cases, whereas supplemental oxygen was required for all patients with severe disease, either at initial presentation or during the course of the illness (38). As the disease progresses, patients develop ARDS and multiorgan failure, including cardiac dysfunction. Other complications that have been reported include pulmonary hemorrhage, pancytopenia, and systemic inflammatory response syndrome without documented bacteremia.

Low white blood cell count, especially lymphopenia, leukopenia, and thrombocytopenia, is a common laboratory finding. Elevated aminotransferases and creatinine can also occur. The chest x-rays are abnormal and may show a variety of patterns. The most common in the Vietnam epidemic was multifocal consolidation. As respiratory failure and ARDS developed, the x-ray took on a diffuse, ground-glass appearance (34).

As the signs and symptoms of avian influenza viral infection are nonspecific, the most important trigger for consideration of the diagnosis is the potential for exposure, including travel to an area where infection is endemic and contact with poultry, ill birds, or another individual with avian influenza. The WHO tracks cases of human and bird infections and their geographic distribution (http://www.who.int/csr/disease/avian_influenza/en/). Additional diagnoses to consider include causes for influenza-like illnesses, ARDS, and severe community-acquired pneumonia. For individuals with severe pneumonia with a history of travel to Southeast Asia, additional infections should be considered, including leptospirosis and melioidosis. For children who are from medically underserved communities, vaccine-preventable infections such as measles and *Haemophilus influenzae* B may occur.

Diagnosis. The preferred method for diagnosis includes oropharyngeal swab specimens and lower respiratory tract specimens for H5N1-specific, reverse-transcriptase PCR testing. Throat swabs have higher yield than nasal swabs (38). Specimens should be placed in viral transport medium. Viral antigen testing may also be conducted. The commonly available kits to identify influenza A may detect the presence of H5/N1 in a minority of cases (34,38). Antigen testing and PCR only require BSL-2 facilities (60).

Viral isolation of specimens from patients who are suspected of having avian influenza should only be processed in a BSL-3+ facility. If avian influenza is suspected, the laboratory must be informed that a specimen is being submitted.

Clinical Management

The H5N1viruses are sensitive to the NA inhibitors oseltamivir and zanamivir, in vitro and in animal models (43,44). In animal models, the optimal timing of the medication to improve survival is within the first 48 hrs. In a series of cases from Thailand, patients who survived received oseltamivir treatment earlier (mean, 4.5 days) than those who did not (mean, 9 days) (20). The standard dose is given for 5 days: 30 mg twice per day for children ≤15 kg, 45 mg twice a day for those >15–23 kg, 60 mg twice a day for those >23–40 kg, and 75 mg twice a day for those >40 kg. Common adverse effects are nausea and vomiting. Anaphylaxis and severe dermatologic reactions have rarely been reported. In mild cases, the standard approved dose can be administered for 5 days. In cases of severe disease, some experts recommend doubling the standard dose. The increased dose has been shown to have improved efficacy in animal models (87) and is well tolerated in adults but does not have superior efficacy against seasonal influenza (77). Oseltamivir prophylaxis is recommended for 7–10 days after the last exposure in cases of high- to moderate-risk exposures.

Although the avian influenza viruses are susceptible to the NA inhibitors, one case of oseltamivir-resistant H5N1 was isolated from a patient in Vietnam who developed clinical illness after receiving oseltamivir post-exposure prophylaxis (42), thus raising the concern that if post-exposure prophylaxis were initiated on a wide scale during a threatened epidemic, drug-resistant strains would be selected and propagated.

Oseltamivir is preferred over zanamivir because it is easier to administer. Zanamivir is administered by oral inhalation of a dry powder, making drug delivery difficult in intubated patients and potentially less effective if distributed unevenly in the respiratory system, as can occur in patients with significant lung disease who may not achieve high enough levels in the blood to treat systemic disease. Zanamivir may be preferable for prophylaxis or for less severely ill patients. Other antivirals, such as the amantadanes and ribavirin, have in vitro activity against H5N1. They are not currently recommended for use against avian influenza but may be considered as components of combination therapy, although this strategy has not been well studied. Both NA inhibitor drug dosages must be adjusted for renal failure, as they are renally excreted. Oseltamivir also undergoes significant hepatic metabolism.

Intensive care management is essential for all cases of severe disease. Respiratory failure requiring intubation occurs in most hospitalized patients. Renal dysfunction occurs commonly, although the etiology is unknown. Inotropic support may also be necessary.

Infection control should be addressed immediately if avian influenza infection is suspected. The appropriate infection control measures (standard, contact, air-borne, and eye) should be instituted. In previous outbreaks, hospital staff did not demonstrate serologic evidence of exposure to the virus (49). However, as a widespread pandemic would likely be caused by a more highly transmissible form of the virus, strict infection control should be instituted immediately.

Outcomes

The case fatality rate for hospitalized patients with A/H5N1 infection is high, with an overall mortality rate reported by the WHO of over 50% of confirmed cases. This illness is more severe than the Hong Kong outbreak in 1997 with a very similar virus, in which the case fatality rate was 33%. Death usually occurs due to progressive respiratory failure and multiple organ dysfunction an average of 9–10 days after onset of illness.

Future Directions—Avian Influenza

The key to preventing an avian influenza pandemic is adequate supply of effective vaccine should a highly transmissible strain emerge. The vaccination production strategies that have been studied thus far are similar to the seasonal influenza vaccinations: inactivated virus and live attenuated virus. Using the current technology, the production of these vaccines requires many months of preparation and may pose a safety risk for those involved in production. Newer technology, including recombinant proteins, DNA vaccines, and vector-based delivery are being developed and tested as vaccines that would be easily produced, safely, on a large scale, and in a timely fashion.

Severe Acute Respiratory Syndrome

Epidemiology

The first documented case of SARS occurred in February 2003 in Hong Kong. The index case was a medical physician who traveled from Guangdong province and stayed in a hotel in Hong Kong and infected 12 guests or visitors. By the time this outbreak ended in the summer of 2003, over 8000 people were infected in multiple countries, including Southeast Asia, Canada, the US, and several European countries, with a significantly high mortality rate in adult cases. New cases of SARS were identified in 2004 but were apparently related to laboratory exposure (16,63). At this writing, no cases have been reported to the CDC or the WHO since 2004. Nonetheless, this section is presented for historic interest and as an example of the rapidity with which an emerging infection can travel worldwide. SARS highlights the potentially disastrous consequences of emerging infections in today's global society.

The disease appears to be transmitted through droplet or fomite contact of the mucous membranes of the respiratory system. The large number of nosocomial cases is thought to be caused by contact with infective droplets generated by the use of respiratory equipment and nebulized medications that would amplify transmission (81). Spread to community occurred through hospital visitors or other healthcare workers, representing the primary mode of transmission. Disease in children during the outbreak occurred through sick household contacts or hospital contacts, with no major spread through schools. Two cases of transmission from children to adults were reported, and no instances of child-child transmission were reported. All children and up to 90% of adults in the 2003 outbreak had a positive contact history (7). Implementation of infection-control procedures has been shown to effectively control the spread of SARS. Quarantine measures have been effective, as no instances of transmission have been reported prior to the onset of symptoms. In some outbreaks, some individuals appear to be "super-spreaders," where a few cases result in a disproportionate number of transmissions. Other factors have been identified to be important contributors to the rapid spread of SARS as well. These factors include long incubation period (4–7 days on average, but up to 14 days), insidious onset of symptoms, and infectivity that appears to increase as symptoms progress (9,16,36,63).

Etiology

The etiology of SARS has now been established to be a novel coronavirus (SARS-CoV). The family of coronaviruses includes enveloped, single-stranded RNA viruses that had previously been known only to cause cold symptoms. SARS-CoV is unrelated to known human or animal coronaviruses but is thought to have arisen from interspecies transmission and adaptation. Specifically, interspecies transmission is thought to have potentially occurred in the game markets in southern China, as coronaviruses similar to SARS-CoV have been isolated in civet cats and other wild animals in that region. Recent epidemiologic evidence suggests that Chinese horseshoe bats may be the natural reservoir for SARS-like coronaviruses. Some cases of SARS have had other coinfections, including human metapneumovirus and *Chlamydia* infections, but it is unclear how these coinfections affect the severity or transmissibility of SARS (16,63).

Presentation and Differential Diagnosis

The disease course in SARS has been described as triphasic. Patients with SARS initially present with myalgia, fever, malaise, and chills/rigors after an incubation period of ~4–7 days (phase I). Upper respiratory tract symptoms such as rhinorrhea and sore throat occur less commonly. This phase is associated with viral replication and is transient, with resolution in approximately one-third of cases. The remaining cases develop persistent fever and may have cough, oxygen desaturation, chest pain, tachypnea, and dyspnea as they develop bronchopneumonia (phase II). This phase has been characterized as an immunopathologic phase and has been thought to be related to an exaggerated host immunologic response. The viral load has been noted to be decreasing during this period. Some patients have also developed a watery diarrhea at this time. The median time from onset of symptoms to hospital admission is 3–5 days (16,47,53,63,84).

During the course of illness, laboratory data may reveal lymphopenia (56%–90%), thrombocytopenia (13%–41%), and elevated transaminases. Chest radiography demonstrates abnormalities in 60%–100% of cases. Findings include a ground-glass appearance or focal consolidation in the lung bases, peripheral, and/or subpleural areas. In those patients with normal chest x-rays, CT scanning demonstrates abnormalities 67% of the time. Also reported is the development of pneumomediastinum without previous positive-pressure ventilation or intubation, but this occurs later in the disease course (3). Some patients may progress to ARDS with diffuse alveolar damage and pulmonary fibrosis (phase III). Most children have relatively mild disease, with the more severe cases in pediatrics being in the adolescent age group (3,7,84).

Others have noted that establishing a diagnosis of SARS during an outbreak can be problematic if using WHO case definitions, as the symptoms of SARS are similar to other frequently encountered respiratory illnesses in children (46). This finding led to a modification of the definition for probable pediatric cases to include a positive test for SARS-CoV. Reverse transcriptase PCR (RT-PCR) analyses of nasopharyngeal or stool specimens have been reported to have 50% sensitivity in pediatric patients. A higher sensitivity and fast turnaround time have been found using one step, real-time RT-PCR to detect viral RNA in plasma. Paired acute and convalescent serology for SARS-CoV is useful for confirmation of infection but not for triage. In addition to specific testing for SARS-CoV, testing for other viral and/or bacterial etiologies for the patient's signs and symptoms should be performed, as coinfection could be present and initial presenting signs may not be reliable to differentiate SARS from non-SARS cases (3,7, 84).

Treatment

A key component of treatment is the use of infection-control procedures to control spread of disease through droplets, aerosolization, and fomites. Effective control also involves successful triage of patients based upon definitions of probable and suspected cases. Antimicrobial therapy should be administered for other bacterial etiologies for the patients' signs and symptoms or atypical pneumonia. This therapy might consist of a third-generation cephalosporin and a macrolide in cases of pneumonia and fever. A temporal relationship has been seen between the administration of corticosteroids and clinical improvement in seriously ill pediatric patients. Immunomodulation during this phase of illness (phase II) is thought to have theoretic benefit. Additionally, ribavirin was administered to patients during the outbreak, but SARS-CoV has not been found to be sensitive to this agent in vitro (16).

Terminal events in adult patients have been associated with progressive respiratory failure, multiple organ dysfunction, or intercurrent illness such as myocardial infarction (9,12,53,63).

Outcomes

Approximately 30% of adult patients with SARS-CoV infection require ICU admission, and the mortality rate has been reported to be as high as 50% in older patients. Fewer than 10% of the reported SARS cases have been in children (16,47,63,88). It has been suggested that children <12 years of age have a less severe course of disease, and to date, no deaths in young children or adolescents have been reported. Approximately 5% of these cases have required PICU admission, and 1% have required mechanical ventilation. In pediatric patients with severe disease, abnormalities in biochemical markers and lymphopenia persist longer. Sore throat and peak neutrophil count have been identified to predict more severe disease in pediatric patients. Most of the pediatric patients treated with steroids have been adolescent patients. In a follow-up study of 47 children (ages 9.8–16 years) 6 months after SARS diagnosis, no child had symptomatic lung disease, and mild lung abnormalities were identified in 34% of patients by high-resolution CT (48). These findings most commonly included residual ground-glass changes and/or air trapping. Two of the 47 children required mechanical ventilation. The need for supplemental oxygen and lymphopenia were identified as risk factors for the noted CT findings. Of 38 patients who underwent pulmonary function testing, only 4 had abnormal findings, all of which all were mild. The findings on high-resolution CT also correlated with diminished aerobic capacity (88).

Future Directions—Severe Acute Respiratory Syndrome

Because the SARS outbreak has not continued, little current research is being conducted concerning the disease. However, SARS taught us major lessons concerning the control of nosocomial outbreaks of respiratory pathogens. Clinicians must be ever-cognizant of the potential for a new, heretofore undescribed viral infection. Participation in reporting systems and cooperation with public health officials are essential to identify and prevent the spread of emerging diseases.

KEY POINTS

International Infections

Malaria

- Most severe infections are caused by *P. falciparum* transmitted by *Anopheles* mosquito.
- Most deaths are in children <5 years of age in sub-Saharan Africa.
- Some signs of severe malaria include lactic acidosis, severe anemia, respiratory distress, hypoglycemia, impaired consciousness, and prostration.
- The level of parasitemia may not reflect true parasite burden, but >5% of parasitized red blood cells suggests severe disease in nonimmune individuals.
- Severe malaria requires intensive care monitoring and antimicrobial treatment with quinidine or quinine and another agent active against *P. falciparum*.
- EKG monitoring is necessary during quinidine or quinine therapy to assess for cardiac toxicity, including widening of the QRS and QT_C prolongation.
- Attention to glucose level is critical, as hypoglycemia frequently complicates severe malaria and may contribute significantly to morbidity and mortality.

Typhoid Fever

- Typhoid fever is a bacterial infection spread by the fecal-oral route without any nonhuman reservoirs.
- Disease is prevalent in most tropical developing countries but highest on the Indian subcontinent.
- Diarrhea is more common among children but does not occur in most cases.
- Diagnosis can be difficult, as blood cultures have a low sensitivity. Bone marrow culture may have a higher yield, especially after the initiation of therapy.
- Empiric therapy should be IV ceftriaxone until susceptibility of the organism is known.
- Fluoroquinolone-resistant infections are increasing in Asia and make the treatment of the disease more complicated.
- Death occurs in cases of complicated disease: gastrointestinal bleeding, perforation, or typhoid encephalopathy.
- Relapse is common.

Chagas Disease

- Infection with *T. cruzi* causes Chagas disease.
- Acute infection is usually nonspecific, but subclinical cardiac involvement may occur.
- Treatment during the acute phase of illness prevents progression to chronic end-organ damage.
- After acute infection, untreated patients enter an indeterminate phase.
- 10%–15% of patients in the indeterminate phase go on to develop the chronic sequelae of infection: cardiomyopathy and megaviscera.

Human African Trypanosomiasis

- HAT is caused by *T. brucei rhodiense* (East) or *T. brucei gambiense* (West) and results in sleeping sickness.
- In children, developmental delay may be more prominent than somnolence.
- Acute and late-stage infections are treated differently. The presence of >5 cells/mm^3 in the CSF defines late-stage infection.
- The disease is fatal if untreated.

Leptospirosis

- Infection with *Leptospira* species causes a chronic low-grade infection in animal hosts who subsequently excrete the organisms into the environment, where they can survive for prolonged periods of time.
- In urban environments, small rodents are important hosts.
- The majority of leptospirosis infections are asymptomatic or mild.
- Icteric leptospirosis (Weil disease) is characterized by renal failure, icterus, and hemorrhagic manifestations.
- Treatment with penicillin, ceftriaxone, or doxycycline is recommended for symptomatic disease, although the role of therapy has not been definitively established.
- Mortality rates have been reported to be 5%–25% in hospitalized patients.

Hantavirus

- Infection with American Hantaviruses can result in HPS.
- HFRS can be seen with other Hantaviruses in Europe and Asia.
- Rodents are the hosts for disease and transmit disease to humans.
- HFRS is characterized by fever, renal failure, and hemorrhage and is classically associated with Hantaan or Dobrava viruses.
- HPS in North America is usually manifest by fever and respiratory disease, but renal failure is not infrequently seen in cases of HPS in South America.
- The overall mortality rate for HPS in North America is 33%. The mortality rate for HFRS is 5%–10%, but varies with infecting serotype.

Polio

- Polio is currently endemic in six countries—Afghanistan, India, Pakistan, Nigeria, Niger, and Egypt, with occasional outbreaks occurring elsewhere in the developing world.
- Most polio infections are unapparent, and paralytic poliomyelitis is seen in only 1% of all infections.
- Patients with the paralytic form often require mechanical ventilation for prolonged periods and may benefit from tracheostomy.
- With no known specific antiviral therapy, care is primarily supportive.

- Patients with mild weakness may have full recovery, although those with flaccid paralysis usually have residual weakness.

Emerging Diseases

West Nile Virus

- WNV is a mosquito-borne infection transmitted to humans from bird hosts.
- Human infection is found throughout the US, except in Alaska and Hawaii, with increasing incidence and severity.
- Most commonly, infection with WNV results in West Nile fever.
- WNND develops in <1% of those infected.
- Weakness commonly occurs with WNND, along with meningitis, encephalitis, or meningoencephalitis.
- The mortality rate is 4%–14%, with a higher mortality rate seen in patients with encephalitis.

Avian Influenza

- Influenza A/H5N1 is associated with severe respiratory failure in Southeast Asia and China.
- Avian influenza is commonly associated with exposure to domestic poultry and wild waterfowl.
- Suspected cases of person-to-person transmission have been reported. A more highly transmissible strain of the virus would be capable of producing a global pandemic.
- Symptoms include fever, diarrhea, lower respiratory tract symptoms, and respiratory failure.
- Treatment with oseltamivir is recommended for treatment and prophylaxis.
- If a suspected case of avian influenza is identified, isolation measures should be taken immediately, and the laboratory that is processing diagnostic specimens should be warned.
- The overall morality is ~50%.

Severe Acute Respiratory Syndrome

- SARS was first identified in 2003, and no cases have been reported since 2004.
- SARS is caused by a novel coronavirus (SARS-CoV), which causes a triphasic course of disease.
- Children are only rarely affected with the severe form of the disease. Only 2 of 47 children reported to have been infected with the SARS virus during the outbreak required mechanical ventilation.
- Infection control practices are effective at preventing transmission, as the disease is not contagious prior to the onset of symptoms.

References

1. Akech S, Gwer S, Idro R, et al. Volume Expansion with albumin compared to gelofusine in children with severe malaria: Results of a controlled trial. *PLoS Clin Trials* 2006;1:e21.
2. Apisarnthanarak A, Erb S, Stephenson I, et al. Seroprevalence of anti-H5 antibody among Thai health care workers after exposure to avian influenza (H5N1) in a tertiary care center. *Clin Infect Dis* 2005;40:e16–8.
3. Babyn PS, Chu WC, Tsou IY, et al. Severe acute respiratory syndrome (SARS): Chest radiographic features in children. *Pediatric Radiology* 2004;34:47–58.
4. Basnyat B. Typhoid and paratyphoid fever. *Lancet* 2005;366:1603.
5. Beigel JH, Farrar J, Han AM, et al. Avian influenza A (H5N1) infection in humans. *N Engl J Med* 1929;353:1374–85.
6. Berkley J, Mwarumba S, Bramham K, et al. Bacteraemia complicating severe malaria in children. *Trans R Soc Trop Med Hyg* 1999;93:283–6.
7. Bitnun A, Allen U, Heurter H, et al. Children hospitalized with severe acute respiratory syndrome-related illness in Toronto. *Pediatrics* 2003;112: e261.
8. Blood donor screening for chagas disease—United States, 2006–2007. *MMWR Morb Mortal Wkly Rep* 2007;56:141–3.
9. Booth CM, Stewart TE. Severe acute respiratory syndrome and critical care medicine: The Toronto experience. *Crit Care Med* 2005;33:S53–S60.
10. Bronzan RN, Taylor TE, Mwenechanya J, et al. Bacteremia in Malawian children with severe malaria: Prevalence, etiology, HIV coinfection, and outcome. *J Infect Dis* 2007;195:895–904.
11. Bruce MG, Sanders EJ, Leake JA, et al. Leptospirosis among patients presenting with dengue-like illness in Puerto Rico. *Acta Trop* 2005;96:36–46.
12. Brun-Buisson C. SARS: The challenge of emerging pathogens to the intensivist. *Intensive Care Med* 2003;29:861–2.
13. Bruneel F, Hocqueloux L, Alberti C, et al. The clinical spectrum of severe imported falciparum malaria in the intensive care unit: Report of 188 cases in adults. *Am J Respir Crit Care Med* 2001;167:684–9.
14. Carter R, Mendis KN. Evolutionary and historical aspects of the burden of malaria. *Clin Microbiol Rev* 2002;15:564–94.
15. Chan PK. Outbreak of avian influenza A(H5N1) virus infection in Hong Kong in 1997. *Clin Infect Dis* 2002;34(Suppl 2):S58–64.
16. Chan PK, Tang JW, Hui DS. SARS: Clinical presentation, transmission, pathogenesis and treatment options. *Clin Sci* 2006;110:193–204.
17. Chart H, Cheesbrough JS, Waghorn DJ. The serodiagnosis of infection with Salmonella typhi. *J Clin Pathol* 2000;53:851–3.
18. Cherry JD. Enteroviruses and Parechoviruses. In: Feigin RD, Cherry JD, Demmler GJ, Kaplan SL, eds. *Textbook of Pediatric Infectious Diseases*. Philadelphia: Saunders, 2004;1984–2034.
19. Chinh NT, Parry CM, Ly NT, et al. A randomized controlled comparison of azithromycin and ofloxacin for treatment of multidrug-resistant or nalidixic acid-resistant enteric fever. *Antimicrob Agents Chemother* 2000;44:1855–9.
20. Chotpitayasunondh T, Ungchusak K, Hanshaoworakul W, et al. Human disease from influenza A (H5N1), Thailand, 2004. *Emerg Infect Dis* 2005;11:201–9.
21. Clinical Trials for Treating West Nile Virus Disease. http://www.cdc.gov/ncidod/dvbid/westnile/clinicalTrials.htm. Accessed 07/10/07.
22. Crump JA, Luby SP, Mintz ED. The global burden of typhoid fever. *Bull World Health Organ* 2004;82:346–53.
23. Day NP, Phu NH, Mai NT, et al. Effects of dopamine and epinephrine infusions on renal hemodynamics in severe malaria and severe sepsis. *Crit Care Med* 2000;28:1353–62.
24. Duchin JS, Koster FT, Peters CJ, et al. Hantavirus pulmonary syndrome: A clinical description of 17 patients with a newly recognized disease. The Hantavirus Study Group. *New Engl J Med* 1994;330:949–55.
25. Eliades MJ, Shah S, Nguyen-Dinh P, et al. Malaria surveillance—United States, 2003. *MMWR Surveill Summ* 2005;54:25–40.
26. Ferreira MS, Nishioka SA, Silvestre MT, et al. Reactivation of Chagas' disease in patients with AIDS: Report of three new cases and review of the literature. *Clin Infect Dis* 1997;25:1397–400.
27. Ferres M, Vial P. Hantavirus infection in children. *Curr Opin Pediatr* 2004;16:70–5.
28. Francisco AM, Glaser C, Frykman E, et al. 2004 California pediatric West Nile virus case series. *Pediatr Infect Dis J* 2006;25:81–4.
29. Freedman DO, Weld LH, Kozarsky PE, et al. Spectrum of disease and relation to place of exposure among ill returned travelers. *N Engl J Med* 2006;354:119–30.
30. Gea-Banacloche J, Johnson RT, Bagic A, et al. West Nile virus: Pathogenesis and therapeutic options. *Ann Intern Med* 2004;140:545–53.
31. Hallin GW, Simpson SQ, Crowell RE, et al. Cardiopulmonary manifestations of Hantavirus pulmonary syndrome. *Crit Care Med* 1996;24:252–8.
32. Hantavirus pulmonary syndrome cases by state of residence. Centers for Disease Control. 2006. http://www.cdc.gov/ncidod/diseases/hanta/hps/noframes/casemap.htm. Accessed 07/10/07.
33. Hayes EB, O'Leary DR. West Nile virus infection: A pediatric perspective. *Pediatrics* 2004;113:1375–81.
34. Hien TT, Liem NT, Dung NT, et al. Avian Influenza A (H5N1) in 10 Patients in Vietnam. *N Engl J Med* 2004;350:1179–88.
35. Hoffman SL, Punjabi NH, Kumala S, et al. Reduction of mortality in chloramphenicol-treated severe typhoid fever by high-dose dexamethasone. *N Engl J Med* 1984;310:82–8.
36. Hui DS, Chan MC, Wu AK, et al. Severe acute respiratory syndrome (SARS): Epidemiology and clinical features. *Postgrad Med J* 2004;80:373–81.
37. Kadhiravan T, Wig N, Kapil A, et al. Clinical outcomes in typhoid fever: Adverse impact of infection with nalidixic acid-resistant Salmonella typhi. *BMC Infect Dis* 2005;5:37.
38. Kandun IN, Wibisono H, Sedyaningsih ER, et al. Three Indonesian clusters of H5N1 virus infection in 2005. *N Engl J Med* 2006;355:2186–94.
39. Ketai LH, Kelsey CA, Jordan K, et al. Distinguishing Hantavirus pulmonary syndrome from acute respiratory distress syndrome by chest radiography: Are there different radiographic manifestations of increased alveolar permeability? *J Thorac Imaging* 1998;13:172–7.

40. Laras K, Cao BV, Bounlu K, et al. The importance of leptospirosis in Southeast Asia. *Am J Trop Med Hyg* 2002;67:278–86.

41. LaRocque RC, Breiman RF, Ari MD, et al. Leptospirosis during dengue outbreak, Bangladesh. *Emerg Infect Dis* 2005;11:766–9.

42. Le QM, Kiso M, Someya K, et al. Avian flu: Isolation of drug-resistant H5N1 virus. *Nature* 2005;437:1108.

43. Leneva IA, Goloubeva O, Fenton RJ, et al. Efficacy of zanamivir against avian influenza A viruses that possess genes encoding H5N1 internal proteins and are pathogenic in mammals. *Antimicrob Agents Chemother* 2001;45:1216–24.

44. Leneva IA, Roberts N, Govorkova EA, et al. The neuraminidase inhibitor GS4104 (oseltamivir phosphate) is efficacious against A/Hong Kong/156/97 (H5N1) and A/Hong Kong/1074/99 (H9N2) influenza viruses. *Antiviral Res* 2000;48:101–15.

45. Levett PN. Leptospirosis. *Clin Microbiol Rev* 2001;14:296–326.

46. Li AM, Hon KL, Cheng WT, et al. Severe acute respiratory syndrome: "SARS" or "not SARS." *J Paediatr Child Health* 2004;40:63–5.

47. Li AM, Ng PC. Severe acute respiratory syndrome (SARS) in neonates and children. *Arch Dis Child Fetal Neonatal Ed* 2005;90:F461–5.

48. Li AM, So HK, Chu W, et al. Radiological and pulmonary function outcomes of children with SARS. *Pediatr Pulmonol* 2004;38:427–33.

49. Liem NT, Lim W. Lack of H5N1 avian influenza transmission to hospital employees, Hanoi, 2004. *Emerg Infect Dis* 2005;11:210–5.

50. MacLennan C, Dunn G, Huissoon AP, et al. Failure to clear persistent vaccine-derived neurovirulent poliovirus infection in an immunodeficient man. *Lancet* 1908;363:1509–13.

51. Maitland K, Nadel S, Pollard AJ, et al. Management of severe malaria in children: Proposed guidelines for the United Kingdom. *Br Med J* 2005;331:337–43.

52. Maitland K, Pamba A, Newton CR, et al. Hypokalemia in children with severe falciparum malaria. *Pediatr Crit Care Med* 2004;5:81–5.

53. Manocha S, Walley KR, Russell JA. Severe acute respiratory distress syndrome (SARS): A critical care perspective. *Crit Care Med* 2003;31:2684–92.

54. Marotto PC, Marotto MS, Santos DL, et al. Outcome of leptospirosis in children. *Am J Trop Med Hygiene* 1997;56:307–10.

55. Martinez VP, Bellomo C, San JJ, et al. Person-to-person transmission of Andes virus. *Emerg Infect Dis* 2005;11:1848–53.

56. Mertz GJ, Hjelle B, Crowley M, et al. Diagnosis and treatment of new world hantavirus infections. *Curr Opin Infect Dis* 2006;19:437–42.

57. Mertz GJ, Miedzinski L, Goade D, et al. Placebo-controlled, double-blind trial of intravenous ribavirin for the treatment of hantavirus cardiopulmonary syndrome in North America. *Clin Infect Dis* 2004;39:1307–13.

58. O'Leary DR, Marfin AA, Montgomery SP, et al. The epidemic of West Nile virus in the United States, 2002. *Vector Borne Zoonotic Dis* 2004;4(1):61–70.

59. Olsen SJ, Pruckler J, Bibb W, et al. Evaluation of rapid diagnostic tests for typhoid fever. *J Clin Microbiol* 2004;42:1885–9.

60. Outbreaks of avian influenza A (H5N1) in Asia and interim recommendations for evaluation and reporting of suspected cases—United States, 2004. *MMWR Morb Mortal Wkly Rep* 2004;53:97–100.

61. Overturf GD. Clinical sin nombre hantaviral infections in children. *Pediatr Infect Dis J* 2005;24:373–4.

62. Parry CM, Ho VA, Phuong T, et al. Randomized controlled comparison of ofloxacin, azithromycin, and an ofloxacin-azithromycin combination for treatment of multidrug-resistant and nalidixic Acid-resistant typhoid Fever. *Antimicrob Agents Chemother* 2007;51:819–25.

63. Peiris JS, Yuen KY, Osterhaus AD, et al. The severe acute respiratory syndrome. [see comment]. [Review] [89 refs]. *N Engl J Med* 1918;349:2431–41.

64. Peters CJ, Khan AS. Hantavirus pulmonary syndrome: The new American hemorrhagic fever. *Clin Infect Dis* 2002;34:1224–31.

65. Phu NH, Hien TT, Mai NT, et al. Hemofiltration and peritoneal dialysis in infection-associated acute renal failure in Vietnam. *N Engl J Med* 2002;347:895–902.

66. Pini N. Hantavirus pulmonary syndrome in Latin America. *Curr Opin Infect Dis* 2004;17:427–31.

67. Pini NC, Resa A, del J, et al. Hantavirus infection in children in Argentina. *Emerg Infect Dis* 1998;4:85–7.

68. Planche T, Krishna S. The relevance of malaria pathophysiology to strategies of clinical management. *Curr Opin Infect Dis* 2005;18:369–75.

69. Poliomyelitis. Centers for Disease Control, http://www.cdc.gov/vaccines/pubs/pinkbook/downloads/polio.pdf. Accessed 07/10/07.

70. Ramos MM, Overturf GD, Crowley MR, et al. Infection with Sin Nombre Hantavirus: Clinical presentation and outcome in children and adolescents. *Pediatrics* 2001;108:E27.

71. Rassi A, Jr., Rassi A, Little WC, et al. Development and validation of a risk score for predicting death in Chagas' heart disease. *N Engl J Med* 2006;355:799–808.

72. Rodriques CJ, de Castro SL. A critical review on Chagas disease chemotherapy. *Mem Inst Oswaldo Cruz* 2002;97:3–24.

73. Seydel KB, Milner DA, Jr., Kamiza SB, et al. The distribution and intensity of parasite sequestration in comatose Malawian children. *J Infect Dis* 2006;194:208–5.

74. Shinya K, Ebina M, Yamada S, et al. Avian flu: Influenza virus receptors in the human airway. *Nature* 2006;440:435–6.

75. Siriwanij T, Suttinont C, Tantawichien T, et al. Haemodynamics in leptospirosis: Effects of plasmapheresis and continuous venovenous haemofiltration. *Nephrology* 2005;10:1–6.

76. Suputtamongkol Y, Niwattayakul K, Suttinont C, et al. An open, randomized, controlled trial of penicillin, doxycycline, and cefotaxime for patients with severe leptospirosis. *Clin Infect Dis* 2004;39:1417–24.

77. Treanor JJ, Hayden FG, Vrooman PS, et al. Efficacy and safety of the oral neuraminidase inhibitor oseltamivir in treating acute influenza: A randomized controlled trial. US Oral Neuraminidase Study Group. *JAMA* 2000;283:1016–24.

78. Truccolo J, Serais O, Merien F, et al. Following the course of human leptospirosis: Evidence of a critical threshold for the vital prognosis using a quantitative PCR assay. *FEMS Microbiol Lett* 2001;204:317–21.

79. Ungchusak K, Auewarakul P, Dowell SF, et al. Probable person-to-person transmission of avian influenza A (H5N1). *N Engl J Med* 2005;352:333–40.

80. van Riel D, Munster VJ, de Wit E, et al. H5N1 Virus attachment to lower respiratory tract. *Science* 2006;312:399.

81. Varia M, Wilson S, Sarwal S, et al. Investigation of a nosocomial outbreak of severe acute respiratory syndrome (SARS) in Toronto, Canada. *CMAJ* 2003;169:285–92.

82. West NS, Riordan FAI. Fever in returned travelers: A prospective review of hospital admissions for a 2 1/2 year period. *Arch Dis Child* 2003;88:432–4.

83. Williams TN. Red blood cell defects and malaria. *Mol Biochem Parasitol* 2006;149:121–7.

84. Wong GW, Li AM, Ng PC, et al. Severe acute respiratory syndrome in children. *Pediatr Pulmonol* 2003;36:261–6.

85. World Health Organization. http://www.who.int/csr/disease/avian_influenza/country/cases_table_2006_11_29/en/index.html. Accessed 07/10/07.

86. Writing Committee of the World Health Organization Consultation on Human Influenza. Avian Influenza A (H5N1) Infection in Humans. *N Engl J Med* 2005;353:1374–85.

87. Yen HL, Monto AS, Webster RG, et al. Virulence may determine the necessary duration and dosage of oseltamivir treatment for highly pathogenic A/Vietnam/1203/04 influenza virus in mice. *J Infect Dis* 2005;192:665–72.

88. Yu CC, Li AM, So RC, et al. Longer term follow up of aerobic capacity in children affected by severe acute respiratory syndrome (SARS). *Thorax* 2006;61:240–6.

CHAPTER 83 ■ TOXIN-RELATED DISEASES

SUNIT C. SINGHI • M. JAYASHREE • JOHN P. STRAUMANIS • KAREN L. KOTLOFF

Several bacterial infections cause illness, not because of direct tissue invasion, but because of toxin(s) released by the bacteria. In most of these diseases, toxin(s) often cause a localized disease, which sometimes may become life-threatening systemic disease that requires admission to the ICU. Examples of such diseases include food poisoning and scalded-skin syndrome caused by *Staphylococcus aureus;* diarrhea caused by enterotoxigenic *Escherichia coli,* Shiga toxin-producing *E. coli, Shigella dysenteriae* type 1, and *Bacteroides fragilis;* anthrax; cholera; gas gangrene; and others. On the other hand, some of the toxin-mediated diseases by their very nature cause life-threatening systemic illnesses that require intensive care. These diseases are associated with localized bacterial infection or, sometimes, just colonization. The toxin produced at the site of infection and/or colonization spreads systemically and causes typical disease. In some instances, infection and/or colonization do not occur. For instance, in botulism, ingestion of toxin present in contaminated food causes the disease. Important toxin-producing bacteria and the life-threatening systemic diseases caused by them are listed in **Table 83.1.**

Rarely, other streptococci, including groups B, C, and G, β-hemolytic streptococci, and *S. viridans* (usually in immunocompromised individuals) and *S. suis.* have been reported to cause toxic shock syndrome (TSS). *Clostridium sordellii* has been reported as a cause of infection of the female genital tract and fatal TSS (22). *C. botulinum* produces most cases of botulism, with a few other strains of *Clostridium (C. butyricum, C. baratii, C. novyi, C. bifermentans,* etc.) accounting for the remainder. Those toxin-related infections that generally require treatment in an ICU are discussed in this chapter.

TETANUS

Tetanus is a potentially fatal disease characterized by hypertonia, muscle spasms, and autonomic instability caused by action of tetanospasmin (commonly called *tetanus toxin*), a potent neurotoxin elaborated by the organism *Clostridium tetani (C. tetani).*

Tetanus was known to Egyptians over 3000 years ago. Hippocrates gave the first detailed description of the disease in 400 BC, Arthur Nicolaier discovered the tetanus bacterium in 1884, and in 1889 Shibasaburo Kitasato at Koch's Institute obtained the first pure culture of tetanus bacilli. German bacteriologist Emil Von Behring developed a toxin-antitoxin mixture that was an effective vaccine against tetanus. In 1893, French scientist Emile Roux, assistant to Louis Pasteur, improved procedures for using serum antitoxin to prevent and to treat tetanus. Tetanus antitoxin was first used during World War I, dramatically reducing the incidence of the disease.

Epidemiology

Tetanus remains a major health problem in the world despite the availability of active and passive immunization. The estimated incidence of tetanus is 700,000–1 million cases per year worldwide (57), the majority of which occur in developing countries. Surveys indicate that only 3% of neonatal tetanus is reported. The World Health Organization (WHO) estimated that ~1.9 million (76%) of the 2.5 million vaccine-preventable deaths among children <5 years of age worldwide occur in Africa and Southeast Asia, with 8% due to tetanus (40).

Worldwide, tetanus affects all age groups, particularly newborns (who account for half of all cases) and younger persons. Tetanus rarely occurs among young persons who have received the primary series of tetanus toxoid vaccine. In industrialized nations such as the US, tetanus is a disease of the elderly; a population that was either born before immunization programs were implemented or have an age-related decline in antitoxin levels. Fewer than 75% of adults were immune or partially immune to tetanus in a recent serosurvey in Australia (26).

The Pathogen

Tetanus is caused by *C. tetani,* a drumstick-shaped, anaerobic, Gram-positive bacillus that forms endospores on maturation. The spores are widely distributed in soil, house and operating room dust, freshwater, and saltwater and may survive for years. They are also present in the feces of a number of animals, including sheep, cattle, dogs, cats, chickens, and horses, and in the intestinal tract of as many as 40% of humans. Soil rich in organic matter or treated with animal manure can therefore be highly infective. The spores are highly resistant to extremes of temperature and moisture, to various disinfectants (ethanol, phenol, and, formalin), and to boiling for 20 mins.

Pathogenesis

Disease is initiated when *C. tetani* spores enter a breach in the skin or mucosa and typically occurs after acute injury to soft tissue, particularly with deep penetrating or puncture wounds or lacerations, in which anaerobic bacterial growth is facilitated. The common portals of infection are wounds on the lower limbs, nonsterile intramuscular (IM) injections, and compound fractures. Tetanus can occur as a result of animal bites, drug injection with dirty needles, dental abscesses, and burns and surgical procedures, and in patients with chronic infections, such as otitis media or decubitus ulcers. The portal of entry may not be apparent in approximately one-third of patients.

TABLE 83.1

COMMON TOXIN-PRODUCING BACTERIA AND THE LIFE-THREATENING SYSTEMIC DISEASES THEY CAUSE

Corynebacterium diphtheria	Diphtheria
Clostridium tetani	Tetanus
Clostridium botulinum	Botulism
Clostridium perfringens	Gas gangrene, food poisoning
Clostridium difficile	Antibiotic-associated colitis
Staphylococcus aureus	Toxic shock syndrome
Streptococcus pyogenes (group A streptococcus)	Toxic shock syndrome

Inside the wound, in an anaerobic environment, the spores transform into vegetative forms and proliferate. The process is facilitated by the presence of a foreign body, necrotic tissue, or suppuration in the wound. Replicating bacteria do not cause inflammation, and the wound appears benign. The vegetative forms produce two toxins under plasmid control: tetanospasmin and tetanolysin. Tetanolysin damages the viable tissue around the infected wound, lowers the redox potential in the wound, and further facilitates growth of anaerobic organisms. Tetanospasmin causes the clinical manifestations of tetanus.

Tetanospasmin is synthesized as a single, 1315-amino-acid polypeptide that acts as a zinc-dependent peptidase. The molecule becomes toxic after being cleaved at serine 458 by a bacterial protease into a heterodimer of a 100-kDa heavy chain and a 50-kDa light chain connected by a disulfide bridge. The heavy chain is further cleaved by pepsin into the B and C fragments. The resulting toxin thus comprises the amino-terminal end of a heavy chain (fragment B) linked with a light chain (fragment A) by a disulfide bridge (fragment A–B) and a heavier carboxyl-terminal polypeptide (fragment C). Fragment C is responsible for attachment to the neuronal cell surface receptors and internalization of toxin, while fragment A–B produces the presynaptic inhibition of neurotransmitter release that results in clinical tetanus.

After entering the body, tetanospasmin spreads via lymphatics and blood vessels to enter the nervous system at the neuromuscular junction of the lower motor neurons. Although its greatest affinity is for inhibitory systems, a small amount of toxin also may enter sensory and autonomic neurons. The receptor to which toxin binds is thought to be membrane gangliosides, but this theory remains contentious. The toxin spreads through the central nervous system (CNS) by retrograde axonal transport to the cell body and migrates transsynaptically to other neurons, particularly the presynaptic inhibitory neurons. The proteins synaptotagmin, syntaxin, and synaptobrevin are involved in docking of synaptic vesicles to presynaptic membrane and release of the contents of synaptic vesicles into the synaptic clefts. Tetanospasmin cleaves peptide bonds of synaptobrevin and inhibits release of neurotransmitters, predominantly glycine, in the spinal cord and γ-aminobutyric acid (GABA) in the brainstem. Once the toxin binds to receptors within neurons, antitoxin therapy is ineffective (12). The loss of inhibition of α-motor neurons and dysfunction of polysynaptic reflexes result in inhibition of antagonists, causing sustained, uninhibited contraction of muscles (tetany). Ex-citatory transmission is also disrupted, causing weakness of muscles.

Blood-borne spread of toxin occurs from the site of entry to the brain at the area postrema of the floor of the fourth ventricle, where the blood-brain barrier (BBB) is nonexistent, possibly explaining the early manifestations of tetanus, such as trismus and nuchal rigidity.

The autonomic dysfunction in tetanus is due to various mechanisms, including the effect of tetanolysin on brainstem and autonomic interneurons, and is a direct effect of the toxin on the myocardium and adrenal inhibition. The loss of glycine inhibition by tetanospasmin affects preganglionic sympathetic neurons in spinal cord and causes increased sympathetic activity and increased catecholamine levels. Tetanospasmin may also interfere with the release of acetylcholine in peripheral somatic and autonomic nerves, producing a progressive interference with the inhibition of nervous transmission. Tetanospasmin probably also has an angiotensin-converting enzyme-like effect that contributes to hypertension; inhibition by captopril of the effect of tetanospasmin on synaptobrevin supports this view.

Clinical Features

The incubation period—the time interval between spore inoculation and symptom onset—may vary from 2 days to months (average 2 weeks). In severe forms, the incubation period is shorter, and the period of onset is <48 hrs. Tetanus typically evolves as one of four clinical forms, generalized, localized, neonatal, or cephalic.

Generalized Tetanus

The most common form of tetanus is generalized tetanus, which manifests with classical trismus or "lockjaw," as tetanus is commonly called (**Fig. 83.1**), followed by *risus sardonicus* (a facial grimace that results from hypertonia of the orbicularis oris), generalized muscle rigidity, hyperreflexia, dysphagia, opisthotonos, and spasms. The body assumes an opisthotonic position that resembles decorticate posturing (without loss of consciousness) with flexion of the arms and extension of the legs. The muscle spasms are caused by a sudden burst of tonic contraction in muscles and are very painful. Pharyngeal spasms lead to severe dysphagia. If prolonged, spasms may lead to rhabdomyolysis and its complications: laryngeal obstruction, acute respiratory failure, and cardiac arrest. Spasms are more prominent in the first 2 weeks, and their severity may increase during this period. Rigidity may last beyond the occurrence of spasms and autonomic disturbances, which usually occur some days after the spasms and reach a peak during the second week of the disease (36). Sympathetic overactivity, associated with elevated plasma norepinephrine and epinephrine concentrations, causes fluctuating heart rate, peripheral pallor, labile hypertension, and fever with profound sweating. Fluctuations in blood pressure and heart rate appear to be related to changes in systemic vascular resistance rather than cardiac output or left-ventricular filling pressure. Sometimes, hypotension and cardiac arrhythmias, such as paroxysmal supraventricular tachycardia, runs of ventricular tachycardia, or ventricular and arterial premature beats, may follow. Parasympathetic involvement may manifest as excessive salivation and increased

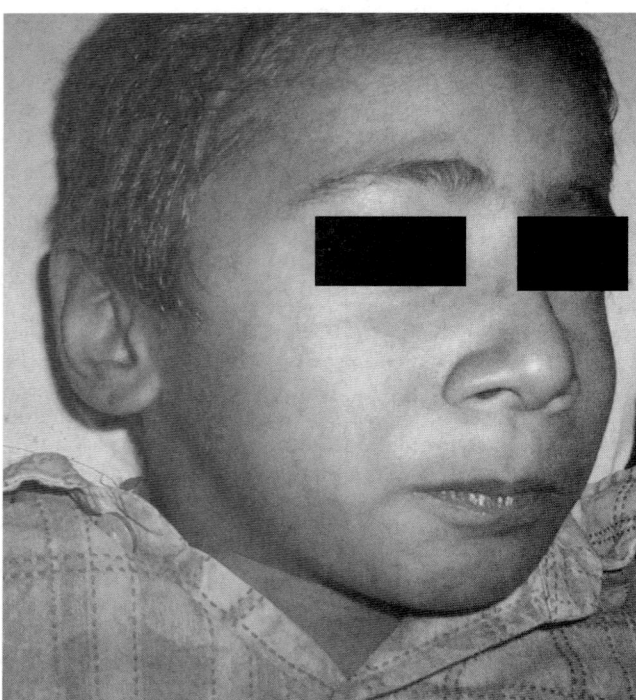

FIGURE 83.1. Typical risus sardonicus in a 9-year-old child with tetanus. Photo used with permission.

bronchial secretions as well as bradycardia and sudden cardiac arrest in severe tetanus. Recovery usually begins after 3 weeks and takes ~4 weeks. However, the clinical course is often unpredictable.

Localized Tetanus

Occasionally, muscle rigidity, often in association with muscle weakness, may remain localized at the site of spore inoculation. Symptoms may be mild and self-limited, persistent (in partially immune hosts), or progress to generalized tetanus.

Neonatal Tetanus

Neonatal tetanus is a generalized form of tetanus that develops through contamination of the umbilical stump in infants born to inadequately immunized mothers. The contamination may be caused by use of unsterile instruments to cut the cord or by unhygienic cord care practices (e.g., applying soil or cow dung dressing to the stump) that are prevalent in certain populations. The first signs are poor sucking and excessive crying, followed by variable degrees of trismus, risus sardonicus, and repeated generalized muscle spasms. Apnea may result from spasm of respiratory muscles. The baby cannot be nursed and, unless appropriate treatment is available, is at high risk for death. If the baby survives, spasms subside by the late second or early third week, and swallowing returns by the end of 4 weeks.

Cephalic Tetanus

Cephalic tetanus is an uncommon localized form of disease that is often associated with otitis media and head injuries and affects the cranial nerves. Facial paresis is usually present. A coexisting aerobic infection, often caused by *S. aureus* may be present. Rarely, extraocular movements are affected, causing "ophthalmologic tetanus."

Diagnosis and Differential Diagnosis

The diagnosis of tetanus is made on clinical grounds alone (**Table 83.2**). Recent history of injury or bites or presence of known portal of entry (such as otitis media, dental abscess, infected wounds) supports the diagnosis. In patients with trismus or neck stiffness, diagnosis may be difficult in the early phase of disease in the absence of clear evidence of injury. A bedside "spatula test," developed by Apte and Karnad, which has 94% sensitivity and 100% specificity, can be helpful. On insertion of a spatula (or tongue blade) that touches the posterior pharyngeal wall, if the patient gags and expels the spatula, the test is negative for tetanus; if the patient bites the spatula because of reflex masseter spasms, the test is positive for tetanus.

No serologic test exists to determine presence of toxin in serum or cerebrospinal fluid (CSF). A confirmed history of full active immunization almost excludes tetanus; the failure rate after a full course of tetanus toxoid in immunocompetent population is 4 per 100 million. Serum antitoxin levels of 0.01 IU/mL are protective, making the diagnosis unlikely. Culture of spores from suspicious wounds is not useful.

The differential diagnoses are few. Trismus caused by peritonsillar and odontogenic abscesses and abdominal rigidity caused by local trauma or peritonitis can be excluded by history and examination. Dystonic reactions to dopamine blockade usually cause torticollis and oculogyric crises. However, spasms are not seen. Benztropine or diphenhydramine can be administered to rule out such a reaction. Meningitis, meningoencephalitis, and tuberculous meningitis, which cause generalized hypertonia, neck rigidity, and tonic seizures, may sometimes mimic tetanus but can be differentiated by the presence of impaired mental status. Hypocalcemic tetany involves limb muscles more than the trunk and is associated with positive Chvostek and Trousseau signs. Poisoning with strychnine, a direct antagonist of glycine receptors, closely resembles generalized tetanus. Trismus is absent and abdominal muscles are less rigid in strychnine poisoning. Stiff-man syndrome has an insidious onset; hypertonia involves face and jaw muscles minimally and improves during sleep.

Entities that cause diffuse muscle spasms, such as toxidromes and encephalopathies, are accompanied by changes in mental status. The authors described a child with Guillain-Barré syndrome who initially had characteristic stimulation-induced opisthotonos and arching, mimicking tetanus (9).

TABLE 83.2

CLINICAL CRITERIA FOR DIAGNOSIS OF TETANUS

1. An illness characterized by the acute onset of hypertonia and/or painful muscle contractions (usually of the jaw and neck) and generalized muscle spasms without other apparent causes, such as drug reactions, other central nervous system disorders, hysteria
2. No history of contact with strychnine
3. Subsequent disease course consistent with tetanus

Adapted from Centers for Disease Control and Prevention (CDC). Epidemiologic notes and reports tetanus—Kansas, 1993. *MMWR* 1994;43:309–11.

Cephalic tetanus without trismus can be easily mistaken for Bell palsy.

Complications of Tetanus

Hypoxemia that leads to respiratory failure is a major cause of death. Cardiovascular consequences of autonomic instability, including cardiac arrhythmias and cardiomyopathy, sometimes occur and may be less amenable to secondary prevention.

Patients who are treated in the ICU are particularly prone to respiratory complications related to the use of mechanical ventilation (pneumothorax, atelectasis, ventilator-associated pneumonia), nosocomial infection, urinary tract infection related to indwelling catheters and wound sepsis, and gastrointestinal hemorrhage. The most common bacteria-causing infections are those that are Gram negative and *S. aureus*.

Rhabdomyolysis may occur in severe generalized tetanus and may lead to acute renal failure. If the serum creatine kinase level is high or myoglobin is detected in the urine, hydration with normal saline and urinary alkalinization with sodium bicarbonate should be considered. Phrenic and laryngeal neuropathies and other mononeuropathies can occur as a consequence of tetanus. Compression of the common peroneal nerve at the fibular head may produce foot drop.

Management

Tetanus at any age is a medical emergency and is best managed in a referral hospital. Availability of intensive care and critical care protocols has made a significant impact on survival of patients with tetanus (13). Grading of tetanus severity on the basis of Ablett criteria (**Table 83.3**) may help in selecting patients who might most benefit from intensive monitoring and care. The following are management goals, and a proposed protocol for management of severe grades of tetanus appears in **Table 83.4**.

1. Neutralization of the unbound toxin
2. Removal of the source of toxin
3. Control of rigidity and muscle spasms
4. Control of autonomic dysfunction
5. Supportive care—airway and ventilation

TABLE 83.3

ABLETT'S CRITERIA FOR CLASSIFICATION OF SEVERITY OF TETANUS

Grade I	Mild or no respiratory involvement and dysphagia
Grade II	Moderate respiratory involvement and trismus
Grade IIIA	Severe respiratory involvement, generalized rigidity, and major spasms, with no autonomic involvement
Grade IIIB	Severe manifestations as above with autonomic dysfunction

Adapted from Ablett JJL, Analysis and main experience in 82 patients treated in the Leeds tetanus unit. In Ellis M, ed. *Symposium on Tetanus in Great Britain*. Boston Spa, UK: National Lending Library, 1967.

Neutralization of the Unbound Toxin

Passive immunization to neutralize circulating (unbound) toxin by using antitoxin shortens the course and reduces the severity of tetanus. Human tetanus immunoglobulin (HTIG) is the preparation of choice. It consists of immunoglobulin G and has a half-life of 25 days. The dose of HTIG is 500 IU given IM, although doses as high as 3000–6000 IU have been used. Where HTIG is unavailable, equine antitetanus serum may be used after testing for hypersensitivity. Equine antitetanus serum has a higher risk of anaphylactic reactions and a short half-life of 2 days but is less expensive. The usual dose of antitetanus serum is 500–1000 U/kg; half of the dose is given IM, and half IV. Although HTIG and antitetanus serum have effect only on the unbound toxin (which is present in serum samples of only 10% of cases), either one of them should be administered as soon as possible in all cases, irrespective of the duration or severity of the disease. Whether antitoxin should also be infiltrated locally at the portal of entry is unclear and needs scrutiny.

Intrathecal Administration of Antitoxin. Antitoxin is administered intrathecally with the assumption that high concentrations of antitoxin in CSF and around the nerve roots will neutralize the toxin bound to neurons in CNS. Some studies have found it effective, whereas others have not. A randomized trial from Brazil found shorter duration of occurrence of spasm, hospital stay, and respiratory assistance in adult patients treated with 1000 IU of intrathecal HTIG (38). A meta-analysis of 12 randomized studies that included 484 patients in the intrathecal group and 458 in the IM group concluded that intrathecal therapy was superior to IM therapy (32). The superiority of intrathecal therapy also emerged when the analysis was performed separately for adults and neonates and for high and low doses.

Removal of the Source of Toxin

Toxin production may continue in suppurated wounds, wounds with retained foreign bodies, persistent otitis, untreated dental abscess, etc. The portal of entry should, therefore, be identified and treated appropriately with IV antibiotics and extensive wound debridement under local anesthesia after spasms are controlled. After debridement, the wound should be kept clean through regular wound care and aseptic dressing changes.

Antibiotic Therapy

Antibiotic therapy should be given to eradicate toxin-producing *C. tetani*. Although in vitro *C. tetani* is sensitive to metronidazole, penicillin, cephalosporins, carbapenems, and macrolides, crystalline penicillin and metronidazole are generally preferred (**Table 83.5**). Some prefer metronidazole to penicillin because the structure of penicillin is similar to GABA, which is the principal inhibitory neurotransmitter in the CNS. It is believed that, in high doses, penicillin may cause competitive antagonism to GABA and act synergistically with tetanospasmin to worsen the spasms. A randomized, controlled study suggests that benzyl penicillin, benzathine penicillin (single IM injection), and metronidazole are equally effective (24). In the authors' experience clinical outcome is similar with either of the antibiotics in severe, generalized tetanus treated in the PICU (53).

TABLE 83.4

SUGGESTED PROTOCOL FOR TETANUS MANAGEMENT (STEPS IN MANAGEMENT)

A. **Stabilization in Emergency Room**
1. Assess airway and ventilation, prepare for endotracheal intubation using rapid-sequence intubation technique, if generalized rigidity or spasm.
2. Obtain samples for electrolytes, blood urea, creatinine, creatinine kinase, and urinary myoglobin. If clinically indicated, perform neuroimaging and a lumbar puncture to rule out other diagnosis.
3. Determine and record the portal of entry, incubation period, period of onset, immunization history, and severity grade.
4. Administer diazepam IV, starting with 0.2 mg/kg to control spasms and decrease rigidity. If this compromises the airway or ventilation, intubate using rapid-sequence induction technique.
5. Transfer the patient to a dark isolated room in the ICU.
B. **Early management in PICU; first week**
1. Administer human tetanus immune globulin (HTIG; 500 units), IM; and tetanus toxoid (0.5 mL) IM, at different sites.
2. Consider intrathecal administration of HTIG (1000 IU).
3. Start crystallin penicillin (100,000 IU/kg/day, q 6 hrs, IV) for 10–14 days or metronidazole (50 mg/kg, IV q 8 hrs) for 7–10 days.
4. Initiate airway management: endotracheal intubation. Perform a tracheostomy if spasms produce any degree of airway compromise or difficulty in managing secretions.
5. Debride the wound under local anesthesia.
6. Establish a nasogastric tube for feeding.
7. Start continuous monitoring of heart rate, blood pressure, and cardiac rhythm.
8. Continue benzodiazepine infusion (in incremental doses as needed) to control spasms and achieve sedation. If adequate control of spasm is not achieved, initiate neuromuscular junction blockade with vecuronium 0.1 mg/kg/hr. Continue benzodiazepine for sedation.
9. Administer magnesium IV to achieve a serum magnesium concentration of 4–8 mEq/L (2–4 mmol/L).
C. **Continuing management in PICU: next 2–3 weeks**
1. Control sympathetic hyperactivity with IV propranolol or labetalol. Administer fluids, dopamine, or norepinephrine as and when needed to maintain hemodynamic stability. Avoid diuretics and blood.
2. With sustained bradycardia, atropine is useful; a pacemaker may be needed.
3. Use water or air mattress, if possible, to prevent skin breakdown.
4. Maintain benzodiazepines until neuromuscular junction blockade is no longer necessary. Taper the dose over 14–21 days.
5. Maintain serum magnesium, if used, until spasms are no longer present.
D. **Convalescent stage**
1. Active physical therapy. Supportive psychotherapy.
2. Administer another dose of the appropriate tetanus toxoid.

Control of Rigidity and Spasms

Even slight external stimuli, such as noise or touch, can trigger muscle spasms. It is therefore essential to keep the patient's external surroundings as quiet and dark as possible. No one drug or group of drugs has been consistently effective in controlling rigidity and spasms in severe tetanus.

Benzodiazepines. Benzodiazepines (diazepam, midazolam, and lorazepam) are commonly used for control of rigidity and spasms, as they are GABA$_A$ agonists and antagonize the effect of toxin on inhibitory receptors. They control spasms by blocking the polysynaptic reflexes, working peripherally, without depressing the cortical centers.

Diazepam is a sedative, anticonvulsant, and a muscle relaxant long used as a therapy for tetanus. It has a wide margin of safety and a rapid onset of action and can be given orally, rectally, or intravenously. A meta-analysis of in-hospital deaths caused by tetanus indicated that children treated with diazepam alone had a better chance of survival than those treated with a combination of phenobarbitone and chlorpromazine (relative risk for death, 0.36; 95% confidence interval, 0.15–0.86) (42). The dose of diazepam required for control of spasms may vary greatly. Initial control is achieved with IV diazepam infusion; enteral administration through a feeding tube may be started once spasms are under control (53). After 2–3 weeks of the full dose, the drug is gradually tapered over 2 weeks. Alternatively infusion of midazolam (0.1–0.3 mg/kg/hr) or lorazepam (0.15 mg/kg loading dose, followed by 1–2 mcg/kg/min) can be used. Midazolam does not require glycols for solubility and is gaining acceptance as the drug of choice. However, data that compare midazolam and lorazepam with diazepam in a randomized, controlled study are not available.

TABLE 83.5

PHARMACOLOGIC TREATMENT OF TETANUS

Drug	Dose	Major side effects	Contraindication	Duration
ANTIBIOTICS				
Penicillin G	100,000–200,000 IU/kg IV in 4 divided doses	Local pain, inflammation at injection site, hypersensitivity, may potentiate effects of tetanus toxin due to its GABA agonist effect.	Documented hypersensitivity	10–14 days
Metronidazole	30–40 mg/kg/day IV every 6 hrs; max, 4 g/day	Neurotoxicity in the form of dizziness, vertigo; rarely, convulsions	Documented hypersensitivity	7–10 days
CONTROL OF SPASMS				
Benzodiazepines				
Diazepam	0.2 mg/kg initial dose through IV infusion, stepped up rapidly in increments until spasms are controlled; usually, 1 mg/kg/hr. Change to enteral route in 4–6 divided doses through nasogastric tube; max. 2 mg/kg/hr	Respiratory depression, hypotension secondary to vasodilation and myocardial depression. Glycols and benzyl alcohol used as preservatives in IV preparation are toxic when very high doses of diazepam are used.	Shock, respiratory depression	Full doses for 2–3 weeks; then, gradually tapered off over 2 weeks
Midazolam	0.1–0.3 mg/kg/hr as IV infusion	Respiratory depression, hypotension	Shock	
Lorazepam	0.15 mg/kg loading dose, followed by 1–2 mcg/kg/min.	Respiratory depression, hypotension, toxic glycols or benzyl alcohol used as preservatives	Hypotension, shock	
Neuromuscular Blocking Agents				
Pancuronium	Initial dose 0.08–0.1 mg/kg; then as IV infusion 0.1 mg/kg/hr or 0.5–1.7 mcg/kg/min	Tachycardia, hypertension, and increased cardiac output due to intrinsic sympathomimetic activity. Delayed recovery from paralysis and need for prolonged ventilation	Known hypersensitivity and lack of access to mechanical ventilation	Shortest possible
Vecuronium	Initial dose 0.08–0.1 mg/kg; then as IV infusion 0.1 mg/kg/hr or 0.5–1.7 mcg/kg/min	Minimal cardiovascular side effects; the drug is considered "cardiovascularly clean." Complications related to prolonged use are similar to pancuronium.	Used cautiously in presence of hepatic or renal disease.	Shortest possible
Atracurium	Initial dose 0.5 mg/kg, followed by infusion of 4–12 mcg/kg/min	Increases bronchial secretions, itching and wheezing due to histamine release	Safe in hepatic and renal disease unlike vecuronium and baclofen.	Shortest possible
Intrathecal baclofen	No definite guidelines. Average bolus dose for patients <55 years is 1000 mcg. Infusion through an epidural catheter placed in the L3–L4 space for prolonged therapy.	Drowsiness, sedation coma, respiratory depression, hypersensitivity. Side effects increase with repeated boluses. Reversible on stopping therapy.	Known hypersensitivity. Used with caution in presence of respiratory depression and altered sensorium.	7–14 days

(Continued)

TABLE 83.5

(CONTINUED)

Drug	Dose	Major side effects	Contraindication	Duration
CONTROL OF AUTONOMIC INSTABILITY				
Propranolol	0.5–1 mg/kg/day in 3–4 divided doses. Increased gradually every 3–5 days to 1–5 mg/kg/day, max. 8 mg/kg/day	Bradycardia, hypotension, congestive heart failure, pulmonary edema, hypoglycemia, hyperglycemia, bronchospasm, agranulocytosis	Known hypersensitivity, asthma/chronic obstructive pulmonary disease, cardiogenic shock, bradycardia, pulmonary edema	6–8 weeks
Labetalol	IV 0.2–0.5 mg/kg/dose, titrated to effect, max 20 mg/dose. Oral 4 mg/kg/day in 2 divided doses, max 20 mg/kg/day	Bradycardia, hypotension, congestive heart failure, bronchospasm, rash, dizziness, reversible myopathy (very rarely)	Known hypersensitivity, asthma, cardiogenic shock, bradycardia, pulmonary edema	6–8weeks
Morphine	0.01–0.1 mcg/kg/min as IV infusion or 0.1 mg/kg IV every 4–6 hrs	Respiratory depression, hence caution in patients with respiratory compromise Bronchoconstriction, vomiting, and hypotension	Used with caution in advanced liver and renal disease and in known asthmatic.	7–10 days
Magnesium sulfate	25–50 mg/kg/dose IV as an hourly infusion, max dose ~2 g/dose, repeated every 6 hrs, depending on the clinical response and serum magnesium	Hypocalcemia, weakness, sedation, paralysis, hypotension, and bradyarrhythmias. Serum magnesium levels must be monitored closely, as clinical signs may be missed in a sedated and paralyzed patient.	Compromised renal function	Maintain serum magnesium at ~4–8 mEq/L
Clonidine	Initial 5–10 mcg/kg/day in divided doses every 8–12 hrs. Increase to 5–25 mcg/kg/day every 6 hrs gradually	Hypotension, bradycardia, headache, dizziness, fatigue, respiratory depression, Raynaud phenomenon		

Neuromuscular Blockade. Neuromuscular blockade is required when sedatives are not fully effective in controlling rigidity and spasms. Long-acting muscle relaxants such as pancuronium have been used. However, pancuronium is an inhibitor of catecholamine uptake (intrinsic sympathomimetic effect) and may cause tachycardia and hypertension and worsen the autonomic instability. Vecuronium and atracurium are neuromuscular blocking agents of choice in ventilated tetanus patients. Vecuronium is "cardiovascularly clean" and induces minimum autonomic instability but is relatively short-acting and requires continuous infusion. During the period of use of neuromuscular blockade, adequate sedation must be ensured.

Other Drugs. Continuous and intermittent intrathecal administration of baclofen (a GABA_B agonist) has been reported to be useful. It reduced the need for sedation and ventilatory support in adult patients (49). The technique is invasive and expensive, and facilities for ventilation must be available. IV infusion of dantrolene, a direct-acting muscle relaxant, may be useful in select cases. The sedative agent propofol has been used for its muscle-relaxing properties, but it should not be used alone, as it does not have any GABA activity or analgesic effect. The drug concentrations required to control spasms are very high; closer to anesthetic rather than sedative doses.

Control of Autonomic Dysfunction

Continuous hemodynamic and electrocardiogram monitoring is essential for timely detection of autonomic dysfunction. As with control of spasms, no one class of drugs or combination has been demonstrated to be consistently effective for management of autonomic dysfunction.

Propranolol, a β-adrenergic blocking agent, is one of the most commonly used drugs for quick control of sympathetic dysfunction; namely tachycardia, hypertension, and supraventricular tachycardia. It should be used in small doses, as it may produce serious side effects. Enteral administration may be dangerous; absorption and response may be erratic because of altered gastrointestinal motility. Labetalol has been used for its combined α and β effect and is currently preferred over other drugs. Esmolol (short-acting β blocker) reduces catecholamine release and may have advantage over other pure β blockers.

Morphine acts centrally to reduce sympathetic tone to the heart and vascular system and reduces heart rate and blood pressure. It also has a sedative effect, which is an added advantage.

Magnesium is a presynaptic neuromuscular blocker, inhibits the release of humoral and neuronal catecholamines, and reduces the sensitivity of α-adrenergic receptors. Magnesium infusion adjusted to maintain a serum magnesium level between 4 and 8 mEq/L reduced extreme variability of heart rate and blood pressure and the need for neuromuscular blocking agents and sedatives in adult patients (7). Successful use of magnesium sulfate infusion for control of muscle rigidity and spasm refractory to moderate sedation has been reported in a 12-year-old child. The patient did not require deep sedation, neuromuscular blockade, or mechanical ventilation (25).

Clonidine is a selective partial agonist for α_2-adrenergic receptors in the CNS. It inhibits sympathetic outflow and potentiates parasympathetic activity, produces marked sedation and anxiolysis, and decreases spontaneous motor activity. Further investigation of clonidine as a treatment modality for autonomic dysfunction in tetanus should be conducted.

Other drugs that have anecdotal evidence of potential benefit in tetanus include atropine for parasympathetic autonomic dysfunction, sodium valproate for sedation, angiotensin-converting enzyme inhibitors for hypertension, and adenosine for arrhythmias. To date, their use in tetanus has been largely experimental. The role of pyridoxine is controversial, and corticosteroids are not advised. Doses and salient features of various drugs commonly used in tetanus are listed in **Table 83.5.**

Supportive Treatment

Supportive treatment in a patient with tetanus should include maintenance of airway and ventilation, proper gastrointestinal function, skin integrity, and prevention of complications of respiratory dysfunction, such as atelectasis.

Airway Management and Ventilatory Support. Patients with tetanus are at risk of hypoxic insult from frequent spasms of laryngeal, diaphragmatic, or respiratory muscles or from drug-induced respiratory failure. Endotracheal intubation should be performed in all patients who have generalized rigidity on arrival, even in absence of frequent spasms, as the disease is likely to progress in severity for 10–14 days after onset. All patients with frequent spasms or those who require high-dose IV diazepam or neuromuscular blockade for uncontrolled spasms must be intubated. An endotracheal tube should be inserted under sedation and neuromuscular blockade using the rapid-sequence induction technique. A nasogastric tube should be inserted concurrently. No consensus exists regarding the role of tracheostomy. It is required in patients who have uncontrolled laryngospasm or who receive prolonged ventilation.

Ventilatory support is needed when neuromuscular blockade or high doses of diazepam are used for poorly controlled rigidity and spasms. Controlled ventilation is used initially; once the spasms and rigidity are controlled and not likely to progress (usually by the end of the second week of illness), weaning gradually is accomplished through the ventilatory modes that allow graded return to spontaneous respiratory effort.

Strict asepsis, meticulous mouth care, chest physiotherapy, and regular endotracheal tube care are essential to prevent atelectasis, lobar collapse, and pneumonia. Suctioning should be done only when necessary. Adequate sedation is mandatory when all of these interventions are performed to minimize the risk of uncontrolled spasms.

Continuous pulse oximetry, respiratory monitoring, and periodic measurements of respiratory dynamics should be undertaken to assess pulmonary functions.

Gastrointestinal and Metabolic Considerations. Energy demand is high in patients with tetanus because of muscular spasms, excessive sweating, and associated sepsis. Therefore, adequate caloric intake should be ensured as early as possible. Enteral feeding, with head elevated to 30–45 degrees, is preferred. Gastrointestinal hypomotility or paralytic ileus may develop as a result of immobility and treatment with morphine. If patients cannot tolerate enteral feedings, parenteral nutrition becomes necessary.

The complications of immobility caused by heavy sedation and paralysis must be minimized. Special water or air mattresses to allow turning the patient with minimal stimulation and to prevent the development of pressure ulcers are preferred. Passive range-of-motion exercises must be instituted early to maintain muscle strength, prevent deformities, and stimulate circulation.

Psychosocial Considerations. Psychosocial care is important for paralyzed patients. It is essential to keep them comfortable and anticipate their needs. Patients who are anxious or in pain have reflex increases in heart rate and blood pressure. Patients' family members should be allowed to participate in the patients' care.

Outcome and Prognosis

Mortality rates are <10% in mild, generalized disease but are as high as 50% in severe disease with frequent spasms, and are up to 90% in neonates. Death results form various complications, such as respiratory failure, pneumonia, septicemia, and cardiovascular instability. Spasm of the glottis can cause immediate death. Availability of intensive care and mechanical ventilation has helped in reducing early deaths caused by acute respiratory failure and uncontrolled spasms. Autonomic disturbances that appear later in the course of the illness and intensive care-related complications (ventilator-associated pneumonia, gastrointestinal hemorrhage) are now major causes of death.

The prognosis is determined by clinical severity at presentation, incubation period, progression of disease (as determined from "period of onset"—the time interval between first symptoms of tetanus and first generalized spasm), patient's age, portal of entry, and autonomic instability. Generally, the longer the incubation period, the milder the illness and the better the prognosis. An incubation period of <1 week tends to be associated with more severe progression of the disease. Tetanus following burns, IM injections, or compound fractures has a poor outcome. Tetanus acquired after IM injection with quinine is associated with a higher mortality than other modes of acquisition.

Poor prognostic factors in neonatal tetanus include age <7 days, symptom duration <5 days, fever, and *risus sardonicus*. Respiratory signs at or within 24 hrs of admission, respiratory failure that requires mechanical ventilation, fever, and tachycardia are poor prognostic signs. Autonomic dysfunction (presence of labile or persistent hypertension or hypotension, sinus tachycardia or tachyarrhythmia, or bradycardia on electrocardiogram) even in patients with mild or moderate tetanus, irrespective of the need for mechanical ventilation, predicted poor outcome in adult patients (59).

Sequelae include enuresis, mild mental retardation, and growth delay in children. Psychologic aftereffects, including a perception of permanent worsening of health, have been reported in adults. Data on this aspect in children are not available.

Prevention

Tetanus is preventable with proper use of tetanus toxoid and HTIG. Active immunization of all survivors of tetanus with tetanus toxoid is imperative to prevent reinfection and further illness. The total amount of toxin produced during disease is inadequate to mount an immune response; therefore, patients with newly diagnosed tetanus must be actively immunized.

Recommendations for primary immunization depend on the age of the patient. A total of five doses of combined diphtheria tetanus-pertussis vaccine at ages 2, 4, 6, 15–18 months, and 5 years is recommended during primary childhood immunization. The vaccine may be given simultaneously with hepatitis-B and *Haemophilus influenzae* type b (Hib) vaccines. The vaccine confers protective antibody levels in 81%–95% of previously unimmunized people after two doses and in 100% after three doses. A booster dose of tetanus toxoid is recommended every 10 years. Protective antibodies develop rapidly after a booster dose.

Postinjury Prophylaxis

Postinjury prophylaxis is not required in people who have received a tetanus toxoid booster dose within the previous 5 years. Children who have received partial immunization need only the remaining doses from the schedule, rather than to restart from the first dose. Although any wound can contain tetanus spores, some wounds are considered to be "tetanus prone." These include wounds that are contaminated with dirt, saliva, or feces, and puncture wounds (including unsterile injections, missile injuries, burns, frostbite, avulsions, and crush injuries). If an individual who sustains a tetanus-prone wound has an uncertain history of vaccination or received the last dose of tetanus toxoid 5 years or more before injury, she should receive one dose of HTIG and three doses of tetanus toxoid—two doses 2 months apart, followed by a third one after 6 months. HTIG should also be given to immunodeficient patients with a tetanus-prone wound. If doubt exists, a wound should be considered to be tetanus prone. In children, the dose of HTIG should be 500 units to achieve adequate antibody concentration (0.1 IU/mL). Tetanus toxoid and HTIG should be administered at different sites in different syringes to avoid interaction between the two.

Conclusions and Future Directions

Severe tetanus remains a clinical challenge. Drugs that can control spasms and rigidity without causing respiratory depression must be evaluated. Failure to identify ideal drug(s) and limited availability of intensive care and ventilation in developing countries are some of the challenges. A bigger challenge is to find ways to achieve universal immunization of the susceptible population for this fully vaccine-preventable disease.

DIPHTHERIA

Diphtheria is an acute localized infection of skin or respiratory mucous membranes caused by toxin-producing strains of *Corynebacterium diphtheriae*. It is characterized by a pseudomembrane in the throat and a systemic illness that results from absorption of toxin. Edwin Klebs and Fredrick Loeffler, both pupils of Robert Koch, discovered the diphtheria bacillus in 1884. Four years later, Emile Roux discovered the diphtheria toxin secreted by *C. diphtheria*. In 1890, Emil Adolf Von Behring at Koch's Institute paved the way for the use of serum therapy, and in 1891, Behring injected the newly prepared protective serum, named "antitoxin," to a severely ill, 8-year-old boy with diphtheria. The boy made a full recovery and became the first human to be cured with specific immunotherapy. The first Nobel Prize in Physiology or Medicine was awarded to Emil Adolf Von Behring in 1901 for developing serum therapy for diphtheria.

Epidemiology

The incidence of diphtheria steadily declined in the developed nations following effective immunization programs introduced in the 1920s. However, in the mid-1990s, large epidemics of diphtheria occurred in Eastern Europe and the former Soviet Union, with case fatality rates as high as 17%–23% in Azerbaijan, Georgia, and Turkmenistan. Resurgence of the disease in these countries was largely attributed to waning vaccine immunity in adults and importation of cases from the endemic developing world (23).

Diphtheria remains endemic in resource-poor countries and caused 5000 deaths in 2002, mainly due to inadequate vaccine coverage (60). An immunization level of 70%–80% in the community is necessary to prevent epidemic spread. The diptheria-tetanus-pertussis-3 coverage in 2004 in Southeast Asia and Africa was 69% and 66%, respectively, compared to more than 90% coverage in the European, Western Pacific, and American regions (40). The case fatality rate, which had improved dramatically after introduction of antitoxin therapy, has subsequently remained constant. Poor socioeconomic standards, overcrowding, delayed reporting to hospital, and nonavailability or delay in antitoxin administration, further contribute to the high mortality in developing countries.

The Pathogen

C. diphtheriae is an aerobic pleomorphic, Gram-positive, non–acid-fast, nonmotile bacillus that appears slightly curved or club-shaped. It has four subspecies: mitis, gravis, intermedius, and belfanti; each can cause the disease. The only known reservoir for C. diphtheriae is man. Transmission of the organism occurs by exposure to respiratory secretions or exudates from the skin lesions. Carriers can transmit the disease, but patients with active infection are more likely to do so. C. diphtheriae has been known to survive for weeks in floor dust, suggesting the potential for indirect transmission of infections. In tropical countries, cutaneous diphtheria is the principal source of infection. It may serve as an important reservoir of infection in epidemics of faucial diphtheria.

Pathogenesis

Both toxigenic and nontoxigenic strains can cause localized mucocutaneous infection, even with bacteremia and seeding of distant sites. However, the strains of C. diphtheriae that are lysogenized with bacteriophages that contain the structural genes encoding for production of the exotoxin (tox+ strains) produce diphtheria toxin. The toxin is the major virulence factor responsible for severe local and systemic effects.

Diphtheria exotoxin is a 62-kDa polypeptide that includes two segments: the active moiety (A) and the binding segment (B). The latter binds to specific receptors on susceptible cells and allows fragment A to enter into the cell. Fragment A then inhibits protein synthesis by inactivation of elongation factor (EF)-2. All human cells are potentially susceptible to the effects of diphtheria toxin because they have receptors for the toxin and its substrate, EF-2. However, differential effects on various tissues, with predilection for myocardium, peripheral nerves, and kidneys, are poorly explained.

The toxin also causes local destruction of the respiratory mucosa at the site of infection, facilitating formation of a dense coagulum of organism, necrotic epithelial cells, fibrin, and pus cells over the mucosa, the so-called *pseudomembrane*. Formation of pseudomembrane further promotes replication and person-person transmission of diphtheria bacillus.

Age and the immunization status of the individual are host factors that are major determinants of disease severity and transmission. Although immunization does not prevent carriage or infection with toxigenic C. diphtheriae, antitoxic immunity decreases local tissue spread and necrosis (and therefore ameliorates the incidence and severity of disease). In addition, it inhibits replication and transmission of the organism, thus providing herd immunity. It is estimated that 70%–80% of a population must be immunized to prevent epidemic spread. Nonetheless, even populations with very high immunization rates remain vulnerable to diphtheria outbreaks if travelers or immigrants introduce toxigenic strains of C. diphtheriae, particularly in crowded conditions with intense exposure (41).

The protective level of serum antitoxin is 0.01 IU/mL. These levels may decline with increasing age and increased vulnerability to the infection. A recent study found that among persons aged ≥50 years fewer than 60% were immune or partially immune to diphtheria (26). Booster doses may succeed in maintaining sustained antitoxin levels and preventing infections.

Clinical Manifestations

Onset of symptoms may be insidious or abrupt following an incubation period of 2–5 days. Both sore throat and fever are almost universal. Cough and stridor may be presenting features in 65%–70% of unimmunized children with an acute fulminant course. Hoarseness of voice and dysphagia may be evident in 30%–40% of patients (43) (**Table 83.6**). Cervical lymphadenopathy with a brawny edema of the cervical region, described as "bull neck," is common in severe cases. Unilateral purulent to blood-tinged nasal discharge is characteristic of nasal diphtheria and is seen in 3%–4% of patients. Nonspecific symptoms, such as nausea, vomiting, malaise, and headache, may precede or coexist with onset of the disease.

TABLE 83.6

SALIENT CLINICAL FEATURES OF DIPHTHERIA

Pseudomembrane	100%
Fever	92.4%
Upper respiratory tract infection	91.6%
Upper airway obstruction	42.3%
Hoarseness	36.7%
Bull neck	11.3%

n = 381.
Data from Pancharoen C, Mekmullica J, Thisyakorn U, et al. Clinical features of diphtheria in Thai children: A historical perspective. *Southeast Asian J Trop Med Public Health* 2002;33:352–4.

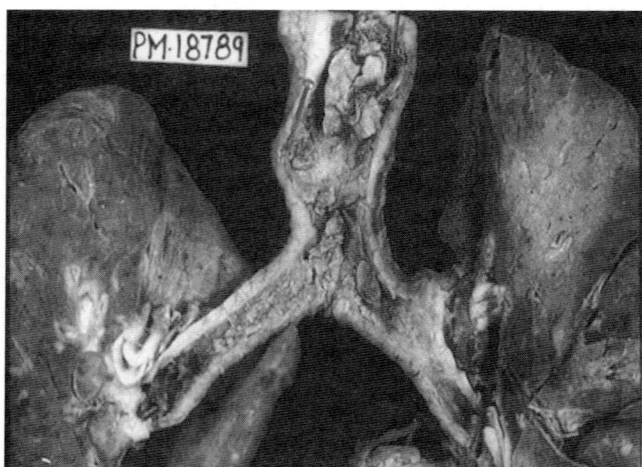

FIGURE 83.2. Gross photograph showing thick diphtheritic membrane on the mucosal aspect of trachea and bronchi. Courtesy Dr. Ashim Dass, Additional Professor, Department of Histopathology, *PGIMER*, Chandigarh.

The hallmark of respiratory diphtheria is the presence of the characteristic thick adherent fibrinous pseudomembrane on the respiratory epithelium. The membrane looks dull and grayish and bleeds easily on touch. It may be found on the palate, pharynx, tonsils, epiglottis, and larynx, or may extend to the tracheobronchial tree (**Fig. 83.2**). Among patients admitted to the PICU, faucial diphtheria (i.e., involvement of the posterior mouth and the proximal pharynx) is most common (~70%), followed by pharyngolaryngeal (25%), laryngeal (2%–3%), and combined faucial and nasal (4.2%) (31). Laryngeal diphtheria is usually secondary to an extension of faucial diphtheria. Isolated laryngeal membrane, nasal diphtheria, or tracheal membrane without pharyngeal involvement is rare.

Other forms of diphtheria may be seen less commonly. Cutaneous diphtheria infection typically presents as a chronic non-healing ulcer with a gray membrane. Etiologic agents of impetigo (*Streptococcus pyogenes* and *S. aureus*) can often be isolated from the same lesion. Infection is most often found in the tropics and in hosts subjected to inadequate hygiene. Clusters of invasive disease, e.g., endocarditis, septic arthritis, and osteomyelitis, have been reported in similar populations.

Complications

Extensive membrane in an unimmunized child who presents within the first 5–6 days of onset of illness with a high leukocyte count should be considered as "severe disease." Delay in initiating treatment in patients with severe disease increases the risk of toxin spread and systemic complications.

Airway Obstruction

Upper airway obstruction is seen in nearly three-fourths of patients with "severe disease." Extension of diphtheritic membrane into the larynx and tracheobronchial tree is the main cause of airway obstruction. Other contributing factors are soft tissue edema and necrosis, dislodgement of pharyngeal membrane, and bleeding into the airway. Stridor, hoarseness, aphonia or dysphonia, and respiratory distress are manifestations of an obstructed airway. Ongoing assessment is essential, and

the airway should be secured early, as rapid progression of the membrane may preclude a later opportunity. Timely intubation or tracheostomy in patients with airway complications carries a good prognosis. In both children and adults, pulmonary aspiration of the membrane that is causing complete airway obstruction is a common cause of death.

Myocarditis

Myocarditis is one of the most serious complications of diphtheria, occurring in 10%–25% of patients, with the incidence being higher (60%–70%) in patients with severe and fulminant disease. On histologic examination, myocardium shows hyaline degeneration and myonecrosis associated with active inflammation in the interstitial spaces and numerous lipid droplets within myofibrils (27) (**Fig. 83.3**).

Independent predictors of development of myocarditis include bull neck, a pseudomembrane score of >2 (0, no membrane; 1, only nose or incomplete tonsillar coverage; 2, confluent coverage of tonsils; 3, as in 2 plus palate and/or pharyngeal wall; 4, as in 3 plus nose and/or larynx), and an elevated aspartate aminotransferase level. Subclinical cardiac damage may be identified by the presence of troponin T (33). Age, fever, shared accommodation, and extensive respiratory tract infection with subcutaneous edema were independent risk factors for cardiac involvement (35). Adequate immunization and early administration of antitoxin may have some role in preventing myocarditis.

Typically, myocarditis is seen at the end of the second week of illness but may be seen as early as 5 days following the onset of upper respiratory disease in unimmunized patients (31,35). It may have a varied presentation, including muffled heart sounds, new or altered murmurs, ectopic beats, cardiac enlargement, arrhythmias, cardiogenic shock, or syncope. At times, only mild electrocardiographic changes, such as ectopic beats and sinus bradycardia, may be indicative of myocarditis. Diphtheria toxin has a high affinity for the conduction system of the heart, and prolonged PR interval is frequent. Bradyarrhythmias in the form of bundle-branch blocks progressing

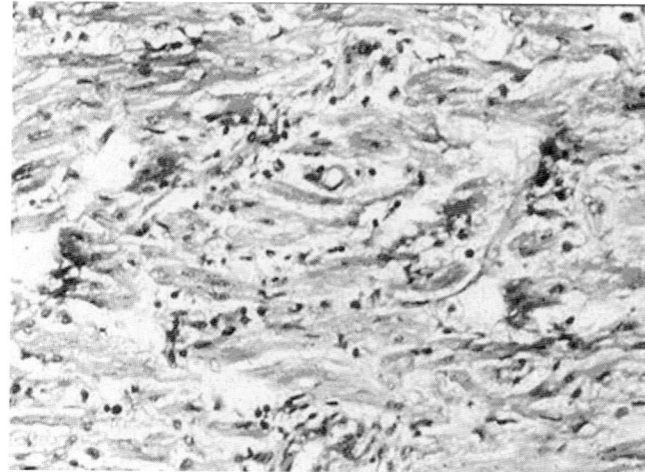

FIGURE 83.3. Microscopy with hematoxylin and eosin (H&E) staining of heart showing foci of necrotic cardiac myocytes with lymphocytic infiltrates in a child with toxic myocarditis caused by diphtheria. Courtesy Dr. Ashim Dass, Additional Professor, Department of Histopathology, *PGIMER*, Chandigarh.

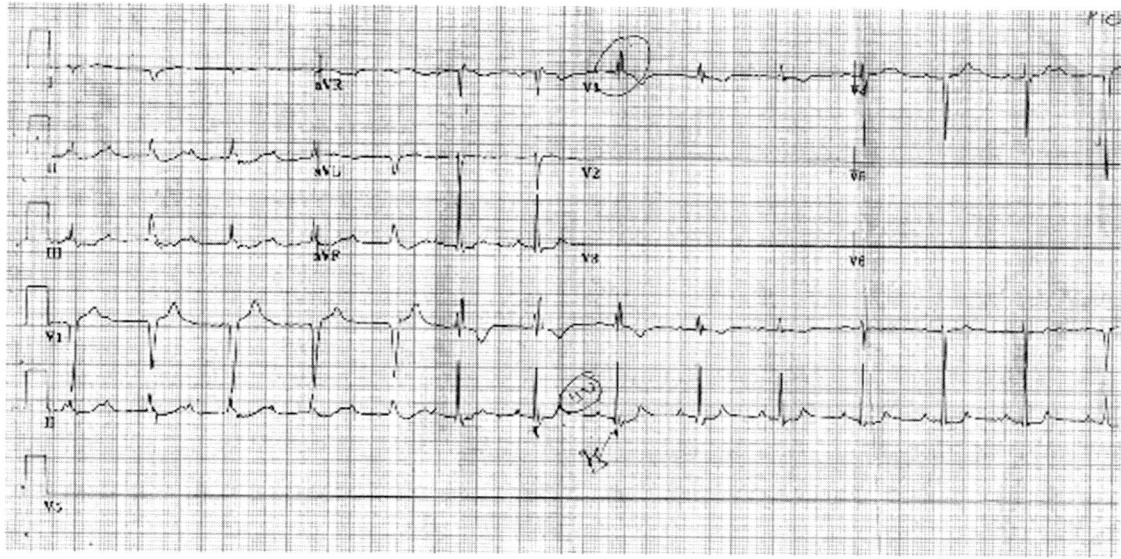

FIGURE 83.4. Electrocardiogram in a patient with diphtheritic myocarditis, showing right bundle-branch block and atrioventricular dissociation.

to complete heart blocks are more common than tachyarrhythmias (**Fig. 83.4**).

Neuropathy

Diphtheritic polyneuropathy usually occurs after a latent period of 3–16 weeks after the onset of acute diphtheria, but this sequence can vary from 4 days to 3–5 weeks. Neuropathy has been variably reported to occur in 3%–43% of patients. The frequency is directly proportional to the severity of diphtheria and timely antitoxin therapy (45). Polyneuropathy was attenuated in patients who were vaccinated according to schedule and had received antitoxin within 2–3 days of the onset of acute respiratory symptoms (34).

The neuropathy involves the motor cranial nerves (III, IV, VI, VII, IX, and XII) and the peripheral nerves and is predominantly motor in character. In severe cases, respiratory and abdominal muscles may be involved. Weakness usually begins proximally and spreads distally. Typically, palatal paralysis (nasal twang, dysphonia, and regurgitation of fluids) occurs in the second week; ocular palsies (loss of accommodation, squint, and diplopia) in the third week, and generalized motor weakness after 3–6 weeks of illness. Autonomic disturbances, such as tachycardia, hypotension, or hypertension and hyperhidrosis may be seen. CSF may show pleocytosis and elevated protein levels. Complete recovery of neurologic function occurs in most survivors. Resolution usually occurs by 5–6 months, but may take as long as 12 months.

Renal Failure

Renal tubular cells are potentially susceptible to the effects of the exotoxin. Renal failure in diphtheria is generally secondary to acute tubular necrosis but may also be a consequence of decreased cardiac output secondary to myocarditis and cardiogenic shock

Thrombocytopenia

Thrombocytopenia and bleeding are considered rare manifestations. However, these have been described in nearly one-third of patients with severe and complicated diphtheria (31).

Diagnosis and Differential Diagnosis

The diagnosis of diphtheria and indication for initiating antitoxin therapy should be based on clinical grounds. The definition recommended by the WHO for a probable clinical case is "an illness characterized by laryngitis or pharyngitis or tonsillitis, *and* an adherent membrane of the tonsils, pharynx, and/or nose."

Diphtheria should be suspected in any patient with membranous tonsillopharyngitis, especially if it extends to the uvula and soft palate, or if bull-neck, hoarseness, stridor, unilateral bloody nasal discharge, or palatal palsy is observed. Other conditions that can give rise to a membranous tonsillopharyngitis should be considered in the differential diagnosis. These include acute streptococcal pharyngitis, candidiasis, Vincent angina, infectious mononucleosis, and agranulocytosis (mucositis). At the beginning of the illness, diphtheria can look like any type of tonsillitis, with only a small spot of membrane on the tonsil. Marked edema of the tonsils, uvula, and pharyngeal wall helps distinguish this condition from other entities that can present as membranous tonsillopharyngitis. Pharyngeal coinfection with group A streptococci (GAS) is common in diphtheria; therefore, identification of streptococcal infection does not exclude diphtheria (46).

Laboratory Diagnosis

Presumptive rapid diagnosis is usually obtained with methylene blue and Gram stain of pharyngeal smear. *C. diphtheriae* is seen as club-shaped, Gram-positive, pleomorphic bacillus with terminal swellings, arranged in a Chinese letter pattern. Diphtheroids that are normal commensals in the throat may give rise to a false-positive test. Isolation of *C. diphtheriae* from a clinical specimen or fourfold or greater rise in serum antibody is necessary for confirmation of diagnosis.

Successful isolation of *C. diphtheriae* depends on proper collection of swabs and transport to the laboratory. The laboratory must be alerted to the suspicion of diphtheria, as routine cultures are not likely to identify the organism. In cases of respiratory diphtheria, culturing of both nasal and pharyngeal sites improves the rate of isolation. Cultures should be obtained from samples of membrane or a submembrane swab, if possible. In cutaneous disease, samples should be obtained from any wound or skin lesions. Swabs should be immediately streaked into proper media, including a selective tellurite-containing medium, such as modified Tinsdale or Hoyle tellurite medium (on which the organism appears as a black colony with a gray-brown halo), blood agar, and a Loeffler slant, and then incubated at 35–37°C. Isolated organisms stained with Loeffler stain give the characteristic appearance of metachromatic granules. Confirmatory biochemical tests are required. If a delay in plating is unavoidable, the swab should be transported dry and then incubated overnight in broth that contains plasma or blood before plating. Suspicious colonies are stained by Gram stain and Albert stain. Prior antibiotic use may substantially reduce the yield of culture. Because most microbiology labs in the US lack the expertise and materials to reliably identify diphtheria, practitioners in the US should contact their local health department or the Centers for Disease Control and Prevention for guidance on correct handling of specimens.

Test for Toxigenicity

Toxigenicity is demonstrated by in vivo and in vitro tests. In vivo tests using guinea pigs are usually slow. In vitro tests are done by immunodiffusion, in which antitoxin-impregnated filter paper is laid over pure growth on solid blood agar culture media (Elek test). Polymerase chain reaction (PCR) detection of sequences from the toxin A subunit and enzyme immunoassay for toxin have also been developed. The results of an Elek test are usually available within 24–36 hrs. Use of an immunochromatographic strip test correlates well with the Elek test and may speed identification (20). The PCR test for the presence of tox$^+$ is the fastest, simplest, and most accurate test for toxigenicity. Because both toxigenic and nontoxigenic organisms may coexist in the same patient, at least 10 colonies from a primary culture plate should be tested for toxigenicity.

Additional tests are often performed to evaluate the extent of multisystem involvement. Cultures of blood or other affected sites should be performed as appropriate. Serial electrocardiograms can detect early changes of myocarditis and monitor conduction abnormalities. Cardiac enzymes may be measured to detect myocarditis; elevations in serum aspartate transaminase closely parallel severity of myocarditis. A chest x-ray and echocardiography should be obtained to assess the cardiac size and contractility, respectively. Platelet counts to detect thrombocytopenia, serum electrolytes, and blood urea nitrogen are obtained to assess renal injury.

Management

Emergency Room Management

Attention must first be given to the airway, breathing, and circulation (ABCs). Once these are stabilized, antitoxin therapy must be initiated immediately after taking appropriate specimens for culture. Airway problems must be anticipated in children who present with extensive disease and bull- neck. Use of accessory muscles of respiration is an indication for immediate

airway management. Airway should be secured early, as rapid progression of membrane may preclude a later opportunity. Tracheostomy serves as a better form of airway (31). Endotracheal intubation is difficult because of a friable upper airway and carries a high risk of dislodgement of the membrane. In patients with severe disease, hemodynamic monitoring should be established to detect early signs of myocarditis.

Indication for Transfer to the ICU

Patients with signs of airway obstruction or myocarditis should be transferred to the ICU immediately. Others who should be transferred to the ICU on priority include unimmunized patients, patients with delayed presentation to hospital (>5 days), delayed antitoxin therapy, or severe pharyngotonsillar disease. These patients are at high risk for systemic complications.

Isolation Policy

Patients with respiratory-tract diphtheria should be placed in strict isolation, which should be maintained until therapy has been completed and two cultures obtained at least 24 hrs apart after completion of antibiotic therapy are both negative. In situations in which initial cultures are negative due to prior antibiotic therapy, patients should be isolated until completion of antibiotic therapy.

Specific Management

The goals of specific therapy are neutralization of the circulating toxin, eradication of residual bacteria to halt further toxin production, and establishment of active immunity to diphtheria toxin.

Antitoxin. Diphtheria antitoxin acts by neutralizing the unbound toxin and prevents its binding to the cell membrane surface receptor cells. The dose of the antitoxin varies from 20,000 to 120,000 units, depending on the site of primary infection, the extent of pseudomembrane, and the delay between onset and seeking of medical advice. The usual recommended dose is 20,000–40,000 units for faucial diphtheria of <48-hr duration, 40,000–80,000 units for faucial diphtheria of >48-hr duration or laryngeal infection, and 60,000–120,000 units for severe toxic state with bull-neck. Therapy is usually given IV over 30–60 mins. Extensive late or complicated disease should always be treated with doses at the higher end of the range. As antitoxin is a horse serum preparation, it may provoke severe hypersensitivity reactions. A test dose of 50–100 units is recommended 30 min prior to giving the therapeutic dose. If any untoward reactions are observed, desensitization must be accomplished before the full dose is given.

Immediate initiation of treatment with antitoxin at the onset of respiratory illness has been shown to decrease mortality by ≥80% when compared with case fatality rates in those who receive antitoxin a week after onset (52). It may also prevent spread to susceptible contacts.

Antibiotics. In tox$^+$ infections, antimicrobial therapy eradicates organism, limits toxin production, and prevents locally invasive disease. However, antibiotics are adjuncts and not a substitute for antitoxin. Although C. *diphtheriae* is susceptible to a variety of antibiotics in vitro, only penicillin and erythromycin are recommended. Acceptable regimens include IV or IM aqueous crystalline penicillin G (100,000–150,000 units/kg/day in four divided doses), IM procaine penicillin G

(300,000 units for patients who weigh <10 kg and 600,000 units for patients who weigh >10 kg every 12 hrs; *OR* 25,000–50,000 units/kg/day in two divided doses), or erythromycin 50 mg/kg/day (maximum 2 g/day, orally or parenterally) in four divided doses. Therapy is given for 10–14 days. Erythromycin is the most effective drug for elimination of the carrier state. Antibiotic treatment usually renders patients noninfectious within 24 hrs. Untreated patients are infectious for 2 to 3 weeks. Elimination of the organism should be documented at a minimum of 2 weeks after completion of therapy with two negative cultures of nose, throat, and skin (as appropriate) 24 hrs apart. A course of erythromycin is given if end-of-treatment cultures remain positive.

Supportive Therapy

Once specific therapy has been started, monitoring and support of ABCs should continue. Complications should be anticipated and treated accordingly.

Of the treatment options available for diphtheritic myocarditis, neither carnitine nor pacing has been conclusively proven to be of any benefit. The importance of carnitine as a therapeutic agent in diphtheritic myocarditis first came to light from animal studies. Carnitine, a cofactor for the transport of fatty acids into the mitochondria, accumulates in the cytoplasm of cardiac cells, with resultant low serum carnitine. Carnitine depletion and fatty acid accumulation have been observed in patients with diphtheria as a consequence of ribosomal damage. Significant reduction in incidence of myocarditis and mortality following DL-carnitine therapy (100 mg/kg/day in two divided doses orally for 4 days) was observed in a large, case-controlled study of 625 patients (47). However, the literature contains no conclusive report regarding its role in prevention of myocarditis.

The severe systolic dysfunction that accompanies bundle branch blocks and complete heart blocks remains refractory to pharmacologic stimulation and inotropes. Benefit of ventricular pacing for advanced atrioventricular block remains doubtful, and mechanical response to electrical stimulation of the ventricle with pacing may be insufficient in patients with atrioventricular blocks. However, a prospective study from Vietnam suggests that temporary insertion of a pacemaker may improve the outcome in children with diphtheritic myocarditis with severe conduction defects (19).

Outcome and Prognosis

Overall, care fatality rate is 5%–10%. Mortality rates are higher at extremes of age, in severe form of disease, in unimmunized patients, and if antitoxin administration is delayed. Airway complications alone carry a good prognosis if managed in time (31). Mortality in diphtheritic myocarditis may be as high as 60%–70%. The need for inotropic support after pacemaker insertion is a poor prognostic sign (19). The risk of death is increased when bleeding occurs secondary to thrombocytopenia or renal failure. Generally, patients who survive diphtheria make a complete recovery. Persistent or progressive cardiac conduction defects have been reported years after the original episode. Some patients die suddenly and unexpectedly weeks after a full recovery. These deaths have been attributed to cardiac arrhythmias secondary to persistent subclinical myocarditis.

Prevention and Treatment of Contacts and Carriers

Clinical diphtheria does not confer natural immunity. Patients who recover from diphtheria should begin or complete active immunization with diphtheria toxoid during convalescence. Persons who have had close contact with diphtheria should have cultures obtained from nose, throat, and skin lesions and receive daily check for development of signs of diphtheria for 7 days. Contacts, regardless of immunization status, and carriers should receive oral erythromycin (40–50 mg/kg/day, maximum 2 g/day) for 7–10 days or IM benzathine penicillin (one dose of 0.6 mega units for patients <5 years of age and 1.2 mega units for those >5 years). The immunization status of the carriers and contacts should be assessed, and booster doses or primary series should be administered as needed. A total of five doses of combined diphtheria-tetanus-pertussis vaccine at ages 2, 4, 6, 15–18 months, and 5 years is recommended during primary immunization. Carriers should be placed in strict isolation (for respiratory tract colonization) or contact isolation (for cutaneous colonization) until at least two cultures taken 24 hrs apart at least 2 weeks after cessation of therapy are negative for *C. diphtheriae*. If cultures remain positive, a course of erythromycin should be repeated.

Conclusions and Future Directions

Early diagnosis, prompt administration of antitoxin and antibiotics, and chemoprophylaxis of close contacts and carriers remain the cornerstone of effective prevention and treatment of diphtheria. The primary focus in the developing world should be to ensure age-appropriate immunization universally. Effective therapy of myocarditis and polyneuropathy remains elusive. The future challenges are to find more effective modalities to prevent and treat these serious complications and to find simpler ways to immunize each and every susceptible host.

HUMAN BOTULISM

Human botulism is caused by the neurotoxin produced by *Clostridium botulinum* and, rarely, by *C. baratii* and *C. butyricum*. These organisms are ubiquitous, anaerobic, spore-forming, Gram-positive bacilli. The organism and its spores are found in all types of soil; in aquatic sediment from streams, lakes, and coastal waters; in the digestive system of fish and mammals; and in the viscera of shellfish and crabs. Once the spores are in a suitable environment, they germinate, begin to multiply, and produce toxin. Seven heat-labile, antigenic toxin subtypes of *C. botulinum* have been identified and are designated by the letters A through G. Types A, B, E, and, rarely, F cause human botulism. Toxin types C and D cause disease in animals. Type G has been isolated in soil but has not been implicated in human disease (4). Purified botulinum toxin type A is commercially available and is used for cosmetic indications, hyperhidrosis, cervical dystonia, and strabismus. Five specific forms of the disease are seen in humans, three of which are infant botulism, food-borne botulism, and wound botulism. The fourth form is thought to be due to intestinal sources and is observed only in patients >12 months of age with symptoms of botulism without a food or wound source of exposure. A fifth form is rarely seen as a complication of therapeutic use. Each form has its own epidemiology, pathogenesis, prognosis, and treatment. Inhalation botulism does not occur naturally but could potentially result from a biologic warfare application.

Toxin Mechanism

All of the toxin types have the same mechanism of action, which is blocking the release of acetylcholine from nerve endings. The toxin does not cross the blood brain barrier but does affect the neuromuscular junction, parasympathetic nerve endings, autonomic ganglia, and acetylcholine sympathetic nerve endings. The toxin enters the body through a wound or mucosal surface. Absorption of the toxin is rapid from the gastrointestinal tract. Toxin type E must first be activated by pancreatic enzymes to cause symptoms. Once in the bloodstream, the toxin enters the neuromuscular junction—specifically, the nerve terminus.

The light chain of the botulinum toxin cleaves one of the soluble N-ethylmaleimide-sensitive factor attachment protein receptor (SNARE) proteins (29). The SNARE proteins form a synaptic fusion complex and allow the acetylcholine-containing synaptic vesicle to fuse with the nerve terminus membrane. Which SNARE protein is cleaved depends upon the toxin type. Toxin types B, D, F, and G cleave synaptobrevin; types A, C, and E cleave SNAP-2; type C cleaves syntaxin. The disruption of any of the SNARE proteins prevents assembly of the synaptic fusion complex. Without this complex, the presynaptic acetylcholine vesicles cannot bind and release acetylcholine into the synaptic cleft, causing paralysis (**Fig. 83.5**). The nerve cell itself is uninjured by the toxin. Although recovery of synaptic function does occur, it may take months and is achieved through sprouting of new presynaptic axons by the nerve cell with the formation of an entirely new neuromuscular junction (4).

Infant Botulism

Infant botulism is due to ingestion of *C. botulinum* spores. Once in the digestive tract, the spores germinate and the bacteria multiply to colonize the intestines. Toxin is then produced and readily absorbed to cause disease. The colonization occurs

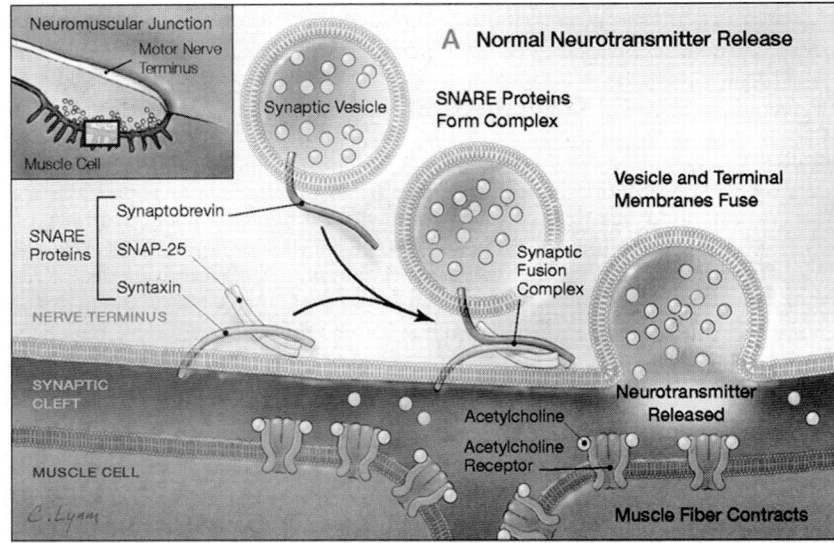

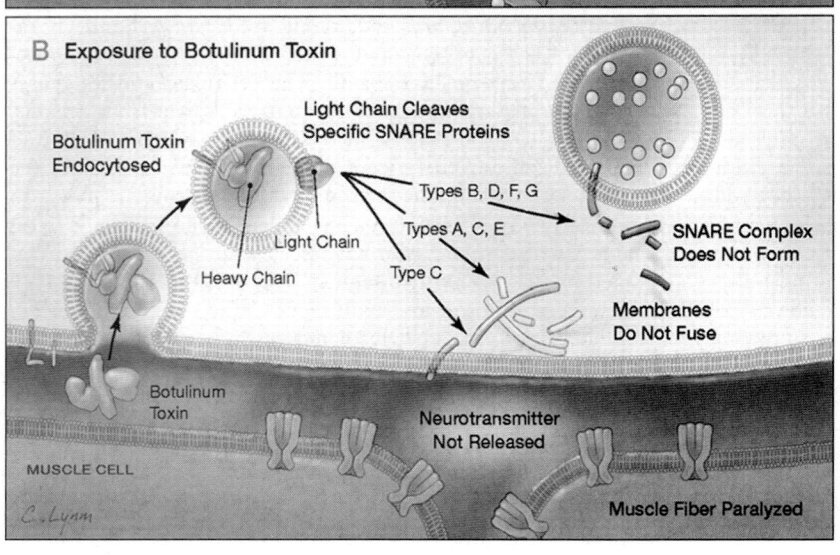

FIGURE 83.5. Mechanism of action of botulinum toxin. **A:** Release of acetylcholine at the neuromuscular junction is mediated by the assembly of a synaptic fusion complex that allows the membrane of the synaptic vesical that contains acetylcholine to fuse with the neuronal cell membrane. The synaptic fusion complex is a set of SNARE proteins, which include synaptobrevin, SNAP-25, and syntaxin. After membrane fusion, acetylcholine is released into the synaptic cleft and bound by receptors on the muscle cell. **B:** Botulinum toxin binds to the neuronal cell membrane at the nerve terminus and enters the neuron by endocytosis. The light chain of botulinum toxin cleaves specific sites on the SNARE proteins, preventing complete assembly of the synaptic fusion complex, thereby blocking acetylcholine release. Botulinum toxin types B, D, F, and G cleave synaptobrevin; types A, C, and E cleave SNAP-25; and type C cleaves syntaxin. Without acetylcholine release, the muscle is unable to contract. SNARE, soluble NSF-attachment protein receptor; NSF, N-ethylmaleimide-sensitive fusion protein; SNAP-25, synaptosomal-associated protein of 25 kd. From Arnon SS, Schechter R, Inglesby TV, et al. Botulinum toxin as a biologic weapon: Medical and public health management. *JAMA* 2001;285:1059–70, with permission.

in infants because the infant digestive tract lacks the normal intestinal flora to compete with and prevent the growth of *C. botulinum*. Older children and adults routinely ingest *C. botulinum* spores without developing disease due to competition from the normal intestinal flora (55). The transition from infant to adult intestinal flora usually occurs at between 6 and 12 months of age with the introduction of foods. For this reason, infant botulism is rarely if ever seen after the age of 1 year.

Epidemiology

Infant botulism is the most common form of disease caused by *C. botulinum* and its toxins, with an annual average of 1.9 reported cases per 100,000 live births in the US (28). Cases of infant botulism have been reported worldwide in all major racial and ethnic groups, with the exception of Africa (37). Given the prevalence of *C. botulinum* in the environment, the global incidence is likely higher than reported. Almost all cases in the US are caused by either toxin A or B, with a distinctive geographic distribution. Type A is more common from the West Coast to the Rocky Mountains, and type B is more common from the Mississippi River to the East Coast (28,37). California and Utah, along with the Mid-Atlantic states, particularly southeastern Pennsylvania and Delaware, have identified the most cases in the US. Approximately 94% of patients are <6 months of age, with equal gender prevalence (6). One study revealed differences in the risk factors based on age. Affected infants <2 months of age were more likely to live in a rural area, whereas those ≥2 months of age were more likely to be breast-fed and to have ingested corn syrup (56). One reason for the older age at presentation for breast-fed infants may be the introduction of solid foods. Feeding of solid foods to breast-fed infants causes a rapid change in the infant intestinal flora, with an increase in the numbers of *Enterobacteriaceae*, enterococci, *Bacteroides* species, *Clostridium* spp., and anaerobic streptococci. Similar changes are not seen with the introduction of solid food to the formula-fed infant's diet (6). In one study, it was found that infants with botulism who died of sudden infant death syndrome (SIDS) were all formula-fed and that breast-fed infants were disproportionately hospitalized. Researchers postulated that breast milk or factors associated with breast-feeding may have lessened the severity of symptoms to allow time to present to the hospital. Potential reasons included the presence of secretory antibodies in breast milk and differences in intestinal microbial flora between breast- and formula-fed infants (2).

The source of the spore exposure is not identified in the majority of cases. Where the source has been identified, it has typically been isolated in soil, honey, or household dust (37). The history at admission should include questions about soil exposure through gardening, construction, or ingestion of honey. Honey was once associated with ~35% of the reported infant botulism cases in the US, but preventive health counseling has diminished the association to less than 5% (3,35); a need for similar warnings to diminish honey-associated botulism in Europe has been noted (8). Changes in processing of corn syrup have been made in the US to eliminate the risk of infant botulism due to spore contamination, and commercial preparations of corn syrup are now considered safe for infants.

Clinical Features

Most cases of infant botulism have an insidious onset. The most common symptom is constipation, which may be iden-

tified only in hindsight after presentation with more severe symptoms. Clinical suspicion and careful physical examination are keys to making the diagnosis. No evidence of infection, such as fever, leukocytosis, or positive cultures in the absence of a complicating infection, is observed. Presenting symptoms are often vague. Most cases of infant botulism are admitted to the PICU. In one series, the frequency of signs noted at admission were weakness/floppiness (88%), poor feeding (79%), constipation (65%), lethargy or decreased activity (60%), poor cry, (18%), irritability (18%), respiratory difficulties (11%), and seizures (2%). Of note, once the diagnosis was suspected, further questioning obtained a history of constipation in all patients (50). The classic presentation is that of cranial nerve palsies associated with symmetric descending weakness in the face of a normal sensorium. Fatigue is noted on repetitive muscle contraction and can be elicited by repeated examination of the pupillary light reflex, with slowing of the pupil's constriction over 2–3 mins. Deep tendon reflexes diminish as the paralysis worsens. Autonomic effects are responsible for the constipation and may occasionally cause hypertension. Affected infants have a characteristic appearance (**Fig. 83.6**).

A subset of infant botulism cases has a more rapid course of progression that has been implicated as one potential cause of SIDS. It was recognized shortly after infant botulism was described that the peak incidence of infant botulism and SIDS closely overlapped (**Fig. 83.7**). Infant botulism as an etiology of SIDS has been further established by the isolation of botulinum toxin in the stool of children who died of SIDS. Typically, symptoms progress gradually over the week prior to presentation. These few rapidly progressive cases begin quickly and can progress over hours rather than days, with ensuing respiratory or cardiac arrest. The diagnosis of infant botulism may be delayed or even prevented due to this atypical presentation (39).

Diagnosis and Differential Diagnosis

Diagnosis leading to treatment must be made on clinical grounds to avoid delays in potential disease-shortening therapies. Electromyography (EMG) may be helpful in confirming the diagnosis. EMG findings consistent with botulism are small amplitude and overly abundant motor endplate potentials. During repetitive nerve stimulation at 20-Hz and 50-Hz stimulation, a staircase phenomenon is seen. EMG results will usually become positive during the course of the disease but may be equivocal or even negative at presentation. Therefore, a negative EMG study should not prevent treatment if the clinical signs and symptoms are compatible with botulism. In most but not all patients, the stool samples will have an assay positive for toxin or a culture positive for *C. botulinum* (50).

With the appearance of lethargy due to hypotonia, sepsis is a common admitting diagnosis. Infectious causes, such as sepsis, pneumonia, meningitis, and encephalitis, can be ruled out quickly due to the lack of fever, leukocytosis, or signs of inflammation. CSF studies will be normal to aid in ruling out meningitis, encephalitis, Guillain-Barré Syndrome, and poliomyelitis. The weakness in polio is usually asymmetric, which further differentiates it from infant botulism. Myasthenia gravis should not be considered without a history of maternal disease. Encephalopathy, as seen in heavy-metal poisoning or metabolic diseases, is not associated with a normal electroencephalogram, as would be expected in botulism. Normal

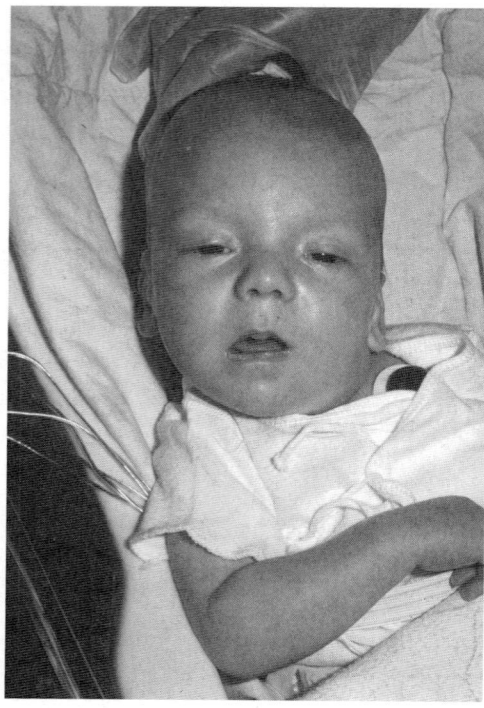
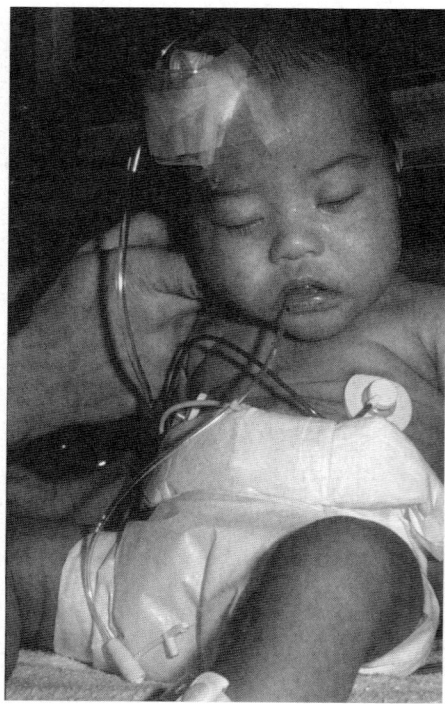

FIGURE 83.6. Photographs showing characteristic appearance of infants affected with botulism. Note the floppy appearance, poor head control, expressionless faces, and ptosis. Left photo is courtesy of Johnson RO, Clay SA, Arnon SS. Diagnosis and management of infant botulism. *Am J Dis Child* 1979;133:586–593. Right photo is courtesy of Infant Botulism Treatment and Prevention Program, California Department of Public Health.

electrolytes, acid-base status, ammonia, and liver transaminases eliminate electrolyte abnormalities, hepatic dysfunction, and metabolic disease from the differential diagnosis. Thyroid function testing will be normal, ruling out hypothy-roidism. Spinal muscular atrophy has a very similar presentation but can be differentiated by the EMG findings, the presence of tongue fasciculations, and definitively, by positive genetic testing.

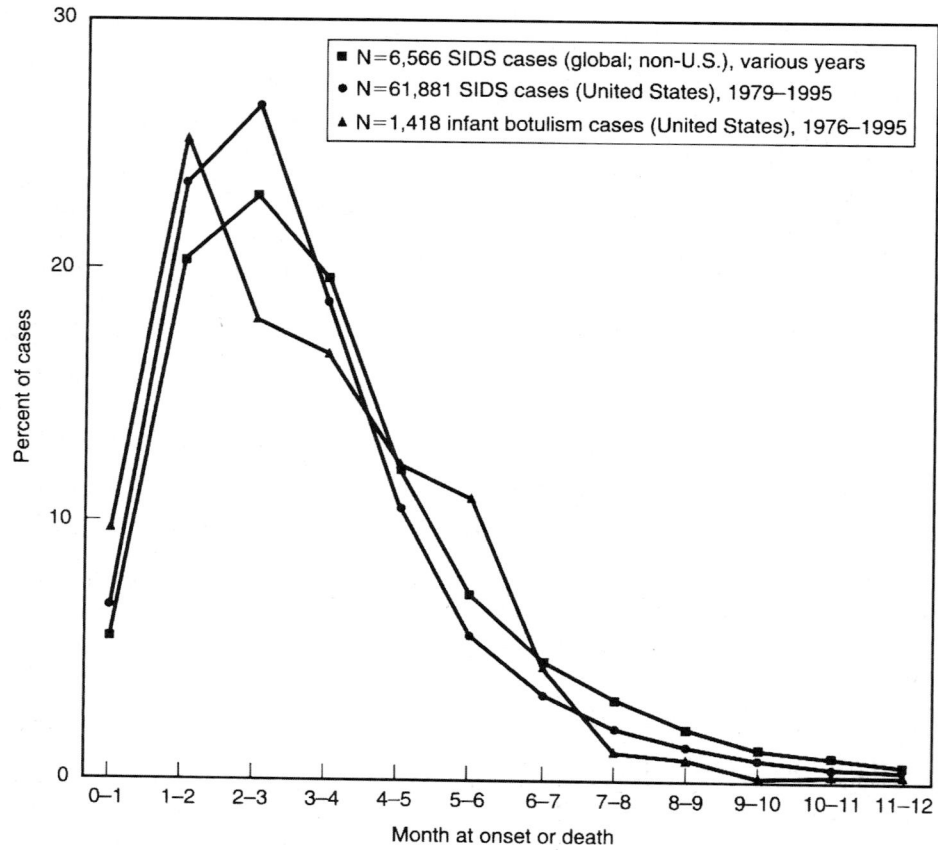

FIGURE 83.7. Epidemiologic data showing closely overlapped peak incidence of infant botulism and SIDS. From Arnon SS. Infant Botulism. In Feigin RD, Cherry J, eds. *Textbook of Pediatric Infectious Diseases, 5th ed.* Philadelphia: WB Saunders, 2003, with permission.

Treatment

Once the diagnosis of infant botulism is clinically made, specific therapy should be given as soon as possible, without delaying for confirmatory testing. Human botulism immune globulin as a single dose of 50 mg/kg is reserved for the treatment of infant botulism. Equine botulinum toxin used in adult forms of botulism should not be given to infants, as it is ineffective and confers a sensitization and anaphylaxis risk. Observations that most infants with botulism have detectable toxin in their serum prompted a placebo-controlled study to evaluate the efficacy of IV human botulism immune globulin derived from pooled plasma of immunized adult volunteers. The study showed that the immune globulin binds to botulinum toxin and prevents action at the neuromuscular junction. No effect was seen on toxin already bound at the neuromuscular junction making early administration crucial. This study demonstrated significant decreases in hospital length of stay and hospitalization costs when therapy was given within the first 3 days of hospitalization. Late administration has less dramatic effects. In the US, information on how to obtain botulism immune globulin can be obtained from the California Department of Health Services' Infant Botulism Treatment and Prevention Program at www.infantbotulism.org or calling 510–231-7600 (available around the clock) (5). Botulism immune globulin is only licensed for use in the US. Arrangements must be made in individual countries in accordance with regulations for acquisition and use of unlicensed medications.

Whether or not the child is treated with botulism immune globulin, the prognosis will be greatly affected by providing meticulous intensive care and preventing potential complications.

The overall goal of supportive treatment is to prevent nosocomial infections, skin breakdown, malnutrition, and airway complications until recovery of the neuromuscular junction is complete. Antibiotics are not indicated unless a complicating infection is involved. If antibiotics are used, aminoglycosides in particular should be avoided due to the risk of worsening the degree of weakness by effects on the neuromuscular junction. The airway and respiratory status should be closely monitored in an ICU until significant signs of improvement are noted. Monitoring of vital capacity, negative inspiratory force, the child's ability to adequately protect the airway, and arterial blood gases will help to determine the need for mechanical ventilation. Once intubation is required, the risks and benefits of tracheotomy must be carefully weighed. Most children can be managed without tracheotomy. Due to weakness, accidental extubation is rare; when it does occur, it is typically when the patient is being bathed, repositioned, etc. Tracheotomy greatly lengthens the duration of ICU admission. Nutrition should be given enterally via nasojejunal or nasogastric feeding tubes, as indicated (50).

Prognosis

In the US, the case-fatality ratio of infants with botulism who are admitted to the hospital is approaching zero. In areas that do not have PICU facilities, this is not the case. The true mortality rate of infant botulism is unknown and is dependent upon the number of SIDS cases that are due to botulinum intoxication. Children hospitalized with access to intensive care have an excellent prognosis for full recovery, as long as complications do not occur. The risk of such complications can be further min-imized by decreasing the length of hospitalization with the use of botulism immune globulin. Use of immune globulin within the first 3 days of hospitalization, compared to treatment during hospital days 4 through 7, and no treatment results in significantly shorter hospital admissions (2 vs. 2.9 vs. 5 weeks, respectively) (10,12).

Food-Borne Botulism

Epidemiology

Unlike infant botulism, food-borne botulism is caused by the ingestion of food contaminated with preformed botulinum toxin. The conditions for germination and growth of *C. botulinum* in food are fairly strict. Anaerobic conditions must exist, with a pH of >4.5, a low sugar and salt content, and a temperature between 4° and 121°C (55). In the US, 9.4–9.7 outbreaks occur annually that average ~2.5 cases per outbreak (28). Toxin types A, B, and E predominate in these cases, with a distinct epidemiologic distribution. Large outbreaks are usually associated with restaurants, whereas small outbreaks or single cases are usually related to home-prepared foods, such as home-canned vegetables, fruits, and fish products. Toxin type E is the most common in Alaskan Natives as a result of fish fermentation (54). The pH of the implicated products is usually >4.6.

Clinical Features

The initial symptoms of food-borne botulism are gastrointestinal. Abdominal pain, nausea, vomiting, and diarrhea occur shortly after ingestion of toxin but are usually not severe enough to cause the victim to seek medical care. Constipation is not seen until after the onset of neurologic symptoms (30,51), which occur 1–5 days after consumption of the toxin but usually within 18–36 hrs. Onset of neurologic symptoms can vary from person to person, even within the same outbreak. However, they do have a typical order of appearance. The first symptoms to occur are dry mouth due to autonomic nervous system involvement, diplopia from cranial nerve paralysis, and dilated pupils. These bulbar palsies progress to involve the facial muscles and then the muscles of the oropharynx, with symptoms of ptosis, facial droop, depressed gag reflex, dysphagia, dysarthria, and dysphonia. Cranial nerve involvement is complete once the neck muscles become involved. The paralysis continues to descend in a proximal-to-distal pattern, with diaphragmatic involvement typically prior to that of the lower extremities (30,51,55). The cranial nerve palsies will result in difficulty or inability to speak or swallow, the diaphragmatic involvement will lead to respiratory distress or failure, and the skeletal muscle involvement will interfere with movement. An important feature to recognize is that CNS and/or sensory function are not impaired. As in infant botulism, no signs of infection are seen, as food-borne botulism is an intoxication.

Diagnosis

The diagnosis of botulism is based on the recognition of the clinical syndrome. An isolated case, as would be seen with the index case or if affected individuals presented to different hospitals, has a limited differential diagnosis. Once a cluster of cases present with pathognomonic symptoms, as in an outbreak of food-borne botulism, the diagnosis should be straightforward because the diseases in the differential diagnosis of a single case do not cause outbreaks. Common diagnoses entertained in botulism cases are Guillain-Barré syndrome, cerebrovascular accident, myasthenia gravis, tick paralysis, and other intoxications, such as carbon monoxide, organophosphates, and mushrooms. The evaluation of these illnesses with CSF studies, cranial imaging, and Tensilon test will be negative in cases of botulism (28,51,55). EMG may be helpful in making the diagnosis of botulism. Important topics to cover when obtaining the patient's history include the presence of gastrointestinal symptoms and a careful food history of the preceding week, paying particularly close attention to use of home-canned foods, situations in which susceptible foods may have been inadequately stored, and ingestion of marine animals. Confirmatory testing is warranted but should not delay treatment with antitoxin. In food-borne botulism, 10 mL of serum, stool samples, suspect foods in their original containers, and vomitus or gastric secretions, especially if symptoms have recently started, should be tested (55).

Treatment

Antitoxin is the most important treatment modality. As the binding of the toxin at the neuromuscular junction is irreversible, the goal is to treat the patient with the equine-derived antitoxin before respiratory symptoms become severe enough to require prolonged ventilation. Late administration of antitoxin does little to shorten the hospital stay and may be of no benefit. In the US, patients are most commonly treated with trivalent antitoxin, which covers serotypes A, B, and E. Bivalent forms against serotypes A and B and a monovalent type E antitoxin are available in Alaska and Canada. The US Army has a heptavalent antitoxin preparation (serotypes A–G), which is indicated for all non-A, -B, and -E serotypes. The dose of the trivalent antitoxin for both adults and children is one vial diluted 1:10 in normal saline and given IV over 30–60 mins. Prior to administration, skin testing with horse serum is recommended. Some authors argue that the risk-benefit ratio favors administration without the skin test, especially if the symptoms are progressing rapidly or if respiratory muscle involvement is beginning. If skin testing is not performed, pretreatment with antihistamines and steroids is recommended. Regardless of whether a skin test has been completed, the antitoxin should be administered in an ICU environment, with the staff prepared to treat anaphylaxis. The incidence of a hypersensitivity reaction to the diluted antitoxin given slowly is 9%, with <1% of the recipients having serious reactions (30,55).

In addition to prompt treatment with antitoxin, patients require close monitoring in an ICU setting. The respiratory status should be closely monitored for deterioration, even after administration of the antitoxin. Vital capacity must be monitored and mechanical ventilation may be necessary. The paralysis associated with botulism can be lengthy; therefore, tracheotomy may be considered for severely affected individuals. Regardless, careful attention must be paid to preventing complications, such as nosocomial infections, skin breakdown, and neuromuscular injury from disuse, which are associated with prolong intensive care admissions.

Prognosis

Prior to the development of critical care as a medical subspecialty, the case fatality rate was >60%, even when high-dose equine antitoxin was used. Between 1950 and 1996, the case fatality rate dropped to 15.5%, and the most recent fatality rates reported are 3%–5% (28,55). Disease caused by type A toxin tends to have more severe symptoms and, as a result, has a higher fatality rate than types B and E (51).

Wound Botulism

Wound botulism is an extremely rare disease, but it has been reported in children. The classic at-risk wound is a crush injury, puncture wound, or gross trauma to an extremity. Toxin is released from bacteria in the wound into the bloodstream, producing neurologic symptoms as described for food-borne botulism. Inflammation, fever, and leukocytosis are often absent in wound botulism, making the diagnosis potentially more difficult. The diagnosis should be considered in a patient who presents with classic symptoms and an at-risk wound. Even wounds that do not appear to be infected should be explored with swabs, and wound exudates and tissue samples should be sent for anaerobic cultures and serum toxin levels. Prompt treatment with antitoxin, as described for food-borne botulism is indicated, even before laboratory results are available. The case fatality rate is estimated to be 15% (30).

Adult (Intestinal) Botulism

Intestinal botulism has a pathophysiology similar to infant botulism and a similar presentation. It is very rare and only occurs in patients with severe alteration of their intestinal bacterial flora, which favors the germination and growth of ingested spores. As a result, the onset of symptoms is more insidious than that seen in infant botulism. The diagnosis should be considered in immunosuppressed patients with the classic neuromuscular findings. Treatment is with botulinum antitoxin, as described in the food-borne botulism section. Confirmatory testing should include stool and serum for toxin, obtained prior to antitoxin administration, as well as stool cultures.

TOXIC SHOCK SYNDROME

TSS is an acute, toxin-mediated, multisystem, febrile illness caused by *S. aureus* and *S. pyogenes* (group A β-hemolytic streptococcus). It is characterized by high fever, hypotension, vomiting, and an erythematous rash that rapidly progress to variable degrees of multiorgan system failure with serious morbidity and mortality. The bacterial toxins that cause the disease have been labeled as "superantigens" due to their ability to bypass usual steps in the antigen-mediated immune response and activate the immune system directly. They bind directly to the major histocompatibility complex (Class II) to trigger a massive activation and expansion of T cells that display a specific β-chain variable region of T-cell receptor (30). Superantigens can stimulate over 20% of all T cells; in contrast, conventional antigen stimulates only 1 in 10,000 T cells. The TSS caused by the toxins of these two bacteria share certain features, but major differences are apparent in clinical signs, symptoms, morbidity, and mortality. Other bacteria that have been reported in association with TSS include non-group A β-hemolytic streptococci and *S. viridans*, *S. suis* (from China), and *Clostridium sordellii*.

Staphylococcal Toxic Shock Syndrome

Staphylococcal TSS has two forms: menstrual and nonmenstrual. More than 99% of menstrual TSS cases are associated with tampon use. Until the early 1980s, menstrual TSS accounted for the vast majority of reported cases; however, by 1990 nonmenstrual TSS exceeded menstrual TSS cases, possibly related to increased awareness and better reporting. Nonmenstrual TSS has been described in nonmenstruating women, children, and men and is associated with *S. aureus* colonization of nasal packing or focal infection, such as wound infection, soft tissue infections, lymphadenitis, sinusitis, tracheitis, empyema, abscesses, infection following burn, abortion, animal and insect bites, osteomyelitis, etc.

The incidence of menstrual TSS in the US is estimated to be ~1 per 100,000, with a case fatality rate of 3.3% (30). Lately, an increase in the incidence of menstrual TSS has been recorded, with the incidence lower in children than in adults (15). Menstrual TSS is caused by TSS toxin (TSST)-1 producing strains of *S. aureus*, which may colonize the vagina. Nonmenstrual TSS is caused by *S. aureus* that cause focal sites of staphylococcal infection (58). Most patients are merely colonized with the offending strain, though some have evidence of *S. aureus* bacteremia or deep tissue infection. The major toxins responsible for all of the manifestations of the disease are TSST-1 and enterotoxins A, B, and C (18). TSST-1 is found in nearly all cases of menstrual TSS and in 50% of nonmenstrual TSS, while enterotoxins are found in the other 50% of nonmenstrual TSS. The toxins act together as superantigens that stimulate the release of various cytokines, prostaglandins, and leukotrienes and are integral in the pathogenesis of the illness. The cytokines cause capillary leak, massive vasodilatation with extravasations of fluids and serum, and consequently, severe hypotension and multiorgan dysfunction. TSST-1 suppresses neutrophil chemotaxis, induces T-suppressor function, and blocks the reticuloendothelial system. Staphylococcal enterotoxins are pyrogenic and enhance susceptibility to lethal shock. Direct toxin-mediated organ injuries to kidney, liver or myocardium cannot be excluded.

Though the association of tampon use and TSS is very strong, the exact role of tampons in the pathogenesis of TSS remains unclear. Epidemiologic and in vitro studies suggest that these toxins are selectively produced in a clinical environment that consists of a neutral pH, a high Pco_2, and an "aerobic" Po_2. Similar conditions are found in the vagina with tampon use during menstruation.

TSST-1 produces an antibody response in vivo that is believed to be protective. A survey of 3012 menstruating women between the ages of 13 and 40 years showed that 81% of teenagers had protective antibody titers ($\geq$1:32) (44). Patients with TSS lack this protective response. A nonimmune host colonized with a toxin-producing organism that is exposed to growth conditions that induce toxin production is at risk for symptomatic disease.

Clinical Features

Menstrual TSS occurs during or within 2 days of onset or termination of menses. Nonmenstrual TSS is encountered in association with focal staphylococcal infections. The onset is abrupt, with high fever ($\geq$39°C), headache, vomiting, diarrhea, and myalgia, rapidly progressing to hypotension and shock. A diffuse erythematous rash that resembles sunburn appears within 24 hrs and may be associated with hyperemia of pharyngeal, conjunctival, and vaginal mucus membrane. Impairment of consciousness can result in somnolence, agitation, disorientation, and obtundation. Gastrointestinal involvement is often pronounced, with diffuse abdominal pain. Diarrhea is watery, without blood or fecal leukocytes. Renal involvement manifests with pyuria, hematuria, oliguria, and in extreme cases with acute renal failure often in combination with profound hypotension. Recovery from TSS starts within 7–10 days. It is associated with desquamation, particularly of palms and soles; hair and nail loss may occur after 1–2 months. Clinicians must remember that desquamation is a feature of convalescence and that its initial absence does not exclude the diagnosis.

Complications of TSS include acute renal failure, acute respiratory distress syndrome (ARDS), disseminated intravascular coagulation, electrolyte imbalance (hypocalcemia, hypophosphatemia, and hypomagnesemia), rhabdomyolysis, cardiomyopathy, and encephalopathy. Nonmenstrual TSS is more likely to cause renal and CNS complications.

Laboratory Investigations

Nonspecific laboratory abnormalities are found in >85% of affected patients. Leukocytosis and moderate thrombocytopenia are common, as are mildly elevated serum transaminase levels. Pyuria, proteinuria, and elevated blood urea nitrogen and creatinine may be seen. These urinary changes are not related to direct infection of the urinary tract by the staphylococci. Approximately 40% of patients may have elevated serum creatine phosphokinase levels more than twice the normal range; a few patients may also have myoglobinuria. Symptomatic hypocalcemia has been observed in a few patients.

Diagnosis and Differential Diagnosis

The diagnosis of TSS is based on clinical signs, and no rapid definitive diagnostic test exists. The Centers for Disease Control and Prevention has established a set of diagnostic criteria based on clinical and laboratory findings (**Table 83.7**). When the illness lacks one of the defining criteria, the term *probable TSS* is used.

The differential diagnosis of TSS is broad (**Table 83.8**). Fever, vomiting, and diarrhea may mimic gastroenteritis. High fever, headache, myalgias, vomiting, and rash may mimic any acute viral infection. Progression to impaired consciousness that results in somnolence, agitation, disorientation, or obtundation may necessitate a lumbar tap to exclude a diagnosis of bacterial meningitis. When headache, disorientation, and thrombocytopenia dominate the clinical picture, the condition may resemble meningococcemia. In its milder forms, TSS may resemble Kawasaki disease because of fever, rash, and desquamation. Hypotension and renal failure are not characteristic of Kawasaki disease. Conversely, lymphadenopathy, a major criterion for diagnosis of Kawasaki disease, is usually absent in TSS. The other diagnosis most commonly entertained in cases of TSS is scarlet fever. The typical epidemiologic setting and the absence of pharyngeal GAS are the most important differential features. The characteristic rash of TSS allows differentiation from all other entities.

TABLE 83.7

CENTERS FOR DISEASE CONTROL AND PREVENTION CLINICAL CASE DEFINITION OF STAPHYLOCOCCAL TOXIC SHOCK SYNDROME

An illness with the following clinical manifestations:
- Fever—temperature $\geq$38.9°C (102°F)
- Rash—diffuse macular erythroderma
- Desquamation—1–2 weeks after onset of illness, particularly palms and soles
- Hypotension—systolic blood pressure $\leq$90 mm Hg for adults or less than fifth percentile by age for children <16 years of age; orthostatic drop in diastolic blood pressure $\geq$15 mm Hg from lying to sitting, orthostatic syncope, or orthostatic dizziness
- Multisystem involvement—three or more of the following:

Gastrointestinal: vomiting or diarrhea at onset of illness

Muscular: severe myalgia or creatine phosphokinase level at least twice the upper limit of normal for laboratory

Mucous membrane: vaginal, oropharyngeal, or conjunctival hyperemia

Renal: blood urea nitrogen or creatinine at least twice the upper limit of normal for laboratory or urinary sediment with pyuria ($\geq$5 leukocytes per high-power field) in the absence of urinary tract infection

Hepatic: total bilirubin, serum alanine aminotransferase (ALT), or serum aspartate aminotransferase (AST), at least twice the upper limit of normal for laboratory

Hematologic: platelets <100,000/mm^3

Central nervous system: disorientation or alterations in consciousness without focal neurologic signs when fever and hypotension are absent
- Negative results on the following tests, if obtained:
  1. Blood, throat, or cerebrospinal fluid cultures (blood culture may be positive for *S. aureus*)
  2. Rise in titer to Rocky Mountain spotted fever, leptospirosis, or measles

Case classification

Probable: A case with five of the six clinical findings described above

Confirmed: A case with all six of the clinical findings described above, including desquamation, unless the patient dies before desquamation occurs.

Adapted from Centers for Disease Control and Prevention. Case definition for public health surveillance *MMWR* 1990;39:38–9.

TABLE 83.8

DIFFERENTIAL DIAGNOSIS IN TOXIC SHOCK SYNDROME

Infectious	Noninfectious
Acute viral syndrome	Kawasaki disease
Acute gastroenteritis	Acute rheumatic fever
Acute pyelonephritis	Systemic lupus
Legionnaire disease	erythematosus
Leptospirosis	Thrombophlebitis
Lyme disease	Tumor
Meningococcemia/	Hematoma
meningococcal meningitis	Hemolytic uremic
Typhus	syndrome
Streptococcal scarlet fever	
Rocky Mountain spotted fever	
Septic shock	

Adapted from Herzer CM. Toxic shock syndrome: Broadening the differential diagnosis. *J Am Board Fam Pract* 2001;14:131–6.

Treatment

Immediate and aggressive management of shock forms the cornerstone of management. To ensure adequate perfusion of vital organs, volume replacement with appropriate crystalloids and colloids is a must. Vasoactive therapy may be required to normalize blood pressure and to improve perfusion once volume repletion is accomplished. Hypoproteinemia may worsen peripheral edema, but colloids should be used with extreme caution in a setting of leaky capillaries. Children are more likely to require respiratory support.

All possible sites of staphylococcal infection must be examined to remove preformed toxin and to stop further toxin production. Infected wounds and necrotizing skin lesions should be debrided immediately. All packings and foreign objects, including retained tampons, should be removed. Abscesses should be drained and irrigated.

Parenteral administration of a β-lactamase-resistant, antistaphylococcal antibiotic is recommended after appropriate cultures have been taken. Cloxacillin, oxacillin, or nafcillin in combination with aminoglycosides are the first-line agents. Clindamycin or vancomycin can be used in patients who are allergic to penicillin. Addition of clindamycin in severe cases will halt toxin production. Therefore, clindamycin should be used in combination with a β-lactamase-resistant, antistaphylococcal antibiotic for the first few days to decrease the synthesis of

TSST-1. No prospective study on antibiotic use in treating TSS has been reported.

Antibiotics do not shorten the duration of acute illness but are useful in decreasing the organism load, the risk of bacteremia, and the rate of relapse. Treatment of an acute episode of TSS with a β-lactamase-resistant antibiotic is believed to decrease the likelihood of recurrent TSS. Eradication of toxigenic strains of *S. aureus* may require prolonged antibiotics (1). Some studies have recommended a 2-week course of antistaphylococcal antibiotic, wherein elimination of carriage is important. Use of combination therapy with rifampicin, mupirocin, or both might decrease the risk of recurrence by eliminating carriage. Further studies should be conducted.

IV immunoglobulin (IVIG), 1 g/kg for 2 days, is suggested for severe cases in which conventional therapies fail to control symptoms, although its efficacy has not been confirmed. As the diseases occur in patients who are seronegative to the implicated staphylococcal toxins, IVIG probably provides the needed antibodies to neutralize the antitoxin. In vitro studies suggest that staphylococcal superantigens are not inhibited as efficiently as streptococcal superantigens by IVIG; hence, a higher dose of IVIG may be required for therapy of staphylococcal TSS (16). Plasma exchange has been found to reduce circulating toxins and mediators of TSS. Corticosteroids are not effective.

Outcome and Prognosis

The overall fatality rate from TSS in children has been reported to be 3%–5% (15). Sequelae include prolonged muscle weakness, abnormal renal function, behavioral changes, and memory impairment.

One of the striking features of TSS is its propensity to recur. Several reports of recurrent menstrual and nonmenstrual TSS can be found in the literature. Failure to eradicate colonization with *S. aureus* predisposes the patient to recurrent nonmenstrual TSS. Women with recurrent menstrual TSS have persistent colonization with a toxigenic strain of *S. aureus* and persistent absence of neutralizing antibody. For women who have recurrent menstrual TSS, tampon use should be discontinued and oral antistaphylococcal antibiotics should be administered before and during each menstrual period until anti-TSST-1 titers rise. Patient education about proper use of tampons and recognition of early signs of disease are important.

Streptococcal Toxic Shock Syndrome

Streptococcal TSS (STSS) is a severe, potentially fatal form of infection caused by invasive GAS. It is characterized by early shock and multiorgan failure. Whereas staphylococcal TSS is often associated with colonization, GAS TSS most often accompanies invasive GAS infection. Population-based studies in Canada and the US have documented an annual incidence of invasive GAS infection of 1.5–5.2 cases/10,000 population, with higher incidence at the extremes of age. Approximately 8%–14% of patients with invasive GAS infection have associated STSS (11), and its presence increases case fatality.

Pathogen and Pathogenesis

GAS is a Gram-positive organism. It is classified by the presence of surface proteins, primarily M and T antigens. The strains that are encapsulated and rich in M protein are more virulent.

Most of the strains responsible for STSS have M protein types 1 and 3. Extracellular products of GAS include the hemolysins streptolysin O and streptolysin S and pyrogenic exotoxins A, B, C, and F. The streptococcal exotoxins possess superantigenic properties and trigger massive T-cell proliferation and cytokine release in the same way as staphylococcal superantigens. A strong association between infection with strains that produce pyrogenic exotoxin A gene and STSS has been reported (21). The factors that determine the severity of infection are not fully understood. Protective antibody levels to specific M protein and streptococcal superantigens are lower in patients with invasive streptococcal infection and STSS as compared to healthy controls (10).

Clinical Features

In children, STSS commonly occurs following varicella or during the use of nonsteroidal anti-inflammatories (15); in others, the focus could be pharyngitis (14). Onset is abrupt with fever, vomiting, diarrhea, and early shock, just as with staphylococcal TSS. In STSS associated with necrotizing fasciitis, pain is the most common initial symptom; it is severe and out of proportion to physical findings and usually involves an extremity or the abdomen. Influenza-like syndrome, consisting of fever, nausea, vomiting, and diarrhea, may occur in 20% of patients. Hypotension may be a presenting sign or develop shortly after presentation. Hypothermia may occur in patients with shock. Confusion is present in more than half of the patients. Erythematous rash, as seen in staphylococcal TSS, is seen only in 10% cases of STSS. Eight percent of patients have clinical signs of soft tissue infection, such as localized swelling and erythema, which often progress to necrotizing fascitis and myositis and require surgical debridement, fasciotomy, or amputation. In 20% of patients without soft tissue infection, clinical symptoms may suggest endophthalmitis, myositis, perihepatitis, peritonitis, myocarditis, or overwhelming sepsis.

The systolic blood pressure normalizes within 4–8 hrs with antibiotics, fluids, and vasoactive agents in 10% of patients only. In most cases, the shock persists and organ dysfunction may progress. Multiorgan dysfunction may precede shock. Renal failure progresses with 48–72 hrs, and many patients may require dialysis. ARDS is seen in nearly half of patients, with the majority requiring mechanical ventilation. Coagulopathy with disseminated intravascular coagulation is frequently present on admission. Rarely severe thrombotic, disseminated, intravascular coagulation in the form of purpura fulminans has been reported.

Diagnosis

The criteria for diagnosis of STSS have been defined (**Table 83.9**). In a child with fever, diarrhea, vomiting, and abdominal pain, rapid onset of septic shock should raise the possibility of STSS. A search for site of infection and early multiorgan dysfunction should be made.

Laboratory Investigation

Renal involvement is indicated by the presence of hemoglobinuria and by serum creatinine values that are usually >2.5 times normal; creatine kinase level is useful in detecting deeper soft-tissue infections. Mild leukocytosis may be seen as in any other infection, but more striking is the left shift. The percentage of immature neutrophils (band forms, metamyelocytes, and myelocytes) can reach 40%–50%.

TABLE 83.9

CASE DEFINITION OF STREPTOCOCCAL TOXIC SHOCK SYNDROME

A. Isolation of group A Streptococcus
  1. From a sterile site
  2. From a nonsterile body site
B. Clinical signs of severity
  1. Hypotension
  2. Clinical and laboratory abnormalities (requires 2 or more of the following):
     a) Renal impairment
     b) Coagulopathy
     c) Liver abnormalities
     d) ARDS
     e) Extensive tissue necrosis, i.e., necrotizing fasciitis
     f) Generalized erythematous rash

Streptococcal toxic shock syndrome is defined as any group A streptococcal infection associated with the early onset of shock and organ failure.
Definite case = A1 + B(1 + 2); Probable case = A2 + B(1 + 2)
Adapted from The Working Group on Severe Streptococcal Infections. Defining the group A streptococcal toxic shock syndrome. Rationale and consensus definition. *JAMA* 1993;269:390–1.

Hypocalcemia, hypoalbuminemia, and elevated liver transaminases are commonly found at the time of admission. Bacteremia is common in STSS (15). Cultures from sites of infection, including tissue taken at surgery, CSF, pleural fluid, and synovial fluid, can yield organism in up to 95% of cases.

Treatment

The goals of management are removal of the source of toxin (appropriate antibiotic therapy and surgical debridement of necrotic tissues), neutralization of toxin (IVIG therapy), and aggressive supportive therapy for shock (fluids and vasopressors) and multiorgan failure.

GAS remains sensitive to penicillin, but aggressive GAS infection responds less well to penicillin. It has been suggested that failure of penicillin is these situations is because of the Eagle effect, wherein a high inoculum of organisms reaches a stationary phase of growth more quickly, making penicillin less effective. Penicillin and other β-lactams are more efficacious against rapidly growing bacteria.

Clindamycin is more efficacious, as it is a potent suppressor of bacterial toxin production and is not affected by the size of the inoculum or stage of growth. It facilitates phagocytosis of streptococcus by inhibiting M-protein synthesis. Clindamycin possesses a longer postantibiotic effect than β-lactams and causes suppression of lipopolysaccharide-induced monocyte synthesis of tumor necrosis factor. Studies have demonstrated a lower fatality rate with clindamycin use in GAS-necrotizing fasciitis. Therefore, an antibiotic combination of high-dose penicillin and clindamycin should be given when concomitant invasive GAS infection is suspected. Depending on the clinical presentation, particularly if it includes necrotizing fasciitis, empirical simultaneous coverage for Gram negatives, anaerobes, and possibly *S. aureus* might be considered until a specific organism is identified.

The presence of necrotizing fasciitis or myositis mandates immediate surgical debridement and constitutes a surgical

emergency. The rapidity with which the infection spreads often outpaces the rate of surgical debridement. Most patients may require a second debridement procedure to ensure that all necrotic, infected, and devitalized tissue is removed

Neutralization of circulating toxin is desirable, and it is in this context that the role of IVIG in TSS has emerged. IVIG has been shown to inhibit the activation of T cells by superantigens and to downregulate the production of tumor necrosis factor-α. Commercial IVIG contains neutralizing antibodies to streptococcal exotoxin. Although inconclusive, evidence suggests that IVIG in STSS confers a survival benefit (17). IVIG is usually given in a dose of 1 g/kg for 2 days at the slightest suspicion of STSS.

Supportive management of shock and multiorgan failure form the main thrust of therapy. Volume deficits are massive due to external and interstitial loss, combined with peripheral vasodilatation and peripheral pooling. Vasopressors are required after adequate volume replenishment as in any septic shock. Frequent hemodynamic monitoring, including urine output, acid-base status, and lactate levels, should be performed to assess organ perfusion. Patients should also be monitored for development and progression of multiorgan dysfunction.

Most patients with STSS require tracheal intubation and mechanical ventilation for septic shock and for complicating ARDS. The role of hyperbaric oxygen in STSS remains uncertain.

Prognosis

Prognosis of STSS is worse than staphylococcal TSS. Mortality associated with STSS in children is 5%–10%, much lower than that in adults (30%–70%) (15). Beneficial effects of prophylactic antibiotics for prevention of STSS in burn patients have been suggested, but no consensus has been reached regarding their use (48).

CONCLUSION AND FUTURE DIRECTIONS

Early diagnosis based on "defined" clinical criteria, antibiotics, supportive fluid, and vasoactive drug therapy remain the mainstay of management of TSS. IVIG is the most successful adjunctive therapy.

A better understanding of the molecular mechanism, pathogenesis, and host characteristics may help in developing more definite rapid diagnostic and therapeutic options for this potentially fatal condition. Development of specific antitoxin(s) that can neutralize the toxins that mediate TSS is necessary. Other priorities include evaluating antibiotic options and defining more precisely the role of IVIG.

KEY POINTS

Tetanus

- Tetanus is caused by infection with *C. tetani, which* elaborates a toxin designated tetanospasmin, which blocks release of inhibitory neurotransmitters, and causes uninhibited sustained muscle contraction.

- Worldwide, between 500,000 and 1 million cases occur per year.
- Trismus and risus sardonicus are most common initial symptoms, progressing gradually to generalized rigidity and muscle spasms. Mental status is not affected. Cranial nerve palsies occur in cephalic tetanus. Signs of autonomic dysfunction, such as hypertension and tachyarrhythmias, occur 5–7 days after the onset of generalized spasms.
- Diagnosis is made on clinical grounds alone: no laboratory test is needed.
- Treatment in the ICU is focused on: neutralization of circulating toxin with HTIG: 500 IU; early intubation/tracheostomy if frequent generalized, pharyngeal or laryngeal spasms occur, penicillin or metronidazole; control of muscle spasms with IV benzodiazepines or with neuromuscular blockade, using vecuronium in severe cases; and control of hypertension and tachycardia with propranolol or labetalol and morphine.
- All survivors must be vaccinated.

Diphtheria

- Diphtheria is a severe, widespread infectious disease that has the potential to reach epidemic proportions. Large epidemics occurred in Eastern Europe and the former Soviet Union in the 1990s. Worldwide, diphtheria caused 5000 deaths in 2002.
- Most infections are localized at a mucocutaneous site and can result in severe disease if produced by a toxigenic strain of *C. diphtheriae*, manifested by tonsillopharyngitis (in 90% cases) and pseudomembrane formation. The toxin also can cause serious systemic toxic effects, including myocarditis and polyneuritis.
- Isolation of *C. diphtheriae* from a clinical specimen or fourfold or greater rise in serum antibody confirms the diagnosis.
- Treatment consists of immediate administration of diphtheria antitoxin and antibiotics (penicillin or erythromycin), admission to an isolation room in the ICU for airway management (intubation/tracheostomy), administration of oxygen, and monitoring of cardiac function (heart rate, blood pressure, electrocardiogram).
- All survivors must be immunized. All close contacts should be cultured, observed daily for signs of diphtheria for 7 days, and given antibiotic regardless of immunization status (oral erythromycin for 7–10 days or 1 dose of IM benzathine penicillin). In addition, immunized household contacts should receive a booster dose of toxoid, and unimmunized household contacts should receive primary immunization.
- Primary control of disease can be achieved with high population immunity (>90%).

Human Botulism

- Botulism is caused by neurotoxin(s) produced by *C. botulinum*.
- Neurologic symptoms start with autonomic signs and oculobulbar muscle weakness, followed by symmetric descending weakness of limbs. Sensory system and mentation are usually spared.
- Diagnosis is based on clinical syndrome to avoid delays in therapy. Detection of toxin in patient's serum, stool, or suspect foods confirms diagnosis.
- Infants should receive human botulism immune globulin; other patients should receive equine botulinum toxin.
- Supportive treatment should include support of airway and respiratory status. Elective intubation should be considered.
- An association exists between infant botulism and SIDS.

Toxic Shock Syndrome

- TSS is an acute, toxin-mediated, multisystem, febrile illness mainly caused by *S. aureus* and GAS.
- TSS is characterized by abrupt onset of high fever, vomiting, and erythematous rash that rapidly progress to hypotension and variable degrees of multiorgan failure.
- The bacterial toxins that cause the disease have been labeled as "superantigens."
- Staphylococcal TSS has two forms: menstrual (associated with tampon use) and nonmenstrual. TSST-1 is found in nearly all cases of menstrual TSS and in 50% of nonmenstrual TSS, while enterotoxins are found in the other 50% of nonmenstrual TSS.
- Streptococcal TSS is characterized by early shock and multiorgan failure and often accompanies invasive infections (e.g., rapidly progressive necrotizing fasciitis), sometimes in previously healthy patients.
- The goals of management are removal of the source of toxin, appropriate antibiotic therapy, surgical debridement of necrotic tissues, neutralization of toxin with IVIG therapy (1 g/kg for 2 days), and aggressive supportive therapy for shock (fluids and vasopressors) and multiorgan failure. Clindamycin is recommended for streptococcal TSS and in combination with a β-lactamase-resistant antistaphylococcal antibiotic (cloxacillin, oxacillin, or nafcillin) for staphylococcal TSS.
- Most patients require tracheal intubation and mechanical ventilation for shock and for complicating ARDS.
- Prognosis of streptococcal TSS is worse than staphylococcal TSS.

References

1. Andrews MM, Parent EM, Barry M, et al. Recurrent non-menstrual toxic shock syndrome: Clinical manifestations, diagnosis and treatment. *CID* 2001;32:1470–9.
2. Arnon SS, Damus K, Thompson B, et al. Protective role of human milk against sudden death from infant botulism. *J Pediatr* 1982;100:568–73.
3. Arnon SS, Midura TF, Damus K, et al. Honey and other environmental risk factors for infant botulism. *J Pediatr* 1979;94:331–6.
4. Arnon SS, Schechter R, Inglesby TV, et al. Botulinum toxin as a biological weapon: Medical and public health management. *JAMA* 2001;285:1059–70.
5. Arnon SS, Schechter R, Maslanka SE, et al. Human botulism immune globulin for the treatment of infant botulism. *N Engl J Med* 2006;354:462–71.
6. Arnon SS. Infant botulism: Anticipating the second decade. *J Infect Dis* 1986; 154:201–6.
7. Attygalle D, Rodrigo N. Magnesium as first line therapy in the management of tetanus: A prospective study of 40 patients. *Anaesthesia* 2002;57:811–17.
8. Aureli P, Franciosa G, Fenicia L. Infant botulism and honey in Europe: A commentary. *Pediatr Infect Dis J* 2002;21:866–8.

9. Baranwal AK, Singhi SC. Hyperextension of spine: Unusual presentation of Guillain Barré syndrome. *Arch Dis Child* 2002;87:359.

10. Basma H, Norrby-Teglund A, Guedez Y, et al. Risk factors in the pathogenesis of invasive Group A streptococcal infections: Role of protective humoral immunity. *Inf Immun* 1999;67:1871–7.

11. Baxter F, McChesney J. Severe Group A Severe streptococcal infection and streptococcal toxic shock syndrome. *Can J Anesth* 2000;47:1129–40.

12. Bleck TP, Brauner JS. Tetanus. In: Scheld WM, Whitley RJ, Durack DT, eds. *Infections of the Central Nervous System*, 3rd ed. Philadelphia: Raven, 2003;625–48.

13. Brauner JS, Vieira SR, Bleck TP. Changes in severe accidental tetanus mortality in the ICU during two decades in Brazil. *Intensive Care Med* 2002;28: 930–5.

14. Chiang MC, Jaing TH, Wu CT, et al. Streptococcal toxic shock syndrome in children without skin and soft tissue infection: Report of four cases. *Acta Paediatr* 2005;94:763–5.

15. Chuang YY, Huang YC, Lin TY. Toxic shock syndrome in children: Epidemiology, pathogenesis, and management. *Paediatr Drugs* 2005;7: 11–25.

16. Darenberg J, Soderquist B, Normark BH, et al. Differences in potency of intravenous polyspecific immunoglobulin G against streptococcal and staphylococcal superantigens: Implications for therapy of toxic shock syndrome. *Clin Infect Dis* 2004;38:836–42.

17. Darenberg J, Ihendyane N, Sjolin J, et al. Intravenous immunoglobulin G therapy for streptococcal toxic shock syndrome: A European randomized double blind placebo controlled trial. *Clin Infect Dis* 2003;37:333–40.

18. Dinges MM, Orwin PM, Schievert PM. Exotoxins of *Staphylococcus aureus*. *Clin Microbiol Rev* 2000;13:16–34.

19. Dung NM, Kneen R, Kiem N, et al. Treatment of severe diphtheritic myocarditis by temporary insertion of a cardiac pacemaker. *Clin Infect Dis* 2002;35:1425–9.

20. Engler KH, Efstratiou A, Norn D, et al. Immunochromatographic strip test for rapid detection of diphtheria toxin: Description and multicenter evaluation in areas of low and high prevalence of diphtheria. *J Clin Microbiol.* 2002;40(1):80–3.

21. Eriksson BKG, Andersson J, Holm SE, et al. Invasive Group A streptococcal infections: TIMI isolates expressing pyrogenic exotoxins A and B in combination with selective lack of toxin-neutralising antibodies are associated with increased risk of streptococcal toxic shock syndrome. *J Infect Dis* 1999;180:410–8.

22. Fischer M, Bhatnagar J, Guarner J, et al. Fatal toxic shock syndrome associated with Clostridium sordellii after medical abortion. *N Engl J Med.* 2005;353(22):2352–60.

23. Galazka A. The changing epidemiology of diphtheria in the vaccine era. *J Infect Dis* 2000;181:S2–9.

24. Ganesh Kumar AV, Kothari VM, Krishnan A, et al. Benzathine penicillin, metronidazole and benzyl penicillin in the treatment of tetanus: A randomized controlled trial. *Ann Trop Med Parasitol* 2004;98:59–63.

25. Geneviva GD, Thomas NJ, Kees-Folts D. Magnesium sulfate for control of muscle rigidity and spasms and avoidance of mechanical ventilation in pediatric tetanus. *Pediatr Crit Care Med* 2003;4:480–4.

26. Gidding HF, Backhouse JL, Burgers MA, et al. Immunity to diphtheria and tetanus in Australia: A national serosurvey. *Med J Aust* 2005;183:301–4.

27. Hadfield TL, McEnvoy P, Polotsky Y, et al. The pathology of diphtheria. *J Infect Dis* 2000;181:S116–20.

28. *Handbook for Epidemiologists, Clinicians, and Laboratory Workers.* Atlanta, GA: Centers for Disease Control and Prevention; 1998.

29. Horowitz BZ. Botulinum toxin. *Crit Care Clin* 2005;21:825–39.

30. Issa NC, Thompson RL. Staphylococcal toxic shock syndrome: Suspicion and prevention are keys to control. *Postgrad Med* 2001;110:55–62.

31. Jayashree M, Shruthi N, Singhi S. Predictors of outcome in patients with diphtheria receiving intensive care. *Indian Pediatr* 2006;43:155–60.

32. Kabura L, Ilibagiza D, Menten J, et al. Intrathecal vs. intramuscular administration of human antitetanus immunoglobulin or equine tetanus antitoxin in the treatment of tetanus: A meta-analysis. *Trop Med Int Health* 2006;11:1075–81.

33. Kneen R, Nguyen MD, Solomon T, et al. Clinical features and predictors of diphtheritic cardiomyopathy in Vietnamese children. *Clin Infect Dis* 2004;39:1591–8.

34. Krumina A, Logina I, Donaghy M, et al. Diphtheria with polyneuropathy in a closed community despite receiving recent booster vaccination. *J Neurol Neurosurg Psychiatr* 2005;76:1555–7.

35. Lumio JT, Groundstroem KW, Huhtala H, et al. Electrocardiographic abnormalities in patients with diphtheria: A prospective study. *Am J Med* 2004;116:78–83.

36. Mazzei de Davila CA, Davila DF, Donis JH, et al. Autonomic nervous system dysfunction in children with severe tetanus: Dissociation of cardiac and vascular sympathetic control. *Braz J Med Biol Res* 2003;36:815–9.

37. Midura TF. Update: Infant botulism. *Clin Microbiol Rev* 1996;9(2):119–25.

38. Miranda-Filho DB, Ximenes RA, Barone AA, et al. Randomized controlled trial of tetanus treatment with antitetanus immunoglobulin by the intrathecal or intramuscular route. *BMJ* 2004;328:615–7.

39. Mitchell WG, Tseng-Ong L. Catastrophic presentation of infant botulism may obscure or delay diagnosis. *Pediatrics* 2005;116:e436–8.

40. MMWR, Morb Mortal Wkly Rep. Vaccine-preventable deaths and the global immunization vision and strategy, 2006–2015. 2006;55:511–15.

41. Ohuabunwo C, Perevoscikovs J, Griskevica A, et al. Respiratory diphtheria among highly vaccinated military trainees in Latvia: Improved protection from DT compared with Td booster vaccination. *Scand J Infect Dis* 2005; 37:813–20.

42. Okoromah CN, Lesi FE. Diazepam for treating tetanus. *Cochrane Database Syst Rev* 2004;(1):CD003954.

43. Pancharoen C, Mekmullica J, Thisyakorn U, et al. Clinical features of diphtheria in Thai children: A historical perspective. *Southeast Asian J Trop Med Public Health* 2002;33:352–4.

44. Personnel J, Hansmann MA, Delaney ML, et al. Prevalence of toxin shock syndrome toxin 1-producing Staphylococcus aureus and the presence of antibodies to this superantigen in menstruating women. *J Clin Microbiol* 2005;43:4628–34.

45. Piradov MA, Pirogov VN, Popova LM, et al. Diphtheritic polyneuropathy. Clinical analysis of severe forms. *Arch Neurol* 2001;58:1438–42.

46. Quick ML, Sutter RW, Kobaidze K, et al. Risk factors for diphtheria: A prospective case control study in the Republic of Georgia, 1995–1996. *J Infect Dis* 2000;181:S 121–9.

47. Ramos A, Barrucand L, Elias PRP, et al. Carnitine supplementation in diphtheria. *Indian Pediatr* 1992;29:1501–5.

48. Rashid A, Brown AP, Khan K. On the use of prophylactic antibiotics in prevention of toxic shock syndrome. *Burns* 2005;31:981–5.

49. Santos ML, Mota-Miranda A, Alves-Pereira A, et al. Intrathecal baclofen for treatment of tetanus. *Clin Infect Dis* 2004;38:321–8.

50. Schreiner MS, Field E, Ruddy R. Infant botulism: A review of 12 years' experience at the Children's Hospital of Philadelphia. *Pediatrics* 1991;87:159–65.

51. Shapiro RL, Hatheway C, Swerdlow DL. Botulism in the United States: A clinical and epidemiologic review. *Ann Intern Med* 1998;129:221–8.

52. Singh J, Harit AK, Jain DC, et al. Diphtheria is declining but continues to kill many children: Analysis of data from a sentinel centre in Delhi, 1997. *Epidemiol Infect* 1999;123:209–15.

53. Singhi S, Jain V, Subramanian C. Postneonatal tetanus: Issues in intensive care management. *Indian J Pediatr* 2001;68:267–72.

54. Sobel J, Tucker N, Sulka A, et al. Foodborne botulism in the United States, 1990–2000. *Emerg Infect Dis* 2004;10(9):1606–11.

55. Sobel J. Botulism. *Clin Infect Dis* 2005;41:1167–73.

56. Spika JS, Shaffer N, Hargrett-Bean N, et al. Risk factors for infant botulism in the United States. *Am J Dis Child* 1989;143:828–32.

57. Thwaites CL and Ferrar JJ. Preventing and treating tetanus. *BMJ* 2003;326:117–118.

58. Todd J, Fishaut M, Kapral F, Welsh T. Toxic shock syndrome associated with phage group I staphylococci. *Lancet* 1978;2:1116–8.

59. Wasay M, Khealani BA, Talati N, et al. Autonomic nervous system dysfunction predicts poor prognosis in patients with mild-to-moderate tetanus. *BMC Neurol* 2005;5:2.

60. World Health Organization. Global immunization data. *WHO report* 2004.

CHAPTER 84 ■ OPPORTUNISTIC INFECTIONS

SUSHIL K. KABRA • MATTHEW B. LAURENS

Opportunistic infections are infections that usually do not cause disease in a person with a healthy immune system but can affect people with a poorly functioning or suppressed immune system because of immunodeficiency or immunosuppression.

The infections can be severe and fatal if they are not recognized early and appropriate treatment is not instituted. The diagnosis of infections in immunocompromised pediatric patients remains a difficult challenge. Immunocompromised children are those with congenital defects of host defense and defects in cell-mediated or humoral immunity, but the major expansion of this population has occurred with increased bone marrow and solid-organ transplantation, successful treatment of childhood malignancy, and increased use of immunomodulatory agents for chronic diseases, such as Crohn disease, rheumatoid arthritis, and acquired immunodeficiency syndrome (AIDS). These developments have significantly increased the population of children at risk for opportunistic infections, and the list of organisms that lead to infections in these groups is extensive and growing. Pediatric intensivists are likely to see increasing numbers of children survive with primary immunodeficiencies or receive immunosuppressive therapy for treatment of malignancy, autoimmune disorders, or transplantation. For this reason, it is critical that all practitioners are able to recognize signs and symptoms of infections in these patients.

Conditions that predispose to opportunistic infections, common opportunistic infections, and their diagnostic approach and management are reviewed in this chapter.

CONDITIONS THAT PREDISPOSE TO OPPORTUNISTIC INFECTIONS

Conditions that predispose an individual to opportunistic infection may be congenital or acquired immune deficiencies. Each of the more than 100 known primary immune deficiency conditions may predispose an individual to particular infections. Knowledge of underlying immune deficiency aids in proper management of infection. Common conditions, organisms that cause infection, and clinical manifestations are summarized in **Table 84.1** (see Chapter 76).

Opportunistic Infections and Pediatric Intensive Care Settings

Patients with opportunistic infections present to PICUs with fulminant infections, such as respiratory infections, sepsis, infections of the central nervous system (CNS), or multiorgan dysfunction. Due to underlying immunodeficiency, the clinical course is fulminant and case fatality is high. Clinical signs and symptoms may provide important clues of immunodeficiency, as well as the possible etiologic agent of the infection, knowledge which is of paramount importance in instituting appropriate treatment.

When to Suspect Immune Deficiency

If a patient presents with fulminant opportunistic infection to the PICU, it is important to define the underlying immunodeficiency disorder, as it provides clues regarding the possible etiology of infection and aids in selection of the appropriate antimicrobial agent and supportive care. Secondary immune deficiency disorders can be suspected upon taking good history in most cases. Primary immune deficiency may be suspected if patients have any of the following:

- Eight or more new ear infections within 1 year
- Two or more serious sinus infections within 1 year
- Two or more months on antibiotics with little effect
- Two or more pneumonias within 1 year
- Failure of an infant to gain weight or grow normally
- Recurrent deep-skin or organ abscesses
- Persistent thrush in mouth or elsewhere on skin after age 1
- Need for IV antibiotics to clear infections
- Two or more deep-seated infections such as meningitis, osteomyelitis, cellulites, or sepsis
- A family history of primary immune deficiency

OPPORTUNISTIC INFECTIONS DUE TO VIRUSES

Cytomegalovirus Infection

Cytomegalovirus (CMV) is in the herpes virus group and is a common infection in immunocompromised children. The incidence has decreased significantly since the introduction of active antiretroviral treatment in patients infected with human immunodeficiency virus (HIV) (53). The organism can be transmitted through an infected birth canal and by breast milk, saliva, and blood (via infected white cells). Both humoral and cellular immune mechanisms are important in protection against CMV. Individuals who are CMV-negative prior to acquired immunosuppression (due to organ or marrow transplantation) and acquire the virus by transfusion are particularly at risk for disease. CMV-positive individuals who receive immunosuppressive therapy are at significant risk for "reactivation" pneumonia. Approximately 50% of patients with aplastic anemia or hematologic malignancy treated by allogeneic marrow transplantation develop CMV infection. CMV may also be a copathogen with other opportunistic organisms,

TABLE 84.1

CONDITIONS PREDISPOSING AN INDIVIDUAL TO OPPORTUNISTIC INFECTIONS

Major defects in immune system	Clinical conditions	Infections/clinical manifestations
B-cell defects (humoral deficiencies)	Agammaglobulinemia, hypogammaglobulinemia, selective IgA deficiency, IgG subclass deficiencies, common variable immune deficiency, hyper-IgM syndrome	Infections with *S. aureus*; encapsulated organisms, such as *S. pneumoniae*, *H. influenzae*; and gram-negative organisms, such as pseudomonas species Arthritis due to echoviruses, coxsackieviruses, adenoviruses, and *U. urealyticum* Infections due to *P. jiroveci* (*P. carinii*) pneumonitis, and *Cryptosporidium*
T-cell defects (cell-mediated immunity)	Thymic dysplasia (DiGeorge syndrome), defective T-cell receptor, defective cytokine production, T-cell activation defects, CD8 lymphocytopenia	Disseminated viral infections due to herpes simplex, varicella-zoster, and CMV Progressive pneumonia caused by parainfluenza, respiratory syncytial virus, cytomegalovirus, varicella, and *P. jiroveci* Superficial and systemic fungal infections and parasitic infections. Severe mucocutaneous candidiasis; disseminated BCG disease after BCG vaccination
Combined B- and T-cell defects	Severe combined immunodeficiency, Omenn syndrome, Wiskott-Aldrich syndrome, ataxia telangiectasia, hyper-IgE syndrome	Infections caused by bacteria, fungi, or viruses Chronic diarrhea, mucocutaneous or systemic candidiasis, *P. jiroveci* pneumonitis, and CMV early in life Infections with *S. pneumoniae* or *H. influenzae* type b, *P. jiroveci* Late-onset recurrent sinopulmonary infections from bacteria and respiratory viruses Recurrent episodes of *S. aureus* abscesses of the skin, lungs, and musculoskeletal system
Abnormalities in phagocytic system	Inadequate numbers (congenital or acquired), Chronic granulomatous disease, leukocyte adhesion deficiency, Chédiak-Higashi syndrome	Recurrent pyogenic and fungal infections due to *Pseudomonas*, *S. marcescens*, and *S. aureus*, and fungi such as *Aspergillus* and *Candida* present as cellulitis, perirectal abscesses, or stomatitis Pulmonary infection, suppurative adenitis, subcutaneous abscess, liver abscess, osteomyelitis, and sepsis due to fungi or bacteria (*Staphylococcus*) Gastric outlet obstruction, urinary tract obstruction, and enteritis or colitis History of delayed cord separation and recurrent infections of the skin, oral mucosa, and genital tract, Predisposed to development of ecthyma gangrenosum and pyoderma gangrenosum
Disorders of the complement system	Disorders involving any one of the complement components, asplenia, splenic dysfunction due to hemoglobinopathies, splenectomy	Infections due to *Salmonella* spp. and encapsulated bacteria including *S. pneumoniae* and *H. influenzae*. These agents can cause sepsis, pneumonia, meningitis, and osteomyelitis
Infections occurring with acquired immunodeficiencies	HIV and other virus infections, cancer chemotherapy, immunosuppressive therapy after organ transplant, diabetes mellitus, sickle cell disease, severe malnutrition	Similar to cell-mediated immune deficiency Neutropenic patients: infections due to gram-positive cocci and gram-negative organisms, such as *P. aeruginosa*, *E. coli*, and *Klebsiella* Fungal infections due to *Candida* and *Aspergillus* in prolonged neutropenia

CMV, cytomegalovirus; BCG, Bacille Calmette-Guérin

including *Pneumocystis jiroveci* and *Aspergillus* spp., especially in AIDS patients and patients following bone marrow transplant (BMT).

Clinical Manifestations

Congenital CMV infection is a well-known clinical entity and is beyond the scope of this chapter. CMV as an opportunistic infection is recognized more commonly and has varying clinical manifestations. It involves almost all organ systems of the body (**Table 84.2**).

Pulmonary involvement due to CMV is a major cause of serious, often fatal, pneumonia in children with congenital immunodeficiency, AIDS, organ or marrow transplantation, or malignancy. It may complicate the course of pediatric heart

TABLE 84.2

CLINICAL MANIFESTATIONS OF CYTOMEGALOVIRUS INFECTION

Organ involved	Susceptible hosts	Clinical features
Mononucleosis syndrome	Immunocompetent and immunosuppressed persons; reactivation infection in immunosuppressed	Fever, severe malaise, headache, myalgia, abdominal pain with diarrhea Less common features: interstitial pneumonitis, myocarditis and pericarditis, arthralgias and arthritis, maculopapular rashes, adrenal insufficiency, splenic infarction, ulcerative colitis, and proctitis, Guillain-Barré syndrome, and meningoencephalitis
Respiratory system	Congenital immunodeficiency, AIDS, organ or marrow transplantation, or malignancy	Fever, dry/nonproductive cough, dyspnea, retractions, wheezing, and hypoxia, which require ventilatory support Coinfection with other pathogens, especially gram-negative enteric bacteria and fungal pathogens in transplant recipients and *P. jiroveci* in patients with AIDS
Eyes	Severe immunosuppression, especially in BMT recipients and patients with AIDS	Rapidly progressive retinitis with white perivascular infiltrates, hemorrhage, with a necrosis Peripheral retinitis Conjunctivitis, corneal epithelial keratitis and disk neovascularization
Liver and hepatobiliary system	Recipients of bone marrow, liver, heart, and lung transplant and patients with cancer or AIDS	Fever, thrombocytopenia, and lymphopenia or lymphocytosis with mild hepatomegaly Occasionally granulomatous hepatitis Jaundice and hyperbilirubinemia usually do not occur
Gastrointestinal system	Patients with AIDS and those with organ transplant	Esophagitis, gastritis, gastroenteritis, pyloric and small-bowel obstruction, duodenitis, colitis, proctitis, pancreatitis, hemorrhage, and acalculous cholecystitis
Central nervous system syndrome	Patients with AIDS and those with organ transplant	Meningoencephalitis headache, photophobia, nuchal rigidity, memory deficits, and inability to concentrate Ascending paralysis caused by myelitis, with or without vasculitis or necrosis Polyradiculopathy in patients with AIDS
Other organs systems	Renal and heart transplant patients AIDS patients	Myocarditis: heart failure, cardiomegaly, electrocardiographic abnormalities, and poor left ventricular function on echocardiography Endocrinopathy: Addison's disease

and lung transplantation. CMV pneumonitis usually occurs 1–3 months following transplantation and begins with symptoms of fever and a dry, nonproductive cough. It can then progress over the course of 1–2 weeks to dyspnea, retractions, wheezing, and hypoxia, which require ventilatory support. It may occur as the only disease manifestation or be part of a disseminated CMV infection. Coinfection with other pathogens, especially gram-negative enteric bacteria and fungal pathogens in transplant recipients and *P. jiroveci* in patients with AIDS, can occur. The differential diagnosis of CMV pneumonitis in immunocompromised patients includes bacterial pneumonia, infection with protozoa (e.g., *P. jiroveci, Toxoplasma gondii, Chlamydia, Mycoplasma)*, and fungal pneumonia caused especially by *Candida* and *Aspergillus*. Noninfectious causes of pneumonitis, such as pulmonary hemorrhage, aspiration pneumonia, and pulmonary damage from chemotherapeutic agents, should also be considered in the differential diagnosis of CMV pneumonia.

A clinical condition called *mononucleosis syndrome* may occur due to CMV infection in both immunocompetent and immunosuppressed persons and, occasionally, as a reactivation infection in immunosuppressed patients. Typical CMV-induced mononucleosis is characterized by fever and strikingly severe malaise of approximately 1–4 weeks' duration, peripheral lymphocytosis with atypical lymphocytes, and mildly elevated liver enzymes. In some patients, headache, myalgias, and abdominal pain with diarrhea are prominent symptoms (28) (**Table 84.2**). The differential diagnosis of CMV-induced mononucleosis includes mononucleosis induced by other viruses, such as Epstein-Barr virus (EBV), hepatitis A or B virus, and HIV.

Over the last 2–3 decades, CMV retinitis has emerged as a common manifestation of CMV disease in patients with severe immunosuppression, especially in BMT recipients and patients with AIDS. CMV produces characteristic white perivascular infiltrates and hemorrhage, with a necrotic, rapidly progressive retinitis. Peripheral retinitis can be asymptomatic, or the complaints may be minimal and nonspecific; it is especially difficult to ascertain in infants and young children. At an advanced stage, it can cause blurred vision, decreased visual acuity, visual field defects, and blindness. Early diagnosis may allow prompt institution of antiviral therapy, which may be sight saving. CMV may also produce conjunctivitis, corneal epithelial keratitis, and disk neovascularization. The differential diagnoses of CMV retinitis include other causes of retinal lesions, such as ocular toxoplasmosis, candidal infection of the retina, syphilis, herpes simplex virus (HSV) infection, lymphocytic choriomeningitis virus infection, and varicella infection.

CMV hepatitis may occur in recipients of bone marrow, liver, heart, or lung transplantation, and in patients with cancer or AIDS (59). It manifests as fever, thrombocytopenia, and lymphopenia or lymphocytosis with mild hepatomegaly. Jaundice and hyperbilirubinemia usually do not occur. Occasionally, it may produce granulomatous hepatitis. Liver transplant may be complicated with CMV hepatitis in children who have received liver from a seropositive donor and in whom OKT3 antibodies are used for severe rejection. CMV hepatitis in liver transplantation recipients is characterized by prolonged fever, leukopenia, thrombocytopenia, elevated liver enzymes, hyperbilirubinemia, and liver failure. Distinguishing between CMV hepatitis and acute rejection is difficult, as both conditions may coexist. CMV infection has also been associated with ascending cholangitis, chronic rejection, and the vanishing bile duct syndrome in liver transplant recipients. The differential diagnoses of CMV hepatitis include other causes of viral hepatitis (EBV, HSV, enterovirus, adenovirus, and hepatitis A, B, and C), toxoplasmosis, bacterial hepatitis (including ascending cholangitis), and noninfectious causes (including ischemic injury, vascular thrombosis, hemolysis, rejection, and hepatitis induced by drugs or toxins).

Gastrointestinal manifestations due to CMV infection in immunocompromised patients (especially those with AIDS and those who have undergone bone marrow, kidney, intestinal, or liver transplantation) include esophagitis, gastritis, gastroenteritis, pyloric and small bowel obstruction, duodenitis, colitis, proctitis, pancreatitis, hemorrhage, and acalculous cholecystitis. The differential diagnosis of CMV colitis includes infection with other viruses, especially HSV and adenovirus, and infection with bacteria, particularly *Salmonella, Shigella, Campylobacter, Yersinia, Clostridium difficile,* and *Mycobacterium avium-intracellulare.* Parasitic infection with *Cryptosporidium, Giardia,* and amebae should also be excluded. The differential diagnoses of CMV esophagitis and gastritis include HSV infection, *Candida* esophagitis, reflux esophagitis, and peptic ulcer disease.

In postnatal life, CMV meningoencephalitis appears to be rare yet well documented. Symptoms include headache, photophobia, nuchal rigidity, memory deficits, and inability to concentrate. Ascending paralysis caused by myelitis, with or without vasculitis or necrosis, can also occur and may appear similar to Guillain-Barré syndrome. In addition, CMV polyradiculopathy has been described in adult patients with AIDS and may occur in older children. This disease usually begins with leg pain and sacral paresthesias and may progress to weakness and flaccid paralysis (58).

CMV myocarditis has been seen in renal and heart transplant recipients, usually as part of a disseminated CMV infection and associated with graft rejection treated with high-dose immunosuppressive therapy. Patients can have heart failure, cardiomegaly, electrocardiographic abnormalities, and poor left ventricular function on echocardiography; cytomegalic inclusion cells and the presence of CMV DNA can be documented by myocardial biopsy.

Immunosuppressed patients, especially those with AIDS, may manifest clinical endocrinopathies caused by CMV infection, such as adrenal insufficiency and adrenal necrosis. Involvement of skin due to CMV may manifest as localized cutaneous ulcers or a widespread exanthematous, maculopapular eruption.

Diagnosis

CMV is diagnosed by serology, polymerase chain reaction (PCR), antigenemia, and viral culture. For suspected CNS infections, PCR of cerebrospinal fluid (CSF) for CMV is the most sensitive diagnostic method (5).

Immunocompetent Hosts. Serology is used primarily in healthy patients to distinguish primary infection from reactivation. Acute serum IgG and IgM titers are obtained at the onset of illness. The presence of CMV IgG titer indicates that the patient has been infected with CMV in the past. The presence of CMV IgG titer indicates that the patient has not been exposed to CMV in the past. Interpretation of CMV IgM antibody requires more careful evaluation, considering other processes that might produce cross-reacting antibody or polyclonal responses (e.g., rheumatoid factor). Presence of CMV IgM indicates current or recent CMV infection. CMV IgM antibody persists for 6 weeks in healthy adults and may be present for 3–6 months after primary infection. CMV IgG avidity index may be helpful to diagnose primary infection. Low avidity index (30%) suggests recent primary infection, and high avidity index (>60%) suggests a past or recurrent CMV infection (17). Primary infection is diagnosed if the patient is CMV IgG negative on acute presentation and becomes positive when convalescent titers are drawn. CMV IgM titers may be low or slightly elevated in the face of acute infection that is primary or reactivated. For previously healthy individuals, serum PCR testing for CMV may not be positive in patients with acute mononucleosis due to CMV (34).

Immunocompromised Hosts. CMV isolated from immunocompromised patients does not equate with CMV disease, but documentation of primary infection (that usually causes disease) by seroconversion or viremia in a previously seronegative patient is important. In transplant recipients, primary CMV infection usually occurs 4–12 weeks after transplant. In immunocompromised children, reactivated CMV cannot reliably be diagnosed in spite of virus in urine, saliva, or respiratory secretions. Among recipients of solid organ transplant, isolation from buffy coat or antigenemia correlates with CMV disease. Both serologic PCR and pp65 antigenemia testing for CMV in these patients appear to be sensitive (>90%) with regard to diagnosing CMV disease; however, neither are very specific (around 60%) (21). Either quantitative serologic PCR for CMV or CMV pp65 antigenemia may be used to monitor viral loads during antiviral therapy. For BMT recipients and patients with AIDS, plasma detection of CMV DNA by PCR tends to correlate with clinical severity of disease. Among immunocompromised patients, quantitative PCR assays also correlate viral load with risk of CMV disease. However, it must be stated that the quantity of CMV DNA in blood that is predictive of disease varies with the method of measurement, type of sample, and the clinical setting. Among recipients of solid organ transplant, 2000–5000 genome copies/mL of plasma is identified as a useful cutoff value to determine significant risk of CMV disease.

Management

In the immunocompetent host, no treatment is indicated. It is suggested only in severe or life-threatening disease. Among the immunocompromised, 85% of patients with AIDS and CMV retinitis improve or show stabilization of lesions after induction therapy with ganciclovir, foscarnet, or cidofovir. Induction followed by continuous maintenance therapy to prevent relapse is indicated in this population. Initially IV antiviral agent (ganciclovir 5–7.5 mg/kg/day) is given for 2–3 weeks, followed by maintenance treatment 3–5 times a week by IV or oral route (5 mg/kg/day). For induction therapy, a survival advantage has been demonstrated of foscarnet over ganciclovir. Combination therapy with ganciclovir and foscarnet is associated with longer time to recurrence, compared with monotherapy. Oral ganciclovir may be considered for patients who are CMV seropositive and have CD4 <50/mm^3.

For transplant recipients, different regimens of antiviral agents, immunoglobulins, and combinations are used at different centers for treatment of CMV. Most include prophylaxis for CMV disease with immunoglobulin (IG) or antiviral agent or some combination before and during the period of highest risk. One of the protocols of combining antiviral agent with IVIG includes administration of ganciclovir, 2.5 mg/kg body weight, three times daily for 20 days, plus IVIG, 500 mg/kg every other day for 10 doses, followed by ganciclovir, 5 mg/kg/day three to five times per week for 20 more doses, and IVIG, 500 mg/kg twice a week for eight more doses.

Preemptive therapy is an alternative in allogeneic BMT recipients, for whom regular lab screening with antigenemia or PCR determines the need for initiation of antiviral therapy. This strategy is associated with a survival advantage. However, autologous and stem cell BMT recipients have lower risk of CMV disease and might not warrant prophylaxis.

In recipients of renal transplant, prophylactic antiviral therapy is recommended (a) when the donor or recipient is seropositive and antilymphocyte treatment is part of the immunosuppressive regimen, and (b) for seronegative recipients of grafts from seropositive donors.

Prevention

Prevention of CMV disease is achieved through screening of donors, use of transfusion filters, consideration of daycare and school avoidance, and good hygienic habits. Seronegative donor blood products should be reserved for seronegative recipients. Additionally, filters that remove leukocytes from blood products should be used, especially in those who are at risk for severe CMV disease. For children with HIV infection, the risk of acquiring CMV disease should be carefully weighed before enrollment in daycare or preschool. To reduce household and community transmission, careful handwashing and hygiene should be observed.

Varicella-zoster Virus Infection

Varicella-zoster virus (VZV) is a DNA virus that typically causes benign infections of the skin and mucous membranes. It may cause both varicella and zoster in the normal host. However, in certain groups, including neonates, cancer and BMT patients, patients with AIDS and congenital defects of cell-mediated immunity, and organ transplant patients, VZV can lead to visceral dissemination and pneumonia. HIV-infected children who develop varicella in the setting of severe immunodeficiency are at an especially high risk to develop zoster (15).

Clinical Features

VZV infection may be confined to skin or may be disseminated. It may be severe and even fatal in immunocompromised patients. In these patients, fever may continue for longer duration. New vesicular lesions may appear over a period of up to 2 weeks or longer. Their skin lesions characteristically are large, umbilicated, and hemorrhagic, and primary varicella pneumonia is a frequent complication. Mucosal surfaces, including gastrointestinal tract, may be involved and may manifest as chest pain, abdominal pain, and bleeding (49).

Most fatalities from varicella are due to primary varicella pneumonia. The clinical presentations of varicella pneumonia are nonspecific and include fever, cough, dyspnea, and chest pain. Other common symptoms and signs are cyanosis, rales, hemoptysis, and chest pain. The chest x-ray typically reveals a diffuse nodular or miliary pattern, most pronounced in the perihilar region (54). Varicella pneumonia may be complicated by acute respiratory distress syndrome, rhabdomyolysis, acute hepatitis, and disseminated intravascular coagulation (30).

CNS complications of VZV include cerebellar ataxia and encephalitis. Patients with varicella may develop ischemic strokes and radiologic and histopathologic evidence of CNS vasculitis. Ocular manifestations of VZV infection include conjunctivitis, keratitis, iridocyclitis, panuveitis, and acute retinal necrosis. Sudden loss of vision due to retrobulbar optic neuritis and retinitis following varicella in a vaccinated child with acute lymphoblastic leukemia has also been reported (55). Other uncommon but important manifestations of varicella infection in immunocompromised hosts include fulminant hepatic failure, myocarditis, arrhythmias, and progression to dilated cardiomyopathy and endocarditis (1).

Diagnosis

Herpes zoster can be diagnosed based on physical findings, vesicle scrapings, serology, or PCR. Scraping of vesicles in the first few days following their appearance is likely to yield identification of the virus. After unroofing a vesicle, the fluid can be sent for viral culture as well as direct fluorescent antibody testing. The direct fluorescent antibody test is advantageous, as the results are more rapidly obtained and can differentiate HSV from VZV. The Tzanck smear of vesicle scrapings will show multinucleated giant cells but is not specific for VZV. Acute and convalescent titers of serum IgG for varicella zoster will show a rise in antibody titer in immunocompetent persons but not in the immunocompromised. Most serum antibody testing methods are not sensitive enough to identify vaccine-induced immunity. Finally, PCR testing for VZV is a very sensitive test and can be performed on body fluid or tissue specimens.

Management

Management of Varicella-zoster Virus Exposure. Susceptible persons exposed to varicella should be given immune globulin (either varicella zoster immune globulin or IVIG up to 92 hrs after exposure). The VZIG dose is 1.25 mL (125 IU) for every 10 kg of body weight, with a maximum dose of 6 mL (625 IU) (up to 72 hrs after exposure). To maximize benefit, immune globulin should be given as soon as possible after exposure. Those who are susceptible include:

- Immunocompromised children without history of varicella or varicella immunization
- Susceptible pregnant women

- Newborn infants whose mothers had onset of chickenpox within 5 days before delivery or within 48 hrs after delivery
- Hospitalized premature infants ≥28 weeks gestation whose mothers lack a history of chickenpox or serologic evidence of protection
- Hospitalized premature infants <28 weeks gestation or ≤1000 g birth weight, regardless of maternal history or serologic status

Significant exposures include:

- Residents of the same household
- Face-to-face indoor playmates
- For varicella, hospital exposure in the same multi-bed room or adjacent beds in a large ward, face-to-face contact with an infectious staff member or patient, or visit by a person deemed contagious
- For zoster, intimate contact (touching or hugging) with a contagious person
- For newborns, onset of maternal chickenpox ≤5 days before delivery or within 48 hrs after delivery; immune globulin is not indicated if the mother has zoster

Exposure to varicella merits airborne and contact precautions from 8 until 21 days after the onset of rash in the index case, and for 28 days after exposure to the index case in those treated with VZIG or IVIG. For those who have received high-dose immune globulin (400 mg/kg or greater) within 3 weeks prior to exposure, a second dose is not indicated.

Management of Varicella-zoster Virus Disease. Treatment of varicella in immunocompetent children is not recommended. However, those with increased risk for moderate-to-severe varicella should be considered candidates for oral therapy with acyclovir. Those at increased risk include people >12 years of age, those with chronic cutaneous or pulmonary disorders, those receiving long-term salicylate therapy, and those receiving short or intermittent courses of corticosteroids. Famciclovir and valacyclovir are licensed (in the US) for treatment of varicella in adults but not in pediatric patients. Pregnant women should not be routinely treated with acyclovir for varicella, as the risks to the fetus are unknown. However, IV acyclovir is indicated for pregnant women with serious complications of varicella. Salicylates should be avoided in children with varicella, as they increase the risk of Reye syndrome.

Immunocompromised patients should receive IV acyclovir. The dose of acyclovir is 1500 mg/m^2/day in three divided doses for children and 30 mg/kg/day for adolescents. Oral, high-dose acyclovir (80 mg/kg/day in four divided doses) can be considered in patients who are mildly immunosuppressed and at lower risk for developing severe varicella. The use of VZIG or IVIG is indicated for immunocompromised persons who are exposed and has not shown benefit in those who have established disease.

Air-borne and contact precautions should be maintained in patients with varicella for 5 days after appearance of the rash and while vesicular lesions are present. For those with disseminated varicella, air-borne and contact precautions should be maintained for the duration of the illness. Children with varicella may return to school when their lesions have crusted over.

Prevention

The mainstay of prevention of varicella includes a combination of vaccination of the general population, proper isolation of suspected and known cases, administration of VZIG or IVIG to those who are immunocompromised, and isolation of susceptible contacts.

Varicella vaccine is a live-attenuated preparation of the varicella virus. A single dose of 0.5 mL is indicated for children aged 12 months to 12 years, while a two-dose regimen separated by at least 4–8 weeks is recommended in those aged 13 and older.

Herpes Virus Type 6

Human herpes virus 6 (HHV-6) is a DNA virus that is the etiologic agent for roseola and is among the most widespread of the human herpesviruses.

Clinical Features

In immunocompetent children, HHV-6 causes exanthem subitum, febrile episodes without skin rash, and non-EBV and non-CMV infectious mononucleosis. HHV-6 has also been associated with clinical disease in recipients of bone marrow and solid organ transplant. Its potential role in HIV-1–associated clinical syndromes is now being recognized and evaluated. Viral reactivation in the immunocompromised host has been linked to a variety of diseases, including encephalitis, and HHV-6 has been tentatively associated with multiple sclerosis (6).

The virus remains latent in the body after primary infection and reactivates in immunocompromised patients. HHV-6 infection occurs in nearly 50% of all recipients of BMT and in 20%–30% of recipients of solid-organ transplant 2–3 weeks following the procedure. It has been suggested that the viral infection and activation result in clinical symptoms, including fever, skin rash, pneumonia, bone marrow suppression, encephalitis, and rejection (56). Most cases of HHV-6–associated pneumonia involve immunocompromised patients, especially those who have received a bone marrow transplant or who have been infected by HIV.

Diagnosis

Testing for HHV-6 includes serology, culture, immunohistochemistry, and nucleic acid assays. Serology testing is usually reserved for the immunocompetent and is not useful in post-transplant patients. PCR testing on tissue samples is a commonly used test for HHV-6. The disadvantage of this method is that it does not differentiate between active and latent infection. Other methods utilized include serum plasma PCR and reverse transcriptase PCR, which detect virus that is circulating and are thought to be indicative of active infection. However, the best method for detection of active HHV-6 is quantitative PCR analysis of body secretions. This method is sensitive and efficient, and allows direct determination of viral burden in the host (11).

Management

While treatment is not indicated in healthy children, those who are immunocompromised may experience severe disease. Antiviral therapies have not been evaluated in randomized clinical trials. Drugs commonly used when indicated are the same as those used for treatment of CMV, including ganciclovir, valganciclovir, acyclovir, valacyclovir, cidofovir, and foscarnet. In vitro studies indicate that ganciclovir is superior to acyclovir in treating HHV-6, and several case reports support treatment with ganciclovir, particularly in HHV-6 encephalitis. Foscarnet is another alternative that shows in vitro activity against HHV-6. Cidofovir is another alternative that shows good activity in vitro, but its use is limited by associated nephrotoxicity and limited experience (11). In addition to these therapies, patients may benefit from a reduction in immunosuppression.

Prevention

Routine prophylaxis or preemptive therapy to prevent HHV-6 infection is not indicated. However, prophylaxis with ganciclovir has proven efficacious in preventing HHV-6 reactivation in BMT patients (42). A potential pitfall is that prophylaxis has been shown to promote resistance of CMV to ganciclovir.

FUNGAL INFECTIONS

Candidiasis

Candida spp. are recognized as a leading contributor to morbidity and mortality in patients with oncohematologic malignancies, HIV infection, primary immunodeficiencies, prolonged neutropenia, diabetes, corticosteroid administration, broad-spectrum antibiotic treatment, IV hyperalimentation, and presence of central venous lines. The frequency of *Candida* species in 64 patients from a PICU was *C. tropicalis* (48.4%), *C. albicans* (29.7%), *C. guilliermondii* (14.1%), *C. krusei* (6.3%), and *C. glabrata* (1.6%) (46).

Intrinsic differences may exist between different populations sampled. For instance, malnutrition may favor the presence of yeast species other than *C. albicans* (22). Neutropenic children colonized with *C. tropicalis* are at higher risk for dissemination compared to those colonized with *C. albicans* (27).

Clinical Features

Acute disseminated candidiasis occurs in immunocompromised hosts. Frequent sites of infection in patients with disseminated candidiasis include lungs, kidneys, liver, spleen, and brain. The portals of entry are usually lesions of the gastrointestinal tract or oral mucosa, skin puncture sites. Organisms may disseminate via the hematogenous route to the tissues of one or more organs. The clinical manifestations depend on the sites that are involved and the extent of involvement. The clinical features are nonspecific in infants and children and are similar to those with sepsis caused by other organisms. Presence of ocular lesions of endophthalmitis and maculopapular rash in an immunocompromised state suggest a possibility of candidal sepsis. The skin lesions consist of generalized rashes or discrete, firm, erythematous papules that measure 0.5–1 cm in diameter. A nodular center is often surrounded by an erythematous halo. Candidiasis may involve bones, joints, heart, and CNS. Osteomyelitis of bones may develop in young infants and children. Cardiac involvement may be in the form of endocarditis, myocarditis, or arrhythmia. CNS involvement may occur in disseminated candidiasis and is more common in preterm infants and young children.

Oral candidiasis can be an early sign of illness or disease progression in HIV/AIDS. The sites commonly involved are buccal mucosa and dorsal and lateral surfaces of tongue. Submucosal edema and bleeding may occur while plaques are removed. Esophageal candidiasis is one of the important clinical manifestations of candidal infection in immunocompromised hosts. Patients may have concurrent oropharyngeal candidiasis, odynophagia, retrosternal pain, fever, nausea/vomiting, drooling, dehydration, hoarseness, and upper gastrointestinal bleeding. *Candida* infection may also manifest as *C. epiglottitis* (31).

Gastrointestinal candidiasis may occur in children with immune deficiency disorders, cancer, and after surgery. It may involve the stomach, intestine, or hepatobiliary system. Peritonitis due to *Candida* spp. may occur secondary to bowel perforation, peritoneal dialysis, or intestinal surgery. Clinical manifestations are nonspecific and include abdominal distention, fever, vomiting, and abdominal pain.

The airway from pharynx to bronchi may be involved. A child may present with hoarseness of voice, low-grade fever, tachypnea, or nonspecific physical examination findings. Pulmonary infection may be complicated by development of abscess and empyema.

Renal involvement in children with candidemia is relatively common and includes renal microabscesses, papillary necrosis, calyceal distortion, and obstruction due to fungal ball or perinephric abscesses.

C. albicans may be associated with vaginitis in immunocompetent as well as immunocompromised host. Clinical features include swelling and erythema of vaginal mucosa with creamy white discharge and involvement of perineal skin.

Diagnosis

Diagnosis of *Candida* infections is based on clinical findings and tissue and body fluid culture. Mucocutaneous candidiasis is diagnosed clinically and can be confirmed with Gram stain and culture. Endoscopy is useful for diagnosis of esophageal candidiasis. Tissue samples can be stained and cultured, and the addition of potassium hydroxide to specimens may help to identify yeast and pseudohyphae. For retinal candidal infections, ophthalmologic examination identifies characteristic findings. Candidal infections in solid organs may be seen on CT or ultrasound studies, but characteristic findings typically occur late in the course of the disease. Four ultrasound patterns of hepatosplenic candidiasis have been described. The first pattern, described as having a "wheel-within-a-wheel" appearance, consists of a central hypoechoic area of necrosis that contains fungi surrounded by an echogenic zone of inflammatory cells. A hypoechoic rim is noted at the periphery. The second pattern is a "bull's-eye" configuration, consisting of a central echogenic nidus surrounded by a hypoechoic rim. In general, this second pattern occurs in patients with active fungal infection and a relatively normal white blood cell count. The third pattern consists of a uniformly hypoechoic nodule and is the most common pattern seen on ultrasound; however, it is the least specific appearance of candidiasis and may simulate metastatic disease or lymphoma. The fourth pattern consists of echogenic foci, with variable degrees of posterior acoustic shadowing. This pattern occurs in later stages of infection and generally indicates early resolution (39). In contrast-enhanced CT, fungal microabscesses usually appear as multiple, round, discrete areas of low attenuation, generally ranging from 2 to 20 mm. Characteristic histopathology may also be useful to diagnose candidal infection. Blood cultures to detect disseminated candidiasis are only 50%–70% sensitive and may not detect active infection.

The advancement of in situ hybridization techniques has permitted rapid detection of *Candida* spp. in a matter of hours. Serologic techniques to detect candidal antigens are being perfected to improve diagnostic methods. Specifically, $(1\rightarrow3)\beta$-D-glucan has shown high sensitivity and specificity as an adjunct for diagnosis of invasive fungal infections (37).

Management

Evidence-based guidelines for the treatment of candidiasis are published by the Infectious Disease Society of America (38). According to the guidelines, first-line therapy includes amphotericin B and fluconazole, which are approved for use in pediatrics. Caspofungin is indicated for first-line treatment in adults, but its safety and efficacy has not been proven in children. Other therapies that have been developed for use in candidiasis include micafungin, anidulafungin, posaconazole, and voriconazole. Safety and efficacy of voriconazole has been established in children >12 years of age. For yeast specimens identified as *C. albicans*, fluconazole therapy should be used. Fluconazole therapy should also be used in clinically stable patients in ICUs where the predominant candidal pathogen is *C. albicans*. For other species of *Candida*, empiric therapy with amphotericin B can be initiated while awaiting culture results (37).

For severe disease, including meningitis, osteomyelitis, and endocarditis, a combination of amphotericin B and flucytosine is an option; however, other combination therapies are not recommended. Studies of combination therapy using amphotericin B and fluconazole to treat candidemia in nonneutropenic patients show improvement in clearance rates of candidemia but no survival benefit due to related toxicity. Other therapies that combine caspofungin with fluconazole or amphotericin B may be beneficial (26). The length of antifungal therapy for candidemia is 14 days, starting from the first negative blood culture. For disseminated disease, patients are treated until clinical, radiologic, or microbiologic resolution is achieved (38).

Another mainstay in the treatment of invasive candidiasis is the removal of infected vascular lines and hardware, which improves morbidity and mortality in this patient population. Special consideration should be given to patients with tunneled catheters, as these are unlikely to be sources of infection, and to febrile neutropenic patients who are more likely to become candidemic due to gut translocation than via central catheter infection. All candidemic patients should have a dilated eye examination by an ophthalmologist to look for signs of invasive ocular disease, as this would require prolonged antifungal therapy (37).

Prevention

Prevention of invasive candidiasis and associated sequelae involves prophylactic therapy. Studies in the adult ICU setting have demonstrated that invasive candidiasis can be prevented by fluconazole prophylaxis, but decreased mortality was not observed. These studies also report no increase in fluconazole-resistant *Candida* species during the study period. Identifying and prescribing prophylaxis in patients at risk for invasive fungal disease, such as the febrile neutropenic population, appears to be appropriate until specific populations at risk for invasive candidemia are identified (37).

Pneumocystis jiroveci

P. jiroveci, earlier known as *P. carinii*, is a eukaryotic microorganism of uncertain taxonomy that can infect numerous mammalian hosts. Developing from a small, unicellular "trophozoite" into a "cyst" that contains eight "sporozoites," its life cycle superficially resembles those seen in both the protozoa and fungi. Morphologic and ultrastructural observations have led some investigators to conclude that the organism is a protozoan, while others feel that it more closely resembles a fungus. Phylogenetic analysis of *Pneumocystis* 16S-like rRNA demonstrates it to be a member of the fungi family.

Patients at higher risk for *P. jiroveci* pneumonia include infants with severe malnutrition and children with primary immunodeficiencies, including combined immune deficiency and hyper-IgM syndrome, hematologic malignancies, HIV infection, and recipients of solid organ or bone marrow transplants. Patients with solid tumors, in particular those who receive high-dose corticosteroids for brain neoplasms, and patients with inflammatory or collagen-vascular disorders, especially those with Wegener granulomatosis who receive immunosuppressive therapy, have been identified as subgroups at increased risk for *P. jiroveci* pneumonia. Other factors associated with *P. jiroveci* pneumonia include the intensity of the immunosuppressive regimen and tapering doses of corticosteroids (43,44).

Clinical Features

The natural course of *P. jiroveci* infection in children varies highly and depends primarily on the status of host defenses and the underlying illness in individual patients. The onset may be insidious, with a clinical course of 3 or more weeks, or it may be fulminant and rapidly progressive over a few days.

The clinical manifestations of *P. jiroveci* pneumonia in HIV-infected and non–HIV-infected children differ. Patients with AIDS typically have a longer duration of symptoms and a more insidious presentation. Hypoxemia may be less intense. Organisms appear to be abundant in AIDS patients and can usually be identified in sputum, bronchoalveolar lavage (BAL) fluid, or even gastric lavage samples. In children with and without AIDS, physical examination at the time of initial evaluation may reveal tachypnea, nasal flaring, and intercostal, subcostal, or supracostal retractions. An ashen color or cyanosis may be present or may develop rapidly. Despite rapid (80–100/min), shallow respirations, auscultation of the chest frequently shows absence of adventitious sounds. Scattered rales, rhonchi, or wheezing most often are detected later in the clinical course as resolution occurs. Apart from variable elevation in temperature, few other physical abnormalities are noted, except those referable to pulmonary disease or secondary to the patient's underlying disease or treatment. Infants with HIV infection may have polymicrobial infections, especially with *P. jiroveci* and CMV, and the manifestations are severe in these patients and are more likely to require ventilatory support.

Though the carriage rates of *P. jiroveci* in children without AIDS is low, their clinical illness due to pneumocystic pneumonia (PCP) may be particularly abrupt in onset and more rapidly progressive. Even within these patients, the course varies widely. In children, fever is generally present and of high grade. It often precedes the onset of nonproductive cough, tachypnea, and severe dyspnea. The time of onset of clinical disease in non-AIDS, high-risk patients is unpredictable, but disease often occurs after discontinuance or a reduction in the dose of corticosteroid therapy (43).

Though pneumocystic infection predominantly causes pneumonia, cases of extrapulmonary or disseminated infection of Pneumocystis have been described. Extrapulmonary pneumocystosis represents <1% of all cases of infection with *P. jiroveci*. Extrapulmonary spread of *P. jiroveci* infection occurs via both lymphatic and hematogenous routes. Several organs or tissues may be involved, but the most common sites are lymph nodes, spleen, liver, and bone marrow. While all patients with disseminated forms of this infection die rapidly, survival for patients with AIDS is possible if systemic treatment is provided, if a single extrapulmonary site is involved, and if no concomitant pneumonia is present.

Diagnosis

PCP is diagnosed through direct identification of organisms from lung tissue or induced sputum specimens. While identification of organisms from lung biopsy specimens is the gold standard for diagnosis, other methods of identification may be adequate. A meta-analysis of diagnostic procedures to identify PCP found that sputum induction in patients with HIV infection is adequate for diagnosis, compared with BAL specimens. The yield was increased with immunofluorescence testing versus cytochemical staining (10). Additionally, PCR testing for PCP using induced sputum or BAL fluid can increase the diagnostic yield for HIV patients with suspected PCP. The value of PCR testing in immunocompetent patients is controversial, however, as it may indicate colonization (51).

Management

Pneumocystis disease can progress quickly, and the success of treatment depends largely on the stage of disease at the time of treatment initiation. Therefore, prompt diagnosis and treatment are essential. The first-line treatment for PCP is with trimethoprim-sulfamethoxazole (TMP-SMZ) given either intravenously or orally, regardless of previous prophylactic regimen. The initial dosage is 15–20 mg/kg/day of the trimethoprim component, divided every 6–8 hrs. With good clinical response, the dosage can be decreased to 10–15 mg/kg/day, divided every 6–8 hrs. Second-line treatments include oral dapsone with oral or IV TMP-SMZ, oral atovaquone, or IV pentamidine isethionate. Treatment duration is 21 days. For extrapulmonary pneumocystosis, IV therapy is preferred for initial treatment. Those with extrapulmonary disease should not be given prophylaxis with aerosolized pentamidine in the future due to the possibility of recurrence of extrapulmonary infection.

For patients who present with moderate-to-severe disease (Po$_2$ <70 mm Hg or Pao$_2$-to-Pao$_2$ gradient >35 mm Hg), early corticosteroid administration is also indicated and should be started within the first 72 hrs of therapy. The recommended regimen is oral prednisone, 40 mg twice daily for days 1–5, then 40 mg daily for days 6–10, and 20 mg daily for days 11–20. Alternatively, IV methylprednisolone can be given at 75% of the recommended prednisone dose if indicated (4).

Treatment failure occurs if no clinical improvement is seen despite 4–8 days of appropriate therapy. For failures related to drug toxicity, changing the regimen to another that is better tolerated is appropriate. It is anticipated that patients will have deterioration after the first 3–5 days of treatment due to the inflammatory response generated (4). Patients who do not tolerate TMP-SMZ may be treated with pentamidine, 4 mg/kg/day

by IV route once daily. Other drugs include trimethoprim/dapsone combination, pyrimethamine/sulfadoxine combination, clindamycin, primaquine, and atovaquone. None of them has been systematically studied in children.

Prevention

Prevention of PCP includes appropriate prophylaxis. For HIV-positive patients with CD4 counts of <200/mm^3, daily prophylaxis with TMP-SMZ is indicated. If this therapy cannot be tolerated, second-line therapies should be used, including dapsone, dapsone and pyrimethamine, atovaquone, or aerosolized pentamidine. Prophylaxis should continue until the CD4 count is >200/mm^3 for 3 months. For patients who became infected while their CD4 counts were >200/mm^3, prophylaxis should continue indefinitely (4).

Invasive Aspergillosis

Aspergillus is a group of ubiquitous fungal organisms found in soil and other settings, including the hospital environment. The pathogenic species include *A. fumigatus*, *A. niger* and *A. flavus*. *A. fumigatus* is the most common species responsible for pneumonia in immunocompromised hosts. In tissue, the organisms form septate hyphae with regular 45-degree dichotomous branching, best seen with methenamine silver staining. The organisms enter the body via the respiratory route. Aspergillosis of the lung is often preceded or accompanied by invasion of the nose and paranasal sinuses in susceptible hosts.

Clinical Features

Susceptible hosts include recipients of lung, bone marrow, and liver transplants; those who have received treatment for malignancy, chronic granulomatous disease, or HIV infection; and those on immunosuppressive chemotherapy. Invasiveness appears to depend on the genetic and immune status of the host, and on the extent and duration of exposure to spores. Disseminated aspergillosis, defined as infection of 2 or more noncontiguous organs, is the most severe form of clinical aspergillosis. Patients usually have pulmonic disease and widespread organ involvement (**Table 84.3**).

Invasive pulmonary aspergillosis is manifested most commonly as necrotizing bronchopneumonia or hemorrhagic infarction, although single or multiple abscesses, granulomata, or lobar infiltrates are occasionally present. Positive-surveillance nasal cultures for *Aspergillus* frequently precede the development of invasive pulmonary aspergillosis. Patients may present with fever, dyspnea, nonproductive cough, mild hemoptysis, and pleuritic chest pain, which may be especially prominent in patients with hemorrhagic pulmonary infarction. Coexisting sinusitis is a common finding in neutropenic children. In children with chronic granulomatous disease, direct extension from the lungs to the chest wall may occur. Several unusual clinical manifestations in children have been reported, including necrotizing bronchitis with pseudomembrane formation, invasive tracheitis, tracheoesophageal fistula, and pleural aspergillosis (33).

Acute, invasive sinusitis is rare in children and occurs almost exclusively in patients with profound neutropenia associated with chemotherapy or following organ transplant. In the setting of profound immunosuppression, the course may be fulminant, with early bone destruction, direct extension to

TABLE 84.3

CLINICAL MANIFESTATIONS OF INVASIVE ASPERGILLOSIS

Organ system	Patients predisposed	Clinical manifestations
Respiratory system	Organ transplant patients, chronic granulomatous disease, HIV infection, and immunosuppressive chemotherapy	Necrotizing bronchopneumonia or hemorrhagic infarction, single or multiple abscesses, granulomata, or lobar infiltrates Patients may present with fever, dyspnea, nonproductive cough, mild hemoptysis, and pleuritic chest pain, necrotizing bronchitis with pseudomembrane formation, invasive tracheitis, tracheoesophageal fistula, and pleural aspergillosis In CGD: direct extension from the lungs to the chest wall
Paranasal sinuses	Profound neutropenia associated with chemotherapy or recipient of organ transplant	Sinusitis: direct extension to the orbit, early bone destruction, fever, cough, epistaxis, headache, sinus pain, periorbital swelling, and nasal congestion; duskiness or necrosis of the nasal septum or inferior turbinates
Eyes	Organ transplant patients, chronic granulomatous disease, HIV infection, and immunosuppressive chemotherapy	Fungal endophthalmitis: pain, photophobia, and diminished visual acuity Retinal hemorrhage, infarction, focal retinitis, and vitreitis Fungal keratitis and episcleritis Orbital cellulites: diplopia, periorbital edema, proptosis, and pain on lateral gaze
Central nervous system	Immunosuppressed patients	Brain abscess: single or multiple in cerebrum or cerebellum Present with neurologic deficits, hemiparesis, cranial nerve palsies, or seizures Meningeal signs may be absent
Bones and joints	Immunosuppressed patients, CGD	Vertebral and rib osteomyelitis: cord compression due to epidural abscess secondary to vertebral osteomyelitis
Heart	Patients with open-heart surgery	Endocarditis: persistent fever, evidence of embolic phenomena, and disseminated intravascular coagulopathy Pericarditis: cardiac tamponade
Genitourinary system	Immunosuppressed patients	Urinary tract infection: fever, chills, and microhematuria Unilateral flank pain may occur with ascending infection
Other organ systems		Abscesses: liver, thyroid, testis, spleen, and adrenals

HIV, human immunodeficiency virus; CGD, chronic granulomatous disease

the orbit and anterior cranial fossa, widespread dissemination, and a high mortality rate. Fever, cough, epistaxis, headache, sinus pain, periorbital swelling, and nasal congestion are the most common clinical signs. Examination typically shows nasal crusting with rhinorrhea, sinus tenderness, nasal or oral ulceration, and duskiness or necrosis of the nasal septum or inferior turbinates. Multiple sinus involvement with opacification or air-fluid levels can be demonstrated radiographically or by CT. Biopsy and culture of the nasal or sinus mucosa demonstrate large numbers of hyphae, and fungal cultures typically yield *A. fumigatus, A. flavus,* or, less often, *Rhizopus* or *Candida.*

Otomycosis may occur in immunosuppressed children due to *A. niger* or *A. fumigatus.* Occasionally, otitis externa and mastoiditis may occur in malnourished children.

Cutaneous aspergillosis is a common manifestation of invasive disease in immunocompromised children secondary to hematogenous dissemination or local spread. Local spread may result either from direct inoculation of the skin at sites of local trauma, such as IV catheter sites or complicating burn wounds, or from diaper dermatitis. Cutaneous lesions progress from erythematous or violaceous papules or plaques through a hemorrhagic bullous stage to a purpuric ulcer with central necrosis and eschar formation, called *ecthyma gangrenosum.*

In disseminated *Aspergillus* infection, fungal endophthalmitis may be an important finding. Patients may have pain, photophobia, and diminished visual acuity. Examination of the retina shows retinal hemorrhage, focal retinitis, and vitreitis. Unusual ocular manifestations include bilateral retinal infarction secondary to disseminated disease and fungal keratosis due to direct inoculation of spores into the eye and episcleritis.

Orbital cellulitis may occur even in immunocompetent patients secondary to invasive sinusitis. Infection spreads locally through destroyed orbital walls and may involve the retro-orbital space. Patients may present with diplopia, periorbital edema, proptosis, and pain on lateral gaze (18).

Aspergillosis of the CNS may result from direct spread from the paranasal sinuses or, more commonly, from widespread dissemination in immunosuppressed patients. CNS aspergillosis is rare but has very high fatality rates. The disease may be associated with single or multiple abscesses in the cerebrum or cerebellum. Patients may present with neurologic deficits, hemiparesis, cranial nerve palsies, or seizures. Meningeal signs may be absent (32).

Involvement of bones due to *Aspergillus* infection is uncommon. It may follow direct extension of infection from lungs,

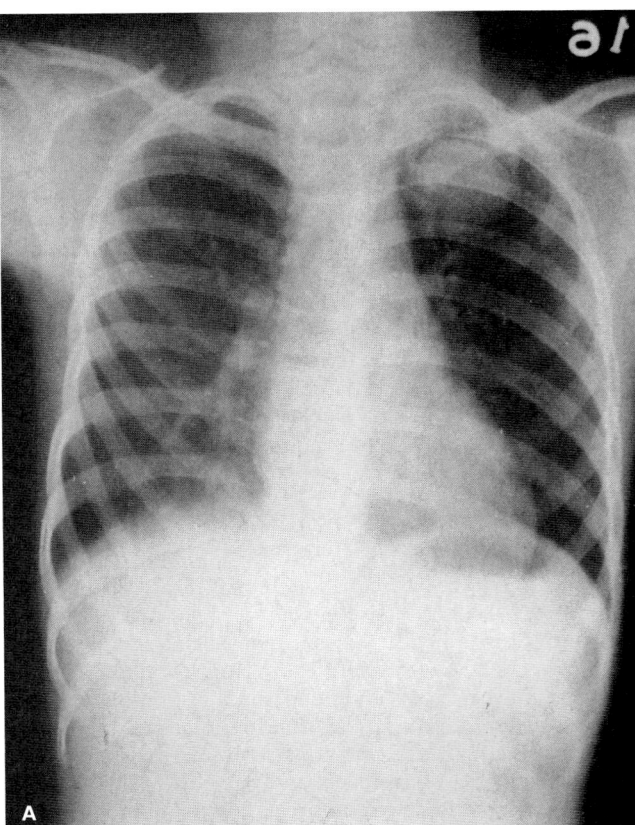
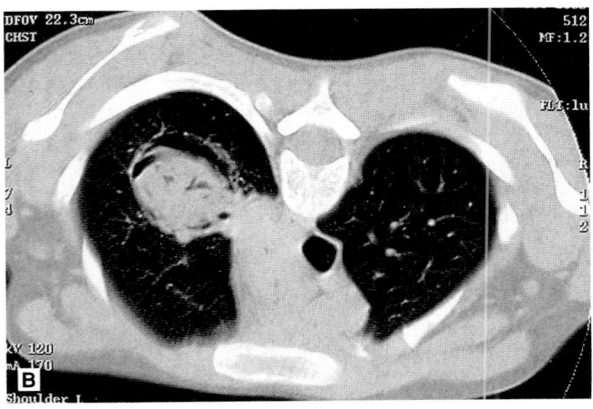
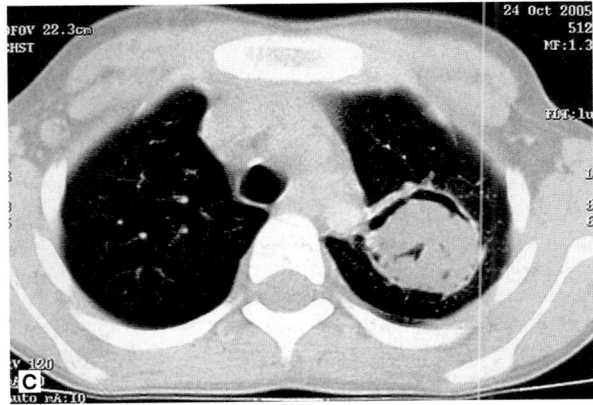

FIGURE 84.1. X-ray and chest CT films of 8-year-old girl suffering from pulmonary aspergillosis. A: X-ray of chest, showing homogenous round shadow in left upper zone. B,C: CT scan of chest, showing a fungal ball in left upper lobe. This patient underwent lobectomy of left upper lobe. Histopathology and culture showed *Aspergillus fumigatus.*

overlying skin, a surgical or traumatic wound, or hematogenous spread. Vertebra and ribs are the commonly involved bones. Invasive aspergillosis may present as cord compression due to epidural abscess secondary to vertebral osteomyelitis in children with chronic granulomatous disease (19).

Aspergillus endocarditis may occur during open heart surgery or as part of disseminated disease. Clinical features include persistent fever, evidence of embolic phenomena, and disseminated intravascular coagulopathy after cardiac surgery. Echocardiography may be useful for the detection of mycotic aneurysms, intracardiac vegetations, or intra-aortic vegetations (41). Pericarditis due to spread from contiguous pleural foci may occur, and these patients may develop cardiac tamponade.

Infection of the genitourinary tract with *Aspergillus* may result from hematogenous spread or ascending infection. Clinical manifestations include fever, chills, and microhematuria. Unilateral flank pain may occur with ascending infection.

Abscesses due to *Aspergillus* species may develop in immunocompromised children in liver, thyroid, testis, spleen, and adrenals. The infection may spread either as part of hematogenous infection or local extension.

Diagnosis

The mainstay for diagnosis of invasive aspergillosis is chest x-ray. Older children and adults are more likely to show the classic cavitation and air crescent formation than young children (**Fig. 84.1**). A diagnostic adjunct is the galactomannan assay, commonly used in adults. This assay is difficult to interpret in children, because of the differences in pediatric and adult values. Pediatric studies have shown a false-positive rate of 40% using the galactomannan assay, as compared to a false-positive rate of 1% in adults. Potential reasons for the age-related difference are (a) pediatric gut flora may contain cross-reactive antigens to the assay, and (b) the antigen may be found in infant formula. Furthermore, patients with chronic granulomatous disease who have positive lung biopsy specimens for aspergillosis have been shown to be galactomannan negative. Therefore, this test should not be used to diagnose invasive aspergillosis in children.

In the laboratory, wet preparations of BAL fluid or tissue specimens can be examined using potassium hydroxide or Gomori methenamine-silver nitrate stain to look for the typical morphologic features of *Aspergillus*. Identification from tissue culture renders a definitive diagnosis and is isolated readily from lung, sinus, and skin biopsy specimens on Sabouraud dextrose agar or brain-heart infusion media. Blood culture specimens rarely yield positive results.

If allergic aspergillosis is suspected clinically, results of *Aspergillus*-specific IgE serology, eosinophilia, and a positive skin test can provide evidence for the diagnosis. As with invasive candidiasis, a potential adjunct for the diagnosis of invasive fungal disease that has been used successfully in adults is the β-D-glucan detection assay (36,37). This assay has not yet been standardized for the pediatric population.

The utility of PCR for the diagnosis of invasive aspergillosis is limited. Assays are not standardized, nor are they commercially available. A positive result from a BAL specimen may indicate colonization with a low positive predictive value. A negative result may be helpful to exclude aspergillosis.

Management

High-dose amphotericin B (1–1.5 mg/kg/day) is the treatment of choice for invasive aspergillosis. The duration of therapy is 4–12 weeks. Lipid formulations of amphotericin B should be considered when the patient is refractory to conventional amphotericin, or when conventional amphotericin causes toxic effects. Itraconazole can also be considered for children whose isolate is susceptible, but safety and toxicity data in children are lacking. Caspofungin is an alternative therapy, but it lacks approval by the US Food and Drug Administration for use in children. Voriconazole is approved for children aged 12 and older for treatment of invasive aspergillosis but not for younger children. Data suggest that the optimal dose of voriconazole in children is much higher than in adults, but the exact pediatric dosage is unknown. However, caution is necessary when using voriconazole to treat invasive aspergillosis as, unlike amphotericin, it does not have activity against zygomycosis. Breakthrough infections with zygomycosis have been reported while treating invasive aspergillosis with voriconazole. At this writing, no prospective, randomized, controlled clinical trial has been conducted to evaluate treatment of invasive aspergillosis in the pediatric population.

Prevention

Outbreaks of *Aspergillus* infection have been reported among immunosuppressed patients at hospitals that are undergoing renovation or construction. Measures to reduce the risk of aspergillosis in this population include the use of containment systems for construction/remodeling of facilities and routine cleaning of air systems, including air filters. Patient rooms equipped with high-efficiency particulate air filters and laminar flow also decrease risk. Though prophylactic regimens exist for prevention of invasive aspergillosis in adults using amphotericin B, itraconazole, caspofungin, and voriconazole, none of these strategies has been tested in children.

Mucormycosis

Mucormycosis is an acute and often fatal infection caused by a fungus of the Mucorales order of the Zygomycetes class. Infections by members of the mucormycosis class of fungi typically arise in patients with substantial underlying immunosuppression, such as critically ill premature newborns and older children with underlying hematopoietic malignancies, organ transplantation, and diabetes.

Clinical Features

The organisms that cause mucormycosis may involve lungs, brain, sinuses, kidneys, and skin. Pulmonary involvement may present with persistent fever, chest pain, hemoptysis, and weight loss. Cavitation may occur. The organism invades blood vessels and may disseminate to the brain and other sites. Sudden death may occur due to massive pulmonary hemorrhage, mediastinitis, or airway obstruction.

Rhinocerebral mucormycosis, though relatively uncommon, may cause fatal infection. Sinusitis may occur in children with underlying diseases such as malignancies. It may progress to involve orbits and brain. Multiple abscesses in brain may manifest as headache, vomiting, fever, focal deficits, loss of vision, and occasionally, seizures.

Primary cutaneous mucormycosis is an uncommon, deep, and aggressive fungal infection that occurs mainly in immunosuppressed or diabetic patients. Skin involvement may begin as a vascular, hemorrhagic, erythematous plaque and rapidly progress to a dark, necrotic, painful ulcer with erythematous border on the extremities or other parts of body (45). Occasionally, gangrenous cellulitis may be one of the serious manifestations in critically ill, premature newborns and older children with underlying hematopoietic malignancies and/or following BMT.

Diagnosis

Diagnosis of zygomycosis is achieved through a high level of suspicion and aggressive pursuit of tissue culture. Often, mucormycosis is not suspected among hematology patients, as most patients are presumed to have aspergillosis. The direct morphologic classification of tissue culture specimens remains the standard for diagnosis. While wet mounts of sputum, sinus secretions, or BAL fluid are often negative, positivity denotes invasive zygomycosis that should be treated. Cultures of blood or urine are also rarely positive. Invasive testing procedures, including fine-needle aspirates of lesions in deep tissue, transbronchial biopsies of pulmonary lesions, sinus tissue samples, scrapings of mucocutaneous lesions, or samples of deep tissue lesions, yield higher results (16).

Various methods can be used to detect Mucorales, including treatment with potassium hydroxide, Gomori's methenamine-silver staining, hematoxylin and eosin staining, and periodic acid-Schiff staining. Histopathologic specimens show evidence of vascular invasion. CT of the chest may identify infiltrates suggestive of Mucorales that are not seen on chest x-ray. PCR methods to detect mucormycosis are being developed and may soon be available for diagnosis (40).

Management

The mainstays of treatment include a combination of early diagnosis, treatment of the underlying medical condition, reduction of immunosuppression, antifungal therapy, and surgical debridement. After the patient is diagnosed, predisposing factors such as hyperglycemia and metabolic acidosis should be corrected to increase survival. Immunosuppressive therapy should be decreased or postponed until the mucormycosis is under control. Improvement of outcomes is related to neutrophil recovery, and antifungal therapy has been ineffective in patients with persistent neutropenia. Granulocyte colony-stimulating factor and granulocyte-macrophage colony-stimulating factor should be considered as adjunct therapy to enhance neutrophil activity against zygomycoses. Amphotericin B is the drug of choice for the treatment of mucormycosis, although higher doses are necessary due to resistance. The duration of therapy is not well established. Lipid formulations of amphotericin B may be preferred due to their lower toxicity profile and the ability to achieve higher serum concentrations while limiting toxicity. Evidence exists for the effectiveness of hyperbaric oxygen therapy against zygomycosis, and it should be considered where available. Lastly, surgical debridement of mucormycosis lesions results in increased survival compared to patients who are treated medically (16). A new, enhanced-spectrum triazole agent, posaconazole, has shown promise in treating zygomycosis that is refractory to amphotericin (52). While its use is not approved in children, it may be used in the future as an alternative to amphotericin for the treatment of zygomycosis.

Prevention

Prophylactic amphotericin is not indicated for prevention of mucormycosis. Prevention strategies include control of underlying predisposing factors, such as diabetes, and judicious use of deferoxamine and corticosteroids (16).

Cryptococcosis

Cryptococcosis is a fungal disease of humans and animals caused by *Cryptococcus neoformans*, a yeast-like encapsulated fungus. Infection is thought to be acquired by inhalation of fungus into lungs, where the infection mostly goes unnoticed, and it has strong predilection for the CNS. The increasing number of cases of HIV-related cryptococcosis over time paralleled the AIDS epidemic. The other conditions that predispose for cryptococcosis include malignancies, organ transplantation, primary immune deficiencies, and corticosteroid therapy. Of the two varieties, *C. neoformans* var. *neoformans* is more common and mainly infects immunocompromised hosts, whereas in immunocompetents, the infection is exclusively caused by var. *gatti* (14).

Clinical Manifestations

The disease primarily presents as subacute or chronic meningitis, although involvement of other organs (liver, spleen, skin, lymph node, eye, bones, adrenals, and ears) is variably seen. Cryptococcal meningitis more frequently occurs in patients with AIDS. These patients commonly present with headache and fever. Other manifestations include nausea and vomiting, neck stiffness, alteration of consciousness, impaired mental function, cranial nerve lesions, visual deficits, papilledema, seizures, diplopia, focal neurologic deficits, photophobia, and abnormal cerebellar signs.

Disseminated cryptococcosis may present with cough or chest pain, weight loss, fever, hemoptysis, hepatosplenomegaly, and cutaneous findings (e.g., ulcers, nodules, vesicles, abscesses, papules, and cellulitis). Occasional cases of cryptococcosis presenting as acute abdomen or mimicking pulmonary metastasis in Wilms tumor have been reported (8,12,25).

Diagnosis

The diagnosis of cryptococcal pulmonary infection is suggested by characteristic clinical and radiographic findings, sputum culture, serologic assays for IgG and IgM, and serologic testing for cryptococcal polysaccharide antigen by latex agglutination. Even in asymptomatic patients, chest x-ray findings of diffuse infiltrations with hilar adenopathy may be seen. Sputum culture results are more likely to be positive in patients with AIDS than in those without severely depressed T-cell function. Furthermore, sputum culture and cryptococcal-specific antibody testing are difficult to interpret, as they may indicate colonization. Latex agglutination studies for cryptococcal anti-

gen in serum are thought to reflect disseminated infection, but may be negative in those with isolated pulmonary disease. The definitive diagnosis of cryptococcus is via biopsy or fine-needle aspiration. The organism is slow-growing in culture, requiring a week to proliferate, making tissue culture slow and difficult. To improve yield and turnaround time, tissue specimens should be tested for cryptococcal antigenemia via in situ hybridization.

Cryptococcal meningitis is suggested by visualization of encapsulated yeast cells in CSF using India ink stain. Serum blood culture may yield the organism if the lysis-centrifugation technique is used. Cryptococcal polysaccharide antigen studies on CSF or serum yield results in 90% of patients infected.

Management

Immunocompetent patients with isolated pulmonary disease usually clear the organism without antifungal agents. However, as a small risk of dissemination is present, these patients should be treated with fluconazole.

For immunocompromised patients with isolated pulmonary disease, CSF and serum should be evaluated for evidence of disseminated disease. Patients with disseminated disease (including meningitis) should be treated with a combination of amphotericin B and flucytosine for at least 2 weeks or until CSF testing is negative, continuing with amphotericin B for an additional 4 weeks of therapy. Patients who are immunosuppressed should be treated with a longer course of therapy. Children who are HIV positive should continue on fluconazole after treatment of their primary infection for life-long suppressive therapy.

Prevention

The mainstay of prevention is chronic suppressive therapy for HIV-positive children who have had cryptococcus in the past. Those who have cellular immunodeficiency, AIDS (especially with CD4 count <100/mm^3), or are on high-dose corticosteroids should avoid contact with birds.

Histoplasmosis

Histoplasmosis is a systemic disease caused by the dimorphic fungus *Histoplasma capsulatum*, which exists as a soil saprophyte and grows best in soil enriched with bird or bat guano. Histoplasmosis occurs throughout the Western hemisphere, but is highly endemic in the Ohio River and Mississippi River valleys of the US. Most outbreaks occur following activities that disturb the soil of old roosting sites for birds or following visits to bat-inhabited caves. Histoplasmosis has been described in travelers returning from several Central American, South American, and Caribbean countries. Cases of histoplasmosis have also been reported from other parts of the world.

Clinical Features

In children, histoplasmosis occurs exclusively as an acute, progressive, life-threatening infection. Most of these infections develop in children with acquired or congenital cellular immune deficiency. Histoplasmosis is an AIDS-defining opportunistic infection and commonly occurs in HIV-infected persons residing in endemic areas. Clinical manifestations of disseminated histoplasmosis include prolonged, unexplained fever, respiratory complaints, abdominal pain, weight loss, and diarrhea. Liver, spleen, and lymph nodes may be enlarged. Skin may show mucocutaneous lesions, maculopapular rash, papules, nodules, pustules, and ulcerative lesions. Children may present with meningitis or encephalitis and focal brain lesions (3,23).

Diagnosis

The diagnosis of histoplasmosis is made via culture, fungal stain, antigen detection, and serologic tests for antibodies. Cultures of lung tissue or BAL specimens are positive in 85% of those with acute pulmonary disease, but much less in those with more limited pulmonary histoplasmosis. Blood cultures are more likely to yield organism if the lysis-centrifugation technique is utilized. The organism requires weeks to grow i+ culture Genitourinary system. Other organ systems, and this method, while the gold standard for identification, is often used in conjunction with antigen testing. Rapid results of antigen testing of pulmonary, CSF, urine, and blood are fairly sensitive for disseminated disease, with sensitivity being higher in urine than blood. The only drawback is that cross-reactivity can occur with penicilliosis, paracoccidioidomycosis, blastomycosis, and African histoplasmosis. Furthermore, antigen levels can be followed as therapy is initiated to determine the success of treatment. Fungal silver or Wright stain can be used on peripheral blood or tissue culture to diagnose histoplasmosis. Serologic tests for histoplasma antibodies typically yield 80%–90% positivity for those with disseminated or acute pulmonary disease, but they may not be useful due to lack of production early in the disease course and in immunosuppressed patients.

Management

No treatment is indicated for immunocompetent children with primary pulmonary histoplasmosis, as the disease usually follows a self-limited course. For complicated disease in children, including those who are immunocompromised, the treatment of histoplasmosis generally follows treatment guidelines for adults. Amphotericin B is the standard therapy for serious infections, followed by itraconazole for long-term suppressive therapy. Those with HIV who become infected with *H. capsulatum* should be placed on itraconazole therapy for life. For isolated pericarditis, drainage of pericardial fluid and nonsteroidal anti-inflammatory drugs are the mainstays of therapy—no antifungals are indicated (2).

Prevention

To prevent histoplasmosis in immunocompromised patients, encourage them to avoid traveling to endemic areas and walking inside caves where bird droppings may aerosolize readily. It is also important to know the serologic status of patients diagnosed with immunodeficiency or in whom transplantation is considered, especially if they spent time in endemic areas, though no recommendations exist for prophylaxis.

MYCOBACTERIAL INFECTIONS

Mycobacterial infections are frequent, opportunistic pathogens associated with the AIDS. With the onset of the AIDS epidemic, disease due to both *Mycobacterium tuberculosis* and atypical strains such as *M. avium-intracellulare* have been increasingly recognized in both AIDS and non-AIDS immunodeficient populations. Those infected with the HIV are particularly susceptible to tuberculosis (TB), either by the reactivation of latent

infection or by a primary infection with rapid progression to active disease (50).

Nontuberculous Mycobacteria

Nontuberculous mycobacteria, ubiquitous organisms in the environment, historically have not caused invasive disease in immunocompetent hosts. However, increasing numbers of case reports document the spectrum of disease caused by these bacteria in otherwise healthy individuals in the past two decades (35).

Clinical Features

Lymphadenitis is the most common manifestation of infection due to nontuberculous mycobacteria. The majority of patients present with an enlarged palpable mass and preceding constitutional symptoms. The lymph node involvement may be multiple, with the most common site being the cervical region. Cases of disseminated *M. avium* complex with gastrointestinal tract involvement have been reported in HIV-infected children, hematopoietic stem cell transplant recipients, and patients with interferon (IFN)-γ receptor-1 deficiency. Common clinical findings include prolonged fever, weight loss, lymphadenopathy, hepatosplenomegaly, diarrhea, anemia, and leukopenia (13).

Diagnosis

If atypical mycobacterial disease is suspected, samples should be sent for acid-fast bacillus (AFB) smear and culture, as well as DNA-probe testing. Rapid identification using DNA-probe analysis can differentiate tuberculous from nontuberculous mycobacteria (9). A positive DNA-probe test can be confirmed by culture, and appropriate therapy based on known susceptibilities can be initiated. Susceptibility testing should be ordered for organisms that are grown in culture, so that therapy can be tailored.

Diagnostic testing for atypical mycobacteria depends on the involved site of infection. For suspected pulmonary disease, three sputum specimens obtained on three different days should be sent for AFB smear and culture. PCR testing is becoming the gold standard for detection of atypical mycobacterial infection and should be performed on at least one sputum specimen and any AFB smear-positive specimen.

Susceptibility testing for atypical mycobacterium is useful for appropriate management of disease, but these results might not correlate with clinical efficacy. In addition to general susceptibility testing, some organism-specific testing recommendations are important to consider. For *M. avium-intracellulare*, susceptibility to clarithromycin should be tested if the patient was previously on macrolide therapy, is currently failing therapy, or is intolerant to current therapy. *M. kansasii* isolates should be tested for susceptibility to rifampin, as resistance does not develop during the course of therapy. Susceptibility testing is recommended only for *M. marinum* if patients fail to respond to initial therapy.

Management

Therapy for atypical mycobacterial infections depends on the organism and the site of involvement. For lymphadenitis due to *M. avium-intracellulare* or other atypical mycobacteria, surgical excision, if complete, is sufficient without antimicrobial therapy. If excision is not possible or incomplete, therapy with clarithromycin or azithromycin should be considered. The appropriate length of therapy, however, is not established (29).

For pulmonary disease due to *M. avium-intracellulare*, the treatment of choice includes clarithromycin or azithromycin, ethambutol, and rifabutin. Amikacin or streptomycin may be added in case of cavitary pulmonary disease. This therapy should be continued until the patient is culture negative for 12 months. For salvage therapy, rifabutin and amikacin and/or levofloxacin should be used.

Disseminated or pulmonary disease due to *M. kansasii* should be treated with rifampin, ethambutol, and isoniazid. Streptomycin or clarithromycin may be added for severe disease. This therapy should be continued for 18 months, provided the patient is culture-negative for at least 12 months. HIV-positive patients with disease due to *M. kansasii* should be given rifabutin instead of rifampin, and clarithromycin should be added to their regimen.

Prevention

Atypical mycobacterial infection is difficult to prevent, as these organisms are ubiquitous in the environment, and immunocompromised populations are particularly susceptible. In patients who are HIV positive, prophylaxis with azithromycin or clarithromycin is indicated for those with a CD4 count of $<100/mm^3$. This prophylaxis should continue for patients who are on antiretroviral therapy until their CD4 count is $>100/mm^3$ for 3–6 months (60).

Mycobacterium Tuberculosis

HIV and TB form a lethal combination, each speeding the other's progress. HIV weakens the immune system. TB, a leading cause of death among people who are HIV positive, accounts for ~13% of AIDS deaths worldwide. In Africa, HIV is the single most important factor that determines the increased incidence of TB in the past 10 years. It is estimated that by the end of 2000, 11.5 million HIV-infected adults worldwide were coinfected with *M. tuberculosis*; Africa and Southeast Asia accounted for 70% and 20%, respectively, of these cases (20).

Clinical Features

TB can occur in HIV-infected individuals at any CD4 count, which is in contrast to other opportunistic infections that generally occur when CD4 counts significantly decline. When children who are infected with HIV develop TB, the clinical picture is similar to TB in the immunocompetent child, although the disease tends to progress more rapidly and the clinical manifestations are more severe. An increased tendency for extrapulmonary disease and dissemination may be seen, as well as involvement of unusual sites and atypical chest x-ray findings. Extrapulmonary involvement occurs in more than 70% of patients with TB and preexisting AIDS or AIDS that is diagnosed soon after TB [0]onset but only in 24%–45% of patients with TB and less-advanced HIV infection (7).

Diagnosis

The diagnosis of TB in an immunocompromised patient requires a heightened suspicion and diagnostic modalities beyond the traditional purified protein derivative skin test. If purified protein derivative testing is utilized, a positive test for those who are immunosuppressed is defined as induration of >5 mm in diameter. While a positive purified protein derivative test without evidence of clinical disease (e.g., absence of pulmonary symptoms or chest x-ray findings) indicates latent TB infection, the additional x-ray findings and pulmonary symptoms are consistent with TB.

Evaluation for pulmonary TB should include a chest x-ray, although some experts would argue that lymphadenopathy characteristic of TB infection is best visualized on CT scan. In addition, sputum or gastric aspirate samples should be sent for AFB smear and culture for patients with pulmonary symptoms, cervical lymphadenopathy, or abnormalities on chest x-ray. For children and adolescents with suspected TB, the best test is the early-morning gastric aspirate, obtained on awakening via a nasogastric tube on 3 separate days, or induced sputum using hypertonic saline inhalation by nebulizer. If a sample returns positive for AFB, confirmation via culture or PCR is required, as other mycobacteria can give positive results for this test.

Evaluation for nonpulmonary TB includes AFB smear and culture of suspected sterile body sites, including CSF and lymph node or other biopsy specimens. PCR testing for mycobacterium TB can also be performed on these specimens to improve diagnostic yield. For patients with suspected disseminated disease, mycobacterial blood cultures can be obtained for diagnosis. Positive cultures for TB should be evaluated for drug sensitivity testing (4).

Management

Latent TB infection is managed with a single drug regimen, depending on the resistance pattern in particular geographic regions or the index case. For isoniazid-susceptible latent TB, the child is treated with isoniazid once daily for 6–9 months. In cases with isoniazid resistance, rifampin may be given once daily for 6 months. A combination of three drugs, including pyrazinamide, was associated with high rates of hepatotoxicity in some studies.

The recommended treatment for TB disease in patients who are HIV-positive includes a 6-month regimen, using isoniazid, rifampin (or rifabutin), pyrazinamide, and ethambutol for the first 2 months, and isoniazid and rifampin for next 4 months. Prolonged therapy for 9 months is indicated for those with delayed clinical or bacteriologic response to therapy. Caution is advised for HIV patients on antiretroviral therapy, as many of these drugs have overlapping toxicities and additive side effects. Substantial pharmacokinetic interactions occur between the rifamycin component of antituberculosis treatment and antiretroviral drugs, especially protease inhibitors and nonnucleoside reverse transcriptase inhibitors. The key therapeutic principles that underlie the treatment of HIV-TB are (a) treatment of TB always takes precedence over the treatment of HIV infection; (b) in patients who are already on highly active antiretroviral therapy (HAART), it must be continued with appropriate modifications in both HAART and antituberculosis treatment; and (c) in patients who are not receiving HAART, the need for, and timing of, initiation of HAART should be decided on an individual basis after assessing the short-term risk of disease progression and death, based on CD4$^+$ count and type of TB. If a child infected with HIV is diagnosed with TB, immunosuppression is not severe (CD4 counts of $>15\%$), and no significant HIV-related illnesses are present, the child should be treated for TB first and monitored carefully for any worsening of immune status. If a child who is infected with HIV is diagnosed to have TB and immunosuppression is severe (CD4

TABLE 84.4

STANDARDIZED TUBERCULOSIS TREATMENT REGIMENS

Categories	Suggested by WHO for adults	Suggested type of tuberculosis in children	Suggested regimens
Category I	New sputum-positive pulmonary TB	PPC, PPD, TBL, pleural effusion, abdominal TB, osteoarticular TB, genitourinary TB, CNS TB	2 HRZE 4 HR **OR** 2 SHRZ 4HR
Category II	Relapse treatment failure; return after adult default (interrupted treatment)	Relapse/treatment failure Interrupted treatment	2 SHRZE 1 HRZE 5 HRE
Category III	Sputum-negative pulmonary with limited parenchymal involvement, extrapulmonary TB (less severe forms)	Single lymph node, small effusion, skin TB	2 HRZ 4 HR

WHO, World Health Organization; TB, tuberculosis; PPC, pulmonary primary complex; PPD, progressive primary disease, TBL, tubercular lymphadenitis, CNS TB, central nervous system tuberculosis. H, isoniazid; R, rifampicin; Z, pyrazinamide; E, ethambutol; S, Streptomycin; 2 HRZE 4 HR, 2 months of 4 drugs (HRZE) followed by 4 months of 2 drugs (HR); 2 SHRZE 1 HRZE, 5 HRE: 2 months of 5 drugs (SHRZE), followed by 1 month of 4 drugs (HRZE), followed by 5 months of 3 drugs (HRE); 2 HRZE 4 HR, 2 months of 3 drugs (HRZ), followed by 4 months of 2 drugs (HR)

counts of <15%) or if he has significant HIV-related illnesses, the child should be treated concurrently with antitubercular therapy and modified efavirenz-based antiretroviral therapy. If a child who is on antiretroviral therapy (protease inhibitor or nevirapine-based regimes) develops TB, the antiretroviral therapy is modified, and efavirenz is used instead of nevirapine or protease inhibitor, and antitubercular therapy is started. After completion of antitubercular therapy, the initial antiretroviral therapy regimen may be restarted.

Treatment of TB that is not associated with HIV infection should be based on drug resistance in the index case, in the local geographic area, or in the country of origin for imported cases. The local health department maintains data on local patterns of TB resistance and can advise if a three- or four-drug regimen should be used. Local health departments should also be notified of any new case of TB so that investigation and testing of contacts can begin. Directly observed therapy is offered in many countries through local health departments/facilities. The World Health Organization has recommended category-based treatment for children in high-endemic areas (24) (**Table 84.4**).

Management of extrapulmonary TB includes chemotherapy and consideration of other therapies. No evidence suggests that surgery in addition to chemotherapy provides added benefit for spinal TB (48). For pericarditis associated with TB, adjunctive corticosteroids should be considered, but not routinely given for treatment, as no advantage has been proven.

Monitoring for treatment success is essential for treatment of TB. For patients with evidence of pulmonary TB, sputum specimens should be obtained monthly until two consecutive specimens are negative. Patients should be followed clinically and radiographically for evidence of treatment success. Routine laboratory testing is not indicated to monitor for adverse medication effects unless elevated transaminase levels are noted at baseline (4).

Prevention

A successful approach to prevention of TB comprises many strategies, including hospital infection control measures, case-finding and managing contacts, pharmacotherapy for contacts,

and consideration for Bacille Calmette-Guérin vaccine in select populations. Though most children with TB are not contagious (except those with cavitary lesions, positive sputum AFB smears, laryngeal involvement, pulmonary infection, or suspected congenital infection), they are often exposed by a visiting family member who is infectious. For this reason, many hospitals attempt to place these children in a negative-pressure room, with caregivers using particulate respirators. The local health department should be immediately informed when a child tests positive for TB. The health department will direct testing of contacts to identify others who have been exposed and, potentially, the index case. Those who test positive should be given appropriate therapy based on their diagnosis of latent infection or TB disease. Bacille Calmette-Guérin vaccination should be considered for children who live in an environment in which they are exposed to TB that is either not being treated or is resistant to isoniazid and rifampin, and from which the child cannot be removed. In countries with universal Bacille Calmette-Guérin vaccination programs, immunocompromised children who are in contact with adults whose sputum smear is positive for TB should be treated with isoniazid prophylaxis for 6–9 months. If the index case has documented isoniazid resistance, the child may be treated with rifampicin for 6 months. If the index case has documented resistance to isoniazid and rifampicin, the child may be treated with two drugs (e.g., ethambutol and fluoroquinolones) for 9–12 months.

PARASITIC INFECTIONS

Toxoplasmosis

Toxoplasmosis is a parasitic infection. *Toxoplasma gondii* infects cats and other animals and secondarily infects man, causing congenital toxoplasmosis during intrauterine infection.

Clinical features

Owing to the increasing number of patients with AIDS and immunosuppressed transplant patients, disseminated *T. gondii* has emerged as a potentially fatal pathogen. Common presentations include fever, encephalitis, pneumonia, myocarditis, and bone marrow suppression.

Diagnosis

The diagnosis of infection due to toxoplasma is made through clinical presentation with confirmation either through serologic methods (reserved for immunocompetent hosts) or molecular methods, such as PCR. In infants and other immunocompromised patients (i.e., HIV patients) with a suspected diagnosis of toxoplasma, sera should be sent for PCR testing.

In immunocompetent patients, toxoplasma-specific IgG will peak in serum 1–2 months after infection and may remain positive for life. A fourfold rise in serum IgG is consistent with infection. A positive IgM titer for *T. gondii* indicates recent or acute infection. IgM titers may not be positive until 1 month after onset of infection, and may take up to 2 years to fall.

Pregnant females who test positive for toxoplasma-specific IgG can be further tested for IgG avidity. During the course of infection with toxoplasma, the production of high-avidity IgG takes 12–16 weeks. Therefore, if a pregnant female has a positive IgG in the first trimester, testing for high-avidity IgG that is positive denotes an infection in the distant past and is not consistent with gestational infection.

HIV-1–infected patients with suspected toxoplasma encephalitis should undergo serologic testing, CSF analysis including PCR testing, and serum PCR testing. They are usually positive for serum toxoplasma IgG. Definitive testing for toxoplasma encephalitis involves a brain biopsy, with organisms seen on hematoxylin and eosin stains. CSF testing for toxoplasma via PCR is highly specific (96%–100%) but is associated with a low sensitivity (50%) (4).

Management

For pregnant females infected during the first trimester or early during the second trimester, spiramycin is recommended for treatment. For females infected late in the second trimester or during the third trimester, a combination of pyrimethamine, sulfadoxine, and folinic acid is recommended.

Infants with toxoplasmosis may be treated with sulfadiazine, pyrimethamine, and folinic acid for a minimum of 12 months. Steroids should be considered for infants with elevated CSF protein and chorioretinitis. Intensive monitoring of ophthalmologic, neuroradiologic, and CSF parameters should be part of their follow-up.

HIV-positive patients with *T. gondii* encephalitis should be treated with pyrimethamine, sulfadiazine, and leucovorin. Pyrimethamine penetrates the brain parenchyma, while leucovorin prevents hematologic toxicities associated with its use. TMP-SMZ is reported to be effective and better tolerated but has less in vitro activity, and practitioners have less experience with its use in the setting of toxoplasma encephalitis. Other regimens include atovaquone, pyrimethamine, and leucovorin; atovaquone with or without sulfadiazine; and azithromycin, pyrimethamine, and leucovorin. Therapy should be given for at least 6 weeks, with longer courses for extensive disease or evidence of incomplete response. Corticosteroids should be considered when a mass effect associated with focal lesions is seen. Patients should be monitored for clinical and radiologic improvement. Leucovorin dosage can be increased if bone marrow suppression develops. Brain biopsy and change in treatment regimen should be considered in patients who deteriorate within the first 2 weeks of therapy (4).

Prevention

Primary prevention efforts designed to educate and increase awareness among pregnant women have resulted in reduction of seroconversion in pregnant women by 60%. Secondary prevention of fetal infection includes diagnosis and treatment of gestational toxoplasmosis. HIV-positive pregnant women with a history of toxoplasma infection and CD4 count of <200/mm^3 should be placed on prophylaxis with TMP-SMZ to prevent reactivation and neonatal infection. HIV-positive patients who have been treated for toxoplasma encephalitis should be placed on life-long prophylaxis with sulfadiazine, pyrimethamine, and folinic acid. Prophylaxis may be discontinued if immune reconstitution occurs with antiretroviral therapy (a sustained CD4 count of >200/mm^3 for 6 months) (4).

Cryptosporidium Infection

Cryptosporidium spp. is a major cause of diarrheal disease in both immunocompetent and immunodeficient individuals. The most severe disease is seen in individuals with defects in the T-cell response. Children with HIV infection, primary immunodeficiencies (most notably severe combined immunodeficiency syndrome), and acute leukemia seem to be most at risk from cryptosporidiosis.

Clinical Features

Immunocompromised patients, including children with severe malnutrition, suffer from severe and prolonged watery diarrhea. Disease may be fatal. In addition, body systems other than the gastrointestinal tract may be affected. Cryptosporidium may cause cholangitis (particularly sclerosing cholangitis), pancreatitis, and respiratory symptoms. Cryptosporidium may also cause respiratory symptoms. In most patients with respiratory symptoms, coinfection with typical or atypical mycobacterium occurs.

Diagnosis

Diagnosis of cryptosporidium is made by examination of stool, which can be performed using a modified acid-fast stain to look for oocysts. However, due to increased sensitivity and specificity, immunofluorescence microscopy and enzyme-linked immunoassays are now the methods of choice for identifying cryptosporidium in stool. Molecular methods for diagnosis are currently being used primarily for research purposes and are not available for clinical use.

Management

Infection in immunocompetent persons is self-limiting and does not require treatment. However, in the immunocompromised, treatment is indicated. The current therapy for immunocompromised children with cryptosporidiosis, in addition to electrolyte management and replacement of fluids, is nitazoxanide. However, the effect of nitazoxanide on the course of cryptosporidiosis has been reported as marginal, with little significant benefit (57). Immunocompromised patients require a different dosing regimen than immunocompetent patients for nitazoxanide (47). The suggested doses of nitazoxanide are 500 mg twice daily for 3 days in adults and adolescents, 200 mg twice daily for 3 days in children aged 4–11 years, and 100-mg doses twice daily for 3 days in children aged 1–3 years.

Prevention

Immune reconstitution is essential to preventing cryptosporidiosis in immunocompromised patients (47). Those with diarrhea should not use public recreational waters until 2 weeks after diarrhea is resolved. In areas where drinking water is contaminated, it should be boiled prior to consumption.

CONCLUSIONS AND FUTURE DIRECTIONS

Opportunistic infections are common causes of morbidity and mortality in children admitted in PICUs. The predisposing conditions include primary or secondary immune deficiencies. The common conditions include primary immune deficiency of T cells and B cells, complement deficiency, or phagocytic defects. Acquired immune deficiencies include children with HIV infections, children on immunosuppressant for organ transplant, collagen vascular diseases, etc.

Patients with opportunistic infections present to PICUs with respiratory infections, sepsis, infections of the CNS, or multiorgan dysfunction. Due to underlying immune deficiency, the clinical course is fulminant, and the case fatality is high. Clinical signs and symptoms may provide important clues of the immune deficiency and the possible etiologic agent of infection. Children with humoral immune deficiency conditions contract infections due to *S. aureus*, encapsulated organisms such as *S. pneumoniae* and *H. influenzae*, and with gram-negative organisms such as *Pseudomonas* spp. These patients may develop arthritis due to echoviruses, coxsackie viruses, adenoviruses, and *Ureaplasma urealyticum*. Some of these patients may develop infections due to *P. jiroveci (P. carinii)* pneumonitis, and *Cryptosporidium*. Children with T-cell deficiency disorders are more prone to disseminated viral infections due to HSV, VZV, and CMV, and may develop progressive pneumonia caused by parainfluenza, respiratory syncytial virus, cytomegalovirus, varicella, and *P. jiroveci*. They may also develop superficial and systemic fungal infections, parasitic infections, and disseminated bacilli Calmette-Guérin disease after vaccination for that disease. Children with phagocytic disorders are more prone for recurrent pyogenic and fungal infections due to *Pseudomonas*, *Serratia marcescens*, and *S. aureus*, and fungi such as *Aspergillus* and *Candida*. Patients may present with cellulitis, perirectal abscesses, stomatitis, pulmonary infection, suppurative adenitis, subcutaneous abscess, liver abscess, osteomyelitis, and sepsis. Early recognition of diagnosis of immune deficiency disorders and etiologic agents with appropriate laboratory tests may help in institution of appropriate treatment.

To make rational use of antibiotics in critically sick children, it is important that PICUs have a surveillance system for etiologic agents and their sensitivity in opportunistic infections. The first-line empirical therapy may be decided on the basis of surveillance data.

Cultures are not a very efficient method by which to diagnosis viruses, fungi, and mycobacterial species. Therefore, future development of noninvasive and rapid diagnostic methods for these infections in children would greatly improve treatment strategies.

KEY POINTS

Cytomegalovirus Infection

- CMV is a virus in the herpes group and a common cause of infection in patients with congenital immune deficiency, HIV infection, and organ transplant and cancer chemotherapy.
- The organism can be transmitted through an infected birth canal and by breast milk, saliva, and blood (via infected white cells) and involve all organ systems.
- CMV pneumonia is a major cause of morbidity and mortality.
- Diagnosis is established by serology, PCR, antigenemia, and viral culture.
- Administration of antiviral drugs (ganciclovir, foscarnet) in immunocompromised hosts improves outcome.
- No randomized clinical trials have been conducted that involve different antiviral drugs.

Varicella-zoster Virus Infection

- VZV is a DNA virus that typically causes benign infections of the skin and mucous membranes.
- VZV can lead to visceral dissemination and pneumonia in children with cancer, AIDS, congenital defects of cell-mediated immunity, or those who have received organ transplantation.
- Varicella can be diagnosed based on physical findings, vesicle scrapings using direct fluorescent antibody, serology, or PCR.
- The high-risk group of susceptible individuals exposed to varicella should be given immune globulin (either VZIG or IVIG up to 92 hrs after exposure).
- Immunocompromised patients should receive IV acyclovir.
- Experience with efficacy of famciclovir and valacyclovir in children is limited.

Herpes Virus Type 6

- HHV-6 is the most widespread among the human herpesviruses and causes exanthem subitum in immunocompetent children.
- HHV-6 has been associated with clinical disease (pneumonia, encephalopathy) in HIV infection and in recipients of bone marrow and solid organ transplant.
- Testing for HHV-6 includes serology, culture, immunohistochemistry, and nucleic acid assays.
- Treatment is not well established, antiviral drugs that can be used are ganciclovir, valganciclovir, acyclovir, valacyclovir, cidofovir, and foscarnet.
- HHV-6 is an emerging pathogen in immunocompromised hosts, and experience is limited concerning its clinical manifestations, diagnosis, and treatment.

Fungal Infections

- *Candida* species are recognized as a leading contributor to morbidity and mortality in patients with oncohematologic malignancies, HIV infection, primary immunodeficiencies, prolonged neutropenia, diabetes, corticosteroid administration, broad-spectrum antibiotic treatment, IV hyperalimentation, and presence of central venous lines.

■ The portals of entry are usually lesions of the gastrointestinal tract, oral mucosa, or skin puncture sites, and organisms disseminated by the hematogenous route to the tissues of one or more organs.

■ Common sites of infection in patients with disseminated candidiasis include lungs, kidneys, liver, spleen, and brain.

■ Diagnosis of *Candida* infections is based on clinical findings and tissue and body fluid culture.

■ First-line therapy includes amphotericin B and fluconazole.

■ Caspofungin is indicated as a first-line treatment in adults, but its safety and efficacy has not been proven in pediatric patients.

Pneumocystis jiroveci

■ *P. jiroveci* (earlier known as *P. carinii*) is a eukaryotic microorganism of uncertain taxonomy.

■ Patients at higher risk for PCP include infants with severe malnutrition, children with primary immunodeficiencies, hematologic malignancies, HIV infection, and recipients of solid organ or bone marrow transplants.

■ PCP is diagnosed through direct identification of organisms from lung tissue or induced sputum specimens.

■ The first-line treatment for PCP is with TMP-SMZ, given either intravenously or orally, regardless of previous prophylactic regimen.

■ No randomized, controlled trials have been conducted to evaluate trimethoprim/dapsone combination, pyrimethamine/sulfadoxine combination, clindamycin, primaquine, or atovaquone in children.

Invasive Aspergillosis

■ *Aspergillus* is a group of ubiquitous fungal organisms found in soil and other settings, including the hospital environment, that enter the body via the respiratory route.

■ Susceptible hosts include recipients of lung, bone marrow, and liver transplants; those who received treatment for malignancy, chronic granulomatous disease, or HIV infection; and those on immunosuppressive chemotherapy.

■ Invasive pulmonary aspergillosis is manifested most commonly as necrotizing bronchopneumonia.

■ Diagnosis is established by demonstration of organisms on body fluids or tissue.

■ High-dose amphotericin B (1–1.5 mg/kg/day) is the treatment of choice for invasive aspergillosis.

■ Diagnosis is difficult, as noninvasive tests (galactomannan assay) are difficult to interpret in children.

Mucormycosis

■ Infections by members of the mucormycosis class of fungi occur in children with hematopoietic malignancies, organ transplantation, and diabetes.

■ Mucormycosis may involve lungs, brain, sinuses, kidneys, and skin.

■ The organism invades blood vessels and may disseminate other sites. Sudden death may occur due to massive pulmonary hemorrhage, mediastinitis, or airway obstruction.

■ Isolation of fungi is difficult; diagnosis is established by histopathology and tissue culture.

■ Treatment consists of prompt management of the underlying medical condition, reduction of immunosuppression, antifungal therapy (amphotericin B), and surgical debridement.

■ A noninvasive method for diagnosis is not available.

Cryptococcus

■ *C. neoformans*, a yeast-like encapsulated fungus, causes disease in immunocompromised patients.

■ The disease primarily presents as subacute or chronic meningitis, and may involve all organ systems in disseminated disease.

■ Diagnosis of cryptococcal pulmonary infection is suggested by characteristic clinical and radiographic findings, sputum culture, serologic assays for IgG and IgM, and serologic testing for cryptococcal polysaccharide antigen by latex agglutination.

■ Treatment consists of combination of amphotericin B and flucytosine.

Histoplasmosis

■ Histoplasmosis is a systemic disease caused by the dimorphic fungus *H. capsulatum*.

■ Histoplasmosis occurs more commonly in children with HIV infection.

■ Clinical manifestations include acute, progressive, life-threatening infection that presents as unexplained fever, weight loss, respiratory complaints, abdominal pain, and diarrhea.

■ Diagnosis is made via culture, fungal stain, antigen detection, and serologic tests for antibodies.

■ Amphotericin B is the standard therapy for serious infections, followed by itraconazole for long-term suppressive therapy.

Nontuberculous Mycobacteria

■ Nontuberculous mycobacterial infections are frequent opportunistic pathogens associated with the AIDS and primary immune deficiency disorders.

■ Clinical manifestations of disseminated disease include lymphadenopathy and gastrointestinal tract involvement.

■ Diagnosis is based on culture and PCR.

■ Treatment depends on organisms and site of infection. Commonly used drugs are azithromycin and clarithromycin, with other antituberculosis drugs in disseminated disease.

■ Epidemiology, clinical features, and management protocols have not been well established.

Mycobacterium Tuberculosis

- HIV and TB form a lethal combination, each speeding the other's progress.
- TB can occur in HIV-infected individuals at any CD4 count.
- TB in children who are infected with HIV children may be more severe, and progress very fast with increased extrapulmonary manifestations.
- Diagnosis is based on demonstration of AFB in sputum or other body fluid. In the absence of AFB, a diagnosis of probable TB can be made on the basis of history of contact with adults with TB, positive tuberculin test, and compatible radiologic findings.
- Treatment consists of antituberculosis drugs for 6–9 months.
- Diagnosis of TB in children is very difficult. No simple test exists for confirmation of diagnosis.

Toxoplasmosis

- Disseminated *T. gondii* infection in immunocompromised patients has emerged as a potentially fatal pathogen.
- Common presentations include fever, encephalitis, pneumonia, myocarditis, and bone marrow suppression.
- Confirmation of diagnosis is either through serologic methods (reserved for immunocompetent hosts) or molecular methods, such as PCR.
- Treatment consists of administration of pyrimethamine, sulfadiazine, and leucovorin.

Cryptosporidium Infection

- *Cryptosporidium* spp. causes severe diarrheal in children with HIV infection, primary immunodeficiencies, or acute leukemia on chemotherapy.
- Diagnosis of cryptosporidium is made by examination of stool.
- Treatment is not satisfactory. The current therapy includes supportive care with administration of nitazoxanide.

References

1. Abrams D, Derrick G, Penny DJ, et al. Cardiac complications in children following infection with varicella zoster virus. *Cardiol Young* 2001;11: 647–52.
2. Adderson E. Histoplasmosis. *Pediatr Infect Dis J* 2006;25:73–4.
3. Adderson EE. Histoplasmosis in a pediatric oncology center. *J Pediatr* 2004;144:100–6.
4. Benson CA, Kaplan JE, Masur H et al. Treating opportunistic infections among HIV-infected adults and adolescents. *MMWR* 2004;53 (RR15):1–112.
5. Boivin G. Diagnosis of herpes virus infections of the central nervous system. *Herpes* 2004;11(Suppl 2):4A–56A.
6. Caserta MT, Mock DJ, Dewhurst S. Human herpesvirus 6. *Clin Infect Dis* 2001;33:829–33.
7. Chan SP, Bimbaum J, Rao M. Clinical manifestation and outcome of tuberculosis in children with AIDS. *Pediatr Infect Dis J* 1996;15:443–7.
8. Chaudhary MW, Sardana K, Kumar P, et al. Disseminated infection with *Cryptococcus neoformans* var neoformans in an 8 years immunocompetent girl. *Indian J Pediatr* 2005;72:85.
9. Chemlal K. Portaels F. Molecular diagnosis of nontuberculous mycobacteria. *Curr Opin Infect Dis* 2003;16:77–83.
10. Cruciani M, Marcati P, Malena M, et al. Meta-analysis of diagnostic procedures for Pneumocystis carinii pneumonia in HIV-1-infected patients. *Eur Respir J* 2002;20:982–9.
11. De Bolle L, Naesens L, Clercq ED. Update on human herpesvirus 6 biology, Clinical Features, and Therapy. *Clin Microbiol Rev* 2005;18:217–245.
12. de Camargo B, Pereira de Carvalho Filho N, Lopes Pinto CA, et al. Cryptococcosis mimicking a pulmonary metastasis in a child with Wilms tumor. *Med Pediatr Oncol* 2003;41:88–9.
13. Ding LW, Lai CC, Lee LN, et al. Lymphadenitis caused by non tuberculous mycobacteria in a university hospital of Taiwan: Predominance of rapidly growing mycobacteria and high recurrence rates. *J Formos Med Assoc* 2005;104:897–904.
14. Dromer F, Mathoulin S, Dupont B, et al. Epidemiology of cryptococcosis in France: A 9-year survey (1985–1993). French Cryptococcosis Study Group. *Clin Infect Dis* 1996;23:82–90.
15. Gershon AA. Prevention and treatment of VZV infections in patients with HIV. *Herpes* 2001;8:32–6.
16. Gonzalez CE, Rinaldi MG, Sugar AM. Zygomycosis. *Infect Dis Clin N Am* 2002;16:895–914.
17. Grangeot-Keros L, Mayaux JF, Lebon P, et al. Value of cytomegalovirus (CMV) IgG avidity index for the diagnosis of primary CMV infection in pregnant women. *J Infect Dis* 1997;175:944–50.
18. Gupta AK, Ghosh S, Gupta AK. Sinonasal aspergillosis in immunocompetent Indian children: An eight-year experience. *Mycoses* 2003;46:455–61.
19. Gupta PK, Mahapatra AK, Gaind R, et al. Aspergillus spinal epidural abscess. *Pediatr Neurosurg* 2001;35:18–23.
20. Harries A, Maher D, Graham S. *TB/HIV: A clinical manual*, 2nd ed. Geneva: World Health Organization, 2004;23–40.
21. Hernando S, Folgueira L, Lumbreras C, et al. Comparison of cytomegalovirus viral load measure by real-time PCR with pp65 antigenemia for the diagnosis of cytomegalovirus disease in solid organ transplant patients. *Transplant Proc* 2005;37:4094–6.
22. Jabra-Rizk MA, Falkler WA Jr, Enwonwu CO, et al. Prevalence of yeast among children in Nigeria and the United States. *Oral Microbiol Immunol* 2001;16:383–5.
23. K Ramdial P, Mosam A, Dlova NC, et al. Disseminated cutaneous histoplasmosis in patients infected with human immunodeficiency virus. *J Cutan Pathol* 2002;29:215–25.
24. Kabra SK, Lodha R, Seth V. Category-based treatment of tuberculosis in children *Indian Pediatrics* 2004;41:927–937
25. Karaguzel G, Kilicarslan-Akkaya B, Melikoglu M, et al. Cryptococcal mesenteric lymphadenitis: An unusual cause of acute abdomen. *Pediatr Surg Int* 2004;20:633–5.
26. Kontoyiannis DP, Lewis RE. Toward more effective antifungal therapy: The prospects of combination therapy. *British J Haematol* 2004;126:165–75.
27. Kumar CP, Sundararajan T, Menon T, et al. Candidosis in children with onco-hematological diseases in Chennai, south India. *Jpn J Infect Dis* 2005;58:218–21.
28. Lajo A, Borque C, Del Castillo F, et al. Mononucleosis caused by Epstein-Barr virus and cytomegalovirus in children: A comparative study of 124 cases. *Pediatr Infect Dis J* 1994;13:56–60.
29. Mandell DL, Wald ER, Michaels MG, et al. Management of nontuberculous mycobacterial cervical lymphadenitis. *Arch Otolaryngol Head Neck Surg* 2003;129:341–4.
30. Mantadakis E, Anagnostatou N, Danilatou V, et al. Fulminant hepatitis due to varicella zoster virus in a girl with acute lymphoblastic leukemia in remission: Report of a case and review. *J Pediatr Hematol Oncol* 2005;27: 551–3.
31. Mathur KK, Mortelliti AJ. Candida epiglottitis. *Ear Nose Throat J* 2004; 83:13.
32. Middelhof CA, Loudon WG, Muhonen MD, et al. Improved survival in central nervous system aspergillosis: A series of immunocompromised children with leukemia undergoing stereotactic resection of aspergillomas. Report of four cases. *J Neurosurg.* 2005;103(4Suppl):374–8.
33. Miyake F, Yoshikawa T, Fujita A, et al. Pneumonia with marked pleural effusion caused by Aspergillus infection. *Pediatr Infect Dis J* 2006;25: 186–7.
34. Navalpotro D, Gimeno C, Navarro D. PCR detection of viral DNA in serum as an ancillary analysis for the diagnosis of acute mononucleosis-like syndrome due to human cytomegalovirus (HCMV) in immunocompetent patients. *J Clin Virol* 2006;35:193–6.
35. Nicholson O, Feja K, LaRussa P, et al. Nontuberculous mycobacterial infections in pediatric hematopoietic stem cell transplant recipients: Case report and review of the literature. *Pediatr Infect Dis J* 2006;25:263–7.
36. Odabasi Z, Mattiuzzi G, Estey E, et al. Beta-D-glucan as a diagnostic adjunct for invasive fungal infections: Validation, cutoff development, and performance in patients with acute myelogenous leukemia and myelodysplastic syndrome. *Clin Infect Dis* 2004;39:199–205.
37. Ostrosky-Zeichner L, Pappas PG. Invasive candidiasis in the intensive care unit. *Crit Care Med* 2006;34:857–63.
38. Pappas PG, Rex JH, Sobel JD, et al. Guidelines for treatment of candidiasis. *Clin Infect Dis* 2004;38:161–189.
39. Pastakia B, Shawker TH, Thaler M, et al. Hepatosplenic candidiasis: Wheels within wheels. *Radiology* 1988;166:417–44.

40. Prabhu RM, Patel R. Mucormycosis and entomophthoramycosis: A review of the clinical manifestations, diagnosis and treatment. *Clin Microbiol Infect* 2004;10(Suppl 1):31–47.

41. Rao K, Saha V. Medical management of Aspergillus flavus endocarditis. *Pediatr Hematol Oncol* 2000;17:425–7.

42. Rapaport D, Engelhard D, Tagger G, et al. Antiviral prophylaxis may prevent human herpesvirus-6 reactivation in bone marrow transplant recipients. *Transplant Infect Dis* 2002;4:10–6.

43. Russian DA, Levine SJ. Pneumocystis carinii pneumonia in patients without HIV infection. *Am J Med Sci* 2001;321:56–65.

44. Sepkowita KA. Opportunistic infections in patients with and patients without acquired immunodeficiency syndrome. *Clin Infect Dis* 2002;34: 1098–107.

45. Shah A, Lagvankar S, Shah A. Cutaneous mucormycosis in children. *Indian Pediatr* 2006;43:167–70.

46. Singhi SC, Reddy TC, Chakrabarti A. Candidemia in a pediatric intensive care unit. *Pediatr Crit Care Med* 2004;5:369–74.

47. Smith HV, Corcoran GD. New drugs and treatment for cryptosporidiosis. *Curr Opin Infect Dis* 2004;7:557–64.

48. Swanson AN, Pappou IP, Cammisa FP, et al. Chronic infections of the spine: Surgical indications and treatments. *Clin Orthop* 2006;444:100–6.

49. Takatoku M, Muroi K, Kawano-Yamamoto C, et al. Involvement of the esophagus and stomach as a first manifestation of varicella zoster virus infection after allogeneic bone marrow transplantation. *Intern Med* 2004;43: 861–4.

50. Tran DQ. Susceptibility to mycobacterial infections due to interferon-gamma and interleukin-12 pathway defects. *Allergy Asthma Proc* 2005;26:418–21.

51. Turner D, Schwarz Y, Yust I. Induced sputum for diagnosing Pneumocystis carinii pneumonia in HIV patients: New data, new issues. *Eur Resp J* 2003;21:204–8.

52. van Burik JA, Hare RS, Solomon HF, et al. Posaconazole is effective as salvage therapy in zygomycosis: A retrospective summary of 91 cases. *Clin Infect Dis* 2006;42 (7):e61–5.

53. Varani S, Spezzacatena P, Manfredi R, et al. The incidence of cytomegalovirus (CMV) antigenemia and CMV disease is reduced by highly active antiretroviral therapy. *Eur J Epidemiol* 2000;16:433–7.

54. Welgama U, Wickramasinghe C, Perera J. Varicella-zoster virus infection in the Infectious Diseases Hospital, Sri Lanka. *Ceylon Med J* 2003;48:119–21.

55. Yoshida M, Hayasaka S, Yamada T, et al. Ocular findings in Japanese patients with varicella-zoster virus infection. *Ophthalmologica* 2005;219: 272–5.

56. Yoshikawa T. Human herpesvirus-6 and -7 infections in transplantation. *Pediatr Transplant* 2003;7:11–7.

57. Zardi EM, Picardi A, Afeltra A. Treatment of cryptosporidiosis in immunocompromised hosts. *Chemotherapy* 2005;51:193–6.

58. Zaucha-Prazmo A, Wojcik B, Drabko K, et al. Neurological manifestation of CMV disease after allogeneic haematopoietic stem cells transplantation–a case report. *Ann Univ Mariae Curie Sklodowska [Med]* 2004;59:198–200.

59. Zekri AR, Mohamed WS, Samra MA, et al. Risk factors for cytomegalovirus, hepatitis B and C virus reactivation after bone marrow transplantation. *Transpl Immunol* 2004;13:305–11.

60. Zeller V, Truffot C, Agher R, et al. Discontinuation of secondary prophylaxis against mycobacterium avium complex infection and toxoplasmic encephalitis. *CID* 2002;34:662–7.

CHAPTER 85 ■ PRINCIPLES OF NUTRITION AND METABOLISM

MURAYA GATHINJI • Z. LEAH HARRIS

Cellular homeostasis relies on a delicate interplay between the metabolic processes that support cell growth and development, those that protect the cell from injury and damage, and those that regulate cell death. Many of these intricate processes rely on vitamins, trace elements, and minerals as cofactors to function. The redox milieu of the cell is determined by the presence of transition metals (Fe^{2+}, Cu^{1+}), antioxidants, reductants, nitric oxide (NO)/nitrites, and oxygen (O_2). These factors are very important for cellular functioning under normal physiologic conditions, and perturbations of the system place an additional need for these substrates. To date, the role of macronutrients and micronutrients in critical illness has yet to be fully evaluated.

Issues with nutrition in the management of critically ill children range from how much to feed (i.e., what is the resting energy expenditure of a critically ill child?) to what to feed, and even how to feed. Significant debate exists as to the role and use of specially supplemented diets, particularly *immunonutrition*, which refers to nutritional supplements that modulate the immune response. Multiple studies have been conducted to determine a role for micronutrient supplementation in acquired immune deficiency syndrome/human immunodeficiency virus, prematurity, lung disease, and cardiovascular disease. Compelling outcomes studies in adult ICUs suggest that implementing an evidence-based nutritional management protocol increases the likelihood that critically ill patients receive enteral feeds and is associated with shortened duration of mechanical ventilation (6).

Controlling for nutrient intake and distinguishing among the effects of various nutrients and vitamins ingested from food complicate the design and interpretation of studies aimed at assessing nutrient-dependent outcomes in both healthy and critically ill populations. Individual nutrient bioavailability adds a further complexity to interpretation of studies of nutrient supplementation and its effect on the development or prevention of disease. The identification of single-nucleotide polymorphisms within populations has led to the concept of "personalized designer medicine" (39). The notion that diets can be customized based on individual genetic profiles to decrease the risk of disease underscores two new areas of nutritional research: *nutrigenomics* and *nutrigenetics*. The future of nutraceuticals may depend upon translating gene-based differences into health outcomes differences.

Currently, $23 billion dollars per year are spent by American adults on multivitamin and dietary supplements. Multivitamin use is highest among women and the children of women who take supplements. The State-of-the-Science Conference panel of the National Institutes of Health concluded that insufficient evidence exists to support or advise against the use of multivitamin and mineral supplements for the prevention of chronic disease in the general population (27). The lack of randomized, controlled trials makes it difficult for those who work in the field of nutrition to form evidence-based recommendations. Potential clearly exists for adverse effects from the consumption of multivitamin supplements, a situation that is quite evident in the current debate regarding vitamin supplementation in the Third World. The World Health Organization and UNICEF has recognized that "although the benefits of iron supplementation have generally been considered to outweigh the putative risks, there is some evidence to suggest that supplementation at levels recommended for otherwise healthy children carries the risk of increased severity of infectious disease in the presence of malaria and/or undernutrition" (34).

The goals of this chapter are to introduce the relevance of nutrition in disease as it relates energy and metabolism to critical illness, review macronutrients and micronutrients and their significance in health, discuss the role of immunonutrition in the management of critically ill children, and present a review of current clinical trials as they relate to best practices in nutrition in the PICU. In presenting the principles of nutrition and metabolism in critically ill children, it is hoped that nutrition will be viewed as adjuvant therapy in combating disease states and that, like pharmaceuticals, nutrition will one day be "personalized" for individualized care and support.

BASIC PRINCIPLES OF ENERGY EXPENDITURE AND METABOLISM

The metabolic response of critically ill individuals, both adult and children, is characterized by an increase in resting energy expenditure (REE). Defined as the amount of calories required by the body during a nonactive, 24-hr period, the REE (calories/day) represents 70%–80% of the calories used by the body. The REE is synonymous to the *resting* metabolic rate, which defines the energy released to maintain normal, basal physiologic functioning. A more sophisticated measurement, the *basal* metabolic rate, represents the amount of energy expended while at rest at a neutral temperature and under fasting conditions (12-hr fast).

The REE is useful in optimizing nutrition management for the patient. While critically ill individuals have a greater REE than healthy controls and have an increased caloric need over their "resting" state, a formula by which to derive REE is

EQUATIONS FOR CALCULATING RESTING ENERGY EXPENDITURE

Harris-Benedict Equations (calories/day)
Male: 66.5 + [13.8 × weight (kg)] + [5.0 × height (cm)] − [6.8 × age (years)]
Female: 655.1 + [9.6 × weight (kg)] + [1.8 × height (cm)] − [4.7 × age (years)]

FAO/WHO/UNU (calories/day)
Male (3–10 years): REE = [22.7 × weight (kg)] + 495
Female (3–10 years): REE = [22.5 × weight (kg)] + 499
Male (10–18 years): REE = [12.2 × weight (kg)] + 746
Female (10–18 years): REE = [17.5 × weight (kg)] + 651

Schofield-HW (calories/day)
Male (3–10 years): REE = [19.6 × weight (kg)] + [1.033 × height (cm)] + 414.9
Female (3–10 years): REE = [16.97 × weight (kg)] + [1.618 × height (cm)] + 371.2
Male (10–18 years): REE = [16.25 × weight (kg)] + [1.372 × height (cm)] + 515.5
Female (10–18 years): REE = [8.365 × weight (kg)] + [4.65 × height (cm)] + 200

useful to prevent the underfeeding or overfeeding of individuals. A common calculation for predicted energy expenditure uses the Harris-Benedict equations, which take into account gender, age, height, and weight.

The Harris-Benedict equations have been found to overestimate the actual energy expenditure measurements calculated by indirect calorimetry by 6%–15% (13). The Harris-Benedict equation is likely the most accurate for use in adult critical care units if an activity factor is taken into account when deriving the predicted energy expenditure (3). The Harris-Benedict equations are only two of many equations available to calculate REE. Others include the Food and Agriculture/World Health Organization/United Nations University equation and the Schofield-height/weight (Schofield-HW) equation (**Table 85.1**). For any of the calculations, a large variation between individuals should be considered, when their measured energy expenditure is compared to the calculated amount.

As the large variations in critically ill children can lead to inaccuracy in predictions when using these equations, the most accurate assessment of REE requires that it be measured. Energy expenditure can be measured indirectly with a metabolic cart, using an analysis of expired gases to derive the volume of air that passes through the lungs, the amount of oxygen extracted from it (V_{O_2}) and the amount of carbon dioxide that is expelled into atmosphere (V_{CO_2}) as a by-product of metabolism. An additional formula to represent V_{O_2} and V_{CO_2} is the respiratory quotient (RQ), which measures the inherent composition and utilization of carbohydrates, fats, and proteins as they are converted to energy substrate units that can be used by the body as energy. The RQ represents the ratio of carbon dioxide produced to the amount of oxygen consumed by the individual.

$$(RQ) = V_{CO_2}/V_{O_2}$$

Respiratory Quotient

As previously defined by the REE, ~70% of total energy expenditure is due to the basal physiologic processes; 20% comes from physical activity, and another 10% from digestion of macronutrients in the form of food. In the Krebs cycle, energy is derived from catabolism of large molecules into smaller molecules. All of these processes require an intake of oxygen and expel carbon dioxide. Hence, the RQ provides a valuable determination of metabolic balance and usually ranges from 1.0 (representing the value expected for pure carbohydrate oxidation) to ~0.7 (the value expected for pure fat oxidation). Interestingly, RQ, as measured, does include a contribution for protein-derived energy, but due to the extreme variability in which complex amino acids are metabolized, no single RQ can be "assigned" to the oxidation of protein. The physiologic range of RQ is 0.67–1.3. An RQ >1.0 indicates a greater oxidation of carbohydrate as compared to fat and a relatively large production of carbon dioxide, and it is recommended to decrease the total calorie intake or decrease the carbohydrate-to-fat ratio in these situations. An RQ of <0.81 indicates a greater oxidation of fat, which may indicate a need to increase the total calorie intake or increase the carbohydrate-to-fat ratio.

Indirect calorimetry or metabolic carts have been avoided in PICUs for a variety of reasons: technical difficulties in performing the technique on mechanically ventilated children, lack of experience in handling expired gases, limitations on the use of high-inspired oxygen, and difficulties controlling for patient temperature, feeding regimens, movement, degree of sedation (too much or too little), and environmental noise. To maximize the results of a metabolic cart and to improve accuracy: (a) infused feeds should be held constant for at least 12 hrs, and intermittent or cyclic feeds should be held for at least 4 hrs; (b) ventilator settings should remain constant for 6 hrs; and (c) no procedures (including dialysis) should be performed 2 hrs prior to testing.

In a study of severely burned children (>40% body surface area), REE was measured by indirect calorimetry and compared with predicted equations when the children were assessed to be their most hypermetabolic. For all children, good agreement was obtained between the three sets of equations used to calculate REE. Unfortunately, the predicted REEs were significantly lower than the measured REEs (mean difference of 635 kcal/day; 95% confidence interval, 525–745 kcal/day; p <0.05). The authors concluded that indirect calorimetry should be used to determine energy expenditure until more accurate equations are developed for this hypermetabolic group of critically ill patients (41). In a study that compared the predictive value of four separate equations to determine REE (as compared to indirect calorimetry) in children with bronchopulmonary dysplasia, the Harris-Benedict equations were the best to predict REE, while the Schofield-HW equations had the best agreement for control children (7). The authors concluded that while all prediction equations underestimated REE in children with a chronic disease (bronchopulmonary dysplasia), the appropriate equation could be a useful tool toward preventing undernutrition and promoting growth.

In critically ill children, the ability to accurately predict energy expenditure is essential. Underfeeding results in nutrient depletion, protein-energy malnutrition, decreased immunocompetence, and increased morbidity and mortality. Overfeeding may induce thermogenesis, hepatic fat deposition, and increased carbon dioxide production. Although it seems intuitive that the severity of illness would affect energy metabolism, this factor was not studied in children until 2000. In a prospective study in critically ill children, investigators hypothesized that measured energy expenditure during critical illness would be lower than predicted energy expenditure and that nutritional and clinical indices would correlate (8). In a group of 37 children (24% with sepsis, 24% with traumatic brain injury, 13% with respiratory failure, 21% with transplant and 16% post-cardiac surgery), measured energy expenditure was found to be significantly lower than predicted energy expenditure. Measured energy expenditure did not differ substantially by disease or by administration of muscle relaxation but was different when protein intake, use of vasoactive agents, and sedation were factored in. A study of energy expenditure in children with severe head injury compared four sets of REE prediction equations to measured energy expenditure and found significant variation between predicted and measured for all equations, with more than half of all children having differences of >10% (19). Indirect calorimetry is necessary to determine the energy expenditure of critically ill children and guide accurate treatment of the metabolic response during critical illness.

KEY NUTRIENTS

The goals of nutrition have changed over the last decade, with a paradigm shift away from maintaining lean body mass to using nutrition as an intervention to modulate the immune response, minimize oxidative stress, normalize gut integrity, and maintain glycemic control. Clinicians need to better understand the components of the nutrition they provide and their contribution as immunomodulators and specific energy sources. As well, it must be determined which patients need active nutritional intervention and which nutrients are optimal to deliver. As a simple, inexpensive indicator of potential morbidity, albumin remains the recommended lab value to obtain for nutritional assessment. In a retrospective cohort study, serum albumin was identified as the single best indicator of outcome in adult surgical patients: a serum albumin <3.25 g/dL was predictive of worse postoperative outcomes (22). With more than 200 enteral formulas available and a growing list of components and their effects, sorting out the macronutrient and micronutrient requirements and deciding upon the optimal nutrient delivery is more complicated than ever before.

Macronutrients

Like adults, infants and children rely on the metabolism of macronutrients—carbohydrates, fats, and protein—to meet their energy demands. Oxidation of carbohydrates usually begins with glycolysis, in which glucose is converted to two molecules of pyruvate. Pyruvate oxidation follows, in which pyruvate is transported to the mitochondria to be converted to acetyl coenzyme A (CoA), followed by the tricarboxylic acid (TCA) cycle, in which acetyl CoA (from many sources) is converted to energy, carbon dioxide, and water. β-oxidation of fatty acids produces acetyl CoA, which again enters into the TCA cycle. The acetyl CoA produced by fat β-oxidation during periods of decreased glucose intake is converted to ketones in the liver and converted by the brain back to acetyl CoA for entry into the TCA cycle. Proteins enter either as precursors for acetyl CoA or as other intermediaries of the TCA cycle.

Energy produced per gram of substrate metabolized is as follows:

- Carbohydrate   4–5 kcal/g
- Protein   4–5 kcal/g
- Fat   9 kcal/g

The most significant difference between children and adults is found in their macronutrient reserves. A review of body composition over age groups (infant, child, and adult) reveals that, whereas the percentage of carbohydrate as a percentage of total body weight is relatively constant (0.4%), differences in fat reserve/composition (infant, 14%; child, 17%; adult, 19%) and protein (infant, 11%; child, 15%; adult, 18%) are substantial (1). Clearly, children have half of the protein stores and a third of the fat stores of adults, and thus have much less available at times of injury or illness. Therefore, the composition of the macronutrients for infants and children must be specialized. Current recommendations for energy and protein requirements in healthy individuals are:

- Infants   2.2 g/kg/day protein, 120 kcal/kg/day total cal
- Children   1.0 g/kg/day protein, 70 kcal/kg/day total cal
- Adults   0.8 g/kg/day protein, 35 kcal/kg/day total cal

Glucose

Glucose production in children is critical to meet their energy demands, especially during illness. It is imperative to provide adequate carbohydrate calories so that autocatabolism and further consumption of depleted carbohydrate stores are minimized. Glucose is the preferred energy substrate for the brain, red blood cells, and renal medulla. It is this increased need for glucose in children that drives the breakdown of skeletal muscle to generate glucose. Without adequate carbohydrate replacement, the catabolism of the diaphragm and intercostal muscles causes additional compromise of respiratory function in an already ill child. Initial attempts at pediatric nutritional support produced regimens that were high in glucose and protein with minimal fat. This unbalanced supplementation caused excess glucose to be converted to fat, with subsequent generation of carbon dioxide, and led to increased respiratory effort. The current goal is to provide a balanced supplementation composed of fat, glucose, and protein. The estimation for carbohydrate requirement is 200–300 g/day, based on a need of 3–6 mg/kg/min in the critically ill (26).

Fats

Fats are listed in six categories: total fat, saturated fatty acid, monounsaturated fatty acid, polyunsaturated fatty acid, trans-fatty acid, and dietary cholesterol. To provide basal, or resting, metabolic needs, saturated fatty acids require more energy to burn than do unsaturated fatty acids. Free fatty acids, released from glycerol in the hydrolysis of triglycerides, are the primary lipid source for energy. The glycerol released following triglyceride breakdown is converted to pyruvate, which is shuttled into glucose metabolism as a gluconeogenic precursor. Critically ill children who do not receive lipids develop essential fatty acid deficiencies within a week (1). To prevent this condition, linoleic acid (4.5% total calories) and linolenic acid (0.5% total calories) are administered. Currently available lipid preparations provide essential free fatty acids but are associated with a risk of an increased incidence of pneumonia in adult intensive care patients. Free fatty acids interfere with leukocyte function, and hyperlipidemia is associated with decreased oxygenation in premature infants who receive IV fat infusions. Neonates have a theoretical risk of IV lipid displacing unconjugated bilirubin and causing kernicterus. Restricting the infusion of lipid to 2–3 g/kg/day protects against bilirubin displacement. (1).

Proteins

Proteins are composed of carbon, hydrogen, oxygen, and nitrogen arranged to form amino acids. Unlike the storage of fat, the body has no storage depots of protein. Approximately 98% of the amino acids are incorporated in proteins, and protein recycling represents the major pathway for amino acid/protein utilization. Newborns have a protein turnover twice as active as adults: 6.7 g/kg/day versus 3.5 g/kg/day. Burns, trauma, and extracorporeal membrane oxygenation (ECMO) cause protein turnover to increase further. A 100% increase in urinary nitrogen excretion is seen with bacterial sepsis in infants, and a 100% increase in protein breakdown is seen if they require ECMO support. Amino acid supplementation has been shown to be successful in restoring negative protein balance, but limited data exist that detail the optimal amount of protein to deliver. To provide adequate amino acids for wound healing, protein synthesis, and preservation of skeletal muscle mass, the quantity of amino acid delivered should be:

- Low-birth-weight infants   3–4 g/kg/day
- Term neonates   2–3 g/kg/day
- Children   1.5 g/kg/day

Protein administration >6 g/kg/day is associated with toxicity to the liver and kidneys and should be avoided. Infants should receive 43% of protein as essential amino acids, and children should receive 36%. While infants should receive a minimum of 30% of their calories from fat, children should receive a maximum of 30% of total calories from fat and no more than 10% of their calories from saturated or unsaturated fats (9).

Micronutrients

Micronutrients are required in small amounts, compared to macronutrients, and are classified as *vitamins* [A (retinol), B_1 (thiamin), B_2 (riboflavin), B_3 (niacin), B_5 (pantothenic acid), B_6 (pyridoxine), B_7 (biotin), B_9 (folate), B_{12} (cobalamin or cyanocobalamin), C, D, E (tocopherol), and K], *trace elements/minerals* (zinc, iron, copper, selenium, fluoride, iodine, chromium, molybdenum, cobalt, and manganese), and *amino acids* (glutamine, arginine, homocysteine). The significance of these micronutrients lies in their unique disease states, discovered as a result of their deficiency. The word *vitamin* is derived from the words "vital" and "amine" because they were originally thought to be amines vital for life. Divided into fat-soluble (vitamins A, D, E, and K) and water-soluble (vitamins B and C), vitamins are organic compounds required by humans in small amounts from the diet. Minerals are elements that originated in the atmosphere and earth's crust and were likely incorporated into energy metabolism secondary to their abundance in the soil.

Vitamin A (retinol) is a member of the family of compounds known as the *retinoids*. β-carotene and other carotenoids that are converted into retinoids are frequently referred to as *provitamin A carotenoids*. Retinol ($C_{20}H_{30}O$) can be oxidized to either of the metabolically active forms retinal ($C_{20}H_{28}O$) or retinoic acid ($C_{20}H_{28}O_2$). Retinoic acid (RA) is integral in regulating gene transcription. Correctly classified as hormones, based on their ability to affect gene expression, retinoic acid and its isomers (all-trans RA and 9-cis RA) are transported to the nucleus via cytoplasmic retinoic acid-binding proteins and participate in an elaborate cascade of nuclear gene regulation via binding to specific retinoic acid receptors (either a retinoic acid receptor, RAR, or a retinoid X receptor, RXR). Once bound, both RAR and RXR are able to form either homodimers or heterodimers and complex to a specific retinoic acid response element that is located on the 5′ end of a host of genes that are critical for cellular differentiation and regulation of embryonic limb development, cardiac development, ocular and otic development, growth hormone expression, development and differentiation of T-lymphocytes, and stem cell differentiation into red blood cell precursors. RAR and RXR are also capable of forming heterodimers with several other nuclear receptors including but not limited to thyroid hormone receptors and vitamin D receptors.

Retinol also plays a unique and essential role in the formation of the visual pigment rhodopsin. Following transport to the retina, retinol is stored as a retinyl ester in the retinal pigment epithelial cells; 11-cis retinal, derived from the retinyl ester, binds to opsin in the interphotoreceptor matrix of the rod cell to form rhodopsin. Vitamin A deficiency leads to decreased retinal and is the leading cause of blindness in developing nations.

Thiamin (Thiamine, B_1) is a water-soluble B vitamin required for the coenzyme thiamin pyrophosphate, which is a critical component of multiple dehydrogenase enzymes—pyruvate dehydrogenase, α-ketoglutarate dehydrogenase, and branched-chain ketoacid dehydrogenase—all located in the mitochondria and required for ATP generation. In addition, thiamine triphosphate is concentrated in both nerve and muscle cells and is believed to activate ion channels. A deficiency of B₁ results in beriberi, which was first described in Chinese literature in 2600 BC and has three forms: (a) dry beriberi, characterized by peripheral neuropathy; (b) wet beriberi, characterized by neurologic and cardiovascular abnormalities (congestive heart failure); and (c) cerebral beriberi, best characterized by Wernicke disease. Thiamine disease is usually associated with either inadequate intake (malnutrition) or alcoholism. Less common causes include a diet high in thiaminase-rich foods (raw fish, ferns) and/or foods high in antithiamine factors (betel nuts). Thiamine loss can also occur during hemodialysis. Thiamine deficiency is easily remedied with thiamine replacement and fortification in diet. The cardiac disease appears somewhat reversible while the neurologic injury remains fixed.

Riboflavin (B₂) is a water-soluble B vitamin essential for the coenzyme, flavin adenine dinucleotide (FAD) and flavin mononucleotide (FMN). Flavins (coenzymes derived from riboflavin) and flavoproteins (proteins that use a flavin coenzyme) participate in numerous redox pathways, in particular glutathione reductase, glutathione peroxidase, and xanthine oxidase. Methylene tetrahydrofolate reductase (MTHFR) is a flavin adenine dinucleotide-dependent enzyme that maintains the folate coenzyme responsible for converting homocysteine to methionine. Cataracts and migraine headaches have been ascribed to decreased levels of riboflavin. Deficiency is usually caused by inadequate intake or, rarely, by impaired absorption.

Niacin (B₃) is an essential ligand for the enzymes nicotinamide adenine dinucleotide (NAD) and nicotinamide adenine dinucleotide phosphate (NADP). The transfer of electrons during oxidation-reduction reactions are predominantly NAD/NADP dependent, and more than 200 enzymes require NAD/NADP. Niacin deficiency is usually secondary to inadequate intake. It may also occur with administration of isoniazid, inadequate absorption of tryptophan (Hartnup disease), or inadequate synthesis of niacin from tryptophan (carcinoid syndrome). The late stage of severe niacin deficiency is known as *pellagra*, the symptoms of which are dermatitis, diarrhea, dementia, and if untreated, death. Niacin can be synthesized from tryptophan and, as such, severe tryptophan deficiencies may also present clinically as pellagra.

Pantothenic acid, B₅, is found in every living cell in the form of CoA, an enzyme critical for glucose metabolism, fat metabolism, protein homeostasis, cholesterol synthesis, steroid synthesis, neurotransmitter synthesis, and heme synthesis. Its ubiquitous expression is due to the acetate group donated by CoA for all acetylation reactions required for life. With the exception of that experimentally induced, pantothenic acid deficiency is unknown.

Vitamin B₆ exists in multiple forms, but pyridoxine and pyridoxal 5′-phosphate are the two most common. Humans cannot synthesize B₆ and thus are susceptible to disease from abnormalities in this class of B vitamin. Infant seizures are associated with pyridoxine deficiency, in which seizures are the final manifestation. Irritability, depression, and confusion can frequently occur with this disorder. Pyridoxal phosphate is linked to nucleic acid synthesis, steroid hormone synthesis, heme-oxygen-carrying capacity, red blood cell formation, and neurotransmitter synthesis and secretion. Homocysteine, an intermediate in the metabolism of methionine, can be metabolized by either a folate/B₁₂ pathway or a B₆ pathway. The risk of cardiovascular disease is significantly increased in patients with elevated homocysteine levels, and trials are underway to examine the risk of cardiovascular disease in relation to B₆ levels. Deficiency can be due to inborn enzyme abnormalities, inadequate intake, or as a complication of administration of either isoniazid or estro-progestational hormones.

Biotin (B₇) (the vitamin formerly known as H) searched for an identity for many decades before being classified as a B-complex vitamin. Biotin is essential for fatty acid metabolism, gluconeogenesis, leucine metabolism, and histone biotinylation/DNA replication and transcription. Fatty acid metabolism requires four separate carboxylases to transfer carbon dioxide, using bicarbonate as its one-carbon substrate. Biotin is the cofactor for each of these carboxylase reactions:

- Acetyl-CoA carboxylase catalyzes the formation of malonyl-CoA.
- Methylcrotonyl-CoA carboxylase catalyzes leucine metabolism.
- Propionyl-CoA carboxylase catalyzes cholesterol and fatty acid metabolism.
- Pyruvate carboxylase is critical for gluconeogenesis.

Once the carboxylase reaction has occurred, biotin is recycled and cleaved from the holocarboxylase by a biotinidase. The biotinidases have been determined to be critical for the selective biotinylation of histones involved in gene transcription and DNA packaging. Biotin deficiency may result from either a biotinidase mutation that interrupts effective biotin recycling or severe dietary restriction. Despite being required by all organisms, biotin is synthesized exclusively by bacteria, yeasts, molds, and select plant species. Bacteria in the human intestine are thought to play a role in biotin homeostasis. The signs and symptoms of biotin deficiency include an erythematous, scaly skin eruption distributed around the eyes, nose, mouth, and perineum, as well as alopecia, conjunctivitis, and neurologic abnormalities. "Biotin deficiency facies" is composed of a rash around the eyes, nose, and mouth, along with an unusual distribution of facial fat. In biotin-deficient infants, the neurologic findings are hypotonia, lethargy, and developmental delay. In adults, the neurologic findings are lethargy, depression, hallucinations, and paresthesias of the extremities. Because biotin requirements are low and it is so readily available, deficiency is rare. One cause is prolonged consumption of raw egg whites. Avidin, a protein in egg whites that is inactivated by cooking, scavenges and binds biotin, leading to deficiency. Other causes of biotin deficiency include genetic inborn errors, extended parenteral nutrition, pregnancy, or long-term anticonvulsant therapy.

Folic acid, B₉ and folate coenzymes are uniquely required to mediate one-carbon unit transfers and may act as both donors and acceptors. Folates are required for methionine synthesis, homocysteine regulation, rapidly dividing cell growth, and DNA methylation. Folate deficiency manifests with bone marrow abnormalities: megaloblastic or macrocytic anemia, hypersegmented neutrophils, and is followed by abnormalities associated with disrupted homocysteine metabolism. The link between rapid cell growth and folates resulted in research that linked neural tube defects with low folate levels. Adequate folate is critical for DNA and RNA synthesis, and the neural tube is most susceptible to injury during the period between gestational days 21 and 27. It is the link with homocysteine metabolism (folate has an effect of lowering elevated homocysteine levels) that suggests that a folate-rich diet is associated with decreased heart disease. Folates also appear to be of benefit in reducing colorectal cancer risk, Alzheimer disease, and cognitive impairment. Folate deficiency can be caused by inadequate intake, malabsorption (celiac disease, alcoholism), pregnancy and lactation, hemodialysis, and medications (methotrexate, phenytoin, primidone, sulfasalazine, triamterene, and trimethoprim-sulfamethoxazole).

Vitamin B$_{12}$ (cobalamin or cyanocobalamin) is the largest and most complex of the vitamins and is unique in that it contains cobalt. Cyanocobalamin and methylcobalamin are required for the function of the folate-dependent enzyme methionine synthase (also known as tetrahydrofolate-methyltransferase or 5′-tetrahydrofolate-homocysteine methyltransferase), which produces methionine from homocysteine. In the acidity of the stomach, B$_{12}$ is released from food stuffs and binds to a family of proteins referred to as *R-proteins* or *R-binders*. In the alkaline environment of the duodenum, the R-proteins are degraded by pancreatic enzymes, B$_{12}$ is released and binds to the intrinsic factor (IF). The B$_{12}$-IF complex then traffics through the enterocyte coupled to calcium metabolism. Deficiency can cause anemia (usually macrocytic megaloblastic anemia) or demyelination (numbness, tingling, ataxia). Deficiency can be seen with abnormalities of the stomach (intact stomach is needed for acid environment and R-protein), pancreas (releases proteolytic enzymes that cleave R-protein), gastric parietal cells (release intrinsic factor), and terminal ileum (where cyanocobalamin is absorbed). The most common causes of B$_{12}$ deficiency are inadequate intake, autoantibodies against gastric parietal cells (pernicious anemia), and malabsorption. It has also been reported with metformin administration.

Vitamin C (L-ascorbate), a potent antioxidant and reductant, must be ingested and obtained from the diet. Vitamin C is required for collagen synthesis, neurotransmitter release, carnitine synthesis, and redox stability. Scurvy, seen in severe vitamin C deficiency, is fatal if left untreated. While many studies reflect on the link between vitamin C and lower rates of heart disease, stroke, and cancer, many of the participants in theses studies were also on a weight-loss program that included increased fruits and vegetables in their diet and decreased meats/fat. It is unclear if vitamin C is truly associated with decreased cardiovascular disease and reduced risk of many cancers. Because the body cannot store vitamin C, ascorbic acid deficiency occurs soon after fresh supply becomes inadequate.

Vitamin D is a group of fat-soluble vitamins essential for maintaining calcium homeostasis. Vitamin D$_3$ (cholecalciferol) is synthesized in the skin after it is consumed in the diet or after exposure to ultraviolet light. It is then transported to the liver, where it is hydroxylated to the form 25-hydroxycholeclaciferol (calcidiol). An additional hydroxylation occurs in the kidneys, producing 1,25-dihydroxycholecalciferol (calcitriol), which is the active form of the vitamin. The biologic effects of vitamin D are mediated through a nuclear transcription factor, the vitamin D receptor, VDR. Upon binding active vitamin D, the complex enters the nucleus and associates with the RXR. The VDR-RXR complex, in the presence of 1,25-dihydroxyvitamin D, binds to the vitamin D response elements and initiates a cascade that modulates the transcription of numerous genes, including gene expression of transport proteins that are responsible for calcium absorption in the intestine. In addition to its presence in the intestine, the VDR is on bone, kidney, and parathyroid cells. The activation of the VDR on these sites is responsible for maintenance of blood levels of calcium and phosphorus and of bone mineral content. Vitamin D is also involved in immune modulation through VDR activation on the surface of T cells and antigen-presenting cells, leading to cell proliferation and differentiation. Severe vitamin D deficiency is seen in the PICU as rickets, osteopenia, or osteoporosis—all due to failure of the bone to mineralize. The main cause of vitamin D deficiency is inadequate intake; rarely, it is secondary to inadequate exposure to ultraviolet light.

Vitamin E is a term that broadly covers eight forms of this fat-soluble antioxidant vitamin: four tocopherols and four tocotrienols. α-tocopherol is the most active form of vitamin E and appears to be an antioxidant that prevents lipid peroxidation and cell membrane destruction. Vitamin E deficiency is seen in children with fat malabsorption syndromes (cystic fibrosis, pancreatic insufficiency, gastrectomy, Crohn disease, and cholestatic liver disease), very low-birth-weight neonates, and abetalipoproteinemia. Vitamin E deficiency presents with ataxia, peripheral neuropathy, myopathy, and a pigmented retinopathy.

Vitamin K represents a group of fat-soluble vitamins that are essential for the normal functioning of a host of clotting factors. This fat-soluble vitamin has a single function: the γ-carboxylation of glutamic acid such that calcium binding occurs and a signaling pathway generates a clot. Vitamin K-dependent coagulation factors are synthesized in the liver. Newborn infants are the most susceptible to vitamin K deficiency and hence bleeding; they therefore receive vitamin K injections shortly after birth. Other causes of vitamin K deficiency include inadequate intake, abnormal intestinal absorption, or administration of vitamin K antagonists.

Trace Elements and Minerals

The trace elements and minerals comprise a long list of compounds found in minute quantities in the body. A micronutrient is considered "essential" if the body maintains homeostatic control over its uptake into the bloodstream or tissue and its elimination. The following are considered essential micronutrients: cobalt, copper, chromium, fluorine, iron, iodine, manganese, molybdenum, selenium, and zinc. Nickel, tin, vanadium, silicon, and boron have been classified as important micronutrients. Aluminum, arsenic, barium, bismuth, bromine, cadmium, germanium, gold, lead, lithium, mercury, rubidium, silver, strontium, titanium, and zirconium are all found in plant and animal tissue; however, their importance is still being determined. A systematic review investigated whether supplementing critically ill patients with trace elements and minerals improved survival (21). Trace elements that appeared to support antioxidant function were the most advantageous. Selenium and zinc were involved the most in studies of 11 eligible papers. Multivitamin supplementation alone was not associated with any benefits.

Selenium is a trace element nutrient that functions as a cofactor for reduction of antioxidant enzymes such as glutathione peroxidases and thioredoxin reductase. Selenium-dependent enzymes are involved in peroxide degradation, cellular redox, transcriptional regulation, cytokine excretion, and thyroid hormone deiodination. Selenoprotein P appears to regulate immune and endothelial cell function. As critically ill patients have been noted to have low glutathione peroxidase activity, it has been hypothesized that low selenium levels are associated with increased mortality. A meta-analysis of critically ill patient outcomes following selenium supplementation revealed a trend toward a reduction in 28-day mortality following sepsis. Further studies are necessary to determine the impact of this trace element in the management of septic patients (4,5).

Many of the trace elements are transition metals with a free electron in their outer valence that can participate as both a reductant and oxidant. The ability of these compounds to participate both as antioxidants and catalysts in oxidative stress injury makes their trafficking and their appropriate cellular compartmentalization essential. In particular, mitochondria are most susceptible to redox injury.

Recent interest has been generated utilizing coenzyme Q_{10} (ubiquinone) in the management of pediatric cardiomyopathy. Coenzyme Q_{10} is a vitamin-like substance present in the mitochondria that is essential for generating ATP. In the role as a substrate to enhance cellular energy production, exogenous coenzyme Q_{10} (idebenone) has been used in adults with promising results with heart failure with or without cardiomyopathy. Studies in 6 children with idiopathic dilated cardiomyopathy (2 months to 11 years) revealed an increase in fractional shortening and ejection fraction in 5 out of 6 cases after 8 months of treatment (17). The topic deserves the design and conduct of a larger trial before a conclusion can be drawn, but the concept is intriguing.

IMMUNONUTRITION

The notions that (a) nutrition is beneficial to critically ill patients, and (b) enteral nutrition is preferred to parenteral nutrition in the critically ill have been well studied. A systematic review of the literature revealed that, indeed, enteral nutrition resulted in a decrease in infectious complications in critically ill adults and reduced hospital costs (18). In a review of 13 studies in which multiple small clinical studies were pooled to allow a more precise estimation of treatment effect, no difference in length of ICU stay, number of ventilator days, or mortality was shown, but enteral nutrition was associated with fewer infectious complications. For many, this single observation is frequently heralded as proof that providing enteral nutrition to the critically ill maintains a normal immunity. Further, the hyperglycemia that occurs more frequently with parenteral than with enteral nutrition is suggested to increase the likelihood for a bacterial bloodstream complication. Thus, nutrition provided to the gut offers both a protective effect on maintaining the mucosal barrier and delivers nutrients critical for normal immune function.

The concept of immunonutrition was born out of the observation that nutritional deficiencies are associated with immunodeficiencies. Protein calorie malnutrition is associated with leukotriene reduction, impaired microbial ingestion, and microbial killing. Cellular immunity is much more sensitive to protein calorie malnutrition: thymus structure and function deteriorates, and T-cell memory response to antigen is reduced. Studies of the mechanisms of nutrient modulation of the immune response provided critical insight as to how general nutrition and immunity are related. However, the corollary to this work has proven controversial, in that some believe that if certain nutrients are required for normal immune functioning,

then certainly diets with enhanced specific nutrients must be more immuno-beneficial. However, a better outcome is not necessarily guaranteed with enhanced nutrient supplementation. The identification of certain nutrients as being immunomodulators has generated significant interest and will be discussed in detail in this section.

Three areas of the immune defense system represent targets for specific nutritional manipulation: the mucosal barrier, cellular immunity, and the inflammatory response. The duality of the small-bowel epithelia is remarkable; the mucosa must be both permeable for nutrient uptake and protective against a wide variety of antigens, resident bacteria, and invading microorganisms. The mucosal surface is coated by mucins that are synthesized and secreted by goblet cells and interspersed among the absorptive enterocytes. The mucous coat provides a layer of protection and acts as a filter, allowing smaller nutrients to pass through and keeping larger molecules (antigens, pathogens) out. The cell surface structure itself acts as a barrier to antigen trafficking: microvilli density, rhythmic movement, and negative charge are combined to repel macromolecules, antigens, and microorganisms. Thus, any disease process that results in altered charge, decreased microvilli number, or microvilli atrophy makes the host imminently susceptible to more disease and antigen and microorganism infiltration.

Antigens pass through the mucosal barrier into the enterocyte and are either taken up via endocytosis and rapidly degraded by lysosomes (major pathway), or they pass through the cell untouched and are released into the systemic circulation (minor pathway). The gastrointestinal tract is composed of a single layer of epithelial cells, and antigens/nutrients can pass through the cell via a transcellular trafficking pathway or between the tight junctions that connect these cells via paracellular transport. Transcellular trafficking involves a clathrin-mediated endocytosis in which a ligand bound to its receptor aggregates in high concentration within a clathrin-coated pit that subsequently invaginates to produce a vesicle. These receptor-rich microdomains are not randomly found along the cell surface but rather are static structures called *caveolae* that are cholesterol- and sphingolipid-rich. Caveolae represent specialized areas on the cell surface where pit-mediated endocytosis takes place. Certain pathogens have adapted to penetrate the cell at the caveolae; Shiga toxin and cholera toxin (a) can bind to lipid-enriched "rafts" that bind the sphingolipid-enriched caveolae, and (b) are internalized via clathrin-mediated endocytosis. Vesicles, with nutrients or pathogens, fuse with an endosome within the cell. In the endosome, an acidification process occurs that results in ligand-receptor uncoupling, with trafficking of the ligand across the endosome membrane and recycling of the receptor back to the cell surface. The acidification process both allows for recycling of the receptor (which avoids limiting transportation of ligands and nutrients by the need for de novo synthesis of receptors) and provides another barrier to infection by killing pathogens trapped in the acidified endosome. Nutrients, antigens, macromolecules, and pathogens that successfully transverse the cell are transported to the systemic circulation (38). Paracellular transport through gaps in tight junctions and pores that open between epithelial cells occurs following activation of certain apical membrane-coupled transport systems (Na^+-glucose-coupled transport), which signals opening a pore in the tight junction. With an average pore radius of 5 nm, many small molecules and proteins can readily pass through. So too can pathogens and cholera toxins readily induce pore opening and cytoskeleton reorganization, allowing for the trafficking of larger macromolecules.

Processed antigens are further presented to T cells within or beneath the enterocyte epithelium by the major histocompatibility complex class I and class II molecules on the enterocyte surface. The role of this antigen presentation in the development of tolerance is critical. Under conditions of infection and inflammation, costimulatory cytokine production in conjunction with antigen presentation by the enterocyte on its cell surface is capable of generating a significant immune response. Ongoing research is directed toward studying how manipulation of the mucosal surface may alter an immune response versus developing tolerance in cases of food allergy, inflammatory bowel disease, and celiac disease.

Glutamine

Glutamine is the most prevalent amino acid in the human body. It serves as a nitrogen donor and is essential for the synthesis of purine, pyrimidines, nucleotides, and glutathione. The high requirement by rapidly proliferating cells for glutamine explains the significant requirement for this amino acid by the intestinal mucosa. In 1991, investigators revealed that glutamine-supplemented enteral or parenteral solutions were associated with increased mucosal thickness, improved integrity of the mucosal barrier, and reduced bacterial translocation across the enterocyte mucosal barrier. Glutamine supplementation has been associated with heat shock protein (hsp70) induction, reduced heat shock-induced cell death, restoration of mucosal immunoglobulin (IgA), enhanced bacterial clearance in peritonitis, and enhanced production of both intestinal and hepatic glutathione stores.

Glutamine supplementation of parenteral nutrition in a double-blinded, randomized, controlled trial did not improve intestinal permeability or nitrogen balance, decrease infection rate, or improve survival in newborn and infant children who underwent digestive-tract surgery (2). These findings are in contrast to those of a prospective, controlled, double-blinded, randomized, multicentered study in critically ill adults from 16 different surgical ICUs, which found that patients who received the glutamine-supplemented parenteral nutrition (0.5 g/kg/day) had fewer bloodstream infections, lower incidence of pneumonia, and a lower rate of requirement for insulin to manage hyperglycemia (15). Whereas no study to date has conclusively confirmed the benefit of glutamine in nutritional supplementation during critical illness, neither risk nor adverse outcome appears to be associated with its delivery either enterally or parenterally.

Arginine

Arginine is a versatile dibasic amino acid that plays many roles in cellular homeostasis. The liver and gut are the two organs that are critical for arginine homeostasis. Hepatic arginase activity rapidly converts the majority of liver arginine to urea. This process is regulated at the level of the intestine, which converts dietary arginine into citrulline, thereby limiting the concentration of arginine presented to the liver. Citrulline is converted back to arginine by argininosuccinate synthetase and argininosuccinate lyase, enzymes that are nearly absent in the enterocyte and liver. Thus, arginine in the form of citrulline passes through the enterocyte, enters the circulation, bypasses the liver, and is captured by the kidneys. Renal citrulline uptake is highly efficient, and the kidney converts 80% of gut citrulline into circulating serum arginine. Thus arginine, the precursor for multiple proteins and signaling molecules, can enter the body as arginine or as citrulline. Concern for increasing hepatic urea stores by supplementing enteral diets with arginine has been studied, and citrulline successfully increased the arginine pool and restored nitrogen balance in rats that underwent intestinal resection (29).

Arginine is metabolized in the liver and gut via the arginase pathway into urea and ornithine. Ornithine is a critical regulator of cell proliferation and differentiation; critical for the formation of proline and hydroxyproline; a precursor for polyamine, histidine, and nucleic acid synthesis; an essential promoter of thymic growth and development; and stimulator of the release of a plethora of hormones, including insulin, prolactin, glucagon, and growth hormone. More importantly, arginine is a unique substrate for the signaling molecule NO, which is formed by the oxidation of L-arginine by NO synthase. Three separate NO isoenzymes have been characterized: inducible NO (iNO), endothelial NO, and neuronal NO. iNO plays a significant role as an immunomodulator. Early studies documented the effect of enteral arginine on increased lymphocyte and monocyte proliferation and enhanced T-helper cell formation. Multiple studies in wound healing have shown a significant improvement in results with patients on arginine supplementation (25–30 g/dose), such as enhanced protein synthesis, improved wound healing, increased nitrogen balance, increased insulin-like growth factor 1 levels, and enhanced immuno-activity (40).

Although it may appear that arginine would enhance immune function, clinical studies suggest that NO potentiates the systemic inflammatory response in patients with sepsis and is associated with worse outcomes (28). The use of a nonselective NO synthase inhibitor is associated with increased mortality (25).

Early clinical trials that studied the benefit of oral citrulline in reducing pulmonary hypertension in children who underwent cardiopulmonary bypass and who were at risk for the development of pulmonary hypertension showed some promising results. In one study, 40 children were randomized to receive five perioperative doses of either oral citrulline or placebo. Postoperative pulmonary hypertension developed in 30% of the placebo group and 15% of the citrulline group. Despite concerns for the study size and design, the conclusion that oral citrulline supplementation may be effective in reducing postoperative pulmonary hypertension is intriguing (37).

Nucleotides

Nucleotides are by definition composed of a heterocyclic base, a sugar, and one or more phosphate groups, and they are the building blocks that compose RNA and DNA. The sugar is usually a five-carbon sugar—either ribose (RNA) or deoxyribose (DNA). The nucleotides/deoxynucleotides can be classified as either purines (adenosine or guanosine) or pyrimidines (thymidine, uridine, cytidine). Nucleotides also are the primary components of CoA, flavin adenine dinucleotide, flavin mononucleotide, nicotinamide adenine dinucleotide, and nicotinamide adenine dinucleotide phosphate. During catabolic stress or protein malnutrition, de novo nucleotide biosynthesis is severely impaired. Rapidly dividing cells are the most sensitive to this loss, and immune cells appear to be exceptionally susceptible. T-helper cells are selectively lost, and IL-2 production is impaired with selective dietary loss of urines and pyrimidines (40). In animal models, an association of increased susceptibility to *Staphylococcus aureus* and *Candida albicans* sepsis is seen during nucleotide deficiency (23). No randomized clinical trial has been conducted to explore whether the demand for nucleotides can exceed the endogenous production or to determine the safety of enhancing nucleotides in either parenteral or enteral nutrition.

Omega-3 Polyunsaturated Fatty Acids

Omega-3 polyunsaturated fatty acids (PUFAs) are metabolized to the 3-series of prostanoids and the 5-series of leukotrienes. As compared to the metabolites of the other subclass of long-chain omega fatty acids (omega-6), these prostanoids and leukotrienes lack the inflammatory and immunosuppressive characteristics, notably vasoconstriction, induced platelet aggregation, impaired cytokine secretion, defective leukocyte migration, and abnormal macrophage function. In fact, evidence suggests that nutritional intervention with omega-3 PUFAs modulates and downregulates inflammatory eicosanoids and prostaglandin E1 production. Omega-3 PUFAs are obtained from fish or canola oils and provide an excellent lipid energy source (23). Fatty acids are characterized by the number of carbon atoms, the number of double bonds, and the position of the first double bond. An omega-3 PUFA has the first double bond at position C-3 from the methyl end. Important examples of the omega-3 PUFAs are α-linolenic acid, eicosapentaenoic acid (EPA), and docosahexaenoic acid (DHA). α-linolenic acid contains 18 carbons, EPA contains 20 carbon atoms, and DHA contains 22. ALA is the precursor to EPA and DHA. Deficiencies of these PUFAs have been associated with delayed growth, skin lesions, decreased visual acuity, delayed learning ability, and mild neuropathology (40). Diets higher in monounsaturated fatty acids and PUFAs are believed to decrease risk of heart disease, in particular because they can lower levels of low-density lipoprotein cholesterol and triglycerides. PUFAs are also called *essential fatty acids* because they are not synthesized by the human body and must be obtained in our diet.

Previous anecdotal studies suggested that omega-3 PUFAs were able to ameliorate the symptoms of multiple inflammatory diseases, such as rheumatoid arthritis, psoriasis, Crohn disease, and ulcerative colitis. Small, randomized, controlled trials that have studied omega-3 PUFAs and clinical improvement in cystic fibrosis, autism, depression and asthma have been encouraging. Considerable interest was generated in the possibility that the 3-omega PUFAs acted in reducing proinflammatory cytokines (IL-1 and IL-6), oxidative injury, and lipid peroxidation. One group showed that the administration of omega-3 PUFAs as part of total parenteral nutrition significantly decreased energy requirements, was well tolerated, and did not downregulate lipogenic genes, plasma triglyceride levels, or lipid oxidation, and did not affect glucose metabolism (42).

In a single-centered, prospective, randomized, controlled, unblended study, 100 patients with acute lung injury were ran-

domized to receive a standard enteral diet versus a standard diet supplemented with EPA and γ-linoleic acid (GLA) for 14 days. EPA/GLA-treated patients had shorter lengths of ventilation and improved respiratory mechanics. However, improvements in oxygenation at days 4 and 7 in the EPA/GLA-enriched group were lost by day 14, and length of stay and survival were the same (36).

Branched-chain Amino Acids

The branched-chain amino acids (BCAA) include leucine, isoleucine, and valine and account for 35%–40% of the dietary essential amino acids in the body's protein pool and 14%–18% of the total amino acids found in muscle proteins. Studies in the 1970s suggested that the exogenous supplemented BCAA had anabolic properties. In a review of all known studies that characterize the effect of the BCAAs as anticatabolic agents under conditions of burns, sepsis, or trauma, investigators concluded that leucine alone possesses protein-regulatory properties and is solely responsible for the decreased protein degradation observed (14). Leucine promotes protein synthesis and inhibits protein degradation via a leucine-specific signaling of mTOR, the mammalian target for rapamycin. Leucine supplementation was associated with improved muscle recovery following rigorous muscle exercise in healthy volunteers (35). Clearly, the "leucine concept" deserves to be evaluated in a randomized, controlled trial prior to endorsing its use.

Immunonutrition and the concept of immuno-enhancing diets remain controversial but represent an important shift in our approach to nutrition; dietary manipulation of the immune system adds yet another therapeutic tool to our armamentarium to fight disease states. A systematic review of 22 randomized trials concluded that while immunonutrition may have decreased infectious disease complications, it was not associated with an overall mortality advantage and that the treatment effect was patient-population specific (20). Advances in basic science and clinical trials are increasing clinicians' understanding of which patients and which diseases are most amenable to adjuvant nutritional therapy. Recognizing the specific patient populations that will benefit from immunonutrition will be the task for the next decade. Current consensus reports on immune-enhancing diets recommend that those who should receive early enteral nutrition with an immuno-enhancing diet are: (a) moderately or severely malnourished patients (albumin <3.5 g/dL) who undergo elective gastrointestinal surgery, (b) severely malnourished patients with albumin <2.8 g/dL who undergo colonic or rectal surgery, and (c) patients who have suffered blunt and penetrating torso trauma (31).

In the first blinded, prospective, randomized, controlled clinical trial to study early enteral administration of immunonutrition in critically ill children, 100 children admitted to a single PICU were randomized within the first 12 hrs to receive either an enteral formula supplemented with glutamine, arginine, omega-3 PUFAs, and antioxidants or a control formula. Randomization, prepared formula masking, and energy calculations were performed by a single, blinded individual. Both formulas provided adequate energy protein balance, with the supplemented immuno-enhancing diet providing more favorable effect on nitrogen balance, decreased gastric colonization rates, and a decreasing trend in nosocomial infections. No difference was observed in length of stay or mortality (12).

However, a more careful analysis of the data suggests a trend for increased mortality among the immunonutrition-fed group. Concern that these deaths may have been in children who were admitted with sepsis sparked an intense debate (24). A clear position on the effectiveness and safety of immuno-enhanced diets for both children and adults has yet to be determined. This topic warrants well-designed, randomized studies as the field of immunonutrition grows.

BEST PRACTICES IN NUTRITION THERAPY

The last two decades have heralded a new commitment to enteral feeding accompanied with an aggressive feeding tube-placement strategy. The recognition that even small feed volumes could significantly maintain a normal gut flora, minimize bacterial overgrowth, decrease the rate of drug-resistant bacteria emergence, and reduce bacterial translocation was accepted by the critical care community, although implementation remains poor. While the importance of calories and maintaining "normal" gut function were recognized, macronutrients and micronutrients were quickly recognized to be essential ligands for the signaling process critical for cellular responses to illness, and macronutrient and micronutrient composition and caloric content became important. Hypermetabolism and skeletal muscle breakdown during critical illness are only a fraction of the documented catabolism that occurs during illness.

Markers of nutritional sufficiency are lacking. Vitamin levels are variable, and micronutrient pools are rapidly depleted. Macronutrient values appear to provide the most accurate serum markers of nutrition status. Albumin, prealbumin, transferrin, and retinol-binding proteins represent the four proteins most commonly measured to assess protein malnutrition and extrapolated to reflect total body nutrient needs. The serum protein half-lives of these proteins are:

Albumin (3.5–5.5 g/dL)	20 days
Transferrin (200–400 mg/dL)	8 days
Pre-albumin (16–35 mg/dL)	2 days
Retinol-binding protein (2.6–7.6 mg/dL)	10 hrs

It is clear that early implementation of a nutritional regimen improves clinical outcomes, decreases infection rate, and reduces hospital stay. A review of adult critical care outcomes studies confirms that malnutrition, defined as inadequate nutritional support to meet metabolic demand, is associated with increased morbidity and mortality, increased dependency on ventilatory support, increased nosocomial infection rates, and impaired wound healing. The adult ICU literature also reveals that enteral feeds are superior to parenteral feeds. Despite providing caloric and substrate support, parenteral nutrition is associated with increased incidence of central-line and wound infections. Secondary hepatobiliary dysfunction is associated with parenteral feeds. Parenteral nutrition does not confer the gastric-stimulated gut peristalsis or neutralization of gastric acid that protects from both ulcer development and bacterial translocation that is accomplished with enteral feeds.

Despite all of the benefits of implementing enteral feeding, delays in initiating feeding regimens are commonplace. An adult study was conducted to examine outcomes in critically ill patients in both medical and surgical ICUs before and after

implementation of an evidence-based nutritional management protocol. Feeding tubes were placed within 24 hrs of admission to the ICU and patients were randomized to a protocolized feeding algorithm by 48 hrs. This approach resulted in fewer days to feed (2.9 ± 1.7 vs. 3.2 ± 2.0) and fewer mechanical ventilation days (11.2 ± 19.5 vs. 17.9 ± 31.3), with no difference in length of stay or mortality between the groups. Not surprising, patients with better premorbid nutritional status and those who tolerated full enteral feeds early were less likely to die than those with poor premorbid nutritional deficiencies and those who had difficulty tolerating or advancing their enteral diet (6).

Whereas adult ICU feeding protocols start at a rate of 25 mL/hr and target a gastric intraluminal volume of <100 mL to indicate an excessive gastric residual after 4 hrs of feeding, pediatric protocols require volume and rate adjustment based on patient size and age. In a retrospective comparison chart review that evaluated the use of a nasogastric feeding protocol in a PICU, time to reach goal feedings was the single most significant difference identified as a result of establishing a protocol. Twenty percent of the patient population was receiving inotropes, and 80% was receiving sedation. While patients enterally fed early had improved tolerance to feeds (less vomiting, less diarrhea, and less constipation), no differences in ICU stay or hospital length of stay were noted (30). While length of stay, days on ventilator, and total hospital days may not differ between the groups, it is interesting to note that surviving children uniformly have prealbumin values on day 5 of feeding that are significantly higher than nonsurvivors (9). Still, the use of feeding protocols in children remains controversial. Splanchnic blood flow and the effect of inotropes and/or sepsis on intestinal mucosal oxygenation remain substantially understudied (33). It is interesting that multiple studies on nasogastric feedings initiated by protocol in critically ill children (sepsis and traumatic brain injury, no cardiovascular postoperative patients or other pediatric surgical patients) have failed to document gut catastrophes associated with intestinal ischemia secondary to feeding (10,11).

The reduction in gastric motility associated with critical illness and an increased risk for pulmonary aspiration appears to be another barrier to early feeding. Transpyloric feeding (placing a tube in the first to fourth segment of the duodenum) was compared with nasogastric feeds in terms of tolerance, complications, and outcomes. Despite the many limitations of the study, the authors were able to conclude that transpyloric feeding was well tolerated, desired calories were reached more rapidly, and the patients required less sedation (32).

CONCLUSIONS AND FUTURE DIRECTIONS

According to the program, the topic of nutrition and nutrition as therapy in the critically ill featured prominently at the Annual Congress of Society of Critical Care Medicine in June 2007. The field is appreciating a new recognition of the roles of nutrition, both as a moderator of outcome in patients who are significantly-to-severely malnourished and as a therapy to deal with increasing rates of polymicrobial antibiotic resistance in the ICU. Clinical studies reveal that patients' nutritional status is related to their immune competence and hence their susceptibility to infection. In the future, single-nucleotide polymorphisms will be used (a) to predict which diseases patients are susceptible to and which drugs are likely to provide benefit, and (b) in the ICU in the form of *individualized, genomic-based nutrigenetics* to determine genetic-based differences that will guide nutritional supplementation. The fields of nutraceuticals, nutrigenomics, and nutrigenetics will be instrumental in guiding the use of nutrition as an immunomodulator. Nutrient modification of genetic susceptibility to disease will be enthusiastically embraced as large, randomized, controlled clinical trials are able to show a specific effect. The use of *probiotics* (which contain microbes) and *prebiotics* (which promote the growth of microbes) in pediatric practice to modify the intestinal environment will increase as we struggle to deal with antibiotic resistance. Our understanding of the role of the intestinal flora as a means to control infectious processes and to modulate the immune response will culminate in the practice of introducing microorganisms into the gut that will either provide health benefits directly or provide substances that will help beneficial intestinal microbiota to grow (16). In the future, "We are what we eat" will take on new significance in the PICU.

KEY POINTS

- Adequate and appropriate nutrition, implemented early, is critical in treating malnutrition in the ICU.
- Malnutrition is associated with increased morbidity and mortality in the ICU.
- Susceptibility to infectious complications is directly related to a patient's nutritional status.
- It is premature to institute immunonutrition routinely for all critically ill patients and yet an understanding and appreciation of the benefits of immune-enhanced diets for specific patient populations is necessary.
- Correcting redox imbalance with vitamins and trace elements may represent the next wave of nutritional supplementation.
- The fields of nutraceuticals, nutrigenomics and nutrigenetics will guide our use of nutrition to modify gene susceptibility to disease.
- Enteral feeding maintains intestinal trophism, stimulates the immune system, reduces bacterial translocation, and is associated with decreased cost.
- Transpyloric feeding is not associated with an increased complication rate, as is nasogastric feeding.
- Disease-related malnutrition occurs rapidly in critically ill children, especially those <2 years of age.
- Protein and fat depletion are the most severe in infants and children.

References

1. Agus MSD, Jaksic T. Nutritional support of the critically ill child. *Curr Opin Pediatr* 2002;14:470–81.
2. Albers MJ, Steyerberg EW, Hazebroek FW, et al. Glutamine supplementation of parenteral nutrition does not improve intestinal permeability, nitrogen balance, or outcome in newborns and infants undergoing digestive-tract surgery: Results from a double-blind, randomized, controlled trial. *Ann Surg* 2005;241:599–606.
3. Alexander E, Susla G, Burstein AH, et al. Retrospective evaluation of commonly used equations to predict energy expenditure in mechanically ventilated, critically ill patients. *Pharmacotherapy* 2004;24:1659–67.

4. Angstwurm MW, Engelmann L, Zimmermann T, et al. Selenium in Intensive Care (SIC): Results of a prospective randomized, placebo-controlled, multiple-center study in patients with severe systemic inflammatory response syndrome, sepsis, and septic shock. *Crit Care Med* 2007;35(1):118–26; comment, 206–7.
5. Angstwurm MW, Gaertner R. Practicalities of selenium supplementation in critically ill patients. *Curr Opin Clin Nutr Metab Care* 2006;9(3):233–8.
6. Barr J, Hecht M, Flavin KE, et al. Outcomes in Critically-ill patients before and after implementation of an evidence-based nutritional management protocol. *Chest* 2004;125:1446–57.
7. Bott L, Béghin L, Marichez C, et al. Comparison of resting energy expenditure in bronchopulmonary dysplasia to predicted equation. *Eur J Clin Nutr.* 2006;60(11):1323–9.
8. Briassoulis G, Venkataraman S, Thompson AE. Energy expenditure in critically ill children. *Crit Care Med* 2000;28:1166–72.
9. Briassoulis G, Zavras N, Hatzis T. Malnutrition, nutritional indices and early enteral feeding in critically ill children. *Nutrition* 2001;17:548–57.
10. Briassoulis G, Zavras NJ, Hatzis TD. Effectiveness and safety of a protocol for promotion of early intragastric feeding in critically ill children. *Pediatr Crit Care Med* 2001;2:113–21.
11. Briassoulis G, Tsorva A, Zavras N, et al. Influence of an aggressive early enteral nutrition protocol on nitrogen balance in critically ill children. *J. Nutr Biochem* 2002;13:560–9.
12. Briassoulis G, Filippou O, Hatzi E, et al. Early enteral administration of immunonutrition in critically ill children: Results of a blinded randomized controlled clinical trial. *Nutrition* 2005;21:799–807.
13. Coss-Bu JA, Jefferson LS, Walding D, et al. Resting energy expenditure and nitrogen balance in critically ill pediatric patients on mechanical ventilation. *Nutrition* 1998;14(9):649–52.
14. De Bandt JP, Cynober L. Therapeutic use of branched-chain amino acids in burn, trauma and sepsis. *J Nutr* 2006;136:308S–13S.
15. Dechelotte P, Hasselmann M, Cynober L, et al. L-alanyl-L-glutamine dipeptide-supplemented total parenteral nutrition reduces infectious complications and glucose intolerance in critically ill patients: The French controlled, randomized, double-blind, multicenter study. *Crit Care Med* 2006;34:598–604.
16. de Morais MB, Jacob CMA. The role of probiotics and prebiotics in pediatric practice. *J Pediatria* 2006;82:S189–97.
17. Elshershari H, Ozer S, Ozkutlu S, et al. Potential usefulness of coenzyme Q$_{10}$ in the treatment of idiopathic dilated cardiomyopathy in children. *Int. J Cardiol* 2003;88:101–2.
18. Gramlich L, Kichian K, Pinilla J, et al. Does enteral nutrition compared to parenteral nutrition result in a better outcomes in critically ill adult patients? *A systematic review of the literature. Nutrition* 2004;20:843–8.
19. Havalad S, Quaid MA, Sapiega V. Energy expenditure in children with severe head injury: Lack of agreement between measured and estimated energy expenditure. *Nutr Clin Pract* 2006;2:175–81.
20. Heyland DK, Novak F, Drover JW, et al. Should immunonutrition become routine in critically ill patients? *A systematic review of the evidence. JAMA* 2001;286:944–53.
21. Heyland D, Dhaliwal R, Suchner U, et al. Antioxidant nutrients: A systematic review of trace elements and vitamins in the critically ill patient. *Int Care Med* 2005;31:327–37.
22. Kudsk KA, Tolley EA, DeWitt RC. Preoperative albumin and surgical site identify surgical risk for major postoperative complications. *J Parenter Enteral Nutr* 2003;27:1–9.
23. Kudsk KA. Immunonutrition in surgery and critical care. *Annu Rev Nutr* 2006;26:463–79.
24. Leite HP, Iglesias SBO. Are immune-enhancing diets safe for critically ill children? *Nutrition* 2006;22:579–80.
25. Lopez A, Lorente JA, Steingrub J. Multiple-center, randomized, placebo-controlled, double-blind study of the nitric oxide synthase inhibitor 546C88: Effect on survival in patients with septic shock. *Crit Care Med* 2004;32:21–30.
26. Martindale RG, Maerz LL. Management of perioperative nutrition support. *Curr Opin Crit Care* 2006;12:290–4.
27. National Institutes of Health (NIH) State-of-the-Science Conference Statement: Multivitamin/mineral supplements and chronic disease prevention. *Ann Int Med* 2006;145:364–71.
28. Ochoa JB, Makarenkova V, Bansal V. A rational use of immune enhancing diets: When should we use arginine supplementation? *Nutrition Clin Pract* 2004;19:216–25.
29. Osowska S, Moinard C, Neveux N, et al. Citrulline increases arginine pool and restores nitrogen balance after massive intestinal resection. *Gut* 2004;53:1781–6.
30. Petrillo-Albarano T, Pettignano R, Asfaw M, et al. Use of feeding protocol to improve nutritional support through early, aggressive enteral nutrition in the pediatric intensive care unit. *Pediatr Crit Care Med* 2006;7:340–4.
31. Sacks GS, Genton L, Kudsk KA. Controversy of immunonutrition for surgical-critical-illness patients. *Curr Op Critical Care* 2003;9:300–5.
32. Sanchez C, Lopez-Herce J, Carrillo A, et al. Early transpyloric enteral nutrition in critically ill children. *Nutrition* 2007;23:16–22.
33. Sasbon JS, Cardigni G. Nutritional support in the critically ill child: Fast food or haute cuisine. *Pediatr Crit Care Med* 2006;7:395–6.

34. Sazawal S, Black RE, Ramsan M, et al. Effects of routine prophylactic supplementation with iron and folic acid on admission to hospital and mortality in preschool children in a high malaria transmission setting: Community-based, randomized, placebo-controlled trial. *Lancet* 2006;367:133–43.

35. Shimomura Y, Yamaoto Y, Bajotta G, et al. Nutraceutical effects of branched-chain amino acids on skeletal muscle. *J Nutr* 2006;136: 529S–32S.

36. Singer P, Theilla M, Fisher H, et al. Benefit of an enteral diet enriched with eicosapentaenoic acid and gamma-linolenic acid in ventilated patients with acute lung injury. *Crit Care Med* 2006;34:1033–8.

37. Smith HAB, Canter JA, Christian KG, et al. Nitric oxide precursors and congenital heart surgery" a randomized controlled trial of oral citrulline. *J. Thoracic Cardiovasc Surgery* 2006;132:58–65.

38. Snoeck V, Goddeeris B, Cox E. The role of enterocytes in the intestinal barrier function and antigen uptake. *Microbes and Infection* 2005;7:997–1004.

39. Subbiah MTR. Nutrigenetics and nutraceuticals: The next wave riding on personalized medicine. *Translational Res* 2007;149:55–61.

40. Suchner U, Kuhn KS, Furst P. The scientific basis of immunonutrition. *Proc Nutr Soc* 2000;59:553–63.

41. Suman OE, Mlcak RP, Chinkes DL, et al. Resting energy expenditure in severely burned children: Analysis of agreement between indirect calorimetry and prediction equations using the Bland-Altman method. *Burns* 2006;32:335–42.

42. Tappy L, Berger MM, Schwarz JM, et al. Metabolic effects of parenteral nutrition enriched with n-3 polyunsaturated fatty acids in critically ill patients. *Clin Nutr* 2006;25:588–95.

CHAPTER 86 ■ NUTRITIONAL SUPPORT IN THE CRITICALLY ILL CHILD

WERTHER BRUNOW DE CARVALHO • HEITOR PONS LEITE

Nutrition in children must ensure maintenance of body mass and normal metabolism and allow for growth. General growth rate is increased both in the first years of life and during adolescence; the brain grows most rapidly between the last 3 months of pregnancy and the first year of life. Malnutrition during these critical phases may compromise both somatic and neurologic growth, impacting the child's future. Hence, proper nutrition should be guaranteed in ill children who are unable to feed normally and who are at risk of malnutrition. Such feeding is achieved through artificial nutritional support, either enterally or parenterally.

Nutrition in children with severe infection or trauma or following major surgery is hampered by the hormonal and metabolic changes associated with the systemic inflammatory response triggered by such conditions. To devise proper nutritional support, these changes and their implications for nutrient use must be well understood.

METABOLIC STRESS

The systemic inflammatory response includes activation of the sympathetic nervous system and the hypothalamic-pituitary-adrenal axis (5). These responses are characterized by changes in glucose metabolism and lipids, along with increased protein turnover and breakdown, which result in increased energy expenditure and a negative nitrogen balance and lead to muscle protein loss. Hypermetabolic and hyperdynamic states are characterized by hyperthermia, tachycardia, tachypnea, hyperglycemia, and an increase in oxygen consumption and in cardiac index (17).

These neurohormonal responses divert substrate from nonvital functions to functions that are essential to survival. Beneficial effects include the supply of alternative energy sources to meet the increased demand and to furnish substrate for the protein synthesis required for wound healing. Hyperglycemia and increased glyconeogenesis most likely occur in response to the elevated need for glucose by injured tissues and vital organs such as the brain. Peripheral resistance to insulin action ensures continued glucose production and reduction in its oxidation within muscle and in its storage as hepatic glycogen. Increased lipolysis provides free fatty acids for energy, and glycerol for gluconeogenesis. Protein hypercatabolism occurs in skeletal muscle, converting branched-chain amino acids into alanine, a precursor of both gluconeogenesis and hepatic protein synthesis, and glutamine, a preferential fuel for cells (e.g., enterocytes and lymphocytes) that have a high rate of cellular division. Deamination of branched-chain amino acids supplies amino acids for the pro-

tein synthesis that occurs in the healing process and in the immunologic response—immunoglobulins and reactants of the acute phase. Cortisol, secreted in response to adrenocorticotropic hormone, activates the aldosterone-angiotensin-renin system. Levels of catecholamines, cortisol, glucagon, growth hormone, aldosterone, and antidiuretic hormone are all increased, and insulin is generally elevated but not sufficiently to impede hyperglycemia. Insulin secretion is initially suppressed by the α-adrenergic mechanism and later increased together with glucagon levels. Peripheral resistance to growth hormone action occurs, with a reduction in insulin-like growth factor (IGF)-1 secretion, while hyperglycemia and lipolytic effects remain. Increased counter-regulating hormone concentrations induce both insulin-resistant and growth hormone-resistant states, a characteristic sign of stress, which results in protein catabolism and the utilization of endogenous carbohydrate and fat stores to meet the increased basal metabolic rate. All of these mechanisms constitute interaction among the nervous, endocrine, and immunologic systems in a bid to mediate stress (5,74).

These changes can be explained by the neuroendocrine reflex comprising afferent and efferent pathways (17,18). Afferent information derived from neurosensorial and visceral receptors, as well as from the cerebral cortex, is integrated in the thorax and hypothalamus, resulting in activation of the sympathetic nervous system and hypothalamic secretion of release factors that stimulate the pituitary. Another pathophysiologic mechanism that is thought to occur is the synthesis and release of inflammatory and metabolic response mediators through monocytes, primarily Kupffer cells and alveolar macrophages. These mediators include cytokines, products of arachidonic acid metabolism, and platelet activation factors. Acting locally or distally, they promote changes in cell function and metabolism. Such mediators also act directly on hypothalamic activity, influencing the release of classic stress hormones.

The stress response peaks on the third or fourth day following injury reversing in 7 to 10 days. Continued hypermetabolism results in a rapid process of malnutrition and immunologic dysfunction, leading to multiorgan dysfunction in some cases (17,19). The standard response depends on the nature, intensity, and duration of the stimulus, as well as the degree of response, which in turn is determined by the nutritional state and genetic factors. Continued hypermetabolism results from complicating factors, such as hypotension or infection, and prolongs alterations in nutrient production, demand, and use in cells, leading to rapid malnutrition and lowering of immunologic function. Loss of body mass may be minimal or of no great consequence in well-nourished patients or those with self-limited disease. In malnourished children, however, already scarce energy reserves, insufficient to promote proper growth, are redirected to meet demands increased by metabolic stress.

MALNOURISHED PATIENTS

Protein-calorie malnutrition is associated with increased duration of hospitalization, morbidity, and mortality among hospitalized patients (21). The prevalence of malnutrition in critically ill children varies among studies from 18% to 65% (47,60).

Children's lower energy reserve in relation to adults shortens their survival time in inanition states. For example, the survival time is 60–90 days in adults, 44 days in 1-year-old children, and falls to 12 days in 2-kg, premature neonates (33). Given that malnutrition in children is associated with increased risk of infection and delayed wound healing, the prompt identification of this condition is essential and even more important due to the growth demands on a child's physiology.

To prevent malnutrition-related complications, a child should be assessed for risk of becoming malnourished or of exacerbated malnourishment during hospitalization, and adequate nutrition must be guaranteed in ill children who are unable to feed normally. When planning nutritional support in severely malnourished children, several limitations must be considered.

Limitations Inherent to Malnourished and Metabolically Stressed Children

Critically ill, malnourished children are less able to handle substrate, liquid, and solute overload. The most common absorptive disturbances involve carbohydrates (particularly lactose) and fats.

The main functional and physiologic alterations that arise from malnutrition are reductions in cardiac output, glomerular filtration rate, renal blood flow, and renal solute excretion capacity. Intracellular potassium and sodium pump activity is lowered.

In view of these limitations, caution is urged in initial phases of treatment, as excessive volume intake of water and nutrients may cause complications or death (7). Well-nourished children who are likely to return to normal feeding within 4–5 days do not generally require artificial nutritional support, whereas malnourished patients with hypermetabolism or hypercatabolism should receive treatment as swiftly as possible.

OBJECTIVES OF NUTRITIONAL SUPPORT

The objective of the initial phases of nutritional support is to attenuate losses due to hypercatabolism, allowing the patient to maintain body mass and organic functions without overloading metabolism, the cardiovascular system, or the respiratory muscles. Once metabolic stress has been resolved, energy supply should be increased to achieve anabolism.

Nutrient Needs and Supply

Fluid Intake

Water needs depend on a patient's clinical picture. Daily assessment of weight, urinary osmolality, diuresis volume, and fluids balance provides a good estimation of hydration state. Fever, increased ambient temperature, hypermetabolism, and liquid loss through diarrhea or digestive juices all imply further water loss and call for increased water intake. A significant weight loss from one day to the next tends to reflect abnormal liquid loss, and conversely, marked weight gain may be the result of excessive water intake. Fluid losses through diarrhea or ileostomy drainage should be replaced daily. Fluid retention that stems from changes in endothelium permeability that occur with the systemic inflammatory response may require fluid restriction. Hypoxia and arterial hypotension may cause cortical or tubular necrosis, compromising renal function. In the presence of acute renal insufficiency, the volume required to supply protein-calorie needs should be administered in association with peritoneal dialysis to remove excess liquid. Having resolved systemic inflammatory response and with no further need to restrict volume, an increase of up to 50% over basal fluid requirements can be made to increase nutrient intake and promote anabolism.

Energy Intake

The main components of energy expenditure in children are base metabolism, growth, and activity. During metabolic stress, no growth or physical activity takes place; therefore, the lack of these elements in conjunction with sedation reduces energy expenditure. Basing the energy intake of a critically ill child on the predicted requirements of a healthy child (90–110 kcal/kg/day) lends to a risk of overfeeding. Overfeeding predisposes to increased respiratory quotient, risk of steatosis and hepatic cholestasis, and increased risk of infection (20). Hence, for sedated infants in intensive care, the caloric requirement during acute metabolic stress is limited to that needed to reach basal metabolic rate plus a stress factor, which, depending on the clinical situation, is between 1.1 and 1.2 (1,20,62).

The basal metabolic rate in newborns and infants is ~50–55 kcal/kg/day and falls steadily until adolescence to 25 kcal/kg/day (70). This calculation represents only an estimate of energy needs, considering that the rules tend to overestimate energy expenditure and that energy expenditure can vary by up to 30% over any given 24-hr period.

Parenteral Nutrition

Parenteral nutrition aims to recuperate or maintain nutritional status while promoting growth and is indicated when the gastrointestinal tract is compromised by disease or treatment or when the enteral route alone is unable to meet nutritional needs. Previously well-nourished patients without likelihood of receiving effective enteral nutrition in 5–7 days are candidates for parenteral nutrition. It is recommended that commencement of parenteral nutrition not be delayed to beyond 48 hrs in severely malnourished patients or neonates who are not receiving enteral nutrition, provided they are hemodynamically and metabolically stable. In this context, parenteral nutrition should be used mainly in chronically malnourished patients, in those at risk of malnutrition due to acute disease or post-surgical complications, in those with syndromes of poor intestinal absorption, and in premature neonates.

Parenteral nutrition is a much more costly procedure than enteral nutrition and is subject to complications. Therefore, in addition to considering the cost-benefit ratio, proper implementation should also consider assessment and monitoring of nutritional and metabolic needs, access route, and formulation.

Access Route and Osmolarity

Nutritional need is the main factor that determines access route, with preference given to the peripheral venous route when use will be <2 weeks. Usually, peripheral veins can support solutions with glucose concentrations of up to 12.5%; this limit does not take into account solution osmolarity and is only valid for IV solutions that contain glucose and electrolytes in quantities equivalent to basal needs.

In parenteral nutrition solutions, amino acids and electrolytes in addition to glucose contribute to the final osmolarity of the solution. Concentrations of glucose higher than 8% generally have osmolarity of >600 mOsm/L, independent of amino acid concentration. In the case of intermediate concentrations between 6% and 8%, raised osmolarities are found when amino acid concentrations are ≥10%. Notably, even infusions of solutions with osmolarity of ~600 mOsm/L have been associated with thrombophlebitis in peripheral veins (69).

Infusion time is another factor to be considered. Data from an experimental study in which parenteral nutrition solutions with increasing osmolarities were given suggest that vein tolerance of increased osmolarity lessens with increased infusion time (69). The tolerated osmolarity by normal-flow peripheral veins was 820 mOsm/kg for 8 hrs, 690 mOsm/kg for 12 hrs, and 550 mOsm/kg for 24 hrs. Superficial veins, due to their low flow, are prone to sclerosis or phlebitis during hypertonic solution infusion, as well as leakage of solution and consequent injury to the subcutaneous tissue. High-osmolarity solutions should be administrated through a central vein.

The osmolarity of the parenteral nutrition solution must be known prior to administration, particularly when the solution is suspected to be hypertonic. The formula below has been validated for estimating parenteral nutrition osmolarity in children (57).

$$\text{Osmolarity (mOsm/L)}$$
$$= (A \times 8) + (G \times 7) + (Na \times 2) + (P \times 0.2) - 50$$

where:

> G = glucose (g/L)
> A = amino acids (mg/L)
> Na = sodium (mEq/L)
> P = phosphorus (mg/L).

This formula is useful in cases in which the final glucose concentration is >7% or when it is <7% and amino acids are >10%, conditions which do not guarantee a final solution osmolarity of <600 mOsm/L.

Those children unable to receive nutrition through the enteral route for 2 weeks or more and whose needs cannot be met by the peripheral route must receive parenteral nutrition through the central vein. To lower the risk of phlebitis secondary to parenteral nutrition solutions, solutions with osmolarity of >600 Osm/L should be administered through the central vein.

Electrolyte Intake

In addition to meeting basal requirements, electrolyte intake must also replace abnormal losses that occur in situations associated with alterations in water and electrolytic balance, such as sepsis, malnutrition, and refeeding syndrome. Malnutrition leads to losses in intracellular potassium, magnesium, and phosphorus and increases in sodium and water. Although monitoring of sodium, potassium, and calcium serum levels is integral to routine care, too little attention has been given to phosphorus in patient follow-up. The demand for phosphorus is greater in children because it is needed for the formation of new tissues, a state that puts a critically ill patient with severe malnutrition at higher risk of developing hypophosphatemia. The recommended amounts of electrolytes by parenteral route are shown in **Table 86.1**.

Glucose

Glucose, the main source of carbohydrate in parenteral nutrition, is vital to fuel the central nervous system, red blood cells, leukocytes, and renal medulla, supplying 3.4 kcal/g of hydrated glucose. The maximum rate of glucose that can be oxidized by adults and adolescents is 5 mg/kg/min.

Excessive intake of calories in the form of glucose can give rise to increased metabolic rate, hyperglycemia, and hepatic alterations. Glucose intake that exceeds 18 g/kg/day (equivalent to a 12.5 mg/kg/min infusion rate) in neonates can lead to lowered energy benefit, increased hepatic lipogenesis, and

---

TABLE 86.1

DAILY ELECTROLYTE REQUIREMENTS BY PARENTERAL ROUTE

Electrolyte	Neonates	Infants/children	Adolescents
Sodium	2–5 mEq/kg	2–6 mEq/kg	Individualized
Chloride	1–5 mEq/kg	2–5 mEq/kg	Individualized
Potassium	1–4 mEq/kg	2–3 mEq/kg	Individualized
Calcium	3–4 mEq/kg	1–2.5 mEq/kg	10–20 mEq
Phosphorus	1–2 mmol/kg	0.5–1 mmol/kg	10–40 mmol
Magnesium	0.3–0.5 mEq/kg	0.3–0.5 mEq/kg	10–30 mEq

Adapted from ASPEN. Board of Directors and The Clinical Guidelines Task Force. Guidelines for the use of parenteral and enteral nutrition in adult and pediatric patients. *JPEN* 2002;26(1):97SA–128SA.

increased CO_2 production (38). However, the clinical significance of such events is not yet fully known.

The glucose infusion rate in full-term newborns required to prevent hypoglycemia is between 3 and 4 mg/kg/min, and these values are generally higher in extremely premature births. Acute stress and corticotherapy are conditions that call for reduced glucose intake. Hyperglycemia may trigger glycosuria with osmotic diuresis, hampering immunologic function and healing, and may be associated with intracranial hemorrhage and worse neurologic prognosis in patients with cranioencephalic trauma. Should hyperglycemia occur, the cause must be treated, and the concentration or rate of glucose infusion reduced.

Lipids

Lipids are the main energy source for most tissues. The main fatty acids are ω-3, ω-6 series polyunsaturated fatty acids (PUFAs), monounsaturated fatty acids belonging to the ω-9 series, and those from medium and short chains.

ω-6 and ω-3 Fatty Acids. Fatty acids from the ω-6 and ω-3 families and their derivatives originate from linoleic acids and α-linolenic acids, respectively, and are considered vital. The ω-6 fatty acids are derived chiefly from animal and vegetable fats, while ω-3 fatty acids are found mainly in deepwater fish oil sources. Endogenous production is insufficient to ensure suitable concentrations of PUFAs. Both ω-6 and ω-3 PUFAs are considered metabolic antagonists. From series 6, linoleic acid (18:2 ω-6) forms γ-linoleic (18:3 ω-6), which converts to arachidonic acid (20:4 ω-6), the precursor of series 2 prostaglandins (PGE_2), thromboxane A_2 (TXA_2), and series 4 leukotrienes (LT4). They are involved in inflammation, modulating the immune system, regulating vascular tonus, and platelet aggregation. From series 3, α-linolenic acid (18:3 ω-3) is converted into eicosapentaenoic acid (20:5 ω-3) and docosahexaenoic acid (22:6 ω-3), which are precursors of series 3 prostaglandins (PGE_3), thromboxane A_3 (TXA_3), and series 5 leukotrienes (LT5). An excess of ω-6 PUFA may elevate the synthesis of proinflammatory eicosanoids, which may depress immune defense and increase the systemic inflammatory response.

Series 3 fatty acids play a key role during pregnancy and in the growth and development of a child in the first years of life. Docosahexaenoic acid, in particular, is incorporated into the brain of the fetus from the first 3 months of pregnancy to the eighth month of postnatal life. As neonates are unable to fully synthesize docosahexaenoic and arachidonic acids from their precursors, these fatty acids must be present in their diet. The ω-3 PUFAs possess few inflammatory properties compared to ω-6 PUFAs, but they inhibit production of inflammatory eicosanoids and decrease production of inflammatory cytokines, providing potential benefit in chronic disease and during the acute stress response.

Medium-Chain Fatty Acids. Medium-chain fatty acids are spontaneously hydrolyzed in intestinal lumen, independent of pancreatic lipase and bile salts for absorption and not dependent on plasma binding with albumin or carnitine for use in mitochondria, representing a rapid-use source.

Lipid Emulsions. IV lipid emulsions ensure provision of essential fatty acids and allow caloric intake to be increased without the need or inconvenience of greater glucose intake. Conventional emulsions are essentially composed of soybean oil and phospholipids from egg yolk as emulsifying agents and are available in 10% and 20% concentrations. They contain excessive quantities of PUFAs (55% linoleic and 9% linolenic acids) and insufficient amounts of α-tocopherol. They all contain long-chain triglycerides (LCTs) or a mixture of these with medium-chain triglycerides (MCTs) in equal ratio, which speeds lipid metabolization. Emulsions of 20% concentrations are more easily cleared in patients receiving high doses of lipids, an advantage over lower-concentration emulsions. Two other types of emulsions have become available: one is an olive oil- and soy oil-based emulsion, which, by virtue of its predominantly monounsaturated fatty acid make-up (80% olive oil), is less subject to lipid peroxidation; the other contains a soy oil and olive oil mix, with MCTs in fish oil that contains the ω-3 eicosapentaenoic and docosahexaenoic acids, with a lower ω-6/ω-3 ratio. It is enriched with α-tocopherol to inhibit lipid peroxidation in cell membranes due to high levels of long-chain PUFAs. This lipid emulsion, besides being a source of energy and essential fatty acids, also has a beneficial effect in reducing inflammation and modulating the immune system, given its balanced level of ω-6 and ω-3 fatty acids (16). With a lower proportion of PUFAs, the olive oil-based lipid emulsion is well tolerated in premature neonates, and may represent a promising alternative to parenteral nutrition in this patient group (42). Nevertheless, the benefit of these new lipid emulsions has yet to be proven in terms of clinical outcome.

Children in metabolic stress have increased serum levels of triglycerides, fatty acids, and glycerol due to increased lipolysis. Elevated concentrations of plasma triglycerides (>200 mg/dL) saturate the lipoprotein lipase system, resulting in clearance through phagocytosis by the liver's endothelial-reticular system and the lungs and possible depression in immunologic function. The immunosuppressive effect of lipid emulsions has yet to be established, as further evidence is needed from in vivo studies.

Infusion of lipid emulsions in high doses has been reported to impair function and hemodynamics, with inflammatory changes, edema, and surfactant alterations in adults with acute lung injury. Adverse effects depend on the mixture of lipid used, with MCT/LCT lipid emulsions causing fewer alterations in respiratory failure than LCT. Given that no studies have been reported in children, it is advisable to closely monitor lipid intake during the acute phase of respiratory failure (30).

Particularities in Premature Neonates. In newborn infants who cannot receive sufficient enteral feeding, IV lipid emulsions should be started no later than on the third day of life, but may be started on the first day of life. Preterm infants who weigh <1000 g deserve special attention because of their limited tolerance to IV lipids. The use of lipid emulsions in newborns—particularly in the premature with sepsis, thrombocytopenia, respiratory discomfort, or jaundice—has been the subject of discussion regarding risk of adverse effects, such as impairment of oxygenation, reduced immunologic function, and increased levels of free bilirubin. Compared with older children, premature and low-weight newborn patients exhibit slower lipid clearance and lower lipoprotein lipase activity, likely due to immaturity of hepatic and reduced adipose tissue mass. The upper limit of triglyceride plasma concentration tolerated by the premature is not well known.

IV lipid infusion can reduce arterial P_{O_2} through the following mechanisms: (a) changes in ventilation:perfusion ratio through eicosanoid production, which alters vascular tone; vasodilation in little ventilated alveoli causes intrapulmonary shunt and hypoxemia; (b) the deposition of fat in the capillary-alveoli membrane. This effect is minimized by slowing the infusion of lipid emulsion over 20–24 hrs.

Hyperlipemia in the premature with jaundice increases the risk of kernicterus with free fatty acid molar:albumin ratio of greater than 6:1 as fatty acids compete with bilirubin for binding sites on albumin. Icteric premature newborns should be started on 0.5 g/kg/day doses, increasing after bilirubin levels fall or on determination of free fatty acid levels. No increase in fatty acid and free bilirubin concentrations have been seen following lipid intake of up to 3 g/kg/day. Liver function tests should be monitored when lipid emulsions are given. If evidence of progressive hepatic dysfunction or cholestasis is seen, a decrease in lipid administration should be considered, especially if other concurrent morbidities (e.g., sepsis, thrombocytopenia) are present. Lipids in amounts that supply at least the minimal essential fatty acid requirements are necessary to maintain normal platelet function. In patients with severe thrombocytopenia, lipid administration can activate mechanisms that contribute to platelet aggregation, reduced lifespan, and hemophagocytosis; serum triglyceride concentrations should be monitored and a reduction of parenteral lipid dosage considered (30).

Carnitine facilitates the transport of long-chain fatty acids through the mitochondrial membrane for later oxidation and energy production. Given the low serum and tissue levels of carnitine in newborns, its administration has been recommended in the presence of persistent hypertriglyceridemia or in infants who are exclusively on parenteral nutrition for >4 weeks. Nevertheless, no clear evidence exists regarding the benefits of carnitine supplementation in neonates who receive parenteral nutrition.

Points Warranting Attention.

- Infant diets should supply 30% of energy in lipid form, where 1%–2% of energy intake is derived from linoleic acid and 0.5% is derived from α-linolenic acid.
- Parenteral lipid intake should usually be limited to a maximum of 3–4 g/kg/day (0.13–0.17 g/kg/hr) in infants and 2–3 g/kg/day (0.08–0.13 g/kg/hr) in older children.
- In premature neonates, lipid emulsion should be started after 24 hrs of life at a dose of 0.5 g/day up to a maximum of 3 g/kg/day.
- Lipid emulsions should be administered over 24 hrs.
- Infusion of lipid emulsions as 3-in-1 solutions (protein, sugar, lipid in same container) is not recommended, particularly when calcium concentrations exceed 8.5 mEq/L, as the mixture is not complete and the stability of the emulsion may be impaired. Administration in the Y- or 3-route tap connection is also not recommended, as the mixture in low-caliber tubes is also incomplete.
- Heparin does not improve utilization of IV lipids and should not be given with lipid infusion on a routine basis, unless indicated for other reasons.
- Lipid emulsions should be protected by validated light-protected tubing during phototherapy to decrease the formation of hydroperoxides.

Amino Acids

Estimates of protein requirements should be made on an individual basis, as these may differ according to the child's age, clinical condition, intake of energy and other nutrients, and quality of the protein given. Protein needs using the parenteral route are lower than through the enteral route: 2.5–3.0 g/kg/day promotes nitrogen retention in newborns and in young infants. Emphasis is generally given to growth in planning protein intake, provided the patient is relatively metabolically stable. However, in hypercatabolic patients, protein intake aims to minimize the effects of nitrogen loss, partially offsetting protein catabolism, thereby calling for different amino acid needs. Increased protein intake does not lower catabolism, nor does it reverse the endocrine alterations that caused it; however, a positive nitrogen balance is needed to enable return to anabolism.

Parenteral protein needs also vary according to age. Recommended intakes are 2.5–3 g/kg/day for neonates, 2–2.5 g/kg/day for infants, 1–1.2 g/kg/day for older children, and 0.8–1 g/kg/day for adolescents. The proportion of protein as caloric source should represent 8%–15% of total energy intake, attaining 20% or more in hypercatabolic states.

Incorporation of protein depends on adequate intake of all essential and nonessential amino acids and intake of nitrogen to synthesize it; it also depends on the minimum quantity of nonprotein energy, equivalent to 25 kcal for every gram of amino acid. To promote anabolism, the nitrogen:nonprotein calorie ratio must lie between 1:150 and 1:250, or between 1:90 and 1:150 in hypercatabolism. One gram of protein provides 4 kcal; 1 g of protein corresponds to 0.16 g of nitrogen, or 1 g nitrogen is contained in 6.25 g of protein.

Parameters for monitoring of protein intake are levels of serum urea, ammonia, total protein, arterial blood gas, and nitrogen balance. Administration of excessive quantities of amino acids can lead to acidosis, respiratory discomfort, uremia, hyperammonemia, hepatic dysfunction, increased oxygen consumption, and cholestatic icterus.

Particularities in Premature Neonates. In premature neonates, the objective of artificial nutritional therapy is to mimic the intrauterine growth pattern for the gestational age. Usual amino acid intake in the postnatal period falls short of this goal and does not prevent proteolysis in premature neonates, resulting in a negative impact on growth and development in such children. At 26 weeks of pregnancy, the supply of amino acids by the placenta is 3.5 g/kg/day and the fetus incorporates 1.8–2.2 g of protein daily. Extremely premature infants who receive only glucose lose protein at ~1.2 g/kg for each day without amino acids, and this loss corresponds to 1%–2% of their endogenous protein stores (58). However, immaturity of hepatic and intestinal metabolism as well as renal function, place them at risk of toxicity through excessive protein intake. No consensus has been reached on the ideal amino acid intake for premature infants. To equilibrate nitrogen balance, the minimum intake would be 1.0–1.5 g/kg/day, while a positive balance has been achieved administering 2.5 g/kg/day. The maximum intake has not been determined but most likely lies between 3.0 and 4.0 g/kg/day. Despite the variations in solution compositions and quantities given, these studies highlight the advantage of early commencement of parenteral amino acid solution—within the first 24 hrs—in limiting catabolism and preserving endogenous reserves (56).

The majority of premature infants tolerate parenteral amino acid intake of 1.5–2.0 g/kg/day in the first day of life, sufficient to avoid protein catabolism. In premature infants who receive parenteral nutrition with solutions standardized for adults, immaturity of metabolic pathways may result in toxic concentrations of plasma amino acids, such as phenylalanine and methionine, along with deficiency in others such as cysteine, tyrosine, and taurine. Parenteral amino acid solutions for neonates have been developed to achieve an amino acid plasma profile akin to that obtained in children with normal growth who are breast-fed. No differences in nitrogen retention, growth, or the incidence of cholestasis are seen between infants who receive pediatric amino acid solutions and those who receive the standard solution. Pediatric solutions appear to be beneficial during the neonatal period in that they include taurine and contain greater amounts of semi-essential amino acids such as cysteine and tyrosine, along with lower quantities of phenylalanine and methionine. However, they are not fully suited for neonates and are even less fully suited for premature infants.

Results of a multicentered, randomized, double-masked, clinical trial performed on 721 infants showed that parenteral glutamine supplementation did not decrease mortality or the incidence of late-onset sepsis in extremely low-birthweight infants. No significant adverse events were observed with glutamine supplementation (59).

Clinical situations associated with hypercatabolism are monitored for specific amino acid deficits in which patients can benefit from selective administration of these. Under these conditions certain amino acids deemed nonessential may be considered *conditionally indispensable*. In this context, L-glutamine is the amino acid which has been most investigated.

Micronutrient Intake

Micronutrients act as cofactors in metabolic processes and in eliminating oxygen free radicals. Besides increasing utilization of micronutrients, disease may affect micronutrient metabolism through (a) reduced intestinal absorption; (b) loss of water-soluble micronutrients (diarrhea, tubes, fistula, dialysis) and increased utilization on the extreme end of the scale results in marked high losses in zinc, copper, and selenium; and (c) intracellular release and excretion in urine, especially zinc, sec-

ondary to increased tissue protein turnover, such as in skeletal muscle, which occurs in the acute-phase response (64).

Scant information is available regarding the needs, bioavailability, and efficacy of micronutrient supplementation during metabolic stress. Most recommendations tend to be based on the needs of stable children and do not pertain to disease (Tables 86.2 and 86.3).

Prior malnutrition, drug use, acute and chronic disease, surgery, trauma, and anabolism increase micronutrient requirements. Actual needs of each patient cannot be determined, and although formulas for IV use are generally adequate, some may be lacking in certain nutrients such as zinc and water-soluble

TABLE 86.3

DAILY VITAMIN REQUIREMENTS BY PARENTERAL ROUTE

Vitamin	Preterm infants (kg/body weight)	Children and full-term infants (total dose)
A (UI)	1640	2300
E (mg)	2.8	7
K (mcg)	80	200
D (UI)	160	400
C (mg)	25	80
Thiamin (mg)	0.35	1.2
Riboflavin (mg)	0.15	1.4
Pyridoxine (mg)	0.18	1.0
Niacin (mg)	6.8	17
Pantothenic acid (mg)	2.0	5
Biotin (mcg)	6.0	20
Folate (mcg)	56	140
B_{12} (mcg)	0.3	1.0
Vitamin K (mcg)	—	200
Carnitine (mg)	20	2–10 mg/kg/day

Adapted from Greene H.L., Hambidge K, Schanler R, et al. Guidelines for the use of vitamins, trace elements, calcium, magnesium and phosphorus in infants and children receiving total parenteral nutrition: Report of the Subcommittee on Clinical Practice Issues of the American Society for Clinical Nutrition. *Am J Clin Nutr* 1988;48: 1324–42.

TABLE 86.2

DAILY TRACE ELEMENT REQUIREMENTS BY PARENTERAL ROUTE

Element	Newborns (mcg/kg) Preterm	Full term	<5 years (mcg/kg)	Older children and adolescents
Zinc	400	300	100	2–5 mg
Copper	20	20	20	200–500 mcg
Selenium	2.0	2.0	2–3	30–40 mcg
Chromium	0.20	0.20	0.14–0.2	5–15 mcg
Manganese	1.0	1.0	2–10	50–150 mcg
Iodine	1.0	1.0	1.0	—

Adapted from Greene HL, Hambidge K, Schanler R, et al. Guidelines for the use of vitamins, trace elements, calcium, magnesium and phosphorus in infants and children receiving total parenteral nutrition: Report of the Subcommittee on Clinical Practice Issues of the American Society for Clinical Nutrition. *Am J Clin Nutr* 1988;48:1324–42.

vitamins. Additional intake is likely needed during the anabolic period following hypercatabolic states. In the absence of consensus on the supplementary quantities needed during stress, administration at levels normally recommended for IV use are indicated (28).

Enteral Nutrition

The enteral route is preferable, as it prevents intestinal atrophy and reduces infectious complications when compared with parenteral nutrition (35). Furthermore, as it is less expensive, its use provides a corresponding reduction in hospital costs (48). Most studies have shown that enteral nutrition in critically ill children is well tolerated and presents a minimal risk of complications. A historic cohort study that spanned a 12-year period found an increase in enteral feeding and a decrease in parenteral nutrition use promoted by an ongoing education program in nutrition support, chiefly when the nutrition-support team began to assume responsibility for the nutrition support. Those infants who received enteral nutrition for longer periods during hospitalization presented an 83% lower risk of death (31). Nevertheless, caution should be exercised to avoid overuse of the digestive route in critical patients; very liberal initial use in patients with mesenteric hypoperfusion may cause intestinal necrosis.

Enteral nutrition is indicated in the presence or risk of malnutrition, when the oral intake proves insufficient to prevent weight loss but when gastrointestinal tract use is viable. In this context, conditions that justify the enteral route include: prematurity, mechanical pulmonary ventilation, severe malnutrition, hypermetabolic states, and neurologic diseases. The best point in time at which to begin enteral nutrition is also a question of debate; although delay can be harmful, very early commencement in cases that evolve to mesenteric hypoperfusion may cause intestinal necrosis.

In patients with functional digestive tracts, enteral nutrition should be started within 24–48 hrs following admission. Parameters that indicate adequate intestinal function are presence of bowel sounds, absent abdominal distension or vomiting, and a small quantity of gastric residue. As measurement of blood perfusion from the digestive tract using gastric tonometry is not routinely performed, signs of adequate intestinal perfusion in the critical patient include stabilized vital signs, no continuous requirement for administration of fluid volume or vasoactive drugs, and a normalized acid-base balance and serum lactate. Enteral use is not advised when high doses of α-adrenergic drugs and neuromuscular blockers are used.

Enteral nutrition intolerance can be a sign of intestinal hypoperfusion due to a worsening clinical picture, which, together with the use of α-adrenergic agonists, indicates discontinuation of enteral nutrition. Those patients who do not tolerate sufficient feeding volume through the enteral route to meet their needs may benefit from a combination of parenteral and enteral nutrition.

Diets

Selection of the most suitable diet to meet the patient's needs requires knowledge of the formula composition, as well as of possible alterations in the physiologic processes of digestion absorption secondary to the disease. The following items should be considered regarding the patient: digestive and absorptive capacity of the gastrointestinal tract; specific nutritional needs, which differ depending on the patient's clinical picture; and the need for fluid or electrolyte restriction.

With regard to the formula, the degree of absorption is determined by the form and concentration of each nutrient (e.g., whole or hydrolyzed protein, lactose or glucose polymers). Severity and variability of disease dictate the metabolic and nutritional profile of each patient, with each case calling for a specific formulation. A number of diets for special situations, mainly formulated for adult use, have high osmolarity levels and excessive concentrations of electrolytes for pediatric age groups; therefore, these are not recommended for children, particularly young infants, owing to their inherent risk of diarrhea and hypertonic dehydration. The main pediatric enteral feeding formulas with their indications and contraindications are listed in **Table 86.4**.

Potential Renal Solute Load

The potential renal solute load (PRSL) is the quantity of endogenous or dietary solutes that must be excreted by urine if none is used in new tissue synthesis or excreted by extrarenal routes. It consists of nonmetabolizable dietary components, especially electrolytes, in excess of needs, and nitrogenous compounds that result from protein metabolism and can be expressed by the following formula:

$$PRSL = Na\ [mEq] + K\ [mEq] + Cl\ [mEq] + Pa\ [mEq] + protein\ [g]/0.175$$

where:

Na = sodium
Cl = chloride
K = potassium
Pa = available phosphorus.

The actual renal solute load (RSL) is PRSL minus the proportion of PRSL excreted by extrarenal routes and nutrients used for new tissue synthesis. Except in the presence of diarrhea, extrarenal losses are nominal and may be ignored. Thus, estimated RSL is calculated as follows:

$$RSL = PRSL - (0.9 \times daily\ weight\ gain\ in\ grams)$$

PRSL is an important consideration in maintaining water balance in the following circumstances: (a) during acute illness, when fluid intake is decreased, especially if the illness is accompanied by fever; (b) when a calorie-dense diet is fed; and (c) when environmental temperature is elevated; or (d) when renal concentrating ability is decreased, as in chronic renal disease and diabetes insipidus (26). An understanding of osmolarity is another key factor, as high-osmolarity formulas may cause diarrhea when administered through duodenal or jejunal routes. The American Academy of Pediatrics recommends that osmolarity of infant formulas for oral or intragastric administration be <460 mOsm/kg (3).

Infants

Maternal milk is indicated as the exclusive food source in infants up to 6 months of age. After 6 months, solid foods are introduced, and maternal milk is continued up to at least the age of 12 months or older. Contraindications of maternal milk are (a) maternal infections caused by passive microorganisms transmittable through maternal milk, a number of innate metabolism errors, or other conditions that cause intolerance to

TABLE 86.4

ENTERAL FEEDING: FORMULAS, INDICATIONS AND CONTRAINDICATIONS

Formula	Indications	Contraindications
Cow's milk–based formulas, iron-fortified	Healthy term infants	Cow's milk protein intolerance; lactose intolerance
Cow's milk–based, lactose-free formulas	Lactase deficiency/lactose intolerance	Cow's milk protein intolerance; galactosemia (enough galactose remains)
Cow's milk–based, low mineral/electrolyte formula	Hypocalcemia/hyperphosphatemia Renal disease	Cow's milk protein intolerance. Note: This is a low-iron formula; iron should be supplied from other sources
Cow's milk–based, high (86%) medium-chain-triglyceride formula	Severe fat malabsorption, chylothorax	Monitor for signs of essential fatty acid deficiency if used for prolonged periods.
Cow's milk–based follow-up formula	Older infants who are eating solid foods	No advantage over breast-feeding or standard infant formula for the first year of life (according to the American Academy of Pediatrics).
Soy-based formula (milk-free, lactose-free)	Galactosemia; hereditary or transient lactase deficiency; documented IgE-mediated allergy to cow's milk; vegetarian-based diet	Birth weight <800 g Prevention of colic or allergy Cow's milk protein-induced enterocolitis or enteropathy
Soy-based formula with fiber	Diarrhea	Constipation
Casein-hydrolysate formulas	Allergies; intact protein sensitivity	Note: Infants with severe cow's milk protein allergies may react to whey-protein hydrolysate formula
Amino acid-based	Malabsorption due to gastrointestinal or hepatobiliary disease and not responsive to hydrolyzed protein formulas	
Human milk fortifiers	Preterm/low-birthweight infants	Fortifiers are low in iron; additional iron should be supplied from other sources.
Preterm formulas	Preterm/low-birthweight infants	
Preterm discharge formulas	Former preterm/low-birthweight infants from hospital discharge through 9 months of age	

Adapted from ASPEN. Board of Directors and The Clinical Guidelines Task Force. Guidelines for the use of parenteral and enteral nutrition in adult and pediatric patients. *JPEN* 2002;26(1):97SA–128SA.

the components of human milk; (b) galactosemia or tyrosinemia; and (c) mother's exposure to foods, drugs, or environmental agents that, when excreted by human milk, can harm the infant (3). Infant formulas are recommended in situations where maternal breast-feeding is precluded. The caloric density of infant formulas is 0.67 kcal/mL, the same as human milk.

Cow's Milk-based Formulas. These fulfill the nutrient needs of healthy children when used exclusively up to the age of 4–6 months. Their main carbohydrate source, as in maternal milk, is lactose. Protein levels are generally 1.5 times that of maternal milk, and the ratio of whey protein to casein is 60:40, similar to human milk. The main whey protein in the formulas is β-lactoglobulin, whereas in human milk, it is α-lactoglobulin. In the preparation process, cow's milk is substituted with polyunsaturated vegetable fat, which improves digestibility and in-creases the concentration of essential fatty acids. Some amino acids, such as taurine are added, as well as micronutrients such as iron. Cow's milk formulas are indicated as a substitute or supplement for maternal milk in children whose mothers are not breast-feeding (or do not do so exclusively), as a substitute for maternal milk in children for whom breast-feeding is contraindicated, and as a supplement for breast-fed children with insufficient weight gain (3).

Soy Formulas. Soy formulas are indicated for children with cow's-milk protein or lactose intolerance. In term infants, soy formulas promote growth and bone mineralization to the same degree as cow's milk-based formulas. They are milk free and have sucrose and hydrolyzed starch carbohydrates. They contain minerals and vitamins in greater quantities than milk-based formulas to compensate for the presence of possible mineral absorption antagonists such as soy phytates (3).

Protein Hydrolysate Formulas. Protein hydrolysate formulas are processed by enzymatic hydrolysis of different protein sources, such as bovine casein/whey and soy, with the hydrolysate consisting of free amino acids, dipeptides, and tripeptides that do not require additional digestion. These formulas are lactose free, and their carbohydrate source is tapioca starch, corn syrup, or corn starch. Fats are provided by a blend of MCTs and LCTs in varying amounts.

Protein hydrolysates are recommended for children who are intolerant to whole-milk formulas because of decreased intestinal length, absorptive capacity, or pancreatic or hepatobiliary diseases (3). These formulas might be considered during the systemic inflammatory response, when alterations in permeability and reduction of the absorptive surface of the intestinal epithelium take place (37). No pediatric studies are available that compare whole diets (breast milk, cow formula, or soy formula) with partially digested formulas in relation to ICU prognoses. The studies that do exist were conducted in heterogenous adult groups and show no evidence of major favorable clinical outcome associated with their use, but they do not take into account the nutritional status of the patients, which represents an important factor for increased intestinal permeability (10).

Amino acid-based formulas are indicated for patients who have protein hypersensitivity unresponsive to hydrolyzed protein formulas.

Immune-enhancing Formulas. Studies have demonstrated immunostimulating properties of nutrients, such as glutamine, arginine, ω-3 chain fatty acids, probiotics, nucleic acids, and antioxidants, used in conjunction or separately in critically ill patients. Given the higher cost of these diets, both safety and cost benefits have been considered in a few studies. Review of these studies reveals conflicting results. Although immunonutrition may reduce the rate of infectious complications in trauma and perioperative adult patients, a clear position on its effectiveness has yet to be established. The only study that demonstrates decreased mortality associated with immunonutrition was not a blinded study, and the treatment benefit of immunonutrition was only evident in the least sick patients; on the other hand, the possibility that immunonutrition may be harmful to some groups of critically ill patients is apparent from the results of some randomized trials on adult patients (9,36). In these studies, deaths were higher in patients who were given enteral immunonutrition than in those who received standard nutrition. It has been suggested that overstimulation of the inflammatory response by an immune-enhancing diet can be harmful for the critically ill.

In the only randomized, controlled trial that examined the effect of an immune-enhancing formula in pediatric patients, beneficial effects on laboratory nutritional indices and a trend toward improving colonization rates were reported, but no effect on mortality and length of stay was observed for the immunonutrition group (11). Given the potential risk of harm reported in some groups of patients, especially those with severe sepsis, and the fact that these formulas have not been designed according to pediatric standards, their recommendation seems to be premature in critically ill children (46).

Nutrition for Premature Newborns

In feeding premature infants, it should be considered that immaturity of the digestive function and increased growth rate together with limited energy reserves make this group partic-

ularly sensitive to overfeeding. Nutrition through enteral tube feeding using expressed breast milk taken from the mother of the premature infant has obvious benefits over artificial formula use, as it is associated with lower risk of necrotizing enteritis and death (61). The use of supplements to maternal milk has been recommended in very-low-weight, premature newborns because they offer increased calcium, phosphorus, proteins, and calorie content and allow for greater weight gain.

Formula for Preterm Infants. When use of maternal breast milk is not possible, a special formula for preterm newborns may be used. These formulas have added nutrients but lack the digestion facilitators and protective factors present in maternal milk.

Low duodenal lipase and biliary acid activity in premature neonates reduce absorption of fats ingested to 65%–70%. In this respect, maternal milk is particularly advantageous because it contains its own lipase, which aids triglyceride digestion. MCTs are added to formulas for premature infants in an attempt to reverse the tendency of poor fat absorption. To compensate for lower carbohydrate absorption and digestion that results from lactase deficiency, these formulas, in addition to lactose, also contain additional glucose polymer, given that active transport of monosaccharides by intestinal mucous is present in premature infants.

Premature infants, due to their needs for higher quantities of protein and owing to their limited metabolizing capacity, run the risk of developing uremia, metabolic acidosis, and neurologic disturbances if protein intake exceeds metabolic capacity. Formulas for premature infants contain greater protein levels (up to 3 g/100 kcal) and higher amounts of cysteine, as premature infants who are enzymatically immature cannot properly convert methionine into cysteine, making this amino acid conditionally essential in this situation. Calcium, phosphorus, and vitamin D are also present in greater concentrations in these formulas, allowing for higher bone incorporation and rates of bone mineralization similar to those in intra-uterine life. Due to their raised concentrations of protein and minerals, these formulas exert a higher renal solute load than formulas for term newborns.

Formulas developed for premature infants yield higher calorie (0.81 kcal/mL), protein, vitamin, and mineral levels, along with lower lactose levels than formulas for term children. Use of these formulas in indicated up to the postnatal age of 9 months.

Children Aged 1 to 10 Years

At an energy density of 1 kcal/mL, formulas for children aged 1–10 years vary in osmolarity from 300 to 650 mOsm/L and are lactose free. Vitamin and trace elements can be met with a total intake of 950–2000 mL. Patients with fluid restriction may require vitamin and trace element supplementation. Isotonic formulas are preferred for pediatric patients because they allow transpyloric tube feeding.

Children Older than 10 Years

Children over the age of 10 years can be fed adult formulas. These formulas are not suitable for young children because of the elevated renal solute load and inadequate vitamin levels. Children whose calorie and protein needs are elevated due to severe trauma or burn injury may receive high-nitrogen and high-calorie formulations (1.5 kcal/mL). Because of their elevated protein and electrolyte levels, the use of these formulas in children requires close monitoring of hydration status.

NUTRITIONAL AND METABOLIC MONITORING

Assessment of nutritional state identifies nutritional alterations, follows response to treatment, and should be an integral part of routine care for all children on nutritional support. Nutrient tolerance must be rigorously monitored to allow for replacement of losses and to recognize excessive substrate intake.

Anthropometric Assessment

Anthropometric measures are useful to assess nutritional alterations prior to hospital admission and to document long-term therapeutic effects, but they do not accurately reflect the acute nutritional alteration present under conditions of metabolic stress. Such alterations may be difficult to interpret in initial phases of illness due to water retention and loss of liquid and protein to the interstice, resulting from capillary permeability changes. Although hypercatabolism leads to reduced cellular mass, absolute expansion of intracellular liquid also occurs, causing weight loss to be underestimated. In fact, weight gain may have been brought on by liquid accumulation in the third space.

Considering the limitations in children who are admitted to the PICU, anthropometric measurements are vital to allow for an objective assessment, enabling the detection of malnutrition and aiding in the planning and monitoring of nutritional support throughout the hospital stay. Weight and height measurements should be set against a reference standard, preferably those by the National Center for Health Statistics of the Centers for Disease Control and Prevention or the World Health Organization, and weight-height charts should be employed as needed. On ascertaining weight, patients should be properly hydrated. Falsely increased weight levels due to fluid retention during the acute phase of severe infections or following resuscitation should be guarded against.

Laboratory Monitoring

Serum levels of electrolytes, urea, lactate, ammonia, proteins, arterial blood gas, glucose, triglycerides, and nitrogen balance are all parameters for monitoring.

Nitrogen Balance

Nitrogen balance is the difference between nitrogen intake and nitrogen excreted. It assesses the suitability of protein intake and degree of hypercatabolism. However, it is not an indicator of protein reserves, showing only metabolism and ingestion over 24 hrs. It can be expressed by the following formula:

$$\frac{\text{ingested protein (g/24 hrs)}}{6.25} - \frac{\text{urinary urea(g/24 hrs)}}{2.14} + 4^*$$

The Wilmore nomogram is used in younger children (75).

---

*estimated value of extraurinary nitrogen losses, used in adolescents and adults only.

This estimate must be made in the absence of diarrhea or abnormal losses. A 24-hr urinary volume is required. The aim is to obtain a positive nitrogen balance as a reflection of anabolism. If the balance proves negative, it could be due to insufficient protein ingestion; or hypercatabolism. Unmeasured losses (burns, renal disease, diarrhea, protein-losing enteropathy) can contribute to a negative nitrogen balance that is not reflected by the calculation.

Serum Proteins

It is not always possible to identify inflammatory response evolution in severely ill children through clinical means. Serial monitoring of proteins such as C-reactive protein in the acute phase may, by identifying return to anabolism, enable timely increase in nutritional supply, thereby avoiding the risks of overfeeding. Falls in serum C-reactive protein levels to <2 mg/dL can be interpreted as resolution of stress and return to anabolism, a change which is also reflected by increased serum levels of albumin and prealbumin (19). Serum levels of transport proteins can fall in response to metabolic stress or rise upon simple resolution of the process. In the presence of inflammation, their measurement is only valuable in conjunction with that of C-reactive protein, as this provides a reference parameter to assess the course of the inflammatory response (43).

C-reactive protein is an acute-phase reactant normally present in minute quantities in the blood of healthy individuals, increasing in concentration in several inflammatory states, and considered a good indicator of bacterial infection and postsurgical complications. It is synthesized in the liver in response to cytokine stimulation, mainly by IL-6. Serum levels increase 6–8 hrs following injury, peaking at 24–48 hrs. It has a short half-life (8–12 hrs) and, in the absence of complications, serum levels return to basal values within ~4 days.

Pro-calcitonin, with its half-life of 24 hrs is advantageous for its greater sensitivity in detecting sepsis and its more rapid elevation than C-reactive protein, although it is associated with a higher cost. Those proteins whose plasma concentrations drop below basal levels in response to inflammatory reaction are known as *acute-phase negative reactants*. Synthesis may be normal or reduced, but both catabolism and flow into extravascular space are increased. The principal proteins are albumin, prealbumin, apolipoprotein A1, retinol-binding protein, transferrin, and fibronectin.

Prealbumin, due to its short half-life and the fact that it is affected by malnutrition, is the most relevant protein as a plasma protein pool marker. It is synthesized by the liver and has a half-life of 2 days. Its serum concentration falls rapidly when calorie and protein intake is below normal but rises soon after the initiation of nutritional support; therefore, it is useful in detecting acute malnutrition. Although normally considered an indicator of nutritional state, it has been better employed in monitoring response to nutritional support in critically ill patients. In practice, interpreting its level during illness can prove difficult, as it may fall in response to metabolic stress or rise upon simple resolution of the process. Ideally, it should be assessed together with C-reactive protein to provide a reference parameter for the magnitude of inflammatory response.

Serum albumin, given its relatively long half-life and redistribution from the extravascular pool, may not accurately reflect protein-calorie malnutrition. Although malnutrition is an important factor in the regulation of albumin production, serum albumin concentration is influenced by various non-nutritional factors such as inflammation, infection, hepatic failure, and dilution from fluid overload, thus impairing its validity as a nutritional parameter in patients who have acute-phase response and metabolic stress. The transcapillary flow of plasma proteins secondary to endothelial lesion is the main underlying mechanism to explain hypoalbuminemia in critically ill patients. Its magnitude may be related to the severity of the metabolic response. In the initial stage of the inflammatory process, an increase in permeability of the microcirculation occurs, allowing greater transcapillary flow of plasma proteins (25). This event may be more important in the postoperative period of cardiac surgery because the contact of blood with the surface of cardiopulmonary bypass tubes may produce an endothelial lesion that, in turn, is a triggering factor of the systemic inflammatory response (72). Data in a pediatric study suggest that concentration of serum albumin may be associated with higher risks of mortality and postsurgical infection and longer periods of hospitalization following cardiac surgery (44). Thus, in critically ill patients, hypoalbuminemia is more indicative of the degree of metabolic stress than are alterations in nutritional state.

Plasma Triglyceride Concentrations

Triglyceride levels in serum or plasma should be monitored in patients who receive lipid emulsions, particularly in those with significant risk for hyperlipidemia (e.g., sepsis, trauma, liver or renal diseases, use of steroids, extremely low-birthweight infants). No data define the triglyceride level at which adverse effects may occur (66). In children with slightly elevated hypertriglyceridemia (175–225 mg/dL), steady increases in infusion rates are recommended. At moderately elevated concentrations (225–275 mg/dL), infusion rates should be reassessed without further increase until levels have normalized. At concentrations that exceed 400 mg/dL, it is recommended that infusion be halted for 12–24 hrs and then resumed at 0.02–0.04 g/kg/hr.

Glycemia

Acute stress and corticotherapy are conditions that require careful glucose monitoring. Hyperglycemia may trigger glycosuria with osmotic diuresis, hamper immunologic function and wound healing, and may possibly be associated with intracranial hemorrhage and a worsened neurologic prognosis in patients with cranioencephalic trauma. It has been demonstrated that tight control of glucose levels (between 80 and 110 mg/dL) using insulin reduced mortality among adults in the ICU (71). Peak blood glucose and duration of hyperglycemia were associated with increased mortality (67). However, in critically ill children, evidence suggests that glycemic control through insulin use is beneficial. Should hyperglycemia occur, the cause must be treated and the concentration or rate of glucose infusion must be reduced.

Measured Energy Expenditure

At present, the only accurate method by which to determine daily energy expenditure in the critical care setting is to measure it with indirect calorimetry, which allows the assessment of energy expenditure for adequate energy supply, monitoring of the volume of oxygen consumption during weaning from mechanical ventilation, and measurement of the respiratory quotient. Moreover, with indirect calorimetry, it is possible to determine the required type and amount of macronutrient substrates. However, it is important to be aware of methodologic pitfalls, when applying indirect calorimetry, to avoid potential inaccuracies (51). Only patients who are hemodynamically stable with an inspired F_{IO_2} of <0.6, no air leaks around the endotracheal tube, adequate sedation, no fever, and no anaerobic metabolism can be adequately measured. In the recovery phase of critical illness, the energy needed can increase to levels above the energy needs for normal, healthy children. Another aspect of energy measurement is the time required to measure the energy expenditure by indirect calorimetry. In a clinical setting, total daily energy expenditure is usually estimated with a 1–2-hr measurement, while energy expenditure can change throughout the day. When it is not possible to perform indirect calorimetry, energy expenditure can be calculated using a predictive formula (see Chapter 85).

COMPLICATIONS OF ENTERAL AND PARENTERAL NUTRITION

Complications of Total Parenteral Nutrition

Mechanical Complications

Mechanical complications may occur when administering total parenteral nutrition (TPN) immediately subsequent to catheter insertion and include pneumothorax, hemothorax, hematoma, and tracheal puncture. Other late complications are linked to catheter blockage, catheter migration, or to vein thrombosis.

Septic Complications

Septic complications may be exogenous in nature (extraluminal, with cutaneous microorganisms, and intraluminal, with microorganisms introduced within the vein) or endogenous, stemming from germ-contaminated intravascular catheters. Exogenous-type infections are the most frequent.

Sepsis in children who receive TPN is a serious risk that may lead to morbidity or death. Infections appear to be more commonplace in parenteral feeding via a central line, although such children are already predisposed to becoming more seriously ill and requiring prolonged parenteral nutrition. The propensity of infections is also linked to glucose overadministration (13,27), with hyperglycemia being an initial risk factor for infectious complications. A child is deemed infected following a shift to an unstable clinical (or metabolic) state, and/or the development of feeding intolerance.

Fluid and Electrolyte Complications

Fluid and electrolyte complications are also related to inadequate intake and/or to severity or instability of the underlying disease (cardiac insufficiency, renal failure, hepatic failure, sepsis or digestive changes, including vomiting, diarrhea, fistula), stemming from changes in the metabolism of sodium, potassium, phosphorus, calcium, and magnesium.

Hypernatremia (sodium >145 mmol/L) is associated with excessive sodium intake and consequent cellular dehydration. Hyponatremia (sodium <135 mmol/L) occurs with sodium depletion or water intoxication.

Hypokalemia may result from insufficient intake or increased losses of potassium (vomiting, diarrhea, digestive fistula, malnutrition). Treatment consists of increased potassium intake. Hyperkalemia is caused by excessive potassium intake coupled with low renal potassium excretion, and treatment consists of reduction in potassium intake and use of ion-exchange resins, diuretics (furosemide), and sodium bicarbonate.

Hypophosphatemia is the result of inadequate phosphorus intake or an increase in phosphorus intracellular shift and uptake during the anabolic protein phase. It represents a frequent complication in malnourished patients during the refeeding process. Treatment consists of increasing phosphorus intake. Osteopenia chiefly results from the inability to supply sufficient quantities of calcium and phosphorus to a patient with a limited volume intake through TPN. Conversely, hyperphosphatemia occurs owing to excessive intake.

Hypocalcemia occurs due to insufficient intake or excessive losses of calcium, or poor intestinal absorption, or it is concomitant with hypomagnesemia.

Osteopenia may occur in 30% of newborns who weigh <1500 g and undergo prolonged TPN without enteral feeding. Other children at risk include those with fluid or protein restrictions treated chronically with diuretics (6). Routine measurement of levels of calcium, phosphorus, and alkaline phosphatase is useful for detecting signs of metabolic bone disease. Generally, alkaline phosphatase serum levels are high and phosphorus levels are low in children with osteopenia. Calcium levels are typically maintained at the expense of bone reabsorption, although the presence of acute and chronic acid-base disturbances may influence this calcium level control. Treatment of hypocalcemia consists of increasing calcium intake and correcting associated fluid and electrolyte disturbances: metabolic or respiratory alkalosis, hypomagnesemia, and hyperkalemia, possibly using vitamin D.

Hypercalcemia occurs due to excessive calcium or vitamin D intake, immobilization, or insufficient intake of phosphates. Treatment involves reducing calcium and vitamin D intake, increasing urinary elimination of calcium, and correction of associated electrolyte disturbances, namely, hypokalemia and hyponatremia.

Hypomagnesemia occurs due to insufficient intake or excessive losses of magnesium (chronic diarrhea, digestive fistula or malnutrition). Hypermagnesemia may occur in the presence of renal insufficiency.

Hypoglycemia/Hyperglycemia

Hypoglycemia is one of the most serious TPN complications, given its neurologic consequences and the fact that premature newborns are high-risk patients due to their limited glycogen reserves. Hyperglycemia is a complication frequent in children who receive TPN and is caused by a drop in the patient's glucose tolerance (resistance to insulin or the presence of the counter-regulating hormones during stress: cortisol and glucagon). Hyperglycemia can provoke glycosuria with osmotic diuresis and dehydration, complicating fluid management. Hyperglycemia control is usually established by reducing glucose concentrations, although adequate supply of calories may be affected. The use of insulin is indicated only in children unresponsive to reduced glucose supply and who continue to present high levels (>145 mg/dL). When using insulin, it is vital to perform close monitoring of glucose and acid-base conditions.

Hyperlipemia

Intolerance to lipid use may occur in children who are preterm, septic, or malnourished; have hepatic or renal insufficiency;

or in those who are receiving steroids (63). The use of some medicines that contain lipids (e.g., propofol and amphotericin B) may contribute a sufficient quantity of energy in relation to total daily intake and may increase the possibility of hyperlipemia. Triglyceride levels must be measured 4 hrs following commencement of IV fat infusion or 4 hrs after any increased infusion rate, given that hypertriglyceridemia tends to occur within this time frame (66). High levels of triglycerides may also be attributed to carnitine deficiency, as premature newborns under 34 weeks have a limited stock of carnitine (50). Interpretation of data concerning IV fat infusion and pulmonary dysfunction is complicated, as adverse effects seem to depend on the dose, administration rate, and the presence of peroxides, and the clinical condition of the lungs. On rare occasions, IV fat infusion has been associated with thrombocytopenia.

Complications Related to Protein Intake

The safety margin for administration of amino acids is wide, having minimal likelihood of causing an impact on blood ammonia levels. However, ammonia levels in children who present with hepatic failure must be carefully monitored and controlled. Preterm newborns have lower levels of albumin, prealbumin, and retinol-binding protein than do full-term newborns (39). When the patient presents with normal renal function and hydration, monitoring blood urea nitrogen levels is adequate on a 3-g/kg/day intake of amino acids. Blood urea can be used as a marker for amino acid intolerance. It has been suggested that an increase in blood urea nitrogen levels is a direct reflection of increased quantities of amino acids being available and is evidence of efficient nitrogen use and retention (22).

Lack of Trace Elements

Patients on TPN at risk of iron deficiency include premature newborns, those with low or no enteral intake, and chiefly, those who present with poor absorption or fluid loss. Iron can be administered using oral, intramuscular, or parenteral routes for prophylaxis or treatment. Iron overload is linked to increased risk of sepsis in malnourished children who have low transferrin levels and is associated with increasing requirements for vitamin E (15).

Zinc deficiency is seen in patients with severe diarrhea, poor absorption, digestive fistula, and insufficient zinc intake present with characteristic cutaneous lesions (enteropathic acrodermatitis) (32). Low selenium can cause cardiomyopathy, whereas excessive intake leads to toxic manifestations, such as alopecia, headache, nausea, and garlic-like breath odor. Manganese is a frequent ingredient in parenteral nutrition solutions and is present in sufficient quantities to meet daily requirements; with long-term administration, it can lead to toxic symptoms from a build up. Manganese intoxication may provoke parkinsonian-like symptoms, with muscle weakness, stiffness, trembling, ataxia, asthenia, and speech difficulties (23).

Several parenteral component-nutrition solutions (albumin, heparin, calcium, phosphate salts) contain aluminium; any additional supply of aluminium raises risk of toxicity in children on TPN, owing to the element's tendency to become incorporated into body tissues.

Cholestasis

If prolonged TPN is predicted (>2 weeks), hepatic function tests should be performed, particularly in very-low-weight neonates, to obtain measurements that might suggest the likelihood of hepatic disease or cholestasis (22). Increased bilirubin and transaminase are late indicators of cholestasis. The earliest indicator, albeit nonspecific, is γ-glutamyl transpeptidase, and its specificity increases when it is used in conjunction with alkaline phosphatase (55). The etiopathogenesis of hepatopathy is multifactorial, and cholestasis-associated risk factors include absence of enteral feeding, immaturity, infection, hypoxia, excessive glucose and caloric intake, and toxicity of amino acids (such as methionine) or trace elements (including copper, chromium, and manganese). TPN light oxidation, medications, and deficit in nutrients such as taurine, choline, fatty acids, and minerals have all been associated with increased incidence of cholestasis (14).

The supply of at least some nutrition enterally is important, especially in children on TPN for long periods, as small quantities of food have trophic effects on the intestine, reduce bacterial translocation, improve gastric motility, and promote biliary flow (24). It has been suggested that TPN cycling for children on prolonged TPN may reduce continuous, nonphysiologic, hepatic stimulation and assist visceral protein synthesis (49).

Overfeeding Syndrome

Overfeeding syndrome occurs when TPN intake exceeds need, resulting in increased fat synthesis (66). Overfeeding is associated with fatty infiltration of the liver, hyperglycemia, hypertriglyceridemia, increased metabolic rate, and electrolyte disturbances (4). Furthermore, in cases with increased glucose and caloric intake, increases in oxygen uptake, in CO_2 production, and in CO_2 retention may be seen in children with pulmonary or cardiac insufficiency. Hypermetabolic and malnourished patients are more susceptible to these respiratory problems (65). Another potential complication of overfeeding with glucose is an increase in infectious complications, as hyperglycemia represents a risk factor for infection (41). To avoid overfeeding, nutritional status must be assessed and monitored to achieve a balanced supply of nutrient needs in accordance with the infant's clinical condition.

Complications of Enteral Nutrition

Enteral nutrition can present a number of practical difficulties. Initial delays are common, owing to reduced bowel motility (34), prescription of inadequate quantities of nutrients (53), and interruptions as a result of nursing interventions (2) or delayed gastric emptying.

The total aspirated gastric volume is considered a simple measure for assessing gastrointestinal motility in critically ill patients. Nevertheless, increased gastric residual volume may not accurately express low gastric emptying. A study in adult patients compared data on gastric residual volume with clinical and radiologic evidence of gastroparesis and found no correlation among the variables (52). High residual volume is not necessarily indicative of intolerance; conversely, low residual volume does not indicate tolerance. The main causes and examples of gastrointestinal intolerance are shown in Table 86.5.

Diarrhea

The general incidence of diarrhea in children in the PICU ranges from 35% to 63% (40,45), but in one pediatric study (12), the incidence was reported as only 5.6%. Diarrhea has been attributed to a series of factors such as food osmolarity, formula

TABLE 86.5

CAUSES OF GASTROINTESTINAL INTOLERANCE

Cause	Examples
Site and speed of nutrition delivery	High delivery speed, post-pyloric feeding
Diet type	Low fiber content, high-osmolarity
Drug-related	Laxatives, antibiotics, proton pump inhibitors, nonsteroidal anti-inflammatory drugs, medications that contain magnesium, antihypertensives
Infectious	Contaminated food, excessive bacterial growth in the small bowel, *Clostridium difficile*
Lactose deficiency	Primary and secondary
Poor fat absorption	Pancreatic dysfunction, hepatic disease, celiac disease

type, low serum albumin concentration, and medication interactions.

Some guidelines for enteral nutrition in hospitalized adults (68) note that simultaneous use of some medications, particularly antibiotics, is often the cause of diarrhea in enteral nutrition. These guidelines recommend reducing suppression of gastric acidity and providing interruption of feeding, thereby allowing pH to fall and helping to prevent excessive bacterial growth during enteral nutrition. It has also been suggested that, occasionally, alimentation-containing fibers may improve enteral nutrition-related diarrhea (68).

The most frequent mechanical, gastrointestinal, and metabolic complications, along with their probable causes and corresponding treatments are summarized in **Tables 86.6, 86.7, and 86.8**, respectively (8).

Interaction among Medications and Nutrients

Pharmacologic implications are associated with enteral nutrition and concomitant medication use, whether via tube feeding or other routes (29,54).

A number of medications are incompatible with enteral diets and may cause tube blockage when given in parallel. Thus, both the benefit and efficacy of the drug given may be affected. The most common example is phenytoin, which, upon continued use, causes deficiencies in folate, vitamin B_{12}, and calcium. Phenytoin also has a reduced absorption by 75% if administered simultaneously with food, leading to inconsistent blood levels. If use of the IV route is not possible, a 2-hr interval should be allowed between administration of this drug and infusion of the diet.

CONCLUSIONS AND FUTURE DIRECTIONS

Deeper knowledge of the physiopathology of metabolic stress, the application of new concepts in nutrition and metabolism (such as tighter control of hyperglycemia), and the deployment of multidisciplinary nutritional therapy teams within the hospital setting can bring about improvements in the quality of nutritional intervention. Furthermore, insights into how

TABLE 86.6

MECHANICAL COMPLICATIONS OF ENTERAL NUTRITION

Complication	Probable cause	Prevention
Tube blockage	Failure to regularly irrigate tube Medication administration via tube Fiber-rich diet	Flush tube with water after each diet infusion. Use medications in liquid form and flush tube with water following administration of medicines. Use a 10-caliber tube to infuse fiber-rich diets.
Pulmonary aspiration	Reduction in protective reflexes of airways, gastric atonia, ileum, badly placed tube	Choose post-pyloric route in patient with reduced level of consciousness or who is on mechanical ventilation. Infuse diet slowly with child in elevated decubitus position; monitor gastric residue.
Poor or shifted-tube position	Incorrect insertion technique Coughing or vomiting	Correct tube insertion technique; monitor position daily.
Accidental tube withdrawal	Agitated patient; inadequate affixation	Correct tube attachment; monitor constantly, sedate when necessary.

TABLE 86.7

GASTROINTESTINAL COMPLICATIONS OF ENTERAL NUTRITION

Complication	Probable cause	Prevention/treatment
Diarrhea	Overly fast infusion High-osmolarity diet Lactose intolerance Formula with high lipid level Food intolerance Medicines (metoclopramide, aminophylline, erythromycin, sorbitol, xylitol, magnesium, phosphorus) Change in intestinal flora due to antibiotic therapy Bacterial and diet contamination	↓ infusion speed. ↑ dilution or change of formula. Use lactose-free formula. ↓ level of fat in the diet. Use hydrolyzed protein formula. Do not use antidiuretics; consider vancomycin or metronidazole orally. Avoid medicine administration via tube. Aseptic preparation and administration technique; infusion flask must not remain exposed to ambient temperature for >8 hrs. Choose ready diets and closed infusion systems.
Abdominal distension	Use of antacids and antibiotics, overly fast infusion; hypertonic formula or with high fat level, narcotic use, ileum.	Consider suspending drugs ↓ flow or volume of infusion; consider formula change; review use of drugs causing gastric atonia.
Nausea and Vomiting	Multifactorial	↓ flow; consider change of formula; exclude infectious process.
Intestinal Obstipation	Diet poor in residues; dehydration	Consider fiber-rich diet; maintain adequate hydration.

TABLE 86.8

METABOLIC COMPLICATIONS OF ENTERAL NUTRITION

Complication	Probable cause	Prevention/treatment
Hyperglycemia	Metabolic stress	↓ infusion rate; monitor glycosuria and glycemia
Dehydration	High-osmolarity diets, inadequate liquid intake	Monitor electrolytes, urea, hematocrit ↓ protein intake ↑ liquid intake
Hypokalemia	Anabolism and intake shortage; losses through diarrhea, digestive juices, or diuretic use	Frequent monitoring of potassium
Hyperkalemia	Renal insufficiency; metabolic acidosis	↓ potassium intake, treat underlying cause
Hypernatremia	Hypertonic formulas; inadequate liquid intake	Consider formula change; ↑ liquid intake
Hypophosphatemia	Refeeding of the severely malnourished; use of antacids	Frequent monitoring of phosphate.
Hypercapnia	Hypercaloric diet with high level of carbohydrates in patients with respiratory insufficiency	↑ proportion of lipids as caloric source

the genotype of the individual influences response to nutrients can enable their efficacy to be assessed more accurately than at present. Nutrigenomics, a science that studies the interface among nutrients and cellular and genetic processes has the potential to make this kind of genotyping a reality. The variability in response to nutrients determined by genetic polymorphism can influence inflammatory mediator production. A field within enteral nutrition that is open to further investigation is that concerning how genetic polymorphism can affect the efficacy of the so-called immunomodulating diets. In practical terms, nutrigenomics emerges with the perspective that future nutritional support, in addition to taking into account nutritional state and individual needs, considers the standard genotypical response to nutrients, with the goal of preventing or curing diseases. Perfecting this science would likely result in lowering the rates of morbidity and mortality of severely malnourished patients who gain greatest benefit from nutritional intervention.

KEY POINTS

- Critically ill patients are at nutritional risk.
- Nutritional support strategies consist of avoiding substrate intake beyond that deemed essential and required to maintain metabolic homeostasis during the metabolic stress phase.
- Overfeeding or nutrient excess predisposes to increased respiratory quotient, risk of steatosis and hepatic cholestasis, and increased risk of infection.
- The digestive route is preferential when nutritional and metabolic monitoring should be frequent.
- Children who receive TPN have an increased risk of sepsis.
- Given that the neurologic consequences of hypoglycemia make it one of the most feared TPN complications. Hyperglycemia is a frequent complication in patients who receive TPN, close attention and monitoring of patient glycemia is of paramount importance to reduce risk of infection and dehydration.
- As early diagnosis of hepatic failure (cholestasis) improves outcome in patients receiving TPN, clinicians should be alert to its signs.
- Enteral nutrition complications can be mechanical, gastrointestinal, or metabolic; each has its own specific therapy.
- Neither low nor high residual volumes are reliable signs of gastrointestinal intolerance in enteral nutrition.
- Diarrhea incidence is variable, and its main causes are high osmolarity, formula type, low serum albumin concentration, and drug interactions.

References

1. ASPEN. Board of Directors and The Clinical Guidelines Task Force. Guidelines for the use of parenteral and enteral nutrition in adult and pediatric patients. *JPEN* 2002;26(1):97SA–128SA.
2. Adams S, Batson AS. Study of problems associated with the delivery of enteral feed in critically ill patients in five ICUs in the UK. *Intensive Care Med* 1997;23:261–6.
3. American Academy of Pediatrics. *Pediatric Nutrition Handbook, 5th ed.* 2003;55–97.
4. American Society of Enteral and Parenteral Nutrition Board of Directors: The Clinical Guidelines Task Force. Guidelines for the use of parenteral and enteral nutrition in adult and pediatric patients. *J Parenter Enteral Nutr* 2002;26 (Suppl 1):1SA–138SA.
5. Anand K. The stress response to surgical trauma: From physiological basis to therapeutic implications. *Prog Food Nutr Sci* 1986;10:67–132.
6. Anderson D. Nutritional assessment and therapeutic interventions for the preterm infant. *Clin Perinatol* 2002;29:313–26.
7. Ashworth A. Treatment of severe malnutrition. *J Pediatr Gastroenterol Nutr* 2001;32:516–8.
8. Baker S. Enteral Nutrition in Pediatrics. In: Rombeau JL, Rollandelli RH, eds. *Enteral and Tube Feeding.* Philadelphia: WB Saunders Co., 1997; 349–67.
9. Bertolini G, Iapichino G, Radrizzani D, et al. Early enteral immunonutrition in patients with severe sepsis: Results of an interim analysis of a randomized multicentre clinical trial. *Intensive Care Med* 2003;2:834–40.
10. Brewster DR, Manary MJ, Menzies IS, et al. Intestinal permeability in kwashiorkor. *Arch Dis Child* 1997;76:236–41.
11. Briassoulis G, Filippou O, Hatzi E, et al. Early enteral administration of immunonutrition in critically ill children: Results of a blinded randomized controlled clinical trial. *Nutrition* 2005; 21:700–807.
12. Briassoulis GC, Zavras NJ, Hartzis TD. Effectiveness and safety of early intragastric feeding in critically ill children. *Ped Crit Care Med* 2001;2: 113–21.
13. Bristrian B. Hyperglycemia and infection: Which is the chicken and which is the egg? *J Parenteral and Enteral Nutr* 2001;25(4):180–1.
14. Buchman A, Ament M, Sohel M, et al. Choline deficiency causes reversible hepatic abnormalities in patients receiving parenteral nutrition: Proof of human choline requirement: A placebo-controlled trial. *JPEN* 2001;25(5): 260–8.
15. Burns D, Mascioli E, Bistrian B. Parenteral iron dextran therapy: A review. *Nutrition* 1995;11:163–8.
16. Carpentier YA, Simoens C, Siderova V, et al. Recent developments in lipid emulsions: Relevance to intensive care. *Nutrition* 1997;13(Suppl):S73–8.
17. Cerra FB. Hypermetabolism, organ failure and metabolic support. *Surgery* 1987;101:1–13.
18. Chwals WJ. Metabolism and nutritional frontiers in pediatric surgical patients. *Pediatric Surg* 1992;72(6):1237–66.
19. Chwals WJ, Fernandez ME, Jamie AC, Charles BJ. Relationship of metabolic indexes to postoperative mortality in surgical infants. *J Pediatr Surg* 1993;28(6):819–22.
20. Chwals WJ. Overfeeding the critically ill child: Fact or fantasy? *New Horizons* 1994;2(2):147–55.
21. Correia MI, Waitzberg DL. The impact of malnutrition on morbidity, mortality, length of hospital stay and costs evaluated through a multivariate model analysis. *Clin Nutr* 2003;22:235–9.
22. Deme S, Poindexter B, Leitch C. Nutrition and metabolism in the high-risk neonate. Part 2;Parenteral Nutrition. In: Fanaroff A, Martin R, eds. *Neonatal-Perinatal Medicine*, 7th ed. St. Louis: Mosby, 2002;598–617.
23. Dickerson RN. Manganese intoxication and parenteral nutrition. *Nutrition* 2001;17:689–93.
24. Dunn L, Hutman S, Weiner, et al. Beneficial effects of early hypocaloric enteral feeding on neonatal gastrointestinal function: Preliminary report of a randomized trial. *J Pediatric* 1988;112:622–9.
25. Fleck A, Raines G, Hawker F, et al. Increased intravascular permeability: A major cause of hypoalbuminaemia in disease and injury. *Lancet* 1985; 1(8432):781–4.
26. Fomon SJ. Potential renal solute load: Considerations relating to complementary feedings of breastfed infants pediatrics. *Pediatrics* 2000;106(5 Suppl):1284.
27. Gore D, Chinkes D, Heggers J. Association of hyperglycemia with increased mortality after severe burn injury. *J Trauma* 2001;51(3):540–4.
28. Greene H. L, Hambidge K, Schanler R, et al. Guidelines for the use of vitamins, trace elements, calcium, magnesium and phosphorus in infants and children receiving total parenteral nutrition: Report of the Subcommittee on Clinical Practice Issues of the American Society for Clinical Nutrition. *Am J Clin Nutr* 1988;48:1324–42.
29. Guidelines for the use of parenteral and enteral nutrition in adult and pediatric patients. *JPEN* 2002;26:42SA–44SA.
30. Guidelines on paediatric parenteral nutrition. 4. Lipids. *J Ped Gastroenterol Nutr* 2005;41:S19–27.
31. Gurgueira GL, Leite HP, Taddei JA. Outcomes in a pediatric intensive care unit before and after the implementation of a nutrition support team. *JPEN* 2005;29:176–85.
32. Hardy G, Reilly C. Technical aspects of trace element supplementation. *Curr Opin Nutr Metab Care* 1999;2:277–85.
33. Heird WC, Driscoll JM Jr., Schullinger JN, et al. Intravenous alimentation in pediatric patients. *J Pediatr* 1972;80(3):351–72.
34. Heyland DK, Cook DJ, Winder B, et al. Enteral nutrition in the critically ill patient: A prospective survey. *Crit Care Med* 1995;23:1055–60.
35. Heyland DK, Dhaliwal R, Drover JW, et al. Canadian Critical Care Clinical Practice Guidelines Committee. Canadian Clinical Practice Guidelines for Nutrition Support in Mechanically Ventilated, Critically ill Adult Patients. *JPEN* 2003;27:355–73.

36. Heyland DK, Novak F, Drover J, et al. Should immunonutrition become routine in critically ill patients? *A systematic review of the evidence. JAMA* 2001;286:944–53.
37. Johnston JD, Harvey CJ, Mengies IS, et al. Gastrointestinal permeability and absorptive capacity in sepsis. *Crit Care Med* 1996;24:1144–9.
38. Jones MO, Pierro A Hammond P, et al. Glucose utilization in the surgical newborn infant receiving total parenteral nutrition. *J Pediatric Surg* 1993;28:1121–5.
39. Kanakoudi F, Drossou V, Tzimouli V. Serum concentration of 10 acute-phase proteins in healthy term and preterm infants from birth to 6 months. *Clin Chem* 1995;41:605–8.
40. Kelly TW, Patrick MR, Hillman KM. Study of diarrhea in critically ill patients. *Crit Care Med* 1983;11:7–9.
41. Khaodhiar L, McCowen K, Bistrian B. Perioperative hyperglycemia, infection or risk? *Curr Opin Clin Nutr Metab Care* 1999;2:79–82.
42. Koletzko B, Göbel Y, Engelsberger I, et al. Parenteral feeding of preterm infants with fat emulsions based on soybean and olive oils: Effects on plasma phospholipid fatty acids. *Clin Nutr* 1998;17(Suppl):25.
43. Leite HP, Fisberg M, Vieira JG, et al. The role of insulin-like growth factor I, growth hormone and plasma proteins in surgical outcome of children with congenital heart disease. *Ped Crit Care Med* 2001;2(1):29–35.
44. Leite HP, Fisberg M, Carvalho WB, et al. Serum albumin and clinical outcome in pediatric cardiac surgery. *Nutrition* 2005;21:553–8.
45. Leite HP, Grandini S, Carvalho WB. Nasoduodenal feeding of the critically ill child. *Rev Paul Med* 1992;110:124–30.
46. Leite HP, Iglesias SB. Are immune-enhancing diets safe for critically ill children? *Nutrition* 2006;22:579–80.
47. Leite HP, Isatugo MKI, Sawaki L, et al. Anthropometric nutritional assessment of critically ill hospitalized children. *Rev Paul Med* 1993;111:309–13.
48. Lucas C, Moreno M, Lopez-Herce J, et al. Transpyloric enteral nutrition reduces the complication rate and cost in the critically ill child. *J Pediatr Gastroenterol Nutr* 2000;30:176–81.
49. Maehan J, Georgeston K. Prevention of liver failure in parenteral nutrition-dependent children with short bowel syndrome. *J Paediatr Surg* 1997;32:473–5.
50. Magnussum G, Bobert M, Cederblad G, et al. Plasma and tissue of lipids, fatty acids and plasma carnitine in neonates receiving a new fat emulsion. *Acta Paediatr* 1997;86:638–44.
51. Martinez JL, Martinez-Romillo PD, Sebastian JD, et al. Predicted versus measured energy expenditure by continuous, online indirect calorimetry in ventilated, critically ill children during the early postinjury period. *Pediatr Crit Care Med* 2004;5:19–27.
52. McClave SA, Snider JL, Lowen CC, et al. Use of residual volume as a marker for enteral feeding intolerance: Prospective blinded comparison with physical examination and radiographic findings. *JPEN* 1992;16:99–105.
53. McClave SA, Sexton L, Spain DA et, al. Enteral tube feeding in the intensive care unit: Factors impeding adequate delivery. *Crit Care Med* 1999;27:1252–6.
54. Melnik G. Pharmacologic Aspects of Enteral Nutrition. In: Rombeau JL, Caldwell MD, eds. *Enteral and Tube Feeding.* Philadelphia: WB Saunders Company; 1990:614.
55. Nanji A, Anderson F. Sensitivity and specificity of liver function tests in detection of parenteral nutrition—associated cholestasis. *J Parenter Enteral Nutr* 1985;9:307–8.
56. Paisley J, Baron KA, Hay WW, et al. Safety and efficacy of low versus high parenteral amino acid intakes in extremely-low-birth-weight neonates (ELBW) immediately after birth. *Pediatr Res* 2000;47:293A.
57. Pereira-da Silva L, Virella D, Henriques G, et al. A simple equation to estimate the osmolarity of neonatal parenteral nutrition solutions. *JPEN* 2004;28:34–7.
58. Poindexter B. Protein needs of the preterm infant. Postgraduate course #5. Changing the Guidelines for Neonatal Nutrition. 25th ASPEN Congress, January 2001, Chicago, IL.
59. Poindexter BB, Ehrenkranz RA, Stoll BJ, et al. Parenteral glutamine supplementation does not reduce the risk of mortality or late-onset sepsis in extremely low birth weight infants. *Pediatrics* 2004;113(5):1209–15.
60. Pollack MM, Wiley JS, Kanter R, et al. Malnutrition in critically ill infants and children. *JPEN J Parenter Enteral Nutr* 982;6:20–4.
61. Schanler RJ. Suitability of human milk for the low-birthweight infant. *Clin Perinatol* 1995;22:207–22.
62. Seashore JH. Nutritional support of children in the intensive care unit. *Yale J Biol Med* 1984;57:111–34.
63. Sentipal-Walerius J, Dolberg S, Mimouni F. Effect of pulsed dexamethasone therapy on tolerance of intravenously administered lipids in extremely low birth weight infants. *J Pediatr* 1999;134:229–32.
64. Shenkin A, Alwood MC. Trace elements in adult intravenous nutrition. In Rombeau JL, Rolandelli RH, eds. *Clinical Nutrition Vol. II: Parenteral Nutrition, 3rd ed.* Philadelphia: WB Saunders Company, 2000.
65. Shulman R. New developments in total parenteral nutrition for children. *Curr Gastroenterol Rep* 2000;2:253–8.
66. Shulman RJ, Phillips S. Parenteral nutrition in infants and children. *J Pediatric Gastroenterol Nut* 2003;36:587–607.
67. Srinivasan V, Spinella PC, Drott HR, et al. Association of timing, duration, and intensity of hyperglycemia with intensive care unit mortality in critically ill children. *Pediatr Crit Care Med* 2004;5:329–36.
68. Stroud M, Duncan H, Nightingale J. Guidelines for enteral feeding in adult hospital patients. *Gut* 2003;52(Suppl VII):vii 1–vii 12.
69. Takashi T, Asanami S, Kubo S. Experimental infusion phlebitis: Tolerance osmolality of peripheral venous endothelial cells. *Nutrition* 1998;14:496–501.
70. Talbot FB. Basal Metabolism standards for children. *Am J Dis Child* 1938;55:455–9.
71. Van den Berghe G, Wouters PJ, Bouillon R, et al. Outcome benefit of intensive insulin therapy in the critically ill: Insulin dose versus glycemic control. *Crit Care Med* 2003;31:359–66.
72. Verrier ED, Boyle EM. Endothelial cell injury in cardiovascular surgery. *Ann Thorac Surg* 1996;62:915–22.
73. Waitzberg DL, Borges VC. Gorduras. In: Waitzberg DL, ed. *Nutrição Oral, Enteral, Parenteral na Prática Clínica, 3rd ed.* São Paulo: Atheneu, 2000;55–78.
74. Watters J.M, Wilmore DW. The metabolic responses to trauma and sepsis. In: Degroot LJ, Jameson JL. *Endocrinology.* Philadelphia: WB Saunders Co., 1989;2367–93.
75. Wilmore DW. The Metabolic Management of the Critically Ill. New York: Plenum Publishing Corporation, 1980;262.

CHAPTER 87 ■ THE ACUTE ABDOMEN

EDUARDO SCHNITZLER • TOMAS IÖLSTER • RICARDO D. RUSSO

The term *acute abdomen* is used to define a clinical syndrome characterized by signs and symptoms of an intra-abdominal disease that usually requires operative treatment. A diverse spectrum of diseases may produce similar signs and symptoms that culminate in abdominal pain. Accurate clinical assessment is essential to diagnose the underlying pathology and begin appropriate medical or surgical treatment (18).

EVALUATION OF THE EVIDENCE

Due to the paucity of medical evidence, most of the decisions related to the critical care management of children with acute abdomen are based mostly on consensus or expert opinion. Conversely, most of the published controlled clinical trials or prospective series are from the adult population, where etiology, complications, and clinical scenarios differ considerably from those found in pediatric intensive care.

The following evidence grading will be considered in this chapter:

Grade A—decisions based on systematic reviews, meta-analysis, or at least one randomized, controlled trial applicable to the adult critical patient (A−) or the pediatric critical patient (A+).

Grade B—evidence based on at least one cohort study or case control studies applicable to the adult critical patient (B−) or the pediatric critical patient (B+). Only recommendations based on this type of evidence (A or B) will be emphasized.

Grade C—remaining references will be those based on case series, consensus, or expert opinion.

CLINICAL ASSESSMENT

The clinical history and physical examination, essential for the diagnosis, together with laboratory tests and imaging studies, will determine the probable diagnosis and guide the initial management. Causes of acute abdomen are listed in **Table 87.1** and are divided into three diagnostic groups:

■ Primary abdominal pathology (caused in the gastrointestinal tract)
■ Abdominal pathology of the critical patient (secondary)
■ Abdominal manifestations in some systemic diseases that may present as acute abdomen

Four basic processes may provoke signs and symptoms of acute abdomen: infection or inflammation, obstruction, perforation, and ischemia. A fifth process, gastrointestinal hemorrhage, may be associated with acute abdomen, but this pathology is described in Chapter 90. Most patients with pri-

mary abdominal pathology do not require PICU admission, provided that diagnosis and treatment (usually surgical) occur promptly. However, if the child's abdominal pathology progresses to ischemia and perforation, severe disease will result and lead to perioperative PICU admission.

The critically ill patient may present with complications that compromise the function of the gastrointestinal tract, adding further critical illness. Intestinal ileus, acute cholecystitis, toxic megacolon, abdominal compartment syndrome, intra-abdominal collections, and tertiary peritonitis are some of the complications of critical illness that increase the patient's morbidity and mortality. These complications may cause progression to multiorgan failure and subsequent death.

Finally, diverse systemic diseases may present situations that generate or simulate an acute surgical abdomen. The history and clinical examination may be suggestive of a systemic disease that presents as an acute abdomen caused by direct or indirect lesions of the gastrointestinal tract.

The causative factor and the time that elapses from initiation of symptoms can explain the condition of the patient. A volvulus-associated bowel ischemia usually progresses quickly to a life-threatening situation. An acute appendicitis, if unrecognized or treated inappropriately, may lead to a critical condition. Any one of the situations assigned to the diagnostic groups (primary abdominal pathology, abdominal pathology of the critical patient, or abdominal compromise in systemic diseases) may necessitate admission to the PICU. Overlap among the three groups may occur. Hence, a strict classification or categorization is not intended. Rather, the goal of this chapter is to distinguish scenarios that allow a better guide to diagnosis and management.

Other diseases, such as pneumonia, gastroenteritis, hepatitis, renal colic, vertebral disk inflammation, pericarditis, and osteoarthritis, may present with abdominal symptoms and should be considered among the differential diagnosis of abdominal pain or acute abdomen in children.

INITIAL MANAGEMENT OF THE CHILD WITH AN ACUTE ABDOMEN

Primary Evaluation and Stabilization

One of the most important initial determinations to be made is whether the patient requires an urgent laparotomy or laparoscopy for diagnosis and treatment. The initial approach, as in any other emergency, includes a quick assessment of the severity of the condition and the potential dangers. Intra-abdominal catastrophe may be suspected based on a clinical examination. If the child is clinically unstable or if an intra-abdominal catastrophe is a possibility, prioritization must

TABLE 87.1

CAUSES OF ACUTE ABDOMEN

Primary abdominal pathology
  Mechanical obstruction
  Acute intestinal ischemia
  Infection/inflammation
  Hollow viscera perforation
  Abdominal trauma
  Diseases linked to the reproductive organs?

Abdominal pathology of the critical patient
  Gastrointestinal hemorrhage
  Ileus
  Acute pancreatitis
  Acute cholecystitis
  Enteritis: pseudomembranous colitis
  Toxic megacolon
  Abdominal compartment syndrome

Abdominal manifestations of systemic diseases
  Diabetic ketoacidosis
  Acute intermittent porphyria
  Henoch-Schönlein purpura
  Kawasaki disease
  Sickle cell crisis

include the establishment of an adequate airway, gas exchange, and circulation. The presence of ecchymoses with discoloration in the periumbilical region (Cullen sign) or a dirty green discoloration in both flanks (Turner sign) has been reported in severe cases of ruptured extrauterine pregnancy and acute pancreatitis, respectively. Other lesions, such as bowel ischemia or retroperitoneal hemorrhage, may have similar findings. The presence of severe abdominal distension or board-like rigidity and the degree of dehydration or the presence of shock will guide the initial resuscitation and will define the need for urgent surgical intervention (**Fig. 87.1**). Monitoring of pulse oximetry, heart rate, electrocardiogram, and noninvasive blood pressure is essential to guide therapy. Two peripheral venous catheters for vascular access should be established as quickly as possible, and blood and urine samples should be obtained for complete blood count, coagulation profile, chemistries, blood typing and crossmatching, blood cultures, and urine studies. Fluid boluses should be administered rapidly until appropriate perfusion has been established, and broad-spectrum IV antibiotic treatment should be initiated whenever sepsis is suspected. Early surgical review and initial imaging studies, such as abdominal x-ray or abdominal ultrasound, will guide the first therapeutic decisions.

If perforation, peritonitis, or ischemic bowel compromise is suspected, immediate surgical intervention is necessary. If the diagnosis is not clear, further options include an abdominal CT scan, an observation period, or an urgent diagnostic surgery (exploratory laparotomy). When bowel obstruction is suspected, initial management will depend on the probable cause and the presence of clinical signs compatible with

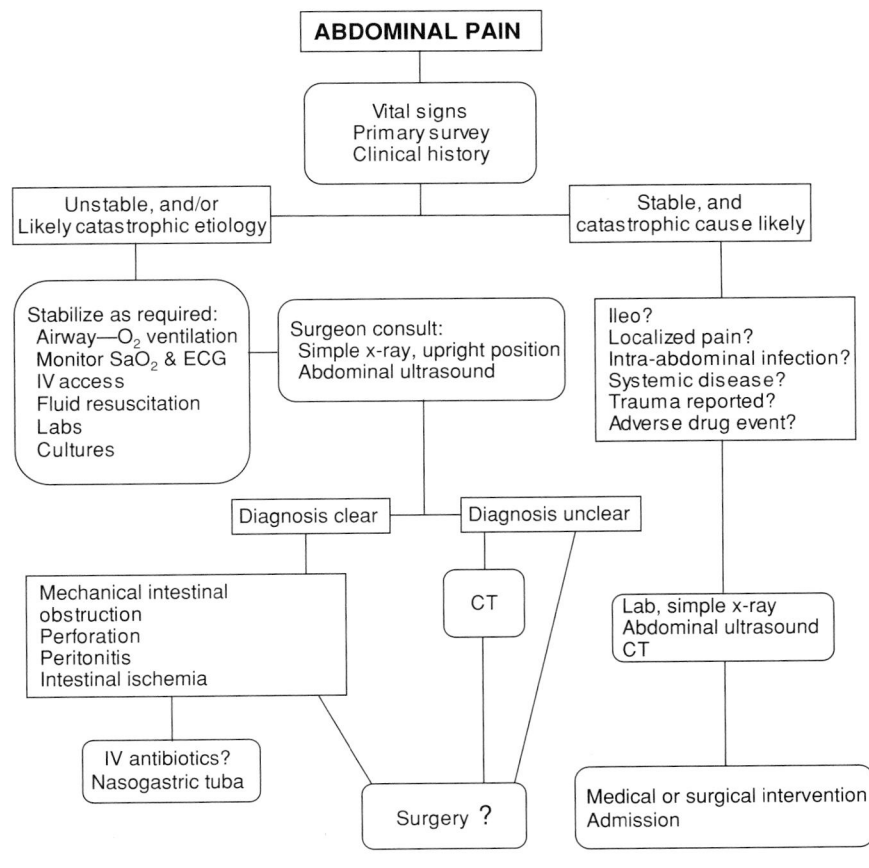

FIGURE 87.1. Initial approach to child with acute abdomen.

ischemia. In these patients, the placement of a nasogastric (NG) tube is mandatory.

History

As soon as the child is stable and intra-abdominal catastrophe is not suspected, a detailed history of the presenting signs and symptoms and sequence of events should be obtained. The presentation and sequence of such symptoms as fever, vomiting, diarrhea, constipation, urinary symptoms, and pelvic symptoms in female teenagers, are important for the diagnosis. When possible, localization and radiation of the pain should be determined. Taking an accurate history is essential for the diagnosis and should include previous medical pathologies, previous surgery, chronic drug therapy, recent trauma, and possibility of accidental ingestion of harmful substances in young children.

Physical Examination

Clinical examination of the abdomen should be thorough and systematic. Inspection may reveal significant findings, such as distension, masses, hernias, surgical scars, or other alterations in the skin. The presence of petechiae, purpura, or rash may be suggestive of a systemic disease. Auscultation should precede palpation to avoid modification of the peristalsis by external stimulation. Bowel sounds are typically altered during abdominal pathology. However, sometimes, findings may not be typical; they may be absent in mild diseases or may be present even during intra-abdominal catastrophes. Abdominal percussion helps to differentiate between gaseous distension (tympanic) and distension due to masses or ascites (dull). Abdominal palpation should be gentle, and the child's attention should be distracted. Palpation should be systematic, beginning with a superficial examination in the most distant quadrant from the site of maximum pain and moving slowly toward the painful area. The interexaminer reliability in physical examination of children with abdominal pain performed by emergency medicine physicians (residents and attendings) and the pediatric surgeon was studied (41). The investigators found less than moderate chance-adjusted agreement (κ range: -0.04 to 0.38) when comparing residents and attending physicians in the evaluation of the presence or absence of abdominal distension, tenderness to percussion, tenderness to abdominal palpation, guarding, rebound tenderness, and bowel sounds. Only the presence of rebound tenderness showed a moderate agreement ($\kappa = 0.54$) when attending physician and surgeon were compared. Because the reliability of the abdominal exam can vary, abdominal x-ray and/or ultrasound are almost always indicated when abdominal pathology is suspected but the diagnosis is not immediately obvious.

Examination of the inguinal and scrotal regions is essential to detect possible hernias or changes in the scrotal filling. Digital rectal examination should not be performed routinely in the evaluation of abdominal pain or acute abdomen. It can be useful for the evaluation of occult blood, local masses, rectal lesions, and peritoneal irritation. Pelvic examination is only indicated for adolescents whose pain is suggestive of gynecologic pathology. Pregnancy tests should be included as part of the laboratory examination for all adolescent females. In cases of suspected sexual abuse of prepubescent girls, the pelvic exam should be performed by very experienced gynecologists after the patient has been deeply sedated or anesthetized.

Once the cause of the acute abdomen has been established, it is necessary to consider its impact and possible complications. The repercussion of a specific diagnosis on a child will be modified by the time that elapses from the beginning of symptoms. Abdominal emergencies are dynamic and will change within hours. The child should be assessed frequently to rule out possible complications and define timely surgical intervention when necessary.

The critically ill child who is receiving mechanical ventilation is usually sedated and may be receiving muscle relaxants. In this situation, physical examination may not reflect the abdominal pathology, and a high degree of suspicion is essential. Clinical worsening, persistence of signs of infection or inflammation, increased nasogastric fluid losses, or persistence of ileus should be considered as possible markers of underlying abdominal pathology. Frequent clinical examination and serial imaging studies will indicate the need for more invasive procedures.

Diagnostic Imaging

The plain abdominal x-ray is useful for the diagnosis of bowel obstruction, renal lithiasis, pneumoperitoneum, and pneumatosis intestinalis (**Fig. 87.2**). In bowel obstruction, the distribution of air may show a few localized loops (sentinel loops) of small intestine and/or cecum, distended loops of small bowel

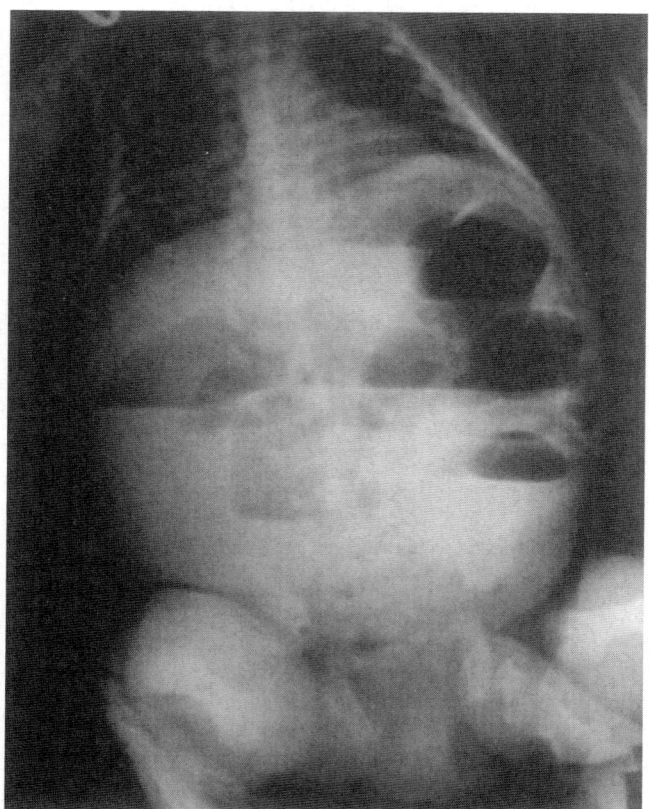

FIGURE 87.2. Paralytic ileus. Enteritis.

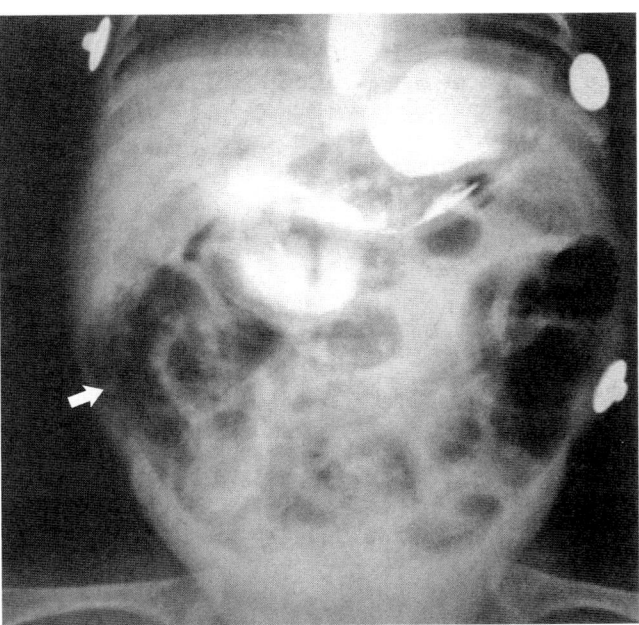

FIGURE 87.3. Abdominal x-ray film showing pneumatosis intestinalis (**arrow**). Image of double wall (**big bubble**).

in an organized, obstructive pattern, or in the upright view, numerous air-fluid levels. Sometimes, the finding of an opacity in the upper abdomen that obscures the caudal border of the liver may help to confirm the diagnosis of intussusception. Conversely, the presence of air or opacities suggestive of feces in the cecum may help to exclude a diagnosis of intestinal pathology, although specificity and sensitivity are low.

The diagnostic and prognostic significance of the presence of pneumatosis (air lining the bowel wall) (**Fig. 87.3**) after the neonatal period has been retrospectively analyzed, and the authors report 37 episodes during an 8-year period (19). The children in the study included those with a previous history of solid-organ or bone-marrow transplantation, congenital heart disease, malformation or pathology of the gastrointesti-

nal tract, or no significant previous pathology. The most frequent immediate precedent was noninfectious colitis (32%), followed by infectious or toxin-linked enteritis (27%), and intestinal ischemia (20%).

Abdominal ultrasound and CT scan are the two principal tools for the assessment of the child with abdominal emergencies. The best options depend on the suspected diagnosis (**Table 87.2**).

Many authors consider the abdominal ultrasound to be the preferred initial study of choice when intussusception is suspected, even though air or barium contrast studies of the colon have been considered the standard diagnostic tests for this diagnosis. Ultrasound has the advantage of a high diagnostic sensitivity (98%–100%) and specificity (88%–100%), with the absence of exposure to radiation and greater comfort for the child (37).

Ultrasound is also the preferred method with which to study the biliary duct, delineate abdominal masses, and distinguish appendix inflammation from other intra-abdominal or pelvic pathology. The diagnostic accuracy in cases of acute abdomen increases when ultrasound is added to the clinical exam and plain abdominal x-ray. Furthermore, ultrasound decreases the need for exploratory laparotomy because of an uncertain diagnosis.

The double-contrast CT scan helps to determine the size and location of an intra-abdominal mass and its relation to other organs, and it is useful to study the cause of an intestinal obstruction and to evaluate pancreatic, retroperitoneal, and pelvic pathology. Compared to serial contrast radiography, the CT scan has a greater sensitivity and requires less time to establish the diagnosis (8). *Recommendation: Grade B–*.

One of the frequent concerns of the pediatric intensivist is how to manage analgesia during the diagnostic phase. The classic decision in adult and pediatric emergency medicine, based on expert opinion, has been to avoid giving analgesia to patients with abdominal pain before the surgeon's evaluation. A double-blinded, randomized, controlled trial evaluated if early morphine administration impeded the diagnosis of appendicitis in children >5 years of age who presented with acute abdominal pain and were thought by the pediatric emergency attending

TABLE 87.2

USEFULNESS OF ABDOMINAL ULTRASOUND (US) AND CT SCAN FOR THE EVALUATION OF ACUTE ABDOMINAL EMERGENCIES

	US sensitivity	US specificity	CT sensitivity	CT specificity
Appendicitis[a]	80%–92%	86%–98%	87%–100%	83%–97%
Intussusception[b]	98%–100%	88%–100%		
Acute pancreatitis[c]	25%–50%	35%	90%	78%
Acute cholecystitis	81%–92%	60%–96%	High	High
Acute small bowel obstruction			87.5%	100%
Bowel ischemia			82%	Unknown
Intra-abdominal abscess[d]	Moderate-High	High	High	High

[a]US can be useful when the diagnosis is in doubt. CT scan with double contrast is rarely justified.
[b]US is used as diagnostic tool and to guide air-contrast reduction.
[c]US is the most sensitive test for diagnosis of gallstones (biliary pancreatitis). CT is the gold standard for diagnosing pancreatic necrosis and for staging after first week (extent of necrosis) and follow-up in severe pancreatitis. CT scan can be helpful when the diagnosis is in doubt.
[d]US can detect abscess but is operator dependent. CT is the most useful radiologic tool, but the IV contrast and transport to the CT room are principal limitations.

physician to require a surgical consultation (13). The sample was small; however, no differences were observed between the groups in the diagnoses of appendicitis or perforated appendicitis or the number of children who underwent laparotomy. The authors concluded that morphine reduced the intensity of the abdominal pain without adversely affecting the diagnosis of appendicitis.

PRIMARY ABDOMINAL PATHOLOGY

Bowel Obstruction

Bowel obstruction is a mechanical blockage to the transit of the intestinal contents that may be either intrinsic (intraluminal or from the bowel wall) or due to extrinsic compression. The former may include obstruction secondary to *Ascaris lumbricoides* (still existent in developing countries) or intussusception, whereas causes of extrinsic compressions may include postsurgical adhesions or incarcerated hernia (**Table 87.3**). Prolonged complete bowel obstruction will usually cause plasma leakage into the extracellular space ("third spacing") and dehydration. It may also lead to intestinal ischemia due to distension, to systemic infections, and finally, to death.

Congenital causes of small-bowel obstruction include annular pancreas, malrotation-volvulus, malrotation-Ladd bands, Meckel diverticulum with volvulus or intussusception, inguinal hernia, and intestinal duplication. Duodenal or ileal atresias are congenital causes diagnosed during the newborn period. The most frequent causes of acquired obstructions are postsurgical adhesions and intussusception. Crohn disease may also be a cause of small bowel obstruction, with less-frequent causes including duodenal hematoma and superior mesenteric artery syndrome.

Congenital obstructions of the colon include Hirschsprung disease, pseudo-obstruction, volvulus, and colonic duplication.

In the immediate neonatal period, imperforate anus or colonic atresia may be diagnosed. As acquired causes, Crohn disease and toxic megacolon associated with ulcerative colitis deserve mention. In patients with cystic fibrosis, obstructive syndromes in the distal ileum or in the colon may be present.

The clinical presentation of bowel obstruction may include cramping abdominal pain, nausea, bilious vomiting, and absence of intestinal transit when the obstruction is complete. Diarrhea, sometimes bloody, may signal the onset of obstruction before intestinal transit ceases. Cramping abdominal pain changes to continuous pain once intestinal ischemia begins to develop. Typically, symptoms are more sudden, intense, and progressive than in ileus, where symptoms are less intense and have a slower progression. The patient with mechanical obstruction presents with severe pain and systemic signs, such as tachycardia, sweating, and occasionally, shock. Abdominal distension may be generalized when the obstruction is in the distal bowel, or it may be absent in proximal obstruction, such as duodenal or jejunal obstruction due to bowel malrotation. Bowel sounds are usually increased. External examination of the abdominal wall may reveal previous scars, implicating postsurgical adhesions as a possible cause of obstruction. Palpation may reveal the presence of intra-abdominal masses or hernias. Signs of peritoneal irritation, such as rebound tenderness or abdominal rigidity, are suggestive of ischemia and perforation. No clinical or laboratory findings can clearly predict the presence of intestinal ischemia during mechanical obstruction; clinical judgment by an experienced surgeon is essential in deciding the best moment for surgical intervention (**Table 87.4**).

Plain abdominal x-rays may reveal air-fluid levels in the small bowel, dilated small bowel, or colon loops, as well as intestinal wall edema or minimal intestinal gas distal to the obstruction. The upright or lateral position is necessary to visualize air-fluid levels (see **Fig. 87.2**). Abdominal CT scan is the study of choice to identify less clear causes of obstruction or to evaluate the presence of ischemia (32), although

---

TABLE 87.3

MECHANICAL OBSTRUCTION

Obstruction due to adhesions
Intussusception
Incarcerated hernia
Tumoral obstruction
Crohn disease
Duodenal hematoma
Obstruction due to *Ascaris lumbricoides*
Malrotation—midgut volvulus
Meckel diverticulum with volvulus or intussusception
Intestinal duplication
Annular pancreas
Duodenal or ileal atresia*
Hirschsprung disease
Toxic megacolon
Chronic intestinal pseudo-obstruction
Imperforate anus*
Colonic atresia*

*Diagnosis can be made in the immediate neonatal period.

TABLE 87.4

BOWEL OBSTRUCTION

Clinical presentation
  Sudden, intense, and progressive symptoms
  Cramping abdominal pain
  Nausea and bilious vomiting
  Diarrhea and enterorrhagia (onset)
  Bowel sound increased (onset)
  Absence of intestinal transit (complete obstruction)
  Continuous pain, peritoneal irritation (ischemia or perforation)
  Tachycardia, sweating, hypovolemia, shock
  Abdominal distension (in relation with level of obstruction)
  Increase nasogastric-tube output

Imaging
  Plain abdominal x-ray
  CT scan
  Bedside ultrasound (useful in diagnosis of intussusception)

Management
  Hydration
  Placement of nasogastric tube
  Evaluation of surgical resolution

most of the evidence is from adult studies. Unnecessary imaging studies should never delay exploratory laparotomy when an urgent indication is clear. Abdominal ultrasound is useful for the diagnosis of intussusception, and the presence of free fluid may suggest a collection secondary to bowel perforation. In the intensive care setting, when the child is ventilated and sedated, the diagnosis of mechanical obstruction may be difficult. Increased NG tube output and the absence of stool output may be key signs for the diagnosis of bowel obstruction. Presurgical insertion of an NG tube is useful to control vomiting, to measure fluid losses, and to control pain. However, the patient should be fully conscious, with intact airway-protective reflexes before any attempt is made to insert the NG tube. If these criteria cannot be satisfied, the airway should be secured first using a rapid-sequence intubation technique.

Surgical resolution of complete obstruction is a priority, and any delay will influence the outcome. An observational study in adults with surgically treated complete small-bowel obstruction found that patients who needed intestinal resection had waited a longer time from symptom onset to surgery (7). When surgery was performed within the first 24 hrs of symptom onset, risk of resection was 4%, whereas risk increased to 10%–14% during the next 96 hrs. In this same study, the authors also found that patients treated first with an NG tube waited longer between first examination and surgery (40.6 hrs vs. 10.2 hrs), but this was not associated with an increased risk of resection. Postponing surgery for >24 hrs in a complete obstruction increases the risk of ischemia and intestinal resection. The recommendation for expeditious surgery in the presence of persistent signs of obstruction or signs of ischemia is based on evidence grade B. *Recommendation: Grade B–.*

A frequent conundrum after surgical resolution of a bowel obstruction with or without anastomosis is the utility of routine NG-tube placement. A systematic review of the routine use of NG tubes after abdominal surgery was conducted in patients who had emergency or elective surgery (27). The patients who did not have an NG tube routinely inserted experienced an earlier return to bowel function and a similar rate of anastomotic leakage, as compared to the patients with routine NG-tube insertion. The conclusion is that routine postoperative NG decompression should be abandoned in favor of selective use in patients with abdominal distension or vomiting or in those at risk of aspiration; or if NG tube is used for other reasons, early removal should be considered. *Recommendation: Grade A–.*

Intussusception

Intussusception represents the most common cause of acute abdomen in infants and preschool children and usually presents within the first 2 years of life, with a peak incidence between 5 months and 9 months of age. It occurs when one segment of the intestine (proximal) is telescoped into the adjacent segment (distal). In most cases, no lead point can be identified, and these cases are regarded as idiopathic, possibly linked to swollen Peyer patches in the terminal ileum (>90% of cases). Lead points may be noted in children <3 months but are especially frequent in children >2 years (2%–8% of cases). Meckel diverticulum, mesenteric lymph nodes, intestinal polyps, hemangioma, mucosal hemorrhage, and lymphoma are all causes of lead points. The most frequent form of intussusception involves the ileocolic region, where the terminal ileum is telescoped into the colon. Less-frequent types of intussusception are ileoileal,

TABLE 87.5

INTUSSUSCEPTION

Clinical presentation
  Severe paroxysmal colicky pain*
  Emesis
  Normal or jelly (red) stools*
  Sausage shaped mass palpable*
  Progressive lethargy
  Late diagnosis (perforation, shock, sepsis)

Imaging
  Ultrasound

Management
  Nonsurgical reduction (when early diagnosis)—air or
    saline-solution enema with ultrasound or fluoroscopic
    guidance
  Surgical reduction or resection (when late diagnosis or lead
    point identified)

*Classic triad is present only in 30% of cases.

cecocolic, or combinations (e.g., ileoileocolic). Ileoileal intussusception may be present after abdominal surgery, usually within the first 5 days. During intussusception, mesenteric venous drainage of the intussusceptum is obstructed, resulting in increased volume of the segment, edema, and mucosal bleeding. The apex of the intussusception may extend and displace itself through the interior of the colon. When intussusception is resolved within the first 24 hrs, most cases do not present with ischemic compromise; however, after 24 hrs, the risk of severe ischemia and intestinal gangrene increases progressively.

The classic clinical picture occurs in a previously healthy infant who presents with severe paroxysmal colicky pain accompanied by drawing up of the legs and intense weeping. Initially, the child recovers between episodes; however, if the diagnosis is delayed, progressive lethargy occurs in most cases. Emesis is usually present, and normal stools may be present during the initial phase. Passage of (red) currant jelly stool or presence of blood on rectal examination may happen in the first 12 hrs but may also occur later. A slightly tender, sausage-shaped mass may be palpable in the subhepatic region of the abdomen (**Table 87.5**). However, the triad of colicky abdominal pain, red currant jelly stools (or hematochezia), and a palpable abdominal mass is present only in 30% of patients. Children with delayed diagnosis or perforation secondary to hydrostatic or pneumatic reduction will develop critical illness with compromised perfusion and sepsis. The initial diagnosis depends on clinical examination and may be confirmed by abdominal ultrasound. In the event that ultrasound is not available, other traditional diagnostic alternatives, include plain abdominal x-ray and contrast enema study, which combines the diagnostic and therapeutic procedures. Ultrasound may show a tubular mass in the longitudinal views or a doughnut or target sign in the transverse images. Other ultrasound findings include multiple hypoechoic and hyperechoic layers and a kidney-like appearance (pseudokidney) in the longitudinal view (**Fig. 87.4**). Although target and pseudokidney signs are the most frequent findings, they are not pathognomonic of intussusception (14). However, ultrasound is a very sensitive test for intussusception. If a competent ultrasonographer has ruled out intussusception

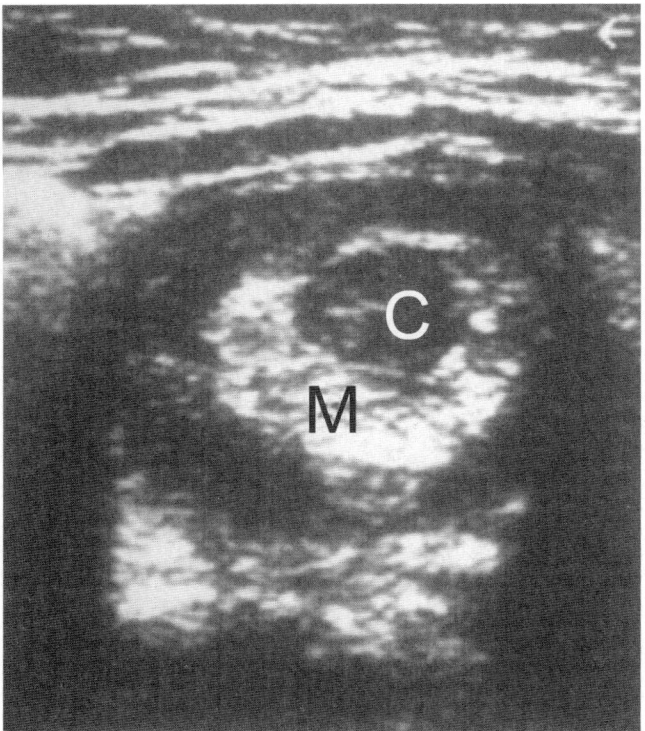

FIGURE 87.4. Ultrasonographic pattern of intussusception. **C,** central bowel; **M,** mesentery ("pseudokidney sign").

using ultrasound, no further imaging tests should be necessary to search for that diagnosis.

For nonsurgical reduction, the use of pneumatic enema or saline-solution enema under ultrasound guidance has a success rate of 70%–90% when performed within the first 48 hrs. Perforation rates during pneumatic reduction have been reported to occur in 0.1%–0.2% of cases. The two most widely used and recommended methods for reducing intussusception are pneumatic enema under fluoroscopic control and saline enema under ultrasound guidance (25). Barium enema may cause perforation and chemical peritonitis and is, therefore, contraindicated.

Nonsurgical reduction is contraindicated when symptoms have been present for >48 hrs or in the presence of shock, peritoneal irritation, perforation, pneumatosis, or ultrasound findings that predict failure of a nonsurgical intervention or are suggestive of the presence of a lead point. When nonsurgical reduction fails or is not possible, urgent laparotomy is the rule. The need for surgical reduction or bowel resection and the risk of complications are directly related to the time that elapses between onset of symptoms and laparotomy. Intussusception may recur within the first 6 months and is more frequent during the first day after reduction.

Peritoneal Adhesions

Fibrous adhesions following abdominal surgery are a frequent cause of bowel obstruction, representing as much as 33% of all cases. The reported incidence in children after abdominal surgery is 2%–3% and may be present as soon as 2 weeks after the procedure. Postsurgical adhesions may produce folding or strangling of the bowel loops or, less frequently, may

predispose to intestinal volvulus secondary to loop distension and peritoneal shortening. The presence of fever, leukocytosis, or peritoneal signs is suggestive of intestinal ischemia. Usual treatment includes NG-tube placement, hydration, and presurgical antibiotic therapy effective against gram-negative aerobic and anaerobic bacteria and enterococci. If ischemia is not associated with bowel obstruction from adhesions, spontaneous recovery without the need for surgery is possible.

Other Causes of Intestinal Obstruction

A child with incarcerated hernia presents with a sudden attack of irritability and refusal to eat. The hernia is obvious as a mass, protruding from the inguinal canal, that cannot be reduced. Once incarceration takes place, bowel ischemia will follow within a matter of hours. Ultrasound with color-flow Doppler will show decreased or absent blood flow to the incarcerated intestine. Urgent surgery is required for the incarcerated hernia.

Patients with Crohn disease may present with signs or symptoms of intestinal obstruction produced by the intestinal strictures that may affect the small bowel or the colon. The challenge in these patients is to determine if the symptoms are linked to chronic inflammatory disease and if they can be resolved by intensifying the treatment or if surgical intervention is necessary. The diagnosis is established with colonoscopy that shows patchy lesions and granulomas. Biopsies of these lesions should be obtained. Abdominal CT scan and MRI may help to identify transmural lesions and to exclude strictures.

Tumors usually present as abdominal masses and not as acute episodes of intestinal obstruction. Neuroblastomas originate in the suprarenal gland and are the most frequent abdominal tumors in infants, usually presenting as large abdominal masses. Rarely, the presence of intratumoral bleeding or intestinal compression may cause an acute abdomen. A Wilms tumor, due to its retroperitoneal origin, may grow significantly without compressing other structures. Lymphomas, the third most frequent tumor in children, are aggressive and diffuse tumors and may present with abdominal pain, vomiting, diarrhea, distension, and, occasionally, intussusception, peritonitis, or ascites. Less frequently, they present with intestinal occlusion or perforation (12).

Meckel diverticulum may cause bowel obstruction by acting as a lead point in intussusception or by causing internal hernias, loop volvulus, or formation of adhesions. More commonly, Meckel diverticulum is the cause of lower gastrointestinal bleeding (see Chapter 90).

Hirschsprung disease, or congenital aganglionic colon, is usually diagnosed during the neonatal period due to the presence of meconium ileus. However, in some cases, this sign may be absent and presentation may occur later with signs of acute enterocolitis, bowel obstruction, or sepsis. The enterocolitis is precipitated by bowel dilation, increased intraluminal pressure, compromise of the intestine blood flow, and alterations in the mucosal barrier added to the bacterial proliferation (38). The diagnosis is established by anorectal manometry and rectal mucosal biopsy. Colonic contrast study shows an area of transition between the colon that is proximal to the obstruction and the distal aganglionic, narrowed segment. Children with chronic intestinal pseudo-obstruction present with symptoms within the first months of life; these include abdominal distension, vomiting, chronic constipation, failure to thrive, diarrheal episodes, and abdominal pain. The diagnosis is usually suspected due to the absence of anatomical causes of obstruction. Diagnosis is confirmed by manometric studies and bowel biopsy, which should reveal muscular fiber involvement or compromise of the enteric nervous system.

Intestinal Ischemia

Bowel ischemia is the final common pathway of many different abdominal pathologies and may arise following progression of anatomical malformations, such as malrotation or intestinal volvulus. It may also develop after delayed management of abdominal pathology, such as intussusception, incarcerated hernia, or any other complete mechanical obstruction that has not been promptly resolved. Bowel ischemia during the postoperative period following repair of a coarctation of the aorta, although infrequent, has been clearly reported. Furthermore, intestinal mucosal ischemia may occur during or after cardiac surgery in children (see Chapter 70). Much less frequently, arterial mesenteric thrombosis and venous occlusive thrombosis are reported as causes of intestinal ischemia or gangrene in the pediatric population. Colonic ischemia may be secondary to such vasculitic processes as the hemolytic uremic syndrome (Table 87.6).

Patients with severe bowel ischemia progress from mucosal ischemia to transmural necrosis and bowel perforation. Combined sepsis and multiorgan failure are frequently present. In nonintubated, conscious children, the apparent lack of proportion between the referred pain and the clinical findings may be suggestive of the diagnosis. The presence of abdominal distension, severe hypovolemia and hemoconcentration, refractory metabolic acidosis, or hematochezia may lead to the diagnosis. During the initial phase in patients with no obvious surgical pathology, useful diagnostic tests include sigmoidoscopy, colonoscopy, and multidetector CT. Whenever signs of perforation are present, surgery must not be delayed.

Midgut volvulus secondary to malrotation of the bowel may cause one of the most severe forms of bowel ischemia in children. The mesenteric vessels and bowel are twisted and fixed in the volvulus, which leads to intestinal ischemia and necrosis (**Figs. 87.5** and **87.6**). This diagnosis should be suspected in infants and children with severe abdominal pain and bilious vomiting. A child admitted with intestinal ischemia or necrosis is usually in shock and may or may not present with abdominal distension (depending on the localization of the volvulus), and the abdominal wall may appear to be blue. Hematochezia is a late sign. The presence of diarrhea does not exclude the diagno-

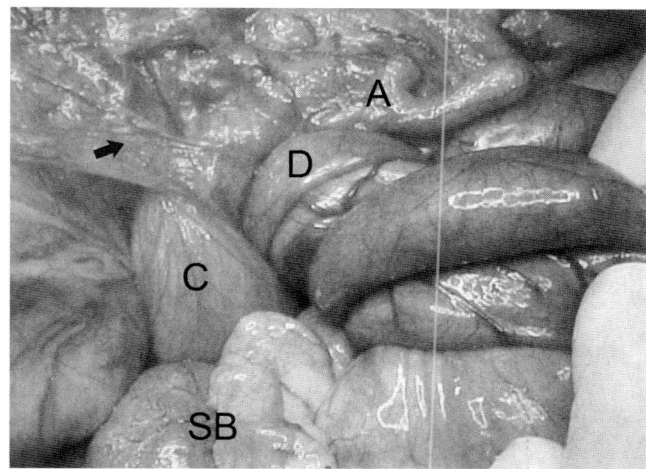

FIGURE 87.5. Operative photograph of midgut volvulus caused by a short mesenteric artery pedicle. **A,** appendix; **D,** duodenum; **C,** colon; **SB,** small bowel; **arrow,** peritoneal bands (Ladd).

sis. Occasionally, the disease may present with less-clear signs or even with a normal abdominal x-ray. The classic radiologic findings are the double-bubble sign (**Fig. 87.7**) that shows an abdomen with scarce intestinal air with two air bubbles, one in the stomach and one in the duodenum, air-fluid levels, abnormal position of the cecum, and absence of distal air. Although ultrasound or abdominal CT may yield the diagnosis, contrast studies under fluoroscopic control (upper gastrointestinal series) remain the diagnostic gold standard. Treatment is always surgical (26).

TABLE 87.6

INTESTINAL ISCHEMIA

Malrotation—midgut volvulus
Intussusception (late diagnosis)
Incarcerated hernia (late diagnosis)
Complete intestinal obstruction
Surgical repair of coarctation of the aorta
Postoperative of cardiac surgery
Arterial mesenteric thrombosis
Venous occlusive thrombosis
Hemolytic uremic syndrome

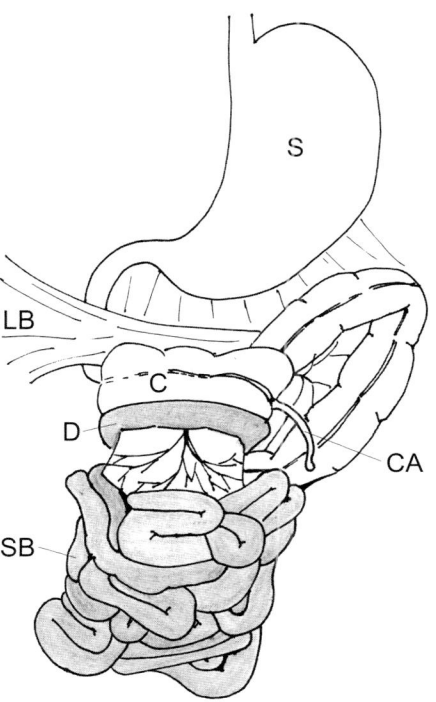

FIGURE 87.6. Volvulus. **S,** stomach; **LB,** Ladd bands; **C,** colon; **CA,** appendix; **D,** duodenum; **SB,** small bowel.

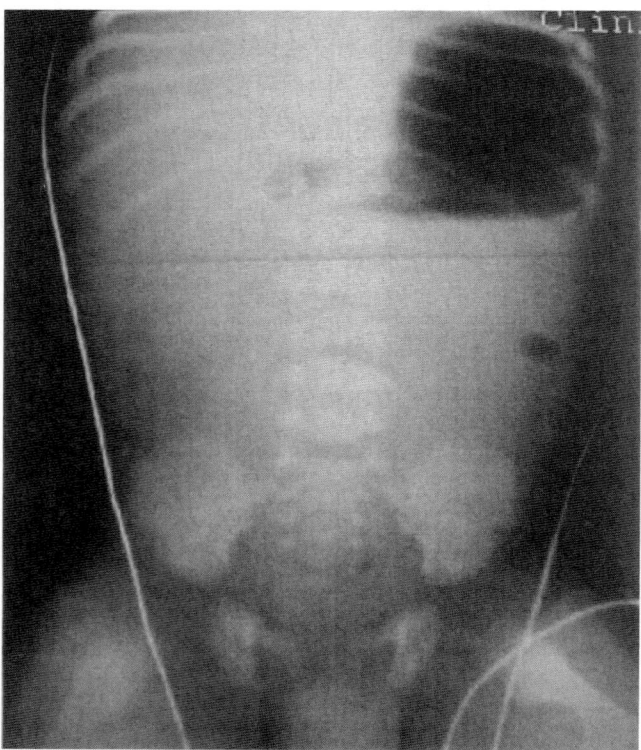

FIGURE 87.7. Abdominal x-ray showing a double bubble (stomach and duodenum) image.

TABLE 87.7

PERITONITIS AND INTRA-ABDOMINAL INFECTIONS

Peritonitis
  Primary peritonitis: no apparent intra-abdominal pathology
    Single organism
    Ascites (cirrhosis, portal hypertension, nephrotic
      syndrome)
    Associated with peritoneal dialysis
  Secondary peritonitis: associated with perforation of
    intestinal wall secondary to obstructive, ischemic, or
    inflammatory process
    Polymicrobial organisms
    Appendiceal perforation, bowel ischemia, Crohn disease
    Gangrenous cholecystitis, dehiscence in enteroanastomosis
  Tertiary peritonitis: peritonitis following failure of more
    than one surgical procedure undertaken to control an
    intra-abdominal focus of infection
    Nosocomial polymicrobial organisms and presence of
      facilitator material

Other intra-abdominal infections
  Intra-abdominal abscess: solid organ, inter-intestinal,
    periappendiceal, subhepatic, subphrenic, pelvic,
    peripancreatic, or retroperitoneal abscess
  Acute cholecystitis
  Fistulae: lateral or partial and complete or terminal
  Enteritis: invasive or cytotoxin-producing organism
  Hemolytic uremic syndrome
  Neutropenic enterocolitis or typhlitis

Peritonitis

Peritonitis is an inflammation of the peritoneal lining of the abdominal cavity that may result from an infectious, chemical, or peritoneal process. The perforation of the appendix is the most frequent cause. In young children, this diagnosis may be difficult or delayed until diffuse peritonitis is present. Primary peritonitis occurs when the source of infection is outside of the abdomen and reaches the peritoneal cavity via hematogenous or lymphatic dissemination. Secondary peritonitis originates from the rupture or extension of an intra-abdominal viscus or abscess (polymicrobial etiology). Other intra-abdominal infections are listed in **Table 87.7.**

Primary Peritonitis

Primary peritonitis is a rare peritoneal infection with no apparent intra-abdominal pathology, such as perforation, abscesses, or other intra-abdominal sources of infection. In previously healthy children, the history and signs are similar to peritonitis due to suspected appendix perforation, and the diagnosis is often intraoperative. Primary peritonitis is usually caused by a single organism, the most frequent being *Streptococcus pneumoniae*, group A streptococci, *Escherichia coli,* or other enteric bacteria. The presence of polymicrobial flora or anaerobes is an indicator of perforation and secondary peritonitis.

In children with ascites caused by cirrhosis, portal hypertension, or nephrotic syndrome, the diagnosis of primary peritonitis should be suspected and should be sought in the presence of fever, increased ascites, or a worsening clinical condition.

The most frequent causative agents are enterococcus, streptococcus, staphylococcus, or enteric bacteria (e.g., *E. coli* or *Klebsiella pneumoniae*).

In children with ascites caused by cirrhosis or nephrotic syndrome, the disease may have an insidious progression, and clinical findings may be similar to those found in children with ascites and without primary peritonitis. At other times, especially in patients with nephrotic syndrome, primary peritonitis may present with severe hypovolemic shock.

In children with ascites, diagnostic paracentesis should be undertaken whenever spontaneous peritonitis is suspected, and the presence of an ascitic fluid neutrophil count >250 cells/m^3 confirms the diagnosis. Gram-stain examination of the ascitic fluid has a low sensitivity, and culture may be negative in up to 50% of cases. Initial empiric antibiotic treatment includes ceftriaxone or cefotaxime in combination with aminoglycosides. The results of the culture's sensitivity will guide the definitive therapy.

The diagnosis of primary peritonitis should be suspected among patients receiving peritoneal dialysis in the presence of fever, local signs at the entry site of the cannula, or changes in the characteristics of the dialysate. Confirmed, probable, or possible diagnosis is defined by the presence of symptoms of peritoneal inflammation and >100 white cells/mcL (polymorphonuclear >50%) with or without organisms on Gram-stain or culture (34). The empiric antibiotic treatment depends on the predominant infections in each center. Some authors consider device-associated peritonitis within secondary peritonitis; however, it shares with primary peritonitis a similar clinical pattern and the attribute that a single species of bacteria causes the infection.

Secondary Peritonitis

Secondary peritonitis is produced by the entrance of bacteria into the peritoneal cavity through a perforation or rupture of the intestinal wall or other viscus as a consequence of an obstructive, ischemic, or inflammatory process. The rupture of an abscess into the peritoneal cavity is another mechanism. This process may develop in previously healthy children as a community-acquired infection, with the progression of appendicitis as the most frequent cause. Appendiceal perforation is more frequent in children than in adults, and an undeveloped omentum in children explains the low incidence of walled-off perforations. Complicated ischemic processes, including intussusception, midgut volvulus, or incarcerated hernias may be other causes. At other times, perforation may be the consequence of the progression of inflammatory diseases, such as Crohn disease, gangrenous cholecystitis, typhlitis, or peripancreatic abscesses. The dehiscence of sutures during the postoperative period of an enteroanastomosis or complications during the course of a traumatic intra-abdominal injury are the most frequent causes of peritonitis produced by nosocomial bacteria that colonize the gastrointestinal tract of hospitalized patients. In postpubertal females, such bacteria as *Neisseria gonorrhoeae* and *Chlamydia trachomatis* may invade the pelvic cavity through the fallopian tubes.

The clinical picture of secondary peritonitis includes high fever, diffuse abdominal pain, and vomiting. The physical findings consist of rebound tenderness, abdominal wall rigidity, and diminished or absent bowel sounds. Most children with peritonitis secondary to appendicular perforation improve with surgical treatment and antibiotic therapy and do not need admission to the PICU. However, a systemic inflammatory response may be severe, and children may develop third-space fluid losses, shock, or acute respiratory distress syndrome. Laboratory tests may show leukocytosis, and the upright abdominal x-ray may show free air in the abdominal cavity, ileus, and signs of obstruction or obliteration of the psoas shadow.

The critically ill child with an abdominal infection is seen frequently in the PICU; the seriousness of illness may be the consequence of the progression of inflammatory, infectious, or mechanical processes and, many times, may be exacerbated by diagnostic delays or delays during initial management.

These children may develop recurrent sepsis and multiorgan failure, with increased risk of mortality (see Chapter 21). Frequent surgical review is essential for determining the need for further diagnostic studies or surgery.

The defense mechanisms of the peritoneal cavity include the lymphatic system, peritoneal macrophage phagocytosis, and the formation of abscesses. The local inflammatory response and the formation of abscesses may impede a generalized peritoneal inflammation, and in a way, this process implies a localization and temporary control of the infection (4). Fluid accumulation caused by submesothelial edema may lead to significant third-spacing and cause hypovolemia. Basal membrane exposure due to inflammatory denudation of mesangial cells and the basal membrane's contact with platelets and fibrin contribute to the formation of the abscess wall and of adherences. Plasminogen activation contributes to peritoneum repair within 1 week. During ischemic or hypoxic conditions, the peritoneal cavity is invaded by fibroblasts and angiogenesis is stimulated, leading to formation of fibrous adhesions and bands.

As secondary peritonitis is caused by rupture of a hollow viscus, the typical microbiologic finding is polymicrobial flora.

The most frequent pathogens include enteric gram-negative bacteria (*E. coli*, *Klebsiella*, *Enterobacter*, etc.) and anaerobes (*Bacteroides fragilis*, *Clostridium* spp., and others) (31). The site of perforation determines the inoculum and type of bacteria. Most secondary peritonitis incidences are a consequence of appendicular inflammation and are caused by community pathogens. Therefore, these infections are usually sensitive to antibiotics that are effective against gram-negative and anaerobic bacteria. The recovery depends on an adequate and timely surgery and the addition of broad-spectrum antibiotic treatment. Ninety percent of children recover adequately and do not require admission to the PICU.

In patients with secondary generalized peritonitis, surgery is mandatory. The type of surgery performed will depend on the cause of the peritonitis and may include different strategies, such as repair and anastomosis in a single procedure or formation of an ileostomy or colostomy with or without anastomosis. Postponing the anastomosis for a later procedure should be considered in situations that involve a high risk of dehiscence, such as low blood flow or ischemia, severe peritoneal inflammation, or intestinal edema.

The peritoneal toilet strategy that includes a washout and irrigation of the peritoneal cavity during the operative procedure has not been proven to be effective and may have adverse effects (30). The efficacy of irrigating the peritoneal cavity with antibiotic solution is not fully supported by the literature. Experimental studies show that the irrigation may contribute to the dissemination of the infection and that bacteria adherent to the peritoneal serous membrane are not removed by low-pressure instillations. Peritoneal irrigation is not a proven method and is not free of risk. *Recommendation: Grade B–*.

Only 11% of adult patients with secondary peritonitis develop severe sepsis, but when this occurs, the risk of mortality is increased up to 19 times (1).

Tertiary Peritonitis

Tertiary peritonitis is defined by the appearance of peritonitis following the failure of one or more surgical procedure undertaken to control an intra-abdominal focus of infection. It is characterized by the presence of nosocomial polymicrobial flora, such as coagulase-negative *Staphylococcus*, *Candida*, *Enterococcus*, *Pseudomonas*, or *Enterobacter*. Many times, it is not possible to differentiate between a colonization of the peritoneal cavity by these pathogens and an invasive infection. These infections occur as a consequence of alterations in the peritoneal defense mechanisms, and the fluid collections may not be clearly purulent. The presence of any material in the peritoneal cavity facilitates local infection and the persistence of a septic focus. The most frequent facilitator is peritoneal blood; however, other frequent predisposing causes include fibrin, biliary salts, necrotic tissue, feces, or the remains of such material as nonabsorbable sutures, drains, gauze fibers, etc.

Intra-abdominal Abscesses

Solid-organ abscesses may be another cause of intra-abdominal infections, and may develop in abdominal viscera, such as liver, spleen, kidneys, pancreas, or uterine adnexa, as well as in the interintestinal, periappendiceal, subhepatic, pelvic, and retroperitoneal spaces. Intra-abdominal abscesses may be caused by community-acquired infections such as those secondary to appendicular infection, or they may be the consequence of complications related to surgical procedures. Periappendicular abscesses may present with prolonged fever, vomiting, deterioration of the patient's clinical condition, leukocytosis, pain in the right lower abdominal quadrant, or a palpable mass in the same area. A periappendicular infection may progress into the pelvis or toward the psoas. Pelvic abscesses may present symptoms such as rectal tenesmus or dysuria, and a rectal digital examination may be useful when this process is suspected.

In pediatric critical care, a clear history of the progression of the disease, of the surgical procedures, and of the probable or confirmed complications is essential for the diagnosis. The finding of more than one bacterial pathogen in blood cultures or the presence of sepsis without a clear source of infection should lead to suspicion of an intra-abdominal infection. Imaging studies may contribute to the diagnosis. A plain abdominal lateral x-ray may show pneumoperitoneum; however, this finding may also be present in patients who receive mechanical ventilation due to air leak from the lungs. Air-fluid levels due to intestinal obstruction may also be present. A chest x-ray may suggest the presence of subdiaphragmatic abscesses in the presence of infradiaphragmatic gas, basal segment collapse, elevated diaphragm, or pleural effusion. Bedside ultrasound helps to evaluate the biliary duct, but the visualization may be limited in the presence of ileus. Abdominal ultrasound is effective to guide percutaneous drainage of intra-abdominal fluid collections. The CT scan is the best diagnostic tool for intra-abdominal or pelvic infections, and the use of oral and IV contrast significantly improves the diagnostic sensitivity during this procedure (**Fig. 87.8**). CT scan allows a clear visualization of extraluminal air, free fluid, and changes in the homogeneity of solid organs, which is suggestive of the presence of an abscess. CT scan is also the best method by which to diagnose the cause of a mechanical intestinal obstruction. The visualization of the gallbladder wall and the intestinal wall may reveal inflammatory processes or mesenteric ischemia. Drawbacks of this study include transport of a critically ill child to the imaging department, the risks of IV contrast solutions, and radiation exposure. A thorough clinical examination of the surgical wounds and drain sites performed by an experienced surgeon, combined

with contrast studies through fistulous conduits, may add useful data. Laparoscopy and bedside mini-laparoscopy have been reported as ways to avoid laparotomies in adult patients.

The treatment of all patients with intra-abdominal sepsis includes respiratory and hemodynamic stabilization. Aggressive resuscitation, with fluid boluses and early use of vasoactive and inotropic drugs, has been shown to improve survival in patients with septic shock. The choice of initial empiric antibiotic therapy depends on the suspicion of a community-acquired or nosocomial infection. No antibiotic scheme has shown to be superior. In a systematic review of antibiotic regimens for secondary peritonitis of gastrointestinal origin in adults, the authors, after comparing 16 different regimens, all of which showed equivocal efficacy, concluded that no specific recommendations exist for the first-line antibiotic treatment in secondary peritonitis (40). The antibiotic regimen should be decided with consideration of local guidelines, preferences, ease of administration, costs, and availability. *Recommendation: Grade A−.*

A combination of an aminoglycoside (amikacin or gentamicin) or a third- or fourth-generation cephalosporin with an antianaerobic antimicrobial (clindamycin or metronidazole) is the most frequently used regimen for intra-abdominal abscesses (24). Single antibiotic regimens with imipenem, meropenem, or piperacillin-tazobactam have not been shown to be superior and are more expensive. Seven days of treatment are sufficient, provided that an appropriate resolution of the intra-abdominal focus has been achieved. Adequate focus control refers to the surgical removal or drainage of the primary cause. The source of infection should be identified with the help of the surgeon and the imaging studies. The elimination of abscesses, the debridement of devitalized tissue, and the removal of contaminants, in conjunction with the appropriate antibiotic treatment, allow resolution of the focus. Abscesses are considered to be at an intermediate point between the progression and the resolution of an infection. Even though the defense mechanisms of the child have controlled a dissemination of the infection, the process has not been resolved. Antibiotic treatment without drainage of the source may be effective only for small abscesses. For a well-circumscribed, accessible abscess that is not loculated, percutaneous drainage is the desired procedure, in conjunction with an adequate antibiotic treatment. A success rate of 85% for this technique is reported in adults. Percutaneous drainage may be the definitive solution, or it may buy time to stabilize the patient before definitive surgery.

Interloop abscesses and fluid collections may be recurrent or persistent sources of infections for which antibiotics have poor penetration. These collections are best treated by ultrasound- or CT-guided needle aspiration or with laparotomy. Possible complications related to failure to control the focus include local complications, such as abdominal wall infection, suture dehiscence, enteric fistulas, or recurrent or tertiary peritonitis. Systemic complications include recurrent sepsis, septic shock, and multiorgan failure.

Fistulae

Fistulae are abnormal epithelialized ducts that connect two hollow viscera or a hollow viscus with the skin. The intestinal wall defects may be partial (lateral fistulae) or complete (terminal fistulae). The presence of a distal obstruction transforms a lateral fistula into a functional terminal fistula. Fistulae may occur in the context of an intestinal operation and in the presence of

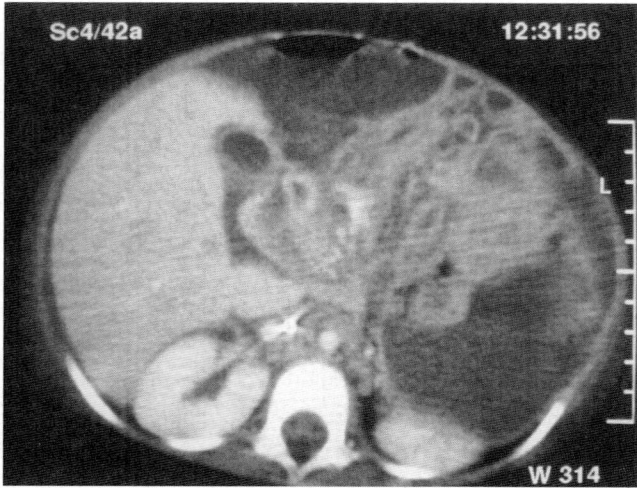

FIGURE 87.8. CT of intra-abdominal fluid collections.

an inflammatory process. During the development of a fistula and before it finally connects to the skin or to another viscus, the conduit may act as an occult source of infection. Fistulae may develop with an abscess in their tract, or they may develop without intraperitoneal collections. Fistulae tracts must be studied to find their origin, even though the clinical picture and recent history may suggest it. The best way to study the tract is by injecting water-soluble contrast material through a catheter that is introduced into the external opening and obtaining a sinogram (fistulogram). Very short fistulae that have a direct contact between the gastrointestinal tract and the skin are the most difficult to close (39). Abdominal and pelvic CT scans are important diagnostic tools for studying fistulae, especially because they may be associated with intra-abdominal infectious foci.

In high-output fistulae, close measurement and replacement of fluid losses and monitoring of electrolytes are essential to avoid severe derangements. The factors that influence the spontaneous closure include the child's nutritional status, the absence of a distal obstruction, and the absence of abscess cavities within the tract. General therapy includes antibiotic treatment until the resolution of the intra-abdominal infection, initial intestinal rest, care of the skin surrounding the external ostium, and parenteral nutritional support. Low-output distal fistulae may be adequately controlled with enteral feeding with elemental diets or partially digested formulae. Fifty percent of enterocutaneous fistulae close spontaneously within the first month. Octreotide or somatostatin can be used to decrease fistula output, but randomized, controlled studies in adults have not shown a significant increase in the spontaneous fistula closure rate when comparing these agents with placebo. When spontaneous closure is not achieved, surgical correction is indicated.

Enteritis

Enteritis is an intestinal infection that may mimic an acute abdomen. Intestinal infections may be caused by a wide variety of enteropathogenic organisms, including bacteria, viruses, and parasites. They often present with fever and such gastrointestinal symptoms as vomiting, bloody diarrhea, severe abdominal pain, and tenesmus. The process may progress to submucosal compromise and complete involvement of the intestinal wall, producing ileus, systemic bacterial migration, and sepsis. The finding of leukocytes in the feces indicates the presence of an invasive or cytotoxin-producing organism, such as *Salmonella*, *Shigella*, *Campylobacter jejuni*, enteroinvasive *E. coli*, *Clostridium difficile*, or *Yersinia enterocolitica*. The specific diagnosis requires culture of the organism and/or immunoassay for toxin. Enteric infections may produce bacteremia, sepsis, and extra-intestinal complications such as seizures (*Shigella*) and extra-intestinal foci of infection, including osteomyelitis, urinary tract infections, meningitis, peritonitis, or soft tissue infections.

Hemolytic Uremic Syndrome

In previously healthy hosts, the presence of bloody diarrhea caused by the verotoxin-producing *E. coli* 0157 may develop into hemolytic uremic syndrome (see Chapter 96). The diagno-

sis is confirmed by the growth of *E. coli* 0157 (or sometimes other serotypes) and the recovery of the verotoxin from the stool using immunoassay. The verotoxin is a Shiga-like toxin that consists of a protein with A and B subunits. The B subunit binds the protein to the cell wall of small-vessel endothelium (particularly in the gastrointestinal tract and the glomerulus). Once inside the cell, the A subunit inactivates ribosomal protein synthesis, which leads to cell death. Bloody diarrhea is usually the first sign of *E. coli* 0157 infection because the toxin is usually ingested with contaminated food.

In this disease, the classic triad that consists of microangiopathic hemolytic anemia, thrombocytopenia, and oliguria may be associated with severe complications of the gastrointestinal tract (mainly severe ischemic lesions in the colon). This complication frequently raises the dilemma of an acute surgical abdomen, which would complicate the placement of a peritoneal catheter for dialysis in a child with acute renal failure. The ischemic lesions may progress to perforation or total segmentary gangrene. Ischemic colitis as a part of the extrarenal involvement of the diarrhea associated with hemolytic uremic syndrome is a major determinant of morbidity and mortality (11).

Neutropenic Enterocolitis and Typhlitis

In children with oncologic diseases who are receiving chemotherapy or bone marrow transplant, the onset of abdominal pain and fever raises the possibility of neutropenic enterocolitis, or typhlitis (see Chapter 100). The presence of an intra-abdominal infectious process in these children, usually localized in the right lower quadrant, implies a therapeutic dilemma for which surgical treatment may engender infectious and hemorrhagic risks due to pancytopenia. Tenderness, presence of peritoneal signs, and absence of exaggerated bowel sounds are the most important clinical signs, but they may be blunted by neutropenia or corticosteroid treatment. The most frequent clinical diagnoses are acute appendicitis, paralytic ileus, and typhlitis. Neutropenic enterocolitis and typhlitis are gastrointestinal complications of chemotherapy that may be life-threatening. They are more frequent during treatment for lymphomas or leukemias and with the use of new chemotherapy drugs for the treatment of solid tumors, bone marrow transplantation conditioning, and immunosuppressive therapy for solid-organ transplants and acquired immunodeficiency syndrome. The term *typhlitis* specifically defines an inflammation of the cecum that may extend to the terminal portion of the ileum and the ascending colon. The pain may be localized in the right iliac fossa or may be diffuse with peritoneal reaction. Other symptoms that may be present include watery or bloody diarrhea, abdominal distension, and vomiting. Symptoms appear between 10 and 14 days after chemotherapy.

The plain abdominal x-ray may show signs compatible with obstruction, but the diagnosis is confirmed by ultrasound or CT scan, which may show a thickening of the walls of the cecum or other involved areas with mucous edema, fat or mesenteric infiltration, pneumatosis, hepatic portal venous gas, and free cavity fluid. Treatment includes broad-spectrum antibiotics, NG-tube drainage, intestinal rest, parenteral nutrition, and close observation. Platelets and red blood cells should be replaced as needed, and recombinant granulocyte colony-stimulating factor should be administered until normalization of the neutrophil count. Signs of perforation, persistent bleeding, or progressive worsening that require hemodynamic or respiratory support indicate the need for surgery. Mortality is high, has historically been reported to be in the range 50%–100%, and is associated with intestinal perforation and sepsis. It is probable that early recognition and the progress in management that are currently possible have contributed to decreased mortality.

Acute Pancreatitis

Inflammation of the pancreas can cause an acute abdomen and life-threatening disease when it is severe or in the presence of local complications, such as necrosis, pseudocysts, or pancreatic abscesses. These cases may develop systemic inflammatory manifestations or multiorgan failure. Approximately 50% of pediatric cases have no identifiable cause, and the remainder of cases are either obstructive (e.g., choledochal cysts, pancreatic duct stricture, or stones) or nonobstructive (e.g., trauma, hemorrhage, infection, or medications) in origin. Among cases of pancreatitis with identifiable causes, trauma, structural anomalies, and multisystemic diseases predominate. Hereditary forms of pancreatitis may arise from mutations in the trypsinogen gene and in the cystic fibrosis transmembrane regulator gene. Genetic assays can detect alterations and help to explain some cases of recurrent pancreatitis, previously categorized as idiopathic. Milder inflammations with only associated abdominal pain and moderate increases of the amylase and lipase levels are usually the consequence of viral infections and some systemic diseases.

The pathogenesis of pancreatitis is not clear. The classic explanation suggests that the inappropriate activation of the digestive proenzymes in the pancreatic glandular cells that is mediated by the lysosomal hydrolases is a consequence of ductal obstruction. A process of autodigestion of the pancreatic tissue is started with the participation of cathepsin, trypsin, phospholipase A2, and lecithin. An alternate explanation proposes a premature activation of the intracellular zymogens, the transcription of nuclear factor (NK)-κB and activator protein-1, and the consequent generation of cytokines and chemokines. This inflammatory cascade leads to a proinflammatory state that produces multiorgan failure and explains early mortality.

Pancreatitis is rare in the previously healthy child. The patient usually presents as acutely ill with nausea, vomiting, and abdominal pain (**Table 87.8**). The pain is usually epigastric and may radiate toward the back. Abdominal distension and muscular guarding are frequent features in children. The child is irritable and may adopt an antalgic position, such as sitting forward with flexed legs or lying in lateral decubitus position. Hemodynamic compromise, fever, jaundice, ascites, hypocalcemia, and pleural effusion may be present. Mortality is high and is linked to the systemic inflammatory response syndrome and multiorgan failure. The diagnosis should be considered in children with acute abdomen and/or systemic inflammatory response syndrome without a clear cause or in the presence of probable etiologic factors (e.g., lithiasic pathology). The diagnosis is confirmed by an increased serum amylase and lipase level of at least three times their normal value (>300 U/l and 900 U/l, respectively). Even though the lipase elevation is sensitive and more specific in adults, this has not been validated in pediatric patients. The enzyme levels diminish progressively

---

TABLE 87.8

SEVERE ACUTE PANCREATITIS

Types
  Obstructive (gallstone, choledochal cyst, pancreatic duct stricture)
  Nonobstructive (trauma, infection, drugs)
  Hereditary forms or idiopathics

Clinical presentation
  Abdominal pain, vomiting, abdominal distension, and guarding
  Systemic inflammatory response syndrome, shock, jaundice, ascites, and pleural effusion
  Labs: Amylase >300 U/L, lipase >900 U/L

Imaging
  Ultrasound to evaluate obstructive causes and pseudocysts control
  CT to confirm diagnosis and evaluation of necrotic areas
  ERCP for suspected or proved lithiasis acute pancreatitis

Treatment
  Fluid resuscitation
  Control of hypocalcemia or hyperglycemia
  Analgesics
  Nasogastric tube
  Nutrition: parenteral (initial) and enteral nutrition (when tolerated)
  Evaluation of antibiotic treatment
  Evaluation of percutaneous draining, fine needle aspiration or laparotomy to resolve the complications (pseudocysts, necrosis, abscess)

ERCP, endoscopic retrograde cholangiopancreatography

---

after the first days; therefore, the time elapsed since the beginning of symptoms will affect the sensitivity of enzyme concentrations as a diagnostic method. British guidelines recommend the use of the serum lipase level as the diagnostic test of choice due to its greater sensitivity and prolonged elevation of up to 2 weeks (36). Pancreatic enzymes may also be elevated in other situations, including perforated gastroduodenal ulcers, intestinal perforation or occlusion, peritonitis, acidosis, and renal failure.

Ultrasound and CT scan are the diagnostic studies that are used to confirm the diagnosis, evaluate the etiology, and search for complications of pancreatitis (**Fig. 87.9**). Ultrasound is helpful in locating gall stones in the pancreatic or common bile ducts. However, as its sensitivity is lower during acute pancreatitis, it is convenient to repeat the ultrasound during the course of the disease. When the pancreas can be visualized, the structural characteristics and the findings in the adjacent tissues contribute to the diagnosis and follow-up. Possible findings include increased size, peripancreatic fluid collections, structural heterogeneity, and abscesses. In 20% of pediatric cases, the initial ultrasound is normal. The plain abdominal x-ray film may reveal indirect signs, such as sentinel loop, ileus, blurring of the psoas, transverse colon dilation, or pancreatic calcification. The chest film may show basal infiltrates, diaphragmatic elevation, pleural effusion, or pulmonary edema. The CT scan is the most useful study to confirm the diagnosis and to exclude other causes of acute abdomen. The use of contrast allows the identification of necrotic areas. When contrast cannot be used,

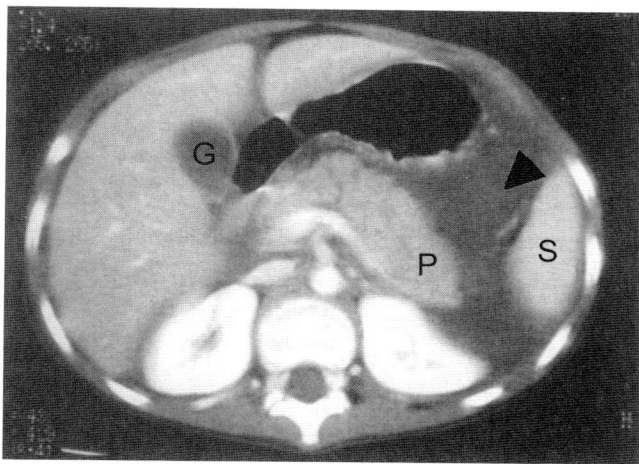

FIGURE 87.9. CT of acute pancreatitis. **P,** inflamed pancreas; **S,** spleen; **G,** gallbladder; **arrow,** free fluid.

MRI is an alternative. MR cholangiopancreatography and endoscopic ultrasonography have been incorporated recently as diagnostic tools in pediatric care. The endoscopic retrograde cholangiopancreatography has been accepted as an essential method in the evaluation of patients with recurrent pancreatitis.

Treatment includes early fluid resuscitation, hemodynamic stabilization, and adequate oxygen administration. An adequate fluid and electrolyte balance should be maintained (2). NG-tube insertion is necessary to relieve symptoms, especially in patients with gastric atony. Patients should receive parenteral nutrition while enteral feedings are being withheld. Analgesics are necessary for pain control, but opioids should be used with caution because of possible biliary spasm. Hypocalcemia and hyperglycemia may require treatment with calcium supplementation and insulin infusion, respectively. Gastric acid secretions should be suppressed

The data on the use of prophylactic antibiotics are contradictory in adults (16). No clear evidence exists to support prophylactic antibiotic treatment in preventing infection of the necrotic areas. However, infection of these necrotic areas is the most severe local complication and is associated with high mortality. When the area of necrosis exceeds 30% of the parenchyma, the risk of infection is increased. Antibiotic treatment may be considered in this group and continued for 1–2 weeks. *A precise recommendation cannot be made due to the contradictory evidence; however, we favor the use of prophylactic antibiotics in this setting.*

Feeding can be started once the symptoms subside and the levels of pancreatic enzymes decrease; however, ~20% of patients will not tolerate feeding. The effects of feeding should be monitored by performing clinical examination and checking serum enzyme levels. A meta-analysis that compared parenteral with enteral nutrition in adult patients with acute pancreatitis described a significantly lower risk of infection [relative risk (RR), 0.45; 95% confidence interval (CI), 0.26–0.78], reduced need for surgery to control pancreatitis (RR, 0.48; 95% CI, 0.22–0.1), and reduced length of hospital stay (mean reduction, 2.9 days; 95% CI, 1.6–4.3 days) in the enteral group (23). However, no differences were found in mortality or noninfectious complications. Enteral nutrition should be introduced early and replace parenteral nutrition as soon as the enteral tolerance is adequate. *Recommendation: Grade A–.*

Endoscopic retrograde cholangiopancreatography should be performed in patients with suspected or proven lithiasic acute pancreatitis, or when acute pancreatitis coexists with cholangitis, jaundice, or dilation of the common bile duct. It is advisable to perform this procedure within the first 72 hrs after the onset of symptoms. The endoscopic procedure includes sphincterotomy, the extraction of gallstones, and the use of stents (2). Patients with mild pancreatitis associated with cholelithiasis should have cholecystectomy performed as part of their treatment.

One of the most frequent complications during the course of the disease is the formation of pseudocysts, named for the capsule that is formed by granulation tissue without an epithelial layer. These are diagnosed by ultrasound studies, are usually asymptomatic, and resolve spontaneously. The term *pseudocyst* is used for the collections that persist for >4 weeks after the initiation of the disease. When pseudocysts are associated with the persistence or recurrence of vomiting, pain, ileus, and elevated enzymes, or if they have an expansive course or jeopardize adjacent structures, a surgeon should be consulted regarding percutaneous drainage or laparotomy. Local infection should be suspected in the presence of fever, leukocytosis, pain, or abdominal guarding. CT scan is useful during follow-up and to guide invasive draining procedures.

In the presence of signs of sepsis and tomographic demonstration of pancreatic or peripancreatic necrosis, a fine-needle aspiration should be performed to obtain material for culture to confirm or exclude the diagnosis of infected necrotic tissue. If the diagnosis is confirmed, surgical drainage or interventional radiology should be considered. If symptoms persist for >7 days, if necrotic area is >30%, or if any necrotic area exists in association with sepsis, cultures should be obtained through guided, fine-needle aspiration. Patients with infected necrosis will require surgical debridement or percutaneous drainage of all of the cavities that contain necrotic material. Surgery is recommended after 2 weeks of disease onset. Patients with noninfected necrosis can usually be managed without surgical treatment (2). The mortality from acute pancreatitis in children is significantly lower than in adults; however, in severe disease, it can be as high as 10%.

ABDOMINAL PATHOLOGY OF THE CRITICAL PATIENT

A dysfunction of the gastrointestinal tract has severe consequences for the critically ill child due to both its negative effect on nutrition and the complications related to bacterial overgrowth and possible bacterial translocation. The gastrointestinal and abdominal complications that may affect a critically ill child include gastrointestinal hemorrhage, ileus, acute cholecystitis, ischemic colitis, pseudomembranous colitis, and toxic megacolon due to *C. difficile* or other bacterial infections, pancreatitis, and abdominal compartment syndrome (**Table 87.1**).

Ileus

Ileus is defined as an intestinal dysmotility in the absence of a mechanical obstruction. Signs and symptoms include diminished or absent bowel sounds, failure to pass stools or flatus, abdominal distension, vomiting or increased drainage through the NG tube, and increased gastric residual volume during enteral feeds. The presence of ileus may provoke severe consequences, such as ischemia, perforation, or compartment syndrome. The three types of ileus are adynamic, spastic, and ischemic. The latter is observed in hemodynamically unstable patients or in patients with nonocclusive mesenteric ischemia. Signs present in the upright abdominal x-ray are nonspecific, and this study is frequently inadequate. Increased air in the small bowel, intestinal distension, or air-fluid levels are signs suggestive of ileus. These signs do not allow for differentiation of a functional ileus from a mechanical obstruction. The abdominal CT has a high sensitivity and specificity to differentiate ileus from mechanical obstruction. The causes of ileus are multiple in the critically ill child, the most frequent being intestinal manipulation during abdominal surgery. The ileus may extend from 3 to 5 days after a major intra-abdominal surgery; the small bowel recovers its motility within the first 24 hrs, whereas the stomach and colon take longer. The presence of ileus predisposes to the following problems: risk of vomiting and aspiration pneumonia, intestinal ischemia, fluid and electrolyte imbalances, sepsis, and difficulty in reestablishing nutrition. Fear of initiating early enteral nutrition is another negative consequence of postoperative ileus. Although pathophysiology is not clearly known, two causes considered to be responsible for its development are an imbalance in the sympathetic and parasympathetic splanchnic innervations and inflammation. Ileus is also a complication of sepsis. Experimental infusion of lipopolysaccharide diminishes visceral muscle contractility in the same way as in cardiac or skeletal muscle. Decrease in intestinal transit, which results in intraluminal bacterial multiplication, may be a cause of sepsis that begins a cycle that leads to recurrent and severe sepsis and results in multiorgan failure. Narcotic administration is another contributing factor for ileus. Narcotics act by stimulating μ-opioid receptors that inhibit peristalsis and diminish visceral smooth muscle tone. The decrease in analgesia seen with opioid tolerance does not correlate with decreased gastrointestinal effects; therefore, higher doses worsen constipation. Severe hypokalemia, exogenous catecholamines, general anesthetics, and a diversity of medicines, such as benzodiazepines, calcium-channel blocking agents, and anticholinergics, may be involved in the development of ileus.

The prevention of ileus includes adequate fluid resuscitation (22), a rational use of vasopressors, the weaning of opioids, and the institution of early enteral feeding. Nutrients help to maintain intestinal mucosa trophism and motility. The advantages of early nutrition in the critically ill child are well known. In a systematic review of adults that compared early postoperative feeding with initial fasting, a decrease in the length of stay and a reduction in the risk of infection were observed in the former (20). *Recommendation: Grade A–.*

The primary treatment for ileus is gastric decompression with an NG tube, which reduces the risk of vomiting and aspiration pneumonia. Data on the pharmacologic management of ileus in children are scarce. The use of epidural anesthesia with bupivacaine is one of the known strategies for adult patients that can also be used in children. Some studies have shown a favorable affect of cisapride on ileus, but this drug has been removed from the US market because of the high incidence of associated dysrhythmias. In adults, the use of neostigmine, a cholinesterase inhibitor that increases acetylcholine concentration in the neuromuscular junction within the intestinal muscular layer, has been described. Alvimopan acts as a selective peripheral μ-opioid receptor antagonist and is being developed for the management of acute postoperative ileus and for reversing delays in the reestablishment of the gastrointestinal transit.

Acute Cholecystitis

Acute cholecystitis is less common in children than in adults, but its incidence in the pediatric population appears to be rising, especially among the critically ill. In children, most cholecystitis is acalculous and frequently related to dehydration, certain infections, or systemic diseases, such as leptospirosis or Kawasaki disease (21). Calculous cholecystitis may present in premature infants, hemolytic diseases, or cystic fibrosis, or it may be associated with total parenteral nutrition irrespective of the underlying clinical disease. Calculous or acalculous cholecystitis is a known complication during the postoperative course of diverse surgical procedures, including cardiovascular, orthopedic, or general surgery. It may also be observed in patients who are admitted to the PICU due to multiple trauma or severe burns (33). It is one of the causes to be ruled out in the septic patient suspected of having an intra-abdominal infection.

The pathogenesis of cholecystitis in the critical patient is triggered by the supersaturation of bile with cholesterol crystals, or calcium bilirubinate, leading to biliary obstruction with or without stone formation. Once functional or physical obstruction of the bile duct has occurred, contractile function of the gallbladder decreases. Bacterial overgrowth occurs as bile stasis worsens. Ultimately, the gallbladder wall becomes edematous and inflamed. Necrosis of the mucosa, perforation, and/or gangrene, and other histologic findings of the gallbladder's wall also suggest an ischemic etiology in the critical patient. Hypoperfusion, due to hypovolemia or distributive shock, which is worsened by the use of vasoconstrictors, and an increase in the intraluminal pressure, produced by fasting or use of opioids, lead to a fall in the gallbladder's perfusion pressure. Bacterial invasion and multiplication in the ischemic tissue worsens the course of the disease.

The classic clinical presentation of cholecystitis, which consists of right upper-quadrant pain, fever, and jaundice (Charcot triad), has a low sensitivity and specificity in critically ill patients (35). The laboratory findings are nonspecific and may include leukocytosis, as well as elevated bilirubin, γ-glutamyl transpeptidase, and other liver enzymes (ALT, AST). Ultrasound is the most useful diagnostic test; compatible findings include thickening of the gallbladder wall and the presence of pericholecystic fluid. Other less-frequent signs are the double wall (edema of the gallbladder wall), the halo sign (intramural gas) (**Fig. 87.10**), and the presence of gallbladder distension. The absence of gallstones does not exclude the diagnosis. False-positive or false-negative ultrasound results may occur; this is clearly an operator-dependent technique. The sensitivity of ultrasound for acalculous cholecystitis is 81%–92%, and the specificity is 60%–96%. Repeated evaluation may increase the diagnostic sensitivity.

Initial treatment of acute cholecystitis consists of supportive care and the administration of antibiotics that are effective against gram-negative strains, enterococcus, and anaerobes.

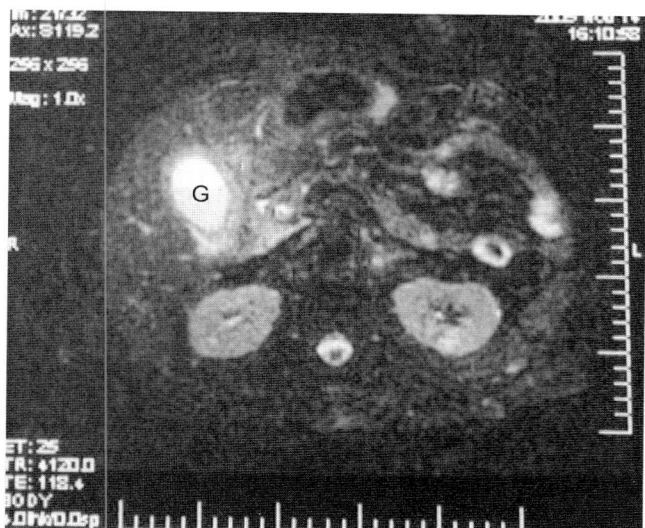

FIGURE 87.10. MRI of halo sign in cholecystitis. **G**, gallbladder.

Ultrasound- or CT-guided percutaneous drainage of the gall-bladder is the recommended treatment in adults, especially when they are clinically unstable (29). The obtained material should be cultured for guidance of antibiotic treatment in accordance with bacterial sensitivities. However, in 50% of cases, the culture may be negative. Cholecystectomy is indicated when the process cannot be resolved by means of percutaneous cholecystostomy or when this procedure is contraindicated. Urgent cholecystectomy may be necessary during complications such as acute cholangitis or gallstone pancreatitis.

Pseudomembranous Colitis

C. difficile is a gram-positive, anaerobic, spore-forming rod that can be responsible for the development of colitis. The pathogenic strains produce two major exotoxins: A and B. The spores must germinate in the anaerobic environment of the colon before toxin can be released. Manifestations of disease range from mild diarrhea to severe pseudomembranous colitis, which occurs in 3%–5% of carriers. An infrequent but very severe complication is toxic megacolon (10).

C. difficile usually affects patients who are receiving or have received antibiotics during the previous 3 weeks. Antibiotics act by altering the indigenous colonic flora (5). The possibility of infection increases, the longer the child stays in the hospital. The diagnosis is confirmed by means of stool culture that grows *C. difficile* and stool assays for toxins using enzyme-linked immunosorbent assay (ELISA), a specific but low-sensitivity method. The cytotoxin test in tissue cultures (to detect toxin B) is more sensitive, but it is also more expensive and requires 24–48 hrs. Positive results may be obtained in asymptomatic carriers, but the presence of compatible clinical signs is sufficient for the diagnosis. Hence, the intensivist must be aware of which test the laboratory is using to identify *C. difficile* toxin, because a negative ELISA test does not exclude the presence of toxin.

The treatment for *C. difficile* infection includes vancomycin via the oral or NG routes (10 mg/kg/dose; maximum dose, 500 mg) every 6 hrs for 7 days. In the presence of toxic megacolon,

the addition of IV metronidazole (every 8 hrs) is recommended. Broad-spectrum antibiotics should be stopped or avoided, if possible, to stimulate the recovery of the endogenous flora. Antidiarrheal medications that decrease intestinal motility are contraindicated. In addition to specific antibiotic therapy and fluid and electrolyte replacement, the patient should be isolated, and caregivers should wear gowns, masks, and gloves. Strict hand-washing precautions should be in effect for every patient in the PICU, but are reinforced for patients with *C. difficile*.

Toxic Megacolon

Toxic megacolon presents as an acute abdomen with abdominal distension, fever, hemodynamic involvement, alterations in the level of consciousness, hypoalbuminemia, electrolyte imbalances, leukocytosis, and thrombocytopenia. It is a serious complication of inflammatory bowel disease and of certain types of infectious colitis, and may progress to septic shock and multiorgan failure. Patients with ulcerative colitis are at greater risk of having this complication, even during the initial presentation. Diverse predisposing factors include treatment interruption, hypokalemia, the use of medication for diarrhea, or colonoscopy. The most frequent causes currently described in adults are *C. difficile* infections; however, other infections have been reported to be the cause as well (28).

The treatment of this critical situation includes circulatory and ventilatory support when necessary, IV antibiotics, hydrocortisone (1.5 mg/kg/dose, up to 100 mg) every 6 hrs, and gastrointestinal decontamination with nonabsorbable antibiotics (polymyxin, tobramycin, amphotericin B) via NG tube. Factors such as hypokalemia or hyperglycemia that favor intestinal hypomotility should be corrected, and the use of drugs that inhibit peristaltic activity, such as α-adrenergic agonists, dopamine, clonidine, opioids, anticholinergics, calcium antagonists, or theophylline, should be discontinued when possible. The utilization of probiotics via enteral feeds that may act by stimulating the immune response, has been recommended for ulcerative colitis. If medical treatment does not produce a rapid response, surgery may be necessary to perform a subtotal colectomy. Indications for surgery include progression to multiorgan failure, tomographic signs of progression, and signs of peritonitis or perforation. Mortality due to toxic megacolon is high, especially when surgery is delayed.

Abdominal Compartment Syndrome

In the adult, abdominal compartment syndrome (ACS) is defined as the combination of an intra-abdominal pressure >25 mm Hg (measured by means of a urinary catheter), progressive organ dysfunction (urinary output <1 mL/kg/hr, PaO_2/FIO_2 <150, peak airway pressure >45 mm Hg, or cardiac index <3 L/min/m², despite resuscitation), and organ function improvement after decompression. ACS associated with intra-abdominal injury is defined as primary, whereas it is labelled as secondary when it happens as a consequence of massive resuscitation in trauma, sepsis, or shock and in the absence of intra-abdominal injury or pathology (3).

ACS has been progressively more recognized in adults, but it has been scarcely reported in children. In a prospective series of 15 episodes in 10 patients admitted to a PICU, the incidence was 0.6% of the total admissions during a period of 5 years (6). In this series, 40% of the ACS incidences were secondary, related to shock-reperfusion or intracranial lesions. The pediatric diagnostic criteria include the presence of abdominal distension with an intra-abdominal pressure >15 mm Hg, accompanied by at least three of the following signs: oliguria or anuria, respiratory decompensation that resulted from a reduction of the thoracic compliance with increased carbon dioxide or decreased PaO_2/FIO_2, hypotension or shock, and metabolic acidosis. The hemodynamic and respiratory functions and the urinary output improve within the first hour after decompressive surgery. Following decompressive surgery, the abdomen is left open and covered with a Dacron mesh or a sterile IV bag (Bogota bag). A negative-pressure wound system may be applied to facilitate continuous drainage.

Measurement of the intra-abdominal pressure is achieved by means of a T-piece with a three-way stopcock placed between the urinary catheter and the pressure tubing. Urine is allowed to empty from the bladder. Thereafter, only sufficient sterile, isotonic sodium chloride solution is injected through the distal stopcock and urinary catheter and into the bladder, to allow for a continuous fluid column in the system. The exact amount of fluid will vary, depending on the length of the tubing and the size of the child. Clinical judgment is always required in the diagnosis of ACS because bladder pressure has not been validated against a measurement of true intra-abdominal pressure in the critically ill child. A comparison of indirect methods for measuring intra-abdominal pressure in children over a normal range of pressures found that the quantification of the bladder pressure via a transurethral urinary catheter using 1 mL/kg of sterile saline was the most accurate method (9).

ACS can develop within 4–6 hrs; therefore, measurements should be frequent. ACS may develop due to an increase in intra-abdominal contents or a decrease in abdominal compartment compliance. An increase of the content may be caused by ascites, hemoperitoneum, visceral edema, abdominal packs, peritonitis, pancreatitis, retroperitoneal hematomas, intestinal obstruction, ileus, gastric distension, or tumoral mass. The speed at which the increase in the content develops is related to abdominal compliance and development of ACS. A diminution in the volume of the cavity may be seen in reduction of voluminous hernias, the closure of an abdominal wall defect, circumferential burns of the abdominal wall, retroperitoneal edema or hematoma, positive-pressure ventilation, and high levels of positive end-expiratory pressure. The prognosis is poor even with decompressive surgery; therefore, the main goal is to prevent ACS from developing by recognizing patients at risk and monitoring their intra-abdominal (bladder) pressure. In the previously mentioned pediatric series, the mortality was 60% (6). Early decompressive surgery is the definitive treatment, and it consists of a complete opening of the medial fascia.

ABDOMINAL MANIFESTATION IN SYSTEMIC DISEASES

Some pediatric patients may present with symptoms of an abdominal surgical emergency in the context of systemic diseases.

Recognizing these situations may avoid unnecessary surgical interventions and allow an appropriate treatment without delays (**Table 87.1**).

Diabetic Ketoacidosis

Insulin-dependent diabetic patients may develop diabetic ketoacidosis during the initial presentation or during subsequent decompensations. A child with diabetic ketoacidosis may present with abdominal pain and vomiting associated with polyuria, glucosuria, ketonuria, acidosis, and hyperglycemia. The child may present with a tense abdomen with guarding and absent bowel sounds, simulating an acute abdomen. The presence of ketotic breath may be helpful for the diagnosis. Occasionally, patients with ketoacidosis may present with normal serum glucose levels. This scenario may occur in known diabetic patients who receive insulin before arrival at the emergency department or in children with diabetic ketoacidosis and persistent vomiting who have not received adequate oral intake. In children with prolonged fasting, relatively low glucose levels may also be observed, whereas dehydration favors elevated serum glucose levels.

Acute Porphyria

Porphyrias are both hereditary and acquired diseases in which the activity of the enzymes responsible for the heme biosynthesis pathways is partially or completely deficient. Acute, intermittent porphyria may present with nausea, vomiting, abdominal pain, diarrhea, constipation, or ileus and may occasionally be confused with an acute surgical abdomen. The presence of other neurologic symptoms, such as hypotonia, peripheral neuropathy, or seizures, is suggestive of this diagnosis. The clinical expression occurs after puberty, is more frequent in females, and is associated with menstrual periods. Abdominal pain, generalized or localized, is the most frequent symptom and is the initial sign of an acute attack. Other frequent symptoms include dysuria, urinary retention, and incontinence. Urine that has a port wine color may be present in severe cases. The Watson-Schwartz test, which is used as urinary screening to detect porphobilinogen, has high sensitivity but low specificity, and the diagnosis should be confirmed by means of chromatography measurement.

Rheumatologic Diseases

Children and adolescents with rheumatologic diseases constitute a small group, but these diseases may present life-threatening situations. Among the abdominal complications, ischemic lesions due to mesenteric vascular compromise may be observed. The clinical manifestations depend on the caliber of the affected vessels and the degree of obstruction. The most severe cases may produce infarct or gangrene. Other complications include perforations, intussusception, intestinal volvulus, and colonic strictures. Episodes of acute pancreatitis have been described in patients with systemic lupus erythematosus (SLE), juvenile rheumatoid arthritis, and Kawasaki disease. Episodes of primary peritonitis without evidence of infection or perforation have been described in patients with familial

Mediterranean fever, SLE, Still disease, and juvenile rheumatoid arthritis (17).

Henoch-Schönlein Purpura

In children, vasculitides are caused by diverse conditions that produce primary inflammation of the vascular wall. Henoch-Schönlein purpura affects small vessels and is the most frequent cause of nonthrombocytopenic purpura in children. The association of colicky abdominal pain, arthralgia or arthritis, edema in dependent or distensible areas, palpable nonthrombocytopenic purpura, and proteinuria is the basis of the diagnosis. Severe abdominal pain may be the only symptom, and recognizing the diagnosis can avoid unnecessary surgery. The pain is usually colicky and may be accompanied by fecal occult blood or hematemesis. Noninfectious peritoneal exudates, enlargement of the mesenteric lymph nodes, intestinal edema, or segmental intramural intestinal hemorrhages may also be present. Occasionally, the intestinal manifestations may be severe, and such complications as intussusception or intestinal perforation may be present. The renal compromise may be demonstrated by the presence of isolated hematuria, proteinuria, or findings compatible with glomerulonephritis. Treatment with steroids has been associated with a rapid improvement of the gastrointestinal or neurologic complications; however, use of steroids with the initial symptoms has not shown to reduce the risk of renal compromise or the frequency of gastrointestinal complications (15). The early use of steroids in uncomplicated Henoch-Schönlein purpura cannot be recommended. *Recommendation: Grade A+.*

Kawasaki Disease

A 4.6% (10 cases) incidence of severe abdominal symptoms was reported in a series of 219 children with Kawasaki disease (42). In most, the presentation of acute abdomen was not accompanied by sufficient signs for the diagnosis of Kawasaki disease. Two to four days after admission, the characteristic signs appeared: maculopapular rash, conjunctivitis, mucositis, cervical adenitis, and edema of the feet and hands. The most frequent abdominal signs were acute abdominal pain, distension, emesis, jaundice, and hepatomegaly. Gallbladder hydrops and cholestasis appeared later during the course of the disease. Exploratory laparotomy or transhepatic biliary drainage was necessary in 8 children. Kawasaki disease should be considered as a differential diagnosis in children with fever, rash, and acute abdominal pain or hematemesis.

Sickle Cell Disease

Sickle cell disease is a hereditary disease that presents with chronic hemolytic anemia and recurrent episodes of pain as cardinal manifestations (see Chapter 104). The hemolytic anemia may be exacerbated by additional events, such as aplastic crisis, acute splenic or hepatic sequestration, bone marrow necrosis, renal failure, and late hemolytic transfusion reactions. The episodes of acute pain, previously called *sickle cell crisis*, are based on the occlusion of the bone marrow vascular bed that leads to bone infarction and release of inflammatory me-

diators. Severe abdominal pain can be one of the clinical manifestations.

CONCLUSIONS AND FUTURE DIRECTIONS

The diagnostic precision of abdominal emergencies continues to improve with the use of new imaging technologies. However, early diagnosis will always depend on the clinical skills of the emergency pediatrician, the intensivist, and the pediatric surgeon. On the other hand, the continuous increase in the costs of medicine makes it essential to carefully evaluate the benefits of diagnostic studies in relation to their cost efficiency. Minimally invasive surgical techniques and laparoscopy are being used more frequently; however, classic surgical skills to resolve abdominal emergencies should not disappear. The improved survival in patients who undergo complex surgery or solid-organ, bone marrow, or intestinal transplantation; in those with acquired immunodeficiency syndrome; and in those with previously fatal oncologic pathology will expose the intensivist to new morbidities that may present as abdominal emergencies. The improvement in respiratory, circulatory, renal, metabolic, and immunologic support techniques will lead to better results in patients who undergo multiple interventions due to complications of gastrointestinal tract surgery. Also, differences in access to adequate care will continue to limit the possibilities of children who reside in areas with poor resources or limited health systems.

KEY POINTS

- The most frequent cause of acute abdomen in previously healthy children is acute appendicitis.
- Acute appendicitis in infants and small children has an initial presentation that is less clear. It is sometimes associated with diarrhea, and the diagnosis is frequently late, once generalized peritonitis has been installed.
- The most frequent cause of intestinal obstruction is acquired adhesions, and adequate treatment may only require decompression and intestinal rest.
- Timely diagnosis of intussusception allows a quick resolution and avoids progression to intestinal ischemia and obstruction.
- Midgut volvulus associated with malrotation is a severe condition with rapid development of ischemia; its suspicion obliges an urgent surgical decision.
- Severe acute pancreatitis is less frequent in the pediatric population; however, it may be a severe illness when accompanied by local and systemic intense inflammatory responses.
- The most frequent abdominal and intestinal complications in a child admitted to the PICU for postoperative controls or for the treatment of other critical pathology include gastrointestinal hemorrhage, postoperative ileus, acalculous cholecystitis, pseudomembranous colitis, toxic megacolon, and abdominal compartment syndrome.
- Recognizing the causes of abdominal pain or of episodes that simulate acute abdomen in systemic illnesses, such as diabetic ketoacidosis, acute porphyria, sickle cell crisis,

Henoch-Schönlein purpura, or Kawasaki disease, is essential for adequate management.

References

1. Anaya DA, Nathens AB. Risk factors for severe sepsis in secondary peritonitis. *Surg Infect (Larchmt)* 2003;4:355–62.
2. Athens A, Curtis R, Beale R, et al. Management of the critically ill patient with severe acute pancreatitis. *Crit Care Med* 2004;32:2524–36.
3. Balogh Z, McKinley BA, Holcomb JB, et al. Both primary and secondary abdominal compartment syndrome can be predicted early and are harbingers of multiple organ failure. *J Trauma* 2003;54:848–61.
4. Barie P, May AK, Malhotra A, et al. Peritonitis and intra-abdominal abscess. In Fink M, Abraham E, Vincent JL, et al., eds. *Textbook of Critical Care, 5th ed.* Philadelphia: WB Saunders, 2005;1033–47 (Chap. 123).
5. Bartlett JG. *Clostridium difficile:* History of its role as an enteric pathogen and the current state of knowledge about the organism. *Clin Infect Dis* 1994;18(Suppl 4):S265–72.
6. Beck R, Halberthal M, Zonis Z, et al. Abdominal compartment syndrome in children. *Pediatr Crit Care Med* 2001;2:51–6.
7. Bickell N, Federman A, Aufses A. Influence of time on risk of bowel resection in complete small bowel obstruction. *J Am Coll Surg* 2005;201:847–54.
8. Bogusevicius A, Maleckas A, Pundzius J, et al. Prospective randomized trial of computer-aided diagnosis and contrast radiography in acute small bowel obstruction. *Eur J Surg* 2002;168:78–83.
9. Davis PJ, Koottayi S, Taylor A, et al. Comparison of indirect methods of measuring intra-abdominal pressure in children. *Intensive Care Med* 2005;31:471–5.
10. Dobson G, Hickey C, Trinder J. *Clostridium difficile* colitis causing toxic megacolon, severe sepsis and multiple organ dysfunction syndrome. *Intensive Care Med* 2003;29:1030.
11. Gallo E, Ginanatonio CA. Extrarenal involvement in diarrhoea-associated haemolytic-uraemic syndrome. *Pediatr Nephrol* 1995;9:117–9.
12. Golden C, Feusner J. Malignant abdominal masses in children: Quick guide to evaluation and diagnosis. *Pediatr Clin N Am* 2002;49:1369–92.
13. Green R, Bulloch B, Kabani A, et al. Early analgesia for children with acute abdominal pain. *Pediatrics* 2005;116:978–83.
14. Henrikson S, Blane CE, Koujok S, et al. The effect of screening sonography on the positive rate of enemas for intussusception. *Pediatr Radiol* 2003;33:190–3.
15. Huber AK, King J, McLaine P, et al. A randomized, placebo-controlled trial of prednisone in early Henoch Schonlein Purpura. *BMC Med* 2004;2:7.
16. Isenmann R, Runzi M, Kron M, et al. Prophylactic antibiotic treatment in patients with predicted severe acute pancreatitis: A placebo-controlled, double-blind trial. *Gastroenterology* 2004;126:997–1004.
17. Janssen N, Karnad D, Guntupalli K. Rheumatologic diseases in the intensive care unit: Epidemiology, clinical approach, management, and outcome. *Crit Care Clin* 2002;18(4):729–48.
18. Jones S, Claridge J. Acute Abdomen. In: Townsend JR, Beauchamp D, Evers BM, et al., eds. *Sabiston Textbook of Surgery, 17th ed.,* Philadelphia: WB Saunders, 2004;1219–35.
19. Kurbegov AC, Sondheimer JM. Pneumatosis intestinalis in non-neonatal pediatric patients. *Pediatrics* 2001;108:402–6.
20. Lewis SJ, Egger M, Sylvester PA, et al. Early enteral feeding versus "nil by mouth" after gastrointestinal surgery: Systematic review and meta-analysis of controlled trials. *Br Med J* 2001;323:773–6.
21. Lobe TE. Cholelithiasis and cholecystitis in children. *Semin Pediatr Surg* 2000;9:170–6.
22. Lobo DN, Bostock KA, Neal KR, et al. Effect of salt and water balance on recovery of gastrointestinal function after elective colonic resection: A randomised controlled trial. *Lancet* 2002;359:1812–8.
23. Marik E, Zaloga G. Meta-analysis of parenteral nutrition versus enteral nutrition in patients with acute pancreatitis. *Br Med J* 2004;328 (7453):1407.
24. Mazuski JE, Sawyer RG, Nathens AB, et al. The Surgical Infection Society guidelines on antimicrobial therapy for intra-abdominal infections: Evidence for the recommendations. *Surg Infect* 2003;3:175–233.
25. Meyer JS, Dangman BC, Buonomo C, et al. Air and liquid contrast agents in the management of intussusception: A controlled, randomized trial. *Radiology* 1993;188:507–11.
26. Millar AJ, Rode H, Cywes S. Malrotation and volvulus in infancy and childhood. *Semin Pediatr Surg* 2003;12:229–36.
27. Nelson R, Tse B, Edwards S. Systematic review of prophylactic nasogastric decompression after abdominal operations. *Br J Surg* 2005;92:673–80.
28. Oudeman-van Straaten HM. Acute Megacolon in Critically Ill Patients. In: Fink M, Abraham E, Vincent JL, et al. eds. *Textbook of Critical Care 5th ed.,* Philadelphia: WB Saunders, 2005;1055–60.
29. Patel M, Miedema BW, James MA, et al. Percutaneous cholecystostomy is an effective treatment for high-risk patients with acute cholecystitis. *Am Surg* 2000;66:33–7.
30. Platell C, Papadimitriou JM, Hall JC. The influence of lavage on peritonitis. *J Am Coll Surg* 2000;191:672–80.
31. Roehrborn A, Thomas L, Potreck O, et al. The microbiology of postoperative peritonitis. *Clin Infect Dis* 2001;33:1513–19.
32. Scaglione M, Romano S, Pinto F, et al. Helical CT diagnosis of small bowel obstruction in the acute clinical setting. *Eur J Radiol* 2004;50:15–22.
33. Shapiro MJ, Luchtefeld WB, Kurzweil S, et al. Acute acalculous cholecystitis in the critically ill. *Am Surg* 1994;60:335–9.
34. Thomson A, Marshall J, Opal S. Intraabdominal infections in infants and children: Descriptions and definitions. *Pediatr Crit Care Med* 2005;6:S30–5.
35. Trowbridge RL, Rutkowski NK, Shojania KG. Does this patient have acute cholecystitis? *JAMA* 2003;289:80–6.
36. UK Working Party on Acute Pancreatitis. UK guidelines for the management of acute pancreatitis. *Gut* 2005;54(Suppl):1–9.
37. Vasavada P. Ultrasound evaluation of acute abdominal emergencies in infants and children. *Radiol Clin N Am* 2004;42:445–6.
38. Vieten D, Spicer R. Enterocolitis complicating Hirschsprung's disease. *Semin Pediatr Surg* 2004;13:263–72.
39. West M. Conservative and operative management of gastrointestinal fistulae in the critically ill patient. *Curr Opin Crit Care* 2000;6:143–7.
40. Wonf PF, Gillian AD, Kumar S, et al. Antibiotic regimens for secondary peritonitis of gastrointestinal origin in adults. *Cochrane Database Syst Rev* 2005;18:CD004539.
41. Yen K, Karpas A, Pinkerton HJ, et al. Interexaminer reliability in physical examination of pediatric patients with abdominal pain. *Arch Pediatr Adolesc Med* 2005;159:373–6.
42. Zulian F, Falcini F, Zancan L, et al. Acute surgical abdomen as presenting manifestation of Kawasaki disease. *J Pediatr* 2003;142:731–5.

CHAPTER 88 ■ FULMINANT HEPATIC FAILURE AND TRANSPLANTATION

PIERRE TISSIÈRES • DENIS J. DEVICTOR

FULMINANT HEPATIC FAILURE

Fulminant hepatic failure (FHF) is a rare disease in most countries but remains endemic in some regions where viral hepatitis is highly prevalent. In the US, the estimated frequency of FHF is 17 cases per 100,000 per year, inclusive of all age groups. The incidence of FHF in the pediatric population is unknown, but accounts for 10%–15% of all pediatric liver transplantations (36,47).

Definition and Classifications

In adults, no standardized definition exists for FHF. One of the most widely used was proposed by Trey and Davidson in 1970, who defined FHF as "a potentially reversible condition, the consequence of severe liver injury, with the onset of hepatic encephalopathy within 8 weeks of the first symptoms and in the absence of pre-existing liver disease" (74). Classification of adult patients according to the delay between jaundice and onset of encephalopathy has been suggested by groups in Paris (fulminant and subfulminant) and in London (hyperacute, acute, and subacute) (5,50). However, these definitions used to describe this disease in adult patients are not applicable to children. For instance, newborns and infants with FHF are known to have nonspecific symptoms, with some failing to show jaundice or encephalopathy. An accepted definition proposed by the King's College group defines FHF in children as "a multi-systemic disorder in which severe impairment of liver function, with or without encephalopathy, occurs in a patient with no recognized underlying chronic liver disease" (6).

Causes

FHF can be schematically classified into seven categories: metabolic, infective, toxic, autoimmune, malignancy-induced, vascular-induced, and undetermined. In infants, metabolic disease is the most frequent cause of FHF, whereas in children, viral FHF is most frequently seen. Whatever the age, undetermined FHF is frequently observed (10,14,22,25,27,44,63,75) (Table 88.1). Speed in determining the etiology of the FHF and providing a diagnosis is essential because instituting specific therapy or determining the potential for liver regeneration has an impact on the need for liver transplantation. Patients with FHF secondary to hepatitis A have a higher chance to recover spontaneously than those with FHF secondary to undetermined cause. Some causes of FHF may be contraindications to liver transplantation (for instance, leukemia and some mitochondrial respiratory chain diseases). Finally, some causes require specific therapy to be administered to the patient's family, such in cases of hepatitis B virus or neonatal herpes infection.

Metabolic Fulminant Hepatic Failure

Galactosemia, hereditary fructose intolerance, tyrosinemia, neonatal hemochromatosis, ornithine transcarbamylase deficiency, and Wilson disease are the main metabolic causes of FHF. Inborn error of bile acid synthesis, fatty-acid oxidation disorders, and mitochondrial respiratory chain disorders can also cause FHF in infants (25). In the newborn, the clinical spectrum of metabolic FHF is characterized by the association of coagulopathy, hypoglycemia, lactic acidosis, failure to thrive, and irritability, but jaundice is frequently lacking at the time of FHF diagnosis.

Mitochondrial respiratory chain disorders that cause FHF are increasingly recognized. Association of hypoglycemia, lactic acidosis, neurologic, muscle, and renal tubular abnormalities in an infant should raise the suspicion for mitochondrial diseases. The mitochondrial disease spectrum is wide and can either be generalized throughout the body or not. Involvement can include muscle, nerve, brain, liver, kidney, and heart (30). Diagnosis is difficult and requires extensive and immediate workup because emergency liver transplantation may be contraindicated, especially when multiple organs are involved (24). Diagnostic testing includes echocardiography, electroencephalography, renal function, serum muscle enzymes, cerebrospinal fluid lactate, liver biopsy, and muscle biopsy [for ultrastructural mitochondrial changes and respiratory chain enzyme activity (complexes I, II, III, IV)].

Fulminant Wilson disease has a mortality reaching 100% without liver transplantation, and is not observed in children <7 years old (23,68). Diagnosis of fulminant Wilson disease is based on the presence of hemolytic anemia, elevated serum and urinary copper levels, low ceruloplasmin (normal in 15% of cases), low alkaline phosphatase in regard to the elevated bilirubin (total bilirubin to alkaline phosphatase <1 mcmol/IU), and the presence of Kayser-Fleischer rings on slit-lamp eye examination (23,68). Renal function is frequently impaired.

Infectious Fulminant Hepatic Failure

Viral hepatitis represents the largest proportion of infective FHF (10,14,48,75). Hepatitis A is the most frequently encountered infective FHF (1.5%–3%) in infants and children and represents a public health challenge in endemic regions (10,18,75). Although hepatitis A infections are usually benign, 0.5% evolve into FHF (18). Hepatitis A can also precipitate the course of other liver disease, such as Wilson disease and hepatitis due to

TABLE 88.1

CAUSES OF FULMINANT HEPATIC FAILURE IN 200 INFANTS AND CHILDREN ADMITTED AT THE
BICÊTRE HOSPITAL PICU (1986–2006)

	Cause	Infants ($n = 82$)	Children ($n = 118$)	Total ($n = 200$)
Metabolic	Galactosemia, tyrosinemia, hemochromatosis, Wilson disease, Reye syndrome, fatty-acid oxidation disorder, mitochondrial cytopathy.	35 (43%)	21 (18%)	56 (28%)
Infectious	HAV, HBV, herpes simplex, HHV6, EBV, enterovirus, adenovirus, parvovirus B19, Dengue fever	19 (23%)	33 (28%)	52 (26%)
Toxic	Acetaminophen, sulfamide, sodium valproate, sulfasalazine, halothane, amanita phalloides	4 (5%)	18 (15%)	22 (11%)
Other	Autoimmune, familial lymphohistiocytosis, macrophage activation syndrome, leukemia, hyperthermia, veno-occlusive disease	13 (16%)	14 (12%)	27 (13%)
Undetermined		11 (13%)	32 (27%)	43 (22%)

HAV, hepatitis A virus; HBV, hepatitis B virus; HHV, human herpes virus; EBV, Epstein-Barr virus

B or E virus (3). Its prevalence should decrease with wide-range vaccination and improved sanitation policies. Hepatitis B may evolve toward FHF in 1% of cases. Although it is infrequent, hepatitis B FHF in children may be endemic (11,14). It can occur at any age, especially in the newborn period following peripartum infection (40-day latency). Intrafamilial contamination can occur and should be always suspected.

Other hepatitis viruses (C, D, E, G) rarely cause FHF in children. Herpesviridae family viruses [HV-1, 2, 6, cytomegalovirus (CMV), Epstein-Barr virus (EBV), and varicella-zoster virus] are known to be highly hepatocytopathic and are all reported to cause FHF but usually in immunocompromised hosts. Neonatal herpes simplex infection is well known to produce devastating FHF associated with encephalitis in the first week following birth.

Other viruses can cause FHF and should be suspected, among them echovirus (serotype 11), adenovirus, enterovirus (Coxsackie), EBV, and parvovirus B19. Bacterial and parasitic infections are usually not associated with FHF, although they may be observed in cases of exotoxin-induced FHF (invasive group A streptococcal infection) or during malignant hyperthermia secondary to malaria. In rare cases, congenital syphilis could cause FHF in infants. Leptospirosis, brucellosis, Q fever, and Dengue fever have been reported to cause FHF.

Toxic Fulminant Hepatic Failure

Drug intoxication leads to FHF in a large number of cases, either directly through hepatotoxicity or indirectly through an idiosyncratic reaction (43). Acetaminophen overdose is the most common cause of toxic FHF. It is more frequently encountered in adults and teenagers (intentional overdosage) than in children (inappropriate dosage regimen). In a large series of 73 children, 39% had severely abnormal liver enzyme levels, and 8% required emergency liver transplantation. Fatality occurred in 2 patients (3%) (55). Children seem to be more resistant to the toxic effect. Sodium valproate can cause acute hepatic necrosis in 1 in 5000 treated children during the first 4–6 months after initiation of therapy. Such toxicity occurs more frequently in younger children or when associated with other seizure treatments. Sodium valproate-induced FHF has a significant resemblance to Reye syndrome and mitochondrial

cytopathy, in which a microvacuolar steatosis associated with centrilobular necrosis is found. In adults, halothane is known to cause FHF in 1 in 35,000 patients receiving halothane anesthetics and to increase in frequency if two exposures to halothane occur within 6 weeks. However, in children incidence has been demonstrated to be <1 in 100,000 patients receiving halothane anesthetics. Its pathogenicity involves an immune reaction with subsequent cellular inflammation and necrosis. Similarly, other volatile anesthetics (enflurane, isoflurane, sevoflurane) have been documented to cause FHF in children (66). Other drugs, such as carbamazepine, sulfasalazine, antituberculosis drugs, and recreational drugs (ecstasy, cocaine), are involved in drug-induced FHF. Mushroom-induced FHF can occur following ingestion of a wide variety of mushrooms, including *Amanita phalloides* and *Lepiotae* species. Phosphorus and carbon tetrachloride intoxication are other potential causes of FHF.

Autoimmune Fulminant Hepatic Failure

In the newborn and infant, giant-cell hepatitis may cause FHF. It is associated with an immune hemolytic anemia (positive Coombs test) and can evolve to FHF if immunosuppressive therapy is not initiated. In older children, autoimmune hepatitis can be diagnosed if autoantibodies (anti-endoplasmic reticulum, anti-smooth muscle, or anti-cytosolic antibodies) are recovered in the plasma. Immunosuppressive therapy (e.g., cyclosporine) may be effective (19).

Malignancy and Hematologic-induced Fulminant Hepatic Failure

Leukemia and other lymphoproliferative syndromes with massive hepatic infiltration may cause FHF in children. In the newborn, familial lymphohistiocytosis may present as FHF with hypofibrinogemia, coagulopathy, elevated liver enzymes, and sometimes jaundice. Associated hyponatremia, hypertriglyceridemia, high ferritin level, pancytopenia, cerebrospinal fluid lymphocytosis, and signs of hemophagocytosis on marrow smear obtained after bone marrow transplantation are highly suggestive. Macrophage activation syndrome is increasingly recognized as a cause of FHF, and an association with a viral trigger should be suspected. These diagnoses should be systematically evoked, as they contraindicate liver transplantation.

Vascular-induced Fulminant Hepatic Failure

In children, as in adults, veno-occlusive disease of the liver (i.e., hepatic vein occlusion following bone marrow transplantation or chemotherapy), Budd-Chiari syndrome (i.e., obstruction of the hepatic venous outflow), or "cardiac liver" (left heart hypoplasia) may initially display a FHF. A reversible hepatic insufficiency occurs frequently after cardiogenic shock, septic shock, multiorgan failure, or any significant hypoperfusion state.

Undetermined Fulminant Hepatic Failure

When all mentioned diagnoses are excluded, undetermined FHF should be considered, and it is called non-A, non-B FHF, or non A–G FHF. Undetermined causes represent 20%–50% of FHF in children (22,36,44,63) (**Table 88.1**).

Diagnostic Criteria

Clinical Manifestations

Clinical symptoms of FHF vary according to the etiology and the age of the patient. In the newborn, symptoms are nonspecific, sometimes only related to an altered general condition, failure to thrive, and vomiting, whereas in older children, most have jaundice associated with hepatic encephalopathy.

In viral-induced FHF, jaundice is preceded by symptoms such as fever, myalgia, arthralgia, and nausea. Thereafter, jaundice worsens, liver enzymes become increasingly elevated, and prothombin time becomes prolonged before hepatic encephalopathy appears, underscoring hepatic dysfunction secondary to significant viral destruction of the liver. In some cases, in which initial viral-induced cytolytic effect and jaundice are minimal, a delayed improvement (days to weeks) is followed by a recurrence secondary to a viral-induced autoimmune response. This is frequently associated with fever, anorexia, abdominal pain, vomiting, and encephalopathy. In some cases, such as after drug-, toxin- or metabolic-induced FHF, encephalopathy or bleeding can occur before the occurrence of the jaundice.

Hepatic encephalopathy is a complex neuropsychiatric syndrome characterized by a reversible chemical and neurophysiologic status that occurs when liver function is altered. Hepatic encephalopathy pathophysiology is complex and multifactorial. Various nonexclusive theories deserve mention: (a) *the hyperammonemia theory*, in which hyperammonemia is thought to have a "direct" effect on neuronal membranes, enhancement of neuroinhibitory γ-aminobutyric acid (GABA)-mediated transmission by direct activation of GABA receptors, and "indirect" effect on neuronal dysfunction due to disturbance of glutamate neurotransmission and plasma amino acid profile; (b) *the false-neurotransmitter theory*, in which liver failure modifies the plasma amino acid profile (increase in aromatic amino acids, decrease in branched-chain amino acids) and results in alterations to brain metabolism; and (c) *the neuroinhibition*, or *GABA-benzodiazepine, theory*, which is characterized by increased levels of neuroinhibitory GABA and a synergistic neuroinhibitory effect with benzodiazepine receptor ligands, explaining why, in some cases, use of flumazenil has been shown to reverse encephalopathy without affecting outcome. It is essential to recognize the difference between hepatic encephalopathy that occurs in chronic liver disease and acute hepatic encephalopathy that occurs during FHF, which

TABLE 88.2	
GRADES OF HEPATIC ENCEPHALOPATHY[a]	
I	Changes in behavior, minimal change in level of consciousness, altered sleep (hypersomnia, insomnia, inversed sleep cycle in the newborn)
II	Spatiotemporal disorientation, drowsiness, inappropriate behavior, obvious asterixis
III	Marked confusion, stuporous, respond or not to auditory stimuli, decerebrate posturing to pain, asterixis usually absent
IV	Comatose, unresponsive to pain, decorticate posturing

[a]Adapted from the West Haven criteria. Atterbury CE, Maddrey WC, Conn HO. Neomycin-sorbitol and lactulose in the treatment of acute portal-systemic encephalopathy. A controlled, double-blind clinical trial. *Am J Dig Dis* 1978;23:398–406.

is often associated with cerebral edema and intracranial hypertension (8,70). Hepatic encephalopathy can occur a few hours to days after jaundice appears. In the newborn, hepatic encephalopathy is nonspecific and can be reflected only by behavioral changes, agitation, and a high-pitched cry. These signs may precede the development of brisk reflexes, clonus, and appearance of a coma with hypertonia, agitation, and pupillary abnormalities (sluggish then fixed), followed by a deeper coma with hypotonia and brainstem coning. In older children, signs and symptoms are identical to those in adults. Hepatic encephalopathy is classified into four grades using a modification of the West Haven criteria (**Table 88.2**). Status epilepticus may complicate hepatic encephalopathy, especially in grade IV. Hepatic encephalopathy may be precipitated by disease progression as well as by infection, metabolic abnormalities, gastrointestinal bleeding, excessive protein load (fresh frozen plasma), and portal vein thrombosis.

Diagnostic Workup

Diagnostic workup is directed toward establishing a diagnosis and characterizing the severity of liver failure (**Table 88.3**). Cholestasis is usually present in viral-induced FHF and may be accompanied by elevated alkaline phosphatase and γ-glutaryl transferase, whereas cholestasis may be moderated in toxic FHF. Absence of hyperbilirubinemia should suggest a Reye syndrome. Increase in serum liver enzyme level is usually proportional to the degree of hepatic necrosis. Marked elevation of liver enzymes (>3000 UI/L) is usually found; however, normal or normalization of liver enzymes could be the result of an end-stage hepatic necrosis. In this case, decreased liver enzymes are accompanied by increased bilirubin and γ-glutaryl transferase. Hemostasis abnormalities are closely correlated with severity of FHF. Prolonged prothrombin time (PT) (INR >2) and decreased factor V activity (<50%) are the most potent abnormalities. Additionally, hypofibrinogenemia and altered factor II, VII, and X activities are found. These alterations in hemostasis factors may be associated with a disseminated intravascular coagulopathy. Therefore, a decreased factor V activity from 50% to 30% or lower underscores a severe liver injury. Other blood abnormalities could be observed: hypoglycemia, hyperammonemia, lactic acidosis, and hypoalbuminemia. Respiratory alkalosis secondary to neurogenic hyperventilation is frequently observed. Renal failure could indicate hepatorenal

TABLE 88.3

DIAGNOSTIC WORKUP

GENERAL WORKUP

Na, K, Cl, Ph, Mg, Ca, BUN, creatinine, LDH, lactate, ammonia, blood gas; complete blood count; Coombs test, blood, urine and CSF culture; blood group determination, AST, ALT, alkaline phosphatase, γ-glutaryl transferase, total and conjugated bilirubin, α-fetoprotein; prothrombin time, partial thrombin time, fibrinogen, factor II, V, VII, IX, X activity, D-dimer

METABOLIC WORKUP

Tyrosinemia	Urine succinyl acetone, wrist radiograph
Galactosemia	Red-cell galactose-1-phosphate uridylyl transferase activity (spot test)
Hemochromatosis	Ferritin level, extrahepatic iron deposition, i.e., salivary gland (biopsy, NMR)
OTC deficiency	Orotic acid
Wilson disease	Serum ceruloplasmin, serum, and urinary copper, Kayser-Fleisher rings
Reye syndrome and fatty-acid oxidation disorders	Urinary and blood organic acid chromatography, carnitine and fatty-acid level
Mitochondrial cytopathy	Mitochondrial DNA, muscle and liver biopsy for quantitative respiratory chain enzyme determination, CSF lactate, creatinine kinase, echocardiography

INFECTIOUS WORKUP

Hepatitis A, B; HHV-1, 2, 6; CMV; EBV; VZV; echovirus; adenovirus; enterovirus; parvovirus B19	Viral serology, keep frozen serum, PCR (blood, CSF), stool culture
Treponema pallidum (syphilis)	VDRL (maternal if newborn)

OTHER

Familial lymphohistiocytosis and macrophage activating syndrome	Blood triglycerides, cholesterol, ferritin, bone marrow analysis
Autoimmune	Coombs test, autoantibodies, biopsy
Intoxication	Acetaminophen level, salicylate level, keep frozen urine and blood
Vascular	Echocardiography

NMR, nuclear magnetic resonance; OTC, ornithine transcarbamylase; HHV, human herpes virus; CMV, cytomegalovirus; EBV, Epstein-Barr virus; VZV, varicella-zoster virus; PCR, polymerase chain reaction; CSF, cerebrospinal fluid; VDRL, venereal disease research laboratory test

syndrome, which is more frequently observed with viral or toxic FHF. Lactic acidosis may indicate tissue hypoxia and severe liver failure. No optimal tool is available for monitoring time-responsive indicators of liver function. Blood lactate and coagulation parameters may be used, but the response time is slow. Preliminary work using kinetics of the indocyanine green elimination rate measured by pulse-dye densitometry (LiMON®, Pulsion Medical Systems AG, Munich, Germany) may prove beneficial at the bedside to identify failing or recovery of the liver function (35).

Abdominal sonography allows the assessment of hepatic size and condition of the parenchyma, observation of occurrence of ascites, and the evaluation of the vascular supply. Liver biopsy should be postponed due to its associated elevated bleeding risk and reduced benefit. In cases of suspected mitochondrial respiratory chain defects, liver and muscle biopsy should be considered. Electroencephalographic abnormalities are associated with the various grades of hepatic encephalopathy. These are characterized by the association of diminished basal activity and the occurrence of characteristic slow triphasic waves that are not found in the youngest child. Five types of electroencephalographic pattern can be associated with prognosis values (**Table 88.4**). Deceleration of the electric frequency below 2 Hz frequently precedes type IV hepatic encephalopathy. However, the EEG pattern may not discriminate brain death from grade IV hepatic encephalopathy. Transcranial-Doppler ultrasound, somatosensory-evoked potential, nuclear brain flow, or cerebral angio scan will be required to diagnose brain death. Electrical seizures usually indicate grade II or higher hepatic encephalopathy. Brain CT has a limited utility in FHF. Although identification of cerebral edema is correlated with poor prognosis, CT scan sensitivity to detect cerebral edema is approximate (2). Repetitive transcranial-Doppler examination of arterial cerebral flow is emerging as a useful tool with which to identify intracranial hypertension (1,54).

TABLE 88.4

ELECTROENCEPHALOGRAPHIC PATTERN OF FULMINANT HEPATIC FAILURE

Type I	Slow polyrhythmic activity associating 5–6 Hz, 3–4 Hz, 1–2 Hz frequencies with a reactive or inconsistently reactive EEG pattern.
Type II	Slow theta-delta (3–4 Hz) activity of 50–100 mcV amplitude. Inconsistent or absent EEG reactivity.
Type III	Large (100–150 mcV) monomorphic delta activity (1–3 Hz). No EEG reactivity.
Type IV	Slow, depressed (<1 Hz) pattern, with decreasing amplitude. No EEG reactivity.
Type V	Progressive disappearance of EEG activity.

EEG, electroencephalogram

FHF etiologic diagnosis remains undetermined in ~30% of cases. Although most cases are related to an acute failure, decompensated, previously unrecognized chronic liver disease may look similar to viral FHF, such as in fulminant Wilson disease, tyrosinemia, or chronic active autoimmune hepatitis. Decompensated, unrecognized chronic liver disease usually displays nodular and hard hepatomegaly and splenomegaly. The diagnostic work-up in infants and children with FHF is summarized in **Table 88.3**.

Complications

Preoperative and early postoperative complications of FHF are listed in **Table 88.5**.

Cerebral Edema

In children, cerebral edema with intracranial hypertension frequently occurs during FHF and is recognized as a major risk for death (2,22,36,44). In the newborn, symptoms include a tense fontanelle, axial hypertonia, oculomotor disturbances, decerebrate posturing, neurovegetative symptoms (apnea, Cushing triad, dysrhythmia), and disappearance of brainstem reflexes. Death following FHF could be attributed to cerebral edema in 40% of cases. Development of cerebral edema is related to two main mechanisms: (a) cytotoxic edema may develop in relation to Na/K-ATPase pump inhibition, ammonium accumulation, and deregulated equilibrium of cerebral osmotic amino acids; and (b) vasogenic edema is secondary to dysfunctional brain perfusion autoregulation mechanisms, which will ultimately result in cerebral hypoxemia. Cerebral hyperemia is described but is less frequent than cerebral hypoxemia. The cerebral hyperemia mechanism, as well as increased permeability of the blood-brain barrier (BBB), may explain the excessive central nervous system (CNS) sensitivity that patients with FHF have to drugs (52,54).

Hemorrhage

Hemorrhage may occur spontaneously in <10% of patients with FHF, and is located mainly in the digestive tract and at the site of insertion of intravascular catheters. Hemorrhage may be associated with disseminated intravascular coagulopathy (22,44).

Renal Failure

Renal failure may be secondary to hypovolemia, acute tubular necrosis, or a functional renal failure, as in hepatorenal syndrome. Hepatorenal syndrome, defined as a progressive renal insufficiency in patients with liver disease, is characterized by a

TABLE 88.5

PREOPERATIVE AND EARLY POSTOPERATIVE COMPLICATIONS OF FULMINANT HEPATIC FAILURE

Preoperative	Postoperative
Cerebral edema	Cerebral edema
Intracranial hypertension	Intracranial hypertension
Circulatory collapse	Hypovolemia, hemorrhage
Dysrhythmia	Myocardial dysfunction
Hypoxemia, ARDS	Hypoxemia, ALI-VILI, ARDS
Renal failure	Renal failure
Hemostasis disorders	Anemia, thrombocytopenia, leucopenia
Disseminated intravascular coagulopathy	Hemostasis disorders
Metabolic and electrolyte disorders (hypoglycemia, hypokalemia, hyponatremia, hypophosphatemia, hypomagnesemia), lactic acidosis, hyperammonemia, kernicterus	Disseminated intravascular disorders, electrolyte disorders
Bleeding disorders (gastrointestinal, cerebral)	Abdominal compartment syndrome, acute pancreatitis, bleeding disorders, hemorrhage (abdominal), primary graft nonfunction, graft vascular anastomosis stenosis/thrombosis, acute graft rejection
Bacterial sepsis	Bacterial and fungal sepsis

ARDS, acute respiratory distress syndrome; ALI, acute lung injury; VILI, ventilator-induced lung injury low urine sodium output and elevated urinary-to-plasma ratios for creatinine and osmolarity. In patients with FHF, type 1 hepatorenal syndrome is found and defined as a rapid and progressive renal impairment. The pathogenesis is poorly understood; however, it is characterized by renal cortical vasoconstriction and corticomedullary redistribution of renal blood flow. Recognized risk factors are low mean arterial blood pressure and dilutional hyponatremia. Hepatorenal syndrome may be precipitated after digestive bleeding, septicemia, and dehydration. Nephrotoxic drugs such as aminoglycosides should be avoided. Tubular nephropathy is frequently observed and results in low blood phosphate, magnesium, and potassium.

Cardiocirculatory and Pulmonary Disorders

Pulmonary edema is an underestimated complication of FHF and occurs in up to 35% of patients. Causes may be related to the development of central neurogenic pulmonary edema coupled with fluid overload (syndrome of inappropriate antidiuretic hormone, hyperaldosteronism). In addition, ventilation-perfusion mismatch (loss of vasoconstrictive hypoxia mechanism due to circulating vasodilatory substances) occurs and results in severe refractory hypoxemia. The hemodynamic profile of FHF patients is characterized by cardiac hyperkinesia with elevated cardiac indices and low systemic vascular resistances (41). Adrenal insufficiency is frequently found in adults with FHF (up to 68% of cases) and is associated with hemodynamic instability (31). Dysrhythmias, such as sinus tachycardia, ectopic rhythms, and atrioventricular conduction block, are less frequent in children than in adults and are usually associated with electrolyte abnormalities.

Systemic Inflammatory Response Syndrome and Sepsis

A systemic inflammatory response syndrome is observed in 57% of adults with FHF, 68% of whom will develop secondary sepsis (57). Severity of systemic inflammatory response syndrome may be correlated with progression of hepatic encephalopathy, development of respiratory failure, disseminated intravascular coagulopathy, renal failure, acute pancreatitis, and multiorgan failure. Risk of developing sepsis in the course of FHF is elevated, which may be related to a decreased immune response to pathogens and may be aggravated by invasive procedures inherent in the critically ill condition. Sepsis was shown to aggravate and worsen the overall prognosis of patients with FHF, and may participate in a quarter of all deaths following FHF. Incriminated pathogens are gram-negative bacteria, cutaneous bacteria, and fungi (which may reach 13%–32% of all infections).

Metabolic Disorders

Severe hypoglycemia frequently occurs in FHF patients as a result of impaired glycogen storage, decreased gluconeogenesis, hyperinsulinism (decreased insulin degradation and increased insulin resistance), and increased glucose use (anaerobic metabolism) and should be recognized early. Fat and protein stores are used, leading to breakdown of muscle and adipose tissue. Glucagon and growth hormone levels are increased, which further increases catabolism. It has been shown that energy expenditure in FHF is elevated. Electrolyte abnormalities, such as hyponatremia, hypokalemia, hypophosphatemia, and hypomagnesemia, can be found in patients with FHF. Kernicterus may precipitate hepatic encephalopathy and appear if

plasma direct bilirubin is >26 mg/dL, especially if BBB permeability is increased (acidosis, hypoxemia). Kernicterus can typically occur in cases of fulminant Wilson disease, with which hemolytic anemia is associated (40,53).

Therapy

Management of FHF should be performed in an ICU within a liver transplantation center, where continuous monitoring and multidisciplinary expertise are available. Patients should be admitted to the ICU if they show signs of clinical or electric hepatic encephalopathy, if factor V activity decreases below 50%, PT index decreases to <50% (PT index = standard PT/observed PT × 100), and/or if significant lactic acidosis (>2.0 mEq/L), and/or renal failure, and/or intractable hypoglycemia occur. Because patients with FHF can deteriorate rapidly, transportation must include (a) appropriate staff that is qualified in advanced airway management, (b) cardiac and respiratory monitoring, and (c) sufficient equipment to initiate new treatment during transfer and to manage airway maintenance, circulatory compromise, or cerebral edema. Because the deterioration may be very rapid, families require early support and should be informed of the severity, prognosis, and therapeutic alternatives, especially liver transplantation, when available.

Medical

General Supportive Care. The mainstay of medical care is to minimize the effect of FHF complications and to limit additional morbidity. Key to managing patients with FHF is avoidance of administering drugs that have no proven beneficial effect. It is essential to understand that pharmacodynamic processes and drug kinetics are modified during FHF and therefore toxic effects, especially on the CNS, as well as systemically, could occur. In addition, in some conditions, such in hepatitis A and hepatitis B infection, community healthcare measures are required.

Specific Therapies. Some causes of FHF, such as galactosemia, fructosemia, tyrosinemia, hemochromatosis, ornithine transcarbamylase defect, Wilson disease, herpetic FHF, acetaminophen or mushroom intoxications, and autoimmune FHF, may respond to a specific therapy (**Table 88.6**).

In the infant, congenital galactosemia and hereditary fructose intolerance can lead to FHF that is reversible within a week if galactose and fructose are removed from the diet. Acute hepatic manifestations of hereditary tyrosinemia can occur early in life and are usually triggered by infection. Although a low-tyrosine diet does not usually reverse FHF, use of nitisinone or NTBC [2-(2-nitro-4-trifluoromethylbenzoil)-1, 3 cyclohexanedione], an inhibitor of the enzyme 4-hydroxyphenylpyruvate dioxygenase, is recommended. NTBC prevents the formation of fumarylacetoacetate from tyrosine—the metabolite toxic to hepatocytes. Results from an international study showed a dramatic improvement in overall survival for patients with hereditary tyrosinemia type I (34). Neonatal hemochromatosis treatment is based on prenatal diagnosis, iron chelation, and aggressive antioxidative drug delivery. A few patients survived under this regimen and underwent transplantation when they were older. However, successful liver transplantation is rare in this disease. The greatest

TABLE 88.6

RECOMMENDED SPECIFIC THERAPIES

Cause	Treatment	Quality of evidence
Hereditary tyrosinemia	Nitisinone (NTBC or 2-(2-nitro-4-trifluoromethylbenzoyl)-1,3-cyclohexanedione) 1 mg/kg/day orally in 2 doses	II-1
Neonatal hemochromatosis	Deferoxamine 30 mg/kg/day IV in 3 doses Selenium 2–3 mcg/kg/day IV N-acetyl-cysteine 140 mg/kg, then 70 mg/kg orally or IV α-tocopherol polyethylene glycol succinate 20 UI/kg/day orally	II-3/III
Herpetic hepatitis	Acyclovir 150 mg/m²/day IV	I
Acetaminophen poisoning	Activated charcoal 1 g/kg orally N-acetylcysteine 150 mg/kg IV in 15 min, then maintenance dose 50 mg/kg over 4 hrs, followed by 100 mg/kg administered over 16 hrs	I II-1
Mushroom poisoning	Penicillin G 300,000–1 million units/kg/day IV Silymarin 30–40 mg/kg/day IV or orally	II-3

Quality of evidence: I, randomized, controlled trials; II-1, controlled trials without randomization, II-2, cohort or case-controlled analytic study; II-3, multiple time series, dramatic uncontrolled experiments; III, expert opinions

predictor for survival is for the infant to be born at, or immediately transferred to, an institution that performs neonatal liver transplants. Implementation of a low-protein diet is the therapy for ornithine transcarbamylase deficiency and can limit neurologic symptoms. However, in some cases, whole-liver transplantation will be required.

Fulminant Wilson disease is considered to be uniformly lethal without transplantation. Its initial treatment is directed toward lowering serum copper and, therefore, limiting further hemolysis; therapy includes albumin dialysis, continuous hemofiltration, plasmapheresis, or plasma exchange. Initiation of treatment with penicillamine is not recommended in FHF, due to the risk of hypersensitivity to this drug (56).

Although rare, herpetic FHF is devastating and is rapidly lethal unless acyclovir is used. Acyclovir should be started preventively in all newborns with FHF, as delayed initiation could be lethal.

Acetaminophen is a dose-related hepatotoxin, with most ingestions that exceed 150 mg/kg leading to FHF. An acetaminophen toxicity nomogram (**Fig. 88.1**) may aid in determining the likelihood of serious liver damage after acute intoxication, but it cannot exclude toxicity due to prolonged administration or in fasting patients. Therefore, if acetaminophen intoxication is suspected, specific therapy should be started without delay. If acetaminophen ingestion is known or suspected to have occurred within a few hours (up to 4 hrs), activated charcoal may be useful for gastrointestinal decontamination. Oral N-acetylcysteine efficiency is not precluded by previous charcoal administration, although the IV route is preferred in patients with FHF and possibly altered mental status or gastrointestinal bleeding (42,53). N-acetylcysteine should be given as soon as possible and may still be useful 48 hrs after ingestion.

If early enough, gastric lavage and activated charcoal administration should be performed in cases of suspected mushroom poisoning. Penicillin G and silibinin (silymarin) are the accepted antidotes. Based on a few case reports,

N-acetylcysteine is sometimes administered with penicillin G and silibinin, the two previously mentioned antidotes. However, mushroom poisoning still has a low transplant-free rate of survival.

Cerebral Edema. Cerebral edema and, ultimately, intracranial hypertension should be aggressively treated. Some interventions are supported by more evidence than others, and no

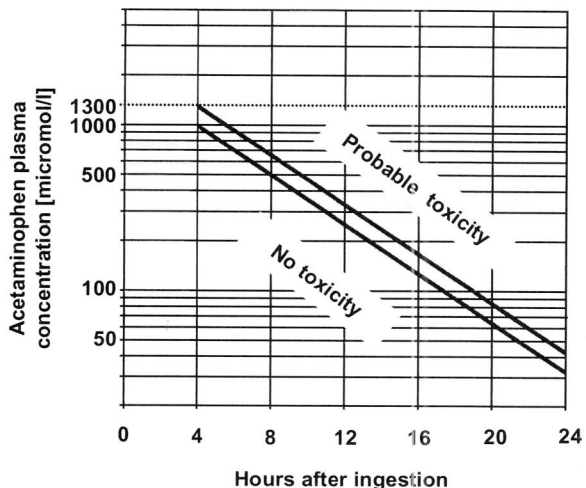

FIGURE 88.1. Acetaminophen intoxication nomogram. The time coordinates refer to time of ingestion. Blood level drawn before 4 hrs may not represent peak value. The graph should be used only in relation to a single, acute ingestion. The lower solid line, 25% below the standard nomogram, is included to allow for possible errors in acetaminophen plasma assays and estimated time from ingestion. Acetaminophen concentration conversion: 1 mg/L = 6.6 mcmol/L. Adapted from Rumack BH. Acetaminophen overdose in young children. Treatment and effects of alcohol and other additional ingestants in 417 cases. *Am J Dis Child* 1984;138:428–33.

uniform protocol has been established. The first line of treatment is to minimize aggravating conditions. Therefore, any precipitating events that can result in hyperammonemia should be avoided. Treatment should include (a) lowering endogenous nitrogen intake (by limiting bleeding and infection and preventing slowed intestinal transit) or exogenous nitrogen intake (by keeping protein delivery below 0.5 g/kg/day and avoiding unjustified fresh frozen plasma administration); and (b) administration of oral or rectal lactulose (10–15 mL/kg, titrated to result in 2–4 daily soft stools), an osmotic cathartic nonabsorbable disaccharide. Lactulose administration is associated with a small increase in survival time, without effect on overall outcome. It lowers colonic pH as a result of production of organic acids by bacterial fermentation, which is hostile to the survival of urease-producing intestinal bacteria. Moreover, the acidic lumen will decrease ammonia absorption by nonionic diffusion and will extract ammonia from the blood to the lumen. However, as hyperammonemia is recognized as a key pathogenic element of cerebral edema (12,15,53), use of lactulose is recommended; concern has been raised about increasing bowel distension during a subsequent transplant procedure. Neomycin is not recommended and should not be used, as it may precipitate renal failure and has not shown a benefit when combined with lactulose (16). Ornithine aspartate and sodium benzoate have been proposed to decrease serum ammonia, as in Reye syndrome and in urea cycle defects, but hemofiltration remains the main treatment of acute hyperammonemia (20,39,67). It is important to consider that minimizing neurosensory and painful stimulation (quiet and darkened room, limited nasopharyngeal aspiration) may help in controlling intracranial pressure (ICP) outburst.

No consensus exists on the use of invasive ICP monitoring. The ultimate goal of this technique is to maintain adequate cerebral perfusion pressure, which may be particularly critical during the anhepatic phase of liver transplantation. However, an effect on mortality has never been shown. The bleeding risk is higher with subdural or intraparenchymal catheter use than with an epidural catheter. In the US, it is estimated that slightly more than half of the adult centers use ICP monitors. Such noninvasive methods as transcranial arterial Doppler monitoring are preferred and certainly will be more widely used in the future (53).

In patients with signs (decerebrate posturing, pupillary abnormalities) or measured intracranial hypertension, treatment with mannitol (0.25–0.5 g/kg bolus) is recommended. This dose can be repeated, provided that serum osmolality does not exceed 320 mOsm/L. However, prophylactic use of mannitol is not recommended. Hyperventilation to reduce $PaCO_2$ to 30 mm Hg is known to quickly lower ICP via decreasing cerebral blood flow and concomitant oxygen delivery and, in patients with FHF, to restore loss of cerebral blood flow autoregulation (65). However, in a randomized trial, prophylactic moderate hyperventilation in patients with FHF did not change the outcome (26). Therefore, besides temporary hyperventilation in an attempt to lower ICP in impending herniation, prolonged hyperventilation is not recommended. A controlled trial of hypertonic sodium chloride use in FHF, with a target plasma natremia of 145–155 mEq/L, was shown to prevent increases in ICP but did not affect mortality. Barbiturate use (thiopental, pentobarbital) may be considered when severe intracranial hypertension does not respond to other therapies; it has been shown to effectively decrease ICP (28). However,

systemic hypotension should be anticipated following barbiturate administration and treated with vasopressors. Moderate hypothermia (32–34°C) has been shown to prevent the development of brain edema in a FHF animal model. Moderate hypothermia prevents increases in ICP during liver transplantation for FHF (37). In addition, in a report of 14 adults with FHF and uncontrolled ICP who awaited liver transplantation, a moderate hypothermia allowed control of the ICP and successfully bridged 13 patients to liver transplantation (38). Corticosteroids and flumazenil are not recommended. Although no controlled data are available, the use of indomethacin and extracorporeal liver-assist devices may soon join the therapeutic arsenal to treat cerebral edema and hepatic encephalopathy (discussed in the section Liver Support Devices).

Hemorrhage and Digestive Tract Bleeding. In the absence of bleeding, it is not recommended to correct homeostasis, because doing so will interfere with the evaluation of liver function (factor V activity, PT). An exception would be if an invasive procedure is planned, such as placement of a central venous catheter. In these cases, procedures can be performed under cover of platelet or administration of activated recombinant factor VII if profound thrombopenia ($<10,000/mm^3$) is observed. Activated recombinant factor VII induces hemostasis at the site of injury independent of the presence of factor VIII or factor IX by forming complexes with exposed tissue factor. It is recommended for the treatment of bleeding episodes and for the prevention of bleeding in patients with congenital factor VII deficiency who are undergoing surgery or an invasive procedure. The recommended dosage is 15–30 mcg/kg every 4–6 hrs until hemostasis is achieved. A nonrandomized trial of 15 patients with FHF showed an effective temporary correction of coagulopathy when activated recombinant factor VII was used in association with fresh frozen plasma, thereby facilitating the invasive procedure (60). Administration of fresh frozen plasma is hampered by the risk of volume and protein overload and should be thoughtfully evaluated. Vitamin K is routinely administered intravenously. Patients with FHF are at risk for gastrointestinal bleeding. Histamine-2 receptor blockers should be avoided because of their effect on the CNS. Sucralfate is therefore preferred. No study has evaluated proton-pump inhibitors for gastrointestinal bleeding prophylaxis in FHF patients.

Renal Failure. Acute renal failure is frequent in FHF. Every effort should be made to protect renal function by maintaining adequate renal perfusion and avoiding nephrotoxic drugs. If renal failure occurs, dialysis should not be delayed. Continuous, rather than discontinuous, renal replacement therapy is preferred. If dialysis is used, hypophosphatemia and hypomagnesemia may be precipitated. Evidence is limited to support the potential utility of N-acetylcysteine in improving renal function as part of the management of FHF. Use of terlipressin, for type I hepatorenal syndrome, even at a low dose, is not recommended due to the risk of increased cerebral blood flow, hyperemia, and intracranial hypertension (61). Hepatorenal syndrome will reverse in most cases after liver transplantation.

Cardiopulmonary Failure. Hypovolemia may be present at admission, but fluid resuscitation should be monitored carefully in regard to volume overload, especially if renal failure occurs. Vasoplegia will generally respond to α-adrenergic agents that should be used as a first-line drug for hypotension once intravascular volume has been restored. As adrenal insufficiency can occur in FHF, hydrocortisone may be beneficial if hemodynamic instability occurs (31). Although myocardial dysfunction is unusual, echocardiographic examination may help to appreciate pulmonary pressure, preload condition, and contractility. Respiratory failure, especially severe hypoxemia, may occur and require mechanical ventilation. Patients with grade III or IV encephalopathy may require secured airways. Noninvasive ventilation (bilevel positive airway pressure) is almost never indicated because of the need for airway protection.

Metabolic Disorders. Continuous glucose administration (frequently up to 1 g/kg/hr) is necessary and often requires a central venous line to deliver high-concentration dextrose in a smaller volume. Phosphate, magnesium, and potassium supplementation is common. Enteral nutrition (gastric, duodenal) is recommended (stress ulcer prevention) and should be initiated early. Protein intake should be limited to 0.5 g/kg/day. Finally, branched-chain amino acids are not recommended.

Liver Support Devices

Liver support devices have been developed for more than 40 years to circumvent the lack of efficient treatment for FHF (68). The latest generation of liver support techniques can be divided into ex vivo whole-organ perfusion (animal or human), bioartificial liver support using hepatocytes, "detoxification" methods, or a combination of these techniques.

Ex vivo whole-organ perfusion has been used by a number of centers, but no improvement in survival has been found. Results of auxiliary liver transplantation for FHF differ significantly between centers, and this procedure is not recommended. Bioartificial liver support incorporates hepatocytes in hollow fibers through which patient blood is filtrated. These systems are either combined with nonbiologic techniques (HepatAssist, MELS) or not (BLSS, Liverx2000, AMC-BAL). Preliminary studies failed to show improved survival. A multicentered, randomized trial that used a HepatAssist device with porcine hepatocytes demonstrated an improvement in patients with FHF of known etiology but not in patients with primary graft dysfunction (21).

Among the nonbiologic detoxification systems, the principal systems are the BioLogicDTBF system (hemodiafiltration associated with high-volume plasma exchange) and albumin dialysis. The molecular absorbent recirculating system (MARS) is currently the most widely used nonbiologic liver support system. In MARS, blood is dialyzed against albumin in a three-step process (hemodialysis circuit, activated charcoal, and anion-exchange membrane) aimed at removing albumin-bound toxins, such as fatty acids, bile acids, and bilirubin. MARS was shown to improve liver function and hepatic encephalopathy in patients with acute decompensation of chronic liver disease and to improve renal function in patients with hepatorenal syndrome (33). Hundreds of patients with FHF have been treated with MARS, with decreases in hepatic encephalopathy and plasma bilirubin levels. However, the plasma ammonia level is less reduced than with high-performance hemofiltration. Of significant interest is that half of the patients with primary graft dysfunction survived without transplantation, although >80% were placed on the list for retransplantation (64). Adult randomized trials on MARS are ongoing. Published experience with MARS and other liver support devices in children is anec-

dotal (62). However, a controlled trial conducted to evaluate the hemodynamic consequences of MARS suggested that the vasoplegic hemodynamic status found during FHF could be reversed by dialysis systems (59). Other important outcomes, such as hemodynamic stabilization and delay between registration and liver transplantation while being on assistance, should also be considered (72). In the authors' practice, high-flow venovenous hemofiltration has replaced MARS because of convincing results obtained in ammonia detoxification, neurologic improvement, electrolyte homeostasis, and hemodynamic stabilization in all pediatric patients, including newborns. It is performed as soon as patients display severe metabolic disturbance (metabolic acidosis, lactic acidosis, hyperammonemia), vasoplegic hemodynamic profile, and hepatic encephalopathy higher than grade II irrespective of the renal function.

Of the 8 published controlled trials that evaluated liver support devices, none showed that liver support devices significantly reduced mortality when compared to standard medical therapy (21,32,72). Controlled data are mandatory before liver support devices can be recommended outside of clinical trials. However, data do suggest that liver support devices may be efficient in other outcomes, such as a bridge to liver transplantation, by controlling cerebral edema and stabilizing hemodynamics, thereby providing time to evaluate spontaneous recovery capacity of the failing liver.

Emergency Liver Transplantation and Outcome

Emergency liver transplantation remains the only treatment of end-stage FHF in children. At our center, liver transplantation is performed in 45% of children admitted for FHF (**Table 88.7**). Transplantation decisions rely on the cause and severity of FHF and the potentialities of spontaneous liver regeneration and the comorbidities, especially the development of permanent neurologic damage. In adults, the most commonly used transplantation criteria are those developed at King's College in London and Beaujon's Hospital in Paris (5,49). However, these criteria fail to be adequate in children, mainly due to a very weak negative predictive value (69). In children, etiology is a critical determinant of outcome. Fulminant Wilson disease and undetermined FHF carry the worst prognosis and require emergency liver transplantation, whereas hepatitis A-induced and acetaminophen-induced FHF have significant spontaneous recovery without transplantation. Other FHF causes have variable outcome, mainly determined by the severity of neurologic involvement. In a large study that analyzed 198 patients with FHF secondary to mushroom poisoning, fatal outcome was accurately predicted if prothrombin index of <25% was combined with a serum creatinine of >1.2 mg/dL from day 3 after intoxication (29). In a prospective trial that involved 81 children with FHF, peak values of total bilirubin, PT, and ammonia were the most predictive of death or a need for liver transplantation, and a simple risk-staging system was developed (45). A large, retrospective study of 94 children with FHF showed that total bilirubin and PT were the factors that predicted outcome (11). As in adult studies that showed that severity of associated organ dysfunction correlated with hepatic encephalopathy and outcome (57,58), the pediatric risk of mortality (PRISM) score was shown to reflect severity of FHF in children (9,71). Although scoring systems may be relevant for epidemiologic purposes, the decision to transplant depends on dynamic clinical and biochemical assessment of patient condition.

TABLE 88.7

OUTCOME OF PEDIATRIC FULMINANT HEPATIC FAILURE AT
BICÊTRE HOSPITAL (1986–2006)

	Number Died/Total Number (%)		
	<1 year old	>1 year old	Total
No criteria for ELT	6/30 (20%)	1/38 (3%)	7/68 (11%)
ELT contraindicated	25/25 (100%)	18/18 (100%)	43/43 (100%)
ELT performed	11/27 (41%)	20/62 (32%)	31/89 (34%)
Overall death	42/82 (51%)	39/118 (33%)	81/200 (40%)

ELT, emergency liver transplantation

Emergency liver transplantation should be discussed if hepatic encephalopathy is higher than grade II associated with factor V activity of <20% or a prothrombin index of <20% (PT index = standard PT/observed PT × 100). These levels should be adjusted for the age of the patient (in infants, encephalopathy could be unapparent). Other criteria that suggest emergency liver transplantation include a rapid decrease in liver size, seizures, ascites, hepatorenal syndrome, a fibrinogen level of <1 g/L, bilirubinemia of >23 mg/dL, worsening lactic acidosis, and hyperammonemia of >150 mmol/L.

Liver transplantation may be contraindicated in 11%–20% of cases (44). For instance, malignant disease, such as leukemia, lymphoproliferative syndrome, lymphohistiocytosis, and some mitochondrial respiratory chain disorders, as well as the patient's end-stage intracranial hypertension or uncontrolled multiorgan failure, are contraindications to transplantation due to poor outcome.

Postoperative Care

Neurologic awakening from coma is the key element in early postoperative evaluation, as it determines the success of overall management (Table 88.5). Although the postoperative period is hallmarked by the restoration of liver function and neurologic improvement, postoperative care of patients with FHF is marked by an elevated incidence of associated multiorgan failure. Early circulatory resuscitation may be required due to bleeding. It is not unusual to have depressed cardiac outflow associated with inadequate preload. Intra-abdominal pressure (IAP) monitoring is required, especially in small receiver-to-donor weight ratio, because intra-abdominal hypertension and/or abdominal compartment syndrome will precipitate vascular thrombosis, liver hypoperfusion, and graft failure. At our institution, IAP monitoring is measured by the means of an intravesical Foley catheter connected through the culture-aspiration port (18-gauge plastic IV infusion catheter) to two three-way stopcocks and a pressure transducer. Before measuring IAP, 1 mL/kg of saline solution is injected into the bladder. Interpretation of IAP measures is based on two important criteria: kinetics of IAP measures and occurrence and/or development of organ failure (oliguria, lactic acidosis, respiratory restrictive syndrome) related to increased IAP. Acute pancreatitis was shown to occur after transplantation in patients with FHF and resulted in a bad prognosis (73). Susceptibility to infection (bacterial, fungal) may lead to sepsis or septic shock. Of significance is posttransplantation generalized edema mainly due to

severe capillary leak syndrome that may be secondary to FHF and the surgical procedure. High ventilatory pressure may alter respiratory function and gas exchange and decrease abdominal wall compliance, increasing intra-abdominal pressure and potentially affecting graft perfusion. Postoperative hemofiltration may effectively control water balance and serve to supplement temporary renal failure. Electrolyte homeostasis is particularly important, as hypophosphatemia may interfere with extubation success.

Outcome

FHF prognosis has significantly improved since the performance of the initial series of emergency liver transplantations, shifting from an overall survival of 15% to >60% (51). In children, published experience of emergency liver transplantation in the setting of FHF shows long-term survival ranging from 52% in infants to 79% in older children (10,14,22,25,27,44,75). In a multicentered observational study of 141 children transplanted for FHF, pretransplant factors associated with poor postoperative outcome were a grade IV encephalopathy, children <1 year of age, and dialysis (4).

TRANSPLANTATION

Historical Perspective

Successful liver transplantation was first attempted in the early 1960s in Paris, Boston, and Denver, and the first successful liver transplantation in a child occurred in 1967. However, the unpredictability of immunosuppression and difficulty of this new surgical procedure led to a 1-year survival rate of only 30% until the use of cyclosporine was introduced in 1978. With that innovation, liver transplantation drastically changed the outcome of FHF and end-stage chronic liver disease and became the mainstay of treatment for these ailments. However, results in small pediatric patients were hampered by shortage of sized-match organs as well as technical problems associated with reconstruction of hepatic vasculature. During the last 15 years, considerable improvements have occurred in both pediatric graft and patient survival that were related to successful harvesting techniques, the introduction of the University of Wisconsin preservation solution, and the development of techniques that allow for the preparation of reduced-size allografts. The anatomic basis of splitting a cadaver organ to transplant two recipients comes from the work of Couinaud, who described the segmental division of the liver in 1957 (17). Bismuth reported the first successful split-liver transplantations in 1989 (7). In the 1990s, experience with adult-to-child split-liver transplantation was increasingly reported with an elevated complication rate (30%), with biliary problems being the most common.

Causes for Liver Transplantation

The most common indication for pediatric liver transplantation is biliary atresia (50%) and, more specifically, patients with progressive disease despite the Kasai procedure. Infants with dysfunctional portoenterostomies may develop recurrent bacterial cholangitis, ascites, portal hypertension, hypersplenism, gastrointestinal bleeding (varices), and liver failure. Other cholestatic conditions, such as Alagille syndrome and progressive familial intrahepatic cholestasis (Byler syndrome), represent 25% of all transplantations, whereas metabolic disease, such as α-1 antitrypsin deficiency, Wilson disease, tyrosinemia, type IV glycogen storage disease, Crigler-Najjar syndrome, inborn errors of bile acid synthesis, and urea cycle defects, account for <10% (36,46) (**Table 88.8**).

Technical Aspects

The limited number of donor organs available for pediatric transplant recipients and the elevated vascular complications associated with whole-organ transplantation using infant donor organs led to the development of reduced-size transplantation. Reduced-size liver graft is most often limited to the left anatomic lobe (segments II, III, IV) or left lateral segment (segments II and III) of the donor liver (**Fig. 88.2**). The development of this procedure improved organ availability for pediatric recipients, especially for the youngest patients. Split-liver trans-

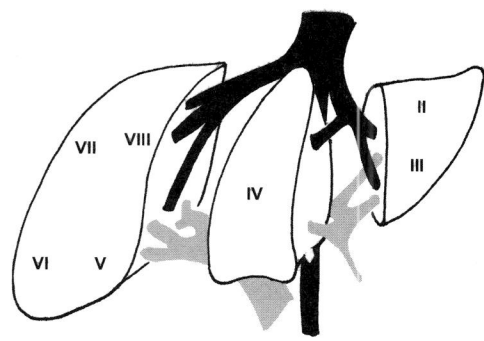

FIGURE 88.2. Couinaud's segmental classification of the liver. Liver segments are determined by portal (**gray**) and hepatic veins (**black**). Adapted from Couinaud C. *Le Foie. Etudes Anatomiques et Chirurgicales.* Paris, Masson, 1957.

plantation further improved organ availability by allowing two functional allografts. To date, whole-organ transplantation is used when a cadaveric donor has an approximate recipient size. When using whole-organ grafts, the donor weight should range 15% above or below that of the recipient. Whereas bigger grafts may result in difficulties during abdominal closure and subsequent risk of abdominal compartment syndrome, undersized grafts are associated with significant risk of hemorrhagic necrosis due to excessive portal flow. Left lateral segments and split livers provide the majority of grafts in infants, whereas left or right lobes are used in older recipients. Estimates of donor graft-to-recipient body weight ratio (optimal between 1.5%–2%, or 150–200 g for a recipient who weighs 10 kg) appear to be the most accurate predictor of adequate graft volume. Because split-liver transplantation may require a prolonged time, selection of donor patients is critical. Hemodynamic stability with limited vasopressor administration is essential.

The operative procedure is marked by several important issues that should be recognized because they may influence postoperative management. Severe portal hypertension may result in critical bleeding during removal of the diseased liver.

TABLE 88.8

PEDIATRIC LIVER TRANSPLANTATION: CAUSES AND OUTCOMES

	Diagnosis	Bicêtre Hospital (1986–2002)	Pittsburgh Children's Hospital[a] (1981–1998)	SPLIT Registry[b] (1995–2002)
Number of patients		568	808	1092
Number of liver transplantations		648	1113	NA
	Biliary atresia	53%	51%	42%
	Chronic cholestasis	25%	11%	14%
	Metabolic disease	8%	15%	12%
	Fulminant hepatic failure	11%	6%	13%
	Others causes	3%	13%	10%
Liver graft survival		65%[†]	52%[†]	75%[‡]
Patient survival		78%[†]	69%[†]	83%[‡]

SPLIT, Studies of pediatric liver transplantation, NA, not available; [†]15-year outcome; [‡]3-year outcome
[a]Jain A, Mazariegos G, Kashyap R, et al. Pediatric liver transplantation. A single-center experience spanning 20 years. *Transplantation* 2002;73:941–7.
[b]Martin SR, Atkison P, Anand R, et al. Studies of pediatric liver transplantation 2002: Patient and graft survival and rejection in pediatric recipients of a first liver transplant in the United States and Canada. *Pediatr Transplant* 2004;8:273–83.

Bleeding may occur during dissection of extensive adherences, such as in children with biliary atresia who underwent previous portoenterostomy surgeries. Assessment of vascular anastomosis is essential; for example, portal anastomosis in children with biliary atresia may be difficult, as portal vessels are frequently hypoplastic. Arterial anastomosis may preclude important dissection along the infrarenal aorta, with subsequent risk of traumatic lesions to the pancreas. The appearance of the liver graft after unclamping may be informative regarding the quality of the graft. Finally, abdominal closure should be performed in a manner to avoid increased IAP.

Postoperative Care and Complications

Immunosuppressive therapy has undergone many changes. Use of calcineurin inhibitors, cyclosporine, sirolimus, tacrolimus, and chimeric humanized monoclonal antibodies (basiliximab and daclizumab) directed at the IL-2 receptor, has drastically improved graft survival. Immunosuppressive protocols vary among centers. However, the degree of immunosuppression will determine the risk of rejection, as well as hematologic, renal, and neurologic complications of overdosage. Daily determination of calcineurin blood level is essential because it will help in dosing immunosuppressive therapy. Multiple commonly used medications interact with calcineurin inhibitor pharmacokinetics, as displayed in **Table 88.9**.

One of the most feared postoperative complications is primary graft nonfunction, which requires emergency retransplantation. It usually occurs within the first 48 hrs, and diagnosis is based on absence of neurologic awakening, hepatic encephalopathy, hemorrhagic diathesis, increasing liver enzymes, lactic acidosis, and vasoplegic shock. In cases of split-liver transplant, information regarding the other liver recipient's postoperative course may help in diagnosing primary graft nonfunction.

Vascular thrombosis is the main postoperative complication that will cause graft loss. Hepatic artery thrombosis occurs in children (10%) three times more frequently than in adults, usually within the first 30 days after transplantation (36,46). Hepatic artery thrombosis can occur with various clinical presentations, which may include fulminant allograft failure, biliary obstruction, or sepsis. Successful thrombectomy is possible if hepatic artery thrombosis diagnosis is made before graft necrosis occurs. Biliary complications are particularly frequent

after hepatic artery thrombosis because the hepatic artery offers most of the vascularization to the bile duct. Early portal vein thrombosis occurs usually within the first week (median, 2 days) after transplantation and requires emergency thrombectomy in most cases (13,36,46). Children with biliary atresia have an increased risk of portal vein thrombosis (20%), and deficiencies of anticoagulant proteins (proteins C and S and antithrombin III) should be excluded (13). A meta-analysis regrouping 1257 pediatric liver transplantations showed an overall risk of portal thrombosis of 2.2% in groups using postoperative aspirin (with or without dipyridamole), compared to 8% when no antiaggregative therapy were given (13). Refractory ascites may indicate a portal thrombosis or stenosis or stenosis of suprahepatic veins. As a minor vascular gradient may precipitate extensive ascites, investigational technical limits as well as high intravascular volume may mask a small but significant vascular stenosis, and this should be considered when vascular investigations of refractory ascites are performed.

Although biliary complications are frequent in pediatric recipients (anastomosis stricture, biliary sludge, and recurrent cholangitis), they do not significantly affect immediate postoperative care. Rising serum bilirubin and alkaline phosphatase may signify acute rejection, although biliary expression of rejection is usually a late event. Despite improved immunosuppressive regimens, acute rejection remains a problem after liver transplantation. Viral infection (CMV, EBV, and adenovirus) should be considered, as it may precipitate liver rejection. Liver biopsy is the key for diagnosis, and histologic findings of acute rejection are a mixed portal inflammatory infiltrate, predominantly mononuclear cells associated with portal and central vein endotheliitis, and bile duct damage. The primary treatment is a short course of high-dose methylprednisolone, which is effective in treating rejection in 80% of cases (20).

Infection is the most common source of morbidity and mortality following transplantation. Patients, due to their immunosuppressed condition, are at risk of developing nosocomial and opportunistic infection. In addition, the patient's preoperative condition may be a risk factor for sepsis. For example, patients with FHF are known to have defective innate immunity, as characterized by hypocomplementemia and phagocytosis alteration, and children with chronic cholestasis have increased risk for bacterial peritonitis and recurrent cholangitis. Bacterial sepsis occurs in the immediate posttransplant period and is more frequently due to gram-negative enteric organisms, *Enterococcus* spp. and *Staphylococcus* spp. Fungal sepsis

---

TABLE 88.9

DRUG INTERACTION WITH CALCINEURIN INHIBITORS

Increase blood level		Decrease blood level	
Increased absorption	Decreased metabolism	Decreased absorption	Increased metabolism
Grapefruit juice	Ketoconazole	Phenytoin	Corticosteroids
Octreotide	Fluconazole	Carbamazepine	
Metoclopramide	Itraconazole	Barbiturates	
	Quinolones	Imipenem	
	Ganciclovir		
	Acyclovir		
	Trimethoprim-sulfamethoxazole		

TABLE 88.10

CAUSES OF RETRANSPLANTATION

	Bicêtre Hospital (1986–2001) ($n = 568$)	Pittsburgh Children's Hospital (1981–1998) ($n = 808$)[a] (52)	SPLIT registry (1995–2002) ($n = 1092$)[b]
# of retransplantation / # of patients (% of all patients)	75/67 (12%)	305/250 (31%)	NA/121 (11%)
Vascular thrombosis	40%	33%	43%
Primary graft nonfunction	28%	17%	25%
Chronic graft rejection	22%	22%	6%
Hyperacute or acute graft rejection	5%	3%	5%
Biliary complications	5%	NA	7%

[a] Jain A, et al. Pediatric liver transplantation. A single-center experience spanning 20 years. *Transplantation* 2002;73:941–7.
[b] Martin SR, et al. Studies of pediatric liver transplantation 2002: Patient and graft survival and rejection in pediatric recipients of a first liver transplant in the United States and Canada. *Pediatr Transplant* 2004;8:273–83.

(*Candida* spp., *Aspergillus* spp.) may occur in the early post-transplant period and hold an elevated mortality if severe infection occurs, making monitoring of colonization index and early treatment mandatory. Frequent postoperative prophylactic regimens include acyclovir, amphotericin B, a β-lactam antibiotic, and trimethoprim-sulfamethoxazole. Although viral and opportunistic infections may occur later after transplantation, EBV, CMV, herpes simplex virus, and adenovirus can cause early infection that must be recognized.

Perioperative trauma may result in digestive perforation in 20% of children with biliary atresia. Acute pancreatitis may occur in <2% of children who undergo liver transplantation but is associated with high mortality (50%) (73). Postoperative cardiopulmonary failure is worth mentioning, as restrictive or obstructive cardiomyopathy (oxalosis, chronic cholestasis) and pulmonary hypertension (hepatopulmonary syndrome, pulmonary vein stenosis in Alagille syndrome) may be encountered.

Results and Outcome

Retransplantation is required in ~11% of children and occurs mainly within the first 30 days following initial transplantation (Table 88.10). Causes of graft failure include vascular thrombosis in ~40% of cases, primary graft nonfunction in 17%–28%, and graft rejection in 11%–27% (36,46).

Although the potential complications are numerous, the overall results of pediatric liver transplantation are good, especially for long-term outcome, as most indications for pediatric liver transplantation do not recur within the transplanted allograft, whereas disease recurrence represents a significant cause of long-term graft loss in adults. Overall survival of children after liver transplantation is 70%–80% in the largest series, and 15-year graft survival is between 52% and 65% (Table 88.8). However, as techniques and patient care improve, actual survival can exceed 85% (46). Although the patient and graft survival are dependent on surgical techniques and patient care, their influence on survival is limited to the initial perioperative period and does not affect long-term outcome. In our experience, posttransplantation survival is lower for FHF (61%) and metabolic disease (61%–53%, depending on age and hepatic lesions), whereas it reaches 90% survival for

Alagille syndrome, α-1-antitrypsin deficiency, and sclerosing cholangitis. Biliary atresia, familial fibrosing cholestasis, and other cholestatic disease have a survival rate of 82%–84%. Early postoperative death is mainly related to sepsis, graft failure, multiorgan failure, and cardiopulmonary and neurologic complications, whereas late mortality is mainly related to sepsis (46). Finally, liver transplantation gives children with a potentially lethal disease an excellent long-term prognosis and quality of life.

CONCLUSIONS AND FUTURE DIRECTIONS

Liver transplantation has drastically changed the prognosis of infants and children with FHF and end-stage liver disease. Thorough knowledge of FHF etiology, pathogenesis, and complications is required to allow efficient management of a complex syndrome. Discussion in this chapter has especially emphasized a rational, therapeutic approach to FHF and its comorbidities, outlining the critical importance of referring infants and children with FHF to centers with high expertise in pediatric liver disease and FHF management. In the future, liver support devices will probably find a position in the therapeutic arsenal against FHF.

KEY POINTS

- Infants and children with FHF should be referred to centers with expertise in pediatric liver disease, as determination of an accurate etiologic diagnosis before encephalopathy occurs is critical.
- Fresh frozen plasma should be avoided as long as no active bleeding is present. It will modify coagulation factors that are important criteria by which to evaluate FHF severity.
- Encephalopathy and coagulation parameter (factor V activity, PT) kinetics are major FHF severity criteria that aid in deciding whether to perform emergency liver transplantation.
- Liver support devices may have found a role in the therapeutic arsenal of FHF treatment; however, its precise indication remains to be determined.

■ Liver transplantation has drastically changed prognosis of pediatric FHF and end-stage liver disease.

References

1. Abdo A, Lopez O, Fernandez A, et al. Transcranial Doppler sonography in fulminant hepatic failure. *Transplant Proc* 2003;35:1859–60.
2. Alper G, Jarjour IT, Reyes JD, et al. Outcome of children with cerebral edema caused by fulminant hepatic failure. *Pediatr Neurol* 1998;18:299–304.
3. Arora NK, Nanda SK, Gulati S, et al. Acute viral hepatitis types E, A, and B singly and in combination in acute liver failure in children in north India. *J Med Virol* 1996;48:215–21.
4. Baliga P, Alvarez S, Lindblad A, et al. Posttransplant survival in pediatric fulminant hepatic failure: The SPLIT experience. *Liver Transpl* 2004;10: 1364–71.
5. Bernuau J, Rueff B, Benhamou JP. Fulminant and subfulminant liver failure: Definitions and causes. *Semin Liver Dis* 1986;6:97–106.
6. Bhaduri BR, Mieli-Vergani G. Fulminant hepatic failure: Pediatric aspects. *Semin Liver Dis* 1996;16:349–55.
7. Bismuth H, Morino M, Castaing D, et al. Emergency orthotopic liver transplantation in two patients using one donor liver. *Br J Surg* 1989;76:722–4.
8. Blei AT. Medical therapy of brain edema in fulminant hepatic failure. *Hepatology* 2000;32:666–9.
9. Carroll CL, Goodman DM, Superina RA, et al. Timed Pediatric Risk of Mortality scores predict outcomes in pediatric liver transplant recipients. *Pediatr Transplant* 2003;7:289–95.
10. Centeno MA, Bes DF, Sasbon JS. Mortality risk factors of a pediatric population with fulminant hepatic failure undergoing orthotopic liver transplantation in a pediatric intensive care unit. *Pediatr Crit Care Med* 2002;3: 227–33.
11. Chan PC, Chen HL, Kong MS, et al. Factors affecting the mortality of pediatric fulminant hepatic failure in relation to hepatitis B virus infection. *J Gastroenterol Hepatol* 2005;20:1223–7.
12. Chan PC, Chen HL, Ni YH, et al. Outcome predictors of fulminant hepatic failure in children. *J Formos Med Assoc* 2004;103:432–6.
13. Chardot C, Herrera JM, Debray D, et al. Portal vein complications after liver transplantation for biliary atresia. *Liver Transpl* 1997;3:351–8.
14. Chen HL, Chang CJ, Kong MS, et al. Pediatric fulminant hepatic failure in endemic areas of hepatitis B infection: 15 years after universal hepatitis B vaccination. *Hepatology* 2004;39:58–63.
15. Clemmesen JO, Larsen FS, Kondrup J, et al. Cerebral herniation in patients with acute liver failure is correlated with arterial ammonia concentration. *Hepatology* 1999;29:648–53.
16. Curioso WH, Monkemuller KE. Neomycin should not be used to treat hepatic encephalopathy. *BMJ*. 2001;323(7306):233.
17. Couinaud C. *Le Foie. Etudes Anatomiques et Chirurgicales*. Paris, Masson, 1957.
18. Debray D, Cullufi P, Devictor D, et al. Liver failure in children with hepatitis A. *Hepatology* 1997;26:1018–22.
19. Debray D, Maggiore G, Girardet JP, et al. Efficacy of cyclosporin A in children with type 2 autoimmune hepatitis. *J Pediatr* 1999;135:111–4.
20. Debray D, Yousef N, Durand P. New management options for end-stage chronic liver disease and acute liver failure: Potential for pediatric patients. *Paediatr Drugs* 2006;8:1–13.
21. Demetriou AA, Brown RS, Jr., Busuttil RW, et al. Prospective, randomized, multicenter, controlled trial of a bioartificial liver in treating acute liver failure. *Ann Surg* 2004;239:660–7; discussion 7–70.
22. Devictor D, Desplanques L, Debray D, et al. Emergency liver transplantation for fulminant liver failure in infants and children. *Hepatology* 1992;16:1156–62.
23. Dhawan A, Taylor RM, Cheeseman P, et al. Wilson's disease in children: 37-year experience and revised King's score for liver transplantation. *Liver Transpl* 2005;11:441–8.
24. Dubern B, Broue P, Dubuisson C, et al. Orthotopic liver transplantation for mitochondrial respiratory chain disorders: A study of 5 children. *Transplantation* 2001;71:633–7.
25. Durand P, Debray D, Mandel R, et al. Acute liver failure in infancy: A 14-year experience of a pediatric liver transplantation center. *J Pediatr* 2001;139:871–6.
26. Ede RJ, Gimson AE, Bihari D, et al. Controlled hyperventilation in the prevention of cerebral oedema in fulminant hepatic failure. *J Hepatol* 1986;2:43–51.
27. Fonseca JC, Souza RA, Brasil LM, et al. Fulminant hepatic failure in children and adolescents in Northern Brazil. *Rev Soc Bras Med Trop* 2004;37:67–9.
28. Forbes A, Alexander GJ, O'Grady JG, et al. Thiopental infusion in the treatment of intracranial hypertension complicating fulminant hepatic failure. *Hepatology* 1989;10:306–10.
29. Ganzert M, Felgenhauer N, Zilker T. Indication of liver transplantation following amatoxin intoxication. *J Hepatol* 2005;42:202–9.
30. Gillis LA, Sokol RJ. Gastrointestinal manifestations of mitochondrial disease. *Gastroenterol Clin North Am* 2003;32:789–817, v.

31. Harry R, Auzinger G, Wendon J. The clinical importance of adrenal insufficiency in acute hepatic dysfunction. *Hepatology* 2002;36:395–402.
32. He JQ, Chen CY, Deng JT, et al. Clinical study on the treatment of fatal hepatitis with artificial liver support system. *Chin Crit Care Med* 2000;12:105–8.
33. Heemann U, Treichel U, Loock J, et al. Albumin dialysis in cirrhosis with superimposed acute liver injury: A prospective, controlled study. *Hepatology* 2002;36:949–58.
34. Holme E, Lindstedt S. Tyrosinaemia type I and NTBC (2-(2-nitro-4-trifluoromethylbenzoyl)-1,3-cyclohexanedione). *J Inherit Metab Dis* 1998;21:507–17.
35. Inderbitzin D, Muggli B, Ringger A, et al. Molecular absorbent recirculating system for the treatment of acute liver failure in surgical patients. *J Gastrointest Surg* 2005;9:1155–61; discussion 1161–2.
36. Jain A, Mazariegos G, Kashyap R, et al. Pediatric liver transplantation. A single-center experience spanning 20 years. *Transplantation* 2002;73:941–7.
37. Jalan R, Olde Damink SW, Deutz NE, et al. Moderate hypothermia prevents cerebral hyperemia and increase in intracranial pressure in patients undergoing liver transplantation for acute liver failure. *Transplantation* 2003;75:2034–9.
38. Jalan R, Olde Damink SWM, Deutz NEP, et al. Moderate hypothermia in patients with acute liver failure and uncontrolled intracranial hypertension. *Gastroenterology* 2004;127:1338–46.
39. Kircheis G, Wettstein M, Dahl S, et al. Clinical efficacy of L-ornithine-L-aspartate in the management of hepatic encephalopathy. *Metab Brain Dis* 2002;17:453–62.
40. Larsen FS. Optimal management of patients with fulminant hepatic failure: Targeting the brain. *Hepatology* 2004;39:299–301.
41. Larsen FS, Strauss G, Knudsen GM, et al. Cerebral perfusion, cardiac output, and arterial pressure in patients with fulminant hepatic failure. *Crit Care Med* 2000;28:996–1000.
42. Larson AM, Polson J, Fontana RJ, et al. Acetaminophen-induced acute liver failure: Results of a United States multicenter, prospective study. *Hepatology* 2005;42:1364–72.
43. Lee WM. Drug-induced hepatotoxicity. *N Engl J Med* 2003;349:474–85.
44. Lee WS, McKiernan P, Kelly DA. Etiology, outcome and prognostic indicators of childhood fulminant hepatic failure in the United Kingdom. *J Pediatr Gastroenterol Nutr* 2005;40:575–81.
45. Liu E, MacKenzie T, Dobyns EL, et al. Characterization of acute liver failure and development of a continuous risk of death staging system in children. *J Hepatol* 2006;44:134–41.
46. Martin SR, Atkison P, Anand R, et al. Studies of pediatric liver transplantation 2002: Patient and graft survival and rejection in pediatric recipients of a first liver transplant in the United States and Canada. *Pediatr Transplant* 2004;8:273–83.
47. McDiarmid SV, Anand R, Lindblad AS. Studies of pediatric liver transplantation: 2002 update. An overview of demographics, indications, timing, and immunosuppressive practices in pediatric liver transplantation in the United States and Canada. *Pediatr Transplant* 2004;8:284–94.
48. Millar AJ, Spearman W, McCulloch M, et al. Liver transplantation for children—the Red Cross Children's Hospital experience. *Pediatr Transplant* 2004;8:136–44.
49. O'Grady JG, Alexander GJ, Hayllar KM, et al. Early indicators of prognosis in fulminant hepatic failure. *Gastroenterology* 1989;97:439–45.
50. O'Grady JG, Schalm SW, Williams R. Acute liver failure: Redefining the syndromes. *Lancet* 1993;342:273–5.
51. Ostapowicz G, Fontana RJ, Schiodt FV, et al. Results of a prospective study of acute liver failure at 17 tertiary care centers in the United States. *Ann Intern Med* 2002;137:947–54.
52. Ott P, Clemmesen O, Larsen FS. Cerebral metabolic disturbances in the brain during acute liver failure: From hyperammonemia to energy failure and proteolysis. *Neurochem Int* 2005;47:13–8.
53. Polson J, Lee WM. AASLD position paper: The management of acute liver failure. *Hepatology* 2005;41:1179–97.
54. Raghavan M, Marik PE. Therapy of intracranial hypertension in patients with fulminant hepatic failure. *Neurocrit Care* 2006;4:179–89.
55. Rivera-Penera T, Gugig R, Davis J, et al. Outcome of acetaminophen overdose in pediatric patients and factors contributing to hepatotoxicity. *J Pediatr* 1997;130:300–4.
56. Roberts EA, Schilsky ML. A practice guideline on Wilson disease. *Hepatology* 2003;37:1475–92.
57. Rolando N, Wade J, Davalos M, et al. The systemic inflammatory response syndrome in acute liver failure. *Hepatology* 2000;32:734–9.
58. Schmidt LE, Larsen FS. Prognostic implications of hyperlactatemia, multiple organ failure, and systemic inflammatory response syndrome in patients with acetaminophen-induced acute liver failure. *Crit Care Med* 2006;34:337–43.
59. Schmidt LE, Wang LP, Hansen BA, et al. Systemic hemodynamic effects of treatment with the molecular adsorbents recirculating system in patients with hyperacute liver failure: A prospective controlled trial. *Liver Transpl* 2003;9:290–7.
60. Shami VM, Caldwell SH, Hespenheide EE, et al. Recombinant activated factor VII for coagulopathy in fulminant hepatic failure compared with conventional therapy. *Liver Transpl* 2003;9:138–43.
61. Shawcross DL, Davies NA, Mookerjee RP, et al. Worsening of cerebral hyperemia by the administration of terlipressin in acute liver failure with severe encephalopathy. *Hepathology* 2004;39:471–5.

62. Singer AL, Olthoff KM, Kim H, et al. Role of plasmapheresis in the management of acute hepatic failure in children. *Ann Surg* 2001;234:418–24.

63. Squires RH, Shneider BL, Bucuvalas J, et al. Acute liver failure in children: The first 348 patients in the pediatric acute liver failure study group. *J Pediatr* 2006;148:652–8.

64. Steiner C, Mitzner S. Experiences with MARS liver support therapy in liver failure: Analysis of 176 patients of the International MARS Registry. *Liver* 2002;22 Suppl 2:20–5.

65. Strauss G, Hansen BA, Knudsen GM, et al. Hyperventilation restores cerebral blood flow autoregulation in patients with acute liver failure. *J Hepatol* 1998;28:199–203.

66. Subcommittee on the National Halothane Study of the Committee on Anesthesia. Summary of the national halothane study. Possible association between halothane anesthesia and postoperative hepatic necrosis. *JAMA* 1966;197(10):775–88.

67. Summar M. Current strategies for the management of neonatal urea cycle disorders. *J Pediatr* 2001;138:S30–9.

68. Tissieres P, Chevret L, Debray D, et al. Fulminant Wilson's disease in children: Appraisal of a critical diagnosis. *Pediatr Crit Care Med* 2003;4:338–43.

69. Tissieres P, Debray D, Dousset B, et al. Are London and Clichy indicators of prognosis accurate in infants and children with fulminant liver failure. [abstract]. *Pediatr Transplant* 1998;2:89.

70. Tissieres P, Devictor D. Drug treatment of encephalopathy associated with fulminant liver failure. *CNS Drugs* 1999;11:335–49.

71. Tissieres P, Prontera W, Chevret L, et al. The pediatric risk of mortality score in infants and children with fulminant liver failure. *Pediatr Transplant* 2003;7:64–8.

72. Tissieres P, Sasbon JS, Devictor D. Liver support for fulminant hepatic failure: Is it time to use the molecular adsorbents recycling system in children? *Pediatr Crit Care Med* 2005;6:585–91.

73. Tissieres P, Simon L, Debray D, et al. Acute pancreatitis after orthotopic liver transplantation in children: Incidence, contributing factors, and outcome. *J Pediatr Gastroenterol Nutr* 1998;26:315–20.

74. Trey C, Davidson CS. The Management of Fulminant Hepatic Failure. In: Popper H, Schaffner F, eds. *Progress in Liver Failure*. New York: Grune and Stratton, 1970;282–98.

75. Uribe M, Buckel E, Ferrario M, et al. Epidemiology and results of liver transplantation for acute liver failure in Chile. *Transplant Proc* 2003;35:2511–2.

CHAPTER 89 ■ INTESTINAL AND MULTIVISCERAL TRANSPLANTATION

GEOFFREY J. BOND • KATHRYN A. FELMET • RONALD JAFFE • KYLE A. SOLTYS • ROBERT H. SQUIRES, JR.
• DOLLY MARTIN • RAKESH SINDHI • KAREEM ABU-ELMAGD • GEORGE V. MAZARIEGOS

Although intestine was one of the first organs attempted to be transplanted (55), early case reports of intestinal transplantation noted a high incidence of graft loss from rejection, infection, and technical complications (23). In 1987, a 3-year-old girl received a multivisceral abdominal graft that included the stomach, duodenum, pancreas, small bowel, colon, and liver; she survived for 6 months with good intestinal graft function (57). A modification of this operation using a "cluster" of organs that consisted of the liver and the pancreaticoduodenal complex (**Fig. 89.1**) was reported in 1989 (58). Until 1990, only 2 patients survived isolated cadaveric intestinal grafts (22,24). The use of the immunosuppressive agent tacrolimus (FK506, Prograf), introduced in 1989, revolutionized the field, permitting successful transplantation of human intestinal grafts (alone or as part of a multivisceral graft) (61).

INDICATIONS

Diseases associated with loss of intestinal function can be divided into surgical and nonsurgical etiologies. Patients with surgical causes generally suffer from loss of bowel length after resections or from strictures and fistulas, as with Crohn disease. With nonsurgical causes of intestinal failure, the anatomic length and gross morphology of the intestine may be normal. Nonsurgical causes of intestinal failure include motility disorders (e.g., intestinal pseudo-obstruction, Hirschsprung disease) (8,38) and absorptive problems (e.g., microvillus inclusion disease) (51). The indications for transplantation in the case experience at the University of Pittsburgh and Children's Hospital of Pittsburgh are listed in **Table 89.1**.

Parenteral nutrition (PN) is the standard of care for patients with intestinal failure who are unable to maintain a normal, nutritional fluid balance and electrolyte state by use of the gastrointestinal tract alone (28). Management of intestinal failure can be medical and/or operative. However, a group of patients persists who develop irreversible intestinal failure and require indefinite PN, only to suffer from the complications of this therapy. Transplantation of the intestine, either alone or accompanied by other intra-abdominal organs (liver, stomach, duodenum, pancreas), may be life-saving in this group of patients.

Decisions regarding the best transplant options are based on the integrity of the remaining gut and other abdominal organs, both functionally and anatomically, as well as on vascular issues. Replacement of the liver in intestinal transplantation candidates is based on biochemical dysfunction (hyperbilirubinemia, transaminase abnormalities, hypoalbuminemia,

thrombocytopenia, and coagulopathy), presence of bridging fibrosis or cirrhosis on liver biopsy, and the presence of portal hypertension. Hypercoagulable patients deficient in protein S, protein C, and antithrombin III (14) may develop diffuse thromboses within the splanchnic system and undergo transplantation for mesenteric venous hypertension, rather than for intestinal failure. Similarly, patients may present requiring a liver transplant that may not be technically feasible due to extensive portomesenteric thrombosis.

In October 2000, the Center for Medicare and Medicaid Services in the US approved intestinal, combined liver/intestine, and multivisceral transplantation (3,30) at centers of excellence as a standard of care for patients with irreversible intestinal failure who could no longer be maintained on parenteral nutrition due to any of the following four criteria: (a) TPN associated liver injury, as manifested by jaundice or elevated liver injury tests, clinical findings (splenomegaly, varices, coagulopathy), history of stomal bleeding, or hepatic cirrhosis on biopsy; (b) loss of major venous access, defined as more than two thromboses in the great vessels (subclavian, jugular, and femoral veins); (c) frequent central line-related sepsis that consists of more than two episodes of systemic sepsis per year, or one episode of line-related fungemia associated with septic shock or acute respiratory distress syndrome; (d) recurrent episodes of severe dehydration despite IV fluid management.

CLINICAL MANAGEMENT OF THE PRETRANSPLANT CHILD IN THE PICU

Intensive care of children with intestinal and combined intestinal and liver failure presents a unique set of challenges that can generally be divided into two categories: (a) need for PN and associated vascular access issues, and (b) development of liver disease. PN dependence requiring long-term central access brings its own set of problems. Additionally, 40%–60% of infants who require long-term PN for intestinal failure will develop liver disease, which may not ultimately require liver transplant but can complicate their management (32). Both problems are compounded by the long wait times that may be encountered before size-appropriate organs can be located (often 6 months to 1 year). For this reason, it is of primary importance that a potential intestinal transplant candidate be referred to a transplant service for evaluation as soon as possible. The success of the intestinal or multivisceral transplantation depends in large measure on the health and nutritional status of the transplant

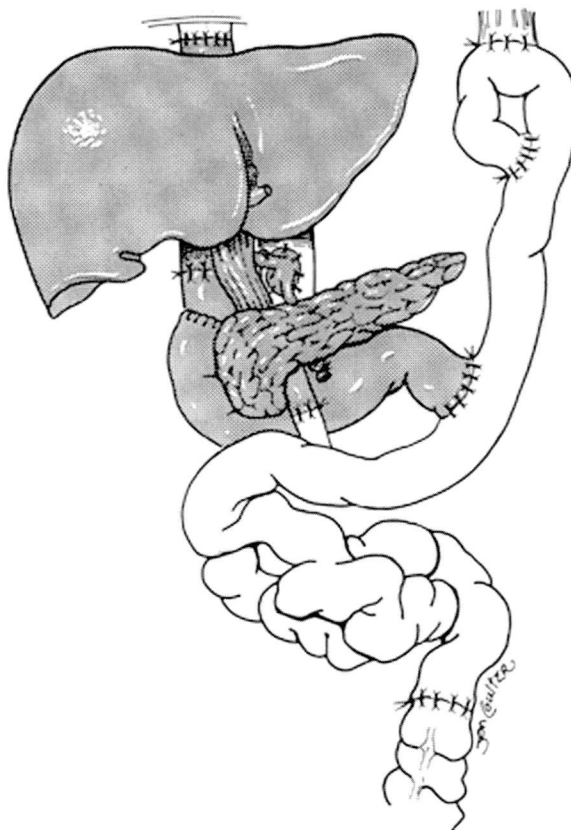

FIGURE 89.1. Cluster allograft (**shaded portion**), including the liver, pancreas, and duodenal segment of small intestine. From Starzl TE, Todo S, Tzakis A, et al. Abdominal organ cluster transplantation for the treatment of upper abdominal malignancies. *Ann Surg* 1989;210: 374–386.

recipient. Even if the child does not ultimately require a transplant, early referral to a center at which the staff is experienced in the management of intestinal failure, including surgical and transplantation options, can dramatically impact outcomes.

TABLE 89.1

INDICATIONS FOR COMPOSITE AND ISOLATED INTESTINAL TRANSPLANTATION

Pediatric patients	Adult patients
Volvulus	Trauma
Gastroschisis	Superior mesenteric artery
Necrotizing enterocolitis	thrombosis
Intestinal atresia	Crohn disease
Pseudo-obstruction	Desmoid tumor
Microvillus inclusion disease	Volvulus
Intestinal polyposis	Familial polyposis
Hirschsprung disease	Gastrinoma
Trauma	Budd-Chiari disease
	Intestinal adhesions
	Pseudo-obstruction
	Inflammatory bowel disease
	Radiation enteritis

The treating physician must be cognizant that the goal of critical care is to keep the child in optimal condition to receive a transplant. For this reason, the intensivist and the transplant surgeon should be in close communication, both to review the patient's status and discuss PICU interventions that may interfere with the patient's candidacy.

Parenteral Nutrition Dependence

PN-dependent patients have chronic problems with venous access; existing central lines often become infected, and line sites may be lost to thrombosis. Any patient with a central line has increased susceptibility to infection, but intestinal transplant candidates are unique in several ways. Prevention of infection is particularly important in this patient population, as episodes of sepsis contribute to deterioration in liver function (31,54). The central lines of patients with short-gut syndrome can become infected by external contamination of the line and by translocation of bacteria across a gut with inadequate barrier function (33). Because patients have been repeatedly exposed to broad-spectrum antibiotics and because intestinal stasis may contribute to bacterial overgrowth, infections that result from bowel translocation may be multiply resistant (46). Fungal infections occur more commonly in this patient group compared to the general population (33). Enteric feedings may help to preserve intestinal mucosal barrier function and decrease infectious complications (46).

Patients with liver failure have impaired immune responses. Impaired neutrophil and Kupffer cell oxidative burst function and reduced complement levels have been documented (33,44). Additionally, adrenal insufficiency with failure of the stress cortisol response is common in patients with acute and chronic liver disease (27,37). The combination of adrenal insufficiency, relative immune deficiency, and the intestinal transplant candidate's requirement for invasive procedures creates a dangerous susceptibility to severe sepsis and septic shock.

Treatment for septic shock should follow established parameters (13), with a few caveats. The cardiac function of intestinal transplant candidates with liver disease is not normal. Patients with severe liver failure may have a hyperdynamic state at baseline but a blunted contractile response to stress. Both systolic and diastolic ventricular function may be impaired (35). Clinical experience indicates that children with cirrhotic cardiomyopathy may not tolerate a large-volume fluid challenge. Resuscitation should be appropriately aggressive, but with careful attention to signs of intravascular volume overload, as patients may have concomitant hepatopulmonary or hepatorenal syndrome. Palpation of the liver may not be a reliable indicator of intravascular volume overload in patients with cirrhosis; instead, clinicians must often rely on changes in central venous pressure, development of rales on lung exam, and changes on chest x-ray. Echocardiogram can be used in difficult cases to assess cardiac filling and function. In patients with advanced liver disease, albumin may be preferable to crystalloid as a resuscitation fluid to avoid worsening anasarca. High salt loads (e.g., normal saline) should be avoided in established liver disease.

Inotropic or vasopressor agents should be used if clinical signs suggest that the child is intravascularly replete. Low diastolic blood pressures are associated with advanced liver disease (35,42). Early septic shock in these children follows a vasodilatory pattern commonly seen in adults and may respond to vasopressor agents. In patients with catecholamine-unresponsive septic shock, adrenal responsiveness should be evaluated with a cortisol level and/or adrenocorticotropic hormone (ACTH)-stimulation test. In some cases, it may be appropriate to treat adrenal insufficiency empirically (hydrocortisone bolus and intermittent dosing or continuous infusion) while results of these tests are pending.

When infections cannot be cleared, it may be necessary to remove and replace lines. As children who await intestinal transplant are dependent on central access, meticulous care must be given to prevention of infection and preservation of line sites when possible. Intestinal transplant candidates are at high risk for forming clots around central lines that can become occlusive and persist after line removal. Although failure of clotting is a more obvious sign of liver dysfunction, patients with liver failure are also unable to synthesize anticoagulating factors, such as protein C, protein S, and antithrombin III (33). The loss of two or more great vessels to thrombosis is part of the criteria for considering transplantation, but clotting in most or all of the available sites for central venous catheterization can make transplantation technically challenging or impossible. When new lines are being placed, care should be taken not to damage the vessel unduly. Before line placement, a careful history should be taken with respect to clot history, and when appropriate, Doppler ultrasound of great vessels should be used to guide the individual performing the procedure. In some cases, especially in older children, venograms of the extremity venous structures are performed as part of the pretransplant workup to better delineate vascular patency that may not be accurately assessed by ultrasound (34,50).

A full discussion of nutritional requirements of children with intestinal failure is beyond the scope of this chapter, but it is important to note that (a) the ability to heal after a major operation is partly dependent on preoperative nutritional status, and (b) the development of liver disease may be influenced by nutritional and metabolic parameters (25,32). A nutritional specialist should routinely be involved in the care of a prospective intestinal transplant patient, whether the patient is at home or in the ICU. In general, attention should be paid to providing PN with adequate calories and an appropriate balance of fats, protein, and carbohydrate calories, with an appropriate complement of trace elements and minerals.

Adequate nutrition is crucial, but clinical experience with preoperative intestinal transplant patients suggests that these patients have a tendency to gain excess adipose tissue. When calculating metabolic requirements of these children in the PICU, it is important to factor in an estimate of their decreased activity on actual caloric expenditure. When possible, delivery of some enteral calories may preserve intestinal epithelial barrier function, may decrease the risk or severity of intestinal failure-associated liver disease, and may improve hospital mortality (4,32,43).

Liver Failure

Isolated intestinal transplant candidates may have mild, reversible liver disease. Patients who await combined liver and small intestine or multivisceral transplants may persistently struggle with all of the problems seen in hepatic failure over a waiting period of several months. Coagulopathy, portal hypertension with ascites and hepatomegaly, variceal bleeding, hypoalbuminemia, hyperbilirubinemia, hyperammonemia with hepatic encephalopathy, and hepatorenal and hepatopulmonary syndrome may all be seen in this patient population. The management of these problems in liver/intestine and candidates for multivisceral transplantation differs from their management in isolated liver candidates only in duration: the wait time for an isolated liver is comparatively brief.

In particular, issues related to the long-term effects of increased abdominal girth, renal dysfunction, and persistent coagulopathy, particularly in combined liver-intestinal transplant and multivisceral transplant candidates, deserve further discussion.

Intestinal transplant candidates with cirrhosis and liver failure have increased abdominal girth due to organomegaly and ascites. In children, particularly infants <1 year of age, the abdominal contents, especially an enlarged liver, may impinge on lung volumes and impede respiration. Although the problem is easily overcome with positive-pressure ventilation, mechanical ventilation should be considered a last resort, as it brings with it the problems of sedation, respiratory muscle deconditioning, and ventilator-associated pneumonia. Due to problems with the risk of bleeding and infection, tracheostomy is usually contraindicated and should only be performed after consultation with the transplant surgeon. If ascites predominates over organomegaly as a cause of increased abdominal girth, drainage of ascitic fluid may relieve symptoms. Relief is usually temporary, as the circumstances that lead to the fluid collection persist. The indications for peritoneal drainage must be weighed against the risk of infection. Additionally, rapid drainage of large volumes of peritoneal fluid may lead to intravascular hypovolemia and shock.

Combined liver and intestinal transplant patients and multivisceral transplant patients often have some degree of renal dysfunction that renders them sensitive to fluid overload. Repeated infections with fungus and gram-negative organisms expose these patients to multiple nephrotoxic agents. Additionally, episodes of septic shock can expose the kidney to low-flow states, causing acute tubular necrosis. Hepatorenal syndrome is a very late finding in liver failure but can contribute to renal insufficiency.

Persistent coagulopathy in combined liver and intestinal transplant candidates is a significant complication. Coagulopathy may be managed with administration of clotting factors. It may be impossible to normalize laboratory indicators of clotting function; instead, clinical evidence of bleeding should guide therapy. Intracranial hemorrhage, though rare, can occur. Correction of disordered coagulation with large volumes of clotting factors can lead to fluid overload, particularly in patients with renal insufficiency. Frequent gram-negative and fungal infections often necessitate exposure to nephrotoxic agents; hence, some degree of renal insufficiency is common in these patients. In cases of severe or recurrent bleeding, plasma exchange (plasmapheresis) and judicious use of recombinant factor 7 have been successful in correcting coagulopathy without fluid overload (11,53). Plasma exchange may also have a role as a liver support therapy (53).

Extracorporeal liver support therapy, though in its infancy, someday may have application in combined liver and intestinal transplant or multivisceral transplant patients. Support systems in use today mimic the liver's detoxifying function, relying on diffusion of molecules across a membrane (dialysis with or without albumin-enriched dialysate), absorption (by charcoal, albumin), or dilution (exchange of plasma volumes) (15). Bioartificial liver systems that use animal or immortalized human cells are under development.

The pathophysiology of liver failure and the resulting brain edema and multiple organ failure is not well understood, and, unfortunately, none of the extracorporeal liver support systems have been rigorously evaluated in children (39). Of the therapies under investigation, molecular adsorbents recirculating system (MARS), a system based on albumin dialysis and plasma exchange, has been most extensively used (53,60). Studies with both systems have documented clinical improvement, but it has been difficult to demonstrate survival benefit. At one center, it has successfully been used in an adult patient to bridge the time until a suitable multivisceral donor could be localized. Someday, these systems may help to keep patients healthy enough to undergo a transplant until appropriate organs become available.

THE TRANSPLANT OPERATION

Abdominal Visceral Procurement

Optimal donor selection is imperative to a successful transplant outcome, especially whenever the intestine is involved. Intestine-containing allografts should be assessed and procured (1,2,6) by surgeons intimately involved in the specialty. A further technical factor is size disparity, especially in recipients in whom the abdominal domain is reduced from prior resec-

tion, particularly pronounced in the very young, among whom size-matched donors are infrequent. Allograft reductions and efforts to provide increased abdominal domain, whether via abdominal wall transplant or delayed closure measures, have been performed to expand the donor pool.

Recipient Operations

Obtaining vascular access, especially when the liver requires transplantation, can be problematic in these patients who have multiple thrombosed veins. Innovative therapies, including reopening venous channels (34) and intra-arterial perfusion (10), may be necessary. Access issues are best determined prior to the patient going to the operating room due to the time constraints involved in minimizing the cold ischemic time of the allograft. Even so, time is often spent at the beginning of the procedure establishing appropriate access. The recipient operation consists of removal of the failed organs after exposure of the vascular anatomy, followed by allograft implantation, as described in the following sections.

Isolated Small Bowel

In cases of surgical short gut, the recipient's diseased small intestine is removed and the superior mesenteric artery of the donor bowel is sewn to the infrarenal aorta (or occasionally the native superior mesenteric artery), and the donor superior mesenteric vein is anastomosed to the recipient superior mesenteric vein or inferior vena cava (**Fig. 89.2A**). The anastomoses are

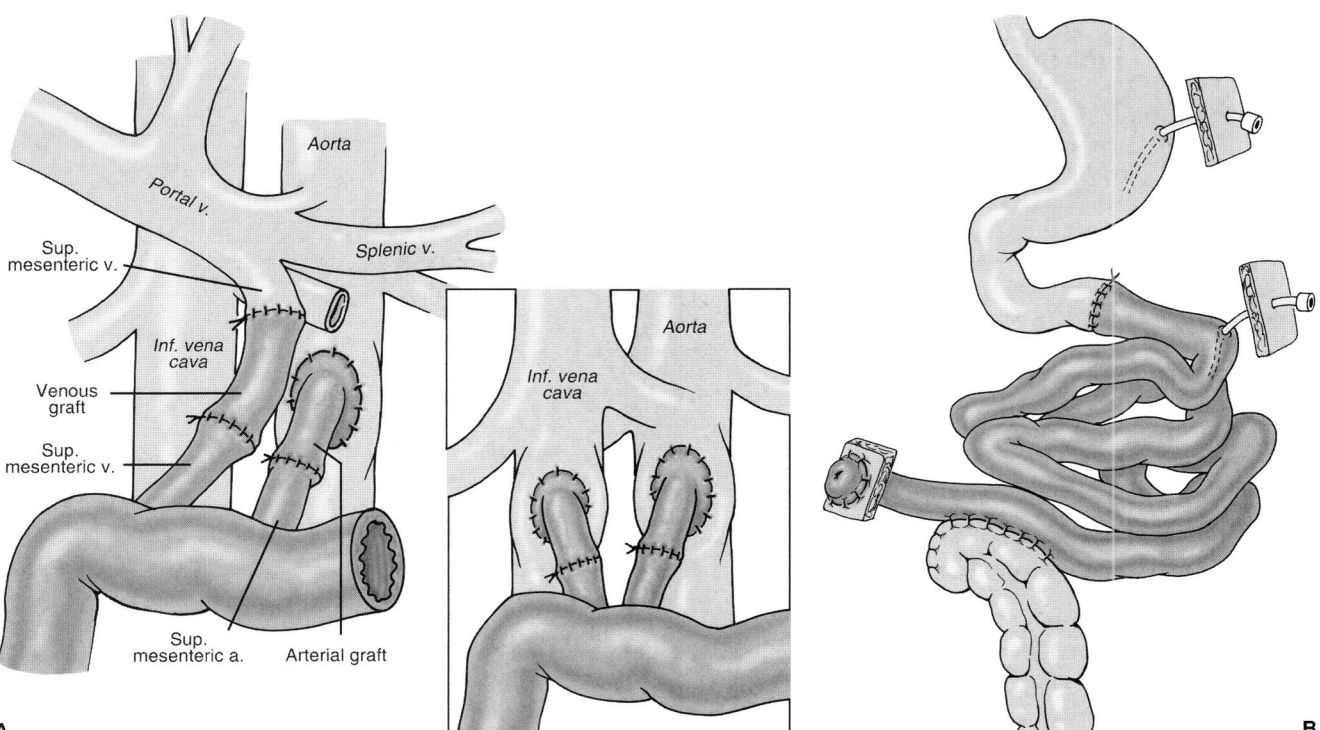

FIGURE 89.2. (**A**) Arterialization and potential venous drainage options of the isolated small intestine allograft. (**B**) Illustration of an isolated small-bowel graft; the distal ileal chimney allows easy access to bowel mucosa.

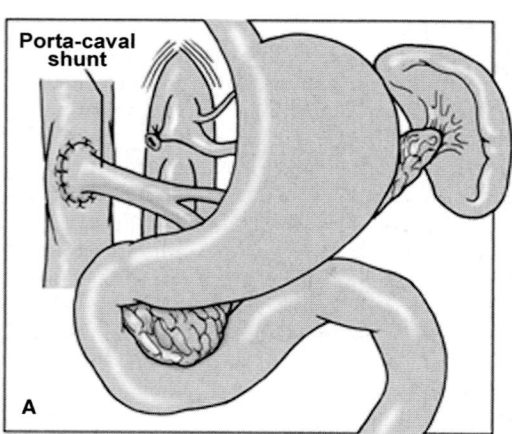

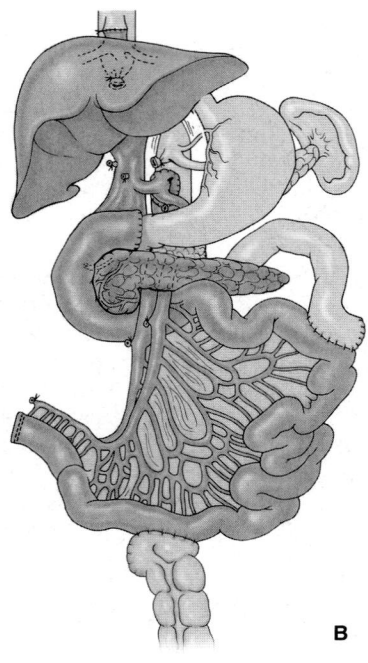

FIGURE 89.3. (A) Combined liver-small intestinal allograft. Systemic porta caval shunt allows venous outflow of retained pancreas and stomach from recipient. (B) Composite liver and intestine graft with preservation of the duodenum in continuity with the graft jejunum and hepatobiliary system.

often facilitated by the use of interposition arterial and venous grafts. Intestinal continuity is completed with proximal and distal gastrointestinal anastomoses, and access to the ileum for endoscopic examination is provided by a temporary chimney ileostomy (**Fig. 89.2B**) (49), except in the case of a permanent end-ileostomy.

Liver-Small Bowel

The diseased liver is removed with the retrohepatic vena cava preserved in situ ("piggyback"), and a permanent portal-caval shunt draining the native stomach and pancreas is performed (**Fig. 89.3A**). Prior to implantation of the allograft (**Fig. 89.3B**), the double arterial stem of the celiac and superior mesenteric arteries (using the Carrel patch technique) is connected to the infrarenal aorta using a donor aortic conduit homograft. A proximal jejunojejunostomy, ileocolostomy, and a temporary distal ileostomy complete the operation. The allograft duodenum remains in continuity with the allograft biliary system (12).

Multivisceral Transplantation

After removal of the native liver, distal stomach, duodenum, pancreas, and intestine, the retroperitoneal aorta is exposed and the multivisceral graft (**Fig. 89.4A**) is connected to its vascular inflow and outflow. With a full multivisceral transplant (liver included), the suprahepatic venous attachment is completed initially, followed by the aorto-aortic anastomosis. No portal vein anastomosis is required in this procedure, as the recipient's portal vein and its inflow native organs (gastrointestinal tract, pancreas, and liver) are removed with the enterectomy. Patients with a normal native liver receive a modified multivisceral procedure in which allograft portal venous return is directed into the recipient's native portal vein (**Fig. 89.4B**), preserving the native liver.

A gastrogastric anastomosis, coloenteric anastomosis, and a chimney ileostomy are routinely performed. A pyloroplasty is also necessary, due to vagal denervation, to avoid gastric outlet obstruction. In all types of intestinal recipients, the ileostomy is primarily placed to allow for ease of allograft monitoring via ileoscopy and ileal allograft biopsies. Takedown of the ileostomy can be performed once oral nutrition is consistently adequate and a stable immunosuppressant regimen has been achieved with less need for frequent endoscopic surveillance.

POSTTRANSPLANTION MANAGEMENT

Immunosuppression

The immunosuppression regimens used at the University of Pittsburgh from 1990–2007 are presented in **Table 89.2**. Currently, Thymoglobulin is given as 7.5 mg/kg in divided doses of 5 mg/kg pre-allograft reperfusion and 2.5 mg/kg post-reperfusion in children. Methylprednisolone is given as a bolus (2 mg/kg/IV) as premedication for the lymphocyte-depleting agent to limit the cytokine reaction, but this drug is not used routinely postoperatively (56). Rejection is treated with optimization of tacrolimus levels, supplemental corticosteroids, and monoclonal or polyclonal antibody if necessary. Additional or alternative agents have occasionally been used, including azathioprine, rapamycin, cyclosporin (at other centers), and mycophenolate mofetil, especially in the face of complications such as renal dysfunction and recurrent rejection, although their efficacy appears to be less than that of the standard agent(s).

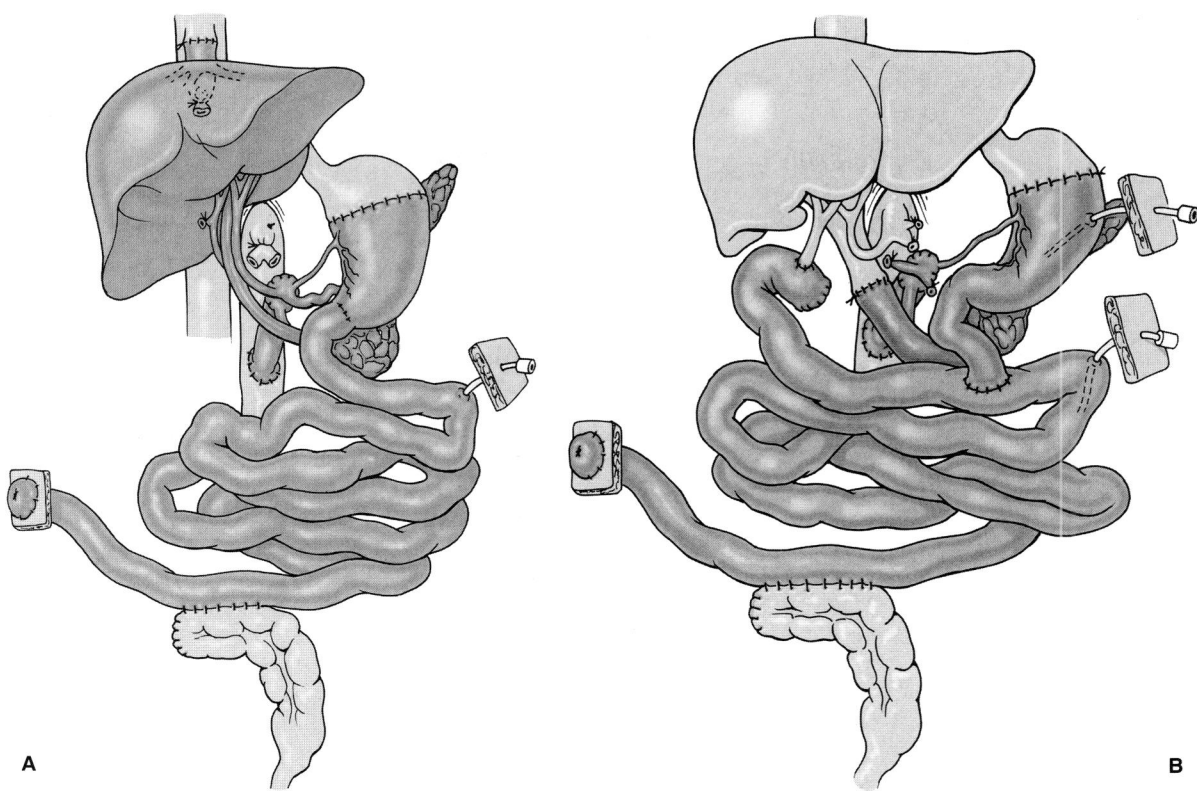

FIGURE 89.4. Diagrams of multivisceral donor organs: (**A**) complete, (**B**) modified multivisceral.

Postoperative Care

For recipients with pretransplant liver failure, postoperative care is similar (although more intense) to that provided for isolated liver transplant recipients. Recipients of isolated small-bowel transplants who have stable liver function usually have a more routine initial ICU course.

Ventilatory Management

Pretransplant status, postoperative graft status, sepsis, inability to close the abdominal wall, and the presence of diaphragmatic

weakness or paralysis, must be considered in formulating a plan for weaning the intestine transplant patient from the ventilator. Pain management is a serious complicating factor, as many chronic patients have been on long-term pain medications, and obtaining the appropriate level of analgesia may be difficult.

Infection Control

Recipients of intestinal grafts receive prophylactic, broad-spectrum IV antibiotics. Antiviral prophylaxis currently includes a 2-week course of IV ganciclovir (5 mg/kg twice daily IV).

Cytomegalovirus (CMV)-specific hyperimmune globulin (Cytogam^R) (150 mg/kg IV at 2, 4, 6, and 8 weeks posttransplant and 100 mg/kg/dose IV at 12 and 16 weeks posttransplant) and oral ganciclovir for 90 days is given in CMV-negative recipients of CMV-positive allografts. Oral administration of trimethoprim-sulfamethoxazole (80 mg orally 3 times weekly) is used for the lifetime of the patient as prophylaxis against *Pneumocystis jiroveci* (formerly *Pneumocystis carinii*) pneumonia.

Bacterial translocation most commonly occurs during episodes of acute rejection, when the mucosal barrier of the allograft has been immunologically damaged, or in enteritis associated with Epstein-Barr virus infection (52).

Gastrointestinal Function and Assessment

The normal intestine is pink and nonedematous and occasionally demonstrates contractions. Changes in the ileal stoma postoperatively should be promptly investigated, and vascular,

TABLE 89.2

INTESTINAL TRANSPLANTATION: IMMUNOSUPPRESSION REGIMENS BY ERA AT THE UNIVERSITY OF PITTSBURGH

Years	Drug	No. of patients
1990–1995	Tacrolimus (T)/Steroids (S)	70
1995–1997	T/S/Cyclophosphamide	24
1997–1998	Tacrolimus/Steroids	13
1998–2001	T/S/Daclizumab	61
2002–2007	Thymoglobulin/Campath preconditioning protocol	172
	Total	340

technical, or immunologic causes ruled out (7). Dramatic and rapid changes may be seen in recipients of a positive tissue typing crossmatch, especially B-cell, which may herald a vascular humoral type of rejection (64).

Routine endoscopic surveillance is used to assess graft integrity and for the diagnosis of intestinal rejection. Zoom endoscopy has been used in some centers in an effort to establish a prompt visual tool to diagnose rejection; however, as the changes are not specific, it has yet to receive widespread application.

Normal stomal output is 40–60 mL/kg/day. No reliable serum tests exist for monitoring function intestinal grafts. Data on prospective markers, such as citrulline, have been inconclusive (20). While PN is continued in the early postoperative weeks, enteral nutrition is introduced once integrity of the gastrointestinal tract has been demonstrated by contrast study, usually at 1 week posttransplant.

Management of Complications

Graft Rejection

Clinically, intestinal allograft rejection may be asymptomatic or present with fever, abdominal pain, distention, nausea, vomiting, and a sudden increase or decrease in stomal output. The stoma may be normal in appearance or lose its normal velvety appearance and become friable or ulcerated. Histologically (63), the rejection is graded by the degree of epithelial damage. In mild rejection, epithelial cell apoptosis leads to epithelial cell loss within the deep crypts (**Fig. 89.5A**). In moderate rejection (**Fig. 89.5B**), more severe crypt damage with focal crypt loss is observed. Severe rejection (**Fig. 89.5C**) leads to denuded mucosa. Regeneration (**Fig. 89.5D**) occurs by re-epithelialization over the surface of a lamina propria devoid of crypts.

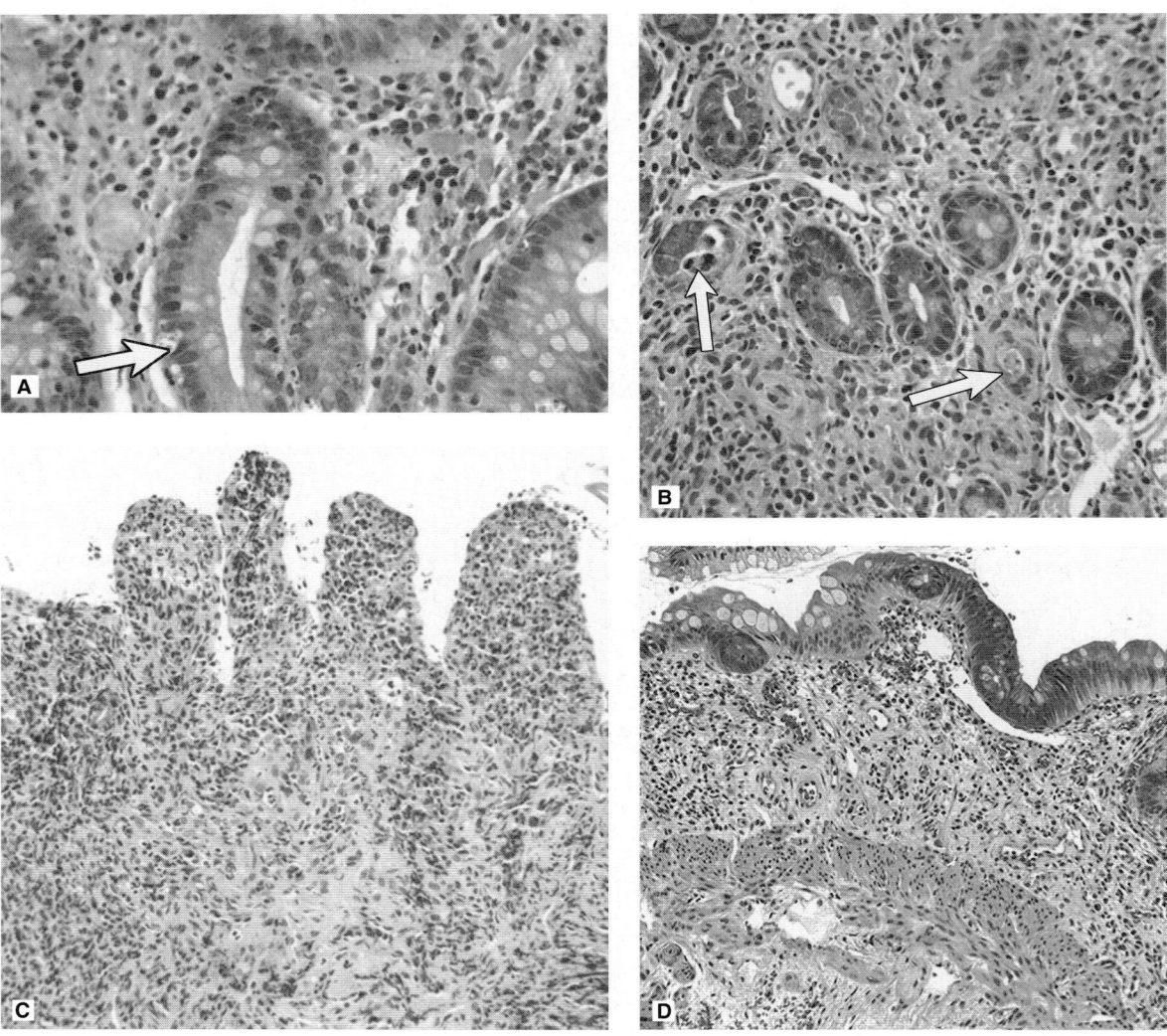

FIGURE 89.5. The rejection is graded by the degree of epithelial damage. In mild rejection (**A**), epithelial cell apoptosis leads to epithelial cell loss within the deep crypts. In moderate rejection (**B**), more severe crypt damage with focal crypt loss is observed. Severe rejection (**C**) leads to denuded mucosa (original magnification ×400 a, b ×200, c). Regeneration (**D**) occurs by re-epithelialization over the surface of a lamina propria devoid of crypts.

TABLE 89.3

PEDIATRIC INTESTINAL TRANSPLANTATION: REJECTION BY ERA

Years	Drug	Rejection rate
1990–1995	Tacrolimus/Steroids	81%
1995–1997	Cyclophosphamide	79%
1998–2001	Daclizumab	79%
2002–2007	Thymoglobulin preconditioning protocol	46%

Chronic rejection has been historically observed in ~15% of patients. The presentation may include weight loss, chronic diarrhea, intermittent fever, or gastrointestinal bleeding. Histologically, villous blunting, focal ulcerations, epithelial metaplasia, and scant cellular infiltrates are present on endoscopic mucosal biopsies (45). Full-thickness intestinal biopsies show obliterative thickening of intestinal arterioles.

Acute rejection occurs in ~50% of patients with the use of a preconditioning protocol (**Table 89.3**). Lower overall immunosuppression use has subsequently resulted in a concomitant reduction in CMV and Epstein-Barr virus disease (**Table 89.4**), especially in pediatric recipients.

Mild graft rejection in most cases responds to IV methylprednisolone, with optimization of tacrolimus levels to 15 ng/mL. Antibody therapy with OKT3 is used when rejection has progressed despite a steroid taper, or as the initial therapeutic agent in cases of severe mucosal injury and crypt damage.

Biliary Complications

With the modification in donor technique, allowing preservation of the donor duodenum and entire pancreas, and maintenance of the hepaticopancreaticobiliary system, biliary and pancreatic complications from leaks and strictures from anastomoses have been avoided. However, a group of these patients has been identified who have signs and radiologic evidence

TABLE 89.4

PEDIATRIC INTESTINAL TRANSPLANTATION: CYTOMEGALOVIRUS DISEASE AND POSTTRANSPLANTATION LYMPHOPROLIFERATIVE DISEASE BY ERA

Years	Drugs	CMV rate	PTLD rate
1990–1995	Tacrolimus/Steroids	25%	43%
1995–1997	Cyclophosphamide	60%	20%
1997–1998	Tacrolimus/Steroids	13%	25%
1998–2001	Daclizumab	4%	22%
2002–2007	Thymoglobulin preconditioning protocol	8%	8%

CMV, cytomegalovirus; PTLD, posttransplantation lymphoproliferative disease

of obstruction, perhaps from ampulla of Vater dysfunction. This obstruction can occur months to years posttransplantation and can be managed via percutaneous transhepatic cholangiography with balloon dilatation and/or endoscopic retrograde cholangiopancreaticogram and stenting or incision of the ampulla.

In modified multivisceral grafts, continuity of the biliary axis is surgically reestablished, either via a Roux-en-Y enteric loop or duct-to-duct in bigger donors and recipients. Correspondingly, these grafts can develop biliary system-related surgical complications (i.e., leaks and obstructions).

Infection

Infectious complications continue to be responsible for significant morbidity and mortality after intestinal transplantation. However, current immunosuppressive modifications have decreased the incidence of life-threatening bacterial complications, and fungal and viral infections are the main source of morbidity in current transplant series.

Fungal infections are more common after heavy treatment for rejection, extensive antibiotic usage, intestinal leaks, and multiple surgical explorations. The current incidence of CMV infection is ~8% (**Table 89.4**). Clinical presentation is usually with enteritis (**Fig. 89.6 A,B**). Successful clinical management has been accomplished in the majority of episodes, using ganciclovir alone or ganciclovir in combination with CMV-specific hyperimmunoglobulin (36). A CMV-positive donor graft transplanted into a CMV-negative recipient is a significant risk factor for CMV disease, but monitoring of CMV polymerase chain reaction with preemptive therapy has allowed the successful use of CMV-mismatched organs.

Presentation of posttransplantation lymphoproliferative disorder (PTLD) may include asymptomatic findings at routine endoscopy, Epstein-Barr virus enteritis (**Fig. 89.7A**) and systemic symptoms, bleeding, lymphadenopathy or tumors (**Fig. 89.7B**). PTLD has decreased in incidence to <10% (**Table 89.4**) under current immunosuppression. Therapy includes reduction of immunosuppression, antiviral therapy using ganciclovir, acyclovir, and/or hyperimmunoglobulin; rituximab (anti-CD20 monoclonal antibody); and chemotherapy.

Graft-versus-Host Disease

Skin changes consistent with graft-versus-host disease GVHD were diagnosed by histopathologic criteria in ~5% of cases and confirmed by immunohistochemical studies visualizing donor cell infiltration into the lesions on two occasions or by flow cytometry detecting elevated donor cell chimerism in peripheral blood. Two children died (one with hereditary IgG and IgM deficiency and one from sepsis), and one adult developed a complex chronic GVHD in association with PTLD (41). All other cases have been treated with optimization of immunosuppression and limited steroid therapy if necessary.

OUTCOMES

Current overall actuarial survival at 1 and 4 years is 94% and 76%, respectively (**Fig. 89.8**), and full nutritional support

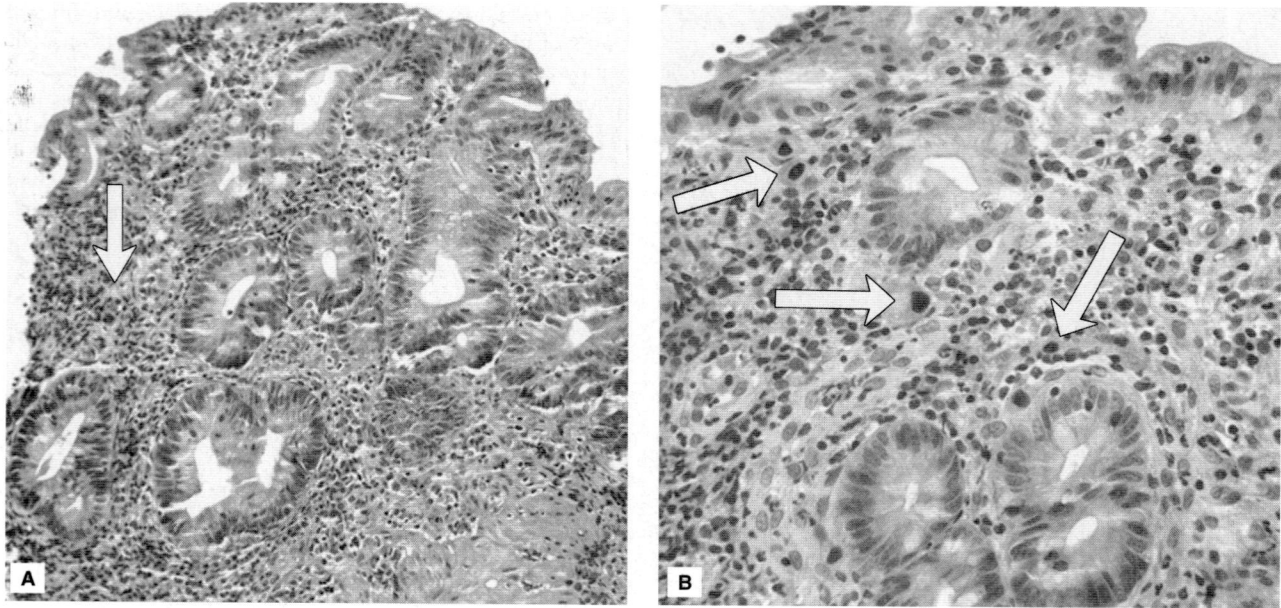

FIGURE 89.6. Cytomegaloviral enteritis is characterized histologically by (**A**) the presence of characteristic inclusions, by (**B**) staining for viral antigens, or both. Note the focal neutrophilic inflammation (immunoperoxidase for cytomegalovirus antigens, 350×).

has been achieved in 91% of surviving patients (48). Optimal donor selection, transplantation of suitable candidates who are free from infection, and attention to detail in the technical performance of the operation are prerequisites for success. However, even under the best of circumstances, the critical care and managing physicians should anticipate potential postoperative difficulties and be prepared to support these patients fully for an extended period of time. Managing the balance between excessive and inadequate immunosuppression in the face of infections or rejection are the most challenging tasks.

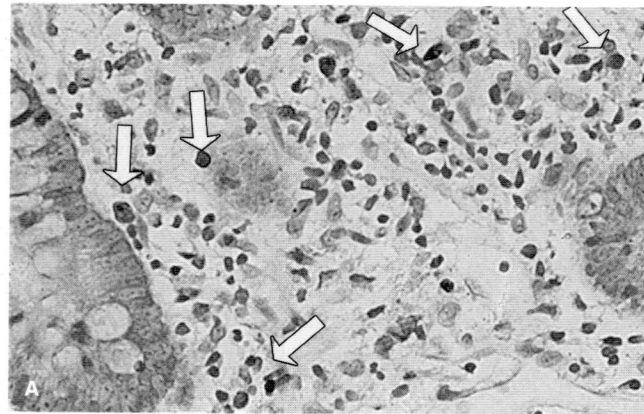

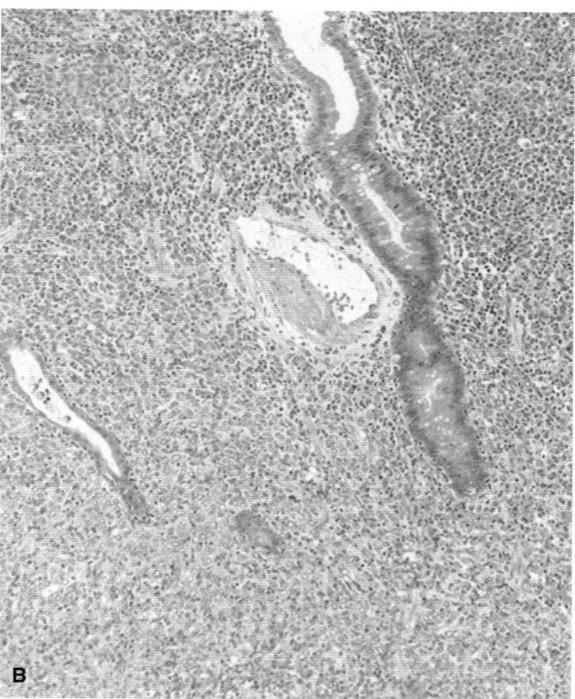

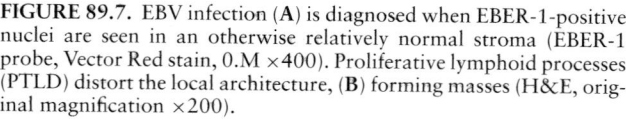

FIGURE 89.7. EBV infection (**A**) is diagnosed when EBER-1-positive nuclei are seen in an otherwise relatively normal stroma (EBER-1 probe, Vector Red stain, 0.M ×400). Proliferative lymphoid processes (PTLD) distort the local architecture, (**B**) forming masses (H&E, original magnification ×200).

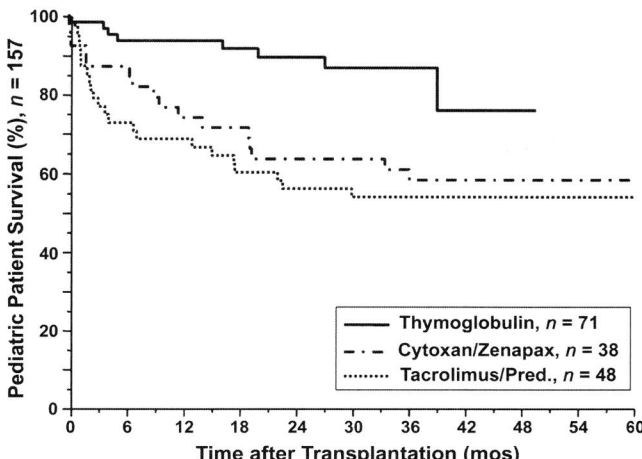

FIGURE 89.8. Patient survival by immunosuppression.

CONCLUSIONS AND FUTURE DIRECTIONS

Although intestinal and multivisceral transplantation has progressed significantly over the last 16 years so that the procedure is more "routine," several issues still challenge the intestinal transplant community and those interested in advancing the field. These include:

Allograft Reduction(s) and Organ Availability

The death rate in pediatric recipients awaiting liver and intestinal transplantation is disproportionately higher than in those requiring intestine alone (19), especially in the very small patient (<1 year), for whom obtaining appropriate size-matched donors is difficult. Attempts at increasing the Model for End-stage Liver disease/Pediatric End-stage Liver Disease (MELD/PELD) score so that these patients can be transplanted earlier has only been marginally successful. To overcome the size disparity, centers at Birmingham (17) and Pittsburgh (47) have undergone a trial of allograft reduction. Although technically successful, the outcomes in some cases have been less than desirable compared to whole transplants, with some recipients still dependent on IV fluids and line access in the long run. Others have adapted poorly after episodes of rejection and required retransplantation.

Live Donor Intestinal and Combined Liver/Intestinal Allografts

Although some of the earliest attempts at intestinal transplantation involved live donors, results were not overly successful, with no long-term survivors and most suffering from chronic rejection (26). Renewed attempts at this procedure appear to be successful, although results are still in their infancy (5). The need for a live-donor isolated intestinal transplant is debatable, as there appears to be little shortage of these organs, except perhaps in the very young. More interesting is the combined liver/intestine live-donor transplant, particularly for the small infant, which may overcome a lack in the appropriate size-matched donor pool (59).

Liver-Alone Transplantation in Patients with Intestinal Failure

The very young infant with gut dysfunction is more susceptible to PN-associated liver failure. These livers may fail before the patient has had time for intestinal adaptation to fully develop. In some recipients, it may not be clear whether, given more time, they may undergo enough further intestinal adaptation to avoid the need for intestinal transplantation. A few centers (9,40) have, in this circumstance, transplanted the failing liver alone, hoping that the intestine would continue to undergo adaptation.

Utility of the Stomach and Colon

Early experience with the use of donor colon as part of the allograft transplant led to an increased incidence of infectious complications. More recently, the colon has been transplanted in some centers (21) without undue increase in morbidity and mortality. Although technically feasible, it is debatable as to whether this procedure significantly increases fluid resorption compared to pharmacologic manipulation with antidiarrheals to warrant the inherent risks.

Another issue is whether to replace the native stomach in cases of chronic intestinal pseudo-obstruction. The authors' experience is that if significant dysmotility exists in the native stomach, it should be replaced. Failure to do so has frequently led to inability to advance oral feeds. Gastrojejunostomy, although successful in some, has not necessarily been the solution, with some patients still suffering ongoing feeding difficulties. In chronic intestinal pseudo-obstruction, the question has also been raised as to whether a small amount of native rectum can be retained and an ileorectal anastomosis performed to avoid committing the patient to a life-long ileostomy. This procedure has successfully been performed with adequate functional outcomes in those patients who did not have associated urologic involvement with the disease process or marked rectal abnormalities on manometry.

Immunosuppression Protocols and Tolerance

Some programs have developed novel strategies in attempts to achieve operational transplant tolerance (56,62). Although drug minimization (steroid-free, spaced monotherapy) has been successfully achieved, the goal of complete immunosuppression avoidance in the intestinal recipient has not been achieved. Considerable work is necessary to identify those in whom immunologic activity may allow for drug weaning and, conversely, those at risk of rejection (65).

Chronic Rejection and Retransplantation: Is the Liver Protective?

Patient and graft survival for intestinal and multivisceral transplantation continues to improve, with results in some experienced centers nearing that of liver transplantation. However, long-term outcomes, in particular with the isolated intestine, are of concern due to chronic rejection being a significant cause of delayed graft loss. Although debated, data suggest that the liver does have a protective effect on the intestinal allograft (29). At present, especially given the lack of donor livers, it is improper to recommend "prophylactically" transplanting the liver with the intestine in a patient who does not have combined liver failure. However, in cases in which the intestine has been lost to chronic rejection, repeated isolated intestinal transplantation has often led to recurrent loss due to immunologic causes. In this situation, consideration should be given to performing a combined liver/intestine retransplant at an appropriate time.

Early Transplantation

As the outcomes for intestinal transplantation continue to improve, matching and often bettering those of nontransplant medical and surgical management, it is now conceivable that in patients with clearly irreversible intestinal failure (extremely short gut, nonreconstructible gastrointestinal tract), intestinal transplantation should be considered earlier rather than later in the disease process. Doing so may avoid problems, such as venous thromboses with loss of access, recurrent line infections, sepsis, and liver dysfunction, let alone the psychological complications (including narcotic dependency) and financial stresses involved with chronic intestinal failure and PN usage.

Bioartificial Neointestine

Although tissue engineering is an exciting advancing field (16,18), as the intestine is a complex functional and highly immunologic organ, significant barriers exist to bringing this concept to a clinical entity. In theory, a neointestine from autologous human tissue would assist in overcoming immunologic issues and provide prompt access to an organ, avoiding the need for live donation.

Continued advancement in the field of intestinal and multivisceral transplantation requires ongoing concerted effort and dedication from a multidisciplinary team of healthcare professionals so that this extremely challenging group of patients can receive optimal care with the best chance of successful long-term outcome.

KEY POINTS

- Causes of irreversible intestinal failure in children are predominantly attributable to surgical conditions (mostly short-gut syndrome from volvulus, necrotizing enterocolitis, gastroschisis, etc). In addition, medical conditions can lead to functional intestinal failure, such as motility disorders (e.g., intestinal pseudo-obstruction), and enterocyte dysfunction, such as microvillus inclusion disease.
- Indications for intestinal transplantation include evidence of liver dysfunction or failure, loss of major venous access, frequent central line-related sepsis, and recurrent episodes of severe dehydration despite IV fluid management.
- Recipient operations should be tailored to the specific indications of each patient and include isolated intestinal transplantation, combined liver-intestinal transplantation, and multivisceral transplantation, including the stomach (with or without the liver).
- Immunosuppression for intestinal transplantation is based on tacrolimus therapy.
- Current modifications in intestinal transplantation include pretreatment of the recipient with antilymphocyte antibodies, such as antithymocyte antibody and alemtuzumab, to allow for the elimination of maintenance steroid use postoperatively.
- Sepsis following intestinal transplantation should prompt a rapid search for technical complications (intra-abdominal abscess, anastomotic dehiscence, etc.) and immunologic causes (rejection may lead to bacterial translocation, overimmunosuppression places the recipient at risk of infection).

References

1. Abu-Elmagd K, Bond G, Reyes J, et al. Intestinal transplantation: A coming of age. *Adv Surg* 2002;36:65–101.
2. Abu-Elmagd K, Fung J, Bueno J, et al. Logistics and technique for procurement of intestinal, pancreatic, and hepatic grafts from the same donor. *Ann Surg* 2000;232(5):680–7.
3. American Gastroenterological Association (AGA). American Gastroenterological Association Medical Position Statement: Short bowel syndrome and intestinal transplantation. *Gastroenterology* 2003;124:1105–10.
4. Artinian V, Krayem H, DiGiovine B. Effects of early enteral feeding on the outcome of critically ill mechanically ventilated medical patients. *Chest* 2006;129(4):960–7.
5. Benedetti E, Testa G, Holterman M, et al. Application of living donor bowel transplantation in pediatric patients. *Clin Transpl* 2004;13:134.
6. Boggi U, Vistoli F, Del Chiaro M, et al. A simplified technique for the en bloc procurement of abdominal organs that is suitable for pancreas and small-bowel transplantation. *J Surg* 2003;10(011):629–41.
7. Bond GJ, Mazariegos GV, Sindhi R, et al. Evolutionary experience with immunosuppression in pediatric intestinal transplantation. *J Pediatr Surg* 2005;40:274–80.
8. Bond GJ, Reyes JD. Intestinal transplantation for total/near-total aganglionosis and intestinal pseudo-obstruction. *Sem Ped Surg* 2004;13:286–92.
9. Botha J, Grant W, Torres C, et al. Isolated liver transplantation in infants with end-stage liver disease due to short bowel syndrome. *Liver Transpl* 2006;12:1062–6.
10. Bouchek C, Abu-Elmagd K. Alternative route transfusion for transplantation surgery in patients lacking accessible veins. *Anesth Analg* 2006;102:1585–98.
11. Brown JB, Emerick KM, Brown DL, et al. Recombinant factor VIIa improves coagulopathy caused by liver failure. *J Pediatr Gastroenterol Nutr* 2003;37(3):268–72.
12. Bueno J, Abu-Elmagd K, Mazariegos G, et al. Composite liver-small bowel allografts with preservation of donor duodenum and hepatic biliary system in children. *Pediatr Surg* 2000;35(2):291–6.
13. Carcillo JA, Fields AI. American College of Critical Care Medicine Task Force Committee Members: Clinical practice parameters for hemodynamic support of pediatric and neonatal patients in septic shock. *Crit Care Med* 2002;30(6):1365–78.
14. Casella JF, Lewis JH, Bontempo FA, et al. Successful treatment for homozygous protein C deficiency by hepatic transplantation. *Lancet* 1988;1:435–438.
15. Chamuleau RA, Poyck PP, van de Kerkhove MP. Bioartificial liver: Its pros and cons. *Ther Apher Dial* 2006;10(2):168–74.
16. Chen MK, Beierle EA. Animal models for intestinal tissue engineering. *Biomaterials* 2004;25:1675–81.
17. de Goyet J, Mitchell A, Mayer AD, et al. En bloc combined reduced-liver and small bowel transplants: From large donors to small children. *Transplantation* 2000;69:555–9.

18. Duxbury MS, Grikscheit TC, Gardner-Thorpe J, et al. Lymphangiogenesis in tissue-engineered small intestine. *Transplantation* 2004;77(8):1162–6.

19. Fryer J, Pellar S, Ormond D, et al. Mortality in candidates waiting for combined liver-intestine transplants exceeds that for other candidates waiting for liver transplants. *Liver Transpl* 2003;9:748–53.

20. Godolesi G, Kaufman S, Sansaricq C, et al. Defining normal plasma citrulline in intestinal transplant recipients. *Am J Transplantation* 2004;4:414–8.

21. Goulet O, Auber F, Fourcade L, et al. Intestinal transplantation including the colon in children. *Transpl Proceed* 2002;34:1885–6.

22. Goulet OK, Revillon Y, Jan D, et al. Small-bowel transplantation in children. *Transplant Proc* 1990;22:2499–500.

23. Grant D. Intestinal transplantation: Current status. *Transplant Proc* 1989;21:2869–71.

24. Grant D, Wall W, Mimeault R, et al. Successful small-bowel/liver transplantation. *Lancet* 1990;335:181–4.

25. Greer R, Lehnert M, Lewindon P, et al. Body composition and components of energy expenditure in children with end-stage liver disease. *J Pediatr Gastroenterol Nutr* 2003;36(3):358–63.

26. Gruessner RW, Sharp HL. Living-related intestinal transplantation: First report of a standardized surgical technique. *Transplantation* 1997;11:271–4.

27. Harry R, Auzinger G, Wendon J. The clinical importance of adrenal insufficiency in acute hepatic dysfunction. *Hepatology* 2002;36(2):395–402.

28. Howard L, Ament M, Fleming RC, et al. Current use and clinical outcome of home parenteral and enteral nutrition therapies in the United States. *Gastroenterology* 1995;109:355–65.

29. Jugie M, Canioni D, LeBihan C, et al. Study of the impact of liver transplantation on the outcome of intestinal grafts in children. *Transplantation* 2006;81(7):992–7.

30. Kaufman SS, Atkinson JB, Bianchi A, et al. Indications for pediatric intestinal transplantation: A position paper of the American Society of Transplantation. *Pediatr Transplant* 2001;5:80–7.

31. Kaufman SS, Loseke CA, Lupo JV, et al. Influence of bacterial overgrowth and intestinal inflammation on duration of PN in children with short bowel syndrome. *J Pediatr* 1997;131:356–61.

32. Kelly D. Intestinal failure-associated liver disease: What do we know today? *Gastroenterology* 2006;130:S70–7.

33. Krasko A, Deshpande K, Bonvino S. Liver failure, transplantation, and critical care. *Crit Care Clin* 2003;19(2):155–83.

34. Lang EV, Reyes J, Faintuch S. Central venous recanalization in patients with short gut syndrome: Restoration of candidacy for intestinal and multivisceral transplantation. *J Vasc Interv Radiol* 2005;16:1203–13.

35. Liu H, Gaskari SA, Lee SS. Cardiac and vascular changes in cirrhosis: Pathogenic mechanisms. *World J Gastroenterol* 2006;12(6):837–42.

36. Manez R, Kusne S, Green M, et al. Incidence and risk factors associated with the development of cytomegalovirus disease after intestinal transplantation. *Transplantation* 1995;59:1110–4.

37. Marik PE, Gayowski T, Starzl TE. Hepatic cortisol research and Adrenal Pathophysiology Study Group. The hepatoadrenal syndrome: A common yet unrecognized clinical condition. *Crit Care Med* 2005;33(6):1254–9.

38. Masetti M, DiBenedetto F, Cautero N, et al. Intestinal transplantation for chronic intestinal pseudo-obstruction in adult patients. *Am J Transpl* 2004;4:826–9.

39. Mazariegos G, Chen Y, Squires R. Biological and artificial liver support system in children: A new perspective. *Pediatr Crit Care Med* 2005;6(5):616–7.

40. Mazariegos G, Soltys K, Bond G, et al. Isolated liver transplantation in infants with short gut syndrome: Is less better? *Liver Transpl* 2006;12:1040–1.

41. Mazariegos GV, Abu-Elmagd K, Jaffe R, et al. Graft versus host disease in intestinal transplantation. *Am J Transplant* 2004;4(9):1459–65.

42. Moller S, Henriksen JH. Cirrhotic cardiomyopathy: A pathophysiological review of circulatory dysfunction in liver disease. *Heart* 2002;87(1):9–15.

43. Moore FA, Feliciano DV, Andrassy RJ, et al. Early enteral feeding, compared with parenteral, reduces postoperative septic complications. The results of a meta-analysis. *Ann Surg* 1992;216(2):172–83.

44. Panasiuk A, Wysocka J, Maciorkowska E, et al. Phagocytic and oxidative burst activity of neutrophils in the end stage of liver cirrhosis. *World J Gastroenterol* 2005;11(48):7661–5.

45. Parizhskaya M, Redondo C, Demetris A, et al. Chronic rejection of small bowel grafts: A pediatric and adult study of risk factors and morphologic progression. *Ped Dev Pathol* 2003;6:240–50.

46. Pierro A, van Saene HK, Jones MO, et al. Clinical impact of abnormal gut flora in infants receiving parenteral nutrition. *Ann Surg* 1998;227:547–52.

47. Reyes J, Fishbein T, Bueno J, et al. Reduced-size orthotopic composite liver-intestinal allograft. *Transplantation* 1998;66(4):489–92.

48. Reyes J, Mazariegos GV, Abu-Elmagd K, et al. Intestinal transplantation under tacrolimus monotherapy after perioperative lymphoid depletion with rabbit anti-thymocyte globulin (thymoglobulin). *Am J Transplant* 2005;5(6):1430–6.

49. Reyes J, Mazariegos GV, Bond GM, et al. Pediatric intestinal transplantation: Historical notes, principles and controversies. *Pediatr Transplant* 2002;6(3):193–207.

50. Rodrigues AF, van Mourik IDM, Sharif K, et al. Management of end-stage central venous access in children referred for possible small bowel transplantation. *J Pediatr Gastroenterol Nutr* 2006;42:427–33.

51. Ruemmele FM, Jan D, Lacaille F, et al. New perspectives for children with microvillous inclusion disease: Early small bowel transplantation. *Transplantation* 2004;77(7):1024–8.

52. Sigurdsson L, Green M, Putnam P, et al. Bacteremia frequently accompanies rejection following pediatric small bowel transplantation. *J Pediatr Gastroenterol Nutr* 1995;21(3):356.

53. Singer AL, Olthoff KM, Kim H, et al. Role of plasmapheresis in the management of acute hepatic failure in children. *Ann Surg* 2001;234(3):418–24.

54. Sondheimer JM, Asturias E, Cadnapaphornchai M. Infection and cholestasis in neonates with intestinal resection and long-term PN. *J Pediatr Gastroenterol Nutr* 1998;27:131–7.

55. Starzl TE, Kaupp HA, Jr., Brock DR, et al. Homotransplantation of multiple visceral organs. *Am J Surg* 1962;103:219–29.

56. Starzl TE, Murase N, Abu-Elmagd K, et al. Tolerogenic immunosuppression for organ transplantation. *Lancet* 2003;361(9368):1502–10.

57. Starzl TE, Rowe M, Todo S, et al. Transplantation of multiple abdominal viscera. *JAMA* 1989;261:1449–57.

58. Starzl TE, Todo S, Tzakis A, et al. Abdominal organ cluster transplantation for the treatment of upper abdominal malignancies. *Ann Surg* 1989;210:374–86.

59. Testa G, Holterman M, John E, et al. Combined living donor liver/small bowel transplantation. *Transplantation* 2005;79(10):1401–04.

60. Tissieres P, Sasbon JS, Devictor D. Liver support for fulminant hepatic failure: Is it time to use the molecular adsorbents recycling system in children? *Pediatr Crit Care Med* 2005;6(5):585–91.

61. Todo S, Tzakis AG, Abu-Elmagd K, et al. Cadaveric small bowel and small bowel-liver transplantation in humans. *Transplantation* 1992;53:369–76.

62. Tzakis AG, Kato T, Nishida S, et al. Alemtuzumab (Campath-1H) combined with tacrolimus in intestinal and multivisceral transplantation. *Transplantation* 2003;75:1512–7.

63. White FV, Reyes J, Jaffe R, et al. Pathology of intestinal transplantation in children. *Am J Surg Pathol* 1995;19:687–98.

64. Wu T, Abu-Elmagd K, Bond G, et al. A clinicopathologic study of isolated allografts with preformed IgG lymphotoxic antibodies. *Human Pathol* 2004;35:1332–9.

65. Zeevi A, Britz JA, Bentlejewski CA, et al. Monitoring immune function during tacrolimus tapering in small bowel transplant recipients. *Transpl Immunol* 2005;15:17–24.

CHAPTER 90 ■ CRITICAL ASPECTS OF INTESTINAL DISORDERS

ARISTIDES BALTODANO • MEHRENGISE K. COOPER

The gastrointestinal (GI) tract serves as the portal of entry for both nutrients and potential pathogens. The GI tract of the infant handles 285 mL/kg/day of dietary and endogenous fluids. In order to absorb nutrients, a large surface area and a thin epithelium are needed, and this has the potential to compromise host defenses. Many infectious diseases involve the gut, and the investment by the gut in protecting itself is evident in the abundant lymphoid tissue and immune cells it harbors. The alimentary tract provides the body with a continual supply of water, electrolytes, and nutrients, a role which requires movement of food through the alimentary tract; secretion of digestive juices and digestion of food; absorption of water, various electrolytes, and digestive products; circulation of blood through the GI organs to carry away the absorbed substances; and control of all these functions by the local nervous and hormonal systems.

Multiple-organ failure is a leading cause of death in ICUs. The GI tract is implicated in the pathogenesis of the systemic inflammatory response syndrome and multiorgan dysfunction syndrome. Therefore, understanding the role of GI perfusion has become an important focus of critical care and anesthesiology research (3).

Diseases of the GI tract may themselves necessitate admission of a patient to the ICU or may complicate disorders of other systems. Some GI complications are avoidable, most are treatable, but all are potentially lethal. Children admitted to the PICU, regardless of their primary illness, may have their course complicated by bleeding, absorption and motility disorders, ischemia and reperfusion disorders, infection, and primary or secondary immunologic compromise. Optimal outcome depends on careful, repeated monitoring, appropriate diagnostic testing, and rapid intervention when required.

OVERVIEW OF INTESTINAL ANATOMY AND PHYSIOLOGY

Small Intestine

The net effect of passage through the small intestine is absorption of most of the water and electrolytes [sodium (Na), chloride (Cl), potassium (K)] and essentially all dietary organic molecules (including glucose, amino acids, and fatty acids). Through these activities, the small intestine not only provides nutrients to the body, but plays a critical role in water and acid-base balance. The absorption of virtually all nutrients into blood entails breaking down large supramolecular aggregates into small molecules that can be transported across the epithelium.

The small intestine incorporates three features that account for its huge absorptive surface area: the mucosal folds, which increase surface area and aid in mixing the ingesta; the villi or mucosal projections, which protrude into the lumen and are covered with epithelial cells; and the microvilli, formed by absorptive epithelial cells. The microvillus border of intestinal epithelial cells is referred to as the *brush border*. The enterocytes are the epithelial cells that mature into absorptive epithelial cells, which cover the villi. These are the cells that take up and deliver into blood virtually all nutrients from the diet (10).

Small-intestinal Motility

Coordinated contractions of smooth muscle facilitate mixing with digestive juices, digestion, and absorption in the small intestine. Following a meal, both propulsive movements and mixing movements predominate. During the interdigestive state, so-called "housekeeping contractions" propagate from the stomach through the entire small intestine, sweeping it clear of debris. Motility in the small intestine, as in all parts of the digestive tube, is controlled predominantly by excitatory and inhibitory signals from the enteric nervous system. However, these local nervous signals are modulated by inputs from the central nervous system (CNS), and a number of GI hormones appear to affect intestinal motility to some degree (10).

Transport across the Intestinal Epithelium

Transport across the epithelium of the gut has two routes: (a) the transcellular route, or across the plasma membrane of the epithelial cells; and (b) the paracellular route, or across tight junctions between epithelial cells. Some molecules, water for instance, are transported by both routes. In contrast, the tight junctions are impermeable to large organic molecules from the diet (e.g., amino acids and glucose). Those types of molecules are transported exclusively by the transcellular route because the plasma membrane of the absorptive enterocytes is equipped with transporter molecules that facilitate entry into and exit out of the cells. The epithelium of the gut is not a monotonous sheet of functionally identical cells. This diversity in function results from differences in phenotype of the enterocytes; that is, the number and type of transporter molecules they express in their plasma membrane and the structure of the tight junctions they form. Even within a given segment, major differences exist, depending on the type of transport that occurs; for example, cells in the crypts transport very differently than cells on the tips of villi. A proximal-to-distal gradient in osmotic permeability exists within the intestine. Water flows across the epithelium more "freely" in the proximal, compared to distal, gut because the effective pore size is larger. The distal intestine actually can absorb water better than the proximal gut. The observed differences in permeability to water across the epithelium are due almost entirely to differences in conductivity across the paracellular path (10).

Secretion in the Small Intestine

Large quantities of water are secreted into the lumen of the small intestine during the digestive process. Almost all of this water is also reabsorbed in the small intestine. Regardless of whether it is being secreted or absorbed, water flows across the mucosa in response to osmotic gradients. In the case of secretion, two distinct processes establish an osmotic gradient that pulls water into the lumen of the intestine: increases in luminal osmotic pressure and the secretion of electrolytes by crypt cells.

- Increases in luminal osmotic pressure result from influx and digestion of foodstuffs. The chyme that floods into the intestine from the stomach typically is not very hyperosmotic, but as its macromolecular components are broken down, osmolarity of that solution increases dramatically. Therefore, water is pulled into the lumen. Then, as the osmotically active molecules are absorbed, osmolarity of the intestinal contents decreases and water can be absorbed.
- Crypt cells actively secrete electrolytes, leading to water secretion. The apical or luminal membrane of crypt epithelial cells contain a cyclic AMP (cAMP)-dependent chloride channel known also as the cystic fibrosis transmembrane conductance regulator. Mutations in the gene for this ion channel result in cystic fibrosis. This channel is responsible for secretion of water by the following steps: (a) Elevated intracellular concentrations of cAMP in crypt cells activate this channel, resulting in secretion of chloride ions into the lumen. Accumulation of negatively charged chloride anions in the crypt creates an electric potential that attracts Na, pulling it into the lumen across the tight junctions; the net result is secretion of NaCl. (b) Secretion of NaCl into the crypt creates an osmotic gradient across the tight junction; therefore, water is drawn into the lumen.

Abnormal activation of the cAMP-dependent chloride channel in crypt cells is a major cause of watery diarrhea. Several types of bacteria produce toxins that strongly, often permanently, activate the adenylate cyclase, leading to elevated levels of cAMP and causing the chloride channels to essentially become stuck in the "open" position. The result is massive secretion of water that is manifested as severe diarrhea. Cholera toxin, produced by cholera bacteria, is the best known example of this phenomenon, but several other bacteria produce toxins that act similarly (10).

Absorption in the Small Intestine: General Mechanisms

Virtually all nutrients from the diet are absorbed into blood across the mucosa of the small intestine. In addition, the intestine absorbs water and electrolytes, thus playing a critical role in maintenance of body water and acid-base balance. To make such a process possible, an electrochemical gradient of Na across the epithelial cell boundary of the lumen must be established. To remain viable, all cells are required to maintain a low intracellular concentration of Na. In polarized epithelial cells such as enterocytes, low intracellular Na is maintained by a large number of Na,K/ATPases, so called *sodium pumps*, embedded in the basolateral membrane. These pumps export

TABLE 90.1

GASTROINTESTINAL FLUIDS IN INFANTS

Source	Amount (mL/kg/day)
INPUT	
Diet	100
Saliva	70
Gastric juice	70
Pancreatic + bile juice	45
Total	285
OUTPUT	
Stool output	5–10 g/kg/day
Stool Na	25 ± 5 mEq/L
Stool K	60 mEq/L
Stool Cl	20 mEq/L

three Na ions from the cell in exchange for two K ions, establishing a gradient of both charge and Na concentration across the basolateral membrane (10).

Absorption of Water and Electrolytes. The small intestine must absorb massive quantities of water. A normal adult consumes roughly 1–2 liters of dietary fluid every day. In addition, another 6–7 liters of fluid are received by the small intestine daily as secretions from salivary glands, stomach, pancreas, liver, and the small intestine itself. In comparison, an infant's small intestine handles up to 285 mL/kg/day (**Table 90.1**). By the time the ingesta enters the large intestine, ~80% of the fluid has been absorbed. Net movement of water across cell membranes always occurs by osmosis; therefore, absorption of water is absolutely dependent on absorption of solutes, particularly Na. Na is absorbed into the cell by several mechanisms but especially by cotransport with glucose and amino acids. Absorbed Na is rapidly exported from the cell via Na pumps, establishing a high osmolarity in the small intercellular spaces between adjacent enterocytes. Water diffuses in response to the osmotic gradient established by Na into the intercellular space. It seems that the bulk of the water absorption is transcellular, but some also diffuses through the tight junctions. Water, as well as Na, then diffuses into capillary blood within the villus. Water is thus absorbed into the intercellular space by diffusion down an osmotic gradient. However, considering the process as a whole, transport of water from lumen to blood is often against an osmotic gradient. This is an important concept because it means that the intestine can absorb water into blood even when the osmolarity in the lumen is higher than osmolarity of blood (10).

Absorption of Monosaccharides. It is beyond the scope of this chapter to discuss absorption of different nutrients. As carbohydrate absorption is linked to Na absorption, the absorption of simple carbohydrates will be briefly discussed. Simple carbohydrates are the predominant carbohydrate absorbed in the digestive tract. However, monosaccharides are only rarely found in normal diets. Rather, they are derived by enzymatic digestion of more complex carbohydrates (starch and disaccharides such as lactose and sucrose) within the digestive tube. None of these molecules can be absorbed for the simple reason that they cannot cross cell membranes unaided and, unlike the situation for monosaccharides, they have no transporters to carry them across. The final enzymatic digestion that liberates monosaccharides is conducted by enzymes that are tethered in the luminal plasma membrane of absorptive enterocytes (*brush border hydrolases*). Polysaccharides and disaccharides must be broken down to monosaccharides prior to absorption by the brush border hydrolases, which include maltase, lactase, and sucrase. Glucose generated by digestion of starch or lactose is absorbed in the small intestine only by cotransport with Na. Glucose and galactose are taken into the enterocytes by cotransport with Na via the same transporter (secondary active transport). Fructose enters the cell from the intestinal lumen via facilitated diffusion through another transporter (10).

Absorption of simple carbohydrates entails transport from the intestinal lumen, across the epithelium, and into the blood. The transporter that carries glucose and galactose into the enterocytes is the Na-dependent hexose transporter, known as SGLUT-1. This molecule transports both glucose and Na into the cell and will not transport either alone. Transport by SGLUT-1 involves a series of conformational changes induced by binding and release of Na and glucose: the transporter is initially oriented facing into the lumen; at this point, it is capable of binding Na but not glucose. Then, Na binds, inducing a conformational change that opens the glucose-binding pocket; glucose binds, and the transporter reorients in the membrane such that the pockets holding Na and glucose are moved inside the cell. Finally, Na dissociates into the cytoplasm, causing glucose binding to destabilize; glucose dissociates into the cytoplasm, and the unloaded transporter reorients back to its original, outward-facing position. Once inside the enterocyte, glucose and Na must be exported from the cell into blood. Na is rapidly exported out in exchange for K by the Na pumps on the basolateral membrane. Glucose is transported out of the enterocyte through a different transporter (GLUT-2) in the basolateral membrane. Glucose then diffuses "down" its concentration gradient into capillary blood within the villus. This mechanism is very important, as it is basic to understanding the rationale of oral rehydrating solutions (10).

Large Intestine

Although the mucosa in the large and small intestines have many histologic similarities, the most obvious difference is that the mucosa of the large intestine is devoid of villi. It has numerous crypts that extend deeply and open onto a flat luminal surface. Another difference is that mucus-secreting goblet cells are also much more abundant in the colonic epithelium than in the small intestine (10).

Absorption, Secretion, and Formation of Feces in the Large Intestine

The large intestine absorbs water, Na ions, and Cl ions and secretes bicarbonate ions and mucus. Water is absorbed in response to an osmotic gradient. The mechanism responsible for generating this osmotic pressure is essentially identical to that of the small intestine (Na pumps). The colonic epithelium is actually more efficient at absorbing water than the small intestine, and Na absorption in the colon is enhanced by aldosterone. Cl is absorbed by exchange with bicarbonate. The resulting secretion of bicarbonate ions into the lumen aids in neutralization of the acids generated by microbial fermentation in the large gut. Goblet cells are abundant in the colonic epithelium, and

they secrete mucus in response to tactile stimuli from luminal contents as well as parasympathetic stimuli from pelvic nerves. Mucus is an important lubricant that protects the epithelium and serves to bind the dehydrated ingesta to form feces (10).

Large-intestinal Motility

Three patterns of motility are observed in the colon: (a) segmentation contractions, which chop and mix the ingesta, presenting it to the mucosa, where absorption occurs; (b) antiperistaltic contractions, which propagate toward the ileum and serve to retard the movement of ingesta through the colon, allowing additional opportunity for absorption of water and electrolytes (peristaltic contractions, in addition to influx from the small intestine, facilitate movement of ingesta through the colon); and (c) mass movements that constitute a type of motility not seen elsewhere in the digestive tube. Also known as *giant migrating contractions*, this pattern of motility is like a very intense and prolonged peristaltic contraction that strips an area of large intestine clear of contents (10).

Microbial Fermentation

Fermentation is the enzymatic decomposition and utilization of foodstuffs, particularly carbohydrates, by microbes. The large intestine does not produce its own digestive enzymes but contains huge numbers of bacteria that have the enzymes to digest and utilize many substrates. In all animals, two processes are attributed to the microbial flora of the large intestine: (a) digestion of carbohydrates not digested in the small intestine, and (b) synthesis of vitamin K and certain B vitamins. Synthesis of vitamin K by colonic bacteria provides a valuable supplement to dietary sources and makes clinical vitamin K deficiency rare. Similarly, formation of B vitamins by the microbial flora in the large intestine is useful to many animals (10).

Neural Control of Gastrointestinal Function—Enteric Nervous System

The GI tract has a nervous system all its own called the *enteric nervous system*. It lies entirely within the wall of the gut, beginning in the esophagus and extending all the way to the anus. The number of neurons in this enteric system is almost exactly equal to the number in the entire spinal cord. This highly developed enteric nervous system is especially important in controlling GI movements and secretion. The enteric nervous system is composed mainly of two plexuses: (a) an outer plexus that lies between the longitudinal and circular muscle layers, called the *myenteric plexus* or Auerbach plexus; and (b) an inner plexus, called the *submucosal plexus* or Meissner plexus, which lies in the submucosa. The myenteric plexus mainly controls GI movements, and the submucosal plexus mainly controls GI secretion and local blood flow (34).

Gastrointestinal Perfusion

Under normal circumstances, in addition to the fundamental role of the splanchnic circulation in maintaining liver and gut perfusion toward maintaining mucosal integrity, the splanchnic bed also acts as a "circulatory sink." The redistribution of blood flow that occurs during feeding and exercise are routine hemodynamic challenges for the splanchnic circulation. The hepatosplanchnic circulation receives 30% of total cardiac output. With increasing age, splanchnic blood flow declines both absolutely and as a fraction of total cardiac output. Resistance arterioles regulate blood flow to the splanchnic bed so that at constant hydrostatic pressure, flow is inversely proportional to resistance. Although these arterioles partake in a markedly less impressive autoregulatory system than in the kidney or brain, they do enable a partial compensation for falls in blood flow. The tone of these vessels depends on the complex balance between neurally mediated sympathetic vasoconstriction, the local action of vasoregulatory substances that are under the influence of the apparently paradoxically named "sensory-motor" nerves, the parasympathetic cholinergic nerve supply, the enteric nervous system, and endothelial-derived agents (3).

Anatomy of the Gastrointestinal Blood Supply

The general distribution of the arterial blood supply to the gut includes the superior mesenteric and inferior mesenteric arteries that supply the walls of the small and large intestines by way of an arching arterial system. On entering the wall of the gut, the arteries branch and send smaller arteries circling in both directions around the gut, with the tips of these arteries meeting on the side of the gut wall opposite the mesenteric attachment. From the circling arteries, still much smaller arteries penetrate into the intestinal wall and spread along the muscle bundles into the intestinal villi and into submucosal vessels beneath the epithelium to serve the secretory and absorptive functions of the gut.

The special organization of the blood flow through an intestinal villus, including a small arteriole and venule that interconnect with a system of multiple looping capillaries, is shown in **Figure 90.1**. The walls of the arterioles are highly muscular and are highly active in controlling villus blood flow (34).

Effect of Gut Activity and Metabolic Factors on Gastrointestinal Blood Flow

Under normal conditions, the blood flow in each area of the GI tract, as well as in each layer of the gut wall, is directly related to the level of local activity. For instance, during active absorption of nutrients, blood flow in the villi and adjacent regions of the submucosa is increased as much as eightfold. Likewise, blood flow in the muscle layers of the intestinal wall increases with increased motor activity in the gut. For instance, after a meal, the motor activity, secretory activity, and absorptive activity all increase; likewise, the blood flow increases greatly but then decreases back to the resting level over another 2–4 hrs (34).

Possible Causes of the Increased Blood Flow during Gastrointestinal Activity

Although the precise cause or causes of the increased blood flow during increased GI activity are still unclear, some facts are known. First, several vasodilator substances are released from the mucosa of the intestinal tract during the digestive process. Most of these are peptide hormones, including cholecystokinin, vasoactive intestinal peptide, gastrin, and secretin. Second, some of the GI glands also release into the gut wall two kinins—kallidin and bradykinin—at the same time that they secrete their secretions into the lumen. These kinins are powerful vasodilators that are believed to cause much of the increased mucosal vasodilation that occurs along with secretion. Third, decreased oxygen concentration in the gut wall can increase intestinal blood flow at least 50%–100%; there-

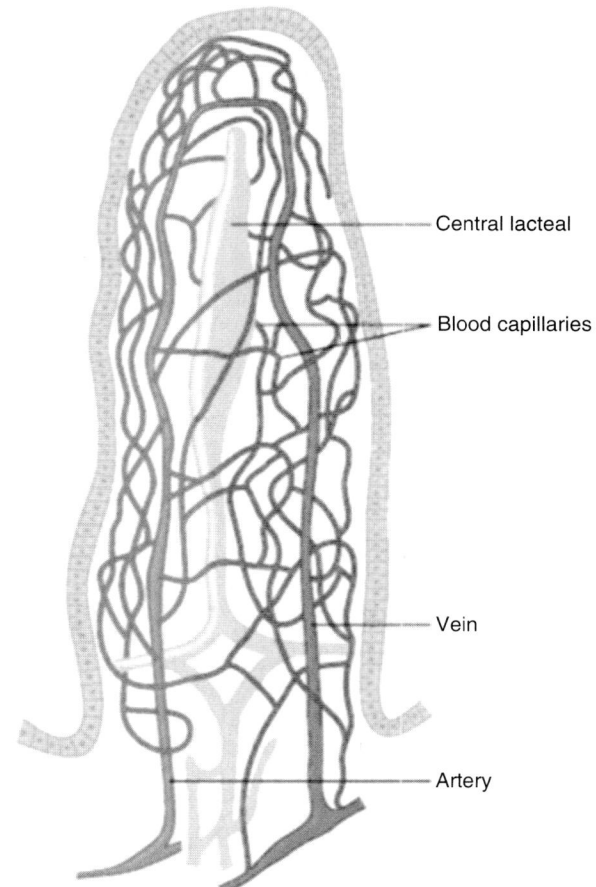

FIGURE 90.1. Special organization of the blood flow through an intestinal villus, including a small arteriole and a venule, which interconnect with a system of multiple looping capillaries. The arterial flow into the villus and the venous flow out of the villus are in directions opposite to each other, and the vessels lie in close apposition to each other. Because of this vascular arrangement, much of the blood oxygen diffuses out of the arterioles directly into the adjacent venules without ever being carried in the blood to the tips of the villi. Under normal conditions, most of the oxygen may take this short-circuit route and may not be available for local metabolic functions of the villi.

fore, the increased mucosal and gut wall metabolic rate during gut activity probably lowers the oxygen concentration enough to cause much of the vasodilation. The decrease in oxygen can also lead to as much as a fourfold increase of adenosine, a well-known vasodilator that could be responsible for much of the increased flow. Thus, the increased blood flow during increased GI activity is probably a combination of many of the aforementioned factors plus still others yet undiscovered (34).

"Countercurrent" Blood Flow in the Villi

The arterial flow into the villus and the venous flow out of the villus are in directions opposite to each other, and the vessels lie in close apposition to each other (**Fig. 90.1**). Because of this vascular arrangement, much of the blood oxygen diffuses out of the arterioles directly into the adjacent venules without ever being carried in the blood to the tips of the villi. As much as 80% of the oxygen may take this short-circuit route and, therefore, not be available for local metabolic functions of the villi. Under normal conditions, this shunting of oxygen from the arterioles to the venules is not harmful to the villi; however, in disease conditions in which blood flow to the gut becomes greatly curtailed, such as in circulatory shock, the oxygen deficit in the tips of the villi can become so great that the villus tip or even the entire villus suffers ischemic death and can disintegrate. For this reason and others, in many GI diseases, the villi become seriously blunted, leading to greatly diminished intestinal absorptive capacity (34).

Nervous Control of Gastrointestinal Blood Flow

Stimulation of the parasympathetic nerves going to the stomach and lower colon increases local blood flow at the same time that it increases glandular secretion. This increased flow probably results secondarily from the increased glandular activity and not as a direct effect of the nervous stimulation. Sympathetic stimulation, by contrast, has a direct effect on essentially the entire GI tract to cause intense vasoconstriction of the arterioles with greatly decreased blood flow. After a few minutes of this vasoconstriction, the flow often returns to almost normal by means of a mechanism called *autoregulatory escape*. That is, the local metabolic vasodilator mechanisms that are elicited by ischemia become prepotent over the sympathetic vasoconstriction and, therefore, redilate the arterioles, thus causing return of necessary nutrient blood flow to the GI glands and muscle (10). A major value of sympathetic vasoconstriction in the gut is that it allows shut-off of GI and other splanchnic blood flow for short periods of time during heavy exercise, when increased flow is needed by the skeletal muscle and heart. Also, in circulatory shock, when all of the body's vital tissues, especially the brain and the heart, are in danger of cellular death for lack of blood flow, sympathetic stimulation can decrease splanchnic blood flow to very little for many hours. Sympathetic stimulation also causes strong vasoconstriction of the large-volume intestinal and mesenteric veins, thereby decreasing the volume of these veins and displacing large amounts of blood into other parts of the circulation. In hemorrhagic shock or other states of low blood volume, this mechanism can provide, in adults, as much as 200–400 mL of extra blood to sustain the general circulation (55).

THE GUT AS AN IMMUNE SYSTEM

To protect the body from its constant exposure to microbes, toxins, and other antigenic stimuli, the gut has developed an intricate array of defenses. Nonimmune defense elements include chemical and mechanical barriers, such as saliva, gastric acid, proteolytic enzymes, bile cryptdins, and the epithelial tight junction (14). Saliva contains peroxidase, which inhibits the growth of bacteria, and lysozyme, which lyses bacteria and enhances phagocytosis. The mucous layer provides a barrier that separates bacteria from the villous surface of the small intestine. The bile acids (chenodeoxycholic and cholic acids) possess antibacterial qualities. Cryptdins are low-molecular-weight proteins that are derived from the Paneth cells in the crypts of Lieberkühn. Preliminary findings suggest that cryptdins may form an antimicrobial barrier in the intestinal tract (55).

The primary cellular barrier of the gut that restricts luminal antigens from encountering the immune system is the single layer of gut epithelium. Each epithelial cell maintains intimate association with its neighbors and seals the surface of the gut with tight junctions. In the upper bowel, the bulk of antigen exposure comes from the diet, whereas in the ileum and colon, the additional antigenic load of an abundant and highly complex commensal microflora exists. Nevertheless, the gut epithelial barrier does not completely prevent luminal antigens from entering the tissues. The gut epithelial barrier therefore represents a highly dynamic structure that limits, but does not exclude, antigens from entering the tissues, whereas the immune system constantly samples gut antigens through the follicle-associated epithelium that overlies the organized lymphoid tissues of the intestinal wall and through the antigen-presenting dendritic cell processes. Follicle-associated epithelium contains specialized epithelial cells, termed *M cells*, whose function is to transport luminal antigens into the dome area of the follicle. Antigen-presenting dendritic cells also sense processes between gut epithelial cells without disturbing tight-junction integrity and sample commensal and pathogenic gut bacteria. The gut epithelium itself can also directly sense commensal bacteria and pathogens; integral to this are the mammalian pattern-recognition receptors, which recognize conserved structures of bacteria and viruses and generally activate proinflammatory pathways, alerting the host to infection. Two different classes of pattern recognition receptors are involved: the Toll-like receptors (TLRs) usually associated with cell membranes and the nucleotide-binding oligomerization domain (Nod) molecules. Signaling through Nod or TLR activates the transcription factor nuclear factor (NF)-κB, leading to proinflammatory gene expression.

TLR1 to TLR9 and Nod1 and Nod2 are all expressed by gut epithelial cells. Nod1 and Nod2 recognize slightly different muropeptide motifs derived from bacterial peptidoglycans, which suggests that they sense intracellular infection or attempted bacterial subversion of epithelial cells. TLRs recognize many different components of bacteria and viruses. For example, TLR4 recognizes lipopolysaccharide from the gram-negative bacterial cell wall, and TLR5 recognizes bacterial flagellin. An unresolved question is how the gut distinguishes between pathogens and commensal bacteria.

Mutualism also appears to exist between the commensal flora and the gut epithelium to maintain epithelial integrity. For example, recognition of TLR2 or TLR9 ligands by epithelial cells increases gut barrier function. The normal flora also induces cytoprotective proteins in colonic epithelial cells. Nonpathogenic microorganisms in the gut have also been shown to regulate inflammation negatively in other ways. For example, avirulent Salmonella inhibits activation of NFκB in epithelial cells by blocking polyubiquitination of phosphorylated IκBa. Overall, substantial evidence suggests that the normal commensal flora exerts an anti-inflammatory influence and protects epithelial cells from toxic insult. Epithelial proinflammatory responses to the commensal flora exist in vitro, but most individuals maintain an abundant intestinal flora without incurring disease (55).

Interactions of Commensal Bacteria with the Mucosal Immune System

Healthy individuals possess an abundant and highly active gut immune system that is tightly regulated to prevent excessive immune responses to foods and gut bacteria. A major difference between the systemic and mucosal immune system is the anatomic separation of the inductive sites of mucosal immunity in the organized lymphoid tissue, such as Peyer patches, from the effector sites in the lamina propria and epithelium. When T and B cells are activated in Peyer patches, they express the $\alpha 4\beta 7$ integrin and migrate to the blood. Gut-specific homing is achieved by expression of the ligand for $\alpha 4\beta 7$, mucosal addressin cell adhesion molecule (MADCAM)-1, on gut endothelial cells, which allows Peyer patch-derived cells to migrate through blood vessels into the lamina propria. Chemokines produced by either colon or small-bowel epithelial cells fine-tune the localization of lymphocytes to these tissues. The lamina propria is filled with antibody-producing plasma cells that secrete 3–5 g of the IgA immunoglobulin isotype into the gut lumen each day. This secretory IgA binds to bacteria in the lumen, thus preventing the microorganisms from attaching to mucosa. Numerous other immune cells also reside in the gut lamina propria, including large numbers of CD4$^+$ T cells, macrophages, dendritic cell, mast cells, and eosinophils. The gut epithelium also contains abundant intraepithelial lymphocytes, an intriguing population comprised of mostly of CD8$^+$ T cells. Compared with other tissues, intraepithelial lymphocytes are enriched in T cells that express the $\gamma\delta$ T-cell receptor and often express the homodimeric form of the CD8α coreceptor. The exact function of intraepithelial lymphocytes is not known, although it has been suggested that they may play a role in epithelial tumor surveillance, protection against epithelial pathogens, or promotion of healing of the gut after injury (55). The presence of an extensive and activated intestinal immune system depends on the commensal flora. The relationship between the immune system and the commensal flora is a precarious one, and perturbations in immune or epithelial homeostasis can lead to gut inflammation.

NEUTROPENIC ENTEROCOLITIS (TYPHLITIS)

Advances in neoplastic treatment modalities for children have greatly increased the cancer survival rate (2); however, cancer continues to be a leading cause of death by disease in children. Typhlitis was initially described as necrotizing colitis (NEC) involving the cecum ("typhlon" in Greek) that occurred in patients with acute leukemia (21). Since then, this entity has been recognized both in patients with advanced malignant tumors and in patients with immunodeficiencies. Typhlitis is a life-threatening oncologic emergency that occurs in the presence of neutropenia, often in the induction phase of chemotherapy for leukemia. It is an inflammatory process of the GI tract that presents as NEC in the cecum and ascending colon.

Pathogenesis

The pathogenesis of typhlitis is poorly understood. The disease appears to be the result of a combination of factors, including mucosal injury by cytotoxic drugs, neutropenia, and impaired host defense to intestinal organisms. It has been postulated that the intact colonic mucosa cannot be maintained due to either leukemic infiltration or direct cytotoxic effect of chemotherapy.

Bacterial invasion of the bowel wall ensues, facilitated by a decreased defense due to neutropenia, followed by production of bacterial endotoxins, with subsequent bacteremia, necrosis, and hemorrhage. The cecum is almost always affected, and the disease can often extend into the terminal ileum, other parts of the small bowel, and right and left colon. The predilection for the cecum may be related to its distensibility and limited blood supply. Pathology may reveal edema of the mucosa or entire intestinal wall, mucosal ulcerations, focal hemorrhage, and mucosal or transmural necrosis. Leukemic or acute inflammatory infiltrates are rarely identified (21).

Diagnosis

Imaging studies can be useful in supporting a diagnosis of neutropenic enterocolitis. Abdominal ultrasound typically reveals a right lower-quadrant inflammatory mass, bowel wall edema, and pericecal fluid or soft-tissue inflammation (70,78). CT may be the preferred diagnostic modality over ultrasound and plain abdominal films, particularly because it helps to differentiate this entity from other potential diagnoses. Barium enema and colonoscopy can be hazardous and may be contraindicated, as they can precipitate perforation. The syndrome is characterized on CT scan by bowel wall thickening, inflammation, and the presence of peritoneal fluid and other areas of edema (66). As chemotherapy can alter the GI mucosa in cases of gastritis and esophagitis, it can also decrease the integrity of the colon, causing tissue alteration and inflammation and precipitating the invasion of bacteria, which results in septicemia. Necrosis can result in bowel perforation, seen as pneumatosis intestinalis on plain x-rays, especially with an infectious process (66).

Various organisms, alone or in combination, have been identified in surgical specimens and peritoneal fluid, including gram-negative rods, gram-positive cocci, enterococci, *Clostridium septicum*, *Candida*, and cytomegalovirus (CMV). *Clostridium difficile* toxin is occasionally detected in the stool; therefore, treatment must be broad-spectrum, encompassing coverage for anaerobes and treatment for fungus. Vascular compromise, mucosal ulceration, and ultimately, tissue perforation lead to a high mortality rate with this illness. In children with leukemia, survival rates from neutropenic enterocolitis have been reported as only 55%–60% (21).

Clinical Presentation

Neutropenic enterocolitis should be suspected in any severely neutropenic patient (absolute neutrophil count <500/mL) who presents with fever and abdominal pain, particularly in the right lower quadrant, with or without rebound tenderness. Symptoms of typhlitis include right-sided abdominal pain; watery, bloody diarrhea; abdominal distention; and fever. Vomiting, anorexia, and possible hematemesis are also hallmark signs, with guarding and positive peritoneal signs found on physical exam. Typhlitis represents an emergency, as it could lead to bowel obstruction or perforation, necessitating an immediate surgical referral. Treatment for the child with typhlitis includes obtaining serial abdominal x-rays, CT, or ultrasounds; ensuring bowel rest; administering broad-spectrum antibiotics; monitoring and managing fluids and electrolytes; and providing nutrition in the form of total parenteral nutrition. Surgical intervention is needed by a significant number of children with this diagnosis. A combination of antibiotics should be used with the goal of broad-spectrum, gram-positive, and gram-negative coverage. Pain management for these children can be a challenge due to the decreased motility associated with the use of opioids, but pain and comfort measures are also an important part of treatment.

In children, neutropenic enterocolitis has been defined as fever, abdominal pain, and abdominal tenderness in an immunosuppressed, neutropenic patient with radiologic evidence of right-side colonic inflammation (78). Diarrhea occurs in 50%–80% of patients, with melena or hematochezia in 25%–40%. Virtually all patients have mucositis.

HYPOMOTILITY

Postoperative ileus, defined as the functional inhibition of propulsive bowel activity after surgery, irrespective of pathogenic mechanism, is common, especially after abdominal laparotomy, and severity is inversely related to the child's age. GI hypomotility manifesting as decreased bowel sounds or abdominal distention is common and has been reported in up to half of patients with respiratory failure. Studies on the frequency of nonhemorrhagic GI complications in adult ICU patients who are receiving enteral feeds indicate that almost two-thirds of subjects develop one or more GI complications; high gastric residuals and constipation are most common. Patients with GI complications have longer ICU stays and higher mortality compared to the group without GI complications (59).

Inflammation and Motility in Experimental Models

Experimental animal models have clearly shown interaction between inflammation and motility (47). Intestinal hypomotility and delayed gastric emptying have been shown to be characteristic in a mouse model of postoperative ileus. The study showed that this condition is the result of intestinal inflammation due to activation of macrophages that are triggered by bowel manipulation and that intestinal inflammation can be prevented by perioperative stimulation of the vagus nerve. Also, vagal stimulation ameliorates postoperative ileus. It has also been shown in this model that leukocyte-derived inducible nitric oxide (NO) plays an important role in the generation of intestinal inflammation and inhibition of GI motility. In the rat model of hemorrhagic shock, it has been shown that induced NO contributes to the inflammatory changes in the gut wall and participates in the activation of cytokine expression that regulates impaired gut motility. These observations clearly suggest that inflammation of the GI tract causes significant alteration in gut motor function, and the immunologic profile of the inflammatory response may be an important determinant of these changes that occur in each model (47).

Using manometric evaluation, it has been reported that the motility of the upper GI tract in patients who receive mechanical ventilation is severely impaired (47). Contractile activity was completely lost in the stomach and diminished to

a lesser degree in the duodenum. These abnormalities may be related to dysfunction of interstitial cells of Cajal that are concentrated in the antrum and act as the pacemaker and controller of GI motor activity. Clinically, most patients with hypomotility present with intolerance to enteral nutrition and high gastric residuals. This contraction abnormality may also favor duodenogastric reflux and colonization of the stomach by enteric gram-negative pathogens. Correction of electrolyte abnormalities (e.g., hypokalemia, hypomagnesemia) and avoidance of medications (particularly opiates) that impair GI motility are important for the prevention of ileus and bowel dilatation.

Like opiates, dopamine has been shown to impair GI motility (50). This negative effect can be seen at doses as low as 5 mcg/kg/min and worsens with increasing rates of infusion. Other commonly used medications that cause GI hypomotility are phenothiazines, diltiazem, verapamil, and drugs with anticholinergic side effects. If necessary, nasogastric suction and/or rectal tubes and, in intractable cases, colonoscopy can be used to decompress the GI tract. Rectal tubes have been associated with complications, including discomfort, local ulceration, infection, and perforation of rectum. Prokinetic agents, such as erythromycin, have been shown to promote gastric emptying in patients receiving mechanical ventilation and should be considered once mechanical obstruction is excluded.

Erythromycin can improve gastric motility in these patients by increasing the amplitude of antral contractions and improving antroduodenal coordination. While erythromycin acts via motilin receptors, an intact vagal pathway has been shown to be necessary for its GI effects (61). While considerable evidence suggests that erythromycin may be a useful prokinetic agent in children, the quality of these data is significantly limited by the lack of randomized, placebo-controlled trials. The optimum dose for prokinetic activity is not known but it appears that low-dose erythromycin (1–3 mg/kg) effectively stimulates gastric antral motility (19). A total daily dose of 20 mg/kg/day divided in 3–4 doses/day, by mouth, is generally used for prokinetic effects. Metoclopramide is another prokinetic agent that is useful in the treatment of gastroduodenal hypomotility. The precise mechanism of action is unclear, but metoclopramide improves antroduodenal coordination and reverses the inhibitory effects of dopamine on GI motility (43,50). Similarly, cisapride stimulates myenteric cholinergic nerves with consequent increase of acetylcholine release and was used extensively in ICU patients to promote motility. However, many reports, both in children and adult populations, which showed its association with cardiac arrhythmia, including many deaths, have led to withdrawal of cisapride from the US and European markets (19). Data that directly compare the relative potency of prokinetics in critically ill patients with GI hypomotility are insufficient (77).

DIARRHEA

Diarrhea is defined as a change in bowel habit for the individual child that results in substantially more frequent and/or looser stools (4). Young children are at great risk for infectious diarrhea and resulting dehydration. Diarrhea is common in critically ill patients, especially when sepsis and hypoalbuminemia are present and during enteral feeding and antibiotic therapy. Up to 50% of critically ill patients develop diarrhea during their ICU stay, and those with acute respiratory failure appear to be particularly at risk (61).

Causes of Diarrhea

Although many factors have been implicated, the etiology of diarrhea in the ICU is unknown and probably multifactorial (61) (**Table 90.2**). Diarrhea may be a reflection of the severity of underlying illness that leads to gut dysmotility. Diarrhea is a frequently reported complication of enteral feeding, affecting up to 12%–25% of adult patients, even in the absence of GI dysfunction (61). The main pathophysiologic mechanisms of diarrhea include osmotic and secretory diarrhea. Malabsorption of nonabsorbable solutes in the GI tract, such as carbohydrates, causes osmotic diarrhea. In addition, bacterial fermentation of a portion of the nonabsorbed carbohydrate reaching the colon results in the formation of short-chain fatty acids, which further contributes to the osmotic load presented to the colon and limits water resolution. In addition, short-chain fatty acids stimulate peristalsis. Abdominal distention ensues because of the large fluid loads in the lumen (67) and the production of gaseous products of fermentation. Injury to the villous surface impairs sugar absorption, resulting in osmotic retention of water in the intestinal lumen. Depletion of carbohydrase may occur as a result of a variety of viral, bacterial, or parasitic injuries (**Table 90.2**). Enzyme depletion is also noted in the critically ill child who is significantly malnourished.

Reducing the rate of tube feeds generally improves diarrhea, probably by reducing the carbohydrate load to the gut. Thus, dilution of enteral formulas may not be helpful, especially if the patient is receiving an iso-osmolar tube feeding. This practice is a misconception that resulted from previous experience with hyperosmolar formulas and should not be expected to decrease the diarrhea seen with iso-osmolar feedings. Interestingly, diluting iso-osmolar tube feedings may be associated with decreased absorption of nutrients. In view of current evidence, there is no need to start enteral nutrition by diluting iso-osmolar tube feeds in an attempt to improve tolerance or prevent diarrhea.

Recently, relative luminal excess of bile acids has been offered as a cause of diarrhea in ICU patients (23). Both animal and human studies have shown that prolonged starvation causes diffuse atrophy of the gut, including the terminal ileum (36). Theoretically, if mucosal damage extends to the terminal ileum, abnormal bile acid homeostasis can occur, leading to five- to tenfold increases in stool bile acid as compared to normal volunteers. The administration of bile acid-binding agents improved the diarrhea (23).

Liberal use of antibiotics in ICU patients predisposes patients to antibiotic-associated diarrhea, which accounts for 20%–50% of all cases of nosocomial diarrhea (52). The incidence has increased fivefold over 10 years, probably because of increasing use of cephalosporins in the early 1990s (61). Approximately 15%–25% of antibiotic-associated diarrhea in adults is caused by *C. difficile* infection. Antibiotic-associated diarrhea that is not due to *C. difficile* is probably caused by the direct effect of the antibiotic on intestinal motility and by a reduction of intestinal carbohydrate fermentation (52). It is usually self-limited and resolves with the discontinuation of antibiotic therapy. *C. difficile*, however, is associated with significant morbidity and even mortality if fulminant colitis or toxic megacolon (TM) develops because of delay in diagnosis (61).

The mechanisms for secretory diarrhea include activation of the intracellular mediators, such as cAMP, cyclic GMP, and intracellular calcium (Ca^{2+}), which stimulate active Cl^- secretion from the crypt cells and inhibit the absorption of neutral, coupled NaCl. These mediators alter the paracellular ion flux because of toxin-mediated injury to the tight junctions. The classic example of secretory diarrhea is that induced by cholera and *Escherichia coli* enterotoxins that bind to a specific enterocyte surface receptor (the monosialoganglioside GM_1); a fragment of the toxin then enters the cell, where it activates adenylate cyclase on the basolateral membrane through interaction with a stimulatory G protein, thereby increasing intracellular cAMP.

It is simple to differentiate osmotic from secretory diarrhea, as osmotic diarrhea has a reduced volume of stool per day, a lower Na content, a pH of <5, tests positive for reducing/nonreducing sugars, and usually responds to fasting (31).

Diarrhea Secondary to Hypoalbuminemia

Hypoalbuminemia has been implicated as a predisposing factor for diarrhea in critically ill patients, especially those with a serum albumin level <2.6 g/dL (11). For the same degree of hypoalbuminemia, subjects with chronic malnutrition had a higher incidence of diarrhea compared to those with acute hypoalbuminemia (e.g., burn patients). These results suggested that it is not the severity, but rather the chronicity of malnutrition, that is more important in the development of diarrhea.

Evaluation of Diarrhea

After documenting increased stool frequency and volume, gross stool examination must be conducted to detect blood, leukocytes, mucus, ova, and parasites. Presence of leukocytes suggests presence of invasive or toxin-producing microorganism

---

TABLE 90.2

CAUSES OF DIARRHEA IN ICU PATIENTS

Enteral nutrition
  Hyperosmolar formulas
  High infusion rates
  Dietary lipids
Infection
  Viruses (*rotavirus, adenovirus, calicivirus, astrovirus*)
  Bacteria (*Salmonella spp., shigella spp., C. difficile,*
    C. jejuni, E coli O157H:, Yersinia spp.)
  Parasites (*Aeromonas spp., G. lamblia,*
    Cryptosporidium spp.)
Medications
  Antacids
  H_2-Receptor antagonists
  Antibiotics
Hypoalbuminemia
  Particularly those with chronic severe hypoalbuminemia
    (<2.6 g/dL)
Prolonged fasting (>5 day)

Adapted from Mutlu GM, MD, Mutlu EA, and Factor P. GI complications in patients receiving mechanical ventilation. *Chest* 2001;119:1222–41.

bacteria in the gut, such as *Shigella, Salmonella, Campylobacter jejuni,* invasive *E. coli, C. difficile, Yersinia enterocolitica, Vibrio parahaemolyticus,* and possibly *Aeromonas* or *Plesiomonas shigelloides.* Cultures for enteric pathogens and enzyme-linked immunosorbent assay (ELISA) for viral pathogens and *C. difficile* toxin are recommended (68). Osmotic or secretory causes of diarrhea must be ascertained.

Management of Diarrhea

Specific treatment depends on the underlying cause. The inability to identify the exact cause often complicates the picture and limits optimal care. Patients should be placed on regimens of enteric precautions and empiric antibiotic therapy while the laboratory tests are pending. If the clinical evolution of the child with diarrhea does not suggest *C. difficile,* other common causes of diarrhea (**Table 90.2**) must be ruled out and treated accordingly.

Fluid Therapy in Diarrhea

Diarrhea is a common cause of fluid loss, dehydration, and electrolyte disorders. In the patient with significant diarrhea and a limited ability to take oral fluid, it is important to devise a treatment that incorporates total deficit, ongoing losses, and maintenance fluids.

Clinical Evaluation of Dehydration. Following are clinical presentations of dehydration.

■ *Mild dehydration* (3% in older children and 5% in infants): normal or increased pulse rate, decreased urinary output, thirst, and normal physical examination.
■ *Moderate dehydration* (6% in older children and 10% in infants): tachycardia, little or no urine output, irritability/lethargy, sunken eyes and fontanelle, decreased tears, dry mucous membranes, mild tenting of the skin, delayed capillary refill, cool and pale skin.
■ *Severe dehydration* (>9% in older children and >15% in infants): rapid and weak pulse, decreased blood pressure, no urine output, very sunken eyes and fontanelle, no tears, parched mucous membranes, tenting of the skin, very delayed capillary refill, cold and mottled skin (5,33).

Calculation of Fluid Deficits. The dehydrated child has lost water, with concurrent loss of Na and K. Most patients have isotonic dehydration and, therefore, have normal serum Na values. The water deficit in liters can be estimated as the percent dehydration multiplied by the patient's weight in kilograms. The Na and K deficits are estimated from the water deficit.

For acute dehydration of <3-day duration, a relatively greater loss of the extracellular fluid (ECF) and electrolyte deficits occurs and can be estimated using:

$$\text{Na deficit (mEq)} = \text{water deficit (L)} \times 110\,\text{mEq/L}$$
$$\text{K deficit (mEq)} = \text{water deficit (L)} \times 30\,\text{mEq/L}$$

For more prolonged dehydration, of >3-day duration, relatively more intracellular fluid is lost, and electrolyte deficits can be estimated using:

$$\text{Na deficit (mEq)} = \text{water deficit (L)} \times 80\,\text{mEq/L}$$
$$\text{K deficit (mEq)} = \text{water deficit (L)} \times 60\,\text{mEq/L}$$

Approach to Dehydration. Initial rapid hydration is necessary for children with clinical signs and symptoms of severe dehydration to ensure adequate tissue perfusion. Initial therapy requires administration of 20–40 mL/kg of 0.9% saline or Ringer's lactate in the first hour to expand the ECF volume. Rapid administration of larger quantities—60–100 mL/kg—may be necessary to restore circulation. Once ECF volume is expanded and renal perfusion is restored, treatment can be changed to a slower rate to replace maintenance requirements, remaining deficit fluids, and any ongoing abnormal losses. Acidosis is readily corrected when circulation is restored. It is important to closely monitor fluid electrolytes and acid-base status after the initial rehydration therapy. Because restoration of volume status usually stops production of metabolic acidosis, correction of pH is rarely needed. If bicarbonate HCO_3 losses are large and need to be corrected, the HCO_3 deficit can be estimated using:

$$HCO_3 \text{ deficit (mEq)} = 0.5\,(\text{L/kg}) \times \text{weight (kg)} \times$$
$$[\text{desired } HCO_3\,(\text{mEq/L}) - \text{current } HCO_3\,(\text{mEq/L})]$$

When the intravascular volume is reestablished, it is appropriate to plan the fluid therapy for the first 24 hrs.

Isonatremic Dehydration. Isonatremic dehydration (serum Na concentration 130–150 mEq/L) is the most common form of diarrheal dehydration in children. In isonatremic dehydration, water and Na are lost in physiologic proportion (isotonic loss), thus maintaining the serum Na concentration within the normal range. In isotonic dehydration, the entire fluid deficit is corrected over 24 hrs.

The normal maintenance fluids and the fluid deficit are given. If possible, oral rehydrating therapy should be started as soon as tolerated, usually 6–12 hrs after parenteral therapy has begun, and continued for the remaining 24 hrs to replace deficit fluids. If IV fluid therapy is warranted, the total amount of water and electrolyte deficits is determined and appropriate fluids are selected. IV fluid administration can then proceed, using three solutions. One of the solutions can contain the "deficit replacement" for water and electrolytes, the second can contain "maintenance" water and electrolyte fluid, and the third, a fluid with the appropriate water and electrolyte concentrations to address the "ongoing" losses. A two-solution strategy combines the fluid and electrolyte needs for both half of the "deficit" and one-third of the "maintenance," and again, a second fluid is used for replacing "ongoing" losses. One-half of the deficit replacement fluid can be administered over the first 8 hrs, along with one-third of the maintenance fluid. Using the two-solution method, adjustments may be necessary for the next 16 hrs, with a combination of water and electrolytes to address the other half of the "deficit" and the other two-thirds of the "maintenance" fluids.

The K concentration of the maintenance solution must be tailored, depending on the clinical situation. K is not usually included in the IV fluids until the patient voids. Half of the total fluid is given over the first 8 hrs; previous boluses are subtracted from this volume. The remainder is given over the next 16 hrs. It is important to consider ongoing fluid losses of the patient. The child with copious diarrhea must receive an additional replacement solution (the "ongoing" loss replacement), or the rehydration will not be complete (5,33). Ongoing losses from diarrhea can vary in their electrolyte concentration. Na losses may range from 10 to 90 mEq/L, and K losses may range from 10 to 80 mEq/L. A solution of half normal saline can be used initially for replacement, and the electrolyte concentration of this solution can be adjusted based on electrolyte concentrations measured in the stool and serum.

Hyponatremic Dehydration. Hyponatremic dehydration (serum Na concentration <130 mEq/L) occurs when Na loss is disproportionately greater than the water loss. Because serum osmolality is low, water shifts from ECF into the intracellular fluid, making the symptoms of ECF volume contraction more severe than in the other forms of dehydration. In addition, some patients develop symptoms, predominantly neurologic, from the hyponatremia. The initial goal in treating hyponatremia is correction of intravascular volume depletion with isotonic fluid (normal saline or Ringer's lactate). Hyponatremic dehydration requires replacement of Na and water losses. The excess Na deficit can be calculated using the following formula:

$$\text{Excess Na deficit (mEq)} = 0.6\,(\text{L/kg}) \times \text{weight (kg)} \times$$

$$[\text{desired Na (mEq/L)} - \text{present Na concentration (mEq/L)}]$$

This is the amount of Na that should be added to the Na deficit calculated from the electrolyte deficits based on the fluid loss (above).

It is not necessary to increase the Na beyond 135 mEq/L, as "overcorrection" is associated with an increased risk of central pontine myelinolysis. The risk of this condition also increases with overly rapid correction of the serum Na concentration. The risk in children is not clear, but it is prudent to avoid increasing the Na by more than 10–20 mEq/L every 24 hrs.

As with isotonic dehydration, half of the deficit replacement fluid can be administered over the first 8 hrs, along with one-third of the maintenance fluid. Again, K delivery is adjusted based on the initial serum K and the patient's renal function. K is not given until the patient voids. The patient's Na concentration should be monitored to ensure appropriate correction and that the Na concentration of the fluid is adjusted appropriately. Patients with ongoing losses require an appropriate replacement solution. Patients with neurologic symptoms (e.g., seizures) from hyponatremia must receive an acute infusion of hypertonic (3%) saline to rapidly increase the serum Na concentration to 120 mEq/L. The above formula for excess Na deficit can be used with 120 mEq as the desired Na concentration. The calculated amount of Na in mEq needed to raise the Na level to 120 mEq/L can be given as a bolus of 3% normal saline, with each 2 mL of 3% normal saline containing 1 mEq of Na (5,33).

Hypernatremic Dehydration. Hypernatremic dehydration (serum Na concentration >150 mEq/L) occurs when the lost fluid contains less Na than water (hypotonic fluid). Because of the ECF hyperosmolality, water is osmotically moved from intracellular fluid into the extracellular space. Hypernatremic dehydration is the most dangerous form of dehydration due to complications of hypernatremia and therapy. Hypernatremia can cause serious neurologic damage, including hemorrhage and thrombosis, which appears to be secondary to movement of water from the brain cells into the hypertonic ECF, causing brain-cell shrinkage and tearing blood vessels within the brain. The movement of water from the intracellular space to the extracellular space during hypernatremic dehydration protects the intravascular volume. Thus, children with hypernatremia often appear less ill than children with a similar degree of

isotonic dehydration. Urine output may be preserved longer, and less tachycardia may occur. Children with hypernatremic dehydration are often lethargic but irritable. Hypernatremia may cause fever, hypertonicity, and hyperreflexia. More severe neurologic symptoms may develop if cerebral bleeding occurs.

Treatment of hypernatremic dehydration may cause significant morbidity and mortality. Generation of idiogenic osmoles occurs within the brain during the development of hypernatremia. These idiogenic osmoles increase the osmolality within the cells of the brain, providing protection against brain-cell shrinkage caused by movement of water out of cells into the hypertonic ECF. However, these idiogenic osmoles dissipate slowly during correction of hypernatremia. With overly rapid lowering of the extracellular osmolality during correction of hypernatremia, an osmotic gradient may be created that causes water movement from the extracellular space into the cells of the brain, producing cerebral edema. Symptoms of the resultant cerebral edema can range from seizures to brain herniation and death. To minimize the risk of cerebral edema during correction of hypernatremic dehydration, the guideline is that serum Na concentration should not decrease more than 12–15 mEq/L every 24 hrs. Severe hypernatremic dehydration may need to be corrected over 3–4 days.

The initial management of hypernatremic dehydration requires restoration of the intravascular volume with normal saline. Ringer's lactate should not be used because it is more hypotonic than normal saline (Ringer's lactate has 100 mL more free water per liter than normal saline) and may cause too rapid a decrease in the serum Na concentration, especially if multiple fluid boluses are necessary. To avoid cerebral edema when correcting hypernatremic dehydration, the fluid deficit is corrected slowly. The rate of correction depends on the initial Na concentration. Under these circumstances, the free water deficit (FWD) can be estimated using an estimate of the total body water (TBW in liters = 0.6 L/kg × weight in kg) and the following equation:

$$\text{FWD in liters} = \text{TBW} - \text{TBW}\,(\text{desired Na/current Na})$$

The FWD is subtracted from estimated total fluid deficit (in liters = % dehydration × wt in kg) to produce the solute fluid deficit (SFD): SFD in liters = Total fluid deficit – FWD.

The SFD is used to calculate the amount of electrolytes that have been lost. All of the SFD (and electrolytes) is replaced in the first 24 hrs, while only one-third of the FWD is replaced in the first 24 hrs and the other two-thirds are replaced in the second 48 hrs. Again, maintenance and ongoing losses must be considered and addressed.

Unlike patients with isotonic or hyponatremic dehydration, the fluid is not run at a faster rate during the first 8 hrs. No general agreement exists on the choice of fluid or the rate of fluid for correcting hypernatremic dehydration. The choice and rate of fluid administration are not nearly as important as vigilant monitoring of the serum Na concentration and adjustment of the therapy based on the result. The rate of decrease of the serum Na concentration is roughly related to the "free water" delivery, although variation between patients is considerable. Adjustment in the Na concentration of the IV fluid is the most common approach for modifying the rate of decrease in the serum concentration (5,33).

C. DIFFICILE AND PSEUDOMEMBRANOUS COLITIS

Numerous studies have implicated *C. difficile* as an etiologic agent of pseudomembranous colitis PMC (12). *C. difficile* infections may affect all age groups, although a lower incidence has been noted in children (73). The antibiotics most frequently implicated in PMC in children are ampicillin, penicillin, cephalosporins, amoxicillin, and clindamycin (12). Those that rarely cause PMC are aminoglycosides, fluorouracil, rifampin, methotrexate, and sulfonamides. Other species of *Clostridium* (*C. innocuum*, *C. oroticum*, and *C. ramosum*), along with *Candida* species and aerobic gram-negative bacilli, have also been implicated in rare cases. Some reports have also described infants and adults with severe PMC associated with *C. difficile* toxin in the stools without previous antibiotic exposure. *C. difficile* can produce at least two toxins, both of which are necessary to produce PMC (46), an enterotoxin (toxin A) and a cytotoxin (toxin B). The cytotoxin is potent in tissue culture assays and is a relatively sensitive and specific marker for *C. difficile*-induced disease, whereas toxin A is significantly more potent in biologic assays of enteric toxins when animal models are used and may be more important in clinical expression of GI complications.

Most stools from patients with antibiotic-associated PMC contain the *C. difficile* organism as well as its cytotoxin (12). Individuals treated with antibiotics can become susceptible to acquiring the organism from an environmental source (12). Nearly 30% of healthy newborns harbor *C. difficile* as a component of the fecal flora, and some also have detectable toxin in their stool without clinically apparent consequences (12). *C. difficile* can be spread in a neonatal nursery, in hospital wards, and in households (12). The organism is transmitted by hands of personnel caring for symptomatic or colonized patients and by fomites. A high incidence of asymptomatic carriage of *C. difficile* has been found in children <2 years of age, particularly those who have received antibiotics (12).

Disruption of the competitive microbial balance in the intestine is an important initiating step of PMC. The ability of *C. difficile* to produce PMC mostly in the presence of antibiotic exposure is explained by its enhanced growth in an environment that has reduced bacterial competition. Animal studies support this hypothesis. The toxin of *C. difficile* has not generally been implicated in the pathogenesis of NEC. It is speculated that infants are generally not as susceptible as older children are to the toxicity of *C. difficile* toxin (12).

Clinical Presentation and Diagnosis

Disease as a result of *C. difficile* represents a wide spectrum, ranging from asymptomatic carriage, asymptomatic cases, mild nonspecific diarrhea, antibiotic-associated colitis without pseudomembrane formation, PMC, and fulminant colitis. Fortunately, the most severe forms are also the least common (12). The extent of other abdominal complaints or systemic symptoms varies from mild to severe. The disease may be fatal. Abdominal pain, cramps, lower-quadrant tenderness, fever, and leukocytosis are common. Severe dehydration and vascular collapse are rare, particularly in children. The duration of symptoms in those with mild disease not requiring specific therapy

usually ranges from 7 to 10 days after discontinuation of the instigating antibiotic. More prolonged symptoms or significant toxicity may indicate the need for specific antimicrobial intervention. The severe form of PMC must be differentiated from other causes of acute intra-abdominal pathology (e.g., appendicitis, perforated viscus, intussusception, or ischemic bowel), whereas the mild, self-limited disease can resemble viral gastroenteritis. Blood in stool out of proportion to diarrhea or systemic illness is a clue to *C. difficile* disease.

Diagnosis of *C. difficile* diarrhea requires a high index of suspicion and is frequently made by detection of cytotoxins in the stool. No rapid test is completely reliable. Several new enzyme immunoassays approach the accuracy of tissue culture assay and can detect toxins A or B, or both. The latex particle agglutination assay is not as reliable. The immunoblot assay and polymerase chain reaction can detect toxin A only (22). The tissue culture assay remains the gold standard, but it is expensive and requires overnight incubation of samples. The rapid enzyme immunoassay can detect *C. difficile* with fair sensitivity (69%–87%) and excellent specificity (99%–100%) (46). Stool cultures for *C. difficile* using selective medium should be attempted, accompanied by a reliable toxin assay. Owing to the lack of sensitivity, it may be necessary to repeat the enzyme immunoassay. While no guidelines have been suggested as to how many assays should be performed before *C. difficile* can be excluded, repeat testing may be helpful when clinical suspicion is high. Clinical and laboratory features that predict a positive assay are the onset of diarrhea 6 days after the administration of antibiotics, hospital stay >15 days, the presence of fecal leukocytes, the presence of semi-formed (as opposed to watery) stools, and cephalosporin use (56).

Endoscopy can detect the typical plaque-like lesions of the pseudomembrane. Sigmoidoscopy may be sufficient when the distal colon is involved, but if the pseudomembrane is restricted to the right colon, colonoscopy is necessary. Findings range from a normal mucosa through a spectrum of changes, including erythema and edema, friability, ulceration, and hemorrhage, as well as PMC. The most useful x-ray study is air-contrast barium enema, which is often nonspecific. However, the demonstration of PMC by either x-rays or endoscopy is an anatomic, not an etiologic, diagnosis (12).

Management of Pseudomembranous Colitis

Supportive therapy only is generally adequate for patients with mild diarrhea and no systemic complications. Those with severe symptoms or persistent diarrhea require aggressive therapy. Vancomycin is effective but is associated with a relapse rate of up to 20%. Cholestyramine, an anion-exchange resin that binds both *C. difficile* toxins, is an alternative to vancomycin. It is more likely to result in primary treatment failure than vancomycin but is less likely to be followed by relapse. Metronidazole and bacitracin can also be used to treat PMC. Oral metronidazole has similar efficacy to oral vancomycin in mild and moderate cases, lower cost, and does not select enterococcal resistance to vancomycin. Disadvantages of metronidazole are occasional resistance to *C. difficile*, rare induction of PMC, absence of convenient preparations for children, and its complete absorption at the upper GI tract so that bactericidal levels are achieved erratically in the lower GI tract. Antimotility agents, including loperamide, diphenoxylate hydrochloride with atropine, and opioids, should be avoided because they can adversely affect the ability to clear the toxins. Fever, systemic manifestations, and severe diarrhea generally improve within 1–2 days of therapy, but diarrhea may last for 4–5 days (12).

Relapses may be caused by reacquisition or persistence of spores in the colon. Most patients with a relapse respond to re-treatment but may experience multiple recurrences. Surgical intervention may be required to manage severe cases of PMC unresponsive to medical therapy or to manage complications such as toxic megacolon or colonic perforation. In fulminate PMC, careful vigilance is necessary to detect early signs of peritonitis and abdominal cellulitis that can indicate underlying intestinal perforation.

Complications

Complications of PMC include dehydration, electrolyte imbalance, hypotension, hypoalbuminemia with anasarca, transverse volvulus, colon perforation, and TM. Severe cases of PMC are prone to secondary systemic infection because of acquired malnutrition, hypogammaglobulinemia, lymphopenia, ascites, pleural effusions, and bacteremia from the intestinal inflammatory process. Recurrent colitis and diarrhea occur in one of five patients 2–8 weeks after completion of therapy; occasionally, more than six episodes might occur.

INTESTINAL ISCHEMIA

Splanchnic hemodynamics may be impaired by mechanical ventilation, particularly when a high level of positive end-expiratory pressure (PEEP) is used, as well as by shock and other hypoperfusion/reperfusion states. Experimental evidence suggests that PEEP decreases mesenteric flow by either increasing vascular resistance or by reducing cardiac output. This effect of PEEP may be partially reversed with IV fluids and dopexamine, a potent β_2-adrenoceptor and dopaminergic agonist, but not with dopamine or dobutamine. Similar effects of mechanical ventilation have been demonstrated on pancreatic and liver perfusion in animals (61).

Abdominal Compartment Syndrome

Abdominal compartment syndrome (ACS) is now a well-recognized but, until recently, uncommon entity that results from intra-abdominal hypertension (IAH). Its main features include abdominal distention and IAH, refractory oliguria or anuria, decreased cardiac output and hypotension secondary to reduced venous return from the lower part of the body, and markedly reduced thoracic compliance (15,72). The effects of IAH have been known for more than a century (72). However, the term *abdominal compartment syndrome* as a clinical entity was coined only in the early 1980s and came to the forefront of medical practice only during the last decade. Most patients with ACS described thus far have been adults and, in almost all cases, ACS developed after a primary abdominal problem—traumatic, surgical, or medical (7). The frequency of IAH and ACS in adult ICUs is unknown; ACS was identified in 14%–

15% of adults with severe abdominal trauma. As the frequency of major abdominal trauma in children and adults is similar, a similar rate of ACS with severe trauma would be expected for children. A 1999 report states that, "Children normally have relative organomegaly, so that their free intra-abdominal space may be relatively small, and they may be less able to accommodate additional intra-abdominal volume. However, less omental fat and a thinner, more compliant abdominal wall may compensate for that" (7). Clinical constellations that can lead to IAH have been well known in children for many years, although they were not categorized under the title of ACS. Life-threatening IAH has been well described in neonates born with gastroschisis and omphalocele, when primary closure of the abdominal defect was attempted, resulting in decreased thoracic compliance and in hemodynamic compromise (7). In fact, the surgical techniques currently used to treat ACS, namely, temporary abdominal closure with synthetic materials and staged abdominal repair, were pioneered in these patients. IAH and its effects have also been described in children with major burns, resulting in poorer prognosis (7). In children, ACS has been associated with primary abdominal problems and primarily extra-abdominal problems (isolated CNS pathology and meningococcemia). The most frequent cause of ACS in pediatric patients in a recent report was bowel ischemia or necrosis, a finding reported rarely in adults (7), and the majority of the other episodes resulted from severe bowel edema and ascites, likely secondary to ischemia-reperfusion injury after shock and fluid resuscitation. However, the 3 patients with primary isolated CNS problems neither had shock nor received fluid resuscitation, and the mechanism leading to bowel ischemia/necrosis was unclear (7). It has been suggested that splanchnic hypoperfusion and mucosal acidosis commence at much lower abdominal pressures and that bowel mucosal ischemia starts long before ACS is clinically recognizable (41).

Signs and symptoms of ACS in pediatric series are similar to those reported for adults; however, ACS develops at a lower intra-abdominal pressure (IAP) (lowest, 17 mm Hg), contrasting with reports in adults, in whom only an IAP >25 mm Hg or even 30 mm Hg is considered severe enough to warrant abdominal decompression (7). Therefore, this finding suggests that children are prone to develop ACS at lower IAP than are adults. This observation is of crucial clinical importance: If signs of IAH are present, even in part, one must not exclude the diagnosis of ACS solely because IAP is not elevated "enough." Such an approach might delay the crucial decompressive laparotomy and might result in disastrous consequences, such as extensive intestinal necrosis.

IAH also can increase intracranial pressure and reduce splanchnic and hepatic perfusion, which may lead to bowel ischemia and refractory metabolic acidosis. The most common causes of ACS are major abdominal surgeries, as in abdominal trauma and aortic aneurysm, but ACS has been reported in a variety of critically ill surgical and medical patients, both adults and children (7). Patients are diagnosed as having ACS when they have increasing abdominal distention with IAP >15 mm Hg, accompanied by at least three of the following major criteria: oliguria (urine output <1 mL/kg/hr) or anuria refractory to volume expanders or diuretics, hemodynamic instability or hypotension refractory to volume expanders, reduced chest compliance leading to increasing $PaCO_2$ and decreasing PO_2/FIO_2 ratio and requiring higher FIO_2 and ventilatory pressures; and metabolic acidosis with a base deficit >6 mmol/L (7).

Intra-abdominal Pressure Measurements

IAP is measured as urinary bladder pressure (15) with the patient supine: 1 mL/kg of sterile saline (maximum of 30 mL) is instilled into the bladder through a Foley catheter; the end of the catheter is connected to transparent, open-ended plastic tubing; and the level of the water column above the symphysis pubis defines IAP. Once the diagnosis is made, the patients must undergo emergency abdominal decompression—if necessary, at the bedside in the PICU if the patient's condition deteriorates rapidly and transport to the operating room is judged to be too risky. Surgical procedures and methods of abdominal-wall closure vary; in some cases, the abdomen is left open after the initial decompressive laparotomy, covered with a Dacron mesh or with a sterile IV bag ("Bogota" bag). If the open incision wound and Dacron cover do not provide enough decompression for the increasing intra-abdominal contents, episodes of ACS may still develop; therefore, close monitoring is mandatory while the abdomen is still "open" (7).

TOXIC MEGACOLON

TM is defined as an acute dilation of the colon due to diffuse inflammation or necrosis of the bowel wall in the absence of mechanical obstruction. The crucial features of this disorder are that the dilatation results from inflammatory colitis and that it is accompanied by systemic manifestations or toxicity. TM is most frequently associated with idiopathic inflammatory bowel disease, including ulcerative colitis, Hirschsprung disease (congenital megacolon), infectious colitis (amebiasis, salmonellosis, shigellosis, *Campylobacter* and *Yersinia* bacteria), chronic constipation (intestinal dysmotility), and antibiotic-associated PMC (75,78).

Etiology

Although TM was thought to be a complication solely of ulcerative colitis, it is now known that almost any inflammatory condition of the colon could predispose patients to toxic dilation (28). In the patients who develop TM, mortality rates are high. In a large review of the early literature, an overall mortality of 19% was found, and mortality in medically managed patients was slightly higher than in those managed with early surgery (27% vs. 19.5%). Mortality was significantly higher if the patients experienced perforation (41.5% vs. 8.8% without perforation) (76). Remarkably, mortality does not seem to be related to the extent of underlying disease. Although TM does indeed tend to occur in patients with pancolitis, mortality is similar in groups with pancolitis or with limited colitis, suggesting that mortality is related more to the process of TM rather than to the colitis itself. In one study, mortality was higher in the group with partial or segmental colitis (55%) than in the group with pancolitis (44%) (28).

Pathogenesis

Although the exact mechanism of TM is not known, a number of reasons for an apparent dysmotility of the colon have been postulated. Several studies have reported abnormal colonic motility in patients with nontoxic colitis. These included findings of defective smooth muscle contraction, lowered basal pressure in the colonic lumen, and an inhibited gastrocolic reflex. Further research suggests that these effects may be the result of changes in colonic response to vasoactive intestinal polypeptide, substance P, neurotensin, leukotrienes, and NO (28).

It has been postulated that severe inflammation and damage to the colonic wall are necessary for the development of TM (28). NO, a known inhibitor of smooth-muscle tone, may be involved in the pathogenesis of TM. NO is generated by macrophages and smooth-muscle cells through the inducible form of NO synthase in the inflamed colon (75).

Clinical Features

TM can occur in any patient with colitis, young or old. The majority of patients present in the midst of an ongoing bout of severe colitis. Signs of colitis, including diarrhea (often bloody), fever, chills, and abdominal cramping, are the predominant clinical features before the onset of TM. The onset of TM is inconsistent but may be heralded by abdominal distension, constipation, obstipation, reduced bowel sounds, and constitutional symptoms such as fever, tachycardia, or hypotension. The abdomen can be extremely tender, either locally or diffusely, but these signs and others may be masked by high-dose corticosteroids or a decreased level of consciousness. Diagnosis of TM is made on the basis of clinical information and plain x-rays of the abdomen. The most widely used criteria for the clinical diagnosis of TM in adults were proposed by Jalan et al. (42) as radiographic evidence of colonic dilation plus any three of the following: fever $>101.5°F$ ($>38.6°C$), heart rate >120 beats/min, white blood cell count >10.5 ($>10^9$/L), or anemia. Patients should furthermore have one of the following criteria: dehydration, mental changes, electrolyte disturbances, or hypotension. Radiological diagnosis (dilation of transverse or ascending colon to >6 cm) is based on consensus and clinical data that suggest that the transverse colon and the ascending colon are usually the most prone to dilation (28). No criteria have been developed for children; however, infants and children with TM seem to be toxic, with fever ($>39°C$), dehydration, and marked colon dilation (diameter of >1.5 times the width of the vertebra body of the first lumbar spine on plain abdominal radiographs) (78).

On physical examination, the patient has altered consciousness, tachycardia, fever, postural hypotension, and abdominal distension and tenderness, with or without signs of local or general peritonitis.

Laboratory studies usually reveal evidence of severe underlying colitis. Patients may be anemic because of blood loss or chronic disease. White blood count may be elevated, often with a left shift, except in patients with sepsis or acquired immunodeficiency syndrome, in whom neutropenia may supervene. Electrolyte abnormalities are very common and multifactorial, and hypokalemia and hypoalbuminemia in particular reflect significant diarrhea and volume depletion. Erythrocyte-sedimentation rate and C-reactive protein concentrations are increased in most cases.

Plain abdominal x-ray is crucial for diagnosis of TM and for following its course. The transverse, or right colon, is usually the most dilated, frequently to >6 cm and sometimes up to 15 cm, on films taken with the patient supine. Distension of the descending colon is less frequent, and that of the sigmoid colon and rectum, rare (75). Endoscopy may be of value in cases when the underlying diagnosis is in question, but extreme caution is advised, as perforation may ensue (28).

Treatment

The main goal of treatment is to reduce the severity of colitis so as to restore normal colonic motility and to decrease the likelihood of perforation. The initial treatment of toxic dilatation should be medical and obviates the need for surgery in ~50% of patients. However, a surgical consultation should be obtained on admission, and the patient should be assessed daily by both medical and surgical teams. The patient should be monitored in the ICU with frequent examinations by nursing and medical staff for signs of deterioration. Complete blood counts, electrolytes, and serial abdominal plain films are reviewed every 12 hrs initially and then daily as the patient improves. Anemia, dehydration, and electrolyte deficits, particularly hypokalemia, may aggravate colonic dysmotility and should be aggressively treated (75). The bowel should be completely rested, and a nasogastric tube (or long intestinal tube) should be placed initially to decompress the GI tract. If the patient shows signs of improvement, enteral feeding is started, as it may hasten mucosal healing and stimulate normal motility. All antimotility agents, narcotics, and anticholinergics should be discontinued. Broad-spectrum antibiotics are recommended to reduce septic complications and in anticipation of peritonitis resulting from perforation (75).

NECROTIZING ENTEROCOLITIS

NEC is the most common acquired abdominal emergency in preterm infants requiring intensive care. It also occurs in term infants; those with congenital heart disease are at particular risk, especially those with the potential for significant runoff from the systemic to pulmonary circulation. Enteric feeding and prematurity, however, remain the most consistent risk factors (78). The characteristic feature of NEC is bowel wall necrosis of variable length and depth, with perforation in up to one-third of infants affected (44).

Epidemiology

NEC mainly affects infants in NICUs, and both sporadic cases and nosocomial outbreaks have been described. The incidence varies among countries, as well as among different centers within the same country. In the US, it has been reported to be 1%–7.7% of all NICU admissions or 1–3 per 1000 live births. Although overall infant mortality has diminished, NEC-associated mortality increased from 11.5 to 12.3/100,000 or 10%–30% of all NEC cases across centers. On the other hand, the surgical mortality rate for this condition has decreased from ~70% to between 20% and 50% over the past decade (44).

Etiology

It seems that NEC is the product of an interaction of numerous factors, with prematurity being the single parameter most frequently encountered. Various other risk factors have been implicated, such as episodes of birth asphyxia, polycythemia, umbilical-vessel catheterization, congenital heart disease, blood transfusions, exchange transfusions, early and rapid feeding, hyperosmolar formulas, maternal cocaine use, medications used in the neonate, hypoalbuminemia, symptomatic or subclinical perinatal infection, respiratory distress syndrome, and hypoxic-ischemic encephalopathy (44).

Pathogenesis

The pathogenesis of NEC is multifactorial: ischemia, infection, and intraluminal injury, and subsequent circulatory, immunologic, and inflammatory host response lead to mucosal injury. Patients with confirmed NEC may or may not have positive blood cultures, but therapy routinely includes broad-spectrum antibiotics (78).

Pathophysiology

According to Kosloske (48), NEC occurs by the coincidence of two of three pathologic events: (a) intestinal ischemia, (b) colonization by pathogenic bacteria, and (c) excess protein substrate in the intestinal lumen.

A large number of inflammatory mediators and molecular mechanisms involved in the pathogenesis of NEC have been studied in an attempt to obtain a clear vision of this disorder and to discover novel preventive measures. Among these, platelet-activating factor (PAF), defensin mRNA, NO and inducible NO synthase, IL-1, IL-6, tumor necrosis factor (TNF)-α, IL-11, magnesium and copper deficiency, oxygen-derived free radicals, epidermal growth factor, heparin-binding hepatocyte growth factor, intestinal trefoil factor, hematopoietic cytokines, and cyclooxygenase-2/NFκB pathway are all worth mentioning (44).

Diagnosis

Diagnosis is based on a combination of clinical, radiologic, and, frequently, surgical findings. Clinical evidence of GI and systemic illness includes temperature instability, poor feeding, increased residuals, abdominal distension, bloody (or guaiac-positive) stools, a palpable abdominal mass, and overlying abdominal wall cellulitis. A decrease in urinary output and poor perfusion may also be noted. Late findings of peritonitis include abdominal wall edema, erythema, and even crepitus (44). Nevertheless, the most common presenting sign is abdominal distension, which is frequently accompanied by bilious vomiting and feeding intolerance with gastric aspirates. Evidence of shock develops in many infants.

Common laboratory findings include an increased white blood cell count with an elevated band count, but as the disease progresses, an absolute neutropenia may develop with a worse prognosis. Thrombocytopenia and metabolic acidosis are also often found. More specifically, the nadir platelet count during the course of the disease was found to be lower in patients at more advanced stage and in those who finally succumbed. A platelet count of <100,000/mcL or a rapid fall represents poor prognostic factors (81). Blood and peritoneal cultures as well as

TABLE 90.3

BELL'S CRITERIA FOR NECROTIZING ENTEROCOLITIS

Stage	Classification	Systemic signs	Intestinal signs	Radiologic signs
I	Suspected	Temperature instability, apnea, bradycardia, lethargy	Increased residuals, mild abdominal distension, emesis, guaiac + stool or bright red rectal bleeding	Normal or intestinal dilation, mild ileus
II	Definite	Mild metabolic acidosis, mild thrombocytopenia	Absent bowel sounds, ± abdominal tenderness, ± abdominal cellulitis, or RLQ mass	Intestinal dilation, ileus, pneumatosis intestinalis, ± portal venous gas
III	Advanced	Hypotension, bradycardia, apnea, respiratory and metabolic acidosis, DIC, neutropenia	Peritonitis, marked abdominal distension, and tenderness	Ascites ± pneumoperitoneum

RLQ, right lower quadrant; DIC, disseminated intravascular coagulation

susceptibility tests are necessary for the appropriate administration of antibiotics.

Radiologic findings include pneumatosis intestinalis, portal venous gas, fixed dilated loop of bowel on serial examinations, and pneumoperitoneum. MRI reveals bubbly gas in the bowel wall. Histologic evidence at surgery or on autopsy of coagulation necrosis, inflammation, and hemorrhage further confirms the diagnosis. Stages of disease with a variety of modifications are commonly used to define severity and guide treatment (Table 90.3) (8,78). Stage I is characterized by abdominal distension, poor feeding, and vomiting and with findings consistent with ileus on plain abdominal x-rays. Stage II includes the same clinical signs and GI bleeding. Pneumatosis or portal venous air is seen on abdominal films. Stage III is characterized by progression into septic shock, with pneumoperitoneum on abdominal films.

The earliest x-ray finding is most commonly a nonspecific intestinal dilation and edema. Intestinal pneumatosis may be either linear (subserosal) or cystic (submucosal) and is present in 70%–80% of cases. However, this finding can appear with a significant delay, transiently, and is often misinterpreted as air mixed with feces, blood, or meconium. Air in the Morison pouch (a recess in the peritoneal cavity with the liver anterior and the kidney and adrenal posterior, which, when containing air, appears as a triangular lucency in the right upper quadrant) represents an early sign of pneumoperitoneum and is thus significant as a clear indication for surgery (44). Portal venous gas is identified on the abdominal x-ray in 25% of NEC cases as a linear branching lucency within the portal venous system. Portal venous gas has been reported often to be associated with panintestinal involvement in the very-low-birth-weight (VLBW) infant. Portal vein ultrasonography appears to be much more sensitive in the detection of portal venous gas compared with plain x-ray and, as a result of its portable nature, is a reliable and readily available tool for the early diagnosis of NEC in any questionable case. Ultrasonography is also used to evaluate the presence and character of ascites (particulate matter probably indicates perforation) and to identify a site for paracentesis (44).

Treatment

The management of infants with NEC is initially medical, consisting of remaining in a nothing-by-mouth status for ~10–14 days, orogastric drainage for decompression, IV fluids, and broad-spectrum antibiotics, as well as blood-product transfusion, if necessary. Careful observation should include repeating physical, laboratory, and radiographic examination of the patient. Absolute indications for operation are considered to be conditions such as pneumoperitoneum, intestinal necrosis, or gangrene obtained on paracentesis. Relative indications include deterioration of clinical condition, oliguria, hypotension, metabolic acidosis, thrombocytopenia, leucopenia, leukocytosis, ventilatory failure, portal venous gas, fixed abdominal masses, persistently dilated bowel loops, or erythema of the abdominal wall (62). Although indications remain the same for both VLBW and full-term infants, the nature of operative management is somewhat different between these groups of patients. More specifically, peritoneal drainage is becoming the method of choice as the primary treatment for infants who weigh <1500 g (VLBW) or who weigh >1500 g but are too unstable to undergo laparotomy. Peritoneal drainage may be applied either as a definitive therapy or as a transitional step toward laparotomy (44). The latter seems to confer greater survival rates for larger infants compared with intraperitoneal drain techniques. Nonetheless, various complications, such as the formation of an enterocolonic fistula and intestinal stenosis, have been reported as a result of either medical or surgical treatment of NEC.

Prevention of Necrotizing Colitis

Prevention of NEC still remains elusive. Avoidance of preterm birth, judicious use of antenatal steroids in preterm deliveries to induce intestinal maturation, breast-milk feedings, and trophic feedings may be reasonable strategies in reducing the incidence of NEC.

GASTROINTESTINAL BLEEDING

GI bleeding is a common occurrence in the PICU; it may be the primary indication for admission or may occur as a complication of the primary illness in a critically ill child. One study to determine the prevalence and the risk factors for the development of upper GI bleeding in critically ill children found that 25% had evidence of upper GI bleeding, with no association between age, weight, race, or sex (16). Increased risks for upper GI bleeding were circulatory shock, a prolonged operative procedure, and trauma. Children who suffer from clinically significant upper-GI bleeding acquired during their intensive care admission are more likely to have a longer length of stay in the ICU, which has a significant impact both clinically and economically (29).

Anatomically, the ligament of Treitz, located at the end of the duodenum and beginning of the jejunum, provides the division between the origins of the upper- and lower-GI tracts; upper bleeds originate proximal to the ligament, and lower bleeds originate distally. It is essential to exclude other, non-GI sites where bleeding may originate, such as from the nose or lungs, as different management is required.

Upper GI tract bleeding typically presents with hematemesis and melena, although with massive acute bleeding, fresh blood may be passed per rectum. Melanotic stools are black, tarry, and contain partially digested blood, giving rise to an offensive smell. When bleeding occurs from the lower GI tract, fresh blood is passed per rectum or mixed in with stools and both melena and hematochezia may be present (maroon-colored stools). Where ischemia has occurred (i.e., intussusception),

red, "currant jelly" stool may be seen, which is stool that consists of mucus (products of inflammation) and blood. Black stools that are negative for occult blood must not be mistaken for melena. Chronic occult bleeding may occur anywhere in the GI tract and can be confirmed by stool analysis. Whenever massive bleeding occurs, hemodynamic instability and circulatory instability are likely to occur, and therapeutic actions must be instituted urgently.

The cause of bleeding in the pediatric population varies with the age of the child and the presence of congenital or inherited abnormalities. The causes of upper- and lower-GI bleeding in children by age category are listed in **Table 90.4**.

Management

Severe GI bleeding that results in shock and the need for resuscitation, continuous monitoring, and intensive care may have several causal factors. Massive upper GI bleeding may arise due to esophageal or gastric varices, vascular anomalies, and gastric or duodenal ulcer disease. Substantial lower-GI bleeding can occur in inflammatory bowel disease, Henoch-Schönlein purpura, intussusception, Meckel diverticulum, vascular anomalies, intestinal duplications, and infectious colitis. Significant bleeding may also arise from GI infections, as a result of critical illness (stress-induced GI bleeding) and as an adverse reaction to drugs, including corticosteroids (more predominantly seen in neonates), nonsteroidal anti-inflammatory drugs (53), and the newer cyclooxygenase (COX)-2 inhibitors (79). The management of each of these will depend upon the cause, although

---

TABLE 90.4

CAUSES OF GASTROINTESTINAL BLEEDING IN CHILDREN

Upper GI Bleeding	*Child*	*Adolescent*
Neonates/Infants	Esophagitis	Esophagitis
Swallowed maternal blood	Mallory-Weiss syndrome	Mallory-Weiss syndrome
Esophagitis	Gastritis	Gastritis
Gastritis	Ulcer—gastric/duodenal	Ulcer—gastric/duodenal
Ulcer/erosions—gastric/duodenal	*Helicobacter pylori* infection	*Helicobacter pylori* infection
Vascular malformation	Arteriovenous malformations	Arteriovenous malformations
Vitamin K deficiency	Esophageal or gastric varices	Esophageal or gastric varices
	Adverse drug reactions—NSAIDs	Adverse drug reactions—NSAIDs
	Portal hypertension	Portal hypertension
	Swallowed epistaxis	
Lower GI Bleeding	*Child*	*Adolescent*
Neonates/Infants	Polyps	Infectious enterocolitis
Swallowed maternal blood	Hereditary illness	Inflammatory bowel disease
Anal fissures	Intussusception	Arteriovenous malformation
Upper-GI bleed	Infectious enterocolitis	Polyps
Milk protein allergy	Meckel diverticulum	Hereditary illness
Necrotizing enterocolitis	Hemolytic uremic syndrome	Hemolytic uremic syndrome
Hirschsprung enterocolitis	Henoch-Schönlein purpura	
Malrotation and volvulus	Inflammatory bowel disease	
Infectious enterocolitis		

NSAID, nonsteroidal anti-inflammatory drugs

general resuscitation and stabilization measures are often needed before specific therapeutic strategies can be instituted.

Continuous observation of vital signs is mandatory, together with meticulous fluid-management regimens. With severe and substantial hemorrhage, the primary goals are resuscitation of the patient from hemodynamic shock, including the administration of blood products and other life-saving therapies as necessary. Some pharmacologic agents (discussed later) have therapeutic benefit in the acute and short-to-medium term and may be used. It is vital to identify the cause of the bleeding and institute appropriate action. In addition, some techniques used in investigating the cause of GI bleeding are therapeutic. Options in the management of acute GI bleeding are summarized in **Table 90.5**.

TABLE 90.5

MANAGEMENT OF ACUTE GASTROINTESTINAL BLEEDING

Stabilization
Airway Breathing Circulation
Continuous monitoring of vital signs
Central venous pressure in severe cases or when volume status unclear or critical

Diagnosis
Source of bleeding
  Nasal, oral, abdominal, and rectal examinations
  Nasogastric aspiration to differentiate upper from lower and to assess for ongoing bleeding
  Emesis or gastric contents and stool tests for blood
Imaging studies
  Plain abdominal film
  Abdominal ultrasound
  Upper endoscopy
  Lower endoscopy
  Contrast CT
  Nuclear medicine studies
  Angiography
Laboratory tests
  Complete blood counts
  Coagulation studies
  Fibrinogen
  D-dimers
  Serum urea nitrogen/creatinine
  Liver function tests
  C-reactive protein
  Stool for white cells
  Stool for culture

Therapeutic Interventions
Stop feeding
Neutralize acid
Institute pharmacotherapy
  Octreotide
  Vasopressin
  Activated factor VII
Invasive techniques
  Endoscopic resection, cautery, sclerosis, or band ligation
  Arteriography and embolization
  Transjugular intrahepatic portosystemic shunt
  Surgery

Investigations

Some invasive investigations may be life-saving and should be instituted while resuscitation is undertaken. Blood tests, such as hemoglobin and coagulation profile may be normal, but in general, most patients will have anemia and thrombocytopenia. With an infectious etiology, leukocytosis and other markers of infection may occur; e.g., C-reactive protein may be increased. Prothrombin time and international normalized ratio may be elevated, which reflects a disseminated intravascular coagulation picture or disturbed synthetic liver function. Blood urea may be elevated, indicating an upper GI source of bleeding. Blood urea may also be elevated in hemolytic uremic syndrome or hepatorenal failure. Nasogastric lavage may be useful to differentiate upper GI bleeding from lower GI bleeding. Lavage may also be useful to determine if bleeding has ceased or continues. Care should be taken when placing a nasogastric tube in patients with suspected varices. Stool should be analyzed both macroscopically and microscopically. More specific investigations will be directed toward the specific etiologies discussed below.

Endoscopy

Where possible, endoscopy is the investigation of choice and may have therapeutic options as well. Massive bleeding may make endoscopy technically difficult, and in general, upper-GI endoscopy (esophagogastroduodenoscopy) has a better yield than lower-GI endoscopy (colonoscopy), as bleeding often obscures the view (39). Wireless capsule endoscopy and double-balloon enteroscopy are new techniques useful in imaging the small intestine when the source of bleeding remains obscure.

Imaging Studies

Plain radiographic studies are often not helpful in determining the cause of acute bleeding. Where NEC is suspected, plain abdominal x-ray will show characteristic features of intramural gas or portal air. For suspected intussusception, ultrasound characteristically shows a target lesion of the telescoping small bowel. Enema studies are not indicated in the presence of shock, peritoneal irritation, perforation, or pneumatosis, as bowel ischemia has taken place and this is a surgical emergency.

Contrast CT scans of the abdomen have been used to localize acute lower-GI bleeding points. In one retrospective review, adult patients who had lower-GI bleeding but whose endoscopy was normal and with no further evidence of bleeding underwent CT scans of the abdomen, which yielded a source for the bleeding in 6 of 7 patients (69). CT may be of benefit to localize the bleeding point for patients whose bleeding appears to have stopped. Arterial-phase, multidetector row helical CT was accurate in identifying bleeding points in 21 of 26 patients, with the location of contrast material corresponding accurately to that of active bleeding on angiography (85).

Mesenteric angiography has been used for many years, with extravasation of contrast making the positive diagnosis. Angiography is a sensitive investigation in the evaluation of patients with a Meckel diverticulum (1,58). Angiography showed a persistent vitellointestinal artery (omphalomesenteric artery remnant) in most patients (11 of 16) with a Meckel diverticulum who presented with a history of chronic GI bleeding. In 88 adults with lower GI bleeding, catheter angiography localized the bleeding point in 50% of cases and was found to be more sensitive in those with hemodynamic instability requiring transfusion (6). Once the bleeding point has been identified, potential angiographic treatment options (e.g., embolization) can take place.

Nuclear medicine techniques allow localization of bleeding points when there is active bleeding in the lower GI tract (38). It can detect bleeding rates as low as 0.1 mL/min. $^{(99m)}$Tc(technium)-labelled red blood cells (TRBC) and $^{(99m)}$Tc-sulphur colloid are two techniques that can identify active bleeding. When imaging is more prolonged or delayed, TRBC may be used, but interpretation requires care, as the radiotracer is likely to be moving away from the bleeding site (64). A retrospective study of adults who underwent TRBC scintigraphy showed that this technique has a low positive yield (65). In patients with significant bleeding who were transfused with at least 2 units of packed red blood cells in the preceding 24 hrs, the scan was more likely to be positive. In children with overt or occult rectal bleeding, its benefit was mixed (35). Sequential subtraction angiography was developed by one group, in both adults and children, to avoid the high background activity, enabling augmentation of the detectability of minimal bleeding on TRBC images (83). This technique was significantly more sensitive in isolating the bleeding point for the detection of early GI bleeding than were standard methods of TRBC.

The use of technetium pertechnetate for Meckel scans can be enhanced and the rate of false negatives decreased with administration of either pentagastrin or an H_2-receptor antagonist. Pentagastrin increases the uptake of pertechnetate into the gastric mucosal cells, while the H_2-receptor antagonist decreases its release so that either or both will increase the sensitivity of the test.

Therapy

When the patient is stable, continued observation of vital signs and fluid status is important. A large amount of bleeding may occur in the bowel lumen and is hidden from direct observation; if clinical deterioration occurs without obvious blood loss, this should be considered. Large-bore IV access is essential, with the ability to use more than one lumen. Saline solution or water at room temperature may be used, via gastric lavage, to determine if bleeding continues or has resolved. Enteral feeding regimens should be stopped and parenteral feeding commenced in acute situations. Gastric-acid prophylaxis should begin when feedings are held, and enteral feeding should be recommenced as soon as possible.

Pharmacotherapeutic Therapies

Transfusion with blood and clotting factors may be necessary for either acute or prolonged chronic bleeding. Recombinant activated factor VII has been used with success as rescue treatment for patients with severe GI bleeding or varices when usual blood and coagulation replacement fails, and further studies are warranted in this area (71,82).

The somatostatin analog octreotide has been widely used to control variceal bleeding due to portal hypertension when administered by continuous IV infusion. It has been reported to inhibit gastric-acid secretion and reduce splanchnic and azygous blood flow in patients with cirrhosis and portal hypertension. Greater bleeding control was achieved with octreotide (1–2 mcg/kg/hr) in children with portal hypertension, compared to those without portal hypertension (27). In this study, bleeding stopped during octreotide infusion in 71% of children with portal hypertension and in 50% of those without portal hypertension. Postinfusion rebleeding occurred in 52% of children with portal hypertension and in 39% of those without portal hypertension. Octreotide's side effect profile includes nausea, abdominal cramps, diarrhea, fat malabsorption, and hyperglycemia. IV vasopressin is another agent that works by reducing splanchnic blood flow and portal venous pressure, and has been used for GI bleeding with good effect at doses of 0.01 U/kg/min; higher doses increase side effects without improving bleeding (80). A Cochrane meta-analysis that compared vasopressin, terlipressin, somatostatin, or octreotide for variceal bleeding in cirrhosis indicated that these pharmacologic agents control bleeding in 83% of patients. They also found that sclerotherapy was not superior to these pharmacologic agents and might be added for pharmacologic treatment failures (20).

Invasive Therapies

Endoscopy provides both diagnostic and therapeutic roles. Bleeding sources such as polyps may be removed using sigmoidoscopy. Thermal or laser coagulation can be applied to lesions with upper GI endoscopy. Endoscopic emergency sclerotherapy and variceal band ligation are useful for acute variceal bleeding (24,87). A beneficial interventional radiology treatment for uncontrolled variceal bleeding in children is the placement of a transjugular intrahepatic portosystemic shunt (TIPS) (37).

Surgery may be indicated in circumstances in which, despite pharmacologic and nonoperative management, bleeding continues. If preoperative diagnostic studies have localized a bleeding point, this area of bowel can be resected. However, when this is not possible and a point is not found intraoperatively, a more extensive resection may be life-saving. The management options available for specific conditions are discussed in the following sections.

Stress-ulcer-induced Bleeding

Stress-ulcer bleeding is a common complication in critically ill patients and is a major factor affecting morbidity and mortality. The incidence in adults ranges from 0.17% to 14%, depending upon underlying illness, patient selection, and investigation. In critically ill children with traumatic brain injury, major organ failure, burns, liver failure, oncologic conditions, or medication exposure, the incidence has been reported to be up to 44% (63). One of the reasons for this high rate of stress-ulcer bleeding is that critically ill children with severe illness or CNS injury have been shown to have gastric pH that is lower and more difficult to control (30).

Multiple mechanisms can lead to stress-ulcer bleeding. Hypotension and metabolic abnormalities are associated with the development of mucosal injury due to increased acid production and reduced gastric blood flow. The mucosa loses its ability to produce mucus and maintain integrity. A mucosal-energy deficit contributes to cell death and backward diffusion of acid, leading to further mucosal injury. Where hypoxia has damaged the mucosal integrity, in an acid pH environment, bile salts lead to further loss of integrity. Where hydrogen ions have penetrated the epithelium, histamine is released, leading to inflammation, edema, and disruption of the upper mucosal layers, erosion, and ultimately, the development of an ulcer.

The risk factors for developing stress-induced upper GI bleeding were examined in 170 children under the age of 15 admitted to a PICU (63). Signs of overt GI bleeding hematemesis, coffee-ground gastric content, or melena were seen in 43%. Clinically significant bleeding (major changes in vital signs: a fall in blood pressure of >20 mm Hg, an increase in heart rate of >20 beats above baseline, or >2-g/dL drop in hemoglobin) was seen in 5%. Only 25 of the 170 children had been prescribed stress-ulcer prophylaxis, with the majority receiving ranitidine and 3 patients receiving antacids. Where stress-ulcer prophylaxis was given, 14 patients suffered with an upper-GI bleed (3 clinically significant), and 60 out of 145 who had not received prophylaxis had upper-GI bleeding episodes (6 clinically significant). Mechanical ventilation was found to be a risk factor for the development of GI bleeding in these critically ill children. Those patients who required transfusion were found to have a higher mortality.

Another study found that 10.2% of critically ill children suffer upper-GI bleeding but that only 1.6% of cases were clinically significant (13). The complications associated with these GI bleeds were a decrease in hemoglobin concentration, need for transfusion, hypotension, and need for surgery. This study determined that three independent risk factors might predict those at risk of clinically significant bleeding: respiratory failure, coagulopathy, and pediatric risk of mortality score ≥ 10.

The data are conflicting concerning the effect of the administration of medications that block histamine H_2 receptors or the effect of cytoprotective agent sucralfate on the rates of GI bleeding and ventilator-associated pneumonia. In adult studies in which stress-ulcer prophylaxis was utilized, gastric pH increased, resulting in the overgrowth of gram-negative bacteria with retrograde colonization, which was associated with ventilator-associated pneumonia (26). Critically ill adult patients who required mechanical ventilation and received stress-ulcer prophylaxis with ranitidine had less clinically significant bleeding than those who received sucralfate (18). In the same study, no differences were found between the two groups in terms of ventilator-associated pneumonia, duration of ICU stay, or mortality. In mechanically ventilated children, no difference in incidence of ventilator-associated pneumonia or stress-ulcer bleeding was found between those treated with H_2-receptor antagonists, omeprazole (proton-pump inhibitor), or sucralfate and those who did not receive prophylaxis (54,84). An adult study showed that the use of an immediate-release omeprazole suspension is as valuable in the prevention of upper-GI bleeding when compared with IV cimetidine (17).

Critically ill children who may benefit from stress-ulcer prophylaxis include those with two of the following: respiratory failure, coagulopathy, and a Pediatric Risk of Mortality score of ≥ 10 (when duration of mechanical ventilation is likely to be ≥ 48 hrs). The prophylactic regimen introduced should take into consideration the underlying disease state of the child in order to provide the most optimum therapy.

Inflammatory Bowel Disease

The incidence of childhood inflammatory bowel disease is increasing. Evidence also suggests that both Crohn disease and ulcerative colitis are more widespread microscopically in children when compared with adults (74). Bleeding is a common occurrence in children with inflammatory bowel disease but usually is not severe. Where colitis is severe and unresponsive to conservative medical management (typically IV corticosteroids and cyclosporin), tacrolimus has been shown to have benefit in the short term (9). When bleeding is acute and severe, it may be possible to identify the bleeding points by colonoscopy or angiography; however, emergency surgery is often inevitable (49).

Liver Disease

Chronic liver disease leads to portal hypertension and can be complicated by life-threatening GI bleeding. Esophageal varices are the major cause of bleeding in this group, with variceal bleeding dependent upon the height of portal pressure. Bleeding duodenal ulcers have been found concurrently in children with portal hypertension, especially in those who have had a previous variceal bleed (40). Therefore, it is important to consider both varices and duodenal ulcers as a source of bleeding in children with liver disease. It is thought that increased portal pressure leads to an alteration in the microcirculation of the gastroduodenal mucosa, making it more susceptible to injury and thereby affecting the capacity to repair. Urgent conservative and invasive options are required to manage bleeding while more definitive procedures are awaited and organized.

Infectious Causes of Gastrointestinal Bleeding

Infectious agents may cause GI bleeding to different degrees. Organisms associated with bloody diarrhea include rotavirus, *Salmonella* spp., *Shigella* spp., *Yersinia*, enterohemorrhagic *E. coli*, and *C. difficile*. An uncommon complication of intestinal tuberculosis is GI bleeding following the formation of ulcers in the small bowel and colon. CMV causes a colitis that may result in severe GI bleeding. The patient's history or isolation of the infecting organism by culture or antigen detection should be used to institute specific antimicrobial therapy.

Helicobacter pylori infection is usually not associated with severe GI side effects. In adults, it is commonly associated with the development of gastric and duodenal ulcers. Gastritis attributed to *H. pylori* is characterized by a mixed infiltrate of plasma cells, lymphocytes, and polymorphonuclear cells, together with the urease-producing, flagellated, gram-negative organisms. Diagnosis is confirmed by *H. pylori*-specific IgG, breath tests for urea production, and endoscopic biopsy. Duodenal ulceration is far less common in children. Contributing factors are the host's genetics and the bacteria's markers of virulence. The risk of duodenal ulcer is increased with the combined presence of the IL-1 receptor antagonist gene (IL1RN*2) allele and an infection by a *cag*A-positive *H. pylori* strain (25). Currently, benefit has not been proven in treating *H. pylori*-infected children with gastritis, unless a peptic ulcer is present. Vaccinating children in early childhood may help prevent peptic ulcer disease and other complications (88).

Enterohemorrhagic Escherichia coli

Young children infected with enterohemorrhagic *E. coli* develop bloody diarrhea and the hemolytic uremic syndrome due to the production of verocytotoxins, in particular after infection with *E. coli* 0157. These patients require resuscitation from GI bleeding and require renal supportive therapy. Continuous veno-venous hemofiltration can be used to provide renal support in critically ill patients.

Clostridium difficile

Children who develop *C. difficile* colitis-associated bloody diarrhea have usually received antibiotics within the previous 1–2 months, described in more detail previously (60). Antibiotic treatment puts critically ill children at a higher risk for *C. difficile* colitis, and although the associated mortality is significantly less than in adults, it is important to screen stools and treat when suspected. Oral metronidazole is the treatment of choice.

Cytomegalovirus

GI bleeding is the most common presentation of GI CMV disease; the majority of patients infected with CMV in the GI tract are immunocompromised. Another associated feature is fever (51). At endoscopy, the abnormalities seen include inflammation of the mucosa, ulceration, a combination of mucosal inflammation and ulcer formation, and submucosal tumor with ulceration. GI involvement varies in site, extent, manifestation, and severity. Infection may be histologically diagnosed by the identification of CMV-inclusion bodies and/or immuno-histochemical stain. Treatment is with ganciclovir as first-line therapy.

Gastrointestinal Bleeding in Immunocompromised Patients

The immunocompromised host is vulnerable to GI bleeding in several circumstances. Immunocompromised patients are more susceptible to infections, including those due to opportunist organisms. CMV is a well-recognized cause of massive lower-GI hemorrhage in patients with HIV infection (86). Bone marrow transplant recipients and those who have received solid-organ transplants are at greater risk of GI complications, including GI bleeding. Hemorrhagic lesions into the wall, not lumen, of the colon have been shown by TRBC in immunocompromised patients (32).

Typhlitis

Typhlitis is an unusual complication of childhood acute leukemia, described previously. GI bleeding may occur and can vary from minor bleeding episodes to severe bleeding requiring transfusion. An arteriogram may reveal a hypervascular cecum with dilatation of the ileocolic branches of the superior mesenteric artery; if an active hemorrhage is present, extravasation of contrast material may be in superficial ulcers or into the cecal lumen.

Management of GI bleeding from typhlitis depends upon its severity, varying from conservative management, including transfusion of blood products, to more intensive therapy, including the administration of granulocyte transfusions (57). Transcatheter embolization may be required as a therapeutic alternative to surgery.

Bleeding Following Bone Marrow Transplant

A retrospective study reviewed hepatic and GI complications in 132 children following bone marrow transplant (6). GI bleeding in the form of melena and hematochezia occurred in 8% of patients, and typhlitis developed in 3.5%. GI bleeding was disproportionately represented in patients who required ICU admission (18.5%) and in 100-day mortality (23.8%), representing an important cause of morbidity and mortality.

Bleeding Following Liver and Intestinal Transplantation

Critically ill children following liver and intestinal transplantation have been found to be a high-risk population for the development of stress-related GI bleeding. Omeprazole suspension delivered by nasogastric instillation was effective at acid neutralization and preventing GI bleeding as a complication in children with liver or intestinal transplants (45).

CONCLUSIONS AND FUTURE DIRECTIONS

It is essential that intensivists understand intestinal physiology because of its role in both health and disease. Normal intestinal function is imperative for nutrition and defense against infection, both elements of vital importance to the recovery of children from critical illness. Knowledge of pathology of intestinal functions is important in the ICU, as the pathology can be a primary source of critical injury and other primary injuries and their management can lead to a secondary intestinal disorder that the intensivist can prevent.

Future directions for improving management of intestinal disorders in critically ill children include determining the effects of mechanical ventilation or administration of PEEP on intestinal motility and perfusion, understanding the role of NO and its promoters or inhibitors in intestinal inflammation and inhibition of GI motility, determining age-related criteria for the level of IAH that leads to ACS in children, and clarifying the role played by stress-ulcer prophylaxis in critically ill children in preventing GI hemorrhage and contributing to VAP.

KEY POINTS

- Virtually all nutrients from the diet are absorbed into blood across the mucosa of the small intestine. The intestine also absorbs water and electrolytes, thus playing a critical role in maintenance of body water and acid-base balance.
- Under normal circumstances, in addition to the fundamental role of the splanchnic circulation in maintaining liver and gut perfusion toward maintaining mucosal integrity, the splanchnic bed also acts as a "circulatory sink."
- To protect the body from its constant exposure to microbes, toxins, and other antigenic stimuli, the gut has developed an intricate array of defenses.
- Typhlitis is a life-threatening oncologic emergency that occurs in the presence of neutropenia, often in the induction phase of chemotherapy for leukemia. It is an inflammatory process of the GI tract that presents as NEC in the cecum and ascending colon.
- Typhlitis should be suspected in any severely neutropenic patient who presents with fever and abdominal pain,

particularly in the right lower quadrant, with or without rebound tenderness.

■ Postoperative ileus, irrespective of pathogenic mechanism, is common, especially after abdominal laparotomy, and severity is inversely related to the child's age.

■ GI hypomotility manifesting as decreased bowel sounds or abdominal distention is common and has been reported in up to half of adult patients with respiratory failure.

■ In diarrhea, after documenting increased stool frequency and volume, gross stool examination must be conducted to detect blood, leukocytes, mucus, ova, and parasites. Presence of leukocytes suggests presence of invasive or toxin-producing microorganisms in the gut. Cultures for enteric pathogens and ELISA for viral pathogens and *C. difficile* toxin are recommended. Osmotic or secretory causes of diarrhea must be ascertained.

■ The antibiotics most frequently implicated in PMC in children are ampicillin, penicillin, cephalosporins, amoxicillin, and clindamycin. Antibiotics that infrequently cause pseudomembranous colitis are other penicillins, first-generation cephalosporins, chloramphenicol, macrolides, quinolones, tetracyclines, and trimethoprim-sulfamethoxazole.

■ Numerous studies have implicated *C. difficile* as an etiologic agent of PMC. Other species of *Clostridium* (*C. innocuum, C. oroticum,* and *C. ramosum*), along with *Candida* species and aerobic gram-negative bacilli, have also been implicated.

■ The main features of ACS include abdominal distention and IAH, refractory oliguria or anuria, decreased cardiac output and hypotension secondary to reduced venous return from the lower part of the body, and markedly reduced thoracic compliance.

■ TM is most frequently associated with idiopathic inflammatory bowel disease, including ulcerative colitis and other inflammation of the colon caused by amebiasis, salmonellosis, shigellosis, *Campylobacter* and *Yersinia* bacteria, and antibiotic-associated PMC.

■ NEC is the most common acquired abdominal emergency in preterm infants requiring intensive care. It also occurs in term infants; those with congenital heart disease are at particular risk, especially those with the potential for significant runoff from the systemic to pulmonary circulation. Enteric feeding and prematurity, however, remain the most consistent risk factors. The characteristic feature of NEC is bowel wall necrosis of variable length and depth, with perforation in up to one-third of infants affected.

■ Upper GI tract bleeding typically presents with hematemesis and melena, although with massive acute bleeding, fresh blood may be passed per rectum. Melanotic stools are black, tarry, and contain partially digested blood, giving rise to an offensive smell.

■ When bleeding occurs from the lower GI tract, fresh blood is passed per rectum or mixed in with stools, and both melena and hematochezia may be present (maroon-colored stools).

■ It is important to consider both varices and duodenal ulcers as a source of bleeding in children with liver disease.

■ Infectious agents may cause GI bleeding to different degrees. Organisms associated with bloody diarrhea include rotavirus, *Salmonella* spp., *Shigella* spp., *Yersinia*, enterohemorrhagic *E. coli*, and *C. difficile*.

References

1. Abbas SM, Bissett IP, Holden A, et al. Clinical variables associated with positive angiographic localization of lower gastrointestinal bleeding. *ANZ J Surg* 2005;75:953–7.
2. Abraham R, Toren A, Ono N, et al. Predictors of outcome in the pediatric intensive care units of children with malignancies. *J Pediatr Hematol/Oncol* 2002;24:23–6.
3. Ackland G, Grocott MPW, Mythe MG. Understanding gastrointestinal perfusion in critical care: So near, and yet so far. *Crit Care* 2000;4:269–81.
4. Armon K, Stephenson T, MacFaul R, et al. An evidence and consensus based guideline for acute diarrhea management. *Arch Dis Child* 2001;85:132–42.
5. Assadi F, Copelovitch L. Simplified treatment strategies to fluid therapy in diarrhea. *Pediatr Nephrol* 2003;18:1152–6.
6. Barker CC, Anderson RA, Sauve RS, et al. GI complications in pediatric patients post-BMT. *BMT* 2005;36:51–8.
7. Beck R, Halberthal M, Zonis Z, et al. Abdominal compartment syndrome in children. *Pediatr Crit Care Med* 2001;2:51–6.
8. Bell MJ. Perforation of the gastrointestinal tract and peritonitis in the neonate. *Surg Gynecol Obstet* 1985;160:20–6.
9. Bousvaros A, Kirschner BS, Werlin SL, et al. Oral tacrolimus treatment of severe colitis in children. *J Pediatr* 2000;137:794–9.
10. Bowen RA, Austgen L, Rouge M. Fundamental Physiology and Anatomy of the Digestive System. In: *Hypertext for Biomedical Sciences.* Fort Collins, CO: Colorado State University, 1998. From http://arbl.cvmbs.colostate.edu/hbooks/pathphys/digestion/basics/index.html, accessed April 2007.
11. Brinson RR, Kolts BE. Hypoalbuminemia as an indicator of diarrheal incidence in critically ill patients. *Crit Care Med* 1987;15:506–9.
12. Brook I. Pseudomembranous colitis in children. *J Gastroenterol Hepatol* 2005;20:182–6.
13. Chaibou M, Tucci M, Dugas MA, et al. Clinically significant upper gastrointestinal bleeding acquired in a pediatric intensive care unit: A prospective study. *Pediatrics* 1998;102:933–8.
14. Char S, Farthing MJG. Bacteria and gut immunity. *Curr Op Gastroenterol* 1994;10:659–63.
15. Cheatham ML. Intra-abdominal hypertension and abdominal compartment syndrome. *New Horiz* 1999;7:96–115.
16. Cochran EB, Phelps SJ, Tolley EA, et al. Prevalence of, and risk factors for, upper gastrointestinal bleeding in critically ill pediatric patients. *Crit Care Med* 1992;20:1519–23.
17. Conrad SA, Gabrielli A, Margolis B, et al. Randomized, double-blind comparison of immediate-release omeprazole oral suspension versus intravenous cimetidine for the prevention of upper gastrointestinal bleeding in critically ill patients. *Crit Care Med* 2005;33:760–5.
18. Cook D, Guyatt G, Marshall J, et al. A comparison of sucralfate and ranitidine for the prevention of upper gastrointestinal bleeding in patients requiring mechanical ventilation. *N Engl J Med* 1998;338:791–7.
19. Curry JI, Lander TD, Stringer MD. Review article: Erythromycin as a prokinetic agent in infants and children. *Aliment Pharmacol Ther* 2001;15:595–603.
20. D'Amico G, Pietrosi G, Tarantino I, et al. Emergency sclerotherapy versus vasoactive drugs for variceal bleeding in cirrhosis: A Cochrane meta-analysis. *Gastroenterology* 2003;124(5):1277–91.
21. Davila MA. Neutropenic colitis. *Curr Opin Gastroenterol* 2006;22:44–7.
22. DeGirolami PC, Hanff PA, Eichelberger K, et al. Multicenter evaluation, of a new enzyme immunoassay for detection of *Clostridium difficile* enterotoxin *Am J Clin Microbiol* 1992;30:1085–8.
23. DeMeo M, Kolli S, Keshavarzian A, et al. Beneficial effect of a bile acid resin binder on enteral feeding induced diarrhea. *Am J Gastroenterol* 1998;93:967–71.
24. Desai CS, Shah SR, Mathur SK. Emergency sclerotherapy for control of acute oesophageal variceal bleeding using 3% aqueous phenol: A 15-year experience. *ANZ J Surg* 2004;74:460–2.
25. Dulcienne M, Magalhaes Q, Bittencourt P, et al. IL1RN polymorphism and cagA-Positive *Helicobacter pylori* strains increase the risk of duodenal ulcer in children. *Pediatr Res* 2005;58:892–6.
26. du Moulin GC, Paterson DG, Hedley-Whyte J, et al. Aspiration of gastric bacteria in antacid-treated patients: A frequent cause of postoperative colonisation of the airway. *Lancet* 1982;1:242–5.
27. Eroglu Y, Emerick KM, Whitington PF, et al. Octreotide therapy for control of acute gastrointestinal bleeding in children. *JPGN* 2004;38:41–7.
28. Gan SI, and Beck PL. A new look at toxic megacolon: An update and review of incidence, etiology, pathogenesis, and management. *Am J Gastroenterol* 2003;98:2363–71.
29. Gauvin F, Dugas MA, Chaibou M, et al. The impact of clinically significant upper gastrointestinal bleeding acquired in a pediatric intensive care unit. *Pediatr Crit Care Med* 2001;2:349–50.
30. Gedeit RG, Weigle CG, Havens PL, et al. Control and variability of gastric pH in critically ill children. *Crit Care Med* 1993;21:1850–5.
31. Ghizan FK. C. Diarrea crónica. In: Behrman RE, Kliegman RM, Jenson HB, eds. *Nelson Tratado de Pediatría, 17th ed.* Madrid: Elsevier España, 2004;1276–81.

32. Goris ML, Licho R. Case report: Diffuse gastrointestinal bleeding. *Am J Physiol Imaging* 1992;7:42–3.

33. Greenbaum LA. Fisiopatología de los líquidos corporales y tratamiento hidroelectrolítico. In: Behrman RE, Kliegman RM, Jenson HB, eds. *Nelson Tratado de Pediatría, 17th ed*. Madrid: Elsevier España, 2004;191–252.

34. Guyton AC, Hall JE. General Principles of Gastrointestinal Function—Motility, Nervous Control, and Blood Circulation. In: Guyton AC, Hall JE, eds. *Textbook of Medical Physiology, 11th ed*. Philadelphia: Elsevier, 2005;771–80.

35. Haluk C, Puntis JWL, Abbott C, et al. Recurrent perianastomotic ileo/jejunocolic ulceration (case reports). *JPGN* 2000;30:450–2.

36. Hernandez G, Velasco N, Wainstein C, et al. Gut mucosal atrophy after a short enteral fasting period in critically ill patients. *J Crit Care* 1999;14:73–7.

37. Heymann MB, LaBerge JM, Somberg KA et al. Transjugular intrahepatic portosystemic shunts (TIPS) in children. *J Pediatr* 1997;131:914–9.

38. Howarth DM. The role of nuclear medicine in the detection of acute gastrointestinal bleeding. *Semin Nucl Med* 2006;36:133–46.

39. Huang IF, Wu TC, Wang KS, et al. Upper gastrointestinal endoscopy in children with upper gastrointestinal bleeding. *J Chin Med Assoc* 2003;66:271–5.

40. Hung PY, Ni YH, Hsu HY, et al. Portal hypertension and duodenal ulcer in children. *JPGN* 2004;39:158–60.

41. Ivatury RR, Diebel L, Porter JM, et al. Intraabdominal hypertension and the abdominal compartment syndrome. *Surg Clin N Am* 1997;77:783–800.

42. Jalan KN, Circus W, Cord WI, et al. An experience with ulcerative colitis: Toxic dilatation in 55 cases. *Gastroenterology* 1969;57:68–82.

43. Jooste CA, Mustoe J, Collee G. Metoclopramide improves gastric motility in critically ill patients. *Intensive Care Med* 1999;25:464–8.

44. Kafetzis DA, Skevaki C, Costalos C. Neonatal necrotizing enterocolitis: An overview. *Curr Opin Infect Dis* 2003;16:349–55.

45. Kaufman SS, Lyden ER, Brown CR et al. Omeprazole therapy in pediatric patients after liver and intestinal transplantation. *JPGN* 2002;34:194–8.

46. Kelly CP, Pothoulakis C, LaMont JT. *Clostridium difficile* colitis: Current concepts. *N Engl J Med* 1994;330:257–62.

47. Khan WI, Collins SM. Gut motor function: Immunological control in enteric infection and inflammation. *Clin Exp Immunol* 2006;143:389–97.

48. Kosloske AM. Pathophysiology and prevention of necrotizing enterocolitis: A hypothesis based on personal observation and a review of the literature. *Pediatrics* 1984;74:1086–92.

49. Kostka R, Lukas M. Massive, life-threatening bleeding in Crohn's disease. *Acta Chir Belg* 2005;105:168–74.

50. Levein NG, Thorn SE, Wattwil M. Dopamine delays gastric emptying and prolongs orocaecal transit time in volunteers. *Eur J Anaesthesiol* 1999;16:246–50.

51. Lin WR, Su MY, Hsu CM, et al. Clinical and endoscopic features for alimentary tract cytomegalovirus disease: Report of 20 cases with gastrointestinal cytomegalovirus disease. *Chang Gung Med J* 2005;28:476–84.

52. Liolios A, Oropello JM, Benjamin E. Gastrointestinal complications in the ICUs. *Clin Chest Med* 1999;20:329–45.

53. Li Voti G, Acierno C, Tulone V, et al. Relationship between upper gastrointestinal bleeding and non-steroidal anti-inflammatory drugs in children. *Pediatr Surg Int* 1997;12:264–5.

54. Lopriore E, Markhorst DG, Gemke RJ. Ventilator-associated pneumonia and upper airway colonisation with gram-negative bacilli: The role of stress-ulcer prophylaxis in children. *Intensive Care Med* 2002;28:763–7.

55. MacDonald TT, Montelone G. Immunity, inflammation, and allergy in the gut. *Science* 2005;307:1920–5.

56. Manabe YC, Vinetz JM, Moore RD, et al. *Clostridium difficile* colitis: An efficient clinical approach to diagnosis. *Ann Intern Med* 1995;123:835–40.

57. Meyerovitz MF, Fellows KE. Typhlitis: A cause of gastrointestinal hemorrhage in children. *AJR* 1984;143:833–5.

58. Mitchell AW, Spencer J, Allison DJ, et al. Meckel's diverticulum: Angiographic findings in 16 Patients. *AJR* 1998;170:1329–33.

59. Montejo JC. Enteral nutrition-related gastrointestinal complications in critically ill patients: A multicenter study. The Nutritional and Metabolic Working Group of the Spanish Society of Intensive Care Medicine and Coronary Units. *Crit Care Med* 1999;27:1447–53.

60. Morinville V, McDonald J. *Clostridium difficile*-associated diarrhea in 200 Canadian children. *Can J Gastroenterol* 2005;19:497–501.

61. Mutlu GM, Mutlu EA, Factor P. GI complications in patients receiving mechanical ventilation. *Chest* 2001;119:1222–41.

62. Ng SCY. Necrotizing enterocolitis in the full-term neonate. *Paediatr Child Health* 2001;37:1–4.

63. Nithiwathanapong C, Reungrongrat S, Ukarapol N. Prevalence and risk factors of stress-induced gastrointestinal bleeding in critically ill children. *World J Gastroenterol* 2005;21:6389.

64. Nwakanma L, Meyerrose G, Kennedy S, et al. Recurrent gastrointestinal bleeding diagnosed by delayed scintigraphy with Tc-99m-labeled red blood cells. *Clin Nucl Med* 2003;28:691–3.

65. Olds GD, Cooper GS, Chak A, et al. The yield of bleeding scans in acute lower gastrointestinal hemorrhage. *J Clin Gastroenterol* 2005;39:273–7.

66. Perkin RM, Sharma RK. Imaging Choices for Specialty Conditions. In: Barkin RM, Swift JD, Newton DA, eds. *Pediatric Hospital Medicine*. Philadelphia: Lippincott, Williams and Wilkins; 2003:48–73.

67. Perman JA. Carbohydrate Intolerance and the Enteric Microflora. In: Lifshitz F, ed. *Carbohydrate Intolerance in Infancy*. New York: Marcel Dekker, 1982;137.

68. Pickering LK, Snyder JD. C. Gastroenteritis. In: Behrman RE, Kliegman RM, Jenson HB, eds. *Nelson Tratado de Pediatría, 17th ed*. Madrid: Elsevier España, 2004;1272–6.

69. Rajan R, Dhar P, Praseedom RK, et al. Role of contrast ct in acute lower gastrointestinal bleeding. *Dig Surg* 2004;21:293–6.

70. Ripolles T, Martinez-Perez MJ, Morote V, et al. Diseases that simulate acute appendicitis. *BJ Radiol* 1998;71:94–8.

71. Romero-Castro R, Jimenez-Saenz M, Pellicer-Bautista F, et al. Recombinant-activated factor VII as hemostatic therapy in eight cases of sever hemorrhage from esophageal varices. *Clin Gastroenterol Hepatol* 2004;2:78–84.

72. Saggi BH, Sugerman HJ, Ivatury RR: Abdominal compartment syndrome. *J Trauma* 1998;45:597–609.

73. Samore MH. Epidemiology of nosocomial *Clostridium difficile* diarrhoea. *J Hosp Infect* 1999;43 (Suppl):S183–90.

74. Sawczenko A, Sanhu BK. Presenting features of inflammatory bowel disease in Great Britain and Ireland. *Arch Dis Child* 2003;88:995–1000.

75. Sheth SG, LaMont JT. Toxic megacolon. *Lancet* 1998;351:509–13.

76. Strauss RJ, Flint GW, Platt N, et al. The surgical management of toxic dilatation of the colon: A report of 28 cases and review of the literature. *Ann Surg* 1976;184:682–8.

77. Sturm A, Holtmann G, Goebell H, et al. Prokinetics in patients with gastroparesis: A systematic analysis. *Digestion* 1999;60:422–7.

78. Thompson AE, Marshall JC, Opal SM. Intraabdominal infections in infants and children: Descriptions and definitions. *Pediatr Crit Care Med* 2005;6(Suppl):S30–5.

79. Titchen T, Cranswick N, Beggs S. Adverse drug reactions to nonsteroidal anti-inflammatory drugs, COX-2 inhibitors, and paracetamol in a pediatric hospital. *Br J Clin Pharmacol* 2005;59:718–23.

80. Tuggle DW, Bennett KG, Scott J, et al. Intravenous vasopressin and gastrointestinal hemorrhage in children. *J Pediatr Surg* 1988;23:627–9.

81. Ververidis M, Kiely EM, Spitz L, et al. The clinical significance of thrombocytopenia in neonates with necrotizing enterocolitis. *J Pediatr Surg* 2001;36:799–803.

82. Vilstrup H, Markiewicz M, Biesma D, et al. Recombinant activated factor VII in an unselected series of cases with upper gastrointestinal bleeding. *Thromb Res* 2006;118(5):595–601.

83. Wu Y, Seto H. Clinical value of sequential subtraction scintigraphy with ^{99m}Tc-RBC for gastrointestinal bleeding. *Chin Med J* 2001;114:69–72.

84. Yildizdas D, Yapicioglu H, Yilmas HL. Occurrence of ventilator-associated pneumonia in mechanically ventilated pediatric intensive care patients during stress-ulcer prophylaxis with sucralfate, ranitidine, and omeprazole. *J Crit Care* 2002;17:240–5.

85. Yoon W, Jeong YY, Shin SS, et al. Acute massive gastrointestinal bleeding: Detection and localization with arterial phase multi-detector row helical CT. *Radiology* 2006;239:160–7.

86. Zanolla G, Resener T, Knebel R, et al. Massive lower gastrointestinal hemorrhage caused by CMV disease as a presentation of HIV in an infant. *Pediatr Surg Int* 2001;17:65–7.

87. Zargar SA, Gul J, Bashir AK et al. Endoscopic ligation compared with sclerotherapy for bleeding esophageal varices in children with extrahepatic portal venous obstruction. *Hepatology* 2002;36:666–72.

88. Zetterstrom R. The Nobel Prize for the discovery of *Helicobacter pylori*: Implications for child health. *Acta Pediatrica* 2006;95:3–5.

CHAPTER 91 ■ ADRENAL DYSFUNCTION

ABEER HASSOUN • SHARON E. OBERFIELD

The pathophysiology and management of adrenal disorders that are relevant to the care of children in the intensive care unit setting are reviewed in this chapter.

MECHANISM OF DISEASE

Four hundred and fifty years ago, Bartholomeo Eustacius described the anatomy of the adrenal gland (24); shortly thereafter, the zonation of the gland and the distinction of the cortex and medulla were described. The human adrenal glands are located superior to the upper pole of each kidney and can be considered as two unique endocrine organs—the adrenal cortex and the adrenal medulla. Thomas Addison defined the function of the adrenal gland in the 1850s (2). However, it was 100 years later, during the 1950s, after performing adrenalectomies in animals, that Brown-Séquard described the adrenal glands as "organs essential for life" (11). Pituitary control of the adrenal function was reported during the 1920s, followed by the isolation of sheep adrenocorticotropic hormone (ACTH) (40). Corticotrophin-releasing hormone (CRH), the hypothalamic releasing factor, was not synthesized until 1981 (68). With respect to the adrenal glomerulosa, primary aldosteronism was described by Conn in the mid-1950s, and the regulation of aldosterone by angiotensin II demonstrated after that (17). It is now known that transcription factors [e.g., steroidogenic factor-1 (SF-1) and *dosage-sensitive sex reversal, adrenal hypoplasia congenita, X-chromosome* (DAX-1)] are essential for the development of the adrenal gland (33).

The size of the adrenal gland differs with age and is predominantly related to changes in the size of the adrenal cortex. During pregnancy and at birth, the adrenal glands are larger relative to body size than during adulthood, and the weight of the gland (7–9 g) is nearly that of the adult adrenal gland. In the newborn, the adrenal glands comprise nearly 0.5% of total body weight, with the fetal cortex comprising 80% of the gland. By 1 month of age, the size of the adrenal cortex is reduced by more than 50%, due to the involution of the fetal component of the adrenal cortex. The adrenal gland then gradually increases in size so that, by adulthood, the average weight of the glands is 8–12 g, but it comprises 0.02% of the lean body weight (9,45,47). The adrenal cortex also shows a gradual regression in size by 41–50 years of age, which is associated with the process of aging (63).

Anatomy and Histology of the Adrenal Gland

The adrenal cortex consists of three zones: the outermost, *zona glomerulosa* (15%), from which there is a gradual transition to the middle, *zona fasciculata* (75%), and then a clear transition to the innermost, *zona reticularis* (10%). The zona glomerulosa contains relatively small cells with a low cytoplasm-to-nuclear ratio. It is the primary site of mineralocorticoid synthesis. The zona fasciculata has large cells with a high cytoplasmic-to-nuclear ratio and a large number of cytoplasmic lipid vacuoles that are arranged in columns directed toward the center of the gland (radial cords). This zone is involved in the production of cortisol. The zona reticularis contains compact, anastomosing cords of cells and an intermediate cytoplasmic-to-nuclear ratio. The zona reticularis produces predominantly androgens.

The adrenal medulla, considered a part of the sympathetic nervous system, is comprised of chromaffin cells that are arranged in nests and cords with sympathetic ganglion cells. In adults, epinephrine is the major catecholamine synthesized and stored in the adrenal medulla; however, this varies with age (e.g., at birth, norepinephrine is the major catecholamine) (22).

Steroid Hormone Synthesis by Age

In umbilical cord blood and in newborns, the concentrations of both cortisol and cortisone are low and approximately equal, 4–10 mcg/100 mL of plasma (7). After 3–4 weeks of life, the cortisol concentration increases in relation to that of cortisone. Little or no diurnal variation of glucocorticoid concentration occurs until ~4–6 months of age (52). Cortisol secretion rates, corrected for body surface area, remain constant during childhood, puberty, and adulthood and maintain a diurnal variation. However, urinary free cortisol excretion may be higher in perimenarcheal females (39). Aldosterone is secreted at a constant rate during infancy, childhood, and adulthood, although the concentrations of aldosterone in infancy tend to be relatively higher than those observed later on in childhood for specific levels of sodium (70). Adrenal androgen secretion is low during childhood. Prior to puberty, with onset of adrenarche (physically noted as the onset of pubic hair), secretions of dehydroepiandrosterone (DHEA), dehydroepiandrosterone sulfate (DHEAS), and androstenedione increase (6). At the same time,

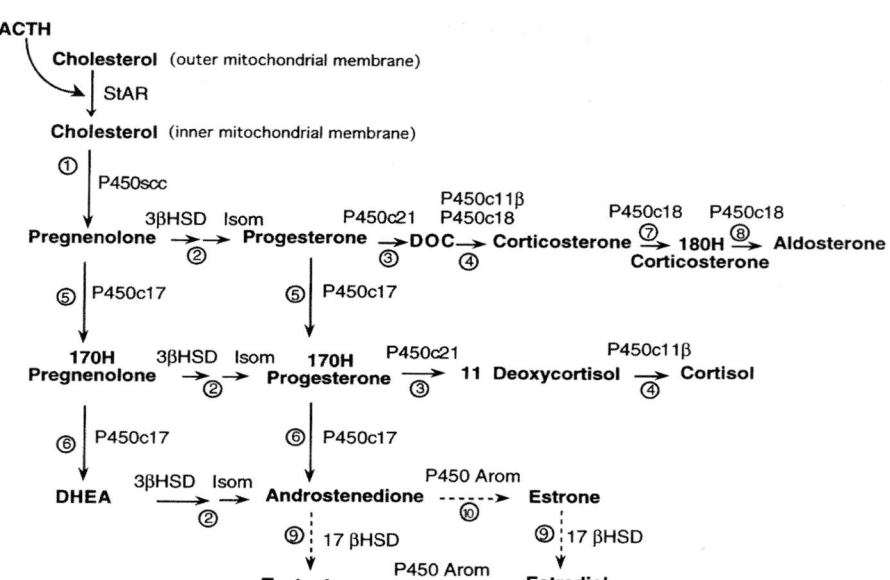

FIGURE 91.1. Steroidogenesis pathways. StAR, steroidogenic acute regulatory protein; DHEA, dehydroepiandrosterone; 3βHSD, 3β-hydroxysteroid dehydrogenase. Adapted from Levine LS, White PC. Disorders of the Adrenal Gland. In: Behrman RE, Kliegman RM, Jenson HB. *Nelson Textbook of Pediatrics, 17th ed.* Philadelphia: Saunders, 2003;1900.

however, no changes occur in ACTH concentrations in blood or in the cortisol secretion rate corrected for body size, provoking a question as to what stimulates the increase in DHEA/DHEAS secretion.

Adrenal Cortex

Steroidogenesis

Three main classes of hormones are produced by the adrenal cortex: glucocorticoids (e.g., cortisol), mineralocorticoids (e.g., aldosterone), and sex steroids (e.g., testosterone, DHEA, and androstenedione). All steroid hormones are derived from the cyclopentanoperhydrophenanthrene structure that is comprised of three cyclohexane rings and a single cyclopentane ring. Although adrenal steroid cells can synthesize cholesterol de novo from acetate, 80% of the cholesterol precursor for adrenal cortex hormone synthesis is provided by circulating plasma lipoproteins.

Cholesterol (mainly low-density lipoprotein in circulation) is the precursor for all adrenal steroidogenesis (29). The biochemical pathways involved in adrenal steroidogenesis are shown in (**Fig. 91.1**), and the adrenal steroidogenic enzymes and cofactors are illustrated in (**Table 91.1**). Conversion of cholesterol to pregnenolone has been described as the rate-limiting step for steroidogenesis, catalyzed by the side-chain cleavage enzyme.

TABLE 91.1

ADRENAL STEROIDOGENIC ENZYMES AND COFACTORS

Name	Cellular location/action	Chromosomal location
StAR	Cholesterol transport to adrenal and gonadal mitochondria	Active gene: 8 Pseudo gene: 13
CYP11A (P450scc)	(Mitochondrial) 20-hydroxylase, 22-hydroxylase, 20,22-desmolase (cholesterol side-chain cleavage)	15q23-q24
3βHSD 2	(Microsomal) 3 β-hydroxysteroid dehydrogenase, $\Delta4$-$\Delta5$-isomerase	1p13.1
CYP17 (P450c17)	(Microsomal) 17α-hydroxylase, 17, 20-lyase	10q24-q25
CYP21 CYP21P (P450c21)	(Microsomal) 21-hydroxylase	6p21-active gene and pseudogene
CYP11B1 (P450c11)	(Mitochondrial) 11β-hydroxylase (Zona fasciculata/reticularis)	8q22-two homologous CYP11B genes
CYP11B2	(Mitochondrial) 11β-hydroxylase, 18-hydroxylase (CMOI), 18-dehydrogenase (CMOII) (Zona glomerulosa)	8q22

StAR, steroidogenic acute regulatory protein; CMO, corticosterone methyloxidase. Adapted from Donohue PA. The Adrenal Gland and Its Disorders. In: Kappy MS, Allen DB, Geffner ME. *Principles and Practice of Pediatric Endocrinology.* Springfield: Charles C. Thomas, 2005:366.

However, the true rate-limiting step of adrenal steroidogenesis is the transfer of cholesterol across the inner mitochondrial membrane, which requires the action of the steroidogenic acute regulatory (StAR) protein. At the mitochondrial inner membrane, the side chain of cholesterol is cleaved to yield pregnenolone, catalyzed by the cholesterol side-chain cleavage enzyme (cholesterol desmolase, P450scc, CYP11A1), a cytochrome P450 (CYP) enzyme (46). Pregnenolone then diffuses out of mitochondria and enters the endoplasmic reticulum. The subsequent reactions that occur are zone dependent. In the zona glomerulosa, pregnenolone is converted to progesterone by 3β-hydroxysteroid dehydrogenase (3βHSD). Progesterone is converted to 11-deoxycorticosterone by steroid 21-hydroxylase (P450c21, CYP21). In the mitochondria, deoxycorticosterone is then converted to aldosterone by aldosterone synthase (P450aldo, CYP11B2). Aldosterone synthase also performs three successive oxidations: 11β-hydroxylation, 18-hydroxylation, and further oxidation of the 18-methyl carbon to an aldehyde. In the zona fasciculata, pregnenolone and progesterone are converted by 17α-hydroxylase (P450c17, CYP17) to 17-hydroxypregnenolone and 17-hydroxyprogesterone, respectively, in the endoplasmic reticulum; CYP17 is not expressed in the zona glomerulosa. 17-hydroxypregenolone is converted to 17-hydroxyprogesterone and 11-deoxycortisol by the same 3β-hydroxysteroid and CYP21 enzymes, respectively, that are active in the zona glomerulosa. 11-deoxycortisol is converted to cortisol in the mitochondria by steroid 11β-hydroxylase (P450c11, CYP11B1). In the zona reticularis and, to some extent, in the zona fasciculata, the CYP17 enzyme has an additional activity, which is the cleavage of the 17,20 carbon-carbon bond. 17-hydroxypregnenolone is converted by 3βHSD to androstenedione (46).

Regulation of the Adrenal Cortex

The major regulator of glucocorticoid secretion is by ACTH, which is a 39-amino acid peptide that is produced in the anterior pituitary (30) and is synthesized as part of a large-molecular-weight precursor, pro-opiomelanocortin (POMC). ACTH is released in bursts that vary in amplitude throughout a 24-hr cycle. The normal diurnal rhythm of cortisol secretion is established after infancy. In children and adults, the pulses of ACTH and cortisol are the highest in the early morning hours, become lower in late afternoon and evening, and reach their nadir 1 or 2 hrs after sleep begins. ACTH secretion from the anterior pituitary is stimulated mainly by CRH, which is synthesized by neurons of the parvocellular division of the hypothalamic paraventricular nucleus (28,61). The secretion of ACTH and CRH is predominantly regulated by cortisol through a negative-feedback effect. ACTH can also inhibit its own secretion.

Aldosterone secretion is regulated mainly by the renin-angiotensin system and by serum potassium levels (34,38); ACTH plays a very small role in the regulation of its synthesis. Predominantly in response to decreased intravascular volume, as in dehydration, renin is secreted by the juxtaglomerular apparatus of the kidney. Renin is a proteolytic enzyme that cleaves an α_2 globulin, which is produced by the liver and called *angiotensinogen*. This cleaving results in the formation of angiotensin I, which is cleaved further by angiotensin-converting enzyme in the lungs and other tissues, yielding the biologically active angiotensin II. Angiotensin II is cleaved further to produce the angiotensin III. Angiotensins II and III are potent stimulators of aldosterone secretion. Angiotensin II occupies a G-protein-coupled receptor and activates phospholipase C. Phospholipase C triggers a cascade that results in a rise in intracellular calcium and activates protein kinase C and calmodulin-activated kinases. Calmodulin-activated kinases increase transcription of CYP11B2, the enzyme needed for aldosterone synthesis (12).

Adrenal Steroid Action

Both cortisol and aldosterone act by binding to the intracellular glucocorticoid receptor and mineralocorticoid receptor, which belong to the super family of nuclear receptors. They have a common structure that contains a C-terminal ligand-binding domain, a central DNA-binding domain, and an N-terminal hypervariable region. The binding of a steroid to its receptor in the cytoplasm results in its dimerization and translocation to the nucleus. In the nucleus, glucocorticoids, for example, bind to the glucocorticoid response element on the glucocorticoid-responsive genes, which results in increased transcription.

Glucocorticoids have regulating effects on carbohydrate, lipid, and protein metabolism. They increase hepatic gluconeogenesis, glycolysis, proteolysis, and lipolysis. Glucocorticoids can result in increased insulin levels, which will inhibit peripheral tissue glucose uptake, leading to hyperglycemia. In addition, glucocorticoids may work in parallel with insulin by stimulating glycogen deposition and production in the liver, which provides protection against starvation. An increase in free fatty acid levels is associated with glucocorticoid administration and results from glucocorticoid enhancement of lipolysis, decrease in cellular glucose uptake, and decrease in glycerol production. In addition, an increase of amino acid substrates occurs, and they are used in gluconeogenesis due to proteolysis in fat, skeletal muscle, bone, lymphoid, and connective tissues.

Glucocorticoid excess can decrease the levels of insulin-like growth factor (IGF)-1 and increase the levels of insulin-like growth factor binding protein-1, resulting in a decrease in free IGF-1. Glucocorticoids also exert a direct inhibitory effect on the epiphyses, which results in delayed skeletal maturation and decreased linear growth in children (10,67). Although excess glucocorticoids can impair growth, they are also essential for normal growth and development. In the fetus and neonate, they accelerate the differentiation and development of various tissues (e.g., the hepatic and gastrointestinal systems) as well as the production of surfactant in the fetal lung.

Glucocorticoids also play a major role in immune regulation. They suppress the inflammatory process. Depletion of monocytes, eosinophils, and lymphocytes (T lymphocytes) is observed with the administration of high doses of glucocorticoids. T lymphocytes are reduced more than are B lymphocytes, leading to a predominantly humoral immune response. Glucocorticoids inhibit immunoglobulin synthesis and stimulation of lymphocyte apoptosis (15). In addition, they block other anti-inflammatory effects, including histamine and the secretion of proinflammatory cytokines such as tumor necrosis factor (TNF)-α, IL-1, and IL-6 (15).

Glucocorticoids have a positive inotropic effect on the heart that leads to an increase in left ventricular output. They also increase blood pressure by a number of mechanisms that involve the vascular system and the kidneys. In the vascular smooth

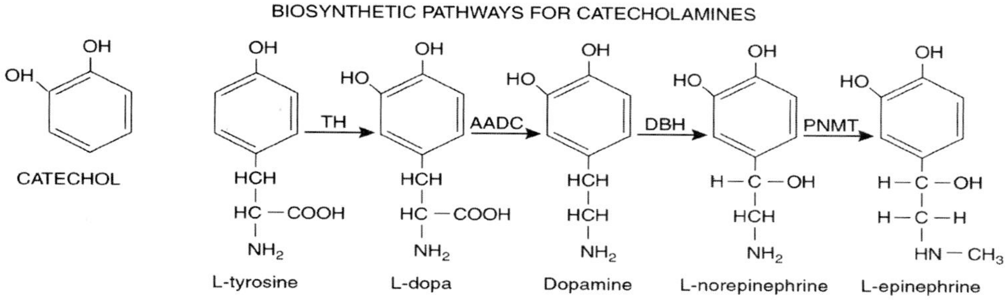

BIOSYNTHETIC PATHWAYS FOR CATECHOLAMINES

FIGURE 91.2. Biosynthetic pathway for catecholamines (left to right). All catecholamines contain the catechol nucleus. L-tyrosine is converted to L-3, 4-dihydroxyphenylalanine (L-dopa) in the rate-limiting step by tyrosine hydroxylase (TH). Aromatic L-amino acid decarboylase converts L-dopa to dopamine. Dopamine is hydroxylated to L-norepinephrine by dopamine β-hydroxylase (DBH). L-Norepinephrine is converted to L-epinephrine by phenylethanolamine N-methyltransferase (PNMT). From Larsen, Kronenberg, Melmed, and Polonasky. (eds.) Williams textbook of Endocrinology, 10e Saunders, Philadelphia, PA. pg 555.

muscles and the heart, glucocorticoids have a permissive effect on the actions of epinephrine and norepinephrine. They also increase the sensitivity to pressor agents such as catecholamines and angiotensin II, while reducing nitric oxide-mediated endothelial dilatation (27). Hypertension is often observed in patients with glucocorticoid excess; it is thought to be due to the activation of the mineralocorticoid receptor.

Glucocorticoids can induce a negative calcium balance by increasing excretion of renal calcium and inhibition of calcium absorption by the intestine. Long-term use of glucocorticoids can lead to osteopenia and osteoporosis, as they also inhibit the osteoblastic activity. Glucocorticoids have direct effects on brain metabolism and, in practice, are used to treat increased intracranial pressure. Their use has also been associated with appetite stimulation, insomnia, and mood changes, such as emotional lability with irritability and euphoria.

The major role of mineralocorticoids is to maintain intravascular volume, which is achieved by sodium retention coupled with the elimination of potassium and hydrogen ions. The main target tissues for the action of mineralocorticoids are the kidney, gut, and salivary and sweat glands. Mineralocorticoids act mainly on the distal convoluted tubules and cortical collecting ducts of the kidney. They stimulate the reabsorption of sodium and the secretion of potassium in the distal convoluted tubules. The mineralocorticoid receptor has a similar affinity for cortisol and aldosterone; yet, glucocorticoids have limited mineralocorticoid activity due to the action of 11β-hydroxysteroid dehydrogenase type 2, which converts cortisol to cortisone. Cortisone does not, under normal circumstances, occupy the mineralocorticoid receptor (57).

The Effect of Stress on Adrenocortical Function

Stress can lead to increased secretion of ACTH, which involves an immune-endocrine cascade that results in the activation of the hypothalamic-pituitary-adrenal (HPA) axis. IL-1 is secreted by macrophages in response to immunologic and inflammatory reactions (21); it also triggers a proinflammatory response that will lead to antibody production. At the same time, the CRH-ACTH-cortisol axis is activated (62), leading to increased plasma cortisol concentration, which then results in a negative feedback on the macrophages. IL-6, TNF-α, and IL-1 are other cytokines that have been shown to stimulate CRH release and

to be inhibited by cortisol (14). It has also been observed that the autonomic nervous system can influence interactions of the endocrine immune system (8).

Altered Cortisol Secretion in Systemic Disease

Disturbance of cortisol metabolism can occur in advanced hepatic failure, but plasma cortisol usually remains normal due to a prolongation of the half-life of cortisol in the blood. On the other hand, renal failure results in a reduced excretion of steroid metabolites despite the normal secretion of cortisol.

Altered Aldosterone Secretion in Systemic Disease

It is important to note that aldosterone secretion is increased in the presence of the hyperkalemia that is associated with renal failure. In patients with heart failure, renin-angiotensin-aldosterone is secreted in response to inadequate systemic perfusion (56). It has also been reported that patients with depression can have a significant increase in aldosterone levels during sleep, which was not reported in healthy controls (48).

Adrenal Medulla

The catecholamines dopamine, norepinephrine, and epinephrine are the main hormones produced by the adrenal medulla. Catecholamine synthesis also occurs in extra-adrenal tissue, including the brain, sympathetic nerve endings, and in chromaffin tissue. The biosynthesis of catecholamines is illustrated in **Figure 91.2**. Catecholamine metabolites are excreted in the urine. They include 3-methoxy-4-hydroxymandelic acid (VMA), metanephrine, and normetanephrine. Epinephrine and norepinephrine levels in the adrenal gland vary with age. No epinephrine is detected in early fetal stages. At birth, norepinephrine is the principal catecholamine and, in adults (22), norepinephrine constitutes up to one-third of the pressor amines in the medulla.

In states of stress, a high concentration of glucocorticoids has been described in the venous drainage of the adrenal cortex; this exposure is required for the release of epinephrine from the medulla. Loss of basal epinephrine secretion, as well as the response to upright posture, cold pressor, and exercise, has been reported in patients with glucocorticoid deficiency due to ACTH unresponsiveness (74).

CLINICAL PRESENTATION AND DIFFERENTIAL DIAGNOSIS OF ADRENAL INSUFFICIENCY

Adrenocortical Insufficiency

Primary adrenal insufficiency (AI) can result from the reduced production of cortisol and occasionally aldosterone that is caused by congenital or acquired lesions of the adrenal cortex. Lesions in the anterior pituitary gland or hypothalamus may cause a deficiency of ACTH (*secondary AI*) or CRH (*tertiary AI*) and lead to insufficient production of cortisol by the adrenal cortex (**Table 91.2**). The signs and symptoms of adrenocortical insufficiency vary, depending on the hormones that are deficient and on the specific steroids that are oversecreted, as in cases of inborn errors of the biosynthesis of cortisol and aldosterone (64) (**Table 91.3**). The clinical features of chronic hypoadrenocorticism may be influenced by additional symptoms caused by the destructive processes that involve the autoimmune system.

Primary Adrenal Insufficiency

Congenital

In infancy, the salt-wasting forms of congenital adrenal hyperplasia are the most common causes. These patients usually have CYP21 deficiency; lipoid adrenal hyperplasia and 3βHSD deficiency are also described. The inability to synthesize cortisol and/or aldosterone is present in these patients and can lead to symptoms of salt-wasting (shock and vascular collapse) in the newborn period. The patients with salt-wasting crisis usually present in the first weeks of life. Females with CYP21 deficiency or 3βHSD deficiency are easier to diagnose due to virilization of the external genitalia, which results from extra-adrenal androgen production in utero. Adrenal hypoplasia congenita with AI also presents in the first few weeks of life. However, the presentation can be delayed into later childhood or may even present in adulthood. This disorder is caused by a mutation of the *DAX 1* gene and primarily affects boys, who can also present with cryptorchidism or hypogonadotropic hypogonadism, and who do not undergo puberty. This disorder also occurs in conjunction with Duchenne muscular dystrophy, glycerol kinase deficiency, and mental retardation. The combination of these conditions has been termed a *contiguous gene defect* (53,72).

Familial glucocorticoid deficiency is another form of inherited AI, and patients present with hypoglycemia, seizures, and increased pigmentation. These symptoms commonly present in the first decade of life, and patients usually have an isolated deficiency of glucocorticoid, elevated levels of ACTH, and normal aldosterone production. Indeed, salt-wasting symptoms are not common in this type of AI. The disorder has an autosomal-recessive mode of inheritance. Some, but not all, of these patients have been shown to have mutations in the gene for the ACTH receptor. Triple A syndrome, an autosomal recessive disorder, is another syndrome of ACTH

TABLE 91.2

ETIOLOGY OF ADRENAL INSUFFICIENCY

Primary adrenal insufficiency
  Adrenal hypoplasia or aplasia
    X-linked
      Duchenne muscular dystrophy and glycerol kinase deficiency (Xp21 deletion)
      Hypogonadotropic hypogonadism (*DAX1* mutation)
    Familial glucocorticoid deficiency
    Corticotrophin-receptor mutations/ACTH unresponsiveness
      Alacrima, achalasia, and neurologic disorders (triple A syndrome)
  Defects of steroid biosynthesis
    Lipoid adrenal hyperplasia (StAR mutation)
    3β-hydroxysteroid dehydrogenase deficiency
    21-hydroxylase (P450C21) deficiency
    Isolated aldosterone (P450C18) deficiency
  Pseudohypoaldosteronism (aldosterone unresponsiveness)
  Adrenoleukodystrophy (peroxisomal membrane protein defect)
  Acid lipase deficiency
    Wolman disease
  Destructive lesions of adrenal cortex
    Granulomatous lesions (e.g., tuberculosis)
  Autoimmune adrenalitis (idiopathic Addison disease)
    Isolated
    Associated with hypoparathyroidism or mucocutaneous candidiasis (type I autoimmune polyglandular syndrome/AIRE gene mutation), or both
    Associated with autoimmune thyroid disease and insulin-dependent diabetes (type II autoimmune polyglandular syndrome)
  Neonatal hemorrhage
  Acute infection (Waterhouse-Friderichsen syndrome)
  Mitochondrial disorders
  Acquired immunodeficiency syndrome

Secondary adrenal insufficiency (ACTH deficiency)
  Isolated
  Autosomal recessive
  Multiple deficiencies
    Pituitary hypoplasia or aplasia
    Destructive lesions (e.g., craniopharyngioma)
    Autoimmune hypophysitis

Tertiary adrenal insufficiency
  Isolated
  Multiple deficiencies
    Congenital defects (e.g., anencephaly, septo-optic dysplasia)
    Destructive lesions (e.g., tumor)
    Idiopathic (e.g., idiopathic hypopituitarism)

Secondary/tertiary/combined forms of adrenal insufficiency
  Iatrogenic
    Abrupt cessation of exogenous corticosteroids or corticotropin
    Removal of functioning adrenal tumor
    Adrenalectomy for Cushing disease
    Drug administration: aminoglutethimide, mitotane (o, p′-DDD), metyrapone, ketoconazole
  Fetal adrenal suppression—maternal hypercortisolism

TABLE 91.3

SIGNS AND SYMPTOMS OF ADRENAL INSUFFICIENCY

Glucocorticoid deficiency	Mineralocorticoid deficiency	Adrenal androgen deficiency
Fasting hypoglycemia Increased insulin sensitivity Nausea Vomiting Fatigue Muscle weakness	Weight loss Fatigue Nausea Vomiting Salt-craving Hypotension Hyperkalemia, hyponatremia, 　metabolic acidosis (normal 　anion gap)	Decreased pubic and axillary 　hair Increased β-lipotropin levels Hyperpigmentation

Adapted from Donohue PA. The Adrenal Gland and Its Disorders. In: Kappy MS, Allen DB, Geffner ME. *Principles and Practice of Pediatric Endocrinology*. Springfield: Charles C. Thomas, 2005;395.

resistance that occurs in association with achalasia of the gastric cardia and alacrima. Deafness, mental retardation, autonomic dysfunction, and motor neuropathy have been described in these patients. Insufficient adrenal cortical function has been described in patients with disorders of cholesterol synthesis or metabolism, such as abetalipoproteinemia and familial hypercholesterolemia. Patients with Smith-Lemli-Optiz syndrome, an autosomal-recessive disorder with multiple congenital anomalies, have also been reported to have AI. Wolman disease is a rare disorder that results from intralysosomal accumulation of cholesterol esters in different body organs; it can lead to hepatosplenomegaly, steatorrhea, abdominal distention, bilateral adrenal calcification with AI, and failure to thrive. Death usually occurs during infancy (5). In steroid sulfatase deficiency, patients can present with ichthyosis, an X-linked recessive disorder of steroid metabolism. This enzyme deficiency results in accumulation of sulfated 3-β hydroxysteroids, particularly DHEAS and cholesterol sulfate.

Acquired Disorders

The term *Addison disease* was historically applied to primary AI due mainly to tuberculosis of the adrenal gland. At the present time, "Addison disease" is used to describe primary AI that is mainly due to autoimmune adrenalitis, the most common cause (90% of the cases) of acquired AI (35). Macroscopically, the glands may be too small to be seen, and often only remnants of tissue are found in microscopic sections. The medulla is preserved, while the cortex is markedly infiltrated with lymphocytes. Antiadrenal cytoplasmic antibodies and anti-CYP21 are the most frequently reported antibodies. Clinically, Addison disease has also been described in association with two syndromes: type I autoimmune polyendocrinopathy (APS-1), which is known as autoimmune polyendocrinopathy/candidiasis/ectodermal dystrophy syndrome, and type II autoimmune polyendocrinopathy (APS-2), which consists of Addison disease associated with autoimmune thyroid disease (Schmidt syndrome) or type 1 diabetes (Carpenter syndrome).

Adrenoleukodystrophy is a potential cause of AI. Patients have demyelination of the central nervous system (CNS) due to the accumulation of high levels of very long-chain fatty acids in different tissues including the adrenal gland, as a result of impaired β-oxidation in the peroxisomes. Although AI can be evident in many patients at the time of neurologic presentation, it may also precede the neurologic symptoms by many years. Therefore, the diagnosis should be considered in all patients with Addison disease of unknown etiology, and screening for very long-fatty acids is advisable (23).

As stated previously, during the last century, tuberculosis was considered a common cause of adrenal destruction; however, it is much less prevalent now. Currently, the most common infection that causes AI is meningococcemia, which can present as adrenal crisis and is referred to as the *Waterhouse-Friderichsen syndrome*. In autoimmune deficiency syndrome, frank AI is rare. However, these patients may show different subclinical abnormalities in the HPA axis. They may have problems with adrenal hormone production and action, which is often related to the medications that are used in treating this condition. Drugs such as rifampicin, and anticonvulsive drugs such as phenytoin and phenobarbital, induce steroid-metabolizing enzymes in the liver and reduce the effectiveness and bioavailability of corticosteroid replacement therapy. Ketoconazole, by inhibiting adrenal enzymes, can cause AI. Mitotane is cytotoxic to the adrenal cortex. It is used in the treatment of refractory Cushing syndrome and adrenal carcinoma. It may also alter extra-adrenal cortisol metabolism.

In children, hypoadrenalism can occur after severe adrenal hemorrhage in the neonatal period, which can be observed after breech presentation and/or difficult labor. These patients may present with an abdominal mass, anemia, unexplained jaundice, or scrotal hematoma. However, most of the time, the hemorrhage is asymptomatic, limited, and may be identified later as an incidental calcification of the adrenal gland noted on sonography.

Clinical Features of Primary Adrenal Insufficiency

In primary adrenal failure, production of one or all three groups of adrenal steroid hormones is decreased or absent (50). Thus, the signs and symptoms will vary, depending on the hormone that is deficient. Usually the signs and symptoms develop slowly (**Table 91.3**). Most patients have fatigue, muscle pain, and weight loss. Gastrointestinal and orthostatic symptoms are common. Children may present with anorexia, nausea, vomiting, and diarrhea, which may result in growth failure. They may also present with signs of acute AI precipitated by a febrile illness. Hyperpigmentation is present in >90% of patients and may develop over a long period of time, sometimes years. Although it may be difficult to appreciate in individuals with dark complexions, the typical distribution of hyperpigmentation is over the extensor surfaces of the extremities, particularly in sun-exposed areas. The mucous membranes (vaginal mucosa, gingival borders), axillae, and palmar creases are involved, and hyperpigmentation of these areas is the hallmark of Addison disease. Sometimes, the skin pigmentation is generalized. The melanocytes are stimulated by excessively high levels of α-melanocyte-stimulating hormone, which is secreted concomitantly with ACTH from the anterior pituitary gland, as both are cleavage products of pro-opiomelanocortin (13,42).

The clinical presentation of AI also depends upon the age of the patient and, to some extent, on the underlying etiology. In early infancy, the most common causes include sepsis, inborn errors of steroid biosynthesis, adrenal hypoplasia congenita, and adrenal hemorrhage. Although infants may present with only a few days of decreased activity with gastrointestinal symptoms, they can become ill very quickly. Infants have a greater requirement for aldosterone than older children; they can deteriorate quickly, with rapid occurrence of dehydration and electrolyte abnormalities. In older children with Addison disease, as previously stated, the onset is usually more gradual and is characterized by muscle weakness, malaise, anorexia, vomiting, weight loss, and orthostatic hypotension. Hyperpigmentation is often but not always present. Hypoglycemia, hyponatremia, and ketosis are common. Hyperkalemia occurs later in the course of the disease, is more frequent in younger than in older children, and may not manifest in patients who also have significant vomiting and diarrhea.

Laboratory Findings

Electrocardiographic signs of hyperkalemia should be sought. The blood urea nitrogen level is elevated if the patient is dehydrated. Cortisol levels may sometimes be at the low end of normal range but are invariably low when the patient's degree of illness and stress are considered. In primary AI, ACTH levels are high. Aldosterone level may be within the normal range but inappropriately low in relation to the level of hyponatremia, hyperkalemia, and hypovolemia, and this is usually associated with markedly elevated levels of plasma renin activity. Hypercalcemia is associated with Addison disease.

Treatment

Immediate and vigorous treatment of acute AI is very important. A blood sample should be obtained before therapy for determination of electrolytes, glucose, ACTH, cortisol, aldosterone, and plasma renin activity to establish the etiology of AI. If possible, specifically in infants, a 17α-hydroxyprogesterone level should be obtained. An ACTH-stimulation test can be performed even while initial fluid resuscitation is under way. A bolus of 20 mL/kg of 5% dextrose with 0.9% sodium chloride should be given, and IV fluid can be continued to correct hypoglycemia, hypovolemia, and hyponatremia. Hyperkalemia can be very severe and may necessitate specific treatment with calcium, sodium bicarbonate, potassium-binding resin (sodium polystyrene sulfonate), or IV infusion of glucose and insulin. Stress doses of hydrocortisone, preferably a water-soluble form, such as hydrocortisone sodium succinate, should be given intravenously. An acute dose of 10 mg for infants, 25 mg for toddlers, 50 mg for older children, and 100 mg

for adolescents should be administered immediately and then every 6 hrs for the first 24 hrs. These doses may be tapered during the next 24 hrs if the patient has satisfactory progress. Fluid and electrolyte balance is typically achieved by continuous IV saline administration, aided by the mineralocorticoid effect of high doses of hydrocortisone. Most patients require chronic replacement therapy for their cortisol and aldosterone deficiencies. Hydrocortisone may be given orally in doses of 10 mg/m²/day in three divided doses. During stressful conditions, such as infection or minor operative procedures, the dose should be increased two- to threefold. Major surgery under general anesthesia requires high IV doses of hydrocortisone similar to those used for acute AI. If aldosterone deficiency is present, fludrocortisone, a mineralocorticoid, is given orally in a doses of 0.05–0.30 mg daily and often is started empirically pending steroid results.

Secondary Adrenal Insufficiency

By definition, secondary AI is due to ACTH deficiency. Pituitary or hypothalamic dysfunction can cause ACTH deficiency, usually associated with deficiencies of other pituitary hormones such as growth hormone and thyrotropin. Craniopharyngioma and germinoma are the most common causes of corticotrophin deficiency in childhood. Surgical removal or radiotherapy of tumors in the midbrain, in most cases, leads to damage of the pituitary and/or the hypothalamus, resulting in secondary AI. Very rarely, autoimmune hypophysitis can be the cause of corticotropin deficiency. Congenital lesions of the pituitary alone or with additional midline structure defect may be involved, as in septo-optic dysplasia. More severe developmental anomalies of the brain, such as anencephaly and holoprosencephaly, can also affect the pituitary. Patients with multiple pituitary hormone deficiencies due to mutations in the *PROP1* gene have been described with progressive ACTH/cortisol deficiency (58).

Tertiary Adrenal Insufficiency

By definition, tertiary AI implies a hypothalamic decrease in CRH secretion or production. Most commonly, it occurs when the HPA axis is suppressed by prolonged administration of high doses of a potent glucocorticoid that is withdrawn suddenly or tapered too rapidly. Patients at risk for this problem are those undergoing treatment for leukemia, asthma, and collagen vascular disease or other autoimmune conditions that require massive doses of potent glucocorticoids, and those who have undergone tissue transplants or neurosurgical procedures. The maximum duration and dose of glucocorticoid that can be administered before encountering this problem is not known, but it is assumed that high-dose glucocorticoids (e.g., prednisone 2 mg/kg/day to a maximum of 60 mg/day) can be administered for up to ~1 week without requiring a subsequent slow taper of dose (73). On the other hand, when high doses of dexamethasone are given to children with leukemia, return of the integrity of the HPA axis may take more than a month after therapy is stopped (25,36,54). These patients, when subsequently subjected to stress such as severe infections or additional surgical procedures, should be presumed adrenally incompetent for up to 1 year unless normal cortisol response to provocative stimulation is documented (e.g., ACTH stimulation test). However, even with a normal peak stimulated cortisol response to ACTH, any sign of vasomotor instability during a surgical procedure warrants immediate glucocorticoid coverage.

Clinical Presentation

Because the adrenal gland is, by definition, intact in secondary and tertiary AI, and the renin angiotensin system is not involved, aldosterone secretion is unaffected. Therefore, the signs and symptoms of secondary and tertiary AI are hypoglycemia, orthostatic hypotension, or weakness. Electrolytes usually remain in the normal range. Hyponatremia may be observed due to the decreased glomerular filtration rate and decreased free water clearance associated with cortisol deficiency. When secondary AI is due to an inborn or acquired anatomic defect that involves the pituitary, signs of associated deficiencies of other pituitary hormones may be seen, including microphallus and jaundice in infancy or poor growth after the first year of life.

Treatment

Iatrogenic AI (caused by chronic glucocorticoid administration) is best avoided by using the smallest effective doses of systemic glucocorticoids for the shortest period of time. When the patient is thought to be at risk, rapid tapering of the dose to a level equivalent to, or slightly less than, physiologic replacement ($\sim$10 mg/m^2/24 hrs) and further tapering over several weeks may allow the adrenal cortex to recover without the development of signs of AI. Patients with anatomic lesions of the pituitary should be treated indefinitely with glucocorticoids. Mineralocorticoid replacement is not required. When a unilateral adrenocortical tumor produces cortisol that, for example, results in Cushing syndrome, steroid secretion is autonomous and does not require ACTH activation. The high concentration of circulating cortisol will suppress endogenous CRH/ACTH secretion and result in atrophy of the contralateral adrenal gland. Following removal of the tumor, the patient is in a condition similar to that of cessation of iatrogenic glucocorticoid therapy. It is therefore appropriate to provide exogenous cortisol during the stress of surgery and during the postsurgical period. Therapy can then be tapered or stopped, depending on the individual's response while under close observation. In these cases, the patient usually requires additional steroid coverage at times of intercurrent stress for the next 6–12 months.

Disorders of Aldosterone Production

Deficiencies in CYP11B2 are associated with two related genetic disorders of aldosterone synthesis. A third genetic disorder of this locus is a rare form of autosomal-dominant hypertension caused by a hybrid CYP11B1/CYP11B2 gene. A genetic defect in the CYP11B2 gene impairs the production of mineralocorticoids without compromising glucocorticoid production. Previously, it was hypothesized that two distinct enzymes performed 18-hydroxylation and 18-oxidation, now known to be performed by CYP11B2, and two deficiencies were clinically characterized—corticosterone methyloxidase I (CMO I) deficiency and corticosterone methyloxidase II (CMO II) deficiency. Subsequent analysis has shown definitively that a single protein, encoded by the CYP11B2 gene, catalyzes both of these reactions, as well as the initial 11β-hydroxylation required for aldosterone production (45). Deficiency of CMO I or CMO II causes elevated renin activity and aldosterone defi-

ciency, with the accumulation of steroid precursors prior to the biosynthetic block: (a) corticosterone and deoxycorticosterone in CMO I deficiency, and (b) corticosterone, deoxycorticosterone, and 18-hydroxycorticosterone in CMO II deficiency. These precursors have some mineralocorticoid activity, which partially compensate for the aldosterone deficiency. Thus, partial salt loss is the usual presentation rather than the typical salt-losing crisis of complete mineralocorticoid deficiency. Renal salt-wasting and decreased growth velocity develop in these patients, while infants may present only with failure to thrive. Laboratory evaluation reveals a low aldosterone level and elevated corticosterone and deoxycorticosterone levels in CMO I deficiency and increased corticosterone concentration and 18-hydroxycortixosterone, accompanied by an increased ratio of 18-hydroxycorticosterone to aldosterone in CMO II deficiency. Treatment consists of giving enough fludrocortisone (0.05–0.3 mg daily), sodium chloride, or both in order to achieve normal plasma renin activity. With increasing age (not fully understood), salt-replacement requirements usually improve, and drug therapy can often be discontinued.

In pseudohypoaldosteronism, the kidneys do not respond to aldosterone. This disorder presents in infancy with dehydration, hyponatremia, and hyperkalemia despite marked elevation of aldosterone and renin levels. The mutations in the gene encoding the mineralocorticoid receptor are autosomal dominant and mild, whereas the mutations in the genes encoding the amiloride-sensitive epithelial sodium channel have been described as autosomal recessive and severe. Treatment with mineralocorticoid is ineffective, and the only effective treatment is with sodium chloride. In acquired hypoaldosteronism, as in hyporeninemic hypoaldosteronism, damage to the juxtaglomerular apparatus and, hence, renin deficiency occur. Patients have hyponatremia, hyperkalemia, normal or elevated blood pressure with both low aldosterone and plasma renin activity. Patients usually have impaired renal function, as seen in diabetes mellitus, systemic lupus erythematosus, myeloma, amyloidosis, autoimmune deficiency syndrome, and as seen with use of nonsteroidal anti-inflammatory drugs, unusual in the pediatric setting. Many patients are asymptomatic, with only mild-to-moderate hyperkalemia. In the ICU, administration of heparin may exacerbate relative hypoaldosteronism by inhibiting its synthesis and thereby precipitating significant salt wasting and volume loss.

Relative Adrenal Insufficiency in the PICU

Critically ill patients may develop glucocorticoid insufficiency at some point in the course of their illness. The diagnosis can be challenging due to the variable changes that normally occur as part of the response of the hypothalamo-pituitary-adrenal axis to severe illness. Critical illness can result in an increase in serum cortisol, changes in the circadian rhythm of serum cortisol, decrease in corticosteroid binding proteins, and changes in the number and sensitivity of tissue glucocorticoid receptors (4,18). Changes in cortisol levels in significant systemic illness are described in **Table 91.4**, and the effects of drugs on total cortisol concentration are described in **Table 91.5** (4). Special consideration regarding etomidate will be discussed in detail later. The initial response to stress is illustrated in **Figure 91.3**, panel B. The early increases in CRH, ACTH, and cortisol levels are usually proportional to the degree of illness. However, due to multiple mechanisms, prolonged illness can lead to

TABLE 91.4

ILLNESSES AFFECTING MEASURED SERUM TOTAL CORTISOL CONCENTRATIONS IN CRITICALLY ILL PATIENTS

Illness	Hepatitis/liver disease	Septic shock	Malnutrition	Nephrotic syndrome	Dilutional	Illness severity
Mechanism	Increased transcortin	Possible glucocorticoid resistance; significant inflammatory response	Lower transcortin and albumin	Lower transcortin and/or albumin	Lower transcortin and albumin	Increased production
Impact	Generally higher levels	Increased levels despite symptoms suggestive of adrenal insufficiency	Relatively lower total but appropriate free cortisol	Relatively lower total but normal free cortisol	Relatively lower total cortisol but normal free cortisol levels	Generally proportionate to stress
Clinical Examples	Patients with hepatitis	Patients with septic shock	Patients with malnutrition	Patients with nephrotic syndrome	Cardiopulmonary bypass, excess IV fluids	Patients with septic shock

Adapted from Arafah BM. Review: hypothalamic pituitary adrenal function during critical illness limitations of current assessment methods. *J Clin Endocr Metab* 2006;91:3725–45.

impairment of the glucocorticoid rise, resulting in acute AI, as illustrated in **Figure 91.3**, panel C. This phenomenon has been called *functional AI* to denote that a "functional" and not a "structural" defect is responsible for the AI. Another term that describes perturbations of the HPA axis during severe illness is "relative" AI, which is used by some to describe situations when, although high absolute cortisol levels are present, they are "relatively" insufficient to overcome the degree of physiologic stress put upon the patient. Moreover, the patient often cannot mount an additional response to subsequent stress (60,66). Attempts to define relative AI may require assessing the response to exogenous administration of ACTH (3). Unfortunately, studies that define relative or functional AI in children are limited. However, assessment of severely ill children with septic shock have begun to show that both absolute and relative AI are common in children with catecholamine-resistant shock and absent in children with fluid-responsive shock (20,55).

Adrenal insufficiency is also common in critical illnesses other than sepsis. Many factors and illnesses in the PICU can contribute to relative AI, including trauma, hemorrhagic shock, and following traumatic brain injury (16,31). In a study in which AI was reported following traumatic brain injury, patients were considered adrenally insufficient if, post-injury, they had an initial cortisol level of <5 mcg/dL or two consecutive cortisol levels of ≤15 mcg/dL. These patients were also found to have considerably lower ACTH levels, suggesting secondary AI. In addition, they had higher injury severity scores, higher frequency of hypotension, and higher probability of etomidate use. The state of AI was found to be transient; most survivors showed a normal response to a 1-mcg ACTH stimulation test 6 months after injury (16). Another factor that may contribute to relative AI is mechanical ventilation. In a study of adult ICU patients who required mechanical ventilation for >24 hrs, 75% were found to have AI. They were considered to have normal adrenal function if they had a plasma cortisol level of

TABLE 91.5

DRUGS THAT AFFECT MEASURED SERUM TOTAL CORTISOL CONCENTRATIONS IN CRITICALLY ILL PATIENTS

Drug	Estrogens	Ketoconazole	Spironolactone	Aminoglutethimide	Etomidate
Mechanism	Increases transcortin	Decreases synthesis of cortisol	Interferes in the assay, depending on antibody specificity	Inhibits cortisol synthesis	Decreases synthesis due to 11β hydroxylase-inhibition
Impact	Higher total cortisol; low free cortisol	Lower serum cortisol levels; low free cortisol	Generally higher cortisol levels; variable influence, depending on assay specificity	Lower serum total and free cortisol	Lower serum cortisol levels; decreased responsiveness to cosyntropin
Clinical Examples	Estrogen, oral contraceptives, pregnancy, hepatitis	Patients receiving the drug	Patients receiving the drug	Patients receiving the drug, e.g., medical adrenalectomy for metastatic breast cancer	Use of the drug

Adapted from Arafah BM. Review: hypothalamic pituitary adrenal function during critical illness limitations of current assessment methods. *J Clin Endocr Metab* 2006;91:3725–45.

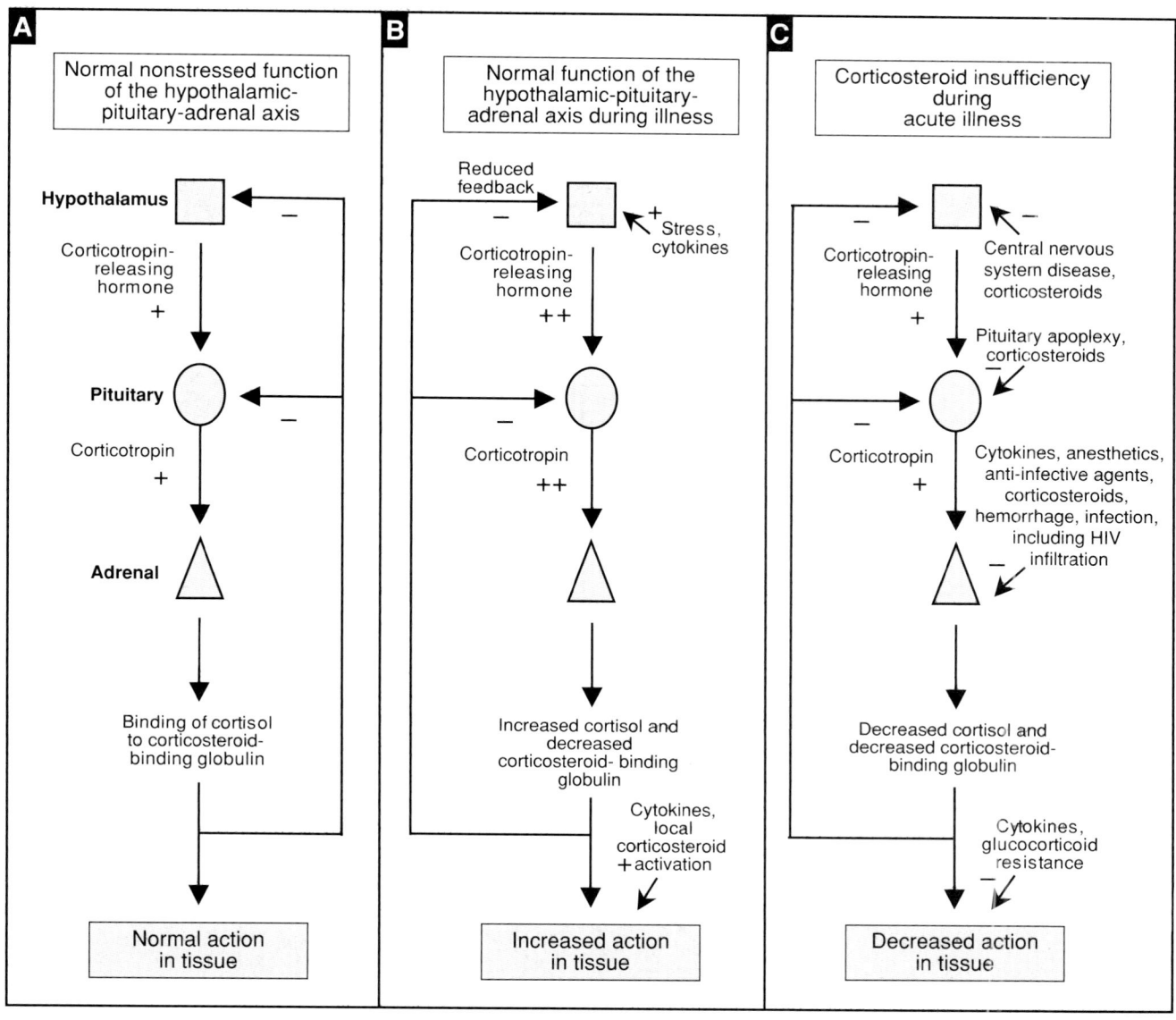

FIGURE 91.3. Activity of the hypothalamic-pituitary-adrenal axis under normal conditions (**A**), during an appropriate response to stress (**B**), and during an inappropriate response to critical illness (**C**). A plus sign indicates a stimulatory effect; a minus sign indicates an inhibitory effect. From Cooper M, Stewart P. Corticosteroid insufficiency in acutely ill patients. *N Engl J Med* 2003;348:727–34, with permission.

>25 mcg/dL or a 9-mcg/dL increase in serum cortisol level after an ACTH stimulation test. Weaning from mechanical ventilation was significantly higher in the group with adequate adrenal reserve than in the hydrocortisone-treated group (32). AI was also described in patients who had end-stage liver disease. Interestingly, the only factor that predicted the development of an adrenal exhaustion syndrome in these patients was a low high-density lipoprotein (HDL) level (43,44).

Clinical Diagnosis of Relative Adrenal Insufficiency in the ICU

Diagnosis of relative AI can be very difficult. Hemodynamic instability in a critically ill patient despite adequate fluid resuscitation can suggest the diagnosis. In addition, an inadequate response to empirical treatment in cases of ongoing inflamma-

tion can provide clues to the diagnosis. Laboratory tests can be confusing and misleading. In an ICU setting, both high and low cortisol levels can be detected. Many levels have been proposed below which the patient may be diagnosed with relative AI. An ACTH stimulation test can be used as a diagnostic tool in the ICU setting and can be performed in the same way as in non-critically ill patients, using 250 mcg of synthetic ACTH. The absolute post-ACTH response is yet to be determined, especially in children. The threshold can be the same as in the noncritical patients or may ultimately be found to be higher, to compensate for the level of stress. Cortisol levels and cortisol response to corticotropin were studied in patients with septic shock (3) (**Fig. 91.4**). A high baseline cortisol level was the most prognostic factor. Investigators considered the absolute cortisol increment of 9 mcg/dL above baseline as having

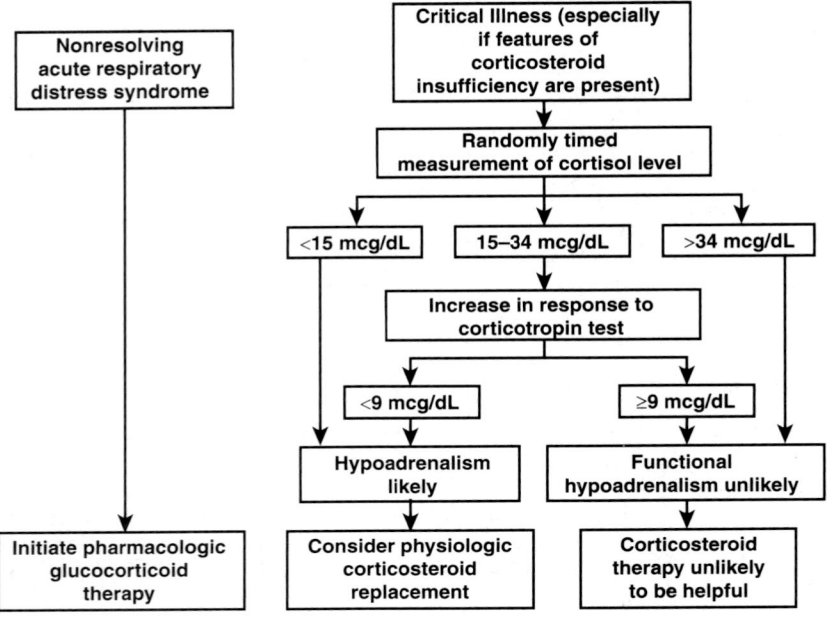

FIGURE 91.4. Investigation of adrenal corticosteroid function in critically ill patients on the basis of cortisol levels and response to the corticotropin stimulation test. The scheme has been evaluated for patients with septic shock. However, it must be remembered that no cut-off value will be entirely reliable. From Cooper M, Stewart P. Corticosteroid insufficiency in acutely ill patients. *N Engl J Med* 2003;348:727–34, with permission.

prognostic implication. It was reported that a <9-mcg/dL increase from the baseline 60 mins after ACTH administration is associated with an increased death risk (3). A high baseline cortisol with low incremental rise probably means that the patient is maximally stressed, and not that the patient has AI, per se. Another group compared a low-dose (1 mcg) corticotropin stimulation test with the standard (250 mcg) test for the diagnosis of relative AI (65). The ACTH stimulation tests were performed consecutively with a minimum of 4 hrs between the low- and the standard-dose tests. Serum cortisol was measured at baseline, 30, 60, and 90 mins post-ACTH administration, and a response was considered adequate if the increment in cortisol response was >9 mcg/dL. Nonresponders to the low-dose test had a higher mortality rate than responders to both tests, which suggests that the low-dose test can identify patients in septic shock with inadequate adrenal function (65). These patients had poorer outcomes and would have been missed by the high-dose test. The authors suggested that this subgroup may benefit from steroid replacement.

Studies are warranted to determine the diagnostic criteria of relative AI and whether corticosteroid use in the PICU in these instances benefits the overall outcome in children with suspected relative AI.

Adrenal Hyperfunction

Cushing Syndrome

The principal causes of Cushing syndrome in childhood are listed in Table 91.6. In the PICU setting, Cushing syndrome is most often seen in children who have received exogenous glucocorticoids. Glucocorticoids can be administered for chronic steroid replacement in states of AI or as a part of high-dose or bolus steroid therapy for renal or rheumatologic disorders. In these instances, the patient may present with physical and biochemical signs of glucocorticoid excess, including cushingoid appearance, with moon-like facies, centripetal obesity, short

stature, thin extremities with fragile capillaries, hirsutism, and acne. They may also present with delayed puberty and amenorrhea. Hypertension, hyperglycemia or glucose intolerance, and osteopenia are also observed. Patients, who receive chronic treatment with glucocorticoid, should not have abrupt cessation of their glucocorticoid therapy and should receive stress doses of glucocorticoid during the peri-, intra- and postoperative periods (see the previous section, Primary Adrenal Insufficiency).

TABLE 91.6

ETIOLOGIES OF DIFFERENT TYPES OF ADRENAL HYPERFUNCTION

Disorder	Etiology
Cushing disease	Pituitary adenoma
Cushing syndrome	Adrenal adenoma
	Bilateral micronodular adrenal hyperplasia (e.g., McCune-Albright syndrome)
	Primary pigmented adrenal hyperplasia (e.g., Carney complex)
	Bilateral macronodular adrenal hyperplasia
	Adrenal carcinoma
	Ectopic ACTH (CRH): non-pituitary ACTH (CRH)-producing tumor
Pseudo-cushing syndrome	Depression, alcoholism (increased CRH secretion)
Iatrogenic Cushing syndrome	Pharmacologic glucocorticoid therapy

ACTH, adrenocorticotropic hormone; CRH, corticotrophin-releasing hormone

Diagnosis and Treatment

The diagnosis of Cushing syndrome can be difficult to make in an ICU setting. Typically, in the ICU, the circadian rhythm of cortisol secretion is lost and cortisol levels at midnight and 8 am are usually comparable (18). Further, diurnal blood samples from patients under conditions of stress in the ICU may demonstrate high levels of cortisol, making it difficult to differentiate these patients from those with Cushing syndrome. Of course, the diagnosis of Cushing syndrome in the ICU can always be made on clinical grounds using the history and the physical examination. The more specific evaluation can be obtained after the patient is discharged from the ICU to a regular hospital ward. The most common cause of Cushing syndrome in children is of adrenal origin. In adolescents who have Cushing disease, a CNS lesion such as an ACTH-secreting pituitary adenoma is most likely the cause of Cushing syndrome.

The treatment of choice for pituitary-related Cushing disease in children is transsphenoidal pituitary microsurgery. Reoperation or pituitary irradiation is performed when a relapse occurs. Long-term remission is predicted by low postoperative serum or urinary cortisol concentrations. Patients with benign cortical adenoma can benefit from adrenalectomy. Such adenomas are occasionally bilateral and may require subtotal adrenalectomy. Adrenocortical carcinomas frequently metastasize, especially to the liver and lungs, and the prognosis may be unfavorable despite removal of the primary lesion (66–68).

Virilizing Tumors

Virilizing tumors of the adrenal gland are the most common adrenal tumors in children. Virilization is the most common presenting symptom, and includes accelerated growth velocity, acne, muscular development, precocious development of axillary and pubic hair, and penile enlargement without testicular enlargement in males. In females, signs include hirsutism, masculinization with clitoral enlargement, and the precocious development of axillary and pubic hair, with rapid growth. In addition to virilization, 20%–40% of patients present with symptoms of cortisol excess. Patients with these tumors have elevated levels of serum DHEA, DHEA sulfate, androstenedione, and testosterone. Cortisol, aldosterone, and serum electrolyte levels are usually within normal limits. Ultrasonography, CT, and MRI can be used to diagnose the tumor and the presence of any metastases. Histologically, it is often difficult to differentiate between benign and malignant tumors. Surgery or laparoscopic removal of the tumor is the treatment of choice. AI may follow the resection of the adrenal tumor if cortisol excess is a manifestation on presentation.

Hyperaldosteronism

The discussion of hyperaldosteronism and associated hypertension will be limited to primary forms of the disease. In adults, this includes patients with hypertension due to adrenal hyperplasia, aldosterone-producing adenomas, or more rarely, adrenocortical carcinoma. Familial forms are also rare. In children, primary hypertension due to hyperaldosteronism is exceedingly rare. It has been described in association with increased aldosterone due to adrenal hyperplasia, as previously mentioned, but can also be of a severe and refractory nature. It may be due to monogenic mutations that are associated with familial forms of low-renin hypertension such as glucocorticoid remediable hyperaldosteronism, now referred to as familial hyperaldosteronism type I. Secondary states of hyperaldosteronism, such as those seen in congestive heart failure, are associated with elevated renin levels and are discussed in Chapter 66.

Simply stated, the hypertension associated with increased aldosterone is due to the increase in sodium, chloride, and water reabsorption in the luminal cells of the cortical-collecting renal tubule and the distal convoluted tubule. With increased levels of aldosterone, epithelial sodium-channel activity occurs, which is responsible for renal sodium reabsorption (49). Screening tests include assessment of plasma renin activity levels and measurement of both urinary and serum levels of aldosterone. Imaging tests, including CT, MRI, and sonography, may be diagnostic but are often not conclusive.

Familial hyperaldosteronism type I has been described to be an autosomal dominant form of low-renin hyperaldosteronism. The genetic abnormality is actually due to the presence of a chimeric gene on chromosome 8, in which the regulatory region of the 11β-hydroxylase gene is coupled with the structural region of the aldosterone synthase gene CY11B2 in the zona glomerulosa. Familial hyperaldosteronism type II is due to a mutation on chromosome 7p22 (37).

Diagnosis and Treatment

In familial hyperaldosteronism type I, secretion of aldosterone and the 18OH corticosteroid metabolites is under ACTH regulation and produced in the zona fasciculata. In this condition, elevated levels of aldosterone suppress renin. Diagnosis can be made with a dexamethasone suppression test, which will cause virtual suppression of urinary aldosterone within 48 hrs. Genetic testing is also available for this disorder (51). Treatment with glucocorticoids will suppress ACTH, allowing for suppression of the aldosterone that is stimulated by ACTH and recovery of the rennin-aldosterone axis, which is evidenced by a sodium diuresis that results in the production of normal levels of aldosterone. Young patients can present with severe hypertension and, although this was initially thought to be a more benign form of hypertensive disease, families have been described with hemorrhagic strokes. Serum potassium levels may be low or normal. Treatment is usually initiated with low-dose glucocorticoids followed by potassium-sparing agents such as spironolactone (26,41,71).

In familial hyperaldosteronism type II, a trial of dexamethasone does not cause aldosterone suppression. Treatment of involves use of potassium-sparing diuretics such as spironolactone.

MANAGEMENT ISSUES DURING ANESTHESIA, INTUBATION, AND THE PERIOPERATIVE PERIOD

General Considerations

In patients with acute glucocorticoid or complete AI, treatment consists of supportive care, treatment of the underlying disease, and hydrocortisone replacement. Supportive care includes administration of fluids, appropriate electrolyte supplementation

TABLE 91.7

PHARMACOLOGIC CHARACTERISTICS OF VARIOUS STEROIDS RELATIVE TO CORTISOL

Steroid	Anti-inflammatory glucocorticoid effect	Salt-retaining mineralocorticoid effect	Growth-retarding glucocorticoid effect	Plasma half-life (min)	Biologic half-life (hrs)
Cortisone (hydrocortisone, cortef)	1.0	1.0	1.0	80–120	8
Cortisone acetate (oral)	0.8	0.8	0.8	80–120	8
Cortisone acetate (intramuscular)	0.8	0.8	1.3		18
Prednisone	3.5–4	0.8	5	200	16–36
Prednisolone	4	0.8		120–300	16–36
Methylprednisolone	5	0.5	7.5		
Dexamethasone	30		80	150–300	36–54
9α-Fluorocortisone		200			
Aldosterone	0.3	200–1000			

Adapted from Miller WL. The Adrenal Cortex. In: Sperling MA, ed. *Pediatric Endocrinology Textbook, 2nd ed.* Philadelphia: Saunders, 2002;413.

(to treat hyponatremia, hyperkalemia, hypercalcemia, and acidosis), nutritional supplements, medications, antibiotics, and organ support. It is important to maintain body temperature and glucose levels. Patients in shock may require little or no anesthesia. Hyperkalemia is a contraindication to the use of succinylcholine. Etomidate, a short-acting IV anesthetic agent used commonly for the induction of general anesthesia in critically ill patients, has an inhibitory effect on adrenal function (1,69). Etomidate use in these patients results in depression of the adrenal cortical stress response, with reduction of cortisol and aldosterone production (69). Thiopental, propofol, and midazolam do not depress the adrenocortical response to stress, but some of these drugs inhibit steroidogenic enzymes in vitro (19,59). In Cushing syndrome, after surgical resection of the pituitary or adrenal tumor, most patients have transient suppression of the normal CRH/ACTH/adrenal axis, necessitating corticosteroid replacement therapy for several months.

Children who have been exposed to high doses of endogenous (Cushing syndrome or disease) or exogenous steroids are susceptible to osteoporosis and may be at risk for pathologic fractures. Therefore, care should be taken during positioning for procedures in the operating room or the PICU. As patients may have muscle weakness, neuromuscular-blocking drugs should be used with caution and at lowerk doses.

Patients who receive long-term steroid therapy need appropriate supplemental glucocorticoid therapy in the perioperative period. During general anesthesia, with or without surgery, the cortisol secretion rate in normal subjects increases greatly. Parenteral steroids are needed. Although protocols vary, the following protocol has been useful: a dose of 25 mg/m^2 of hydrocortisone sodium succinate given IV immediately prior to anesthesia, followed by a dose of ~50 mg/m^2 as a constant infusion for the period of the surgical procedure; finally, a third dose of ~25–50 mg/m^2 hydrocortisone sodium succinate given as a constant IV infusion for the remainder of the first 24 hrs of the surgical day. These doses total 100–125 mg/m^2 over a 24-hr period, or ~10 times replacement therapy, and should be followed on the first postoperative day by three to four times replacement therapy (50 mg/m^2/day) of constant IV infusion. Eventually, oral therapy is resumed as tolerated.

Therapeutic Guidelines/Steroid Preparations

Various derivatives of steroids are available and can be given via multiple routes. To choose the appropriate product, the clinician must to realize that, by convention, glucocorticoid potency is described according to its anti-inflammatory potency. Further, different glucocorticoid preparations have different plasma and biologic half-lives, with various growth-suppressant effects. These actions can differ significantly from their established anti-inflammatory effect. Additionally, the mineralocorticoid activity of glucocorticoids varies widely among the different preparations. In patients who receive phenobarbital or phenytoin, cortisone and prednisolone are cleared rapidly, whereas in hepatic failure, glucocorticoid clearance is decreased. In general, the rapidly absorbed steroids are orally administered (they are usually incompletely absorbed) while intramuscular administered steroids are absorbed slowly but more completely (Table 91.7).

In the ICU setting, the most commonly used corticosteroids are those that are administered intravenously and include dexamethasone, methylprednisolone, prednisolone, and hydrocortisone. Hydrocortisone has the highest mineralocorticoid activity, whereas dexamethasone has none. Thus, in patients with adrenal crisis and hypovolemia, hydrocortisone is the favored steroid, whereas in patients with intracranial tumors or increased intracranial pressure, dexamethasone (which has no mineralocorticoid activity) is the most appropriate steroid to be used.

OUTCOME

Maintenance of normal adrenal function is essential in patients treated in the ICU, as they have higher plasma levels of cortisol. In some instances, patients develop relative AI. Few studies have demonstrated that treatment with steroids improves outcome in patients with sepsis and septic shock. For patients with respiratory failure, it was demonstrated that early identification of AI with stress steroid dose replacement can result in a shorter and more successful weaning from the ventilator (32). In an ICU setting, it has also been shown—in patients with chronic liver failure or in those following liver transplantation with AI—that treatment with a steroid can decrease the requirement for vasopressor therapy. These patients also had a significantly lower mortality rate than those who were not treated (44); however, studies of this sort are rare in children.

CONCLUSIONS AND FUTURE DIRECTIONS

At this time, research studies are critically needed to determine what defines relative AI in the PICU. Further protocols for early steroid use in critically ill patients that are designed to achieve better long-term results should also be developed.

K E Y P O I N T S

- Management of adrenal disorders in the PICU is challenging
- Stress affects the adrenocortical function by increasing the concentration of plasma cortisol.
- Cortisol and aldosterone secretion can be altered in systemic diseases.
- Signs of steroid insufficiency are similar to those of sepsis and shock in children.
- Iatrogenic AI secondary to chronic glucocorticoid administration is a common clinical problem that can be avoided by using the smallest effective doses of glucocorticoids for the shortest period of time.
- Relative AI, especially in children, is a clinical problem that requires further definition and clarification.

ACKNOWLEDGMENT

The authors would like to thank C. Pomeranz, BA, for her assistance with this chapter.

References

1. Absalom A, Pledger D, Kong A. Adrenocortical function in critically ill patients 24 h after a single dose of etomidate. *Anesthesia* 1999;54:861–7.
2. Addison T. *On the constitutional and local effects of disease of the suprarenal capsules.* London: Highley, 1855.
3. Annane D, Sebille V, Troche G, et al. A 3-level prognostic classification in septic shock based on cortisol levels and cortisol response to corticotrophin. *JAMA* 2000;283:1038–45.
4. Arafah BM. Review: Hypothalamic pituitary adrenal function during critical illness limitations of current assessment methods. *J Clin Endocr Metab* 2006;91:3725–45.
5. Assmann G, Seedorf U. Acid Lipase Deficiency: Wolman disease and cholesterol ester storage disease. In: Scriver CR, Beaudet AL, Sly WS, et al., eds. *The Metabolic and Molecular Bases of Inherited Diseases, 8th ed., vol. 3.* New York: McGraw-Hill, 2001;3551–72.
6. Auchus RJ, Rainey WE. Adrenarche—physiology, biochemistry, and human disease. *Clin Endocrinol* 2004;60:288–96.
7. Beitins IZ, Bayard F, Anecs IG, et al. The metabolic clearance rate, blood production, interconversion and transplacental passage of cortisol and cortisone in pregnancy near term. *Ped Res* 1973;7:509–19.
8. Besedovsky HO, De Ray A. Immune-neuro-endocrine interactions: Facts and hypotheses. *Endocr Rev* 1996;17:64–102.
9. Bethune JE. *The Adrenal Cortex. A Scope Monograph.* Kalamazoo: The Upjohn Company, 1975.
10. Blodgett FM, Burgin L, Lezzoni D, et al. Effects of prolonged cortisone ther-
11. apy on the structural growth, skeletal maturation, and metabolic status of children. *N Engl J Med* 1956;254:636–41.
11. Brown-Séquard CE. Recherches experimentales sur la physiologie et la pathologie des capsules surrenales. *Arch Gen Med* 1856;ser 5, no 8:385–401.
12. Burnay M, Python C, Vallotton M, et al. Role of the capacitative calcium influx in the activation of steroidogenesis by angiotensin-II in adrenal glomerulosa cells. *Endocrinol* 1994;135:751–8.
13. Chang AC, Cochet M, Cohen SN. Structural organization of human genomic DNA encoding the pro-opiomelanocortin peptide. *Proc Natl Acad Sci USA* 1980;77:4890–4.
14. Chroousos GP. The hypothalamic-pituitary-adrenal axis and immune-mediated inflammation. *N Engl J Med* 1995;332:1351–62.
15. Cidlowski JA, King KL, Evans-Storms RB, et al. The biochemistry and molecular biology of glucocorticoid-induced apoptosis in the immune system. *Recent Prog Horm Res* 1996;51:457–91.
16. Cohan P, Wang C, McArthur DL, et al. Acute secondary adrenal insufficiency after traumatic brain injury: A prospective study. *Crit Care Med* 2005;33:2358–66.
17. Conn JW. Primary aldosteronism: a new clinical entity. *J Lab Clin Med* 1955;45:3–17.
18. Cooper MS, Stewart PM. Corticosteroid insufficiency in acutely ill patients. *N Engl J Med* 2003;348:727–34.
19. Crozier TA, Beck D, Schlaeger M, et al. Endocrinological changes following etomidate, midazolam, or methohexital for minor surgery. *Anesthesiol* 1987;66:628–35.
20. Den Brinker M, Joosten K, Liem O, et al. Adrenal Insufficiency in meningococcal sepsis: Bioavailable cortisol levels and impact of interleukin-6 levels and intubation with etomidate on adrenal function and mortality. *J Clin Endocrinol Metab* 2005;90:5110–7.
21. Dinarello CA, Mier JW. Current concepts-Lymphokines. *N Engl J Med* 1987;317:940–5.
22. Donohue PA. The Adrenal Gland and Its Disorders. In: Kappy MS, Allen DB, Geffner ME, eds. *Principles and Practice of Pediatric Endocrinology.* Springfield: Charles C. Thomas, 2005;357–485.
23. Dubey P, Raymond GV, Moser AB, et al. Adrenal insufficiency in asymptomatic adrenoleukodystrophy patients identified by very long-chain fatty acid screening. *J Pediatr* 2005;146:528–32.
24. Eustachius B. *Tabulae Anatomicae.* Amsterdam: Amstelaedami, apud R & G Wetstenios, 1774.
25. Felner EI, Thompson MT, Ratliff AF, et al. Time course of recovery of adrenal function in children treated for leukemia. *J Pediatr* 2000;137:21–4.
26. Garovic V, Hilliard A, Turner S. Monogenic forms of low renin hypertension. *Nature Clin Prac Nephr* 2006;2:624–30.
27. Grunfeld J-P, Eloy L. Glucocorticoids modulates vascular reactivity in the rat. *Hypertension* 1987;10:608–18.
28. Guillemin R, Rosenberg B. Humoral hypothalamic control of anterior pituitary: A study with combined tissue cultures. *Endocrinology* 1955;57:599–607.
29. Gwynne JT, Strauss JF III. The role of lipoprotein in steroidogenesis and cholesterol metabolism in steroidogenic glands. *Endocr Rev* 1982;3:299–329.
30. Hale AC, Rees LH. ACTH and Related Peptides. In: De Groot LJ, Besser GM, Marshall JC, et al, eds. *Endocrinology, 2nd ed.,* vol. 1. Philadelphia: WB Saunders, 1989;363–76.
31. Hoen S, Asehnoune K, Brailly-Tabard S, et al. Cortisol response to corticotrophin stimulation in trauma patients: Influence of hemorrhagic shock. *Anesthesiology* 2002;97:807–13.
32. Huang CJ, Lin HC. Association between adrenal insufficiency and failed ventilator weaning. *Am J Respir Crit Care Med* 2006;173:276–80.
33. Ikeda Y, Swain A, Weber T, et al. Steroidogenic factor 1 and DAX 1 colocalize in multiple cell lineages: Potential links in endocrine development. *Mol Endocrinol* 1996;10:1261–72.
34. Kaplan NM. The biosynthesis of adrenal steroids. Effects of angiotensin II, adrenocorticotropin and potassium. *J Clin Invest* 1965;44:2029–39.
35. Kong M, Jeffcoate W. Eighty-six cases of Addison's disease. *Clin Endocrinol* 1994;41:757–61.
36. Kuperman H, Damiani D, Chrousos GP, et al. Evaluation of the hypothalamic-pituitary-adrenal axis in children with leukemia before and after 6 weeks of high-dose glucocorticoid therapy. *J Clin Endocrinol Metab* 2001;86:2993–6.
37. Lafferty AR, Torpy DJ, Stowasser M, et al. A novel genetic locus for low renin hypertension: Familial hyperaldosteronism type II maps to chromosome 7. *J Med Genet* 2000;37:831–5.
38. Laragh JH, Angers M, Kelly WG, et al. Hypotensive agents and pressor substances. The effects of epinephrine, norepinephrine, angiotensin II and others on the secretion rate of aldosterone in man. *JAMA* 1960;174:234–40.
39. Legro RS, Lin HM, Demers LM, et al. Urinary free cortisol increases in adolescent Caucasian females during perimenarche. *J Clin Endocrinol Metab* 2003;88:215–9.
40. Li CH. Lipotropin, a new active peptide from pituitary glands. *Nature* 1964;201:924.
41. Li CH, Simpson ME, Evans HM. Adrenocorticotrophic hormone. *J Biol Chem* 1943;149:413–24.

42. Lifton RP, Dluhy RG, Powers M, et al. Hereditary hypertension caused by chimaeric gene duplications and ectopic expression of aldosterone synthase. *Nat Genet* 1992;2:66–74.

43. Marik PE. Adrenal-exhaustion syndrome in patients with liver disease. *Intensive Care Med* 2006;32:275–80.

44. Marik PE, Gayowski T, Starlz TE. The hepato-adrenal syndrome: A common yet unrecognized clinical condition. *Crit Care Med* 2005;33:1254–9.

45. Migeon CJ. Physiology and pathology of adrenocortical function in infancy and childhood. In: Collu R, Ducharme JR, Guyda H, eds. *Pediatric Endocrinology*. New York: Raven Press, 1981;465.

46. Miller WL. Molecular biology of steroid hormone synthesis. *Endocr Rev* 1988;9:295–318.

47. Moore M, Amberson JB, Kazam E, et al. Anatomy, histology, embryology. In: Vaughan EE Jr., Carey RM, eds. *Adrenal Disorders*. New York: Thieme, 1989;1–11.

48. Murck H, Held K, Ziegenbein M, et al. The Renin-angiotensin-aldosterone system in patients with depression compared to controls—a sleep endocrine study. *BMC Psychiatry* 2003;3:15.

49. Naray-Fejes-Toth A, Canessa C, Cleaveland ES, et al. SGK is an aldosterone-induced kinase in the renal collecting duct. Effects on epithelial Na+ channels. *J Biol Chem* 1999;274:16973–8.

50. Nerupt J. Addison syndrome—clinical studies: A report of 108 cases. *Acta Endocrinologica* 1974;76:127–41.

51. Oberfield SE, Levine LS, Stoner E, et al. Adrenal glomerulosa function in patients with dexamethasone suppressible hyperaldosteronism. *J Clin Endocrinol Metab* 1981;53:158–64.

52. Onishi S, Miyazawa G, Nishimura Y, et al. Postnatal development of circadian rhythm in serum cortisol levels in children. *Pediatrics* 1983;72:399–404.

53. Patil S, Bartley JA, Murray JC, et al. X-linked glycerol kinase, adrenal hypoplasia, and myopathy maps to Xq21. *Cytogenet* 1985;40:720–1.

54. Petersen K, Muller J, Rasmussen M, et al. Impaired adrenal function after glucocorticoid therapy in children with acute lymphoblastic leukemia. *Med Pediatr Oncol* 2003;41:110–4.

55. Pizarro C, Troster E, Damiani D, et al. Absolute and relative adrenal insufficiency in children with septic shock. *Crit Care Med* 2005;33:855–9.

56. Pratt, NG. Pathophysiology of heart failure: Neuroendocrine response. *Crit Care Nurs Q* 1995;18:22–31.

57. Quinkler H, Stewart PM. Hypertension and the cortisol-cortisone shuttle. *J Clin Endocrinol Metab* 2003;88:2384–92.

58. Reynaud R, Chadli-Chaieb M, Vallette-Kasic S, et al. A familial form of congenital hypopituitarism due to a PROP1 mutation in large kindred: Phenotypic and in vitro functional studies. *J Clin Endocrinol Metab* 2004;89:5779–86.

59. Robertson WR, Reader SC, Davidson B, et al. On the biopotency and site of action of drugs affecting endocrine tissues with specific reference to the antisteroidogenic effect of anesthetic agents. *Postgrad Med J* 1985;61(Suppl 3):145–51.

60. Rothwell PM, Udwadia ZF, Lawler PG. Cortisol response to corticotrophin and survival in septic shock. *Lancet* 1991;337:582–3.

61. Saffran M, Schally AV, Benfey BG. Stimulation of the release of corticotrophin from the adenohypophysis by neurohypophysial factor. *Endocrinology* 1955;57:439–44.

62. Sapolsky R, Rivier C, Yamamoto G, et al. Interleukin-1 stimulates the secretion of hypothalamic corticotrophin-releasing factor. *Science* 1987;238:522–4.

63. Sasano N, Sasano H. The Adrenal Cortex. In: Kovacs K, Asa SL, eds. *Functional Endocrine Pathology*. Boston: Blackwell Scientific, 1991;546–92.

64. Shizuta Y, Kawamoto T, Mitsuuchi Y, et al. Molecular genetic studies on the biosynthesis of aldosterone in humans. *J Steroid Biochem* 1992;43:981–7.

65. Siraux V, De Backer D, Yalavatti G, et al. Relative adrenal insufficiency in patients with septic shock: Comparison of low-dose and conventional corticotrophin test. *Crit Care Med* 2005;33:2479–86.

66. Soni A, Pepper GM, Wyrwinski PM, et al. Adrenal insufficiency occurring during septic shock: Incidence, outcome, and relationship to peripheral cytokine levels. *Am J Med* 1995;98:266–71.

67. Stickland AL, Underwood LE, Voina SJ. Growth retardation in Cushing's syndrome. *Am J Dis Child* 1972;123:207–13.

68. Vale W, Spiess J, Rivier C, et al. Characterization of a 41-residue ovine hypothalamic peptide that stimulates secretion of corticotrophin and β-endorphin. *Science* 1981;213:1394–7.

69. Wagner RL, White PF. Etomide inhibits adrenocortical function in surgical patients. *Anesthesiol* 1984;61:652–6.

70. Weldon VV, Kowarski A, Migeon CJ. Aldosterone secretion rates in normal subjects from infancy to adulthood. *Pediatrics* 1967;39:713–23.

71. White PC. Inherited forms of mineralcorticoid hypertension. *Hypertension* 1996;28:927–36.

72. Wise J, Matalon R, Morgan AM, et al. Phenotypic features of patients with congenital adrenal hypoplasia and glycerol kinase deficiency. *Am J Dis Child* 1987;141:744–7.

73. Zora JA, Zimmerman TL, Carey EJ, et al. Hypothalamic-pituitary-adrenal axis suppression after short-term, high-dose glucocorticoid therapy in children with asthma. *J Allergy Clin Immuno* 1986;17:9–13.

74. Zuckerman-Levin N, Tiosano D, Eisenhofer G, et al. The importance of adrenocortical glucocorticoids for adrenomedullary and physiological response to stress: A study in isolated glucocorticoid deficiency. *J Clin Endocrinol Metab* 2001;86:5920–4.

CHAPTER 92 ■ DISORDERS OF GLUCOSE HOMEOSTASIS

STUART A. WEINZIMER • MICHAEL F. CANARIE • EDWARD VINCENT S. FAUSTINO
• WILLIAM V. TAMBORLANE • CLIFFORD W. BOGUE

DIABETIC KETOACIDOSIS IN CHILDREN

Diabetic ketoacidosis (DKA) is a life-threatening, preventable complication of diabetes mellitus that is characterized by inadequate insulin action, hyperglycemia, dehydration, electrolyte loss, metabolic acidosis, and ketosis. It is associated with a significant mortality rate and is the most frequent cause of death in children with type 1 diabetes mellitus. As type 1 diabetes is one of the most common chronic illnesses in children, occurring in ~1 in every 350 children by age 18 in the US (71), DKA is one of the most common reasons for admission to the ICU in pediatrics. DKA occurs in ~15%–70% of children with diabetes at disease onset and in 1%–10% of children with a previous diagnosis of diabetes due to infection or other intercurrent illness, insulin pump malfunction, or purposeful insulin omission (73). DKA at diagnosis of type 1 diabetes occurs more commonly in very young children, children without a prior family history of type 1 diabetes, and in families from lower socioeconomic backgrounds. Likewise, the risk of DKA in established type 1 diabetes is associated with children with a history of prior poor metabolic control, concomitant psychiatric disease, adolescent girls, and lower socioeconomic background (55).

Definition and Pathophysiology

Diabetic ketoacidosis is defined as a blood glucose concentration >200 mg/dL, with ketonemia/ketonuria, and a pH of <7.3. The primary abnormality is insulin deficiency, which results in hyperglycemia by three mechanisms: increased gluconeogenesis, accelerated glycogenolysis, and impaired peripheral glucose utilization. Early in the progression of type 1 diabetes, the defects in peripheral glucose uptake predominate over the abnormalities in hepatic glucose production, such that postprandial glucose levels are elevated while fasting glucose levels are normal. However, as insulin deficiency becomes progressively more severe and absolute, fasting hyperglycemia occurs. As serum glucose levels exceed the renal threshold of 180 mg/dL, an osmotic diuresis occurs, resulting in the loss of extracellular water and electrolytes.

Although insulin deficiency is the primary defect, physiologic stress caused by acidosis and progressive dehydration, as well as coexistent infection or illness, stimulate the release of counter-regulatory hormones (glucagon, catecholamines, cortisol), which further exacerbate hyperglycemia by increasing hepatic glucose production and further impairing peripheral glucose uptake. Counter-regulatory hormones, particularly epinephrine, also promote lipolysis and free fatty acid release through the activation of adipose tissue hormone-sensitive lipase and, subsequently, ketoacidosis through the activation of hepatic β-oxidation of free fatty acids to ketone bodies, predominantly β-hydroxybutyrate and acetoacetate. Accumulation of ketoacids is the primary cause of the metabolic acidosis in DKA. Acetone is also formed and gives a fruity odor to the breath, but it does not contribute to the acidosis.

The increasing levels of hyperglycemia and acidosis contribute to a vicious cycle: osmotic diuresis leads to intravascular volume depletion, which decreases renal blood flow and glomerular perfusion, limiting the body's ability to excrete glucose and worsening the hyperglycemia. Likewise, progressive dehydration and acidosis further stimulate the release of counter-regulatory hormones, which accelerates the production of glucose and ketoacids (**Fig. 92.1**). More severe dehydration then leads to poor peripheral tissue perfusion, with resultant increases in lactic acidosis. Abdominal pain and vomiting, which occur as a result of the intestinal ileus brought on by ketoacids and dehydration, then prevents patients from maintaining hydration with oral fluids. In the setting of metabolic acidosis, potassium (K), primarily an intracellular ion, is transported out of the cell into the plasma in exchange for hydrogen and is lost in the urine. Thus, virtually all patients with DKA develop a "total-body" deficiency of K, regardless of their serum K level. Phosphate, another predominantly intracellular ion, is handled similarly. Deficiency of 2,3-diphosphoglycerate, a phosphate-containing glycolytic intermediate in red blood cells that facilitates release of oxygen from hemoglobin, may also contribute to the development of lactic acidosis, complicating the ketoacidosis. As sodium (Na) and K are excreted in the urine with lactate and the ketoacids, hyperchloremia occurs. Electrolyte deficits of up to 5–10 mEq/kg Na, 3–5 mEq/kg K, and 0.5–1.5 mmol/kg phosphate (PO_4) in DKA are not uncommon.

Clinical Presentation and Differential Diagnosis

Diabetic ketoacidosis is not difficult to recognize in a child with known diabetes who is dehydrated, hyperventilating, and obtunded. In the child whose diabetes has not yet been diagnosed, however, it may be confused with gastroenteritis, pneumonia, sepsis, toxic ingestion, or a central nervous system (CNS) lesion. The diagnosis of diabetes (if not already established) is suggested by a history of polyuria, polydipsia, polyphagia,

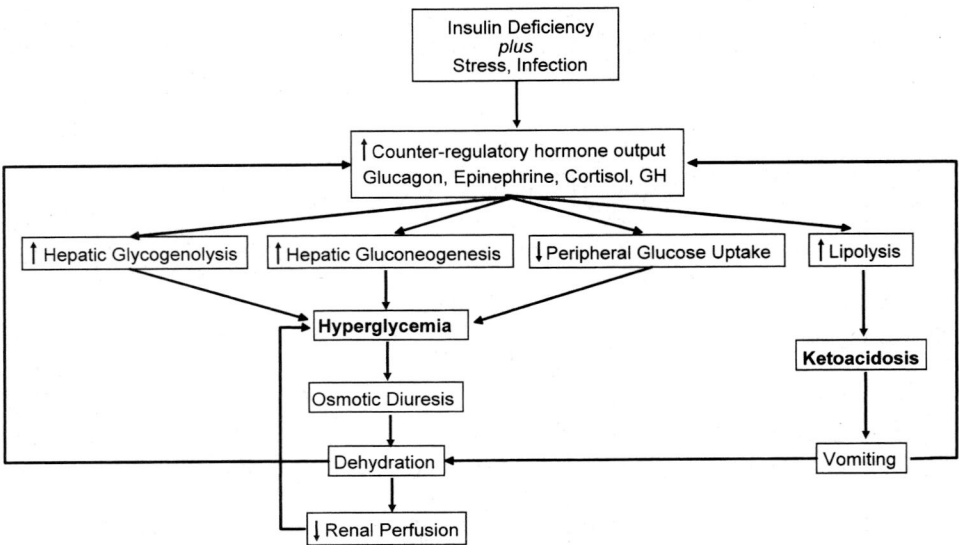

FIGURE 92.1. Pathophysiology of diabetic ketoacidosis.

nocturia, or enuresis in a previously toilet-trained child. Weakness and unexplained weight loss may also be presenting features. Abdominal pain, tenderness, and guarding is frequently present in DKA and may be of sufficient intensity to mimic an acute surgical abdomen. Other nonspecific symptoms of DKA, such as mental obtundation, vomiting, and abnormal breathing, are related to the dehydration and acidosis.

DKA in children must be differentiated from such commonly occurring childhood illnesses as urinary tract infection, gastroenteritis, more severe conditions that result in a "surgical abdomen," asthma, and pneumonia. In all of these conditions, symptoms and signs may overlap with diabetes: urinary frequency, polyuria, nocturia, abdominal pain, vomiting, changes in breathing, and dehydration. In particular, extreme hyperglycemia, due to stress hormone excess, and acidosis, due to dehydration and/or fasting, may closely mimic DKA in infants and toddlers with a febrile illness associated with poor oral intake. However, in these children the absence of polyuria, and polydipsia and the rapid clinical improvement with rehydration alone (without insulin) easily differentiate these episodes of stress hyperglycemia from true DKA, although hospital admission and serial measurement of glucose values and electrolytes are often warranted.

The physical examination findings in DKA are predominantly those of dehydration: tachycardia, delayed capillary refill, dry mucous membranes, and poor skin turgor. Severe acidosis and dehydration may impair cardiac contractility, resulting in hypotension. Respiratory compensation for the metabolic acidosis induces hyperventilation, which may appear as deep sighing respirations (Kussmaul breathing) and may initially suggest a primary respiratory illness. Acetone on the breath yielding a fruity odor may be present but is not always reliably detected. Mental status may vary from full alertness to frank coma; most patients with severe metabolic derangements are lethargic but do not have severe CNS depression and are able to protect their own airway.

The primary survey should focus initially on the adequacy of the airway, breathing, a thorough assessment of the circulatory status (heart rate, blood pressure, description of mucous membranes, capillary refill, distal pulses, and warmth of extremities), degree of dehydration (including weight if possible), and mental status. A rough estimation of degree of dehydration should be made to calculate the fluid deficit and facilitate rehydration therapy, although studies have shown such clinical approximations typically overestimate the actual degree of dehydration (38). Furthermore, the dehydration of DKA is hyperosmolar, resulting in a translocation of intracellular water to the extracellular compartment; significant total-body fluid losses can occur before evidence of changes in vital signs or physical examination. A careful examination and written documentation of the neurologic status is critical to serve as a baseline in case of deterioration in neurologic status later in therapy. General physical examination should include respiratory and abdominal examinations, as well as a search for an intercurrent illness that may have served as the precipitating factor for the episode of DKA.

Laboratory Findings

The laboratory evaluation of patients suspected to have DKA includes determination of the blood glucose, plasma or urinary ketones, serum electrolyte concentration, blood urea nitrogen (BUN), creatinine, osmolarity, baseline calcium and phosphorus, and, if infection is suspected, complete blood count and blood culture. Bedside determination of the blood glucose with a glucose monitoring device and evaluation of the urine for glucose and ketones should be performed as quickly as possible, and treatment should be initiated without waiting for the results of the laboratory assessment to become available. A baseline blood gas measurement should also be made to determine the pH and Pco_2. While venous blood gas measurements may suffice in most episodes of DKA, an arterial blood gas measurement should be considered in patients who are suspected to have incomplete respiratory compensation and/or those expected to require bicarbonate therapy (see later discussion).

The initial blood glucose level is characteristically but not invariably elevated. Hyperglycemia beyond the renal threshold for glucose filtration indicates reduced glomerular filtration. Although the definition of DKA presupposes hyperglycemia, ketoacidosis with normal or even low glucose levels may occur in patients with known diabetes who have taken insulin recently. Poor oral intake and/or vomiting may also present with near-normal glucose concentrations.

Measurement of serum electrolytes in DKA reveals a low bicarbonate level and increased anion-gap metabolic acidosis, primarily due to the unmeasured ketoacids, including β-hydroxybutyrate and acetoacetate, as well as lactate in situations of severe tissue hypoxia. Most urine dipsticks that utilize a nitroprusside reaction to measure ketones detect only acetoacetate. In normal individuals, the ratio of β-hydroxybutyrate to acetoacetate is ~1:1; in DKA, however, this ratio may increase to 10:1 or more. Therefore, while useful to diagnose ketosis, these strips are not helpful in gauging the severity of DKA or response to treatment. End-tidal CO_2 measurements, or more recently, newer home glucose meters with the ability to measure blood β-hydroxybutyrate concentrations, have been shown to be accurate and may be beneficial in guiding therapy in DKA (18,56).

Serum electrolyte concentrations are almost always abnormal in DKA and may not accurately reflect total body electrolyte disturbances. Due to the osmotic flux of water from the intracellular space to the extracellular space in the presence of hyperglycemia, the serum Na will be reduced. The actual Na may be determined by adding 1.6 mEq/L for each 100 mg/dL rise in glucose concentration greater than 100 mg/dL (35). Furthermore, extreme hypertriglyceridemia may cause the serum Na concentration to be spuriously lowered (pseudohyponatremia) (34). A normal or elevated Na level in the setting of severe DKA suggests extreme free water losses. The degree of elevation of the BUN and creatinine, as well as the hematocrit, may also indicate the extent of dehydration (and the possibility of renal damage).

The initial serum K may be low, normal, or high, depending on the degree of acidosis and the quantitative urinary losses. K moves from the intracellular to extracellular and intravascular compartments in exchange for hydrogen ion in the setting of metabolic acidosis, typically leading to elevated serum K levels. However, total-body K stores are almost always depleted from excessive urinary losses, and normal or low K levels at presentation may be associated with severe hypokalemia once treatment for DKA is initiated. Phosphate, like K, is depleted in the setting of DKA, and serum phosphate levels may not accurately reflect total body stores. Serum phosphate level may also decrease during therapy.

Clinical Management

The acute management of DKA is directed at correction of the dehydration, electrolyte deficits, hyperglycemia, and acidosis. Initial fluid therapy is aimed at rapid stabilization of the circulation to correct impending shock, but as in other forms of hypertonic dehydration, too rapid fluid administration should be avoided. Fluid replacement in excess of 4 L/m²/24 hrs has been associated with the development of potentially fatal cerebral edema in DKA (12). For this reason, an initial fluid bolus is usually advised to expand the vascular compartment and improve peripheral circulation, but once the patient has been stabilized, subsequent rehydration is accomplished with caution. Typically, the fluid defect should be corrected gradually, over 36–48 hrs. Serial calculations of actual (as opposed to measured) serum Na concentrations are recommended, as Na levels that fail to rise with treatment may signify excessive free

water accumulation and an increased risk of cerebral edema (22,28). Rehydration fluids should contain at least 115–135 mEq/L sodium chloride (NaCl) to ensure a gradual decline in serum osmolarity and prevent excessive free water accumulation (30). Generally, fluid replacement with 0.9% normal saline is provided for at least the first 6 hrs; the development of hyperchloremic metabolic acidosis with continued use of large volumes of normal saline may require a switch to 0.45% saline.

Early K replacement is also important to correct the K depletion; with the initiation of insulin therapy and correction of acidosis, serum K levels may drop precipitously as K shifts back from the extracellular to the intracellular compartment. K should be administered only after adequate renal function is determined. Electrocardiographic monitoring facilitates early recognition of either hyperkalemia (peaked T waves) or hypokalemia (flat or inverted T waves) and the development of potentially dangerous cardiac dysrhythmias. K is usually given at a dose of 30–40 mEq/L of fluid, either as potassium chloride (KCl) or in combination with potassium phosphate, which has the additional advantage of replacing the phosphate deficit. It can also be repleted as potassium acetate, which may theoretically provide buffering equivalents for the metabolic acidosis; however, the relative risks and benefits of these infusion alternatives in the treatment of DKA in children have not been rigorously studied (13). It should be noted that while hypophosphatemia in DKA may predispose to rhabdomyolysis and hemolysis and while low 2,3-diphosphoglycerate levels in DKA may impair tissue delivery of oxygen, complications of hypophosphatemia in DKA are rare, and phosphate replacement may precipitate acute hypocalcemia. Serum calcium should be monitored if phosphate is given.

Insulin therapy should be initiated immediately after the patient has been stabilized with an initial fluid bolus, at a dose of 0.1 U/kg/hr. As with fluid replacement, the aim of therapy is gradual correction: reduction of the blood glucose by 50–100 mg/dL/hr. However, the serum glucose concentration often falls significantly with initial rehydration alone due to increased glomerular filtration from improved renal perfusion. Because continuous insulin infusion often results in lowering of the blood glucose concentration before the decrease in ketoacidosis, it is important to add dextrose to the rehydration fluids, not to decrease the rate of insulin infusion, but to prevent hypoglycemia. Dextrose should be added to the IV solution when the serum glucose level falls below 300 mg/dL and should then be titrated to provide a continued gradual decline in blood glucose to target levels; this may be easily accomplished with the simultaneous use of two IV solutions that differ only in the dextrose concentration (10% and 0%); independent manipulation of each infusion allows the dextrose infusion to be varied quickly and efficiently (the so-called "two-bag" system) (27).

Bicarbonate, once considered routine therapy in severe DKA, is no longer thought to be beneficial and is no longer recommended in the treatment of uncomplicated DKA. Frequently, dramatic clinical improvement results simply from initial expansion of extracellular fluid volume, reestablishment of adequate peripheral perfusion, and prompt insulin administration. An elevation in blood pH following bicarbonate administration may lead to a paradoxical worsening of CNS acidosis because carbon dioxide (but not bicarbonate) diffuses across the blood-brain barrier. Bicarbonate administration may also be associated with hypokalemia, Na overload, late alkalosis, and theoretically, impaired tissue perfusion due to leftward shift of the oxyhemoglobin dissociation curve. Finally, bicarbonate has been associated, in multivariate analysis, with a higher risk of development of cerebral edema (22). Bicarbonate may still be considered in the setting of severe acidosis with impaired cardiac contractility and vasomotor tone, given in a slow infusion of 1–2 mmol/kg over 1–2 hrs.

Successful management of DKA requires meticulous attention to clinical and laboratory changes. Most children with DKA should be treated in a PICU. Clinical monitoring is essential: vital signs, perfusion, input/output balance, and neurologic status should be documented at least hourly. Cardiac monitoring is recommended due to the risk of dysrhythmia. Laboratory monitoring should include venous blood sugar concentrations hourly and electrolytes and venous pH every 2–4 hrs until normal. BUN and creatinine levels should be followed until they are normal, and calcium should be monitored, particularly if K is given with phosphate. Lack of improvement in clinical and biochemical parameters with time suggests an occult infection or inadequate insulin or fluid replacement. Several clinical consensus documents among leading pediatric endocrinologists on the treatment of DKA in children have been published and are recommended (13,14,73).

Outcomes

DKA is the most frequent diabetes-related cause of death in children, with a mortality rate of ~0.15%–0.3% across many centers and geographic regions (14). With appropriate treatment, complications of DKA are uncommon. However, the most common complication of DKA, acute cerebral edema, is also the most serious, and accounts for 75%–87% of the mortality in DKA. Cerebral edema occurs in ~0.5%–1% of episodes of pediatric DKA and carries a mortality rate of over 20% and a rate of permanent neurologic disability of over 25% (21). Cerebral edema is more likely to occur in patients at the time of first diagnosis of diabetes, younger children, and those presenting with the most severe degree of dehydration and metabolic derangement. It typically develops within the first 24 hrs of treatment of DKA; symptoms and signs include headache, confusion, slurred speech, bradycardia, hypertension, and other signs of increased intracranial pressure.

Although a number of causes of acute cerebral edema have been suggested from uncontrolled, retrospective studies, the etiology in many cases is not known. A common proposed mechanism involves a rapid decline in serum osmolality with treatment of DKA. During the hyperosmolar state of DKA, the brain produces "idiogenic osmoles" as a compensatory measure to increase intracellular osmotic pressure and prevent cerebral dehydration. If these idiogenic osmoles dissipate from the brain parenchyma at a slower rate than the plasma osmolality is being reduced by the treatment for DKA, the osmotic pressure gradient will favor fluid reaccumulation in the brain, leading to cellular swelling and increased intracranial pressure. This theory is supported by animal and human studies that document increased intracranial pressure during treatment for DKA (29,31). To that end, previous recommendations for treatment advised limiting the rate of fluid administration of rehydration fluids to <4 L/m²/day (12) and avoiding hypotonic rehydration fluids (30).

However, using multivariate statistics, no association was found between the rate of fluid administration, tonicity of fluids, or rate of fall of glucose and the risk for development of cerebral edema (22). Furthermore, subclinical brain swelling (39) and more serious clinical manifestations of cerebral edema (7,24) have been reported at presentation even before initiation of treatment for DKA. Other mechanisms for fluid accumulation have been proposed, including swelling due to cerebral hypoperfusion and hypoxia, activation of ion transporters in the brain, and direct effects of ketoacidosis and/or cytokines on endothelial function (23). Demographic factors associated with greater risk of cerebral edema included younger age, new onset, and longer duration of symptoms. Laboratory factors associated with greater risk included lower PCO_2, more severe acidosis, increased BUN, use of bicarbonate, greater volumes of rehydration fluids, and failure of serum Na to rise with treatment (22). However, a subsequent population-based, case-controlled study of cerebral edema complicating DKA found that early administration of insulin and high volumes of fluid, not bicarbonate therapy, were important predictors of cerebral edema (15). Therefore, until the precise mechanisms that underlie the development and progression of cerebral edema are elucidated, it appears prudent to avoid hypotonic fluids, correct dehydration evenly over 48 hrs, and monitor clinical and laboratory parameters closely, particularly as failure of Na levels to rise with treatment was associated in the multivariate analysis with an increased risk of cerebral edema.

Treatment of cerebral edema is aimed at lowering intracranial pressure: prompt administration of IV mannitol (0.25–1 g/kg), an osmotic diuretic, may be beneficial if given early in the course of cerebral edema. Tracheal intubation to mechanically hyperventilate and surgical decompression with ventriculostomy are less successful at preventing mortality or severe disability. Intracranial imaging to exclude other pathologies, such as cerebral infarction or thrombosis, should be obtained but not at the expense of timely therapeutic interventions.

Other less common complications of DKA include thrombosis, a particular concern in children who require a central venous catheter for access; cardiac arrhythmias, usually related to electrolyte disturbances; pulmonary edema; renal failure; pancreatitis; rhabdomyolysis; and infection, such as aspiration pneumonia, sepsis, and mucormycosis. Frequent iatrogenic complications include hypoglycemia and hypokalemia, which are rarely problematic if detected and treated promptly.

Conclusions and Future Directions—Diabetic Ketoacidosis

One of the most important areas for further investigation in the management of DKA is in improving prevention strategies: all episodes of DKA are theoretically preventable. Many unanswered questions remain in the management of DKA; future research endeavors should address the basic pathophysiologic mechanisms of cerebral edema so that treatment algorithms may be optimized to reduce or eliminate this main complication of DKA. Differentiation of hyperosmolar coma from DKA and management of DKA in children with type 2 diabetes are areas that require more attention, as increasing numbers of pediatric patients with type 2 diabetes are being recognized. Lastly, the use of continuous glucose-monitoring systems that track glucose values and trends in real time to facilitate clinical management of DKA have yet to be fully explored.

HYPERGLYCEMIA HYPEROSMOLAR SYNDROME

The hyperglycemic hyperosmolar syndrome (HHS) is a potentially lethal disorder of decompensated glucose homeostasis. Patients with this syndrome, known formerly as HONK (hyperosmolar, nonketotic crisis) or HHNS (hyperglycemic, hyperosmolar nonketotic syndrome), suffer from the dangerous consequences of marked hyperglycemia and hyperosmolarity. Once thought limited to the adult population, an increasing incidence in younger patients is now of concern.

Epidemiology

Cases of extreme hyperglycemia without significant ketosis have been described in adults for more than 100 years (2). Currently, the adult literature cites the rate of HHS as 17.5 per 100,000, with a greater distribution in the elderly and disabled (9). The syndrome affects known diabetics (particularly type 2) but may also herald its onset. In addition, precipitating factors associated with HHS include infections, coexisting medical problems (e.g., renal failure, pancreatitis), medications (notably, diuretics, steroids, anticonvulsants, and psychotropic drugs), and total parenteral nutrition, as well as other conditions that lead to dehydration, such as burns and heat stroke (9).

The syndrome of hyperglycemic hyperosmolarity was first described in children in 1951, followed by sporadic case reports that involved patients from infancy through adolescence over the succeeding decades (49). Often depicted as idiopathic, various triggers akin to those in adults have also been ascribed to the syndrome. In addition, concerns about an underlying incipient diabetes mellitus ("pseudodiabetes of infancy") or impaired osmoregulatory function have been considered (58). Unfortunately, the lack of data has precluded any reasonable attempt at estimating the syndrome's prevalence. Nonetheless, a review of the English language literature reveals an increasing number of reported cases (44 in the past 10 years), compared to the handful that appeared in the preceding decade (5,20,33,51). These reports noted a high degree of morbidity and mortality (i.e., 15 deaths in 44 cases) and, in contrast to the various etiologies described in the past, pointed to a trend of new-onset type 2 diabetes presenting as HHS. In fact, 75% of the recently described patients had either a confirmed or presumptive diagnosis of type 2 diabetes or a ketotic variant. The epidemic of pediatric obesity and its strong association with altered glucose metabolism, insulin resistance, and ultimately, type 2 diabetes creates the potential for an explosion in the number of cases of HHS (4,36). This risk is magnified in certain ethnic groups. Numerous studies have shown that African Americans and Latinos, representing 75% of the above cohort, are at greater risk of developing type 2 diabetes compared with whites (36,44).

Pathophysiology

HHS and DKA are often depicted as opposite extremes along the spectrum of decompensated diabetes. In HHS, insulin levels may be sufficient to suppress the full-blown lipolysis and ketogenesis seen in DKA, but they are inadequate to promote normal anabolic function and inhibit the creation of glucose through gluconeogenesis and glycogenolysis. Thus, HHS can be seen as the combustion of a smoldering relative insulin deficiency that may be ignited by intercurrent illness or medication. The hyperbolic shape of the insulin sensitivity curve may help to explain the seemingly acute decompensation. Regardless of the proximal cause, once initiated, the cells' privation of glucose triggers a counter-regulatory surge, further raising glucose levels both by enhanced hepatic glucose generation and worsening insulin resistance. Hyperglycemia itself triggers a heightened inflammatory state, which, in turn, exacerbates glucose dysregulation (66). This maladaptive milieu can precipitate a massive osmotic diuresis and, ultimately, dehydration. The resultant volume contraction reduces the glomerular filtration rate, further elevating glucose levels, and may lead to the monumental hyperosmolarity of the syndrome. In short, the disorder "begins" with elevated blood glucose and "progresses with varying degrees of speed toward the development of profound dehydration" (2).

The risks related to the hyperglycemic hyperosmolar state extend beyond the effects of volume contraction and circulatory compromise. The long-term ill effects of hyperglycemia on the microcirculation and macrocirculation have been well described, but evidence shows an association between acute hyperglycemia itself and morbidity and mortality in critically ill patients (59,68). Through a variety of mechanisms, hyperglycemia can cause vascular injury and thrombus formation; it also disrupts the phagocytic and oxidative burst functions of the innate immune system (6,16,23,64,66). Finally, hyperglycemia has been shown to disrupt the blood-brain barrier and metabolism of the CNS and worsen the effects of ischemia on brain tissue (59).

Although it may be fitting to place HHS and DKA on a continuum of perturbed glucose homeostasis, from a critical care perspective, important distinctions exist. For example, in HHS, ketoacidemia is generally neither the underlying nor most extreme pathophysiologic disturbance. Second, due to the duration of symptoms and the extreme hyperosmolarity of patients with HHS, a much greater degree of volume depletion may be present. Thus, it is estimated that DKA patients are 10% dehydrated, whereas patients with HHS are felt to be 15%–20% volume depleted (45). In fact, an early study estimated patients with HHS and coma to be 24% dehydrated (2). Greater electrolyte loss may also be present in HHS as compared with DKA (37). Finally, the scant, existing data suggest that HHS may pose a more serious threat to pediatric patients than does DKA.

Clinical Presentation and Diagnosis

One case series suggests that a failure to consider the diagnosis of HHS greatly contributes to morbidity and mortality (42). Patients with HHS commonly present with a history of weight loss, complaints of polydipsia/polyuria of variable duration, and gastrointestinal distress. On exam, patients are lethargic and often present with neurologic impairments that range from slightly altered sensoria, to focal neurologic deficits, to frank coma. These patients are dehydrated and in varying—and often tenuous—states of cardiovascular compensation. The duration of these symptoms and the ability of the patient to compensate for the prodigious osmotic diuresis dictate how they ultimately present. However, the diagnosis and treatment of HHS can be clouded by a number of factors. First, the onset of symptoms is likely insidious, with an indolent prelude to decompensation and a correspondingly vague history. An altered sensorium may further shroud the history (and a workup for mental status changes may not include HHS). Second, the frequent absence of the symptomologic and objective hallmarks of ketoacidemia may obscure the diagnosis; the abdominal discomfort and nausea and vomiting have been reported to be less severe, and acetone breath and Kussmaul breathing pattern are not present. Lastly, assessing the volume status of an obese patient can be difficult, which may obscure both the correct diagnosis, and gravity of illness.

Lab findings should confirm the presence of a possibly extreme hyperosmolarity and hyperglycemia. The classic diagnostic criteria for HHS complement those for DKA, namely, a glucose of >600 mg/dL, $HCO_3 \geq 15$ mEq/L, serum osmolarity of >320 mOsm/L, and a pH ≥ 7.3 without evidence of significant ketosis (37). However, clinical experience shows that the level of acidemia is influenced by the severity of shock and starvation with concomitant varying degrees of lactic acidosis and moderate ketonuria described in reports over the years (1,2,5,37,58). In fact, overlap or "mixed" syndromes are not uncommon (65,70). Lab evidence of end-organ hypoperfusion or injury, particularly acute renal failure, is typically found, as are rhabdomyolysis and pancreatitis. Finally, patients with this disorder may have significant electrolyte imbalance, although depending on the degree of acidemia, serum K may be elevated (45).

Treatment

Experience in treating pediatric HHS is limited, and existing recommendations are adapted largely from the treatment of either children with DKA or adults with HHS. Nonetheless, given the potential for life-threatening complications, HHS must be viewed as a matter of medical urgency, if not emergency. As such, it is prudent for patients with HHS to be monitored in an ICU until they are stabilized—even in the absence of significant acidemia. Initial management, as dictated by the degree of hemodynamic compromise and complications on presentation, should emphasize the essentials of ICU care. Accordingly, the early goals of treatment should target airway protection and mechanical ventilation based on Glasgow Coma Scale and compensatory response and the restoration of hemodynamic stability and tissue perfusion. The placement of appropriate cardiovascular monitoring (including arterial and central venous pressure monitoring as indicated) may be required. Electrolytes should be rigorously repleted based on frequent sampling and conservative correction of hyperglycemia. Finally, vigilant monitoring for neurologic or other complications, detection and treatment of precipitat-

ing causes, and appropriate prophylactic measures should be undertaken.

Volume resuscitation is the mainstay of therapy for HHS (42,45,63). The American Diabetes Association guidelines for the management of DKA and HHS in patients <20 years old suggest boluses of normal saline at 10–20 mL/kg (repeating as necessary to reverse shock), with replacement of the remaining volume deficit over 48 hrs (37). The adult critical care literature advocates a more aggressive degree of volume resuscitation (2–3 liters of normal saline over the first 2 hrs) with replacement of 50% of the deficits in the first 12 hrs (45). Similar recommendations appear in the pediatric and adult emergency medicine literature (26,52). As poor outcomes have been associated with failure to recognize and aggressively treat, a timely and appropriate response is essential (45,63). In areas of ambiguity, central venous monitoring may assure objective and adequate volume repletion. Normal saline is generally recommended for the resuscitative phase of treatment, with half-normal saline employed later to complete rehydration.

Although insulin may have salutary, anti-inflammatory benefits, in the absence of significant ketoacidemia, it is felt by many to play a secondary role in the initial management of HHS (26,63). In fact, hyperglycemia can often be corrected by reestablishing renal perfusion and glomerular filtration rate and thereby ensuring a more gradual correction of hyperosmolarity without rapid fluid and electrolyte shifts (26,52,72). The American Diabetes Association currently recommends an insulin infusion at 0.1 Units/kg/hr without initial bolus, then titrating and transitioning as clinically indicated (37).

Theoretically, the absence of a large ketotic diuresis should lessen the cationic urinary loss; nevertheless, the duration of illness may lead to total-body depletion. Estimated electrolyte deficit ranges in adults with HHS are 3–7 mmol/kg for phosphate, 4–6 mEq/kg for K, and 5–13 mEq/kg for Na (37). Electrolytes should be monitored carefully and replaced as indicated, with particular attention to K shifts with the initiation of insulin therapy.

Although current research suggests that hyperglycemia predisposes to thrombogenesis and that HHS in particular predisposes to deep vein thromboses in patients with central venous catheters, the degree of risk of thromboembolism has not been formally assessed. Therefore, current evidence does not support the use of anticoagulation in HHS. Nonetheless, appropriate prophylaxis for deep vein thromboses should be employed.

Outcomes

In the adult population, complications and fatalities associated with HHS are most often due to comorbid conditions (45). The recent pediatric literature describes deaths in HHS caused by cardiac arrest and refractory dysrhythmias, pulmonary thromboemboli, circulatory collapse and refractory shock, and multisystem organ failure. Morbidity includes acute renal failure, rhabdomyolysis, coma, and significant electrolyte disturbances. Neurologic findings are common in HHS, and earlier case series have attributed demise to "diabetic coma" and cerebral edema (1,58). Yet, a parallel to the more isolated and devastating intracerebral events (cerebral edema) of DKA has not been established. In the more recent cases, positive autopsy or CT findings of cerebral edema are rare and consistently described in the context of multisystem organ failure or sudden cardiac death (5,33,51).

Historically, the adult mortality rate has been cited to be between 15%–60%, with newer estimates suggesting a rate closer to 15% (37). In children, as the prevalence of the disorder is unknown, only crude approximations of mortality are possible. One case series cited a mortality rate of 14%, while as discussed previously, an estimate based on the past 10 years of case reports has more than double that number (20).

Conclusions and Future Directions—Hyperglycemia Hyperosmolar Syndrome

Aside from epidemiologic gaps in our knowledge, a great deal more remains to be explained regarding HHS, including clarification of the underlying pathophysiology, with attention to the role of obesity and its relationship with inflammatory mediators; the role of hyperglycemia-induced inflammation in the complications of HHS; a clear understanding of those patients most at risk for HHS, as well as a method for determining the degree of that risk; and finally and perhaps most importantly, data that evaluate the optimal treatment for this syndrome.

HYPERGLYCEMIA IN CRITICALLY ILL CHILDREN

Hyperglycemia in the sick, nondiabetic patient was first described in the 19th century by Claude Bernard (66). "Stress diabetes," "traumatic diabetes," or "diabetes of injury," as it was previously called, was thought of as an adaptive response, and the rise in glucose was thought to represent the body's attempt to provide an adequate energy source to combat the stress. Previously, hyperglycemia was considered simply a marker of illness severity that required no significant intervention unless glucosuria occurred. However, with the publication of the landmark study by Van den Berghe et al. in 2001 (69), compelling data suggest that high glucose levels are deleterious, and strict glycemic control is warranted to improve outcome in critically ill patients.

Epidemiology of Hyperglycemia

The prevalence of hyperglycemia among critically ill, nondiabetic children ranges from 16.7% to 75.0% (17,59), a rate not significantly different from the 3%–71% cited for adults (50). The wide range reflects the lack of standard diagnostic criteria for this selected population of patients. According to the World Health Organization and the American Diabetes Association, diabetic hyperglycemia is defined as a fasting blood glucose level of ≥110 mg/dL. Adult studies of hyperglycemia in critically ill patients utilize this threshold because of a demonstrated decrease in morbidity and mortality in this population in those whose serum glucose is controlled to a level ≤110 mg/dL (69). In contrast, pediatric intensivists do not have a consensus as to the therapeutic threshold for treating hyperglycemia. Thresh-

old values used for the initiation of insulin therapy in children range from 110 mg/dL to >200 mg/dL.

Despite the lack of uniformity in defining hyperglycemia, elevated glucose levels have consistently been associated with increased morbidity and mortality in children. Among all admissions to a general PICU, serum glucose >150 mg/dL was associated with at least a 2.5-fold increase in mortality (17). The association holds true for different subsets of critically ill children, including patients who are mechanically ventilated, in septic shock, with massive burns, severe traumatic brain injury, and near drowning. In these groups of patients, nonsurvivors consistently have higher glucose levels compared to survivors (25,59). In addition to an increase in mortality, hyperglycemic patients also have prolonged ICU stays, poorer neurodevelopmental outcomes, and higher infection rates (25). The intensity, timing, and duration of hyperglycemia substantially affects outcome (59).

In adults, high blood glucose concentration is similarly associated with elevated morbidity and mortality. Tight control of glucose between 80 and 110 mg/dL resulted in a reduced risk of mortality by as much as 34% in mechanically ventilated adults admitted to a surgical ICU (69). The intervention, likewise, significantly lowered the rate of bloodstream infection, acute renal failure requiring dialysis or hemofiltration, median number of red cell transfusions, and critical illness polyneuropathy in this selected group of patients. Among adult patients in a medical ICU, tight glycemic control prevented the development of kidney injury, accelerated weaning from mechanical ventilation, and accelerated discharge from the ICU and the hospital (67).

Normal Glucose Homeostasis

Maintenance of normoglycemia, a complex process that involves the removal and addition of glucose to the bloodstream, is tightly regulated by neurohormonal and autoregulatory mechanisms. An excellent review of normal glucose homeostasis can be found in the article by Mizock (50) and is summarized here.

Noninsulin-mediated uptake of glucose by the CNS accounts for 80% of glucose utilization during basal conditions. Skeletal muscles remove the remaining 20%, half of which is insulin-mediated. After a meal, glucose is cleared in nearly equal amounts by the muscle, fat, hepatosplanchnic bed, and noninsulin-requiring tissues, including the CNS. As much as 40% of ingested glucose can be extracted by the liver for conversion to glycogen.

Cellular glucose transport is facilitated by the glut proteins (41,50,66). Five isoforms have been identified, of which glut1, glut2, and glut4 are thought to play major roles in glucose metabolism. Found in nearly all cells, glut1 is most abundant and is important in basal glucose uptake. Glut2, on the other hand, is found mainly in hepatocytes, where it transports glucose into and out of the hepatocytes. Glut4 facilitates glucose absorption in insulin-responsive cells in the presence of the hormone (62).

While nearly all cells are involved in glucose uptake, glucose production occurs only in the liver and the kidneys (47,50). Two processes contribute to glucose formation: breakdown of glycogen in the liver and production of new glucose molecules from both liver and kidneys. Glycogenolysis provides most of the glucose after an overnight fast. However, with prolonged starvation, glycogen stores become depleted and other sources of energy are utilized.

The balance of uptake and production of glucose is the result of an interaction between a number of hormonal, neural, and hepatic autoregulatory mechanisms (50). Insulin, glucagon, catecholamines, cortisol, and growth hormone are the major hormones involved in glucose metabolism (41,47,50). Insulin decreases blood glucose levels by enhancing glucose uptake and glycogenesis and conversely inhibiting gluconeogenesis. In contrast, the other hormones, which are also known as *counter-regulatory hormones*, have the opposite effect of elevating blood glucose by inhibiting glucose uptake and enhancing glycogenolysis and gluconeogenesis.

Different sites within the brain affect glucose control (50). These centers, which include various nuclei in the brainstem and the hypothalamus, affect sympathetic and parasympathetic outflow to the liver, pancreas, and splanchnic circulation to adjust the amount of insulin secreted and the amount of glycogen cleaved into glucose. Peripherally, glucose sensors found in the portal vein and the intestines relay glycemic levels to the brainstem and the hypothalamus. Effectors of these pathways include the pancreas and the adrenal glands, which respond by changing insulin and catecholamine secretion.

The liver also has an intrinsic autoregulatory ability to respond to changing glucose levels (50). The major step in this process is the interconversion of glucose to glucose-6-phosphate, and vice versa, which is mediated by glucokinase and glucose-6-phosphatase. Autoregulation enables the liver to adjust glucose production based on glucose levels and availability of the requisite glucose precursors.

Glucose Control during Critical Illness

Hyperglycemia results from the body's systemic response to stress. During stress, the hypothalamic-pituitary-adrenal axis and sympathetic system are activated, leading to increased cortisol and catecholamine secretion (**Fig. 92.1**). Other counter-regulatory hormones and cytokines are secreted as well. The combination of these factors leads to insulin resistance and elevated blood glucose.

Most studies indicate that stress hyperglycemia is a result of glucose overproduction rather than impairment of glucose uptake (47,50,62). The orchestrated rise in the counter-regulatory hormones leads to enhanced hepatic gluconeogenesis and glycogenolysis (**Table 92.1**), which in this abnormal setting, are not inhibited by increased blood glucose levels or by increased insulin secretion. Insulin resistance in the liver ensues. Among the stress hormones, catecholamines and glucagon are responsible for an initial transient rise in glucose. Epinephrine and norepinephrine promote gluconeogenesis via a cAMP-dependent mechanism. Glucagon, also working through a cAMP-mediated mechanism, increases the activity of hepatic enzymes involved in gluconeogenesis and inhibits the enzymes of glycogenesis. Sustaining hyperglycemia requires the action of cortisol and growth hormone on mRNA transcription. Cytokines such as tumor necrosis factor (TNF)-α, IL-1, and IL-6 worsen hyperglycemia by promoting the secretion of counter-regulatory hormones both centrally and peripherally.

In addition to the effect of increased counter-regulatory hormones on circulating glucose levels, other gluconeogenic precursors, including lactate, alanine, glycerol, and glutamine, are produced during stress (47,50). Major sources of lactate are the lungs (in acute lung injury), intestines, and wounds—a

TABLE 92.1

MAJOR ACTIONS OF COUNTER-REGULATORY HORMONES AND CYTOKINES IN MEDIATING STRESS HYPERGLYCEMIA

Hormone	Mechanism
Glucagon	Increased gluconeogenesis Increased hepatic glycogenolysis
Epinephrine	Skeletal muscle insulin resistance by altering postreceptor signaling Increased gluconeogenesis Increased skeletal muscle and hepatic glycogenolysis Increased lipolysis, increased free fatty acids Direct suppression of insulin secretion
Norepinephrine	Increased lipolysis Increased gluconeogenesis, but hyperglycemia not marked except at high concentrations
Glucocorticoids	Skeletal muscle insulin resistance Increased lipolysis Gluconeogenesis increased through provision of substrate
Growth hormone	Skeletal muscle insulin resistance Increased lipolysis Increased gluconeogenesis
Tumor necrosis factor	Skeletal muscle insulin resistance, altered post-receptor signaling Hepatic insulin resistance

Reprinted from Critical Care Clinics, Vol 17(1), McCowen KC, Malhotra A, Bistrian BR, Stress-induced hyperglycemia. *Crit Care Clin* 2001;107–24.

reflection of increased rates of glycolysis and possible down-regulation of pyruvate dehydrogenase. The liver avidly extracts lactate from the circulation and converts it to glucose via the Cori cycle. The principal source of alanine is de novo synthesis from pyruvate in skeletal muscle rather than muscle breakdown, whereas glycerol is a by-product of adipocyte lipolysis. Fat mobilization significantly increases during stress. Lastly, glutamine provides the primary source of carbon for glucose production in the kidneys.

Glucose uptake during stress is significantly higher than during basal conditions (50,66). Cytokines and hypoxia are some of the factors shown to upregulate glut1 expression and its translocation to the membrane. However, the majority of glucose removal occurs in noninsulin-dependent tissues such as the CNS and red blood cells as a result of the insulin resistance that develops.

Counter-regulatory hormones and cytokines are responsible for the impaired glucose uptake in insulin-dependent tissues (62) (**Table 92.1**). Catecholamines inhibit glucose utilization by increasing glucose-6-phosphate from glycogen in the skeletal muscles. In turn, the phosphorylated form of glucose negatively inhibits hexokinase, the rate-limiting step in glucose catabolism, by decreasing its uptake from the blood. Epinephrine has also been shown to blunt the insulin-induced autophosphorylation of glut4, whereas glucocorticoids and growth hormone attenuate glucose uptake through their effects on glut4 processing. Glucocorticoids prevent the translocation of the protein through the plasma membrane, while growth hormone interferes with phosphorylation of the transporter. The latter also inhibits the insulin-signaling cascade. Cytokines are thought to confer peripheral insulin resistance through their interference with the tyrosine phosphorylation and mRNA expression of glut4 (64).

In addition to the direct effects on the glut4 protein, epinephrine, cortisol, growth hormone, and TNF-α stimulate lipase activity in the adipocytes, leading to increased levels of free fatty acids (47,64). Strong evidence suggests that free fatty acids themselves augment insulin resistance through inhibition of the insulin-signaling pathway.

A number of other factors also contribute to hyperglycemia among critically ill patients (47,54). Obesity, even in the absence of diabetes, is associated with insulin resistance. Hypothermia and hypoxemia can lead to insulin deficiency, while uremia and cirrhosis can increase insulin resistance. Glucocorticoid therapy and exogenous catecholamines produce hyperglycemia through a mechanism similar to their endogenous counterparts. Other underappreciated sources of hyperglycemia in the ICU are hypercaloric nutrition, infusion of dextrose-diluted medications, and the use of high glucose-containing dialysis solutions.

Pathologic Effects of Hyperglycemia

The detrimental effects of hyperglycemia were previously thought to be limited to osmotic diuresis (leading to dehydration and electrolyte imbalance) and hyperosmolar nonketotic coma (50). However, recent studies show that the effects of elevated glucose levels, even of short duration, are more profound (66). Broadly, the adverse effects of hyperglycemia can be attributed to endothelial dysfunction (47,54,66) and impaired immune response (47,50,62,64).

The data on the deleterious effect of hyperglycemia on the vasculature are derived mainly from adult studies (48,54). Hyperglycemic patients, both diabetic and nondiabetic, have a worse outcome after an acute cardiac or cerebral ischemic event, compared to normoglycemic patients. This finding is attributed to a number of causes, including impaired cardiac contractility, increased frequency of dysrhythmias, disruption of the blood-brain barrier, impaired endothelium-dependent vasorelaxation, and a prothrombotic state. Hyperglycemia, especially when prolonged, leads to nephropathy, neuropathy, and retinopathy.

The mechanism behind these events is unknown. However, it is speculated that they are, at least in part, due to endothelial dysfunction (66). Endothelial cells, like neurons and red blood cells, do not require insulin for glucose uptake. In the presence of hyperglycemia and upregulated glut1 transporters, the endothelium is confronted with an intracellular glucose load. Normally, when glucose enters the cell, it is diverted to the Krebs cycle to produce ATP. Production of reactive oxygen species accompanies this process, which is easily detoxified by manganese superoxide dismutase. However, with the high intracellular glucose concentration, superoxide is overproduced and interacts with nitric oxide to form peroxynitrite. The latter compound is capable of nitrating intracellular proteins, including those in the mitochondrial electron transport chain, manganese superoxide dismutase, glyceraldehyde-3-phosphate dehydrogenase, and voltage-dependent anion channels. Theoretically, nitration of these compounds would suppress electron transport chain activity, impair superoxide detoxification, shuttle glucose into toxic pathways, or induce advanced glycation end-product formation and increased apoptosis. Interestingly, inhibition of glyceraldehyde-3-phosphate dehydrogenase has been linked to vascular damage in organs and tissues of diabetic patients (66).

High glucose concentrations also alter various components of the immune response (64). Normally, in response to injury, vasoactive substances and chemotactic factors from the complement cascade, mast cells, and the kininogen-bradykinin system are released at the site of injury, resulting in increased blood flow and capillary permeability. Neutrophils and, later, macrophages migrate to the area, with resultant phagocytosis and lysis of the offending agent. During hyperglycemia, vasodilation is decreased secondary to impaired endothelial nitric oxide generation, a dysfunctional kininogen-bradykinin system, and reduced mast cell secretion. Hyperglycemia-induced expression of adhesion molecules enhances the interaction between leukocytes and endothelium, preventing the white blood cells from migrating to the area of injury. The interaction is further augmented by activation of nuclear factor-$\kappa\beta$, downregulation of the inhibitory protein I-$\kappa\beta$, and activation of protein kinase C. Concentrations of complement cascade components increase with hyperglycemia. However, complement-mediated functions such as phagocytosis and opsonization are depressed. Chemotaxis, phagocytosis, and generation of reactive oxygen species, which are all functions of neutrophils, are likewise attenuated, with elevated glucose levels impairing clearance of microorganisms.

Clinically, hyperglycemia is associated with increased risk of infection (47,48,62,64). In pediatric burn patients, for example, sustained glucose levels of 140 mg/dL resulted in a higher rate of positive blood cultures and less skin engraftment (25). In adults, nosocomial infections and sternal wound infections are higher in the hyperglycemic population. Furthermore, in the Leuven study in 2001, the 46% reduction in bacteremia significantly contributed to the decrease in mortality (67).

Management of Hyperglycemia

Historically, insulin therapy was initiated at the onset of glucosuria because of the belief that osmotic diuresis was the sole adverse effect of a high serum glucose. However, with a deeper understanding of the pathologic effects of hyperglycemia, tight control of glucose with insulin infusion has become usual care in adults.

The landmark prospective, randomized trial by Van den Berghe et al. was published in 2001 (69). In this study, 1548 mechanically ventilated adults admitted to a surgical ICU were randomized to receive either intensive insulin therapy (with a blood glucose goal of 80–110 mg/dL) or conventional treatment (with a blood glucose goal of 180–200 mg/dL). Less than 6% of the included patients had a history of diabetes mellitus. Intensive insulin therapy significantly reduced mortality in the ICU from all causes from 8.0% to 4.6%. A similar reduction in hospital mortality was noted in the treatment group (33.9% reduction from 10.9% to 7.2%). The biggest decrease in mortality was seen in patients with ICU length of stay longer than 5 days and in patients with multiple organ failure and a proven focus of infection. In terms of morbidity, bloodstream infections dropped by 46%, acute renal failure requiring dialysis or hemofiltration by 41%, median number of red cell transfusions by 50%, and critical illness neuropathy by 44%. Patients in the intensive insulin therapy arm were less likely to require prolonged mechanical ventilation and extended stay in the ICU.

The survival benefit of the Van den Berghe surgical ICU trial was corroborated by Krinsley's study, in which a total of 800 patients (18.1% diabetics) admitted to a medical-surgical ICU were treated with insulin infusion to maintain glucose levels below 140 mg/dL (40). Compared to historic controls (16.4% diabetics), the treatment group had a 29.3% reduction in hospital mortality (20.9% vs. 14.8%), a result comparable to the Leuven study of 2001. Furthermore, length of stay in the ICU was decreased by 10.8%, development of renal insufficiency dropped by 75%, and the number of patients who required red cell transfusion decreased by 18.7%.

In a follow-up to their initial study, Van den Berghe's group investigated the benefits of aggressive glucose control in a medical ICU (67). Critically ill adults predicted to remain in the ICU for at least 3 days were randomized to strict glycemic control (80–110 mg/dL) or conventional treatment (180–200 mg/dL). Analysis of the 1200 patients (16.9% with history of diabetes) included in the study demonstrated no significant difference in hospital mortality (40.0% in the conventional treatment vs. 37.3% in the intensive-treatment group). In contrast, morbidity was decreased in the intensive-treatment group. A reduction in newly acquired kidney injury, decrease in the number of days of mechanical ventilation, and decrease in both ICU and total hospital days were reported. A subset analysis of all patients who actually stayed in the unit for at least 3 days showed a significant reduction in hospital mortality by 18.1% (52.5% vs. 43.0%).

At this writing, no randomized controlled trials have been conducted to evaluate a survival benefit with strict glucose control among critically ill children. In the absence of data in pediatrics, management of hyperglycemia ranges from the conservative approach of starting insulin with glucosuria to strict glycemic control at 80–110 mg/dL with insulin infusion therapy. Until a prospective, randomized trial is performed, the benefits of tight glucose control in critically ill children remains speculative.

Conclusions and Future Directions—Hyperglycemia

Many unanswered questions remain regarding the management of hyperglycemia in children. The central question is whether a benefit is derived from strict glycemic control in critically ill children. The retrospective data in children coupled with the initial Leuven study would argue for a similar survival benefit in children. Yet, based on the results of the Van den Berghe trial on medical ICU patients (67), even the advantage of intensive insulin treatment in adults is questionable. The theoretical advantages of strictly controlling blood glucose in children must be tempered by the higher risk of hypoglycemia with insulin use. Timing of the therapy may also be important. In both the surgical and medical ICU patients of the two Van den Berghe trials, survival was higher in patients who stayed in the unit for at least 3 days. The rationale behind the improved survival is unclear. The pathologic effects of hyperglycemia have been fully discussed, but insulin per se has anti-inflammatory and metabolic effects that can decrease the risk of infection and possibly mortality (41). Multivariate logistic regression analysis of the data from the Leuven study on surgical ICU patients indicated that control of glucose, and not the insulin dose, was related to reduced mortality, bacteremia, critical illness polyneuropathy, and inflammation (68). Insulin dose, on the other hand, was associated with prevention of acute renal failure. In an attempt to answer these questions, a multicentered trial is being planned that will involve various PICUs in North America.

HYPOGLYCEMIA IN CHILDREN

Glucose serves as the body's predominant fuel, responsible for at least half of basal energy requirements and almost all of the basal energy needs of the neonate. The brain in particular utilizes glucose at a rate, per gram, that is 20 times that of the rest of the body, primarily because it cannot use free fatty acids as a fuel source. The brain, therefore, derives >99% of its energy from glucose metabolism, and in neonates, whose brain comprises a relatively greater proportion of body weight, glucose requirements are 5- to 10-fold greater than in older children and adults (8–10 mg/kg/min vs. 1–2 mg/kg/min) (3,32).

The definition of "normal" blood glucose itself is controversial. Historically, the parameters for hypoglycemia were based on statistical rather than physiologic grounds. Delayed first feeding of infants commonly resulted in hypoglycemia in the first hours after birth, which may have led physicians to accept lower thresholds of blood glucose as "normal" (60). In the absence of evidence that the infant brain is less sensitive to hypoglycemia than is the brain of an older child or adult, and given that it may indeed be more vulnerable to hypoglycemic injury, the same, if not more, rigorous therapeutic standards should be maintained for an infant as those maintained for an adult. Therefore, we agree with recommendations that consider any blood glucose <55–60 mg/dL as abnormal and deserving of further attention (61).

Pathophysiology

With rare exceptions, hypoglycemia in infants and children is a failure of fasting adaptation. An understanding of normal fasting physiology can provide a framework for diagnosing and treating the various disorders of hypoglycemia. The elements of fasting include the four alternative fuel pathways: (a) hepatic glycogenolysis, (b) hepatic gluconeogenesis, (c) adipose tissue lipolysis, and (d) hepatic fatty acid oxidation and ketogenesis. These systems are under hormonal control, primarily by insulin, which suppresses the fasting systems, and the "counter-regulatory" hormones glucagon, cortisol, epinephrine, and growth hormone, which act to stimulate them.

The first phase of normal fasting occurs 2–3 hrs after a meal; thereafter, circulating glucose that is derived from intestinal absorption of carbohydrates dissipates (**Fig. 92.2A**). Insulin secretion is suppressed (**X**), and counter-regulatory hormones increase (+), allowing glucose to be released from hepatic glycogen stores (**B**). By 12–16 hrs of fasting (and even earlier in sick or premature newborns), these glycogen stores are depleted; muscle and adipose tissue stores are then mobilized during this second phase of fasting. Amino acids derived from muscle breakdown (**C**) are the primary substrates for the production of new glucose by hepatic gluconeogenesis (**D**). Fatty acids released from lipolysis of adipose tissue (**E**) are utilized either directly as a fuel (particularly in muscle) or further oxidized in the liver, generating the energy required for the process of hepatic gluconeogenesis and the formation of ketones (**F**), an alternate fuel for the brain, which cannot utilize fatty acids as an energy source. Hepatic glycogenolysis is primarily stimulated by glucagon and epinephrine, lipolysis is stimulated by increases in epinephrine and growth hormone, and gluconeogenesis is stimulated by glucagon and cortisol.

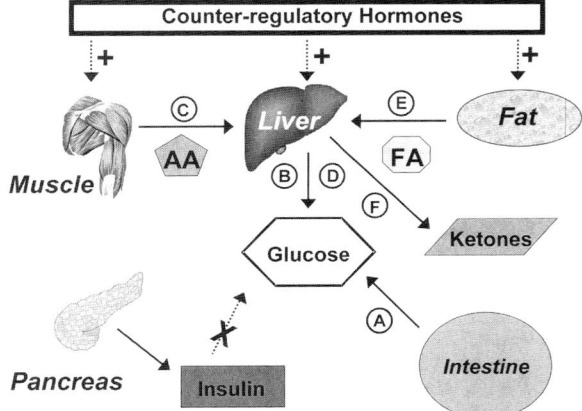

FIGURE 92.2. Pathways of fasting adaptation. See text for details. AA, amino acids; FA, fatty acids. Adapted from Louis CA, Weinzimer SA. A 12-day-old infant with hypoglycemia: Case report. *Curr Opin Pediatr* 2003;15:333–7.

Although the physiology of fasting adaptation in infants is similar to that of older children and adults, the neonate is more susceptible to hypoglycemia due to its greater metabolic demands. Hepatic glycogenolysis is sufficient to meet energy requirements for only a few hours, due to diminished glycogen stores. The production of new glucose is also limited by the relatively low body stores of protein and the developmental immaturity of several key enzymes in the gluconeogenesis and ketogenesis pathways.

Clinical Presentation

Symptoms and signs of hypoglycemia can be divided into those that arise from autonomic responses to hypoglycemia (adrenergic) and those that arise from neurologic dysfunction (neuroglycopenic). Adrenergic symptoms/signs include tremors, diaphoresis, tachycardia, hunger, weakness, and nervousness. Neuroglycopenic symptoms/signs include lethargy, confusion, unusual behavior, and with more severe decrements in blood glucose, seizures and coma. Autonomic activation usually occurs earlier and at a glucose threshold higher than would cause neuroglycopenia, although with repeated episodes of hypoglycemia, the threshold for adrenergic responses decreases, leading eventually to the development of serious neurologic symptoms with little or no warning. This "hypoglycemia unawareness" or "hypoglycemia-associated autonomic failure" is more frequently encountered in patients with insulin-treated diabetes, and its mechanism is unknown (8).

Both autonomic and neuroglycopenic symptoms and signs of hypoglycemia are less obvious, or even absent, in infants and young children with hypoglycemia. Alternative manifestations of hypoglycemia in infants include apnea, pallor, cyanosis, feeding difficulties, tachypnea, respiratory distress, hypothermia, or sepsis-like state. Thus, a high index of suspicion must be maintained. Other clinical features are specific to the etiology of hypoglycemia and are discussed individually here.

Diagnosis and Classification of Hypoglycemic Disorders

A normal child should not become hypoglycemic until all available fuel sources are depleted and counter-regulatory hormone stimulation is maximized, at which time (a) glycogen stores will be depleted and no glycemic response to glucagon will occur; (b) lactate will be low, reflecting exhaustion of gluconeogenic stores; (c) free fatty acids and ketones will be elevated; and (d) insulin will be undetectable in the serum. Therefore, in the child with a disorder of hypoglycemia, in whom at least one control system is defective, analysis of the integrity of all of the control systems at the time of hypoglycemia is required to determine the etiology of the disorder, the so-called "critical sample." The critical sample, which should be obtained prior to treating the hypoglycemia, consists of the primary fuel glucose, alternate fuels (lactate, ketones, free fatty acids), and controlling hormones (insulin, cortisol, growth hormone). Administration of glucagon, intravenously or intramuscularly, at the time of hypoglycemia provides valuable information, as a hyperglycemic response to glucagon signifies persistent hepatic glycogen stores, which is abnormal in the face of hypoglycemia

TABLE 92.2

CRITICAL SAMPLE FOR EVALUATION OF HYPOGLYCEMIA IN CHILDREN

Test	Sample requirements	Normal values @ Hypoglycemia (Glu <55)
Glucose	1 mL serum or plasma	
Electrolytes	1 mL serum	Bicarbonate >18 mEq/L
Lactate	1 mL plasma	<2.5 mmol
Insulin	1 mL serum	<2 mcU/mL
Cortisol	1 mL serum	>20 mcg/dL
Growth hormone	1 mL serum	>7–10 ng/mL
Free fatty acids	1 mL plasma	>1.5 mmol/L
β-Hydroxybutyrate	1 mL plasma	>2 mmol/L
Acetoacetate	1 mL plasma	>2 mmol/L
Ammonia	1 mL plasma	<35 mcmol/L
C-peptide	1 mL EDTA plasma	<0.5 ng/mL
Acylcarnitine profile	1 mL EDTA plasma	
Urine organic acids	5–10 mL urine, frozen stat	
Urine ketones	1–2 mL	Positive

Requires specialist interpretation.

(19). Additional studies to be obtained include electrolytes, ammonia, lactate, acylcarnitine and organic acid profiles, and urinalysis for ketones (**Table 92.2**).

The duration of fasting tolerance (i.e., time to hypoglycemia from last carbohydrate consumed), amount of glucose required to restore and maintain euglycemia, serum bicarbonate, urinary ketones, and response to glucagon suggest the etiology of the hypoglycemia until the confirmatory critical sample results are known. The presence of acidosis with hypoglycemia indicates an accumulation of either ketones or lactate. Ketoacidosis is a normal response to prolonged fasting, while lactic acidosis generally indicates a block in the gluconeogenic pathway (failure to convert lactate to glucose). However, fasting tolerance of <4–6 hrs, significant ketosis, and fatty acid breakdown in a child with hepatomegaly suggest one of the glycogen-storage diseases (GSDs), which are all characterized by the absence of glycemic response to glucagon (<30 mg/dL rise in blood glucose) and normal parenteral glucose requirements to restore and maintain euglycemia. Supraphysiologic glucose requirement, low or absent ketones, and glycemic response to glucagon (>30 mg/dL) are the hallmarks of hyperinsulinism (HI), in which excessive insulin action inhibits glycogenolysis and promotes excessive peripheral glucose uptake. Disorders of fatty acid oxidation are also associated with low or absent ketones, but glucose requirements are normal and glycemic response to glucagon is absent. Hypopituitarism, either simple growth hormone deficiency or multiple pituitary hormone deficiency, is difficult to classify in this framework, as glucose requirements may be supraphysiologic and glycemic response to glucagon inconclusive.

Disorders of Glycogen Storage

The GSDs are a family of autosomal recessively inherited disorders characterized by defects in the formation and/or degradation of glycogen. Certain subtypes of GSD are associated with hypoglycemia: debranching enzyme deficiency (type III GSD), liver phosphorylase deficiency (type VI), and phosphorylase kinase deficiency (type IX). Other associated features include hepatomegaly and failure to thrive. As hepatic gluconeogenesis is intact and some functional glycogenolysis occurs, these forms of GSD are typically associated with only mild defects in fasting tolerance. Muscle-specific forms of GSD, while associated with myopathy, do not cause hypoglycemia. Glycogen synthetase deficiency (GSD type 0) is a very rare form of GSD that is associated with fasting hypoglycemia and postprandial hyperglycemia and lactic acidosis. Glucose-6-phosphatase deficiency, while known as GSD type I, is more appropriately considered a disorder of gluconeogenesis and, as such, will be discussed below.

Disorders of Gluconeogenesis

Defects in gluconeogenesis are characterized by hypoglycemia, hepatomegaly, lactic acidosis, and hyperlipidemia. The most severe disorder of gluconeogenesis is glucose-6-phosphatase deficiency (GSD type I); this enzyme catalyzes the hepatic release of glucose and is required not only for the last step in gluconeogenesis, but also for glycogenolysis. Therefore, glycogen breakdown does not provide glucose, and fasting tolerance is extremely short—only 2–4 hrs. Other disorders of gluconeogenesis, such as fructose-1,6-diphosphatase deficiency, hereditary fructose intolerance, and galactosemia, are distinguished from GSD type I by a longer fasting tolerance, as glycogenolysis is intact.

Fatty Acid Oxidation Disorders

Defects in fatty acid oxidation manifest when the fasting tolerance of ~12 hrs is exceeded or when a significant stress calls upon adipose tissue stores. Under normal fasting conditions, free fatty acids are mobilized by the hormone-sensitive adipose tissue lipase and utilized as alternative fuel, as a substrate for the production of ketone bodies, and as an energy source for gluconeogenesis. Children with a disorder of fatty acid oxidation have impairments either in transport of fatty acids across the mitochondrial membrane or metabolism within the mitochondrial β-oxidation cycle. The most common fatty acid oxidation disorder, medium-chain acyl-coenzyme A deficiency (MCAD), occurs in ~1 in 10,000 Caucasians of Northern European ancestry. In addition to hypoglycemia, fatty acid oxidation disorders may present with hyperammonemia, liver dysfunction, myopathy, coma, and sudden death. Because fatty acid oxidation disorders are life threatening and account for some cases of sudden death, their identification and appropriate management are crucial. Definitive diagnosis may be made by the demonstration of an abnormal acylcarnitine profile by mass spectrometry.

Hormone Deficiencies

Hypoglycemia may occur in children with hypopituitarism, as both growth hormone and cortisol are required for optimal counter-regulation and fasting adaptation. Most commonly, hypoglycemia in adrenal insufficiency occurs during periods of intercurrent illness with vomiting or poor oral intake and inadequate replacement of cortisol. Hypoglycemia with isolated growth hormone deficiency is limited primarily to newborns.

Hyperinsulinism

HI may be transient or permanent. Transient dysregulated insulin secretion occurs in the newborn period, typically in the setting of some physiologic perinatal stress such as asphyxia, maternal hypertension, or precipitous delivery. Such hypoglycemia occurs within the first few hours of life and can last weeks unless treated. More familiar is the infant of the diabetic mother, in which the fetus upregulates insulin secretion in response to maternal hyperglycemia. At birth, the infant is large for gestational age due to the growth factor effects of insulin and suffers from hypoglycemia when the excessive glucose supply is acutely withdrawn. The time course to normalization of blood glucose in an infant of a diabetic mother may be several days to several weeks.

Although the persistent forms of HI can resemble the large-for-gestational-age infant of a diabetic mother, recent insights into the genetic defects responsible for congenital HI have greatly expanded our appreciation of various, including more subtle, forms of HI (11). The severe phenotype is typical of genetic defects of the β-cell sulfonylurea receptor/K channel complex (SUR1/Kir6.2), which transduces the energy state of the β cell to the cell membrane to effect insulin release. The autosomal recessive form effects the endocrine pancreas diffusely. More commonly, focal lesions expressing a SUR1 mutation can arise by loss of heterozygosity mechanism; loss of the normal maternal SUR1 allele and tumor suppressor genes on chromosome 11p15.1 in a child who inherits an abnormal paternal SUR1 mutation permits the clonal expansion of an abnormal β-cell lesion with dysregulated insulin secretion. Other genetic forms of HI include (a) dominantly inherited defects in glucokinase that lower the glycemic threshold for insulin secretion to cause milder degrees of hypoglycemia, and (b) gain-of-function mutations in glutamate dehydrogenase, characterized by protein-sensitive hypoglycemia and asymptomatic hyperammonemia.

Drug-induced/Iatrogenic Causes

One of the most common causes of hypoglycemia in hospitalized children is the acute interruption of high-concentration IV dextrose infusion, particularly seen in sick newborns who are treated with total parenteral nutrition. It is thought that supraphysiologic insulin secretion cannot be downregulated quickly enough when the infusion is abruptly stopped or accidentally blocked or removed. Inappropriate elevated insulin levels at the time of hypoglycemia, along with suppression of free fatty acids and ketones, are consistent with this phenomenon of transient iatrogenic HI.

Certain drugs and medications are known to be associated with hypoglycemia. By far the most common cause of drug-induced hypoglycemia in children (aside from insulin in diabetics) is alcohol. Sources of alcohol include parents' supply, mouthwash, and transdermal exposure of rubbing alcohol. The amount of alcohol required to induce hypoglycemia is frequently less than that required to cause drunkenness. Alcohol causes hypoglycemia by impairing gluconeogenesis, blocking hepatic lactate uptake, and inhibiting counter-regulatory hormone release. Thus, the risks of alcohol-induced hypoglycemia are highest when alcohol is ingested at night before the child goes to sleep.

Other drugs/medications that may induce hypoglycemia include sulfonylureas and other antidiabetic drugs, by stimulating insulin release; quinine, pentamidine, and disopyramide, also through augmentation of insulin secretion; β-blockers, by blunting adrenergic response to hypoglycemia; and salicylates, whose mechanism is unknown. Ingestion of the unripe *ackee* fruit is associated with hypoglycemia due to the naturally occurring toxin hypoglycin (46). Lastly, factitious hypoglycemia due to Munchausen syndrome, in which children or their caregivers surreptitiously administer insulin or an oral secretagogue, may mimic true HI.

Other Causes of Hypoglycemia

Transient hypoglycemia is frequently seen in newborn infants; 30% of normal newborn infants and an even greater percentage of infants born prematurely or small for gestational age have been shown to have hypoglycemia in the first few hours of life (43), as glycogen stores are not yet replete and several key enzymes in the gluconeogenic and fatty acid oxidation pathways are not fully expressed. Similarly, ketotic hypoglycemia is a poorly understood condition of blunted fasting tolerance that generally occurs in underweight children who are 1–6 years of age. Symptoms occur after a prolonged overnight fast or during intercurrent illness with vomiting or poor feeding. The cause of ketotic hypoglycemia is unknown, but it has been proposed to result from a decreased muscle mass, which limits the gluconeogenic substrate supply, as demonstrated by low alanine levels during fasting (53). Reactive (or postprandial) hypoglycemia, either alone or in conjunction with other symptoms of the dumping syndrome, may rarely be seen in children with dysregulated intestinal transit or after fundoplication (57). Last, neonatal disorders such as sepsis (74) and hyperviscosity syndrome (10) are noted to cause hypoglycemia in sick newborns by an uncharacterized mechanism.

Treatment of Hypoglycemia

In the acute setting, the immediate goal in the treatment of hypoglycemia is to increase the plasma glucose to at least 70 mg/dL. The critical sample should be drawn prior to treatment, if tolerated by the patient. Rapid improvement in blood sugar is normally seen after administration of 10% dextrose, 2 mL/kg by IV push, followed by continuous IV dextrose at a rate of at least 8 mg/kg/min. Glucose levels should be repeated frequently; for continuing hypoglycemia, additional boluses should be given, and the basal glucose infusion should be increased in 10%–15% increments. Some infants with HI require 20 mg/kg/min dextrose to maintain euglycemia; in fact, the requirement of supraphysiologic amounts of glucose indicates elevated glucose utilization, a reliable sign for HI.

Definitive treatment of hypoglycemia depends on the underlying condition. Withdrawal of medications that cause hypoglycemia usually results in prompt improvement; likewise, children with hormone deficiencies (e.g., growth hormone deficiency or hypoadrenalism) usually respond well to appropriate hormonal supplementation. The GSDs and disorders of fatty acid oxidation respond well to avoidance of long fasts. In patients with very poor fasting tolerance, home nasogastric or gastrostomy feeding is required. Uncooked cornstarch feedings, as a long-acting source of glucose overnight, have also been used effectively for a number of hypoglycemic conditions.

Treatment of true congenital HI is more challenging. Children with mutations in glucokinase or glutamate dehydrogenase may respond well to diazoxide, given at a dose of 5–15 mg/kg/day. Diazoxide inhibits insulin secretion by opening β-cell K channels. However, children with defects in the K channel or sulfonylurea receptor will typically not respond to diazoxide; octreotide, a long-acting somatostatin analog, may be administered subcutaneously every 6–8 hrs at a dose of 5–20 mcg/kg/day. However, tachyphylaxis frequently develops to octreotide, so that most children with K channel-sulfonylurea receptor complex mutations require subtotal or complete pancreatectomy for long-term control of hypoglycemia. Continuous IV infusion of glucagon, 1 mg/day, may be used to stabilize the glucose levels prior to surgery.

Outcomes

The long-term outcome for children with hypoglycemia depends primarily on the underlying etiology. The primary risk of hypoglycemia in infants and young children relates to neurodevelopmental sequelae. The precise level and duration of hypoglycemia required to cause permanent neurologic dysfunction is unknown. Of the hypoglycemic disorders, children with HI appear to be most vulnerable, with neurodevelopmental complications reported in 26%–44% (11). Younger age at presentation, longer duration of hypoglycemia, and unresponsiveness to medical therapy are associated with greater risk of neurologic sequelae. Post-pancreatectomy diabetes mellitus may occur transiently or may be a permanent complication of surgical resection. The risk of diabetes mellitus has been reported to be ~27% in children who require one surgery but increases to over 70% in children in whom repeated surgical resections are required to remove residual islet tissue (11).

Conclusions and Future Directions—Hypoglycemia

Difficulties in differentiating focal from diffuse lesions and localizing small pancreatic lesions that are readily amenable to surgical resection have led researchers to investigate whether newer modalities of pancreatic imaging hold potential for improving the diagnostic and therapeutic modalities available for the management of HI. Current imaging techniques such as spiral CT and MRI are of limited use; newer technologies such as PET scanning have demonstrated compelling early results and warrant further study (11). Laparoscopic surgical techniques to enucleate smaller pancreatic lesions hold the promise to minimize the risk of postoperative diabetes.

KEY POINTS

- DKA is the most frequent cause of diabetes-related death in children, with a mortality rate of 0.2%–0.3%. Over 75% of the mortality in DKA can be attributed to cerebral edema.
- Prompt volume resuscitation with isotonic fluids and insulin replacement are necessary for optimal management of DKA. Once the plasma volume has been restored, however, subsequent fluid therapy should be gradual.
- The risk of cerebral edema may be minimized by slow volume replacement, use of isotonic fluids, and frequent monitoring of the serum Na, fluid balance, and neurologic status.
- The use of sodium bicarbonate is no longer warranted, except in situations of extreme acidosis with cardiovascular instability; and should be given gradually.
- HHS is under-recognized in children and may be mistaken for DKA.
- Early and aggressive fluid therapy is critical for effective management of HHS.
- Mortality in HHS is high, 15% or higher, attributable to circulatory collapse, thrombotic complications, and multisystem organ failure.
- Hyperglycemia commonly occurs in critically ill nondiabetic children and is associated with increased morbidity and mortality.
- Neurohormonal factors that accompany stress response lead to insulin resistance, increased glucose production, and hyperglycemia.
- Elevated blood glucose levels, even if brief, can result in detrimental effects, including endothelial dysfunction and immunologic compromise.
- Data in adults suggest that aggressive glycemic control with insulin infusion improves outcome. However, its benefit in children is unknown. A multicentered pediatric trial is planned to address this issue.
- Hypoglycemia is, except in rare circumstances, a defect in fasting adaptation. Understanding the ordered responses to fasting provides the framework for differentiating among the various causes of hypoglycemia and making a prompt diagnosis.
- Infants and young children may not present with typical adrenergic symptoms. Such nonspecific manifestations as apnea, cyanosis, feeding difficulties, tachypnea, and hypothermia, may be the early signs.
- Collection of the appropriate alternate fuels and hormones at the time of hypoglycemia provides the most efficient opportunity for determining the etiology of hypoglycemia.

References

1. Arieff AI. Cerebral edema complicating nonketotic hyperosmolar coma. *Miner Electrolyte Metab* 1986;12:383–9.

2. Arieff AI, Carroll HJ. Nonketotic hyperosmolar coma with hyperglycemia: Clinical features, pathophysiology, renal function, acid-base balance, plasma-cerebrospinal fluid equilibria and the effects of therapy in 37 cases. *Medicine (Baltimore)* 1972;51:73–94.

3. Bier DM, Leaker RD, Haymond MW, et al. Measurement of "true" glucose production rates in infancy and childhood with 6,6-dideuteroglucose. *Diabetes* 1977;26:1016–23.

4. Bloomgarden ZT. Type 2 diabetes in the young: The evolving epidemic. *Diabetes Care* 2004;27:998–1010.

5. Carchman RM, Dechert-Zeger M, Calikoglu AS, et al. A new challenge in pediatric obesity: Pediatric hyperglycemic hyperosmolar syndrome. *Pediatr Crit Care Med* 2005;6:20–4.

6. Carl GF, Hoffman WH, Passmore GG, et al. Diabetic ketoacidosis promotes a prothrombotic state. *Endocr Res* 2003;29:73–82.

7. Couch RM, Acott PD, Wong GW. Early onset fatal cerebral edema in diabetic ketoacidosis. *Diabetes Care* 1991;14:78–9.

8. Cryer PE. Mechanisms of hypoglycemia-associated autonomic failure and its component syndromes in diabetes. *Diabetes* 2005;54:3592–601.

9. Delaney MF, Zisman A, Kettyle WM. Diabetic ketoacidosis and hyperglycemic hyperosmolar nonketotic syndrome. *Endocrinol Metab Clin North Am* 2000;29(4):683–705.

10. Delaney-Black V, Camp BW, Lubchenko, et al. Neonatal hyperviscosity association with lower achievement and IQ scores at school age. *Pediatrics* 1989;83:662–7.

11. De Leon DD, Stanley CA. Mechanisms of disease: Advances in diagnosis and treatment of hyperinsulinism in neonates. *Nat Clin Pract Endocrinol Metab* 2007;3:57–68.

12. Duck SC, Wyatt DT. Factors associated with brain herniation in the treatment of diabetic ketoacidosis. *J Pediatr* 1988;113:10–4.

13. Dunger DB, Sperling MA, Acerini CL, et al. European Society for Paediatric Endocrinology/Lawson Wilkins Pediatric Endocrine Society consensus statement on diabetic ketoacidosis in children and adolescents. *Pediatriatrics* 2004;113:e133–40.

14. Dunger DB, Sperling MA, Acerini CL, et al. ESPE/LWPES consensus statement on diabetic ketoacidosis in children and adolescents. *Arch Dis Child* 2004;89:188–94.

15. Edge JA, Jakes RW, Roy Y, et al. The UK case-control study of cerebral oedema complicating diabetic ketoacidosis in children. *Diabetologia* 2006;49:2002–9.

16. Evan-Wong LA, Davidson RJ, Stowers JM. Alterations in erythrocytes in hyperosmolar diabetic decompensation: A pathophysiological basis for impaired blood flow and for an improved design of fluid therapy. *Diabetologia* 1985;28:739–42.

17. Faustino EV, Apkon M. Persistent hyperglycemia in critically ill children. *J Pediatr* 2005;146:30–4.

18. Fearon DM, Steele DW. End-tidal carbon dioxide predicts the presence and severity of acidosis in children with diabetes. *Acad Emerg Med* 2002;9:1373–8.

19. Finegold D, Stanley CA, Baker L. Glycemic response to glucagon during fasting hypoglycemia: An aid in the diagnosis of hyperinsulinism. *J Pediatr* 1980;96:257–9.

20. Fourtner SH, Weinzimer SA, Levitt Katz LE. Hyperglycemic hyperosmolar non-ketotic syndrome in children with type 2 diabetes. *Pediatr Diabetes* 2005;6:129–35.

21. Glaser N. Pediatric diabetic ketoacidosis and hyperglycemic hyperosmolar state. *Pediatr Clin N Am* 2005;52:1611–35.

22. Glaser N, Barnett P, McCaslin I, et al. Risk factors for cerebral edema in children with diabetic ketoacidosis. The Pediatric Emergency Medicine Collaborative Research Committee of the American Academy of Pediatrics. *N Engl J Med* 2001;344:264–9.

23. Glaser N, Gorges S, Marcin J, et al. Mechanism of cerebral edema in children with diabetic ketoacidosis. *J Pediatr* 2004;145:164–71.

24. Glasgow AM. Devastating cerebral edema in diabetic ketoacidosis before therapy. *Diabetes Care* 1991;14:77–78.

25. Gore DC, Chinkes D, Heggers J, et al. Association of hyperglycemia with increased mortality after severe burn injury. *J Trauma* 2001;51:540–4.

26. Gottschalk ME, Ros SP, Zeller WP. The emergency management of hyperglycemic-hyperosmolar nonketotic coma in the pediatric patient. *Pediatr Emerg Care* 1996;12:48–51.

27. Grimberg A Cerri RW, Satin-Smith M, et al. The "two bag system" for variable intravenous dextrose and fluid administration: Benefits in diabetic ketoacidosis management. *J Pediatr* 1999;134:376–8.

28. Harris GD, Fiordalisi I, Harris W, et al. Minimizing the risk of brain herniation during treatment of diabetic ketoacidemia: A retrospective and prospective study. *J Pediatr* 1990;117:22–31.

29. Harris GD, Lohr JW, Fiordalisi I, et al. Brain osmoregulation during extreme and moderate dehydration in a rat model of severe DKA. *Life Sci* 1993;53:185–91.

30. Harris GD, Fiordalisi I. Physiological management of diabetic ketoacidemia: A 5-year prospective pediatric experience in 231 episodes. *Arch Pediatr Adolesc Med* 1994;148:1046–52.

31. Harris GD, Fiordalisi I, Yu C. Maintaining normal intracranial pressure in a rabbit model during treatment of severe diabetic ketoacidemia. *Life Sci* 1996;59:1695–702.

32. Haymond MW, Sunehag A. Controlling the sugar bowl: Regulation of glucose homeostasis in children. *Endocrinol Metab Clin North Am* 1999;28:663–9.

33. Hollander AS, Olney RC, Blackett PR, et al. Fatal malignant hyperthermia-like syndrome with rhabdomyolysis complicating the presentation of diabetes mellitus in adolescent males. *Pediatrics* 2003;111:1447–52.

34. Kaminska E, Pourmotabbed G. Spurious laboratory values in diabetic ketoacidosis and hyperlipidemia. *Am J Emerg Med* 1993;11:77–80.

35. Katz M. Hyperglycemia-induced hyponatremia: Calculation of expected serum sodium depression. *N Engl J Med* 1973;289:843–4.

36. Kaufman FR. Type 2 diabetes in children and youth. *Endocrinol Metab Clin North Am* 2005;34:659–76, ix–x.

37. Kitabchi AE, Umpierrez GE, Murphy MB, et al. Hyperglycemic crises in diabetes. *Diabetes Care* 2004;27 Suppl 1:S94–102.

38. Koves IH, Neutze J, Donath S, et al. The accuracy of clinical assessment of dehydration during diabetic ketoacidosis in childhood. *Diabetes Care* 2004;27:2485–7.

39. Krane EJ, Rockoff MA, Wallman JK, et al. Subclinical brain swelling in children during treatment of diabetic ketoacidosis. *N Engl J Med* 1985;312:1147–51.

40. Krinsley JS. Effect of an intensive glucose management protocol on the mortality of critically ill adult patients. *Mayo Clin Proc* 2004;79:992–1000.

41. Langouche L, Van den Berghe G. Glucose metabolism and insulin therapy. *Crit Care Clin* 2006;22:119–29, vii.

42. Lorber D. Nonketotic hypertonicity in diabetes mellitus. *Med Clin North Am* 1995;79:39–52.

43. Lubchenko LO, Bard H. Incidence of hypoglycemia in newborn infants classified by birth weight and gestational age. *Pediatrics* 1971;47:831–8.

44. Macaluso CJ, Bauer UE, Deeb LC, et al. Type 2 diabetes mellitus among Florida children and adolescents, 1994 through 1998. *Public Health Rep* 2002;117:373–9.

45. Magee MF, Bhatt BA. Management of decompensated diabetes. Diabetic ketoacidosis and hyperglycemic hyperosmolar syndrome. *Crit Care Clin* 2001;17:75–106.

46. Marks V, Teale JD. Drug-induced hypoglycemia. *Endocrinol Metab Clin North Am* 1999;28:555–77.

47. McCowen KC, Malhotra A, Bistrian BR. Stress-induced hyperglycemia. *Crit Care Clin* 2001;17:107–24.

48. Mesotten D, Van den Berghe G. Clinical potential of insulin therapy in critically ill patients. *Drugs* 2003;63:625–36.

49. Meyer PC, Salt HB. Unusually high blood sugar in a boy. *Br Med J* 1951;4699:171–2.

50. Mizock BA. Alterations in fuel metabolism in critical illness: Hyperglycaemia. *Best Pract Res Clin Endocrinol Metab* 2001;15:533–51.

51. Morales AE, Rosenbloom AL. Death caused by hyperglycemic hyperosmolar state at the onset of type 2 diabetes. *J Pediatr* 2004;144:270–3.

52. Nugent BW. Hyperosmolar hyperglycemic state. *Emerg Med Clin North Am* 2005;23:629–48, vii.

53. Pagliara AS, Karl IE, DeVito DC, et al. Hypoalaninemia: A concomitant of ketotic hypoglycemia. *J Clin Invest* 1972;51:1440–9.

54. Preiser JC, Devos P, Van den Berghe G. Tight control of glycaemia in critically ill patients. *Curr Opin Clin Nutr Metab Care* 2002;5:533–7.

55. Rewers A, Chase HP, Mackenzie T, et al. Predictors of acute complications in children with type 1 diabetes. *JAMA* 2002;287:2511–8.

56. Rewers A, McFann K, Chase HP. Bedside monitoring of blood β-hydroxybutyrate levels in the management of diabetic ketoacidosis in children. *Diab Technol Ther* 2006;8:671–6.

57. Rivkees SA, Crawford JD. Hypoglycemia pathogenesis in children with dumping syndrome. *Pediatrics* 1987;80:937–42.

58. Rubin HM, Kramer R, Drash A. Hyperosmolality complicating diabetes mellitus in childhood. *J Pediatr* 1969;74:177–86.

59. Srinivasan V, Spinella PC, Drott HR, et al. Association of timing, duration, and intensity of hyperglycemia with intensive care unit mortality in critically ill children. *Pediatr Crit Care Med* 2004;5:329–36.

60. Stanley CA. Hypoglycemia. In: Radovick S, MacGillivray MH, eds. *Pediatric Endocrinology: A Practical Clinical Guide*. Totowa: Humana Press, 2003;511–21.

61. Stanley CA, Baker L. The causes of neonatal hypoglycemia. *N Engl J Med* 1999;340:1200–1.

62. Taylor JH, Beilman GJ. Hyperglycemia in the intensive care unit: No longer just a marker of illness severity. *Surg Infect (Larchmt)* 2005;6:233–45.

63. Trence DL, Hirsch IB. Hyperglycemic crises in diabetes mellitus type 2. *Endocrinol Metab Clin North Am* 2001;30:817–31.

64. Turina M, Fry DE, Polk HC, Jr. Acute hyperglycemia and the innate immune system: Clinical, cellular, and molecular aspects. *Crit Care Med* 2005;33:1624–33.

65. Umpierrez GE, Smiley D, Kitabchi AE. Narrative review: Ketosis-prone type 2 diabetes mellitus. *Ann Intern Med* 2006;144:350–7.

66. Van den Berghe G. How does blood glucose control with insulin save lives in intensive care? *J Clin Invest* 2004;114:1187–95.

67. Van den Berghe G, Wilmer A, Hermans G, et al. Intensive insulin therapy in the medical ICU. *N Engl J Med* 2006;354:449–61.

68. Van den Berghe G, Wouters PJ, Bouillon R, et al. Outcome benefit of intensive insulin therapy in the critically ill: Insulin dose versus glycemic control. *Crit Care Med* 2003;31:359–66.

69. Van den Berghe G, Wouters P, Weekers F, et al. Intensive insulin therapy in the critically ill patients. *N Engl J Med* 2001;345:1359–67.

70. Wachtel TJ, Tetu-Mouradjian LM, Goldman DL, et al. Hyperosmolarity and acidosis in diabetes mellitus: A three-year experience in Rhode Island. *J Gen Intern Med* 1991;6:495–502.

71. Weinzimer SA, Tamborlane WV. Diabetes mellitus in children and adolescents. In: Fonseca VA, ed. *Clinical Diabetes: Translating Research into Practice.* Philadelphia: Saunders Elsevier, 2006;505–21.

72. West ML, Marsden PA, Singer GG, et al. Quantitative analysis of glucose loss during acute therapy for hyperglycemic hyperosmolar syndrome. *Diabetes Care* 1986;9:465–71.

73. Wolfsdorf J, Craig ME, Daneman D , etc. Diabetic ketoacidosis: IS-PAD clinical practice guidelines 2006–2007. *Pediatr Diabetes* 2007;8: 28–42.

74. Yeung CY. Hypoglycemia in neonatal sepsis. *J Pediatr* 1970;77:812.

CHAPTER 93 ■ DISORDERS OF WATER, SODIUM, AND POTASSIUM HOMEOSTASIS

ANDREA KELLY • THOMAS MOSHANG, JR.

A disorder of water, sodium (Na^+), or potassium (K^+) in the critically ill child frequently requires superb clinical judgment, an expeditious needs assessment based upon history and clinical examination without guidance from extensive laboratory data, and minute-to-minute alterations in therapy. This patient often has little leeway in either body reserves or time for prolonged evaluations by laboratory measures or consultations. Discussion in this chapter focus on the evaluation and management of water, Na^+, and K^+ disorders as they pertain to the critically ill child and will not attempt to be inclusive of all such disorders in less critical settings. Although mentioned in various sections, molecular mechanisms, genetic alterations, animal models, and similar information will not be discussed in detail. Further, sophisticated laboratory studies not generally immediately available to the intensivist will be discussed to only a limited degree. Specifically, discussions will focus on paradigms regarding the clinical evaluation and management of fluid disorders, as appropriate correction of fluid disturbances in the critically ill child is often paramount for resuscitation and survival.

To provide the foundation for an understanding of the pathophysiologic disturbances, this chapter will include a review of normal physiology and the mechanisms that regulate water, Na^+, and K^+ balance. The disorders of water, Na^+, and K^+ will be discussed as to etiology and most common presentations in the critical care setting. As to the differential diagnosis of the various conditions, the discussions will focus upon the most probable causes that result in admission to a critical care unit. Fluid management will emphasize the differences in initial therapies involving resuscitation, as opposed to maintenance of hydration and electrolyte control. A review of outcomes that have resulted due to either inappropriate resuscitation or maintenance fluid treatment or drug therapy will be presented as a basis for discussion of potential sources of error.

NORMAL PHYSIOLOGY AND PATHOPHYSIOLOGY

Strict regulation of total body water, Na^+, and K^+ occurs through multiple, often redundant, pathways. Regulation of Na^+ is critical for maintaining extracellular fluid (ECF) volume, while regulation of K^+ is vital for maintaining cellular electrophysiology. Superimposed upon regulation of these electrolytes is water metabolism, which is primarily influenced by changes in serum osmolality and, to a lesser extent, volume status. The kidney is the primary site for disposal of Na^+, K^+, and water; several hormonal pathways converge at the level of the kidney to further regulate their disposal (**Fig. 93.1**).

Renal Handling of Water and Solutes—An Overview

A number of renal factors influence the dilution and concentration of urine. First, the glomerular filtration rate, the amount of renal blood flow that enters the nephron, dictates the maximum amount of fluid that can be delivered to the tubules. The glomerular filtration rate is heavily influenced by renal blood flow through the afferent and efferent arterioles. Vasoconstriction of afferent arterioles decreases glomerular blood flow, thereby decreasing glomerular pressure and filtration, while vasoconstriction of efferent arterioles, to an extent, increases glomerular pressure and filtration. A feedback mechanism, mediated by the macula densa, controls the vasoconstriction and vasodilation of the afferent and efferent arterioles to autoregulate the glomerular filtration rate. When the macula densa "senses" a low glomerular filtration rate, vasodilatation of afferent arterioles (and vasoconstriction of efferent arterioles mediated by angiotensin II) increases glomerular perfusion, thereby increasing the glomerular filtration rate to effect urine output. Conversely, with increased glomerular filtration, the macula densa again provides negative feedback to the afferent and efferent arterioles: vasoconstriction of afferent arterioles (and vasodilatation of efferent arterioles) occurs, decreasing glomerular filtration, slowing fluid transport through the nephron, and allowing increased filtrate reabsorption and, ultimately, decreased urine output. Afferent and efferent arterioles are regulated by the sympathetic nervous system and angiotensin II, as described later.

Following filtration at the level of the glomerulus, the fluid is delivered to the tubules, where solute absorption varies depending upon the segment. The proximal tubule accounts for 65% of filtrate reabsorption, including that of Na^+, K^+, and water. The descending thin limb of the loop of Henle is permeable to water, urea, and other solutes, while the ascending thin limb is relatively impermeable to water. The thick ascending limb and the initial segment of the distal tubule avidly absorb Na^+ and other solutes but are impermeable to water regardless of the status of vasopressin and, hence, are referred to as the *diluting segment* of the kidney. Here, tubular fluid osmolality falls below that of the glomerular filtrate. The late distal tubule and cortical collecting duct mediate the Na^+-retaining and K^+-wasting effects of aldosterone. In addition, like the collecting duct, they are permeable to water only in the presence of vasopressin.

Na^+ absorption occurs through an active process and facilitates the absorption of many other solutes. Na/K-ATPase, expressed on the basolateral membrane of tubular epithelium,

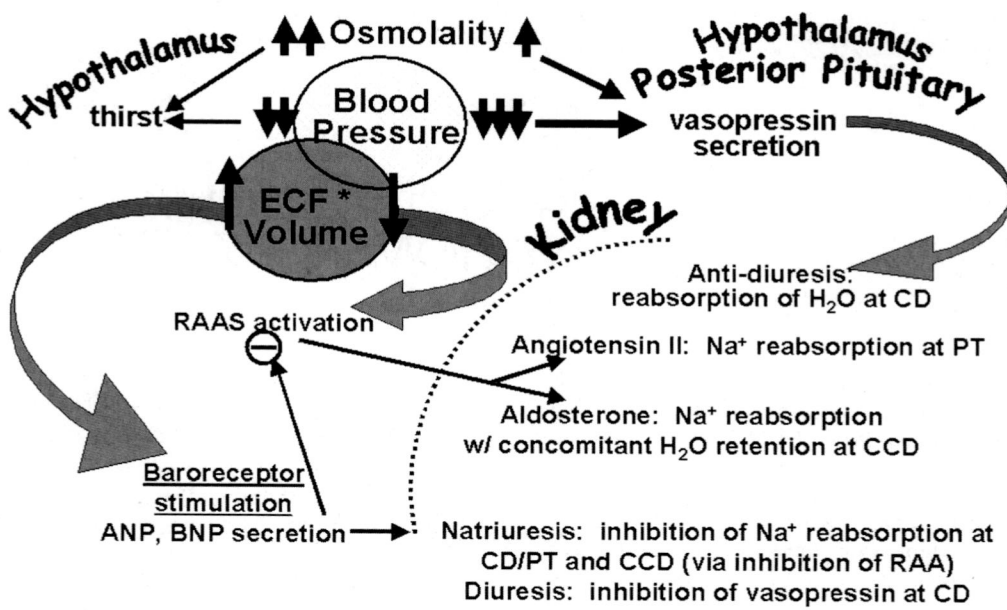

FIGURE 93.1. Regulation of extracellular fluid osmolality and volume. Vasopressin secretion is primarily responsible for preserving plasma osmolality. Secretion of vasopressin by the hypothalamus occurs with as little as a 1% increase in plasma osmolality. Much larger increases in plasma osmolality are required to trigger thirst, the center for which is also located in the hypothalamus. This offsetting likely occurs to avoid simultaneously activating thirst and vasopressin secretion at the lower end of normal plasma osmolality, which would result in overcorrection. Significant decreases in blood pressure/effective extracellular fluid (ECF) volume, communicated to the hypothalamus via cardiovascular baroreceptors, are required to trigger vasopressin secretion. Vasopressin recruits aquoporin-2 water channels in the renal collecting ducts (CD) to promote reabsorption of water and concentration of urine. ECF volume is primarily maintained through Na^+ homeostasis. Decreases in blood pressure/effective ECF volume also activate the renin angiotensin aldosterone system (RAAS). Aldosterone promotes reabsorption of Na^+ and water at the renal cortical collecting duct (CCD), and angiotensin II stimulates Na^+ reabsorption at the proximal tubules (PT). Hypertension/fluid overload activate cardiovascular baroreceptors, leading to atrial natriuretic peptide (ANP) and brain natriuretic peptide (BNP) release. These peptides promote Na^+ and water excretion at the level of the kidney.

pumps Na^+ into the renal interstitium and ultimately to the peritubular capillaries (**Fig. 93.2**). Activity of this enzyme generates a Na^+ concentration gradient and an electrochemical gradient between the tubule lumen and the tubular cell. These gradients facilitate Na^+ transport from tubular fluid into the tubular epithelium, further supplying Na^+ for the Na/K-ATPase pump. In addition, these gradients drive water reabsorption. Because the cellular concentration of K^+ is already high relative to interstitial fluid, and because the tubular epithelial basolateral membrane is readily permeable to K^+, K^+ driven into the cell by Na/K-ATPase diffuses easily into the interstitium for reabsorption from the filtrate.

From this discussion, it can be concluded that water, Na^+, and K^+ homeostasis are not completely independent. A disorder that primarily affects one of these important body constituents can have a significant impact on another.

Water Homeostasis

The human body is composed of 42%–75% water, with the exact content dependent upon age, sex, and amount of body fat. Approximately two-thirds of the water is located intracellularly. The remaining estimated one-third is located extracellularly and is divided between the interstitium (three-fourths) and plasma (one-fourth). The solute content of these fluid

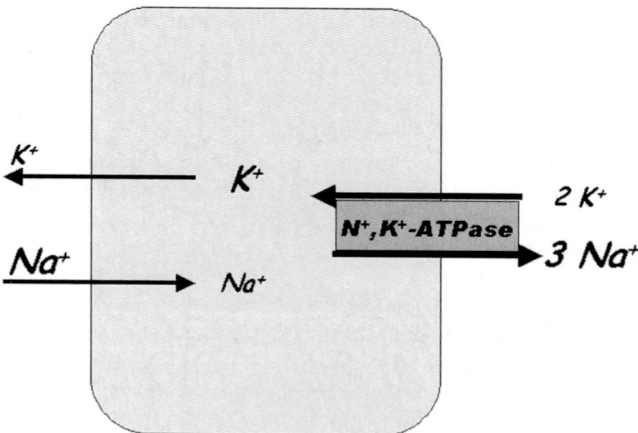

FIGURE 93.2. Na/K-ATPase activity. Na/K-ATPase is ubiquitously expressed on the plasma cell membrane. Via an ATP-consuming process, this enzyme exchanges 3 intracellular Na^+ cations for two extracellular K^+ cations to maintain the intracellular-to-extracellular gradients for these two cations. Na^+ can pass down this concentration gradient from the ECF to the ICF, whereas K^+ diffuses down its concentration gradient from the ICF to the ECF. The location of these pumps varies depending upon the cell type; they may be distributed evenly along the cell membrane or localized to the basolateral membranes as in renal epithelial cells.

compartments differs significantly, with K^+ being the primary constituent of intracellular fluid (ICF) and Na^+ being the major electrolyte in ECF. Na/K-ATPase, a plasma membrane enzyme expressed on most cells, is responsible for maintaining this discordant distribution of Na^+ and K^+ in body fluids (**Fig. 93.2**). It plays a key role in maintaining cellular volume: through its active transport of Na^+ extracellularly, it prevents accumulation of intracellular water that would arise from the significant intracellular concentrations of impermeable proteins and organic compounds. Na/K-ATPase maintains this transcellular gradient through an energy-expending process: Na/K-ATPase exchanges three molecules of intracellular Na^+ for every two molecules of extracellular K^+ (**Fig. 93.2**) (27).

Strict regulation of body water is critical for preserving ECF osmolality within a narrow range. The normal range for blood osmolality is 280–290 mOsm/kg H_2O. Cell membranes are freely water permeable. As a result, when a concentration gradient develops between ECF and ICF, water passively moves from the compartment with the lower to the higher gradient, thus restoring equilibrium. ECF osmolality can be estimated based upon the equation:

$$2 \times Na^+ + [ureanitrogen(mg/dL)]/2.8 + [glucose(mg/dL)]/18$$

Urea nitrogen and glucose (in the absence of hyperglycemia/insulin deficiency) freely permeate most cell membranes, with the exception of the blood-brain barrier (BBB), and are considered ineffective osmoles because they do not influence transcellular water flux. Because Na^+ is the prevailing extracellular cation, it and its companion anions largely determine ECF osmolality; that is, plasma Na^+ effectively drives water homeostasis.

Maintenance of body water and, hence, osmolality occurs despite potentially large variations at the sites of regulation: intake and output. Fluid intake is regulated by thirst. However, other unregulated factors play a large role in determining fluid intake in the absence of thirst, such as the consumption of beverages socially and the ingestion of water-containing foods.

Water output is primarily regulated by vasopressin at the level of the kidney. In fact, over 99% of water in the glomerular filtrate is reabsorbed by the renal tubules. However, unregulated (and potentially substantial) water loss can occur through the skin, gastrointestinal tract, and lungs. In addition, obligate water loss occurs via the kidney in the elimination of solutes. In general, the kidney disposes of 500 mOsm solute/m²/day. The amount of solute to be excreted by the kidney can vary considerably (high-salt diet, normal saline solution), and thus, obligate water losses can vary significantly.

Vasopressin

Vasopressin is a peptide hormone encoded on chromosome 20, and it is referred to as antidiuretic hormone. Magnocellular neurons located in the hypothalamus produce vasopressin. Their distal axons store vasopressin until its release and, together with the terminal axons of oxytocin-producing hypothalamic neurons, constitute the posterior pituitary (**Fig. 93.3**). The posterior pituitary has been reported in animals to store vasopressin in amounts sufficient for maximal diuresis for a week. As detailed later, vasopressin production and secretion are regulated by serum osmolality, ECF volume, and blood pressure (**Fig. 93.4**).

Plasma osmotic pressure is the major determinant of vasopressin release (**Fig. 93.4**). Osmotically responsive vasopressin

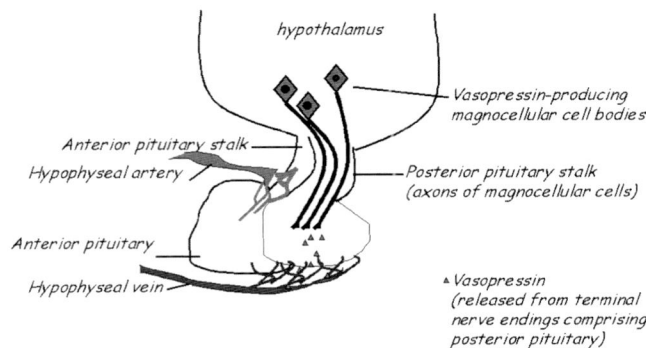

FIGURE 93.3. Anatomy of the hypothalamic-pituitary axis. The pituitary is composed of two embryologically distinct subdivisions. The anterior pituitary is one of several distinct neuroendocrine cell types that produce and secrete growth hormone, adrenocorticotropic hormone, prolactin, thyroid-stimulating hormone, or gonadotropins. It is regulated by the hypothalamus through axons that traverse the anterior pituitary stalk and by the peripheral milieu through the hypophyseal artery. Vasopressin and oxytocin are produced by distinct cell bodies located in the hypothalamus. The axons of these cells compose the posterior pituitary stalk, while the posterior pituitary houses their terminal endings, the storage sites for vasopressin and oxytocin. Hormones from both the anterior and posterior pituitaries are transported to the periphery via the hypophyseal veins.

release is believed to occur through a threshold effect: below a certain osmotic threshold, vasopressin release is suppressed; above this threshold, vasopressin release increases in a linear fashion with osmolarity. Individual differences in vasopressin release exist. In general, the threshold for vasopressin release is 280–285 mOsm/kg H_2O and for every 1 mOsm/kg H_2O increase in plasma osmolality, plasma vasopressin increases by 0.4–1 pg/mL to a maximum of 4–5 pg/mL for maximal urinary concentration (41). Individual thresholds for vasopressin release and vasopressin responsiveness are at least partly determined by genetics, but these can be altered by nonosmotic inputs, such as blood pressure and drugs, as well as by chronic perturbations in plasma osmolality. This fine-tuning of responsiveness is mediated through inhibitory and excitatory inputs that include angiotensin II.

Plasma osmolality is "monitored" via stretch-sensitive channels in osmo-sensitive cells. Changes in plasma osmotic

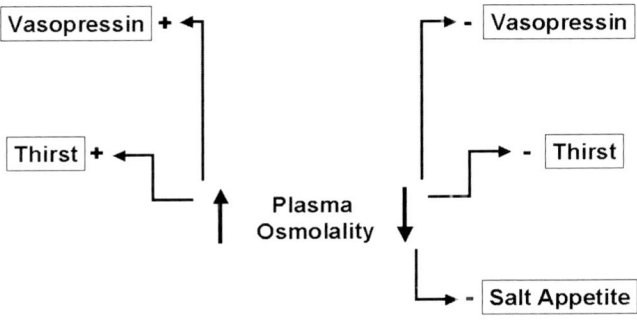

FIGURE 93.4. Responses to changes in plasma osmolality. Slight increases in plasma osmolality stimulate vasopressin secretion; further increases are required to stimulate thirst. Increases in plasma osmolality also suppress salt intake. Decreases in plasma osmolality suppress vasopressin secretion and thirst while activating the salt appetite.

pressure lead to changes in cell volume; stretch-inactivated channels transduce this volume by altering the plasma membrane potential and the likelihood of depolarization. For instance, hyperosmolality leads to cell shrinkage, activation of stretch-inactivated channels, membrane depolarization, and excitation of the neurosecretory cell. This osmotic-sensing capability is intrinsic to vasopressin-producing cells. Local glial cells and neurons in the anterior hypothalamus are also osmosensors and participate in regulating vasopressin release by magnocellular cells (42). Not all osmotically active solutes stimulate vasopressin release, highlighting the role of changes in cell volume in transducing the signal for change in plasma osmolality. Na^+ and mannitol are "effective" solutes because they do not freely permeate the cell membrane, leading to an osmotic gradient, shifts in osmosensor water content, and alterations in vasopressin release. On the other hand, despite their osmotic properties, urea and glucose freely permeate the cell membrane (in the absence of the BBB) and do not generate an osmotic gradient to induce cellular volume changes and vasopressin release. In the absence of insulin (as occurs in diabetic ketoacidosis, DKA), glucose entry into osmosensing cells is impaired, and glucose becomes a stimulant for vasopressin release.

Nonosmotic regulators of vasopressin release include blood pressure, ECF volume (**Fig. 93.5**), pain, nausea, and hypoglycemia. Normally, pressure receptors tonically inhibit vasopressin secretion. In contrast to the small increases in osmolality that stimulate vasopressin release, relatively large decreases in blood pressure (effective ECF volume) are required to mount a vasopressin response. However, unlike the relationship between osmolality and vasopressin, which is linear, the

relationship between blood pressure (volume) and vasopressin is exponential: blood pressure decreases of 5%–10% are required to evoke vasopressin release while decreases of 20%–30% prompt vasopressin secretion many times above that required for maximal antidiuresis. Smaller changes in blood pressure (ECF volume) modulate vasopressin responsiveness, with modest decreases in blood pressure sensitizing vasopressin release to changes in osmolality and increases in blood pressure potentially blunting responses (35).

These responses to blood pressure and ECF volume are mediated through baroreceptors in the cardiovascular system. Activation of neural stretch-sensitive sensors in the cardiac atria, aorta, and carotid arteries leads to tonic inhibition of vasopressin secretion. Pathways for baroreceptor-mediated vasopressin secretion are distinct from those of osmoreceptors; these pathways converge at the level of the vasopressin-secreting cells (6). Angiotensin II, both directly and through neural pathways, has also been implicated in vasopressin release (6). Additional nonosmotic stimuli of vasopressin release are stress, hypoglycemia, and nausea, with the latter being extremely potent—generating vasopressin concentrations 20–40 times that of hyperosmolality.

Multiple pharmacologic agents can either stimulate (isoproterenol, vincristine) or inhibit (opioids, alcohol, carbamazepine) vasopressin release. These agents do not appear to have clinical significance in the absence of pathologic conditions.

The primary antidiuretic activity of vasopressin occurs through recruitment of renal water channels (aquaporin-2) in the collecting duct (35) (**Fig. 93.6**). These collecting ducts traverse the medullary interstitium of the kidney, the site of an increasing concentration gradient, ranging from ~50–60 to 1100–1200 mOsm/kg H_2O. In infants, this range is narrower—200–600 mOsm/kg H_2O. In the absence of vasopressin/aquaporin channels, urine is dilute—~50 mOsm/kg H_2O—reflecting the obligate solute losses by the kidney. With the provision of aquaporin along the tubular side of the collecting ducts, water is absorbed along the concentration gradient. Urine concentration increases linearly with increasing plasma vasopressin concentrations until a maximum above which urine can no longer be further concentrated. This maximum reflects the greatest concentration of the medullary interstitium

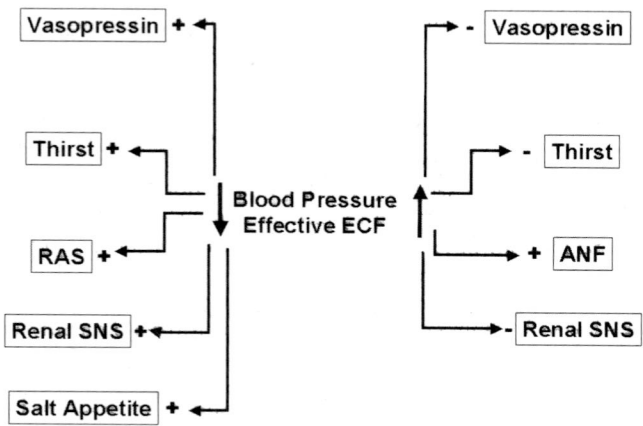

FIGURE 93.5. Responses to changes in blood pressure and effective extracellular fluid volume. Detection of increased blood pressure or effective ECF volume by baroreceptors triggers suppression of vasopressin secretion, thirst, and the renal sympathetic nervous system, while stimulating secretion of A-type natriuretic peptide (ANP). Together, these mechanisms work to lower ECF volume and blood pressure. In contrast, detection of decreased blood pressure or effective ECF volume by baroreceptors triggers secretion of vasopressin, thirst, salt appetite, the rennin angiotensin system, and the renal sympathetic nervous system to effect water and salt retention and, ultimately, an increase in ECF volume. Discrepancies in blood pressure and effective ECF volume do occur; e.g., an increased ECF volume is ineffective, such as occurs with congestive heart failure, and causes additional fluid retention. RAS, renin-angiotensin system; renal SNS, sympathetic nervous system.

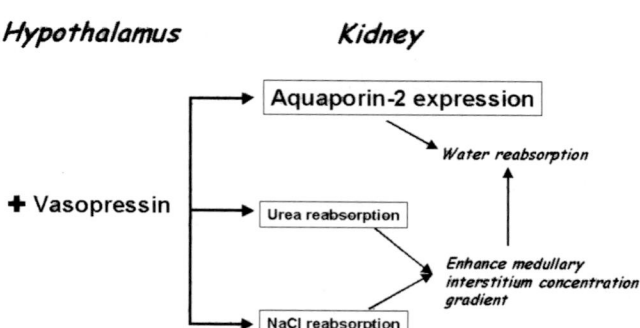

FIGURE 93.6. Effects of vasopressin. Vasopressin secretion by the hypothalamus stimulates fluid retention by increasing aquaporin-2 expression in the renal tubules to promote water absorption from urine. By promoting, to a lesser extent, Na^+ and urea reabsorption in the collecting tubules, vasopressin secretion helps to maintain the concentration gradient of the medullary interstitium and the kidney's ability to concentrate urine.

TABLE 93.1

URINE EXCRETION

Urine concentration (mOsm/kg/H_2O)	Solute for excretion (mOsm)	Urine volume required for solute excretion (L)
50	500	10
1200		0.42
50	1000	20
1200		0.83

and is ~1100–1200 mOsm/kg. This maximum is achieved with plasma vasopressin concentrations of ~4–5 pg/mL, levels achieved with hyperosmolality but much lower than those attained with hypotension and nausea. An example of the amount of urine required to dispose of a normal solute load during various states is presented in **Table 93.1**, emphasizing the importance of vasopressin in maintaining water balance.

The concentration gradient of the corticomedullary interstitium that is responsible for osmotic withdrawal of water from urine in the collecting ducts is achieved through the accumulation of a number of solutes, including Na^+ chloride and urea. Vasopressin may contribute to this gradient by regulating delivery of urea to the medullary interstitium (36) and increasing Na^+ chloride channel expression. Chronic polyuria can "wash out" this concentration gradient, preventing maximum concentration of urine despite adequate amounts of vasopressin. This dilution of the medullary interstitium can occur with excessive fluid intake, such as occurs with primary polydipsia and diabetes insipidus, and can impact the results of a water deprivation test. Vasopressin is important for transcription of aquaporin-2; chronic deficits could conceivably also impact urine-concentrating ability during water deprivation.

Thirst

Thirst is the sensation aroused by the need to replenish body water and is distinguished from an "appetite for water," in which fluid-seeking behaviors occur not because of a physiologic water shortage but to serve other purposes including social and habitual. The thirst center is located in the preoptic medial nucleus in the anterior hypothalamus. As with vasopressin, thirst is regulated by plasma osmolality and blood pressure/volume status. The osmosensors that trigger the preoptic nucleus to trigger the thirst sensation are located in the anterior hypothalamus, specifically the organum vasculosum and subfornical organ, and are outside the BBB (25,39).

Cardiovascular baroreceptors transmit their signals to the thirst center through the vagal and glossopharyngeal nerves via the medulla, while angiotensin II directly stimulates thirst. Hypoosmolality, increased arterial blood pressure, and increased gastric water all inhibit thirst (15,25).

The threshold for activating thirst may be higher than that for vasopressin secretion, ~295 mOsm/kg H_2O. This offsetting is hypothesized to occur to prevent simultaneous activation of thirst and vasopressin secretion, which would obligate frequent water consumption to maintain the set plasma osmolality. In addition, the simultaneous activation of these two mechanisms would predispose to hypo-osmolality, as antidiuresis would be occurring with concomitant water intake. Instead, follow-

ing activation of thirst and consumption of fluids, vasopressin secretion is suppressed. This suppression occurs prior to decreases in osmolality and is thought to occur to minimize the risk of overcorrection of plasma osmolality.

Sodium Homeostasis

Na^+ plays a key role in maintaining ECF volume and blood pressure. Hence, the mechanisms that regulate its abundance primarily revolve around changes in fluid volume/blood pressure and include natriuretic factors, the renin-angiotensin aldosterone system (RAAS), and the sympathetic nervous system.

Salt Appetite

Like the thirst center, the salt appetite center is located in the hypothalamus. It, too, is regulated by ECF Na^+ concentration and effective blood volume. In contrast, however, the desire for salt occurs much more slowly (hours to days) than that for thirst (6).

Renin-Angiotensin System

Two distinct renin-angiotensin systems exist: one in the brain and the other in the periphery, the latter of which only has access to the central nervous system (CNS) at sites where the BBB is absent, such as the posterior pituitary and the circumventricular structures: the vascular organ of the laminar terminalis, the subfornical organ, area postrema, median eminence, and neurohypophysis. Both systems play a role in maintaining fluid status, although data is limited in humans with respect to the brain system (6) (**Fig. 93.7**).

Decreases in circulating blood volume/blood pressure detected by baroreceptors in the renal arterioles, extrarenal baroreceptors, and the renal macula densa stimulate renin release from the renal juxtaglomerular cells. Renin release is inhibited by angiotensin II, vasopressin, and atrial natriuretic factor. A proteolytic enzyme, renin converts hepatically derived angiotensinogen to angiotensin I. Angiotensin-converting enzyme, located throughout the vasculature endothelium (particularly the lung), then converts angiotensin I to the active hormone angiotensin II.

Angiotensin II serves a number of roles in maintaining ECF volume. Circulating angiotensin II has access to brain osmoreceptors in the organum vasculosum and subfornical organ. Activation of these receptors stimulates thirst and vasopressin secretion. Angiotensin II-mediated thirst activation is blunted by increased blood pressure. At the level of the kidney, angiotensin II stimulates Na^+ and water reabsorption (a) directly, by renal proximal tubules, and (b) indirectly, through presynaptic stimulation of intrarenal norepinephrine release and stimulation of adrenal aldosterone secretion (13). Angiotensin II is a potent vasoconstrictor. In the kidney, this vasoconstriction is more potent for the efferent than for the afferent arterioles, thus maintaining glomerular filtration despite decreased renal perfusion; the decreased renal perfusion, nonetheless, contributes to increased filtrate reabsorption.

Angiotensin II derived from the brain contributes to ECF fluid homeostasis through a variety of mechanisms: (a) by increasing thirst, Na^+ appetite, vasopressin and adrenocorticotropic hormone (ACTH) release, and sympathetic output; and (b) by decreasing baroreceptor responsiveness (6).

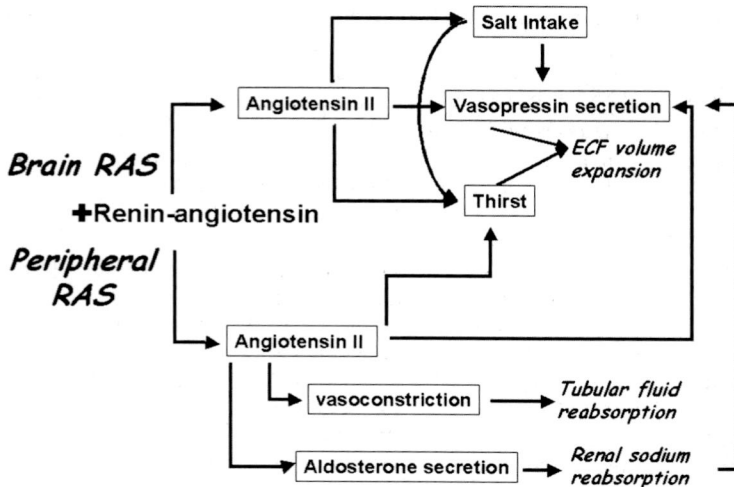

FIGURE 93.7. Effect of the renin-angiotensin system. Both brain and peripheral renin angiotensin systems exist, and both act to preserve ECF volume. Stimulation of both of the systems generates angiotensin II. In the brain, angiotensin II stimulates thirst, salt appetite, and vasopressin secretion. An increase in salt further stimulates thirst and vasopressin secretion. Angiotensin II, generated in the periphery, stimulates thirst, vasopressin secretion, vasoconstriction, which stimulates fluid absorption from the renal tubules, and aldosterone secretion, which promotes renal salt retention. The ultimate result of these intertwined and redundant pathways is an expansion of ECF volume. RAS, renin-angiotensin system; ECF, extracellular fluid.

Aldosterone

Angiotensin II stimulates aldosterone secretion by the adrenal zona glomerulosa, the outermost zone of the adrenal cortex. In addition to angiotensin II, the major regulator for aldosterone secretion, increased plasma K^+ and decreased plasma Na^+ also stimulates aldosterone release.

Like other adrenal steroid hormones, aldosterone is synthesized from cholesterol through the action of a series of enzymes. Steroidogenic acute regulatory protein (StAR) transports cholesterol into the cells of the adrenal cortex. Following entry into the cell, cholesterol is converted to pregnenolone by cytochrome P450 side chain cleavage enzyme. 3-β-hydroxysteroid dehydrogenase then converts pregnenolone to progesterone. 21-α hydroxylase converts progesterone to 11-deoxycorticosterone, an aldosterone precursor with mineralocorticoid activity. Through the action of 11-hydroxylase, this precursor is converted to corticosterone, which is ultimately converted to aldosterone through the activity of aldosterone synthase. Although the three zones of the adrenal cortex (glomerulosa, fasciculata, reticularis) have similar enzymatic machinery, differential expression of specific enzymes imparts the restriction of specific hormones to the various zones: mineralocorticoids to the glomerulosa, glucocorticoids to the fasciculata, and androgens to the reticularis.

The mineralocorticoid properties of aldosterone are imparted through its actions on the principal cells of the cortical ducts, where it increases Na^+ channel expression in the luminal membrane and Na/K-ATPase expression in the basolateral membrane, leading to enhanced Na^+ reabsorption and K^+ excretion (**Fig. 93.8**). Coupled with vasopressin, aldosterone increases ECF: aldosterone-mediated Na^+ reabsorption increases plasma osmolality, triggering vasopressin secretion, and, hence, water reabsorption. In addition, aldosterone increases Na^+/H^+ antiporter activity in renal intercalated cells to enhance hydrogen (H^+) excretion in the urine. These mineralocorticoid effects occur through the interaction of aldosterone with a specific

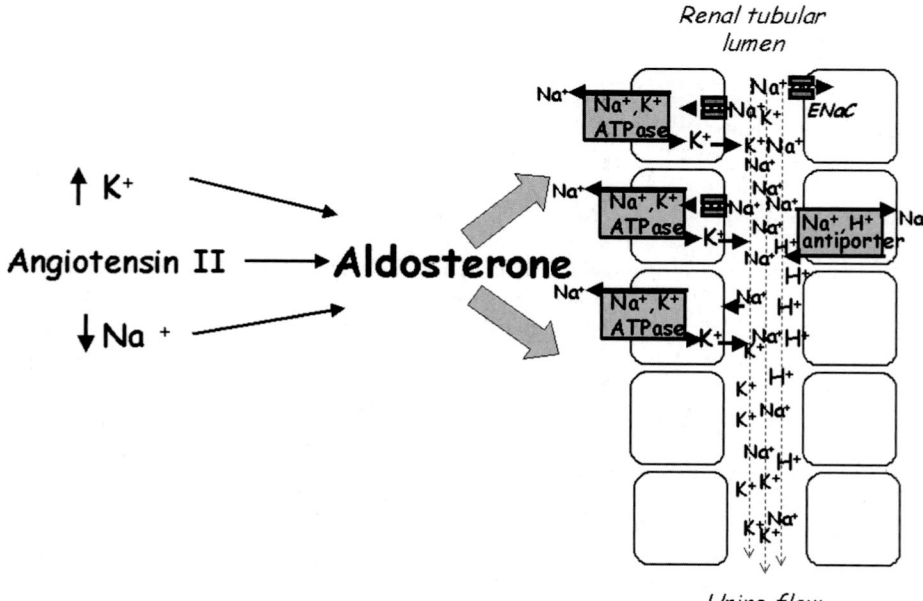

FIGURE 93.8. Stimulants and effects of aldosterone secretion. Hyperkalemia, angiotensin II, and hyponatremia all stimulate aldosterone secretion. Aldosterone then interacts with the mineral corticoid receptors in the distal tubules to effect Na^+ reabsorption by increasing expression of amiloride-sensitive epithelial Na^+ channels (ENaC) in the apical membrane and Na/K-ATPase activity in the basal membrane. Increased Na^+ reabsorption drives K^+ and hydrogen excretion, but aldosterone also directly stimulates excretion of these ions through as yet poorly defined pathways.

receptor. Other adrenal hormones, such as cortisol and deoxy-corticosterone, also bind the mineralocorticoid receptor to affect salt retention. Despite the many-fold higher plasma concentrations of cortisol over aldosterone, cortisol displays significantly lower levels of mineralocorticoid activity. This specificity is conferred through renal expression of 11-β-hydroxysteroid dehydrogenase type 2, an enzyme that inactivates cortisol to cortisone.

Although only 2%–4% of filtered Na⁺ reaches the collecting duct, over a 24-hr period, this amount is substantial. In a 30-kg child (approximate body surface area = 1 m²) with normal renal function (glomerular filtration rate = 110 mL/min/1.73 m²), the kidney filters 90 L/day. With a plasma Na⁺ level of 140 mEq/L, ~12,600 mEq of Na⁺ will be filtered and 252 mEq (2%) will be delivered to the collecting ducts. The 252 mEq represents ~1.8 L ECF—almost one-third of the total ECF in a 30-kg child. Hence, aldosterone plays a key role in maintaining fluid homeostasis.

Natriuretic Peptides

A number of natriuretic peptides have been identified, the prototype of which is A-type natriuretic peptide (ANP); these peptides also include B-type natriuretic peptide (BNP), C-type natriuretic peptide (CNP), and urodilatin. These peptides have a similar 17-amino acid ring structure; their activity spectrum is conferred by their affinity for specific natriuretic receptors. Both CNS and peripheral natriuretic systems exist (**Fig. 93.9**) (6).

ANP, previously referred to as atrial natriuretic peptide, is a 28-amino acid hormone produced both by the hypothalamus and the cardiac atrial myocytes. Atrial myocytes release ANP in response to distention of the cardiac atria, as occurs in the setting of fluid overload. β-adrenergic stimulation also promotes ANP release. ANP lowers circulating volume and, hence, blood pressure through a variety of mechanisms. Through its effects on the renal vasculature, ANP increases the glomerular filtration rate, thereby promoting fluid excretion. It decreases renal Na⁺ reabsorption by the distal convoluted tubules and collecting ducts, thereby promoting natriuresis. In addition, it inhibits renin secretion. Given that angiotensin II stimulates ANP secretion, ANP provides negative feedback for the renin-angiotensin system. ANP also directly inhibits aldosterone secretion by the adrenal glomerulosa and relaxes vascular smooth muscle. Hypothalamic ANP may potentiate ANP secretion by the cardiac atria. In addition, ANP participates in water metabolism by inhibiting thirst (6,40).

BNP, formerly referred to as brain natriuretic peptide, is a 32-amino acid peptide secreted by the ventricular myocardium in response to excessive stretching (i.e., fluid overload). Its mode of action is similar to that of ANP, although it binds to the natriuretic peptide receptor with much lower affinity. Its half-life is only 22 mins, allowing it to dynamically reflect the state of the heart. Consequently, plasma BNP concentrations are used in the diagnosis and management of heart failure (6,40).

CNP is produced by vascular endothelial cells. Although a member of the natriuretic peptide family, CNP does not directly induce natriuresis and is thought to have an autocrine/paracrine effect at the level of the endothelium. This difference between ANP/BNP and CNP arises from selective affinities for the natriuretic receptors (type A for the former and type B for the latter).

Cellular Responses to Disturbances in Plasma Osmolality

Proper cellular function depends upon preservation of ICF osmolality. Because changes in ECF osmolality elicit transmembrane cellular shifts in water and solute, the mechanisms previously described are critical for preserving both ECF and ICF homeostasis. In addition, cellular mechanisms exist to maintain ICF osmolality in the face of chronic perturbations in ECF osmolality. These compensatory mechanisms, however, can

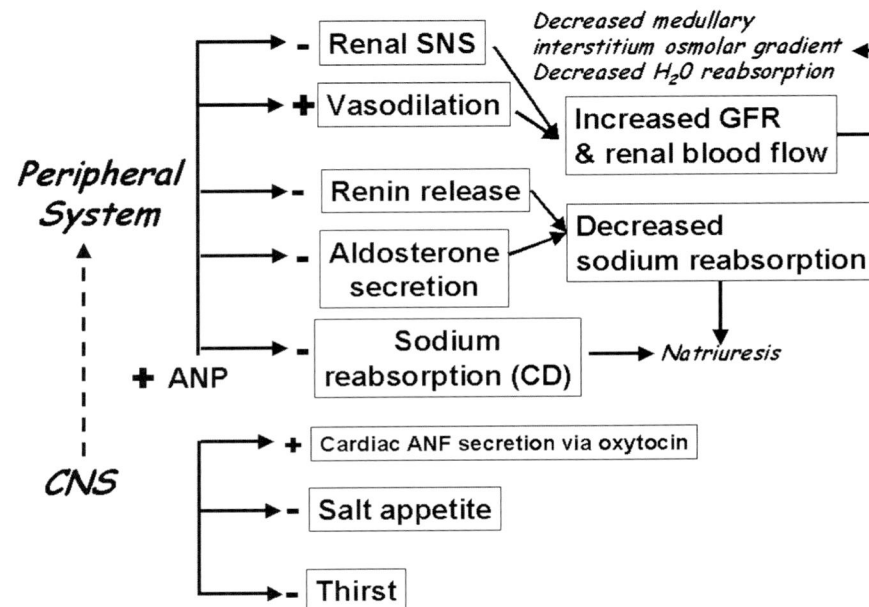

FIGURE 93.9. Activities of A-type natriuretic peptide (ANP). ANP acts both centrally and peripherally to mediate its effects. Centrally, ANP suppresses thirst and salt appetite while promoting additional ANP release by the heart. Peripherally, ANP promotes vasodilation and inhibits the renal sympathetic nervous system (SNS) to increase glomerular filtration (GFR) and, ultimately, urine output. In addition, it directly inhibits renin and aldosterone secretion and Na⁺ reabsorption at the collecting duct (CD), to promote natriuresis.

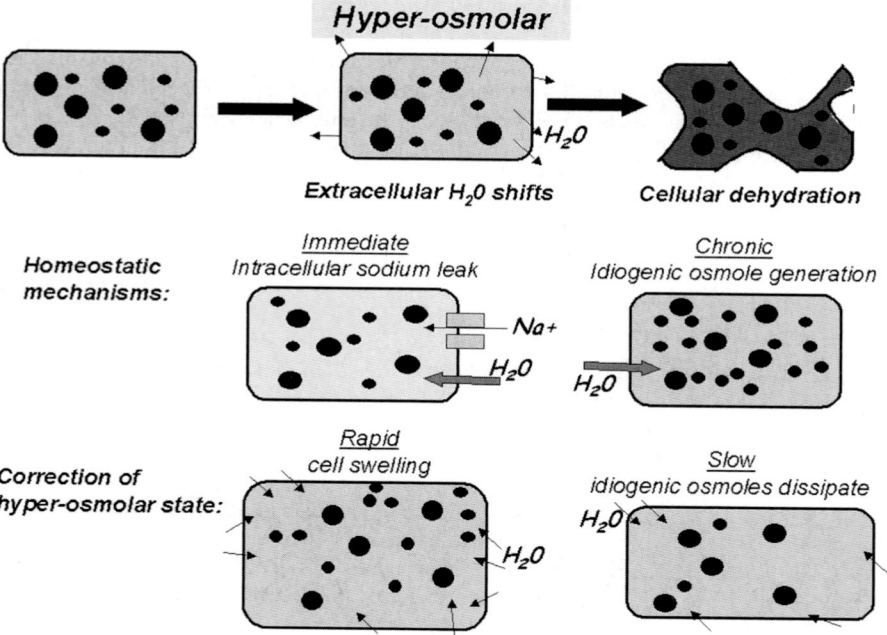

FIGURE 93.10. Cellular responses to hyperosmolality. Hyperosmolar ECF promotes movement of water from the ICF to the ECF and, thus, cell shrinkage. To preserve cell volume, Na$^+$ leakage into the cell occurs; water accompanies this movement to the intracellular space. The cellular response to chronic hyperosmolality is the generation of "idiogenic osmoles," which shifts water from the ECF to the ICF, preserving cell volume. Rapid correction of the chronic hyperosmolar state causes excessive shifts of water into the ICF because idiogenic osmoles persist intracellularly.

predispose to significant disturbances in ICF during therapeutic interventions and, thus, frequently dictate our delivery of fluid and solute to patients.

In response to an increase in plasma osmolality, water is shifted from the ICF to ECF in an attempt to maintain a balance in osmolality (**Fig. 93.10**). An intracellular leak of Na$^+$ is accompanied by a shift of water to the ICF to help prevent cellular dehydration. Additionally, hypothalamic, pituitary, and renal mechanisms are invoked to preserve body water. Significant hyperosmolality occurring abruptly can be accompanied by cellular shrinkage and likely accounts for the abrupt clinical symptomatology that accompanies such perturbations. On the other hand, for many cell types, additional mechanisms operate in response to chronic hyperosmolar states. For instance, in the brain, idiogenic osmoles are generated to offset increased plasma osmolality and reestablish normal intracellular volume without further increasing intracellular Na$^+$ and chloride that can interrupt normal metabolism (32). These "compatible" (idiogenic) osmoles include inositol, glycine, and taurine, and do not interfere with cellular metabolism. However, the generation

of these osmoles presents a therapeutic dilemma for clinicians, as rapid correction of the hyperosmolar state in their presence can lead to cellular swelling (i.e., cerebral edema).

In response to a decrease in plasma osmolality, water is shifted to the intracellular compartment, thereby reestablishing the equilibrium between ECF and ICF (**Fig. 93.11**). The increase in cellular volume that accompanies these shifts activates Na/K-ATPase: Na$^+$ is exported extracellularly and is accompanied by water, minimizing the risk of cellular swelling. To compensate for chronic hypoosmolality, idiogenic osmoles are extruded and normal cell volume preserved (31).

Potassium Homeostasis

K$^+$ plays a key role in creating the resting membrane potential of the cell and does so because of the significant transcellular concentration gradient maintained through the activity of Na/K-ATPase. The ICF contains nearly 98% of total body (40–50 mEq/kg) K$^+$ and has a K$^+$ concentration of 140–150 mEq/L.

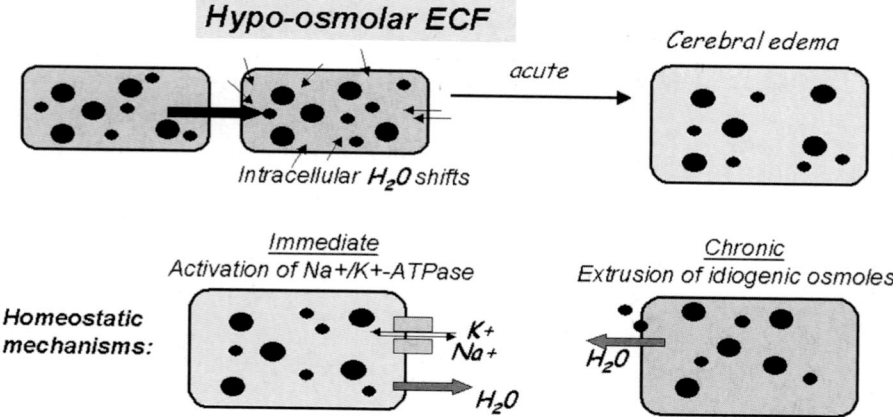

FIGURE 93.11. Cellular responses to hypoosmolality. Hypo-osmolar ECF promotes water shifts from the ECF to the ICF. Acutely, large shifts cause cellular edema. To minimize cellular swelling, Na/K-ATPase is activated and water is shunted with Na$^+$ to the extracellular space. The cell adapts to chronic hypo-osmolality by extruding idiogenic osmoles, thus lowering the gradient between the ICF and the ECF.

The concentration of K^+ in the ECF, the site of the remaining 2% of total body K^+, ranges from 3.5–5.5 mEq/L. Because K^+ is primarily located intracellularly, plasma K^+ concentration may not accurately reflect changes in total body stores.

As occurs with Na^+ and water, the kidneys play a large role in responding to variable inputs of K^+ to ensure total body K^+ homeostasis. Transport of K^+ with Na^+ occurs in the proximal tubule and thick ascending limb and accounts for over 90% of K^+ reabsorbed from glomerular filtrate. The distal tubules and cortical-collecting ducts can then reabsorb the majority of the remaining K^+, if necessary.

Dietary intake frequently exceeds the amount of K^+ available for excretion following the initial reabsorption phase, and secretion of K^+ must occur in the distal tubules and cortical collecting ducts to prevent a positive K^+ balance. Hence, K^+ regulation largely occurs in the distal tubules and cortical-collecting ducts. With increased plasma K^+ concentration, K^+ directly stimulates its secretion by activating Na/K-ATPase and luminal Na^+ and K^+ channels.

In addition, increases in ECF K^+ stimulate aldosterone secretion, thereby indirectly stimulating K^+ excretion in urine. Aldosterone interacts with the mineralocorticoid receptor in renal principal cells, which comprise the majority of the tubular epithelium in the late distal tubules and cortical-collecting ducts. Stimulation of the mineralocorticoid receptor upregulates Na/K-ATPase activity at the basolateral membrane, thereby effecting an increase in intracellular K^+ (**Fig. 93.8**). Because the luminal border of the principal cells is highly permeable to K^+ (unlike other renal tubular cells), K^+ can flow down its concentration gradient into the tubular lumen for excretion. Aldosterone also acts upon the colon to stimulate Na^+ reabsorption and K^+ secretion.

Other nonrenal regulators of K^+ include insulin, catecholamines, and acid-base balance. Insulin promotes intracellular K^+ uptake through direct stimulation of Na/K-ATPase; the importance of basal insulin in maintaining plasma K^+ within a normal range is highlighted by insulin-deficient states, which are characterized by hyperkalemia.

The sympathetic nervous system regulates the transcellular K^+ gradient through opposing mechanisms. Stimulation of β_2-adrenergic receptors activates Na/K-ATPase, thereby lowering plasma K^+ concentrations. This activity may prevent excessive ECF K^+ concentrations due to exercise-induced K^+ release by muscles. Stimulation of α-adrenergic receptors triggers movement of K^+ to the ECF.

Metabolic acidosis caused by mineral acids triggers a shift in K^+ to the extracellular space in exchange for hydrogen ions. Respiratory acidosis and metabolic organic acidosis less consistently cause these shifts because blood pH is not the sole determinant of K^+ shifts. Studies suggest that these differences in the setting of metabolic acidoses may arise from the different hormonal responses evoked by organic versus mineral acids, with ketoacids stimulating an insulin response and hydrogen chloride stimulating a glucagon response (4).

CLINICAL PRESENTATION AND DIFFERENTIAL DIAGNOSIS

Many of the disorders resulting in disturbances of Na^+ and K^+ frequently do not cause clinical symptoms unless accompanied by disturbances of hydration. However, children admitted to the PICU frequently have associated ventilatory difficulties, severe muscle weakness, neurologic symptoms (including seizures, coma, tremors, and disorientation), nausea, vomiting, and even cardiac arrhythmias. Disturbances in Na^+ or K^+ are commonly coincident to other serious comorbidities (such as a child admitted for a head injury and found to have unrelated hyponatremia due to diuretics) and may be confusing to the medical staff, raising issues of pituitary stalk injury. More likely, however, a clear association exists between the biochemical findings and preceding medical events in the critically ill child. Hence, a complete past medical history, including medications, family history as to a potential genetic disorder, and the events antecedent to the PICU admission, are essential for narrowing the differential diagnosis of the biochemical abnormality.

Disorders of Sodium Balance

Differential Diagnosis of Hypernatremic Conditions

The disorders that can result in hypernatremic states (as noted in **Table 93.2**) include some that are only infrequent problems of management in the intensive care setting. The more common disorders are associated with dehydration. Nevertheless, the differential diagnosis of even those disorders uncommon in the ICU will be included for completeness.

Hypernatremic Disorders Generally Associated with Normal Hydration. Hypothalamic hypodipsia arises from loss of function of the hypothalamic thirst center incurred by brain injury or, less commonly, acquired congenitally. This brain insult may be due to head trauma, brain tumor, or injury sustained during surgery for a CNS abnormality. Affected children often have elevated Na^+ levels but remain asymptomatic. Such children are not likely to be admitted to the PICU for hypernatremic dehydration unless a comorbid condition results in critical illness. History of known insufficient fluid intake, brain injury or developmental delay, lack of polyuria, and previous findings of asymptomatic hypernatremia will distinguish such patients from those with acute hypernatremia. Central hypoventilation syndrome is associated with hypothalamic hypodipsia and can be both congenital and late-onset, although the

TABLE 93.2

HYPERNATREMIC CONDITIONS

Clinically normal hydration (or mild hypervolemia)
  Hypothalamic hypodipsia
  Iatrogenic
  Hyperaldosteronism
  Cushing syndrome

Clinically dehydrated (or mild dehydration to normal hydration)
  Diabetes insipidus (central or nephrogenic)
  Hypertonic dehydration—gastrointestinal losses (infection, fistulas)
  Skin loss—burns, fever, excessive sweating (over heating)
  Drugs—alcohol ingestion, diuretics

congenital form is less likely to be associated with hypothalamic problems. The major issues in children with central hypoventilation syndromes are, in fact, due to hypoventilation; therefore, these children might be admitted to the PICU for care because of their need for mechanical respiratory support.

Congenital central hypoventilation syndrome (CCHS) generally presents in the newborn period with periodic apnea and hypoventilation. This condition is often associated with Hirschsprung disease (20% of patients with congenital hypoventilation syndrome) and other autonomic nervous dysfunction, as well as tumors of the neural crest. This condition arises from mutations of the *PHOX 2B* gene that encodes a transcription factor in the developing hindbrain and peripheral nervous system (44). The main issue with children with CCHS is hypoventilation during sleep, which results in hypercapnia and hypoxemia. Affected infants often die with cor pulmonale, respiratory failure, sepsis, and aspiration. However, since identification of mutations in *PHOX 2B* in this syndrome, variable expression of this disorder has been appreciated. In fact, patients with *PHOX 2B* mutations may present later in life, with one such patient identified at 35 years of age following a history of "snoring" throughout life. The genetic pattern of inheritance is autosomal dominant with variable penetrance and expression and with many mutations arising de novo. In general, children with CCHS have normal growth and have intact hypothalamic function, including that of the thirst center (unlike late-onset central hypoventilation syndrome).

Late-onset central hypoventilation syndrome (LOCHS) overlaps with CCHS because the latter is also associated with neural crest tumors and central hypoventilation during sleep. However, LOCHS is frequently associated with hypothalamic dysfunction, including hypothalamic obesity, variable degrees of hypopituitarism, and hypernatremia secondary to hypodipsia, as well as some degree of vasopressin deficiency (but generally without polyuria) (21). Many children with LOCHS have asymptomatic hypernatremia, with a Na+ concentration of 145 mEq/L–155 mEq/L, but they develop somnolence when Na+ levels exceed these values. *PHOX2B* mutations have not been associated with the majority of LOCHS patients despite the commonality of sleep-associated central hypoventilation and neural crest tumors (as well as Hirschsprung disease). This is especially true of the LOCHS patients with the phenotype of obesity and hypothalamic-pituitary dysfunction.

Iatrogenic causes of hypernatremia are generally recognizable because such children are invariably being treated with IV solutions or tube feedings. Clearly, the prolonged use of hypertonic saline or even continued use of normal saline in certain states, such as diabetes ketoacidosis after correction of hyperglycemia and hydration, can result in hypernatremia.

Primary hyperaldosteronism is unlikely to occur in children, whereas Cushing syndrome may occur (often due to primary adrenal tumors and less commonly due to pituitary adenoma). The more common cause of Cushing syndrome in PICU patients is iatrogenic, due to prolonged use of high-dose glucocorticoids in patients admitted because of worsening of the primary morbidity for which they are receiving glucocorticoid treatment. In glucocorticoid excess (iatrogenic or otherwise), Na+ is only modestly elevated at best.

Hypernatremic Conditions Associated with Dehydration (or Normal Hydration). Many of the disorders that result in free water loss can be overcome with water intake, and relatively

TABLE 93.3

CAUSES OF CENTRAL DIABETES INSIPIDUS

Genetic
  Autosomal dominant inheritance
  Autosomal recessive inheritance
  Wolfram syndrome (DIDMOAD syndrome) autosomal recessive
  X-linked recessive inherited (associated with Xq2B)

Anatomic congenital malformation
  Septo-optic dysplasia
  Holoprosencephaly
  Pituitary agenesis

Acquired
  CNS tumors that involve hypothalamus or pituitary stalk (germinoma, craniopharyngioma)
  Trauma—severing pituitary stalk
  Surgery involving pituitary stalk (removal of craniopharyngioma or optic glioma)
  Hypophysitis
  Granulomatous disease—histiocytosis, sarcoid
  Infection—meningitis, encephalitis
  Vascular injury

DIDMOAD—DI, diabetes insipidus; DM, diabetes mellitus; OA, optic atrophy; D, deafness; CNS, central nervous system

normal Na+ levels and normal hydration can be preserved. However, if the fluid intake in response to free water loss contains significant electrolytes, hypernatremia is the outcome, despite normal hydration. Conversely, loss of free water without replacement will result in dehydration as well as hypernatremia.

Diabetes insipidus (DI) can arise from vasopressin deficiency (central DI) or vasopressin insensitivity (nephrogenic DI). The various causes of central DI are listed in **Table 93.3.** Children with congenital forms of DI, both central and nephrogenic variants, rarely are admitted to the PICU unless an intercurrent illness interferes with their routine management. The most common reason for children with DI to be admitted to the PICU is for postoperative management of resection of a craniopharyngioma or other midline intracranial tumors such as astrocytoma. These resections frequently require severing of the pituitary stalk, although they may be accompanied by reversible injury/edema to the area. Vasopressin deficiency follows severing of the pituitary stalk/injury. In some children, a phase of excessive, although temporary, vasopressin release can follow this initial deficient state. This second phase reflects release of stored vasopressin from necrotic vasopressin-secreting neurons. Varying degrees of vasopressin deficiency then ensue, reflecting the extent of retrograde neuronal degeneration of vasopressin-secreting neurons. In general, the higher the injury to the pituitary stalk, the greater the number of vasopressin-secreting axons that will be damaged (as the axons terminate at different levels along the stalk) and the greater the loss of vasopressin-secreting neurons. During this second phase of stored vasopressin release, hyponatremia can occur if fluid management is not curbed and/or vasopressin administration is continued. Following this brief period of vasopressin release, permanent DI is the usual outcome. DI can also result from head trauma, which can manifest this "triple phase" as well. Profuse polyuria is evident during the initial phase, but urine output diminishes when stored vasopressin is released. Because the patient is often being managed with aggressive fluid replacement, the intensivist must monitor Na^+ often, being cognizant of this second phase that can result in sudden profound hyponatremia. Hypothalamic brain tumors, such as a germinoma or ependymoma, or pituitary stalk lesions, such as histiocytosis, will often present with central DI. Generally, ICU physicians are aware of the presence of these lesions.

Severe diarrhea or other forms of gastrointestinal loss of water, especially in very young children being treated with oral electrolyte fluid, can result in hypertonic dehydration. The child will be often be obtunded, with a doughy-like skin that will "tent" when pinched during assessment for degree of dehydration. The history of profuse watery diarrhea and oral electrolyte replacement should alert the admitting physician to administer fluids judiciously.

The loss of free water due to injury to the skin (as in burns), excessive heat, or fever with profuse sweating is a relatively rare situation in children, except in the well-publicized cases of children locked inside automobiles or enclosed rooms without ventilation during extremely hot weather. Fluid and electrolyte management of children with burns is discussed in the section Hyponatremia with Clinically Normal Hydration.

Diuretics that affect the loop of Henle in the kidney can result in mild hypernatremia. In addition, the accidental (or intentional) ingestion of alcohol will inhibit vasopressin release and cause excessive loss of free water. In an adolescent, the history of excessive alcohol intake and the clinical findings of vomiting and disturbed mental status with disorientation are indicative of this cause of hypernatremia. Historical information regarding medications, including diuretics or alcohol ingestion, provides the explanation of the cause of hypernatremia and directs the management as needed. The clinical management of the obtunded adolescent or child due to alcohol exposure is dictated by the dehydration and hypernatremia as well as by the seriousness of alcohol poisoning of brain function.

Differential Diagnosis of Hyponatremic Conditions

Disorders associated with hyponatremia can be separated into those with clinically normal hydration (or mild overhydration) and those with clinical dehydration as outlined in **Table 93.4**.

TABLE 93.4

HYPONATREMIC CONDITIONS

Associated with clinically normal hydration (or mild hypervolemia)
SIADH
Iatrogenic—water overload
Protein loss
Renal disease
Skin loss
Central adrenal insufficiency
Hypothyroidism
Associated with clinical dehydration
Salt-wasting (cerebral, renal tubular)
Primary adrenal insufficiency
Non-ketotic hyperosmolar coma
Drugs—diuretics

Hyponatremia with Clinically Normal Hydration. Syndrome of inappropriate antidiuretic hormone (SIADH) is actually a clinical description of a critically ill child with profound hyponatremia in the face of normal hydration (and even perhaps evidence of mild overhydration) and lack of polyuria. SIADH is one of the most common causes of hyponatremia in the ICU. The urinary Na^+ is disproportionately elevated for the degree of hyponatremia. The plasma concentration of vasopressin is elevated or at least relatively elevated for the degree of hyponatremia. SIADH may arise through multiple mechanisms, but the exact CNS pathophysiologic mechanisms are not completely characterized. SIADH is associated with a number of conditions, especially brain injury due to CNS radiation and surgery, as well as congenital malformations. Mechanical ventilation can cause SIADH. A number of chemotherapeutic agents used to treat childhood cancer, including vincristine and cyclophosphamide, have also been implicated as causing SIADH. Parenthetically, as discussed later, some of these same chemotherapeutic agents cause renal tubular injury, resulting in salt and water wasting (causing hyponatremia and raising diagnostic and, therefore, management issues). As a result of plasma expansion during SIADH, ANP may be elevated and exacerbate the hyponatremic condition by causing renal salt wasting. This compensatory response has led to the misdiagnosis of SIADH as cerebral salt wasting, a hyponatremic condition associated with polyuria and natriuresis from inappropriate secretion of BNP, as discussed later. These salt-wasting conditions are part of the major diagnostic dilemmas in managing SIADH, especially in that the primary causes of the conditions overlap.

Hyponatremia due to excessive free water ingestion is extremely uncommon because of the number of endogenous counter-regulatory mechanisms available to prevent such an event from occurring. In critically ill children, free water overload can occur from resuscitation efforts using hypotonic solutions or from excessive free water administered to patients with central diabetes insipidus on vasopressin therapy. In otherwise healthy infants, excessive free water intake due to overdilution of formula or excessive administration of tap/bottled water can also cause hyponatremia. The inability of the infant to handle the free water load has been attributed to immaturity of the kidney, including a low glomerular filtration rate.

In protein-losing disorders, such as in nephrotic syndrome, interstitial fluid volume expansion often results in symptoms of fluid overload, such as edema or ascites, but also may result in intravascular hypovolemia due to these fluid shifts. Counter-regulatory Na^+-retaining mechanisms are stimulated, resulting in increased total body Na^+ and water but mild hyponatremia. Urinary Na^+ excretion is low.

Renal disease, both acute and chronic renal failure, with reduced glomerular filtration and loss of tubular function, is a known cause of hyponatremia. Hyponatremia is also associated with postrenal transplant. Multiple mechanisms exist and involve many of the factors discussed previously in the physiology section, including water retention, unresponsiveness to aldosterone, tubular loss of Na^+, and hyperkalemic metabolic acidosis. This form of hyponatremia is easily recognizable by history, the elevated K^+, elevated phosphorus levels, azotemia, and elevated creatinine levels. The management is more complex and often requires therapeutic measures such as dialysis.

Loss of Na^+ through skin can be substantial, especially in patients with cystic fibrosis or adrenal insufficiency during periods of excessive heat, or in very febrile patients, or those with significant burns. As mentioned previously, water is also lost during these circumstances, but salt loss is especially concerning in patients with cystic fibrosis, salt-wasting congenital adrenal hyperplasia, and other forms of adrenal insufficiency. Furthermore, hyponatremia can develop if thirst is treated by ingestion of nonelectrolyte fluids during periods of excessive heat and excessive perspiration.

Central adrenal insufficiency (i.e., secondary or tertiary corticotrophin-releasing hormone or ACTH deficiency) results in insufficient glucocorticoid production, especially during stress. Because glucocorticoids (a) have an adjunctive role in aldosterone production, (b) suppress production of nitric oxide (nitric oxide causes vasopressin-independent insertion of aquaporin-2 into renal tubules), and (c) suppress vasopressin production, mild hyponatremia without hyperkalemia can occur with central adrenal insufficiency; this is true as well in the syndromes of ACTH insensitivity. Affected patients do not have the marked water and electrolyte problems of primary adrenal insufficiency because the adrenal zona glomerulosa is regulated by the renin-angiotensin system and not affected by ACTH deficiency. These conditions are discussed in more detail in the chapter concerning adrenal function (Chapter 91).

Thyroid hormone deficiency results in a decreased glomerular filtration rate and decreased renal plasma blood flow, but patients have no difficulty in excreting a salt load. Very rarely, a severely myxedematous patient can have profound hyponatremia. The edema is nonpitting, and the patients are sallow in complexion and carotinemic in appearance. Hypothyroidism is an extremely unlikely cause of hyponatremia in children, as growth failure occurs years earlier before such a profound state of hyponatremia and myxedema occur.

Hyponatremia Associated with Clinical Dehydration. Salt wasting can occur at the level of the renal tubules either from a primary tubular defect or through medication or a hormone-mediated process. Because salt wasting is associated with simultaneous water loss, it can result in severe hyponatremia and clinical dehydration. In patients with brain tumor-related DI, chemotherapeutic treatment with salt-wasting agents such as cisplatin can make management difficult. In addition, natriuretic peptide-mediated cerebral salt wasting secondary to brain injury, surgery, radiation, or infection can complicate management and diagnosis in the same patient with central DI. Severe hyponatremia in the setting of persistent urine output

raises questions as to whether the patient has (a) SIADH and compensatory ANP production from fluid overload, (b) cerebral salt wasting, or (c) vasopressin insufficiency in the setting of a salt-losing process. The clue to differentiating CSW from SIADH is hydration status. The child with CSW will be dehydrated; the child with SIADH has normal-to-expanded blood volume. The clinical picture becomes more complicated in the child with DI who also develops CSW as a result of underlying CNS pathology or radiation therapy. The finding of a coexisting salt-losing process in the patient with central DI requires vasopressin administration to be withheld; Na^+ concentrations are normalized with salt replacement while intravascular volume is repleted. The clinical and biochemical differences between these often coexisting conditions are listed in **Table 93.5**.

Primary adrenal crisis causes the characteristic findings of hyponatremia and severe hyperkalemia and metabolic acidosis. The condition is generally associated with shock, hypotension, tachycardia, cardiac arrhythmias, and severe obtundation. The patient may be hyperpigmented. This condition is discussed fully in Chapter 91.

The patient with type 2 diabetes who presents in the nonketotic hyperosmolar state can have significant urinary Na^+ loss from the osmotic diuresis and can have additional salt loss in vomitus. Although the patient is total-body Na^+ depleted, the degree of hyponatremia is more reflective of an osmotic shift in intracellular water, with some degree of spurious hyponatremia. This cause of hyponatremia and the clinical manifestations of nonketotic hyperosmolar coma are discussed more fully in the section on glucose homeostasis (Chapter 92).

Prolonged use of diuretics, especially in the presence of concomitant salt restriction, can cause volume-contracted hyponatremia. The loop diuretics, such as furosemide, inhibit salt absorption in the medullary ascending limb of the loop of Henle, causing Na^+ loss but rarely causing hyponatremia. The thiazide diuretics inhibit the sodium chloride (NaCl) cotransporter reabsorption at the cortical diluting segments (the early distal convoluted tubule), but evidence also suggests that thiazides promote retention of free water by upregulation of aquaporin channels in the renal tubule collecting ducts. Therefore, thiazides are associated with greater risk, and studies suggest that hyponatremia is more common and more severe with the thiazides. It is important to note that diuretics are K^+-depleting as well, and correction requires both Na^+ and K^+ replacement.

TABLE 93.5

CLINICAL AND BIOCHEMICAL FINDINGS IN PATIENTS WITH DI AND INADEQUATELY TREATED DIABETES INSIPIDUS, IATROGENIC FLUID OVERLOAD OR VASOPRESSIN EXCESS, SIADH, AND SALT WASTING

| Disorder | Clinical and biochemical findings | | | |
	Serum sodium	Urine sodium	Urine output	Hydration
DI—inadequate treatment	High	Low	High	Dehydrated
Excess DDAVP or water excess	Low	Low	Normal or Low	Normal or mild edema
SIADH	Low	High	Low	Normal or mild edema
Salt wasting	Low	High	High	Dehydrated

DI, diabetes insipidus; DDAVP, 1-deamino(8-D-arginine) vasopressin; SIADH, syndrome of inappropriate antidiuretic hormone

Disorders of Potassium Balance

Differential Diagnosis of Hyperkalemic Disorders

Although the disorders of hyperkalemia are separated into mild, moderate, and severe hyperkalemia in **Table 93.6**, the clinical disturbances might not be reflected by serum concentrations of K^+. In general, mild hyperkalemia refers to plasma K^+ in the 5–6 mE/L range, without ECG changes or with only tall T waves; moderate hyperkalemia refers to plasma K^+ in the 6–7 mE/L range, with ECG changes that reveal absent P waves and wide QRS complexes; and severe hyperkalemia refers to plasma K^+ levels of >7–8 and ventricular arrhythmias. It is the intracellular content of K^+ that is of major concern. The acid-base status, serum calcium and Na^+ concentrations, and rate of change in K^+ concentrations all influence the clinical threat of hyperkalemia. The complaints vary from fatigue to muscle weakness, disorientation, paresthesias, and palpitations. The major concern is cardiac dysfunction due to the hyperkalemia, with asystole being the most serious outcome. Initially, hyperkalemia is demonstrated by tall-peaked T waves, then by a prolonged P-R interval, and then flattened or absent P waves. Concern for major cardiac disturbances and asystole is heightened by ECG findings that demonstrate widening QRS intervals, merging ST waves, and then bradycardia, all of which precede ventricular tachycardia. As an example, in salt-losing congenital adrenal hyperplasia, patients occasionally have serum concentrations of K^+ of 9 or 10 mEq/L without any cardiac manifestations or ECG changes.

Mild Elevations of Potassium Level. Routine serum electrolyte determinations often find mild elevations of K^+ secondary to hemolysis of red blood cells during the blood sampling. A form of spurious hyperkalemia (also referred to as *pseudohyperkalemia*) may be found, especially in hyperviscosity syndromes. No ECG abnormalities are present with spurious hyperkalemia.

Dietary ingestion of high K^+-containing foods or K^+ salt substitutes rarely causes hyperkalemia, but such cases with mild elevation of serum K^+ concentration have been reported. Fasting or chronic starvation, such as occurs in anorexia nervosa, can result in suppression of insulin production and mild hyperkalemia. The list of drugs that have resulted in mild hyperkalemia is extensive and includes β-blockers, angiotensin-converting enzyme inhibitors, and nonsteroidal anti-inflammatory drugs.

Moderate to Occasionally Severe Elevation of Potassium Levels. A number of drugs, including K^+-sparing diuretics, such as spironolactone, can raise K^+ levels. Other drugs that interfere with the renin-angiotensin system (including losartan) may cause hyperkalemia.

Massive cell death, such as occurs with tumor lysis or rhabdomyolysis, can cause hyperkalemia. Massive blood transfusion and red cell lysis during mechanical dialysis can similarly cause red cell breakdown and increase serum K^+ levels. Rhabdomyolysis that results in cell death and hyperkalemia has occurred during treatment of DKA because of prolonged use of isotonic saline in the hypernatremic patient after restoration of hydration and fluid volume, as noted by normal glucose levels and normal acid-base balance.

An interesting cause of hyperkalemia is the genetic form of hyperkalemic periodic paralysis. Periodic paralysis includes a group of genetic disorders with mutations in Na^+, calcium, and K^+ channels. Hyperkalemic periodic paralysis presents with attacks of disabling weakness and elevated serum K^+ levels. In a large study of kindreds, mutations of the Na^+ channel were found in 64%, and none were found in 36% (26). The onset was young (approximately age 2 years) in those in whom mutations were found and much older (approximately age 14) in those in whom no mutations were found. Attacks were more frequent in those with mutations. The average serum K^+ levels ranged between 4.9 and 6.1 mEq/L, with the lower levels in those patients in whom no mutations were found. A number of precipitants for these attacks are known, including cold, exercise, and hunger. Occasionally, cardiac arrhythmias are found, especially in the form of hyperkalemic periodic paralysis, referred to as Andersen-Tawil syndrome, which arises from mutations in a gene encoding a K^+ channel; the phenotype includes cardiac arrhythmias, dysmorphia, and periodic paralysis, in the setting of elevated, normal, or low K^+.

Potassium Disorders with Marked Elevation of Potassium. Renal disease, including chronic renal insufficiency, acute renal failure, and end-stage renal failure can be associated with significant hyperkalemia. In acute renal failure, the increase in K^+ levels may be rapid and tolerated poorly. In more chronic situations, despite K^+ levels of 7 to 8 mEq/L, cardiac function and ECG findings remain normal. Chronicity of renal failure often leads to tolerance of even moderately severe hyperkalemia.

Patients with primary adrenal crisis present in shock, dehydration, and often, with cardiac arrhythmias. The biochemical abnormalities include hyponatremia, severe hyperkalemia, and a nonanion gap metabolic acidosis.

Type IV renal tubular acidosis occurs in states of aldosterone deficiency or insensitivity and manifests as persistent hyperkalemia, reduced bicarbonate reabsorption, and potentially mild-to-moderate glomerular insufficiency. One form of type IV renal tubular acidosis is associated with an obstructive uropathy that damages the juxtaglomerular apparatus, leading to hyporeninemia and subsequent hypoaldosteronism. However, in the setting of primary aldosterone deficiency or resistance, renin will be elevated.

TABLE 93.6

HYPERKALEMIC CONDITIONS

Mild increase
  Spurious hyperkalemia
  Dietary intake of potassium
  Fasting

Moderate (to severe) increase
  Drugs
  Cell death—tumor lysis
  Hyperkalemic periodic paralysis

Severe hyperkalemia
  Chronic and acute renal failure
  Adrenal insufficiency
  Low-renin hyperkalemia

Differential Diagnosis of the Hypokalemic Disorders

Hypokalemia is generally less threatening than hyperkalemia. Nevertheless, low K^+ levels can be associated with cardiac arrhythmias, particularly in the setting of preexisting cardiac problems. In general, no symptoms or only mild weakness are present. Certainly, muscular weakness can be associated with ileus or respiratory difficulties. The disorders of hypokalemia are listed in **Table 93.7**.

Drugs, such as K^+-losing diuretics, are a frequent cause of mild hypokalemia. Generally, patients are asymptomatic, although complaints of muscle spasms or cramps are common. Other drugs responsible for hypokalemia, especially in the intensive care setting, include glucocorticoids, cancer chemotherapeutic agents, and laxatives used chronically. Chronic ingestion of licorice can also cause hypokalemia. Licorice (glycyrrhizic acid, specifically) inhibits the steroidogenic enzyme, 11-β-hydroxysteroid dehydrogenase-2 and suppresses the renin-angiotensin system, resulting in hypertension, hypokalemia and "pseudohyperaldosteronism."

Gastrointestinal disease with loss of K^+ in stool is also a frequent cause of mild hypokalemia. Children with malignancy are at particular risk for loss of K^+ due to gastrointestinal losses, either due to chemotherapy or due to the malignant process.

Primary adrenal cortical disease (adrenal tumors or Cushing disease) occurs frequently in children, and the signs and symptoms are generally quite evident. The incidence and findings are discussed in Chapter 81. Sporadic primary aldosteronism, which includes benign aldosterone-secreting tumors and bilateral adrenal hyperplasia, is unlikely to occur in childhood. However, inherited disorders in the mineralcorticoid pathway are recognized. For instance, recessively inherited defects in 11-β-hydroxysteroid dehydrogenase type 2 cause low-renin hypertension and hypokalemia by interfering with inactivation of cortisol. Failure to inactivate cortisol to cortisone leads to excessive stimulation of the mineralcorticoid receptor by cortisol. In addition, defects in 11-β-hydroxylase cause a form of congenital adrenal hyperplasia that is associated not only with excessive androgen production but accumulation of deoxycorticosterone, a precursor to aldosterone. Deoxycorticosterone has significant mineralcorticoid activity and its accumulation leads to low-renin hypertension and hypokalemia.

Hypokalemic periodic paralysis arises from mutations in either the calcium (more common) or the Na^+ channel (26). Attacks are characterized by intermittent muscular weakness (particularly of the shoulders and hips) or generalized paralysis that lasts <24 hrs; weakness that compromises breathing and swallowing has also been described. In those families with documented genetic mutations, the frequency of attacks was greater, and the patients tended to present at a younger age. Those with calcium channel defects presented earlier and had more frequent attacks than those with mutations of the Na^+ channel.

Bartter syndrome is clinically recognized by failure to thrive, developmental delay, increased renin levels, hypokalemia, and alkalosis. Muscle weakness, muscle cramps, and salt craving may also be present. Hypertension and edema are absent. Hyperplasia of the juxtaglomerular cells, with elevated urinary excretion of prostaglandin E_2 is present. Genetic studies have identified four subtypes (34), with the most serious presenting before birth with polyhydramnios and premature delivery, and, immediately after birth, Na^+ chloride loss. All subtypes of Bartter syndrome are autosomal recessive in inheritance and are characterized by abnormal $NaCl$ reabsorption in the ascending limb of the loop of Henle. A number of children with all of the characteristics of genetically confirmed Bartter syndrome (including urinary $NaCl$ loss) have been described in whom genetic mutations have not been identified.

Pseudo-Bartter syndrome describes those children with hypokalemic alkalosis, normotensive hyperreninism, and hyperaldosteronism, in whom these abnormalities arise as a result of chronic loop diuretic use or $NaCl$ loss by other means, such as vomiting.

Gitelman syndrome was considered a variant of Bartter syndrome. Genetic studies now clearly define an autosomally inherited disorder that is distinct from Bartter syndrome. Gitelman syndrome arises from mutations in the thiazide-sensitive Na^+ chloride cotransporter. Affected children do not have growth failure or developmental delay. This condition often presents later in childhood with hypokalemia, hypocalciuria, and, frequently hypomagnesemia. Prostaglandin E_2 excretion is normal. These children characteristically have carpopedal spasm.

ASSESSMENT AND MANAGEMENT OF SODIUM AND POTASSIUM DISORDERS

In the pediatric critical care setting, the assessment and management of disorders of Na^+ and K^+ rely on timely clinical evaluations that utilize readily available laboratory tests and other technologies that will provide information rapidly. Genetic studies and the measurement of various hormones, peptides, and urinary metabolites, although important to obtain, often will not be immediately useful in the management of the critically ill child. Detailed and complete histories and physical examinations will often provide the information needed to judge the cause of the electrolyte disturbance and initiate resuscitation.

Assessment

History

The information pertaining to the changes that prompted the admission will often lead to an appreciation of the etiology of the electrolyte abnormality. Ascertaining whether the child had a rapid onset of gastrointestinal difficulties, has known

TABLE 93.7

HYPOKALEMIC CONDITIONS

Drugs—diuretics, chemotherapeutic agents (cis-platinum), amphotericin B, penicillin derivatives and licorice
Gastrointestinal disease—severe diarrhea
Adrenal cortical excess, primary aldosteronism, and other hyporeninemic syndromes
Hypokalemic periodic paralysis
Bartter syndrome
Pseudo-Bartter syndrome
Gitelman syndrome

central DI, or has a history of head injury is crucial in determining the rate of onset of the abnormality. As an example, the child with rapid onset of hyponatremia due to severe burn or head injury is at greater risk for cerebral edema, seizures, and coma than the child with chronic hyponatremia. A detailed review of systems must be obtained, including onset of mental changes, gastrointestinal changes (diarrhea or vomiting), appetite or eating alterations, weight loss, changes in skin color or skin tone, and urinary output. Patients and their families must be queried as to the presence of muscle cramps, weakness, or paresthesias. Recent medications, including the use of "natural supplements" or laxatives must be reviewed.

Physical Examination

The physical examination must include degree of hydration as judged by vital signs (especially repeated measures of blood pressure and heart rate), skin tone, and perfusion. An accurate weight must be obtained, although this is often overlooked in the critically ill child. Respiratory rate and respiratory function might suggest the possibility of pulmonary edema or impending heart failure. Examination should include a search for the possibility of physical abuse, i.e., bruising or burns that might raise the possibility of head trauma (even in those children with a known previous morbidity). Abuse of a child with a chronic illness has been known to occur.

Laboratory and Technical Studies

In addition to a basic metabolic panel, laboratory studies should include ionized calcium, serum magnesium, and studies of acid-base balance. Blood urea nitrogen and creatinine help to evaluate both the potential degree of dehydration and renal function. A spot urinary Na^+ is extremely useful, with urinary Na^+ >30 mmol/L indicative of high urinary Na^+ excretion. Direct measurements of plasma and urine osmolalities can be extremely useful in DI and helpful in documenting salt-wasting polyuria. Urine output must be measured and recorded. Dependent upon a number of variables, including age, urine output >2–3 mL/kg/hr in children (outside of infancy) is excessive.

CT scan of the brain in those patients with potential cerebral edema or brain injury may be indicated. ECG, especially in those patients with disorders of K^+, is necessary for evaluation and for monitoring progress of all patients with water and electrolyte disturbances. Central venous pressure determination might be indicated in assessing the degree of dehydration in certain patients.

Management

Management of these disorders depends upon the severity of patient compromise and the duration of the water or electrolyte abnormality. Management can be divided into resuscitation and maintenance therapies. In addition, management includes addressing the specific electrolyte/water abnormality, while also attending to the underlying cause of the abnormality. In the PICU setting, the intensivist is likely to be confronted with cardiovascular and neurologic compromise as a result of water and electrolyte disorders and be forced to address these issues while minimizing the risk of treatment-incurred complications.

Regardless of the underlying electrolyte abnormality (hypo- or hypernatremia, hypo- or hyperkalemia), the dehydrated child requires fluid resuscitation. The initial volume to be ad-

ministered will depend upon the extent of cardiovascular compromise and generally consists of 0.9% NaCl solution. While a mildly dehydrated child may only require a 20 mL/kg bolus of normal saline solution, repeated boluses may be required for the severely dehydrated child. Isotonic saline is continued until the cardiovascular status is stabilized. Continued fluid therapy will then depend upon the child's cardiovascular status, remaining fluid deficit, and nature of the electrolyte abnormality. Based upon the studies of Holliday et al., maintenance fluid therapy has been indexed to metabolic rate: 100 mL water/100 kcal/day (19). In general, 1000 mL is required for the first 10 kg, 500 mL for the next 10 kg, and 500 mL for the next 25 kg.

Hypernatremia

Hypernatremia with Dehydration. Hypernatremic dehydration arises from excessive free water loss, as occurs with DI, or water loss that is disproportionate to electrolyte loss. Following initial resuscitation with boluses and continuous infusions administered to restore perfusion and correct volume depletion, replacement therapy is required and must address the free water deficit in the child with persistent hypernatremia due to pure water loss or the Na^+ and water deficit, as occurs with hypotonic Na^+ loss. With the use of typical resuscitation fluids (0.9% NaCl), the plasma Na^+ is likely only to decrease slightly [for example, 1 L of 0.9% NaCl in a 30-kg child with total body water of 18 L (30 × 0.6) and plasma Na^+ of 165 will decrease the plasma Na^+ by $(165 - 154)/(18 + 1) = 0.6$ mEq/L]. Continued use of isotonic saline will not correct the hypernatremia, and a hypotonic solution must be introduced. In the child with known or presumed chronic hypernatremia, the subsequent goal of therapy is to decrease plasma Na^+ by ~0.5 mEq/L every hour (12 mEq/L/24 hrs) to reduce the risk of cerebral edema (2).

For patients with pure water loss (DI), included in the calculations are (a) daily water and electrolyte requirements, (b) the free water deficit, and (c) on-going losses. For patients with pure water loss, the free water deficit can generally be calculated with the following equation:

$$Free\ water\ deficit = Total\ body\ water$$
$$- Total\ body\ water\ at\ time\ of\ hypernatremia$$
$$= (TBWD) \times (weight\ kg)$$
$$- \frac{[(normal\ P_{Na} = 140\ mEq/L) \times (TBWD) \times (weight\ kg)]}{(current\ P_{Na}\ mEq/L)}$$

where TBWD = total body water distribution and P_{Na} = plasma Na^+.

The TBWD depends upon the age, sex, and weight of the child. An extremely obese adolescent may have a water distribution of 0.5; 0.6 is frequently used for the adult male, 0.5 for the adult female, 0.7 for infants. The free water deficit can then be used to calculate the rate of free water replacement over the desired correction period. If possible, this free water should be delivered via the gastrointestinal tract. IV administration will require it to be administered with dextrose or a minimal amount of Na^+; this Na^+ may reflect the daily requirement infused in the water replacement plus the daily water requirement. For acutely acquired hypernatremia (over a few hours), the correction can occur more rapidly, as accumulation of "idiogenic" osmoles has not occurred. Large and rapid shifts occur commonly in the hospitalized child with DI, in whom vasopressin/1-deamino(8-D-arginine) vasopressin (DDAVP) administration is delayed.

Continued losses must also be addressed. For the child with untreated DI, urine output will essentially reflect free water loss, which can be voluminous unless treated. For the child with central DI, institution of vasopressin by continuous infusion (starting dose 0.5 mU/kg/hr) will curb excessive losses. The continuous vasopressin infusion allows quick titration and avoids excessive urine output associated with "breakthroughs." DDAVP is avoided in the initial management because of its long half-life, preventing fine-tuning of fluid therapy. The use of vasopressin may dictate a recalculation of replacement fluids based upon either 1) normal maintenance fluids of 1500 cc/m²/day or 2) the previously outlined formula by Holliday et al. (19), both of which reflect insensible losses as well as normal urinary losses, not urinary losses under maximally anti-diuresed states. In the completely antidiuresed state, maintenance fluid may be less than 50% of normal. For these reasons, calculating the fluid deficit, determining the amount to be replaced over a 24-hr period, establishing the desired positive fluid balance over 6–8-hr intervals, and examining the "ins and outs" and plasma Na⁺ over these individual time frames will allow adequate fluid replacement and avoidance of overshooting the goal. For some patients, vasopressin is not an option (for example, the child with central DI undergoing chemotherapy that mandates dilute urine to minimize bladder toxicity). In such circumstances, urine output must be replaced with water. Again, fluid calculations must consider that usual maintenance fluid (1500 mL/m²) covers urine output and insensible losses. If all urine output is to be replaced, then the maintenance component of the calculations must reflect insensible water losses only (30–50% of normal maintenance) and daily electrolyte requirements. Also, additional sources of fluid should be considered; for instance, in the PICU, antibiotics and other medications can be significant sources of fluid.

For the postoperative patient in whom DI is anticipated, urine output and plasma Na⁺ are closely monitored. As patients frequently receive significant amounts of fluid intraoperatively, initial urine output often represents mobilization of these fluids rather than DI. Additionally, patients commonly receive high-dose glucocorticoids, which can provoke hyperglycemia and diuresis; thus, urine and blood glucose should be monitored. Once the diagnosis of DI is established postoperatively based upon excessive urine output and increasing serum Na⁺, a vasopressin drip can be initiated, as described previously. Again, fluid administration must be tailored to restore insensible fluid losses, replace ongoing urinary losses, and meet daily electrolyte requirements.

For children with hypotonic Na⁺ loss, the just-mentioned free water deficit formula may underestimate their losses. The Adrogue-Madias formula calculates the amount that plasma Na⁺ will drop following infusion of 1 liter of fluid of varying components (2):

$$\frac{(NaCl \text{ of infusate}) - (current \; P_{Na} \; mEq/L)}{TBWD \times WT(kg) + \text{infusate volume}}$$

For a 30-kg child with a total body water distribution of 0.6 and plasma Na⁺ of 170 receiving 600 mL (0.6 L) of normal saline solution: $(154 - 170)/[(0.6 \times 30) + 0.6] = -0.86$; the plasma Na⁺ will decrease by 0.86 mEq/L, whereas use of 600 nL of half-normal saline solution (77 mEq/L) will decrease plasma Na⁺ by 5 mEq/L. Additional loss must be addressed. For the child with severe diarrhea, vomitus, or nasogastric output, these losses will include water and other electrolytes, and

additional fluid supplementation should reflect this fluid composition.

Hypernatremia with Normal or Overhydration. Hypernatremia with normal or overhydration arises from salt loading, as might occur in the infant who receives a concentrated formula preparation or in the child who receives excessive NaCl or sodium bicarbonate during resuscitation. Treatment requires the withdrawal of the Na⁺ source and the addition of water. For more severely compromised patients with fluid overload, the addition of furosemide to increase Na⁺ excretion and water may be indicated. The Adrogue-Madias formula, as detailed previously, has its limits but does provide a target for initiating fluid replacement therapy. For patients with renal failure, dialysis may be indicated.

Hyponatremia

Hyponatremia with Dehydration. With hyponatremic dehydration, the Na⁺ deficit exceeds the free water deficit. The clinical presentation may largely reflect CNS irritability from hyponatremia or dehydration, and initial management should reflect attention to the clinical situation. CNS findings, such as seizure, frequently reflect an acute decrease in plasma Na⁺. Treatment considerations should include administration of 3% NaCl to raise plasma Na⁺ by ~3–5 mEq/L over several hours. If symptoms primarily reflect dehydration, normal saline solution should be administered; the plasma Na⁺ will also increase with this step but to a much lesser extent. Again, following initial resuscitation, further correction of the fluid and Na⁺ deficits must be addressed. Additionally, sources of free water should be discontinued. In general, a conservative approach is to assume that the development of hyponatremia has occurred over an extended period of time and thus should be corrected slowly (0.5 mEq/L/hr). Maintenance Na⁺ and water requirements should be calculated; Na⁺ and water deficits should be estimated. The total Na⁺ deficit can be calculated as (3):

$$(140 \; mEq/L - P_{Na} \; mEq/L) \times (TBWD \times WT \text{ in kg})$$

Generally, half of the deficit is replaced at a rate of 0.5 mEq/hr. Thus, the 30-kg child with a P_{Na} of 120 and a distribution of water of 0.6 will have a Na⁺ deficit of $(140 - 120) \times (0.6 \times 30) = 360$ mEq. The initial correction of 10 mEq/L will be replaced at a rate of 0.5 mEq/hr; that is, over 20 hrs. If 0.9% NaCl solution is used (154 mEq/L = 0.154 mEq/mL), the infusion rate necessary to correct half of the deficit is (360 mEq/0.154 mEq/mL)/20hr = 117 mL/hr. Following institution of specific fluid rates and types, the effect of these therapies upon hydration and biochemical parameters must be reviewed every 6–8 hrs and, as always, the child's clinical status must be continuously evaluated. Sources of continued salt loss should be investigated. For instance, the child with excessive salt losses from cerebral salt wasting may require additional salt replacement (which can be estimated from the amount of urinary Na⁺ × the volume of urine). Plasma Na⁺ in the child with adrenal insufficiency will improve with administration of salt-containing fluids, but initiation of glucocorticoids (which have mineralocorticoid activity at "stress" doses of 100 mg/m²) and/or mineralocorticoids is also important for stabilization of the patient.

Hyponatremia with Salt-wasting and Known Central Diabetes Insipidus. Hyponatremia with salt-wasting and known central

DI can be both a diagnostic and a therapeutic challenge. For the child with DI who has been overtreated with vasopressin and water, the salt wasting reflects a normal response to fluid overload, and withholding of fluids and additional vasopressin will permit diuresis and correction of the hyponatremic state. For the child with DI and either concomitant cerebral salt wasting or natriuresis due to drug toxicity, the approach to hyponatremia can be more problematic. After initial resuscitation, the Na^+ deficit should be determined and ongoing urinary Na^+ losses should be calculated by measuring urine Na^+ and volume. Vasopressin is withheld because it can potentiate hyponatremia. However, a vasopressin drip should be readily available at the bedside, as the waning effect of previously administered vasopressin/DDAVP and resolution of the salt-wasting state may be accompanied by excessive free water losses and rapid increases in plasma Na^+.

Hyponatremia with Normal or Overhydration. As with hyponatremic dehydration, initial management depends upon clinical symptoms. The child with symptomatic hyponatremia, such as significant lethargy, seizures, or coma, will require infusion of hypertonic saline. Following initial resuscitation in the symptomatic child, water restriction alone or in combination with hypertonic Na^+ chloride and furosemide, will increase Na^+ without exacerbating the fluid overloaded state. In addition, the underlying cause of the hyponatremia must be addressed. Excessive free water intake due to primary polydipsia or to overdiluted infant formula may respond to fluid restriction. However, caution must be taken so that withdrawal of the free water source does not cause over-rapid correction of the plasma Na^+. In such cases, it may be necessary to administer hypotonic fluids to control the rate of plasma Na^+ rise (3).

Hyperkalemia

Hyperkalemia brings the cell membrane potential closer to the threshold for cell membrane depolarization and thus is a significant risk for cardiac conduction abnormalities and muscle weakness/paralysis. Treatment of hyperkalemia in the setting of these emergencies is two-pronged: stabilize the cell membrane electrical potential and acutely lower the plasma K^+ through redistribution. The former is achieved through administration of 10% calcium gluconate, 1 mg/kg IV over 2–3 mins (and has been suggested to occur over 20–30 mins in the setting of digitalis toxicity). Calcium infusion can be repeated in 5 mins if ECG abnormalities persist. As to the second prong, rapid IV infusion of glucose (0.25–0.5 g/kg, 2–5 mL/kg of 10% dextrose solution) and regular insulin (0.3 units/g glucose) will lower plasma K^+ within 10–20 mins, with a peak effect between 30 and 60 mins. IV dextrose should be continued and blood glucose tested to monitor for the development of hypoglycemia or hyperglycemia. Treatment with inhaled β-adrenergic agonists is recommended in adults, and some centers follow this recommendation; however, data are limited in children. Additionally, removal of plasma K^+ with Kayexalate, 1 g/kg orally or by rectum in sorbitol solution is indicated if not contraindicated by bowel pathology. In the setting of renal failure, dialysis may be required. K^+ administration and medications that interfere with K^+ excretion should be discontinued if possible. Treatment of hyperkalemia with Na^+ bicarbonate has recently been revisited, and the adult literature recommends that it not be used as initial or monotherapy, although it may have a role in the setting of severe metabolic acidosis (14).

Hypokalemia

Management of hypokalemia depends upon the acuity of symptoms and the underlying etiology. The child with hypokalemia-induced paralysis or with hypokalemia-induced ECG changes requires urgent IV treatment (0.5 mEq/kg over 30–60 mins), continuous IV infusion, and frequent assessments to monitor the response. The child who is on digoxin or has an underlying cardiac defect is at increased risk of arrhythmias and may require IV treatment at higher doses (1 mEq/kg) and at higher plasma K+ concentrations. Magnesium replacement may also be necessary to treat hypokalemia.

The child with hypokalemia in the setting of DKA also requires aggressive attention, as glucose and insulin administration will drive K+ intracellularly and aggravate hypokalemia. In fact, the child in DKA represents a special situation that the intensivist will frequently encounter. K+ is delivered at higher-than-usual rates (provided that the child is urinating) in the setting of normal plasma K+ concentrations because, despite significant total body K+ deficits, the plasma K+ is normal or elevated as a result of insulin deficiency. The K+ can be administered as a combination of K+ chloride and K+ phosphate, as the child with DKA also has a phosphorus deficit. If hypokalemia develops during the course of DKA treatment, and hyperglycemia and acidosis have nearly resolved, lowering the insulin infusion rate will help to address the hypokalemia.

In the PICU setting, mild, asymptomatic deficits are treated slowly with increased IV K+ supplementation or, if possible, oral replacement. The child on chronic diuretics may need to have these reassessed or have chronic K+ supplementation initiated.

OUTCOMES: MORBIDITY AND MORTALITY

A discussion of morbidity and mortality is an important exercise as a means by which to determine how clinicians can improve outcome. However, the disorders of water, Na^+, and K^+ do not occur without underlying processes that alter the protective physiologic homeostatic mechanisms meant to prevent dehydration and electrolyte disturbance, and the underlying disease process is often a major contributor to outcome data. Examples of such conditions include DKA, adrenal crisis, acute renal failure, severe burns, or cystic fibrosis. Cerebral edema, as an example, still occurs in young children with DKA despite reducing fluid flow rates, avoidance of hypotonic solutions during resuscitation, and restraint of bicarbonate use because all of the multiple factors that cause cerebral edema during resuscitation of DKA are not fully elucidated. The outcome in many conditions, therefore, is often related to the homeostatic disturbances of water and electrolytes and to a number of other factors related to the underlying disease. The mortality and morbidity of the various specific conditions that commonly present with disturbed fluid and electrolyte homeostasis are discussed in the chapters pertaining to the respective diseases.

The studies that document outcomes of fluid and electrolyte disturbances generally do not exclude underlying diseases, but they review the outcomes in particular settings, such as intensive care, postoperative care, or inpatient care. The study by Arieff (7) evaluated healthy children admitted for elective surgery to one center over a 6-year period and ascertained that the incidence of hyponatremia was 0.34% (83 of 24,412 consecutively admitted patients), and, of these patients, 7 children (8.4%) died. This study concluded, based upon a prospectively studied group of 16 hyponatremic patients (evaluated by the authors from multiple centers), that the hyponatremia was caused by extrarenal losses and replacement with hypotonic saline. However, this study further suggested that in children with no underlying threatening conditions except surgery alone, the incidence of hyponatremia during postoperative fluid management is relatively low, i.e., 0.34%. This study, therefore, indicates that the higher incidence of hyponatremia seen in the hospital setting also reflects the morbidity associated with underlying conditions. A study of 11,702 admissions to one pediatric center over 1 year found that the incidence of hyponatremia was 1.38%; 37 of these 161 cases were otherwise previously healthy children (43). The authors concluded that adverse outcomes, neurologic deficits (3.7%), and death (12%, but many deaths occurred some time after correction of hyponatremia) in their study were more closely related to the underlying condition rather than to hyponatremia or its correction. Unfortunately, this study did not provide sufficient information as to the underlying conditions or sufficient data to support the reasoning as to why they suggested that the underlying conditions dictated prognosis. However, multiple studies that have evaluated hyponatremia indicate that hyponatremia in the hospital setting occurs "commonly," a finding no doubt related to the fact that children are admitted to the hospital (and especially the PICU) because of associated severe acute and chronic disease and exposure to drugs, which frequently cause disturbances of water, Na^+, and K^+. Therefore, the incidence of hyponatremia in the hospital setting, and especially in the PICU, is certainly greater than the 1% of children cited in the previously mentioned studies.

A review of Na^+ disturbances emphasizes that the more common underlying conditions that predispose to hyponatremia during fluid therapy are those with impaired renal water excretion; and, therefore, the use of hypotonic saline solution for resuscitation and maintenance frequently results in hyponatremia (30). The morbidity from hyponatremia is such that >50% (with serum Na^+ <125 mEq/L) will develop encephalopathy. Postoperative patients have a number of factors predisposing to hyponatremia during fluid therapy, including pain, subclinical hypovolemia, and medications that stimulate vasopressin release, and therefore, are susceptible to development of hyponatremia with hypotonic fluid administration. However, although strong proponents of isotonic saline (and even hypertonic saline in certain conditions, such as cerebral salt wasting) for resuscitation and maintenance, the authors also note that hypernatremia is not without neurologic sequelae and death (28,30). The mortality attributed to hypernatremia was 16%, and neurologic complications were noted in 15% of patients (28). This review allows for the use of hypotonic solutions in certain circumstances, especially when fluid volume has been restored and maintained in patients but hypernatremia persists. The consequences of prolonged hypernatremia include shrinkage of brain volume that can result in cerebral demyelinating lesions, cavernous sinus thrombosis, and rhabdomyolysis. Although demyelinating lesions have generally been associated with hyponatremia, the finding of central pontine myelinolysis in severely burned patients who had suffered hyperosmolality, including hypernatremia, suggested that hypernatremia could lead to this neurologic lesion

(24). Although uncommon, additional cases of myelinolysis in adults (9,22) and children (5,8,37) in association with hypernatremia, make this neurologic insult a real concern in the setting of hypernatremia. Demyelinization of brain due to prolonged hypernatremia has been demonstrated in rats and has been attributed to hyperosmolality, although the underlying pathology for this condition remains unclear (38).

Much less pediatric data in terms of incidence, morbidity, and mortality are available for disorders of K^+ in children, as compared with Na^+ disturbances. A study of hospitalized adult and pediatric patients in a university hospital suggested that severe hypokalemia occurred in 2.6% of yearly hospitalizations and that the death rate was 20.4% or 10-fold greater than that of the entire hospitalized population (33). However, only 11.2% of the patients with hypokalemia were pediatric patients, and the odds ratio for death in children from hypokalemia was 1.00.

It is estimated that the incidence of hyperkalemia in hospitalized patients is 1%–10%, but to what degree spurious hyperkalemia influences the estimate of incidence is not clear. Several older studies estimated that mortality due to hyperkalemia is 1.9% and higher. However, very little information about children is available, and certainly no studies have been devoted to incidence of hyperkalemia focused only on the pediatric population. A study from Pittsburgh in adult patients estimated the incidence of hyperkalemia to be ~2.3% of hospitalized patients over a 4-month period in 1996 (1). Although ECG abnormalities were noted, no deaths occurred. In children, it is likely that the highest risk for morbidity and mortality would be in those children with underlying cardiac conditions.

The question of whether outcome can be improved by retrospective evaluation of therapy and morbidity and mortality is standard medical practice. In disorders of water and electrolytes, the evaluation therapy in terms of morbidity and mortality is no minor issue. The general consensus is that resuscitation, especially in the dehydrated state, requires careful fluid management and avoidance of the use of hypotonic fluid replacement to prevent iatrogenic hyponatremia. However, a degree of controversy exists as to the appropriate use of hypotonic fluid for maintenance fluid therapy, as originally described by Holliday et al. (19). For instance, Moritz and Ayus suggested that use of isotonic saline rather than hypotonic fluids for maintenance therapy may prevent hyponatremia in hospitalized children (29). Nevertheless, hypernatremia, especially after fluid volume has been restored, is also life- and brain-threatening and cannot be ignored (28,30). Holiday et al. would argue that a physiologic approach to maintenance therapy is still appropriate (18). The therapeutic management discussed previously is an attempt to approach resuscitation and maintenance therapy, allowing for some clinical judgment and interventions that are not simply based upon formulas or dogmatic algorithms.

CONCLUSIONS AND FUTURE DIRECTIONS

In conclusion, disorders of water, Na^+, and K^+ homeostasis occur commonly in children in the PICU. Often, these disturbances are associated with underlying conditions that perturb the mechanisms that regulate water and electrolyte homeostasis. At present, the evaluation, management, and therapeutic modalities rely on knowledge of the physiology and potential pathology, with superb clinical judgment and the use of relatively few technical or biochemical modalities. As well, newer pharmacologic therapies based upon even better understanding of mechanisms that regulate water, Na^+, and K^+ homeostasis will allow newer therapeutic strategies.

The new information regarding water, Na^+, and K^+ abnormalities will provide further recognition of the underlying biochemical and genetic disturbances responsible for, or contributing to, these abnormalities. The identification of additional pathways will then provide the foundation for development of diagnostic and therapeutic strategies that may apply to numerous other disease states.

As an example, in congestive heart failure, coactivation of volume overload and volume depleted response mechanisms occurs: cardiac release of ANP and BNP in response to atrial stretch are accompanied by baroreceptor-mediated activation of vasopressin secretion, the sympathetic nervous system, and RAAS. As congestive heart failure progresses, the "volume-depleted" antinatriuretic and vasoconstrictive responses predominate, and fluid overload ensues. However, traditional treatment of the fluid-overloaded state with diuretics can (a) further activate the sympathetic nervous system and RAAS, and (b) exacerbate hyponatremia. Thus, alternative medications for the treatment are being sought (10).

For instance, potentiation of natriuretic peptide activity in congestive heart failure has received attention. Administration of natriuretic peptide in the form of nesiritide (a synthetic BNP) has been approved for the treatment of congestive heart failure, and treatment with natriuretic peptide agonists and inhibitors of natriuretic peptide degradation are being entertained (10). Moreover, the measurement of BNP is being increasingly used in the diagnosis, prognosis, and assessment of treatment response in patients with congestive heart failure (23). Limited data for the use of this assay in children are available (11).

The development of vasopressin-2 receptor antagonists, such as conivaptan and tolvaptan, has a potentially important role in hyponatremia. These agents prevent water reabsorption at the level of the kidney without natriuresis, thus offering removal of excessive water without the hyponatremia that frequently accompanies diuresis. These agents may have a role in the treatment of congestive heart failure and chronic SIADH (16,17).

Experience with these newer medications in children is lacking, but with increased use and experience in adults, they are likely to be tested in children. For example, based upon adult data from the 1980s (12), oral urea has been successfully used to treat the hyponatremia associated with chronic SIADH in children (20).

While much has been learned about the genetics and pathophysiology of disturbances of water, Na^+, and K^+ homeostasis, the challenge remains to understand the development and prevention of their complications.

KEY POINTS

- Disorders of water, Na^+, and K^+ occur commonly in the PICU, and these disturbances of fluid and electrolyte homeostasis are generally associated with underlying comorbidities, such as renal dysfunction, DKA, DI, chemotherapy, brain tumors, and brain surgery.

- Evaluation, assessment, and management of fluid and electrolyte disorders require an understanding of those basic factors that regulate homeostasis as well as the differential diagnosis of the underlying conditions that predispose to altering water, Na^+, and K^+ homeostasis.

- Therapeutic management requires both managing the underlying condition appropriately and being aware that inappropriate therapeutic measures can be an iatrogenic cause of disturbance of fluid and electrolyte homeostasis.

- In the clinical acute care setting, careful historic information and physical examination are the cornerstone of therapy; however, it must be stressed that physical assessment of the degree of dehydration or hydration is, at best, only an initial estimation; that vital signs, clinical improvement, and biochemical parameters must be monitored closely; and that changes in fluid therapy must be allowed for as necessary.

- Often, the most complicated disorders of water, Na^+, and K^+ to manage are those in which the basic underlying conditions are changing, such as in SIADH, postoperative craniopharyngioma patients, or patients with known central diabetes subsequently developing a salt-wasting condition.

- Clear potential for morbidity and mortality exists with any disturbance of water, Na^+, and K^+ homeostasis, but perhaps the most common abnormality that results in injury and death is hyponatremia. It must be stressed, however, that prolonged and untreated hypernatremia is also associated with significant injury and death.

- Recent studies stressed the need to avoid the use of hypotonic fluids during resuscitation, as they are a major cause of iatrogenic hyponatremia. However, some controversy remains as to continued use of isotonic fluids long after correction of disordered volume and electrolyte balance. The fear of inducing hyponatremia has led to prolonged hypernatremia in certain conditions.

- Management of fluid and electrolyte disturbance requires therapeutic flexibility because dogmatic approaches can often lead to undesirable outcomes.

ACKNOWLEDGMENTS

Andrea Kelly, MD is supported by NIH-K23 RR021973.

References

1. Acher CG, Johnson JP, Palevsky PM, et al. Hyperkalemia in hospitalized patients. *Arch Intern Med* 1998;158:917–924.
2. Adrogue H, Madias N. Hypernatremia. *N Engl J Med* 2000;342:1493–9.
3. Adrogue H, Madias N. Hyponatremia. *N Engl J Med* 2000;342:1581–9.
4. Adrogue H, Chap Z, Ishida T, et al. Role of the endocrine pancreas in the kalemic response to acute metabolic acidosis in conscious dogs. *J Clin Invest* 1985;5:798–808.
5. Al-Orainy IA, O'Gorman AM, Decell MK. Cerebral bleeding, infarcts, and presumed extrapontine myelinolysis in hypernatremic dehydration. *Neuroradiology* 1999;41(2):144–6.
6. Antunes-Rodrigues J, deCastro M, Elias L, et al. Neuroendocrine control of body fluid metabolism. *Physiol Rev* 2004;84:169–208.
7. Arieff AI, Ayus JC, Fraser CL. Hyponatraemia and death or permanent brain damage in healthy children. *BMJ* 1992;304:218–22.
8. Brown WD and Caruso JM. Extrapontine myelinolysis with involvement of the hippocampus in three children with severe hypernatremia. *J Child Neurol* 1999;14:428–33.

9. Clark WR. Diffuse demyelinating lesions of the brain after the rapid development of hypernatremia. *West J Med* 1992;157:571–3.

10. Costello-Boerrigter L, Boerrigter G, Burnett J. Revisiting salt and water retention: New diuretics, aquaretics, and natriuretics. *Med Clin North Am* 2003;87:475–91.

11. Davis G, Bamforth F, Sarpal A, et al. B-type natriuretic peptide in pediatrics. *Clin Biochem* 2006;39:600–5.

12. Decaux G, Genette F. Urea for long-term treatment of syndrome of inappropriate secretion of antidiuretic hormone. *Be Med J* 1981;283:1081–1083.

13. DiBona G. Nervous kidney. Interaction between renal sympathetic nerves and the renin-angiotensin system in the control of renal function. *Hypertension* 2000;36:1083–8.

14. Evans K, Greenberg A. Hyperkalemia: A review. *J Intensive Care Med* 2005;20:279–90.

15. Fitzsimons J. Angiotensin, thirst, and sodium appetite. *Physiol Rev* 1998;78:583–686.

16. Ghali J, Koren M, Taylor J, et al. Efficacy and safety of oral conivaptan: A V1A/V2 vasopressin receptor antagonist, assessed in a randomized, placebo-controlled trial in patients with euvolemic or hypervolemic hyponatremia. *J Clin Endocrinol Metab* 2006;91:2145–52.

17. Gheorghiade M, Gottlieb S, Udelson J, et al. Vasopressin v(2) receptor blockade with tolvaptan versus fluid restriction in the treatment of hyponatremia. *Am J Cardiol* 2006;97:1064–7.

18. Holliday MA, Friedman Al, Segar WE, et al. Acute hospital-induced hyponatremia in children: A physiologic approach. *J Pediatr* 2004;145:584–7.

19. Holliday MA, Segar WE. The maintenance need for water in parenteral fluid therapy. *Pediatrics* 1957;19:823–2.

20. Huang E, Feldman B, Schwartz I, et al. Oral urea for the treatment of chronic syndrome of inappropriate antidiuresis in children. *J Pediatr* 2006;148:128–31.

21. Katz ES, McGrath S, Marcus CL. Late-onset hypoventilation with hypothalamic dysfunction: A distinct Clinical Syndrome. *Pediatr Pulmonol* 2000;29:62–68.

22. McComb RD, Pfeiffer RI, Casey JH, et al. Lateral pontine and extrapontine myelinolysis with hypernatremia and hyperglycemia. *Clin Neuropathol* 1989;8:284–8.

23. McCullough P. Clinical applications of B-type natriuretic peptide levels in the care of cardiovascular patients. *Minerva Cardioangiol* 2004;52:479–89.

24. McKee AC, Winkelman MD, Banker BQ. Central pontine myelinolysis in severely burned patients: Relationship to serum hyperosmolality. *Neurology* 1988;38:1211–7.

25. McKinley M, Johnson A. The physiological regulation of thirst and fluid intake. *News Physiol Sci* 2004;19:1–6.

26. Miller TM, de Silva D, Miller HA, et al. Correlating phenotype and genotype in the periodic paralyses. *Neurology* 2004;63:1657–1655.

27. Mobasheri A, Avila J, Cozar-Castellano I, et al. Na/K-ATPase isozyme diversity: Comparative biochemistry and physiological implications of novel functional interactions. *Biosci Rep* 2000;20:51–91.

28. Moritz ML, Ayus JC. The changing pattern of hypernatremia in hospitalized children. *Pediatrics* 1999;104:435–439.

29. Moritz ML, Ayus JL. Prevention of hospital acquired hyponatremia: a case for using isotonic saline in maintenance fluid therapy, *Pediatrics* 2003; 111:227–30.

30. Moritz ML, Ayus JL. Preventing neurological complications from dysnatremias in children. *Pediatr Nephrol* 2005;20:1687–1700.

31. Ordaz B, Tuz K, Ochoa L, et al. Osmolytes and mechanisms involved in regulatory volume decrease under conditions of sudden or gradual osmolarity decrease. *Neurochem Res* 2004;65–72.

32. Pasantes-Morales H, Franco R, Torres-Marquez M, et al. Amino acid osmolytes in regulatory volume decrease and isovolumetric regulation in brain cells: Contribution and mechanisms. *Cell Physiol Biochem* 2000;10:361–70.

33. Patiel O, Salakhov E, Ronen I, et al. Management of severe hypokalemia in hospitalized patients. *Arch Intern Med* 2001;161:1089–1095.

34. Proesmans W. Threading through the mizmaze of Bartter Syndrome. *Pediatr Nephrol* 2006;7:896–902.

35. Robertson G. Antidiuretic hormone. Normal and disordered function. *Endocrinol Metab Clin North Am* 2001;30:671–94.

36. Sands J. Mammalian urea transporters. *Annu Rev Physiol* 2003;65:543–66.

37. Shah B, Tobias JD. Osmotic demyelination and hypertonic dehydration in a 9-year-old girl: Changes in cerebrospinal fluid myelin basic protein. *J Intensive Care Med* 2006;21:372–6.

38. Soupart A, Pennickx R, Namias B, et al. Brain myelinolysis following hypernatremia in rats. *J Neuropathol Exp Neurol* 1996;55:106–13.

39. Stricker E, Sved A. Thirst. *Nutrition* 2000;16:821–6.

40. Suttner S, Boldt J. Natriuretic peptide system: Physiology and clinical utility. *Curr Opin Crit Care* 2004;10:336–41.

41. Verbalis J. Disorders of body water homeostasis. *Best Pract Res Clin Endocrinol Metab* 2003;17:471–503.

42. Voisin D, Bourque C. Integration of sodium and osmosensory signals in vasopressin neurons. *Trends Neurosci* 2002;25:199–205.

43. Wattad A., Chiang ML, Hill LL. Hyponatremia in hospitalized children. *Clin Pediatr* 1992;31:153–157.

44. Weese-Mayer DE, Berry-Kravis EM, Marazita ML. In pursuit (and discovery) of a genetic basis for congenital central hypoventilation syndrome. *Resp Physiol Neurobiol* 2005;149:73–82.

CHAPTER 94 ■ DISORDERS OF CALCIUM, MAGNESIUM, AND PHOSPHATE

KENNETH J. BANASIAK • THOMAS O. CARPENTER

Calcium, magnesium, and phosphate are critical regulators of cellular and organ function. These substances act as enzyme cofactors and regulators of metabolic function within cells. The distribution of magnesium and phosphate is represented by a substantial intracellular concentration component. Calcium, however, is largely excluded from the intracellular space, but extracellular calcium is a major determinant of neuromuscular stability. For the clinician, it is important to understand the regulation of these divalent ions, as disruption in this regulation adversely impacts a variety of physiologic functions.

REGULATION OF EXTRACELLULAR CALCIUM, MAGNESIUM, AND PHOSPHATE HOMEOSTASIS

Calcium and magnesium exist in the body as the divalent cations, Ca^{2+} and Mg^{2+}, respectively. Approximately 99% of the total body calcium resides in the skeleton, whereas the remaining 1% is found in the soft tissues and extracellular spaces. Approximately 40%–50% of magnesium lies within bone. While 40%–50% of magnesium resides in the intracellular space, only 1% is found in the extracellular space. Approximately 40% of plasma calcium is bound to protein, principally albumin, 10% is complexed with anions, and the remaining 50% exists in the unbound, or ionized, form. The unbound calcium is the physiologically important circulating form of calcium within the body. While 20%–30% of plasma magnesium is bound to protein, chiefly albumin (27), the remaining 70%–80% exists in the ionized form or is complexed to citrate, bicarbonate, and phosphate. As with calcium, the ionized form is the most physiologically significant circulating form of magnesium.

Phosphorus is predominantly found in bones and teeth (~85% of total body phosphorus). The remaining total body phosphorus is distributed in the soft tissues (14%) and the extracellular space (1%). Approximately 60% of plasma phosphorous exists in the ionized forms of phosphate, HPO_4^{2-} and $H_2PO_4^-$. The remaining plasma phosphate is complexed to cations, primarily Ca^{2+}, Mg^{2+}, and Na^+, or is bound to plasma proteins.

REGULATION OF CALCIUM, MAGNESIUM, AND PHOSPHATE

The extracellular concentrations of calcium, magnesium, and phosphate are maintained within a normal range through (a) absorption of ingested calcium, magnesium, and phosphate through the intestinal tract; (b) absorption and excretion via the kidney; and (c) mobilization from the bone. All of these processes are regulated by hormonal action.

Intestinal Absorption

Dietary calcium is passively absorbed in a concentration-dependent fashion throughout the small intestine and is actively transported in the duodenum and upper jejunum by mechanisms regulated by 1, 25-dihydroxyvitamin D. The efficiency of calcium absorption is increased with reduced dietary intake, rapid growth during childhood, pregnancy, and lactation. Dietary magnesium is principally absorbed in the jejunum and the ileum by both active and passive mechanisms. Magnesium absorption is enhanced during reduced dietary intake. Phosphate is absorbed in the duodenum and jejunum by passive processes and active mechanisms regulated by 1, 25-dihydroxyvitamin D. Absorption of phosphate is impeded by the presence of polyvalent cations (e.g., Ca^{2+}, Mg^{2+}, and Al^{3+}) in the intestinal lumen or by deficiency of vitamin D. A small proportion of calcium, magnesium, and phosphate is secreted in digestive juices and excreted via stool. Intestinal absorption is the main site of regulation of total body calcium.

Renal Handling

Approximately 60%–70% of total plasma calcium, chiefly in its ionized and complexed forms, is filtered by the kidneys. Most (~70%) of filtered calcium is reabsorbed along with sodium and water in the proximal convoluted tubule by a concentration-dependent mechanism. An additional 15%–20% of calcium is reabsorbed in the thick ascending limb of the loop of Henle. The action of the Na^+-K^+-$2Cl^-$ cotransporter in the thick ascending limb creates a potential difference that favors voltage-dependent absorption of calcium. The remaining 10%–15% of filtered calcium is reabsorbed in the distal convoluted tubule by active mechanisms that are poorly understood and that are regulated by parathyroid hormone (PTH) and cyclic AMP. Usually less than 5% of filtered calcium is excreted in the urine.

Approximately 70%–80% of plasma magnesium, in its ionized or complex forms is filtered in the glomerulus; 5%–15% of the filtered magnesium is reabsorbed in the proximal convoluted tubule by an undefined passive mechanism. The majority of filtered magnesium (60%–70%) is reabsorbed in the thick ascending limb of the loop of Henle as the consequence of a voltage-dependent gradient generated by action of the Na^+-K^+-$2Cl^-$ cotransporter. The remaining 5%–10% of magnesium is reabsorbed in the distal convoluted tubule by an unknown mechanism that is stimulated by PTH (6). Approximately 3% of filtered magnesium is excreted in the urine.

As with calcium and magnesium, the ionized and complexed forms of phosphate are filtered in the glomerulus and accounts for ultrafiltration of 85%–90% of the total plasma phosphate. Nearly 80% of the filtered phosphate is reabsorbed in the proximal convoluted tubule through the action of sodium-phosphate (Na-P) cotransporters, which are regulated by PTH. An additional 5% of phosphate is reabsorbed in the distal convoluted tubule by an unknown active mechanism (11). The amount of phosphate excreted in the urine ranges from 3% to 20% of the filtered load. Thus, the kidney is the major site of regulation of total body phosphorous.

Multiple factors can alter renal reabsorption or excretion of calcium, magnesium, and phosphate (27) (**Table 94.1**). Administration of a saline infusion for volume expansion leads to increased calcium, magnesium, and phosphate excretion primarily due to decreased proximal tubular reabsorption. Hypercalcemia decreases renal blood flow and glomerular filtration rate and simultaneously increases excretion of calcium due to decreased reabsorption of calcium in the proximal tubule, loop of Henle, and distal convoluted tubule. The net effect of these two potentially opposing mechanisms is enhanced calcium excretion. These actions are due to suppression of PTH release by elevated serum calcium levels. The effects of hypercalcemia on phosphate excretion are determined by the duration of the hypercalcemic state. During acute hypercalcemia, reduction in glomerular filtration rate, formation of calcium-phosphate-protein complexes (which prevents ultrafiltration of phosphate), and suppression of PTH release (which prevents phosphate reabsorption in the proximal tubule) contribute to decreased phosphate excretion. In contrast, during chronic hypercalcemia, phosphate excretion increases due to decreased reabsorption via unknown mechanisms. Hypocalcemia induces PTH secretion, which in turn, reduces renal excretion of calcium by enhancing reabsorption in the distal convoluted tubule. Hypocalcemia contributes to reduced excretion of magnesium and phosphate by increasing magnesium absorption in the thick ascending limb of the loop of Henle and by increasing phosphate absorption by an unknown mechanism. Hypermagnesemia has no clear effect on calcium or phosphate excretion but increases magnesium excretion by reducing the fractional reabsorption of magnesium in the proximal tubule and inhibiting reabsorption in the loop of Henle. Conversely, during hypomagnesemia, magnesium excretion is decreased due to increased reabsorption in the loop of Henle by an unclear mechanism. Hyperphosphatemia induces PTH secretion, thereby reducing calcium excretion through increased uptake in the distal convoluted tubule. In contrast, hypophosphatemia increases Na-P-cotransporter-mediated reabsorption in the proximal tubule, thereby decreasing phosphate excretion. Hyperphosphatemia has no clearly defined effect on magnesium excretion; it does reduce the tubular absorption of both calcium and magnesium, enhancing their excretion.

Acid-base disturbances have significant effects on renal handling of calcium, magnesium, and phosphate. Both acute and chronic metabolic acidosis induce calciuria by inhibiting epithelial calcium channel type 1 (ECaC1)-mediated uptake of calcium in the distal tubule (33). On the other hand, metabolic alkalosis enhances conductance of calcium through the ECaC1, leading to reduced calcium excretion (33). The effect of metabolic acidosis on magnesium excretion has not been delineated, but it is known that metabolic alkalosis reduces renal losses of magnesium by increasing absorption in the loop of Henle. Acute metabolic acidosis does not seem to have any significant effect on phosphate excretion, while chronic metabolic acidosis causes phosphaturia by reducing Na-P cotransporter expression at the tubular cell surface, resulting in decreased absorption in the proximal tubule (1). Respiratory acidosis enhances both calcium and phosphate excretion. Respiratory alkalosis decreases renal phosphate excretion but has no effect on calcium excretion. Respiratory acid-base disturbances do not appear to have any significant effect on magnesium excretion.

Multiple medications, in particular diuretics, have a major impact on renal excretion of calcium, magnesium, and phosphate. Thiazide diuretics enhance calcium reabsorption in the distal convoluted tubule. In contrast, thiazide diuretics cause a modest increase in magnesium excretion via inhibition of the Na^+-Cl^- cotransporter. Thiazides induce phosphaturia by inhibiting carbonic anhydrase. Loop diuretics augment calcium and magnesium excretion through inhibition of the Na^+-K^+-Cl^- cotransporter in the thick ascending limb of the loop of Henle, which reduces voltage-dependent absorption of both calcium and magnesium. Similar to thiazides, loop diuretics slightly enhance phosphate excretion through inhibition of carbonic anhydrase (31). Other medications such as aminoglycosides, cisplatin, and cyclosporine have been shown to increase magnesium excretion by inhibiting magnesium reabsorption in the loop of Henle (31). These medications generally do not affect calcium or phosphate excretion.

Hormonal Regulation

The plasma concentrations of calcium, phosphate, and to a lesser degree, magnesium are precisely regulated by several hormones (**Table 94.2**). The key hormones in calcium regulation are parathyroid hormone, 1,25-dihydroxyvitamin D, and calcitonin.

Parathyroid Hormone

PTH tightly regulates ionized calcium and, to a lesser degree, phosphate levels in the blood and extracellular fluids. PTH is synthesized in the parathyroid gland and is enzymatically cleaved from the prohormone prior to its secretion. The signal sequences contained in this pre-prohormone are critical to hormone processing, as mutations at these sites have been seen in hereditary forms of hypoparathyroidism.

PTH binds to cell surface receptors linked to adenyl cyclase within the kidney and bone (17). In the kidney, PTH enhances transcellular reabsorption of calcium in the distal convoluted tubule and paracellular reabsorption in the cortical thick ascending loop of Henle. In contrast, PTH inhibits phosphate reabsorption in the proximal and distal tubules by inducing cellular uptake and proteolytic degradation of the Na-P cotransporters (16). Furthermore, PTH stimulates the conversion of 25-hydroxyvitamin D to $1,25(OH)_2D_3$ in the proximal tubule via induction of transcription of the 25-hydroxyvitamin D 1α-hydroxylase gene (20). PTH enhances release of calcium from bone by increasing expression of the surface protein RANK

TABLE 94.1

FACTORS AFFECTING RENAL EXCRETION OF CALCIUM, MAGNESIUM AND PHOSPHATE

Factor affecting excretion	Calcium — Effect on renal excretion	Calcium — Mechanism(s)	Magnesium — Effect on renal excretion	Magnesium — Mechanism(s)	Phosphate — Effect on renal excretion	Phosphate — Mechanism(s)
Volume expansion	↑	↓ reabsorption in PCT	↑	↓ reabsorption in PCT	↑	↓ reabsorption in PCT
ELECTROLYTE DISTURBANCES						
Hypercalcemia	↑	↓ reabsorption in PCT, TALH, DCT (↓ PTH)	↑	↓ tubular reabsorption	↓ (acute) ↑ (chronic)	↓ ultrafiltration, ↓ GFR and ↓ PTH (acute); ↓ tubular reabsorption via unknown mechanism (chronic)
Hypocalcemia	↓	↑ reabsorption in DCT due to ↑ PTH	↓	↑ reabsorption TALH	↑ or ↓ (chronic hypocalcemia)	↓ tubular reabsorption secondary to ↑ PTH
Hypermagnesemia	—	—	↑	↓ reabsorption in TALH	—	—
Hypomagnesemia	—	—	↓	↑ reabsorption in TALH	—	—
Hyperphosphatemia	↓	↑ reabsorption in DCT due to ↑ PTH	—	—	↑	↑ tubular reabsorption due to ↓ Na-P activity
Hypophosphatemia	↑	↓ reabsorption in DCT	↑	↓ reabsorption in TALH	↓	↑ tubular reabsorption due to ↑ Na-P activity
ACID-BASE DISTURBANCES						
Metabolic acidosis	↑	↓ reabsorption in DCT due to ↓ ECaC1 conductance	—	—	↑ (chronic metabolic acidosis)	↓ tubular reabsorption due to ↓ Na-P activity
Metabolic alkalosis	↓	↑ reabsorption in DCT due to ↑ ECaC1 conductance	↓	↓ reabsorption in TALH	↓	↑ tubular reabsorption due to ↑ Na-P activity
Respiratory acidosis	↑	—	↑	—	↓	—
Respiratory alkalosis	—	—	↑	—	↓	—
MEDICATIONS						
Thiazide diuretics	↓		minimal ↑	↓ reabsorption in DCT due to inhibition of Na-Cl cotransporter	↑	—
Loop diuretics	↑	↓ reabsorption in DCT due to altered inhibition of Na-K-2Cl cotransporter	↑	↓ reabsorption in DCT due to altered inhibition of Na-K-2Cl cotransporter	↑	—
Aminoglycosides	↑	—	↑	↓ reabsorption in TALH	—	—
Cisplatin	↑	—	↑	↓ reabsorption in TALH	—	—
Cyclosporine	↑	—	↑	↓ reabsorption in TALH	—	—

PCT, proximal convoluted tubule; TALH, thick ascending limb of the loop of Henle; DCT, distal convoluted tubule; PTH, parathyroid hormone; GFR, glomerular filtration rate

Modified from Suki WN, Lederer ED, Rouse D. Renal Transport of Calcium, Magnesium, and Phosphate. In: Brenner BM, ed. Brenner and Rector's The Kidney, 6th ed. Philadelphia: WB Saunders, 2000;520–74.

TABLE 94.2

HORMONAL REGULATION OF CALCIUM AND PHOSPHATE

Hormone	Effect on serum level			
	Calcium	Mechanism of action	Phosphate	Mechanism of action
PTH	↑	↑ reabsorption in DCT and TALH	↓	↓ reabsorption in PCT and DCT
Vitamin D	↑	↑ absorption in intestine and reabsorption in DCT	↑	↑ absorption in intestine and reabsorption in DCT
Calcitonin	↓	↓ bone reabsorption ↓ reabsorption in renal tubules	—	—

PTH, parathyroid hormone; DCT, distal convoluted tubule; TALH, thick ascending limb of the loop of Henle; PCT, proximal convoluted tubule

ligand, which stimulates osteoclast maturation and activity, leading to bone resorption (26).

Blood concentration of ionized calcium is the chief regulator of PTH secretion. PTH secretion is decreased in response to high blood concentrations of ionized calcium and, conversely, increased in response to low concentrations. The dose-response relationship of PTH secretion to blood ionized calcium is sigmoidal in nature. In addition, the greater the rate of fall in blood ionized calcium, the greater the rise in PTH secretion. From the teleologic standpoint, these two properties protect against abrupt falls in blood ionized calcium.

The signal for regulation of PTH secretion by ionized calcium is transduced through G-protein-coupled, calcium-sensing receptors on the parathyroid cell surface. When extracellular ionized calcium increases, binding of calcium to these receptors through unknown mechanisms leads to an increase in intracellular calcium with a consequent decrease in PTH secretion. As extracellular ionized calcium falls, binding to the calcium-sensing receptor decreases, intracellular ionized calcium concentration falls, and PTH secretion increases.

Calcium can also directly affect the biosynthesis of PTH. Although the precise mechanism is unknown, hypocalcemia has been shown to enhance PTH gene transcription, enhance PTH mRNA stability, and stimulate PTH mRNA translation. In contrast, hypercalcemia has no affect on production of PTH mRNA. Phosphate has also been shown to effect PTH synthesis. Elevated blood phosphate indirectly stimulates PTH secretion by reducing blood calcium and 1,25-dihydroxyvitamin D levels (7). PTH secretion can be stimulated directly by markedly elevated levels of phosphate, but the precise mechanism is unknown. 1,25-dihydroyvitamin D, although having no direct effect on PTH synthesis, has been shown to inhibit PTH gene transcription.

Vitamin D

Vitamin D is obtained from two primary sources: the skin and dietary supplementation. In the skin, the precursor of vitamin D, 7-dehydrochesterol, undergoes photochemical cleavage to form previtamin D. Previtamin D then undergoes a temperature-dependent molecular rearrangement to form vitamin D. Vitamin D consumed in the diet is absorbed by the lymphatics and enters the circulation, where it is bound to vitamin D-binding protein and, to a lesser extent, albumin. Vitamin D-binding protein serves to act as a serum reservoir for vitamin D precursors and to modulate serum levels of vi-

tamin D metabolites. In the liver, vitamin D undergoes 25-hydroxylation. Subsequently, the 25-hydroxyvitamin D undergoes 1-hydroxylation by a cytochrome P450 enzyme in the kidney to form the biologically active 1,25-dihydroxyvitamin D (29). 1,25-dihydroxyvitamin D is metabolized to inactive forms by 24- or 26-hydroxylation side-chain oxidation and cleavage, and is then excreted into bile.

1,25-dihydroxyvitamin D acts via nuclear receptors to enhance calcium and phosphate absorption primarily in the intestine and, to some extent, in distal renal tubules. 1,25-dihydroxyvitamin D also functions to promote osteoclast differentiation and bone resorption and to stimulate the synthesis of matrix proteins integral to normal bone mineralization (37). In addition, 1,25-dihydroxyvitamin D has been shown to decrease transcription of PTH. It is unclear whether this effect is critical to PTH regulation under normal conditions, but it has been used as a therapeutic strategy in the treatment of secondary hyperparathyroidism.

Calcitonin

Calcitonin is a 32-amino-acid polypeptide secreted and stored in the C cells of the thyroid gland. Calcitonin has been shown to inhibit renal tubular reabsorption of calcium and osteoclast-mediated bone resorption. The secretion of calcitonin is stimulated by increased blood calcium levels and by glucocorticoids, calcitonin gene-related peptide, glucagon, enteroglucagon, gastrin, pentagastrin, pancreozymin, and β-adrenergic agents. Although calcitonin is known to be important in regulating calcium blood levels in other species, its importance in the human physiologic regulation of calcium is unclear.

DISORDERS OF CALCIUM, MAGNESIUM, AND PHOSPHATE HOMEOSTASIS

Normal Values

Published normal values for total serum calcium range from 8.8–10.8 mg/dL (23). Although measurement of total calcium is a well-accepted means of monitoring calcium levels in healthy patients, this measurement may be inaccurate in critically ill patients. Because critically ill patients frequently are hypoalbuminemic and because ~40% of calcium is predominantly bound to albumin, it is not infrequent to encounter low total calcium levels in the critically ill. One approach has been to calculate the corrected calcium level using the following equation (11):

$$Ca_{corrected} = Ca_{measured}$$
$$+ [0.8 (4.0 - serum\ albumin_{measured}\ mg/dL)]$$

However, it may be useful for the clinician to obtain measurements of ionized calcium in critically ill patients if the technology necessary to make these measurements is readily available and the measurements can be performed accurately and in a timely fashion. Normal values for ionized calcium range between 4.2 and 5.5 mg/dL (1.0–1.4 mmol/dL) (23). Reported normal values of magnesium are 1.5–2.3 mg/dL (23). Normal phosphate levels vary with age, with values ranging from 4.8–8.2 mg/dL in newborns to 2.7–4.7 mg/dL in older adolescents (23).

Hypocalcemia

Causes

Hypocalcemia can occur as the consequence of inadequate calcium intake or malabsorption, hormonal imbalance or dysfunction, chelation by anions, or other causes (**Table 94.3**). PTH-deficient hypocalcemia may be due to impaired synthesis of PTH (either primary dysfunction or hypoplasia or agenesis of the parathyroid glands), inappropriate suppression of PTH secretion, or target organ resistance to PTH. Physiologic deficiency of PTH secretion occurs in neonates ("early neonatal hypocalcemia") during the first 4 days of life. This disorder most commonly occurs in premature infants, low-birth-weight infants, infants of diabetic mothers, and infants born after prolonged, difficult deliveries. Patients recover after several days of nutritional supplementation. Congenital agenesis or dysgenesis of the parathyroid glands has been observed in a number of inherited genetic defects. The most notable is the family of disorders that are associated with deletions in the chromosome 22q11 region, the locus for DiGeorge syndrome, velocardiofacial syndrome, and conotruncal face syndromes (10). Embryologically, these disorders result as a consequence of maldevelopment of the third and fourth branchial pouches, resulting in thymic aplasia, facial anomalies (hypertelorism, antimongoloid slant of the eyes, short philtrum, low set ears, micrognathia), and aortocardiac anomalies (right-sided aortic arch, tetralogy of Fallot, truncus arteriosus). On occasion, neonatal hypoparathyroidism may be the only presenting symptom of DiGeorge syndrome. Defects in the PTH signal peptide site have been detected in rare cases of congenital hypoparathyroidism (28). Antibody-mediated destruction of the parathyroid glands has been detected in autoimmune polyglandular syndrome type 1 (APS1), also known as the autoimmune polyendocrinopathy-candidiasis-ectodermal dystrophy (APECED) syndrome, which is caused by mutations in the autoimmune regulator gene (*AIRE*), resulting in hypoparathyroidism, primary adrenal insufficiency, and mucocutaneous candidiasis. The candidiasis is usually the first presenting symptom and is followed by hypoparathyroidism as early as 3 years of age and subsequently adrenal insufficiency. Postsurgical destruction of the parathyroid glands is the most common cause of hypoparathyroidism and occurs as a complication of thyroidectomy, radical neck dissection for malignancies, or after inadvertent interruption

TABLE 94.3

CAUSES OF HYPOCALCEMIA

Inadequate intake or malabsorption

PTH-related
  Impaired parathyroid gland formation
    Congenital agenesis or dysgenesis of the parathyroid glands
      DiGeorge syndrome
      X-linked hypoparathyroidism
  PTH gene mutations
  Parathyroid gland destruction
    Autoimmune polyglandular syndrome type 1
    Inadvertent surgical destruction
    Hemochromatosis
    Thalassemia major
    Wilson disease
  Impaired secretion of PTH
    Hypomagnesemia
    Maternal hypercalcemia
    Calcium-sensing receptor mutations
    Cytokine release
    Respiratory alkalosis
  End-organ resistance to PTH (pseudohypoparathyroidism)

Vitamin D related
  Inadequate intake or absorption
    Breast-feeding (without vitamin D supplementation)
    Gastrectomy
    Small-bowel surgery
    Celiac disease
    Inflammatory bowel disease
    Cystic fibrosis
  Increased catabolism
    Phenobarbital
    Phenytoin
    Carbamazepine
    Isoniazid
    Rifampin
    Theophylline
  Decreased 25-hydroxylation (hepatic disease)
  Decreased 1-hydroxylation (renal disease)
  Vitamin D resistance

Chelation by anions
  Hyperphosphatemia
  Red blood cell transfusions (citrate)
  Lipid administration
  Pancreatitis (fatty acids)

Other
  Fluoride intoxication
  "Hungry-bone" syndrome
  Critical illness

of the blood supply to the parathyroid glands during head and neck surgery. Destruction of the parathyroid glands is a rare complication of radioablative iodine therapy for Graves disease. In addition, parathyroid destruction has rarely occurred as the consequence of (a) deposition of iron in patients with hemochromatosis, and (b) thalassemia major and copper deposition in patients with Wilson disease.

Impaired secretion is observed in hypomagnesemia. In the initial stages of hypomagnesemia, PTH secretion is increased. However, as the hypomagnesemia persists, intracellular depletion of magnesium develops and impairs PTH secretion.

Pronounced suppression of PTH occurs in neonates of mothers with hyperparathyroidism. The resultant maternal hypercalcemia suppresses PTH secretion in the fetus and the responsiveness of the parathyroid glands to hypocalcemia following birth. Autosomal-dominant activating mutations in the gene encoding the calcium-sensing receptor (*CASR*) cause impaired PTH secretion. With activating mutations, PTH secretion is decreased because the receptor falsely detects low serum calcium concentrations as being normal. Patients with this disorder have mild-to-moderate hypocalcemia and are generally asymptomatic. However, under stress conditions, such as a febrile illness, they can present with seizures or tetany. Disorders that contribute to macrophage-mediated cytokine release, such as gram-negative sepsis and toxic shock syndrome, have also been found to impair PTH secretion.

End-organ resistance to the action of PTH, or pseudohypoparathyroidism, results from defects in the PTH receptor-adenyl cyclase system (22). Specifically in the α subunit of the GTP binding protein G_s. In these disorders, PTH levels are high in the face of hypocalcemia. The disorders are classified by the urinary excretion of cyclic AMP (cAMP) and phosphate in response to PTH administration. In type 1 pseudohypoparathyroidism, decreased urinary excretion of cAMP and phosphate occurs in response to PTH. The type 1 disorders have been divided into three subtypes. In type 1a, an autosomally inherited mutation of the *GNAS1* gene occurs, leading to an inability to activate adenyl cyclase when PTH binds to its receptor. Patients with this defect present with Albright hereditary osteodystrophy, characterized by round facies, short stature, short fourth metacarpal bones, obesity, subcutaneous ossifications, and developmental delay. Patients with type 1b pseudohypoparathyroidism have mutations that affect regulatory elements of *GNAS1* but do not exhibit the Albright phenotype. It is believed that PTH resistance is confined to the kidneys in this disorder. Patients have been described with normal cAMP excretion and decreased phosphate excretion in response to PTH administration (13) and were said to have pseudohypoparathyroidism type 2. This disorder has been seen in some patients with myotonic dystrophy.

Hypocalcemia as the result of low 1,25-dihydroxyviatmin D can occur due to inadequate vitamin D intake or production, increased vitamin D catabolism, decreased 25-hydroxylation in the liver, decreased 1-hydroxylation in the kidney, and vitamin D resistance. Inadequate intake of fatty fishes, milk or other vitamin D-containing foods, exclusive breast-feeding (without vitamin D supplementation), and inadequate sun exposure can lead to vitamin D deficiency and rickets. Inadequate intestinal absorption of vitamin D has been observed in patients with gastrectomy, celiac disease, extensive bowel surgery, inflammatory bowel disease, or pancreatic insufficiency due to cystic fibrosis. Enhanced catabolism of 1,25-dihydroxyvitamin D by activation of the cytochrome P450 system has been reported in patients receiving phenobarbital, phenytoin, carbamazepine, isoniazid, theophylline, rifampin, primidone, and glutethimide. Hepatic 25-hydroxylation of vitamin D is mildly impaired in severe liver disease or dysfunction. Decreased 1-hydroxylation of 25-hydroxyvitamin D occurs in patients with renal disease due to decreased 1-hydroxlase synthesis. Vitamin D resistance occurs as the consequence of mutations that involve the vitamin D receptor gene. These mutations result in impaired signal transduction associated with the vitamin D-receptor interaction producing clinical rickets.

Chelation of ionized calcium by anions is seen in a number of clinical situations. Hyperphosphatemia as a consequence of massive tissue lysis (e.g., tumor lysis syndrome and rhabdomyolysis), or phosphate administration can induce hypocalcemia due to formation of calcium phosphate precipitates in soft tissues. Hypocalcemia due to complex formation with citrate present in packed red blood cells is typically transient and not clinically significant unless large volumes (>5 units of packed red blood cells in adults) are given. EDTA-containing radiocontrast dyes have been shown to cause hypocalcemia. Administration of lipids or excess release of free fatty acids, as seen in pancreatitis, may also cause hypocalcemia. Other unclassified causes of hypocalcemia include the "hungry-bone syndrome" and fluoride intoxication. The "hungry-bone syndrome" occurs following parathyroidectomy in patients with primary hyperparathyroidism. Persistently high PTH levels result in prolonged bone resorption. Following parathyroid gland resection, the acute drop in PTH leads to pronounced uptake of calcium, leading to hypocalcemia. Excessive fluoride intake has been shown to inhibit bone resorption. The hypocalcemia that has been observed in critically ill patients is poorly understood and is likely the consequence of multiple factors. Potential mechanisms for the suppression of hypocalcemia during critical illness include suppression of PTH secretion by cytokines, increase calcium binding to albumin, PTH deficiency, impaired renal hydroxylation of vitamin D, calcium chelation, and hypomagnesemia. Hypocalcemia has been associated with increased mortality in critically ill patients but was found to be a poor independent predictor of mortality (12,35).

Signs and Symptoms

The signs and symptoms of hypocalcemia are most commonly the manifestations of altered function of calcium-dependent excitable tissues such as nerves and skeletal and cardiac muscle (**Table 94.4**). Patients may report myoclonic jerks and paresthesias of the perioral region, fingers, and toes. In more severe cases, patients may present with seizures, apnea, cyanosis, laryngospasm, tachypnea, tachycardia, and vomiting. On physical examination, percussion of the facial nerve below the zygomatic arch may result in facial muscle contraction

TABLE 94.4

SIGNS AND SYMPTOMS OF HYPOCALCEMIA

Neuromuscular
  Paresthesias
  Chvostek sign (facial muscle spasm with percussion of nerve)
  Trousseau sign (carpopedal spasm with ischemia)
  Bronchospasm
  Laryngospasm
  Apnea
  Seizures

Cardiac
  Prolonged QT interval
  Nonspecific ST-T wave changes

Rickets (radiographic findings)
  Epiphyseal widening
  Costochondral widening ("rachitic rosary")
  Genu varum or valgum
  Osteopenia

(Chvostek sign). Compression of the arm or leg with a blood pressure cuff may result in carpopedal spasm (Trousseau sign). On electrocardiogram, prolongation of the QT interval and nonspecific ST-T-wave changes may be observed. Hypocalcemia may rarely causes ventricular arrhythmias.

Deficiency of vitamin D due to inadequate intake, 1-α-hydroxylase deficiency (vitamin D dependency type I), and resistance to vitamin D (vitamin D dependency type II) result in rickets. Rickets is characterized by abnormal mineralization of bone and growth-plate cartilage, resulting in widening, cupping, and fraying of the bone metaphysis. On clinical exam, skeletal changes include widened wrists, swelling of the costochondral junctions of the ribs (the "rachitic rosary"), and bowing of the legs. In more severe cases of hypocalcemic rickets, symptoms of hypocalcemia may manifest.

Diagnosis and Treatment

Diagnosis of the patient with hypocalcemia should begin with a thorough history of dietary intake (concentrating on sources of calcium and vitamin D). It should also include an investigation of family history of rickets, hypocalcemia, and endocrine disorders. Physical examination should include a close evaluation of the bones and joints.

For most patients, the clinical history may provide a clear etiology, obviating the need for extensive evaluation; this also applies to most critically ill patients in the ICU. For those patients with no clear etiology or suspected rickets, a more extensive evaluation should be performed. Total serum calcium and, often, ionized calcium and albumin are useful. Other recommended laboratory studies include assessments of circulating levels of phosphorus, magnesium, blood urea nitrogen, creatinine, alkaline phosphatase activity, PTH, 1,25-dihydroxyvitamin D, and 25-hydroxyvitamin D. On a random "spot" urine collection, urinary calcium excretion is best interpreted as a calcium/creatinine (mg/mg) ratio.

Urinary phosphorous excretion is very dependent upon diet and body phosphorous status. The ideal assessment is obtained with a fasting 2-hr urine collection, with a concomitant serum sample obtained midway through the urine collection. The tubular reabsorption of phosphate (TRP) is expressed as a percentage of the filtered phosphate load and is calculated by the formula:

$$TRP = 1 - \left[\frac{[P]u \times [Cr]s}{[P]s \times [Cr]u} \right] \times 100\%$$

where [P]u is the concentration of phosphate in urine, [P]s is the concentration of phosphate in serum, [Cr]u is the concentration of creatinine in urine, and [Cr]s is the concentration of creatinine in serum. All units should be identical (e.g., mg/dL).

Serum phosphorus is usually low in patients with vitamin D deficiency and is elevated in renal failure, hypoparathyroidism, and pseudohypoparathyroidism. In vitamin D-dependent rickets type I, the serum 25-hydroxyvitamin D level is normal and the 1,25-dihydroxyvitamin D is low. Serum alkaline phosphatase activity may be elevated in patients with long-standing vitamin D deficiency but usually not in early disease. A low or normal circulating PTH in the presence of hypocalcemia indicates an inappropriate parathyroid response to hypocalcemia or, therefore, functional hypoparathyroidism. Increased PTH secretion is a normal physiologic response to hypocalcemia, so that elevated serum PTH would occur in nonparathyroid-related hypocalcemia, such as in vitamin D deficiency or impaired vitamin D action. Increased PTH levels are usually seen in pseudohypoparathyroidism.

A primary tenet in the treatment of hypocalcemia is to tailor the therapy to the cause of hypocalcemia. Calcium may be given intravenously or orally. For patients who present with acute symptomatic hypocalcemia, (i.e., tetany, muscle twitching, carpopedal spasm, laryngospasm, or seizures), a bolus dose of calcium gluconate (100–200 mg/kg or 9–18 mg/kg elemental calcium to a maximum of 1–3 g in adults) should be administered over 10–20 mins (5,11). A continuous infusion of calcium gluconate infusion may be administered at starting dose of 10–30 mg/kg/hr in order to maintain adequate calcium levels to prevent symptoms. The rate of the infusion can then be titrated based on serial calcium measurements (or ionized calcium if necessary). Much controversy has existed concerning the use of calcium chloride as a better alternative to calcium gluconate for the correction of ionized hypocalcemia. To date, published studies that compare calcium chloride to calcium gluconate show that they have similar bioavailability and are equally effective in correcting ionized hypocalcemia (18,32). We recommend administering IV calcium through a central venous catheter because of a significant risk of tissue necrosis with peripheral administration (9). Calcification of soft tissue may result if extravasation of the infusion occurs (5). All patients receiving IV calcium require close monitoring of total or ionized calcium levels. Cardiac telemetry or electrocardiograms should be used during IV calcium administration to detect cardiac rhythm disturbances. In hypocalcemic patients with hypomagnesemia, magnesium should be replenished with IV magnesium sulfate or oral magnesium oxide. In patients with concurrent hyperphosphatemia, the elevated phosphate should be corrected with phosphate binders, due to the risk of tissue deposition of calcium phosphate if the calcium-phosphate product [(Ca)s × (PO$_4$)s] exceeds 80. This figure is the product of total serum calcium (mg/dL) and the serum phosphorous levels (mg/dL).

Once tetany resolves in symptomatic patients receiving IV calcium or in asymptomatic patients who can take enteral calcium, a variety of oral preparations are available, including calcium carbonate (400 mg of elemental calcium/g), calcium glubionate (64 mg of elemental calcium/g), and calcium gluconate (90 mg of elemental calcium/g). A recommended starting dose is 50 mg/kg body weight/24 hrs of elemental calcium divided into three to four doses. The dose is then titrated based on serum calcium levels (11).

In patients with hypocalcemia secondary to vitamin D deficiency or resistance, vitamin D replacement and adequate dietary calcium intake are the mainstays of therapy. The formulation and dosage of vitamin D required are dependent on the cause of the disorder. Children with deficiency of vitamin D due to poor dietary intake or malabsorption will typically respond to oral vitamin D therapy. Children with nutritional rickets will typically require 1000–5000 IU/day of vitamin D (11). Patients for whom medication compliance is a concern may be treated with a single dose of 600,000 IU of vitamin D. Patients with malabsorption require doses of vitamin D as high as 25,000–50,000 IU/day to correct the deficiency (11). Similarly, patients on phenytoin therapy may require vitamin D supplementation. In patients with renal failure, vitamin D-dependent rickets type 1, hypoparathyroidism, or pseudohypoparathyroidism, reduced 1,25 (OH)$_2$ D synthesis may occur, requiring replacement with 1,25-dihydroxyvitamin D itself (calcitriol; 0.01–0.08 mcg/kg/day in children up to 10 kg; 0.25–1.0 mcg/day in adults) (5,11). Calcium levels should be monitored during the course of therapy.

At the time of this writing, no evidence exists that correction of hypocalcemia in critically ill patients has any clear benefit (5,35). Furthermore, data obtained from hypocalcemic animals in sepsis indicate that calcium supplementation may actually increase mortality. Although these data have not been borne out in humans, it has been suggested that hypocalcemia should be corrected in critically ill patients with symptomatic hypocalcemia or hemodynamic instability.

Hypercalcemia

Causes

Hypercalcemia generally occurs as the consequence of excessive dietary calcium intake or increased intestinal absorption. These alterations may be related to hormonal imbalance or dysfunction, increased renal reabsorption, or increased bone resorption (**Table 94.5**). One of the earliest descriptions of hypercalcemia due to excessive calcium intake is the milk-alkali syndrome, a disorder that was first reported in the early 20th century in patients who ingested excessive amounts of milk and related dairy products and sodium bicarbonate for treatment

TABLE 94.5

CAUSES OF HYPERCALCEMIA

Excessive intake
    "Milk-alkali syndrome"
    Oral calcium supplements
    Parenteral nutrition

PTH-related
    Calcium-sensing receptor mutations
    Multiple endocrine neoplasia type 1
    Multiple endocrine neoplasia type 2a
    Parathyroid adenoma
    Transient neonatal hyperparathyroidism (parathyroid gland hyperplasia)
    Chronic lithium toxicity
    Chronic renal failure
    Hyperparathyroid-jaw tumor syndrome

Humoral hypercalcemia of malignancy (PTHrP-, TNF-, cytokine-mediated)

Vitamin D intoxication

Increased renal reabsorption
    Thiazide diuretics
    Calcium-sensing receptor mutations

Increased bone resorption
    Thyrotoxicosis
    Vitamin A intoxication
    Primary and metastatic tumors
    Cytokine release
    Immobilization

Other
    Williams syndrome
    Subcutaneous fat necrosis

of peptic ulcer disease. These patients presented with the classic triad of hypercalcemia, metabolic alkalosis, and renal failure. Changes in therapy for peptic ulcer disease led to a significant reduction in the incidence of this disorder, but a resurgence of this disorder has been seen in the past 20 years in patients receiving calcium carbonate as part of their therapy for chronic renal failure. Children who receive oral calcium supplementation for other hypocalcemic disorders or parenteral nutrition are at risk for hypercalcemia.

The most common hormonal imbalance contributing to hypercalcemia is hyperparathyroidism. Primary hyperparathyroidism may occur as the result of mutations in *CASR* or defects in tumor-suppressor genes in parathyroid cells (2). Familial hypocalciuric hypercalcemia is the consequence of heterozygous mutations in the *CASR* gene. Parathyroid cells are stimulated and secrete relatively large amounts of PTH in the setting of normal calcium levels (2). When mutations in *CASR* are homozygous, severe neonatal hyperparathyroidism ensues. This rare autosomal-recessive disorder presents in the neonatal period and can be fatal if diagnosis and treatment are delayed. Parathyroid adenomas that produce excess PTH can be seen as part of multiple endocrine neoplasia type 1 (hyperparathyroidism, tumors of the anterior pituitary and pancreatic islets) and multiple endocrine neoplasia type 2a (hyperparathyroidism, medullary carcinoma of the thyroid, pheochromocytoma) (19). Transient neonatal secondary hyperparathyroidism occurs in infants of mothers with hypoparathyroidism due to prolonged fetal exposure to hypocalcemia, which stimulates hyperplasia of the parathyroid glands (25). In older children, somatic mutations in parathyroid tumor suppressor genes may lead to the development of pituitary adenomas (2). A mild form of secondary hyperparathyroidism can be seen in patients with chronic lithium toxicity. It is believed that lithium interferes with signaling by the calcium-sensing receptor, leading to excess PTH production. "Tertiary" hyperparathyroidism is seen in children with chronic renal failure. This entity refers to the development of autonomous PTH secretion following chronic "secondary" or physiologic parathyroid gland hyperfunction, for example, due to prolonged hypocalcemia.

A number of childhood malignancies, including rhabdoid tumors of the kidney, congenital mesoblastic nephroma, neuroblastoma, medulloblastoma, leukemia, Burkitt lymphoma, dysgerminoma, and rhabdomyosarcoma, are associated with hypercalcemia of malignancy. Similarly, in adults, squamous cell, breast, renal cell, and bladder cancers may manifest hypercalcemia as a paraneoplastic phenomenon. PTH-related peptide (PTHrP) mediates this hypercalcemia commonly in adults and rarely in children. PTHrP has been shown in vitro and in vivo to stimulate the PTH1 receptor (4). Vitamin D intoxication, typically seen with ingestions of >100,000 units/day of vitamin D, and malignant lymphomas that produce 1,25-dihydroxyvitamin D are uncommon causes of hypercalcemia. Variably elevated circulating levels of $1,25(OH)_2$ have been reported in subcutaneous fat necrosis in infants.

Increased renal absorption of calcium that leads to hypercalcemia can be seen with thiazide therapy and with inactivating mutations of *CASR*. Thiazide diuretics stimulate calcium reabsorption in the distal convoluted tubule.

Hypercalcemia secondary to increased bone resorption may rarely accompany thyrotoxicosis and excess vitamin A ingestion. Tumors that cause bone osteolysis and hypercalcemia (e.g., multiple myeloma and breast cancer) are seen in adults and, rarely, in children. It is believed that tumor necrosis factor-β, IL-1β, and IL-6 released from these tumors stimulate bone resorption. Other causes of hypercalcemia include Williams syndrome and immobilization.

Signs and Symptoms

Signs and symptoms of hypercalcemia are varied, and the severity of the symptoms is correlated with the degree of hypercalcemia (**Table 94.6**). Severe symptoms are observed in patients with serum calcium levels >15 mg/dL. Patients with serum levels of <15 mg/dL may be asymptomatic. Infants tend to present with gastrointestinal symptoms such as poor feeding, emesis, and failure to thrive. In older children, neurologic symptoms such as altered mental status, psychosis, and hallucinations may be present. Severe hypercalcemia contributes to hyperpolarization across myocardial membranes, leading to shortening of the QT interval and ventricular dysrhythmias. Hypercalcemia impairs the renal response to antidiuretic hormone (ADH), causing nephrogenic diabetes insipidus and resulting in an inability to concentrate urine and polyuria.

Diagnosis and Treatment

Hypercalcemia in children is uncommon. The diagnosis of the patient with hypercalcemia should begin with a thorough history of dietary intake, medications, vitamin intake, renal function, and familial disorders, including sarcoidosis and other granulomatous diseases, endocrine disorders, and hypercalcemia.

Laboratory investigation should include total serum calcium, serum phosphorus, blood urea nitrogen, creatinine, alkaline phosphatase, urinary calcium, urinary phosphorus,

urinary creatinine (for calculation of the calcium/creatinine ratio and the tubular reabsorption of phosphorus), PTH, 1,25-dihydroxyvitamin D, and 25-hydroxyvitamin D. If malignancy is suspected as a cause, a PTHrP level may be useful. An elevated PTH in the presence of hypercalcemia is diagnostic for primary hyperparathyroidism, unless the history and physical examination suggest familial hypocalciuric hypercalcemia, malignancy, or lithium therapy. When distinguishing between primary hyperparathyroidism and familial hypocalciuric hypercalcemia, a urinary calcium:creatinine ratio of <0.01 (mg/mg) raises suspicion for the familial disorder, although the distinction may be difficult to make on clinical grounds (5). A low or normal PTH level should prompt investigation of malignancy-related or other non-PTH-dependent causes of hypercalcemia.

The treatment of hypercalcemia is dependent on its severity. The initial basic tenets of therapy are to restore intravascular volume (as hypercalcemic patients are typically dehydrated) and to enhance renal excretion, which can be accomplished by administration of normal saline at two to three times maintenance fluid rate. If the patient is adequately rehydrated and calcium levels do not decrease, loop diuretics may be administered to enhance renal excretion of calcium but should be done judiciously to avoid intravascular volume depletion. Calcitonin and bisphosphonates, which inhibit bone resorption, are useful adjuncts in severe hypercalcemia (5). Patients with malignancy-related hypercalcemia also have been successfully treated with bisphosphonate. Reasonable success has been achieved with IV pamidronate in treating selected cases of childhood hypercalcemia. In severe cases in which hydration and medications fail to reduce serum calcium levels, hemodialysis using a low-calcium dialysate can be performed. Glucocorticoids have been useful in treating hypercalcemia secondary to sarcoidosis and vitamin D deficiency (through inhibition of intestinal actions of vitamin D) (5).

Indications for surgery for primary hyperparathyroidism include total calcium level >12 mg/dL, hyperparathyroid crisis (discrete episode of life-threatening hypercalcemia), marked hypercalciuria, nephrolithiasis, impaired renal function, osteitis fibrosa cystica, reduced cortical bone density (measured with dual x-ray absorptiometry or similar technique), bone mass greater than two standard deviations below age-matched controls, classic neuromuscular symptoms, proximal muscle weakness and atrophy, hyperreflexia, gait disturbance, and age <50 years (21).

TABLE 94.6

SIGNS AND SYMPTOMS OF HYPERCALCEMIA

Neuromuscular
  Fatigue
  Weakness
  Lethargy
  Confusion
  Coma
  Hallucinations
  Psychosis

Gastrointestinal
  Poor feeding
  Failure to thrive
  Nausea
  Vomiting
  Constipation
  Pancreatitis (rare)

Cardiac
  Shortened QT interval
  Ventricular dysrhythmias

Renal
  Polyuria
  Hyposthenuria
  Dehydration
  Hypernatremia
  Renal stone formation
  Renal failure

Hypomagnesemia

Causes

Hypomagnesemia generally occurs as the consequence of decreased dietary magnesium intake or malabsorption, its decreased renal reabsorption, or its redistribution from the extracellular to the intracellular space (**Table 94.7**). Dietary deficiency of magnesium is exceedingly uncommon due to the presence of magnesium in a wide variety of foods. The three most common scenarios in which nutritional magnesium deficiency can be seen are protein-calorie malnutrition, parenteral nutrition, and alcoholism. In patients with fat malabsorption, free fatty acids in the intestinal lumen chelate magnesium, preventing its absorption. Intestinal malabsorption or syndromes that are characterized by significant diarrhea (e.g., celiac

CAUSES OF HYPOMAGNESEMIA

Decreased dietary intake or malabsorption
    Protein-calorie malnutrition
    Parenteral nutrition
    Alcoholism
    Diarrhea
    Celiac disease
    Inflammatory bowel disease
Decreased renal reabsorption
    Inherited disorders
        Isolated familial hypomagnesemia
        Primary hypomagnesemia with hypercalciuria
        Primary hypomagnesemia with hypocalcemia
        Bartter syndrome
        Gitelman syndrome
    Medications
        Loop diuretics
        Cisplatin
        Pentamidine
        Cyclosporine
        Aminoglycosides
        Foscarnet
        Amphotericin
Redistribution from the extracellular to the intracellular space
    Insulin therapy
    Hyperinsulinism
    Pancreatitis
    Hyperaldosteronism
    Respiratory alkalosis
    Catecholamines

disease, inflammatory bowel disease, and Whipple disease) are associated with increased magnesium loss in the stool. Decreased renal reabsorption of magnesium may occur as the consequence of congenital or acquired renal disorders, certain medications (loop diuretics, cisplatin, cyclosporine, amphotericin B, aminoglycosides), or with metabolic abnormalities. Inherited disorders associated with renal magnesium wasting include (a) isolated familial hypomagnesemia, (b) familial hypomagnesemia with hypercalciuria [associated with mutations in the paracellin (*PCLN1*) gene], (c) primary hypomagnesemia with hypocalcemia (associated with defects in the TRP gene family), (d) Bartter syndrome [associated with mutations in the genes for the apical sodium-potassium-chloride cotransporter (*BSC1*), the apical inwardly rectifying potassium channel (*ROMK1*), or the basolateral chloride channel (*CLC-Kb*)], and (e) Gitelman syndrome [associated with mutations in the DCT electroneutral thiazide-sensitive sodium-chloride cotransporter (*TSC*)] (3,14,34,36).

Patients with isolated familial hypomagnesemia present with hypomagnesemia and hypermagnesuria but no other electrolyte disturbances. Familial hypomagnesemia with hypercalciuria is characterized by hypomagnesemia, hypermagnesuria, and marked hypercalciuria, contributing to hypocalcemia and nephrocalcinosis. Primary hypomagnesemia with hypocalcemia is an autosomal-recessive disorder found in Bedouin kindreds; affected patients typically present with hypocalcemia-induced seizures. Bartter syndrome is an autosomal recessive disorder that presents in infancy or early childhood. Patients

typically present with sodium wasting, hypokalemic metabolic alkalosis, and hypercalciuria. Gitelman syndrome presents after age 6, and is differentiated from Bartter syndrome by the presence of hypocalciuria. Impaired renal reabsorption of magnesium occurs as a side effect of various medications, including diuretics (most commonly of the loop type), cisplatin, pentamidine, cyclosporine, aminoglycosides, foscarnet, and amphotericin. Typically, renal magnesium wasting resolves within several days of discontinuation of the medication. One exception is cisplatin, with which renal magnesium loss may persist for several months. Intravascular volume expansion, osmotic diuresis (as seen in diabetic ketoacidosis), and polyuria during the recovery phase of acute renal failure have been reported as causes of hypomagnesemia due to renal loss.

The movement of magnesium from the extracellular to the intracellular compartment occurs in a variety of disorders, including insulin therapy for diabetic ketoacidosis and hyperinsulinism associated with the "refeeding syndrome" in chronically malnourished children. Enhanced intracellular uptake of magnesium has also been observed in pancreatitis, hyperaldosteronism, respiratory alkalosis, and elevation in plasma catecholamines. Hypomagnesemia has been observed in patients who undergo cardiopulmonary bypass or require massive transfusion and in those with extensive burn injury or excessive sweating.

Signs and Symptoms

The signs and symptoms of hypomagnesemia do not typically manifest until serum levels fall below 1 mg/dL. The imbalance in serum magnesium typically affects the neuromuscular system and heart. Symptoms are often due to the hypocalcemia from impaired PTH release and hypokalemia, which are also associated with hypomagnesemia. Presenting neurologic signs include muscle weakness and tremors, tetany, Chvostek sign, Trousseau sign, and seizures. Hypokalemia consequent to hypomagnesemia lowers the myocardial action potential threshold, manifesting in nonspecific T-wave changes, U waves, a prolonged QT interval, and ventricular arrhythmias. Hypomagnesemia per se can predispose to cardiac dysrhythmias, particularly those of ventricular origin. However, the degree of risk for dysrhythmias in patients with hypomagnesemia in general and the relative importance of Mg^{2+} deficiency alone versus hypomagnesemia with coexisting hypokalemia or intrinsic cardiac disease in the pathogenesis of the dysrhythmia remain controversial.

Diagnosis and Treatment

The diagnosis of hypomagnesemia can frequently be determined by the clinical history, which should explore dietary intake, gastrointestinal disorders, medications, renal function, and familial disorders. In addition to serum magnesium, serum calcium and potassium levels should be measured. If the cause of hypomagnesemia is unknown, measurement of plasma and urinary magnesium and creatinine concentrations and calculation of the fractional excretion of magnesium (FE_{Mg}) using the equation below can assist in the differentiation between renal and nonrenal causes of hypomagnesemia (11).

$$FE_{Mg} = [(U_{Mg} \times P_{creatinine})/(0.7 \times P_{Mg} \times U_{creatinine})] \times 100$$

Normal values for the fractional excretion of magnesium range from 1% to 8%. In patients with hypomagnesemia due to nonrenal causes, the FE_{Mg} is <2%. In patients with renal magnesium wasting, the FE_{Mg} is >4%. If a renal cause of hypomagnesemia is suspected, an arterial blood gas should be obtained to assess for metabolic alkalosis.

Symptomatic patients or asymptomatic patients with magnesium levels <1 mg/dL require IV replacement with a magnesium salt (11,12). Magnesium sulfate at a dose of 25–50 mg/kg (2.5–5.0 mg/kg of elemental magnesium) given as a slow IV infusion is recommended. Serum magnesium levels should be closely monitored, and the dose should be repeated every 6 hrs until levels stabilize. For patients who require long-term therapy or for mild-to-moderate hypomagnesemia, oral supplementation with agents such as magnesium gluconate (5.4 mg elemental magnesium/100 mg), magnesium oxide (60 mg elemental magnesium/100 mg), and magnesium sulfate (10 mg elemental magnesium/100 mg) at doses of 20–40 mg/kg of elemental magnesium per day can be instituted. Patients with hypocalcemia and hypokalemia require replenishment of these minerals.

Hypermagnesemia

Causes

Hypermagnesemia can be the consequence of increased intake or administration of magnesium, decreased renal excretion, massive cellular release, or other causes (**Table 94.8**). Hypermagnesemia most commonly occurs in the setting of excess administration of medications that contain magnesium, such as cathartics and antacids or parenteral administration of magnesium for patients with preeclampsia. Patients with renal failure have impaired renal excretion of magnesium, but hypermagnesemia is uncommon unless the patient is receiving magnesium supplementation. Significant cellular lysis with release of intracellular magnesium and consequent hypermagnesemia has been reported in the setting of shock, trauma, and burns. Hypothyroidism and hypoaldosteronism are rare causes of hypermagnesemia.

TABLE 94.8

CAUSES OF HYPERMAGNESEMIA

Increased intake
Laxatives
Enemas
Parenteral administration
Magnesium supplementation
Decreased renal excretion (renal failure)
Cellular release
Shock
Trauma
Burns
Other
Hypothyroidism
Hypoaldosteronism

Modified from Hastbacka J, Petilla V. Prevalence and predictive value of ionized hypocalcemia among critically ill patients. *Acta Anesthesiol Scand* 2003;47:1264–9.

TABLE 94.9

SIGNS AND SYMPTOMS OF HYPERMAGNESEMIA

Neuromuscular
Muscle weakness
Muscle paralysis
Respiratory depression
Lethargy
Coma
Cardiac
Prolonged PR interval
Prolonged QT interval

Signs and Symptoms

The signs and symptoms of hypermagnesemia usually do not manifest until the serum level is >4.0 mg/dL. The manifestations of hypermagnesemia are attributable, in part, to impaired release and binding of acetylcholine at the neuromuscular junction (**Table 94.9**). Patients may develop muscle weakness, loss of deep tendon reflexes, lethargy, progression to coma, and respiratory failure. Magnesium-induced vasodilatation contributes to the genesis of hypotension. Ileus or decreased gastrointestinal motility may be a presenting sign. Hypermagnesemia also induces significant cardiac effects, including bradycardia, prolongation of the PR and QT intervals, heart block, and cardiac arrest.

Diagnosis and Treatment

The diagnosis of hypermagnesemia may be suggested by the clinical history, which should explore medications and symptoms of renal dysfunction. The basic tenets of therapy for hypermagnesemia are to interrupt magnesium intake and promote magnesium excretion (5,11). Because hypermagnesemia may contribute to hypocalcemia, serum calcium levels should be measured and followed closely during therapy.

Patients with mild, asymptomatic hypermagnesemia and good renal function can be safely treated by stopping the magnesium-containing agent. Patients with significant neuromuscular or cardiac toxicity require measures to enhance magnesium excretion, which can be achieved by hydration with normal saline and administration of a loop diuretic. Alternatively, non-magnesium-containing enemas or a cathartic may be administered. Patients with refractory hypermagnesemia or with renal failure and severe hypermagnesemia may require hemodialysis or peritoneal dialysis to effectively reduce serum magnesium levels. Hypocalcemia should be corrected by calcium replacement.

Hypophosphatemia

Causes

Hypophosphatemia occurs as the consequence of (a) decreased dietary phosphate intake or malabsorption, (b) decreased renal reabsorption, (c) increased bone formation, or (d) redistribution of phosphate from the extracellular to the intracellular space (**Table 94.10**). Hypophosphatemia due to poor intake is uncommon because of the abundance of phosphate in foodstuffs and compensatory ability of the renal tubule to enhance reabsorption of phosphate when supply

CAUSES OF HYPOPHOSPHATEMIA

Decreased dietary intake or malabsorption
    Protein calorie malnutrition
    Disorders of the duodenum and jejunum
    Chronic diarrhea

Decreased renal reabsorption
    PTH-dependent mechanisms
        Hyperparathyroidism
        Tumor release of PTH-related peptide
    PTH/PTH-related peptide-independent mechanisms
        X-linked hyperphosphatemic rickets and other
            FGF23-related disorders
        Intravascular volume expansion
        Fanconi syndrome
        Vitamin D deficiency
        Medications/toxins
            Acetazolamide
            Glucocorticoids
            Ifosfamide
            Cisplatin
            Pamidronate
            Heavy-metal ingestion

Increased bone formation ("hungry-bone" syndrome)

Redistribution from the extracellular to the intracellular space
    Insulin therapy
    Catecholamine administration
    Theophylline
    Respiratory alkalosis

PTH, parathyroid hormone; FGF, fibroblast growth factor. Modified from Hastbacka J, Petilla V. Prevalence and predictive value of ionized hypocalcemia among critically ill patients. *Acta Anesthesiol Scand* 2003;47:1264–9.

is low. Children with severe protein-calorie malnutrition and premature infants who ingest unsupplemented breast milk (which is low in phosphate content) may develop hypophosphatemia. Critically ill, malnourished patients, in particular those who require mechanical ventilation, may develop hypophosphatemia during refeeding. Administration of carbohydrate in these patients enhances insulin release, which stimulates intracellular uptake of phosphate. The combination of phosphate depletion from their baseline poor nutritional state, along with cellular uptake of phosphate, may contribute to symptomatic hypophosphatemia—most commonly muscle weakness—impairing the ability to wean from mechanical ventilation. Malabsorption due to intestinal disorders that affect the duodenum and jejunum (the primary sites for phosphate absorption) and ingestion of phosphate-binding acids are more frequently encountered causes of hypophosphatemia.

Increased renal excretion of phosphate may occur by PTH-dependent and PTH-independent mechanisms. Hyperparathyroidism (and tumor secretion of PTHrP, as described previously) decreases renal tubular reabsorption of phosphate. PTH-independent mechanisms of hypophosphatemia include intravascular volume expansion, renal tubular disorders (such as X-linked hypophosphatemia and Fanconi syndrome), various medications, and toxins. The Fanconi syndrome is a generalized renal tubular wasting of solutes that typically include phosphate, amino acids, glucose, and bicarbonate. Fanconi

syndrome may be inherited or acquired; renal tubular acidosis and hypophosphatemia are usually the most clinically significant features, although hypokalemia may also ensue. Acetazolamide, glucocorticoids, bicarbonate, ifosfamide, cisplatin, pamidronate, ethanol, and heavy metals enhance renal excretion of phosphate.

X-linked hypophosphatemia, which usually presents as a rachitic disorder in early childhood, is due to mutations in *PHEX*, a gene encoding an enzyme of the neuropeptidase family (15,24). For reasons that are not clear, elevated serum levels of a novel member of the fibroblast growth factor family, FGF23, are characteristic of X-linked hypophosphatemia and are thought to mediate the renal phosphate wasting.

Elevated FGF23 levels are typical of other related causes of hypophosphatemic rickets. These include (a) autosomal-dominant hypophosphatemic rickets (due to specific *FGF23* mutation that prevent its breakdown), (b) autosomal-recessive hypophosphatemic rickets (due to mutations in *DMP1*, dentine matrix protein), and (c) oncogenic osteomalacia, in which FGF23 is overproduced by tumors (38).

Other causes of redistribution of phosphate from the extracellular to the intracellular space with resultant hypophosphatemia include increased endogenous insulin production following glucose infusion, insulin therapy for treatment of diabetic ketoacidosis, catecholamine administration, theophylline, and respiratory alkalosis.

Signs and Symptoms

Signs and symptoms of severe hypophosphatemia occur when serum phosphate levels are <1–1.5 mg/dL. The signs and symptoms are believed to be the consequence of intracellular ATP and resultant cellular energy depletion (**Table 94.11**). The signs and symptoms are variable. Patients may present with hemolysis, leukocyte dysfunction, platelet dysfunction, muscle weakness and paralysis, muscle atrophy, respiratory failure, rhabdomyolysis, and lethargy.

Diagnosis and Treatment

The diagnosis of hypophosphatemia may be suspected from elements of the clinical history, which should explore dietary intake, medications, renal function, and family history of renal tubular disorders or hyperparathyroidism. Measurement of serum phosphate, total serum calcium, circulating PTH, and vitamin D levels is usually helpful. Patients with serum phosphate levels >2.2 mg/dL do not require aggressive therapy and can be treated with an increased intake of milk (5,11). Patients with serum phosphate levels <1.5 mg/dL and/or symptomatic

SIGNS AND SYMPTOMS OF HYPOPHOSPHATEMIA

Muscle weakness
Paralysis
Coma
Seizures
Respiratory depression
Hemolysis
Leukocyte dysfunction
Platelet dysfunction
Rhabdomyolysis

hypophosphatemia may require treatment with IV phosphate. It has been recommended that patients with severe asymptomatic hypophosphatemia should receive 2.5 mg/kg body mass of elemental phosphorus over a 6-hr period, while symptomatic patients should receive 5 mg/kg body mass of elemental phosphorus over a 6-hr period (5,11).

Hyperphosphatemia

Causes

Hyperphosphatemia is the result of increased intake of phosphate, or its decreased renal excretion or redistribution from the extracellular to the intracellular space. Increased intake is an uncommon cause of hyperphosphatemia (**Table 94.12**), reported in patients with renal failure who are receiving phosphate supplementation and in children receiving phosphate enemas. Acute and chronic renal failure is the most common cause of hyperphosphatemia due to limitations of phosphate excretion, with progressive nephron impairment or loss. Other indications associated with impaired renal phosphate excretion include acromegaly and tumoral calcinosis, a rare disease characterized by hyperphosphatemia, increased 1,25-dihydroxyvitamin D levels, and low or normal PTH levels. More common in African Americans, tumoral calcinosis presents with focal hyperostosis and large, lobulated periarticular ectopic calcifications. It may result from loss of function mutations in *FGF23*, or *GALNT3*, a gene encoding an *N*-acetylgalactosaminyltransferase (GalNAc-transferase) that is thought to be important in the posttranslational modification of FGF23 (30). Respiratory acidosis, metabolic acidosis, tumor lysis syndrome, rhabdomyolysis, hemolysis, crush injuries, and hyperthermia are also associated with hyperphosphatemia.

TABLE 94.12

CAUSES OF HYPERPHOSPHATEMIA

Increased intake
Phosphate supplements
Phosphate-containing enemas
Decreased renal excretion
Acute and chronic renal failure
Hypoparathyroidism
Acromegaly
Heparin
Tumoral calcinosis
Vitamin D intoxication
Redistribution from the extracellular to the intracellular space
Tumor lysis syndrome
Rhabdomyolysis
Hemolysis
Crush injuries
Hyperthermia
Respiratory acidosis
Metabolic acidosis

Modified from Hastbacka J, Petilla V. Prevalence and predictive value of ionized hypocalcemia among critically ill patients. *Acta Anesthesiol Scand* 2003;47:1264–9.

Signs, Symptoms, Diagnosis, and Treatment

Hyperphosphatemia, in and of itself, generally does not result in acute physiologic manifestations. Hyperphosphatemia, however, may serve to increase the Ca × P product, which when >80 mg/dL in infants (>60 in small children and >40 in older children and adults), promotes soft tissue calcification. Acute increases in serum phosphate levels will also result in a hypocalcemic response. Supportive history for the finding of hypophosphatemia should include a review of dietary intake, medications, and renal function. The basic tenets of treatment are to improve renal filtration and excretion of phosphate through intravascular volume expansion with normal saline and to stop intake of excess phosphate (5,11). Dialysis is effective in decreasing phosphate in renal failure patients with severe hyperphosphatemia.

CONCLUSIONS AND FUTURE DIRECTIONS

Many disorders of calcium, magnesium, and phosphate result from disruptions in their supply and demand. Hormonal signalling pathways that regulate these minerals may be disrupted. As these pathways and the genetic mutations that alter them are more clearly delineated, tailored therapies will likely be developed that are directed toward molecular targets within the various biochemical pathways. For example, identification of the calcium-sensing receptor as central to regulation of PTH secretion has resulted in "calcimimetic" medications. These compounds increase the sensitivity of the calcium-sensing receptor to circulating ionized calcium concentrations and have been employed as a medical treatment for selected cases of hyperparathyroidism (8).

KEY POINTS

- Regulation of serum concentrations of calcium is the net sum of the interface between the circulating compartment with three tissues: the intestines, bone, and kidneys.
- The primary site of regulation of calcium is at the level of the intestine.
- The primary site of regulation of phosphorus is the kidney.
- Total serum calcium concentration ranges between 8.8 and 10.8 mg/dL and is 40% protein bound, 50% in a free ionized form, and 5%–10% complexed to small anions.
- The ionized fraction of calcium is relevant with respect to clinical symptomatology and can be measured directly in the settings of hypoalbuminemia and acid-base disturbances.
- Parathyroid hormone and 1,25-dihydroxyvitamin D are the major hormonal regulators of calcium and phosphorus homeostasis.
- Hypocalcemia may be manifest by neuromuscular irritability, tetany, seizures, and coma. Symptoms include lethargy, constipation, bone pain, and features of hypercalciuria (hematuria, dysuria, renal stones, hyposthenuria). In infants, signs of hypocalcemia may be nonspecific, such as poor feeding.
- Clinical findings of hypocalcemia include Chvostek and Trousseau signs.

■ The initial step in assessment of calcium disorders is to determine whether they are PTH-dependent or -independent.

■ Phosphate is ubiquitous in the diet, and hypophosphatemia due to dietary causes is uncommon, except in breast-fed premature infants.

■ Hypophosphatemia is often due to primary renal losses or intracellular-extracellular compartmental shifts.

References

1. Ambuhl PM, Zajicek HK, Wang H, et al. Regulation of renal phosphate transport by acute and chronic metabolic acidosis in the rat. *Kidney Int* 1998;53:1288–98.

2. Beall DP, Henslee HB, Webb HR, et al. Milk alkali syndrome: A historical review and description of the modern version of the syndrome. *Am J Med Sci* 2006;331:233–42.

3. Blostein R, Pu HX, Scanzano R, Zouzoulas A. Structure/function studies of the gamma subunit of the Na,K-ATPase. *Ann New York Acad Sci* 2003;986:420–7.

4. Body JJ. Hypercalcemia of malignancy. *Semin Nephrol* 2004;24:48–54.

5. Bringhurst FR, Demay MB, Kronenberg HM. Hormones and disorders of mineral metabolism. In: Larsen PR, Kronenberg HM, Melmed S, et al., eds. *Williams Textbook of Endocrinology, 10th ed.* St. Louis: WB Saunders, 2003 (MD Consult version).

6. Dai LJ, Ritchie G, Kerstan D, et al. Magnesium transport in the renal distal convoluted tubule. *Physiol Rev* 2001;81:51–84.

7. Estepa JC, Aguilera-Tejero E, Lopez I, et al. Effect of phosphate on parathyroid hormone secretion in vivo. *J Bone Miner Res* 1999;14:1848–54.

8. Falchetti A. Calcium agonists in hyperparathyroidism. *Expert Opin Investig Drugs* 2004;14:229–44.

9. Ford DC, Leist ER, Algren JR, et al. *Guidelines for Administration of Intravenous Medications to Pediatric Patients, 2nd ed.* Bethesda, MD: American Society of Health-System Pharmacists, 1984

10. Garabedian M. Hypocalcemia and chromosome 22q11 microdeletion. *Genet Couns* 1999;10:389–94.

11. Greenbaum LA. Pathophysiology of Body Fluids and Fluid Therapy. In: Behrman RE, Kliegman RM, Jensen HB, eds. *Nelson Textbook of Pediatrics, 17th ed.* St. Louis: WB Saunders, 2004 (MD consult version).

12. Hastbacka J, Petilla V. Prevalence and predictive value of ionized hypocalcemia among critically ill patients. *Acta Anesthesiol Scand* 2003;47:1264–9.

13. Jüppner H, Schipani E, Bastepe. M, et al. The gene responsible for pseudohypoparathyroidism type Ib is paternally imprinted and maps in four unrelated kindreds to chromosome 20q13.3. *Proc Natl Acad Sci USA* 1998;95:11798–803.

14. Konrad M, Schlingmann KP, Gudermann T. Insights into the molecular nature of magnesium homeostasis. *Am J Physiol Renal Physiol* 2004;286:F599–605.

15. Liu S, Guo R, Simpson LG, et al. Regulation of fibroblastic growth factor 23 expression but not degradation by PHEX. *J Biol Chem* 2003;278(39):37419–26.

16. Lotscher M, Scarpetta Y, Levi M, et al. Rapid downregulation of rat renal Na/P(i) cotransporter in response to parathyroid hormone involves microtubule rearrangement. *J Clin Invest* 1999;104:483–494.

17. Mannstadt M, Juppner H, Gardella TJ. Receptors for PTH and PTHrP: Their biological importance and functional properties. *Am J Physiol* 1999;277:F665–75.

18. Martin TJ, Kang Y, Robertson KM, et al. Ionization and hemodynamic effects of calcium chloride and calcium gluconate in the absence of hepatic function. *Anesthesiology* 1990;73:62–5.

19. Marx SJ, Agarwal SK, Kester MB, et al. Multiple endocrine neoplasia type 1: Clinical and genetic features of the hereditary endocrine neoplasias. *Recent Prog Horm Res* 1999;54:397–439.

20. Murayama A, Takeyama K, Kitanaka S, et al. Positive and negative regulations of the renal 25-hydroxyvitamin D3 1a-hydroxylase gene by parathyroid hormone, calcitonin, and 1a,25(OH)2D3 in intact animals. *Endocrinology* 1999;140:2224–31.

21. NIH conference. Diagnosis and management of asymptomatic primary hyperparathyroidism: Consensus development conference statement. *Ann Intern Med* 1991;114:593–7.

22. Pearce SH, Williamson C, Kifor O, et al. A familial syndrome of hypocalcemia with hypercalciuria due to mutations in the calcium-sensing receptor. *N Engl J Med* 1996;335:1115–22.

23. Price PA. Blood Chemistries and Body Fluids. In: Robertson J, Shilkofski N, eds. *Johns Hopkins: The Harriet Lane Handbook: A Manual for Pediatric House Officers, 17th ed.* St. Louis: Mosby, 2005 (MD Consult version).

24. Sabbagh Y, Boileau G, Campos M, et al. Structure and function of disease-causing missense mutations in the PHEX gene. *J Clin Endocrinol Metab* 2003;88(5):2213–22

25. Schuffenecker I, Virally-Monod M, Brohet R, et al. Risk and penetrance of primary hyperparathyroidism in multiple endocrine neoplasia type 2A families with mutations at codon 634 of the RET proto-oncogene. *J Clin Endocrinol Metab* 1998;83:487–91.

26. Suda T, Takahashi N, Udagawa N, et al. Modulation of osteoclast differentiation and function by the new members of the tumor necrosis factor receptor and ligand families. *Endocr Rev* 1999;20:345–57.

27. Suki WN, Lederer ED, Rouse D. Renal Transport of Calcium, Magnesium, and Phosphate. In: Brenner BM, ed. *Brenner and Rector's The Kidney, 6th ed.* Philadelphia: WB Saunders, 2000;520–74.

28. Sunthornthepvarakul T, Churesigaew S, Ngowngarmratana S. A novel mutation of the signal peptide of the preproparathyroid hormone gene associated with autosomal recessive familial isolated hypoparathyroidism. *J Clin Endocrinol Metab* 1999;84:3792–6.

29. Takeyama K, Kitanaka S, Sato T, et al. 25-Hydroxyvitamin D3 1α-hydroxylase and vitamin D synthesis. *Science* 1997;277:1827–30.

30. Topaz O, Shurman DL, Bergman R, et al. Mutations in GALNT3, encoding a protein involved in O-linked glycosylation, cause familial tumoral calcinosis. *Nature Genetics* 2004;36(6):579–81.

31. Topf JM, Murray PT. Hypomagnesemia and hypermagnesemia. *Rev Endocrinol Metab Dis* 2003;4:195–206.

32. Umpaichitra V, Bastian W, Castells S. Hypocalcemia in children: Pathogenesis and management. *Clin Pediatr* 2001;40:305–12.

33. VennekensR, Prenen J, Hoenderop JG, et al. Modulation of the epithelial Ca^{2+} channel ECaC by extracellular pH. *Pflugers Arch* 2001;442:237–42.

34. Walder RY, Landau D, Meyer P, et al. Mutation of TRPM6 causes familial hypomagnesemia with secondary hypocalcemia. *Nat Genet* 2002;31:171–174.

35. Ward, RT, Colton, DM, Meade PC, et al. Serum levels of calcium and albumin in survivors after critical injury. *J Crit Care* 2004;19:54–64.

36. Wolf MT, Dotsch J, Konrad M, et al. Follow-up of five patients with FHHNC due to mutations in the paracellin-1 gene. *Pediatr Nephrol* 2002;17:602–8.

37. Yasuda H, Shima N, Nakagawa N, et al. Osteoclast differentiation factor is a ligand for osteoprotegerin/osteoclastogenesis-inhibitory factor and is identical to TRANCE/RANKL. *Proc Natl Acad Sci USA* 1998;95:3597–602.

38. Yu X, White KE. FGF23 and disorders of phosphate homeostasis. *Cytokine Growth Factor Rev* 2005;16(2):221–32.

CHAPTER 95 ■ THYROID DISEASE

ORI EYAL • SUSAN R. ROSE

NORMAL PHYSIOLOGY

Thyroid hormones play a key role in the regulation of energy expenditure and substrate metabolism and are essential for normal growth and development. A classic feedback control loop exists between the thyroid gland and the hypothalamus and pituitary (**Fig. 95.1**). Thyrotropin-releasing hormone (TRH) is expressed in the hypothalamus and regulates thyroid-stimulating hormone (TSH) synthesis and secretion by the thyrotroph cells in the pituitary. Serum TSH concentration exhibits a circadian pattern. After it reaches its nadir in the late afternoon, the serum TSH concentration rises to a peak around midnight, remains on a plateau for several hours, and then declines (29). TSH is the major regulator of the morphologic and functional states of the thyroid gland. In addition, an inverse relationship exists between the thyroid organic iodine and the rate of hormone formation.

The substrate for the synthesis of thyroid hormone is circulating iodide. The thyroid gland is able to trap iodide from the circulation by an energy-requiring mechanism. The trapped iodide is oxidized by the enzyme peroxidase. The next step in the synthesis of triiodothyronine (T_3) and tetraiodothyronine (T_4) is iodination of tyrosine to monoiodotyrosine (MIT) and to diiodotyrosine (DIT). Coupling of two DIT molecules results in the formation of T_4. Some T_3 is also formed within the thyroid gland by condensation of one molecule of MIT and DIT. The formed T_3 and T_4 are stored in the thyroid gland in combination with thyroglobulin. Release of T_3 and T_4 from thyroglobulin in the colloid occurs by proteolysis and is regulated by TSH (36).

Under normal conditions, 10%–20% of T_3 and 100% of T_4 in the serum are directly secreted by the thyroid gland. The remaining 80%–90% of T_3 is derived from peripheral monodeiodination of T_4 by the enzyme 5'-monodeiodinase. Thyroxine may also be metabolized peripherally by the enzyme 5'-monodeiodinase to reverse T_3 (rT_3), which is largely metabolically inactive. Three types of monodeiodinase have been described: Type I 5'-monodeiodinase predominantly is expressed in the liver and kidney and accounts for most circulating T_3. Type II 5'-monodeiodinase is located predominantly in the brain, pituitary, and brown adipose tissue, and acts primarily to increase intracellular levels of T_3 in these tissues. Circulating T_3 is not active in the brain, and T_4 is not active in the brain without this enzyme. Type III 5'-monodeiodinase catalyzes the conversion of T_4 to rT_3 and of T_3 to T_2 (diiodothyronine).

In the blood, thyroid hormones are mainly associated with carrier proteins: thyroxine-binding globulin (TBG), prealbumin or transthyretin, and albumin. The prolonged half-life of thyroid hormone is related to its protein binding. The bound form is in equilibrium with free hormones. The most important carrier protein for T_4 is TBG. TBG and albumin seem equally important as carrier proteins for T_3. The concentration of free T_4 and free T_3 approximate 0.03% and 0.30%, respectively, of the total serum thyroid hormone concentration (9). The bound hormone acts merely as a serum reservoir. It is the free hormone that is available to the tissues for intracellular transport and feedback regulation. The free hormones penetrate the cell membrane by carrier-mediated, energy-dependent transport. The carrier-transport system for T_3 and T_4 is saturable, stereospecific, and requires ATP. The two iodothyronines typically do not compete for uptake (19). T_4 is monodeiodinated to T_3 in the cell cytoplasm.

The cellular cytoplasmic T_3 diffuses into the nucleus and initiates its actions by binding to one of two groups of nuclear DNA-bound thyroid hormone receptors (TR), $TR\alpha$ or $TR\beta$. After binding, the T_3/TR complex either homodimerizes with a second TR or heterodimerizes to a retinoid x receptor. These complexes directly bind to consensus DNA sequences, resulting in either activation or inhibition of gene transcription (**Fig. 95.2**). The thyroid hormone nuclear receptors are members of the steroid hormone/retinoic acid receptor superfamily and function as DNA transcription factors. The gene for $TR\alpha$ is located on chromosome 17, and the gene for $TR\beta$ is on chromosome 3. Each gene is translated to several mRNA species, including $TR\alpha1$, $TR\alpha2$, $TR\beta1$, and $TR\beta2$. $TR\alpha1$ and $TR\beta1$ are the major nuclear receptors present in most tissues. $TR\alpha2$ is present in developing brain tissue. $TR\beta2$ is present in pituitary and selected brain tissues (9). T_3 is the active hormone and has a 15-fold higher binding affinity for the DNA-receptor than does T_4.

A number of assays have been developed for TSH and free T_4 (FT_4). One should be aware of the specific assays being used at one's own institution, the normal ranges in these assays, and the possible factors that may interfere with each assay and cause falsely elevated or falsely lowered results. The ultrasensitive TSH immunoassay uses monoclonal antibodies. With the availability of third- and fourth-generation ultrasensitive assays, TSH can now be measured quickly and with more accuracy than with previous assays. Estimates of the FT_4 concentration in serum can be generated by direct and indirect assay. Analog indirect assays for FT_4 employ radioimmunoassay. The gold standard for measurement of FT_4 uses equilibrium dialysis, which is the most accurate and direct measurement of the concentrations of FT_4. FT_4 can be measured indirectly by using radiolabeled T_4; the proportion that is unbound by protein is determined by dialysis, and the concentration of FT_4 can then be calculated as the product of the total hormone concentration and the fraction that is free (19).

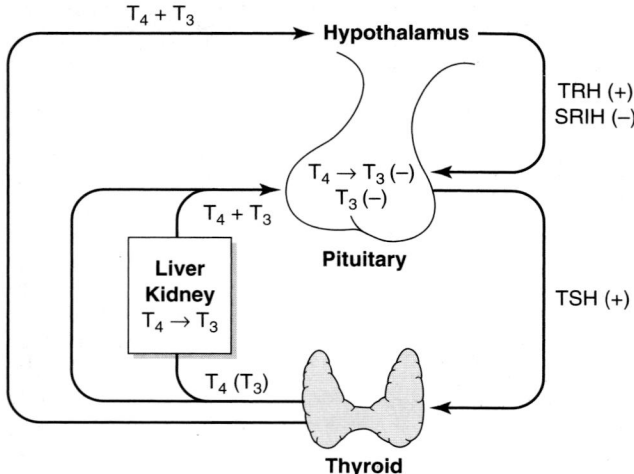

FIGURE 95.1. Basic elements in the regulation of thyroid function. Thyrotropin-releasing hormone (TRH) stimulates thyroid-stimulating hormone (TSH) synthesis and release. TRH synthesis is regulated directly by thyroid hormones. TSH stimulates the thyroid gland to synthesize and secret thyroid hormones. T_4 is the predominant secretory product of the thyroid gland, with peripheral deiodination of tetraiodothyronine (T_4) to triiodothyronine (T_3) in the liver and kidney, supplying approximately 80% of the circulating T_3. Both circulating T_3 and T_4 inhibit TSH synthesis and release independently; T_4 via its rapid conversion to T_3. SRIH, somatostatin. (Adapted from www.thyroidmanager.org.)

CRITICAL NONTHYROIDAL ILLNESS

A decrease in serum T_3 and an increase in rT_3 levels are characteristic of the fasting state. These are also the most common changes in nonthyroidal illness (NTI) in response to a variety of acute and chronic illnesses, a condition that is referred to

as the euthyroid sick syndrome, NTI, or the low-T_3 syndrome. The most rapid and consistent findings in NTI are decline in circulating total T_3 and free T_3 and an increase in the inactivated rT_3 concentrations. A major contributing factor to the decrease in the peripheral production of T_3 is the decreased conversion of T_4 into T_3 by type I enzyme 5'-monodeiodinase. The concomitant rise of rT_3 appears to be attributable to impaired rT_3 clearance secondary to decreased 5'-monodeiodinase activity during illness, and not so much to an increase of rT_3 production by type III monodeiodinase. The greater the severity of the disease, the lower the serum T_3 levels become (21,38).

The majority of patients with NTI have normal or slightly decreased serum FT_4 levels. Most commonly, serum total and free T_3 concentrations are low, while serum T_4 concentrations remain within the normal range. However, with increasing severity of illness, serum T_4 levels, as well as those of T_3 decrease. In severely ill patients, an additional suppression of the hypothalamic-pituitary hormone release is often observed (21). The concentrations of TSH typically remain within the low-to-normal range, but the circadian variation of TSH may be lost, and response of TSH to TRH is blunted. Low TSH levels during critical illness are associated with poorer prognosis. Various agents, such as dopamine and steroids, may further decrease TSH levels (**Table 95.1**). Patients with prolonged critical illness show diminished TSH pulsatility, as if progressive dysfunction of the hypothalamus is involved, characterized by an absent nocturnal TSH surge and decreased TSH pulse amplitude. The changes in nocturnal TSH secretion in NTI resemble those found in central hypothyroidism, suggesting that hypothalamic changes are involved in this condition. In severe prolonged illness, the changes in thyroid function may be accompanied by decline in secretion of growth hormone, gonadotropins, and adrenocorticotropic hormone (ACTH) (21,24,38). During the recovery phase, the TSH levels may rise slightly above the normal range. Whether these alternations serve as physiologic

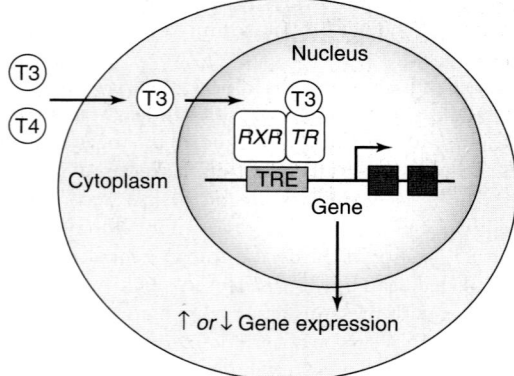

FIGURE 95.2. Thyroid hormones exhibit their action through binding to nuclear receptors. T_3 and T_4 (the major circulating thyroid hormone) are transported across plasma membranes into peripheral cells, where T_4 is monodeiodinated to T_3. The cytoplasmic T_3 diffuses into the nucleus, where it binds to the thyroid hormone receptors, which in turn, bind to DNA at RXR. The hormone-activated receptor binds to thyroid hormone response elements (TRE) and regulates gene transcription and, thus, levels of mRNA. (Adapted from www.thyroidmanager.org.)

TABLE 95.1
MEDICATIONS ASSOCIATED WITH HYPOTHYROIDISM
Decreased TSH secretion
Dopamine
Glucocorticoids
Octreotide
Decreased thyroid hormone secretion
Lithium
Iodide
Amiodarone
Decreased T_4 absorption
Colestipol
Cholestyramine
Aluminum hydroxide
Ferrous sulfate
Sucralfate
Increased thyroid hormone metabolism
Phenobarbital
Rifampin
Phenytoin
Carbamazepine

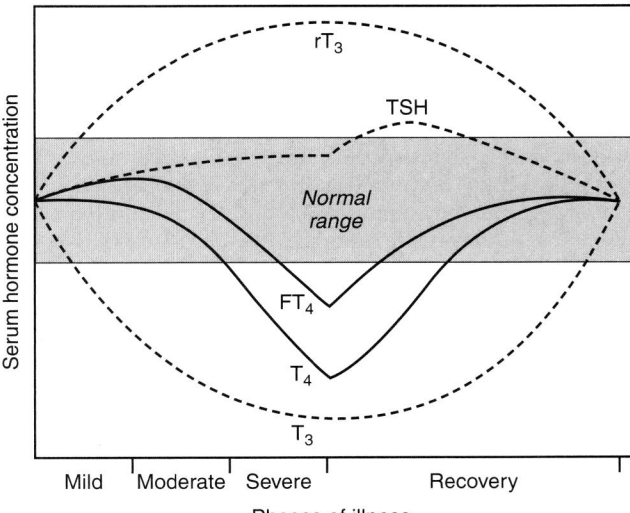

FIGURE 95.3. Changes in thyroid function during critical illness. In the acute phase of illness, the following are observed: reduction in circulating T_3, increase in serum rT_3, and no change in serum FT_4, total T_4, or TSH. In stage 2: modest increase in FT_4 and further decrease in T_3 and increase in rT_3. In phase 3: a loss of pulsatile secretion of TSH; decrease in T_4, T_3, and FT_4; and an increase—followed by a decrease—in serum rT_3. In the recovery phase: a gradual normalization of parameters; TSH can be elevated in this stage. From Brent GA, Hershman JM. Effects of nonthyroidal illness on thyroid function tests. In: Van Middlesworth L. ed. *The Thyroid Gland: A Practical Clinical Treatise.* Chicago: Year Book Medical, 1986;83–110.

adaptation or contribute to further deterioration remains an intriguing question (**Fig. 95.3**).

The treatment of NTI is controversial. Multiple studies have addressed this issue in patients with cardiac disease, sepsis, pulmonary disease, burn, and trauma. Brent et al. found no difference in mortality between critically ill patients with NTI who were treated with T_4 and the control group (critically ill patients with NTI who were not treated with T_4) (4). Treatment with T_4 delayed the normalization of thyroid function during recovery. An argument may be made for using T_3 therapy rather than T_4 because of the decreased conversion of T_4 into T_3 by type I enzyme 5′-monodeiodinase that occurs in NTI. However, administration of T_3 alone will not have an effect on the brain, as the cells in the brain depend on T_4 uptake and intracellular conversion of T_4 to T_3. In addition, treatment of critically ill

patients with T_3 has the potential hazardous effect of increasing metabolic rate and energy expenditure. In spite of these studies, it is very difficult to form clear recommendations for treatment with thyroid hormone in the ICU (24).

In view of the argument that the downregulation in NTI is part of energy-saving neuroendocrine adaptation to disease, attempts to increase and thereby restore thyroid hormone concentrations may be disadvantageous. At the current time, thyroid hormone therapy should not be initiated in the critical care setting in the absence of clear clinical and laboratory evidence for hypothyroidism (33). However, it is important to distinguish between patients with primary hypothyroidism and patients with NTI (**Table 95.2**). The former will benefit from therapy, and the latter will not. Patients with primary hypothyroidism almost always have TSH levels above 10 mU/L in parallel with decreased T_4 levels. In more severe stages, they also have decreased T_3 levels. Although elevated TSH may also occur in NTI upon recovery, it rarely exceeds 10 mU/L. In a situation in which TSH is mildly elevated (TSH 5–20 mU/L), with a low serum concentration of rT_3, a low thyroid hormone binding ratio (the ratio between the result of T_3 resin uptake for the unknown sample and the result of T_3 resin uptake simultaneously obtained in the same assay for standard control sera), and especially a high ratio of serum T_3 to FT_4 of >100, the patient is more likely to have hypothyroidism with or without NTI. It is particularly difficult to distinguish between central hypothyroidism and NTI because, in both conditions, the TSH tends to be low-normal, and the FT_4 low (24). However, if the FT_4 is <0.4 ng/dL in conjunction with normal TSH, central hypothyroidism is more likely, as only a small percentage of patients with NTI would have such a low FT_4. T_4 therapy could be considered in such a case.

HYPOTHYROIDISM

Congenital hypothyroidism might be due to (in descending order of frequency) thyroid dysgenesis, thyroid dyshormonogenesis, and hypothalamic-pituitary hypothyroidism. In parts of the world where salt is not iodized, iodine deficiency may be the most common cause. Hashimoto (autoimmune) thyroiditis is the most common cause of acquired hypothyroidism in children >6 years of age in North America. Hashimoto thyroiditis occurs in a genetically predisposed population. A family history of thyroid disease is seen in 30%–40% of patients with Hashimoto thyroiditis (9). The disease has also marked

TABLE 95.2

CHANGES IN THYROID FUNCTION TESTS IN HYPOTHYROIDISM AND DURING CRITICAL ILLNESS

	TSH	T_4	FT_4	T_3	rT_3
Primary hypothyroidism	↑↑	↓	↓	↓ or =	↓
Central hypothyroidism	= or ↓	↓ or =	↓ or =	=	↓
NTI, acute phase	=	= or ↑	= or ↑	↓	↑
NTI, prolonged phase	↓	↓	↓	↓↓	↑ or =
NTI, recovery phase	= or ↑	↓ or =	↓ or =	↓ or =	V

V, variable; ↑, increased; ↓, decreased; =, normal range

predilection for females. Usually, the onset of the disease is insidious, with the thyroid gland enlarged and firm (goiter). Occasionally, the goiter causes local pressure and difficulty in swallowing. Most patients have detectable circulating autoantibodies against the thyroid (**Fig. 95.4**).

Hypothalamic or pituitary disorders are frequently associated with TSH deficiency, producing central hypothyroidism. All patients with hypothalamic or pituitary disease should have thyroid function tests performed (8). Isolated central hypothyroidism is uncommon and associated with subclinical hypothyroidism and short stature (27). In central hypothyroidism, the TSH is inappropriately low (below normal range, within normal range, or only slightly above normal) in relationship to low thyroid hormone concentrations. In children with central hypothyroidism, the FT_4 concentrations are below the normal range or in the lowest third of the normal range. These children manifest an abnormal circadian pattern of TSH concentrations, with absence or blunting of the normal nocturnal TSH surge (14,27,29).

An increased frequency of primary hypothyroidism is associated with several chromosomal disorders, including Turner syndrome, Down syndrome, Klinefelter syndrome, and 18p or 18q deletions (22,31). The most common cause of hypothyroidism in these disorders is autoimmune thyroiditis.

Clinical Manifestations

Hypothyroidism should be considered in any child with subnormal growth and delayed bone age. In most children with hypothyroidism, pubertal development is delayed. Affected girls may present with primary or secondary amenorrhea. The onset of hypothyroidism is usually insidious. Signs and symptoms include lethargy; cold intolerance; bradycardia; weight gain; slow and husky speech; dry, coarse skin; sparse, dry, and coarse hair; constipation; muscle pain; anorexia; and delayed deep tendon reflexes (**Table 95.3**). In severe cases, the patient may exhibit myxedematous features that consist of edema of periorbital tissues and hands and feet, macroglossia, and cool and dry skin. In addition, pleural effusion, pericardial effusion, or bowel obstruction may be the first presenting symptom in previously unrecognized long-standing severe hypothyroidism.

Diagnosis

In primary hypothyroidism, serum TSH is usually elevated (>3 mU/mL) (28) and is often the earliest laboratory finding. In secondary or tertiary (central) hypothyroidism, the TSH levels are low, normal, or slightly elevated (<10 mU/L). T_4 and FT_4 concentrations are low or low-normal (it is not useful to measure T_3, as levels are preserved). When the FT_4 is in the lowest third of the normal range and the TSH is low or normal, a TSH surge test is needed to confirm the diagnosis of central hypothyroidism. In central hypothyroidism, the TSH surge test shows blunting of the normal nocturnal surge.

Treatment

Most children require therapy with ~100 mcg/m² body surface levothyroxine. Thyroid function tests should be checked

4–6 weeks after initiation of treatment and after a dose change has been made (sooner in newborn and infants), and the dose should be adjusted accordingly. In addition, thyroid function tests should be taken semiannually in children and annually in adolescents (more often in infants). A child with hypothyroidism who is admitted to the ICU should continue thyroid hormone therapy. If the patient cannot take oral medication, T_4 should be given intravenously in a dose that is approximately two-thirds of the oral dose (if the patient is unable to take oral intake for only 1 or 2 days, thyroid treatment can be omitted for this short period).

HYPERTHYROIDISM (THYROTOXICOSIS)

The term *thyrotoxicosis* is often used to describe the hypermetabolic state that results from elevated circulating levels of thyroid hormones. Hyperthyroidism in childhood and adolescence is most commonly the result of Graves disease (**Fig. 95.5**). Graves disease is an autoimmune disease. Autoantibodies against the thyroid gland can be found in the majority of the patients, of which the autoantibodies against the TSH receptor play a key role. In this case, antibody binding to the receptor mimics TSH binding. Graves disease involves hyperthyroidism, elevated metabolic rate, eye manifestations, and dermopathy. The disease has a genetic predisposition and is more prevalent in females.

Other causes of hyperthyroidism include toxic multinodular goiter, toxic nodular goiter, exogenous thyroid hormone, iodine-induced thyrotoxicosis, excess release of thyroid hormone, struma ovarii, molar pregnancy, thyroid adenoma, destruction of thyroid tissue with excess hormone release as a result of trauma, subacute thyroiditis, chronic thyroiditis, or post-radiation thyroiditis. In rare cases, hyperthyroidism can be caused by increased TSH secretion as a result of pituitary adenoma (8).

Generalized resistance to thyroid hormone (RTH) involves tissues throughout the body being resistant to the effects of thyroid hormone. In RTH, T_4 is high, TSH is normal, and the patients are euthyroid with a small goiter. Pituitary resistance to thyroid hormone (PRTH) is a rare nonneoplastic disorder caused by inherited mutations in the gene for the $TR\beta1$. In this syndrome, T_4 is high, TSH is high, and patients are clinically hyperthyroid. The pituitary gland may be resistant to the feedback inhibitory effects of circulating thyroid hormones, whereas peripheral tissues respond normally, causing patients to experience hyperthyroidism (23).

Clinical Manifestations

The onset of thyrotoxicosis is usually insidious, with a period of increasing nervousness, palpitations, increased appetite, and muscle weakness. A cardinal sign is loss of weight in the face of increased appetite. Other symptoms include fatigue with sleep disturbance, emotional instability, heat intolerance, excessive sweating, tremor, diarrhea, dyspnea, tachycardia, and atrial arrhythmia (**Table 95.4**). On physical examination, findings may include thyroid enlargement; thyroid bruit; ophthalmopathy; retraction of the eyelids and lid lag; tremor; hyperactive reflexes; increased precordial activity; tachycardia; atrial

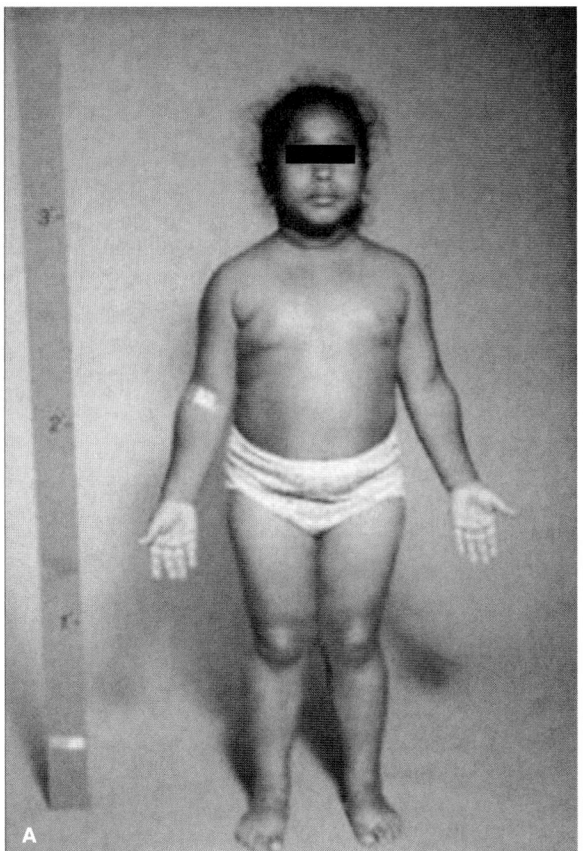

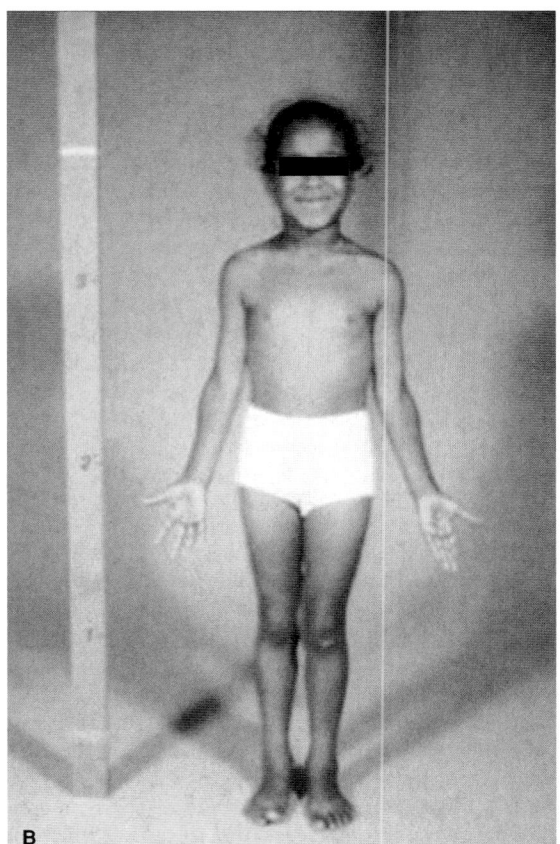

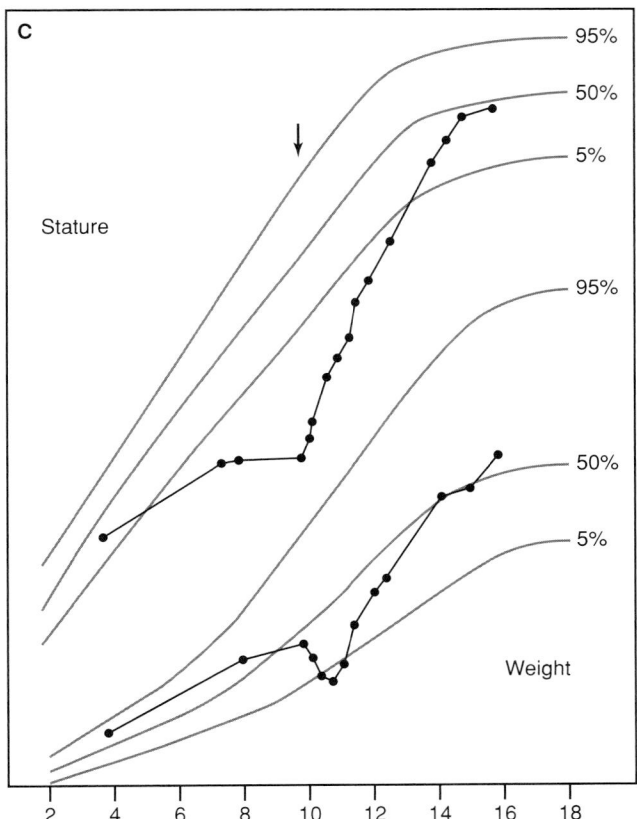

FIGURE 95.4. A 10-year-old girl with severe primary hypothyroidism before (**A**) and after (**B**) treatment. Presenting complaint was poor growth. Note the dull facies, relative obesity, and immature body proportions prior to treatment. At age 10, she had not lost a single deciduous tooth. After treatment was initiated (indicated by the arrow in **C**), she lost 6 teeth in 10 months and had striking catch-up growth. Bone age was 5 years at a chronologic age of 10. From www.thyroidmanager.org.

TABLE 95.3

MANIFESTATIONS OF HYPOTHYROIDISM

Symptoms	Signs
Fatigue	Thyroid enlargement
Lethargy	Cool, pale skin
Headache	Brittle nails
Weight gain	Bleeding tendencies
Cold intolerance	Alopecia; coarse, sparse hair
Somnolence	Macroglossia
Decreased appetite	Bradycardia
Dry skin	Constipation
Hoarseness of voice	Muscle hypertrophy
Constipation	Slowed speech
Menstrual irregularities	Dementia
Myalgias	Slowed reflexes (with delayed
Paresthesias	relaxation phase)
Depression	Psychosis
	Diminished libido
	Memory defects

TABLE 95.4

MANIFESTATIONS OF HYPERTHYROIDISM

Symptoms	Signs
Nervousness	Tachycardia
Anxiety	Thyroid enlargement[2]
Heat intolerance	Tremor
Palpitations	Thyroid bruit
Fatigue	Eye signs[1]
Weight loss	Hyperactive reflexes
Tachycardia	Atrial fibrillation
Dyspnea	Hot and moist skin
Weakness	Thin and fine hair
Increased appetite	Onycholysis
Eye complaints[1]	Muscle weakness
Swelling legs	Hyperactive precordial pulse
Hyperdefecation	Splenomegaly[3]
(without diarrhea)	Gynecomastia
Diarrhea	Liver palms
Anorexia	
Personality change	
Emotional lability	
Impaired concentration	
Insomnia	
Difficulty swallowing	
Menstrual irregularities	

[1]These manifestations are much more common in patients with Graves disease.
[2] Enlargement of the thyroid may be lacking in fewer than 5% of patients with thyrotoxicosis.
[3] Exclusively present in patients with Graves disease.

fibrillation; warm, smooth, and moist skin; separation of the end of the fingernail from the nail bed (onycholysis). Proximal muscle weakness is common and may be the dominant manifestation in some individuals (25). Cardiovascular manifestations of thyrotoxicosis are common. The hemodynamic changes of thyrotoxicosis mimic a hyperadrenergic state. These changes are caused by an increase in myocardial β receptors, which is induced by excessive thyroid hormone. Supraventricular tachyarrhythmias are common. Severe hyperthyroidism may lead to cardiac failure secondary to atrial fibrillation, which causes a decrease in cardiac output in the face of increased circulatory demand. Such cardiac failure usually occurs in patients with underlying heart disease (6). Uncontrolled hyperthyroidism with large goiter secondary to Graves disease may cause edema of the upper airway, a potentially life-threatening situation that requires a high degree of vigilance (20).

Diagnosis

Laboratory findings in patients with hyperthyroidism include increased serum concentrations of T_3 and T_4 because of increased production of these hormones. Occasionally, only the serum T_3 concentration is increased (T_3 toxicosis). Conversely, it is possible that only the serum T_4 concentration is increased (T_4 toxicosis). It is more valuable to measure the active thyroid hormone concentrations, free T_3 (FT_3) and FT_4, and to verify that either or both are elevated. The TSH is low and usually undetectable (except in the extremely rare cases of TSH-secreting tumors, TRH-secreting tumors, and selective pituitary resistance to thyroid hormone). Quantitative human chorionic gonadotropin (hCG), which can cross-react at the TSH receptor level, is elevated in molar pregnancy.

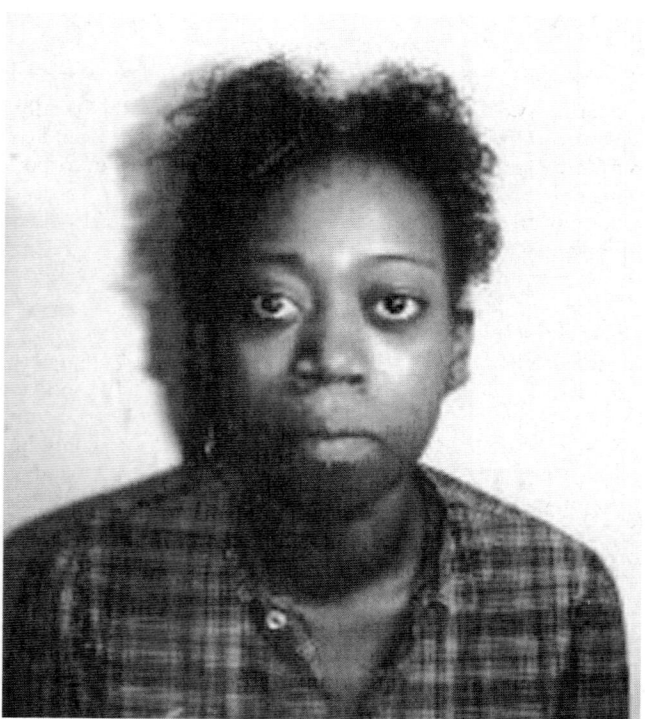

FIGURE 95.5. A 16-year-old girl with Graves disease. Note the exophthalmos, stare, asymmetry of the eyes, and thyroid enlargement. From www.emedicine.com with permission.

Treatment

Management of hyperthyroidism includes medical treatment, radioactive iodine, or surgery. Most children with hyperthyroidism would initially be treated with an antithyroid agent, such as propylthiouracil, methimazole, or carbimazole (used in Europe but not in the US). These agents block synthesis of the thyroid hormone by inhibiting oxidation of iodide. In addition, propylthiouracil impairs the conversion of T_4 to T_3 by inhibiting type I 5'-monodeiodinase. The initial dose of propylthiouracil (PTU) varies from 300 to 600 mg (4–6 mg/kg) daily, divided into three to four doses. An initial dose of methimazole or carbimazole varies from 30 to 60 mg (0.4–0.6 mg/kg) daily, divided into two to three doses. In the initial state (before a euthyroid state is achieved), a β-adrenergic blocking agent, such as propranolol, may be added (10–40 mg/dose orally every 6 hours) (see the later section on thyroid storm). After a euthyroid state is achieved, the PTU dose should be decreased to maintenance dose (usually one-third to two-thirds of the initial dose). PTU is given in two to four divided doses, while methimazole or carbimazole is given once or twice daily. The doses should be adjusted according to the FT_4 concentration, as TSH may remain suppressed for months.

A small percentage of patients develop hypersensitivity reactions to these drugs; they are usually mild and resolve when the drug is withdrawn, but a severe reaction may occur (**Table 95.5**). The most common hypersensitivity reaction, occurring in as many as 10% of patients, is a rash that can take many forms, including hives. Among the serious reactions, agranulocytosis is the most common, occurring in fewer than 1% of the patients and is accompanied by fever and sore throat. Hypersensitivity reaction usually occurs within the first few weeks of treatment. As these medications can affect blood count and liver function tests, it is advisable to perform complete blood count and liver function tests before initiation of an antithyroid drug treatment and to repeat them after the first few weeks of treatment, to help recognize these potential side effects. Suspicion of any serious manifestation should be an indication for discontinuation of antithyroid drug therapy and recourse to surgery or radioactive iodine (6). Usually, it is necessary to continue medical treatment for 2 years before the patient achieves remission.

Patients with hyperthyroidism admitted to the ICU should be monitored carefully for possible development of thyroid storm. Medical treatment should be continued and adjusted according to the thyroid function tests. As no parenteral preparations of these drugs are available, they must be administered orally or via a nasogastric tube. Rectal administration has also been used.

Radioactive iodine has been used relatively infrequently in childhood due to the potential risks of leukemia, thyroid cancer in the patient, and genetic mutations in the offspring of the patient. However, a number of recent reports show that this approach is not associated with an increased risk of these complications and is safe enough to be considered as treatment, particularly in adolescents (3,7,32). Radioactive iodine is used for treatment of older children and adolescents who fail medical treatment or in whom medical treatment is contraindicated due to severe side effects. The main complication is primary hypothyroidism. Radioactive iodine may cause thyroid storm.

Surgical treatment is used less often now, but it is still an effective treatment option for hyperthyroidism (39). With proper preparation and if performed by an experienced surgeon, the complication rate is relatively low (see the later section on thyroidectomy). Surgery should be considered in patients with a large thyroid gland, severe ophthalmopathy, and a lack of remission with medical treatment. With proper surgical management, most patients achieve a rapid remission; some may have recurrence of thyrotoxicosis or may develop hypothyroidism.

CRITICAL HYPOTHYROIDISM: "MYXEDEMA COMA"

The term *myxedema coma* is often used to describe clinically severe hypothyroidism. However, this term is a misnomer, because most patients who have severe hypothyroidism do not present with myxedema or in a comatose state. Critical hypothyroidism is characterized by progressive dysfunction of the cardiovascular, respiratory, and central nervous systems. Myxedema is related to organ hypofunction (e.g., cardiac, gastrointestinal, skin, renal) and occurs with prolonged or severe hypothyroidism. If not recognized and treated, the mortality rate is exceedingly high. Myxedema coma is rare in the pediatric population. Typically, patients are older and have known hypothyroidism; however, it can be the initial presentation of hypothyroidism. Myxedema coma occurs most commonly in winter. Common precipitants include infection, trauma, hypothermia, and medications (**Table 95.6**).

Clinical Manifestations

Cardinal findings include hypothermia and altered mental status. Additional features include bradycardia, hypotension, and hypoventilation. A reduction in hypoxic ventilatory drive causes a reduction in respiratory rate, leading to carbon dioxide narcosis and progressive somnolence, which compound the slow mental status of the patient. Respiratory muscle weakness may also occur, further compromising the ability to

TABLE 95.5

HYPERSENSITIVITY REACTIONS TO ANTITHYROID DRUGS

Rash
Agranulocytosis (accompanied by fever and sore throat)
Arthralgia
Myalgia
Neuritis
Hepatitis (with PTU)
Cholestasis (with methimazole)
Liver necrosis
Thrombocytopenia
Loss of or abnormal pigmentation of the hair
Loss of sensation
Enlargement of lymph nodes or salivary glands
Edema
A lupus-like syndrome
Toxic psychosis

TABLE 95.6

PRECIPITATING FACTORS FOR MYXEDEMA COMA

Infections
  Pneumonia
  Sepsis
  Urinary infections
  Influenza
Surgery
Burns
Trauma
Hypothermia
Drugs
  Sedatives (narcotics, tranquilizers, barbiturates)
  Cardiac medications (amiodarone, β blockers)
  Lithium
  Phenytoin
  Rifampin
Stroke
Gastrointestinal bleeding
Congestive heart failure

TABLE 95.7

CLINICAL MANIFESTATIONS OF MYXEDEMA COMA

Organ system	Clinical features
Skin and soft tissues	Generalized swelling Edema Periorbital edema Ptosis Cool, dry skin Coarse, sparse hair Macroglossia; hoarseness
Neurologic	Hypothermia Lethargy Altered mental status Psychosis Seizures Delayed reflex relaxation
Cardiovascular	Bradycardia Hypotension
Respiratory	Depressed ventilatory drive Hypoventilation Hypoxia Hypercapnia
Gastrointestinal	Constipation Abdominal distention Paralytic ileus Megacolon
Hematologic	Anemia Leukopenia
Renal	Decreased glomerular filtration rate

ventilate. Presence of ascites, pleural effusion, or pericardial effusion may further impede effective ventilation (26). Cardiac contractility is reduced, resulting in a reduction of stroke volume and cardiac output. Cardiac output can be further limited by significant pericardial effusion. If present, myxedema is characterized by decreased metabolic clearance of all substances, reduced intravascular volume with fluid retention in tissues, generalized skin and soft tissue swelling, often with associated periorbital edema, ptosis, macroglossia, and cool, dry skin (**Table 95.7**).

Diagnosis

The diagnosis of myxedema coma requires low levels of T_3 and of T_4 (total and free). TSH levels are usually elevated, but may be normal or low in the setting of hypothalamic-pituitary disease or critical illness. Additional laboratory findings include anemia, hyponatremia, hypoglycemia, azotemia, elevated liver enzymes, hypercholesterolemia, and elevated creatine phosphokinase (CPK) levels. Hypoxia, hypercapnia, and respiratory acidosis are common.

The occurrence of pericardial effusion in hypothyroidism appears to be dependent on the severity of the disease. Pericardial effusion may be a frequent manifestation in myxedema at an advanced severe stage, but it is rare in hypothyroidism at an early mild stage (17). A chest radiograph may reveal cardiomegaly and pleural effusions. Echocardiography can reveal septal hypertrophy and hypertrophic subaortic stenosis in addition to the pericardial effusion. Echocardiographic findings include sinus bradycardia, decreased voltage with electrical alternans if a pericardial effusion is present, and nonspecific ST- and T-wave abnormalities. Other echocardiographic abnormalities include prolongation of the QT interval and conduction abnormalities of varying degrees (36).

A lumbar puncture may be indicated to exclude meningitis. An increased opening pressure and elevated protein levels in the cerebral spinal fluid are nonspecific findings associated with myxedema coma (36).

Treatment

The treatment of myxedema coma involves general supportive measures, correction of physiologic derangements, and immediate intravenous replacement of thyroid hormone (11). Patients should be treated in the ICU setting with careful monitoring. In patients who have severe hypotension, vasopressor therapy should be considered. Warm room temperature, blankets, and/or heating pad should be used to correct hypothermia. Rapid correction of hypothermia may cause hypotension and cardiovascular collapse due to peripheral dilatation. Severe hyponatremia may be treated with hypertonic saline. Hypoglycemia should be treated with continuous dextrose infusion. Precipitating factors should be pursued and treated. Broad-spectrum antibiotics should be considered until infection has been excluded.

The proper initiation of thyroid hormone therapy in myxedema is controversial (11,30). Enteral absorption of T_4 may be disrupted by edema of intestinal villi. Most investigators recommend initiating therapy with intravenous T_4 alone, with a loading dose of 200–500 mcg (4 mcg/kg), followed by 50–100 mcg/day (1–2 mcg/kg). We recommend using doses in parentheses for children who weigh <50 kg. Using T_4 alone allows a slow conversion of T_4 to T_3 in the periphery, thereby reducing the possible adverse cardiac effects that may occur with a large dose of T_3, especially in those with preexisting heart disease (36). If the combination of T_3/T_4 is used, a loading dose of 4 mcg/kg of T_4 and 10 mcg of T_3 (0.2 mcg/kg) may be used, followed by maintenance doses of T$_4$ (50–100 mcg daily; 1–2 mcg/kg) and T$_3$ (10 mcg; 0.2 mcg/kg) every 8 hrs until oral therapy is initiated. If intravenous T$_3$ alone is used, initial dose should be 10–20 mcg (0.2–0.4 mcg/kg), followed by 10 mcg (0.2 mcg/kg) every 4 hrs for the first 24 hrs, then 10 mcg (0.2 mcg/kg) every 6 hrs for another 1–2 days. Then, depending on the clinical response, the patient may be converted to oral T$_4$ therapy. Rapid onset of action of T$_3$ can lead to adverse cardiovascular effects. A study that compared the response of thyroid hormones between intravenous high-dose T$_4$ and oral T$_4$ in affected adults found that with oral administration of 500 mcg of T$_4$ on the first day, followed by 100 mcg of T$_4$ daily by mouth, plasma T$_3$ and T$_4$ increased slowly, remaining in the hypothyroid range, but clinical response occurred within 24–72 hrs (1). The intravenous route involved high peaks of plasma T$_3$ and T$_4$ within 3 hrs. IV administration of T$_4$ at the proposed doses causes an abrupt rise in serum T$_4$ to a supraphysiologic level, and then a fall to the normal range in 24 hrs. Serum T$_3$ levels rise slightly, and serum TSH levels fall sharply and substantially (30). Whatever the regimen, subsequent thyroid hormone dosing should be guided by frequent measurement of FT$_4$ concentrations. With the IV route, the peak level is reached within 3 hrs, with subsequent gradual decline over a few days (1). Thus, we recommend checking FT$_4$ twice daily when using the IV route to ensure that most levels are within the normal range. When the patient is converted to oral T$_4$, FT$_4$ can be measured once or twice per week.

Cortisol response to stress is blunted during severe hypothyroidism. Most investigators recommend the concurrent administration of "stress dose" corticosteroid therapy, in case of concurrent adrenal insufficiency. Hydrocortisone, 100 mg/m^2 IV, should be administered initially, followed by 25 mg/m^2 IV every 6 hrs. Cortisol levels should be drawn before initiation of corticosteroid therapy. If the levels are appropriately elevated, the steroid therapy may be safely discontinued. If the cortisol levels are low (<25 micrograms/dL), steroid therapy should be continued until the critical illness phase is resolved. At a later time, an ACTH stimulation test can be performed to exclude persistence of hypoadrenalism.

CRITICAL HYPERTHYROIDISM: "THYROID STORM"

Thyroid storm (or thyrotoxic crisis) is a life-threatening condition caused by the exaggeration of clinical manifestations of thyrotoxicosis. Thyroid storm most commonly occurs in Graves disease. The progression from thyrotoxicosis to life-threatening thyroid storm involves high fever, mental status changes, and evidence of multiorgan dysfunction, including adrenergic crisis (tachycardia, hypertension) and gastrointestinal hypermotility. Early diagnosis and intervention are crucial to prevent morbidity and mortality. Precipitating factors include thyroid surgery, withdrawal of antithyroid drugs, radioiodine therapy, or the administration of iodinated radiocontrast dyes (**Table 95.8**). In patients who have preexisting thyrotoxicosis, thyroid storm can also be precipitated by systemic insults, including surgery, trauma, severe infection, and diabetic ketoacidosis.

Thyroid storm may be less frequent now than in the past due to the earlier diagnosis and management of hyperthyroidism

TABLE 95.8

PRECIPITATING FACTORS FOR THYROID STORM

Infection
Surgery (thyroidal and nonthyroidal)
Therapy with radioactive iodine
Administration of iodinated contrast dyes or ingestion of
   large, stable iodine loads
Withdrawal of antithyroid medication
Amiodarone therapy
Ingestion of excessive amounts of exogenous thyroid hormone
Diabetic ketoacidosis
Congestive cardiac failure
Hypoglycemia
Toxemia of pregnancy
Parturition and the immediate postpartum state
Severe emotional stress
Acute manic crisis
Pulmonary embolism
Cerebral vascular accident
Bowel infarction
Acute trauma
Tooth extraction
Vigorous palpation of thyroid gland

(30). If left untreated, the mortality rate ranges between 20% and 30% (37). Thus, prevention, early diagnosis, and aggressive management of thyroid storm are extremely important.

Most studies have not found a significant difference in serum thyroid hormonal levels between uncomplicated hyperthyroidism and thyroid storm (37). Acute and rapid increase in serum levels of thyroid hormones might be the cause of thyroid storm, as evidenced by cases of thyroid storm that present following thyroid surgery, administration of radioactive iodine, and abrupt discontinuation of antithyroid medication. The sympathetic nervous system has been implicated in the pathogenesis of thyroid storm, as many of the manifestations are similar to those seen in conditions of catecholamine excess; administration of β-blockers causes a marked relief of these signs and symptoms. Although the catecholamine levels are within the normal range, thyroid hormones upregulate adrenergic receptor expression and thus affect tissue responsiveness to catecholamines. Another mechanism might be enhancement of cellular response to thyroid hormones as seen in conditions that precipitate thyroid storm, such as infection, hypoxemia, hypovolemia, and diabetic ketoacidosis.

Clinical Manifestations

Thyroid storm is characterized by four major features: fever, tachycardia, central nervous system dysfunction, and gastrointestinal symptoms. The fever can progress to frank hyperpyrexia. Sinus tachycardia is usually seen, although a variety of supraventricular arrhythmias may also be present, such as atrial fibrillation. Central nervous system manifestations can range from agitation, restlessness, and emotional lability, to confusion, frank psychosis, and coma. GI symptoms include nausea, vomiting, and diarrhea. A useful scoring system for recognition of thyroid storm is presented in **Table 95.9** (30).

TABLE 95.9

THE PREDICTIVE CLINICAL SCALE FOR THYROID STORM (BURCH AND WARTOFSKY)

Parameter taken into consideration		Scoring points
Thermoregulatory dysfunction, Temperature (oral)		
99–99.9°F	37.2–37.7°C	5
100–100.9°F	37.8–38.2°C	10
101–101.9°F	38.3–38.8°C	15
102–102.9°F	38.9–39.3°C	20
103–103.9°F	39.4–39.9°C	25
≥104°F	≥40°C	30
CNS effects		
Absent		0
Mild (agitation)		10
Moderate (delirium, psychosis, extreme lethargy)		20
Severe (seizures, coma)		30
GI-hepatic dysfunction		
Absent		0
Moderate (diarrhea, nausea/vomiting, abdominal pain)		10
Severe (unexplained jaundice)		20
Tachycardia (beats/min)		
99–109		5
110–119		10
120–129		15
130–139		20
≥140		25
Congestive cardiac failure		
Absent		0
Mild (pedal edema)		5
Moderate (bibasal rales)		10
Severe (pulmonary edema)		15
Atrial fibrillation		
Absent		0
Present		10
Precipitating event		
Absent		0
Present		10

A cumulative score of ≥45 is highly suggestive of thyroid storm, 25–44 is suggestive of "impeding" storm, and <25 is unlikely to represent thyroid storm.
From Sarlis NJ, Gourgiotis L. Thyroid emergencies. *Rev Endocr Metab Disord* 2003;4:129–36.

Diagnosis

Laboratory findings include elevated serum total and free thyroid hormonal levels (free T_3 and/or free T_4), with undetectable TSH. Serum electrolytes are usually normal. Liver function abnormalities, leukocytosis, or leucopenia may also be present.

Treatment

The management of thyroid storm is complicated. Patients with thyroid storm should be monitored and treated in the ICU. The aims of the treatment are to reduce the production and secretion of thyroid hormones, antagonize the peripheral action of the thyroid hormones, alleviate signs and symptoms, and treat the precipitating factor. Supportive therapy includes respiratory support and management of hyperthermia. Phenobarbital may be used for sedation because it stimulates metabolic clearance of thyroid hormone by the liver. Hyperthermia may be treated with cool IV fluids, antipyretics, or cooling blankets.

An early step in the treatment must include complete blockade of new thyroid hormone synthesis. PTU is the drug of choice because of its inhibition of peripheral conversion of T_4 to T_3 in addition to its inhibition of synthesis of thyroid hormone. PTU is administered as a 600–1000 mg (12–20 mg/kg) loading dose, followed by 200–300 mg (4–6 mg/kg) every 4–6 hrs orally. Methimazole is an acceptable alternative and is given as a loading dose of 60–100 mg (1.2–2 mg/kg), followed by 20–30 mg (0.4–0.7 mg/kg) every 6–8 hrs orally, but it does not provide inhibition of conversion of T_4 to T_3. Both PTU and methimazole can be administered rectally, but no parenteral preparation for these drugs is available. As thyrotoxicosis improves, the doses should be gradually lowered to the standard dose ranges (see the previous discussion on the medical treatment of hyperthyroidism).

In order to block the release of preformed thyroid hormone from the thyroid gland, inorganic iodine should be used. Ideally, iodine therapy should be administered 2 hrs after initial thiourea dosing, to allow for initial blockade of iodine organification. Formulations for oral inorganic iodine that can be used include saturated solution of potassium iodide (children, 5 drops, 250 mg, 2–4 times/day, infants 2 drops 4 times/day) and Lugol solution (4–8 drops 3 times/day). Iodinated contrast dyes given intravenously, including ipodate and iohexol, are also effective. In addition to blocking thyroid hormone release, these radiocontrast agents interfere with peripheral conversion of T_4 to T_3 and may antagonize the binding of thyroid hormone to its receptors (11).

Lithium therapy (300 mg or 6 mg/kg every 6 hrs) may be used in addition to iodine to block thyroid hormone release. High-dose corticosteroids (hydrocortisone 50–100 mg, IV, every 6–8 hrs or 25–50 mg/m^2 body surface) are also effective in blocking peripheral conversion of T_4 to T_3. Blocking the action of thyroid hormone is another mainstay of the treatment. In the absence of cardiac failure, a β-adrenergic blocking agent should be added. β blockers (e.g., propranolol, 40–80 mg, 0.5 mg/kg, orally, or 1–3 mg/dose IV, every 4–8 hrs) are effective in reducing tachycardia, hypertension, and adrenergic symptoms associated with thyrotoxicosis (11). However, a short-acting β blocker such as esmolol given IV may be safer in the critically ill patient by minimizing the risk of cardiovascular collapse and allowing better titration of the medication's effects because of the short half-life (6,18). In life-threatening cases in which medical therapy has been proven ineffective, plasmapheresis, plasma exchange, charcoal plasma perfusion, and peritoneal dialysis have all been used successfully to remove circulating thyroid hormone (2,5,16,35).

Following initiation of therapy for thyroid storm, clinical and biochemical improvement should occur within 24 hrs, although full recovery may take several days to weeks. In most cases, medical therapy should be used for weeks to months before definitive treatment with radioactive iodine or thyroidectomy. In rare cases, definitive therapy with thyroidectomy may be considered during the acute phase of thyroid storm. Radioactive iodine has no role in the acute management due

TABLE 95.10

INDICATIONS FOR THYROIDECTOMY

Thyroid cancer
Prophylactic thyroidectomy in children with MEN-2
A large multinodular goiter
Graves disease
(including young children, not responding to antithyroid
drugs, in whom radioactive iodine is contraindicated)

to therapeutic administration of inorganic iodine, antithyroid drugs, and concerns over excess thyroid hormone release.

THYROIDECTOMY

Children and adolescents who undergo thyroid surgery commonly are admitted to PICU postoperatively for treatment and observation. Among children who underwent head and neck endocrine surgery in 1997 and 2000 in the US, the most common procedure was thyroglossal duct cyst excision. Thyroid lobectomy was the second most common procedure. Thyroid malignant neoplasm (usually treated by total thyroidectomy) was the second most common diagnosis (after thyroglossal duct cyst) (15). One study found that the main postoperative complications of thyroidectomy consisted of transient hypocalcemia (13.1%), permanent hypocalcemia (2.5%), transient vocal cord palsy (1.4%), and permanent vocal cord palsy (0.4%) (12). According to this study, performance of neck and paratracheal lymph node dissections was the most significant predictor of hypocalcemia (the most common complication) in patients who underwent total thyroidectomy.

Thyroidectomy may be indicated in children and adolescents with Graves disease who have had adverse reaction to antithyroid drugs or who relapse after antithyroid drug therapy (Table 95.10). Surgical complications were more frequently observed in children than in adolescents (34) (Table 95.11). In a study that investigated the complications after subtotal or total thyroidectomy for hyperthyroidism, 2.6% of patients had transient effect on the vocal cords. Prolonged postoperative hypocalcemia occurred in 3.1%, and permanent hypothyroidism in 1%. One of the potential risks of thyroidectomy for Graves disease is the development of intraoperative thyroid storm (13).

After thyroid surgery, it is crucial to monitor serum calcium by frequent measurements of ionized calcium (every few hours), to monitor for signs and symptoms of hypocalcemia

TABLE 95.11

COMPLICATIONS OF THYROIDECTOMY

Transient hypocalcemia
Permanent hypocalcemia
Transient recurrent laryngeal nerve palsy
Permanent recurrent laryngeal nerve palsy
Thyroid storm
Hemorrhage

(Chapter 94), and to begin IV administration of calcium gluconate as soon as indicated. After the acute phase, calcitriol (20–60 ng/kg/day) and supplemental calcium may be needed (for treatment of hypoparathyroidism, see Chapter 94). In addition, it is crucial to watch for upper airway obstruction that may occur secondary to edema, hemorrhage, or vocal cord paralysis.

CONCLUSIONS AND FUTURE DIRECTIONS

NTI occurs in most patients admitted to the ICU. At this point, it is not clear whether thyroid hormone administration is beneficial or detrimental. Further large-scale prospective studies are required to determine when such a treatment could be beneficial, based on the clinical presentation, laboratory evaluation, and the primary condition. In addition, these studies should determine the correct treatment (T_3 and/or T_4) and doses to be used.

Myxedema coma and thyroid storm are extremely rare in the pediatric population. Current treatment has significantly reduced the mortality rate associated with these conditions. However, better understanding of the physiology may enable us to anticipate the development of these complications and prevent them. Improvement in treatment may further decrease the morbidity and mortality. Our recommendations regarding the treatment of these conditions are adopted from the adult literature due to the rarity of these conditions in the pediatric population and may need further adjustments in order to achieve a optimal outcome.

KEY POINTS

- To understand the effects of critical illness on thyroid function, it is necessary to understand normal physiology of thyroid hormone secretion and action.
- Most patients in the ICU will exhibit NTI, which probably reflects physiologic adaptation to disease.
- Currently, treatment of NTI with thyroid hormone therapy is not recommended, nor is thyroid function testing during intercurrent illness. However, if clinical suspicion for hypothyroidism arises, thyroid function tests should be checked; if hypothyroidism is confirmed, thyroid treatment should be initiated.
- The two thyroid emergencies, myxedema coma and thyroid storm, are extremely rare in the pediatric population (myxedema coma occurs typically in older patients). However, it is important to recognize the diagnostic features and the precipitating factors and to initiate treatment as soon as possible, as both are life-threatening conditions with high mortality rates if left untreated.

References

1. Arlot S, Debussche X, Lalau JD, et al. Myxoedema coma: Response of thyroid hormones with oral and intravenous high-dose L-thyroxine treatment. *Intensive Care Med* 1991;17:16–8.
2. Ashkar FS, Katims RB, Smoak WM, 3rd, et al. Thyroid storm treatment with blood exchange and plasmapheresis. *JAMA* 1970;214:1275–9.

3. Barrio R, Lopez-Capape M, Martinez-Badas I, et al. Graves' disease in children and adolescents: Response to long-term treatment. *Acta Paediatr* 2005;94:1583–9.
4. Brent GA, Hershman JM. Thyroxine therapy in patients with severe nonthyroidal illnesses and low serum thyroxine concentration. *J Clin Endocrinol Metab* 1986;63:1–8.
5. Candrina R, Di Stefano O, Spandrio S, et al. Treatment of thyrotoxic storm by charcoal plasma perfusion. *J Endocrinol Invest* 1989;12:133–4.
6. Davies TF, Larsen PR. Thyrotoxicosis. In: Larsen PR, Kronenberg HM, Melmed SM, KS Polonsky, eds. *Williams Textbook of Endocrinology, 10th ed.* Philadelphia: Saunders, 2003;374–421.
7. Dotsch J, Rascher W, Dorr HG. Graves disease in childhood: A review of the options for diagnosis and treatment. *Paediatr Drugs* 2003;5:95–102.
8. Emerson CH. Central hypothyroidism and hyperthyroidism. *Med Clin North Am* 1985;69:1019–34.
9. Fisher DA. Thyroid Disorder in Childhood and Adolescence. In: Sperling MA, ed. *Pediatric Endocrinology.* Philadelphia: Saunders, 2002;187–209.
10. Fraser T, Green D. Weathering the storm: Beta-blockade and potential for disaster in severe hypothyroidism. *Emerg Med* 2001;13:376–80.
11. Goldberg PA, Inzucchi SE. Critical issues in endocrinology. *Clin Chest Med* 2003;24:583–606, vi.
12. Goncalves Filho J, Kowalski LP. Surgical complications after thyroid surgery performed in a cancer hospital. *Otolaryngol Head Neck Surg* 2005;132:490–4.
13. Grimes CM, Muniz H, Montgomery WH, et al. Intraoperative thyroid storm: A case report. *Aana J* 2004;72:53–5.
14. Gruneiro-Papendieck L, Chiesa A, Martinez A, et al. Nocturnal TSH surge and TRH test response in the evaluation of thyroid axis in hypothalamic pituitary disorders in childhood. *Horm Res* 1998;50:252–7.
15. Harsha WJ, Perkins JA, Lewis CW, et al. Head and neck endocrine surgery in children: 1997 and 2000. *Arch Otolaryngol Head Neck Surg* 2005;131:564–70.
16. Herrmann J, Schmidt HJ, Kruskemper HL. Thyroxine elimination by peritoneal dialysis in experimental thyrotoxicosis. *Horm Metab Res* 1973;5:180–3.
17. Kabadi UM, Kumar SP. Pericardial effusion in primary hypothyroidism. *Am Heart J* 1990;120:1393–5.
18. Knighton JD, Crosse MM. Anaesthetic management of childhood thyrotoxicosis and the use of esmolol. *Anaesthesia* 1997;52:67–70.
19. Larsen PR, Davies TF, Schlumberger M-J, et al. Thyroid physiology and diagnostic evaluation of patients with thyroid disorders. In: Larsen PR, Kronenberg HM, Melmed SM, KS Polonsky, eds. *Williams Textbook of Endocrinology, 10th ed.* Philadelphia: Saunders, 2003;331–73.
20. Li Pi Shan W, Hatzakorzian R, Sherman M, et al. Upper airway compromise secondary to edema in Graves' disease. *Can J Anaesth* 2006;53:183–7.
21. Ligtenberg JJ, Girbes AR, Beentjes JA, et al. Hormones in the critically ill patient: To intervene or not to intervene? *Intensive Care Med* 2001;27:1567–77.
22. Lomenick JP, Smith WJ, Rose SR. Autoimmune thyroiditis in 18q deletion syndrome. *J Pediatr* 2005;147:541–3.
23. McDermott MT, Ridgway EC. Central hyperthyroidism. *Endocrinol Metab Clin North Am* 1998;27:187–203.
24. Nylen ES, Muller B. Endocrine changes in critical illness. *J Intensive Care Med* 2004;19:67–82.
25. Reasner CA, Isley WL. Thyrotoxicosis in the critically ill. *Crit Care Clin* 1991;7:57–74.
26. Ringel MD. Management of hypothyroidism and hyperthyroidism in the intensive care unit. *Crit Care Clin* 2001;17:59–74.
27. Rose SR. Isolated central hypothyroidism in short stature. *Pediatr Res* 1995;38:967–73.
28. Rose SR. Thyrotropin above 3 is not usually normal. *Endocrinologist* 2006;16:189–90.
29. Rose SR, Nisula BC. Circadian variation of thyrotropin in childhood. *J Clin Endocrinol Metab* 1989;68:1086–90.
30. Sarlis NJ, Gourgiotis L. Thyroid emergencies. *Rev Endocr Metab Disord* 2003;4:129–36.
31. Schaub RL, Hale DE, Rose SR, et al. The spectrum of thyroid abnormalities in individuals with 18q deletions. *J Clin Endocrinol Metab* 2005;90:2259–63.
32. Segni M, Gorman CA. The aftermath of childhood hyperthyroidism. *J Pediatr Endocrinol Metab* 2001;14 Suppl 5:1277–82; discussion 1297–8.
33. Stathatos N, Levetan C, Burman KD, et al. The controversy of the treatment of critically ill patients with thyroid hormone. *Best Pract Res Clin Endocrinol Metab* 2001;15:465–78.
34. Sugino K, Ito K, Mimura T, et al. Surgical treatment of Graves' disease in children. *Thyroid* 2004;14:447–52.
35. Tajiri J, Katsuya H, Kiyokawa T, et al. Successful treatment of thyrotoxic crisis with plasma exchange. *Crit Care Med* 1984;12:536–7.
36. Tews MC, Shah SM, Gossain VV. Hypothyroidism: mimicker of common complaints. *Emerg Med Clin North Am* 2005;23:649–67, vii.
37. Tietgens ST, Leinung MC. Thyroid storm. *Med Clin North Am* 1995;79:169–84.
38. Vanhorebeek I, Van den Berghe G. The neuroendocrine response to critical illness is a dynamic process. *Crit Care Clin* 2006;22:1–15, v.
39. Weber KJ, Solorzano CC, Lee JK, et al. Thyroidectomy remains an effective treatment option for Graves' disease. *Am J Surg* 2006;191:400–5.

CHAPTER 96 ■ ACUTE RENAL FAILURE AND END-STAGE RENAL DISEASE

RICHARD M. HACKBARTH • NORMA J. MAXVOLD • TIMOTHY E. BUNCHMAN

Renal failure is a common problem in the PICU. Whether it is the primary reason for admission to the PICU or secondary to the underlying disease process, knowledge of the underlying causes, diagnosis, and management of acute or chronic renal failure is essential to the intensivist. In addition to the evaluation and treatment of renal failure and its sequelae, drug dosing and nutritional management are extremely important considerations in children with impaired renal function. Furthermore, the intensivist must have an understanding of end-stage renal disease (ESRD) and management of the posttransplant patient. This chapter will provide an overview of the spectrum of renal pathology, from acute renal failure (ARF) to ESRD and its management, short of renal replacement therapy (RRT), which is covered in considerable detail in Chapter 37.

ACUTE RENAL FAILURE

Incidence

ARF is defined as an abrupt reduction in glomerular filtration rate (GFR) of at least 50% from baseline that is characterized by $\geq 50\%$ increase in serum creatinine, rising levels of nitrogenous wastes, and disturbances in the regulation of fluid, electrolyte, and acid-base homeostasis by the kidney. ARF may affect individuals with chronic renal insufficiency and those with previously normal renal function. Although oliguria is not a part of the definition of ARF, it is present in 30%–70% of patients; the remaining children have normal or increased urine output. The incidence of ARF in the pediatric population is difficult to determine, as not all cases are reported; however, it is thought to be 3.9 per 100,000 children annually. An important component of pathology in the critical care environment, ARF was shown to have a prevalence of ~6% in a multinational study of adult ICU patients (57). In children, 3%–10% of NICU admissions have ARF as a part of their pathology, but data for PICU patients are sparse. A recent query of the Virtual PICU (performance) System database for pediatric critical care patients with primary or secondary diagnosis of ARF or acute tubular necrosis (ATN) from January 2004 through September 2005 showed a period prevalence of 1.2% for ARF in the PICU. This data set contained a total of 52,644 patients, encompassing all patients admitted to 31 PICUs in the US during the 21-month period of the query (unpublished data; Virtual PICU System data were provided from VPS, LLC. No endorsement or editorial restriction of the interpretation of these data or opinions of the authors has been implied or stated). Al-

though reporting by diagnosis may be somewhat subjective and these data may under-report the true prevalence of ARF in the PICU, it may well be the best available estimate of prevalence in a multi-institutional sample. The overall mortality of pediatric ARF is 25%–40% or more in the ICU population, and >50% for patients who require RRT or who are <1 year of age (33,61).

Etiology

The etiology of ARF can be classified as primary, when the kidney is the intended victim of the insult, or secondary, when the kidney is more the innocent bystander. Perhaps the more clinically useful classification is to divide causality into prerenal, renal, and postrenal categories (Table 96.1). Prerenal ARF is a secondary insult to the kidney due to factors that alter renal perfusion. Processes that decrease extracellular fluid volume or cause extravascular redistribution of that fluid (dehydration, burns, nephrotic syndrome), processes associated with decreased cardiac output (cardiogenic shock, myocarditis, tamponade), or those associated with vasodilatation or renal vasoconstriction (sepsis, drugs, anaphylaxis) are all causes of prerenal ARF. Regardless of cause, if the perfusion alteration persists long enough, prerenal ARF will be converted to renal ARF in the form of ATN. Worldwide, the most common cause of prerenal ARF is gastroenteritis. Renal causes of ARF can be either primary or secondary insults and are processes that affect the renal parenchymal structures. ATN, rhabdomyolysis, hemolysis, tumor lysis syndrome, interstitial nephritis, acute glomerulonephritis, and renal vascular occlusion are all causes of renal ARF. Globally, hemolytic uremic syndrome (HUS) is the most common renal cause of ARF, but ischemic causes account for most of the intrinsic renal ARF in many ICUs in North America. Finally, postrenal causes of ARF affect the outflow of urine from the kidney and are all either congenital or acquired forms of obstructive uropathy.

Although the most common causes of ARF worldwide are gastroenteritis, HUS, and other infectious entities, the most common causes of ARF among hospitalized children in North America are HUS, renal ischemia, nephrotoxic drugs, and sepsis (33,61). The relative contribution of each cause varies based on patient population and geographic location of the individual studies; however, it seems clear that a significant amount of the ARF seen in the PICU is a comorbidity of the patient's underlying disease process, consequent interventions, and resulting sequelae (e.g., chemotherapy, bone marrow transplant, postoperative complex congenital heart repair, to name a few) (27).

TABLE 96.1

CATEGORIES OF ACUTE RENAL FAILURE IN CHILDREN

Prerenal causes	Intrinsic renal causes	Postrenal (obstructive) causes
Intravascular volume depletion	**Acute tubular necrosis (ATN)**	Posterior urethral valves
Dehydration	**Ischemic Injury**	Obstruction of a solitary kidney
Gastroenteritis	Prerenal causes	Bilateral ureteral obstruction
Hemorrhage	**Exogenous toxins**	Neurogenic bladder
Diabetes Insipidus	Nephrotoxic antibiotics	Trauma
Burns	Chemotherapeutic agents	
Diuretics	NSAIDs	
Redistribution of fluid/vasodilation	ACE inhibitors and ARBs	
Sepsis	Radiographic contrast	
Pancreatitis	Venoms	
Intestinal obstruction	Heavy metals	
Peritonitis	Ethylene glycol	
Nephrotic syndrome	**Endogenous toxins**	
Hepatic failure	Myoglobinuria/hemoglobinuria	
Decreased Cardiac Output	Tumor lysis syndrome	
Congenital heart failure	**Acute interstitial nephritis**	
Cardiogenic shock	Drug-induced or idiopathic	
Myocarditis	**Acute glomerulonephritis**	
Cardiac tamponade	Postinfectious (Streptococcal)	
	HSP, SLE, Goodpasture syndrome	
	Vascular Pathology	
	Renal artery/vein thrombosis	
	HUS/TTP	
	Cortical necrosis	
	Congenital	
	Renal dysplasia/hypoplasia	
	Polycystic kidney disease	

NSAIDs, nonsteroidal anti-inflammatories; ACE, angiotensin-converting enzyme; ARBs, adrenergic receptor binders; HSP, Henoch-Schönlein purpura; SLE, systemic lupus erythematosus; HUS, hemolytic-uremic syndrome; TTP, thrombotic thrombocytopenic purpura

Renal Physiology and the Pathophysiology of ARF

To understand the treatment or prevention of ARF, it is first necessary to appreciate the pathophysiology of renal injury and how it is affected by predisposing factors such as the underlying disease process, drug effects, and genetic predisposition to renal insult.

Normal Regulation of Renal Blood Flow and Glomerular Filtration

Renal blood flow is ~25% of total cardiac output. Approximately 90% of renal blood flow is to the renal cortex and, hence, the glomeruli. A considerable step-down occurs in hydrostatic pressure from the renal artery to the afferent arteriole of the glomerulus to less than half of systemic pressure, which is still roughly twice the hydrostatic pressure found in other capillary beds; therefore, the transcapillary pressure gradient (ΔP) is the main force that drives glomerular filtration. Single-nephron GFR (SNGFR) can be expressed as

$$SNGFR = K_f(\Delta P - \pi_{GC})$$

where:

K_f = ultrafiltration constant
π_{GC} = oncotic pressure of the glomerular capillary.

The contribution of oncotic pressure of Bowman's capsule is negligible, as permeability of macromolecules should normally be nil. The ultrafiltration constant K_f can vary, depending on changes in glomerular capillary surface area and permeability changes. The mesangial cells of the glomerulus are functionally and structurally similar to vascular smooth muscle and can contract with vasogenic stimuli to reduce the glomerular surface area available for filtration. Renal blood flow is autoregulated between mean arterial blood pressures of 80 mm Hg and 180 mm Hg in adults, likely due to a mechanism intrinsic to the kidney, as the phenomenon is preserved in the isolated, perfused kidney. Referred to as the *myogenic reflex*, changes in hydrostatic pressure in the preglomerular arteriolar circulation affect the amount of cytosolic calcium present in the vascular smooth muscle and thereby maintain a constant glomerular blood flow. Autoregulation of GFR is accomplished by altering afferent and efferent arteriolar tone. As renal artery pressure falls, the afferent arteriole vasodilates and the efferent arteriole vasoconstricts, allowing the glomerular capillary hydrostatic pressure to be maintained and the GFR to remain constant. The dilation of the afferent arteriole is mediated by prostacyclin or endothelium-derived nitric oxide (NO). The vasoconstriction of the efferent arteriole is controlled by local production of angiotensin II. This low-level production of angiotensin II appears to affect the efferent arteriole selectively. Obviously, drugs such as nonsteroidal anti-inflammatories can

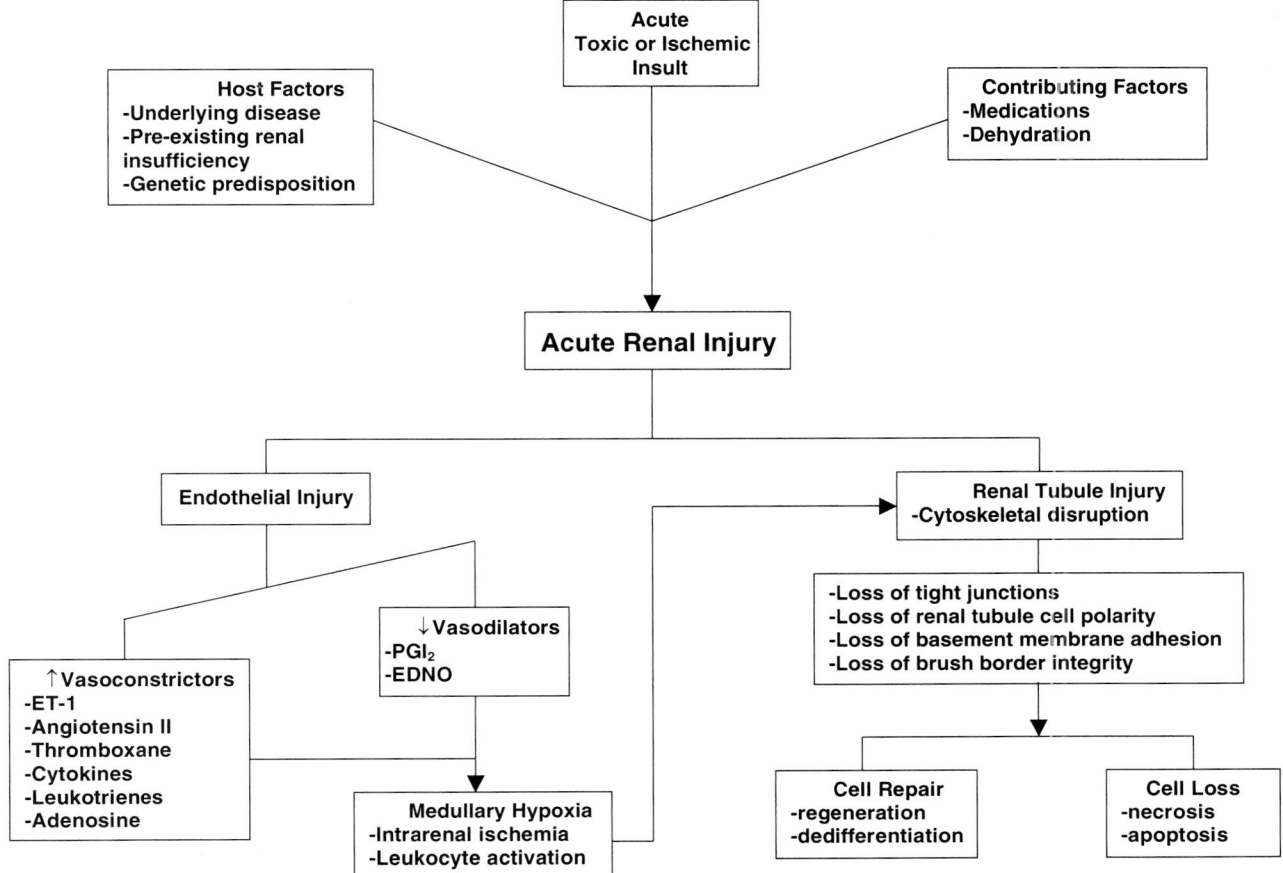

FIGURE 96.1. Changes in renal vascular pressure will trigger compensatory mechanisms to maintain a constant glomerular filtration rate by modifying afferent and efferent arteriolar tone. Decreased renal perfusion pressure leads to afferent arteriole dilation via prostacyclin or EDNO. Efferent arteriole tone is increased by angiotensin II. The combined effect is to maintain the transcapillary hydrostatic pressure and, therefore, glomerular filtration rate. EG-1, endothelin-1; EDNO, endothelium-derived nitric oxide.

adversely affect this compensatory mechanism. A third mechanism for maintaining GFR is tubuloglomerular feedback. If GFR increases above the normal rate, which in turn increases solute delivery to the distal tubule, the juxtaglomerular apparatus is stimulated to produce rennin; angiotensin II is released locally and, in turn, causes mesangial cell contraction and afferent arteriolar constriction, which reduces GFR to normal levels (Fig. 96.1).

Pathophysiology of Acute Tubular Necrosis

ATN is really a misnomer, as the renal histology of ATN is tubular cell injury and rarely necrosis. A more apt term for the process would be *acute tubular dysfunction*, but ATN seems too ingrained in our consciousness to be changed. An isolated, brief ischemic insult is unlikely to cause ATN; rather, a more sustained insult or an insult to a patient with predisposing factors, such as hypovolemia, nephrotoxic drugs, or preexisting renal insufficiency, is probably necessary for significant renal tubular injury to occur. The same series of events can be triggered by ischemia, rhabdomyolysis, hemolysis, etc. The process can be divided into three phases: initiation, maintenance, and recovery. The initiation phase entails the time period in which the ischemic or toxic insult occurs, as well as the postischemic-reperfusion period. The next phase is a protracted period of

maintenance in which ongoing inflammation causes further injury, cell necrosis, and apoptosis. Finally, the third phase is a recovery period in which tubular cell regeneration and clearance of tubular debris take place (5).

The pathophysiology of ATN can be divided into two processes: microvascular pathology and renal tubular pathology (**Fig. 96.2**). Each one affects the other, and both impair GFR. The hallmark of microvascular pathology is vasoconstriction. The ischemic process causes increased sympathetic tone and an increase in the production of angiotensin II, leukotrienes, thromboxane A_2, and cytokines. Renal vascular endothelial injury also leads to an increase in endothelin-1 production. Endothelin-1 is a very potent vasoconstrictor and has even more potent activity in the renal vascular bed than elsewhere (42). Simultaneously, endothelial injury suppresses production of endothelium-derived NO due to decreased activity of endothelial NO synthase (eNOS). Endothelium-derived NO normally downregulates endothelin production and modulates its activity at the endothelin receptor. Furthermore, adenosine liberated from ATP depletion can also cause vasoconstriction. This extreme imbalance of vasoconstrictors to vasodilators causes a decrease in overall renal blood flow and glomerular blood flow. The endothelial injury and cytokinemia also activates leukocytes and promotes leukocyte adhesion, causing

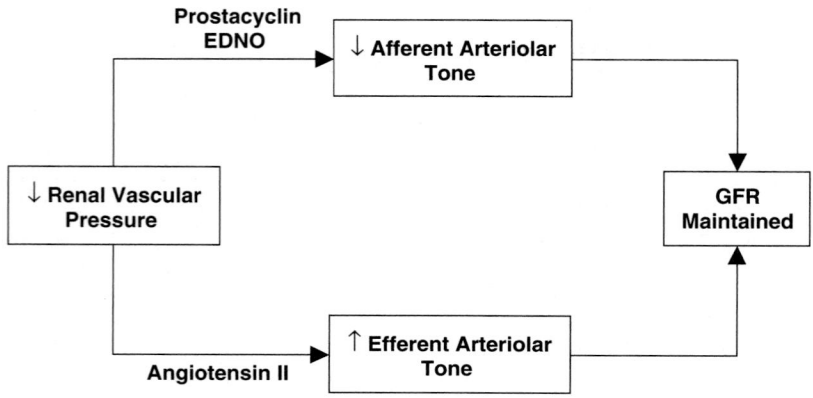

FIGURE 96.2. A schematic diagram of the pathophysiology of ATN. Host factors and other contributing factors can prime the kidney for injury from an acute insult. Endothelial injury, with subsequent stimulation of the inflammatory cascade, contributes to direct renal tubule cell damage from the acute injury. The end result is either cell repair or loss through necrosis or apoptosis. EDNO, endothelium-derived nitric oxide; GFR, glomerular filtration rate.

microvascular congestion and thrombosis, which further exacerbates tissue ischemia and promotes inflammation. GFR is compromised by the overall reduction in renal perfusion pressure and by constriction of the afferent and efferent arterioles, causing a decrease in capillary hydrostatic pressure and, therefore, decreased filtration. GFR is also reduced by vasoconstrictor-mediated mesangial contraction, which reduces the capillary surface area so that filtration occurs.

The medulla of the kidney normally functions at a lower oxygen tension than does the cortex due to the countercurrent arrangement of the arterial and venous vasa rectae. The oxygen delivery and content in the deep medulla, coupled with the significant energy requirements of cellular pumps engaged in active solute transport, make the outer medullary region of the kidney a high-risk area for ischemic injury (42). The cells of the S3 segment of the proximal tubule are the most susceptible to injury. Injury to renal tubular cells results in disruption of the actin cytoskeleton, which, in turn, leads to loss of cell polarity, brush-border integrity, cellular adhesion to the basement membrane, and tight-junction integrity. When the cell loses polarity, Na/K-ATPase complexes that are normally found on the basolateral portion of the cell membrane can migrate to the apical membrane, causing loss of unidirectional salt and water transport and increased solute load in the tubule. Through the tubuloglomerular feedback mechanism, afferent arteriolar tone is increased, adversely affecting GFR. Loss of cell-to-basement membrane adhesion causes shedding of tubular cells into the tubular lumen, thereby obstructing the flow of ultrafiltrate and increasing intraluminal pressure, which, in turn, decreases the transcapillary pressure gradient in the glomerulus and further decreases GFR. Loss of tight-junction integrity causes back leak of glomerular filtrate into the interstitial space and subsequently into the vasculature. In addition to the reduction in GFR and tubular function brought about by structural changes, adenosine is released by tubular cells due to ATP depletion. These cells are also capable of producing cytokines, such as IL-6 and tumor necrosis factor (TNF)-α (5). Tubular cells can also produce NO via inducible NOS (iNOS). In contrast to the low-level, transient production of NO by eNOS, iNOS causes sustained production of NO. Systemic production causes hypotension and worsens renal ischemia; in the renal tubule, it may produce oxidative cellular damage during reperfusion by formation of peroxynitrite (28).

Once the insult on the injured renal tubular cells has abated, one of four fates awaits the cell. If the injury is mild, it may return to its preinjury state. Alternatively, the cell may dedif-

ferentiate and proliferate to regenerate the tubular epithelium. The injury may also prove fatal, and the cell may undergo either necrosis or apoptosis. If ATP depletion is severe enough, necrosis can take place in very severely injured cells or very early in the ischemic process, even before the injury would be considered irreversible (5). The energy-depleted cell cannot regulate sodium (Na$^+$), potassium (K$^+$), or calcium (Ca$^+$) balance, nor can it regulate its volume. Cellular swelling and disruption ensue, and proteolytic enzymes spill into the extracellular space causing further inflammation. In contrast to the very chaotic and unregulated process of necrosis, apoptosis is highly regulated, requires energy, and leads to involution and eventual clearance of the cells by phagocytosis (42). Triggers of apoptosis may include TNF-α, sublethal ischemia, toxin exposure, or deficiency of renal growth factors.

Repair of the tubular epithelium, as alluded to previously, occurs either by healing of the injured cell or by dedifferentiation and replication of existing renal tubular cells. Normal renal tubular cells do not tend to divide in response to growth factors. After ischemic or nephrotoxic injury, however, gene expression that promotes cellular regeneration is induced. The medullary, thick, ascending limb of the loop of Henle (mTAL) appears to be a major site for this activity. This segment, along with the S3 segment of the proximal tubule, are the two areas of the renal tubule most susceptible to ischemic injury and are also in close anatomic proximity to each other. The regenerative activity in the mTAL has been postulated to have a paracrine effect on tubular cell regeneration in the proximal tubule (42). Growth factors such as epidermal growth factor, insulin-like growth factor (IGF), and hepatocyte growth factor have all been shown to have a therapeutic effect in animal models of renal tubular regeneration following ARF. The application of growth factors to human therapy is uncertain at this time (15). Following ARF from ischemic or toxin-induced ATN, the usual end result of these regenerative processes is recovery of normal tubular structure and function.

Genetic Predisposition to Acute Renal Failure

Whether the inciting event of ARF is sepsis, ischemia, or exposure to a nephrotoxic agent, it is clear that inflammation has a central role in the pathology of the disease process. The interaction of certain host factors with the insult may result in either suppression or promotion of the inflammatory process and protect or predispose the host to the development of ARF. Gene polymorphisms are likely relevant to the pathophysiology of ARF, just as they are in sepsis or systemic inflammatory response syndrome. Polymorphisms that either promote or inhibit the production of inflammatory cytokines, reactive oxygen species, neutrophil activation, or iNOS activity are all potentially important to the development of ARF. Certain TNF-α high-producer alleles have been associated with an increased risk of mortality in adults with ARF who require dialysis (34). This same TNF-α genotype, in combination with a low IL-6-producer genotype, was shown to have a higher prevalence among neonates with ARF than in those without ARF (60). The IL-1 receptor antagonist polymorphic allele-2 has been associated with the severity of nephritis in Henoch-Schönlein purpura (34). Polymorphism in the IL-8 gene has been associated with an increased severity of lupus nephritis. Neonates carrying the heat shock protein genotype that codes for low inducibility of the HSP70-2 protein are at greater risk for the development of ARF (60). These are just a few of the many genetic polymorphisms that may play a role in the development or modulation of ARF (34). It is as yet unclear how this rapidly expanding area of investigation will impact our understanding of ARF and our ability to affect its course.

Evaluation and Treatment of Acute Renal Failure

Evaluation

Just as the etiology of ARF can be categorized into prerenal, intrarenal, and postrenal causes, the evaluation of ARF can be approached using the same classification system.

Prerenal. Prerenal failure occurs in clinical conditions associated with intravascular volume depletion or inadequate cardiac output. Underlying disease states or clinical exam findings that are compatible with low perfusion states should heighten suspicion for prerenal failure. The definitive laboratory diagnosis of prerenal azotemia is based on the fractional excretion of Na^+ (FE_{Na}):

$$FE_{Na} = (U_{Na}/P_{Cr})/(P_{Na}/U_{Cr}) \times 100$$

where:

U_{Na} = urine Na^+ concentration
P_{Cr} = plasma creatinine concentration
P_{Na} = plasma Na^+ concentration
U_{Cr} = urine creatinine concentration.

The calculation requires simultaneous urine and plasma values to be meaningful. As a rule, an FE_{Na} of <1% is compatible with prerenal azotemia. However, the accuracy of this assay can be influenced by confounding therapies, the most common being diuretic use. In this situation, one can have an inappropriately high urinary excretion of Na^+ despite a true decrease in renal blood flow. Fractional excretion of urea (FE_{UN}) has been found to be a more sensitive and specific assay to distinguish between prerenal and intrarenal pathology without being influenced by other common therapies, including diuretics. It is calculated in the same manner

as FE_{Na}:

$$FE_{UN} = [(\text{urine urea nitrogen/blood urea nitrogen})/ \\ (\text{urine creatinine/blood creatinine})] \times 100\%$$

Prerenal oliguria and azotemia are associated with an FE_{UN} of <35%; intrarenal disease, including ATN, produces an FE_{UN} of >50%. This effect may be influenced by the use of diuretics but should be considered, even if diuretics are being used. An alternative method by which to differentiate between prerenal and intrarenal processes is Doppler ultrasound, which, in addition to being noninvasive, is unaffected by changes in Na^+ or creatinine after diuretics or hemodialysis and can be formed in complete anuria.

Intrarenal. The intrarenal causes of ARF are numerous, as mentioned previously. Throughout the world, the primary cause of ARF is HUS. The classic presentation is a triad of microangiopathic-hemolytic anemia, thrombocytopenia, and ARF. In most children, HUS is preceded by a diarrheal prodrome. Once HUS has been excluded as a cause, the evaluation should be methodical, starting with the urinalysis. If the urine is bland without any evidence of protein, hemoglobin, concentrating defect, or white cells, acute interstitial nephritis should be considered. If the urine contains eosinophils, the cause may be drug related. If the urine contains protein, the protein should be quantified using either a spot urinary protein/creatinine ratio, or a 24-hr urine collection. The two measures can be correlated to each other. For example, a protein/creatinine ratio of 2 is equivalent to a 2-g collection in 24 hrs. Although urinary protein is presumed to be glomerular in origin, it can be tubular interstitial as well. A urine protein electrophoresis can be used to distinguish the source of the urinary protein if necessary.

If the urinary sediment contains blood and protein, and hypertension is present, glomerulonephritis (GN) should be suspected. Blood work should include electrolytes, blood urea nitrogen (BUN), creatinine, Ca^+, phosphorus, and albumin. The albumin is imperative when proteinuria is present to exclude hypoalbuminemia. Further workup includes complement C3 and C4 levels. A low C3 and abnormal urine sediment suggest the differential diagnosis of postinfectious GN, systemic lupus erythematosus (SLE), or membranoproliferative GN. The C4 level is equivocal in membranoproliferative GN, low in SLE, and usually normal in postinfectious GN. If the C3 is normal, all other forms of GN should be considered. Obtaining other serology, including antinuclear antibody (ANA, which may be positive in up to 30% of normal children), antiDNA (more specific), and antineutrophil cytoplasmic antibody (ANCA) may be helpful. In the event of a concomitant finding of pulmonary involvement, especially pulmonary hemorrhage, Wegener granulomatosis, SLE, Churg-Strauss syndrome, and Goodpasture syndrome should be considered. Churg-Strauss disease is associated with peripheral eosinophilia, and antiglomerular basement antibodies are found in Goodpasture syndrome. Immunoglobin levels, erythrocyte sedimentation rate, and C-reactive protein are not definitive and, therefore, not helpful in making a diagnosis. In the case of a normal complementemic GN or an unknown etiology of ARF, a renal biopsy is in order to obtain a definitive diagnosis and assess disease activity and chronicity. Currently, analysis of the renal histology is often the fastest means of diagnosing intrarenal pathology. Many nephrologists prefer to biopsy early while awaiting supporting laboratory tests. When immunologically based renal disease

TABLE 96.2

COMPLEMENT PATTERNS IN GLOMERULAR NEPHRITIS

Diagnosis	C3	C4
Postinfectious glomerular nephritis	Decreased	Normal Limits
Systemic lupus erythematous	Decreased	Decreased
Membranoproliferative glomerular nephritis	Decreased	Decreased or Normal Limits
IgA nephropathy	Normal Limits	Normal Limits
Henoch Schönlein purpura	Normal Limits	Normal Limits
Anti-GBM disease	Normal Limits	Normal Limits
Insulin-dependent diabetes mellitus	Normal Limits	Normal Limits
Membranous nephropathy	Normal Limits	Normal Limits
Focal segmental glomerulosclerosis	Normal Limits	Normal Limits
Wegener granulomatosis	Normal Limits	Normal Limits
Churg-Strauss syndrome	Normal Limits	Normal Limits

is suspected, immunosuppression may be started, if necessary, before the renal biopsy is obtained, without effecting renal histology (**Table 96.2**).

Postrenal. The causes of postrenal failure are related to urinary tract obstruction. It is imperative to obtain some sort of renal imaging to assess the location of the obstruction. Renal ultrasound, IV pyelogram, CT imaging with and without contrast, and radioisotope studies have all been used. The problem with IV pyelogram and CT scan is the potential for contrast nephropathy. The contrast itself, as well as the contrast used in MRIs, is a tubular toxin. Nuclear medicine studies do not show anatomic detail well. Therefore, the standard diagnostic imaging modality is bedside ultrasound. Ultrasound evaluates kidney size and assesses for hydronephrosis, ureteral or bladder dilatation, and the presence of debris or echogenicity in the kidneys or bladder.

Growth grids for kidneys correlate with patient age. If the kidneys are small for the patient's age and body size, the ultrasound suggests chronic renal failure. Conversely, if the kidneys are large for age and size, it implies that the process is acute and potentially reversible. If hydronephrosis is bilateral, blockage at or distal to the level of the bladder (i.e., posterior urethral valve in males), bilateral ureteropelvic junction, or the ureterovesical junction must be considered. If urinary tract obstruction is unilateral, obstructive renal failure should not occur.

Treatment of Acute Renal Failure

Prevention of Acute Renal Failure and Renal Protection Strategies. Early recognition of renal dysfunction and prompt treatment to limit further injury to the kidney are the keys to successful management of ARF. Prerenal causes of renal insufficiency should be aggressively treated by optimizing intravascular volume and cardiac output. The treatment of hypovolemia, cardiogenic shock, and septic shock are covered in great detail elsewhere in this text. Relief of obstructive uropathy can be expected to precipitate fluid and electrolyte losses due to renal dysfunction and loss of concentrating ability. Careful management of fluid and electrolyte balance is necessary to avoid further renal dysfunction.

Beyond these general guidelines for management of prerenal and postrenal failure, this section will focus on renal protection strategies, drug clearance considerations in ARF, and the importance of nutritional support to the overall management of the renal failure patient. (RRT is covered in Chapter 37.) Specific causes of renal disease common to the ICU are addressed in a later section of this chapter.

Regardless of the cause of renal insufficiency, ensuring adequate perfusion pressure to the kidney is key to supporting the renal function. Many vasoactive agents have been used to support renal perfusion. Interest has resurfaced in vasopressin as a vascular tone agent in refractory shock. Although vasopressin enhances systemic perfusion, it has not been shown to improve the renal-perfusion gradient (24). In animal studies, low-dose vasopressin has been found to increase urine output but has no effect on renal blood flow and actually causes a decrease in mesenteric blood flow and conductance. Due to the microcirculatory effects to vital organs, no evidence of improved outcome has been shown to date (18).

The use of "renal dose" dopamine (0.5–3 mcg/kg/min) has found wide acceptance for decades despite poor evidence of any real advantage in patients with ARF. Although well-documented evidence exists for intrarenal vasodilatation mediated by DA_1 and DA_2 receptor stimulation, no evidence exists for improvement of renal function in patients who have already experienced renal injury (1). When no preexisting renal dysfunction is present, an increase in urine output and renal blood flow has been documented in the "low-dose" dopamine concentrations in animals. Early implementation of low-dose dopamine prior to the development of renal insufficiency may ease management of fluid balance in patients (19).

Fenoldopam, a DA_1 receptor agonist, has recently been evaluated in patients with renal insufficiency as a renal protective therapy for IV contrast administration. Although fenoldopam does increase GFR by renal vasodilatation, extensive systemic metabolism occurs during IV administration, resulting in an inadequate amount of the drug being delivered to the kidney and, therefore, a minimal actual increase in GFR. A study that compared IV infusion and direct delivery of the drug to the renal vasculature found that if the drug is able to reach the kidney at an appropriate level, GRF and renal plasma flow do increase (55). Whether this drug will prove useful in the treatment of ARF remains to be determined.

Investigation of atrial natriuretic peptide (ANP) and its synthetic analogs has found that ANP does cause vasodilatation of the afferent glomerular arteriole and constriction of the efferent arteriole, thereby increasing GFR independent of the renal blood flow. ANP also increases tubular flow rate and natriuresis. However, protection of renal function has not been demonstrated. In a multicentered study, no beneficial effect of ANP was found in patients who suffered from acute, oliguric renal failure (41).

Of all of the agents that affect vascular tone, only norepinephrine has been shown to improve GFR under the circumstances of experimentally compromised renal perfusion (17).

For many decades, diuretics have been used in the treatment of ARF. Mannitol has been widely used in the critical care setting. Theoretically, it exerts its beneficial effects by inducing an osmotic diuresis, which clears tubular debris and prevents the compensatory preglomerular vasoconstriction that accompanies tubular congestion, in turn, helping to maintain GFR. Other potential renal-protective mechanisms of mannitol include its acting as a free radical scavenger and inducing the osmotic limitation of intracellular swelling after an ischemic insult. Evidence of increased urine output in response to mannitol is well documented, but few studies have found actual protection of GFR.

Furosemide has likewise been used to induce diuresis and protect against preglomerular vasoconstriction. It has also been proposed that, as an inhibitor of active transport in the ascending thick limb, furosemide lessens the energy expenditure of injured cells, thus reducing substrate depletion and tubular damage in the ischemic kidney. As is the case with mannitol, urine output improves, but no change in the GFR can be demonstrated. Loop diuretics carry the risks of ototoxicity and nephrotoxicity, which can be potentiated by other agents (e.g., aminoglycosides) that may be used concurrently. Care should be taken not to "over-diuresis" the patient and further impede renal plasma flow. Limited studies have been completed that compare continuous versus intermittent dosing of loop diuretics, and greater effectiveness and less toxicity appear to be associated with continuous infusion of diuretics. Patients who are severely hypoalbuminemic have a diminished response to loop diuretics due to a decrease in effective renal blood flow from third-spacing of intravascular fluid. They also have diminished plasma protein binding; therefore, a larger free fraction of the loop diuretic is available to be metabolized and inactivated. With this in mind, improved response to diuretics can be seen when hypoalbuminemia is corrected.

Regardless of the cause of ischemia to the kidney, normal cellular Ca^+ homeostasis is disrupted, leading to an abnormal accumulation of free intracellular Ca^+. This finding has stimulated interest in using Ca^+-channel blockers for renal protection. Most of the investigations of this therapeutic intervention have involved renal transplantation. In these studies, a Ca^+-channel blocker was added to the infusate of the donor kidney prior to transplant and given to the recipient as well. The result was a significant drop in posttransplant ATN (45). Further investigation of Ca^+-channel blockers in patients with established ARF may help to define whether they offer renal protection under these circumstances.

Estimation of Glomerular Filtration Rate by Creatinine Clearance and the Impact of Acute Renal Failure on Drug Dosing. Assessment of the extent of the ARF during critical illness in children is desirable both for the hour-to-hour management of the patient and for any potential modulation and, if possible, lessening of the already present renal dysfunction. Avoidance of further injury to the kidneys and awareness of all medications that are primarily cleared by the kidneys are vital for safe and effective overall treatment of the critically ill child.

The most utilized and accurate measurement of renal dysfunction is the GFR. Basic knowledge of normal GFR for age and the associated renal development is essential for proper interpretation of the measurement. The preterm infant at 30-week gestation has a GFR of <10 mL/min/1.73 m^2; at term, the GFR is $\sim$10–40 mL/min/1.73 m^2, and by 2 years of age, the GFR reaches adult levels of 110–120 mL/min/1.73 m^2 (7,13).

Although multiple methods for calculating GFR are available, the most commonly used is creatinine clearance (CrCl). Creatinine is produced in the muscle as a byproduct of creatine during protein metabolism and is proportional to the body's muscle mass. Creatinine is readily water soluble and distributed throughout total body water compartments. In addition to being filtrated at the glomerulus, it is secreted by the tubules. Therefore, CrCl gives somewhat of an overestimation of the GFR (23,37,50). For this reason, some centers prefer to use a filtered substance (e.g., inulin) that is neither secreted nor absorbed further along the nephron, thus providing a more accurate measurement of GFR (36).

Most centers still use the CrCl, which is readily calculated from equations. The Traub equation is most commonly used for children 1–18 years of age (56):

$$CrCl\,(mL/min/1.73\,m^2\,BSA) = (0.48)(H)/S_{Cr}$$

where:

$\quad$ BSA = body surface area
$\quad$ H = height (cm)
$\quad$ S_{Cr} = measured serum creatinine.

For infants <1 year old, the following adjustment in the equation is made for the proportionately lower muscle mass-to-surface area ratio in this age group (52):

$$CrCl\,(mL/min/1.73\,m^2\,BSA) = (0.45)(H)/S_{Cr}$$

The above equation expresses the CrCl in terms of the standard adult BSA (1.73 m^2), but to obtain the actual clearance in a child, the result must be multiplied by the patient's actual BSA (30):

$$BSA = W^{0.5378} \times H^{0.3864} \times 0.024265$$

where W = weight (kg).

In the critically ill child, the severity of renal dysfunction is changing, often worsening, and CrCl calculated based on more than one creatinine measurement is preferable (40).

$$CrCl\,(males)(mLs/min) = [293 - 2.03(age)] \times 1.035$$
$$- [0.01685(S_{Cr1} + S_{Cr2})] + 49(S_{Cr1} - S_{Cr2})/\Delta t$$

where Δt = change in time in days between the S_{Cr1} and $S_{Cr2.}$

$$CrCl\,(females) = CrCl\,(males) \times 0.86$$

It is important to note that creatinine is also secreted, not just filtered, especially as renal dysfunction worsens. The more impaired kidney function becomes, the greater the error in the equation's estimates of GFR. Active tubular secretion of creatinine gives an exaggerated estimate of GFR when CrCl equations are used. When the GFR is actually 100 mL/min, the CrCl will overestimate it by only $\sim$20% (i.e., calculated as 120 mL/min). At a GFR of 60 mL/min, the CrCl will produce $\sim$60% overestimate, giving a value of near-normal range (i.e., 96 mL/min). At very low GFR (20 mL/min), the CrCl can overestimate by 100%, giving a 40 mL/min estimate (23,50).

To attempt a more accurate assessment of GFR, a timed CrCl can be measured, the standard interval being a 24-hr collection (38,23).

$$CrCl = U_{Cr} \times V_U/S_{Cr} \times t$$

where:

U_{Cr} = urine creatinine concentration (mg/dL)
V_U = urine volume (mL)
S_{Cr} = serum creatinine concentration (mg/dL) at the midpoint of the collection
t = time interval of the collection.

During acute renal dysfunction, other methods of GFR assessment are helpful. An accurate assessment can be attained by measuring a low protein-binding substance that is primarily eliminated through the kidney via passive glomerular filtration without significant secretion or absorption by the kidney. Aminoglycosides are antibiotics that fit these specifications. Measuring these drug levels provides both help in pharmacokinetic dosing based on the elimination half-life of the drug in patients with renal dysfunction and a greater appreciation of the true degree of GFR impairment (4). In a trial designed to compare methods of estimating GFR in critically ill patients, the GFR calculated from aminoglycoside measurements correlated well with inulin clearance data (62).

The following equation has been used to relate clearance of aminoglycosides (CL_{ag}) to CrCl (35,62):

$$CL_{ag} = CrCl$$

In renal dysfunction, altered renal clearance impacts on all drugs primarily eliminated by the kidneys; therefore, the elimination half-lives are also affected in proportion to the altered clearance and can be calculated from the Dettli method:

$$t\,{}^{1}\!/_{2} = 0.693/K$$

where $K = k_r + k_{nr}$.

In other words, the total elimination rate constant (K) is equal to the sum of the elimination rate constant of renal excretion (k_r) and the elimination rate constant of the nonrenal processes (k_{nr}).

Renal elimination (k_r) can also be expressed as a function of CrCl:

$$k_r = \alpha\,(CrCl)$$

where α is the linear relationship between CrCl and the renal elimination rate constant.

When both k_r and k_{nr} are known, the patient's half-life ($t\,{}^{1}\!/_{2}$) for a drug can be found using the Dettli method (16,35).

To individualize a drug dosage during renal failure, calculations are based on the drug's half-life or clearance adjustment related to the patient's $CrCl_r$ (reduced) relative to the normal $CrCl_n$ (120 mL/min/1.73 m^2). KF expresses this ratio:

$$KF = CrCl_r/CrCl_n$$

From this relationship, a dosage adjustment factor (DF) can be calculated as:

$$DF = 1 - [f(1 - KF)]$$

where f is the fraction of drug that is renally eliminated unchanged in normal kidney function (16,35).

The above adjustment calculations assume that (a) the decrease in total body clearance and elimination rate constant are proportional to the CrCl, (b) the renal disease itself does not significantly alter the drug's metabolism, (c) drug metabolites are inactive, and (d) that the drug follows linear kinetics. From the estimated dosage adjustment factor (DF), the individualized drug dose (D_r) or interval (τ_r) or both can be calculated as:

Adjusted dose: $\quad D_r = D_n \times DF$

Adjusted interval: $\quad \tau_r = \tau_n/DF$

where D_n is the dose and τ_n is the interval for patients with normal renal function.

This adjustment's accuracy depends on the volume of distribution, bioavailability, and protein binding remaining unchanged. Multiple tables with renal-adjustment recommendations for commonly used drugs in the PICU are available in most pharmacologic texts (12).

Nutrition and Energy Requirements in Acute Renal Failure. Our understanding of changes that occur in the neuroendocrine axis during acute illness has focused attention on the influence of growth factors on cellular stability. Thus far, investigations of a possible application of IGF-1 to help protect the cellular integrity and deter accelerated catabolism in ARF have not shown benefit (31). A multifactorial approach with combinations of growth factors has yet to be well studied. This area is still early in its investigations of potential applications.

In addition to drug pharmacokinetic alterations during acute renal dysfunction, specific nutritional metabolism changes also occur and require attention. The ability to handle nitrogenous waste, measured most commonly as BUN, is adversely affected. In addition to an impaired renal clearance of nitrogen, the rate of protein catabolism is exceptionally high in children with ARF, on the order of 180–250 mg/kg/day, which further exacerbates uremia (37,43). The amino acid profile is abnormal in ARF, with alterations in the clearance of specific amino acids as well as impairment of the normal interconversion (glycine to serine, citrulline to arginine, phenylalanine to tyrosine) of amino acids by the kidneys (22). Glutamine balance in ARF is critical in that this amino acid is the primary metabolite for ammonia genesis by the kidney and accounts for >50% of total renal amino acid metabolism. In all critical illness, a great efflux of glutamine from muscle occurs, which provides the amino acid substrate for gluconeogenesis in the liver due to altered substrate utilization (46,59). This shifting away from the kidney and high turnover of glutamine further stresses the kidney's ability to continue its normal function. Glutamine is also used as a substrate for cellular energy by renal tubular cells, immune cells, and gastrointestinal mucosa cells (46). In ARF, plasma glutamine falls and, when any form of renal support (dialysis) is begun, the glutamine efflux increases (43).

It is now well recognized that glutamine becomes a conditionally essential amino acid during critical illness or catabolic stress and that glutamine supplementation limits nitrogen loss (47,64). Altering the standard amino acid composition during ARF or supplementing with arginine have not found clear clinical benefit, although arginine appears to improve the ischemic recovery phase (11). Certainly during acute renal dysfunction the catabolic state must be recognized, and an attempt must be made to adequately support the protein requirements, which are often >2 gm/kg/day (2), in an effort to limit the large nitrogen losses, even if a net positive nitrogen balance cannot be achieved (3).

Providing optimal nonprotein calories is a necessary component of nutrition during any acute illness, and this is especially true of ARF. Multiple studies have shown a maximum rate of glucose utilization in the early phase of critical illness (~4–5 mg/kg/min), and exceeding this rate will only cause additional metabolism, as excess amounts are stored as fat (53,54). Energy needs during acute illness change as the process evolves. Early on in critical illness, alterations in the neuroendocrine axis cause altered carbohydrate metabolism, resulting in hyperglycemia (9). The use of insulin during this insulin-resistant period (glycemic control in the 80–110 mg/dL range) has been shown to improve survival, decrease morbidity, and help to deter the development of renal dysfunction (58).

Overfeeding is detrimental during acute illness, and multiple studies utilizing indirect calorimetry have been conducted to help guide nutritional support by measuring the energy expenditure in children. Estimated patient energy requirements of 0.20–0.26 mJ/kg/day, or 50–60 kcal/kg/day, have been shown to agree within 10%–20% with measured energy expenditure by multiple investigators (6,14). Whenever the clinical course does not appear to match what was estimated to be adequate, obtaining a resting energy expenditure by indirect calorimetry is helpful in objectively assessing nutritional needs.

Lipid metabolism is likewise altered in ARF, with total cholesterol and high-density lipoprotein cholesterol being decreased and low-density lipoprotein being increased. These abnormalities are a result of impaired lipolysis; both hepatic triglyceride lipase and lipoprotein lipase are diminished resulting in a total lipase activity of only ~50% of normal (21). In a study that evaluated whether cholesterol becomes a conditionally essential nutrient during ARF, free cholesterol was added to the 20% lipid emulsions. Improved lipid oxidation, shortened plasma half-life of triglycerides, a reduction in plasma triglyceride levels, and increased total body clearance of triglycerides were demonstrated (20).

Other conditional nutrients might be advantageous during ARF, one of which is biotin. As a cofactor for the carboxylation of pyruvate, acetyl CoA, and propionyl CoA, biotin plays an important role in carbohydrate and lipid metabolism. Recent work in patients with type II diabetes showed that supplementation with 15 mg/day of biotin improved hypertriglyceridemia, and hyperglycemia, and decreased insulin requirements.

Electrolyte disorders due to impaired renal clearance include those of K^+, magnesium, Ca^+, and phosphorus. K^+ is filtered from the glomerulus, and normally all but 10% of it is reabsorbed. Farther along, in the distal tubule, K^+ is primarily secreted. When oliguria develops in ARF, a significant decrease in distal tubular flow occurs, resulting in impaired secretion of K^+. Ca^+ and phosphate metabolism are both altered in ARF by the decrease in GFR, resulting in a decrease filtration of phosphate from the plasma and, therefore, decreased excretion of phosphate. Rising plasma phosphate levels further inhibit the renal production of calcitriol, which then leads to secondary hyperparathyroidism in an attempt to enhance excretion of phosphate and correct the hypocalcemia that is present. All of these electrolytes must be monitored and adjusted daily as part of the nutritional support of acute renal dysfunction.

Dietary vitamins and trace elements are also altered by renal dysfunction. In ARF, plasma levels of water-soluble vitamins are often low due, early on, to a larger volume of distribution associated with fluid overload and, later, from removal by RRT. Additional supplementation of these vitamins is often necessary if the ARF becomes extended. Ascorbic acid is an exception;

the intake recommended for vitamin C is to be no more than 200 mg/day due to the risk of causing oxalosis.

Although renal catabolism of retinol-binding globulin decreases and, over time, vitamin A excess can occur, this rarely is the case in ARF. In fact, vitamin A and vitamin E are often low during ARF. As renal failure extends beyond the acute phase (>4 weeks), adjustment of vitamin A to prevent accumulation may be necessary. Vitamin K seems to be stable during ARF. Vitamin D activation in the kidney is severely depressed in ARF; therefore, supplementation is required as the active form—calcitriol. Likewise, it may be necessary to adjust trace minerals during ARF. Selenium concentrations are often low in critically ill patients, and this is also seen in ARF. Additional supplementation with selenium has been found to reduce the severity of ARF (44). Another trace element that may need adjustment in ARF is chromium, as it tends to be elevated in uremia. As trace elements tend to be highly protein bound, supplementation with them will not be eliminated by dialytic therapies; therefore, supplementation with trace elements should be accompanied by caution for potential accumulation.

Specific Diseases That Lead to or Present with Acute Renal Failure

ARF has many causes; however, a few are especially common in children and are frequently seen in the PICU.

Glomerulonephritis

The glomerulonephritides are a group of diseases characterized by an immune-mediated injury to the glomerulus. Usually, this injury is in the form of immune complex formation and deposition within the glomerulus with subsequent inflammation. Poststreptococcal GN, Henoch-Schönlein purpura nephritis, and lupus nephritis are examples. Alternatively, antibody production may be directed against the glomerular basement membrane (as in Goodpasture syndrome), or immune complexes may not be discernible (Wegener granulomatosis). GN can lead to ARF, or it can follow a more indolent course and lead to chronic renal insufficiency and ESRD. Any GN, regardless of cause, is characterized by hematuria and proteinuria, which is often accompanied by oliguria, hypertension, and fluid overload. Depending on the underlying pathology, pulmonary edema or pulmonary hemorrhage may also be present in critically ill patients. Though somewhat less common, hypertensive encephalopathy can occur in these patients. This discussion will focus only on the more common causes of acute GN seen in pediatric patients.

Postinfectious Glomerulonephritis. Postinfectious GN is the most common cause of GN in children and can follow a previous illness. These children usually present with symptoms of GN ~7–21 days following the initial insult. The most common cause of postinfectious GN is due to group A β-hemolytic streptococci. Less common causes include atypical mycobacteria, mycoplasma, staphylococci, and viruses. The urine is often described as smoky or cola-colored. Nephrotic range proteinuria is rare, and 90% of patients have depressed C3 levels. The diagnosis is usually made clinically without need for biopsy. Treatment is primarily supportive, with fluid and salt restriction and diuresis as needed. Antihypertensive medications are frequently required to control blood pressure. Prognosis is very good and <1% of cases progress to renal failure.

Henoch-Schönlein Nephritis. Henoch-Schönlein nephritis is a vasculitic process characterized by a purpuric rash mostly on the lower extremities and buttock, abdominal pain, and arthritis. Peak age of onset is 4–6 years and the renal pathology manifests within a month of diagnosis. Renal biopsy shows crescent formation with mesangial IgA deposition. The pathology is very similar in appearance to IgA nephropathy. Approximately 30% of patients with Henoch-Schönlein purpura with renal pathology present with acute nephritic syndrome, which consists of hematuria and two out of three of the following: hypertension, oliguric renal failure, or nephrotic syndrome. Over 80% of children without acute nephritic syndrome will have normal long-term renal function, versus 56% of those with the syndrome. Treatment includes corticosteroids and other immunosuppressive agents. Angiotensin-converting enzyme (ACE) inhibitors and angiotensin receptor blockers may also be useful (49).

Systemic Lupus Erythematosus. Rare in the first decade of life, SLE is more often seen in teenagers in the pediatric age group, with a 5–10:1 ratio of female to male. Renal disease occurs in as many as 82% of affected individuals, is a major cause of morbidity and, without control, can progress to ESRD. Serology showing markedly decreased C3 and C4 in a patient with GN is highly suggestive of lupus nephritis. Treatment includes corticosteroids and other immunosuppressive agents, such as cyclophosphamide, azathioprine, or mycophenolate mofetil, as well as control of hypertension and management of fluid overload.

Hemolytic Uremic Syndrome

HUS is the most common cause of intrinsic ARF in children worldwide. The syndrome is manifest by microangiopathic hemolytic anemia, thrombocytopenia, and acute, usually oliguric, renal failure. HUS in children most commonly follows a diarrheal prodrome often due to toxin-producing *Escherichia coli*, but it can be associated with other bacterial pathogens, bone marrow transplant, SLE, hereditary factor H deficiency, or certain drugs. An atypical form also exists that is uncommon in children, has no clear etiology, and tends to have a relapsing course with a worse long-term prognosis than postinfectious HUS. The following discussion will concentrate on the diarrheal form, which is by far the most common, accounting for more than 90% of cases in children. The incidence is ~2.1/100,000 children/year, with a peak age of onset of <5 years. In North America, the most common cause is the verotoxin-producing strain of *E. coli* 0157:H7. Other pathogenic strains are more common in other areas of the world. The illness typically starts as hemorrhagic colitis that precedes HUS by several days. Only ~5%–8% of children with toxin-associated colitis will develop HUS. The toxin is essentially the same as Shiga toxin (*Shigella dysenteriae* serotype 1). Several subtypes of the toxin have been characterized, and the Stx-2 form seems to carry the highest risk for progression to HUS. The Shiga toxin (verotoxin) inhibits protein synthesis and binds to the glycolipid Gb3 on renal tubular cells and the vascular endothelium of the kidney and other organs. Gb3 expression in the kidney may be greater in infants than in adults and may help to explain the increased susceptibility of young

children to the development of HUS. Renal histology shows the characteristic capillary endothelial swelling and intravascular platelet thrombi of the microangiopathic process. Aside from the gut and kidney, other organ systems can be affected. Neurologic involvement occurs in 20%–30% of patients and manifests as seizures, altered mental status, or cerebral infarction. Pancreatic insufficiency can develop, and cardiomyopathy also occurs.

HUS can also be seen with neuraminidase-producing organisms. Although an uncommon occurrence, when seen, it is usually associated with *Streptococcus pneumoniae* infections. The neuraminidase cleaves sialic acid on cell membranes, exposing the Thomsen-Friedenreich antigen on platelets, red cells, and vascular endothelium. This form of HUS is usually quite severe and often associated with neurologic involvement.

The management of HUS consists of control of fluid overload and hypertension, which is common, and nutritional support and dialysis if uremia or fluid and electrolyte abnormalities cannot be controlled with more conservative measures. Red cell transfusions may be necessary for symptomatic anemia. Platelet transfusion may promote the pathologic process and should be reserved for procedures associated with significant bleeding risk or for profound thrombocytopenia. Corticosteroids, prostacyclin, anticoagulants, and thrombolytics have not been shown to be helpful. Plasmapheresis is usually unnecessary in the diarrheal form of HUS but may be helpful in the nondiarrheal (atypical) form of HUS, HUS following bone marrow transplant, or the adult counterpart of HUS, namely, thrombotic thrombocytopenic purpura.

Prognosis is generally good in the short term, with a mortality of 3%–5% and an additional 5% needing prolonged dialysis. However, as many as 30%–50% of patients will later be found to have hypertension or some degree of renal dysfunction. In long-term follow-up studies, 10%–15% of patients progress to ESRD; therefore, extended outpatient follow-up is advisable, even if resolution of the acute process seems complete (51).

Contrast Medium-induced Nephropathy

An estimated 60 million doses of radiologic contrast medium are given annually (48). Contrast medium-induced nephropathy (CIN) has been reported to account for 12% of ARF in hospitalized patients. Over the years, radiographic contrast has evolved from high-osmolar compounds (2000 mOsm/L), to low-osmolar compounds (600–900 mOsm/L), to the current nonionic iso-osmolar dimers. Although the incidence of CIN has fallen with newer contrast formulations, it continues to be a significant concern. CIN is defined as a 25% rise in creatinine 48–72 hrs following contrast that has no alternative explanation. Renal function usually returns to baseline within 2 weeks of the insult. Although the incidence is low in normal individuals, it is much higher in patients with preexisting renal insufficiency, dehydration, or diabetes mellitus. The mechanism of injury is probably multifactorial and relates to the viscosity of the contrast agent, its effect on renal perfusion and GFR, and predisposing host factors. Contrast agents exacerbate the relative hypoxic environment that normally exists in the outer medullary region of the kidney, probably an effect of the viscosity of the contrast increasing resistance to blood flow in the vasa rectae, as well as contrast-induced renal vasoconstriction. Increased viscosity in the tubular lumen may increase intraluminal pressure and, therefore, decrease GFR.

In addition, reactive oxygen species are produced in response to reperfusion oxidative stress, causing further tubular injury. The vasoconstriction and free radical production may be particularly prominent in diabetic nephropathy, where endothelial function is already impaired.

The treatment of CIN should focus on prevention and is threefold. First, predisposing host risk factors for CIN must be recognized. For patients at risk, the clinician should determine if the desired information can be acquired by an alternate method of imaging that does not require iodinated contrast. Nonionic iso-osmolar contrast should be used in the minimum volume necessary to achieve a quality study. Hydration is the only therapeutic intervention proven to minimize the risk of developing CIN (48). Many regimens have been suggested, but data are insufficient to determine which is best. As a general guideline, hydration with IV isotonic saline beginning 6–12 hrs prior to contrast injection at 1 mL/kg/hr and continued for 4–12 hrs after the study can be used. Some studies have advocated the use of sodium bicarbonate-containing fluids as superior to saline, but data are insufficient to recommend this solution above isotonic saline alone. N-acetylcysteine has been promoted as a preventative agent for its antioxidant properties, but it is not clear from currently available data that using N-acetylcysteine with IV hydration is superior to hydration alone. It may be that N-acetylcysteine has a place in prevention of CIN when emergent imaging is necessary, precluding preprocedure hydration; however, further study is necessary. Agents such as mannitol, fenoldopam, furosemide, and dopamine have not been shown to reduce the risk of CIN. Prophylactic hemofiltration has been used and may be effective, but it is invasive and, for most patients, the risk outweighs the benefits.

Acute Renal Failure Secondary to Rhabdomyolysis

Rhabdomyolysis is responsible for ~5%–7% of all cases of ARF in the US. The causes are numerous, including trauma, hyperosmolar diabetic coma, drugs, malignant hyperthermia, infection, certain inherited metabolic disorders, and autoimmune diseases such as polymyositis (32). Rhabdomyolysis results from myocyte injury that causes a rapid influx of Ca^+, Na^+, and fluid into the cytoplasm. Myoglobin, K^+, phosphate, and lactate are released to the extracellular fluid space, resulting in hypocalcemia, hyperkalemia, and acidosis. Approximately one-third of individuals with rhabdomyolysis will develop ARF. Three mechanisms are involved with the development of renal failure in rhabdomyolysis. The first is decreased renal perfusion from intravascular volume depletion that occurs due to movement of fluid into damaged muscle tissue. Renal vasoconstriction due to increased platelet activating factor and endothelin-1 production exacerbates the renal ischemia. The second mechanism of renal injury is tubular obstruction. Myoglobin is a 17,800-dalton molecule that is freely filtered by the kidney. In the renal tubule, myoglobin increases in concentration because it cannot be reabsorbed. The myoglobin reacts with Tamm-Horsfall protein and precipitates forming casts, which can obstruct the tubules. The cast formation is enhanced by an acidic pH and can be inhibited by alkalinization of the urine with sodium bicarbonate. The third mechanism of injury is the direct toxic effect of myoglobin on the kidney, and this is probably the major cause of renal failure in rhabdomyolysis. Myoglobin breaks down into protein and a heme-iron moiety under acidic conditions. The iron catalyzes free radical formation that, in turn, leads to lipid peroxidation of the tubular cells. Myoglobin itself may be able to catalyze lipid peroxidation by redox cycling between oxidation states. Both of these processes are attenuated in an alkaline environment.

The diagnosis of rhabdomyolysis requires a high index of clinical suspicion and is supported by high serum creatine kinase (CK) levels and dark, tea-colored urine that tests heme positive without evidence of red blood cells. Although a urine myoglobin level may be helpful, it is often not readily available, and the diagnosis and treatment should not be delayed while awaiting the result.

The treatment of rhabdomyolysis first involves prevention of ARF. Patients with CK levels of >20,000 ng/mL are likely to be at greatest risk of developing ARF. Vigorous hydration with IV fluids to maintain intravascular volume and urine output is the mainstay of therapy. Bicarbonate-containing fluids, although not shown to be superior to saline alone, theoretically offer the advantage of decreasing systemic acidosis and facilitating urine alkalinization. Using these fluids will help to treat hyperkalemia that may be present, discourage myoglobin cast formation, and inhibit free radical formation and lipid peroxidation. Using mannitol as an osmotic diuretic with IV hydration may be a helpful adjunct therapy but has not been proven to be superior to hydration alone (32). Compartment syndrome may develop from muscle injury and additional tissue swelling due to hydration; the intensivist must be wary of this, and monitoring of compartment pressures may become necessary. The primary causes of early mortality in rhabdomyolysis are hyperkalemia and hypovolemia. Intractable hyperkalemia and acidosis unresponsive to hydration and alkalinization requires RRT. Most survivors will recover normal renal function within 3 months of the acute insult.

Tumor Lysis Syndrome

Although an important cause of ARF in the PICU, tumor lysis syndrome is covered in detail in Chapter 100.

END-STAGE RENAL DISEASE IN THE PICU

In contrast to the patient with ARF who is admitted to the PICU, the patient with ESRD who requires critical care poses a different level of complexity. Patients with ESRD, by definition, are those who either have irreversible renal failure that requires chronic dialysis or are going on to kidney transplantation. ESRD patients warrant admission to the PICU in three different situations: (a) the patient who has progressive loss of renal function and is admitted to the PICU either for stabilization of electrolytes prior to placement of a chronic dialysis catheter or because of concerns for potential complications during the initial dialysis therapy with new-onset ESRD, (b) the patient who already carries the diagnosis of ESRD and has complications related to the dialysis access or has sepsis, or (c) the patient with ESRD who has just undergone a kidney transplant.

New-onset End-stage Renal Disease

The causes of ESRD in the pediatric patient are often quite different than in the adult. Ninety percent of adults develop ESRD secondary to glomerular renal disease, whereas 70%–80% of children develop ESRD related to tubular interstitial renal disease. Glomerular-based renal disease is associated with fluid retention, hypertension, and blood and protein in the urine (25). Therefore, the patient will often seek medical care because of overt clinical symptoms. Tubular interstitial renal disease is often associated with polyuria and polydipsia. Classically, these children have a history of recurrent dehydration, for they have no ability to concentrate their urine. Therefore, at the time of progressive loss of kidney function or at the time of intercurrent illness (i.e., vomiting, diarrhea), new-onset ESRD may be discovered. The peak times for onset of ESRD in children are in the first 5 years of life and at puberty, corresponding with the peak times of rapid growth (25).

Tubular interstitial disease is a silent yet progressive loss of kidney function. It is not unusual for patients to present first with signs and symptoms of tiredness, yet have no previous overt symptoms of renal failure. Their only symptom over time may be a loss of growth parameters that may or may not be noticed. It is not at all uncommon for these patients to present with volume depletion, hyperosmolality secondary to elevated BUN, hypernatremia, and other complications of ESRD, including Ca^+/phosphorous imbalance and anemia. Patients with uremia and hypernatremia present a very unique problem in terms of hyperosmolality. Osmolality can be calculated as

$$Osms = 2 \times Na + (BUN/2.8) + (glucose/18)$$

In a dialysis setting, the osmolality of a dialysate bath is roughly 280 mOsm. Therefore, in patients with osmolality ≥350 mOsm, if aggressive dialysis (such as with hemodialysis) is begun, a rapid osmolar shift could occur, which may result in seizures, referred to *dialysis disequilibrium*. Therefore, improving hydration status and electrolyte imbalance prior to dialysis will lower BUN, Na^+, and, consequently, osmolality, which will often make the first dialysis less problematic. Any form of dialysis can be used: hemodialysis (less aggressive), peritoneal dialysis, or hemofiltration in order to attain a slow improvement of osmolality with less risk of dialysis disequilibrium. Recent work by our group demonstrates the preferential use of hemofiltration to avoid complications due to hyperosmolality (8).

As with other forms of ESRD, patients often will have a combination of hypocalcemia and hyperphosphatemia due to secondary hyperparathyroidism. They also present with anemia secondary to loss of their natural erythropoiesis compounded by iron deficiency. Hyperphosphatemia is often unrecognized in children because, in 1997, the US government assigned panels of lab work throughout the US that excluded the phosphorous analysis from a routine analysis. Therefore, unless phosphorous analysis is specifically requested, hyperphosphatemia will not be recognized at the onset.

Low Ca^+ is often seen in the absence of hypomagnesemia or hypoalbuminemia. In this setting, typically the therapy, if hyperphosphatemia coexists, is to reduce phosphate by use of phosphate binders, phosphorous restriction, or dialysis. Of these, dialysis is least efficient. Phosphate binders prior to 1984 were aluminum based, but because of risk of dementia as well as bone disease, these are no longer recommended for use. During the late 1990s, calcium carbonate was the preferred phosphorous binder, but it has since been found to cause Ca^+ deposition later in life (29). Therefore, a newer generation of phosphate binders, including sevelamer (rINN), is the current therapeutic choice. Phosphate binders are used at the end of meals to bind the phosphate load during the time of dietary intake. Ca^+ stores are improved with Ca^+ supplementation and vitamin D. Vitamin D can be given orally as 25-hydroxy D3 or 1,25-dihydroxy D3, or it can be given IV as 1,25-dihyroxy D3. The regulation of Ca^+ and phosphorous is done slowly over time to minimize the risk of seizures and to prevent ongoing metabolic bone disease.

The anemia of ESRD is twofold. The target level of hemoglobin in ESRD is 12–13 g/dL. Classically, these patients are iron deficient and lack natural erythropoiesis. Iron can be supplemented either orally or intravenously. The standard of care that has been adopted throughout nephrology programs is to use IV iron. The newer forms of IV iron are safe, with a very low incidence of systemic side effects. In combination with short-acting erythropoietics (erythropoietin) or long-acting erythropoietics [darbepoetin alfa (rINN)], IV iron can improve the hemoglobin levels in these patients. Erythropoietin products will not work effectively in the face of inflammation, such as infection or severe secondary hyperparathyroidism.

Avoidance of blood transfusion is considered the standard of care with ESRD. Data suggest that the use of blood transfusions has a negative impact upon future renal transplants (10). If transfusion becomes necessary, the standard of care at many institutions is to leukoreduce the transfused blood by using either leuko-poor cells or frozen diglyceride cells. This approach is not universally accepted and does not offer 100% protection against forming antibodies.

End-stage Renal Disease with Acute Illness

The second group of patients with ESRD who may require admission to the ICU includes those on established hemodialysis or peritoneal dialysis therapy. Classically, the patients would be admitted secondary to either a hypertensive crisis or overwhelming infection. In patients with ESRD, the primary cause of hypertension is fluid retention, and one of the causes of fluid retention in ESRD is overestimation of dry weight in malnourished patients. In this case, very aggressive dialysis to achieve the true dry weight and eliminate volume overload will result in improved blood pressure control. A vast number of antihypertensives is available. Certain antihypertensives may cause hyperkalemia (ACEs, adrenergic receptor binders, β-blockers); therefore, in situations that are risky for hyperkalemia, these should be avoided. Further, certain medications, such as sodium nitroprusside, are contraindicated in ESRD due to poor renal clearance and the potential for thiocyanate toxicity. Ca^+-channel blockers, either orally or intravenously, offer a safe method of blood pressure control with minimal side effects.

Infectious complications are not infrequent in the ESRD population and may require care in the ICU. In hemodialysis patients, infectious complications are usually related to vascular access. Access in the majority of children is an external double-lumen venous access, despite very clear data that an arteriovenous fistula offers better dialysis and fewer complications (29). External access accounts for one or two bouts of systemic sepsis per year in patients. The vast majority of these patients can be treated as outpatients or, at worst, as inpatients on the regular pediatric ward. In patients with severe sepsis that is unrelenting, removal of the vascular access may be in order; however, removal must be balanced against the ongoing need for vascular access necessary for ESRD therapy. Typically, gram-positive bacteria account for 60%–80% of all venous access infections. Therefore, broad-spectrum antibiotics such as vancomycin and aminoglycosides should be used in ESRD patients. The advantage of using these medications is that a single dose can be given initially, with subsequent doses based on dialysis clearance. In patients on peritoneal dialysis, peritonitis can account for worsening illness and transfer to the ICU. Approximately 65%–70% of peritonitis is due to gram-positive bacteria. These cases can typically be treated with intraperitoneal instillment of antibiotics and show rapid improvement. Occasionally, patients with many exposures to antibiotics may develop fungal peritonitis. The risk of fungal peritonitis is particularly high in patients who are malnourished, and morbidity and mortality are high. The therapy of choice for fungal peritonitis is removal of the peritoneal dialysis catheter, treatment with antifungal medications, and converting the patient to hemodialysis.

The third cause of admission to the ICU for ESRD patients is related to malnutrition. Morbidity and mortality in patients with ESRD are often related to the patient's nutritional state. An adult with an albumin of <2.5 has a 100% mortality rate within 5 years. Although data are limited, the rate is thought to be similar in the pediatric population (10). Patients with ESRD may become malnourished as a result of numerous causes. Malnutrition is often related to the anorexia of chronic illness, certain food restrictions by the medical service, and lack of taste sensation by the patient. The malnutrition may be exacerbated in patients on peritoneal dialysis who are typically in negative nitrogen balance because of protein losses across the peritoneal membrane. The typical patient on peritoneal dialysis may lose 0.5–1 g/kg/day of protein. It is not unusual for these patients to have albumin levels of <3 g/dL secondary to negative nitrogen balance, resulting in severe protein malnutrition, which constitutes a medical emergency and requires either transpyloric feedings or, less preferably, total parenteral nutrition. The advantage of enteral feeding is the number of excellent formulas that can be used in the pediatric ESRD. These include infant formulas such as Similac PM 60/40 (Ross, Abbott Park, IL) and, for older children, Suplena (Ross, Abbott Park, IL), Renalcal® (Nestle Nutrition, Glendale, CA), Nepro® (Ross Abbott Park, IL), or Nutren® Renal (Nestle Nutrition, Glendale, CA). In patients with severe electrolyte disturbances who cannot be dialyzed but require ongoing nutritional support, formulas such as Renalcal® can be used. Renalcal® is a very unique formula that has a 2-cal/mL concentration, 8 g of protein per 240 mL, yet has no electrolytes. This formula may be used for the short term in patients, but its long-term use should be avoided. In other ESRD patients, Suplena (8 g of protein in 8 oz) or Nepro® (16 g of protein in 8 oz) can offer high calories and varying amounts of protein, with minimal volume. In the setting of the malnourished ESRD patient on phosphate binders, the clinician should very wary of the potential for refeeding syndrome with low-phosphate formulas. It is not unusual that these patients will present with normal-to-high phosphorus levels, and once adequate nutrition is established, the phosphorous will plummet. Monitoring the phosphorous level routinely in this patient population is an essential component of management.

Outcome of End-stage Renal Disease

The mortality risk for children with ESRD varies by age and treatment modality. One-year mortality rates for children <2 years old on dialysis are 7%–40%, depending on comorbidities, and 3%–7% for older children and adolescents. The mortality rate drops to <5% posttransplant. Therefore, any child who requires chronic dialysis should be considered for renal transplantation.

Transplantation in End-stage Renal Disease

The ultimate goal for all ESRD patients is renal transplantation. Kidneys can be obtained from living or deceased donors. In the era of the newer generation of immunosuppressive agents, data have shown that both types of transplants are very successful. Living donors are preferred over cadaver donors because of ready availability and convenience, but they offer little advantage in terms of long-term graft survival (39).

Preoperative Care of End-stage Renal Disease

The preoperative patient must be carefully managed in the 24 hrs prior to transplantation. Some patients with ESRD are still polyuric, and other patients are anuric. It is important to optimize the volume status of all patients so that they are euvolemic or hypervolemic at the time of surgery. If these patients are on dialysis, the nephrologist must ensure that they are dialyzed preprocedure for solute clearance, avoiding hypovolemia from excessive fluid removal. Careful attention to the patient's volume status in the preoperative period will help avoid hypotension during anesthesia. Optimum hemodynamic status at the time of anastomosis of the transplanted kidney is essential to good graft perfusion. The typical blood volume of a transplanted kidney is ~250 mL. In a child who weights ≥40 kg, this volume is insignificant. In a 10-kg child, whose intravascular blood volume is roughly 1400 mL, shifting 250 mL of blood into the kidney is significant and can result in under perfusion if the child is not adequately volume expanded before allograft perfusion.

Intraoperative Care of End-stage Renal Disease

A patient who is hypovolemic at the time of transplantation will experience hypotension and have suboptimal allograft perfusion. It is imperative that the anesthesiologist, the transplant physician, and the transplant surgeon have a high level of communication during and after the case. Many programs would prefer a postoperative patient to be intubated and hypervolemic after transplant, as opposed to extubated and dehydrated. Whereas the latter approach may appear to facilitate postoperative pulmonary management, it may also result in poor allograft perfusion and potentially adversely affect graft survival.

Urine output in the first 1–2 hrs after the transplant can be reflective of allograft function but can be reflective of native urine output. Therefore, a patient who produces a liter of urine per day from the native kidney (40 mL/hr) pretransplant and 200–300 mL/hr posttransplant shows evidence of immediate allograft function.

In the face of no urine output or low urine output, urgent assessment of the cause is essential. The most important determination to be made is whether blood flow is reaching the kidney, which can be evaluated either by Doppler flow ultrasound or a nuclear medicine renal blood flow study. The advantage of the Doppler flow study is that it can be performed immediately at bedside. Many transplant physicians now perform their own Doppler ultrasounds to make rapid assessments. Ultrasonography can assess for both vascular flow to the kidney and the presence of fluid around the kidney. Furthermore, an ultrasound allows for bladder evaluation. If the bladder is full, the Foley catheter is blocked. Foley patency is often an issue after kidney transplant because the urine is usually bloody. Gently flushing the Foley with 20–30 mL of either sterile saline or sterile water will maintain patency and may be necessary every 1–2 hrs until consistent urine flow is achieved. If the catheter cannot be cleared, it must be replaced. If the bladder is empty, it must be determined if blood flow to the kidney is compromised or if urine is leaking outside the bladder or the kidney.

Urine Leak

Urinary leak is a rare complication, usually related to a ureter slipping out of the anastomosis to the bladder or related to distal ureter necrosis. It may be associated with abdominal pain, fevers, or decreased urine output, and increasing ascites. A simultaneous analysis of urinary creatinine, plasma creatinine, and the perinephric fluid for creatinine will help to discriminate the source of the fluid. If the perinephric fluid's creatinine is closer to that of plasma, it is not a urine leak. If the perinephric fluid's creatinine is closer to that of urine, then most likely it is urinary leak. Urinary leaks must be immediately fixed surgically, and prolonged Foley drainage maintained.

Fluid Management

Fluid management in the immediate postoperative period is crucial and has three components. The first is maintenance IV fluids, typically D5/0.45% normal saline with or without sodium bicarbonate and with or without K^+, based on the patient's needs. The second is urine replacement with 0.45% normal saline without dextrose. Many programs would use one-to-one urine output replacement for the first 6 hrs to maintain euvolemia. Thus, if the patient makes 400 mL of urine in 1 hr, in the next hour, the patient should receive 400 mL of 0.45% normal saline above their maintenance fluid requirement. The final component would be any sort of bolus fluid, whether normal saline, Ringer's lactate, or 5% albumin used to optimize preload. In the face of a low CVP and low urine output, it is imperative to improve the CVP and establish adequate urine output. Conversely, a low CVP and good urine output is reassuring that the transplanted kidney is doing well. High CVP with poor urine output warrants diuretic therapy. Finally, if CVP is high and urine output is good, reducing the replacement fluid is in order. This component of fluid management will result in a net positive fluid balance in the patient in the first 24-hr postoperative period.

Typically, 36 hrs after surgery, extravascular volume will recirculate into the intravascular space. If the patient is making good urine, spontaneous diuresis will occur. If, however, the patient is oliguric or anuric, development of pulmonary edema and hypertension should be considered. Hypertension in this setting can best be treated with antihypertensives and either (a) with diuretics if the patient is making urine, or (b) dialysis if the patient is anuric. Ca^+-channel blockers are the preferred drugs of choice in transplant patients because of the renal pro-

tective mechanisms they offer in the face of the patient being on calcineurin inhibitors (tacrolimus, cyclosporin, sirolimus) (26).

Immunosuppressive Agents

T-cell induction is used at many programs immediately after transplant. T-cell induction agents, such as antithymocyte globulin, lymphocyte immune globulin, basiliximab, and daclizumab, as well as other agents, can be used at the time of induction. These drugs have a very low risk of causing anaphylaxis. The polyclonal agents (e.g., antithymocyte globulin, lymphocyte immune globulin) should be infused through a central venous catheter in order to avoid peripheral vessel irritation. Other drugs (e.g., basiliximab and daclizumab) can easily be administered by either central or peripheral venous access.

Other immunosuppressive regimens often employ a combination of steroids (prednisone or methylprednisolone), calcineurin inhibitors (tacrolimus or cyclosporin), an antiproliferative agent (mycophenolate or azathioprine), and, in some cases, sirolimus as an alternative to either the calcineurin inhibitors or to the antiproliferative agent. The side effects of these drugs are primarily related to fluid retention and hypertension (steroids and calcineurin agents) and hyperkalemia (calcineurin inhibitor agents). Other preventative therapies are often used in the posttransplant period. These include the use of trimethoprim sulfa for both *Pneumocystis carinii* pneumonia and urinary tract prophylaxis, antifungal agents, and antiviral agents, depending on the patient's cytomegalovirus (CMV) or Epstein-Barr virus (EPV).

Patients who are CMV- or EPV-naïve and receive a CMV- or EBV-positive kidney may be at risk for infection from these viruses. The peak time of onset of CMV or EBV disease is roughly 8–12 weeks after transplant. Therefore, prophylactic antivirals are used for the first 3 months posttransplant. Some programs will also use immunoglobulin products such as CMV immune globulin IV for additional antiviral protection. Antifungal prophylaxis is often used, which would typically include nystatin swish and swallow. Many of the newer-generation antifungals interfere with calcineurin-inhibitor kinetics and may cause calcineurin-inhibitor toxicity. Therefore, it is imperative to understand all of the drug interactions that may occur.

Fever in the Immediate Posttransplant Period

Evaluation of fever in the patient who is 0–7 days posttransplant includes assessment in three areas: (a) exclusion of atelectasis or other pulmonary pathology is necessary, but may not be the only cause; (b) evaluation for urinary tract infection; and (c) assessment of the wound. In the first week after transplant, fever is often related to bacterial infection. Fungal and viral infections typically occur later (6 and 12 weeks posttransplant, respectively) (63).

Rejection

Rejection is a very rare event in the immediate posttransplant period. In the last 20 years, advancements in immunologic crossmatch prior to transplantation and advancements in immunosuppressive agents have made acute rejection quite rare. Acute rejection can either be humoral- or T-cell-mediated. Humoral or T-cell rejection can be treated with the use of polyclonal agents, plasmapheresis, or an increase in the total amount of immunosuppression. Rejection that occurs in the first week after transplant has a very profound negative impact upon long-term allograft function.

In the face of concerns about rejection, the clinician should look for unrecognized antibodies in the serum of the patient by repetitive crossmatch between the donor and recipient and by looking at an allograft renal biopsy for histologic changes. The use of noninvasive therapies such as ultrasound or scan is not diagnostic and may lead to either over- or undertreatment with immunosuppression. Biopsy of the kidney in the first weeks posttransplant is very safe in the hands of a skilled transplant physician. The procedure can be performed easily at bedside with very low morbidity, and with a high yield for identifying the cause of allograft dysfunction.

CONCLUSIONS AND FUTURE DIRECTIONS

Acute and chronic renal failure is commonly found in PICU patients. ARF in the PICU population is often secondary to the underlying disease process, and patient outcome is, therefore, related more to the primary disease than to ARF itself. Aggressive therapy of prerenal insufficiency, proper supportive care of the patient, and conscious avoidance or minimization of therapies that would exacerbate ARF are the mainstays of treatment. Patients with ESRD in the PICU are complex and require careful, collaborative management by the nephrology and critical care services. The outcome of these patients ultimately depends on the ability to see them through to successful renal transplantation.

Looking to the future, three areas are ripe for further exploration. Specifically, these are early detection of renal failure, renal preservation therapy, and an expanded role for RRT in the PICU. More sensitive laboratory methods (i.e., micro albumin in urine, cystatin C levels, etc.) of detecting renal injury early in its course are needed. Identification of patients who are genetically predisposed to renal failure and the ability to tailor therapy for these patients would offer a huge advantage to early recognition and treatment of ARF. Severity-of-illness scoring systems that are better suited to assessing risk of mortality in renal disease are also needed.

Pharmacologic means of renal protection or preservation have been disappointing to date. Dopamine and other pressors (with the possible exception of norepinephrine), fenoldopam, and nesiritide have all proven ineffective as renal-protective agents. The pathophysiology of ARF is analogous to that seen in sepsis and ischemia-reperfusion injury elsewhere. It is likely that therapies developed to attenuate the consequences of the processes will benefit ARF patients as well.

Finally, data suggest that early intervention with RRT in septic or fluid-overloaded ICU patients may improve outcome. Further studies, to better define which modality, which patients, and at what point in the disease process RRT is appropriate are needed, and they must be multicentered studies, as it is unlikely that single-centered studies will have the patient numbers to be adequately powered for meaningful conclusions. Groups such as the pediatric prospective continuous RRT (ppCRRT) registry can serve as a model for the type of multi-institutional collaboration necessary to successfully address these and other questions.

KEY POINTS

- ARF is an abrupt decrease in GFR of at least 50% from baseline with a corresponding 50% or greater increase in serum creatinine. Not uncommon in the PICU population, ARF carries a mortality of up to 25%–40% in these children.

- The etiology if ARF can be categorized as pre-, intra-, or postrenal. Worldwide, the most common cause is HUS. Much of the ARF in the PICU is a comorbidity of the underlying disease, and outcome depends on successful treatment of the inciting illness more than on ARF itself.

- The evaluation of ARF includes a good history and physical, urinalysis, FE_{Na}, and renal ultrasound. Although serologic tests and 24-hr urine collection may be useful in diagnosing intrinsic renal disease, renal biopsy for histology offers the fastest means of diagnosis and is relatively safe in experienced hands.

- Adjusting the dosage of renally cleared drugs for changing CrCl is essential in ARF. Aminoglycoside kinetics correlate well with other estimates of GFR and can be used to estimate CrCl in patients receiving these medications.

- ARF is a highly catabolic state and protein losses are exacerbated by RRT. Protein requirements can exceed 2 g/kg/day, and total caloric needs are ~50–60 kcal/kg/day. Careful attention to electrolyte balance and to vitamin and trace metal supplementation is necessary for patients with ARF and patients with ESRD.

- HUS, the most common cause of ARF in children, usually has a diarrheal prodrome. Many organ systems can be affected by the microangiopathy, and as many as 20%–30% of children will have neurologic involvement. Long-term follow-up is essential, as some patients develop late hypertension and a few develop ESRD.

- ESRD can be glomerular or tubular interstitial in origin. The former presents with fluid overload and hypertension; the latter may be silent and present much later.

- Anemia is common in ESRD due to iron deficiency and impaired erythropoiesis. Iron supplementation and erythropoietin administration are used to manage anemia. Transfusion should be avoided, if possible, as it can negatively impact future transplantation.

- Proper management of the posttransplant patient requires good communication between the critical care and nephrology services. Aggressive hydration is necessary to establish and maintain good graft perfusion. Low urine output posttransplant requires emergent assessment of the problem. Ultrasound is useful in distinguishing between renal vascular compromise, bladder obstruction, and urinary leak.

References

1. Bellomo R, Chapman M, Finfer S, et al. Low-dose dopamine in patients with early renal dysfunction: A placebo-controlled randomized trial. Australian and New Zealand Intensive Care Society (ANZICS) Clinical Trials Group. *Lancet* 2000;356:2139–43.
2. Bellomo R, Seacombe J, Daskalakis M, et al. A prospective comparative study of moderate versus high protein intake for critically ill patients with acute renal failure. *Ren Fail* 1997;19:111–20.
3. Bellomo R, Tan HK, Bhonagiri S, et al. High protein intake during continuous hemodiafiltration: Impact on amino acids and nitrogen balance. *Int J Artif Organs* 2002;25:261–8.

4. Blakey S. Dosing concepts in renal dysfunction. In: Murphy JE, ed. *Clinical Pharmacokinetics, 2nd ed.* Bethesda, MD: American Journal of Health-System Pharmacy; 2001:510–3.

5. Bonventre JV, Weinberg JM. Recent advances in the pathophysiology of ischemic acute renal failure. *J Am Soc Nephrol* 2003;14:2199–210.

6. Briassoulis G, Venkataraman S, Thompson AE. Energy expenditure in critically ill children. *Crit Care Med* 2000;28:1166–72.

7. Bueva A, Guighard JP. Renal function in preterm neonates. *Pediatr Res* 1994;36:572–7.

8. Bunchman TE, Hackbarth RM, Maxvold NJ, et al. Prevention of dialysis disequilibrium by use of CVVH. *Int J Artif Organs* 2007; in press.

9. Callahan LA, Supinski GS. Down regulation of diaphragm electron transport chain and glycolytic enzyme gene expression is sepsis. *J Appl Physiol* 2005;99:1120–6.

10. Chavers BM, Sullivan EK, Tejani A, Harmon WE. Pre-transplant blood transfusion and renal allograft outcome: A report of the North American Pediatric Renal Transplant Cooperative Study. *Pediatr Transplant* 1997;1:22–8.

11. Cherla G, Jaimes EA. Role of L-arginine in the pathogenesis and treatment of renal disease. *J Nutr* 2004;134:2801S–6S.

12. Chernow B, ed. *The Pharmacologic Approach to the Critically Ill Patient, 3rd ed.* Baltimore, MD: Williams and Wilkins; 1994:56–74.

13. Chevalier RL. Developmental renal physiology of the low birth weight preterm newborn. *J Urol* 1996;156(2 pt 2):714–9.

14. Coss-Bu JA, Klish WJ, Walding D, et al. Energy metabolism, nitrogen balance and substrate utilization in critically ill children. *Am J Clin Nutr* 2001;74:664–9.

15. De Vriese AS. Prevention and treatment of acute renal failure in sepsis. *J Am Soc Nephrol* 2003;14:792–805.

16. Dettli L. Drug dosage in renal disease. *Clin Pharmacokinet* 1976;1:126–34.

17. DiGiantomasso D, May CN, Bellomo R. Norepinephrine and vital organ blood flow during experimental hyperdynamic sepsis. *Intensive Care Med* 2003;29:1774–81.

18. DiGiantomasso D, Morimatsu H, Bellomo R, et al. Effect of low dose vasopressin infusion on vital organ blood flow in the conscious normal and septic sheep. *Anaesth Intensive Care* 2006;34(4):427–33.

19. Di Giantomasso D, Morimatsu H, May CN, et al. Increasing renal blood flow: Low-dose dopamine or medium-dose norepinephrine. *Chest* 2004;125(6):2260–7.

20. Druml W, Fischer M. Cholesterol improves the utilization of parenteral lipid emulsions. *Wien Klin Wochenschr* 2003;115:767–74.

21. Druml W, Fischer M, Sertle S, et al. Fat elimination in acute renal failure: Long-chain versus medium-chain triglycerides. *Am J Clin Nutr* 1992;55:368–72.

22. Druml W, Kleinberger G, Burger V, et al. Elimination of amino acids in acute renal failure. *Nephron* 1986;42(1):62–7.

23. Duarte CG, Preuss HG. Assessment of renal function: Glomerular and tubular. *Clin Lab Med* 1993;13:33–52.

24. Ertmer C, Sielen Kamper AW, VanAken H, et al. Vasopressin and terlipressin in sepsis and system inflammatory response syndrome. Effects on microcirculation, oxygen transport, metabolism and organ function. *Anaesthesist* 2005;54:346–56.

25. Ferris ME, Gipson DS, Kimmel PL, Eggers PW. Trends in treatment and outcomes of survival of adolescents initiating end-stage renal disease in the United States of America. *Pediatr Nephrology* 2006;21:1020–6.

26. Fung F, Sherrard DJ, Gillen DL, et al. Increased risk for cardiovascular mortality among malnourished end-stage renal disease patients. *Am J Kidney Dis* 2002;40:307–14.

27. Goldstein SL. Pediatric acute renal failure: Demographics and treatment. *Contrib Nephrol* 2004;144:284–90.

28. Goligorsky MS, Noiri E. Duality of nitric oxide in acute renal injury. *Semin Nephrol* 1999;19:263–71.

29. Goodman WG, London G, Amann K, et al. Vascular calcification in chronic kidney disease. *Am J Kidney Dis* 2004;43:572–9.

30. Haycock GB, Schwartz GJ, Wisotsky DH. Geometric method for measuring body surface area: A height-weight formula validated in infants, children, and adults. *J Pediatr* 1978;93:62–6.

31. Hirschberg R, Kopple J, Lipsett P, et al. Multicenter clinical trial of recombinant human insulin-like growth factor I in patients with acute renal failure. *Kidney Int* 1999;55:2423–32.

32. Holt SG, Moore KP. Pathogenesis and treatment of renal dysfunction in rhabdomyolysis. *Intensive Care Med* 2001;27:803–11.

33. Hui-Stickle S, Brewer ED, Goldstein SL. Pediatric ARF epidemiology at a tertiary care center from 1999 to 2001. *Am J Kidney Dis* 2005;45:96–101.

34. Jaber BL, Pereira BJ, Bonventre JV, et al. Polymorphism of host response genes: Implications in the pathogenesis and treatment of acute renal failure. *Kidney Int* 2005;67:14–33.

35. Karen G, James A, Perlman R. A simple method for the estimation of glomerular filtration rate by gentamicin pharmacokinetics during routine drug monitoring in newborns. *Clin Pharmacol Ther* 1985;38:680–5.

36. Kim KE, Onesti G, Ramirez O, et al. Creatinine clearance in renal disease. A reappraisal. *Br Med J* 1969;4(5674):11–4.

37. Kittnig M, Zobel G, Ring E, et al. Nitrogen and amino acid balance during total parenteral nutrition and continuous arteriovenous hemofiltration in critically ill anuric children. *Child Nephrol Urol* 1991;118:74–8.

38. Lam YW, Banerji S, Hatfield C, et al. Principles of drug administration in renal insufficiency. *Clin Pharmacokinet* 1997;32:30–57.

39. Leonard MB, Donaldson LA, Ho M, Geary DF. A prospective cohort study of incident maintenance dialysis in children: An NAPRTC study. *Kidney Int* 2003;63:744–55.

40. Levey AS, Bosch JP, Lewis JB, et al. A more accurate method to estimate glomerular filtration rate from serum creatinine: A new prediction equation. *Ann Intern Med* 1999;130:461–70.

41. Lewis J, Salem MM, Chertow GM, et al. Atrial natriuretic factor in oliguric acute renal failure. Anaritide acute renal failure study group. *Am J Kidney Dis* 2000;36:767–74.

42. Lieberthal W. Biology of acute renal failure: Therapeutic implications. *Kidney Int* 1997;21:1102–15.

43. Maxvold NJ, Smoyer WE, Custer JR, et al. Amino acid loss and nitrogen balance in critically ill children with acute renal failure: A prospective comparison between classic hemofiltration and hemofiltration with dialysis. *Crit Care Med* 2000;28:1161–5.

44. Metnitz GH, Fischer M, Bartens S, et al. Impact of acute renal failure on antioxidant status in patients with multiple organ failure. *Acta Anaesthesiol Scand* 2000;44:236–40.

45. Neumayer HH, Kunzendorf V, Schreiber M. Protective effects of calcium antagonists in human renal transplantation. *Kidney Int* 1992;41:S87–93.

46. Newsholme P, Procopio J, Lima MM, et al. Glutamine and glutamate—their central role in cell metabolism and function. *Cell Biochem Funct* 2003;21:1–9.

47. Nolin F, Beaumier L. Parenteral G/n supplementation decreases whole body protein breakdown and improves net balance in surgical neonates. *Pediatr Research* 2001;49:349A.

48. Persson PB, Hansell P, Liss P. Pathophysiology of contrast medium-induced nephropathy. *Kid Int* 2005;68:14–22.

49. Rieu P, Noël L. Henoch-Schönlein nephritis in children and adults: Morphological features and clinicopathological correlations. *Ann Med Intern* 1999;150:151–8.

50. Robert S, Zarowitch BJ. Is there a reliable index of glomerular filtration rate in critically ill patients? *DICP* 1991;25:169–78.

51. Ruggenenti P, Noris M, Remuzzi G. Thrombotic microangiopathy, hemolytic uremic syndrome, and thrombotic thrombocytopenic purpura. *Kidney Int* 2001;60:831–46.

52. Schwartz GJ, Feld LG, Langford DJ. A simple estimate of glomerular filtration rate in full-term infants during the first year of life. *J Pediatr* 1984;104:849–54.

53. Sheridan RL, Yu YM, Prelack K, et al. Maximal parenteral glucose oxidation in hypermetabolic young children: A stable isotope study. *JPEN* 1998;22:212–6.

54. Tappy L, Schwarz JM, Schneiter P, et al. Effects of isoenergetic glucose-based or lipid-based parenteral nutrition on glucose metabolism, de novo lipogenesis and respiratory gas exchanges in critically ill patients. *Crit Care Med* 1998;26:860–7.

55. Teirstein RS, Price MJ, Mathur VS, et al. Differential effects between intravenous and targeted renal delivery of fenoldopam on renal function and blood pressure in patients undergoing cardiac catheterization. *Am J Cardiol* 2006;97:1076–81.

56. Traub SL, Johnson CE. Comparison of methods of estimating creatinine clearance in children. *Am J Hosp Pharm* 1980;37:195–201.

57. Uchino S, Bellomo R, Morimatsu H, et al. External validation of severity scoring systems for acute renal failure using a multinational database. *Crit Care Med* 2005;33:1961–7.

58. Van den Berghe G, Wouters PJ, Bouillon R, et al. Outcome benefit of intensive insulin therapy in the critically ill: Insulin dose versus glycemia control. *Crit Care Med* 2003;31:359–366.

59. VanAcker BA, vonMeyenfeldt MF, vanderHulst RR, et al. Glutamine: The pivot of our nitrogen economy. *JPEN* 1999;23:545–8.

60. Vasarhelyi B, Toth-Heyn P, Treszl A, et al. Genetic polymorphisms and risk for acute renal failure in preterm neonates. *Pediatr Nephrol* 2005;20:132–5.

61. Williams DM, Sreedhar SS, Mickell JJ, et al. Acute kidney failure: A pediatric experience over 20 years. *Arch Pediatr Adolesc Med* 2002;156:893–900.

62. Winter ME. Aminoglycoside Antibiotics. In: Winter ME, ed. *Basic Clinical Pharmacokinetics, 3rd ed.* Vancouver, WA: Applied Therapeutics 1994;128–38.

63. Wong CS, Hingorani S, Gillen DL, et al. Hypoalbuminemia and risk of death in pediatric patients with end-stage renal disease. *Kidney Int* 2002;61:630–7.

64. Ziegler TR, Young LS, Benfell K, et al. Clinical and metabolic efficacy of glutamine supplemented parenteral nutrition after bone marrow transplantation. *Ann Intern Med* 1992;116:831–8.

CHAPTER 97 ■ HYPERTENSIVE CRISES

GEORGE OFORI-AMANFO • ARTHUR SMERLING

Blood pressure (BP) homeostasis is achieved by a fine relationship between blood flow and resistance across the vascular bed. This relationship is defined as:

$$Pressure = Flow \times Resistance$$

This relationship is the hemodynamic extrapolation of Ohm's Law, defined as:

$$Voltage\,(V) = Current\,(I) \times Resistance\,(R)$$

Hypertension occurs when flow or resistance (or both) increase without appropriate autoregulatory compensation. Therapy can, therefore, be targeted at the specific derangement.

Severe acute hypertension is uncommon in the pediatric population, but when it occurs, it may cause life-threatening consequences. It represents two pathophysiologically distinct groups of hypertensive crises: hypertensive emergencies and hypertensive urgencies. *Hypertensive emergency* is defined as sudden, severe hypertension complicated by acute end-organ damage; *hypertensive urgency* is characterized by severely elevated BP without end-organ damage. The clinical distinction between these two groups is the *presence* or *absence* of target organ damage—not the absolute level of the BP. The organ systems most frequently involved are those that maintain strict autoregulation to sustain physiologic function, and these include the central nervous system (CNS), cardiovascular system, and kidneys. Involvement of these organ systems results in specific clinical syndromes (**Table 97.1**). Some patients may have an acute onset and extraordinary elevation of BP without end-organ injury but may experience severe headache, altered sensorium, anxiety, or epistaxis. Such patients are judged to be in imminent hypertensive crisis and are treated as true emergencies.

Malignant hypertension has been used to describe a syndrome of severe hypertension associated with encephalopathy or acute nephropathy, but this condition is best referred to and treated as a hypertensive crisis. The diagnosis of this entity requires the presence of papilledema on funduscopy (4).

PATHOPHYSIOLOGY

Hypertensive crisis can develop either de novo or as a complication of preexisting essential or secondary hypertension (**Table 97.2**). Any disorder that causes hypertension can give rise to hypertensive crisis. Because of the rapidity of onset of hypertensive crisis, a trigger factor may be implicated; this trigger effect may either be superimposed on a preexisting hypertension or act de novo in a previously normotensive individual. The endothelium in resistance vessels plays a central role in BP homeostasis, as it attempts to compensate for changes in vascular resistance through increased autocrine and paracrine release of vasodilator molecules, such as nitric ox-

ide (NO) and prostacyclin. With sustained severe hypertension, these compensatory endothelium-mediated vasodilator responses are overwhelmed, which leads to endothelial decompensation, endothelial failure, and vasoconstriction. Although the detailed pathophysiology of hypertensive crisis remains to be elucidated, an initial abrupt increase in vascular resistance seems to be a necessary step (38).

The pathophysiologic basis of hypertensive crisis is characterized by severe BP elevation combined with malignant vascular injury and the consequent failure of hemodynamic control. Although the vascular lesions have been well recognized (2), the understanding of the molecular pathogenesis is still evolving. The characteristic vascular injury falls into two categories. The first type is *transmural smooth muscle cell necrosis* that affects the afferent arterioles combined with fibrin and platelet deposition and intramural hemorrhage. The endothelial cells in these vessels appear to remain viable. Healing occurs by fibrous replacement of the arterial wall, with consequent loss of autoregulation. The second type of injury is one of *malignant vascular injury*, characterized by proliferative endarteritis that affects small-to-medium sized resistance arteries. The ramifications of these pathologic changes are narrowing of the vessel lumen, tissue ischemia, and failure of local autoregulation (9). Endothelial damage causes local activation of the clotting cascade, further fibrinoid necrosis of the small blood vessels, and release of vasoconstrictor substances, all of which result in a vicious cycle of worsening vascular injury, tissue ischemia, and further release of vasoconstrictor substances (36) (**Fig. 97.1**). Local endothelial dysfunction also induces platelet activation, intravascular hemolysis, and consequent microangiopathic anemia (35). Because of the acute onset and rapid perpetuation of crises, the release of humoral vasoconstrictor substances from the stressed vessel wall seems to be a plausible pathophysiologic explanation for hypertensive crises.

Although the factors that trigger the acute BP elevation are not well understood, neurohormonal factors have been heavily implicated. Activation of the rennin-angiotensin system (29), NO (16), endothelin (39), vasopressin (34), and catecholamines (16) all have been postulated to play important roles in the pathophysiology of hypertensive crises. These mechanisms alter systemic and renal hemodynamics and culminate in end-organ injury.

Of these trigger factors, the role of the renin-angiotensin system in the pathogenesis of end-organ injury has been the most studied. In humans, a rapid elevation of circulating renin levels occurs during transition to malignant hypertension (6); in transgenic mice, evidence suggests that the renin-angiotensin system is important for transformation to malignant hypertension and lethality, independent of BP (19). Mice that express the mouse renin gene, *Ren-2*, develop severe hypertension compared to controls (22). Moreover, rats that are

TABLE 97.1

MANIFESTATIONS OF HYPERTENSIVE CRISES

Hypertensive crises
Hypertensive encephalopathy
Acute stroke
Retinopathy
Acute myocardial ischemia
Acute left ventricular failure with pulmonary edema
Dissecting aortic aneurysm
Acute renal failure
Microangiopathic hemolytic anemia

double-transgenic for human renin and human angiotensinogen genes develop not only severe hypertension, but also an inflammatory vasculopathy similar to that seen in human severe hypertension (12). Angiotensin II has direct cytotoxic effects on the vessel wall, some of which seem to be mediated through activation of expression of genes for proinflammatory cytokines (e.g., IL-6) and activation of the transcription factor, nuclear factor (NF)-κB (11,21). Furthermore, inhibition of angiotensin-converting enzyme (ACE) prevents the development of malignant hypertension in transgenic rats that express the murine renin gene (19). Activation of the renin-angiotensin-aldosterone system may be primary or secondary to renal ischemia produced by arteriolar occlusion. The BP elevation may induce pressure natriuresis, intravascular volume depletion, and a further increase in renin secretion. Increased

TABLE 97.2

CAUSES OF HYPERTENSIVE CRISIS

Disorder	Associated clinical conditions and drugs
Essential hypertension	
Renal parenchymal disorders	Glomerulonephritis Interstitial nephritis Hemolytic uremic syndrome Systemic lupus erythematosus Vasculitides
Renovascular disorders	Fibromuscular dysplasia Acute renal artery occlusion Polyarteritis nodosa
Endocrine disorders	Renin secreting tumors Pheochromocytoma Thyroid crisis Cushing syndrome Conn disease
Ingestions/Drugs	Cocaine Amphetamines Phencyclidine Cyclosporine Tacrolimus
Cardiovascular disorder	Coarctation of the aorta Midaortic syndrome
Preeclampsia/Eclampsia	Pregnancy

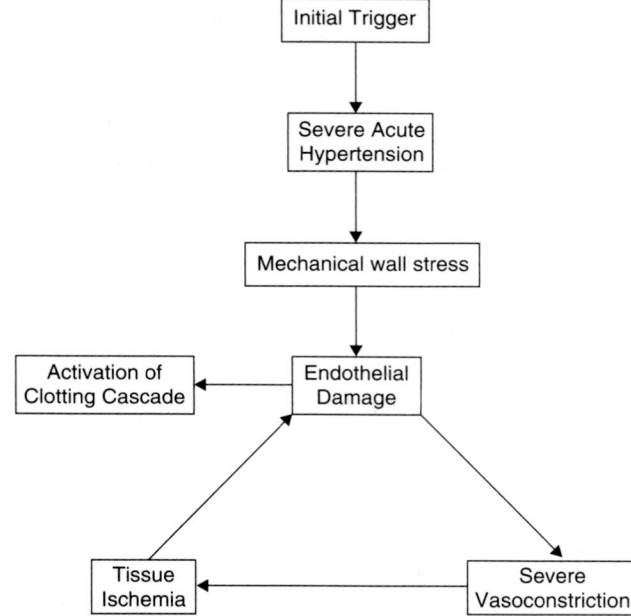

FIGURE 97.1. Pathophysiology of hypertensive crisis.

angiotensin II causes further renal vasoconstriction and, hence, worsening hypertension.

NO, formed by the action of endothelial nitric oxide synthase (NOS) on L-arginine, diffuses from the endothelial cells to activate soluble guanylate cyclase, resulting in an increase of cyclic guanosine monophosphate (cGMP) in vascular smooth muscle cells, thus causing vasodilation. Other agents that cause vasodilation include endothelial-derived hyperpolarizing factor, and prostacyclin (PGI_2). Endothelin is also an endothelium-derived agent with potent vasoconstrictor effects. It may act alone or in concert with other agents, such as thromboxane A_2, prostaglandin ($PGF_{2\alpha}$), or endothelial-derived constrictor factor to cause vasoconstriction. The relative amounts of the various factors released by the endothelial cell are kept in tight equilibrium and are dependent on the physiologic circumstance and pathophysiologic status. Appropriate disturbance of this equilibrium can result in an acute hypertensive episode.

It is important to note that patients with chronic hypertension may have arterial wall hypertrophy and, therefore, may be relatively protected from the effects of acute BP elevation (26). Conversely, in patients without preexisting chronic hypertension, a hypertensive emergency can develop at substantially lower BPs (38).

Cerebral Autoregulation

The pathophysiologic mechanism of development of hypertensive encephalopathy, though controversial, deserves mention. Autoregulation of cerebral blood flow (CBF) is governed by the relationship between cerebral perfusion pressure (CPP) and cerebrovascular resistance (CVR).

$$CBF = CPP/CVR$$

CPP is defined as mean arterial pressure (MAP) – cerebral venous pressure (CVP).

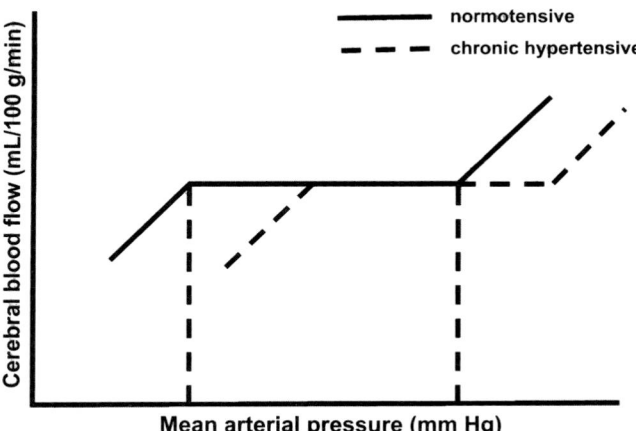

FIGURE 97.2. Chronic hypertension is associated with a rightward displacement of the cerebral autoregulation curve.

Under normal conditions, CVP is negligible; therefore, CBF maintains a reciprocal relationship with CVR. In normotensive adults, CBF is maintained over a wide BP range (MAP between 60 and 150 mm Hg). The range of autoregulation shifts to the right in chronically hypertensive patients (31) (**Fig. 97.2**), a phenomenon that is reversible with long-term BP control (30). This autoregulation is maintained by the appropriate adjustments in CVR. Hypertensive encephalopathy occurs when MAP exceeds the upper limit autoregulation. One suggested pathophysiologic mechanism of hypertensive encephalopathy is failure of autoregulation, which is characterized by profound cerebral vasodilation, inappropriately increased CBF, the subsequent dysfunction of the blood-brain barrier (BBB) and vascular endothelium, and cerebral edema (18). Decreased CBF from severe cerebral vasoconstriction in response to acute hypertension is another suggested mechanism of hypertensive encephalopathy, but this hypothesis has been heavily disputed (28). Other proposed mechanisms include cerebrovascular endothelial dysfunction, disruption of the BBB with increased permeability, cerebral edema, elevated intracranial pressure, and microhemorrhage (38).

CLINICAL PRESENTATION

The risk of development of hypertensive crisis is greater in patients with secondary hypertension than in patients with essential hypertension. The absolute BP is often not as important as the rate of elevation. Acute elevations in BP are less well tolerated and more likely to produce symptoms than are chronic elevations. Clinical manifestations may be divided into features related to hypertension and features related to target organ injury. In the neonate, symptoms and signs related to hypertension are lethargy and irritability, whereas in the older child, they include severe headache, dizziness, blurred vision, and epistaxis. Typically, the headache is occipital and more prominent in patients with hypertensive encephalopathy.

Blood Pressure

It is difficult to apply an absolute BP level to define hypertensive emergencies and urgencies. Normal and abnormal BPs vary widely with age and body size. The Fourth Task Force has defined stage II hypertension as systolic or diastolic BP that is >5 mm Hg greater than the 99th percentile for age and height, and this condition requires prompt evaluation and pharmacologic therapy (24). Systolic and diastolic BP levels for children and adolescents by age and height percentiles are defined in the Fourth Report on the Diagnosis, Evaluation, and Treatment of High Blood Pressure in Children and Adolescents, published in *Pediatrics* (24).

Neurologic Manifestations

Hypertensive Encephalopathy

Hypertensive encephalopathy is defined as an acute, organic brain syndrome characterized by profound headache, severe nausea and vomiting, blurred vision, and altered mental status. These symptoms may progress to focal or generalized seizures, focal neurologic deficits, and cortical blindness. If not appropriately treated, hypertensive encephalopathy may progress rapidly to cerebral hemorrhage, coma, and death. It occurs as a result of failure of the upper limit of cerebral vascular autoregulation (autoregulation breakthrough), cerebrovascular endothelial dysfunction, microhemorrhage, or BBB disruption, with cerebral edema and intracranial hypertension. It is associated with untreated or inadequately treated hypertension and other known causes and associations of severe hypertension, such as renal disease, immunosuppressive therapy (e.g., tacrolimus, cyclosporine) (33), erythropoietin administration (7), and thrombotic thrombocytopenic purpura. In the pregnant adolescent, hypertensive encephalopathy may occur in the setting of preeclampsia and eclampsia. Physical examination findings are consistent with the neurologic symptoms. In some cases, funduscopy may reveal evidence of malignant hypertension: papilledema, retinal hemorrhages, and exudates. These manifestations occur as a result of failure of cerebral autoregulation and are completely reversible with appropriate BP management. In chronic hypertensive patients, adaptive mechanisms allow cerebral autoregulation to occur at relatively higher MAPs and thereby provide some protection against the development of hypertensive encephalopathy during sudden increases in BP (15) (**Fig. 97.2**).

Acute Stroke

Acute stroke with concomitant severe hypertension poses a diagnostic and management dilemma. The hypertension may be a reflex response to maintain cerebral perfusion, or it may be the cause of the stroke. Careful assessment and management of such patients are imperative. In many patients in whom hypertension is secondary to stroke, the BP tends to resolve spontaneously within 48 hrs. The clinical presentation includes acute onset of severe headache, altered mental status, or loss of consciousness associated with focal neurologic findings (e.g., hemiparesis, hemiplegia). The distribution of the focal findings depends on the extent of cerebral vascular involvement.

Cardiovascular Manifestations

Myocardial Ischemia

Acute hypertensive crisis subjects the left ventricle to a sudden increase in afterload, intraventricular pressure, and myocardial oxygen demand. Ischemia results if an increase in myocardial blood flow does not occur in parallel (1). Sustained increase in myocardial work load leads to failure of the left ventricle, elevated left ventricle end-diastolic pressure, and pulmonary edema. These pathophysiologic events manifest as acute chest pain, tachypnea, dyspnea, orthopnea, cough, and hemoptysis. Physical examination reveals diffuse, fine crackles at the lung bases, and possibly an S_3 gallop on cardiac auscultation.

Aortic Dissection

Severe acute hypertension can cause aortic dissection, especially in patients with predisposing syndromes such as Marfan syndrome. Severe chest or abdominal pain is the most common symptom of acute aortic dissection. The precise location of the pain depends on the site and extent of the dissecting process. Syncope, paralysis, and blindness may result from carotid or innominate artery involvement. Dissection of the thoracic aorta may be associated with hemoptysis, orthopnea, and dyspnea, while involvement of the abdominal aorta may cause a variety of gastrointestinal and genitourinary disturbances. The diagnosis of acute aortic dissection should be suspected in a hypertensive patient with abrupt onset of pain, pulse deficits, and signs of end-organ circulatory compromise. Mortality from acute aortic dissection is not from the intimal disruption per se; rather, it is the result of the course taken by the dissecting hematoma, which may rupture or interrupt blood supply to a major organ.

Renal Manifestations

The most common etiology of severe hypertension in pediatric patients is renal or renovascular disorders. Renal diseases, such as poststreptococcal glomerulonephritis and hemolytic uremic syndrome, are common causes of de novo acute hypertension. Mild proteinuria and elevated serum creatinine can be the result of a primary renal disease or may be secondary manifestations of severe hypertension, and such cases may be difficult to differentiate. In cases in which the kidneys are the target organs of severe acute hypertension, the injury may manifest as multiple intraparenchymal hemorrhages with many areas of renal destruction and, eventually, kidney failure, uremia, and death.

CLINICAL EVALUATION

The goal of initial clinical evaluation is to differentiate hypertensive emergency from urgency. All organ systems at risk of involvement in hypertensive emergencies must be critically assessed. The presence of one organ dysfunction at presentation does not preclude evaluation of others. The history and physical examination must determine the nature, severity, and subsequent management of the hypertensive syndrome. The duration and severity of preexisting hypertension and the presence of previous end-organ damage must be ascertained. History of antihypertensive drug therapy, degree of BP control, and use of any other drugs, including illicit drugs (e.g., cocaine), must be determined. A focused examination to identify any evidence of end-organ injury is imperative.

BP should be obtained in all four extremities to exclude coarctation of the aorta. Funduscopic examination is particularly useful because it can distinguish a true hypertensive emergency from hypertensive urgency (the presence of new

hemorrhages, exudates, or papilledema, indicating hypertensive emergency). The cardiovascular assessment should focus on the presence of heart failure, and neurologic examination should evaluate level of consciousness, signs of meningeal irritation, visual fields, and focal neurologic deficits.

Initial laboratory investigations include serum electrolytes, urea, and creatinine, full blood count with peripheral smear (for evidence of hemolysis), urinalysis, electrocardiogram, and chest x-ray. Measurement of plasma renin and aldosterone activity may be helpful in making a retrospective diagnosis of hypertension. Once the patient is stabilized, investigations for secondary causes of severe hypertension should be performed, as guided by clinical presentation and laboratory findings (Table 97.2). Brain MRI, though not part of the initial workup, may reveal the characteristic posterior leukoencephalopathy that predominantly (but not exclusively) affects the white matter of the parieto-occipital regions, which are best appreciated on T2-weighted images (27). Pregnancy must be ruled out in female adolescents who present with hypertensive crisis, as this may impact on the approach to treatment and the choice of antihypertensive agents.

DIFFERENTIAL DIAGNOSES

Hypertensive encephalopathy must be differentiated from other acute neurologic events that may be associated with hypertension, such as cerebral infarct or hemorrhage. Reflex elevation of systemic BP in response to cerebral ischemia (e.g., brainstem ischemia can induce hypertension) or hypertension as a component of the Cushing triad must be recognized. Pseudotumor cerebri, when associated with severe hypertension, may mimic hypertensive encephalopathy. Other differential diagnoses to be considered include primary renal disease with severe hypertension and uremic encephalopathy, as well as hepatic encephalopathy with hepatorenal syndrome and hypertension.

Post-coarctectomy Hypertension

Severe paradoxic hypertension commonly occurs in the first week after relief of coarctation of the aorta. An incidence of 56% has been reported following surgical repair in the pediatric population (10), and a few cases have been reported following balloon angioplasty (5). Provided the repair is satisfactory, the hypertension usually resolves after several days, though intensive antihypertensive therapy during the early postoperative period is frequently required. Both the sympathetic and renin-angiotensin systems have been implicated in the pathogenesis of paradoxic hypertension (17). Aggressive treatment of the hypertension is crucial if end-organ damage and risk of rupture of surgical suture lines are to be avoided. Treatment with esmolol infusion or sodium nitroprusside has been successful.

TREATMENT

General Principles

While it is important to establish the distinction between hypertensive emergency and hypertensive urgency, the treatment algorithm is the same for either condition. Management requires the immediate assessment of the airway, breathing, and circulation and initiation of appropriate interventions. The patient must be admitted to the PICU, and an arterial line must be placed for continuous, invasive BP monitoring. However, it is imperative that specific antihypertensive therapy is not delayed while these measures are being implemented. The primary goal of therapy is to prevent end-organ injury, not solely to restore BP to normal. Reversible causes must be identified and treated appropriately. The recommended aim is to reduce MAP by 20%–25% within a period of 15 mins to 2 hrs. Subsequent rate of reduction of the BP is dictated by clinical status and the rapidity with which the hypertension may have evolved. Too rapid a reduction in BP is to be avoided, as that can worsen end-organ dysfunction. An exception to this guideline is the treatment of hypertensive crisis associated with aortic dissection. Aortic dissection is the most dramatic and most rapidly fatal complication of severe hypertension. Appropriate treatment requires rapid reduction of systolic BP. Rapid minimization of aortic wall stress is imperative and can be accomplished by lowering both BP and heart rate and, consequently, the dP/dt (change in BP/change in time). Volume depletion is common in patients with hypertensive crises and may lead to excessive fall in BP during treatment. Volume repletion with IV crystalloid often restores organ perfusion.

Pharmacologic Therapy

The aim of drug therapy is to reduce BP in a controlled, predictable, and safe manner, which is best achieved with continuous infusion of pharmacologic agents that have rapid onset, short half-life, and ease of titration. However, oral agents have been used to treat some cases of hypertensive urgencies. These antihypertensive agents act by inducing vascular smooth muscle relaxation and vasodilation. They enhance organ perfusion and minimize end-organ dysfunction. The choice of drug must take into consideration the nature and extent of target-organ involvement. For example, such drugs as clonidine and methyldopa that significantly affect the CNS should be avoided in patients with hypertensive encephalopathy. Also, drugs that act by predominant β-receptor blockade must be avoided in pheochromocytoma crisis, as unopposed α-receptor stimulation may cause a paradoxic worsening of the hypertension. From the wide array of IV antihypertensive drugs available, the most commonly used in the pediatric population are sodium nitroprusside (SNP), fenoldopam, labetalol, and nicardipine, although esmolol has been favored in post-coarctectomy hypertension. Oral agents have an important place in the management of hypertensive crisis. The most commonly used oral agents are the calcium-channel blockers (e.g., nifedipine), ACE inhibitors (enalapril, captopril), and ganglion blockers (clonidine).

PARENTERAL ANTIHYPERTENSIVE AGENTS

Sodium Nitroprusside

SNP has been used as first-line medication in most cases of hypertensive crisis. A nonselective vasodilator that affects both ar-

terioles and venules, it decreases both systemic and pulmonary vascular resistance. Once infused, SNP interacts with oxyhemoglobin, dissociating immediately to form methemoglobin, while releasing free cyanide and NO. This process is independent of enzyme activity. NO activates guanylate cyclase in the vascular smooth muscle, triggering an increase in intracellular cGMP, followed by relaxation of vascular smooth muscle and vasodilation. The free cyanide radicals (CN^-) bind to methemoglobin to form cyanomethemoglobin. Each molecule of SNP metabolized results in the release of five cyanide radicals, some of which bind to methemoglobin, with the remainder available to be converted to thiocyanate by rhodanase enzyme in the liver and kidneys. Any free cyanide that is not rapidly converted to thiocyanate can bind to and inactivate tissue cytochrome oxidase and manifest as tissue hypoxia. Because the conversion of SNP to cyanide is a nonenzymatic process, the amount of CN^- released from SNP depends entirely on the total dose of the drug administered. The subsequent rate at which CN^- is converted to the less toxic thiocyanate by rhodanase enzyme is dependent on the availability of a sulfur donor for the enzyme, usually endogenous thiosulfate derived from the amino acid cysteine. Thiocyanate is cleared by the kidneys with an elimination half-life of 4–7 days. The presence of renal failure or prolonged SNP therapy can cause accumulation of thiocyanate.

SNP has been favored in the management of hypertensive crises because of its rapid onset of action, ease of titration, rapid dissipation of its effects after discontinuation, and almost universal efficacy. It acts within 30 secs, peak antihypertensive effect occurs within 2 mins, and its effects persist for 2–4 mins after cessation of infusion. Most patients respond to a starting dose of 0.3–0.5 mcg/kg/min, and the dose may be escalated as needed to rates not exceeding 5 mcg/kg/min. Occasionally, doses as high as 10 mcg/kg/min may be necessary for adequate BP response, but they must be administered for no longer than 10 mins to minimize toxicity. Reflex tachycardia can occur with SNP therapy, which may be accompanied by inadequate BP response. In such situations, the addition of a small dose of β-blocker will result in significant improvement in BP control. When used in the treatment of aortic dissection, prior institution of β-blocking agent is imperative, as the reflex tachycardia could be extremely deleterious in such patients.

The most common adverse effect of SNP is precipitous hypotension, with or without reflex tachycardia, due to its potent vasodilator effect on both the venous and arterial beds. This reaction is accentuated in the hypovolemic patient. SNP has been shown to cause increased intracranial pressure (13).

Cyanide accumulation, i.e., cyanide poisoning, accounts for the rare but fatal toxic effects of SNP. Free cyanide radicals bind and inactivate tissue cytochrome oxidase, leading to tissue anoxia, anaerobic metabolism, and lactic acidosis. Toxic accumulation of cyanide that leads to severe lactic acidosis can occur if SNP is infused at a rate >5 mcg/kg/min over a period of hours to days, assuming normal rhodanase activity. Patients receiving SNP who demonstrate any evidence of tissue hypoxia must be investigated for methemoglobinemia and cyanide poisoning. Antidotes for cyanide poisoning include sodium thiosulfate and hydroxocobalamin (vitamin B_{12}).

Methemoglobinemia is another important toxic effect of SNP. Severe methemoglobinemia causes tissue hypoxia and subsequent acidosis. The total SNP required to generate 10% methemoglobinemia exceeds 10 mg/kg (~10 mcg/kg/min for >16 hrs).

The most common clinically observed toxicity of SNP is thiocyanate accumulation, which results in nausea, confusion, and muscle weakness. This toxicity occurs predominantly in patients with concomitant renal dysfunction.

Fenoldopam

Fenoldopam is a benzapine derivative of dopamine and a selective dopamine agonist that interacts with DA_1 receptor without significant interaction with DA_2, α_1-adrenergic, or β-adrenergic receptors. Stimulation of the receptor results in vasodilation and, in the kidneys, induces diuresis and natriuresis. During reduction of severely elevated BP, fenoldopam significantly increased creatinine clearance, urinary flow, and sodium and potassium excretion (3). These unique effects on the kidneys make fenoldopam a particularly attractive drug in the treatment of hypertensive emergencies with renal impairment.

Peripheral DA_1 receptors are located postsynaptically in the systemic and renal vasculature and at various sites in the nephrons, parathyroid gland, and the gastrointestinal tract (25). DA_1 receptors are also present in the brain, but fenoldopam does not cross the BBB. It is not metabolized by the cytochrome P450 pathway and, therefore, has no significant drug interactions; furthermore, its pharmacokinetics is not altered by hepatic or renal insufficiency. Fenoldopam has a short half-life (5 mins) and predictable dose response, is easily titrated, and is not associated with precipitous decline in BP. The onset of BP response occurs within 15 mins of initiation (3 half-lives); therefore, it is recommended that the drug be titrated no more frequently than every 15 mins. Steady state is reached within 30 mins, and elimination half-life is about 10 mins. The recommended starting dose is 0.1 mcg/kg/min, titrated to effect to a maximum of 1.6 mcg/kg/min (23). In one pediatric case series, doses up to 2.5 mcg/kg/min were successfully without excessive hypotension or clinically significant adverse effects (32).

Most adverse effects associated with fenoldopam are attributable to the vasodilator action of the drug. These include headache, flushing, dizziness, and reflex tachycardia. Most of the adverse effects occur in the first 24 hrs of treatment. Electrocardiographic changes (flattening T waves in anterior and lateral leads) have been reported with fenoldopam, but these have not been shown to have any clinical significance. Elevation of intraocular pressure has also been reported (8). Fenoldopam must be used with caution in patients with increased intracranial pressure because of the risk of worsening intracranial hypertension (14).

Nicardipine

Nicardipine is a nondihydropyridine-derivative calcium-channel blocker. It differs from nifedipine by the addition of tertiary amine moiety to the ester side-chain pyridine ring and movement of the nitro group to the meta position of the phenyl ring, making it 100 times more water soluble than nifedipine. Nicardipine acts by blocking calcium influx through voltage-sensitive channels in vascular smooth muscle cells, resulting in smooth muscle relaxation and vasodilation. It can be given as a continuous IV infusion and is easily titratable. The pharma-

cokinetic characteristics of nicardipine include onset of action of 5–15 mins, peak hypotensive effect at 30 mins to 2 hrs, half-life of 2–4 hrs, and duration of action of 4–6 hrs. It is administered as a loading dose of 5–10 mcg/kg, given over 1 minute, followed by a continuous infusion of 1–3 mcg/kg/min. Adverse effects include orthostatic hypotension, tachycardia (reflex), and peripheral edema. It can be used alone or in conjunction with other antihypertensive agents.

Labetalol

Labetalol is a competitive α_1-adrenergic and β-adrenergic receptor antagonist. When given intravenously, the α-blocker effect is seven times greater than the β-blocker effect. The α_1 receptor blockade causes arterial smooth muscle relaxation and vasodilation, and the β-receptor antagonism contributes to the fall in BP by blocking reflex sympathetic stimulation of the heart. In addition, labetalol has intrinsic sympathomimetic activity at β_2 receptors, which may contribute further to the peripheral vasodilation. The hypotensive effect of labetalol begins 2–5 mins after an IV dose, peaks at 5–15 mins, and persists for ~2–4 hrs (37). The recommended dose in children is an initial dose of 0.25 mg/kg bolus, followed by continuous infusion of 0.25 mg/kg/hr, titrated up to 3 mg/kg/hr (20). The most common adverse effects associated with labetalol are precipitous hypotension and orthostatic hypotension. Bradycardia, heart block, and bronchospasm may also complicate its use.

Esmolol

Esmolol is an IV, ultra-short-acting, selective, β_1-adrenergic antagonist. It has virtually no intrinsic sympathomimetic activity; therefore, significant bradycardia can be associated with its administration. Peak hemodynamic effect occurs in 6–10 mins following an appropriate loading dose; it has a half-life of 8 mins, and a rapid offset of effect occurs within 15–30 mins following discontinuation. Esmolol is administered as a bolus of 300–500 mcg/kg IV over 1–3 mins, then 25–200 mcg/kg/min. An infusion dose may be titrated by 25–50 mcg/kg/min every 5–10 min for optimal antihypertensive effect to a maximum infusion dose of 1000 mcg/kg/min. Adverse effects include bradycardia, hypotension, congestive heart failure, and bronchoconstriction. Esmolol is contraindicated in second- or third-degree heart block and in cardiogenic shock.

ORAL ANTIHYPERTENSIVE AGENTS

Nifedipine

Nifedipine is a dihydropyridine calcium-channel blocking agent that induces peripheral vasodilation. It is administered either orally or sublingually. Following its administration, nifedipine reduces BP abruptly and therefore has an important role in the management of hypertensive urgencies. The usual dose is 0.25–0.5 mg/kg/dose; however, the lower end of this range is the preferred starting dose due to the risk of precipitous hypotension. The dose may be repeated as needed to a daily maximum of 3 mg/kg. Absorption is nearly complete, but bioavailability is 45%–75% due to first-pass effect. Onset of action is observed within 15–30 mins, and the elimination half-life may be as short as 1.5 hrs. Even though its rapid onset of action is viewed as a major advantage, nifedipine must be used with caution, as the peripheral vasodilation that follows its administration can trigger an intense reflex adrenergic stimulation with tachycardia, as well as activation of the renin-angiotensin system.

Captopril

Captopril, an ACE inhibitor, which works by reducing the levels of circulating angiotensin II, represents an important component of the treatment of hypertensive crises. Captopril lowers BP promptly without causing tachycardia and, therefore, offers distinct hemodynamic advantage over other vasodilator drugs. Captopril is very well absorbed, and its antihypertensive effect can be witnessed within 15 min of administration and can last for up to 2 hrs. Elimination half-life is 4–6 hrs. The initial dose of 0.3–0.5 mg/kg and may be repeated to a maximum daily dose of 6 mg/kg. Patients must be closely monitored after the first dose, as an exaggerated hypotensive effect may be observed in patients who present with acute severe hypertension associated with a high renin state. Adverse effects include cough, hyperkalemia, neutropenia, and rarely, angioedema. In patients with renovascular hypertension, the glomerular filtration rate is maintained by an increased postglomerular arteriolar resistance caused by angiotensin II. Therefore, in patients with bilateral renal artery stenosis or stenosis in a solitary kidney, captopril and other ACE inhibitors are contraindicated. Autoimmune renal disease with hypertension (e.g., scleroderma) is often associated with high renin states, and ACE inhibitors are to be used with utmost caution. Captopril is also contraindicated in severe renal failure.

CONCLUSION AND FUTURE DIRECTIONS

Hypertensive crisis is a medical emergency that continue to afflict children. Although advances have been made in the therapeutic options available for lowering BP, more advanced treatments are necessary to prevent and treat end-organ damage. More is yet to be learned about the pathophysiology of hypertensive crisis and the molecular mechanisms that mediate target organ injury. With the elucidation of these molecular mechanisms, translational studies in humans may lead to additional therapeutic options that are directed at both tight BP control and prevention of target organ injury.

KEY POINTS

- Hypertensive crisis is characterized by severe hypertension associated with end-organ damage (hypertensive emergency) or impending end-organ damage (hypertensive urgency).
- Hypertensive crisis can develop either de novo or as a complication of preexisting essential or secondary hypertension. Any disorder that causes hypertension can give rise to a hypertensive crisis.

- Hypertensive crisis is a rapid onset, acute disease; therefore, a trigger factor (including neurohormonal factors such as the renin-angiotensin system, endothelin, vasopressin, and catecholamines) may be implicated in its pathogenesis.
- The endothelium in resistance vessels plays a central role in BP homeostasis, as it attempts to compensate for changes in vascular resistance through increased autocrine and paracrine release of vasodilator molecules, such as NO and prostacyclin.
- In sustained, severe hypertension, these compensatory endothelium-mediated vasodilator responses are overwhelmed, which leads to endothelial decompensation, endothelial failure, and vasoconstriction.
- Clinical manifestations consist of features related to hypertension and those related to target organ injury. The absolute BP is often not as important as the rate of elevation. Acute elevations in BP are less well tolerated and more likely to produce symptoms than are chronic elevations.
- Clinical distinction between hypertensive emergency and hypertensive urgency is crucial; however, the principles of treatment are the same.
- The principal goals of treatment are tightly controlled BP reduction and prevention of end-organ injury. The recommended aim is to reduce MAP by 20%–25% within a period of 15 mins to 2 hrs. Subsequent rate of reduction of the BP is dictated by clinical status and the rapidity with which the hypertension may have evolved. A too-rapid reduction in BP is to be avoided, as that can worsen end-organ dysfunction, *except* in the treatment of hypertensive crisis associated with aortic dissection, where appropriate treatment requires rapid reduction of systolic BP to minimize aortic wall stress.
- Choice of drugs must take into account organs involved in the disease process and the adverse-effect profile.
- Although IV antihypertensive infusions are preferred in the treatment of hypertensive crisis, oral agents may be used in a select group of patients with hypertensive urgency.

References

1. Angel Gomez-Sanchez M, Saenz De La Calzada C, Escribano Subias P, et al. Pilot assessment of the response of several pulmonary hemodynamic variables to sublingual sildenafil in candidates for heart transplantation. *Eur J Heart Fail* 2004;6(5):615–7.
2. Bales A. Hypertensive crisis. How to tell if it's an emergency or an urgency. *Postgrad Med* 1999;105(5):119–26.
3. Brogden RN, Markham A. Fenoldopam: A review of its pharmacodynamic and pharmacokinetic properties and intravenous clinical potential in the management of hypertensive urgencies and emergencies. *Drugs* 1997;54(4):634–50.
4. Chobanian AV, Bakris GL, Black HR, et al. Seventh report of the Joint National Committee on Prevention, Detection, Evaluation, and Treatment of High Blood Pressure. *Hypertension* 2003;42(6):1206–52.
5. Choy M, Rocchini AP, Beekman RH, et al. Paradoxical hypertension after repair of coarctation of the aorta in children: Balloon angioplasty versus surgical repair. *Circulation* 1987;75(6):1186–91.
6. Collidge TA, Lammie GA, Fleming S, et al. The role of the renin-angiotensin system in malignant vascular injury affecting the systemic and cerebral circulations. *Prog Biophys Mol Biol* 2004;84(2–3):301–19.
7. Delanty N, Vaughan C, Frucht S, et al. Erythropoietin-associated hypertensive posterior leukoencephalopathy. *Neurology* 1997;49(3):686–9 [see comment, Neurology 1998;51(2):651].
8. Everitt DE, Boike SC, Piltz-Seymour JR, et al. Effect of intravenous fenoldopam on intraocular pressure in ocular hypertension. *J Clin Pharmacol* 1997;37(4):312–20.
9. Fleming S. Malignant hypertension: The role of the paracrine renin-angiotensin system. *J Pathol* 2000;192(2):135–9.

10. Fox S, Pierce WS, Waldhausen JA. Pathogenesis of paradoxical hypertension after coarctation repair. *Ann Thor Surg* 1980;29(2):135–41.

11. Funakoshi Y, Ichiki T, Ito K, et al. Induction of interleukin-6 expression by angiotensin II in rat vascular smooth muscle cells. *Hypertension* 1999;34(1):118–25.

12. Ganten D, Wagner J, Zeh K, et al. Species specificity of renin kinetics in transgenic rats harboring the human renin and angiotensinogen genes. *Proc Natl Acad Sci U S A* 1992;89(16):7806–10.

13. Hartmann A, Buttinger C, Rommel T, et al. Alteration of intracranial pressure, cerebral blood flow, autoregulation and carbon dioxide-reactivity by hypotensive agents in baboons with intracranial hypertension. *Neurochirurgia* 1989;32(2):37–43.

14. Hennes HJ, Jantzen JP. Effects of fenoldopam on intracranial pressure and hemodynamic variables at normal and elevated intracranial pressure in anesthetized pigs. *J Neurosurg Anesthesiol* 1994;6(3):175–81.

15. Immink RV, van den Born BJ, van Montfrans GA, et al. Impaired cerebral autoregulation in patients with malignant hypertension. *Circulation* 2004;110(15):2241–5.

16. Kitiyakara C, Guzman NJ. Malignant hypertension and hypertensive emergencies. *J Am Soc Nephrol* 1998;9(1):133–42.

17. Leenen FH, Balfe JA, Pelech AN, et al. Postoperative hypertension after repair of coarctation of aorta in children: Protective effect of propranolol? *Am Heart J* 1987;113(5):1164–73.

18. MacKenzie ET, Strandgaard S, Graham DI, et al. Effects of acutely induced hypertension in cats on pial arteriolar caliber, local cerebral blood flow, and the blood-brain barrier. *Circulation Research* 1976;39(1):33–41.

19. Montgomery HE, Kiernan LA, Whitworth CE, et al. Inhibition of tissue angiotensin-converting enzyme activity prevents malignant hypertension in TGR(mREN2)27. *J Hypertension* 1998;16(5):635–43.

20. Morgenstern BZ. Dosage guidelines for pediatric hypertension. *Mayo Clin Proc* 1995;70(4):406–7 [see comment, *Mayo Clin Proc.* 1994;69(11):1098–107].

21. Muller DN, Dechend R, Mervaala EM, et al. NF-kappaB inhibition ameliorates angiotensin II-induced inflammatory damage in rats. *Hypertension* 2000;35(1 Pt 2):193–201.

22. Mullins JJ, Peters J, Ganten D, Fulminant hypertension in transgenic rats harbouring the mouse Ren-2 gene. *Nature* 1990;344(6266):541–4.

23. Murphy MB, Murray C, Shorten GD. Fenoldopam: A selective peripheral dopamine-receptor agonist for the treatment of severe hypertension. *New Engl J Med* 2001;345(21):1548–57.

24. National High Blood Pressure Education Program Working Group on High Blood Pressure in Children. The fourth report on the diagnosis, evaluation, and treatment of high blood pressure in children and adolescents. *Pediatrics* 2004;114(2 Suppl 4th Report):555–76.

25. Oparil S, Aronson S, Deeb GM, et al. Fenoldopam: A new parenteral antihypertensive: Consensus roundtable on the management of perioperative hypertension and hypertensive crises. *Am J Hypertension* 1999;12(7):653–64.

26. Rey E, LeLorier J, Burgess E, et al. Report of the Canadian Hypertension Society Consensus Conference: 3. Pharmacologic treatment of hypertensive disorders in pregnancy. *CMAJ* 1997;157(9):1245–54.

27. Schwartz RB, Mulkern RV, Gudbjartsson H, et al. Diffusion-weighted MR imaging in hypertensive encephalopathy: Clues to pathogenesis. *Am J Neuroradiol* 1998;19(5):859–62.

28. Smeda JS, Payne GW. Alterations in autoregulatory and myogenic function in the cerebrovasculature of Dahl salt-sensitive rats. *Stroke* 2003;34(6):1484–90.

29. Stefansson B, Ricksten A, Rymo L, et al. Angiotensin-converting enzyme gene I/D polymorphism in malignant hypertension. *Blood Press* 2000;9(2–3):104–9.

30. Strandgaard S. Autoregulation of cerebral blood flow in hypertensive patients. The modifying influence of prolonged antihypertensive treatment on the tolerance to acute, drug-induced hypotension. *Circulation* 1976;53(4):720–7.

31. Strandgaard S, Paulson OB. Cerebral blood flow in untreated and treated hypertension. *Nether J Med* 1995;47(4):180–4.

32. Tobias JD. Fenoldopam for controlled hypotension during spinal fusion in children and adolescents. *Paediatr Anaesth* 2000;10(3):261–6.

33. Torocsik HV, Curless RG, Post J, et al. FK506-induced leukoencephalopathy in children with organ transplants. *Neurology* 1999;52(7):1497–500.

34. Vacher E, Richer C, Cazaubon C, et al. Are vasopressin peripheral V1 receptors involved in the development of malignant hypertension and stroke in SHR-SPs? *Fundam Clin Pharmacol* 1995;9(5):469–78.

35. van den Born BJ, Honnebier UP, Koopmans RP, et al. Microangiopathic hemolysis and renal failure in malignant hypertension. *Hypertension* 2005;45(2):246–51.

36. Varon J, Marik PE. Clinical review: The management of hypertensive crises. *Crit Care (London)* 2003;7(5):374–84.

37. Varon J, Marik PE. The diagnosis and management of hypertensive crises. *Chest* 2000;118(1):214–27.

38. Vaughan CJ, Delanty N. Hypertensive emergencies. *Lancet* 2000;356(9227):411–7 [see comments, *Lancet* 2000;356(9239):1442–3].

39. Yoshida M, Nonoguchi H, Owada A, et al. Three cases of malignant hypertension: The roles of endothelin-1 and the renin-angiotensin-aldosterone system. *Clin Nephrol* 1994;42(5):295–9.

CHAPTER 98 ■ INBORN ERRORS OF METABOLISM

MICHAEL WILHELM • WENDY CHUNG

Inborn errors of metabolism (IEMs) result from the deficiency of any one of over 400 enzymes involved in intermediary metabolism. Although individually rare, collectively, they are common in pediatrics. Many children with previously diagnosed IEMs will come to the PICU postoperatively or during an acute metabolic decompensation and require specialized cardiorespiratory management that will be dictated by their underlying IEM. Other children with previously unrecognized IEMs will present with a variety of symptoms, including change in mental status, shock, metabolic acidosis, vomiting, failure to thrive, developmental delay, intractable seizures, liver failure, and cardiomyopathy. Therefore, pediatric intensivists must have a fundamental understanding of these conditions, including when to suspect an IEM and how to initially manage these patients. This chapter provides a basic framework for approaching the patient with a suspected IEM, with particular focus on management issues confronted by the pediatric intensivist. Because of the large number of IEMs, some general concepts are presented initially, followed by specific discussions of the more important individual presentations and diseases.

GENERAL APPROACH TO INBORN ERRORS OF METABOLISM

Pathophysiology of Inborn Errors of Metabolism

Inborn errors often present with nonspecific manifestations that may culminate in critical illness, particularly in the young infant or neonate. Because these disorders result from enzyme deficiencies for which 50% of normal activity is usually adequate, they are inherited predominantly in an autosomal recessive fashion. In that the mitochondrial genome is maternally inherited, some mitochondrial disorders are matrilineally transmitted. Furthermore, many mitochondrial diseases depend upon the percentage of the mitochondrial population that carries the mutation (heteroplasmy); therefore, manifestations depend on the load of mutant mitochondria in each tissue. Thus, a given mutation may produce varying manifestations in different family members. Specific disorders with X-linked inheritance that predominantly affect males are identified in the appropriate sections of this chapter.

IEMs manifest either as a result of the lack of products of the deficient enzyme, accumulation of upstream metabolites, shunting of accumulated metabolites into other pathways, or some combination thereof. Pathophysiologically, IEMs presenting in the PICU can be categorized into one of the following processes: (a) intoxication from a metabolite such as ammonia, amino acid derivatives, or ketoacids; (b) reduced fasting tolerance; (c) derangements of energy metabolism; (d) derangement of neurotransmission; or (e) storage of nonmetabolizable substrates in vital organs or tissues. Disorders associated with each of these categories are listed in **Table 98.1**.

Clinical Presentation and Differential Diagnosis

Historical Clues

The history and physical examination may provide clues that a patient has an IEM. Commonly, IEMs present with changes in mental status (lethargy, irritability, seizures, and coma) with or without overt cardiorespiratory compromise and can be easily confused with sepsis. Furthermore, infection often exacerbates metabolic derangements and precipitates metabolic decompensation due to increased energy requirements and the frequent association with decreased food intake. Finally, certain IEMs make patients more susceptible to infection, such as *Escherichia coli* sepsis in galactosemia, and neutropenia associated with many organic acidurias. Therefore, empiric treatment for suspected sepsis should be initiated after obtaining appropriate cultures. The history may reveal decreased oral intake, often associated with an intercurrent infection or with fasting, as occurs when infants begin to sleep through the night. Neonates may present with failure to regain birth weight by the second week of life. The older child may present with recurrent episodes of lethargy and difficulty in recovering from minor illnesses. Children of all ages often demonstrate failure to thrive.

In rare cases, the specific dietary intake may suggest the diagnosis. Particular foods, such as a high-protein meal, may induce symptoms, including nausea in urea cycle defects. Children with partial enzymatic deficiencies and milder disorders may even unknowingly alter their diet to avoid foods that make them feel lethargic or ill.

A history of developmental delay, hypotonia, and/or seizures is associated with many IEMs. A history of developmental regression is particularly concerning and should prompt a careful search for an IEM, particularly the lysosomal storage disorders and mitochondrial disorders.

Metabolic disease may be suggested by features of the family history, including parental consanguinity, ethnicity of the patient (hepatorenal tyrosinemia in French Canadians and maple syrup urine disease, MSUD, in Pennsylvania Amish); history of sudden, unexplained death (e.g., sudden infant death

TABLE 98.1

CATEGORIES OF INBORN ERRORS OF METABOLISM WITH ACUTE PRESENTATIONS

Pathophysiology	Likely disorders
Intoxication (Encephalopathy)	Urea cycle*, organic acidemias*, aminoacidopathies*
Reduced fasting tolerance	Glycogen storage disease type 1, disorders of gluconeogenesis, fatty acid oxidation defects
Impaired Energy Production	Mitochondrial disorders, fatty acid oxidation disorders, and disorders of the pyruvate dehydrogenase complex
Altered neurotransmission	Pyridoxine- or folinic acid-dependent epilepsy, nonketotic hyperglycinemia, sulfite oxidase deficiency
Storage disorders/complex macromolecules	Mucopolysaccharidoses, sphingolipidoses, glycogen storage diseases, peroxisomal biogenesis disorders, congenital disorders of glycosylation

*Denotes diseases that may require emergent dialysis.

syndrome); developmental delay; seizures; failure to thrive; or other unexplained chronic illness in a sibling or other family member. Although the prenatal history is often unremarkable, a history of maternal liver disease or HELLP (hemolysis, elevated liver enzymes, and low platelets) syndrome may suggest a long-chain fatty acid oxidation disorder. The sex of the patient is relevant in a small number of IEMs that are X-linked, such as the urea cycle defect ornithine transcarbamylase deficiency, the carbohydrate defect pyruvate dehydrogenase deficiency E1α, and the defect of the nucleotide salvage pathway, Lesch-Nyhan disease.

Findings on Physical Examination

On physical examination, the presence of an unusual body or urine odor might suggest a specific organic acidemia (Table 98.2), but these odors can be subtle and their absence should not dissuade pursuit of an IEM. Careful attention should be paid to the respiratory pattern; although tachypnea may herald sepsis with acute respiratory distress syndrome, Kussmaul respirations occur with metabolic acidosis. Hypothermia may be associated with metabolic decompensation, especially in the urea cycle defects.

Progressive hepatosplenomegaly occurs in a number of IEMs as nonmetabolizable substrate accumulates in glycogen storage disorders and lysosomal storage disorders. Dysmorphic features are present at birth in a number of peroxisomal biogenesis disorders, fatty acid oxidation disorders, congenital disorders of glycosylation, and pyruvate dehydrogenase deficiency,

while they develop over time in the mucopolysaccharidoses (MPS) because storage material progressively accumulates in the soft tissues and bones. Smith-Lemli-Opitz syndrome, a defect in sterol biosynthesis, may present with ambiguous genitalia. Ophthalmologic examination may also provide clues to an IEM, with cataracts observed in galactosemia and other disorders, and retinal pigmentary changes appearing in Tay-Sachs disease and some mitochondrial disorders.

Myopathy demonstrated by hypotonia or cardiomyopathy (hypertrophic or dilated), possibly detected by heart murmur or signs of heart failure, may herald a disorder of fatty acid oxidation, mitochondrial derangement, glycogen storage disorder, or, rarely, a congenital disorder of glycosylation. As they can be treated and, in some cases, cured, it is important to exclude IEMs as causes of cardiomyopathy in children.

Laboratory Findings

Routine laboratory test results may also suggest an IEM (Tables 98.3 and 98.4). A primary respiratory alkalosis may be found with hyperammonemia caused by a urea cycle defect. A metabolic acidosis, particularly with an elevated anion gap (AG) or elevated lactate, also occurs in certain IEMs, though it may also occur in other diseases, such as sepsis or hypoperfusion. However, while patients with elevated lactate due to hypoperfusion appear quite ill, a patient with an IEM may have lactate elevations out of proportion to the degree of illness. Subtracting the lactate level (in mMol/L) from the AG (the lactate-adjusted AG) can provide further clues as to the etiology. In diseases of energy metabolism or hypoperfusion, the lactate-adjusted AG is normal, while it is elevated in the organic acidemias due to the presence of anions other than lactate. The lactate-to-pyruvate ratio is also helpful, with normal levels being about 20 when both concentrations are expressed in mMol/L. A consistent ratio of <10 suggests a pyruvate dehydrogenase deficiency, which has important therapeutic implications, while a consistent ratio of >25 occurs in tissue hypoxia, pyruvate carboxylase deficiency, and mitochondrial disorders.

Hypoglycemia may also occur in sepsis, liver disease, or any other severe illness, particularly in the neonate in whom the ability to mobilize glycogen stores is limited. However, in the setting of other clinical and laboratory findings listed here, hypoglycemia is much more likely to indicate an IEM. The

TABLE 98.2

ODORS ASSOCIATED WITH METABOLIC DISEASES

Odor	Associated inborn error(s)
Sweaty feet	Glutaric acidemia (type II), isovaleric academia
Maple syrup	Maple syrup urine disease
Mousy	Phenylketonuria
Boiled cabbage	Hypermethioninemia, tyrosinemia type I
Swimming pool	Hawkinsinuria
Rotten fish	Trimethylaminuria, dimethylglycinuria

TABLE 98.3

LABORATORY EVALUATION OF A SUSPECTED IEM

	Blood tests	Urine tests	CSF tests
Initial studies	Blood gas, dextrose stick, electrolytes, basic metabolic panel, ammonia, lactate, pyruvate, β-hydroxybutyrate, transaminases, blood count, coagulation profile, creatinine kinase	Ketones, pH, reducing substances	As indicated
Further workup	Plasma amino acids, plasma acylcarnitine profile, carnitine	Organic acids, amino acids	

relationship of hypoglycemia to feeding can be helpful in identifying a specific disease. Hypoglycemia that occurs immediately after ingestion of fructose (fruits or sweet foods containing sucrose), usually when an infant begins eating solid foods, suggests hereditary fructose intolerance. Hereditary fructose intolerance can be further suggested by the presence of reducing substance in the urine. In most other IEMs, including the glycogen storage diseases, fatty acid oxidation defects, disorders of gluconeogenesis, and some organic acidemias, hypoglycemia occurs with fasting.

The presence or absence of ketones can further narrow the differential diagnosis. Normally, in the setting of hypoglycemia, the liver mobilizes ketone bodies as an alternative energy substrate. Therefore, nonketotic hypoglycemia suggests a defect in fatty acid oxidation or ketogenesis. Although normal neonates effectively generate 3-hydroxybutyrate, they have a limited capacity to generate acetoacetate. Because urine dipsticks detect only acetoacetate, serum 3–hydroxybutyrate levels must be evaluated in the hypoglycemic infant. Conversely, a positive urine dip for ketones in the first month is always abnormal and suggests an organic acidemia or inability to utilize ketone bodies (13). Elevated ketone levels in the nonfasting/nonhypoglycemic patient suggest an organic acidemia or MSUD.

Evidence of hepatic injury or dysfunction provides another clue to a possible IEM. This includes elevation of transaminases, as well as hyperammonemia and coagulopathy. Although hyperammonemia may occur in liver injury, including that due to sepsis and toxins, levels greater than 400 μmol/L suggest a urea cycle defect and require swift and aggressive intervention to prevent irreversible brain damage. Disorders of mitochondrial metabolism, fatty acid oxidation disorders, and the organic acidemias may all cause secondary hyperammonemia due to interactions between these pathways and the urea cycle within the mitochondria. However, in these disorders, ammonia is elevated to a much lesser degree than in the urea cycle defects. In the setting of severe decompensation, a number of IEMs may present with elevated transaminases and coagulopathy. Mitochondrial disorders, neonatal hemochromatosis, Wilson disease, hepatorenal tyrosinemia, galactosemia, Crigler-Najjar syndrome, and Niemann-Pick disease may all present with prominent liver injury.

Although individually, each of the above historical, physical, or laboratory findings may occur in a number of disease states, the combination of several of these features increases the likelihood that a patient has an IEM. In addition to supporting the diagnosis of an IEM, the initial lab studies help to point to specific etiologies (**Fig. 98.1**). Once an IEM is suspected, specific metabolic tests should be performed, including urine organic acids, plasma amino acids, the plasma carnitine levels, and acylcarnitine profile, as well as other specific tests dictated by the suggested diagnoses. These samples should preferably be obtained before therapy, because pathognomonic metabolites may clear rapidly with resuscitative therapy. Definitive diagnosis, beginning with the biochemical signature of the tests just mentioned, often requires tissue for enzymatic assays and/or

TABLE 98.4

RESULTS OF INITIAL LABORATORY TESTS IN IEMS

	Urea cycle defect	Amino acidopathy	Organic aciduria	Fatty acid oxidation disorder	Carbohydrate metabolism	Electron transport chain
Blood pH	↑	↓/–	↓	↓/–	↓	↓
Anion gap	WNL	↑/–	↑	↑/–	↑	↑
Glucose	WNL	+/–	WNL	↓↓	↓↓	+/–
Ammonia	↑↑	WNL	↑	↑	WNL	WNL
Lactate	WNL	WNL	↑/–	WNL	↑	↑↑
Ketones	Neg	↑	↑	↓↓	↑	Neg
LFTs	WNL	WNL	WNL	↑	↑	WNL
Serum amino acids	Abnormal	Abnormal	Abnormal	WNL	WNL	Alanine high
Urine organic acids	Some abnormal	Abnormal	Abnormal	Abnormal	WNL	Lactate in urine
Urine reducing substances	–	–	–	–	+/–	–

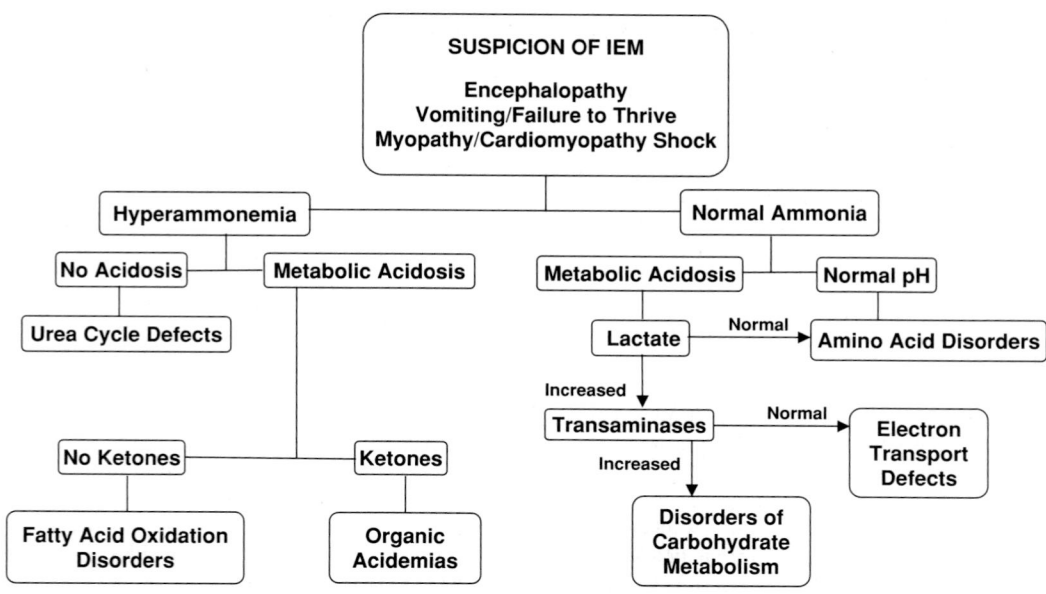

FIGURE 98.1.

molecular genetic testing, and may require several weeks to months for complete evaluation.

Clinical Management Principles

As in all cases, initial management begins with provision of adequate respiratory and circulatory support. As will be discussed later in this chapter, securing the airway may require advanced techniques in certain patients with storage diseases (e.g., MPS). A number of complications of IEMs may require respiratory support. Encephalopathy may render a patient unable to protect her airway. With profound metabolic acidosis, even with adequate energy production, patients may not maintain an adequate minute ventilation, particularly during infancy. In older children who are capable of generating large tidal volumes, it may be difficult to maintain an equivalent minute ventilation after administration of neuromuscular blockade. Acute worsening of acidosis may necessitate treatment of further complications (i.e., hyperkalemia, worsened cardiovascular function).

Because many of these diseases are associated with emesis and anorexia, patients often present with dehydration. However, care must be exerted in volume resuscitation of patients who may have a complicating cardiomyopathy or cerebral edema. Obviously, rapid correction of hypoglycemia requires a bolus of dextrose (2–4 cc/kg of 25% dextrose solution). Furthermore, if an IEM is strongly suspected, all patients should be placed in NPO status and given sufficient intravenous glucose (~10 mg/kg/min) to prevent catabolism of amino acids and fatty acids, which may increase the production of abnormal metabolic products. Rarely, glucose will exacerbate lactic acidosis, suggesting an error in the pyruvate dehydrogenase complex, in which case, changing to a ketogenic diet will improve the metabolic acidosis. Older patients with intoxication syndromes may present with cerebral edema and, because their sutures are closed, are at greater risk for intracranial hypertension during therapy than are neonates. Management of the cerebral edema is discussed more extensively in Chapter 56. IV

fluids must provide adequate sodium to prevent hyponatremia, which could exacerbate this situation.

Disease-specific therapies must sometimes be initiated empirically prior to obtaining a specific metabolic diagnosis, which will be discussed in their respective sections in this chapter. However, in diseases in which symptoms result from toxic metabolic intermediates (**Table 98.1**), specifically in the setting of hyperammonemia in urea cycle defects or elevated plasma leucine levels in MSUD, direct elimination of these toxins is crucial and must be accomplished quickly to prevent irreversible brain damage. Initial approaches included exchange transfusion with or without peritoneal dialysis, with peritoneal dialysis superior to exchange transfusion alone (4,28). However, with the advent of effective continuous venovenous hemofiltration and dialysis (CVVHD) in children, this has become the method of choice when available (10,36). CVVHD has been shown to clear ammonia more rapidly than peritoneal dialysis in neonates and is particularly more rapid at clearing elevated leucine levels (29). Optimal clearance depends on high blood flow rates (and hence catheter size) and dialysis rate (29). Many patients were able to achieve clearance rates similar to those seen with intermittent hemodialysis without the associated rebound hyperammonemia. Importantly, it was also shown that rapid elimination of ammonia or leucine correlated with improved neurodevelopmental outcome. Hemofiltration and dialysis have even been used successfully in patients with IEMs that required extracorporeal membrane oxygenation support (33).

Those diseases that produce neonatal epileptic encephalopathy are another category that deserve brief mention here. In this setting, a trial of intravenous pyridoxine and folinic acid may produce rapid and dramatic improvement. A number of metabolic diseases require supplementation of specific vitamins or cofactors, as listed elsewhere in this chapter. Given the low toxicity of these agents, they should be initiated before confirmation of a definitive diagnosis if the specific disease is within the differential diagnosis. General recommendations for empiric therapy based on suspected disease category are provided

TABLE 98.5

SUPPLEMENTAL THERAPY FOR METABOLIC EMERGENCIES

Suspected category of IEM	Empiric therapy	Rationale
Urea cycle	L-Arginine 600 mg/kg over 90 mins and 200–600 mg/kg/24 hr	Essential amino acid in all but arginase deficiency
	Sodium benzoate 250 mg/kg over 90 mins and 250 mg/kg/day	Condenses with glycine to enhance nitrogen excretion
	Sodium phenylacetate 250 mg/kg over 90 mins and 250 mg/kg/day	Condenses with glutamine to enhance nitrogen excretion
	Sodium phenylbutyrate 100–200 mg/kg PO TID	Source of phenylacetate to enhance nitrogen excretion once patient is stabilized
Biotinidase deficiency and multiple carboxylase deficiency	Biotin 10–15 mg/kg/d PO	Replace biotin that is not adequately recycled
Methylmalonic academia and methionine synthase deficiency	Hydroxycobalamin 1–5 mg/d IM/IV	Enzymatic cofactor
Organic acidurias, carnitine transport defects, and fatty acid oxidation disorders	L-Carnitine 50–100 mg/d divided b.i.d. IV/PO	Replace carnitine losses
Propionic acidemia	Metronidazole 15 mg/kg q 8–12 hr PO/IV	Inhibit production of propionate by intestinal bacteria
MSUD	Thiamine 150 mg/d IV/PO; >3 years 300 mg/d	Enzymatic cofactor
Mitochondrial disorders	Coenzyme Q10 25 mg t.i.d. Carnitine 50 mg/kg b.i.d. α lipoic acid 100 mg q.d. B complex vitamins (100 mg each q.d.) Vitamin E 50 units q.d.	Cofactors and antioxidants
Ketotic hyperglycinemia	Sodium benzoate 250 mg/kg over 90 mins and 250 mg/kg/day	Condenses with glycine to enhance nitrogen excretion

in **Table 98.5.** In all cases, early involvement of a metabolic disease specialist ensures optimal management of these complex patients.

Postmortem Evaluation

Unfortunately, some patients with a suspected IEM will die, despite aggressive therapy, prior to a specific diagnosis being established. In this setting, the postmortem diagnosis can have significant implications for the patient's siblings and for genetic counseling. Therefore, obtaining appropriate specimens for analysis is crucial. Approximately 5–10 mL of plasma should be collected in a lithium or sodium heparin tube, separated, and frozen at –70°C. An additional sample of blood should be collected in EDTA and stored at room temperature for up to several days for DNA extraction for future genetic analysis. The earliest sample of urine obtained during the illness should be frozen, as should several milliliters of cerebrospinal fluid. Tissue samples should ideally be obtained as part of a complete autopsy. However, selected tissues can be helpful if the family refuses autopsy. A punch skin biopsy should be obtained pre- or postmortem for a fibroblast culture for enzymatic testing. Postmortem kidney, liver, muscle, and cardiac biopsies should also be performed. Tissues should ideally be obtained as soon as possible after death to preserve enzymatic activity, and they should be immediately frozen in liquid nitrogen and stored at –70°C. Samples of bile may also provide important information. Again, consultation with a metabolic specialist and careful discussion with the pathologist are extremely important.

Impact of Neonatal Screening

Newborn screening programs have existed in the US for more than 40 years and are administered on a state level. Although dramatic differences in the disorders screened can be noted from state to state, in accordance with the consensus recommendation of the American College of Medical Genetics, over two-thirds of all babies born in the US are screened for the minimum 29 recommended disorders (http://www.mchb.hrsa.gov/screening). A number of online resources will identify the tests currently performed in any given state (http://genes-r-us.uthscsa.edu). With the widespread use of tandem mass spectrometry in the last 5 years, the number of identifiable IEMs has increased dramatically. The results of the child's newborn screening should be obtained if an IEM is suspected. At the same time, however, a normal neonatal screening test does not exclude the possibility of an IEM in a critically ill patient since not all IEMs can be screened by this methodology and, in some cases, deranged metabolism will be episodic with fluctuations in energy requirements.

DISORDERS ASSOCIATED WITH LACTIC ACIDOSIS

Symptoms of lactic acidosis include poor feeding, failure to thrive, lethargy, change in mental status, seizures, hypotonia, ataxia, developmental delay, optic nerve atrophy, deafness, and dysfunction of the most energy-dependent organs, including the brain, heart, muscle, kidney, and liver. As a general rule, the greater the number of systems involved, the greater the likelihood of a mitochondrial disorder of oxidative phosphorylation. The family history may suggest an IEM when children within the nuclear family have been previously affected or when individuals on the maternal side of the family have been similarly, but more or less severely, affected due to mutations in the maternally transmitted, mitochondrial-encoded genes.

Lactic acidosis results from accumulation of pyruvate, which is converted into lactic acid and alanine. *Primary* lactic acidemia results from defects in gluconeogenesis or in oxidative phosphorylation. Definitive diagnoses of the IEMs that cause primary lactic acidosis are often challenging and frequently require tissue biopsies for enzymatic analysis in specialized laboratories and/or genetic testing. Treatment in these cases is often started empirically prior to a definitive diagnosis.

Secondary lactic acidemia results from either anaerobic metabolism or other IEMs that produce less significant degrees of lactic acidosis, often only detectable during an acute metabolic crisis. Secondary lactic academia is a consequence of decreased flux through oxidative phosphorylation due to tissue hypoxia or hypoperfusion. Within the intensive care setting, causes of secondary lactic academia are much more common than primary etiologies. Many conditions in the PICU promote tissue hypoxia or hypoperfusion sufficient to cause lactic acidosis. In addition, liver injury or malperfusion prevents the normal conversion of lactate into pyruvate. However, one must be cautious, because severe metabolic decompensation due to an IEM can also be associated with cardiopulmonary failure. Therefore, IEMs should always be considered when the underlying cause of tissue hypoxia is unknown. The differential diagnosis of IEMs causing secondary lactic acidosis includes many of the organic acidemias (propionic and methylmalonic acidemia), which are associated with accumulation of other acids to a greater extent than lactate and can be readily identified by analyzing urine for organic acids.

The first step in investigating lactic acidemia is to ensure that the lactic acid is truly elevated. The levels of lactic acid can be artifactually elevated by use of a tourniquet, difficulty obtaining the blood sample, or prolonged time between sample collection and analysis. If a primary lactic acidemia is strongly suggested by a significant elevation of lactate of greater than twice the normal level (3 mol/L), arterial or free-flowing venous blood from a catheter should be obtained. Consideration should be given to measuring lactic acid from the cerebrospinal fluid if any neurologic symptoms are present, even without elevated plasma lactate. Fluctuations in levels of lactate with feeding may suggest the underlying etiology. Lactate is most elevated after a prolonged fast in disorders of gluconeogenesis (fructose bisphosphatase deficiency), and provocative, carefully monitored fasting studies may be necessary to evaluate these diagnoses. In the setting of fasting lactic acidosis, measurement of biotinidase can identify readily treatable cases of biotinidase deficiency. In other cases of gluconeogenic defects, the patient should be treated by avoiding fasting.

In defects of oxidative phosphorylation, lactate levels may fluctuate significantly in the blood or may only be elevated in the cerebrospinal fluid. Simultaneous measurement of pyruvate allows determination of the lactate to pyruvate ratio, which reflects the redox potential of the cell, and ratios greater than 25 suggest a defect in mitochondrial oxidative phosphorylation.

Repeated simultaneous measurement of lactate and pyruvate and their relative ratios is often helpful to establish a consistent ratio. Measuring alanine in the blood and cerebrospinal fluid also allows for an independent, indirect measurement of defective pyruvate metabolism and is not subject to the same difficulties in measurement as lactate. If a defect in mitochondrial oxidative phosphorylation is suspected, a muscle biopsy should be performed to search for ragged red fibers, as well as to biochemically assess the respiratory chain complexes. In addition, specific genetic testing for conditions such as MELAS (*m*itochondrial *e*ncephalopathy, *l*actic *a*cidosis, and *s*troke) and MERRF (*m*itochondrial *e*ncephalopathy with *r*agged *r*ed *f*ibers) are available. Defects of the pyruvate dehydrogenase complex should be treated with a high-fat, low-carbohydrate diet and supplementation with thiamine and lipoic acid. Most of the other mitochondrial defects of oxidative phosphorylation are difficult to treat but can be empirically treated with thiamine, riboflavin, nicotinamide, vitamin K, and co-enzyme Q10 while a definitive diagnosis is being established (**Table 98.5**). Sodium bicarbonate can be used to correct the metabolic acidosis, but it will not decrease lactic acid production. Experimentally, dichloroacetate has been used to treat lactic acidosis; it works by activating the pyruvate dehydrogenase complex (30). In most cases, however, dichloroacetate is not appropriate for long-term clinical care outside of study protocols, because it is still under investigation and has been associated with toxic neuropathy.

METABOLIC ACIDOSIS WITHOUT INCREASED LACTATE

Although any metabolic disease may present with modest lactic acidosis during an acute decompensation because of the associated dehydration or hypoperfusion, the organic acidemias and aminoacidopathies typically present with an AG acidosis due to accumulation of the abnormal organic acids or ketoacids, but the AG is *not* predominantly due to elevated lactate. As mentioned previously, the lactate-adjusted AG is abnormal in these conditions. Many of these disorders present with significant ketoacidosis, though some (3-hydroxy-3-methylglutaric aciduria and acyl CoA dehydrogenase deficiency) do not. Classically, the organic acidurias present as massive ketosis and metabolic acidosis in a vomiting or lethargic neonate. Establishing a specific etiology typically depends upon determination, often by mass spectrometry, of urine organic acids and serum amino acids. These disorders are included in the recommended list of IEMs for inclusion in newborn screening programs, and chronic treatment of most of them requires carefully balanced protein intake to provide an adequate supply of essential amino acids and minimization of the load of precursors that cannot be metabolized.

Most disorders of metabolic acidosis without increased lactate present as intoxication syndromes with episodes of encephalopathy and vomiting, particularly during periods of catabolic stress. Thus, they tend to present during the early neonatal period in an infant who initially appears well or during an intercurrent illness. The most common disorders within this category are MSUD, methylmalonic academia. and propionic acidemia. The age-specific differential diagnoses for metabolic acidosis without elevated plasma lactate are listed in

TABLE 98.6

AGE-SPECIFIC DIFFERENTIAL DIAGNOSIS OF METABOLIC ACIDOSIS WITHOUT INCREASED LACTATE

Age at presentation	Metabolic derangement
Neonate	MSUD, isovaleric acidemia, glutaric acidemia type II, multiple carboxylase deficiency
Infant	MSUD, methylmalonic acidemia, propionic acidemia, ketotic hyperglycinemia, biotinidase deficiency
Older children	Biotinidase deficiency, dietary biotin deficiency

MSUD, maple syrup urine disease

Table 98.6. Because intoxication plays a central role, extracorporeal toxin removal with hemodialysis or hemofiltration may be useful in the acute management of some of these conditions, including MSUD.

MSUD is a disorder of metabolism of the essential, branched-chain amino acids: valine, leucine, and isoleucine. Normally, the enzyme complex branched-chain α-ketoacid dehydrogenase, which requires thiamine pyrophosphate as a coenzyme, decarboxylates all three branched-chain amino acids. Infants with the classic form present in the first few days of life with vomiting, encephalopathy, and severe metabolic acidosis. The characteristic odor of urine, sweat, and cerumen can provide an important clue to the diagnosis. MSUD has an increased incidence in the Old Order Amish and Mennonites (27) and Ashkenazi Jewish populations (11). Milder forms, with greater residual enzyme activity, may present in older children during stress (e.g., infection, surgery) and may be associated with a history of mild developmental delay or failure to thrive. Acute episodes in these nonclassical forms are indistinguishable from those of classic MSUD. Some patients respond dramatically to thiamine supplementation, which should be started empirically in all patients upon presentation.

Isovaleric acidemia results from a deficiency of isovaleryl CoA dehydrogenase, which is further down the leucine degradative pathway. The acute form presents much like MSUD, though patients have a characteristic odor of sweaty socks and may have associated neutropenia.

Propionic acid and methylmalonic acid are sequential catabolic products of isoleucine and valine, as well as threonine, methionine, cholesterol, and odd-chain fatty acids. Deficiency of the enzymes responsible for their catabolism (propionyl CoA carboxylase and methylmalonyl CoA mutase, respectively) results in ketotic hyperglycinemia. Because methylmalonyl CoA mutase requires adenosylcobalamin (a metabolite of vitamin B_{12}) as a coenzyme, disorders of cobalamin metabolism may also result in secondary methylmalonic acidemia. These conditions all present with vomiting, severe ketoacidosis, encephalopathy that progresses to coma, and neutropenia. Because of secondary inhibition of the urea cycle, moderate to severe hyperammonemia may also occur. In addition to supportive care, constipation should be prevented or treated and sterilization of the intestinal tract with metronidazole should be initiated to minimize production of propionic acid by intestinal bacteria. Carnitine supplementation

(50–100 mg/kg/24 hr IV or orally) replaces losses due to propionyl-carnitine formation and hastens resolution of metabolic acidosis. Because propionic acidemia may occur as part of multiple carboxylase deficiency (see later discussion), biotin (10 mg/24 hrs) should be provided until a definitive diagnosis is established. Similarly, large doses of cobalamin (1–2 mg IV/24 hr) should be provided to patients with suspected methylmalonic acidemia.

Several other IEMs, including disorders that affect the four biotin-dependent carboxylases, may present primarily with metabolic acidosis, ketosis, and an intoxication syndrome. Deficiency of holocarboxylase synthetase, which catalyzes the binding of biotin to all of the carboxylases, results in the most severe disorder and presents in the first few weeks of life. These patients have rashes that mimic eczema and a tomcat urine odor in addition to the already mentioned metabolic derangements. Biotinidase deficiency presents similarly in older infants and children and may be associated with an eczematoid rash. Dietary biotin deficiency may occur in short-gut syndrome, inadequate supplementation in parenteral nutrition, prolonged anticonvulsant therapy (23), and significant raw egg consumption. Biotinidase deficiency and acquired biotin deficiency both respond well to biotin supplementation (10 mg/24 hr) and can be cured with this simple therapy.

Novel Therapies

Liver transplantation has been performed in more than 10 patients with MSUD (3) and provides improved dietary protein tolerance and apparent elimination of episodic decompensations (6). Insufficient long-term follow-up exists to determine whether the risks and costs of this procedure outweigh the benefits. Liver transplantation (with simultaneous renal transplant in methylmalonic academia) (26) has been performed in a small number of patients with other organic acidemias (10). Although initial results suggested an improvement, long-term prognosis remains guarded. Unfortunately, many children develop irreversible neurocognitive deficits prior to transplantation.

HYPOGLYCEMIA

Children with hypoglycemia may present with diaphoresis, pallor, irritability, decreased feeding, jitteriness, temperature instability, lethargy, coma, or seizure. Hypoglycemia must be promptly recognized and treated to prevent damage to the brain. Severe and/or recurrent hypoglycemia can result in permanent brain damage, producing a range of injuries that include global mental retardation, behavioral problems, attention deficit disorder, and occipital blindness.

Hypoglycemia is defined as a serum concentration of less than 50 mg/dL or a whole blood concentration of less than 45 mg/dL. Historically, some neonatologists defined hypoglycemia as <35 mg/dL in a term infant, or <25 mg/dL in the preterm infant. However, it is advisable to maintain glucose concentrations greater than at least 40 mg/dL even in a neonate. A patient can appear artifactually hypoglycemic if the blood has been sitting for several hours. Therefore, hypoglycemia should be confirmed with the bedside glucometer reading and a stat measurement.

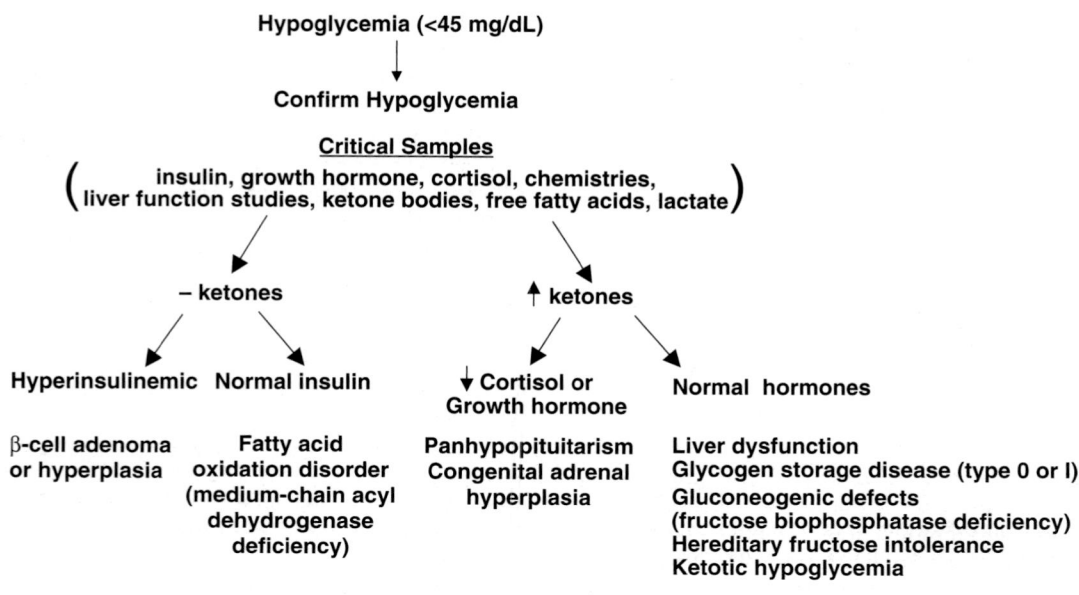

FIGURE 98.2. Etiology at the time of hypoglycemia.

Hypoglycemia must be treated promptly and continuously reassessed. Recurrent hypoglycemia is more likely to suggest a serious underlying disorder that will require definitive diagnosis and treatment. Acute treatment in the intensive care setting consists of a bolus of intravenous dextrose, 0.5–1 g/kg given as a 10%–25% solution, followed by continuous dextrose infusion to maintain a glucose concentration >70 mg/dL (usually 3–5 mg/kg/min in older children and 5–10 mg/kg/min in neonates). An IV line should be in place at all times, and glucose should be monitored at least every 4 hrs to ensure normoglycemia.

Although sometimes difficult, it is diagnostically ideal to evaluate the etiology at the time of hypoglycemia (**Fig. 98.2**). Common etiologies of hypoglycemia are listed in **Table 98.7**. Evaluation of the metabolic status during the time of derangement is essential to produce the maximal diagnostic yield. If it is not possible to obtain the critical samples at the time of hypoglycemia, carefully monitored fasting and glucagon challenge studies can be performed later to attempt to replicate the hypoglycemia and obtain critical samples. At the time of hypoglycemia, it is necessary to evaluate the hormonal response, including insulin, growth hormone, and cortisol as well as alternate metabolic substrates, including the appropriate production of ketone bodies. The critical sample should consist of glucose, insulin, growth hormone, cortisol, serum chemistries, liver function tests, ammonia, β-hydroxybutyrate, acetoacetate, free fatty acids, and lactate. Insulin measured at the time of hypoglycemia should normally be extremely low or undetectable. Additionally, ketone bodies and free fatty acids should be extremely elevated in the normal physiologic response to hypoglycemia. Failure to appropriately produce ketone bodies during hypoglycemia suggests either inappropriate hyperinsulinemia or a defect in the oxidation of fatty acids or ketone body production. Fatty acid oxidation disorders can then be further evaluated with an acylcarnitine profile, free and total carnitines, urine organic acids, and urine acylglycines.

The timing of the hypoglycemia in relationship to meals may offer clues to the etiology. Hypoglycemia immediately after a meal suggests provocation by some component of the ingested substance. Infants with hereditary fructose intolerance

TABLE 98.7

COMMON CATEGORIES AND CAUSES OF HYPOGLYCEMIA

Endocrinopathies
  Growth hormone deficiency
  Cortisol deficiency
  Hyperinsulinism
  • Infants of diabetic mothers
  • Beckwith-Wiedemann syndrome
  • Surreptitious insulin

Defective hepatic glucose release and/or utilization of available gluconeogenic substrate
  Ketotic hypoglycemia
  Enzymatic defects
  • Glycogen storage diseases (glycogen synthetase deficiency, glucose-6-phosphatase deficiency)
  • Galactosemia (galactose-1-phosphate uridyltransferase deficiency)
  • Hereditary fructose intolerance (fructose-1-phosphate aldolase)

Fatty acid oxidation or ketogenesis disorders
  Carnitine acyl transferase deficiency
  Long-chain fatty acid acyl-CoA dehydrogenase deficiency
  Medium-chain fatty acid acyl-CoA dehydrogenase deficiency
  Short-chain fatty acid acyl-CoA dehydrogenase deficiency
  Hydroxymethylglutaryl CoA lyase deficiency

Toxic
  Salicylate
  Acetaminophen
  Alcohol
  Oral hypoglycemic agents (biguanides, sulfonylureas)

typically present at ~6 months of age, when transitioning from breast milk or formula to solid foods, including fruits and vegetables. Within ~30 mins of ingesting foods that contain fructose or sucrose, patients will become acutely hypoglycemic and have transient elevations of transaminases and lactic acid. Treatment for hereditary fructose intolerance consists solely of eliminating fructose and sucrose from the diet and is compatible with normal health, growth, and development. Hypoglycemia associated with a high-protein diet can be provoked by high levels of leucine in disorders such as a deficiency of glutamate dehydrogenase, which results in hyperinsulinemic hyperammonemia. Hypoglycemia and liver dysfunction in infancy can also be caused by ingestion of breast milk or cow's milk-based formulas in galactosemia, but most cases are now diagnosed by newborn screening and readily treated with a soy-based formula.

Hypoglycemia can also be associated with ingestion of toxins or medications. Oral hypoglycemic agents, such as the sulfonylureas, can produce acute, rapid hypoglycemia. Other agents, such as aspirin, acetaminophen, ethanol, and any hepatotoxic agent, can cause hypoglycemia. Generally, the age of the patient and a thorough history will suggest this etiology.

Hypoglycemia associated with fasting for ~8 hrs is most characteristic of glycogen storage disorders, such as glycogen storage disorder type I (glucose-6-phosphatase deficiency) or glycogen storage disorder type 0 (glycogen synthase deficiency). These disorders frequently present as infants begin to sleep through the night, with increased fasting intervals and/or during periods of intercurrent illness associated with anorexia or vomiting. Children with type I glycogen storage disease also have an associated biochemical profile of lactic acidosis, hyperalaninemia, hyperuricemia, and hyperlipidemia. Hypoglycemia associated with fasting for ~16 hrs is more characteristic of defects in gluconeogenesis (fructose-1,6-bisphosphatase deficiency, glycerol kinase deficiency, pyruvate carboxylase deficiency, or pyruvate kinase deficiency) or fatty acid oxidation disorders. After ~16–24 hrs, all of the glycogen reserves have been utilized and the body begins to rely on gluconeogenesis and fatty acid oxidation. Definitive diagnosis of all of these conditions requires genetic testing or enzyme assays in leukocytes, fibroblasts, or, in some cases, liver. Treatment for these disorders consists of avoiding fasting and dietary modifications.

Hyperinsulinemia that causes hypoglycemia can be due to exogenous or endogenous insulin. An insulin value of greater than 10 U/mL simultaneous with hypoglycemia is always abnormal. Levels of C-peptide can differentiate the source of insulin because C-peptide is produced only with endogenous insulin. Endogenous hyperinsulinemia typically presents within the neonatal period and can produce the most severe, persistent, and difficult-to-manage hypoglycemia. Persistent dextrose requirements of 10 mg/kg/min suggest underlying hyperinsulinemia. Hyperinsulinemia may ultimately require treatment with diazoxide to inhibit insulin secretion, partial pancreatectomy if evidence is seen of an islet cell adenoma, or near complete pancreatectomy for diffuse islet cell hyperplasia. More extensive discussion of hyperinsulinemia is presented in Chapter 92.

Hypoglycemia is more common in neonates who are small for gestational age or in preterm infants in the first few days of life. Additionally, maternal diabetes may lead to perina-tal hyperinsulinemia and hypoglycemia in the neonate. Hypoglycemia in these situations is always associated with ketosis and usually resolves within the first few days to weeks of life.

Patients with liver disease are also more prone to hypoglycemia due to the decreased capacity of the liver to supply glucose through glycogenolysis and gluconeogenesis. Though other causes of hypoglycemia must be excluded, these patients respond to symptomatic treatment with IV glucose.

Physical examination may also provide useful clues as to the etiology of hypoglycemia. A baby who is large for gestational age and hypoglycemic suggests an infant of a diabetic mother. Macrosomia, hemihypertrophy, macroglossia, umbilical hernia, and ear pits or creases in a neonate suggest Beckwith-Wiedemann syndrome. Midline defects with a cleft lip and/or palate or a small penis may suggest panhypopituitarism. Hepatomegaly suggests a glycogen storage disorder or nonspecific liver disease. Inverted nipples and decreased gluteal fat suggest a congenital disorder of glycosylation that may be associated with hyperinsulinemia.

A common and relatively benign cause of hypoglycemia is ketotic hypoglycemia, often seen in toddlers and young children. These children appropriately mobilize fats and have massive ketosis during periods of hypoglycemia and are most often symptomatic during an intercurrent illness associated with anorexia or a vomiting. Ketotic hypoglycemia can be treated simply by avoiding fasting for more than 12 hrs at a time and is usually outgrown by the age of 5 to 10 years.

HYPERAMMONEMIA

Severe hyperammonemia represents one of the most emergent metabolic conditions. Newborns often present with rapidly progressive decreased feeding, hypothermia, lethargy, apnea, coma, and death within a period of hours in the most severe cases. Elevated concentrations of ammonia are extremely toxic to the brain and cause permanent brain damage, even when rapidly corrected. Therefore, it is imperative to suspect and diagnose hyperammonemia early in the clinical course and immediately institute therapy. Severe hyperammonemia can be rapidly progressive and associated with respiratory depression. Therefore, prophylactic intubation is indicated with ammonia levels >500 μM/L.

Hyperammonemia is defined as an ammonia level higher than 150 μM/L in the neonate or higher than 100 μM/L in the older child. Blood samples should be placed on ice and analyzed immediately to avoid artifactual elevations. Mild hyperammonemia (less than ~300 μM/L) can be associated with transient hyperammonemia of the newborn, as well as with several IEMs, including the organic acidurias, fatty acid oxidation defects, lysinuric protein intolerance, and hyperammonemia, hyperornithinemia, and homocitrullinuria syndrome. More severe degrees of hyperammonemia are typically observed with urea cycle defects. Such cases are often associated with depression of blood urea nitrogen due to the inability to produce urea. These patients often demonstrate a respiratory alkalosis on their initial arterial blood gas. Secondary hyperammonemia can also be associated with liver failure and/or overwhelming viral hepatitis.

The sex of the patient is sometimes helpful. Ornithine transcarbamylase deficiency is an X-linked disorder that usually presents in males in the neonatal period. A family history of neonatal deaths of unknown etiology is always suspicious.

The various causes of hyperammonemia are metabolically diverse, each requiring specific treatment. Therefore, it is imperative to act quickly to obtain the results of the necessary biochemical diagnostic studies within 24–48 hrs. Initial treatment should consist of making the child NPO and keeping the child anabolic, with infusion of only dextrose and electrolytes to meet the age-dependent metabolic demands. Diagnostic laboratory tests should include arterial blood gas, serum chemistries, liver function studies, urine organic acids (specifically tested for orotic acid), urinalysis, serum amino acids, acylcarnitine profile, and repeated and frequent measures of ammonia until the rate of rise can be determined. Metabolic acidosis or an increased AG suggests that the diagnosis is not a urea cycle defect. Urinary ketosis with mild hyperammonemia suggests an organic aciduria. Fatty acid oxidation disorders should not be associated with urinary ketones, but they are often associated with hypoglycemia and elevated creatine phosphokinase with mild hyperammonemia.

Urea cycle defects are associated with the greatest and most rapid rise in ammonia. Elevations of ammonia rapidly rising beyond 500 μM/L should be treated with some form of hemodialysis (including CVVHD), if available. Peritoneal dialysis and exchange transfusion with such severe hyperammonemia are much less efficacious. The specific defect in the urea cycle is important to establish for definitive therapy. However, while awaiting the results of diagnostic studies, in addition to initiation of hemodialysis, patients with suspected urea cycle disorders should be started on intravenous L-arginine (to maintain the urea cycle) and given loading doses and continuous infusions of sodium benzoate and phenylacetate (to remove ammonia via alternative metabolic pathways that utilize glycine and glutamine to eliminate nitrogen) (**Table 98.5**). Sodium benzoate and phenylacetate are approved by the US Food and Drug Administration and can be stocked; however, they are expensive, rarely used, and may not be available except in tertiary neonatal and PICUs unless specifically requested. Mannitol should be utilized to decrease cerebral edema, if present. Definitive diagnoses of urea cycle defects ultimately depend on biochemical analysis of liver tissue and/or molecular genetic testing. To date, the best long-term treatment for children with urea cycle defects has been liver transplant (24). However, if significant hyperammonemia has occurred prior to transplant, permanent and irreversible brain damage should be carefully considered by parents prior to pursuing transplantation. For some urea cycle defects in which enzymes are also active outside the liver, dietary treatment and arginine supplementation in addition to liver transplantation may be necessary. In cases in which the diagnosis was known or suspected prenatally because of a previously affected sibling, neonatal metabolic management and liver transplant can enable children to avoid neurocognitive damage. Furthermore, neonatal liver transplants have required minimal long-term immunosuppression.

Notably, females heterozygous for the X-linked ornithine transcarbamylase deficiency or patients with partial urea cycle defects may demonstrate only periodic metabolic crises with normal intervening metabolic evaluations. In these cases, metabolic crises are associated with ingestion of large amounts of protein and/or a catabolic state induced by an intercurrent illness. Metabolic crises should be managed as outlined previously.

LIVER FAILURE

Liver failure associated with elevated transaminases, jaundice, bleeding, and edema and/or hepatomegaly is a common presentation for IEMs. Because the liver is the metabolic center of the body, most processes causing severe hepatic impairment can also cause alterations in metabolic pathways and produce mild hyperammonemia or hypoglycemia. Some inherited disorders, including hepatorenal tyrosinemia, galactosemia, Wilson disease, α_1-antitrypsin deficiency, peroxisomal disorders (Zellweger syndrome and Refsum disease), cause direct hepatocyte damage and defects in cholesterol and bile acid synthesis. Initially, it may be difficult to distinguish these IEMs from infectious causes, such as sepsis; hepatitis A, B, or C; cytomegalovirus; Epstein-Barr virus; herpes simplex; toxoplasmosis; or human immunodeficiency virus. The size of the liver may aid in differentiation between IEMs and infectious etiologies; hepatomegaly occurs more commonly with IEMs.

Liver function should be assessed with a liver function panel that includes albumin, transaminases, direct and indirect bilirubin, alkaline phosphatase, γ-glutamyltranspeptidase, α-fetoprotein, glucose, ammonia, blood urea nitrogen, prothrombin time, and partial thromboplastin time. If liver disease is suspected, titers and viral cultures of stool and urine should be performed to exclude viral etiologies of hepatitis. Once an IEM is suspected, specialized testing may be necessary, including lactate, pyruvate, serum amino acids, urine organic acids (succinylacetone in hepatorenal tyrosinemia, dicarboxylic acids in fatty acid oxidation disorders, and orotic acid in urea cycle defects), bile acids, urinary reducing substances (galactose and fructose), α_1-antitrypsin activity and Pi phenotyping, very long-chain fatty acids for peroxisomal biogenesis disorders, iron and ferritin for hemochromatosis, galactose-1-phosphate uridyl transferase activity for galactosemia, and transferrin isoelectric focusing for congenital disorders of glycosylation. Many hepatic processes will produce a pattern of tyrosyluria and elevated tyrosine and methionine in the serum amino acids. This pattern is usually not diagnostic of hepatorenal tyrosinemia but simply indicates liver dysfunction. A liver biopsy may be necessary to identify storage material within the liver, followed by specific enzymatic testing with fibroblasts or liver tissue used for definitive diagnosis.

Many children with liver disease present initially with jaundice. As neonates, most babies with inborn errors of hepatic metabolism present with conjugated hyperbilirubinemia. Unconjugated hyperbilirubinemia, in contrast, suggests the diagnosis of Crigler-Najjar syndrome or a hemolytic anemia. Crigler-Najjar syndrome is treated with phototherapy and plasmapheresis acutely and, ultimately, by liver transplantation. α_1-antitrypsin deficiency presents as cholestasis in a minority of infants with the Pi-ZZ phenotype. Progressive familial intrahepatic cholestasis, Dubin-Johnson, and Rotor syndromes usually present as conjugated hyperbilirubinemia after 3 months of age. Hepatorenal tyrosinemia, Niemann-Pick disease type C, and peroxisomal disorders can also initially present as conjugated hyperbilirubinemia, but all usually progress rapidly to severe liver failure.

Liver failure associated with hepatocellular necrosis can be observed in the neonatal period and in the older infant. Neonatal liver failure can be caused by infectious etiologies as well as neonatal hemochromatosis, galactosemia, hepatorenal tyrosinemia, urea cycle defects, defects in oxidative phosphorylation, long-chain fatty acid oxidation disorders, and Niemann-Pick disease types A and B. Galactosemia is suggested by reducing substance in the urine if the infant has ingested lactose within the previous 24 hrs. Galactosemia may be associated with cataracts and *Escherichia coli* sepsis. Definitive diagnosis is based on enzymatic testing of blood and is part of newborn screening panels in most states. Neonatal hemochromatosis is a rare cause of acute liver dysfunction of largely unknown etiology. Diagnosis is largely by exclusion, demonstration of increased concentrations of serum iron and ferritin, and decreased concentrations of transferrin. Abdominal MRI may also be useful to demonstrate increased liver iron stores. Hepatorenal tyrosinemia is suggested by rapid hepatic decompensation and greatly elevated α-fetoprotein and is confirmed by demonstration of succinylacetone in the urine. Defects of long-chain fatty acid oxidation are suggested by the combination of hepatic necrosis, myopathy, and cardiomyopathy, which may occur in the neonatal period and/or intermittently throughout infancy. Biochemically, these disorders are most specifically associated with elevations in creatine phosphokinase and abnormal acylcarnitine profiles that suggest the specific enzymatic deficiency. Defects in oxidative phosphorylation characteristically have multisystem involvement and are associated with increased levels of lactic acid. Definitive diagnosis often rests on a liver biopsy to demonstrate mitochondrial DNA depletion.

In the older child, hepatocellular necrosis and encephalopathy suggest a Reye-like syndrome that may be due to an underlying IEM, chronic viral hepatitis, autoimmune disease, or acute intoxication. The differential diagnoses of IEMs presenting with Reye-like syndrome include fatty acid oxidation disorders, urea cycle disorders, hepatorenal tyrosinemia, hereditary fructose intolerance, Wilson disease, and α_1-antitrypsin deficiency. Wilson disease is characterized by choreoathetoid movements and dystonia, Kayser-Fleischer rings around the cornea, reduced levels of serum ceruloplasmin, and increased urinary copper. The age of presentation for some of these disorders depends on the degree of the enzymatic deficiency, with less severe deficiencies presenting at older ages.

Hepatomegaly is often observed in IEMs, especially those associated with storage of nonmetabolizable large molecules. The combination of splenomegaly with hepatomegaly is more specific for storage disorders. In many of the lysosomal storage disorders, liver function is intact, although the liver can become extremely enlarged. Lysosomal storage disorders are further suggested by short stature, failure to thrive, or coarse facial features, and developmental delay, hypotonia, or seizures. Many of the glycogen storage diseases can also produce hepatomegaly with or without associated hypoglycemia and are often diagnosed by findings of abnormal quantity and/or quality of glycogen on a liver biopsy. Hemochromatosis is a rare cause of hepatomegaly that results from excess storage of iron.

Treatment for many liver diseases caused by IEMs is supportive therapy to treat associated coagulopathies with vitamin K and fresh frozen plasma, edema due to hypoalbuminemia with diuretics and albumin infusion, and unconjugated hyperbilirubinemia with phototherapy. Deranged metabolism that produces hypoglycemia and hyperammonemia must also be treated. Diet should be carefully considered and, in the cases of severe liver dysfunction, the child should be made NPO and receive only intravenous dextrose and electrolytes until initial

metabolic labs have been evaluated. A growing number of these disorders can ultimately be treated by liver transplant from either a cadaveric liver or living, related donor (22). Disease-specific treatments are available for a few IEMs that cause liver dysfunction. A lactose-free, soy-based diet is a simple cure in galactosemia. A diet free of fructose and sucrose is curative for hereditary fructose intolerance. A low phenylalanine and tyrosine metabolic formula and administration of 2(2-nitro-4-trifluoro-methyl-benzoyl)-1,3-cyclohexanedione (NTBC) have revolutionized treatment for hepatorenal tyrosinemia and can allow normalization of hepatic and renal function. Long-chain fatty acid oxidation disorders remain problematic to treat, but current treatment relies on a low-fat diet, with the majority of fat supplied as medium-chain triglycerides and supplementation of carnitine. Copper chelation is effective treatment for Wilson disease, and phlebotomy for hemochromatosis.

NONMETABOLIC CRITICAL ILLNESS IN INBORN ERRORS OF METABOLISM

Many IEMs present in the PICU not due to metabolic crisis, but due to their effects on specific vital organ systems. Effects on the hepatic, renal, pulmonary, cardiovascular, and hematologic systems may all have significant implications for the pediatric intensivist. Any disorder that produces hepatic or renal insufficiency requires careful dose adjustments of medications cleared by these organs. Because of the rarity of individual IEMs, many recommendations are based on retrospective data, case reports, and anecdotal experience, rather than on randomized clinical trials. Lactate-containing fluids should not be administered to patients who may not metabolize exogenous lactate [as in mitochondrial disorders (35) and pyruvate dehydrogenase complex deficiency]. Though propofol has been used successfully in mitochondrial disorders, it should probably be avoided in fatty acid oxidation defects because of possible predisposition to propofol infusion syndrome (32,35). Following use of depolarizing neuromuscular blockers, several IEMs, including glycogen storage diseases V (McArdle disease) and VII (Tauri disease), place patients at significant risk for rhabdomyolysis leading to myoglobinuria and for hyperkalemia. The absence of acidosis distinguishes this phenomenon from malignant hyperthermia. The mitochondrial disorders, however, may predispose to true malignant hyperthermia following use of depolarizing agents and volatile anesthetics (12).

IEMs may affect many aspects of the cardiovascular system, including the vessels themselves, the coagulation system, myocardium, endocardium, and pericardium. Extensive reviews of these diseases are outside the scope of this text and can be found elsewhere (14). An increasing number of known abnormalities of proteins involved in the contractile machinery cause cardiomyopathy, and these disorders are covered in detail in Chapter 66. Any IEM that impairs energy metabolism, particularly disorders of the mitochondrial respiratory chain and fatty acid oxidation defects may also present with cardiomyopathy, usually dilated rather than hypertrophic. The fatty acid oxidation disorders (including fatty acyl-CoA dehydrogenase deficiencies and glutaric acidemia type II) may present with arrhythmias in addition to neonatal cardiomyopathy (7). They are treated primarily with a low-fat diet with minimal amounts of essential fatty acids and supplementation with medium-chain triglycerides and carnitine replacement. Primary carnitine deficiency, due to a defect in the carnitine transporter in the heart, liver and kidneys, presents with cardiomyopathy, with or without skeletal myopathy, beginning in late infancy or early childhood. Carnitine-acylcarnitine translocase deficiency and the severe form of carnitine palmitoyltransferase-2 deficiency also present with dilated cardiomyopathy. Treatment with high doses of oral carnitine can be curative for primary carnitine deficiency.

IEMs also affect cardiovascular function in the PICU through their effects on coagulation and microvascular physiology. The hyperlipoproteinemias increase cardiovascular risk through atherogenesis. Only type II (familial hypercholesterolemia) has consequences in children (2). When hypertriglyceridemia occurs (type IIB), homozygous children can have severe atherosclerotic disease and dilated cardiomyopathy out of proportion to the degree of ischemia. Homocystinuria predisposes patients to thromboembolic disease. In the classic form (cystathionine synthase deficiency), patients typically present with ectopia lentis after 3 years of age, a Marfanoid habitus, and developmental delay. On the other hand, IEMs may promote a bleeding diathesis due to hypersplenism in a number of storage diseases or due to decreased liver synthetic function.

The lysosomal storage diseases often involve both the cardiovascular and respiratory systems, providing a number of challenges for the intensivist and anesthesiologist. Perioperative considerations are reviewed more extensively in other texts (19). Type II glycogen storage disease (Pompe disease) results from deficiency of the enzyme α-1,4 glucosidase (acid maltase) and causes a hypertrophic cardiomyopathy syndrome with a short P-R interval. These patients also have glycogen storage in other organs, which causes hypotonia and macroglossia. The X-linked disorder Fabry disease (lysosomal α-galactosidase A deficiency) causes disseminated glycosphingolipid deposition. Angiokeratomas are characteristic and result from deposition in the skin, typically in a "bathing suit distribution." The cardiovascular manifestations result from deposition causing obstructive vasculopathy, mitral valve thickening, and hypertrophic (progressing to dilated) cardiomyopathy. Mutations of the γ subunit of AMP-activated protein kinase (PRKAG2) and X-linked lysosome-associated membrane protein (LAMP2, Danon disease) result in hypertrophic cardiomyopathy due to glycogen accumulation in the heart and are associated with ventricular preexcitation (1).

The MPS can affect both the myocardium and the endocardium (valvular disease). Type I (Hunter/Scheie) and type II (Hurler) MPS result in varying degrees of myocardial and valvular disease. Although the mucolipidoses I-cell disease and pseudo-Hurler polydystrophy share many features with the MPS, such as valvular disease, reports of cardiomyopathy are rare (25,31). Together with Pompe disease, these lysosomal storage disorders also affect a variety of systems involved in respiratory management in the PICU. The associated dysmorphisms and tracheal narrowing can make endotracheal intubation extremely challenging; a view of the larynx may be unobtainable with direct laryngoscopy. Atlanto-axial instability, particularly in MPS IV (Morquio syndrome), must be considered during laryngoscopy as well. These patients are also at high risk for airway obstruction during induction. Therefore, they may require fiberoptic intubation or even tracheotomy,

and should be intubated awake whenever possible. Muscle relaxants are contraindicated before successful intubation, unless an easy-mask airway can be established.

Novel Therapies

Enzyme replacement therapy is available for a growing number of lysosomal storage disorders, including Gaucher disease (8), Pompe disease (20), Fabry disease (8), MPS I (18,37), and MPS VI (15). None of these enzymes are able to cross the blood-brain barrier, and therapy is, therefore, only effective at treating the systemic disease, not the neurologic components. Furthermore, though in most cases enzyme replacement therapy effectively prevents further accumulation of material, it may not effectively reverse organ damage already sustained. Several problems exist with this therapy, including the high cost, need for biweekly intravenous infusions and, in rare cases, development of neutralizing antibodies (17). Small-molecule inhibitors of substrate accumulation and chaperones to rescue patients' endogenous misfolded proteins are being explored as alternative therapies. Direct intracerebroventricular infusion of enzyme is currently being considered for clinical trials to treat the neurologic symptoms.

Hobbs first reported improvement in a patient with Hurler syndrome following bone marrow transplantation in 1981 (16). Since then, several other storage disorders, including Krabbe disease (21), metachromatic leukodystrophy (21), and Niemann-Pick disease type B (34), have been treated with bone marrow transplantation with at least partial success. By replacing resident macrophages [or microglia in the central nervous system (CNS)] with donor-derived cells, stored material may be cleared, even in the CNS. However, stabilization or improvement in organ function can occur slowly (in the CNS) or not at all (in bone/heart valves) due to poor penetration of donor macrophages into these tissues. Early treatment (even neonatally) of appropriate patients without severe organ dysfunction dramatically improves outcome. Fortunately, even with obtaining only modest levels of sustained enzyme production and mixed chimerism, clinical improvement or stabilization has been noted (9). Ongoing investigations should determine the optimal ablative regimens and immunosuppression in these patients, as well as which other diseases are amenable to this therapy. Some patients may even benefit from combinations of enzyme replacement therapy, substrate inhibitors, and bone marrow transplantation, either sequentially or simultaneously (5).

CONCLUSIONS AND FUTURE DIRECTIONS

Patients with IEMs frequently present with critical illnesses. Although, individually, IEMs are rare, collectively, they are not infrequent; therefore intensivists are virtually certain to care for such patients. With advances in diagnosis, particularly, improved neonatal screening with tandem mass spectroscopy, many patients will be diagnosed before their first metabolic decompensation. However, a normal newborn screen does not rule out all IEMs. A systematic approach to the diagnosis and initial treatment of these disorders is imperative, as is early involvement of a metabolic disease specialist. Early recognition of an IEM and appropriate therapy, including dietary management, cofactor supplementation, and removal of toxic metabolites, improves neurologic outcome. Additionally, enzyme replacement therapy, substrate inhibitors, and liver and bone marrow transplantation are now being used to treat many of these diseases. With improvements in gene delivery, enzyme delivery across the blood-brain barrier and chaperoning misfolded endogenous proteins, we should be able to improve the treatment for many of these conditions.

KEY POINTS

- Although individually rare, IEMs are collectively common in pediatrics.
- A high index of suspicion should exist in patients with encephalopathy, (cardio)myopathy, hyperammonemia, hypoglycemia, or refractory metabolic acidosis.
- Prompt initiation of specific therapy can prevent irreversible brain injury.
- Patients with IEMs may have a number of nonmetabolic complications that require pediatric intensive care.
- With advances in therapy (enzyme replacement, transplantation), the long-term prognosis of many of these patients is likely to continue to improve.

References

1. Arad M, Maron BJ, Gorham JM, et al. Glycogen storage diseases presenting as hypertrophic cardiomyopathy. *N Engl J Med* 2005;352:362–72.
2. Barness LA. An approach to the diagnosis of metabolic diseases. *Fetal Pediat Pathol* 2004;23:3–10.
3. Barshop BA, Khanna A. Domino hepatic transplantation in maple syrup urine disease. *N Engl J Med* 2005;353:2410–1.
4. Batshaw ML, Brusilow SW. Treatment of hyperammonemic coma caused by inborn errors of urea synthesis. *J Pediatr* 1980;97:893–900.
5. Biswas S, LeVine SM. Substrate-reduction therapy enhances the benefits of bone marrow transplantation in young mice with globoid cell leukodystrophy. *Pediatr Res* 2002;51:40–7.
6. Bodner-Leidecker A, Wendel U, Saudubray JM, et al. Branched-chain L-amino acid metabolism in classical maple syrup urine disease after orthotopic liver transplantation. *J Inherit Metab Dis* 2000;23:805–18.
7. Bonnet D, Martin D, Pascale De L, et al. Arrhythmias and conduction defects as presenting symptoms of fatty acid oxidation disorders in children. *Circulation* 1999;100:2248–53.
8. Brady RO. Enzyme replacement therapy: Conception, chaos and culmination. *Philos Trans R Soc Lond B Biol Sci* 2003;358:915–9.
9. Conway J, Dyack S, Crooks BNA, et al. Mixed donor chimerism and low level iduronidase expression may be adequate for neurodevelopmental protection in Hurler Syndrome. *J Pediatr* 2005;147:106–8.
10. de Baulny HO, Benoist JF, Rigal O, et al. Methylmalonic and propionic acidaemias: Management and outcome. *J Inherit Metab Dis* 2005;28:415–23.
11. Edelmann L, Wasserstein MP, Kornreich R, et al. Maple syrup urine disease: Identification and carrier-frequency determination of a novel founder mutation in the Ashkenazi Jewish population. *Am J Hum Genet* 2001;69:863–8.
12. Fricker RM, Raffelsberger T, Rauch-Shorny S, et al. Positive malignant hyperthermia susceptibility in vitro test in a patient with mitochondrial myopathy and myoadenylate deaminase deficiency. *Anesthesiology* 2002;97:1635–7.
13. Garganta CL, Smith WE. Metabolic evaluation of the sick neonate. *Semin Perinatol* 2005;29:164–72.
14. Gilbert-Barness E. Cardiovascular involvement in metabolic diseases. *Pediatr Pathol Mol Med* 2002;21:93–136.
15. Harmatz P, Whitley CB, Waber L, et al. Enzyme replacement therapy in mucopolysaccharidosis VI (Maroteaux-Lamy syndrome). *J Pediatr* 2004;144:574–80.
16. Hobbs JR, Hugh-Jones K, Barrett AJ, et al. Reversal of clinical features of Hurler's disease and biochemical improvement after treatment by bone-marrow transplantation. *Lancet* 1981;2:709–12.
17. Kakavanos R, Turner CT, Hopwood JJ, et al. Immune tolerance after long-term enzyme-replacement therapy among patients who have mucopolysaccharidosis I. *Lancet* 2003;361:1608–13.
18. Kakkis ED, Muenzer J, Tiller GE, et al. Enzyme-replacement therapy in mucopolysaccharidosis I. *N Engl J Med* 2001;344:182–8.
19. Katz JAS, David J (eds.). *Anesthesia and Uncommon Pediatric Diseases, 1st ed.* Philadelphia: WB Saunders Company, 1987.
20. Klinge L, Straub V, Neudorf U, et al. Enzyme replacement therapy in classical infantile Pompe disease: Results of a ten-month follow-up study. *Neuropediatrics* 2005;36:6–11.
21. Krivit W, Aubourg P, Shapiro E, et al. Bone marrow transplantation for globoid cell leukodystrophy, adrenoleukodystrophy, metachromatic leukodystrophy, and Hurler syndrome. *Curr Opin Hematol* 1999;6:377–82.
22. Meyburg J, Hoffmann GF. Liver transplantation for inborn errors of metabolism. *Transplantation* 2005;80:S135–S7.
23. Mock DM, Mock NI, Nelson RP, et al. Disturbances in biotin metabolism in children undergoing long-term anticonvulsant therapy. *J Pediatr Gastroenterol Nutr* 1998;26:245–50.
24. Morioka D, Kasahara M, Takada Y, et al. Current role of liver transplantation for the treatment of urea cycle disorders: A review of the worldwide English literature and 13 cases at Kyoto University. *Liver Transpl* 2005;11:1332–42.
25. Muller P, Reichenbach H, Mockel A, et al. I-cell disease complicated by unusual dilatative cardiomyopathy. *J Inherit Metab Dis* 2000;23:514–6.
26. Nagarajan S, Enns GM, Millan MT, et al. Management of methylmalonic acidaemia by combined liver-kidney transplantation. *J Inherit Metab Dis* 2005;28:517–24.
27. Puffenberger EG. Genetic heritage of the Old Order Mennonites of southeastern Pennsylvania. *Am J Med Genet C Semin Med Genet* 2003;121:18–31.
28. Saudubray JM, Ogier H, Charpentier C, et al. Hudson memorial lecture. Neonatal management of organic acidurias. Clinical update. *J Inherit Metab Dis* 1984;7(Suppl 1):2–9.
29. Schaefer F, Straube E, Oh J, et al. Dialysis in neonates with inborn errors of metabolism. *Nephrol Dial Transplant* 1999;14:910–8.
30. Stacpoole PW, Nagaraja NV, Hutson AD. Efficacy of dichloroacetate as a lactate-lowering drug. *J Clin Pharmacol* 2003;43:683–91.
31. Steet RA, Hullin R, Kudo M, et al. A splicing mutation in the alpha/beta GlcNAc-1-phosphotransferase gene results in an adult onset form of mucolipidosis III associated with sensory neuropathy and cardiomyopathy. *Am J Med Genet A* 2005;132:369–75.
32. Steiner LA, Studer W, Baumgartner ER, et al. Perioperative management of a child with very-long-chain acyl-coenzyme A dehydrogenase deficiency. *Paediatr Anaesth* 2002;12:187–91.
33. Summar M, Pietsch J, Deshpande J, et al. Effective hemodialysis and hemofiltration driven by an extracorporeal membrane oxygenation pump in infants with hyperammonemia. *J Pediatr* 1996;128:379–82.
34. Vellodi A, Hobbs JR, O'Donnell NM, et al. Treatment of Niemann-Pick disease type B by allogeneic bone marrow transplantation. *Br Med J (Clin Res Ed)* 1987;295:1375–6.
35. Vilela H, Garcia-Fernandez J, Parodi E, et al. Anesthetic management of a patient with MERRF syndrome. *Paediatr Anaesth* 2005;15:77–9.
36. Wong KY, Wong SN, Lam SY, et al. Ammonia clearance by peritoneal dialysis and continuous arteriovenous hemodiafiltration. *Pediatr Nephrol* 1998;12:589–91.
37. Wraith JE, Clarke LA, Beck M, et al. Enzyme replacement therapy for mucopolysaccharidosis I: a randomized, double-blinded, placebo-controlled, multinational study of recombinant human alpha-L-iduronidase (laronidase). *J Pediatr* 2004;144:581–8.

CHAPTER 99 ■ CANCER THERAPY: MECHANISMS, TOXICITY, AND ETHICS IN THE PICU

DAVID M. LOEB • DAVID G. NICHOLS

MECHANISMS

Most pediatric malignancies are treated with multimodal therapy, traditionally consisting of chemotherapy, radiation therapy, and surgery. More recently, biologically based therapies have been developed, including small-molecule kinase inhibitors, cytokine therapies, differentiation therapies, and antiangiogenic therapies. Some of these treatments have entered the realm of standard of care, while others remain available only in the context of a clinical trial. A clear understanding of the mechanism of action of each of these modalities, along with an understanding of the most common toxicities, is essential to the delivery of optimal critical care to pediatric oncology patients. This chapter discusses the mechanism of action of the major classes of chemotherapeutic agents, the distinctions between different radiation therapy modalities, and the most common side effects that might be encountered in the critical care setting. A comprehensive discussion of the mechanism of action of each available chemotherapy drug is beyond the scope of this chapter. We will focus on the most commonly used agents in pediatric oncology practice, with an emphasis on discussion of classes of drugs, rather than focusing on individual compounds. The reader is referred to any of several excellent textbooks for a more comprehensive discussion of individual chemotherapy drugs (10,38). In addition to material on therapeutic modalities, we will discuss some ethical concepts important in dealing with oncology patients in the PICU.

Mechanism of Action of Chemotherapeutics

Chemotherapy drugs are classified by their mechanism of action. **Table 99.1** lists the commonly used constituents of each major drug class. **Table 99.2** lists some regimens commonly used to treat certain pediatric malignancies. The mechanism of action of each class of drug is discussed in more detail below.

Alkylating Agents

The oldest class of chemotherapeutic drugs is the alkylating agents. Mechlorethamine, also known as nitrogen mustard, was the first nonhormonal drug successfully given to a patient for the explicit purpose of treating cancer (18). A number of related agents have subsequently been developed for clinical use. Most alkylating agents commonly used in pediatric oncology are derivatives of nitrogen mustard, including cyclophosphamide and ifosfamide, or derivatives of methylnitrosourea, such as lomustine (CCNU) and carmustine (BCNU). These drugs contain highly reactive alkyl groups that form covalent bonds with DNA and other intracellular macromolecules. Both nitrogen mustard derivatives and nitrosoureas primarily modify the N-7 position of guanine (32); nitrosoureas also alkylate the N-3 position on cytidine (26) or the O-6 position on guanine (37). Following this initial alkylation reaction, the remaining reactive group can interact with a second macromolecule, resulting in either intrastrand or interstrand DNA cross-links. It has been suggested that these cross-links are the events that lead to cytotoxicity, perhaps by impeding DNA replication or by direct mutagenesis (19). While compelling arguments exist to support this hypothesis, direct proof remains lacking.

In addition to the nitrogen mustard and nitrosourea derivatives, platinum-based antitumor compounds also create DNA cross-links. While not true alkylating agents, these compounds have a similar mechanism of action and are therefore sometimes referred to as "nonclassical alkylating agents." The two commonly used platinum-based compounds are cisplatin and carboplatin, which, like the classical alkylating agents, form adducts at the N-7 position of guanine (57). These drugs can form both intrastrand and interstrand cross-links, and these cross-links are correlated with cytotoxicity (15). As with the classical alkylating agents, the relationship between DNA cross-links and cytotoxicity remains correlative, with definitive proof of causality lacking.

Antimetabolites

Antimetabolites are commonly used by both medical and pediatric oncologists to treat a variety of tumor types. The several classes of antimetabolites are classified based on the metabolic pathways with which they interfere. In pediatric oncology, antifolates and purine antimetabolites are most commonly used; therefore, they will be discussed here to the exclusion of other types of antimetabolites.

Antifolates. In the early 1940s, it was recognized that patients with acute leukemia were folate deficient. This observation prompted a series of investigations culminating in the use of aminopterin by Farber to induce temporary remissions in children with acute lymphoblastic leukemia (ALL). Methotrexate was eventually developed as a clinically useful

TABLE 99.1

CHEMOTHERAPEUTICS ORGANIZED BY CLASS

Class	Drugs
Alkylating agents	Cyclophosphamide, ifosfamide, BCNU, CCNU, cisplatin, carboplatin
Antimetabolites	Methotrexate, 6-mercaptopurine, 6-thioguanine
Topoisomerase inhibitors	Etoposide (VP16) and teniposide (VM26) inhibit Topo II
	Irinotecan and topotecan inhibit Topo I
Anthracyclines	Doxorubicin, daunorubicin, idarubicin
Antimicrotubule agents	Vincristine, vinblastine, vinorelbine, paclitaxel, docetaxel

chemotherapeutic agent because it has a more favorable therapeutic index than does aminopterin. Methotrexate acts by competitively inhibiting the enzyme dihydrofolate reductase. Inhibition of this key enzyme required for synthesis of thymidine leads to depletion of intracellular thymidine triphosphate and eventually to arrest of DNA synthesis (17). It has also been reported that high doses of methotrexate lead to decreased purine synthesis and ultimately to cell death (24). Another potential mechanism of action of methotrexate is its toxicity to endothelial cells (23). Mounting evidence supports methotrexate as an effective therapy for autoimmune diseases, in part, through inhibition of angiogenesis (8)—although the antiangiogenic mechanism is unclear—and this inhibition may play a role in the antineoplastic effects of methotrexate as well.

Purine Antimetabolites. Purine biosynthesis is critical for DNA synthesis and, therefore, for cell replication. The development of drugs that interfere with purine biosynthesis was a major focus during the 1950s, ultimately leading to the awarding of the Nobel Prize to Gertrude Elion and George Hitchings (along with James Black) in 1988 for the development of, among other drugs, 6-mercaptopurine and 6-thioguanine. These drugs are thought to act primarily by being incorporated into growing DNA strands, thereby inhibiting DNA synthesis. Other mechanisms by which these drugs exert their cytotoxicity include inhibition of the activity of enzymes that are necessary for the synthesis of natural purines (adenine and guanine).

Topoisomerase Inhibitors

Topoisomerases are enzymes involved in the maintenance of supercoiling of the DNA double helix (12). They are essential for DNA replication, transcription, and chromosomal segregation—critical processes for cell division and, therefore, for tumor growth. Two classes of topoisomerase inhibitors are type I enzymes, which make single-strand cuts in DNA, and type II enzymes, which make double-strand cuts. Inhibitors of each type of topoisomerase are in common use in pediatric oncology.

Inhibitors of Topoisomerase II. The two types of topoisomerase II inhibitors are podophyllotoxins and anthracyclines. Etoposide (VP16) is the more commonly used podophyllotoxin, and teniposide (VM26) is rarely used. Etoposide was approved by the US food and Drug Administration (FDA) in 1983, but it was not clear until 1984 that this drug functioned by inhibiting topoisomerase II. This enzyme modulates DNA topology by passing an intact DNA helix through a transient

TABLE 99.2

COMMONLY USED CHEMOTHERAPY REGIMENS IN PEDIATRIC ONCOLOGY

Diagnosis	Chemotherapy
Acute lymphoblastic leukemia (induction only)	Prednisone or dexamethasone, vincristine, L-asparaginase (and daunorubicin for high-risk patients)
Acute myelogenous leukemia (induction only)	Daunorubicin, cytarabine, etoposide
Osteosarcoma	Methotrexate, cisplatin, doxorubicin (ifosfamide and etoposide added for some patients with poor response to neoadjuvant therapy)
Ewing sarcoma	Vincristine, doxorubicin, cyclophosphamide, alternating with ifosfamide and etoposide
Rhabdomyosarcoma	Vincristine, dactinomycin, cyclophosphamide
Hodgkin disease	**Low risk:** Doxorubicin, prednisone, vincristine, cyclophosphamide **Intermediate and high risk:** Doxorubicin, bleomycin, vincristine, etoposide, prednisone, cyclophosphamide
Neuroblastoma	**Intermediate risk:** Carboplatin, etoposide, cyclophosphamide, doxorubicin **High risk:** Cyclophosphamide, topotecan, cisplatin, etoposide, doxorubicin, vincristine
Wilms tumor	**Low risk:** Vincristine, dactinomycin **Intermediate risk:** Vincristine, dactinomycin, doxorubicin **High risk:** Vincristine, doxorubicin, cyclophosphamide, etoposide

double-stranded break in the DNA backbone (12). Etoposide poisons topoisomerase II by increasing the steady-state concentration of DNA cleavage complexes (20)—in essence by gluing the enzyme to the broken strand of DNA and preventing repair of the cleaved helix.

In addition to podophyllotoxins, anthracycline antibiotics, such as doxorubicin, daunorubicin, and idarubicin, also inhibit topoisomerase II. First isolated from fermentation products of *Streptomyces peucetius*, anthracycline antibiotics were originally thought to act primarily by virtue of their ability to intercalate between DNA base pairs in the intact double helix. In the 1980s it was recognized that these compounds are also inhibitors of topoisomerase II (51). Other activities of anthracycline antibiotics include effects on nuclear helicases and the generation of iron free radicals. At present, it is unclear whether the cytotoxicity of these drugs is a result of just one mechanism (inhibition of topoisomerase II), or a combination of all of these activities.

Inhibitors of Topoisomerase I. Inhibitors of topoisomerase I represent a newer class of chemotherapeutic agents. The agents in common use, irinotecan and topotecan, are derivatives of camptothecin, a plant alkaloid obtained from the *Camptotheca acuminata* tree. These drugs target the DNA-topoisomerase I complex, preventing the reannealing of the nicked DNA strand, which leads to the accumulation of drug-stabilized, nicked DNA strands, causing an arrest of DNA replication and subsequent cell death (39). Other agents in this class are under development.

Antimicrotubule Agents

Vinca Alkaloids. All vinca alkaloids are derived from compounds originally identified in the pink periwinkle plant (older scientific name *Vinca rosea Linn*). Three related compounds are commonly used in the US: vincristine, vinblastine, and vinorelbine. Vinca alkaloids are thought to produce cytotoxicity through interaction with tubulin, the major protein component of microtubules (21), an interaction that disrupts the structure of the microtubules and leads to dissolution of the mitotic spindle and metaphase arrest of dividing cells. The importance of microtubules in other cellular functions explains the noncytotoxic effects of these compounds. In particular, neurons require intact microtubules for axonal transport, and disruption of this function causes the well-known peripheral neuropathy associated with vincristine treatment (40).

Taxanes. The original taxane, paclitaxel, was found through a National Cancer Institute program that screened plant extracts for anticancer activity (42), and it was initially isolated from the bark of the Pacific yew tree. The major source of taxanes today is a semisynthetic derivative of the needles and other components of more abundant trees, such as the European yew. Docetaxel and paclitaxel are the two most commonly used taxanes, and they act by binding to tubulin at sites distinct from those bound by the vinca alkaloids. Taxanes function by stabilizing microtubules against depolymerization, primarily through an effect on tubulin dissociation rates at both ends of the microtubule (43), affecting dynamic instability of the microtubules, which is critical for normal microtubule dynamics during both mitotic and nonmitotic phases of the cell cycle. Ultimately, this disruption of microtubule dynamics leads to induction of apoptosis. Interestingly, taxanes also inhibit an-

giogenesis at concentrations below those that are cytotoxic (7). The contribution of this and other effects to the cytotoxicity of taxanes is as yet unclear.

Other Cytotoxic Drugs

Asparaginase. L-Asparaginase hydrolyzes asparagines to aspartic acid and ammonia. In sensitive tumor cells that lack adequate levels of asparagine synthetase, this enzyme depletes the cells of a critical amino acid, thus rapidly inhibiting protein synthesis. DNA and RNA synthesis are eventually also inhibited, and cell death ensues. Asparaginase is particularly used to treat pediatric ALL and, as a single agent, is able to induce complete remission in 50%–60% of patients (9). Interestingly, relapsed patients will achieve a second complete remission with asparaginase alone in 30%–50% of cases. Remissions induced by a single agent are short lived, however; therefore, ALL is always treated with combination chemotherapy.

Cytarabine. Cytarabine (araC) differs from cytidine by the substitution of arabinose for ribose. Uptake into the cell is via the same transport mechanisms that are responsible for uptake of other nucleosides. Once internalized, cytarabine is serially phosphorylated to generate araCTP by deoxycytidine kinase. Cytarabine decreases intracellular concentrations of deoxycytidine by competition for enzymes that are responsible for the activation of cytidine and, thereby, inhibits DNA synthesis. DNA polymerase is also inhibited by incorporation of araCTP into nascent DNA strands, and incorporation of araCTP into DNA correlates with cytotoxicity (27). In addition to these effects, araC also causes cells to synthesize small reduplicated segments of DNA, increasing the possibility of crossovers and recombination (56). Chromosome fragmentation has been observed in cells cultured with araC, possibly reflecting the effects of these small reduplications. The importance of this finding to the cytotoxic effects of the drug remains unclear.

Gemcitabine is another cytidine analog that has recently been introduced into pediatric oncology practice. Like araC, gemcitabine is phosphorylated by nucleoside kinases. Gemcitabine triphosphate competes with dCTP for incorporation into DNA and inhibits DNA polymerase, thus inhibiting DNA synthesis.

The Basics of Radiation Therapy

In pediatric oncology, radiation therapy is primarily used in the treatment of solid tumors, as a means of local control. For some tumor types, such as Wilms tumor and most central nervous system (CNS) malignancies, radiation is a standard part of therapy. For others, such as Ewing sarcoma, radiation is used to treat patients for whom surgery is not an option or patients who have an inadequate resection. In the past, radiation was used for CNS prophylaxis for all leukemia patients, but modern regimens reserve radiation for patients at high risk for CNS involvement. In addition, radiation therapy is sometimes incorporated into bone marrow transplant (BMT) preparative regimens and in treatment of patients with leukemia who have CNS involvement.

General Principles of Radiation Therapy

Radiation therapy is the delivery of packets of energy to a target tissue with the intention of causing lethal damage to malignant cells while minimizing damage to normal cells. Radiation energy comes in different packets, the most commonly used being photons (for example, from x-rays), although other particles (e.g., protons or electrons) are also used. Different packets of energy possess different properties, including the amount of energy per packet and depth of tissue penetration, and these properties determine the mode of treatment. As the packets deposit their energy, ionization events occur in biologically important molecules, and it is these events that lead to tissue damage and death. These events can occur directly (as when a photon causes the release of an electron from a target biological molecule, and this electron directly damages the molecule) or indirectly (as when a released electron interacts with a neighboring water molecule to generate free radicals, which then damage macromolecules). The dose of energy delivered is measured in Grays (Gy), and 1 Gy = 1 J/kg. An older dose term, rad, is still sometimes used, and 1 rad = 1 cGy = 0.01 Gy. While multiple biological macromolecules can be affected by ionizing radiation, it is thought that induction of double-strand DNA breaks is the proximate cause of cell death. It is estimated that a 1-Gy dose of x-rays will result in 40 double-strand DNA breaks per cell (41).

Because double-stranded DNA breaks cause cell death in irradiated tissue, understanding the response to DNA damage is necessary in order to understand the toxicities of radiation. Ionizing radiation initiates a complex cascade of cellular responses that can result in cell-cycle arrest, induction of stress-response genes, induction of apoptosis, or repair of DNA damage. These responses are not mutually exclusive. For example, transient cell-cycle arrest allows time for DNA damage repair prior to mitosis initiation, potentially triggering apoptosis as a result of unrepaired double-strand breaks. The response to DNA damage is a very active field of research, but the details are beyond the scope of this chapter.

Several biologic characteristics of a tumor modify its sensitivity to radiation. Oxygenation status of target tissue is a critical factor. It is clear that hypoxic tumors are more resistant to ionizing radiation than are normally oxygenated tumors (6). As cancer cells die within the tumor mass, anoxic regions can "reoxygenate," and cells that had been relatively protected can become more sensitive. Another important determinant of radiosensitivity is position in the cell cycle. Cells in the G2 and M phases of the cell cycle are most sensitive to radiation, while cells in late S phase are relatively resistant (11). This differential sensitivity can lead to a relative synchronization of tumor cells. These factors (oxygenation status and fluxes related to irradiation as well as cell cycle and tumor synchronization) are taken into account when developing treatment plans.

Types of External-Beam Radiation

Typical external beam radiotherapy is delivered from a ^{60}Co source and is composed of photons. To minimize dose delivery to normal tissue, perpendicular beams are used to deliver the radiation, with the area of overlap corresponding to the target. Because the beams are rectangular, but most tumors are irregularly shaped, devices known as *collimators* in the head of the radiation source shape the beam to more closely conform to the shape of the tumor as determined by CT scan. The beam can be further shaped with the use of individually constructed blocks, which shield body regions that are not in the target area. Modern, multileaf collimators provide additional precision to the shape of the beam.

Photons typically deposit energy relatively deep into tissue, with higher-energy photons penetrating deeper than lower-energy photons. Electrons, in contrast, deposit their energy in a relatively shallow range, with a rapid drop-off of energy with increasing depth. Thus, a superficial tumor (such as leukemia cutis) will be more appropriately treated with electron-beam therapy, rather than standard photons.

Like electrons, protons have a very rapid drop-off of energy in the last few millimeters of penetration. Unlike electrons, protons penetrate relatively deeply into tissue. Thus, a proton beam can treat a target deeper than can an electron beam, but with similar precision in the deposition of energy. Thus, proton-beam radiation is valuable when the target is located deep but adjacent to particularly sensitive normal tissue. Whereas photons and electrons are commonly available, a limited number of centers are capable of delivering proton-beam radiotherapy, including only four sites in the US (Loma Linda University Health Sciences Center, the University of California at San Francisco Medical Center, Massachusetts General Hospital Cancer Center, and Indiana University Medical Center). Indications for, and results of, proton-beam radiotherapy, with particular reference to pediatric malignancies, have recently been reviewed (33).

Targeted Radiation Therapy

Other means of delivering radiation therapy, aside from external beam, are brachytherapy and targeted radiation therapy. Because brachytherapy is unlikely to result in complications requiring critical care, it will not be discussed further. In pediatric oncology, interest is growing in physiologic targeting of radiation. Examples of physiologic targeting include the use of ^{131}I-metaiodobenzylguanidine (MIBG) to treat neuroblastoma and samarium-153 ethylene diamine tetramethylene phosphonate (^{153}Sm-EDTMP) to treat osteosarcoma. MIBG is a catecholamine precursor that, when labeled with ^{123}I, has been used as a diagnostic imaging tool for neural crest tumors, such as neuroblastoma. Oncologists are exploring the use of ^{131}I-MIBG as a therapeutic tool, based on the concept that neuroblastoma cells concentrate MIBG, allowing the delivery of potentially cytotoxic doses of ^{131}I to the tumor, while sparing normal tissue. The feasibility of this approach in the setting of an autologous peripheral blood stem cell transplant has recently been demonstrated (35). ^{153}Sm-EDTMP is a bone-seeking radiopharmaceutical that has been used to treat high-risk osteosarcoma (3). Just as the MIBG targets ^{131}I to neuroblastoma cells, EDTMP targets ^{153}Sm to osteosarcoma cells, essentially sparing surrounding normal tissue. Like ^{131}I-MIBG, ^{153}Sm-EDTMP is sometimes delivered in the context of autologous peripheral blood stem cell support, making it possible that such patients will require critical care.

Biologic Therapy

As our understanding of the biology of pediatric tumors improves, biologically based therapy is becoming a reality. Biologic therapies currently in clinical use include differentiation therapy, immunotherapy, small-molecule kinase inhibitors, and monoclonal antibody therapies. A full review of biologically based anticancer therapy is beyond the scope of this chapter, but we will discuss examples of each type of biologic therapy, with an emphasis on agents that have significant enough toxicities that patients run a reasonable risk of needing critical care.

Differentiation Therapy

The best-known example of differentiation therapy is the use of all-trans retinoic acid (ATRA) in the treatment of acute promyelocytic leukemia (APL). APL is well known to the intensivist because of the characteristic profound bleeding diathesis seen at presentation. Prior to the routine use of ATRA, APL was associated with a very poor prognosis, with an overall survival rate of ~20% and 10%–20% of patients dying of hemorrhage during induction therapy. Molecular research into the pathogenesis of this disease revealed that the malignant cells are characterized by the presence of a translocation between chromosomes 15 and 17 that causes the production of a fusion protein that combines the retinoic acid receptor RARα with a nuclear protein called PML. Pharmacologic doses of ATRA overcome the block to differentiation caused by PML-RARα, and the malignant promyelocytes differentiate into granulocytes (54). The advent of ATRA therapy has improved the remission induction rate from 62% to greater than 90% and has significantly decreased the rate of hemorrhagic death.

A second common example of differentiation therapy in pediatric oncology is the use of 13-cis-retinoic acid to treat neuroblastoma. As laboratory work demonstrated that retinoids induce the differentiation of neuroblastoma cells, a large-scale trial was performed that randomized patients with high-risk neuroblastoma to receive either 13-cis-retinoic acid or nothing following a randomization to autologous peripheral blood stem cell transplant or intensive chemotherapy. Because this study showed a clear survival advantage for patients who were treated with 13-cis-retinoic acid (34), this therapy is now the standard of care in the US.

Immunotherapy

Like differentiation therapy, immunotherapy is gaining acceptance in the treatment of pediatric malignancies. Under the broad category of immunotherapy are classified such diverse treatments as allogeneic hematopoietic stem cell transplantation, with or without infusion of donor lymphocytes, and treatment with various recombinant cytokines. Stem cell transplantation and donor lymphocyte infusions are covered in depth in Chapter 102. Cytokine administration remains a rare event in pediatric oncology, but this approach was pioneered by the National Cancer Institute's efforts at inducing an immune response to metastatic melanoma and to renal cell carcinoma by infusions of IL-2. Similar protocols are being explored by the Children's Oncology Group and, over time, manipulation of the immune system via cytokine administration will become a more frequent event.

Small-Molecule Kinase Inhibitors

The advent of Gleevec for the treatment of chronic myelogenous leukemia (CML) heralded the era of targeted therapy based on a molecular understanding of tumorigenesis. CML is defined by the presence of a distinctive chromosomal translocation, t(9;22), or the Philadelphia chromosome. This translocation leads to the production of a fusion protein tyrosine kinase called BCR-ABL, and this kinase drives the neoplastic process. Gleevec is a competitive inhibitor of the BCR-ABL tyrosine kinase and causes complete hematologic response as a single agent in 95% of CML patients (25). Given the dramatic success with Gleevec, a host of similar small-molecule inhibitors are being developed, both for leukemias and for solid tumors.

Monoclonal Antibodies

Monoclonal antibody therapy is also finding expanded use in pediatric oncology. Two frequently used monoclonal antibodies target antigens on the surface of lymphocytes. Rituximab is an antibody against CD20, a marker of B lymphocytes, and is seeing increased use in treating non-Hodgkin lymphoma and autoimmune disorders, such as immune thrombocytopenic purpura (ITP) and hemolytic anemia. Response to rituximab can be monitored indirectly by measuring CD20$^+$ cells in the circulation, and they often become undetectable within a day of only one dose of the antibody. Clearance of circulating CD20$^+$ cells does not necessarily correlate with efficacy, unfortunately, because most CD20$^+$ cells do not circulate, but are found in spleen and lymph nodes, where they are not easily measured. Another commonly used monoclonal antibody is alemtuzumab, which is anti-CD52. CD52 is a pan-lymphocyte marker, and treatment with alemtuzumab results in a rapid, profound, and long-lasting depletion of circulating T cells, B cells, natural killer (NK) cells, and monocytes. Patients become lymphopenic within 2 weeks and remain lymphopenic for as long as a year after treatment (52). In adult oncology, alemtuzumab is primarily used as therapy for lymphomas, but in pediatric oncology, its primary use is in the context of BMT—either as part of an immunoablative preparative regimen or in the prevention or treatment of graft-versus-host disease. An appreciation of the profoundly immunosuppressive nature of this drug is critical to appropriately evaluating BMT patients who have received the drug.

TOXICITIES

The management of acute toxicities of cancer therapy often falls to a partnership between the pediatric oncologist and the pediatric intensivist. Understanding the unique toxicities experienced by the pediatric oncology patient is critical to the successful management of the critically ill child with cancer. This section will outline the common therapy-related toxicities that may be experienced by a pediatric oncology patient. Some of these toxicities are covered more extensively in other chapters (e.g., graft-versus-host disease, GVHD, is covered in Chapter 102), and the reader is referred to those chapters for more detail. Typical toxicities that are caused by the commonly used chemotherapy drugs are listed in **Table 99.3**. The following discussion is organized by organ system, rather than by individual drug.

Fever in the Neutropenic Patient

The most common side effect of cytotoxic chemotherapy is myelosuppression, which leads to periods of absolute neutropenia. A fever in a neutropenic cancer patient represents a true emergency due to the significant rate of gram-negative bacteremia in such patients, which can rapidly lead to septic shock. Because of the emergent nature of febrile neutropenia, this topic is dealt with in Chapter 100.

TYPICAL TOXICITIES OF COMMONLY USED
CHEMOTHERAPY DRUGS

Drug	Toxicities
Ifosfamide	Renal tubular dysfunction, encephalopathy, hemorrhagic cystitis
Cyclophosphamide	Renal tubular dysfunction, hemorrhagic cystitis, myocardial necrosis
Cytarabine	Cerebellar syndrome, myelopathy, leukoencephalopathy, pulmonary edema, pneumonitis
Methotrexate	Skin sloughing, nephrotoxicity, seizures, hepatic dysfunction
Anthracyclines	Severe mucositis, congestive heart failure
Bleomycin	Pneumonitis
ATRA	Capillary leak syndrome
L-asparaginase	Pancreatitis
Cisplatin	Renal tubular dysfunction, cardiotoxicity
Vincristine	Peripheral neuropathy, ileus, neuropathic pain

Most chemotherapeutic agents cause nausea, vomiting, mucositis, and pancytopenia; therefore, these are not included in the table above. This table is *not* intended to be a comprehensive listing of chemotherapy side effects, but rather a list of the most common toxicities that may be encountered by the pediatric intensivist.

Toxicities Related to Bone Marrow Transplantation

Children who have undergone BMT are subject to a number of unique toxicities, including veno-occlusive disease, cytokine storm/engraftment syndrome, and GVHD. BMT patients may also develop fever while they are neutropenic, and many of the immunosuppressive drugs used as prophylaxis or in treatment of GVHD can cause significant, difficult-to-control hypertension. Finally, pneumonitis is a common problem encountered in the post-BMT setting. These topics are covered extensively in other chapters in this text.

Toxicities of the Central Nervous System

A number of commonly used chemotherapeutic drugs cause distinct CNS toxicities. The greatest culprit in the pediatric population is ifosfamide. Ifosfamide causes encephalopathy in 10%–30% of patients, with onset of symptoms, which can range from mild (somnolence) to severe (coma or seizure), occurring between 2 and 48 hrs after drug administration (13). The mechanism for this toxicity is unclear, although several potential pathophysiologic explanations have been proposed, including accumulation of glutaric acid, which can lead to disturbances in the mitochondrial respiratory chain, ultimately leading to high levels of the ifosfamide metabolite chloroacetaldehyde, which is neurotoxic (29). David and Picus investigated risk factors for the development of ifosfamide-induced encephalopathy and found no correlation with renal function or dose of drug. They did, however, find a statistically signifi-

cant association between encephalopathy and hypoalbuminemia (13). The management of ifosfamide-induced encephalopathy includes discontinuation of the drug and standard supportive measures (discussed in more detail elsewhere in this text). Several groups have reported of the use of methylene blue for the treatment of ifosfamide-induced encephalopathy, but the lack of any controlled trials (and reports of spontaneous resolution) makes it impossible to determine if this agent is helpful (36). The mechanism by which methylene blue might treat this encephalopathy is also unclear.

The other chemotherapy drug that commonly causes acute CNS toxicity is araC (5). The neurologic toxicities depend on dose and route of administration. Intrathecal araC has been associated with a rapid-onset myelopathy (although this might be related to the use of benzyl alcohol as a diluent) or a slower-onset myelopathy, with symptoms beginning 2 days to 6 months after treatment. On autopsy in many of these patients, correlative evidence of demyelination was observed. Other CNS toxicities have also been reported more rarely after intrathecal araC, including seizures and leukoencephalopathy. Seizures have also been described in patients being treated with IV high-dose araC. In general, these have been self-limited and do not recur once therapy is stopped. Cerebral dysfunction, usually accompanying cerebellar syndrome, has also been described and usually takes the form of generalized encephalopathy. Cerebral dysfunction also usually resolves spontaneously.

The acute cerebellar syndrome is the most prominent and common neurologic toxicity associated with cytarabine (5). The syndrome is only seen after treatment with high-dose systemic cytarabine and occurs at an incidence of at least 10%. Onset of symptoms is 3–8 days after treatment, and manifestations include dysarthria, dysdiadochokinesia, dysmetria, and ataxia. The outcome is variable, with complete resolution of symptoms common, but ~30% of adults never regain normal function. Diagnostic evaluation is unrevealing. Risk factors include age (with incidence increasing from 3% in patients who are <40 years of age to 30% in patients who are >60 years of age). Other possible risk factors include renal dysfunction and cumulative exposure to drug, although these are not completely agreed upon. The neuropathology of cerebellar syndrome has been extensively investigated, and findings consistently include the loss of Purkinje cells in the cerebellar hemispheres and vermis with a reactive gliosis. The only effective therapy for this disorder is discontinuation of the drug and institution of supportive care as indicated.

Cardiac Toxicities

The best-known cardiotoxic chemotherapy drugs are the anthracyclines: doxorubicin, daunorubicin, and idarubicin. The mechanism of cardiotoxicity involves the generation of O_2 free radicals, which ultimately lead to irreversible loss of myocardiocytes and the development of cardiomyopathy. Anthracycline cardiotoxicity can be acute or delayed. Acute effects include transient arrhythmias and acute left ventricular failure (46). The acute effects are usually transient and will attenuate after discontinuation of therapy (44). Cardiac injury can also present in a delayed fashion, years or decades after treatment, as new-onset congestive heart failure. The most significant risk factor for serious cardiotoxicity is cumulative dose. Many approaches to minimizing the risk of cardiotoxicity have been investigated. Other than limiting total exposure, measures that have been investigated include the administration of liposome-encapsulated anthracyclines and the use of cardioprotectants, such as dexrazoxane (Zinecard). Dexrazoxane acts as an iron chelator; it prevents the formation of an anthracycline-iron complex that is thought to be a critical mediator of myocardiocyte injury and thus prevent cardiac damage. Clinical evidence suggests that dexrazoxane does, in fact, reduce cardiotoxicity caused by doxorubicin. Once patients exhibit symptoms of cardiotoxicity, standard treatments should be administered, aimed at decreasing afterload and increasing contractility. Anticoagulation is useful in the setting of severe left ventricular dysfunction and persistent dysrhythmia. Cardiac transplantation remains an option for end-stage cardiomyopathy.

Cyclophosphamide has also been associated with severe cardiotoxicity at high doses, such as are employed in BMT. The estimated incidence in children is 5% in patients treated with marrow ablative doses (46). Risk factors include prior anthracycline chemotherapy and chest irradiation. Clinically, cardiotoxicity presents as congestive heart failure or myocarditis. Severe hemorrhagic cardiac necrosis has been reported as well. Symptoms may be delayed by up to 2 weeks after administration, but can be rapidly fatal, with a 10% mortality rate. With no specific treatment available for cyclophosphamide-induced cardiotoxicity, standard supportive measures are indicated.

Paclitaxel has been associated with asymptomatic bradycardia in up to 29% of treated patients (46). Second- and third-degree heart blocks are also seen, though less frequently. These bradyarrhythmias are reversible. Several cases of acute myocardial infarction after cisplatin therapy have also been reported (44).

Several other drugs have been associated with cardiac toxicities. Amsacrine, an acridine derivative with activity against hematologic malignancies (not commercially available in the US), can affect cardiac electrophysiology and cause a wide range of EKG changes, including ventricular tachycardia. The arrhythmias can occur within minutes of treatment. More rare are reports of delayed (days after treatment) cardiomyopathy. 5-fluorouracil has also been reported to induce cardiotoxicity (including arrhythmias, silent ischemia, and even sudden death) in up to 18% of treated patients, occurring mostly in the setting of continuous infusion, rather than bolus dosing. Risk factors include pre-existing coronary artery disease and concurrent radiotherapy. The mechanism of this toxicity is unknown.

Pulmonary Toxicities

Bleomycin is the chemotherapeutic most frequently thought of in the context of pulmonary toxicity, but other cytotoxic treatments can cause pulmonary fibrosis or edema, including gemcitabine, cytarabine, and radiation therapy. Additionally, a number of drugs (including carmustine, methotrexate, procarbazine, and bleomycin) have been linked with a hypersensitivity pneumonitis syndrome. Also referred to as inflammatory interstitial pneumonitis, this syndrome is characterized by an insidious progression of nonproductive cough, dyspnea, and low-grade fevers. Eosinophilia is noted in the peripheral blood and on lung biopsy, which often also reveals bronchiolitis obliterans with organizing pneumonia (BOOP). This syndrome resolves with removal of the offending agent, although sometimes oral corticosteroids speed recovery.

Bleomycin toxicity is primarily limited to lungs and skin because these organs lack bleomycin hydrolase. Most commonly, bleomycin causes an interstitial pneumonitis (bleomycin-induced pneumonitis, BIP) and has been reported in up to 46% of patients treated with bleomycin (depending on diagnostic criteria), with mortality seen in 3%. BIP usually begins during therapy and is initially indolent, with a cough and dyspnea on exertion as the primary symptoms. The disorder can progress to dyspnea at rest, tachypnea, and cyanosis. Radiographic findings are nonspecific and may be focal or diffuse, unilateral or bilateral. Interstitial or alveolar infiltrates can be seen on plain film, and CT scan often shows small linear and subpleural nodular lesions in the lung bases. Lung biopsy may show characteristic lesions, such as squamous metaplasia of bronchiolar epithelium, inflammatory cells infiltrating into alveoli and alveolar septa, edema plus focal collagen depositions in these septa, and fibrotic areas. In animal models, the pathogenesis appears to be related to initial endothelial damage, probably mediated through free radical production and release of cytokines, followed by an influx of inflammatory cells, ultimately leading to pulmonary fibrosis. Decrease in diffusion capacity is seen in patients with BIP, although this finding is nonspecific. Decreased vital capacity is also seen and was noted in patients who received combination therapy with bleomycin, etoposide, and cisplatin, but not in patients treated with etoposide and cisplatin alone (50), suggesting that decreased vital capacity may be a more specific indicator of BIP. High-dose corticosteroids (60–100 mg/day in adults) are frequently used to treat clinically significant BIP but, as yet, no randomized studies demonstrate the efficacy of steroids in this setting. Also of importance to the intensivist is the acute onset of pulmonary edema, often mimicking adult respiratory distress syndrome, in patients previously treated with bleomycin who are exposed to high concentrations of inspired oxygen, as may occur in conjunction with a surgical procedure, even years after chemotherapy is completed. This complication can be minimized by administering the lowest possible concentration of O_2 to patients with a history of treatment with bleomycin.

A vascular leak syndrome, leading to significant, sometimes life-threatening, pulmonary edema has also been described with infusions of araC or IL-2 (1). The vascular leak is usually reversible with discontinuation of therapy and is treated with diuresis and oxygen. Prostaglandins or cyclooxygenase-2 may attenuate IL-2–induced vascular leak. Vascular leak has also been reported in patients treated with ATRA for acute promyelocytic leukemia. The leukemia itself is probably involved in this process, because vascular leak has not been reported in patients treated with ATRA for other disorders.

Other chemotherapeutic agents associated with pulmonary toxicity include Mitomycin-C, which causes a delayed-onset interstitial pneumonitis that is symptomatic in ~5% of treated patients; actinomycin D, which acts as a radiation sensitizer; and, rarely, cyclophosphamide or ifosfamide, which can cause pulmonary fibrosis in less than 1% of treated patients.

Radiation therapy can damage capillary endothelial cells and type I pneumocytes, eventually leading to a pneumonitis syndrome. Incidence and severity are primarily related to the amount of lung volume irradiated, total dose delivered, and the fractions into which the total dose is divided. Radiation pneumonitis is rare in patients treated with <20 Gy, but is highly likely in patients who receive >60 Gy. Symptoms become evident 2–3 months following completion of therapy, and primarily include complaints of dyspnea and a nonproductive cough. Physical findings are usually minimal. Permanent changes of fibrosis evolve over 6–24 months, but usually stabilize after this time period. No controlled trials of treatment have been conducted for radiation pneumonitis, but objective responses to corticosteroids are seen. Once fibrosis develops, most experts believe corticosteroids have no further therapeutic role. Clinical symptomatic relief has been reported in patients with pulmonary fibrosis who were treated with pentoxifylline and vitamin E (14).

Retinoic Acid Syndrome

The advent of ATRA for the treatment of APL has transformed this disease from one that carried a grave prognosis into one that is frequently curable. The major complication of ATRA treatment is the retinoic acid syndrome, which occurs in as many as 25% of patients with APL who are treated with ATRA. Improvements in recognition and treatment have decreased the mortality of retinoic acid syndrome from 30% to 5%. The diagnosis is established by the presence of at least three of the following signs and/or symptoms in the absence of alternative explanations: fever, weight gain, respiratory distress, pulmonary infiltrates, pleural or pericardial effusions, hypotension, and renal failure (31). The syndrome most commonly manifests ~10 days after the start of chemotherapy, but has been reported as soon as 2 days into treatment. The pathogenesis is related to tissue infiltration with newly differentiated granulocytes and cytokine production by these cells. The final pathway is endothelial damage leading to edema, hemorrhage, fibrinous exudates, and respiratory failure. The only specific therapy available for retinoic acid syndrome is dexamethasone. As noted, improved recognition of the syndrome and prompt institution of steroid therapy has dramatically improved prognosis.

Pancreatitis

It has long been recognized that treatment with L-asparaginase may cause acute pancreatitis. Management of asparaginase-induced pancreatitis is identical to the management of idiopathic pancreatitis, including gut rest. Asparaginase-induced acute pancreatitis can progress to hemorrhagic pancreatitis, and chronic pancreatitis is also seen in some patients.

Urinary Tract Toxicities

Both ifosfamide and cyclophosphamide can cause hemorrhagic cystitis. Ifosfamide is a more potent urotoxin than cyclophosphamide. Both drugs are broken down to produce, among other degradation products, acrolein. Acrolein has been incriminated as the major cause of hemorrhagic cystitis after treatment with these drugs, but the difference between ifosfamide and cyclophosphamide is not accounted for entirely by increased production of acrolein; therefore, other metabolites are probably also involved. Prophylaxis against hemorrhagic cystitis includes aggressive hydration (alkaline intravenous fluids at twice maintenance) and the use of mesna (sodium-2-mercaptoethanesulfonate). Mesna can be administered either orally or intravenously and is rapidly oxidized to dimesna,

which is filtered and excreted by the kidneys. Between 30% and 50% of glomerularly filtered dimesna is reduced back to mesna in the renal tubular epithelium by glutathione reductase. Mesna collects in the bladder, where it detoxifies acrolein and other oxazaphosphorine metabolites. Mesna is superior to placebo or to hydration alone in the prevention of hemorrhagic cystitis (48). Uncontrolled hemorrhagic cystitis can be life-threatening, and exsanguination can occur. If prophylaxis fails, management includes cystoscopy and clot evacuation, aggressive bladder irrigation, and intravesical instillation of formalin.

In addition to cystitis, cyclophosphamide and ifosfamide can also cause renal dysfunction, both tubular and glomerular. Ifosfamide is a far more potent nephrotoxin, although nephrotoxicity is seen after very high doses of cyclophosphamide. Proximal tubular dysfunction is the most common form of nephrotoxicity observed and frequently manifests as Fanconi syndrome, with hypophosphatemia, renal tubular acidosis, hypokalemia, hypocalcemia, or hypomagnesemia. Any of these can be quite severe and require aggressive replacement therapy. Distal tubular dysfunction is less common, but nephrogenic diabetes insipidus has been reported. Glomerular toxicity, though more rare, can be severe enough to require dialysis and may become chronic. Hypertension is also seen. The specific mechanism of renal tubular damage caused by these drugs is unknown. Risk factors for ifosfamide nephrotoxicity include age (increased risk in children <5 years old), total dose of ifosfamide (increased risk with total dose >60 g/m^2), prior or concurrent treatment with cisplatin (which increases the risk), and preexisting renal impairment (49). A theoretical basis exists for the belief that very high doses of mesna might protect against renal tubular damage caused by ifosfamide, but no clinical studies have been conducted to support this theory. Thus, currently, the only available preventive measures are careful screening of patients and limiting treatment in patients with the risk factors described previously.

Cisplatin is also nephrotoxic. Cisplatin accumulates in the proximal tubules, with intracellular concentrations fivefold higher than plasma concentrations (28). Through inhibition of protein synthesis and depletion of glutathione, cisplatin causes the tubular necrosis that underlies its renal toxicity. Cisplatin administration results in a dose-dependent reduction of glomerular filtration rate, hypomagnesemia, hypokalemia, and polyuria. Evidence suggests that aggressive hydration, including the use of mannitol, can attenuate the toxicity of cisplatin. The renal toxicity of cisplatin is usually reversible, but can become chronic and progressive.

Radiation Recall

Radiation recall is an inflammatory reaction in a previously irradiated body area. Most commonly, radiation recall manifests as an acute dermatitis. Reactions can range from a mild maculopapular erythematous skin rash to severe necrosis and occurs in a sharply demarcated area corresponding to the prior radiation field. The reaction can occur weeks to years after radiation exposure, and the mechanism of this reaction is unclear. First described in patients treated with actinomycin D, radiation recall has subsequently been described with numerous other antineoplastic drugs and, more recently, even in patients treated with other classes of pharmacologic agents (4).

Although skin is the most common organ involved, radiation recall has been reported in lung, esophagus, gut, and the CNS. In visceral organs, it manifests as inflammation of the target organ within a previous radiation field. Numerous hypotheses have been proposed to explain the phenomenon of radiation recall, but none have been proven to explain the process. The most reasonable current explanation is an idiosyncratic drug reaction in a tissue with an altered inflammatory response ratio induced by prior irradiation (4). A dose-response phenomenon is suggested, in that radiation recall is more frequent in areas that receive higher doses of radiation. Also, while numerous drugs have been implicated in radiation recall, nearly 50% of reported cases have been associated with the use of taxanes or anthracyclines. Treatment is straightforward, with the mainstays of therapy being corticosteroids and withdrawal of the offending agent. Topical steroids are appropriate for skin reactions, but clearly systemic steroids are necessary for visceral involvement.

Management of Chemotherapy Overdose

As chemotherapeutic agents can cause life-threatening complications when dosed appropriately, a chemotherapy overdose is certainly an indication for careful evaluation and will likely lead to a need for critical care. The literature contains few reports of the effects of accidental chemotherapy overdose, and even fewer reports of successful specific treatments. Most reports document the efficacy of aggressive supportive care allowing the patient to recover. Others report specific therapies administered to patients who received an overdose of cisplatin, including plasmapheresis and the administration of sodium thiosulfate. Hemodialysis has not been found to be effective, probably because cisplatin is extensively protein bound and deposits in tissues from which it is unable to be cleared by hemodialysis. Plasmapheresis is expected to be more effective by virtue of removing circulating plasma proteins to which cisplatin is bound. In 1 patient who was accidentally given a threefold overdose of cisplatin, at the time of overt renal failure, sodium thiosulfate was administered (loading dose of 4 g/m^2, followed by 2.7 g/m^2/day in three divided doses of 0.9 g/m^2/dose for 13 days) based on the assumption that this compound would bind the platinum and remove it from circulation (16). An increase in urinary platinum levels was seen after initiation of this therapy. The other reported specific treatment for cisplatin overdose is the administration of N-acetylcysteine to replenish glutathione and allow the usual detoxification reactions to function (45).

Ifosfamide overdose has been treated with the use of methylene blue. A patient who was accidentally given an overdose of ifosfamide was found to have excessive urinary excretion of glutaric acid and sarcosine, which is compatible with glutaric aciduria type II, a defect in mitochondrial fatty acid oxidation that results from defective electron transfer to flavoproteins (30). This observation led to the administration of 50 mg of methylene blue intravenously, based on the function of methylene blue as an electron acceptor. The severe neurotoxicity experienced by that patient rapidly reversed.

Carboxypeptidase G2 is another recently developed "antidote" to chemotherapy overdose. It is a bacterial enzyme that hydrolyzes methotrexate to its inactive metabolites, 4-deoxy-4-amino-N10-methylpteroic acid and glutamate. Carboxypep-

TABLE 99.4

USE OF HEMODIALYSIS FOR OVERDOSE OF CHEMOTHERAPY

Readily cleared by hemodialysis	Not cleared by hemodialysis
Ifosfamide Methotrexate Cyclophosphamide	Etoposide Dactinomycin Vinca alkaloids Anthracyclines

Platinum agents are cleared only if dialysis is initiated rapidly after drug administration. These drugs become protein-bound (carboplatin) or distribute into tissue (cisplatin) quickly and are no longer dialyzable. Paclitaxel pharmacokinetics is unaltered in anephric patients undergoing hemodialysis.

tidase G2 has been administered intravenously to patients with delayed methotrexate clearance after they were given appropriate high-dose methotrexate therapy, and more recently, it has been given intrathecally with good results to patients with an accidental intrathecal methotrexate overdose (55).

Hemodialysis is a nonspecific intervention often employed in the treatment of drug overdose. The effects of hemodialysis on the pharmacokinetics of antineoplastic drugs have been recently reviewed (53) and are summarized in **Table 99.4.** Paclitaxel pharmacokinetics is unaltered in anephric patients who are undergoing hemodialysis. Dialysis is effective in clearing cisplatin and carboplatin only within a relatively short time after drug administration due to rapid and stable binding to proteins in serum (carboplatin) or peripheral tissues (cisplatin). Methotrexate and cyclophosphamide are readily dialyzable, with an increased rate of elimination, compared to renal clearance. Ifosfamide is also readily removed by hemodialysis, while etoposide, dactinomycin, vinca alkaloids, and anthracyclines are rapidly and extensively protein bound and not cleared effectively by hemodialysis.

ETHICAL CONSIDERATIONS

Pediatric cancer patients represent a distinct population within the PICU, presenting with a specific set of ethical and decision-making challenges. For these reasons, we have chosen to address some of these issues here. For a more complete discussion of ethics in the PICU, please refer to Chapter 14.

Clinical Trials in Pediatric Oncology

Application of the therapies discussed in this chapter often occurs through national, cooperative clinical trials. In 1997, 81% of children treated for cancer at a center with membership in the Pediatric Oncology Group were enrolled in clinical trials, compared to a rate of 5% for adults with cancer. It has therefore been argued that being treated within a clinical trial can represent the "standard of care" for a child with cancer. This concept is important for the nononcologist to understand, because in many other branches of pediatrics, clinical trials reflect significant deviations from standard care or represent treatment options in the situation in which no standard of care exists.

Clinical trials are classified by "phase," with different phases having different study goals. For example, a phase I study is designed to establish a tolerable dose of a new drug. Such studies are not designed to test efficacy. A phase II study is designed to determine types of cancer that may respond to a new agent, and phase III studies are designed to determine which of two (or more) treatments is more effective. Because of these differing goals, the population of patients who may be eligible for a particular trial phase will differ. In general, phase III studies are limited to patients with a new diagnosis who were previously untreated. Phase II studies often enroll patients whose disease did not respond to standard therapy, but who have not yet received more than one or two treatment regimens. Phase I studies, in contrast, are usually open to patients whose disease has failed to respond to multiple attempts at treatment and for whom no potentially curative therapy is available. Because these studies are designed to determine the toxicity of the treatment, rather than its effectiveness, enrollment is usually limited to patients who have not yet suffered severe end-organ damage and who have a long enough life expectancy (typically 8 weeks or more) for treatment-related toxicities to become evident, but enrollment may not require the patient to have measurable disease.

Decision-making in Pediatric Oncology

The pediatric oncology population represents a unique group of PICU patients. Many critically ill children are otherwise healthy and are experiencing a singular event (trauma or surgery) from which they are likely to recover and which is unlikely to be repeated. The oncology patient, in contrast, may have been ill and under treatment for years, and the family has been told repeatedly about the life-threatening nature of their child's condition even during periods of relative health. In contrast to other patients with chronic illnesses, pediatric cancer patients are offered treatment on clinical trials, with the implication of participating in experimental therapy from the time of initial diagnosis. Also, unlike other patients with chronic illnesses, these patients are treated with modalities that themselves can cause significant morbidity and even mortality, and the families are made aware of this from the beginning as well. These experiences will engender a different approach to decision making than that taken by the parent of a child who is acutely ill but otherwise has a normal life expectancy or by the parent of a patient whose treatment itself is not likely to cause death.

When the oncologist and intensivist disagree about prognosis or the appropriateness of specific further therapeutic interventions, it is helpful to keep in mind the potential biases that frame each specialist's perspective (2). Parents and patients suffer from poor communication among specialists. Much of the tension and inaccuracy in communication can be avoided when all sides are fully aware of the potential for bias.

Timing Bias

Timing bias involves the change in perception that occurs depending on the immediacy of death or complication. Oncologists and the parents of cancer patients have faced the possibility of the patient's death at some ill-defined point in the future from the moment the diagnosis was established. Even though admission to the PICU may heighten the sense of immediacy of death or severe morbidity, it may not change the oncologist's perception of an ill-defined event in the future of a chronically life-threatening disease. Conversely, the intensivist may perceive the timing of the patient's admission to the PICU as a sudden life-threatening deterioration in a previously stable patient for whom specific curative therapy is unlikely.

Exposure Bias

Exposure bias involves the change in perception that occurs depending on how readily the specialist recalls the outcome of similar patients. For instance, if a patient is admitted to the PICU with methotrexate-induced bronchiolitis obliterans 1 day after another patient dies of the same complication, the PICU team is likely to perceive a heightened risk of mortality in the new patient, although the outcome of the previous admission has no a priori effect on the outcome of the current one. The admitting oncologist may lack this perception if he was not involved in the previous case.

Miscalibration Bias

Miscalibration bias involves the tendency of physicians to be overconfident in the extent of their knowledge. Each specialist is likely to be very knowledgeable in his field and less knowledgeable in the other's, and problems may arise from the failure of a specialist to acknowledge his knowledge limitations.

Frame Bias

Frame bias can lead to an entirely different perception of risk, especially when parents are involved in the conversation. For instance, the oncologist's statement that the patient has a 10% chance of survival (positive framing) is perceived entirely differently from the intensivist's statement that the patient has a 90% chance of death (negative framing), even though both specialists have quoted the same numerical probabilities.

Denominator Bias

Denominator bias arises from imprecision in the description of the population sample used for comparisons. When quoting probabilities about future events, it is vital that both specialties draw their conclusions based on population samples that were similar to the patient under treatment. It is helpful to stipulate the risk category (cancer grade), severity score, and other measures of severity adjustment so that the quoted data apply to the present patient. If the data result from studies with small sample sizes, one should acknowledge the increasing uncertainty in applying those conclusions to the present patient.

One issue that often arises in the care of critically ill pediatric cancer patients is the question of how informed the patient and the family are about prognosis and about the toxicity of treatment being offered. A recent study compared the informed consent process in pediatric and adult oncology and found that pediatric oncology decision-makers (parents or legal guardians) tended to be given more information about prognosis, randomization, and voluntariness than adult oncology patients were (47). Because all clinical trials require a signed consent form that has been approved by the Institutional Review Board, the families of most patients have at least had the opportunity to hear about the risks and benefits of enrollment. The consent forms suggested for use by the Children's Oncology Group list treatment side effects by drug in tabular form, with columns indicating the likelihood of each side effect, ranging from rare (<5%) to common (>20%), as well as the time frame in which the side effect is expected, ranging from immediate (within 1–2 days of receiving the drug) through delayed/late (more than 3 weeks after treatment). These documents are usually given to the family for future reference, because most families will not retain the enormous amount of information presented during a typical informed-consent conference.

The other major challenge that frequently arises in critically ill pediatric oncology patients involves end-of-life decisions. In that this process is inadequately studied, few data are available to guide the physician. A review all of the available studies of pediatric oncology family decision making at the end of life reported several interesting findings: (a) patients, when included in the discussions, most frequently made the final decisions regarding end-of-life care, (b) patients with cystic fibrosis were more eager to participate in medical decision-making than were patients with scoliosis about to undergo corrective surgery, (c) parents of recently deceased children emphasized the importance of avoiding pain and suffering and considerations of quality of life in their decision-making processes, and (d) families strongly desire that physicians share information with parents, regardless of how upsetting the information may be (22). The reviewers then combined this information with that gleaned from a review of the recommendations of professional societies and their own unpublished institutional studies to develop a set of guidelines to assist parents, adolescent patients, and healthcare providers in making end-of-life decisions (22).

CONCLUSIONS AND FUTURE DIRECTIONS

The future of pediatric oncology therapy lies not with the development of improved cytotoxic drugs, but rather with the expansion of biologically based therapies and targeted therapies. The prototype for the potential of these approaches remains the astounding success of ATRA in the treatment of APL. The profound efficacy of Gleevec for the treatment of CML in the absence of significant toxicity further emphasizes the power of biologically based therapies. It is hoped that the future will see the expansion of this type of treatment and the disappearance of highly toxic, highly nonspecific cytotoxic chemotherapy.

KEY POINTS

- Modern cancer therapy is often multimodal, including chemotherapy, surgery, and radiotherapy.
- Chemotherapeutics can be categorized based on structure and function:
  - Alkylating agents, such as nitrogen mustard derivatives and nitrosoureas, contain highly reactive alkyl groups that form covalent bonds with DNA, resulting in cross-linking events that lead to cell death by impeding DNA replication.
  - Antimetabolites, such as the antifolate methotrexate and the purine analogs, induce cell death predominantly through interference with DNA synthesis.
  - Topoisomerase inhibitors, such as podophyllotoxins and anthracyclines, induce cell death by interfering with the maintenance of DNA supercoiling.

- Antimicrotubule agents, such as vinca alkaloids and taxanes, interfere with the function of the mitotic spindle.
- Radiation therapy can be delivered as either photons or protons, and causes cytotoxicity predominantly through the induction of DNA damage.
- More recently, biologic therapies, such as immunotherapy, small-molecule kinase inhibitors, cytokine therapies, and antiangiogenic therapies, are being actively developed.
- Toxicities of cancer therapies are usually related to interference with the function or survival of normal cell types.
  - Central nervous system toxicities include ifosfamide-induced encephalopathy and the araC acute cerebellar syndrome.
  - Anthracyclines cause a cumulative dose-dependent cardiotoxicity, due to O_2 free radicals and characterized primarily by cardiomyopathy, resulting in congestive heart failure.
  - Bleomycin and radiation therapy are the primary agents that cause pulmonary toxicity. This toxicity is predominantly fibrotic and is worsened by high O_2 tension.
  - The most common genitourinary toxicities of chemotherapy are the renal tubular dysfunction associated with ifosfamide and cisplatin and the hemorrhagic cystitis caused by cyclophosphamide and ifosfamide.
- Radiation recall is an inflammatory reaction in a previously irradiated body area. Most commonly, it manifests as an acute dermatitis, but visceral involvement has also been reported.
- Options for the management of chemotherapy overdose are limited. Some agents can be removed by hemodialysis or plasmapheresis. Carboxypeptidase G2, a bacterial enzyme that hydrolyzes methotrexate to inactive metabolites extremely rapidly, is an "antidote" to methotrexate. Methylene blue has been administered to treat ifosfamide overdose.
- Most pediatric oncology therapy is administered in the context of a clinical trial. Phase I trials are designed to establish a tolerable dose of a new drug. Phase II trials are designed to determine which types of cancer respond to a new agent, and phase III studies are designed to determine which of two or more treatments is more effective.

References

1. Abid SH, Malhotra V, Perry MC. Radiation-induced and chemotherapy-induced pulmonary injury. *Curr Opin Oncol* 2001;13:242–8.
2. Adams AM, Smith AF. Risk perception and communication: Recent developments and implications for anaesthesia. *Anaesthesia* 2001;56:745–55.
3. Anderson PM, Wiseman GA, Dispenzieri A, et al. High-dose samarium-153 ethylene diamine tetramethylene phosphonate: low toxicity of skeletal irradiation in patients with osteosarcoma and bone metastases. *J Clin Oncol* 2002;20:189–96.
4. Azria D, Magne N, Zouhair A, et al. Radiation recall: A well recognized but neglected phenomenon. *Cancer Treat Rev* 2005;31:555–70.
5. Baker WJ, Royer GL, Jr., Weiss RB. Cytarabine and neurologic toxicity. *J Clin Oncol* 1991;9:679–93.
6. Belli JA, Dicus GJ, Bonte FJ. Radiation response of mammalian tumor cells. I. Repair of sublethal damage in vivo. *J Natl Cancer Inst* 1967;38:673–82.
7. Belotti D, Vergani V, Drudis T, et al. The microtubule-affecting drug paclitaxel has antiangiogenic activity. *Clin Cancer Res* 1996;2:1843–9.
8. Billington DC. Angiogenesis and its inhibition: Potential new therapies in oncology and non-neoplastic diseases. *Drug Des Discov* 1991;8:3–35.

9. Capizzi RL, Bertino JR, Handschumacher RE. L-asparaginase. *Annu Rev Med* 1970;21:433–44.
10. Chabner B, Longo DL. *Cancer Chemotherapy and Biotherapy: Principles and Practice, 3rd edition.* Philadelphia: Lippincott Williams & Wilkins, 2001.
11. Chaffey JT, Hellman S. Differing responses to radiation of murine bone marrow stem cells in relation to the cell cycle. *Cancer Res* 1971;31:1613–5.
12. Chen AY, Liu LF. DNA topoisomerases: Essential enzymes and lethal targets. *Annu Rev Pharmacol Toxicol* 1994;34:191–218.
13. David KA, Picus J. Evaluating risk factors for the development of ifosfamide encephalopathy. *Am J Clin Oncol* 2005;28:277–80.
14. Delanian S, Balla-Mekias S, Lefaix JL. Striking regression of chronic radiotherapy damage in a clinical trial of combined pentoxifylline and tocopherol. *J Clin Oncol* 1999;17:3283–90.
15. Eastman A. Reevaluation of interaction of cis-dichloro(ethylenediamine) platinum(II) with DNA. *Biochemistry* 1986;25:3912–5.
16. Erdlenbruch B, Pekrun A, Schiffmann H, et al. Topical topic: Accidental cisplatin overdose in a child: Reversal of acute renal failure with sodium thiosulfate. *Med Pediatr Oncol* 2002;38:349–52.
17. Fridland A. Effect of methotrexate on deoxyribonucleotide pools and DNA synthesis in human lymphocytic cells. *Cancer Res* 1974;34:1883–8.
18. Gilman A. The initial clinical trial of nitrogen mustard. *Am J Surg* 1963;105: 574–8.
19. Hall AG, Tilby MJ. Mechanisms of action of, and modes of resistance to, alkylating agents used in the treatment of haematological malignancies. *Blood Rev* 1992;6:163–73.
20. Hande KR. Etoposide: Four decades of development of a topoisomerase II inhibitor. *Eur J Cancer* 1998;34:1514–21.
21. Himes RH. Interactions of the catharanthus (Vinca) alkaloids with tubulin and microtubules. *Pharmacol Ther* 1991;51:257–67.
22. Hinds PS, Oakes L, Furman W, et al. End-of-life decision making by adolescents, parents, and healthcare providers in pediatric oncology: Research to evidence-based practice guidelines. *Cancer Nurs* 2001;24:122–34.
23. Hirata S, Matsubara T, Saura R, et al. Inhibition of in vitro vascular endothelial cell proliferation and in vivo neovascularization by low-dose methotrexate. *Arthritis Rheum* 1989;32:1065–73.
24. Hryniuk WM. Pureless death as a link between growth rate and cytotoxicity by methotrexate. *Cancer Res* 1972;32:1506–11.
25. Kantarjian H, Sawyers C, Hochhaus A, et al. Hematologic and cytogenetic responses to imatinib mesylate in chronic myelogenous leukemia. *N Engl J Med* 2002;346:645–52.
26. Kohn KW. Interstrand cross-linking of DNA by 1,3-bis(2-chloroethyl)-1-nitrosourea and other 1-(2-haloethyl)-1-nitrosoureas. *Cancer Res* 1977;37: 1450–4.
27. Kufe DW, Major PP, Egan EM, et al. Correlation of cytotoxicity with incorporation of ara-C into DNA. *J Biol Chem* 1980;255:8997–900.
28. Kuhlmann MK, Burkhardt G, Kohler H. Insights into potential cellular mechanisms of cisplatin nephrotoxicity and their clinical application. *Nephrol Dial Transplant* 1997;12:2478–80.
29. Kupfer A, Aeschlimann C, Cerny T. Methylene blue and the neurotoxic mechanisms of ifosfamide encephalopathy. *Eur J Clin Pharmacol* 1996;50: 249–52.
30. Kupfer A, Aeschlimann C, Wermuth B, et al. Prophylaxis and reversal of ifosfamide encephalopathy with methylene-blue. *Lancet* 1994;343: 763–4.
31. Larson RS, Tallman MS. Retinoic acid syndrome: Manifestations, pathogenesis, and treatment. *Best Pract Res Clin Haematol* 2003;16:453–61.
32. Lawley PD, Brookes P. Acidic dissociation of 7:9-dialkylguanines and its possible relation to mutagenic properties of alkylating agents. *Nature* 1961;192: 1081–2.
33. Levin WP, Kooy H, Loeffler JS, et al. Proton beam therapy. *Br J Cancer* 2005; 93:849–54.
34. Matthay KK. Intensification of therapy using hematopoietic stem-cell support for high-risk neuroblastoma. *Pediatr Transplant* 1999;3 Suppl 1:72–7.
35. Matthay KK, Tan JC, Villablanca JG, et al. Phase I dose escalation of iodine-131-metaiodobenzylguanidine with myeloablative chemotherapy and autologous stem-cell transplantation in refractory neuroblastoma: A new approaches [sic] to Neuroblastoma Therapy Consortium Study. *J Clin Oncol* 2006;24:500–6.
36. Patel PN. Methylene blue for management of Ifosfamide-induced encephalopathy. *Ann Pharmacother* 2006;40:299–303.
37. Pegg AE. Mammalian O6-alkylguanine-DNA alkyltransferase: Regulation and importance in response to alkylating carcinogenic and therapeutic agents. *Cancer Res* 1990;50:6119–29.
38. Perry MC, ed. *The Chemotherapy Source Book, 3rd edition.* Philadelphia: Lippincott Williams & Wilkins, 2001.
39. Pommier Y. Eukaryotic DNA topoisomerase I: Genome gatekeeper and its intruders, camptothecins. *Semin Oncol* 1996;23:3–10.
40. Quasthoff S, Hartung HP. Chemotherapy-induced peripheral neuropathy. *J Neurol* 2002;249:9–17.
41. Radford IR. The level of induced DNA double-strand breakage correlates with cell killing after X-irradiation. *Int J Radiat Biol Relat Stud Phys Chem Med* 1985;48:45–54.
42. Rowinsky EK, Donehower RC. Paclitaxel (Taxol). *N Engl J Med* 1995;332: 1004–14.
43. Schiff PB, Fant J, Horwitz SB. Promotion of microtubule assembly in vitro by taxol. *Nature* 1979;277:665–7.
44. Schimmel KJ, Richel DJ, van den Brink RB, et al. Cardiotoxicity of cytotoxic drugs. *Cancer Treat Rev* 2004;30:181–91.
45. Sheikh-Hamad D, Timmins K, Jalali Z. Cisplatin-induced renal toxicity: possible reversal by N-acetylcysteine treatment. *J Am Soc Nephrol* 1997;8: 1640–4.
46. Simbre VC, Duffy SA, Dadlani GH, et al. Cardiotoxicity of cancer chemotherapy: implications for children. *Paediatr Drugs* 2005;7:187–202.
47. Simon CM, Siminoff LA, Kodish ED, et al. Comparison of the informed consent process for randomized clinical trials in pediatric and adult oncology. *J Clin Oncol* 2004;22:2708–17.
48. Siu LL, Moore MJ. Use of mesna to prevent ifosfamide-induced urotoxicity. *Support Care Cancer* 1998;6:144–54.
49. Skinner R, Sharkey IM, Pearson AD, et al. Ifosfamide, mesna, and nephrotoxicity in children. *J Clin Oncol* 1993;11:173–90.
50. Sleijfer S. Bleomycin-induced pneumonitis. *Chest* 2001;120:617–24.
51. Tewey KM, Rowe TC, Yang L, et al. Adriamycin-induced DNA damage mediated by mammalian DNA topoisomerase II. *Science* 1984;226:466–8.
52. Thursky KA, Worth LJ, Seymour JF, et al. Spectrum of infection, risk and recommendations for prophylaxis and screening among patients with lymphoproliferative disorders treated with alemtuzumab. *Br J Haematol* 2006; 132:3–12.
53. Tomita M, Aoki Y, Tanaka K. Effect of haemodialysis on the pharmacokinetics of antineoplastic drugs. *Clin Pharmacokinet* 2004;43:515–27.
54. Warrell RP, Jr., de The H, Wang ZY, et al. Acute promyelocytic leukemia. *N Engl J Med* 1993;329:177–89.
55. Widemann BC, Balis FM, Shalabi A, et al. Treatment of accidental intrathecal methotrexate overdose with intrathecal carboxypeptidase G2. *J Natl Cancer Inst* 2004;96:1557–9.
56. Woodcock DM, Fox RM, Cooper IA. Evidence for a new mechanism of cytotoxicity of 1-beta-D arabinofuranosylcytosine. *Cancer Res* 1979;39: 1418–24.
57. Zwelling LA, Kohn KW. Mechanism of action of cis-dichlorodiammineplatinum(II). *Cancer Treat Rep* 1979;63:1439–44.

CHAPTER 100 ■ ONCOLOGIC EMERGENCIES AND COMPLICATIONS

RODRIGO MEJIA • JOSE A. CORTES • DEBORAH L. BROWN • GERARDO QUEZADA • MICHAEL E. RYTTING • CARROLL J. KING • ALAN I. FIELDS

The prognosis and outcome for pediatric cancer patients have steadily improved over recent decades, except for those patients admitted to the PICU (13,19,20,23,25). Outcomes for these patients showed little progress until the last decade. Earlier published reports indicated poor outcomes, and some even questioned if oncology patients should be admitted to the PICU at all, as treatment was frequently viewed as futile. More recent studies have noted improved outcomes and suggest that a more aggressive therapeutic approach, with earlier application of invasive therapies, may be responsible. Studies by Hallahan and Rossi suggest that early intervention for patients with lower Pediatric Risk of Mortality (PRISM) scores upon PICU admission are associated with better outcomes (20). Although inclusion of less severely ill patients could not be ruled out, these studies consistently show that mortality increases as more organ systems fail. It seems reasonable that intervention before end-organ failure has occurred is a prudent therapeutic goal, as once three or more organ systems fail, survival markedly decreases (23), and this finding has changed little in the past two decades. We include in this earlier intervention one of the "Holy Grails" of challenges for the intensive care team—the patient who has received stem cell transplantation. A review of recent literature on this population indicates improved PICU and short-term hospital outcomes (19).

This chapter is designed to provide the pediatric intensive care team with basic information on aspects of care that may be critical to this patient population early in the admission and treatment phase. The special complications encountered by the patient after hematopoietic stem cell transplant are discussed in Chapter 102. Because cancer patients often encounter the same critical illnesses as noncancer patients, the reader will be referred to other chapters in the text where these illnesses are discussed in greater detail.

Based on current knowledge, consideration for admission to the PICU and application of aggressive supportive therapies should occur as early as possible in the context of a child's declining clinical course. However, the goals of therapy should be discussed with the oncology team, the caregivers, and the patient, if applicable, when the intensivist is first alerted to the possibility of an admission. Decisions regarding therapy should be continuously reevaluated based on the patient's clinical course to ensure an informed discussion among caregivers, patients, and families concerning the continuation, limitations, or even withdrawal of PICU care.

SHOCK IN THE CHILD WITH CANCER

It is not uncommon for the pediatric cancer patient to present in shock, and these patients are subject to the same differential diagnosis as children who do not carry a diagnosis of cancer. It is our experience that rapid recognition of shock physiology, along with aggressive treatment, both to stabilize the patient and to address the underlying physiology, are critical to obtaining good outcomes. However, this may prove to be a challenge to the intensivist not familiar with these patients, as those who have undergone chemotherapy may exhibit lower baseline blood pressures than children of a similar age who have not been exposed to these agents. Thus, a patient with a lower blood pressure (especially diastolic), if not accompanied by changes in perfusion or a compensatory tachycardia, may only need a fluid challenge and evaluation of the patient's response. Thus, reviewing the patient's medical record to ascertain a baseline blood pressure may be important in helping to assess the need for therapy.

Septic Shock

In a large retrospective study of outcomes for severe sepsis in pediatric cancer patients, 446 PICU admissions that occurred over a 13-year period were reviewed. The study revealed 6-month survival of 69% among patients who had not received bone marrow transplants and 39% among patients who had undergone transplantation (16). Although the survival rates are still well below those reported for severe sepsis in the general pediatric population, they are better than rates previously reported and provide support for aggressive ICU management in such patients (16).

The general features of sepsis and septic shock, as well as their management, have been discussed at length in Chapter 26. The development of sepsis or septic shock in the pediatric patient with cancer presents special challenges because these patients are usually immune compromised and frequently profoundly neutropenic, with impaired mucosal barriers and possible preexisting end-organ dysfunction, and they are more vulnerable to multiple organ system failure (MOSF). Their care should be meticulously directed to avoid organ failure, as they have substantially greater mortality from MOSF than other patients (50). Aggressive fluid resuscitation, prompt administration of appropriate antibiotics and antifungals, use of inotropic support, and ventilator strategy designed to minimize lung injury and optimize oxygenation are critical. Renal replacement therapies should be applied early to maintain fluid balance, avoiding the lung injury and breakdown of integument that are associated with fluid overload and diminished renal function. In addition to providing for the aggressive fluid resuscitation (60 mL/kg in the first hour) and goal-directed therapy that are commonly employed in critically ill patients with sepsis syndrome, physicians who care for cancer patients with sepsis should be mindful that preexisting complications of chemotherapy present special risks, especially chemotherapy-related cardiomyopathy and opportunities for intervention (Table 100.1). They should also be aware that steroids are used frequently in these patients as part of their chemotherapy and for control of complications, such as vomiting and graft-versus-host disease (GVHD). The American College of Critical Care Medicine's *Practice Parameters for Pediatric Shock* suggests that the use of steroids be limited to patients with catecholamine-resistant shock and proven or suspected adrenal insufficiency (7). The neutropenia common in PICU patients with cancer predisposes them to acquire sepsis or septic shock, as well as to have a longer and potentially more complicated course than other children. Cultures should be frequently reviewed and antibiotics tailored appropriately. Consultation with an infectious disease specialist is often very helpful.

Two strategies have emerged that attempt to ameliorate neutropenia in septic shock; each shows some promise, but neither has been adequately studied in children. The *transfusion of granulocytes* has been used in the treatment of disseminated infection in neutropenic patients. A meta-analysis published in 2005 evaluated 8 randomized, controlled trials in which granulocyte infusions were administered to patients with neutropenia and disseminated infection (45). Although the procedure was generally well tolerated, the reviewer concluded that evidence was insufficient to support or refute the use of granulocyte infusions for these patients. No study yet undertaken has been adequately powered to address the effect on mortality. The reviewer did note a trend that suggested increased efficacy at doses of 1×10^{10}. *Colony-stimulating factors* are used by oncologists primarily to shorten the duration of neutropenia so that chemotherapy can progress, and they have been very successful in that setting. These agents are also being utilized with

increasing frequency for patients who have neutropenia and MOSF, sepsis or septic shock, or invasive fungal disease.

Granulocyte colony-stimulating factor (GCSF) stimulates the release of neutrophils, while granulocyte-macrophage colony-stimulating factor (GM-CSF) enhances the release of both neutrophils and macrophages. Bone pain and myalgia are the most commonly reported side effects of these agents; however, increased uric acid and lactate dehydrogenase (LDH) levels have also been noted, and these levels should be monitored in the PICU patient. Exacerbation of existing inflammatory conditions, such as vasculitis or psoriasis, has also been reported. GCSF is generally given subcutaneously in a dose of 5–10 mcg/kg/day. GM-CSF, also administered subcutaneously, is dosed at 5 mcg/kg/day. During treatment, white cell count should be monitored daily, and the medication should be continued until neutrophil counts have recovered to >1000 for 3 consecutive days. The agents may then be discontinued or weaned by half and stopped if no significant drop in counts is seen for 3 days following the dose reduction. Although no large trial has been conducted that includes children (47), a large study has been conducted of adult patients with solid tumors and high-risk neutropenia and infections treated with GCSF and antibiotics or antibiotics alone. Findings included significant reductions in duration of neutropenia, length of antibiotic treatment, and number of hospital days (10). Hence, GCSF should be considered for the neutropenic patient with bacterial sepsis. In general, the use of GCSF in patients with neutropenia and life-threatening infection has been better studied than has the use of GM-CSF. However, GM-CSF should be considered for patients in whom fungal disease is confirmed or strongly suspected.

Cardiogenic Shock

When evaluating a child with cancer who presents in shock, the intensivist must review the patient history and actively seek physical signs of a cardiogenic component. PICU patients with cancer may have received cardiotoxic treatment regimens (see Chapter 99). Specifically, anthracyclines, high-dose cyclophosphamide, 5-FU, and radiation therapy are known to cause injury to the cardiac myocytes. Patients, especially those with lymphoma or thoracic tumors, can present with or develop pericardial effusions that may progress to tamponade physiology. Stem cell transplant patients, particularly those with acute or chronic GVHD, are also at risk for developing this complication.

Cardiac Tamponade

Cardiac tamponade is defined as the significant compression of the heart by accumulating pericardial contents, including effusion fluid, blood clot, pus, or air. In cancer patients, such effusions are most frequently either malignant or hemorrhagic (as the result of erosion of pericardial vessels by tumor or secondary to thrombocytopenia). If the reserve pericardial volume is exceeded, cardiac tamponade is life-threatening. Classic signs of cardiac tamponade include tachycardia, jugular venous distension, pulsus paradoxus, Kussmaul sign (respiratory variation of jugular venous distension), muffled heart sounds

TABLE 100.2

PULMONARY COMPLICATIONS AFTER BONE MARROW TRANSPLANT

Phase	Infectious	Noninfectious
Neutropenic phase (0–30 days)	Bacteria (20%–50%) Fungal (12%–45%)	Pulmonary edema Drug toxicity DAH
Early phase (30–100 days)	CMV pneumonitis (40%) PCP	Idiopathic pneumonia syndrome
Late phase (>100 days)	Uncommon except in GVHD	Bronchiolitis obliterans Cryptogenic organizing pneumonia Chronic GVHD

DAH, diffuse alveolar hemorrhage; CMV, cytomegalovirus; PCP, *Pneumocystis carinii* pneumonia; GVHD, graft-versus-host disease

on auscultation, electrical alternans on electrocardiogram, and findings on chest x-ray of cardiomegaly.

Malignant pericardial effusion in the pediatric cancer patient may result from direct extension of a regional tumor or metastatic spread of a remote tumor, probably via lymphatic vessels. In addition, the treatment regimens used in oncology, such as radiation and bone marrow or stem cell transplantation, may cause inflammation and lead to the accumulation of pericardial fluid. Hemorrhagic effusions are common as well and may result from the progression of angioinvasive tumors, such as sarcomas, or from thrombocytopenia or the coagulopathy noted in acute myelogenous leukemia (AML). Lymphatic congestion in patients with mediastinal lymphomas or other thoracic tumors may also result in the accumulation of pericardial fluid.

The evaluation of any patient in whom a pericardial effusion is suspected should include an echocardiograph. The diagnosis cannot be excluded on the basis of a normal chest x-ray, and electrocardiographic changes may be nonspecific. A cardiac echocardiograph, however, is both sensitive and specific in diagnosing the presence or absence of a pericardial effusion and is also helpful in assessing both the extent of hemodynamic compromise and the effectiveness of interventions.

The management of cardiac tamponade may include the use of inotropes to support cardiac output, but careful attention should be given to fluid status, as hypovolemia will exacerbate the pathophysiology of this condition and lead to a relatively greater reduction in cardiac output. Definitive treatment for tamponade requires the removal of the pericardial accumulation, usually via emergency pericardiocentesis following echocardiograph-guided placement of a percutaneous pericardial catheter. Drainage may also be accomplished by surgical pericardiotomy.

RESPIRATORY EMERGENCIES

Respiratory emergencies are frequent in the pediatric cancer patient and may have a dramatic presentation in patients after bone marrow transplantation. The immune deficiency that results from the primary disease, the toxicity of the therapy, or both, make these patients susceptible to a wide range of infectious and noninfectious problems that may progress rapidly to

respiratory failure (**Table 100.2**). Patients should be fully evaluated to rule out a treatable infectious illness. Initiation of broad-spectrum antimicrobial therapy (to address *Pseudomonas*, cytomegalovirus [CMV], *Pneumocystis*, and *Aspergillus*) is often indicated in patients with rapid clinical or radiologic deterioration. Bronchoscopy with bronchoalveolar lavage or open lung biopsy should be performed early in the course of the illness. The former may help differentiate infection from diffuse alveolar hemorrhage, a common complication after stem cell transplantation. High-resolution CT to identify fungal lesions should be considered in all patients with respiratory symptomatology, irrespective of the plain radiograph findings.

Stem cell transplant recipients with respiratory failure that requires endotracheal intubation, especially in the presence of pneumonia or diffuse alveolar hemorrhage, present the greatest challenge to the intensivist. Traditionally, these patients have had poor outcomes. A lung-protective strategy that employs conventional mechanical ventilation has shown better outcomes in this group of patients, whereas a late rescue therapy with high-frequency oscillatory ventilation has seemed ineffective. However, in a recent study, mechanically ventilated, pediatric stem cell recipients placed on high-frequency oscillatory ventilation within the first 6 hrs of mechanical ventilation had better outcomes, indicating potential for improved outcome with earlier intervention in the acute lung injury process (19).

Massive Hemoptysis

Massive hemoptysis is defined as a volume of blood >240 mL (in adults). Massive hemoptysis is a rare but dramatic finding in children that can lead to rapid asphyxiation and death.

The most common cause of massive hemoptysis in the pediatric cancer patient is invasive pulmonary aspergillosis (IPA) (40). IPA usually presents after myeloablative chemotherapy for bone marrow transplantation or during the recovery phase of prolonged neutropenia after chemotherapy. Other infections to be considered in the differential in this patient population include mucormycosis, tuberculosis, and bacterial necrotizing pneumonia secondary to *Staphylococcus aureus*, *Pseudomonas aeruginosa*, or *Klebsiella* (17). Noninfectious etiologies may include primary endobronchial tumors, diffuse alveolar hemorrhage, bronchiectasis, and foreign bodies. Bronchiectasis is often the result of a chronic inflammatory process caused by the accumulation of purulent secretions and obstruction of the airways, leading to chronic atelectasis. The internal digestion of bronchial structural proteins by lytic enzymes released by activated neutrophils, in combination with the traction on the airway wall, results in distension of the airways, fibrosis, and ulceration. These ulcerations may erode into an underlying blood vessel wall, causing hemoptysis. Hemoptysis is rarely found in foreign-body aspiration; when present, it is generally connected with the existence of bronchiectasis. Neutropenic patients with fever >96 hrs despite adequate antibiotic therapy should be evaluated for IPA. Chest pain and cough are common symptoms. The highest risk for hemoptysis occurs during recovery from prolonged neutropenia. The inflammatory process includes a focal cavitary lesion surrounded by collateral vessels. The presence of increasing neutrophils leads to focal necrosis and enhanced risk for vessel perforation and bleeding (38).

CT scan is the most sensitive radiologic test available for the early diagnosis of IPA. The *halo sign*, a dense nodular lesion surrounded by ground-glass attenuation (>180 degrees) is consistent with IPA. The *air crescent sign* indicates necrosis and cavitation. Tissue diagnosis is required to conclusively confirm or exclude IPA. Tissue may be obtained by CT-guided percutaneous lung biopsy, transbronchial biopsy, or open lung biopsy.

The treatment of massive hemoptysis should be directed at the prevention of asphyxia. Early intubation and mechanical ventilation should be considered. Aggressive treatment of any associated coagulopathy, thrombocytopenia, and anemia is warranted. Nonsurgical mortality risk in patients with invasive pulmonary aspergillosis ranges between 30%–90% (31). Combination antifungal therapy with Caspofungin [loading dose of 70 mg/m^2 (maximum loading dose, 70 mg), followed by 50 mg/m^2/d (maximum daily dose, 50 mg)] and liposomal amphotericin B (5–6 mg/kg/day) with voriconazole rescue (loading dose of 6 mg/kg every 12 hr IV on day 1, followed by 4 mg/kg every 12 hr IV) has proven to be a safe alternative for immunosuppressed children with invasive mycosis (9). Bronchoscopy should be considered in patients in whom endoluminal therapy for control of the bleeding is feasible. Fiberoptic bronchoscopy is helpful as a diagnostic tool for confirmation of the bleeding site only when radiologic confirmation cannot be obtained. Bronchial arteriography with transcatheter embolization may be effective in nonsurgical candidates. Wedge resection of the affected lung segment or lobectomy carries a low mortality risk and offers a lower recurrence rate when compared with nonsurgical options (31).

Superior Mediastinal Syndrome

Superior mediastinal syndrome (SMS) results from the compression of the superior mediastinum structures. SMS is almost synonymous with superior vena cava syndrome (SVCS), which refers to the symptoms that result from compression or obstruction from invasion or thrombus of the superior vena cava's normal venous flow. SVCS and SMS are particularly rare in children. When present, most cases are attributed to congenital heart lesions or lymphomas. A review of the records of children who presented to St. Jude Children's Research Hospital during a 16-year period reported that 16 of the 24 patients described presented with SVCS. Non-Hodgkin lymphoma was the most frequent diagnosis (50%), followed by T-cell acute lymphoblastic leukemia (ALL) (25%) and Hodgkin disease (12.5%). Five of 8 patients with solid tumors (sarcomas) developed SVCS later in the course of their disease treatment. Dyspnea, orthopnea, and wheezing were the most common symptoms. Pleural and pericardial effusions were also noted at presentation (22).

Progressive venous congestion and airway compression will lead to the usual symptoms found in SVCS and SMS: facial engorgement, headache, plethora, cyanotic facies, cough, dyspnea, orthopnea, hoarseness, and dysphagia. Less common symptoms include pleural and/or pericardial effusions. Most patients at this stage may not tolerate the supine position. Chest x-ray and CT scan may confirm distortion of the superior mediastinal structures. Echocardiography is indicated in patients with suspected thrombus or pericardial effusion. Pulmonary function tests may also be obtained to evaluate pulmonary reserve. Elevation of serum markers may be helpful in identifying the possible etiology of the underlying tumor that causes the SMS. Elevation of lactate dehydrogenase may be present in 75% of patients with non-Hodgkin lymphoma and leukemia. α-fetoprotein may be elevated in yolk sac tumors (22).

Anterior Mediastinal Masses

Patients with anterior mediastinal masses are at particular risk of rapid cardiopulmonary collapse when sedated or placed under general anesthesia. Bone marrow biopsy, lymph node biopsy, or CT-guided percutaneous mediastinal biopsies may be safely performed with local anesthesia, if tolerated. Pericardial and/or pleural collections should be drained under ultrasound or CT guidance for therapeutic and diagnostic purposes (40). General anesthesia should not be administered, even in asymptomatic patients, if the tracheal cross-section area, as measured by CT scan, and the peak expiratory flow rate are less than 50% of predicted values (41). In rare situations, it is impossible to obtain a tissue diagnosis before beginning treatment. Most of these tumors, particularly lymphomas, may prove to be very sensitive to radiation or chemotherapy and will dissolve rather quickly (40). Surgical resection may be unavoidable in patients with tumors not sensitive to cytoreductive therapy (e.g., large-cell lymphomas, teratomas, germ-cell tumors).

NEUROLOGIC EMERGENCIES

Increased Intracranial Pressure

Increased intracranial pressure (ICP) may occur in pediatric cancer patients as a result of a mass effect from a tumor (primary or metastatic) on normal brain structures, spontaneous bleeding of a tumor mass, intracerebral bleeding from a coagulopathy, or obstruction of normal cerebrospinal fluid flow, which causes hydrocephalus that frequently requires early ventricular drainage. The intensivist plays an important role in the early diagnosis and treatment of children with increased ICP. Early management will include conventional ICP measures (see Chapter 56). When the increased ICP is secondary to a brain tumor, the use of dexamethasone (2 mg/kg followed by 0.5 mg/kg every 6 hrs) is helpful in reducing the edema surrounding the tumor. In fact, brain tumors represent the only current indication for the use of steroids in the management of increased ICP. It has been reported that dexamethasone reduces peritumoral water content and local tissue pressure without affecting cerebral blood flow and cerebral blood volume (4). Even though the precise mode of action of dexamethasone is unclear, it might be achieved by decreasing the blood-tumor barrier permeability or increasing parenchymal resistance to fluid transport.

Spinal Cord Compression

Spinal cord compression is a common presenting symptom in children with cancer, occurring in 3%–5% of patients. Spinal cord compression most frequently results from metastatic spread of sarcomas, neuroblastomas, germ-cell tumors, lymphoma/leukemia, or metastatic central nervous system (CNS) tumors.

Back pain is a red flag. The greater majority of patients with spinal cord compression may present with localized back pain. The pain can start weeks to months before the diagnosis is made, but once neurologic signs appear, the progression is rapid and may be irreversible. Other common symptoms include lower extremity weakness (67%), sphincter dysfunction (57%), and sensory abnormality (14%).

All patients with progressive neurologic signs or symptoms should be treated with high-dose steroids (dexamethasone 1–2 mg/kg). Craniospinal T1- and T2-weighted MR imaging allows demonstration of epidural involvement, intraparenchymal spread, and compression of nerve roots. Cerebrospinal fluid studies are necessary to evaluate for subarachnoid disease, CNS leukemia, or carcinomatosis. Further treatment encompasses three different scenarios: (a) radiation therapy, if the diagnosis is known and the tumor is radiosensitive (27); (b) chemotherapy, if the diagnosis is leukemia/lymphoma or neuroblastoma; or (c) surgery, if the diagnosis of the tumor is unknown or if symptoms progress despite radiation therapy (27). The prognosis depends on the severity of the neurologic findings at presentation and the time interval to definitive treatment.

Convulsions

The pediatric cancer patient is at greater risk for seizures than are other pediatric patients, perhaps due to the cancer itself (e.g., primary CNS tumors, metastatic CNS lesions, or CNS leukemia) or from complications arising from its treatment (e.g., antineoplastic therapy, metabolic abnormalities, hemorrhage, or infection). Seizures account for up to 60% of all neurologic consults in oncology patients. Although the pediatric cancer patient may have a more complex differential diagnosis, the management and workup of new-onset seizures in this group are similar to the standard pediatric approach (see Chapter 57). The intensivist should treat the seizure and provide supportive care, and conduct appropriate studies, including blood tests, an electroencephalogram, and CT or MRI scan. Specific abnormal findings should be addressed where applicable. It may be wise to avoid starting valproic acid or carbamazepine, as these agents are known to cause marrow suppression.

Stroke

Children with leukemia and hyperleukocytosis (white blood cell count, WBC >100,000/mm^3) are at increased risk for stroke due to leukostasis (microcirculatory dysfunction with sludging of leukemic cells in capillary vessels). The majority of strokes in children with cancer are due to arterial or venous thrombosis, intraparenchymal hemorrhage, local or metastatic tumor spread, or hematologic abnormalities. Embolic events are uncommon.

The etiology of the stroke in relation to the stage of the oncologic process is listed in **Table 100.3**. Patients with any form of leukemia and hyperleukocytosis are at high risk for stroke at diagnosis and early in the treatment phase. Clinically significant hyperleukocytosis occurs with WBC of >200,000/mm^3 in AML and in excess of 300,000/mm^3 in ALL and chronic myelocytic leukemia (CML). These differences are due to the size of the leukemic cells. Myeloblasts are larger (350–450 mm^3) compared to lymphoblasts (250–350 mm^3). Hyperleukocytosis occurs in 9%–13% of children with ALL, 5%–22% of children with AML, and in almost all patients with CML in chronic phase. In acute promyelocytic leukemia (APL), stroke may result from enhanced thrombin activation and increased production of plasmin secondary to annexin II expression (32). L-asparaginase, alone or in combination with vincristine and prednisone, is associated with an increased risk of venous thrombosis (acquired antithrombin III, protein S, and protein C deficiency). Radiation therapy may cause stroke, even years after treatment, and the risk is related to the total dose of radiation. Large-vessel occlusions are associated with doses in excess of 50 gray. The adjuvant use of intrathecal or parenteral methotrexate and cytosine arabinoside potentiates this risk.

CT or MRI with and without contrast is useful in evaluating the nature and extent of a stroke. The general management of stroke is supportive (see Chapter 58). If stroke is the presenting symptom in childhood cancer, treating the underlying malignancy with cytotoxic therapy may prevent additional strokes. In hemorrhagic stroke, platelet levels should be maintained above 50–75 thousand/mm^3.

TABLE 100.3

ETIOLOGY OF STROKE

Time of presentation	Likely diagnosis
At presentation of malignancy	Malignancy Coagulopathy Intratumoral hemorrhage
During treatment of malignancy	Drug toxicity Malignancy
At the end stage of the malignancy	Infection Disseminated intravascular coagulation Progressive malignancy
Months to years after therapy	Radiation-induced vascular damage

Coma

Occasionally, a pediatric cancer patient may present with significant obtundation or in coma. Common causes of coma in the pediatric oncology patient include mass effect from a primary or metastatic brain tumor, obstructive hydrocephalus, bleeding (tumor-related or secondary to treatment), infection, therapeutic agents (vincristine and methotrexate), and other causes (postictal state, metabolic disorders, etc). Infratentorial tumors, in particular, can produce obstructive hydrocephaly, elevated ICP, and herniation. Chapter 53 provides a detailed discussion of the diagnosis and management of coma, which also applies to the cancer patient. The intensivist should focus on the stabilization of the patient's airway, breathing, and circulation, and on the management of impending herniation (see previous section). A contrast/noncontrast CT or MRI is often helpful in determining the etiology.

METABOLIC EMERGENCIES

Water and electrolyte disorders are commonplace in the pediatric cancer patient admitted to the PICU. Glomerular and/or tubular disorders may arise as a result of the tumor's direct renal involvement (Wilms tumor), metastatic infiltration of the renal parenchyma (leukemia, neuroblastoma), compression of the urinary tract (sarcomas), or as a consequence of the toxic properties of the chemotherapy on the kidney. Water and sodium (Na) balance disturbances in particular are frequently found in this patient population.

Syndrome of Inappropriate Antidiuretic Hormone Secretion

Syndrome of inappropriate antidiuretic hormone secretion (SIADH) is an excessive secretion of antidiuretic hormone in the presence of low Na levels and normal or low plasma osmolality. SIADH may occur in the pediatric cancer patient (medulloblastoma, lymphoma, ovarian teratoma) and in the setting of cerebral insults (intracranial surgery, trauma), neck surgery, mechanical ventilation, infections, and lung disease. SIADH has been recognized to occur with several medications, including anticonvulsants (carbamazepine) and chemotherapeutic agents (vincristine, ifosfamide, cyclophosphamide) (42). SIADH-related hyponatremia may be aggravated by the aggressive fluid hydration strategy used in patients who receive chemotherapy. The late manifestations of SIADH (confusion, seizures, coma) are usually the reason for admission to the PICU. Confirmation of the diagnosis is based on the presence of increased total body water and hyponatremia in the setting of low serum osmolality (<280 mOsm/L) with an elevated urine osmolality, usually >500 mOsm/L (urine-to-serum osmolality ratio >1), elevated urinary Na concentration, and decreased urine output (<1 mL/kg/hr). The treatment of SIADH should include fluid restriction to 30%–50% maintenance until the serum Na levels normalize. Hypertonic saline (3% saline solution) is indicated in severely symptomatic patients with coma and/or seizures until symptoms resolve. The dose of hypertonic saline can be calculated using the formula:

$$\text{Na deficit (mEq)} = [\text{Desired Na} - \text{Actual Na}] \times 0.5 \text{ body weight (kg)}$$

Hypertonic saline should be given acutely to raise the serum Na concentration to >120 mEq/L and then more gradually to 130 mEq/L. A rate of rise of 0.5 mEq/L/hr is considered safe after the serum Na concentration has reached 120 mEq/L and symptoms have subsided. Rapid correction of hyponatremia may lead to central pontine myelinolysis (1).

Cerebral Salt-Wasting Syndrome

Patients with cerebral salt-wasting syndrome (CSW) may share similar intracerebral diseases and laboratory criteria with those patients with SIADH (Table 100.4). CSW in children typically occurs 2–7 days post-CNS injury and is probably the result of abnormal secretion of natriuretic peptides. Patients with cerebral salt-wasting syndrome have volume contraction and hyponatremia in the setting of polyuria and increased urine Na losses. The differentiation between SIADH and CSW is made by observing urine volume patterns during the development of hyponatremia and natriuresis (5). The treatment of CSW should be directed to vigorous extracellular fluid and Na replacement. Treatment with high-dose fludrocortisone (0.2–0.4 mg/day) has proven to be beneficial in some patients (1).

TABLE 100.4

DIAGNOSIS OF SIADH, CSW, AND DI

	SIADH	CSW	DI (central)
Body water	Increased	Decreased	Decreased
Sodium	Low	Low	High
Serum osmolality	<280 mOsm/L	Decreased	>300 mOsm/L
Urine osmolality	>500 mOsm/L	Increased	Low
Urine to serum osmolality ratio	>1	>1	<1.5
Urine output	Low	High	High
Urine sodium concentration	Increased	Increased	Decreased

SIADH, Syndrome of inappropriate antidiuretic hormone secretion; CSW, cerebral salt wasting; DI, diabetes insipidus

Diabetes Insipidus

Central diabetes insipidus (DI) typically presents in the pediatric cancer patient as a result of a direct injury, or compression or infiltration of the hypothalamic supraoptic or paraventricular nuclei or of the supraoptic-hypophyseal tract. DI is most often caused by surgical resection of a hypothalamic-pituitary tumor (craniopharyngioma, germinoma) or by local tumor infiltration or destruction (histiocytosis, leukemia, lymphoma). The diagnostic confirmation is based on the presence of hypernatremia (or rapidly rising serum Na), elevated serum osmolality >300 mOsm/L, low urine osmolality (urine-to-serum osmolality ratio <1.5), low urine specific gravity ($\leq$1.005), and increased urine output. DI most often presents in a triphasic pattern after surgical resection of a suprasellar mass. During the initial phase, typically lasting 2–5 days, the patient may develop DI as a consequence of a deficient secretion of arginine vasopressin or secretion of a biologically inactive form. The second phase is characterized by an inappropriate arginine vasopressin (AVP) release that lasts 1–14 days (1), during which time the signs and symptoms of DI may disappear. A recurrent and very often permanent form of DI characterizes the third phase.

The treatment of DI should be directed to fluid and AVP replacement. Patients in shock should receive fluid replacement with large volumes of isotonic solutions in order to reverse the shock state. Once the hemodynamics have been stabilized and the child remains hypernatremic, normal saline should be infused over 48–72 hrs at a rate designed to meet maintenance requirements and replace any existing water deficit. Ongoing urinary losses should be replaced milliliter for milliliter with 0.45% normal saline until AVP replacement has been effective in decreasing urine output to 3–4 mL/kg/hr. Thereafter, the replacement of ongoing urinary losses can be weaned to 0.5 mL with 0.45% normal saline per mL urine output and, finally, discontinued altogether once urine output equals 2–3 mL/kg/hr and serum Na concentration has normalized. The possibility of rapid osmolar shifts mandates very close monitoring of the serum Na (every 1–4 hrs), urine output (every hour), urine-specific gravity (every 1–2 hrs), and serum and urine osmolality (every 4–6 hrs). Hypernatremia should be corrected over 48–72 hrs. Desmopressin acetate or AVP should be used cautiously, with consideration for the risk of hyponatremia development. The recommended dose for desmopressin acetate is 2–4 mcg/day IV or subcutaneous in two divided doses. Recommended doses for AVP start at 0.5 mU/kg/hr, with a 30-min titration interval to a maximum of 10 mU/kg/hr.

Hypercalcemia

Hypercalcemia is a rare finding in children in the PICU. The incidence in children with cancer is ~0.4%, compared to 5%–20% in the adult population. Malignancy-associated hypercalcemia can be found in patients with leukemia, lymphoma, hepatoblastoma, rhabdomyosarcoma, Ewing sarcoma, or brain tumors. The most common cause of malignancy-associated hypercalcemia is a humoral hypercalcemia, caused by solid tumor production of a parathyroid hormone-related peptide (PTHrP), resulting in a systemic osteoclast-mediated bone resorption, increased renal calcium resorption, and increased renal phospho-

rus excretion (44). The second most common cause of hypercalcemia is osteolysis secondary to cytokine-mediated osteoclast activation at the site of bone metastasis. The third category and most frequent form of hypercalcemia in Hodgkin and non-Hodgkin disease is calcitriol-mediated hypercalcemia, which results from dysregulated renal production of 1α-hydroxylase secondary to PTHrP stimulation. Patients with malignant hypercalcemia will usually present with bradyarrhythmias, coma, muscle weakness, and renal insufficiency.

Management of severe hypercalcemia (>14 mg/dL) includes the basic principles of monitoring of electrocardiographic changes (prolonged PR, broad T waves), vigorous hydration with saline solution (10–20 mL/kg/bolus), forced diuresis with furosemide (1–2 mg/kg/dose) to induce calciuresis, reduction of calcium mobilization with calcitonin 4 IU/kg intramuscularly or subcutaneously every 24 hrs in combination with prednisone 1 mg/kg/day IV, and treatment of the underlying malignancy. Pamidronate, a bisphosphonate, binds hydroxyapatite crystals and blocks osteoclast-mediated resorption. The recommended dose is 1 mg/kg/dose IV. The side effects include hypocalcemia, hypophosphatemia, and hypomagnesemia (52). Combined treatment with calcitonin and pamidronate may be used in refractory cases that do not respond to conventional treatment with hydration and forced diuresis with loop diuretics (30).

Tumor Lysis Syndrome

Tumor lysis syndrome (TLS) is a constellation of metabolic abnormalities that result from the rapid destruction of tumor cells overwhelming usual metabolic pathways. TLS usually occurs after chemotherapy administration but may also occur after administration of steroids, hormones, or radiation therapy. TLS most often develops ~12–72 hrs after the initiation of cytolytic therapy and is typically characterized by hyperuricemia, hyperkalemia, and hyperphosphatemia. Precipitation of calcium phosphate in the microvasculature results in symptomatic hypocalcemia. If left untreated, the precipitation of the urate crystals and calcium phosphate crystals in the renal tubules may rapidly lead to acute intrarenal failure (42).

Frequency

TLS occurs most frequently in patients with a large tumor burden or in those whose tumors are widely disseminated, rapidly proliferating, or highly sensitive to chemotherapy. TLS has been observed primarily following the treatment of Burkitt lymphoma, lymphoblastic lymphoma, and leukemia. Nonetheless, TLS can present in other forms of cancer, including Hodgkin lymphoma, neuroblastoma, medulloblastoma, and in non-Hodgkin lymphoma (40). TLS is rare in AML and in the chronic leukemias. The incidence of TLS is unknown. Patients with B-cell ALL and Burkitt lymphoma with elevated LDH (>500 U/L) had the highest risk of developing TLS or anuria (51). Laboratory evidence of TLS is far more frequent than the actual symptomatic clinical syndrome.

TLS affects children of all ages, with no gender discrimination. Older children seem to be at higher risk of severe complications due to the progressive decline with age of the fractional excretion and clearance of uric acid. The patient's symptomatology at the time of diagnosis reflects the severity of the primary tumor extension. Symptoms are directly related to the metabolic abnormalities found in TLS and may include anorexia, malaise, weakness, vomiting, hiccups, paresthesia, tetany, carpopedal spasm, and seizures.

Pathophysiology

The high cell turnover results in an increase of the different byproducts of cellular breakdown, including proteins, nucleic acids, cations, and anions. Brisk cellular breakdown that results from cytolytic therapy causes a dramatic rise in plasma levels of uric acid, urea nitrogen, phosphorus, and potassium (K^+), overwhelming the normal homeostatic mechanisms. A rapid rise in serum K^+ levels may result in severe arrhythmias and death. Uric acid is in the ionized form at normal serum concentrations and normal pH. The presence of metabolic acidosis and high uric acid plasma concentrations increases the risk of uric acid crystal formation and precipitation in the renal collecting ducts and tubules (sites of urinary acidification). Metabolic acidosis exacerbates the already elevated serum phosphate concentration by shifting intracellular phosphate to the extracellular space. Secondary hypocalcemia results from calcium phosphate precipitation when the solubility product factor is reached (Ca $\times$ P = 60). The glomerular filtration rate declines and progresses to renal failure as a result of calcium phosphate and uric acid crystal precipitation in the renal tubules. The risk of acute renal failure will increase if the primary tumor infiltrates or obstructs the normal flow of urine. Other risk factors for acute renal failure include preexisting renal pathology and dehydration.

Risk factors for TLS are Burkitt lymphoma/leukemia (B-ALL), acute leukemias (ALL, AML), non-Hodgkin lymphoma, tumors with rapid growth rate, large tumor burden, elevated serum LDH (>500 U/L), dehydration, and elevated uric acid.

Treatment

Early diagnosis of the primary condition, recognition of the risk factors, and aggressive management of symptoms and abnormalities are key to the management of TLS. It is essential to monitor the electrocardiographic changes associated with hyperkalemia (prolonged PR, flattened P, widened QRS, peaked T wave) and/or hypocalcemia (prolonged QT interval). A summary of TLS treatment is presented in **Table 100.5**.

Early and aggressive hydration is crucial in the prevention and management of TLS. The expansion of the intravascular blood volume increases renal blood flow and glomerular filtration rate, thus decreasing the concentration of solutes in the distal tubules. IV hydration should begin at least 24 hrs before the initiation of cytoreductive therapy. Infusion rates are usu-

ally 2–4 times maintenance unless volume overload is of particular concern. Alkalinization is also recommended. Typical solutions are 5% dextrose in 0.25% normal saline/L with 60–100 mEq of sodium bicarbonate/L. The goal is to increase the urinary pH to 7–7.5 and to keep the specific gravity at ~1.010, thereby promoting uric acid (pKa 5.4) solubility. Rapid and aggressive alkalinization should be discouraged, as it may worsen the ionized hypocalcemia by shifting the calcium from its ionized form to a nonionized form. Restriction of K^+ and phosphorus is essential. Urine flow should be maintained at about 100–200 mL/hr. Diuretic use is discouraged in the volume-depleted patient, as it may worsen urate and phosphate precipitation. Osmotic diuretics and/or furosemide may be beneficial in normovolemic patients with poor urine output or fluid overload.

Uric acid control can be achieved with a recombinant urate oxidase (rasburicase) or with a xanthine oxidase inhibitor (allopurinol). Urate oxidase catalyzes the enzymatic oxygen-dependent conversion of poorly soluble urate to allantoin, a highly water-soluble product easily excreted in the urine. This enzyme is absent in humans. The usual dose of rasburicase in children of 0.15 or 0.2 mg/kg/day, once daily in a 30-min IV infusion for 5 days, produces a sharp and sustained drop in uric acid levels (36). Urate oxidase infusion is contraindicated in patients with glucose-6-phosphate dehydrogenase (G6PD) deficiency, and high-risk patients (African or Mediterranean descent) should be screened for G6PD deficiency before urate oxidase is infused (24). Xanthine oxidase catalyzes the oxidation of hypoxanthine to xanthine and the oxidation of xanthine to uric acid. Allopurinol reduces the conversion of nucleic acids to uric acid but will not affect existing uric acids levels. The initial oral dose is 10 mg/kg/day or 200 mg/m²/day, starting 24–48 hrs prior to initiation of chemotherapy. In a recent randomized, multicentered, comparative trial that compared allopurinol to rasburicase in children with cancer at high risk for TLS, a more rapid reduction of uric acid and lower plasma levels were demonstrated in the group of children randomized to rasburicase when compared to the group randomized to allopurinol (18).

Management of Severe Electrolyte Disturbances

Patients with hyperkalemia should be aggressively monitored and treated. Dietary and supplemental K^+ should be restricted. Patients with K^+ levels >6.5 mEq/L or with electrocardiographic alterations should receive insulin, glucose, bicarbonate, and calcium. Diuretics (K^+ wasting) should be used with caution in volume-depleted patients. Kayexalate (sodium polystyrene sulfonate), a K^+ exchange resin, should be given early to help control the K^+ rebound after the transient effect of the acute hyperkalemia treatment. The usual dose is 1 g/kg orally, mixed in water or sorbitol. Renal replacement therapy should be considered early in patients with rapid renal deterioration or in those with refractory hyperkalemia. Calcium replacement during TLS is indicated only in patients with neuromuscular irritability secondary to hypocalcemia: seizures, arrhythmias, or positive Chvostek or Trousseau signs. Calcium replacement in hyperphosphatemic, nonsymptomatic, hypocalcemic patients may aggravate calcium phosphate precipitation in the renal tubules. Hyperphosphatemia is managed with oral phosphate binders, such as sevelamer hydrochloride, calcium carbonate, calcium acetate, or aluminum hydroxide (29).

TABLE 100.5

TREATMENT OF TUMOR LYSIS SYNDROME

5% dextrose in 0.25% normal saline +60–100 mEq sodium bicarbonate/L at 2–4 times maintenance

Keep urinary pH 7–7.5 and specific gravity ~1.010

Restrict potassium and phosphorus. Replace calcium in symptomatic patients only.

Urate oxidase (rasburicase): 0.15 or 0.2 mg/kg once daily in a 30-min IV infusion for 5 days

Allopurinol: 10 mg/kg/day or 200 mg/m²/day starting 24–48 hrs prior to initiation of chemotherapy

Renal Replacement Therapy

Renal replacement therapy (see Chapter 37) is indicated in patients in whom aggressive interventions to reestablish normal urine flow or to correct metabolic abnormalities are unsuccessful (24). The goals of dialysis are treatment of obstructive nephropathy by rapid removal of uric acid and phosphorus, treatment of acute renal failure and the associated metabolic abnormalities, and facilitation of earlier chemotherapy in the oliguric patient. Some practitioners institute continuous venovenous hemofiltration (CVVH) in addition to conventional preventive measures in high-risk children before the initiation of chemotherapy, as they feel that this may prevent further renal dysfunction, although no objective data support this practice. Cytoreductive chemotherapy should be delayed if indicated in patients with high risk of TLS until the preventive treatment measures are initiated.

HEMATOLOGIC EMERGENCIES

Febrile Neutropenia in the Critical Care Setting

Febrile neutropenia is a common complication of the treatment of pediatric malignancies. The intensification of chemotherapy regimens over the past 50 years has not only improved survival in children with cancer, but also increased the risk from infections in certain high-risk groups, for which fever may be the only presenting sign. The current standard of care involves hospitalization with empiric antimicrobial therapy during the febrile neutropenic state. This approach has resulted in a lower mortality rate. Nevertheless, complications that require admission to the ICU do exist. Febrile neutropenia risk factors and complications that may require critical care intervention are discussed here.

Fever is defined as a single oral temperature $\geq 38.3°C$ or a temperature of $\geq 38°C$ that persists for more than 1 hr. A rectal temperature should never be taken in a neutropenic pediatric patient, as doing so may disrupt the mucosal barrier and create a nidus for infection. Neutropenia is defined as an absolute neutrophil count of either <500 cells/mm^3 or of <1000 cells/mm^3 with a downward trend of the absolute neutrophil count on two separate peripheral blood counts (21).

Certain patients are at a higher risk for complications due to the intensive nature of their chemotherapy regimens and may require the ICU during the course of their hospitalization (2). Identification of these patients is important for the early implementation of life-saving strategies. The risk of sepsis or invasive bacterial infections increases with the degree and duration of neutropenia. The risk of bacteremia and septicemia increases with an absolute neutrophil count of <200 cells/mm^3. Neutropenia that lasts >7 days results in a worse outcome. Certain populations in pediatric oncology, including those with hematologic malignancies (including relapsed leukemia) and those who have undergone an allogeneic hematopoietic stem cell transplant (HSCT), are at increased risk for prolonged periods of neutropenia due to the intensity and timing of their treatment regimens.

Multiple clinical- and laboratory-based criteria for identifying high-risk febrile neutropenic patients have been validated in various prospective clinical trials (37,43). The clinical and

CLINICAL AND LABORATORY HIGH-RISK FACTORS IN FEBRILE NEUTROPENIA

Clinical risk factors	Laboratory-based risk factors
Evidence of shock	Elevated C-reactive protein
Near-myeloablative	>10 mg/L
chemotherapy (leukemia	Absolute neutrophil count
induction or delayed	<200 cells/mm^3
intensification)	Absolute monocyte count
Allogeneic hematopoietic	<100 cells/mm^3
stem cell transplant	Gram-negative bacteremia
recipient	
Relapsed leukemia	
Pneumonia	
Neutropenic enterocolitis	
Invasive fungal infection	
Oropharyngeal mucositis	
Prolonged neutropenia	
(>7 days)	
High presenting temperature	
($>39°C$)	

laboratory risk factors that may place a pediatric cancer patient at a higher risk for a serious infection are listed in **Table 100.6**. Furthermore, a presenting temperature of $>39.5°C$, capillary refill time of >3 seconds, a low diastolic blood pressure (defined as DBP <2 standard deviations below the mean), and the presence of oral mucositis were identified retrospectively on multivariate analysis as variables that were significantly associated with implementation of critical care therapies in febrile neutropenic children with cancer (48).

Specific Complications

Bacteremia. Improved management and antimicrobial prophylaxis have led to a shift in pathogens that complicate the neutropenic state. Overall, 13%–36% of febrile neutropenic patients will have documented bacteremia (3). Patients who are not at high risk for a serious infection (those who do not have any of the risk factors listed in **Table 100.6**) have an incidence of ~10% (37). Catheter-related infections are the most common cause of bacteremia. While the rate of gram-positive infections has increased, the rate of infections caused by gram-negative organisms has remained unchanged. Even though most gram-positive infections are less virulent than gram-negative infections, an exception is α-hemolytic streptococcal infections. Certain groups, such as AML patients, are at a higher risk. Mucositis also places these patients at risk for *Streptococcus viridans* infections (26). For this reason, adequate antimicrobial coverage for *S. viridans* should be instituted for any AML patient admitted with fever and neutropenia.

Commonly used antimicrobials for the management of febrile neutropenia are listed in **Table 100.7**. The evidence is strong that monotherapy with a broad-spectrum antimicrobial with antipseudomonal coverage, such as cefepime or ceftazidime, is appropriate for the neutropenic patient presenting with a fever without infectious focus (21). Even though supportive evidence is lacking, the addition of vancomycin to the initial regimen is a common practice for high-risk patients (11,21). Additional antibiotic agents for suspected or documented bacteremia should be tailored to cover for the most

TABLE 100.7

SELECT ANTIMICROBIALS FOR MANAGEMENT OF FEBRILE NEUTROPENIA

Broad-spectrum antibiotics	Gram-positive coverage	Gram-negative coverage	Anaerobic coverage
Cefepime Ceftazidime Carbapenems (Meropenem, Imipenem)	Vancomycin Ampicillin/Sulbactam Linezolid	Aminoglycoside (Gentamicin, Tobramycin) Aztreonam	Metronidazole Clindamycin

likely organisms, subsequent susceptibility results, as well as resistance patterns in the institution.

Neutropenic Enterocolitis. Neutropenic enterocolitis is a complication seen in patients with prolonged neutropenia. It is referred to as *typhlitis* when it involves the cecum. The pathogenesis is poorly understood, but it appears to be a combination of factors, including direct cytotoxic effect of chemotherapy combined with bacterial invasion that results in bacteremia, necrosis, and hemorrhage. The incidence in adult cancer patients is ~5%, with the incidence in children falling between 2%–3%. The classic triad of fever, abdominal pain, and diarrhea may not always be present and is not highly specific, making the clinical diagnosis difficult. Imaging with either ultrasonography or abdominal CT is essential. CT allows for differentiation of other diagnoses and is usually the modality of choice. Ultrasonography may also prove useful as a prognostic tool, based on the degree of bowel thickness. It is also easily performed at the bedside of even the most critically ill patients. Bowel wall thickness >4 mm, along with clinical symptoms, confirms the diagnosis. Sepsis and perforation are the most common complications. To date, no prospective, randomized trials have been conducted to study the management of this disease. A conservative approach in patients without perforation includes bowel rest until the patient has active bowel sounds, nasogastric suction in patients actively vomiting, total parenteral nutrition while fasting, and broad antimicrobial coverage if appropriate (8). Surgical intervention may be needed in some cases but is not universally recommended and may be unnecessary even in high-risk pediatric patients.

Invasive Fungal Infections. Periods of prolonged neutropenia and steroid use are well-known risk factors for the development of invasive fungal infections. Populations at risk include patients with an acute leukemia and those patients who have undergone an allogeneic HSCT. The immunosuppression involved in treating graft-versus-host disease also places the transplant population at high risk for invasive fungal infections. Mortality from disseminated fungal infections is high. Historically, *Candida albicans*, non-albicans species, and *Aspergillus fumigatus* have been the most frequently isolated organisms. In recent years, with the advent of fluconazole prophylaxis, the incidence of invasive candidiasis has dropped to less than 5%, with a shift toward non-albicans species. Another trend seen from the advent of fluconazole prophylaxis is that of invasive aspergillosis slowly becoming the most predominant invasive fungal infection. Due to the nonspecific symptoms, a high index of suspicion for fungal infections is appropriate in

any patient with persistent fever and a prolonged neutropenic state. A 2002 international consensus to define invasive fungal infections in cancer patients emphasized the need for early diagnosis and treatment (2). The neutropenic patient with persistent fever for longer than 3–5 days should have empiric coverage expanded to include fungal organisms (43). For many years, amphotericin has been the gold standard in the treatment of fungal infections. Fluconazole is an appropriate empiric option when it is not being used as a prophylactic agent. Newer agents, such as caspofungin and voriconazole, have shown similar efficacy in the empiric management of fungal infections (48,49). As with bacterial organisms, therapy should be tailored to specific infection and resistance patterns in the institution so that the most likely fungal organisms are covered.

Lower Respiratory Tract Infections. Pneumonia is an uncommon complication of febrile neutropenia. Although routine chest radiography is not warranted, febrile neutropenic patients who present with cough or respiratory distress require immediate imaging due to the potential for rapid progression of infection.

Pneumocystis (carinii) jiroveci pneumonia is now rare due to widespread use of trimethoprim-sulfamethoxazole prophylaxis in immunosuppressed patients; however, it should be in the differential of any immunocompromised patient who presents with respiratory symptoms and diffuse patchy infiltrates on chest x-ray. First-line treatment is with IV trimethoprim-sulfamethoxazole (pentamidine is an alternative). Corticosteroids should be initiated within 72 hrs of initiating therapy for any patient with moderate or severe *P. jiroveci* pneumonia (Pao$_2$ <70 mm Hg on room air).

Community-acquired infections well known to the general pediatric population (influenza, respiratory syncytial virus, and parainfluenza) can have devastating effects in immunocompromised hosts, especially in transplant patients. While therapy is available for influenza (neuraminidase and M2 inhibitors), no effective therapy exists for parainfluenza pneumonia. Ribavirin, palivizumab, and respiratory syncytial virus immune globulin have been shown in small, uncontrolled trials to be of some benefit in the management of HSCT patients with respiratory syncytial virus pneumonia.

Mortality from CMV pneumonitis in HSCT patients is high. Preemptive therapy is the ideal, when a patient has an active (CMV antigenemia in peripheral blood) but asymptomatic CMV infection. Either IV ganciclovir or foscarnet is adequate for preemptive therapy, depending on which prophylactic agent was used prior to detection of CMV antigenemia (39). Although based on uncontrolled studies, current recommended treatment of CMV pneumonia is with a combination of IV ganciclovir and immune globulin.

The unique and fragile nature of the pediatric cancer patient requires a truly multidisciplinary approach in the management of infectious complications in the intensive care setting. The intensivist should work in conjunction with the pediatric oncology and infectious disease teams to develop the best management strategy for each patient hospitalized with complications from febrile neutropenia.

Hyperleukocytosis

Hyperleukocytosis is defined as a WBC of $\geq 100,000/mm^3$ in the peripheral blood. In children, it is mainly seen in patients with acute leukemia, though an occasional patient with CML may present with hyperleukocytosis.

Children with hyperleukocytosis often develop a consumptive coagulopathy, likely through activation of the extrinsic pathway by tumor cells. The platelet count, prothrombin time, partial thromboplastin time, fibrinogen, and D-dimers should be evaluated at diagnosis and followed for abnormalities. To avoid bleeding problems once a consumptive coagulopathy has been diagnosed, the fibrinogen should be maintained at >100 g/dL, if possible, and the platelet count should be maintained at >50,000/mm^3 until the patient is stable.

Finally, hyperleukocytosis can lead to hyperviscosity and microvascular complications, involving most prominently the lungs and the CNS. Complications from leukostasis can be seen with WBC as low as 50,000/mm^3. CNS hemorrhage or stroke is rare in pediatric ALL patients until the WBC reaches very high numbers, such as 400,000/mm^3. At present, leukapheresis or exchange transfusion should be implemented, if available, in patients with symptoms of leukostasis or with very high WBC. However, more invasive interventions may not be superior to hydration, alkalinization, and allopurinol. Equally important to any of these listed therapies is the prompt initiation of cytotoxic therapy. In patients with AML, the occurrence of microvascular complications is more frequent and occurs at lower WBC. Adult centers often apheresis patients at a WBC of 100,000/mm^3, and this may be a reasonable threshold for pediatric patients. The WBC at which to start and stop apheresis remains empiric (35). If apheresis is not available, exchange transfusion may be attempted. As patients with hyperleukocytosis may have problems with blood viscosity, infusions of packed red blood cells should be avoided.

In summary:

- The symptoms of leukostasis may occur at WBC <100,000/mm^3.
- The lungs and CNS are most often involved.
- Prompt initiation of therapy is recommended.
- Pheresis therapy is empiric but may be helpful initially.
- Conservative therapy with allopurinol, hydration, and alkalinization may be effective.

Hemorrhage and Thrombosis in Childhood Malignancy

Hemorrhage and thrombosis are potentially life-threatening complications of cancer treatment for patients who may oth-

erwise be cured of their disease. Up to 10% of patients with APL die from bleeding complications during the first 2 weeks of therapy. Recognition and treatment of hemostatic abnormalities is an important component of supportive care that has contributed to improved long-term survival in cancer patients. Major bleeding events, which occur frequently in oncology patients, include intracranial and retinal hemorrhages, gastrointestinal bleeding, pulmonary alveolar hemorrhage, and hemorrhagic cystitis. In addition, severe localized bleeding may be caused by tumor invasion, chemotherapy-induced mucositis or cystitis, radiation toxicity, infection, or surgery.

The etiology of hemorrhage in oncology patients is often multifactorial, as cancer patients are susceptible to tissue destruction, thrombocytopenia, coagulopathy, and fibrinolytic disorders. Treatment must be targeted to each deficit. Evaluation of each component is required so that targeted therapies can be applied (**Table 100.8**). Localization of bleeding vessels or mucosal injury is important to identify potential surgical or mechanical remedies. Topical treatment of bleeding is an important first-line approach to mucosal or cutaneous bleeding sites. Topical thrombin or tissue sealants applied with pressure dressings to bleeding sites in the oral cavity or nasopharynx may lessen the requirement for transfusions. Severe thrombocytopenia is caused by myelosuppressive chemotherapy, and up to 60% of patients with leukemia and 90% of aplastic anemia patients will become refractory to platelet transfusions after a limited number of exposures. One-hour and 6-hr post-transfusion platelet counts can differentiate between immune and nonimmune causes of a poor response to platelet transfusion. Platelet refractoriness due to alloimmune or autoimmune antibodies will prevent an immediate response to transfusion, while sepsis and disseminated intravascular coagulopathy (DIC) lead to decreased survival of transfused platelets, with a rapid fall in platelet count. If random donor platelet transfusions are no longer achieving a therapeutic goal, ABO-type specific or human leukocyte antigen-matched single donor units may be requested from the blood bank.

Coagulopathy in oncology patients may result from the primary disease, infection and DIC, hepatic dysfunction, chemotherapy-associated toxicity, or vitamin K deficiency. Patients with ALL who present with DIC are at increased risk of early mortality and decreased long-term survival. Acute promyelocytic leukemia (AML-M3 or APL) is associated with DIC in over 50% of patients at diagnosis, and up to 40% of patients with DIC develop CNS or pulmonary hemorrhage in the first few weeks of treatment. Promyelocytic blasts contain granules that carry the procoagulants *tissue factor, cancer procoagulant,* and *annexin II,* which are released upon cytolysis, a process that is accelerated once treatment has begun. Induction treatment with *all*-trans retinoic acid shortens the duration of DIC from 7 to 3 days, but has not been shown to decrease the overall rate of hemorrhage in pediatric patients. A prolonged prothrombin time with elevated D-dimer or fibrin degradation products and low fibrinogen is suggestive of DIC and should be treated with replacement therapy of fresh frozen plasma, cryoprecipitate, and platelet transfusions prior to onset of major bleeding symptoms. APL is also associated with hyperfibrinolysis, which may accelerate bleeding symptoms, although use of antifibrinolytic therapy (aminocaproic acid 100 mg/kg, maximum dose 3 g orally or IV) should be reserved for use in life-threatening bleeding because of the potential to cause thrombosis and exacerbate DIC. The role of heparin for

TABLE 100.8

CAUSES OF BLEEDING IN PEDIATRIC CANCER PATIENTS

Cause	Diagnostic test	Treatment	Monitoring
Local anatomic causes	Visual inspection Unexplained drop in hemoglobin	Surgical control and pressure dressings	Hemoglobin, dressing inspection
Thrombocytopenia: chemotherapy-induced	Post-transfusion platelet increase	1 RDP unit/10 kg of body weight or 1 SDP unit/50 kg will increase platelets by 40,000	Platelet count daily
Thrombocytopenia with alloimmunization	No increase with 1 hr post-transfusion platelet count	ABO-type specific or HLA-matched platelets	1 hr post-transfusion platelet count
Thrombocytopenia with sepsis	Drop in platelet count between 1 and 6 hrs post-transfusion	1 RDP unit/10 kg of body weight as often as needed to maintain platelets >20,000/mm^3	Platelet count 6 hrs posttransfusion
Coagulopathy: DIC	Prolonged PT/INR Elevated d-dimer or FDPs Low fibrinogen	FFP to control bleeding. Cryoprecipitate for fibrinogen <100 ng/mL.	PT/INR, fibrinogen, D-dimer every 6 hrs
Coagulopathy: Hepatic dysfunction	Prolonged PT/INR Factors II, V, VII, IX, X are low. Factor VIII and fibrinogen are normal.	FFP to maintain INR <1.5	PT/INR 6 hrs after FFP and daily
Coagulopathy: Vitamin K deficiency	Prolonged PT/INR Factors II, VII, IX, X are low. Factors V and VIII are normal.	FFP if bleeding Vitamin K orally/SC	PT/INR 6 hrs after vitamin K and daily
Fibrinolytic disorder	Consider if bleeding out of proportion to coagulopathy in appropriate clinical setting (APL, ALL). Diagnostic laboratory tests of limited utility: Euglobulin lysis test TAT/roTEG (research).	Consider antifibrinolytic therapy for life-threatening bleeding.	None

RDP, random donor platelet; SDP, single donor platelet; HLA, human leukocyte antigen; DIC, disseminated intravascular coagulopathy; PT/INR, prothrombin/International Normalized Ratio; FDP, fibrin degradation products; FFP, fresh frozen plasma; SC, subcutaneously; APL, acute promyelocytic leukemia; ALL, acute lymphoblastic leukemia; TAT, thrombin-antithrombin complex; roTEG, rotational thromboelastography

APL-associated coagulopathy is controversial, as with DIC in general, as randomized, controlled trials and meta-analyses fail to confirm a benefit for anticoagulation in DIC.

Antineoplastic agents may also induce coagulopathies. L-asparaginase significantly decreases plasma concentrations of coagulation proteins, although it does not appear to impair thrombin generation. Methotrexate-associated hepatotoxicity may reduce synthesis of factors II, V, VII, IX, and X, while factor VIII and fibrinogen are usually spared. Prednisone use has been associated with hypofibrinogenemia. Vitamin K deficiency as a result of inadequate dietary intake, malabsorption, or prolonged antibiotic use will cause decrements in factors II, VII, IX, and X, sparing factor V, which is made in the liver but does not require vitamin K for carboxylation. Replacement therapy with fresh frozen plasma and/or cryoprecipitate is necessary to treat bleeding symptoms associated with hepatic dysfunction and vitamin K deficiency, as specific factor concentrates are not available for most coagulation factors. Recombinant factor VIIa (rFVIIa) has been used for bleeding patients with liver failure when volume restrictions impose limitations on factor VII replacement through plasma, but rFVIIa should be used guardedly in patients with DIC and malignancy, as thrombotic complications have been described. Dosing of rFVIIa for liver failure should not exceed 25 mcg/kg/3 hrs, unlike the supraphysiologic levels that the USFDA has approved for use in hemophilia patients. A randomized trial of 40, 80, or 160 mcg/kg of rFVIIa as a hemostatic agent in stem cell transplant recipients with gastrointestinal, pulmonary, or genitourinary hemorrhage failed to demonstrate improvement in bleeding or transfusion requirement (34).

Thromboembolic complications are becoming increasingly more common in pediatric cancer patients, as treatment regimens have intensified and long-term survival has improved. Central venous catheters are the primary risk factor for thrombosis during treatment for cancer. The chemotherapeutic agent L-asparaginase, which is used during induction therapy for ALL, causes reduction of the endogenous anticoagulants antithrombin, protein C, and protein S, which leads to an 11% risk of symptomatic thromboembolic events during the first 30 days of ALL induction therapy with BFM-93/98 protocols

(12). Asymptomatic thrombosis detected by screening venography, ultrasound of the upper body, echocardiogram, and MRI of the head occurs in 37% (33). Symptomatic thrombosis most often occurs in the CNS or upper central venous system. Headaches, seizures, and a decreased level of consciousness, with papilledema or cranial nerve palsies, are presenting signs and symptoms of cerebral venous thrombosis in children. Asymptomatic thrombosis occurs predominantly in the upper central venous system and may result in extensive collateralization or symptoms of the post-phlebitic syndrome, as well as limit future sites for venous access. An open-label, randomized, placebo-controlled treatment trial of antithrombin replacement therapy to prevent thrombosis during ALL induction therapy showed a trend to safety and efficacy, but the study was underpowered to prove superiority of treatment over placebo (33). Patients who had central venous catheters placed during induction therapy had a much higher risk of thrombosis in both treatment arms, leading to the suggestion that insertion of indwelling catheters should be delayed until after induction therapy whenever practical. Thromboprophylaxis for adult cancer patients with indwelling catheters has been shown to reduce the incidence of thrombosis, but these studies have not been replicated in children. Although retrospective surveys have shown an increased risk of thrombosis among children with inherited prothrombotic risk factors, such as the prothrombin G20210A mutation, available evidence does not support the routine screening of pediatric cancer patients for thrombophilia at this time.

ABDOMINAL EMERGENCIES

Acute Abdomen

Abdominal emergencies in pediatric cancer patients arise most commonly due to hemorrhage, mechanical obstruction, perforation, or inflammation. The development of abdominal pathology in the neutropenic or immunocompromised patient presents a special diagnostic and treatment challenge, when compared to immunologically normal hosts. The presence of pain, a generally reliable sign of acute abdomen, may be less useful in a patient with abnormal sensation, spinal cord pathology, or recent treatment with high-dose steroids.

Acute Appendicitis

Appendicitis is one of the most common abdominal surgical conditions in childhood, with a peak incidence at age 12; the incidence in children with cancer is between 2%–4%, which parallels the general population. The use of steroids may mask the symptoms of appendicitis in some patients, making the diagnosis more difficult.

The differential diagnosis of appendicitis includes typhlitis, abdominal obstruction, intussusception, gastroenteritis, constipation, urinary tract infection, renal colic, pelvic inflammatory disease, and lower lobe pneumonia.

Studies in oncology patients have shown that the diagnosis of appendicitis was delayed in 37.5% of children in whom typhlitis was primarily suspected. We recommend the use of CT or ultrasound in all pediatric cancer patients suspected of typhlitis. Appendectomy is the definitive treatment, but associ-

ated mortality among pediatric cancer patients is higher than for other children due to immunosuppression, opportunistic infections, and delayed diagnosis.

Bowel Obstruction

Bowel obstruction is a considerable source of morbidity and mortality in the patient with cancer. Bowel obstruction from primary malignancy is not as common in children as it is in adults because of a lower frequency of these tumors (colon and ovarian cancer). It may be the presenting symptom of certain diseases, such as non-Hodgkin lymphoma, rhabdomyosarcoma, and colonic neoplasias. Bowel obstruction may also be present in metastatic disease. It is almost always found in carcinomatosis. It is most commonly seen in children who have received adjuvant therapy for their primary malignancy and/or have had abdominal surgery. Many conditions that increase the risk of bowel obstruction are encountered in children who are being treated for cancer. These include surgery, radiation therapy, narcotic use, prolonged bed rest, malnutrition, and electrolyte abnormalities. CT is superior to plain x-rays in identifying the level and, sometimes, the cause of the obstruction (28).

Patients with partial obstruction (i.e., those with plain x-rays showing the presence of intraluminal air in the small and large bowel) and those without mechanical obstruction may be managed medically. Surgery is indicated for patients with complete mechanical obstruction, partial mechanical obstruction not responding to medical treatment, or developing signs of peritonitis and frank perforation. Palliative measures, such as the use of a venting gastrostomy or jejunostomy, are appropriate in patients with end-stage disease who present with inoperable bowel obstruction.

Intussusception

Primary intestinal neoplasms or intestinal metastatic tumors, such as carcinomas or lymphomas, may serve as lead points for intussusception. These occur most commonly in the jejunum and the ileum. Nausea, vomiting, abdominal distension, and lethargy are the most consistent presenting symptoms. A high index of suspicion and the use of appropriate imaging are required to make the correct diagnosis in a timely manner. Ultrasonography is more accurate than abdominal x-rays and can detect the lead point and other intra-abdominal pathology. The treatment of choice in the cancer patient is surgical reduction of the intussusception and resection of the inciting pathology rather than radiologic reduction using contrast enema.

Abdominal Compartment Syndrome

Abdominal compartment syndrome is a life-threatening condition characterized by elevation of intra-abdominal pressure (IAP).

$$APP = MAP - IAP$$

where APP is abdominal perfusion pressure and MAP is mean arterial pressure.

Normal IAP is ~5–7 mm Hg. Intra-abdominal hypertension is defined by a sustained or repeated pathologic elevation of IAP ≥12 mm Hg. Abdominal compartment syndrome is defined as a sustained IAP ≥20 mm Hg (with or without an APP <60 mm Hg) that is associated with new organ dysfunction/failure. Organ dysfunction may occur with abdominal pressure as low as 10 mm Hg. Higher pressures (15–25 mm Hg) are associated with a further decrease in perfusion and cardiopulmonary dysfunction. Sustained increases in IAP cause a marked decrease in blood flow and oxygen delivery to the mesenteric, celiac, and renal arteries, affecting the viability and function of the tissues within (15,46). This hypoxic-ischemic event has been implicated in the release of cytokines from the Kupffer cells of the liver and bacterial translocation from the gut to the mesenteric lymph nodes (14). Intestinal ischemia plays an important role in the development of multiorgan dysfunction. With increasing IAP, compression of the inferior vena cava and other large veins occurs, resulting in decreased preload (IAP > central venous pressure) and decreased cardiac output. Increased IAP also causes elevation of the diaphragm, which increases intrathoracic pressure causing further depression of cardiac function. The diagnosis of abdominal compartment syndrome should be considered in any patient in whom tense abdominal distention develops. Possible precipitating factors include septic shock, requiring large volume resuscitation; bowel distension from ileus or mechanical obstruction; ascites/peritonitis or peritoneal bleeding; high tumor load; and complications from surgery.

Britt showed that time to diagnosis and management had an impact on outcome; the diagnosis in the nonsurvivor group was made in an average of 26.7 hrs versus 10.5 hrs in the survivor group (6). The diagnosis can be confirmed by measuring bladder pressure by instilling 1 mL/kg of sterile saline (maximum of 25 mL) into a Foley catheter placed in a patient in a complete supine position at the end of expiration and connecting the catheter to a pressure transducer via a three-way stopcock. The transducer is zeroed at the level of the mid-axillary line (15). Timely surgical decompression of abdominal compartment syndrome using a prosthetic silo, mesh, or plastic bag will produce an immediate improvement of cardiopulmonary and renal function. A prophylactic prosthetic mesh may be indicated in high-risk surgical patients to prevent abdominal compartment syndrome.

CONCLUSION AND FUTURE DIRECTIONS

Recent experience with pediatric cancer patients in the PICU suggests that outcomes are improved with early and aggressive interventions that are targeted to preventing or avoiding organ damage or failure, as survival for these patients is markedly reduced once three or more systems are implicated. It is important that critical care professionals be aware of the effects of new chemotherapeutic agents and treatment strategies and that they be attentive to the special challenges posed by immune compromise. A dynamic and vigorous partnership with the oncology team will help to ensure that these patients receive timely physiologic support as they undergo treatment. Future directions may include the use of less-toxic cancer therapies and the potential earlier use of therapies available to the intensivist

to prevent end-organ dysfunction. Further investigation is necessary to determine if several promising therapies, including the early institution of noninvasive modes of ventilation, therapeutic immune modulation, and renal or plasma replacement therapies, will have a further positive effect on outcomes.

KEY POINTS

- The survival of pediatric cancer patients admitted to the PICU is profoundly affected by the incidence and severity of organ system failure. End-organ protection should be a primary goal of treatment.
- Fever in neutropenic patients should be treated with aggressive and early institution of broad-spectrum antibiotics and aggressive fluid resuscitation, if necessary.
- Infection and neutropenia contribute substantially to mortality among these patients. Careful attention to antibiotic sensitivities and frequent surveillance are necessary. Disseminated or resistant infection in a neutropenic patient should trigger consideration of colony-stimulating factors and granulocyte transfusion.
- Respiratory distress in the pediatric cancer patient may reflect bacterial, fungal, and viral infection or toxicity. Bronchoalveolar lavage and high-resolution CT should be considered to clarify etiology. If invasive ventilation is indicated for any reason, early institution of a lung-protective strategy, including the use of high-frequency oscillatory ventilation, seems to improve outcome in these patients.
- Metabolic derangements are common in pediatric cancer patients and may be life-threatening. TLS, characterized by hyperuricemia, hyperkalemia, and hyperphosphatemia and most often triggered by chemotherapy, can result in renal failure and potentially fatal cardiac arrhythmias. Frequent laboratory studies, aggressive hydration, and alkalinization are helpful in reducing these risks.
- Hyperleukocytosis, a common presentation of patients with leukemia, can cause coagulopathy and hyperviscosity, leading to lung injury and stroke. Prompt initiation of cancer therapy is recommended. Apheresis may be considered if the WBC is >100,000/mm^3.

References

1. Albanese A, Hindmarsh P, Stanhope R. Management of hyponatraemia in patients with acute cerebral insults. *Arch Dis Child* 2001;85:246–51.
2. Ascioglu S, Rex JH, de Pauw B, et al. Defining opportunistic invasive fungal infections in immunocompromised patients with cancer and hematopoietic stem cell transplants: An international consensus. *Clin Infect Dis* 2002; 34:7–14.
3. Baorto EP, Aquino VM, Mullen CA, et al. Clinical parameters associated with low bacteremia risk in 1100 pediatric oncology patients with fever and neutropenia. *Cancer* 2001;92:909–13.
4. Bastin ME, Carpenter TK, Armitage PA, et al. Effects of dexamethasone on cerebral perfusion and water diffusion in patients with high-grade glioma. *Am J Neuroradiol* 2006;27:402–8.
5. Berkenbosch JW, Lentz CW, Jimenez DF, et al. Cerebral salt wasting syndrome following brain injury in three pediatric patients: Suggestions for rapid diagnosis and therapy. *Pediatr Neurosurg* 2002;36:75–9.
6. Britt RC, Gannon T, Collins JN, et al. Secondary abdominal compartment syndrome: Risk factors and outcomes. *Am Surg* 2005;71:982–5.
7. Carcillo JA, Fields AI, American College of Critical Care Medicine Task Force Committee M. Clinical practice parameters for hemodynamic support of pediatric and neonatal patients in septic shock. *Crit Care Med* 2002;30: 1365–78.
8. Cartoni C, Dragoni F, Micozzi A, et al. Neutropenic enterocolitis in patients with acute leukemia: Prognostic significance of bowel wall thickening detected by ultrasonography. *J Clin Oncol* 2001;19:756–61.

9. Cesaro S, Toffolutti T, Messina C, et al. Safety and efficacy of caspofungin and liposomal amphotericin B, followed by voriconazole in young patients affected by refractory invasive mycosis. *Eur J Haematol* 2004;73:50–5.

10. Clark OA, Lyman G, Castro AA, et al. Colony-stimulating factors for chemotherapy-induced febrile neutropenia. *Cochrane Database Syst Rev* 2003;CD003039.

11. Cometta A, Kern WV, De Bock R, et al. Vancomycin versus placebo for treating persistent fever in patients with neutropenic cancer receiving piperacillin-tazobactam monotherapy. *Clin Infect Dis* 2003;37:382–9.

12. Creutzig U, Zimmermann M, Reinhardt D, et al. Early deaths and treatment-related mortality in children undergoing therapy for acute myeloid leukemia: Analysis of the multicenter clinical trials AML-BFM 93 and AML-BFM 98. *J Clin Oncol* 2004;22:4384–93.

13. Diaz MA, Vicent MG, Prudencio M, et al. Predicting factors for admission to an intensive care unit and clinical outcome in pediatric patients receiving hematopoietic stem cell transplantation. *Haematologica* 2002;87:292–8.

14. Diebel LN, Dulchavsky SA, Brown WJ. Splanchnic ischemia and bacterial translocation in the abdominal compartment syndrome. *J Trauma* 1997;43:852–5.

15. Epelman M, Soudack M, Engel A, et al. Abdominal compartment syndrome in children: CT findings. *Pediatr Radiol* 2002;32:319–22.

16. Fiser RT, West NK, Bush AJ, et al. Outcome of severe sepsis in pediatric oncology patients. *Pediatr Crit Care Med* 2005;6:531–6.

17. Gillet Y, Issartel B, Vanhems P, et al. [Severe staphylococcal pneumonia in children]. *Arch Pediatr* 2001;8(Suppl 4):742s–6s.

18. Goldman SC, Holcenberg JS, Finklestein JZ, et al. A randomized comparison between rasburicase and allopurinol in children with lymphoma or leukemia at high risk for tumor lysis. *Blood* 2001;97:2998–3003.

19. Hagen SA, Craig DM, Martin PL, et al. Mechanically ventilated pediatric stem cell transplant recipients: Effect of cord blood transplant and organ dysfunction on outcome. *Pediatr Crit Care Med* 2003;4:206–13.

20. Hallahan AR, Shaw PJ, Rowell G, et al. Improved outcomes of children with malignancy admitted to a pediatric intensive care unit. *Crit Care Med* 2000;28:3718–21.

21. Hughes WT, Armstrong D, Bodey GP, et al. 2002 guidelines for the use of antimicrobial agents in neutropenic patients with cancer. *Clin Infect Dis* 2002;34:730–51.

22. Ingram L, Rivera GK, Shapiro DN. Superior vena cava syndrome associated with childhood malignancy: Analysis of 24 cases. *Med Pediatr Oncol* 1990;18:476–81.

23. Jacobe SJ, Hassan A, Veys P, et al. Outcome of children requiring admission to an intensive care unit after bone marrow transplantation. *Crit Care Med* 2003;31:1299–305.

24. Jones DP, Mahmoud H, Chesney RW. Tumor lysis syndrome: Pathogenesis and management. *Pediatr Nephrol* 1995;9:206–12.

25. Keenan HT, Bratton SL, Martin LD, et al. Outcome of children who require mechanical ventilatory support after bone marrow transplantation. *Crit Care Med* 2000;28:830–5.

26. Lehrnbecher T, Varwig D, Kaiser J, et al. Infectious complications in pediatric acute myeloid leukemia: Analysis of the prospective multi-institutional clinical trial AML-BFM 93. *Leukemia* 2004;18:72–7.

27. Loblaw DA, Laperriere NJ. Emergency treatment of malignant extradural spinal cord compression: An evidence-based guideline. *J Clin Oncol* 1998;16:1613–24.

28. Maglinte DD, Kelvin FM, Rowe MG, et al. Small-bowel obstruction: Optimizing radiologic investigation and nonsurgical management. *Radiology* 2001;218:39–46.

29. Mahdavi H, Kuizon BD, Gales B, et al. Sevelamer hydrochloride: An effective phosphate binder in dialyzed children. *Pediatr Nephrol* 2003;18:1260–4.

30. Mathur M, Sykes JA, Saxena VR, et al. Treatment of acute lymphoblastic leukemia-induced extreme hypercalcemia with pamidronate and calcitonin. *Pediatr Crit Care Med* 2003;4:252–5.

31. Matt P, Bernet F, Habicht J, et al. Predicting outcome after lung resection for invasive pulmonary aspergillosis in patients with neutropenia. *Chest* 2004;126:1783–8.

32. Menell JS, Cesarman GM, Jacovina AT, et al. Annexin II and bleeding in acute promyelocytic leukemia. *N Engl J Med* 1999;340:994–1004.

33. Mitchell L, Andrew M, Hanna K, et al. Trend to efficacy and safety using antithrombin concentrate in prevention of thrombosis in children receiving L-asparaginase for acute lymphoblastic leukemia. Results of the PAARKA study. *Thromb Haemost* 2003;90:235–44.

34. Pihusch M, Bacigalupo A, Szer J, et al. Recombinant activated factor VII in treatment of bleeding complications following hematopoietic stem cell transplantation. *J Thromb Haemost* 2005;3:1935–44.

35. Porcu P, Cripe LD, Ng EW, et al. Hyperleukocytic leukemias and leukostasis: A review of pathophysiology, clinical presentation and management. *Leuk Lymphoma* 2000;39:1–18.

36. Pui CH, Mahmoud HH, Wiley JM, et al. Recombinant urate oxidase for the prophylaxis or treatment of hyperuricemia in patients With leukemia or lymphoma. *J Clin Oncol* 2001;19:697–704.

37. Quezada G, Sunderland T, Chan KW, et al. Medical and non-medical barriers to outpatient treatment of fever and neutropenia in children with cancer. *Pediatr Blood Cancer* 2007; 48(3):273–7.

38. Reichenberger F, Habicht JM, Gratwohl A, et al. Diagnosis and treatment of invasive pulmonary aspergillosis in neutropenic patients. *Eur Respir J* 2002;19:743–55.

39. Reusser P, Einsele H, Lee J, et al. Randomized multicenter trial of foscarnet versus ganciclovir for preemptive therapy of cytomegalovirus infection after allogeneic stem cell transplantation. *Blood* 2002;99:1159–64.

40. Rheingold SR. LB. *Oncologic Emergencies, 5th ed.* Philadelphia: Lippincott Williams & Wilkins; 2006:1202–30.

41. Ricketts RR. Clinical management of anterior mediastinal tumors in children. *Semin Pediatr Surg* 2001;10:161–8.

42. Rossi R, Kleta R, Ehrich JH. Renal involvement in children with malignancies. *Pediatric Nephrology* 1999;13:153–62.

43. Santolaya ME, Alvarez AM, Aviles CL, et al. Prospective evaluation of a model of prediction of invasive bacterial infection risk among children with cancer, fever, and neutropenia. *Clin Infect Dis* 2002;35:678–83.

44. Seymour JF, Gagel RF. Calcitriol: The major humoral mediator of hypercalcemia in Hodgkin's disease and non-Hodgkin's lymphomas. *Blood* 1993; 82:1383–94.

45. Stanworth SJ, Massey E, Hyde C, et al. Granulocyte transfusions for treating infections in patients with neutropenia or neutrophil dysfunction. *Cochrane Database of Syst Rev* 2005;CD005339.

46. Sugerman HJ, Bloomfield GL, Saggi BW. Multisystem organ failure secondary to increased intraabdominal pressure. *Infection* 1999;27:61–6.

47. Sung L, Nathan PC, Lange B, et al. Prophylactic granulocyte colony-stimulating factor and granulocyte-macrophage colony-stimulating factor decrease febrile neutropenia after chemotherapy in children with cancer: A meta-analysis of randomized controlled trials. *J Clin Oncol* 2004;22:3350–6.

48. Walsh TJ, Pappas P, Winston DJ, et al. Voriconazole compared with liposomal amphotericin B for empirical antifungal therapy in patients with neutropenia and persistent fever. *N Engl J Med* 2002;346:225–34.

49. Walsh TJ, Teppler H, Donowitz GR, et al. Caspofungin versus liposomal amphotericin B for empirical antifungal therapy in patients with persistent fever and neutropenia. *N Engl J Med* 2004;351:1391–402.

50. Watson RS, Carcillo JA. Scope and epidemiology of pediatric sepsis. *Pediatr Crit Care Med* 2005;6:S3–5.

51. Wossmann W, Schrappe M, Meyer U, et al. Incidence of tumor lysis syndrome in children with advanced stage Burkitt lymphoma/leukemia before and after introduction of prophylactic use of urate oxidase. *Ann Hematol* 2003;82:160–5.

52. Young G, Shende A. Use of pamidronate in the management of acute cancer-related hypercalcemia in children. *Med Pediatr Oncol* 1998;30:117–21.

CHAPTER 101 ■ HEMATOLOGIC EMERGENCIES

R. BLAINE EASLEY • KENNETH M. BRADY • JOSEPH D. TOBIAS

The pediatric critical care clinician is constantly evaluating infants and children who experience nonmalignant "blood test" abnormalities. Often, these hematologic issues are secondary to another process, such as trauma, infection, or chronic illness. However, primary abnormalities will present in previously healthy children or may be contributing to the complexity those with significant medical or surgical illness. The challenge is differentiating between a normal variation and a potentially life-threatening disease on routine hematologic testing. The goal of this chapter is to review the common causes and treatments for pediatric patients in the critical care unit who have quantitative and qualitative hematologic abnormalities. Many of the primary hematologic problems and oncology-related issues are addressed elsewhere in this text. We will focus on selected nonmalignant, hematologic disorders and review the pathophysiology and management of these processes when caring for a critically ill child. In most cases, the intensivist should seek collaboration with a pediatric hematologist in the management of these disorders.

A discussion of hematologic and coagulation disorders in children requires an understanding of the normal complete blood count (CBC) clotting function. The normal pediatric ranges for red cell, white cell, platelet, and coagulation values in children are detailed, respectively, in **Tables 101.1, 101.2, and 101.3**. The common causes of erroneous values on routine CBC testing are identified in **Table 101.4**. These should always be considered when investigating spurious values, whether abnormally low or high.

RED BLOOD CELL ABNORMALITIES IN INFANTS AND CHILDREN

Anemia

Anemia, or erythropenia, is the most common hematologic abnormality diagnosed and managed in the PICU. The most common anemia etiologies that require emergent evaluation and care are acute blood loss, acute hemolysis, and acute splenic sequestration. With acute blood loss (whether traumatic, surgical, or gastrointestinal), the approach is uniform—identify the potential source of bleeding, develop a diagnostic and/or therapeutic plan, and maintain intravascular volume with red blood cell (RBC) transfusion and crystalloid until the plan can be implemented. However, when an acutely ill child presents with anemia among other symptoms and problems, the critical care provider must work through the primary and secondary causes for the anemia, which involves evaluating the potential etiologies by considering the different mechanisms: (a) conditions of failed RBC production, (b) conditions of increased RBC destruction, and (c) conditions of abnormal RBC maturation (**Fig. 101.1**).

Anemia, regardless of etiology, results in a decreased O_2-carrying capacity; when severe, anemia can result in decreased O_2 delivery. Physical symptoms are extremely variable and not predictive of anemia severity (41). Common symptoms of anemia are pallor, nausea, vomiting, weakness, fatigue, irritability, tachycardia, tachypnea, and edema. It has been determined that anemia is only one of the leading determinates for RBC transfusion in the PICU (8). In addition, comorbid conditions that may contribute directly to the anemic state are both acute and chronic in nature. Chronic illnesses with anemia as a feature often have adaptive pathophysiology that alters vascular perfusion and diphosphoglycerate (2,3-DPG) levels, expands plasma volume, and lowers blood viscosity.

Anemia secondary to sickle cell disease (SCD) and acute hemorrhage are discussed in Chapters 26, 39, and 104. The differential diagnoses of anemia based on mean corpuscular volume (MCV) are summarized in **Figure 101.2**. Following are some of the most commonly encountered causes for reduction in RBC number and function in children.

Iron-deficiency anemia is the most common nutritional abnormality worldwide and is the leading cause of anemia in early childhood. When iron-deficiency anemia severe (e.g., hemoglobin, Hb, is <4 g/dL), children can be symptomatic with cardiac and respiratory instability. Iron-deficiency anemia characteristically has a low Hb, low RBC count, low MCV, and low reticulocyte count, with elevated free erythrocyte protoporphyrin and red-cell distribution width measurements. The peripheral blood smear in iron deficiency typically demonstrates microcytic and hypochromic erythrocytes. During the first 4–6 months of life, most full-term infants are iron sufficient owing to transplacental passage of iron during the last trimester of pregnancy. Iron deficiency occurs most frequently in children <3 years of age and results from inadequate iron intake during this period of rapid growth. Poor iron intake is often complicated by other clinical findings of poor nutrition, neglect, and/or excess intake of dietary cow's milk. Diets high in whole milk result in additional comorbidities of an increased incidence of colitis and gastrointestinal bleeding. In older children and adults with iron deficiency, occult blood loss should be suspected and should prompt a gastrointestinal evaluation. Differentiating between the two most common causes of microcytic anemia (iron deficiency vs. thalassemia) can be challenging, and the Mentzer index (MCV/RBC count) can be a useful bedside tool. When applied to conditions of microcytic anemia, Mentzer index values of >13.5 suggest iron deficiency,

TABLE 101.1

NORMAL VALUES AND RANGES FOR RED BLOOD CELL INDICES

Age	Hemoglobin (g/dL) Mean	Hemoglobin (g/dL) ± 2SD	Hematocrit (%) Mean	Hematocrit (%) ± 2SD	Reticulocytes (%) range	MCV (fL)
Cord	16.8	13.7–20.1	55	45–65	3.0–7.0	110
2 wk	16.5	13.0–20.0	50	42–66	0.1–1.7	98–116
3 mo	12.0	9.5–14.5	36	31–41	0.7–2.3	*
6 mo–6 yr	12.0	10.5–14.0	37	33–42	0.5–1.0	70–74
7–12 yr	13.0	11.0–16.0	38	34–40	0.5–1.0	76–80
12–18 yr						
Female	14.0	12.0–16.0	42	37–47	1.6	80–96
Male	14.5	14.0–18.0	43	36–50		80–96
Adult						
Female	14.0	12.0–16.0	42	36–47	1.6	80–96
Male	16.0	14.0–18.0	47	42–52		80–96

MCV, mean corpuscular volume; fL, femtoliters
*Approximate MCV ranges in ages >1 month to ≤9 years: low MCV = 70+ (age in years), high MCV = 90 – (age in years). Adapted from Dallman PR, Siimes MA. Percentile curves for hemoglobin and red cell volume in infancy and childhood. *J Pediatr* 1979;94(1):26–31.

TABLE 101.2

NORMAL VALUES AND RANGES FOR WHITE BLOOD CELL COUNT AND DIFFERENTIAL

Age	Leukocytes (WBC/mm³) Mean	Leukocytes (WBC/mm³) Range	Neutrophils (%) Mean	Neutrophils (%) Range	Lymphocytes (%) Mean	Eosinophils (%) Mean	Monocytes (%) Mean
Cord	18,000	9000–30,000	61	40–80	31	2	6
2 wks	12,000	5000–21,000	40		63	3	9
3 mos	12,000	6000–18,000	30		48	2	5
6 mos–6 yrs	10,000	6000–15,000	45		48	2	5
7–12 yrs	8,000	4500–13,500	55		38	2	5
Adult	7,500	5000–10,000	55	35–70	35	3	7

*Relatively wide range. WBC, white blood cell. Adapted from Cranendonk E, van Gennip AH, Abeling NG, et al. Reference values for automated cytochemical differential count of leukocytes in children 0–16 years old: Comparison with manually obtained counts from Wright-stained smears. *J Clin Chem Clin Biochem* 1985;23(10):663–7.

TABLE 101.3

NORMAL VALUE AND RANGE FOR PLATELET COUNT AND COAGULATION PARAMETERS

Age	Platelets (10³/mm³)	PT (sec)	aPTT (sec)	Fibrinogen (g/dL)	BT (min)
Preterm	180–327	15.4 (14.6–16.9)	108 (80–168)	243 (150–373)	–
Birth	290	13.0 (10.1–15.9)	42.9 (31.3–54.3)	283 (167–309)	–
1 mo	252				
1 yr–7 yrs	150–350	11 (10.6–11.4)	30 (24–36)	276 (170–405)	6 (2.5–10)
7 yrs–18yrs	150–350	11.2 (10.2–12.0)	32 (26–37)	300 (154–448)	5 (3–8)

PT, prothrombin time (extrinsic pathway); aPTT, activated partial thromboplastin time (intrinsic pathway); BT, bleeding time (clot formation)
Adapted from Andrew M, Paes B, Milner R, et al. Development of the human coagulation system in the full-term infant. *Blood* 1987;70(1):165–72; Andrew M, Paes B, Milner R, et al. Development of the human coagulation system in the healthy premature infant. *Blood* 1988;72(5):1651–7; Andrew M, Vegh P, Johnston M, Bowker J, et al. Maturation of the hemostatic system during childhood. *Blood* 1992;80(8):1998–2005.

TABLE 101.4

COMMON SOURCES OF SPURIOUS RESULTS WITH AUTOMATED CELL COUNTERS

CBC parameter	Causes of increase	Causes of decrease
WBC	Cryoglobulin, cryofibrinogen Heparin Monoclonal proteins Nucleated red cells Platelet clumping Unlysed red cells	Clotting Smudge cells Uremia Immunosuppressants
RBC	Cryoglobulin, cryofibrinogen Giant platelets High WBC (>50,000/μL)	Autoagglutination Clotting Hemolysis (*in vitro*) Microcytic red cells
Hemoglobin	Carboxyhemoglobin (>10%) Cryoglobulin, cryofibrinogen Hemolysis (in vitro) Heparin High WBC (>50,000/μL) Hyperbilirubinemia Lipemia Monoclonal proteins	Clotting Sulfhemoglobin (?)
Hematocrit (automated)	Cryoglobulin, cryofibrinogen Giant platelets High WBC (>50,000/μL) Hyperglycemia (>600 mg/dL) Hyponatremia Plasma trapping	Autoagglutination Clotting Hemolysis (*in vitro*) Microcytic red cells Excess EDTA Hemolysis (*in vitro*) Hypernatremia
Mean corpuscular volume	Autoagglutination High WBC (>50,000/μL) Hyperglycemia Reduced red cell deformability	Cryoglobulin, Cryofibrinogen Giant platelets Hemolysis (*in vitro*) Microcytic red cells Swollen red cells
Platelets	Cryoglobulin, cryofibrinogen Hemolysis (*in vitro* and *in vivo*) Microcytic red cells Red cell inclusions White cell fragments	Clotting Giant platelets Heparin Platelet clumping Platelet satellitosis

CBC, complete blood count; WBC, white blood cell count; RBC, red blood cell count; EDTA, ethylenediaminetetraacetic acid
Adapted from Cornbleet J, Kessinger S. Evaluation of Coulter S-Plus three-part differential in population with a high prevalence of abnormalities. *Am J Clin Pathol* 1985;84(5):620–6.

while a value of <11.5 suggests thalassemia minor. Differential diagnosis for microcytic anemia also includes lead poisoning, chronic inflammation, copper deficiency, and thalassemia (**Fig. 101.2**).

Perhaps the most conclusive evidence of iron-deficiency anemia is the incremental rise in Hb concentration during therapeutic iron supplementation. Optimal response is obtained with 3–6 mg/kg/day of elemental iron. Ferrous sulfate is the preferred form. Routine enteral administration is adequate, although parenteral administration (with iron dextran) is an option if compliance or tolerance of the oral preparation is an issue. Following iron repletion, the reticulocyte count increases within 1 week, and gradual correction of Hb occurs over 4 weeks. In most patients, the treatment should continue for ~3

months. Additional iron studies (serum iron, ferritin, total iron-binding capacity, and transferrin) are rarely necessary in young children with a typical history and characteristic CBC findings. Recommendations to prevent iron-deficiency anemia include iron supplementation (1–2 mg/kg/day) for all breast-fed infants after 3 months of age, use of iron-fortified formulas (containing 12 mg iron as ferrous sulfate per liter) and cereals, iron supplement (2–3 mg/kg/day) to preterm infants after the first month of life, and delaying the introduction of cow's milk until after 1 year of age. Blood transfusion is rarely needed (75). Studies of children with multifactorial anemia (nutritional, malaria, hemoglobinopathy, etc.) in Africa have demonstrated significant improvements in mortality with blood transfusion therapy, regardless of age. This data, along with published clinical

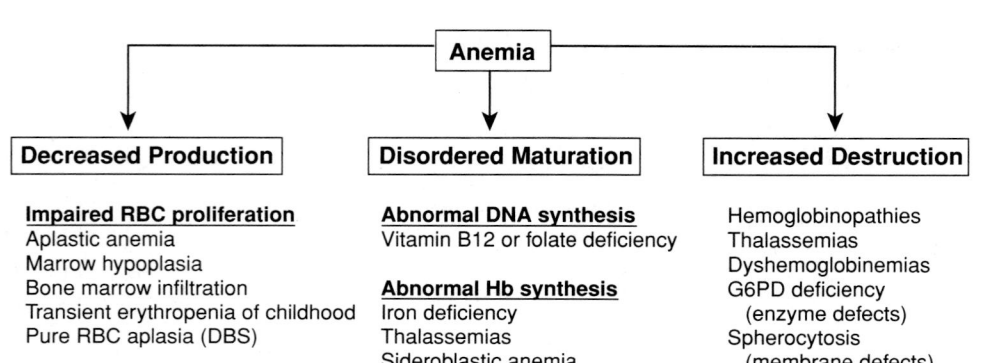

FIGURE 101.1. The etiology of anemia. TEC, transient erythropenia of childhood; RBC, red blood cell; DBS, Diamond-Blackfan syndrome; EPO, erythropoietin; Hb, hemoglobin. Adapted from Sadowitz PD, Amanullah S, Souid AK. Hematologic emergencies in the pediatric emergency room. *Emerg Med Clin North Am* 2002; 20(1):177–98, vii.

practice, supports transfusing children with or without cardiorespiratory symptoms when Hb is ≤4 g/dL (15). In infants and children who have Hb values >4 and ≤6 g/dL, treatment practices vary worldwide and the decision to transfuse is largely based on symptoms, available resources, and comorbid conditions (malaria, fever, hypotension). If transfusion therapy is undertaken in either severe or moderate anemia, slow, monitored transfusion of packed RBCs should be performed, with continuous cardiorespiratory monitoring to avoid congestive heart failure from the adaptive changes of prolonged anemia (76). Typically, 5 mL/kg over 4 hrs, followed by another 5 mL/kg transfusion over 4 hrs is adequate. Note that diuretics may also be required to avoid volume overload in an anemic patient's volume-expanded state.

Hemolytic anemia can be caused by either intracellular or extracellular disorders. Intracellular disorders consist of RBC membrane defects, abnormal erythrocyte metabolism, or hemoglobinopathies. Extracorpuscular disorders include immune-mediated destruction, mechanical fragmentation, infections, drugs, chemicals, and venoms. Inherent red cell susceptibilities, such as enzyme disorders and unstable hereditary hemoglobinopathies, enhance the ability of certain agents to produce damage. For instance, the hexose-monophosphate shunt and the glutathione pathways are the predominant mechanisms by which the erythrocyte handles oxidative stress. Disorders of either of these pathways can result in oxidative damage to the RBC and lysis (82). Discussion will focus on the most common intracellular disorder [glucose-6-phosphate

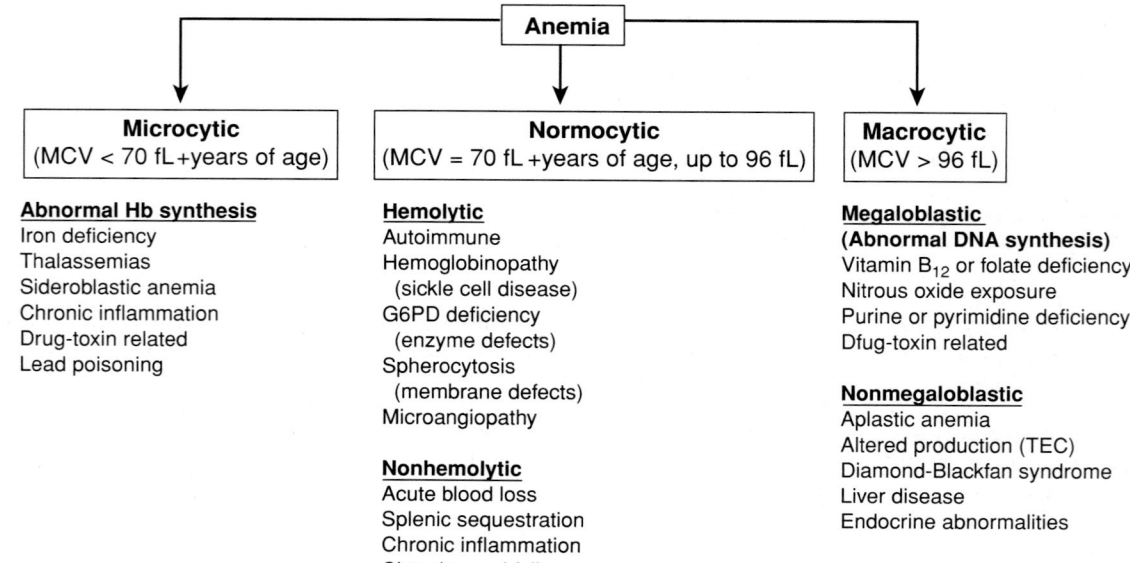

FIGURE 101.2. The differential diagnosis of anemia. MCV, mean corpuscular volume; fL, femtoliter; TEC, transient erythropenia of childhood. Adapted from Sadowitz PD, Amanullah S, Souid AK. Hematologic emergencies in the pediatric emergency room. *Emerg Med Clin North Am* 2002;20(1):177–98, vii.

dehydrogenase (G6PD) deficiency], and the most common extracellular disorder (autoimmune hemolytic anemia). Hemolytic uremic syndrome (HUS) is an important cause of hemolytic anemia in the PICU and is discussed in Chapter 96. Tests that are useful in the diagnosis of a hemolytic process include evaluation of peripheral blood smear for Heinz bodies (denatured Hb) or irregular RBCs (spherocytes), elevated reticulocyte count, positive Coombs test (direct and indirect), elevated serum aspartate aminotransferase (AST), lactate dehydrogenase (LDH), and serum bilirubin, with lowered serum haptoglobin.

G6PD deficiency is the most common RBC-associated enzyme disorder and is genetically determined by X-linked inheritance. Children and adults prone to this disorder include Africans, Asians, and those of Mediterranean descent. The Mediterranean variety is the classic form and is the most severe, as it results from the lowest G6PD activity. The African variety is unique because only the mature RBCs are enzyme-deficient. The incidence of G6PD deficiency in African American males is ~11% (12). The susceptibility of a patient with G6PD deficiency to drug-induced oxidative stress depends on the phenotype of the enzyme disorder and on drug metabolism and excretion. G6PD catalyzes the reduction of nicotinamide adenine dinucleotide phosphate (NADP) to NADPH in the hexosemonophosphate shunt. NADPH converts glutathione disulfide to reduced glutathione. Glutathione, in turn, inactivates hydrogen peroxide (H_2O_2) and protects protein sulfhydryl groups from oxidation. Lack of this enzyme allows for the rapid depletion of protective antioxidants and subsequent denaturation of the Hb unit. Oxidative stressors attack Hb sulfhydryl groups, releasing heme, the protein chain of which then unfolds and precipitates as insoluble aggregates (Heinz bodies). Unripened peaches, fava beans, methylene blue, naphthalene, phenazopyridine, and sulfamethoxazole are just a few of the agents that result in hemolysis for G6PD-deficient patients. Salicylates do not pose a risk for hemolysis, except in high doses. Avoidance of oxidants (e.g., sulfa drugs) and careful observation during stress (e.g., infection and surgery) are necessary. Patients with a diagnosis of G6PD deficiency who develop severe pallor or abdominal pain require immediate evaluation. Other patients who develop hemolytic symptoms of unknown etiology should have a G6PD assay performed. Identification of possible sources that trigger hemolysis and the elimination of continued exposure are crucial to the patient's recovery. RBC transfusion is sometimes necessary during episodes of severe hemolysis.

Antibody-mediated (autoimmune) hemolytic anemia is an extracellular process of RBC destruction. Typically, this disorder manifests as sudden pallor and fatigue, often following a viral illness. Because of the rapid onset, jaundice, hyperbilirubinemia, and reticulocytosis might not be present initially. The laboratory findings reveal a rapidly falling Hb, low haptoglobin, increased bilirubin metabolites in the urine, positive Coombs tests, and abundant spherocytes on the smear. The direct Coombs test confirms the diagnosis of antibody bound to the patient's RBCs. The indirect Coombs test detects free antibody in the patient's serum. Hemolysis can occur with either IgG or IgM antibodies. Typically, IgG antibodies do not agglutinate RBC in vitro and react at 37°C; therefore, they are termed *warm (incomplete) antibodies*. In contrast, IgM antibodies cause in vitro agglutination at ≤20°C and are termed *cold (complete) antibodies*. The antibody-coated RBCs are de-

stroyed in the reticuloendothelial system of the spleen, making intravascular hemolysis rare. The treatment involves hospitalization, careful observation, high-dose steroids, and if necessary, RBC transfusion using the most compatible blood.

Transient erythrocytopenia of childhood is characterized by gradual onset of a normocytic anemia and reticulocytopenia caused by temporary suppression of RBC production. It usually occurs in children between 1 month and 6 years of age and is commonly preceded by a viral illness. Full recovery usually occurs in 4–6 weeks. Blood transfusions are necessary if Hb concentration is <5 g/dL. Follow-up studies are necessary until the Hb concentration and reticulocyte count recover. In ~25% of patients, the anemia is associated with mild neutropenia. Transient erythrocytopenia of childhood must be distinguished from a rare disease, termed *pure red cell aplasia* or *Diamond-Blackfan syndrome*. Patients with Diamond-Blackfan syndrome typically have macrocytic erythrocytes (elevated MCV), dysmorphic features, and persistent anemia. Bone marrow recovery is the hallmark of transient erythrocytopenia of childhood and rules out Diamond-Blackfan syndrome.

Bone marrow infiltration can result from malignant cells or be the result of other processes such as inherited metabolic disorders or infections (fungus, tuberculosis). Regardless of the primary process, the result is a normocytic anemia (normal MCV) with a low reticulocyte count. These patients can have lymphadenopathy, hepatomegaly, and splenomegaly on physical examination, although laboratory abnormalities can include reticulocytopenia, neutropenia, thrombocytopenia, and circulating immature cells (e.g., nucleated RBCs, promyelocytes, metamyelocytes, and myelocytes). Bone marrow examination is essential in this setting to establish the correct diagnosis.

Acquired aplastic anemia is defined as peripheral blood pancytopenia with variable bone marrow hypocellularity in the absence of underlying malignant or myeloproliferative disease (18). Pathophysiologic mechanisms include maturation failure of pluripotent stem cells, failure of the stromal microenvironment of the marrow, impaired production and/or release of hematopoietic growth factors, and cellular or humoral immune suppression of the marrow. The incidence of acquired aplastic anemia increases with age and is attributed to the exposure to and accumulation of toxins over time. The incidence is low for patients <1 year of age, slowly increases to an intermediate level by the age of 50 years, and has its highest occurrence in older adults (>50 years of age). Drug-induced causes account for 50% of all cases (19).

Drug-induced aplastic anemia can result from either toxic effects or immune-mediated phenomena. Progenitor stem cells are most commonly affected. Common toxic agents include ionizing radiation, chemotherapeutic drugs, antibiotics (chloramphenicol), hydrocarbons (benzene), anti-inflammatory medications (phenylbutazone, indomethacin), and metals (gold) (**Table 101.5**). Other drugs with a relatively high risk for aplastic anemia are anticonvulsants (mephenytoin, phenytoin, carbamazepine), and quinacrine (52). Phenytoin and carbamazepine result in the production of toxic arene-oxide intermediate metabolites in vivo that bind covalently to macromolecules of marrow stem cells and lymphocytes. Supportive care is typically required, with recovery of the RBC counts occurring over time once the causative agent is discontinued.

Megaloblastic anemias result from decreased vitamin absorption, impaired metabolism, or both. Vitamin B_{12} and folate

COMMON AGENTS THAT CAUSE APLASTIC ANEMIA

Acetazolamide	Ibuprofen
Antineoplastic*	Mephenytoin
Alkylating	Oxyphenbutazone*
Antimetabolite	Paramethadione
Antibiotics	Phenothiazines
Benzene*	Phenylbutazone*
Captopril	Phenytoin
Carbamazepine	Propylthiouracil
Chloramphenicol*	Quinacrine
Chlorpheniramine	Radiation (ionizing)*
Colchicine*	Sulfonamides*
Gold salts*	

*Toxic mechanism.

deficiencies selectively impair cellular DNA synthesis. Because RNA protein production is maintained, an increased ratio of cytoplasmic-to-nucleic mass results, creating megaloblastic red cells. All cells are affected, including red cells, granulocytes, and megakaryocytes (20). Abnormal cellular maturation leads to premature cellular death. Decreased vitamin B_{12} absorption usually results from limited nutritional intake or intestinal malabsorptive diseases. Agents that impair vitamin B_{12} gut absorption include metformin, colchicine, neomycin, para-aminosalicylic acid, and slow-release potassium chloride. Causes of folate deficiency include sepsis, pregnancy, malignancy, chronic hemodialysis, and drugs.

Chronic ethanol ingestion interferes with folic acid intestinal absorption and metabolism. Some anticonvulsant drugs can also lower serum folate concentrations by limiting gut absorption. Approximately 50% of patients on long-term phenytoin therapy have low serum folate concentrations, and ~30% have red cell macrocytosis and early megaloblastic changes in the bone marrow. Folate replacement therapy improves the anemia. Methotrexate, trimethoprim, triamterene, and pyrimethamine inhibit dihydrofolate reductase, and megaloblastic anemia can develop during long-term and high-dose therapy. Lack of dihydrofolate reductase activity causes uridine substitution for thymidine in DNA synthesis, resulting in an unstable DNA strand. Antineoplastic agents that inhibit pyrimidine and purine synthesis also can cause megaloblastosis, which is not folate responsive.

Acute megaloblastic anemia may also be caused by prolonged nitrous oxide anesthesia (37). This gas inactivates vitamin B_{12} through oxidation, and this effect on RBCs is usually observed after a cumulative 5-hr exposure to $\geq$50% nitrous oxide. Case reports have also suggested that nitrous oxide exposure contributed to acute megaloblastic anemia and neuropathy in susceptible patients with comorbid illnesses such as viral infections, poor nutrition, alcoholism, malignancy, and sepsis (51).

Hemoglobinopathies

Primary hemoglobinopathies is a term that describes structural abnormalities of Hb that are often inherited. The globin genes are found in clusters on chromosomes 11 (β-globin chain) and 16 (α-globin chain). Point mutations and deletions in the genes for the Hb molecule result in alterations and production of functionally abnormal Hb. In normal human maturation, HbA ($\alpha 2 \beta 2$) becomes the dominant form, taking over from the HbF ($\alpha 2 \gamma 2$) during the first year of life. Presence of abnormal Hb species, as in SCD (HbS) and its variants (HbSC, HbAS, etc.), can result in persistence of HbF. The thalassemias are the most common worldwide genetic disorder. Though thalassemias represent a larger number of specific gene mutations, the end result is overexpression of one of the structurally normal Hb chains. β-thalassemias (excess of α-globin chain production) are more common than α-thalassemias (abnormalities that decrease α-globin chain production). However, the specific population statistic varies widely between different ethnicities and regions of the world. Approximately 700 structural variants of Hb have been described, and most are extremely rare and asymptomatic. More unstable Hb forms result in denaturation and formation of Heinz bodies on peripheral smear in the RBC. Again, most aberrant forms of Hb are asymptomatic; however, some will present with mild, chronic anemia and others with increased levels of chronic and episodic hemolysis. Detection on routine Hb electrophoresis is difficult, and specialized testing is often required to detect these abnormalities. Other structurally abnormal Hbs result in increased O_2 affinity and relative tissue hypoxia, which leads to polycythemia. Erythropoietin levels are often elevated and diagnosis is difficult. Those Hb abnormalities that result in decreased O_2 binding result in cyanosis. A complete review is beyond the scope of this chapter; however, *familial methemoglobinemia* (HbM) deserves comment.

HbM is a rare autosomal-dominant disorder, and affected individuals often present with cyanosis at birth. The structural abnormality results in stabilization of the iron heme moiety in the ferric (Fe^{3+}) form. As "secondary" causes of methemoglobinemia are more common, diagnosis of HbM was classically found when individuals failed to respond to methylene blue therapy for their methemoglobinemia. HbM and the other clinically significant hemoglobinopathies are detectable by newborn screening utilizing high-performance liquid chromatography or electrophoresis (as in HbS). Chronic complications from HbM are rare. However, if hemolysis is chronic or acute, it can cause jaundice, cardiomegaly, hepatosplenomegaly, neurologic impairment, nephropathy, retinopathy, impaired growth and development, gallbladder stones, and skin ulcers. Diagnostic evaluation should include CBC and reticulocyte count, bilirubin, pulse oximetry, blood pressure, growth and development, academic performance, biliary ultrasonography, and renal and pulmonary function studies.

Secondary hemoglobinopathies result from conditions that either induce abnormal Hb production or adversely affect Hb function. Dyshemoglobinemias are conditions that produce abnormal O_2 binding of structurally normal Hb. Disorders of heme moiety oxidation occur in both genetically susceptible and unsusceptible individuals. Environmental and iatrogenic causes of methemoglobinemia, carboxyhemoglobinemia, cyanohemoglobinemia, and sulfhemoglobinemia have been reported. Both chronic and acute forms have been described, with anemia, decreased O_2 delivery, and functional hypoxia as commonly associated features. Toxic exposures, such as cyanide and carbon monoxide, resulting in abnormal Hb function are discussed in Chapter 31.

All dyshemoglobinemias result in shifting of the oxygen disassociation curve, impairment of binding of O_2 by Hb, and impairment of O_2 delivery to the tissues. Diagnosis is often made with routine co-oximetry, which measures the elevated fraction of the abnormal Hb. Iatrogenic causes of dyshemoglobinemia in the PICU may result from inhaled nitric oxide therapy (methemoglobinemia) and nitroprusside infusions (cyanohemoglobinemia). If the dyshemoglobinemia is acute and potentially life-threatening (typically from a toxic exposure), treatment should involve removal of the offending cause and consideration of antidote treatment when appropriate. Exchange transfusion and hyperbaric oxygen therapy are considerations for acute and life-threatening causes of dyshemoglobinemia with clinically impaired O_2 delivery. Outcomes from hyperbaric therapy and other treatments for acquired dyshemoglobinemias have not been clearly delineated. Treatment for toxic gas exposures is reviewed in Chapter 31.

Medications and common environmental factors that cause dyshemoglobinemia in children are listed in **Table 101.6**. A normal individual has up to 1.5% methemoglobin (MetHb), and <1% of sulfhemoglobin (SulfHb), cyanohemoglobin (CyanoHb), and carboxyhemoglobin (COHb). MetHb and COHb are the most common acquired dyshemoglobinemias and are detectable on routine co-oximetry. Commonly encountered dyshemoglobinemias and current treatment options are listed in **Table 101.7**. Of these, MetHb has the greatest risk to result from therapeutics in the critical care environment. MetHb will cause chocolate-brown discoloration of blood, cyanosis, and functional "anemia" if present in high enough concentrations. Cyanosis becomes obvious at a concentration of MetHb of 1.5 g/dL (~10% of total Hb). The degree of cyanosis, however, does not necessarily correlate with the concentration of acquired MetHb. Normally, a small amount of MetHb is continuously being formed but is reduced by enzyme systems within the RBC. The most important is the NADH-dependent MetHb reductase system (NADH-cytochrome-b5 reductase). Infants are thought to be at a greater risk to the toxic effects of MetHb because they have lower MetHb-reductase levels and altered oxygen-Hb dissociation properties (44).

Whether acquired or congenital, MetHb concentrations of 10%–25% may give no apparent symptoms; levels of 35%–50% result in mild symptoms, such as exertional dyspnea and headaches; and levels exceeding 70% are probably lethal. Therapy with ascorbic acid or methylthioninium chloride (methylene blue) will reduce the level of oxidized Hb, the latter apparently by activation of the NADPH-MetHb reductase system. Heterozygotes for this enzyme have intermediate levels of NADH-cytochrome-b5 reductase activity and normal blood levels of MetHb. They may become cyanotic because of methemoglobinemia after exposure to oxidizing chemicals or drugs in amounts that will not affect normal individuals (61).

SulfHb is a mixture of oxidized and partially denatured Hb that forms during oxidative hemolysis (79). The normal Hb concentration of SulfHb in vivo is ≤1% and, in diseases, seldom exceeds 10%. During oxidation of Hb, sulfur (from some source, which may vary) is incorporated into heme rings, resulting in a green hemochrome. Continued oxidation can result in the denaturation and precipitation of Hb in the RBC (Heinz bodies). SulfHb cannot transport O_2, but it can combine with carbon monoxide (CO) to form carboxysulfhemoglobin (COSulfHb). Unlike MetHb, SulfHb cannot be reduced back to Hb, and it remains in the cells until they break down, typically

resulting in a mild, asymptomatic cyanosis; blood samples are typically mauve-lavender color. SulfHb has been reported in patients receiving treatment with sulfonamides or aromatic amine drugs (phenacetin, acetanilide), as well as in patients with severe constipation who develop bacteremia due to *Clostridium perfringens*, resulting in a condition called, "enterogenous cyanosis." The reason some patients develop methemoglobinemia, some sulfhemoglobinemia, and others form Heinz bodies and experience hemolysis is not well understood. SulfHb cannot be detected on routine co-oximetry, as it will be incorrectly measured as MetHb. SulfHb is best detected and quantitated by more complex techniques using differential Hb spectrophotometry or gas chromatography. Sulfhemoglobinemia should be suspected in cases of environmentally acquired cyanosis that fails to respond to conventional MetHb therapy.

CyanoHb forms when Hb combines with cyanide. Cyanide is present in many forms and can be inhaled, absorbed transcutaneously, or ingested. Most pathology in humans is related to toxic exposures from ingestions and inhalation. However, low levels of cyanide exposure are present from environmental and dietary sources. Toxic effects of cyanide arise because of the greater affinity of Hb for cyanide than for O_2, which leads to decreased O_2 delivery, and because of the inhibition of mitochondrial cytochrome oxidase, which leads to decreased cellular oxidative metabolism. In pediatric patients, CyanoHb formation and toxicity have been reported in children from holistic drugs (laetrile), ingestion of cyanogenic foods (fava beans, apricot pits), and administration of medications (nitroprusside infusions) (35). CyanoHb and O_2Hb are responsible for the "cherry red" appearance of mucous membranes in cyanide poisoning. Neither CyanoHb nor RBC cyanide levels have been found to correlate with the severity of cellular asphyxia in children; however, their abnormal elevation should raise suspicion, and an explanation should be sought. Other laboratory test results (high anion gap metabolic acidosis, elevated lactate, elevated venous O_2) can support the diagnosis of cyanide toxicity but do not provide specific evidence.

Toxicity related to nitroprusside infusions deserves special comment. Sodium nitroprusside contains an iron molecule bound to five cyanide molecules and one molecule of nitric oxide. The nitric oxide molecule is rapidly released during infusion from the iron moiety, creating significant arteriolar dilatation, whereas the cyanide molecules are liberated gradually. In most patients, cyanide release from sodium nitroprusside is slow enough that the body's innate detoxification mechanisms (thiosulfate to thiocyanate formation via the rhodanase enzyme) can eliminate the poison before it interferes with cellular respiration. However, critically ill children and those receiving very rapid infusions of sodium nitroprusside may not be able to eliminate the cyanide quickly enough to avert toxic effects. In rare cases, excessive light exposure of the nitroprusside leads to a premature and excessive release of cyanide. Normal nitroprusside infusions release ~44 mg of free cyanide per 100 mg nitroprusside infused.

Treatment for cyanide toxicity has classically involved inducing MetHb (with nitrites) to attract the cyanide ion from cytochrome oxidase, as MetHb has a high affinity for cyanide and readily combines to form CyanoMetHb, a safe but non-oxygen-carrying form of Hb. Because of reduced MetHb-reductase activity in children and concern about their susceptibility to thiocyanate toxicity, alternative strategies for the treatment of cyanide toxicity, such as hydroxycoalbumin and

TABLE 101.6

REPORTED CAUSES OF ACQUIRED DYSHEMOGLOBINEMIAS IN CHILDREN

	Met	Sulf	Cyano	CO
Drugs				
Acetanilide	+	+		
Aminophenol		+		
Alloxan	+			
Ammonium nitrate		+		
Amyl nitrite		+		
Aniline	+	+		
Arsine	+			
Arsenic			+	
Benzine derivative	+			
Benzocaine	+			
Bivalent copper	+			
Bismuth subnitrates	+	+		
Bupivacaine HCl	+			
Chlorates	+			
Chloroquine	+			
Chromates	+			
Clofazimine	+			
Dapsone	+	+		
Dimethylamine		+		
Dimethyl sulfoxide	+			
Dinitrobenzene		+		
Dinitrophenol	+			
Ethyl nitrite		+		
Ferricyanide	+			
Flutamide	+			
Hydroxylamine	+	+		
Lidocaine HCl	+			
Methylene Blue		+		
Metoclopramide with N-acetylcysteine		+		
Naphthalene	+	+		
Nitrates	+	+		
Nitric oxide	+			
Nitrofuran	+			
Nitroglycerin	+	+		
Sodium nitroprusside	+		+	
Paraquat	+			
Phenacetin	+	+		
Phenazopyridine HCl	+	+		
Phenol	+	+		
Phenytoin	+			
Prilocaine HCl	+			
Primaquine	+			
Rifampin	+			
Silver nitrate	+			
Sodium valproate	+			
Sulfasalazine	+			
Sulfonamides	+			
Trinitrotoluene	+	+		
Environmental Exposures				
Combustible Exhaust Fumes	+		+	+
House Fire	+	+	+	+
Foods and well water—almonds, sorghum, cassava (tapioca), beans, pits, bamboo shoots	+		+	
Soap enemas	+			
Laetrile enemas			+	

Met, methemoglobinemia; Sulf, sulfhemoglobinemia; Cyano, cyanohemoglobinemia; CO, carboxyhemoglobinemia

TABLE 101.7

TABLE 101.7

TREATMENT OF ACQUIRED DYSHEMOGLOBINEMIAS

Hb variant	Measurement	Treatment
MetHb	Routine co-oximetry	1) determine source 2) IV methylene blue 3) consider SulfHb if fails to resolve with treatment
SulfHb	Hb spectrophotometry Gas chromatography	1) determine source 2) irreversible 3) consider exchange transfusion if severe
CyanoHb	Hb spectrophotometry RBC cyanide level	1) determine source 2) IV sodium nitrate or inhaled amyl nitrate with IV thiosulfate 3) IV hydroxycoalbumin 4) IV dicobalt edetate 5) consider exchange transfusion if severe
COHb	Routine co-oximetry	1) determine source 2) provide F_{IO_2} 1.0 via non-rebreather/high-flow breathing mask 3) consider HBO_2 therapy, if severe 4) consider exchange transfusion if HBO_2 unavailable

MetHb, methemoglobin; SulfHb, sulfhemoglobin; Hb, hemoglobin; CyanoHb, cyanohemoglobin; RBC, red blood cell; COHb, carboxyhemoglobin; HBO_2, hyperbaric oxygen
HBO_2 and/or exchange transfusion may be useful treatments if severe impairment to O_2 delivery is present.
Note: Contacting local poison control authorities will help to identify local resources and latest treatment information.

dicobalt edentate, are being investigated (67). A more complete discussion of cyanide toxicity and treatment is reviewed in Chapter 31.

Endogenous CO produced in the degradation of heme to bilirubin normally accounts for about 0.5% COHb in the blood and is increased in hemolytic anemia. Hb has the capacity to combine with CO with an affinity 210 times greater than for O_2, which means that CO will bind with Hb even if its concentration in the air is extremely low (0.02%–0.04%). In those scenarios, COHb will build up until typical symptoms of CO poisoning appear (headache, dizziness, muscular weakness, and nausea). COHb cannot bind to O_2. Furthermore, increasing concentrations of COHb shift the Hb-oxygen dissociation curve increasingly to the left, thus adding to the anoxia. If a patient poisoned with CO receives pure O_2, the conversion of COHb to O_2Hb is greatly enhanced. COHb is light sensitive and has a typical "cherry red" color, and patients demonstrate high values on pulse oximetry. Healthy adults with limited exposure to CO do not experience symptoms unless the concentration of COHb reaches 20%–30%. However, the effects in children may result in severe symptoms at lower concentrations (31). COHb may be quantitated with most routine co-oximetry monitors.

Erythrocytosis

The term *polycythemia* is derived from the classical Greek, meaning "many cells in the blood" and is used synonymously with *erythrocytosis*. Apparent increases in red cell mass and Hb content (>2 SD of appropriate normal) treated in the PICU can occur from a variety of causes, such as dehydration, chronic hypoxia, and overtransfusion in surgical patients. Relative or "spurious" causes of erythrocytosis are the result of serum volume loss, such as in dehydration from diarrhea or aggressive diuretic therapy. These causes of polycythemia are often the consequence of an identifiable process. The absolute red cell mass and erythropoietin levels are within normal range, and Hb/hematocrit (Hct) will normalize rapidly following hydration therapy. However, the clinician should be vigilant for other less obvious etiologies and for the possible direct and indirect complications of elevated RBC mass, such as hyperviscosity, hypercoagulability, and thrombosis.

Polycythemia can be divided between primary and secondary causes based on the respective low or high levels of erythropoietin (**Table 101.8**). Primary causes such as *primary absolute erythrocytosis* and *polycythemia vera* are rare in children. Treatment for primary erythrocytosis varies depending on the underlying etiology. Sometimes phlebotomy in conjunction with suppressive therapies utilizing hydroxyurea and interferon-α, have been beneficial. If other cell lines are affected, additional antiplatelet therapy (e.g., aspirin) may be necessary to reduce thrombotic events. Though acute intervention is often phlebotomy, maintenance treatment and evaluation should be undertaken with a pediatric hematologist.

Secondary Absolute Erythrocytosis

Secondary absolute erythrocytosis is more common in the pediatric population but remains relatively rare in critically ill patients. Increase in erythropoietin production results in an

DIFFERENTIAL DIAGNOSIS OF ERYTHROCYTOSIS IN CHILDREN

Primary Erythrocytosis (Epo level normal or low)	
Congenital	Epo receptor mutations (primary familial congenital erythrocytosis)
Acquired	Polycythemia vera
Secondary Erythrocytosis (Epo level elevated)	
Congenital	Hemoglobinopathy with increased O_2 affinity
	2,3-DPG deficiency
	Chuvash polycythemia (rare VHL mutation)
	Sporadic or familial erythrocytosis secondary to VHL mutation
Acquired	Physiologic elevation of Epo secondary to:
	Right-to-left shunting cardiac lesion
	Pulmonary disease
	Renal disease
	Hepatic disease
	Abnormal elevation in Epo synthesis:
	Renal: malignancy
	Liver: malignancy
	CNS: hemangioblastoma
	Endocrine tumor: pheochromocytoma
	Uterine tumor

Epo, erythropoietin; VHL, von Hippel-Lindau disease; CNS, central nervous system

elevation of the RBC mass; elevation of other cell lines is rarely associated. This condition can be seen as an appropriate response to hypoxia, as in cyanotic congenital heart disease, chronic pulmonary disease, severe obstructive sleep apnea (Pickwickian syndrome), and hemoglobinopathies with increased O_2 affinity. However, inappropriate overproduction of erythropoietin is also a consideration. In evaluating these children, routine hemogram with red cell parameters, measurement of serum and urine erythropoietin levels, and arterial oxygen content (PaO_2) is indicated (**Table 101.9**). If the tests are normal, other causes, such as renal abnormalities or tumors,

SEQUENTIAL EVALUATION OF ERYTHROCYTOSIS

1. CBC, including differential WBC count
2. Rule out plasma volume decrease
3. Diagnose *Secondary Erythrocytosis*:
   Arterial oxygen saturation (rule out hypoxia)
   Co-oximetry (rule out dyshemoglobinemias)
   Renal ultrasonography
   Abdominal/cranial CT
   Erythropoietin level (if elevated suggests secondary etiology)
4. Special studies for *Primary Erythrocytosis*:
   (See **Table 101.8** for diagnostic evaluation for *polycythemia vera*)
   Leukocyte alkaline phosphatase
   Serum vitamin B_{12} level and binding capacity
   Red blood cell colony formation

CBC, complete blood count; WBC, white blood cell

should be sought. Treatment often involves management of the underlying cause, e.g., increased ventilatory support, oxygen supplementation, and surgical repair of congenital heart lesions. However, in the setting of uncorrectable causes of erythrocytosis, chronic phlebotomy to keep Hct <60% has been used to prevent hyperviscosity and microcirculatory congestion. Unfortunately, experimental data in support of this practice are limited.

Neonatal Polycythemia and Hyperviscosity

Approximately 1%–5% of all newborns in the US are polycythemic. As the venous Hct rises above 65%, the thickness or viscosity of whole blood also increases, potentially compromising blood flow to a variety of organs. Fortunately, relatively few infants who have neonatal polycythemia or hyperviscosity develop complications attributable to their thick blood. Infants who have polycythemia often show increased whole-blood viscosity. Hyperviscosity refers to an increase in the internal friction of blood or the force required to achieve flow. The viscosity of whole blood is affected by numerous factors, including the red cell mass, the plasma components, and the interaction of cellular elements with the vessel wall. When the Hct is between 65% and 70%, an increased tendency for diminished blood flow may occur, especially in the cerebral, hepatic, renal, and mesenteric microcirculations. Clinical symptoms may include lethargy, cyanosis, respiratory distress, jitteriness, hypotonia, feeding intolerance, hypoglycemia, and hyperbilirubinemia.

Treatment of neonatal polycythemia and hyperviscosity remains controversial. The debate lies in whether this care should involve symptomatic therapy or routine partial exchange transfusion (PET) to replace the infant's blood with a plasma substitute. Although PET is recommended for symptomatic infants, outcome data do not show clear long-term benefits. Undoubtedly, infants who have clinical manifestations should receive care aimed at alleviating their symptoms. In the polycythemic newborn, the total exchange volume for PET is generally calculated using the following formula:

$$PET\ volume = Circulating\ blood\ volume \times [(Hct\ current - Hct\ desired)/Hct\ current]$$

In this equation, the circulating blood volume refers to the infant's weight in kilograms multiplied by the expected intravascular volume in milliliter per kilogram of body weight. In term infants, it is usually estimated at 80–90 mL/kg; in preterm infants, intravascular volume is usually estimated at 100 mL/kg. In clinical practice, the exchange procedure is performed through removal and administration of 5–10 mL aliquots, depending on the infant's weight and response to treatment. Typically, arterial and venous line access is required. Careful planning is important and can reduce the number of complications and adverse reactions. Attention to thermoregulation, glucose homeostasis, and vital signs is imperative. Resuscitation equipment, medications, and IV dextrose should be readily available. Both during and up to 4 hrs following PET, feedings should be withheld. In addition, monitoring should be continued until the infant is asymptomatic. Typical Hct goals from PET are <55%.

Reported complications from PET include vessel perforation, vasospasm, thrombosis, infarction, electrolyte abnormalities, arrhythmias, bleeding, infection, hypothermia and hyperthermia, and necrotizing enterocolitis. Moreover, the replacement fluid selected may impact the procedure's risk. For instance, the use of fresh frozen plasma is associated with increased risk of viral and bacterial infections, anaphylactic reactions, metabolic acidosis, and hypocalcemia.

WHITE BLOOD CELL ABNORMALITIES (NONMALIGNANT) IN INFANTS AND CHILDREN

Leukopenia

Leukopenia is defined as a total white blood cell (WBC) count <4000/mm^3. However, in children a WBC count 2 SDs below an age-appropriate mean is often used (**Table 101.2**). Evaluation of patients with leukopenia requires a careful history, physical examination, and review of the CBC count with differential. Often, critically ill children will have significant abnormalities in the WBC differential count that will reflect lymphopenia and/or neutropenia. The discussion here will focus on common etiologies of lymphopenia, neutropenia, and hemophagocytic lymphohistiocytosis (HLH).

Lymphopenia

Lymphopenia is characterized by a decline in total lymphocytes below the lower range of normal (1000/mm^3 in adults and 4500/ mm^3 in infants). Lymphopenia usually has no specific symptoms and is often found in the context of evaluating another illness. Most often, it results transiently from viral, fungal, or parasitic infections. However, it can result from chronic illness or reflect more serious inherited or acquired disease. Clinicians should be cognizant that human immunodeficiency virus (HIV), with or without AIDS, is the most common globally relevant infectious disease associated with lymphopenia (**Table 101.10**). The majority of children with isolated lymphopenia typically have spontaneous recovery and require only careful observation and follow-up while their primary disease process undergoes treatment. If the condition persists, multiple cell lines are deficient, or common transiently acquired etiologies are not found, flow cytology and CD4 and CD8 T-lymphocyte quantification are warranted.

Neutropenia

Neutropenia is defined as a decreased number of circulating neutrophils in the peripheral blood. An absolute neutrophil count <1500/mm^3 is defined as neutropenia. The lower limit for African American patients can be 200–600/mm^3 less than the figure cited for Caucasians. Increased risk for a life-threatening infection occurs when the absolute neutrophil count is <500/mm^3. This susceptibility varies from patient to patient, depending on the clinical state. Patients with an underlying malignancy and neutropenia tend to have more infections than do those patients with congenital defects in neutrophil production. Children with fever and neutropenia require

TABLE 101.10

DIFFERENTIAL DIAGNOSIS OF LYMPHOPENIA IN CHILDREN

Infections	Mycobacteria	*Mycobacterium tuberculosis*
		Atypical mycobacteria
	Viral	Cytomegalovirus
		Epstein-Barr virus
		Hepatitis B virus
		Human immunodeficiency virus
		Human T-cell lymphotropic virus 1 and 2
		Influenza
		Respiratory syncytial virus
Malignancy		Non-Hodgkin lymphoma
		Mycosis fungoides
		Aplastic anemia
		Myelodysplastic syndrome
Autoimmune diseases		Sjögren syndrome
		Systemic lupus erythematosus
		Rheumatoid arthritis
Drugs		Corticosteroids
		Chemotherapy and cytotoxic immunosuppressants (cyclophosphamide, azathioprine, methotrexate)
		Others (cephalosporin, IFN-α)
Primary immunodeficiency		Common variable immunodeficiency
		Severe combined immunodeficiency
		Bare lymphocyte syndrome, type I
Miscellaneous conditions		Severe burns
		Radiation therapy
		Malnutrition

TABLE 101.11

DIFFERENTIAL DIAGNOSIS OF NEUTROPENIA

Congenital Neutropenic Disorders
Kostmann's agranulocytosis-severe congenital neutropenia
Reticular dysgenesis (absence of thymus, lymphocytes, and neutrophils)
Cyclic neutropenia (autosomal dominant)
Shwachman syndrome (neutropenia, pancreatic insufficiency, growth failure, and skeletal anomalies)
Neutropenia with abnormal B or T lymphocytes (e.g., X-linked agammaglobulinemia)

Transient Neonatal Neutropenia
Prematurity/sepsis/asphyxia
Pregnancy-induced maternal hypertension
Periventricular hemorrhage
Congenital cytomegalovirus infection
Maternal antineutrophil antibodies (alloimmune-isoimmune neutropenia)

Immune-mediated Destruction
Autoimmune neutropenia

Postinfectious
Influenza A, Hepatitis A and B, varicella, respiratory syncytial virus, Epstein-Barr Virus, cytomegalovirus (counts recover spontaneously over several days)

Drug-induced
Chemotherapy, anticonvulsants, cimetidine, ranitidine, phenothiazines, semisynthetic penicillins, cephalosporins, NSAIDs

Acquired/Decreased Production
Aplastic anemia
Marrow infiltration (malignant cells, inborn metabolic errors)

Sequestration
Splenomegaly

prompt evaluation and institution of appropriate antibiotic therapy. A careful physical examination is needed, with special attention to those areas most susceptible to bacterial infection in the neutropenic patients (oral mucosa, skin, ears, lungs, and perianal area). Digital rectal examination and rectal temperatures should never be done in a patient with neutropenia to avoid bloodstream seeding of gram-negative organisms, although visual inspection of the anus and gentle examination of the area is acceptable. In addition, phenotypic abnormalities (i.e., cartilage-hair hypoplasia syndrome) associated with neutropenia should be noted (**Table 101.11**). A brief review of nonmalignant neutropenia in children and the treatment strategies for them is summarized below.

General Management of Nonmalignant Neutropenia

Regardless of etiology, children with neutropenia are at increased risk for infectious complications because of their weakened host defense system. The type and pattern of infection vary according to the degree of immune suppression and potential cause of the neutropenia (discussed later). Most infections result from organisms that are part of the normal flora of healthy patients (gram-negative bacteria, *Candida albicans*, varicella, and *Pneumocystis*). When the host immune system is weak-

ened, these organisms proliferate and produce life-threatening infections. Other exogenously acquired infective agents are *Pseudomonas* or *Aspergillus* species.

Most infections in immunocompromised children result from bacterial pathogens. *Escherichia coli*, *Pseudomonas*, and *Klebsiella* species represent the most common gram-negative organisms that produce infections in immunocompromised children, whereas coagulase-negative staphylococci represent the predominant gram-positive organisms that cause infection, especially in patients who have central venous catheters (CVCs). Anaerobic infections are uncommon. *Candida* and *Aspergillus* species compose most fungal infections. The most common viral pathogens include herpes simplex, varicella zoster, cytomegalovirus (CMV), Epstein-Barr virus (EBV), and adenovirus. *Pneumocystis* and *Toxoplasma* represent the major protozoan infections in this group of patients.

The standard approach for managing a neutropenic patient who develops fever with no discernible focus of infection has been combination therapy to cover gram-positive and gram-negative bacteria. Ceftazidime and vancomycin are often used as initial therapy (especially in patients with a CVC). Other centers choose to use an aminoglycoside in combination with a β-lactam antibiotic. Children with pneumonia or perirectal infections sometimes require antibiotics designed to cover pathogens such as *Pneumocystis* and *Clostridium*. Each hospital can have a specific profile of documented infections and antibiotic susceptibility that must be considered in selecting appropriate therapy in these settings. Culturing strategies are also controversial. We advocate culturing from all central-line ports, as well as percutaneously ("peripheral blood culture"). Additional tests include a CBC with differential, urine analysis with Gram stain and culture, and chest x-ray. Consultation with a pediatric hematologist, pediatric infectious disease specialist, and/or pediatric immunology specialist is also useful to direct further diagnostic evaluation (bone marrow biopsy, peripheral blood smear evaluation, additional WBC studies) and customize antibiotic coverage, especially if the neutropenia and fevers become persistent (>3 days).

Catheter-related infections are a significant problem in this population. Although coagulase-negative staphylococcal infections are most prevalent, other organisms can be responsible (gram-negative organisms, fungi, *Bacteroides* species, and *Corynebacterium*). Most simple catheter infections can be cleared with antibiotics without catheter removal. Tunnel-site infections (infections where the catheter enters the skin) represent a more difficult problem. Despite appropriate antibiotics, many catheters must be removed to clear the infection.

In a neutropenic patient without evidence of fever or focus of infection, prophylactic antibiotic treatment and surveillance cultures have not proven to be beneficial in preventing or detecting infectious disease. However, treatment to stimulate neutrophil recovery should be considered. Recombinant human granulocyte colony-stimulating factor (rhGCSF or GCSF) stimulates the production of neutrophils from committed progenitor cells in the marrow. The dose is 5–10 mcg/kg (maximum dose = 480 mcg) administered subcutaneously, with an improvement in 10–14 days to an absolute neutrophil count above 1500/mm^3. This medication is routinely started following chemotherapy-related neutropenia (see Chapter 100). However, the long-term effects of GCSF treatment on children with episodic and recurrent, nonmalignant neutropenia remain controversial.

Autoimmune Neutropenia

Autoimmune neutropenia is caused by the production of antibodies against neutrophil antigens. The physical examination and laboratory findings are normal, except for isolated neutropenia. The bone marrow shows a normal myeloid proliferation and maturation. This entity is usually self-limited, with return of a normal neutrophil count over a 5–7-week period. Appropriate antibiotics and rhGCSF should be given to febrile, neutropenic patients, as noted previously. Aggressive treatment of asymptomatic patients remains controversial. With clear fever or infection, the duration of treatment depends on the site and nature of the infection. Alternative treatments with corticosteroids (prednisone, 1–2 mg/kg/day for 1 week) and IV immunoglobulin (IVIG) (a single dose of 1 g/kg over 3 hrs) have been shown to hasten recovery of the absolute neutrophil count; however, the decision to use these therapeutic modalities should be individualized and made in consultation with a pediatric hematologist.

Congenital Cyclical Neutropenia

Congenital cyclical neutropenia is characterized by chronic periodic oscillations in the neutrophil count from normal to profound neutropenia. The disease is caused by a defect in stem cell development, more pronounced in the late myeloid precursors. The duration of each cycle is usually 21 days (range, 14–36 days). The nadir of neutrophil counts ranges from low normal to zero and usually lasts 3–10 days. The most common manifestations of this entity are oral ulcers, stomatitis, pharyngitis, tonsillitis, lymphadenitis, cellulitis, otitis media, and sinusitis. All infectious episodes should be treated promptly with appropriate antibiotics and rhGCSF (5 mcg/kg daily subcutaneous injections until WBC count is $\geq$10,000/mm^3).

Hemophagocytic Lymphohistiocytosis (HLH)

HLH is a multisystem disease process that results from hyperinflammation from the phagocytosis of blood cells and their precursors. The initiating events and exact disease mechanisms behind this life-threatening disease process are unknown, but HLH (and closely related "hemophagocytic syndromes") have been associated with infectious, genetic, autoimmune, and neoplastic disorders. The reported incidence of HLH is 1.2 cases per million per year. There are case reports of HLH or hemophagocytic syndromes in all age groups, though the familial and sporadic cases are reported primarily in children. It is unclear whether this syndrome is associated with a seasonal variability that favors summer.

Clinical features of HLH are very general and can be present in many critically ill children. Diagnostic guidelines were established to help to direct the study and treatment of this often lifethreatening condition. Common clinical features that should prompt consideration of HLH in a child include fever (60%–100%), hepatosplenomegaly (65%–100%), and cytopenia, involving two or more cell lines (100%). Other physical exam findings associated with HLH are rash, lymphadenopathy, and jaundice. Biochemical abnormalities occur from the consumption of the various blood cell lines with resulting hypertriglyceridemia, hypertransferrinemia, and hypofibrinogenemia (**Table 101.12**). Other findings that are supportive of the diagnosis but not part of current diagnostic criteria are CSF pleocytosis and/or elevated protein, elevated serum transaminases, elevated bilirubin, and elevated LDH ($\geq$1000 U/L) (45).

TABLE 101.12

DIAGNOSTIC GUIDELINES FOR HEMOPHAGOCYTIC LYMPHOHISTIOCYTOSIS

The diagnosis of HLH requires either criteria 1 or 2 to be present:
1. A molecular diagnosis consistent with HLH (e.g., *PRF* gene mutations, *SAP* gene mutations, etc.)

OR

2. Having 5 out of 8 of the following findings:
   a. Fever
   b. Splenomegaly
   c. Cytopenia ($\geq$2 cell lines)
   d. Hypertriglyceridemia ($\geq$265 mg/dL) and/or Hypofibrinogenemia ($\leq$150 mg/dL)
   e. Hyperferritinemia ($\geq$500 ng/mL)
   f. Hemophagocytosis in the bone marrow, lymph node, spleen, or CSF
   g. Low or absent NK cell cytotoxicity
   h. Elevated soluble CD25 ($\geq$2400 U/mL)

HLH, hemophagocytic lymphohistiocytosis; CSF, cerebrospinal fluid; NK, natural killer
Adapted from Treatment Protocol of the 2nd International HLH Study, 2004.

Originally treated by clinicians as a diagnosis of exclusion, the coexistence of HLH with other disease processes necessitates its prompt recognition and treatment. Bone marrow aspiration and lumbar puncture are recommended early in the evaluation. The bone marrow aspirate is often required to differentiate this process from a neoplastic process (though it is an insensitive test for HLH). Many times, bone marrow aspirates will be negative for evidence of hemophagocytosis and will only demonstrate nonspecific findings. Lumbar puncture is often performed in those patients with altered mental status, though increased cellularity is a commonly reported finding in both neurologically symptomatic and asymptomatic patients. Two highly diagnostic tests with limited availability are elevated serum test for the soluble subunit of the IL-2 receptor (sCD 25) and decreased activity of natural killer cells. Genetic evaluation for susceptible gene mutations in the perforin gene and SLAM-associated protein is essential to recognize familial forms of HLH. Because of the evolution of HLH is often multifactorial and many cases originally thought to be secondary in etiology have later demonstrated primary defects in perforin/granulocyte pathways, early genetic evaluation and follow-up are indicated. Further, individuals with identifiable gene defects may benefit from bone marrow transplant, stem cell therapy and direct anticytokine treatments. Consultation with a pediatric hematologist and/or oncologist is often required to effectively complete the evaluation and determine the best treatment regimen.

Prognosis and Therapy

During the late 1980s, prior to the development of aggressive chemotherapeutic and immunosuppressive regimens, 1-year survival following diagnosis of HLH was ~5%. Today, with early recognition and treatment of children with HLH, survival and recovery rates have improved to 60%–70%. Unfortunately, HLH associated with EBV continues to have a high incidence of mortality (50%–60%), thought to result from the high rate of complications, such as hemorrhage, multisystem organ failure, and secondary bacterial infections. In genetic (or familial) HLH, stem cell transplant can be curative. This therapeutic option is guided by the severity of symptoms and other factors.

The Histiocyte Society (www.histio.org) helped to establish the current diagnostic guidelines and treatment protocol for HLH (HLH-2004), which includes dexamethasone, etoposide, cyclosporine A, and intrathecal methotrexate (in select cases). Hyperinflammation is treated with immunosuppression. The goal is to inhibit cytokine release via steroid suppression with dexamethasone. Cyclosporine A prevents T-cell activation and immunoglobulin infusions are thought to provide additional anticytokine activity and pathogen-specific antibodies. Etoposide may have significant benefit in EBV-associated HLH (46).

Leukocytosis

Abnormally high (>2 SDs) circulating levels of age-appropriate WBCs counts are regarded as "leukocytosis." Leukocytosis results from either the increased release of cellular elements from the storage pool or alterations in the rate at which these cells are removed from the blood. Various causes of leukocytosis are characterized by the class/subtype of WBC that is increased and whether the elevation is chronic, acute, or persistent (sustained or life-long). Primary leukocytosis is an extremely rare event and is often hereditary. Secondary leukocytosis may occur from stress, infections, inflammation, endocrinopathies, drugs, and toxins. As a group, these disorders are most often caused by malignancy. However, nonmalignant etiologies frequently occur in critically ill children. WBC counts >50,000/mm^3 are classified as *leukemoid reactions* because of the similarity of features to leukemia.

Leukocytosis after exercise, seizures, and pain results from demargination of mature granulocytes from the pulmonary circulation. Toxicity from drugs (iron, theophylline, cocaine) and envenomation (black widow spider, cobra) causes a sympathetic stress that elevates the WBC count by similar mechanisms. Regardless of the etiology, the resulting leukocyte elevation is the result of multiple factors, including decreased neutrophil adhesiveness, shearing from altered blood flow, and stimulation of β-adrenergic receptors located on the lymphocytes and granulocytes.

WBC subtypes from the CBC can be useful in creating a differential diagnosis and suggesting an underlying cause for the leukocytosis. Stress-induced demargination in the setting of trauma, burns, surgery, hemolysis, and hemorrhage will typically result in an elevation of multiple WBC subtypes (neutrophils, monocytes, lymphocytes). However, acute leukocytosis with a neutrophil predominance is highly suggestive of a serious bacterial infection, while elevation in WBC with a majority of eosinophils is suggestive of an allergic reaction or parasitic infection. The following discussion will focus on specific WBC subtype elevations associated with common disease processes in critically ill children.

Neutrophilia

Neutrophilia is an elevation in the age-appropriate amount of neutrophils in the serum. In adults and older children, neutrophil counts >8000/mm^3 are usually significant for neutrophilia (**Table 101.2**). A transient increase in the number of circulating neutrophils can result acutely from inflammation,

stress, infection, or injury. Common intensive care medications found to induce neutrophilia are epinephrine, corticosteroids, and rhGCSF. Chronic inflammatory diseases (autoimmune, tuberculosis, sarcoidosis, etc.), and chronic drug exposure (corticosteroids) can result in a more chronic neutrophilia. However, both the acquired and chronic forms will return to normal with treatment of the disease or removal of the stimulating agent. Persistent or life-long neutrophilia represents a rare cause of elevated neutrophils in the serum. Evaluation of persistent neutrophilia requires a careful history, physical exam, and thorough diagnostic evaluation to exclude infectious, inflammatory, and malignant conditions. Potential nonmalignant causes of persistent neutrophilia include congenital asplenia, familial myeloproliferative disease, and genetic disorders of leukocyte adhesion.

Eosinophilia

Eosinophilia has been related to a number of acute and chronic disease processes in adults and children and is arbitrarily classified as mild (351–1500/mm^3), moderate (>1500–5000/mm^3), or severe (>5000/mm^3). The most common cause of eosinophilia worldwide is helminthic infections, and the most common cause in industrialized nations is atopic disease. Eosinophilia occurs as a result of one or more of the following processes: differentiation of progenitor cells and proliferation of eosinophils in bone marrow, chemoattraction and endothelial interactions directing eosinophils to a specific location, and increased activation and/or decreased destruction of eosinophils (71).

Eosinophilic disorders can be clinically divided into reactive, disease associated, clonal, or idiopathic (**Table 101.13**). Common reactive causes of eosinophilia are life-threatening allergic reactions (anaphylaxis and status asthmaticus), parasitic infections (acute and chronic infections such as helminths and other parasites), and drug reactions. Diagnosis of reactive eosinophilia is typically made by history (drug exposure, foreign travel, allergic symptoms) and/or physical findings (urticarial rash, worms in stool). Tests should be disease- and history-focused (with drug exposure and sudden onset of symptoms, serum should be sent for mast cell tryptase testing; if history of travel is involved, stool should be sent for ova and parasite, blood for bacterial culture, etc.). Reactive eosinophilia is often acute and limited to the course of the accompanying disease. Secondary or disease-associated eosinophilia occurs in gastroenteritis/esophagitis, autoimmune (connective tissue diseases), paraneoplastic (Hodgkin lymphoma), immunologic (hyper-IgA syndrome), vasculitis (Churg-Strauss syndrome, Wegener granulomatosis), pulmonary (Loeffler syndrome, cystic fibrosis), and endocrine (adrenal insufficiency) disorders. These associated disorders may result in acute and chronic eosinophilia and must be monitored for possible malignancy. Clonal disease is either malignant or myeloproliferative (premalignant). Clonal eosinophilia is diagnosed by the presence of cytogenetic abnormalities. Treatment for clonal eosinophilia will involve gene-specific chemotherapeutics and, potentially, bone marrow transplant. *Idiopathic hypereosinophilia syndrome* is a diagnosis of exclusion. It has been described in critically ill adults and children and is a rare but life-threatening cause of eosinophilia. This disorder results from abnormal immunologic signaling and occurs predominantly in adult males (peak incidence between 20 and 50 years of age) and is usually a progressive, fatal disease in the absence of effective

TABLE 101.13

CAUSES OF EOSINOPHILIA

Differential diagnosis	Examples
Reactive Eosinophilia	
Allergic	Rhinoconjunctivitis, asthma, eczema
Infection	Bacterial and fungal
Parasitic infection	Helminth
Drug reaction (iatrogenic)	Granulocyte colony-stimulating factor
Secondary (Disease-associated) Eosinophilia	
Autoimmune disorders	Rheumatoid arthritis, eosinophilic fasciitis
Vasculitis	Polyarteritis nodosa, Wegner granulomatosis
Gastrointestinal disorders	Inflammatory bowel disease, eosinophilic
	Gastroenteritis, eosinophilic esophagitis, allergic colitis
Pulmonary disorders	Churg-Strauss syndrome, Loeffler syndrome
Endocrine disorders	Adrenal insufficiency (Addison Disease)
Clonal Eosinophilia	
Cytogenetic	FIP1L1-PDGFRA fusion gene positive
Leukemia	Acute and chronic eosinophilic leukemia
Mastocytosis	Systemic mastocytosis with eosinophilia, Myeloproliferative disorder
Idiopathic Persistent Eosinophilia (Diagnosis of Exclusion)	
Idiopathic	Idiopathic hypereosinophilia syndrome

medical management. Bone marrow biopsy and consultation with a pediatric hematologist and/or immunologist is necessary to evaluate all cases of nonreactive or persistent eosinophilia. In cases of secondary or disease-associated eosinophilia, specific tissue diagnosis may be required (lung, renal, or myocardial biopsy) and should be performed in conjunction with a multispecialty evaluation.

In the cases of reactive or secondary eosinophilia (which represent the majority of eosinophilia cases in children), these episodes resolve spontaneously or with treatment of the underlying condition. In other scenarios when a diagnosis cannot be found, clonal causes have been excluded, and eosinophilia persists, treatment remains controversial. Some authors advocate a brief course of antiparasitic treatment, especially when persistent eosinophilia occurs in a patient who either lives or has traveled to an endemic area for parasitic infection. Others advocate a short trial of steroids (prednisone 1 mg/kg body weight per day for 3–5 days). This approach is advocated to help define the persistent eosinophilia as steroid-responsive or -resistant. In this approach, steroid-resistant cases may be candidates for additional drug therapy (anti-IL-5 agent, mepolizumab). Regardless, patients with persistent eosinophilia should have periodic clinical evaluations, including pulmonary, cardiac (echocardiographic), and ophthalmologic examinations to detect eosinophil-mediated tissue damage. Clinicians should be aware that insidious end-organ damage can occur at any time and may not correlate with the severity of persistent eosinophilia (81).

Lymphocytosis

As lymphocytes compose 20%–40% of the circulating WBC count, lymphocytosis is typically associated with leukocytosis. Leukemia and lymphoma are the most common cause in children. However, the most common, isolated, nonmalignant elevation is related to an acute transient increase of circulating T cells (lymphocytes) brought on by a viral infection. Many viral infections, such as EBV, CMV, and viral hepatitis, have lymphocytosis as a feature. Bacterial infections (tuberculosis, brucellosis, histoplasmosis) can result in chronic or sustained lymphocytosis. Notably, pertussis infections result in lymphocytosis in up to 25% of infants <6 months of age. Endocrinologic abnormalities such as hyperthyroidism and adrenal insufficiency have been associated with lymphocytosis in critically ill adults and children. Often, lymphocytosis represents a diagnostic clue to the underlying source of a patient's illness, and more persistent and chronic forms deserve a careful evaluation for myeloproliferative disorders and malignancy.

Monocytosis. Monocytosis, the rarest form of leukocytosis, must be evaluated within the age-specific variation of this WBC-count subpopulation. Monocytes play a crucial role in antigen presentation and cytokine signaling. Monocytosis is most often described in children recovering from myelosuppressive chemotherapy and can precede recovery from neutropenia. However, bacterial infections and parasitic infections have been described with associated monocytosis. In addition, chronic neutropenia and post-splenectomy patients can have sustained monocytosis.

PLATELET ABNORMALITIES IN INFANTS AND CHILDREN

Thrombocytosis

Thrombocytosis in children, as in adults, is defined by an elevated platelet count. The definition of normal platelet counts in the range of 150,000–350,000/mm^3 is generally accepted for healthy neonates, infants, children, and adolescents. However, the definition of thrombocytosis varies between platelet counts of 400,000–1,000,000/mm^3 (80). To consider the characteristics and clinical implications of thrombocytosis and to compare published data, the following arbitrary classifications are often used: mild thrombocytosis, if the platelet count is 500,000–700,000/mm^3; moderate thrombocytosis, if the platelet count is between 700,000 and 900,000/mm^3; severe thrombocytosis, if the platelet count is >900,000/mm^3–1,000,000/mm^3; and extreme thrombocytosis, if the platelet count is >1,000,000/mm^3 (80).

Essential (or Primary) Thrombocytosis

Essential (or primary) thrombocytosis is extremely rare in children. This disorder is a form of myeloproliferative disease resulting from either monoclonal/polyclonal expansion of megakaryocytes or abnormalities in thrombopoietin. Acquired and familial forms of essential thrombocytosis have been reported, with much of the genetic and chronic determination made in adult patients. Typical features of essential thrombocytosis are outlined in **Table 101.14**.

TABLE 101.14

ESSENTIAL AND REACTIVE THROMBOCYTOSIS IN CHILDREN

Criteria	Essential thrombocytosis	Reactive thrombocytosis
Age-dependent occurrence	>11 years* or adult	Mostly <2 years*
Incidence per year	1 per 1 million children	>600 per 1 million children
Duration of thrombocytosis	Months, years, or permanent	Days, weeks, or months, temporary
Splenomegaly	Often	Rare
Fever	No	Often
Bleeding disorders and thrombosis	Often in monoclonal ET, rare in familiar thrombocythemia	Extremely rare
Frequent laboratory findings	Prolonged bleeding time, increased PT and PTT in 20%; increased prevalence of anti-phospholipid antibodies and proinflammatory cytokines	Increased vWF, fibrinogen, C-reactive protein if RT is caused by infection
Platelet count	Mostly >1,000,000/mm^3	Typically <800,000/mm^3
Platelet morphology	Large or small, dysmorphic	Large, but normal morphology
Platelet function	Abnormal	Normal
Bone marrow	Increased megakaryocyte number with abnormal morphology	Increased megakaryocyte number with normal morphology
Pathogenic mechanisms	Clonal defect in hematopoietic or megakaryopoietic progenitors, decreased c-mpl expression, and/or hyper-reactivity to Tpo. In some familial forms: mutations in the Tpo or c-mpl gene locus	Increased Tpo production or released megakaryopoietic growth factors, in particular IL-6

Tpo, thrombopoietin; vWF, von Willebrand factor; PT, partial prothrombin time; PTT, partial thromboplastin time
*This number is relevant only for differentiating primary thrombocytosis in childhood. Adapted from Dror Y, Blanchette VS. Essential thrombocythaemia in children. *Br J Haematol* 1999;107(4):691–8.

Reactive (or Secondary) Thrombocytosis

Reactive (or secondary) thrombocytosis (RT) causes are the most common. Current reports suggest an estimated incidence of RT in 6%–15% of hospitalized children. Biochemical profiles typically demonstrate an elevation in thrombopoietin and IL-6 (a pro-megakaryocyte growth factor). Most children with RT have viral or bacterial respiratory illness (**Table 101.14**). However, RT has been reported following gastroenteritis, urinary tract infection, autoimmune disorders, surgery, trauma, and several pharmacologic interventions. Pharmacotherapy that creates or contributes to RT in children includes epinephrine, corticosteroids, vinca-alkaloids, penicillamine, imipenem, and meropenem. Complications are rare, but risk factors for thromboembolic disease in children are young age (neonate/infant), CVC, cardiac malformations, and septicemia (32). Treatment should focus on diagnosis and management of the underlying disease process. Prophylactic treatment with antiplatelet drugs (e.g., aspirin) has not proven beneficial in preventing thromboembolic complications in asymptomatic children with RT. In those children who become symptomatic or have evidence of thrombosis, consultation with a hematologist and consideration for patient-specific platelet inhibition and/or reduction therapy may be considered, but these therapies have not been proven to be beneficial.

Thrombocytopenia

For most critically ill children, relatively low platelet counts are usually well tolerated. Patients will not typically develop bleeding symptoms until platelet counts are <50,000/mm^3. Spontaneous bleeding rarely occurs until the platelet count is <10,000/mm^3. Further, laboratory studies of hemostasis have demonstrated that platelet counts of ~7000/mm^3 are necessary for microvascular integrity. However, with comorbid medical illness, trauma, or surgery, maintaining higher platelet counts is often clinically indicated to reduce bleeding risk and assist in promoting patient stability. We typically transfuse platelets to maintain platelet counts at >50,000/mm^3 in the presence of an associated risk of bleeding. In surgical patients, especially with post-bypass bleeding, we will attempt to keep the count >100,000/mm^3. Medical history of children with low platelet counts should include family history and past medical history of bleeding/bruising problems. Common clinical symptoms associated with thrombocytopenia are petechiae (periarticular and mucosal), excessive bruising, epistaxis, menorrhagia, and gastrointestinal hemorrhage. Pseudothrombocytopenia can result from platelet clumping in EDTA anticoagulation tubes. Repeating the test in a citrate collection tube and/or reviewing the smear for evidence of platelet clumping should clarify if

TABLE 101.15

PREVALENT INHERITED THROMBOCYTOPENIAS

Syndrome	Inheritance	Gene mutation (chromosome)	Associated findings
Bernard-Soulier syndrome	AR	*GP1BA, GP1BB* (17pter-p12)	none
TAR syndrome	AR	unknown	shortened or absent radii, bilaterally
DiGeorge syndrome/ Velocardiofacial Association/ CATCH 22	AD	*GP1BB* (22q11)	cardiac, facial, and parathyroid anomalies and immune dysfunction
Paris-Trousseau syndrome/ Jacobsen syndrome	AD	*FLI1* (11q23)	mental retardation, cardiac and facial anomalies
May-Hegglin anomaly	AD	*MYH9* (22q11)	neutrophil inclusions (Döhle bodies), nephritis, cataracts, and sensorineural hearing loss
Familial platelet disorder	AD	*AML1* (21q22.2)	myelodysplasia, AML
Grey platelet syndrome	AD	unknown	none
Wiskott-Aldrich syndrome	X-linked	*WAS* (Xp11.23)	immunodeficiency, eczema, lymphoma

Differentiation based on platelet features

Small Platelets (MPV <7 fL)	Normal Platelets (MPV 7–11 fL)	Large/giant platelets (MPV >11 fL)
Wiskott-Aldrich syndrome	Familial platelet disorder	Bernard-Soulier syndrome
X-linked thrombocytopenia	Congenital amegakaryocytic thrombocytopenia	DiGeorge syndrome
	TAR syndrome	Grey platelet syndrome
		GATA 1 mutation
		Paris-Trousseau thrombocytopenia

AR, autosomal recessive; AD, autosomal dominant; TAR, thrombocytopenia and absent radii; AML, acute myeloid leukemia; MPV, mean platelet volume

Adapted from Drachman JG. Inherited thrombocytopenia: When a low platelet count does not mean ITP. *Blood* 2004;103(2):390–8.

artificial thrombocytopenia is the cause. True thrombocytopenia can be characterized by inherited or acquired causes of thrombocytopenia. Primary (or inherited) thrombocytopenia (**Table 101.15**) is often associated with genetic disorders and results in abnormal platelet number and function. These disorders are significantly less common than acquired platelet disorders in children.

Secondary (or Acquired) Thrombocytopenia

Secondary (or acquired) thrombocytopenia is the most common cause diagnosed in the PICU population. These low platelet counts are typically acute in onset and are best described by their underlying mechanism: (a) impaired production, (b) increased destruction, (c) dilution, or (d) sequestration. The differential diagnosis of acquired thrombocytopenia is summarized in **Figure 101.3**, and the most common entities are discussed below. Disseminated intravascular coagulopathy is discussed in detail in Chapter 103.

Medication (Iatrogenic) Thrombocytopenia

Medication (iatrogenic) thrombocytopenia represents impairment in platelet production. Drug-induced thrombocytopenia occurs most often in adults and children who have a routine illness (viral or bacterial) and are undergoing treatment. Often, the occurrence of the decreased platelet count is an incidental finding, diagnosed on a follow-up CBC to evaluate WBC. On rare occasions, bleeding symptoms will result in an evaluation that demonstrates decreased platelet count. Often, these bleeding symptoms are related to accompanying abnormalities in platelet function (thrombocytopathy), which may or may not be medication related. Although medications can cause other hematologic abnormalities (agranulocytosis, aplastic anemia, hemolytic anemia), thrombocytopenia is the most common drug-induced hematologic abnormality. A more comprehensive list is provided in **Table 101.16**. When thrombocytopenia is detected in the course of providing critical care, investigating possible pharmacologic causes is important. In healthy subjects who develop a drug-induced decrease in platelet counts, discontinuation of the medication is often curative. However, in critically ill adults and children, identifying the source of drug-induced thrombocytopenia is often confounded by treatment with multiple agents that can lower platelet counts, as well as the underlying illness. In these patients, changing current treatments to alternative drugs or other agents known to have lesser platelet effects may be beneficial but is not always possible.

Common ICU medications, such as cardiovascular drugs, antibiotics, and sedative/anesthetics, have been implicated in iatrogenic thrombocytopenia. In addition, many of the neuroleptics/antiepileptics and mood stabilizers, such as carbamazepine, valproate, and phenytoin, and the antidepressants,

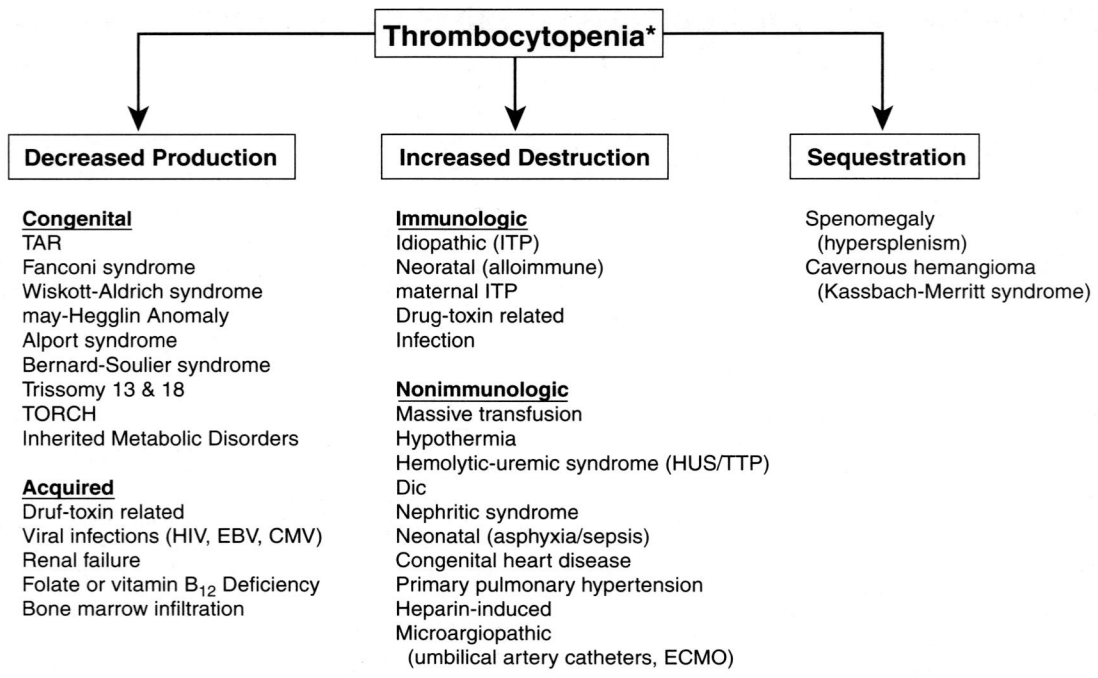

FIGURE 101.3. Differential diagnosis of thrombocytopenia. *Note*: "Pseudo-thrombocytopenia" occurs with platelet clumping, either spontaneously or from collection-tube preservatives (EDTA or citrate). TAR, thrombocytopenia with absent radius; TORCH, toxoplasmosis, other infections, rubella, cytomegalovirus infection, and herpes simplex; HIV, human immunodeficiency virus; EBV, Epstein-Barr virus; CMV, cytomegalovirus; ITP, idiopathic thrombocytopenic purpura; DIC, disseminated intravascular coagulopathy; ECMO, extracorporeal membrane oxygenation. Adapted from Sadowitz PD, Amanullah S, Souid AK. Hematologic emergencies in the pediatric emergency room. *Emerg Med Clin North Am.* 2002;20(1):177–98, vii.

such as lithium, fluoxetine, sertraline, paroxetine, and citalopram, can cause thrombocytopenia. More prevalent in adults and increasingly used in pediatric patients, serotonin reuptake inhibitors have been associated with bleeding diathesis with and without thrombocytopenia (84). The commonly used medications that result in abnormalities of platelet number are listed in **Table 101.16.**

Heparin is a very common, very severe cause of drug-induced immune thrombocytopenia in critically ill infants and children. Although the incidence is higher in adults, heparin-induced thrombocytopenia (HIT) is an important phenomenon to recognize. The diagnosis and treatment of HIT are discussed in a separate section of this chapter. Other medications such as quinidine result in a similar pattern of thrombocytopenia. Whether quinidine or heparin, the drug acts as a hapten to stimulate antibody binding to the platelet surface, resulting in autoantibody formation, subsequent platelet lysis, and a falling platelet count (10). Treatment for this type of immune-related process should involve stopping the offending agent as soon as thrombocytopenia develops, even if it is mild. Thromboembolic complications of HIT are discussed here.

Idiopathic Thrombocytopenic Purpura

Idiopathic thrombocytopenic purpura (ITP) is caused by the production of antibodies against platelet antigens. These antibody-coated platelets are trapped and destroyed in the reticuloendothelial system (primarily the spleen), resulting in thrombocytopenia. The typical history is sudden onset of petechiae and bruising in a previously healthy child; often, the child has a history of a preceding viral illness. Fever, bone or joint pain, weight loss, pallor, fatigue, weakness, and other complaints are typically lacking. Physical examination is usually normal except for mucocutaneous bleeding. Physical findings of lymphadenopathy and/or hepatosplenomegaly are atypical of ITP and should prompt investigation for a marrow infiltrative process. In the diagnostic evaluation of ITP, the CBC and blood smear are normal except for isolated thrombocytopenia. Additional laboratory tests for antinuclear antibody, anti-DNA antibody, and HIV tests are sometimes necessary because these entities can present initially with isolated thrombocytopenia. The need for bone marrow examination to confirm the diagnosis is controversial; many specialists perform this test before initiating prednisone therapy. Typically, the bone marrow shows a normal hematopoietic system with increased number of megakaryocytes. In many children with ITP, the thrombocytopenia resolves within 6 weeks. Although the incidence of life-threatening hemorrhages is reported at <1%, intracranial, pulmonary, upper-airway, and gastrointestinal bleedings have all been observed in children with acute ITP (47). Children with excessive skin and mucosal bleeding or with platelet counts of <10,000/mm³ are especially at risk for life-threatening bleeding. A careful evaluation and appropriate treatment are essential in the child with newly diagnosed ITP.

Treatment for ITP remains controversial. Current reported treatment options include corticosteroids, IVIG, and anti-Rh (D) immunoglobulin (**Table 101.17**). Corticosteroids (e.g., prednisone 2 mg/kg/day) remain the treatment of choice for most patients. Corticosteroids increase vascular stability,

TABLE 101.16

COMMON AGENTS THAT CAUSE THROMBOCYTOPENIA

Increased destruction or usage	Decreased production
Amitriptyline	Alkylating agents
Amphotericin B	Anthracyclines
Amrinone	Antimetabolite agents
Asparaginase	Cytarabine
Benzene	Epipodophyllotoxins
Bleomycin	Ethanol
Carbamazepine	Procarbazine
Chloroquine	Radiation, ionizing
Chlorpheniramine	Thiazides
Cimetidine	Vinblastine
Cocaine (i.e., DIC)	
Colchicine	
Crotalidae envenomation (i.e., DIC)	
Cyclosporine	
Furosemide	
Ganciclovir	
Glyburide	
Gold salts	
Heparin	
Indomethacin	
Meprobamate	
Mesoridazine	
Methyldopa	
Penicillin	
Pentamidine	
Quinidine	
Quinine	
Rifampin	
Sulfonamides	

DIC, disseminated intravascular coagulation
Adapted Drachman JG. Inherited thrombocytopenia: When a low platelet count does not mean ITP. *Blood* 2004;103(2):390–8.

TABLE 101.17

TREATMENT OF ACUTE CHILDHOOD IDIOPATHIC THROMBOCYTOPENIA PURPURA

Corticosteroids – one of the following:
Prednisone, 1–5 mg/kg/day in 3 divided doses for 1–2 weeks, followed by tapering and discontinuation by day 21
OR
Methylprednisolone, 30 mg/kg (maximum, 1 g/dose) IV over 30 mins every 24 hrs for 3 doses. Then return to maintenance steroid therapy. This option is reserved for hospitalized patients with severe bleeding.

IgG Concentrates
IVIG 1 g/kg/day for 2 consecutive days
Anti-D (for Rh-positive patients)
IV anti-D, single dose of 40–80 mcg/kg IV over 5 mins

Combination Therapy
Corticosteroids in combination with either IgG or anti-D (using the previously cited dosages). This option is used for patients with significant mucocutaneous bleeding in a hospital setting in consultation with a pediatric hematologist.

Platelet Transfusion
Not routinely needed. Indicated for life-threatening hemorrhage and in conjunction with above medical management.

enhance platelet production, decrease antibody production, and impair clearance of antibody-coated platelets, thus immediately reducing the risk of bleeding before any rise in the platelet count occurs. IVIG (1 g/kg/day infused over 3 hrs for 2 consecutive days) binds to receptors in the reticuloendothelial system, preventing platelet destruction. Typically, platelet counts will increase in 1 to 2 days following IVIG therapy. IV anti-D (a single dose of 40–80 mg/kg over 5 mins) is effective in Rh-positive patients. The anti-D antibodies saturate the reticuloendothelial sites with anti-D-coated RBC, preventing platelet destruction. Side effects associated with IV anti-D include chills and a slight drop in Hb concentration by 1 to 2 g/dL, secondary to hemolysis. Prophylactic treatment with acetaminophen, diphenhydramine, and prednisone can reduce these symptoms. Emergency splenectomy and platelet transfusion are reserved for severe and refractory ITP with life-threatening bleeding. Aspirin and nonsteroidal anti-inflammatories (NSAIDs) should be avoided in all thrombocytopenic patients (62).

Idiopathic Splenic Sequestration

Almost all conditions that lead to portal hypertension and enlargement of the spleen have been associated with reduction of circulating platelet counts. The spleen serves a combined immunologic, reservoir, and filtering function. The spleen can empty its reservoir to create a transient thrombocytosis; however, the filtering and immunologic functions of the spleen underlie its association with thrombocytopenia. Conditions of hypersplenism (accessory spleens and idiopathic enlargement of the spleen) have demonstrated thrombocytopenia secondary to sequestration or destruction of circulating cells. Normally, these events occur secondary to another disease process, and multiple hematologic cell lines are involved. Thus, idiopathic splenic sequestration is a diagnosis of exclusion, and unlike other etiologies of hypersplenism, thrombocytopenia is usually the isolated hematologic finding and bleeding problems are rarely reported. Peripheral smears may demonstrate burr cells but are typically normal except for thrombocytopenia. Management is typically observational, though long-term implications for future spleen trauma and bleeding risk remain unknown. Certainly any evidence of increased bleeding or bruising should prompt evaluation by a pediatric hematologist and reconsideration of an "idiopathic sequestration" diagnosis.

Postoperative (Dilutional) Thrombocytopenia

Postoperative (dilutional) thrombocytopenia occurs whenever massive blood loss and volume replacement take place. Timing of treatment is controversial. A study of traumatized adults demonstrates no prophylactic benefit to early platelet transfusion. However, in pediatric patients the need for treatment depends on the starting platelet count and on the clinical scenario. It was demonstrated that those patients with low starting platelet ($\sim$100,000/mm^3) counts developed dilutional thrombocytopenia and bleeding after blood loss of only 1–2 blood volumes (23). In this scenario, patients often require platelet treatment at $\leq$50,000/mm^3. In addition, certain surgeries associated with higher bleeding complications (e.g., neurosurgery, cardiac surgery, or organ transplantation), may require a higher threshold for treatment (see Chapter 38).

Neonatal Thrombocytopenia

Neonatal thrombocytopenia that occurs in patients from birth to 2 months of age represents a unique group and warrants special consideration. The incidence of thrombocytopenia is high in this group; it is estimated to occur in ~2%–3% of healthy term infants and increases to 20%–30% in all sick neonates, whether born prematurely or at term. In general, the thrombocytopenia seen in a sick infant is likely related to the primary disease process and will resolve as the primary process improves. Most of these infants develop platelet counts of <50,000 at >48 hrs of age. Causes include abnormalities of decreased production, increased consumption, and immune-mediated destruction. Often, altered production results in the most common late (>72 hrs of life) presentation of neonatal thrombocytopenia. Common neonatal conditions that impact platelet production are infectious processes (viral, bacterial, fungal), stress (necrotizing enterocolitis, surgery), medication (ranitidine, milrinone), hepatic disease, respiratory distress syndrome, maternal factors (pregnancy-induced hypertension and gestational diabetes), leukemia, and intrauterine growth retardation. Consumptive processes are variable in their timing of presentation and can present early or late, depending on severity and on the presence of in utero insults to the neonate. Common neonatal diseases that create consumption of platelets are thrombosis (catheter-related), infections (disseminated intravascular coagulopathy), vascular malformations (cavernous hemangiomas), and hypoxia/asphyxia. Finally, presentation with low platelet counts within <24 hrs of birth often represents immune-mediated destruction or inherited platelet abnormality. Immune-mediated processes are related to IgG or complement attachment to the platelets and their subsequent elimination. Autoimmune (ITP), alloimmune (maternal factors), congenital infections (TORCH—toxoplasmosis, other infections, rubella, CMV infection, and herpes simplex), and inborn platelet abnormalities can be the source. Regardless of the early or late timing, diagnosis and treatment of the underlying disease, with increased vigilance for hemorrhagic complications from neonatal thrombocytopenia, is always important.

As the etiology can be multifactorial, the diagnostic approach to neonatal thrombocytopenia should be broad enough to safely detect common treatable causes and identify complications of neonatal thrombocytopenia, such as bleeding and intraventricular hemorrhage. Careful family history that evaluates for bleeding problems and/or platelet abnormalities should be obtained. Review of the maternal smear and platelet count can also be informative, as some infectious, inherited, and immune-mediated causes may give the mother a low platelet count with abnormal platelet morphology. Physical exam should focus on careful neurologic examination and evaluation for evidence of bruising or abnormal bleeding. Size of the liver and spleen should be noted and examined daily. In the critically ill neonate, daily platelet counts are a minimum requirement, with more frequent assessment if bleeding symptoms or complications are present. When platelet counts are <30,000/mm^3, head ultrasounds to evaluate and monitor for intraventricular hemorrhage are common practice. For persistent and prolonged cases of neonatal thrombocytopenia, additional imaging with ultrasound, CT, and even angiography of the head, chest, and abdomen may be necessary to evaluate

for cavernous hemangiomas and/or arteriovenous malformations. Rarely, bone marrow aspiration will be required, except in those patients with persistent and otherwise unexplained thrombocytopenia.

Of these various neonatal causes, alloimmune thrombocytopenia represents a unique and potentially treatable newborn cause of low platelets. The incidence is thought to be 1 per 1000 live births and may be more common. In this disease, maternal antibodies are attacking and destroying the neonatal platelets. This process often begins in utero and may necessitate fetal therapy in future pregnancies. Though platelet counts can improve over 2–3 days as maternal antibody levels lower, during this period, infants are at a much higher risk for intraventricular hemorrhage and severe thrombocytopenia (<20,000/mm^3). For these neonates, transfusion of matched (antigen-negative) platelets is the treatment of choice. Prompt recognition and consultation with a pediatric hematologist to facilitate appropriate treatment is crucial. In addition, infants with alloimmune thrombocytopenia should undergo urgent neuroimaging studies to evaluate for intracranial bleeding. If platelets cannot be maintained at >20,000/mm^3 with platelet transfusion, consideration should be given to IVIG (1 g/kg/day) and/or methylprednisone (1 mg/kg IV every 8 hours) therapy until the platelet counts improve (>30–50,000/mm^3). If an intracranial bleed is detected, random platelet transfusions should be performed emergently until antigen-negative platelets are available. Treatment, whether conservative or aggressive, is usually required only for 2–3 days.

Thrombocytopathy

Described functional abnormalities of platelets are both inherited and acquired. Thrombocytopathy implies a normal number of platelets with impairment in their biochemical functionality. These disorders may result in either increased bleeding or hypercoagulability, depending on the relative impairment to platelet function. Inherited forms, such as gray platelet syndrome (reduction or absence of platelet α granules) and Paris-Trousseau syndrome, are rare causes of functional platelet abnormalities. Often, with these genetic disorders, other associated clinical (immunologic dysfunction) and dysmorphic features are present. Histologic evaluation of the blood smear often demonstrates unusual platelet morphology and number (**Table 101.15**).

The most common problems with platelet function are the acquired forms (**Table 101.18**). Causes of acquired functional platelet disorders include uremia, autoimmune disorders, infections, liver disease, nutritional deficiencies, and drugs. Salicylates, NSAIDs, and antibiotics are common medications that affect platelet function. Aspirin, with its permanent inhibition of cyclooxygenase (COX), is perhaps the most well known. Salicylates prevent thromboxane A$_2$ synthesis by acetylating COX, thus inhibiting platelet and megakaryocyte activities. The resulting decreased platelet aggregation causes a prolonged bleeding time. This process is irreversible, but recovery occurs in 7–10 days with the production and release of new platelets. Salicylates can precipitate hemorrhage in patients with pre-existing hemostatic defects such as von Willebrand disease, hemophilia A, warfarin ingestion, or uremia. NSAIDs also inhibit platelet COX. However, in contrast to salicylates, their effects are reversible and generally last <4 hrs (36).

High-dose penicillin and cephalosporin antibiotics can prolong the bleeding time by reducing platelet adhesion and

TABLE 101.18

DRUGS THAT INHIBIT PLATELET FUNCTION (THROMBOCYTOPATHY)

Nonsteroidal anti-inflammatory drugs
  Aspirin, ibuprofen, indomethacin, naproxen, and others
Antibiotics
  Penicillins, cephalosporins, nitrofurantoin
Cardiovascular drugs
  Amrinone/milrinone, dipyridamole, diltiazem,
    propranolol, nitroprusside, nifedipine, nitroglycerin,
    procainamide, verapamil
Anticoagulants, fibrinolytics, and anti-fibrinolytics
  Aprotinin, ε-aminocaproic acid, heparin, protamine,
    alteplase
Anesthetics
  Propofol, ketamine, benzocaine, cocaine, lidocaine,
    procaine, tetracaine, halothane, heroin
Anticonvulsants/psychotropic drugs
  Valproate, amitriptyline, haloperidol, imipramine,
    nortriptyline, chlorpromazine
Chemotherapy
  Carmustine, daunorubicin, vincristine, L-asparaginase
Antihistamines
  Chlorpheniramine, diphenhydramine, ranitidine,
    cimetidine
Herbal/alternative medicines
  Garlic, ginseng, gingko biloba
Other drugs/toxins
  Guaifenesin, dextran, pseudoephedrine, hetastarch,
    mustard gas

activation (33). The serum concentration, drug potency, and lipid solubility of the specific antibiotic will determine the degree of platelet impairment. This impairment is maximal after 1–3 days of drug administration and may last for several days after therapy. The penicillins may impair the interaction of von Willebrand factor (vWF) with the platelet membrane. Patients with coexisting hemostatic defects such as thrombocytopenia and vitamin K deficiency are at risk for bleeding with use of these antibiotics.

Other agents that affect platelet function include heparin, organic nitrates such as nitroprusside and nitroglycerin, and fish oils. Heparin's effects on platelets are multiple, and they can prolong the bleeding time by inhibiting thrombin, a potent platelet agonist (10). Organic nitrates are converted to nitric oxide, which activates guanylate cyclase, resulting in increased intracellular cyclic guanosine monophosphate (cGMP), which inhibits platelet aggregation. Fish oils that contain eicosapentaenoic acid (ω-3 fatty acid) prolong bleeding time through competitive inhibition of COX by reducing the formation of thromboxane A_2. Black tree fungus, garlic, gingko balboa, and ginseng cumin have similar antiplatelet effects and have been associated with increased perioperative bleeding (84).

Common medical conditions associated with impaired platelet function are renal failure, hepatic failure, and autoimmune disorders. Medical conditions can create thrombocytopathies through a variety of mechanisms, including reduced degranulation, impaired signaling, and decreased surface expression of binding receptors. Treatment for most functional platelet abnormalities is often discontinuation of the problematic agent and transfusion of functional platelets. However, in other conditions (uremia, alcohol toxicity, hepatic dysfunction, congenital platelet abnormalities), newly transfused platelets may develop similar dysfunction. In this setting, treatment with desmopressin may be beneficial, as desmopressin increases vWF levels and promotes platelet aggregation.

Clinically available quantitative tests to assess platelet function are available but are typically specialized and not immediately available at all centers. Though a bleeding test is often recommended, it is often not practical in the pediatric population and, like a thromboelastogram, it is only a qualitative measure. As qualitative and quantitative functional platelet tests are more widely available, they may help guide future treatment strategies to assess multifactorial platelet dysfunction in critically ill children who are bleeding following trauma, multisystem organ failure, cardiopulmonary bypass, and chemotherapy.

THROMBOTIC DISEASES IN INFANTS AND CHILDREN

The Coagulation Cascade—Antithrombotic Mechanisms

Normal coagulation function involves not only the production of adequate amounts of thrombin and fibrin to stop bleeding, but also mechanisms to prevent pathologic clot formation. Through these processes, the coagulation process attempts to confine thrombin generation to the site of the injury and avoid thrombotic events. The classic description of Virchow, which still holds true, stated that thrombi form due to (a) changes in the vessel wall, (b) changes in blood flow, and (c) changes in the blood composition. Although inherited disorders of coagulation that leads to excessive bleeding have been recognized and studied for centuries, inherited defects that predispose to thrombosis have only recently been identified. As in other physiologic and biochemical processes throughout the body, the coagulation system has both natural agonists and inhibitors. The latter can be divided into two general categories based on their site of production and/or action: endothelial and hepatic.

Endothelial-dependent inhibition of coagulation includes protein C (and its co-factor, protein S) and tissue factor pathway inhibitor (TFPI). The interactions of the coagulation cascade with its checks and balances are illustrated by the antithrombotic factor, protein C, which is directly activated by thrombin. Although protein C is a vitamin K-dependent serine protease produced by the liver, its conversion to activated protein C (APC) is dependent on an interaction that occurs on the endothelial surface. Thrombin formed either on the surface of platelets or at the site of tissue injury binds to the endothelium via thrombomodulin. The proteolytic site of thrombin cleaves a peptide from the protein C molecule, converting it to APC. APC acts by the enzymatic removal of a peptide from factors V and VIII. This alteration of the factor V molecule prevents its participation with activated factor Xa as part of the prothrombinase complex and the subsequent conversion of factor II (prothrombin) to IIa (thrombin). The alteration of factor VIII prevents its participation with activated factor IX as part of the tenase (X-ase) complex, which converts factor X to activated factor X. The function of APC in the inactivation of factors

V and VIII is facilitated by protein S, another member of the antithrombotic cascade, first identified in 1984.

A more recently described component of the antithrombotic pathway is TFPI (69). TFPI is produced and released from the vascular endothelium. It is the major inhibitor of the tissue factor pathway that regulates the conversion of factor VII to VIIa after tissue factor has been exposed at the site of tissue injury. Eighty to 90% of TFPI is bound to the endothelium, while the remainder is bound to plasma lipoproteins. Although currently named TFPI, its original isolation from the plasma as a factor bound to plasma lipoproteins led to its initial title of *lipoprotein-associated coagulation inhibitor*. The antithrombotic effects of TFPI include the inhibition of the tissue factor-VIIa complex and reversible binding to the active, proteolytic site of Xa (39). Animal studies have demonstrated that a homozygous state that results in deficient TFPI function is not compatible with life and results in in utero death (85). Given its key role in the control of thrombosis, a deficiency state in humans has not been reported.

Hepatic-dependent aspects of the antithrombotic cascade include antithrombin III (AT-III), heparin cofactor (HC) II, and plasminogen. AT-III is an hepatic, synthesized, serine, protease inhibitor, is not vitamin K-dependent, and has been estimated to account for more than 50% of the endogenous plasma anticoagulant activity. It irreversibly inhibits the function of several activated coagulation factors, including IXa, Xa, XIa, and XIIa. The activity of AT-III is greatly enhanced by the exogenous administration of therapeutic heparin concentrations and by endogenous glycosaminoglycans, such as heparin sulfate, which are found on the endothelial surface (58). Although AT-III is produced by the liver and circulates in the plasma, its activity is greatest after its interaction with endothelial-bound molecules such as heparin sulfate. AT-III has an effective plasma half-life of 3–5 days. Deficiency states may be acquired or congenital, as described later.

The other major plasma thrombin inhibitor is HC-II, a plasma protein that inhibits thrombin by formation of a covalent 1:1 complex to thrombin. Unlike AT-III, it has no activity against other activated coagulation factors. Endogenous compounds (dermatan sulfate, heparan sulfate) as well as exogenous heparin bind to HC-II and increase the rate of thrombin inhibition by more than 1000-fold. HC-II is unique among the serine protease inhibitors in its ability to be stimulated by dermatan sulfate. It has been estimated that HC-II accounts for ~30% of the total plasma anticoagulant activity. Both acquired and inherited deficiency states have been reported, although their association with clinical disease remains controversial.

The final major component of the antithrombotic cascade is the plasminogen system. A major part of its mechanism comes into play after the formation of the thrombus. As such, it is a key component of the fibrinolytic system that acts to dissolve fibrin clots and restore patency to the vascular system. However, it is also part of the antithrombotic cascade as it inhibits the ongoing coagulation process by degradation of fibrinogen as well as inhibition of activated factors Va and VIIIa. Plasminogen is a glycoprotein, produced by the liver, with a molecular weight of 92 kilodaltons. Its plasma half-life is 2 days. Plasminogen is converted to the proteolytic enzyme plasmin by cleavage of a single peptide bond. The two physiologic activators of plasminogen are tissue plasminogen activator (tPA) and urinary-type plasminogen activator, also known as *urokinase*. Thrombin generated from the coagulation cascade stimulates the release of tPA from endothelial cells. tPA forms a complex with fibrin and converts plasminogen to plasmin. Kallikrein, a protein component of the plasma contact activation system, stimulates the release of urokinase from the kidney. In the normal state, the majority of the released urokinase is bound to the endothelial tissue via the urokinase plasminogen activator receptor. Exogenously produced forms of tPA, urokinase, and streptokinase (another plasminogen activator, produced by α-hemolytic streptococci), have been used as therapeutic agents in the treatment of thrombotic disease.

The plasminogen cascade, similar to the other limbs of the antithrombotic process, is regulated by other endogenous factors. The two principal inhibitors of fibrinolysis in the circulation are plasminogen activator inhibitor (PAI)-1, which inhibits both urinary-type plasminogen activator (urokinase) tPA and α_2-antiplasmin, a specific plasmin inhibitor. PAI-1, produced by the endothelial cells, provides an important mechanism for controlling the activity of tPA and urokinase. The specific plasmin inhibitor, α_2-antiplasmin, is covalently bound to polymerizing fibrin by activated factor XIII. Deficiencies of PAI-1 and α_2-antiplasmin may play a role in both acquired and inherited prothrombotic states.

Disorders and Situations That Predispose to Thrombosis

Although recognized for decades as a significant cause of morbidity and mortality in the adult population, the potential deleterious effects of thrombotic disease in infants and children have been relatively overlooked. The incidence of deep vein thrombosis (DVT) when effective prophylaxis is not employed following lower extremity surgery has been estimated at 40%–60% in adults versus 1% in infants and children. However, various acquired or inherited disorders may place the pediatric patient at risk for thrombotic diseases. When compared with adults, the epidemiology of thrombotic diseases is quite different in children. The majority of children have one or more comorbid or associated features that place them at risk, whereas ~50% of such problems in adults are idiopathic. Additionally, 95% of thrombotic problems affect the lower venous system in adults, whereas the distribution of upper versus lower venous system issues is evenly distributed in infants and children. A summary of some of the commonly encountered risk factors for thrombosis in children is presented in **Table 101.19**.

The potential impact of thrombotic disease in infants and children is demonstrated by a Canadian registry that demonstrates that incidence in the general pediatric inpatient hospital population is 5.3 per 10,000 hospital admissions, or 0.07 per 10,000 children, with a mortality rate of 2.2% (3,21). Although the physiologic differences between the pediatric and adult population result in an overall reduction in the risk of thrombotic disease in children (26), in various clinical scenarios or with associated comorbid features, thrombotic disease impacts on morbidity and mortality. The latter may be especially true in the PICU arena.

Acquired Diseases

In the majority of infants and children who present with thrombotic events, some underlying comorbid disease or provocative factor is present. In an analysis of children with DVT or

TABLE 101.19

RISK FACTORS FOR HYPERCOAGULABILITY IN CHILDREN

Physiologic alterations	Clinical conditions
Blood Flow	
Hypovolemia	Shock, dehydration
Hyperviscosity	Erythrocytosis, leukocytosis, thrombocytosis, sickle cell disease
Mechanical stasis	Immobilization after surgery
Foreign body	CVC, cardiac prosthesis
Vasculature	
Anatomic defects	Congenital heart disease, arteriovenous malformation
Endothelial disorders	Vasculitis, inflammation, trauma
Blood coagulation	
Increased and/or abnormal	Malignancy, dysfibrinogenemias, procoagulants, inflammatory bowel disease
Decreased anticoagulants	AT-III deficiency, protein S or C deficiency, APC resistance (factor V Leiden)
Decreased fibrinolysis	Hereditary defects
Increased platelet-vessel reactivity	atherosclerotic disease, inherited dyslipidemia, diabetes mellitus
Mixed or idiopathic syndrome, recurrent idiopathic DVT	HIT, HUS, TTP, oral contraceptives, nephrotic

CVC, central venous catheter; APC, activated protein C; HIT, heparin-induced thrombocytopenia; HUS, hemolytic uremic syndrome; TTP, thrombotic thrombocytopenic purpura; DVT, deep vein thrombosis
Adapted from Hathaway WE. Congenital and acquired defects in coagulation: Diagnosis and treatment. *Mead Johnson Symp Perinat Dev Med* 1986;(28):45–54.

pulmonary embolism (PE) identified from a comprehensive literature study, 98% had a comorbid feature or predisposing factor (26). The predisposing factor was the presence of a central venous catheter (CVC) in more than 20% of the patients, while associated conditions were less likely and included a history of recent surgery (13%) or trauma (8.8%). Other risk factors included collagen vascular disorders (systemic lupus erythematosus, SLE, in 7.5%), infection (6.2%), oncologic diseases (5.8%), or use of parenteral nutrition (5.5%). Inherited prothrombotic states were identified in only 3.9% of the patients, while an acquired prothrombotic state due to nephrotic syndrome was present in 2.9%. Similar findings were reported in the subsequent Canadian registry of pediatric patients with thromboembolic events in 96% of children (oncologic diseases, presence of a central venous line), with many having more than 1 risk factor and only 4% having no identifiable predisposing factor (3). In addition, they reported a bimodal occurrence rate, with the highest rates of thrombotic disease occurring in infants <1 year of age and a secondary, albeit lower, peak during the teenage years. These studies reflect the fact that comorbid processes responsible for thrombotic disease have changed. Before the 1970s, identified risk factors included ventriculoatrial shunts, infection, and congenital heart disease (CHD), whereas the current literature demonstrates that the presence of a CVC, oncologic diseases, collagen vascular diseases, and inherited prothrombotic conditions lead the comorbid disease list. Recent data from the Canadian registry during the follow-up period of 6 months to 3 years, suggests 2.2% of the children died as a direct result of their thrombotic disease, while 18.5% developed recurrent disease (16, or 70%, of these patients were receiving anticoagulant therapy at the time of recurrence).

Central Venous Catheters. CVCs represent the single most commonly identified acquired risk factor for thrombotic events in infants and children. Many of these children may have other acquired (oncologic) or inherited diseases that act as additional comorbid features. CVCs are thrombogenic because their foreign, nonendothelial surfaces act as a nidus for activation of the coagulation cascade. Two variants of thrombi have been identified in association with CVCs: (a) a fibrin sleeve that forms around the catheter, is not adherent to the wall, and does not occlude the vessel, and (b) a thrombus around the tip of the catheter that adheres to the wall and obstructs the vessel. Although symptomatic occlusion of the CVC is common and easily treated by a thrombolytic agent, catheter-related thrombi can result in significant morbidity and even mortality; problems include pulmonary emboli, superior vena cava syndrome, chylothorax, and post-phlebitic syndrome with pain, discoloration, swelling, and ulceration of the affected extremity. The latter is being recognized as a more common long-term effect of CVCs, with an incidence as high as 20%. Although it may appear early in the course of catheter use, it has also been reported years following catheter removal. The potential morbidity and even mortality associated with such problems is illustrated by reports in the literature of fatal pulmonary embolic disease associated with CVC use.

Temporary central venous access is frequently required in the care of critically ill children. In this setting, coexisting comorbid disease processes may place these patients at risk for thrombotic disease. In a prospective study, consecutive children admitted to the PICU who required placement of a CVC for more than 48 hrs were screened using Doppler ultrasonography at days 2, 4, 6, 7, and weekly thereafter (9). A diagnosis of thrombus was made by Doppler ultrasonography if two of four of the following features were identified: (a) an echogenic filling defect, (b) noncompressibility of the vein, (c) loss of respiratory variability and vessel pulsation, and (d) no flow detected or abnormal Doppler waveforms distal to the occluded segment. The incidence of CVC-related thrombosis was 18.3% (17 of 93 patients). In the majority of patients (15 of 17), the diagnosis was made within 4 days of catheter placement. Only 7 of 17 patients manifested clinical signs and symptoms at the time that the Doppler study was first positive. The sites of catheter placement affected by thrombosis included external jugular (3), internal jugular (4), subclavian (2), and femoral (11). Risk factors for thrombus formation determined by multivariate analysis included the presence of an oncologic disease and young age. Although symptomatic thrombosis was found more frequently in the femoral vein, statistical analysis did not demonstrate that the catheter site was a risk factor. Therapy was not controlled by the study. One patient with an asymptomatic thrombus in the subclavian vein received no therapy. In 4 patients (2 with clinical symptoms), the catheter was removed without further therapy. In the remaining 12 patients, treatment with low-molecular-weight heparin (LMWH) or standard heparin was administered, either with (9 of 12) or without (3 of 12) catheter removal. No significant morbidity or mortality related to the thrombi were noted other than persistent leg edema in 2 patients.

Total Parenteral Nutrition. The risk of CVC-thrombotic disease may be further increased by the presence of other comorbid features or therapeutic interventions. The administration of total parenteral nutrition, especially long-term use, has been identified as a risk factor for the development of thrombotic complications. A retrospective review of silastic catheters for home total parenteral nutrition demonstrated that 25 (68%) were removed because of blockage that did not resolve with urokinase instillation—9 due to sepsis, 2 due to dislodgement, and 1 due to leakage. Among the patients, 8 had extensive thrombotic disease diagnosed by venography, and 5 had signs and symptoms of superior vena cava obstruction. The authors concluded that flushing catheters with heparin, the most common form of prophylaxis, was insufficient in their patients (4). They suggest that in this population the efficacy of prophylactic warfarin therapy should be investigated in a prospective, randomized trial, as such therapy in adults has been shown to reduce CVC-related DVT diagnosed by venography from 37.5% to 9.5% (11).

Oncologic Diseases. Patients with oncologic diseases may be predisposed to thrombotic events because of the prothrombotic changes induced by the malignancy itself, chemotherapy-related issues, and/or changes in the vessel wall related to acute/chronic infectious disease issues or the oncologic process. One example of such problems is the prothrombotic state produced by the effects of the chemotherapeutic agent, L-asparaginase, by depressing AT-III levels. Additionally, these patients frequently require placement of a CVC and/or the administration of total parenteral nutrition. A prospective study that evaluated the incidence of thrombotic disease associated with CVCs in children with malignancies reported an incidence of 8.8% (13 of 156 patients) (50). Of the 13 thrombi, 6 were adherent to the right atrial wall. In 2 of these patients, clinical symptoms of obstruction to venous return necessitated

operative intervention with the use of cardiopulmonary bypass (CPB). Further comparison of children with thrombi with those without thrombi demonstrated no difference in age, duration of catheter use, administration of L-asparaginase, or use of total parenteral nutrition. However, a higher incidence of thrombotic disease was noted in children with acute lymphocytic leukemia and when the tip of the catheter was in the right atrium compared to the superior vena cava. This finding agrees with prior studies, confirming an association of acute lymphocytic leukemia with the risk of thrombotic disease not observed with acute myelogenous leukemia. Thromboses may occur in association with CVC or at distal sites, the most common site being the venous drainage of the central nervous system. The incidence is relatively low (1%–10%) when clinical signs and symptoms are used, but increases to 30% with ultrasound evaluation. The risk of thrombosis in acute lymphocytic leukemia relates to several factors, including an acquired AT-III deficiency from L-asparaginase, in vivo activation of the coagulation cascade due to the disease, and hyperleukocytosis (63).

Nephrotic Syndrome. The association of thrombotic disease and nephrotic syndrome was first identified in the 18th century. Although thought to be a less significant risk factor than in adults, nephrotic syndrome is recognized as a risk factor for thrombotic disease in infants and children, with an incidence ranging from 3% to 30% (2). The most common thrombotic events include renal vein thrombosis and PE. Coagulation studies performed in children with steroid-resistant nephritic syndrome demonstrated an inverse correlation between serum albumin levels versus fibrinogen and α_2-macroglobulin concentrations. Conversely, a direct correlation exists between serum albumin levels and AT-III levels. Ventilation-perfusion scans in the same cohort of children demonstrated a pattern consistent with PE in 27.9%, residual changes suggestive of PE in 38.5%, and normal findings in 34.9%. The authors concluded that the incidence of thromboembolic events is high in children with severe nephrotic syndrome and similar to that reported in adults. They suggest that pulmonary symptoms in patients with nephrotic syndrome may be due to PE. Hematologic abnormalities in nephrotic syndrome include increased plasma concentrations of factors I, V, and VIII; increased vWF; low AT-III levels; increased platelet aggregation; and depressed fibrinolysis. These effects relate not only to renal losses of protein, but also to nonspecific increases in hepatic protein synthesis in an attempt to maintain oncotic homeostasis (73). The severity of the changes follows the severity of the nephrotic syndrome and serum albumin concentrations.

Autoimmune Disorders and Antiphospholipid Antibody Syndrome. SLE and other autoimmune disorders may predispose patients to thromboembolic diseases regardless of their association with the antiphospholipid antibody syndrome (APAS). The APAS is characterized by the formation of autoantibodies to phospholipids. Antiphospholipid antibodies (APA) are immunoglobulins (IgG, IgA, IgM) directed against negatively charged phospholipids. The prothrombotic effects of these autoantibodies may relate to their effects on phospholipids located on the vascular endothelium and/or the surface of platelets. APAs can be separated into two distinct groups: the lupus anticoagulant and the anticardiolipin antibody.

The first work regarding APAs began in the early 1950s with the discovery of altered in vitro coagulation function in patients with SLE. Because of its effects on laboratory measurements of coagulation function with prolongation of the prothrombin time (PT) and partial thromboplastin time (PTT), it was originally termed "the lupus anticoagulant." Further laboratory investigation demonstrated that the inhibitor was an immunoglobulin directed against the prothrombin activator complex. Although it prolonged the in vitro measurement of clotting function, it was subsequently shown to have the opposite effect in vivo, with a predisposition to thrombotic complications. A mixing test can be conducted to identify whether the prolongation of the PT/PTT is a true clinical effect or the result of the lupus anticoagulant. If the prolongation of the PT/PTT is due to a factor deficiency, the PT/PTT will be corrected by the addition of normal plasma, while no effect is seen with the presence of the lupus anticoagulant. In the 1960s, additional clinical work demonstrated that patients with SLE who manifested APAs or the lupus anticoagulant had an increased thrombotic tendency (16). It was also documented that patients without autoimmune disorders could develop the APAS with the same predisposition to thrombotic complications. Patients without an associated collage vascular disorder were said to have primary APAS, while patients with SLE or other collagen vascular disorders were said to have secondary APAS. Anticardiolipin antibodies have been shown to be relatively common in the pediatric population on chronic hemodialysis and may predispose these patients to thrombotic complications, including fistula thrombosis (74). The constellation of clinical findings, including recurrent arterial or venous thrombosis, recurrent fetal losses, thrombocytopenia, and APAs, became known as the APAS. Patients with APAS may manifest recurrent thrombotic events, typically on the venous side. The most likely sites of thrombosis include DVT of the lower extremities, although other sites may be involved, including retinal, hepatic, renal, and even the coronary or cerebral vasculature (14).

The first reports of thrombotic complications in pediatric patients with APAs were published in 1981. In general, the incidence of thrombotic complications in children is less than in adults due to a decreased incidence of comorbid prothrombotic factors, such as smoking, hypertension, hyperlipidemia, diabetes, and underlying atherosclerotic disease. In a review of 50 pediatric patients with APAS, a male:female ratio of 2:1, with a mean age of presentation of 10.2 years (range of 8 months to 16 years) was demonstrated (70). Each child had one or more thrombotic complication, with a greater risk of arterial involvement in younger patients. The incidence of arterial involvement was 62% in patients <10 years of age, compared to 28% in those >10 years of age. As in the adult population, DVT of the lower extremity was the most likely site of involvement, although the risk of subsequent PE was lower in children. Additionally, as in adults, the most likely site of arterial involvement was the cerebral vasculature.

The coexistence of SLE and APAS remains a significant risk factor for thrombotic complications in both adults and children. In a retrospective study of pediatric SLE patients, a total of 16 thrombotic episodes occurred in 11 of the 120 children (9%). Thrombosis was a presenting sign of the disease in 7 patients. Of the 16 thrombotic episodes, 14 involved the leg, 2 involved the cerebral vasculature, and 4 were associated with PE. The presence of the lupus anticoagulant was a risk factor for the occurrence of thrombotic complications. The lupus anticoagulant was present in 8 of 11 patients with thrombotic events, versus 10 of 74 without thrombosis (66).

Treatment of APAS remains controversial, with limited prospective data on which to base clinical decisions. As with any of the prothrombotic states reviewed in this chapter, reduction or control of associated risk factors, such as smoking, hyperlipidemia, and diabetes mellitus, may be helpful. Other treatment strategies aimed at reducing the antiphospholipid antibody levels include the administration of corticosteroids, immunosuppressive agents, IVIG, and plasmapheresis. Perioperative measures may include the use of low-dose heparin protocols, maintenance of adequate hydration, early ambulation, and anti-embolic intermittent compression devices for the lower extremities.

Heparin-induced Thrombocytopenia. Although HIT in the adult population has received significant attention, much less information is available regarding this disorder in infants and children (68). Following the introduction in the 1930s of heparin for clinical use, reports of thrombocytopenia associated with heparin therapy began to appear, although its clinical implications were not appreciated. In 1958, the first reports of the potential morbidity and mortality from HIT appeared in the literature, with Weisman and Tobin reporting arterial thrombosis in 10 patients who received heparin. The incidence of HIT varies widely in the literature, ranging from 1% to as high as 30%.

HIT can develop after exposure to unfractionated heparin or LMWH, although the incidence is highest with unfractionated heparin. Exposure to heparin can occur from a bolus or an infusion, through the IV or subcutaneous route, as a flush solution for invasive monitors, or on heparin-impregnated catheters. In most cases, the platelet count decreases 7–14 days after exposure to heparin. If circulating antiheparin IgG antibody from a previous exposure is already present, the platelet count may fall immediately on re-exposure to heparin. In the adult population, thrombotic complications are primarily arterial and tend to involve the extremities, although cerebral, myocardial, and mesenteric thromboses have also been reported. A propensity to develop thrombotic complications in vessels with endothelial damage has been reported (53). Venous thrombosis and PE are less frequent, and their association with HIT is less clearly defined. Thrombotic complications may occur at multiple anatomic sites and can result in significant morbidity, including loss of limb and even mortality (rates up to 30% in the adult population).

The incidence and associated morbidity and mortality from HIT are less well defined in pediatric patients. Literature review of neonates and children demonstrates a high incidence of thrombotic complications from HIT. As opposed to the adult experience, the thrombotic complication included the venous system in two-thirds of the patients. Arterial involvement was reported, including CNS involvement, an intracardiac thrombus, and thrombosis of the femoral/tibial artery. The true incidence is unknown, but data suggest an incidence of 1.5% in neonates who are exposed to heparin. Information concerning morbidity and mortality is also limited. However, mortality in neonates with HIT has been reported as high as 21%, which was not statistically different from the mortality rate of 35% in neonates with thrombocytopenia from other etiologies.

The mechanisms that result in thrombocytopenia with HIT are not completely understood. Antibodies are formed against an antigenic compound composed of heparin and platelet factor 4. Platelet factor 4, a protein stored in the α-granule, binds heparin. The platelet factor 4/heparin complex binds heparin antibodies and activates platelets, leading to their clearance from the circulation (1). HIT is subclassified into types 1 and 2. HIT type 1 is a less severe form of the disease in which patients experience a mild, early decrease in platelet count that improves even with the ongoing administration of heparin. Thrombotic complications generally do not occur. HIT type 2 results in a more severe degree of thrombocytopenia, which does not resolve without cessation of heparin therapy and includes the potential for thrombotic complications that involve both the arterial and venous vasculature. Differentiating between these two forms of HIT is not possible with current laboratory testing.

The diagnosis of HIT is based on the identification of heparin antibodies by detecting the activation and aggregation of platelets incubated with the patient's serum. Two basic assays are available. In most centers, a heparin-induced platelet aggregation study is used. The patient's serum is mixed with a platelet suspension, and the aggregation of platelets is determined by a change in optical density of the solution (a greater than 20% change is considered positive). Results are reported as negative, weakly positive, positive, or strongly positive. A second test assesses platelet aggregation by the identification of a substance released from platelets during activation, such as adenosine diphosphate (identified by chemiluminescence) or a ^{14}C-serotonin release assay. The latter test is considered the gold standard for heparin antibody assays but is also more cumbersome and time consuming.

Common treatment of HIT includes the immediate cessation of heparin administration of any type or route, including LMWH, heparin-coated catheters, and heparin flushes of invasive catheters. Several alternative anticoagulants are available for patients with HIT who require ongoing anticoagulation. Studies are limited, but use of alternative anticoagulation with danaparoid sodium, warfarin, and even LMWH have been reported in pediatric patients (68). Although cross-reactivity occurs with LMWH in 80%–90% of cases, these medications have been safely used provided that *in vitro* testing fails to demonstrate platelet aggregation. A lower incidence of cross-reactivity (10%–20%) is seen with danaparoid, a factor Xa-inhibiting heparinoid. Other nonheparin anticoagulants include the glycoprotein IIb/IIIa inhibitors, the direct thrombin inhibitors (hirudin, recombinant hirudin-lepirudin and bivalirudin, and argatroban), and the defibrinogenating enzyme (ancrod). However, experience is limited with these agents in the pediatric population.

Hemoglobinopathies. Both venous and arterial thrombotic events are recognized sequelae of SCD and other hemoglobinopathies. Although generally attributed to the vascular occlusion by the abnormal hemoglobin species, several other factors have been subsequently recognized as contributing to the prothrombotic state of the hemoglobinopathies, including activation of the coagulation cascade and deficiencies in antithrombotic mechanisms. Although these processes may occur in all hemoglobinopathies, their magnitude appears to be greatest in SCD. Patients with SCD have depressed levels of protein S and C, elevated plasma concentrations of vWF factor and factor VIII, and depressed levels of factor V and VII (65). Endothelial interactions have also been shown to play a potential role in the thrombotic tendency of SCD, with increased adherence of sickle cells to the endothelium,

an increased number of activated endothelial cells, chronic endothelial damage with cell adhesion molecule activation, and platelet activation due to abnormal endothelial cell function. In addition, APAs are found in higher concentrations in patients with SCD. All of these processes combine to increase the risk of thrombotic disease in patients with SCD.

Congenital Heart Disease. Various factors, including altered or sluggish blood flow, polycythemia, or the presence of grafts, valves, or patches composed of foreign materials, may explain the increased tendency of patients with cyanotic CHD to develop thrombotic events. In addition to these structural abnormalities, coexisting disorders of the coagulation system with enhanced coagulation function or depressed antithrombotic function may further increase the incidence of thrombotic complications in patients with CHD. A study that evaluated children with CHD and thrombotic events to assess prothrombotic risk factors found some underlying predisposition for thrombotic events, including factor V Leiden, protein C deficiency, and elevated levels of lipoprotein A. The authors concluded that secondary or comorbid diseases are frequently present, although nongenetic risk factors are generally thought to be the contributing variable in infants and children with CHD who ultimately experience a thrombotic event (49).

Miscellaneous Factors. Various other situations or disease processes have been clearly or anecdotally linked to thrombotic complications. In some, such as meningitis, mastoiditis, or otitis media, the thrombotic complications occur in the direct vicinity of the disease process, resulting from a localized vasculitis associated with the infection. In such cases, vasculitis and small-vessel occlusion may lead to arterial or venous infarction and CNS sequelae. In other infectious situations, the thrombotic process may occur at sites distal to the infection or as in a patient with systemic bacteremia. In this setting, thrombosis becomes one component of multisystem organ failure and the systemic inflammatory response syndrome. Other than SLE, other disease processes (Takayasu arteritis, Kawasaki disease) that result in vasculitis may also lead to thrombotic complications. Various prothrombotic changes have been reported in patients with inflammatory bowel disease (ulcerative colitis), including increased factor I and VIII concentrations, accelerated thromboplastin generation, and decreased protein C concentrations (17). These thrombotic problems may predate the gastrointestinal symptoms.

Severe dehydration or shock may predispose the pediatric patient to thrombotic sequelae. In the adult population, the postoperative period is recognized as a period in which thrombotic complications, most commonly DVT, may occur. In contrast, such problems are generally not encountered in the pediatric population; however, following puberty, the risk increases, especially following abdominal or long-bone procedures. Additionally, as with adults, pregnancy, smoking, or various medications, including oral contraceptives, may be risk factors. Metabolic diseases, either acquired or inherited, including diabetes mellitus, homocystinuria, increased lipoprotein A, and galactosemia, may also be associated with an increased risk of thrombotic complications.

Inherited/Congenital Diseases

The inherited disorders that result in a prothrombotic state are relatively uncommon; however, when routine screening is performed, they have a disproportionately high incidence in patients with what is assumed to be a spontaneous thrombotic event. Although the thrombotic event may be attributed to one of the many acquired disease processes or comorbid diseases listed previously, it is also recognized that the presence of any of a number of inherited deficiencies of the antithrombotic cascade may facilitate an acute thrombotic event in a patient who experiences a comorbid disease process such as trauma or a surgical procedure.

Protein S/C and Resistance to Activate Protein C (Factor V Leiden). Protein C and its cofactor, protein S, cleave a peptide from activated factors V and VIII, thereby preventing their participation in the X-ase and prothrombinase complex. Defects in this system may involve protein S, protein C, or a mutation in the amino acid sequence of factor V, which confers resistance to the effects of APC. Protein S and C deficiency are inherited as simple Mendelian traits. Homozygous states of S and C deficiency result in severe disease, including purpura fulminans, during infancy, while the heterozygous state increases the risk of spontaneous thrombotic events alone (with an annual thrombotic event rate of 1 per 1000 patients) or in association with comorbid diseases (78). Protein C deficiency may result from a low concentration of normally functioning protein C (type I) or a normal concentration of a defective protein C molecule (type II). Protein C deficiency (heterozygous state) is present in ~0.2% of the general population. Treatment is divided into therapy for acute thrombotic complications, including heparin, LMWH, or thrombolytic agents, and consideration of prophylactic therapy to prevent recurrent thrombotic complications. In the homozygous state, the risk of death from thrombosis is imminent. As a result, treatment necessitates providing a source of protein C by the administration of fresh frozen plasma. In addition, a form of human protein C concentrate is available, although no studies have compared the efficacy of fresh frozen plasma versus the protein C concentrates in severe protein C deficiency-related thrombosis.

Like protein C, its cofactor, protein S, is inherited as a simple Mendelian trait, with the homozygous state resulting in severe thrombotic disease (purpura fulminans) in the neonatal period. Protein S exists in the body in a free form and protein-bound form. Only the free form of protein S is able to interact with protein C and participate in its antithrombotic effects. Three classifications of protein S deficiency have been characterized. Type I deficiency results from an inadequate amount of both the free and protein-bound forms. Although the protein S that is present functions normally, its amount is insufficient to control the coagulation cascade. Type II deficiency results from a defective protein S molecule. The amount of protein S present is normal, but it is unable to interact normally with the other molecules involved in coagulation. Type III protein S deficiency is characterized by a low amount of free protein S but an overall normal amount of total protein S. The incidence of protein S deficiency in the general population is not known. In the adult Caucasian population, protein S deficiency is present in 1%–5% of patients who have a thrombotic event. Like protein C deficiency, the presence of the heterozygous state for protein S deficiency is thought to confer an increased relative risk of thrombotic disease, estimated at six to eight times that of the general adult population, in which the risk of thrombotic complications is estimated to be 1 per 1000 patients per year. This relative risk may increase with other comorbid disease

processes. Treatment is similar to that described for protein C deficiency; however, no purified protein-S concentration is commercially available (59).

In addition to dysfunction or deficiencies of the protein S and C system, a prothrombotic state may be the result of alterations in the amino acid sequence of the factor-V molecule, thereby making it resistant to the actions of protein C or protein S; this is commonly known as *resistance to APC*. Most cases are related to a single amino acid change in the factor V molecule (arginine to glutamine at position 506, otherwise known as factor V Leiden). Factor V Leiden is more common in the northern European populations. It is estimated that ~4%–7% of the general population is heterozygous for factor V Leiden, while 0.06%–0.25% of the population is homozygous for it. The factor V Leiden mutation is relatively uncommon in the native populations of Asia, Africa, and North America. In contrast, in Greece and southern Sweden, rates above 10% have been reported. The relative risk of thrombotic complications for the heterozygous state is five to eight times that of the general adult population, a rate similar to the heterozygous state of protein S and C deficiency. However, the risk of thrombotic complications increases significantly when other comorbid diseases are present. For example, in the heterozygous state, the relative risk may be 100 times that of the general population in a person who is placed on oral contraceptive medications. Although reports vary, factor V Leiden is considered the most prevalent of the prothrombotic conditions identified in the adult population.

Antithrombin III Deficiency. AT-III deficiency may be an acquired or inherited defect. Acquired AT-III deficiency can result from various medications (L-asparaginase) or comorbid disease processes, including hepatic failure, nephrotic syndrome, preeclampsia, shock, disseminated intravascular coagulation, and the use of extracorporeal circulation. AT-III levels that are <50% of normal during septic shock are associated with increased morbidity and mortality with overall hospital mortality approaching 100% when AT-III levels are <20% (34). As with many of the inherited prothrombotic states, AT-III issues can be classified as (a) type I AT-III deficiency, with a low plasma concentration of the enzyme, or (b) type II disease when the concentration is normal but the enzyme is dysfunctional. The latter case may result from defective binding to heparin, thereby affecting the efficiency of the enzyme. The disorder is carried as a simple Mendelian trait, with an estimated incidence of the heterozygous state of ~0.02%–1.0% in the general adult population. The homozygous state is not compatible with life. Treatment includes standard therapy for the prothrombotic states, including elimination of risk factors and consideration for long-term anticoagulation in patients with recurrent thrombotic disease. Antithrombin concentrates are available, and their use is considered when oral anticoagulants are not feasible (prior to a major surgery and during pregnancy). AT-III concentrates may also be used to allow for therapeutic heparinization during cardiopulmonary bypass.

Heparin Cofactor Deficiency. Knock-out mice have recently been developed as a tool to investigate the physiologic function of HC-II and its role in prothrombotic states. Unlike AT-III-deficient mice, which die in utero with extensive fibrin deposition in the liver and myocardium (43), HC-II-deficient mice undergo normal fetal development, with normal growth and survival up to at least 1 year of age. They do not appear to have spontaneous thrombosis, and they develop normal hematopoiesis, liver, and kidney function. Homozygous mice, produced from crosses in which both parents are HC-II-deficient, also demonstrate normal development without increased in utero death rates. However, HC-II-deficient mice are more likely to develop a thrombotic occlusion of the carotid artery after photochemically induced damage to the endothelium. These observations suggest that HC-II may place a role in vessel protection in response to chemical or traumatic injury. To date, limited information is available to define the role of HC-II deficiency in the pathogenesis of thrombotic complications in humans (83).

Plasminogen Deficiency. Plasminogen deficiency is a risk factor for thrombosis. Hereditary deficiencies in plasminogen activity are rare and include type 1 deficiency, characterized by decreased plasminogen levels, and type II deficiency, characterized by normal levels of dysfunctional plasminogen (57). Plasminogen deficiency is transmitted as an autosomal-recessive defect. Homozygous plasminogen deficiency can result in ligneous conjunctivitis with conjunctival fibrin deposition. Plasminogen deficiency has been noted in 2%–3% of patients with thrombotic events; however, its role in such complications has not been inconclusively established. Likewise, although it is postulated that abnormalities in inhibitors of the plasminogen pathway, such as PAI-1, may also be involved in thrombotic disease, their exact role remains to be clearly defined (48).

Homocystinuria. Homocystinuria is an inherited defect of amino acid metabolism that results in a syndrome of mental retardation, skeletal involvement, and visual problems related to lens dislocation and arterial/venous thrombosis. Elevated plasma concentrations of homocysteine may result from defective function of one of three enzymatic processes: cystathionine synthase (type I disease), methylcobalamin formation (type II disease), or methylenetetrahydrofolate reductase (type III disease). The homozygous state is characterized by the full phenotypic expression of the disorder, while the heterozygous state may be associated with a prothrombotic tendency without the other phenotypic changes of the disorder. Many of the studies to date have included the adult population in which elevated plasma concentrations of homocysteine have been linked to an increased risk of coronary artery disease and DVT. However, the increased risk may occur only in association with other risk factors for arterial disease, including smoking, hypertension, hyperlipidemia, obesity, and sedentary lifestyle. A unique feature of homocystinuria is that, depending on the enzymatic defect involved, the administration of pharmacologic doses of vitamin B_{12} or B_6 may provide effective therapy and control plasma levels.

Prothrombin Gene Mutation. Prothrombin gene mutation, also known as the *prothrombin mutation*, the *prothrombin variant*, *prothrombin G20210A*, or *factor II mutation*, results in the increased production of prothrombin. Approximately 2% of the Caucasian population in the US is heterozygous for the prothrombin mutation, with a much lower incidence (∼0.5%) in African Americans. It is rare in Asians, Africans, and Native Americans. It is inherited as a simple Mendelian trait. The heterozygous carrier state results in a relative risk of thrombotic disease (DVT or PE) of three to four times that

of the general population. The risk of the homozygous state, although assumed to be greater than the heterozygous state, has not been determined due to its relative rarity in the general population. Although the exact mechanism by which the prothrombin gene mutation results in a prothrombotic state is unclear, it is thought that the increased amount of circulating prothrombin acts to amplify the normal clotting cascade after initiation. The potential sequelae of the prothrombin mutation were investigated through a survey of pediatric hematologists. Data were collected on 38 pediatric patients with a thrombotic event and the prothrombin mutation. Thrombotic events involved both the arterial and venous circulations. Children with arterial thrombosis were younger, fewer than half had additional risk factors at the time of the event, and they had a high frequency of CNS involvement. Children with venous thrombosis were older, had additional risk factors, and had thrombosis most commonly in the extremities, although a significant number of events also occurred in the central venous and cerebral circulations. A striking predilection for CNS involvement (30% of all events and 67% of the arterial events) was noted. Fourteen of 38 children (37%) had CNS thrombosis. Unlike factor V Leiden and deficiencies of proteins C and S, which tend to lead to venous thrombotic disease, the prothrombin mutation in children is often associated with arterial thrombosis and CNS events (86).

Lipoprotein A. Lipoprotein A is a cholesterol-containing protein with a composition similar to that of low-density lipoproteins. Various studies have demonstrated an increased risk of coronary artery disease and stroke in adults with elevated lipoprotein A concentrations. Its role in venous and arterial thrombotic disease in children has also recently been suggested, with increased lipoprotein A concentrations (≥50 mg/dL) noted in 22% of children with arterial disease and 13.8% of children with venous involvement in one series (64).

Platelet Disorders. Although more commonly associated with a bleeding diathesis, rare platelet disorders may manifest as a prothrombotic state. They may manifest as peripheral venous/arterial thrombosis, but more commonly result in early myocardial infarction in otherwise normal coronary arteries. In the congenital Wein-Penzing defect, a defect in the lipoxygenase pathway leads to a compensatory increase in the COX pathway, with increased production of thromboxane, prostaglandin E_2, and prostaglandin D_2, thereby augmenting platelet aggregation. A second disorder, sticky platelet syndrome, may also be associated with premature coronary artery occlusion. Platelets from patients affected with this autosomal-dominant disorder show increased aggregation at lower concentrations of various factors (epinephrine, ADP) that promote platelet aggregation (13).

Diagnosis: Clinical Signs, Radiologic Imaging, Laboratory Studies

The clinical manifestations of thrombotic disease in infants and children vary depending on the site of involvement, the amount of the vessel occluded, whether the clot has resulted in embolic sequelae, and the vasculature affected (arterial versus venous). On the arterial side, the clinical signs and symptoms are relatively straightforward when total occlusion is present and include a painful, cold, pulseless extremity. When clinical signs and symptoms are apparent, they depend on the site of involvement, with the unilateral extremity swelling with extremity involvement, superior vena cava syndrome or chylothorax with superior vena cava involvement, and hepatomegaly and ascites with inferior vena cava involvement. When the vasculature of the CNS is involved (arterial or venous), the CNS manifestations may be subtle, as the classic manifestations of a stroke may not be initially evident. Loss of patency of a CVC may be the first indication of thrombotic disease. The development of collateral circulation may be the primary manifestation of the disease process when bleeding occurs from esophageal varices with splenic, portal, or hepatic vein thrombosis.

Radiologic Imaging

On the venous side, the manifestations are frequently more subtle and may remain asymptomatic, with the diagnosis made only by radiologic imaging. Although the venogram remains the gold standard for the diagnosis of thrombotic disease, it is invasive, difficult to perform in small infants and children with poor peripheral venous access, requires patient transportation to the radiologic site, and may require sedation or general anesthesia to perform. Additionally, various factors may account for a false-negative test. A partially recanalized vein filled with a thrombus may opacify normally with contrast even when the cross-sectional area of the lumen is markedly decreased. Mural thrombi may be missed in views taken perpendicular to the vessel wall to which the thrombus is attached.

Given their noninvasive nature and portability, ultrasound or echocardiography remain the primary techniques used to identify thrombotic disease, especially in the PICU population. A diagnosis of thrombus is made using Doppler ultrasonography to identify the following features: an echogenic filling defect, noncompressibility of the vein, loss of respiratory variability and vessel pulsation, and lack of flow or abnormal Doppler waveforms distal to the occluded segment. However, false negatives may occur, especially when the thrombus does not totally occlude the vein. The problems of diagnosing thrombi, especially when they involve the upper venous system, has led some authors to recommend ultrasound to evaluate the venous system of the neck and venography to evaluate the central venous system (60).

Given the drawbacks of the currently available techniques, alternative diagnostic tests are necessary to improve the diagnosis of thrombotic disease in infants and children. MRI, or more specifically, MR venography has become the most sensitive and specific test, especially for venous disease of the lower extremities and pelvis. An additional advantage of the MRI is that it frequently provides an alternative diagnosis for nonvascular causes of leg pain and edema. However, its utility is limited by its lack of portability, patient monitoring issues during scanning, and the requirement for sedation/general anesthesia to ensure a motionless patient.

Laboratory Evaluation for a Prothrombotic State

A high index of suspicion for an underlying prothrombotic condition should be entertained in patients who lack associated risk factors or comorbid diseases when thrombotic disease involves unusual locations (CNS, mesentery), with arterial occlusion, recurrent thrombotic events, and a family history of thrombotic disease in first-degree relatives. One study that eval-

uated the etiology of thrombotic events in children found that the incidence of protein S deficiency, protein C deficiency, or lupus anticoagulant was ~90% in children without an identifiable comorbid process or risk factor for thrombosis, compared with 50% in patients with identifiable risk factors (66). This study not only demonstrates the importance of screening for potential prothrombotic states in patients without apparent risk factors, but also stresses the potential role that the prothrombotic state may have on further increasing the incidence of a thrombotic event in patients with other risk factors.

Routine laboratory screening is rarely helpful in identifying a prothrombotic state; however, the presence of anticardiolipin antibodies or the lupus anticoagulant may be suspected when an elevated prothrombin or partial thromboplastin time do not respond to the addition of normal plasma (mixing test). The coexistence of thrombocytopenia in a patient on heparin therapy may suggest HIT. Thrombotic disease may be the first manifestation of a hemoglobinopathy, oncologic disease, or autoimmune disorder. When an inherited prothrombotic state is suspected, consultation with the hematology service may be helpful to arrange for the appropriate screening tests to identify specific reference laboratories that are able to identify specific molecular defects responsible for prothrombotic states. Many hospital laboratories offer a hypercoagulable panel, which includes the most commonly diagnosed prothrombotic states, including factor V Leiden, protein C/S deficiency, AT-III deficiency, prothrombin gene mutation, antiphospholipid antibodies, and elevated plasma homocysteine or lipoprotein A concentrations. The basic diagnostic approach to thrombosis in children is summarized in **Table 101.20.** For further information regarding the laboratory evaluation of a prothrombotic state, the reader is referred to the web site of the International Society of Thrombosis and Haemostasis and its link to Scientific and Standardizations Committee (www.med.unc.edu/isth/).

Treatment Strategies

Regardless of the disease process (inherited or acquired) responsible for the thrombotic disorder, primary therapy must include the elimination of comorbid diseases or associated conditions that exacerbate the prothrombotic state. In the perioperative period or in the PICU patient, these may include early ambulation, maintenance of adequate hydration, or the use of physical maneuvers such as sequential lower extremity compression devices. Additionally, elimination of medications such as oral contraceptive pills, avoidance of provocative factors (e.g., heparin in patients with HIT), avoidance of hyperlipidemia, and weight reduction may be beneficial. In the perioperative period, the use of adjunctive regional anesthetic techniques may be considered, although unlike in the adult population, their efficacy in reducing thromboembolic events has not been established in infants and children. Likewise, no guidelines exist for the use of intravascular coagulation filters in pediatric patients with risk factors that preclude anticoagulation.

Additional treatment options can be divided into acute treatment regimens in patients who manifest a thrombotic condition (these strategies are generally aimed at preventing thrombus extension and embolization), prophylactic strategies to reduce the recurrence of thrombotic events, and fibrinolytic therapies to dissolve a thrombus. When these therapies are used in

TABLE 101.20

DIAGNOSTIC EVALUATION OF
HYPERCOAGULABILITY IN CHILDREN

LEVEL I—Basic Evaluation
Basic hematologic test
  CBC with differential
    PT, PTT, fibrinogen
    Antithrombin III activity*
    Protein C activity*
    Protein S – free and total antigen*
    Anti-cardiolipin (anti-phospholipid) antibodies*
    APC resistance (factor V Leiden)+
    Homocysteine level*
    Lupus anticoagulant*
    Lipoprotein (a)+
    [HIT type 2*]

LEVEL II—Extended Evaluation
  Dysfibrinogenemia evaluation+
  (FDP, fibrinogen activity, thrombin and reptilase time,
    consider immunoelectrophoresis)
  Heparin cofactor II++
  Plasminogen activity++
  PAI: plasminogen activator inhibitor++
  If not previously performed:
    ESR, CRP
    Hemoglobin electrophoresis
    Fasting homocysteine level
    Functional APC resistance (modified assay for factor V
    Leiden)

LEVEL III—Under Investigation
  Factor VIII+
  Factor XII++
  Factor XI++
  Von Willebrand factor level++ and multimers
    [ADAMTS13*]
  Spontaneous platelet aggregation
  Tissue plasminogen activity
  Tissue factor pathway inhibitor

Level I tests are recommended in all children with thrombosis. Level II
tests are recommended in those children with normal Level I values
and/or in the settings of recurrent thrombosis or strong family history
of thrombotic disease. Level III tests are recommended in those
patients with normal Level I and Level II tests with a history of
recurrent thrombosis. [], indicates studies to be done when clinical
scenarios implicate their involvement; *, indicates high risk factors
with therapeutic and/or prognostic relevance; +, indicates lower risk
factors; ++, potential thrombotic risk factors.
CBC, complete blood count; PT, prothrombin time; PTT, partial
thromboplastin time; APC, activated protein C; HIT, heparin-induced
thrombocytopenia; FDP, fibrin degradation products; ESR, erythrocyte
sedimentation rate; CRP, C reactive protein
Adapted from Manco-Johnson MJ, Grabowski EF, Hellgreen M, et al.
Laboratory testing for thrombophilia in pediatric patients. On behalf
of the Subcommittee for Perinatal and Pediatric Thrombosis of the
Scientific and Standardization Committee of the International Society
of Thrombosis and Haemostasis (ISTH). *Thromb Haemost*
2002;88(1):155–6; and Schneppenheim R, Greiner J. Thrombosis in
infants and children. *Hematology Am Soc Hematol Educ Program*
2006;86–96.

the pediatric population, the risks of therapy must be weighed
against the risk of the disease itself. In the adult population,
therapeutic anticoagulation with Coumadin carries the risk of
hemorrhage of ~3% per year, with one-fifth of the hemorrhages being fatal. Although fatalities from thrombotic disease

(most commonly PE) have been anecdotally reported, the incidence and risk factors for such problems have not been clearly
defined in the pediatric population, and therefore, arriving at
definite recommendations for long-term therapy is problematic.

Prophylactic and long-term therapies include heparin and
warfarin preparations. Additionally, in specific inherited deficiencies (protein C or AT-III deficiency), replacement therapy may be indicated, especially in patients with homozygous disease in whom mortality is imminent without such interventions. Recommendations from the International Society
on Thrombosis and Haemostasis for the treatment of venous
thromboembolic disease in infants and children is similar to
that recommended for adults and includes unfractionated heparin (bolus dose of 75 U/kg, followed by a continuous infusion of 20 U/kg/hr for children and 28 U/kg/hr for infants).
The PTT is measured 4–6 hrs following the initiation of therapy and maintained at 1.5–2.5 times the normal range. When
long-term anticoagulation therapy is planned, oral Coumadin
is started at 0.2 mg/kg (maximum dose of 10 mg) and adjusted
according to the International Normalized Ratio (INR) of the
PT. Once a therapeutic level is achieved with warfarin (INR
= 2–3), heparin is discontinued. The effect of various anticoagulants on the coagulation cascade is demonstrated in **Figure
101.4.**

Heparin and Low-molecular-weight Heparin

Problems with unfractionated heparin include variability
in bioavailability and age-related pharmacokinetics, requirements for ongoing IV access for administration, delays in
achieving the desired level of anticoagulation, repeated blood
draws to monitor the PTT, and adverse effects, including hemorrhage. Given these problems, the trend has been toward the
use of LMWH in the adult population. LMWHs are prepared
by chemical or enzymatic treatment of unfractionated heparin.
Unlike unfractionated heparin, which acts against both Xa and
thrombin, the anticoagulant effect of LMWH is mediated only
via its anti-Xa activity. The initial data regarding the use of
LMWH in the pediatric population have demonstrated efficacy in the treatment of thromboembolic events, with reported
benefits over unfractionated heparin that include the option
of subcutaneous administration, predictable pharmacokinetics, a decreased incidence of HIT, minimal monitoring, and a
decreased risk of bleeding (27).

Heparin Alternatives

The most commonly used of the alternative anticoagulants
are the direct thrombin inhibitors (argatroban, lepirudin, bivalirudin). Argatroban is a synthetic molecule that binds reversibly to the active site of the thrombin molecule. It is primarily metabolized in the liver, with an elimination half-life
of 40–60 mins. Significant increases in the elimination half-life
are seen in patients with hepatic dysfunction. Unlike other direct thrombin inhibitors, argatroban undergoes minimal renal
clearance, and the plasma half-life is not prolonged in patients
with renal dysfunction. No reversal agent is available; therefore, argatroban's effects must dissipate gradually, which may
increase bleeding following procedures that use CPB. To date,
data are limited regarding the use of argatroban in infants and
children (30,54).

Hirudin is a direct thrombin inhibitor that is derived from
the medicinal leech *Hirudo medicinalis.* It is a 65-amino-acid

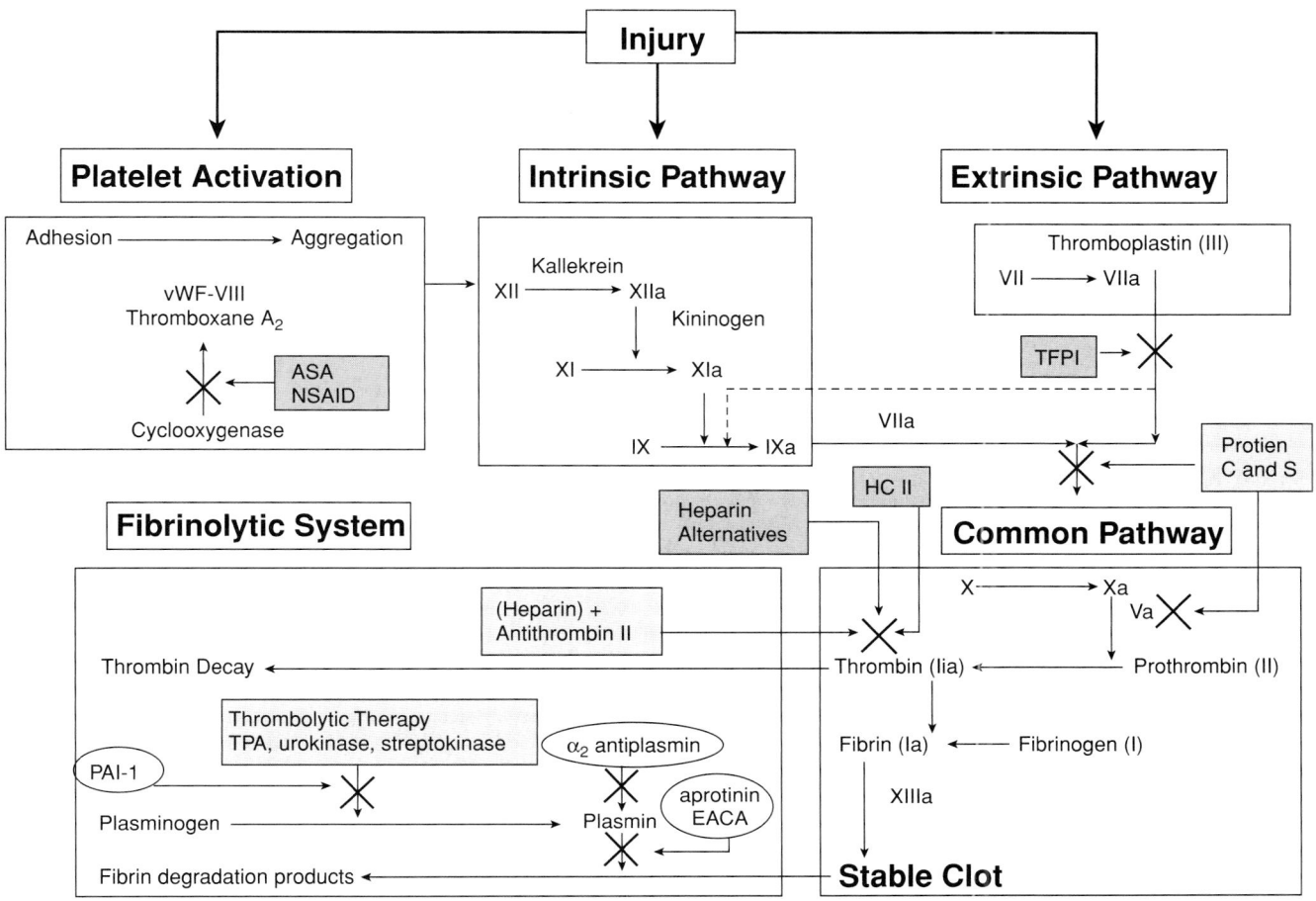

FIGURE 101.4. Coagulation cascade. "X" indicate sites of inhibition/inactivation. Anti-coagulants are indicated in gray. Protein C & S, antithrombin III, HC II, and TFPI are considered "natural anti-coagulants" (inhibitors). Anti-fibrinolytics are indicated in circles. PAI-1 and α_2 antiplasmin are "natural anti-fibrinolytics." vWF, von Willebrand factor; ASA, aspirin; NSAID, nonsteroidal anti-inflammatory drug; TFPI, tissue factor pathway inhibitor; tPA, tissue plasminogen activator; EACA, ϵ-aminocaproic acid.

polypeptide that forms an irreversible 1:1 complex with thrombin. Although originally isolated from the medicinal leech, hirudin is now produced by using recombinant technology, resulting in the r-hirudins, including lepirudin and desirudin. Only the former is routinely used in clinical practice. Lepirudin was the first direct thrombin inhibitor approved for use in Europe and the US for the treatment of HIT complicated by thrombosis. It undergoes renal clearance with an elimination half-life of ~80 mins in normal subjects, with significant prolongations in patients with renal insufficiency or failure. No reversal agent exists, although modified ultrafiltration has been used to enhance its elimination. Monitoring of its anticoagulant effect may be somewhat problematic, as the activated clotting time, PT, PTT, and thrombin time are all prolonged; however, the correlation between these tests and plasma concentrations of lepirudin is poor when larger doses are used, as for CPB. Current recommendations for monitoring include the ecarin clotting time. As with argatroban, information on lepirudin's use in pediatric patients is limited to case reports (42).

Bivalirudin is a drug modeled after the structure of hirudin. It is a synthetic 20-amino-acid peptide that consists of two hirudin peptide fragments joined together. Unlike lepirudin, the

binding of bivalirudin to thrombin is reversible. Bivalirudin has a short plasma half-life of ~25 mins and is cleared from the blood primarily by enzymatic breakdown by plasma proteases as well as renal clearance, with 20% of an administered dose recovered in the urine. Reduced clearance with renal failure mandates dose adjustments in such patients. As with the other direct thrombin inhibitors, no reversal agent exists. Hemofiltration has been used to reduce plasma concentrations of bivalirudin in cardiac patients after CPB. The most appropriate monitoring strategy for bivalirudin anticoagulation has not been established. The PT, PTT, INR, thrombin time, and activated clotting time all increase after the bolus administration of bivalirudin.

Fibrinolytic Therapy

The currently available thrombolytic agents include tissue plasminogen activator (tPA), streptokinase, and urokinase. These agents act by activating plasminogen to plasmin and augmenting the fibrinolytic system, which results in the degradation of fibrin. Given the high probability of recent streptococcal infections in pediatric patients and the risk of allergic phenomena, streptokinase is rarely used in infants and children. Although

TABLE 101.21

TREATMENT OF CENTRAL CATHETER OCCLUSION

Age/weight	Type of catheter and no. of lumens	Urokinase dose and volume	Alteplase (tPA) dose and volume
Newborn (birth–4 weeks)	Single-lumen Hickman	0.5 mL/2500 U	0.5 mg/0.5 mL
≤10 kg	Single-lumen Hickman	1 mL/5000 U	1 mg/L mL
≤10 kg	Double-lumen Hickman	1 mL/5000 U each lumen	1 mg/1 mL each lumen
≥10 kg	Single-lumen Hickman	1.5 mL/7500 U	1.5 mg/1.5 mL
≥10 kg	Double-lumen Hickman	1 ml/5000 U each lumen	1 mg/1 mL small lumen
		1.5 mL/7500 U in large lumen	1.5 mg/1.5 mL large lumen
Any weight	Small/low-volume Infusaport	1.5 mL/7,500 U	1.5 mg/1.5 mL
Any weight	Large/high-volume Infusaport	3 mL/15,000 U	3 mg/3 mL
Any weight	3.0 & 4.0 Fr. PICC	1 mL/5,000 U	1 mg/1 mL
Any weight	≤2.0 Fr. PICC	Manufacturer does not recommend declotting	

General Recommendations:
Urokinase or Alteplase (tPA) are the drugs of choice for bolus administration to indwell in the catheter. Length of time urokinase or tPA should indwell in catheter: 1st dose of urokinase or tPA should indwell for at least 2 hrs before blood withdrawal is attempted. After 2 hrs, attempts to withdraw blood may be made every 2 hrs for 3 attempts. The 2nd dose of urokinase or tPA should indwell in the catheter for 3–4 hrs before blood withdrawal is attempted. After 3–4 hrs, blood withdrawal should be attempted every 2 hrs for 3 attempts. If the catheter remains difficult to flush after 2 bolus urokinase doses or 2 bolus tPA doses, a 24-hr continuous urokinase infusion can be considered.
Urokinase and streptokinase continuous infusion doses:
a) The dose of streptokinase for a continuous infusion is 80 U/kg/hr (per lumen)
b) The dose of urokinase for a continuous infusion is 200 U/kg/hr (per lumen)
Note: tPA is not routinely utilized as a continuous infusion for catheter clearance due to limited data in pediatrics. The urokinase and streptokinase should be mixed in solutions of normal saline or dextrose and water for IV infusion. In patients with a recent streptococcal infection or signs and symptoms of an allergic response to streptokinase, an alternative agent is selected. Unsuccessfully declotted catheters should be considered for removal.
PICC, peripherally inserted central catheter
Adapted from Children's Center Care Protocol, Johns Hopkins Hospital.

urokinase found some utility in the pediatric population, its prolonged unavailability related to manufacturing issues led to the development of clinical experience with tPA and, although urokinase is now available in a recombinant form, it has seen little use other than for clearing of central-line occlusions (**Table 101.21**). Additionally, tPA only activates plasminogen that is bound to fibrin and, therefore, limits the fibrinolytic effect to the surface of the clot.

Experience with tPA in children is limited. A retrospective study reviewed the use of tPA for thrombolytic therapy in 80 children (65 arterial and 15 venous thrombi) (38). Dosing included 0.5 mg/kg/hr and was limited to 6 hrs in the majority of patients. tPA resulted in complete resolution of the clot in 65% of the patients, partial resolution in 20%, and no effect in 15%. Complications were noted in 40% of patients and included bleeding with the need for transfusion in 39%. Two patients suffered intracranial hemorrhage. Complications were more common in smaller patients, those with longer durations of therapy, those with a greater decrease in fibrinogen levels, and those who failed to have clot dissolution. No randomized trials have been conducted in the pediatric population on which to base decisions regarding the most appropriate applications of these medications. In general, thrombolytic therapy may be indicated when the risks of morbidity and morality from the thrombotic process outweigh the risks of thrombolytic therapy. Such instances may include arterial occlusions, especially in the CNS or where loss of limb is imminent, and thrombi within the cardiac chambers, which may necessitate a major surgical intervention with CPB for removal (56).

CONCLUSIONS AND FUTURE DIRECTIONS

Hematologic abnormalities are a common occurrence in the practice of critical care medicine. Recent clinical studies have improved our understanding and recognition of developmental and age-specific changes in the hematologic system. Although these age-specific parameters are complex, hospitals and clinicians should continue to make them readily available to assist in the recognition and diagnosis of common hematologic abnormalities such as anemia, thrombocytopenia, and low/high WBC counts. Future clinical and basic science research will continue to improve our understanding and recognition of relatively new disease processes (HLH and eosinophilic syndromes) and should provide for new and improved treatment strategies for affected children. Perhaps the greatest increase in our knowledge has occurred in the recognition of thromboembolic disease in children. Though recent consensus meetings have provided definitions and guidelines, continued research into the genetics, molecular basis, and pathophysiology of arterial and venous thrombosis in children will result in evolving recommendations and treatment approaches, especially for those with genetic predisposition and/or associated risk factors.

KEY POINTS

■ It is essential that the clinician understand the normal pediatric hemogram and common nonmalignant hematologic abnormalities in children with critical illness.

■ Most patients in the PICU will exhibit abnormalities of one or more cell lines, resulting in anemia, thrombocytopenia, and/or coagulopathy. Early recognition and consultation with a pediatric hematologist is prudent for directed evaluation, care plans, and follow-up beyond the ICU stay.

■ Treatment of common hematologic emergencies in the PICU is based on recognition of the underlying cause of these abnormalities, providing supportive care, and using clinical judgment on the initial therapeutic approach—whether pharmacologic, transfusion, or observation.

■ Clinicians should be aware of the increasing recognition, diagnosis, and treatment of HLH and eosinophilic disorders in critically ill children.

■ Thromboembolic events in children are attributable to genetic, disease, and risk factors that are associated with care of critical illness (HIT, CVCs, etc). PICU physicians should be familiar with the evolving recommendations for the detection and treatment of thromboembolism in children.

References

1. Amiral J, Bridey F, Dreyfus M, et al. Platelet factor 4 complexed to heparin is the target for antibodies generated in heparin-induced thrombocytopenia. *Thromb Haemost* 1992;68(1):95–6.
2. Andrew M, Brooker LA. Hemostatic complications in renal disorders of the young. *Pediatr Nephrol* 1996;10(1):88–99.
3. Andrew M, David M, Adams M, et al. Venous thromboembolic complications (VTE) in children: first analyses of the Canadian Registry of VTE. *Blood* 1994;83(5):1251–7.
4. Andrew M, Marzinotto V, Pencharz P, et al. A cross-sectional study of catheter-related thrombosis in children receiving total parenteral nutrition at home. *J Pediatr* 1995;126(3):358–63.
5. Andrew M, Paes B, Milner R, et al. Development of the human coagulation system in the full-term infant. *Blood* 1987;70(1):165–72.
6. Andrew M, Paes B, Milner R, et al. Development of the human coagulation system in the healthy premature infant. *Blood* 1988;72(5):1651–7.
7. Andrew M, Vegh P, Johnston M, et al. Maturation of the hemostatic system during childhood. *Blood* 1992;80(8):1998–2005.
8. Armano R, Gauvin F, Ducruet T, et al. Determinants of red blood cell transfusions in a pediatric critical care unit: A prospective, descriptive epidemiological study. *Crit Care Med* 2005;33(11):2637–44.
9. Beck C, Dubois J, Grignon A, et al. Incidence and risk factors of catheter-related deep vein thrombosis in a pediatric intensive care unit: A prospective study. *J Pediatr* 1998;133(2):237–41.
10. Bell WR. Heparin-associated thrombocytopenia and thrombosis. *J Lab Clin Med* 1988;111(6):600–5.
11. Bern MM, Lokich JJ, Wallach SR, et al. Very low doses of warfarin can prevent thrombosis in central venous catheters. A randomized prospective trial. *Ann Intern Med* 1990;112(6):423–8.
12. Beutler E. Glucose-6-phosphate dehydrogenase deficiency. *N Engl J Med* 1991;324(3):169–74.
13. Bick RL. Platelet function defects associated with hemorrhage or thrombosis. *Med Clin North Am* 1994;78(3):577–607.
14. Bick RL, Pegram M. Syndromes of hypercoagulability and thrombosis: a review. *Semin Thromb Hemost* 1994;20(1):109–32.
15. Blackman S, Ray JGD. Hematologic Emergencies: Acute anemia. *Clin Pediatr Emerg Med* 2005;6:124–37.
16. Bowie EJ, Thompson JH, Jr., PascuzziCA, et al. Thrombosis in systemic lupus erythematosus despite circulating anticoagulants. *J Lab Clin Med* 1963;62:416–30.
17. Calderon A, Wong JW, Becker LE. Multiple cerebral venous thromboses in a child with ulcerative colitis. *Clin Pediatr (Phila)* 1993;32(3):169–71.
18. Camitta BM, Storb R, Thomas ED. Aplastic anemia (first of two parts): Pathogenesis, diagnosis, treatment, and prognosis. *N Engl J Med* 1982;306(11):645–52.
19. Camitta BM, Storb R, Thomas ED. Aplastic anemia (second of two parts): pathogenesis, diagnosis, treatment, and prognosis. *N Engl J Med* 1982;306(12):712–8.
20. Chanarin I. Pernicious anaemia. *BMJ* 1992;304(6842):1584–5.
21. Clark DJ. Venous thromboembolism in paediatric practice. *Paediatr Anaesth* 1999;9(6):475–84.
22. Cornbleet J, Kessinger S. Evaluation of Coulter S-Plus three-part differential in population with a high prevalence of abnormalities. *Am J Clin Pathol* 1985;84(5):620–6.
23. Cote CJ, Liu LM, Szyfelbein SK, et al. Changes in serial platelet counts following massive blood transfusion in pediatric patients. *Anesthesiology* 1985;62(2):197–201.
24. Cranendonk E, van Gennip AH, Abeling NG, et al. Reference values for automated cytochemical differential count of leukocytes in children 0-16 years old: Comparison with manually obtained counts from Wright-stained smears. *J Clin Chem Clin Biochem* 1985;23(10):663–7.
25. Dallman PR, Siimes MA. Percentile curves for hemoglobin and red cell volume in infancy and childhood. *J Pediatr* 1979;94(1):26–31.
26. David M, Andrew M. Venous thromboembolic complications in children. *J Pediatr* 1993;123(3):337–46.
27. Dix D, Andrew M, Marzinotto V, et al. The use of low molecular weight heparin in pediatric patients: a prospective cohort study. *J Pediatr* 2000;136(4):439–45.
28. Drachman JG. Inherited thrombocytopenia: when a low platelet count does not mean ITP. *Blood* 2004;103(2):390–8.
29. Dror Y, Blanchette VS. Essential thrombocythaemia in children. *Br J Haematol* 1999;107(4):691–8.
30. Dyke PC, Russo P, Mureebe L, et al. Argatroban for anticoagulation during cardiopulmonary bypass in an infant. *Paediatr Anaesth* 2005;15(4):328–33.
31. Easley RB. Open air carbon monoxide poisoning in a child swimming behind a boat. *South Med J* 2000;93(4):430–2.
32. Edstrom CS, Christensen RD. Evaluation and treatment of thrombosis in the neonatal intensive care unit. *Clin Perinatol* 2000;27(3):623–41.
33. Fass RJ, Copelan EA, Brandt JT, et al. Platelet-mediated bleeding caused by broad-spectrum penicillins. *J Infect Dis* 1987;155(6):1242–8.
34. Fourrier F, Chopin C, Huart JJ, et al. Double-blind, placebo-controlled trial of antithrombin III concentrates in septic shock with disseminated intravascular coagulation. *Chest* 1993;104(3):882–8.
35. Geller RJ, Barthold C, Saiers JA, et al. Pediatric cyanide poisoning: Causes, manifestations, management, and unmet needs. *Pediatrics* 2006;118(5):2146–58.
36. George JN, Shattil SJ. The clinical importance of acquired abnormalities of platelet function. *N Engl J Med* 1991;324(1):27–39.
37. Gillman MA. Folinic acid prevents megaloblastic changes associated with nitrous oxide. *Anesth Analg* 1988;67(10):1018–9.
38. Gupta AA, Leaker M, Andrew M, et al. Safety and outcomes of thrombolysis with tissue plasminogen activator for treatment of intravascular thrombosis in children. *J Pediatr* 2001;139(5):682–8.
39. Hamamoto T, Yamamoto M, Nordfang O, et al. Inhibitory properties of full-length and truncated recombinant tissue factor pathway inhibitor (TFPI). Evidence that the third Kunitz-type domain of TFPI is not essential for the inhibition of factor VIIa-tissue factor complexes on cell surfaces. *J Biol Chem* 1993;268(12):8704–10.
40. Hathaway WE. Congenital and acquired defects in coagulation: diagnosis and treatment. *Mead Johnson Symp Perinat Dev Med* 1986;(28):45–54.
41. Hung OL, Kwon NS, Cole AE, et al. Evaluation of the physician's ability to recognize the presence or absence of anemia, fever, and jaundice. *Acad Emerg Med* 2000;7(2):146–56.
42. Iannoli ED, Eaton MP, Shapiro JR. Bidirectional Glenn shunt surgery using lepirudin anticoagulation in an infant with heparin-induced thrombocytopenia with thrombosis. *Anesth Analg* 2005;101(1):74–6.
43. Ishiguro K, Kojima T, Kadomatsu K, et al. Complete antithrombin deficiency in mice results in embryonic lethality. *J Clin Invest* 2000;106(7):873–8.
44. Jaffe ER. Enzymopenic hereditary methemoglobinemia. *Haematologia (Budap)* 1982;15(4):389–99.
45. Janka G, Zur Stadt U. Familial and acquired hemophagocytic lymphohistiocytosis. *Hematology Am Soc Hematol Educ Program* 2005:82–8.
46. Janka GE. Hemophagocytic lymphohistiocytosis. *Hematology* 2005;10(Suppl 1):104–7.
47. Kirchner JT. Acute and chronic immune thrombocytopenic purpura. Disorders that differ in more than duration. *Postgrad Med* 1992;92(6):112–8, 25–6.
48. Kohler HP, Grant PJ. Plasminogen-activator inhibitor type 1 and coronary artery disease. *N Engl J Med* 2000;342(24):1792–801.
49. Kohlhase B, Vielhaber H, Kehl HG, et al. Thromboembolism and resistance to activated protein C in children with underlying cardiac disease. *J Pediatr* 1996;129(5):677–9.
50. Korones DN, Buzzard CJ, Asselin BL, Harris JP. Right atrial thrombi in children with cancer and indwelling catheters. *J Pediatr* 1996;128(6):841–6.
51. Litman RS. Nitrous oxide: The passing of a gas? *Curr Opin Anaesthesiol* 2004;17(3):207–9.
52. Lubran MM. Hematologic side effects of drugs. *Ann Clin Lab Sci* 1989;19(2):114–21.
53. Makhoul RG, Greenberg CS, McCann RL. Heparin-associated thrombocytopenia and thrombosis: a serious clinical problem and potential solution. *J Vasc Surg* 1986;4(5):522–8.
54. Malherbe S, Tsui BC, Stobart K, et al. Argatroban as anticoagulant in cardiopulmonary bypass in an infant and attempted reversal with recombinant activated factor VII. *Anesthesiology* 2004;100(2):443–5.
55. Manco-Johnson MJ, Grabowski EF, Hellgreen M, et al. Laboratory testing for thrombophilia in pediatric patients. On behalf of the Subcommittee

for Perinatal and Pediatric Thrombosis of the Scientific and Standardization Committee of the International Society of Thrombosis and Haemostasis (ISTH). *Thromb Haemost* 2002;88(1):155–6.

56. Manco-Johnson MJ, Grabowski EF, Hellgreen M, et al. Recommendations for tPA thrombolysis in children. On behalf of the Scientific Subcommittee on Perinatal and Pediatric Thrombosis of the Scientific and Standardization Committee of the International Society of Thrombosis and Haemostasis. *Thromb Haemost* 2002;88(1):157–8.

57. Mannucci PM, Boyer C, Tripodi A, et al. Multicenter comparison of five functional and two immunological assays for protein C. *Thromb Haemost* 1987;57(1):44–8.

58. Marcum JA, Rosenberg RD. Anticoagulantly active heparin-like molecules from vascular tissue. *Biochemistry* 1984;23(8):1730–7.

59. Marlar RA, Adcock DM. Clinical evaluation of protein C: A comparative review of antigenic and functional assays. *Hum Pathol* 1989;20(11):1040–7.

60. Massicotte MP. Low-molecular-weight heparin therapy in children. *J Pediatr Hematol Oncol* 2001;23(3):189–94.

61. McDonald MJ, Turci SM, Bunn HF. Subunit assembly of normal and variant human hemoglobins. *Prog Clin Biol Res* 1984;165:3–15.

62. Medeiros D, Buchanan GR. Current controversies in the management of idiopathic thrombocytopenic purpura during childhood. *Pediatr Clin North Am* 1996;43(3):757–72.

63. Nguyen LT, Laberge JM, Guttman FM, et al. Spontaneous deep vein thrombosis in childhood and adolescence. *J Pediatr Surg* 1986;21(7):640–3.

64. Nowak-Gottl U, Debus O, Findeisen M, et al. Lipoprotein (a): Its role in childhood thromboembolism. *Pediatrics* 1997;99(6):E11.

65. Nsiri B, Gritli N, Bayoudh F, et al. Abnormalities of coagulation and fibrinolysis in homozygous sickle cell disease. *Hematol Cell Ther* 1996;38(3):279–84.

66. Nuss R, Hays T, Chudgar U. Antiphospholipid antibodies and coagulation regulatory protein abnormalities in children with pulmonary emboli. *J Pediatr Hematol Oncol* 1997;19:202–7.

67. Peddy SB, Rigby MR, Shaffner DH. Acute cyanide poisoning. *Pediatr Crit Care Med* 2006;7(1):79–82.

68. Ranze O, Ranze P, Magnani HN, et al. Heparin-induced thrombocytopenia in paediatric patients—a review of the literature and a new case treated with danaparoid sodium. *Eur J Pediatr* 1999;158(Suppl 3):S130–3.

69. Rapaport E. Thrombolysis, anticoagulation, and reocclusion. *Am J Cardiol* 1991;68(16):17E–22E.

70. Ravelli A, Martini A. Antiphospholipid antibody syndrome in pediatric patients. *Rheum Dis Clin North Am* 1997;23(3):657–76.

71. Rothenberg ME. Eosinophilia. *N Engl J Med* 1998;338(22):1592–600.

72. Sadowitz PD, Amanullah S, Souid AK. Hematologic emergencies in the pediatric emergency room. *Emerg Med Clin North Am* 2002;20(1):177–98.

73. Sagripanti A, Barsotti G. Hypercoagulability, intraglomerular coagulation, and thromboembolism in nephrotic syndrome. *Nephron* 1995;70(3):271–81.

74. Sallam S, Wafa E, el-Gayar A, et al. Anticardiolipin antibodies in children on chronic haemodialysis. *Nephrol Dial Transplant* 1994;9(9):1292–4.

75. Sandoval C. Thrombocytosis in children with iron deficiency anemia: Series of 42 children. *J Pediatr Hematol Oncol* 2002;24(7):593.

76. Sandoval C, Berger E, Ozkaynak MF, et al. Severe iron deficiency anemia in 42 pediatric patients. *Pediatr Hematol Oncol* 2002;19(3):157–61.

77. Schneppenheim R, Greiner J. Thrombosis in infants and children. *Hematology Am Soc Hematol Educ Program* 2006;86–96.

78. Seligsohn U, Berger A, Abend M, et al. Homozygous protein C deficiency manifested by massive venous thrombosis in the newborn. *N Engl J Med* 1984;310(9):559–62.

79. Smith RP. Chemicals reacting with various forms of hemoglobin: Biological significance, mechanisms, and determination. *J Forensic Sci* 1991;36(3):662–72.

80. Sutor AH. Thrombocytosis in childhood. *Semin Thromb Hemost* 1995;21(3):330–9.

81. Sutton SA, Assa'ad AH, Rothenberg ME. Anti-IL-5 and hypereosinophilic syndromes. *Clin Immunol* 2005;115(1):51–60.

82. Tabbara IA. Hemolytic anemias. Diagnosis and management. *Med Clin North Am* 1992;76(3):649–68.

83. Tollefsen DM. Heparin cofactor II deficiency. *Arch Pathol Lab Med* 2002;126(11):1394–400.

84. Vandendries ER, Drews RE. Drug-associated disease: Hematologic dysfunction. *Crit Care Clin* 2006;22(2):347–55, viii.

85. Walker ID. Prothrombotic genotypes and pre-eclampsia. *Thromb Haemost* 2002;87(5):777–8.

86. Young G, Krohn KA, Packer RJ. Prothrombin G20210A mutation in a child with spinal cord infarction. *J Pediatr* 1999;134(6):777–9.

CHAPTER 102 ■ BONE MARROW AND STEM CELL TRANSPLANTATION

KATHERINE BIAGAS • M. BRIGID BRADLEY • MITCHELL S. CAIRO

Transplantation of hematopoietic progenitor cells (HPCs) has been used increasingly for treatment of malignant and non-malignant conditions. For the pediatric intensivist, familiarity with the types of transplantation, preparative regimens, common complications, comorbidities, and medical emergencies that can occur is imperative. Transplantation patients may be brought to the ICU for commonly occurring critical conditions: respiratory failure, fluid and electrolyte disturbances, life-threatening infections, renal failure, and multiorgan dysfunction syndrome (MODS). Usual principles of management for these conditions apply, but additional factors that result from the transplantation or the underlying condition should be appreciated. Conditions more unique to the therapy, such as veno-occlusive disease (VOD) and graft-versus-host disease (GVHD), may result. Lastly, improved survival of patients after transplantation means that some complications will present long after the procedure and include infections, chronic organ failure, relapse of primary disease, or more severe courses of common medical conditions. The types of blood and HPC transplantations and the medical conditions that are associated with them will be reviewed in this chapter, with a focus on management of critical illnesses.

OVERVIEW OF BLOOD AND MARROW TRANSPLANTATION IN CHILDREN AND ADOLESCENTS

Blood and marrow transplantation has been successfully utilized in a variety of childhood and adolescent diseases, including malignant conditions, immune deficiencies, inborn errors of metabolism, genetic disorders, hematopoietic disorders, and autoimmune conditions. The most common childhood and adolescent malignant conditions treated with blood and marrow transplantation include acute lymphoblastic leukemia, acute nonlymphoblastic leukemia, chronic myelogenous leukemia, neuroblastoma, non-Hodgkin lymphoma, Hodgkin disease, and poor-risk brain tumors (**Table 102.1**). The most common nonmalignant conditions that have been successfully cured with HPC transplantation include sickle cell disease, homozygous β thalassemia, severe combined immune deficiency, Wiskott-Aldrich syndrome, and severe aplastic anemia (**Table 102.1**).

Hematopoietic-committed progenitor cells and their progeny are used in a variety of ways depending on the underlying malignant or nonmalignant conditions. HPCs have been used for therapeutic intent in at least six potential applications. Autologous HPCs have been successfully utilized to (a) rescue patients from prolonged bone marrow (BM) pancytopenia in a subset of children with malignant tumors following myeloablative therapy, (b) correct BM aplasia, (c) induce a graft-versus-tumor effect, (d) induce a graft-versus-autoimmune effect, (d) as gene replacement therapy for genetic disorders, and (f) as a vehicle for gene transfection and gene therapy (**Table 102.2**). Cure rates have varied from 10% to 80%, depending on the disease, type of HPC, condition and performance status of the patient, specific conditioning regimen, and comorbidities.

Sources of Hematopoietic Progenitor Cells

HPCs may be collected and obtained from BM, peripheral blood, or cord blood (CB). Three donor sources of HPCs exist, and the risks and benefits of each of the three subtypes are derived from the origin of the HPCs. Autologous HPCs are progenitor cells obtained from the recipient (self). Syngeneic HPCs are obtained from an identical twin and, therefore, are genetically identical between the donor and the recipient. Allogeneic HPCs are cells obtained from a human being other than a genetically identical twin (**Table 102.3**). Selection of allogeneic donors is determined by histocompatibility testing between the donor and the recipient.

Histocompatibility leukocyte antigens (HLAs) comprise a highly polymorphic, closely linked group of genes located on the short arm of chromosome 6 that regulate T-cell recognition and are critical to both immunocompetence and self-tolerance. The two major classes of HLA antigens include HLA class I antigens (A, B, C) and class II antigens (DR, DQ, DP). The preferred allogeneic donor source is a genotypic-matched sibling donor who usually matches at HLA A, B, and DR (six out of six match). Additional good allogeneic donor sources include related mismatched family members, including parents and other siblings who match at six out of six or five out of six antigens at HLA A, B, and DRB1. If a closely matched family donor is not available, two large sources of unrelated donors exist—unrelated adult donors and unrelated CB donors.

Only 25% of potential recipients have an HLA-identical related sibling or parental donor. Therefore, efforts have been made to develop alternative sources of HPCs for allogeneic stem cell transplantation (AlloSCT). The National Marrow Donor Program has established a computerized registry of potential volunteer adult donors and has over 8 million potential adult donors currently available for unrelated donor HPC transplantation. Additionally, a number of umbilical CB banks have been established throughout the world, and over 200,000 CB donor units have been cryopreserved and are currently available for unrelated CB donor transplantation. Recent

TABLE 102.1

CHILDHOOD AND ADOLESCENT DISEASES SUCCESSFULLY TREATED WITH BLOOD AND MARROW TRANSPLANTATION

Malignant diseases	Nonmalignant diseases
ALL, ANLL, CML	SAA, FA, SCID, WAS
Neuroblastoma, brain tumors	SCD, BT
NHL, HD, Wilms tumor	ALD, Hurler disease

ALL, acute lymphoblastic leukemia; ANLL, acute non-lymphoblastic leukemia; CML, chronic myelogenous leukemia; NHL, non-Hodgkin lymphoma; HD, Hodgkin disease; SAA, severe aplastic anemia; FA, Fanconi anemia; SCID, severe combined immunodeficiency disorder; WAS, Wiskott-Aldrich syndrome; SCD, sickle cell disease; BT, β thalassemia; ALD, adrenoleukodystrophy

results with unrelated CB donor transplantation have suggested that cell dose and HLA disparity are the most important predictors for outcome following unrelated CB donor transplantation. To date, the use of unrelated CB donor transplantation has been associated with delayed hematopoietic reconstitution, decreased severe acute GVHD (aGVHD), and decreased chronic GVHD (cGVHD) in children and adolescents (13,54).

Preparative Therapy or Conditioning

Prior to infusion of HPCs, most patients receive some form of conditioning or preparative therapy, usually consisting of myeloablative therapy, which commonly includes total-body irradiation with additional high-dose chemotherapy (chemoradiotherapy). Alternatively, in some settings of AlloSCT, a fludarabine-based nonmyeloablative conditioning regimen may be used (17,46). Myeloablative conditioning is uniform for autologous transplantation, in large part because of the need to eradicate any remaining tumor cells. The HPC infusion is usually used to rescue the patient from hematopoietic toxicity and to reduce the time to hematopoietic reconstitution. Common acute complications following myeloablative conditioning include mucositis, infection, bleeding, pain, nausea and vomiting, and aggravation of GVHD. However, some centers have initiated the use of nonmyeloablative conditioning to reduce the acute and long-term effects that usually follow the myeloablative approach. The practice of nonmyeloablative conditioning followed by AlloSCT is to provide enough immunosuppression to allow the allogeneic graft to be accepted

TABLE 102.2

RATIONALE FOR HEMATOPOIETIC PROGENITOR CELL TRANSPLANTATION

Dose Intensity for malignant tumor
Graft versus tumor
Gene replacement
Graft versus autoimmune
Gene therapy
Marrow failure

TABLE 102.3

SOURCES OF HEMATOPOIETIC PROGENITOR CELLS

Type	Source	Location
Autologous	Self (recipient)	BM, PB, CB
Syngeneic	Identical twin	BM, PB, CB
Allogeneic	Human other than identical twin	BM, PB, CB

BM, bone marrow; PB, peripheral blood; CB, cord blood

while decreasing the associated morbidities that commonly occur following myeloablative conditioning. This type of nonmyeloablative conditioning works best in selected diseases that have an unusual sensitivity to a graft-versus-tumor effect, diseases with a genetic defect, and diseases that may benefit from a graft-versus-autoimmune effect (17,46).

Collection of Hematopoietic Progenitor Cells

HPCs can be obtained from the BM, peripheral blood, or placental CB. BM HPCs are collected by BM harvesting, in which either the patient (autologous) or the donor undergoes general or regional anesthesia. Multiple BM aspirations are obtained from the posterior iliac crest (bilaterally) or, on occasion, from the anterior iliac crest. Each percutaneous BM aspiration is ~2–10 mL in volume, depending on the size of the donor. The total amount collected from a BM-harvesting procedure is usually dependent on the size of the recipient. Most autologous collections, which historically had been performed following BM harvesting, are now performed by apheresis. However, HPC collection from allogeneic donors still utilizes, to a great extent, BM harvesting.

Peripheral blood HPCs are harvested after the patient's or the donor's white cells are mobilized with cytokines, most commonly granulocyte colony-stimulating factor (GCSF) or, in the case of autologous collection, during recovery from chemotherapy combined with cytokine administration. Collection is performed by apheresis, in which multiple blood volumes are processed to extract a buffy coat layer that is rich in HPCs. Apheresis has the advantage of not requiring anesthesia and has a low rate of serious complications, although electrolyte disturbances and exacerbation of thrombocytopenia may result.

The third source of HPCs can be obtained at the time of delivery from placental CB. In the past, placentas and their associated umbilical cords were discarded after delivery. However, the umbilical CB is rich in HPCs, and a minimum volume of 60 mL may contain enough HPCs to engraft a recipient following myeloablative therapy. Today, over 200,000 CB units have been collected, screened for infectious diseases, HLA typed, and cryopreserved, and they are available for CB transplantation (9). Cell dose and HLA disparity are the two primary factors in the success following CB transplantation. Data suggest that two CB units can be combined to circumvent a low CB-cell dose from a single unit. Outcomes appear to be similar or better using two CB units as compared with a single, low-CB dose unit.

Processing Hematopoietic Progenitor Cells

HPCs sometimes require processing before infusion into the recipient. All autologous stem cell transplantation (AutoSCT) requires previous collection of HPCs from the recipient before myeloablation. As mentioned previously, HPCs may be collected by BM harvesting, peripheral-blood apheresis, or, on occasion, CB collection for future autologous use. To preserve autologous HPCs, cell processing must be performed for long-term cryopreservation. In the case of autologous BM or peripheral blood, the HPC product may be purged of potential tumor cell contamination. Purging may involve positive selection of early HPCs through CD34 selection, the use of monoclonal antibody with or without complement, or the use of chemotherapy. These purging techniques theoretically preserve the healthy HPCs and eliminate any microscopic residual tumor cell contamination. However, this processing may result in a decrease in total HPC count, thereby causing a delay in hematopoietic reconstitution. Autologous HPCs also require cryopreservation, which normally consists of 5%–10% dimethyl sulfoxide (DMSO) to protect cells during the freezing period and to ensure their viability during long-term cryopreservation. However, the addition of DMSO to autologous HPCs results in an increased risk of infusion-related reactions with anaphylaxis or even death.

Allogeneic HPCs usually do not require significant processing prior to infusion; however, under certain conditions, they do. On the rare occasion that infusion of the transplant is delayed from the time of collection, allogeneic HPCs may be cryopreserved and infusion may result in the same DMSO-related reactions. Additionally, allogeneic HPCs may require red blood cell depletion because of ABO incompatibility between the donor-allogeneic HPCs and the recipient. Depleting ABO-mismatched red blood cells from the allogeneic HPCs may prevent an ABO-related hemolytic reaction and may be life-saving. Lastly, allogeneic HPCs may be depleted of T cells to reduce the incidence of aGVHD. Transplants from haploidentical donors and/or HLA-disparate, unrelated adult donors are associated with a high incidence of serious aGVHD. Some require a depletion of total or subpopulations of T cells from the allogeneic HPC aliquot to prevent severe aGVHD. T-cell depletion, however, may result in a decreased incidence of or delay in hematopoietic reconstitution and is commonly associated with a delay in immunologic reconstitution and an increased incidence of Epstein-Barr virus (EBV)-related posttransplantion lymphoproliferative syndrome (PTLD).

HPCs derived from CB almost always require prior cell processing and cryopreservation, as they are most commonly collected from unrelated maternal donors who are located at distant sites. Traditionally, CB HPCs are depleted of red blood cells and then incubated with DMSO for long-term cryopreservation.

Infusion of Hematopoietic Progenitor Cells

Most recipients are premedicated with diphenhydramine and acetaminophen prior to HPC infusion. Usually, HPCs are in-fused through a central venous catheter. Infusion of HPCs may result in acute reactions, including fever, chills, tachycardia, bradycardia, hypotension, respiratory distress, allergic reactions, and on rare occasions, anaphylaxis. Furthermore, if the HPCs are contaminated with microbial organisms, HPC infusion may result in overwhelming infection. In the setting of ABO incompatibility, hemolytic reactions may occur. Patients who receive HPC products are closely monitored with vital signs at a minimum of every 5 mins during the infusion and are under the care of both a physician and nurse at the bedside.

Graft-versus-host Disease Prophylaxis

The setting of AlloSCT is associated with a measurable risk of the patient developing acute and/or chronic GVHD. GVHD most commonly occurs after AlloSCT; however, it can develop following AutoSCT, although the incidence is well under 10%. In the case of an AlloSCT, the development of GVHD requires the following three underlying risk factors: the recipient must have a depressed or abnormal immune system, the donor cells must be immunocompetent, and an HLA disparity must exist between the donor and the recipient.

Additional factors can contribute to the risk of developing GVHD, including type of allogeneic donor source, T-cell dose administered, age of the donor, age of the recipient, type of GVHD prophylaxis, underlying disease, type of conditioning therapy, associated comorbidities, risk of developing cytomegalovirus (CMV) disease, and many other minor factors. In general, the highest risk of developing GVHD occurs following mismatched or haploidentical family donor transplants. Adult donor transplants and unrelated CB transplants have a lower risk. The least risk occurs with transplants from matched, related family donors. Prevention of GVHD involves careful selection of family and unrelated donor sources and prophylactic therapies with carefully selected combinations of immunosuppressive medications. Previous GVHD prophylaxis regimens have utilized cyclosporine and methotrexate, and more recent regimens incorporate tacrolimus, mycophenolate mofetil, and sirolimus. Many combinations of prophylactic immunosuppressive therapies exist. While the administration of immunosuppressive medications may result in a decreased incidence or decreased severity of GVHD, such therapies also increase the risk of serious opportunistic infections. The delicate balance between the prevention of GVHD and an increased risk of developing serious opportunistic infections presents a serious challenge. Another GVHD prophylactic approach is T-cell depletion of allogeneic HPC donor sources, which results in extremely low incidence of GVHD after significant T-cell depletion. However, this type of cell processing also results in a delay or reduction in allogeneic HPC engraftment and, more importantly, a delay in immune reconstitution, with attendant increase in opportunistic infections and/or malignant relapse. It should be stressed that a delicate balance exists between overzealous T-cell depletion, which may eliminate the GVHD risk, and a less vigorous T-cell depletion, which may result in GVHD of reduced severity without a significant increase in serious opportunistic infections (11).

Supportive Care

Reconstitution of Hematopoietic Cells

Supportive care regimens are employed post-HPC transplantation to accelerate HPC reconstitution and prevent serious opportunistic infection. Hematopoietic reconstitution is accelerated using hematopoietic growth factors, either GCSF or granulocyte macrophage colony-stimulating factor (GM-CSF), and is performed after AutoSCT and AlloSCT. They are administered starting on day +1 after HPC infusion. While hematopoietic growth factors probably enhance the time to neutrophil reconstitution, it is not certain that the improvement in neutrophil recovery results in improved survival or decreased morbidity (12).

Preemptive or Prophylactic Treatment of Infections

The most common opportunistic infections that occur post-HPC transplantation include herpes simplex virus (HSV), CMV, *Candida* and *Aspergillus spp.*, and *Pneumocystis jiroveci* (formerly *Pneumocystis carinii*) pneumonia (PCP). Preemptive or prophylactic strategies are required. Prevention of HSV infections is dependent on the immunologic status of the recipient toward HSV and the use of acyclovir prophylaxis. Commonly, acyclovir is administered until the time of neutrophil reconstitution and recovery from mucositis. Fungal prophylaxis usually requires the use of fluconazole in AlloSCT recipients. Recent practice favors the use of liposomal amphotericin products to avoid possible nephrotoxicity. Two approaches have been utilized for the prevention of serious CMV infections. The preemptive approach uses CMV screening techniques with CMV antigen or determination of CMV DNA burden by polymerase chain reaction (PCR) and the administration of ganciclovir or foscarnet at the time of a rising CMV antigen load or DNA titer. An alternative approach has been the use of chemoprophylaxis with ganciclovir alone or ganciclovir alternating with foscarnet during the period of highest risk of CMV reconversion. Recipients who are CMV negative and who receive CMV-negative blood products do not require chemoprophylaxis but must receive leukodepleted or CMV-negative blood products post-HPC transplantation. However, patients who are CMV-positive and/or those whose donors are CMV positive require either a preemptive or prophylactic strategy. PCP prophylaxis is achieved with trimethoprim-sulfamethoxazole (TMP-SMX), starting at the time of hematopoietic reconstitution and continuing during the highest risk period of immunosuppression. A more thorough discussion of the treatment of infections, as well as additional comments on prophylactic or preemptive approaches, is discussed in later sections.

Additional Support

Additional supportive care includes the use of irradiated blood products, nutrition, IV γ-globulin supplementation, good oral hygiene and catheter care protocols, protective isolation, and other infection-preventive methods. A multidisciplinary team that includes pediatric bone marrow transplant (BMT) physicians, nurses, BMT coordinators, clinical pharmacists, nurse practitioners, dieticians, psychologists, social workers, child-life therapists, occupational therapists, physical therapists, and pediatric intensivists is required to provide supportive care throughout the pre- and post-BMT period. Moreover, when pediatric BMT recipients require intensive care, psychosocial support is required by patients and their families to help them cope during this stressful period.

RESPIRATORY FAILURE ASSOCIATED WITH TRANSPLANTATION

Clinical Presentation

Pulmonary complications represent a major cause of morbidity and mortality in patients who undergo HPC transplantation. Dyspnea, impaired gas exchange, and respiratory system dysfunction are common presenting signs in an HPC recipient who is admitted to the PICU. The many possible causes are generally classified as infectious and noninfectious etiologies (Table 102.4). Pulmonary function testing usually reveals that the dysfunction is restrictive in nature, often with a reduction in diffusion capacity and sometimes obstruction to ventilation. An estimated 40%–60% of the HPC transplantation population has demonstrable pulmonary dysfunction, with some patients remaining asymptomatic and others having long-term impairment (36). Risk factors for development of transplantation-related pulmonary dysfunction are listed in Table 102.5.

Mechanisms of Disease

Infections that Cause Respiratory Failure

Early Recovery Period. Pulmonary infections tend to occur in specific epochs. In the early posttransplant period, usually up to 3 weeks, patients are neutropenic and susceptible to bacterial and fungal infections, especially *Aspergillus* and *Candida* species. *Aspergillus* infections in this early phase may be particularly severe, with angioinvasive disease. Isolation from respiratory specimens, including bronchoalveolar lavage (BAL) is

TABLE 102.4

CAUSES OF PULMONARY DISEASE

Early recovery period
 Bacterial and fungal infections
 Sepsis
 Mucositis and upper airway obstruction
 Acute pulmonary edema
 Pulmonary vascular disease
  Diffuse alveolar hemorrhage

Mid-recovery period
 Cytomegalovirus pneumonitis
  Primary or reactivation
 Opportunistic infections
 Interstitial pneumonitis

Late recovery period
 Common childhood infections
 Cytomegalovirus reactivation
 Adenovirus infection
 Chronic graft-versus-host disease
 Bronchiolitis obliterans

TABLE 102.5

RISK FACTORS FOR DEVELOPMENT OF PULMONARY
DISEASE WITH HEMATOPOIETIC PROGENITOR CELL
TRANSPLANTATION

Transplantation after >1 year complete remission
Transplantation performed in advanced disease
Allogeneic stem cell transplantation
Cytomegalovirus seropositivity
Graft-versus-host disease
New intercurrent pulmonary infection with underlying
   lung disease

specific but not sensitive (57). BAL has a positive predictive
value of 82% (29). High-resolution CT is usually the study
of choice. If CT lesions are peripheral, a lung biopsy may be
considered.

Noninfectious complications of this early posttransplantation period, such as pulmonary edema and fluid overload, drug
reactions, and diffuse alveolar hemorrhage, may be superimposed on infection and worsen pulmonary function. Clinical
presentations of transplant-associated pulmonary infections
are similar to those of patients without transplantation—fever,
increased work of breathing, progressive respiratory insufficiency, and progressive hypoxemia with eventual respiratory
acidosis—however, the progression to respiratory failure is often quite rapid, and the severity of disease extreme.

Mid-recovery Period. In the second posttransplantation phase,
usually 3 weeks to 3 months post-HPC transplantation, viral infections predominate, particularly CMV infection. CMV
pneumonitis has a very high fatality rate that is higher in recipients of HPC than in those with solid-organ transplants.
Increased incidence of the disease is seen in certain subpopulations, namely, patients who are seropositive, are older, have
received total-body irradiation, or suffer from more severe
GVHD. Approximately 20%–30% of patients with GVHD
develop CMV pneumonitis. The use of leukocyte-depleted,
seronegative blood products has reduced the incidence of the
disease. Prophylaxis with ganciclovir or preemptive treatment
based on results of regular screening for pp65 antigenemia or
DNA detection in high-risk patients has decreased disease incidence. For demonstrated cases, the combination of ganciclovir
and CMV-specific immunoglobulin has reduced mortality dramatically.

Patients are also at risk for infections with other opportunistic organisms, particularly *P. jiroveci* in the first few posttransplantation months. The use of low-dose TMP-SMX (5
mg TMP/kg/day in divided doses every 12 hrs, 3 days/week
on consecutive days) or pentamidine (4 mg/kg given IV every
14 days) provides effective prophylaxis and greatly reduces the
incidence of PCP in this patient population. Actual PCP has become an infrequent event. For true infection, TMP-SMX is the
treatment of choice (15–20 mg TMP/kg/day in divided doses
every 6–8 hrs) (57). Pentamidine can be used in patients unable
to tolerate TMP-SMX. Confirmed cases of PCP should be investigated for antimicrobial resistance or noncompliance with
the prophylaxis regimen.

Late Recovery Period. In the late posttransplantation phase,
>100 days post-HPC infusion, noninfectious pulmonary com-
plications predominate, such as bronchiolitis obliterans (BO)
and cGVHD. Pulmonary infections in this phase tend to be
those that are more common in childhood. However, late CMV
infections may be seen, particularly in recipients of reduced-
intensity conditioning supported with peripheral-blood allografts or with the use of T-cell-depleting monoclonal antibodies and reduced-intensity regimens. CMV reactivation, as well
as adenovirus infection, should be considered in children who
have received these preparative regimens with late-onset, progressive, respiratory insufficiency.

Respiratory Failure from Noninfectious Causes

The hallmarks of noninfectious pulmonary diseases are interstitial disease, restrictive changes of respiratory system components, and chronic airflow obstruction consistent with BO.
These result from host responses to radiation and previous
cytotoxic therapy, especially as a consequence of the same
techniques used at the time of transplantation. Noninfectious
respiratory diseases include mucositis with upper airway inflammation and obstruction, pulmonary edema, pulmonary
vascular disease, interstitial pneumonitis, and BO. The first of
these will be discussed in greater detail later; however, it should
be noted here that extreme cases of oropharyngeal mucositis
may result in laryngeal edema, which may require tracheal intubation to maintain patency. Additionally, copious oral secretions and bleeding may occur and aspirate into the respiratory tree.

Pulmonary Edema. Pulmonary edema is one of the most common early complications of HPC transplantation and is associated with several causes. Large volumes of fluids are often needed to administer medications, minimize their toxicity,
and provide parenteral nutrition. Renal dysfunction is common. Additionally, cardiac dysfunction may be present, including congestive cardiomyopathy associated with the use
of anthracyclines and mediastinal irradiation. The necessary use of large fluid volumes in patients with such dysfunctions is often poorly tolerated, and pulmonary edema
results. Last, patients may have concurrent processes that promote systemic inflammatory response syndrome, such as systemic infection, pneumonia, or recent irradiation, exacerbating
pulmonary edema. The clinical manifestations are impaired
gas exchange, especially hypoxemia, and increased work of
breathing.

**Pulmonary Vascular Disease and Diffuse Alveolar Hemor-
rhage.** Clinically important pulmonary vascular disease is
rare, although many patients have subclinical abnormalities.
Pulmonary vascular involvement includes thromboembolism,
thrombus in situ, pulmonary VOD, and diffuse alveolar hemorrhage. Clinical signs are those of acute, congestive right heart
failure with hepatic engorgement, jugular venous distention,
tachycardia, and right ventricular heave. Pulmonary vascular
disease with diffuse alveolar hemorrhage may be especially severe and is an important cause of early morbidity and mortality. Diffuse alveolar hemorrhage occurs with reconstitution
of peripheral white blood cells, usually 1–3 weeks after transplantation. In addition to the clinical signs noted above, patients with diffuse alveolar hemorrhage present with progressive hypoxemia, dyspnea, and diffuse infiltrates on chest x-ray.
Hemoptysis is rare, although examination of BAL fluid demonstrates hemosiderin-laden macrophages and fluid that becomes

progressively bloodier with successive normal saline aliquots. High doses of corticosteroids (>100 mg/day of methylprednisolone or equivalent) may be effective in reducing mortality from diffuse alveolar hemorrhage.

Interstitial Pneumonitis. Interstitial pneumonitis is an important complication of HPC transplantation, usually developing 45–75 days after engraftment. In fact, interstitial pneumonitis is a major limiting factor of the success of transplantation and a major contributor to mortality in patients who have successful engraftment. Interstitial pneumonitis occurs predominately in patients who undergo total-body irradiation, although it may occur with conditioning regimens that do not contain total-body irradiation at all. Additional contributing factors include the use of methotrexate or cyclophosphamide (especially in combination with irradiation), severe aGVHD, longer interval between initial disease and transplantation, and preexisting lung injury, especially of the restrictive type. Concurrent infection, especially with CMV and, occasionally, bacterial or fungal species may contribute as well. The clinical hallmarks are fever, restrictive lung disease (tachypnea, dyspnea, retractions and grunting, and gas exchange abnormalities), and diffuse interstitial infiltrates on chest x-ray. Dose-response effects for both lung radiation and cyclophosphamide have been demonstrated. Reduction in the incidence of interstitial pneumonitis has been achieved with the use of fractionated radiation regimens (45).

Bronchiolitis Obliterans. Chronic GVHD plays an important role in the development of BO and is estimated to affect 10% of transplant recipients (31). In fact, BO occurs almost exclusively in this population, suggesting that the pathophysiologic mechanism is chronic rejection of transplanted cells by the lung. However, other nonimmunologic factors such as concurrent respiratory infection and prolonged methotrexate administration may contribute. Moreover, BO has been reported in autologous transplant patients and HLA-matched recipients, supporting the possibility of mechanisms other than rejection. Patients present with progressive dyspnea on exertion, nonproductive cough, and breathing patterns of obstructive disease, so-called *braking respirations* or *pursed-lipped breathing*. Pulmonary function tests reveal nonreversible obstructive airflow. Chest x-ray shows hyperinflation with or without infiltrates. Biopsy material shows occlusion of the lumens of respiratory and terminal bronchioles with inflammatory and fibrous material. In extreme cases, termed *constrictive obliterative bronchiolitis*, cicatricial scarring is present, with obliteration of distal airways. As disease may be patchy, transbronchial lung biopsies may not demonstrate the pathology. Open biopsy is required for pathologic confirmation of BO. However, most centers consider compatible history and symptoms, chest x-ray findings, and consistent findings on pulmonary function test to be sufficient in making the diagnosis. BAL is generally performed to rule out associated infection and confirm the presence of airway-infiltrating lymphocytes. Therapy consists of augmented immunosuppression and bronchodilators. Reversal of airway obstruction is usually only partial, and associated lung infection may worsen with the increase in immunosuppressive therapy. BAL is necessary to target antimicrobial therapy appropriately. Repeated studies may be required to follow the course of disease in severe cases.

Outcomes from Respiratory Failure

As stated previously, pulmonary complications of HPC transplantation are common. The final common pathways for severe restrictive lung disease of both infectious and noninfectious etiologies are acute lung injury and acute respiratory distress syndrome (ARDS). Obstructive lung disease may be superimposed, as with BO. Disease severe enough to result in respiratory failure tends to occur early in the posttransplantation phase. White cell reconstitution, especially with administration of GCSF, may increase the risk of developing ARDS (56). Patients present with fluid overload and weight gain, specific clinical signs of respiratory failure, and often, liver and/or renal dysfunction. In adults, the need for mechanical ventilation is associated with total-body irradiation and treatment with amphotericin B (47). Survival of patients requiring intubation and mechanical ventilation is uniformly low, ≤20% (30). Death comes from MODS. The likelihood of survival is nearly 0% in children who have dysfunction of more than one organ system after 7 days of mechanical ventilation (30).

Management of Respiratory Failure

Noninvasive Ventilation

The need for mechanical ventilation is a marker of illness severity. It is also, no doubt, a contributor to respiratory failure and death. Volutrauma, barotrauma, and oxygen toxicity add to lung injury. Ventilator-associated pneumonia, especially in the setting of profound immunosuppression, contributes to mortality. Advances in noninvasive ventilatory support, with either continuous positive-airway pressure or bilevel positive-airway pressure, may avoid some of these complications by avoiding endotracheal intubation. Normalization of gas exchange is not necessary; respiratory acidosis (generally pH ≥7.15) and moderate hypoxemia (SaO_2 ≥90) are usually tolerated. Close observation for worsened condition is an absolute. Intubation is reserved for patients with severe or progressive respiratory failure. Intubation may also be required to safely perform diagnostic studies such as BAL. In such cases, the need for the procedure should be carefully considered, and attempts should be made to extubate patients quickly, if possible.

Mechanical Ventilation

For patients who require intubation, aggressive measures should be used to quickly make a diagnosis. Empiric therapy for likely specific causes should begin immediately and be revised according to findings. Treatment of cardiac failure, supportive care for renal and liver failure, and management of fluid overload are important adjunctive therapies. Fluid management should be targeted to render the patient 10% dehydrated as long as cardiac output is maintained. Prone positioning and alternating prone-supine positions, may improve oxygenation. An "open-lung" strategy that limits ventilator peak pressures to 25 torr and tidal volumes to 6–8 mL/kg should be employed to minimize ventilator-induced injury. Positive end-expiratory pressure should be used liberally, and the fraction of inspired oxygen should be limited to ≤0.60, if possible. Again, permissive hypercapnia with respiratory acidosis and moderate hypoxemia (SaO_2 ≥80%) are tolerated. If adequate oxygenation cannot be achieved with such measures, consideration should be given to the use of high-frequency oscillatory ventilation, which may lessen ventilator-induced lung injury. Liberal use of high mean airway pressures, in this modality, may greatly improve oxygenation. Irrespective of the mode of delivery, the duration of mechanical ventilation should be as short as possible to minimize toxicity and the risk of ventilator-associated pneumonia; "pushing" patients off of such support to noninvasive ventilatory support should be an interim goal.

Controversies

Controversy surrounds the use of some of the more novel respiratory support modes in patients with severe ARDS, given their poor prognosis. As stated, mortality in such patients may be nearly 100%. No biomarkers or clinical signs allow clinicians to reliably predict those patients who will survive ARDS. Accordingly, some of the more novel modes of respiratory support have been tried in individual cases. No mode has been studied exclusively in children with HPC transplantation, and no mode has been adopted per se.

Alternative modes include surfactant, nitric oxide, and extracorporeal membrane oxygenation (ECMO). A clinical trial of the use of a modified bovine surfactant for patients with an oxygenation index of >7 included patients with HPC transplantation (see Chapter 46). Patients who received surfactant had lower risk of mortality and improved short-term oxygenation (61). Data in the subgroup of immunocompromised patients (10 of 22 with HPC transplantation and treatment with surfactant) suggested a lower mortality without statistical significance. Inhaled nitric oxide should be considered for patients with likely reversible, pulmonary vascular disease and demonstration of right heart dysfunction or failure.

A third modality is the use of ECMO, although few would advocate its use in this population. Generally accepted indications for ECMO are a transpulmonary shunt of >30% despite optimal ventilatory management or successive oxygenation index determinations suggestive of ≥50% risk of mortality. Contraindications for ECMO include those commonly found in patients who undergo HPC transplantation, namely, the presence of irreversible lung disease, terminal disease or poor functional status, or important ventilator-induced lung injury, generally considered to occur with 7–9 days of positive-pressure ventilation. Given the potential for serious complications, the expectation is that appropriate ECMO candidates have severe lung disease but not disease that is so advanced as to consist of end-stage pulmonary fibrosis or the inability of the patient to wean from this support. Few recipients of HPC transplantation meet such standards. Rather than such novel modalities, therapy for patients with ARDS after HPC transplantation remains largely supportive, with efforts focused on minimizing ventilator-associated damage, diagnosing and treating respiratory pathology, controlling fluid overload, and managing MODS.

RENAL FAILURE ASSOCIATED WITH TRANSPLANTATION

Clinical Presentation

Renal dysfunction and acute renal failure (ARF) are common sequelae after HPC transplantation. Approximately 25%–

50% of children have renal dysfunction in the first 3 months after transplantation, and ≥10% require renal replacement therapy (RRT), usually to control fluid imbalance. ARF contributes to mortality. An increase of serum creatinine by twofold or greater is associated with doubling of mortality for all types of HPC transplantation. Mortality is ≥80% in patients who require dialysis for correction of severe acidosis or electrolyte disturbances.

Early Renal Dysfunction

The causes of ARF in the early period (first 3 months) are numerous (**Table 102.6**). Often, multiple factors influence patient renal function. It may be difficult to determine the contribution of a single factor to the patient's overall ARF. Preexisting renal dysfunction may be present in children who have had cytotoxic therapy for their primary disease. Conditioning regimens may be additionally nephrotoxic. Special note should be made of patients with reduced glomerular filtration rate (GFR) and preexisting Fanconi syndrome or previous unilateral nephrectomy, as these patients do have a poorer prognosis. For the majority, reduction in GFR is the chief dysfunction, although specific correlation between pretransplant GFR and ARF has not been found (37).

Mechanisms of Disease

Nephrotoxicity with Infusion of Hematopoietic Progenitor Cells. In a few cases, nephrotoxicity is seen with HPC infusion. The mechanisms of injury are not fully known. Some speculate that release of free hemoglobin and cytotoxic products from cellular lysis during storage of HPC causes tubular obstruction and damage. The proximal tubules are particularly affected. In addition, infusion of the cryoprotectant DMSO has been implicated as a cause of hemoglobinuria, contributing to pigment-induced nephropathy. These insults occur on the background of preexisting injury and recent conditioning and may result in dramatic and immediate onset of ARF with acute tubular necrosis.

Sepsis and Acute Renal Failure. Sepsis, with or without hypotension, is a common cause of ARF. As many as 25%–40% of patients with sepsis in the early posttransplant phase develop

---

TABLE 102.6

CAUSES OF ACUTE RENAL FAILURE

Early period
  Preexisting renal disease
    Previous nephrectomy
    Preexisting Fanconi syndrome
  Nephrotoxic agents
  Infusion of preserved hematopoietic progenitor cells
  Sepsis
    Shock
    Hepatitis B or C infection
    Adenovirus infection
  Hepatorenal syndrome
    Hepatic veno-occlusive disease
  Indirect effects
    Obstructive hemorrhagic nephritis
    Treatment of acute graft-versus-host disease

Late period
  "Bone marrow transplant nephropathy"

ARF. The incidence is even higher in patients with culture-proven infection and requirement for RRT (37). Impairment of GFR results from maldistribution of blood flow, impaired cardiac output, and vasoparesis of the renal efferent arterioles. Frank shock may ensue with further reductions in GFR. Direct glomerular and tubular injury may be induced by cytokines and other inflammatory cascades. Although infection of the kidney is rare, renal abscesses, with fungal or gram-negative bacterial species, occur. And, infection with adenoviruses, especially BK virus, can cause primary nephritis. Hepatitis B or C infection may cause membranous glomerulonephropathy. Additional deleterious effects on the kidney are seen with nephrotoxic side effects of antimicrobial therapies. Although often required, antimicrobials such as vancomycin, aminoglycosides, amphotericin B, and β-lactam antibiotics require careful consideration when used in patients with already reduced renal function. Empiric courses of these antibiotics should be as short as possible. Medication doses and dosing regimens should be adjusted for the patient's creatinine clearance. Other conditions of sepsis may contribute. Hepatic dysfunction with CMV infection, sepsis, or hepatic VOD may lead to hepatorenal syndrome.

Hepatorenal Syndrome. The most severe form of renal disease in the early phase of transplantation is hepatorenal syndrome, characterized by hepatic dysfunction with poor GFR and sodium retention, with peripheral edema, weight gain, and ascites. Hepatic failure usually accompanies sepsis, GVHD, or VOD and is heralded by hyperbilirubinemia with mild elevations in serum transaminase levels. Patients also demonstrate a high urea:creatinine ratio. Patients are fluid overloaded with urinary excretion of small glycoproteins, suggesting proximal tubule and prerenal injury. Clinically, patients have pulmonary edema, hypotension, and preserved urine output, especially in the early phase of the condition. Urine output falls later and hypotension worsens. Severe hepatorenal syndrome is associated with a very high risk of mortality.

Rarely, other conditions may indirectly cause renal dysfunction. Hemorrhagic cystitis, although not generally nephrotoxic, may cause bladder obstruction and postrenal failure. Maintenance of brisk urine output is essential in such cases, and aGVHD, while not involving the kidney primarily, may require treatment, which may be nephrotoxic.

Late Renal Dysfunction

Late renal dysfunction, termed "BMT nephropathy," occurs more than 3 months after HPC transplantation and is especially found in patients with history of total-body irradiation. The incidence may be higher in young children than in adults, as the developing kidney may have less tolerance for total-body irradiation. BMT nephropathy is similar to hemolytic uremic syndrome or thrombotic thrombocytopenic purpura syndrome, with hypertension, peripheral edema, and microangiopathic hemolytic anemia. Renal dysfunction may be rapidly progressive with accompanying proteinuria and, sometimes, hematuria. Plasma exchange and immunoadsorption have been attempted for fulminant cases of BMT nephropathy (37), although the efficacy of such therapies has not been proved.

Management of Renal Failure

Therapeutic approaches for ARF are few. Care for the kidney is largely supportive. Prevention of injury or slowing injury

progression is important. The use of nephrotoxic antibiotics must be carefully considered, their use must be monitored, and choices must be made for less toxic preparations, such as the liposomal form of amphotericin B, when applicable. Chemotherapy should be adjusted in children with reduced GFR, as with the use of less toxic platinum derivatives, and renal perfusion should be preserved. Intravascular volume must be maintained, despite losses from vomiting, diarrhea, or "third spacing" of fluids. IV administration of fluid in excess of maintenance requirements, sometimes $\geq$2-fold greater than maintenance, may be required. The use of angiotensin-converting enzyme inhibitors, which can reduce GFR, should be avoided unless specifically indicated, as with BMT nephropathy. Heart failure should be treated, and hypertension controlled. Vigorous efforts should be made to identify underlying treatable conditions, such as sepsis, GVHD, or VOD.

Renal Replacement Therapy

RRT is a frequent component of the care of the critically ill child with HPC transplantation. The simplest RRT is vigorous use of diuretics with or without hyperhydration. In patients with normal urine output, especially those with requirements for large volumes of IV fluids, frequent doses of diuretics may diminish fluid overload while maintaining normal intravascular volume. Usual diuretics are the loop agents, such as bumetanide or furosemide, but others may be effective (**Table 102.7**). Both bolus administration and continuous infusion may be used. The latter is better tolerated in patients with hemodynamic compromise. In the oliguric patient, a trial of larger-than-standard-dose furosemide (2–4 mg/kg to a maximum dose of 200 mg) may be made; however, the potential for toxicity is greater (**Table 102.7**). Loop diuretics may improve renal blood flow and may reestablish adequate urine flow. However, if a single, larger dose of a furosemide is not effective, additional large doses are not warranted. Moreover, no indication exists for the use of diuretics—usual doses or larger doses—in the anuric patient.

A rarely used form of RRT is dialysis. Both peritoneal dialysis and intermittent hemodialysis are possible but not popular. Peritoneal dialysis requires placement of a peritoneal catheter, which is a port of entry for infection in immunocompromised patients. Hemodialysis usually requires that the patient be transported to an unmonitored dialysis unit, an undesirable move. Moreover, the rapid removal of large volumes of fluid with hemodialysis is rarely well tolerated.

In recent years, widespread use of extracorporeal continuous venovenous hemofiltration (CVVH) has been adopted for RRT (see Chapter 37). The therapy is easy to administer and flexible. Therapy can be tailored to achieve primarily fluid removal, hemofiltration, dialysis, some degree of solute removal, or any combination of these goals. Indications for CVVH in this population are anuria or severe oliguria, severe metabolic acidemia (pH <7.1), hyperkalemia (serum K >6.5 mmol/dL or rapidly rising), progressive dysnatremia, or coagulopathy that requires administration of large volumes of blood products. Early initiation of CVVH should be considered for patients with underlying electrolyte disorders, anuric ARF, Fanconi syndrome, or renal tubular acidosis.

Controversies

Controversy surrounds the use of CVVH as a treatment for sepsis and to improve survival from MODS. It is clear that this form of RRT is particularly effective at removing water.

TABLE 102.7

INTRAVENOUS DIURETIC THERAPY IN FLUID OVERLOAD STATES

Medication	Dose	Comment
Furosemide	Intermittent dosing: 0.5–1.0 mg/kg/dose every 6–12 hrs Trial of extremely large dose: 50–200 mg/dose Infusion: 0.3–1.0 mg/kg/hrs	May be ototoxic, especially at extremely large doses noted here. May increase RBF.
Bumetanide	Intermittent dosing: 0.5–2.0 mg/dose every 6–12 hrs	Similar to furosemide.
Ethacrynic Acid	Intermittent dosing: 0.5–1.0 mg/kg/dose every 8–12 hrs	Increases RBF and venous capacitance. Potentially ototoxic.
Chlorothiazide	Intermittent dosing: 1.0–2.0 mg/kg/dose every 12 hrs	Usually not useful when GFR <30 mL/min.

RBF, renal blood flow; GFR, glomerular filtration rate

Many centers use this modality almost routinely for early treatment of fluid overload states (8%–10% fluid overload). It is not clear that the attendant risks of extracorporeal circulation (heparinization, need for central vascular access, clot embolization, and blood loss with circuit thrombosis) are justified if fluid removal is the sole therapeutic benefit anticipated. Such risks are certainly in question when the same result can be achieved with diuretics. A rational approach would seem to reserve the use of CVVH for fluid control (a) to situations in which orderly fluid removal is advantageous, such as in the patient with compensated shock, or (b) to allow for more adequate support (blood product administration, parenteral nutrition, etc.) in patients who would otherwise require fluid restriction.

Based on evidence in preclinical investigations and a small case series (18), some have advocated the use of CVVH for its possible immunomodulatory effects—either from filtration of inflammatory constituents or mobilization of metabolic by-products and deleterious mediators. In such therapy, the goal is high-volume hemofiltration with total clearance rates of 4–6 L/hr. Clearance of small- and middle-molecular-weight substances is desired. While the presence of adverse biomarkers such as inflammatory cytokines can be measured in the ultrafiltrates of patients on such regimens, little evidence suggests that their overall outcome is changed. Given the risks of the therapy, such practice remains controversial.

FLUID AND ELECTROLYTE PROBLEMS

Mechanisms of Disease

Fluid Overload

Patients with HPC transplantation frequently have problems with fluids, electrolytes, and nutrition. Children may present to the PICU with ≥10% body weight gain due to fluid overload. As discussed, the causes are generally a combination of need for excess IV fluid combined with some degree of systemic inflammatory response syndrome, cardiac failure, and/or renal failure. Such fluid overload contributes to MODS, particularly to respiratory failure with pulmonary edema and effusions, and to congestive heart failure.

Electrolyte Disorders

Several disorders of serum electrolytes are seen in HPC transplantation. Electrolyte disorders can be seen without ARF, and certain abnormalities are common. Sodium overloading is a frequent occurrence, with the need for normal saline as a medication diluent or administration with total parenteral nutrition. Hyponatremia may be seen in patients with congestive heart failure due to activation of the renin-angiotensin system and release of atrial natriuretic factor. Treatment consists of reduction of fluid intake, rather than sodium supplementation. Hyponatremia and hyperkalemia may be seen with the use of tacrolimus, presumed to result from altered renal handling of univalent cations. Ifosfamide may induce phosphate wasting and Fanconi syndrome. Foscarnet can cause losses of all cations and phosphate.

Nutritional Disease

Parenteral nutrition is frequently given to patients in the peritransplant period. Reasons include anorexia, mucositis, and enteritis, which make ingestion difficult, and aGVHD, which causes gut dysfunction and loss of mucosal integrity. Patients may suffer from extended periods of vomiting and diarrhea. The use of total parenteral nutrition is associated with high cost, need for ongoing central venous access, fluid overload, hyperglycemia, biliary stasis and hepatic dysfunction, and enterocyte atrophy with loss of gut mucosal barrier. Even small-volume, non-nutritive feedings may ameliorate barrier dysfunction. Patients should resume enteral intake as soon as possible; generally, this is not accomplished until engraftment occurs.

With the association between hyperglycemia and poorer outcomes in some critically ill patients, relatively tight control of serum glucose levels is generally recommended. Insulin infusion is often required while patients are on total parenteral nutrition, with a target range of serum glucose levels of 90–130 mg/dL.

Nutritional supplementation with glutamine to preserve the gut barrier or enhance its function has been proposed. Glutamine is an essential component in the synthesis of the antioxidant glutathione. In non-cancer patients, glutamine administration has demonstrated improvement in gut integrity. Studies in patients who undergo HPC transplantation are limited in number and conflicting in results. While parenteral administration of glutamine decreased infectious complications and length of hospital stay in AlloSCT patients, poorer survival rates were seen in AutoSCT patients who received glutamine (4). Others have postulated that lipid supplementation is desirable to prevent essential fatty acid deficiencies secondary to malabsorption, while minimizing the use of carbohydrates and the risk of hyperglycemia and favorably altering immunologic responses in GVHD. Last, infusions of specific substrates to minimize intestinal toxicity have been proposed. Palifermin, a recombinant human growth factor, has shown promise in reducing severity of oral mucositis. Preliminary results with use of a glucagon-like peptide 2 analog suggest decreased gut breakdown in other intestinal conditions.

GRAFT-VERSUS-HOST DISEASE

Mechanisms of Disease

The incidence and severity of GVHD following AlloSCT depends on donor source, HLA disparity between donor and recipient, type of graft-versus-host prophylaxis, CMV status of donor and recipient, and age of donor, among others. The pathophysiology of aGVHD following AlloSCT is a three-step process in which interaction between innate and adaptive immunity occurs (22). Following intensive conditioning therapy, significant host tissue damage, usually in the gastrointestinal (GI) tract, leads to activation of host antigen-presenting cells by local release of inflammatory mediators and cytokines. During the second part of the process, host antigen-presenting cells present alloantigen to resting donor T cells, leading to donor T-cell proliferation, activation, and the secretion of inflammatory cytokines, including IL-2 and interferon-γ. In the final stage, donor mononuclear phagocytes and neutrophils induce systemic inflammation, which is triggered by mediators such as lipopolysaccharide that leak through the damaged intestinal mucosa. This inflammation promotes recruitment of donor effector cells into target organs, amplifying tissue injury with additional release of inflammatory cytokines and promotion of target tissue destruction by cytotoxic T lymphocytes (**Fig. 102.1**).

Clinical Presentation

GVHD is subdivided into hyperacute, acute, and chronic GVHD. Hyperacute GVHD usually occurs within the first

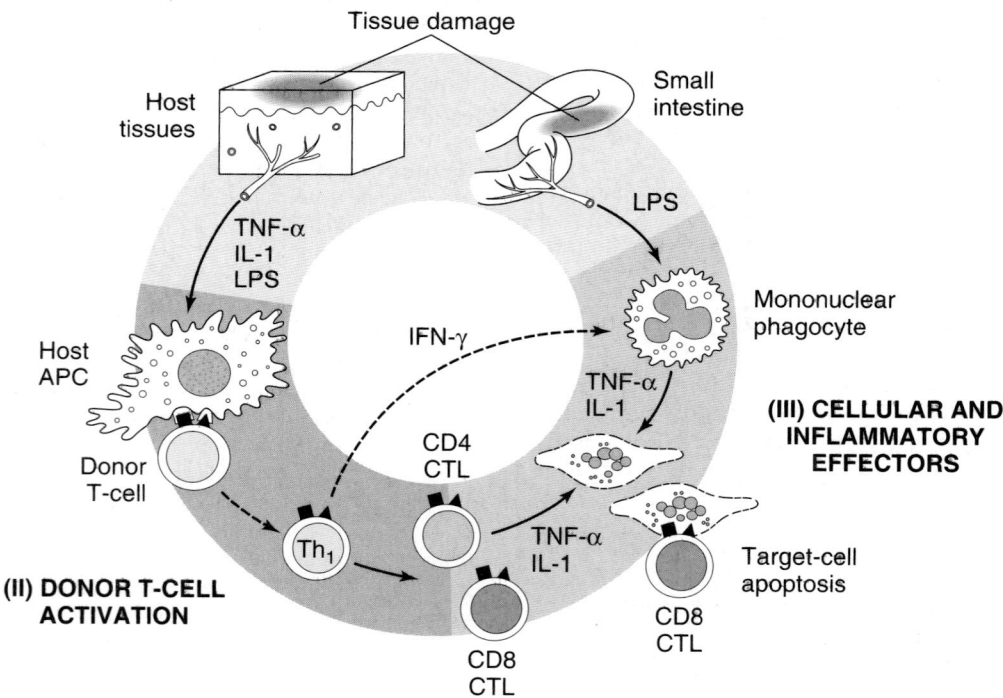

FIGURE 102.1. The pathophysiology of acute graft-versus-host disease (GVHD). GVHD is a three-step process: (**I**) Conditioning regimens (irradiation, chemotherapy, or both) lead to damage and activation of host tissues, especially the intestinal mucosa, allowing the translocation of lipopolysaccharide (LPS) and stimulating the secretion of the inflammatory cytokines TNF-α and IL-1 from host tissues, particularly macrophages. These cytokines increase the expression of MHC antigens and adhesion molecules on host tissues. (**II**) Donor T-cell activation is characterized by the predominance of Th1 cells and the secretion of interferon (IFN)-γ, which activates mononuclear phagocytes. (**III**) Effector functions of activated mononuclear phagocytes are triggered by LPS and other stimulatory molecules. Activated macrophages, along with CTL, secrete inflammatory cytokines that cause target cell apoptosis. CD8-CTL also lyse target cells directly. Damage to the gastrointestinal tract in this phase, principally by inflammatory cytokines, amplifies LPS release and leads to the "cytokine storm" characteristic of severe acute GVHD. This damage results in the amplification of local tissue injury and further promotes an inflammatory response. From Ferrara JLM, Reddy P. Pathophysiology of graft-versus-host disease. *Semin Hematol* 2006;43(1):3–10, with permission.

week after AlloSCT and before full HPC engraftment, but with early engraftment of donor T cells into targeted affected tissues, most commonly the upper and lower GI tract. Acute GVHD commonly develops between day +7 and day +100 following AlloSCT. Chronic GVHD is defined as GVHD occurring after day +100, and may be diagnosed as long as 2–3 years post-AlloSCT. Severe aGVHD (usually ≥ grade II) is a common cause of admission to the PICU for AlloSCT recipients.

Acute Graft-versus-Host Disease

Skin Graft-versus-host Disease. Acute GVHD involves three target organs: skin, liver, and GI tract. Skin aGVHD usually presents as a macular-papular rash that commonly involves the palms and soles and may be asymptomatic, pruritic, or even painful. The rash usually begins in the upper body on the face, arms, behind the ears, and shoulders in sun-exposed areas. It is graded into four stages, using the "rule of nines" to determine body surface area involvement for stages 1 through 3. Stage 4 is defined as generalized erythroderma with bulla formation (**Table 102.8**). Rarely is skin aGVHD, by itself, sufficient to require admission to the PICU; however, stage 4 disease requires management using burn protocols with support of fluids, electrolytes, and cardiovascular function.

The differential diagnosis of skin GVHD includes skin reactions secondary to (a) conditioning regimens or antibiotics, or (b) histopathologic skin manifestations of disseminated infections. In fact, severe skin aGVHD may be difficult to distinguish from Stevens-Johnson syndrome and/or toxic epidermal necrolysis. A major difference is the lack of involvement of the conjunctiva in skin aGVHD. A skin biopsy is required to document dermal-epidermal junction damage with evidence of epidermal and basal cell vascular degeneration, disorganization of epidermal cell maturation, or evidence of apoptosis.

Hepatic GVHD. The biomarker of acute hepatic GVHD is an increase in the serum bilirubin level, with staging based entirely on this level (**Table 102.8**). Patients with acute hepatic GVHD, particularly those with disease stages 2 through 4, commonly require intensive care monitoring and specific therapy (see later discussion). Hepatic GVHD is the most difficult form of aGVHD to treat.

The differential diagnosis of acute hepatic GVHD includes a number of diseases also associated with increases in serum bilirubin. During the first 30 days post-AlloSCT, hepatic VOD secondary to intensive conditioning may be difficult to distinguish from hepatic GVHD. Other diagnoses include drug toxicity, infection, cholelithiasis, and other sinusoidal obstructive syndromes. On occasion, a liver biopsy is required to distinguish hepatic aGVHD from these listed conditions. The biopsy usually demonstrates segmental destruction of small bile ducts, injury to periductular epithelium, cellular degeneration, and cholestasis.

Gastrointestinal Graft-versus-host Disease. Gastrointestinal GVHD presents as secretory or watery diarrhea, abdominal pain, nausea, vomiting, and anorexia. Severe intestinal GVHD may lead to significant mucosal damage with electrolyte abnormalities, protein-losing enteropathy, bloody diarrhea, and massive losses of fluid to the extravascular space. In stages 1–3, staging of GI GVHD is based on the amount of diarrhea per day (**Table 102.8**). Stage 4 GI GVHD is defined as severe abdominal pain with or without ileus and large amounts of secretory diarrhea.

Acute intestinal GVHD may be confused with a number of other conditions, including conditioning-related toxicity, infection (particularly with CMV), lactose intolerance, and other causes of damage to the intestinal tract. Biopsy may be required

---

TABLE 102.8

CONSENSUS GRADING OF ACUTE GRAFT VERSUS HOST DISEASE

	Organ/extent of involvement		
	Skin	**Liver**	**Intestinal tract**
Stage			
1	Rash on <25% of skin[a]	Bilirubin 2–3 mg/dL[b]	Diarrhea >500 mL/day[c] or persistent nausea[d]
2	Rash on 25%–50% of skin	Bilirubin 3–6 mg/dL	Diarrhea >1,000 mL/day
3	Rash on >50% of skin	Bilirubin 6–15 mg/dL	Diarrhea >1,500 mL/day
4	Generalized erythroderma with bulla formation	Bilirubin >15 mg/dL	Severe abdominal pain with or without ileus
Grade			
0	None	None	None
I	Stage 1–2	None	None
II	Stage 3	or Stage 1	or Stage 1
III	—	Stage 2–3	or Stage 2–4
IV[e]	Stage 4	or Stage 4	—

[a]Use the "rule of nines" to determine body surface area involvement.
[b]Range given as total bilirubin. Downgrade one stage if an additional cause of elevated bilirubin has been documented.
[c]Volume of diarrhea applies to adults. For pediatric patients, the volume of diarrhea should be based on body surface area.
[d]Persistent nausea with histologic evidence of GVHD in the stomach or duodenum.
[e]Grade IV may also include lesser organ involvement but with extreme decrease in performance status.
From Przepiorka D, Weisdorf D, Martin P, et al. 1994. Consensus Conference on Acute GVHD Grading. *Bone Marrow Transplant* 1995;15(6):825–8, with permission.

for diagnosis; usually, a rectal biopsy is performed. On occasion, gastric/duodenal mucosal biopsies are required to demonstrate upper GI tract involvement. Pathology includes mucosal ulceration, crypt destruction, crypt cell apoptosis, and flattening of the villous architecture.

Management of Severe Acute Graft-versus-Host Disease

The best strategy for severe aGVHD is preemptive—the best donor source should be identified and GVHD prophylaxis measures should be employed. Despite this approach, between 40% and 60% of patients will develop severe aGVHD ($\geq$ grade II). Most admissions to the PICU for severe aGVHD are for hepatic or GI tract involvement. In addition to supportive care, specific treatment usually requires systemic immunosuppression, most commonly with systemic corticosteroids. Additional immunosuppression directed against cytotoxic T lymphocytes and their inflammatory mediators (tumor necrosis factor-α), may be required. With severe intestinal aGVHD, patients may develop dehydration and electrolyte disorders. Managing fluids and maintaining electrolyte balance is crucial. With severe hepatic aGVHD, patients have progressive hepatic failure with ascites, poor nutrition, and coagulopathy. Therapy includes replacement of coagulation factors, treatment of hyperammonemia, portal venous shunting, and other hepatic support, as well as aggressive systemic immunosuppression (see Chapter 88).

Outcomes of Severe Acute Graft-versus-Host Disease

Grades III and IV aGVHD are associated with a high degree of morbidity and mortality, such that treatment with corticosteroids results in complete or partial response in only 50%–60% of patients. Only 25%–35% of patients develop complete resolution of aGVHD, even with therapy. Another 15%–20% improve, although usually with multiple exacerbations. Patients with aGVHD resistant to corticosteroids have poor long-term survival. Only 5%–30% of these patients will have a long-term cure (34,59) and will require increasing amounts of immunosuppressives, usually leading to serious opportunistic infections and death.

VENO-OCCLUSIVE DISEASE

Clinical Presentation

VOD usually presents with the triad of hepatomegaly, weight gain, and jaundice. It is heralded with the appearance of right upper-quadrant tenderness and hepatomegaly within 7–20 days after myeloablative HPC transplantation. Fluid retention usually manifests as peripheral edema, ascites, pleural or pericardial effusions, and measurable weight gain. Additional signs of liver dysfunction include hyperbilirubinemia, portal hypertension, and clotting abnormalities. Ultrasound and CT of the liver demonstrate hepatomegaly, ascites, and, most importantly, attenuated hepatic venous flow.

VOD should be differentiated from direct drug toxicity, liver failure from parenteral nutrition or infection, cholelithiasis, and systemic conditions such as sepsis. If symptoms are severe, or when the diagnosis is uncertain, liver biopsy may be helpful in differentiating the etiology. However, percutaneous

liver biopsy is associated with a high risk of bleeding due to the usual coagulopathy. Transjugular biopsy has a lower morbidity and is the procedure of choice, especially in the early posttransplant period.

Mechanisms of Disease

Chemo/radiotherapy injury to hepatic sinusoidal/venous endothelium and zone 3 hepatocytes induces the release of cytokines and other inflammatory mediators, resulting in the activation of clotting factors. Factor VIII, von Willebrand factor, and fibrinogen are deposited in the subendothelial zone of small venules, causing intravascular microvessel thrombosis. Thrombosis leads to hepatic congestion and ischemia, with additional hepatocyte damage and necrosis and a cycle of additional microvascular thrombosis. As the process continues, collagen deposition within the sinusoids, sclerosis of venule walls that progresses to obliteration of the venules, and further hepatocyte necrosis occur. Early microscopic findings in the liver include narrowing of terminal hepatic venules, subendothelial edema, necrosis of endothelium, engorgement and dilatation of sinusoids, and necrosis of centrizonal hepatocytes. In the most advanced stage, extensive necrosis and progressive fibrosis occur. The term *defrayed sinusoidal obstruction syndrome*, rather than VOD, has been used to describe this process.

Management of Hepatic Veno-occlusive Disease

Identification of high-risk patients and the initiation of prophylactic measures are important in the prevention and amelioration of hepatic VOD. Pretransplant risk factors include a previous history of elevated liver transaminases, poor performance status, active or advanced disease, prior hepatic radiation, prior myeloablative HPC transplantation, or previous treatment with amphotericin B, vancomycin, or acyclovir. When significant comorbidities and high risk of hepatic VOD exist, nonmyeloablative or reduced-intensity conditioning regimens are preferred. Pharmacokinetic monitoring of cytotoxic therapy, especially of busulfan, is important in VOD prevention. Close monitoring of fluid and electrolytes in the first 2 weeks after HPC transplantation and the avoidance of significant weight gain may prevent additional complications. Other prophylactic therapies include the use of ursodeoxycholic acid, a hydrophilic water-soluble bile acid, to prevent bilirubin and stone formation, and low-dose, low-molecular-weight heparin to treat microthrombosis.

The treatment for hepatic VOD, in large part, depends on disease severity. Mild VOD does not require medical intervention. Moderate VOD requires medical intervention but is reversible with little serious systemic toxicity. Severe VOD is associated with important systemic complications and a high mortality rate. The risk of developing severe VOD is based on the percent of weight gain, total serum bilirubin, and day posttransplant (5) (**Fig. 102.2**). For example, a 10% weight gain and a serum bilirubin of 6 mg/dL on day +1 is associated with a 60% risk of developing severe VOD versus a 10% weight gain and a serum bilirubin of 6 on day +10, which is associated with only a 30% risk (**Fig. 102.2**). The treatment for moderate and severe VOD includes close fluid and electrolyte

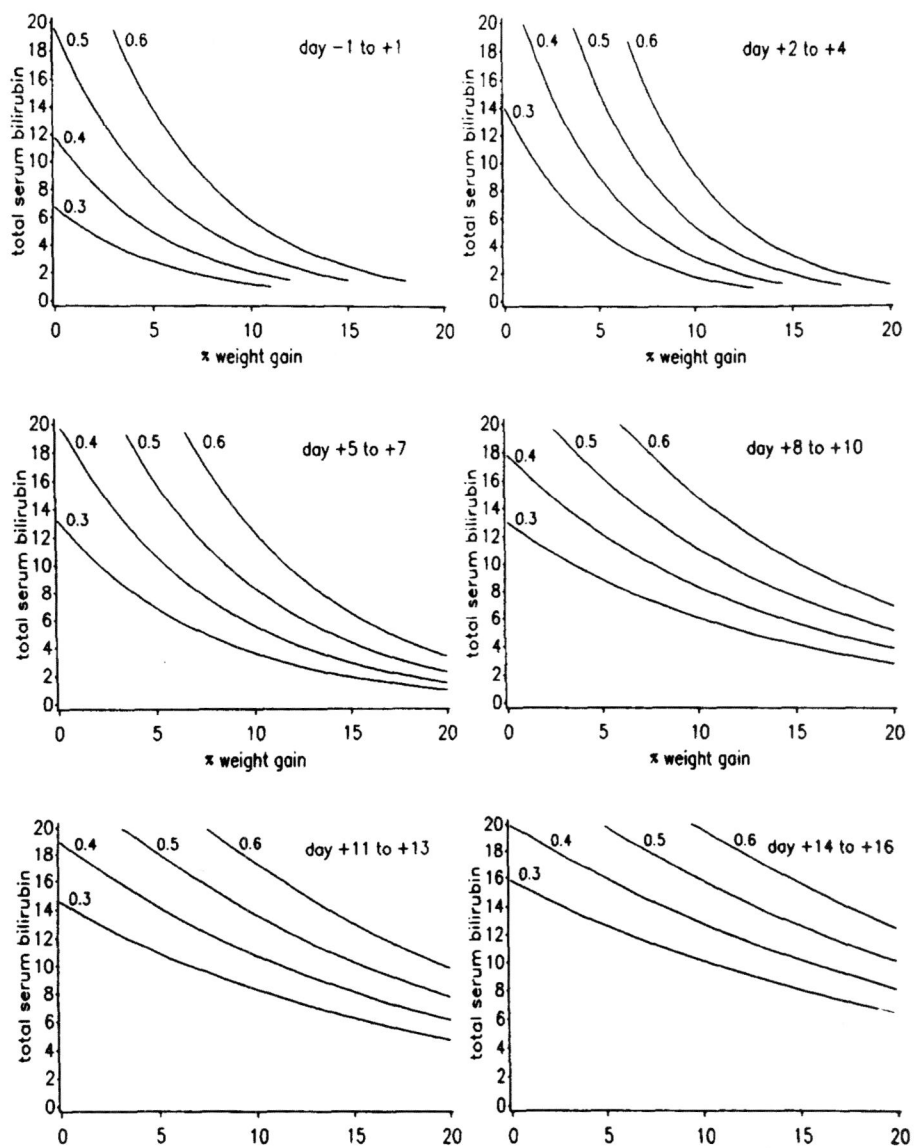

FIGURE 102.2. Risk of severe veno-occlusive disease based on percent weight gain, total serum bilirubin, and day posttransplant. Contour lines estimate probability of developing severe VOD as ≥30, ≥40%, ≥50%, and ≥60% using total serum bilirubin (mg/dL) and percent weight gain above baseline. If the plotted point lies above the probability line, the probability of severe VOD is or exceeds the probability of that line. From Bearman SI, Anderson GL, Mori M, et al. Venoocclusive disease of the liver: Development of a model for predicting fatal outcome after marrow transplantation. *J Clin Oncol* 1993;11:1729–36, with permission.

monitoring, aggressive use of diuretics, reduction of weight gain, and nutritional support. Thrombolytic therapies with recombinant human tissue plasminogen activator and heparin have shown some efficacy in treating patients with moderate-to-severe VOD. These therapies are frequently limited by the risk of severe or fatal bleeding, especially in patients with disordered coagulation. Other anticoagulant therapies have included human antithrombin III concentrate or activated protein C. Defibrotide, a single-stranded polydeoxyribonucleotide, has been used with moderate success in patients with moderate-to-severe VOD. Defibrotide binds to adenine C receptors A_1 and A_2 on the surface of vascular endothelium, thereby altering endothelial cell regulation and response to injury. Additionally, defibrotide has been demonstrated to increase prostacyclin, prostaglandin E_2 and thrombomodulin, and may decrease thrombin generation and inhibit fibrin deposition.

Patients who require transfer to the ICU for severe hepatic VOD usually have significant ascites with abdominal compart-

ment syndrome, weight gain, jaundice, portal venous hypertension, and hyperbilirubinemia. Other treatments with surgically or radiologically placed peritoneal venous shunts or transhepatic and intrahepatic portal systemic shunting have had some success. The shunting procedure, which creates a channel between the hepatic vein and the portal vein by percutaneous catheter insertion, has resulted in significant improvement in patients with severe ascites and coagulopathy. Occasionally, liver transplantation has been required to treat severe hepatic failure.

Outcomes of Veno-occlusive Disease

Nearly 100% of patients with mild VOD are cured and do not develop serious systemic toxicity. However, severe VOD has a high mortality rate, with as many as 30%–70% of patients dying. Severe VOD usually leads to renal and respiratory failure and MODS. However, patients with moderate-to-severe VOD who receive aggressive medical or surgical management usually do quite well, with almost 80%–100% being cured.

INFECTIONS

Clinical Presentation

Infection is a major cause of morbidity and mortality after HPC transplantation. The risk of developing infection is influenced by the type of transplantation, conditioning regimen, donor source, underlying disease, intensity of previous therapy, and other complications. Clinical examination, history, and microbial findings are important. Yet, diagnosis of an infection, especially opportunistic infections, may be difficult because of a lack of usual clinical signs and symptoms. Fever, usually the main indicator of infection, may be blunted by immunomodulatory treatment. Other signs, such as tachycardia, tachypnea, and organ dysfunction, should be considered as signs of possible infection. Sites with known risk, such as the perianal area, lungs, skin, central venous catheter exit sites, and oropharynx, should be assessed for any sign of infection. Workup should include blood cultures and cultures from any suspected site of infection.

Mechanisms of Disease

As discussed previously, three different risk periods are associated with post-HPC transplantation, each with its own unique immunodeficient predisposition: (a) early recovery (preengraftment phase, corresponding to the first several weeks after transplantation), (b) mid-recovery (early post engraftment phase, corresponding to the second and third months after transplantation), and (c) late recovery (the period beyond 3 months). In the early recovery period, neutropenia and alteration of mucosal and integument barriers make the patient susceptible to bacterial infections, which predominate in this period. In the mid-recovery period, the patient is susceptible to infection because of decreased cellular immunity, skin barriers compromised by central venous catheters, and disruption of the GI mucosal barrier due to GVHD. In the late recovery period, impaired mucosal defenses, chemotactic defects, functional asplenia, and qualitative and quantitative B- and T-cell abnormalities associated with cGVHD are seen. During the mid- and late-recovery phases, with recovery of the neutrophil count, bacterial infections are less common, and viral and fungal infections predominate. The spectrum of infections post-HPC transplantation and how they vary over time as the patient's immune status changes are shown in **Fig. 102.3.**

Bacterial Infections

The source of infection is usually from the patient's own colonized flora or from hospital- acquired bacteria. Bacteria account for >90% of infections during the neutropenic phase (62). Infections with gram-positive organisms are mainly associated with central venous catheters and severe mucositis; infections with gram-negative organisms occur with severe GI mucosal damage. In the neutropenic patient, infections with *Staphylococcus epidermidis*, *Staphylococcus aureus*, streptococcus species, *Pseudomonas aeruginosa*, *Escherichia*

coli, *Klebsiella* spp., *Corynebacterium jeikeium*, and *Bacillus* spp. often lead to serious sepsis. α-Hemolytic streptococci are increasingly recognized as a cause of sepsis in the neutropenic patient. *Streptococcus mitis* is associated with ARDS and septic shock (20). Infection caused by aerobic gram-negative bacilli, such as *Enterobacteriaceae* and *P. aeruginosa*, can cause overwhelming sepsis and toxemia in the neutropenic patient. The most serious localized infection in the HPC recipient is ecthyma gangrenosum, often caused by *P. aeruginosa* (40).

Viral Infections

Herpes Simplex Virus Infections. Viral infection is the leading cause of morbidity and mortality following HPC transplantation. Patients encounter viruses through exposure to the environment or reactivation of latent virus. The herpesviruses, including HSV, CMV, varicella-zoster virus, EBV, and human herpesvirus 6 (HHV-6), account for the majority of posttransplant viral infection (8). Pretransplant serology helps to identify patients at risk for HSV reactivation, which typically occurs up to 2 months after transplantation. Dissemination can occur, and mortality varies from 10% to 50%. Skin lesions may be atypical and present in unusual sites. Esophagitis is common, and pneumonia can develop. Isolation of the virus or positive direct immunofluorescence using monoclonal antibodies leads to diagnosis and aids in management (10).

Cytomegalovirus Infections. CMV commonly occurs 4–10 weeks after transplantation and can be life-threatening. With preemptive therapy, the disease is also seen after day +100. Pretransplant serology helps to identify patients at risk for CMV reactivation, but diagnosis is made by isolation of the virus or by detection of viral DNA by PCR. CMV infection occurs in ~60%–70% of CMV-seropositive patients or in seronegative patients who receive a transplant from a seropositive donor. Transplant recipients can have latent infection, active infection with replicating virus found in monocytes, or CMV disease with tissue damage. Active CMV infection manifests as fever, fatigue, leukopenia, hepatitis, colitis, myelitis, chorioretinitis, or pneumonia. CMV disease, particularly CMV pneumonia, is often fatal (39,64). The mortality rate for patients with untreated CMV pneumonia is as high as 85% and is 30%–50% in patients who receive specific therapy (64).

Other Viral Infections. Varicella-zoster virus infection, which can be seen from 4 months to 1 year after transplantation, develops as a primary infection or as reactivation of latent virus and is potentially lethal (10). Reactivation of latent virus can present as shingles or as disseminated disease. HHV-6 infection, although rare, manifests as encephalitis, pneumonitis, or graft suppression (63). Infection with EBV, typically in the first 6 months, also develops as either primary disease or reactivation and can cause B-cell PTLD (2), often a life-threatening disease. Patients with mismatched, unrelated, or T-cell-depleted transplants and those who receive antithymocyte globulin, alemtuzumab, or other anti-T-cell monoclonal antibodies are at a higher risk of developing PTLD (2). Patients present with high fever, lymphadenopathy, and sometimes diarrhea or elevated liver enzymes, depending on organ involvement. Adenovirus infection presents with diarrhea, hemorrhagic cystitis, and pneumonia and, when disseminated to cause hepatitis or MODS, is associated with a high mortality rate (55). Severity of infection correlates with the degree of immune dysfunction.

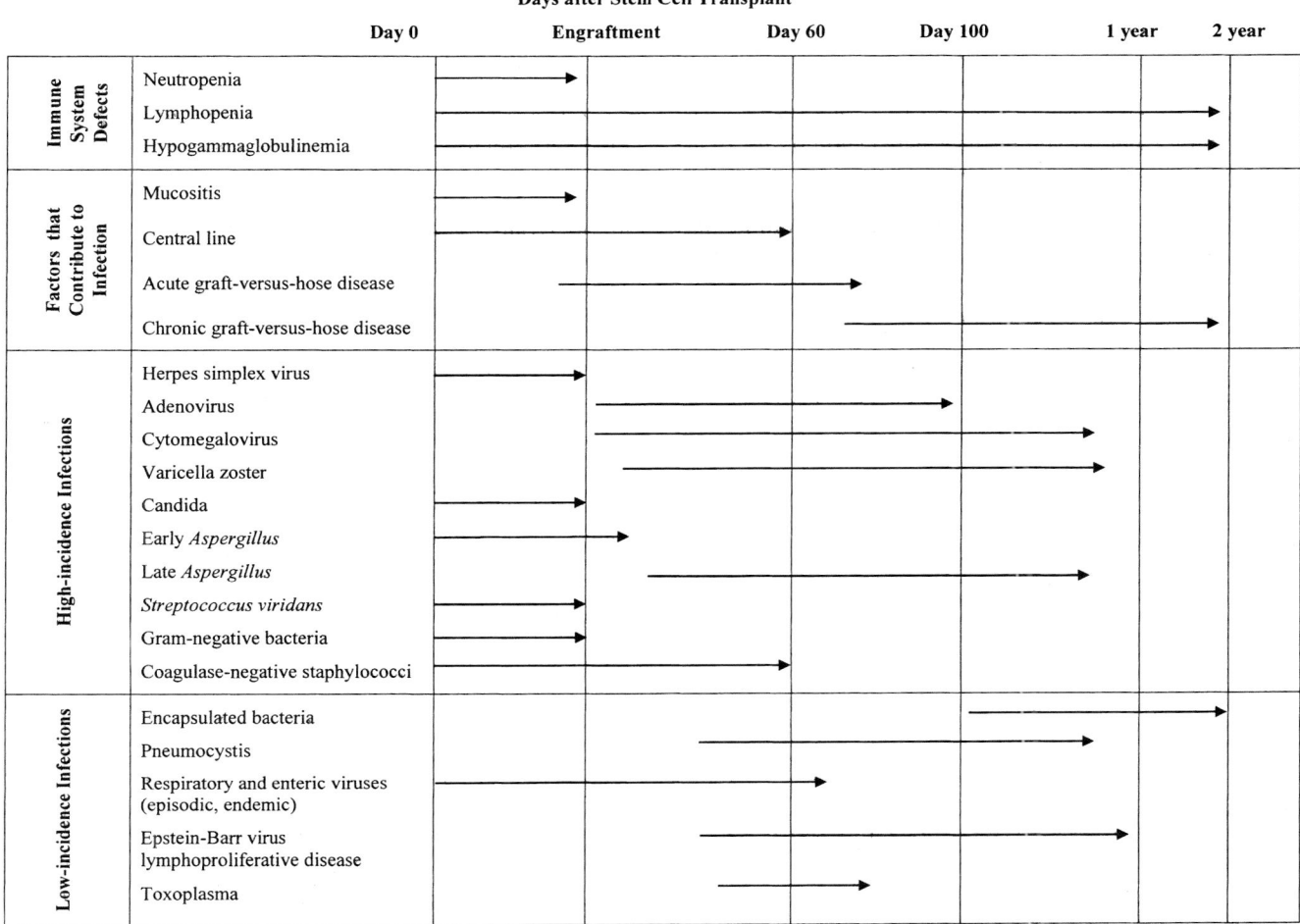

FIGURE 102.3. Types of opportunistic infections occurring in stem cell transplant recipients and the time period they are at the highest risk for these infections. Immune system defects and transplant-related factors occur at these time periods to contribute to infection. Adapted from Van Burik J, Weisdorf D. Infections in recipients of hematopoietic stem cell transplantation. In: Mandell GL, Bennett JE, Dolin R, eds. *Mandell, Douglas, and Bennett's Principles and Practice of Infectious Diseases, 6th ed.*, Philadelphia: Elsevier Churchill Livingstone, 2005;3486–97.

Diagnosis is made by viral culture from infected body fluids or tissue (excluding the GI tract) by direct antigen detection or by molecular methods (55). Viremia strongly predicts disseminated disease (55). Adenovirus infection develops from reactivation of latent virus or, commonly, in young children with primary infection contracted by contact. Infections with respiratory syncytial virus, influenza A and B, or parainfluenza infection occur seasonally and coincide with community outbreaks. Respiratory syncytial virus affects up to 1%–3% of transplant recipients (60) and carries a mortality rate as high as 50% in patients who develop lower-tract disease (60).

Fungal Infections

Risk factors for invasive fungal disease include neutropenia, HLA-mismatched transplant, GVHD or its treatment, steroid therapy, and graft failure. Signs and symptoms of fungal infection are often absent or nonspecific and include fever unresponsive to antibiotics. Making the diagnosis of invasive fungal infection is the single most important limitation to successful treatment. Diagnosis relies on culture of the organism from a sterile site or identification by histologic methods. Serum anti-gens can be detected in select situations, such as detection of cryptococcal antigen. Galactomannan antigen can be detected in *Aspergillus* infection (57).

Candida and *Aspergillus* are the most common opportunistic fungal organisms isolated, but other emerging pathogens have been reported (57). A shift has occurred in the incidence of *Candida* infections, with a decrease in *Candida albicans* and an emergence of non-albicans species, such as *C. tropicalis, C. parapsilosis, C. glabrata,* and *C. krusei* (57). *Candida* infections may be superficial, mucocutaneous, or deep-seated. *C. albicans* and *C. tropicalis* are known causes of disseminated candidiasis and are associated with high mortality (57). *C. parapsilosis,* a catheter-associated yeast, rarely disseminates systemically (57). Hepatosplenic candidiasis commonly presents during neutrophil regeneration. *Aspergillus* is the leading cause of death from infection after AlloSCT. *Aspergillus* species such as *A. fumigatus, A. flavus,* and *A. niger,* cause invasive disease, predominately during the neutropenic period (7). The primary site for *Aspergillus* infection is the lung. Such infection often presents as invasive, pulmonary aspergillosis with thrombotic and hemorrhagic lung disease. Dissemination to the brain, liver, and skin is common. Cutaneous lesions, also known as ecthyma gangrenosum, are a common manifestation of disseminated disease that carries a high mortality. Serious infections with other fungal species may be seen as well in transplant recipients. Cryptococcosis is rare and most often results in meningitis or pulmonary infection (57). Zygomycosis or mucormycosis often present as sinusoidal disease, but pulmonary and disseminated disease may occur (7,57). Corticosteroid use and active GVHD increase the risk of opportunistic fungal infections.

Pneumocystis jiroveci (P. carinii) Infections

Pneumocystis jiroveci (formerly known as *P. carinii*) pneumonia, a protozoan infection, occurs postengraftment. Patients present with progressive dyspnea with a dry cough but can also present with a fulminant course. Hypoxia is present in >90% of patients at presentation (57). Chest x-ray often show interstitial acinar infiltrates. BAL is the preferred diagnostic test. Giemsa and Gomori methenamine silver staining, although simple to perform, is relatively insensitive. Molecular diagnosis by PCR is highly sensitive and specific and should be used when available.

Mycobacterium Infections

Tuberculous and nontuberculous *Mycobacterium* infections, although infrequent in HPC transplantation recipients, are being identified and reported more commonly. Increased recognition may be due to better detection methods or increased susceptibility of recipients because of greater use of alternate donors, necessitating increased immunosuppression (16). Diagnosis is difficult because of the lag in development of symptoms and isolation of the organism. *Mycobacterium* infection can occur at any time after transplantation. Patients often present with fever, pneumonia, and in some instances, diarrhea. Primary skin infection and central nervous system disease have been reported (16).

Differential Diagnosis

Correct identification of an infection in an HPC-transplantation recipient is a critical management issue. Early identification of the specific infection and institution of appropriate therapy may greatly decrease a patient's risk of mortality and serious morbidity; alternatively, determination of the absence of infection and appropriate discontinuation of empiric antimicrobial therapies minimizes drug toxicity and the presence of resistant organisms. Clinical signs and symptoms of infection in the HPC-transplantation patient are numerous and often nonspecific. Fever, sometimes the only sign of infection in this patient population, can also result from medication reactions, systemic inflammatory response syndrome, or ARDS. Diarrhea, a common manifestation of intestinal infection, is also the common presenting symptom of intestinal GVHD, drug toxicities, and mucositis/enteritis. Hyperbilirubinemia and elevation of serum transaminase levels, a common manifestation of many infections, also occurs with VOD, medication toxicity, cholelithiasis, and GVHD. Rash or skin lesions may also be due to drug reactions or GVHD. Even sepsis, which often presents with high spiking fevers, tachycardia, and hypotension, shares symptoms with infusion reactions or engraftment syndrome, in which patients have a release of cytokines at the time of engraftment.

Management of Infections

A number of advances in infection control and supportive care have improved outcome. Prophylactic or preemptive therapies have reduced the incidence, morbidity, and mortality associated with most infections. Empiric therapy started at the onset of fever and new antimicrobial agents improve outcome. The choice of antibacterial regimen depends on the presentation of infection and the resistance patterns of the organism in a particular institution. When the infecting organism is identified and sensitivities are available, treatment should be tailored to treat the specific infection. While a complete discussion of the use of antimicrobials in HPC recipients is beyond the scope of this chapter, some specific recommendations should be noted.

Treatment of Viral Infections

Acyclovir is the drug of choice in the treatment of HSV and varicella-zoster virus infections. The value of oral or IV acyclovir prophylaxis in HSV seropositive patients is well established. Immunocompromised patients exposed to varicella-zoster virus should receive zoster immunoglobulin to confer passive immunity (57). Ganciclovir, foscarnet, and cidofovir have all been reported as effective therapies against infection with HHV-6 (63). No controlled, randomized studies have been conducted that demonstrate that one therapy is more effective than any other (63). Treatment of EBV PTLD involves antibody therapy with rituximab and donor-derived cytotoxic T cells (2). No specific therapy has been identified for adenovirus infection; however, some have reported that cidofovir is successful (32,55). Reports have shown that 20 of 29 HPC transplantation patients with adenovirus disease responded to cidofovir therapy (32).

Some specific issues should be noted with respect to CMV exposure and disease. Prophylactic or preemptive approaches to those patients at risk for CMV reactivation has reduced the incidence of infection and disease and resulted in a significant reduction in mortality (57). For seronegative patients who receive transplants from seronegative donors, the use of CMV-negative blood products will suffice. For seropositive patients or seronegative patients who receive a transplant from a seropositive donor, intervention is required. CMV disease can be prevented by prophylactic administration of antiviral medication or preemptive early intervention in which treatment is started when antigenemia or evidence of viral replication is observed (57,64). Ganciclovir and foscarnet are effective in preventing and treating CMV. The use of ganciclovir in combination with foscarnet and high-dose IV immune globulin was associated with a 50% survival rate in patients with acute CMV infection (26). Prophylaxis with either ganciclovir or foscarnet has reduced the incidence and severity of CMV infection in CMV-seropositive patients (57,64). Lastly, it is the lack of CMV specific T-cell responses that places the patient at risk for recurrence of CMV disease or persistent disease. Some centers have shown that the adoptive transfer of CMV-specific T cells restores immunity and is effective treatment (19).

Adenovirus infection is associated with almost uniformly fatal disease. Adenovirus reactivates without clinical symptoms. With newer methods for rapid, early detection, some investigators believe that preemptive treatment will be most effective. Others are investigating an immunotherapeutic approach using adenoviral-specific cytotoxic T-cell therapy (55).

Treatment of Fungal Infections

With fungal infection, prevention is the goal. Treatment of established infection remains difficult and depends on recovery of neutrophils and phagocytic and cellular immunity. Prevention consists of the use of laminar flow rooms, prophylaxis with antifungal agents, and reduced-intensity conditioning or reduced immunosuppressive therapies. Empiric therapy should be started if fungal infection is suspected. Historically, amphotericin B, which has broad antifungal activity, was the only parenteral agent available (7). Newer preparations, such as the liposomal amphotericin, show equal efficacy and reduced toxicity as compared with standard amphotericin (27). The azoles have broad antimycotic activity. Fluconazole, used prophylactically, protects against candidiasis and improves overall survival. However, its spectrum of activity is limited. It has no activity against some of the non-albicans species (57). Voriconazole has activity against *Aspergillus* species and is considered the treatment of choice in patients with proven *Aspergillus* (28), although it lacks activity against newer, emerging molds. The echinocandins, caspofungin and micofungin, are as effective as amphotericin B for the treatment of invasive candidiasis and have shown efficacy as salvage therapy in patients with invasive aspergillosis (48). The combination of caspofungin with a broad-spectrum azole or amphotericin B is effective. Additional support with granulocyte transfusions may be required for treatment of invasive fungal infections in neutropenic patients (44).

Treatment of Mycobacterium Infections

Treatment of *Mycobacterium* infection requires multidrug therapy. Testing for organism sensitivity is recommended to better tailor therapy, as resistant strains are seen. The usual course of recommended treatment is 3–6 months and should continue until evidence of immune reconstitution is observed (16).

Outcomes from Infection

Although infection remains a serious complication following HPC transplantation, a better understanding of the pathogenesis of infection, the development of better diagnostic techniques to detect infection early, and the use of prophylactic/preemptive therapy has dramatically reduced the associated morbidity and mortality. Once disseminated disease develops, the risk of mortality increases significantly despite appropriate therapy. The patient's immune status plays an important role. A current focus of care is to improve immune function of the recipient by using a reduced-intensity preparative regimen, withdrawing immune suppression earlier, and administering immunoregulatory therapy in the form of donor lymphocytes or specific cytotoxic T cells.

MUCOSITIS

Clinical Presentation

Oral and GI mucositis contributes significantly to morbidity and mortality and is a severe complication of treatment. Approximately 75%–90% of HPC-transplantation recipients experience mucositis, with 50% developing grade III–IV mucositis (21) (**Fig. 102.3**). For some, oral mucositis is the most common and most debilitating side effect reported (21). Mucositis presents in varying degrees and is multifactorial in origin (6,58). Disease severity is related to the type of conditioning regimen used, the degree of match between the donor and patient, the severity of GVHD, the presence of infection (i.e., HSV), and the use of methotrexate for GVHD prophylaxis (6,51). Severe mucositis causes pain and bleeding. Patients experience prolonged hospitalization, increased need for analgesics, increased need for total parenteral nutrition, reduced quality of life, and episodes of infection, especially bacteremia, invasive fungal disease, and typhlitis associated with mucosal-barrier breakdown. Mortality at day +100 is increased in this population. Severe grade IV mucositis can cause airway obstruction that necessitates endotracheal intubation. Bacteremia caused by *Streptococcus viridans* is related to mucosal damage and can be associated with serious complications such as sepsis and ARDS, with a mortality rate as high as 80% (43). Bloodstream infections with *S. aureus*, *P. aeruginosa*, *Clostridium* species, and *Candida* occur and are associated with typhlitis.

Mechanisms of Disease

Mucositis involves the entire GI tract. Oral mucositis typically develops 5–10 days after initiation of myeloablative therapy. It is a self-limited process. Initially, mucosal atrophy is associated with erythema. Ulceration develops 7–11 days after transplantation. The mucosa then gradually heals over the next 2 weeks. The small intestine is the second most common area affected and usually exhibits changes within a few days after the administration of myeloablative chemoradiotherapy. Involvement of the large intestine follows a short time later. Mucosal injury is the consequence of several biologic processes that begin in the submucosa and target the epithelium. It was believed that chemotherapy and radiation therapy directly damaged the basal epithelium. Mucosal barrier injury is now viewed as a complex biologic process that consists of five phases (49) (**Fig. 102.4**). Injury begins with the initiation phase, which is characterized by the generation of reactive oxygen species and transcription factors that produce injury to the submucosa with changes in the endothelium, connective tissue, and extracellular matrix. This leads to the messaging, signalling, and amplification phases, which involve the production of transcription factors and proinflammatory cytokines, resulting in tissue injury and apoptosis. Epithelial apoptosis and necrosis then give rise to the ulcerative phase. Ultimately, healthy epithelium migrates from the wound margins (49). Clinical assessment scales have been developed to classify the severity of mucosal damage. No single mucositis assessment scale is universally accepted. Most combine both subjective and objective measures of appearance, patient pain, and functional capabilities. One of these is depicted in **Table 102.9**.

Differential Diagnosis

Differential diagnosis of mucositis includes oral hemorrhage, infection, GVHD, and local viral infections. Infection with HSV is often accompanied by extensive and deep ulcerations. Although not common, CMV infection can lead to mucosal tissue injury. It is important to distinguish mucosal tissue injury

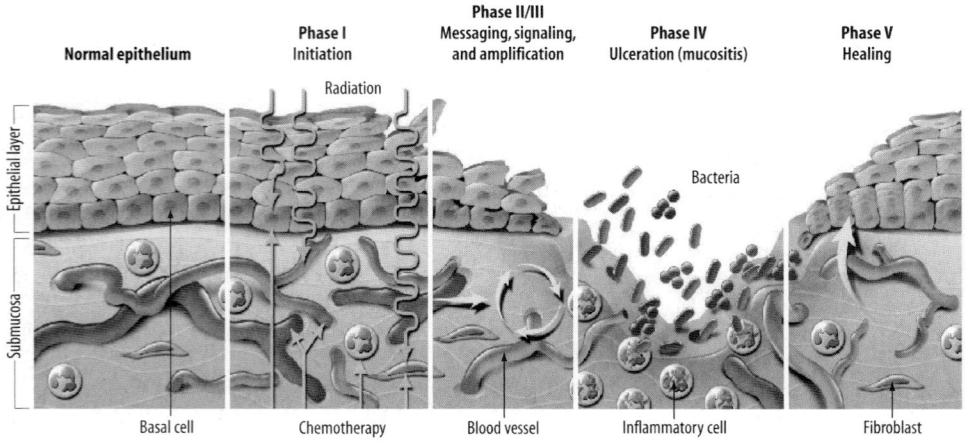

Normal epithelium   **Phase I** Initiation   **Phase II/III** Messaging, signaling, and amplification   **Phase IV** Ulceration (mucositis)   **Phase V** Healing

Radiation — Bacteria

Epithelial layer — Submucosa

Basal cell — Chemotherapy — Blood vessel — Inflammatory cell — Fibroblast

FIGURE 102.4. Pathobiology of mucositis: a five-stage process. The biologic sequence of mucositis can be arbitrarily divided into five stages or phases: initiation, upregulation and message generation, amplification and signaling, ulceration, and healing. From Sonis ST. A biological approach to mucositis. *J Support Oncol* 2004;2: 21–32, with permission.

that results from infection so that appropriate antiviral therapy will be used. Biopsy may be required to make this determination.

Management of Mucositis

Management can be challenging. The focus is largely on supportive care to control symptoms. Basic oral care is important to reduce oral microbial flora, reduce symptoms of pain and bleeding, and prevent soft tissue infections (42). Most oral regimens incorporate a combination of agents that collectively serve to coat and anesthetize the mucosa and to reduce the risk for mucosal infection. Saline and sodium bicarbonate rinses or mucosal coating agents can provide symptomatic relief for mild mucositis. As mucosal breakdown and pain increase, topical anesthetics, such as viscous lidocaine and benzocaine, and analgesics are added. Additional ingredients in topical oral solutions include diphenhydramine, magnesium hydroxide/aluminum hydroxide, pectin, sucralfate, nystatin, chlorhexidine, and corticosteroids (14). IV pain medication, especially with patient-controlled analgesia, may be required. For patients with severe grade III/IV mucositis who are also often neutropenic and thrombocytopenic, treatment focuses on control of severe bleeding, tissue desquamation, and infection. Protection of the airway with either an oral airway or intu-

bation may be required until the patient reaches the healing phase.

Controversies

Some controversy surrounds more recently used approaches for the prevention and treatment of mucositis. One approach to reduce regimen-related morbidity is with the use of nonmyeloablative preparative regimens. With better understanding of the pathobiology of mucositis, targeted therapeutic agents are being developed. Amifostine, which was originally developed as a free radical scavenger, has been shown to reduce proinflammatory cytokine levels (33). In patients with refractory hematologic malignancies who undergo AutoSCT, amifostine reduced the incidence and severity of mucositis compared with historic controls, resulting in a reduction in the need for nutritional support and the median duration of narcotic use (23). In a randomized trial of patients who received an AutoSCT, amifostine reduced the incidence of mucositis (25). Other studies have found no benefit from amifostine prophylaxis (15). Nutritional supplementation with oral glutamine, an essential amino acid for enterocytes, showed a trend toward reducing the severity of mucositis in children who underwent HPC transplantation (3). The use of AES-14 L-glutamine, a carrier molecule designed to aid in the delivery of L-glutamine to the epithelial oral mucosa, is in experimental stages. In a multicentered, randomized, double-blinded, placebo-controlled study, AES-14 reduced the incidence of grades II–IV mucositis by 22%, compared with placebo (1,38). Studies have shown that growth factors such as GM-CSF, epidermal growth factor, and transforming growth factor-$\beta3$ may protect the mucosa from damage. These may reduce the incidence and decrease the duration of mucositis (24,52). GM-CSF, applied systemically or locally, has demonstrated mixed results and may work best in radiotherapy-induced mucositis (35,41). The keratinocyte growth factor (KGF), a member of the fibroblast growth factor (FGF) superfamily, is the newest class of agents being investigated, which includes FGF-7 (palifermin or KGF-1) and FGF-20 (CG53135, velafermin) (49,50). KGF agents aid in the proliferation of mucosal epithelium, stimulate epithelial cell division, decrease inflammation by reducing the production of proinflammatory cytokines, and decrease epithelial apoptosis through upregulation of BCL-2 (49,50). In 2004, palifermin was approved for use in patients with mucositis and hematologic malignancies who require myeloablative therapy. In a

---

TABLE 102.9

WORLD HEALTH ORGANIZATION MUCOSITIS SCALE

Grade 0	No mucositis.
Grade 1	Irritation of the oral mucosa with pain; no overt ulceration; patient is able to eat a normal diet.
Grade 2	Sores are evident in the oral mucosa, but patient is still able to swallow solid food.
Grade 3	Patients need to be on a liquid diet, as they experience extreme sensitivity on swallowing solid food.
Grade 4	Patients are not able to swallow. Total parenteral nutrition or tube feeding is necessary.

phase III randomized, placebo-controlled trial, palifermin was well tolerated and effective in reducing the incidence and duration of severe oral mucositis in AutoSCT patients (53). Fewer patients experienced febrile neutropenia after palifermin, and fewer episodes of bacteremia were reported, suggesting that palifermin is effective in maintaining mucosal barrier function (53).

Outcomes from Mucositis

With a better understanding of the pathobiology of mucositis, a focus on prevention, and the development of targeted therapies, the incidence of severe mucositis in patients who undergo HPC transplantation should be reduced, which should result in fewer patients requiring intensive care for this complication of therapy. The publication of evidence-based clinical practice guidelines for mucositis should also help to reduce the incidence of severe mucositis requiring intensive care management. These guidelines provide a more standardized approach for the transplant clinician on how to prevent mucositis and recommendations for therapy based on the chemotherapy given (42).

CONCLUSIONS AND FUTURE DIRECTIONS

The field of HPC transplantation is evolving. A therapy that was once applied only to a select group of relatively young people with hematologic malignancies and a matched sibling donor has grown to uses in other malignant and nonmalignant conditions. Modifications that allow for the use of grafts from mismatched or unrelated donors have resulted in application to a much larger population. The many efforts to minimize the toxicity of HPC transplantation have been quite successful, translating into the treatment of patients with serious, preexisting comorbidities. In short, centers are reshaping their ideas of suitable donors and recipients. Such evolution will challenge the pediatric intensivist, as these patients possess clinical conditions that are among the most difficult to treat. As care of all patients improves, no doubt, lessons will be learned that will be applicable to the care of critically ill recipients of HPC transplantation. However, the major hurdles faced in the care of these children—the elimination of death and serious morbidity from MODS and ARDS—remain among the most difficult challenges in critical care medicine.

KEY POINTS

- Transplantation of HPCs, derived from bone marrow, peripheral blood, or cord blood, is used for malignant and nonmalignant conditions.
- Specialized preparation of the recipient, including myeloablation or partial ablation, and processing of HPCs is required for transplantation.
- Posttransplantation supportive care includes preemptive or prophylactic antimicrobials, treatment for GVHD, treatment for VOD, nutritional support, and protective isolation and minimization of opportunistic infections.
- Critical illness may occur in these patients with respiratory failure—severe infection, including opportunistic infections, ARF, dyselectrolytemias, severe GVHD, or severe

VOD—all necessitating PICU care. The pediatric intensivist should be familiar with management of all of these conditions.
- Respiratory failure may be life-threatening. Noninvasive modes of ventilation are preferred, if possible.
- ARF is often multifactorial. Management consists of supportive care. RRTs have greatly assisted in the management of fluids and electrolytes in these patients.
- Patients who are prone to life-threatening infections, especially opportunistic infections, require aggressive management with appropriate workup and antimicrobials.
- GVHD is unique to this treatment and results in important morbid conditions of the skin, GI tract, and liver.
- Veno-occlusive disease, induced by chemotherapeutic and radiation injuries, contributes to hepatic failure, hepatorenal syndrome, and sometimes, death.

ACKNOWLEDGMENTS

This work was supported in part by the Pediatric Cancer Research Foundation, Scaramella Fund, Brittany Barron Fund, and Marisa Fund.

References

1. Anonymous. Experimental L-glutamine agent shown effective in oral mucositis. *J Support Oncol* 2005;3:414.
2. Ambinder R. Epstein-Barr virus infections. In: Thomas E, Forman SJ, Appelbaum FR, et al., eds. *Hematopoietic Cell Transplantation*. Malden, Massachusetts: Blackwell Science, Ltd., 1999.
3. Aquino VM, Harvey AR, Garvin JH, et al. A double-blind, randomized, placebo-controlled study of oral glutamine in the prevention of mucositis in children undergoing hematopoietic stem cell transplantation: A pediatric blood and marrow transplant consortium study. *Bone Marrow Transplant* 2005;36:611–6.
4. Arfons LM, Lazarus HM. Total parenteral nutrition and hematopoietic stem cell transplantation: An expensive placebo? *Bone Marrow Transplant* 2005;36:281–8.
5. Bearman SI, Anderson GL, Mori M, et al. Venoocclusive disease of the liver: Development of a model for predicting fatal outcome after marrow transplantation. *J Clin Oncol* 1993;11:1729–36.
6. Blijlevens NM, Donnelly JP, De Pauw BE. Mucosal barrier injury: Biology, pathology, clinical counterparts and consequences of intensive treatment for haematological malignancy: An overview. *Bone Marrow Transplant* 2000;25:1269–78.
7. Bowden R. Fungal Infection after Hematopoietic Cell Transplantation. In: Thomas E, Forman SJ, Appelbaum FR, et al., eds. *Hematopoietic Cell Transplantation*. Malden, Massachusetts: Blackwell Science, Ltd., 1999.
8. Bowden RA. Other viruses after hematopoietic cell transplantation. In: Thomas E, Forman SJ, Appelbaum FR, et al., eds. *Hematopoietic Cell Transplantation*. Malden, Massachusetts: Blackwell Science, Ltd., 1999;618–26.
9. Bradley MB, Cairo MS. Cord blood immunology and stem cell transplantation. *Hum Immunol* 2005;66:431–46.
10. Burns WH. Herpes simplex virus infections. In: Thomas E, Forman SJ, Appelbaum FR, et al., eds. *Hematopoietic Cell Transplantation*. Malden, Massachusetts: Blackwell Science, Ltd., 1999;584–90.
11. Cairo MS. Graft-versus-host disease: Pathophysiology and therapy. In: Pochedly C, ed. *Neoplastic Diseases in Childhood*. London: Harwood Academic Publishers, 1994;833–37.
12. Cairo MS. Myelopoietic growth factors after stem cell transplantation: Does it pay. *J Pediatr Hematol Oncol* 2001;23:2–6.
13. Cairo MS, Wagner JE. Placental and/or umbilical cord blood: An alternative source of hematopoietic stem cells for transplantation. *Blood* 1997;90:4665–78.
14. Chan A, Ignoffo RJ. Survey of topical oral solutions for the treatment of chemo-induced oral mucositis. *J Oncol Pharm Pract* 2005;11:139–43.
15. Chauncey TR, Gooley TA, Lloid ME, et al. Pilot trial of cytoprotection with amifostine given with high-dose chemotherapy and autologous peripheral blood stem cell transplantation. *Am J Clin Oncol* 2000;23:406–11.
16. Cordonnier C, Martino R, Trabasso P, et al. Mycobacterial infection: A difficult and late diagnosis in stem cell transplant recipients. *Clin Infect Dis* 2004;38:1229–36.

17. Del Toro G, Satwani P, Harrison L, et al. A pilot study of reduced intensity conditioning and allogeneic stem cell transplantation from unrelated cord blood and matched family donors in children and adolescent recipients. *Bone Marrow Transplant* 2004;33:613–22.

18. DiCarlo JV, Alexander SR, Agarwal R, et al. Continuous venovenous hemofiltration may improve survival from acute respiratory distress syndrome after bone marrow transplantation or chemotherapy. *J Pediatr Hematol Oncol* 2003;25:801–5.

19. Einsele H, Hebart H. CMV-specific immunotherapy. *Hum Immunol* 2004;65:558–64.

20. Elting LS, Bodey GP, Keefe BH. Septicemia and shock syndrome due to viridans streptococci: A case-control study of predisposing factors. *Clin Infect Dis* 1992;14:1201–7.

21. Elting LS, Cooksley C, Chambers M, et al. The burdens of cancer therapy. Clinical and economic outcomes of chemotherapy-induced mucositis. *Cancer* 2003;98:1531–9.

22. Ferrara JL, Reddy P. Pathophysiology of graft-versus-host disease. *Semin Hematol* 2006;43:3–10.

23. Gabriel DA, Shea TC, Serody JS, et al. Cytoprotection by amifostine during autologous stem cell transplantation for advanced refractory hematologic malignancies. *Biol Blood Marrow Transplant* 2005;11:1022–30.

24. Girdler NM, McGurk M, Aqual S, et al. The effect of epidermal growth factor mouthwash on cytotoxic-induced oral ulceration. A phase I clinical trial. *Am J Clin Oncol* 1995;18:403–6.

25. Hartmann JT, von Vangerow A, Fels LM, et al. A randomized trial of amifostine in patients with high-dose VIC chemotherapy plus autologous blood stem cell transplantation. *Br J Cancer* 2001;84:313–20.

26. Hebart H, Einsele H. Clinical aspects of CMV infection after stem cell transplantation. *Hum Immunol* 2004;65:432–6.

27. Hebart H, Einsele H. Specific infectious complications after stem cell transplantation. *Support Care Cancer* 2004;12:80–5.

28. Herbrecht R, Denning DW, Patterson TF, et al. Voriconazole versus amphotericin B for primary therapy of invasive aspergillosis. *N Engl J Med* 2002;347:408–15.

29. Horvath JA, Dummer S. The use of respiratory-tract cultures in the diagnosis of invasive pulmonary aspergillosis. *Am J Med* 1996;100:171–8.

30. Keenan HT, Bratton SL, Martin LD, et al. Outcome of children who require mechanical ventilatory support after bone marrow transplantation. *Crit Care Med* 2000;28:830–5.

31. Kurland G, Michelson P. Bronchiolitis obliterans in children. *Pediatr Pulmonol* 2005;39:193–208.

32. Ljungman P, Ribaud P, Eyrich M, et al. Cidofovir for adenovirus infections after allogeneic hematopoietic stem cell transplantation: A survey by the Infectious Diseases Working Party of the European Group for Blood and Marrow Transplantation. *Bone Marrow Transplant* 2003;31:481–6.

33. Mantovani G, Maccio A, Madeddu C, et al. Reactive oxygen species, antioxidant mechanisms, and serum cytokine levels in cancer patients: Impact of an antioxidant treatment. *J Environ Pathol Toxicol Oncol* 2003;22:17–28.

34. Martin PJ, Schoch G, Fisher L, et al. A retrospective analysis of therapy for acute graft-versus-host disease: Initial treatment. *Blood* 1990;76:1464–72.

35. Masucci G, Broman P, Kelly C, et al. Therapeutic efficacy by recombinant human granulocyte/monocyte-colony stimulating factor on mucositis occurring in patients with oral and oropharynx tumors treated with curative radiotherapy: A multicenter open randomized phase III study. *Med Oncol* 2005;22:247–56.

36. Meyer S, Reinhard H, Gottschling S, et al. Pulmonary dysfunction in pediatric oncology patients. *Pediatr Hematol Oncol* 2004;21:175–95.

37. Patzer L, Kentouche K, Ringelmann F, et al. Renal function following hematological stem cell transplantation in childhood. *Pediatr Nephrol* 2003;18:623–35.

38. Peterson D PR. Phase III study: AES-14 in chemotherapy patients at risk for mucositis. *Prog Proc Am Soc Clin Oncol* 2003;22:725.

39. Prentice G, Grundy J, Kho P. Cytomegalovirus. In: Barret J, Treleaven J, eds. *The Clinical Practice of Stem Cell Transplantation*. Oxford, UK: Isis Medical Media, Ltd., 1998.

40. Riley U. Bacterial Infections. In: Barret J, Treleaven J, eds. *The Clinical Practice of Stem Cell Transplantation*. Oxford, UK: Isis Medical Media, Ltd., 1998.

41. Rosso M, Blasi G, Gherlone E, et al. Effect of granulocyte-macrophage colony-stimulating factor on prevention of mucositis in head and neck cancer patients treated with chemo-radiotherapy. *J Chemother* 1997;9:382–5.

42. Rubenstein EB, Peterson DE, Schubert M, et al. Clinical practice guidelines for the prevention and treatment of cancer therapy-induced oral and gastrointestinal mucositis. *Cancer* 2004;100:2026–46.

43. Ruescher TJ, Sodeifi A, Scrivani SJ, et al. The impact of mucositis on alpha-hemolytic streptococcal infection in patients undergoing autologous bone marrow transplantation for hematologic malignancies. *Cancer* 1998;82:2275–81.

44. Safdar A, Hanna HA, Boktour M, et al. Impact of high-dose granulocyte transfusions in patients with cancer with candidemia: Retrospective case-control analysis of 491 episodes of *Candida* species bloodstream infections. *Cancer* 2004;101:2859–65.

45. Sampath S, Schultheiss TE, Wong J. Dose response and factors related to interstitial pneumonitis after bone marrow transplant. *Int J Radiat Oncol Biol Phys* 2005;63:876–84.

46. Satwani P, Harrison L, Morris E, et al. Reduced-intensity allogeneic stem cell transplantation in adults and children with malignant and nonmalignant diseases: End of the beginning and future challenges. *Biol Blood Marrow Transplant* 2005;11:403–22.

47. Shorr AF, Moores LK, Edenfield WJ, et al. Mechanical ventilation in hematopoietic stem cell transplantation: Can we effectively predict outcomes? *Chest* 1999;116:1012–8.

48. Singh N, Paterson DL. Aspergillus infections in transplant recipients. *Clin Microbiol Rev* 2005;18:44–69.

49. Sonis ST. A biological approach to mucositis. *J Support Oncol* 2004;2:21–32; discussion 35–6.

50. Sonis ST. The pathobiology of mucositis. *Nat Rev Cancer* 2004;4:277–84.

51. Sonis ST, Elting LS, Keefe D, et al. Perspectives on cancer therapy-induced mucosal injury: Pathogenesis, measurement, epidemiology, and consequences for patients. *Cancer* 2004;100:1995–2025.

52. Sonis ST, Lindquist L, Van Vugt A, et al. Prevention of chemotherapy-induced ulcerative mucositis by transforming growth factor beta 3. *Cancer Res* 1994;54:1135–8.

53. Spielberger R, Stiff P, Bensinger W, et al. Palifermin for oral mucositis after intensive therapy for hematologic cancers. *N Engl J Med* 2004;351:2590–8.

54. Styczynski J, Cheung YK, Garvin J, et al. Outcomes of unrelated cord blood transplantation in pediatric recipients. *Bone Marrow Transplant* 2004;34:129–36.

55. Suparno C, Milligan DW, Moss PA, et al. Adenovirus infections in stem cell transplant recipients: Recent developments in understanding of pathogenesis, diagnosis, and management. *Leuk Lymphoma* 2004;45:873–85.

56. Takatsuka H, Takemoto Y, Mori A, et al. Common features in the onset of ARDS after administration of granulocyte colony-stimulating factor. *Chest* 2002;121:1716–20.

57. Van Burik J-A, Weisdorf D. Infections in Recipients of Hematopoietic Stem Cell Transplantation. In: Mandell GL, Bennett JE, Dolin R, ed. *Mandell, Douglas and Bennett's Principles and Practice of Infectious Diseases*, 6th ed. Philadelphia: Elsevier Churchill Livingstone, 2005;3486–98.

58. Wardley AM, Jayson GC, Swindell R, et al. Prospective evaluation of oral mucositis in patients receiving myeloablative conditioning regimens and haemopoietic progenitor rescue. *Br J Haematol* 2000;110:292–9.

59. Weisdorf D, Haake R, Blazar B, et al. Treatment of moderate/severe acute graft-versus-host disease after allogeneic bone marrow transplantation: An analysis of clinical risk features and outcome. *Blood* 1990;75:1024–30.

60. Westmoreland D. Other Viral Infections. In: Barret J, Treleaven J, eds. *The Clinical Practice of Stem Cell Transplantation*. Oxford, UK: Isis Medical Media, Ltd., 1998.

61. Willson DF, Thomas NJ, Markovitz BP, et al. Effect of exogenous surfactant (calfactant) in pediatric acute lung injury: A randomized controlled trial. *JAMA* 2005;293:470–6.

62. Wingard J. Bacterial infection. In: Thomas E, Forman SJ, Appelbaum FR, et al., eds. *Hematopoietic Cell Transplantation*. Malden, Massachusetts: Blackwell Science, Ltd., 1999.

63. Yoshikawa T. Human herpesvirus 6 infection in hematopoietic stem cell transplant patients. *Br J Haematol* 2004;124:421–32.

64. Zaia J. Cytomegalovirus. In: Thomas E, Forman SJ, Appelbaum FR, et al., eds. *Hematopoietic Cell Transplantation*. Malden, Massachusetts: Blackwell Science, Ltd., 1999.

CHAPTER 103 ■ COAGULATION ISSUES IN THE PICU

ROBERT I. PARKER • JAN A. HAZELZET

The focus of this chapter is on the variety of pathophysiologic conditions that are associated with abnormal hemostasis or abnormal laboratory measurements of hemostasis. However, appropriate management of a patient with a bleeding problem requires a basic understanding of the processes involved in regulating blood coagulation. Therefore, the current understanding of coagulation will be reviewed, including a brief discussion of the interactions of coagulation and inflammation.

The coagulopathic conditions frequently encountered in the PICU can be arbitrarily divided into three categories: conditions associated with serious bleeding or a high probability of bleeding, thrombotic syndromes or conditions associated with a higher probability of thrombosis, and systemic diseases associated with acquired selective coagulation factor deficiencies (**Table 103.1**). These categories are prioritized to suggest their relative importance to the critical care practitioner. While space constraints do not allow a comprehensive discussion of all aspects of pathophysiology, clinical presentation, and management of hemorrhagic and thrombotic disorders encountered in the PICU, a framework is provided that will allow the reader to garner a basic understanding of the issues and direct him toward additional sources of information.

OVERVIEW OF COAGULATION

Because medical students have traditionally been taught that the process of blood clotting is divided into the "intrinsic," "extrinsic," and "common" pathways (**Fig. 103.1**), many think that clotting occurs as the result of an orderly, sequential process. While this arbitrary segmentation of the clotting process may allow for a basic level of understanding, it obscures the fact that, once initiated, clot production and clot destruction (fibrinolysis) occur simultaneously and minimize the roles of platelets and the endothelium in the overall process. Some of the newer thoughts on coagulation are clarified below.

While it was previously thought that the "intrinsic" pathway, beginning with the activation of factor XII to activated factor XII in contact with some biologic or foreign surface was physiologically the most important in the initiation of clot formation, it is now known that the activation of factor X to factor Xa through the action of the factor VIIa/tissue factor (TF) complex is paramount in this regard (22,38). It is also evident that the various elements of the clotting cascade frequently act in concert; hence, the use of the term *tenase* to describe the action of factor VIIa /TF complex, along with the

factor IXa/factor VIIIa complex on the activation of factor X to factor Xa, and the use of the term *prothrombinase* to describe the factor Xa/factor Va complex, which cleaves prothrombin (factor II) to form thrombin (factor IIa). In addition, it is now known that "cross-talk" occurs between the two arms of the clotting cascade, with factor VIIa being able to enhance the activation of factor IX (to factor IXa) and factor XI (to factor XIa), further highlighting the central role of factor VIIa and TF in vivo (**Fig. 103.2**). Furthermore, various positive feedback loops that principally involve thrombin enhance the upstream activation of the clotting process.

The activation of coagulation is initiated from TF, which is found not only in the subendothelial matrix but also on cellular elements (e.g., as monocytes) and circulating freely in plasma as soluble TF. However, clotting does not occur in free-flowing blood but rather on surfaces. Platelets, endothelial cells, the subendothelial matrix, and biologic polymers (e.g., catheters, grafts, stents, etc.,) provide these surfaces for clot formation, and they all play a critical role in clot formation.

Platelets not only initiate the clot formation through the formation of a platelet plug, but more importantly, they bring specialized proteins that regulate the clotting response (e.g., factor VIII, inhibitors of fibrinolysis, etc.) to the area of bleeding and provide a surface for the colocalization of clotting factors for efficient clot formation (**Fig. 103.3**). Platelets do not ordinarily adhere to the vascular endothelium, but when the endothelium is mechanically disrupted (e.g., cut) or activated by inflammation, platelets will bind to the endothelial cell or subendothelial matrix via a von Willebrand factor (vWF)-dependent mechanism. Once adherent, the platelets become activated and secrete various molecules that further enhance platelet adherence and aggregation, vascular contraction, clot formation, and wound healing (34).

The endothelium is a specialized organ that is integral to the regulation of clot formation (i.e., hemostasis), as it presents a nonthrombogenic surface to flowing blood and enhances clot formation when the endothelium is disrupted by trauma or injured by infection or inflammation (2,42) (**Fig. 103.4**). The normal endothelium produces inhibitors of blood coagulation and platelet activation and modulates vascular tone and permeability. Endothelial cells also synthesize and secrete the components of the subendothelial extracellular matrix, including adhesive glycoproteins, collagen, fibronectin, and vWF. When this system is disrupted, bleeding occurs. However, when injured, the endothelium often becomes a prothrombotic rather than an antithrombotic organ, and unwanted clot formation may occur.

TABLE 103.1

OVERVIEW OF COAGULATION DISORDERS SEEN
IN THE ICU

**Conditions associated with serious bleeding or a high
probability of bleeding**
Disseminated intravascular coagulation
Liver disease/hepatic insufficiency
Vitamin K deficiency/depletion
Massive transfusion syndrome
Anticoagulant overdose (heparin, warfarin)
Thrombocytopenia (drug induced, immunologic)
Acquired platelet defects (drug induced, uremia)

Thrombotic clinical syndromes
Thrombotic thrombocytopenia purpura/hemolytic uremic
  syndrome
Deep venous thrombosis
Pulmonary embolism
Coronary thrombosis/acute myocardial infarction

Laboratory abnormalities not associated with clinical bleeding
Lupus anticoagulant
Reactive hyperfibrinogenemia

Other selected clinical syndromes
Hemophilia (A and B)
Specific factor deficiencies associated with specific diseases
  Amyloidosis-factor X, Gaucher disease-factor IX,
    nephritic syndrome-factor IX, antithrombin III
  Cyanotic congenital heart disease (polycythemia,
    qualitative platelet defect)
Depressed clotting factor levels (newborns)

Interaction of Coagulation and Inflammation

The response of the coagulation system during acute inflammation has received wider attention due to the recognition that coagulation is an integral part of the host immune response. In addition, the recognition that disseminated intravascular coagulation (DIC), when accompanied by sepsis and a systemic inflammatory response, results in a more severe clinical picture, higher degree of organ dysfunction, and a higher mortality, further supports the presumed importance of the interaction of coagulation and inflammation. In DIC, coagulation pathways are activated, natural inhibitory pathways are dysfunctional, and the fibrinolytic system is dysregulated—all direct or indirect consequences of an inflammatory response. The natural inhibitory pathways of coagulation are of particular interest in this intersection of coagulation and inflammation, as potential therapies have been based around these systems (19,26). Coagulation may be initiated in the flowing blood, on the endothelial surface, at endothelial lesions, in the perivascular tissues, and in areas not directly linked to the vascular bed, and it may or may not be associated with the formation of fibrin clots (19).

During sepsis, TF expression is upregulated in activated monocytes and endothelial cells as a response to endotoxin and other pathogen-associated molecular patterns, with the consequence being the secretion of proinflammatory cytokines and activation of coagulation. This process leads to an increased production of thrombin. While thrombin is a short-lived intermediate, owing to its neutralization by antithrombin, it plays a central role in coagulation and inflammation through the induction of procoagulant, anticoagulant, inflammatory, and mitogenic responses (25). The presence of thrombin will result in the activation, aggregation, and lysis of leukocytes and platelets, in the activation of endothelial adhesion molecules, and in the expression of a proinflammatory cytokine (IL-6). Thrombin increases endothelial permeability by causing contraction of endothelial cells; it also stimulates cellular proliferation. The net result of thrombin generation is production of a procoagulant state; it leads to the formation of fibrin, activates coagulation factors V, VIII, IX, XI, and leads to the expression of TF and vWF and the aggregation of platelets. However, thrombin also has anti-inflammatory effects through the production of activated protein C (APC) (25) (**Fig. 103.4**). Besides coagulation activation, two other crucial mechanisms occur during sepsis. One is the depression of natural anticoagulant systems, involving antithrombin and protein C (PC), and the second is the inhibition of fibrinolysis through the production of plasminogen activator inhibitor type (PAI)-1 and thrombin-activatable fibrinolysis inhibitor (TAFI) (**Fig. 103.5**).

Reduced levels of antithrombin III and PC may result from decreased production secondary to impaired liver function, loss from the vascular space in the case of capillary leakage, age dependency (antithrombin III and PC levels are normally decreased at birth and do not achieve "near-adult" levels until 3–6 months of age), and consumption (e.g., the conversion of PC to APC).

The PC system has been extensively studied, both because the decreased function of this natural anticoagulant pathway may result in pathologic thrombosis and because of the immunomodulating properties of the PC system (**Fig. 103.5**). In vitro, APC inhibits tumor necrosis factor-α elaboration from monocytes, blocks leukocyte adhesion to selectins, and influences apoptosis (25). The PC pathway is engaged when thrombin binds to thrombomodulin on the surface of the endothelium. Binding of PC to the endothelial cell PC receptor augments PC activation by the thrombin-thrombomodulin complex more than 10-fold in vivo. This receptor is shed from the endothelium by inflammatory mediators and thrombin, thereby downregulating PC activation in sepsis and inflammation; it can also undergo translocation from the plasma membrane to the nucleus, where it redirects gene expression. During translocation, it can carry APC to the nucleus, possibly accounting for the ability of APC to modulate inflammatory mediator responses in the endothelium (25).

The third important property of APC is its influence on fibrinolysis. APC is capable of neutralizing the fibrinolysis inhibitors PAI-1 and TAFI. PAI-1 is a 50-kDa glycoprotein of the serine protease inhibitor family. Its primary role in vivo is the inhibition of both tissue- and urokinase-type plasminogen activators. PAI-1 is an acute-phase protein that can dramatically increase during acute inflammation. In patients with sepsis, increased levels of PAI-1 are associated with increased levels of various cytokines and acute-phase proteins, abnormal coagulation parameters, increased severity of disease, and poorer outcomes. The regulation of the production of PAI-1 is multifactorial (**Fig. 103.6**). The 4G/5G insertion/deletion promoter polymorphism, which leads to differences in PAI-1 production, has been demonstrated to affect the risk of developing severe complications and death from sepsis during meningococcal infection and multiple trauma (36,37,46). The highest plasma levels of PAI-1 have been described in patients with

INTRINSIC PATHWAY

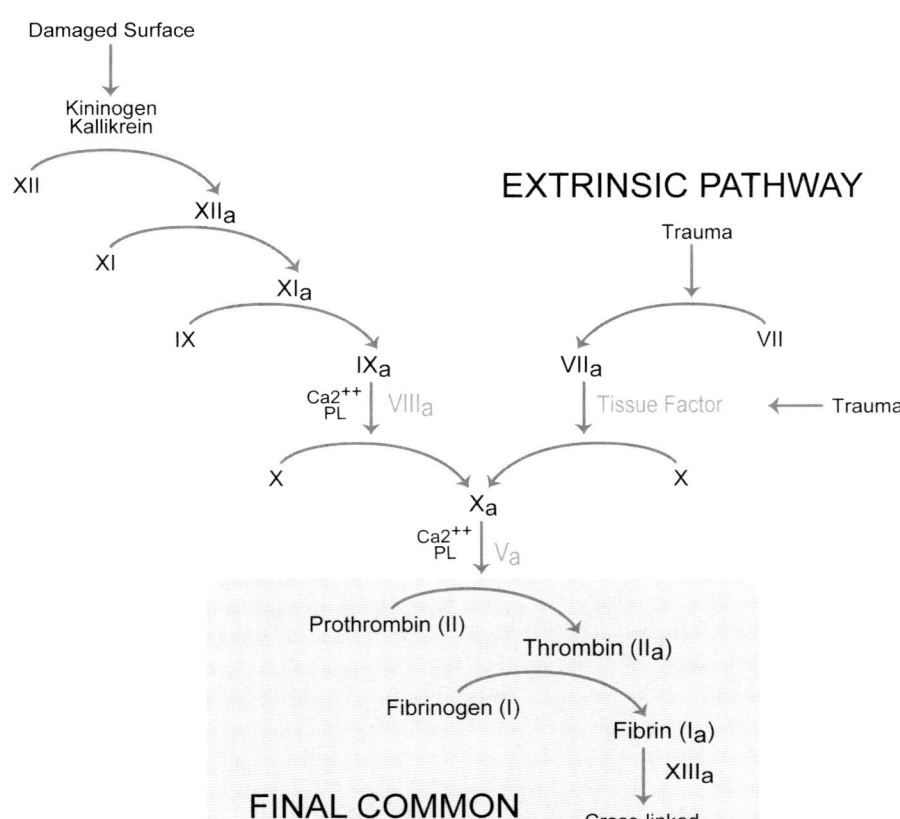

FIGURE 103.1. Coagulation is initiated either through the "intrinsic" pathway by activation of factor XII by the generation of high-molecular-weight kininogen and kallikrein or through activation of the "extrinsic" pathway by tissue factor. Roman numerals indicate zymogen clotting factors; "a" indicates activated forms of the clotting factors. Parker RI. Coagulation Disorders. In: Civetta JM, Taylor RW, Kirby RR. *Critical Care, 4th ed.* Philadelphia: Lippincott Williams & Wilkins, 2008, with permission.

meningococcal sepsis. APC can stimulate fibrinolysis by forming a tight 1:1 complex with PAI-1, leading to inactivation of this fibrinolysis inhibitor. High levels of thrombin lead to increased levels of activated protein, which can complex to PAI-1. This complex is subsequently cleared from the circulation, resulting in PC depletion (36).

Thrombin generation also increases the levels of TAFI, also known as carboxypeptidase R. TAFI is an important negative regulator of the fibrinolytic system and has been shown to inactivate inflammatory peptides such as complement factors C3a and C5a, which can play a role in the contact activation of coagulation. The full role of TAFI in the hemostatic and innate immune response to sepsis is still under active investigation.

APPROACH TO THE PATIENT WITH AN ACTUAL OR SUSPECTED COAGULATION DISORDER

Clinical History

Diagnostic assessment begins at the bedside. The medical history, both past and present, may lend some insight into the risk for significant bleeding (40,43). A prior history of prolonged or excessive bleeding or of recurrent thrombosis is important. Specific questions regarding bleeding should investigate the oc-

currence of any of the following: spontaneous, easy, or disproportionately severe bruising; intramuscular hematoma formation (either spontaneous or related to trauma); spontaneous or trauma-induced hemarthrosis; spontaneous mucous membrane bleeding; prior problems with bleeding related to surgery (including dental extractions, tonsillectomy, and circumcision); the need for transfusions in the past; menstrual history; and, finally, current medications.

The innumerable aspirin-containing medications that are available to the consumer can potentially interfere with platelet-mediated primary hemostasis. Many other drugs used in the ICU are also associated with bleeding abnormalities and are discussed later. In trauma situations (either surgical or accidental), it is important to determine the severity of injury relative to the magnitude of bleeding that follows. A prior history of significant thrombosis (e.g., deep venous thrombosis, pulmonary embolus, stroke) also suggests the possibility of the presence of a hypercoagulable condition. As thrombotic events are generally uncommon in children, the occurrence of thrombotic events, particularly early cardiovascular events such as myocardial infarction, in young adult relatives should cause the clinician to consider the presence of a congenital thrombophilic abnormality in the patient. These abnormalities include antithrombin-III deficiency, PC or S deficiency, presence of the factor V Leiden R506Q mutation, the prothrombin G20210A polymorphism/mutation, and the C677T mutation/polymorphism of the methylenetetrahydrofolate

Intrinsic Pathway

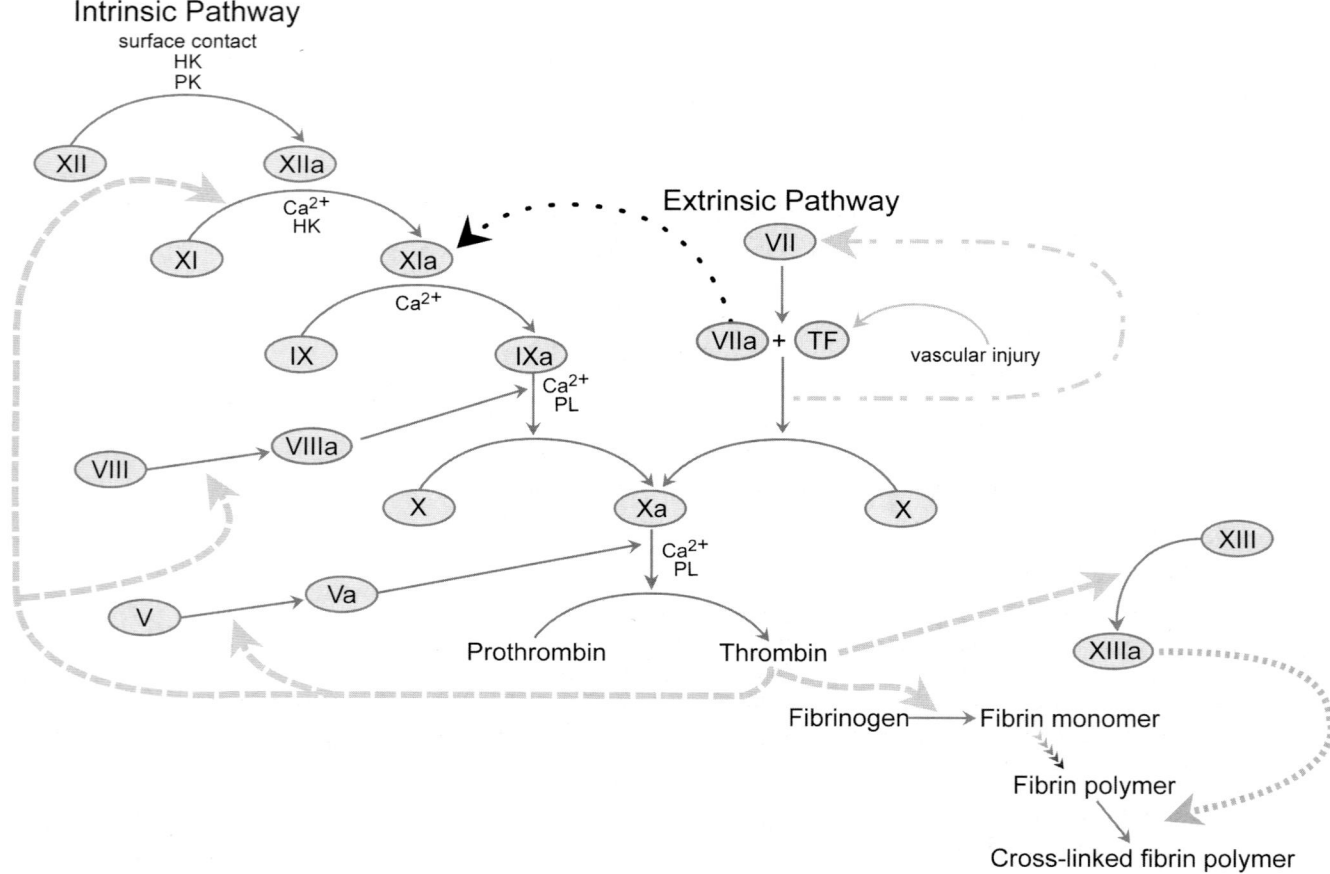

FIGURE 103.2. Modified clotting cascade indicating cross-talk between the intrinsic and extrinsic pathways by the action of factor VIIa/tissue factor (TF) enhancing the conversion of factor XI to activated factor XI (XIa) (*dotted lines*). HK, high-molecular-weight kininogen; PK, prekallikrein; PL, phospholipid. Parker RI. Coagulation Disorders. In: Civetta JM, Taylor RW, Kirby RR. *Critical Care, 4th ed.* Philadelphia: Lippincott Williams & Wilkins, 2008, with permission.

reductase (MTHFR) gene. In addition, vasculitis associated with an autoimmune disorder such as systemic lupus erythematosus (SLE) must always be considered in the evaluation of a child with an unexplained pathologic clot. In all cases, the family history is important in attempting to separate congenital from acquired disorders.

In a general sense, defects in primary or secondary hemostasis can be separated according to the nature of the bleeding. Patients with primary hemostatic defects tend to manifest "capillary-type bleeding"—oozing from cuts or incisions, mucous membrane bleeding, or excessive bruising. This type of bleeding is seen in patients with quantitative or qualitative platelet defects or von Willebrand disease. In contrast, patients with dysfunction of secondary hemostasis tend to display "large-vessel bleeding," characterized by hemarthrosis, intramuscular hematomas, and the like. This type of bleeding is most often associated with specific coagulation factor deficiencies or inhibitors.

Physical Examination

Development of generalized bleeding in critically ill patients in the ICU presents a special problem. Such bleeding is often

a marker of severe underlying multiorgan system dysfunction. Thus, correction of the coagulopathy usually requires improvement in the patient's overall clinical status. Supportive evidence or physical findings of other concurrent organ system dysfunction (e.g., renal failure, respiratory failure, hypotension) often are readily apparent. With the exception of massive transfusion syndrome (discussed later), generalized bleeding in critically ill children and infants is often caused by sepsis related DIC (15,51). However, the clinician must also consider the coagulopathy of severe liver dysfunction, undiagnosed hemophilia, battered-child syndrome, or, in newborns, vitamin K deficiency in the differential diagnosis (15,21,31,51). In young infants (<3 months of age), the coagulation system is often not yet mature, and abnormalities of the prothrombin time (PT) or activated partial thromboplastin time (aPTT) may not reflect an abnormality in hemostasis (1). Consequently, the intensivist must also take this into consideration when interpreting "abnormal" results. In these cases, consultation with a pediatric hematologist may be indicated.

The physical examination of the patient with a bleeding disorder should answer several basic questions. Is the process localized or diffuse? Is it related to an anatomic or surgical lesion? Is mucosal bleeding present? Finally, when appropriate, are there signs of thrombosis (either arterial or venous)? The

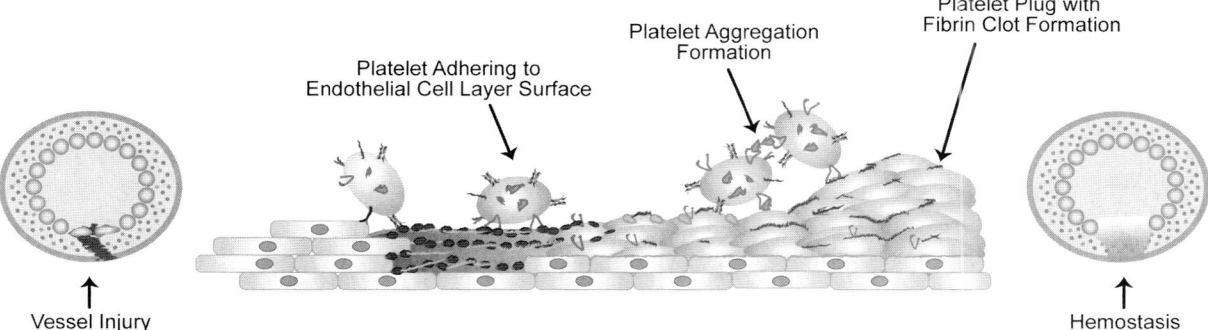

FIGURE 103.3. The role of platelets in mediating primary hemostasis at sites of vascular injury. Platelets are initially activated and express specific adhesion receptors on their surface, followed by adhesion to activated endothelial cells and exposed subendothelial components (e.g., collagen, vWF). Subsequent platelet aggregation occurs with the development of a primary platelet plug. Coagulation occurs on the developing platelet plug with the creation of a fibrin clot. Parker RI. Coagulation Disorders. In: Civetta JM, Taylor RW, Kirby RR. *Critical Care, 4th ed.* Philadelphia: Lippincott Williams & Wilkins, 2008, with permission.

answers to these questions may provide clues to the cause of the problem (primary versus secondary hemostatic dysfunction).

During the general examination, particular attention should be paid to the presence of several specific physical findings that may be helpful in determining the etiology of a suspected hemostatic abnormality. For example, the presence of an enlarged spleen coupled with thrombocytopenia suggests that splenic sequestration may be a contributor to the observed thrombocytopenia. Further, evidence of liver disease (e.g., portal hypertension, ascites), points to decreased factor synthesis as a possible etiology of a prolonged PT or aPTT. When lymphadenopathy, splenomegaly, or other findings suggestive of disseminated malignancy are detected, acute or chronic DIC should be suspected as the cause of prolonged coagulation times, hypofibrinogenemia, and/or thrombocytopenia. Purpura that are palpable suggest capillary leak from vasculitis, whereas purpura associated with thrombocytopenia or qualitative platelet de-

fects are generally not elevated and cannot be distinguished by touch. Finally, venous and arterial telangiectasia may be seen in von Willebrand disease and liver disease, respectively. When selective pressure is centrally applied to an arterial telangiectasia, the entire lesion fades, whereas a venous telangiectasia requires confluent pressure across the entire lesion (as with a glass slide) for blanching to occur.

Diagnostic Laboratory Evaluation

Before discussion of the appropriate tests that enable the clinician to interpret information from the history, physical examination, or previously obtained (and often confusing) laboratory data, the importance of correct specimen collection for hemostatic evaluation must be emphasized. In the PICU, it is common for laboratory samples to be drawn through an indwelling

Protein C Pathway

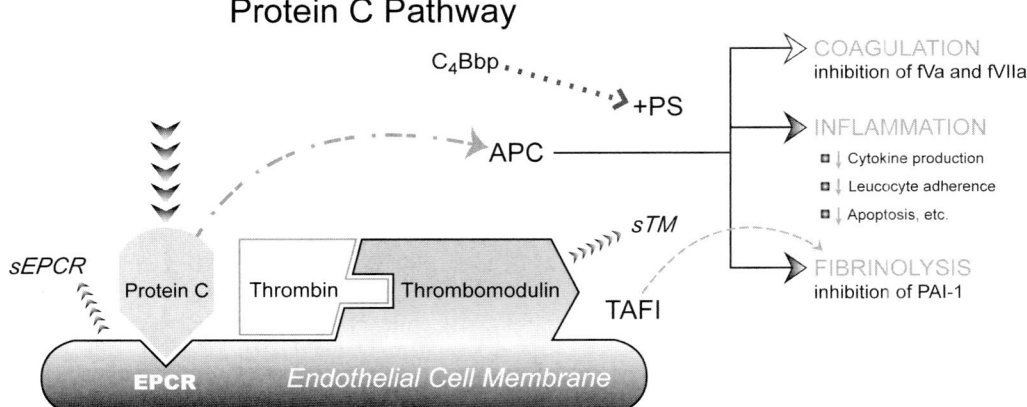

FIGURE 103.4. The interaction of the protein C system with the endothelium: thrombin bound to thrombomodulin (TM) modifies protein C bound to the endothelial protein C receptor on the cell surface to generate activated protein C (APC). APC acts as a natural anticoagulant by inactivating activated factors V (fVa) and VIII (fVIIIa), modulating inflammation by downregulating the synthesis of proinflammatory cytokines, leukocyte adherence, and apoptosis, and enhancing fibrinolysis by inhibiting thrombin-activatable fibrinolysis inhibitor (TAFI) and plasminogen activator inhibitor type-1 (PAI-1). C4Bbp, C4b binding protein; +PS, in the presence of protein S; sTM, soluble thrombomodulin; sEPCR, soluble endothelial cell protein C receptor. Parker RI. Coagulation Disorders. In: Civetta JM, Taylor RW, Kirby RR. *Critical Care, 4th ed.* Philadelphia: Lippincott Williams & Wilkins, 2008, with permission.

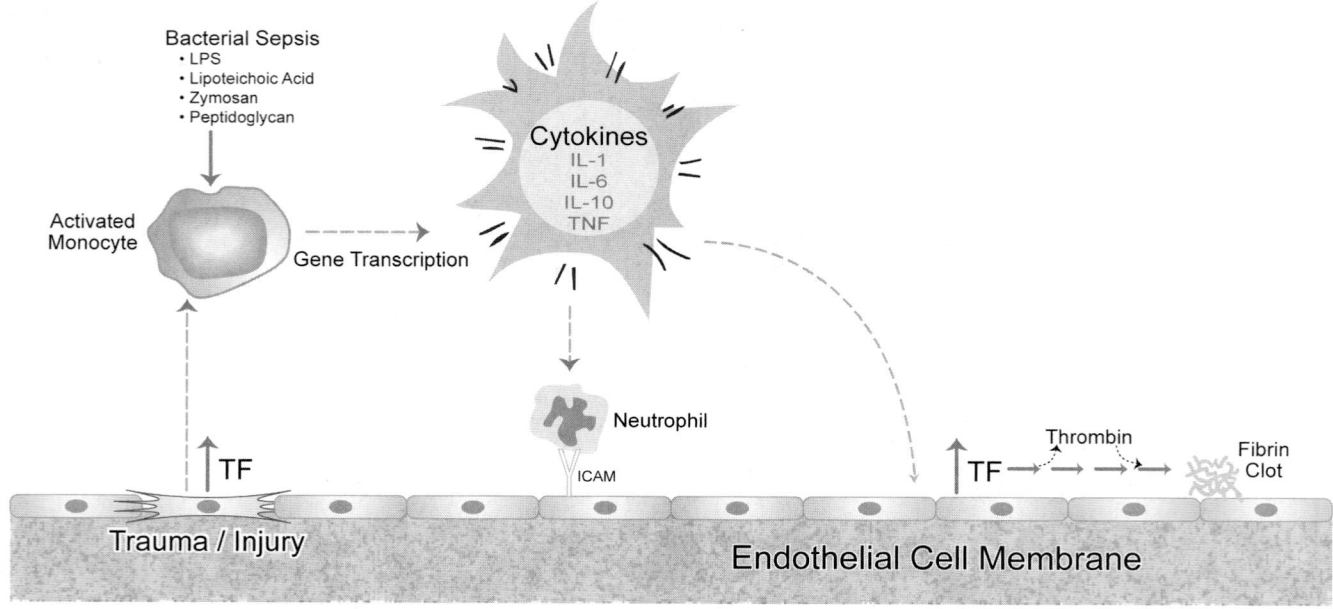

FIGURE 103.5. Inflammation enhances coagulation through the induction of proinflammatory cytokines that induce tissue factor formation, which in turn decreases activated protein C (APC) formation, leading to enhanced thrombin and fibrin generation. In addition, the decrease in APC allows for greater inhibition of fibrinolysis through the action of plasminogen activator inhibitor type-1 (PAI-1). Parker RI. Coagulation Disorders. In: Civetta JM, Taylor RW, Kirby RR. *Critical Care, 4th ed.* Philadelphia: Lippincott Williams & Wilkins, 2008, with permission.

arterial or central venous cannula, often because other access is no longer available. Therefore, heparin is commonly present, either in solutions used to flush the cannula, to transduce a waveform, or as a component of the IV infusion. Depending on the concentration of heparin in the infusing fluid and the volume of blood withdrawn, several tests can be influenced. Fibrin degradation products (FDPs) can be falsely elevated and fibrinogen levels shown as falsely low. Likewise, the PT, aPTT, and thrombin time (TT) can be spuriously prolonged. Therefore, a minimum of 20 mL of blood in adolescents and adults (10 mL of blood in younger children) should be withdrawn through the cannula and either discarded or used for other purposes before obtaining a specimen for laboratory hemostasis analysis (5). This practice should minimize any influence of heparin on the results. In young children and infants, it may not be reasonable to withdraw this volume of blood, and a peripheral venipuncture may be necessary. Because the aPTT is sensitive to the presence of small amounts of heparin, the presence of an unexpected prolonged aPTT obtained through a heparinized catheter should raise the suspicion of sample contamination. In this setting, the TT will also be prolonged but will normalize if the contaminating heparin is neutralized (e.g., with toluidine blue or Hepasorb™).

The presence of most suspected bleeding disorders can be confirmed using routinely available tests, including evaluation of the peripheral blood smear (including an estimate of the platelet count and platelet and red blood cell morphologic features); measurement of the PT, aPTT, and the TT; and, assays for fibrinogen, the presence of FDPs, or the D-dimer fragment of polymerized fibrin. This latter test is more specific for the fibrinolytic fragment produced when polymerized fibrin monomer, produced through the action of thrombin on fibrinogen, is cleaved by the proteolytic enzyme plasmin. In contrast, the older assays for FDPs or fibrin split products will be positive,

even if fibrin is not produced and the fragments are the result of proteolytic degradation of native fibrinogen. Discretion should be used in determining which of these tests is most appropriate for assessment; they need not be ordered as a blanket panel on all patients with known or suspected bleeding disorders. Several major categories of hemorrhagic disorders and the tests that are characteristically abnormal in each are summarized in **Table 103.2.** In most instances, measurement of the platelet count, fibrinogen level, PT, aPTT, and TT should provide sufficient information for determining the correct diagnosis—or at least for making an educated guess. By using these five screening tests and assessing other, more specific tests only when an absolute diagnosis is necessary, inappropriate use of laboratory resources may be avoided.

Patients who present with a thrombotic event will generally not display abnormalities of usual "clotting" studies; that is, their PT, aPTT, TT, and fibrinogen will usually be within normal ranges. While hyperfibrinogenemia and persistent elevations of factor VIII have been associated with an increased risk of thrombosis, both may be elevated by acute inflammation; consequently, the finding of elevations of these clotting factors is generally not helpful in the evaluation of a thrombotic event in an acutely ill child.

Several inherited or acquired abnormalities that place an individual at increased risk for thrombosis have been identified, and determination of these factors should be undertaken when a thrombotic event is suspected or documented. Prior to initiation of anticoagulation, plasma levels of PC (antigen and activity), protein S (antigen and activity; total and free), and anti-thrombin III (antigen and activity) should be obtained. In addition, PCR analysis for mutations in the factor V [factor V Leiden; R(Arg)506Q(Gln)], prothrombin [G(Gly)20210A (Ala)], and MTHFR; [C(Cys)677T(Thr)] genes should be performed. In addition, a baseline serum homocysteine may be

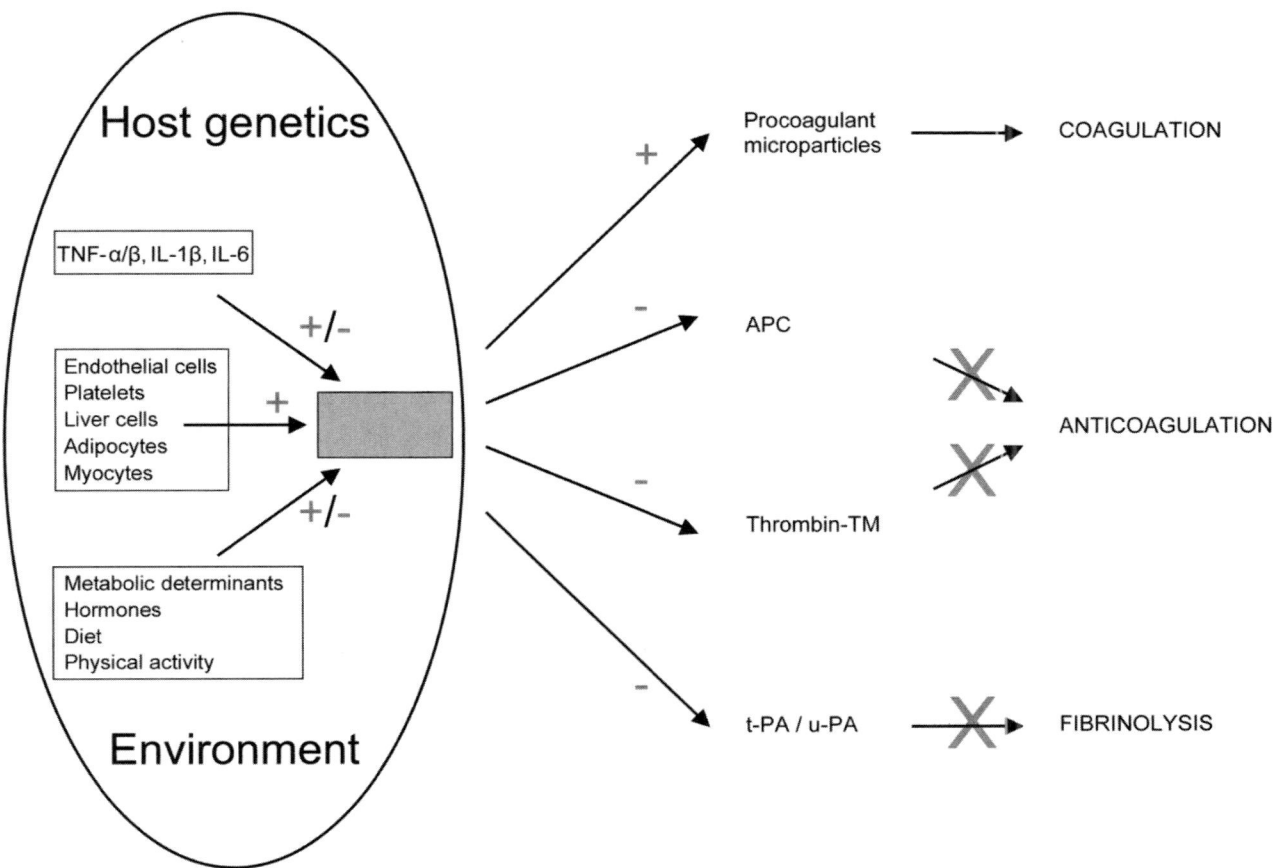

FIGURE 103.6. Genetic and environmental influences on the expression of plasminogen activator inhibitor type 1 (PAI-1) and the importance of PAI-1 in the coagulation and fibrinolysis pathways. TNF-α, tumor necrosis factor-α; APC, activated protein C; TM, thrombomodulin; tPA, tissue-type plasminogen activator; u-PA, urokinase-type plasminogen activator. From Hermans PW, Hazelzet JA. Plasminogen activator inhibitor type 1 gene polymorphism and sepsis. *Clin Infect Dis* 2005;41(Suppl 7):S453–8, with permission.

obtained, as the thrombosis risk of the MTHFR mutation may be related to elevations of homocysteine caused by alterations in the metabolism of folic acid rather than the mutation per se. In adult populations, ~40% of patients with thrombosis will not display one of the known thrombophilic risk factors, and it is likely that the percentage in children who are negative for these abnormalities is higher. The intensivist must look for confounding clinical conditions, such as dehydration (in the case of central venous sinus thrombosis), indwelling catheters, vascular compression (e.g., cervical ribs), type-II heparin-induced thrombocytopenia (see later discussion), etc., in evaluating a patient with thrombosis.

CONDITIONS ASSOCIATED WITH SERIOUS BLEEDING OR A HIGH PROBABILITY OF BLEEDING

Disseminated Intravascular Coagulation

Pathogenesis

Because it often occurs in conjunction with more serious, life-threatening disorders, DIC is one of the most serious hemo-static abnormalities seen in the PICU. The clinical syndrome itself results from the activation of blood coagulation, which then leads to excessive thrombin generation. The final result of this process is the widespread formation of fibrin thrombi in the microcirculation, with resultant consumption of certain clotting factors and platelets. Ultimately, this consumption is largely responsible for the development of significant bleeding, as the rate of consumption outpaces the rate at which the clotting factors and platelets are produced (7). Several specific conditions associated with the development of DIC are presented in **Table 103.3.** In general, the conditions associated with DIC are the same in adults and children and include a wide variety of disorders, the common feature of which is their ability to initiate coagulation to varying degrees. The mechanisms involved generally can be considered in two categories: (a) those intrinsic processes that enzymatically activate procoagulant proteins, and (b) those that cause the release of TF, which then triggers coagulation. These are complex events that can lead to significant bleeding and often complicate the management of an already critically ill child.

Fibrinolysis invariably accompanies thrombin formation in DIC (7), and thrombin generation or release of tissue plasminogen activator usually initiates this process. Plasmin is generated and then digests fibrinogen and fibrin clots as they form.

TABLE 103.2

HEMORRHAGIC SYNDROMES AND ASSOCIATED LABORATORY FINDINGS

Clinical syndrome	Screening tests	Supportive tests
Disseminated intravascular coagulation	Prolonged PT, aPTT, TT; decreased fibrinogen, platelets; microangiopathy	(+) FDPs, D-dimer; decreased factors V, VIII, and II (late)
Massive transfusion	Prolonged PT, aPTT; decreased fibrinogen, platelets ± prolonged TT	All factors decreased; (−) FDPs, D-dimer (unless DIC develops); (+) transfusion history
Anticoagulant overdose		
Heparin	Prolonged aPTT, TT; ± prolonged PT	Toluidine blue/protamine corrects TT; reptilase time normal
Warfarin (same as vitamin K deficiency)	Prolonged PT; ± prolonged aPTT (severe); normal TT, fibrinogen, platelets	Vitamin K-dependent factors decreased; factors V, VIII normal
Liver disease		
Early	Prolonged PT	Decreased factor VII
Late	Prolonged PT, aPTT; decreased fibrinogen (terminal liver failure); normal platelet count (if splenomegaly absent)	Decreased factors II, V, VII, IX, and X; decreased plasminogen; ± FDPs unless DIC develops
Primary fibrinolysis	Prolonged PT, aPTT, TT; decreased fibrinogen ± platelets decreased	(+) FDPs, (−) D-dimer; short euglobulin clot lysis time
Thrombotic thrombocytopenic purpura	Thrombocytopenia, microangiopathy with mild anemia; PT, aPTT, fibrinogen generally within normal limits/mildly abnormal	ADAMTS13 deficiency/inhibitor, unusually large von Willebrand factor multimers between episodes; mild increase in FDPs or D-dimer
Hemolytic uremic syndrome	Microangiopathic hemolytic anemia, ± thrombocytopenia; PT, aPTT generally within normal limits	Renal insufficiency; FDPs and D-dimer generally (−)

PT, prothrombin time; aPTT, activated partial thromboplastin time; TT, thrombin time; FDPs, fibrin degradation products.

Plasmin also inactivates several activated coagulation factors and impairs platelet aggregation. As such, DIC represents an imbalance between the activity of thrombin, which leads to microvascular thrombi with coagulation factor and platelet consumption, and plasmin, which degrades these fibrin-based clots as they form. Therefore, thrombin-induced coagulation factor consumption, thrombocytopenia, and plasmin generation contribute to the presence of bleeding.

In addition to bleeding complications, the presence of fibrin thrombi in the microcirculation can lead to ischemic tissue injury. Pathologic data indicate that renal failure, acrocyanosis, multifocal pulmonary emboli, and transient cerebral ischemia may be related clinically to the presence of such thrombi. The presence of fibrinopeptides A and B (resulting from enzymatic cleavage of fibrinogen) leads to pulmonary and systemic vasoconstriction, which can potentiate an existing ischemic injury. In a given patient with DIC, either bleeding or thrombotic tendencies may predominate; in most patients, bleeding is usually the predominant problem. However, in up to 10% of patients with DIC, the presentation is exclusively thrombotic (e.g., pulmonary emboli with pulmonary hypertension, renal insufficiency, altered mental status, acrocyanosis) without hemorrhage. Whether the presentation of DIC is thrombotic, hemorrhagic, or "compensated" (that is, laboratory results consistent with DIC without overt bleeding), microthrombosis probably contributes to the development and progression of multiorgan failure.

TABLE 103.3

UNDERLYING DISEASES ASSOCIATED WITH DISSEMINATED INTRAVASCULAR COAGULATION

Sepsis	Retained placenta
Liver disease	Hypertonic saline abortion
Shock	Amniotic fluid embolus
Penetrating brain injury	Retention of a dead fetus
Necrotizing pneumonitis	Eclampsia
Tissue necrosis/crush injury	Localized endothelial injury
Intravascular hemolysis	(aortic aneurysm, giant
Acute promyelocytic leukemia	hemangiomata,
Thermal injury	angiography)
Freshwater drowning	Disseminated malignancy
Fat embolism syndrome	(prostate, pancreatic)

Clinical Presentation and Diagnosis

The suspicion that DIC is present usually stems from one of two conditions: (a) unexplained, generalized oozing or bleeding, or (b) unexplained, abnormal laboratory parameters of hemostasis. This usually occurs in the context of a suggestive clinical scenario or associated disease (Table 103.3). Although infection and multiple trauma are the most common underlying conditions associated with the development of DIC, certain other organ system dysfunctions predispose to DIC, including hepatic insufficiency and splenectomy (15,51). Both of these conditions are associated with impaired reticuloendothelial

TABLE 103.4

LABORATORY TESTS FOR THE DIAGNOSIS OF
DISSEMINATED INTRAVASCULAR COAGULATION

Test	Discriminator value
Platelet count	<80–100,000 mcL or a decrease of >50% from baseline
Fibrinogen	<100 mg/dL or a decrease of >50% from baseline
Prothrombin time	>3-sec prolongation above upper limit of normal
Fibrin degradation products	>80 mg/dL
D-dimer	"moderate" increase

system function and consequent impaired clearance of activated coagulation proteins and fibrin/fibrinogen degradation fragments, which may inhibit fibrin polymerization and clot formation.

The clinical severity of DIC frequently has traditionally been assessed by the severity of bleeding and coagulation abnormalities. Scoring tools that employ a panel of laboratory tests along with severity-of-illness scores to assess the likelihood and severity of DIC have been proposed in an attempt to determine prognosis at the time of diagnosis to better direct initial therapy. The tests most commonly employed in many of these scoring systems for the diagnosis of DIC are listed in **Table 103.4**. While no data exist for pediatric patients, this approach does have prognostic value, particularly in patients with sepsis (14,29,60). Two of the more commonly employed scoring systems may serve as a template for the diagnosis of DIC; one (41) involves a qualitative score, the other (59), a quantitative score, both strongly suggestive of a diagnosis of DIC. Limited studies have shown that early identification of DIC, before the onset of a gross hemorrhagic diathesis, improves survival in critically ill children (23).

The combination of a prolonged PT, hypofibrinogenemia, and thrombocytopenia in the appropriate clinical setting is sufficient to suspect the diagnosis of DIC in most instances. Severe hepatic insufficiency (with splenomegaly and splenic sequestration of platelets) can yield a similar laboratory profile and must be ruled out. In addition to liver disease, several other conditions have presentations similar to DIC and must be considered in the differential diagnosis; they include liver disease, massive transfusion, primary fibrinolysis, thrombotic thrombocytopenic purpura (TTP)/hemolytic uremic syndrome (HUS), heparin therapy, and dysfibrinogenemia.

With the exception of massive transfusion syndrome, these disorders generally have only two of the three characteristic laboratory findings of DIC; a comparison of the laboratory findings in these disorders is noted in **Table 103.2**.

To confirm a diagnosis of suspected DIC, tests that indicate increased fibrinogen turnover (i.e., elevated FDPs or D-dimer assay) may be necessary. The D-dimer assay for the D-dimer fragment of polymerized fibrin has been shown to be both highly sensitive and specific for proteolytic degradation of polymerized fibrin (fibrin clot that has been produced in the presence of thrombin). Consequently, this test is employed with increasing frequency in patients with suspected DIC. However, remembering that thrombin is produced whenever coagulation

is activated in the presence of bleeding, the clinician must interpret a modest elevation of D-dimer in a postoperative or trauma patient with some degree of caution. The presence of a marked elevation of D-dimer in a nonbleeding patient essentially excludes primary fibrinogenolysis as the sole cause of measurable FDPs in the serum. The TT is a less sensitive test for DIC, but may be useful in cases of suspected heparin overdose, because it corrects in the test tube with the addition of protamine sulfate or toluidine blue. Similarly, the euglobulin clot lysis time may not be sensitive to fibrinolysis associated with DIC but is significantly shortened in most cases of primary fibrinolysis. Other tests of purported value, such as soluble fibrin monomer or thrombin-antithrombin complex formation, either have problems with sensitivity or are impractical for widespread use outside of a research setting.

Meningococcal Purpura Fulminans

Purpura fulminans is a systemic coagulopathy similar, if not identical, to DIC that classically accompanies meningococcal sepsis and is sporadically noted with other similarly severe infections. The hallmark of this syndrome is tissue ischemia and necrosis due to marked microvascular thrombosis. Patients are generally noted to have severely depressed levels of PC, with a degree of suppression that correlates with mortality. The highest plasma levels of PAI-1 have been described in patients with meningococcal sepsis. As mentioned before, APC can stimulate fibrinolysis by forming a tight 1:1 complex with PAI-1, which leads to inactivation of this fibrinolysis inhibitor. Thus, because APC complexes to PAI-1, these findings of increased PAI-1 and decreased PC are probably interrelated. High levels of thrombin lead to high levels of APC, APC complexes to PAI-1, and finally, PC is depleted (37). This mechanism is possibly the explanation for the extremely low levels of PC found in meningococcal disease. The purpura seen in this disease is similar to that seen in congenital PC deficiency. From a therapeutic point of view, meningococcal sepsis has been considered as a model for sepsis-associated PC deficiency, and many open-label studies of PC-concentrate therapy have been published in this patient population. The suggestion of one study—that a disturbed activation process of PC on the basis of semi-quantitative analysis of expression of thrombomodulin and the endothelial PC receptor in the dermal microvasculature of children with severe meningococcemia and purpuric or petechial lesions (27)—calls into question the benefit of PC concentrates. A randomized, placebo-controlled, dose-finding study of PC concentrate in the same patient population demonstrated adequate activation of PC to APC, even in the most severely ill patients, with a dose-dependent improvement in coagulation parameters (18). However, because of the positive effects of recombinant APC in baboons (58), the use of recombinant human APC (rhAPC) in sepsis has been the focus of study, despite the fact that APC is an anticoagulant and can theoretically lead to bleeding. These efforts resulted in a large, randomized, controlled trial in adults with sepsis, which showed a positive result on mortality (6). The pediatric trial for this agent was stopped because of futility and an unacceptably high incidence of bleeding in infants. In addition, small series have suggested benefit from antithrombin III supplementation (49) but not from tissue plasminogen activator (62).

Thrombocytopenic Purpura and Hemolytic Uremic Syndrome

While neither TTP nor HUS generally produces a coagulopathic state, both are characterized by marked microangiopathy and microvascular thrombosis. These two diseases are felt to represent different ends of the spectrum of end-organ dysfunction possible in microangiopathic states. HUS is more commonly seen in children and is characterized by a prodrome of fever and diffuse diarrhea (often bloody). Endemic cases of HUS are generally caused by verotoxin-expressing enteropathic strains of *Escherichia coli* (O157:H7) or shigatoxin-expressing strains of *Shigella*. Sporadic cases are generally not associated with diarrhea and may represent variant TTP or familial defects in complement factor H. Therapy is supportive, including renal replacement measures when indications exist. Neither plasma infusion nor plasma exchange appears to be beneficial. TTP is characterized by the pentad of microangiopathic hemolytic anemia, thrombocytopenia, neurologic symptoms, fever, and renal dysfunction. While only 40% of patients will display the full pentad, up to 75% will manifest a triad of microangiopathic hemolytic anemia, neurologic symptoms, and thrombocytopenia. This disorder is felt to be due to the absence of a vWF-cleaving protease (ADAMTS13), resulting in the circulation of unusually large vWF multimers that can induce or enhance the pathologic adhesion of platelets to the endothelium. The therapy of choice for TTP is plasma exchange by apheresis. Platelet transfusions are generally not recommended, except in the case of major bleeding.

Management

The primary treatment for DIC is correction of the underlying problem that led to its development. Specific therapy for DIC should not be undertaken unless the patient has significant bleeding or organ dysfunction secondary to DIC, significant thrombosis has occurred, or treatment of the underlying disorder (i.e., acute promyelocytic leukemia) is likely to increase the severity of DIC.

Supportive therapy for DIC includes the use of several component blood products (24,32). Packed red blood cells are given according to accepted guidelines in the face of active bleeding. Fresh whole blood (i.e., <24–48 hrs old) may be given to replete both volume and oxygen-carrying capacity, with the potential additional benefit of providing coagulation proteins, including fibrinogen and platelets. Cryoprecipitate contains a much higher concentration of fibrinogen than does whole blood or fresh frozen plasma (FFP) and therefore is more likely to provide the quantity of fibrinogen necessary to replace fibrinogen that is consumed by DIC. In this regard, FFP is of limited value for the treatment of significant hypofibrinogenemia because of the inordinate volumes required to make any meaningful contribution to plasma fibrinogen concentration. FFP infusions may effectively replete other coagulation factors consumed with DIC, such as PC, although the increase in these proteins may be quite small unless large volumes of FFP are infused. The use of cryoprecipitate or FFP in the treatment of DIC has been open to debate in the past because of concern that these products merely provide further substrate for ongoing DIC and thus increase the amount of fibrin thrombi formed. However, clinical (autopsy) studies have failed to confirm this concern.

The goal of blood component therapy is not to produce normal "numbers" but rather to produce clinical stability. If the serum fibrinogen level is <75–50 mg/dL, repletion with cryoprecipitate to raise plasma levels to ≥100 mg/dL is the goal. A reasonable starting dose is one bag of cryoprecipitate for every 10 kg of body weight every 8–12 hrs. As cryoprecipitate is not a standardized component (i.e., its content varies from bag to bag), the fibrinogen level should be rechecked after an infusion to document the increase. The amount and timing of the next infusion is then adjusted according to the results. Platelet transfusions also may be used when thrombocytopenia is thought to contribute to ongoing bleeding. Many of the fibrin/fibrinogen fragments produced in DIC have the potential to impair platelet function by inhibiting fibrinogen binding to platelets, which may be clinically significant at the concentration of FDPs achieved with DIC. Platelet transfusions in patients with DIC should be considered to maintain platelet counts up to 40,000 to 80,000/μL depending on the clinical specifics of the patient.

Pharmacologic therapy for DIC has two primary aims: to "turn off" ongoing coagulation so that repletion of coagulation factors may begin and to impede thrombus formation and ensuing ischemic injury. Two recombinant blood products have been developed that have some usefulness in the treatment of DIC. The first, recombinant APC, was shown to result in a 6% reduction in sepsis mortality in adults and possibly a reduction in the incidence of DIC (6). However, its use was associated with an increase in intracranial bleeding in older adults. The pediatric experience with recombinant APC is limited. A multi-institutional trial in pediatric sepsis failed to result in a recommendation for its use and was stopped because of a significant incidence of severe bleeding, particularly in infants and young children. Consequently, the use of recombinant APC is decided on a case-by-case basis and should be used with some caution. The second new agent for the treatment of severe bleeding, including DIC, is activated recombinant human factor VII (rhFVIIa). While only a limited number of controlled trials have been conducted to explore its use in adults and none have been conducted in children, with the exception of those patients with acquired inhibitors to factor VIII, rhFVIIa has been shown to be a potent agent for the control of bleeding from a number of medical and surgical causes, including DIC and other consumptive coagulopathies (9,45,55,56). This agent has also been shown to correct the hemostatic defect caused by the antiplatelet agents aspirin and clopidogrel (4). Reports have noted that use of rhFVIIa may result in an increase in thrombosis and thromboembolic events, although the incidence appears to be small and the severity of most events mild (50). In addition to APC, other anticoagulant molecules (e.g., heparin and antithrombin III), and thrombolytic agents continue to be studied as therapy for DIC and sepsis (17,39).

Liver Disease and Hepatic Insufficiency

Abnormal Hemostasis in Liver Disease

Liver disease is a common cause of abnormal hemostasis in patients in the ICU, with abnormal coagulation studies or overt bleeding occurring in ~15% of patients who have either clinical or laboratory evidence of hepatic dysfunction. It is a common cause of a prolonged PT or aPTT, often without any clinical sequelae. The hemostatic defect associated with liver disease is multifactorial, with multiple aspects of hemostasis being affected (3,44).

In liver disease, synthesis of several plasma coagulation proteins, including factors II, V, VII, IX, and X, is impaired. Fibrinogen synthesis by the liver usually can be maintained at levels that prevent bleeding until terminal liver failure supervenes. However, the physiologic action of fibrinogen synthesized by a diseased liver is suspect because it has been shown to have increased carbohydrate content (sialic acid) in its structure and may be dysfunctional (i.e., a dysfibrinogen). Factor XIII activity also is often decreased in the setting of hepatocellular disease. However, the clinical significance of this decrease is uncertain because levels as low as 3% provide for normal fibrin clot stabilization. Although it is apparently synthesized by the liver, factor VIII (i.e., factor VIII:C, antihemophilic factor) synthesis seems to be independent of the state of hepatic function. Indeed, factor VIII levels may be increased in some types of liver disease. Plasma PC and antithrombin III levels are low in many conditions of hepatic insufficiency, with variable effects.

In addition to these deficiencies in plasma coagulation protein synthesis, many patients with liver disease, particularly cirrhosis, have increased fibrinolytic activity. The mechanism for this heightened fibrinolytic state is not clear, although increased amounts of plasminogen activator can often be demonstrated. It may be difficult to discern whether fibrinolysis occurs solely because of underlying severe liver disease or as a result of concurrent DIC, as patients with cirrhosis are at increased risk for the development of DIC. The clinical distinction can be virtually impossible if active bleeding is present. In liver disease, levels of FDPs can be increased by increased fibrinolysis and by decreased hepatic clearance. Finally, clinically significant fibrinolysis is a frequent occurrence in patients who undergo portacaval shunt procedures.

Thrombocytopenia may be present to a variable degree in patients with hepatic dysfunction—usually ascribed to splenic sequestration. It is rarely profound and generally does not produce clinically significant bleeding as a solitary defect. In vitro platelet aggregation is often affected, however. Increased plasma concentrations of FDPs are a possible cause of these abnormalities. The thrombocytopenia of liver disease in conjunction with other coagulation/hemostatic defects secondary to liver disease may result in bleeding that is difficult to manage clinically, particularly if all aspects of the problem are not addressed.

Patients with synthetic liver disease may also exhibit decreased synthesis of the vitamin K-dependent anticoagulant proteins PC and protein S, as well as antithrombin III (44). Decreased levels of these natural anticoagulants may increase the risk of thrombosis. The PT, aPTT, and TT will not be affected by the levels of any of these naturally occurring anticoagulants.

Presentation

The hemostatic defect in liver disease is multifactorial, and each patient should be approached accordingly. The most common scenario is a patient with liver disease and a prolonged PT without overt bleeding in whom the potential for bleeding is a concern. In patients with liver disease and impaired synthetic capabilities, particularly those who are critically ill, factor VII activity levels are usually the first to decrease due to its short half-life of 4–6 hrs and increased turnover, which results in

a prolonged PT and can be noted even when usual markers of hepatocellular injury/hepatic insufficiency remain relatively normal (3,44). A prolonged TT in the setting of liver disease may indicate the presence of dysfibrinogenemia as a result of altered hepatic fibrinogen synthesis. As the severity of liver disease increases, the aPTT may also be affected, reflecting more severely impaired synthetic function. In this setting, plasma concentrations of the vitamin K-dependent coagulation proteins decrease, as do those of factor V (which is not vitamin K dependent). Although fibrinogen synthesis occurs in the liver, its plasma level is maintained until the disease approaches end stage. When fibrinogen levels are severely depressed, liver failure has typically reached the terminal phase.

In more severe forms of liver disease, fibrinolysis may complicate clinical management. The differentiation between concomitant DIC and fibrinolysis attributable to liver disease alone may be difficult. The D-dimer assay result should be negative in the patient who has liver disease and elevated FDPs but no active bleeding. Further clinical distinction usually is not possible.

Management

If the patient is not actively bleeding, no specific therapy is required, with certain provisos. In patients with a prolonged PT who are in a postoperative state or are scheduled for an invasive procedure, correction of the PT should be attempted. FFP provides the most immediate source of specific coagulation factors (i.e., factor VII) and usually corrects an isolated mild PT prolongation. Cryoprecipitate is required only if fibrinogen levels are <50–100 mg/dL or if significant dysfibrinogenemia is documented. Vitamin K deficiency also is relatively common in this patient population, and replacement may be necessary. In contrast to children with dietary vitamin K deficiency and normal liver function, correction of the PT in vitamin K-responsive critically ill patients typically requires longer than 12–24 hrs. Patients with significant hepatic impairment may manifest a partial response or may not respond at all. The immediate use of FFP is therefore appropriate when rapid correction is necessary. rhFVIIa infusions have been shown to control bleeding in severe liver disease, although reduced mortality does not necessarily result (30,53).

When the synthetic capability of the liver becomes more profoundly impaired and the aPTT is prolonged, greater volumes of FFP or more specific therapy may be necessary. The use of factor IX concentrates (prothrombin complex concentrates) or rhFVIIa has been advocated, particularly if bleeding is present. However, their use remains controversial. The products produced from plasma pooled from multiple donors carry a significant risk of hepatitis (both types B and C). In addition, they may provoke DIC and actually worsen hemostasis. The use of prothrombin complex concentrates or rhFVIIa should be reserved for patients with poorly controlled bleeding that is unresponsive to other, more established therapeutic modalities such as infusion of FFP.

A comprehensive therapeutic approach is required in the patient with active bleeding as a result of liver disease. Initially, FFP, 10–15 mL/kg body weight, may be given every 6–8 hrs until bleeding slows significantly; it should then be continued at maintenance levels as dictated by clinical status and coagulation studies. Continuous infusions of FFP (starting dose 2–4 mL/kg/hr) have also been used with success to control bleeding following a bolus infusion (21). rhFVIIa or prothrombin complex concentrates may be used in those patients who are unresponsive to FFP infusions (12,53). Cryoprecipitate should be infused for fibrinogen levels <50–100 mg/dL. Platelet transfusions also may be required if the platelet count is <40–80,000/μL, depending on the clinical situation. Vitamin K should be empirically administered on the presumption that part of the synthetic defect may result from a lack of this cofactor. However, a poor response to vitamin K in the presence of severe liver disease should be anticipated. Transfusions of packed cells are administered as deemed appropriate by the clinician.

Vitamin K Deficiency

The most common cause of a prolonged PT in the ICU is vitamin K deficiency. Vitamin K is necessary for the γ-carboxylation of factors II, VII, IX, and X, without which these factors cannot bind calcium and are not efficiently converted into their activated forms. Factor VII has the shortest half-life of these coagulation proteins; accordingly, the PT is the most sensitive early indicator of vitamin K deficiency.

Vitamin K deficiency is relatively common in critically ill patients for several reasons, including the use of broad-spectrum antibiotics, poor nutrition preceding or subsequent to ICU admission, and the use of parenteral nutrition without vitamin K supplementation. Many of the second- and third-generation cephalosporins directly interfere with vitamin K absorption from the gut lumen. The metabolites of these antibiotics may even act as competitive inhibitors of vitamin K. In addition, these and other antibiotics may kill or inhibit the growth of gut bacteria and limit the amounts of vitamin K that they normally produce and excrete into the gut lumen. While malnutrition also may contribute to the development of vitamin K deficiency, it usually requires 1–2 weeks to develop in the complete absence of vitamin K intake. However, the use of parenteral alimentation without vitamin K supplementation coupled with antibiotic use may result in rapid vitamin K depletion, and prolongation of the PT can occur within only 2–3 days. Finally, fat malabsorption states, including cystic fibrosis, may be associated with vitamin K deficiency. Vitamin K is fat soluble and is not absorbed well in some conditions of biliary tract and intrinsic small-bowel disease. In the ICU, vitamin K deficiency usually results from the interaction of several of these factors and is rarely limited to one of the conditions mentioned. It is the responsibility of the clinician to maintain an awareness of the potential for vitamin K deficiency and to treat accordingly.

The differential diagnosis of an isolated prolongation of the PT, with or without bleeding, includes both vitamin K deficiency and liver disease. The clinical presentation of these patients is often quite similar. In fact, the distinction sometimes can be made only on the basis of the response (or lack thereof) to empirical vitamin K therapy. Warfarin administration (either overt or covert) also should be excluded as a cause of a prolonged PT. Newer, long-acting vitamin K antagonist rodenticides (so-called "superwarfarin"), which, when ingested, produce a profound, prolonged, vitamin K-resistant reduction in vitamin K-dependent clotting factors, may produce an isolated prolongation of the PT initially. Treatment of poisoning with these agents requires aggressive, prolonged use of vitamin K and, in the bleeding patient, FFP infusions or rhFVIIa. Confirmation of warfarin exposure as the cause of a prolonged PT

is possible by toxicologic methods to detect the drug and/or its metabolites, or the presence of noncarboxylated forms of vitamin K-dependent clotting factors in plasma (*proteins induced by vitamin K antagonist*; PIVKAs) can be identified. In addition, the presence of a specific inhibitor or congenital deficiency of factor VII will also result in an isolated prolongation of the PT. Acquired inhibitors of factor VII are rare, and homozygous deficiency of factor VII has not been described. Individuals who are heterozygous for factor VII deficiency and those with certain polymorphisms of the promoter region of the factor VII gene tend to have factor VII levels in the 25%–35% range and do not appear to be at significant increased risk for bleeding. Lupus-like anticoagulants that result from inflammation may also lead to an isolated prolongation of the PT; these are generally of no clinical significance and are not associated with an increased risk of bleeding.

Infants who fail to receive vitamin K in the immediate postnatal period may develop a systemic coagulopathy manifested by bruising and gastrointestinal bleeding, generally occurring between 1 and 2 weeks of age. The first manifestation is often prolonged bleeding following circumcision. Infants with malabsorption or breast-fed infants who ingest medications that interfere with vitamin K in breast milk may develop similar manifestations beyond 2 weeks of age.

The laboratory findings of an isolated vitamin K deficiency, in addition to a prolonged PT, include a normal fibrinogen level, platelet count, and factor V level. Factor V is not a vitamin K-dependent protein and should therefore be normal, except in cases of DIC (consumption) or severe liver disease (decreased production). Prolongation of the aPTT from vitamin K deficiency, warfarin therapy, or liver disease is a relatively late event and occurs initially as a result of factor IX depletion.

Management

The management of vitamin K deficiency consists primarily of its repletion, usually by IV or subcutaneous routes in critically ill patients. Therapy should not await the development of bleeding or oozing but should be administered when the PT abnormality is detected and vitamin K deficiency is thought to be responsible. As with other drugs administered subcutaneously (e.g., insulin), adequate blood pressure and subcutaneous perfusion are necessary to ensure reliable absorption from the soft tissues. Concern exists regarding the possibility of anaphylactoid reactions with the IV use of vitamin K. This risk is minimized when the drug is given as a piggyback infusion over 30–45 mins in a small volume of fluid rather than as a bolus or "slow-push" dose; the former is the preferred method of drug administration in hemodynamically unstable patients. The usual dose of vitamin K in children is 1–5 mg IV or subcutaneously (up to 10 mg in larger children). In an otherwise healthy person, the PT should correct within 12–24 hrs after this dose. However, serial dosing of critically ill patients is often utilized, and the PT may require up to 72 hrs to normalize. If the PT does not correct within 72 hrs after three daily doses of vitamin K, intrinsic liver disease should be suspected. Further administration of vitamin K is of no additional benefit in this setting.

When the patient is actively bleeding, it is not sufficient to give vitamin K alone. A more immediate restoration of coagulation is required. FFP has traditionally been employed in this setting. To restore hemostasis to an acceptable level (30%–50%) of normal enzyme activity, 10–15 mL/kg body weight of FFP is typically required. A similar approach is used in patients who were previously given warfarin. rhFVIIa has been used with success to reverse the bleeding noted in vitamin K deficiency and in warfarin overdose (12,20,45,53).

Massive Transfusion Syndrome

Transfusion of large quantities of blood can result in a multifactorial hemostatic defect. The genesis of this problem is related to the "washout" of plasma coagulation proteins and platelets, and it may be exacerbated by the development of DIC with consequent factor consumption, hypothermia, acidosis, or rarely, by citrate toxicity or hypocalcemia. These variables often act in combination to cause a coagulopathic state (33).

A washout syndrome can result from the transfusion of large amounts of stored blood products that are devoid of clotting factors and platelets and develops exclusively in patients who receive large volumes of packed red blood cells (e.g., trauma victims, patients with massive gastrointestinal hemorrhage or hepatectomy, or those undergoing cardiopulmonary bypass) without also receiving FFP and platelets. Factors V and VII have short shelf half-lives and are often deficient in blood that has been banked longer than 48 hrs. In addition, a qualitative platelet defect can be demonstrated in whole blood within hours of its storage, especially if an acid-citrate-dextrose solution is used. Consequently, transfusion of large quantities of stored whole blood may produce limited improvement in the bleeding that results from decreased clotting factors and platelets. The development of a washout coagulopathy is directly dependent on the volume of blood transfused relative to the blood volume of the patient. As a general rule, residual plasma clotting activity after single-blood-volume exchange falls to 18%–37% of normal; after a double-blood-volume exchange, residual activity is only 3%–14% of normal; and after a triple-blood-volume exchange, <5% of normal clotting function remains.

As previously discussed, DIC may develop in many clinical settings, including some associated with major hemorrhage or massive transfusion. In the presence of hypotension associated with hypovolemia or hemorrhagic shock, DIC is a common sequela. Major trauma itself, especially with the release of TFs into the plasma, also can result in the development of DIC. Exsanguinating hemorrhage sometimes requires blood replacement faster than a type and cross-match of each unit can be performed, and unmatched blood is given as a life-saving measure. Donor-recipient incompatibility—even when the mismatch is only of the minor blood group systems—can lead to DIC. Human error that results in major incompatibility can produce lethal hemorrhage. Finally, microaggregates of blood cells that form within stored blood products can also cause DIC; however, the advent of smaller-pore, more effective filtering systems for blood product administration has essentially eliminated this as a source of problems.

The patient who is bleeding as a consequence of massive transfusion or washout presents with diffuse oozing and bleeding from all surgical wounds and puncture sites. Laboratory abnormalities include prolonged PT, aPTT, and TT. Fibrinogen levels and platelet counts are typically decreased; FDPs are not usually increased unless concurrent DIC is present (**Table 103.2**). The likelihood that the clinicolaboratory picture is a direct result of the massive transfusion can be estimated from the amount of bleeding that has occurred and the blood volume that has been administered relative to the patient's blood volume (i.e., the number of blood volume exchanges that have been given). The more stored blood (e.g., packed red blood cells) transfused relative to the patient's blood volume, the greater the chance of the development of coagulopathy due to massive transfusion.

Management

The therapeutic approach to patients who develop a coagulopathy from massive transfusion is supportive. Platelets and FFP are given to replete the components of coagulation that are typically lacking (35). Platelet administration may help to stem bleeding from anatomic wounds. Severe bleeding associated with thrombocytopenia alone is uncommon, unless counts fall below 20,000–30,000μL of blood. Because of the complex nature of bleeding seen with massive transfusion, patients may benefit from platelet transfusion at counts even as high as 80,000– 100,000/μL. FFP is preferred over cryoprecipitate because it has a more complete coagulation protein composition. However, cryoprecipitate may be specifically given when fibrinogen depletion is thought to be a major contributor to the observed bleeding.

Prospective identification of those at risk to develop a coagulopathy from massive transfusion is important. When the magnitude of the insult and the anticipated need for blood are large, both platelets and FFP should be given before a coagulopathy develops. In larger children (e.g., weight $\geq$30–40 kg or body surface area $\geq$1.0 m^2), 4 units of platelets (or half of a unit of apheresis-collected platelets) and 1 unit of FFP should be given for each 5 units of whole blood or packed cells transfused. In smaller children, 10 mL/kg of platelets and 10–15 mL/kg FFP should be given for each 40–50 mL/kg of blood transfused. These amounts should prevent washout and its attendant bleeding.

If the patient continues to bleed despite what should be adequate therapy for massive transfusion syndrome, other causes should be considered. Specifically, anatomic bleeding and the possibility of DIC should be investigated. Therapy in this setting may include rhFVIIa infusion (9).

Anticoagulant Overdose

Anticoagulant therapy is not unusual in the PICU, and the possibility of errors in administration exists. Methods of prophylactic anticoagulant use, systemic anticoagulation, and thrombolytic therapy are sometimes poorly standardized and can lead to overdose.

Heparin

Heparin is a repeating polymer of two disaccharide glycosaminoglycans and is commercially prepared from either porcine intestinal mucosa or bovine lung. Heparin is currently found in two forms: unfractionated heparin (UH) and low-molecular-weight heparin (LMWH). It is important to understand the differences between these two forms of the drug, as they have different mechanisms of action and associated precautions. UH has an immediate effect on coagulation that is mediated primarily through its interaction with antithrombin III. The resulting heparin-antithrombin III complex possesses a much greater affinity for thrombin than does antithrombin III alone, and it inactivates thrombin, thereby damping down clot formation. In addition, heparin has a direct effect by inhibiting activated factor X (factor Xa). As this anticoagulant effect of UH is relatively minor, achieving a therapeutic aPTT with UH is very difficult in the face of low levels of antithrombin III. The degree of anticoagulation produced by heparin is monitored by the prolongation of the aPTT. In contrast, LMWH, produced by controlled enzymatic cleavage of heparin polymers, effects anticoagulation almost exclusively through inhibition of factor Xa, which produces a more stable degree of anticoagulation. Due to its longer half-life (~3–5 hrs) and biologic activity (~24 hrs), LMWH allows for intermittent bolus therapy (i.e., every 12 or 24 hrs) while maintaining a steady-state effect. However, LMWH does not produce consistent prolongation of the aPTT and requires assay of anti-Xa activity for monitoring (if desired).

Heparin is metabolized in the liver by the "heparinase" enzyme in a dose-dependent fashion, with excess heparin then being excreted through the kidneys. As the rate of heparin administration is increased, the half-life of the drug is prolonged because of the increased percentage of the drug being excreted by the kidney. For example, when a 100-U/kg bolus of heparin is infused IV, the average half-life of the drug is 1 hr. If the bolus is increased to 400 or 800 U/kg, the half-life is prolonged to 2.5 and 5 hrs, respectively. The nonlinear response results in greater drug effects on coagulation with smaller dosage increments. When one "re-boluses" or increases a heparin infusion rate in response to insufficient anticoagulation (i.e., inadequate prolongation of the aPTT), a point will be reached when further small increments in the heparin infusion rate may result in a substantially greater prolongation of the aPTT. The risk of pathologic bleeding associated with heparin increases when the prolongation of the aPTT is beyond the therapeutic window (generally considered to be 1.5–2.5 times the patient's baseline aPTT, corresponding to a plasma heparin concentration of 0.2–0.4 units/mL). As a corollary, administration of heparin as a continuous infusion rather than in an intermittent bolus dose regimen is less likely to be associated with pathologic bleeding.

Management

Serious bleeding associated with heparin overdose can be rapidly reversed by protamine sulfate. Protamine binds ionically with heparin to form a complex that lacks any anticoagulant activity. As a general rule, 1 mg of protamine neutralizes ~100 U of heparin (specifically, 90 USP units of bovine heparin or 115 USP units of porcine heparin). The dose of protamine required is calculated from the number of units of active heparin remaining in the patient's system. This, in turn, is estimated from the original heparin dose and the typical half-life for that infusion rate. The aPTT is used to gauge the residual effects of heparin. During and after cardiopulmonary bypass surgery, the activated clotting time is frequently used to measure heparin effect and to judge the effectiveness of and need for protamine neutralization. This methodology is sometimes employed in the ICU. However, the equipment used for this measurement is poorly standardized, with different systems giving different results (11). Consequently, care must be taken when employing one of these methods in the ICU.

Protamine itself potentially has anticoagulant effects, and precautions are necessary during its administration. The drug should be given by slow IV push over 8–10 mins. A single dose should not exceed 1 mg/kg (50 mg maximum dose). This dose

may be repeated, but no more than 2 mg/kg (100 mg maximum dose) should be given as a cumulative dose without rechecking coagulation parameters. The dose of protamine should always be monitored by coagulation studies. Significant side effects are most commonly seen in situations of overly rapid drug administration and include hypotension and anaphylactoid-like reactions. The allergic reactions to protamine represent type I anaphylactic reactions between an antigen (protamine) and antibody (IgE or IgG) and result in histamine release. Consequently, H_2 blockers have been shown to be effective in treating and minimizing these reactions. In addition, complement activation, thromboxane, and nitric oxide production have all been shown to play some role in the pathogenesis of these reactions (13,52). Risk factors for protamine hypersensitivity reactions include prior exposure to protamine, insulin-dependent diabetes (with NPH exposure), fish allergy, and vasectomy. In that LMWH is not consistently neutralized by protamine, invasive procedures should not be performed within 24 hrs of administration. Bleeding following LMWH therapy has been treated effectively with rhFVIIa.

Warfarin

Warfarin and vitamin K are structurally similar in their respective 4-hydroxycoumarin nucleus and naphthoquinone ring. The mechanism of action of warfarin is through competitive binding at the vitamin K receptor site, where postribosomal modification, through γ-carboxylation, of the vitamin K-dependent coagulation proteins (factors II, VII, IX, and X) occurs. This postsynthetic modification is necessary to produce a calcium-binding site on the molecule, which, when occupied, allows for the efficient activation of the zymogen clotting factor into its enzymatically active form. When warfarin is present in sufficient plasma concentrations, the active forms of vitamin K-dependent factors are depleted.

The PT is an accurate indicator of the effects of warfarin when its use has continued beyond 2 or 3 days. Factor VII (the active form) has a half-life of only 4–6 hrs and is rapidly depleted after one or two doses of warfarin. The remainder of the vitamin K-dependent factors may take up to a week to become depleted. The PT becomes prolonged with factor VII depletion alone but does not reflect an overall state of anticoagulation until an equilibrium period of several days has passed. Over this time, the other vitamin K-dependent factors are depleted, and PT prolongation can then be used to assess the anticoagulant effects of warfarin. In severe cases of warfarin overdose, the aPTT also becomes prolonged as a result of depletion of the active forms of factors II, IX, and X.

Several drugs and pathophysiologic conditions are associated with potentiation of warfarin's effects on coagulation. Many of the drugs known to prolong the effects of warfarin are listed in **Table 103.5**. These drugs have a variety of mechanisms that generally include either inhibition of function or competitive binding of the enzymes that are responsible for active warfarin metabolism. Aspirin does not seem to have any direct influence on warfarin metabolism but so profoundly influences qualitative platelet function that it must be considered as a potentiator of warfarin's anticoagulant effects. The same is true for clofibrate. Large ingestion of aspirin may also impair prothrombin (factor II) synthesis, further increasing the effects of warfarin administration. Warfarin is metabolized by the liver. Conditions of acute and chronic hepatic dysfunction can alter warfarin metabolism and vitamin

TABLE 103.5

DRUGS THAT POTENTIATE THE ANTICOAGULANT EFFECTS OF WARFARIN

Antibiotics
  Broad-spectrum antibiotics (especially cephalosporins)
  Griseofulvin (oral)
  Metronidazole
  Sulfonamides
  Trimethoprim-sulfamethoxazole

Anti-inflammatory Drugs
  Steroids (anabolic, in particular)
  Acetylated salicylates
  Phenylbutazone (oxyphenbutazone)
  Sulfinpyrazone

Other Drugs
  Clofibrate
  Disulfiram
  Phenytoin
  Thyroxine (both D- and L-isomers)
  Tolbutamide

K-mediated γ-carboxylation of the vitamin K-dependent coagulation proteins. Broad-spectrum antibiotics also may limit vitamin K availability through their alteration of the gut flora (in addition to any direct effect on vitamin K metabolism). All of these factors may ultimately influence a patient's response to warfarin.

A clinical syndrome referred to as "warfarin (Coumadin) necrosis" has been noted during the initial stages of anticoagulation with a vitamin-K antagonist. It is characterized clinically by the development of skin and subcutaneous necrosis, particularly in areas of subcutaneous fat, and pathologically by the thrombosis of small blood vessels in the fat and subcutaneous tissues. This syndrome is caused by the rapid depletion of the vitamin K-dependent, anticoagulant PC prior to achieving depletion of procoagulant proteins and occurs predominantly in individuals who are heterozygous for PC deficiency. While anticoagulation generally requires a decrease in procoagulant protein levels to ~20%–25%, a prothrombotic milieu is created with PC levels of ≤40%. Consequently, individuals who are heterozygous for PC deficiency and have baseline PC levels of 50%–60% may develop a prothrombotic environment during the first few days of warfarin therapy. The risk of developing warfarin necrosis appears to be greater when an initial dose of warfarin >10–15 mg is administered. The development of this syndrome generally can be avoided if heparin and warfarin therapy are overlapped until "Coumadinization" is complete and if large loading doses of warfarin are avoided.

Management

When over-anticoagulation with warfarin presents with bleeding, immediate reversal is usually mandated (20). The treatment of choice is FFP, which provides prompt restoration of the deficient vitamin K-dependent coagulation proteins, along with restoration of hemostatic function. Ten to 15 mL/kg of FFP is usually sufficient to produce significant correction of the PT, although repeat infusions of FFP may be necessary to effect continued correction of the PT due to the short half-life of factor VII (35). Vitamin K also may be administered, particularly in situations that are less acute (see the previous section, Vita-

min K Deficiency), although this will make it more difficult to "re-Coumadinization" the patient afterward. For severe bleeding or bleeding not controlled by FFP infusions, rhFVIIa has been used successfully.

Platelet Disorders

Platelets are necessary for efficient clot formation. They not only produce a physical barrier at the site of vascular injury (the so-called "platelet plug"); they also serve to focus the clotting process at the point of bleeding by delivering vasoconstrictors, clotting factors, and a surface on which clot development occurs to the bleeding site (**Fig. 103.3**). Quantitative and qualitative platelet disorders are a common cause of clinical bleeding in the PICU. An overview of platelet disorders based on this classification scheme is presented in **Table 103.6**.

Quantitative Platelet Disorders

A decrease in the number of circulating platelets reflects the presence of increased peripheral destruction/sequestration, decreased marrow production, or a combination of these factors. Examples of increased peripheral destruction include immune-mediated processes (both autoimmune and drug induced), abnormal consumption (as in DIC), and mechanical destruction (e.g., cardiopulmonary bypass, hyperthermia). Autoimmune processes such as idiopathic thrombocytopenic purpura (ITP), SLE, or acquired immunodeficiency syndrome can result in increased peripheral destruction and increased splenic sequestration of platelets. Autoimmune destruction also may occur in conjunction with lymphocytic leukemia or lymphoma.

The prototypic example of immune thrombocytopenia is ITP, in which immunoglobin (generally IgG) directed against specific platelet antigens is thought to be responsible for platelet destruction. Acute ITP is usually self-limited, with life-threatening bleeding occurring only rarely. In contrast, chronic ITP generally requires immunosuppressive therapy. Steroids may be given (2–4 mg/kg day of prednisone or its equivalent). High doses of IV γ-globulin (1–2 g/kg given over 2–5 days) and infusions of anti-RhD antigen antibody (WinRho; 25–60 mcg/kg) are equally efficacious in producing at least transient elevations in platelet counts. Agents such as vincristine/vinblastine, cyclophosphamide, and rituximab (anti-CD20 monoclonal antibody) also have been used as immunosuppressants, with variable success, although responses are generally not immediate. Splenectomy may be required to avert serious bleeding complications in patients who do not respond to medical management, although this approach is chosen much less often in children than in adults. In ITP, the degree of bleeding attributed to thrombocytopenia is generally less than that noted when thrombocytopenia results from decreased production. In general, severe bleeding is not noted until the platelet count is <10,000/mcL, although levels below 40,000–50,000/mcL may increase the risk of bleeding associated with invasive procedures.

Drug-induced, immune-mediated platelet destruction is the cause of thrombocytopenia that is frequently considered in the thrombocytopenic PICU patient. When it is present, it is usually reversible; withdrawal of the offending drug prevents further immune-mediated platelet destruction. The exact mechanism of platelet destruction seems to be related to the binding of a drug to the platelet membrane, with subsequent binding to

TABLE 103.6

PLATELET DISORDERS SEEN IN THE ICU

Quantitative	Qualitative

Increased destruction
  Immune
    Idiopathic thrombocytopenic purpura
    Systemic lupus erythematosus
    Acquired immunodeficiency syndrome
    Drugs (gold salts, heparin, sulfonamides,
      quinidine, quinine)
    Sepsis
  Nonimmune
    Thrombotic thrombocytopenic purpura/
      hemolytic uremic syndrome
    Mechanical destruction (e.g.,
      cardiopulmonary bypass, hyperthermia)
    Consumption (i.e., disseminated
      intravascular coagulation)
 	
Decreased production
  Marrow suppression
    Chemotherapy
    Viral illness (e.g., cytomegalovirus,
      Epstein-Barr virus, herpes simplex,
      parvovirus)
    Drugs (thiazides, ethanol, cimetidine)
  Marrow replacement
    Tumor
    Myelofibrosis
  Other conditions
    Splenic sequestration
    Dilution (see massive transfusion
      syndrome)
	Drugs
	  Antiinflammatory agents
	    Aspirin (irreversible)
	    Nonsteroidal anti-inflammatory agents
	    Corticosteroids
	  Antibiotics
	    Penicillins (e.g., ampicillin,
	      carbenicillin, ticarcillin, penicillin-G)
	    Cephalosporins (e.g., cephalothin)
	    Nitrofurantoin
	    Chloroquine, hydroxychloroquine
	  Phosphodiesterase inhibitors
	    Dipyridamole
	    Methylxanthines (e.g., theophylline)
	
	Other drugs
	  Antihistamines
	  α-blockers (e.g., phentolamine)
	  β-blockers (e.g., propranolol)
	  Dextran
	  Ethanol
	  Furosemide
	  Heparin
	  Local anesthetics (e.g., lidocaine)
	  Phenothiazines
	  Tricyclic antidepressants
	  Nitrates (e.g., sodium nitroprusside,
	    nitroglycerin)
	
	Metabolic causes
	  Uremia
	  Stored whole blood
	  Disseminated intravascular coagulation
	    (i.e., fibrin degradation product-
	    mediated inhibition)
	  Hypothyroidism

the platelet, platelet-drug complex, or both, of a specific antibody. The resulting platelet-drug-antibody complexes are then cleared by the reticuloendothelial system (e.g., the spleen), and thrombocytopenia develops. Drugs used in the ICU that are most commonly associated with this clinical picture include quinidine, quinine, heparin, gold salts, various penicillin and cephalosporin antibiotics, and the sulfonamides. The anticonvulsant valproic acid frequently produces a dose-dependent thrombocytopenia that is, at least in part, immunologic in nature.

A variety of drugs are associated with the nonimmune development of thrombocytopenia by bone marrow suppression. Most commonly, most cancer chemotherapeutic agents produce thrombocytopenia as a consequence of marrow suppression. The thiazide diuretics, cimetidine, ethanol, and several of the cephalosporin and penicillin antibiotics may suppress platelet production. Generalized infection (such as bacterial sepsis) and many viral illnesses are also associated with bone marrow suppression and thrombocytopenia, even if an element of immune platelet destruction is present. Disorders such as Gaucher disease may produce a mild-to-moderate thrombocytopenia as a result of marrow replacement by nonhematopoietic cells.

Consumption of platelets can also cause thrombocytopenia. Mechanical destruction invariably occurs during the use of cardiopulmonary bypass machines, and it is not uncommon to note a 50% drop in platelet count post-bypass, when compared to preoperative platelet levels. Platelet counts generally recover toward preoperative levels by 48–72 hrs after bypass. Platelets may also be destroyed by the high body temperatures seen in severe hyperthermic syndromes, and they are consumed during microvascular coagulation in DIC. In many of these circumstances, the thrombocytopenia may be the sole or a contributing cause of significant bleeding.

Heparin-induced Thrombocytopenia

As heparin use is ubiquitous in the ICU, the special problems associated with it merit emphasis. Heparin-induced thrombocytopenia (HIT) may develop in one of two ways. Acute, nonidiosyncratic HIT is seen in 10%–15% of patients who receive heparin. The degree of thrombocytopenia is usually mild and usually remits despite continued use of the drug (type I HIT), and the thrombocytopenia that develops has no clinical significance. Heparin need not be stopped in these patients. Idiosyncratic HIT is of much greater clinical consequence. Although it is a less frequent occurrence (typically seen in <5% of patients who receive heparin), it has a much greater potential for clinical morbidity. Arterial thrombosis is the most significant risk of this form of HIT (type II HIT) and may be life threatening, causing myocardial infarction, cerebrovascular accident, pulmonary embolism, or renal infarction. The mechanism of thrombosis is thought to be a consequence of the deposition of platelet aggregates in the microcirculation (28,61). Thrombocytopenia, like other immune-mediated drug reactions, seems to involve the formation of platelet aggregates mediated by the binding of a specific antibody, directed against a heparin-platelet factor 4 complex, to platelets in the presence of heparin. This process seems to require minuscule amounts of heparin. Clinical bleeding is an infrequent problem in these patients.

From a practical perspective, the diagnosis of HIT is usually one of exclusion. Diagnostic markers do exist (e.g., heparin-dependent platelet antibodies, aggregation or serotonin release), but these tests are best considered confirmatory and not exclusionary. An enzyme-linked immunoabsorbent assay (ELISA) test for heparin-dependent platelet antibodies is the most common test obtained to investigate a possible diagnosis of HIT, but because of a relatively high false-positive rate, it is generally recommended that a more specific heparin-induced platelet injury assay, such as a serotonin release assay, be performed for confirmation. The diagnosis may be difficult to confirm because coexisting clinical illnesses with the potential to cause thrombocytopenia also may be present. While HIT may be more likely to be associated with the use of bovine lung heparin, it can occur after exposure to porcine heparin or, much less commonly, LMWH. When type II HIT is suspected or confirmed, all exposure to heparin, including heparin flushes, heparin in total parenteral nutrition, and heparin-coated catheters, must be removed, and anticoagulation with an alternate agent must be initiated because of the risk of delayed thrombosis, which can occur up to 30 days after removal of heparin exposure (54,61). Patients with type II HIT should receive continued anticoagulation with direct thrombin inhibitors (argatroban, lepirudin) or with the heparinoid danaparoid. The direct thrombin inhibitors are preferred, as they carry no risk of cross-reacting with the heparin-dependent antibodies already present (16,54). Argatroban is cleared by the liver and lepirudin by the kidney. Consequently, the choice and dose of drug may be affected by the presence of hepatic or renal insufficiency. Warfarin alone is not adequate therapy for suspected type II HIT because of the risk of thrombosis from depression of PC levels. However, warfarins can be utilized in conjunction with a direct thrombin inhibitor and subsequently continued as a single agent once therapeutic suppression of vitamin K-dependent clotting factors has been achieved.

Qualitative Platelet Disorders

Many of the drugs frequently used in the ICU have the potential to impair platelet function. Frequently, the sicker the patient, the greater the likelihood that she will be exposed to one of these drugs. These patients often have other underlying pathophysiologic conditions that, in and of themselves, can predispose to bleeding. An abbreviated list of the drugs that can affect at least in vitro platelet function is presented in **Table 103.6**.

All unnecessary drugs should be viewed as suspect and discontinued in patients with evidence of qualitative platelet dysfunction or in those in whom it is strongly suspected. In most cases, terminating the offending drugs usually results in a

restoration of normal platelet functional activity. Aspirin is the notable exception, as it irreversibly inhibits platelet cyclooxygenase, resulting in a defect that lasts for the duration of the platelet lifespan (8–9 days). The effect is profound: a single 325-mg aspirin tablet results in a qualitative platelet defect that remains in 50% of the circulating platelets 5 days after its ingestion. Ideally, all aspirin ingestion should be avoided for at least 7 days prior to an elective invasive procedure.

Nonsteroidal anti-inflammatory agents similarly affect the platelet cyclooxygenase enzyme. However, their effects are reversible, and normal platelet function is usually restored within 24 hours of the last dose. Under most circumstances, the degree of platelet inhibition produced by these agents is not clinically significant, and patients can receive these drugs for analgesia and fever control. However, it is reasonable to minimize their use in the severely bleeding thrombocytopenic patient. The β-lactam antibiotics can stearically hinder the binding of a platelet aggregation agonist (e.g., ADP) to its specific platelet receptor, resulting in impaired platelet aggregation under circumstances of normal physiologic stimulation. This, too, is reversed on removal of the drug. Fortunately, only a minority of patients exposed to these antibiotics will exhibit clinically significant platelet inhibition.

In the PICU, the possibility must always be considered that a patient with bleeding suggestive of a platelet defect might have an inherited disorder of platelet function. While rare, these disorders are encountered from time to time and include Glanzmann thrombasthenia (abnormal platelet GPIIb/IIIa), Bernard-Soulier syndrome (abnormal GP Ib/IX), Wiskott-Aldrich syndrome, platelet storage pool deficiency (abnormal platelet-dense bodies), and the Gray platelet disorder (abnormal platelet α-granules).

Management

Because many of the adverse drug-related platelet effects are reversible, all unnecessary medications should be discontinued promptly when platelet function seems impaired. The more controversial issue is deciding whether platelet transfusions are warranted in a particular patient. The relationship of thrombocytopenia to clinical bleeding is relative; that is, it is difficult to identify a specific, arbitrary platelet count (threshold) below which bleeding is likely to occur. Several conditions, such as massive transfusion syndrome and DIC, may respond to empirical platelet transfusion at counts as high as 80,000 or even 100,000 platelets/μL, although bleeding in the presence of a platelet count of 80,000/mcL (or greater) is unlikely to be a result of the thrombocytopenia. With other causes such as thrombocytopenia seen with cancer chemotherapy and bone marrow aplasia, therapy may not be required until counts fall below 10,000–20,000/mcL. As previously stated, rhFVIIa has been used to reverse the hemostatic defect caused by aspirin or clopidogrel (4).

The morbidity and mortality related to bleeding increase measurably in patients who undergo induction chemotherapy for acute leukemia when the platelet count falls below 10,000–20,000/mcL. Empirical administration of platelets to these patients significantly limits both morbidity and mortality. However, this finding has been generalized to virtually all patients with platelet counts in this range, and the appropriateness of this approach is unclear. A major concern that should temper the empirical use of platelet transfusion is the development of alloimmunization to transfused platelets, potentially negating any future benefit from platelet transfusion in a time of need. Patients with acute leukemia typically have self-limited marrow aplasia as a result of chemotherapy. Therefore, the need for platelet transfusion is also limited, and the chances for development of antiplatelet antibodies are greatly decreased. However, as patients with aplastic anemia have an ongoing need for platelet transfusion, their risk of alloimmunization is high. Autoimmune disorders associated with increased peripheral platelet destruction, disorders of splenic sequestration, and drug-related thrombocytopenia are unlikely to benefit from platelet transfusion. An exception is related to planned, invasive procedures with an increased risk of bleeding. In this situation, empirical platelet transfusion immediately before the procedure may be reasonable.

Uremia

Uremia is commonly seen in the ICU and is associated with an increased risk of bleeding (8,57). Uremia has been shown to cause a reversible impairment of platelet function, although the "toxin" responsible for this defect is not well defined. Some studies have demonstrated an impairment of platelet-vessel wall interactions and suggest defects in vWF. The degree of platelet impairment appears to be related to the severity of uremia for a given patient. In addition, thrombotic events are also increased in patients with uremia. These, too, appear to be multifactorial in etiology but in part reflect the increased renal loss of antithrombin III and protein S in nephritic-range proteinuria (47).

Several therapeutic approaches may modulate the qualitative platelet defect associated with uremia. The primary therapy in this setting is dialysis. Cryoprecipitate, 1-deamino-8-D-arginine vasopressin (DDAVP; 0.3 mcg/kg, maximum dose 21 mcg), and conjugated estrogens (10 mg/day in adult patients) have been given with good results to patients with severe uremia and an acquired defect in primary hemostasis. The benefit derived by treatment with cryoprecipitate or DDAVP appears to be related to the consequent increase in the plasma concentration of the large multimeric forms of vWF, thus greatly improving platelet adhesion. However, the durations of action of these agents are limited, with them reaching their zenith at between 2 and 6 hrs. Additional doses of DDAVP during the same 24-hr period may result in a diminished response to the drug (tachyphylaxis) with little or no further benefit. Patients who exhibit tachyphylaxis to DDAVP may require 48–72 hrs before again responding to this agent. The mechanism of action of the conjugated estrogens is not known. In contrast to the first two therapies described, the effect of estrogen is more protracted and does not diminish with repeat dosing, although a benefit is not noted until 3–5 days after therapy is started.

THROMBOTIC SYNDROMES

While thrombosis is not a common feature of pediatric illness, several thrombotic syndromes are seen with some degree of frequency in the PICU and include deep venous thrombosis (specifically in association with a central venous catheter), HIT, pulmonary embolism syndrome, TTP/HUS, thrombotic DIC, stroke, and central nervous system venous sinus thrombosis (most commonly seen in infants in association with marked dehydration).

Many of these conditions, particularly venous thromboembolic events, often develop while the patient is in the PICU and may be preventable. While young children often do not require prophylactic treatment to prevent deep vein thrombosis, the pediatric critical care physician should evaluate the risk for it and for thromboprophylaxis in older and/or larger patients and institute appropriate therapy on a case-by-case basis. In general, thromboprophylaxis measures should be considered for postpubertal pediatric patients, as their risk of thrombosis may more closely conform to that of the adult population.

Management

The initial management approach for a child with a documented (or highly suspected) thrombotic event is generally anticoagulation with either UH or LMWH. Their efficacy appears to be equivalent, although some studies (in adult populations) suggest that the incidence of severe bleeding is less with LMWH. The use of LMWH may produce a more stable level of anticoagulation, which may result in fewer laboratory tests and dose adjustments. The choice of agent is at the discretion of the intensivist. However, if repeated invasive procedures are anticipated, UH may be the preferred agent, owing to its shorter half-life. Infants tend to require relatively more heparin (UH) than do young children, who in turn, require more than older children and adults due to an apparent greater volume of distribution. While an adult or older child might be started on UH with a bolus dose of 50 U/kg followed by a continuous infusion of 10 U/kg/hr, the dose for a young child is a bolus of 75 units/kg followed by 15–20 U/kg/hr, and the dose for an infant is 100 U/kg bolus followed by a continuous infusion of 25 U/kg/hr (48). Irrespective of the age of the patient, anticoagulation is adjusted to keep the aPTT roughly 1.5–2.5 times baseline values (corresponding to a plasma heparin concentration of 0.2–0.4 units/mL in adult plasma). Dosing of LMWH does not appear to be age related. Warfarin (Coumadin) therapy is weight-related, with a loading dose of ~0.2 mg/kg/day for 2–3 days followed by a maintenance dose of ~0.1 mg/kg/day (10). The dose of warfarin is titrated to maintain an international normalized ratio of the PT between 1.5 and 4.0, depending on the intensity of anticoagulation desired. Thrombolytic therapy is generally not recommended as first-line therapy for thrombosis in newborn infants because of the high risk of hemorrhage; however, thrombolytic therapy may be appropriate in older infants and children, depending on the clinical presentation (48). No large, randomized trials of thrombolytic therapy in children have been conducted; consequently, adult dosing guidelines are generally followed. In general, thrombolytic therapy would generally be administered in consultation with pediatric hematology.

SELECTED DISORDERS

Systemic Diseases Associated with Factor Deficiencies

Amyloidosis, Gaucher disease, and the nephrotic syndrome are occasionally seen in the ICU. Each may have one or more associated factor deficiencies that may complicate patient management and result in bleeding. Patients with either amyloidosis or Gaucher disease may develop factor IX deficiency. Factor X deficiency has also been associated with amyloidosis. These deficiencies generally result from the absorption of the specific clotting factor onto the abnormal proteins present with each disorder. In the nephrotic syndrome, factor IX deficiency may develop. Although it was originally thought that proteinuria was responsible for the development of factor IX deficiency, this does not appear to be the case. The deficiency typically remits with corticosteroid therapy. Finally, antithrombin III deficiency can be seen along with the nephrotic syndrome and may lead to thrombosis. The loss of antithrombin III does appear to be related to proteinuria.

CONCLUSIONS AND FUTURE DIRECTIONS

Much attention is being given to elucidating the interplay of coagulation and inflammation and how the inflammatory state triggers a chain reaction that results in microvascular thrombosis and multiorgan dysfunction/failure. Complete characterization of these interactions will require a better understanding of the normal function of the endothelium and how this function is disrupted in sepsis and severe acute illness, as well as a better understanding of the specific host factors that regulate the balance between too little and too much thrombosis (**Fig. 103.6**). As the clinician's ability to treat the acute event that brings a child to the PICU improves, a better understanding of the processes that increase the potential for end-organ failure and of the best methods with which to treat them proactively will also be necessary.

Old and newer drugs are being tested in the setting of sepsis to prevent DIC and microvascular thrombosis; if successful, these tests may lead to improved survival with decreased morbidity. Although some of these strategies will involve ways to better regulate the coagulation process, a means by which to protect the endothelium must also be developed. While waiting for these scientific and therapeutic advances, clinicians must work to recognize disease processes (e.g., DIC) earlier so that they can determine how to best utilize those treatments already available (e.g., APC, thrombolytics, anticoagulants, etc.) in a more precise, cost effective, and safe manner.

KEY POINTS

- Hemostasis is a dynamic process; once bleeding occurs, clot formation, and degradation (fibrinolysis) are also initiated.
- Coagulation is an integral part of inflammation and usually will lead to microvascular thrombosis.
- A consumptive coagulopathy should always be considered in a patient with diffuse or generalized bleeding; however, liver disease and vitamin K deficiency are much more common.
- Localized bleeding in a trauma or postoperative patient is generally the result of an anatomic lesion rather than a systemic coagulopathy.
- Thrombotic events are being recognized with increased frequency in the PICU; no more than 60% of children with documented thromboses will be found to have an identifiable underlying hematologic abnormality.

- rhFVIIa is effective in controlling bleeding unresponsive to other measures, but its use has not yet been shown to improve outcome.

References

1. Abshire TC. An approach to the diagnosis and treatment of bleeding disorders in infants. *Int J Hematol* 2002;76(Suppl 2):265–70.
2. Aird WC. The role of the endothelium in severe sepsis and the multiple organ dysfunction syndrome. *Blood* 2003;101(10):3765–77.
3. Al Ghumias AK, Gader A, Faleh FZ. Haemostatic abnormalities in liver disease: Could some haemostatic tests be useful as liver function tests? *Blood Coagul Fibrinolysis* 2005;16(5):329–35.
4. Altman R, Scazziota A, De Lourdes Herrera M, et al. Recombinant factor VIIa reverses the inhibitory effect of aspirin or aspirin plus clopidogrel on in vivo thrombin generation. *J Thromb Haemost* 2006;4(9):2022–7.
5. Barton JC, Poon MC. Coagulation testing of the Hickmann catheter blood in patients with acute leukemia. *Arch Intern Med* 1986;146(11):2165–9.
6. Bernard GR, Vincent JL, Laterre PF, et al. Efficacy and safety of recombinant human activated protein C for severe sepsis. *New Engl J Med* 2001;344:699–709.
7. Bick RL, Arun B, Frenkel EP. Disseminated intravascular coagulation. Clinical and pathophysiological mechanisms and manifestations. *Haemostasis* 1999;29(2-3):111–34.
8. Boccardo P, Remuzzi G, Galbusera M. Platelet dysfunction in renal failure. *Semin Thromb Hemost* 2004;30 (5):579–89.
9. Boffard KD, Riou B, Warren B, et al. Recombinant factor VIIa as adjunctive therapy for bleeding control in severely injured trauma patients: Two parallel randomized, placebo-controlled, double blind clinical trials. *J Trauma* 2005;59(1):8–15;discussion 15–8.
10. Bonduel MM. Oral anticoagulation therapy in children. *Thromb Res* 2006;118(1):85–94.
11. Bosch YP, Ganushchak YM, de Jong DS. Comparison of ACT point-of-care measurements: Repeatability and agreement. *Perfusion* 2006;21(1):27–31.
12. Brady KM, Easley RB, Tobias JD. Recombinant activated factor VII (rFVIIa) treatment in infants with hemorrhage. *Paediatr Anaesth* 2006;16(10):1042–6.
13. Carr JA, Silverman N. The heparin-protamine interaction: A review. *J Cardiovasc Surg (Torino)*. 1999;40(5):659–66.
14. Cauchie P, Cauchie Ch, Boudjeltia KZ, C et al. Diagnosis and prognosis of overt disseminated intravascular coagulation in a general hospital—meaning of the ISTH score system, fibrin monomers, and lipoprotein-C-reactive protein complex formation. *Am J Hematol* 2006;81(6):414–9.
15. Chuansumrit A, Hotrakitya S, Sirinavin S, et al. Disseminated intravascular coagulation findings in 100 patients. *J Med Assoc Thai* 1999;82(Suppl 1):S63–8.
16. Dager WE, White RH. Pharmacotherapy of heparin-induced thrombocytopenia. *Expert Opin Pharmacother* 2003;4(6):919–40.
17. Davis-Jackson R, Correa H, Horswell R, et al. Antithrombin III (AT) and recombinant tissue plasminogen activator (R-TPA) used singly and in combination versus supportive care as treatment of endotoxin-induced disseminated intravascular coagulation (DIC) in the neonatal pig. *Thromb J* 2006;4:7.
18. De Kleijn ED, De Groot R, Hack CE, et al. Activation of protein C following infusion of protein C concentrate in children with severe meningococcal sepsis and purpura fulminans: A randomized, double-blinded, placebo-controlled, dose-finding study. *Crit Care Med* 2003;31(6):1839–47.
19. Dempfle CE. Coagulopathy and sepsis. *Thromb Haemost* 2004;91(2):213–24.
20. Dentali F, Ageno W, Crowther M. Treatment of coumarin-associated coagulopathy: A systemic review and proposed treatment algorithms. *J Thromb Haemost* 2006;4(9):1853–63.
21. Drews RE. Critical issues in hematology, anemia, thrombocytopenia, coagulopathy, and blood product transfusion in critically ill patients. *Clin Chest Med* 2003;24(4):607–22.
22. Eilertsen KE, Osterud B. Tissue factor: (patho)physiology and cellular biology. *Blood Coagul Fibrinolysis* 2004;15(7):521–38.
23. El-Nawawy A, Abbassy AA, El-Bordiny M, et al. Evaluation of early detection and management of disseminated intravascular coagulation among Alexandria University pediatric intensive care patients. *J Trop Pediatr* 2004;50(6):339–47.
24. Erber WN. Plasma and plasma products in the treatment of massive haemorrhage. *Best Prac Resch Clin Haematol* 2005;19(1):97–112.
25. Esmon CT. Crosstalk between inflammation and thrombosis. *Maturitas* 2004;47(4):305–14.
26. Faust SN, Heyderman RS, Levin M. Disseminated intravascular coagulation and purpura fulminans secondary to infection. *Baillieres Best Prac Rec Clin Haematol* 2000;13(2):179–97.
27. Faust SN, Levin M, Harrison OB, et al. Dysfunction of endothelial protein C activation in severe meningococcal sepsis. *N Engl J Med* 2001;345(6):408–16.

28. Frost J, Mureebe L, Russo P, et al. Heparin-induced thrombocytopenia in the pediatric intensive care unit population. *Pediatr Crit Care Med* 2005; 6(2):216–9.

29. Gando S, Iba T, Eguchi Y, et al. A multicenter, prospective validation of disseminated intravascular coagulation diagnostic criteria for critically ill patients: Comparing current criteria. *Crit Care Med* 2006;34(3):625–31.

30. Ganguly S, Spengel K, Tilzer LL, et al. Recombinant factor VIIa: Unregulated continuous use in patients with bleeding and coagulopathy does not alter mortality and outcome. *Clin Lab Haematol* 2006;28(5):309–12.

31. Girolami A, Luzzatto G, Varvarikis C, et al. Main clinical manifestations of a bleeding diathesis: An often disregarded aspect of medical and surgical history taking. *Hemophilia* 2005;11(3):193–202.

32. Goldenberg NA, Manco-Johnson MJ. Pediatric hemostasis and use of plasma components. *Best Prac Res Clin Haematol* 2005;19(1):143–55.

33. Hardy JF, de Moerloose P, Samama CM, et al. Massive transfusion and coagulopathy: Pathophysiology and implications for clinical management. *Can J Anaesth* 2006;53(6 Suppl):S40–58.

34. Hayward CP, Rao AK, Cattaneo M. Congenital platelet disorders: Overview of their mechanisms, diagnostic evaluation and treatment. *Haemophilia* 2006;12(Suppl 3):128–36.

35. Hellerstern P, Muntean W, Schramm W, et al. Practical guidelines for the clinical use of plasma. *Thromb Res* 2002;107(Suppl 1):S53–8.

36. Hermans PW, Hazelzet JA. Plasminogen activator inhibitor type 1 gene polymorphism and sepsis. *Clin Infect Dis* 2005;41(Suppl 7):S453–8.

37. Hermans PW, Hibberd ML, Booy R, et al. 4G/5G promoter polymorphism in the plasminogen-activator-inhibitor-1 gene and outcome in meningococcal disease. Meningococcal Research Group. *Lancet* 1999;354(9178): 556–60.

38. Horne M. Overview of hemostasis and thrombosis;current status of antithrombotic therapies. *Thromb Res* 2005;117(1-2):15–7;discussion 39–42.

39. Jaimes F, de la Rosa G, Arango C, et al. A randomized clinical trial of unfractionated heparin for treatment of sepsis (the HETRASE study): Design and rationale. *Trials* 2006;7:19.

40. Khair K, Liesner R. Bruising and bleeding in infants and children—a practical approach. *British J Haematol* 2006;133(3):221–31.

41. Leclerc F, Hazelzet J, Jude B, et al. Protein C and S deficiency in severe infectious purpura of children: A collaborative study of 40 cases. *Intensive Care Med* 1992;18(4):202–5.

42. Levi M, ten Cate H, van der Poll T. Endothelium: Interface between coagulation and inflammation. *Crit Care Med* 2002;30(5 Suppl):S220–4.

43. Lillicrap D, Nair SC, Srivastava A. Laboratory issues in bleeding disorders. *Hemophilia* 2006;12 (Suppl 3):68–75.

44. Lisman T, Caldwell SH, Leebeck FWG, et al. Hemostasis in chronic liver disease. *J Thromb Haemost* 2006;4:2059.

45. Mathew P, Young G. Recombinant factor VIIa in paediatric bleeding disorders—a 2006 review. *Haemophilia* 2006;12(5):457–72.

46. Menges T, Hermans PW, Little SG, et al. Plasminogen-activator-inhibitor-1

47. Molino D, DeLucia D, Gaspare de Santo N. Coagulation disorders in uremia. *Semin Nephrol* 2006;26(1):46–51.

48. Monagle P, Chan A, Massicotte P, et al. Antithrombotic Therapy in Children: The Seventh ACCP Conference on Antithrombotic and Thrombolytic Therapy. *Chest* 2004;126(3 Suppl):645S–87S.

49. Munteanu C, Bloodworth LL, Korn TH. Antithrombin concentrate with plasma exchange in purpura fulminans. *Pediatr Crit Care Med* 2000;1:84–7.

50. O'Connell KA, Wood JJ, Wise RP, et al. Thromboembolic adverse events after use of recombinant human coagulation factor VIIa. *JAMA* 2006;295(3): 293–8.

51. Oren H, Cingoz I, Duman M, et al. Disseminated intravascular coagulation in pediatric patients: Clinical and laboratory features and prognostic factors influencing survival. *Pediatr Hematol Oncol* 2005;22(8):679–88.

52. Park KW. Protamine and protamine reactions. *Int Anesthesiol Clin* 2004; 42(3):135–45.

53. Ramsey G. Treating coagulopathy in liver disease with plasma transfusions or recombinant factor VIIa: An evidence based review. *Best Prac Res Clin Haematol* 2005;19(1):113–26.

54. Risch L, Huber AR, Schmugge M. Diagnosis and treatment of heparin-induced thrombocytopenia in neonates and children. *Thromb Res* 2006; 118(1):123–35.

55. Sallah S, Husain A, Nguyen NP. Recombinant activated factor VII in patients with cancer and hemorrhagic disseminated intravascular coagulation. *Blood Coagul Fibrinolysis* 2004;15(7):577–82.

56. Scarpelini S, Rizoli S. Recombinant factor VIIa and the surgical patient. *Curr Opin Crit Care* 2006;12(4):351–6.

57. Sohal AS, Gangji AS, Crowther MA, et al. Uremic bleeding: Pathophysiology and clinical risk factors. *Thromb Res* 2006;118(3):417–22.

58. Taylor FB, ChangA, EsmonCT, et al. Protein C prevents the coagulopathic and lethal effects of Escherichia coli infusion in the baboon. *J Clin Invest* 1987;79(3):918–25.

59. Taylor FB, Jr., Toh CH, Hoots WK, et al. Scientific Subcommittee on Disseminated Intravascular Coagulation (DIC) of the International Society on Thrombosis and Haemostasis (ISTH): Towards definition, clinical and laboratory criteria, and a scoring system for disseminated intravascular coagulation. *Thromb Haemost* 2001;86(5):1327–30.

60. Voves C, Wuillemin WA, Zeerleder S. International Society on Thrombosis and Haemostasis score for overt disseminated intravascular coagulation predicts organ dysfunction and fatality in sepsis patients. *Blood Coagul Fibrinolysis* 2006;17(6):445–51.

61. Warkentin TE, Kelton JG. A 14-year study of heparin-induced thrombocytopenia. *Am J Med* 1996;101:502–7.

62. Zenz W, Zoehrer B, Levin M, et al. Use of recombinant tissue plasminogen activator in children with meningococcal purpura fulminans: A retrospective study. *Crit Care Med* 2004;32:1777–80.

4G/5G promoter polymorphism and prognosis of severely injured patients. *Lancet* 2001;357(9262):1096–7.

KEVIN J. SULLIVAN • NIRANJAN "TEX" KISSOON • SALVATORE R. GOODWIN

Sickle hemoglobinopathies are characterized by the formation of sickled erythrocytes in response to deoxygenation of hemoglobin and are responsible for substantial morbidity and mortality among those afflicted. In this chapter, the normal structure and function of hemoglobin, the pathophysiology of sickle cell disease (SCD), and the diagnosis and management of the complications of SCD that commonly require PICU admission are discussed.

Normal Hemoglobin

Normal hemoglobin quantity, structure, and function are essential for adequate oxygen delivery to tissues. Normal human hemoglobin is a tetrameric protein composed of two α chains and two β chains. Each chain consists of an iron-containing protoheme moiety, which binds oxygen, as well as a globin chain of amino acids arranged in a specific sequential and spatial pattern. Each chain contains an identical heme group, but the amino acid sequence of the globin chain imparts unique chemical and functional characteristics, including oxygen affinity. The primary structure of a globin chain refers to the specific amino acid sequence, the secondary structure refers to the helical structure of the resulting chains, the tertiary structure refers to the three-dimensional configuration of the globin chain, and the quaternary structure refers to the overall structure created by the interaction of the four subunits.

With the exception of hemoglobin expressed early in embryologic development, hemoglobin consists of two α and two non-α chains attached to four iron-containing heme complexes. α-chain production is genetically coded for by four alleles present on chromosome 16, and non-α-chain production is coded by two alleles on present on chromosome 11. α and β chains are the subunits that comprise normal hemoglobin, or hemoglobin A (HbA, α_2, β_2). Hemoglobin A_2 is a component of normal adult hemoglobin and is composed of two α and two δ chains (HbA$_2$, $\alpha_2\delta_2$). Fetal hemoglobin, which is the predominant hemoglobin in fetal development, gradually declines during the first 6 months of life and is composed of two α and two γ chains (HbF, α_2, γ_2). At birth, human erythrocytes contain 70%–90% HbF, which predominates until 2–4 months of age in normal patients. The persistence of HbF production exists in many conditions and offers a protective effect when present in patients with certain hemoglobinopathies.

Abnormal Hemoglobin

SCD refers not to a specific disease, but to a variety of genotypes that share a common phenotype that is characterized by the production of sickled erythrocytes upon hemoglobin deoxygenation, chronic hemolysis, recurrent vaso-occlusion, and ischemic end-organ injury to virtually every organ system. All patients with an SCD phenotype inherit of a mutant β-globin allele in which the sixth codon is altered, resulting in the substitution of valine for glutamine at the sixth amino acid position of the β-globin chain. Hemoglobin that incorporates this mutant β^S-globin chain is referred to as *sickle hemoglobin* (HbS), and homozygotes for the β^S allele are said to have *sickle cell anemia* (SCA, HbSS), while heterozygotes for the β^S allele are said to have *sickle cell trait* (HbAS). Patients with sickle cell trait do not express the SCD phenotype because of the protective effects of HbA, which is produced in sufficient quantities to prevent sickling under most circumstances.

Heterozygous genotypes coding for HbS, together with other alterations in β-chain expression, can also result in the expression of the SCD phenotype, occasionally leading to SCD complications that require pediatric critical care. The most common heterozygous SCD genotypes are hemoglobin SC disease (HbSC) and the sickle-β thalassemias. Approximately 70% of the SCD population in the US is homozygous for β^S (SCA), while HbSC (~20%) and sickle β-thalassemias (10%) comprise the remainder (45). Patients with HbSC or HbS-β^+-thalassemia demonstrate less severe symptoms than patients with HbSS due to the protective effects of HbF (in patients with HbSC) or hemoglobins A and F (in patients with HbS-β^+-thalassemia). Patients with HbS-β^{0-}thalassemia exhibit a clinical course similar in severity to that of patients with HbSS, as neither group produces HbA (**Table 104.1**).

As a result of global migration, SCD now has worldwide distribution. Sickle cell trait (HbAS) is estimated to be present in 8%–9% of African Americans (12,51), and SCA (HbSS) occurs in ~0.2%–0.4% of this population (12,51). SCD is inherited in an autosomal recessive fashion, with standard Mendelian inheritance, so that heterozygote (HbAS) parents will have a 25% chance of producing either a normal (HbAA) or abnormal (SCA, HbSS) homozygote offspring and a 50% chance of producing a heterozygote offspring (sickle cell trait, HbAS).

In addition to understanding of the basic genetic modes of transmission of SCD, understanding the modifiers of the disease that regulate the severity of phenotypic expression is also important. It is not clear why different patients who share the same genotype exhibit vastly different severities of clinical course. For instance, it is recognized that haplotypes of the β^S allele exist that differ in genetic sequences around the mutant β^S allele. These haplotypes of the β^S gene are specific to geographic regions in equatorial Africa and parts of Asia and have been correlated with varying degrees of clinical severity within the SCD population. Similarly, it is possible that other genetic modifiers may exist that significantly influence the basic genetic hemoglobin defect. An example of genetic modification is the fact that, among patients afflicted with the acute

TABLE 104.1

SEVERITY AND DIAGNOSTIC TESTING FOR RELEVANT SICKLE CELL SYNDROMES

Syndrome	Genotype	Severity	Neonatal screening[a]	Hemoglobin electrophoresis in older children (%)				
				HbA	HbS	Hb F	HbA$_2$	HbC
Sickle cell anemia (HbSS)	S-S	++++	FS	0	80–95	2–20	<3.5	0
Sickle β^{0}-thalassemia[b]	S-β^{0}	+++	FS	0	80–92	2–15	3.5–7	0
Hemoglobin SC disease (HbSC)	S-C	++	FSC	0	45–50	1–5	NA[c]	45–50
Sickle β^{+}-thalassemia[b]	S-β^{+}	+	FSA or FS[d]	5–30	65–90	2–10	3.5–6	0
Sickle cell trait (HbAS)	A-S	0	FAS	50–60	35–45	<2	<3.5	0

[a]Hemoglobins reported in order of decreasing quantity (e.g., FS = F>S); F, fetal hemoglobin; S, sickle hemoglobin; C, hemoglobin C; A, hemoglobin A
[b]β^{0} indicates thalassemia mutation with absent production of β-globin; β^{+} indicates thalassemia mutation with reduced production of β-globin.
[c]Quantity of HbA2 cannot be measured in the presence of HbC.
[d]Quantity of HbA at birth sometimes insufficient for detection.
Adapted from Lane PA. Sickle cell disease. *Pediatr Clin N Am* 1996;43:639–664, with permission.

chest syndrome (ACS), many will develop recurrent episodes, while others will never suffer from this complication. Whether identified abnormalities in endothelial and neuronal nitric oxide synthase (NOS) underlie this predilection, or there exists another co-linked genetic locus that predisposes to the development of ACS is not known (50,54). Investigation into the genetic modifiers of SCD remains a fertile field for investigation as exploration of the human genome progresses.

Relevance to Pediatric Critical Care

The common acute complications of SCD that require the attention of the pediatric intensivist include splenic sequestration, aplastic crisis, sepsis, ACS, and stroke. Additionally, the intensivist may be called upon to manage patients with SCD who require exchange transfusion to ameliorate refractory vaso-occlusive crisis, priapism, or orbital infarction. Finally, intensivists and anesthesiologist are often involved in the perioperative management of patients with SCD and may be asked to assist with pain management of patients with refractory vaso-occlusive crisis (VOC).

SCD represents a spectrum of disease severity that is characterized by repetitive injuries to virtually every organ system in the body. Therefore, chronic injury to the circulatory, respiratory, nervous, renal, and immune systems may already be present in children with SCD who present to the PICU. SCD is of special interest to pediatric and adult subspecialists alike, as it represents a disease process that begins in infancy and culminates in multiorgan dysfunction in young adults. As such, therapeutic interventions in childhood may improve both quality of life and life expectancy for adult patients.

CORE PATHOPHYSIOLOGY

The fundamental defect in SCD is an abnormality of the β-globin gene that results in a tendency for hemoglobin to irreversibly polymerize and form a gel that decreases the flexibility of the erythrocyte, resulting in microvascular occlusion, hemolysis, and chronic anemia. While it is clear that hemoglobin abnormalities play a major role, many other factors contribute

to the pathogenesis of SCD-related complications. The contributions to the pathogenesis of SCD of hemoglobin and erythrocytes, platelets, coagulation cascade, endothelium, nitric oxide (NO), systemic oxidant-mediated injury, and environmental factors are discussed here (**Tables 104.2** and **104.3**).

The Erythrocyte

Erythrocytes in patients with SCD have a tendency to change their shape and flexibility (i.e., "sickle") when hemoglobin deoxygenation occurs. The consequence of erythrocyte sickling is occlusion of the microvasculature of every organ system, resulting in ischemic injury or death of cells in the involved vascular distribution.

Two consequences arise as a result of the amino acid substitution at the sixth position of the β chain. First, oxygenated hemoglobin is significantly destabilized, resulting in accelerated denaturation and breakdown (49). Second, the solubility of deoxygenated hemoglobin is dramatically reduced when the valine at β-6 bonds with the β-85 phenylalanine and β-88 leucine of an adjacent tetramer (13). Aggregation of HbS in this fashion causes large-scale polymerization and results in

TABLE 104.2

PRECIPITANTS OF COMPLICATIONS OF SICKLE CELL ANEMIA

Intrinsic patient factors
Erythrocytes
Endothelial cells
Platelets
Leukocytes
    Lymphocytes
    Neutrophils
Coagulation cascade
Aberrations in NO metabolism
Oxidant mediated injury
Systemic inflammation

TABLE 104.3

FACTORS THAT MAY PROMOTE SICKLING

1. Hemoglobin desaturation
    a. Failure to oxygenate in the lungs
        i. Atelectasis
        ii. Infection
            1. Bacterial
            2. Viral
        iii. Chronic lung disease
        iv. Pulmonary vascular disease
        v. High altitude
    b. Diminished tissue oxygen delivery
        i. Diminished cardiac output
            1. Hypovolemia (dehydration, sequestration, sepsis)
            2. Septic shock
            3. Diminished cardiac contractility
            4. Pericardial disease
            5. Increased systemic vascular resistance
            6. Anesthetics/drugs
        ii. Severe anemia
        iii. Hypoxemic cardiac output (see 1.a.)
    c. Increased tissue extraction of oxygen
        i. Increased tissue demands
            1. Vigorous exercise
            2. Thyrotoxicosis
            3. Malignant hyperthermia
            4. Seizures
            5. Sepsis
            6. Shivering
        ii. Factors accelerating tissue oxygen extraction
            1. Acidosis
            2. Hyperthermia
2. Increased microvascular transit time
    a. Increased viscosity
        i. Excessive transfusion
        ii. Dehydration
    b. Vasoconstriction
        i. Hypothermia
        ii. Vasoconstrictor drugs
        iii. Tourniquet use (orthopedic surgery)

precipitation of deoxygenated HbS to form an erythrocyte-deforming gel.

Globin chains shield the intracellular milieu from heme moieties, preventing oxidant injury within the erythrocyte. In sickle erythrocytes, accelerated destruction of the globin chains results in accelerated oxidation of iron to the ferric state and increased generation of superoxide, hydrogen peroxide, and hydroxyl radical (3,28,48). These potent oxidant compounds, in combination with liberated iron inside the erythrocyte, cause denaturation and abnormal distribution of erythrocyte surface proteins, abnormal cation permeability, and disruption of normal phospholipid membrane structure. Transmembrane ion transport mechanisms are also disrupted, resulting in erythrocyte dehydration and consequent increased corpuscular hemoglobin concentration, which accelerates hemoglobin polymerization and potentiates intracellular oxidant injury. Thus, a vicious cycle is initiated within the erythrocyte that leads to increased hemoglobin gelation, oxidative injury to the erythrocyte membrane, cellular deformation, and intracellular dehydration. Acquired changes in erythrocyte cell membranes alter the flexibility and normal flow characteristics of the erythrocyte, which results in stagnant microvascular blood flow, blood vessel obstruction, and distal tissue ischemia.

The Endothelium

The endothelium, once thought to be a passive bystander during intravascular events, is recognized to be an active participant in the pathogenesis of SCD. Adhesion between the endothelium and erythrocytes is mediated by membrane-bound adhesion molecules expressed on the surfaces of endothelial cells and circulating components of the blood (26). Vascular cell adhesion molecule (VCAM)-1 is an endothelial membrane protein that facilitates sickle cell erythrocyte adherence to the endothelium (15). The production of VCAM-1 is increased in the presence of systemic inflammation, allowing sickle reticulocytes to adhere to the endothelium with greater avidity through interaction with the sickle reticulocyte membrane integrin very late activation antigen-4 (15). The degree of affinity between erythrocytes and endothelium has been shown to correlate with clinical severity of illness in sickle cell patients (27). Finally, endothelin-1, an extremely potent vasoconstrictor, is produced in activated endothelial cells in increased quantities in patients with SCD (19), and it has been implicated in the production of pulmonary artery hypertension (PAH) in the ACS (19,24).

Platelets

Platelets and vascular endothelium in patients with SCD are in a chronic state of heightened activity (31). Diminished platelet life and rapid platelet turnover support the notion that platelets are in a constant state of destruction and turnover. Platelets in these patients are less responsive in vitro when incubated with proaggregatory compounds due to chronic in vivo stimulation resulting in fatiguing of the platelet response (33). Finally, circulating platelet-derived factors such as thrombospondin facilitate erythrocyte adherence to the endothelial cell (8,15).

Leukocytes

Leukocyte adherence to endothelial cells and subsequent release of destructive proteolytic enzymes are thought to propagate vascular injury in SCD. Indeed, monocytes from patients with SCD are potent inducers of endothelial activation and contain more IL-1β and tumor necrosis factor (TNF)-α than do monocytes from non-SCD patients. Monocytes from SCD patients have been shown to cause cytoplasmic-to-nuclear translocation of nuclear factor-κB in endothelial cells (a phenomenon seen during upregulation of the inflammatory response) (6). In addition, neutrophils from these patients demonstrate increased endothelial cell adhesion when compared with neutrophils from healthy controls after incubation with proinflammatory cytokines (4).

Coagulation Cascade

The coagulation cascade has also been implicated as a contributor to the pathogenesis of SCD. Investigators have noted enhanced thrombin generation, reduced protein C, reduced protein S activity, diminished factor V, elevated factor VIII, diminished plasminogen levels, shorter thrombin times, and higher serum fibrinogen degradation products in SCD patients, when compared with controls (22,32,43). The role of accelerated endothelial injury and intravascular thrombosis is underscored by autopsy studies of SCD patients who demonstrated diffuse arteriolar thrombosis and interstitial fibrotic lesions not related to large-vessel thrombotic or embolic disease.

Nitric Oxide and Oxidant-Mediated Injury

NO is a poorly water-soluble gas produced in, among other places, the vascular endothelial cell, where it is free to diffuse into the vascular smooth muscle, causing increased levels of cyclic guanosine monophosphate. Elevated levels of cyclic guanosine monophosphate cause intracellular calcium levels to decrease, resulting in smooth muscle relaxation and vasodilation. In the presence of oxygen and hemoglobin, NO produced in endothelial cells may be oxidized to nitrite or bound by hemoglobin, forming S-nitrosohemoglobin (11,40). NO bioactivity is thus transported to peripheral tissues, where decreases in peripheral oxygen tension cause release of oxygen from hemoglobin, triggering an allosteric transformation of hemoglobin and concomitant delivery of NO, to produce vasodilation in the microcirculation (40).

In the setting of hemolysis, as is seen in SCD, free hemoglobin and arginase liberated from erythrocyte scavenge NO and prevent the production of NO from arginine, while diminished erythrocyte mass limits the delivery of NO to the tissues. Plasma from patients with VOC and ACS has been found to be oxidative in nature, depleting cellular glutathione and promoting the formation of injurious peroxynitrite from NO (23). Additionally, consumption of NO by xanthine oxidase via superoxide-dependent pathways limits NO bioavailability and promotes oxidant injury at the endothelial level. Disruption of NO regulation can result in exacerbation of SCD vaso-occlusion via several mechanisms: (a) diminished inhibitory effects of NO on vascular cell adhesion molecule expression, (b) diminished inhibitory effect of NO on leukocyte adhesion, (c) diminished inhibitory effect of NO on platelet activation, and (d) diminished NO-mediated vasodilation of tissue beds, promoting vasoconstriction, ischemia, and further erythrocyte sickling.

In children, levels of both arginine and NO metabolites (nitrite and nitrate, collectively referred to as NO_x) were noted to decrease dramatically during progression of VOC (37). Patients who developed ACS presented to the hospital with significantly lower NO_x levels than did VOC patients or SCD patients at steady state, reached lower levels during ACS than VOC, and were discharged with significantly lower NO_x levels than those of VOC patients (37). The lowest NO_x values correlated temporally with the lowest serum arginine values (37). Another group noted decreased arginine levels and elevated NO_x levels in SCD patients at steady state, when compared with normal controls (36). With oral arginine supplementation, plasma arginine levels increased in SCD patients and healthy controls, but NO_x levels paradoxically decreased in SCD patients at steady state, increased in healthy controls, and increased in SCD patients during VOC (36). The authors concluded that the inability of arginine supplementation to consistently increase NO_x

levels in SCD patients at steady state rendered pure arginine depletion as an incomplete explanation for their observations. They hypothesized a "threshold dose" or "threshold plasma arginine level" that was required to be present to induce NO_x production (36).

Diminished levels of NO have also been described in the exhaled breath (FE_{NO}) of children and adults with SCD and may be responsible for the promotion of ventilation-perfusion mismatch, regional hypoxemia, and intrapulmonary erythrocyte sickling. It has been demonstrated that children with SCD and history of ACS at steady state had significantly lower FE_{NO} levels when compared with SCD patients without ACS history and healthy controls, despite similar arginine, citrulline, and NO_x concentrations in the plasma (54). They also noted that the number of intron sequences in the *NOS 1* gene of the patients was inversely correlated with the FE_{NO} values, suggesting a possible genetic basis for low FE_{NO} and ACS susceptibility (54). Another group found that adults with SCD and history of ACS had lower FE_{NO} values than adult SCA patients without history of ACS, and that the severity of clinical dyspnea experienced by these patients correlated well with severity of FE_{NO} reduction (17).

Physiologic Aggravating Factors in Sickle Cell Disease

Hemoglobin deoxygenation has classically been described as a potent precipitant of vaso-occlusive phenomena. However, reports in the medical literature describe examples of patients with SCD and cyanotic congenital heart disease, occlusive operative tourniquet use, experimental inhalation of hypoxic gas mixtures, as well as chronic hypoxemia in patients with end-stage sickle cell chronic lung disease, none of whom suffered immediate SCD-related complications. Similarly, postoperative SCD-related complications continue to occur despite the avoidance of hypoxemia intraoperatively, and no reports in the anesthesia or surgical literature have definitively linked intraoperative hypoxemia to the development of postoperative complications related to SCD. Nevertheless, close monitoring of arterial oxygenation and administration of supplemental oxygen are recommended to keep arterial oxygen saturation in the normal range.

The consequences of hemoglobin deoxygenation may be mitigated if the transit time of the erythrocyte through the microcirculation to the pulmonary circulation is rapid. As such, avoidance of clinical circumstances in which both significant desaturation and slow transit time to the lungs are present is critical. Significant hemoglobin desaturation occurs when oxygen delivery to the tissues is impaired by diminished cardiac output, severe anemia, or arterial hypoxemia. Patients with SCD are accustomed to moderately severe anemia and preserve oxygen delivery by increasing cardiac output, increasing erythrocytic 2,3-diphosphoglycerate concentrations, and preserving arterial oxygenation. Transit time through the circulation is adversely affected by dehydration, systemic hypotension, occlusive tourniquet use, and physiologic or pharmacologically induced vasoconstriction. Preservation of arterial oxygenation, oxygen-carrying capacity, and cardiac output are essential to minimize excessive and prolonged hemoglobin deoxygenation.

Dehydration has also been classically described as a precipitant of SCD-related complications. Despite this belief, SCD patients with neurosurgical and cardiac disease have been subjected to water deprivation, diuresis, and hypertonic contrast media administration without precipitation of SCD-related complications, but the presence of intracellular erythrocyte dehydration appears to promote hemoglobin polymerization and gel formation, especially in the presence of the cellular, inflammatory, oxidant, and NO abnormalities already discussed. It is therefore prudent to tailor perioperative fluid management to provide generous intravascular hydration that at least preserves euvolemia.

Hypothermia restricts oxygen unloading, promotes cutaneous vasoconstriction, increases red cell tissue-lung transit time, and may promote erythrocyte sickling. Despite the fact that patients with SCD have safely undergone anesthetics and surgeries for cardiac and neurosurgical procedures that require deep hypothermic circulatory arrest, it is a basic tenet of anesthetic and critical care management to attempt to preserve normothermia in these patients in the perioperative period. The benefits of mild, therapeutically induced hypothermia used in the critical care setting for neurologic protection must be weighed against the potential for hypothermia to work synergistically with other physiologic and environmental perturbations to promote SCD-related complications.

Hyperthermia also occurs in critical illness and may be due to many causes, including atelectasis, infection, and systemic inflammation. Hyperthermia shifts the hemoglobin-oxygen dissociation curve to the right, favoring release of oxygen to the tissues and hemoglobin desaturation, and it may be associated with vasoconstriction or vasodilation in core and peripheral compartments. As such, it could theoretically promote vaso-occlusive phenomena, though no definitive work has related the presence of pyrexia to the development of SCD-related complications.

Systemic acidosis shifts the hemoglobin-oxygen dissociation curve to the right, facilitating oxygen delivery and hemoglobin desaturation, and it may potentiate erythrocyte deformation in the microvasculature. Clinical evidence linking systemic acidosis to the development of SCD-related complications is lacking, and administration of sodium bicarbonate has not been shown to be effective in the prevention of perioperative pain crises in SCD patients. In the perioperative and critical care environments, it can be difficult to separate the effects of acidosis from the underlying causes of acidosis when attempting to establish causality between acid-base derangement and development of SCD complications. It is probably prudent, however, to maintain acid-base status in a reasonable physiologic range when caring for critically ill patients with SCD.

SICKLE CELL DISEASE COMPLICATIONS: PRESENTATION, DIFFERENTIAL DIAGNOSIS, AND MANAGEMENT

Patients with SCD suffer a lifetime of indolent, ischemic injury to every organ system in the body. Additionally, their clinical course is marked by periodic acute crises that represent a source of considerable morbidity or premature mortality. The following SCD-related complications are discussed here: vaso-occlusive crisis, ACS, stroke, acute splenic sequestration crisis (ASC), aplastic crisis, sepsis, and the chronic complications of SCD relevant to the practice of pediatric critical care medicine, including sickle cell chronic lung disease and PAH.

Identification of patients with SCD is usually accomplished in most states in the US through perinatal hemoglobin electrophoresis. In rare instances, an undiagnosed child with a sickle hemoglobinopathy may present for elective surgery or with critical illness. Therefore, critical care physicians should be familiar with a suitable algorithm for the diagnosis of the sickle hemoglobinopathies in children of all ages. Further discussion of this topic is provided in the discussion on perioperative management of patients with SCD.

Vaso-occlusive Crisis

The most common crisis seen in pediatric patients with SCD is painful VOC, a condition that usually does not require PICU admission but may precede the development of more serious complications. The most common type of VOC is bony crisis, affecting the long bones, ribs, and vertebrae. Patients with bony VOC will present with symptoms of ischemic pain from the bony cortex or marrow compartment of the extremities, chest, and back and is often associated with fever, leukocytosis, and malaise. In children <3 years old, the distribution of VOC may be confined to the small bones of the hands and feet and is referred to as hand-foot syndrome, or dactylitis. The clinical presentation of bony VOC is fairly characteristic and usually very familiar to the patient and physician. The differential diagnosis of bony VOC, when accompanied by fever, focal bone tenderness, or overlying erythema and tenderness, includes local trauma and osteomyelitis, a condition common in SCD patients due to their susceptibility to bacteremia. Differentiation of the two conditions can be difficult but can be aided by cultures of the blood and involved bone and by a combination of plain x-rays, MRIs, and bone scans. The white blood cell count and differential are not helpful in making the distinction between infection and infarction. If osteomyelitis is suspected on clinical grounds, therapy should be initiated with antimicrobials effective against *Staphylococcus aureus* and *Salmonella* species while arrangements are made for bone biopsy, if necessary.

VOC that involves the abdominal vasculature (mesenteric vessels and blood vessels supplying the solid abdominal organs) produces abdominal pain, fever, malaise, anorexia, and nausea. Patients will demonstrate diminished bowel sounds and nonspecific abdominal tenderness, making differentiation of VOC from a surgical cause of abdominal symptoms difficult. As noted for bone VOC, the nature and distribution of the abdominal crisis pain may be typical of previous crises, but other causes for abdominal pain should always be considered. Children with SCD have an increased frequency of cholelithiasis and cholecystitis due to chronic hemolysis. On the basis of history and physical examination, the clinician may elect to exclude non-SCD abdominal pathology through plain x-ray, CT of the abdomen, and liver function tests, including total and fractionated bilirubin, amylase, lipase, and urinalysis. Serial examinations of the abdomen and surgical consultation are recommended if the diagnosis remains in question after initial evaluation.

Treatment of Vaso-occlusive Crisis

Treatment is largely supportive, with emphasis placed on the provision of adequate analgesia, supplemental oxygen, antibiotics to treat any precipitating infections, and hydration provided liberally (at 1.5 times maintenance fluid requirements). For refractory crisis, many pediatric hematologists will provide simple transfusion to break the VOC cycle. When severe or refractory pain is associated with VOC, anesthesiologists, intensivists, and pain specialists may be called upon to assist in optimizing pain control. In such instances, pain management modalities, including the use of nonsteroidal anti-inflammatory medications, intermittent injection of opioid medications, patient-controlled analgesia with or without continuous basal infusion rates, and regional anesthesia techniques (epidural analgesia and regional nerve blocks) have been utilized with success. When appropriate, clinical psychology and psychiatry services may also be required to assist with identification and treatment of depression, and development of pain coping strategies.

Transfusion Therapy in Sickle Cell Disease Patients

Erythrocyte transfusion is a cornerstone of medical therapy for the treatment of medical complications of SCD and remains a controversial therapy when used in the perioperative period to prevent SCD-related complications. Transfusion therapy is usually employed in the treatment of critically ill children (**Table 104.4**). The decision to employ transfusion therapy in the management of patients with ACS or other complications of SCD is made for two reasons. First (and most commonly), transfusion therapy is used to decrease the percentage of erythrocytes in the circulation, which contains HbS, so that vaso-occlusion can be minimized. Second, improvement in hemoglobin concentration is used to restore reduced oxygen delivery due to decreased cardiac output or impaired hemoglobin oxygenation.

Transfusion therapy can be administered in the form of simple transfusion or exchange transfusion. *Simple transfusion* refers to the IV administration of sickle-free, packed red blood cells, while *exchange transfusion* involves the IV administration of sickle-free packed red blood cells with simultaneous

TABLE 104.4

INDICATIONS FOR TRANSFUSION THERAPY IN CHILDREN WITH SICKLE CELL DISEASE

Prophylactic
Preoperative
Post-stroke
Abnormal transcranial Doppler flow rates
Therapeutic
Acute chest syndrome
Transient ischemic attack
Stroke
Spinal cord infarct
Persistent priapism
Aplastic crisis
Splenic sequestration crisis
Refractory vaso-occlusive crisis

removal of the patient's whole blood. Selection of type of transfusion used is made on the basis of which beneficial effects are desired—increased hematocrit, decreased HbS percentage, or both. During transfusions, the hemoglobin concentration and hematocrit should be monitored closely, as abrupt elevations in hematocrit of >33% are associated with increase in blood viscosity and potential for central nervous system (CNS) ischemic injury.

Effective exchange transfusion therapy is designed to achieve a decreased percentage of sickle erythrocytes to the desired level, maintain a constant circulating blood volume during the procedure, prevent sudden and excessive increases in blood viscosity, achieve an acceptable final hematocrit, and limit exposure to the smallest number of blood units. Exchange transfusion therapy can be accomplished in infants after placement of an arterial catheter for blood withdrawal and suitable venous access for infusion of blood. Alternatively, a large-bore central venous catheter can be used for both withdrawal and infusion of blood during exchange transfusion.

Exchange transfusion can be performed manually or, in larger children, by automated erythrocytapheresis. To quickly reduce HbS percentage to <30% in smaller infants and children, roughly twice the circulating blood volume is replaced with a solution of reconstituted sickle-free erythrocytes and fresh frozen plasma over 4–6 hrs, while the hematocrit is closely monitored. If the hematocrit increases to >30%–33% at any time during the transfusion, a nonerythrocyte volume expander (i.e., fresh frozen plasma) is substituted for the packed red blood cells until the hematocrit falls to an acceptable level. With rapid transfusions and in the setting of hepatic dysfunction, ionized hypocalcemia may result from citrate toxicity and must be closely monitored and treated when necessary.

Exchange transfusion can also be accomplished using an automated process known as *erythrocytapheresis*. In erythrocytapheresis, sickle erythrocytes are separated from the patient's circulating blood volume and replaced with sickle-free erythrocytes. A complete discussion of the factors and calculations required for planning and execution of a safe exchange transfusion has been described in excellent reviews (44).

The decision to employ exchange transfusion versus simple transfusion depends greatly on the clinical scenario encountered, the relative stability of the patient, and the judgment of the intensivist and hematologists involved. For medical complications of SCD, such as VOC, ACS, and ASC, simple transfusion is usually offered, and more aggressive transfusion is reserved for patients who are not improving, deteriorating at a rapid rate or in extremis. For patients with an acute cerebrovascular accident, the goal is to restore cerebral circulation as quickly as possible to minimize irreversible CNS injury. A complete discussion of the role of perioperative transfusion medicine is provided in the discussion of perioperative management of SCD patients.

SCD Crises Specifically Associated with ICU Admission

The Acute Chest Syndrome

The ACS is a clinical syndrome characterized by fever, cough, pleuritic chest pain, tachypnea, hypoxemia, and a new or rapidly progressive pulmonary infiltrate on chest x-ray. It is not uncommon for a patient with ACS to also demonstrate an abrupt decrease in platelet count and hematocrit. ACS may develop de novo, in the perioperative period, or in the setting of VOC or an otherwise innocuous pulmonary infection. Risk factors for the development of ACS include younger age, higher steady-state Hb level, lower fetal Hb percentage, and increased neutrophil count (9). ACS is of clinical significance to hematologists and intensivists because the mortality associated with an episode of ACS has been reported to be as high as 25%, representing a leading cause of premature demise among patients with SCA.

The cause of ACS is often difficult to discern and may be related to acute pulmonary infection, vaso-occlusion in the pulmonary vasculature, or both. Additionally, cases of ACS may be precipitated by bone marrow emboli, in situ pulmonary vascular thrombosis, and fat emboli. ACS occurs more commonly in children in whom an infectious etiology is more likely to be found and in whom episodes are less likely to be fatal (9). The finding that many children who experience a first episode of ACS suffer repeated episodes of ACS suggests the presence of an acquired or inherited predisposition to this affliction (9,50,54). While our earliest pathophysiologic models of SCA emphasized the importance of hemoglobin desaturation, erythrocyte deformation, and consequent microvascular occlusion, more contemporary paradigms recognize the additional contributions of platelets, leukocytes, endothelial cells, vascular adhesion molecules, and inflammatory mediators.

Other mechanisms for the development of ACS are also well described and include acute viral and bacterial infections of the respiratory tract and atelectasis secondary to acute pain associated with VOC or the perioperative setting. In all of these settings, regional hypoxemia occurs and promotes intravascular erythrocyte deformation (34,56). Release of fat emboli from necrotic bone and subsequent release of proinflammatory mediators (e.g., phospholipase A_2) have also been demonstrated in patients suffering from ACS and in autopsies of nonsurvivors (14,52,57). Finally, abnormalities in the production and metabolism of NO are very well described in children with ACS.

Treatment of Acute Chest Syndrome. Although the cause of the ACS is often not known in an individual patient, it is most commonly believed to be related to acute pulmonary infection, pulmonary vaso-occlusion, or both. Although it is not possible to tell which of these etiologies underlies the development of ACS in a given patient, therapy is directed at both infection and vaso-occlusion.

Treatment of patients with ACS begins with general supportive care. Hydration is instituted liberally and modified as clinically indicated on the basis of cardiovascular status, renal function, and measured atrial filling pressures. Supplemental oxygen is administered with a goal of keeping Pao_2 and hemoglobin Sao_2 in an acceptable range (Pao_2 >80–100 mm Hg, Sao_2 >95%). For milder disease, incentive spirometry and ambulation can be encouraged, as it improves ventilation-perfusion matching, prevents atelectasis, and may slow the progression of pulmonary injury. Analgesia should also be provided to minimize pleuritic chest pain, and exercises that promote pulmonary toilet are encouraged. Pain relief is commonly provided with patient-controlled analgesia for older children, and in toddlers and infants, continuous infusions of opioid (morphine or fentanyl) are titrated to comfort level

while respiratory rate and effort are monitored. Analgesia can be augmented through the administration of scheduled acetaminophen doses during the acute illness; in the absence of significant renal disease or gastrointestinal bleeding, nonsteroidal anti-inflammatory medications, such as ibuprofen or ketorolac, may be offered as well. In the absence of specific contraindications (coagulopathy and infection overlying the needle placement site), regional anesthetic techniques, including central neuraxial blockade and continuous nerve block techniques have also been employed with good results. Finally, dexamethasone (0.3 mg/kg/dose every 12 hrs for 4 doses) has been administered in mild and moderate ACS with beneficial results (7).

ACS can progress in severity to severe acute lung injury or acute respiratory distress syndrome, requiring positive-pressure airway support in the form of noninvasive continuous positive airway pressure, bilevel positive airway pressure, or, more commonly, with standard endotracheal intubation. In keeping with minimizing pulmonary injury secondary to mechanical ventilation, efforts should be made to minimize plateau pressure and tidal volume while positive end-expiratory pressure is adjusted to provide optimal lung compliance and inflation. To minimize iatrogenic lung injury while optimizing ventilation-perfusion matching, the pressure-limited or airway pressure-release modes of mechanical ventilation and high-frequency oscillatory ventilation can be used for children and adolescents with severe lung injury. Case reports that describe the administration of inhaled NO to patients with severe ACS have resulted in favorable outcomes, presumably by improving PAH, right ventricular function, severe ventilation-perfusion mismatch, and systemic oxygenation (5,53).

Children with SCD are very susceptible to infection due to deficiencies in splenic function and opsonization of bacterial pathogens. Therefore, broad-spectrum antibiotic therapy should be instituted while the appropriate culture and serology samples are being evaluated. Blood should be sent for bacterial culture and *Mycoplasma* serologies, sputum should be sent for bacterial and viral culture, and nasopharyngeal aspirates should be sent for detection of viral antigens of common respiratory pathogens (respiratory syncytial virus, adenovirus, parainfluenza virus, and influenza viruses). In critically ill patients with extensive lung disease, bronchoalveolar lavage should be performed, and specimens should be sent for opportunistic pathogens (fungi, protozoa) in addition to the more commonly encountered pathogens.

Aggressive empiric antibiotic therapy is instituted, with consideration given to local antibiotic resistance patterns of commonly encountered pathogens. Empiric antibiotic therapy with a third-generation cephalosporin and a macrolide antibiotic is provided to cover for common causes of community-acquired pneumonia, including *Streptococcus pneumoniae*, *Mycoplasma pneumoniae*, and *Chlamydia pneumoniae*. In those patients considered to be at risk for infection with nosocomial or resistant pathogens, antistaphylococcal and antipseudomonal antibiotics (nafcillin or vancomycin, ceftazidime, and an aminoglycoside) are added. When culture results are known, the spectrum of antibiotic coverage can be appropriately narrowed.

The most effective therapeutic modality available to the intensivist in the treatment of ACS is transfusion therapy. Blood transfusion is not offered to correct anemia, as SCD patients have a well-compensated chronic anemia that provides adequate systemic oxygen delivery during steady-state conditions. Transfusion therapy is offered in the setting of ACS to dilute the HbS-containing erythrocytes with HbA-containing erythrocytes in the hope that microvascular occlusion of the pulmonary circulation will be attenuated. Additionally, during critical illness, systemic oxygen delivery may be compromised by impaired cardiac output or decreased arterial oxygen saturation. Improved oxygen-carrying capacity from packed erythrocyte transfusion will offset decreased oxygen delivery due to these causes. For mild-to-moderate ACS, many clinicians provide simple transfusion to increase the hemoglobin concentration to 10 g/dL. For more severe disease or disease that is rapidly progressive, exchange transfusion is provided to rapidly decrease the percentage of HbS to <30%, with total hemoglobin and hematocrit of 10 g/dL and 30%, respectively. Detailed discussion of the indications and techniques for exchange transfusion is provided elsewhere in this chapter.

Case reports have described the use of inhaled NO and extracorporeal membrane oxygenation as a therapeutic modality in severe ACS in children and adolescents with ACS (5,42,53). In these cases, beneficial effects of NO have included improved ventilation-perfusion matching, improved systemic oxygenation, decreased intrapulmonary shunting, and improved hemodynamics. Additional benefits of inhaled NO that are pertinent to the pathophysiology of SCD include its antiplatelet and anti-inflammatory properties, as well as the purported effect of NO to increase the affinity of HbS for oxygen (25).

Stroke

Stroke, or cerebrovascular accident (CVA), is a poorly understood complication of SCD that frequently presents to the PICU staff for management and monitoring. Angiographic and pathologic studies of SCD patients with CVA have demonstrated proximal intracranial arterial stenosis, particularly of the internal carotid artery, and histopathologic studies have demonstrated segmental thickening of the vessel walls and intimal hyperplasia. Occlusion of the vessel may, therefore, result from intimal hyperplasia, secondary thrombosis, distal thromboembolization, or any combination of these factors. Additionally, a subset of SCD patients exists that may present with predominantly small-vessel disease in the CNS vasculature. The tendency for intimal hyperplasia to develop at sites of arterial bifurcation suggests that repeated endothelial injury might underlie this process. Most CVAs in children are due to ischemic infarcts, but as many as one-third of CVAs in adults with SCD are hemorrhagic in nature (39).

While SCD patients with CVA may present to the PICU with sudden onset of neurologic symptoms, it is now known that subclinical CNS injury occurs more commonly in the SCD patient than previously appreciated. Silent cerebral infarction is the most common form of CNS injury seen in patients with SCD, and it is increasingly recognized as a source of cognitive deficits, diminished intelligence quotient, poor school performance, and a risk factor for progressive CNS injury, including subsequent CVA.

Silent cerebral infarction is prevalent in the SCD population, occurring in 15%–25% of children <14 years of age (29,41). The presence of silent cerebral infarction in children with SCD is of great clinical relevance, as it is a potent predictor of proba-

bility of subsequent neurologic injury. It is now common practice in pediatric hematology clinics to measure flow velocity in the middle cerebral and terminal internal carotid arteries, utilizing transcranial Doppler ultrasonography (TCD). Elevated flow velocity in the middle cerebral artery or internal carotid artery results from local stenosis in the blood vessels and is associated with increased risk for CVA (2). Patients with abnormally elevated TCD flow velocities are now offered the choice of chronic erythrocyte transfusion or stem cell transplantation to prevent subsequent CVA. Other risk factors for development of CVA include a recent acute decrease in hemoglobin concentration, as seen in aplastic crises due to parvovirus B19, although neurologic injury has been described to occur weeks after the aplastic crisis.

The diagnosis of CVA is made on the basis of the usual clinical signs and symptoms of CVA. In the presence of acute contralateral hemiplegia and aphasia (left-sided CVA), the diagnosis is clear. However, in many cases, the presentation may not be straightforward and stroke may present simply as altered or depressed mental status. In these cases, in addition to stroke, other causes for acute alteration in mental status must be considered. Focal seizures may be the presenting symptom of focal cerebral ischemia and may progress to a generalized tonic-clonic convulsion. In patients with SCD, the new onset of seizure activity should be considered to be indicative of cerebral ischemic injury until proven otherwise. Seizure control should be implemented as described for status epilepticus, with particular care taken to ensure arterial oxygenation. In the appropriate age groups, acute alteration in mental status may be secondary to toxic ingestion and should be pursued and treated accordingly. In the presence of fever, acute alteration in mental status may also be indicative of meningitis due to bacterial or viral pathogens. Lumbar puncture should be performed, and antibiotics should be implemented if the clinical picture suggests meningitis, and physical examination and imaging studies have excluded intracranial hypertension or neurosurgical catastrophes.

SCD patients who present with signs or symptoms of CVA or other intracranial pathology should undergo emergent CT scan or MRI of the brain to define any CNS abnormalities and to exclude the presence of lesions amenable to neurosurgical intervention (parenchymal, epidural, or subdural hematoma). Advantages of MRI over CT scan in acute CVA include the ability to clearly define the CNS vasculature using MR angiography and increased sensitivity of MRI for early detection of ischemic parenchymal changes. When selecting the most appropriate neuroimaging procedure for a given patient, the clinician must weigh the benefits of increased diagnostic potential of MRI against the need for sedation to facilitate longer MRI studies in uncooperative or physiologically unstable pediatric patients.

Treatment of Stroke

The most urgent therapeutic intervention for the SCD patient who presents with CVA is an immediate exchange transfusion to reverse or prevent progression of ischemic CNS injury. Exchange transfusion is provided to decrease the HbS percentage to <30% while the hemoglobin concentration is maintained at or around 10 g/dL. Therapy for children with SCD and CVA is otherwise supportive, with careful attention to protection of the airway, suppression of seizure activity, and preservation of respiratory and hemodynamic function. In the setting of a large cerebral infarction, the patient is monitored for the development of intracranial hypertension, and neurosurgical consultation is obtained when clinically indicated.

While it is also standard practice to maintain normothermia and euglycemia in SCD patients with CVA to prevent secondary neuronal ischemic injury, these practices will require ongoing critical appraisal as the critical care community examines the beneficial effects of glycemic control and therapeutic hypothermia in patients with ischemic brain injury. In particular, the safety of moderate hypothermia in patients with sickle hemoglobinopathies should be considered, as peripheral vasoconstriction may promote vascular stasis and erythrocyte sickling, although the protective effects of aggressive exchange transfusion therapy may mitigate the potential for erythrocyte sickling under conditions of moderate hypothermia. Finally, to date, no study has demonstrated the efficacy or safety of thrombolytic therapy in patients with CVA and SCD.

The natural history of patients with SCD and CVA is one of recurrent CNS ischemic injury. After a CVA, or ideally before a CVA in the setting of increased TCD flow rates, patients are maintained on a regime of chronic blood transfusion ("hypertransfusion program") designed to keep the HbS <30%, often for a period of 10 years, which requires monthly transfusions and chelation therapy with deferoxamine to slow the progression of systemic iron overload. Transfusion therapy is effective at correcting elevated TCD flow rates and preventing recurrent stroke, but the necessary duration of therapy is unclear, as cessation of transfusion is associated with recurrence of TCD abnormalities and CVA (1). Hematopoietic stem cell transplantation represents an alternative to chronic transfusion but is associated with obvious morbidity and the need for a suitable marrow donor.

Splenic Sequestration and Aplastic Crisis

Patients with SCD occasionally suffer from life-threatening decreases in hemoglobin concentration as a result of splenic sequestration or acute bone marrow aplasia. Under normal circumstances, SCD patients demonstrate brisk reticulocytosis to offset accelerated red blood cell destruction. Viral suppression of bone marrow function may result in severe anemia that prevents adequate systemic oxygen delivery. The most common cause of aplastic crisis among SCD patients is viral infection, particularly with parvovirus B19.

ASC refers to a sudden drop in hemoglobin concentration associated with development of splenomegaly, reticulocytosis, intravascular volume depletion, and shock. Platelet and leukocyte counts may decrease as well. ASC is a disease of toddlers and infants and is not seen in older children, presumably due to autosplenectomy. Patients with other SCD genotypes, such as HbSC disease and HbS-β thalassemia, may undergo autosplenectomy later in childhood and consequently may experience ASC later in childhood as well. Children with ASC are anemic, pale, and may demonstrate signs of inadequate systemic oxygen delivery. In severe cases, shock is present and patients may present in extremis.

Treatment of Aplastic Crisis and Acute Sequestration Crisis

Treatment of aplastic crisis is supportive, with erythrocyte transfusion to restore hemoglobin concentration to levels suf-

ficient to support systemic oxygen delivery until marrow function recovers and reticulocytosis resumes. The specific hemoglobin level to target for ASC and aplastic crisis depends upon the balance between oxygen supply and demand and can be monitored with serial measurements of lactic acid concentration, oxygen saturation in the superior vena cava or pulmonary artery, and arteriovenous oxygen content gradient. In general, however, these patients are accustomed to a moderately severe chronic anemia, and restoration of a hemoglobin level to 7–9 g/dL is usually adequate.

Therapy of ASC involves restoration of circulating blood volume with crystalloid solutions and sickle-free packed red blood cells. In severe shock, rapid exchange transfusion may be necessary to rapidly restore adequate oxygen-carrying capacity. For patients who do not respond to aggressive medical therapy, splenectomy may be considered as a life-saving surgical intervention. With resolution of ASC, spleen size decreases and sequestered blood elements may return to the circulation. Patients with SCD who experience a first episode of ASC often experience recurrent episodes of sequestration. Due to the risk of recurrence of ASC, pediatric hematologists in some centers recommend splenectomy after a first episode of ASC. The risk of ASC recurrence must be weighed against the detrimental effects of splenectomy on immune function, even in this patient population with impaired and short-lived splenic function.

Sepsis

Due to impaired splenic function and decreased opsonic activity, children with SCD are at increased risk for serious bacterial infections with a variety of bacterial pathogens, especially encapsulated organisms, such as *Streptococcus pneumoniae* and *Neisseria meningitidis*. Early identification of at-risk patients through newborn sickle cell screening programs, use of penicillin prophylaxis, availability of vaccinations against *S. pneumoniae*, *N. meningitidis*, and *Haemophilus influenzae*, and aggressive antibiotic therapy in febrile SCD patients have had a beneficial effect on sepsis-related mortality in SCD patients (47).

Therapy for patients with sepsis includes early, aggressive administration of broad-spectrum antibiotics in all febrile SCD patients and in afebrile SCD patients who demonstrate other clinical signs of systemic bacterial infection. In patients with infection, hypotension, and organ dysfunction, supportive therapies, including early goal-directed therapy, mechanical ventilation, vasopressor support, steroid therapy (when appropriate), and other sepsis therapies outlined elsewhere in this text, are implemented as indicated.

Chronic Organ System Dysfunction

By the time older children and adolescents present with critical complications of SCD, incremental, subclinical damage to major organ systems has already occurred over time. As such, patients who present for critical care services for acute complications of sickle cell disease may do so with significant preexisting dysfunction of the respiratory, cardiovascular, and renal systems.

Chronic Lung Disease

Sickle cell chronic lung disease has been well documented in SCA, but its etiology is not completely understood. It is marked by progressive episodes of chest pain, progressive dyspnea, and progressive pulmonary fibrosis on chest x-ray (46). The mechanism that underlies the development of disabling lung disease in SCA is not clear but is thought to involve repetitive episodes of pulmonary injury that result in pulmonary parenchymal fibrosis and/or an ongoing obliterative pulmonary vasculitis. A recent study designed to examine the relationship between hemolysis-mediated erythrocyte arginase release and activity in the plasma of SCD patients demonstrated that increased plasma arginase activity was associated with decreased arginine bioavailability and increased risk for the development of PAH (35). In addition to diminished arginine levels, the amino acid profiles in this study in patients with SCD and PAH demonstrated increased ornithine and proline levels, which are known to be precursors required for collagen deposition and smooth muscle proliferation responsible for pulmonary vascular, airway, and pulmonary parenchymal remodeling and fibrosis. The clinician should be aware that SCD patients may present to the PICU with preexisting pulmonary abnormalities that include restrictive lung disease, obstructive lung disease, airway smooth-muscle hyperreactivity, and significant ventilation-perfusion mismatch. Preexisting respiratory system injury may compromise the physiologic reserve of the SCD patient.

Cardiovascular System

Cardiac dysfunction is well described in the setting of SCD and affects both the left and right ventricles. Patients with long-standing chronic anemia augment systemic oxygen delivery by increasing stroke volume and, to a much smaller degree, heart rate. Stroke volume is increased on a chronic basis by increasing end-diastolic volume and preserving ejection fraction. As such, it is common for SCD patients to demonstrate cardiomegaly on chest x-ray and left ventricular dilatation and, to a lesser degree, increased wall thickness, on echocardiography.

More ominous, however, is the presence of PAH, a significant source of disability and premature demise among older patients (10,55). Indeed, in one series of 60 patients with SCA who were undergoing echocardiography for a variety of indications, 20% were found to have pulmonary hypertension and the majority were asymptomatic from a cardiovascular viewpoint (55). PAH is suggested by prominence of the right heart border on chest x-ray and the development of right ventricular hypertrophy and tricuspid regurgitation on echocardiographic examination. More recently, echocardiographic evidence of pulmonary hypertension was demonstrated in 32% of a large series of adults with SCA (18). PAH has not been commonly seen in children outside of the realm of severe acute lung injury but has been noted in adolescent SCD patients (38). The mechanism(s) for the development of pulmonary hypertension in patients with SCA is not clear but has been proposed to include diffuse pulmonary arteriolar thrombosis, scavenging of NO by free hemoglobin, arginase-mediated consumption of circulating arginine (limiting NO availability), increased oxidant production, and upregulation of expression of cellular adhesion molecules.

Renal

Repeated infarctions of the viscera may result in significant deterioration of organ system function over time. Like the de-terioration in splenic function that occurs over time, the kidney is affected by repeated ischemic insults, resulting in significant functional impairment. While rare in children, older patients may suffer anatomic and functional impairment of renal function, requiring dialysis or renal transplantation. Patients with SCD and sickle cell trait demonstrate isosthenuria, a progressive impairment in the ability to concentrate urine and preserve free water, making the SCD patient more susceptible to dehydration. The potential for presence of renal dysfunction in SCD patients must be considered for fluid management, acid-base, electrolyte, and pharmacologic considerations.

Perioperative Management of the SCD Patient

Optimal perioperative care necessarily includes the accurate identification of patients at risk, appropriate preoperative preparation of the patient with SCD, optimal anesthetic management, and appropriate postoperative care. Attention to all aspects of perioperative care is required to optimize outcomes of SCD patients who undergo surgical intervention.

Patient Identification

In most states in the US, patients with the SCD phenotype will have been previously identified as a result of newborn screening hemoglobin electrophoresis. Unfortunately, this is not always true, and children may elude neonatal detection with catastrophic results. Therefore, it is important that the healthcare provider (a) be cognizant that lack of knowledge of an SCD diagnosis on the part of the patient's caretaker does not exclude SCD as a diagnostic possibility, and (b) be familiar with the limitations of testing modalities for the detection of SCD.

A suitable screening algorithm is necessary for those children who present for medical care for whom neonatal screening has not been done or for whom the results are not known. Patients may be screened for the presence of a sickle cell hemoglobinopathy with a "sickle prep" examination, in which sickle hemoglobin production is provoked in vitro. Patients with a positive screening solubility test require hemoglobin electrophoresis to precisely delineate the specific sickle cell hemoglobinopathy present. In the presence of high concentrations of HbF, solubility testing lacks the sensitivity required to detect HbS and cannot be relied upon for screening in children <6 months old. Hb electrophoresis is required in this age group to exclude the presence of a sickle hemoglobinopathy.

Preoperative Preparation

Once the diagnosis of an SCD phenotype is made, it is appropriate to obtain pediatric hematology consultation for longitudinal follow-up. Additionally, the pediatric hematologists may help the pediatrician or intensivist in the preoperative preparation of the SCD patient. Preoperative preparation includes careful attention to preoperative hydration, optimization of vital organ function, and consideration of administrating prophylactic preoperative packed red blood cell transfusion. Patients with SCD should be well hydrated, and it is customary to hydrate the patient on the night prior to surgery with IV fluids administered at a rate of 1.5 times maintenance. The patient should be screened and treated for infection, a potent stimulus for many systemic inflammatory complications. Major organ systems should be evaluated for dysfunction that may adversely impact the intraoperative and postoperative course. Finally, a thorough preoperative evaluation and discussion with the parents are required to delineate risks, explain the anesthetic plan, and provide for postoperative analgesia and prevention of postoperative SCD complications.

Perioperative transfusion therapy is a common, sometimes controversial topic of discussion among surgeons, anesthesiologists, hematologists, and intensivists. The reasons for provision of perioperative transfusion therapy are usually to correct anemia and improve oxygen-carrying capacity. However, this is an uncommon indication in the SCD patient who is not going to surgery, as the anemia associated with SCD is a chronic, compensated anemia. The other reason for the provision of preoperative transfusion therapy is to dilute the erythrocytes that contain HbS with erythrocytes that contain HbA to minimize the extent of hemoglobin gel formation and erythrocyte sludging in the microvasculature. Prophylactic therapy of this nature should be effective in decreasing postoperative SCD complications, and evidence exists as to its efficacy.

In a report on 54 pediatric patients who underwent 66 surgical procedures without the benefit of preoperative transfusion, most did not receive packed red blood cell transfusion at any time during the perioperative course (20). Postoperative complications were observed in 26% of the cases and were usually minor and self-limited. Complications were most common after thoracotomy, laparotomy, and tonsillectomy and adenoidectomy. The authors recommended prospective, randomized studies to confirm the safety of anesthesia and surgery for minor surgical procedures without the benefit of preoperative transfusion, and recognized that the type of surgical procedure has significant impact on the frequency of postoperative complications (20).

In a retrospective study of 1079 procedures in adults and children, authors found that perioperative blood transfusion conferred a protective effect against SCD complications in low-risk procedures in HbSS patients, and low- and moderate-risk procedures in patients with HbSC (30). In neither retrospective study was an attempt made to stratify enrolled patients according to overall disease severity, recent disease activity, or changing anesthetic and surgical techniques. As such, the results of these studies must be extrapolated to the clinical setting with caution. Of note, however, the authors found a mortality rate of 1:100 for all patients within 30 days of surgery, emphasizing the increased perioperative risk incurred by SCD patients, when compared with the general population (1:300,000 in adults, 1:80,000 children).

Members of the Preoperative Transfusion in Sickle Cell Disease Study Group published their results of a prospective, randomized trial that examined the effects of conservative and aggressive transfusion strategies on perioperative outcome in SCD patients (58). In the aggressive transfusion arm, patients were transfused to a target HbS of 30% by either serial transfusion or exchange transfusion, while the patients in the conservative transfusion arm were transfused to a hemoglobin concentration of 10 g/dL. This study demonstrated similar rates of perioperative SCD complications in both arms, with increased frequency of transfusion-related complications in the aggressive transfusion arm. A nontransfusion arm was not included in this study. The authors concluded that a conservative transfusion strategy, using simple transfusion, was as effective as aggressive transfusion in the prevention of SCD complications but resulted in less transfusion-related complications.

In 1997, utilizing a subset of the database of the Preoperative Transfusion in Sickle Cell Disease Study Group, other investigators examined outcomes of 364 SCD patients who underwent cholecystectomy (21). In this study, the findings of equivalence of aggressive and conservative transfusion strategies with respect to prevention of postoperative SCD complications were confirmed. Interestingly, a group of patients that was not randomized and did not receive preoperative transfusion was followed in this study (most demonstrated healthier American Society of Anesthesiologist class scores). This nonrandomized, nontransfusion group demonstrated a 32% frequency of sickle cell-related complications, including an ACS incidence double that of the next highest group in the report. Disturbingly, a 1% perioperative mortality rate was again noted in the patients who underwent cholecystectomy. Extrapolation about the hazards of undergoing elective surgery without preoperative transfusion should be made cautiously, as the only group in this study who did not receive blood transfusion was nonrandomized.

Finally, in 1999, a study of 138 orthopedic procedures from the Preoperative Transfusion in Sickle Cell Disease Study Group was reported, which again confirmed the lack of superiority of aggressive transfusion, when compared with conservative transfusion, in the prevention of SCD-related complications and, surprisingly, demonstrated an ACS frequency of 14% and a mortality rate of ~1%. As with the previous studies by this group of investigators, a randomized, nontransfusion group was not included in the study; therefore, a direct comparison between simple transfusion and nontransfusion could not be made.

SCD patients present difficult management decisions for physicians involved in their perioperative care. In aggregate, the literature to date would support the presence of a protective effect upon postoperative SCD complications through the application of a conservative transfusion strategy to most SCD patients undergoing most surgical procedures. The benefit from such a strategy must be weighed against the potential for transfusion-related complications, which include hemolytic reactions, transfusion-associated acute lung injury, alloimmunization, iron overload, allergic reaction to leukocyte antigens, and transmission of viral pathogens. While it might seem excessive to transfuse a patient for myringotomy tube placement or foreign-body removal from the finger, the literature does not strongly support the acceptability of a nontransfusion approach to any surgical procedure and certainly not to moderate- or high-risk procedures. For patients with aggressive SCD and those undergoing procedures with high potential for CNS injury and ACS (i.e., cardiac surgery with cardiopulmonary bypass, deep hypothermia with circulatory arrest, and neurosurgical procedures), consultation with their hematologists is recommended, and consideration should be given to more aggressive transfusion preparation of the patient. Until such time as these comparisons are made in large, well-controlled, prospective, randomized trials, a prudent approach to preoperative preparation is recommended, with consideration of the patient, comorbidities, SCD severity, contemplated operative procedure, and the opinions of the anesthesiologist, surgeon, and hematologists caring for the patient.

Operative Management

Operative management of the SCD patient involves careful attention to the precipitants of SCD complications and mitigation of their impact. Factors to be considered include oxygenation, hydration status, acid-base balance, and thermoregulation.

These were discussed previously in the section on core pathophysiology.

The type of surgery and anesthetic technique employed to facilitate surgery have been examined as potential factors in the development of SCD-related complications. Reported incidences of SCD-related complications in the perioperative period vary widely, and an individual patient's risk of developing SCD complications is probably determined by many factors. The type of operation performed has been described to impact the probability of development of SCD complications in the perioperative period, with high-risk procedures variously described as obstetrical procedures, thoracotomy/laparotomy, intracranial procedures, and operations related to the airway. Other considerations in operative management of SCD patients include the presence or absence of significant major organ system dysfunction, recent patterns of SCD-related activity, and precipitants of SCD complications, particularly infection. Anesthetic technique has not been shown to be related to the development of perioperative SCD complications, with successful application of general anesthesia, regional anesthesia, or combined techniques in the care of these patients. Additionally, regional anesthetic techniques have been safely employed with variable efficacy to assist in the management of SCD crises, including refractory vaso-occlusive crisis and priapism.

Postoperative Management

The postoperative management of the SCD patient represents a continuation of the principles and practices applied in the preparation and operative management of these patients. In some institutions, patients are admitted to the ward for perioperative management, and aggressive analgesia is provided in the form of peripheral nerve blocks, neuraxial blockade, patient-controlled opioid analgesia, and nonsteroidal anti-inflammatory drugs (when not contraindicated). Analgesia is optimized to facilitate respiratory function without excessively depressing respiratory drive. Pulmonary toilet is optimized with incentive spirometry for older children, bubble-blowing games for younger children, supplemental oxygen administration when it is required, moving from bed to chair, and early ambulation whenever possible. IV hydration is continued postoperatively, with careful attention to fluid intake and output, including insensible losses, urine output, and all losses from drains and catheters. Whether patients with SCD should be managed as outpatients for surgery is a controversial issue that engenders passionate views on both sides.

Outcomes

Patients with SCD are living longer than they have ever lived at any time in history. Thirty years ago, only one-half of children with SCD were expected to survive until adulthood. In 1994, the National Institutes of Health-sponsored Cooperative Study of Sickle Cell Disease estimated that the median survival for SCD patients was 42 years for men and 48 years for women. Therefore, SCD patients are more often surviving into adulthood and bringing with them chronic organ system dysfunction of the central nervous, cardiovascular, pulmonary, and renal systems. The overall incidence of death in SCD patients has been described to range between 0.59–1.1 per 100 patient years, with recent studies demonstrating decreased childhood mortality when compared with earlier studies (16,47). The im-

proved trend in mortality in SCD has been attributed to the routine administration of penicillin prophylaxis; availability of vaccinations against *H. influenzae* and *S. pneumoniae*; surveillance measures, including echocardiography and transcranial Doppler studies, against catastrophic complications of SCD; and disease-altering therapies, such as hydroxyurea, stem cell transplantation, and chronic transfusion therapy.

As a result of these advancements in therapy, fewer children die of infection and early childhood complications of the disease. As such, pulmonary complications in general and ACS in particular remain leading causes of morbidity and mortality among patients with SCD. Stroke, often with debilitating residual sequelae is becoming an increasingly important cause of morbidity and mortality among patients with SCD, with peak incidence occurring between 2 and 8 years of age. A child with SCD is estimated to have a 20% probability of suffering from stroke by the age of 20. A significant percentage of SCD patients will develop dysfunction of the lung and pulmonary vasculature, manifest as sickle cell chronic lung disease and PAH. The presence of the latter is a potent independent risk factor for early mortality, and it is not known how to predict which patients will develop this complication.

CONCLUSIONS AND FUTURE DIRECTIONS

Children with four principal genotypes, (sickle cell anemia, hemoglobin SC disease, sickle β^0-thalassemia, and sickle β^+-thalassemia) are prone to the development of a clinical course marked by chronic end-organ dysfunction punctuated by episodes of acute, life-threatening deterioration due to splenic sequestration, aplastic crisis, ACS, sepsis, and stroke. Critical care of patients with the SCD phenotype involves meticulous basic supportive care of the major organ systems and the application of transfusion therapy to ameliorate the severity of SCD complications.

Whereas the role of hemoglobin desaturation and subsequent polymerization was emphasized as central to the pathophysiology of SCD, it is now recognized that SCD is more accurately depicted as a global disease marked by endothelial dysfunction and inflammation. Specifically, it is now appreciated that vascular injury is exacerbated by significant contributions from platelets, leukocytes, erythrocytes, endothelial expression of adhesion molecules, endothelial secretion of vasoconstrictor hormones, aberrations in NO production and consumption, and oxidant-mediated injury.

Children with SCA are living longer, often into early adulthood and middle age. Clinicians have made considerable therapeutic progress in preventing early mortality in children with SCD due to infectious complications and have had some success in attenuating the severity of the disease through the administration of chronic transfusion therapy, hydroxyurea, and, in select circumstances, the provision of hematopoietic stem cell transplantation. Chronic care issues relevant to the SCD patient in the next century will focus on attempts to limit or severely delay the cumulative end-organ injury. Identification of patients at risk for CVA and determination of the optimal transfusion therapy to maximize protection against CVA, while minimizing transfusion-related morbidity will be essential. Similarly, determination of the risk factors and mechanisms of development of

PAH and lung disease is necessary to prevent the progression of these debilitating and life-limiting complications. Additionally, the optimal therapies available to treat these complications, which include IV and inhaled prostaglandin compounds, NO donors and their precursors (sildenafil and arginine supplementation), and endothelin-1 antagonist medications will need to be elucidated. Finally, randomized, controlled trials are needed to clarify whether transfusion therapy is necessary for low-risk SCD patients who undergo low-risk surgical procedures.

Advances in our understanding of the human genome and the ability of investigators to manipulate it hold the greatest hope for curing patients of SCD without incurring the complications associated with hematopoietic stem cell transplantation. A recent study demonstrated the ability of a viral vector to be used to introduce a construct of the β^A globin gene into transgenic mice with SCD, effectively curing the disease. Until genetic therapies are available for the treatment of human SCD, hematopoietic stem cell transplantation, with its treatment-associated morbidity, represents the best hope for curative therapy for this disease.

SCD patients are surviving into adulthood with cumulative disease and therapy-related injuries to every organ system. The challenge for clinicians in the future will be to implement evidence-based practices that address the expanded fundamental pathophysiology of the disease in all aspects of patient treatment, including prophylactic treatment, management of chronic complications, and treatment of acute life-threatening complications of SCD in the PICU.

KEY POINTS

- Sickle hemoglobinopathies are characterized by the formation of sickled erythrocytes in response to deoxygenation of hemoglobin and are responsible for substantial morbidity and mortality among those afflicted.

- SCD refers not to a specific disease, but to a variety of genotypes that share a common phenotype that is characterized by the production of sickled erythrocytes upon hemoglobin deoxygenation, chronic hemolysis, recurrent vaso-occlusion, and ischemic end-organ injury to virtually every organ system.

- Whereas the role of hemoglobin desaturation and subsequent polymerization was emphasized as central to the pathophysiology of SCD, it is now recognized that SCD is more accurately depicted as a global disease marked by endothelial dysfunction and inflammation.

- The fundamental defect in SCD is an abnormality of the β-globin gene that results in a tendency for hemoglobin to irreversibly polymerize and form a gel that decreases the flexibility of the erythrocyte, resulting in microvascular occlusion, hemolysis, and chronic anemia.

- While it is clear that hemoglobin abnormalities play a major role, many other factors, including hemoglobin and erythrocytes, platelets, coagulation cascade, endothelium, NO, systemic oxidant-mediated injury, and environmental factors, contribute to the pathogenesis of SCD-related complications.

- SCD-related complications include VOC, ACS, stroke, acute splenic sequestration crisis, aplastic crisis, sepsis, and the chronic complications of SCD relevant to the practice of pediatric critical care medicine, including sickle cell chronic lung disease and PAH.

- Optimal perioperative care necessarily includes the accurate identification of patients at risk, appropriate preoperative preparation of the patient with SCD, optimal anesthetic management, and appropriate postoperative care.

- Patients with SCD are living longer than they have ever lived at any time in history. Therefore, SCD patients are more often surviving into adulthood and bringing with them chronic organ system dysfunction of the central nervous, cardiovascular, pulmonary, and renal systems.

- A significant percentage of SCD patients will develop dysfunction of the lung and pulmonary vasculature, manifest as sickle cell chronic lung disease and PAH.

- Until genetic therapies are available for the treatment of human SCD, hematopoietic stem cell transplantation, with its treatment-associated morbidity, represents the best hope for curative therapy for this disease.

References

1. Adams RJ, Brambilla D. Discontinuing prophylactic transfusions used to prevent stroke in sickle cell disease. *N Engl J Med* 2005;353:2769–78.
2. Adams RJ, McKie VC, Hsu L, et al. Prevention of a first stroke by transfusions in children with sickle cell anemia and abnormal results on transcranial Doppler ultrasonography. *N Engl J Med* 1998;339:5–11.
3. Aslan M, Thornley-Brown D, Freeman BA. Reactive species in sickle cell disease. *Ann N Y Acad Sci* 2000;899:375–91.
4. Assis A, Conran N, Canalli AA, et al. Effect of cytokines and chemokines on sickle neutrophil adhesion to fibronectin. *Acta Haematol* 2005;113:130–6.
5. Atz AM, Wessel DL. Inhaled nitric oxide in sickle cell disease with acute chest syndrome. *Anesthesiology* 1997;87:988–90.
6. Belcher JD, Marker PH, Weber JP, et al. Activated monocytes in sickle cell disease: Potential role in the activation of vascular endothelium and vaso-occlusion. *Blood* 2000;96:2451–9.
7. Bernini JC, Rogers ZR, Sandler ES, et al. Beneficial effect of intravenous dexamethasone in children with mild to moderately severe acute chest syndrome complicating sickle cell disease. *Blood* 1998;92:3082–9.
8. Brittain HA, Eckman JR, Swerlick RA, et al. Thrombospondin from activated platelets promotes sickle erythrocyte adherence to human microvascular endothelium under physiologic flow: A potential role for platelet activation in sickle cell vaso-occlusion. *Blood* 1993;81:2137–43.
9. Castro O, Brambilla DJ, Thorington B, et al. The acute chest syndrome in sickle cell disease: Incidence and risk factors. The Cooperative Study of Sickle Cell Disease. *Blood* 1994;84:643–9.
10. Castro O, Hoque M, Brown BD. Pulmonary hypertension in sickle cell disease: Cardiac catheterization results and survival. *Blood* 2003;101:1257–61.
11. Cosby K, Partovi KS, Crawford JH, et al. Nitrite reduction to nitric oxide by deoxyhemoglobin vasodilates the human circulation. *Nat Med* 2003;9:1498–505.
12. Dean J, Schechter AN. Sickle-cell anemia: Molecular and cellular bases of therapeutic approaches (third of three parts). *N Engl J Med* 1978;299:863–70.
13. Eaton WA, Hofrichter J. Hemoglobin S gelation and sickle cell disease. *Blood* 1987;70:1245–66.
14. Garza JA. Massive fat and necrotic bone marrow embolization in a previously undiagnosed patient with sickle cell disease. *Am J Forensic Med Pathol* 1990;11:83–8.
15. Gee BE, Platt OS. Sickle reticulocytes adhere to VCAM-1. *Blood* 1995;85:268–74.
16. Gill FM, Sleeper LA, Weiner SJ, et al. Clinical events in the first decade in a cohort of infants with sickle cell disease. Cooperative Study of Sickle Cell Disease. *Blood* 1995;86:776–83.
17. Girgis RE, Qureshi MA, Abrams J, et al. Decreased exhaled nitric oxide in sickle cell disease: Relationship with chronic lung involvement. *Am J Hematol* 2003;72:177–84.
18. Gladwin MT, Sachdev V, Jison ML, et al. Pulmonary hypertension as a risk factor for death in patients with sickle cell disease. *N Engl J Med* 2004;350:886–95.
19. Graido-Gonzalez E, Doherty JC, Bergreen EW, et al. Plasma endothelin-1, cytokine, and prostaglandin E2 levels in sickle cell disease and acute vaso-occlusive sickle crisis. *Blood* 1998;92:2551–5.
20. Griffin TC, Buchanan GR. Elective surgery in children with sickle cell disease without preoperative blood transfusion. *J Pediatr Surg* 1993;28:681–5.

21. Haberkern CM, Neumayr LD, Orringer EP, et al. Cholecystectomy in sickle cell anemia patients: Perioperative outcome of 364 cases from the National Preoperative Transfusion Study. Preoperative Transfusion in Sickle Cell Disease Study Group. *Blood* 1997;89:1533–42.

22. Hagger D, Wolff S, Owen J, et al. Changes in coagulation and fibrinolysis in patients with sickle cell disease compared with healthy black controls. *Blood Coagul Fibrinolysis* 1995;6:93–9.

23. Hammerman SI, Klings ES, Hendra KP, et al. Endothelial cell nitric oxide production in acute chest syndrome. *Am J Physiol* 1999;277:H1579–92.

24. Hammerman SI, Kourembanas S, Conca TJ, et al. Endothelin-1 production during the acute chest syndrome in sickle cell disease. *Am J Respir Crit Care Med* 1997;156:280–5.

25. Head CA, Brugnara C, Martinez-Ruiz R, et al. Low concentrations of nitric oxide increase oxygen affinity of sickle erythrocytes in vitro and in vivo. *J Clin Invest* 1997;100:1193–8.

26. Hebbel RP. Adhesive interactions of sickle erythrocytes with endothelium. *J Clin Invest* 1997;100:S83–6.

27. Hebbel RP, Boogaerts MA, Eaton JW, et al. Erythrocyte adherence to endothelium in sickle-cell anemia. A possible determinant of disease severity. *N Engl J Med* 1980;302:992–5.

28. Hebbel RP, Morgan WT, Eaton JW, et al. Accelerated autoxidation and heme loss due to instability of sickle hemoglobin. *Proc Natl Acad Sci U S A* 1988; 85:237–41.

29. Kirkham FJ, Prengler M, Hewes DK, et al. Risk factors for arterial ischemic stroke in children. *J Child Neurol* 2000;15:299–307.

30. Koshy M, Weiner SJ, Miller ST, et al. Surgery and anesthesia in sickle cell disease. Cooperative Study of Sickle Cell Diseases. *Blood* 1995;86:3676–84.

31. Kurantsin-Mills J, Ibe BO, Natta CL, et al. Elevated urinary levels of thromboxane and prostacyclin metabolites in sickle cell disease reflects activated platelets in the circulation. *Br J Haematol* 1994;87:580–5.

32. Liesner R, Mackie I, Cookson J, et al. Prothrombotic changes in children with sickle cell disease: Relationships to cerebrovascular disease and transfusion. *Br J Haematol* 1998;103:1037–44.

33. Mehta P, Mehta J. Abnormalities of platelet aggregation in sickle cell disease. *J Pediatr* 1980;96:209–13.

34. Miller ST, Hammerschlag MR, Chirgwin K, et al. Role of Chlamydia pneumoniae in acute chest syndrome of sickle cell disease. *J Pediatr* 1991;118: 30–3.

35. Morris CR, Kato GJ, Poljakovic M, et al. Dysregulated arginine metabolism, hemolysis-associated pulmonary hypertension, and mortality in sickle cell disease. *JAMA* 2005;294:81–90.

36. Morris CR, Kuypers FA, Larkin S, et al. Arginine therapy: A novel strategy to induce nitric oxide production in sickle cell disease. *Br J Haematol* 2000;111: 498–500.

37. Morris CR, Kuypers FA, Larkin S, et al. Patterns of arginine and nitric oxide in patients with sickle cell disease with vaso-occlusive crisis and acute chest syndrome. *J Pediatr Hematol Oncol* 2000;22:515–20.

38. Morris CR, Morris SM, Jr., Hagar W, et al. Arginine therapy: A new treatment for pulmonary hypertension in sickle cell disease? *Am J Respir Crit Care Med* 2003;168:63–9.

39. Pavlakis SG, Prohovnik I, Piomelli S, et al. Neurologic complications of sickle cell disease. *Adv Pediatr* 1989;36:247–76.

40. Pawloski JR, Hess DT, Stamler JS. Export by red blood cells of nitric oxide bioactivity. *Nature* 2001;409:622–6.

41. Pegelow CH, Macklin EA, Moser FG, et al. Longitudinal changes in brain magnetic resonance imaging findings in children with sickle cell disease. *Blood* 2002;99:3014–8.

42. Pelidis MA, Kato GJ, Resar LM, et al. Successful treatment of life-threatening acute chest syndrome of sickle cell disease with venovenous extracorporeal membrane oxygenation. *J Pediatr Hematol Oncol* 1997;19:459–61.

43. Peters M, Plaat BE, ten Cate H, et al. Enhanced thrombin generation in children with sickle cell disease. *Thromb Haemost* 1994;71: 169–72.

44. Piomelli S, Seaman C, Ackerman K, et al. Planning an exchange transfusion in patients with sickle cell syndromes. *Am J Pediatr Hematol Oncol* 1990;12: 268–76.

45. Platt OS, Brambilla DJ, Rosse WF, et al. Mortality in sickle cell disease. Life expectancy and risk factors for early death. *N Engl J Med* 1994;330: 1639–44.

46. Powars D, Weidman JA, Odom-Maryon T, et al. Sickle cell chronic lung disease: Prior morbidity and the risk of pulmonary failure. *Medicine (Baltimore)* 1988;67:66–76.

47. Quinn CT, Rogers ZR, Buchanan GR. Survival of children with sickle cell disease. *Blood* 2004;103:4023–7.

48. Repka T, Hebbel RP. Hydroxyl radical formation by sickle erythrocyte membranes: Role of pathologic iron deposits and cytoplasmic reducing agents. *Blood* 1991;78:2753–8.

49. Roth EF, Jr., Elbaum D, Bookchin RM, et al. The conformational requirements for the mechanical precipitation of hemoglobin S and other mutants. *Blood* 1976;48:265–71.

50. Sharan K, Surrey S, Ballas S, et al. Association of T-786C eNOS gene polymorphism with increased susceptibility to acute chest syndrome in females with sickle cell disease. *Br J Haematol* 2004;124:240–3.

51. Steinberg M. Management of sickle cell disease. *N Engl J Med* 1999;340: 1021–30.

52. Styles LA, Schalkwijk CG, Aarsman AJ, et al. Phospholipase A2 levels in acute chest syndrome of sickle cell disease. *Blood* 1996;87:2573–8.

53. Sullivan KJ, Goodwin SR, Evangelist J, et al. Nitric oxide successfully used to treat acute chest syndrome of sickle cell disease in a young adolescent. *Crit Care Med* 1999;27:2563–8.

54. Sullivan KJ, Kissoon N, Duckworth LJ, et al. Low exhaled nitric oxide and a polymorphism in the NOS I gene is associated with acute chest syndrome. *Am J Respir Crit Care Med* 2001;164:2186–90.

55. Sutton LL, Castro O, Cross DJ, et al. Pulmonary hypertension in sickle cell disease. *Am J Cardiol* 1994;74:626–8.

56. Vichinsky E, Styles L. Pulmonary complications. *Hematol Oncol Clin North Am* 1996;10:1275–87.

57. Vichinsky E, Williams R, Das M, et al. Pulmonary fat embolism: A distinct cause of severe acute chest syndrome in sickle cell anemia. *Blood* 1994;83: 3107–12.

58. Vichinsky EP, Haberkern CM, Neumayr L, et al. A comparison of conservative and aggressive transfusion regimens in the perioperative management of sickle cell disease. The Preoperative Transfusion in Sickle Cell Disease Study Group. *N Engl J Med* 1995;333:206–13.

Note: Page numbers followed by f indicate figures; page numbers followed by t indicate tabular material.